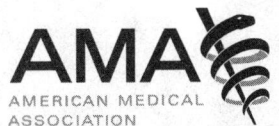

AMA|store

IMMEDIATE. INTERACTIVE. FACE-TO-FACE.
That's AMA's live Training & Events.

DATES & LOCATIONS

Experience one or two days of code training in December at locations throughout the country.

Dec. 8–9: Georgia

Dec. 8–9: New Jersey

Dec. 11–12: Maryland

Dec. 11–12: Nevada

Dec. 15–16: Texas

One-day experience: $545
Two-day experience: $900

Sign up before Oct. 25 and save $50 to $100 with early-bird rates.

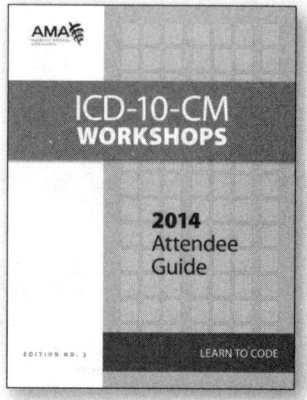

CPT® CHANGES WORKSHOPS
Day 1

A practical explanation of the changes in the 2015 CPT® code set. If you can't attend Symposium, then you want to attend this workshop.

ICD-10-CM WORKSHOPS
Day 2

Make use of the ICD-10 delay and train. Learn to transition to and code for ICD-10-CM with the help of our coding experts.

To learn more and register, visit
"Training & Events" at **amastore.com**.

Special group rate pricing available for three or more coworkers! Call (800) 882-3000 for details.

AMA
AMERICAN MEDICAL
ASSOCIATION

AMERICAN MEDICAL
ASSOCIATION

ICD-10-CM

The Complete Official Draft Codebook

2015

Publisher's Notice

The *ICD-10-CM The Complete Official Draft Codebook* is designed to be an accurate and authoritative source regarding coding and every reasonable effort has been made to ensure accuracy and completeness of the content. However, the AMA makes no guarantee, warranty, or representation that this publication is accurate, complete or without errors. It is understood that the AMA is not rendering any legal or other professional services or advice in this publication and that the AMA bears no liability for any results or consequences that may arise from the use of this book.

Our Commitment to Accuracy

The AMA is committed to producing accurate and reliable materials.

To report corrections, please call the AMA Unified Service Center at (800) 621-8335.

Acknowledgments

Lauri Gray, RHIT, CPC, AHIMA-Approved ICD-10-CM/PCS Trainer, *Product Manager*

Karen Schmidt, BSN, *Technical Director*

Anita Schmidt, BS, RHIT, *Clinical Technical Editor*

Peggy Willard, CCS, AHIMA-Approved ICD-10-CM/PCS Trainer, *Clinical Technical Editor*

Stacy Perry, *Manager, Desktop Publishing*

Lisa Singley, *Project Manager*

Tracy Betzler, *Senior Desktop Publishing Specialist*

Hope M. Dunn, *Senior Desktop Publishing Specialist*

Katie Russell, *Desktop Publishing Specialist*

Kate Holden, *Editor*

Anita Schmidt, BS, RHIT

Ms. Schmidt has expertise in level I adult and pediatric trauma hospital coding, specializing in ICD-9-CM, DRG, and CPT coding. Her experience includes analysis of medical record documentation and assignment of ICD-9-CM codes and DRGs, and CPT code assignments for same-day surgery cases. She has conducted coding training and auditing, including DRG validation; conducted electronic health record training; and worked with clinical documentation specialists to identify documentation needs and potential areas for physician education. Ms. Schmidt is an active member of the American Health Information Management Association (AHIMA) and the Minnesota Health Information Management Association (MHIMA).

Karen Schmidt, BSN

Ms. Schmidt has more than 25 years of health care experience, beginning with a strong clinical background in critical care nursing and later functioning as director of case management, including the components of quality assurance, utilization management, concurrent coding, case-mix analysis, and discharge planning. Her areas of expertise include ICD-9-CM/DRG coding, outpatient observation, billing compliance, implementation of concurrent coding methodology, and physician documentation education. She is an active member of the American Health Information Management Association (AHIMA).

Peggy Willard, CCS, AHIMA-Approved ICD10-CM/PCS Trainer

Ms. Willard has several years of experience in Level I Adult and Pediatric Trauma hospital coding, specializing in ICD-9-CM, DRG, and CPT coding. She has been extensively trained in ICD-10-CM and PCS. Her recent experience includes in-depth analysis of medical record documentation, ICD-10-CM code assignment, and DRG shifts based on ICD-10-CM code assignment. Ms. Willard's expertise includes conducting coding audits, conducting coding training for coding staff and clinical documentation specialists, and creating internal ICD-10-CM coding guidelines/tips. Ms. Willard is an active member of the American Health Information Management Association (AHIMA) and the Minnesota Health Information Management Association (MHIMA).

Contents

Preface iii

Introduction v
History and Future of ICD-10-CM v

How to Use ICD-10-CM for Physicians (Draft 2015) vi
Steps to Correct Coding vi
Organization vi

ICD-10-CM Draft Official Conventions vii
Format vii
Punctuation vii
Abbreviations vii
General Notes vii

Additional Conventions ix
Additional Characters Required ix
Boldface ix
Color Coding ix
Other Notations in the Tabular ix
Other Notations in the Alphabetic Indexes x

ICD-10-CM Draft Official Guidelines for Coding and Reporting .... Coding Guidelines – 1

ICD-10-CM Index to Diseases and Injuries 1

ICD-10-CM Neoplasm Table 321

ICD-10-CM Table of Drugs and Chemicals 339

ICD-10-CM Index to External Causes................................ 387

ICD-10-CM Tabular List of Diseases and Injuries 423
Chapter 1   Certain Infectious and Parasitic Diseases (A00-B99) 423
Chapter 2   Neoplasms (C00-D49) 441
Chapter 3   Diseases of the Blood and Blood-forming Organs (D50-D89) 472
Chapter 4   Endocrine, Nutritional and Metabolic Diseases (E00-E89) 479
Chapter 5   Mental, Behavioral, and Neurodevelopmental Disorders (F01-F99) 495
Chapter 6   Diseases of the Nervous System (G00-G99) 512
Chapter 7   Diseases of the Eye and Adnexa (H00-H59) 528
Chapter 8   Diseases of the Ear and Mastoid Process (H60-H95) 559
Chapter 9   Diseases of the Circulatory System (I00-I99) 569
Chapter 10 Diseases of the Respiratory System (J00-J99) 601
Chapter 11 Diseases of the Digestive System (K00-K95) 612
Chapter 12 Diseases of the Skin and Subcutaneous Tissue (L00-L99) 629
Chapter 13 Diseases of the Musculoskeletal System and Connective Tissue (M00-M99) 645
Chapter 14 Diseases of the Genitourinary System (N00-N99) ...721
Chapter 15 Pregnancy, Childbirth and the Puerperium (O00-O9A) 734
Chapter 16 Certain Conditions Originating in the Perinatal Period (P00-P96) 765
Chapter 17 Congenital Malformations, Deformations and Chromosomal Abnormalities (Q00-Q99) 774
Chapter 18 Symptoms, Signs and Abnormal Clinical and Laboratory Findings (R00-R99) 789
Chapter 19 Injury, Poisoning and Certain Other Consequences of External Causes (S00-T88) 804
Chapter 20 External Causes of Morbidity (V00-Y99)....................991
Chapter 21 Factors Influencing Health Status and Contact With Health Services (Z00-Z99) 1058

Illustrations Illustrations-1

Preface

ICD-10-CM Official Preface

This 2015 update of the International Classification of Diseases, 10th revision, Clinical Modification (ICD-10-CM) is being published by the United States government in recognition of its responsibility to promulgate this classification throughout the United States for morbidity coding. The International Statistical Classification of Diseases and Related Health Problems, 10th Revision (ICD-10), published by the World Health Organization (WHO), is the foundation of ICD-10-CM. ICD-10 continues to be the classification used in cause-of-death coding in the United States. The ICD-10-CM is comparable with the ICD-10. The WHO Collaborating Center for the Family of International Classifications in North America, housed at the National Center for Health Statistics (NCHS), has responsibility for the implementation of ICD and other WHO-FIC classifications and serves as a liaison with the WHO, fulfilling international obligations for comparable classifications and the national health data needs of the United States. The historical background of ICD and ICD-10 can be found in the Introduction to the International Classification of Diseases and Related Health Problems (ICD-10), 2008, World Health Organization, Geneva, Switzerland.

ICD-10-CM is the United States' clinical modification of the World Health Organization's ICD-10. The term clinical is used to emphasize the modification's intent: to serve as a useful tool in the area of classification of morbidity data for indexing of medical records, medical care review, and ambulatory and other medical care programs, as well as for basic health statistics. To describe the clinical picture of the patient the codes must be more precise than those needed only for statistical groupings and trend analysis.

Characteristics of ICD-10-CM

ICD-10-CM far exceeds its predecessors in the number of concepts and codes provided. The disease classification has been expanded to include health-related conditions and to provide greater specificity at the sixth and seventh character level. The sixth and seventh characters are not optional and are intended for use in recording the information documented in the clinical record.

Introduction

History and Future of ICD-10-CM

The ICD-10-CM classification system was developed by the National Center for Health Statistics (NCHS) as a clinical modification to the ICD-10 system developed by the World Health Organization (WHO), primarily as a unique system for use in the United States for morbidity and mortality reporting. Although ICD-10-CM has not yet been implemented for use in the United States, ICD-10 has been adopted for use in the coding and classification of mortality data from death certificates. ICD-10 replaced ICD-9 for this purpose as of January 1, 1999. Upon legislative approval, ICD-10-CM is planned as the replacement for ICD-9-CM, volumes 1 and 2.

ICD-10 is the copyrighted product of the World Health Organization (WHO), which has authorized the development of a clinical modification (CM) of ICD-10 for use in the United States. However, all modifications to the ICD-10 must conform to WHO conventions for ICD. The development of ICD-10-CM included comprehensive evaluation by a Technical Advisory Panel and extensive consultation with physician groups, clinical coders, and other industry experts.

The ICD-10-CM draft and crosswalk between ICD-9-CM and ICD-10-CM were made available on the Centers for Medicare and Medicaid Services (CMS) website for public comment. The initial public comment period extended from December 1997 through February 1998. A field test for ICD-10-CM was conducted in the summer of 2003 jointly by The American Hospital Association (AHA) and the American Health Information Management Association (AHIMA). Public comments and suggestions were reviewed and additional modifications to ICD-10-CM were made. Revisions were made to ICD-10-CM based on the established update process for ICD-9-CM (the ICD-9-CM Coordination and Maintenance Committee) and the World Health Organization's ICD-10 (the Update and Revision Committee).

These revisions to ICD-10-CM have included:

- information relevant to ambulatory and managed care encounters
- expanded injury codes
- creation of combination diagnosis/symptom codes to reduce the number of codes needed to fully describe a condition
- the addition of 6th and 7th character classifications
- incorporation of common 4th and 5th character classifications
- classifications specific to laterality
- classification refinement for increased data granularity

This new structure allows for further expansion than was possible with the ICD-9-CM classification system.

This new 2015 draft update release is available for public viewing. ICD-10-CM codes are not currently valid for any purpose or use other than the reporting of mortality data for death certificates.

The Department of Health and Human Services (HHS) published the final rule regarding the adoption of both ICD-10-CM and ICD-10-PCS in the January 16, 2009, Federal Register (45 CFR part 162 [CMS—0013—F]). The initial compliance date for implementation of ICD-10-CM and ICD-10-PCS as a replacement for ICD-9-CM was set at October 1, 2013. On April 17, 2012, the Department of Health and Human Services (HHS) released a notice to postpone the date by which certain health care entities have to comply with International Classification of Diseases, 10th Revision diagnosis and procedure codes (ICD-10). The compliance date for implementation of ICD-10-CM and ICD-10-PCS as a replacement for

ICD-9-CM was changed to October 1, 2014. On April 1, 2014, Congress enacted the Protecting Access to Medicare Act of 2014, which contained a provision to delay the implementation of ICD-10-CM/PCS by a least one year. The act prohibits the Department of Health and Human Services (HHS) from adopting the ICD-10-CM/PCS code sets as the mandatory standard until at least October 1, 2015.

ICD-10-CM: The Complete Official Draft Codebook

ICD-10-CM: The Complete Official Draft Codebook 2015 edition includes many of the enhancements described below in direct response to requests from our subscribers. Users will find many of the conventions, icons, color bars, and other enhancements familiar since many of these features are similar to the hallmark color coding and symbols of our ICD-9-CM codebooks.

As you review the content, you will find the following:

- Exclusive feature — Check XTension Alert symbol, indicating the need for one or more "filler" x character assignments in the 5th and/or 6th character position, in order to appropriately assign a required character in the 7th character position

- Exclusive feature — Key word differentiation by the use of a green font that highlights the differentiating terms in similar code descriptions in a given category

- Exclusive color coding, symbols, and footnotes that alert coders to coding and reimbursement issues, including the majority of the Medicare code edits

- Exclusive feature — Exclusive *following* references and Check Additional Character symbol in the indexes. The *following* references help coders locate those alphanumeric codes that are out of sequence in the tabular section.

- Exclusive feature — Exclusive shaded guides in the index help users easily follow the indent levels for the subterms under a main term.

- Illustrations at the back of the book feature anatomy and terminology included in the ICD-10-CM classification system

- The complete ICD-10-CM official guidelines for coding and reporting, published by the U.S. Department of Health and Human Services and approved by the cooperating parties (American Health Information Management Association, National Center for Health Statistics, Centers for Medicare and Medicaid Services, American Hospital Association)

- All the official ICD-10-CM codes, indexes, notes, footnotes, and symbols

- Icons and definitions to differentiate between the two types of Excludes notes

- Check 4th, 5th, 6th, and 7th character symbols identify codes that require the addition of a 4th, 5th, 6th, or 7th character for code specificity and validity

- Color coding and symbol legend at the bottom of each page

Please review "How to Use *ICD-10-CM for Physicians*" in this section to learn about the features that will help you assign and report correct codes, ensuring appropriate reimbursement.

How to Use ICD-10-CM for Physicians (Draft 2015)

This draft of the International Classification of Diseases, 10th Revision, Clinical Modification (ICD-10-CM) is being published by the United States Government in recognition of its responsibility to promulgate this classification throughout the United States for morbidity coding. This code book represents an adaptation of ICD-10 which was created specifically for use in the United States. Future revisions to ICD-10-CM will be made based on the established update process for ICD-9-CM (the ICD-9-CM Coordination and Maintenance Committee) and the World Health Organization's ICD-10 (the Update and Revision Committee). ICD-10-CM has been approved for implementation on October 1, 2015.

Steps to Correct Coding

1. Before beginning to use this code book, review section 1.A., "Conventions for the ICD-10-CM" and section 1.B., "General Coding Guidelines" of the ICD-10-CM Draft Official Guidelines for Coding and Reporting 2014.

2. Look up the main term in the alphabetic index and scan the subterm entries as appropriate. Review continued lines and additional subterms that may appear in the next column or on the next page.

3. Note all parenthetical terms (nonessential modifiers) that help in code selection but do not affect code assignment. Shaded vertical guidelines in the Index are provided to help determine the indentation level for each subterm in relation to the main terms.

4. Pay close attention to the following instructions in the Index:
   - "see," "see also," and "see category" cross-references
   - "with"/"without" notes
   - "omit code" notes
   - "due to" subterms
   - other instructions found in note boxes, such as "code by site"
   - *Following* references and Check Additional Character symbol in the indexes. The *following* references help coders locate those alphanumeric codes that are out of sequence in the tabular section.

5. Do not code from the alphabetic index without verifying the accuracy of the code in the tabular list. Locate the code in the alphanumerically arranged tabular list.

6. To determine the appropriateness of the code selection and proper coding, read all instructional material:
   - "includes" and both types of "excludes" notes
   - "use additional code" and "code first underlying disease" instructions
   - "code also"
   - 4th, 5th, and 6th character requirements and 7th character extension requirements
   - age and sex symbols

7. Consult the official Draft ICD-10-CM guidelines, which govern the use of specific codes. These guidelines provide both general and chapter-specific coding guidance.

8. Confirm and assign the correct code.

Organization
This book is organized in the following manner:

Introduction
The introductory material in this book includes the ICD-10-CM Official Preface, the history and future of ICD-10-CM as well as an overview of the classification system.

Draft Official ICD-10-CM Conventions and Guidelines
This section provides an explanation of the conventions and guidelines regulating the appropriate assignment and reporting of ICD-10-CM codes. This coding guidance is presented by the National Center for Health Statistics (NCHS), a governmental agency of the Centers for Disease Control and Prevention (CDC), within the United States Department of Health and Human Services (DHHS).

Alphabetic Index to Diseases
The alphabetic index to diseases is arranged in alphabetic order by disease — by specific illness, injury, eponym, abbreviation, or other descriptive diagnostic term. The Index also lists diagnostic terms for other reasons for encounters with health care professionals.

Neoplasm Table
The Neoplasm Table provides the proper code based upon histology of the neoplasm and site.

Table of Drugs and Chemicals
The Table of Drugs and Chemicals is also included within the alphabetic index.

The Table of Drugs and Chemicals lists the drug and the specific codes that identify the drug and the intent. No additional external cause of injury and poisoning code is assigned in ICD-10-CM.

Index to External Causes
The alphabetic index to external causes of injuries is arranged in alphabetic order by main term indicating the event.

Tabular List of Diseases
ICD-10-CM codes and descriptors are arranged numerically within the tabular list of diseases within 21 separate chapters according to body system or nature of injury and disease. Classifications which were previously considered supplemental to ICD-9-CM (e.g., V codes and E codes) are incorporated into the tabular listing of ICD-10-CM as individual chapters. Chapters 20 External Causes of Morbidity and 21 Factors Influencing Health Status and Contact with Health Services include chapter-specific guidelines.

Illustrations
This section includes illustrations of normal anatomy with ICD-10-CM specific terminology.

Use of Official Sources
The *ICD-10-CM for Physicians* contains the official U.S. Department of Health and Human Services, Tenth Revision, Clinical Modification, ICD-10-CM codes, effective for the current year.

The color-coding, footnotes and symbols, which identify coding and reimbursement issues, are derived from official federal government sources, including the Medicare Code Edits (MCE), version 31R.

ICD-10-CM Draft Official Conventions

The ICD-10-CM conventions are general rules for the use of the classification system, independent of the guidelines. These conventions are incorporated within the Index and tabular list as instructional notes and are applicable regardless of the health care setting.

Format

ICD-10-CM is divided into two main parts: the Index, an alphabetical list of terms and their corresponding code, and the tabular list, a sequential, alphanumeric list of codes divided into chapters based on body system or condition. The Index contains the Index to Diseases and Injuries (main index) and the Index to External Causes of Injury. Also included in the main Index is the Neoplasm Table and a Table of Drugs and Chemicals.

The tabular list contains categories, subcategories, and valid codes. ICD-10-CM is an alphanumeric classification system. The 1st character of a three-character category is a letter. The 2nd and 3rd characters may be numbers or alpha characters. A three-character category without further subclassification is equivalent to a valid three-character code. Subcategories are either four or five characters. Subcategory characters include either letters or numbers. Codes may be four, five, or six characters in length, in which each level of subdivision after a category is a subcategory. The final level of subdivision is a valid code. The final character in a code may be either a letter or a number.

The ICD-10-CM uses the letter "X" as a place-holder. A placeholder "X" is used as a 5th character place-holder at certain six-character codes to allow for future expansion, without disturbing the 6th character structure. For instance, an initial encounter for accidental poisoning by penicillin is coded to T36.0X1A. The "X" in the 5th character position is a place-holder, or filler character.

Similarly, certain categories have applicable 7th character extensions. In these cases, the 7th character extension is required for all codes within the category, or as otherwise instructed in the tabular list notations. 7th character extensions must always be the last character in the data field. If a code is not a full six characters in length, a dummy place-holder "X" must be used to fill in the empty characters when a 7th character extension is required.

Punctuation

[ ]   In the tabular list, brackets are used to enclose synonyms, alternative wording, or explanatory phrases. In the Index, brackets are used to identify manifestation codes.

( )   Parentheses are used in both the Index and tabular list to enclose nonessential modifiers; supplementary words that may be present or absent in the statement of a disease or procedure without affecting the code number to which it is assigned.

:   Colons are used in the tabular list after an incomplete term that needs one or more of the modifiers following the colon to make it assignable to a given category.

Abbreviations

NEC

The abbreviation NEC, "Not elsewhere classifiable" represents "other specified" in the ICD-10-CM. An index entry that states NEC directs the coder to an "other specified" code in the tabular list. Codes titled "Other" or "Other specified" in the tabular list (usually a code with a 4th or 6th character 8 and 5th character 9) are for use when the information in the medical record provides detail for which a specific code does not exist.

NOS

The abbreviation NOS, "Not otherwise specified," in the tabular list may be interpreted as "unspecified." Codes in the tabular list with "Unspecified" in the title (usually a code with a 4th or 6th character 9 and 5th character 0) are for use when the information in the medical record is insufficient to assign a more specific code.

Typeface

Boldface

Boldface type is used for main term entries in the alphabetic index, and all codes and descriptions in the tabular list.

Italicized

Italicized type is used for all exclusion notes and to identify manifestation codes, those codes that should not be reported as first-listed (principal) diagnoses.

General Notes

The following conventions and notes appear only in the tabular list of diseases:

Includes Notes

The word "Includes" appears immediately under certain categories to further define, clarify, or give examples of the content of a code category.

Inclusion Terms

Lists of inclusion terms are included under certain codes. These terms indicate some of the conditions for which that code number may be used. Inclusion terms may be synonyms with the code title, or, in the case of "other specified" codes, the terms may also provide a list of various conditions included within a classification code. The inclusion terms are not exhaustive. The Index may provide additional terms that may also be assigned to a given code.

Excludes Notes

ICD-10-CM has two types of excludes notes. Each note has a different definition for use. However, they are similar in that they both indicate that codes excluded from each other are independent of each other.

Excludes1

An Excludes1 note is a "pure" excludes. It means "NOT CODED HERE!" An Excludes1 note indicates mutually exclusive codes; two conditions that cannot be reported together. For example, a congenital form of a disease may not be reported with the acquired form of the same condition. The code excluded should never be reported with the applicable codes listed above the excludes notation.

Excludes2

An Excludes2 note means "NOT INCLUDED HERE." An Excludes2 note indicates that although the excluded condition is not part of the condition it is excluded from, a patient may have both conditions at the same time. Therefore, when an Excludes2 note appears under a code, it may be acceptable to use both the code and the excluded code together if supported by the medical documentation.

Default Codes

In the index, the default code is the code listed next to the main term. The default code represents the condition most commonly associated with the main term. This code may be assigned when documentation does not facilitate reporting a more specific code. Alternately, it may provide an unspecified code for the condition.

Syndromes

Follow the alphabetic index guidance when coding syndromes. In the absence of index guidance, assign codes for the documented manifestations of the syndrome.

And

When the term "and" is used in a narrative statement it may be interpreted as "and/or."

With/Without

When "with" and "without" are the two options for the final character of a set of codes, the default is always "without." For five-character codes, a "Ø" as the 5th position character represents "without", and "1" represents "with." For six-character codes, the 6th position character "1" represents "with" and "9" represents "without."

Instructional Notes Used in the Tabular List

In the tabular section, the following instructional notes appear in red type for emphasis:

Code First/Use additional code:

These instructional notes are in red type and provide sequencing instruction. They may appear independently of each other or to designate certain etiology/manifestation paired codes. These instructions signal the coder that an additional code should be reported to provide a more complete picture of that diagnosis.

In etiology/manifestation coding, ICD-1Ø-CM requires the underlying condition to be sequenced first, followed by the manifestation. In these situations, codes with "In diseases classified elsewhere" in the code description are never permitted as a first-listed or principal diagnosis code and must be sequenced following the underlying condition code.

Code Also:

A code also note alerts the coder that more than one code may be required to fully describe the condition. Code sequencing is discretionary. Factors that may determine sequencing include severity and reason for the encounter. These coding notes appear in red type.

Additional Conventions

Color-coding and symbols are included to alert the coder to important reimbursement issues affected by the diagnosis code assignment. Some codes may carry more than one color and/or symbol. For a quick reference to the color codes and their meanings, refer to the color/symbol legend located at the bottom of each page in the tabular listing.

Additional Characters Required

✓4ᵗʰ This symbol indicates that the code requires a 4th character.

✓5ᵗʰ This symbol indicates that the code requires a 5th character.

✓6ᵗʰ This symbol indicates that the code requires a 6th character.

✓7ᵗʰ This symbol indicates that the code requires a 7th character.

✓x7ᵗʰ This symbol indicates that the code requires a 7th character following the placeholder X. Codes with fewer than six characters that require a 7th character must contain placeholder "X" to fill in the empty character(s).

Boldface

Note

The term "Note" appears enclosed within a red icon and precedes the instructional information. These notes function as an alert, to highlight coding instruction within the text.

Key Word

Green font is used throughout the tabular list of diseases to differentiate the key words that appear in similar code descriptions in a given category or subcategory.

For example, refer to the list of codes below from category C7A:

C7A.Ø2Ø   Malignant carcinoid tumor of the **appendix**

C7A.Ø21   Malignant carcinoid tumor of the **cecum**

C7A.Ø22   Malignant carcinoid tumor of the **ascending colon**

C7A.Ø23   Malignant carcinoid tumor of the **transverse colon**

C7A.Ø24   Malignant carcinoid tumor of the **descending colon**

C7A.Ø25   Malignant carcinoid tumor of the **sigmoid colon**

C7A.Ø29   Malignant carcinoid tumor of the large intestine, unspecified portion

The portion of the code description that appears in bold font above appears in green font in the tabular list, to assist the coder in quickly identifying the key terms and in identifying the correct code. This convention is especially useful when the codes describe laterality, such as the following codes from category H4Ø.22:

H4Ø.221   Chronic angle-closure glaucoma, **right** eye

H4Ø.222   Chronic angle-closure glaucoma, **left** eye

H4Ø.223   Chronic angle-closure glaucoma, **bilateral**

H4Ø.229   Chronic angle-closure glaucoma, unspecified eye

The key word convention is only used in those categories in which there are multiple codes with very similar descriptions with only a few words that differentiate them.

Color Coding

Medicare administrative contractors and many payers use Medicare code edits to check the coding accuracy on claims. The coding edit information in this manual, effective from October 1, 2014, to September 30, 2015, reflect those edits used for physician office encounters. This ICD-10 version of the Medicare Code Editor (MCE) is version 31R. However, the MCE is not intended to be used to process claims since the ICD-10 code set will not be mandated for use until the implementation of ICD-10 beginning no sooner than October 1, 2015.

Manifestation Code

These codes appear in italic type, with a blue color bar over the title. A manifestation code cannot be reported as a first-listed or principal diagnosis. By definition, a manifestation code represents a demonstration of some aspect of an underlying disease, which is separately classifiable. In the alphabetic index, these codes are listed as the secondary code in brackets. The underlying disease code is listed first.

Age and Sex Edit Symbols

The age edits below are used to detect inconsistencies between the patient's age and diagnosis. The following edit symbols appear in the tabular list of diseases to the right of the code description.

Newborn Age: Ø   **N**
These diagnoses are intended for newborns and neonates and the patient's age must be Ø years.

Pediatric Age: Ø-17   **P**
These diagnoses are intended for children and the patient's age must between Ø and 17 years.

Maternity Age: 12-55   **M**
These diagnoses are intended for childbearing patients between the age of 12 and 55 years.

Adult Age: 15-124   **A**
These diagnoses are intended for the patients between the age of 15 and 124 years.

The sex symbols below are used to detect inconsistencies between the patient's sex and diagnosis. These symbols appear in the tabular list of diseases to the right of the code description.

♂   **Male diagnosis only**
This symbol appears to the right of the code description. This reference appears in the disease and procedure tabular list.

♀   **Female diagnosis only**
This symbol appears to the right of the code description. This reference appears in the disease and procedure tabular list.

Other Notations in the Tabular

Other Specified Code

These codes will appear with a gray color bar over the code description. Use these codes when the documentation indicates a specified diagnosis, but the ICD-10-CM system does not have a specific code that describes the condition. These codes may be stated as "Other" or "Not elsewhere classified (NEC)."

Unspecified Code

These codes will have a yellow color bar over the code description. Use these codes when neither the diagnostic statement nor the documentation provides enough information to assign a more specific diagnosis code. These codes may be stated as "Unspecified" or "Not otherwise specified (NOS)." Note: Do not assign these codes when a more specific diagnosis has been determined.

PDx Symbol

This symbol identifies a Z code that generally is for use as a first-listed (or primary) diagnosis only but may be used as an additional diagnosis if the patient has more than one encounter on the same day or there is more than one reason for the encounter.

The instructions for Z code use contained in the ICD-10-CM official coding guidelines identify those Z codes that can only be used as a PDx. All other Z codes may either be SDx or PDx, depending upon circumstances of the encounter, by meeting the definition of first-listed or principal diagnosis, and by following any specific Z code guidelines in section I.C.21 a-c. The responsibility of those assigning the Z codes as PDx is to make sure the circumstances of the encounter meet the definition of first-listed or principal diagnosis, follow all coding instructions, and follow the Z code specific guidelines. Codebook does not include any SDx edit since there is no official source for it and the Z code use is determined by circumstances of the encounter.

Note: Please note that the symbols indicating the Z code "principal or first-listed only" designation and the Z codes that may be principal or first-listed diagnoses included in the official coding guidelines [Section 1.C.21.c.16] are consistent with reporting guidelines for health care encounters *excluding acute care inpatient admissions.* These Z code edits are often in conflict with the inpatient prospective payment system (IPPS) edits. For example, code Z34.90 Encounter for supervision of normal pregnancy, unspecified, unspecified trimester, may be an appropriate primary reason for an outpatient encounter. However, supervision for a normal pregnancy is not an acceptable principal diagnosis or reason for an inpatient admission and will have an unacceptable principal diagnosis edit under inpatient prospective payment system (IPPS).

Other Notations in the Alphabetic Indexes

▽ Subterms under main terms may continue to next column or page. This warning statement is a reminder to always check for additional subterms and information that may continue onto the next page or column before making a final selection.

Following References

The index includes *following* references to assist in locating "out-of-sequence" codes in the tabular list. "Out-of-sequence" codes contain an alphabetic character (letter) in the 3rd or 4th character position. These codes are placed according to the classification rules — the placement of the codes according to condition — not according to alphabetic or numeric sequencing rules.

Example:

Carcinoma (malignant) (*see also,* Neoplasm, by site, malignant)
   neuroendocrine (*see also* Tumor, neuroendocrine)
      high grade, any site C7A.1 (*following* C75)
      poorly differentiated, any site C7A.1 (*following* C75)

In the tabular rubric, C7A is included after rubric C75 and before C76.

Gout, chronic (*see also* Gout, gouty) M1A.9
   drug-induced M1A.20 (*following* M08)
      ankle M1A.27-(*following* M08)
      elbow M1A.22-(*following* M08)

In the tabular rubric, MIA is included after rubric M08 and before M10.

ICD-10-CM Draft Official Guidelines for Coding and Reporting 2014

Narrative changes appear in **bold** text.

Items <u>underlined</u> have been moved within the guidelines since the 2013 version.

Italics are used to indicate revisions to heading changes.

The Centers for Medicare and Medicaid Services (CMS) and the National Center for Health Statistics (NCHS), two departments within the U.S. Federal Government's Department of Health and Human Services (DHHS) provide the following guidelines for coding and reporting using the International Classification of Diseases, 10th Revision, Clinical Modification (ICD-10-CM). These guidelines should be used as a companion document to the official version of the ICD-10-CM as published on the NCHS website. The ICD-10-CM is a morbidity classification published by the United States for classifying diagnoses and reason for visits in all health care settings. The ICD-10-CM is based on the ICD-10, the statistical classification of disease published by the World Health Organization (WHO).

These guidelines have been approved by the four organizations that make up the Cooperating Parties for the ICD-10-CM: the American Hospital Association (AHA), the American Health Information Management Association (AHIMA), CMS, and NCHS.

These guidelines are a set of rules that have been developed to accompany and complement the official conventions and instructions provided within the ICD-10-CM itself. The instructions and conventions of the classification take precedence over guidelines. These guidelines are based on the coding and sequencing instructions in the Tabular List and Alphabetic Index of ICD-10-CM, but provide additional instruction. Adherence to these guidelines when assigning ICD-10-CM diagnosis codes is required under the Health Insurance Portability and Accountability Act (HIPAA). The diagnosis codes (Tabular List and Alphabetic Index) have been adopted under HIPAA for all healthcare settings. A joint effort between the healthcare provider and the coder is essential to achieve complete and accurate documentation, code assignment, and reporting of diagnoses and procedures. These guidelines have been developed to assist both the healthcare provider and the coder in identifying those diagnoses and procedures that are to be reported. The importance of consistent, complete documentation in the medical record cannot be overemphasized. Without such documentation accurate coding cannot be achieved. The entire record should be reviewed to determine the specific reason for the encounter and the conditions treated.

The term encounter is used for all settings, including hospital admissions. In the context of these guidelines, the term provider is used throughout the guidelines to mean physician or any qualified health care practitioner who is legally accountable for establishing the patient's diagnosis. Only this set of guidelines, approved by the Cooperating Parties, is official.

The guidelines are organized into sections. Section I includes the structure and conventions of the classification and general guidelines that apply to the entire classification, and chapter-specific guidelines that correspond to the chapters as they are arranged in the classification. Section II includes guidelines for selection of principal diagnosis for non-outpatient settings. Section III includes guidelines for reporting additional diagnoses in non-outpatient settings. Section IV is for outpatient coding and reporting. It is necessary to review all sections of the guidelines to fully understand all of the rules and instructions needed to code properly.

Section I. Conventions, general coding guidelines and chapter specific guidelines 3
- A. Conventions for the ICD-10-CM 3
  1. The Alphabetic Index and Tabular List 3
  2. Format and Structure 3
  3. Use of codes for reporting purposes 3
  4. Placeholder character 3
  5. 7th Characters 3
  6. Abbreviations 3
     a. Alphabetic Index abbreviations 3
     b. Tabular List abbreviations 3
  7. Punctuation 3
  8. Use of "and" 3
  9. Other and Unspecified codes 3
     a. "Other" codes 3
     b. "Unspecified" codes 3
  10. Includes Notes 3
  11. Inclusion Terms 3
  12. Excludes Notes 3
     a. Excludes1 3
     b. Excludes2 3
  13. Etiology/manifestation convention ("code first", "use additional code" and "in diseases classified elsewhere" notes) 3
  14. "And" 4
  15. "With" 4
  16. "See" and "See Also" 4
  17. "Code also note" 4
  18. Default codes 4
- B. General Coding Guidelines 4
  1. Locating a code in the ICD-10-CM 4
  2. Level of Detail in Coding 4
  3. Code or codes from A00.0 through T88.9, Z00-Z99.8 4
  4. Signs and symptoms 4
  5. Conditions that are an integral part of a disease process 4
  6. Conditions that are not an integral part of a disease process 4
  7. Multiple coding for a single condition 4
  8. Acute and Chronic Conditions 5
  9. Combination Code 5
  10. Sequela (Late Effects) 5
  11. Impending or Threatened Condition 5
  12. Reporting Same Diagnosis Code more than Once 5
  13. Laterality 5
  14. Documentation for BMI, Non-pressure Ulcers and Pressure Ulcer Stages 5
  15. Syndromes 5
  16. Documentation of Complications of Care 5
  17. Borderline Diagnosis 5
  18. Use of Sign/Symptom/Unspecified Codes 5
- C. Chapter-Specific Coding Guidelines 6
  1. Chapter 1: Certain Infectious and Parasitic Diseases (A00-B99) 6
     a. Human immunodeficiency virus (HIV) infections 6
     b. Infectious agents as the cause of diseases classified to other chapters 6
     c. Infections resistant to antibiotics 6
     d. Sepsis, severe sepsis, and septic shock 6
     e. Methicillin resistant *Staphylococcus aureus* (MRSA) conditions 7
  2. Chapter 2: Neoplasms (C00-D49) 8
     a. Treatment directed at the malignancy 8
     b. Treatment of secondary site 8
     c. Coding and sequencing of complications 8
     d. Primary malignancy previously excised 8
     e. Admissions/Encounters involving chemotherapy, immunotherapy and radiation therapy 8
     f. Admission/encounter to determine extent of malignancy 9
     g. Symptoms, signs, and abnormal findings listed in Chapter 18 associated with neoplasms 9
     h. Admission/encounter for pain control/management 9
     i. Malignancy in two or more noncontiguous sites 9
     j. Disseminated malignant neoplasm, unspecified 9
     k. Malignant neoplasm without specification of site 9
     l. Sequencing of neoplasm codes 9
     m. Current malignancy versus personal history of malignancy 9
     n. Leukemia, multiple myeloma, and malignant plasma cell neoplasms in remission versus personal history 9
     o. Aftercare following surgery for neoplasm 9
     p. Follow-up care for completed treatment of a malignancy 9
     q. Prophylactic organ removal for prevention of malignancy 9
     r. Malignant neoplasm associated with transplanted organ 9
  3. Chapter 3: Disease of the Blood and Blood-forming Organs and Certain Disorders Involving the Immune Mechanism (D50-D89) .. 9
  4. Chapter 4: Endocrine, Nutritional, and Metabolic Diseases (E00-E89) 10
     a. Diabetes mellitus 10
  5. Chapter 5: Mental, Behavioral and Neurodevelopmental Disorders (F01 – F99) 10
     a. Pain disorders related to psychological factors 10
     b. Mental and behavioral disorders due to psychoactive substance use 10
  6. Chapter 6: Diseases of Nervous System (G00-G99) 10
     a. Dominant/nondominant side 10
     b. Pain - Category G89 11
  7. Chapter 7: Diseases of Eye and Adnexa (H00-H59) 11
     a. Glaucoma 11
  8. Chapter 8: Diseases of Ear and Mastoid Process (H60-H95) 12
  9. Chapter 9: Diseases of Circulatory System (I00-I99) 12

a. Hypertension 12
b. Atherosclerotic coronary artery disease and angina 12
c. Intraoperative and postprocedural cerebrovascular accident 12
d. Sequelae of cerebrovascular disease 13
e. Acute myocardial infarction (AMI) 13

10. Chapter 10: Diseases of *the* Respiratory System (J00-J99) 13
a. Chronic Obstructive Pulmonary Disease [COPD] and Asthma 13
b. Acute Respiratory Failure 13
c. Influenza due to certain identified influenza viruses ... 13
d. Ventilator associated pneumonia 13

11. Chapter 11: Diseases of the Digestive System (K00-K95) 14

12. Chapter 12: Diseases of the Skin and Subcutaneous Tissue (L00-L99) 14
a. Pressure ulcer stage codes 14

13. Chapter 13: Diseases of the Musculoskeletal System and Connective Tissue (M00-M99) 14
a. Site and laterality 14
b. Acute traumatic versus chronic or recurrent musculoskeletal conditions 14
c. Coding of Pathologic Fractures 14
d. Osteoporosis 14

14. Chapter 14: Diseases of Genitourinary System (N00-N99) 15
a. Chronic kidney disease 15

15. Chapter 15: Pregnancy, Childbirth, and the Puerperium (O00-O9A) 15
a. General Rules for Obstetric Cases 15
b. Selection of OB principal or first-listed diagnosis 15
c. Pre-existing conditions versus conditions due to the pregnancy 16
d. Pre-existing hypertension in pregnancy 16
e. Fetal conditions affecting the management of the mother 16
f. HIV Infection in pregnancy, childbirth and the puerperium ... 16
g. Diabetes mellitus in pregnancy 16
h. Long term use of insulin 16
i. Gestational (pregnancy induced) diabetes ... 16
j. Sepsis and septic shock complicating abortion, pregnancy, childbirth and the puerperium 16
k. Puerperal sepsis 16
l. Alcohol and tobacco use during pregnancy, childbirth and the puerperium 16
m. Poisoning, toxic effects, adverse effects and underdosing in a pregnant patient 16
n. Normal delivery, code O80 16
o. The peripartum and postpartum periods 17
p. Code O94, Sequelae of complication of pregnancy, childbirth, and the puerperium 17
q. Termination of Pregnancy and Spontaneous Abortions 17
r. Abuse in a pregnant patient 17

16. Chapter 16: Certain Conditions Origination in the Perinatal Period (P00-P96) 17
a. General Perinatal Rules 17
b. Observation and evaluation of newborns for suspected conditions not found 18
c. Coding Additional Perinatal Diagnoses 18
d. Prematurity and fetal growth retardation 18
e. Low birth weight and immaturity status 18
f. Bacterial sepsis of newborn 18
g. Stillbirth 18

17. Chapter 17: Congenital Malformations, Deformations, and Chromosomal Abnormalities (Q00-Q99) 18

18. Chapter 18: Symptoms, Signs, and Abnormal Clinical and Laboratory Findings, Not Elsewhere Classified (R00-R99) 18
a. Use of symptom codes 18
b. Use of a symptom code with a definitive diagnosis code 18
c. Combination codes that include symptoms 18
d. Repeated falls 18
e. Coma scale 18
f. Functional quadriplegia 18
g. SIRS due to non-infectious process 18
h. Death NOS 19

19. Chapter 19: Injury, Poisoning, and Certain Other Consequences of External Causes (S00-T88) 19
a. Application of 7th Characters in Chapter 19 ... 19

b. Coding of injuries 19
c. Coding of traumatic fractures 19
d. Coding of burns and corrosions 19
e. Adverse effects, poisoning, underdosing and toxic effects 20
f. Adult and child abuse, neglect and other maltreatment 21
g. Complications of care 21

20. Chapter 20: External Causes of Morbidity (V00-Y99) 21
a. General external cause coding guidelines 21
b. Place of occurrence guideline 22
c. Activity code 22
d. Place of occurrence, activity, and status codes used with other external cause code 22
e. If the reporting format limits the number of external cause codes 22
f. Multiple external cause coding guidelines 22
g. Child and adult abuse guideline 22
h. Unknown or undetermined intent guideline ... 22
i. Sequelae (Late Effects) of external cause guidelines 22
j. Terrorism guidelines 22
k. External cause status 22

21. Chapter 21: Factors Influencing Health Status and Contact with Health Services (Z00-Z99) 23
a. Use of Z codes in any healthcare setting 23
b. Z Codes indicate a reason for an encounter ... 23
c. Categories of Z codes 23

Section II. Selection of Principal Diagnosis 27
A. Codes for symptoms, signs, and ill-defined conditions 27
B. Two or more interrelated conditions, each potentially meeting the definition for principal diagnosis 27
C. Two or more diagnoses that equally meet the definition for principal diagnosis 27
D. Two or more comparative or contrasting conditions 27
E. A symptom(s) followed by contrasting/ comparative diagnoses 27
F. Original treatment plan not carried out 28
G. Complications of surgery and other medical care 28
H. Uncertain diagnosis 28
I. Admission from observation unit 28
   1. Admission Following Medical Observation 28
   2. Admission Following Post-Operative Observation 28
J. Admission from outpatient surgery 28
K. Admissions/Encounters for Rehabilitation 28
Section III. Reporting Additional Diagnoses 28
A. Previous conditions 28
B. Abnormal findings 28
C. Uncertain Diagnosis 28

Section IV. Diagnostic Coding and Reporting Guidelines for Outpatient Services 29
A. Selection of first-listed condition 29
   1. Outpatient surgery 29
   2. Observation stay 29
B. Codes from A00.0 through T88.9, Z00-Z99 29
C. Accurate reporting of ICD-10-CM diagnosis codes 29
D. Codes that describe symptoms and signs 29
E. Encounters for circumstances other than a disease or injury 29
F. Level of Detail in Coding 29
   1. ICD-10-CM codes with 3, 4, 5, 6 or 7 characters 29
   2. Use of full number of characters required for a code ... 29
G. ICD-10-CM code for the diagnosis, condition, problem, or other reason for encounter/visit 29
H. Uncertain diagnosis 29
I. Chronic diseases 29
J. Code all documented conditions that coexist 29
K. Patients receiving diagnostic services only 29
L. Patients receiving therapeutic services only 29
M. Patients receiving preoperative evaluations only 30
N. Ambulatory surgery 30
O. Routine outpatient prenatal visits 30
P. Encounters for general medical examinations with abnormal findings 30
Q. Encounters for routine health screenings 30

Appendix I. Present on Admission Reporting Guidelines 30
Categories and Codes Exempt from Diagnosis Present on Admission Requirement 31

Section I. Conventions, general coding guidelines and chapter specific guidelines

The conventions, general guidelines and chapter-specific guidelines are applicable to all health care settings unless otherwise indicated. The conventions and instructions of the classification take precedence over guidelines.

A. Conventions for the ICD-10-CM

The conventions for the ICD-10-CM are the general rules for use of the classification independent of the guidelines. These conventions are incorporated within the Alphabetic Index and Tabular List of the ICD-10-CM as instructional notes.

1. **The Alphabetic Index and Tabular List**
    The ICD-10-CM is divided into the Alphabetic Index, an alphabetical list of terms and their corresponding code, and the Tabular List, a structured chronological list of codes divided into chapters based on body system or condition. The Alphabetic Index consists of the following parts: the Index of Diseases and Injury, the Index of External Causes of Injury, the Table of Neoplasms and the Table of Drugs and Chemicals.

    See Section I.C2. General guidelines

    See Section I.C.19. Adverse effects, poisoning, underdosing and toxic effects

2. **Format and Structure**
    The ICD-10-CM Tabular List contains categories, subcategories and codes. Characters for categories, subcategories and codes may be either a letter or a number. All categories are 3 characters. A three-character category that has no further subdivision is equivalent to a code. Subcategories are either 4 or 5 characters. Codes may be 3, 4, 5, 6 or 7 characters. That is, each level of subdivision after a category is a subcategory. The final level of subdivision is a code. Codes that have applicable 7th characters are still referred to as codes, not subcategories. A code that has an applicable 7th character is considered invalid without the 7th character.

    The ICD-10-CM uses an indented format for ease in reference.

3. **Use of codes for reporting purposes**
    For reporting purposes only codes are permissible, not categories or subcategories, and any applicable 7th character is required.

4. **Placeholder character**
    The ICD-10-CM utilizes a placeholder character "X". The "X" is used as a placeholder at certain codes to allow for future expansion. An example of this is at the poisoning, adverse effect and underdosing codes, categories T36-T50.

    Where a placeholder exists, the X must be used in order for the code to be considered a valid code.

5. **7th Characters**
    Certain ICD-10-CM categories have applicable 7th characters. The applicable 7th character is required for all codes within the category, or as the notes in the Tabular List instruct. The 7th character must always be the 7th character in the data field. If a code that requires a 7th character is not 6 characters, a placeholder X must be used to fill in the empty characters.

6. **Abbreviations**
    a. **Alphabetic Index abbreviations**
        NEC   "Not elsewhere classifiable"
        This abbreviation in the Alphabetic Index represents "other specified". When a specific code is not available for a condition, the Alphabetic Index directs the coder to the "other specified" code in the Tabular List.
        NOS   "Not otherwise specified"
        This abbreviation is the equivalent of unspecified.
    b. **Tabular List abbreviations**
        NEC   "Not elsewhere classifiable"
        This abbreviation in the Tabular List represents "other specified". When a specific code is not available for a condition the Tabular List includes an NEC entry under a code to identify the code as the "other specified" code.
        NOS   "Not otherwise specified"
        This abbreviation is the equivalent of unspecified.

7. **Punctuation**
    [ ]   Brackets are used in the Tabular List to enclose synonyms, alternative wording or explanatory phrases. Brackets are used in the Alphabetic Index to identify manifestation codes.
    ( )   Parentheses are used in both the Alphabetic Index and Tabular List to enclose supplementary words that may be present or absent in the statement of a disease or procedure without affecting the code number to which it is assigned. The terms within the parentheses are referred to as nonessential modifiers. **The nonessential modifiers in the Alphabetic Index to Diseases apply to subterms following a main term except when a nonessential modifier and a subentry are mutually exclusive, the subentry takes precedence. For example, in the ICD-10-CM Alphabetic Index under the main term Enteritis, "acute" is a nonessential modifier and "chronic" is a subentry. In this case, the nonessential modifier "acute" does not apply to the subentry "chronic".**
    :   Colons are used in the Tabular List after an incomplete term which needs one or more of the modifiers following the colon to make it assignable to a given category.

8. **Use of "and"**
    See Section I.A.14. Use of the term "And"

9. **Other and Unspecified codes**
    a. **"Other" codes**
        Codes titled "other" or "other specified" are for use when the information in the medical record provides detail for which a specific code does not exist. Alphabetic Index entries with NEC in the line designate "other" codes in the Tabular List. These Alphabetic Index entries represent specific disease entities for which no specific code exists so the term is included within an "other" code.
    b. **"Unspecified" codes**
        Codes titled "unspecified" are for use when the information in the medical record is insufficient to assign a more specific code. For those categories for which an unspecified code is not provided, the "other specified" code may represent both other and unspecified.
        See Section I.B.18 Use of Signs/Symptom/Unspecified Codes

10. **Includes Notes**
    This note appears immediately under a three character code title to further define, or give examples of, the content of the category.

11. **Inclusion Terms**
    List of terms is included under some codes. These terms are the conditions for which that code is to be used. The terms may be synonyms of the code title, or, in the case of "other specified" codes, the terms are a list of the various conditions assigned to that code. The inclusion terms are not necessarily exhaustive. Additional terms found only in the Alphabetic Index may also be assigned to a code.

12. **Excludes Notes**
    The ICD-10-CM has two types of excludes notes. Each type of note has a different definition for use but they are all similar in that they indicate that codes excluded from each other are independent of each other.
    a. **Excludes1**
        A type 1 Excludes note is a pure excludes note. It means "NOT CODED HERE!" An Excludes1 note indicates that the code excluded should never be used at the same time as the code above the Excludes1 note. An Excludes1 is used when two conditions cannot occur together, such as a congenital form versus an acquired form of the same condition.
    b. **Excludes2**
        A type 2 Excludes note represents "Not included here". An excludes2 note indicates that the condition excluded is not part of the condition represented by the code, but a patient may have both conditions at the same time. When an Excludes2 note appears under a code, it is acceptable to use both the code and the excluded code together, when appropriate.

13. **Etiology/manifestation convention ("code first", "use additional code" and "in diseases classified elsewhere" notes)**
    Certain conditions have both an underlying etiology and multiple body system manifestations due to the underlying etiology. For such conditions, the ICD-10-CM has a coding convention that requires the underlying condition be sequenced first followed by the manifestation.

Wherever such a combination exists, there is a "use additional code" note at the etiology code, and a "code first" note at the manifestation code. These instructional notes indicate the proper sequencing order of the codes, etiology followed by manifestation.

In most cases the manifestation codes will have in the code title, "in diseases classified elsewhere." Codes with this title are a component of the etiology/ manifestation convention. The code title indicates that it is a manifestation code. "In diseases classified elsewhere" codes are never permitted to be used as first-listed or principal diagnosis codes. They must be used in conjunction with an underlying condition code and they must be listed following the underlying condition. See category F02, Dementia in other diseases classified elsewhere, for an example of this convention.

There are manifestation codes that do not have "in diseases classified elsewhere" in the title. For such codes, there is a "use additional code" note at the etiology code and a "code first" note at the manifestation code and the rules for sequencing apply.

In addition to the notes in the Tabular List, these conditions also have a specific Alphabetic Index entry structure. In the Alphabetic Index both conditions are listed together with the etiology code first followed by the manifestation codes in brackets. The code in brackets is always to be sequenced second.

An example of the etiology/manifestation convention is dementia in Parkinson's disease. In the Alphabetic Index, code G20 is listed first, followed by code F02.80 or F02.81 in brackets. Code G20 represents the underlying etiology, Parkinson's disease, and must be sequenced first, whereas codes F02.80 and F02.81 represent the manifestation of dementia in diseases classified elsewhere, with or without behavioral disturbance.

"Code first" and "Use additional code" notes are also used as sequencing rules in the classification for certain codes that are not part of an etiology/ manifestation combination.

See Section I.B.7. Multiple coding for a single condition.

14. "And"

The word "and" should be interpreted to mean either "and" or "or" when it appears in a title.

For example, cases of "tuberculosis of bones", "tuberculosis of joints" and "tuberculosis of bones and joints" are classified to subcategory A18.0, Tuberculosis of bones and joints.

15. "With"

The word "with" should be interpreted to mean "associated with" or "due to" when it appears in a code title, the Alphabetic Index, or an instructional note in the Tabular List.

The word "with" in the Alphabetic Index is sequenced immediately following the main term, not in alphabetical order.

16. "See" and "See Also"

The "see" instruction following a main term in the Alphabetic Index indicates that another term should be referenced. It is necessary to go to the main term referenced with the "see" note to locate the correct code.

A "see also" instruction following a main term in the Alphabetic Index instructs that there is another main term that may also be referenced that may provide additional Alphabetic Index entries that may be useful. It is not necessary to follow the "see also" note when the original main term provides the necessary code.

17. "Code also note"

A "code also" note instructs that two codes may be required to fully describe a condition, but this note does not provide sequencing direction.

18. Default codes

A code listed next to a main term in the ICD-10-CM Alphabetic Index is referred to as a default code. The default code represents that condition that is most commonly associated with the main term, or is the unspecified code for the condition. If a condition is documented in a medical record (for example, appendicitis) without any additional information, such as acute or chronic, the default code should be assigned.

B. General Coding Guidelines

1. Locating a code in the ICD-10-CM

To select a code in the classification that corresponds to a diagnosis or reason for visit documented in a medical record, first locate the term in the Alphabetic Index, and then verify the code in the Tabular List. Read and be guided by instructional notations that appear in both the Alphabetic Index and the Tabular List.

It is essential to use both the Alphabetic Index and Tabular List when locating and assigning a code. The Alphabetic Index does not always provide the full code. Selection of the full code, including laterality and any applicable 7th character can only be done in the Tabular List. A dash (-) at the end of an Alphabetic Index entry indicates that additional characters are required. Even if a dash is not included at the Alphabetic Index entry, it is necessary to refer to the Tabular List to verify that no 7th character is required.

2. Level of Detail in Coding

Diagnosis codes are to be used and reported at their highest number of characters available.

ICD-10-CM diagnosis codes are composed of codes with 3, 4, 5, 6 or 7 characters. Codes with three characters are included in ICD-10-CM as the heading of a category of codes that may be further subdivided by the use of fourth and/or fifth characters and/or sixth characters, which provide greater detail.

A three-character code is to be used only if it is not further subdivided. A code is invalid if it has not been coded to the full number of characters required for that code, including the 7th character, if applicable.

3. Code or codes from A00.0 through T88.9, Z00-Z99.8

The appropriate code or codes from A00.0 through T88.9, Z00-Z99.8 must be used to identify diagnoses, symptoms, conditions, problems, complaints or other reason(s) for the encounter/visit.

4. Signs and symptoms

Codes that describe symptoms and signs, as opposed to diagnoses, are acceptable for reporting purposes when a related definitive diagnosis has not been established (confirmed) by the provider. Chapter 18 of ICD-10-CM, Symptoms, Signs, and Abnormal Clinical and Laboratory Findings, Not Elsewhere Classified (codes R00.0 - R99) contains many, but not all codes for symptoms.

See Section I.B.18 Use of Signs/Symptom/Unspecified Codes

5. Conditions that are an integral part of a disease process

Signs and symptoms that are associated routinely with a disease process should not be assigned as additional codes, unless otherwise instructed by the classification.

6. Conditions that are not an integral part of a disease process

Additional signs and symptoms that may not be associated routinely with a disease process should be coded when present.

7. Multiple coding for a single condition

In addition to the etiology/manifestation convention that requires two codes to fully describe a single condition that affects multiple body systems, there are other single conditions that also require more than one code. "Use additional code" notes are found in the Tabular List at codes that are not part of an etiology/manifestation pair where a secondary code is useful to fully describe a condition. The sequencing rule is the same as the etiology/manifestation pair, "use additional code" indicates that a secondary code should be added.

For example, for bacterial infections that are not included in chapter 1, a secondary code from category B95, Streptococcus, Staphylococcus, and Enterococcus, as the cause of diseases classified elsewhere, or B96, Other bacterial agents as the cause of diseases classified elsewhere, may be required to identify the bacterial organism causing the infection. A "use additional code" note will normally be found at the infectious disease code, indicating a need for the organism code to be added as a secondary code.

"Code first" notes are also under certain codes that are not specifically manifestation codes but may be due to an underlying cause. When there is a "code first" note and an underlying condition is present, the underlying condition should be sequenced first.

"Code, if applicable, any causal condition first", notes indicate that this code may be assigned as a principal diagnosis when the causal condition is unknown or not applicable. If a causal condition is known, then the code for that condition should be sequenced as the principal or first-listed diagnosis.

Multiple codes may be needed for sequela, complication codes and obstetric codes to more fully describe a condition. See the specific guidelines for these conditions for further instruction.

8. Acute and Chronic Conditions

If the same condition is described as both acute (subacute) and chronic, and separate subentries exist in the Alphabetic Index at the same indentation level, code both and sequence the acute (subacute) code first.

9. Combination Code

A combination code is a single code used to classify:

> Two diagnoses, or
>> A diagnosis with an associated secondary process (manifestation)
>> A diagnosis with an associated complication

Combination codes are identified by referring to subterm entries in the Alphabetic Index and by reading the inclusion and exclusion notes in the Tabular List.

Assign only the combination code when that code fully identifies the diagnostic conditions involved or when the Alphabetic Index so directs. Multiple coding should not be used when the classification provides a combination code that clearly identifies all of the elements documented in the diagnosis. When the combination code lacks necessary specificity in describing the manifestation or complication, an additional code should be used as a secondary code.

10. Sequela (Late Effects)

A sequela is the residual effect (condition produced) after the acute phase of an illness or injury has terminated. There is no time limit on when a sequela code can be used. The residual may be apparent early, such as in cerebral infarction, or it may occur months or years later, such as that due to a previous injury. Coding of sequela generally requires two codes sequenced in the following order: The condition or nature of the sequela is sequenced first. The sequela code is sequenced second.

An exception to the above guidelines are those instances where the code for the sequela is followed by a manifestation code identified in the Tabular List and title, or the sequela code has been expanded (at the fourth, fifth or sixth character levels) to include the manifestation(s). The code for the acute phase of an illness or injury that led to the sequela is never used with a code for the late effect.

See Section I.C.9. Sequelae of cerebrovascular disease

See Section I.C.15. Sequelae of complication of pregnancy, childbirth and the puerperium

See Section I.C.19. Application of 7th characters for Chapter 19

11. Impending or Threatened Condition

Code any condition described at the time of discharge as "impending" or "threatened" as follows:

> If it did occur, code as confirmed diagnosis.
> If it did not occur, reference the Alphabetic Index to determine if the condition has a subentry term for "impending" or "threatened" and also reference main term entries for "Impending" and for "Threatened."
> If the subterms are listed, assign the given code.
> If the subterms are not listed, code the existing underlying condition(s) and not the condition described as impending or threatened.

12. Reporting Same Diagnosis Code More than Once

Each unique ICD-10-CM diagnosis code may be reported only once for an encounter. This applies to bilateral conditions when there are no distinct codes identifying laterality or two different conditions classified to the same ICD-10-CM diagnosis code.

13. Laterality

Some ICD-10-CM codes indicate laterality, specifying whether the condition occurs on the left, right or is bilateral. If no bilateral code is provided and the condition is bilateral, assign separate codes for both the left and right side. If the side is not identified in the medical record, assign the code for the unspecified side.

14. Documentation for BMI, Non-pressure Ulcers and Pressure Ulcer Stages

For the Body Mass Index (BMI), depth of non-pressure chronic ulcers and pressure ulcer stage codes, code assignment may be based on medical record documentation from clinicians who are not the patient's provider (i.e., physician or other qualified healthcare practitioner legally accountable for establishing the patient's diagnosis), since this information is typically documented by other clinicians involved in the care of the patient (e.g., a dietitian often documents the BMI and nurses often documents the pressure ulcer stages). However, the associated diagnosis (such as overweight, obesity, or pressure ulcer) must be documented by the patient's provider. If there is conflicting medical record documentation, either from the same clinician or different clinicians, the patient's attending provider should be queried for clarification.

The BMI codes should only be reported as secondary diagnoses. As with all other secondary diagnosis codes, the BMI codes should only be assigned when they meet the definition of a reportable additional diagnosis (see Section III, Reporting Additional Diagnoses).

15. Syndromes

Follow the Alphabetic Index guidance when coding syndromes. In the absence of Alphabetic Index guidance, assign codes for the documented manifestations of the syndrome.

Additional codes for manifestations that are not an integral part of the disease process may also be assigned when the condition does not have a unique code.

16. Documentation of Complications of Care

Code assignment is based on the provider's documentation of the relationship between the condition and the care or procedure. The guideline extends to any complications of care, regardless of the chapter the code is located in. It is important to note that not all conditions that occur during or following medical care or surgery are classified as complications. There must be a cause-and-effect relationship between the care provided and the condition, and an indication in the documentation that it is a complication. Query the provider for clarification, if the complication is not clearly documented.

17. Borderline Diagnosis

If the provider documents a "borderline" diagnosis at the time of discharge, the diagnosis is coded as confirmed, unless the classification provides a specific entry (e.g., borderline diabetes). If a borderline condition has a specific index entry in ICD-10-CM, it should be coded as such. Since borderline conditions are not uncertain diagnoses, no distinction is made between the care setting (inpatient versus outpatient). Whenever the documentation is unclear regarding a borderline condition, coders are encouraged to query for clarification.

18. Use of Sign/Symptom/Unspecified Codes

Sign/symptom and "unspecified" codes have acceptable, even necessary, uses. While specific diagnosis codes should be reported when they are supported by the available medical record documentation and clinical knowledge of the patient's health condition, there are instances when signs/symptoms or unspecified codes are the best choices for accurately reflecting the healthcare encounter. Each healthcare encounter should be coded to the level of certainty known for that encounter.

If a definitive diagnosis has not been established by the end of the encounter, it is appropriate to report codes for sign(s) and/or symptom(s) in lieu of a definitive diagnosis. When sufficient clinical information isn't known or available about a particular health condition to assign a more specific code, it is acceptable to report the appropriate "unspecified" code (e.g., a diagnosis of pneumonia has been determined, but not the specific type). Unspecified codes should be reported when they are the codes that most accurately reflects what is known about the patient's condition at the time of that particular encounter. It would be inappropriate to select a specific code that is not supported by the medical record documentation or conduct medically unnecessary diagnostic testing in order to determine a more specific code.

C. Chapter-Specific Coding Guidelines

In addition to general coding guidelines, there are guidelines for specific diagnoses and/or conditions in the classification. Unless otherwise indicated, these guidelines apply to all health care settings. Please refer to Section II for guidelines on the selection of principal diagnosis.

1. **Chapter 1: Certain Infectious and Parasitic Diseases (A00-B99)**
   a. **Human immunodeficiency virus (HIV) infections**
      1) **Code only confirmed cases**

         Code only confirmed cases of HIV infection/illness. This is an exception to the hospital inpatient guideline Section II, H.

         In this context, "confirmation" does not require documentation of positive serology or culture for HIV; the provider's diagnostic statement that the patient is HIV positive, or has an HIV-related illness is sufficient.

      2) **Selection and sequencing of HIV codes**
         (a) **Patient admitted for HIV-related condition**

            If a patient is admitted for an HIV-related condition, the principal diagnosis should be B20, Human immunodeficiency virus [HIV] disease followed by additional diagnosis codes for all reported HIV-related conditions.

         (b) **Patient with HIV disease admitted for unrelated condition**

            If a patient with HIV disease is admitted for an unrelated condition (such as a traumatic injury), the code for the unrelated condition (e.g., the nature of injury code) should be the principal diagnosis. Other diagnoses would be B20 followed by additional diagnosis codes for all reported HIV-related conditions.

         (c) **Whether the patient is newly diagnosed**

            Whether the patient is newly diagnosed or has had previous admissions/encounters for HIV conditions is irrelevant to the sequencing decision.

         (d) **Asymptomatic human immunodeficiency virus**

            Z21, Asymptomatic human immunodeficiency virus [HIV] infection status, is to be applied when the patient without any documentation of symptoms is listed as being "HIV positive," "known HIV," "HIV test positive," or similar terminology. Do not use this code if the term "AIDS" is used or if the patient is treated for any HIV-related illness or is described as having any condition(s) resulting from his/her HIV positive status; use B20 in these cases.

         (e) **Patients with inconclusive HIV serology**

            Patients with inconclusive HIV serology, but no definitive diagnosis or manifestations of the illness, may be assigned code R75, Inconclusive laboratory evidence of human immunodeficiency virus [HIV].

         (f) **Previously diagnosed HIV-related illness**

            Patients with any known prior diagnosis of an HIV-related illness should be coded to B20. Once a patient has developed an HIV-related illness, the patient should always be assigned code B20 on every subsequent admission/encounter. Patients previously diagnosed with any HIV illness (B20) should never be assigned to R75 or Z21, Asymptomatic human immunodeficiency virus [HIV] infection status.

         (g) **HIV infection in pregnancy, childbirth and the puerperium**

            During pregnancy, childbirth or the puerperium, a patient admitted (or presenting for a health care encounter) because of an HIV-related illness should receive a principal diagnosis code of O98.7-, Human immunodeficiency [HIV] disease complicating pregnancy, childbirth and the puerperium, followed by B20 and the code(s) for the HIV-related illness(es). Codes from Chapter 15 always take sequencing priority.

            Patients with asymptomatic HIV infection status admitted (or presenting for a health care encounter) during pregnancy, childbirth, or the puerperium should receive codes of O98.7- and Z21.

      (h) **Encounters for testing for HIV**

         If a patient is being seen to determine his/her HIV status, use code Z11.4, Encounter for screening for human immunodeficiency virus [HIV]. Use additional codes for any associated high risk behavior.

         If a patient with signs or symptoms is being seen for HIV testing, code the signs and symptoms. An additional counseling code Z71.7, Human immunodeficiency virus [HIV] counseling, may be used if counseling is provided during the encounter for the test.

         When a patient returns to be informed of his/her HIV test results and the test result is negative, use code Z71.7, Human immunodeficiency virus [HIV] counseling.

         If the results are positive, see previous guidelines and assign codes as appropriate.

   b. **Infectious agents as the cause of diseases classified to other chapters**

      Certain infections are classified in chapters other than Chapter 1 and no organism is identified as part of the infection code. In these instances, it is necessary to use an additional code from Chapter 1 to identify the organism. A code from category B95, Streptococcus, Staphylococcus, and Enterococcus as the cause of diseases classified to other chapters, B96, Other bacterial agents as the cause of diseases classified to other chapters, or B97, Viral agents as the cause of diseases classified to other chapters, is to be used as an additional code to identify the organism. An instructional note will be found at the infection code advising that an additional organism code is required.

   c. **Infections resistant to antibiotics**

      Many bacterial infections are resistant to current antibiotics. It is necessary to identify all infections documented as antibiotic resistant. Assign a code from category Z16, Resistance to antimicrobial drugs, following the infection code only if the infection code does not identify drug resistance.

   d. **Sepsis, severe sepsis, and septic shock**
      1) **Coding of sepsis and severe sepsis**
         (a) **Sepsis**

            For a diagnosis of sepsis, assign the appropriate code for the underlying systemic infection. If the type of infection or causal organism is not further specified, assign code A41.9, Sepsis, unspecified organism.

            A code from subcategory R65.2, Severe sepsis, should not be assigned unless severe sepsis or an associated acute organ dysfunction is documented.

            (i) Negative or inconclusive blood cultures and sepsis
               Negative or inconclusive blood cultures do not preclude a diagnosis of sepsis in patients with clinical evidence of the condition, however, the provider should be queried.

            (ii) Urosepsis
               The term urosepsis is a nonspecific term. It is not to be considered synonymous with sepsis. It has no default code in the Alphabetic Index. Should a provider use this term, he/she must be queried for clarification.

            (iii) Sepsis with organ dysfunction
               If a patient has sepsis and associated acute organ dysfunction or multiple organ dysfunction (MOD), follow the instructions for coding severe sepsis.

            (iv) Acute organ dysfunction that is not clearly associated with the sepsis
               If a patient has sepsis and an acute organ dysfunction, but the medical record documentation indicates that the acute organ dysfunction is related to a medical condition other than the sepsis, do not assign a code from subcategory R65.2, Severe sepsis. An acute organ dysfunction must be associated with the sepsis in order to assign the severe sepsis code. If the documentation is not clear as to whether an acute organ dysfunction is related to the sepsis or another medical condition, query the provider.

(b) Severe sepsis

The coding of severe sepsis requires a minimum of 2 codes: first a code for the underlying systemic infection, followed by a code from subcategory R65.2, Severe sepsis. If the causal organism is not documented, assign code A41.9, Sepsis, unspecified organism, for the infection. Additional code(s) for the associated acute organ dysfunction are also required.

Due to the complex nature of severe sepsis, some cases may require querying the provider prior to assignment of the codes.

2) Septic shock

(a) Septic shock generally refers to circulatory failure associated with severe sepsis, and therefore, it represents a type of acute organ dysfunction.

For cases of septic shock, the code for the systemic infection should be sequenced first, followed by code R65.21, Severe sepsis with septic shock or code T81.12, Postprocedural septic shock. Any additional codes for the other acute organ dysfunctions should also be assigned. As noted in the sequencing instructions in the Tabular List, the code for septic shock cannot be assigned as a principal diagnosis.

3) Sequencing of severe sepsis

If severe sepsis is present on admission, and meets the definition of principal diagnosis, the underlying systemic infection should be assigned as principal diagnosis followed by the appropriate code from subcategory R65.2 as required by the sequencing rules in the Tabular List. A code from subcategory R65.2 can never be assigned as a principal diagnosis.

When severe sepsis develops during an encounter (it was not present on admission) the underlying systemic infection and the appropriate code from subcategory R65.2 should be assigned as secondary diagnoses.

Severe sepsis may be present on admission but the diagnosis may not be confirmed until sometime after admission. If the documentation is not clear whether severe sepsis was present on admission, the provider should be queried.

4) Sepsis and severe sepsis with a localized infection

If the reason for admission is both sepsis or severe sepsis and a localized infection, such as pneumonia or cellulitis, a code(s) for the underlying systemic infection should be assigned first and the code for the localized infection should be assigned as a secondary diagnosis. If the patient has severe sepsis, a code from subcategory R65.2 should also be assigned as a secondary diagnosis. If the patient is admitted with a localized infection, such as pneumonia, and sepsis/severe sepsis doesn't develop until after admission, the localized infection should be assigned first, followed by the appropriate sepsis/severe sepsis codes.

5) Sepsis due to a postprocedural infection

(a) Documentation of causal relationship

As with all postprocedural complications, code assignment is based on the provider's documentation of the relationship between the infection and the procedure.

(b) Sepsis due to a postprocedural infection

For such cases, the postprocedural infection code, such as, T80.2, Infections following infusion, transfusion, and therapeutic injection, T81.4, Infection following a procedure, T88.0, Infection following immunization, or O86.0, Infection of obstetric surgical wound, should be coded first, followed by the code for the specific infection. If the patient has severe sepsis the appropriate code from subcategory R65.2 should also be assigned with the additional code(s) for any acute organ dysfunction.

(c) Postprocedural infection and postprocedural septic shock

In cases where a postprocedural infection has occurred and has resulted in severe sepsis and postprocedural septic shock, the code for the precipitating complication such as code T81.4, Infection following a procedure, or O86.0, Infection of obstetrical surgical wound should be coded first followed by

code R65.21, Severe sepsis with septic shock and a code for the systemic infection.

6) Sepsis and severe sepsis associated with a noninfectious process (condition)

In some cases a noninfectious process (condition), such as trauma, may lead to an infection which can result in sepsis or severe sepsis. If sepsis or severe sepsis is documented as associated with a noninfectious condition, such as a burn or serious injury, and this condition meets the definition for principal diagnosis, the code for the noninfectious condition should be sequenced first, followed by the code for the resulting infection. If severe sepsis, is present a code from subcategory R65.2 should also be assigned with any associated organ dysfunction(s) codes. It is not necessary to assign a code from subcategory R65.1, Systemic inflammatory response syndrome (SIRS) of non-infectious origin, for these cases.

If the infection meets the definition of principal diagnosis it should be sequenced before the non-infectious condition. When both the associated non-infectious condition and the infection meet the definition of principal diagnosis either may be assigned as principal diagnosis.

Only one code from category R65, Symptoms and signs specifically associated with systemic inflammation and infection, should be assigned. Therefore, when a non-infectious condition leads to an infection resulting in severe sepsis, assign the appropriate code from subcategory R65.2, Severe sepsis. Do not additionally assign a code from subcategory R65.1, Systemic inflammatory response syndrome (SIRS) of non-infectious origin.

See Section I.C.18. SIRS due to non-infectious process

7) Sepsis and septic shock complicating abortion, pregnancy, childbirth, and the puerperium

See Section I.C.15. Sepsis and septic shock complicating abortion, pregnancy, childbirth and the puerperium

8) Newborn sepsis

See Section I.C.16. f. Bacterial sepsis of Newborn

e. Methicillin resistant *Staphylococcus aureus* (MRSA) conditions

1) Selection and sequencing of MRSA codes

(a) Combination codes for MRSA infection

When a patient is diagnosed with an infection that is due to methicillin resistant *Staphylococcus aureus* (MRSA), and that infection has a combination code that includes the causal organism (e.g., sepsis, pneumonia) assign the appropriate combination code for the condition (e.g., code A41.02, Sepsis due to Methicillin resistant *Staphylococcus aureus* or code J15.212, Pneumonia due to Methicillin resistant *Staphylococcus aureus*). Do not assign code B95.62, Methicillin resistant *Staphylococcus aureus* infection as the cause of diseases classified elsewhere, as an additional code because the combination code includes the type of infection and the MRSA organism. Do not assign a code from subcategory Z16.11, Resistance to penicillins, as an additional diagnosis.

See Section C.1. for instructions on coding and sequencing of sepsis and severe sepsis.

(b) Other codes for MRSA infection

When there is documentation of a current infection (e.g., wound infection, stitch abscess, urinary tract infection) due to MRSA, and that infection does not have a combination code that includes the causal organism, assign the appropriate code to identify the condition along with code B95.62, Methicillin resistant *Staphylococcus aureus* infection as the cause of diseases classified elsewhere for the MRSA infection. Do not assign a code from subcategory Z16.11, Resistance to penicillins.

(c) Methicillin susceptible *Staphylococcus aureus* (MSSA) and MRSA colonization

The condition or state of being colonized or carrying MSSA or MRSA is called colonization or carriage, while an individual person is described as being colonized or being a carrier. Colonization means that MSSA or MSRA is present on or in the body without necessarily causing illness. A positive MRSA colonization test might be documented by the provider as "MRSA screen positive" or "MRSA nasal swab positive".

Assign code Z22.322, Carrier or suspected carrier of Methicillin resistant *Staphylococcus aureus*, for patients documented as having MRSA colonization. Assign code Z22.321, Carrier or suspected carrier of Methicillin susceptible *Staphylococcus aureus*, for patient documented as having MSSA colonization. Colonization is not necessarily indicative of a disease process or as the cause of a specific condition the patient may have unless documented as such by the provider.

(d) MRSA colonization and infection

If a patient is documented as having both MRSA colonization and infection during a hospital admission, code Z22.322, Carrier or suspected carrier of Methicillin resistant *Staphylococcus aureus*, and a code for the MRSA infection may both be assigned.

2. Chapter 2: Neoplasms (C00-D49)

General guidelines

Chapter 2 of the ICD-10-CM contains the codes for most benign and all malignant neoplasms. Certain benign neoplasms, such as prostatic adenomas, may be found in the specific body system chapters. To properly code a neoplasm it is necessary to determine from the record if the neoplasm is benign, in-situ, malignant, or of uncertain histologic behavior. If malignant, any secondary (metastatic) sites should also be determined.

Primary malignant neoplasms overlapping site boundaries

A primary malignant neoplasm that overlaps two or more contiguous (next to each other) sites should be classified to the subcategory/code .8 ('overlapping lesion'), unless the combination is specifically indexed elsewhere. For multiple neoplasms of the same site that are not contiguous such as tumors in different quadrants of the same breast, codes for each site should be assigned.

Malignant neoplasm of ectopic tissue

Malignant neoplasms of ectopic tissue are to be coded to the site of origin mentioned, e.g., ectopic pancreatic malignant neoplasms involving the stomach are coded to pancreas, unspecified (C25.9).

The neoplasm table in the Alphabetic Index should be referenced first. However, if the histological term is documented, that term should be referenced first, rather than going immediately to the Neoplasm Table, in order to determine which column in the Neoplasm Table is appropriate. For example, if the documentation indicates "adenoma," refer to the term in the Alphabetic Index to review the entries under this term and the instructional note to "see also neoplasm, by site, benign." The table provides the proper code based on the type of neoplasm and the site. It is important to select the proper column in the table that corresponds to the type of neoplasm. The Tabular List should then be referenced to verify that the correct code has been selected from the table and that a more specific site code does not exist.

See Section I.C.21. Factors influencing health status and contact with health services, Status, for information regarding Z15.0, codes for genetic susceptibility to cancer.

a. Treatment directed at the malignancy

If the treatment is directed at the malignancy, designate the malignancy as the principal diagnosis.

The only exception to this guideline is if a patient admission/encounter is solely for the administration of chemotherapy, immunotherapy or radiation therapy, assign the appropriate Z51.- code as the first-listed or principal diagnosis, and the diagnosis or problem for which the service is being performed as a secondary diagnosis.

b. Treatment of secondary site

When a patient is admitted because of a primary neoplasm with metastasis and treatment is directed toward the secondary site only, the secondary neoplasm is designated as the principal diagnosis even though the primary malignancy is still present.

c. Coding and sequencing of complications

Coding and sequencing of complications associated with the malignancies or with the therapy thereof are subject to the following guidelines:

1) Anemia associated with malignancy

When admission/encounter is for management of an anemia associated with the malignancy, and the treatment is only for anemia, the appropriate code for the malignancy is sequenced as the principal or first-listed diagnosis followed by the appropriate code for the anemia (such as code D63.0, Anemia in neoplastic disease).

2) Anemia associated with chemotherapy, immunotherapy and radiation therapy

When the admission/encounter is for management of an anemia associated with an adverse effect of the administration of chemotherapy or immunotherapy and the only treatment is for the anemia, the anemia code is sequenced first followed by the appropriate codes for the neoplasm and the adverse effect (T45.1X5, Adverse effect of antineoplastic and immunosuppressive drugs).

When the admission/encounter is for management of an anemia associated with an adverse effect of radiotherapy, the anemia code should be sequenced first, followed by the appropriate neoplasm code and code Y84.2, Radiological procedure and radiotherapy as the cause of abnormal reaction of the patient, or of later complication, without mention of misadventure at the time of the procedure.

3) Management of dehydration due to the malignancy

When the admission/encounter is for management of dehydration due to the malignancy and only the dehydration is being treated (intravenous rehydration), the dehydration is sequenced first, followed by the code(s) for the malignancy.

4) Treatment of a complication resulting from a surgical procedure

When the admission/encounter is for treatment of a complication resulting from a surgical procedure, designate the complication as the principal or first-listed diagnosis if treatment is directed at resolving the complication.

d. Primary malignancy previously excised

When a primary malignancy has been previously excised or eradicated from its site and there is no further treatment directed to that site and there is no evidence of any existing primary malignancy, a code from category Z85, Personal history of malignant neoplasm, should be used to indicate the former site of the malignancy. Any mention of extension, invasion, or metastasis to another site is coded as a secondary malignant neoplasm to that site. The secondary site may be the principal or first-listed with the Z85 code used as a secondary code.

e. Admissions/Encounters involving chemotherapy, immunotherapy and radiation therapy

1) Episode of care involves surgical removal of neoplasm

When an episode of care involves the surgical removal of a neoplasm, primary or secondary site, followed by adjunct chemotherapy or radiation treatment during the same episode of care, the code for the neoplasm should be assigned as principal or first-listed diagnosis.

2) Patient admission/encounter solely for administration of chemotherapy, immunotherapy and radiation therapy

If a patient admission/encounter is solely for the administration of chemotherapy, immunotherapy or radiation therapy assign code Z51.0, Encounter for antineoplastic radiation therapy, or Z51.11, Encounter for antineoplastic chemotherapy, or Z51.12, Encounter for antineoplastic immunotherapy as the first-listed or principal diagnosis. If a patient receives more than one of these therapies during the same admission more than one of these codes may be assigned, in any sequence.

The malignancy for which the therapy is being administered should be assigned as a secondary diagnosis.

3) **Patient admitted for radiation therapy, chemotherapy or immunotherapy and develops complications**
When a patient is admitted for the purpose of radiotherapy, immunotherapy or chemotherapy and develops complications such as uncontrolled nausea and vomiting or dehydration, the principal or first-listed diagnosis is Z51.Ø, Encounter for antineoplastic radiation therapy, or Z51.11, Encounter for antineoplastic chemotherapy, or Z51.12, Encounter for antineoplastic immunotherapy followed by any codes for the complications.

f. **Admission/encounter to determine extent of malignancy**
When the reason for admission/encounter is to determine the extent of the malignancy, or for a procedure such as paracentesis or thoracentesis, the primary malignancy or appropriate metastatic site is designated as the principal or first-listed diagnosis, even though chemotherapy or radiotherapy is administered.

g. **Symptoms, signs, and abnormal findings listed in Chapter 18 associated with neoplasms**
Symptoms, signs, and ill-defined conditions listed in Chapter 18 characteristic of, or associated with, an existing primary or secondary site malignancy cannot be used to replace the malignancy as principal or first-listed diagnosis, regardless of the number of admissions or encounters for treatment and care of the neoplasm.

See section I.C.21. Factors influencing health status and contact with health services, Encounter for prophylactic organ removal.

h. **Admission/encounter for pain control/management**
See Section I.C.6. for information on coding admission/encounter for pain control/management.

i. **Malignancy in two or more noncontiguous sites**
A patient may have more than one malignant tumor in the same organ. These tumors may represent different primaries or metastatic disease, depending on the site. Should the documentation be unclear, the provider should be queried as to the status of each tumor so that the correct codes can be assigned.

j. **Disseminated malignant neoplasm, unspecified**
Code C8Ø.Ø, Disseminated malignant neoplasm, unspecified, is for use only in those cases where the patient has advanced metastatic disease and no known primary or secondary sites are specified. It should not be used in place of assigning codes for the primary site and all known secondary sites.

k. **Malignant neoplasm without specification of site**
Code C8Ø.1, Malignant (primary) neoplasm, unspecified, equates to Cancer, unspecified. This code should only be used when no determination can be made as to the primary site of a malignancy. This code should rarely be used in the inpatient setting.

l. **Sequencing of neoplasm codes**

1) **Encounter for treatment of primary malignancy**
If the reason for the encounter is for treatment of a primary malignancy, assign the malignancy as the principal/first-listed diagnosis. The primary site is to be sequenced first, followed by any metastatic sites.

2) **Encounter for treatment of secondary malignancy**
When an encounter is for a primary malignancy with metastasis and treatment is directed toward the metastatic (secondary) site(s) only, the metastatic site(s) is designated as the principal/first-listed diagnosis. The primary malignancy is coded as an additional code.

3) **Malignant neoplasm in a pregnant patient**
When a pregnant woman has a malignant neoplasm, a code from subcategory O9A.1-, Malignant neoplasm complicating pregnancy, childbirth, and the puerperium, should be sequenced first, followed by the appropriate code from Chapter 2 to indicate the type of neoplasm.

4) **Encounter for complication associated with a neoplasm**
When an encounter is for management of a complication associated with a neoplasm, such as dehydration, and the treatment is only for the complication, the complication is coded first, followed by the appropriate code(s) for the neoplasm.

The exception to this guideline is anemia. When the admission/encounter is for management of an anemia associated with the malignancy, and the treatment is only for anemia, the appropriate code for the malignancy is sequenced as the principal or first-listed diagnosis followed by code D63.Ø, Anemia in neoplastic disease.

5) **Complication from surgical procedure for treatment of a neoplasm**
When an encounter is for treatment of a complication resulting from a surgical procedure performed for the treatment of the neoplasm, designate the complication as the principal/first-listed diagnosis. See guideline regarding the coding of a current malignancy versus personal history to determine if the code for the neoplasm should also be assigned.

6) **Pathologic fracture due to a neoplasm**
When an encounter is for a pathological fracture due to a neoplasm, and the focus of treatment is the fracture, a code from subcategory M84.5, Pathological fracture in neoplastic disease, should be sequenced first, followed by the code for the neoplasm.

If the focus of treatment is the neoplasm with an associated pathological fracture, the neoplasm code should be sequenced first, followed by a code from M84.5 for the pathological fracture.

m. **Current malignancy versus personal history of malignancy**
When a primary malignancy has been excised but further treatment, such as an additional surgery for the malignancy, radiation therapy or chemotherapy is directed to that site, the primary malignancy code should be used until treatment is completed.

When a primary malignancy has been previously excised or eradicated from its site, there is no further treatment (of the malignancy) directed to that site, and there is no evidence of any existing primary malignancy, a code from category Z85, Personal history of malignant neoplasm, should be used to indicate the former site of the malignancy.

See Section I.C.21. Factors influencing health status and contact with health services, History (of)

n. **Leukemia, multiple myeloma, and malignant plasma cell neoplasms in remission versus personal history**
The categories for leukemia, and category C9Ø, Multiple myeloma and malignant plasma cell neoplasms, have codes indicating whether or not the leukemia has achieved remission. There are also codes Z85.6, Personal history of leukemia, and Z85.79, Personal history of other malignant neoplasms of lymphoid, hematopoietic and related tissues. If the documentation is unclear, as to whether the leukemia has achieved remission, the provider should be queried.

See Section I.C.21. Factors influencing health status and contact with health services, History (of)

o. **Aftercare following surgery for neoplasm**
See Section I.C.21. Factors influencing health status and contact with health services, Aftercare

p. **Follow-up care for completed treatment of a malignancy**
See Section I.C.21. Factors influencing health status and contact with health services, Follow-up

q. **Prophylactic organ removal for prevention of malignancy**
See Section I.C. 21, Factors influencing health status and contact with health services, Prophylactic organ removal

r. **Malignant neoplasm associated with transplanted organ**
A malignant neoplasm of a transplanted organ should be coded as a transplant complication. Assign first the appropriate code from category T86.-, Complications of transplanted organs and tissue, followed by code C8Ø.2, Malignant neoplasm associated with transplanted organ. Use an additional code for the specific malignancy.

3. **Chapter 3: Disease of the Blood and Blood-forming Organs and Certain Disorders Involving the Immune Mechanism (D5Ø-D89)**
Reserved for future guideline expansion

4. **Chapter 4: Endocrine, Nutritional, and Metabolic Diseases (E00-E89)**

    a. **Diabetes mellitus**

    The diabetes mellitus codes are combination codes that include the type of diabetes mellitus, the body system affected, and the complications affecting that body system. As many codes within a particular category as are necessary to describe all of the complications of the disease may be used. They should be sequenced based on the reason for a particular encounter. Assign as many codes from categories E08 – E13 as needed to identify all of the associated conditions that the patient has.

    1) **Type of diabetes**

    The age of a patient is not the sole determining factor, though most type 1 diabetics develop the condition before reaching puberty. For this reason type 1 diabetes mellitus is also referred to as juvenile diabetes.

    2) **Type of diabetes mellitus not documented**

    If the type of diabetes mellitus is not documented in the medical record the default is E11.-, Type 2 diabetes mellitus.

    3) **Diabetes mellitus and the use of insulin**

    If the documentation in a medical record does not indicate the type of diabetes but does indicate that the patient uses insulin, code E11, Type 2 diabetes mellitus, should be assigned. Code Z79.4, Long-term (current) use of insulin, should also be assigned to indicate that the patient uses insulin. Code Z79.4 should not be assigned if insulin is given temporarily to bring a type 2 patient's blood sugar under control during an encounter.

    4) **Diabetes mellitus in pregnancy and gestational diabetes**

    See Section I.C.15. Diabetes mellitus in pregnancy.

    See Section I.C.15. Gestational (pregnancy induced) diabetes

    5) **Complications due to insulin pump malfunction**

    (a) **Underdose of insulin due to insulin pump failure**

    An underdose of insulin due to an insulin pump failure should be assigned to a code from subcategory T85.6, Mechanical complication of other specified internal and external prosthetic devices, implants and grafts, that specifies the type of pump malfunction, as the principal or first-listed code, followed by code T38.3x6-, Underdosing of insulin and oral hypoglycemic [antidiabetic] drugs. Additional codes for the type of diabetes mellitus and any associated complications due to the underdosing should also be assigned.

    (b) **Overdose of insulin due to insulin pump failure**

    The principal or first-listed code for an encounter due to an insulin pump malfunction resulting in an overdose of insulin, should also be T85.6-, Mechanical complication of other specified internal and external prosthetic devices, implants and grafts, followed by code T38.3X1-, Poisoning by insulin and oral hypoglycemic [antidiabetic] drugs, accidental (unintentional).

    6) **Secondary diabetes mellitus**

    Codes under categories E08, Diabetes mellitus due to underlying condition, E09, Drug or chemical induced diabetes mellitus, and E13, Other specified diabetes mellitus, identify complications/manifestations associated with secondary diabetes mellitus. Secondary diabetes is always caused by another condition or event (e.g., cystic fibrosis, malignant neoplasm of pancreas, pancreatectomy, adverse effect of drug, or poisoning).

    (a) **Secondary diabetes mellitus and the use of insulin**

    For patients who routinely use insulin, code Z79.4, Long-term (current) use of insulin, should also be assigned. Code Z79.4 should not be assigned if insulin is given temporarily to bring a patient's blood sugar under control during an encounter.

    (b) **Assigning and sequencing secondary diabetes codes and its causes**

    The sequencing of the secondary diabetes codes in relationship to codes for the cause of the diabetes is based on the Tabular List instructions for categories E08, E09 and E13.

    (i) **Secondary diabetes mellitus due to pancreatectomy**

    For postpancreatectomy diabetes mellitus (lack of insulin due to the surgical removal of all or part of the pancreas), assign code E89.1, Postprocedural hypoinsulinemia. Assign a code from category E13 and a code from subcategory Z90.41-, Acquired absence of pancreas, as additional codes.

    (ii) **Secondary diabetes due to drugs**

    Secondary diabetes may be caused by an adverse effect of correctly administered medications, poisoning or sequela of poisoning.

    See section I.C.19.e for coding of adverse effects and poisoning, and section I.C.20 for external cause code reporting.

5. **Chapter 5: Mental, Behavioral and Neurodevelopmental Disorders (F01 – F99)**

    a. **Pain disorders related to psychological factors**

    Assign code F45.41, for pain that is exclusively related to psychological disorders. As indicated by the Excludes 1 note under category G89, a code from category G89 should not be assigned with code F45.41

    Code F45.42, Pain disorders with related psychological factors, should be used with a code from category G89, Pain, not elsewhere classified, if there is documentation of a psychological component for a patient with acute or chronic pain.

    See Section I.C.6. Pain

    b. **Mental and behavioral disorders due to psychoactive substance use**

    1) **In remission**

    Selection of codes for "in remission" for categories F10-F19, Mental and behavioral disorders due to psychoactive substance use (categories F10-F19 with -.21) requires the provider's clinical judgment. The appropriate codes for "in remission" are assigned only on the basis of provider documentation (as defined in the Official Guidelines for Coding and Reporting).

    2) **Psychoactive substance use, abuse and dependence**

    When the provider documentation refers to use, abuse and dependence of the same substance (e.g. alcohol, opioid, cannabis, etc.), only one code should be assigned to identify the pattern of use based on the following hierarchy:

    • If both use and abuse are documented, assign only the code for abuse

    • If both abuse and dependence are documented, assign only the code for dependence

    • If use, abuse and dependence are all documented, assign only the code for dependence

    • If both use and dependence are documented, assign only the code for dependence.

    3) **Psychoactive substance use**

    As with all other diagnoses, the codes for psychoactive substance use (F10.9-, F11.9-, F12.9-, F13.9-, F14.9-, F15.9-, F16.9-) should only be assigned based on provider documentation and when they meet the definition of a reportable diagnosis (see Section III, Reporting Additional Diagnoses). The codes are to be used only when the psychoactive substance use is associated with a mental or behavioral disorder, and such a relationship is documented by the provider.

6. **Chapter 6: Diseases of Nervous System (G00-G99)**

    a. **Dominant/nondominant side**

    Codes from category G81, Hemiplegia and hemiparesis, and subcategories, G83.1, Monoplegia of lower limb, G83.2, Monoplegia of upper limb, and G83.3, Monoplegia, unspecified, identify whether the dominant or nondominant side is affected. Should the affected side be documented, but not specified as dominant or nondominant, and the classification system does not indicate a default, code selection is as follows:

    • For ambidextrous patients, the default should be dominant.

    • If the left side is affected, the default is non-dominant.

- If the right side is affected, the default is dominant.

b. Pain - Category G89

1) General coding information

Codes in category G89, Pain, not elsewhere classified, may be used in conjunction with codes from other categories and chapters to provide more detail about acute or chronic pain and neoplasm-related pain, unless otherwise indicated below.

If the pain is not specified as acute or chronic, post-thoracotomy, postprocedural, or neoplasm-related, do not assign codes from category G89.

A code from category G89 should not be assigned if the underlying (definitive) diagnosis is known, unless the reason for the encounter is pain control/ management and not management of the underlying condition.

When an admission or encounter is for a procedure aimed at treating the underlying condition (e.g., spinal fusion, kyphoplasty), a code for the underlying condition (e.g., vertebral fracture, spinal stenosis) should be assigned as the principal diagnosis. No code from category G89 should be assigned.

(a) Category G89 codes as principal or first-listed diagnosis

Category G89 codes are acceptable as principal diagnosis or the first-listed code:

- When pain control or pain management is the reason for the admission/encounter (e.g., a patient with displaced intervertebral disc, nerve impingement and severe back pain presents for injection of steroid into the spinal canal). The underlying cause of the pain should be reported as an additional diagnosis, if known.

- When a patient is admitted for the insertion of a neurostimulator for pain control, assign the appropriate pain code as the principal or first-listed diagnosis. When an admission or encounter is for a procedure aimed at treating the underlying condition and a neurostimulator is inserted for pain control during the same admission/encounter, a code for the underlying condition should be assigned as the principal diagnosis and the appropriate pain code should be assigned as a secondary diagnosis.

(b) Use of category G89 codes in conjunction with site specific pain codes

(i) Assigning category G89 and site-specific pain codes

Codes from category G89 may be used in conjunction with codes that identify the site of pain (including codes from chapter 18) if the category G89 code provides additional information. For example, if the code describes the site of the pain, but does not fully describe whether the pain is acute or chronic, then both codes should be assigned.

(ii) Sequencing of category G89 codes with site-specific pain codes

The sequencing of category G89 codes with site-specific pain codes (including chapter 18 codes), is dependent on the circumstances of the encounter/admission as follows:

- If the encounter is for pain control or pain management, assign the code from category G89 followed by the code identifying the specific site of pain (e.g., encounter for pain management for acute neck pain from trauma is assigned code G89.11, Acute pain due to trauma, followed by code M54.2, Cervicalgia, to identify the site of pain).

- If the encounter is for any other reason except pain control or pain management, and a related definitive diagnosis has not been established (confirmed) by the provider, assign the code for the specific site of pain first, followed by the appropriate code from category G89.

2) Pain due to devices, implants and grafts

See Section I.C.19. Pain due to medical devices

3) Postoperative pain

The provider's documentation should be used to guide the coding of postoperative pain, as well as *Section III. Reporting Additional Diagnoses* and *Section IV. Diagnostic Coding and Reporting in the Outpatient Setting.*

The default for post-thoracotomy and other postoperative pain not specified as acute or chronic is the code for the acute form.

Routine or expected postoperative pain immediately after surgery should not be coded.

(a) Postoperative pain not associated with specific postoperative complication

Postoperative pain not associated with a specific postoperative complication is assigned to the appropriate postoperative pain code in category G89.

(b) Postoperative pain associated with specific postoperative complication

Postoperative pain associated with a specific postoperative complication (such as painful wire sutures) is assigned to the appropriate code(s) found in Chapter 19, Injury, poisoning, and certain other consequences of external causes. If appropriate, use additional code(s) from category G89 to identify acute or chronic pain (G89.18 or G89.28).

4) Chronic pain

Chronic pain is classified to subcategory G89.2. There is no time frame defining when pain becomes chronic pain. The provider's documentation should be used to guide use of these codes.

5) Neoplasm related pain

Code G89.3 is assigned to pain documented as being related, associated or due to cancer, primary or secondary malignancy, or tumor. This code is assigned regardless of whether the pain is acute or chronic.

This code may be assigned as the principal or first-listed code when the stated reason for the admission/encounter is documented as pain control/pain management. The underlying neoplasm should be reported as an additional diagnosis.

When the reason for the admission/encounter is management of the neoplasm and the pain associated with the neoplasm is also documented, code G89.3 may be assigned as an additional diagnosis. It is not necessary to assign an additional code for the site of the pain.

See Section I.C.2 for instructions on the sequencing of neoplasms for all other stated reasons for the admission/encounter (except for pain control/pain management).

6) Chronic pain syndrome

Central pain syndrome (G89.0) and chronic pain syndrome (G89.4) are different than the term "chronic pain," and therefore codes should only be used when the provider has specifically documented this condition.

See Section I.C.5. Pain disorders related to psychological factors

7. Chapter 7: Diseases of Eye and Adnexa (H00-H59)

a. Glaucoma

1) Assigning glaucoma codes

Assign as many codes from category H40, Glaucoma, as needed to identify the type of glaucoma, the affected eye, and the glaucoma stage.

2) Bilateral glaucoma with same type and stage

When a patient has bilateral glaucoma and both eyes are documented as being the same type and stage, and there is a code for bilateral glaucoma, report only the code for the type of glaucoma, bilateral, with the seventh character for the stage.

When a patient has bilateral glaucoma and both eyes are documented as being the same type and stage, and the classification does not provide a code for bilateral glaucoma (i.e. subcategories H40.10, H40.11 and H40.20) report only one code for the type of glaucoma with the appropriate seventh character for the stage.

3) Bilateral glaucoma stage with different types or stages

When a patient has bilateral glaucoma and each eye is documented as having a different type or stage, and the classification distinguishes laterality, assign the appropriate code for each eye rather than the code for bilateral glaucoma.

When a patient has bilateral glaucoma and each eye is documented as having a different type, and the classification does not distinguish laterality (i.e. subcategories H40.10, H40.11 and H40.20), assign one code for each type of glaucoma with the appropriate seventh character for the stage.

When a patient has bilateral glaucoma and each eye is documented as having the same type, but different stage, and the classification does not distinguish laterality (i.e. subcategories H40.10, H40.11 and H40.20), assign a code for the type of glaucoma for each eye with the seventh character for the specific glaucoma stage documented for each eye.

4) Patient admitted with glaucoma and stage evolves during the admission

If a patient is admitted with glaucoma and the stage progresses during the admission, assign the code for highest stage documented.

5) Indeterminate stage glaucoma

Assignment of the seventh character "4" for "indeterminate stage" should be based on the clinical documentation. The seventh character "4" is used for glaucomas whose stage cannot be clinically determined. This seventh character should not be confused with the seventh character "0", unspecified, which should be assigned when there is no documentation regarding the stage of the glaucoma.

8. Chapter 8: Diseases of Ear and Mastoid Process (H60-H95)
Reserved for future guideline expansion

9. Chapter 9: Diseases of Circulatory System (I00-I99)

a. Hypertension

1) Hypertension with heart disease

Heart conditions classified to I50.- or I51.4-I51.9, are assigned to, a code from category I11, Hypertensive heart disease, when a causal relationship is stated (due to hypertension) or implied (hypertensive). Use an additional code from category I50, Heart failure, to identify the type of heart failure in those patients with heart failure.

The same heart conditions (I50.-, I51.4-I51.9) with hypertension, but without a stated causal relationship, are coded separately. Sequence according to the circumstances of the admission/encounter.

2) Hypertensive chronic kidney disease

Assign codes from category I12, Hypertensive chronic kidney disease, when both hypertension and a condition classifiable to category N18, Chronic kidney disease (CKD), are present. Unlike hypertension with heart disease, ICD-10-CM presumes a cause-and-effect relationship and classifies chronic kidney disease with hypertension as hypertensive chronic kidney disease.

The appropriate code from category N18 should be used as a secondary code with a code from category I12 to identify the stage of chronic kidney disease.

See Section I.C.14. Chronic kidney disease.

If a patient has hypertensive chronic kidney disease and acute renal failure, an additional code for the acute renal failure is required.

3) Hypertensive heart and chronic kidney disease

Assign codes from combination category I13, Hypertensive heart and chronic kidney disease, when both hypertensive kidney disease and hypertensive heart disease are stated in the diagnosis. Assume a relationship between the hypertension and the chronic kidney disease, whether or not the condition is so designated. If heart failure is present, assign an additional code from category I50 to identify the type of heart failure.

The appropriate code from category N18, Chronic kidney disease, should be used as a secondary code with a code from category I13 to identify the stage of chronic kidney disease.

See Section I.C.14. Chronic kidney disease.

The codes in category I13, Hypertensive heart and chronic kidney disease, are combination codes that include hypertension, heart disease and chronic kidney disease. The Includes note at I13 specifies that the conditions included at I11 and I12 are included together in I13. If a patient has hypertension, heart disease and chronic kidney disease then a code from I13 should be used, not individual codes for hypertension, heart disease and chronic kidney disease, or codes from I11 or I12.

For patients with both acute renal failure and chronic kidney disease an additional code for acute renal failure is required.

4) Hypertensive cerebrovascular disease

For hypertensive cerebrovascular disease, first assign the appropriate code from categories I60-I69, followed by the appropriate hypertension code.

5) Hypertensive retinopathy

Subcategory H35.0, Background retinopathy and retinal vascular changes, should be used with a code from category I10 – I15, Hypertensive disease to include the systemic hypertension. The sequencing is based on the reason for the encounter.

6) Hypertension, secondary

Secondary hypertension is due to an underlying condition. Two codes are required: one to identify the underlying etiology and one from category I15 to identify the hypertension. Sequencing of codes is determined by the reason for admission/encounter.

7) Hypertension, transient

Assign code R03.0, Elevated blood pressure reading without diagnosis of hypertension, unless patient has an established diagnosis of hypertension. Assign code O13.-, Gestational [pregnancy-induced] hypertension without significant proteinuria, or O14.-, Pre-eclampsia, for transient hypertension of pregnancy.

8) Hypertension, controlled

This diagnostic statement usually refers to an existing state of hypertension under control by therapy. Assign the appropriate code from categories I10-I15, Hypertensive diseases.

9) Hypertension, uncontrolled

Uncontrolled hypertension may refer to untreated hypertension or hypertension not responding to current therapeutic regimen. In either case, assign the appropriate code from categories I10-I15, Hypertensive diseases.

b. Atherosclerotic coronary artery disease and angina

ICD-10-CM has combination codes for atherosclerotic heart disease with angina pectoris. The subcategories for these codes are I25.11, Atherosclerotic heart disease of native coronary artery with angina pectoris and I25.7, Atherosclerosis of coronary artery bypass graft(s) and coronary artery of transplanted heart with angina pectoris.

When using one of these combination codes it is not necessary to use an additional code for angina pectoris. A causal relationship can be assumed in a patient with both atherosclerosis and angina pectoris, unless the documentation indicates the angina is due to something other than the atherosclerosis.

If a patient with coronary artery disease is admitted due to an acute myocardial infarction (AMI), the AMI should be sequenced before the coronary artery disease.

See Section I.C.9. Acute myocardial infarction (AMI)

c. Intraoperative and postprocedural cerebrovascular accident

Medical record documentation should clearly specify the cause-and-effect relationship between the medical intervention and the cerebrovascular accident in order to assign a code for intraoperative or postprocedural cerebrovascular accident.

Proper code assignment depends on whether it was an infarction or hemorrhage and whether it occurred intraoperatively or postoperatively. If it was a cerebral hemorrhage, code assignment depends on the type of procedure performed.

d. Sequelae of cerebrovascular disease

1) Category I69, sequelae of cerebrovascular disease
Category I69 is used to indicate conditions classifiable to categories I6Ø-I67 as the causes of sequela (neurologic deficits), themselves classified elsewhere. These "late effects" include neurologic deficits that persist after initial onset of conditions classifiable to categories I6Ø-I67. The neurologic deficits caused by cerebrovascular disease may be present from the onset or may arise at any time after the onset of the condition classifiable to categories I6Ø-I67.

Codes from category I69, Sequelae of cerebrovascular disease, that specify hemiplegia, hemiparesis and monoplegia identify whether the dominant or nondominant side is affected. Should the affected side be documented, but not specified as dominant or nondominant, and the classification system does not indicate a default, code selection is as follows:

- For ambidextrous patients, the default should be dominant.
- If the left side is affected, the default is non-dominant.
- If the right side is affected, the default is dominant.

2) Codes from category I69 with codes from I6Ø-I67
Codes from category I69 may be assigned on a health care record with codes from I6Ø-I67, if the patient has a current cerebrovascular disease and deficits from an old cerebrovascular disease.

3) Codes from category I69 and Personal history of transient ischemic attack (TIA) and cerebral infarction (Z86.73)
Codes from category I69 should not be assigned if the patient does not have neurologic deficits.

See Section I.C.21. 4. History (of) for use of personal history codes

e. Acute myocardial infarction (AMI)

1) ST elevation myocardial infarction (STEMI) and non ST elevation myocardial infarction (NSTEMI)
The ICD-1Ø-CM codes for acute myocardial infarction (AMI) identify the site, such as anterolateral wall or true posterior wall. Subcategories I21.Ø-I21.2 and code I21.3 are used for ST elevation myocardial infarction (STEMI). Code I21.4, Non-ST elevation (NSTEMI) myocardial infarction, is used for non ST elevation myocardial infarction (NSTEMI) and nontransmural MIs.

If NSTEMI evolves to STEMI, assign the STEMI code. If STEMI converts to NSTEMI due to thrombolytic therapy, it is still coded as STEMI.

For encounters occurring while the myocardial infarction is equal to, or less than, four weeks old, including transfers to another acute setting or a postacute setting, and the patient requires continued care for the myocardial infarction, codes from category I21 may continue to be reported. For encounters after the 4 week time frame and the patient is still receiving care related to the myocardial infarction, the appropriate aftercare code should be assigned, rather than a code from category I21. For old or healed myocardial infarctions not requiring further care, code I25.2, Old myocardial infarction, may be assigned.

2) Acute myocardial infarction, unspecified
Code I21.3, ST elevation (STEMI) myocardial infarction of unspecified site, is the default for the unspecified term acute myocardial infarction. If only STEMI or transmural MI without the site is documented, query the provider as to the site, or assign code I21.3.

3) AMI documented as nontransmural or subendocardial but site provided
If an AMI is documented as nontransmural or subendocardial, but the site is provided, it is still coded as a subendocardial AMI.

See Section I.C.21.3 for information on coding status post administration of tPA in a different facility within the last 24 hrs.

4) Subsequent acute myocardial infarction
A code from category I22, Subsequent ST elevation (STEMI) and non ST elevation (NSTEMI) myocardial infarction, is to be used when a patient who has suffered an AMI has a new AMI within the 4 week time frame of the initial AMI. A code from category I22 must be used in conjunction with a code from category I21.

The sequencing of the I22 and I21 codes depends on the circumstances of the encounter.

1Ø. Chapter 1Ø: Diseases of the Respiratory System (JØØ-J99)

a. Chronic Obstructive Pulmonary Disease [COPD] and Asthma

1) Acute exacerbation of chronic obstructive bronchitis and asthma
The codes in categories J44 and J45 distinguish between uncomplicated cases and those in acute exacerbation. An acute exacerbation is a worsening or a decompensation of a chronic condition. An acute exacerbation is not equivalent to an infection superimposed on a chronic condition, though an exacerbation may be triggered by an infection.

b. Acute Respiratory Failure

1) Acute respiratory failure as principal diagnosis
A code from subcategory J96.Ø, Acute respiratory failure, or subcategory J96.2, Acute and chronic respiratory failure, may be assigned as a principal diagnosis when it is the condition established after study to be chiefly responsible for occasioning the admission to the hospital, and the selection is supported by the Alphabetic Index and Tabular List. However, chapter-specific coding guidelines (such as obstetrics, poisoning, HIV, newborn) that provide sequencing direction take precedence.

2) Acute respiratory failure as secondary diagnosis
Respiratory failure may be listed as a secondary diagnosis if it occurs after admission, or if it is present on admission, but does not meet the definition of principal diagnosis.

3) Sequencing of acute respiratory failure and another acute condition
When a patient is admitted with respiratory failure and another acute condition, (e.g., myocardial infarction, cerebrovascular accident, aspiration pneumonia), the principal diagnosis will not be the same in every situation. This applies whether the other acute condition is a respiratory or nonrespiratory condition. Selection of the principal diagnosis will be dependent on the circumstances of admission. If both the respiratory failure and the other acute condition are equally responsible for occasioning the admission to the hospital, and there are no chapter-specific sequencing rules, the guideline regarding two or more diagnoses that equally meet the definition for principal diagnosis (Section II, C.) may be applied in these situations.

If the documentation is not clear as to whether acute respiratory failure and another condition are equally responsible for occasioning the admission, query the provider for clarification.

c. Influenza due to certain identified influenza viruses
Code only confirmed cases of influenza due to certain identified influenza viruses (category JØ9), and due to other identified influenza virus (category J1Ø). This is an exception to the hospital inpatient guideline Section II, H. (Uncertain Diagnosis).

In this context, "confirmation" does not require documentation of positive laboratory testing specific for avian or other novel influenza A or other identified influenza virus. However, coding should be based on the provider's diagnostic statement that the patient has avian influenza, or other novel influenza A, for category JØ9, or has another particular identified strain of influenza, such as H1N1 or H3N2, but not identified as novel or variant, for category J1Ø.

If the provider records "suspected" or "possible" or "probable" avian influenza, or novel influenza, or other identified influenza, then the appropriate influenza code from category J11, Influenza due to unidentified influenza virus, should be assigned. A code from category JØ9, Influenza due to certain identified influenza viruses, should not be assigned nor should a code from category J1Ø, Influenza due to other identified influenza virus.

d. Ventilator associated pneumonia

1) Documentation of ventilator associated pneumonia
As with all procedural or postprocedural complications, code assignment is based on the provider's documentation of the relationship between the condition and the procedure.

Code J95.851, Ventilator associated pneumonia, should be assigned only when the provider has documented ventilator associated pneumonia (VAP). An additional code to identify the organism (e.g., Pseudomonas aeruginosa, code B96.5) should also be assigned. Do not assign an additional code from categories J12-J18 to identify the type of pneumonia.

Code J95.851 should not be assigned for cases where the patient has pneumonia and is on a mechanical ventilator and the provider has not specifically stated that the pneumonia is ventilator-associated pneumonia. If the documentation is unclear as to whether the patient has a pneumonia that is a complication attributable to the mechanical ventilator, query the provider.

2) Ventilator associated pneumonia develops after admission

A patient may be admitted with one type of pneumonia (e.g., code J13, Pneumonia due to Streptococcus pneumonia) and subsequently develop VAP. In this instance, the principal diagnosis would be the appropriate code from categories J12-J18 for the pneumonia diagnosed at the time of admission. Code J95.851, Ventilator associated pneumonia, would be assigned as an additional diagnosis when the provider has also documented the presence of ventilator associated pneumonia.

11. Chapter 11: Diseases of the Digestive System (K00-K95)

Reserved for future guideline expansion

12. Chapter 12: Diseases of the Skin and Subcutaneous Tissue (L00-L99)

a. Pressure ulcer stage codes

1) Pressure ulcer stages

Codes from category L89, Pressure ulcer, are combination codes that identify the site of the pressure ulcer as well as the stage of the ulcer.

The ICD-10-CM classifies pressure ulcer stages based on severity, which is designated by stages 1-4, unspecified stage and unstageable.

Assign as many codes from category L89 as needed to identify all the pressure ulcers the patient has, if applicable.

2) Unstageable pressure ulcers

Assignment of the code for unstageable pressure ulcer (L89.--0) should be based on the clinical documentation. These codes are used for pressure ulcers whose stage cannot be clinically determined (e.g., the ulcer is covered by eschar or has been treated with a skin or muscle graft) and pressure ulcers that are documented as deep tissue injury but not documented as due to trauma. This code should not be confused with the codes for unspecified stage (L89.--9). When there is no documentation regarding the stage of the pressure ulcer, assign the appropriate code for unspecified stage (L89.--9).

3) Documented pressure ulcer stage

Assignment of the pressure ulcer stage code should be guided by clinical documentation of the stage or documentation of the terms found in the Alphabetic Index. For clinical terms describing the stage that are not found in the Alphabetic Index, and there is no documentation of the stage, the provider should be queried.

4) Patients admitted with pressure ulcers documented as healed

No code is assigned if the documentation states that the pressure ulcer is completely healed.

5) Patients admitted with pressure ulcers documented as healing

Pressure ulcers described as healing should be assigned the appropriate pressure ulcer stage code based on the documentation in the medical record. If the documentation does not provide information about the stage of the healing pressure ulcer, assign the appropriate code for unspecified stage.

If the documentation is unclear as to whether the patient has a current (new) pressure ulcer or if the patient is being treated for a healing pressure ulcer, query the provider.

6) Patient admitted with pressure ulcer evolving into another stage during the admission

If a patient is admitted with a pressure ulcer at one stage and it progresses to a higher stage, assign the code for the highest stage reported for that site.

13. Chapter 13: Diseases of the Musculoskeletal System and Connective Tissue (M00-M99)

a. Site and laterality

Most of the codes within Chapter 13 have site and laterality designations. The site represents the bone, joint or the muscle involved. For some conditions where more than one bone, joint or muscle is usually involved, such as osteoarthritis, there is a "multiple sites" code available. For categories where no multiple site code is provided and more than one bone, joint or muscle is involved, multiple codes should be used to indicate the different sites involved.

1) Bone versus joint

For certain conditions, the bone may be affected at the upper or lower end, (e.g., avascular necrosis of bone, M87, Osteoporosis, M80, M81). Though the portion of the bone affected may be at the joint, the site designation will be the bone, not the joint.

b. Acute traumatic versus chronic or recurrent musculoskeletal conditions

Many musculoskeletal conditions are a result of previous injury or trauma to a site, or are recurrent conditions. Bone, joint or muscle conditions that are the result of a healed injury are usually found in chapter 13. Recurrent bone, joint or muscle conditions are also usually found in chapter 13. Any current, acute injury should be coded to the appropriate injury code from chapter 19. Chronic or recurrent conditions should generally be coded with a code from chapter 13. If it is difficult to determine from the documentation in the record which code is best to describe a condition, query the provider.

c. Coding of Pathologic Fractures

7th character A is for use as long as the patient is receiving active treatment for the fracture. Examples of active treatment are: surgical treatment, emergency department encounter, evaluation and treatment by a new physician. 7th character, D is to be used for encounters after the patient has completed active treatment. The other 7th characters, listed under each subcategory in the Tabular List, are to be used for subsequent encounters for treatment of problems associated with the healing, such as malunions, nonunions, and sequelae.

Care for complications of surgical treatment for fracture repairs during the healing or recovery phase should be coded with the appropriate complication codes.

See Section I.C.19. Coding of traumatic fractures.

d. Osteoporosis

Osteoporosis is a systemic condition, meaning that all bones of the musculoskeletal system are affected. Therefore, site is not a component of the codes under category M81, Osteoporosis without current pathological fracture. The site codes under category M80, Osteoporosis with current pathological fracture, identify the site of the fracture, not the osteoporosis.

1) Osteoporosis without pathological fracture

Category M81, Osteoporosis without current pathological fracture, is for use for patients with osteoporosis who do not currently have a pathologic fracture due to the osteoporosis, even if they have had a fracture in the past. For patients with a history of osteoporosis fractures, status code Z87.310, Personal history of (healed) osteoporosis fracture, should follow the code from M81.

2) Osteoporosis with current pathological fracture

Category M80, Osteoporosis with current pathological fracture, is for patients who have a current pathologic fracture at the time of an encounter. The codes under M80 identify the site of the fracture. A code from category M80, not a traumatic fracture code, should be used for any patient with known osteoporosis who suffers a fracture, even if the patient had a minor fall or trauma, if that fall or trauma would not usually break a normal, healthy bone.

14. **Chapter 14: Diseases of Genitourinary System (N00-N99)**
    a. **Chronic kidney disease**
       1) **Stages of chronic kidney disease (CKD)**
          The ICD-10-CM classifies CKD based on severity. The severity of CKD is designated by stages 1-5. Stage 2, code N18.2, equates to mild CKD; stage 3, code N18.3, equates to moderate CKD; and stage 4, code N18.4, equates to severe CKD. Code N18.6, End stage renal disease (ESRD), is assigned when the provider has documented end-stage-renal disease (ESRD).

          If both a stage of CKD and ESRD are documented, assign code N18.6 only.

       2) **Chronic kidney disease and kidney transplant status**
          Patients who have undergone kidney transplant may still have some form of chronic kidney disease (CKD) because the kidney transplant may not fully restore kidney function. Therefore, the presence of CKD alone does not constitute a transplant complication. Assign the appropriate N18 code for the patient's stage of CKD and code Z94.0, Kidney transplant status. If a transplant complication such as failure or rejection or other transplant complication is documented, see section I.C.19.g for information on coding complications of a kidney transplant. If the documentation is unclear as to whether the patient has a complication of the transplant, query the provider.

       3) **Chronic kidney disease with other conditions**
          Patients with CKD may also suffer from other serious conditions, most commonly diabetes mellitus and hypertension. The sequencing of the CKD code in relationship to codes for other contributing conditions is based on the conventions in the Tabular List.

          See I.C.9. Hypertensive chronic kidney disease.

          See I.C.19. Chronic kidney disease and kidney transplant complications.

15. **Chapter 15: Pregnancy, Childbirth, and the Puerperium (O00-O9A)**
    a. **General Rules for Obstetric Cases**
       1) **Codes from chapter 15 and sequencing priority**
          Obstetric cases require codes from chapter 15, codes in the range O00-O9A, Pregnancy, Childbirth, and the Puerperium. Chapter 15 codes have sequencing priority over codes from other chapters. Additional codes from other chapters may be used in conjunction with chapter 15 codes to further specify conditions. Should the provider document that the pregnancy is incidental to the encounter, then code Z33.1, Pregnant state, incidental, should be used in place of any chapter 15 codes. It is the provider's responsibility to state that the condition being treated is not affecting the pregnancy.

       2) **Chapter 15 codes used only on the maternal record**
          Chapter 15 codes are to be used only on the maternal record, never on the record of the newborn.

       3) **Final character for trimester**
          The majority of codes in Chapter 15 have a final character indicating the trimester of pregnancy. The timeframes for the trimesters are indicated at the beginning of the chapter. If trimester is not a component of a code it is because the condition always occurs in a specific trimester, or the concept of trimester of pregnancy is not applicable. Certain codes have characters for only certain trimesters because the condition does not occur in all trimesters, but it may occur in more than just one.

          Assignment of the final character for trimester should be based on the provider's documentation of the trimester (or number of weeks) for the current admission/encounter. This applies to the assignment of trimester for pre-existing conditions as well as those that develop during or are due to the pregnancy. The provider's documentation of the number of weeks may be used to assign the appropriate code identifying the trimester.

          Whenever delivery occurs during the current admission, and there is an "in childbirth" option for the obstetric complication being coded, the "in childbirth" code should be assigned.

       4) **Selection of trimester for inpatient admissions that encompass more than one trimesters**
          In instances when a patient is admitted to a hospital for complications of pregnancy during one trimester and remains in the hospital into a subsequent trimester, the trimester character for the antepartum complication code should be assigned on the basis of the trimester when the complication developed, not the trimester of the discharge. If the condition developed prior to the current admission/encounter or represents a pre-existing condition, the trimester character for the trimester at the time of the admission/encounter should be assigned.

       5) **Unspecified trimester**
          Each category that includes codes for trimester has a code for "unspecified trimester." The "unspecified trimester" code should rarely be used, such as when the documentation in the record is insufficient to determine the trimester and it is not possible to obtain clarification.

       6) **7th character for fetus identification**
          Where applicable, a 7th character is to be assigned for certain categories (O31, O32, O33.3 - O33.6, O35, O36, O40, O41, O60.1, O60.2, O64, and O69) to identify the fetus for which the complication code applies.

          Assign 7th character "0":
          - For single gestations
          - When the documentation in the record is insufficient to determine the fetus affected and it is not possible to obtain clarification.
          - When it is not possible to clinically determine which fetus is affected.

    b. **Selection of OB principal or first-listed diagnosis**
       1) **Routine outpatient prenatal visits**
          For routine outpatient prenatal visits when no complications are present, a code from category Z34, Encounter for supervision of normal pregnancy, should be used as the first-listed diagnosis. These codes should not be used in conjunction with chapter 15 codes.

       2) **Prenatal outpatient visits for high-risk patients**
          For routine prenatal outpatient visits for patients with high-risk pregnancies, a code from category O09, Supervision of high-risk pregnancy, should be used as the first-listed diagnosis. Secondary chapter 15 codes may be used in conjunction with these codes if appropriate.

       3) **Episodes when no delivery occurs**
          In episodes when no delivery occurs, the principal diagnosis should correspond to the principal complication of the pregnancy which necessitated the encounter. Should more than one complication exist, all of which are treated or monitored, any of the complications codes may be sequenced first.

       4) **When a delivery occurs**
          When a delivery occurs, the principal diagnosis should correspond to the main circumstances or complication of the delivery. In cases of cesarean delivery, the selection of the principal diagnosis should be the condition established after study that was responsible for the patient's admission. If the patient was admitted with a condition that resulted in the performance of a cesarean procedure, that condition should be selected as the principal diagnosis. If the reason for the admission/encounter was unrelated to the condition resulting in the cesarean delivery, the condition related to the reason for the admission/encounter should be selected as the principal diagnosis.

       5) **Outcome of delivery**
          A code from category Z37, Outcome of delivery, should be included on every maternal record when a delivery has occurred. These codes are not to be used on subsequent records or on the newborn record.

c. **Pre-existing conditions versus conditions due to the pregnancy**

Certain categories in Chapter 15 distinguish between conditions of the mother that existed prior to pregnancy (pre-existing) and those that are a direct result of pregnancy. When assigning codes from Chapter 15, it is important to assess if a condition was pre-existing prior to pregnancy or developed during or due to the pregnancy in order to assign the correct code.

Categories that do not distinguish between pre-existing and pregnancy-related conditions may be used for either. It is acceptable to use codes specifically for the puerperium with codes complicating pregnancy and childbirth if a condition arises postpartum during the delivery encounter.

d. **Pre-existing hypertension in pregnancy**

Category O10, Pre-existing hypertension complicating pregnancy, childbirth and the puerperium, includes codes for hypertensive heart and hypertensive chronic kidney disease. When assigning one of the O10 codes that includes hypertensive heart disease or hypertensive chronic kidney disease, it is necessary to add a secondary code from the appropriate hypertension category to specify the type of heart failure or chronic kidney disease.

See Section I.C.9. Hypertension.

e. **Fetal conditions affecting the management of the mother**

1) **Codes from categories O35 and O36**

Codes from categories O35, Maternal care for known or suspected fetal abnormality and damage, and O36, Maternal care for other fetal problems, are assigned only when the fetal condition is actually responsible for modifying the management of the mother, i.e., by requiring diagnostic studies, additional observation, special care, or termination of pregnancy. The fact that the fetal condition exists does not justify assigning a code from this series to the mother's record.

2) **In utero surgery**

In cases when surgery is performed on the fetus, a diagnosis code from category O35, Maternal care for known or suspected fetal abnormality and damage, should be assigned identifying the fetal condition. Assign the appropriate procedure code for the procedure performed.

No code from Chapter 16, the perinatal codes, should be used on the mother's record to identify fetal conditions. Surgery performed in utero on a fetus is still to be coded as an obstetric encounter.

f. **HIV Infection in pregnancy, childbirth and the puerperium**

During pregnancy, childbirth or the puerperium, a patient admitted because of an HIV-related illness should receive a principal diagnosis from subcategory O98.7-, Human immunodeficiency [HIV] disease complicating pregnancy, childbirth and the puerperium, followed by the code(s) for the HIV-related illness(es).

Patients with asymptomatic HIV infection status admitted during pregnancy, childbirth, or the puerperium should receive codes of O98.7- and Z21, Asymptomatic human immunodeficiency virus [HIV] infection status.

g. **Diabetes mellitus in pregnancy**

Diabetes mellitus is a significant complicating factor in pregnancy. Pregnant women who are diabetic should be assigned a code from category O24, Diabetes mellitus in pregnancy, childbirth, and the puerperium, first, followed by the appropriate diabetes code(s) (E08-E13) from Chapter 4.

h. **Long term use of insulin**

Code Z79.4, Long-term (current) use of insulin, should also be assigned if the diabetes mellitus is being treated with insulin.

i. **Gestational (pregnancy induced) diabetes**

Gestational (pregnancy induced) diabetes can occur during the second and third trimester of pregnancy in women who were not diabetic prior to pregnancy. Gestational diabetes can cause complications in the pregnancy similar to those of pre-existing diabetes mellitus. It also puts the woman at greater risk of developing diabetes after the pregnancy. Codes for gestational diabetes are in subcategory O24.4, Gestational diabetes mellitus. No

other code from category O24, Diabetes mellitus in pregnancy, childbirth, and the puerperium, should be used with a code from O24.4.

The codes under subcategory O24.4 include diet controlled and insulin controlled. If a patient with gestational diabetes is treated with both diet and insulin, only the code for insulin-controlled is required.

Code Z79.4, Long-term (current) use of insulin, should not be assigned with codes from subcategory O24.4.

An abnormal glucose tolerance in pregnancy is assigned a code from subcategory O99.81, Abnormal glucose complicating pregnancy, childbirth, and the puerperium.

j. **Sepsis and septic shock complicating abortion, pregnancy, childbirth and the puerperium**

When assigning a chapter 15 code for sepsis complicating abortion, pregnancy, childbirth, and the puerperium, a code for the specific type of infection should be assigned as an additional diagnosis. If severe sepsis is present, a code from subcategory R65.2, Severe sepsis, and code(s) for associated organ dysfunction(s) should also be assigned as additional diagnoses.

k. **Puerperal sepsis**

Code O85, Puerperal sepsis, should be assigned with a secondary code to identify the causal organism (e.g., for a bacterial infection, assign a code from category B95-B96, Bacterial infections in conditions classified elsewhere). A code from category A40, Streptococcal sepsis, or A41, Other sepsis, should not be used for puerperal sepsis. If applicable, use additional codes to identify severe sepsis (R65.2-) and any associated acute organ dysfunction.

l. **Alcohol and tobacco use during pregnancy, childbirth and the puerperium**

1) **Alcohol use during pregnancy, childbirth and the puerperium**

Codes under subcategory O99.31, Alcohol use complicating pregnancy, childbirth, and the puerperium, should be assigned for any pregnancy case when a mother uses alcohol during the pregnancy or postpartum. A secondary code from category F10, Alcohol related disorders, should also be assigned to identify manifestations of the alcohol use.

2) **Tobacco use during pregnancy, childbirth and the puerperium**

Codes under subcategory O99.33, Smoking (tobacco) complicating pregnancy, childbirth, and the puerperium, should be assigned for any pregnancy case when a mother uses any type of tobacco product during the pregnancy or postpartum. A secondary code from category F17, Nicotine dependence, or code Z72.0, Tobacco use, should also be assigned to identify the type of nicotine dependence.

m. **Poisoning, toxic effects, adverse effects and underdosing in a pregnant patient**

A code from subcategory O9A.2, Injury, poisoning and certain other consequences of external causes complicating pregnancy, childbirth, and the puerperium, should be sequenced first, followed by the appropriate injury, poisoning, toxic effect, adverse effect or underdosing code, and then the additional code(s) that specifies the condition caused by the poisoning, toxic effect, adverse effect or underdosing.

See Section I.C.19. Adverse effects, poisoning, underdosing and toxic effects.

n. **Normal delivery, code O80**

1) **Encounter for full term uncomplicated delivery**

Code O80 should be assigned when a woman is admitted for a full-term normal delivery and delivers a single, healthy infant without any complications antepartum, during the delivery, or postpartum during the delivery episode. Code O80 is always a principal diagnosis. It is not to be used if any other code from chapter 15 is needed to describe a current complication of the antenatal, delivery, or perinatal period. Additional codes from other chapters may be used with code O80 if they are not related to or are in any way complicating the pregnancy.

2) Uncomplicated delivery with resolved antepartum complication

Code O80 may be used if the patient had a complication at some point during the pregnancy, but the complication is not present at the time of the admission for delivery.

3) Outcome of delivery for O80

Z37.0, Single live birth, is the only outcome of delivery code appropriate for use with O80.

o. The peripartum and postpartum periods

1) Peripartum and postpartum periods

The postpartum period begins immediately after delivery and continues for six weeks following delivery. The peripartum period is defined as the last month of pregnancy to five months postpartum.

2) Peripartum and postpartum complication

A postpartum complication is any complication occurring within the six-week period.

3) Pregnancy-related complications after 6 week period

Chapter 15 codes may also be used to describe pregnancy-related complications after the peripartum or postpartum period if the provider documents that a condition is pregnancy related.

4) Admission for routine postpartum care following delivery outside hospital

When the mother delivers outside the hospital prior to admission and is admitted for routine postpartum care and no complications are noted, code Z39.0, Encounter for care and examination of mother immediately after delivery, should be assigned as the principal diagnosis.

5) Pregnancy associated cardiomyopathy

Pregnancy associated cardiomyopathy, code O90.3, is unique in that it may be diagnosed in the third trimester of pregnancy but may continue to progress months after delivery. For this reason, it is referred to as peripartum cardiomyopathy. Code O90.3 is only for use when the cardiomyopathy develops as a result of pregnancy in a woman who did not have pre-existing heart disease.

p. Code O94, Sequelae of complication of pregnancy, childbirth, and the puerperium

1) Code O94

Code O94, Sequelae of complication of pregnancy, childbirth, and the puerperium, is for use in those cases when an initial complication of a pregnancy develops a sequelae requiring care or treatment at a future date.

2) After the initial postpartum period

This code may be used at any time after the initial postpartum period.

3) Sequencing of code O94

This code, like all late effect codes, is to be sequenced following the code describing the sequelae of the complication.

q. Termination of Pregnancy and Spontaneous Abortions

1) Abortion with liveborn fetus

When an attempted termination of pregnancy results in a liveborn fetus, assign code Z33.2, Encounter for elective termination of pregnancy and a code from category Z37, Outcome of Delivery.

2) Retained products of conception following an abortion

Subsequent encounters for retained products of conception following a spontaneous abortion or elective termination of pregnancy are assigned the appropriate code from category O03, Spontaneous abortion, or codes O07.4, Failed attempted termination of pregnancy without complication and Z33.2, Encounter for elective termination of pregnancy. This advice is appropriate even when the patient was discharged previously with a discharge diagnosis of complete abortion.

3) Complications leading to abortion

Codes from Chapter 15 may be used as additional codes to identify any documented complications of the pregnancy in conjunction with codes in categories in O07 and O08.

r. Abuse in a pregnant patient

For suspected or confirmed cases of abuse of a pregnant patient, a code(s) from subcategories O9A.3, Physical abuse complicating pregnancy, childbirth, and the puerperium, O9A.4, Sexual abuse complicating pregnancy, childbirth, and the puerperium, and O9A.5, Psychological abuse complicating pregnancy, childbirth, and the puerperium, should be sequenced first, followed by the appropriate codes (if applicable) to identify any associated current injury due to physical abuse, sexual abuse, and the perpetrator of abuse.

See Section I.C.19.f. Adult and child abuse, neglect and other maltreatment.

16. Chapter 16: Certain Conditions Origination in the Perinatal Period (P00-P96)

For coding and reporting purposes the perinatal period is defined as before birth through the 28th day following birth. The following guidelines are provided for reporting purposes

a. General Perinatal Rules

1) Use of Chapter 16 codes

Codes in this chapter are <u>never</u> for use on the maternal record. Codes from Chapter 15, the obstetric chapter, are never permitted on the newborn record. Chapter 16 codes may be used throughout the life of the patient if the condition is still present.

2) Principal diagnosis for birth record

When coding the birth episode in a newborn record, assign a code from category Z38, Liveborn infants according to place of birth and type of delivery, as the principal diagnosis. A code from category Z38 is assigned only once, to a newborn at the time of birth. If a newborn is transferred to another institution, a code from category Z38 should not be used at the receiving hospital.

A code from category Z38 is used only on the newborn record, not on the mother's record.

3) Use of codes from other chapters with codes from Chapter 16

Codes from other chapters may be used with codes from chapter 16 if the codes from the other chapters provide more specific detail. Codes for signs and symptoms may be assigned when a definitive diagnosis has not been established. If the reason for the encounter is a perinatal condition, the code from chapter 16 should be sequenced first.

4) Use of Chapter 16 codes after the perinatal period

Should a condition originate in the perinatal period, and continue throughout the life of the patient, the perinatal code should continue to be used regardless of the patient's age.

5) Birth process or community acquired conditions

If a newborn has a condition that may be either due to the birth process or community acquired and the documentation does not indicate which it is, the default is due to the birth process and the code from Chapter 16 should be used. If the condition is community-acquired, a code from Chapter 16 should not be assigned.

6) Code all clinically significant conditions

All clinically significant conditions noted on routine newborn examination should be coded. A condition is clinically significant if it requires:

- clinical evaluation; or
- therapeutic treatment; or
- diagnostic procedures; or
- extended length of hospital stay; or
- increased nursing care and/or monitoring; or
- has implications for future health care needs

Note: The perinatal guidelines listed above are the same as the general coding guidelines for "additional diagnoses", except for the final point regarding implications for future health care needs. Codes should be assigned for conditions that have been specified by the provider as having implications for future health care needs.

b. **Observation and evaluation of newborns for suspected conditions not found**
   Reserved for future expansion

c. **Coding Additional Perinatal Diagnoses**

   1) **Assigning codes for conditions that require treatment**
      Assign codes for conditions that require treatment or further investigation, prolong the length of stay, or require resource utilization.

   2) **Codes for conditions specified as having implications for future health care needs**
      Assign codes for conditions that have been specified by the provider as having implications for future health care needs.

      Note: This guideline should not be used for adult patients.

d. **Prematurity and fetal growth retardation**
   Providers utilize different criteria in determining prematurity. A code for prematurity should not be assigned unless it is documented. Assignment of codes in categories P05, Disorders of newborn related to slow fetal growth and fetal malnutrition, and P07, Disorders of newborn related to short gestation and low birth weight, not elsewhere classified, should be based on the recorded birth weight and estimated gestational age. Codes from category P05 should not be assigned with codes from category P07.

   When both birth weight and gestational age are available, two codes from category P07 should be assigned, with the code for birth weight sequenced before the code for gestational age.

e. **Low birth weight and immaturity status**
   Codes from category P07, Disorders of newborn related to short gestation and low birth weight, not elsewhere classified, are for use for a child or adult who was premature or had a low birth weight as a newborn and this is affecting the patient's current health status.

   See Section I.C.21. Factors influencing health status and contact with health services, Status.

f. **Bacterial sepsis of newborn**
   Category P36, Bacterial sepsis of newborn, includes congenital sepsis. If a perinate is documented as having sepsis without documentation of congenital or community acquired, the default is congenital and a code from category P36 should be assigned. If the P36 code includes the causal organism, an additional code from category B95, Streptococcus, Staphylococcus, and Enterococcus as the cause of diseases classified elsewhere, or B96, Other bacterial agents as the cause of diseases classified elsewhere, should not be assigned. If the P36 code does not include the causal organism, assign an additional code from category B96. If applicable, use additional codes to identify severe sepsis (R65.2-) and any associated acute organ dysfunction.

g. **Stillbirth**
   Code P95, Stillbirth, is only for use in institutions that maintain separate records for stillbirths. No other code should be used with P95. Code P95 should not be used on the mother's record.

17. **Chapter 17: Congenital Malformations, Deformations, and Chromosomal Abnormalities (Q00-Q99)**
    Assign an appropriate code(s) from categories Q00-Q99, Congenital malformations, deformations, and chromosomal abnormalities when a malformation/deformation or chromosomal abnormality is documented. A malformation/deformation/or chromosomal abnormality may be the principal/first-listed diagnosis on a record or a secondary diagnosis.

    When a malformation/deformation/or chromosomal abnormality does not have a unique code assignment, assign additional code(s) for any manifestations that may be present.

    When the code assignment specifically identifies the malformation/deformation/or chromosomal abnormality, manifestations that are an inherent component of the anomaly should not be coded separately. Additional codes should be assigned for manifestations that are not an inherent component.

    Codes from Chapter 17 may be used throughout the life of the patient. If a congenital malformation or deformity has been corrected, a personal history code should be used to identify the history of the malformation or deformity. Although present at birth, malformation/deformation/or chromosomal abnormality may not be identified until later in life.

Whenever the condition is diagnosed by the physician, it is appropriate to assign a code from codes Q00-Q99.

For the birth admission, the appropriate code from category Z38, Liveborn infants, according to place of birth and type of delivery, should be sequenced as the principal diagnosis, followed by any congenital anomaly codes, Q00- Q99.

18. **Chapter 18: Symptoms, Signs, and Abnormal Clinical and Laboratory Findings, Not Elsewhere Classified (R00-R99)**
    Chapter 18 includes symptoms, signs, abnormal results of clinical or other investigative procedures, and ill-defined conditions regarding which no diagnosis classifiable elsewhere is recorded. Signs and symptoms that point to a specific diagnosis have been assigned to a category in other chapters of the classification.

a. **Use of symptom codes**
   Codes that describe symptoms and signs are acceptable for reporting purposes when a related definitive diagnosis has not been established (confirmed) by the provider.

b. **Use of a symptom code with a definitive diagnosis code**
   Codes for signs and symptoms may be reported in addition to a related definitive diagnosis when the sign or symptom is not routinely associated with that diagnosis, such as the various signs and symptoms associated with complex syndromes. The definitive diagnosis code should be sequenced before the symptom code.

   Signs or symptoms that are associated routinely with a disease process should not be assigned as additional codes, unless otherwise instructed by the classification.

c. **Combination codes that include symptoms**
   ICD-10-CM contains a number of combination codes that identify both the definitive diagnosis and common symptoms of that diagnosis. When using one of these combination codes, an additional code should not be assigned for the symptom.

d. **Repeated falls**
   Code R29.6, Repeated falls, is for use for encounters when a patient has recently fallen and the reason for the fall is being investigated.

   Code Z91.81, History of falling, is for use when a patient has fallen in the past and is at risk for future falls. When appropriate, both codes R29.6 and Z91.81 may be assigned together.

e. **Coma scale**
   The coma scale codes (R40.2-) can be used in conjunction with traumatic brain injury codes, acute cerebrovascular disease or sequelae of cerebrovascular disease codes. These codes are primarily for use by trauma registries, but they may be used in any setting where this information is collected. The coma scale codes should be sequenced after the diagnosis code(s).

   These codes, one from each subcategory, are needed to complete the scale. The 7th character indicates when the scale was recorded. The 7th character should match for all three codes.

   At a minimum, report the initial score documented on presentation at your facility. This may be a score from the emergency medicine technician (EMT) or in the emergency department. If desired, a facility may choose to capture multiple Glasgow coma scale scores.

   Assign code R40.24, Glasgow coma scale, total score, when only the total score is documented in the medical record and not the individual score(s).

f. **Functional quadriplegia**
   Functional quadriplegia (code R53.2) is the lack of ability to use one's limbs or to ambulate due to extreme debility. It is not associated with neurologic deficit or injury, and code R53.2 should not be used for cases of neurologic quadriplegia. It should only be assigned if functional quadriplegia is specifically documented in the medical record.

g. **SIRS due to non-infectious process**
   The systemic inflammatory response syndrome (SIRS) can develop as a result of certain non-infectious disease processes, such as trauma, malignant neoplasm, or pancreatitis. When SIRS is documented with a noninfectious condition, and no subsequent infection is documented, the code for the underlying condition, such as an injury, should be assigned, followed by code R65.10, Systemic inflammatory response syndrome (SIRS) of non-infectious origin without acute organ dysfunction, or code R65.11, Systemic inflammatory response syndrome (SIRS) of non-infectious origin

with acute organ dysfunction. If an associated acute organ dysfunction is documented, the appropriate code(s) for the specific type of organ dysfunction(s) should be assigned in addition to code R65.11. If acute organ dysfunction is documented, but it cannot be determined if the acute organ dysfunction is associated with SIRS or due to another condition (e.g., directly due to the trauma), the provider should be queried.

h. Death NOS

Code R99, Ill-defined and unknown cause of mortality, is only for use in the very limited circumstance when a patient who has already died is brought into an emergency department or other healthcare facility and is pronounced dead upon arrival. It does not represent the discharge disposition of death.

19. Chapter 19: Injury, Poisoning, and Certain Other Consequences of External Causes (S00-T88)

a. Application of 7th Characters in Chapter 19

Most categories in chapter 19 have a 7th character requirement for each applicable code. Most categories in this chapter have three 7th character values (with the exception of fractures): A, initial encounter, D, subsequent encounter and S, sequela. Categories for traumatic fractures have additional 7th character values.

7th character "A", initial encounter is used while the patient is receiving active treatment for the condition. Examples of active treatment are: surgical treatment, emergency department encounter, and evaluation and treatment by a new physician.

7th character "D" subsequent encounter is used for encounters after the patient has received active treatment of the condition and is receiving routine care for the condition during the healing or recovery phase. Examples of subsequent care are: cast change or removal, removal of external or internal fixation device, medication adjustment, other aftercare and follow up visits following treatment of the injury or condition.

The aftercare Z codes should not be used for aftercare for conditions such as injuries or poisonings, where 7th characters are provided to identify subsequent care. For example, for aftercare of an injury, assign the acute injury code with the 7th character "D" (subsequent encounter).

7th character "S", sequela, is for use for complications or conditions that arise as a direct result of a condition, such as scar formation after a burn. The scars are sequelae of the burn. When using 7th character "S", it is necessary to use both the injury code that precipitated the sequela and the code for the sequela itself. The "S" is added only to the injury code, not the sequela code. The 7th character "S" identifies the injury responsible for the sequela. The specific type of sequela (e.g. scar) is sequenced first, followed by the injury code.

b. Coding of injuries

When coding injuries, assign separate codes for each injury unless a combination code is provided, in which case the combination code is assigned. Code T07, Unspecified multiple injuries should not be assigned in the inpatient setting unless information for a more specific code is not available. Traumatic injury codes (S00-T14.9) are not to be used for normal, healing surgical wounds or to identify complications of surgical wounds.

The code for the most serious injury, as determined by the provider and the focus of treatment, is sequenced first.

1) Superficial injuries

Superficial injuries such as abrasions or contusions are not coded when associated with more severe injuries of the same site.

2) Primary injury with damage to nerves/blood vessels

When a primary injury results in minor damage to peripheral nerves or blood vessels, the primary injury is sequenced first with additional code(s) for injuries to nerves and spinal cord (such as category S04), and/or injury to blood vessels (such as category S15). When the primary injury is to the blood vessels or nerves, that injury should be sequenced first.

c. Coding of traumatic fractures

The principles of multiple coding of injuries should be followed in coding fractures. Fractures of specified sites are coded individually by site in accordance with both the provisions within categories S02, S12, S22, S32, S42, S49, S52, S59, S62, S72, S79, S82, S89, S92 and the level of detail furnished by medical record content.

A fracture not indicated as open or closed should be coded to closed. A fracture not indicated whether displaced or not displaced should be coded to displaced.

More specific guidelines are as follows:

1) Initial vs. subsequent encounter for fractures

Traumatic fractures are coded using the appropriate 7th character extension for initial encounter (A, B, C) while the patient is receiving active treatment for the fracture. Examples of active treatment are: surgical treatment, emergency department encounter, and evaluation and treatment by a new physician. The appropriate 7th character for initial encounter should also be assigned for a patient who delayed seeking treatment for the fracture or nonunion.

Fractures are coded using the appropriate 7th character extension for subsequent care for encounters after the patient has completed active treatment of the fracture and is receiving routine care for the fracture during the healing or recovery phase. Examples of fracture aftercare are: cast change or removal, removal of external or internal fixation device, medication adjustment, and follow-up visits following fracture treatment.

Care for complications of surgical treatment for fracture repairs during the healing or recovery phase should be coded with the appropriate complication codes.

Care of complications of fractures, such as malunion and nonunion, should be reported with the appropriate 7th character extensions for subsequent care with nonunion (K, M, N,) or subsequent care with malunion (P, Q, R).

A code from category M80, not a traumatic fracture code, should be used for any patient with known osteoporosis who suffers a fracture, even if the patient had a minor fall or trauma, if that fall or trauma would not usually break a normal, healthy bone.

See Section I.C.13. Osteoporosis.

The aftercare Z codes should not be used for aftercare for traumatic fractures. For aftercare of a traumatic fracture, assign the acute fracture code with the appropriate 7th character.

2) Multiple fractures sequencing

Multiple fractures are sequenced in accordance with the severity of the fracture.

d. Coding of burns and corrosions

The ICD-10-CM makes a distinction between burns and corrosions. The burn codes are for thermal burns, except sunburns, that come from a heat source, such as a fire or hot appliance. The burn codes are also for burns resulting from electricity and radiation. Corrosions are burns due to chemicals. The guidelines are the same for burns and corrosions.

Current burns (T20-T25) are classified by depth, extent and by agent (X code). Burns are classified by depth as first degree (erythema), second degree (blistering), and third degree (full-thickness involvement). Burns of the eye and internal organs (T26-T28) are classified by site, but not by degree.

1) Sequencing of burn and related condition codes

Sequence first the code that reflects the highest degree of burn when more than one burn is present.

a. When the reason for the admission or encounter is for treatment of external multiple burns, sequence first the code that reflects the burn of the highest degree.

b. When a patient has both internal and external burns, the circumstances of admission govern the selection of the principal diagnosis or first-listed diagnosis.

c. When a patient is admitted for burn injuries and other related conditions such as smoke inhalation and/or respiratory failure, the circumstances of admission govern the selection of the principal or first-listed diagnosis.

2) **Burns of the same local site**

Classify burns of the same local site (three-character category level, T20-T28) but of different degrees to the subcategory identifying the highest degree recorded in the diagnosis.

3) **Non-healing burns**

Non-healing burns are coded as acute burns.

Necrosis of burned skin should be coded as a non-healed burn.

4) **Infected burn**

For any documented infected burn site, use an additional code for the infection.

5) **Assign separate codes for each burn site**

When coding burns, assign separate codes for each burn site. Category T30, Burn and corrosion, body region unspecified is extremely vague and should rarely be used.

6) **Burns and corrosions classified according to extent of body surface involved**

Assign codes from category T31, Burns classified according to extent of body surface involved, or T32, Corrosions classified according to extent of body surface involved, when the site of the burn is not specified or when there is a need for additional data. It is advisable to use category T31 as additional coding when needed to provide data for evaluating burn mortality, such as that needed by burn units. It is also advisable to use category T31 as an additional code for reporting purposes when there is mention of a third-degree burn involving 20 percent or more of the body surface.

Categories T31 and T32 are based on the classic "rule of nines" in estimating body surface involved: head and neck are assigned nine percent, each arm nine percent, each leg 18 percent, the anterior trunk 18 percent, posterior trunk 18 percent, and genitalia one percent. Providers may change these percentage assignments where necessary to accommodate infants and children who have proportionately larger heads than adults, and patients who have large buttocks, thighs, or abdomen that involve burns.

7) **Encounters for treatment of sequela of burns**

Encounters for the treatment of the late effects of burns or corrosions (i.e., scars or joint contractures) should be coded with a burn or corrosion code with the 7th character "S" for sequela.

8) **Sequelae with a late effect code and current burn**

When appropriate, both a code for a current burn or corrosion with 7th character "A" or "D" and a burn or corrosion code with 7th character "S" may be assigned on the same record (when both a current burn and sequelae of an old burn exist). Burns and corrosions do not heal at the same rate and a current healing wound may still exist with sequela of a healed burn or corrosion.

9) **Use of an external cause code with burns and corrosions**

An external cause code should be used with burns and corrosions to identify the source and intent of the burn, as well as the place where it occurred.

e. **Adverse effects, poisoning, underdosing and toxic effects**

Codes in categories T36-T65 are combination codes that include the substance that was taken as well as the intent. No additional external cause code is required for poisonings, toxic effects, adverse effects and underdosing codes.

1) **Do not code directly from the Table of Drugs**

Do not code directly from the Table of Drugs and Chemicals. Always refer back to the Tabular List.

2) **Use as many codes as necessary to describe**

Use as many codes as necessary to describe completely all drugs, medicinal or biological substances.

3) **If the same code would describe the causative agent**

If the same code would describe the causative agent for more than one adverse reaction, poisoning, toxic effect or underdosing, assign the code only once.

4) **If two or more drugs, medicinal or biological substances**

If two or more drugs, medicinal or biological substances are reported, code each individually unless a combination code is listed in the Table of Drugs and Chemicals.

5) **The occurrence of drug toxicity is classified in ICD-10-CM as follows:**

(a) **Adverse effect**

When coding an adverse effect of a drug that has been correctly prescribed and properly administered, assign the appropriate code for the nature of the adverse effect followed by the appropriate code for the adverse effect of the drug (T36-T50). The code for the drug should have a 5th or 6th character "5" (for example T36.0X5-) Examples of the nature of an adverse effect are tachycardia, delirium, gastrointestinal hemorrhaging, vomiting, hypokalemia, hepatitis, renal failure, or respiratory failure.

(b) **Poisoning**

When coding a poisoning or reaction to the improper use of a medication (e.g., overdose, wrong substance given or taken in error, wrong route of administration), first assign the appropriate code from categories T36-T50. The poisoning codes have an associated intent as their 5th or 6th character (accidental, intentional self-harm, assault and undetermined. Use additional code(s) for all manifestations of poisonings.

If there is also a diagnosis of abuse or dependence of the substance, the abuse or dependence is assigned as an additional code.

Examples of poisoning include:

(i) Error was made in drug prescription

Errors made in drug prescription or in the administration of the drug by provider, nurse, patient, or other person.

(ii) Overdose of a drug intentionally taken

If an overdose of a drug was intentionally taken or administered and resulted in drug toxicity, it would be coded as a poisoning.

(iii) Nonprescribed drug taken with correctly prescribed and properly administered drug

If a nonprescribed drug or medicinal agent was taken in combination with a correctly prescribed and properly administered drug, any drug toxicity or other reaction resulting from the interaction of the two drugs would be classified as a poisoning.

(iv) Interaction of drug(s) and alcohol

When a reaction results from the interaction of a drug(s) and alcohol, this would be classified as poisoning.

See Section I.C.4. if poisoning is the result of insulin pump malfunctions.

(c) **Underdosing**

Underdosing refers to taking less of a medication than is prescribed by a provider or a manufacturer's instruction. For underdosing, assign the code from categories T36-T50 (fifth or sixth character "6").

Codes for underdosing should never be assigned as principal or first-listed codes. If a patient has a relapse or exacerbation of the medical condition for which the drug is prescribed because of the reduction in dose, then the medical condition itself should be coded.

Noncompliance (Z91.12-, Z91.13-) or complication of care (Y63.6-Y63.9) codes are to be used with an underdosing code to indicate intent, if known.

(d) **Toxic effects**

When a harmful substance is ingested or comes in contact with a person, this is classified as a toxic effect. The toxic effect codes are in categories T51-T65.

Toxic effect codes have an associated intent: accidental, intentional self-harm, assault and undetermined.

f. **Adult and child abuse, neglect and other maltreatment**

Sequence first the appropriate code from categories T74.- (Adult and child abuse, neglect and other maltreatment, confirmed) or T76.- (Adult and child abuse, neglect and other maltreatment, suspected) for abuse, neglect and other maltreatment, followed by any accompanying mental health or injury code(s).

If the documentation in the medical record states abuse or neglect it is coded as confirmed (T74.-). It is coded as suspected if it is documented as suspected (T76.-).

For cases of confirmed abuse or neglect an external cause code from the assault section (X92-Y08) should be added to identify the cause of any physical injuries. A perpetrator code (Y07) should be added when the perpetrator of the abuse is known. For suspected cases of abuse or neglect, do not report external cause or perpetrator code.

If a suspected case of abuse, neglect or mistreatment is ruled out during an encounter code Z04.71, Encounter for examination and observation following alleged physical adult abuse, ruled out, or code Z04.72, Encounter for examination and observation following alleged child physical abuse, ruled out, should be used, not a code from T76.

If a suspected case of alleged rape or sexual abuse is ruled out during an encounter code Z04.41, Encounter for examination and observation following alleged physical adult abuse, ruled out, or code Z04.42, Encounter for examination and observation following alleged rape or sexual abuse, ruled out, should be used, not a code from T76.

See Section I.C.15. Abuse in a pregnant patient.

g. **Complications of care**

1) **General guidelines for complications of care**

(a) **Documentation of complications of care**

See Section I.B.16. for information on documentation of complications of care.

2) **Pain due to medical devices**

Pain associated with devices, implants or grafts left in a surgical site (for example painful hip prosthesis) is assigned to the appropriate code(s) found in Chapter 19, Injury, poisoning, and certain other consequences of external causes. Specific codes for pain due to medical devices are found in the T code section of the ICD-10-CM. Use additional code(s) from category G89 to identify acute or chronic pain due to presence of the device, implant or graft (G89.18 or G89.28).

3) **Transplant complications**

(a) **Transplant complications other than kidney**

Codes under category T86, Complications of transplanted organs and tissues, are for use for both complications and rejection of transplanted organs. A transplant complication code is only assigned if the complication affects the function of the transplanted organ. Two codes are required to fully describe a transplant complication: the appropriate code from category T86 and a secondary code that identifies the complication.

Pre-existing conditions or conditions that develop after the transplant are not coded as complications unless they affect the function of the transplanted organs.

See I.C.21. for transplant organ removal status

See I.C.2. for malignant neoplasm associated with transplanted organ.

(b) **Kidney transplant complications**

Patients who have undergone kidney transplant may still have some form of chronic kidney disease (CKD) because the kidney transplant may not fully restore kidney function. Code T86.1- should be assigned for documented complications of a kidney transplant, such as transplant failure or rejection or other transplant complication. Code T86.1- should not be assigned for post kidney transplant patients who have chronic kidney (CKD) unless a transplant complication such as transplant failure or rejection is documented. If the documentation is unclear as to whether the patient has a complication of the transplant, query the provider.

Conditions that affect the function of the transplanted kidney, other than CKD, should be assigned a code from subcategory T86.1, Complications of transplanted organ, Kidney, and a secondary code that identifies the complication.

For patients with CKD following a kidney transplant, but who do not have a complication such as failure or rejection, *see section I.C.14. Chronic kidney disease and kidney transplant status.*

4) **Complication codes that include the external cause**

As with certain other T codes, some of the complications of care codes have the external cause included in the code. The code includes the nature of the complication as well as the type of procedure that caused the complication. No external cause code indicating the type of procedure is necessary for these codes.

5) **Complications of care codes within the body system chapters**

Intraoperative and postprocedural complication codes are found within the body system chapters with codes specific to the organs and structures of that body system. These codes should be sequenced first, followed by a code(s) for the specific complication, if applicable.

20. **Chapter 20: External Causes of Morbidity (V00-Y99)**

The external causes of morbidity codes should never be sequenced as the first-listed or principal diagnosis.

External cause codes are intended to provide data for injury research and evaluation of injury prevention strategies. These codes capture how the injury or health condition happened (cause), the intent (unintentional or accidental; or intentional, such as suicide or assault), the place where the event occurred the activity of the patient at the time of the event, and the person's status (e.g., civilian, military).

There is no national requirement for mandatory ICD-10-CM external cause code reporting. Unless a provider is subject to a state-based external cause code reporting mandate or these codes are required by a particular payer, reporting of ICD-10-CM codes in Chapter 20, External Causes of Morbidity, is not required. In the absence of a mandatory reporting requirement, providers are encouraged to voluntarily report external cause codes, as they provide valuable data for injury research and evaluation of injury prevention strategies.

a. **General external cause coding guidelines**

1) **Used with any code in the range of A00.0-T88.9, Z00-Z99**

An external cause code may be used with any code in the range of A00.0-T88.9, Z00-Z99, classification that is a health condition due to an external cause. Though they are most applicable to injuries, they are also valid for use with such things as infections or diseases due to an external source, and other health conditions, such as a heart attack that occurs during strenuous physical activity.

2) **External cause code used for length of treatment**

Assign the external cause code, with the appropriate 7th character (initial encounter, subsequent encounter or sequela) for each encounter for which the injury or condition is being treated.

3) **Use the full range of external cause codes**

Use the full range of external cause codes to completely describe the cause, the intent, the place of occurrence, and if applicable, the activity of the patient at the time of the event, and the patient's status, for all injuries, and other health conditions due to an external cause.

4) **Assign as many external cause codes as necessary**

Assign as many external cause codes as necessary to fully explain each cause. If only one external code can be recorded, assign the code most related to the principal diagnosis.

5) **The selection of the appropriate external cause code**

The selection of the appropriate external cause code is guided by the Alphabetic Index of External Causes and by Inclusion and Exclusion notes in the Tabular List.

6) **External cause code can never be a principal diagnosis**
An external cause code can never be a principal (first-listed) diagnosis.

7) **Combination external cause codes**
Certain of the external cause codes are combination codes that identify sequential events that result in an injury, such as a fall which results in striking against an object. The injury may be due to either event or both. The combination external cause code used should correspond to the sequence of events regardless of which caused the most serious injury.

8) **No external cause code needed in certain circumstances**
No external cause code from Chapter 20 is needed if the external cause and intent are included in a code from another chapter (e.g. T36.0x1- Poisoning by penicillins, accidental (unintentional)).

b. **Place of occurrence guideline**
Codes from category Y92, Place of occurrence of the external cause, are secondary codes for use after other external cause codes to identify the location of the patient at the time of injury or other condition.

A place of occurrence code is used only once, at the initial encounter for treatment. No 7th characters are used for Y92. Only one code from Y92 should be recorded on a medical record.

Do not use place of occurrence code Y92.9 if the place is not stated or is not applicable.

c. **Activity code**
Assign a code from category Y93, Activity code, to describe the activity of the patient at the time the injury or other health condition occurred.

An activity code is used only once, at the initial encounter for treatment. Only one code from Y93 should be recorded on a medical record.

The activity codes are not applicable to poisonings, adverse effects, misadventures or sequela.

Do not assign Y93.9, Unspecified activity, if the activity is not stated.

A code from category Y93 is appropriate for use with external cause and intent codes if identifying the activity provides additional information about the event.

d. **Place of occurrence, activity, and status codes used with other external cause code**
When applicable, place of occurrence, activity, and external cause status codes are sequenced after the main external cause code(s). Regardless of the number of external cause codes assigned, there should be only one place of occurrence code, one activity code, and one external cause status code assigned to an encounter.

e. **If the reporting format limits the number of external cause codes**
If the reporting format limits the number of external cause codes that can be used in reporting clinical data, report the code for the cause/intent most related to the principal diagnosis. If the format permits capture of additional external cause codes, the cause/intent, including medical misadventures, of the additional events should be reported rather than the codes for place, activity, or external status.

f. **Multiple external cause coding guidelines**
More than one external cause code is required to fully describe the external cause of an illness or injury. The assignment of external cause codes should be sequenced in the following priority:

If two or more events cause separate injuries, an external cause code should be assigned for each cause. The first-listed external cause code will be selected in the following order:

External codes for child and adult abuse take priority over all other external cause codes.

See Section I.C.19., Child and Adult abuse guidelines.

External cause codes for terrorism events take priority over all other external cause codes except child and adult abuse.

External cause codes for cataclysmic events take priority over all other external cause codes except child and adult abuse and terrorism.

External cause codes for transport accidents take priority over all other external cause codes except cataclysmic events, child and adult abuse and terrorism.

Activity and external cause status codes are assigned following all causal (intent) external cause codes.

The first-listed external cause code should correspond to the cause of the most serious diagnosis due to an assault, accident, or self-harm, following the order of hierarchy listed above.

g. **Child and adult abuse guideline**
Adult and child abuse, neglect and maltreatment are classified as assault. Any of the assault codes may be used to indicate the external cause of any injury resulting from the confirmed abuse.

For confirmed cases of abuse, neglect and maltreatment, when the perpetrator is known, a code from Y07, Perpetrator of maltreatment and neglect, should accompany any other assault codes.

See Section I.C.19. Adult and child abuse, neglect and other maltreatment

h. **Unknown or undetermined intent guideline**
If the intent (accident, self-harm, assault) of the cause of an injury or other condition is unknown or unspecified, code the intent as accidental intent. All transport accident categories assume accidental intent.

1) **Use of undetermined intent**
External cause codes for events of undetermined intent are only for use if the documentation in the record specifies that the intent cannot be determined.

i. **Sequelae (Late Effects) of external cause guidelines**
1) **Sequelae external cause codes**
Sequela are reported using the external cause code with the 7th character extension "S" for sequela. These codes should be used with any report of a late effect or sequela resulting from a previous injury.

2) **Sequela external cause code with a related current injury**
A sequela external cause code should never be used with a related current nature of injury code.

3) **Use of sequela external cause codes for subsequent visits**
Use a late effect external cause code for subsequent visits when a late effect of the initial injury is being treated. Do not use a late effect external cause code for subsequent visits for follow-up care (e.g., to assess healing, to receive rehabilitative therapy) of the injury when no late effect of the injury has been documented.

j. **Terrorism guidelines**
1) **Cause of injury identified by the Federal Government (FBI) as terrorism**
When the cause of an injury is identified by the Federal Government (FBI) as terrorism, the first-listed external cause code should be a code from category Y38, Terrorism. The definition of terrorism employed by the FBI is found at the inclusion note at the beginning of category Y38. Use additional code for place of occurrence (Y92.-). More than one Y38 code may be assigned if the injury is the result of more than one mechanism of terrorism.

2) **Cause of an injury is suspected to be the result of terrorism**
When the cause of an injury is suspected to be the result of terrorism a code from category Y38 should not be assigned. Suspected cases should be classified as assault.

3) **Code Y38.9, terrorism, secondary effects**
Assign code Y38.9, Terrorism, secondary effects, for conditions occurring subsequent to the terrorist event. This code should not be assigned for conditions that are due to the initial terrorist act.

It is acceptable to assign code Y38.9 with another code from Y38 if there is an injury due to the initial terrorist event and an injury that is a subsequent result of the terrorist event.

k. **External cause status**
A code from category Y99, External cause status, should be assigned whenever any other external cause code is assigned for an encounter, including an Activity code, except for the events noted below. Assign a code from category Y99, External cause status, to

indicate the work status of the person at the time the event occurred. The status code indicates whether the event occurred during military activity, whether a non-military person was at work, whether an individual including a student or volunteer was involved in a non-work activity at the time of the causal event.

A code from Y99, External cause status, should be assigned, when applicable, with other external cause codes, such as transport accidents and falls. The external cause status codes are not applicable to poisonings, adverse effects, misadventures or late effects.

Do not assign a code from category Y99 if no other external cause codes (cause, activity) are applicable for the encounter.

An external cause status code is used only once, at the initial encounter for treatment. Only one code from Y99 should be recorded on a medical record.

Do not assign code Y99.9, Unspecified external cause status, if the status is not stated.

21. **Chapter 21: Factors Influencing Health Status and Contact with Health Services (Z00-Z99)**
    Note: The chapter specific guidelines provide additional information about the use of Z codes for specified encounters.

    a. **Use of Z codes in any healthcare setting**
       Z codes are for use in any healthcare setting. Z codes may be used as either a first-listed (principal diagnosis code in the inpatient setting) or secondary code, depending on the circumstances of the encounter. Certain Z codes may only be used as first-listed or principal diagnosis.

    b. **Z Codes indicate a reason for an encounter**
       Z codes are not procedure codes. A corresponding procedure code must accompany a Z code to describe any procedure performed.

    c. **Categories of Z codes**
       1) **Contact/exposure**
          Category Z20 indicates contact with, and suspected exposure to, communicable diseases. These codes are for patients who do not show any sign or symptom of a disease but are suspected to have been exposed to it by close personal contact with an infected individual or are in an area where a disease is epidemic.

          Category Z77, indicates contact with and suspected exposures hazardous to health.

          Contact/exposure codes may be used as a first-listed code to explain an encounter for testing, or, more commonly, as a secondary code to identify a potential risk.

       2) **Inoculations and vaccinations**
          Code Z23 is for encounters for inoculations and vaccinations. It indicates that a patient is being seen to receive a prophylactic inoculation against a disease. Procedure codes are required to identify the actual administration of the injection and the type(s) of immunizations given. Code Z23 may be used as a secondary code if the inoculation is given as a routine part of preventive health care, such as a well-baby visit.

       3) **Status**
          Status codes indicate that a patient is either a carrier of a disease or has the sequelae or residual of a past disease or condition. This includes such things as the presence of prosthetic or mechanical devices resulting from past treatment. A status code is informative, because the status may affect the course of treatment and its outcome. A status code is distinct from a history code. The history code indicates that the patient no longer has the condition.

          A status code should not be used with a diagnosis code from one of the body system chapters, if the diagnosis code includes the information provided by the status code. For example, code Z94.1, Heart transplant status, should not be used with a code from subcategory T86.2, Complications of heart transplant. The status code does not provide additional information. The complication code indicates that the patient is a heart transplant patient.

          For encounters for weaning from a mechanical ventilator, assign a code from subcategory J96.1, Chronic respiratory

failure, followed by code Z99.11, Dependence on respirator [ventilator] status.

The status Z codes/categories are:

Z14   Genetic carrier

      Genetic carrier status indicates that a person carries a gene, associated with a particular disease, which may be passed to offspring who may develop that disease. The person does not have the disease and is not at risk of developing the disease.

Z15   Genetic susceptibility to disease

      Genetic susceptibility indicates that a person has a gene that increases the risk of that person developing the disease.

      Codes from category Z15 should not be used as principal or first-listed codes. If the patient has the condition to which he/she is susceptible, and that condition is the reason for the encounter, the code for the current condition should be sequenced first. If the patient is being seen for follow-up after completed treatment for this condition, and the condition no longer exists, a follow-up code should be sequenced first, followed by the appropriate personal history and genetic susceptibility codes. If the purpose of the encounter is genetic counseling associated with procreative management, code Z31.5, Encounter for genetic counseling, should be assigned as the first-listed code, followed by a code from category Z15. Additional codes should be assigned for any applicable family or personal history.

Z16   Resistance to antimicrobial drugs

      This code indicates that a patient has a condition that is resistant to antimicrobial drug treatment. Sequence the infection code first.

Z17   Estrogen receptor status

Z18   Retained foreign body fragments

Z21   Asymptomatic HIV infection status

      This code indicates that a patient has tested positive for HIV but has manifested no signs or symptoms of the disease.

Z22   Carrier of infectious disease

      Carrier status indicates that a person harbors the specific organisms of a disease without manifest symptoms and is capable of transmitting the infection.

Z28.3 Underimmunization status

Z33.1 Pregnant state, incidental

      This code is a secondary code only for use when the pregnancy is in no way complicating the reason for visit. Otherwise, a code from the obstetric chapter is required.

Z66   Do not resuscitate

      This code may be used when it is documented by the provider that a patient is on do not resuscitate status at any time during the stay.

Z67   Blood type

Z68   Body mass index (BMI)

Z74.01 Bed confinement status

Z76.82 Awaiting organ transplant status

Z78   Other specified health status

      Code Z78.1, Physical restraint status, may be used when it is documented by the provider that a patient has been put in restraints during the current encounter. Please note that this code should not be reported when it is documented by the provider that a patient is temporarily restrained during a procedure.

Z79   Long-term (current) drug therapy

      Codes from this category indicate a patient's continuous use of a prescribed drug (including such things as aspirin therapy) for the long-term treatment of a condition or for prophylactic use. It is not for use for patients who have addictions to drugs. This subcategory is not for use of medications for detoxification or maintenance programs to prevent withdrawal symptoms in patients with drug dependence (e.g., methadone maintenance for opiate dependence). Assign the appropriate code for the drug dependence instead.

Assign a code from Z79 if the patient is receiving a medication for an extended period as a prophylactic measure (such as for the prevention of deep vein thrombosis) or as treatment of a chronic condition (such as arthritis) or a disease requiring a lengthy course of treatment (such as cancer). Do not assign a code from category Z79 for medication being administered for a brief period of time to treat an acute illness or injury (such as a course of antibiotics to treat acute bronchitis).

Z88   Allergy status to drugs, medicaments and biological substances

     Except: Z88.9, Allergy status to unspecified drugs, medicaments and biological substances status

Z89   Acquired absence of limb

Z90   Acquired absence of organs, not elsewhere classified

Z91.0- Allergy status, other than to drugs and biological substances

Z92.82 Status post administration of tPA (rtPA) in a different facility within the last 24 hours prior to admission to a current facility

     Assign code Z92.82, Status post administration of tPA (rtPA) in a different facility within the last 24 hours prior to admission to current facility, as a secondary diagnosis when a patient is received by transfer into a facility and documentation indicates they were administered tissue plasminogen activator (tPA) within the last 24 hours prior to admission to the current facility.

     This guideline applies even if the patient is still receiving the tPA at the time they are received into the current facility.

     The appropriate code for the condition for which the tPA was administered (such as cerebrovascular disease or myocardial infarction) should be assigned first.

     Code Z92.82 is only applicable to the receiving facility record and not to the transferring facility record.

Z93   Artificial opening status

Z94   Transplanted organ and tissue status

Z95   Presence of cardiac and vascular implants and grafts

Z96   Presence of other functional implants

Z97   Presence of other devices

Z98   Other postprocedural states

     Assign code Z98.85, Transplanted organ removal status, to indicate that a transplanted organ has been previously removed. This code should not be assigned for the encounter in which the transplanted organ is removed. The complication necessitating removal of the transplant organ should be assigned for that encounter.

     See section I.C19.g.3. for information on the coding of organ transplant complications.

Z99   Dependence on enabling machines and devices, not elsewhere classified

     Note: Categories Z89-Z90 and Z93-Z99 are for use only if there are no complications or malfunctions of the organ or tissue replaced, the amputation site or the equipment on which the patient is dependent.

4) History (of)
There are two types of history Z codes, personal and family. Personal history codes explain a patient's past medical condition that no longer exists and is not receiving any treatment, but that has the potential for recurrence, and therefore may require continued monitoring.

Family history codes are for use when a patient has a family member(s) who has had a particular disease that causes the patient to be at higher risk of also contracting the disease.

Personal history codes may be used in conjunction with follow-up codes and family history codes may be used in conjunction with screening codes to explain the need for a test or procedure. History codes are also acceptable on any medical record regardless of the reason for visit. A history of an illness, even if no longer present, is important information that may alter the type of treatment ordered.

The history Z code categories are:

Z80   Family history of primary malignant neoplasm

Z81   Family history of mental and behavioral disorders

Z82   Family history of certain disabilities and chronic diseases (leading to disablement)

Z83   Family history of other specific disorders

Z84   Family history of other conditions

Z85   Personal history of malignant neoplasm

Z86   Personal history of certain other diseases

Z87   Personal history of other diseases and conditions

Z91.4- Personal history of psychological trauma, not elsewhere classified

Z91.5   Personal history of self-harm

Z91.8- Other specified personal risk factors, not elsewhere classified

     Exception: Z91.83, Wandering in diseases classified elsewhere

Z92   Personal history of medical treatment

     Except: Z92.0, Personal history of contraception

     Except: Z92.82, Status post administration of tPA (rtPA) in a different facility within the last 24 hours prior to admission to a current facility

5) Screening
Screening is the testing for disease or disease precursors in seemingly well individuals so that early detection and treatment can be provided for those who test positive for the disease (e.g., screening mammogram).

The testing of a person to rule out or confirm a suspected diagnosis because the patient has some sign or symptom is a diagnostic examination, not a screening. In these cases, the sign or symptom is used to explain the reason for the test.

A screening code may be a first-listed code if the reason for the visit is specifically the screening exam. It may also be used as an additional code if the screening is done during an office visit for other health problems. A screening code is not necessary if the screening is inherent to a routine examination, such as a pap smear done during a routine pelvic examination.

Should a condition be discovered during the screening then the code for the condition may be assigned as an additional diagnosis.

The Z code indicates that a screening exam is planned. A procedure code is required to confirm that the screening was performed.

The screening Z codes/categories:

Z11   Encounter for screening for infectious and parasitic diseases

Z12   Encounter for screening for malignant neoplasms

Z13   Encounter for screening for other diseases and disorders

     Except: Z13.9, Encounter for screening, unspecified

Z36   Encounter for antenatal screening for mother

6) Observation
There are two observation Z code categories. They are for use in very limited circumstances when a person is being observed for a suspected condition that is ruled out. The observation codes are not for use if an injury or illness or any signs or symptoms

related to the suspected condition are present. In such cases the diagnosis/symptom code is used with the corresponding external cause code.

The observation codes are to be used as principal diagnosis only. Additional codes may be used in addition to the observation code but only if they are unrelated to the suspected condition being observed.

Codes from subcategory Z03.7, Encounter for suspected maternal and fetal conditions ruled out, may either be used as a first-listed or as an additional code assignment depending on the case. They are for use in very limited circumstances on a maternal record when an encounter is for a suspected maternal or fetal condition that is ruled out during that encounter (for example, a maternal or fetal condition may be suspected due to an abnormal test result). These codes should not be used when the condition is confirmed. In those cases, the confirmed condition should be coded. In addition, these codes are not for use if an illness or any signs or symptoms related to the suspected condition or problem are present. In such cases the diagnosis/symptom code is used.

Additional codes may be used in addition to the code from subcategory Z03.7, but only if they are unrelated to the suspected condition being evaluated.

Codes from subcategory Z03.7 may not be used for encounters for antenatal screening of mother. *See Section I.C.21.c.5, Screening.*

For encounters for suspected fetal condition that are inconclusive following testing and evaluation, assign the appropriate code from category O35, O36, O40 or O41.

The observation Z code categories:

Z03   Encounter for medical observation for suspected diseases and conditions ruled out

Z04   Encounter for examination and observation for other reasons

  Except: Z04.9, Encounter for examination and observation for unspecified reason

7) **Aftercare**

Aftercare visit codes cover situations when the initial treatment of a disease has been performed and the patient requires continued care during the healing or recovery phase, or for the long-term consequences of the disease. The aftercare Z code should not be used if treatment is directed at a current, acute disease. The diagnosis code is to be used in these cases. Exceptions to this rule are codes Z51.0, Encounter for antineoplastic radiation therapy, and codes from subcategory Z51.1, Encounter for antineoplastic chemotherapy and immunotherapy. These codes are to be first-listed, followed by the diagnosis code when a patient's encounter is solely to receive radiation therapy, chemotherapy, or immunotherapy for the treatment of a neoplasm. If the reason for the encounter is more than one type of antineoplastic therapy, code Z51.0 and a code from subcategory Z51.1 may be assigned together, in which case one of these codes would be reported as a secondary diagnosis.

The aftercare Z codes should also not be used for aftercare for injuries. For aftercare of an injury, assign the acute injury code with the appropriate 7th character (for subsequent encounter).

The aftercare codes are generally first-listed to explain the specific reason for the encounter. An aftercare code may be used as an additional code when some type of aftercare is provided in addition to the reason for admission and no diagnosis code is applicable. An example of this would be the closure of a colostomy during an encounter for treatment of another condition.

Aftercare codes should be used in conjunction with other aftercare codes or diagnosis codes to provide better detail on the specifics of an aftercare encounter visit, unless otherwise directed by the classification. Should a patient receive multiple types of antineoplastic therapy during the same encounter, code Z51.0, Encounter for antineoplastic radiation therapy, and codes from subcategory Z51.1, Encounter for antineoplastic

chemotherapy and immunotherapy, may be used together on a record. The sequencing of multiple aftercare codes depends on the circumstances of the encounter.

Certain aftercare Z code categories need a secondary diagnosis code to describe the resolving condition or sequelae. For others, the condition is included in the code title.

Additional Z code aftercare category terms include fitting and adjustment, and attention to artificial openings.

Status Z codes may be used with aftercare Z codes to indicate the nature of the aftercare. For example code Z95.1, Presence of aortocoronary bypass graft, may be used with code Z48.812, Encounter for surgical aftercare following surgery on the circulatory system, to indicate the surgery for which the aftercare is being performed. A status code should not be used when the aftercare code indicates the type of status, such as using Z43.0, Encounter for attention to tracheostomy, with Z93.0, Tracheostomy status.

The aftercare Z category/codes:

Z42   Encounter for plastic and reconstructive surgery following medical procedure or healed injury

Z43   Encounter for attention to artificial openings

Z44   Encounter for fitting and adjustment of external prosthetic device

Z45   Encounter for adjustment and management of implanted device

Z46   Encounter for fitting and adjustment of other devices

Z47   Orthopedic aftercare

Z48   Encounter for other postprocedural aftercare

Z49   Encounter for care involving renal dialysis

Z51   Encounter for other aftercare

8) **Follow-up**

The follow-up codes are used to explain continuing surveillance following completed treatment of a disease, condition, or injury. They imply that the condition has been fully treated and no longer exists. They should not be confused with aftercare codes, or injury codes with a 7th character for subsequent encounter, that explain ongoing care of a healing condition or its sequelae. Follow-up codes may be used in conjunction with history codes to provide the full picture of the healed condition and its treatment. The follow-up code is sequenced first, followed by the history code.

A follow-up code may be used to explain multiple visits. Should a condition be found to have recurred on the follow-up visit, then the diagnosis code for the condition should be assigned in place of the follow-up code.

The follow-up Z code categories:

Z08   Encounter for follow-up examination after completed treatment for malignant neoplasm

Z09   Encounter for follow-up examination after completed treatment for conditions other than malignant neoplasm

Z39   Encounter for maternal postpartum care and examination

9) **Donor**

Codes in category Z52, Donors of organs and tissues, are used for living individuals who are donating blood or other body tissue. These codes are only for individuals donating for others, not for self-donations. They are not used to identify cadaveric donations.

10) **Counseling**

Counseling Z codes are used when a patient or family member receives assistance in the aftermath of an illness or injury, or when support is required in coping with family or social problems. They are not used in conjunction with a diagnosis code when the counseling component of care is considered integral to standard treatment.

The counseling Z codes/categories:

Z30.0- Encounter for general counseling and advice on contraception

Z31.5   Encounter for genetic counseling

Z31.6-   Encounter for general counseling and advice on procreation

Z32.2   Encounter for childbirth instruction

Z32.3   Encounter for childcare instruction

Z69   Encounter for mental health services for victim and perpetrator of abuse

Z70   Counseling related to sexual attitude, behavior and orientation

Z71   Persons encountering health services for other counseling and medical advice, not elsewhere classified

Z76.81   Expectant mother prebirth pediatrician visit

11) Encounters for obstetrical and reproductive services
See Section I.C.15. Pregnancy, Childbirth, and the Puerperium, for further instruction on the use of these codes.

Z codes for pregnancy are for use in those circumstances when none of the problems or complications included in the codes from the Obstetrics chapter exist (a routine prenatal visit or postpartum care). Codes in category Z34, Encounter for supervision of normal pregnancy, are always first-listed and are not to be used with any other code from the OB chapter.

Codes in category Z3A, Weeks of gestation, may be assigned to provide additional information about the pregnancy. **The date of the admission should be used to determine weeks of gestation for inpatient admissions that encompass more than one gestational week.**

The outcome of delivery, category Z37, should be included on all maternal delivery records. It is always a secondary code. Codes in category Z37 should not be used on the newborn record.

Z codes for family planning (contraceptive) or procreative management and counseling should be included on an obstetric record either during the pregnancy or the postpartum stage, if applicable.

Z codes/categories for obstetrical and reproductive services:

Z30   Encounter for contraceptive management

Z31   Encounter for procreative management

Z32.2   Encounter for childbirth instruction

Z32.3   Encounter for childcare instruction

Z33   Pregnant state

Z34   Encounter for supervision of normal pregnancy

Z36   Encounter for antenatal screening of mother

Z3A   Weeks of gestation

Z37   Outcome of delivery

Z39   Encounter for maternal postpartum care and examination

Z76.81   Expectant mother prebirth pediatrician visit

12) Newborns and Infants
See Section I.C.16. Newborn (Perinatal) Guidelines, for further instruction on the use of these codes.

Newborn Z codes/categories:

Z76.1   Encounter for health supervision and care of foundling

Z00.1-   Encounter for routine child health examination

Z38   Liveborn infants according to place of birth and type of delivery

13) Routine and administrative examinations
The Z codes allow for the description of encounters for routine examinations, such as, a general check-up, or, examinations for administrative purposes, such as, a pre-employment physical. The codes are not to be used if the examination is for diagnosis of a suspected condition or for treatment purposes. In such cases the diagnosis code is used. During a routine exam, should a diagnosis or condition be discovered, it should be coded as an additional code. Pre-existing and chronic conditions and history codes may also be included as additional codes as long as the examination is for administrative purposes and not focused on any particular condition.

Some of the codes for routine health examinations distinguish between "with" and "without" abnormal findings. Code assignment depends on the information that is known at the time the encounter is being coded. For example, if no abnormal findings were found during the examination, but the encounter is being coded before test results are back, it is acceptable to assign the code for "without abnormal findings." When assigning a code for "with abnormal findings," additional code(s) should be assigned to identify the specific abnormal finding(s).

Pre-operative examination and pre-procedural laboratory examination Z codes are for use only in those situations when a patient is being cleared for a procedure or surgery and no treatment is given.

The Z codes/categories for routine and administrative examinations:

Z00   Encounter for general examination without complaint, suspected or reported diagnosis

Z01   Encounter for other special examination without complaint, suspected or reported diagnosis

Z02   Encounter for administrative examination

        Except: Z02.9, Encounter for administrative examinations, unspecified

Z32.0-   Encounter for pregnancy test

14) Miscellaneous Z codes
The miscellaneous Z codes capture a number of other health care encounters that do not fall into one of the other categories. Certain of these codes identify the reason for the encounter; others are for use as additional codes that provide useful information on circumstances that may affect a patient's care and treatment.

Prophylactic Organ Removal
For encounters specifically for prophylactic removal of an organ (such as prophylactic removal of breasts due to a genetic susceptibility to cancer or a family history of cancer), the principal or first-listed code should be a code from category Z40, Encounter for prophylactic surgery, followed by the appropriate codes to identify the associated risk factor (such as genetic susceptibility or family history).

If the patient has a malignancy of one site and is having prophylactic removal at another site to prevent either a new primary malignancy or metastatic disease, a code for the malignancy should also be assigned in addition to a code from subcategory Z40.0, Encounter for prophylactic surgery for risk factors related to malignant neoplasms. A Z40.0 code should not be assigned if the patient is having organ removal for treatment of a malignancy, such as the removal of the testes for the treatment of prostate cancer.

Miscellaneous Z codes/categories:

Z28   Immunization not carried out

        Except: Z28.3, Underimmunization status

Z40   Encounter for prophylactic surgery

Z41   Encounter for procedures for purposes other than remedying health state

        Except: Z41.9, Encounter for procedure for purposes other than remedying health state, unspecified

Z53   Persons encountering health services for specific procedures and treatment, not carried out

Z55   Problems related to education and literacy

Z56   Problems related to employment and unemployment

Z57   Occupational exposure to risk factors

Z58   Problems related to physical environment

Z59   Problems related to housing and economic circumstances

Z60   Problems related to social environment

Z62   Problems related to upbringing

Z63   Other problems related to primary support group, including family circumstances

Z64	Problems related to certain psychosocial circumstances
Z65	Problems related to other psychosocial circumstances
Z72	Problems related to lifestyle
Z73	Problems related to life management difficulty
Z74	Problems related to care provider dependency
	Except: Z74.01, Bed confinement status
Z75	Problems related to medical facilities and other health care
Z76.0	Encounter for issue of repeat prescription
Z76.3	Healthy person accompanying sick person
Z76.4	Other boarder to healthcare facility
Z76.5	Malingerer [conscious simulation]
Z91.1-	Patient's noncompliance with medical treatment and regimen
Z91.83	Wandering in diseases classified elsewhere
Z91.89	Other specified personal risk factors, not elsewhere classified

15) Nonspecific Z codes

Certain Z codes are so non-specific, or potentially redundant with other codes in the classification, that there can be little justification for their use in the inpatient setting. Their use in the outpatient setting should be limited to those instances when there is no further documentation to permit more precise coding. Otherwise, any sign or symptom or any other reason for visit that is captured in another code should be used.

Nonspecific Z codes/categories:

Z02.9	Encounter for administrative examinations, unspecified
Z04.9	Encounter for examination and observation for unspecified reason
Z13.9	Encounter for screening, unspecified
Z41.9	Encounter for procedure for purposes other than remedying health state, unspecified
Z52.9	Donor of unspecified organ or tissue
Z86.59	Personal history of other mental and behavioral disorders
Z88.9	Allergy status to unspecified drugs, medicaments and biological substances status
Z92.0	Personal history of contraception

16) Z codes that may only be principal/first-listed diagnosis

The following Z codes/categories may only be reported as the principal/first-listed diagnosis, except when there are multiple encounters on the same day and the medical records for the encounters are combined:

Z00	Encounter for general examination without complaint, suspected or reported diagnosis
Z01	Encounter for other special examination without complaint, suspected or reported diagnosis
Z02	Encounter for administrative examination
Z03	Encounter for medical observation for suspected diseases and conditions ruled out
Z04	Encounter for examination and observation for other reasons
Z31.81	Encounter for male factor infertility in female patient
Z31.82	Encounter for Rh incompatibility status
Z31.83	Encounter for assisted reproductive fertility procedure cycle
Z31.84	Encounter for fertility preservation procedure
Z33.2	Encounter for elective termination of pregnancy
Z34	Encounter for supervision of normal pregnancy
Z38	Liveborn infants according to place of birth and type of delivery
Z39	Encounter for maternal postpartum care and examination
Z42	Encounter for plastic and reconstructive surgery following medical procedure or healed injury
Z51.0	Encounter for antineoplastic radiation therapy

Z51.1-	Encounter for antineoplastic chemotherapy and immunotherapy
Z52	Donors of organs and tissues
	Except: Z52.9, Donor of unspecified organ or tissue
Z76.1	Encounter for health supervision and care of foundling
Z76.2	Encounter for health supervision and care of other healthy infant and child
Z99.12	Encounter for respirator [ventilator] dependence during power failure

Section II. Selection of Principal Diagnosis

The circumstances of inpatient admission always govern the selection of principal diagnosis. The principal diagnosis is defined in the Uniform Hospital Discharge Data Set (UHDDS) as "that condition established after study to be chiefly responsible for occasioning the admission of the patient to the hospital for care."

The UHDDS definitions are used by hospitals to report inpatient data elements in a standardized manner. These data elements and their definitions can be found in the July 31, 1985, Federal Register (Vol. 50, No, 147), pp. 31038-40.

Since that time the application of the UHDDS definitions has been expanded to include all non-outpatient settings (acute care, short term, long term care and psychiatric hospitals; home health agencies; rehab facilities; nursing homes, etc).

In determining principal diagnosis the coding conventions in the ICD-10-CM, the Tabular List and Alphabetic Index take precedence over these official coding guidelines.

(See Section I.A., Conventions for the ICD-10-CM)

The importance of consistent, complete documentation in the medical record cannot be overemphasized. Without such documentation the application of all coding guidelines is a difficult, if not impossible, task.

A. Codes for symptoms, signs, and ill-defined conditions

Codes for symptoms, signs, and ill-defined conditions from Chapter 18 are not to be used as principal diagnosis when a related definitive diagnosis has been established.

B. Two or more interrelated conditions, each potentially meeting the definition for principal diagnosis

When there are two or more interrelated conditions (such as diseases in the same ICD-10-CM chapter or manifestations characteristically associated with a certain disease) potentially meeting the definition of principal diagnosis, either condition may be sequenced first, unless the circumstances of the admission, the therapy provided, the Tabular List, or the Alphabetic Index indicate otherwise.

C. Two or more diagnoses that equally meet the definition for principal diagnosis

In the unusual instance when two or more diagnoses equally meet the criteria for principal diagnosis as determined by the circumstances of admission, diagnostic workup and/or therapy provided, and the Alphabetic Index, Tabular List, or another coding guidelines does not provide sequencing direction, any one of the diagnoses may be sequenced first.

D. Two or more comparative or contrasting conditions

In those rare instances when two or more contrasting or comparative diagnoses are documented as "either/or" (or similar terminology), they are coded as if the diagnoses were confirmed and the diagnoses are sequenced according to the circumstances of the admission. If no further determination can be made as to which diagnosis should be principal, either diagnosis may be sequenced first.

E. A symptom(s) followed by contrasting/comparative diagnoses

When a symptom(s) is followed by contrasting/comparative diagnoses, the symptom code is sequenced first. **However, if the symptom code is integral to the conditions listed, no code for the symptom is reported.** All the contrasting/comparative diagnoses should be coded as additional diagnoses.

F. Original treatment plan not carried out

Sequence as the principal diagnosis the condition, which after study occasioned the admission to the hospital, even though treatment may not have been carried out due to unforeseen circumstances.

G. Complications of surgery and other medical care

When the admission is for treatment of a complication resulting from surgery or other medical care, the complication code is sequenced as the principal diagnosis. If the complication is classified to the T80-T88 series and the code lacks the necessary specificity in describing the complication, an additional code for the specific complication should be assigned.

H. Uncertain diagnosis

If the diagnosis documented at the time of discharge is qualified as "probable", "suspected", "likely", "questionable", "possible", or "still to be ruled out", or other similar terms indicating uncertainty, code the condition as if it existed or was established. The bases for these guidelines are the diagnostic workup, arrangements for further workup or observation, and initial therapeutic approach that correspond most closely with the established diagnosis.

Note: This guideline is applicable only to inpatient admissions to short-term, acute, long-term care and psychiatric hospitals.

I. Admission from observation unit

1. **Admission Following Medical Observation**

   When a patient is admitted to an observation unit for a medical condition, which either worsens or does not improve, and is subsequently admitted as an inpatient of the same hospital for this same medical condition, the principal diagnosis would be the medical condition which led to the hospital admission.

2. **Admission Following Post-Operative Observation**

   When a patient is admitted to an observation unit to monitor a condition (or complication) that develops following outpatient surgery, and then is subsequently admitted as an inpatient of the same hospital, hospitals should apply the Uniform Hospital Discharge Data Set (UHDDS) definition of principal diagnosis as "that condition established after study to be chiefly responsible for occasioning the admission of the patient to the hospital for care."

J. Admission from outpatient surgery

When a patient receives surgery in the hospital's outpatient surgery department and is subsequently admitted for continuing inpatient care at the same hospital, the following guidelines should be followed in selecting the principal diagnosis for the inpatient admission:

- If the reason for the inpatient admission is a complication, assign the complication as the principal diagnosis.

- If no complication, or other condition, is documented as the reason for the inpatient admission, assign the reason for the outpatient surgery as the principal diagnosis.

- If the reason for the inpatient admission is another condition unrelated to the surgery, assign the unrelated condition as the principal diagnosis.

K. Admissions/Encounters for Rehabilitation

When the purpose for the admission/encounter is rehabilitation, sequence first the code for the condition for which the service is being performed. For example, for an admission/encounter for rehabilitation for right-sided dominant hemiplegia following a cerebrovascular infarction, report code I69.351, Hemiplegia and hemiparesis following cerebral infarction affecting right dominant side, as the first-listed or principal diagnosis.

If the condition for which the rehabilitation service is no longer present, report the appropriate aftercare code as the first-listed or principal diagnosis. For example, if a patient with severe degenerative osteoarthritis of the hip, underwent hip replacement and the current encounter/admission is for rehabilitation, report code Z47.1, Aftercare following joint replacement surgery, as the first-listed or principal diagnosis.

See Section I.C.21.c.7, Factors influencing health states and contact with health services, Aftercare.

Section III. Reporting Additional Diagnoses

GENERAL RULES FOR OTHER (ADDITIONAL) DIAGNOSES

For reporting purposes the definition for "other diagnoses" is interpreted as additional conditions that affect patient care in terms of requiring:

> clinical evaluation; or
>
> therapeutic treatment; or
>
> diagnostic procedures; or
>
> extended length of hospital stay; or
>
> increased nursing care and/or monitoring.

The UHDDS item #11-b defines Other Diagnoses as "all conditions that coexist at the time of admission, that develop subsequently, or that affect the treatment received and/or the length of stay. Diagnoses that relate to an earlier episode which have no bearing on the current hospital stay are to be excluded." UHDDS definitions apply to inpatients in acute care, short-term, long term care and psychiatric hospital setting. The UHDDS definitions are used by acute care short-term hospitals to report inpatient data elements in a standardized manner. These data elements and their definitions can be found in the July 31, 1985, Federal Register (Vol. 50, No, 147), pp. 31038-40.

Since that time the application of the UHDDS definitions has been expanded to include all non-outpatient settings (acute care, short term, long term care and psychiatric hospitals; home health agencies; rehab facilities; nursing homes, etc).

The following guidelines are to be applied in designating "other diagnoses" when neither the Alphabetic Index nor the Tabular List in ICD-10-CM provide direction. The listing of the diagnoses in the patient record is the responsibility of the attending provider.

A. Previous conditions

If the provider has included a diagnosis in the final diagnostic statement, such as the discharge summary or the face sheet, it should ordinarily be coded. Some providers include in the diagnostic statement resolved conditions or diagnoses and status-post procedures from previous admission that have no bearing on the current stay. Such conditions are not to be reported and are coded only if required by hospital policy.

However, history codes (categories Z80-Z87) may be used as secondary codes if the historical condition or family history has an impact on current care or influences treatment.

B. Abnormal findings

Abnormal findings (laboratory, x-ray, pathologic, and other diagnostic results) are not coded and reported unless the provider indicates their clinical significance. If the findings are outside the normal range and the attending provider has ordered other tests to evaluate the condition or prescribed treatment, it is appropriate to ask the provider whether the abnormal finding should be added.

Please note: This differs from the coding practices in the outpatient setting for coding encounters for diagnostic tests that have been interpreted by a provider.

C. Uncertain Diagnosis

If the diagnosis documented at the time of discharge is qualified as "probable", "suspected", "likely", "questionable", "possible", or "still to be ruled out" or other similar terms indicating uncertainty, code the condition as if it existed or was established. The bases for these guidelines are the diagnostic workup, arrangements for further workup or observation, and initial therapeutic approach that correspond most closely with the established diagnosis.

Note: This guideline is applicable only to inpatient admissions to short-term, acute, long-term care and psychiatric hospitals.

Section IV. Diagnostic Coding and Reporting Guidelines for Outpatient Services

These coding guidelines for outpatient diagnoses have been approved for use by hospitals/ providers in coding and reporting hospital-based outpatient services and provider-based office visits.

Information about the use of certain abbreviations, punctuation, symbols, and other conventions used in the ICD-1Ø-CM Tabular List (code numbers and titles), can be found in Section IA of these guidelines, under "Conventions Used in the Tabular List." **Section I.B. contains general guidelines that apply to the entire classification. Section I.C. contains chapter-specific guidelines that correspond to the chapters as they are arranged in the classification.** Information about the correct sequence to use in finding a code is also described in Section I.

The terms encounter and visit are often used interchangeably in describing outpatient service contacts and, therefore, appear together in these guidelines without distinguishing one from the other.

Though the conventions and general guidelines apply to all settings, coding guidelines for outpatient and provider reporting of diagnoses will vary in a number of instances from those for inpatient diagnoses, recognizing that:

> The Uniform Hospital Discharge Data Set (UHDDS) definition of principal diagnosis applies only to inpatients in acute, short-term, long-term care and psychiatric hospitals.

> Coding guidelines for inconclusive diagnoses (probable, suspected, rule out, etc.) were developed for inpatient reporting and do not apply to outpatients.

A. Selection of first-listed condition

In the outpatient setting, the term first-listed diagnosis is used in lieu of principal diagnosis.

In determining the first-listed diagnosis the coding conventions of ICD-1Ø-CM, as well as the general and disease specific guidelines take precedence over the outpatient guidelines.

Diagnoses often are not established at the time of the initial encounter/visit. It may take two or more visits before the diagnosis is confirmed.

The most critical rule involves beginning the search for the correct code assignment through the Alphabetic Index. Never begin searching initially in the Tabular List as this will lead to coding errors.

1. Outpatient surgery

When a patient presents for outpatient surgery (same day surgery), code the reason for the surgery as the first-listed diagnosis (reason for the encounter), even if the surgery is not performed due to a contraindication.

2. Observation stay

When a patient is admitted for observation for a medical condition, assign a code for the medical condition as the first-listed diagnosis.

When a patient presents for outpatient surgery and develops complications requiring admission to observation, code the reason for the surgery as the first reported diagnosis (reason for the encounter), followed by codes for the complications as secondary diagnoses.

B. Codes from AØØ.Ø through T88.9, ZØØ-Z99

The appropriate code(s) from AØØ.Ø through T88.9, ZØØ-Z99 must be used to identify diagnoses, symptoms, conditions, problems, complaints, or other reason(s) for the encounter/visit.

C. Accurate reporting of ICD-1Ø-CM diagnosis codes

For accurate reporting of ICD-1Ø-CM diagnosis codes, the documentation should describe the patient's condition, using terminology which includes specific diagnoses as well as symptoms, problems, or reasons for the encounter. There are ICD-1Ø-CM codes to describe all of these.

D. Codes that describe symptoms and signs

Codes that describe symptoms and signs, as opposed to diagnoses, are acceptable for reporting purposes when a diagnosis has not been established (confirmed) by the provider. Chapter 18 of ICD-1Ø-CM, Symptoms, Signs, and Abnormal Clinical and Laboratory Findings Not Elsewhere Classified (codes RØØ-R99) contain many, but not all codes for symptoms.

E. Encounters for circumstances other than a disease or injury

ICD-1Ø-CM provides codes to deal with encounters for circumstances other than a disease or injury. The Factors Influencing Health Status and Contact with Health Services codes (ZØØ-Z99) are provided to deal with occasions when circumstances other than a disease or injury are recorded as diagnosis or problems.

See Section I.C.21. Factors influencing health status and contact with health services.

F. Level of Detail in Coding

1. ICD-1Ø-CM codes with 3, 4, 5, 6 or 7 characters

ICD-1Ø-CM is composed of codes with 3, 4, 5, 6 or 7 characters. Codes with three characters are included in ICD-1Ø-CM as the heading of a category of codes that may be further subdivided by the use of fourth, fifth, sixth or seventh characters to provide greater specificity.

2. Use of full number of characters required for a code

A three-character code is to be used only if it is not further subdivided. A code is invalid if it has not been coded to the full number of characters required for that code, including the 7th character extension, if applicable.

G. ICD-1Ø-CM code for the diagnosis, condition, problem, or other reason for encounter/visit

List first the ICD-1Ø-CM code for the diagnosis, condition, problem, or other reason for encounter/visit shown in the medical record to be chiefly responsible for the services provided. List additional codes that describe any coexisting conditions. In some cases the first-listed diagnosis may be a symptom when a diagnosis has not been established (confirmed) by the physician.

H. Uncertain diagnosis

Do not code diagnoses documented as "probable", "suspected," "questionable," "rule out," or "working diagnosis" or other similar terms indicating uncertainty. Rather, code the condition(s) to the highest degree of certainty for that encounter/visit, such as symptoms, signs, abnormal test results, or other reason for the visit.

Please note: This differs from the coding practices used by short-term, acute care, long-term care and psychiatric hospitals.

I. Chronic diseases

Chronic diseases treated on an ongoing basis may be coded and reported as many times as the patient receives treatment and care for the condition(s)

J. Code all documented conditions that coexist

Code all documented conditions that coexist at the time of the encounter/visit, and require or affect patient care treatment or management. Do not code conditions that were previously treated and no longer exist. However, history codes (categories Z8Ø-Z87) may be used as secondary codes if the historical condition or family history has an impact on current care or influences treatment.

K. Patients receiving diagnostic services only

For patients receiving diagnostic services only during an encounter/visit, sequence first the diagnosis, condition, problem, or other reason for encounter/visit shown in the medical record to be chiefly responsible for the outpatient services provided during the encounter/visit. Codes for other diagnoses (e.g., chronic conditions) may be sequenced as additional diagnoses.

For encounters for routine laboratory/radiology testing in the absence of any signs, symptoms, or associated diagnosis, assign ZØ1.89, Encounter for other specified special examinations. If routine testing is performed during the same encounter as a test to evaluate a sign, symptom, or diagnosis, it is appropriate to assign both the Z code and the code describing the reason for the non-routine test.

For outpatient encounters for diagnostic tests that have been interpreted by a physician, and the final report is available at the time of coding, code any confirmed or definitive diagnosis(es) documented in the interpretation. Do not code related signs and symptoms as additional diagnoses.

Please note: This differs from the coding practice in the hospital inpatient setting regarding abnormal findings on test results.

L. Patients receiving therapeutic services only

For patients receiving therapeutic services only during an encounter/visit, sequence first the diagnosis, condition, problem, or other reason for encounter/visit shown in the medical record to be chiefly responsible for the outpatient services provided during the encounter/visit. Codes for other diagnoses (e.g., chronic conditions) may be sequenced as additional diagnoses.

The only exception to this rule is that when the primary reason for the admission/encounter is chemotherapy or radiation therapy, the appropriate Z code for the service is listed first, and the diagnosis or problem for which the service is being performed listed second.

M. Patients receiving preoperative evaluations only

For patients receiving preoperative evaluations only, sequence first a code from subcategory Z01.81, Encounter for pre-procedural examinations, to describe the pre-op consultations. Assign a code for the condition to describe the reason for the surgery as an additional diagnosis. Code also any findings related to the pre-op evaluation.

N. Ambulatory surgery

For ambulatory surgery, code the diagnosis for which the surgery was performed. If the postoperative diagnosis is known to be different from the preoperative diagnosis at the time the diagnosis is confirmed, select the postoperative diagnosis for coding, since it is the most definitive.

O. Routine outpatient prenatal visits

See Section I.C.15. Routine outpatient prenatal visits.

P. Encounters for general medical examinations with abnormal findings

The subcategories for encounters for general medical examinations, Z00.0-, provide codes for with and without abnormal findings. Should a general medical examination result in an abnormal finding, the code for general medical examination with abnormal finding should be assigned as the first-listed diagnosis. A secondary code for the abnormal finding should also be coded.

Q. Encounters for routine health screenings

See Section I.C.21. Factors influencing health status and contact with health services, Screening

Appendix I. Present on Admission Reporting Guidelines

Introduction

These guidelines are to be used as a supplement to the *ICD-10-CM Official Guidelines for Coding and Reporting* to facilitate the assignment of the Present on Admission (POA) indicator for each diagnosis and external cause of injury code reported on claim forms (UB-04 and 837 Institutional).

These guidelines are not intended to replace any guidelines in the main body of the *ICD-10-CM Official Guidelines for Coding and Reporting*. The POA guidelines are not intended to provide guidance on when a condition should be coded, but rather, how to apply the POA indicator to the final set of diagnosis codes that have been assigned in accordance with Sections I, II, and III of the official coding guidelines. Subsequent to the assignment of the ICD-10-CM codes, the POA indicator should then be assigned to those conditions that have been coded.

As stated in the Introduction to the *ICD-10-CM Official Guidelines for Coding and Reporting*, a joint effort between the healthcare provider and the coder is essential to achieve complete and accurate documentation, code assignment, and reporting of diagnoses and procedures. The importance of consistent, complete documentation in the medical record cannot be overemphasized. Medical record documentation from any provider involved in the care and treatment of the patient may be used to support the determination of whether a condition was present on admission or not. In the context of the official coding guidelines, the term "provider" means a physician or any qualified healthcare practitioner who is legally accountable for establishing the patient's diagnosis.

These guidelines are not a substitute for the provider's clinical judgment as to the determination of whether a condition was/was not present on admission. The provider should be queried regarding issues related to the linking of signs/symptoms, timing of test results, and the timing of findings.

General Reporting Requirements

All claims involving inpatient admissions to general acute care hospitals or other facilities that are subject to a law or regulation mandating collection of present on admission information.

Present on admission is defined as present at the time the order for inpatient admission occurs -- conditions that develop during an

outpatient encounter, including emergency department, observation, or outpatient surgery, are considered as present on admission.

POA indicator is assigned to principal and secondary diagnoses (as defined in Section II of the Official Guidelines for Coding and Reporting) and the external cause of injury codes.

Issues related to inconsistent, missing, conflicting or unclear documentation must still be resolved by the provider.

If a condition would not be coded and reported based on UHDDS definitions and current official coding guidelines, then the POA indicator would not be reported.

Reporting Options

Y – Yes
N – No
U – Unknown
W – Clinically undetermined
Unreported/Not used (or "1" for Medicare usage) – (Exempt from POA reporting)

Reporting Definitions

Y – present at the time of inpatient admission
N – not present at the time of inpatient admission
U – documentation is insufficient to determine if condition is present on admission
W – provider is unable to clinically determine whether condition was present on admission or not

Timeframe for POA Identification and Documentation

There is no required timeframe as to when a provider (per the definition of "provider" used in these guidelines) must identify or document a condition to be present on admission. In some clinical situations, it may not be possible for a provider to make a definitive diagnosis (or a condition may not be recognized or reported by the patient) for a period of time after admission. In some cases it may be several days before the provider arrives at a definitive diagnosis. This does not mean that the condition was not present on admission. Determination of whether the condition was present on admission or not will be based on the applicable POA guideline as identified in this document, or on the provider's best clinical judgment.

If at the time of code assignment the documentation is unclear as to whether a condition was present on admission or not, it is appropriate to query the provider for clarification.

Assigning the POA Indicator

Condition is on the "Exempt from Reporting" list

Leave the "present on admission" field blank if the condition is on the list of ICD-10-CM codes for which this field is not applicable. This is the only circumstance in which the field may be left blank.

POA Explicitly Documented

Assign "Y" for any condition the provider explicitly documents as being present on admission.

Assign "N" for any condition the provider explicitly documents as not present at the time of admission.

Conditions diagnosed prior to inpatient admission

Assign "Y" for conditions that were diagnosed prior to admission (example: hypertension, diabetes mellitus, asthma).

Conditions diagnosed during the admission but clearly present before admission

Assign "Y" for conditions diagnosed during the admission that were clearly present but not diagnosed until after admission occurred.

Diagnoses subsequently confirmed after admission are considered present on admission if at the time of admission they are documented as suspected, possible, rule out, differential diagnosis, or constitute an underlying cause of a symptom that is present at the time of admission.

Condition develops during outpatient encounter prior to inpatient admission

Assign "Y" for any condition that develops during an outpatient encounter prior to a written order for inpatient admission.

Documentation does not indicate whether condition was present on admission

Assign "U" when the medical record documentation is unclear as to whether the condition was present on admission. "U" should not be routinely assigned and used only in very limited circumstances. Coders are encouraged to query the providers when the documentation is unclear.

Documentation states that it cannot be determined whether the condition was or was not present on admission

Assign "W" when the medical record documentation indicates that it cannot be clinically determined whether or not the condition was present on admission.

Chronic condition with acute exacerbation during the admission

If a single code identifies both the chronic condition and the acute exacerbation, see POA guidelines pertaining to combination codes.

If a single code only identifies the chronic condition and not the acute exacerbation (e.g., acute exacerbation of chronic leukemia), assign "Y."

Conditions documented as possible, probable, suspected, or rule out at the time of discharge

If the final diagnosis contains a possible, probable, suspected, or rule out diagnosis, and this diagnosis was based on signs, symptoms or clinical findings suspected at the time of inpatient admission, assign "Y."

If the final diagnosis contains a possible, probable, suspected, or rule out diagnosis, and this diagnosis was based on signs, symptoms or clinical findings that were not present on admission, assign "N".

Conditions documented as impending or threatened at the time of discharge

If the final diagnosis contains an impending or threatened diagnosis, and this diagnosis is based on symptoms or clinical findings that were present on admission, assign "Y".

If the final diagnosis contains an impending or threatened diagnosis, and this diagnosis is based on symptoms or clinical findings that were not present on admission, assign "N".

Acute and Chronic Conditions

Assign "Y" for acute conditions that are present at time of admission and N for acute conditions that are not present at time of admission.

Assign "Y" for chronic conditions, even though the condition may not be diagnosed until after admission.

If a single code identifies both an acute and chronic condition, see the POA guidelines for combination codes.

Combination Codes

Assign "N" if any part of the combination code was not present on admission (e.g., COPD with acute exacerbation and the exacerbation was not present on admission; gastric ulcer that does not start bleeding until after admission; asthma patient develops status asthmaticus after admission).

Assign "Y" if all parts of the combination code were present on admission (e.g., patient with acute prostatitis admitted with hematuria).

If the final diagnosis includes comparative or contrasting diagnoses, and both were present, or suspected, at the time of admission, assign "Y".

For infection codes that include the causal organism, assign "Y" if the infection (or signs of the infection) was present on admission, even though the culture results may not be known until after admission (e.g., patient is admitted with pneumonia and the provider documents pseudomonas as the causal organism a few days later).

Same Diagnosis Code for Two or More Conditions

When the same ICD-10-CM diagnosis code applies to two or more conditions during the same encounter (e.g. two separate conditions classified to the same ICD-10-CM diagnosis code):

> Assign "Y" if all conditions represented by the single ICD-10-CM code were present on admission (e.g. bilateral unspecified age-related cataracts).

Assign "N" if any of the conditions represented by the single ICD-10-CM code was not present on admission (e.g. traumatic secondary and recurrent hemorrhage and seroma is assigned to a single code T79.2, but only one of the conditions was present on admission).

Obstetrical conditions

Whether or not the patient delivers during the current hospitalization does not affect assignment of the POA indicator. The determining factor for POA assignment is whether the pregnancy complication or obstetrical condition described by the code was present at the time of admission or not.

If the pregnancy complication or obstetrical condition was present on admission (e.g., patient admitted in preterm labor), assign "Y".

If the pregnancy complication or obstetrical condition was not present on admission (e.g., 2nd degree laceration during delivery, postpartum hemorrhage that occurred during current hospitalization, fetal distress develops after admission), assign "N".

If the obstetrical code includes more than one diagnosis and any of the diagnoses identified by the code were not present on admission assign "N". (e.g., Category O11, Pre-existing hypertension with pre-eclampsia).

Perinatal conditions

Newborns are not considered to be admitted until after birth. Therefore, any condition present at birth or that developed in utero is considered present at admission and should be assigned "Y". This includes conditions that occur during delivery (e.g., injury during delivery, meconium aspiration, exposure to streptococcus B in the vaginal canal).

Congenital conditions and anomalies

Assign "Y" for congenital conditions and anomalies except for categories Q00-Q99, Congenital anomalies, which are on the exempt list. Congenital conditions are always considered present on admission.

External cause of injury codes

Assign "Y" for any external cause code representing an external cause of morbidity that occurred prior to inpatient admission (e.g., patient fell out of bed at home, patient fell out of bed in emergency room prior to admission).

Assign "N" for any external cause code representing an external cause of morbidity that occurred during inpatient hospitalization (e.g., patient fell out of hospital bed during hospital stay, patient experienced an adverse reaction to a medication administered after inpatient admission).

Categories and Codes Exempt from Diagnosis Present on Admission Requirement

Note: "Diagnosis present on admission" for these code categories are exempt because they represent circumstances regarding the healthcare encounter or factors influencing health status that do not represent a current disease or injury or are always present on admission.

B90–B94	Sequelae of infectious and parasitic diseases
E64	Sequelae of malnutrition and other nutritional deficiencies
I25.2	Old myocardial infarction
I69	Sequelae of cerebrovascular disease
O09	Supervision of high risk pregnancy
O66.5	Attempted application of vacuum extractor and forceps
O80	Encounter for full-term uncomplicated delivery
O94	Sequelae of complication of pregnancy, childbirth, and the puerperium
P00	Newborn (suspected to be) affected by maternal conditions that may be unrelated to present pregnancy
Q00 – Q99	Congenital malformations, deformations and chromosomal abnormalities
S00-T88.9	Injury, poisoning and certain other consequences of external causes with 7th character representing subsequent encounter or sequela
V00- V09	Pedestrian injured in transport accident
	Except: V00.81-, Accident with wheelchair (powered) V00.83-, Accident with motorized mobility scooter
V10-V19	Pedal cycle rider injured in transport accident
V20-V29	Motorcycle rider injured in transport accident

V30-V39	Occupant of three-wheeled motor vehicle injured in transport accident
V40-V49	Car occupant injured in transport accident
V50-V59	Occupant of pick-up truck or van injured in transport accident
V60-V69	Occupant of heavy transport vehicle injured in transport accident
V70-V79	Bus occupant injured in transport accident
V80-V89	Other land transport accidents
V90-V94	Water transport accidents
V95-V97	Air and space transport accidents
V98-V99	Other and unspecified transport accidents
W09	Fall on and from playground equipment
W14	Fall from tree
W15	Fall from cliff
W17.0	Fall into well
W17.1	Fall into storm drain or manhole
W18.01	Striking against sports equipment with subsequent fall
W21	Striking against or struck by sports equipment
W30	Contact with agricultural machinery
W31	Contact with other and unspecified machinery
W32-W34	Accidental handgun discharge and malfunction
W35- W40	Exposure to inanimate mechanical forces
W52	Crushed, pushed or stepped on by crowd or human stampede
W56	Contact with nonvenomous marine animal
W58	Contact with crocodile or alligator
W61	Contact with birds (domestic) (wild)
W62	Contact with nonvenomous amphibians
W89	Exposure to man-made visible and ultraviolet light
X02	Exposure to controlled fire in building or structure
X03	Exposure to controlled fire, not in building or structure
X04	Exposure to ignition of highly flammable material
X52	Prolonged stay in weightless environment
X71	Intentional self-harm by drowning and submersion
	Except: X71.0-, Intentional self-harm by drowning and submersion while in bath tub
X72	Intentional self-harm by handgun discharge
X73	Intentional self-harm by rifle, shotgun and larger firearm discharge
X74	Intentional self-harm by other and unspecified firearm and gun discharge
X75	Intentional self-harm by explosive material
X76	Intentional self-harm by smoke, fire and flames
X77	Intentional self-harm by steam, hot vapors and hot objects
X81	Intentional self-harm by jumping or lying in front of moving object
X82	Intentional self-harm by crashing of motor vehicle
X83	Intentional self-harm by other specified means
Y03	**Assault by crashing of motor vehicle**
Y07	**Perpetrator of assault, maltreatment and neglect**
Y08.8	**Assault by strike by sports equipment**
Y21	Drowning and submersion, undetermined intent
Y22	Handgun discharge, undetermined intent
Y23	Rifle, shotgun and larger firearm discharge, undetermined intent
Y24	Other and unspecified firearm discharge, undetermined intent
Y30	Falling, jumping or pushed from a high place, undetermined intent
Y32	**Assault by crashing of motor vehicle, undetermined intent**
Y36	Operations of war
Y37	Military operations
Y92	Place of occurrence of the external cause
Y93	Activity code
Y99	External cause status
Z00	Encounter for general examination without complaint, suspected or reported diagnosis
Z01	Encounter for other special examination without complaint, suspected or reported diagnosis
Z02	Encounter for administrative examination
Z03	Encounter for medical observation for suspected diseases and conditions ruled out

Z08	Encounter for follow-up examination following completed treatment for malignant neoplasm
Z09	Encounter for follow-up examination after completed treatment for conditions other than malignant neoplasm
Z11	Encounter for screening for infectious and parasitic diseases
Z11.8	Encounter for screening for other infectious and parasitic diseases
Z12	Encounter for screening for malignant neoplasms
Z13	Encounter for screening for other diseases and disorders
Z13.4	Encounter for screening for certain developmental disorders in childhood
Z13.5	Encounter for screening for eye and ear disorders
Z13.6	Encounter for screening for cardiovascular disorders
Z13.83	Encounter for screening for respiratory disorder NEC
Z13.89	Encounter for screening for other disorder
Z14	Genetic carrier
Z15	Genetic susceptibility to disease
Z17	Estrogen receptor status
Z18	Retained foreign body fragments
Z22	Carrier of infectious disease
Z23	Encounter for immunization
Z28	Immunization not carried out and underimmunization status
Z28.3	Underimmunization status
Z30	Encounter for contraceptive management
Z31	Encounter for procreative management
Z34	Encounter for supervision of normal pregnancy
Z36	Encounter for antenatal screening of mother
Z37	Outcome of delivery
Z38	Liveborn infants according to place of birth and type of delivery
Z39	Encounter for maternal postpartum care and examination
Z41	Encounter for procedures for purposes other than remedying health state
Z42	Encounter for plastic and reconstructive surgery following medical procedure or healed injury
Z43	Encounter for attention to artificial openings
Z44	Encounter for fitting and adjustment of external prosthetic device
Z45	Encounter for adjustment and management of implanted device
Z46	Encounter for fitting and adjustment of other devices
Z47.8	Encounter for other orthopedic aftercare
Z49	Encounter for care involving renal dialysis
Z51	Encounter for other aftercare
Z51.5	Encounter for palliative care
Z51.8	Encounter for other specified aftercare
Z52	Donors of organs and tissues
Z59	Problems related to housing and economic circumstances
Z63	Other problems related to primary support groupincluding family circumstances
Z65	Problems related to other psychosocial circumstances
Z65.8	Other specified problems related to psychosocial circumstances
Z67.1-Z67.9	Blood type
Z68	Body mass index (BMI)
Z72	Problems related to lifestyle
Z74.01	Bed confinement status
Z76	Persons encountering health services in other circumstances
Z77.110- Z77.128	Environmental pollution and hazards in the physical environment
Z78	Other specified health status
Z79	Long term (current) drug therapy
Z80	Family history of primary malignant neoplasm
Z81	Family history of mental and behavioral disorders
Z82	Family history of certain disabilities and chronic diseases (leading to disablement)
Z83	Family history of other specific disorders
Z84	Family history of other conditions
Z85	Personal history of primary malignant neoplasm
Z86	Personal history of certain other diseases
Z87	Personal history of other diseases and conditions
Z87.828	Personal history of other (healed) physical injury and trauma
Z87.891	Personal history of nicotine dependence

Z88	Allergy status to drugs, medicaments and biological substances	Z92	Personal history of medical treatment
Z89	Acquired absence of limb	Z93	Artificial opening status
Z90.710	Acquired absence of both cervix and uterus	Z94	Transplanted organ and tissue status
Z91.0	Allergy status, other than to drugs and biological substances	Z95	Presence of cardiac and vascular implants and grafts
Z91.4	Personal history of psychological trauma, not elsewhere classified	Z97	Presence of other devices
Z91.5	Personal history of self-harm	Z98	Other postprocedural states
Z91.8	Other specified risk factors, not elsewhere classified	Z99	Dependence on enabling machines and devices, not elsewhere classified

ICD-10-CM Index to Diseases and Injuries

A

Aarskog's syndrome Q87.1
Abandonment — *see* Maltreatment
Abasia (-astasia) (hysterical) F44.4
Abderhalden-Kaufmann-Lignac syndrome (cystinosis) E72.04
Abdomen, abdominal (*see also* condition)
  acute R10.0
  angina K55.1
  muscle deficiency syndrome Q79.4
Abdominalgia — *see* Pain, abdominal
Abduction contracture, hip or other joint — *see* Contraction, joint
Aberrant (congenital) (*see also* Malposition, congenital)
  adrenal gland Q89.1
  artery (peripheral) Q27.8
    basilar NEC Q28.1
    cerebral Q28.3
    coronary Q24.5
    digestive system Q27.8
    eye Q15.8
    lower limb Q27.8
    precerebral Q28.1
    pulmonary Q25.79
    renal Q27.2
    retina Q14.1
    specified site NEC Q27.8
    subclavian Q27.8
    upper limb Q27.8
    vertebral Q28.1
  breast Q83.8
  endocrine gland NEC Q89.2
  hepatic duct Q44.5
  pancreas Q45.3
  parathyroid gland Q89.2
  pituitary gland Q89.2
  sebaceous glands, mucous membrane, mouth, congenital Q38.6
  spleen Q89.09
  subclavian artery Q27.8
  thymus (gland) Q89.2
  thyroid gland Q89.2
  vein (peripheral) NEC Q27.8
    cerebral Q28.3
    digestive system Q27.8
    lower limb Q27.8
    precerebral Q28.1
    specified site NEC Q27.8
    upper limb Q27.8
Aberration
  distantial — *see* Disturbance, visual
  mental F99
Abetalipoproteinemia E78.6
Abiotrophy R68.89
Ablatio, ablation
  retinae — *see* Detachment, retina
Ablepharia, ablepharon Q10.3
Abnormal, abnormality, abnormalities (*see also* Anomaly)
  acid-base balance (mixed) E87.4
  albumin R77.0
  alphafetoprotein R77.2
  alveolar ridge K08.9
  anatomical relationship Q89.9
  apertures, congenital, diaphragm Q79.1
  auditory perception H93.29- ☑
    diplacusis — *see* Diplacusis
    hyperacusis — *see* Hyperacusis
    recruitment — *see* Recruitment, auditory
    threshold shift — *see* Shift, auditory threshold
  autosomes Q99.9
    fragile site Q95.5
  basal metabolic rate R94.8
  biosynthesis, testicular androgen E29.1
  bleeding time R79.1
  blood level (of)
    cobalt R79.0
    copper R79.0
    iron R79.0
    lithium R78.89

Abnormal, abnormality, abnormalities — *continued*
  blood level — *continued*
    magnesium R79.0
    mineral NEC R79.0
    zinc R79.0
  blood pressure
    elevated R03.0
    low reading (nonspecific) R03.1
  blood sugar R73.09
  blood-gas level R79.81
  bowel sounds R19.15
    absent R19.11
    hyperactive R19.12
  brain scan R94.02
  breathing R06.9
  caloric test R94.138
  cerebrospinal fluid R83.9
    cytology R83.6
    drug level R83.2
    enzyme level R83.0
    hormones R83.1
    immunology R83.4
    microbiology R83.5
    nonmedicinal level R83.3
    specified type NEC R83.8
  chemistry, blood R79.9
    C-reactive protein R79.82
    drugs — *see* Findings, abnormal, in blood
    gas level R79.81
    minerals R79.0
    pancytopenia D61.818
    PTT R79.1
    specified NEC R79.89
    toxins — *see* Findings, abnormal, in blood
  chest sounds (friction) (rales) R09.89
  chromosome, chromosomal Q99.9
    with more than three X chromosomes, female Q97.1
    analysis result R89.8
      bronchial washings R84.8
      cerebrospinal fluid R83.8
      cervix uteri NEC R87.89
      nasal secretions R84.8
      nipple discharge R89.8
      peritoneal fluid R85.89
      pleural fluid R84.8
      prostatic secretions R86.8
      saliva R85.89
      seminal fluid R86.8
      sputum R84.8
      synovial fluid R89.8
      throat scrapings R84.8
      vagina R87.89
      vulva R87.89
      wound secretions R89.8
    dicentric replacement Q93.2
    ring replacement Q93.2
    sex Q99.8
      female phenotype Q97.9
        specified NEC Q97.8
      male phenotype Q98.9
        specified NEC Q98.8
      structural male Q98.6
    specified NEC Q99.8
  clinical findings NEC R68.89
  coagulation D68.9
    newborn, transient P61.6
    profile R79.1
    time R79.1
  communication — *see* Fistula
  conjunctiva, vascular H11.41- ☑
  coronary artery Q24.5
  cortisol-binding globulin E27.8
  course, eustachian tube Q17.8
  creatinine clearance R94.4
  cytology
    anus R85.619
      atypical squamous cells cannot exclude high grade squamous intraepithelial lesion (ASC-H) R85.611
      atypical squamous cells of undetermined significance (ASC-US) R85.610

Abnormal, abnormality, abnormalities — *continued*
  cytology — *continued*
    anus — *continued*
      cytologic evidence of malignancy R85.614
      high grade squamous intraepithelial lesion (HGSIL) R85.613
      human papillomavirus (HPV) DNA test
        high risk positive R85.81
        low risk postive R85.82
      inadequate smear R85.615
      low grade squamous intraepithelial lesion (LGSIL) R85.612
      satisfactory anal smear but lacking transformation zone R85.616
      specified NEC R85.618
      unsatisfactory smear R85.615
    female genital organs — *see* Abnormal, Papanicolaou (smear)
  dark adaptation curve H53.61
  dentofacial NEC — *see* Anomaly, dentofacial
  development, developmental Q89.9
    central nervous system Q07.9
  diagnostic imaging
    abdomen, abdominal region NEC R93.5
    biliary tract R93.2
    breast R92.8
    central nervous system NEC R90.89
    cerebrovascular NEC R90.89
    coronary circulation R93.1
    digestive tract NEC R93.3
    gastrointestinal (tract) R93.3
    genitourinary organs R93.8
    head R93.0
    heart R93.1
    intrathoracic organ NEC R93.8
    limbs R93.6
    liver R93.2
    lung (field) R91.8
    musculoskeletal system NEC R93.7
    retroperitoneum R93.5
    site specified NEC R93.8
    skin and subcutaneous tissue R93.8
    skull R93.0
    urinary organs R93.4
  direction, teeth, fully erupted M26.30
  ear ossicles, acquired NEC H74.39- ☑
    ankylosis — *see* Ankylosis, ear ossicles
    discontinuity — *see* Discontinuity, ossicles, ear
    partial loss — *see* Loss, ossicles, ear (partial)
  Ebstein Q22.5
  echocardiogram R93.1
  echoencephalogram R90.81
  echogram — *see* Abnormal, diagnostic imaging
  electrocardiogram [ECG] [EKG] R94.31
  electroencephalogram [EEG] R94.01
  electrolyte — *see* Imbalance, electrolyte
  electromyogram [EMG] R94.131
  electro-oculogram [EOG] R94.110
  electrophysiological intracardiac studies R94.39
  electroretinogram [ERG] R94.111
  erythrocytes
    congenital, with perinatal jaundice D58.9
  feces (color) (contents) (mucus) R19.5
  finding — *see* Findings, abnormal, without diagnosis
  fluid
    amniotic — *see* Abnormal, specimen, specified
    cerebrospinal — *see* Abnormal, cerebrospinal fluid
    peritoneal — *see* Abnormal, specimen, digestive organs
    pleural — *see* Abnormal, specimen, respiratory organs
    synovial — *see* Abnormal, specimen, specified
    thorax (bronchial washings) (pleural fluid) — *see* Abnormal, specimen, respiratory organs
    vaginal — *see* Abnormal, specimen, female genital organs
  form
    teeth K00.2
    uterus — *see* Anomaly, uterus
  function studies
    auditory R94.120
    bladder R94.8

Abnormal, abnormality, abnormalities — *continued*
function studies — *continued*
brain R94.09
cardiovascular R94.30
ear R94.128
endocrine NEC R94.7
eye NEC R94.118
kidney R94.4
liver R94.5
nervous system
central NEC R94.09
peripheral NEC R94.138
pancreas R94.8
placenta R94.8
pulmonary R94.2
special senses NEC R94.128
spleen R94.8
thyroid R94.6
vestibular R94.121
gait — *see* Gait
hysterical F44.4
gastrin secretion E16.4
globulin R77.1
cortisol-binding E27.8
thyroid-binding E07.89
glomerular, minor (*see also* N00-N07 with fourth character .0) N05.0
glucagon secretion E16.3
glucose tolerance (test) (non-fasting) R73.09
gravitational (G) forces or states (effect of) T75.81 ☑
hair (color) (shaft) L67.9
specified NEC L67.8
hard tissue formation in pulp (dental) K04.3
head movement R25.0
heart
rate R00.9
specified NEC R00.8
shadow R93.1
sounds NEC R01.2
hemoglobin (disease) (*see also* Disease, hemoglobin) D58.2
trait — *see* Trait, hemoglobin, abnormal
histology NEC R89.7
immunological findings R89.4
in serum R76.9
specified NEC R76.8
increase in appetite R63.2
involuntary movement — *see* Abnormal, movement, involuntary
jaw closure M26.51
karyotype R89.8
kidney function test R94.4
knee jerk R29.2
leukocyte (cell) (differential) NEC D72.9
liver
loss of
height R29.890
weight R63.4
mammogram NEC R92.8
calcification (calculus) R92.1
microcalcification R92.0
Mantoux test R76.11
movement (disorder) (*see also* Disorder, movement)
head R25.0
involuntary R25.9
fasciculation R25.3
of head R25.0
spasm R25.2
specified type NEC R25.8
tremor R25.1
myoglobin (Aberdeen) (Annapolis) R89.7
neonatal screening P09
oculomotor study R94.113
palmar creases Q82.8
Papanicolaou (smear)
anus R85.619
atypical squamous cells cannot exclude high grade squamous intraepithelial lesion (ASC-H) R85.611
atypical squamous cells of undetermined significance (ASC-US) R85.610
cytologic evidence of malignancy R85.614
high grade squamous intraepithelial lesion (HGSIL) R85.613
human papillomavirus (HPV) DNA test
high risk positive R85.81
low risk positve R85.82

Abnormal, abnormality, abnormalities — *continued*
Papanicolaou — *continued*
anus — *continued*
inadequate smear R85.615
low grade squamous intraepithelial lesion (LGSIL) R85.612
satisfactory anal smear but lacking transformation zone R85.616
specified NEC R85.618
unsatisfactory smear R85.615
bronchial washings R84.6
cerebrospinal fluid R83.6
cervix R87.619
atypical squamous cells cannot exclude high grade squamous intraepithelial lesion (ASC-H) R87.611
atypical squamous cells of undetermined significance (ASC-US) R87.610
cytologic evidence of malignancy R87.614
high grade squamous intraepithelial lesion (HGSIL) R87.613
inadequate smear R87.615
low grade squamous intraepithelial lesion (LGSIL) R87.612
non-atypical endometrial cells R87.618
satisfactory cervical smear but lacking transformation zone R87.616
specified NEC R87.618
thin preparaton R87.619
unsatisfactory smear R87.615
nasal secretions R84.6
nipple discharge R89.6
peritoneal fluid R85.69
pleural fluid R84.6
prostatic secretions R86.6
saliva R85.69
seminal fluid R86.6
sites NEC R89.6
sputum R84.6
synovial fluid R89.6
throat scrapings R84.6
vagina R87.629
atypical squamous cells cannot exclude high grade squamous intraepithelial lesion (ASC-H) R87.621
atypical squamous cells of undetermined significance (ASC-US) R87.620
cytologic evidence of malignancy R87.624
high grade squamous intraepithelial lesion (HGSIL) R87.623
inadequate smear R87.625
low grade squamous intraepithelial lesion (LGSIL) R87.622
specified NEC R87.628
thin preparation R87.629
unsatisfactory smear R87.625
vulva R87.69
wound secretions R89.6
partial thromboplastin time (PTT) R79.1
pelvis (bony) — *see* Deformity, pelvis
percussion, chest (tympany) R09.89
periods (grossly) — *see* Menstruation
phonocardiogram R94.39
plantar reflex R29.2
plasma
protein R77.9
specified NEC R77.8
viscosity R70.1
pleural (folds) Q34.0
posture R29.3
product of conception O02.9
specified type NEC O02.89
prothrombin time (PT) R79.1
pulmonary
artery, congenital Q25.79
function, newborn P28.89
test results R94.2
pulsations in neck R00.2
pupillary H21.56- ☑
function (reaction) (reflex) — *see* Anomaly, pupil, function
radiological examination — *see* Abnormal, diagnostic imaging
red blood cell(s) (morphology) (volume) R71.8
reflex — *see* Reflex
renal function test R94.4
response to nerve stimulation R94.130

Abnormal, abnormality, abnormalities — *continued*
retinal correspondence H53.31
retinal function study R94.111
rhythm, heart (*see also* Arrhythmia)
saliva — *see* Abnormal, specimen, digestive organs
scan
kidney R94.4
liver R93.2
thyroid R94.6
secretion
gastrin E16.4
glucagon E16.3
semen, seminal fluid — *see* Abnormal, specimen, male genital organs
serum level (of)
acid phosphatase R74.8
alkaline phosphatase R74.8
amylase R74.8
enzymes R74.9
specified NEC R74.8
lipase R74.8
triacylglycerol lipase R74.8
shape
gravid uterus — *see* Anomaly, uterus
sinus venosus Q21.1
size, tooth, teeth K00.2
spacing, tooth, teeth, fully erupted M26.30
specimen
digestive organs (peritoneal fluid) (saliva) R85.9
cytology R85.69
drug level R85.2
enzyme level R85.0
histology R85.7
hormones R85.1
immunology R85.4
microbiology R85.5
nonmedicinal level R85.3
specified type NEC R85.89
female genital organs (secretions) (smears) R87.9
cytology R87.69
cervix R87.619
human papillomavirus (HPV) DNA test
high risk positive R87.810
low risk positive R87.820
inadequate (unsatisfactory) smear R87.615
non-atypical endometrial cells R87.618
specified NEC R87.618
vagina R87.629
human papillomavirus (HPV) DNA test
high risk positive R87.811
low risk positive R87.821
inadequate (unsatisfactory) smear R87.625
vulva R87.69
drug level R87.2
enzyme level R87.0
histological R87.7
hormones R87.1
immunology R87.4
microbiology R87.5
nonmedicinal level R87.3
specified type NEC R87.89
male genital organs (prostatic secretions) (semen) R86.9
cytology R86.6
drug level R86.2
enzyme level R86.0
histological R86.7
hormones R86.1
immunology R86.4
microbiology R86.5
nonmedicinal level R86.3
specified type NEC R86.8
nipple discharge — *see* Abnormal, specimen, specified
respiratory organs (bronchial washings) (nasal secretions) (pleural fluid) (sputum) R84.9
cytology R84.6
drug level R84.2
enzyme level R84.0
histology R84.7
hormones R84.1
immunology R84.4
microbiology R84.5
nonmedicinal level R84.3
specified type NEC R84.8

Abnormal, abnormality, abnormalities — *continued*

specimen — *continued*
  specified organ, system and tissue NOS R89.9
    cytology R89.6
    drug level R89.2
    enzyme level R89.0
    histology R89.7
    hormones R89.1
    immunology R89.4
    microbiology R89.5
    nonmedicinal level R89.3
    specified type NEC R89.8
  synovial fluid — *see* Abnormal, specimen, specified
  thorax (bronchial washings) (pleural fluids) — *see* Abnormal, specimen, respiratory organs
  vagina (secretion) (smear) R87.629
  vulva (secretion) (smear) R87.69
  wound secretion — *see* Abnormal, specimen, specified
spermatozoa — *see* Abnormal, specimen, male genital organs
sputum (amount) (color) (odor) R09.3
stool (color) (contents) (mucus) R19.5
  bloody K92.1
  guaiac positive R19.5
synchondrosis Q78.8
thermography (*see also* Abnormal, diagnostic imaging) R93.8
thyroid-binding globulin E07.89
tooth, teeth (form) (size) K00.2
toxicology (findings) R78.9
transport protein E88.09
tumor marker NEC R97.8
ultrasound results — *see* Abnormal, diagnostic imaging
umbilical cord complicating delivery O69.9 ☑
urination NEC R39.19
urine (constituents) R82.90
  bile R82.2
  cytological examination R82.8
  drugs R82.5
  fat R82.0
  glucose R81
  heavy metals R82.6
  hemoglobin R82.3
  histological examination R82.8
  ketones R82.4
  microbiological examination (culture) R82.7
  myoglobin R82.1
  positive culture R82.7
  protein — *see* Proteinuria
  specified substance NEC R82.99
    chromoabnormality NEC R82.91
  substances nonmedical R82.6
uterine hemorrhage — *see* Hemorrhage, uterus
vectorcardiogram R94.39
visually evoked potential (VEP) R94.112
white blood cells D72.9
  specified NEC D72.89
X-ray examination — *see* Abnormal, diagnostic imaging

Abnormity (any organ or part) — *see* Anomaly
Abocclusion M26.29
  hemolytic disease (newborn) P55.1
  incompatibility reaction ABO — *see* Complication(s), transfusion, incompatibility reaction, ABO
Abolition, language R48.8
Aborter, habitual or recurrent — *see* Loss (of), pregnancy, recurrent
Abortion (complete) (spontaneous) O03.9
  with
    retained products of conception — *see* Abortion, incomplete
  attempted (elective) (failed) O07.4
    complicated by O07.30
      afibrinogenemia O07.1
      cardiac arrest O07.36
      chemical damage of pelvic organ(s) O07.34
      circulatory collapse O07.31
      cystitis O07.38
      defibrination syndrome O07.1
      electrolyte imbalance O07.33
      embolism (air) (amniotic fluid) (blood clot) (fat) (pulmonary) (septic) (soap) O07.2
      endometritis O07.0
      genital tract and pelvic infection O07.0
      hemolysis O07.1

Abortion — *continued*

attempted — *continued*
  complicated by — *continued*
    hemorrhage (delayed) (excessive) O07.1
    infection
      genital tract or pelvic O07.0
      urinary tract tract O07.38
    intravascular coagulation O07.1
    laceration of pelvic organ(s) O07.34
    metabolic disorder O07.33
    oliguria O07.32
    oophoritis O07.0
    parametritis O07.0
    pelvic peritonitis O07.0
    perforation of pelvic organ(s) O07.34
    renal failure or shutdown O07.32
    salpingitis or salpingo-oophoritis O07.0
    sepsis O07.37
    shock O07.31
    specified condition NEC O07.39
    tubular necrosis (renal) O07.32
    uremia O07.32
    urinary tract infection O07.38
    venous complication NEC O07.35
      embolism (air) (amniotic fluid) (blood clot) (fat) (pulmonary) (septic) (soap) O07.2
complicated (by) (following) O03.80
  afibrinogenemia O03.6
  cardiac arrest O03.86
  chemical damage of pelvic organ(s) O03.84
  circulatory collapse O03.81
  cystitis O03.88
  defibrination syndrome O03.6
  electrolyte imbalance O03.83
  embolism (air) (amniotic fluid) (blood clot) (fat) (pulmonary) (septic) (soap) O03.7
  endometritis O03.5
  genital tract and pelvic infection O03.5
  hemolysis O03.6
  hemorrhage (delayed) (excessive) O03.6
  infection
    genital tract or pelvic O03.5
    urinary tract O03.88
  intravascular coagulation O03.6
  laceration of pelvic organ(s) O03.84
  metabolic disorder O03.83
  oliguria O03.82
  oophoritis O03.5
  parametritis O03.5
  pelvic peritonitis O03.5
  perforation of pelvic organ(s) O03.84
  renal failure or shutdown O03.82
  salpingitis or salpingo-oophoritis O03.5
  sepsis O03.87
  shock O03.81
  specified condition NEC O03.89
  tubular necrosis (renal) O03.82
  uremia O03.82
  urinary tract infection O03.88
  venous complication NEC O03.85
    embolism (air) (amniotic fluid) (blood clot) (fat) (pulmonary) (septic) (soap) O03.7
failed — *see* Abortion, attempted
habitual or recurrent N96
  with current abortion — *see* categories O03-O06
  without current pregnancy N96
  care in current pregnancy O26.2- ☑
incomplete (spontaneous) O03.4
  complicated (by) (following) O03.30
    afibrinogenemia O03.1
    cardiac arrest O03.36
    chemical damage of pelvic organ(s) O03.34
    circulatory collapse O03.31
    cystitis O03.38
    defibrination syndrome O03.1
    electrolyte imbalance O03.33
    embolism (air) (amniotic fluid) (blood clot) (fat) (pulmonary) (septic) (soap) O03.2
    endometritis O03.0
    genital tract and pelvic infection O03.0
    hemolysis O03.1
    hemorrhage (delayed) (excessive) O03.1
    infection
      genital tract or pelvic O03.0
      urinary tract O03.38
    intravascular coagulation O03.1
    laceration of pelvic organ(s) O03.34
    metabolic disorder O03.33

Abortion — *continued*

incomplete — *continued*
  complicated — *continued*
    oliguria O03.32
    oophoritis O03.0
    parametritis O03.0
    pelvic peritonitis O03.0
    perforation of pelvic organ(s) O03.34
    renal failure or shutdown O03.32
    salpingitis or salpingo-oophoritis O03.0
    sepsis O03.37
    shock O03.31
    specified condition NEC O03.39
    tubular necrosis (renal) O03.32
    uremia O03.32
    urinary infection O03.38
    venous complication NEC O03.35
      embolism (air) (amniotic fluid) (blood clot) (fat) (pulmonary) (septic) (soap) O03.2
induced (encounter for) Z33.2
  complicated by O04.80
    afibrinogenemia O04.6
    cardiac arrest O04.86
    chemical damage of pelvic organ(s) O04.84
    circulatory collapse O04.81
    cystitis O04.88
    defibrination syndrome O04.6
    electrolyte imbalance O04.83
    embolism (air) (amniotic fluid) (blood clot) (fat) (pulmonary) (septic) (soap) O04.7
    endometritis O04.5
    genital tract and pelvic infection O04.5
    hemolysis O04.6
    hemorrhage (delayed) (excessive) O04.6
    infection
      genital tract or pelvic O04.5
      urinary tract O04.88
    intravascular coagulation O04.6
    laceration of pelvic organ(s) O04.84
    metabolic disorder O04.83
    oliguria O04.82
    oophoritis O04.5
    parametritis O04.5
    pelvic peritonitis O04.5
    perforation of pelvic organ(s) O04.84
    renal failure or shutdown O04.82
    salpingitis or salpingo-oophoritis O04.5
    sepsis O04.87
    shock O04.81
    specified condition NEC O04.89
    tubular necrosis (renal) O04.82
    uremia O04.82
    urinary tract infection O04.88
    venous complication NEC O04.85
      embolism (air) (amniotic fluid) (blood clot) (fat) (pulmonary) (septic) (soap) O04.7
missed O02.1
spontaneous — *see* Abortion (complete) (spontaneous)
  threatened O20.0
threatened (spontaneous) O20.0
tubal O00.1

Abortus fever A23.1
Aboulomania F60.7
Abrami's disease D59.8
Abramov-Fiedler myocarditis (acute isolated myocarditis) I40.1
Abrasion T14.8
  abdomen, abdominal (wall) S30.811 ☑
  alveolar process S00.512 ☑
  ankle S90.51- ☑
  antecubital space — *see* Abrasion, elbow
  anus S30.817 ☑
  arm (upper) S40.81- ☑
  auditory canal — *see* Abrasion, ear
  auricle — *see* Abrasion, ear
  axilla — *see* Abrasion, arm
  back, lower S30.810 ☑
  breast S20.11- ☑
  brow S00.81 ☑
  buttock S30.810 ☑
  calf — *see* Abrasion, leg
  canthus — *see* Abrasion, eyelid
  cheek S00.81 ☑
    internal S00.512 ☑
  chest wall — *see* Abrasion, thorax
  chin S00.81 ☑
  clitoris S30.814 ☑

Abrasion — *continued*
- cornea S05.0- ☑
- costal region — *see* Abrasion, thorax
- dental K03.1
- digit(s)
  - foot — *see* Abrasion, toe
  - hand — *see* Abrasion, finger
- ear S00.41- ☑
- elbow S50.31- ☑
- epididymis S30.813 ☑
- epigastric region S30.811 ☑
- epiglottis S10.11 ☑
- esophagus (thoracic) S27.818 ☑
  - cervical S10.11 ☑
- eyebrow — *see* Abrasion, eyelid
- eyelid S00.21- ☑
- face S00.81 ☑
- finger(s) S60.41- ☑
  - index S60.41- ☑
  - little S60.41- ☑
  - middle S60.41- ☑
  - ring S60.41- ☑
- flank S30.811 ☑
- foot (except toe(s) alone) S90.81- ☑
  - toe — *see* Abrasion, toe
- forearm S50.81- ☑
  - elbow only — *see* Abrasion, elbow
- forehead S00.81 ☑
- genital organs, external
  - female S30.816 ☑
  - male S30.815 ☑
- groin S30.811 ☑
- gum S00.512 ☑
- hand S60.51- ☑
- head S00.91 ☑
  - ear — *see* Abrasion, ear
  - eyelid — *see* Abrasion, eyelid
  - lip S00.511 ☑
  - nose S00.31 ☑
  - oral cavity S00.512 ☑
  - scalp S00.01 ☑
  - specified site NEC S00.81 ☑
- heel — *see* Abrasion, foot
- hip S70.21- ☑
- inguinal region S30.811 ☑
- interscapular region S20.419 ☑
- jaw S00.81 ☑
- knee S80.21- ☑
- labium (majus) (minus) S30.814 ☑
- larynx S10.11 ☑
- leg (lower) S80.81- ☑
  - knee — *see* Abrasion, knee
  - upper — *see* Abrasion, thigh
- lip S00.511 ☑
- lower back S30.810 ☑
- lumbar region S30.810 ☑
- malar region S00.81 ☑
- mammary — *see* Abrasion, breast
- mastoid region S00.81 ☑
- mouth S00.512 ☑
- nail
  - finger — *see* Abrasion, finger
  - toe — *see* Abrasion, toe
- nape S10.81 ☑
- nasal S00.31 ☑
- neck S10.91 ☑
  - specified site NEC S10.81 ☑
  - throat S10.11 ☑
- nose S00.31 ☑
- occipital region S00.01 ☑
- oral cavity S00.512 ☑
- orbital region — *see* Abrasion, eyelid
- palate S00.512 ☑
- palm — *see* Abrasion, hand
- parietal region S00.01 ☑
- pelvis S30.810 ☑
- penis S30.812 ☑
- perineum
  - female S30.814 ☑
  - male S30.810 ☑
- periocular area — *see* Abrasion, eyelid
- phalanges
  - finger — *see* Abrasion, finger
  - toe — *see* Abrasion, toe
- pharynx S10.11 ☑
- pinna — *see* Abrasion, ear

Abrasion — *continued*
- popliteal space — *see* Abrasion, knee
- prepuce S30.812 ☑
- pubic region S30.810 ☑
- pudendum
  - female S30.816 ☑
  - male S30.815 ☑
- sacral region S30.810 ☑
- scalp S00.01 ☑
- scapular region — *see* Abrasion, shoulder
- scrotum S30.813 ☑
- shin — *see* Abrasion, leg
- shoulder S40.21- ☑
- skin NEC T14.8
- sternal region S20.319 ☑
- submaxillary region S00.81 ☑
- submental region S00.81 ☑
- subungual
  - finger(s) — *see* Abrasion, finger
  - toe(s) — *see* Abrasion, toe
- supraclavicular fossa S10.81 ☑
- supraorbital S00.81 ☑
- temple S00.81 ☑
- temporal region S00.81 ☑
- testis S30.813 ☑
- thigh S70.31- ☑
- thorax, thoracic (wall) S20.91 ☑
  - back S20.41- ☑
  - front S20.31- ☑
- throat S10.11 ☑
- thumb S60.31- ☑
- toe(s) (lesser) S90.416 ☑
  - great S90.41- ☑
- tongue S00.512 ☑
- tooth, teeth (dentifrice) (habitual) (hard tissues) (occupational) (ritual) (traditional) K03.1
- trachea S10.11 ☑
- tunica vaginalis S30.813 ☑
- tympanum, tympanic membrane — *see* Abrasion, ear
- uvula S00.512 ☑
- vagina S30.814 ☑
- vocal cords S10.11 ☑
- vulva S30.814 ☑
- wrist S60.81- ☑

Abrism — *see* Poisoning, food, noxious, plant
Abruptio placentae O45.9- ☑
- with
  - afibrinogenemia O45.01- ☑
  - coagulation defect O45.00- ☑
    - specified NEC O45.09- ☑
  - disseminated intravascular coagulation O45.02- ☑
  - hypofibrinogenemia O45.01- ☑
- specified NEC O45.8- ☑
Abruption, placenta — *see* Abruptio placentae
Abscess (connective tissue) (embolic) (fistulous) (infective) (metastatic) (multiple) (pernicious) (pyogenic) (septic) L02.91
- with
  - diverticular disease (intestine) K57.80
    - with bleeding K57.81
    - large intestine K57.20
      - with
        - bleeding K57.21
        - small intestine K57.40
          - with bleeding K57.41
    - small intestine K57.00
      - with
        - bleeding K57.01
        - large intestine K57.40
          - with bleeding K57.41
  - lymphangitis — *code by* site under Abscess
- abdomen, abdominal
  - cavity K65.1
  - wall L02.211
- abdominopelvic K65.1
- accessory sinus — *see* Sinusitis
- adrenal (capsule) (gland) E27.8
- alveolar K04.7
  - with sinus K04.6
- amebic A06.4
  - brain (and liver or lung abscess) A06.6
  - genitourinary tract A06.82
  - liver (without mention of brain or lung abscess) A06.4
  - lung (and liver) (without mention of brain abscess) A06.5
  - specified site NEC A06.89

Abscess — *continued*
- amebic — *continued*
  - spleen A06.89
- anerobic A48.0
- ankle — *see* Abscess, lower limb
- anorectal K61.2
- antecubital space — *see* Abscess, upper limb
- antrum (chronic) (Highmore) — *see* Sinusitis, maxillary
- anus K61.0
- apical (tooth) K04.7
  - with sinus (alveolar) K04.6
- appendix K35.3
- areola (acute) (chronic) (nonpuerperal) N61
  - puerperal, postpartum or gestational — *see* Infection, nipple
- arm (any part) — *see* Abscess, upper limb
- artery (wall) I77.89
- atheromatous I77.2
- auricle, ear — *see* Abscess, ear, external
- axilla (region) L02.41- ☑
  - lymph gland or node L04.2
- back (any part, except buttock) L02.212
- Bartholin's gland N75.1
  - with
    - abortion — *see* Abortion, by type complicated by, sepsis
    - ectopic or molar pregnancy O08.0
    - following ectopic or molar pregnancy O08.0
- Bezold's — *see* Mastoiditis, acute
- bilharziasis B65.1
- bladder (wall) — *see* Cystitis, specified type NEC
- bone (subperiosteal) (*see also* Osteomyelitis, specified type NEC)
  - accessory sinus (chronic) — *see* Sinusitis
  - chronic or old — *see* Osteomyelitis, chronic
  - jaw (lower) (upper) M27.2
  - mastoid — *see* Mastoiditis, acute, subperiosteal
  - petrous — *see* Petrositis
  - spinal (tuberculous) A18.01
    - nontuberculous — *see* Osteomyelitis, vertebra
- bowel K63.0
- brain (any part) (cystic) (otogenic) G06.0
  - amebic (with abscess of any other site) A06.6
  - gonococcal A54.82
  - pheomycotic (chromomycotic) B43.1
  - tuberculous A17.81
- breast (acute) (chronic) (nonpuerperal) N61
  - newborn P39.0
  - puerperal, postpartum, gestational — *see* Mastitis, obstetric, purulent
- broad ligament N73.2
  - acute N73.0
  - chronic N73.1
- Brodie's (localized) (chronic) M86.8X- ☑
- bronchi J98.09
- buccal cavity K12.2
- bulbourethral gland N34.0
- bursa M71.00
  - ankle M71.07- ☑
  - elbow M71.02- ☑
  - foot M71.07- ☑
  - hand M71.04- ☑
  - hip M71.05- ☑
  - knee M71.06- ☑
  - multiple sites M71.09
  - pharyngeal J39.1
  - shoulder M71.01- ☑
  - specified site NEC M71.08
  - wrist M71.03- ☑
- buttock L02.31
- canthus — *see* Blepharoconjunctivitis
- cartilage — *see* Disorder, cartilage, specified type NEC
- cecum K35.3
- cerebellum, cerebellar G06.0
  - sequelae G09
- cerebral (embolic) G06.0
  - sequelae G09
- cervical (meaning neck) L02.11
  - lymph gland or node L04.0
- cervix (stump) (uteri) — *see* Cervicitis
- cheek (external) L02.01
  - inner K12.2
- chest J86.9
  - with fistula J86.0
  - wall L02.213
- chin L02.01
- choroid — *see* Inflammation, chorioretinal

Abscess — continued
  circumtonsillar J36
  cold (lung) (tuberculous) (see also Tuberculosis, abscess, lung)
    articular — see Tuberculosis, joint
  colon (wall) K63.0
  colostomy K94.02
  conjunctiva — see Conjunctivitis, acute
  cornea H16.31- ☑
  corpus
    cavernosum N48.21
    luteum — see Oophoritis
  Cowper's gland N34.0
  cranium G06.0
  cul-de-sac (Douglas') (posterior) — see Peritonitis, pelvic, female
  cutaneous — see Abscess, by site
  dental K04.7
    with sinus (alveolar) K04.6
  dentoalveolar K04.7
    with sinus K04.6
  diaphragm, diaphragmatic K65.1
  Douglas' cul-de-sac or pouch — see Peritonitis, pelvic, female
  Dubois A50.59
  ear (middle) (see also Otitis, media, suppurative)
    acute — see Otitis, media, suppurative, acute
    external H60.0- ☑
  entamebic — see Abscess, amebic
  enterostomy K94.12
  epididymis N45.4
  epidural G06.2
    brain G06.0
    spinal cord G06.1
  epiglottis J38.7
  epiploon, epiploic K65.1
  erysipelatous — see Erysipelas
  esophagus K20.8
  ethmoid (bone) (chronic) (sinus) J32.2
  external auditory canal — see Abscess, ear, external
  extradural G06.2
    brain G06.0
      sequelae G09
    spinal cord G06.1
  extraperitoneal K68.19
  eye — see Endophthalmitis, purulent
  eyelid H00.03- ☑
  face (any part, except ear, eye and nose) L02.01
  fallopian tube — see Salpingitis
  fascia M72.8
  fauces J39.1
  fecal K63.0
  femoral (region) — see Abscess, lower limb
  filaria, filarial — see Infestation, filarial
  finger (any) (see also Abscess, hand)
    nail — see Cellulitis, finger
  foot L02.61- ☑
  forehead L02.01
  frontal sinus (chronic) J32.1
  gallbladder K81.0
  genital organ or tract
    female (external) N76.4
    male N49.9
      multiple sites N49.8
      specified NEC N49.8
  gestational mammary O91.11- ☑
  gestational subareolar O91.11- ☑
  gingival K05.21
  gland, glandular (lymph) (acute) — see Lymphadenitis, acute
  gluteal (region) L02.31
  gonorrheal — see Gonococcus
  groin L02.214
  gum K05.21
  hand L02.51- ☑
  head NEC L02.811
    face (any part, except ear, eye and nose) L02.01
  heart — see Carditis
  heel — see Abscess, foot
  helminthic — see Infestation, helminth
  hepatic (cholangitic) (hematogenic) (lymphogenic) (pylephlebitic) K75.0
    amebic A06.4
  hip (region) — see Abscess, lower limb
  ileocecal K35.3
  ileostomy (bud) K94.12
  iliac (region) L02.214

Abscess — continued
  iliac — continued
    fossa K35.3
  infraclavicular (fossa) — see Abscess, upper limb
  inguinal (region) L02.214
    lymph gland or node L04.1
  intestine, intestinal NEC K63.0
    rectal K61.1
  intra-abdominal (see also Abscess, peritoneum) K65.1
    postoperative T81.4 ☑
      retroperitoneal K68.11
  intracranial G06.0
  intramammary — see Abscess, breast
  intraorbital — see Abscess, orbit
  intraperitoneal K65.1
  intrasphincteric (anus) K61.4
  intraspinal G06.1
  intratonsillar J36
  ischiorectal (fossa) K61.3
  jaw (bone) (lower) (upper) M27.2
  joint — see Arthritis, pyogenic or pyemic
    spine (tuberculous) A18.01
      nontuberculous — see Spondylopathy, infective
  kidney N15.1
    with calculus N20.0
      with hydronephrosis N13.6
    puerperal (postpartum) O86.21
  knee (see also Abscess, lower limb)
    joint M00.9
  labium (majus) (minus) N76.4
  lacrimal
    caruncle — see Inflammation, lacrimal, passages, acute
    gland — see Dacryoadenitis
    passages (duct) (sac) — see Inflammation, lacrimal, passages, acute
  lacunar N34.0
  larynx J38.7
  lateral (alveolar) K04.7
    with sinus K04.6
  leg (any part) — see Abscess, lower limb
  lens H27.8
  lingual K14.0
    tonsil J36
  lip K13.0
  Littre's gland N34.0
  liver (cholangitic) (hematogenic) (lymphogenic) (pylephlebitic) (pyogenic) K75.0
    amebic (due to Entamoeba histolytica) (dysenteric) (tropical) A06.4
    with
      brain abscess (and liver or lung abscess) A06.6
      lung abscess A06.5
  loin (region) L02.211
  lower limb L02.41- ☑
  lumbar (tuberculous) A18.01
    nontuberculous L02.212
  lung (miliary) (putrid) J85.2
    with pneumonia J85.1
      due to specified organism (see Pneumonia, in (due to))
    amebic (with liver abscess) A06.5
    with
      brain abscess A06.6
      pneumonia A06.5
  lymph, lymphatic, gland or node (acute) (see also Lymphadenitis, acute)
    mesentery I88.0
  malar M27.2
  mammary gland — see Abscess, breast
  marginal, anus K61.0
  mastoid — see Mastoiditis, acute
  maxilla, maxillary M27.2
    molar (tooth) K04.7
      with sinus K04.6
    premolar K04.7
    sinus (chronic) J32.0
  mediastinum J85.3
  meibomian gland — see Hordeolum
  meninges G06.2
  mesentery, mesenteric K65.1
  mesosalpinx — see Salpingitis
  mons pubis L02.215
  mouth (floor) K12.2
  muscle — see Myositis, infective
  myocardium I40.0

Abscess — continued
  nabothian (follicle) — see Cervicitis
  nasal J32.9
  nasopharyngeal J39.1
  navel L02.216
    newborn P38.9
      with mild hemorrhage P38.1
      without hemorrhage P38.9
  neck (region) L02.11
    lymph gland or node L04.0
  nephritic — see Abscess, kidney
  nipple N61
    associated with
      lactation — see Pregnancy, complicated by, pregnancy — see Pregnancy, complicated by
  nose (external) (fossa) (septum) J34.0
    sinus (chronic) — see Sinusitis
  omentum K65.1
  operative wound T81.4 ☑
  orbit, orbital — see Cellulitis, orbit
  otogenic G06.0
  ovary, ovarian (corpus luteum) — see Oophoritis
  oviduct — see Oophoritis
  palate (soft) K12.2
    hard M27.2
  palmar (space) — see Abscess, hand
  pancreas (duct) — see Pancreatitis, acute
  parafrenal N48.21
  parametric, parametrium N73.2
    acute N73.0
    chronic N73.1
  paranephric N15.1
  parapancreatic — see Pancreatitis, acute
  parapharyngeal J39.0
  pararectal K61.1
  parasinus — see Sinusitis
  parauterine (see also Disease, pelvis, inflammatory) N73.2
  paravaginal — see Vaginitis
  parietal region (scalp) L02.811
  parodontal K05.21
  parotid (duct) (gland) K11.3
    region K12.2
  pectoral (region) L02.213
  pelvis, pelvic
    female — see Disease, pelvis, inflammatory
    male, peritoneal K65.1
  penis N48.21
    gonococcal (accessory gland) (periurethral) A54.1
  perianal K61.0
  periapical K04.7
    with sinus (alveolar) K04.6
  periappendicular K35.3
  pericardial I30.1
  pericecal K35.3
  pericemental K05.21
  pericholecystic — see Cholecystitis, acute
  pericoronal K05.21
  peridental K05.21
  perimetric (see also Disease, pelvis, inflammatory) N73.2
  perinephric, perinephritic — see Abscess, kidney
  perineum, perineal (superficial) L02.215
    urethra N34.0
  periodontal (parietal) K05.21
    apical K04.7
  periosteum, periosteal (see also Osteomyelitis, specified type NEC)
    with osteomyelitis (see also Osteomyelitis, specified type NEC)
      acute — see Osteomyelitis, acute
      chronic — see Osteomyelitis, chronic
  peripharyngeal J39.0
  peripleuritic J86.9
    with fistula J86.0
  periprostatic N41.2
  perirectal K61.1
  perirenal (tissue) — see Abscess, kidney
  perisinuous (nose) — see Sinusitis
  peritoneum, peritoneal (perforated) (ruptured) K65.1
    with appendicitis K35.3
    pelvic
      female — see Peritonitis, pelvic, female
      male K65.1
    postoperative T81.4 ☑
    puerperal, postpartum, childbirth O85
    tuberculous A18.31
  peritonsillar J36

Abscess — *continued*
  perityphlic K35.3
  periureteral N28.89
  periurethral N34.0
    gonococcal (accessory gland) (periurethral) A54.1
  periuterine (*see also* Disease, pelvis, inflammatory) N73.2
  perivesical — *see* Cystitis, specified type NEC
  petrous bone — *see* Petrositis
  phagedenic NOS L02.91
    chancroid A57
  pharynx, pharyngeal (lateral) J39.1
  pilonidal L05.01
  pituitary (gland) E23.6
  pleura J86.9
    with fistula J86.0
  popliteal — *see* Abscess, lower limb
  postcecal K35.3
  postlaryngeal J38.7
  postnasal J34.0
  postoperative (any site) T81.4 ☑
    retroperitoneal K68.11
  postpharyngeal J39.0
  posttonsillar J36
  post-typhoid A01.09
  pouch of Douglas — *see* Peritonitis, pelvic, female
  premammary — *see* Abscess, breast
  prepatellar — *see* Abscess, lower limb
  prostate N41.2
    gonococcal (acute) (chronic) A54.22
  psoas muscle K68.12
  puerperal — *code by* site under Puerperal, abscess
  pulmonary — *see* Abscess, lung
  pulp, pulpal (dental) K04.0
  rectovaginal septum K63.0
  rectovesical — *see* Cystitis, specified type NEC
  rectum K61.1
  renal — *see* Abscess, kidney
  retina — *see* Inflammation, chorioretinal
  retrobulbar — *see* Abscess, orbit
  retrocecal K65.1
  retrolaryngeal J38.7
  retromammary — *see* Abscess, breast
  retroperitoneal NEC K68.19
    postprocedural K68.11
  retropharyngeal J39.0
  retrouterine — *see* Peritonitis, pelvic, female
  retrovesical — *see* Cystitis, specified type NEC
  root, tooth K04.7
    with sinus (alveolar) K04.6
  round ligament (*see also* Disease, pelvis, inflammatory) N73.2
  rupture (spontaneous) NOS L02.91
  sacrum (tuberculous) A18.01
    nontuberculous M46.28
  salivary (duct) (gland) K11.3
  scalp (any part) L02.811
  scapular — *see* Osteomyelitis, specified type NEC
  sclera — *see* Scleritis
  scrofulous (tuberculous) A18.2
  scrotum N49.2
  seminal vesicle N49.0
  septal, dental K04.7
    with sinus (alveolar) K04.6
  serous — *see* Periostitis
  shoulder (region) — *see* Abscess, upper limb
  sigmoid K63.0
  sinus (accessory) (chronic) (nasal) (*see also* Sinusitis)
    intracranial venous (any) G06.0
  Skene's duct or gland N34.0
  skin — *see* Abscess, by site
  specified site NEC L02.818
  spermatic cord N49.1
  sphenoidal (sinus) (chronic) J32.3
  spinal cord (any part) (staphylococcal) G06.1
    tuberculous A17.81
  spine (column) (tuberculous) A18.01
    epidural G06.1
    nontuberculous — *see* Osteomyelitis, vertebra
  spleen D73.3
    amebic A06.89
  stitch T81.4 ☑
  subarachnoid G06.2
    brain G06.0
    spinal cord G06.1
  subareolar — *see* Abscess, breast
  subcecal K35.3
  subcutaneous (*see also* Abscess, by site)

Abscess — *continued*
  subcutaneous (*see also* Abscess, by site) — *continued*
    pheomycotic (chromomycotic) B43.2
  subdiaphragmatic K65.1
  subdural G06.2
    brain G06.0
      sequelae G09
    spinal cord G06.1
  subgaleal L02.811
  subhepatic K65.1
  sublingual K12.2
    gland K11.3
  submammary — *see* Abscess, breast
  submandibular (region) (space) (triangle) K12.2
    gland K11.3
  submaxillary (region) L02.01
    gland K11.3
  submental L02.01
    gland K11.3
  subperiosteal — *see* Osteomyelitis, specified type NEC
  subphrenic K65.1
    postoperative T81.4 ☑
  suburethral N34.0
  sudoriparous L75.8
  supraclavicular (fossa) — *see* Abscess, upper limb
  suprapelvic, acute N73.0
  suprarenal (capsule) (gland) E27.8
  sweat gland L74.8
  tear duct — *see* Inflammation, lacrimal, passages, acute
  temple L02.01
  temporal region L02.01
  temporosphenoidal G06.0
  tendon (sheath) M65.00
    ankle M65.07- ☑
    foot M65.07- ☑
    forearm M65.03- ☑
    hand M65.04- ☑
    lower leg M65.06- ☑
    pelvic region M65.05- ☑
    shoulder region M65.01- ☑
    specified site NEC M65.08
    thigh M65.05- ☑
    upper arm M65.02- ☑
  testis N45.4
  thigh — *see* Abscess, lower limb
  thorax J86.9
    with fistula J86.0
  throat J39.1
  thumb (*see also* Abscess, hand)
    nail — *see* Cellulitis, finger
  thymus (gland) E32.1
  thyroid (gland) E06.0
  toe (any) (*see also* Abscess, foot)
    nail — *see* Cellulitis, toe
  tongue (staphylococcal) K14.0
  tonsil(s) (lingual) J36
  tonsillopharyngeal J36
  tooth, teeth (root) K04.7
    with sinus (alveolar) K04.6
    supporting structures NEC K05.21
  trachea J39.8
  trunk L02.219
    abdominal wall L02.211
    back L02.212
    chest wall L02.213
    groin L02.214
    perineum L02.215
    umbilicus L02.216
  tubal — *see* Salpingitis
  tuberculous — *see* Tuberculosis, abscess
  tubo-ovarian — *see* Salpingo-oophoritis
  tunica vaginalis N49.1
  umbilicus L02.216
  upper
    limb L02.41- ☑
    respiratory J39.8
  urethral (gland) N34.0
  urinary N34.0
  uterus, uterine (wall) (*see also* Endometritis)
    ligament (*see also* Disease, pelvis, inflammatory) N73.2
    neck — *see* Cervicitis
  uvula K12.2
  vagina (wall) — *see* Vaginitis
  vaginorectal — *see* Vaginitis

Abscess — *continued*
  vas deferens N49.1
  vermiform appendix K35.3
  vertebra (column) (tuberculous) A18.01
    nontuberculous — *see* Osteomyelitis, vertebra
  vesical — *see* Cystitis, specified type NEC
  vesico-uterine pouch — *see* Peritonitis, pelvic, female
  vitreous (humor) — *see* Endophthalmitis, purulent
  vocal cord J38.3
  von Bezold's — *see* Mastoiditis, acute
  vulva N76.4
  vulvovaginal gland N75.1
  web space — *see* Abscess, hand
  wound T81.4 ☑
  wrist — *see* Abscess, upper limb
Absence (of) (organ or part) (complete or partial)
  adrenal (gland) (congenital) Q89.1
    acquired E89.6
  albumin in blood E88.09
  alimentary tract (congenital) Q45.8
    upper Q40.8
  alveolar process (acquired) — *see* Anomaly, alveolar
  ankle (acquired) Z89.44- ☑
  anus (congenital) Q42.3
    with fistula Q42.2
  aorta (congenital) Q25.4
  appendix, congenital Q42.8
  arm (acquired) Z89.20- ☑
    above elbow Z89.22- ☑
      congenital (with hand present) — *see* Agenesis, arm, with hand present
      and hand — *see* Agenesis, forearm, and hand
    below elbow Z89.21- ☑
      congenital (with hand present) — *see* Agenesis, arm, with hand present
      and hand — *see* Agenesis, forearm, and hand
    congenital — *see* Defect, reduction, upper limb
    shoulder (following explantation of shoulder joint prosthesis) (joint) (with or without presence of antibiotic-impregnated cement spacer) Z89.23- ☑
    congenital (with hand present) — *see* Agenesis, arm, with hand present
  artery (congenital) (peripheral) Q27.8
    brain Q28.3
    coronary Q24.5
    pulmonary Q25.79
    specified NEC Q27.8
    umbilical Q27.0
  atrial septum (congenital) Q21.1
  auditory canal (congenital) (external) Q16.1
  auricle (ear), congenital Q16.0
  bile, biliary duct, congenital Q44.5
  bladder (acquired) Z90.6
    congenital Q64.5
  bowel sounds R19.11
  brain Q00.0
    part of Q04.3
  breast(s) (and nipple(s)) (acquired) Z90.1- ☑
    congenital Q83.8
  broad ligament Q50.6
  bronchus (congenital) Q32.4
  canaliculus lacrimalis, congenital Q10.4
  cerebellum (vermis) Q04.3
  cervix (acquired) (with uterus) Z90.710
    with remaining uterus Z90.712
    congenital Q51.5
  chin, congenital Q18.8
  cilia (congenital) Q10.3
    acquired — *see* Madarosis
  clitoris (congenital) Q52.6
  coccyx, congenital Q76.49
  cold sense R20.8
  congenital
    lumen — *see* Atresia
    organ or site NEC — *see* Agenesis
    septum — *see* Imperfect, closure
  corpus callosum Q04.0
  cricoid cartilage, congenital Q31.8
  diaphragm (with hernia), congenital Q79.1
  digestive organ(s) or tract, congenital Q45.8
    acquired NEC Z90.49
    upper Q40.8
  ductus arteriosus Q28.8
  duodenum (acquired) Z90.49
    congenital Q41.0

Absence — *continued*
- ear, congenital Q16.9
  - acquired H93.8- ☑
  - auricle Q16.0
  - external Q16.0
  - inner Q16.5
  - lobe, lobule Q17.8
  - middle, except ossicles Q16.4
    - ossicles Q16.3
  - ossicles Q16.3
- ejaculatory duct (congenital) Q55.4
- endocrine gland (congenital) NEC Q89.2
  - acquired E89.89
- epididymis (congenital) Q55.4
  - acquired Z90.79
- epiglottis, congenital Q31.8
- esophagus (congenital) Q39.8
  - acquired (partial) Z90.49
- eustachian tube (congenital) Q16.2
- extremity (acquired) Z89.9
  - congenital Q73.0
  - knee (following explantation of knee joint prosthesis) (joint) (with or without presence of antibiotic-impregnated cement spacer) Z89.52- ☑
  - lower (above knee) Z89.619
    - below knee Z89.51- ☑
  - upper — *see* Absence, arm
- eye (acquired) Z90.01
  - congenital Q11.1
  - muscle (congenital) Q10.3
- eyeball (acquired) Z90.01
- eyelid (fold) (congenital) Q10.3
  - acquired Z90.01
- face, specified part NEC Q18.8
- fallopian tube(s) (acquired) Z90.79
  - congenital Q50.6
- family member (causing problem in home) NEC (*see also* Disruption, family) Z63.32
- femur, congenital — *see* Defect, reduction, lower limb, longitudinal, femur
- fibrinogen (congenital) D68.2
  - acquired D65
- finger(s) (acquired) Z89.02- ☑
  - congenital — *see* Agenesis, hand
- foot (acquired) Z89.43- ☑
  - congenital — *see* Agenesis, foot
- forearm (acquired) — *see* Absence, arm, below elbow
- gallbladder (acquired) Z90.49
  - congenital Q44.0
- gamma globulin in blood D80.1
  - hereditary D80.0
- genital organs
  - acquired (female) (male) Z90.79
  - female, congenital Q52.8
    - external Q52.71
    - internal NEC Q52.8
  - male, congenital Q55.8
- genitourinary organs, congenital NEC
  - female Q52.8
  - male Q55.8
- globe (acquired) Z90.01
  - congenital Q11.1
- glottis, congenital Q31.8
- hand and wrist (acquired) Z89.11- ☑
  - congenital — *see* Agenesis, hand
- head, part (acquired) NEC Z90.09
- heat sense R20.8
- hip (following explantation of hip joint prosthesis) (joint) (with or without presence of antibiotic-impregnated cement spacer) Z89.62- ☑
- hymen (congenital) Q52.4
- ileum (acquired) Z90.49
  - congenital Q41.2
- immunoglobulin, isolated NEC D80.3
  - IgA D80.2
  - IgG D80.3
  - IgM D80.4
- incus (acquired) — *see* Loss, ossicles, ear
  - congenital Q16.3
- inner ear, congenital Q16.5
- intestine (acquired) (small) Z90.49
  - congenital Q41.9
    - specified NEC Q41.8
  - large Z90.49
    - congenital Q42.9
      - specified NEC Q42.8
- iris, congenital Q13.1

Absence — *continued*
- jejunum (acquired) Z90.49
  - congenital Q41.1
- joint
  - acquired
    - hip (following explantation of hip joint prosthesis) (with or without presence of antibiotic-impregnated cement spacer) Z89.62- ☑
    - knee (following explantation of knee joint prosthesis) (with or without presence of antibiotic-impregnated cement spacer) Z89.52- ☑
    - shoulder (following explantation of shoulder joint prosthesis) (with or without presence of antibiotic-impregnated cement spacer) Z89.23- ☑
  - congenital NEC Q74.8
- kidney(s) (acquired) Z90.5
  - congenital Q60.2
    - bilateral Q60.1
    - unilateral Q60.0
- knee (following explantation of knee joint prosthesis) (joint) (with or without presence of antibiotic-impregnated cement spacer) Z89.52- ☑
- labyrinth, membranous Q16.5
- larynx (congenital) Q31.8
  - acquired Z90.02
- leg (acquired) (above knee) Z89.61- ☑
  - below knee (acquired) Z89.51- ☑
  - congenital — *see* Defect, reduction, lower limb
- lens (acquired) (*see also* Aphakia)
  - congenital Q12.3
  - post cataract extraction Z98.4- ☑
- limb (acquired) — *see* Absence, extremity
- lip Q38.6
- liver (congenital) Q44.7
- lung (fissure) (lobe) (bilateral) (unilateral) (congenital) Q33.3
  - acquired (any part) Z90.2
- menstruation — *see* Amenorrhea
- muscle (congenital) (pectoral) Q79.8
  - ocular Q10.3
- neck, part Q18.8
- neutrophil — *see* Agranulocytosis
- nipple(s) (with breast(s)) (acquired) Z90.1- ☑
  - congenital Q83.2
- nose (congenital) Q30.1
  - acquired Z90.09
- organ
  - of Corti, congenital Q16.5
  - or site, congenital NEC Q89.8
    - acquired NEC Z90.89
- osseous meatus (ear) Q16.4
- ovary (acquired)
  - bilateral Z90.722
  - congenital
    - bilateral Q50.02
    - unilateral Q50.01
  - unilateral Z90.721
- oviduct (acquired)
  - bilateral Z90.722
  - congenital Q50.6
  - unilateral Z90.721
- pancreas (congenital) Q45.0
  - acquired Z90.410
    - complete Z90.410
    - partial Z90.411
    - total Z90.410
- parathyroid gland (acquired) E89.2
  - congenital Q89.2
- patella, congenital Q74.1
- penis (congenital) Q55.5
  - acquired Z90.79
- pericardium (congenital) Q24.8
- pituitary gland (congenital) Q89.2
  - acquired E89.3
- prostate (acquired) Z90.79
  - congenital Q55.4
- pulmonary valve Q22.0
- punctum lacrimale (congenital) Q10.4
- radius, congenital — *see* Defect, reduction, upper limb, longitudinal, radius
- rectum (congenital) Q42.1
  - with fistula Q42.0
  - acquired Z90.49
- respiratory organ NOS Q34.9
- rib (acquired) Z90.89

Absence — *continued*
- rib — *continued*
  - congenital Q76.6
- sacrum, congenital Q76.49
- salivary gland(s), congenital Q38.4
- scrotum, congenital Q55.29
- seminal vesicles (congenital) Q55.4
  - acquired Z90.79
- septum
  - atrial (congenital) Q21.1
  - between aorta and pulmonary artery Q21.4
  - ventricular (congenital) Q20.4
- sex chromosome
  - female phenotype Q97.8
  - male phenotype Q98.8
- skull bone (congenital) Q75.8
  - with
    - anencephaly Q00.0
    - encephalocele — *see* Encephalocele
    - hydrocephalus Q03.9
      - with spina bifida — *see* Spina bifida, by site, with hydrocephalus
    - microcephaly Q02
- spermatic cord, congenital Q55.4
- spine, congenital Q76.49
- spleen (congenital) Q89.01
  - acquired Z90.81
- sternum, congenital Q76.7
- stomach (acquired) (partial) Z90.3
  - congenital Q40.2
- superior vena cava, congenital Q26.8
- teeth, tooth (congenital) K00.0
  - acquired (complete) K08.109
    - class I K08.101
    - class II K08.102
    - class III K08.103
    - class IV K08.104
    - due to
      - caries K08.139
        - class I K08.131
        - class II K08.132
        - class III K08.133
        - class IV K08.134
      - periodontal disease K08.129
        - class I K08.121
        - class II K08.122
        - class III K08.123
        - class IV K08.124
      - specified NEC K08.199
        - class I K08.191
        - class II K08.192
        - class III K08.193
        - class IV K08.194
      - trauma K08.119
        - class I K08.111
        - class II K08.112
        - class III K08.113
        - class IV K08.114
    - partial K08.409
      - class I K08.401
      - class II K08.402
      - class III K08.403
      - class IV K08.404
      - due to
        - caries K08.439
          - class I K08.431
          - class II K08.432
          - class III K08.433
          - class IV K08.434
        - periodontal disease K08.429
          - class I K08.421
          - class II K08.422
          - class III K08.423
          - class IV K08.424
        - specified NEC K08.499
          - class I K08.491
          - class II K08.492
          - class III K08.493
          - class IV K08.494
        - trauma K08.419
          - class I K08.411
          - class II K08.412
          - class III K08.413
          - class IV K08.414
- tendon (congenital) Q79.8
- testis (congenital) Q55.0
  - acquired Z90.79
- thumb (acquired) Z89.01- ☑

Absence — continued
- thumb — continued
  - congenital — see Agenesis, hand
- thymus gland Q89.2
- thyroid (gland) (acquired) E89.0
  - cartilage, congenital Q31.8
  - congenital E03.1
- toe(s) (acquired) Z89.42- ☑
  - with foot — see Absence, foot and ankle
  - congenital — see Agenesis, foot
  - great Z89.41- ☑
- tongue, congenital Q38.3
- trachea (cartilage), congenital Q32.1
- transverse aortic arch, congenital Q25.4
- tricuspid valve Q22.4
- umbilical artery, congenital Q27.0
- upper arm and forearm with hand present, congenital — see Agenesis, arm, with hand present
- ureter (congenital) Q62.4
  - acquired Z90.6
- urethra, congenital Q64.5
- uterus (acquired) Z90.710
  - with cervix Z90.710
  - with remaining cervical stump Z90.711
  - congenital Q51.0
- uvula, congenital Q38.5
- vagina, congenital Q52.0
- vas deferens (congenital) Q55.4
  - acquired Z90.79
- vein (peripheral) congenital NEC Q27.8
  - cerebral Q28.3
  - digestive system Q27.8
  - great Q26.8
  - lower limb Q27.8
  - portal Q26.5
  - precerebral Q28.1
  - specified site NEC Q27.8
  - upper limb Q27.8
- vena cava (inferior) (superior), congenital Q26.8
- ventricular septum Q20.4
- vertebra, congenital Q76.49
- vulva, congenital Q52.71
- wrist (acquired) Z89.12- ☑

Absorbent system disease I87.8
Absorption
- carbohydrate, disturbance K90.4
- chemical — see Table of Drugs and Chemicals
  - through placenta (newborn) P04.9
    - environmental substance P04.6
    - nutritional substance P04.5
    - obstetric anesthetic or analgesic drug P04.0
- drug NEC — see Table of Drugs and Chemicals
  - addictive
    - through placenta (newborn) P04.49
      - cocaine P04.41
  - medicinal
    - through placenta (newborn) P04.1
  - through placenta (newborn) P04.1
    - obstetric anesthetic or analgesic drug P04.0
- fat, disturbance K90.4
  - pancreatic K90.3
- noxious substance — see Table of Drugs and Chemicals
- protein, disturbance K90.4
- starch, disturbance K90.4
- toxic substance — see Table of Drugs and Chemicals
- uremic — see Uremia

Abstinence symptoms, syndrome
- alcohol F10.239
  - with delirium F10.231
- cocaine F14.23
- neonatal P96.1
- nicotine — see Dependence, drug, nicotine, with, withdrawal
- opioid F11.93
  - with dependence F11.23
- psychoactive NEC F19.939
  - with
    - delirium F19.931
    - dependence F19.239
      - with
        - delirium F19.231
        - perceptual disturbance F19.232
      - uncomplicated F19.230
    - perceptual disturbance F19.932
  - uncomplicated F19.930
- sedative F13.939

Abstinence symptoms, syndrome — continued
- sedative — continued
  - with
    - delirium F13.931
    - dependence F13.239
      - with
        - delirium F13.231
        - perceptual disturbance F13.232
      - uncomplicated F13.230
    - perceptual disturbance F13.932
  - uncomplicated F13.930
- stimulant NEC F15.93
  - with dependence F15.23

Abulia R68.89
Abulomania F60.7
Abuse
- adult — see Maltreatment, adult
  - as reason for
    - couple seeking advice (including offender) Z63.0
- alcohol (non-dependent) F10.10
  - with
    - anxiety disorder F10.180
    - intoxication F10.129
      - with delirium F10.121
      - uncomplicated F10.120
    - mood disorder F10.14
    - other specified disorder F10.188
    - psychosis F10.159
      - delusions F10.150
      - hallucinations F10.151
    - sexual dysfunction F10.181
    - sleep disorder F10.182
    - unspecified disorder F10.19
  - counseling and surveillance Z71.41
- amphetamine (or related substance) — see Abuse, drug, stimulant NEC
- analgesics (non-prescribed) (over the counter) F55.8
- antacids F55.0
- antidepressants — see Abuse, drug, psychoactive NEC
- anxiolytic — see Abuse, drug, sedative
- barbiturates — see Abuse, drug, sedative
- caffeine — see Abuse, drug, stimulant NEC
- cannabis, cannabinoids — see Abuse, drug, cannabis
- child — see Maltreatment, child
- cocaine — see Abuse, drug, cocaine
- drug NEC (non-dependent) F19.10
  - with sleep disorder F19.182
  - amphetamine type — see Abuse, drug, stimulant NEC
  - analgesics (non-prescribed) (over the counter) F55.8
  - antacids F55.0
  - antidepressants — see Abuse, drug, psychoactive NEC
  - anxiolytics — see Abuse, drug, sedative
  - barbiturates — see Abuse, drug, sedative
  - caffeine — see Abuse, drug, stimulant NEC
  - cannabis F12.10
    - with
      - anxiety disorder F12.180
      - intoxication F12.129
        - with
          - delirium F12.121
          - perceptual disturbance F12.122
        - uncomplicated F12.120
      - other specified disorder F12.188
      - psychosis F12.159
        - delusions F12.150
        - hallucinations F12.151
      - unspecified disorder F12.19
  - cocaine F14.10
    - with
      - anxiety disorder F14.180
      - intoxication F14.129
        - with
          - delirium F14.121
          - perceptual disturbance F14.122
        - uncomplicated F14.120
      - mood disorder F14.14
      - other specified disorder F14.188
      - psychosis F14.159
        - delusions F14.150
        - hallucinations F14.151
      - sexual dysfunction F14.181
      - sleep disorder F14.182
      - unspecified disorder F14.19
  - counseling and surveillance Z71.51

Abuse — continued
- drug — continued
  - hallucinogen F16.10
    - with
      - anxiety disorder F16.180
      - flashbacks F16.183
      - intoxication F16.129
        - with
          - delirium F16.121
          - perceptual disturbance F16.122
        - uncomplicated F16.120
      - mood disorder F16.14
      - other specified disorder F16.188
      - perception disorder, persisting F16.183
      - psychosis F16.159
        - delusions F16.150
        - hallucinations F16.151
      - unspecified disorder F16.19
  - hashish — see Abuse, drug, cannabis
  - herbal or folk remedies F55.1
  - hormones F55.3
  - hypnotics — see Abuse, drug, sedative
  - inhalant F18.10
    - with
      - anxiety disorder F18.180
      - dementia, persisting F18.17
      - intoxication F18.129
        - with delirium F18.121
        - uncomplicated F18.120
      - mood disorder F18.14
      - other specified disorder F18.188
      - psychosis F18.159
        - delusions F18.150
        - hallucinations F18.151
      - unspecified disorder F18.19
  - laxatives F55.2
  - LSD — see Abuse, drug, hallucinogen
  - marihuana — see Abuse, drug, cannabis
  - morphine type (opioids) — see Abuse, drug, opioid
  - opioid F11.10
    - with
      - intoxication F11.129
        - with
          - delirium F11.121
          - perceptual disturbance F11.122
        - uncomplicated F11.120
      - mood disorder F11.14
      - other specified disorder F11.188
      - psychosis F11.159
        - delusions F11.150
        - hallucinations F11.151
      - sexual dysfunction F11.181
      - sleep disorder F11.182
      - unspecified disorder F11.19
  - PCP (phencyclidine) (or related substance) — see Abuse, drug, hallucinogen
  - psychoactive NEC F19.10
    - with
      - amnestic disorder F19.16
      - anxiety disorder F19.180
      - dementia F19.17
      - intoxication F19.129
        - with
          - delirium F19.121
          - perceptual disturbance F19.122
        - uncomplicated F19.120
      - mood disorder F19.14
      - other specified disorder F19.188
      - psychosis F19.159
        - delusions F19.150
        - hallucinations F19.151
      - sexual dysfunction F19.181
      - sleep disorder F19.182
      - unspecified disorder F19.19
  - sedative, hypnotic or anxiolytic F13.10
    - with
      - anxiety disorder F13.180
      - intoxication F13.129
        - with delirium F13.121
        - uncomplicated F13.120
      - mood disorder F13.14
      - other specified disorder F13.188
      - psychosis F13.159
        - delusions F13.150
        - hallucinations F13.151
      - sexual dysfunction F13.181
      - sleep disorder F13.182
      - unspecified disorder F13.19

Abuse — *continued*
  drug — *continued*
    solvent — *see* Abuse, drug, inhalant
    steroids F55.3
    stimulant NEC F15.10
      with
        anxiety disorder F15.180
        intoxication F15.129
          with
            delirium F15.121
            perceptual disturbance F15.122
          uncomplicated F15.120
        mood disorder F15.14
        other specified disorder F15.188
        psychosis F15.159
          delusions F15.150
          hallucinations F15.151
        sexual dysfunction F15.181
        sleep disorder F15.182
        unspecified disorder F15.19
    tranquilizers — *see* Abuse, drug, sedative
    vitamins F55.4
  hallucinogens — *see* Abuse, drug, hallucinogen
  hashish — *see* Abuse, drug, cannabis
  herbal or folk remedies F55.1
  hormones F55.3
  hypnotic — *see* Abuse, drug, sedative
  inhalant — *see* Abuse, drug, inhalant
  laxatives F55.2
  LSD — *see* Abuse, drug, hallucinogen
  marihuana — *see* Abuse, drug, cannabis
  morphine type (opioids) — *see* Abuse, drug, opioid
  non-psychoactive substance NEC F55.8
    antacids F55.0
    folk remedies F55.1
    herbal remedies F55.1
    hormones F55.3
    laxatives F55.2
    steroids F55.3
    vitamins F55.4
  opioids — *see* Abuse, drug, opioid
  PCP (phencyclidine) (or related substance) — *see* Abuse, drug, hallucinogen
  physical (adult) (child) — *see* Maltreatment
  psychoactive substance — *see* Abuse, drug, psychoactive NEC
  psychological (adult) (child) — *see* Maltreatment
  sedative — *see* Abuse, drug, sedative
  sexual — *see* Maltreatment
  solvent — *see* Abuse, drug, inhalant
  steroids F55.3
  vitamins F55.4
Acalculia R48.8
  developmental F81.2
Acanthamebiasis (with) B60.10
  conjunctiva B60.12
  keratoconjunctivitis B60.13
  meningoencephalitis B60.11
  other specified B60.19
Acanthocephaliasis B83.8
Acanthocheilonemiasis B74.4
Acanthocytosis E78.6
Acantholysis L11.9
Acanthosis (acquired) (nigricans) L83
  benign Q82.8
  congenital Q82.8
  seborrheic L82.1
    inflamed L82.0
  tongue K14.3
Acapnia E87.3
Acarbia E87.2
Acardia, acardius Q89.8
Acardiacus amorphus Q89.8
Acardiotrophia I51.4
Acariasis B88.0
  scabies B86
Acarodermatitis (urticarioides) B88.0
Acarophobia F40.218
Acatalasemia, acatalasia E80.3
Acathisia (drug induced) G25.71
Accelerated atrioventricular conduction I45.6
Accentuation of personality traits (type A) Z73.1
Accessory (congenital)
  adrenal gland Q89.1
  anus Q43.4
  appendix Q43.4
  atrioventricular conduction I45.6

Accessory — *continued*
  auditory ossicles Q16.3
  auricle (ear) Q17.0
  biliary duct or passage Q44.5
  bladder Q64.79
  blood vessels NEC Q27.9
    coronary Q24.5
  bone NEC Q79.8
  breast tissue, axilla Q83.1
  carpal bones Q74.0
  cecum Q43.4
  chromosome(s) NEC (nonsex) Q92.9
    with complex rearrangements NEC Q92.5
      seen only at prometaphase Q92.8
    13 — *see* Trisomy, 13
    18 — *see* Trisomy, 18
    21 — *see* Trisomy, 21
    partial Q92.9
    sex
      female phenotype Q97.8
  coronary artery Q24.5
  cusp(s), heart valve NEC Q24.8
    pulmonary Q22.3
  cystic duct Q44.5
  digit(s) Q69.9
  ear (auricle) (lobe) Q17.0
  endocrine gland NEC Q89.2
  eye muscle Q10.3
  eyelid Q10.3
  face bone(s) Q75.8
  fallopian tube (fimbria) (ostium) Q50.6
  finger(s) Q69.0
  foreskin N47.8
  frontonasal process Q75.8
  gallbladder Q44.1
  genital organ(s)
    female Q52.8
      external Q52.79
      internal NEC Q52.8
    male Q55.8
  genitourinary organs NEC Q89.8
    female Q52.8
    male Q55.8
  hallux Q69.2
  heart Q24.8
    valve NEC Q24.8
      pulmonary Q22.3
  hepatic ducts Q44.5
  hymen Q52.4
  intestine (large) (small) Q43.4
  kidney Q63.0
  lacrimal canal Q10.6
  leaflet, heart valve NEC Q24.8
  ligament, broad Q50.6
  liver Q44.7
    duct Q44.5
  lobule (ear) Q17.0
  lung (lobe) Q33.1
  muscle Q79.8
  navicular of carpus Q74.0
  nervous system, part NEC Q07.8
  nipple Q83.3
  nose Q30.8
  organ or site not listed — *see* Anomaly, by site
  ovary Q50.31
  oviduct Q50.6
  pancreas Q45.3
  parathyroid gland Q89.2
  parotid gland (and duct) Q38.4
  pituitary gland Q89.2
  preauricular appendage Q17.0
  prepuce N47.8
  renal arteries (multiple) Q27.2
  rib Q76.6
    cervical Q76.5
  roots (teeth) K00.2
  salivary gland Q38.4
  sesamoid bones Q74.8
    foot Q74.2
    hand Q74.0
  skin tags Q82.8
  spleen Q89.09
  sternum Q76.7
  submaxillary gland Q38.4
  tarsal bones Q74.2
  teeth, tooth K00.1
  tendon Q79.8
  thumb Q69.1

Accessory — *continued*
  thymus gland Q89.2
  thyroid gland Q89.2
  toes Q69.2
  tongue Q38.3
  tooth, teeth K00.1
  tragus Q17.0
  ureter Q62.5
  urethra Q64.79
  urinary organ or tract NEC Q64.8
  uterus Q51.2
  vagina Q52.10
  valve, heart NEC Q24.8
    pulmonary Q22.3
  vertebra Q76.49
  vocal cords Q31.8
  vulva Q52.79
Accident
  birth — *see* Birth, injury
  cardiac — *see* Infarct, myocardium
  cerebral I63.9
  cerebrovascular (embolic) (ischemic) (thrombotic) I63.9
    aborted I63.9
    hemorrhagic — *see* Hemorrhage, intracranial, intracerebral
    old (without sequelae) Z86.73
      with sequelae (of) — *see* Sequelae, infarction, cerebral
  coronary — *see* Infarct, myocardium
  craniovascular I63.9
  vascular, brain I63.9
Accidental — *see* condition
Accommodation (disorder) (*see also* condition)
  hysterical paralysis of F44.89
  insufficiency of H52.4
  paresis — *see* Paresis, of accommodation
  spasm — *see* Spasm, of accommodation
Accouchement — *see* Delivery
Accreta placenta O43.21- ☑
Accretio cordis (nonrheumatic) I31.0
Accretions, tooth, teeth K03.6
Acculturation difficulty Z60.3
Accumulation secretion, prostate N42.89
Acephalia, acephalism, acephalus, acephaly Q00.0
Acephalobrachia monster Q89.8
Acephalochirus monster Q89.8
Acephalogaster Q89.8
Acephalostomus monster Q89.8
Acephalothorax Q89.8
Acerophobia F40.298
Acetonemia R79.89
  in Type 1 diabetes E10.10
    with coma E10.11
Acetonuria R82.4
Achalasia (cardia) (esophagus) K22.0
  congenital Q39.5
  pylorus Q40.0
  sphincteral NEC K59.8
Ache(s) — *see* Pain
Acheilia Q38.6
Achillobursitis — *see* Tendinitis, Achilles
Achillodynia — *see* Tendinitis, Achilles
Achlorhydria, achlorhydric (neurogenic) K31.83
  anemia D50.8
  diarrhea K31.83
  psychogenic F45.8
  secondary to vagotomy K91.1
Achluophobia F40.228
Acholia K82.8
Acholuric jaundice (familial) (splenomegalic) (*see also* Spherocytosis)
  acquired D59.8
Achondrogenesis Q77.0
Achondroplasia (osteosclerosis congenita) Q77.4
Achroma, cutis L80
Achromat (ism), achromatopsia (acquired) (congenital) H53.51
Achromia, congenital — *see* Albinism
Achromia parasitica B36.0
Achylia gastrica K31.89
  psychogenic F45.8
Acid
  burn — *see* Corrosion
  deficiency
    amide nicotinic E52
    ascorbic E54
    folic E53.8

Acid — *continued*
deficiency — *continued*
nicotinic E52
pantothenic E53.8
intoxication E87.2
peptic disease K30
phosphatase deficiency E83.39
stomach K30
psychogenic F45.8
Acidemia E87.2
argininosuccinic E72.22
isovaleric E71.110
metabolic (newborn) P19.9
first noted before onset of labor P19.0
first noted during labor P19.1
noted at birth P19.2
methylmalonic E71.120
pipecolic E72.3
propionic E71.121
Acidity, gastric (high) K30
psychogenic F45.8
Acidocytopenia — *see* Agranulocytosis
Acidocytosis D72.1
Acidopenia — *see* Agranulocytosis
Acidosis (lactic) (respiratory) E87.2
in Type 1 diabetes E10.10
with coma E10.11
kidney, tubular N25.89
lactic E87.2
metabolic NEC E87.2
with respiratory acidosis E87.4
late, of newborn P74.0
mixed metabolic and respiratory, newborn P84
newborn P84
renal (hyperchloremic) (tubular) N25.89
respiratory E87.2
complicated by
metabolic
acidosis E87.4
alkalosis E87.4
Aciduria
argininosuccinic E72.22
glutaric (type I) E72.3
type II E71.313
type III E71.5- ☑
orotic (congenital) (hereditary) (pyrimidine deficiency)
E79.8
anemia D53.0
Acladiosis (skin) B36.0
Aclasis, diaphyseal Q78.6
Acleistocardia Q21.1
Aclusion — *see* Anomaly, dentofacial, malocclusion
Acne L70.9
artificialis L70.8
atrophica L70.2
cachecticorum (Hebra) L70.8
conglobata L70.1
cystic L70.0
decalvans L66.2
excoriée des jeunes filles L70.5
frontalis L70.2
indurata L70.0
infantile L70.4
keloid L73.0
lupoid L70.2
necrotic, necrotica (miliaris) L70.2
neonatal L70.4
nodular L70.0
occupational L70.8
picker's L70.5
pustular L70.0
rodens L70.2
rosacea L71.9
specified NEC L70.8
tropica L70.3
varioliformis L70.2
vulgaris L70.0
Acnitis (primary) A18.4
Acosta's disease T70.29 ☑
Acoustic — *see* condition
Acousticophobia F40.298
Acquired (*see also* condition)
immunodeficiency syndrome (AIDS) B20
Acrania Q00.0
Acroangiodermatitis I78.9
Acroasphyxia, chronic I73.89
Acrobystitis N47.7
Acrocephalopolysyndactyly Q87.0

Acrocephalosyndactyly Q87.0
Acrocephaly Q75.0
Acrochondrohyperplasia — *see* Syndrome, Marfan's
Acrocyanosis I73.8 ☑
newborn P28.2
meaning transient blue hands and feet — *omit code*
Acrodermatitis L30.8
atrophicans (chronica) L90.4
continua (Hallopeau) L40.2
enteropathica (hereditary) E83.2
Hallopeau's L40.2
infantile papular L44.4
perstans L40.2
pustulosa continua L40.2
recalcitrant pustular L40.2
Acrodynia — *see* Poisoning, mercury
Acromegaly, acromegalia E22.0
Acromelalgia I73.81
Acromicria, acromikria Q79.8
Acronyx L60.0
Acropachy, thyroid — *see* Thyrotoxicosis
Acroparesthesia (simple) (vasomotor) I73.89
Acropathy, thyroid — *see* Thyrotoxicosis
Acrophobia F40.241
Acroposthitis N47.7
Acroscleriasis, acroscleroderma, acrosclerosis — *see*
Sclerosis, systemic
Acrosphacelus I96
Acrospiroma, eccrine — *see* Neoplasm, skin, benign
Acrostealgia — *see* Osteochondropathy
Acrotrophodynia — *see* Immersion
ACTH ectopic syndrome E24.3
Actinic — *see* condition
Actinobacillosis, actinobacillus A28.8
mallei A24.0
muris A25.1
Actinomyces israelii (infection) — *see* Actinomycosis
Actinomycetoma (foot) B47.1
Actinomycosis, actinomycotic A42.9
with pneumonia A42.0
abdominal A42.1
cervicofacial A42.2
cutaneous A42.89
gastrointestinal A42.1
pulmonary A42.0
sepsis A42.7
specified site NEC A42.89
Actinoneuritis G62.82
Action, heart
disorder I49.9
irregular I49.9
psychogenic F45.8
Activated protein C resistance D68.51
Active — *see* condition
Acute (*see also* condition)
abdomen R10.0
gallbladder — *see* Cholecystitis, acute
Acyanotic heart disease (congenital) Q24.9
Acystia Q64.5
Adair-Dighton syndrome (brittle bones and blue sclera, deafness) Q78.0
Adamantinoblastoma — *see* Ameloblastoma
Adamantinoma (*see also* Cyst, calcifying odontogenic)
long bones C40.90
lower limb C40.2- ☑
upper limb C40.0- ☑
malignant C41.1
jaw (bone) (lower) C41.1
upper C41.0
tibial C40.2- ☑
Adamantoblastoma — *see* Ameloblastoma
Adams-Stokes (-Morgagni) disease or syndrome I45.9
Adaption reaction — *see* Disorder, adjustment
Addiction (*see also* Dependence) F19.20
alcohol, alcoholic (ethyl) (methyl) (wood) (without re-mission) F10.20
with remission F10.21
drug — *see* Dependence, drug
ethyl alcohol (without remission) F10.20
with remission F10.21
heroin — *see* Dependence, drug, opioid
methyl alcohol (without remission) F10.20
with remission F10.21
methylated spirit (without remission) F10.20
with remission F10.21

Addiction — *continued*
morphine (-like substances) — *see* Dependence, drug, opioid
nicotine — *see* Dependence, drug, nicotine
opium and opioids — *see* Dependence, drug, opioid
tobacco — *see* Dependence, drug, nicotine
Addison-Biermer anemia (pernicious) D51.0
Addisonian crisis E27.2
Addison's
anemia (pernicious) D51.0
disease (bronze) or syndrome E27.1
tuberculous A18.7
keloid L94.0
Addison-Schilder complex E71.528
Additional (*see also* Accessory)
chromosome(s) Q99.8
21 — *see* Trisomy, 21
sex — *see* Abnormal, chromosome, sex
Adduction contracture, hip or other joint — *see*
Contraction, joint
Adenitis (*see also* Lymphadenitis)
acute, unspecified site L04.9
axillary I88.9
acute L04.2
chronic or subacute I88.1
Bartholin's gland N75.8
bulbourethral gland — *see* Urethritis
cervical I88.9
acute L04.0
chronic or subacute I88.1
chancroid (Hemophilus ducreyi) A57
chronic, unspecified site I88.1
Cowper's gland — *see* Urethritis
due to Pasteurella multocida (p. septica) A28.0
epidemic, acute B27.09
gangrenous L04.9
gonorrheal NEC A54.89
groin I88.9
acute L04.1
chronic or subacute I88.1
infectious (acute) (epidemic) B27.09
inguinal I88.9
acute L04.1
chronic or subacute I88.1
lymph gland or node, except mesenteric I88.9
acute — *see* Lymphadenitis, acute
chronic or subacute I88.1
mesenteric (acute) (chronic) (nonspecific) (subacute)
I88.0
parotid gland (suppurative) — *see* Sialoadenitis
salivary gland (any) (suppurative) — *see* Sialoadenitis
scrofulous (tuberculous) A18.2
Skene's duct or gland — *see* Urethritis
strumous, tuberculous A18.2
subacute, unspecified site I88.1
sublingual gland (suppurative) — *see* Sialoadenitis
submandibular gland (suppurative) — *see* Sialoadeni-tis
submaxillary gland (suppurative) — *see* Sialoadenitis
tuberculous — *see* Tuberculosis, lymph gland
urethral gland — *see* Urethritis
Wharton's duct (suppurative) — *see* Sialoadenitis
Adenoacanthoma — *see* Neoplasm, malignant, by site
Adenoameloblastoma — *see* Cyst, calcifying odonto-genic
Adenocarcinoid (tumor) — *see* Neoplasm, malignant, by site
Adenocarcinoma (*see also* Neoplasm, malignant, by site)
acidophil
specified site — *see* Neoplasm, malignant, by site
unspecified site C75.1
adrenal cortical C74.0- ☑
alveolar — *see* Neoplasm, lung, malignant
apocrine
breast — *see* Neoplasm, breast, malignant
in situ
breast D05.8- ☑
specified site NEC — *see* Neoplasm, skin, in situ
unspecified site D04.9
specified site NEC — *see* Neoplasm, skin, malignant
unspecified site C44.99
basal cell
specified site — *see* Neoplasm, skin, malignant
unspecified site C08.9
basophil
specified site — *see* Neoplasm, malignant, by site

Adenocarcinoma — *continued*
  basophil — *continued*
    unspecified site C75.1
  bile duct type C22.1
    liver C22.1
    specified site NEC — *see* Neoplasm, malignant, by site
    unspecified site C22.1
  bronchiolar — *see* Neoplasm, lung, malignant
  bronchioloalveolar — *see* Neoplasm, lung, malignant
  ceruminous C44.29- ☑
  cervix, in situ (*see also* Carcinoma, cervix uteri, in situ) D06.9
  chromophobe
    specified site — *see* Neoplasm, malignant, by site
    unspecified site C75.1
  diffuse type
    specified site — *see* Neoplasm, malignant, by site
    unspecified site C16.9
  duct
    infiltrating
      with Paget's disease — *see* Neoplasm, breast, malignant
      specified site — *see* Neoplasm, malignant, by site
      unspecified site (female) C50.91- ☑
        male C50.92- ☑
    specified site — *see* Neoplasm, malignant, by site
    unspecified site
      female C56.9
      male C61
  eosinophil
    specified site — *see* Neoplasm, malignant, by site
    unspecified site C75.1
  follicular
    with papillary C73
    moderately differentiated C73
    specified site — *see* Neoplasm, malignant, by site
    trabecular C73
    unspecified site C73
    well differentiated C73
  Hurthle cell C73
  in
    adenomatous
      polyposis coli C18.9
  infiltrating duct
    with Paget's disease — *see* Neoplasm, breast, malignant
    specified site — *see* Neoplasm, by site, malignant
    unspecified site (female) C50.91- ☑
      male C50.92- ☑
  inflammatory
    specified site — *see* Neoplasm, by site, malignant
    unspecified site (female) C50.91- ☑
      male C50.92- ☑
  intestinal type
    specified site — *see* Neoplasm, by site, malignant
    unspecified site C16.9
  intracystic papillary
  intraductal
    breast D05.1- ☑
    noninfiltrating
      breast D05.1- ☑
      papillary
        with invasion
          specified site — *see* Neoplasm, by site, malignant
          unspecified site (female) C50.91- ☑
            male C50.92- ☑
        breast D05.1- ☑
        specified site NEC — *see* Neoplasm, in situ, by site
        unspecified site D05.1- ☑
      specified site NEC — *see* Neoplasm, in situ, by site
      unspecified site D05.1- ☑
    papillary
      with invasion
        specified site — *see* Neoplasm, malignant, by site
        unspecified site (female) C50.91- ☑
          male C50.92- ☑
      breast D05.1- ☑
      specified site — *see* Neoplasm, in situ, by site
      unspecified site D05.1- ☑
    specified site NEC — *see* Neoplasm, in situ, by site
    unspecified site D05.1- ☑

Adenocarcinoma — *continued*
  islet cell
    with exocrine, mixed
      specified site — *see* Neoplasm, malignant, by site
      unspecified site C25.9
    pancreas C25.4
    specified site NEC — *see* Neoplasm, malignant, by site
    unspecified site C25.4
  lobular
    in situ
      breast D05.0- ☑
      specified site NEC — *see* Neoplasm, in situ, by site
      unspecified site D05.0- ☑
    specified site — *see* Neoplasm, malignant, by site
    unspecified site (female) C50.91- ☑
      male C50.92- ☑
  mucoid (*see also* Neoplasm, malignant, by site)
    cell
      specified site — *see* Neoplasm, malignant, by site
      unspecified site C75.1
  nonencapsulated sclerosing C73
  papillary
    with follicular C73
    follicular variant C73
    intraductal (noninfiltrating)
      with invasion
        specified site — *see* Neoplasm, malignant, by site
        unspecified site (female) C50.91- ☑
          male C50.92- ☑
      breast D05.1- ☑
      specified site NEC — *see* Neoplasm, in situ, by site
      unspecified site D05.1- ☑
    serous
      specified site — *see* Neoplasm, malignant, by site
      unspecified site C56.9
  papillocystic
    specified site — *see* Neoplasm, malignant, by site
    unspecified site C56.9
  pseudomucinous
    specified site — *see* Neoplasm, malignant, by site
    unspecified site C56.9
  renal cell C64- ☑
  sebaceous — *see* Neoplasm, skin, malignant
  serous (*see also* Neoplasm, malignant, by site)
    papillary
      specified site — *see* Neoplasm, malignant, by site
      unspecified site C56.9
  sweat gland — *see* Neoplasm, skin, malignant
  water-clear cell C75.0
Adenocarcinoma-in-situ (*see also* Neoplasm, in situ, by site)
  breast D05.9- ☑
Adenofibroma
  clear cell — *see* Neoplasm, benign, by site
  endometrioid D27.9
    borderline malignancy D39.10
    malignant C56- ☑
  mucinous
    specified site — *see* Neoplasm, benign, by site
    unspecified site D27.9
  papillary
    specified site — *see* Neoplasm, benign, by site
    unspecified site D27.9
  prostate — *see* Enlargement, enlarged, prostate
  serous
    specified site — *see* Neoplasm, benign, by site
    unspecified site D27.9
  specified site — *see* Neoplasm, benign, by site
  unspecified site D27.9
Adenofibrosis
  breast — *see* Fibroadenosis, breast
  endometrioid N80.0
Adenoiditis (chronic) J35.02
  with tonsillitis J35.03
  acute J03.90
    recurrent J03.91
    specified organism NEC J03.80
      recurrent J03.81
    staphylococcal J03.80

Adenoiditis — *continued*
  acute — *continued*
    staphylococcal — *continued*
      recurrent J03.81
    streptococcal J03.00
      recurrent J03.01
Adenoids — *see* condition
Adenolipoma — *see* Neoplasm, benign, by site
Adenolipomatosis, Launois-Bensaude E88.89
Adenolymphoma
  specified site — *see* Neoplasm, benign, by site
  unspecified site D11.9
Adenoma (*see also* Neoplasm, benign, by site)
  acidophil
    specified site — *see* Neoplasm, benign, by site
    unspecified site D35.2
  acidophil-basophil, mixed
    specified site — *see* Neoplasm, benign, by site
    unspecified site D35.2
  adrenal (cortical) D35.00
    clear cell D35.00
    compact cell D35.00
    glomerulosa cell D35.00
    heavily pigmented variant D35.00
    mixed cell D35.00
  alpha-cell
    pancreas D13.7
    specified site NEC — *see* Neoplasm, benign, by site
    unspecified site D13.7
  alveolar D14.30
  apocrine
    breast D24- ☑
    specified site NEC — *see* Neoplasm, skin, benign, by site
    unspecified site D23.9
  basal cell D11.9
  basophil
    specified site — *see* Neoplasm, benign, by site
    unspecified site D35.2
  basophil-acidophil, mixed
    specified site — *see* Neoplasm, benign, by site
    unspecified site D35.2
  beta-cell
    pancreas D13.7
    specified site NEC — *see* Neoplasm, benign, by site
    unspecified site D13.7
  bile duct D13.4
    common D13.5
    extrahepatic D13.5
    intrahepatic D13.4
    specified site NEC — *see* Neoplasm, benign, by site
    unspecified site D13.4
  black D35.00
  bronchial D38.1
    cylindroid type — *see* Neoplasm, lung, malignant
  ceruminous D23.2- ☑
  chief cell D35.1
  chromophobe
    specified site — *see* Neoplasm, benign, by site
    unspecified site D35.2
  colloid
    specified site — *see* Neoplasm, benign, by site
    unspecified site D34
  duct
  eccrine, papillary — *see* Neoplasm, skin, benign
  endocrine, multiple
    single specified site — *see* Neoplasm, uncertain behavior, by site
    two or more specified sites D44- ☑
    unspecified site D44.9
  endometrioid (*see also* Neoplasm, benign)
    borderline malignancy — *see* Neoplasm, uncertain behavior, by site
  eosinophil
    specified site — *see* Neoplasm, benign, by site
    unspecified site D35.2
  fetal
    specified site — *see* Neoplasm, benign, by site
    unspecified site D34
  follicular
    specified site — *see* Neoplasm, benign, by site
    unspecified site D34
  hepatocellular D13.4
  Hurthle cell D34
  islet cell
    pancreas D13.7
    specified site NEC — *see* Neoplasm, benign, by site
    unspecified site D13.7

Adenoma — *continued*
liver cell D13.4
macrofollicular
specified site — *see* Neoplasm, benign, by site
unspecified site D34
malignant, malignum — *see* Neoplasm, malignant, by site
microcystic
pancreas D13.7
specified site NEC — *see* Neoplasm, benign, by site
unspecified site D13.7
microfollicular
specified site — *see* Neoplasm, benign, by site
unspecified site D34
mucoid cell
specified site — *see* Neoplasm, benign, by site
unspecified site D35.2
multiple endocrine
single specified site — *see* Neoplasm, uncertain behavior, by site
two or more specified sites D44- ☑
unspecified site D44.9
nipple D24- ☑
papillary (*see also* Neoplasm, benign, by site)
eccrine — *see* Neoplasm, skin, benign, by site
Pick's tubular
specified site — *see* Neoplasm, benign, by site
unspecified site
female D27.9
male D29.20
pleomorphic
carcinoma in — *see* Neoplasm, salivary gland, malignant
specified site — *see* Neoplasm, malignant, by site
unspecified site C08.9
polypoid (*see also* Neoplasm, benign)
adenocarcinoma in — *see* Neoplasm, malignant, by site
adenocarcinoma in situ — *see* Neoplasm, in situ, by site
prostate — *see* Neoplasm, benign, prostate
rete cell D29.20
sebaceous — *see* Neoplasm, skin, benign
Sertoli cell
specified site — *see* Neoplasm, benign, by site
unspecified site
female D27.9
male D29.20
skin appendage — *see* Neoplasm, skin, benign
sudoriferous gland — *see* Neoplasm, skin, benign
sweat gland — *see* Neoplasm, skin, benign
testicular
specified site — *see* Neoplasm, benign, by site
unspecified site
female D27.9
male D29.20
tubular (*see also* Neoplasm, benign, by site)
adenocarcinoma in — *see* Neoplasm, malignant, by site
adenocarcinoma in situ — *see* Neoplasm, in situ, by site
Pick's
specified site — *see* Neoplasm, benign, by site
unspecified site
female D27.9
male D29.20
tubulovillous (*see also* Neoplasm, benign, by site)
adenocarcinoma in — *see* Neoplasm, malignant, by site
adenocarcinoma in situ — *see* Neoplasm, in situ, by site
villous — *see* Neoplasm, uncertain behavior, by site
adenocarcinoma in — *see* Neoplasm, malignant, by site
adenocarcinoma in situ — *see* Neoplasm, in situ, by site
water-clear cell D35.1
Adenomatosis
endocrine (multiple) E31.20
single specified site — *see* Neoplasm, uncertain behavior, by site
erosive of nipple D24- ☑
pluriendocrine — *see* Adenomatosis, endocrine
pulmonary D38.1
malignant — *see* Neoplasm, lung, malignant
specified site — *see* Neoplasm, benign, by site

Adenomatosis — *continued*
unspecified site D12.6
Adenomatous
goiter (nontoxic) E04.9
with hyperthyroidism — *see* Hyperthyroidism, with, goiter, nodular
toxic — *see* Hyperthyroidism, with, goiter, nodular
Adenomyoma (*see also* Neoplasm, benign, by site)
prostate — *see* Enlarged, prostate
Adenomyometritis N80.0
Adenomyosis N80.0
Adenopathy (lymph gland) R59.9
generalized R59.1
inguinal R59.0
localized R59.0
mediastinal R59.0
mesentery R59.0
syphilitic (secondary) A51.49
tracheobronchial R59.0
tuberculous A15.4
primary (progressive) A15.7
tuberculous (*see also* Tuberculosis, lymph gland)
tracheobronchial A15.4
primary (progressive) A15.7
Adenosalpingitis — *see* Salpingitis
Adenosarcoma — *see* Neoplasm, malignant, by site
Adenosclerosis I88.8
Adenosis (sclerosing) breast — *see* Fibroadenosis, breast
Adenovirus, as cause of disease classified elsewhere B97.0
Adentia (complete) (partial) — *see* Absence, teeth
Adherent (*see also* Adhesions)
labia (minora) N90.89
pericardium (nonrheumatic) I31.0
rheumatic I09.2
placenta (with hemorrhage) O72.0
without hemorrhage O73.0
prepuce, newborn N47.0
scar (skin) L90.5
tendon in scar L90.5
Adhesions, adhesive (postinfective) K66.0
with intestinal obstruction K56.5
abdominal (wall) — *see* Adhesions, peritoneum
appendix K38.8
bile duct (common) (hepatic) K83.8
bladder (sphincter) N32.89
bowel — *see* Adhesions, peritoneum
cardiac I31.0
rheumatic I09.2
cecum — *see* Adhesions, peritoneum
cervicovaginal N88.1
congenital Q52.8
postpartal O90.89
old N88.1
cervix N88.1
ciliary body NEC — *see* Adhesions, iris
clitoris N90.89
colon — *see* Adhesions, peritoneum
common duct K83.8
congenital (*see also* Anomaly, by site)
fingers — *see* Syndactylism, complex, fingers
omental, anomalous Q43.3
peritoneal Q43.3
tongue (to gum or roof of mouth) Q38.3
conjunctiva (acquired) H11.21- ☑
congenital Q15.8
cystic duct K82.8
diaphragm — *see* Adhesions, peritoneum
due to foreign body — *see* Foreign body
duodenum — *see* Adhesions, peritoneum
ear
middle H74.1- ☑
epididymis N50.8
epidural — *see* Adhesions, meninges
epiglottis J38.7
eyelid H02.59
female pelvis N73.6
gallbladder K82.8
globe H44.89
heart I31.0
rheumatic I09.2
ileocecal (coil) — *see* Adhesions, peritoneum
ileum — *see* Adhesions, peritoneum
intestine (*see also* Adhesions, peritoneum)
with obstruction K56.5
intra-abdominal — *see* Adhesions, peritoneum
iris H21.50- ☑

Adhesions, adhesive — *continued*
iris — *continued*
anterior H21.51- ☑
goniosynechiae H21.52- ☑
posterior H21.54- ☑
to corneal graft T85.89 ☑
joint — *see* Ankylosis
knee M23.8X ☑
temporomandibular M26.61
labium (majus) (minus), congenital Q52.5
liver — *see* Adhesions, peritoneum
lung J98.4
mediastinum J98.5
meninges (cerebral) (spinal) G96.12
congenital Q07.8
tuberculous (cerebral) (spinal) A17.0
mesenteric — *see* Adhesions, peritoneum
nasal (septum) (to turbinates) J34.89
ocular muscle — *see* Strabismus, mechanical
omentum — *see* Adhesions, peritoneum
ovary N73.6
congenital (to cecum, kidney or omentum) Q50.39
paraovarian N73.6
pelvic (peritoneal)
female N73.6
postprocedural N99.4
male — *see* Adhesions, peritoneum
postpartal (old) N73.6
tuberculous A18.17
penis to scrotum (congenital) Q55.8
periappendiceal (*see also* Adhesions, peritoneum)
pericardium (nonrheumatic) I31.0
focal I31.8
rheumatic I09.2
tuberculous A18.84
pericholecystic K82.8
perigastric — *see* Adhesions, peritoneum
periovarian N73.6
periprostatic N42.89
perirectal — *see* Adhesions, peritoneum
perirenal N28.89
peritoneum, peritoneal (postinfective) (postprocedural) K66.0
with obstruction (intestinal) K56.5
congenital Q43.3
pelvic, female N73.6
postprocedural N99.4
postpartal, pelvic N73.6
to uterus N73.6
peritubal N73.6
periureteral N28.89
periuterine N73.6
perivesical N32.89
perivesicular (seminal vesicle) N50.8
pleura, pleuritic J94.8
tuberculous NEC A15.6
pleuropericardial J94.8
postoperative (gastrointestinal tract) K66.0
with obstruction K91.3
due to foreign body accidentally left in wound — *see* Foreign body, accidentally left during a procedure
pelvic peritoneal N99.4
urethra — *see* Stricture, urethra, postprocedural
vagina N99.2
postpartal, old (vulva or perineum) N90.89
preputial, prepuce N47.5
pulmonary J98.4
pylorus — *see* Adhesions, peritoneum
sciatic nerve — *see* Lesion, nerve, sciatic
seminal vesicle N50.8
shoulder (joint) — *see* Capsulitis, adhesive
sigmoid flexure — *see* Adhesions, peritoneum
spermatic cord (acquired) N50.8
congenital Q55.4
spinal canal G96.12
stomach — *see* Adhesions, peritoneum
subscapular — *see* Capsulitis, adhesive
temporomandibular M26.61
tendinitis (*see also* Tenosynovitis, specified type NEC)
shoulder — *see* Capsulitis, adhesive
testis N44.8
tongue, congenital (to gum or roof of mouth) Q38.3
acquired K14.8
trachea J39.8
tubo-ovarian N73.6
tunica vaginalis N44.8
uterus N73.6

Adhesions, adhesive — *continued*
  uterus — *continued*
    internal N85.6
    to abdominal wall N73.6
  vagina (chronic) N89.5
    postoperative N99.2
  vitreomacular H43.82- ☑
  vitreous H43.89
  vulva N90.89
Adiaspiromycosis B48.8
Adie (-Holmes) **pupil or syndrome** — *see* Anomaly, pupil, function, tonic pupil
Adiponecrosis neonatorum P83.8
Adiposis (*see also* Obesity)
  cerebralis E23.6
  dolorosa E88.2
Adiposity (*see also* Obesity)
  heart — *see* Degeneration, myocardial
  localized E65
Adiposogenital dystrophy E23.6
Adjustment
  disorder — *see* Disorder, adjustment
  implanted device — *see* Encounter (for), adjustment (of)
  prosthesis, external — *see* Fitting
  reaction — *see* Disorder, adjustment
Administration of tPA (rtPA) in a different facility within the last 24 hours prior to admission to current facility Z92.82
Admission (for) (*see also* Encounter (for))
  adjustment (of)
    artificial
      arm Z44.00- ☑
        complete Z44.01- ☑
        partial Z44.02- ☑
      eye Z44.2 ☑
      leg Z44.10- ☑
        complete Z44.11- ☑
        partial Z44.12- ☑
    brain neuropacemaker Z46.2
      implanted Z45.42
    breast
      implant Z45.81 ☑
      prosthesis (external) Z44.3 ☑
    colostomy belt Z46.89
    contact lenses Z46.0
    cystostomy device Z46.6
    dental prosthesis Z46.3
    device NEC
      abdominal Z46.89
      implanted Z45.89
        cardiac Z45.09
          defibrillator (with synchronous cardiace pacemaker) Z45.02
          pacemaker Z45.018
            pulse generator Z45.010
        hearing device Z45.328
          bone conduction Z45.320
          cochlear Z45.321
        infusion pump Z45.1
        nervous system Z45.49
          CSF drainage Z45.41
          hearing device — *see* Admission, adjustment, device, implanted, hearing device
          neuropacemaker Z45.42
          visual substitution Z45.31
        specified NEC Z45.89
        vascular access Z45.2
        visual substitution Z45.31
    nervous system Z46.2
      implanted — *see* Admission, adjustment, device, implanted, nervous system
    orthodontic Z46.4
    prosthetic Z44.9
      arm — *see* Admission, adjustment, artificial, arm
      breast Z44.3 ☑
      dental Z46.3
      eye Z44.2 ☑
      leg — *see* Admission, adjustment, artificial, leg
      specified type NEC Z44.8
    substitution
      auditory Z46.2

Admission — *continued*
  adjustment — *continued*
    device — *continued*
      substitution — *continued*
        auditory — *continued*
          implanted — *see* Admission, adjustment, device, implanted, hearing device
        nervous system Z46.2
          implanted — *see* Admission, adjustment, device, implanted, nervous system
        visual Z46.2
          implanted Z45.31
      urinary Z46.6
    hearing aid Z46.1
      implanted — *see* Admission, adjustment, device, implanted, hearing device
    ileostomy device Z46.89
    intestinal appliance or device NEC Z46.89
    neuropacemaker (brain) (peripheral nerve) (spinal cord) Z46.2
      implanted Z45.42
    orthodontic device Z46.4
    orthopedic (brace) (cast) (device) (shoes) Z46.89
    pacemaker
      cardiac Z45.018
        pulse generator Z45.010
      nervous system Z46.2
        implanted Z45.42
    portacath (port-a-cath) Z45.2
    prosthesis Z44.9
      arm — *see* Admission, adjustment, artificial, arm
      breast Z44.3 ☑
      dental Z46.3
      eye Z44.2 ☑
      leg — *see* Admission, adjustment, artificial, leg
      specified NEC Z44.8
    spectacles Z46.0
  aftercare (*see also* Aftercare) Z51.89
    postpartum
      immediately after delivery Z39.0
      routine follow-up Z39.2
    radiation therapy (antineoplastic) Z51.0
  attention to artificial opening (of) Z43.9
    artificial vagina Z43.7
    colostomy Z43.3
    cystostomy Z43.5
    enterostomy Z43.4
    gastrostomy Z43.1
    ileostomy Z43.2
    jejunostomy Z43.4
    nephrostomy Z43.6
    specified site NEC Z43.8
      intestinal tract Z43.4
      urinary tract Z43.6
    tracheostomy Z43.0
    ureterostomy Z43.6
    urethrostomy Z43.6
  breast augmentation or reduction Z41.1
  breast reconstruction following mastectomy Z42.1
  change of
    dressing (nonsurgical) Z48.00
    neuropacemaker device (brain) (peripheral nerve) (spinal cord) Z46.2
      implanted Z45.42
    surgical dressing Z48.01
  circumcision, ritual or routine (in absence of diagnosis) Z41.2
  clinical research investigation (control) (normal comparison) (participant) Z00.6
  contraceptive management Z30.9
  cosmetic surgery NEC Z41.1
  counseling (*see also* Counseling)
    dietary Z71.3
    HIV Z71.7
    human immunodeficiency virus Z71.7
    nonattending third party Z71.0
    procreative management NEC Z31.69
  delivery, full-term, uncomplicated O80
    cesarean, without indication O82
  dietary surveillance and counseling Z71.3
  ear piercing Z41.3
  examination at health care facility (adult) (*see also* Examination) Z00.00
    with abnormal findings Z00.01

Admission — *continued*
  examination at health care facility (*see also* Examination) — *continued*
    clinical research investigation (control) (normal comparison) (participant) Z00.6
    dental Z01.20
      with abnormal findings Z01.21
    donor (potential) Z00.5
    ear Z01.10
      with abnormal findings NEC Z01.118
    eye Z01.00
      with abnormal findings Z01.01
    general, specified reason NEC Z00.8
    hearing Z01.10
      with abnormal findings NEC Z01.118
    postpartum checkup Z39.2
    psychiatric (general) Z00.8
      requested by authority Z04.6
    vision Z01.00
      with abnormal findings Z01.01
  fitting (of)
    artificial
      arm — *see* Admission, adjustment, artificial, arm
      eye Z44.2 ☑
      leg — *see* Admission, adjustment, artificial, leg
    brain neuropacemaker Z46.2
      implanted Z45.42
    breast prosthesis (external) Z44.3 ☑
    colostomy belt Z46.89
    contact lenses Z46.0
    cystostomy device Z46.6
    dental prosthesis Z46.3
    dentures Z46.3
    device NEC
      abdominal Z46.89
      nervous system Z46.2
        implanted — *see* Admission, adjustment, device, implanted, nervous system
      orthodontic Z46.4
      prosthetic Z44.9
        breast Z44.3 ☑
        dental Z46.3
        eye Z44.2 ☑
      substitution
        auditory Z46.2
          implanted — *see* Admission, adjustment, device, implanted, hearing device
        nervous system Z46.2
          implanted — *see* Admission, adjustment, device, implanted, nervous system
        visual Z46.2
          implanted Z45.31
    hearing aid Z46.1
    ileostomy device Z46.89
    intestinal appliance or device NEC Z46.89
    neuropacemaker (brain) (peripheral nerve) (spinal cord) Z46.2
      implanted Z45.42
    orthodontic device Z46.4
    orthopedic device (brace) (cast) (shoes) Z46.89
    prosthesis Z44.9
      arm — *see* Admission, adjustment, artificial, arm
      breast Z44.3 ☑
      dental Z46.3
      eye Z44.2 ☑
      leg — *see* Admission, adjustment, artificial, leg
      specified type NEC Z44.8
    spectacles Z46.0
  follow-up examination Z09
  intrauterine device management Z30.431
    initial prescription Z30.014
  mental health evaluation Z00.8
    requested by authority Z04.6
  observation — *see* Observation
  Papanicolaou smear, cervix Z12.4
    for suspected malignant neoplasm Z12.4
  plastic and reconstructive surgery following medical procedure or healed injury NEC Z42.8
  plastic surgery, cosmetic NEC Z41.1
  postpartum observation
    immediately after delivery Z39.0
    routine follow-up Z39.2
  poststerilization (for restoration) Z31.0
    aftercare Z31.42

Admission — *continued*
  procreative management Z31.9
  prophylactic (measure)
    organ removal Z40.00
      breast Z40.01
      ovary Z40.02
      specified organ NEC Z40.09
      testes Z40.09
    vaccination Z23
  psychiatric examination (general) Z00.8
    requested by authority Z04.6
  radiation therapy (antineoplastic) Z51.0
  reconstructive surgery following medical procedure
    or healed injury NEC Z42.8
  removal of
    cystostomy catheter Z43.5
    drains Z48.03
    dressing (nonsurgical) Z48.00
    intrauterine contraceptive device Z30.432
    neuropacemaker (brain) (peripheral nerve) (spinal
      cord) Z46.2
      implanted Z45.42
    staples Z48.02
    surgical dressing Z48.01
    sutures Z48.02
    ureteral stent Z46.6
  respirator [ventilator] use during power failure Z99.12
  restoration of organ continuity (poststerilization) Z31.0
    aftercare Z31.42
  sensitivity test (*see also* Test, skin)
    allergy NEC Z01.82
    Mantoux Z11.1
  tuboplasty following previous sterilization Z31.0
    aftercare Z31.42
  vasoplasty following previous sterilization Z31.0
    aftercare Z31.42
  vision examination Z01.00
    with abnormal findings Z01.01
  waiting period for admission to other facility Z75.1
Adnexitis (suppurative) — *see* Salpingo-oophoritis
Adolescent X-linked adrenoleukodystrophy E71.521
Adrenal (gland) — *see* condition
Adrenalism, tuberculous A18.7
Adrenalitis, adrenitis E27.8
  autoimmune E27.1
  meningococcal, hemorrhagic A39.1
Adrenarche, premature E27.0
Adrenocortical syndrome — *see* Cushing's, syndrome
Adrenogenital syndrome E25.9
  acquired E25.8
  congenital E25.0
  salt loss E25.0
Adrenogenitalism, congenital E25.0
Adrenoleukodystrophy E71.529
  neonatal E71.511
  X-linked E71.529
    Addison only phenotype E71.528
    Addison-Schilder E71.528
    adolescent E71.521
    adrenomyeloneuropathy E71.522
    childhood cerebral E71.520
    other specified E71.528
Adrenomyeloneuropathy E71.522
Adventitious bursa — *see* Bursopathy, specified type
  NEC
Adverse effect — *see* Table of Drugs and Chemicals,
  categories T36-T50, with 6th character 5
Advice — *see* Counseling
Adynamia (episodica) (hereditary) (periodic) G72.3
Aeration lung imperfect, newborn — *see* Atelectasis
Aerobullosis T70.3 ☑
Aerocele — *see* Embolism, air
Aerodermectasia
  subcutaneous (traumatic) T79.7 ☑
Aerodontalgia T70.29 ☑
Aeroembolism T70.3 ☑
Aerogenes capsulatus infection A48.0
Aero-otitis media T70.0 ☑
Aerophagy, aerophagia (psychogenic) F45.8
Aerophobia F40.228
Aerosinusitis T70.1 ☑
Aerotitis T70.0 ☑
Affection — *see* Disease
Afibrinogenemia (*see also* Defect, coagulation) D68.8
  acquired D65
  congenital D68.2
    following ectopic or molar pregnancy O08.1

Afibrinogenemia — *continued*
  in abortion — *see* Abortion, by type, complicated by,
    afibrinogenemia
  puerperal O72.3
African
  sleeping sickness B56.9
  tick fever A68.1
  trypanosomiasis B56.9
    gambian B56.0
    rhodesian B56.1
Aftercare (*see also* Care) Z51.89
  following surgery (for) (on)
    amputation Z47.81
    attention to
      drains Z48.03
      dressings (nonsurgical) Z48.00
        surgical Z48.01
      sutures Z48.02
    circulatory system Z48.812
    delayed (planned) wound closure Z48.1
    digestive system Z48.815
    explantation of joint prosthesis (staged procedure)
      hip Z47.32
      knee Z47.33
      shoulder Z47.31
    genitourinary system Z48.816
    joint replacement Z47.1
    neoplasm Z48.3
    nervous system Z48.811
    oral cavity Z48.814
    organ transplant
      bone marrow Z48.290
      heart Z48.21
      heart-lung Z48.280
      kidney Z48.22
      liver Z48.23
      lung Z48.24
      multiple organs NEC Z48.288
      specified NEC Z48.298
    orthopedic NEC Z47.89
    planned wound closure Z48.1
    removal of internal fixation device Z47.2
    respiratory system Z48.813
    scoliosis Z47.82
    sense organs Z48.810
    skin and subcutaneous tissue Z48.817
    specified body system
      circulatory Z48.812
      digestive Z48.815
      genitourinary Z48.816
      nervous Z48.811
      oral cavity Z48.814
      respiratory Z48.813
      sense organs Z48.810
      skin and subcutaneous tissue Z48.817
      teeth Z48.814
    specified NEC Z48.89
    spinal Z48.89
    teeth Z48.814
  fracture — *code to* fracture with seventh character D
  involving
    removal of
      drains Z48.03
      dressings (nonsurgical) Z48.00
      staples Z48.02
      surgical dressings Z48.01
      sutures Z48.02
    neuropacemaker (brain) (peripheral nerve) (spinal
      cord) Z46.2
      implanted Z45.42
    orthopedic NEC Z47.89
  postprocedural — *see* Aftercare, following surgery
After-cataract — *see* Cataract, secondary
Agalactia (primary) O92.3
  elective, secondary or therapeutic O92.5
Agammaglobulinemia (acquired (secondary)) (nonfamilial) D80.1
  with
    immunoglobulin-bearing B-lymphocytes D80.1
    lymphopenia D81.9
  autosomal recessive (Swiss type) D80.0
  Bruton's X-linked D80.0
  common variable (CVAgamma) D80.1
  congenital sex-linked D80.0
  hereditary D80.0
  lymphopenic D81.9
  Swiss type (autosomal recessive) D80.0

Agammaglobulinemia — *continued*
  X-linked (with growth hormone deficiency)(Bruton)
    D80.0
Aganglionosis (bowel) (colon) Q43.1
Age (old) — *see* Senility
Agenesis
  adrenal (gland) Q89.1
  alimentary tract (complete) (partial) NEC Q45.8
    upper Q40.8
  anus, anal (canal) Q42.3
    with fistula Q42.2
  aorta Q25.4
  appendix Q42.8
  arm (complete) Q71.0- ☑
    with hand present Q71.1- ☑
  artery (peripheral) Q27.9
    brain Q28.3
    coronary Q24.5
    pulmonary Q25.79
    specified NEC Q27.8
    umbilical Q27.0
  auditory (canal) (external) Q16.1
  auricle (ear) Q16.0
  bile duct or passage Q44.5
  bladder Q64.5
  bone Q79.9
  brain Q00.0
    part of Q04.3
  breast (with nipple present) Q83.8
    with absent nipple Q83.0
  bronchus Q32.4
  canaliculus lacrimalis Q10.4
  carpus — *see* Agenesis, hand
  cartilage Q79.9
  cecum Q42.8
  cerebellum Q04.3
  cervix Q51.5
  chin Q18.8
  cilia Q10.3
  circulatory system, part NOS Q28.9
  clavicle Q74.0
  clitoris Q52.6
  coccyx Q76.49
  colon Q42.9
    specified NEC Q42.8
  corpus callosum Q04.0
  cricoid cartilage Q31.8
  diaphragm (with hernia) Q79.1
  digestive organ(s) or tract (complete) (partial) NEC
    Q45.8
    upper Q40.8
  ductus arteriosus Q28.8
  duodenum Q41.0
  ear Q16.9
    auricle Q16.0
    lobe Q17.8
  ejaculatory duct Q55.4
  endocrine (gland) NEC Q89.2
  epiglottis Q31.8
  esophagus Q39.8
  eustachian tube Q16.2
  eye Q11.1
    adnexa Q15.8
  eyelid (fold) Q10.3
  face
    bones NEC Q75.8
    specified part NEC Q18.8
  fallopian tube Q50.6
  femur — *see* Defect, reduction, lower limb, longitudi-
    nal, femur
  fibula — *see* Defect, reduction, lower limb, longitudi-
    nal, fibula
  finger (complete) (partial) — *see* Agenesis, hand
  foot (and toes) (complete) (partial) Q72.3- ☑
  forearm (with hand present) — *see* Agenesis, arm,
    with hand present
    and hand Q71.2- ☑
  gallbladder Q44.0
  gastric Q40.2
  genitalia, genital (organ(s))
    female Q52.8
      external Q52.71
      internal NEC Q52.8
    male Q55.8
  glottis Q31.8
  hair Q84.0
  hand (and fingers) (complete) (partial) Q71.3- ☑
  heart Q24.8

Agenesis — *continued*
  heart — *continued*
    valve NEC Q24.8
      pulmonary Q22.0
  hepatic Q44.7
  humerus — *see* Defect, reduction, upper limb
  hymen Q52.4
  ileum Q41.2
  incus Q16.3
  intestine (small) Q41.9
    large Q42.9
      specified NEC Q42.8
  iris (dilator fibers) Q13.1
  jaw M26.09
  jejunum Q41.1
  kidney(s) (partial) Q60.2
    bilateral Q60.1
    unilateral Q60.0
  labium (majus) (minus) Q52.71
  labyrinth, membranous Q16.5
  lacrimal apparatus Q10.4
  larynx Q31.8
  leg (complete) Q72.0- ☑
    with foot present Q72.1- ☑
    lower leg (with foot present) — *see* Agenesis, leg,
      with foot present
      and foot Q72.2- ☑
  lens Q12.3
  limb (complete) Q73.0
    lower — *see* Agenesis, leg
    upper — *see* Agenesis, arm
  lip Q38.0
  liver Q44.7
  lung (fissure) (lobe) (bilateral) (unilateral) Q33.3
  mandible, maxilla M26.09
  metacarpus — *see* Agenesis, hand
  metatarsus — *see* Agenesis, foot
  muscle Q79.8
    eyelid Q10.3
    ocular Q15.8
  musculoskeletal system NEC Q79.8
  nail(s) Q84.3
  neck, part Q18.8
  nerve Q07.8
  nervous system, part NEC Q07.8
  nipple Q83.2
  nose Q30.1
  nuclear Q07.8
  organ
    of Corti Q16.5
    or site not listed — *see* Anomaly, by site
  osseous meatus (ear) Q16.1
  ovary
    bilateral Q50.02
    unilateral Q50.01
  oviduct Q50.6
  pancreas Q45.0
  parathyroid (gland) Q89.2
  parotid gland(s) Q38.4
  patella Q74.1
  pelvic girdle (complete) (partial) Q74.2
  penis Q55.5
  pericardium Q24.8
  pituitary (gland) Q89.2
  prostate Q55.4
  punctum lacrimale Q10.4
  radioulnar — *see* Defect, reduction, upper limb
  radius — *see* Defect, reduction, upper limb, longitudi-
    nal, radius
  rectum Q42.1
    with fistula Q42.0
  renal Q60.2
    bilateral Q60.1
    unilateral Q60.0
  respiratory organ NEC Q34.8
  rib Q76.6
  roof of orbit Q75.8
  round ligament Q52.8
  sacrum Q76.49
  salivary gland Q38.4
  scapula Q74.0
  scrotum Q55.29
  seminal vesicles Q55.4
  septum
    atrial Q21.1
    between aorta and pulmonary artery Q21.4
    ventricular Q20.4
  shoulder girdle (complete) (partial) Q74.0

Agenesis — *continued*
  skull (bone) Q75.8
    with
      anencephaly Q00.0
      encephalocele — *see* Encephalocele
      hydrocephalus Q03.9
        with spina bifida — *see* Spina bifida, by site,
          with hydrocephalus
      microcephaly Q02
  spermatic cord Q55.4
  spinal cord Q06.0
  spine Q76.49
  spleen Q89.01
  sternum Q76.7
  stomach Q40.2
  submaxillary gland(s) (congenital) Q38.4
  tarsus — *see* Agenesis, foot
  tendon Q79.8
  testicle Q55.0
  thymus (gland) Q89.2
  thyroid (gland) E03.1
    cartilage Q31.8
  tibia — *see* Defect, reduction, lower limb, longitudinal,
    tibia
  tibiofibular — *see* Defect, reduction, lower limb,
    specified type NEC
  toe (and foot) (complete) (partial) — *see* Agenesis,
    foot
  tongue Q38.3
  trachea (cartilage) Q32.1
  ulna — *see* Defect, reduction, upper limb, longitudinal,
    ulna
  upper limb — *see* Agenesis, arm
  ureter Q62.4
  urethra Q64.5
  urinary tract NEC Q64.8
  uterus Q51.0
  uvula Q38.5
  vagina Q52.0
  vas deferens Q55.4
  vein(s) (peripheral) Q27.9
    brain Q28.3
    great NEC Q26.8
    portal Q26.5
  vena cava (inferior) (superior) Q26.8
  vermis of cerebellum Q04.3
  vertebra Q76.49
  vulva Q52.71
Ageusia R43.2
Agitated — *see* condition
Agitation R45.1
Aglossia (congenital) Q38.3
Aglossia-adactylia syndrome Q87.0
Aglycogenosis E74.00
Agnosia (body image) (other senses) (tactile) R48.1
  developmental F88
  verbal R48.1
    auditory R48.1
      developmental F80.2
    developmental F80.2
  visual (object) R48.3
Agoraphobia F40.00
  with panic disorder F40.01
  without panic disorder F40.02
Agrammatism R48.8
Agranulocytopenia — *see* Agranulocytosis
Agranulocytosis (chronic) (cyclical) (genetic) (infantile)
  (periodic) (pernicious) (*see also* Neutropenia) D70.9
  congenital D70.0
  cytoreductive cancer chemotherapy sequela D70.1
  drug-induced D70.2
    due to cytoreductive cancer chemotherapy D70.1
  due to infection D70.3
  secondary D70.4
    drug-induced D70.2
      due to cytoreductive cancer chemotherapy
        D70.1
Agraphia (absolute) R48.8
  with alexia R48.0
  developmental F81.81
Ague (dumb) — *see* Malaria
Agyria Q04.3
Ahumada-del Castillo syndrome E23.0
Aichomophobia F40.298
AIDS (related complex) B20
Ailment heart — *see* Disease, heart
Ailurophobia F40.218
Ainhum (disease) L94.6

AIPHI (acute idiopathic pulmonary hemorrhage in infants
  (over 28 days old)) R04.81
Air
  anterior mediastinum J98.2
  compressed, disease T70.3 ☑
  conditioner lung or pneumonitis J67.7
  embolism (artery) (cerebral) (any site) T79.0 ☑
    with ectopic or molar pregnancy O08.2
    due to implanted device NEC — *see* Complications,
      by site and type, specified NEC
    following
      abortion — *see* Abortion by type, complicated
        by, embolism
      ectopic or molar pregnancy O08.2
    infusion, therapeutic injection or transfusion
      T80.0 ☑
    in pregnancy, childbirth or puerperium — *see*
      Embolism, obstetric
    traumatic T79.0 ☑
  hunger, psychogenic F45.8
  rarefied, effects of — *see* Effect, adverse, high altitude
  sickness T75.3 ☑
Airplane sickness T75.3 ☑
Akathisia (drug-induced) (treatment-induced) G25.71
  neuroleptic induced (acute) G25.71
Akinesia R29.898
Akinetic mutism R41.89
Akureyri's disease G93.3
Alactasia, congenital E73.0
Alagille's syndrome Q44.7
Alastrim B03
Albers-Schönberg syndrome Q78.2
Albert's syndrome — *see* Tendinitis, Achilles
Albinism, albino E70.30
  with hematologic abnormality E70.339
    Chédiak-Higashi syndrome E70.330
    Hermansky-Pudlak syndrome E70.331
    other specified E70.338
  I E70.320
  II E70.321
  ocular E70.319
    autosomal recessive E70.311
    other specified E70.318
    X-linked E70.310
  oculocutaneous E70.329
    other specified E70.328
    tyrosinase (ty) negative E70.320
    tyrosinase (ty) positive E70.321
  other specified E70.39
Albinismus E70.30
Albright (-McCune)(-Sternberg) syndrome Q78.1
Albuminous — *see* condition
Albuminuria, albuminuric (acute) (chronic) (subacute)
  (*see also* Proteinuria) R80.9
  complicating pregnancy — *see* Proteinuria, gestational
    with
      gestational hypertension — *see* Pre-eclampsia
      pre-existing hypertension — *see* Hypertension,
        complicating pregnancy, pre-existing,
        with, pre-eclampsia
    gestational — *see* Proteinuria, gestational
    with
      gestational hypertension — *see* Pre-eclampsia
      pre-existing hypertension — *see* Hypertension,
        complicating pregnancy, pre-existing,
        with, pre-eclampsia
  orthostatic R80.2
  postural R80.2
  pre-eclamptic — *see* Pre-eclampsia
  scarlatinal A38.8
Albuminurophobia F40.298
Alcaptonuria E70.29
Alcohol, alcoholic, alcohol-induced
  addiction (without remission) F10.20
    with remission F10.21
  amnestic disorder, persisting F10.96
    with dependence F10.26
  brain syndrome, chronic F10.97
    with dependence F10.27
  cardiopathy I42.6
  counseling and surveillance Z71.41
    family member Z71.42
  delirium (acute) (tremens) (withdrawal) F10.231
    with intoxication F10.921
      in
        abuse F10.121
        dependence F10.221

Alcohol, alcoholic, alcohol-induced — continued
  dementia F10.97
    with dependence F10.27
  deterioration F10.97
    with dependence F10.27
  hallucinosis (acute) F10.951
    in
      abuse F10.151
      dependence F10.251
  insanity F10.959
  intoxication (acute) (without dependence) F10.129
    with
      delirium F10.121
      dependence F10.229
        with delirium F10.221
        uncomplicated F10.220
      uncomplicated F10.120
  jealousy F10.988
  Korsakoff's, Korsakov's, Korsakow's F10.26
  liver K70.9
    acute — see Disease, liver, alcoholic, hepatitis
  mania (acute) (chronic) F10.959
  paranoia, paranoid (type) psychosis F10.950
  pellagra E52
  poisoning, accidental (acute) NEC — see Table of Drugs
    and Chemicals, alcohol, poisoning
  psychosis — see Psychosis, alcoholic
  withdrawal (without convulsions) F10.239
    with delirium F10.231
Alcoholism (chronic) (without remission) F10.20
  with
    psychosis — see Psychosis, alcoholic
    remission F10.21
  Korsakov's F10.96
    with dependence F10.26
Alder (-Reilly) **anomaly or syndrome** (leukocyte granulation) D72.0
Aldosteronism E26.9
  familial (type I) E26.02
  glucocorticoid-remediable E26.02
  primary (due to (bilateral) adrenal hyperplasia) E26.09
  primary NEC E26.09
  secondary E26.1
  specified NEC E26.89
Aldosteronoma D44.10
Aldrich (-Wiskott) **syndrome** (eczema-thrombocytopenia) D82.0
Alektorophobia F40.218
Aleppo boil B55.1
Aleukemic — see condition
Aleukia
  congenital D70.0
  hemorrhagica D61.9
    congenital D61.09
  splenica D73.1
Alexia R48.0
  developmental F81.0
  secondary to organic lesion R48.0
Algoneurodystrophy M89.00
  ankle M89.07- ☑
  foot M89.07- ☑
  forearm M89.03- ☑
  hand M89.04- ☑
  lower leg M89.06- ☑
  multiple sites M89.0- ☑
  shoulder M89.01- ☑
  specified site NEC M89.08
  thigh M89.05- ☑
  upper arm M89.02- ☑
Algophobia F40.298
Alienation, mental — see Psychosis
Alkalemia E87.3
Alkalosis E87.3
  metabolic E87.3
    with respiratory acidosis E87.4
  respiratory E87.3
Alkaptonuria E70.29
Allen-Masters syndrome N83.8
Allergy, allergic (reaction) (to) T78.40 ☑
  air-borne substance NEC (rhinitis) J30.89
  alveolitis (extrinsic) J67.9
    due to
      Aspergillus clavatus J67.4
      Cryptostroma corticale J67.6
      organisms (fungal, thermophilic actinomycete)
        growing in ventilation (air conditioning)
        systems J67.7

Allergy, allergic — continued
  alveolitis — continued
    specified type NEC J67.8
  anaphylactic reaction or shock T78.2 ☑
  angioneurotic edema T78.3 ☑
  animal (dander) (epidermal) (hair) (rhinitis) J30.81
  bee sting (anaphylactic shock) — see Toxicity, venom,
    arthropod, bee
  biological — see Allergy, drug
  colitis K52.2
  dander (animal) (rhinitis) J30.81
  dandruff (rhinitis) J30.81
  dental restorative material (existing) K08.55
  dermatitis — see Dermatitis, contact, allergic
  diathesis — see History, allergy
  drug, medicament & biological (any) (external) (internal) T78.40 ☑
    correct substance properly administered — see
      Table of Drugs and Chemicals, by drug, adverse effect
    wrong substance given or taken NEC (by accident)
      — see Table of Drugs and Chemicals, by
      drug, poisoning
  due to pollen J30.1
  dust (house) (stock) (rhinitis) J30.89
    with asthma — see Asthma, allergic extrinsic
  eczema — see Dermatitis, contact, allergic
  epidermal (animal) (rhinitis) J30.81
  feathers (rhinitis) J30.89
  food (any) (ingested) NEC T78.1 ☑
    anaphylactic shock — see Shock, anaphylactic, due
      to food
    dermatitis — see Dermatitis, due to, food
    dietary counseling and surveillance Z71.3
    in contact with skin L23.6
    rhinitis J30.5
    status (without reaction) Z91.018
      eggs Z91.012
      milk products Z91.011
      peanuts Z91.010
      seafood Z91.013
      specified NEC Z91.018
  gastrointestinal K52.2
  grain J30.1
  grass (hay fever) (pollen) J30.1
    asthma — see Asthma, allergic extrinsic
  hair (animal) (rhinitis) J30.81
  history (of) — see History, allergy
  horse serum — see Allergy, serum
  inhalant (rhinitis) J30.89
    pollen J30.1
  kapok (rhinitis) J30.89
  medicine — see Allergy, drug
  milk protein K52.2
  nasal, seasonal due to pollen J30.1
  pneumonia J82
  pollen (any) (hay fever) J30.1
    asthma — see Asthma, allergic extrinsic
  primrose J30.1
  primula J30.1
  purpura D69.0
  ragweed (hay fever) (pollen) J30.1
    asthma — see Asthma, allergic extrinsic
  rose (pollen) J30.1
  seasonal NEC J30.2
  Senecio jacobae (pollen) J30.1
  serum (see also Reaction, serum) T80.69 ☑
    anaphylactic shock T80.59 ☑
  shock (anaphylactic) T78.2 ☑
    due to
      administration of blood and blood products
        T80.51 ☑
      adverse effect of correct medicinal substance
        properly administered T88.6 ☑
      immunization T80.52 ☑
      serum NEC T80.59 ☑
      vaccination T80.52 ☑
  specific NEC T78.49 ☑
  tree (any) (hay fever) (pollen) J30.1
    asthma — see Asthma, allergic extrinsic
  upper respiratory J30.9
  urticaria L50.0
  vaccine — see Allergy, serum
  wheat — see Allergy, food
Allescheriasis B48.2
Alligator skin disease Q80.9
Allocheiria, allochiria R20.8

Almeida's disease — see Paracoccidioidomycosis
Alopecia (hereditaria) (seborrheica) L65.9
  androgenic L64.9
    drug-induced L64.0
    specified NEC L64.8
  areata L63.9
    ophiasis L63.2
    specified NEC L63.8
    totalis L63.0
    universalis L63.1
  cicatricial L66.9
    specified NEC L66.8
  circumscripta L63.9
  congenital, congenitalis Q84.0
  due to cytotoxic drugs NEC L65.8
  mucinosa L65.2
  postinfective NEC L65.8
  postpartum L65.0
  premature L64.8
  specific (syphilitic) A51.32
  specified NEC L65.8
  syphilitic (secondary) A51.32
  totalis (capitis) L63.0
  universalis (entire body) L63.1
  X-ray L58.1
Alpers' disease G31.81
Alpine sickness T70.29 ☑
Alport syndrome Q87.81
ALTE (apparent life threatening event) **in newborn and
  infant** R68.13
Alteration (of), **Altered**
  awareness, transient R40.4
  mental status R41.82
  pattern of family relationships affecting child Z62.898
  sensation
    following
      cerebrovascular disease I69.998
        cerebral infarction I69.398
        intracerebral hemorrhage I69.198
        nontraumatic intracranial hemorrhage NEC
          I69.298
        specified disease NEC I69.898
        subarachnoid hemorrhage I69.098
Alternating — see condition
Altitude, high (effects) — see Effect, adverse, high altitude
Aluminosis (of lung) J63.0
Alveolitis
  allergic (extrinsic) — see Pneumonitis, hypersensitivity
  due to
    Aspergillus clavatus J67.4
    Cryptostroma corticale J67.6
  fibrosing (cryptogenic) (idiopathic) J84.112
  jaw M27.3
  sicca dolorosa M27.3
Alveolus, alveolar — see condition
Alymphocytosis D72.810
  thymic (with immunodeficiency) D82.1
Alymphoplasia, thymic D82.1
Alzheimer's disease or sclerosis — see Disease,
  Alzheimer's
Amastia (with nipple present) Q83.8
  with absent nipple Q83.0
Amathophobia F40.228
Amaurosis (acquired) (congenital) (see also Blindness)
  fugax G45.3
  hysterical F44.6
  Leber's congenital H35.50
  uremic — see Uremia
Amaurotic idiocy (infantile) (juvenile) (late) E75.4
Amaxophobia F40.248
Ambiguous genitalia Q56.4
Amblyopia (congenital) (ex anopsia) (partial) (suppression) H53.00- ☑
  anisometropic — see Amblyopia, refractive
  deprivation H53.01- ☑
  hysterical F44.6
  nocturnal (see also Blindness, night)
    vitamin A deficiency E50.5
  refractive H53.02- ☑
  strabismic H53.03- ☑
  tobacco H53.8
  toxic NEC H53.8
  uremic — see Uremia
Ameba, amebic (histolytica) (see also Amebiasis)
  abscess (liver) A06.4
Amebiasis A06.9

16

☑ Additional Character Required — Refer to the Tabular List for Character Selection   ▽ Subterms under main terms may continue to next column or page

Amebiasis — *continued*
　with abscess — *see* Abscess, amebic
　acute A06.0
　chronic (intestine) A06.1
　　with abscess — *see* Abscess, amebic
　cutaneous A06.7
　cutis A06.7
　cystitis A06.81
　genitourinary tract NEC A06.82
　hepatic — *see* Abscess, liver, amebic
　intestine A06.0
　nondysenteric colitis A06.2
　skin A06.7
　specified site NEC A06.89
Ameboma (of intestine) A06.3
Amelia Q73.0
　lower limb — *see* Agenesis, leg
　upper limb — *see* Agenesis, arm
Ameloblastoma (*see also* Cyst, calcifying odontogenic)
　long bones C40.9- ☑
　　lower limb C40.2- ☑
　　upper limb C40.0- ☑
　malignant C41.1
　　jaw (bone) (lower) C41.1
　　　upper C41.0
　tibial C40.2- ☑
Amelogenesis imperfecta K00.5
　nonhereditaria (segmentalis) K00.4
Amenorrhea N91.2
　hyperhormonal E28.8
　primary N91.0
　secondary N91.1
Amentia — *see* Disability, intellectual
　Meynert's (nonalcoholic) F04
American
　leishmaniasis B55.2
　mountain tick fever A93.2
Ametropia — *see* Disorder, refraction
Amianthosis J61
Amimia R48.8
Amino-acid disorder E72.9
　anemia D53.0
Aminoacidopathy E72.9
Aminoaciduria E72.9
Amnesia R41.3
　anterograde R41.1
　auditory R48.8
　dissociative F44.0
　hysterical F44.0
　postictal in epilepsy — *see* Epilepsy
　psychogenic F44.0
　retrograde R41.2
　transient global G45.4
Amnes(t)ic syndrome (post-traumatic) F04
　induced by
　　alcohol F10.96
　　　with dependence F10.26
　　psychoactive NEC F19.96
　　　with
　　　　abuse F19.16
　　　　dependence F19.26
　　sedative F13.96
　　　with dependence F13.26
Amnion, amniotic — *see* condition
Amnionitis — *see* Pregnancy, complicated by
Amok F68.8
Amoral traits F60.89
Ampulla
　lower esophagus K22.8
　phrenic K22.8
Amputation (*see also* Absence, by site, acquired)
　neuroma (postoperative) (traumatic) — *see* Complications, amputation stump, neuroma
　stump (surgical)
　　abnormal, painful, or with complication (late) — *see* Complications, amputation stump
　　healed or old NOS Z89.9
　traumatic (complete) (partial)
　　arm (upper) (complete) S48.91- ☑
　　　at
　　　　elbow S58.01- ☑
　　　　　partial S58.02- ☑
　　　　shoulder joint (complete) S48.01- ☑
　　　　　partial S48.02- ☑
　　　　between
　　　　　elbow and wrist (complete) S58.11- ☑
　　　　　　partial S58.12- ☑

Amputation — *continued*
　traumatic — *continued*
　　arm — *continued*
　　　between — *continued*
　　　　shoulder and elbow (complete) S48.11- ☑
　　　　　partial S48.12- ☑
　　　partial S48.92- ☑
　　breast (complete) S28.21- ☑
　　　partial S28.22- ☑
　　clitoris (complete) S38.211 ☑
　　　partial S38.212 ☑
　　ear (complete) S08.11- ☑
　　　partial S08.12- ☑
　　finger (complete) (metacarpophalangeal) S68.11- ☑
　　　index S68.11- ☑
　　　little S68.11- ☑
　　　middle S68.11- ☑
　　　partial S68.12- ☑
　　　　index S68.12- ☑
　　　　little S68.12- ☑
　　　　middle S68.12- ☑
　　　　ring S68.12- ☑
　　　ring S68.11- ☑
　　　thumb — *see* Amputation, traumatic, thumb
　　　transphalangeal (complete) S68.61- ☑
　　　　index S68.61- ☑
　　　　little S68.61- ☑
　　　　middle S68.61- ☑
　　　　partial S68.62- ☑
　　　　　index S68.62- ☑
　　　　　little S68.62- ☑
　　　　　middle S68.62- ☑
　　　　　ring S68.62- ☑
　　　　ring S68.61- ☑
　　foot (complete) S98.91- ☑
　　　at ankle level S98.01- ☑
　　　　partial S98.02- ☑
　　　midfoot S98.31- ☑
　　　　partial S98.32- ☑
　　　partial S98.92- ☑
　　forearm (complete) S58.91- ☑
　　　at elbow level (complete) S58.01- ☑
　　　　partial S58.02- ☑
　　　between elbow and wrist (complete) S58.11- ☑
　　　　partial S58.12- ☑
　　　partial S58.92- ☑
　　genital organ(s) (external)
　　　female (complete) S38.211 ☑
　　　　partial S38.212 ☑
　　　male
　　　　penis (complete) S38.221 ☑
　　　　　partial S38.222 ☑
　　　　scrotum (complete) S38.231 ☑
　　　　　partial S38.232 ☑
　　　　testes (complete) S38.231 ☑
　　　　　partial S38.232 ☑
　　hand (complete) (wrist level) S68.41- ☑
　　　finger(s) alone — *see* Amputation, traumatic, finger
　　　partial S68.42- ☑
　　　thumb alone — *see* Amputation, traumatic, thumb
　　　transmetacarpal (complete) S68.71- ☑
　　　　partial S68.72- ☑
　　head
　　　ear — *see* Amputation, traumatic, ear
　　　nose (partial) S08.812 ☑
　　　　complete S08.811 ☑
　　　part S08.89 ☑
　　　　scalp S08.0 ☑
　　hip (and thigh) (complete) S78.91- ☑
　　　at hip joint (complete) S78.01- ☑
　　　　partial S78.02- ☑
　　　between hip and knee (complete) S78.11- ☑
　　　　partial S78.12- ☑
　　　partial S78.92- ☑
　　labium (majus) (minus) (complete) S38.21- ☑
　　　partial S38.21- ☑
　　leg (lower) S88.91- ☑
　　　at knee level S88.01- ☑
　　　　partial S88.02- ☑
　　　between knee and ankle S88.11- ☑
　　　　partial S88.12- ☑
　　　partial S88.92- ☑
　　nose (partial) S08.812 ☑

Amputation — *continued*
　traumatic — *continued*
　　nose — *continued*
　　　complete S08.811 ☑
　　　penis (complete) S38.221 ☑
　　　　partial S38.222 ☑
　　　scrotum (complete) S38.231 ☑
　　　　partial S38.232 ☑
　　　shoulder — *see* Amputation, traumatic, arm
　　　　at shoulder joint — *see* Amputation, traumatic, arm, at shoulder joint
　　　testes (complete) S38.231 ☑
　　　　partial S38.232 ☑
　　　thigh — *see* Amputation, traumatic, hip
　　　thorax, part of S28.1 ☑
　　　　breast — *see* Amputation, traumatic, breast
　　　thumb (complete) (metacarpophalangeal) S68.01- ☑
　　　　partial S68.02- ☑
　　　　transphalangeal (complete) S68.51- ☑
　　　　　partial S68.52- ☑
　　　toe (lesser) S98.13- ☑
　　　　great S98.11- ☑
　　　　　partial S98.12- ☑
　　　　more than one S98.21- ☑
　　　　　partial S98.22- ☑
　　　　partial S98.14- ☑
　　　vulva (complete) S38.211 ☑
　　　　partial S38.212 ☑
Amputee (bilateral) (old) Z89.9
Amsterdam dwarfism Q87.1
Amusia R48.8
　developmental F80.89
Amyelencephalus, amyelencephaly Q00.0
Amyelia Q06.0
Amygdalitis — *see* Tonsillitis
Amygdalolith J35.8
Amyloid heart (disease) E85.4 [I43]
Amyloidosis (generalized) (primary) E85.9
　with lung involvement E85.4 [J99]
　familial E85.2
　genetic E85.2
　heart E85.4 [I43]
　hemodialysis-associated E85.3
　liver E85.4 [K77]
　localized E85.4
　neuropathic heredofamilial E85.1
　non-neuropathic heredofamilial E85.0
　organ limited E85.4
　Portuguese E85.1
　pulmonary E85.4 [J99]
　secondary systemic E85.3
　skin (lichen) (macular) E85.4 [L99]
　specified NEC E85.8
　subglottic E85.4 [J99]
Amylopectinosis (brancher enzyme deficiency) E74.03
Amylophagia — *see* Pica
Amyoplasia congenita Q79.8
Amyotonia M62.89
　congenita G70.2
Amyotrophia, amyotrophy, amyotrophic G71.8
　congenita Q79.8
　diabetic — *see* Diabetes, amyotrophy
　lateral sclerosis G12.21
　neuralgic G54.5
　spinal progressive G12.21
Anacidity, gastric K31.83
　psychogenic F45.8
Anaerosis of newborn P28.89
Analbuminemia E88.09
Analgesia — *see* Anesthesia
Analphalipoproteinemia E78.6
Anaphylactic
　purpura D69.0
　shock or reaction — *see* Shock, anaphylactic
Anaphylactoid shock or reaction — *see* Shock, anaphylactic
Anaphylactoid syndrome of pregnancy O88.01- ☑
Anaphylaxis — *see* Shock, anaphylactic
Anaplasia cervix (*see also* Dysplasia, cervix) N87.9
Anaplasmosis, human A77.49
Anarthria R47.1
Anasarca R60.1
　cardiac — *see* Failure, heart, congestive
　lung J18.2
　newborn P83.2
　nutritional E43

Anasarca — *continued*
pulmonary J18.2
renal N04.9
Anastomosis
aneurysmal — *see* Aneurysm
arteriovenous ruptured brain I60.8
intestinal K63.89
complicated NEC K91.89
involving urinary tract N99.89
retinal and choroidal vessels (congenital) Q14.8
Anatomical narrow angle H40.03- ☑
Ancylostoma, ancylostomiasis (braziliense) (caninum)
(ceylanicum) (duodenale) B76.0
Necator americanus B76.1
Andersen's disease (glycogen storage) E74.09
Anderson-Fabry disease E75.21
Andes disease T70.29 ☑
Andrews' disease (bacterid) L08.89
Androblastoma
benign
specified site — *see* Neoplasm, benign, by site
unspecified site
female D27.9
male D29.20
malignant
specified site — *see* Neoplasm, malignant, by site
unspecified site
female C56.9
male C62.90
specified site — *see* Neoplasm, uncertain behavior,
by site
tubular
with lipid storage
specified site — *see* Neoplasm, benign, by site
unspecified site
female D27.9
male D29.20
specified site — *see* Neoplasm, benign, by site
unspecified site
female D27.9
male D29.20
unspecified site
female D39.10
male D40.10
Androgen insensitivity syndrome (*see also* Syndrome,
androgen insensitivity) E34.50
Androgen resistance syndrome (*see also* Syndrome,
androgen insensitivity) E34.50
Android pelvis Q74.2
with disproportion (fetopelvic) O33.3 ☑
causing obstructed labor O65.3
Androphobia F40.290
Anectasis, pulmonary (newborn) — *see* Atelectasis
Anemia (essential) (general) (hemoglobin deficiency)
(infantile) (primary) (profound) D64.9
with (due to) (in)
disorder of
anaerobic glycolysis D55.2
pentose phosphate pathway D55.1
koilonychia D50.9
achlorhydric D50.8
achrestic D53.1
Addison (-Biermer) (pernicious) D51.0
agranulocytic — *see* Agranulocytosis
amino-acid-deficiency D53.0
aplastic D61.9
congenital D61.09
drug-induced D61.1
due to
drugs D61.1
external agents NEC D61.2
infection D61.2
radiation D61.2
idiopathic D61.3
red cell (pure) D60.9
chronic D60.0
congenital D61.01
specified type NEC D60.8
transient D60.1
specified type NEC D61.89
toxic D61.2
aregenerative
congenital D61.09
asiderotic D50.9
atypical (primary) D64.9
Baghdad spring D55.0
Balantidium coli A07.0
Biermer's (pernicious) D51.0

Anemia — *continued*
blood loss (chronic) D50.0
acute D62
bothriocephalus B70.0 [D63.8]
brickmaker's B76.9 [D63.8]
cerebral I67.89
childhood D58.9
chlorotic D50.8
chronic
blood loss D50.0
hemolytic D58.9
idiopathic D59.9
simple D53.9
chronica congenita aregenerativa D61.09
combined system disease NEC D51.0 [G32.0]
due to dietary vitamin B12 deficiency D51.3 [G32.0]
complicating pregnancy, childbirth or puerperium —
see Pregnancy, complicated by (management
affected by), anemia
congenital P61.4
aplastic D61.09
due to isoimmunization NOS P55.9
dyserythropoietic, dyshematopoietic D64.4
following fetal blood loss P61.3
Heinz body D58.2
hereditary hemolytic NOS D58.9
pernicious D51.0
spherocytic D58.9
Cooley's (erythroblastic) D56.1
cytogenic D51.0
deficiency D53.9
6-PGD D55.1
2, 3 diphosphoglycurate mutase D55.2
2, 3 PG D55.2
6 phosphogluconate dehydrogenase D55.1
amino-acid D53.0
combined B12 and folate D53.1
enzyme D55.9
drug-induced (hemolytic) D59.2
glucose-6-phosphate dehydrogenase (G6PD)
D55.0
glycolytic D55.2
nucleotide metabolism D55.3
related to hexose monophosphate (HMP) shunt
pathway NEC D55.1
specified type NEC D55.8
erythrocytic glutathione D55.1
folate D52.9
dietary D52.0
drug-induced D52.1
folic acid D52.9
dietary D52.0
drug-induced D52.1
G SH D55.1
G6PD D55.0
GGS-R D55.1
glucose-6-phosphate dehydrogenase D55.0
glutathione reductase D55.1
glyceraldehyde phosphate dehydrogenase D55.2
hexokinase D55.2
iron D50.9
secondary to blood loss (chronic) D50.0
nutritional D53.9
with
poor iron absorption D50.8
specified deficiency NEC D53.8
phosphofructo-aldolase D55.2
phosphoglycerate kinase D55.2
PK D55.2
protein D53.0
pyruvate kinase D55.2
transcobalamin II D51.2
triose-phosphate isomerase D55.2
vitamin B12 NOS D51.9
dietary D51.3
due to
intrinsic factor deficiency D51.0
selective vitamin B12 malabsorption with
proteinuria D51.1
pernicious D51.0
specified type NEC D51.8
Diamond-Blackfan (congenital hypoplastic) D61.01
dibothriocephalus B70.0 [D63.8]
dimorphic D53.1
diphasic D53.1
Diphyllobothrium (Dibothriocephalus) B70.0 [D63.8]
due to (in) (with)
antineoplastic chemotherapy D64.81

Anemia — *continued*
due to — *continued*
blood loss (chronic) D50.0
acute D62
chemotherapy, antineoplastic D64.81
chronic disease classified elsewhere NEC D63.8
chronic kidney disease D63.1
deficiency
amino-acid D53.0
copper D53.8
folate (folic acid) D52.9
dietary D52.0
drug-induced D52.1
molybdenum D53.8
protein D53.0
zinc D53.8
dietary vitamin B12 deficiency D51.3
disorder of
glutathione metabolism D55.1
nucleotide metabolism D55.3
drug — *see* Anemia, by type (*see also* Table of
Drugs and Chemicals)
end stage renal disease D63.1
enzyme disorder D55.9
fetal blood loss P61.3
fish tapeworm (D.latum) infestation B70.0 [D63.8]
hemorrhage (chronic) D50.0
acute D62
impaired absorption D50.9
loss of blood (chronic) D50.0
acute D62
myxedema E03.9 [D63.8]
Necator americanus B76.1 [D63.8]
prematurity P61.2
selective vitamin B12 malabsorption with proteinuria D51.1
transcobalamin II deficiency D51.2
Dyke-Young type (secondary) (symptomatic) D59.1
dyserythropoietic (congenital) D64.4
dyshematopoietic (congenital) D64.4
Egyptian B76.9 [D63.8]
elliptocytosis — *see* Elliptocytosis
enzyme-deficiency, drug-induced D59.2
epidemic (*see also* Ancylostomiasis) B76.9 [D63.8]
erythroblastic
familial D56.1
newborn (*see also* Disease, hemolytic) P55.9
of childhood D56.1
erythrocytic glutathione deficiency D55.1
erythropoietin-resistant anemia (EPO resistant anemia)
D63.1
Faber's (achlorhydric anemia) D50.9
factitious (self-induced blood letting) D50.0
familial erythroblastic D56.1
Fanconi's (congenital pancytopenia) D61.09
favism D55.0
fish tapeworm (D. latum) infestation B70.0 [D63.8]
folate (folic acid) deficiency D52.9
glucose-6-phosphate dehydrogenase (G6PD) deficiency D55.0
glutathione-reductase deficiency D55.1
goat's milk D52.0
granulocytic — *see* Agranulocytosis
Heinz body, congenital D58.2
hemolytic D58.9
acquired D59.9
with hemoglobinuria NEC D59.6
autoimmune NEC D59.1
infectious D59.4
specified type NEC D59.8
toxic D59.4
acute D59.9
due to enzyme deficiency specified type NEC
D55.8
Lederer's D59.1
autoimmune D59.1
drug-induced D59.0
chronic D58.9
idiopathic D59.9
cold type (secondary) (symptomatic) D59.1
congenital (spherocytic) — *see* Spherocytosis
due to
cardiac conditions D59.4
drugs (nonautoimmune) D59.2
autoimmune D59.0
enzyme disorder D55.9
drug-induced D59.2

☑ **Additional Character Required** — Refer to the Tabular List for Character Selection   ⬥ Subterms under main terms may continue to next column or page

Anemia — *continued*
  hemolytic — *continued*
    due to — *continued*
      presence of shunt or other internal prosthetic device D59.4
    familial D58.9
    hereditary D58.9
      due to enzyme disorder D55.9
        specified type NEC D55.8
      specified type NEC D58.8
    idiopathic (chronic) D59.9
    mechanical D59.4
    microangiopathic D59.4
    nonautoimmune D59.4
      drug-induced D59.2
    nonspherocytic
      congenital or hereditary NEC D55.8
        glucose-6-phosphate dehydrogenase deficiency D55.0
        pyruvate kinase deficiency D55.2
        type
          I D55.1
          II D55.2
      type
        I D55.1
        II D55.2
    secondary D59.4
      autoimmune D59.1
    specified (hereditary) type NEC D58.8
    Stransky-Regala type (*see also* Hemoglobinopathy) D58.8
    symptomatic D59.4
      autoimmune D59.1
    toxic D59.4
    warm type (secondary) (symptomatic) D59.1
  hemorrhagic (chronic) D50.0
    acute D62
  Herrick's D57.1
  hexokinase deficiency D55.2
  hookworm B76.9 [D63.8]
  hypochromic (idiopathic) (microcytic) (normoblastic) D50.9
    due to blood loss (chronic) D50.0
      acute D62
    familial sex-linked D64.0
    pyridoxine-responsive D64.3
    sideroblastic, sex-linked D64.0
  hypoplasia, red blood cells D61.9
    congenital or familial D61.01
  hypoplastic (idiopathic) D61.9
    congenital or familial (of childhood) D61.01
  hypoproliferative (refractive) D61.9
  idiopathic D64.9
    aplastic D61.3
    hemolytic, chronic D59.9
  in (due to) (with)
    chronic kidney disease D63.1
    end stage renal disease D63.1
    failure, kidney (renal) D63.1
    neoplastic disease (*see also* Neoplasm) D63.0
  intertropical (*see also* Ancylostomiasis) D63.8
  iron deficiency D50.9
    secondary to blood loss (chronic) D50.0
      acute D62
    specified type NEC D50.8
  Joseph-Diamond-Blackfan (congenital hypoplastic) D61.01
  Lederer's (hemolytic) D59.1
  leukoerythroblastic D61.82
  macrocytic D53.9
    nutritional D52.0
    tropical D52.8
  malarial (*see also* Malaria) B54 [D63.8]
  malignant (progressive) D51.0
  malnutrition D53.9
  marsh (*see also* Malaria) B54 [D63.8]
  Mediterranean (with other hemoglobinopathy) D56.9
  megaloblastic D53.1
    combined B12 and folate deficiency D53.1
    hereditary D51.1
    nutritional D52.0
    orotic aciduria D53.0
    refractory D53.1
    specified type NEC D53.1
  megalocytic D53.1
  microcytic (hypochromic) D50.9
    due to blood loss (chronic) D50.0
      acute D62

Anemia — *continued*
  microcytic — *continued*
    familial D56.8
  microdrepanocytosis D57.40
  microelliptopoikilocytic (Rietti-Greppi- Micheli) D56.9
  miner's B76.9 [D63.8]
  myelodysplastic D46.9
  myelofibrosis D75.81
  myelogenous D64.89
  myelopathic D64.89
  myelophthisic D61.82
  myeloproliferative D47.Z9 (*following* D47.4)
  newborn P61.4
    due to
      ABO (antibodies, isoimmunization, maternal/fetal incompatibility) P55.1
      Rh (antibodies, isoimmunization, maternal/fetal incompatibility) P55.0
    following fetal blood loss P61.3
    posthemorrhagic (fetal) P61.3
  nonspherocytic hemolytic — *see* Anemia, hemolytic, nonspherocytic
  normocytic (infectional) D64.9
    due to blood loss (chronic) D50.0
      acute D62
    myelophthisic D61.82
  nutritional (deficiency) D53.9
    with
      poor iron absorption D50.8
      specified deficiency NEC D53.8
      megaloblastic D52.0
  of prematurity P61.2
  orotaciduric (congenital) (hereditary) D53.0
  osteosclerotic D64.89
  ovalocytosis (hereditary) — *see* Elliptocytosis
  paludal (*see also* Malaria) B54 [D63.8]
  pernicious (congenital) (malignant) (progressive) D51.0
  pleochromic D64.89
    of sprue D52.8
  posthemorrhagic (chronic) D50.0
    acute D62
    newborn P61.3
  postoperative (postprocedural)
    due to (acute) blood loss D62
      chronic blood loss D50.0
    specified NEC D64.9
  postpartum O90.81
  pressure D64.89
  progressive D64.9
    malignant D51.0
    pernicious D51.0
  protein-deficiency D53.0
  pseudoleukemica infantum D64.89
  pure red cell D60.9
    congenital D61.01
  pyridoxine-responsive D64.3
  pyruvate kinase deficiency D55.2
  refractory D46.4
    with
      excess of blasts D46.20
        1 (RAEB 1) D46.21
        2 (RAEB 2) D46.22
        in transformation (RAEB T) — *see* Leukemia, acute myeloblastic
      hemochromatosis D46.1
      sideroblasts (ring) (RARS) D46.1
    without ring sideroblasts, so stated D46.0
    without sideroblasts without excess of blasts D46.0
    megaloblastic D53.1
    sideroblastic D46.1
    sideropenic D50.9
  Rietti-Greppi-Micheli D56.9
  scorbutic D53.2
  secondary to
    blood loss (chronic) D50.0
      acute D62
    hemorrhage (chronic) D50.0
      acute D62
  semiplastic D61.89
  sickle-cell — *see* Disease, sickle-cell
  sideroblastic D64.3
    hereditary D64.0
    hypochromic, sex-linked D64.0
    pyridoxine-responsive NEC D64.3
    refractory D46.1
    secondary (due to)
      disease D64.1
      drugs and toxins D64.2

Anemia — *continued*
  sideroblastic — *continued*
    specified type NEC D64.3
  sideropenic (refractory) D50.9
    due to blood loss (chronic) D50.0
      acute D62
  simple chronic D53.9
  specified type NEC D64.89
  spherocytic (hereditary) — *see* Spherocytosis
  splenic D64.89
  splenomegalic D64.89
  stomatocytosis D58.8
  syphilitic (acquired) (late) A52.79 [D63.8]
  target cell D64.89
  thalassemia D56.9
  thrombocytopenic — *see* Thrombocytopenia
  toxic D61.2
  tropical B76.9 [D63.8]
    macrocytic D52.8
  tuberculous A18.89 [D63.8]
  vegan D51.3
  vitamin
    B6-responsive D64.3
    B12 deficiency (dietary) pernicious D51.0
  von Jaksch's D64.89
  Witts' (achlorhydric anemia) D50.8
Anemophobia F40.228
Anencephalus, anencephaly Q00.0
Anergasia — *see* Psychosis, organic
Anesthesia, anesthetic R20.0
  complication or reaction NEC (*see also* Complications, anesthesia) T88.59 ☑
    due to
      correct substance properly administered — *see* Table of Drugs and Chemicals, by drug, adverse effect
      overdose or wrong substance given — *see* Table of Drugs and Chemicals, by drug, poisoning
  cornea H18.81- ☑
  dissociative F44.6
  functional (hysterical) F44.6
  hyperesthetic, thalamic G89.0
  hysterical F44.6
  local skin lesion R20.0
  sexual (psychogenic) F52.1
  shock (due to) T88.2 ☑
  skin R20.0
  testicular N50.9
Anetoderma (maculosum) (of) L90.8
  Jadassohn-Pellizzari L90.2
  Schweniger-Buzzi L90.1
Aneurin deficiency E51.9
Aneurysm (anastomotic) (artery) (cirsoid) (diffuse) (false) (fusiform) (multiple) (saccular) I72.9
  abdominal (aorta) I71.4
    ruptured I71.3
    syphilitic A52.01
  aorta, aortic (nonsyphilitic) I71.9
    abdominal I71.4
      ruptured I71.3
    arch I71.2
      ruptured I71.1
    arteriosclerotic I71.9
      ruptured I71.8
    ascending I71.2
      ruptured I71.1
    congenital Q25.4
    descending I71.9
      abdominal I71.4
        ruptured I71.3
      ruptured I71.8
      thoracic I71.2
        ruptured I71.1
    ruptured I71.8
    sinus, congenital Q25.4
    syphilitic A52.01
    thoracic I71.2
      ruptured I71.1
    thoracoabdominal I71.6
      ruptured I71.5
    thorax, thoracic (arch) I71.2
      ruptured I71.1
    transverse I71.2
      ruptured I71.1
    valve (heart) (*see also* Endocarditis, aortic) I35.8
  arteriosclerotic I72.9
    cerebral I67.1

Aneurysm — *continued*
  arteriosclerotic — *continued*
    cerebral — *continued*
      ruptured — *see* Hemorrhage, intracranial, subarachnoid
    arteriovenous (congenital) (*see also* Malformation, arteriovenous)
      acquired I77.0
        brain I67.1
        coronary I25.41
        pulmonary I28.0
      brain Q28.2
        ruptured I60.8
      peripheral — *see* Malformation, arteriovenous, peripheral
      precerebral vessels Q28.0
      specified site NEC (*see also* Malformation, arteriovenous)
        acquired I77.0
  basal — *see* Aneurysm, brain
  berry (congenital) (nonruptured) I67.1
    ruptured I60.7
  brain I67.1
    arteriosclerotic I67.1
      ruptured — *see* Hemorrhage, intracranial, subarachnoid
    arteriovenous (congenital) (nonruptured) Q28.2
      acquired I67.1
        ruptured I60.8
      ruptured I60.8
    berry (congenital) (nonruptured) I67.1
      ruptured (*see also* Hemorrhage, intracranial, subarachnoid) I60.7
    congenital Q28.3
      ruptured I60.7
    meninges I67.1
      ruptured I60.8
    miliary (congenital) (nonruptured) I67.1
      ruptured (*see also* Hemorrhage, intracranial, subarachnoid) I60.7
    mycotic I33.0
    ruptured — *see* Hemorrhage, intracranial, subarachnoid
    syphilitic (hemorrhage) A52.05
  cardiac (false) (*see also* Aneurysm, heart) I25.3
  carotid artery (common) (external) I72.0
    internal (intracranial) I67.1
      extracranial portion I72.0
    ruptured into brain I60.0- ☑
    syphilitic A52.09
      intracranial A52.05
  cavernous sinus I67.1
    arteriovenous (congenital) (nonruptured) Q28.3
      ruptured I60.8
  celiac I72.8
  central nervous system, syphilitic A52.05
  cerebral — *see* Aneurysm, brain
  chest — *see* Aneurysm, thorax
  circle of Willis I67.1
    congenital Q28.3
      ruptured I60.6
    ruptured I60.6
  common iliac artery I72.3
  congenital (peripheral) Q27.8
    brain Q28.3
      ruptured I60.7
    coronary Q24.5
    digestive system Q27.8
    lower limb Q27.8
    pulmonary Q25.79
    retina Q14.1
    specified site NEC Q27.8
    upper limb Q27.8
  conjunctiva — *see* Abnormality, conjunctiva, vascular
  conus arteriosus — *see* Aneurysm, heart
  coronary (arteriosclerotic) (artery) I25.41
    arteriovenous, congenital Q24.5
    congenital Q24.5
    ruptured — *see* Infarct, myocardium
    syphilitic A52.06
    vein I25.89
  cylindroid (aorta) I71.9
    ruptured I71.8
    syphilitic A52.01
  ductus arteriosus Q25.0
  endocardial, infective (any valve) I33.0
  femoral (artery) (ruptured) I72.4
  gastroduodenal I72.8

Aneurysm — *continued*
  gastroepiploic I72.8
  heart (wall) (chronic or with a stated duration of over 4 weeks) I25.3
    valve — *see* Endocarditis
  hepatic I72.8
  iliac (common) (artery) (ruptured) I72.3
  infective I72.9
    endocardial (any valve) I33.0
  innominate (nonsyphilitic) I72.8
    syphilitic A52.09
  interauricular septum — *see* Aneurysm, heart
  interventricular septum — *see* Aneurysm, heart
  intrathoracic (nonsyphilitic) I71.2
    ruptured I71.1
    syphilitic A52.01
  lower limb I72.4
  lung (pulmonary artery) I28.1
  mediastinal (nonsyphilitic) I72.8
    syphilitic A52.09
  miliary (congenital) I67.1
    ruptured — *see* Hemorrhage, intracerebral, subarachnoid, intracranial
  mitral (heart) (valve) I34.8
  mural — *see* Aneurysm, heart
  mycotic I72.9
    endocardial (any valve) I33.0
    ruptured, brain — *see* Hemorrhage, intracerebral, subarachnoid
  myocardium — *see* Aneurysm, heart
  neck I72.0
  pancreaticoduodenal I72.8
  patent ductus arteriosus Q25.0
  peripheral NEC I72.8
    congenital Q27.8
      digestive system Q27.8
      lower limb Q27.8
      specified site NEC Q27.8
      upper limb Q27.8
  popliteal (artery) (ruptured) I72.4
  precerebral, congenital (nonruptured) Q28.1
  pulmonary I28.1
    arteriovenous Q25.72
      acquired I28.0
    syphilitic A52.09
    valve (heart) — *see* Endocarditis, pulmonary
  racemose (peripheral) I72.9
    congenital — *see* Aneurysm, congenital
  radial I72.1
  Rasmussen NEC A15.0
  renal (artery) I72.2
  retina (*see also* Disorder, retina, microaneurysms)
    congenital Q14.1
    diabetic — *see* Diabetes, microaneurysms, retinal
  sinus of Valsalva Q25.4
  specified NEC I72.8
  spinal (cord) I72.8
    syphilitic (hemorrhage) A52.09
  splenic I72.8
  subclavian (artery) (ruptured) I72.8
    syphilitic A52.09
  superior mesenteric I72.8
  syphilitic (aorta) A52.01
    central nervous system A52.05
    congenital (late) A50.54 [I79.0]
    spine, spinal A52.09
  thoracoabdominal (aorta) I71.6
    ruptured I71.5
    syphilitic A52.01
  thorax, thoracic (aorta) (arch) (nonsyphilitic) I71.2
    ruptured I71.1
    syphilitic A52.01
  traumatic (complication) (early), specified site — *see* Injury, blood vessel
  tricuspid (heart) (valve) I07.8
  ulnar I72.1
  upper limb (ruptured) I72.1
  valve, valvular — *see* Endocarditis
  venous (*see also* Varix) I86.8
    congenital (nonruptured) Q27.8
      digestive system Q27.8
      lower limb Q27.8
      specified site NEC Q27.8
      upper limb Q27.8
  ventricle — *see* Aneurysm, heart
  visceral NEC I72.8
Angelman syndrome Q93.5
Anger R45.4

Angiectasis, angiectopia I99.8
Angiitis I77.6
  allergic granulomatous M30.1
  hypersensitivity M31.0
  necrotizing M31.9
    specified NEC M31.8
  nervous system, granulomatous I67.7
Angina (attack) (cardiac) (chest) (heart) (pectoris) (syndrome) (vasomotor) I20.9
  with
    atherosclerotic heart disease — *see* Arteriosclerosis, coronary (artery),
    documented spasm I20.1
  abdominal K55.1
  accelerated — *see* Angina, unstable
  agranulocytic — *see* Agranulocytosis
  angiospastic — *see* Angina, with documented spasm
  aphthous B08.5
  crescendo — *see* Angina, unstable
  croupous J05.0
  cruris I73.9
  de novo effort — *see* Angina, unstable
  diphtheritic, membranous A36.0
  equivalent I20.8
  exudative, chronic J37.0
  following acute myocardial infarction I23.7
  gangrenous diphtheritic A36.0
  intestinal K55.1
  Ludovici K12.2
  Ludwig's K12.2
  malignant diphtheritic A36.0
  membranous J05.0
    diphtheritic A36.0
    Vincent's A69.1
  mesenteric K55.1
  monocytic — *see* Mononucleosis, infectious
  of effort — *see* Angina, specified NEC
  phlegmonous J36
    diphtheritic A36.0
  post-infarctional I23.7
  pre-infarctional — *see* Angina, unstable
  Prinzmetal — *see* Angina, with documented spasm
  progressive — *see* Angina, unstable
  pseudomembranous A69.1
  pultaceous, diphtheritic A36.0
  spasm-induced — *see* Angina, with documented spasm
  specified NEC I20.8
  stable I20.9
  stenocardia — *see* Angina, specified NEC
  stridulous, diphtheritic A36.2
  tonsil J36
  trachealis J05.0
  unstable I20.0
  variant — *see* Angina, with documented spasm
  Vincent's A69.1
  worsening effort — *see* Angina, unstable
Angioblastoma — *see* Neoplasm, connective tissue, uncertain behavior
Angiocholecystitis — *see* Cholecystitis, acute
Angiocholitis (*see also* Cholecystitis, acute) K83.0
Angiodysgenesis spinalis G95.19
Angiodysplasia (cecum) (colon) K55.20
  with bleeding K55.21
  duodenum (and stomach) K31.819
    with bleeding K31.811
  stomach (and duodenum) K31.819
    with bleeding K31.811
Angioedema (allergic) (any site) (with urticaria) T78.3 ☑
  hereditary D84.1
Angioendothelioma — *see* Neoplasm, uncertain behavior, by site
  benign D18.00
    intra-abdominal D18.03
    intracranial D18.02
    skin D18.01
    specified site NEC D18.09
  bone — *see* Neoplasm, bone, malignant
  Ewing's — *see* Neoplasm, bone, malignant
Angioendotheliomatosis C85.8- ☑
Angiofibroma (*see also* Neoplasm, benign, by site)
  juvenile
    specified site — *see* Neoplasm, benign, by site
    unspecified site D10.6
Angiohemophilia (A) (B) D68.0
Angioid streaks (choroid) (macula) (retina) H35.33
Angiokeratoma — *see* Neoplasm, skin, benign

Angiokeratoma — *continued*
corporis diffusum E75.21
Angioleiomyoma — *see* Neoplasm, connective tissue,
benign
Angiolipoma (*see also* Lipoma)
infiltrating — *see* Lipoma
Angioma (*see also* Hemangioma, by site)
capillary I78.1
hemorrhagicum hereditaria I78.0
intra-abdominal D18.03
intracranial D18.02
malignant — *see* Neoplasm, connective tissue, malignant
plexiform D18.00
intra-abdominal D18.03
intracranial D18.02
skin D18.01
specified site NEC D18.09
senile I78.1
serpiginosum L81.7
skin D18.01
specified site NEC D18.09
spider I78.1
stellate I78.1
venous Q28.3
Angiomatosis Q82.8
bacillary A79.89
encephalotrigeminal Q85.8
hemorrhagic familial I78.0
hereditary familial I78.0
liver K76.4
Angiomyolipoma — *see* Lipoma
Angiomyoliposarcoma — *see* Neoplasm, connective
tissue, malignant
Angiomyoma — *see* Neoplasm, connective tissue, benign
Angiomyosarcoma — *see* Neoplasm, connective tissue,
malignant
Angiomyxoma — *see* Neoplasm, connective tissue, uncertain behavior
Angioneurosis F45.8
Angioneurotic edema (allergic) (any site) (with urticaria)
T78.3 ☑
hereditary D84.1
Angiopathia, angiopathy I99.9
cerebral I67.9
amyloid E85.4 [I68.0]
diabetic (peripheral) — *see* Diabetes, angiopathy
peripheral I73.9
diabetic — *see* Diabetes, angiopathy
specified type NEC I73.89
retinae syphilitica A52.05
retinalis (juvenilis)
diabetic — *see* Diabetes, retinopathy
proliferative — *see* Retinopathy, proliferative
Angiosarcoma (*see also* Neoplasm, connective tissue,
malignant)
liver C22.3
Angiosclerosis — *see* Arteriosclerosis
Angiospasm (peripheral) (traumatic) (vessel) I73.9
brachial plexus G54.0
cerebral G45.9
cervical plexus G54.2
nerve
arm — *see* Mononeuropathy, upper limb
axillary G54.0
median — *see* Lesion, nerve, median
ulnar — *see* Lesion, nerve, ulnar
axillary G54.0
leg — *see* Mononeuropathy, lower limb
median — *see* Lesion, nerve, median
plantar — *see* Lesion, nerve, plantar
ulnar — *see* Lesion, nerve, ulnar
Angiospastic disease or edema I73.9
Angiostrongyliasis
due to
Parastrongylus
cantonensis B83.2
costaricensis B81.3
intestinal B81.3
Anguillulosis — *see* Strongyloidiasis
Angulation
cecum — *see* Obstruction, intestine
coccyx (acquired) (*see also* subcategory) M43.8 ☑
congenital NEC Q76.49
femur (acquired) (*see also* Deformity, limb, specified
type NEC, thigh)

Angulation — *continued*
femur (*see also* Deformity, limb, specified type, thigh)
— *continued*
congenital Q74.2
intestine (large) (small) — *see* Obstruction, intestine
sacrum (acquired) (*see also* subcategory) M43.8 ☑
congenital NEC Q76.49
sigmoid (flexure) — *see* Obstruction, intestine
spine — *see* Dorsopathy, deforming, specified NEC
tibia (acquired) (*see also* Deformity, limb, specified
type NEC, lower leg)
congenital Q74.2
ureter N13.5
with infection N13.6
wrist (acquired) (*see also* Deformity, limb, specified
type NEC, forearm)
congenital Q74.0
Angulus infectiosus (lips) K13.0
Anhedonia R45.84
Anhidrosis L74.4
Anhydration, anhydremia E86.0
with
hypernatremia E87.0
hyponatremia E87.1
Anhydremia E86.0
with
hypernatremia E87.0
hyponatremia E87.1
Anidrosis L74.4
Aniridia (congenital) Q13.1
Anisakiasis (infection) (infestation) B81.0
Anisakis larvae infestation B81.0
Aniseikonia H52.32
Anisocoria (pupil) H57.02
congenital Q13.2
Anisocytosis R71.8
Anisometropia (congenital) H52.31
Ankle — *see* condition
Ankyloblepharon (eyelid) (acquired) (*see also* Blepharophimosis)
filiforme (adnatum) (congenital) Q10.3
total Q10.3
Ankyloglossia Q38.1
Ankylosis (fibrous) (osseous) (joint) M24.60
ankle M24.67- ☑
arthrodesis status Z98.1
cricoarytenoid (cartilage) (joint) (larynx) J38.7
dental K03.5
ear ossicles H74.31- ☑
elbow M24.62- ☑
foot M24.67- ☑
hand M24.64- ☑
hip M24.65- ☑
incostapedial joint (infectional) — *see* Ankylosis, ear
ossicles
jaw (temporomandibular) M26.61
knee M24.66- ☑
lumbosacral (joint) M43.27
postoperative (status) Z98.1
produced by surgical fusion, status Z98.1
sacro-iliac (joint) M43.28
shoulder M24.61- ☑
spine (joint) (*see also* Fusion, spine)
spondylitic — *see* Spondylitis, ankylosing
surgical Z98.1
temporomandibular M26.61
tooth, teeth (hard tissues) K03.5
wrist M24.63- ☑
Ankylostoma — *see* Ancylostoma
Ankylostomiasis — *see* Ancylostomiasis
Ankylurethria — *see* Stricture, urethra
Annular (*see also* condition)
detachment, cervix N88.8
organ or site, congenital NEC — *see* Distortion
pancreas (congenital) Q45.1
Anodontia (complete) (partial) (vera) K00.0
acquired K08.10 ☑
Anomaly, anomalous (congenital) (unspecified type)
Q89.9
abdominal wall NEC Q79.59
acoustic nerve Q07.8
adrenal (gland) Q89.1
Alder (-Reilly) (leukocyte granulation) D72.0
alimentary tract Q45.9
upper Q40.9
alveolar M26.70
hyperplasia M26.79

Anomaly, anomalous — *continued*
alveolar — *continued*
hyperplasia — *continued*
mandibular M26.72
maxillary M26.71
hypoplasia M26.79
mandibular M26.74
maxillary M26.73
ridge (process) M26.79
specified NEC M26.79
ankle (joint) Q74.2
anus Q43.9
aorta (arch) NEC Q25.4
coarctation (preductal) (postductal) Q25.1
aortic cusp or valve Q23.9
appendix Q43.8
apple peel syndrome Q41.1
aqueduct of Sylvius Q03.0
with spina bifida — *see* Spina bifida, with hydrocephalus
arm Q74.0
arteriovenous NEC
coronary Q24.5
gastrointestinal Q27.33
acquired — *see* Angiodysplasia
artery (peripheral) Q27.9
basilar NEC Q28.1
cerebral Q28.3
coronary Q24.5
digestive system Q27.8
eye Q15.8
great Q25.9
specified NEC Q25.8
lower limb Q27.8
peripheral Q27.9
specified NEC Q27.8
pulmonary NEC Q25.79
renal Q27.2
retina Q14.1
specified site NEC Q27.8
subclavian Q27.8
umbilical Q27.0
upper limb Q27.8
vertebral NEC Q28.1
aryteno-epiglottic folds Q31.8
atrial
bands or folds Q20.8
septa Q21.1
atrioventricular
excitation I45.6
septum Q21.0
auditory canal Q17.8
auricle
ear Q17.8
causing impairment of hearing Q16.9
heart Q20.8
Axenfeld's Q15.0
back Q89.9
band
atrial Q20.8
heart Q24.8
ventricular Q24.8
Bartholin's duct Q38.4
biliary duct or passage Q44.5
bladder Q64.70
absence Q64.5
diverticulum Q64.6
exstrophy Q64.10
cloacal Q64.12
extroversion Q64.19
specified type NEC Q64.19
supravesical fissure Q64.11
neck obstruction Q64.31
specified type NEC Q64.79
bone Q79.9
arm Q74.0
face Q75.9
leg Q74.2
pelvic girdle Q74.2
shoulder girdle Q74.0
skull Q75.9
with
anencephaly Q00.0
encephalocele — *see* Encephalocele
hydrocephalus Q03.9
with spina bifida — *see* Spina bifida, by
site, with hydrocephalus
microcephaly Q02

Anomaly, anomalous — *continued*
brain (multiple) Q04.9
　vessel Q28.3
breast Q83.9
broad ligament Q50.6
bronchus Q32.4
bulbus cordis Q21.9
bursa Q79.9
canal of Nuck Q52.4
canthus Q10.3
capillary Q27.9
cardiac Q24.9
　chambers Q20.9
　　specified NEC Q20.8
　septal closure Q21.9
　　specified NEC Q21.8
　valve NEC Q24.8
　　pulmonary Q22.3
cardiovascular system Q28.8
carpus Q74.0
caruncle, lacrimal Q10.6
cascade stomach Q40.2
cauda equina Q06.3
cecum Q43.9
cerebral Q04.9
　vessels Q28.3
cervix Q51.9
Chédiak-Higashi (-Steinbrinck) (congenital gigantism
　of peroxidase granules) E70.330
cheek Q18.9
chest wall Q67.8
　bones Q76.9
chin Q18.9
chordae tendineae Q24.8
choroid Q14.3
　plexus Q07.8
chromosomes, chromosomal Q99.9
　D (1) — *see* condition, chromosome 13
　E (3) — *see* condition, chromosome 18
　G — *see* condition, chromosome 21
　sex
　　female phenotype Q97.8
　　gonadal dysgenesis (pure) Q99.1
　　Klinefelter's Q98.4
　　male phenotype Q98.9
　　Turner's Q96.9
　specified NEC Q99.8
cilia Q10.3
circulatory system Q28.9
clavicle Q74.0
clitoris Q52.6
coccyx Q76.49
colon Q43.9
common duct Q44.5
communication
　coronary artery Q24.5
　left ventricle with right atrium Q21.0
concha (ear) Q17.3
connection
　portal vein Q26.5
　pulmonary venous Q26.4
　　partial Q26.3
　　total Q26.2
　renal artery with kidney Q27.2
cornea (shape) Q13.4
coronary artery or vein Q24.5
cranium — *see* Anomaly, skull
cricoid cartilage Q31.8
cystic duct Q44.5
dental
　alveolar — *see* Anomaly, alveolar
　arch relationship M26.20
　　specified NEC M26.29
dentofacial M26.9
　alveolar — *see* Anomaly, alveolar
　dental arch relationship M26.20
　　specified NEC M26.29
　functional M26.50
　　specified NEC M26.59
　jaw size M26.00
　　macrogenia M26.05
　　mandibular
　　　hyperplasia M26.03
　　　hypoplasia M26.04
　　maxillary
　　　hyperplasia M26.01
　　　hypoplasia M26.02
　　microgenia M26.06

Anomaly, anomalous — *continued*
dentofacial — *continued*
　jaw size — *continued*
　　specified type NEC M26.09
　jaw-cranial base relationship M26.10
　　asymmetry M26.12
　　　maxillary M26.11
　　specified type NEC M26.19
　malocclusion M26.4
　　dental arch relationship NEC M26.29
　　jaw size — *see* Anomaly, dentofacial, jaw size
　　jaw-cranial base relationship — *see* Anomaly,
　　　dentofacial, jaw-cranial base relationship
　specified type NEC M26.89
　temporomandibular joint M26.60
　　adhesions M26.61
　　ankylosis M26.61
　　arthralgia M26.62
　　articular disc M26.63
　　specified type NEC M26.69
　tooth position, fully erupted M26.30
　　specified NEC M26.39
dermatoglyphic Q82.8
diaphragm (apertures) NEC Q79.1
digestive organ(s) or tract Q45.9
　lower Q43.9
　upper Q40.9
distance, interarch (excessive) (inadequate) M26.25
distribution, coronary artery Q24.5
ductus
　arteriosus Q25.0
　botalli Q25.0
duodenum Q43.9
dura (brain) Q04.9
　spinal cord Q06.9
ear (external) Q17.9
　causing impairment of hearing Q16.9
　inner Q16.5
　middle (causing impairment of hearing) Q16.4
　ossicles Q16.3
Ebstein's (heart) (tricuspid valve) Q22.5
ectodermal Q82.9
Eisenmenger's (ventricular septal defect) Q21.8
ejaculatory duct Q55.4
elbow Q74.0
endocrine gland NEC Q89.2
epididymis Q55.4
epiglottis Q31.8
esophagus Q39.9
eustachian tube Q17.8
eye Q15.9
　anterior segment Q13.9
　　specified NEC Q13.89
　posterior segment Q14.9
　　specified NEC Q14.8
　ptosis (eyelid) Q10.0
　specified NEC Q15.8
eyebrow Q18.8
eyelid Q10.3
　ptosis Q10.0
face Q18.9
　bone(s) Q75.9
fallopian tube Q50.6
fascia Q79.9
femur NEC Q74.2
fibula NEC Q74.2
finger Q74.0
fixation, intestine Q43.3
flexion (joint) NOS Q74.9
　hip or thigh Q65.89
foot NEC Q74.2
　varus (congenital) Q66.3
foramen
　Botalli Q21.1
　ovale Q21.1
forearm Q74.0
forehead Q75.8
form, teeth K00.2
fovea centralis Q14.1
frontal bone — *see* Anomaly, skull
gallbladder (position) (shape) (size) Q44.1
Gartner's duct Q52.4
gastrointestinal tract Q45.9
genitalia, genital organ(s) or system
　female Q52.9
　　external Q52.70
　　internal NOS Q52.9
　male Q55.9

Anomaly, anomalous — *continued*
genitalia, genital organ(s) or system — *continued*
　male — *continued*
　　hydrocele P83.5
　　specified NEC Q55.8
genitourinary NEC
　female Q52.9
　male Q55.9
Gerbode Q21.0
glottis Q31.8
granulation or granulocyte, genetic (constitutional)
　(leukocyte) D72.0
gum Q38.6
gyri Q07.9
hair Q84.2
hand Q74.0
hard tissue formation in pulp K04.3
head — *see* Anomaly, skull
heart Q24.9
　auricle Q20.8
　bands or folds Q24.8
　fibroelastosis cordis I42.4
　obstructive NEC Q22.6
　patent ductus arteriosus (Botalli) Q25.0
　septum Q21.9
　　auricular Q21.1
　　interatrial Q21.1
　　interventricular Q21.0
　　　with pulmonary stenosis or atresia, dextra-
　　　　position of aorta and hypertrophy of
　　　　right ventricle Q21.3
　　specified NEC Q21.8
　　ventricular Q21.0
　　　with pulmonary stenosis or atresia, dextra-
　　　　position of aorta and hypertrophy of
　　　　right ventricle Q21.3
　tetralogy of Fallot Q21.3
　valve NEC Q24.8
　　aortic
　　　bicuspid valve Q23.1
　　　insufficiency Q23.1
　　　stenosis Q23.0
　　　　subaortic Q24.4
　　mitral
　　　insufficiency Q23.3
　　　stenosis Q23.2
　　pulmonary Q22.3
　　　atresia Q22.0
　　　insufficiency Q22.2
　　　stenosis Q22.1
　　　　infundibular Q24.3
　　　　subvalvular Q24.3
　　tricuspid
　　　atresia Q22.4
　　　stenosis Q22.4
　ventricle Q20.8
heel NEC Q74.2
Hegglin's D72.0
hemianencephaly Q00.0
hemicephaly Q00.0
hemicrania Q00.0
hepatic duct Q44.5
hip NEC Q74.2
hourglass stomach Q40.2
humerus Q74.0
hydatid of Morgagni
　female Q50.5
　male (epididymal) Q55.4
　　testicular Q55.29
hymen Q52.4
hypersegmentation of neutrophils, hereditary D72.0
hypophyseal Q89.2
ileocecal (coil) (valve) Q43.9
ileum Q43.9
ilium NEC Q74.2
integument Q84.9
　specified NEC Q84.8
interarch distance (excessive) (inadequate) M26.25
intervertebral cartilage or disc Q76.49
intestine (large) (small) Q43.9
　with anomalous adhesions, fixation or malrotation
　　Q43.3
iris Q13.2
ischium NEC Q74.2
jaw — *see* Anomaly, dentofacial
　alveolar — *see* Anomaly, alveolar
jaw-cranial base relationship — *see* Anomaly, dento-
　facial, jaw-cranial base relationship

Anomaly, anomalous — *continued*
- jejunum Q43.8
- joint Q74.9
  - specified NEC Q74.8
- Jordan's D72.0
- kidney(s) (calyx) (pelvis) Q63.9
  - artery Q27.2
  - specified NEC Q63.8
- Klippel-Feil (brevicollis) Q76.1
- knee Q74.1
- labium (majus) (minus) Q52.70
- labyrinth, membranous Q16.5
- lacrimal apparatus or duct Q10.6
- larynx, laryngeal (muscle) Q31.9
  - web (bed) Q31.0
- lens Q12.9
- leukocytes, genetic D72.0
  - granulation (constitutional) D72.0
- lid (fold) Q10.3
- ligament Q79.9
  - broad Q50.6
  - round Q52.8
- limb Q74.9
  - lower NEC Q74.2
    - reduction deformity — *see* Defect, reduction, lower limb
  - upper Q74.0
- lip Q38.0
- liver Q44.7
  - duct Q44.5
- lower limb NEC Q74.2
- lumbosacral (joint) (region) Q76.49
  - kyphosis — *see* Kyphosis, congenital
  - lordosis — *see* Lordosis, congenital
- lung (fissure) (lobe) Q33.9
- mandible — *see* Anomaly, dentofacial
- maxilla — *see* Anomaly, dentofacial
- May (-Hegglin) D72.0
- meatus urinarius NEC Q64.79
- meningeal bands or folds Q07.9
  - constriction of Q07.8
  - spinal Q06.9
- meninges Q07.9
  - cerebral Q04.8
  - spinal Q06.9
- meningocele Q05.9
- mesentery Q45.9
- metacarpus Q74.0
- metatarsus NEC Q74.2
- middle ear Q16.4
  - ossicles Q16.3
- mitral (leaflets) (valve) Q23.9
  - insufficiency Q23.3
  - specified NEC Q23.8
  - stenosis Q23.2
- mouth Q38.6
- Müllerian (*see also* Anomaly, by site)
  - uterus NEC Q51.818
- multiple NEC Q89.7
- muscle Q79.9
  - eyelid Q10.3
- musculoskeletal system, except limbs Q79.9
- myocardium Q24.8
- nail Q84.6
- narrowness, eyelid Q10.3
- nasal sinus (wall) Q30.8
- neck (any part) Q18.9
- nerve Q07.9
  - acoustic Q07.8
  - optic Q07.8
- nervous system (central) Q07.9
- nipple Q83.9
- nose, nasal (bones) (cartilage) (septum) (sinus) Q30.9
  - specified NEC Q30.8
- ocular muscle Q15.8
- omphalomesenteric duct Q43.0
- opening, pulmonary veins Q26.4
- optic
  - disc Q14.2
  - nerve Q07.8
- opticociliary vessels Q13.2
- orbit (eye) Q10.7
- organ Q89.9
  - of Corti Q16.5
- origin
  - artery
    - innominate Q25.8
    - pulmonary Q25.79

Anomaly, anomalous — *continued*
- origin — *continued*
  - artery — *continued*
    - renal Q27.2
    - subclavian Q25.8
- osseous meatus (ear) Q16.1
- ovary Q50.39
- oviduct Q50.6
- palate (hard) (soft) NEC Q38.5
- pancreas or pancreatic duct Q45.3
- papillary muscles Q24.8
- parathyroid gland Q89.2
- paraurethral ducts Q64.79
- parotid (gland) Q38.4
- patella Q74.1
- Pelger-Huët (hereditary hyposegmentation) D72.0
- pelvic girdle NEC Q74.2
- pelvis (bony) NEC Q74.2
  - rachitic E64.3
- penis (glans) Q55.69
- pericardium Q24.8
- peripheral vascular system Q27.9
- Peter's Q13.4
- pharynx Q38.8
- pigmentation L81.9
  - congenital Q82.8
- pituitary (gland) Q89.2
- pleural (folds) Q34.0
- portal vein Q26.5
  - connection Q26.5
- position, tooth, teeth, fully erupted M26.30
  - specified NEC M26.39
- precerebral vessel Q28.1
- prepuce Q55.69
- prostate Q55.4
- pulmonary Q33.9
  - artery NEC Q25.79
  - valve Q22.3
    - atresia Q22.0
    - insufficiency Q22.2
    - specified type NEC Q22.3
    - stenosis Q22.1
      - infundibular Q24.3
      - subvalvular Q24.3
  - venous connection Q26.4
    - partial Q26.3
    - total Q26.2
- pylorus Q40.3
- pupil Q13.2
  - function H57.00
    - anisocoria H57.02
    - Argyll Robertson pupil H57.01
    - miosis H57.03
    - mydriasis H57.04
    - specified type NEC H57.09
    - tonic pupil H57.05- ☑
- pylorus Q40.3
- radius Q74.0
- rectum Q43.9
- reduction (extremity) (limb)
  - femur (longitudinal) — *see* Defect, reduction, lower limb, longitudinal, femur
  - fibula (longitudinal) — *see* Defect, reduction, lower limb, longitudinal, fibula
  - lower limb — *see* Defect, reduction, lower limb
  - radius (longitudinal) — *see* Defect, reduction, upper limb, longitudinal, radius
  - tibia (longitudinal) — *see* Defect, reduction, lower limb, longitudinal, tibia
  - ulna (longitudinal) — *see* Defect, reduction, upper limb, longitudinal, ulna
  - upper limb — *see* Defect, reduction, upper limb
- refraction — *see* Disorder, refraction
- renal Q63.9
  - artery Q27.2
  - pelvis Q63.9
    - specified NEC Q63.8
- respiratory system Q34.9
  - specified NEC Q34.8
- retina Q14.1
- rib Q76.6
  - cervical Q76.5
- Rieger's Q13.81
- rotation — *see* Malrotation
  - hip or thigh Q65.89
- round ligament Q52.8
- sacroiliac (joint) NEC Q74.2
- sacrum NEC Q76.49
  - kyphosis — *see* Kyphosis, congenital

Anomaly, anomalous — *continued*
- sacrum — *continued*
  - lordosis — *see* Lordosis, congenital
- saddle nose, syphilitic A50.57
- salivary duct or gland Q38.4
- scapula Q74.0
- scrotum — *see* Malformation, testis and scrotum
- sebaceous gland Q82.9
- seminal vesicles Q55.4
- sense organs NEC Q07.8
- sex chromosomes NEC (*see also* Anomaly, chromosomes)
  - female phenotype Q97.8
  - male phenotype Q98.9
- shoulder (girdle) (joint) Q74.0
- sigmoid (flexure) Q43.9
- simian crease Q82.8
- sinus of Valsalva Q25.4
- skeleton generalized Q78.9
- skin (appendage) Q82.9
- skull Q75.9
  - with
    - anencephaly Q00.0
    - encephalocele — *see* Encephalocele
    - hydrocephalus Q03.9
      - with spina bifida — *see* Spina bifida, by site, with hydrocephalus
    - microcephaly Q02
- specified organ or site NEC Q89.8
- spermatic cord Q55.4
- spine, spinal NEC Q76.49
  - column NEC Q76.49
    - kyphosis — *see* Kyphosis, congenital
    - lordosis — *see* Lordosis, congenital
  - cord Q06.9
  - nerve root Q07.8
- spleen Q89.09
  - agenesis Q89.01
- stenonian duct Q38.4
- sternum NEC Q76.7
- stomach Q40.3
- submaxillary gland Q38.4
- tarsus NEC Q74.2
- tendon Q79.9
- testis — *see* Malformation, testis and scrotum
- thigh NEC Q74.2
- thorax (wall) Q67.8
  - bony Q76.9
- throat Q38.8
- thumb Q74.0
- thymus gland Q89.2
- thyroid (gland) Q89.2
  - cartilage Q31.8
- tibia NEC Q74.2
  - saber A50.56
- toe Q74.2
- tongue Q38.3
- tooth, teeth K00.9
  - eruption K00.6
  - position, fully erupted M26.30
  - spacing, fully erupted M26.30
- trachea (cartilage) Q32.1
- tragus Q17.9
- tricuspid (leaflet) (valve) Q22.9
  - atresia or stenosis Q22.4
  - Ebstein's Q22.5
- Uhl's (hypoplasia of myocardium, right ventricle) Q24.8
- ulna Q74.0
- umbilical artery Q27.0
- union
  - cricoid cartilage and thyroid cartilage Q31.8
  - thyroid cartilage and hyoid bone Q31.8
  - trachea with larynx Q31.8
- upper limb Q74.0
- urachus Q64.4
- ureter Q62.8
  - obstructive NEC Q62.39
    - cecoureterocele Q62.32
    - orthotopic ureterocele Q62.31
- urethra Q64.70
  - absence Q64.5
  - double Q64.74
  - fistula to rectum Q64.73
  - obstructive Q64.39
    - stricture Q64.32
  - prolapse Q64.71
  - specified type NEC Q64.79
- urinary tract Q64.9

Anomaly, anomalous — continued
 uterus Q51.9
  with only one functioning horn Q51.4
 uvula Q38.5
 vagina Q52.4
 valleculae Q31.8
 valve (heart) NEC Q24.8
  coronary sinus Q24.5
  inferior vena cava Q24.8
  pulmonary Q22.3
  sinus coronario Q24.5
  venae cavae inferioris Q24.8
 vas deferens Q55.4
 vascular Q27.9
  brain Q28.3
  ring Q25.4
 vein(s) (peripheral) Q27.9
  brain Q28.3
  cerebral Q28.3
  coronary Q24.5
  developmental Q28.3
  great Q26.9
   specified NEC Q26.8
 vena cava (inferior) (superior) Q26.9
 venous — see Anomaly, vein(s)
 venous return Q26.8
 ventricular
  bands or folds Q24.8
  septa Q21.0
 vertebra Q76.49
  kyphosis — see Kyphosis, congenital
  lordosis — see Lordosis, congenital
 vesicourethral orifice Q64.79
 vessel(s) Q27.9
  optic papilla Q14.2
  precerebral Q28.1
 vitelline duct Q43.0
 vitreous body or humor Q14.0
 vulva Q52.70
 wrist (joint) Q74.0
Anomia R48.8
Anonychia (congenital) Q84.3
 acquired L60.8
Anophthalmos, anophthalmus (congenital) (globe)
  Q11.1
 acquired Z90.01
Anopia, anopsia H53.46- ☑
 quadrant H53.46- ☑
Anorchia, anorchism, anorchidism Q55.0
Anorexia R63.0
 hysterical F44.89
 nervosa F50.00
  atypical F50.9
  binge-eating type F50.2
   with purging F50.02
  restricting type F50.01
Anorgasmy, psychogenic (female) F52.31
 male F52.32
Anosmia R43.0
 hysterical F44.6
 postinfectional J39.8
Anosognosia R41.89
Anosteoplasia Q78.9
Anovulatory cycle N97.0
Anoxemia R09.02
 newborn P84
Anoxia (pathological) R09.02
 altitude T70.29 ☑
 cerebral G93.1
  complicating
   anesthesia (general) (local) or other sedation
    T88.59 ☑
    in labor and delivery O74.3
    in pregnancy O29.21- ☑
    postpartum, puerperal O89.2
   delivery (cesarean) (instrumental) O75.4
  during a procedure G97.81
  newborn P84
  resulting from a procedure G97.82
 due to
  drowning T75.1 ☑
  high altitude T70.29 ☑
 heart — see Insufficiency, coronary
 intrauterine P84
 myocardial — see Insufficiency, coronary
 newborn P84
 spinal cord G95.11

Anoxia — continued
 systemic (by suffocation) (low content in atmosphere)
  — see Asphyxia, traumatic
Anteflexion — see Anteversion
Antenatal
 care (normal pregnancy) Z34.90
 screening (encounter for) of mother Z36
Antepartum — see condition
Anterior — see condition
Antero-occlusion M26.220
Anteversion
 cervix — see Anteversion, uterus
 femur (neck), congenital Q65.89
 uterus, uterine (cervix) (postinfectional) (postpartal,
  old) N85.4
  congenital Q51.818
  in pregnancy or childbirth — see Pregnancy,
   complicated by
Anthophobia F40.228
Anthracosilicosis J60
Anthracosis (lung) (occupational) J60
 lingua K14.3
Anthrax A22.9
 with pneumonia A22.1
 cerebral A22.8
 colitis A22.2
 cutaneous A22.0
 gastrointestinal A22.2
 inhalation A22.1
 intestinal A22.2
 meningitis A22.8
 pulmonary A22.1
 respiratory A22.1
 sepsis A22.7
 specified manifestation NEC A22.8
Anthropoid pelvis Q74.2
 with disproportion (fetopelvic) O33.0
Anthropophobia F40.10
 generalized F40.11
Antibodies, maternal (blood group) — see Isoimmunization, affecting management of pregnancy
 anti-D — see Isoimmunization, affecting management
  of pregnancy, Rh
 newborn P55.0
Antibody
 anticardiolipin R76.0
  with
   hemorrhagic disorder D68.312
   hypercoagulable state D68.61
 antiphosphatidylglycerol R76.0
  with
   hemorrhagic disorder D68.312
   hypercoagulable state D68.61
 antiphosphatidylinositol R76.0
  with
   hemorrhagic disorder D68.312
   hypercoagulable state D68.61
 antiphosphatidylserine R76.0
  with
   hemorrhagic disorder D68.312
   hypercoagulable state D68.61
 antiphospholipid R76.0
  with
   hemorrhagic disorder D68.312
   hypercoagulable state D68.61
Anticardiolipin syndrome D68.61
Anticoagulant, circulating (intrinsic) (see also Disorder,
  hemorrhagic) D68.318
 drug-induced (extrinsic) (see also Disorder, hemorrhagic) D68.32
Antidiuretic hormone syndrome E22.2
Antimonial cholera — see Poisoning, antimony
Antiphospholipid
 antibody
  with hemorrhagic disorder D68.312
  syndrome D68.61
Antisocial personality F60.2
Antithrombinemia — see Circulating anticoagulants
Antithromboplastinemia D68.318
Antithromboplastinogenemia D68.318
Antitoxin complication or reaction — see Complications, vaccination
Antlophobia F40.228
Antritis J32.0
 maxilla J32.0
  acute J01.00
   recurrent J01.01
 stomach K29.60

Antritis — continued
 stomach — continued
  with bleeding K29.61
Antrum, antral — see condition
Anuria R34
 calculus (impacted) (recurrent) (see also Calculus,
  urinary) N20.9
 following
  abortion — see Abortion by type complicated by,
   renal failure
  ectopic or molar pregnancy O08.4
 newborn P96.0
 postprocedural N99.0
 postrenal N13.8
 traumatic (following crushing) T79.5 ☑
Anus, anal — see condition
Anusitis K62.89
Anxiety F41.9
 depression F41.8
 episodic paroxysmal F41.0
 generalized F41.1
 hysteria F41.8
 neurosis F41.1
 panic type F41.0
 reaction F41.1
 separation, abnormal (of childhood) F93.0
 specified NEC F41.8
 state F41.1
Aorta, aortic — see condition
Aortectasia — see Ectasia, aorta
 with aneurysm — see Aneurysm, aorta
Aortitis (nonsyphilitic) (calcific) I77.6
 arteriosclerotic I70.0
 Doehle-Heller A52.02
 luetic A52.02
 rheumatic — see Endocarditis, acute, rheumatic
 specific (syphilitic) A52.02
 syphilitic A52.02
  congenital A50.54 [I79.1]
Apathetic thyroid storm — see Thyrotoxicosis
Apathy R45.3
Apeirophobia F40.228
Apepsia K30
 psychogenic F45.8
Aperistalsis, esophagus K22.0
Apertognathia M26.29
Apert's syndrome Q87.0
Aphagia R13.0
 psychogenic F50.9
Aphakia (acquired) (postoperative) H27.0- ☑
 congenital Q12.3
Aphasia (amnestic) (global) (nominal) (semantic) (syntac-
  tic) R47.01
 acquired, with epilepsy (Landau-Kleffner syndrome)
  — see Epilepsy, specified NEC
 auditory (developmental) F80.2
 developmental (receptive type) F80.2
  expressive type F80.1
  Wernicke's F80.2
 following
  cerebrovascular disease I69.920
   cerebral infarction I69.320
   intracerebral hemorrhage I69.120
   nontraumatic intracranial hemorrhage NEC
    I69.220
   specified disease NEC I69.820
   subarachnoid hemorrhage I69.020
 primary progressive G31.01 [F02.80]
  with behavioral disturbance G31.01 [F02.81]
 progressive isolated G31.01 [F02.80]
  with behavioral disturbance G31.01 [F02.81]
 sensory F80.2
 syphilis, tertiary A52.19
 Wernicke's (developmental) F80.2
Aphonia (organic) R49.1
 hysterical F44.4
 psychogenic F44.4
Aphthae, aphthous (see also condition)
 Bednar's K12.0
 cachectic K14.0
 epizootic B08.8
 fever B08.8
 oral (recurrent) K12.0
 stomatitis (major) (minor) K12.0
 thrush B37.0
 ulcer (oral) (recurrent) K12.0
  genital organ(s) NEC
   female N76.6

Aphthae, aphthous — continued
- ulcer — continued
  - genital organ(s) — continued
    - male N50.8
  - larynx J38.7

Apical — see condition

Apiphobia F40.218

Aplasia (see also Agenesis)
- abdominal muscle syndrome Q79.4
- alveolar process (acquired) — see Anomaly, alveolar
  - congenital Q38.6
- aorta (congenital) Q25.4
- axialis extracorticalis (congenita) E75.29
- bone marrow (myeloid) D61.9
  - congenital D61.01
- brain Q00.0
  - part of Q04.3
- bronchus Q32.4
- cementum K00.4
- cerebellum Q04.3
- cervix (congenital) Q51.5
- congenital pure red cell D61.01
- corpus callosum Q04.0
- cutis congenita Q84.8
- erythrocyte congenital D61.01
- extracortical axial E75.29
- eye Q11.1
- fovea centralis (congenital) Q14.1
- gallbladder, congenital Q44.0
- iris Q13.1
- labyrinth, membranous Q16.5
- limb (congenital) Q73.8
  - lower — see Defect, reduction, lower limb
  - upper — see Agenesis, arm
- lung, congenital (bilateral) (unilateral) Q33.3
- pancreas Q45.0
- parathyroid-thymic D82.1
- Pelizaeus-Merzbacher E75.29
- penis Q55.5
- prostate Q55.4
- red cell (with thymoma) D60.9
  - acquired D60.9
    - due to drugs D60.9
  - adult D60.9
  - chronic D60.0
  - congenital D61.01
  - constitutional D61.01
  - due to drugs D60.9
  - hereditary D61.01
  - of infants D61.01
  - primary D61.01
  - pure D61.01
    - due to drugs D60.9
  - specified type NEC D60.8
  - transient D60.1
- round ligament Q52.8
- skin Q84.8
- spermatic cord Q55.4
- spleen Q89.01
- testicle Q55.0
- thymic, with immunodeficiency D82.1
- thyroid (congenital) (with myxedema) E03.1
- uterus Q51.0
- ventral horn cell Q06.1

Apnea, apneic (of) (spells) R06.81
- newborn NEC P28.4
  - obstructive P28.4
  - sleep (central) (obstructive) (primary) P28.3
- prematurity P28.4
- sleep G47.30
  - central (primary) G47.31
    - in conditions classified elsewhere G47.37
  - obstructive (adult) (pediatric) G47.33
  - primary central G47.31
  - specified NEC G47.39

Apneumatosis, newborn P28.0

Apocrine metaplasia (breast) — see Dysplasia, mammary, specified type NEC

Apophysitis (bone) (see also Osteochondropathy)
- calcaneus M92.8
- juvenile M92.9

Apoplectiform convulsions (cerebral ischemia) I67.82

Apoplexia, apoplexy, apoplectic
- adrenal A39.1
- heart (auricle) (ventricle) — see Infarct, myocardium
- heat T67.0 ☑
- hemorrhagic (stroke) — see Hemorrhage, intracranial

Apoplexia, apoplexy, apoplectic — continued
- meninges, hemorrhagic — see Hemorrhage, intracranial, subarachnoid
- uremic N18.9 [I68.8]

Appearance
- bizarre R46.1
- specified NEC R46.89
- very low level of personal hygiene R46.0

Appendage
- epididymal (organ of Morgagni) Q55.4
- intestine (epiploic) Q43.8
- preauricular Q17.0
- testicular (organ of Morgagni) Q55.29

Appendicitis (pneumococcal) (retrocecal) K37
- with
  - perforation or rupture K35.2
  - peritoneal abscess K35.3
  - peritonitis NEC K35.3
    - generalized (with perforation or rupture) K35.2
    - localized (with perforation or rupture) K35.3
- acute (catarrhal) (fulminating) (gangrenous) (obstructive) (retrocecal) (suppurative) K35.80
  - with
    - peritoneal abscess K35.3
    - peritonitis NEC K35.3
      - generalized (with perforation or rupture) K35.2
      - localized (with perforation or rupture) K35.3
    - specified NEC K35.89
- amebic A06.89
- chronic (recurrent) K36
- exacerbation — see Appendicitis, acute
- gangrenous — see Appendicitis, acute
- healed (obliterative) K36
- interval K36
- neurogenic K36
- obstructive K36
- recurrent K36
- relapsing K36
- subacute (adhesive) K36
- subsiding K36
- suppurative — see Appendicitis, acute
- tuberculous A18.32

Appendicopathia oxyurica B80

Appendix, appendicular (see also condition)
- epididymis Q55.4
- Morgagni
  - female Q50.5
  - male (epididymal) Q55.4
    - testicular Q55.29
- testis Q55.29

Appetite
- depraved — see Pica
- excessive R63.2
- lack or loss (see also Anorexia) R63.0
  - nonorganic origin F50.8
  - psychogenic F50.8
- perverted (hysterical) — see Pica

Apple peel syndrome Q41.1

Apprehension state F41.1

Apprehensiveness, abnormal F41.9

Approximal wear K03.0

Apraxia (classic) (ideational) (ideokinetic) (ideomotor) (motor) (verbal) R48.2
- following
  - cerebrovascular disease I69.990
    - cerebral infarction I69.390
    - intracerebral hemorrhage I69.190
    - nontraumatic intracranial hemorrhage NEC I69.290
    - specified disease NEC I69.890
    - subarachnoid hemorrhage I69.090
- oculomotor, congenital H51.8

Aptyalism K11.7

Apudoma — see Neoplasm, uncertain behavior, by site

Aqueous misdirection H40.83- ☑

Arabicum elephantiasis — see Infestation, filarial

Arachnitis — see Meningitis

Arachnodactyly — see Syndrome, Marfan's

Arachnoiditis (acute) (adhesive) (basal) (brain) (cerebrospinal) — see Meningitis

Arachnophobia F40.210

Arboencephalitis, Australian A83.4

Arborization block (heart) I45.5

ARC (AIDS-related complex) B20

Arches — see condition

Arcuate uterus Q51.810

Arcuatus uterus Q51.810

Arcus (cornea) senilis — see Degeneration, cornea, senile

Arc-welder's lung J63.4

Areflexia R29.2

Areola — see condition

Argentaffinoma (see also Neoplasm, uncertain behavior, by site)
- malignant — see Neoplasm, malignant, by site
- syndrome E34.0

Argininemia E72.21

Arginosuccinic aciduria E72.22

Argyll Robertson phenomenon, pupil or syndrome (syphilitic) A52.19
- atypical H57.09
- nonsyphilitic H57.09

Argyria, argyriasis
- conjunctival H11.13- ☑
- from drug or medicament — see Table of Drugs and Chemicals, by substance

Argyrosis, conjunctival H11.13- ☑

Arhinencephaly Q04.1

Ariboflavinosis E53.0

Arm — see condition

Arnold-Chiari disease, obstruction or syndrome (type II) Q07.00
- with
  - hydrocephalus Q07.02
    - with spina bifida Q07.03
  - spina bifida Q07.01
    - with hydrocephalus Q07.03
- type III — see Encephalocele
- type IV Q04.8

Aromatic amino-acid metabolism disorder E70.9
- specified NEC E70.8

Arousals, confusional G47.51

Arrest, arrested
- cardiac I46.9
  - complicating
    - abortion — see Abortion, by type, complicated by, cardiac arrest
    - anesthesia (general) (local) or other sedation — see Table of Drugs and Chemicals, by drug
      - in labor and delivery O74.2
      - in pregnancy O29.11- ☑
      - postpartum, puerperal O89.1
    - delivery (cesarean) (instrumental) O75.4
  - due to
    - cardiac condition I46.2
    - specified condition NEC I46.8
  - intraoperative I97.71- ☑
  - newborn P29.81
  - postprocedural I97.12- ☑
    - obstetric procedure O75.4
- cardiorespiratory — see Arrest, cardiac
- circulatory — see Arrest, cardiac
- deep transverse O64.0 ☑
- development or growth
  - bone — see Disorder, bone, development or growth
  - child R62.50
  - tracheal rings Q32.1
- epiphyseal
  - complete
    - femur M89.15- ☑
    - humerus M89.12- ☑
    - tibia M89.16- ☑
    - ulna M89.13- ☑
    - forearm M89.13- ☑
      - specified NEC M89.13- ☑
      - ulna — see Arrest, epiphyseal, by type, ulna
    - lower leg M89.16- ☑
      - specified NEC M89.168
      - tibia — see Arrest, epiphyseal, by type, tibia
  - partial
    - femur M89.15- ☑
    - humerus M89.12- ☑
    - tibia M89.16- ☑
    - ulna M89.13- ☑
  - specified NEC M89.18
- granulopoiesis — see Agranulocytosis
- growth plate — see Arrest, epiphyseal
- heart — see Arrest, cardiac
- legal, anxiety concerning Z65.3
- physeal — see Arrest, epiphyseal
- respiratory R09.2
  - newborn P28.81

Arrest, arrested — *continued*
  sinus I45.5
  spermatogenesis (complete) — *see* Azoospermia
    incomplete — *see* Oligospermia
  transverse (deep) O64.0 ☑

Arrhenoblastoma
  benign
    specified site — *see* Neoplasm, benign, by site
    unspecified site
      female D27.9
      male D29.20
  malignant
    specified site — *see* Neoplasm, malignant, by site
    unspecified site
      female C56.9
      male C62.90
  specified site — *see* Neoplasm, uncertain behavior,
    by site
  unspecified site
    female D39.10
    male D40.10

Arrhythmia (auricle) (cardiac) (juvenile) (nodal) (reflex)
    (sinus) (supraventricular) (transitory) (ventricle) I49.9
  block I45.9
  extrasystolic I49.49
  newborn
    bradycardia P29.12
    occurring before birth P03.819
      before onset of labor P03.810
      during labor P03.811
    tachycardia P29.11
  psychogenic F45.8
  specified NEC I49.8
  vagal R55
  ventricular re-entry I47.0

Arrillaga-Ayerza syndrome (pulmonary sclerosis with
    pulmonary hypertension) I27.0

Arsenical pigmentation L81.8
  from drug or medicament — *see* Table of Drugs and
    Chemicals

Arsenism — *see* Poisoning, arsenic

Arterial — *see* condition

Arteriofibrosis — *see* Arteriosclerosis

Arteriolar sclerosis — *see* Arteriosclerosis

Arteriolith — *see* Arteriosclerosis

Arteriolitis I77.6
  necrotizing, kidney I77.5
  renal — *see* Hypertension, kidney

Arteriolosclerosis — *see* Arteriosclerosis

Arterionephrosclerosis — *see* Hypertension, kidney

Arteriopathy I77.9

Arteriosclerosis, arteriosclerotic (diffuse) (obliterans)
    (of) (senile) (with calcification) I70.90
  aorta I70.0
  arteries of extremities — *see* Arteriosclerosis, extrem-
    ities
  brain I67.2
  bypass graft
    coronary — *see* Arteriosclerosis, coronary, bypass
      graft
    extremities — *see* Arteriosclerosis, extremities,
      bypass graft
  cardiac — *see* Disease, heart, ischemic, atherosclerotic
  cardiopathy — *see* Disease, heart, ischemic,
    atherosclerotic
  cardiorenal — *see* Hypertension, cardiorenal
  cardiovascular — *see* Disease, heart, ischemic,
    atherosclerotic
  carotid (*see also* Occlusion, artery, carotid) I65.2- ☑
  central nervous system I67.2
  cerebral I67.2
  cerebrovascular I67.2
  coronary (artery) I25.10
    bypass graft I25.810
      with
        angina pectoris I25.709
          with documented spasm I25.701
          specified type NEC I25.708
          unstable I25.700
        ischemic chest pain I25.709
      autologous artery I25.810
        with
          angina pectoris I25.729
            with documented spasm I25.721
            specified type I25.728
            unstable I25.720
          ischemic chest pain I25.729
      autologous vein I25.810

Arteriosclerosis, arteriosclerotic — *continued*
  coronary — *continued*
    bypass graft — *continued*
      autologous vein — *continued*
        with
          angina pectoris I25.719
            with documented spasm I25.711
            specified type I25.718
            unstable I25.710
          ischemic chest pain I25.719
        nonautologous biological I25.810
          with
            angina pectoris I25.739
              with documented spasm I25.731
              specified type I25.738
              unstable I25.730
            ischemic chest pain I25.739
        specified type NEC I25.810
          with
            angina pectoris I25.799
              with documented spasm I25.791
              specified type I25.798
              unstable I25.790
            ischemic chest pain I25.799
    due to
      calcified coronary lesion (severely) I25.84
      lipid rich plaque I25.83
    native vessel
      with
        angina pectoris I25.119
          with documented spasm I25.111
          specified type NEC I25.118
          unstable I25.110
        ischemic chest pain I25.119
    transplanted heart I25.811
      bypass graft I25.812
        with
          angina pectoris I25.769
            with documented spasm I25.761
            specified type I25.768
            unstable I25.760
          ischemic chest pain I25.769
      native coronary artery I25.811
        with
          angina pectoris I25.759
            with documented spasm I25.751
            specified type I25.758
            unstable I25.750
          ischemic chest pain I25.759
  extremities (native arteries) I70.209
    bypass graft I70.309
      autologous vein graft I70.409
        leg I70.409
          with
            gangrene (and intermittent claudica-
              tion, rest pain and ulcer)
              I70.469
            intermittent claudication I70.419
            rest pain (and intermittent claudica-
              tion) I70.429
          bilateral I70.403
            with
              gangrene (and intermittent clau-
                dication, rest pain and ul-
                cer) I70.463
              intermittent claudication I70.463
              rest pain (and intermittent claudi-
                cation) I70.423
              specified type NEC I70.493
          left I70.402
            with
              gangrene (and intermittent clau-
                dication, rest pain and ul-
                cer) I70.462
              intermittent claudication I70.412
              rest pain (and intermittent claudi-
                cation) I70.422
              ulceration (and intermittent
                claudication and rest pain)
                I70.449
              ankle I70.443
              calf I70.442
              foot site NEC I70.445
              heel I70.444
              lower leg NEC I70.448
              midfoot I70.444
              thigh I70.441
              specified type NEC I70.492

Arteriosclerosis, arteriosclerotic — *continued*
  extremities — *continued*
    bypass graft — *continued*
      autologous vein graft — *continued*
        leg — *continued*
          right I70.401
            with
              gangrene (and intermittent clau-
                dication, rest pain and ul-
                cer) I70.461
              intermittent claudication I70.411
              rest pain (and intermittent claudi-
                cation) I70.421
              ulceration (and intermittent
                claudication and rest pain)
                I70.439
              ankle I70.433
              calf I70.432
              foot site NEC I70.435
              heel I70.434
              lower leg NEC I70.438
              midfoot I70.434
              thigh I70.431
            specified type NEC I70.491
          specified type NEC I70.499
        specified NEC I70.408
          with
            gangrene (and intermittent claudica-
              tion, rest pain and ulcer)
              I70.468
            intermittent claudication I70.418
            rest pain (and intermittent claudica-
              tion) I70.428
            ulceration (and intermittent claudica-
              tion and rest pain) I70.45
            specified type NEC I70.498
      leg I70.309
        with
          gangrene (and intermittent claudication,
            rest pain and ulcer) I70.369
          intermittent claudication I70.319
          rest pain (and intermittent claudication)
            I70.329
        bilateral I70.303
          with
            gangrene (and intermittent claudica-
              tion, rest pain and ulcer)
              I70.363
            intermittent claudication I70.313
            rest pain (and intermittent claudica-
              tion) I70.323
            specified type NEC I70.393
        left I70.302
          with
            gangrene (and intermittent claudica-
              tion, rest pain and ulcer)
              I70.362
            intermittent claudication I70.312
            rest pain (and intermittent claudica-
              tion) I70.322
            ulceration (and intermittent claudica-
              tion and rest pain) I70.349
            ankle I70.343
            calf I70.342
            foot site NEC I70.345
            heel I70.344
            lower leg NEC I70.348
            midfoot I70.344
            thigh I70.341
          specified type NEC I70.392
        right I70.301
          with
            gangrene (and intermittent claudica-
              tion, rest pain and ulcer)
              I70.361
            intermittent claudication I70.311
            rest pain (and intermittent claudica-
              tion) I70.321
            ulceration (and intermittent claudica-
              tion and rest pain I70.339
            ankle I70.333
            calf I70.332
            foot site NEC I70.335
            heel I70.334
            lower leg NEC I70.338
            midfoot I70.334
            thigh I70.331
          specified type NEC I70.391

☑ **Additional Character Required — Refer to the Tabular List for Character Selection**   ▽ Subterms under main terms may continue to next column or page

Arteriosclerosis, arteriosclerotic — *continued*
  extremities — *continued*
    bypass graft — *continued*
      leg — *continued*
        specified type NEC I70.399
      nonautologous biological graft I70.509
        leg I70.509
          with
            gangrene (and intermittent claudication, rest pain and ulcer) I70.569
            intermittent claudication I70.519
            rest pain (and intermittent claudication) I70.529
          bilateral I70.503
            with
              gangrene (and intermittent claudication, rest pain and ulcer) I70.563
              intermittent claudication I70.513
              rest pain (and intermittent claudication) I70.523
            specified type NEC I70.593
          left I70.502
            with
              gangrene (and intermittent claudication, rest pain and ulcer) I70.562
              intermittent claudication I70.512
              rest pain (and intermittent claudication) I70.522
              ulceration (and intermittent claudication and rest pain) I70.549
                ankle I70.543
                calf I70.542
                foot site NEC I70.545
                heel I70.544
                lower leg NEC I70.548
                midfoot I70.544
                thigh I70.541
            specified type NEC I70.592
          right I70.501
            with
              gangrene (and intermittent claudication, rest pain and ulcer) I70.561
              intermittent claudication I70.511
              rest pain (and intermittent claudication) I70.521
              ulceration (and intermittent claudication and rest pain) I70.539
                ankle I70.533
                calf I70.532
                foot site NEC I70.535
                heel I70.534
                lower leg NEC I70.538
                midfoot I70.534
                thigh I70.531
            specified type NEC I70.591
          specified type NEC I70.599
        specified NEC I70.508
          with
            gangrene (and intermittent claudication, rest pain and ulcer) I70.568
            intermittent claudication I70.518
            rest pain (and intermittent claudication) I70.528
            ulceration (and intermittent claudication and rest pain) I70.55
          specified type NEC I70.598
      nonbiological graft I70.609
        leg I70.609
          with
            gangrene (and intermittent claudication, rest pain and ulcer) I70.669
            intermittent claudication I70.619
            rest pain (and intermittent claudication) I70.629
          bilateral I70.603
            with
              gangrene (and intermittent claudication, rest pain and ulcer) I70.663
              intermittent claudication I70.613

Arteriosclerosis, arteriosclerotic — *continued*
  extremities — *continued*
    bypass graft — *continued*
      nonbiological graft — *continued*
        leg — *continued*
          bilateral — *continued*
            with — *continued*
              rest pain (and intermittent claudication) I70.623
            specified type NEC I70.693
          left I70.602
            with
              gangrene (and intermittent claudication, rest pain and ulcer) I70.662
              intermittent claudication I70.612
              rest pain (and intermittent claudication) I70.622
              ulceration (and intermittent claudication and rest pain) I70.649
                ankle I70.643
                calf I70.642
                foot site NEC I70.645
                heel I70.644
                lower leg NEC I70.648
                midfoot I70.644
                thigh I70.641
            specified type NEC I70.692
          right I70.601
            with
              gangrene (and intermittent claudication, rest pain and ulcer) I70.661
              intermittent claudication I70.611
              rest pain (and intermittent claudication) I70.621
              ulceration (and intermittent claudication and rest pain) I70.639
                ankle I70.633
                calf I70.632
                foot site NEC I70.635
                heel I70.634
                lower leg NEC I70.638
                midfoot I70.634
                thigh I70.631
            specified type NEC I70.691
        specified NEC I70.608
          with
            gangrene (and intermittent claudication, rest pain and ulcer) I70.668
            intermittent claudication I70.618
            rest pain (and intermittent claudication) I70.628
            ulceration (and intermittent claudication and rest pain) I70.65
          specified type NEC I70.698
      specified graft NEC I70.709
        leg I70.709
          with
            gangrene (and intermittent claudication, rest pain and ulcer) I70.769
            intermittent claudication I70.719
            rest pain (and intermittent claudication) I70.729
          bilateral I70.703
            with
              gangrene (and intermittent claudication, rest pain and ulcer) I70.763
              intermittent claudication I70.713
              rest pain (and intermittent claudication) I70.723
            specified type NEC I70.793
          left I70.702
            with
              gangrene (and intermittent claudication, rest pain and ulcer) I70.762
              intermittent claudication I70.712
              rest pain (and intermittent claudication) I70.722

Arteriosclerosis, arteriosclerotic — *continued*
  extremities — *continued*
    bypass graft — *continued*
      specified graft — *continued*
        leg — *continued*
          left — *continued*
            with — *continued*
              ulceration (and intermittent claudication and rest pain) I70.749
                ankle I70.743
                calf I70.742
                foot site NEC I70.745
                heel I70.744
                lower leg NEC I70.748
                midfoot I70.744
                thigh I70.741
            specified type NEC I70.792
          right I70.701
            with
              gangrene (and intermittent claudication, rest pain and ulcer) I70.761
              intermittent claudication I70.711
              rest pain (and intermittent claudication) I70.721
              ulceration (and intermittent claudication and rest pain) I70.739
                ankle I70.733
                calf I70.732
                foot site NEC I70.735
                heel I70.734
                lower leg NEC I70.738
                midfoot I70.734
                thigh I70.731
            specified type NEC I70.791
          specified type NEC I70.799
        specified NEC I70.708
          with
            gangrene (and intermittent claudication, rest pain and ulcer) I70.768
            intermittent claudication I70.718
            rest pain (and intermittent claudication) I70.728
            ulceration (and intermittent claudication and rest pain) I70.75
          specified type NEC I70.798
      specified NEC I70.308
        with
          gangrene (and intermittent claudication, rest pain and ulcer) I70.368
          intermittent claudication I70.318
          rest pain (and intermittent claudication) I70.328
          ulceration (and intermittent claudication and rest pain) I70.35
        specifiec type NEC I70.398
    leg I70.209
      with
        gangrene (and intermittent claudication, rest pain and ulcer) I70.269
        intermittent claudication I70.219
        rest pain (and intermittent claudication) I70.229
      bilateral I70.203
        with
          gangrene (and intermittent claudication, rest pain and ulcer) I70.263
          intermittent claudication I70.213
          rest pain (and intermittent claudication) I70.223
        specified type NEC I70.293
      left I70.202
        with
          gangrene (and intermittent claudication, rest pain and ulcer) I70.262
          intermittent claudication I70.212
          rest pain (and intermittent claudication) I70.222
          ulceration (and intermittent claudication and rest pain) I70.249
            ankle I70.243
            calf I70.242
            foot site NEC I70.245
            heel I70.244
            lower leg NEC I70.248

Arteriosclerosis, arteriosclerotic — *continued*
  extremities — *continued*
    leg — *continued*
      left — *continued*
        with — *continued*
          ulceration — *continued*
            midfoot I70.244
            thigh I70.241
          specified type NEC I70.292
      right I70.201
        with
          gangrene (and intermittent claudication, rest pain and ulcer) I70.261
          intermittent claudication I70.211
          rest pain (and intermittent claudication) I70.221
          ulceration (and intermittent claudication and rest pain) I70.239
            ankle I70.233
            calf I70.232
            foot site NEC I70.235
            heel I70.234
            lower leg NEC I70.238
            midfoot I70.234
            thigh I70.231
          specified type NEC I70.291
      specified type NEC I70.299
    specified site NEC I70.208
      with
        gangrene (and intermittent claudication, rest pain and ulcer) I70.268
        intermittent claudication I70.218
        rest pain (and intermittent claudication) I70.228
        ulceration (and intermittent claudication and rest pain) I70.25
        specified type NEC I70.298
  generalized I70.91
  heart (disease) — *see* Arteriosclerosis, coronary (artery),
  kidney — *see* Hypertension, kidney
  medial — *see* Arteriosclerosis, extremities
  mesenteric (artery) K55.1
  Mönckeberg's — *see* Arteriosclerosis, extremities
  myocarditis I51.4
  peripheral (of extremities) — *see* Arteriosclerosis, extremities
  pulmonary (idiopathic) I27.0
  renal (arterioles) (*see also* Hypertension, kidney)
    artery I70.1
  retina (vascular) I70.8 [H35.0-] ✓
  specified artery NEC I70.8
  spinal (cord) G95.19
  vertebral (artery) I67.2
Arteriospasm I73.9
Arteriovenous — *see* condition
Arteritis I77.6
  allergic M31.0
  aorta (nonsyphilitic) I77.6
    syphilitic A52.02
  aortic arch M31.4
  brachiocephalic M31.4
  brain I67.7
    syphilitic A52.04
  cerebral I67.7
    in systemic lupus erythematosus M32.19
    listerial A32.89
    syphilitic A52.04
    tuberculous A18.89
  coronary (artery) I25.89
    rheumatic I01.8
      chronic I09.89
    syphilitic A52.06
  cranial (left) (right), giant cell M31.6
  deformans — *see* Arteriosclerosis
  giant cell NEC M31.6
    with polymyalgia rheumatica M31.5
  necrosing or necrotizing M31.9
    specified NEC M31.8
  nodosa M30.0
  obliterans — *see* Arteriosclerosis
  pulmonary I28.8
  rheumatic — *see* Fever, rheumatic
  senile — *see* Arteriosclerosis
  suppurative I77.2
  syphilitic (general) A52.09
    brain A52.04
    coronary A52.06

Arteritis — *continued*
  syphilitic — *continued*
    spinal A52.09
  temporal, giant cell M31.6
  young female aortic arch syndrome M31.4
Artery, arterial (*see also* condition)
  abscess I77.89
  single umbilical Q27.0
Arthralgia (allergic) (*see also* Pain, joint)
  in caisson disease T70.3 ✓
  temporomandibular M26.62
Arthritis, arthritic (acute) (chronic) (nonpyogenic) (subacute) M19.90
  allergic — *see* Arthritis, specified form NEC
  ankylosing (crippling) (spine) (*see also* Spondylitis, ankylosing)
    sites other than spine — *see* Arthritis, specified form NEC
  atrophic — *see* Osteoarthritis
    spine — *see* Spondylitis, ankylosing
  back — *see* Spondylopathy, inflammatory
  blennorrhagic (gonococcal) A54.42
  Charcot's — *see* Arthropathy, neuropathic
    diabetic — *see* Diabetes, arthropathy, neuropathic
    syringomyelic G95.0
  chylous (filarial) (*see also* category M01) B74.9
  climacteric (any site) NEC — *see* Arthritis, specified form NEC
  crystal (-induced) — *see* Arthritis, in, crystals
  deformans — *see* Osteoarthritis
  degenerative — *see* Osteoarthritis
  due to or associated with
    acromegaly E22.0
    brucellosis — *see* Brucellosis
    caisson disease T70.3
    diabetes — *see* Diabetes, arthropathy
    dracontiasis (*see also* category M01) B72
    enteritis NEC
      regional — *see* Enteritis, regional
    erysipelas (*see also* category M01) A46
    erythema
      epidemic A25.1
      nodosum L52
    filariasis NOS B74.9
    glanders A24.0
    helminthiasis (*see also* category M01) B83.9
    hemophilia D66 [M36.2]
    Henoch- (Schönlein) purpura D69.0 [M36.4]
    human parvovirus (*see also* category M01) B97.6
    infectious disease NEC M01 ✓
    leprosy (*see also* category M01) (*see also* Leprosy) A30.9
    Lyme disease A69.23
    mycobacteria (*see also* category M01) A31.8
    parasitic disease NEC (*see also* category M01) B89
    paratyphoid fever (*see also* category M01) (*see also* Fever, paratyphoid) A01.4
    rat bite fever (*see also* category M01) A25.1
    regional enteritis — *see* Enteritis, regional
    respiratory disorder NOS J98.9
    serum sickness (*see also* Reaction, serum) T80.69 ✓
    syringomyelia G95.0
    typhoid fever A01.04
  epidemic erythema A25.1
  febrile — *see* Fever, rheumatic
  gonococcal A54.42
  gouty (acute) — *see* Gout, idiopathic
  in (due to)
    acromegaly (*see also* subcategory M14.8-) E22.0
    amyloidosis (*see also* subcategory M14.8-) E85.4
    bacterial disease (*see also* subcategory M01) A49.9
    Behçet's syndrome M35.2
    caisson disease (*see also* subcategory M14.8-) T70.3 ✓
    coliform bacilli (Escherichia coli) — *see* Arthritis, in, pyogenic organism NEC
    crystals M11.9
      dicalcium phosphate — *see* Arthritis, in, crystals, specified type NEC
      hydroxyapatite M11.0- ✓
      pyrophosphate — *see* Arthritis, in, crystals, specified type NEC
      specified type NEC M11.80
        ankle M11.87- ✓
        elbow M11.82- ✓
        foot joint M11.87- ✓
        hand joint M11.84- ✓

Arthritis, arthritic — *continued*
  in — *continued*
    crystals — *continued*
      specified type — *continued*
        hip M11.85- ✓
        knee M11.86- ✓
        multiple sites M11.8- ✓
        shoulder M11.81- ✓
        vertebrae M11.88
        wrist M11.83- ✓
    dermatoarthritis, lipoid E78.81
    dracontiasis (dracunculiasis) (*see also* category M01) B72
    endocrine disorder NEC (*see also* subcategory M14.8-) E34.9
    enteritis, infectious NEC (*see also* category M01) A09
      specified organism NEC (*see also* category M01) A08.8
    erythema
      multiforme (*see also* subcategory M14.8-) L51.9
      nodosum (*see also* subcategory M14.8-) L52
    gout — *see* Gout, idiopathic
    helminthiasis NEC (*see also* category M01) B83.9
    hemochromatosis (*see also* subcategory M14.8-) E83.118
    hemoglobinopathy NEC D58.2 [M36.3]
    hemophilia NEC D66 [M36.2]
    Hemophilus influenzae M00.8- ✓ [B96.3]
    Henoch (-Schönlein) purpura D69.0 [M36.4]
    hyperparathyroidism NEC (*see also* subcategory M14.8-) E21.3
    hypersensitivity reaction NEC T78.49 ✓ [M36.4]
    hypogammaglobulinemia (*see also* subcategory M14.8-) D80.1
    hypothyroidism NEC (*see also* subcategory M14.8-) E03.9
    infection — *see* Arthritis, pyogenic or pyemic
      spine — *see* Spondylopathy, infective
    infectious disease NEC M01
    leprosy (*see also* category M01) A30.9
    leukemia NEC C95.9- ✓ [M36.1]
    lipoid dermatoarthritis E78.81
    Lyme disease A69.23
    Mediterranean fever, familial (*see also* subcategory M14.8-) E85.0
    Meningococcus A39.83
    metabolic disorder NEC (*see also* subcategory M14.8-) E88.9
    multiple myelomatosis C90.0- ✓ [M36.1]
    mumps B26.85
    mycosis NEC (*see also* category M01) B49
    myelomatosis (multiple) C90.0- ✓ [M36.1]
    neurological disorder NEC G98.0
    ochronosis (*see also* subcategory M14.8-) E70.29
    O'nyong-nyong (*see also* category M01) A92.1
    parasitic disease NEC (*see also* category M01) B89
    paratyphoid fever (*see also* category M01) A01.4
    Pseudomonas — *see* Arthritis, pyogenic, bacterial NEC
    psoriasis L40.50
    pyogenic organism NEC — *see* Arthritis, pyogenic, bacterial NEC
    Reiter's disease — *see* Reiter's disease
    respiratory disorder NEC (*see also* subcategory M14.8-) J98.9
    reticulosis, malignant (*see also* subcategory M14.8-) C86.0
    rubella B06.82
    Salmonella (arizonae) (cholerae-suis) (enteritidis) (typhimurium) A02.23
    sarcoidosis D86.86
    specified bacteria NEC — *see* Arthritis, pyogenic, bacterial NEC
    sporotrichosis B42.82
    syringomyelia G95.0
    thalassemia NEC D56.9 [M36.3]
    tuberculosis — *see* Tuberculosis, arthritis
    typhoid fever A01.04
    urethritis, Reiter's — *see* Reiter's disease
    viral disease NEC (*see also* category M01) B34.9
  infectious or infective (*see also* Arthritis, pyogenic or pyemic)
    spine — *see* Spondylopathy, infective
  juvenile M08.90
    with systemic onset — *see* Still's disease
    ankle M08.97- ✓

✓ **Additional Character Required — Refer to the Tabular List for Character Selection**   ▽ **Subterms under main terms may continue to next column or page**

Arthritis, arthritic — *continued*
  juvenile — *continued*
    elbow M08.92- ☑
    foot joint M08.97- ☑
    hand joint M08.94- ☑
    hip M08.95- ☑
    knee M08.96- ☑
    multiple site M08.99
    pauciarticular M08.40
      ankle M08.47- ☑
      elbow M08.42- ☑
      foot joint M08.47- ☑
      hand joint M08.44- ☑
      hip M08.45- ☑
      knee M08.46- ☑
      shoulder M08.41- ☑
      vertebrae M08.48
      wrist M08.43- ☑
    psoriatic L40.54
    rheumatoid — *see* Arthritis, rheumatoid, juvenile
    shoulder M08.91- ☑
    specified type NEC M08.80
      ankle M08.87- ☑
      elbow M08.82- ☑
      foot joint M08.87- ☑
      hand joint M08.84- ☑
      hip M08.85- ☑
      knee M08.86- ☑
      multiple site M08.89
      shoulder M08.81- ☑
      specified joint NEC M08.88
      vertebrae M08.88
      wrist M08.83- ☑
    wrist M08.93- ☑
  meaning osteoarthritis — *see* Osteoarthritis
  meningococcal A39.83
  menopausal (any site) NEC — *see* Arthritis, specified form NEC
  mutilans (psoriatic) L40.52
  mycotic NEC (*see also* category M01) B49
  neuropathic (Charcot) — *see* Arthropathy, neuropathic
    diabetic — *see* Diabetes, arthropathy, neuropathic
    nonsyphilitic NEC G98.0
    syringomyelic G95.0
  ochronotic (*see also* subcategory M14.8-) E70.29
  palindromic (any site) — *see* Rheumatism, palindromic
  pneumococcal M00.10
    ankle M00.17- ☑
    elbow M00.12- ☑
    foot joint — *see* Arthritis, pneumococcal, ankle
    hand joint M00.14- ☑
    hip M00.15- ☑
    knee M00.16- ☑
    multiple site M00.19
    shoulder M00.11- ☑
    vertebra M00.18
    wrist M00.13- ☑
  postdysenteric — *see* Arthropathy, postdysenteric
  postmeningococcal A39.84
  postrheumatic, chronic — *see* Arthropathy, postrheumatic, chronic
  primary progressive (*see also* Arthritis, specified form NEC)
    spine — *see* Spondylitis, ankylosing
  psoriatic L40.50
  purulent (any site except spine) — *see* Arthritis, pyogenic or pyemic
    spine — *see* Spondylopathy, infective
  pyogenic or pyemic (any site except spine) M00.9
    bacterial NEC M00.80
      ankle M00.87- ☑
      elbow M00.82- ☑
      foot joint — *see* Arthritis, pyogenic, bacterial NEC, ankle
      hand joint M00.84- ☑
      hip M00.85- ☑
      knee M00.86- ☑
      multiple site M00.89
      shoulder M00.81- ☑
      vertebra M00.88
      wrist M00.83- ☑
    pneumococcal — *see* Arthritis, pneumococcal
    spine — *see* Spondylopathy, infective
    staphylococcal — *see* Arthritis, staphylococcal
    streptococcal — *see* Arthritis, streptococcal NEC
      pneumococcal — *see* Arthritis, pneumococcal

Arthritis, arthritic — *continued*
  reactive — *see* Reiter's disease
  rheumatic (*see also* Arthritis, rheumatoid)
    acute or subacute — *see* Fever, rheumatic
  rheumatoid M06.9
    with
      carditis — *see* Rheumatoid, carditis
      endocarditis — *see* Rheumatoid, carditis
      heart involvement NEC — *see* Rheumatoid, carditis
      lung involvement — *see* Rheumatoid, lung
      myocarditis — *see* Rheumatoid, carditis
      myopathy — *see* Rheumatoid, myopathy
      pericarditis — *see* Rheumatoid, carditis
      polyneuropathy — *see* Rheumatoid, polyneuropathy
      rheumatoid factor — *see* Arthritis, rheumatoid, seropositive
      splenoadenomegaly and leukopenia — *see* Felty's syndrome
      vasculitis — *see* Rheumatoid, vasculitis
      visceral involvement NEC — *see* Rheumatoid, arthritis, with involvement of organs NEC
    juvenile (with or without rheumatoid factor) M08.00
      ankle M08.07- ☑
      elbow M08.02- ☑
      foot joint M08.07- ☑
      hand joint M08.04- ☑
      hip M08.05- ☑
      knee M08.06- ☑
      multiple site M08.09
      shoulder M08.01- ☑
      vertebra M08.08
      wrist M08.03- ☑
    seronegative M06.00
      ankle M06.07- ☑
      elbow M06.02- ☑
      foot joint M06.07- ☑
      hand joint M06.04- ☑
      hip M06.05- ☑
      knee M06.06- ☑
      multiple site M06.09
      shoulder M06.01- ☑
      vertebra M06.08
      wrist M06.03- ☑
    seropositive M05.9
      without organ involvement M05.70
        ankle M05.77- ☑
        elbow M05.72- ☑
        foot joint M05.77- ☑
        hand joint M05.74- ☑
        hip M05.75- ☑
        knee M05.76- ☑
        multiple sites M05.79
        shoulder M05.71- ☑
        vertebra — *see* Spondylitis, ankylosing
        wrist M05.73- ☑
      specified NEC M05.80
        ankle M05.87- ☑
        elbow M05.82- ☑
        foot joint M05.87- ☑
        hand joint M05.84- ☑
        hip M05.85- ☑
        knee M05.86- ☑
        multiple sites M05.89
        shoulder M05.81- ☑
        vertebra — *see* Spondylitis, ankylosing
        wrist M05.83- ☑
    specified type NEC M06.80
      ankle M06.87- ☑
      elbow M06.82- ☑
      foot joint M06.87- ☑
      hand joint M06.84- ☑
      hip M06.85- ☑
      knee M06.86- ☑
      multiple site M06.89
      shoulder M06.81- ☑
      vertebra M06.88
      wrist M06.83- ☑
    spine — *see* Spondylitis, ankylosing
  rubella B06.82
  scorbutic (*see also* subcategory M14.8-) E54
  senile or senescent — *see* Osteoarthritis
  septic (any site except spine) — *see* Arthritis, pyogenic or pyemic

Arthritis, arthritic — *continued*
  septic — *see* Arthritis, pyogenic or pyemic — *continued*
    spine — *see* Spondylopathy, infective
  serum (nontherapeutic) (therapeutic) — *see* Arthropathy, postimmunization
  specified form NEC M13.80
    ankle M13.87- ☑
    elbow M13.82- ☑
    foot joint M13.87- ☑
    hand joint M13.84- ☑
    hip M13.85- ☑
    knee M13.86- ☑
    multiple site M13.89
    shoulder M13.81- ☑
    specified joint NEC M13.88
    wrist M13.83- ☑
  spine (*see also* Spondylopathy, inflammatory)
    infectious or infective NEC — *see* Spondylopathy, infective
    Marie-Strümpell — *see* Spondylitis, ankylosing
    pyogenic — *see* Spondylopathy, infective
    rheumatoid — *see* Spondylitis, ankylosing
    traumatic (old) — *see* Spondylopathy, traumatic
    tuberculous A18.01
  staphylococcal M00.00
    ankle M00.07- ☑
    elbow M00.02- ☑
    foot joint — *see* Arthritis, staphylococcal, ankle
    hand joint M00.04- ☑
    hip M00.05- ☑
    knee M00.06- ☑
    multiple site M00.09
    shoulder M00.01- ☑
    vertebra M00.08
    wrist M00.03- ☑
  streptococcal NEC M00.20
    ankle M00.27- ☑
    elbow M00.22- ☑
    foot joint — *see* Arthritis, streptococcal, ankle
    hand joint M00.24- ☑
    hip M00.25- ☑
    knee M00.26- ☑
    multiple site M00.29
    shoulder M00.21- ☑
    vertebra M00.28
    wrist M00.23- ☑
  suppurative — *see* Arthritis, pyogenic or pyemic
  syphilitic (late) A52.16
    congenital A50.55 [M12.80]
  syphilitica deformans (Charcot) A52.16
  temporomandibular M26.69
  toxic of menopause (any site) — *see* Arthritis, specified form NEC
  transient — *see* Arthropathy, specified form NEC
  traumatic (chronic) — *see* Arthropathy, traumatic
  tuberculous A18.02
    spine A18.01
  uratic — *see* Gout, idiopathic
  urethritica (Reiter's) — *see* Reiter's disease
  vertebral — *see* Spondylopathy, inflammatory
  villous (any site) — *see* Arthropathy, specified form NEC
Arthrocele — *see* Effusion, joint
Arthrodesis status Z98.1
Arthrodynia (*see also* Pain, joint)
Arthrodysplasia Q74.9
Arthrofibrosis, joint — *see* Ankylosis
Arthrogryposis (congenital) Q68.8
  multiplex congenita Q74.3
Arthrokatadysis M24.7
Arthropathy (*see also* Arthritis) M12.9
  Charcot's — *see* Arthropathy, neuropathic
    diabetic — *see* Diabetes, arthropathy, neuropathic
    syringomyelic G95.0
  cricoarytenoid J38.7
  crystal (-induced) — *see* Arthritis, in, crystals
  diabetic NEC — *see* Diabetes, arthropathy
  distal interphalangeal, psoriatic L40.51
  enteropathic M07.60
    ankle M07.67- ☑
    elbow M07.62- ☑
    foot joint M07.67- ☑
    hand joint M07.64- ☑
    hip M07.65- ☑
    knee M07.66- ☑

Arthropathy — *continued*
　enteropathic — *continued*
　　multiple site M07.69
　　shoulder M07.61- ☑
　　vertebra M07.68
　　wrist M07.63- ☑
　following intestinal bypass M02.00
　　ankle M02.07- ☑
　　elbow M02.02- ☑
　　foot joint M02.07- ☑
　　hand joint M02.04- ☑
　　hip M02.05- ☑
　　knee M02.06- ☑
　　multiple site M02.09
　　shoulder M02.01- ☑
　　vertebra M02.08
　　wrist M02.03- ☑
　gouty (*see also* Gout, idiopathic)
　　in (due to)
　　　Lesch-Nyhan syndrome E79.1 [M14.8-] ☑
　　　sickle-cell disorders D57- ☑ [M14.8-] ☑
　hemophilic NEC D66 [M36.2]
　　in (due to)
　　　hyperparathyroidism NEC E21.3 [M14.8-] ☑
　　　metabolic disease NOS E88.9 [M14.8-] ☑
　in (due to)
　　acromegaly E22.0 [M14.8-] ☑
　　amyloidosis E85.4 [M14.8-] ☑
　　blood disorder NOS D75.9 [M36.3]
　　diabetes — *see* Diabetes, arthropathy
　　endocrine disease NOS E34.9 [M14.8-] ☑
　　erythema
　　　multiforme L51.9 [M14.8-] ☑
　　　nodosum L52 [M14.8-] ☑
　　hemochromatosis E83.118 [M14.8-] ☑
　　hemoglobinopathy NEC D58.2 [M36.3]
　　hemophilia NEC D66 [M36.2]
　　Henoch-Schönlein purpura D69.0 [M36.4]
　　hyperthyroidism E05.90 [M14.8-] ☑
　　hypothyroidism E03.9 [M14.8-] ☑
　　infective endocarditis I33.0 [M12.80]
　　leukemia NEC C95.9- ☑ [M36.1]
　　malignant histiocytosis C96.A [M36.1]
　　metabolic disease NOS E88.9 [M14.8-] ☑
　　multiple myeloma C90.0- ☑ [M36.1]
　　neoplastic disease NOS (*see also* Neoplasm)
　　　D49.9 [M36.1]
　　nutritional deficiency (*see also* subcategory
　　　M14.8-) E63.9
　　psoriasis NOS L40.50
　　sarcoidosis D86.86
　　syphilis (late) A52.77
　　　congenital A50.55 [M12.80]
　　thyrotoxicosis (*see also* subcategory M14.8-) E05.90
　　ulcerative colitis K51.90 [M07.60]
　　viral hepatitis (postinfectious) NEC B19.9 [M12.80]
　　Whipple's disease (*see also* subcategory M14.8-)
　　　K90.81
　Jaccoud — *see* Arthropathy, postrheumatic, chronic
　juvenile — *see* Arthritis, juvenile
　　psoriatic L40.54
　mutilans (psoriatic) L40.52
　neuropathic (Charcot) M14.60
　　ankle M14.67- ☑
　　diabetic — *see* Diabetes, arthropathy, neuropathic
　　elbow M14.62- ☑
　　foot joint M14.67- ☑
　　hand joint M14.64- ☑
　　hip M14.65- ☑
　　knee M14.66- ☑
　　multiple site M14.69
　　nonsyphilitic NEC G98.0
　　shoulder M14.61- ☑
　　syringomyelic G95.0
　　vertebra M14.68
　　wrist M14.63- ☑
　osteopulmonary — *see* Osteoarthropathy, hyper-
　　trophic, specified NEC
　postdysenteric M02.10
　　ankle M02.17- ☑
　　elbow M02.12- ☑
　　foot joint M02.17- ☑
　　hand joint M02.14- ☑
　　hip M02.15- ☑
　　knee M02.16- ☑
　　multiple site M02.19
　　shoulder M02.11- ☑

Arthropathy — *continued*
　postdysenteric — *continued*
　　vertebra M02.18
　　wrist M02.13- ☑
　postimmunization M02.20
　　ankle M02.27- ☑
　　elbow M02.22- ☑
　　foot joint M02.27- ☑
　　hand joint M02.24- ☑
　　hip M02.25- ☑
　　knee M02.26- ☑
　　multiple site M02.29
　　shoulder M02.21- ☑
　　vertebra M02.28
　　wrist M02.23- ☑
　postinfectious NEC B99 ☑ [M12.80]
　　in (due to)
　　　enteritis due to Yersinia enterocolitica
　　　　A04.6 [M12.80]
　　　syphilis A52.77
　　　viral hepatitis NEC B19.9 [M12.80]
　postrheumatic, chronic (Jaccoud) M12.00
　　ankle M12.07- ☑
　　elbow M12.02- ☑
　　foot joint M12.07- ☑
　　hand joint M12.04- ☑
　　hip M12.05- ☑
　　knee M12.06- ☑
　　multiple site M12.09
　　shoulder M12.01- ☑
　　specified joint NEC M12.08
　　vertebrae M12.08
　　wrist M12.03- ☑
　psoriatic NEC L40.59
　　interphalangeal, distal L40.51
　reactive M02.9
　　in (due to)
　　　infective endocarditis I33.0 [M02.9]
　　specified type NEC M02.80
　　　ankle M02.87- ☑
　　　elbow M02.82- ☑
　　　foot joint M02.87- ☑
　　　hand joint M02.84- ☑
　　　hip M02.85- ☑
　　　knee M02.86- ☑
　　　multiple site M02.89
　　　shoulder M02.81- ☑
　　　vertebra M02.88
　　　wrist M02.83- ☑
　specified form NEC M12.80
　　ankle M12.87- ☑
　　elbow M12.82- ☑
　　foot joint M12.87- ☑
　　hand joint M12.84- ☑
　　hip M12.85- ☑
　　knee M12.86- ☑
　　multiple site M12.89
　　shoulder M12.81- ☑
　　specified joint NEC M12.88
　　vertebrae M12.88
　　wrist M12.83- ☑
　syringomyelic G95.0
　tabes dorsalis A52.16
　tabetic A52.16
　transient — *see* Arthropathy, specified form NEC
　traumatic M12.50
　　ankle M12.57- ☑
　　elbow M12.52- ☑
　　foot joint M12.57- ☑
　　hand joint M12.54- ☑
　　hip M12.55- ☑
　　knee M12.56- ☑
　　multiple site M12.59
　　shoulder M12.51- ☑
　　specified joint NEC M12.58
　　vertebrae M12.58
　　wrist M12.53- ☑
Arthropyosis — *see* Arthritis, pyogenic or pyemic
Arthrosis (deformans) (degenerative) (localized) (*see also*
　Osteoarthritis) M19.90
　spine — *see* Spondylosis
Arthus' phenomenon or reaction T78.41 ☑
　due to
　　drug — *see* Table of Drugs and Chemicals, by drug
Articular — *see* condition
Articulation, reverse (teeth) M26.24

Artificial
　insemination complication — *see* Complications, arti-
　　ficial, fertilization
　opening status (functioning) (without complication)
　　Z93.9
　　anus (colostomy) Z93.3
　　colostomy Z93.3
　　cystostomy Z93.50
　　　appendico-vesicostomy Z93.52
　　　cutaneous Z93.51
　　　specified NEC Z93.59
　　enterostomy Z93.4
　　gastrostomy Z93.1
　　ileostomy Z93.2
　　intestinal tract NEC Z93.4
　　jejunostomy Z93.4
　　nephrostomy Z93.6
　　specified site NEC Z93.8
　　tracheostomy Z93.0
　　ureterostomy Z93.6
　　urethrostomy Z93.6
　　urinary tract NEC Z93.6
　　vagina Z93.8
　vagina status Z93.8
Arytenoid — *see* condition
Asbestosis (occupational) J61
Ascariasis B77.9
　with
　　complications NEC B77.89
　　intestinal complications B77.0
　　pneumonia, pneumonitis B77.81
Ascaridosis, ascaridiasis — *see* Ascariasis
Ascaris (infection) (infestation) (lumbricoides) — *see*
　Ascariasis
Ascending — *see* condition
ASC-H (atypical squamous cells cannot exclude high
　grade squamous intraepithelial lesion on cytologic
　smear)
　anus R85.611
　cervix R87.611
　vagina R87.621
Aschoff's bodies — *see* Myocarditis, rheumatic
Ascites (abdominal) R18.8
　cardiac I50.9
　chylous (nonfilarial) I89.8
　　filarial — *see* Infestation, filarial
　due to
　　cirrhosis, alcoholic K70.31
　　hepatitis
　　　alcoholic K70.11
　　　chronic active K71.51
　　S. japonicum B65.2
　heart I50.9
　malignant R18.0
　pseudochylous R18.8
　syphilitic A52.74
　tuberculous A18.31
ASC-US (atypical squamous cells of undetermined signif-
　icance on cytologic smear)
　anus R85.610
　cervix R87.610
　vagina R87.620
Aseptic — *see* condition
Asherman's syndrome N85.6
Asialia K11.7
Asiatic cholera — *see* Cholera
Asimultagnosia (simultanagnosia) R48.3
Askin's tumor — *see* Neoplasm, connective tissue, ma-
　lignant
Asocial personality F60.2
Asomatognosia R41.4
Aspartylglucosaminuria E77.1
Asperger's disease or syndrome F84.5
Aspergilloma — *see* Aspergillosis
Aspergillosis (with pneumonia) B44.9
　bronchopulmonary, allergic B44.81
　disseminated B44.7
　generalized B44.7
　pulmonary NEC B44.1
　　allergic B44.81
　　invasive B44.0
　specified NEC B44.89
　tonsillar B44.2
Aspergillus (flavus) (fumigatus) (infection) (terreus) —
　see Aspergillosis
Aspermatogenesis — *see* Azoospermia
Aspermia (testis) — *see* Azoospermia
Asphyxia, asphyxiation (by) R09.01

Asphyxia, asphyxiation — *continued*
　antenatal P84
　birth P84
　bunny bag — *see* Asphyxia, due to, mechanical threat to breathing, trapped in bed clothes
　crushing S28.0 ☑
　drowning T75.1 ☑
　gas, fumes, or vapor — *see* Table of Drugs and Chemicals
　inhalation — *see* Inhalation
　intrauterine P84
　local I73.00
　　with gangrene I73.01
　mucus (*see also* Foreign body, respiratory tract, causing asphyxia)
　newborn P84
　pathological R09.01
　postnatal P84
　　mechanical — *see* Asphyxia, due to, mechanical threat to breathing
　prenatal P84
　reticularis R23.1
　strangulation — *see* Asphyxia, due to, mechanical threat to breathing
　submersion T75.1 ☑
　traumatic T71.9 ☑
　　due to
　　　crushed chest S28.0 ☑
　　　foreign body (in) — *see* Foreign body, respiratory tract, causing asphyxia
　　　low oxygen content of ambient air T71.20 ☑
　　　　due to
　　　　　being trapped in
　　　　　　low oxygen environment T71.29 ☑
　　　　　　　in car trunk T71.221 ☑
　　　　　　　　circumstances undetermined T71.224 ☑
　　　　　　　　done with intent to harm by
　　　　　　　　　another person T71.223 ☑
　　　　　　　　　self T71.222 ☑
　　　　　　　in refrigerator T71.231 ☑
　　　　　　　　circumstances undetermined T71.234 ☑
　　　　　　　　done with intent to harm by
　　　　　　　　　another person T71.233 ☑
　　　　　　　　　self T71.232 ☑
　　　　　cave-in T71.21 ☑
　　　mechanical threat to breathing (accidental) T71.191 ☑
　　　　circumstances undetermined T71.194 ☑
　　　　done with intent to harm by
　　　　　another person T71.193 ☑
　　　　　self T71.192 ☑
　　　　hanging T71.161 ☑
　　　　　circumstances undetermined T71.164 ☑
　　　　　done with intent to harm by
　　　　　　another person T71.163 ☑
　　　　　　self T71.162 ☑
　　　　plastic bag T71.121 ☑
　　　　　circumstances undetermined T71.124 ☑
　　　　　done with intent to harm by
　　　　　　another person T71.123 ☑
　　　　　　self T71.122 ☑
　　　　smothering
　　　　　in furniture T71.151 ☑
　　　　　　circumstances undetermined T71.154 ☑
　　　　　　done with intent to harm by
　　　　　　　another person T71.153 ☑
　　　　　　　self T71.152 ☑
　　　　　under
　　　　　　another person's body T71.141 ☑
　　　　　　　circumstances undetermined T71.144 ☑
　　　　　　　done with intent to harm T71.143 ☑
　　　　　　pillow T71.111 ☑
　　　　　　　circumstances undetermined T71.114 ☑
　　　　　　　done with intent to harm by
　　　　　　　　another person T71.113 ☑
　　　　　　　　self T71.112 ☑
　　　　　trapped in bed clothes T71.131 ☑
　　　　　　circumstances undetermined T71.134 ☑
　　　　　　done with intent to harm by
　　　　　　　another person T71.133 ☑
　　　　　　　self T71.132 ☑

Asphyxia, asphyxiation — *continued*
　vomiting, vomitus — *see* Foreign body, respiratory tract, causing asphyxia
Aspiration
　amniotic (clear) fluid (newborn) P24.10
　　with
　　　pneumonia (pneumonitis) P24.11
　　　respiratory symptoms P24.11
　blood
　　newborn (without respiratory symptoms) P24.20
　　　with
　　　　pneumonia (pneumonitis) P24.21
　　　　respiratory symptoms P24.21
　　　specified age NEC — *see* Foreign body, respiratory tract
　bronchitis J69.0
　food or foreign body (with asphyxiation) — *see* Asphyxia, food
　liquor (amnii) (newborn) P24.10
　　with
　　　pneumonia (pneumonitis) P24.11
　　　respiratory symptoms P24.11
　meconium (newborn) (without respiratory symptoms) P24.00
　　with
　　　pneumonitis (pneumonitis) P24.01
　　　respiratory symptoms P24.01
　milk (newborn) (without respiratory symptoms) P24.30
　　with
　　　pneumonia (pneumonitis) P24.31
　　　respiratory symptoms P24.31
　　specified age NEC — *see* Foreign body, respiratory tract
　mucus (*see also* Foreign body, by site, causing asphyxia)
　　newborn P24.10
　　　with
　　　　pneumonia (pneumonitis) P24.11
　　　　respiratory symptoms P24.11
　neonatal P24.9
　　specific NEC (without respiratory symptoms) P24.80
　　　with
　　　　pneumonia (pneumonitis) P24.81
　　　　respiratory symptoms P24.81
　newborn P24.9
　　specific NEC (without respiratory symptoms) P24.80
　　　with
　　　　pneumonia (pneumonitis) P24.81
　　　　respiratory symptoms P24.81
　pneumonia J69.0
　pneumonitis J69.0
　syndrome of newborn — *see* Aspiration, by substance, with pneumonia
　vernix caseosa (newborn) P24.80
　　with
　　　pneumonia (pneumonitis) P24.81
　　　respiratory symptoms P24.81
　vomitus (*see also* Foreign body, respiratory tract)
　　newborn (without respiratory symptoms) P24.30
　　　with
　　　　pneumonia (pneumonitis) P24.31
　　　　respiratory symptoms P24.31
Asplenia (congenital) Q89.01
　postsurgical Z90.81
Assam fever B55.0
Assault, sexual — *see* Maltreatment
Assmann's focus NEC A15.0
Astasia (-abasia) (hysterical) F44.4
Asteatosis cutis L85.3
Astereognosia, astereognosis R48.1
Asterixis R27.8
　in liver disease K71.3
Asteroid hyalitis — *see* Deposit, crystalline
Asthenia, asthenic R53.1
　cardiac (*see also* Failure, heart) I50.9
　　psychogenic F45.8
　cardiovascular (*see also* Failure, heart) I50.9
　　psychogenic F45.8
　heart (*see also* Failure, heart) I50.9
　　psychogenic F45.8
　hysterical F44.4
　myocardial (*see also* Failure, heart) I50.9
　　psychogenic F45.8
　nervous F48.8
　neurocirculatory F45.8
　neurotic F48.8
　psychogenic F48.8
　psychoneurotic F48.8

Asthenia, asthenic — *continued*
　psychophysiologic F48.8
　reaction (psychophysiologic) F48.8
　senile R54
Asthenopia (*see also* Discomfort, visual)
　hysterical F44.6
　psychogenic F44.6
Asthenospermia — *see* Abnormal, specimen, male genital organs
Asthma, asthmatic (bronchial) (catarrh) (spasmodic) J45.909
　with
　　chronic obstructive bronchitis J44.9
　　　with
　　　　acute lower respiratory infection J44.0
　　　　exacerbation (acute) J44.1
　　chronic obstructive pulmonary disease J44.9
　　　with
　　　　acute lower respiratory infection J44.0
　　　　exacerbation (acute) J44.1
　　exacerbation (acute) J45.901
　　hay fever — *see* Asthma, allergic extrinsic
　　rhinitis, allergic — *see* Asthma, allergic extrinsic
　　status asthmaticus J45.902
　allergic extrinsic J45.909
　　with
　　　exacerbation (acute) J45.901
　　　status asthmaticus J45.902
　atopic — *see* Asthma, allergic extrinsic
　cardiac — *see* Failure, ventricular, left
　cardiobronchial I50.1
　childhood J45.909
　　with
　　　exacerbation (acute) J45.901
　　　status asthmaticus J45.902
　chronic obstructive J44.9
　　with
　　　acute lower respiratory infection J44.0
　　　exacerbation (acute) J44.1
　collier's J60
　cough variant J45.991
　detergent J69.8
　due to
　　detergent J69.8
　　inhalation of fumes J68.3
　eosinophilic J82
　extrinsic, allergic — *see* Asthma, allergic extrinsic
　grinder's J62.8
　hay — *see* Asthma, allergic extrinsic
　heart I50.1
　idiosyncratic — *see* Asthma, nonallergic
　intermittent (mild) J45.20
　　with
　　　exacerbation (acute) J45.21
　　　status asthmaticus J45.22
　intrinsic, nonallergic — *see* Asthma, nonallergic
　Kopp's E32.8
　late-onset J45.909
　　with
　　　exacerbation (acute) J45.901
　　　status asthmaticus J45.902
　mild intermittent J45.20
　　with
　　　exacerbation (acute) J45.21
　　　status asthmaticus J45.22
　mild persistent J45.30
　　with
　　　exacerbation (acute) J45.31
　　　status asthmaticus J45.32
　Millar's (laryngismus stridulus) J38.5
　miner's J60
　mixed J45.909
　　with
　　　exacerbation (acute) J45.901
　　　status asthmaticus J45.902
　moderate persistent J45.40
　　with
　　　exacerbation (acute) J45.41
　　　status asthmaticus J45.42
　nervous — *see* Asthma, nonallergic
　nonallergic (intrinsic) J45.909
　　with
　　　exacerbation (acute) J45.901
　　　status asthmaticus J45.902
　persistent
　　mild J45.30
　　　with
　　　　exacerbation (acute) J45.31

Index

Asthma, asthmatic — Atresia, atretic

Asthma, asthmatic — *continued*
  persistent — *continued*
    mild — *continued*
      with — *continued*
        status asthmaticus J45.32
    moderate J45.40
      with
        exacerbation (acute) J45.41
        status asthmaticus J45.42
    severe J45.50
      with
        exacerbation (acute) J45.51
        status asthmaticus J45.52
  platinum J45.998
  pneumoconiotic NEC J64
  potter's J62.8
  predominantly allergic J45.909
  psychogenic F54
  pulmonary eosinophilic J82
  red cedar J67.8
  Rostan's I50.1
  sandblaster's J62.8
  sequoiosis J67.8
  severe persistent J45.50
    with
      exacerbation (acute) J45.51
      status asthmaticus J45.52
  specified NEC J45.998
  stonemason's J62.8
  thymic E32.8
  tuberculous — *see* Tuberculosis, pulmonary
  Wichmann's (laryngismus stridulus) J38.5
  wood J67.8
Astigmatism (compound) (congenital) H52.20- ☑
  irregular H52.21- ☑
  regular H52.22- ☑
Astraphobia F40.220
Astroblastoma
  specified site — *see* Neoplasm, malignant, by site
  unspecified site C71.9
Astrocytoma (cystic)
  anaplastic
    specified site — *see* Neoplasm, malignant, by site
    unspecified site C71.9
  fibrillary
    specified site — *see* Neoplasm, malignant, by site
    unspecified site C71.9
  fibrous
    specified site — *see* Neoplasm, malignant, by site
    unspecified site C71.9
  gemistocytic
    specified site — *see* Neoplasm, malignant, by site
    unspecified site C71.9
  juvenile
    specified site — *see* Neoplasm, malignant, by site
    unspecified site C71.9
  pilocytic
    specified site — *see* Neoplasm, malignant, by site
    unspecified site C71.9
  piloid
    specified site — *see* Neoplasm, malignant, by site
    unspecified site C71.9
  protoplasmic
    specified site — *see* Neoplasm, malignant, by site
    unspecified site C71.9
  specified site NEC — *see* Neoplasm, malignant, by site
  subependymal D43.2
    giant cell
      specified site — *see* Neoplasm, uncertain behavior, by site
      unspecified site D43.2
    specified site — *see* Neoplasm, uncertain behavior, by site
    unspecified site D43.2
  unspecified site C71.9
Astroglioma
  specified site — *see* Neoplasm, malignant, by site
  unspecified site C71.9
Asymbolia R48.8
Asymmetry (*see also* Distortion)
  between native and reconstructed breast N65.1
  face Q67.0
  jaw (lower) — *see* Anomaly, dentofacial, jaw-cranial base relationship, asymmetry
Asynergia, asynergy R27.8
  ventricular I51.89
Asystole (heart) — *see* Arrest, cardiac

At risk
  for falling Z91.81
Ataxia, ataxy, ataxic R27.0
  acute R27.8
  brain (hereditary) G11.9
  cerebellar (hereditary) G11.9
    with defective DNA repair G11.3
    alcoholic G31.2
    early-onset G11.1
    in
      alcoholism G31.2
      myxedema E03.9 [G13.2]
      neoplastic disease (*see also* Neoplasm) D49.9 [G13.1]
      specified disease NEC G32.81
    late-onset (Marie's) G11.2
  cerebral (hereditary) G11.9
  congenital nonprogressive G11.0
  family, familial — *see* Ataxia, hereditary
  following
    cerebrovascular disease I69.993
      cerebral infarction I69.393
      intracerebral hemorrhage I69.193
      nontraumatic intracranial hemorrhage NEC I69.293
      specified disease NEC I69.893
      subarachnoid hemorrhage I69.093
  Friedreich's (heredofamilial) (cerebellar) (spinal) G11.1
  gait R26.0
    hysterical F44.4
  general R27.8
  gluten M35.9 [G32.81]
    with celiac disease K90.0 [G32.81]
  hereditary G11.9
    with neuropathy G60.2
    cerebellar — *see* Ataxia, cerebellar
    spastic G11.4
    specified NEC G11.8
    spinal (Friedreich's) G11.1
  heredofamilial — *see* Ataxia, hereditary
  Hunt's G11.1
  hysterical F44.4
  locomotor (progressive) (syphilitic) (partial) (spastic) A52.11
  diabetic — *see* Diabetes, ataxia
  Marie's (cerebellar) (heredofamilial) (late- onset) G11.2
  nonorganic origin F44.4
  nonprogressive, congenital G11.0
  psychogenic F44.4
  Roussy-Lévy G60.0
  Sanger-Brown's (hereditary) G11.2
  spastic hereditary G11.4
  spinal
    hereditary (Friedreich's) G11.1
    progressive (syphilitic) A52.11
  spinocerebellar, X-linked recessive G11.1
  telangiectasia (Louis-Bar) G11.3
Ataxia-telangiectasia (Louis-Bar) G11.3
Atelectasis (massive) (partial) (pressure) (pulmonary) J98.11
  newborn P28.10
    due to resorption P28.11
    partial P28.19
    primary P28.0
    secondary P28.19
  primary (newborn) P28.0
  tuberculous — *see* Tuberculosis, pulmonary
Atelocardia Q24.9
Atelomyelia Q06.1
Atheroembolism
  of
    extremities
      lower I75.02- ☑
      upper I75.01- ☑
    kidney I75.81
    specified NEC I75.89
Atheroma, atheromatous (*see also* Arteriosclerosis) I70.90
  aorta, aortic I70.0
    valve (*see also* Endocarditis, aortic) I35.8
  aorto-iliac I70.0
  artery — *see* Arteriosclerosis
  basilar (artery) I67.2
  carotid (artery) (common) (internal) I67.2
  cerebral (arteries) I67.2
  coronary (artery) I25.10
    with angina pectoris — *see* Arteriosclerosis, coronary (artery),

Atheroma, atheromatous — *continued*
  degeneration — *see* Arteriosclerosis
  heart, cardiac — *see* Disease, heart, ischemic, atherosclerotic
  mitral (valve) I34.8
  myocardium, myocardial — *see* Disease, heart, is-chemic, atherosclerotic
  pulmonary valve (heart) (*see also* Endocarditis, pulmonary) I37.8
  tricuspid (heart) (valve) I36.8
  valve, valvular — *see* Endocarditis
  vertebral (artery) I67.2
Atheromatosis — *see* Arteriosclerosis
Atherosclerosis (*see also* Arteriosclerosis)
  coronary
    artery I25.10
      with angina pectoris — *see* Arteriosclerosis, coronary (artery),
      due to
        calcified coronary lesion (severely) I25.84
        lipid rich plaque I25.83
    transplanted heart I25.811
      bypass graft I25.812
        with angina pectoris — *see* Arteriosclerosis, coronary (artery),
      native coronary artery I25.811
        with angina pectoris — *see* Arteriosclerosis, coronary (artery),
Athetosis (acquired) R25.8
  bilateral (congenital) G80.3
  congenital (bilateral) (double) G80.3
  double (congenital) G80.3
  unilateral R25.8
Athlete's
  foot B35.3
  heart I51.7
Athrepsia E41
Athyrea (acquired) (*see also* Hypothyroidism)
  congenital E03.1
Atonia, atony, atonic
  bladder (sphincter) (neurogenic) N31.2
  capillary I78.8
  cecum K59.8
    psychogenic F45.8
  colon — *see* Atony, intestine
  congenital P94.2
  esophagus K22.8
  intestine K59.8
    psychogenic F45.8
  stomach K31.89
    neurotic or psychogenic F45.8
  uterus (during labor) O62.2
    with hemorrhage (postpartum) O72.1
    postpartum (with hemorrhage) O72.1
      without hemorrhage O75.89
Atopy — *see* History, allergy
Atransferrinemia, congenital E88.09
Atresia, atretic
  alimentary organ or tract NEC Q45.8
    upper Q40.8
  ani, anus, anal (canal) Q42.3
    with fistula Q42.2
  aorta (arch) (ring) Q25.2
  aortic (orifice) (valve) Q23.0
    arch Q25.2
    congenital with hypoplasia of ascending aorta and defective development of left ventricle (with mitral stenosis) Q23.4
    in hypoplastic left heart syndrome Q23.4
  aqueduct of Sylvius Q03.0
    with spina bifida — *see* Spina bifida, with hydro-cephalus
  artery NEC Q27.8
    cerebral Q28.3
    coronary Q24.5
    digestive system Q27.8
    eye Q15.8
    lower limb Q27.8
    pulmonary Q25.5
    specified site NEC Q27.8
    umbilical Q27.0
    upper limb Q27.8
  auditory canal (external) Q16.1
  bile duct (common) (congenital) (hepatic) Q44.2
    acquired — *see* Obstruction, bile duct
  bladder (neck) Q64.39
    obstruction Q64.31
  bronchus Q32.4

Atresia, atretic — *continued*
 cecum Q42.8
 cervix (acquired) N88.2
  congenital Q51.828
  in pregnancy or childbirth — *see* Anomaly, cervix, in pregnancy or childbirth
   causing obstructed labor O65.5
 choana Q30.0
 colon Q42.9
  specified NEC Q42.8
 common duct Q44.2
 cricoid cartilage Q31.8
 cystic duct Q44.2
  acquired K82.8
   with obstruction K82.0
 digestive organs NEC Q45.8
 duodenum Q41.0
 ear canal Q16.1
 ejaculatory duct Q55.4
 epiglottis Q31.8
 esophagus Q39.0
  with tracheoesophageal fistula Q39.1
 eustachian tube Q17.8
 fallopian tube (congenital) Q50.6
  acquired N97.1
 follicular cyst N83.0
 foramen of
  Luschka Q03.1
   with spina bifida — *see* Spina bifida, with hydrocephalus
  Magendie Q03.1
   with spina bifida — *see* Spina bifida, with hydrocephalus
 gallbladder Q44.1
 genital organ
  external
   female Q52.79
   male Q55.8
  internal
   female Q52.8
   male Q55.8
 glottis Q31.8
 gullet Q39.0
  with tracheoesophageal fistula Q39.1
 heart valve NEC Q24.8
  pulmonary Q22.0
  tricuspid Q22.4
 hymen Q52.3
  acquired (postinfective) N89.6
 ileum Q41.2
 intestine (small) Q41.9
  large Q42.9
   specified NEC Q42.8
 iris, filtration angle Q15.0
 jejunum Q41.1
 lacrimal apparatus Q10.4
 larynx Q31.8
 meatus urinarius Q64.33
 mitral valve Q23.2
  in hypoplastic left heart syndrome Q23.4
 nares (anterior) (posterior) Q30.0
 nasopharynx Q34.8
 nose, nostril Q30.0
  acquired J34.89
 organ or site NEC Q89.8
 osseous meatus (ear) Q16.1
 oviduct (congenital) Q50.6
  acquired N97.1
 parotid duct Q38.4
  acquired K11.8
 pulmonary (artery) Q25.5
  valve Q22.0
 pulmonic Q22.0
 pupil Q13.2
 rectum Q42.1
  with fistula Q42.0
 salivary duct Q38.4
  acquired K11.8
 sublingual duct Q38.4
  acquired K11.8
 submandibular duct Q38.4
  acquired K11.8
 submaxillary duct Q38.4
  acquired K11.8
 thyroid cartilage Q31.8
 trachea Q32.1
 tricuspid valve Q22.4
 ureter Q62.10

Atresia, atretic — *continued*
 ureter — *continued*
  pelvic junction Q62.11
  vesical orifice Q62.12
 ureteropelvic junction Q62.11
 ureterovesical orifice Q62.12
 urethra (valvular) Q64.39
  stricture Q64.32
 urinary tract NEC Q64.8
 uterus Q51.818
  acquired N85.8
 vagina (congenital) Q52.4
  acquired (postinfectional) (senile) N89.5
 vas deferens Q55.3
 vascular NEC Q27.8
  cerebral Q28.3
  digestive system Q27.8
  lower limb Q27.8
  specified site NEC Q27.8
  upper limb Q27.8
 vein NEC Q27.8
  digestive system Q27.8
  great Q26.8
  lower limb Q27.8
  portal Q26.5
  pulmonary Q26.3
  specified site NEC Q27.8
  upper limb Q27.8
 vena cava (inferior) (superior) Q26.8
 vesicourethral orifice Q64.31
 vulva Q52.79
  acquired N90.5
Atrichia, atrichosis — *see* Alopecia
Atrophia (*see also* Atrophy)
 cutis senilis L90.8
  due to radiation L57.8
 gyrata of choroid and retina H31.23
 senilis R54
  dermatological L90.8
   due to radiation (nonionizing) (solar) L57.8
 unguium L60.3
  congenita Q84.6
Atrophie blanche (en plaque) (de Milian) L95.0
Atrophoderma, atrophodermia (of) L90.9
 diffusum (idiopathic) L90.4
 maculatum L90.8
  et striatum L90.8
   due to syphilis A52.79
  syphilitic A51.39
 neuriticum L90.8
 Pasini and Pierini L90.3
 pigmentosum Q82.1
 reticulatum symmetricum faciei L66.4
 senile L90.8
  due to radiation (nonionizing) (solar) L57.8
 vermiculata (cheeks) L66.4
Atrophy, atrophic (of)
 adrenal (capsule) (gland) E27.49
  primary (autoimmune) E27.1
 alveolar process or ridge (edentulous) K08.20
 anal sphincter (disuse) N81.84
 appendix K38.8
 arteriosclerotic — *see* Arteriosclerosis
 bile duct (common) (hepatic) K83.8
 bladder N32.89
  neurogenic N31.8
 blanche (en plaque) (of Milian) L95.0
 bone (senile) NEC (*see also* Disorder, bone, specified type NEC)
  due to
   tabes dorsalis (neurogenic) A52.11
 brain (cortex) (progressive) G31.9
  frontotemporal circumscribed G31.01 [F02.80]
   with behavioral disturbance G31.01 [F02.81]
  senile NEC G31.1
 breast N64.2
  obstetric — *see* Disorder, breast, specified type NEC
 buccal cavity K13.79
 cardiac — *see* Degeneration, myocardial
 cartilage (infectional) (joint) — *see* Disorder, cartilage, specified NEC
 cerebellar — *see* Atrophy, brain
 cerebral — *see* Atrophy, brain
 cervix (mucosa) (senile) (uteri) N88.8
  menopausal N95.8
 Charcot-Marie-Tooth G60.0
 choroid (central) (macular) (myopic) (retina) H31.10- ☑

Atrophy, atrophic — *continued*
 choroid — *continued*
  diffuse secondary H31.12- ☑
  gyrate H31.23
  senile H31.11- ☑
 ciliary body — *see* Atrophy, iris
 conjunctiva (senile) H11.89
 corpus cavernosum N48.89
 cortical — *see* Atrophy, brain
 cystic duct K82.8
 Déjérine-Thomas G23.8
 disuse NEC — *see* Atrophy, muscle
 Duchenne-Aran G12.21
 ear H93.8- ☑
 edentulous alveolar ridge K08.20
 endometrium (senile) N85.8
  cervix N88.8
 enteric K63.89
 epididymis N50.8
 eyeball — *see* Disorder, globe, degenerated condition, atrophy
 eyelid (senile) — *see* Disorder, eyelid, degenerative
 facial (skin) L90.9
 fallopian tube (senile) N83.32
  with ovary N83.33
 fascioscapulohumeral (Landouzy- Déjérine) G71.0
 fatty, thymus (gland) E32.8
 gallbladder K82.8
 gastric K29.40
  with bleeding K29.41
 gastrointestinal K63.89
 glandular I89.8
 globe H44.52- ☑
 gum K06.0
 hair L67.8
 heart (brown) — *see* Degeneration, myocardial
 hemifacial Q67.4
  Romberg G51.8
 infantile E41
  paralysis, acute — *see* Poliomyelitis, paralytic
 intestine K63.89
 iris (essential) (progressive) H21.26- ☑
  specified NEC H21.29
 kidney (senile) (terminal) (*see also* Sclerosis, renal) N26.1
  congenital or infantile Q60.5
   bilateral Q60.4
   unilateral Q60.3
  hydronephrotic — *see* Hydronephrosis
 lacrimal gland (primary) H04.14- ☑
  secondary H04.15- ☑
 Landouzy-Déjérine G71.0
 laryngitis, infective J37.0
 larynx J38.7
 Leber's optic (hereditary) H47.22
 lip K13.0
 liver (yellow) K72.90
  with coma K72.91
  acute, subacute K72.00
   with coma K72.01
  chronic K72.10
   with coma K72.11
 lung (senile) J98.4
 macular (dermatological) L90.8
  syphilitic, skin A51.39
   striated A52.79
 mandible (edentulous) K08.20
  minimal K08.21
  moderate K08.22
  severe K08.23
 maxilla K08.20
  minimal K08.24
  moderate K08.25
  severe K08.26
 muscle, muscular (diffuse) (general) (idiopathic) (primary) M62.50
  ankle M62.57- ☑
  Duchenne-Aran G12.21
  foot M62.57- ☑
  forearm M62.53- ☑
  hand M62.54- ☑
  infantile spinal G12.0
  lower leg M62.56- ☑
  multiple sites M62.59
  myelopathic — *see* Atrophy, muscle, spinal
  myotonic G71.11
  neuritic G58.9
  neuropathic (peroneal) (progressive) G60.0

Atrophy, atrophic — *continued*
  muscle, muscular — *continued*
    pelvic (disuse) N81.84
    peroneal G60.0
    progressive (bulbar) G12.21
      adult G12.1
      infantile (spinal) G12.0
      spinal G12.9
        adult G12.1
        infantile G12.0
    pseudohypertrophic G71.0
    shoulder region M62.51- ☑
    specified site NEC M62.58
    spinal G12.9
      adult form G12.1
      Aran-Duchenne G12.21
      childhood form, type II G12.1
      distal G12.1
      hereditary NEC G12.1
      infantile, type I (Werdnig-Hoffmann) G12.0
      juvenile form, type III (Kugelberg- Welander) G12.1
      progressive G12.21
      scapuloperoneal form G12.1
      specified NEC G12.8
    syphilitic A52.78
    thigh M62.55- ☑
    upper arm M62.52- ☑
  myocardium — *see* Degeneration, myocardial
  myometrium (senile) N85.8
    cervix N88.8
  myopathic NEC — *see* Atrophy, muscle
  myotonia G71.11
  nail L60.3
  nasopharynx J31.1
  nerve (*see also* Disorder, nerve)
    abducens — *see* Strabismus, paralytic, sixth nerve
    accessory G52.8
    acoustic or auditory H93.3 ☑
    cranial G52.9
      eighth (auditory) H93.3 ☑
      eleventh (accessory) G52.8
      fifth (trigeminal) G50.8
      first (olfactory) G52.0
      fourth (trochlear) — *see* Strabismus, paralytic, fourth nerve
      second (optic) H47.20
      sixth (abducens) — *see* Strabismus, paralytic, sixth nerve
      tenth (pneumogastric) (vagus) G52.2
      third (oculomotor) — *see* Strabismus, paralytic, third nerve
      twelfth (hypoglossal) G52.3
    hypoglossal G52.3
    oculomotor — *see* Strabismus, paralytic, third nerve
    olfactory G52.0
    optic (papillomacular bundle)
      syphilitic (late) A52.15
        congenital A50.44
    pneumogastric G52.2
    trigeminal G50.8
    trochlear — *see* Strabismus, paralytic, fourth nerve
    vagus (pneumogastric) G52.2
  neurogenic, bone, tabetic A52.11
  nutritional E41
  old age R54
  olivopontocerebellar G23.8
  optic (nerve) H47.20
    glaucomatous H47.23- ☑
    hereditary H47.22
    primary H47.21- ☑
    specified type NEC H47.29- ☑
    syphilitic (late) A52.15
      congenital A50.44
  orbit H05.31- ☑
  ovary (senile) N83.31
    with fallopian tube N83.33
  oviduct (senile) — *see* Atrophy, fallopian tube
  palsy, diffuse (progressive) G12.22
  pancreas (duct) (senile) K86.8
  parotid gland K11.0
  pelvic muscle N81.84
  penis N48.89
  pharynx J39.2
  pluriglandular E31.8
    autoimmune E31.0
  polyarthritis M15.9

Atrophy, atrophic — *continued*
  prostate N42.89
  pseudohypertrophic (muscle) G71.0
  renal (*see also* Sclerosis, renal) N26.1
  retina, retinal (postinfectional) H35.89
  rhinitis J31.0
  salivary gland K11.0
  scar L90.5
  sclerosis, lobar (of brain) G31.09 [F02.80]
    with behavioral disturbance G31.09 [F02.81]
  scrotum N50.8
  seminal vesicle N50.8
  senile R54
    due to radiation (nonionizing) (solar) L57.8
  skin (patches) (spots) L90.9
    degenerative (senile) L90.8
    due to radiation (nonionizing) (solar) L57.8
    senile L90.8
  spermatic cord N50.8
  spinal (acute) (cord) G95.89
    muscular — *see* Atrophy, muscle, spinal
    paralysis G12.20
      acute — *see* Poliomyelitis, paralytic
      meaning progressive muscular atrophy G12.21
  spine (column) — *see* Spondylopathy, specified NEC
  spleen (senile) D73.0
  stomach K29.40
    with bleeding K29.41
  striate (skin) L90.6
    syphilitic A52.79
  subcutaneous L90.9
  sublingual gland K11.0
  submandibular gland K11.0
  submaxillary gland K11.0
  Sudeck's — *see* Algoneurodystrophy
  suprarenal (capsule) (gland) E27.49
    primary E27.1
  systemic affecting central nervous system in
      myxedema E03.9 [G13.2]
      neoplastic disease (*see also* Neoplasm) D49.9 [G13.1]
      specified disease NEC G13.8
  tarso-orbital fascia, congenital Q10.3
  testis N50.0
  thenar, partial — *see* Syndrome, carpal tunnel
  thymus (fatty) E32.8
  thyroid (gland) (acquired) E03.4
    with cretinism E03.1
    congenital (with myxedema) E03.1
  tongue (senile) K14.8
    papillae K14.4
  trachea J39.8
  tunica vaginalis N50.8
  turbinate J34.89
  tympanic membrane (nonflaccid) H73.82- ☑
    flaccid H73.81- ☑
  upper respiratory tract J39.8
  uterus, uterine (senile) N85.8
    cervix N88.8
    due to radiation (intended effect) N85.8
      adverse effect or misadventure N99.89
  vagina (senile) N95.2
  vas deferens N50.8
  vascular I99.8
  vertebra (senile) — *see* Spondylopathy, specified NEC
  vulva (senile) N90.5
  Werdnig-Hoffmann G12.0
  yellow — *see* Failure, hepatic
Attack, attacks
  with alteration of consciousness (with automatisms) — *see* Epilepsy, localization-related, symptomatic, with complex partial seizures
  without alteration of consciousness — *see* Epilepsy, localization-related, symptomatic, with simple partial seizures
  Adams-Stokes I45.9
  akinetic — *see* Epilepsy, generalized, specified NEC
  angina — *see* Angina
  atonic — *see* Epilepsy, generalized, specified NEC
  benign shuddering G25.83
  cataleptic — *see* Catalepsy
  coronary — *see* Infarct, myocardium
  cyanotic, newborn P28.2
  drop NEC R55
  epileptic — *see* Epilepsy
  heart — *see* infarct, myocardium
  hysterical F44.9

Attack, attacks — *continued*
  jacksonian — *see* Epilepsy, localization-related, symptomatic, with simple partial seizures
  myocardium, myocardial — *see* Infarct, myocardium
  myoclonic — *see* Epilepsy, generalized, specified NEC
  panic F41.0
  psychomotor — *see* Epilepsy, localization-related, symptomatic, with complex partial seizures
  salaam — *see* Epilepsy, spasms
  schizophreniform, brief F23
  shuddering, benign G25.83
  Stokes-Adams I45.9
  syncope R55
  transient ischemic (TIA) G45.9
    specified NEC G45.8
  unconsciousness R55
    hysterical F44.89
  vasomotor R55
  vasovagal (paroxysmal) (idiopathic) R55
Attention (to)
  artificial
    opening (of) Z43.9
      digestive tract NEC Z43.4
        colon Z43.3
        ilium Z43.2
        stomach Z43.1
      specified NEC Z43.8
      trachea Z43.0
      urinary tract NEC Z43.6
        cystostomy Z43.5
        nephrostomy Z43.6
        ureterostomy Z43.6
        urethrostomy Z43.6
      vagina Z43.7
  colostomy Z43.3
  cystostomy Z43.5
  deficit disorder or syndrome F98.8
    with hyperactivity — *see* Disorder, attention-deficit hyperactivity
  gastrostomy Z43.1
  ileostomy Z43.2
  jejunostomy Z43.4
  nephrostomy Z43.6
  surgical dressings Z48.01
  sutures Z48.02
  tracheostomy Z43.0
  ureterostomy Z43.6
  urethrostomy Z43.6
Attrition
  gum K06.0
  tooth, teeth (excessive) (hard tissues) K03.0
Atypical, atypism (*see also* condition)
  cells (on cytolgocial smear) (endocervical) (endometrial) (glandular)
    cervix R87.619
    vagina R87.629
  cervical N87.9
  endometrium N85.9
    hyperplasia N85.00
  parenting situation Z62.9
Auditory — *see* condition
Aujeszky's disease B33.8
Aurantiasis, cutis E67.1
Auricle, auricular (*see also* condition)
  cervical Q18.2
Auriculotemporal syndrome G50.8
Austin Flint murmur (aortic insufficiency) I35.1
Australian
  Q fever A78
  X disease A83.4
Autism, autistic (childhood) (infantile) F84.0
  atypical F84.9
Autodigestion R68.89
Autoerythrocyte sensitization (syndrome) D69.2
Autographism L50.3
Autoimmune
  disease (systemic) M35.9
  inhibitors to clotting factors D68.311
  lymphoproliferative syndrome [ALPS] D89.82
  thyroiditis E06.3
Autointoxication R68.89
Automatism G93.89
  with temporal sclerosis G93.81
  epileptic — *see* Epilepsy, localization-related, symptomatic, with complex partial seizures
  paroxysmal, idiopathic — *see* Epilepsy, localization-related, symptomatic, with complex partial seizures

Autonomic, autonomous
  bladder (neurogenic) N31.2
  hysteria seizure F44.5
Autosensitivity, erythrocyte D69.2
Autosensitization, cutaneous L30.2
Autosome — *see* condition by chromosome involved
Autotopagnosia R48.1
Autotoxemia R68.89
Autumn — *see* condition
Avellis' syndrome G46.8
Aversion
  oral R63.3
    newborn P92.- ☑
    nonorganic origin F98.2 ☑
  sexual F52.1
Aviator's
  disease or sickness — *see* Effect, adverse, high altitude
  ear T70.0 ☑
Avitaminosis (multiple) (*see also* Deficiency, vitamin)
  E56.9
  B E53.9
    with
      beriberi E51.11
      pellagra E52
  B2 E53.0
  B6 E53.1
  B12 E53.8
  D E55.9
    with rickets E55.0
  G E53.0
  K E56.1
  nicotinic acid E52
AVNRT (atrioventricular nodal re-entrant tachycardia)
  I47.1
AVRT (atrioventricular nodal re-entrant tachycardia) I47.1
Avulsion (traumatic)
  blood vessel — *see* Injury, blood vessel
  bone — *see* Fracture, by site
  cartilage (*see also* Dislocation, by site)
    symphyseal (inner), complicating delivery O71.6
  external site other than limb — *see* Wound, open, by
    site
  eye S05.7- ☑
  head (intracranial)
    external site NEC S08.89 ☑
    scalp S08.0 ☑
  internal organ or site — *see* Injury, by site
  joint (*see also* Dislocation, by site)
    capsule — *see* Sprain, by site
  kidney S37.06- ☑
  ligament — *see* Sprain, by site
  limb (*see also* Amputation, traumatic, by site)
    skin and subcutaneous tissue — *see* Wound, open,
      by site
  muscle — *see* Injury, muscle
  nerve (root) — *see* Injury, nerve
  scalp S08.0 ☑
  skin and subcutaneous tissue — *see* Wound, open, by
    site
  spleen S36.032 ☑
  symphyseal cartilage (inner), complicating delivery
    O71.6
  tendon — *see* Injury, muscle
  tooth S03.2 ☑
Awareness of heart beat R00.2
Axenfeld's
  anomaly or syndrome Q15.0
  degeneration (calcareous) Q13.4
Axilla, axillary (*see also* condition)
  breast Q83.1
Axonotmesis — *see* Injury, nerve
Ayerza's disease or syndrome (pulmonary artery sclerosis with pulmonary hypertension) I27.0
Azoospermia (organic) N46.01
  due to
    drug therapy N46.021
    efferent duct obstruction N46.023
    infection N46.022
    radiation N46.024
    specified cause NEC N46.029
    systemic disease N46.025
Azotemia R79.89
  meaning uremia N19
Aztec ear Q17.3
Azygos
  continuation inferior vena cava Q26.8
  lobe (lung) Q33.1

B

Baastrup's disease — *see* Kissing spine
Babesiosis B60.0
Babington's disease (familial hemorrhagic telangiecta-
  sia) I78.0
Babinski's syndrome A52.79
Baby
  crying constantly R68.11
  floppy (syndrome) P94.2
Bacillary — *see* condition
Bacilluria N39.0
Bacillus (*see also* Infection, bacillus)
  abortus infection A23.1
  anthracis infection A22.9
  coli infection (*see also* Escherichia coli) B96.20
  Flexner's A03.1
  mallei infection A24.0
  Shiga's A03.0
  suipestifer infection — *see* Infection, salmonella
Back — *see* condition
Backache (postural) M54.9
  sacroiliac M53.3
  specified NEC M54.89
Backflow — *see* Reflux
Backward reading (dyslexia) F81.0
Bacteremia R78.81
  with sepsis — *see* Sepsis
Bactericholia — *see* Cholecystitis, acute
Bacterid, bacteride (pustular) L40.3
Bacterium, bacteria, bacterial
  agent NEC, as cause of disease classified elsewhere
    B96.89
  in blood — *see* Bacteremia
  in urine — *see* Bacteriuria
Bacteriuria, bacteruria N39.0
  asymptomatic N39.0
Bacteroides
  fragilis, as cause of disease classified elsewhere B96.6
Bad
  heart — *see* Disease, heart
  trip
    due to drug abuse — *see* Abuse, drug, hallucino-
      gen
    due to drug dependence — *see* Dependence, drug,
      hallucinogen
Baelz's disease (cheilitis glandularis apostematosa) K13.0
Baerensprung's disease (eczema marginatum) B35.6
Bagasse disease or pneumonitis J67.1
Bagassosis J67.1
Baker's cyst — *see* Cyst, Baker's
Bakwin-Krida syndrome (craniometaphyseal dysplasia)
  Q78.5
Balancing side interference M26.56
Balanitis (circinata) (erosiva) (gangrenosa) (phagedenic)
  (vulgaris) N48.1
  amebic A06.82
  candidal B37.42
  due to Haemophilus ducreyi A57
  gonococcal (acute) (chronic) A54.09
  xerotica obliterans N48.0
Balanoposthitis N47.6
  gonococcal (acute) (chronic) A54.09
  ulcerative (specific) A63.8
Balanorrhagia — *see* Balanitis
Balantidiasis, balantidiosis A07.0
Bald tongue K14.4
Baldness (*see also* Alopecia)
  male-pattern — *see* Alopecia, androgenic
Balkan grippe A78
Balloon disease — *see* Effect, adverse, high altitude
Balo's disease (concentric sclerosis) G37.5
Bamberger-Marie disease — *see* Osteoarthropathy,
  hypertrophic, specified type NEC
Bancroft's filariasis B74.0
Band(s)
  adhesive — *see* Adhesions, peritoneum
  anomalous or congenital (*see also* Anomaly, by site)
    heart (atrial) (ventricular) Q24.8
    intestine Q43.3
    omentum Q43.3
  cervix N88.1
  constricting, congenital Q79.8
  gallbladder (congenital) Q44.1
  intestinal (adhesive) — *see* Adhesions, peritoneum

Band(s) — *continued*
  obstructive
    intestine K56.5
    peritoneum K56.5
  periappendiceal, congenital Q43.3
  peritoneal (adhesive) — *see* Adhesions, peritoneum
  uterus N73.6
    internal N85.6
  vagina N89.5
Bandemia D72.825
Bandl's ring (contraction), complicating delivery O62.4
Bangkok hemorrhagic fever A91
Bang's disease (brucella abortus) A23.1
Bankruptcy, anxiety concerning Z59.8
Bannister's disease T78.3 ☑
  hereditary D84.1
Banti's disease or syndrome (with cirrhosis) (with portal
  hypertension) K76.6
Bar, median, prostate — *see* Enlargement, enlarged,
  prostate
Barcoo disease or rot — *see* Ulcer, skin
Barlow's disease E54
Barodontalgia T70.29 ☑
Baron Münchausen syndrome — *see* Disorder, facti-
  tious
Barosinusitis T70.1 ☑
Barotitis T70.0 ☑
Barotrauma T70.29 ☑
  odontalgia T70.29 ☑
  otitic T70.0 ☑
  sinus T70.1 ☑
Barraquer (-Simons) **disease or syndrome** (progressive
  lipodystrophy) E88.1
Barré-Guillain disease or syndrome G61.0
Barrel chest M95.4
Barré-Liéou syndrome (posterior cervical sympathetic)
  M53.0
Barrett's
  disease — *see* Barrett's, esophagus
  esophagus K22.70
    with dysplasia K22.719
      high grade K22.711
      low grade K22.710
    without dysplasia K22.70
  syndrome — *see* Barrett's, esophagus
  ulcer K22.10
    with bleeding K22.11
    without bleeding K22.10
Bársony (-Polgár) (-Teschendorf) **syndrome** (corkscrew
  esophagus) K22.4
Barth syndrome E78.71
Bartholinitis (suppurating) N75.8
  gonococcal (acute) (chronic) (with abscess) A54.1
Bartonellosis A44.9
  cutaneous A44.1
  mucocutaneous A44.1
  specified NEC A44.8
  systemic A44.0
Barton's fracture S52.56- ☑
Bartter's syndrome E26.81
Basal — *see* condition
Basan's (hidrotic) ectodermal dysplasia Q82.4
Baseball finger — *see* Dislocation, finger
Basedow's disease (exophthalmic goiter) — *see* Hyper-
  thyroidism, with, goiter
Basic — *see* condition
Basilar — *see* condition
Bason's (hidrotic) ectodermal dysplasia Q82.4
Basopenia — *see* Agranulocytosis
Basophilia D72.824
Basophilism (cortico-adrenal) (Cushing's) (pituitary)
  E24.0
Bassen-Kornzweig disease or syndrome E78.6
Bat ear Q17.5
Bateman's
  disease B08.1
  purpura (senile) D69.2
Bathing cramp T75.1 ☑
Bathophobia F40.248
Batten (-Mayou) **disease** E75.4
  retina E75.4 [H36]
Batten-Steinert syndrome G71.11
Battered — *see* Maltreatment
Battey Mycobacterium infection A31.0
Battle exhaustion F43.0
Battledore placenta O43.19- ☑

Baumgarten-Cruveilhier cirrhosis, disease or syndrome K74.69
Bauxite fibrosis (of lung) J63.1
Bayle's disease (general paresis) A52.17
Bazin's disease (primary) (tuberculous) A18.4
Beach ear — *see* Swimmer's, ear
Beaded hair (congenital) Q84.1
Béal conjunctivitis or syndrome B30.2
Beard's disease (neurasthenia) F48.8
Beat(s)
  atrial, premature I49.1
  ectopic I49.49
  elbow — *see* Bursitis, elbow
  escaped, heart I49.49
  hand — *see* Bursitis, hand
  knee — *see* Bursitis, knee
  premature I49.40
    atrial I49.1
    auricular I49.1
    supraventricular I49.1
Beau's
  disease or syndrome — *see* Degeneration, myocardial
  lines (transverse furrows on fingernails) L60.4
Bechterev's syndrome — *see* Spondylitis, ankylosing
Becker's
  cardiomyopathy I42.8
  disease
    idiopathic mural endomyocardial disease I42.3
    myotonia congenita, recessive form G71.12
  dystrophy G71.0
  pigmented hairy nevus D22.5
Beck's syndrome (anterior spinal artery occlusion) I65.8
Beckwith-Wiedemann syndrome Q87.3
Bed confinement status Z74.01
Bed sore — *see* Ulcer, pressure, by site
Bedbug bite(s) — *see* Bite(s), by site, superficial, insect
Bedclothes, asphyxiation or suffocation by — *see* Asphyxia, traumatic, due to, mechanical, trapped
Bednar's
  aphthae K12.0
  tumor — *see* Neoplasm, malignant, by site
Bedridden Z74.01
Bedsore — *see* Ulcer, pressure, by site
Bedwetting — *see* Enuresis
Bee sting (with allergic or anaphylactic shock) — *see* Toxicity, venom, arthropod, bee
Beer drinker's heart (disease) I42.6
Begbie's disease (exophthalmic goiter) — *see* Hyperthyroidism, with, goiter
Behavior
  antisocial
    adult Z72.811
    child or adolescent Z72.810
  disorder, disturbance — *see* Disorder, conduct
  disruptive — *see* Disorder, conduct
  drug seeking Z72.89
  inexplicable R46.2
  marked evasiveness R46.5
  obsessive-compulsive R46.81
  overactivity R46.3
  poor responsiveness R46.4
  self-damaging (life-style) Z72.89
  sleep-incompatible Z72.821
  slowness R46.4
  specified NEC R46.89
  strange (and inexplicable) R46.2
  suspiciousness R46.5
  type A pattern Z73.1
  undue concern or preoccupation with stressful events R46.6
  verbosity and circumstantial detail obscuring reason for contact R46.7
Behçet's disease or syndrome M35.2
Behr's disease — *see* Degeneration, macula
Beigel's disease or morbus (white piedra) B36.2
Bejel A65
Bekhterev's syndrome — *see* Spondylitis, ankylosing
Belching — *see* Eructation
Bell's
  mania F30.8
  palsy, paralysis G51.0
    infant or newborn P11.3
  spasm G51.3
Bence Jones albuminuria or proteinuria NEC R80.3
Bends T70.3 ☑
Benedikt's paralysis or syndrome G46.3

Benign (*see also* condition)
  prostatic hyperplasia — *see* Hyperplasia, prostate
Bennett's fracture (displaced) S62.21- ☑
Benson's disease — *see* Deposit, crystalline
Bent
  back (hysterical) F44.4
  nose M95.0
    congenital Q67.4
Bereavement (uncomplicated) Z63.4
Bergeron's disease (hysterical chorea) F44.4
Berger's disease — *see* Nephropathy, IgA
Beriberi (dry) E51.11
  heart (disease) E51.12
  polyneuropathy E51.11
  wet E51.12
    involving circulatory system E51.11
Berlin's disease or edema (traumatic) S05.8X- ☑
Berlock (berloque) **dermatitis** L56.2
Bernard-Horner syndrome G90.2
Bernard-Soulier disease or thrombopathia D69.1
Bernhardt (-Roth) **disease** — *see* Mononeuropathy, lower limb, meralgia paresthetica
Bernheim's syndrome — *see* Failure, heart, congestive
Bertielliasis B71.8
Berylliosis (lung) J63.2
Besnier-Boeck (-Schaumann) **disease** — *see* Sarcoidosis
Besnier's
  lupus pernio D86.3
  prurigo L20.0
Bestiality F65.89
Best's disease H35.50
Betalipoproteinemia, broad or floating E78.2
Beta-mercaptolactate-cysteine disulfiduria E72.09
Betting and gambling Z72.6
  pathological (compulsive) F63.0
Bezoar T18.9 ☑
  intestine T18.3 ☑
  stomach T18.2 ☑
Bezold's abscess — *see* Mastoiditis, acute
Bianchi's syndrome R48.8
Bicornate or bicornis uterus Q51.3
  in pregnancy or childbirth O34.59- ☑
    causing obstructed labor O65.5
Bicuspid aortic valve Q23.1
Biedl-Bardet syndrome Q87.89
Bielschowsky (-Jansky) **disease** E75.4
Biermer's (pernicious) anemia or disease D51.0
Biett's disease L93.0
Bifid (congenital)
  apex, heart Q24.8
  clitoris Q52.6
  kidney Q63.8
  nose Q30.2
  patella Q74.1
  scrotum Q55.29
  toe NEC Q74.2
  tongue Q38.3
  ureter Q62.8
  uterus Q51.3
  uvula Q35.7
Biforis uterus (suprasimplex) Q51.3
Bifurcation (congenital)
  gallbladder Q44.1
  kidney pelvis Q63.8
  renal pelvis Q63.8
  rib Q76.6
  tongue, congenital Q38.3
  trachea Q32.1
  ureter Q62.8
  urethra Q64.74
  vertebra Q76.49
Big spleen syndrome D73.1
Bigeminal pulse R00.8
Bilateral — *see* condition
Bile
  duct — *see* condition
  pigments in urine R82.2
Bilharziasis (*see also* Schistosomiasis)
  chyluria B65.0
  cutaneous B65.3
  galacturia B65.0
  hematochyluria B65.0
  intestinal B65.1
  lipemia B65.9
  lipuria B65.0
  oriental B65.2
  piarhemia B65.9

Bilharziasis — *continued*
  pulmonary NOS B65.9 [J99]
    pneumonia B65.9 [J17]
  tropical hematuria B65.0
  vesical B65.0
Biliary — *see* condition
Bilirubin metabolism disorder E80.7
  specified NEC E80.6
Bilirubinemia, familial nonhemolytic E80.4
Bilirubinuria R82.2
Biliuria R82.2
Bilocular stomach K31.2
Binswanger's disease I67.3
Biparta, bipartite
  carpal scaphoid Q74.0
  patella Q74.1
  vagina Q52.10
Bird
  face Q75.8
  fancier's disease or lung J67.2
Birth
  complications in mother — *see* Delivery, complicated
  compression during NOS P15.9
  defect — *see* Anomaly
  immature (less than 37 completed weeks) — *see* Preterm, newborn
    extremely (less than 28 completed weeks) — *see* Immaturity, extreme
  inattention, at or after — *see* Maltreatment, child, neglect
  injury NOS P15.9
    basal ganglia P11.1
    brachial plexus NEC P14.3
    brain (compression) (pressure) P11.2
    central nervous system NOS P11.9
    cerebellum P11.1
    cerebral hemorrhage P10.1
    external genitalia P15.5
    eye P15.3
    face P15.4
    fracture
      bone P13.9
        specified NEC P13.8
      clavicle P13.4
      femur P13.2
      humerus P13.3
      long bone, except femur P13.3
      radius and ulna P13.3
      skull P13.0
      spine P11.5
      tibia and fibula P13.3
    intracranial P11.2
      laceration or hemorrhage P10.9
        specified NEC P10.8
    intraventricular hemorrhage P10.2
    laceration
      brain P10.1
      by scalpel P15.8
      peripheral nerve P14.9
    liver P15.0
    meninges
      brain P11.1
      spinal cord P11.5
    nerve
      brachial plexus P14.3
      cranial NEC (except facial) P11.4
      facial P11.3
      peripheral P14.9
      phrenic (paralysis) P14.2
    paralysis
      facial nerve P11.3
      spinal P11.5
    penis P15.5
    rupture
      spinal cord P11.5
    scalp P12.9
    scalpel wound P15.8
    scrotum P15.5
    skull NEC P13.1
      fracture P13.0
    specified type NEC P15.8
    spinal cord P11.5
    spine P11.5
    spleen P15.1
    sternomastoid (hematoma) P15.2
    subarachnoid hemorrhage P10.3
    subcutaneous fat necrosis P15.6
    subdural hemorrhage P10.0

☑ **Additional Character Required** — Refer to the Tabular List for Character Selection   ▽ Subterms under main terms may continue to next column or page

Birth — *continued*
  injury — *continued*
    tentorial tear P10.4
    testes P15.5
    vulva P15.5
  lack of care, at or after — *see* Maltreatment, child, neglect
  neglect, at or after — *see* Maltreatment, child, neglect
  palsy or paralysis, newborn, NOS (birth injury) P14.9
  premature (infant) — *see* Preterm, newborn
  shock, newborn P96.89
  trauma — *see* Birth, injury
  weight
    4000 grams to 4499 grams P08.1
    4500 grams or more P08.0
    low (2499 grams or less) — *see* Low, birthweight
      extremely (999 grams or less) — *see* Low, birthweight, extreme
Birthmark Q82.5
Birt-Hogg-Dube syndrome Q87.89
Bisalbuminemia E88.09
Biskra's button B55.1
Bite(s) (animal) (human)
  abdomen, abdominal
    wall S31.159 ☑
      with penetration into peritoneal cavity S31.659 ☑
      epigastric region S31.152 ☑
        with penetration into peritoneal cavity S31.652 ☑
      left
        lower quadrant S31.154 ☑
          with penetration into peritoneal cavity S31.654 ☑
        upper quadrant S31.151 ☑
          with penetration into peritoneal cavity S31.651 ☑
      periumbilic region S31.155 ☑
        with penetration into peritoneal cavity S31.655 ☑
      right
        lower quadrant S31.153 ☑
          with penetration into peritoneal cavity S31.653 ☑
        upper quadrant S31.150 ☑
          with penetration into peritoneal cavity S31.650 ☑
      superficial NEC S30.871 ☑
        insect S30.861 ☑
  alveolar (process) — *see* Bite, oral cavity
  amphibian (venomous) — *see* Venom, bite, amphibian
  animal (*see also* Bite, by site)
    venomous — *see* Venom
  ankle S91.05- ☑
    superficial NEC S90.57- ☑
      insect S90.56- ☑
  antecubital space — *see* Bite, elbow
  anus S31.835 ☑
    superficial NEC S30.877 ☑
      insect S30.867 ☑
  arm (upper) S41.15- ☑
    lower — *see* Bite, forearm
    superficial NEC S40.87- ☑
      insect S40.86- ☑
  arthropod NEC — *see* Venom, bite, arthropod
  auditory canal (external) (meatus) — *see* Bite, ear
  auricle, ear — *see* Bite, ear
  axilla — *see* Bite, arm
  back (*see also* Bite, thorax, back)
    lower S31.050 ☑
      with penetration into retroperitoneal space S31.051 ☑
      superficial NEC S30.870 ☑
        insect S30.860 ☑
  bedbug — *see* Bite(s), by site, superficial, insect
  breast S21.05- ☑
    superficial NEC S20.17- ☑
      insect S20.16- ☑
  brow — *see* Bite, head, specified site NEC
  buttock S31.805 ☑
    left S31.825 ☑
    right S31.815 ☑
    superficial NEC S30.870 ☑
      insect S30.860 ☑
  calf — *see* Bite, leg
  canaliculus lacrimalis — *see* Bite, eyelid

Bite(s) — *continued*
  canthus, eye — *see* Bite, eyelid
  centipede — *see* Toxicity, venom, arthropod, centipede
  cheek (external) S01.45- ☑
    internal — *see* Bite, oral cavity
    superficial NEC S00.87 ☑
      insect S00.86 ☑
  chest wall — *see* Bite, thorax
  chigger B88.0
  chin — *see* Bite, head, specified site NEC
  clitoris — *see* Bite, vulva
  costal region — *see* Bite, thorax
  digit(s)
    hand — *see* Bite, finger
    toe — *see* Bite, toe
  ear (canal) (external) S01.35- ☑
    superficial NEC S00.47- ☑
      insect S00.46- ☑
  elbow S51.05- ☑
    superficial NEC S50.37- ☑
      insect S50.36- ☑
  epididymis — *see* Bite, testis
  epigastric region — *see* Bite, abdomen
  epiglottis — *see* Bite, neck, specified site NEC
  esophagus, cervical S11.25 ☑
    superficial NEC S10.17 ☑
      insect S10.16 ☑
  eyebrow — *see* Bite, eyelid
  eyelid S01.15- ☑
    superficial NEC S00.27- ☑
      insect S00.26- ☑
  face NEC — *see* Bite, head, specified site NEC
  finger(s) S61.259 ☑
    with
      damage to nail S61.359 ☑
    index S61.258 ☑
      with
        damage to nail S61.358 ☑
      left S61.251 ☑
        with
          damage to nail S61.351 ☑
      right S61.250 ☑
        with
          damage to nail S61.350 ☑
      superficial NEC S60.478 ☑
        insect S60.46- ☑
    little S61.25- ☑
      with
        damage to nail S61.35- ☑
      superficial NEC S60.47- ☑
        insect S60.46- ☑
    middle S61.25- ☑
      with
        damage to nail S61.35- ☑
      superficial NEC S60.47- ☑
        insect S60.46- ☑
    ring S61.25- ☑
      with
        damage to nail S61.35- ☑
      superficial NEC S60.47- ☑
        insect S60.46- ☑
    superficial NEC S60.479 ☑
      insect S60.469 ☑
    thumb — *see* Bite, thumb
  flank — *see* Bite, abdomen, wall
  flea — *see* Bite, by site, superficial, insect
  foot (except toe(s) alone) S91.35- ☑
    superficial NEC S90.87- ☑
      insect S90.86- ☑
    toe — *see* Bite, toe
  forearm S51.85- ☑
    elbow only — *see* Bite, elbow
    superficial NEC S50.87- ☑
      insect S50.86- ☑
  forehead — *see* Bite, head, specified site NEC
  genital organs, external
    female S31.552 ☑
      superficial NEC S30.876 ☑
        insect S30.866 ☑
      vagina and vulva — *see* Bite, vulva
    male S31.551 ☑
      penis — *see* Bite, penis
      scrotum — *see* Bite, scrotum
      superficial NEC S30.875 ☑
        insect S30.865 ☑

Bite(s) — *continued*
  genital organs, external — *continued*
    male — *continued*
      testes — *see* Bite, testis
  groin — *see* Bite, abdomen, wall
  gum — *see* Bite, oral cavity
  hand S61.45- ☑
    finger — *see* Bite, finger
    superficial NEC S60.57- ☑
      insect S60.56- ☑
    thumb — *see* Bite, thumb
  head S01.95 ☑
    cheek — *see* Bite, cheek
    ear — *see* Bite, ear
    eyelid — *see* Bite, eyelid
    lip — *see* Bite, lip
    nose — *see* Bite, nose
    oral cavity — *see* Bite, oral cavity
    scalp — *see* Bite, scalp
    specified site NEC S01.85 ☑
      superficial NEC S00.87 ☑
        insect S00.86 ☑
    superficial NEC S00.97 ☑
      insect S00.96 ☑
    temporomandibular area — *see* Bite, cheek
  heel — *see* Bite, foot
  hip S71.05- ☑
    superficial NEC S70.27- ☑
      insect S70.26- ☑
  hymen S31.45 ☑
  hypochondrium — *see* Bite, abdomen, wall
  hypogastric region — *see* Bite, abdomen, wall
  inguinal region — *see* Bite, abdomen, wall
  insect — *see* Bite, by site, superficial, insect
  instep — *see* Bite, foot
  interscapular region — *see* Bite, thorax, back
  jaw — *see* Bite, head, specified site NEC
  knee S81.05- ☑
    superficial NEC S80.27- ☑
      insect S80.26- ☑
  labium (majus) (minus) — *see* Bite, vulva
  lacrimal duct — *see* Bite, eyelid
  larynx S11.015 ☑
    superficial NEC S10.17 ☑
      insect S10.16 ☑
  leg (lower) S81.85- ☑
    ankle — *see* Bite, ankle
    foot — *see* Bite, foot
    knee — *see* Bite, knee
    superficial NEC S80.87- ☑
      insect S80.86- ☑
    toe — *see* Bite, toe
    upper — *see* Bite, thigh
  lip S01.551 ☑
    superficial NEC S00.571 ☑
      insect S00.561 ☑
  lizard (venomous) — *see* Venom, bite, reptile
  loin — *see* Bite, abdomen, wall
  lower back — *see* Bite, back, lower
  lumbar region — *see* Bite, back, lower
  malar region — *see* Bite, head, specified site NEC
  mammary — *see* Bite, breast
  marine animals (venomous) — *see* Toxicity, venom, marine animal
  mastoid region — *see* Bite, head, specified site NEC
  mouth — *see* Bite, oral cavity
  nail
    finger — *see* Bite, finger
    toe — *see* Bite, toe
  nape — *see* Bite, neck, specified site NEC
  nasal (septum) (sinus) — *see* Bite, nose
  nasopharynx — *see* Bite, head, specified site NEC
  neck S11.95 ☑
    involving
      cervical esophagus — *see* Bite, esophagus, cervical
      larynx — *see* Bite, larynx
      pharynx — *see* Bite, pharynx
      thyroid gland S11.15 ☑
      trachea — *see* Bite, trachea
    specified site NEC S11.85 ☑
      superficial NEC S10.87 ☑
        insect S10.86 ☑
    superficial NEC S10.97 ☑
      insect S10.96 ☑
  throat S11.85 ☑

Bite(s) — *continued*
  neck — *continued*
    throat — *continued*
      superficial NEC S10.17 ☑
        insect S10.16 ☑
  nose (septum) (sinus) S01.25 ☑
    superficial NEC S00.37 ☑
      insect S00.36 ☑
  occipital region — *see* Bite, scalp
  oral cavity S01.552 ☑
    superficial NEC S00.572 ☑
      insect S00.562 ☑
  orbital region — *see* Bite, eyelid
  palate — *see* Bite, oral cavity
  palm — *see* Bite, hand
  parietal region — *see* Bite, scalp
  pelvis S31.050 ☑
    with penetration into retroperitoneal space
      S31.051 ☑
    superficial NEC S30.870 ☑
      insect S30.860 ☑
  penis S31.25 ☑
    superficial NEC S30.872 ☑
      insect S30.862 ☑
  perineum
    female — *see* Bite, vulva
    male — *see* Bite, pelvis
  periocular area (with or without lacrimal passages) —
      see Bite, eyelid
  phalanges
    finger — *see* Bite, finger
    toe — *see* Bite, toe
  pharynx S11.25 ☑
    superficial NEC S10.17 ☑
      insect S10.16 ☑
  pinna — *see* Bite, ear
  poisonous — *see* Venom
  popliteal space — *see* Bite, knee
  prepuce — *see* Bite, penis
  pubic region — *see* Bite, abdomen, wall
  rectovaginal septum — *see* Bite, vulva
  red bug B88.0
  reptile NEC (*see also* Venom, bite, reptile)
    nonvenomous — *see* Bite, by site
    snake — *see* Venom, bite, snake
  sacral region — *see* Bite, back, lower
  sacroiliac region — *see* Bite, back, lower
  salivary gland — *see* Bite, oral cavity
  scalp S01.05 ☑
    superficial NEC S00.07 ☑
      insect S00.06 ☑
  scapular region — *see* Bite, shoulder
  scrotum S31.35 ☑
    superficial NEC S30.873 ☑
      insect S30.863 ☑
  sea-snake (venomous) — *see* Toxicity, venom, snake,
      sea snake
  shin — *see* Bite, leg
  shoulder S41.05- ☑
    superficial NEC S40.27- ☑
      insect S40.26- ☑
  snake (*see also* Venom, bite, snake)
    nonvenomous — *see* Bite, by site
  spermatic cord — *see* Bite, testis
  spider (venomous) — *see* Toxicity, venom, spider
    nonvenomous — *see* Bite, by site, superficial, insect
  sternal region — *see* Bite, thorax, front
  submaxillary region — *see* Bite, head, specified site
      NEC
  submental region — *see* Bite, head, specified site NEC
  subungual
    finger(s) — *see* Bite, finger
    toe — *see* Bite, toe
  superficial — *see* Bite, by site, superficial
  supraclavicular fossa S11.85 ☑
  supraorbital — *see* Bite, head, specified site NEC
  temple, temporal region — *see* Bite, head, specified
      site NEC
  temporomandibular area — *see* Bite, cheek
  testis S31.35 ☑
    superficial NEC S30.873 ☑
      insect S30.863 ☑
  thigh S71.15- ☑
    superficial NEC S70.37- ☑
      insect S70.36- ☑
  thorax, thoracic (wall) S21.95 ☑

Bite(s) — *continued*
  thorax, thoracic — *continued*
    back S21.25- ☑
      with penetration into thoracic cavity S21.45- ☑
    breast — *see* Bite, breast
    front S21.15- ☑
      with penetration into thoracic cavity S21.35- ☑
    superficial NEC S20.97 ☑
      back S20.47- ☑
      front S20.37- ☑
      insect S20.96 ☑
        back S20.46- ☑
        front S20.36- ☑
  throat — *see* Bite, neck, throat
  thumb S61.05- ☑
    with
      damage to nail S61.15- ☑
    superficial NEC S60.37- ☑
      insect S60.36- ☑
  thyroid S11.15 ☑
    superficial NEC S10.87 ☑
      insect S10.86 ☑
  toe(s) S91.15- ☑
    with
      damage to nail S91.25- ☑
    great S91.15- ☑
      with
        damage to nail S91.25- ☑
    lesser S91.15- ☑
      with
        damage to nail S91.25- ☑
    superficial NEC S90.47- ☑
      great S90.47- ☑
      insect S90.46- ☑
        great S90.46- ☑
  tongue S01.552 ☑
  trachea S11.025 ☑
    superficial NEC S10.17 ☑
      insect S10.16 ☑
  tunica vaginalis — *see* Bite, testis
  tympanum, tympanic membrane — *see* Bite, ear
  umbilical region S31.155 ☑
  uvula — *see* Bite, oral cavity
  vagina — *see* Bite, vulva
  venomous — *see* Venom
  vocal cords S11.035 ☑
    superficial NEC S10.17 ☑
      insect S10.16 ☑
  vulva S31.45 ☑
    superficial NEC S30.874 ☑
      insect S30.864 ☑
  wrist S61.55- ☑
    superficial NEC S60.87- ☑
      insect S60.86- ☑
Biting, cheek or lip K13.1
Biventricular failure (heart) I50.9
Björck (-Thorson) **syndrome** (malignant carcinoid) E34.0
Black
  death A20.9
  eye S00.1- ☑
  hairy tongue K14.3
  heel (foot) S90.3- ☑
  lung (disease) J60
  palm (hand) S60.22- ☑
Blackfan-Diamond anemia or syndrome (congenital
      hypoplastic anemia) D61.01
Blackhead L70.0
Blackout R55
Bladder — *see* condition
Blast (air) (hydraulic) (immersion) (underwater)
  blindness S05.8X- ☑
  injury
    abdomen or thorax — *see* Injury, by site
    ear (acoustic nerve trauma) — *see* Injury, nerve,
        acoustic, specified type NEC
    syndrome NEC T70.8
Blastoma — *see* Neoplasm, malignant, by site
  pulmonary — *see* Neoplasm, lung, malignant
Blastomycosis, blastomycotic B40.9
  Brazilian — *see* Paracoccidioidomycosis
  cutaneous B40.3
  disseminated B40.7
  European — *see* Cryptococcosis
  generalized B40.7
  keloidal B48.0
  North American B40.9

Blastomycosis, blastomycotic — *continued*
  primary pulmonary B40.0
  pulmonary B40.2
    acute B40.0
    chronic B40.1
  skin B40.3
  South American — *see* Paracoccidioidomycosis
  specified NEC B40.89
Bleb(s) R23.8
  emphysematous (lung) (solitary) J43.9
  endophthalmitis H59.43
  filtering (vitreous), after glaucoma surgery Z98.83
  inflamed (infected), postprocedural H59.40
    stage 1 H59.41
    stage 2 H59.42
    stage 3 H59.43
  lung (ruptured) J43.9
    congenital — *see* Atelectasis
    newborn P25.8
  subpleural (emphysematous) J43.9
Blebitis, postprocedural H59.40
  stage 1 H59.41
  stage 2 H59.42
  stage 3 H59.43
Bleeder (familial) (hereditary) — *see* Hemophilia
Bleeding (*see also* Hemorrhage)
  anal K62.5
  anovulatory N97.0
  atonic, following delivery O72.1
  capillary I78.8
    puerperal O72.2
  contact (postcoital) N93.0
  due to uterine subinvolution N85.3
  ear — *see* Otorrhagia
  excessive, associated with menopausal onset N92.4
  familial — *see* Defect, coagulation
  following intercourse N93.0
  gastrointestinal K92.2
  hemorrhoids — *see* Hemorrhoids
  intermenstrual (regular) N92.3
    irregular N92.1
  intraoperative — *see* Complication, intraoperative,
      hemorrhage
  irregular N92.6
  menopausal N92.4
  newborn, intraventricular — *see* Newborn, affected
      by, hemorrhage, intraventricular
  nipple N64.59
  nose R04.0
  ovulation N92.3
  postclimacteric N95.0
  postcoital N93.0
  postmenopausal N95.0
  postoperative — *see* Complication, postprocedural,
      hemorrhage
  preclimacteric N92.4
  puberty (excessive, with onset of menstrual periods)
      N92.2
  rectum, rectal K62.5
    newborn P54.2
  tendencies — *see* Defect, coagulation
  throat R04.1
  tooth socket (post-extraction) K91.840
  umbilical stump P51.9
  uterus, uterine NEC N93.9
    climacteric N92.4
    dysfunctional of functional N93.8
    menopausal N92.4
    preclimacteric or premenopausal N92.4
    unrelated to menstrual cycle N93.9
  vagina, vaginal (abnormal) N93.9
    dysfunctional or functional N93.8
    newborn P54.6
  vicarious N94.89
Blennorrhagia, blennorrhagic — *see* Gonorrhea
Blennorrhea (acute) (chronic) (*see also* Gonorrhea)
  inclusion (neonatal) (newborn) P39.1
  lower genitourinary tract (gonococcal) A54.00
  neonatorum (gonococcal ophthalmia) A54.31
Blepharelosis — *see* Entropion
Blepharitis (angularis) (ciliaris) (eyelid) (marginal)
      (nonulcerative) H01.009
  herpes zoster B02.39
  left H01.006
    lower H01.005
    upper H01.004
  right H01.003
    lower H01.002

Blepharitis — *continued*
right — *continued*
upper H01.001
squamous H01.029
left H01.026
lower H01.025
upper H01.024
right H01.023
lower H01.022
upper H01.021
ulcerative H01.019
left H01.016
lower H01.015
upper H01.014
right H01.013
lower H01.012
upper H01.011
Blepharochalasis H02.30
congenital Q10.0
left H02.36
lower H02.35
upper H02.34
right H02.33
lower H02.32
upper H02.31
Blepharoclonus H02.59
Blepharoconjunctivitis H10.50- ☑
angular H10.52- ☑
contact H10.53- ☑
ligneous H10.51- ☑
Blepharophimosis (eyelid) H02.529
congenital Q10.3
left H02.526
lower H02.525
upper H02.524
right H02.523
lower H02.522
upper H02.521
Blepharoptosis H02.40- ☑
congenital Q10.0
mechanical H02.41- ☑
myogenic H02.42- ☑
neurogenic H02.43- ☑
paralytic H02.43- ☑
Blepharopyorrhea, gonococcal A54.39
Blepharospasm G24.5
drug induced G24.01
Blighted ovum O02.0
Blind (*see also* Blindness)
bronchus (congenital) Q32.4
loop syndrome K90.2
congenital Q43.8
sac, fallopian tube (congenital) Q50.6
spot, enlarged — *see* Defect, visual field, localized, scotoma, blind spot area
tract or tube, congenital NEC — *see* Atresia, by site
Blindness (acquired) (congenital) (both eyes) H54.0
blast S05.8X- ☑
color — *see* Deficiency, color vision
concussion S05.8X- ☑
cortical H47.619
left brain H47.612
right brain H47.611
day H53.11
due to injury (current episode) S05.9- ☑
sequelae — *code to* injury with seventh character S
eclipse (total) — *see* Retinopathy, solar
emotional (hysterical) F44.6
face H53.16
hysterical F44.6
legal (both eyes) (USA definition) H54.8
mind R48.8
night H53.60
abnormal dark adaptation curve H53.61
acquired H53.62
congenital H53.63
specified type NEC H53.69
vitamin A deficiency E50.5
one eye (other eye normal) H54.40
left (normal vision on right) H54.42
low vision on right H54.12
low vision, other eye H54.10
right (normal vision on left) H54.41
low vision on left H54.11
psychic R48.8
river B73.01
snow — *see* Photokeratitis

Blindness — *continued*
sun, solar — *see* Retinopathy, solar
transient — *see* Disturbance, vision, subjective, loss, transient
traumatic (current episode) S05.9- ☑
word (developmental) F81.0
acquired R48.0
secondary to organic lesion R48.0
Blister (nonthermal)
abdominal wall S30.821 ☑
alveolar process S00.522 ☑
ankle S90.52- ☑
antecubital space — *see* Blister, elbow
anus S30.827 ☑
arm (upper) S40.82- ☑
auditory canal — *see* Blister, ear
auricle — *see* Blister, ear
axilla — *see* Blister, arm
back, lower S30.820 ☑
beetle dermatitis L24.89
breast S20.12- ☑
brow S00.82 ☑
calf — *see* Blister, leg
canthus — *see* Blister, eyelid
cheek S00.82 ☑
internal S00.522 ☑
chest wall — *see* Blister, thorax
chin S00.82 ☑
costal region — *see* Blister, thorax
digit(s)
foot — *see* Blister, toe
hand — *see* Blister, finger
due to burn — *see* Burn, by site, second degree
ear S00.42- ☑
elbow S50.32- ☑
epiglottis S10.12 ☑
esophagus, cervical S10.12 ☑
eyebrow — *see* Blister, eyelid
eyelid S00.22- ☑
face S00.82 ☑
fever B00.1
finger(s) S60.429 ☑
index S60.42- ☑
little S60.42- ☑
middle S60.42- ☑
ring S60.42- ☑
foot (except toe(s) alone) S90.82- ☑
toe — *see* Blister, toe
forearm S50.82- ☑
elbow only — *see* Blister, elbow
forehead S00.82 ☑
fracture — *omit code*
genital organ
female S30.826 ☑
male S30.825 ☑
gum S00.522 ☑
hand S60.52- ☑
head S00.92 ☑
ear — *see* Blister, ear
eyelid — *see* Blister, eyelid
lip S00.521 ☑
nose S00.32 ☑
oral cavity S00.522 ☑
scalp S00.02 ☑
specified site NEC S00.82 ☑
heel — *see* Blister, foot
hip S70.22- ☑
interscapular region S20.429 ☑
jaw S00.82 ☑
knee S80.22- ☑
larynx S10.12 ☑
leg (lower) S80.82- ☑
knee — *see* Blister, knee
upper — *see* Blister, thigh
lip S00.521 ☑
malar region S00.82 ☑
mammary — *see* Blister, breast
mastoid region S00.82 ☑
mouth S00.522 ☑
multiple, skin, nontraumatic R23.8
nail
finger — *see* Blister, finger
toe — *see* Blister, toe
nasal S00.32 ☑
neck S10.92 ☑
specified site NEC S10.82 ☑

Blister — *continued*
neck — *continued*
throat S10.12 ☑
nose S00.32 ☑
occipital region S00.02 ☑
oral cavity S00.522 ☑
orbital region — *see* Blister, eyelid
palate S00.522 ☑
palm — *see* Blister, hand
parietal region S00.02 ☑
pelvis S30.820 ☑
penis S30.822 ☑
periocular area — *see* Blister, eyelid
phalanges
finger — *see* Blister, finger
toe — *see* Blister, toe
pharynx S10.12 ☑
pinna — *see* Blister, ear
popliteal space — *see* Blister, knee
scalp S00.02 ☑
scapular region — *see* Blister, shoulder
scrotum S30.823 ☑
shin — *see* Blister, leg
shoulder S40.22- ☑
sternal region S20.329 ☑
submaxillary region S00.82 ☑
submental region S00.82 ☑
subungual
finger(s) — *see* Blister, finger
toe(s) — *see* Blister, toe
supraclavicular fossa S10.82 ☑
supraorbital S00.82 ☑
temple S00.82 ☑
temporal region S00.82 ☑
testis S30.823 ☑
thermal — *see* Burn, second degree, by site
thigh S70.32- ☑
thorax, thoracic (wall) S20.92 ☑
back S20.42- ☑
front S20.32- ☑
throat S10.12 ☑
thumb S60.32- ☑
toe(s) S90.42- ☑
great S90.42- ☑
tongue S00.522 ☑
trachea S10.12 ☑
tympanum, tympanic membrane — *see* Blister, ear
upper arm — *see* Blister, arm (upper)
uvula S00.522 ☑
vagina S30.824 ☑
vocal cords S10.12 ☑
vulva S30.824 ☑
wrist S60.82- ☑
Bloating R14.0
Bloch-Sulzberger disease or syndrome Q82.3
Block, blocked
alveolocapillary J84.10
arborization (heart) I45.5
arrhythmic I45.9
atrioventricular (incomplete) (partial) I44.30
with atrioventricular dissociation I44.2
complete I44.2
congenital Q24.6
congenital Q24.6
first degree I44.0
second degree (types I and II) I44.1
specified NEC I44.39
third degree I44.2
types I and II I44.1
auriculoventricular — *see* Block, atrioventricular
bifascicular (cardiac) I45.2
bundle-branch (complete) (false) (incomplete) I45.4
bilateral I45.2
left I44.7
with right bundle branch block I45.2
hemiblock I44.60
anterior I44.4
posterior I44.5
incomplete I44.7
with right bundle branch block I45.2
right I45.10
with
left bundle branch block I45.2
left fascicular block I45.2
specified NEC I45.19
Wilson's type I45.19
cardiac I45.9

Block, blocked — *continued*
  conduction I45.9
    complete I44.2
  fascicular (left) I44.60
    anterior I44.4
    posterior I44.5
    right I45.0
    specified NEC I44.69
  foramen Magendie (acquired) G91.1
    congenital Q03.1
      with spina bifida — *see* Spina bifida, by site, with hydrocephalus
  heart I45.9
    bundle branch I45.4
      bilateral I45.2
    complete (atrioventricular) I44.2
    congenital Q24.6
    first degree (atrioventricular) I44.0
    second degree (atrioventricular) I44.1
    specified type NEC I45.5
    third degree (atrioventricular) I44.2
  hepatic vein I82.0
  intraventricular (nonspecific) I45.4
    bundle branch
      bilateral I45.2
  kidney N28.9
    postcystoscopic or postprocedural N99.0
  Mobitz (types I and II) I44.1
  myocardial — *see* Block, heart
  nodal I45.5
  organ or site, congenital NEC — *see* Atresia, by site
  portal (vein) I81
  second degree (types I and II) I44.1
  sinoatrial I45.5
  sinoauricular I45.5
  third degree I44.2
  trifascicular I45.3
  tubal N97.1
  vein NOS I82.90
  Wenckebach (types I and II) I44.1
Blockage — *see* Obstruction
Blocq's disease F44.4
Blood
  constituents, abnormal R78.9
  disease D75.9
  donor — *see* Donor, blood
  dyscrasia D75.9
    with
      abortion — *see* Abortion, by type, complicated by, hemorrhage
      ectopic pregnancy O08.1
      molar pregnancy O08.1
    following ectopic or molar pregnancy O08.1
    newborn P61.9
    puerperal, postpartum O72.3
  flukes NEC — *see* Schistosomiasis
  in
    feces K92.1
      occult R19.5
    urine — *see* Hematuria
  mole O02.0
  occult in feces R19.5
  pressure
    decreased, due to shock following injury T79.4 ☑
    examination only Z01.30
    fluctuating I99.8
    high — *see* Hypertension
      borderline R03.0
      incidental reading, without diagnosis of hypertension R03.0
    low (*see also* Hypotension)
      incidental reading, without diagnosis of hypotension R03.1
  spitting — *see* Hemoptysis
  staining cornea — *see* Pigmentation, cornea, stromal
  transfusion
    reaction or complication — *see* Complications, transfusion
  type
    A (Rh positive) Z67.10
      Rh negative Z67.11
    AB (Rh positive) Z67.30
      Rh negative Z67.31
    B (Rh positive) Z67.20
      Rh negative Z67.21
    O (Rh positive) Z67.40
      Rh negative Z67.41
    Rh (positive) Z67.90

Blood — *continued*
  type — *continued*
    Rh — *continued*
      negative Z67.91
  vessel rupture — *see* Hemorrhage
  vomiting — *see* Hematemesis
Blood-forming organs, disease D75.9
Bloodgood's disease — *see* Mastopathy, cystic
Bloom (-Machacek)(-Torre) **syndrome** Q82.8
Blount's disease or osteochondrosis — *see* Osteochondrosis, juvenile, tibia
Blue
  baby Q24.9
  diaper syndrome E72.09
  dome cyst (breast) — *see* Cyst, breast
  dot cataract Q12.0
  nevus D22.9
  sclera Q13.5
    with fragility of bone and deafness Q78.0
  toe syndrome I75.02- ☑
Blueness — *see* Cyanosis
Blues, postpartal O90.6
  baby O90.6
Blurring, visual H53.8
Blushing (abnormal) (excessive) R23.2
BMI — *see* Body, mass index
Boarder, hospital NEC Z76.4
  accompanying sick person Z76.3
  healthy infant or child Z76.2
    foundling Z76.1
Bockhart's impetigo L01.02
Bodechtel-Guttman disease (subacute sclerosing panencephalitis) A81.1
Boder-Sedgwick syndrome (ataxia-telangiectasia) G11.3
Body, bodies
  Aschoff's — *see* Myocarditis, rheumatic
  asteroid, vitreous — *see* Deposit, crystalline
  cytoid (retina) — *see* Occlusion, artery, retina
  drusen (degenerative) (macula) (retinal) (*see also* Degeneration, macula, drusen)
    optic disc — *see* Drusen, optic disc
  foreign — *see* Foreign body
  loose
    joint, except knee — *see* Loose, body, joint
      knee M23.4- ☑
    sheath, tendon — *see* Disorder, tendon, specified type NEC
  mass index (BMI)
    adult
      19 or less Z68.1
      20.0-20.9 Z68.20
      21.0-21.9 Z68.21
      22.0-22.9 Z68.22
      23.0-23.9 Z68.23
      24.0-24.9 Z68.24
      25.0-25.9 Z68.25
      26.0-26.9 Z68.26
      27.0-27.9 Z68.27
      28.0-28.9 Z68.28
      29.0-29.9 Z68.29
      30.0-30.9 Z68.30
      31.0-31.9 Z68.31
      32.0-32.9 Z68.32
      33.0-33.9 Z68.33
      34.0-34.9 Z68.34
      35.0-35.9 Z68.35
      36.0-36.9 Z68.36
      37.0-37.9 Z68.37
      38.0-38.9 Z68.38
      39.0-39.9 Z68.39
      40.0-44.9 Z68.41
      45.0-49.9 Z68.42
      50.0-59.9 Z68.43
      60.0-69.9 Z68.44
      70 and over Z68.45
    pediatric
      5th percentile to less than 85th percentile for age Z68.52
      85th percentile to less than 95th percentile for age Z68.53
      less than fifth percentile for age Z68.51
      greater than or equal to ninety-fifth percentile for age Z68.54
  Mooser's A75.2
  rice (*see also* Loose, body, joint)
    knee M23.4- ☑
  rocking F98.4

Boeck's
  disease or sarcoid — *see* Sarcoidosis
  lupoid (miliary) D86.3
Boerhaave's syndrome (spontaneous esophageal rupture) K22.3
Boggy
  cervix N88.8
  uterus N85.8
Boil (*see also* Furuncle, by site)
  Aleppo B55.1
  Baghdad B55.1
  Delhi B55.1
  lacrimal
    gland — *see* Dacryoadenitis
    passages (duct) (sac) — *see* Inflammation, lacrimal, passages, acute
  Natal B55.1
  orbit, orbital — *see* Abscess, orbit
  tropical B55.1
Bold hives — *see* Urticaria
Bombé, iris — *see* Membrane, pupillary
Bone — *see* condition
Bonnevie-Ullrich syndrome Q87.1
Bonnier's syndrome H81.8 ☑
Bonvale dam fever T73.3 ☑
Bony block of joint — *see* Ankylosis
BOOP (bronchiolitis obliterans organized pneumonia) J84.89
Borderline
  diabetes mellitus R73.09
  hypertension R03.0
  osteopenia M85.8- ☑
  pelvis, with obstruction during labor O65.1
  personality F60.3
Borna disease A83.9
Bornholm disease B33.0
Boston exanthem A88.0
Botalli, ductus (patent) (persistent) Q25.0
Bothriocephalus latus infestation B70.0
Botulism (foodborne intoxication) A05.1
  infant A48.51
  non-foodborne A48.52
  wound A48.52
Bouba — *see* Yaws
Bouchard's nodes (with arthropathy) M15.2
Bouffée délirante F23
Bouillaud's disease or syndrome (rheumatic heart disease) I01.9
Bourneville's disease Q85.1
Boutonniere deformity (finger) — *see* Deformity, finger, boutonniere
Bouveret (-Hoffmann) **syndrome** (paroxysmal tachycardia) I47.9
Bovine heart — *see* Hypertrophy, cardiac
Bowel — *see* condition
Bowen's
  dermatosis (precancerous) — *see* Neoplasm, skin, in situ
  disease — *see* Neoplasm, skin, in situ
  epithelioma — *see* Neoplasm, skin, in situ
  type
    epidermoid carcinoma-in-situ — *see* Neoplasm, skin, in situ
    intraepidermal squamous cell carcinoma — *see* Neoplasm, skin, in situ
Bowing
  femur (*see also* Deformity, limb, specified type NEC, thigh)
    congenital Q68.3
  fibula (*see also* Deformity, limb, specified type NEC, lower leg)
    congenital Q68.4
  forearm — *see* Deformity, limb, specified type NEC, forearm
  leg(s), long bones, congenital Q68.5
  radius — *see* Deformity, limb, specified type NEC, forearm
  tibia (*see also* Deformity, limb, specified type NEC, lower leg)
    congenital Q68.4
Bowleg(s) (acquired) M21.16- ☑
  congenital Q68.5
  rachitic E64.3
Boyd's dysentery A03.2
Brachial — *see* condition
Brachycardia R00.1
Brachycephaly Q75.0

40

☑ **Additional Character Required** — **Refer to the Tabular List for Character Selection** ▽ **Subterms under main terms may continue to next column or page**

Bradley's disease A08.19
Bradyarrhythmia, cardiac I49.8
Bradycardia (sinoatrial) (sinus) (vagal) R00.1
  neonatal P29.12
  reflex G90.09
  tachycardia syndrome I49.5
Bradykinesia R25.8
Bradypnea R06.89
Bradytachycardia I49.5
Brailsford's disease or osteochondrosis — see Osteo-
  chondrosis, juvenile, radius
Brain (see also condition)
  death G93.82
  syndrome — see Syndrome, brain
Branched-chain amino-acid disorder E71.2
Branchial — see condition
  cartilage, congenital Q18.2
Branchiogenic remnant (in neck) Q18.0
Brandt's syndrome (acrodermatitis enteropathica) E83.2
Brash (water) R12
Bravais-jacksonian epilepsy — see Epilepsy, localiza-
  tion-related, symptomatic, with simple partial
  seizures
Braxton Hicks contractions — see False, labor
Brazilian leishmaniasis B55.2
BRBPR K62.5
Break, retina (without detachment) H33.30- ☑
  with retinal detachment — see Detachment, retina
  horseshoe tear H33.31- ☑
  multiple H33.33-
  round hole H33.32- ☑
Breakdown
  device, graft or implant (see also Complications, by
    site and type, mechanical) T85.618 ☑
    arterial graft NEC — see Complication, cardiovas-
      cular device, mechanical, vascular
    breast (implant) T85.41 ☑
    catheter NEC T85.618 ☑
      cystostomy T83.010 ☑
      dialysis (renal) T82.41 ☑
        intraperitoneal T85.611 ☑
      infusion NEC T82.514 ☑
        spinal (epidural) (subdural) T85.610 ☑
      urinary (indwelling) T83.018 ☑
    electronic (electrode) (pulse generator) (stimulator)
      bone T84.310 ☑
      cardiac T82.119 ☑
        electrode T82.110 ☑
        pulse generator T82.111 ☑
        specified type NEC T82.118 ☑
      nervous system — see Complication, prosthetic
        device, mechanical, electronic nervous
        system stimulator
    urinary — see Complication, genitourinary,
      device, urinary, mechanical
    fixation, internal (orthopedic) NEC — see Compli-
      cation, fixation device, mechanical
    gastrointestinal — see Complications, prosthetic
      device, mechanical, gastrointestinal device
    genital NEC T83.418 ☑
      intrauterine contraceptive device T83.31 ☑
      penile prosthesis T83.410 ☑
    heart NEC — see Complication, cardiovascular de-
      vice, mechanical
    joint prosthesis — see Complications..., joint pros-
      thesis,internal, mechanical, by site
    ocular NEC — see Complications, prosthetic device,
      mechanical, ocular device
    orthopedic NEC — see Complication, orthopedic,
      device, mechanical
    specified NEC T85.618 ☑
    sutures, permanent T85.612 ☑
      used in bone repair — see Complications, fixa-
        tion device, internal (orthopedic), me-
        chanical
    urinary NEC (see also Complication, genitourinary,
      device, urinary, mechanical)
      graft T83.21 ☑
    vascular NEC — see Complication, cardiovascular
      device, mechanical
    ventricular intracranial shunt T85.01 ☑
  nervous F48.8
  perineum O90.1
  respirator J95.850
    specified NEC J95.859
  ventilator J95.850

Breakdown — continued
  ventilator — continued
    specified NEC J95.859
Breast (see also condition)
  buds E30.1
    in newborn P96.89
  dense R92.2
  nodule N63
Breath
  foul R19.6
  holder, child R06.89
  holding spell R06.89
  shortness R06.02
Breathing
  labored — see Hyperventilation
  mouth R06.5
    causing malocclusion M26.5 ☑
  periodic R06.3
    high altitude G47.32
Breathlessness R06.81
Breda's disease — see Yaws
Breech presentation (mother) O32.1 ☑
  causing obstructed labor O64.1 ☑
  footling O32.8 ☑
    causing obstructed labor O64.8 ☑
  incomplete O32.8 ☑
    causing obstructed labor O64.8 ☑
Breisky's disease N90.4
Brennemann's syndrome I88.0
Brenner
  tumor (benign) D27.9
    borderline malignancy D39.1- ☑
    malignant C56 ☑
    proliferating D39.1- ☑
Bretonneau's disease or angina A36.0
Breus' mole O02.0
Brevicollis Q76.49
Brickmakers' anemia B76.9 [D63.8]
Bridge, myocardial Q24.5
Bright red blood per rectum (BRBPR) K62.5
Bright's disease (see also Nephritis)
  arteriosclerotic — see Hypertension, kidney
Brill (-Zinsser) **disease** (recrudescent typhus) A75.1
  flea-borne A75.2
  louse-borne A75.1
Brill-Symmers' disease C82.90
Brion-Kayser disease — see Fever, parathyroid
Briquet's disorder or syndrome F45.0
Brissaud's
  infantilism or dwarfism E23.0
  motor-verbal tic F95.2
Brittle
  bones disease Q78.0
  nails L60.3
    congenital Q84.6
Broad (see also condition)
  beta disease E78.2
  ligament laceration syndrome N83.8
Broad- or floating-betalipoproteinemia E78.2
Brock's syndrome (atelectasis due to enlarged lymph
  nodes) J98.19
Brocq-Duhring disease (dermatitis herpetiformis) L13.0
Broken
  arches (see also Deformity, limb, flat foot)
  arm (meaning upper limb) — see Fracture, arm
  back — see Fracture, vertebra
  bone — see Fracture
  implant or internal device — see Complications, by
    site and type, mechanical
  leg (meaning lower limb) — see Fracture, leg
  nose S02.2 ☑
  tooth, teeth — see Fracture, tooth
Bromhidrosis, bromidrosis L75.0
Bromidism, bromism G92
  chronic (dependence) F13.20
  due to
    correct substance properly administered — see
      Table of Drugs and Chemicals, by drug, ad-
      verse effect
    overdose or wrong substance given or taken —
      see Table of Drugs and Chemicals, by drug,
      poisoning
Bromidrosiphobia F40.298
Bronchi, bronchial — see condition
Bronchiectasis (cylindrical) (diffuse) (fusiform) (localized)
  (saccular) J47.9

Bronchiectasis — continued
  with
    acute
      bronchitis J47.0
      lower respiratory infection J47.0
    exacerbation (acute) J47.1
  congenital Q33.4
  tuberculous NEC — see Tuberculosis, pulmonary
Bronchiolectasis — see Bronchiectasis
Bronchiolitis (acute) (infective) (subacute) J21.9
  with
    bronchospasm or obstruction J21.9
    influenza, flu or grippe — see Influenza, with, res-
      piratory manifestations NEC
  chemical (chronic) J68.4
    acute J68.0
  chronic (fibrosing) (obliterative) J44.9
  due to
    external agent — see Bronchitis, acute, due to
    human metapneumovirus J21.1
    respiratory syncytial virus J21.0
    specified organism NEC J21.8
  fibrosa obliterans J44.9
  influenzal — see Influenza, with, respiratory manifes-
    tations NEC
  obliterans J42
    with organizing pneumonia (BOOP) J84.89
  obliterative (chronic) (subacute) J44.9
    due to chemicals, gases, fumes or vapors (inhala-
      tion) J68.4
    due to fumes or vapors J68.4
  respiratory, interstitial lung disease J84.115
Bronchitis (diffuse) (fibrinous) (hypostatic) (infective)
  (membranous) J40
  with
    influenza, flu or grippe — see Influenza, with, res-
      piratory manifestations NEC
    obstruction (airway) (lung) J44.9
    tracheitis (I5 years of age and above) J40
      acute or subacute J20.9
      chronic J42
      under I5 years of age J20.9
  acute or subacute (with bronchospasm or obstruction)
    J20.9
    with
      bronchiectasis J47.0
      chronic obstructive pulmonary disease J44.0
    chemical (due to gases, fumes or vapors) J68.0
    due to
      fumes or vapors J68.0
      Haemophilus influenzae J20.1
      Mycoplasma pneumoniae J20.0
      radiation J70.0
      specified organism NEC J20.8
      Streptococcus J20.2
      virus
        coxsackie J20.3
        echovirus J20.7
        parainfluenzae J20.4
        respiratory syncytial J20.5
        rhinovirus J20.6
    viral NEC J20.8
  allergic (acute) J45.909
    with
      exacerbation (acute) J45.901
      status asthmaticus J45.902
  arachidic T17.528 ☑
  aspiration (due to fumes or vapors) J68.0
  asthmatic J45.9 ☑
    chronic J44.9
      with
        acute lower respiratory infection J44.0
        exacerbation (acute) J44.1
  capillary — see Pneumonia, broncho
  caseous (tuberculous) A15.5
  Castellani's A69.8
  catarrhal (I5 years of age and above) J40
    acute — see Bronchitis, acute
    chronic J41.0
    under I5 years of age J20.9
  chemical (acute) (subacute) J68.0
    chronic J68.4
    due to fumes or vapors J68.0
      chronic J68.4
  chronic J42
    with
      airways obstruction J44.9
      tracheitis (chronic) J42

Bronchitis — *continued*
  chronic — *continued*
    asthmatic (obstructive) J44.9
    catarrhal J41.0
    chemical (due to fumes or vapors) J68.4
    due to
      chemicals, gases, fumes or vapors (inhalation) J68.4
      radiation J70.1
      tobacco smoking J41.0
    emphysematous J44.9
    mucopurulent J41.1
    non-obstructive J41.0
    obliterans J44.9
    obstructive J44.9
    purulent J41.1
    simple J41.0
  croupous — *see* Bronchitis, acute
  due to gases, fumes or vapors (chemical) J68.0
  emphysematous (obstructive) J44.9
  exudative — *see* Bronchitis, acute
  fetid J41.1
  grippal — *see* Influenza, with, respiratory manifestations NEC
  in those under 15 years age — *see* Bronchitis, acute
    chronic — *see* Bronchitis, chronic
  influenzal — *see* Influenza, with, respiratory manifestations NEC
  mixed simple and mucopurulent J41.8
  moulder's J62.8
  mucopurulent (chronic) (recurrent) J41.1
    acute or subacute J20.9
    simple (mixed) J41.8
  obliterans (chronic) J44.9
  obstructive (chronic) (diffuse) J44.9
  pituitous J41.1
  pneumococcal, acute or subacute J20.2
  pseudomembranous, acute or subacute — *see* Bronchitis, acute
  purulent (chronic) (recurrent) J41.1
    acute or subacute — *see* Bronchitis, acute
  putrid J41.1
  senile (chronic) J42
  simple and mucopurulent (mixed) J41.8
  smokers' J41.0
  spirochetal NEC A69.8
  subacute — *see* Bronchitis, acute
  suppurative (chronic) J41.1
    acute or subacute — *see* Bronchitis, acute
  tuberculous A15.5
  under 15 years of age — *see* Bronchitis, acute
    chronic — *see* Bronchitis, chronic
  viral NEC, acute or subacute (*see also* Bronchitis, acute) J20.8
Bronchoalveolitis J18.0
Bronchoaspergillosis B44.1
Bronchocele meaning goiter E04.0
Broncholithiasis J98.09
  tuberculous NEC A15.5
Bronchomalacia J98.09
  congenital Q32.2
Bronchomycosis NOS B49 [J99]
  candidal B37.1
Bronchopleuropneumonia — *see* Pneumonia, broncho
Bronchopneumonia — *see* Pneumonia, broncho
Bronchopneumonitis — *see* Pneumonia, broncho
Bronchopulmonary — *see* condition
Bronchopulmonitis — *see* Pneumonia, broncho
Bronchorrhagia (*see* Hemoptysis)
Bronchorrhea J98.09
  acute J20.9
  chronic (infective) (purulent) J42
Bronchospasm (acute) J98.01
  with
    bronchiolitis, acute J21.9
    bronchitis, acute (conditions in J20) — *see* Bronchitis, acute
  due to external agent — *see* condition, respiratory, acute, due to
  exercise induced J45.990
Bronchospirochetosis A69.8
  Castellani A69.8
Bronchostenosis J98.09
Bronchus — *see* condition
Brontophobia F40.220
Bronze baby syndrome P83.8
Brooke's tumor — *see* Neoplasm, skin, benign

Brown enamel of teeth (hereditary) K00.5
Brown's sheath syndrome H50.61- ☑
Brown-Séquard disease, paralysis or syndrome G83.81
Bruce sepsis A23.0
Brucellosis (infection) A23.9
  abortus A23.1
  canis A23.3
  dermatitis A23.9
  melitensis A23.0
  mixed A23.8
  sepsis A23.9
    melitensis A23.0
    specified NEC A23.8
  suis A23.2
Bruck-de Lange disease Q87.1
Bruck's disease — *see* Deformity, limb
Brugsch's syndrome Q82.8
Bruise (skin surface intact) (*see also* Contusion)
  with
    open wound — *see* Wound, open
  internal organ — *see* Injury, by site
  newborn P54.5
  scalp, due to birth injury, newborn P12.3
  umbilical cord O69.5 ☑
Bruit (arterial) R09.89
  cardiac R01.1
Brush burn — *see* Abrasion, by site
Bruton's X-linked agammaglobulinemia D80.0
Bruxism
  psychogenic F45.8
  sleep related G47.63
Bubbly lung syndrome P27.0
Bubo I88.8
  blennorrhagic (gonococcal) A54.89
  chancroidal A57
  climatic A55
  due to Haemophilus ducreyi A57
  gonococcal A54.89
  indolent (nonspecific) I88.8
  inguinal (nonspecific) I88.8
    chancroidal A57
    climatic A55
    due to H. ducreyi A57
    infective I88.8
  scrofulous (tuberculous) A18.2
  soft chancre A57
  suppurating — *see* Lymphadenitis, acute
  syphilitic (primary) A51.0
    congenital A50.07
  tropical A55
  virulent (chancroidal) A57
Bubonic plague A20.0
Bubonocele — *see* Hernia, inguinal
Buccal — *see* condition
Buchanan's disease or osteochondrosis M91.0
Buchem's syndrome (hyperostosis corticalis) M85.2
Bucket-handle fracture or tear (semilunar cartilage) — *see* Tear, meniscus
Budd-Chiari syndrome (hepatic vein thrombosis) I82.0
Budgerigar fancier's disease or lung J67.2
Buds
  breast E30.1
    in newborn P96.89
Buerger's disease (thromboangiitis obliterans) I73.1
Bulbar — *see* condition
Bulbus cordis (left ventricle) (persistent) Q21.8
Bulimia (nervosa) F50.2
  atypical F50.9
  normal weight F50.9
Bulky
  stools R19.5
  uterus N85.2
Bulla (e) R23.8
  lung (emphysematous) (solitary) J43.9
    newborn P25.8
Bullet wound (*see also* Wound, open)
  fracture — *code as* Fracture, by site
  internal organ — *see* Injury, by site
Bundle
  branch block (complete) (false) (incomplete) — *see* Block, bundle-branch
  of His — *see* condition
Bunion — *see* Deformity, toe, hallux valgus
Buphthalmia, buphthalmos (congenital) Q15.0
Burdwan fever B55.0
Bürger-Grütz disease or syndrome E78.3

Buried
  penis (congenital) Q55.64
    acquired N48.83
  roots K08.3
Burke's syndrome K86.8
Burkitt
  cell leukemia C91.0- ☑
  lymphoma (malignant) C83.7- ☑
    small noncleaved, diffuse C83.7- ☑
    spleen C83.77
    undifferentiated C83.7- ☑
  tumor C83.7- ☑
  type
    acute lymphoblastic leukemia C91.0- ☑
    undifferentiated C83.7- ☑
Burn (electricity) (flame) (hot gas, liquid or hot object) (radiation) (steam) (thermal)
  abdomen, abdominal (muscle) (wall) T21.02 ☑
    first degree T21.12 ☑
    second degree T21.22 ☑
    third degree T21.32 ☑
  above elbow T22.039 ☑
    first degree T22.139 ☑
    left T22.032 ☑
      first degree T22.132 ☑
      second degree T22.232 ☑
      third degree T22.332 ☑
    right T22.031 ☑
      first degree T22.131 ☑
      second degree T22.231 ☑
      third degree T22.331 ☑
    second degree T22.239 ☑
    third degree T22.339 ☑
  acid (caustic) (external) (internal) — *see* Corrosion, by site
  alimentary tract NEC T28.2 ☑
    esophagus T28.1 ☑
    mouth T28.0 ☑
    pharynx T28.0 ☑
  alkaline (caustic) (external) (internal) — *see* Corrosion, by site
  ankle T25.019 ☑
    first degree T25.119 ☑
    left T25.012 ☑
      first degree T25.112 ☑
      second degree T25.212 ☑
      third degree T25.312 ☑
    multiple with foot — *see* Burn, lower, limb, multiple, ankle and foot
    right T25.011 ☑
      first degree T25.111 ☑
      second degree T25.211 ☑
      third degree T25.311 ☑
    second degree T25.219 ☑
    third degree T25.319 ☑
  anus — *see* Burn, buttock
  arm (lower) (upper) — *see* Burn, upper, limb
  axilla T22.049 ☑
    first degree T22.149 ☑
    left T22.042 ☑
      first degree T22.142 ☑
      second degree T22.242 ☑
      third degree T22.342 ☑
    right T22.041 ☑
      first degree T22.141 ☑
      second degree T22.241 ☑
      third degree T22.341 ☑
    second degree T22.249 ☑
    third degree T22.349 ☑
  back (lower) T21.04 ☑
    first degree T21.14 ☑
    second degree T21.24 ☑
    third degree T21.34 ☑
    upper T21.03 ☑
      first degree T21.13 ☑
      second degree T21.23 ☑
      third degree T21.33 ☑
  blisters — *code as* Burn, second degree, by site
  breast(s) — *see* Burn, chest wall
  buttock(s) T21.05 ☑
    first degree T21.15 ☑
    second degree T21.25 ☑
    third degree T21.35 ☑
  calf T24.039 ☑
    first degree T24.139 ☑
    left T24.032 ☑

Burn — *continued*
  calf — *continued*
    left — *continued*
      first degree T24.132 ☑
      second degree T24.232 ☑
      third degree T24.332 ☑
    right T24.031 ☑
      first degree T24.131 ☑
      second degree T24.231 ☑
      third degree T24.331 ☑
    second degree T24.239 ☑
    third degree T24.339 ☑
  canthus (eye) — *see* Burn, eyelid
  caustic acid or alkaline — *see* Corrosion, by site
  cervix T28.3 ☑
  cheek T20.06 ☑
    first degree T20.16 ☑
    second degree T20.26 ☑
    third degree T20.36 ☑
  chemical (acids) (alkalines) (caustics) (external) (internal) — *see* Corrosion, by site
  chest wall T21.01 ☑
    first degree T21.11 ☑
    second degree T21.21 ☑
    third degree T21.31 ☑
  chin T20.03 ☑
    first degree T20.13 ☑
    second degree T20.23 ☑
    third degree T20.33 ☑
  colon T28.2 ☑
  conjunctiva (and cornea) — *see* Burn, cornea
  cornea (and conjunctiva) T26.1- ☑
    chemical — *see* Corrosion, cornea
  corrosion (external) (internal) — *see* Corrosion, by site
  deep necrosis of underlying tissue — *code as* Burn, third degree, by site
  dorsum of hand T23.069 ☑
    first degree T23.169 ☑
    left T23.062 ☑
      first degree T23.162 ☑
      second degree T23.262 ☑
      third degree T23.362 ☑
    right T23.061 ☑
      first degree T23.161 ☑
      second degree T23.261 ☑
      third degree T23.361 ☑
    second degree T23.269 ☑
    third degree T23.369 ☑
  due to ingested chemical agent — *see* Corrosion, by site
  ear (auricle) (external) (canal) T20.01 ☑
    first degree T20.11 ☑
    second degree T20.21 ☑
    third degree T20.31 ☑
  elbow T22.029 ☑
    first degree T22.129 ☑
    left T22.022 ☑
      first degree T22.122 ☑
      second degree T22.222 ☑
      third degree T22.322 ☑
    right T22.021 ☑
      first degree T22.121 ☑
      second degree T22.221 ☑
      third degree T22.321 ☑
    second degree T22.229 ☑
    third degree T22.329 ☑
  epidermal loss — *code as* Burn, second degree, by site
  erythema, erythematous — *code as* Burn, first degree, by site
  esophagus T28.1 ☑
  extent (percentage of body surface)
    less than 10 percent T31.0 ☑
    10-19 percent T31.10 ☑
      with 0-9 percent third degree burns T31.10
      with 10-19 percent third degree burns T31.11
    20-29 percent T31.20 ☑
      with 0-9 percent third degree burns T31.20
      with 10-19 percent third degree burns T31.21
      with 20-29 percent third degree burns T31.22
    30-39 percent T31.30 ☑
      with 0-9 percent third degree burns T31.30
      with 10-19 percent third degree burns T31.31
      with 20-29 percent third degree burns T31.32
      with 30-39 percent third degree burns T31.33
    40-49 percent T31.40 ☑
      with 0-9 percent third degree burns T31.40

Burn — *continued*
  extent — *continued*
    40-49 percent — *continued*
      with 10-19 percent third degree burns T31.41
      with 20-29 percent third degree burns T31.42
      with 30-39 percent third degree burns T31.43
      with 40-49 percent third degree burns T31.44
    50-59 percent T31.50 ☑
      with 0-9 percent third degree burns T31.50
      with 10-19 percent third degree burns T31.51
      with 20-29 percent third degree burns T31.52
      with 30-39 percent third degree burns T31.53
      with 40-49 percent third degree burns T31.54
      with 50-59 percent third degree burns T31.55
    60-69 percent T31.60 ☑
      with 0-9 percent third degree burns T31.60
      with 10-19 percent third degree burns T31.61
      with 20-29 percent third degree burns T31.62
      with 30-39 percent third degree burns T31.63
      with 40-49 percent third degree burns T31.64
      with 50-59 percent third degree burns T31.65
      with 60-69 percent third degree burns T31.66
    70-79 percent T31.70 ☑
      with 0-9 percent third degree burns T31.70
      with 10-19 percent third degree burns T31.71
      with 20-29 percent third degree burns T31.72
      with 30-39 percent third degree burns T31.73
      with 40-49 percent third degree burns T31.74
      with 50-59 percent third degree burns T31.75
      with 60-69 percent third degree burns T31.76
      with 70-79 percent third degree burns T31.77
    80-89 percent T31.80 ☑
      with 0-9 percent third degree burns T31.80
      with 10-19 percent third degree burns T31.81
      with 20-29 percent third degree burns T31.82
      with 30-39 percent third degree burns T31.83
      with 40-49 percent third degree burns T31.84
      with 50-59 percent third degree burns T31.85
      with 60-69 percent third degree burns T31.86
      with 70-79 percent third degree burns T31.87
      with 80-89 percent third degree burns T31.88
    90 percent or more T31.90 ☑
      with 0-9 percent third degree burns T31.90
      with 10-19 percent third degree burns T31.91
      with 20-29 percent third degree burns T31.92
      with 30-39 percent third degree burns T31.93
      with 40-49 percent third degree burns T31.94
      with 50-59 percent third degree burns T31.95
      with 60-69 percent third degree burns T31.96
      with 70-79 percent third degree burns T31.97
      with 80-89 percent third degree burns T31.98
      with 90 percent or more third degree burns T31.99
  extremity — *see* Burn, limb
  eye(s) and adnexa T26.4- ☑
    with resulting rupture and destruction of eyeball T26.2- ☑
    conjunctival sac — *see* Burn, cornea
    cornea — *see* Burn, cornea
    lid — *see* Burn, eyelid
    periocular area — *see* Burn, eyelid
    specified site NEC T26.3- ☑
  eyeball — *see* Burn, eye
  eyelid(s) T26.0- ☑
    chemical — *see* Corrosion, eyelid
  face — *see* Burn, head
  finger T23.029 ☑
    first degree T23.129 ☑
    left T23.022 ☑
      first degree T23.122 ☑
      second degree T23.222 ☑
      third degree T23.322 ☑
    multiple sites (without thumb) T23.039 ☑
      with thumb T23.049 ☑
        first degree T23.149 ☑
        left T23.042 ☑
          first degree T23.142 ☑
          second degree T23.242 ☑
          third degree T23.342 ☑
        right T23.041 ☑
          first degree T23.141 ☑
          second degree T23.241 ☑
          third degree T23.341 ☑
        second degree T23.249 ☑
        third degree T23.349 ☑
      first degree T23.139 ☑
      left T23.032 ☑

Burn — *continued*
  finger — *continued*
    multiple sites — *continued*
      left — *continued*
        first degree T23.132 ☑
        second degree T23.232 ☑
        third degree T23.332 ☑
      right T23.031 ☑
        first degree T23.131 ☑
        second degree T23.231 ☑
        third degree T23.331 ☑
      second degree T23.239 ☑
      third degree T23.339 ☑
    right T23.021 ☑
      first degree T23.121 ☑
      second degree T23.221 ☑
      third degree T23.321 ☑
    second degree T23.229 ☑
    third degree T23.329 ☑
  flank — *see* Burn, abdominal wall
  foot T25.029 ☑
    first degree T25.129 ☑
    left T25.022 ☑
      first degree T25.122 ☑
      second degree T25.222 ☑
      third degree T25.322 ☑
    multiple with ankle — *see* Burn, lower, limb, multiple, ankle and foot
    right T25.021 ☑
      first degree T25.121 ☑
      second degree T25.221 ☑
      third degree T25.321 ☑
    second degree T25.229 ☑
    third degree T25.329 ☑
  forearm T22.019 ☑
    first degree T22.119 ☑
    left T22.012 ☑
      first degree T22.112 ☑
      second degree T22.212 ☑
      third degree T22.312 ☑
    right T22.011 ☑
      first degree T22.111 ☑
      second degree T22.211 ☑
      third degree T22.311 ☑
    second degree T22.219 ☑
    third degree T22.319 ☑
  forehead T20.06 ☑
    first degree T20.16 ☑
    second degree T20.26 ☑
    third degree T20.36 ☑
  fourth degree — *code as* Burn, third degree, by site
  friction — *see* Burn, by site
  from swallowing caustic or corrosive substance NEC — *see* Corrosion, by site
  full thickness skin loss — *code as* Burn, third degree, by site
  gastrointestinal tract NEC T28.2 ☑
    from swallowing caustic or corrosive substance T28.7 ☑
  genital organs
    external
      female T21.07 ☑
        first degree T21.17 ☑
        second degree T21.27 ☑
        third degree T21.37 ☑
      male T21.06 ☑
        first degree T21.16 ☑
        second degree T21.26 ☑
        third degree T21.36 ☑
    internal T28.3 ☑
      from caustic or corrosive substance T28.8 ☑
  groin — *see* Burn, abdominal wall
  hand(s) T23.009 ☑
    back — *see* Burn, dorsum of hand
    finger — *see* Burn, finger
    first degree T23.109 ☑
    left T23.002 ☑
      first degree T23.102 ☑
      second degree T23.202 ☑
      third degree T23.302 ☑
    multiple sites with wrist T23.099 ☑
      first degree T23.199 ☑
      left T23.092 ☑
        first degree T23.192 ☑
        second degree T23.292 ☑
        third degree T23.392 ☑

Burn — *continued*
  hand(s) — *continued*
    multiple sites with wrist — *continued*
      right T23.091 ☑
        first degree T23.191 ☑
        second degree T23.291 ☑
        third degree T23.391 ☑
      second degree T23.299 ☑
      third degree T23.399 ☑
    palm — *see* Burn, palm
    right T23.001 ☑
      first degree T23.101 ☑
      second degree T23.201 ☑
      third degree T23.301 ☑
    second degree T23.209 ☑
    third degree T23.309 ☑
    thumb — *see* Burn, thumb
  head (and face) (and neck) T20.00 ☑
    cheek — *see* Burn, cheek
    chin — *see* Burn, chin
    ear — *see* Burn, ear
    eye(s) only — *see* Burn, eye
    first degree T20.10 ☑
    forehead — *see* Burn, forehead
    lip — *see* Burn, lip
    multiple sites T20.09 ☑
      first degree T20.19 ☑
      second degree T20.29 ☑
      third degree T20.39 ☑
    neck — *see* Burn, neck
    nose — *see* Burn, nose
    scalp — *see* Burn, scalp
    second degree T20.20 ☑
    third degree T20.30 ☑
  hip(s) — *see* Burn, lower, limb
  inhalation — *see* Burn, respiratory tract
    caustic or corrosive substance (fumes) — *see* Corrosion, respiratory tract
  internal organ(s) T28.40 ☑
    alimentary tract T28.2 ☑
      esophagus T28.1 ☑
    eardrum T28.41 ☑
    esophagus T28.1 ☑
    from caustic or corrosive substance (swallowing) NEC — *see* Corrosion, by site
    genitourinary T28.3 ☑
    mouth T28.0 ☑
    pharynx T28.0 ☑
    respiratory tract — *see* Burn, respiratory tract
    specified organ NEC T28.49 ☑
  interscapular region — *see* Burn, back, upper
  intestine (large) (small) T28.2 ☑
  knee T24.029 ☑
    first degree T24.129 ☑
    left T24.022 ☑
      first degree T24.122 ☑
      second degree T24.222 ☑
      third degree T24.322 ☑
    right T24.021 ☑
      first degree T24.121 ☑
      second degree T24.221 ☑
      third degree T24.321 ☑
    second degree T24.229 ☑
    third degree T24.329 ☑
  labium (majus) (minus) — *see* Burn, genital organs, external, female
  lacrimal apparatus, duct, gland or sac — *see* Burn, eye, specified site NEC
  larynx T27.0 ☑
    with lung T27.1 ☑
  leg(s) (lower) (upper) — *see* Burn, lower, limb
  lightning — *see* Burn, by site
  limb(s)
    lower (except ankle or foot alone) — *see* Burn, lower, limb
    upper — *see* Burn, upper limb
  lip(s) T20.02 ☑
    first degree T20.12 ☑
    second degree T20.22 ☑
    third degree T20.32 ☑
  lower
    back — *see* Burn, back
    limb T24.009 ☑
      ankle — *see* Burn, ankle
      calf — *see* Burn, calf
        first degree T24.109 ☑

Burn — *continued*
  lower — *continued*
    limb — *continued*
      foot — *see* Burn, foot
      hip — *see* Burn, thigh
      knee — *see* Burn, knee
      left T24.002 ☑
        first degree T24.102 ☑
        second degree T24.202 ☑
        third degree T24.302 ☑
      multiple sites, except ankle and foot T24.099 ☑
        ankle and foot T25.099 ☑
          first degree T25.199 ☑
          left T25.092 ☑
            first degree T25.192 ☑
            second degree T25.292 ☑
            third degree T25.392 ☑
          right T25.091 ☑
            first degree T25.191 ☑
            second degree T25.291 ☑
            third degree T25.391 ☑
          second degree T25.299 ☑
          third degree T25.399 ☑
        first degree T24.199 ☑
        left T24.092 ☑
          first degree T24.192 ☑
          second degree T24.292 ☑
          third degree T24.392 ☑
        right T24.091 ☑
          first degree T24.191 ☑
          second degree T24.291 ☑
          third degree T24.391 ☑
        second degree T24.299 ☑
        third degree T24.399 ☑
      right T24.001 ☑
        first degree T24.101 ☑
        second degree T24.201 ☑
        third degree T24.301 ☑
      second degree T24.209 ☑
      thigh — *see* Burn, thigh
      third degree T24.309 ☑
      toe — *see* Burn, toe
  lung (with larynx and trachea) T27.1 ☑
  mouth T28.0 ☑
  neck T20.07 ☑
    first degree T20.17 ☑
    second degree T20.27 ☑
    third degree T20.37 ☑
  nose (septum) T20.04 ☑
    first degree T20.14 ☑
    second degree T20.24 ☑
    third degree T20.34 ☑
  ocular adnexa — *see* Burn, eye
  orbit region — *see* Burn, eyelid
  palm T23.059 ☑
    first degree T23.159 ☑
    left T23.052 ☑
      first degree T23.152 ☑
      second degree T23.252 ☑
      third degree T23.352 ☑
    right T23.051 ☑
      first degree T23.151 ☑
      second degree T23.251 ☑
      third degree T23.351 ☑
    second degree T23.259 ☑
    third degree T23.359 ☑
  partial thickness — *code as* Burn, unspecified degree, by site
  pelvis — *see* Burn, trunk
  penis — *see* Burn, genital organs, external, male
  perineum
    female — *see* Burn, genital organs, external, female
    male — *see* Burn, genital organs, external, male
  periocular area — *see* Burn, eyelid
  pharynx T28.0 ☑
  rectum T28.2 ☑
  respiratory tract T27.3 ☑
    larynx — *see* Burn, larynx
    specified part NEC T27.2 ☑
    trachea — *see* Burn, trachea
  sac, lacrimal — *see* Burn, eye, specified site NEC
  scalp T20.05 ☑
    first degree T20.15 ☑
    second degree T20.25 ☑
    third degree T20.35 ☑

Burn — *continued*
  scapular region T22.069 ☑
    first degree T22.169 ☑
    left T22.062 ☑
      first degree T22.162 ☑
      second degree T22.262 ☑
      third degree T22.362 ☑
    right T22.061 ☑
      first degree T22.161 ☑
      second degree T22.261 ☑
      third degree T22.361 ☑
    second degree T22.269 ☑
    third degree T22.369 ☑
  sclera — *see* Burn, eye, specified site NEC
  scrotum — *see* Burn, genital organs, external, male
  shoulder T22.059 ☑
    first degree T22.159 ☑
    left T22.052 ☑
      first degree T22.152 ☑
      second degree T22.252 ☑
      third degree T22.352 ☑
    right T22.051 ☑
      first degree T22.151 ☑
      second degree T22.251 ☑
      third degree T22.351 ☑
    second degree T22.259 ☑
    third degree T22.359 ☑
  stomach T28.2 ☑
  temple — *see* Burn, head
  testis — *see* Burn, genital organs, external, male
  thigh T24.019 ☑
    first degree T24.119 ☑
    left T24.012 ☑
      first degree T24.112 ☑
      second degree T24.212 ☑
      third degree T24.312 ☑
    right T24.011 ☑
      first degree T24.111 ☑
      second degree T24.211 ☑
      third degree T24.311 ☑
    second degree T24.219 ☑
    third degree T24.319 ☑
  thorax (external) — *see* Burn, trunk
  throat (meaning pharynx) T28.0 ☑
  thumb(s) T23.019 ☑
    first degree T23.119 ☑
    left T23.012 ☑
      first degree T23.112 ☑
      second degree T23.212 ☑
      third degree T23.312 ☑
    multiple sites with fingers T23.049 ☑
      first degree T23.149 ☑
      left T23.042 ☑
        first degree T23.142 ☑
        second degree T23.242 ☑
        third degree T23.342 ☑
      right T23.041 ☑
        first degree T23.141 ☑
        second degree T23.241 ☑
        third degree T23.341 ☑
      second degree T23.249 ☑
      third degree T23.349 ☑
    right T23.011 ☑
      first degree T23.111 ☑
      second degree T23.211 ☑
      third degree T23.311 ☑
    second degree T23.219 ☑
    third degree T23.319 ☑
  toe T25.039 ☑
    first degree T25.139 ☑
    left T25.032 ☑
      first degree T25.132 ☑
      second degree T25.232 ☑
      third degree T25.332 ☑
    right T25.031 ☑
      first degree T25.131 ☑
      second degree T25.231 ☑
      third degree T25.331 ☑
    second degree T25.239 ☑
    third degree T25.339 ☑
  tongue T28.0 ☑
  tonsil(s) T28.0 ☑
  trachea T27.0 ☑
    with lung T27.1 ☑
  trunk T21.00 ☑

☑ Additional Character Required — Refer to the Tabular List for Character Selection   ▽ Subterms under main terms may continue to next column or page

Burn — continued
  trunk — continued
    abdominal wall — see Burn, abdominal wall
    anus — see Burn, buttock
    axilla — see Burn, upper limb
    back — see Burn, back
    breast — see Burn, chest wall
    buttock — see Burn, buttock
    chest wall — see Burn, chest wall
    first degree T21.10 ☑
    flank — see Burn, abdominal wall
    genital
      female — see Burn, genital organs, external, female
      male — see Burn, genital organs, external, male
    groin — see Burn, abdominal wall
    interscapular region — see Burn, back, upper
    labia — see Burn, genital organs, external, female
    lower back — see Burn, back
    penis — see Burn, genital organs, external, male
    perineum
      female — see Burn, genital organs, external, female
      male — see Burn, genital organs, external, male
    scapula region — see Burn, scapular region
    scrotum — see Burn, genital organs, external, male
    second degree T21.20 ☑
    specified site NEC T21.09 ☑
      first degree T21.19 ☑
      second degree T21.29 ☑
      third degree T21.39 ☑
    testes — see Burn, genital organs, external, male
    third degree T21.30 ☑
    upper back — see Burn, back, upper
    vulva — see Burn, genital organs, external, female
  unspecified site with extent of body surface involved
    specified
      less than 10 percent T31.0
      10-19 percent (0-9 percent third degree) T31.10
        with 10-19 percent third degree T31.11
      20-29 percent (0-9 percent third degree) T31.20
        with
          10-19 percent third degree T31.21
          20-29 percent third degree T31.22
      30-39 percent (0-9 percent third degree) T31.30
        with
          10-19 percent third degree T31.31
          20-29 percent third degree T31.32
          30-39 percent third degree T31.33
      40-49 percent (0-9 percent third degree) T31.40
        with
          10-19 percent third degree T31.41
          20-29 percent third degree T31.42
          30-39 percent third degree T31.43
          40-49 percent third degree T31.44
      50-59 percent (0-9 percent third degree) T31.50
        with
          10-19 percent third degree T31.51
          20-29 percent third degree T31.52
          30-39 percent third degree T31.53
          40-49 percent third degree T31.54
          50-59 percent third degree T31.55
      60-69 percent (0-9 percent third degree) T31.60
        with
          10-19 percent third degree T31.61
          20-29 percent third degree T31.62
          30-39 percent third degree T31.63
          40-49 percent third degree T31.64
          50-59 percent third degree T31.65
          60-69 percent third degree T31.66
      70-79 percent (0-9 percent third degree) T31.70
        with
          10-19 percent third degree T31.71
          20-29 percent third degree T31.72
          30-39 percent third degree T31.73
          40-49 percent third degree T31.74
          50-59 percent third degree T31.75
          60-69 percent third degree T31.76
          70-79 percent third degree T31.77
      80-89 percent (0-9 percent third degree) T31.80
        with
          10-19 percent third degree T31.81
          20-29 percent third degree T31.82
          30-39 percent third degree T31.83
          40-49 percent third degree T31.84
          50-59 percent third degree T31.85
          60-69 percent third degree T31.86
          70-79 percent third degree T31.87

Burn — continued
  unspecified site with extent of body surface involved
    specified — continued
      80-89 percent — continued
        with — continued
          80-89 percent third degree T31.88
      90 percent or more (0-9 percent third degree) T31.90
        with
          10-19 percent third degree T31.91
          20-29 percent third degree T31.92
          30-39 percent third degree T31.93
          40-49 percent third degree T31.94
          50-59 percent third degree T31.95
          60-69 percent third degree T31.96
          70-79 percent third degree T31.97
          80-89 percent third degree T31.98
          90-99 percent third degree T31.99
  upper limb T22.00 ☑
    above elbow — see Burn, above elbow
    axilla — see Burn, axilla
    elbow — see Burn, elbow
    first degree T22.10 ☑
    forearm — see Burn, forearm
    hand — see Burn, hand
    interscapular region — see Burn, back, upper
    multiple sites T22.099 ☑
      first degree T22.199 ☑
      left T22.092 ☑
        first degree T22.192 ☑
        second degree T22.292 ☑
        third degree T22.392 ☑
      right T22.091 ☑
        first degree T22.191 ☑
        second degree T22.291 ☑
        third degree T22.391 ☑
      second degree T22.299 ☑
      third degree T22.399 ☑
    scapular region — see Burn, scapular region
    second degree T22.20 ☑
    shoulder — see Burn, shoulder
    third degree T22.30 ☑
    wrist — see Burn, wrist
  uterus T28.3 ☑
  vagina T28.3 ☑
  vulva — see Burn, genital organs, external, female
  wrist T23.079 ☑
    first degree T23.179 ☑
    left T23.072 ☑
      first degree T23.172 ☑
      second degree T23.272 ☑
      third degree T23.372 ☑
    multiple sites with hand T23.099 ☑
      first degree T23.199 ☑
      left T23.092 ☑
        first degree T23.192 ☑
        second degree T23.292 ☑
        third degree T23.392 ☑
      right T23.091 ☑
        first degree T23.191 ☑
        second degree T23.291 ☑
        third degree T23.391 ☑
      second degree T23.299 ☑
      third degree T23.399 ☑
    right T23.071 ☑
      first degree T23.171 ☑
      second degree T23.271 ☑
      third degree T23.371 ☑
    second degree T23.279 ☑
    third degree T23.379 ☑
Burnett's syndrome E83.52
Burning
  feet syndrome E53.9
  sensation R20.8
  tongue K14.6
Burn-out (state) Z73.0
Burns' disease or osteochondrosis — see Osteochondrosis, juvenile, ulna
Bursa — see condition
Bursitis M71.9
  Achilles — see Tendinitis, Achilles
  adhesive — see Bursitis, specified NEC
  ankle — see Enthesopathy, lower limb, ankle, specified type NEC
  calcaneal — see Enthesopathy, foot, specified type NEC

Bursitis — continued
  collateral ligament, tibial — see Bursitis, tibial collateral
  due to use, overuse, pressure (see also Disorder, soft tissue, due to use, specified type NEC)
    specified NEC — see Disorder, soft tissue, due to use, specified NEC
  Duplay's M75.0 ☑
  elbow NEC M70.3- ☑
    olecranon M70.2- ☑
  finger — see Disorder, soft tissue, due to use, specified type NEC, hand
  foot — see Enthesopathy, foot, specified type NEC
  gonococcal A54.49
  gouty — see Gout, idiopathic
  hand M70.1- ☑
  hip NEC M70.7- ☑
    trochanteric M70.6- ☑
  infective NEC M71.10
    abscess — see Abscess, bursa
    ankle M71.17- ☑
    elbow M71.12- ☑
    foot M71.17- ☑
    hand M71.14- ☑
    hip M71.15- ☑
    knee M71.16- ☑
    multiple sites M71.19
    shoulder M71.11- ☑
    specified site NEC M71.18
    wrist M71.13- ☑
  ischial — see Bursitis, hip
  knee NEC M70.5- ☑
    prepatellar M70.4- ☑
  occupational NEC (see also Disorder, soft tissue, due to, use)
  olecranon — see Bursitis, elbow, olecranon
  pharyngeal J39.1
  popliteal — see Bursitis, knee
  prepatellar M70.4- ☑
  radiohumeral M77.8
  rheumatoid M06.20
    ankle M06.27- ☑
    elbow M06.22- ☑
    foot joint M06.27- ☑
    hand joint M06.24- ☑
    hip M06.25- ☑
    knee M06.26- ☑
    multiple site M06.29
    shoulder M06.21- ☑
    vertebra M06.28
    wrist M06.23- ☑
  scapulohumeral — see Bursitis, shoulder
  semimembranous muscle (knee) — see Bursitis, knee
  shoulder M75.5- ☑
    adhesive — see Capsulitis, adhesive
  specified NEC M71.50
    ankle M71.57- ☑
    due to use, overuse or pressure — see Disorder, soft tissue, due to, use
    elbow M71.52- ☑
    foot M71.57- ☑
    hand M71.54- ☑
    hip M71.55- ☑
    knee M71.56- ☑
    shoulder — see Bursitis, shoulder
    specified site NEC M71.58
    tibial collateral M76.4- ☑
    wrist M71.53- ☑
  subacromial — see Bursitis, shoulder
  subcoracoid — see Bursitis, shoulder
  subdeltoid — see Bursitis, shoulder
  syphilitic A52.78
  Thornwaldt, Tornwaldt J39.2
  tibial collateral — see Bursitis, tibial collateral
  toe — see Enthesopathy, foot, specified type NEC
  trochanteric (area) — see Bursitis, hip, trochanteric
  wrist — see Bursitis, hand
Bursopathy M71.9
  specified type NEC M71.80
    ankle M71.87- ☑
    elbow M71.82- ☑
    foot M71.87- ☑
    hand M71.84- ☑
    hip M71.85- ☑
    knee M71.86- ☑
    multiple sites M71.89
    shoulder M71.81- ☑

Bursopathy — continued
  specified type — continued
    specified site NEC M71.88
    wrist M71.83- ☑
Burst stitches or sutures (complication of surgery)
    T81.31 ☑
    external operation wound T81.31 ☑
    internal operation wound T81.32 ☑
Buruli ulcer A31.1
Bury's disease L95.1
Buschke's
    disease B45.3
    scleredema — see Sclerosis, systemic
Busse-Buschke disease B45.3
Buttock — see condition
Button
    Biskra B55.1
    Delhi B55.1
    oriental B55.1
Buttonhole deformity (finger) — see Deformity, finger, boutonniere
Bwamba fever A92.8
Byssinosis J66.0
Bywaters' syndrome T79.5 ☑

C

Cachexia R64
    cancerous R64
    cardiac — see Disease, heart
    dehydration E86.0
      with
        hypernatremia E87.0
        hyponatremia E87.1
    due to malnutrition R64
    exophthalmic — see Hyperthyroidism
    heart — see Disease, heart
    hypophyseal E23.0
    hypopituitary E23.0
    lead — see Poisoning, lead
    malignant R64
    marsh — see Malaria
    nervous F48.8
    old age R54
    paludal — see Malaria
    pituitary E23.0
    renal N28.9
    saturnine — see Poisoning, lead
    senile R54
    Simmonds' E23.0
    splenica D73.0
    strumipriva E03.4
    tuberculous NEC — see Tuberculosis
Café, au lait spots L81.3
Caffey's syndrome Q78.8
Caisson disease T70.3 ☑
Cake kidney Q63.1
Caked breast (puerperal, postpartum) O92.79
Calabar swelling B74.3
Calcaneal spur — see Spur, bone, calcaneal
Calcaneo-apophysitis M92.8
Calcareous — see condition
Calcicosis J62.8
Calciferol (vitamin D) deficiency E55.9
    with rickets E55.0
Calcification
    adrenal (capsule) (gland) E27.49
      tuberculous E35 [B90.8]
    aorta I70.0
    artery (annular) — see Arteriosclerosis
    auricle (ear) — see Disorder, pinna, specified type NEC
    basal ganglia G23.8
    bladder N32.89
      due to Schistosoma hematobium B65.0
    brain (cortex) — see Calcification, cerebral
    bronchus J98.09
    bursa M71.40
      ankle M71.47- ☑
      elbow M71.42- ☑
      foot M71.47- ☑
      hand M71.44- ☑
      hip M71.45- ☑
      knee M71.46- ☑
      multiple sites M71.49
      shoulder M75.3- ☑
      specified site NEC M71.48
      wrist M71.43- ☑

Calcification — continued
    cardiac — see Degeneration, myocardial
    cerebral (cortex) G93.89
      artery I67.2
    cervix (uteri) N88.8
    choroid plexus G93.89
    conjunctiva — see Concretion, conjunctiva
    corpora cavernosa (penis) N48.89
    cortex (brain) — see Calcification, cerebral
    dental pulp (nodular) K04.2
    dentinal papilla K00.4
    fallopian tube N83.8
    falx cerebri G96.19
    gallbladder K82.8
    general E83.59
    heart (see also Degeneration, myocardial)
      valve — see Endocarditis
    idiopathic infantile arterial (IIAC) Q28.8
    intervertebral cartilage or disc (postinfective) — see Disorder, disc, specified NEC
    intracranial — see Calcification, cerebral
    joint — see Disorder, joint, specified type NEC
    kidney N28.89
      tuberculous N29 [B90.1]
    larynx (senile) J38.7
    lens — see Cataract, specified NEC
    lung (active) (postinfectional) J98.4
      tuberculous B90.9
    lymph gland or node (postinfectional) I89.8
      tuberculous (see also Tuberculosis, lymph gland) B90.8
    mammographic R92.1
    massive (paraplegic) — see Myositis, ossificans, in, quadriplegia
    medial — see Arteriosclerosis, extremities
    meninges (cerebral) (spinal) G96.19
    metastatic E83.59
    Mönckeberg's — see Arteriosclerosis, extremities
    muscle M61.9
      due to burns — see Myositis, ossificans, in, burns
      paralytic — see Myositis, ossificans, in, quadriplegia
      specified type NEC M61.40
        ankle M61.47- ☑
        foot M61.47- ☑
        forearm M61.43- ☑
        hand M61.44- ☑
        lower leg M61.46- ☑
        multiple sites M61.49
        pelvic region M61.45- ☑
        shoulder region M61.41- ☑
        specified site NEC M61.48
        thigh M61.45- ☑
        upper arm M61.42- ☑
    myocardium, myocardial — see Degeneration, myocardial
    ovary N83.8
    pancreas K86.8
    penis N48.89
    periarticular — see Disorder, joint, specified type NEC
    pericardium (see also Pericarditis) I31.1
    pineal gland E34.8
    pleura J94.8
      postinfectional J94.8
      tuberculous NEC B90.9
    pulpal (dental) (nodular) K04.2
    sclera H15.89
    spleen D73.89
    subcutaneous L94.2
    suprarenal (capsule) (gland) E27.49
    tendon (sheath) (see also Tenosynovitis, specified type NEC)
      with bursitis, synovitis or tenosynovitis — see Tendinitis, calcific
    trachea J39.8
    ureter N28.89
    uterus N85.8
    vitreous — see Deposit, crystalline
Calcified — see Calcification
Calcinosis (interstitial) (tumoral) (universalis) E83.59
    with Raynaud's phenomenon, esophageal dysfunction, sclerodactyly, telangiectasia (CREST syndrome) M34.1
    circumscripta (skin) L94.2
    cutis L94.2
Calciphylaxis (see also Calcification, by site) E83.59
Calcium
    deposits — see Calcification, by site

Calcium — continued
    metabolism disorder E83.50
    salts or soaps in vitreous — see Deposit, crystalline
Calciuria R82.99
Calculi — see Calculus
Calculosis, intrahepatic — see Calculus, bile duct
Calculus, calculi, calculous
    ampulla of Vater — see Calculus, bile duct
    anuria (impacted) (recurrent) (see also Calculus, urinary) N20.9
    appendix K38.1
    bile duct (common) (hepatic) K80.50
      with
        calculus of gallbladder — see Calculus, gallbladder and bile duct
        cholangitis K80.30
          with
            cholecystitis — see Calculus, bile duct, with cholecystitis
            obstruction K80.31
          acute K80.32
            with
              chronic cholangitis K80.36
                with obstruction K80.37
              obstruction K80.33
          chronic K80.34
            with
              acute cholangitis K80.36
                with obstruction K80.37
              obstruction K80.35
        cholecystitis (with cholangitis) K80.40
          with obstruction K80.41
          acute K80.42
            with
              chronic cholecystitis K80.46
                with obstruction K80.47
              obstruction K80.43
          chronic K80.44
            with
              acute cholecystitis K80.46
                with obstruction K80.47
              obstruction K80.45
        obstruction K80.51
    biliary (see also Calculus, gallbladder)
      specified NEC K80.80
        with obstruction K80.81
    bilirubin, multiple — see Calculus, gallbladder
    bladder (encysted) (impacted) (urinary) (diverticulum) N21.0
    bronchus J98.09
    calyx (kidney) (renal) — see Calculus, kidney
    cholesterol (pure) (solitary) — see Calculus, gallbladder
    common duct (bile) — see Calculus, bile duct
    conjunctiva — see Concretion, conjunctiva
    cystic N21.0
      duct — see Calculus, gallbladder
    dental (subgingival) (supragingival) K03.6
    diverticulum
      bladder N21.0
      kidney N20.0
    epididymis N50.8
    gallbladder K80.20
      with
        bile duct calculus — see Calculus, gallbladder and bile duct
        cholecystitis K80.10
          with obstruction K80.11
          acute K80.00
            with
              chronic cholecystitis K80.12
                with obstruction K80.13
              obstruction K80.01
          chronic K80.10
            with
              acute cholecystitis K80.12
                with obstruction K80.13
              obstruction K80.11
        specified NEC K80.18
          with obstruction K80.19
        obstruction K80.21
    gallbladder and bile duct K80.70
      with
        cholecystitis K80.60
          with obstruction K80.61
          acute K80.62
            with
              chronic cholecystitis K80.66
                with obstruction K80.67

☑ **Additional Character Required** — Refer to the Tabular List for Character Selection   ▽ **Subterms under main terms may continue to next column or page**

Calculus, calculi, calculous — *continued*
  gallbladder and bile duct — *continued*
    with — *continued*
      cholecystitis — *continued*
        acute — *continued*
          with — *continued*
            obstruction K80.63
          chronic K80.64
            with
              acute cholecystitis K80.66
                with obstruction K80.67
              obstruction K80.65
        obstruction K80.71
  hepatic (duct) — *see* Calculus, bile duct
  ileal conduit N21.8
  intestinal (impaction) (obstruction) K56.49
  kidney (impacted) (multiple) (pelvis) (recurrent)
      (staghorn) N20.0
    with calculus, ureter N20.2
      congenital Q63.8
  lacrimal passages — *see* Dacryolith
  liver (impacted) — *see* Calculus, bile duct
  lung J98.4
  mammographic R92.1
  nephritic (impacted) (recurrent) — *see* Calculus, kidney
  nose J34.89
  pancreas (duct) K86.8
  parotid duct or gland K11.5
  pelvis, encysted — *see* Calculus, kidney
  prostate N42.0
  pulmonary J98.4
  pyelitis (impacted) (recurrent) N20.0
    with hydronephrosis N13.2
  pyelonephritis (impacted) (recurrent) N20 ☑
    with hydronephrosis N13.2
  renal (impacted) (recurrent) — *see* Calculus, kidney
  salivary (duct) (gland) K11.5
  seminal vesicle N50.8
  staghorn — *see* Calculus, kidney
  Stensen's duct K11.5
  stomach K31.89
  sublingual duct or gland K11.5
    congenital Q38.4
  submandibular duct, gland or region K11.5
  submaxillary duct, gland or region K11.5
  suburethral N21.8
  tonsil J35.8
  tooth, teeth (subgingival) (supragingival) K03.6
  tunica vaginalis N50.8
  ureter (impacted) (recurrent) N20.1
    with calculus, kidney N20.2
      with hydronephrosis N13.2
        with infection N13.6
  urethra (impacted) N21.1
  urinary (duct) (impacted) (passage) (tract) N20.9
    with hydronephrosis N13.2
      with infection N13.6
    in (due to)
      lower N21.9
        specified NEC N21.8
  vagina N89.8
  vesical (impacted) N21.0
  Wharton's duct K11.5
  xanthine E79.8 [N22]
Calicectasis N28.89
Caliectasis N28.89
California
  disease B38.9
  encephalitis A83.5
Caligo cornea — *see* Opacity, cornea, central
Callositas, callosity (infected) L84
Callus (infected) L84
  bone — *see* Osteophyte
  excessive, following fracture — *code as* Sequelae
      of fracture
Calorie deficiency or malnutrition (*see also* Malnutrition) E46
Calvé-Perthes disease — *see* Legg-Calvé-Perthes disease
Calvé's disease — *see* Osteochondrosis, juvenile, spine
Calvities — *see* Alopecia, androgenic
Cameroon fever — *see* Malaria
Camptocormia (hysterical) F44.4
Camurati-Engelmann syndrome Q78.3
Canal (*see also* condition)
  atrioventricular common Q21.2
Canaliculitis (lacrimal) (acute) (subacute) H04.33- ☑
  Actinomyces A42.89

Canaliculitis — *continued*
  chronic H04.42-
Canavan's disease E75.29
Canceled procedure (surgical) Z53.9
  because of
    contraindication Z53.09
      smoking Z53.01
    left against medical advice (AMA) Z53.21
    patient's decision Z53.20
      for reasons of belief or group pressure Z53.1
      specified reason NEC Z53.29
    specified reason NEC Z53.8
Cancer (*see also* Neoplasm, by site, malignant)
  bile duct type liver C22.1
  blood — *see* Leukemia
  breast (*see also* Neoplasm, breast, malignant)
      C50.91- ☑
  hepatocellular C22.0
  lung (*see also* Neoplasm, lung, malignant) C34.90
  ovarian (*see also* Neoplasm ovary, malignant) C56.9
  unspecified site (primary) C80.1
Cancer (o)**phobia** F45.29
Cancerous — *see* Neoplasm, malignant, by site
Cancrum oris A69.0
Candidiasis, candidal B37.9
  balanitis B37.42
  bronchitis B37.1
  cheilitis B37.83
  congenital P37.5
  cystitis B37.41
  disseminated B37.7
  endocarditis B37.6
  enteritis B37.82
  esophagitis B37.81
  intertrigo B37.2
  lung B37.1
  meningitis B37.5
  mouth B37.0
  nails B37.2
  neonatal P37.5
  onychia B37.2
  oral B37.0
  osteomyelitis B37.89
  otitis externa B37.84
  paronychia B37.2
  perionyxis B37.2
  pneumonia B37.1
  proctitis B37.82
  pulmonary B37.1
  pyelonephritis B37.49
  sepsis B37.7
  skin B37.2
  specified site NEC B37.89
  stomatitis B37.0
  systemic B37.7
  urethritis B37.41
  urogenital site NEC B37.49
  vagina B37.3
  vulva B37.3
  vulvovaginitis B37.3
Candidid L30.2
Candidosis — *see* Candidiasis
Candiru infection or infestation B88.8
Canities (premature) L67.1
  congenital Q84.2
Canker (mouth) (sore) K12.0
  rash A38.9
Cannabinosis J66.2
Canton fever A75.9
Cantrell's syndrome Q87.89
Capillariasis (intestinal) B81.1
  hepatic B83.8
Capillary — *see* condition
Caplan's syndrome — *see* Rheumatoid, lung
Capsule — *see* condition
Capsulitis (joint) (*see also* Enthesopathy)
  adhesive (shoulder) M75.0- ☑
  hepatic K65.8
  labyrinthine — *see* Otosclerosis, specified NEC
  thyroid E06.9
Caput
  crepitus Q75.8
  medusae I86.8
  succedaneum P12.81
Car sickness T75.3 ☑
Carapata (disease) A68.0
Carate — *see* Pinta

Carbon lung J60
Carbuncle L02.93
  abdominal wall L02.231
  anus K61.0
  auditory canal, external — *see* Abscess, ear, external
  auricle ear — *see* Abscess, ear, external
  axilla L02.43- ☑
  back (any part) L02.232
  breast N61
  buttock L02.33
  cheek (external) L02.03
  chest wall L02.233
  chin L02.03
  corpus cavernosum N48.21
  ear (any part) (external) (middle) — *see* Abscess, ear, external
  external auditory canal — *see* Abscess, ear, external
  eyelid — *see* Abscess, eyelid
  face NEC L02.03
  femoral (region) — *see* Carbuncle, lower limb
  finger — *see* Carbuncle, hand
  flank L02.231
  foot L02.63- ☑
  forehead L02.03
  genital — *see* Abscess, genital
  gluteal (region) L02.33
  groin L02.234
  hand L02.53- ☑
  head NEC L02.831
  heel — *see* Carbuncle, foot
  hip — *see* Carbuncle, lower limb
  kidney — *see* Abscess, kidney
  knee — *see* Carbuncle, lower limb
  labium (majus) (minus) N76.4
  lacrimal
    gland — *see* Dacryoadenitis
    passages (duct) (sac) — *see* Inflammation, lacrimal, passages, acute
  leg — *see* Carbuncle, lower limb
  lower limb L02.43- ☑
  malignant A22.0
  navel L02.236
  neck L02.13
  nose (external) (septum) J34.0
  orbit, orbital — *see* Abscess, orbit
  palmar (space) — *see* Carbuncle, hand
  partes posteriores L02.33
  pectoral region L02.233
  penis N48.21
  perineum L02.235
  pinna — *see* Abscess, ear, external
  popliteal — *see* Carbuncle, lower limb
  scalp L02.831
  seminal vesicle N49.0
  shoulder — *see* Carbuncle, upper limb
  specified site NEC L02.838
  temple (region) L02.03
  thumb — *see* Carbuncle, hand
  toe — *see* Carbuncle, foot
  trunk L02.239
    abdominal wall L02.231
    back L02.232
    chest wall L02.233
    groin L02.234
    perineum L02.235
    umbilicus L02.236
  umbilicus L02.236
  upper limb L02.43- ☑
  urethra N34.0
  vulva N76.4
Carbunculus — *see* Carbuncle
Carcinoid (tumor) — *see* Tumor, carcinoid
Carcinoidosis E34.0
Carcinoma (malignant) (*see also* Neoplasm, by site, malignant)
  acidophil
    specified site — *see* Neoplasm, malignant, by site
    unspecified site C75.1
  acidophil-basophil, mixed
    specified site — *see* Neoplasm, malignant, by site
    unspecified site C75.1
  adnexal (skin) — *see* Neoplasm, skin, malignant
  adrenal cortical C74.0- ☑
  alveolar — *see* Neoplasm, lung, malignant
    cell — *see* Neoplasm, lung, malignant
  ameloblastic C41.1
    upper jaw (bone) C41.0

Carcinoma — *continued*
  apocrine
    breast — *see* Neoplasm, breast, malignant
    specified site NEC — *see* Neoplasm, skin, malignant
    unspecified site C44.99
  basal cell (pigmented) (*see also* Neoplasm, skin, malignant) C44.91
    fibro-epithelial — *see* Neoplasm, skin, malignant
    morphea — *see* Neoplasm, skin, malignant
    multicentric — *see* Neoplasm, skin, malignant
  basaloid
  basal-squamous cell, mixed — *see* Neoplasm, skin, malignant
  basophil
    specified site — *see* Neoplasm, malignant, by site
    unspecified site C75.1
  basophil-acidophil, mixed
    specified site — *see* Neoplasm, malignant, by site
    unspecified site C75.1
  basosquamous — *see* Neoplasm, skin, malignant
  bile duct
    with hepatocellular, mixed C22.0
    liver C22.1
    specified site NEC — *see* Neoplasm, malignant, by site
    unspecified site C22.1
  branchial or branchiogenic C10.4
  bronchial or bronchogenic — *see* Neoplasm, lung, malignant
  bronchiolar — *see* Neoplasm, lung, malignant
  bronchioloalveolar — *see* Neoplasm, lung, malignant
  C cell
    specified site — *see* Neoplasm, malignant, by site
    unspecified site C73
  ceruminous C44.29- ☑
  cervix uteri
    in situ D06.9
      endocervix D06.0
      exocervix D06.1
      specified site NEC D06.7
  chorionic
    specified site — *see* Neoplasm, malignant, by site
    unspecified site
      female C58
      male C62.90
  chromophobe
    specified site — *see* Neoplasm, malignant, by site
    unspecified site C75.1
  cloacogenic
    specified site — *see* Neoplasm, malignant, by site
    unspecified site C21.2
  diffuse type
    specified site — *see* Neoplasm, malignant, by site
    unspecified site C16.9
  duct (cell)
    with Paget's disease — *see* Neoplasm, breast, malignant
    infiltrating
      with lobular carcinoma (in situ)
        specified site — *see* Neoplasm, malignant, by site
        unspecified site (female) C50.91- ☑
          male C50.92- ☑
      specified site — *see* Neoplasm, malignant, by site
      unspecified site (female) C50.91- ☑
        male C50.92- ☑
  ductal
    with lobular
      specified site — *see* Neoplasm, malignant, by site
      unspecified site (female) C50.91- ☑
        male C50.92- ☑
    ductular, infiltrating
      specified site — *see* Neoplasm, malignant, by site
      unspecified site (female) C50.91- ☑
        male C50.92- ☑
  embryonal
    liver C22.7
  endometrioid
    specified site — *see* Neoplasm, malignant, by site
    unspecified site
      female C56.9
      male C61
  eosinophil
    specified site — *see* Neoplasm, malignant, by site
    unspecified site C75.1

Carcinoma — *continued*
  epidermoid (*see also* Neoplasm, skin, malignant)
    in situ, Bowen's type — *see* Neoplasm, skin, in situ
  fibroepithelial, basal cell — *see* Neoplasm, skin, malignant
  follicular
    with papillary (mixed) C73
    moderately differentiated C73
    pure follicle C73
    specified site — *see* Neoplasm, malignant, by site
    trabecular C73
    unspecified site C73
    well differentiated C73
  generalized, with unspecified primary site C80.0
  glycogen-rich — *see* Neoplasm, breast, malignant
  granulosa cell C56- ☑
  hepatic cell C22.0
  hepatocellular C22.0
    with bile duct, mixed C22.0
    fibrolamellar C22.0
  hepatocholangiolitic C22.0
  Hurthle cell C73
  in
    adenomatous
      polyposis coli C18.9
    pleomorphic adenoma — *see* Neoplasm, salivary glands, malignant
    situ — *see* Carcinoma-in-situ
  infiltrating
    duct
      with lobular
        specified site — *see* Neoplasm, malignant, by site
        unspecified site (female) C50.91- ☑
          male C50.92- ☑
      with Paget's disease — *see* Neoplasm, breast, malignant
      specified site — *see* Neoplasm, malignant
      unspecified site (female) C50.91- ☑
        male C50.92- ☑
    ductular
      specified site — *see* Neoplasm, malignant
      unspecified site (female) C50.91- ☑
        male C50.92- ☑
    lobular
      specified site — *see* Neoplasm, malignant
      unspecified site (female) C50.91- ☑
        male C50.92- ☑
  inflammatory
    specified site — *see* Neoplasm, malignant
    unspecified site (female) C50.91- ☑
      male C50.92- ☑
  intestinal type
    specified site — *see* Neoplasm, malignant, by site
    unspecified site C16.9
  intracystic
    noninfiltrating — *see* Neoplasm, in situ, by site
  intraductal (noninfiltrating)
    with Paget's disease — *see* Neoplasm, breast, malignant
    breast D05.1- ☑
    papillary
      with invasion
        specified site — *see* Neoplasm, malignant, by site
        unspecified site (female) C50.91- ☑
          male C50.92- ☑
      breast D05.1- ☑
      specified site NEC — *see* Neoplasm, in situ, by site
      unspecified site (female) D05.1- ☑
    specified site NEC — *see* Neoplasm, in situ, by site
    unspecified site (female) D05.1- ☑
  intraepidermal — *see* Neoplasm, in situ
    squamous cell, Bowen's type — *see* Neoplasm, skin, in situ
  intraepithelial — *see* Neoplasm, in situ, by site
    squamous cell — *see* Neoplasm, in situ, by site
  intraosseous C41.1
    upper jaw (bone) C41.0
  islet cell
    with exocrine, mixed
      specified site — *see* Neoplasm, malignant, by site
      unspecified site C25.9
    pancreas C25.4

Carcinoma — *continued*
  islet cell — *continued*
    specified site NEC — *see* Neoplasm, malignant, by site
    unspecified site C25.4
  juvenile, breast — *see* Neoplasm, breast, malignant
  large cell
    small cell
      specified site — *see* Neoplasm, malignant, by site
      unspecified site C34.90
  Leydig cell (testis)
    specified site — *see* Neoplasm, malignant, by site
    unspecified site
      female C56.9
      male C62.90
  lipid-rich (female) C50.91- ☑
    male C50.92- ☑
  liver cell C22.0
  liver NEC C22.7
  lobular (infiltrating)
    with intraductal
      specified site — *see* Neoplasm, malignant, by site
      unspecified site (female) C50.91- ☑
        male C50.92- ☑
    noninfiltrating
      breast D05.0- ☑
      specified site NEC — *see* Neoplasm, in situ, by site
      unspecified site D05.0- ☑
    specified site — *see* Neoplasm, malignant, by site
    unspecified site (female) C50.91- ☑
      male C50.92- ☑
  medullary
    with
      amyloid stroma
        specified site — *see* Neoplasm, malignant, by site
        unspecified site C73
      lymphoid stroma
        specified site — *see* Neoplasm, malignant, by site
        unspecified site (female) C50.91- ☑
          male C50.92- ☑
  Merkel cell C4A.9 (*following* C43)
    anal margin C4A.51 (*following* C43)
    anal skin C4A.51 (*following* C43)
    canthus C4A.1- ☑ (*following* C43)
    ear and external auricular canal C4A.2- ☑ (*following* C43)
    external auricular canal C4A.2- ☑ (*following* C43)
    eyelid, including canthus C4A.1- ☑ (*following* C43)
    face C4A.30 (*following* C43)
      specified NEC C4A.39 (*following* C43)
    hip C4A.7- ☑ (*following* C43)
    lip C4A.0 (*following* C43)
    lower limb, including hip C4A.7- ☑ (*following* C43)
    neck C4A.4 (*following* C43)
    nodal presentation C7B.1 (*following* C75)
    nose C4A.31 (*following* C43)
    overlapping sites C4A.8 (*following* C43)
    perianal skin C4A.51 (*following* C43)
    scalp C4A.4 (*following* C43)
    secondary C7B.1 (*following* C75)
    shoulder C4A.6- ☑ (*following* C43)
    skin of breast C4A.52 (*following* C43)
    trunk NEC C4A.59 (*following* C43)
    upper limb, including shoulder C4A.6- ☑ (*following* C43)
    visceral metastatic C7B.1 (*following* C75)
  metastatic — *see* Neoplasm, secondary, by site
  metatypical — *see* Neoplasm, skin, malignant
  morphea, basal cell — *see* Neoplasm, skin, malignant
  mucoid
    cell
      specified site — *see* Neoplasm, malignant, by site
      unspecified site C75.1
  neuroendocrine (*see also* Tumor, neuroendocrine)
    high grade, any site C7A.1 (*following* C75)
    poorly differentiated, any site C7A.1 (*following* C75)
  nonencapsulated sclerosing C73
  noninfiltrating
    intracystic — *see* Neoplasm, in situ, by site
    intraductal
      breast D05.1- ☑

☑ **Additional Character Required — Refer to the Tabular List for Character Selection**   ▼ Subterms under main terms may continue to next column or page

Carcinoma — *continued*
  noninfiltrating — *continued*
    intraductal — *continued*
      papillary
        breast D05.1- ☑
        specified site NEC — *see* Neoplasm, in situ, by site
        unspecified site D05.1- ☑
      specified site — *see* Neoplasm, in situ, by site
      unspecified site D05.1- ☑
      lobular
        breast D05.0- ☑
        specified site NEC — *see* Neoplasm, in situ, by site
        unspecified site (female) D05.0- ☑
  oat cell
    specified site — *see* Neoplasm, malignant, by site
    unspecified site C34.90
  odontogenic C41.1
    upper jaw (bone) C41.0
  papillary
    with follicular (mixed) C73
    follicular variant C73
    intraductal (noninfiltrating)
      with invasion
        specified site — *see* Neoplasm, malignant, by site
        unspecified site (female) C50.91- ☑
          male C50.92- ☑
      breast D05.1- ☑
      specified site NEC — *see* Neoplasm, in situ, by site
      unspecified site D05.1- ☑
    serous
      specified site — *see* Neoplasm, malignant, by site
      surface
        specified site — *see* Neoplasm, malignant, by site
        unspecified site C56.9
      unspecified site C56.9
  papillocystic
    specified site — *see* Neoplasm, malignant, by site
    unspecified site C56.9
  parafollicular cell
    specified site — *see* Neoplasm, malignant, by site
    unspecified site C73
  pilomatrix — *see* Neoplasm, skin, malignant
  pseudomucinous
    specified site — *see* Neoplasm, malignant, by site
    unspecified site C56.9
  renal cell C64- ☑
  Schmincke — *see* Neoplasm, nasopharynx, malignant
  Schneiderian
    specified site — *see* Neoplasm, malignant, by site
    unspecified site C30.0
  sebaceous — *see* Neoplasm, skin, malignant
  secondary (*see also* Neoplasm, secondary, by site)
    Merkel cell C7B.1 (*following* C75)
  secretory, breast — *see* Neoplasm, breast, malignant
  serous
    papillary
      specified site — *see* Neoplasm, malignant, by site
      unspecified site C56.9
    surface, papillary
      specified site — *see* Neoplasm, malignant, by site
      unspecified site C56.9
  Sertoli cell
    specified site — *see* Neoplasm, malignant, by site
    unspecified site C62.90
      female C56.9
      male C62.90
  skin appendage — *see* Neoplasm, skin, malignant
  small cell
    fusiform cell
      specified site — *see* Neoplasm, malignant, by site
      unspecified site C34.90
    intermediate cell
      specified site — *see* Neoplasm, malignant, by site
      unspecified site C34.90
    large cell
      specified site — *see* Neoplasm, malignant, by site

Carcinoma — *continued*
  small cell — *continued*
    large cell — *continued*
      unspecified site C34.90
    solid
      with amyloid stroma
        specified site — *see* Neoplasm, malignant, by site
        unspecified site C73
    microinvasive
      specified site — *see* Neoplasm, malignant, by site
      unspecified site C53.9
  sweat gland — *see* Neoplasm, skin, malignant
  theca cell C56.- ☑
  thymic C37
  unspecified site (primary) C80.1
  water-clear cell C75.0
Carcinoma-in-situ (*see also* Neoplasm, in situ, by site)
  breast NOS D05.9- ☑
    specified type NEC D05.8- ☑
  epidermoid (*see also* Neoplasm, in situ, by site)
    with questionable stromal invasion
      cervix D06.9
      specified site NEC — *see* Neoplasm, in situ, by site
      unspecified site D06.9
    Bowen's type — *see* Neoplasm, skin, in situ
  intraductal
    breast D05.1- ☑
    specified site NEC — *see* Neoplasm, in situ, by site
    unspecified site D05.1- ☑
  lobular
    with
      infiltrating duct
        breast (female) C50.91- ☑
          male C50.92- ☑
        specified site NEC — *see* Neoplasm, malignant
        unspecified site (female) C50.91- ☑
          male C50.92- ☑
      intraductal
        breast D05.8- ☑
        specified site NEC — *see* Neoplasm, in situ, by site
        unspecified site (female) D05.8- ☑
    breast D05.0- ☑
    specified site NEC — *see* Neoplasm, in situ, by site
    unspecified site D05.0- ☑
  squamous cell (*see also* Neoplasm, in situ, by site)
    with questionable stromal invasion
      cervix D06.9
      specified site NEC — *see* Neoplasm, in situ, by site
      unspecified site D06.9
Carcinomaphobia F45.29
Carcinomatosis C80.0
  peritonei C78.6
  unspecified site (primary) (secondary) C80.0
Carcinosarcoma — *see* Neoplasm, malignant, by site
  embryonal — *see* Neoplasm, malignant, by site
Cardia, cardial — *see* condition
Cardiac (*see also* condition)
  death, sudden — *see* Arrest, cardiac
  pacemaker
    in situ Z95.0
    management or adjustment Z45.018
  tamponade I31.4
Cardialgia — *see* Pain, precordial
Cardiectasis — *see* Hypertrophy, cardiac
Cardiochalasia K21.9
Cardiomalacia I51.5
Cardiomegalia glycogenica diffusa E74.02 [I43]
Cardiomegaly (*see also* Hypertrophy, cardiac)
  congenital Q24.8
  glycogen E74.02 [I43]
  idiopathic I51.7
Cardiomyoliposis I51.5
Cardiomyopathy (familial) (idiopathic) I42.9
  alcoholic I42.6
  amyloid E85.4 [I43]
  arteriosclerotic — *see* Disease, heart, ischemic, atherosclerotic
  beriberi E51.12
  cobalt-beer I42.6
  congenital I42.4
  congestive I42.0

Cardiomyopathy — *continued*
  constrictive NOS I42.5
  dilated I42.0
  due to
    alcohol I42.6
    beriberi E51.12
    cardiac glycogenosis E74.02 [I43]
    drugs I42.7
    external agents NEC I42.7
    Friedreich's ataxia G11.1
    myotonia atrophica G71.11 [I43]
    progressive muscular dystrophy G71.0
  glycogen storage E74.02 [I43]
  hypertensive — *see* Hypertension, heart
  hypertrophic (nonobstructive) I42.2
    obstructive I42.1
      congenital Q24.8
  in
    Chagas' disease (chronic) B57.2
      acute B57.0
    sarcoidosis D86.85
  ischemic I25.5
  metabolic E88.9 [I43]
    thyrotoxic E05.90 [I43]
      with thyroid storm E05.91 [I43]
  newborn I42.8
    congenital I42.4
  nutritional E63.9 [I43]
    beriberi E51.12
  obscure of Africa I42.8
  peripartum O90.3
  postpartum O90.3
  restrictive NEC I42.5
  rheumatic I09.0
  secondary I42.9
  stress induced I51.81
  takotsubo I51.81
  thyrotoxic E05.90 [I43]
    with thyroid storm E05.91 [I43]
  toxic NEC I42.7
  tuberculous A18.84
  viral B33.24
Cardionephritis — *see* Hypertension, cardiorenal
Cardionephropathy — *see* Hypertension, cardiorenal
Cardionephrosis — *see* Hypertension, cardiorenal
Cardiopathia nigra I27.0
Cardiopathy (*see also* Disease, heart) I51.9
  idiopathic I42.9
  mucopolysaccharidosis E76.3 [I52]
Cardiopericarditis — *see* Pericarditis
Cardiophobia F45.29
Cardiorenal — *see* condition
Cardiorrhexis — *see* Infarct, myocardium
Cardiosclerosis — *see* Disease, heart, ischemic, atherosclerotic
Cardiosis — *see* Disease, heart
Cardiospasm (esophagus) (reflex) (stomach) K22.0
  congenital Q39.5
  with megaesophagus Q39.5
Cardiostenosis — *see* Disease, heart
Cardiosymphysis I31.0
Cardiovascular — *see* condition
Carditis (acute) (bacterial) (chronic) (subacute) I51.89
  meningococcal A39.50
  rheumatic — *see* Disease, heart, rheumatic
  rheumatoid — *see* Rheumatoid, carditis
  viral B33.20
Care (of) (for) (following)
  child (routine) Z76.2
  family member (handicapped) (sick)
    creating problem for family Z63.6
    provided away from home for holiday relief Z75.5
    unavailable, due to
      absence (person rendering care) (sufferer) Z74.2
      inability (any reason) of person rendering care Z74.2
  foundling Z76.1
  holiday relief Z75.5
  improper — *see* Maltreatment
  lack of (at or after birth) (infant) — *see* Maltreatment, child, neglect
  lactating mother Z39.1
  palliative Z51.5
  postpartum
    immediately after delivery Z39.0
    routine follow-up Z39.2
  respite Z75.5

Care — *continued*
  unavailable, due to
    absence of person rendering care Z74.2
    inability (any reason) of person rendering care Z74.2
  well-baby Z76.2
Caries
  bone NEC A18.03
  dental K02.9
    arrested (coronal) (root) K02.3
    chewing surface
      limited to enamel K02.51
      penetrating into dentin K02.52
      penetrating into pulp K02.53
    coronal surface
      chewing surface
        limited to enamel K02.51
        penetrating into dentin K02.52
        penetrating into pulp K02.53
      pit and fissure surface
        limited to enamel K02.51
        penetrating into dentin K02.52
        penetrating into pulp K02.53
      smooth surface
        limited to enamel K02.61
        penetrating into dentin K02.62
        penetrating into pulp K02.63
    pit and fissure surface
      limited to enamel K02.51
      penetrating into dentin K02.52
      penetrating into pulp K02.53
    root K02.7
    smooth surface
      limited to enamel K02.61
      penetrating into dentin K02.62
      penetrating into pulp K02.63
  external meatus — *see* Disorder, ear, external, specified type NEC
  hip (tuberculous) A18.02
  initial (tooth)
    chewing surface K02.51
    pit and fissure surface K02.51
    smooth surface K02.61
  knee (tuberculous) A18.02
  labyrinth H83.8 ☑
  limb NEC (tuberculous) A18.03
  mastoid process (chronic) — *see* Mastoiditis, chronic tuberculous A18.03
  middle ear H74.8 ☑
  nose (tuberculous) A18.03
  orbit (tuberculous) A18.03
  ossicles, ear — *see* Abnormal, ear ossicles
  petrous bone — *see* Petrositis
  root (dental) (tooth) K02.7
  sacrum (tuberculous) A18.01
  spine, spinal (column) (tuberculous) A18.01
  syphilitic A52.77
    congenital (early) A50.02 [M90.80]
  tooth, teeth — *see* Caries, dental
  tuberculous A18.03
  vertebra (column) (tuberculous) A18.01
Carious teeth — *see* Caries, dental
Carneous mole O02.0
Carnitine insufficiency E71.40
Carotid body or sinus syndrome G90.01
Carotidynia G90.01
Carotinemia (dietary) E67.1
Carotinosis (cutis) (skin) E67.1
Carpal tunnel syndrome — *see* Syndrome, carpal tunnel
Carpenter's syndrome Q87.0
Carpopedal spasm — *see* Tetany
Carr-Barr-Plunkett syndrome Q97.1
Carrier (suspected) of
  amebiasis Z22.1
  bacterial disease NEC Z22.39
    diphtheria Z22.2
    intestinal infectious NEC Z22.1
      typhoid Z22.0
    meningococcal Z22.31
    sexually transmitted Z22.4
    specified NEC Z22.39
    staphylococcal (Methicillin susceptible) Z22.321
      Methicillin resistant Z22.322
    streptococcal Z22.338
      group B Z22.330
    typhoid Z22.0
  cholera Z22.1
  diphtheria Z22.2

Carrier of — *continued*
  gastrointestinal pathogens NEC Z22.1
  genetic Z14.8
    cystic fibrosis Z14.1
    hemophilia A (asymptomatic) Z14.01
      symptomatic Z14.02
  gonorrhea Z22.4
  HAA (hepatitis Australian-antigen) Z22.59
  HB (c)(s)-AG Z22.51
  hepatitis (viral) Z22.50
    Australia-antigen (HAA) Z22.59
    B surface antigen (HBsAg) Z22.51
      with acute delta- (super)infection B17.0
    C Z22.52
    specified NEC Z22.59
  human T-cell lymphotropic virus type-1 (HTLV-1) infection Z22.6
  infectious organism Z22.9
    specified NEC Z22.8
  meningococci Z22.31
  Salmonella typhosa Z22.0
  serum hepatitis — *see* Carrier, hepatitis
  staphylococci (Methicillin susceptible) Z22.321
    Methicillin resistant Z22.322
  streptococci Z22.338
    group B Z22.330
  syphilis Z22.4
  typhoid Z22.0
  venereal disease NEC Z22.4
Carrion's disease A44.0
Carter's relapsing fever (Asiatic) A68.1
Cartilage — *see* condition
Caruncle (inflamed)
  conjunctiva (acute) — *see* Conjunctivitis, acute
  labium (majus) (minus) N90.89
  lacrimal — *see* Inflammation, lacrimal, passages
  myrtiform N89.8
  urethral (benign) N36.2
Cascade stomach K31.2
Caseation lymphatic gland (tuberculous) A18.2
Cassidy (-Scholte) syndrome (malignant carcinoid) E34.0
Castellani's disease A69.8
Castration, traumatic, male S38.231 ☑
Casts in urine R82.99
Cat
  cry syndrome Q93.4
  ear Q17.3
  eye syndrome Q92.8
Catabolism, senile R54
Catalepsy (hysterical) F44.2
  schizophrenic F20.2
Cataplexy (idiopathic) — *see* Narcolepsy
Cataract (cortical) (immature) (incipient) H26.9
  with
    neovascularization — *see* Cataract, complicated
  age-related — *see* Cataract, senile
  anterior
    and posterior axial embryonal Q12.0
    pyramidal Q12.0
  associated with
    galactosemia E74.21 [H28]
    myotonic disorders G71.19 [H28]
  blue Q12.0
  central Q12.0
  cerulean Q12.0
  complicated H26.20
    with
      neovascularization H26.21- ☑
      ocular disorder H26.22- ☑
    glaucomatous flecks H26.23- ☑
  congenital Q12.0
  coraliform Q12.0
  coronary Q12.0
  crystalline Q12.0
  diabetic — *see* Diabetes, cataract
  drug-induced H26.3- ☑
  due to
    ocular disorder — *see* Cataract, complicated
    radiation H26.8
  electric H26.8
  extraction status Z98.4- ☑
  glass-blower's H26.8
  heat ray H26.8
  heterochromic — *see* Cataract, complicated
  hypermature — *see* Cataract, senile, morgagnian type
  in (due to)
    chronic iridocyclitis — *see* Cataract, complicated

Cataract — *continued*
  in — *continued*
    diabetes — *see* Diabetes, cataract
    endocrine disease E34.9 [H28]
    eye disease — *see* Cataract, complicated
    hypoparathyroidism E20.9 [H28]
    malnutrition-dehydration E46 [H28]
    metabolic disease E88.9 [H28]
    myotonic disorders G71.19 [H28]
    nutritional disease E63.9 [H28]
  infantile — *see* Cataract, presenile
  irradiational — *see* Cataract, specified NEC
  juvenile — *see* Cataract, presenile
  malnutrition-dehydration E46 [H28]
  morgagnian — *see* Cataract, senile, morgagnian type
  myotonic G71.19 [H28]
  myxedema E03.9 [H28]
  nuclear
    embryonal Q12.0
    sclerosis — *see* Cataract, senile, nuclear
  presenile H26.00- ☑
    combined forms H26.06- ☑
    cortical H26.01- ☑
    lamellar — *see* Cataract, presenile, cortical
    nuclear H26.03- ☑
    specified NEC H26.09
    subcapsular polar (anterior) H26.04- ☑
      posterior H26.05- ☑
    zonular — *see* Cataract, presenile, cortical
  secondary H26.40
    Soemmering's ring H26.41- ☑
    specified NEC H26.49- ☑
    to eye disease — *see* Cataract, complicated
  senile H25.9
    brunescens — *see* Cataract, senile, nuclear
    combined forms H25.81- ☑
    coronary — *see* Cataract, senile, incipient
    cortical H25.01- ☑
    hypermature — *see* Cataract, senile, morgagnian type
    incipient (mature) (total) H25.09- ☑
      cortical — *see* Cataract, senile, cortical
      subcapsular — *see* Cataract, senile, subcapsular
    morgagnian type (hypermature) H25.2- ☑
    nuclear (sclerosis) H25.1- ☑
    polar subcapsular (anterior) (posterior) — *see* Cataract, senile, incipient
    punctate — *see* Cataract, senile, incipient
    specified NEC H25.89
    subcapsular polar (anterior) H25.03- ☑
      posterior H25.04- ☑
  snowflake — *see* Diabetes, cataract
  specified NEC H26.8
  toxic — *see* Cataract, drug-induced
  traumatic H26.10- ☑
    localized H26.11- ☑
    partially resolved H26.12- ☑
    total H26.13- ☑
  zonular (perinuclear) Q12.0
Cataracta (*see also* Cataract)
  brunescens — *see* Cataract, senile, nuclear
  centralis pulverulenta Q12.0
  cerulea Q12.0
  complicata — *see* Cataract, complicated
  congenita Q12.0
  coralliformis Q12.0
  coronaria Q12.0
  diabetic — *see* Diabetes, cataract
  membranacea
    accreta — *see* Cataract, secondary
    congenita Q12.0
  nigra — *see* Cataract, senile, nuclear
  sunflower — *see* Cataract, complicated
Catarrh, catarrhal (acute) (febrile) (infectious) (inflammation) (*see also* condition) J00
  bronchial — *see* Bronchitis
  chest — *see* Bronchitis
  chronic J31.0
  due to congenital syphilis A50.03
  enteric — *see* Enteritis
  eustachian H68.009
  fauces — *see* Pharyngitis
  gastrointestinal — *see* Enteritis
  gingivitis K05.00
    nonplaque induced K05.01
    plaque induced K05.00
  hay — *see* Fever, hay

Catarrh, catarrhal — *continued*
  intestinal — *see* Enteritis
  larynx, chronic J37.0
  liver B15.9
    with hepatic coma B15.0
  lung — *see* Bronchitis
  middle ear, chronic — *see* Otitis, media, nonsuppurative, chronic, serous
  mouth K12.1
  nasal (chronic) — *see* Rhinitis
  nasobronchial J31.1
  nasopharyngeal (chronic) J31.1
    acute J00
  pulmonary — *see* Bronchitis
  spring (eye) (vernal) — *see* Conjunctivitis, acute, atopic
  summer (hay) — *see* Fever, hay
  throat J31.2
  tubotympanal (*see also* Otitis, media, nonsuppurative)
    chronic — *see* Otitis, media, nonsuppurative, chronic, serous
Catatonia (schizophrenic) F20.2
Catatonic
  disorder due to known physiologic condition F06.1
  schizophrenia F20.2
  stupor R40.1
Cat-scratch (*see also* Abrasion)
  disease or fever A28.1
Cauda equina — *see* condition
Cauliflower ear M95.1-
Causalgia (upper limb) G56.4- ☑
  lower limb G57.7- ☑
Cause
  external, general effects T75.89 ☑
Caustic burn — *see* Corrosion, by site
Cavare's disease (familial periodic paralysis) G72.3
Cave-in, injury
  crushing (severe) — *see* Crush
  suffocation — *see* Asphyxia, traumatic, due to low oxygen, due to cave-in
Cavernitis (penis) N48.29
Cavernositis N48.29
Cavernous — *see* condition
Cavitation of lung (*see also* Tuberculosis, pulmonary)
  nontuberculous J98.4
Cavities, dental — *see* Caries, dental
Cavity
  lung — *see* Cavitation of lung
  optic papilla Q14.2
  pulmonary — *see* Cavitation of lung
Cavovarus foot, congenital Q66.1
Cavus foot (congenital) Q66.7
  acquired — *see* Deformity, limb, foot, specified NEC
Cazenave's disease L10.2
Cecitis K52.9
  with perforation, peritonitis, or rupture K65.8
Cecum — *see* condition
Celiac
  artery compression syndrome I77.4
  disease K90.0
  infantilism K90.0
Cell(s), **cellular** (*see also* condition)
  in urine R82.99
Cellulitis (diffuse) (phlegmonous) (septic) (suppurative) L03.90
  abdominal wall L03.311
  anaerobic A48.0
  ankle — *see* Cellulitis, lower limb
  anus K61.0
  arm — *see* Cellulitis, upper limb
  auricle (ear) — *see* Cellulitis, ear
  axilla L03.11- ☑
  back (any part) L03.312
  broad ligament
    acute N73.0
  buttock L03.317
  cervical (meaning neck) L03.221
  cervix (uteri) — *see* Cervicitis
  cheek (external) L03.211
    internal K12.2
  chest wall L03.313
  chronic L03.90
  clostridial A48.0
  corpus cavernosum N48.22
  digit
    finger — *see* Cellulitis, finger
    toe — *see* Cellulitis, toe

Cellulitis — *continued*
  Douglas' cul-de-sac or pouch
    acute N73.0
  drainage site (following operation) T81.4 ☑
  ear (external) H60.1- ☑
  eosinophilic (granulomatous) L98.3
  erysipelatous — *see* Erysipelas
  external auditory canal — *see* Cellulitis, ear
  eyelid — *see* Abscess, eyelid
  face NEC L03.211
  finger (intrathecal) (periosteal) (subcutaneous) (subcuticular) L03.01- ☑
  foot — *see* Cellulitis, lower limb
  gangrenous — *see* Gangrene
  genital organ NEC
    female (external) N76.4
    male N49.9
      multiple sites N49.8
      specified NEC N49.8
  gluteal (region) L03.317
  gonococcal A54.89
  groin L03.314
  hand — *see* Cellulitis, upper limb
  head NEC L03.811
    face (any part, except ear, eye and nose) L03.211
  heel — *see* Cellulitis, lower limb
  hip — *see* Cellulitis, lower limb
  jaw (region) L03.211
  knee — *see* Cellulitis, lower limb
  labium (majus) (minus) — *see* Vulvitis
  lacrimal passages — *see* Inflammation, lacrimal, passages
  larynx J38.7
  leg — *see* Cellulitis, lower limb
  lip K13.0
  lower limb L03.11- ☑
    toe — *see* Cellulitis, toe
  mouth (floor) K12.2
  multiple sites, so stated L03.90
  nasopharynx J39.1
  navel L03.316
    newborn P38.9
      with mild hemorrhage P38.1
      without hemorrhage P38.9
  neck (region) L03.221
  nose (septum) (external) J34.0
  orbit, orbital H05.01- ☑
  palate (soft) K12.2
  pectoral (region) L03.313
  pelvis, pelvic (chronic)
    female (*see also* Disease, pelvis, inflammatory) N73.2
      acute N73.0
      following ectopic or molar pregnancy O08.0
    male K65.0
  penis N48.22
  perineal, perineum L03.315
  perirectal K61.1
  peritonsillar J36
  periurethral N34.0
  periuterine (*see also* Disease, pelvis, inflammatory) N73.2
    acute N73.0
  pharynx J39.1
  rectum K61.1
  retroperitoneal K68.9
  round ligament
    acute N73.0
  scalp (any part) L03.811
  scrotum N49.2
  seminal vesicle N49.0
  shoulder — *see* Cellulitis, upper limb
  specified site NEC L03.818
  submandibular (region) (space) (triangle) K12.2
    gland K11.3
  submaxillary (region) K12.2
    gland K11.3
  thigh — *see* Cellulitis, lower limb
  thumb (intrathecal) (periosteal) (subcutaneous) (subcuticular) — *see* Cellulitis, finger
  toe (intrathecal) (periosteal) (subcutaneous) (subcuticular) L03.03- ☑
  tonsil J36
  trunk L03.319
    abdominal wall L03.311
    back (any part) L03.312
    buttock L03.317
    chest wall L03.313

Cellulitis — *continued*
  trunk — *continued*
    groin L03.314
    perineal, perineum L03.315
    umbilicus L03.316
    tuberculous (primary) A18.4
    umbilicus L03.316
    upper limb L03.11- ☑
      axilla — *see* Cellulitis, axilla
      finger — *see* Cellulitis, finger
      thumb — *see* Cellulitis, finger
    vaccinal T88.0 ☑
    vocal cord J38.3
    vulva — *see* Vulvitis
    wrist — *see* Cellulitis, upper limb
Cementoblastoma, benign — *see* Cyst, calcifying odontogenic
Cementoma — *see* Cyst, calcifying odontogenic
Cementoperiostitis — *see* Periodontitis
Cementosis K03.4
Central auditory processing disorder H93.25
Central pain syndrome G89.0
Cephalematocele, cephal (o)hematocele
  newborn P52.8
    birth injury P10.8
  traumatic — *see* Hematoma, brain
Cephalematoma, cephalhematoma (calcified)
  newborn (birth injury) P12.0
  traumatic — *see* Hematoma, brain
Cephalgia, cephalalgia (*see also* Headache)
  histamine G44.009
    intractable G44.001
    not intractable G44.009
  trigeminal autonomic (TAC) NEC G44.099
    intractable G44.091
    not intractable G44.099
Cephalic — *see* condition
Cephalitis — *see* Encephalitis
Cephalocele — *see* Encephalocele
Cephalomenia N94.89
Cephalopelvic — *see* condition
Cerclage (with cervical incompetence) in pregnancy — *see* Incompetence, cervix, in pregnancy
Cerebellitis — *see* Encephalitis
Cerebellum, cerebellar — *see* condition
Cerebral — *see* condition
Cerebritis — *see* Encephalitis
Cerebro-hepato-renal syndrome Q87.89
Cerebromalacia — *see* Softening, brain
  sequelae of cerebrovascular disease I69.398
Cerebroside lipidosis E75.22
Cerebrospasticity (congenital) G80.1
Cerebrospinal — *see* condition
Cerebrum — *see* condition
Ceroid-lipofuscinosis, neuronal E75.4
Cerumen (accumulation) (impacted) H61.2- ☑
Cervical (*see also* condition)
  auricle Q18.2
  dysplasia in pregnancy — *see* Abnormal, cervix, in pregnancy or childbirth
  erosion in pregnancy — *see* Abnormal, cervix, in pregnancy or childbirth
  fibrosis in pregnancy — *see* Abnormal, cervix, in pregnancy or childbirth
  fusion syndrome Q76.1
  rib Q76.5
  shortening (complicating pregnancy) O26.87- ☑
Cervicalgia M54.2
Cervicitis (acute) (chronic) (nonvenereal) (senile (atrophic)) (subacute) (with ulceration) N72
  with
    abortion — *see* Abortion, by type complicated by genital tract and pelvic infection
    ectopic pregnancy O08.0
    molar pregnancy O08.0
  chlamydial A56.09
  gonococcal A54.03
  herpesviral A60.03
  puerperal (postpartum) O86.11
  syphilitic A52.76
  trichomonal A59.09
  tuberculous A18.16
Cervicocolpitis (emphysematosa) (*see also* Cervicitis) N72
Cervix — *see* condition
Cesarean delivery, previous, affecting management of pregnancy O34.21

Céstan (-Chenais) paralysis or syndrome G46.3
Céstan-Raymond syndrome I65.8
Cestode infestation B71.9
  specified type NEC B71.8
Cestodiasis B71.9
Chabert's disease A22.9
Chacaleh E53.8
Chafing L30.4
Chagas' (-Mazza) disease (chronic) B57.2
  with
    cardiovascular involvement NEC B57.2
    digestive system involvement B57.30
      megacolon B57.32
      megaesophagus B57.31
      other specified B57.39
    megacolon B57.32
    megaesophagus B57.31
    myocarditis B57.2
    nervous system involvement B57.40
      meningitis B57.41
      meningoencephalitis B57.42
      other specified B57.49
    specified organ involvement NEC B57.5
  acute (with) B57.1
    cardiovascular NEC B57.0
    myocarditis B57.0
Chagres fever B50.9
Chairridden Z74.09
Chalasia (cardiac sphincter) K21.9
Chalazion H00.19
  left H00.16
    lower H00.15
    upper H00.14
  right H00.13
    lower H00.12
    upper H00.11
Chalcosis (see also Disorder, globe, degenerative, chalcosis)
  cornea — see Deposit, cornea
  crystalline lens — see Cataract, complicated
  retina H35.89
Chalicosis (pulmonum) J62.8
Chancre (any genital site) (hard) (hunterian) (mixed) (primary) (seronegative) (seropositive) (syphilitic) A51.0
  congenital A50.07
  conjunctiva NEC A51.2
  Ducrey's A57
  extragenital A51.2
  eyelid A51.2
  lip A51.2
  nipple A51.2
  Nisbet's A57
  of
    carate A67.0
    pinta A67.0
    yaws A66.0
  palate, soft A51.2
  phagedenic A57
  simple A57
  soft A57
    bubo A57
    palate A51.2
  urethra A51.2
  yaws A66.0
Chancroid (anus) (genital) (penis) (perineum) (rectum) (urethra) (vulva) A57
Chandler's disease (osteochondritis dissecans, hip) — see Osteochondritis, dissecans, hip
Change(s) (in) (of) (see also Removal)
  arteriosclerotic — see Arteriosclerosis
  bone (see also Disorder, bone)
    diabetic — see Diabetes, bone change
  bowel habit R19.4
  cardiorenal (vascular) — see Hypertension, cardiorenal
  cardiovascular — see Disease, cardiovascular
  circulatory I99.9
  cognitive (mild) (organic) R41.89
  color, tooth, teeth
    during formation K00.8
    posteruptive K03.7
  contraceptive device Z30.433
  corneal membrane H18.30
    Bowman's membrane fold or rupture H18.31- ☑
    Descemet's membrane
      fold H18.32- ☑
      rupture H18.33- ☑
  coronary — see Disease, heart, ischemic

Change(s) — continued
  degenerative, spine or vertebra — see Spondylosis
  dental pulp, regressive K04.2
  dressing (nonsurgical) Z48.00
    surgical Z48.01
  heart — see Disease, heart
  hip joint — see Derangement, joint, hip
  hyperplastic larynx J38.7
  hypertrophic
    nasal sinus J34.89
    turbinate, nasal J34.3
    upper respiratory tract J39.8
  indwelling catheter Z46.6
  inflammatory (see also Inflammation)
    sacroiliac M46.1
  job, anxiety concerning Z56.1
  joint — see Derangement, joint
  life — see Menopause
  mental status R41.82
  minimal (glomerular) (see also N00-N07 with fourth character .0) N05.0
  myocardium, myocardial — see Degeneration, myocardial
  of life — see Menopause
  pacemaker Z45.018
    pulse generator Z45.010
  personality (enduring) F68.8
    due to (secondary to)
      general medical condition F07.0
    secondary (nonspecific) F60.89
  regressive, dental pulp K04.2
  renal — see Disease, renal
  retina H35.9
    myopic H44.2- ☑
  sacroiliac joint M53.3
  senile (see also condition) R54
  sensory R20.8
  skin R23.9
    acute, due to ultraviolet radiation L56.9
      specified NEC L56.8
    chronic, due to nonionizing radiation L57.9
      specified NEC L57.8
    cyanosis R23.0
    flushing R23.2
    pallor R23.1
    petechiae R23.3
    specified change NEC R23.8
    swelling — see Mass, localized
    texture R23.4
  trophic
    arm — see Mononeuropathy, upper limb
    leg — see Mononeuropathy, lower limb
  vascular I99.9
  vasomotor I73.9
  voice R49.9
    psychogenic F44.4
    specified NEC R49.8
Changing sleep-work schedule, affecting sleep G47.26
Changuinola fever A93.1
Chapping skin T69.8 ☑
Charcot-Marie-Tooth disease, paralysis or syndrome G60.0
Charcot's
  arthropathy — see Arthropathy, neuropathic
  cirrhosis K74.3
  disease (tabetic arthropathy) A52.16
  joint (disease) (tabetic) A52.16
    diabetic — see Diabetes, with, arthropathy
    syringomyelic G95.0
  syndrome (intermittent claudication) I73.9
CHARGE association Q89.8
Charley-horse (quadriceps) M62.831
  traumatic (quadriceps) S76.11- ☑
Charlouis' disease — see Yaws
Cheadle's disease E54
Checking (of)
  cardiac pacemaker (battery) (electrode(s)) Z45.018
    pulse generator Z45.010
  intrauterine contraceptive device Z30.431
Check-up — see Examination
Chédiak-Higashi (-Steinbrinck) **syndrome** (congenital gigantism of peroxidase granules) E70.330
Cheek — see condition
Cheese-washer's lung J67.8
Cheese-worker's lung J67.8

Cheilitis (acute) (angular) (catarrhal) (chronic) (exfoliative) (gangrenous) (glandular) (infectional) (suppurative) (ulcerative) (vesicular) K13.0
  actinic (due to sun) L56.8
    other than from sun L59.8
  candidal B37.83
Cheilodynia K13.0
Cheiloschisis — see Cleft, lip
Cheilosis (angular) K13.0
  with pellagra E52
  due to
    vitamin B2 (riboflavin) deficiency E53.0
Cheiromegaly M79.89
Cheiropompholyx L30.1
Cheloid — see Keloid
Chemical burn — see Corrosion, by site
Chemodectoma — see Paraganglioma, nonchromaffin
Chemosis, conjunctiva — see Edema, conjunctiva
Chemotherapy (session) (for)
  cancer Z51.11
  neoplasm Z51.11
Cherubism M27.8
Chest — see condition
Cheyne-Stokes breathing (respiration) R06.3
Chiari's
  disease or syndrome (hepatic vein thrombosis) I82.0
  malformation
    type I G93.5
    type II — see Spina bifida
    net Q24.8
Chicago disease B40.9
Chickenpox — see Varicella
Chiclero ulcer or sore B55.1
Chigger (infestation) B88.0
Chignon (disease) B36.8
  newborn (from vacuum extraction) (birth injury) P12.1
Chilaiditi's syndrome (subphrenic displacement, colon) Q43.3
Chilblain(s) (lupus) T69.1 ☑
Child
  custody dispute Z65.3
Childbirth — see Delivery
Childhood
  cerebral X-linked adrenoleukodystrophy E71.520
  period of rapid growth Z00.2
Chill(s) R68.83
  with fever R50.9
  without fever R68.83
  congestive in malarial regions B54
Chilomastigiasis A07.8
Chimera 46,XX/46,XY Q99.0
Chin — see condition
Chinese dysentery A03.9
Chionophobia F40.228
Chitral fever A93.1
Chlamydia, chlamydial A74.9
  cervicitis A56.09
  conjunctivitis A74.0
  cystitis A56.01
  endometritis A56.11
  epididymitis A56.19
  female
    pelvic inflammatory disease A56.11
    pelviperitonitis A56.11
  orchitis A56.19
  peritonitis A74.81
  pharyngitis A56.4
  proctitis A56.3
  psittaci (infection) A70
  salpingitis A56.11
  sexually-transmitted infection NEC A56.8
  specified NEC A74.89
  urethritis A56.01
  vulvovaginitis A56.02
Chlamydiosis — see Chlamydia
Chloasma (skin) (idiopathic) (symptomatic) L81.1
  eyelid H02.719
    hyperthyroid E05.90 [H02.719]
      with thyroid storm E05.91 [H02.719]
    left H02.716
      lower H02.715
      upper H02.714
    right H02.713
      lower H02.712
      upper H02.711
Chloroma C92.3- ☑
Chlorosis D50.9

Chlorosis — *continued*
　Egyptian B76.9 [D63.8]
　miner's B76.9 [D63.8]
Chlorotic anemia D50.8
Chocolate cyst (ovary) N80.1
Choked
　disc or disk — *see* Papilledema
　on food, phlegm, or vomitus NOS — *see* Foreign body,
　　by site
　while vomiting NOS — *see* Foreign body, by site
Chokes (resulting from bends) T70.3 ☑
Choking sensation R09.89
Cholangiectasis K83.8
Cholangiocarcinoma
　with hepatocellular carcinoma, combined C22.0
　liver C22.1
　specified site NEC — *see* Neoplasm, malignant, by site
　unspecified site C22.1
Cholangiohepatitis K83.8
　due to fluke infestation B66.1
Cholangiohepatoma C22.0
Cholangiolitis (acute) (chronic) (extrahepatic) (gan-
　grenous) (intrahepatic) K83.0
　paratyphoidal — *see* Fever, paratyphoid
　typhoidal A01.09
Cholangioma D13.4
　malignant — *see* Cholangiocarcinoma
Cholangitis (ascending) (primary) (recurrent) (sclerosing)
　(secondary) (stenosing) (suppurative) K83.0
　with calculus, bile duct — *see* Calculus, bile duct, with
　　cholangitis
　chronic nonsuppurative destructive K74.3
Cholecystectasia K82.8
Cholecystitis K81.9
　with
　　calculus, stones in
　　　bile duct (common) (hepatic) — *see* Calculus,
　　　　bile duct, with cholecystitis
　　　cystic duct — *see* Calculus, gallbladder, with
　　　　cholecystitis
　　　gallbladder — *see* Calculus, gallbladder, with
　　　　cholecystitis
　　　choledocholithiasis — *see* Calculus, bile duct, with
　　　　cholecystitis
　　　cholelithiasis — *see* Calculus, gallbladder, with
　　　　cholecystitis
　acute (emphysematous) (gangrenous) (suppurative)
　　K81.0
　　with
　　　calculus, stones in
　　　　cystic duct — *see* Calculus, gallbladder, with
　　　　　cholecystitis, acute
　　　　gallbladder — *see* Calculus, gallbladder,
　　　　　with cholecystitis, acute
　　　　choledocholithiasis — *see* Calculus, bile duct,
　　　　　with cholecystitis, acute
　　　　cholelithiasis — *see* Calculus, gallbladder, with
　　　　　cholecystitis, acute
　　　chronic cholecystitis K81.2
　　　　with gallbladder calculus K80.12
　　　　　with obstruction K80.13
　chronic K81.1
　　with acute cholecystitis K81.2
　　　with gallbladder calculus K80.12
　　　　with obstruction K80.13
　emphysematous (acute) — *see* Cholecystitis, acute
　gangrenous — *see* Cholecystitis, acute
　paratyphoidal, current A01.4
　suppurative — *see* Cholecystitis, acute
　typhoidal A01.09
Cholecystolithiasis — *see* Calculus, gallbladder
Choledochitis (suppurative) K83.0
Choledocholith — *see* Calculus, bile duct
Choledocholithiasis (common duct) (hepatic duct) —
　see Calculus, bile duct
　cystic — *see* Calculus, gallbladder
　typhoidal A01.09
Cholelithiasis (cystic duct) (gallbladder) (impacted)
　(multiple) — *see* Calculus, gallbladder
　bile duct (common) (hepatic) — *see* Calculus, bile duct
　hepatic duct — *see* Calculus, bile duct
　specified NEC K80.80
　　with obstruction K80.81
Cholemia (*see also* Jaundice)
　familial (simple) (congenital) E80.4
　Gilbert's E80.4
Choleperitoneum, choleperitonitis K65.3

Cholera (Asiatic) (epidemic) (malignant) A00.9
　antimonial — *see* Poisoning, antimony
　classical A00.0
　due to Vibrio cholerae 01 A00.9
　　biovar cholerae A00.0
　　biovar eltor A00.1
　　el tor A00.1
　el tor A00.1
Cholerine — *see* Cholera
Cholestasis NEC K83.1
　with hepatocyte injury K71.0
　due to total parenteral nutrition (TPN) K76.89
　pure K71.0
Cholesteatoma (ear) (middle) (with reaction) H71.9- ☑
　attic H71.0- ☑
　external ear (canal) H60.4- ☑
　mastoid H71.2- ☑
　postmastoidectomy cavity (recurrent) — *see* Compli-
　　cations, postmastoidectomy, recurrent
　　cholesteatoma
　recurrent (postmastoidectomy) — *see* Complications,
　　postmastoidectomy, recurrent cholesteatoma
　tympanum H71.1- ☑
Cholesteatosis, diffuse H71.3- ☑
Cholesteremia E78.0
Cholesterin in vitreous — *see* Deposit, crystalline
Cholesterol
　deposit
　　retina H35.89
　　vitreous — *see* Deposit, crystalline
　elevated (high) E78.0
　　with elevated (high) triglycerides E78.2
　　screening for Z13.220
　imbibition of gallbladder K82.4
Cholesterolemia (essential) (familial) (hereditary) (pure)
　E78.0
Cholesterolosis, cholesterosis (gallbladder) K82.4
　cerebrotendinous E75.5
Cholocolic fistula K82.3
Choluria R82.2
Chondritis M94.8X9
　aurical H61.03- ☑
　costal (Tietze's) M94.0
　external ear H61.03- ☑
　patella, posttraumatic — *see* Chondromalacia, patella
　pinna H61.03- ☑
　purulent M94.8X- ☑
　tuberculous NEC A18.02
　　intervertebral A18.01
Chondroblastoma (*see also* Neoplasm, bone, benign)
　malignant — *see* Neoplasm, bone, malignant
Chondrocalcinosis M11.20
　ankle M11.27- ☑
　elbow M11.22- ☑
　familial M11.10
　　ankle M11.17- ☑
　　elbow M11.12- ☑
　　foot joint M11.17- ☑
　　hand joint M11.14- ☑
　　hip M11.15- ☑
　　knee M11.16- ☑
　　multiple site M11.19
　　shoulder M11.11- ☑
　　vertebrae M11.18
　　wrist M11.13- ☑
　foot joint M11.27- ☑
　hand joint M11.24- ☑
　hip M11.25- ☑
　knee M11.26- ☑
　multiple site M11.29
　shoulder M11.21- ☑
　specified type NEC M11.20
　　ankle M11.27- ☑
　　elbow M11.22- ☑
　　foot joint M11.27- ☑
　　hand joint M11.24- ☑
　　hip M11.25- ☑
　　knee M11.26- ☑
　　multiple site M11.29
　　shoulder M11.21- ☑
　　vertebrae M11.28
　　wrist M11.23- ☑
　vertebrae M11.28
　wrist M11.23- ☑
Chondrodermatitis nodularis helicis or anthelicis
　— *see* Perichondritis, ear

Chondrodysplasia Q78.9
　with hemangioma Q78.4
　calcificans congenita Q77.3
　fetalis Q77.4
　metaphyseal (Jansen's) (McKusick's) (Schmid's) Q78.5
　punctata Q77.3
Chondrodystrophy, chondrodystrophia (familial)
　(fetalis) (hypoplastic) Q78.9
　calcificans congenita Q77.3
　myotonic (congenital) G71.13
　punctata Q77.3
Chondroectodermal dysplasia Q77.6
Chondrogenesis imperfecta Q77.4
Chondrolysis M94.35- ☑
Chondroma (*see also* Neoplasm, cartilage, benign)
　juxtacortical — *see* Neoplasm, bone, benign
　periosteal — *see* Neoplasm, bone, benign
Chondromalacia (systemic) M94.20
　acromioclavicular joint M94.21- ☑
　ankle M94.27- ☑
　elbow M94.22- ☑
　foot joint M94.27- ☑
　glenohumeral joint M94.21- ☑
　hand joint M94.24- ☑
　hip M94.25- ☑
　knee M94.26- ☑
　　patella M22.4- ☑
　multiple sites M94.29
　patella M22.4- ☑
　rib M94.28
　sacroiliac joint M94.259
　shoulder M94.21- ☑
　sternoclavicular joint M94.21- ☑
　vertebral joint M94.28
　wrist M94.23- ☑
Chondromatosis (*see also* Neoplasm, cartilage, uncertain
　behavior)
　internal Q78.4
Chondromyxosarcoma — *see* Neoplasm, cartilage,
　malignant
Chondro-osteodysplasia (Morquio-Brailsford type)
　E76.219
Chondro-osteodystrophy E76.29
Chondro-osteoma — *see* Neoplasm, bone, benign
Chondropathia tuberosa M94.0
Chondrosarcoma — *see* Neoplasm, cartilage, malignant
　juxtacortical — *see* Neoplasm, bone, malignant
　mesenchymal — *see* Neoplasm, connective tissue,
　　malignant
　myxoid — *see* Neoplasm, cartilage, malignant
Chordee (nonvenereal) N48.89
　congenital Q54.4
　gonococcal A54.09
Chorditis (fibrinous) (nodosa) (tuberosa) J38.2
Chordoma — *see* Neoplasm, vertebral (column), malig-
　nant
Chorea (chronic) (gravis) (posthemiplegic) (senile)
　(spasmodic) G25.5
　with
　　heart involvement I02.0
　　　active or acute (conditions in I01-) I02.0
　　　rheumatic I02.9
　　　　with valvular disorder I02.0
　　　rheumatic heart disease (chronic) (inactive)(quies-
　　　　cent) — *code to* rheumatic heart condition
　　　　involved
　drug-induced G25.4
　habit F95.8
　hereditary G10
　Huntington's G10
　hysterical F44.4
　minor I02.9
　　with heart involvement I02.0
　progressive G25.5
　　hereditary G10
　rheumatic (chronic) I02.9
　　with heart involvement I02.0
　Sydenham's I02.9
　　with heart involvement — *see* Chorea, with
　　　rheumatic heart disease
　　nonrheumatic G25.5
Choreoathetosis (paroxysmal) G25.5
Chorioadenoma (destruens) D39.2
Chorioamnionitis O41.12- ☑
Chorioangioma D26.7
Choriocarcinoma — *see* Neoplasm, malignant, by site
　combined with

Choriocarcinoma — *continued*
  combined with — *continued*
    embryonal carcinoma — *see* Neoplasm, malignant, by site
    other germ cell elements — *see* Neoplasm, malignant, by site
    teratoma — *see* Neoplasm, malignant, by site
  specified site — *see* Neoplasm, malignant, by site
  unspecified site
    female C58
    male C62.90
Chorioencephalitis (acute) (lymphocytic) (serous) A87.2
Chorioepithelioma — *see* Choriocarcinoma
Choriomeningitis (acute) (lymphocytic) (serous) A87.2
Chorionepithelioma — *see* Choriocarcinoma
Chorioretinitis (*see also* Inflammation, chorioretinal)
  disseminated (*see also* Inflammation, chorioretinal, disseminated)
    in neurosyphilis A52.19
  Egyptian B76.9 [D63.8]
  focal (*see also* Inflammation, chorioretinal, focal)
  histoplasmic B39.9 [H32]
  in (due to)
    histoplasmosis B39.9 [H32]
    syphilis (secondary) A51.43
      late A52.71
    toxoplasmosis (acquired) B58.01
      congenital (active) P37.1 [H32]
    tuberculosis A18.53
  juxtapapillary, juxtapapillaris — *see* Inflammation, chorioretinal, focal, juxtapapillary
  leprous A30.9 [H32]
  miner's B76.9 [D63.8]
  progressive myopia (degeneration) H44.2- ☑
  syphilitic (secondary) A51.43
    congenital (early) A50.01 [H32]
      late A50.32
    late A52.71
  tuberculous A18.53
Chorioretinopathy, central serous H35.71- ☑
Choroid — *see* condition
Choroideremia H31.21
Choroiditis — *see* Chorioretinitis
Choroidopathy — *see* Disorder, choroid
Choroidoretinitis — *see* Chorioretinitis
Choroidoretinopathy, central serous — *see* Chorioretinopathy, central serous
Christian-Weber disease M35.6
Christmas disease D67
Chromaffinoma (*see also* Neoplasm, benign, by site)
  malignant — *see* Neoplasm, malignant, by site
Chromatopsia — *see* Deficiency, color vision
Chromhidrosis, chromidrosis L75.1
Chromoblastomycosis — *see* Chromomycosis
Chromoconversion R82.91
Chromomycosis B43.9
  brain abscess B43.1
  cerebral B43.1
  cutaneous B43.0
  skin B43.0
  specified NEC B43.8
  subcutaneous abscess or cyst B43.2
Chromophytosis B36.0
Chromosome — *see* Anomaly, by chromosome involved
  D (1) — *see* Anomaly, chromosome 13
  E (3) — *see* Anomaly, chromosome 18
  G — *see* Anomaly, chromosome 21
Chromotrichomycosis B36.8
Chronic — *see* condition
  fracture — *see* Fracture, pathological
Churg-Strauss syndrome M30.1
Chyle cyst, mesentery I89.8
Chylocele (nonfilarial) I89.8
  filarial (*see also* Infestation, filarial) B74.9 [N51]
  tunica vaginalis N50.8
    filarial (*see also* Infestation, filarial) B74.9 [N51]
Chylomicronemia (fasting) (with hyperprebetalipoproteinemia) E78.3
Chylopericardium I31.3
  acute I30.9
Chylothorax (nonfilarial) I89.8
  filarial (*see also* Infestation, filarial) B74.9 [J91.8]
Chylous — *see* condition
Chyluria (nonfilarial) R82.0
  due to
    bilharziasis B65.0
    Brugia (malayi) B74.1

Chyluria — *continued*
  due to — *continued*
    Brugia — *continued*
      timori B74.2
    schistosomiasis (bilharziasis) B65.0
    Wuchereria (bancrofti) B74.0
  filarial — *see* Infestation, filarial
Cicatricial (deformity) — *see* Cicatrix
Cicatrix (adherent) (contracted) (painful) (vicious) (*see also* Scar) L90.5
  adenoid (and tonsil) J35.8
  alveolar process M26.79
  anus K62.89
  auricle — *see* Disorder, pinna, specified type NEC
  bile duct (common) (hepatic) K83.8
  bladder N32.89
  bone — *see* Disorder, bone, specified type NEC
  brain G93.89
  cervix (postoperative) (postpartal) N88.1
  common duct K83.8
  cornea H17.9
    tuberculous A18.59
  duodenum (bulb), obstructive K31.5
  esophagus K22.2
  eyelid — *see* Disorder, eyelid function
  hypopharynx J39.2
  lacrimal passages — *see* Obstruction, lacrimal
  larynx J38.7
  lung J98.4
  middle ear H74.8 ☑
  mouth K13.79
  muscle M62.89
    with contracture — *see* Contraction, muscle NEC
  nasopharynx J39.2
  palate (soft) K13.79
  penis N48.89
  pharynx J39.2
  prostate N42.89
  rectum K62.89
  retina — *see* Scar, chorioretinal
  semilunar cartilage — *see* Derangement, meniscus
  seminal vesicle N50.8
  skin L90.5
    infected L08.89
    postinfective L90.5
    tuberculous B90.8
  specified site NEC L90.5
  throat J39.2
  tongue K14.8
  tonsil (and adenoid) J35.8
  trachea J39.8
  tuberculous NEC B90.9
  urethra N36.8
  uterus N85.8
  vagina N89.8
    postoperative N99.2
  vocal cord J38.3
  wrist, constricting (annular) L90.5
CIDP (chronic inflammatory demyelinating polyneuropathy) G61.81
CIN — *see* Neoplasia, intraepithelial, cervix
Cinchonism — *see* Deafness, ototoxic
  correct substance properly administered — *see* Table of Drugs and Chemicals, by drug, adverse effect
  overdose or wrong substance given or taken — *see* Table of Drugs and Chemicals, by drug, poisoning
Circle of Willis — *see* condition
Circular — *see* condition
Circulating anticoagulants (*see also* Disorder, hemorrhagic) D68.318
  due to drugs (*see also* Disorder, hemorrhagic) D68.32
  following childbirth O72.3
Circulation
  collateral, any site I99.8
  defective (lower extremity) I99.8
    congenital Q28.9
  embryonic Q28.9
  failure (peripheral) R57.9
    newborn P29.89
  fetal, persistent P29.3
  heart, incomplete Q28.9
Circulatory system — *see* condition
Circulus senilis (cornea) — *see* Degeneration, cornea, senile
Circumcision (in absence of medical indication) (ritual) (routine) Z41.2
Circumscribed — *see* condition

Circumvallate placenta O43.11- ☑
Cirrhosis, cirrhotic (hepatic) (liver) K74.60
  alcoholic K70.30
    with ascites K70.31
  atrophic — *see* Cirrhosis, liver
  Baumgarten-Cruveilhier K74.69
  biliary (cholangiolitic) (cholangitic) (hypertrophic) (obstructive) (pericholangiolitic) K74.5
    due to
      Clonorchiasis B66.1
      flukes B66.3
    primary K74.3
    secondary K74.4
  cardiac (of liver) K76.1
  Charcot's K74.3
  cholangiolitic, cholangitic, cholostatic (primary) K74.3
  congestive K76.1
  Cruveilhier-Baumgarten K74.69
  cryptogenic (liver) K74.69
  due to
    hepatolenticular degeneration E83.01
    Wilson's disease E83.01
    xanthomatosis E78.2
  fatty K76.0
    alcoholic K70.0
  Hanot's (hypertrophic) K74.3
  hepatic — *see* Cirrhosis, liver
  hypertrophic K74.3
  Indian childhood K74.69
  kidney — *see* Sclerosis, renal
  Laennec's K70.30
    with ascites K70.31
    alcoholic K70.30
      with ascites K70.31
    nonalcoholic K74.69
  liver K74.60
    alcoholic K70.30
      with ascites K70.31
      fatty K70.0
    congenital P78.81
    syphilitic A52.74
  lung (chronic) J84.10
  macronodular K74.69
    alcoholic K70.30
      with ascites K70.31
  micronodular K74.69
    alcoholic K70.30
      with ascites K70.31
  mixed type K74.69
  monolobular K74.3
  nephritis — *see* Sclerosis, renal
  nutritional K74.69
    alcoholic K70.30
      with ascites K70.31
  obstructive — *see* Cirrhosis, biliary
  ovarian N83.8
  pancreas (duct) K86.8
  pigmentary E83.110
  portal K74.69
    alcoholic K70.30
      with ascites K70.31
  postnecrotic K74.69
    alcoholic K70.30
      with ascites K70.31
  pulmonary J84.10
  renal — *see* Sclerosis, renal
  spleen D73.2
  stasis K76.1
  Todd's K74.3
  unilobar K74.3
  xanthomatous (biliary) K74.5
    due to xanthomatosis (familial) (metabolic) (primary) E78.2
Cistern, subarachnoid R93.0
Citrullinemia E72.23
Citrullinuria E72.23
Civatte's disease or poikiloderma L57.3
Clam digger's itch B65.3
Clammy skin R23.1
Clap — *see* Gonorrhea
Clarke-Hadfield syndrome (pancreatic infantilism) K86.8
Clark's paralysis G80.9
Clastothrix L67.8
Claude Bernard-Horner syndrome G90.2
  traumatic — *see* Injury, nerve, cervical sympathetic
Claude's disease or syndrome G46.3
Claudicatio venosa intermittens I87.8

☑ **Additional Character Required** — Refer to the Tabular List for Character Selection   ▼ **Subterms under main terms may continue to next column or page**

Claudication, intermittent I73.9
 cerebral (artery) G45.9
 spinal cord (arteriosclerotic) G95.19
  syphilitic A52.09
 venous (axillary) I87.8
Claustrophobia F40.240
Clavus (infected) L84
Clawfoot (congenital) Q66.89
 acquired — *see* Deformity, limb, clawfoot
Clawhand (acquired) (*see also* Deformity, limb, clawhand)
 congenital Q68.1
Clawtoe (congenital) Q66.89
 acquired — *see* Deformity, toe, specified NEC
Clay eating — *see* Pica
Cleansing of artificial opening — *see* Attention to, artificial, opening
Cleft (congenital) (*see also* Imperfect, closure)
 alveolar process M26.79
 branchial (cyst) (persistent) Q18.2
 cricoid cartilage, posterior Q31.8
 lip (unilateral) Q36.9
  with cleft palate Q37.9
   hard Q37.1
    with soft Q37.5
   soft Q37.3
    with hard Q37.5
  bilateral Q36.0
   with cleft palate Q37.8
    hard Q37.0
     with soft Q37.4
    soft Q37.2
     with hard Q37.4
  median Q36.1
 nose Q30.2
 palate Q35.9
  with cleft lip (unilateral) Q37.9
   bilateral Q37.8
  hard Q35.1
   with
    cleft lip (unilateral) Q37.1
     bilateral Q37.0
    soft Q35.5
     with cleft lip (unilateral) Q37.5
      bilateral Q37.4
  medial Q35.5
  soft Q35.3
   with
    cleft lip (unilateral) Q37.3
     bilateral Q37.2
    hard Q35.5
     with cleft lip (unilateral) Q37.5
      bilateral Q37.4
 penis Q55.69
 scrotum Q55.29
 thyroid cartilage Q31.8
 uvula Q35.7
Cleidocranial dysostosis Q74.0
Cleptomania F63.2
Clicking hip (newborn) R29.4
Climacteric (female) (*see also* Menopause)
 arthritis (any site) NEC — *see* Arthritis, specified form NEC
 depression (single episode) F32.8
 male (symptoms) (syndrome) NEC N50.8
 paranoid state F22
 polyarthritis NEC — *see* Arthritis, specified form NEC
 symptoms (female) N95.1
Clinical research investigation (clinical trial) (control subject) (normal comparison) (participant) Z00.6
Clitoris — *see* condition
Cloaca (persistent) Q43.7
Clonorchiasis, clonorchis infection (liver) B66.1
Clonus R25.8
Closed bite M26.29
Clostridium (C.) **perfringens, as cause of disease classified elsewhere** B96.7
Closure
 congenital, nose Q30.0
 cranial sutures, premature Q75.0
 defective or imperfect NEC — *see* Imperfect, closure
 fistula, delayed — *see* Fistula
 foramen ovale, imperfect Q21.1
 hymen N89.6
 interauricular septum, defective Q21.1
 interventricular septum, defective Q21.0
 lacrimal duct (*see also* Stenosis, lacrimal, duct)
  congenital Q10.5
 nose (congenital) Q30.0

Closure — *continued*
 nose — *continued*
  acquired M95.0
 of artificial opening — *see* Attention to, artificial, opening
 vagina N89.5
 valve — *see* Endocarditis
 vulva N90.5
Clot (blood) (*see also* Embolism)
 artery (obstruction) (occlusion) — *see* Embolism
 bladder N32.89
 brain (intradural or extradural) — *see* Occlusion, artery, cerebral
 circulation I74.9
 heart (*see also* Infarct, myocardium)
  not resulting in infarction I24.0
 vein — *see* Thrombosis
Clouded state R40.1
 epileptic — *see* Epilepsy, specified NEC
 paroxysmal — *see* Epilepsy, specified NEC
Cloudy antrum, antra J32.0
Clouston's (hidrotic) **ectodermal dysplasia** Q82.4
Clubbed nail pachydermoperiostosis M89.40 [L62]
Clubbing of finger(s) (nails) R68.3
Clubfinger R68.3
 congenital Q68.1
Clubfoot (congenital) Q66.89
 acquired — *see* Deformity, limb, clubfoot
 equinovarus Q66.0
 paralytic — *see* Deformity, limb, clubfoot
Clubhand (congenital) (radial) Q71.4- ☑
 acquired — *see* Deformity, limb, clubhand
Clubnail R68.3
 congenital Q84.6
Clump, kidney Q63.1
Clumsiness, clumsy child syndrome F82
Cluttering F80.81
Clutton's joints A50.51 [M12.80]
Coagulation, intravascular (diffuse) (disseminated) (*see also* Defibrination syndrome)
 complicating abortion — *see* Abortion, by type, complicated by, intravascular coagulation
 following ectopic or molar pregnancy O08.1
Coagulopathy (*see also* Defect, coagulation)
 consumption D65
 intravascular D65
 newborn P60
Coalition
 calcaneo-scaphoid Q66.89
 tarsal Q66.89
Coalminer's
 elbow — *see* Bursitis, elbow, olecranon
 lung or pneumoconiosis J60
Coalworker's lung or pneumoconiosis J60
Coarctation
 aorta (preductal) (postductal) Q25.1
 pulmonary artery Q25.71
Coated tongue K14.3
Coats' disease (exudative retinopathy) — *see* Retinopathy, exudative
Cocainism — *see* Dependence, drug, cocaine
Coccidioidomycosis B38.9
 cutaneous B38.3
 disseminated B38.7
 generalized B38.7
 meninges B38.4
 prostate B38.81
 pulmonary B38.2
  acute B38.0
  chronic B38.1
 skin B38.3
 specified NEC B38.89
Coccidioidosis — *see* Coccidioidomycosis
Coccidiosis (intestinal) A07.3
Coccydynia, coccygodynia M53.3
Coccyx — *see* condition
Cochin-China diarrhea K90.1
Cockayne's syndrome Q87.1
Cocked up toe — *see* Deformity, toe, specified NEC
Cock's peculiar tumor L72.3
Codman's tumor — *see* Neoplasm, bone, benign
Coenurosis B71.8
Cogan's syndrome H16.32- ☑
 oculomotor apraxia H51.8
Coitus, painful (female) N94.1
 male N53.12

Coitus, painful — *continued*
 psychogenic F52.6
Cold J00
 with influenza, flu, or grippe — *see* Influenza, with, respiratory manifestations NEC
 agglutinin disease or hemoglobinuria (chronic) D59.1
 bronchial — *see* Bronchitis
 chest — *see* Bronchitis
 common (head) J00
 effects of T69.9 ☑
  specified effect NEC T69.8 ☑
 excessive, effects of T69.9 ☑
  specified effect NEC T69.8 ☑
 exhaustion from T69.8 ☑
 exposure to T69.9 ☑
  specified effect NEC T69.8 ☑
 head J00
 injury syndrome (newborn) P80.0
 on lung — *see* Bronchitis
 rose J30.1
 sensitivity, auto-immune D59.1
 virus J00
Coldsore B00.1
Colibacillosis A49.8
 as the cause of other disease (*see also* Escherichia coli) B96.20
 generalized A41.50
Colic (bilious) (infantile) (intestinal) (recurrent) (spasmodic) R10.83
 abdomen R10.83
  psychogenic F45.8
 appendix, appendicular K38.8
 bile duct — *see* Calculus, bile duct
 biliary — *see* Calculus, bile duct
 common duct — *see* Calculus, bile duct
 cystic duct — *see* Calculus, gallbladder
 Devonshire NEC — *see* Poisoning, lead
 gallbladder — *see* Calculus, gallbladder
 gallstone — *see* Calculus, gallbladder
  gallbladder or cystic duct — *see* Calculus, gallbladder
 hepatic (duct) — *see* Calculus, bile duct
 hysterical F45.8
 kidney N23
 lead NEC — *see* Poisoning, lead
 mucous K58.9
  with diarrhea K58.0
  psychogenic F54
 nephritic N23
 painter's NEC — *see* Poisoning, lead
 pancreas K86.8
 psychogenic F45.8
 renal N23
 saturnine NEC — *see* Poisoning, lead
 ureter N23
 urethral N36.8
  due to calculus N21.1
 uterus NEC N94.89
  menstrual — *see* Dysmenorrhea
 worm NOS B83.9
Colicystitis — *see* Cystitis
Colitis (acute) (catarrhal) (chronic) (noninfective) (hemorrhagic) (*see also* Enteritis) K52.9
 allergic K52.2
 amebic (acute) (*see also* Amebiasis) A06.0
  nondysenteric A06.2
 anthrax A22.2
 bacillary — *see* Infection, Shigella
 balantidial A07.0
 Clostridium difficile A04.7
 coccidial A07.3
 collagenous K52.89
 cystica superficialis K52.89
 dietary counseling and surveillance (for) Z71.3
 dietetic K52.2
 drug-induced K52.1
 due to radiation K52.0
 eosinophilic K52.82
 food hypersensitivity K52.2
 giardial A07.1
 granulomatous — *see* Enteritis, regional, large intestine
 infectious — *see* Enteritis, infectious
 ischemic K55.9
  acute (fulminant) (subacute) K55.0
  chronic K55.1
  due to mesenteric artery insufficiency K55.1

Colitis — *continued*
  ischemic — *continued*
    fulminant (acute) K55.0
  left sided K51.50
    with
      abscess K51.514
      complication K51.519
        specified NEC K51.518
      fistula K51.513
      obstruction K51.512
      rectal bleeding K51.511
  lymphocytic K52.89
  membranous
    psychogenic F54
  microscopic (collagenous) (lymphocytic) K52.89
  mucous — *see* Syndrome, irritable, bowel
    psychogenic F54
  noninfective K52.9
    specified NEC K52.89
  polyposa — *see* Polyp, colon, inflammatory
  protozoal A07.9
  pseudomembranous A04.7
  pseudomucinous — *see* Syndrome, irritable, bowel
  regional — *see* Enteritis, regional, large intestine
  segmental — *see* Enteritis, regional, large intestine
  septic — *see* Enteritis, infectious
  spastic K58.9
    with diarrhea K58.0
    psychogenic F54
  staphylococcal A04.8
    foodborne A05.0
  subacute ischemic K55.0
  thromboulcerative K55.0
  toxic NEC K52.1
    due to Clostridium difficile A04.7
  transmural — *see* Enteritis, regional, large intestine
  trichomonal A07.8
  tuberculous (ulcerative) A18.32
  ulcerative (chronic) K51.90
    with
      complication K51.919
        abscess K51.914
        fistula K51.913
        obstruction K51.912
        rectal bleeding K51.911
        specified complication NEC K51.918
    enterocolitis — *see* Enterocolitis, ulcerative
    ileocolitis — *see* Ileocolitis, ulcerative
    mucosal proctocolitis — *see* Proctocolitis, mucosal
    proctitis — *see* Proctitis, ulcerative
    pseudopolyposis — *see* Polyp, colon, inflammatory
    psychogenic F54
    rectosigmoiditis — *see* Rectosigmoiditis, ulcerative
    specified type NEC K51.80
      with
        complication K51.819
          abscess K51.814
          fistula K51.813
          obstruction K51.812
          rectal bleeding K51.811
          specified complication NEC K51.818
Collagenosis, collagen disease (nonvascular) (vascular) M35.9
  cardiovascular I42.8
  reactive perforating L87.1
  specified NEC M35.8
Collapse R55
  adrenal E27.2
  cardiorespiratory R57.0
  cardiovascular R57.0
    newborn P29.89
  circulatory (peripheral) R57.9
    during or after labor and delivery O75.1
    following ectopic or molar pregnancy O08.3
    newborn P29.89
  during or
    after labor and delivery O75.1
    resulting from a procedure, not elsewhere classified T81.10 ☑
  external ear canal — *see* Stenosis, external ear canal
  general R55
  heart — *see* Disease, heart
  heat T67.1 ☑
  hysterical F44.89
  labyrinth, membranous (congenital) Q16.5
  lung (massive) (*see also* Atelectasis) J98.19
    pressure due to anesthesia (general) (local) or other sedation T88.2 ☑

Collapse — *continued*
  lung (*see also* Atelectasis) — *continued*
    pressure due to anesthesia or other sedation — *continued*
      during labor and delivery O74.1
      in pregnancy O29.02- ☑
      postpartum, puerperal O89.09
  myocardial — *see* Disease, heart
  nervous F48.8
  neurocirculatory F45.8
  nose M95.0
  postoperative T81.10 ☑
  pulmonary (*see also* Atelectasis) J98.19
    newborn — *see* Atelectasis
  trachea J39.8
  tracheobronchial J98.09
  valvular — *see* Endocarditis
  vascular (peripheral) R57.9
    during or after labor and delivery O75.1
    following ectopic or molar pregnancy O08.3
    newborn P29.89
  vertebra M48.50- ☑
    cervical region M48.52- ☑
    cervicothoracic region M48.53- ☑
    in (due to)
      metastasis — *see* Collapse, vertebra, in, specified disease NEC
      osteoporosis (*see also* Osteoporosis) M80.88 ☑
        cervical region M80.88 ☑
        cervicothoracic region M80.88 ☑
        lumbar region M80.88 ☑
        lumbosacral region M80.88 ☑
        multiple sites M80.88 ☑
        occipito-atlanto-axial region M80.88 ☑
        sacrococcygeal region M80.88 ☑
        thoracic region M80.88 ☑
        thoracolumbar region M80.88 ☑
      specified disease NEC M48.50- ☑
        cervical region M48.52- ☑
        cervicothoracic region M48.53- ☑
        lumbar region M48.56- ☑
        lumbosacral region M48.57- ☑
        occipito-atlanto-axial region M48.51- ☑
        sacrococcygeal region M48.58- ☑
        thoracic region M48.54- ☑
        thoracolumbar region M48.55- ☑
    lumbar region M48.56- ☑
    lumbosacral region M48.57- ☑
    occipito-atlanto-axial region M48.51- ☑
    sacrococcygeal region M48.58- ☑
    thoracic region M48.54- ☑
    thoracolumbar region M48.55- ☑
Collateral (*see also* condition)
  circulation (venous) I87.8
  dilation, veins I87.8
Colles' fracture S52.53- ☑
Collet (-Sicard) syndrome G52.7
Collier's asthma or lung J60
Collodion baby Q80.2
Coloboma (iris) Q13.0
  eyelid Q10.3
  fundus Q14.8
  lens Q12.2
  optic disc (congenital) Q14.2
    acquired H47.31- ☑
Coloenteritis — *see* Enteritis
Colon — *see* condition
Colonization
  MRSA (Methicillin resistant Staphylococcus aureus) Z22.322
  MSSA (Methicillin susceptible Staphylococcus aureus) Z22.321
  status — *see* Carrier (suspected) of
Coloptosis K63.4
Color blindness — *see* Deficiency, color vision
Colostomy
  attention to Z43.3
  fitting or adjustment Z46.89
  malfunctioning K94.03
  status Z93.3
Colpitis (acute) — *see* Vaginitis
Colpocele N81.5
Colpocystitis — *see* Vaginitis
Colpospasm N94.2
Column, spinal, vertebral — *see* condition

Coma R40.20
  with
    motor response (none) R40.231 ☑
      abnormal R40.233 ☑
      extension R40.232 ☑
      flexion withdrawal R40.234 ☑
      localizes pain R40.235 ☑
      obeys commands R40.236 ☑
    opening of eyes (never) R40.211 ☑
      in response to
        pain R40.212 ☑
        sound R40.213 ☑
      spontaneous R40.214 ☑
    verbal response (none) R40.221 ☑
      confused conversation R40.224 ☑
      inappropriate words R40.223 ☑
      incomprehensible words R40.222 ☑
      oriented R40.225 ☑
  eclamptic — *see* Eclampsia
  epileptic — *see* Epilepsy
  Glasgow, scale score — *see* Glasgow coma scale
  hepatic — *see* Failure, hepatic, by type, with coma
  hyperglycemic (diabetic) — *see* Diabetes, coma
  hyperosmolar (diabetic) — *see* Diabetes, coma
  hypoglycemic (diabetic) — *see* Diabetes, coma, hypoglycemic
    nondiabetic E15
  in diabetes — *see* Diabetes, coma
  insulin-induced — *see* Coma, hypoglycemic
  myxedematous E03.5
  newborn P91.5
  persistent vegetative state R40.3
  specified NEC, without documented Glasgow coma scale score, or with partial Glasgow coma scale score reported R40.244
Comatose — *see* Coma
Combat fatigue F43.0
Combined — *see* condition
Comedo, comedones (giant) L70.0
Comedocarcinoma (*see also* Neoplasm, breast, malignant)
  noninfiltrating
    breast D05.8- ☑
    specified site — *see* Neoplasm, in situ, by site
    unspecified site D05.8- ☑
Comedomastitis — *see* Ectasia, mammary duct
Comminuted fracture — *code as* Fracture, closed
Common
  arterial trunk Q20.0
  atrioventricular canal Q21.2
  atrium Q21.1
  cold (head) J00
  truncus (arteriosus) Q20.0
  variable immunodeficiency — *see* Immunodeficiency, common variable
  ventricle Q20.4
Commotio, commotion (current)
  brain — *see* Injury, intracranial, concussion
  cerebri — *see* Injury, intracranial, concussion
  retinae S05.8X- ☑
  spinal cord — *see* Injury, spinal cord, by region
  spinalis — *see* Injury, spinal cord, by region
Communication
  between
    base of aorta and pulmonary artery Q21.4
    left ventricle and right atrium Q20.5
    pericardial sac and pleural sac Q34.8
    pulmonary artery and pulmonary vein, congenital Q25.72
  congenital between uterus and digestive or urinary tract Q51.7
Compartment syndrome (deep) (posterior) (traumatic) T79.A0 ☑ (*following* T79.7)
  abdomen T79.A3 ☑ (*following* T79.7)
  lower extremity (hip, buttock, thigh, leg, foot, toes) T79.A2 ☑ (*following* T79.7)
  nontraumatic
    abdomen M79.A3 (*following* M79.7)
    lower extremity (hip, buttock, thigh, leg, foot, toes) M79.A2- ☑ (*following* M79.7)
    specified site NEC M79.A9 (*following* M79.7)
    upper extremity (shoulder, arm, forearm, wrist, hand, fingers) M79.A1- ☑ (*following* M79.7)
  specified site NEC T79.A9 ☑ (*following* T79.7)
  upper extremity (shoulder, arm, forearm, wrist, hand, fingers) T79.A1- ☑ (*following* T79.7)

☑ Additional Character Required — Refer to the Tabular List for Character Selection   ◹ Subterms under main terms may continue to next column or page

Compensation
  failure — *see* Disease, heart
  neurosis, psychoneurosis — *see* Disorder, factitious
Complaint (*see also* Disease)
  bowel, functional K59.9
    psychogenic F45.8
  intestine, functional K59.9
    psychogenic F45.8
  kidney — *see* Disease, renal
  miners' J60
Complete — *see* condition
Complex
  Addison-Schilder E71.528
  cardiorenal — *see* Hypertension, cardiorenal
  Costen's M26.69
  disseminated mycobacterium avium- intracellulare (DMAC) A31.2
  Eisenmenger's (ventricular septal defect) I27.89
  hypersexual F52.8
  jumped process, spine — *see* Dislocation, vertebra
  primary, tuberculous A15.7
  Schilder-Addison E71.528
  subluxation (vertebral) M99.19
    abdomen M99.19
    acromioclavicular M99.17
    cervical region M99.11
    cervicothoracic M99.11
    costochondral M99.18
    costovertebral M99.18
    head region M99.10
    hip M99.15
    lower extremity M99.16
    lumbar region M99.13
    lumbosacral M99.13
    occipitocervical M99.10
    pelvic region M99.15
    pubic M99.15
    rib cage M99.18
    sacral region M99.14
    sacrococcygeal M99.14
    sacroiliac M99.14
    specified NEC M99.19
    sternochondral M99.18
    sternoclavicular M99.17
    thoracic region M99.12
    thoracolumbar M99.12
    upper extremity M99.17
  Taussig-Bing (transposition, aorta and overriding pulmonary artery) Q20.1
Complication(s) (from) (of)
  accidental puncture or laceration during a procedure (of) — *see* Complications, intraoperative (intraprocedural), puncture or laceration
  amputation stump (surgical) (late) NEC T87.9
    dehiscence T87.81
    infection or inflammation T87.40
      lower limb T87.4- ☑
      upper limb T87.4- ☑
    necrosis T87.50
      lower limb T87.5- ☑
      upper limb T87.5- ☑
    neuroma T87.30
      lower limb T87.3- ☑
      upper limb T87.3- ☑
    specified type NEC T87.89
  anastomosis (and bypass) (*see also* Complications, prosthetic device or implant)
    intestinal (internal) NEC K91.89
      involving urinary tract N99.89
    urinary tract (involving intestinal tract) N99.89
    vascular — *see* Complications, cardiovascular device or implant
  anesthesia, anesthetic (*see also* Anesthesia, complication) T88.59 ☑
    brain, postpartum, puerperal O89.2
    cardiac
      in
        labor and delivery O74.2
        pregnancy O29.19- ☑
      postpartum, puerperal O89.1
    central nervous system
      in
        labor and delivery O74.3
        pregnancy O29.29- ☑
      postpartum, puerperal O89.2
    difficult or failed intubation T88.4 ☑
      in pregnancy O29.6- ☑

Complication(s) — *continued*
  anesthesia, anesthetic (*see also* Anesthesia, complication) — *continued*
    failed sedation (conscious) (moderate) during procedure T88.52 ☑
    hyperthermia, malignant T88.3 ☑
    hypothermia T88.51 ☑
    intubation failure T88.4 ☑
    malignant hyperthermia T88.3 ☑
    pulmonary
      in
        labor and delivery O74.1
        pregnancy NEC O29.09- ☑
      postpartum, puerperal O89.09
    shock T88.2 ☑
    spinal and epidural
      in
        labor and delivery NEC O74.6
          headache O74.5
        pregnancy NEC O29.5X- ☑
      postpartum, puerperal NEC O89.5
        headache O89.4
  anti-reflux device — *see* Complications, esophageal anti-reflux device
  aortic (bifurcation) graft — *see* Complications, graft, vascular
  aortocoronary (bypass) graft — *see* Complications, coronary artery (bypass) graft
  aortofemoral (bypass) graft — *see* Complications, extremity artery (bypass) graft
  arteriovenous
    fistula, surgically created T82.9 ☑
      embolism T82.818 ☑
      fibrosis T82.828 ☑
      hemorrhage T82.838 ☑
      infection or inflammation T82.7 ☑
      mechanical
        breakdown T82.510 ☑
        displacement T82.520 ☑
        leakage T82.530 ☑
        malposition T82.520 ☑
        obstruction T82.590 ☑
        perforation T82.590 ☑
        protrusion T82.590 ☑
      pain T82.848 ☑
      specified type NEC T82.898 ☑
      stenosis T82.858 ☑
      thrombosis T82.868 ☑
    shunt, surgically created T82.9 ☑
      embolism T82.818 ☑
      fibrosis T82.828 ☑
      hemorrhage T82.838 ☑
      infection or inflammation T82.7 ☑
      mechanical
        breakdown T82.511 ☑
        displacement T82.521 ☑
        leakage T82.531 ☑
        malposition T82.521 ☑
        obstruction T82.591 ☑
        perforation T82.591 ☑
        protrusion T82.591 ☑
      pain T82.848 ☑
      specified type NEC T82.898 ☑
      stenosis T82.858 ☑
      thrombosis T82.868 ☑
  arthroplasty — *see* Complications, joint prosthesis
  artificial
    fertilization or insemination N98.9
      attempted introduction (of)
        embryo in embryo transfer N98.3
        ovum following in vitro fertilization N98.2
      hyperstimulation of ovaries N98.1
      infection N98.0
      specified NEC N98.8
    heart T82.9 ☑
      embolism T82.817 ☑
      fibrosis T82.827 ☑
      hemorrhage T82.837 ☑
      infection or inflammation T82.7 ☑
      mechanical
        breakdown T82.512 ☑
        displacement T82.522 ☑
        leakage T82.532 ☑
        malposition T82.522 ☑
        obstruction T82.592 ☑
        perforation T82.592 ☑

Complication(s) — *continued*
  artificial — *continued*
    heart — *continued*
      mechanical — *continued*
        protrusion T82.592 ☑
      pain T82.847 ☑
      specified type NEC T82.897 ☑
      stenosis T82.857 ☑
      thrombosis T82.867 ☑
    opening
      cecostomy — *see* Complications, colostomy
      colostomy — *see* Complications, colostomy
      cystostomy — *see* Complications, cystostomy
      enterostomy — *see* Complications, enterostomy
      gastrostomy — *see* Complications, gastrostomy
      ileostomy — *see* Complications, enterostomy
      jejunostomy — *see* Complications, enterostomy
      nephrostomy — *see* Complications, stoma, urinary tract
      tracheostomy — *see* Complications, tracheostomy
      ureterostomy — *see* Complications, stoma, urinary tract
      urethrostomy — *see* Complications, stoma, urinary tract
  balloon implant or device
    gastrointestinal T85.9 ☑
      embolism T85.81 ☑
      fibrosis T85.82 ☑
      hemorrhage T85.83 ☑
      infection and inflammation T85.79 ☑
      pain T85.84 ☑
      specified type NEC T85.89 ☑
      stenosis T85.85 ☑
      thrombosis T85.86 ☑
    vascular (counterpulsation) T82.9 ☑
      embolism T82.818 ☑
      fibrosis T82.828 ☑
      hemorrhage T82.838 ☑
      infection or inflammation T82.7 ☑
      mechanical
        breakdown T82.513 ☑
        displacement T82.523 ☑
        leakage T82.533 ☑
        malposition T82.523 ☑
        obstruction T82.593 ☑
        perforation T82.593 ☑
        protrusion T82.593 ☑
      pain T82.848 ☑
      specified type NEC T82.898 ☑
      stenosis T82.858 ☑
      thrombosis T82.868 ☑
  bariatric procedure
    gastric band procedure K95.09
      infection K95.01
    specified procedure NEC K95.89
      infection K95.81
  bile duct implant (prosthetic) T85.9 ☑
    embolism T85.81 ☑
    fibrosis T85.82 ☑
    hemorrhage T85.83 ☑
    infection and inflammation T85.79 ☑
    mechanical
      breakdown T85.510 ☑
      displacement T85.520 ☑
      malfunction T85.510 ☑
      malposition T85.520 ☑
      obstruction T85.590 ☑
      perforation T85.590 ☑
      protrusion T85.590 ☑
      specified NEC T85.590 ☑
    pain T85.84 ☑
    specified type NEC T85.89 ☑
    stenosis T85.85 ☑
    thrombosis T85.86 ☑
  bladder device (auxiliary) — *see* Complications, genitourinary, device or implant, urinary system
  bleeding (postoperative) — *see* Complication, postoperative, hemorrhage
    intraoperative — *see* Complication, intraoperative, hemorrhage
  blood vessel graft — *see* Complications, graft, vascular
  bone
    device NEC T84.9 ☑
      embolism T84.81 ☑

Complication(s) — *continued*
  bone — *continued*
    device — *continued*
      fibrosis T84.82 ☑
      hemorrhage T84.83 ☑
      infection or inflammation T84.7 ☑
      mechanical
        breakdown T84.318 ☑
        displacement T84.328 ☑
        malposition T84.328 ☑
        obstruction T84.398 ☑
        perforation T84.398 ☑
        protrusion T84.398 ☑
      pain T84.84 ☑
      specified type NEC T84.89 ☑
      stenosis T84.85 ☑
      thrombosis T84.86 ☑
    graft — *see* Complications, graft, bone
    growth stimulator (electrode) — *see* Complications, electronic stimulator device, bone
    marrow transplant — *see* Complications, transplant, bone, marrow
  brain neurostimulator (electrode) — *see* Complications, electronic stimulator device, brain
  breast implant (prosthetic) T85.9 ☑
    capsular contracture T85.44 ☑
    embolism T85.81 ☑
    fibrosis T85.82 ☑
    hemorrhage T85.83 ☑
    infection and inflammation T85.79 ☑
    mechanical
      breakdown T85.41 ☑
      displacement T85.42 ☑
      leakage T85.43 ☑
      malposition T85.42 ☑
      obstruction T85.49 ☑
      perforation T85.49 ☑
      protrusion T85.49 ☑
      specified NEC T85.49 ☑
    pain T85.84 ☑
    specified type NEC T85.89 ☑
    stenosis T85.85 ☑
    thrombosis T85.86 ☑
  bypass (*see also* Complications, prosthetic device or implant)
    aortocoronary — *see* Complications, coronary artery (bypass) graft
    arterial (*see also* Complications, graft, vascular)
      extremity — *see* Complications, extremity artery (bypass) graft
  cardiac (*see also* Disease, heart)
    device, implant or graft T82.9 ☑
      embolism T82.817 ☑
      fibrosis T82.827 ☑
      hemorrhage T82.837 ☑
      infection or inflammation T82.7 ☑
        valve prosthesis T82.6 ☑
      mechanical
        breakdown T82.519 ☑
          specified device NEC T82.518 ☑
        displacement T82.529 ☑
          specified device NEC T82.528 ☑
        leakage T82.539 ☑
          specified device NEC T82.538 ☑
        malposition T82.529 ☑
          specified device NEC T82.528 ☑
        obstruction T82.599 ☑
          specified device NEC T82.598 ☑
        perforation T82.599 ☑
          specified device NEC T82.598 ☑
        protrusion T82.599 ☑
          specified device NEC T82.598 ☑
      pain T82.847 ☑
      specified type NEC T82.897 ☑
      stenosis T82.857 ☑
      thrombosis T82.867 ☑
  cardiovascular device, graft or implant T82.9 ☑
    aortic graft — *see* Complications, graft, vascular
    arteriovenous
      fistula, artificial — *see* Complication, arteriovenous, fistula, surgically created
      shunt — *see* Complication, arteriovenous, shunt, surgically created
    artificial heart — *see* Complication, artificial, heart
    balloon (counterpulsation) device — *see* Complication, balloon implant, vascular

Complication(s) — *continued*
  cardiovascular device, graft or implant — *continued*
    carotid artery graft — *see* Complications, graft, vascular
    coronary bypass graft — *see* Complication, coronary artery (bypass) graft
    dialysis catheter (vascular) — *see* Complication, catheter, dialysis
    electronic T82.9 ☑
      electrode T82.9 ☑
        embolism T82.817 ☑
        fibrosis T82.827 ☑
        hemorrhage T82.837 ☑
        infection T82.7 ☑
        mechanical
          breakdown T82.110 ☑
          displacement T82.120 ☑
          leakage T82.190 ☑
          obstruction T82.190 ☑
          perforation T82.190 ☑
          protrusion T82.190 ☑
          specified type NEC T82.190 ☑
        pain T82.847 ☑
        specified NEC T82.897 ☑
        stenosis T82.857 ☑
        thrombosis T82.867 ☑
      embolism T82.817 ☑
      fibrosis T82.827 ☑
      hemorrhage T82.837 ☑
      infection T82.7 ☑
      mechanical
        breakdown T82.119 ☑
        displacement T82.129 ☑
        leakage T82.199 ☑
        obstruction T82.199 ☑
        perforation T82.199 ☑
        protrusion T82.199 ☑
        specified type NEC T82.199 ☑
      pain T82.847 ☑
      pulse generator T82.9 ☑
        embolism T82.817 ☑
        fibrosis T82.827 ☑
        hemorrhage T82.837 ☑
        infection T82.7 ☑
        mechanical
          breakdown T82.111 ☑
          displacement T82.121 ☑
          leakage T82.191 ☑
          obstruction T82.191 ☑
          perforation T82.191 ☑
          protrusion T82.191 ☑
          specified type NEC T82.191 ☑
        pain T82.847 ☑
        specified NEC T82.897 ☑
        stenosis T82.857 ☑
        thrombosis T82.867 ☑
      specified condition NEC T82.897 ☑
      specified device NEC T82.9 ☑
        embolism T82.817 ☑
        fibrosis T82.827 ☑
        hemorrhage T82.837 ☑
        infection T82.7 ☑
        mechanical
          breakdown T82.118 ☑
          displacement T82.128 ☑
          leakage T82.198 ☑
          obstruction T82.198 ☑
          perforation T82.198 ☑
          protrusion T82.198 ☑
          specified type NEC T82.198 ☑
        pain T82.847 ☑
        specified NEC T82.897 ☑
        stenosis T82.857 ☑
        thrombosis T82.867 ☑
      stenosis T82.857 ☑
      thrombosis T82.867 ☑
    extremity artery graft — *see* Complication, extremity artery (bypass) graft
    femoral artery graft — *see* Complication, extremity artery (bypass) graft
    heart
      transplant — *see* Complication, transplant, heart
      valve — *see* Complication, prosthetic device, heart valve

Complication(s) — *continued*
  cardiovascular device, graft or implant — *continued*
    heart — *continued*
      valve — *see* Complication, prosthetic device, heart valve — *continued*
        graft — *see* Complication, heart, valve, graft
    heart-lung transplant — *see* Complication, transplant, heart, with lung
    infection or inflammation T82.7 ☑
    umbrella device — *see* Complication, umbrella device, vascular
    vascular graft (or anastomosis) — *see* Complication, graft, vascular
  carotid artery (bypass) graft — *see* Complications, graft, vascular
  catheter (device) NEC (*see also* Complications, prosthetic device or implant)
    cystostomy T83.9 ☑
      embolism T83.81 ☑
      fibrosis T83.82 ☑
      hemorrhage T83.83 ☑
      infection and inflammation T83.59 ☑
      mechanical
        breakdown T83.010 ☑
        displacement T83.020 ☑
        leakage T83.030 ☑
        malposition T83.020 ☑
        obstruction T83.090 ☑
        perforation T83.090 ☑
        protrusion T83.090 ☑
        specified NEC T83.090 ☑
      pain T83.84 ☑
      specified type NEC T83.89 ☑
      stenosis T83.85 ☑
      thrombosis T83.86 ☑
    dialysis (vascular) T82.9 ☑
      embolism T82.818 ☑
      fibrosis T82.828 ☑
      hemorrhage T82.838 ☑
      infection and inflammation T82.7 ☑
      intraperitoneal — *see* Complications, catheter, intraperitoneal
      mechanical
        breakdown T82.41 ☑
        displacement T82.42 ☑
        leakage T82.43 ☑
        malposition T82.42 ☑
        obstruction T82.49 ☑
        perforation T82.49 ☑
        protrusion T82.49 ☑
      pain T82.848 ☑
      specified type NEC T82.898 ☑
      stenosis T82.858 ☑
      thrombosis T82.868 ☑
    epidural infusion T85.9 ☑
      embolism T85.81 ☑
      fibrosis T85.82 ☑
      hemorrhage T85.83 ☑
      infection and inflammation T85.79 ☑
      mechanical
        breakdown T85.610 ☑
        displacement T85.620 ☑
        leakage T85.630 ☑
        malfunction T85.610 ☑
        malposition T85.620 ☑
        obstruction T85.690 ☑
        perforation T85.690 ☑
        protrusion T85.690 ☑
        specified NEC T85.690 ☑
      pain T85.84 ☑
      specified type NEC T85.89 ☑
      stenosis T85.85 ☑
      thrombosis T85.86 ☑
    intraperitoneal dialysis T85.9 ☑
      embolism T85.81 ☑
      fibrosis T85.82 ☑
      hemorrhage T85.83 ☑
      infection and inflammation T85.71 ☑
      mechanical
        breakdown T85.611 ☑
        displacement T85.621 ☑
        leakage T85.631 ☑
        malfunction T85.611 ☑
        malposition T85.621 ☑
        obstruction T85.691 ☑

Complication(s) — *continued*
catheter (*see also* Complications, prosthetic device or implant) — *continued*
 intraperitoneal dialysis — *continued*
  mechanical — *continued*
   perforation T85.691 ☑
   protrusion T85.691 ☑
   specified NEC T85.691 ☑
  pain T85.84 ☑
  specified type NEC T85.89 ☑
  stenosis T85.85 ☑
  thrombosis T85.86 ☑
 intravenous infusion T82.9 ☑
  embolism T82.818 ☑
  fibrosis T82.828 ☑
  hemorrhage T82.838 ☑
  infection or inflammation T82.7 ☑
  mechanical
   breakdown T82.514 ☑
   displacement T82.524 ☑
   leakage T82.534 ☑
   malposition T82.524 ☑
   obstruction T82.594 ☑
   perforation T82.594 ☑
   protrusion T82.594 ☑
  pain T82.848 ☑
  specified type NEC T82.898 ☑
  stenosis T82.858 ☑
  thrombosis T82.868 ☑
 subdural infusion T85.9 ☑
  embolism T85.81 ☑
  fibrosis T85.82 ☑
  hemorrhage T85.83 ☑
  infection and inflammation T85.79 ☑
  mechanical
   breakdown T85.610 ☑
   displacement T85.620 ☑
   leakage T85.630 ☑
   malfunction T85.610 ☑
   malposition T85.620 ☑
   obstruction T85.690 ☑
   perforation T85.690 ☑
   protrusion T85.690 ☑
   specified NEC T85.690 ☑
  pain T85.84 ☑
  specified type NEC T85.89 ☑
  stenosis T85.85 ☑
  thrombosis T85.86 ☑
 urethral, indwelling T83.9 ☑
  displacement T83.028 ☑
  embolism T83.81 ☑
  fibrosis T83.82 ☑
  hemorrhage T83.83 ☑
  infection and inflammation T83.51 ☑
  leakage T83.038 ☑
  malposition T83.028 ☑
  mechanical
   breakdown T83.018 ☑
  obstruction (mechanical) T83.098 ☑
  pain T83.84 ☑
  perforation T83.098 ☑
  protrusion T83.098 ☑
  specified type NEC T83.098 ☑
  stenosis T83.85 ☑
  thrombosis T83.86 ☑
 urinary (indwelling) — *see* Complications, catheter, urethral, indwelling
cecostomy (stoma) — *see* Complications, colostomy
cesarean delivery wound NEC O90.89
 disruption O90.0
 hematoma O90.2
 infection (following delivery) O86.0
chemotherapy (antineoplastic) NEC T88.7 ☑
chin implant (prosthetic) — *see* Complication, prosthetic device or implant, specified NEC
circulatory system I99.8
 intraoperative I97.88
 postprocedural I97.89
  following cardiac surgery I97.19- ☑
   postcardiotomy syndrome I97.0
  hypertension I97.3
  lymphedema after mastectomy I97.2
  postcardiotomy syndrome I97.0
  specified NEC I97.89
colostomy (stoma) K94.00
 hemorrhage K94.01

Complication(s) — *continued*
colostomy — *continued*
 infection K94.02
 malfunction K94.03
 mechanical K94.03
 specified complication NEC K94.09
contraceptive device, intrauterine — *see* Complications, intrauterine, contraceptive device
cord (umbilical) — *see* Complications, umbilical cord
corneal graft — *see* Complications, graft, cornea
coronary artery (bypass) graft T82.9
 atherosclerosis — *see* Arteriosclerosis, coronary (artery),
 embolism T82.818 ☑
 fibrosis T82.828 ☑
 hemorrhage T82.838 ☑
 infection and inflammation T82.7 ☑
 mechanical
  breakdown T82.211 ☑
  displacement T82.212 ☑
  leakage T82.213 ☑
  malposition T82.212 ☑
  obstruction T82.218 ☑
  perforation T82.218 ☑
  protrusion T82.218 ☑
  specified NEC T82.218 ☑
 pain T82.848 ☑
 specified type NEC T82.897 ☑
 stenosis T82.858 ☑
 thrombosis T82.868 ☑
counterpulsation device (balloon), intra-aortic — *see* Complications, balloon implant, vascular
cystostomy (stoma) N99.518
 catheter — *see* Complications, catheter, cystostomy
 hemorrhage N99.510
 infection N99.511
 malfunction N99.512
 specified type NEC N99.518
delivery (*see also* Complications, obstetric) O75.9
 procedure (instrumental) (manual) (surgical) O75.4
 specified NEC O75.89
dialysis (peritoneal) (renal) (*see also* Complications, infusion)
 catheter (vascular) — *see* Complication, catheter, dialysis
  peritoneal, intraperitoneal — *see* Complications, catheter, intraperitoneal
dorsal column (spinal) neurostimulator — *see* Complications, electronic stimulator device, spinal cord
drug NEC T88.7 ☑
ear procedure (*see also* Disorder, ear)
 intraoperative H95.88
  hematoma — *see* Complications, intraoperative, hemorrhage (hematoma) (of), ear
  hemorrhage — *see* Complications, intraoperative, hemorrhage (hematoma) (of), ear
  laceration — *see* Complications, intraoperative, puncture or laceration..., ear
  specified NEC H95.88
 postoperative H95.89
  external ear canal stenosis H95.81- ☑
  hematoma — *see* Complications, postprocedural, hemorrhage (hematoma) (of), ear
  hemorrhage — *see* Complications, postprocedural, hemorrhage (hematoma) (of), ear
  postmastoidectomy — *see* Complications, postmastoidectomy
  specified NEC H95.89
ectopic pregnancy O08.9
 damage to pelvic organs O08.6
 embolism O08.2
 genital infection O08.0
 hemorrhage (delayed) (excessive) O08.1
 metabolic disorder O08.5
 renal failure O08.4
 shock O08.3
 specified type NEC O08.0
 venous complication NEC O08.7
electronic stimulator device
 bladder (urinary) — *see* Complications, electronic stimulator device, urinary
 bone T84.9 ☑
  breakdown T84.310 ☑
  displacement T84.320 ☑
  embolism T84.81 ☑
  fibrosis T84.82 ☑

Complication(s) — *continued*
electronic stimulator device — *continued*
 bone — *continued*
  hemorrhage T84.83 ☑
  infection or inflammation T84.7 ☑
  malfunction T84.310 ☑
  malposition T84.320 ☑
  mechanical NEC T84.390 ☑
  obstruction T84.390 ☑
  pain T84.84 ☑
  perforation T84.390 ☑
  protrusion T84.390 ☑
  specified type NEC T84.89 ☑
  stenosis T84.85 ☑
  thrombosis T84.86 ☑
 brain T85.9 ☑
  embolism T85.81 ☑
  fibrosis T85.82 ☑
  hemorrhage T85.83 ☑
  infection and inflammation T85.79 ☑
  mechanical
   breakdown T85.110 ☑
   displacement T85.120 ☑
   leakage T85.190 ☑
   malposition T85.120 ☑
   obstruction T85.190 ☑
   perforation T85.190 ☑
   protrusion T85.190 ☑
   specified NEC T85.190 ☑
  pain T85.84 ☑
  specified type NEC T85.89 ☑
  stenosis T85.85 ☑
  thrombosis T85.86 ☑
 cardiac (defibrillator) (pacemaker) — *see* Complications, cardiovascular device or implant, electronic
 muscle T84.9 ☑
  breakdown T84.418 ☑
  displacement T84.428 ☑
  embolism T84.81 ☑
  fibrosis T84.82 ☑
  hemorrhage T84.83 ☑
  infection or inflammation T84.7 ☑
  mechanical NEC T84.498 ☑
  pain T84.84 ☑
  specified type NEC T84.89 ☑
  stenosis T84.85 ☑
  thrombosis T84.86 ☑
 nervous system T85.9 ☑
  brain — *see* Complications, electronic stimulator device, brain
  embolism T85.81 ☑
  fibrosis T85.82 ☑
  hemorrhage T85.83 ☑
  infection and inflammation T85.79 ☑
  mechanical
   breakdown T85.118 ☑
   displacement T85.128 ☑
   leakage T85.199 ☑
   malposition T85.128 ☑
   obstruction T85.199 ☑
   perforation T85.199 ☑
   protrusion T85.199 ☑
   specified NEC T85.199 ☑
  pain T85.84 ☑
  peripheral nerve — *see* Complications, electronic stimulator device, peripheral nerve
  specified type NEC T85.89 ☑
  spinal cord — *see* Complications, electronic stimulator device, spinal cord
  stenosis T85.85 ☑
  thrombosis T85.86 ☑
 peripheral nerve T85.9 ☑
  embolism T85.81 ☑
  fibrosis T85.82 ☑
  hemorrhage T85.83 ☑
  infection and inflammation T85.79 ☑
  mechanical
   breakdown T85.111 ☑
   displacement T85.121 ☑
   leakage T85.191 ☑
   malposition T85.121 ☑
   obstruction T85.191 ☑
   perforation T85.191 ☑
   protrusion T85.191 ☑
   specified NEC T85.191 ☑

▽ **Subterms under main terms may continue to next column or page** ☑ **Additional Character Required — Refer to the Tabular List for Character Selection**

Complication(s) — *continued*
electronic stimulator device — *continued*
peripheral nerve — *continued*
pain T85.84 ☑
specified type NEC T85.89 ☑
stenosis T85.85 ☑
thrombosis T85.86 ☑
spinal cord T85.9 ☑
embolism T85.81 ☑
fibrosis T85.82 ☑
hemorrhage T85.83 ☑
infection and inflammation T85.79 ☑
mechanical
breakdown T85.112 ☑
displacement T85.122 ☑
leakage T85.192 ☑
malposition T85.122 ☑
obstruction T85.192 ☑
perforation T85.192 ☑
protrusion T85.192 ☑
specified NEC T85.192 ☑
pain T85.84 ☑
specified type NEC T85.89 ☑
stenosis T85.85 ☑
thrombosis T85.86 ☑
urinary T83.9 ☑
embolism T83.81 ☑
fibrosis T83.82 ☑
hemorrhage T83.83 ☑
infection and inflammation T83.59 ☑
mechanical
breakdown T83.110 ☑
displacement T83.120 ☑
malposition T83.120 ☑
perforation T83.190 ☑
protrusion T83.190 ☑
specified NEC T83.190 ☑
pain T83.84 ☑
specified type NEC T83.89 ☑
stenosis T83.85 ☑
thrombosis T83.86 ☑
electroshock therapy T88.9 ☑
specified NEC T88.8 ☑
endocrine E34.9
postprocedural
adrenal hypofunction E89.6
hypoinsulinemia E89.1
hypoparathyroidism E89.2
hypopituitarism E89.3
hypothyroidism E89.0
ovarian failure E89.40
asymptomatic E89.40
symptomatic E89.41
specified NEC E89.89
testicular hypofunction E89.5
endodontic treatment NEC M27.59
enterostomy (stoma) K94.10
hemorrhage K94.11
infection K94.12
malfunction K94.13
mechanical K94.13
specified complication NEC K94.19
episiotomy, disruption O90.1
esophageal anti-reflux device T85.9 ☑
embolism T85.81 ☑
fibrosis T85.82 ☑
hemorrhage T85.83 ☑
infection and inflammation T85.79 ☑
mechanical
breakdown T85.511 ☑
displacement T85.521 ☑
malfunction T85.511 ☑
malposition T85.521 ☑
obstruction T85.591 ☑
perforation T85.591 ☑
protrusion T85.591 ☑
specified NEC T85.591 ☑
pain T85.84 ☑
specified type NEC T85.89 ☑
stenosis T85.85 ☑
thrombosis T85.86 ☑
esophagostomy K94.30
hemorrhage K94.31
infection K94.32
malfunction K94.33
mechanical K94.33

Complication(s) — *continued*
esophagostomy — *continued*
specified complication NEC K94.39
extracorporeal circulation T80.90 ☑
extremity artery (bypass) graft T82.9 ☑
arteriosclerosis — *see* Arteriosclerosis, extremities,
bypass graft
embolism T82.818 ☑
fibrosis T82.828 ☑
hemorrhage T82.838 ☑
infection and inflammation T82.7 ☑
mechanical
breakdown T82.318 ☑
femoral artery T82.312 ☑
displacement T82.328 ☑
femoral artery T82.322 ☑
leakage T82.338 ☑
femoral artery T82.332 ☑
malposition T82.328 ☑
femoral artery T82.322 ☑
obstruction T82.398 ☑
femoral artery T82.392 ☑
perforation T82.398 ☑
femoral artery T82.392 ☑
protrusion T82.398 ☑
femoral artery T82.392 ☑
pain T82.848 ☑
specified type NEC T82.898 ☑
stenosis T82.858 ☑
thrombosis T82.868 ☑
eye H57.9
corneal graft — *see* Complications, graft, cornea
implant (prosthetic) T85.9 ☑
embolism T85.81 ☑
fibrosis T85.82 ☑
hemorrhage T85.83 ☑
infection and inflammation T85.79 ☑
mechanical
breakdown T85.318 ☑
displacement T85.328 ☑
leakage T85.398 ☑
malposition T85.328 ☑
obstruction T85.398 ☑
perforation T85.398 ☑
protrusion T85.398 ☑
specified NEC T85.398 ☑
pain T85.84 ☑
specified type NEC T85.89 ☑
stenosis T85.85 ☑
thrombosis T85.86 ☑
intraocular lens — *see* Complications, intraocular
lens
orbital prosthesis — *see* Complications, orbital
prosthesis
female genital N94.9
device, implant or graft NEC — *see* Complications,
genitourinary, device or implant, genital tract
femoral artery (bypass) graft — *see* Complication, extremity artery (bypass) graft
fixation device, internal (orthopedic) T84.9 ☑
infection and inflammation T84.60 ☑
arm T84.61- ☑
humerus T84.61- ☑
radius T84.61- ☑
ulna T84.61- ☑
leg T84.629 ☑
femur T84.62- ☑
fibula T84.62- ☑
tibia T84.62- ☑
specified site NEC T84.89 ☑
spine T84.63 ☑
mechanical
breakdown
limb T84.119 ☑
carpal T84.210 ☑
femur T84.11- ☑
fibula T84.11- ☑
humerus T84.11- ☑
metacarpal T84.210 ☑
metatarsal T84.213 ☑
phalanx
foot T84.213 ☑
hand T84.210 ☑
radius T84.11- ☑
tarsal T84.213 ☑
tibia T84.11- ☑

Complication(s) — *continued*
fixation device, internal — *continued*
mechanical — *continued*
breakdown — *continued*
limb — *continued*
ulna T84.11- ☑
specified bone NEC T84.218 ☑
spine T84.216 ☑
displacement
limb T84.129 ☑
carpal T84.220 ☑
femur T84.12- ☑
fibula T84.12- ☑
humerus T84.12- ☑
metacarpal T84.220 ☑
metatarsal T84.223 ☑
phalanx
foot T84.223 ☑
hand T84.220 ☑
radius T84.12- ☑
tarsal T84.223 ☑
tibia T84.12- ☑
ulna T84.12- ☑
specified bone NEC T84.228 ☑
spine T84.226 ☑
malposition — *see* Complications, fixation device, internal, mechanical, displacement
obstruction — *see* Complications, fixation device, internal, mechanical, specified type
NEC
perforation — *see* Complications, fixation device, internal, mechanical, specified type
NEC
protrusion — *see* Complications, fixation device, internal, mechanical, specified type
NEC
specified type NEC
limb T84.199 ☑
carpal T84.290 ☑
femur T84.19- ☑
fibula T84.19- ☑
humerus T84.19- ☑
metacarpal T84.290 ☑
metatarsal T84.293 ☑
phalanx
foot T84.293 ☑
hand T84.290 ☑
radius T84.19- ☑
tarsal T84.293 ☑
tibia T84.19- ☑
ulna T84.19- ☑
specified bone NEC T84.298 ☑
vertebra T84.296 ☑
specified type NEC T84.89 ☑
embolism T84.81 ☑
fibrosis T84.82 ☑
hemorrhage T84.83 ☑
pain T84.84 ☑
specified complication NEC T84.89 ☑
stenosis T84.85 ☑
thrombosis T84.86 ☑
following
acute myocardial infarction NEC I23.8
aneurysm (false) (of cardiac wall) (of heart wall)
(ruptured) I23.3
angina I23.7
atrial
septal defect I23.1
thrombosis I23.6
cardiac wall rupture I23.3
chordae tendinae rupture I23.4
defect
septal
atrial (heart) I23.1
ventricular (heart) I23.2
hemopericardium I23.0
papillary muscle rupture I23.5
rupture
cardiac wall I23.3
with hemopericardium I23.0
chordae tendineae I23.4
papillary muscle I23.5
specified NEC I23.8
thrombosis
atrium I23.6
auricular appendage I23.6
ventricle (heart) I23.6

Complication(s) — *continued*
  following — *continued*
    acute myocardial infarction — *continued*
      ventricular
        septal defect I23.2
        thrombosis I23.6
    ectopic or molar pregnancy O08.9
      cardiac arrest O08.81
      sepsis O08.82
      specified type NEC O08.89
      urinary tract infection O08.83
    termination of pregnancy — *see* Abortion
  gastrointestinal K92.9
    bile duct prosthesis — *see* Complications, bile duct implant
    esophageal anti-reflux device — *see* Complications, esophageal anti-reflux device
    postoperative
      colostomy — *see* Complications, colostomy
      dumping syndrome K91.1
      enterostomy — *see* Complications, enterostomy
      gastrostomy — *see* Complications, gastrostomy
      malabsorption NEC K91.2
      obstruction K91.3
      postcholecystectomy syndrome K91.5
      specified NEC K91.89
      vomiting after GI surgery K91.0
    prosthetic device or implant
      bile duct prosthesis — *see* Complications, bile duct implant
      esophageal anti-reflux device — *see* Complications, esophageal anti-reflux device
      specified type NEC
        embolism T85.81 ☑
        fibrosis T85.82 ☑
        hemorrhage T85.83 ☑
        mechanical
          breakdown T85.518 ☑
          displacement T85.528 ☑
          malfunction T85.518 ☑
          malposition T85.528 ☑
          obstruction T85.598 ☑
          perforation T85.598 ☑
          protrusion T85.598 ☑
          specified NEC T85.598 ☑
        pain T85.84 ☑
        specified complication NEC T85.89 ☑
        stenosis T85.85 ☑
        thrombosis T85.86 ☑
  gastrostomy (stoma) K94.20
    hemorrhage K94.21
    infection K94.22
    malfunction K94.23
    mechanical K94.23
    specified complication NEC K94.29
  genitourinary
    device or implant T83.9 ☑
      genital tract T83.9 ☑
        infection or inflammation T83.6 ☑
        intrauterine contraceptive device — *see* Complications, intrauterine, contraceptive device
        mechanical — *see* Complications, by device, mechanical
        mesh — *see* Complications, mesh
        penile prosthesis — *see* Complications, prosthetic device, penile
        specified type NEC T83.89 ☑
          embolism T83.81 ☑
          fibrosis T83.82 ☑
          hemorrhage T83.83 ☑
          pain T83.84 ☑
          specified complication NEC T83.89 ☑
          stenosis T83.85 ☑
          thrombosis T83.86 ☑
      vaginal mesh — *see* Complications, mesh
      urinary system T83.9 ☑
        cystostomy catheter — *see* Complication, catheter, cystostomy
        electronic stimulator — *see* Complications, electronic stimulator device, urinary
        indwelling urethral catheter — *see* Complications, catheter, urethral, indwelling
        infection or inflammation T83.59 ☑
          indwelling urinary catheter T83.51 ☑

Complication(s) — *continued*
  genitourinary — *continued*
    device or implant — *continued*
      urinary system — *continued*
        kidney transplant — *see* Complication, transplant, kidney
        organ graft — *see* Complication, graft, urinary organ
        specified type NEC T83.89 ☑
          embolism T83.81 ☑
          fibrosis T83.82 ☑
          hemorrhage T83.83 ☑
          mechanical T83.198 ☑
            breakdown T83.118 ☑
            displacement T83.128 ☑
            malfunction T83.118 ☑
            malposition T83.128 ☑
            obstruction T83.198 ☑
            perforation T83.198 ☑
            protrusion T83.198 ☑
            specified NEC T83.198 ☑
          pain T83.84 ☑
          specified complication NEC T83.89 ☑
          stenosis T83.85 ☑
          thrombosis T83.86 ☑
        sphincter implant — *see* Complications, implant, urinary sphincter
    postprocedural
      pelvic peritoneal adhesions N99.4
      renal failure N99.0
      specified NEC N99.89
      stoma — *see* Complications, stoma, urinary tract
      urethral stricture — *see* Stricture, urethra, postprocedural
      vaginal
        adhesions N99.2
        vault prolapse N99.3
  graft (bypass) (patch) (*see also* Complications, prosthetic device or implant)
    aorta — *see* Complications, graft, vascular
    arterial — *see* Complication, graft, vascular
    bone T86.839
      failure T86.831
      infection T86.832
      mechanical T84.318 ☑
        breakdown T84.318 ☑
        displacement T84.328 ☑
        protrusion T84.398 ☑
        specified type NEC T84.398 ☑
      rejection T86.830
      specified type NEC T86.838
    carotid artery — *see* Complications, graft, vascular
    cornea T86.849
      failure T86.841
      infection T86.842
      mechanical T85.398 ☑
        breakdown T85.318 ☑
        displacement T85.328 ☑
        protrusion T85.398 ☑
        specified type NEC T85.398 ☑
      rejection T86.840
      retroprosthetic membrane T85.398 ☑
      specified type NEC T86.848
    femoral artery (bypass) — *see* Complication, extremity artery (bypass) graft
    genital organ or tract — *see* Complications, genitourinary, device or implant, genital tract
    muscle T84.9 ☑
      breakdown T84.410 ☑
      displacement T84.420 ☑
      embolism T84.81 ☑
      fibrosis T84.82 ☑
      hemorrhage T84.83 ☑
      infection and inflammation T84.7 ☑
      mechanical NEC T84.490 ☑
      pain T84.84 ☑
      specified type NEC T84.89 ☑
      stenosis T84.85 ☑
      thrombosis T84.86 ☑
    nerve — *see* Complication, prosthetic device or implant, specified NEC
    skin — *see* Complications, prosthetic device or implant, skin graft
    tendon T84.9 ☑
      breakdown T84.410 ☑

Complication(s) — *continued*
  graft (*see also* Complications, prosthetic device or implant) — *continued*
    tendon — *continued*
      displacement T84.420 ☑
      embolism T84.81 ☑
      fibrosis T84.82 ☑
      hemorrhage T84.83 ☑
      infection and inflammation T84.7 ☑
      mechanical NEC T84.490 ☑
      pain T84.84 ☑
      specified type NEC T84.89 ☑
      stenosis T84.85 ☑
      thrombosis T84.86 ☑
    urinary organ T83.9 ☑
      embolism T83.81 ☑
      fibrosis T83.82 ☑
      hemorrhage T83.83 ☑
      infection and inflammation T83.59 ☑
        indwelling urinary catheter T83.51 ☑
      mechanical
        breakdown T83.21 ☑
        displacement T83.22 ☑
        leakage T83.23 ☑
        malposition T83.22 ☑
        obstruction T83.29 ☑
        perforation T83.29 ☑
        protrusion T83.29 ☑
        specified NEC T83.29 ☑
      pain T83.84 ☑
      specified type NEC T83.89 ☑
      stenosis T83.85 ☑
      thrombosis T83.86 ☑
    vascular T82.9 ☑
      embolism T82.818 ☑
      femoral artery — *see* Complication, extremity artery (bypass) graft
      fibrosis T82.828 ☑
      hemorrhage T82.838 ☑
      mechanical
        breakdown T82.319 ☑
          aorta (bifurcation) T82.310 ☑
          carotid artery T82.311 ☑
          specified vessel NEC T82.318 ☑
        displacement T82.329 ☑
          aorta (bifurcation) T82.320 ☑
          carotid artery T82.321 ☑
          specified vessel NEC T82.328 ☑
        leakage T82.339 ☑
          aorta (bifurcation) T82.330 ☑
          carotid artery T82.331 ☑
          specified vessel NEC T82.338 ☑
        malposition T82.329 ☑
          aorta (bifurcation) T82.320 ☑
          carotid artery T82.321 ☑
          specified vessel NEC T82.328 ☑
        obstruction T82.399 ☑
          aorta (bifurcation) T82.390 ☑
          carotid artery T82.391 ☑
          specified vessel NEC T82.398 ☑
        perforation T82.399 ☑
          aorta (bifurcation) T82.390 ☑
          carotid artery T82.391 ☑
          specified vessel NEC T82.398 ☑
        protrusion T82.399 ☑
          aorta (bifurcation) T82.390 ☑
          carotid artery T82.391 ☑
          specified vessel NEC T82.398 ☑
      pain T82.848 ☑
      specified complication NEC T82.898 ☑
      stenosis T82.858 ☑
      thrombosis T82.868 ☑
  heart I51.9
    assist device
      infection and inflammation T82.7 ☑
    following acute myocardial infarction — *see* Complications, following, acute myocardial infarction
    postoperative — *see* Complications, circulatory system
    transplant — *see* Complication, transplant, heart and lung(s) — *see* Complications, transplant, heart, with lung
    valve
      graft (biological) T82.9 ☑
        embolism T82.817 ☑

Complication(s) — *continued*
  heart — *continued*
    valve — *continued*
      graft — *continued*
        fibrosis T82.827 ☑
        hemorrhage T82.837 ☑
        infection and inflammation T82.7 ☑
        mechanical T82.228 ☑
          breakdown T82.221 ☑
          displacement T82.222 ☑
          leakage T82.223 ☑
          malposition T82.222 ☑
          obstruction T82.228 ☑
          perforation T82.228 ☑
          protrusion T82.228 ☑
        pain T82.847 ☑
        specified type NEC T82.897 ☑
        stenosis T82.857 ☑
        thrombosis T82.867 ☑
      prosthesis T82.9 ☑
        embolism T82.817 ☑
        fibrosis T82.827 ☑
        hemorrhage T82.837 ☑
        infection or inflammation T82.6 ☑
        mechanical T82.09 ☑
          breakdown T82.01 ☑
          displacement T82.02 ☑
          leakage T82.03 ☑
          malposition T82.02 ☑
          obstruction T82.09 ☑
          perforation T82.09 ☑
          protrusion T82.09 ☑
        pain T82.847 ☑
        specified type NEC T82.897 ☑
          mechanical T82.09 ☑
        stenosis T82.857 ☑
        thrombosis T82.867 ☑
  hematoma
    intraoperative — *see* Complication, intraoperative, hemorrhage
    postprocedural — *see* Complication, postprocedural, hemorrhage
  hemodialysis — *see* Complications, dialysis
  hemorrhage
    intraoperative — *see* Complication, intraoperative, hemorrhage
    postprocedural — *see* Complication, postprocedural, hemorrhage
  ileostomy (stoma) — *see* Complications, enterostomy
  immunization (procedure) — *see* Complications, vaccination
  implant (*see also* Complications, by site and type)
    urinary sphincter T83.9 ☑
      embolism T83.81 ☑
      fibrosis T83.82 ☑
      hemorrhage T83.83 ☑
      infection and inflammation T83.59 ☑
      mechanical
        breakdown T83.111 ☑
        displacement T83.121 ☑
        leakage T83.191 ☑
        malposition T83.121 ☑
        obstruction T83.191 ☑
        perforation T83.191 ☑
        protrusion T83.191 ☑
        specified NEC T83.191 ☑
      pain T83.84 ☑
      specified type NEC T83.89 ☑
      stenosis T83.85 ☑
      thrombosis T83.86 ☑
  infusion (procedure) T80.90 ☑
    air embolism T80.0 ☑
    blood — *see* Complications, transfusion
    catheter — *see* Complications, catheter
    infection T80.29 ☑
    pump — *see* Complications, cardiovascular, device or implant
    sepsis T80.29 ☑
    serum reaction (*see also* Reaction, serum) T80.69 ☑
      anaphylactic shock (*see also* Shock, anaphylactic) T80.59 ☑
    specified type NEC T80.89 ☑
  inhalation therapy NEC T81.81 ☑
  injection (procedure) T80.90 ☑
    drug reaction — *see* Reaction, drug
    infection T80.29 ☑

Complication(s) — *continued*
  injection –– *continued*
    sepsis T80.29 ☑
    serum (prophylactic) (therapeutic) — *see* Complications, vaccination
    specified type NEC T80.89 ☑
    vaccine (any) — *see* Complications, vaccination
  inoculation (any) — *see* Complications, vaccination
  insulin pump
    infection and inflammation T85.72 ☑
    mechanical
      breakdown T85.614 ☑
      displacement T85.624 ☑
      leakage T85.633 ☑
      malposition T85.624 ☑
      obstruction T85.694 ☑
      perforation T85.694 ☑
      protrusion T85.694 ☑
      specified NEC T85.694 ☑
  intestinal pouch NEC K91.858
  intraocular lens (prosthetic) T85.9 ☑
    embolism T85.81 ☑
    fibrosis T85.82 ☑
    hemorrhage T85.83 ☑
    infection and inflammation T85.79 ☑
    mechanical
      breakdown T85.21 ☑
      displacement T85.22 ☑
      malposition T85.22 ☑
      obstruction T85.29 ☑
      perforation T85.29 ☑
      protrusion T85.29 ☑
      specified NEC T85.29 ☑
    pain T85.84 ☑
    specified type NEC T85.89 ☑
    stenosis T85.85 ☑
    thrombosis T85.86 ☑
  intraoperative (intraprocedural)
    cardiac arrest
      during cardiac surgery I97.710
      during other surgery I97.711
    cardiac functional disturbance NEC
      during cardiac surgery I97.790
      during other surgery I97.791
    hemorrhage (hematoma) (of)
      circulatory system organ or structure
        during cardiac bypass I97.411
        during cardiac catheterization I97.410
        during other circulatory system procedure I97.418
        during other procedure I97.42
      digestive system organ
        during procedure on digestive system K91.61
        during procedure on other organ K91.62
      ear
        during procedure on ear and mastoid process H95.21
        during procedure on other organ H95.22
      endocrine system organ or structure
        during procedure on endocrine system organ or structure E36.01
        during procedure on other organ E36.02
      eye and adnexa
        during ophthalmic procedure H59.11- ☑
        during other procedure H59.12- ☑
      genitourinary organ or structure
        during procedure on genitourinary organ or structure N99.61
        during procedure on other organ N99.62
      mastoid process
        during procedure on ear and mastoid process H95.21
        during procedure on other organ H95.22
      musculoskeletal structure
        during musculoskeletal surgery M96.810
        during non-orthopedic surgery M96.811
        during orthopedic surgery M96.810
      nervous system
        during a nervous system procedure G97.31
        during other procedure G97.32
      respiratory system
        during other procedure J95.62
        during procedure on respiratory system organ or structure J95.61
      skin and subcutaneous tissue
        during a dermatologic procedure L76.01

Complication(s) — *continued*
  intraoperative — *continued*
    hemorrhage — *continued*
      skin and subcutaneous tissue — *continued*
        during a procedure on other organ L76.02
      spleen
        during a procedure on other organ D78.02
        during a procedure on the spleen D78.01
    puncture or laceration (accidental) (unintentional) (of)
      brain
        during a nervous system procedure G97.48
        during other procedure G97.49
      circulatory system organ or structure
        during circulatory system procedure I97.51
        during other procedure I97.52
      digestive system
        during procedure on digestive system K91.71
        during procedure on other organ K91.72
      ear
        during procedure on ear and mastoid process H95.31
        during procedure on other organ H95.32
      endocrine system organ or structure
        during procedure on endocrine system organ or structure E36.11
        during procedure on other organ E36.12
      eye and adnexa
        during ophthalmic procedure H59.21- ☑
        during other procedure H59.22- ☑
      genitourinary organ or structure
        during procedure on genitourinary organ or structure N99.71
        during procedure on other organ N99.72
      mastoid process
        during procedure on ear and mastoid process H95.31
        during procedure on other organ H95.32
      musculoskeletal structure
        during musculoskeletal surgery M96.820
        during non-orthopedic surgery M96.821
        during orthopedic surgery M96.820
      nervous system
        during a nervous system procedure G97.48
        during other procedure G97.49
      respiratory system
        during other procedure J95.72
        during procedure on respiratory system organ or structure J95.71
      skin and subcutaneous tissue
        during a dermatologic procedure L76.11
        during a procedure on other organ L76.12
      spleen
        during a procedure on other organ D78.12
        during a procedure on the spleen D78.11
    specified NEC
      circulatory system I97.88
      digestive system K91.81
      ear H95.88
      endocrine system E36.8
      eye and adnexa H59.88
      genitourinary system N99.81
      mastoid process H95.88
      musculoskeletal structure M96.89
      nervous system G97.81
      respiratory system J95.88
      skin and subcutaneous tissue L76.81
      spleen D78.81
  intraperitoneal catheter (dialysis) (infusion) — *see* Complications, catheter, intraperitoneal
  intrauterine
    contraceptive device
      embolism T83.81 ☑
      fibrosis T83.82 ☑
      hemorrhage T83.83 ☑
      infection and inflammation T83.6 ☑
      mechanical
        breakdown T83.31 ☑
        displacement T83.32 ☑
        malposition T83.32 ☑
        obstruction T83.39 ☑
        perforation T83.39 ☑
        protrusion T83.39 ☑
        specified NEC T83.39 ☑
      pain T83.84 ☑
      specified type NEC T83.89 ☑
      stenosis T83.85 ☑

☑ **Additional Character Required** — Refer to the Tabular List for Character Selection   ▼ **Subterms under main terms may continue to next column or page**

Complication(s) — *continued*
 intrauterine — *continued*
  contraceptive device — *continued*
   thrombosis T83.86 ☑
  procedure (fetal), to newborn P96.5
 jejunostomy (stoma) — *see* Complications, enterostomy
 joint prosthesis, internal T84.9 ☑
  breakage (fracture) T84.01- ☑
  dislocation T84.02- ☑
  fracture T84.01- ☑
  infection or inflammation T84.50 ☑
   hip T84.5- ☑
   knee T84.5- ☑
   specified joint NEC T84.59 ☑
  instability T84.02- ☑
  malposition — *see* Complications, joint prosthesis, mechanical, displacement
  mechanical
   breakage, broken T84.01- ☑
   dislocation T84.02- ☑
   fracture T84.01- ☑
   instability T84.02- ☑
   leakage — *see* Complications, joint prosthesis, mechanical, specified NEC
   loosening T84.039 ☑
    hip T84.03- ☑
    knee T84.03- ☑
    specified joint NEC T84.038 ☑
   obstruction — *see* Complications, joint prosthesis, mechanical, specified NEC
   perforation — *see* Complications, joint prosthesis, mechanical, specified NEC
   periprosthetic
    fracture T84.049 ☑
     hip T84.04- ☑
     knee T84.04- ☑
     other specified joint T84.048 ☑
    osteolysis T84.059 ☑
     hip T84.05- ☑
     knee T84.05- ☑
     other specified joint T84.058 ☑
   protrusion — *see* Complications, joint prosthesis, mechanical, specified NEC
   specified complication NEC T84.099 ☑
    hip T84.09- ☑
    knee T84.09- ☑
    other specified joint T84.098 ☑
   subluxation T84.02- ☑
   wear of articular bearing surface T84.069 ☑
    hip T84.06- ☑
    knee T84.06- ☑
    other specified joint T84.068 ☑
  specified joint NEC T84.89 ☑
   embolism T84.81 ☑
   fibrosis T84.82 ☑
   hemorrhage T84.83 ☑
   pain T84.84 ☑
   specified complication NEC T84.89 ☑
   stenosis T84.85 ☑
   thrombosis T84.86 ☑
  subluxation T84.02- ☑
 kidney transplant — *see* Complications, transplant, kidney
 labor O75.9
  specified NEC O75.89
 liver transplant (immune or nonimmune) — *see* Complications, transplant, liver
 lumbar puncture G97.1
  cerebrospinal fluid leak G97.0
  headache or reaction G97.1
 lung transplant — *see* Complications, transplant, lung
  and heart — *see* Complications, transplant, lung, with heart
 male genital N50.9
  device, implant or graft — *see* Complications, genitourinary, device or implant, genital tract
  postprocedural or postoperative — *see* Complications, genitourinary, postprocedural
  specified NEC N99.89
 mastoid (process) procedure
  intraoperative H95.88
   hematoma — *see* Complications, intraoperative, hemorrhage (hematoma) (of), mastoid process

Complication(s) — *continued*
 mastoid procedure — *continued*
  intraoperative — *continued*
   hemorrhage — *see* Complications, intraoperative, hemorrhage (hematoma) (of), mastoid process
   laceration — *see* Complications, intraoperative, puncture or laceration, mastoid process
   specified NEC H95.88
  postmastoidectomy — *see* Complications, postmastoidectomy
  postoperative H95.89
   external ear canal stenosis H95.81 ☑
   hematoma — *see* Complications, postprocedural, hemorrhage (hematoma) (of), mastoid process
   hemorrhage — *see* Complications, postprocedural, hemorrhage (hematoma) (of), mastoid process
   postmastoidectomy — *see* Complications, postmastoidectomy
   specified NEC H95.89
 mastoidectomy cavity — *see* Complications, postmastoidectomy
 mechanical — *see* Complications, by site and type, mechanical
 medical procedures (*see also* Complication(s), intraoperative) T88.9 ☑
 metabolic E88.9
  postoperative E89.89
   specified NEC E89.89
 molar pregnancy NOS O08.9
  damage to pelvic organs O08.6
  embolism O08.2
  genital infection O08.0
  hemorrhage (delayed) (excessive) O08.1
  metabolic disorder O08.5
  renal failure O08.4
  shock O08.3
  specified type NEC O08.0
  venous complication NEC O08.7
 musculoskeletal system (*see also* Complication, intraoperative (intraprocedural), by site)
  device, implant or graft NEC — *see* Complications, orthopedic, device or implant
  internal fixation (nail) (plate) (rod) — *see* Complications, fixation device, internal
  joint prosthesis — *see* Complications, joint prosthesis
  post radiation M96.89
   kyphosis M96.3
   scoliosis M96.5
   specified complication NEC M96.89
  postoperative (postprocedural) M96.89
   with osteoporosis — *see* Osteoporosis
   fracture following insertion of device — *see* Fracture, following insertion of orthopedic implant, joint prosthesis or bone plate
   joint instability after prosthesis removal M96.89
   lordosis M96.4
   postlaminectomy syndrome NEC M96.1
    kyphosis M96.3
   pseudarthrosis M96.0
   specified complication NEC M96.89
 nephrostomy (stoma) — *see* Complications, stoma, urinary tract, external NEC
 nervous system G98.8
  central G96.9
  device, implant or graft (*see also* Complication, prosthetic device or implant, specified NEC)
   electronic stimulator (electrode(s)) — *see* Complications, electronic stimulator device
   ventricular shunt — *see* Complications, ventricular shunt
  electronic stimulator (electrode(s)) — *see* Complications, electronic stimulator device
  postprocedural G97.82
   intracranial hypotension G97.2
   specified NEC G97.82
   spinal fluid leak G97.0
 newborn, due to intrauterine (fetal) procedure P96.5
 nonabsorbable (permanent) sutures — *see* Complication, sutures, permanent
 obstetric O75.9
  procedure (instrumental) (manual) (surgical)
   specified NEC O75.4
  specified NEC O75.89

Complication(s) — *continued*
 obstetric — *continued*
  surgical wound NEC O90.89
   hematoma O90.2
   infection O86.0
  ocular lens implant — *see* Complications, intraocular lens
 ophthalmologic
  postprocedural bleb — *see* Blebitis
 orbital prosthesis T85.9 ☑
  embolism T85.81 ☑
  fibrosis T85.82 ☑
  hemorrhage T85.83 ☑
  infection and inflammation T85.79 ☑
  mechanical
   breakdown T85.31- ☑
   displacement T85.32- ☑
   malposition T85.32- ☑
   obstruction T85.39- ☑
   perforation T85.39- ☑
   protrusion T85.39- ☑
   specified NEC T85.39- ☑
  pain T85.84 ☑
  specified type NEC T85.89 ☑
  stenosis T85.85 ☑
  thrombosis T85.86 ☑
 organ or tissue transplant (partial) (total) — *see* Complications, transplant
 orthopedic (*see also* Disorder, soft tissue)
  device or implant T84.9 ☑
   bone
    device or implant — *see* Complication, bone, device NEC
    graft — *see* Complication, graft, bone
   breakdown T84.418 ☑
   displacement T84.428 ☑
   electronic bone stimulator — *see* Complications, electronic stimulator device, bone
   embolism T84.81 ☑
   fibrosis T84.82 ☑
   fixation device — *see* Complication, fixation device, internal
   hemorrhage T84.83 ☑
   infection or inflammation T84.7 ☑
   joint prosthesis — *see* Complication, joint prosthesis, internal
   malfunction T84.418 ☑
   malposition T84.428 ☑
   mechanical NEC T84.498 ☑
   muscle graft — *see* Complications, graft, muscle
   obstruction T84.498 ☑
   pain T84.84 ☑
   perforation T84.498 ☑
   protrusion T84.498 ☑
   specified complication NEC T84.89 ☑
   stenosis T84.85 ☑
   tendon graft — *see* Complications, graft, tendon
   thrombosis T84.86 ☑
  fracture (following insertion of device) — *see* Fracture, following insertion of orthopedic implant, joint prosthesis or bone plate
  postprocedural M96.89
   fracture — *see* Fracture, following insertion of orthopedic implant, joint prosthesis or bone plate
   postlaminectomy syndrome NEC M96.1
    kyphosis M96.3
    lordosis M96.4
   postradiation
    kyphosis M96.2
    scoliosis M96.5
   pseudarthrosis post-fusion M96.0
   specified type NEC M96.89
 pacemaker (cardiac) — *see* Complications, cardiovascular device or implant, electronic
 pancreas transplant — *see* Complications, transplant, pancreas
 penile prosthesis (implant) — *see* Complications, prosthetic device, penile
 perfusion NEC T80.90 ☑
 perineal repair (obstetrical) NEC O90.89
  disruption O90.1
  hematoma O90.2
  infection (following delivery) O86.0
 phototherapy T88.9 ☑
  specified NEC T88.8 ☑

Complication(s) — continued
  postmastoidectomy NEC H95.19- ☑
    cyst, mucosal H95.13- ☑
    granulation H95.12- ☑
    inflammation, chronic H95.11- ☑
    recurrent cholesteatoma H95.Ø- ☑
  postoperative — see Complications, postprocedural
    circulatory — see Complications, circulatory system
    ear — see Complications, ear
    endocrine — see Complications, endocrine
    eye — see Complications, eye
    lumbar puncture G97.1
      cerebrospinal fluid leak G97.Ø
    nervous system (central) (peripheral) — see Complications, nervous system
    respiratory system — see Complications, respiratory system
  postprocedural (see also Complications, surgical procedure)
    cardiac arrest
      following cardiac surgery I97.12Ø
      following other surgery I97.121
    cardiac functional disturbance NEC
      following cardiac surgery I97.19Ø
      following other surgery I97.191
    cardiac insufficiency
      following cardiac surgery I97.11Ø
      following other surgery I97.111
    chorioretinal scars following retinal surgery H59.81- ☑
    following cataract surgery
      cataract (lens) fragments H59.Ø2- ☑
      cystoid macular edema H59.Ø3- ☑
      specified NEC H59.Ø9- ☑
      vitreous (touch) syndrome H59.Ø1- ☑
    heart failure
      following cardiac surgery I97.13Ø
      following other surgery I97.131
    hemorrhage (hematoma) (of)
      circulatory system organ or structure
        following a cardiac bypass I97.611
        following a cardiac catheterization I97.61Ø
        following other circulatory system procedure I97.618
        following other procedure I97.62
      digestive system
        following procedure on digestive system K91.84Ø
        following procedure on other organ K91.841
      ear
        following other procedure H95.42
        following procedure on ear and mastoid process H95.41
      endocrine system
        following endocrine system procedure E89.81Ø
        following other procedure E89.811
      eye and adnexa
        following ophthalmic procedure H59.31- ☑
        following other procedure H59.32- ☑
      genitourinary organ or structure
        following procedure on genitourinary organ or structure N99.82Ø
        following procedure on other organ N99.821
      mastoid process
        following other procedure H95.42
        following procedure on ear and mastoid process H95.41
      musculoskeletal structure
        following musculoskeletal surgery M96.83Ø
        following non-orthopedic surgery M96.831
        following orthopedic surgery M96.83Ø
      nervous system
        following a nervous system procedure G97.51
        following other procedure G97.52
      respiratory system
        following a respiratory system procedure J95.83Ø
        following other procedure J95.831
      skin and subcutaneous tissue
        following a dermatologic procedure L76.21
        following a procedure on other organ L76.22
      spleen
        following procedure on other organ D78.22
        following procedure on the spleen D78.21

Complication(s) — continued
  postprocedural (see also Complications, surgical procedure) — continued
    specified NEC
      circulatory system I97.89
      digestive K91.89
      ear H95.89
      endocrine E89.89
      eye and adnexa H59.89
      genitourinary N99.89
      mastoid process H95.89
      metabolic E89.89
      musculoskeletal structure M96.89
      nervous system G97.82
      respiratory system J95.89
      skin and subcutaneous tissue L76.82
      spleen D78.89
  pregnancy NEC — see Pregnancy, complicated by
  prosthetic device or implant T85.9 ☑
    bile duct — see Complications, bile duct implant
    breast — see Complications, breast implant
    cardiac and vascular NEC — see Complications, cardiovascular device or implant
    corneal transplant — see Complications, graft, cornea
    electronic nervous system stimulator — see Complications, electronic stimulator device
    epidural infusion catheter — see Complications, catheter, epidural
    esophageal anti-reflux device — see Complications, esophageal anti-reflux device
    genital organ or tract — see Complications, genitourinary, device or implant, genital tract
    heart valve — see Complications, heart, valve, prosthesis
    infection or inflammation T85.79 ☑
      intestine transplant T86.892
      liver transplant T86.43
      lung transplant T86.812
      pancreas transplant T86.892
      skin graft T86.822
    intraocular lens — see Complications, intraocular lens
    intraperitoneal (dialysis) catheter — see Complications, catheter, intraperitoneal
    joint — see Complications, joint prosthesis, internal
    mechanical NEC T85.698 ☑
      dialysis catheter (vascular) (see also Complication, catheter, dialysis, mechanical)
        peritoneal — see Complication, catheter, intraperitoneal, mechanical
      gastrointestinal device T85.598 ☑
      ocular device T85.398 ☑
      subdural (infusion) catheter T85.69Ø ☑
      suture, permanent T85.692 ☑
        that for bone repair — see Complications, fixation device, internal (orthopedic), mechanical
      ventricular shunt
        breakdown T85.Ø1 ☑
        displacement T85.Ø2 ☑
        leakage T85.Ø3 ☑
        malposition T85.Ø2 ☑
        obstruction T85.Ø9 ☑
        perforation T85.Ø9 ☑
        protrusion T85.Ø9 ☑
        specified NEC T85.Ø9 ☑
    mesh
      erosion (to surrounding organ or tissue) T83.718 ☑
        vaginal (into pelvic floor muscles) T83.711 ☑
      exposure (into surrounding organ or tissue) T83.728 ☑
        vaginal (into vagina) (through vaginal wall) T83.721 ☑
    orbital — see Complications, orbital prosthesis
    penile T83.9 ☑
      embolism T83.81 ☑
      fibrosis T83.82 ☑
      hemorrhage T83.83 ☑
      infection and inflammation T83.6 ☑
      mechanical
        breakdown T83.41Ø ☑
        displacement T83.42Ø ☑
        leakage T83.49Ø ☑
        malposition T83.42Ø ☑

Complication(s) — continued
  prosthetic device or implant — continued
    penile — continued
      mechanical — continued
        obstruction T83.49Ø ☑
        perforation T83.49Ø ☑
        protrusion T83.49Ø ☑
        specified NEC T83.49Ø ☑
      pain T83.84 ☑
      specified type NEC T83.89 ☑
      stenosis T83.85 ☑
      thrombosis T83.86 ☑
    prosthetic materials NEC
      erosion (to surrounding organ or tissue) T83.718 ☑
        vaginal (into pelvic floor muscles) T83.711 ☑
      exposure (into surrounding organ or tissue) T83.728 ☑
        vaginal (into vagina) (through vaginal wall) T83.721 ☑
    skin graft T86.829
      artificial skin or decellularized allodermis
        embolism T85.81 ☑
        fibrosis T85.82 ☑
        hemorrhage T85.83 ☑
        infection and inflammation T85.79 ☑
        mechanical
          breakdown T85.613 ☑
          displacement T85.623 ☑
          malfunction T85.613 ☑
          malposition T85.623 ☑
          obstruction T85.693 ☑
          perforation T85.693 ☑
          protrusion T85.693 ☑
          specified NEC T85.693 ☑
        pain T85.84 ☑
        specified type NEC T85.89 ☑
        stenosis T85.85 ☑
        thrombosis T85.86 ☑
      failure T86.821
      infection T86.822
      rejection T86.82Ø
      specified NEC T86.828
    specified NEC T85.9 ☑
      embolism T85.81 ☑
      fibrosis T85.82 ☑
      hemorrhage T85.83 ☑
      infection and inflammation T85.79 ☑
      mechanical
        breakdown T85.618 ☑
        displacement T85.628 ☑
        leakage T85.638 ☑
        malfunction T85.618 ☑
        malposition T85.628 ☑
        obstruction T85.698 ☑
        perforation T85.698 ☑
        protrusion T85.698 ☑
        specified NEC T85.698 ☑
      pain T85.84 ☑
      specified type NEC T85.89 ☑
      stenosis T85.85 ☑
      thrombosis T85.86 ☑
    subdural infusion catheter — see Complications, catheter, subdural
    sutures — see Complications, sutures
    urinary organ or tract NEC — see Complications, genitourinary, device or implant, urinary system
    vascular — see Complications, cardiovascular device or implant
    ventricular shunt — see Complications, ventricular shunt (device)
  puerperium — see Puerperal
  puncture, spinal G97.1
    cerebrospinal fluid leak G97.Ø
    headache or reaction G97.1
  pyelogram N99.89
  radiation
    kyphosis M96.2
    scoliosis M96.5
  reattached
    extremity (infection) (rejection)
      lower T87.1X- ☑
      upper T87.ØX- ☑
    specified body part NEC T87.2

Complication(s) — *continued*
  reconstructed breast
    asymmetry between native and reconstructed
      breast N65.1
    deformity N65.Ø
    disproportion between native and reconstructed
      breast N65.1
    excess tissue N65.Ø
    misshappen N65.Ø
  reimplant NEC (*see also* Complications, prosthetic de-
    vice or implant)
    limb (infection) (rejection) — *see* Complications,
      reattached, extremity
    organ (partial) (total) — *see* Complications, trans-
      plant
    prosthetic device NEC — *see* Complications, pros-
      thetic device
  renal N28.9
    allograft — *see* Complications, transplant, kidney
    dialysis — *see* Complications, dialysis
  respirator
    mechanical J95.85Ø
      specified NEC J95.859
  respiratory system J98.9
    device, implant or graft — *see* Complication,
      prosthetic device or implant, specified NEC
    lung transplant — *see* Complications, prosthetic
      device or implant, lung transplant
    postoperative J95.89
      air leak J95.812
      Mendelson's syndrome (chemical pneumonitis)
        J95.4
      pneumothorax J95.811
      pulmonary insufficiency (acute) (after nontho-
        racic surgery) J95.2
        chronic J95.3
        following thoracic surgery J95.1
      respiratory failure (acute) J95.821
        acute and chronic J95.822
      specified NEC J95.89
      subglottic stenosis J95.5
      tracheostomy complication — *see* Complica-
        tions, tracheostomy
    therapy T81.89 ☑
  sedation during labor and delivery O74.9
    cardiac O74.2
    central nervous system O74.3
    pulmonary NEC O74.1
  shunt (*see also* Complications, prosthetic device or
    implant)
    arteriovenous — *see* Complications, arteriovenous,
      shunt
    ventricular (communicating) — *see* Complications,
      ventricular shunt
  skin
    graft T86.829
      failure T86.821
      infection T86.822
      rejection T86.820
      specified type NEC T86.828
  spinal
    anesthesia — *see* Complications, anesthesia, spinal
    catheter (epidural) (subdural) — *see* Complications,
      catheter
    puncture or tap G97.1
      cerebrospinal fluid leak G97.Ø
      headache or reaction G97.1
  stent
    bile duct — *see* Complications, bile duct prosthesis
    urinary T83.9 ☑
      embolism T83.81 ☑
      fibrosis T83.82 ☑
      hemorrhage T83.83 ☑
      infection and inflammation T83.59 ☑
      mechanical
        breakdown T83.112 ☑
        displacement T83.122 ☑
        leakage T83.192 ☑
        malposition T83.122 ☑
        obstruction T83.192 ☑
        perforation T83.192 ☑
        protrusion T83.192 ☑
        specified NEC T83.192 ☑
      pain T83.84 ☑
      specified type NEC T83.89 ☑
      stenosis T83.85 ☑
      thrombosis T83.86 ☑

Complication(s) — *continued*
  stoma
    digestive tract
      colostomy — *see* Complications, colostomy
      enterostomy — *see* Complications, enterosto-
        my
      esophagostomy — *see* Complications,
        esophagostomy
      gastrostomy — *see* Complications, gastrostomy
    urinary tract N99.538
      cystostomy — *see* Complications, cystostomy
      external NOS N99.528
        hemorrhage N99.52Ø
        infection N99.521
        malfunction N99.522
        specified type NEC N99.528
      hemorrhage N99.53Ø
      infection N99.531
      malfunction N99.532
      specified type NEC N99.538
  stomach banding — *see* Complication(s), bariatric
    procedure
  stomach stapling — *see* Complication(s), bariatric
    procedure
  surgical material, nonabsorbable — *see* Complication,
    suture, permanent
  surgical procedure (on) T81.9 ☑
    amputation stump (late) — *see* Complications,
      amputation stump
    cardiac — *see* Complications, circulatory system
    cholesteatoma, recurrent — *see* Complications,
      postmastoidectomy, recurrent
      cholesteatoma
    circulatory (early) — *see* Complications, circulatory
      system
    digestive system — *see* Complications, gastroin-
      testinal
    dumping syndrome (postgastrectomy) K91.1
    ear — *see* Complications, ear
    elephantiasis or lymphedema I97.89
      postmastectomy I97.2
    emphysema (surgical) T81.82 ☑
    endocrine — *see* Complications, endocrine
    eye — *see* Complications, eye
    fistula (persistent postoperative) T81.83 ☑
    foreign body inadvertently left in wound (sponge)
      (suture) (swab) — *see* Foreign body, acciden-
      tally left during a procedure
    gastrointestinal — *see* Complications, gastrointesti-
      nal
    genitourinary NEC N99.89
    hematoma
      intraoperative — *see* Complication, intraopera-
        tive, hemorrhage
      postprocedural — *see* Complication, postpro-
        cedural, hemorrhage
    hemorrhage
      intraoperative — *see* Complication, intraopera-
        tive, hemorrhage
      postprocedural — *see* Complication, postpro-
        cedural, hemorrhage
    hepatic failure K91.82
    hyperglycemia (postpancreatectomy) E89.1
    hypoinsulinemia (postpancreatectomy) E89.1
    hypoparathyroidism (postparathyroidectomy)
      E89.2
    hypopituitarism (posthypophysectomy) E89.3
    hypothyroidism (post-thyroidectomy) E89.Ø
    intestinal obstruction K91.3
    intracranial hypotension following ventricular
      shunting (ventriculostomy) G97.2
    lymphedema I97.89
      postmastectomy I97.2
    malabsorption (postsurgical) NEC K91.2
      osteoporosis — *see* Osteoporosis, postsurgical
        malabsorption
    mastoidectomy cavity NEC — *see* Complications,
      postmastoidectomy
    metabolic E89.89
      specified NEC E89.89
    musculoskeletal — *see* Complications, muscu-
      loskeletal system
    nervous system (central) (peripheral) — *see* Com-
      plications, nervous system
    ovarian failure E89.4Ø
      asymptomatic E89.4Ø
      symptomatic E89.41

Complication(s) — *continued*
  surgical procedure — *continued*
    peripheral vascular — *see* Complications, surgical
      procedure, vascular
    postcardiotomy syndrome I97.Ø
    postcholecystectomy syndrome K91.5
    postcommissurotomy syndrome I97.Ø
    postgastrectomy dumping syndrome K91.1
    postlaminectomy syndrome NEC M96.1
      kyphosis M96.3
    postmastectomy lymphedema syndrome I97.2
    postmastoidectomy cholesteatoma — *see* Compli-
      cations, postmastoidectomy, recurrent
      cholesteatoma
    postvagotomy syndrome K91.1
    postvalvulotomy syndrome I97.Ø
    pulmonary insufficiency (acute) J95.2
      chronic J95.3
      following thoracic surgery J95.1
    reattached body part — *see* Complications, reat-
      tached
    respiratory — *see* Complications, respiratory sys-
      tem
    shock (hypovolemic) T81.19 ☑
    spleen (postoperative) D78.89
      intraoperative D78.81
    stitch abscess T81.4 ☑
    subglottic stenosis (postsurgical) J95.5
    testicular hypofunction E89.5
    transplant — *see* Complications, organ or tissue
      transplant
    urinary NEC N99.89
    vaginal vault prolapse (posthysterectomy) N99.3
    vascular (peripheral)
      artery T81.719 ☑
        mesenteric T81.71Ø ☑
        renal T81.711 ☑
        specified NEC T81.718 ☑
      vein T81.72 ☑
    wound infection T81.4 ☑
  suture, permanent (wire) NEC T85.9 ☑
    with repair of bone — *see* Complications, fixation
      device, internal
    embolism T85.81 ☑
    fibrosis T85.82 ☑
    hemorrhage T85.83 ☑
    infection and inflammation T85.79 ☑
    mechanical
      breakdown T85.612 ☑
      displacement T85.622 ☑
      malfunction T85.612 ☑
      malposition T85.622 ☑
      obstruction T85.692 ☑
      perforation T85.692 ☑
      protrusion T85.692 ☑
      specified NEC T85.692 ☑
    pain T85.84 ☑
    specified type NEC T85.89 ☑
    stenosis T85.85 ☑
    thrombosis T85.86 ☑
  tracheostomy J95.ØØ
    granuloma J95.Ø9
    hemorrhage J95.Ø1
    infection J95.Ø2
    malfunction J95.Ø3
    mechanical J95.Ø3
    obstruction J95.Ø3
    specified type NEC J95.Ø9
    tracheo-esophageal fistula J95.Ø4
  transfusion (blood) (lymphocytes) (plasma) T8Ø.92 ☑
    air emblism T8Ø.Ø
    circulatory overload E87.71
    febrile nonhemolytic transfusion reaction R5Ø.84
    hemochromatosis E83.111
    hemolysis T8Ø.89 ☑
    hemolytic reaction (antigen unspecified)
      T8Ø.919 ☑
    incompatibility reaction (antigen unspecified)
      T8Ø.919 ☑
      ABO T8Ø.3Ø ☑
        delayed serologic (DSTR) T8Ø.39 ☑
        hemolytic transfusion reaction (HTR) (un-
          specified time after transfusion)
          T8Ø.319 ☑
          acute (AHTR) (less than 24 hours after
            transfusion) T8Ø.31Ø ☑

Complication(s) — continued
transfusion — continued
incompatibility reaction — continued
ABO — continued
hemolytic transfusion reaction — continued
delayed (DHTR) (24 hours or more after transfusion) T80.311 ☑
specified NEC T80.39 ☑
acute (antigen unspecified) T80.910 ☑
delayed (antigen unspecified) T80.911 ☑
delayed serologic (DSTR) T80.89 ☑
non-ABO (minor antigens (Duffy) (Kell) (Kidd) (Lewis) (M) (N) (P) (S)) T80.A0 ☑ (following T80.4)
delayed serologic (DSTR) T80.A9 ☑ (following T80.4)
hemolytic transfusion reaction (HTR) (unspecified time after transfusion) T80.A19 ☑ (following T80.4)
acute (AHTR) (less than 24 hours after transfusion) T80.A10 ☑ (following T80.4)
delayed (DHTR) (24 hours or more after transfusion) T80.A11 ☑ (following T80.4)
specified NEC T80.A9 ☑ (following T80.4)
Rh (antigens (C) (c) (D) (E) (e)) (factor) T80.40 ☑
delayed serologic (DSTR) T80.49 ☑
hemolytic transfusion reaction (HTR) (unspecified time after transfusion) T80.419 ☑
acute (AHTR) (less than 24 hours after transfusion) T80.410 ☑
delayed (DHTR) (24 hours or more after transfusion) T80.411 ☑
specified NEC T80.49 ☑
infection T80.29 ☑
reaction NEC T80.89 ☑
sepsis T80.29 ☑
shock T80.89 ☑
transplant T86.90
bone T86.839
failure T86.831
infection T86.832
rejection T86.830
specified type NEC T86.838
bone marrow T86.00
failure T86.02
infection T86.03
rejection T86.01
specified type NEC T86.09
cornea T86.849
failure T86.841
infection T86.842
rejection T86.840
specified type NEC T86.848
failure T86.92
heart T86.20
with lung T86.30
cardiac allograft vasculopathy T86.290
failure T86.32
infection T86.33
rejection T86.31
specified type NEC T86.39
failure T86.22
infection T86.23
rejection T86.21
specified type NEC T86.298
infection T86.93
intestine T86.859
failure T86.851
infection T86.852
rejection T86.850
specified type NEC T86.858
kidney T86.10
failure T86.12
infection T86.13
rejection T86.11
specified type NEC T86.19
liver T86.40
failure T86.42
infection T86.43
rejection T86.41
specified type NEC T86.49
lung T86.819
with heart T86.30
failure T86.32

Complication(s) — continued
transplant — continued
lung — continued
with heart — continued
infection T86.33
rejection T86.31
specified type NEC T86.39
failure T86.811
infection T86.812
rejection T86.810
specified type NEC T86.818
malignant neoplasm C80.2
pancreas T86.899
failure T86.891
infection T86.892
rejection T86.890
specified type NEC T86.898
peripheral blood stem cells T86.5
post-transplant lymphoproliferative disorder (PTLD) D47.Z1 (following D47.4)
rejection T86.91
skin T86.829
failure T86.821
infection T86.822
rejection T86.820
specified type NEC T86.828
specified
tissue T86.899
failure T86.891
infection T86.892
rejection T86.890
specified type NEC T86.898
type NEC T86.99
stem cell (from peripheral blood) (from umbilical cord) T86.5
umbilical cord stem cells T86.5
trauma (early) T79.9 ☑
specified NEC T79.8 ☑
ultrasound therapy NEC T88.9 ☑
umbilical cord NEC
complicating delivery O69.9 ☑
specified NEC O69.89 ☑
umbrella device, vascular T82.9 ☑
embolism T82.818 ☑
fibrosis T82.828 ☑
hemorrhage T82.838 ☑
infection or inflammation T82.7 ☑
mechanical
breakdown T82.515 ☑
displacement T82.525 ☑
leakage T82.535 ☑
malposition T82.525 ☑
obstruction T82.595 ☑
perforation T82.595 ☑
protrusion T82.595 ☑
pain T82.848 ☑
specified type NEC T82.898 ☑
stenosis T82.858 ☑
thrombosis T82.868 ☑
urethral catheter — see Complications, catheter, urethral, indwelling
vaccination T88.1 ☑
anaphylaxis NEC T80.52 ☑
arthropathy — see Arthropathy, postimmunization
cellulitis T88.0 ☑
encephalitis or encephalomyelitis G04.02
infection (general) (local) NEC T88.0 ☑
meningitis G03.8
myelitis G04.89
protein sickness T80.62 ☑
rash T88.1 ☑
reaction (allergic) T88.1 ☑
serum T80.62 ☑
sepsis T88.0 ☑
serum intoxication, sickness, rash, or other serum reaction NEC T80.62 ☑
anaphylactic shock T80.52 ☑
shock (allergic) (anaphylactic) T80.52 ☑
vaccinia (generalized) (localized) T88.1 ☑
vas deferens device or implant — see Complications, genitourinary, device or implant, genital tract
vascular I99.9
device or implant T82.9 ☑
embolism T82.818 ☑
fibrosis T82.828 ☑
hemorrhage T82.838 ☑
infection or inflammation T82.7 ☑

Complication(s) — continued
vascular — continued
device or implant — continued
mechanical
breakdown T82.519 ☑
specified device NEC T82.518 ☑
displacement T82.529 ☑
specified device NEC T82.528 ☑
leakage T82.539 ☑
specified device NEC T82.538 ☑
malposition T82.529 ☑
specified device NEC T82.528 ☑
obstruction T82.599 ☑
specified device NEC T82.598 ☑
perforation T82.599 ☑
specified device NEC T82.598 ☑
protrusion T82.599 ☑
specified device NEC T82.598 ☑
pain T82.848 ☑
specified type NEC T82.898 ☑
stenosis T82.858 ☑
thrombosis T82.868 ☑
dialysis catheter — see Complication, catheter, dialysis
following infusion, therapeutic injection or transfusion T80.1 ☑
graft T82.9 ☑
embolism T82.818 ☑
fibrosis T82.828 ☑
hemorrhage T82.838 ☑
mechanical
breakdown T82.319 ☑
aorta (bifurcation) T82.310 ☑
carotid artery T82.311 ☑
specified vessel NEC T82.318 ☑
displacement T82.329 ☑
aorta (bifurcation) T82.320 ☑
carotid artery T82.321 ☑
specified vessel NEC T82.328 ☑
leakage T82.339 ☑
aorta (bifurcation) T82.330 ☑
carotid artery T82.331 ☑
specified vessel NEC T82.338 ☑
malposition T82.329 ☑
aorta (bifurcation) T82.320 ☑
carotid artery T82.321 ☑
specified vessel NEC T82.328 ☑
obstruction T82.399 ☑
aorta (bifurcation) T82.390 ☑
carotid artery T82.391 ☑
specified vessel NEC T82.398 ☑
perforation T82.399 ☑
aorta (bifurcation) T82.390 ☑
carotid artery T82.391 ☑
specified vessel NEC T82.398 ☑
protrusion T82.399 ☑
aorta (bifurcation) T82.390 ☑
carotid artery T82.391 ☑
specified vessel NEC T82.398 ☑
pain T82.848 ☑
specified complication NEC T82.898 ☑
stenosis T82.858 ☑
thrombosis T82.868 ☑
postoperative — see Complications, postoperative, circulatory
vena cava device (filter) (sieve) (umbrella) — see Complications, umbrella device, vascular
ventilation therapy NEC T81.81 ☑
ventilator
mechanical J95.850
specified NEC J95.859
ventricular (communicating) shunt (device) T85.9 ☑
embolism T85.81 ☑
fibrosis T85.82 ☑
hemorrhage T85.83 ☑
infection and inflammation T85.79 ☑
mechanical
breakdown T85.01 ☑
displacement T85.02 ☑
leakage T85.03 ☑
malposition T85.02 ☑
obstruction T85.09 ☑
perforation T85.09 ☑
protrusion T85.09 ☑
specified NEC T85.09 ☑
pain T85.84 ☑

☑ Additional Character Required — Refer to the Tabular List for Character Selection   ▽ Subterms under main terms may continue to next column or page

Complication(s) — *continued*
  ventricular shunt — *continued*
    specified type NEC T85.89 ☑
    stenosis T85.85
    thrombosis T85.86 ☑
  wire suture, permanent (implanted) — *see* Complications, suture, permanent
Compressed air disease T70.3 ☑
Compression
  with injury — *code by* Nature of injury
  artery I77.1
    celiac, syndrome I77.4
  brachial plexus G54.0
  brain (stem) G93.5
    due to
      contusion (diffuse) — *see* Injury, intracranial, diffuse
        focal — *see* Injury, intracranial, focal
      injury NEC — *see* Injury, intracranial, diffuse
      traumatic — *see* Injury, intracranial, diffuse
  bronchus J98.09
  cauda equina G83.4
  celiac (artery) (axis) I77.4
  cerebral — *see* Compression, brain
  cervical plexus G54.2
  cord
    spinal — *see* Compression, spinal
    umbilical — *see* Compression, umbilical cord
  cranial nerve G52.9
    eighth H93.3 ☑
    eleventh G52.8
    fifth G50.8
    first G52.0
    fourth — *see* Strabismus, paralytic, fourth nerve
    ninth G52.1
    second — *see* Disorder, nerve, optic
    seventh G52.8
    sixth — *see* Strabismus, paralytic, sixth nerve
    tenth G52.2
    third — *see* Strabismus, paralytic, third nerve
    twelfth G52.3
  diver's squeeze T70.3 ☑
  during birth (newborn) P15.9
  esophagus K22.2
  eustachian tube — *see* Obstruction, eustachian tube, cartilaginous
  facies Q67.1
  fracture — *see* Fracture
  heart — *see* Disease, heart
  intestine — *see* Obstruction, intestine
  laryngeal nerve, recurrent G52.2
    with paralysis of vocal cords and larynx J38.00
      bilateral J38.02
      unilateral J38.01
  lumbosacral plexus G54.1
  lung J98.4
  lymphatic vessel I89.0
  medulla — *see* Compression, brain
  nerve (*see also* Disorder, nerve) G58.9
    arm NEC — *see* Mononeuropathy, upper limb
    axillary G54.0
    cranial — *see* Compression, cranial nerve
    leg NEC — *see* Mononeuropathy, lower limb
    median (in carpal tunnel) — *see* Syndrome, carpal tunnel
    optic — *see* Disorder, nerve, optic
    plantar — *see* Lesion, nerve, plantar
    posterior tibial (in tarsal tunnel) — *see* Syndrome, tarsal tunnel
    root or plexus NOS (in) G54.9
      intervertebral disc disorder NEC — *see* Disorder, disc, with, radiculopathy
      with myelopathy — *see* Disorder, disc, with, myelopathy
      neoplastic disease (*see also* Neoplasm) D49.9 [G55]
      spondylosis — *see* Spondylosis, with radiculopathy
    sciatic (acute) — *see* Lesion, nerve, sciatic
    sympathetic G90.8
    traumatic — *see* Injury, nerve
    ulnar — *see* Lesion, nerve, ulnar
    upper extremity NEC — *see* Mononeuropathy, upper limb
  spinal (cord) G95.20
    by displacement of intervertebral disc NEC (*see also* Disorder, disc, with, myelopathy)

Compression — *continued*
  spinal — *continued*
    nerve root NOS G54.9
      due to displacement of intervertebral disc NEC — *see* Disorder, disc, with, radiculopathy
      with myelopathy — *see* Disorder, disc, with, myelopathy
    specified NEC G95.29
    spondylogenic (cervical) (lumbar, lumbosacral) (thoracic) — *see* Spondylosis, with myelopathy NEC
    anterior — *see* Syndrome, anterior, spinal artery, compression
    traumatic — *see* Injury, spinal cord, by region
  subcostal nerve (syndrome) — *see* Mononeuropathy, upper limb, specified NEC
  sympathetic nerve NEC G90.8
  syndrome T79.5 ☑
  trachea J39.8
  ulnar nerve (by scar tissue) — *see* Lesion, nerve, ulnar
  umbilical cord
    complicating delivery O69.2 ☑
      cord around neck O69.1 ☑
      prolapse O69.0 ☑
      specified NEC O69.2 ☑
  ureter N13.5
  vein I87.1
  vena cava (inferior) (superior) I87.1
Compulsion, compulsive
  gambling F63.0
  neurosis F42
  personality F60.5
  states F42
  swearing F42
    in Gilles de la Tourette's syndrome F95.2
  tics and spasms F95.9
Concato's disease (pericardial polyserositis) A19.9
  nontubercular I31.1
  pleural — *see* Pleurisy, with effusion
Concavity chest wall M95.4
Concealed penis Q55.69
Concern (normal) **about sick person in family** Z63.6
Concrescence (teeth) K00.2
Concretio cordis I31.1
  rheumatic I09.2
Concretion (*see also* Calculus)
  appendicular K38.1
  canaliculus — *see* Dacryolith
  clitoris N90.89
  conjunctiva H11.12-
  eyelid — *see* Disorder, eyelid, specified type NEC
  lacrimal passages — *see* Dacryolith
  prepuce (male) N47.8
  salivary gland (any) K11.5
  seminal vesicle N50.8
  tonsil J35.8
Concussion (brain) (cerebral) (current) S06.0X- ☑
  blast (air) (hydraulic) (immersion) (underwater)
    abdomen or thorax — *see* Injury, blast, by site
    ear with acoustic nerve injury — *see* Injury, nerve, acoustic, specified type NEC
  cauda equina S34.3 ☑
  conus medullaris S34.02 ☑
  ocular S05.8X- ☑
  spinal (cord)
    cervical S14.0 ☑
    lumbar S34.01 ☑
    sacral S34.02 ☑
    thoracic S24.0 ☑
  syndrome F07.81
Condition — *see* Disease
Conditions arising in the perinatal period — *see* Newborn, affected by
Conduct disorder -- *see* Disorder, conduct
Condyloma A63.0
  acuminatum A63.0
  gonorrheal A54.09
  latum A51.31
  syphilitic A51.31
    congenital A50.07
  venereal, syphilitic A51.31
Conflagration (*see also* Burn)
  asphyxia (by inhalation of gases, fumes or vapors) (*see also* Table of Drugs and Chemicals) T59.9- ☑
Conflict (with) (*see also* Discord)
  family Z73.9
  marital Z63.0

Conflict — *continued*
  marital — *continued*
    involving divorce or estrangement Z63.5
  parent-child Z62.820
    parent-adopted child Z62.821
    parent-biological child Z62.820
    parent-foster child Z62.822
  social role NEC Z73.5
Confluent — *see* condition
Confusion, confused R41.0
  epileptic F05
  mental state (psychogenic) F44.89
  psychogenic F44.89
  reactive (from emotional stress, psychological trauma) F44.89
Confusional arousals G47.51
Congelation T69.9 ☑
Congenital (*see also* condition)
  aortic septum Q25.4
  intrinsic factor deficiency D51.0
  malformation — *see* Anomaly
Congestion, congestive
  bladder N32.89
  bowel K63.89
  brain G93.89
  breast N64.59
  bronchial J98.09
  catarrhal J31.0
  chest R09.89
  chill, malarial — *see* Malaria
  circulatory NEC I99.8
  duodenum K31.89
  eye — *see* Hyperemia, conjunctiva
  facial, due to birth injury P15.4
  general R68.89
  glottis J37.0
  heart — *see* Failure, heart, congestive
  hepatic K76.1
  hypostatic (lung) — *see* Edema, lung
  intestine K63.89
  kidney N28.89
  labyrinth H83.8 ☑
  larynx J37.0
  liver K76.1
  lung R09.89
    active or acute — *see* Pneumonia
  malaria, malarial — *see* Malaria
  nasal R09.81
  nose R09.81
  orbit, orbital (*see also* Exophthalmos)
    inflammatory (chronic) — *see* Inflammation, orbit
  ovary N83.8
  pancreas K86.8
  pelvic, female N94.89
  pleural J94.8
  prostate (active) N42.1
  pulmonary — *see* Congestion, lung
  renal N28.89
  retina H35.81
  seminal vesicle N50.1
  spinal cord G95.19
  spleen (chronic) D73.2
  stomach K31.89
  trachea — *see* Tracheitis
  urethra N36.8
  uterus N85.8
    with subinvolution N85.3
  venous (passive) I87.8
  viscera R68.89
Congestive — *see* Congestion
Conical
  cervix (hypertrophic elongation) N88.4
  cornea — *see* Keratoconus
  teeth K00.2
Conjoined twins Q89.4
Conjugal maladjustment Z63.0
  involving divorce or estrangement Z63.5
Conjunctiva — *see* condition
Conjunctivitis (staphylococcal) (streptococcal) NOS H10.9
  Acanthamoeba B60.12
  acute H10.3- ☑
    atopic H10.1- ☑
    chemical (*see also* Corrosion, cornea) H10.21- ☑
    mucopurulent H10.02- ☑
      follicular H10.01- ☑
    pseudomembranous H10.22- ☑

Conjunctivitis — *continued*
  acute — *continued*
    serous except viral H10.23- ☑
      viral — *see* Conjunctivitis, viral
    toxic H10.21- ☑
  adenoviral (acute) (follicular) B30.1
  allergic (acute) — *see* Conjunctivitis, acute, atopic
    chronic H10.45
      vernal H10.44
  anaphylactic — *see* Conjunctivitis, acute, atopic
  Apollo B30.3
  atopic (acute) — *see* Conjunctivitis, acute, atopic
  Béal's B30.2
  blennorrhagic (gonococcal) (neonatorum) A54.31
  chemical (acute) (*see also* Corrosion, cornea)
      H10.21- ☑
  chlamydial A74.0
    due to trachoma A71.1
    neonatal P39.1
  chronic (nodosa) (petrificans) (phlyctenular) H10.40- ☑
    allergic H10.45
      vernal H10.44
    follicular H10.43- ☑
    giant papillary H10.41- ☑
    simple H10.42- ☑
    vernal H10.44
  coxsackievirus 24 B30.3
  diphtheritic A36.86
  due to
    dust — *see* Conjunctivitis, acute, atopic
    filariasis B74.9
    mucocutaneous leishmaniasis B55.2
  enterovirus type 70 (hemorrhagic) B30.3
  epidemic (viral) B30.9
    hemorrhagic B30.3
  gonococcal (neonatorum) A54.31
  granular (trachomatous) A71.1
    sequelae (late effect) B94.0
  hemorrhagic (acute) (epidemic) B30.3
  herpes zoster B02.31
  in (due to)
    Acanthamoeba B60.12
    adenovirus (acute) (follicular) B30.1
    Chlamydia A74.0
    coxsackievirus 24 B30.3
    diphtheria A36.86
    enterovirus type 70 (hemorrhagic) B30.3
    filariasis B74.9
    gonococci A54.31
    herpes (simplex) virus B00.53
      zoster B02.31
    infectious disease NEC B99 ☑
    meningococci A39.89
    mucocutaneous leishmaniasis B55.2
    rosacea L71.9
    syphilis (late) A52.71
    zoster B02.31
  inclusion A74.0
  infantile P39.1
    gonococcal A54.31
  Koch-Weeks' — *see* Conjunctivitis, acute, mucopuru-
      lent
  light — *see* Conjunctivitis, acute, atopic
  ligneous — *see* Blepharoconjunctivitis, ligneous
  meningococcal A39.89
  mucopurulent — *see* Conjunctivitis, acute, mucopuru-
      lent
  neonatal P39.1
    gonococcal A54.31
  Newcastle B30.8
  of Béal B30.2
  parasitic
    filariasis B74.9
    mucocutaneous leishmaniasis B55.2
  Parinaud's H10.89
  petrificans H10.89
  rosacea L71.9
  specified NEC H10.89
  swimming-pool B30.1
  trachomatous A71.1
    acute A71.0
    sequelae (late effect) B94.0
  traumatic NEC H10.89
  tuberculous A18.59
  tularemic A21.1
  tularensis A21.1
  viral B30.9

Conjunctivitis — *continued*
  viral — *continued*
    due to
      adenovirus B30.1
      enterovirus B30.3
    specified NEC B30.8
Conjunctivochalasis H11.82- ☑
Connective tissue — *see* condition
Conn's syndrome E26.01
Conradi (-Hunermann) **disease** Q77.3
Consanguinity Z84.3
  counseling Z71.89
Conscious simulation (of illness) Z76.5
Consecutive — *see* condition
Consolidation lung (base) — *see* Pneumonia, lobar
Constipation (atonic) (neurogenic) (simple) (spastic)
    K59.00
  drug-induced — *see* Table of Drugs and Chemicals
  outlet dysfunction K59.02
  psychogenic F45.8
  slow transit K59.01
  specified NEC K59.09
Constitutional (*see also* condition)
  substandard F60.7
Constitutionally substandard F60.7
Constriction (*see also* Stricture)
  auditory canal — *see* Stenosis, external ear canal
  bronchial J98.09
  duodenum K31.5
  esophagus K22.2
  external
    abdomen, abdominal (wall) S30.841 ☑
    alveolar process S00.542 ☑
    ankle S90.54- ☑
    antecubital space — *see* Constriction, external,
        forearm
    arm (upper) S40.84- ☑
    auricle — *see* Constriction, external, ear
    axilla — *see* Constriction, external, arm
    back, lower S30.840 ☑
    breast S20.14- ☑
    brow S00.84 ☑
    buttock S30.840 ☑
    calf — *see* Constriction, external, leg
    canthus — *see* Constriction, external, eyelid
    cheek S00.84 ☑
      internal S00.542 ☑
    chest wall — *see* Constriction, external, thorax
    chin S00.84 ☑
    clitoris S30.844 ☑
    costal region — *see* Constriction, external, thorax
    digit(s)
      foot — *see* Constriction, external, toe
      hand — *see* Constriction, external, finger
    ear S00.44- ☑
    elbow S50.34- ☑
    epididymis S30.843 ☑
    epigastric region S30.841 ☑
    esophagus, cervical S10.14 ☑
    eyebrow — *see* Constriction, external, eyelid
    eyelid S00.24- ☑
    face S00.84 ☑
    finger(s) S60.44- ☑
      index S60.44- ☑
      little S60.44- ☑
      middle S60.44- ☑
      ring S60.44- ☑
    flank S30.841 ☑
    foot (except toe(s) alone) S90.84- ☑
      toe — *see* Constriction, external, toe
    forearm S50.84- ☑
      elbow only — *see* Constriction, external, elbow
    forehead S00.84 ☑
    genital organs, external
      female S30.846 ☑
      male S30.845 ☑
    groin S30.841 ☑
    gum S00.542 ☑
    hand S60.54- ☑
    head S00.94 ☑
      ear — *see* Constriction, external, ear
      eyelid — *see* Constriction, external, eyelid
      lip S00.541 ☑
      nose S00.34 ☑
      oral cavity S00.542 ☑
      scalp S00.04 ☑

Constriction — *continued*
  external — *continued*
    head — *continued*
      specified site NEC S00.84 ☑
    heel — *see* Constriction, external, foot
    hip S70.24- ☑
    inguinal region S30.841 ☑
    interscapular region S20.449 ☑
    jaw S00.84 ☑
    knee S80.24- ☑
    labium (majus) (minus) S30.844 ☑
    larynx S10.14 ☑
    leg (lower) S80.84- ☑
      knee — *see* Constriction, external, knee
      upper — *see* Constriction, external, thigh
    lip S00.541 ☑
    lower back S30.840 ☑
    lumbar region S30.840 ☑
    malar region S00.84 ☑
    mammary — *see* Constriction, external, breast
    mastoid region S00.84 ☑
    mouth S00.542 ☑
    nail
      finger — *see* Constriction, external, finger
      toe — *see* Constriction, external, toe
    nasal S00.34 ☑
    neck S10.94 ☑
      specified site NEC S10.84 ☑
      throat S10.14 ☑
    nose S00.34 ☑
    occipital region S00.04 ☑
    oral cavity S00.542 ☑
    orbital region — *see* Constriction, external, eyelid
    palate S00.542 ☑
    palm — *see* Constriction, external, hand
    parietal region S00.04 ☑
    pelvis S30.840 ☑
    penis S30.842 ☑
    perineum
      female S30.844 ☑
      male S30.840 ☑
    periocular area — *see* Constriction, external, eyelid
    phalanges
      finger — *see* Constriction, external, finger
      toe — *see* Constriction, external, toe
    pharynx S10.14 ☑
    pinna — *see* Constriction, external, ear
    popliteal space — *see* Constriction, external, knee
    prepuce S30.842 ☑
    pubic region S30.840 ☑
    pudendum
      female S30.846 ☑
      male S30.845 ☑
    sacral region S30.840 ☑
    scalp S00.04 ☑
    scapular region — *see* Constriction, external,
        shoulder
    scrotum S30.843 ☑
    shin — *see* Constriction, external, leg
    shoulder S40.24- ☑
    sternal region S20.349 ☑
    submaxillary region S00.84 ☑
    submental region S00.84 ☑
    subungual
      finger(s) — *see* Constriction, external, finger
      toe(s) — *see* Constriction, external, toe
    supraclavicular fossa S10.84 ☑
    supraorbital S00.84 ☑
    temple S00.84 ☑
    temporal region S00.84 ☑
    testis S30.843 ☑
    thigh S70.34- ☑
    thorax, thoracic (wall) S20.94 ☑
      back S20.44- ☑
      front S20.34- ☑
    throat S10.14 ☑
    thumb S60.34- ☑
    toe(s) (lesser) S90.44- ☑
      great S90.44- ☑
    tongue S00.542 ☑
    trachea S10.14 ☑
    tunica vaginalis S30.843 ☑
    uvula S00.542 ☑
    vagina S30.844 ☑
    vulva S30.844 ☑
    wrist S60.84- ☑

☑ **Additional Character Required** — Refer to the Tabular List for Character Selection   **Subterms under main terms may continue to next column or page**

Constriction — *continued*
- gallbladder — *see* Obstruction, gallbladder
- intestine — *see* Obstruction, intestine
- larynx J38.6
  - congenital Q31.8
    - specified NEC Q31.8
    - subglottic Q31.1
- organ or site, congenital NEC — *see* Atresia, by site
- prepuce (acquired) (congenital) N47.1
- pylorus (adult hypertrophic) K31.1
  - congenital or infantile Q40.0
  - newborn Q40.0
- ring dystocia (uterus) O62.4
- spastic (*see also* Spasm)
  - ureter N13.5
- ureter N13.5
  - with infection N13.6
- urethra — *see* Stricture, urethra
- visual field (peripheral) (functional) — *see* Defect, visual field

Constrictive — *see* condition

Consultation
- without complaint or sickness Z71.9
  - feared complaint unfounded Z71.1
  - specified reason NEC Z71.89
- medical — *see* Counseling, medical
- religious Z71.81
- specified reason NEC Z71.89
- spiritual Z71.81

Consumption — *see* Tuberculosis

Contact (with) (*see also* Exposure (to))
- acariasis Z20.7
- AIDS virus Z20.6
- air pollution Z77.110
- algae and algae toxins Z77.121
- algae bloom Z77.121
- anthrax Z20.810
- aromatic amines Z77.020
- aromatic (hazardous) compounds NEC Z77.028
- aromatic dyes NOS Z77.028
- arsenic Z77.010
- asbestos Z77.090
- bacterial disease NEC Z20.818
- benzene Z77.021
- blue-green algae bloom Z77.121
- body fluids (potentially hazardous) Z77.21
- brown tide Z77.121
- chemicals (chiefly nonmedicinal) (hazardous) NEC Z77.098
- cholera Z20.09
- chromium compounds Z77.018
- communicable disease Z20.9
  - bacterial NEC Z20.818
  - specified NEC Z20.89
  - viral NEC Z20.828
- cyanobacteria bloom Z77.121
- dyes Z77.098
- Escherichia coli (E. coli) Z20.01
- fiberglass — *see* Table of Drugs and Chemicals, fiberglass
- German measles Z20.4
- gonorrhea Z20.2
- hazardous metals NEC Z77.018
- hazardous substances NEC Z77.29
- hazards in the physical environment NEC Z77.128
- hazards to health NEC Z77.9
- HIV Z20.6
- HTLV-III/LAV Z20.6
- human immunodeficiency virus (HIV) Z20.6
- infection Z20.9
  - specified NEC Z20.89
- infestation (parasitic) NEC Z20.7
- intestinal infectious disease NEC Z20.09
  - Escherichia coli (E. coli) Z20.01
- lead Z77.011
- meningococcus Z20.811
- mold (toxic) Z77.120
- nickel dust Z77.018
- noise Z77.122
- parasitic disease Z20.7
- pediculosis Z20.7
- pfiesteria piscicida Z77.121
- poliomyelitis Z20.89
- pollution
  - air Z77.110
  - environmental NEC Z77.118
  - soil Z77.112
  - water Z77.111

Contact — *continued*
- polycyclic aromatic hydrocarbons Z77.028
- rabies Z20.3
- radiation, naturally occurring NEC Z77.123
- radon Z77.123
- red tide (Florida) Z77.121
- rubella Z20.4
- sexually-transmitted disease Z20.2
- smallpox (laboratory) Z20.89
- syphilis Z20.2
- tuberculosis Z20.1
- uranium Z77.012
- varicella Z20.820
- venereal disease Z20.2
- viral disease NEC Z20.828
- viral hepatitis Z20.5
- water pollution Z77.111

Contamination, food — *see* Intoxication, foodborne

Contraception, contraceptive
- advice Z30.09
- counseling Z30.09
- device (intrauterine) (in situ) Z97.5
  - causing menorrhagia T83.83 ☑
  - checking Z30.431
  - complications — *see* Complications, intrauterine, contraceptive device
  - in place Z97.5
  - initial prescription Z30.014
  - reinsertion Z30.433
  - removal Z30.432
  - replacement Z30.433
- emergency (postcoital) Z30.012
- initial prescription Z30.019
  - injectable Z30.013
  - intrauterine device Z30.014
  - pills Z30.011
  - postcoital (emergency) Z30.012
  - specified type NEC Z30.018
  - subdermal implantable Z30.019
- maintenance Z30.40
  - examination Z30.8
  - injectable Z30.42
  - intrauterine device Z30.431
  - pills Z30.41
  - specified type NEC Z30.49
  - subdermal implantable Z30.49
- management Z30.9
  - specified NEC Z30.8
- postcoital (emergency) Z30.012
- prescription Z30.019
  - repeat Z30.40
- sterilization Z30.2
- surveillance (drug) — *see* Contraception, maintenance

Contraction(s), contracture, contracted
- Achilles tendon (*see also* Short, tendon, Achilles)
  - congenital Q66.89
- amputation stump (surgical) (flexion) (late) (next proximal joint) T87.89
- anus K59.8
- bile duct (common) (hepatic) K83.8
- bladder N32.89
  - neck or sphincter N32.0
- bowel, cecum, colon or intestine, any part — *see* Obstruction, intestine
- Braxton Hicks — *see* False, labor
- breast implant, capsular T85.44 ☑
- bronchial J98.09
- burn (old) — *see* Cicatrix
- cervix — *see* Stricture, cervix
- cicatricial — *see* Cicatrix
- conjunctiva, trachomatous, active A71.1
  - sequelae (late effect) B94.0
- Dupuytren's M72.0
- eyelid — *see* Disorder, eyelid function
- fascia (lata) (postural) M72.8
  - Dupuytren's M72.0
  - palmar M72.0
  - plantar M72.2
- finger NEC (*see also* Deformity, finger)
  - congenital Q68.1
  - joint — *see* Contraction, joint, hand
- flaccid — *see* Contraction, paralytic
- gallbladder K82.0
- heart valve — *see* Endocarditis
- hip — *see* Contraction, joint, hip
- hourglass
  - bladder N32.89
    - congenital Q64.79

Contraction(s), contracture, contracted — *continued*
- hourglass — *continued*
  - gallbladder K82.0
    - congenital Q44.1
  - stomach K31.89
    - congenital Q40.2
    - psychogenic F45.8
  - uterus (complicating delivery) O62.4
- hysterical F44.4
- internal os — *see* Stricture, cervix
- joint (abduction) (acquired) (adduction) (flexion) (rotation) M24.50
  - ankle M24.57- ☑
  - congenital NEC Q68.8
    - hip Q65.89
  - elbow M24.52- ☑
  - foot joint M24.57- ☑
  - hand joint M24.54- ☑
  - hip M24.55- ☑
    - congenital Q65.89
  - hysterical F44.4
  - knee M24.56- ☑
  - shoulder M24.51- ☑
  - wrist M24.53- ☑
- kidney (granular) (secondary) N26.9
  - congenital Q63.8
  - hydronephritic — *see* Hydronephrosis Page N26.2
  - pyelonephritic — *see* Pyelitis, chronic
  - tuberculous A18.11
- ligament (*see also* Disorder, ligament)
  - congenital Q79.8
- muscle (postinfective) (postural) NEC M62.40
  - with contracture of joint — *see* Contraction, joint
  - ankle M62.47- ☑
  - congenital Q79.8
    - sternocleidomastoid Q68.0
  - extraocular — *see* Strabismus
  - eye (extrinsic) — *see* Strabismus
  - foot M62.47- ☑
  - forearm M62.43- ☑
  - hand M62.44- ☑
  - hysterical F44.4
  - ischemic (Volkmann's) T79.6 ☑
  - lower leg M62.46- ☑
  - multiple sites M62.49
  - pelvic region M62.45- ☑
  - posttraumatic — *see* Strabismus, paralytic
  - psychogenic F45.8
    - conversion reaction F44.4
  - shoulder region M62.41- ☑
  - specified site NEC M62.48
  - thigh M62.45- ☑
  - upper arm M62.42- ☑
- neck — *see* Torticollis
- ocular muscle — *see* Strabismus
- organ or site, congenital NEC — *see* Atresia, by site
- outlet (pelvis) — *see* Contraction, pelvis
- palmar fascia M72.0
- paralytic
  - joint — *see* Contraction, joint
  - muscle (*see also* Contraction, muscle NEC)
    - ocular — *see* Strabismus, paralytic
- pelvis (acquired) (general) M95.5
  - with disproportion (fetopelvic) O33.1
    - causing obstructed labor O65.1
    - inlet O33.2
    - mid-cavity O33.3 ☑
    - outlet O33.3 ☑
- plantar fascia M72.2
- premature
  - atrium I49.1
  - auriculoventricular I49.49
  - heart I49.49
  - junctional I49.2
  - supraventricular I49.1
  - ventricular I49.3
- prostate N42.89
- pylorus NEC (*see also* Pylorospasm)
  - psychogenic F45.8
- rectum, rectal (sphincter) K59.8
- ring (Bandl's) (complicating delivery) O62.4
- scar — *see* Cicatrix
- spine — *see* Dorsopathy, deforming
- sternocleidomastoid (muscle), congenital Q68.0
- stomach K31.89
  - hourglass K31.89

Contraction(s), contracture, contracted — *continued*
 stomach — *continued*
  hourglass — *continued*
   congenital Q40.2
   psychogenic F45.8
  psychogenic F45.8
 tendon (sheath) M62.40
  with contracture of joint — *see* Contraction, joint
  Achilles — *see* Short, tendon, Achilles
  ankle M62.47- ☑
   Achilles — *see* Short, tendon, Achilles
  foot M62.47- ☑
  forearm M62.43- ☑
  hand M62.44- ☑
  lower leg M62.46- ☑
  multiple sites M62.49
  neck M62.48
  pelvic region M62.45- ☑
  shoulder region M62.41- ☑
  specified site NEC M62.48
  thigh M62.45- ☑
  thorax M62.48
  trunk M62.48
  upper arm M62.42- ☑
 toe — *see* Deformity, toe, specified NEC
 ureterovesical orifice (postinfectional) N13.5
  with infection N13.6
 urethra (*see also* Stricture, urethra)
  orifice N32.0
 uterus N85.8
  abnormal NEC O62.9
  clonic (complicating delivery) O62.4
  dyscoordinate (complicating delivery) O62.4
  hourglass (complicating delivery) O62.4
  hypertonic O62.4
  hypotonic NEC O62.2
  inadequate
   primary O62.0
   secondary O62.1
  incoordinate (complicating delivery) O62.4
  poor O62.2
  tetanic (complicating delivery) O62.4
 vagina (outlet) N89.5
 vesical N32.89
  neck or urethral orifice N32.0
 visual field — *see* Defect, visual field, generalized
 Volkmann's (ischemic) T79.6-
Contusion (skin surface intact) T14.8
 abdomen, abdominal (muscle) (wall) S30.1 ☑
 adnexa, eye NEC S05.8X- ☑
 adrenal gland S37.812 ☑
 alveolar process S00.532 ☑
 ankle S90.0- ☑
 antecubital space — *see* Contusion, forearm
 anus S30.3 ☑
 arm (upper) S40.02- ☑
  lower (with elbow) — *see* Contusion, forearm
 auditory canal — *see* Contusion, ear
 auricle — *see* Contusion, ear
 axilla — *see* Contusion, arm, upper
 back (*see also* Contusion, thorax, back)
  lower S30.0 ☑
 bile duct S36.13 ☑
 bladder S37.22 ☑
 bone NEC T14.8
 brain (diffuse) — *see* Injury, intracranial, diffuse
  focal — *see* Injury, intracranial, focal
 brainstem S06.38- ☑
 breast S20.0- ☑
 broad ligament S37.892 ☑
 brow S00.83 ☑
 buttock S30.0 ☑
 canthus, eye S00.1- ☑
 cauda equina S34.3 ☑
 cerebellar, traumatic S06.37- ☑
 cerebral S06.33- ☑
  left side S06.32- ☑
  right side S06.31- ☑
 cheek S00.83 ☑
  internal S00.532 ☑
 chest (wall) — *see* Contusion, thorax
 chin S00.83 ☑
 clitoris S30.23 ☑
 colon — *see* Injury, intestine, large, contusion
 common bile duct S36.13 ☑
 conjunctiva S05.1- ☑

Contusion — *continued*
 conjunctiva — *continued*
  with foreign body (in conjunctival sac) — *see* Foreign body, conjunctival sac
 conus medullaris (spine) S34.139 ☑
 cornea — *see* Contusion, eyeball
  with foreign body — *see* Foreign body, cornea
 corpus cavernosum S30.21 ☑
 cortex (brain) (cerebral) — *see* Injury, intracranial, diffuse
  focal — *see* Injury, intracranial, focal
 costal region — *see* Contusion, thorax
 cystic duct S36.13 ☑
 diaphragm S27.802 ☑
 duodenum S36.420 ☑
 ear S00.43- ☑
 elbow S50.0- ☑
  with forearm — *see* Contusion, forearm
 epididymis S30.22 ☑
 epigastric region S30.1 ☑
 epiglottis S10.0 ☑
 esophagus (thoracic) S27.812 ☑
  cervical S10.0 ☑
 eyeball S05.1- ☑
 eyebrow S00.1- ☑
 eyelid (and periocular area) S00.1- ☑
 face NEC S00.83 ☑
 fallopian tube S37.529 ☑
  bilateral S37.522 ☑
  unilateral S37.521 ☑
 femoral triangle S30.1 ☑
 finger(s) S60.00 ☑
  with damage to nail (matrix) S60.10 ☑
  index S60.02- ☑
   with damage to nail S60.12- ☑
  little S60.05- ☑
   with damage to nail S60.15- ☑
  middle S60.03- ☑
   with damage to nail S60.13- ☑
  ring S60.04- ☑
   with damage to nail S60.14- ☑
  thumb — *see* Contusion, thumb
 flank S30.1 ☑
 foot (except toe(s) alone) S90.3- ☑
  toe — *see* Contusion, toe
 forearm S50.1- ☑
  elbow only — *see* Contusion, elbow
 forehead S00.83 ☑
 gallbladder S36.122 ☑
 genital organs, external
  female S30.202 ☑
  male S30.201 ☑
 globe (eye) — *see* Contusion, eyeball
 groin S30.1 ☑
 gum S00.532 ☑
 hand S60.22- ☑
  finger(s) — *see* Contusion, finger
  wrist — *see* Contusion, wrist
 head S00.93 ☑
  ear — *see* Contusion, ear
  eyelid — *see* Contusion, eyelid
  lip S00.531 ☑
  nose S00.33 ☑
  oral cavity S00.532 ☑
  scalp S00.03 ☑
  specified part NEC S00.83 ☑
 heel — *see* Contusion, foot
 hepatic duct S36.13 ☑
 hip S70.0- ☑
 ileum S36.428 ☑
 iliac region S30.1 ☑
 inguinal region S30.1 ☑
 interscapular region S20.229 ☑
 intra-abdominal organ S36.92 ☑
  colon — *see* Injury, intestine, large, contusion
  liver S36.112 ☑
  pancreas — *see* Contusion, pancreas
  rectum S36.62 ☑
  small intestine — *see* Injury, intestine, small, contusion
  specified organ NEC S36.892 ☑
  spleen — *see* Contusion, spleen
  stomach S36.32 ☑
 iris (eye) — *see* Contusion, eyeball
 jaw S00.83 ☑
 jejunum S36.428 ☑

Contusion — *continued*
 kidney S37.01- ☑
  major (greater than 2 cm) S37.02- ☑
  minor (less than 2 cm) S37.01- ☑
 knee S80.0- ☑
 labium (majus) (minus) S30.23 ☑
 lacrimal apparatus, gland or sac S05.8X- ☑
 larynx S10.0 ☑
 leg (lower) S80.1- ☑
  knee — *see* Contusion, knee
 lens — *see* Contusion, eyeball
 lip S00.531 ☑
 liver S36.112 ☑
 lower back S30.0 ☑
 lumbar region S30.0 ☑
 lung S27.329 ☑
  bilateral S27.322 ☑
  unilateral S27.321 ☑
 malar region S00.83 ☑
 mastoid region S00.83 ☑
 membrane, brain — *see* Injury, intracranial, diffuse
  focal — *see* Injury, intracranial, focal
 mesentery S36.892 ☑
 mesosalpinx S37.892 ☑
 mouth S00.532 ☑
 muscle — *see* Contusion, by site
 nail
  finger — *see* Contusion, finger, with damage to nail
  toe — *see* Contusion, toe, with damage to nail
 nasal S00.33 ☑
 neck S10.93 ☑
  specified site NEC S10.83 ☑
  throat S10.0 ☑
 nerve — *see* Injury, nerve
 newborn P54.5
 nose S00.33 ☑
 occipital
  lobe (brain) — *see* Injury, intracranial, diffuse
   focal — *see* Injury, intracranial, focal
  region (scalp) S00.03 ☑
 orbit (region) (tissues) S05.1- ☑
 ovary S37.429 ☑
  bilateral S37.422 ☑
  unilateral S37.421 ☑
 palate S00.532 ☑
 pancreas S36.229 ☑
  body S36.221 ☑
  head S36.220 ☑
  tail S36.222 ☑
 parietal
  lobe (brain) — *see* Injury, intracranial, diffuse
   focal — *see* Injury, intracranial, focal
  region (scalp) S00.03 ☑
 pelvic organ S37.92 ☑
  adrenal gland S37.812 ☑
  bladder S37.22 ☑
  fallopian tube — *see* Contusion, fallopian tube
  kidney — *see* Contusion, kidney
  ovary — *see* Contusion, ovary
  prostate S37.822 ☑
  specified organ NEC S37.892 ☑
  ureter S37.12 ☑
  urethra S37.32 ☑
  uterus S37.62 ☑
 pelvis S30.0 ☑
 penis S30.21 ☑
 perineum
  female S30.23 ☑
  male S30.0 ☑
 periocular area S00.1- ☑
 peritoneum S36.81 ☑
 periurethral tissue — *see* Contusion, urethra
 pharynx S10.0 ☑
 pinna — *see* Contusion, ear
 popliteal space — *see* Contusion, knee
 prepuce S30.21 ☑
 prostate S37.822 ☑
 pubic region S30.1 ☑
 pudendum
  female S30.202 ☑
  male S30.201 ☑
 quadriceps femoris — *see* Contusion, thigh
 rectum S36.62 ☑
 retroperitoneum S36.892 ☑
 round ligament S37.892 ☑

☑ **Additional Character Required** — Refer to the Tabular List for Character Selection   ▽ **Subterms under main terms may continue to next column or page**

Contusion — *continued*
  sacral region S30.0 ☑
  scalp S00.03 ☑
    due to birth injury P12.3
  scapular region — *see* Contusion, shoulder
  sclera — *see* Contusion, eyeball
  scrotum S30.22 ☑
  seminal vesicle S37.892 ☑
  shoulder S40.01- ☑
  skin NEC T14.8
  small intestine — *see* Injury, intestine, small, contusion
  spermatic cord S30.22 ☑
  spinal cord — *see* Injury, spinal cord, by region
    cauda equina S34.3 ☑
    conus medullaris S34.139 ☑
  spleen S36.029 ☑
    major S36.021 ☑
    minor S36.020 ☑
  sternal region S20.219 ☑
  stomach S36.32 ☑
  subconjunctival S05.1- ☑
  subcutaneous NEC T14.8
  submaxillary region S00.83 ☑
  submental region S00.83 ☑
  subperiosteal NEC T14.8
  subungual
    finger — *see* Contusion, finger, with damage to nail
    toe — *see* Contusion, toe, with damage to nail
  supraclavicular fossa S10.83 ☑
  supraorbital S00.83 ☑
  suprarenal gland S37.812 ☑
  temple (region) S00.83 ☑
  temporal
    lobe (brain) — *see* Injury, intracranial, diffuse
      focal — *see* Injury, intracranial, focal
    region S00.83 ☑
  testis S30.22 ☑
  thigh S70.1- ☑
  thorax (wall) S20.20 ☑
    back S20.22- ☑
    front S20.21- ☑
  throat S10.0 ☑
  thumb S60.01- ☑
    with damage to nail S60.11- ☑
  toe(s) (lesser) S90.12- ☑
    with damage to nail S90.22- ☑
    great S90.11- ☑
      with damage to nail S90.21- ☑
      specified type NEC S90.221 ☑
  tongue S00.532 ☑
  trachea (cervical) S10.0 ☑
    thoracic S27.52 ☑
  tunica vaginalis S30.22 ☑
  tympanum, tympanic membrane — *see* Contusion, ear
  ureter S37.12 ☑
  urethra S37.32 ☑
  urinary organ NEC S37.892 ☑
  uterus S37.62 ☑
  uvula S00.532 ☑
  vagina S30.23 ☑
  vas deferens S37.892 ☑
  vesical S37.22 ☑
  vocal cord(s) S10.0 ☑
  vulva S30.23 ☑
  wrist S60.21- ☑
Conus (congenital) (any type) Q14.8
  cornea — *see* Keratoconus
  medullaris syndrome G95.81
Conversion hysteria, neurosis or reaction F44.9
Converter, tuberculosis (test reaction) R76.11
Conviction (legal), **anxiety concerning** Z65.0
  with imprisonment Z65.1
Convulsions (idiopathic) (*see also* Seizure(s)) R56.9
  apoplectiform (cerebral ischemia) I67.82
  benign neonatal (familial) — *see* Epilepsy, generalized, idiopathic
  dissociative F44.5
  epileptic — *see* Epilepsy
  epileptiform, epileptoid — *see* Seizure, epileptiform
  ether (anesthetic) — *see* Table of Drugs and Chemicals, by drug
  febrile R56.00
    with status epilepticus G40.901
    complex R56.01

Convulsions — *continued*
  febrile — *continued*
    complex — *continued*
      with status epilepticus G40.901
    simple R56.00
  hysterical F44.5
  infantile P90
    epilepsy — *see* Epilepsy
  jacksonian — *see* Epilepsy, localization-related, symptomatic, with simple partial seizures
  myoclonic G25.3
  neonatal, benign (familial) — *see* Epilepsy, generalized, idiopathic
  newborn P90
  obstetrical (nephritic) (uremic) — *see* Eclampsia
  paretic A52.17
  post traumatic R56.1
  psychomotor — *see* Epilepsy, localization-related, symptomatic, with complex partial seizures
  recurrent R56.9
  reflex R25.8
  scarlatinal A38.8
  tetanus, tetanic — *see* Tetanus
  thymic E32.8
Convulsive (*see also* Convulsions)
Cooley's anemia D56.1
Coolie itch B76.9
Cooper's
  disease — *see* Mastopathy, cystic
  hernia — *see* Hernia, abdomen, specified site NEC
Copra itch B88.0
Coprophagy F50.8
Coprophobia F40.298
Coproporphyria, hereditary E80.29
Cor
  biloculare Q20.8
  bovis, bovinum — *see* Hypertrophy, cardiac
  pulmonale (chronic) I27.81
    acute I26.09
  triatriatum, triatrium Q24.2
  triloculare Q20.8
    biatrium Q20.4
    biventriculare Q21.1
Corbus' disease (gangrenous balanitis) N48.1
Cord (*see also* condition)
  around neck (tightly) (with compression)
    complicating delivery O69.1 ☑
  bladder G95.89
    tabetic A52.19
Cordis ectopia Q24.8
Corditis (spermatic) N49.1
Corectopia Q13.2
Cori's disease (glycogen storage) E74.03
Corkhandler's disease or lung J67.3
Corkscrew esophagus K22.4
Corkworker's disease or lung J67.3
Corn (infected) L84
Cornea (*see also* condition)
  donor Z52.5
  plana Q13.4
Cornelia de Lange syndrome Q87.1
Cornu cutaneum L85.8
Cornual gestation or pregnancy O00.8
Coronary (artery) — *see* condition
Coronavirus, as cause of disease classified elsewhere B97.29
  SARS-associated B97.21
Corpora (*see also* condition)
  amylacea, prostate N42.89
  cavernosa — *see* condition
Corpulence — *see* Obesity
Corpus — *see* condition
Corrected transposition Q20.5
Corrosion (injury) (acid) (caustic) (chemical) (lime) (external) (internal) T30.4
  abdomen, abdominal (muscle) (wall) T21.42 ☑
    first degree T21.52 ☑
    second degree T21.62 ☑
    third degree T21.72 ☑
  above elbow T22.439 ☑
    first degree T22.539 ☑
    left T22.432 ☑
      first degree T22.532 ☑
      second degree T22.632 ☑
      third degree T22.732 ☑
    right T22.431 ☑
      first degree T22.531 ☑

Corrosion — *continued*
  above elbow — *continued*
    right — *continued*
      second degree T22.631 ☑
      third degree T22.731 ☑
    second degree T22.639 ☑
    third degree T22.739 ☑
  alimentary tract NEC T28.7 ☑
  ankle T25.419 ☑
    first degree T25.519 ☑
    left T25.412 ☑
      first degree T25.512 ☑
      second degree T25.612 ☑
      third degree T25.712 ☑
    multiple with foot — *see* Corrosion, lower, limb, multiple, ankle and foot
    right T25.411 ☑
      first degree T25.511 ☑
      second degree T25.611 ☑
      third degree T25.711 ☑
    second degree T25.619 ☑
    third degree T25.719 ☑
  anus — *see* Corrosion, buttock
  arm(s) (meaning upper limb(s)) — *see* Corrosion, upper limb
  axilla T22.449 ☑
    first degree T22.549 ☑
    left T22.442 ☑
      first degree T22.542 ☑
      second degree T22.642 ☑
      third degree T22.742 ☑
    right T22.441 ☑
      first degree T22.541 ☑
      second degree T22.641 ☑
      third degree T22.741 ☑
    second degree T22.649 ☑
    third degree T22.749 ☑
  back (lower) T21.44 ☑
    first degree T21.54 ☑
    second degree T21.64 ☑
    third degree T21.74 ☑
    upper T21.43 ☑
      first degree T21.53 ☑
      second degree T21.63 ☑
      third degree T21.73 ☑
  blisters — *code as* Corrosion, second degree, by site
  breast(s) — *see* Corrosion, chest wall
  buttock(s) T21.45 ☑
    first degree T21.55 ☑
    second degree T21.65 ☑
    third degree T21.75 ☑
  calf T24.439 ☑
    first degree T24.539 ☑
    left T24.432 ☑
      first degree T24.532 ☑
      second degree T24.632 ☑
      third degree T24.732 ☑
    right T24.431 ☑
      first degree T24.531 ☑
      second degree T24.631 ☑
      third degree T24.731 ☑
    second degree T24.639 ☑
    third degree T24.739 ☑
  canthus (eye) — *see* Corrosion, eyelid
  cervix T28.8 ☑
  cheek T20.46 ☑
    first degree T20.56 ☑
    second degree T20.66 ☑
    third degree T20.76 ☑
  chest wall T21.41 ☑
    first degree T21.51 ☑
    second degree T21.61 ☑
    third degree T21.71 ☑
  chin T20.43 ☑
    first degree T20.53 ☑
    second degree T20.63 ☑
    third degree T20.73 ☑
  colon T28.7 ☑
  conjunctiva (and cornea) — *see* Corrosion, cornea
  cornea (and conjunctiva) T26.6- ☑
  deep necrosis of underlying tissue — *code as* Corrosion, third degree, by site
  dorsum of hand T23.469 ☑
    first degree T23.569 ☑
    left T23.462 ☑

Corrosion — *continued*
  dorsum of hand — *continued*
    left — *continued*
      first degree T23.562 ☑
      second degree T23.662 ☑
      third degree T23.762 ☑
    right T23.461 ☑
      first degree T23.561 ☑
      second degree T23.661 ☑
      third degree T23.761 ☑
    second degree T23.669 ☑
    third degree T23.769 ☑
  ear (auricle) (external) (canal) T20.41 ☑
    drum T28.91 ☑
    first degree T20.51 ☑
    second degree T20.61 ☑
    third degree T20.71 ☑
  elbow T22.429 ☑
    first degree T22.529 ☑
    left T22.422 ☑
      first degree T22.522 ☑
      second degree T22.622 ☑
      third degree T22.722 ☑
    right T22.421 ☑
      first degree T22.521 ☑
      second degree T22.621 ☑
      third degree T22.721 ☑
    second degree T22.629 ☑
    third degree T22.729 ☑
  entire body — *see* Corrosion, multiple body regions
  epidermal loss — *code as* Corrosion, second degree, by site
  epiglottis T27.4 ☑
  erythema, erythematous — *code as* Corrosion, first degree, by site
  esophagus T28.6 ☑
  extent (percentage of body surface)
    less than 10 percent T32.0
    10-19 percent (0-9 percent third degree) T32.10
      with 10-19 percent third degree T32.11
    20-29 percent (0-9 percent third degree) T32.20
      with
        10-19 percent third degree T32.21
        20-29 percent third degree T32.22
    30-39 percent (0-9 percent third degree) T32.30
      with
        10-19 percent third degree T32.31
        20-29 percent third degree T32.32
        30-39 percent third degree T32.33
    40-49 percent (0-9 percent third degree) T32.40
      with
        10-19 percent third degree T32.41
        20-29 percent third degree T32.42
        30-39 percent third degree T32.43
        40-49 percent third degree T32.44
    50-59 percent (0-9 percent third degree) T32.50
      with
        10-19 percent third degree T32.51
        20-29 percent third degree T32.52
        30-39 percent third degree T32.53
        40-49 percent third degree T32.54
        50-59 percent third degree T32.55
    60-69 percent (0-9 percent third degree) T32.60
      with
        10-19 percent third degree T32.61
        20-29 percent third degree T32.62
        30-39 percent third degree T32.63
        40-49 percent third degree T32.64
        50-59 percent third degree T32.65
        60-69 percent third degree T32.66
    70-79 percent (0-9 percent third degree) T32.70
      with
        10-19 percent third degree T32.71
        20-29 percent third degree T32.72
        30-39 percent third degree T32.73
        40-49 percent third degree T32.74
        50-59 percent third degree T32.75
        60-69 percent third degree T32.76
        70-79 percent third degree T32.77
    80-89 percent (0-9 percent third degree) T32.80
      with
        10-19 percent third degree T32.81
        20-29 percent third degree T32.82
        30-39 percent third degree T32.83
        40-49 percent third degree T32.84
        50-59 percent third degree T32.85
        60-69 percent third degree T32.86

Corrosion — *continued*
  extent — *continued*
    80-89 percent — *continued*
      with — *continued*
        70-79 percent third degree T32.87
        80-89 percent third degree T32.88
    90 percent or more (0-9 percent third degree) T32.90
      with
        10-19 percent third degree T32.91
        20-29 percent third degree T32.92
        30-39 percent third degree T32.93
        40-49 percent third degree T32.94
        50-59 percent third degree T32.95
        60-69 percent third degree T32.96
        70-79 percent third degree T32.97
        80-89 percent third degree T32.98
        90-99 percent third degree T32.99
  extremity — *see* Corrosion, limb
  eye(s) and adnexa T26.9- ☑
    with resulting rupture and destruction of eyeball T26.7- ☑
    conjunctival sac — *see* Corrosion, cornea
    cornea — *see* Corrosion, cornea
    lid — *see* Corrosion, eyelid
    periocular area — *see* Corrosion eyelid
    specified site NEC T26.8- ☑
  eyeball — *see* Corrosion, eye
  eyelid(s) T26.5- ☑
  face — *see* Corrosion, head
  finger T23.429 ☑
    first degree T23.529 ☑
    left T23.422 ☑
      first degree T23.522 ☑
      second degree T23.622 ☑
      third degree T23.722 ☑
    multiple sites (without thumb) T23.439 ☑
      with thumb T23.449 ☑
        first degree T23.549 ☑
        left T23.442 ☑
          first degree T23.542 ☑
          second degree T23.642 ☑
          third degree T23.742 ☑
        right T23.441 ☑
          first degree T23.541 ☑
          second degree T23.641 ☑
          third degree T23.741 ☑
        second degree T23.649 ☑
        third degree T23.749 ☑
      first degree T23.539 ☑
      left T23.432 ☑
        first degree T23.532 ☑
        second degree T23.632 ☑
        third degree T23.732 ☑
      right T23.431 ☑
        first degree T23.531 ☑
        second degree T23.631 ☑
        third degree T23.731 ☑
      second degree T23.639 ☑
      third degree T23.739 ☑
    right T23.421 ☑
      first degree T23.521 ☑
      second degree T23.621 ☑
      third degree T23.721 ☑
    second degree T23.629 ☑
    third degree T23.729 ☑
  flank — *see* Corrosion, abdomen
  foot T25.429 ☑
    first degree T25.529 ☑
    left T25.422 ☑
      first degree T25.522 ☑
      second degree T25.622 ☑
      third degree T25.722 ☑
    multiple with ankle — *see* Corrosion, lower, limb, multiple, ankle and foot
    right T25.421 ☑
      first degree T25.521 ☑
      second degree T25.621 ☑
      third degree T25.721 ☑
    second degree T25.629 ☑
    third degree T25.729 ☑
  forearm T22.419 ☑
    first degree T22.519 ☑
    left T22.412 ☑
      first degree T22.512 ☑
      second degree T22.612 ☑

Corrosion — *continued*
  forearm — *continued*
    left — *continued*
      third degree T22.712 ☑
    right T22.411 ☑
      first degree T22.511 ☑
      second degree T22.611 ☑
      third degree T22.711 ☑
    second degree T22.619 ☑
    third degree T22.719 ☑
  forehead T20.46 ☑
    first degree T20.56 ☑
    second degree T20.66 ☑
    third degree T20.76 ☑
  fourth degree — *code as* Corrosion, third degree, by site
  full thickness skin loss — *code as* Corrosion, third degree, by site
  gastrointestinal tract NEC T28.7 ☑
  genital organs
    external
      female T21.47 ☑
        first degree T21.57 ☑
        second degree T21.67 ☑
        third degree T21.77 ☑
      male T21.46 ☑
        first degree T21.56 ☑
        second degree T21.66 ☑
        third degree T21.76 ☑
    internal T28.8 ☑
  groin — *see* Corrosion, abdominal wall
  hand(s) T23.409 ☑
    back — *see* Corrosion, dorsum of hand
    finger — *see* Corrosion, finger
    first degree T23.509 ☑
    left T23.402 ☑
      first degree T23.502 ☑
      second degree T23.602 ☑
      third degree T23.702 ☑
    multiple sites with wrist T23.499 ☑
      first degree T23.599 ☑
      left T23.492 ☑
        first degree T23.592 ☑
        second degree T23.692 ☑
        third degree T23.792 ☑
      right T23.491 ☑
        first degree T23.591 ☑
        second degree T23.691 ☑
        third degree T23.791 ☑
      second degree T23.699 ☑
      third degree T23.799 ☑
    palm — *see* Corrosion, palm
    right T23.401 ☑
      first degree T23.501 ☑
      second degree T23.601 ☑
      third degree T23.701 ☑
    second degree T23.609 ☑
    third degree T23.709 ☑
    thumb — *see* Corrosion, thumb
  head (and face) (and neck) T20.40 ☑
    cheek — *see* Corrosion, cheek
    chin — *see* Corrosion, chin
    ear — *see* Corrosion, ear
    eye(s) only — *see* Corrosion, eye
    first degree T20.50 ☑
    forehead — *see* Corrosion, forehead
    lip — *see* Corrosion, lip
    multiple sites T20.49 ☑
      first degree T20.59 ☑
      second degree T20.69 ☑
      third degree T20.79 ☑
    neck — *see* Corrosion, neck
    nose — *see* Corrosion, nose
    scalp — *see* Corrosion, scalp
    second degree T20.60 ☑
    third degree T20.70 ☑
  hip(s) — *see* Corrosion, lower, limb
  inhalation — *see* Corrosion, respiratory tract
  internal organ(s) (*see also* Corrosion, by site) T28.90 ☑
    alimentary tract T28.7 ☑
      esophagus T28.6 ☑
    esophagus T28.6 ☑
    genitourinary T28.8 ☑
    mouth T28.5 ☑
    pharynx T28.5 ☑
    specified organ NEC T28.99 ☑

Corrosion — *continued*
  interscapular region — *see* Corrosion, back, upper
  intestine (large) (small) T28.7 ☑
  knee T24.429 ☑
    first degree T24.529 ☑
    left T24.422 ☑
      first degree T24.522 ☑
      second degree T24.622 ☑
      third degree T24.722 ☑
    right T24.421 ☑
      first degree T24.521 ☑
      second degree T24.621 ☑
      third degree T24.721 ☑
    second degree T24.629 ☑
    third degree T24.729 ☑
  labium (majus) (minus) — *see* Corrosion, genital organs, external, female
  lacrimal apparatus, duct, gland or sac — *see* Corrosion, eye, specified site NEC
  larynx T27.4 ☑
    with lung T27.5 ☑
  leg(s) (meaning lower limb(s)) — *see* Corrosion, lower limb
  limb(s)
    lower — *see* Corrosion, lower, limb
    upper — *see* Corrosion, upper limb
  lip(s) T20.42 ☑
    first degree T20.52 ☑
    second degree T20.62 ☑
    third degree T20.72 ☑
  lower
    back — *see* Corrosion, back
    limb T24.409 ☑
      ankle — *see* Corrosion, ankle
      calf — *see* Corrosion, calf
      first degree T24.509 ☑
      foot — *see* Corrosion, foot
      knee — *see* Corrosion, knee
      left T24.402 ☑
        first degree T24.502 ☑
        second degree T24.602 ☑
        third degree T24.702 ☑
      multiple sites, except ankle and foot T24.499 ☑
        ankle and foot T25.499 ☑
          first degree T25.599 ☑
          left T25.492 ☑
            first degree T25.592 ☑
            second degree T25.692 ☑
            third degree T25.792 ☑
          right T25.491 ☑
            first degree T25.591 ☑
            second degree T25.691 ☑
            third degree T25.791 ☑
          second degree T25.699 ☑
          third degree T25.799 ☑
        first degree T24.599 ☑
        left T24.492 ☑
          first degree T24.592 ☑
          second degree T24.692 ☑
          third degree T24.792 ☑
        right T24.491 ☑
          first degree T24.591 ☑
          second degree T24.691 ☑
          third degree T24.791 ☑
        second degree T24.699 ☑
        third degree T24.799 ☑
      right T24.401 ☑
        first degree T24.501 ☑
        second degree T24.601 ☑
        third degree T24.701 ☑
      second degree T24.609 ☑
      thigh — *see* Corrosion, thigh
      third degree T24.709 ☑
  lung (with larynx and trachea) T27.5 ☑
  mouth T28.5 ☑
  neck T20.47 ☑
    first degree T20.57 ☑
    second degree T20.67 ☑
    third degree T20.77 ☑
  nose (septum) T20.44 ☑
    first degree T20.54 ☑
    second degree T20.64 ☑
    third degree T20.74 ☑
  ocular adnexa — *see* Corrosion, eye
  orbit region — *see* Corrosion, eyelid

Corrosion — *continued*
  palm T23.459 ☑
    first degree T23.559 ☑
    left T23.452 ☑
      first degree T23.552 ☑
      second degree T23.652 ☑
      third degree T23.752 ☑
    right T23.451 ☑
      first degree T23.551 ☑
      second degree T23.651 ☑
      third degree T23.751 ☑
    second degree T23.659 ☑
    third degree T23.759 ☑
  partial thickness — *code as* Corrosion, unspecified degree, by site
  pelvis — *see* Corrosion, trunk
  penis — *see* Corrosion, genital organs, external, male
  perineum
    female — *see* Corrosion, genital organs, external, female
    male — *see* Corrosion, genital organs, external, male
  periocular area — *see* Corrosion, eyelid
  pharynx T28.5 ☑
  rectum T28.7 ☑
  respiratory tract T27.7 ☑
    larynx — *see* Corrosion, larynx
    specified part NEC T27.6 ☑
    trachea — *see* Corrosion, larynx
  sac, lacrimal — *see* Corrosion, eye, specified site NEC
  scalp T20.45 ☑
    first degree T20.55 ☑
    second degree T20.65 ☑
    third degree T20.75 ☑
  scapular region T22.469 ☑
    first degree T22.569 ☑
    left T22.462 ☑
      first degree T22.562 ☑
      second degree T22.662 ☑
      third degree T22.762 ☑
    right T22.461 ☑
      first degree T22.561 ☑
      second degree T22.661 ☑
      third degree T22.761 ☑
    second degree T22.669 ☑
    third degree T22.769 ☑
  sclera — *see* Corrosion, eye, specified site NEC
  scrotum — *see* Corrosion, genital organs, external, male
  shoulder T22.459 ☑
    first degree T22.559 ☑
    left T22.452 ☑
      first degree T22.552 ☑
      second degree T22.652 ☑
      third degree T22.752 ☑
    right T22.451 ☑
      first degree T22.551 ☑
      second degree T22.651 ☑
      third degree T22.751 ☑
    second degree T22.659 ☑
    third degree T22.759 ☑
  stomach T28.7 ☑
  temple — *see* Corrosion, head
  testis — *see* Corrosion, genital organs, external, male
  thigh T24.419 ☑
    first degree T24.519 ☑
    left T24.412 ☑
      first degree T24.512 ☑
      second degree T24.612 ☑
      third degree T24.712 ☑
    right T24.411 ☑
      first degree T24.511 ☑
      second degree T24.611 ☑
      third degree T24.711 ☑
    second degree T24.619 ☑
    third degree T24.719 ☑
  thorax (external) — *see* Corrosion, trunk
  throat (meaning pharynx) T28.5 ☑
  thumb(s) T23.419 ☑
    first degree T23.519 ☑
    left T23.412 ☑
      first degree T23.512 ☑
      second degree T23.612 ☑
      third degree T23.712 ☑
    multiple sites with fingers T23.449 ☑

Corrosion — *continued*
  thumb(s) — *continued*
    multiple sites with fingers — *continued*
      first degree T23.549 ☑
      left T23.442 ☑
        first degree T23.542 ☑
        second degree T23.642 ☑
        third degree T23.742 ☑
      right T23.441 ☑
        first degree T23.541 ☑
        second degree T23.641 ☑
        third degree T23.741 ☑
      second degree T23.649 ☑
      third degree T23.749 ☑
    right T23.411 ☑
      first degree T23.511 ☑
      second degree T23.611 ☑
      third degree T23.711 ☑
    second degree T23.619 ☑
    third degree T23.719 ☑
  toe T25.439 ☑
    first degree T25.539 ☑
    left T25.432 ☑
      first degree T25.532 ☑
      second degree T25.632 ☑
      third degree T25.732 ☑
    right T25.431 ☑
      first degree T25.531 ☑
      second degree T25.631 ☑
      third degree T25.731 ☑
    second degree T25.639 ☑
    third degree T25.739 ☑
  tongue T28.5 ☑
  tonsil(s) T28.5 ☑
  total body — *see* Corrosion, multiple body regions
  trachea T27.4 ☑
    with lung T27.5 ☑
  trunk T21.40 ☑
    abdominal wall — *see* Corrosion, abdominal wall
    anus — *see* Corrosion, buttock
    axilla — *see* Corrosion, upper limb
    back — *see* Corrosion, back
    breast — *see* Corrosion, chest wall
    buttock — *see* Corrosion, buttock
    chest wall — *see* Corrosion, chest wall
    first degree T21.50 ☑
    flank — *see* Corrosion, abdominal wall
    genital
      female — *see* Corrosion, genital organs, external, female
      male — *see* Corrosion, genital organs, external, male
    groin — *see* Corrosion, abdominal wall
    interscapular region — *see* Corrosion, back, upper
    labia — *see* Corrosion, genital organs, external, female
    lower back — *see* Corrosion, back
    penis — *see* Corrosion, genital organs, external, male
    perineum
      female — *see* Corrosion, genital organs, external, female
      male — *see* Corrosion, genital organs, external, male
    scapular region — *see* Corrosion, upper limb
    scrotum — *see* Corrosion, genital organs, external, male
    second degree T21.60 ☑
    shoulder — *see* Corrosion, upper limb
    specified site NEC T21.49 ☑
      first degree T21.59 ☑
      second degree T21.69 ☑
      third degree T21.79 ☑
    testes — *see* Corrosion, genital organs, external, male
    third degree T21.70 ☑
    upper back — *see* Corrosion, back, upper
    vagina T28.8 ☑
    vulva — *see* Corrosion, genital organs, external, female
  unspecified site with extent of body surface involved specified
    less than 10 percent T32.0
    10-19 percent (0-9 percent third degree) T32.10
      with 10-19 percent third degree T32.11
    20-29 percent (0-9 percent third degree) T32.20

Corrosion — *continued*
unspecified site with extent of body surface involved specified — *continued*
20-29 percent — *continued*
with
10-19 percent third degree T32.21
20-29 percent third degree T32.22
30-39 percent (0-9 percent third degree) T32.30
with
10-19 percent third degree T32.31
20-29 percent third degree T32.32
30-39 percent third degree T32.33
40-49 percent (0-9 percent third degree) T32.40
with
10-19 percent third degree T32.41
20-29 percent third degree T32.42
30-39 percent third degree T32.43
40-49 percent third degree T32.44
50-59 percent (0-9 percent third degree) T32.50
with
10-19 percent third degree T32.51
20-29 percent third degree T32.52
30-39 percent third degree T32.53
40-49 percent third degree T32.54
50-59 percent third degree T32.55
60-69 percent (0-9 percent third degree) T32.60
with
10-19 percent third degree T32.61
20-29 percent third degree T32.62
30-39 percent third degree T32.63
40-49 percent third degree T32.64
50-59 percent third degree T32.65
60-69 percent third degree T32.66
70-79 percent (0-9 percent third degree) T32.70
with
10-19 percent third degree T32.71
20-29 percent third degree T32.72
30-39 percent third degree T32.73
40-49 percent third degree T32.74
50-59 percent third degree T32.75
60-69 percent third degree T32.76
70-79 percent third degree T32.77
80-89 percent (0-9 percent third degree) T32.80
with
10-19 percent third degree T32.81
20-29 percent third degree T32.82
30-39 percent third degree T32.83
40-49 percent third degree T32.84
50-59 percent third degree T32.85
60-69 percent third degree T32.86
70-79 percent third degree T32.87
80-89 percent third degree T32.88
90 percent or more (0-9 percent third degree) T32.90
with
10-19 percent third degree T32.91
20-29 percent third degree T32.92
30-39 percent third degree T32.93
40-49 percent third degree T32.94
50-59 percent third degree T32.95
60-69 percent third degree T32.96
70-79 percent third degree T32.97
80-89 percent third degree T32.98
90-99 percent third degree T32.99
upper limb (axilla) (scapular region) T22.40 ☑
above elbow — *see* Corrosion, above elbow
axilla — *see* Corrosion, axilla
elbow — *see* Corrosion, elbow
first degree T22.50 ☑
forearm — *see* Corrosion, forearm
hand — *see* Corrosion, hand
interscapular region — *see* Corrosion, back, upper
multiple sites T22.499 ☑
first degree T22.599 ☑
left T22.492 ☑
first degree T22.592 ☑
second degree T22.692 ☑
third degree T22.792 ☑
right T22.491 ☑
first degree T22.591 ☑
second degree T22.691 ☑
third degree T22.791 ☑
second degree T22.699 ☑
third degree T22.799 ☑
scapular region — *see* Corrosion, scapular region
second degree T22.60 ☑
shoulder — *see* Corrosion, shoulder
third degree T22.70 ☑

Corrosion — *continued*
upper limb — *continued*
wrist — *see* Corrosion, hand
uterus T28.8 ☑
vagina T28.8 ☑
vulva — *see* Corrosion, genital organs, external, female
wrist T23.479 ☑
first degree T23.579 ☑
left T23.472 ☑
first degree T23.572 ☑
second degree T23.672 ☑
third degree T23.772 ☑
multiple sites with hand T23.499 ☑
first degree T23.599 ☑
left T23.492 ☑
first degree T23.592 ☑
second degree T23.692 ☑
third degree T23.792 ☑
right T23.491 ☑
first degree T23.591 ☑
second degree T23.691 ☑
third degree T23.791 ☑
second degree T23.699 ☑
third degree T23.799 ☑
right T23.471 ☑
first degree T23.571 ☑
second degree T23.671 ☑
third degree T23.771 ☑
second degree T23.679 ☑
third degree T23.779 ☑
Corrosive burn — *see* Corrosion
Corsican fever — *see* Malaria
Cortical — *see* condition
Cortico-adrenal — *see* condition
Coryza (acute) J00
with grippe or influenza — *see* Influenza, with, respiratory manifestations NEC
syphilitic
congenital (chronic) A50.05
Costen's syndrome or complex M26.69
Costiveness — *see* Constipation
Costochondritis M94.0
Cot death R99
Cotard's syndrome F22
Cotia virus B08.8
Cotton wool spots (retinal) H35.81
Cotungo's disease — *see* Sciatica
Cough (affected) (chronic) (epidemic) (nervous) R05
with hemorrhage — *see* Hemoptysis
bronchial R05
with grippe or influenza — *see* Influenza, with, respiratory manifestations NEC
functional F45.8
hysterical F45.8
laryngeal, spasmodic R05
psychogenic F45.8
smokers' J41.0
tea taster's B49
Counseling (for) Z71.9
abuse NEC
perpetrator Z69.82
victim Z69.81
alcohol abuser Z71.41
family Z71.42
child abuse
nonparental
perpetrator Z69.021
victim Z69.020
parental
perpetrator Z69.011
victim Z69.010
consanguinity Z71.89
contraceptive Z30.09
dietary Z71.3
drug abuser Z71.51
family member Z71.52
family Z71.89
fertility preservation (prior to cancer therapy) (prior to removal of gonads) Z31.62
for non-attending third party Z71.0
related to sexual behavior or orientation Z70.2
genetic NEC Z31.5
health (advice) (education) (instruction) — *see* Counseling, medical
human immunodeficiency virus (HIV) Z71.7
impotence Z70.1
insulin pump use Z46.81

Counseling — *continued*
medical (for) Z71.9
boarding school resident Z59.3
consanguinity Z71.89
feared complaint and no disease found Z71.1
human immunodeficiency virus (HIV) Z71.7
institutional resident Z59.3
on behalf of another Z71.0
related to sexual behavior or orientation Z70.2
person living alone Z60.2
specified reason NEC Z71.89
natural family planning
procreative Z31.61
to avoid pregnancy Z30.02
perpetrator (of)
abuse NEC Z69.82
child abuse
non-parental Z69.021
parental Z69.011
rape NEC Z69.82
spousal abuse Z69.12
procreative NEC Z31.69
fertility preservation (prior to cancer therapy) (prior to removal of gonads) Z31.62
using natural family planning Z31.61
promiscuity Z70.1
rape victim Z69.81
religious Z71.81
sex, sexual (related to) Z70.9
attitude(s) Z70.0
behavior or orientation Z70.1
combined concerns Z70.3
non-responsiveness Z70.1
on behalf of third party Z70.2
specified reason NEC Z70.8
specified reason NEC Z71.89
spiritual Z71.81
spousal abuse (perpetrator) Z69.12
victim Z69.11
substance abuse Z71.89
alcohol Z71.41
drug Z71.51
tobacco Z71.6
tobacco use Z71.6
use (of)
insulin pump Z46.81
victim (of)
abuse Z69.81
child abuse
by parent Z69.010
non-parental Z69.020
rape NEC Z69.81
Coupled rhythm R00.8
Couvelaire syndrome or uterus (complicating delivery) O45.8X- ☑
Cowperitis — *see* Urethritis
Cowper's gland — *see* condition
Cowpox B08.010
due to vaccination T88.1 ☑
Coxa
magna M91.4- ☑
plana M91.2- ☑
valga (acquired) (*see also* Deformity, limb, specified type NEC, thigh)
congenital Q65.81
sequelae (late effect) of rickets E64.3
vara (acquired) (*see also* Deformity, limb, specified type NEC, thigh)
congenital Q65.82
sequelae (late effect) of rickets E64.3
Coxalgia, coxalgic (nontuberculous) (*see also* Pain, joint, hip)
tuberculous A18.02
Coxitis — *see* Monoarthritis, hip
Coxsackie (virus) (infection) B34.1
as cause of disease classified elsewhere B97.11
carditis B33.20
central nervous system NEC A88.8
endocarditis B33.21
enteritis A08.39
meningitis (aseptic) A87.0
myocarditis B33.22
pericarditis B33.23
pharyngitis B08.5
pleurodynia B33.0
specific disease NEC B33.8
Crabs, meaning pubic lice B85.3
Crack baby P04.41

Index

Corrosion — Crack baby

Cracked nipple N64.0
　associated with
　　lactation O92.13
　　pregnancy O92.11- ☑
　　puerperium O92.12
Cracked tooth K03.81
Cradle cap L21.0
Craft neurosis F48.8
Cramp(s) R25.2
　abdominal — see Pain, abdominal
　bathing T75.1 ☑
　colic R10.83
　　psychogenic F45.8
　due to immersion T75.1 ☑
　fireman T67.2 ☑
　heat T67.2 ☑
　immersion T75.1 ☑
　intestinal — see Pain, abdominal
　　psychogenic F45.8
　leg, sleep related G47.62
　limb (lower) (upper) NEC R25.2
　　sleep related G47.62
　linotypist's F48.8
　　organic G25.89
　muscle (limb) (general) R25.2
　　due to immersion T75.1 ☑
　　psychogenic F45.8
　occupational (hand) F48.8
　　organic G25.89
　salt-depletion E87.1
　sleep related, leg G47.62
　stoker's T67.2 ☑
　swimmer's T75.1 ☑
　telegrapher's F48.8
　　organic G25.89
　typist's F48.8
　　organic G25.89
　uterus N94.89
　　menstrual — see Dysmenorrhea
　writer's F48.8
　　organic G25.89
Cranial — see condition
Craniocleidodysostosis Q74.0
Craniofenestria (skull) Q75.8
Craniolacunia (skull) Q75.8
Craniopagus Q89.4
Craniopathy, metabolic M85.2
Craniopharyngeal — see condition
Craniopharyngioma D44.4
Craniorachischisis (totalis) Q00.1
Cranioschisis Q75.8
Craniostenosis Q75.0
Craniosynostosis Q75.0
Craniotabes (cause unknown) M83.8
　neonatal P96.3
　rachitic E64.3
　syphilitic A50.56
Cranium — see condition
Craw-craw — see Onchocerciasis
Creaking joint — see Derangement, joint, specified type NEC
Creeping
　eruption B76.9
　palsy or paralysis G12.22
Crenated tongue K14.8
Creotoxism A05.9
Crepitus
　caput Q75.8
　joint — see Derangement, joint, specified type NEC
Crescent or conus choroid, congenital Q14.3
CREST syndrome M34.1
Cretin, cretinism (congenital) (endemic) (nongoitrous) (sporadic) E00.9
　pelvis
　　with disproportion (fetopelvic) O33.0
　　　causing obstructed labor O65.0
　type
　　hypothyroid E00.1
　　mixed E00.2
　　myxedematous E00.1
　　neurological E00.0
Creutzfeldt-Jakob disease or syndrome (with dementia) A81.00
　familial A81.09
　iatrogenic A81.09
　specified NEC A81.09
　sporadic A81.09

Creutzfeldt-Jakob disease or syndrome — continued
　variant (vCJD) A81.01
Crib death R99
Cribriform hymen Q52.3
Cri-du-chat syndrome Q93.4
Crigler-Najjar disease or syndrome E80.5
Crime, victim of Z65.4
Crimean hemorrhagic fever A98.0
Criminalism F60.2
Crisis
　abdomen R10.0
　acute reaction F43.0
　addisonian E27.2
　adrenal (cortical) E27.2
　celiac K90.0
　Dietl's N13.8
　emotional (see also Disorder, adjustment)
　　acute reaction to stress F43.0
　　specific to childhood and adolescence F93.8
　glaucomatocyclitic — see Glaucoma, secondary, inflammation
　heart — see Failure, heart
　nitritoid I95.2
　　correct substance properly administered — see Table of Drugs and Chemicals, by drug, adverse effect
　　overdose or wrong substance given or taken — see Table of Drugs and Chemicals, by drug, poisoning
　oculogyric H51.8
　　psychogenic F45.8
　Pel's (tabetic) A52.11
　psychosexual identity F64.2
　renal N28.0
　sickle-cell D57.00
　　with
　　　acute chest syndrome D57.01
　　　splenic sequestration D57.02
　state (acute reaction) F43.0
　tabetic A52.11
　thyroid — see Thyrotoxicosis with thyroid storm
　thyrotoxic — see Thyrotoxicosis with thyroid storm
Crocq's disease (acrocyanosis) I73.89
Crohn's disease — see Enteritis, regional
Crooked septum, nasal J34.2
Cross syndrome E70.328
Crossbite (anterior) (posterior) M26.24
Cross-eye — see Strabismus, convergent concomitant
Croup, croupous (catarrhal) (infectious) (inflammatory) (nondiphtheritic) J05.0
　bronchial J20.9
　diphtheritic A36.2
　false J38.5
　spasmodic J38.5
　　diphtheritic A36.2
　stridulous J38.5
　　diphtheritic A36.2
Crouzon's disease Q75.1
Crowding, tooth, teeth, fully erupted M26.31
CRST syndrome M34.1
Cruchet's disease A85.8
Cruelty in children (see also Disorder, conduct)
Crural ulcer — see Ulcer, lower limb
Crush, crushed, crushing T14.8
　abdomen S38.1 ☑
　ankle S97.0- ☑
　arm (upper) (and shoulder) S47.- ☑
　axilla — see Crush, arm
　back, lower S38.1 ☑
　buttock S38.1 ☑
　cheek S07.0 ☑
　chest S28.0 ☑
　cranium S07.1 ☑
　ear S07.0 ☑
　elbow S57.0- ☑
　extremity
　　lower
　　　ankle — see Crush, ankle
　　　below knee — see Crush, leg
　　　foot — see Crush, foot
　　　hip — see Crush, hip
　　　knee — see Crush, knee
　　　thigh — see Crush, thigh
　　　toe — see Crush, toe
　　upper
　　　below elbow S67.9- ☑

Crush, crushed, crushing — continued
　extremity — continued
　　upper — continued
　　　elbow — see Crush, elbow
　　　finger — see Crush, finger
　　　forearm — see Crush, forearm
　　　hand — see Crush, hand
　　　thumb — see Crush, thumb
　　　upper arm — see Crush, arm
　　　wrist — see Crush, wrist
　face S07.0 ☑
　finger(s) S67.1- ☑
　　with hand (and wrist) — see Crush, hand, specified site NEC
　　index S67.19- ☑
　　little S67.19- ☑
　　middle S67.19- ☑
　　ring S67.19- ☑
　　thumb — see Crush, thumb
　foot S97.8- ☑
　　toe — see Crush, toe
　forearm S57.8- ☑
　genitalia, external
　　female S38.002 ☑
　　　vagina S38.03 ☑
　　　vulva S38.03 ☑
　　male S38.001 ☑
　　　penis S38.01 ☑
　　　scrotum S38.02 ☑
　　　testis S38.02 ☑
　hand (except fingers alone) S67.2- ☑
　　with wrist S67.4- ☑
　head S07.9 ☑
　　specified NEC S07.8 ☑
　heel — see Crush, foot
　hip S77.0- ☑
　　with thigh S77.2- ☑
　internal organ (abdomen, chest, or pelvis) NEC T14.8
　knee S87.0- ☑
　labium (majus) (minus) S38.03 ☑
　larynx S17.0 ☑
　leg (lower) S87.8- ☑
　　knee — see Crush, knee
　lip S07.0 ☑
　lower
　　back S38.1 ☑
　　leg — see Crush, leg
　neck S17.9 ☑
　nerve — see Injury, nerve
　nose S07.0 ☑
　pelvis S38.1 ☑
　penis S38.01 ☑
　scalp S07.8 ☑
　scapular region — see Crush, arm
　scrotum S38.02 ☑
　severe, unspecified site T14.8
　shoulder (and upper arm) — see Crush, arm
　skull S07.1 ☑
　syndrome (complication of trauma) T79.5 ☑
　testis S38.02 ☑
　thigh S77.1- ☑
　　with hip S77.2- ☑
　throat S17.8 ☑
　thumb S67.0- ☑
　　with hand (and wrist) — see Crush, hand, specified site NEC
　toe(s) S97.10- ☑
　　great S97.11- ☑
　　lesser S97.12- ☑
　trachea S17.0 ☑
　vagina S38.03 ☑
　vulva S38.03 ☑
　wrist S67.3- ☑
　　with hand S67.4- ☑
Crusta lactea L21.0
Crusts R23.4
Crutch paralysis — see Injury, brachial plexus
Cruveilhier-Baumgarten cirrhosis, disease or syndrome K74.69
Cruveilhier's atrophy or disease G12.8
Crying (constant) (continuous) (excessive)
　child, adolescent, or adult R45.83
　infant (baby) (newborn) R68.11
Cryofibrinogenemia D89.2
Cryoglobulinemia (essential) (idiopathic) (mixed) (primary) (purpura) (secondary) (vasculitis) D89.1

Cryoglobulinemia — *continued*
  with lung involvement D89.1 [J99]
Cryptitis (anal) (rectal) K62.89
Cryptococcosis, cryptococcus (infection) (neoformans)
      B45.9
  bone B45.3
  cerebral B45.1
  cutaneous B45.2
  disseminated B45.7
  generalized B45.7
  meningitis B45.1
  meningocerebralis B45.1
  osseous B45.3
  pulmonary B45.0
  skin B45.2
  specified NEC B45.8
Cryptopapillitis (anus) K62.89
Cryptophthalmos Q11.2
  syndrome Q87.0
Cryptorchid, cryptorchism, cryptorchidism Q53.9
  bilateral Q53.20
      abdominal Q53.21
      perineal Q53.22
  unilateral Q53.10
      abdominal Q53.11
      perineal Q53.12
Cryptosporidiosis A07.2
  hepatobiliary B88.8
  respiratory B88.8
Cryptostromosis J67.6
Crystalluria R82.99
Cubitus
  congenital Q68.8
  valgus (acquired) M21.0- ☑
      congenital Q68.8
      sequelae (late effect) of rickets E64.3
  varus (acquired) M21.1- ☑
      congenital Q68.8
      sequelae (late effect) of rickets E64.3
Cultural deprivation or shock Z60.3
Curling esophagus K22.4
Curling's ulcer — *see* Ulcer, peptic, acute
Curschmann (-Batten) (-Steinert) **disease or syndrome**
      G71.11
Curse, Ondine's — *see* Apnea, sleep
Curvature
  organ or site, congenital NEC — *see* Distortion
  penis (lateral) Q55.61
  Pott's (spinal) A18.01
  radius, idiopathic, progressive (congenital) Q74.0
  spine (acquired) (angular) (idiopathic) (incorrect)
      (postural) — *see* Dorsopathy, deforming
      congenital Q67.5
      due to or associated with
         Charcot-Marie-Tooth disease (*see also* subcate-
            gory M49.8) G60.0
         osteitis
            deformans M88.88
            fibrosa cystica (*see also* subcategory M49.8)
               E21.0
         tuberculosis (Pott's curvature) A18.01
      sequelae (late effect) of rickets E64.3
      tuberculous A18.01
Cushingoid due to steroid therapy E24.2
  correct substance properly administered — *see* Table
      of Drugs and Chemicals, by drug, adverse effect
  overdose or wrong substance given or taken — *see*
      Table of Drugs and Chemicals, by drug, poison-
      ing
Cushing's
  syndrome or disease E24.9
      drug-induced E24.2
      iatrogenic E24.2
      pituitary-dependent E24.0
      specified NEC E24.8
  ulcer — *see* Ulcer, peptic, acute
Cusp, Carabelli — *omit code*
Cut (external) (*see also* Laceration)
  muscle — *see* Injury, muscle
Cutaneous (*see also* condition)
  hemorrhage R23.3
  larva migrans B76.9
Cutis (*see also* condition)
  hyperelastica Q82.8
      acquired L57.4
  laxa (hyperelastica) — *see* Dermatolysis
  marmorata R23.8

Cutis — *continued*
  osteosis L94.2
  pendula — *see* Dermatolysis
  rhomboidalis nuchae L57.2
  verticis gyrata Q82.8
      acquired L91.8
Cyanosis R23.0
  due to
      patent foramen botalli Q21.1
      persistent foramen ovale Q21.1
  enterogenous D74.8
  paroxysmal digital — *see* Raynaud's disease
      with gangrene I73.01
  retina, retinal H35.89
Cyanotic heart disease I24.9
  congenital Q24.9
Cycle
  anovulatory N97.0
  menstrual, irregular N92.6
Cyclencephaly Q04.9
Cyclical vomiting (*see also* Vomiting, cyclical) G43.A0
      (*following* G43.7)
  psychogenic F50.8
Cyclitis (*see also* Iridocyclitis) H20.9
  chronic — *see* Iridocyclitis, chronic
  Fuchs' heterochromic H20.81- ☑
  granulomatous — *see* Iridocyclitis, chronic
  lens-induced — *see* Iridocyclitis, lens-induced
  posterior H30.2- ☑
Cycloid personality F34.0
Cyclophoria H50.54
Cyclopia, cyclops Q87.0
Cyclopism Q87.0
Cyclosporiasis A07.4
Cyclothymia F34.0
Cyclothymic personality F34.0
Cyclotropia H50.41- ☑
Cylindroma (*see also* Neoplasm, malignant, by site)
  eccrine dermal — *see* Neoplasm, skin, benign
  skin — *see* Neoplasm, skin, benign
Cylindruria R82.99
Cynanche
  diphtheritic A36.2
  tonsillaris J36
Cynophobia F40.218
Cynorexia R63.2
Cyphosis — *see* Kyphosis
Cyprus fever — *see* Brucellosis
Cyst (colloid) (mucous) (simple) (retention)
  adenoid (infected) J35.8
  adrenal gland E27.8
      congenital Q89.1
  air, lung J98.4
  allantoic Q64.4
  alveolar process (jaw bone) M27.40
  amnion, amniotic O41.8X- ☑
  anterior
      chamber (eye) — *see* Cyst, iris
      nasopalatine K09.1
  antrum J34.1
  anus K62.89
  apical (tooth) (periodontal) K04.8
  appendix K38.8
  arachnoid, brain (acquired) G93.0
      congenital Q04.6
  arytenoid J38.7
  Baker's M71.2- ☑
      ruptured M66.0
      tuberculous A18.02
  Bartholin's gland N75.0
  bile duct (common) (hepatic) K83.5
  bladder (multiple) (trigone) N32.89
  blue dome (breast) — *see* Cyst, breast
  bone (local) NEC M85.60
      aneurysmal M85.50
         ankle M85.57- ☑
         foot M85.57- ☑
         forearm M85.53- ☑
         hand M85.54- ☑
         jaw M27.49
         lower leg M85.56- ☑
         multiple site M85.59
         neck M85.58
         rib M85.58
         shoulder M85.51- ☑
         skull M85.58
         specified site NEC M85.58

Cyst — *continued*
  bone — *continued*
      aneurysmal — *continued*
         thigh M85.55- ☑
         toe M85.57- ☑
         upper arm M85.52- ☑
         vertebra M85.58
      solitary M85.40
         ankle M85.47- ☑
         fibula M85.46- ☑
         foot M85.47- ☑
         hand M85.44- ☑
         humerus M85.42- ☑
         jaw M27.49
         neck M85.48
         pelvis M85.45- ☑
         radius M85.43- ☑
         rib M85.48
         shoulder M85.41- ☑
         skull M85.48
         specified site NEC M85.48
         tibia M85.46- ☑
         toe M85.47- ☑
         ulna M85.43- ☑
         vertebra M85.48
      specified type NEC M85.60
         ankle M85.67- ☑
         foot M85.67- ☑
         forearm M85.63- ☑
         hand M85.64- ☑
         jaw M27.40
            developmental (nonodontogenic) K09.1
            odontogenic K09.0
            latent M27.0
         lower leg M85.66- ☑
         multiple site M85.69
         neck M85.68
         rib M85.68
         shoulder M85.61- ☑
         skull M85.68
         specified site NEC M85.68
         thigh M85.65- ☑
         toe M85.67- ☑
         upper arm M85.62- ☑
         vertebra M85.68
  brain (acquired) G93.0
      congenital Q04.6
      hydatid B67.99 [G94]
      third ventricle (colloid), congenital Q04.6
  branchial (cleft) Q18.0
  branchiogenic Q18.0
  breast (benign) (blue dome) (pedunculated) (solitary)
      N60.0- ☑
      involution — *see* Dysplasia, mammary, specified
         type NEC
      sebaceous — *see* Dysplasia, mammary, specified
         type NEC
  broad ligament (benign) N83.8
  bronchogenic (mediastinal) (sequestration) J98.4
      congenital Q33.0
  buccal K09.8
  bulbourethral gland N36.8
  bursa, bursal NEC M71.30
      with rupture — *see* Rupture, synovium
      ankle M71.37- ☑
      elbow M71.32- ☑
      foot M71.37- ☑
      hand M71.34- ☑
      hip M71.35- ☑
      multiple sites M71.39
      pharyngeal J39.2
      popliteal space — *see* Cyst, Baker's
      shoulder M71.31- ☑
      specified site NEC M71.38
      wrist M71.33- ☑
  calcifying odontogenic D16.5
      upper jaw (bone) (maxilla) D16.4
  canal of Nuck (female) N94.89
      congenital Q52.4
  canthus — *see* Cyst, conjunctiva
  carcinomatous — *see* Neoplasm, malignant, by site
  cauda equina G95.89
  cavum septi pellucidi — *see* Cyst, brain
  celomic (pericardium) Q24.8
  cerebellopontine (angle) — *see* Cyst, brain
  cerebellum — *see* Cyst, brain
  cerebral — *see* Cyst, brain

☑ **Additional Character Required** — **Refer to the Tabular List for Character Selection**   🔻 **Subterms under main terms may continue to next column or page**

Cyst — *continued*
  cervical lateral Q18.1
  cervix NEC N88.8
    embryonic Q51.6
    nabothian N88.8
  chiasmal optic NEC — *see* Disorder, optic, chiasm
  chocolate (ovary) N80.1
  choledochus, congenital Q44.4
  chorion O41.8X- ☑
  choroid plexus G93.0
  ciliary body — *see* Cyst, iris
  clitoris N90.7
  colon K63.89
  common (bile) duct K83.5
  congenital NEC Q89.8
    adrenal gland Q89.1
    epiglottis Q31.8
    esophagus Q39.8
    fallopian tube Q50.4
    kidney Q61.00
      more than one (multiple) Q61.02
        specified as polycystic Q61.3
          adult type Q61.2
          infantile type NEC Q61.19
            collecting duct dilation Q61.11
      solitary Q61.01
    larynx Q31.8
    liver Q44.6
    lung Q33.0
    mediastinum Q34.1
    ovary Q50.1
    oviduct Q50.4
    periurethral (tissue) Q64.79
    prepuce Q55.69
    salivary gland (any) Q38.4
    sublingual Q38.6
    submaxillary gland Q38.6
    thymus (gland) Q89.2
    tongue Q38.3
    ureterovesical orifice Q62.8
    vulva Q52.79
  conjunctiva H11.44- ☑
  cornea H18.89- ☑
  corpora quadrigemina G93.0
  corpus
    albicans N83.29
    luteum (hemorrhagic) (ruptured) N83.1
  Cowper's gland (benign) (infected) N36.8
  cranial meninges G93.0
  craniobuccal pouch E23.6
  craniopharyngeal pouch E23.6
  cystic duct K82.8
  Cysticercus — *see* Cysticercosis
  Dandy-Walker Q03.1
    with spina bifida — *see* Spina bifida
  dental (root) K04.8
    developmental K09.0
    eruption K09.0
    primordial K09.0
  dentigerous (mandible) (maxilla) K09.0
  dermoid — *see* Neoplasm, benign, by site
    with malignant transformation C56.- ☑
    implantation
      external area or site (skin) NEC L72.0
      iris — *see* Cyst, iris, implantation
      vagina N89.8
      vulva N90.7
    mouth K09.8
    oral soft tissue K09.8
    sacrococcygeal — *see* Cyst, pilonidal
  developmental K09.1
    odontogenic K09.0
    oral region (nonodontogenic) K09.1
    ovary, ovarian Q50.1
  dura (cerebral) G93.0
    spinal G96.19
  ear (external) Q18.1
  echinococcal — *see* Echinococcus
  embryonic
    cervix uteri Q51.6
    fallopian tube Q50.4
    vagina Q51.6
  endometrium, endometrial (uterus) N85.8
    ectopic — *see* Endometriosis
  enterogenous Q43.8
  epidermal, epidermoid (inclusion) (*see also* Cyst, skin) L72.0
    mouth K09.8

Cyst — *continued*
  epidermal, epidermoid (*see also* Cyst, skin) — *continued*
    oral soft tissue K09.8
  epididymis N50.3
  epiglottis J38.7
  epiphysis cerebri E34.8
  epithelial (inclusion) L72.0
  epoophoron Q50.5
  eruption K09.0
  esophagus K22.8
  ethmoid sinus J34.1
  external female genital organs NEC N90.7
  eyelid (sebaceous) H02.829
    infected — *see* Hordeolum
    left H02.826
      lower H02.825
      upper H02.824
    right H02.823
      lower H02.822
      upper H02.821
  eye NEC H57.8
    congenital Q15.8
  fallopian tube N83.8
    congenital Q50.4
  fimbrial (twisted) Q50.4
  fissural (oral region) K09.1
  follicle (graafian) (hemorrhagic) N83.0
    nabothian N88.8
  follicular (atretic) (hemorrhagic) (ovarian) N83.0
    dentigerous K09.0
    odontogenic K09.0
    skin L72.9
      specified NEC L72.8
  frontal sinus J34.1
  gallbladder K82.8
  ganglion — *see* Ganglion
  Gartner's duct Q52.4
  gingiva K09.0
  gland of Moll — *see* Cyst, eyelid
  globulomaxillary K09.1
  graafian follicle (hemorrhagic) N83.0
  granulosal lutein (hemorrhagic) N83.1
  hemangiomatous D18.00
    intra-abdominal D18.03
    intracranial D18.02
    skin D18.01
    specified site NEC D18.09
  hydatid (*see also* Echinococcus) B67.90
    brain B67.99 [G94]
    liver (*see also* Cyst, liver, hydatid) B67.8
    lung NEC B67.99 [J99]
    Morgagni
      female Q50.5
      male (epididymal) Q55.4
        testicular Q55.29
    specified site NEC B67.99
  hymen N89.8
    embryonic Q52.4
  hypopharynx J39.2
  hypophysis, hypophyseal (duct) (recurrent) E23.6
    cerebri E23.6
  implantation (dermoid)
    external area or site (skin) NEC L72.0
    iris — *see* Cyst, iris, implantation
    vagina N89.8
    vulva N90.7
  incisive canal K09.1
  inclusion (epidermal) (epithelial) (epidermoid) (squamous) L72.0
    not of skin — *code under* Cyst, by site
  intestine (large) (small) K63.89
  intracranial — *see* Cyst, brain
  intraligamentous (*see also* Disorder, ligament)
    knee — *see* Derangement, knee
  intrasellar E23.6
  iris H21.309
    exudative H21.31- ☑
    idiopathic H21.30- ☑
    implantation H21.32- ☑
    parasitic H21.33- ☑
    pars plana (primary) H21.34- ☑
      exudative H21.35- ☑
  jaw (bone) M27.40
    aneurysmal M27.49
    developmental (odontogenic) K09.0
    fissural K09.1
    hemorrhagic M27.49

Cyst — *continued*
  jaw — *continued*
    traumatic M27.49
  joint NEC — *see* Disorder, joint, specified type NEC
  kidney (acquired) N28.1
    calyceal — *see* Hydronephrosis
    congenital Q61.00
      more than one (multiple) Q61.02
        specified as polycystic Q61.3
          adult type (autosomal dominant) Q61.2
          infantile type (autosomal recessive) NEC Q61.19
            collecting duct dilation Q61.11
    pyelogenic — *see* Hydronephrosis
    simple N28.1
    solitary (single) Q61.01
      acquired N28.1
  labium (majus) (minus) N90.7
    sebaceous N90.7
  lacrimal (*see also* Disorder, lacrimal system, specified NEC)
    gland H04.13- ☑
    passages or sac — *see* Disorder, lacrimal system, specified NEC
  larynx J38.7
  lateral periodontal K09.0
  lens H27.8
    congenital Q12.8
  lip (gland) K13.0
  liver (idiopathic) (simple) K76.89
    congenital Q44.6
    hydatid B67.8
      granulosus B67.0
      multilocularis B67.5
  lung J98.4
    congenital Q33.0
    giant bullous J43.9
  lutein N83.1
  lymphangiomatous D18.1
  lymphoepithelial, oral soft tissue K09.8
  macula — *see* Degeneration, macula, hole
  malignant — *see* Neoplasm, malignant, by site
  mammary gland — *see* Cyst, breast
  mandible M27.40
    dentigerous K09.0
    radicular K04.8
  maxilla M27.40
    dentigerous K09.0
    radicular K04.8
  medial, face and neck Q18.8
  median
    anterior maxillary K09.1
    palatal K09.1
  mediastinum, congenital Q34.1
  meibomian (gland) — *see* Chalazion
    infected — *see* Hordeolum
  membrane, brain G93.0
  meninges (cerebral) G93.0
    spinal G96.19
  meniscus, knee — *see* Derangement, knee, meniscus, cystic
  mesentery, mesenteric K66.8
    chyle I89.8
  mesonephric duct
    female Q50.5
    male Q55.4
  milk N64.89
  Morgagni (hydatid)
    female Q50.5
    male (epididymal) Q55.4
      testicular Q55.29
  mouth K09.8
  Müllerian duct Q50.4
    appendix testis Q55.29
    cervix Q51.6
    fallopian tube Q50.4
    female Q50.4
    male Q55.29
    prostatic utricle Q55.4
    vagina (embryonal) Q52.4
  multilocular (ovary) D39.10
    benign — *see* Neoplasm, benign, by site
  myometrium N85.8
  nabothian (follicle) (ruptured) N88.8
  nasoalveolar K09.1
  nasolabial K09.1
  nasopalatine (anterior) (duct) K09.1
  nasopharynx J39.2

Index

Cyst — Cystadenofibroma

Cyst — *continued*
- neoplastic — *see* Neoplasm, uncertain behavior, by site
  - benign — *see* Neoplasm, benign, by site
- nervous system NEC G96.8
- neuroenteric (congenital) Q06.8
- nipple — *see* Cyst, breast
- nose (turbinates) J34.1
  - sinus J34.1
- odontogenic, developmental K09.0
- omentum (lesser) K66.8
  - congenital Q45.8
- ora serrata — *see* Cyst, retina, ora serrata
- oral
  - region K09.9
    - developmental (nonodontogenic) K09.1
    - specified NEC K09.8
  - soft tissue K09.9
    - specified NEC K09.8
- orbit H05.81- ☑
- ovary, ovarian (twisted) N83.20
  - adherent N83.20
  - chocolate N80.1
  - corpus
    - albicans N83.29
    - luteum (hemorrhagic) N83.1
  - dermoid D27.9
  - developmental Q50.1
  - due to failure of involution NEC N83.20
  - endometrial N80.1
  - follicular (graafian) (hemorrhagic) N83.0
  - hemorrhagic N83.20
  - in pregnancy or childbirth O34.8- ☑
    - with obstructed labor O65.5
  - multilocular D39.10
  - pseudomucinous D27.9
  - retention N83.29
  - serous N83.20
  - specified NEC N83.29
  - theca lutein (hemorrhagic) N83.1
  - tuberculous A18.18
- oviduct N83.8
- palate (median) (fissural) K09.1
- palatine papilla (jaw) K09.1
- pancreas, pancreatic (hemorrhagic) (true) K86.2
  - congenital Q45.2
  - false K86.3
- paralabral
  - hip M24.85- ☑
  - shoulder S43.43- ☑
- paramesonephric duct Q50.4
  - female Q50.4
  - male Q55.29
- paranephric N28.1
- paraphysis, cerebri, congenital Q04.6
- parasitic B89
- parathyroid (gland) E21.4
- paratubal N83.8
- paraurethral duct N36.8
- paroophoron Q50.5
- parotid gland K11.6
- parovarian Q50.5
- pelvis, female N94.89
  - in pregnancy or childbirth O34.8- ☑
    - causing obstructed labor O65.5
- penis (sebaceous) N48.89
- periapical K04.8
- pericardial (congenital) Q24.8
  - acquired (secondary) I31.8
- pericoronal K09.0
- periodontal K04.8
  - lateral K09.0
- peripelvic (lymphatic) N28.1
- peritoneum K66.8
  - chylous I89.8
- periventricular, acquired, newborn P91.1
- pharynx (wall) J39.2
- pilar L72.11
- pilonidal (infected) (rectum) L05.91
  - with abscess L05.01
  - malignant C44.59- ☑
- pituitary (duct) (gland) E23.6
- placenta O43.19- ☑
- pleura J94.8
- popliteal — *see* Cyst, Baker's
- porencephalic Q04.6
  - acquired G93.0
- postanal (infected) — *see* Cyst, pilonidal

Cyst — *continued*
- postmastoidectomy cavity (mucosal) — *see* Complications, postmastoidectomy, cyst
- preauricular Q18.1
- prepuce N47.4
  - congenital Q55.69
- primordial (jaw) K09.0
- prostate N42.83
- pseudomucinous (ovary) D27.9
- pupillary, miotic H21.27- ☑
- radicular (residual) K04.8
- radiculodental K04.8
- ranular K11.8
- Rathke's pouch E23.6
- rectum (epithelium) (mucous) K62.89
- renal — *see* Cyst, kidney
- residual (radicular) K04.8
- retention (ovary) N83.29
  - salivary gland K11.6
- retina H33.19- ☑
  - ora serrata H33.11- ☑
  - parasitic H33.12- ☑
- retroperitoneal K68.9
- sacrococcygeal (dermoid) — *see* Cyst, pilonidal
- salivary gland or duct (mucous extravasation or retention) K11.6
- Sampson's N80.1
- sclera H15.89
- scrotum L72.9
  - sebaceous L72.3
- sebaceous (duct) (gland) L72.3
  - breast — *see* Dysplasia, mammary, specified type NEC
  - eyelid — *see* Cyst, eyelid
  - genital organ NEC
    - female N94.89
    - male N50.8
  - scrotum L72.3
- semilunar cartilage (knee) (multiple) — *see* Derangement, knee, meniscus, cystic
- seminal vesicle N50.8
- serous (ovary) N83.20
- sinus (accessory) (nasal) J34.1
- Skene's gland N36.8
- skin L72.9
  - breast — *see* Dysplasia, mammary, specified type NEC
  - epidermal, epidermoid L72.0
  - epithelial L72.0
  - eyelid — *see* Cyst, eyelid
  - genital organ NEC
    - female N90.7
    - male N50.8
  - inclusion L72.0
  - scrotum L72.9
  - sebaceous L72.3
  - sweat gland or duct L74.8
- solitary
  - bone — *see* Cyst, bone, solitary
  - jaw M27.40
  - kidney N28.1
- spermatic cord N50.8
- sphenoid sinus J34.1
- spinal meninges G96.19
- spleen NEC D73.4
  - congenital Q89.09
  - hydatid (*see also* Echinococcus) B67.99 [D77]
- Stafne's M27.0
- subarachnoid intrasellar R93.0
- subcutaneous, pheomycotic (chromomycotic) B43.2
- subdural (cerebral) G93.0
  - spinal cord G96.19
- sublingual gland K11.6
- submandibular gland K11.6
- submaxillary gland K11.6
- suburethral N36.8
- suprarenal gland E27.8
- suprasellar — *see* Cyst, brain
- sweat gland or duct L74.8
- synovial (*see also* Cyst, bursa)
  - ruptured — *see* Rupture, synovium
- tarsal — *see* Chalazion
- tendon (sheath) — *see* Disorder, tendon, specified type NEC
- testis N44.2
  - tunica albuginea N44.1
- theca lutein (ovary) N83.1
- Thornwaldt's J39.2

Cyst — *continued*
- thymus (gland) E32.8
- thyroglossal duct (infected) (persistent) Q89.2
- thyroid (gland) E04.1
- thyrolingual duct (infected) (persistent) Q89.2
- tongue K14.8
- tonsil J35.8
- tooth — *see* Cyst, dental
- Tornwaldt's J39.2
- trichilemmal (proliferating) L72.12
- trichodermal L72.12
- tubal (fallopian) N83.8
  - inflammatory — *see* Salpingitis, chronic
- tubo-ovarian N83.8
  - inflammatory N70.13
- tunica
  - albuginea testis N44.1
  - vaginalis N50.8
- turbinate (nose) J34.1
- Tyson's gland N48.89
- urachus, congenital Q64.4
- ureter N28.89
- ureterovesical orifice N28.89
- urethra, urethral (gland) N36.8
- uterine ligament N83.8
- uterus (body) (corpus) (recurrent) N85.8
  - embryonic Q51.818
    - cervix Q51.6
- vagina, vaginal (implantation) (inclusion) (squamous cell) (wall) N89.8
  - embryonic Q52.4
- vallecula, vallecular (epiglottis) J38.7
- vesical (orifice) N32.89
- vitreous body H43.89
- vulva (implantation) (inclusion) N90.7
  - congenital Q52.79
  - sebaceous gland N90.7
- vulvovaginal gland N90.7
- wolffian
  - female Q50.5
  - male Q55.4

Cystadenocarcinoma — *see* Neoplasm, malignant, by site
- bile duct C22.1
- endometrioid — *see* Neoplasm, malignant, by site
- specified site — *see* Neoplasm, malignant, by site
- unspecified site
  - female C56.9
  - male C61
- mucinous
  - papillary
    - specified site — *see* Neoplasm, malignant, by site
    - unspecified site C56.9
  - specified site — *see* Neoplasm, malignant, by site
  - unspecified site C56.9
- papillary
  - mucinous
    - specified site — *see* Neoplasm, malignant, by site
    - unspecified site C56.9
  - pseudomucinous
    - specified site — *see* Neoplasm, malignant, by site
    - unspecified site C56.9
  - serous
    - specified site — *see* Neoplasm, malignant, by site
    - unspecified site C56.9
  - specified site — *see* Neoplasm, malignant, by site
  - unspecified site C56.9
- pseudomucinous
  - papillary
    - specified site — *see* Neoplasm, malignant, by site
    - unspecified site C56.9
  - specified site — *see* Neoplasm, malignant, by site
  - unspecified site C56.9
- serous
  - papillary
    - specified site — *see* Neoplasm, malignant, by site
    - unspecified site C56.9
  - specified site — *see* Neoplasm, malignant, by site
  - unspecified site C56.9

Cystadenofibroma
- clear cell — *see* Neoplasm, benign, by site
- endometrioid D27.9

Cystadenofibroma — *continued*
  endometrioid — *continued*
    borderline malignancy D39.1- ☑
    malignant C56.- ☑
  mucinous
    specified site — *see* Neoplasm, benign, by site
    unspecified site D27.9
  serous
    specified site — *see* Neoplasm, benign, by site
    unspecified site D27.9
  specified site — *see* Neoplasm, benign, by site
  unspecified site D27.9
Cystadenoma (*see also* Neoplasm, benign, by site)
  bile duct D13.4
  endometrioid — *see* Neoplasm, benign, by site
    borderline malignancy — *see* Neoplasm, uncertain
        behavior, by site
  malignant — *see* Neoplasm, malignant, by site
  mucinous
    borderline malignancy
      ovary C56.- ☑
      specified site NEC — *see* Neoplasm, uncertain
          behavior, by site
      unspecified site C56.9
    papillary
      borderline malignancy
        ovary C56.- ☑
        specified site NEC — *see* Neoplasm, uncer-
            tain behavior, by site
        unspecified site C56.9
      specified site — *see* Neoplasm, benign, by site
      unspecified site D27.9
    specified site — *see* Neoplasm, benign, by site
    unspecified site D27.9
  papillary
    borderline malignancy
      ovary C56.- ☑
      specified site NEC — *see* Neoplasm, uncertain
          behavior, by site
      unspecified site C56.9
    lymphomatosum
      specified site — *see* Neoplasm, benign, by site
      unspecified site D11.9
    mucinous
      borderline malignancy
        ovary C56.- ☑
        specified site NEC — *see* Neoplasm, uncer-
            tain behavior, by site
        unspecified site C56.9
      specified site — *see* Neoplasm, benign, by site
      unspecified site D27.9
    pseudomucinous
      borderline malignancy
        ovary C56.- ☑
        specified site NEC — *see* Neoplasm, uncer-
            tain behavior, by site
        unspecified site C56.9
      specified site — *see* Neoplasm, benign, by site
      unspecified site D27.9
    serous
      borderline malignancy
        ovary C56.- ☑
        specified site NEC — *see* Neoplasm, uncer-
            tain behavior, by site
        unspecified site C56.9
      specified site — *see* Neoplasm, benign, by site
      unspecified site D27.9
    specified site — *see* Neoplasm, benign, by site
    unspecified site D27.9
  pseudomucinous
    borderline malignancy
      ovary C56.- ☑
      specified site NEC — *see* Neoplasm, uncertain
          behavior, by site
      unspecified site C56.9
    papillary
      borderline malignancy
        ovary C56.- ☑
        specified site NEC — *see* Neoplasm, uncer-
            tain behavior, by site
        unspecified site C56.9
      specified site — *see* Neoplasm, benign, by site
      unspecified site D27.9
    specified site — *see* Neoplasm, benign, by site

Cystadenoma — *continued*
  pseudomucinous — *continued*
    unspecified site D27.9
  serous
    borderline malignancy
      ovary C56.- ☑
      specified site NEC — *see* Neoplasm, uncertain
          behavior, by site
      unspecified site C56.9
    papillary
      borderline malignancy
        ovary C56.- ☑
        specified site NEC — *see* Neoplasm, uncer-
            tain behavior, by site
        unspecified site C56.9
      specified site — *see* Neoplasm, benign, by site
      unspecified site D27.9
    specified site — *see* Neoplasm, benign, by site
    unspecified site D27.9
Cystathionine synthase deficiency E72.11
Cystathioninemia E72.19
Cystathioninuria E72.19
Cystic (*see also* condition)
  breast (chronic) — *see* Mastopathy, cystic
  corpora lutea (hemorrhagic) N83.1
  duct — *see* condition
  eyeball (congenital) Q11.0
  fibrosis — *see* Fibrosis, cystic
  kidney (congenital) Q61.9
    adult type Q61.2
    infantile type NEC Q61.19
      collecting duct dilatation Q61.11
    medullary Q61.5
  liver, congenital Q44.6
  lung disease J98.4
    congenital Q33.0
  mastitis, chronic — *see* Mastopathy, cystic
  medullary, kidney Q61.5
  meniscus — *see* Derangement, knee, meniscus, cystic
  ovary N83.20
Cysticercosis, cysticerciasis B69.9
  with
    epileptiform fits B69.0
    myositis B69.81
  brain B69.0
  central nervous system B69.0
  cerebral B69.0
  ocular B69.1
  specified NEC B69.89
Cysticercus cellulose infestation — *see* Cysticercosis
Cystinosis (malignant) E72.04
Cystinuria E72.01
Cystitis (exudative) (hemorrhagic) (septic) (suppurative)
      N30.90
  with
    fibrosis — *see* Cystitis, chronic, interstitial
    hematuria N30.91
    leukoplakia — *see* Cystitis, chronic, interstitial
    malakoplakia — *see* Cystitis, chronic, interstitial
    metaplasia — *see* Cystitis, chronic, interstitial
    prostatitis N41.3
  acute N30.00
    with hematuria N30.01
    of trigone N30.30
      with hematuria N30.31
  allergic — *see* Cystitis, specified type NEC
  amebic A06.81
  bilharzial B65.9 [N33]
  blennorrhagic (gonococcal) A54.01
  bullous — *see* Cystitis, specified type NEC
  calculous N21.0
  chlamydial A56.01
  chronic N30.20
    with hematuria N30.21
    interstitial N30.10
      with hematuria N30.11
    of trigone N30.30
      with hematuria N30.31
    specified NEC N30.20
      with hematuria N30.21
  cystic (a) — *see* Cystitis, specified type NEC
  diphtheritic A36.85
  echinococcal
    granulosus B67.39

Cystitis — *continued*
  echinococcal — *continued*
    multilocularis B67.69
  emphysematous — *see* Cystitis, specified type NEC
  encysted — *see* Cystitis, specified type NEC
  eosinophilic — *see* Cystitis, specified type NEC
  follicular — *see* Cystitis, of trigone
  gangrenous — *see* Cystitis, specified type NEC
  glandularis — *see* Cystitis, specified type NEC
  gonococcal A54.01
  incrusted — *see* Cystitis, specified type NEC
  interstitial (chronic) — *see* Cystitis, chronic, interstitial
  irradiation N30.40
    with hematuria N30.41
  irritation — *see* Cystitis, specified type NEC
  malignant — *see* Cystitis, specified type NEC
  of trigone N30.30
    with hematuria N30.31
  panmural — *see* Cystitis, chronic, interstitial
  polyposa — *see* Cystitis, specified type NEC
  prostatic N41.3
  puerperal (postpartum) O86.22
  radiation — *see* Cystitis, irradiation
  specified type NEC N30.80
    with hematuria N30.81
  subacute — *see* Cystitis, chronic
  submucous — *see* Cystitis, chronic, interstitial
  syphilitic (late) A52.76
  trichomonal A59.03
  tuberculous A18.12
  ulcerative — *see* Cystitis, chronic, interstitial
Cystocele (-urethrocele)
  female N81.10
    with prolapse of uterus — *see* Prolapse, uterus
    lateral N81.12
    midline N81.11
    paravaginal N81.12
  in pregnancy or childbirth O34.8- ☑
    causing obstructed labor O65.5
  male N32.89
Cystolithiasis N21.0
Cystoma (*see also* Neoplasm, benign, by site)
  endometrial, ovary N80.1
  mucinous
    specified site — *see* Neoplasm, benign, by site
    unspecified site D27.9
  serous
    specified site — *see* Neoplasm, benign, by site
    unspecified site D27.9
  simple (ovary) N83.29
Cystoplegia N31.2
Cystoptosis N32.89
Cystopyelitis — *see* Pyelonephritis
Cystorrhagia N32.89
Cystosarcoma phyllodes D48.6- ☑
  benign D24- ☑
  malignant — *see* Neoplasm, breast, malignant
Cystostomy
  attention to Z43.5
  complication — *see* Complications, cystostomy
  status Z93.50
    appendico-vesicostomy Z93.52
    cutaneous Z93.51
    specified NEC Z93.59
Cystourethritis — *see* Urethritis
Cystourethrocele (*see also* Cystocele)
  female N81.10
    with uterine prolapse — *see* Prolapse, uterus
    lateral N81.12
    midline N81.11
    paravaginal N81.12
  male N32.89
Cytomegalic inclusion disease
  congenital P35.1
Cytomegalovirus infection B25.9
Cytomycosis (reticuloendothelial) B39.4
Cytopenia D75.9
  refractory
    with multilineage dysplasia D46.A (*following* D46.2)
      and ring sideroblasts (RCMD RS) D46.B (*follow-
        ing* D46.2)
Czerny's disease (periodic hydrarthrosis of the knee) —
      see Effusion, joint, knee

D

Da Costa's syndrome F45.8
Daae (-Finsen) **disease** (epidemic pleurodynia) B33.0
Dabney's grip B33.0
Dacryoadenitis, dacryadenitis H04.00- ☑
  acute H04.01- ☑
  chronic H04.02- ☑
Dacryocystitis H04.30- ☑
  acute H04.32- ☑
  chronic H04.41- ☑
  neonatal P39.1
  phlegmonous H04.31- ☑
  syphilitic A52.71
    congenital (early) A50.01
  trachomatous, active A71.1
    sequelae (late effect) B94.0
Dacryocystoblenorrhea — see Inflammation, lacrimal, passages, chronic
Dacryocystocele — see Disorder, lacrimal system, changes
Dacryolith, dacryolithiasis H04.51- ☑
Dacryoma — see Disorder, lacrimal system, changes
Dacryopericystitis — see Dacryocystitis
Dacryops H04.11- ☑
Dacryostenosis (see also Stenosis, lacrimal)
  congenital Q10.5
Dactylitis
  bone — see Osteomyelitis
  sickle-cell D57.00
    Hb C D57.219
    Hb SS D57.00
    specified NEC D57.819
  skin L08.9
  syphilitic A52.77
  tuberculous A18.03
Dactylolysis spontanea (ainhum) L94.6
Dactylosymphysis Q70.9
  fingers — see Syndactylism, complex, fingers
  toes — see Syndactylism, complex, toes
Damage
  arteriosclerotic — see Arteriosclerosis
  brain (nontraumatic) G93.9
    anoxic, hypoxic G93.1
      resulting from a procedure G97.82
    child NEC G80.9
    due to birth injury P11.2
  cardiorenal (vascular) — see Hypertension, cardiorenal
  cerebral NEC — see Damage, brain
  coccyx, complicating delivery O71.6
  coronary — see Disease, heart, ischemic
  eye, birth injury P15.3
  liver (nontraumatic) K76.9
    alcoholic K70.9
    due to drugs — see Disease, liver, toxic
    toxic — see Disease, liver, toxic
  medication T88.7 ☑
  pelvic
    joint or ligament, during delivery O71.6
    organ NEC
      during delivery O71.5
      following ectopic or molar pregnancy O08.6
  renal — see Disease, renal
  subendocardium, subendocardial — see Degeneration, myocardial
  vascular I99.9
Dana-Putnam syndrome (subacute combined sclerosis with pernicious anemia) — see Degeneration, combined
Danbolt (-Cross) **syndrome** (acrodermatitis enteropathica) E83.2
Dandruff L21.0
Dandy-Walker syndrome Q03.1
  with spina bifida — see Spina bifida
Danlos' syndrome Q79.6
Darier (-White) **disease** (congenital) Q82.8
  meaning erythema annulare centrifugum L53.1
Darier-Roussy sarcoid D86.3
Darling's disease or histoplasmosis B39.4
Darwin's tubercle Q17.8

Dawson's (inclusion body) **encephalitis** A81.1
De Beurmann (-Gougerot) **disease** B42.1
De la Tourette's syndrome F95.2
De Lange's syndrome Q87.1
De Morgan's spots (senile angiomas) I78.1
De Quervain's
  disease (tendon sheath) M65.4
  syndrome E34.51
  thyroiditis (subacute granulomatous thyroiditis) E06.1
De Toni-Fanconi (-Debré) **syndrome** E72.09
  with cystinosis E72.04
Dead
  fetus, retained (mother) O36.4 ☑
    early pregnancy O02.1
  labyrinth H83.2 ☑
  ovum, retained O02.0
Deaf nonspeaking NEC H91.3
Deafmutism (acquired) (congenital) NEC H91.3
  hysterical F44.6
  syphilitic, congenital (see also subcategory) H94.8 A50.09
Deafness (acquired) (complete) (hereditary) (partial) H91.9- ☑
  with blue sclera and fragility of bone Q78.0
  auditory fatigue — see Deafness, specified type NEC
  aviation T70.0 ☑
    nerve injury — see Injury, nerve, acoustic, specified type NEC
  boilermaker's H83.3 ☑
  central — see Deafness, sensorineural
  conductive H90.2
    and sensorineural, mixed H90.8
      bilateral H90.6
    bilateral H90.0
    unilateral H90.1- ☑
  congenital H90.5
    with blue sclera and fragility of bone Q78.0
  due to toxic agents — see Deafness, ototoxic
  emotional (hysterical) F44.6
  functional (hysterical) F44.6
  high frequency H91.9- ☑
  hysterical F44.6
  low frequency H91.9- ☑
  mental R48.8
  mixed conductive and sensorineural H90.8
    bilateral H90.6
    unilateral H90.7- ☑
  nerve — see Deafness, sensorineural
  neural — see Deafness, sensorineural
  noise-induced (see also subcategory) H83.3 ☑
    nerve injury — see Injury, nerve, acoustic, specified type NEC
  nonspeaking H91.3
  ototoxic H91.0 ☑
  perceptive — see Deafness, sensorineural
  psychogenic (hysterical) F44.6
  sensorineural H90.5
    and conductive, mixed H90.8
      bilateral H90.6
    bilateral H90.3
    unilateral H90.4- ☑
  sensory — see Deafness, sensorineural
  specified type NEC H91.8 ☑
  sudden (idiopathic) H91.2- ☑
  syphilitic A52.15
  transient ischemic H93.01- ☑
  traumatic — see Injury, nerve, acoustic, specified type NEC
  word (developmental) H93.25
Death (cause unknown) (of) (unexplained) (unspecified cause) R99
  brain G93.82
  cardiac (sudden) (with successful resuscitation) — code to underlying disease
    family history of Z82.41
    personal history of Z86.74
  family member (assumed) Z63.4
Debility (chronic) (general) (nervous) R53.81
  congenital or neonatal NOS P96.9
  nervous R53.81
  old age R54
  senile R54

Débove's disease (splenomegaly) R16.1
Decalcification
  bone — see Osteoporosis
  teeth K03.89
Decapsulation, kidney N28.89
Decay
  dental — see Caries, dental
  senile R54
  tooth, teeth — see Caries, dental
Deciduitis (acute)
  following ectopic or molar pregnancy O08.0
Decline (general) — see Debility
  cognitive, age-associated R41.81
Decompensation
  cardiac (acute) (chronic) — see Disease, heart
  cardiovascular — see Disease, cardiovascular
  heart — see Disease, heart
  hepatic — see Failure, hepatic
  myocardial (acute) (chronic) — see Disease, heart
  respiratory J98.8
Decompression sickness T70.3 ☑
Decrease (d)
  absolute neutrophile count — see Neutropenia
  blood
    platelets — see Thrombocytopenia
    pressure R03.1
      due to shock following
        injury T79.4 ☑
        operation T81.19 ☑
  estrogen E28.39
    postablative E89.40
      asymptomatic E89.40
      symptomatic E89.41
  fragility of erythrocytes D58.8
  function
    lipase (pancreatic) K90.3
    ovary in hypopituitarism E23.0
    parenchyma of pancreas K86.8
    pituitary (gland) (anterior) (lobe) E23.0
      posterior (lobe) E23.0
  functional activity R68.89
  glucose R73.09
  hematocrit R71.0
  hemoglobin R71.0
  leukocytes D72.819
    specified NEC D72.818
  libido R68.82
  lymphocytes D72.810
  platelets D69.6
  respiration, due to shock following injury T79.4 ☑
  sexual desire R68.82
  tear secretion NEC — see Syndrome, dry eye
  tolerance
    fat K90.4
    glucose R73.09
    pancreatic K90.3
    salt and water E87.8
  vision NEC H54.7
  white blood cell count D72.819
    specified NEC D72.818
Decubitus (ulcer) — see Ulcer, pressure, by site
  cervix N86
Deepening acetabulum — see Derangement, joint, specified type NEC, hip
Defect, defective Q89.9
  3-beta-hydroxysteroid dehydrogenase E25.0
  11-hydroxylase E25.0
  21-hydroxylase E25.0
  abdominal wall, congenital Q79.59
  antibody immunodeficiency D80.9
  aorticopulmonary septum Q21.4
  atrial septal (ostium secundum type) Q21.1
    following acute myocardial infarction (current complication) I23.1
    ostium primum type Q21.2
  atrioventricular
    canal Q21.2
    septum Q21.2
  auricular septal Q21.1
  bilirubin excretion NEC E80.6
  biosynthesis, androgen (testicular) E29.1
  bulbar septum Q21.0

☑ **Additional Character Required** — Refer to the Tabular List for Character Selection

▽ **Subterms under main terms may continue to next column or page**

Defect, defective — *continued*
catalase E80.3
cell membrane receptor complex (CR3) D71
circulation I99.9
  congenital Q28.9
  newborn Q28.9
coagulation (factor) (*see also* Deficiency, factor) D68.9
  with
    ectopic pregnancy O08.1
    molar pregnancy O08.1
  acquired D68.4
  antepartum with hemorrhage — *see* Hemorrhage, antepartum, with coagulation defect
  due to
    liver disease D68.4
    vitamin K deficiency D68.4
  hereditary NEC D68.2
  intrapartum O67.0
  newborn, transient P61.6
  postpartum O72.3
  specified type NEC D68.8
complement system D84.1
conduction (heart) I45.9
  bone — *see* Deafness, conductive
congenital, organ or site not listed — *see* Anomaly, by site
coronary sinus Q21.1
cushion, endocardial Q21.2
degradation, glycoprotein E77.1
dental bridge, crown, fillings — *see* Defect, dental restoration
dental restoration K08.50
  specified NEC K08.59
dentin (hereditary) K00.5
Descemet's membrane, congenital Q13.89
developmental (*see also* Anomaly)
  cauda equina Q06.3
diaphragm
  with elevation, eventration or hernia — *see* Hernia, diaphragm
  congenital Q79.1
    with hernia Q79.0
    gross (with hernia) Q79.0
ectodermal, congenital Q82.9
Eisenmenger's Q21.8
enzyme
  catalase E80.3
  peroxidase E80.3
esophagus, congenital Q39.9
extensor retinaculum M62.89
fibrin polymerization D68.2
filling
  bladder R93.4
  kidney R93.4
  stomach R93.3
  ureter R93.4
Gerbode Q21.0
glycoprotein degradation E77.1
Hageman (factor) D68.2
hearing — *see* Deafness
high grade F70
interatrial septal Q21.1
interauricular septal Q21.1
interventricular septal Q21.0
  with dextroposition of aorta, pulmonary stenosis and hypertrophy of right ventricle Q21.3
  in tetralogy of Fallot Q21.3
learning (specific) — *see* Disorder, learning
lymphocyte function antigen-1 (LFA-1) D84.0
lysosomal enzyme, post-translational modification E77.0
major osseous M89.70
  ankle M89.77- ☑
  carpus M89.74- ☑
  clavicle M89.71- ☑
  femur M89.75- ☑
  fibula M89.76- ☑
  fingers M89.74- ☑
  foot M89.77- ☑
  forearm M89.73- ☑
  hand M89.74- ☑
  humerus M89.72- ☑
  lower leg M89.76- ☑
  metacarpus M89.74- ☑
  metatarsus M89.77- ☑
  multiple sites M89.79
  pelvic region M89.75- ☑
  pelvis M89.75- ☑

Defect, defective — *continued*
major osseous — *continued*
  radius M89.73- ☑
  scapula M89.71- ☑
  shoulder region M89.71- ☑
  specified NEC M89.78
  tarsus M89.77- ☑
  thigh M89.75- ☑
  tibia M89.76- ☑
  toes M89.77- ☑
  ulna M89.73- ☑
mental — *see* Disability, intellectual
modification, lysosomal enzymes, post-translational E77.0
obstructive, congenital
  renal pelvis Q62.39
  ureter Q62.39
    atresia — *see* Atresia, ureter
    cecoureterocele Q62.32
    megaureter Q62.2
    orthotopic ureterocele Q62.31
osseous, major M89.70
  ankle M89.77- ☑
  carpus M89.74- ☑
  clavicle M89.71- ☑
  femur M89.75- ☑
  fibula M89.76- ☑
  fingers M89.74- ☑
  foot M89.77- ☑
  forearm M89.73- ☑
  hand M89.74- ☑
  humerus M89.72- ☑
  lower leg M89.76- ☑
  metacarpus M89.74- ☑
  metatarsus M89.77- ☑
  multiple sites M89.9
  pelvic region M89.75- ☑
  pelvis M89.75- ☑
  radius M89.73- ☑
  scapula M89.71- ☑
  shoulder region M89.71- ☑
  specified NEC M89.78
  tarsus M89.77- ☑
  thigh M89.75- ☑
  tibia M89.76- ☑
  toes M89.77- ☑
  ulna M89.73- ☑
osteochondral NEC (*see also* Deformity) M95.8
ostium
  primum Q21.2
  secundum Q21.1
peroxidase E80.3
placental blood supply — *see* Insufficiency, placental
platelets, qualitative D69.1
  constitutional D68.0
postural NEC, spine — *see* Dorsopathy, deforming
reduction
  limb Q73.8
    lower Q72.9- ☑
      absence — *see* Agenesis, leg
        foot — *see* Agenesis, foot
      longitudinal
        femur Q72.4- ☑
        fibula Q72.6- ☑
        tibia Q72.5- ☑
      specified type NEC Q72.89- ☑
      split foot Q72.7- ☑
    specified type NEC Q73.8
    upper Q71.9- ☑
      absence — *see* Agenesis, arm
        forearm — *see* Agenesis, forearm
        hand — *see* Agenesis, hand
      lobster-claw hand Q71.6- ☑
      longitudinal
        radius Q71.4- ☑
        ulna Q71.5- ☑
      specified type NEC Q71.89- ☑
renal pelvis Q63.8
  obstructive Q62.39
respiratory system, congenital Q34.9
restoration, dental K08.50
  specified NEC K08.59
retinal nerve bundle fibers H35.89
septal (heart) NOS Q21.9
  acquired (atrial) (auricular) (ventricular) (old) I51.0
  atrial Q21.1

Defect, defective — *continued*
septal — *continued*
  atrial — *continued*
    concurrent with acute myocardial infarction — *see* Infarct, myocardium
    following acute myocardial infarction (current complication) I23.1
    ventricular (*see also* Defect, ventricular septal) Q21.0
sinus venosus Q21.1
speech R47.9
  developmental F80.9
  specified NEC R47.89
Taussig-Bing (aortic transposition and overriding pulmonary artery) Q20.1
teeth, wedge K03.1
vascular (local) I99.9
  congenital Q27.9
ventricular septal Q21.0
  concurrent with acute myocardial infarction — *see* Infarct, myocardium
  following acute myocardial infarction (current complication) I23.2
  in tetralogy of Fallot Q21.3
vision NEC H54.7
visual field H53.40
  bilateral
    heteronymous H53.47
    homonymous H53.46- ☑
  generalized contraction H53.48- ☑
  localized
    arcuate H53.43- ☑
    scotoma (central area) H53.41- ☑
      blind spot area H53.42- ☑
    sector H53.43- ☑
    specified type NEC H53.45- ☑
voice R49.9
  specified NEC R49.8
wedge, tooth, teeth (abrasion) K03.1

Deferentitis N49.1
gonorrheal (acute) (chronic) A54.23
Defibrination (syndrome) D65
antepartum — *see* Hemorrhage, antepartum, with coagulation defect, disseminated intravascular coagulation
following ectopic or molar pregnancy O08.1
intrapartum O67.0
newborn P60
postpartum O72.3

Deficiency, deficient
3-beta hydroxysteroid dehydrogenase E25.0
5-alpha reductase (with male pseudo-hermaphroditism) E29.1
11-hydroxylase E25.0
21-hydroxylase E25.0
abdominal muscle syndrome Q79.4
AC globulin (congenital) (hereditary) D68.2
  acquired D68.4
accelerator globulin (Ac G) (blood) D68.2
acid phosphatase E83.39
activating factor (blood) D68.2
adenosine deaminase (ADA) D81.3
aldolase (hereditary) E74.19
alpha-1-antitrypsin E88.01
amino-acids E72.9
anemia — *see* Anemia
aneurin E51.9
antibody with
  hyperimmunoglobulinemia D80.6
  near-normal immunoglobins D80.6
antidiuretic hormone E23.2
anti-hemophilic
  factor (A) D66
    B D67
    C D68.1
  globulin (AHG) NEC D66
antithrombin (antithrombin III) D68.59
ascorbic acid E54
attention (disorder) (syndrome) F98.8
  with hyperactivity — *see* Disorder, attention-deficit hyperactivity
autoprothrombin
  C D68.2
  I D68.2
  II D67
beta-glucuronidase E76.29
biotin E53.8
biotin-dependent carboxylase D81.819

☑ Subterms under main terms may continue to next column or page   ☑ Additional Character Required — Refer to the Tabular List for Character Selection   81

Defect, defective — Deficiency, deficient

Deficiency, deficient — *continued*
- biotinidase D81.810
- brancher enzyme (amylopectinosis) E74.03
- C1 esterase inhibitor (C1-INH) D84.1
- calciferol E55.9
  - with
    - adult osteomalacia M83.8
    - rickets — *see* Rickets
- calcium (dietary) E58
- calorie, severe E43
  - with marasmus E41
    - and kwashiorkor E42
- cardiac — *see* Insufficiency, myocardial
- carnitine E71.40
  - due to
    - hemodialysis E71.43
    - inborn errors of metabolism E71.42
    - Valproic acid therapy E71.43
  - iatrogenic E71.43
  - muscle palmityltransferase E71.314
  - primary E71.41
  - secondary E71.448
- carotene E50.9
- central nervous system G96.8
- ceruloplasmin (Wilson) E83.01
- choline E53.8
- Christmas factor D67
- chromium E61.4
- clotting (blood) (*see also* Deficiency, coagulation factor) D68.9
- clotting factor NEC (hereditary) (*see also* Deficiency, factor) D68.2
- coagulation NOS D68.9
  - with
    - ectopic pregnancy O08.1
    - molar pregnancy O08.1
  - acquired (any) D68.4
  - antepartum hemorrhage — *see* Hemorrhage, antepartum, with coagulation defect
  - clotting factor NEC (*see also* Deficiency, factor) D68.2
  - due to
    - hyperprothrombinemia D68.4
    - liver disease D68.4
    - vitamin K deficiency D68.4
  - newborn, transient P61.6
  - postpartum O72.3
  - specified NEC D68.8
- cognitive F09
- color vision H53.50
  - achromatopsia H53.51
  - acquired H53.52
  - deuteranomaly H53.53
  - protanomaly H53.54
  - specified type NEC H53.59
  - tritanomaly H53.55
- combined glucocorticoid and mineralocorticoid E27.49
- contact factor D68.2
- copper (nutritional) E61.0
- corticoadrenal E27.40
  - primary E27.1
- craniofacial axis Q75.0
- cyanocobalamin E53.8
- debrancher enzyme (limit dextrinosis) E74.03
- dehydrogenase
  - long chain/very long chain acyl CoA E71.310
  - medium chain acyl CoA E71.311
  - short chain acyl CoA E71.312
- diet E63.9
- dihydropyrimidine dehydrogenase (DPD) E88.89
- disaccharidase E73.9
- edema — *see* Malnutrition, severe
- endocrine E34.9
- energy-supply — *see* Malnutrition
- enzymes, circulating NEC E88.09
- ergosterol E55.9
  - with
    - adult osteomalacia M83.8
    - rickets — *see* Rickets
- essential fatty acid (EFA) E63.0
- factor (*see also* Deficiency, coagulation)
  - Hageman D68.2
  - I (congenital) (hereditary) D68.2
  - II (congenital) (hereditary) D68.2
  - IX (congenital) (functional) (hereditary) (with functional defect) D67
  - multiple (congenital) D68.8
    - acquired D68.4

Deficiency, deficient — *continued*
- factor (*see also* Deficiency, coagulation) — *continued*
  - V (congenital) (hereditary) D68.2
  - VII (congenital) (hereditary) D68.2
  - VIII (congenital) (functional) (hereditary) (with functional defect) D66
    - with vascular defect D68.0
  - X (congenital) (hereditary) D68.2
  - XI (congenital) (hereditary) D68.1
  - XII (congenital) (hereditary) D68.2
  - XIII (congenital) (hereditary) D68.2
- femoral, proximal focal (congenital) — *see* Defect, reduction, lower limb, longitudinal, femur
- fibrinase D68.2
- fibrinogen (congenital) (hereditary) D68.2
  - acquired D65
- fibrin-stabilizing factor (congenital) (hereditary) D68.2
  - acquired D68.4
- folate E53.8
- folic acid E53.8
- foreskin N47.3
- fructokinase E74.11
- fructose 1,6-diphosphatase E74.19
- fructose-1-phosphate aldolase E74.19
- galactokinase E74.29
- galactose-1-phosphate uridyl transferase E74.29
- gammaglobulin in blood D80.1
  - hereditary D80.0
- glass factor D68.2
- glucocorticoid E27.49
  - mineralocorticoid E27.49
- glucose-6-phosphatase E74.01
- glucose-6-phosphate dehydrogenase anemia D55.0
- glucuronyl transferase E80.5
- glycogen synthetase E74.09
- gonadotropin (isolated) E23.0
- growth hormone (idiopathic) (isolated) E23.0
- Hageman factor D68.2
- hemoglobin D64.9
- hepatophosphorylase E74.09
- homogentisate 1,2-dioxygenase E70.29
- hormone
  - anterior pituitary (partial) NEC E23.0
    - growth E23.0
  - growth (isolated) E23.0
  - pituitary E23.0
  - testicular E29.1
- hypoxanthine- (guanine)-phosphoribosyltransferase (HG- PRT) (total H-PRT) E79.1
- immunity D84.9
  - cell-mediated D84.8
    - with thrombocytopenia and eczema D82.0
  - combined D81.9
  - humoral D80.9
  - IgA (secretory) D80.2
  - IgG D80.3
  - IgM D80.4
- immuno — *see* Immunodeficiency
- immunoglobulin, selective
  - A (IgA) D80.2
  - G (IgG) (subclasses) D80.3
  - M (IgM) D80.4
- inositol (B complex) E53.8
- intrinsic
  - factor (congenital) D51.0
  - sphincter N36.42
    - with urethral hypermobility N36.43
- iodine E61.8
  - congenital syndrome — *see* Syndrome, iodine-deficiency, congenital
- iron E61.1
  - anemia D50.9
- kalium E87.6
- kappa-light chain D80.8
- labile factor (congenital) (hereditary) D68.2
  - acquired D68.4
- lacrimal fluid (acquired) (*see also* Syndrome, dry eye)
  - congenital Q10.6
- lactase
  - congenital E73.0
  - secondary E73.1
- Laki-Lorand factor D68.2
- lecithin cholesterol acyltransferase E78.6
- lipocaic K86.8
- lipoprotein (familial) (high density) E78.6
- liver phosphorylase E74.09
- lysosomal alpha-1, 4 glucosidase E74.02

Deficiency, deficient — *continued*
- magnesium E61.2
- major histocompatibility complex
  - class I D81.6
  - class II D81.7
- manganese E61.3
- menadione (vitamin K) E56.1
  - newborn P53
- mental (familial) (hereditary) — *see* Disability, intellectual
- methylenetetrahydrofolate reductase (MTHFR) E72.12
- mineralocorticoid E27.49
  - with glucocorticoid E27.49
- mineral NEC E61.8
- molybdenum (nutritional) E61.5
- moral F60.2
- multiple nutrient elements E61.7
- muscle
  - carnitine (palmityltransferase) E71.314
  - phosphofructokinase E74.09
- myoadenylate deaminase E79.2
- myocardial — *see* Insufficiency, myocardial
- myophosphorylase E74.04
- NADH diaphorase or reductase (congenital) D74.0
- NADH-methemoglobin reductase (congenital) D74.0
- natrium E87.1
- niacin (amide) (-tryptophan) E52
- nicotinamide E52
- nicotinic acid E52
- number of teeth — *see* Anodontia
- nutrient element E61.9
  - multiple E61.7
  - specified NEC E61.8
- nutrition, nutritional E63.9
  - sequelae — *see* Sequelae, nutritional deficiency
  - specified NEC E63.8
- ornithine transcarbamylase E72.4
- ovarian E28.39
- oxygen — *see* Anoxia
- pantothenic acid E53.8
- parathyroid (gland) E20.9
- perineum (female) N81.89
- phenylalanine hydroxylase E70.1
- phosphoenolpyruvate carboxykinase E74.4
- phosphofructokinase E74.19
- phosphomannomutuse E74.8
- phosphomannose isomerase E74.8
- phosphomannosyl mutase E74.8
- phosphorylase kinase, liver E74.09
- pituitary hormone (isolated) E23.0
- plasma thromboplastin
  - antecedent (PTA) D68.1
  - component (PTC) D67
- platelet NEC D69.1
  - constitutional D68.0
- polyglandular E31.8
  - autoimmune E31.0
- potassium (K) E87.6
- prepuce N47.3
- proaccelerin (congenital) (hereditary) D68.2
  - acquired D68.4
- proconvertin factor (congenital) (hereditary) D68.2
  - acquired D68.4
- protein (*see also* Malnutrition) E46
  - anemia D53.0
  - C D68.59
  - S D68.59
- prothrombin (congenital) (hereditary) D68.2
  - acquired D68.4
- Prower factor D68.2
- pseudocholinesterase E88.09
- PTA (plasma thromboplastin antecedent) D68.1
- PTC (plasma thromboplastin component) D67
- purine nucleoside phosphorylase (PNP) D81.5
- pyracin (alpha) (beta) E53.1
- pyridoxal E53.1
- pyridoxamine E53.1
- pyridoxine (derivatives) E53.1
- pyruvate
  - carboxylase E74.4
  - dehydrogenase E74.4
- riboflavin (vitamin B2) E53.0
- salt E87.1
- secretion
  - ovary E28.39
  - salivary gland (any) K11.7
  - urine R34
- selenium (dietary) E59

Deficiency, deficient — *continued*
serum antitrypsin, familial E88.01
short stature homeobox gene (SHOX)
   with
      dyschondrosteosis Q78.8
      short stature (idiopathic) E34.3
      Turner's syndrome Q96.9
sodium (Na) E87.1
SPCA (factor VII) D68.2
sphincter, intrinsic N36.42
   with urethral hypermobility N36.43
stable factor (congenital) (hereditary) D68.2
   acquired D68.4
Stuart-Prower (factor X) D68.2
sucrase E74.39
sulfatase E75.29
sulfite oxidase E72.19
thiamin, thiaminic (chloride) E51.9
   beriberi (dry) E51.11
      wet E51.12
thrombokinase D68.2
   newborn P53
thyroid (gland) — *see* Hypothyroidism
tocopherol E56.0
tooth bud K00.0
transcobalamine II (anemia) D51.2
vanadium E61.6
vascular I99.9
vasopressin E23.2
viosterol — *see* Deficiency, calciferol
vitamin (multiple) NOS E56.9
   A E50.9
      with
         Bitot's spot (corneal) E50.1
         follicular keratosis E50.8
         keratomalacia E50.4
         manifestations NEC E50.8
         night blindness E50.5
         scar of cornea, xerophthalmic E50.6
         xeroderma E50.8
         xerophthalmia E50.7
         xerosis
            conjunctival E50.0
               and Bitot's spot E50.1
            cornea E50.2
               and ulceration E50.3
      sequelae E64.1
   B (complex) NOS E53.9
      with
         beriberi (dry) E51.11
            wet E51.12
         pellagra E52
   B1 NOS E51.9
      beriberi (dry) E51.11
         with circulatory system manifestations
            E51.11
         wet E51.12
   B2 (riboflavin) E53.0
   B6 E53.1
   B12 E53.8
   C E54
      sequelae E64.2
   D E55.9
      with
         adult osteomalacia M83.8
         rickets — *see* Rickets
      25-hydroxylase E83.32
   E E56.0
   folic acid E53.8
   G E53.0
   group B E53.9
      specified NEC E53.8
   H (biotin) E53.8
   K E56.1
      of newborn P53
   nicotinic E52
   P E56.8
   PP (pellagra-preventing) E52
   specified NEC E56.8
   thiamin E51.9
      beriberi — *see* Beriberi
zinc, dietary E60
Deficit (*see also* Deficiency)
attention and concentration R41.840
   disorder — *see* Attention, deficit
cognitive communication R41.841
cognitive NEC R41.89

Deficit — *continued*
cognitive — *continued*
   following
      cerebral infarction I69.31
      cerebrovascular disease I69.91
         specified disease NEC I69.81
      intracerebral hemorrhage I69.11
      nontraumatic intracranial hemorrhage NEC
         I69.21
      subarachnoid hemorrhage I69.01
concentration R41.840
executive function R41.844
frontal lobe R41.844
neurologic NEC R29.818
   ischemic
      reversible (RIND) I63.9
         prolonged (PRIND) I63.9
oxygen R09.02
prolonged reversible ischemic neurologic (PRIND) I63.9
psychomotor R41.843
visuospatial R41.842
Deflection
radius — *see* Deformity, limb, specified type NEC,
   forearm
septum (acquired) (nasal) (nose) J34.2
spine — *see* Curvature, spine
turbinate (nose) J34.2
Defluvium
capillorum — *see* Alopecia
ciliorum — *see* Madarosis
unguium L60.8
Deformity Q89.9
abdomen, congenital Q89.9
abdominal wall
   acquired M95.8
   congenital Q79.59
acquired (unspecified site) M95.9
adrenal gland Q89.1
alimentary tract, congenital Q45.9
   upper Q40.9
ankle (joint) (acquired) (*see also* Deformity, limb, lower
   leg)
   abduction — *see* Contraction, joint, ankle
   congenital Q68.8
   contraction — *see* Contraction, joint, ankle
   specified type NEC — *see* Deformity, limb, foot,
      specified NEC
anus (acquired) K62.89
   congenital Q43.9
aorta (arch) (congenital) Q25.4
   acquired I77.89
aortic
   arch, acquired I77.89
   cusp or valve (congenital) Q23.8
      acquired (*see also* Endocarditis, aortic) I35.8
arm (acquired) (upper) (*see also* Deformity, limb, upper
   arm)
   congenital Q68.8
   forearm — *see* Deformity, limb, forearm
artery (congenital) (peripheral) NOS Q27.9
   acquired I77.89
   coronary (acquired) I25.9
      congenital Q24.5
   umbilical Q27.0
atrial septal Q21.1
auditory canal (external) (congenital) (*see also* Malformation, ear, external)
   acquired — *see* Disorder, ear, external, specified
      type NEC
auricle
   ear (congenital) (*see also* Malformation, ear, exter-
      nal)
      acquired — *see* Disorder, pinna, deformity
back — *see* Dorsopathy, deforming
bile duct (common) (congenital) (hepatic) Q44.5
   acquired K83.8
biliary duct or passage (congenital) Q44.5
   acquired K83.8
bladder (neck) (trigone) (sphincter) (acquired) N32.89
   congenital Q64.79
bone (acquired) NOS M95.9
   congenital Q79.9
   turbinate M95.0
brain (congenital) Q04.9
   acquired G93.89
   reduction Q04.3
breast (acquired) N64.89
   congenital Q83.9

Deformity — *continued*
breast — *continued*
   reconstructed N65.0
bronchus (congenital) Q32.4
   acquired NEC J98.09
bursa, congenital Q79.9
canaliculi (lacrimalis) (acquired) (*see also* Disorder,
   lacrimal system, changes)
   congenital Q10.6
canthus, acquired — *see* Disorder, eyelid, specified
   type NEC
capillary (acquired) I78.8
cardiovascular system, congenital Q28.9
caruncle, lacrimal (acquired) (*see also* Disorder,
   lacrimal system, changes)
   congenital Q10.6
cascade, stomach K31.2
cecum (congenital) Q43.9
   acquired K63.89
cerebral, acquired G93.89
   congenital Q04.9
cervix (uterus) (acquired) NEC N88.8
   congenital Q51.9
cheek (acquired) M95.2
   congenital Q18.9
chest (acquired) (wall) M95.4
   congenital Q67.8
   sequelae (late effect) of rickets E64.3
chin (acquired) M95.2
   congenital Q18.9
choroid (congenital) Q14.3
   acquired H31.8
   plexus Q07.8
      acquired G96.19
cicatricial — *see* Cicatrix
cilia, acquired — *see* Disorder, eyelid, specified type
   NEC
clavicle (acquired) M95.8
   congenital Q68.8
clitoris (congenital) Q52.6
   acquired N90.89
clubfoot — *see* Clubfoot
coccyx (acquired) — *see* subcategory M43.8 ☑
colon (congenital) Q43.9
   acquired K63.89
concha (ear), congenital (*see also* Malformation, ear,
   external)
   acquired — *see* Disorder, pinna, deformity
cornea (acquired) H18.70
   congenital Q13.4
   descemetocele — *see* Descemetocele
   ectasia — *see* Ectasia, cornea
   specified NEC H18.79- ☑
   staphyloma — *see* Staphyloma, cornea
coronary artery (acquired) I25.9
   congenital Q24.5
cranium (acquired) — *see* Deformity, skull
cricoid cartilage (congenital) Q31.8
   acquired J38.7
cystic duct (congenital) Q44.5
   acquired K82.8
Dandy-Walker Q03.1
   with spina bifida — *see* Spina bifida
diaphragm (congenital) Q79.1
   acquired J98.6
digestive organ NOS Q45.9
ductus arteriosus Q25.0
duodenal bulb K31.89
duodenum (congenital) Q43.9
   acquired K31.89
dura — *see* Deformity, meninges
ear (acquired) (*see also* Disorder, pinna, deformity)
   congenital (external) Q17.9
      internal Q16.5
      middle Q16.4
         ossicles Q16.3
      ossicles Q16.3
ectodermal (congenital) NEC Q84.9
ejaculatory duct (congenital) Q55.4
   acquired N50.8
elbow (joint) (acquired) (*see also* Deformity, limb, upper arm)
   congenital Q68.8
   contraction — *see* Contraction, joint, elbow
endocrine gland NEC Q89.2
epididymis (congenital) Q55.4
   acquired N50.8
epiglottis (congenital) Q31.8

Deformity — continued

epiglottis — continued
  acquired J38.7
esophagus (congenital) Q39.9
  acquired K22.8
eustachian tube (congenital) NEC Q17.8
eye, congenital Q15.9
eyebrow (congenital) Q18.8
eyelid (acquired) (<i>see also</i> Disorder, eyelid, specified type NEC)
  congenital Q10.3
face (acquired) M95.2
  congenital Q18.9
fallopian tube, acquired N83.8
femur (acquired) — see Deformity, limb, specified type NEC, thigh
fetal
  with fetopelvic disproportion O33.7
    causing obstructed labor O66.3
finger (acquired) M20.00- ☑
  boutonniere M20.02- ☑
  congenital Q68.1
  flexion contracture — see Contraction, joint, hand
  mallet finger M20.01- ☑
  specified NEC M20.09- ☑
  swan-neck M20.03- ☑
flexion (joint) (acquired) (see also Deformity, limb, flexion) M21.20
  congenital NOS Q74.9
    hip Q65.89
foot (acquired) (see also Deformity, limb, lower leg)
  cavovarus (congenital) Q66.1
  congenital NOS Q66.9
    specified type NEC Q66.89
  specified type NEC — see Deformity, limb, foot, specified NEC
  valgus (congenital) Q66.6
    acquired — see Deformity, valgus, ankle
  varus (congenital) NEC Q66.3
    acquired — see Deformity, varus, ankle
forearm (acquired) (see also Deformity, limb, forearm)
  congenital Q68.8
forehead (acquired) M95.2
  congenital Q75.8
frontal bone (acquired) M95.2
  congenital Q75.8
gallbladder (congenital) Q44.1
  acquired K82.8
gastrointestinal tract (congenital) NOS Q45.9
  acquired K63.89
genitalia, genital organ(s) or system NEC
  female (congenital) Q52.9
    acquired N94.89
    external Q52.70
  male (congenital) Q55.9
    acquired N50.8
globe (eye) (congenital) Q15.8
  acquired H44.89
gum, acquired NEC K06.8
hand (acquired) — see Deformity, limb, hand
  congenital Q68.1
head (acquired) M95.2
  congenital Q75.8
heart (congenital) Q24.9
  septum Q21.9
    auricular Q21.1
    ventricular Q21.0
  valve (congenital) NEC Q24.8
    acquired — see Endocarditis
heel (acquired) — see Deformity, foot
hepatic duct (congenital) Q44.5
  acquired K83.8
hip (joint) (acquired) (see also Deformity, limb, thigh)
  congenital Q65.9
  due to (previous) juvenile osteochondrosis — see Coxa, plana
  flexion — see Contraction, joint, hip
hourglass — see Contraction, hourglass
humerus (acquired) M21.82- ☑
  congenital Q74.0
hypophyseal (congenital) Q89.2
ileocecal (coil) (valve) (acquired) K63.89
  congenital Q43.9
ileum (congenital) Q43.9
  acquired K63.89
ilium (acquired) M95.5
  congenital Q74.2
integument (congenital) Q84.9

Deformity — continued

intervertebral cartilage or disc (acquired) — see Disorder, disc, specified NEC
intestine (large) (small) (congenital) NOS Q43.9
  acquired K63.89
intrinsic minus or plus (hand) — see Deformity, limb, specified type NEC, forearm
iris (acquired) H21.89
  congenital Q13.2
ischium (acquired) M95.5
  congenital Q74.2
jaw (acquired) (congenital) M26.9
joint (acquired) NEC M21.90
  congenital Q68.8
  elbow M21.92- ☑
  hand M21.94- ☑
  hip M21.95- ☑
  knee M21.96- ☑
  shoulder M21.92- ☑
  wrist M21.93- ☑
kidney(s) (calyx) (pelvis) (congenital) Q63.9
  acquired N28.89
  artery (congenital) Q27.2
    acquired I77.89
Klippel-Feil (brevicollis) Q76.1
knee (acquired) NEC (see also Deformity, limb, lower leg)
  congenital Q68.2
labium (majus) (minus) (congenital) Q52.79
  acquired N90.89
lacrimal passages or duct (congenital) NEC Q10.6
  acquired — see Disorder, lacrimal system, changes
larynx (muscle) (congenital) Q31.8
  acquired J38.7
  web (glottic) Q31.0
leg (upper) (acquired) NEC (see also Deformity, limb, thigh)
  congenital Q68.8
  lower leg — see Deformity, limb, lower leg
lens (acquired) H27.8
  congenital Q12.9
lid (fold) (acquired) (see also Disorder, eyelid, specified type NEC)
  congenital Q10.3
ligament (acquired) — see Disorder, ligament
  congenital Q79.9
limb (acquired) M21.90
  clawfoot M21.53- ☑
  clawhand M21.51- ☑
  clubfoot M21.54- ☑
  clubhand M21.52- ☑
  congenital, except reduction deformity Q74.9
  flat foot M21.4- ☑
  flexion M21.20
    ankle M21.27- ☑
    elbow M21.22- ☑
    finger M21.24- ☑
    hip M21.25- ☑
    knee M21.26- ☑
    shoulder M21.21- ☑
    toe M21.27- ☑
    wrist M21.23- ☑
  foot
    claw — see Deformity, limb, clawfoot
    club — see Deformity, limb, clubfoot
    drop M21.37- ☑
    flat — see Deformity, limb, flat foot
    specified NEC M21.6X- ☑
  forearm M21.93- ☑
  hand M21.94- ☑
  lower leg M21.96- ☑
  specified type NEC M21.80
    forearm M21.83- ☑
    lower leg M21.86- ☑
    thigh M21.85- ☑
    upper arm M21.82- ☑
  thigh M21.95- ☑
  unequal length M21.70
    short site is
      femur M21.75- ☑
      fibula M21.76- ☑
      humerus M21.72- ☑
      radius M21.73- ☑
      tibia M21.76- ☑
      ulna M21.73- ☑
  upper arm M21.92- ☑
  valgus — see Deformity, valgus

Deformity — continued

limb — continued
  varus — see Deformity, varus
  wrist drop M21.33- ☑
lip (acquired) NEC K13.0
  congenital Q38.0
liver (congenital) Q44.7
  acquired K76.89
lumbosacral (congenital) (joint) (region) Q76.49
  acquired — see subcategory M43.8 ☑
  kyphosis — see Kyphosis, congenital
  lordosis — see Lordosis, congenital
lung (congenital) Q33.9
  acquired J98.4
lymphatic system, congenital Q89.9
Madelung's (radius) Q74.0
mandible (acquired) (congenital) M26.9
maxilla (acquired) (congenital) M26.9
meninges or membrane (congenital) Q07.9
  cerebral Q04.8
    acquired G96.19
  spinal cord (congenital) G96.19
    acquired G96.19
metacarpus (acquired) — see Deformity, limb, forearm
  congenital Q74.0
metatarsus (acquired) — see Deformity, foot
  congenital Q66.9
middle ear (congenital) Q16.4
  ossicles Q16.3
mitral (leaflets) (valve) I05.8
  parachute Q23.2
  stenosis, congenital Q23.2
mouth (acquired) K13.79
  congenital Q38.6
multiple, congenital NEC Q89.7
muscle (acquired) M62.89
  congenital Q79.9
  sternocleidomastoid Q68.0
musculoskeletal system (acquired) M95.9
  congenital Q79.9
  specified NEC M95.8
nail (acquired) L60.8
  congenital Q84.6
nasal — see Deformity, nose
neck (acquired) M95.3
  congenital Q18.9
  sternocleidomastoid Q68.0
nervous system (congenital) Q07.9
nipple (congenital) Q83.9
  acquired N64.89
nose (acquired) (cartilage) M95.0
  bone (turbinate) M95.0
  congenital Q30.9
    bent or squashed Q67.4
  saddle M95.0
    syphilitic A50.57
  septum (acquired) J34.2
    congenital Q30.8
  sinus (wall) (congenital) Q30.8
    acquired M95.0
  syphilitic (congenital) A50.57
    late A52.73
ocular muscle (congenital) Q10.3
  acquired — see Strabismus, mechanical
opticociliary vessels (congenital) Q13.2
orbit (eye) (acquired) H05.30
  atrophy — see Atrophy, orbit
  congenital Q10.7
  due to
    bone disease NEC H05.32- ☑
    trauma or surgery H05.33- ☑
  enlargement — see Enlargement, orbit
  exostosis — see Exostosis, orbit
organ of Corti (congenital) Q16.5
ovary (congenital) Q50.39
  acquired N83.8
oviduct, acquired N83.8
palate (congenital) Q38.5
  acquired M27.8
  cleft (congenital) — see Cleft, palate
pancreas (congenital) Q45.3
  acquired K86.8
parathyroid (gland) Q89.2
parotid (gland) (congenital) Q38.4
  acquired K11.8
patella (acquired) — see Disorder, patella, specified NEC
pelvis, pelvic (acquired) (bony) M95.5

84

☑ Additional Character Required — Refer to the Tabular List for Character Selection   ▽ Subterms under main terms may continue to next column or page

Deformity — *continued*
  pelvis, pelvic — *continued*
    with disproportion (fetopelvic) O33.0
      causing obstructed labor O65.0
    congenital Q74.2
    rachitic sequelae (late effect) E64.3
  penis (glans) (congenital) Q55.69
    acquired N48.89
  pericardium (congenital) Q24.8
    acquired — *see* Pericarditis
  pharynx (congenital) Q38.8
    acquired J39.2
  pinna, acquired (*see also* Disorder, pinna, deformity)
    congenital Q17.9
  pituitary (congenital) Q89.2
  posture — *see* Dorsopathy, deforming
  prepuce (congenital) Q55.69
    acquired N47.8
  prostate (congenital) Q55.4
    acquired N42.89
  pupil (congenital) Q13.2
    acquired — *see* Abnormality, pupillary
  pylorus (congenital) Q40.3
    acquired K31.89
  rachitic (acquired), old or healed E64.3
  radius (acquired) (*see also* Deformity, limb, forearm)
    congenital Q68.8
  rectum (congenital) Q43.9
    acquired K62.89
  reduction (extremity) (limb), congenital (*see also* condition and site) Q73.8
    brain Q04.3
    lower — *see* Defect, reduction, lower limb
    upper — *see* Defect, reduction, upper limb
  renal — *see* Deformity, kidney
  respiratory system (congenital) Q34.9
  rib (acquired) M95.4
    congenital Q76.6
    cervical Q76.5
  rotation (joint) (acquired) — *see* Deformity, limb, specified site NEC
    congenital Q74.9
    hip — *see* Deformity, limb, specified type NEC, thigh
      congenital Q65.89
  sacroiliac joint (congenital) — *see* subcategory Q74.2
    acquired — *see* subcategory M43.8 ☑
  sacrum (acquired) — *see* subcategory M43.8 ☑
  saddle
    back — *see* Lordosis
    nose M95.0
      syphilitic A50.57
  salivary gland or duct (congenital) Q38.4
    acquired K11.8
  scapula (acquired) M95.8
    congenital Q68.8
  scrotum (congenital) (*see also* Malformation, testis and scrotum)
    acquired N50.8
  seminal vesicles (congenital) Q55.4
    acquired N50.8
  septum, nasal (acquired) J34.2
  shoulder (joint) (acquired) — *see* Deformity, limb, upper arm
    congenital Q74.0
    contraction — *see* Contraction, joint, shoulder
  sigmoid (flexure) (congenital) Q43.9
    acquired K63.89
  skin (congenital) Q82.9
  skull (acquired) M95.2
    congenital Q75.8
      with
        anencephaly Q00.0
        encephalocele — *see* Encephalocele
        hydrocephalus Q03.9
          with spina bifida — *see* Spina bifida, by site, with hydrocephalus
        microcephaly Q02
  soft parts, organs or tissues (of pelvis)
    in pregnancy or childbirth NEC O34.8- ☑
      causing obstructed labor O65.5
  spermatic cord (congenital) Q55.4
    acquired N50.8
    torsion — *see* Torsion, spermatic cord
  spinal — *see* Dorsopathy, deforming
    column (acquired) — *see* Dorsopathy, deforming
    congenital Q67.5
    cord (congenital) Q06.9

Deformity — *continued*
  spinal — *see* Dorsopathy, deforming — *continued*
    cord — *continued*
      acquired G95.89
    nerve root (congenital) Q07.9
  spine (acquired) (*see also* Dorsopathy, deforming)
    congenital Q67.5
    rachitic E64.3
    specified NEC — *see* Dorsopathy, deforming, specified NEC
  spleen
    acquired D73.89
    congenital Q89.09
  Sprengel's (congenital) Q74.0
  sternocleidomastoid (muscle), congenital Q68.0
  sternum (acquired) M95.4
    congenital NEC Q76.7
  stomach (congenital) Q40.3
    acquired K31.89
  submandibular gland (congenital) Q38.4
  submaxillary gland (congenital) Q38.4
    acquired K11.8
  talipes — *see* Talipes
  testis (congenital) (*see also* Malformation, testis and scrotum)
    acquired N44.8
    torsion — *see* Torsion, testis
  thigh (acquired) (*see also* Deformity, limb, thigh)
    congenital NEC Q68.8
  thorax (acquired) (wall) M95.4
    congenital Q67.8
    sequelae of rickets E64.3
  thumb (acquired) (*see also* Deformity, finger)
    congenital NEC Q68.1
  thymus (tissue) (congenital) Q89.2
  thyroid (gland) (congenital) Q89.2
    cartilage Q31.8
      acquired J38.7
  tibia (acquired) (*see also* Deformity, limb, specified type NEC, lower leg)
    congenital NEC Q68.8
    saber (syphilitic) A50.56
  toe (acquired) M20.6- ☑
    congenital Q66.9
    hallux rigidus M20.2- ☑
    hallux valgus M20.1- ☑
    hallux varus M20.3- ☑
    hammer toe M20.4- ☑
    specified NEC M20.5X- ☑
  tongue (congenital) Q38.3
    acquired K14.8
  tooth, teeth K00.2
  trachea (rings) (congenital) Q32.1
    acquired J39.8
  transverse aortic arch (congenital) Q25.4
  tricuspid (leaflets) (valve) I07.8
    atresia or stenosis Q22.4
    Ebstein's Q22.5
  trunk (acquired) M95.8
    congenital Q89.9
  ulna (acquired) (*see also* Deformity, limb, forearm)
    congenital NEC Q68.8
  urachus, congenital Q64.4
  ureter (opening) (congenital) Q62.8
    acquired N28.89
  urethra (congenital) Q64.79
    acquired N36.8
  urinary tract (congenital) Q64.9
    urachus Q64.4
  uterus (congenital) Q51.9
    acquired N85.8
  uvula (congenital) Q38.5
  vagina (acquired) N89.8
    congenital Q52.4
  valgus NEC M21.00
    ankle M21.07- ☑
    elbow M21.02- ☑
    hip M21.05- ☑
    knee M21.06- ☑
  valve, valvular (congenital) (heart) Q24.8
    acquired — *see* Endocarditis
  varus NEC M21.10
    ankle M21.17- ☑
    elbow M21.12- ☑
    hip M21.15 ☑
    knee M21.16- ☑
    tibia — *see* Osteochondrosis, juvenile, tibia

Deformity — *continued*
  vas deferens (congenital) Q55.4
    acquired N50.8
  vein (congenital) Q27.9
    great Q26.9
  vertebra — *see* Dorsopathy, deforming
  vertical talus Q66.80
    left foot Q66.82
    right foot Q66.81
  vesicourethral orifice (acquired) N32.89
    congenital NEC Q64.79
  vessels of optic papilla (congenital) Q14.2
  visual field (contraction) — *see* Defect, visual field
  vitreous body, acquired H43.89
  vulva (congenital) Q52.79
    acquired N90.89
  wrist (joint) (acquired) (*see also* Deformity, limb, forearm)
    congenital Q68.8
    contraction — *see* Contraction, joint, wrist

Degeneration, degenerative
  adrenal (capsule) (fatty) (gland) (hyaline) (infectional) E27.8
  amyloid (*see also* Amyloidosis) E85.9
  anterior cornua, spinal cord G12.29
  anterior labral S43.49- ☑
  aorta, aortic I70.0
    fatty I77.89
  aortic valve (heart) — *see* Endocarditis, aortic
  arteriovascular — *see* Arteriosclerosis
  artery, arterial (atheromatous) (calcareous) (*see also* Arteriosclerosis)
    cerebral, amyloid E85.4 [I68.0]
    medial — *see* Arteriosclerosis, extremities
  articular cartilage NEC — *see* Derangement, joint, articular cartilage, by site
  atheromatous — *see* Arteriosclerosis
  basal nuclei or ganglia G23.9
    specified NEC G23.8
  bone NEC — *see* Disorder, bone, specified type NEC
  brachial plexus G54.0
  brain (cortical) (progressive) G31.9
    alcoholic G31.2
    arteriosclerotic I67.2
    childhood G31.9
      specified NEC G31.89
    cystic G31.89
      congenital Q04.6
    in
      alcoholism G31.2
      beriberi E51.2
      cerebrovascular disease I67.9
      congenital hydrocephalus Q03.9
        with spina bifida (*see also* Spina bifida)
      Fabry-Anderson disease E75.21
      Gaucher's disease E75.22
      Hunter's syndrome E76.1
      lipidosis
        cerebral E75.4
        generalized E75.6
      mucopolysaccharidosis — *see* Mucopolysaccharidosis
      myxedema E03.9 [G32.89]
      neoplastic disease (*see also* Neoplasm) D49.6 [G32.89]
      Niemann-Pick disease E75.249 [G32.89]
      sphingolipidosis E75.3 [G32.89]
      vitamin B12 deficiency E53.8 [G32.89]
    senile NEC G31.1
  breast N64.89
  Bruch's membrane — *see* Degeneration, choroid
  capillaries (fatty) I78.8
    amyloid E85.8 [I79.8]
  cardiac (*see also* Degeneration, myocardial)
    valve, valvular — *see* Endocarditis
  cardiorenal — *see* Hypertension, cardiorenal
  cardiovascular (*see also* Disease, cardiovascular)
    renal — *see* Hypertension, cardiorenal
  cerebellar NOS G31.9
    alcoholic G31.2
    primary (hereditary) (sporadic) G11.9
  cerebral — *see* Degeneration, brain
  cerebrovascular I67.9
    due to hypertension I67.4
  cervical plexus G54.2
  cervix N88.8
    due to radiation (intended effect) N88.8
      adverse effect or misadventure N99.89

Degeneration, degenerative — *continued*
  chamber angle H21.21- ☑
  changes, spine or vertebra — *see* Spondylosis
  chorioretinal (*see also* Degeneration, choroid)
    hereditary H31.2Ø
  choroid (colloid) (drusen) H31.1Ø- ☑
    atrophy — *see* Atrophy, choroidal
    hereditary — *see* Dystrophy, choroidal, hereditary
  ciliary body H21.22- ☑
  cochlear — *see* subcategory H83.8 ☑
  combined (spinal cord) (subacute) E53.8 [G32.Ø]
    with anemia (pernicious) D51.Ø [G32.Ø]
      due to dietary vitamin B12 deficiency
        D51.3 [G32.Ø]
    in (due to)
      vitamin B12 deficiency E53.8 [G32.Ø]
        anemia D51.9 [G32.Ø]
  conjunctiva H11.1Ø
    concretions — *see* Concretion, conjunctiva
    deposits — *see* Deposit, conjunctiva
    pigmentations — *see* Pigmentation, conjunctiva
    pinguecula — *see* Pinguecula
    xerosis — *see* Xerosis, conjunctiva
  cornea H18.4Ø
    calcerous H18.43
      band keratopathy H18.42- ☑
    familial, hereditary — *see* Dystrophy, cornea
    hyaline (of old scars) H18.49
    keratomalacia — *see* Keratomalacia
    nodular H18.45- ☑
    peripheral H18.46- ☑
    senile H18.41- ☑
    specified type NEC H18.49
  cortical (cerebellar) (parenchymatous) G31.89
    alcoholic G31.2
    diffuse, due to arteriopathy I67.2
  corticobasal G31.85
  cutis L98.8
    amyloid E85.4 [L99]
  dental pulp KØ4.2
  disc disease — *see* Degeneration, intervertebral disc
    NEC
  dorsolateral (spinal cord) — *see* Degeneration, combined
  extrapyramidal G25.9
  eye, macular (*see also* Degeneration, macula)
    congenital or hereditary — *see* Dystrophy, retina
  facet joints — *see* Spondylosis
  fatty
    liver NEC K76.Ø
      alcoholic K7Ø.Ø
  grey matter (brain) (Alpers') G31.81
  heart (*see also* Degeneration, myocardial)
    amyloid E85.4 [I43]
    atheromatous — *see* Disease, heart, ischemic, atherosclerotic
    ischemic — *see* Disease, heart, ischemic
  hepatolenticular (Wilson's) E83.Ø1
  hepatorenal K76.7
  hyaline (diffuse) (generalized)
    localized — *see* Degeneration, by site
  infrapatellar fat pad M79.4
  intervertebral disc NOS
    with
      myelopathy — *see* Disorder, disc, with, myelopathy
      radiculitis or radiculopathy — *see* Disorder, disc, with, radiculopathy
    cervical, cervicothoracic — *see* Disorder, disc, cervical, degeneration
      with
        myelopathy — *see* Disorder, disc, cervical, with myelopathy
        neuritis, radiculitis or radiculopathy — *see* Disorder, disc, cervical, with neuritis
    lumbar region M51.36
      with
        myelopathy M51.Ø6
        neuritis, radiculitis, radiculopathy or sciatica M51.16
    lumbosacral region M51.37
      with
        neuritis, radiculitis, radiculopathy or sciatica M51.17
    sacrococcygeal region M53.3
    thoracic region M51.34

Degeneration, degenerative — *continued*
  intervertebral disc — *continued*
    thoracic region — *continued*
      with
        myelopathy M51.Ø4
        neuritis, radiculitis, radiculopathy M51.14
    thoracolumbar region M51.35
      with
        myelopathy M51.Ø5
        neuritis, radiculitis, radiculopathy M51.15
  intestine, amyloid E85.4
  iris (pigmentary) H21.23- ☑
  ischemic — *see* Ischemia
  joint disease — *see* Osteoarthritis
  kidney N28.89
    amyloid E85.4 [N29]
    cystic, congenital Q61.9
    fatty N28.89
    polycystic Q61.3
      adult type (autosomal dominant) Q61.2
      infantile type (autosomal recessive) NEC Q61.19
        collecting duct dilatation Q61.11
  Kuhnt-Junius (*see also* Degeneration, macula) H35.32
  lens — *see* Cataract
  lenticular (familial) (progressive) (Wilson's) (with cirrhosis of liver) E83.Ø1
  liver (diffuse) NEC K76.89
    amyloid E85.4 [K77]
    cystic K76.89
      congenital Q44.6
    fatty NEC K76.Ø
      alcoholic K7Ø.Ø
    hypertrophic K76.89
    parenchymatous, acute or subacute K72.ØØ
      with coma K72.Ø1
    pigmentary K76.89
    toxic (acute) K71.9
  lung J98.4
  lymph gland I89.8
    hyaline I89.8
  macula, macular (acquired) (age-related) (senile) H35.3Ø
    angioid streaks H35.33
    atrophic age-related H35.31
    congenital or hereditary — *see* Dystrophy, retina
    cystoid H35.35- ☑
    drusen H35.36- ☑
    exudative H35.32
    hole H35.34- ☑
    nonexudative H35.31
    puckering H35.37- ☑
    toxic H35.38- ☑
  membranous labyrinth, congenital (causing impairment of hearing) Q16.5
  meniscus — *see* Derangement, meniscus
  mitral — *see* Insufficiency, mitral
  Mönckeberg's — *see* Arteriosclerosis, extremities
  motor centers, senile G31.1
  multi-system G90.3
  mural — *see* Degeneration, myocardial
  muscle (fatty) (fibrous) (hyaline) (progressive) M62.89
    heart — *see* Degeneration, myocardial
  myelin, central nervous system G37.9
  myocardial, myocardium (fatty) (hyaline) (senile) I51.5
    with rheumatic fever (conditions in IØØ) IØ9.Ø
      active, acute or subacute IØ1.2
        with chorea IØ2.Ø
      inactive or quiescent (with chorea) IØ9.Ø
    hypertensive — *see* Hypertension, heart
    rheumatic — *see* Degeneration, myocardial, with rheumatic fever
    syphilitic A52.Ø6
  nasal sinus (mucosa) J32.9
    frontal J32.1
    maxillary J32.Ø
  nerve — *see* Disorder, nerve
  nervous system G31.9
    alcoholic G31.2
    amyloid E85.4 [G99.8]
    autonomic G90.9
    fatty G31.89
    specified NEC G31.89
  nipple N64.89
  olivopontocerebellar (hereditary) (familial) G23.8
  osseous labyrinth — *see* subcategory H83.8 ☑
  ovary N83.8
    cystic N83.2Ø
    microcystic N83.2Ø

Degeneration, degenerative — *continued*
  pallidal pigmentary (progressive) G23.Ø
  pancreas K86.8
    tuberculous A18.83
  penis N48.89
  pigmentary (diffuse) (general)
    localized — *see* Degeneration, by site
    pallidal (progressive) G23.Ø
  pineal gland E34.8
  pituitary (gland) E23.6
  popliteal fat pad M79.4
  posterolateral (spinal cord) — *see* Degeneration, combined
  pulmonary valve (heart) I37.8
  pulp (tooth) KØ4.2
  pupillary margin H21.24- ☑
  renal — *see* Degeneration, kidney
  retina H35.9
    hereditary (cerebroretinal) (congenital) (juvenile) (macula) (peripheral) (pigmentary) — *see* Dystrophy, retina
    Kuhnt-Junius (*see also* Degeneration, macula) H35.32
    macula (cystic) (exudative) (hole) (nonexudative) (pseudohole) (senile) (toxic) — *see* Degeneration, macula
    peripheral H35.4Ø
      lattice H35.41- ☑
      microcystoid H35.42- ☑
      paving stone H35.43- ☑
      secondary
        pigmentary H35.45- ☑
        vitreoretinal H35.46- ☑
      senile reticular H35.44- ☑
    pigmentary (primary) (*see also* Dystrophy, retina)
      secondary — *see* Degeneration, retina, peripheral, secondary
    posterior pole — *see* Degeneration, macula
  saccule, congenital (causing impairment of hearing) Q16.5
  senile R54
    brain G31.1
    cardiac, heart or myocardium — *see* Degeneration, myocardial
    motor centers G31.1
    vascular — *see* Arteriosclerosis
  sinus (cystic) (*see also* Sinusitis)
    polypoid J33.1
  skin L98.8
    amyloid E85.4 [L99]
    colloid L98.8
  spinal (cord) G31.89
    amyloid E85.4 [G32.89]
    combined (subacute) — *see* Degeneration, combined
    dorsolateral — *see* Degeneration, combined
    familial NEC G31.89
    fatty G31.89
    funicular — *see* Degeneration, combined
    posterolateral — *see* Degeneration, combined
    subacute combined — *see* Degeneration, combined
    tuberculous A17.81
  spleen D73.Ø
    amyloid E85.4 [D77]
  stomach K31.89
  striatonigral G23.2
  suprarenal (capsule) (gland) E27.8
  synovial membrane (pulpy) — *see* Disorder, synovium, specified type NEC
  tapetoretinal — *see* Dystrophy, retina
  thymus (gland) E32.8
    fatty E32.8
  thyroid (gland) EØ7.89
  tricuspid (heart) (valve) IØ7.9
  tuberculous NEC — *see* Tuberculosis
  turbinate J34.89
  uterus (cystic) N85.8
  vascular (senile) — *see* Arteriosclerosis
    hypertensive — *see* Hypertension
  vitreoretinal, secondary — *see* Degeneration, retina, peripheral, secondary, vitreoretinal
  vitreous (body) H43.81- ☑
  Wallerian — *see* Disorder, nerve
  Wilson's hepatolenticular E83.Ø1

Deglutition
  paralysis
    hysterical F44.4
    pneumonia J69.0
Degos' disease I77.89
Dehiscence (of)
  amputation stump T87.81
  cesarean wound O90.0
  closure of
    cornea T81.31 ☑
    craniotomy T81.32 ☑
    fascia (muscular) (superficial) T81.32 ☑
    internal organ or tissue T81.32 ☑
    laceration (external) (internal) T81.33 ☑
    ligament T81.32 ☑
    mucosa T81.31 ☑
    muscle or muscle flap T81.32 ☑
    ribs or rib cage T81.32 ☑
    skin and subcutaneous tissue (full-thickness) (superficial) T81.31 ☑
    skull T81.32 ☑
    sternum (sternotomy) T81.32 ☑
    tendon T81.32 ☑
    traumatic laceration (external) (internal) T81.33 ☑
  episiotomy O90.1
  operation wound NEC T81.31 ☑
    external operation wound (superficial) T81.31 ☑
    internal operation wound (deep) T81.32 ☑
  perineal wound (postpartum) O90.1
  traumatic injury wound repair T81.33 ☑
  wound T81.30 ☑
    traumatic repair T81.33 ☑
Dehydration E86.0
  hypertonic E87.0
  hypotonic E87.1
  newborn P74.1
Déjérine-Roussy syndrome G89.0
Déjérine-Sottas disease or neuropathy (hypertrophic) G60.0
Déjérine-Thomas atrophy G23.8
Delay, delayed
  any plane in pelvis
    complicating delivery O66.9
  birth or delivery NOS O63.9
  closure, ductus arteriosus (Botalli) P29.3
  coagulation — see Defect, coagulation
  conduction (cardiac) (ventricular) I45.9
  delivery, second twin, triplet, etc O63.2
  development R62.50
    global F88
    intellectual (specific) F81.9
    language F80.9
      due to hearing loss F80.4
    learning F81.9
    pervasive F84.9
    physiological R62.50
      specified stage NEC R62.0
    reading F81.0
    sexual E30.0
    speech F80.9
      due to hearing loss F80.4
    spelling F81.81
  gastric emptying K30
  menarche E30.0
  menstruation (cause unknown) N91.0
  milestone R62.0
  passage of meconium (newborn) P76.0
  primary respiration P28.9
  puberty (constitutional) E30.0
  separation of umbilical cord P96.82
  sexual maturation, female E30.0
  sleep phase syndrome G47.21
  union, fracture — see Fracture, by site
  vaccination Z28.9
Deletion(s)
  autosome Q93.9
    identified by fluorescence in situ hybridization (FISH) Q93.89
    identified by in situ hybridization (ISH) Q93.89
  chromosome
    with complex rearrangements NEC Q93.7
    part of NEC Q93.5
    seen only at prometaphase Q93.89
    short arm
      22q11.2 Q93.81
      4 Q93.3
      5p Q93.4

Deletion(s) — continued
  chromosome — continued
    specified NEC Q93.89
  long arm chromosome 18 or 21 Q93.89
    with complex rearrangements NEC Q93.7
  microdeletions NEC Q93.88
Delhi boil or button B55.1
Delinquency (juvenile) (neurotic) F91.8
  group Z72.810
Delinquent immunization status Z28.3
Delirium, delirious (acute or subacute) (not alcohol- or drug-induced) (with dementia) R41.0
  alcoholic (acute) (tremens) (withdrawal) F10.921
    with intoxication F10.921
      in
        abuse F10.121
        dependence F10.221
    due to (secondary to)
      alcohol
        intoxication F10.921
          in
            abuse F10.121
            dependence F10.221
        withdrawal F10.231
      amphetamine intoxication F15.921
        in
          abuse F15.121
          dependence F15.221
      anxiolytic
        intoxication F13.921
          in
            abuse F13.121
            dependence F13.221
        withdrawal F13.231
      cannabis intoxication (acute) F12.921
        in
          abuse F12.121
          dependence F12.221
      cocaine intoxication (acute) F14.921
        in
          abuse F14.121
          dependence F14.221
      general medical condition F05
      hallucinogen intoxication F16.921
        in
          abuse F16.121
          dependence F16.221
      hypnotic
        intoxication F13.921
          in
            abuse F13.121
            dependence F13.221
        withdrawal F13.231
      inhalant intoxication (acute) F18.921
        in
          abuse F18.121
          dependence F18.221
      multiple etiologies F05
      opioid intoxication (acute) F11.921
        in
          abuse F11.121
          dependence F11.221
      phencyclidine intoxication (acute) F16.921
        in
          abuse F16.121
          dependence F16.221
      psychoactive substance NEC intoxication (acute) F19.921
        in
          abuse F19.121
          dependence F19.221
      sedative
        intoxication F13.921
          in
            abuse F13.121
            dependence F13.221
        withdrawal F13.231
      unknown etiology F05
  exhaustion F43.0
  hysterical F44.89
  postprocedural (postoperative) F05
  puerperal F05
  thyroid — see Thyrotoxicosis with thyroid storm
  traumatic — see Injury, intracranial
  tremens (alcohol-induced) F10.231
    sedative-induced F13.231
Delivery (childbirth) (labor)
  arrested active phase O62.1

Delivery — continued
  cesarean (for)
    without indication O82
    abnormal
      pelvis (bony) (deformity) (major) NEC with disproportion (fetopelvic) O33.0
        with obstructed labor O65.0
      presentation or position O32.9 ☑
    abruptio placentae (see also Abruptio placentae) O45.9- ☑
    acromion presentation O32.2 ☑
    atony, uterus O62.2
    breech presentation O32.1 ☑
      incomplete O32.8 ☑
    brow presentation O32.3 ☑
    cephalopelvic disproportion O33.9
    cerclage O34.3- ☑
    chin presentation O32.3 ☑
    cicatrix of cervix O34.4- ☑
    contracted pelvis (general)
      inlet O33.2
      outlet O33.3 ☑
    cord presentation or prolapse O69.0 ☑
    cystocele O34.8- ☑
    deformity (acquired) (congenital)
      pelvic organs or tissues NEC O34.8- ☑
      pelvis (bony) NEC O33.0
    disproportion NOS O33.9
    eclampsia — see Eclampsia
    face presentation O32.3 ☑
    failed
      forceps O66.5
      induction of labor O61.9
        instrumental O61.1
        mechanical O61.1
        medical O61.0
        specified NEC O61.8
        surgical O61.1
      trial of labor NOS O66.40
        following previous cesarean delivery O66.41
      vacuum extraction O66.5
      ventouse O66.5
    fetal-maternal hemorrhage O43.01- ☑
    hemorrhage (intrapartum) O67.9
      with coagulation defect O67.0
      specified cause NEC O67.8
    high head at term O32.4 ☑
    hydrocephalic fetus O33.6 ☑
    incarceration of uterus O34.51- ☑
    incoordinate uterine action O62.4
    increased size, fetus O33.5 ☑
    inertia, uterus O62.2
      primary O62.0
      secondary O62.1
    lateroversion, uterus O34.59- ☑
    mal lie O32.9 ☑
    malposition
      fetus O32.9 ☑
      pelvic organs or tissues NEC O34.8- ☑
      uterus NEC O34.59- ☑
    malpresentation NOS O32.9 ☑
    oblique presentation O32.2 ☑
    occurring after 37 completed weeks of gestation but before 39 completed weeks gestation due to (spontaneous) onset of labor O75.82
    oversize fetus O33.5 ☑
    pelvic tumor NEC O34.8- ☑
    placenta previa O44.1- ☑
      without hemorrhage O44.0- ☑
    placental insufficiency O36.51- ☑
    planned, occurring after 37 completed weeks of gestation but before 39 completed weeks gestation due to (spontaneous) onset of labor O75.82
    polyp, cervix O34.4- ☑
      causing obstructed labor O65.5
    poor dilatation, cervix O62.0
    pre-eclampsia O14.9- ☑
      mild O14.0- ☑
      moderate O14.0- ☑
      severe
        with hemolysis, elevated liver enzymes and low platelet count (HELLP) O14.2- ☑
    previous
      cesarean delivery O34.21
      surgery (to)
        cervix O34.4- ☑

Delivery — continued
  cesarean — continued
    previous — continued
      surgery — continued
        gynecological NEC O34.8- ☑
          rectum O34.7- ☑
          uterus O34.29
          vagina O34.6- ☑
    prolapse
      arm or hand O32.2 ☑
      uterus O34.52- ☑
    prolonged labor NOS O63.9
    rectocele O34.8- ☑
    retroversion
      uterus O34.53- ☑
    rigid
      cervix O34.4- ☑
      pelvic floor O34.8- ☑
      perineum O34.7- ☑
      vagina O34.6- ☑
      vulva O34.7- ☑
    sacculation, pregnant uterus O34.59- ☑
    scar(s)
      cervix O34.4- ☑
      cesarean delivery O34.21
      uterus O34.29
    Shirodkar suture in situ O34.3- ☑
    shoulder presentation O32.2 ☑
    stenosis or stricture, cervix O34.4- ☑
    streptococcus B carrier state O99.824
    transverse presentation or lie O32.2 ☑
    tumor, pelvic organs or tissues NEC O34.8- ☑
      cervix O34.4- ☑
    umbilical cord presentation or prolapse O69.0 ☑
  completely normal case O80
  complicated O75.9
    by
      abnormal, abnormality (of)
        forces of labor O62.9
          specified type NEC O62.8
        glucose O99.814
        uterine contractions NOS O62.9
      abruptio placentae (see also Abruptio placentae) O45.9- ☑
      abuse
        physical O9A.32 (following O99)
        psychological O9A.52 (following O99)
        sexual O9A.42 (following O99)
      adherent placenta O72.0
        without hemorrhage O73.0
      alcohol use O99.314
      anemia (pre-existing) O99.02
      anesthetic death O74.8
      annular detachment of cervix O71.3
      atony, uterus O62.2
      attempted vacuum extraction and forceps O66.5
      Bandl's ring O62.4
      bariatric surgery status O99.844
      biliary tract disorder O26.62
      bleeding — see Delivery, complicated by, hemorrhage
      blood disorder NEC O99.12
      cervical dystocia (hypotonic) O62.2
        primary O62.0
        secondary O62.1
      circulatory system disorder O99.42
      compression of cord (umbilical) NEC O69.2 ☑
      condition NEC O99.89
      contraction, contracted ring O62.4
      cord (umbilical)
        around neck
          with compression O69.1 ☑
          without compression O69.81 ☑
        bruising O69.5 ☑
        complication O69.9 ☑
          specified NEC O69.89 ☑
        compression NEC O69.2 ☑
        entanglement O69.2 ☑
          without compression O69.82 ☑
        hematoma O69.5 ☑
        presentation O69.0 ☑
        prolapse O69.0 ☑
        short O69.3 ☑
        thrombosis (vessels) O69.5 ☑
        vascular lesion O69.5 ☑
      Couvelaire uterus O45.8X- ☑

Delivery — continued
  complicated — continued
    by — continued
      damage to (injury to) NEC
        perineum O71.82
        periurethral tissue O71.82
        vulva O71.82
      delay following rupture of membranes (spontaneous) — see Pregnancy, complicated by, premature rupture of membranes
      depressed fetal heart tones O76
      diabetes O24.92
        gestational O24.429
          diet controlled O24.420
          insulin controlled O24.424
        pre-existing O24.32
          specified NEC O24.82
          type 1 O24.02
          type 2 O24.12
      diastasis recti (abdominis) O71.89
      dilatation
        bladder O66.8
        cervix incomplete, poor or slow O62.0
      disease NEC O99.89
      disruptio uteri — see Delivery, complicated by, rupture, uterus
      drug use O99.324
      dysfunction, uterus NOS O62.9
        hypertonic O62.4
        hypotonic O62.2
          primary O62.0
          secondary O62.1
        incoordinate O62.4
      eclampsia O15.1
      embolism (pulmonary) — see Embolism, obstetric
      endocrine, nutritional or metabolic disease NEC O99.284
      failed
        attempted vaginal birth after previous cesarean delivery O66.41
        induction of labor O61.9
          instrumental O61.1
          mechanical O61.1
          medical O61.0
          specified NEC O61.8
          surgical O61.1
        trial of labor O66.40
      female genital mutilation O65.5
      fetal
        abnormal acid-base balance O68
        acidemia O68
        acidosis O68
        alkalosis O68
        death, early O02.1
        deformity O66.3
        heart rate or rhythm (abnormal) (non-reassuring) O76
        hypoxia O77.8
        stress O77.9
          due to drug administration O77.1
          electrocardiographic evidence of O77.8
          specified NEC O77.8
          ultrasound evidence of O77.8
      fever during labor O75.2
      gastric banding status O99.844
      gastric bypass status O99.844
      gastrointestinal disease NEC O99.62
      gestational diabetes O24.429
        diet controlled O24.420
        insulin (and diet) controlled O24.424
      gonorrhea O98.22
      hematoma O71.7
        ischial spine O71.7
        pelvic O71.7
        vagina O71.7
        vulva or perineum O71.7
      hemorrhage (uterine) O67.9
        associated with
          afibrinogenemia O67.0
          coagulation defect O67.0
          hyperfibrinolysis O67.0
          hypofibrinogenemia O67.0
        due to
          low-lying placenta O44.1- ☑
          placenta previa O44.1- ☑

Delivery — continued
  complicated — continued
    by — continued
      hemorrhage — continued
        due to — continued
          premature separation of placenta (normally implanted) (see also Abruptio placentae) O45.9- ☑
          retained placenta O72.0
          uterine leiomyoma O67.8
        placenta NEC O67.8
        postpartum NEC (atonic) (immediate) O72.1
          with retained or trapped placenta O72.0
          delayed O72.2
          secondary O72.2
          third stage O72.0
      hourglass contraction, uterus O62.4
      hypertension, hypertensive (pre-existing) — see Hypertension, complicated by, childbirth (labor)
      hypotension O26.5-
      incomplete dilatation (cervix) O62.0
      incoordinate uterus contractions O62.4
      inertia, uterus O62.2
        during latent phase of labor O62.0
        primary O62.0
        secondary O62.1
      infection (maternal) O98.92
        carrier state NEC O99.834
        gonorrhea O98.22
        human immunodeficiency virus (HIV) O98.72
        sexually transmitted NEC O98.32
        specified NEC O98.82
        syphilis O98.12
        tuberculosis O98.02
        viral hepatitis O98.42
        viral NEC O98.52
      injury (to mother) (see also Delivery, complicated, by, damage to) O71.9
        nonobstetric O9A.22 (following O99)
        caused by abuse — see Delivery, complicated by, abuse
      intrauterine fetal death, early O02.1
      inversion, uterus O71.2
      laceration (perineal) O70.9
        anus (sphincter) O70.4
          with third degree laceration O70.2
            with mucosa O70.3
          without third degree laceration O70.4
        bladder (urinary) O71.5
        bowel O71.5
        cervix (uteri) O71.3
        fourchette O70.0
        hymen O70.0
        labia O70.0
        pelvic
          floor O70.1
          organ NEC O71.5
        perineum, perineal O70.9
          first degree O70.0
          fourth degree O70.3
          muscles O70.1
          second degree O70.1
          skin O70.0
          slight O70.0
          third degree O70.2
        peritoneum (pelvic) O71.5
        rectovaginal (septum) (without perineal laceration) O71.4
          with perineum O70.2
            with anal or rectal mucosa O70.3
        specified NEC O71.89
        sphincter ani — see Delivery, complicated, by, laceration, anus (sphincter)
        urethra O71.5
        uterus O71.81
          before labor O71.81
        vagina, vaginal (deep) (high) (without perineal laceration) O71.4
          with perineum O70.0
          muscles, with perineum O70.1
        vulva O70.0
      liver disorder O26.62
      malignancy O9A.12 (following O99)
      malnutrition O25.2

☑ Additional Character Required — Refer to the Tabular List for Character Selection   ▽ Subterms under main terms may continue to next column or page

Delivery — *continued*
  complicated — *continued*
    by — *continued*
      malposition, malpresentation
        without obstruction (*see also* Delivery,
          complicated by, obstruction) O32.9 ☑
          breech O32.1 ☑
          compound O32.6 ☑
          face (brow) (chin) O32.3 ☑
          footling O32.8 ☑
          high head O32.4 ☑
          oblique O32.2 ☑
          specified NEC O32.8 ☑
          transverse O32.2 ☑
          unstable lie O32.0 ☑
      placenta (with hemorrhage) O44.1- ☑
        without hemorrhage O44.0- ☑
      uterus or cervix O65.5
      meconium in amniotic fluid O77.0
      mental disorder NEC O99.344
      metrorrhexis — *see* Delivery, complicated by,
        rupture, uterus
      nervous system disorder O99.354
      obesity (pre-existing) O99.214
      obesity surgery status O99.844
      obstetric trauma O71.9
        specified NEC O71.89
      obstructed labor
        due to
          breech (complete) (frank) presentation
            O64.1 ☑
            incomplete O64.8 ☑
          brow presenation O64.3 ☑
          buttock presentation O64.1 ☑
          chin presentation O64.2 ☑
          compound presentation O64.5 ☑
          contracted pelvis O65.1
          deep transverse arrest O64.0 ☑
          deformed pelvis O65.0
          dystocia (fetal) O66.9
            due to
              conjoined twins O66.3
              fetal
                abnormality NEC O66.3
                ascites O66.3
                hydrops O66.3
                meningomyelocele O66.3
                sacral teratoma O66.3
                tumor O66.3
              hydrocephalic fetus O66.3
            shoulder O66.0
          face presentation O64.2 ☑
          fetopelvic disproportion O65.4
          footling presentation O64.8 ☑
          impacted shoulders O66.0
          incomplete rotation of fetal head
            O64.0 ☑
          large fetus O66.2
          locked twins O66.1
          malposition O64.9 ☑
            specified NEC O64.8 ☑
          malpresentation O64.9 ☑
            specified NEC O64.8 ☑
          multiple fetuses NEC O66.6
          pelvic
            abnormality (maternal) O65.9
              organ O65.5
              specified NEC O65.8
            contraction
              inlet O65.2
              mid-cavity O65.3
              outlet O65.3
          persistent (position)
            occipitoiliac O64.0 ☑
            occipitoposterior O64.0 ☑
            occipitosacral O64.0 ☑
            occipitotransverse O64.0 ☑
          prolapsed arm O64.4 ☑
          shoulder presentation O64.4 ☑
        specified NEC O66.8
      pathological retraction ring, uterus O62.4
      penetration, pregnant uterus by instrument
        O71.1
      perforation — *see* Delivery, complicated by,
        laceration

Delivery — *continued*
  complicated — *continued*
    by — *continued*
      placenta, placental
        ablatio (*see also* Abruptio placentae)
          O45.9- ☑
        abnormality O43.9- ☑
          specified NEC O43.89- ☑
        abruptio (*see also* Abruptio placentae)
          O45.9- ☑
        accreta O43.21- ☑
        adherent (with hemorrhage) O72.0
          without hemorrhage O73.0
        detachment (premature) (*see also* Abruptio
          placentae) O45.9- ☑
        disorder O43.9- ☑
          specified NEC O43.89- ☑
        hemorrhage NEC O67.8
        increta O43.22- ☑
        low (implantation) O44.1- ☑
          without hemorrhage O44.0- ☑
        malformation O43.10- ☑
        malposition O44.1- ☑
          without hemorrhage O44.0- ☑
        percreta O43.23- ☑
        previa (central) (lateral) (low) (marginal)
          (partial) (total) O44.1- ☑
          without hemorrhage O44.0- ☑
        retained (with hemorrhage) O72.0
          without hemorrhage O73.0
        separation (premature) O45.9- ☑
          specified NEC O45.8X- ☑
        vicious insertion O44.1- ☑
      precipitate labor O62.3
      premature rupture, membranes (*see also* Preg-
        nancy, complicated by, premature rup-
        ture of membranes) O42.90
      prolapse
        arm or hand O32.2 ☑
        cord (umbilical) O69.0 ☑
        foot or leg O32.8 ☑
        uterus O34.52- ☑
      prolonged labor O63.9
        first stage O63.0
        second stage O63.1
      protozoal disease (maternal) O98.62
      respiratory disease NEC O99.52
      retained membranes or portions of placenta
        O72.2
        without hemorrhage O73.1
      retarded birth O63.9
      retention of secundines (with hemorrhage)
        O72.0
        without hemorrhage O73.0
        partial O72.2
          without hemorrhage O73.1
      rupture
        bladder (urinary) O71.5
        cervix O71.3
        pelvic organ NEC O71.5
        urethra O71.5
        uterus (during or after labor) O71.1
          before labor O71.0- ☑
      separation, pubic bone (symphysis pubis) O71.6
      shock O75.1
      shoulder presentation O64.4 ☑
      skin disorder NEC O99.72
      spasm, cervix O62.4
      stenosis or stricture, cervix O65.5
      streptococcus B carrier state O99.824
      subluxation of symphysis (pubis) O26.72
      syphilis (maternal) O98.12
      tear — *see* Delivery, complicated by, laceration
      tetanic uterus O62.4
      trauma (obstetrical) (*see also* Delivery, compli-
        cated, by, damage to) O71.9
        non-obstetric O9A.22 (*following* O99)
        periurethral O71.82
        specified NEC O71.89
      tuberculosis (maternal) O98.02
      tumor, pelvic organs or tissues NEC O65.5
      umbilical cord around neck
        with compression O69.1 ☑
        without compression O69.81 ☑
      uterine inertia O62.2
        during latent phase of labor O62.0
        primary O62.0

Delivery — *continued*
  complicated — *continued*
    by — *continued*
      uterine inertia — *continued*
        secondary O62.1
      vasa previa O69.4 ☑
      velamentous insertion of cord O43.12- ☑
    specified complication NEC O75.89
  delayed NOS O63.9
    following rupture of membranes
      artificial O75.5
    second twin, triplet, etc. O63.2
  forceps, low following failed vacuum extraction O66.5
  missed (at or near term) O36.4 ☑
  normal O80
  obstructed — *see* Delivery, complicated by, obstruc-
    tion
  precipitate O62.3
  preterm (*see also* Pregnancy, complicated by, preterm
    labor) O60.10 ☑
  spontaneous O80
  term pregnancy NOS O80
  uncomplicated O80
  vaginal, following previous cesarean delivery O34.21
Delusions (paranoid) — *see* Disorder, delusional
Dementia (degenerative (primary)) (old age) (persisting)
  F03.90
  with
    aggressive behavior F03.91
    behavioral disturbance F03.91
    combative behavior F03.91
    Lewy bodies G31.83 [F02.80]
      with behavioral disturbance G31.83 [F02.81]
    Parkinsonism G31.83 [F02.80]
      with behavioral disturbance G31.83 [F02.81]
    Parkinson's disease G20 [F02.80]
      with behavioral disturbance G20 [F02.81]
    violent behavior F03.91
  alcoholic F10.97
    with dependence F10.27
  Alzheimer's type — *see* Disease, Alzheimer's
  arteriosclerotic — *see* Dementia, vascular
  atypical, Alzheimer's type — *see* Disease, Alzheimer's,
    specified NEC
  congenital — *see* Disability, intellectual
  frontal (lobe) G31.09 [F02.80]
    with behavioral disturbance G31.09 [F02.81]
  frontotemporal G31.09 [F02.80]
    with behavioral disturbance G31.09 [F02.81]
    specified NEC G31.09 [F02.80]
      with behavioral disturbance G31.09 [F02.81]
  in (due to)
    with behavioral disturbance G31.83 [F02.81]
    alcohol F10.97
      with dependence F10.27
    Alzheimer's disease — *see* Disease, Alzheimer's
    arteriosclerotic brain disease — *see* Dementia,
      vascular
    cerebral lipidoses E75.- ☑ [F02.80]
      with behavioral disturbance E75.- ☑ [F02.81]
    Creutzfeldt-Jakob disease (*see also* Creutzfeldt-
      Jakob disease or syndrome (with dementia))
      A81.00
    epilepsy G40.- ☑ [F02.80]
      with behavioral disturbance G40.- ☑ [F02.81]
    hepatolenticular degeneration E83.01 [F02.80]
      with behavioral disturbance E83.01 [F02.81]
    human immunodeficiency virus (HIV) disease
      B20 [F02.80]
      with behavioral disturbance B20 [F02.81]
    Huntington's disease or chorea G10
    hypercalcemia E83.52 [F02.80]
      with behavioral disturbance E83.52 [F02.81]
    hypothyroidism, acquired E03.9 [F02.80]
      with behavioral disturbance E03.9 [F02.81]
      due to iodine deficiency E01.8 [F02.80]
        with behavioral disturbance E01.8 [F02.81]
    inhalants F18.97
      with dependence F18.27
    multiple
      etiologies F03 ☑
      sclerosis G35 [F02.80]
        with behavioral disturbance G35 [F02.81]
    neurosyphilis A52.17 [F02.80]
      with behavioral disturbance A52.17 [F02.81]
      juvenile A50.49 [F02.80]
        with behavioral disturbance A50.49 [F02.81]
    niacin deficiency E52 [F02.80]

Dementia — continued
  in — continued
    niacin deficiency — continued
      with behavioral disturbance E52 [F02.81]
    paralysis agitans G20 [F02.80]
      with behavioral disturbance G20 [F02.81]
    Parkinson's disease G20 [F02.80]
    pellagra E52 [F02.80]
      with behavioral disturbance E52 [F02.81]
    Pick's G31.01 [F02.80]
      with behavioral disturbance G31.01 [F02.81]
    polyarteritis nodosa M30.0 [F02.80]
      with behavioral disturbance M30.0 [F02.81]
    psychoactive drug F19.97
      with dependence F19.27
      inhalants F18.97
        with dependence F18.27
      sedatives, hypnotics or anxiolytics F13.97
        with dependence F13.27
    sedatives, hypnotics or anxiolytics F13.97
      with dependence F13.27
    systemic lupus erythematosus M32.- ☑ [F02.80]
      with behavioral disturbance M32.- ☑ [F02.81]
    trypanosomiasis
      African B56.9 [F02.80]
        with behavioral disturbance B56.9 [F02.81]
    unknown etiology F03 ☑
    vitamin B12 deficiency E53.8 [F02.80]
      with behavioral disturbance E53.8 [F02.81]
    volatile solvents F18.97
      with dependence F18.27
  infantile, infantilis F84.3
  Lewy body G31.83 [F02.80]
    with behavioral disturbance G31.83 [F02.81]
  multi-infarct — see Dementia, vascular
  paralytica, paralytic (syphilitic) A52.17 [F02.80]
    with behavioral disturbance A52.17 [F02.81]
    juvenilis A50.45
  paretic A52.17
  praecox — see Schizophrenia
  presenile F03 ☑
    Alzheimer's type — see Disease, Alzheimer's, early onset
  primary degenerative F03 ☑
  progressive, syphilitic A52.17
  senile F03 ☑
    with acute confusional state F05
    Alzheimer's type — see Disease, Alzheimer's, late onset
    depressed or paranoid type F03 ☑
  vascular (acute onset) (mixed) (multi-infarct) (subcortical) F01.50
    with behavioral disturbance F01.51
Demineralization, bone — see Osteoporosis
Demodex folliculorum (infestation) B88.0
Demophobia F40.248
Demoralization R45.3
Demyelination, demyelinization
  central nervous system G37.9
    specified NEC G37.8
  corpus callosum (central) G37.1
  disseminated, acute G36.9
    specified NEC G36.8
  global G35
  in optic neuritis G36.0
Dengue (classical) (fever) A90
  hemorrhagic A91
  sandfly A93.1
Dennie-Marfan syphilitic syndrome A50.45
Dens evaginatus, in dente or invaginatus K00.2
Dense breasts R92.2
Density
  increased, bone (disseminated) (generalized) (spotted) — see Disorder, bone, density and structure, specified type NEC
  lung (nodular) J98.4
Dental (see also condition)
  examination Z01.20
    with abnormal findings Z01.21
  restoration
    aesthetically inadequate or displeasing K08.56
    defective K08.50
      specified NEC K08.59
    failure of marginal integrity K08.51
    failure of periodontal anatomical integrity K08.54
Dentia praecox K00.6
Denticles (pulp) K04.2
Dentigerous cyst K09.0

Dentin
  irregular (in pulp) K04.3
  opalescent K00.5
  secondary (in pulp) K04.3
  sensitive K03.89
Dentinogenesis imperfecta K00.5
Dentinoma — see Cyst, calcifying odontogenic
Dentition (syndrome) K00.7
  delayed K00.6
  difficult K00.7
  precocious K00.6
  premature K00.6
  retarded K00.6
Dependence (on) (syndrome) F19.20
  with remission F19.21
  alcohol (ethyl) (methyl) (without remission) F10.20
    with
      amnestic disorder, persisting F10.26
      anxiety disorder F10.280
      dementia, persisting F10.27
      intoxication F10.229
        with delirium F10.221
        uncomplicated F10.220
      mood disorder F10.24
      psychotic disorder F10.259
        with
          delusions F10.250
          hallucinations F10.251
      remission F10.21
      sexual dysfunction F10.281
      sleep disorder F10.282
      specified disorder NEC F10.288
      withdrawal F10.239
        with
          delirium F10.231
          perceptual disturbance F10.232
          uncomplicated F10.230
    counseling and surveillance Z71.41
  amobarbital — see Dependence, drug, sedative
  amphetamine(s) (type) — see Dependence, drug, stimulant NEC
  amytal (sodium) — see Dependence, drug, sedative
  analgesic NEC F55.8
  anesthetic (agent) (gas) (general) (local) NEC — see Dependence, drug, psychoactive NEC
  anxiolytic NEC — see Dependence, drug, sedative
  barbital(s) — see Dependence, drug, sedative
  barbiturate(s) (compounds) (drugs classifiable to T42) — see Dependence, drug, sedative
  benzedrine — see Dependence, drug, stimulant NEC
  bhang — see Dependence, drug, cannabis
  bromide(s) NEC — see Dependence, drug, sedative
  caffeine — see Dependence, drug, stimulant NEC
  cannabis (sativa) (indica) (resin) (derivatives) (type) — see Dependence, drug, cannabis
  chloral (betaine) (hydrate) — see Dependence, drug, sedative
  chlordiazepoxide — see Dependence, drug, sedative
  coca (leaf) (derivatives) — see Dependence, drug, cocaine
  cocaine — see Dependence, drug, cocaine
  codeine — see Dependence, drug, opioid
  combinations of drugs F19.20
  dagga — see Dependence, drug, cannabis
  demerol — see Dependence, drug, opioid
  dexamphetamine — see Dependence, drug, stimulant NEC
  dexedrine — see Dependence, drug, stimulant NEC
  dextromethorphan — see Dependence, drug, opioid
  dextromoramide — see Dependence, drug, opioid
  dextro-nor-pseudo-ephedrine — see Dependence, drug, stimulant NEC
  dextrorphan — see Dependence, drug, opioid
  diazepam — see Dependence, drug, sedative
  dilaudid — see Dependence, drug, opioid
  D-lysergic acid diethylamide — see Dependence, drug, hallucinogen
  drug NEC F19.20
    with sleep disorder F19.282
    cannabis F12.20
      with
        anxiety disorder F12.280
        intoxication F12.229
          with
            delirium F12.221
            perceptual disturbance F12.222
          uncomplicated F12.220

Dependence — continued
  drug — continued
    cannabis — continued
      with — continued
        other specified disorder F12.288
        psychosis F12.259
          delusions F12.250
          hallucinations F12.251
        unspecified disorder F12.29
      in remission F12.21
    cocaine F14.20
      with
        anxiety disorder F14.280
        intoxication F14.229
          with
            delirium F14.221
            perceptual disturbance F14.222
          uncomplicated F14.220
        mood disorder F14.24
        other specified disorder F14.288
        psychosis F14.259
          delusions F14.250
          hallucinations F14.251
        sexual dysfunction F14.281
        sleep disorder F14.282
        unspecified disorder F14.29
        withdrawal F14.23
      in remission F14.21
      withdrawal symptoms in newborn P96.1
    counseling and surveillance Z71.51
    hallucinogen F16.20
      with
        anxiety disorder F16.280
        flashbacks F16.283
        intoxication F16.229
          with delirium F16.221
          uncomplicated F16.220
        mood disorder F16.24
        other specified disorder F16.288
        perception disorder, persisting F16.283
        psychosis F16.259
          delusions F16.250
          hallucinations F16.251
        unspecified disorder F16.29
      in remission F16.21
    in remission F19.21
    inhalant F18.20
      with
        anxiety disorder F18.280
        dementia, persisting F18.27
        intoxication F18.229
          with delirium F18.221
          uncomplicated F18.220
        mood disorder F18.24
        other specified disorder F18.288
        psychosis F18.259
          delusions F18.250
          hallucinations F18.251
        unspecified disorder F18.29
      in remission F18.21
    nicotine F17.200
      with disorder F17.209
        remission F17.201
        specified disorder NEC F17.208
        withdrawal F17.203
      chewing tobacco F17.220
        with disorder F17.229
          remission F17.221
          specified disorder NEC F17.228
          withdrawal F17.223
      cigarettes F17.210
        with disorder F17.219
          remission F17.211
          specified disorder NEC F17.218
          withdrawal F17.213
      specified product NEC F17.290
        with disorder F17.299
          remission F17.291
          specified disorder NEC F17.298
          withdrawal F17.293
    opioid F11.20
      with
        intoxication F11.229
          with
            delirium F11.221
            perceptual disturbance F11.222
          uncomplicated F11.220
        mood disorder F11.24

☑ Additional Character Required — Refer to the Tabular List for Character Selection   ▽ Subterms under main terms may continue to next column or page

Dependence — *continued*
  drug — *continued*
    opioid — *continued*
      with — *continued*
        other specified disorder F11.288
        psychosis F11.259
          delusions F11.250
          hallucinations F11.251
        sexual dysfunction F11.281
        sleep disorder F11.282
        unspecified disorder F11.29
        withdrawal F11.23
      in remission F11.21
    psychoactive NEC F19.20
      with
        amnestic disorder F19.26
        anxiety disorder F19.280
        dementia F19.27
        intoxication F19.229
          with
            delirium F19.221
            perceptual disturbance F19.222
          uncomplicated F19.220
        mood disorder F19.24
        other specified disorder F19.288
        psychosis F19.259
          delusions F19.250
          hallucinations F19.251
        sexual dysfunction F19.281
        sleep disorder F19.282
        unspecified disorder F19.29
        withdrawal F19.239
          with
            delirium F19.231
            perceptual disturbance F19.232
          uncomplicated F19.230
    sedative, hypnotic or anxiolytic F13.20
      with
        amnestic disorder F13.26
        anxiety disorder F13.280
        dementia, persisting F13.27
        intoxication F13.229
          with delirium F13.221
          uncomplicated F13.220
        mood disorder F13.24
        other specified disorder F13.288
        psychosis F13.259
          delusions F13.250
          hallucinations F13.251
        sexual dysfunction F13.281
        sleep disorder F13.282
        unspecified disorder F13.29
        withdrawal F13.239
          with
            delirium F13.231
            perceptual disturbance F13.232
          uncomplicated F13.230
      in remission F13.21
    stimulant NEC F15.20
      with
        anxiety disorder F15.280
        intoxication F15.229
          with
            delirium F15.221
            perceptual disturbance F15.222
          uncomplicated F15.220
        mood disorder F15.24
        other specified disorder F15.288
        psychosis F15.259
          delusions F15.250
          hallucinations F15.251
        sexual dysfunction F15.281
        sleep disorder F15.282
        unspecified disorder F15.29
        withdrawal F15.23
      in remission F15.21
    ethyl
      alcohol (without remission) F10.20
        with remission F10.21
      bromide — *see* Dependence, drug, sedative
    carbamate F19.20
    chloride F19.20
    morphine — *see* Dependence, drug, opioid
  ganja — *see* Dependence, drug, cannabis
  glue (airplane) (sniffing) — *see* Dependence, drug,
    inhalant
  glutethimide — *see* Dependence, drug, sedative

Dependence — *continued*
  hallucinogenics — *see* Dependence, drug, hallucino-
    gen
  hashish — *see* Dependence, drug, cannabis
  hemp — *see* Dependence, drug, cannabis
  heroin (salt) (any) — *see* Dependence, drug, opioid
  hypnotic NEC — *see* Dependence, drug, sedative
  Indian hemp — *see* Dependence, drug, cannabis
  inhalants — *see* Dependence, drug, inhalant
  khat — *see* Dependence, drug, stimulant NEC
  laudanum — *see* Dependence, drug, opioid
  LSD (-25) (derivatives) — *see* Dependence, drug, hal-
    lucinogen
  luminal — *see* Dependence, drug, sedative
  lysergic acid — *see* Dependence, drug, hallucinogen
  maconha — *see* Dependence, drug, cannabis
  marihuana — *see* Dependence, drug, cannabis
  meprobamate — *see* Dependence, drug, sedative
  mescaline — *see* Dependence, drug, hallucinogen
  methadone — *see* Dependence, drug, opioid
  methamphetamine(s) — *see* Dependence, drug,
    stimulant NEC
  methaqualone — *see* Dependence, drug, sedative
  methyl
    alcohol (without remission) F10.20
      with remission F10.21
    bromide — *see* Dependence, drug, sedative
    morphine — *see* Dependence, drug, opioid
    phenidate — *see* Dependence, drug, stimulant
      NEC
    sulfonal — *see* Dependence, drug, sedative
  morphine (sulfate) (sulfite) (type) — *see* Dependence,
    drug, opioid
  narcotic (drug) NEC — *see* Dependence, drug, opioid
  nembutal — *see* Dependence, drug, sedative
  neraval — *see* Dependence, drug, sedative
  neravan — *see* Dependence, drug, sedative
  neurobarb — *see* Dependence, drug, sedative
  nicotine — *see* Dependence, drug, nicotine
  nitrous oxide F19.20
  nonbarbiturate sedatives and tranquilizers with similar
    effect — *see* Dependence, drug, sedative
  on
    artificial heart (fully implantable) (mechanical)
      Z95.812
    aspirator Z99.0
    care provider (because of) Z74.9
      impaired mobility Z74.09
      need for
        assistance with personal care Z74.1
        continuous supervision Z74.3
      no other household member able to render
        care Z74.2
      specified reason NEC Z74.8
    machine Z99.89
      enabling NEC Z99.89
      specified type NEC Z99.89
    renal dialysis (hemodialysis) (peritoneal) Z99.2
    respirator Z99.11
    ventilator Z99.11
    wheelchair Z99.3
  opiate — *see* Dependence, drug, opioid
  opioids — *see* Dependence, drug, opioid
  opium (alkaloids) (derivatives) (tincture) — *see* Depen-
    dence, drug, opioid
  oxygen (long-term) (supplemental) Z99.81
  paraldehyde — *see* Dependence, drug, sedative
  paregoric — *see* Dependence, drug, opioid
  PCP (phencyclidine) (*see also* Abuse, drug, hallucino-
    gen) F16.20
  pentobarbital — *see* Dependence, drug, sedative
  pentobarbitone (sodium) — *see* Dependence, drug,
    sedative
  pentothal — *see* Dependence, drug, sedative
  peyote — *see* Dependence, drug, hallucinogen
  phencyclidine (PCP) (and related substances) (*see also*
    Abuse, drug, hallucinogen) F16.20
  phenmetrazine — *see* Dependence, drug, stimulant
    NEC
  phenobarbital — *see* Dependence, drug, sedative
  polysubstance F19.20
  psilocibin, psilocin, psilocyn, psilocyline — *see* Depen-
    dence, drug, hallucinogen
  psychostimulant NEC — *see* Dependence, drug, stim-
    ulant NEC
  secobarbital — *see* Dependence, drug, sedative
  seconal — *see* Dependence, drug, sedative

Dependence — *continued*
  sedative NEC — *see* Dependence, drug, sedative
  specified drug NEC — *see* Dependence, drug
  stimulant NEC — *see* Dependence, drug, stimulant
    NEC
  substance NEC — *see* Dependence, drug
  supplemental oxygen Z99.81
  tobacco — *see* Dependence, drug, nicotine
    counseling and surveillance Z71.6
  tranquilizer NEC — *see* Dependence, drug, sedative
  vitamin B6 E53.1
  volatile solvents — *see* Dependence, drug, inhalant
Dependency
  care-provider Z74.9
  passive F60.7
  reactions (persistent) F60.7
Depersonalization (in neurotic state) (neurotic) (syndrome) F48.1
Depletion
  extracellular fluid E86.9
  plasma E86.1
  potassium E87.6
    nephropathy N25.89
  salt or sodium E87.1
    causing heat exhaustion or prostration T67.4 ☑
    nephropathy N28.9
  volume NOS E86.9
Deployment (current) (military) status Z56.82
  in theater or in support of military war, peacekeeping
    and humanitarian operations Z56.82
  personal history of Z91.82
    military war, peacekeeping and humanitarian de-
      ployment (current or past conflict) Z91.82
  returned from Z91.82
Depolarization, premature I49.40
  atrial I49.1
  junctional I49.2
  specified NEC I49.49
  ventricular I49.3
Deposit
  bone in Boeck's sarcoid D86.89
  calcareous, calcium — *see* Calcification
  cholesterol
    retina H35.89
    vitreous (body) (humor) — *see* Deposit, crystalline
  conjunctiva H11.11- ☑
  cornea H18.00- ☑
    argentous H18.02- ☑
    due to metabolic disorder H18.03- ☑
    Kayser-Fleischer ring H18.04- ☑
    pigmentation — *see* Pigmentation, cornea
  crystalline, vitreous (body) (humor) H43.2- ☑
  hemosiderin in old scars of cornea — *see* Pigmenta-
    tion, cornea, stromal
  metallic in lens — *see* Cataract, specified NEC
  skin R23.8
  tooth, teeth (betel) (black) (green) (materia alba) (or-
    ange) (tobacco) K03.6
  urate, kidney — *see* Calculus, kidney
Depraved appetite — *see* Pica
Depressed
  HDL cholesterol E78.6
Depression (acute) (mental) F32.9
  agitated (single episode) F32.2
  anaclitic — *see* Disorder, adjustment
  anxiety F41.8
    persistent F34.1
  arches (*see also* Deformity, limb, flat foot)
  atypical (single episode) F32.8
  basal metabolic rate R94.8
  bone marrow D75.89
  central nervous system R09.2
  cerebral R29.818
    newborn P91.4
  cerebrovascular I67.9
  chest wall M95.4
  climacteric (single episode) F32.8
  endogenous (without psychotic symptoms) F33.2
    with psychotic symptoms F33.3
  functional activity R68.89
  hysterical F44.89
  involutional (single episode) F32.8
  major F32.9
    with psychotic symptoms F32.3
    recurrent — *see* Disorder, depressive, recurrent
  manic-depressive — *see* Disorder, depressive, recur-
    rent

Depression — *continued*
masked (single episode) F32.8
medullary G93.89
menopausal (single episode) F32.8
metatarsus — *see* Depression, arches
monopolar F33.9
nervous F34.1
neurotic F34.1
nose M95.0
postnatal F53
postpartum F53
post-psychotic of schizophrenia F32.8
post-schizophrenic F32.8
psychogenic (reactive) (single episode) F32.9
psychoneurotic F34.1
psychotic (single episode) F32.3
   recurrent F33.3
reactive (psychogenic) (single episode) F32.9
   psychotic (single episode) F32.3
recurrent — *see* Disorder, depressive, recurrent
respiratory center G93.89
seasonal — *see* Disorder, depressive, recurrent
senile F03 ☑
severe, single episode F32.2
situational F43.21
skull Q67.4
specified NEC (single episode) F32.8
sternum M95.4
visual field — *see* Defect, visual field
vital (recurrent) (without psychotic symptoms) F33.2
   with psychotic symptoms F33.3
    single episode F32.2

Deprivation
cultural Z60.3
effects NOS T73.9 ☑
   specified NEC T73.8 ☑
emotional NEC Z65.8
   affecting infant or child — *see* Maltreatment, child, psychological
food T73.0 ☑
protein — *see* Malnutrition
sleep Z72.820
social Z60.4
   affecting infant or child — *see* Maltreatment, child, psychological
specified NEC T73.8 ☑
vitamins — *see* Deficiency, vitamin
water T73.1 ☑

Derangement
ankle (internal) — *see* Derangement, joint, ankle
cartilage (articular) NEC — *see* Derangement, joint, articular cartilage, by site
   recurrent — *see* Dislocation, recurrent
cruciate ligament, anterior, current injury — *see* Sprain, knee, cruciate, anterior
elbow (internal) — *see* Derangement, joint, elbow
hip (joint) (internal) (old) — *see* Derangement, joint, hip
joint (internal) M24.9
   ankylosis — *see* Ankylosis
   articular cartilage M24.10
    ankle M24.17- ☑
    elbow M24.12- ☑
    foot M24.17- ☑
    hand M24.14- ☑
    hip M24.15- ☑
    knee NEC M23.9- ☑
    loose body — *see* Loose, body
    shoulder M24.11- ☑
    wrist M24.13- ☑
   contracture — *see* Contraction, joint
   current injury (*see also* Dislocation)
    knee, meniscus or cartilage — *see* Tear, meniscus
   dislocation
    pathological — *see* Dislocation, pathological
    recurrent — *see* Dislocation, recurrent
   knee — *see* Derangement, knee
   ligament — *see* Disorder, ligament
   loose body — *see* Loose, body
   recurrent — *see* Dislocation, recurrent
   specified type NEC M24.80
    ankle M24.87- ☑
    elbow M24.82- ☑
    foot joint M24.87- ☑
    hand joint M24.84- ☑
    hip M24.85- ☑

Derangement — *continued*
joint — *continued*
   specified type — *continued*
    shoulder M24.81- ☑
    wrist M24.83- ☑
   temporomandibular M26.69
knee (recurrent) M23.9- ☑
   ligament disruption, spontaneous M23.60- ☑
    anterior cruciate M23.61- ☑
    capsular M23.67- ☑
    instability, chronic M23.5- ☑
    lateral collateral M23.64- ☑
    medial collateral M23.63- ☑
    posterior cruciate M23.62- ☑
   loose body M23.4- ☑
   meniscus M23.30- ☑
    cystic M23.00- ☑
     lateral M23.002
      anterior horn M23.04- ☑
      posterior horn M23.05- ☑
      specified NEC M23.06- ☑
     medial M23.005
      anterior horn M23.01- ☑
      posterior horn M23.02- ☑
      specified NEC M23.03- ☑
    degenerate — *see* Derangement, knee, meniscus, specified NEC
    detached — *see* Derangement, knee, meniscus, specified NEC
    due to old tear or injury M23.20- ☑
     lateral M23.20- ☑
      anterior horn M23.24- ☑
      posterior horn M23.25- ☑
      specified NEC M23.26- ☑
     medial M23.20- ☑
      anterior horn M23.21- ☑
      posterior horn M23.22- ☑
      specified NEC M23.23- ☑
    retained — *see* Derangement, knee, meniscus, specified NEC
    specified NEC M23.30- ☑
     lateral M23.30- ☑
      anterior horn M23.34- ☑
      posterior horn M23.35- ☑
      specified NEC M23.36- ☑
     medial M23.30- ☑
      anterior horn M23.31- ☑
      posterior horn M23.32- ☑
      specified NEC M23.33- ☑
   old M23.8X- ☑
   specified NEC — *see* subcategory M23.8 ☑
   low back NEC — *see* Dorsopathy, specified NEC
   meniscus — *see* Derangement, knee, meniscus
   mental — *see* Psychosis
   patella, specified NEC — *see* Disorder, patella, derangement NEC
   semilunar cartilage (knee) — *see* Derangement, knee, meniscus, specified NEC
   shoulder (internal) — *see* Derangement, joint, shoulder

Dercum's disease E88.2
Derealization (neurotic) F48.1
Dermal — *see* condition
Dermaphytid — *see* Dermatophytosis
Dermatitis (eczematous) L30.9
ab igne L59.0
acarine B88.0
actinic (due to sun) L57.8
   other than from sun L59.8
allergic — *see* Dermatitis, contact, allergic
ambustionis, due to burn or scald — *see* Burn
amebic A06.7
ammonia L22
arsenical (ingested) L27.8
artefacta L98.1
   psychogenic F54
atopic L20.9
   psychogenic F54
   specified NEC L20.89
autoimmune progesterone L30.8
berlock, berloque L56.2
blastomycotic B40.3
blister beetle L24.89
bullous, bullosa L13.9
   mucosynechial, atrophic L12.1
   seasonal L30.8

Dermatitis — *continued*
bullous, bullosa — *continued*
   specified NEC L13.8
calorica L59.0
   due to burn or scald — *see* Burn
caterpillar L24.89
cercarial B65.3
combustionis L59.0
   due to burn or scald — *see* Burn
congelationis T69.1 ☑
contact (occupational) L25.9
   allergic L23.9
    due to
     adhesives L23.1
     cement L23.5
     chemical products NEC L23.5
     chromium L23.0
     cosmetics L23.2
     dander (cat) (dog) L23.81
     drugs in contact with skin L23.3
     dyes L23.4
     food in contact with skin L23.6
     hair (cat) (dog) L23.81
     insecticide L23.5
     metals L23.0
     nickel L23.0
     plants, non-food L23.7
     plastic L23.5
     rubber L23.5
     specified agent NEC L23.89
   due to
    cement L25.3
    chemical products NEC L25.3
    cosmetics L25.0
    dander (cat) (dog) L23.81
    drugs in contact with skin L25.1
    dyes L25.2
    food in contact with skin L25.4
    hair (cat) (dog) L23.81
    plants, non-food L25.5
    specified agent NEC L25.8
   irritant L24.9
    due to
     cement L25.3
     chemical products NEC L24.5
     cosmetics L24.3
     detergents L24.0
     drugs in contact with skin L24.4
     food in contact with skin L24.6
     oils and greases L24.1
     plants, non-food L24.7
     solvents L24.2
     specified agent NEC L24.89
contusiformis L52
diabetic — *see* E08-E13 with .620
diaper L22
diphtheritica A36.3
dry skin L85.3
due to
   acetone (contact) (irritant) L24.2
   acids (contact) (irritant) L24.5
   adhesive(s) (allergic) (contact) (plaster) L23.1
    irritant L24.5
   alcohol (irritant) (skin contact) (substances in category T51) L24.2
    taken internally L27.8
   alkalis (contact) (irritant) L24.5
   arsenic (ingested) L27.8
   carbon disulfide (contact) (irritant) L24.2
   caustics (contact) (irritant) L24.5
   cement (contact) L25.3
   cereal (ingested) L27.2
   chemical(s) NEC L25.3
    taken internally L27.8
   chlorocompounds L24.2
   chromium (contact) (irritant) L24.81
   coffee (ingested) L27.2
   cold weather L30.8
   cosmetics (contact) L25.0
    allergic L23.2
    irritant L24.3
   cyclohexanes L24.2
   dander (cat) (dog) L23.81
   Demodex species B88.0
   Dermanyssus gallinae B88.0
   detergents (contact) (irritant) L24.0
   dichromate L24.81

☑ **Additional Character Required** — Refer to the Tabular List for Character Selection   ▽ Subterms under main terms may continue to next column or page

Dermatitis — *continued*
　due to — *continued*
　　drugs and medicaments (generalized) (internal use) L27.Ø
　　　external — *see* Dermatitis, due to, drugs, in contact with skin
　　　in contact with skin L25.1
　　　　allergic L23.3
　　　　irritant L24.4
　　　localized skin eruption L27.1
　　　specified substance — *see* Table of Drugs and Chemicals
　　dyes (contact) L25.2
　　　allergic L23.4
　　　irritant L24.89
　　epidermophytosis — *see* Dermatophytosis
　　esters L24.2
　　external irritant NEC L24.9
　　fish (ingested) L27.2
　　flour (ingested) L27.2
　　food (ingested) L27.2
　　　in contact with skin L25.4
　　fruit (ingested) L27.2
　　furs (allergic) (contact) L23.81
　　glues — *see* Dermatitis, due to, adhesives
　　glycols L24.2
　　greases NEC (contact) (irritant) L24.1
　　hair (cat) (dog) L23.81
　　hot
　　　objects and materials — *see* Burn
　　　weather or places L59.Ø
　　hydrocarbons L24.2
　　infrared rays L59.8
　　ingestion, ingested substance L27.9
　　　chemical NEC L27.8
　　　drugs and medicaments — *see* Dermatitis, due to, drugs
　　　food L27.2
　　　specified NEC L27.8
　　insecticide in contact with skin L24.5
　　internal agent L27.9
　　　drugs and medicaments (generalized) — *see* Dermatitis, due to, drugs
　　　food L27.2
　　irradiation — *see* Dermatitis, due to, radioactive substance
　　ketones L24.2
　　lacquer tree (allergic) (contact) L23.7
　　light (sun) NEC L57.8
　　　acute L56.8
　　　other L59.8
　　Liponyssoides sanguineus B88.Ø
　　low temperature L3Ø.8
　　meat (ingested) L27.2
　　metals, metal salts (contact) (irritant) L24.81
　　milk (ingested) L27.2
　　nickel (contact) (irritant) L24.81
　　nylon (contact) (irritant) L24.5
　　oils NEC (contact) (irritant) L24.1
　　paint solvent (contact) (irritant) L24.2
　　petroleum products (contact) (irritant) (substances in T52.Ø) L24.2
　　plants NEC (contact) L25.5
　　　allergic L23.7
　　　irritant L24.7
　　plasters (adhesive) (any) (allergic) (contact) L23.1
　　　irritant L24.5
　　plastic (contact) L25.3
　　preservatives (contact) — *see* Dermatitis, due to, chemical, in contact with skin
　　primrose (allergic) (contact) L23.7
　　primula (allergic) (contact) L23.7
　　radiation L59.8
　　　nonionizing (chronic exposure) L57.8
　　　sun NEC L57.8
　　　　acute L56.8
　　radioactive substance L58.9
　　　acute L58.Ø
　　　chronic L58.1
　　radium L58.9
　　　acute L58.Ø
　　　chronic L58.1
　　ragweed (allergic) (contact) L23.7
　　Rhus (allergic) (contact) (diversiloba) (radicans) (toxicodendron) (venenata) (verniciflua) L23.7
　　rubber (contact) L24.5
　　Senecio jacobaea (allergic) (contact) L23.7

Dermatitis — *continued*
　due to — *continued*
　　solvents (contact) (irritant) (substances in category T52) L24.2
　　specified agent NEC (contact) L25.8
　　　allergic L23.89
　　　irritant L24.89
　　sunshine NEC L57.8
　　　acute L56.8
　　tetrachlorethylene (contact) (irritant) L24.2
　　toluene (contact) (irritant) L24.2
　　turpentine (contact) L24.2
　　ultraviolet rays (sun NEC) (chronic exposure) L57.8
　　　acute L56.8
　　vaccine or vaccination L27.Ø
　　　specified substance — *see* Table of Drugs and Chemicals
　　varicose veins — *see* Varix, leg, with, inflammation
　　X-rays L58.9
　　　acute L58.Ø
　　　chronic L58.1
　dyshydrotic L3Ø.1
　dysmenorrheica N94.6
　escharotica — *see* Burn
　exfoliative, exfoliativa (generalized) L26
　　neonatorum LØØ
　eyelid (*see also* Dermatosis, eyelid)
　　allergic HØ1.119
　　　left HØ1.116
　　　　lower HØ1.115
　　　　upper HØ1.114
　　　right HØ1.113
　　　　lower HØ1.112
　　　　upper HØ1.111
　　contact — *see* Dermatitis, eyelid, allergic
　　due to
　　　Demodex species B88.Ø
　　　herpes (zoster) BØ2.39
　　　　simplex BØØ.59
　　eczematous HØ1.139
　　　left HØ1.136
　　　　lower HØ1.135
　　　　upper HØ1.134
　　　right HØ1.133
　　　　lower HØ1.132
　　　　upper HØ1.131
　facta, factitia, factitial L98.1
　　psychogenic F54
　flexural NEC L2Ø.82
　friction L3Ø.4
　fungus B36.9
　　specified type NEC B36.8
　gangrenosa, gangrenous infantum LØ8.Ø
　harvest mite B88.Ø
　heat L59.Ø
　herpesviral, vesicular (ear) (lip) BØØ.1
　herpetiformis (bullous) (erythematous) (pustular) (vesicular) L13.Ø
　　juvenile L12.2
　　senile L12.Ø
　hiemalis L3Ø.8
　hypostatic, hypostatica — *see* Varix, leg, with, inflammation
　infectious eczematoid L3Ø.3
　infective L3Ø.3
　irritant — *see* Dermatitis, contact, irritant
　Jacquet's (diaper dermatitis) L22
　Leptus B88.Ø
　lichenified NEC L28.Ø
　medicamentosa (generalized) (internal use) — *see* Dermatitis, due to drugs
　mite B88.Ø
　multiformis L13.Ø
　　juvenile L12.2
　napkin L22
　neurotica L13.Ø
　nummular L3Ø.Ø
　papillaris capillitii L73.Ø
　pellagrous E52
　perioral L71.Ø
　photocontact L56.2
　polymorpha dolorosa L13.Ø
　pruriginosa L13.Ø
　pruritic NEC L3Ø.8
　psychogenic F54
　purulent LØ8.Ø
　pustular
　　contagious BØ8.Ø2

Dermatitis — *continued*
　pustular — *continued*
　　subcorneal L13.1
　pyococcal LØ8.Ø
　pyogenica LØ8.Ø
　repens L4Ø.2
　Ritter's (exfoliativa) LØØ
　Schamberg's L81.7
　schistosome B65.3
　seasonal bullous L3Ø.8
　seborrheic L21.9
　　infantile L21.1
　　specified NEC L21.8
　sensitization NOS L23.9
　septic LØ8.Ø
　solare L57.8
　specified NEC L3Ø.8
　stasis I87.2
　　with varicose ulcer — *see* Varix, leg, with ulcer, with inflammation
　　due to postthrombotic syndrome — *see* Syndrome, postthrombotic
　suppurative LØ8.Ø
　traumatic NEC L3Ø.4
　trophoneurotica L13.Ø
　ultraviolet (sun) (chronic exposure) L57.8
　　acute L56.8
　varicose — *see* Varix, leg, with, inflammation
　vegetans L1Ø.1
　verrucosa B43.Ø
　vesicular, herpesviral BØØ.1
Dermatoarthritis, lipoid E78.81
Dermatochalasis, eyelid HØ2.839
　left HØ2.836
　　lower HØ2.835
　　upper HØ2.834
　right HØ2.833
　　lower HØ2.832
　　upper HØ2.831
Dermatofibroma (lenticulare) — *see* Neoplasm, skin, benign
　protuberans — *see* Neoplasm, skin, uncertain behavior
Dermatofibrosarcoma (pigmented) (protuberans) — *see* Neoplasm, skin, malignant
Dermatographia L5Ø.3
Dermatolysis (exfoliativa) (congenital) Q82.8
　acquired L57.4
　eyelids — *see* Blepharochalasis
　palpebrarum — *see* Blepharochalasis
　senile L57.4
Dermatomegaly NEC Q82.8
Dermatomucosomyositis M33.1Ø
　with
　　myopathy M33.12
　　respiratory involvement M33.11
　　specified organ involvement NEC M33.19
Dermatomycosis B36.9
　furfuracea B36.Ø
　specified type NEC B36.8
Dermatomyositis (acute) (chronic) (*see also* Dermatopolymyositis)
　in (due to) neoplastic disease (*see also* Neoplasm) D49.9 [M36.Ø]
Dermatoneuritis of children — *see* Poisoning, mercury
Dermatophilosis A48.8
Dermatophytid L3Ø.2
Dermatophytide — *see* Dermatophytosis
Dermatophytosis (epidermophyton) (infection) (Microsporum) (tinea) (Trichophyton) B35.9
　beard B35.Ø
　body B35.4
　capitis B35.Ø
　corporis B35.4
　deep-seated B35.8
　disseminated B35.8
　foot B35.3
　granulomatous B35.8
　groin B35.6
　hand B35.2
　nail B35.1
　perianal (area) B35.6
　scalp B35.Ø
　specified NEC B35.8
Dermatopolymyositis M33.9Ø
　with
　　myopathy M33.92
　　respiratory involvement M33.91
　　specified organ involvement NEC M33.99

Dermatopolymyositis — *continued*
  in neoplastic disease (*see also* Neoplasm)
    D49.9 [M36.0]
  juvenile M33.00
    with
      myopathy M33.02
      respiratory involvement M33.01
      specified organ involvement NEC M33.09
  specified NEC M33.10
    myopathy M33.12
    respiratory involvement M33.11
    specified organ involvement NEC M33.19
Dermatopolyneuritis — *see* Poisoning, mercury
Dermatorrhexis Q79.6
  acquired L57.4
Dermatosclerosis (*see also* Scleroderma)
  localized L94.0
Dermatosis L98.9
  Andrews' L08.89
  Bowen's — *see* Neoplasm, skin, in situ
  bullous L13.9
    specified NEC L13.8
  exfoliativa L26
  eyelid (noninfectious)
    dermatitis — *see* Dermatitis, eyelid
    discoid lupus erythematosus — *see* Lupus, erythe-
      matosus, eyelid
    xeroderma — *see* Xeroderma, acquired, eyelid
  factitial L98.1
  febrile neutrophilic L98.2
  gonococcal A54.89
  herpetiformis L13.0
    juvenile L12.2
  linear IgA L13.8
  menstrual NEC L98.8
  neutrophilic, febrile L98.2
  occupational — *see* Dermatitis, contact
  papulosa nigra L82.1
  pigmentary L81.9
    progressive L81.7
    Schamberg's L81.7
  psychogenic F54
  purpuric, pigmented L81.7
  pustular, subcorneal L13.1
  transient acantholytic L11.1
Dermographia, dermographism L50.3
Dermoid (cyst) (*see also* Neoplasm, benign, by site)
  with malignant transformation C56- ☑
  due to radiation (nonionizing) L57.8
Dermopathy
  infiltrative with thyrotoxicosis — *see* Thyrotoxicosis
  nephrogenic fibrosing L90.8
Dermophytosis — *see* Dermatophytosis
Descemetocele H18.73- ☑
Descemet's membrane — *see* condition
Descending — *see* condition
Descensus uteri — *see* Prolapse, uterus
Desert
  rheumatism B38.0
  sore — *see* Ulcer, skin
Desertion (newborn) — *see* Maltreatment
Desmoid (extra-abdominal) (tumor) — *see* Neoplasm,
    connective tissue, uncertain behavior
  abdominal D48.1
Despondency F32.9
Desquamation, skin R23.4
Destruction, destructive (*see also* Damage)
  articular facet (*see also* Derangement, joint, specified
    type NEC)
    knee M23.8X- ☑
    vertebra — *see* Spondylosis
  bone (*see also* Disorder, bone, specified type NEC)
    syphilitic A52.77
  joint (*see also* Derangement, joint, specified type NEC)
    sacroiliac M53.3
  rectal sphincter K62.89
  septum (nasal) J34.89
  tuberculous NEC — *see* Tuberculosis
  tympanum, tympanic membrane (nontraumatic) —
    see Disorder, tympanic membrane, specified
    NEC
  vertebral disc — *see* Degeneration, intervertebral disc
Destructiveness (*see also* Disorder, conduct)
  adjustment reaction — *see* Disorder, adjustment
Desultory labor O62.2
Detachment
  cartilage — *see* Sprain

Detachment — *continued*
  cervix, annular N88.8
    complicating delivery O71.3
  choroid (old) (postinfectional) (simple) (spontaneous)
    H31.40- ☑
    hemorrhagic H31.41- ☑
    serous H31.42- ☑
  ligament — *see* Sprain
  meniscus (knee) (*see also* Derangement, knee, menis-
    cus, specified NEC)
    current injury — *see* Tear, meniscus
    due to old tear or injury — *see* Derangement, knee,
      meniscus, due to old tear
  retina (without retinal break) (serous) H33.2- ☑
    with retinal:
      break H33.00- ☑
        giant H33.03- ☑
        multiple H33.02- ☑
        single H33.01- ☑
      dialysis H33.04- ☑
    pigment epithelium — *see* Degeneration, retina,
      separation of layers, pigment epithelium
      detachment
    rhegmatogenous — *see* Detachment, retina, with
      retinal break
    specified NEC H33.8
    total H33.05- ☑
    traction H33.4- ☑
  vitreous (body) H43.81 ☑
Detergent asthma J69.8
Deterioration
  epileptic F06.8
  general physical R53.81
  heart, cardiac — *see* Degeneration, myocardial
  mental — *see* Psychosis
  myocardial, myocardium — *see* Degeneration, myocar-
    dial
  senile (simple) R54
Deuteranomaly (anomalous trichromat) H53.53
Deuteranopia (complete) (incomplete) H53.53
Development
  abnormal, bone Q79.9
  arrested R62.50
    bone — *see* Arrest, development or growth, bone
    child R62.50
    due to malnutrition E45
  defective, congenital (*see also* Anomaly, by site)
    cauda equina Q06.3
    left ventricle Q24.8
      in hypoplastic left heart syndrome Q23.4
    valve Q24.8
      pulmonary Q22.3
  delayed (*see also* Delay, development) R62.50
    arithmetical skills F81.2
    language (skills) (expressive) F80.1
    learning skill F81.9
    mixed skills F88
    motor coordination F82
    reading F81.0
    specified learning skill NEC F81.89
    speech F80.9
    spelling F81.81
    written expression F81.81
  imperfect, congenital (*see also* Anomaly, by site)
    heart Q24.9
    lungs Q33.6
  incomplete
    bronchial tree Q32.4
    organ or site not listed — *see* Hypoplasia, by site
    respiratory system Q34.9
  sexual, precocious NEC E30.1
  tardy, mental (*see also* Disability, intellectual) F79
Developmental — *see* condition
  testing, child — *see* Examination, child
Devergie's disease (pityriasis rubra pilaris) L44.0
Deviation (in)
  conjugate palsy (eye) (spastic) H51.0
  esophagus (acquired) K22.8
  eye, skew H51.8
  midline (jaw) (teeth) (dental arch) M26.29
    specified site NEC — *see* Malposition
  nasal septum J34.2
    congenital Q67.4
  opening and closing of the mandible M26.53
  organ or site, congenital NEC — *see* Malposition,
    congenital
  septum (nasal) (acquired) J34.2

Deviation — *continued*
  septum — *continued*
    congenital Q67.4
  sexual F65.9
    bestiality F65.89
    erotomania F52.8
    exhibitionism F65.2
    fetishism, fetishistic F65.0
      transvestism F65.1
    frotteurism F65.81
    masochism F65.51
    multiple F65.89
    necrophilia F65.89
    nymphomania F52.8
    pederosis F65.4
    pedophilia F65.4
    sadism, sadomasochism F65.52
    satyriasis F52.8
    specified type NEC F65.89
    transvestism F64.1
    voyeurism F65.3
  teeth, midline M26.29
  trachea J39.8
  ureter, congenital Q62.61
Device
  cerebral ventricle (communicating) in situ Z98.2
  contraceptive — *see* Contraceptive, device
  drainage, cerebrospinal fluid, in situ Z98.2
Devic's disease G36.0
Devil's
  grip B33.0
  pinches (purpura simplex) D69.2
Devitalized tooth K04.99
Devonshire colic — *see* Poisoning, lead
Dextraposition, aorta Q20.3
  in tetralogy of Fallot Q21.3
Dextrinosis, limit (debrancher enzyme deficiency)
  E74.03
Dextrocardia (true) Q24.0
  with
    complete transposition of viscera Q89.3
    situs inversus Q89.3
Dextrotransposition, aorta Q20.3
d-glycericacidemia E72.59
Dhat syndrome F48.8
Dhobi itch B35.6
Di George's syndrome D82.1
Di Guglielmo's disease C94.0- ☑
Diabetes, diabetic (mellitus) (sugar) E11.9
  with
    amyotrophy E11.44
    arthropathy NEC E11.618
    autonomic (poly)neuropathy E11.43
    cataract E11.36
    Charcot's joints E11.610
    chronic kidney disease E11.22
    circulatory complication NEC E11.59
    complication E11.8
      specified NEC E11.69
    dermatitis E11.620
    foot ulcer E11.621
    gangrene E11.52
    gastroparesis E11.43
    glomerulonephrosis, intracapillary E11.21
    glomerulosclerosis, intercapillary E11.21
    hyperglycemia E11.65
    hyperosmolarity E11.00
      with coma E11.01
    hypoglycemia E11.649
      with coma E11.641
    kidney complications NEC E11.29
    Kimmelstiel-Wilson disease E11.21
    loss of protective sensation (LOPS) — *see* Diabetes,
      by type, with neuropathy
    mononeuropathy E11.41
    myasthenia E11.44
    necrobiosis lipoidica E11.620
    nephropathy E11.21
    neuralgia E11.42
    neurologic complication NEC E11.49
    neuropathic arthropathy E11.610
    neuropathy E11.40
    ophthalmic complication NEC E11.39
    oral complication NEC E11.638
    periodontal disease E11.630
    peripheral angiopathy E11.51
      with gangrene E11.52
    polyneuropathy E11.42

Diabetes, diabetic — *continued*
with — *continued*
  renal complication NEC E11.29
  renal tubular degeneration E11.29
  retinopathy E11.319
    with macular edema E11.311
    nonproliferative E11.329
      with macular edema E11.321
      mild E11.329
        with macular edema E11.321
      moderate E11.339
        with macular edema E11.331
      severe E11.349
        with macular edema E11.341
    proliferative E11.359
      with macular edema E11.351
  skin complication NEC E11.628
  skin ulcer NEC E11.622
bronzed E83.110
complicating pregnancy — *see* Pregnancy, complicated by, diabetes
dietary counseling and surveillance Z71.3
due to drug or chemical E09.9
  with
    amyotrophy E09.44
    arthropathy NEC E09.618
    autonomic (poly)neuropathy E09.43
    cataract E09.36
    Charcot's joints E09.610
    chronic kidney disease E09.22
    circulatory complication NEC E09.59
    complication E09.8
      specified NEC E09.69
    dermatitis E09.620
    foot ulcer E09.621
    gangrene E09.52
    gastroparesis E09.43
    glomerulonephrosis, intracapillary E09.21
    glomerulosclerosis, intercapillary E09.21
    hyperglycemia E09.65
    hyperosmolarity E09.00
      with coma E09.01
    hypoglycemia E09.649
      with coma E09.641
    ketoacidosis E09.10
      with coma E09.11
    kidney complications NEC E09.29
    Kimmelstiel-Wilson disease E09.21
    mononeuropathy E09.41
    myasthenia E09.44
    necrobiosis lipoidica E09.620
    nephropathy E09.21
    neuralgia E09.42
    neurologic complication NEC E09.49
    neuropathic arthropathy E09.610
    neuropathy E09.40
    ophthalmic complication NEC E09.39
    oral complication NEC E09.638
    periodontal disease E09.630
    peripheral angiopathy E09.51
      with gangrene E09.52
    polyneuropathy E09.42
    renal complication NEC E09.29
    renal tubular degeneration E09.29
    retinopathy E09.319
      with macular edema E09.311
      nonproliferative E09.329
        with macular edema E09.321
        mild E09.329
          with macular edema E09.321
        moderate E09.339
          with macular edema E09.331
        severe E09.349
          with macular edema E09.341
      proliferative E09.359
        with macular edema E09.351
    skin complication NEC E09.628
    skin ulcer NEC E09.622
due to underlying condition E08.9
  with
    amyotrophy E08.44
    arthropathy NEC E08.618
    autonomic (poly)neuropathy E08.43
    cataract E08.36
    Charcot's joints E08.610
    chronic kidney disease E08.22
    circulatory complication NEC E08.59
    complication E08.8

Diabetes, diabetic — *continued*
due to underlying condition — *continued*
  with — *continued*
    complication — *continued*
      specified NEC E08.69
    dermatitis E08.620
    foot ulcer E08.621
    gangrene E08.52
    gastroparesis E08.43
    glomerulonephrosis, intracapillary E08.21
    glomerulosclerosis, intercapillary E08.21
    hyperglycemia E08.65
    hyperosmolarity E08.00
      with coma E08.01
    hypoglycemia E08.649
      with coma E08.641
    ketoacidosis E08.10
      with coma E08.11
    kidney complications NEC E08.29
    Kimmelsteil-Wilson disease E08.21
    mononeuropathy E08.41
    myasthenia E08.44
    necrobiosis lipoidica E08.620
    nephropathy E08.21
    neuralgia E08.42
    neurologic complication NEC E08.49
    neuropathic arthropathy E08.610
    neuropathy E08.40
    ophthalmic complication NEC E08.39
    oral complication NEC E08.638
    periodontal disease E08.630
    peripheral angiopathy E08.51
      with gangrene E08.52
    polyneuropathy E08.42
    renal complication NEC E08.29
    renal tubular degeneration E08.29
    retinopathy E08.319
      with macular edema E08.311
      nonproliferative E08.329
        with macular edema E08.321
        mild E08.329
          with macular edema E08.321
        moderate E08.339
          with macular edema E08.331
        severe E08.349
          with macular edema E08.341
      proliferative E08.359
        with macular edema E08.351
    skin complication NEC E08.628
    skin ulcer NEC E08.622
gestational (in pregnancy) O24.419
  affecting newborn P70.0
  diet controlled O24.410
  in childbirth O24.429
    diet controlled O24.420
    insulin (and diet) controlled O24.424
    insulin (and diet) controlled O24.414
  puerperal O24.439
    diet controlled O24.430
    insulin (and diet) controlled O24.434
hepatogenous E13.9
inadequately controlled — *code to* Diabetes, by type, with hyperglycemia
insipidus E23.2
  nephrogenic N25.1
  pituitary E23.2
  vasopressin resistant N25.1
insulin dependent — *code to* type of diabetes
juvenile-onset — *see* Diabetes, type 1
ketosis-prone — *see* Diabetes, type 1
latent R73.09
neonatal (transient) P70.2
non-insulin dependent — *code to* type of diabetes
out of control — *code to* Diabetes, by type, with hyperglycemia
phosphate E83.39
poorly controlled — *code to* Diabetes, by type, with hyperglycemia
postpancreatectomy — *see* Diabetes, specified type NEC
postprocedural — *see* Diabetes, specified type NEC
secondary diabetes mellitus NEC — *see* Diabetes, specified type NEC
specified type NEC E13.9
  with
    amyotrophy E13.44
    arthropathy NEC E13.618
    autonomic (poly)neuropathy E13.43

Diabetes, diabetic — *continued*
specified type — *continued*
  with — *continued*
    cataract E13.36
    Charcot's joints E13.610
    chronic kidney disease E13.22
    circulatory complication NEC E13.59
    complication E13.8
      specified NEC E13.69
    dermatitis E13.620
    foot ulcer E13.621
    gangrene E13.52
    gastroparesis E13.43
    glomerulonephrosis, intracapillary E13.21
    glomerulosclerosis, intercapillary E13.21
    hyperglycemia E13.65
    hyperosmolarity E13.00
      with coma E13.01
    hypoglycemia E13.649
      with coma E13.641
    ketoacidosis E13.10
      with coma E13.11
    kidney complications NEC E13.29
    Kimmelsteil-Wilson disease E13.21
    mononeuropathy E13.41
    myasthenia E13.44
    necrobiosis lipoidica E13.620
    nephropathy E13.21
    neuralgia E13.42
    neurologic complication NEC E13.49
    neuropathic arthropathy E13.610
    neuropathy E13.40
    ophthalmic complication NEC E13.39
    oral complication NEC E13.638
    periodontal disease E13.630
    peripheral angiopathy E13.51
      with gangrene E13.52
    polyneuropathy E13.42
    renal complication NEC E13.29
    renal tubular degeneration E13.29
    retinopathy E13.319
      with macular edema E13.311
      nonproliferative E13.329
        with macular edema E13.321
        mild E13.329
          with macular edema E13.321
        moderate E13.339
          with macular edema E13.331
        severe E13.349
          with macular edema E13.341
      proliferative E13.359
        with macular edema E13.351
    skin complication NEC E13.628
    skin ulcer NEC E13.622
steroid-induced — *see* Diabetes, due to, drug or chemical
type 1 E10.9
  with
    amyotrophy E10.44
    arthropathy NEC E10.618
    autonomic (poly)neuropathy E10.43
    cataract E10.36
    Charcot's joints E10.610
    chronic kidney disease E10.22
    circulatory complication NEC E10.59
    complication E10.8
      specified NEC E10.69
    dermatitis E10.620
    foot ulcer E10.621
    gangrene E10.52
    gastroparesis E10.43
    glomerulonephrosis, intracapillary E10.21
    glomerulosclerosis, intercapillary E10.21
    hyperglycemia E10.65
    hypoglycemia E10.649
      with coma E10.641
    ketoacidosis E10.10
      with coma E10.11
    kidney complications NEC E10.29
    Kimmelstiel-Wilson disease E10.21
    mononeuropathy E10.41
    myasthenia E10.44
    necrobiosis lipoidica E10.620
    nephropathy E10.21
    neuralgia E10.42
    neurologic complication NEC E10.49
    neuropathic arthropathy E10.610
    neuropathy E10.40

Diabetes, diabetic — continued
  type 1 — continued
    with — continued
      ophthalmic complication NEC E10.39
      oral complication NEC E10.638
      periodontal disease E10.630
      peripheral angiopathy E10.51
        with gangrene E10.52
      polyneuropathy E10.42
      renal complication NEC E10.29
      renal tubular degeneration E10.29
      retinopathy E10.319
        with macular edema E10.311
        nonproliferative E10.329
          with macular edema E10.321
          mild E10.329
            with macular edema E10.321
          moderate E10.339
            with macular edema E10.331
          severe E10.349
            with macular edema E10.341
        proliferative E10.359
          with macular edema E10.351
      skin complication NEC E10.628
      skin ulcer NEC E10.622
  type 2 E11.9
    with
      amyotrophy E11.44
      arthropathy NEC E11.618
      autonomic (poly)neuropathy E11.43
      cataract E11.36
      Charcot's joints E11.610
      chronic kidney disease E11.22
      circulatory complication NEC E11.59
      complication E11.8
        specified NEC E11.69
      dermatitis E11.620
      foot ulcer E11.621
      gangrene E11.52
      gastroparesis E11.43
      glomerulonephrosis, intracapillary E11.21
      glomerulosclerosis, intercapillary E11.21
      hyperglycemia E11.65
      hyperosmolarity E11.00
        with coma E11.01
      hypoglycemia E11.649
        with coma E11.641
      kidney complications NEC E11.29
      Kimmelstiel-Wilson disease E11.21
      mononeuropathy E11.41
      myasthenia E11.44
      necrobiosis lipoidica E11.620
      nephropathy E11.21
      neuralgia E11.42
      neurologic complication NEC E11.49
      neuropathic arthropathy E11.610
      neuropathy E11.40
      ophthalmic complication NEC E11.39
      oral complication NEC E11.638
      periodontal disease E11.630
      peripheral angiopathy E11.51
        with gangrene E11.52
      polyneuropathy E11.42
      renal complication NEC E11.29
      renal tubular degeneration E11.29
      retinopathy E11.319
        with macular edema E11.311
        nonproliferative E11.329
          with macular edema E11.321
          mild E11.329
            with macular edema E11.321
          moderate E11.339
            with macular edema E11.331
          severe E11.349
            with macular edema E11.341
        proliferative E11.359
          with macular edema E11.351
      skin complication NEC E11.628
      skin ulcer NEC E11.622

Diacyclothrombopathia D69.1
Diagnosis deferred R69
Dialysis (intermittent) (treatment)
  noncompliance (with) Z91.15
  renal (hemodialysis) (peritoneal), status Z99.2
  retina, retinal — see Detachment, retina, with retinal, dialysis
Diamond-Blackfan anemia (congenital hypoplastic) D61.01

Diamond-Gardener syndrome (autoerythrocyte sensitization) D69.2
Diaper rash L22
Diaphoresis (excessive) R61
Diaphragm — see condition
Diaphragmalgia R07.1
Diaphragmatitis, diaphragmitis J98.6
Diaphysial aclasis Q78.6
Diaphysitis — see Osteomyelitis, specified type NEC
Diarrhea, diarrheal (disease) (infantile) (inflammatory) R19.7
  achlorhydric K31.83
  allergic K52.2
  amebic (see also Amebiasis) A06.0
    with abscess — see Abscess, amebic
    acute A06.0
    chronic A06.1
    nondysenteric A06.2
  bacillary — see Dysentery, bacillary
  balantidial A07.0
  cachectic NEC K52.89
  Chilomastix A07.8
  choleriformis A00.1
  chronic (noninfectious) K52.9
  coccidial A07.3
  Cochin-China K90.1
    strongyloidiasis B78.0
  Dientamoeba A07.8
  dietetic K52.2
  drug-induced K52.1
  due to
    bacteria A04.9
      specified NEC A04.8
    Campylobacter A04.5
    Capillaria philippinensis B81.1
    Clostridium difficile A04.7
    Clostridium perfringens (C) (F) A04.8
    Cryptosporidium A07.2
    drugs K52.1
    Escherichia coli A04.4
      enteroaggregative A04.4
      enterohemorrhagic A04.3
      enteroinvasive A04.2
      enteropathogenic A04.0
      enterotoxigenic A04.1
      specified NEC A04.4
    food hypersensitivity K52.2
    Necator americanus B76.1
    S. japonicum B65.2
    specified organism NEC A08.8
      bacterial A04.8
      viral A08.39
    Staphylococcus A04.8
    Trichuris trichiuria B79
    virus — see Enteritis, viral
    Yersinia enterocolitica A04.6
  dysenteric A09
  endemic A09
  epidemic A09
  flagellate A07.9
  Flexner's (ulcerative) A03.1
  functional K59.1
    following gastrointestinal surgery K91.89
    psychogenic F45.8
  Giardia lamblia A07.1
  giardial A07.1
  hill K90.1
  infectious A09
  malarial — see Malaria
  mite B88.0
  mycotic NEC B49
  neonatal (noninfectious) P78.3
  nervous F45.8
  neurogenic K59.1
  noninfectious K52.9
  postgastrectomy K91.1
  postvagotomy K91.1
  protozoal A07.9
    specified NEC A07.8
  psychogenic F45.8
  specified
    bacterium NEC A04.8
    virus NEC A08.39
  strongyloidiasis B78.0
  toxic K52.1
  trichomonal A07.8
  tropical K90.1
  tuberculous A18.32

Diarrhea, diarrheal — continued
  viral — see Enteritis, viral
Diastasis
  cranial bones M84.88
    congenital NEC Q75.8
  joint (traumatic) — see Dislocation
  muscle M62.00
    ankle M62.07- ☑
    congenital Q79.8
    foot M62.07- ☑
    forearm M62.03- ☑
    hand M62.04- ☑
    lower leg M62.06- ☑
    pelvic region M62.05- ☑
    shoulder region M62.01- ☑
    specified site NEC M62.08
    thigh M62.05- ☑
    upper arm M62.02- ☑
  recti (abdomen)
    complicating delivery O71.89
    congenital Q79.59
Diastema, tooth, teeth, fully erupted M26.32
Diastematomyelia Q06.2
Diataxia, cerebral G80.4
Diathesis
  allergic — see History, allergy
  bleeding (familial) D69.9
  cystine (familial) E72.00
  gouty — see Gout
  hemorrhagic (familial) D69.9
    newborn NEC P53
  spasmophilic R29.0
Diaz's disease or osteochondrosis (juvenile) (talus) — see Osteochondrosis, juvenile, tarsus
Dibothriocephalus, dibothriocephaliasis (latus) (infection) (infestation) B70.0
  larval B70.1
Dicephalus, dicephaly Q89.4
Dichotomy, teeth K00.2
Dichromat, dichromatopsia (congenital) — see Deficiency, color vision
Dichuchwa A65
Dicroceliasis B66.2
Didelphia, didelphys — see Double uterus
Didymytis N45.1
  with orchitis N45.3
Dietary
  inadequacy or deficiency E63.9
  surveillance and counseling Z71.3
Dietl's crisis N13.8
Dieulafoy lesion (hemorrhagic)
  duodenum K31.82
  esophagus K22.8
  intestine (colon) K63.81
  stomach K31.82
Difficult, difficulty (in)
  acculturation Z60.3
  feeding R63.3
    newborn P92.9
      breast P92.5
      specified NEC P92.8
    nonorganic (infant or child) F98.29
  intubation, in anesthesia T88.4 ☑
  mechanical, gastroduodenal stoma K91.89
    causing obstruction K91.3
  reading (developmental) F81.0
    secondary to emotional disorders F93.9
  spelling (specific) F81.81
    with reading disorder F81.89
    due to inadequate teaching Z55.8
  swallowing — see Dysphagia
  walking R26.2
  work
    conditions NEC Z56.5
    schedule Z56.3
Diffuse — see condition
Digestive — see condition
Dihydropyrimidine dehydrogenase disease (DPD) E88.89
Diktyoma — see Neoplasm, malignant, by site
Dilaceration, tooth K00.4
Dilatation
  anus K59.8
    venule — see Hemorrhoids
  aorta (focal) (general) — see Ectasia, aorta
    with aneurysm — see Aneurysm, aorta
  artery — see Aneurysm

Dilatation — *continued*
bladder (sphincter) N32.89
 congenital Q64.79
blood vessel I99.8
bronchial J47.9
 with
  exacerbation (acute) J47.1
  lower respiratory infection J47.0
calyx (due to obstruction) — *see* Hydronephrosis
capillaries I78.8
cardiac (acute) (chronic) (*see also* Hypertrophy, cardiac)
 congenital Q24.8
  valve NEC Q24.8
   pulmonary Q22.3
 valve — *see* Endocarditis
cavum septi pellucidi Q06.8
cervix (uteri) (*see also* Incompetency, cervix)
 incomplete, poor, slow complicating delivery O62.0
colon K59.3
 congenital Q43.1
 psychogenic F45.8
common duct (acquired) K83.8
 congenital Q44.5
cystic duct (acquired) K82.8
 congenital Q44.5
duct, mammary — *see* Ectasia, mammary duct
duodenum K59.8
esophagus K22.8
 congenital Q39.5
 due to achalasia K22.0
eustachian tube, congenital Q17.8
gallbladder K82.8
gastric — *see* Dilatation, stomach
heart (acute) (chronic) (*see also* Hypertrophy, cardiac)
 congenital Q24.8
 valve — *see* Endocarditis
ileum K59.8
 psychogenic F45.8
jejunum K59.8
 psychogenic F45.8
kidney (calyx) (collecting structures) (cystic)
 (parenchyma) (pelvis) (idiopathic) N28.89
lacrimal passages or duct — *see* Disorder, lacrimal
 system, changes
lymphatic vessel I89.0
mammary duct — *see* Ectasia, mammary duct
Meckel's diverticulum (congenital) Q43.0
 malignant — *see* Table of Neoplasms, small intestine, malignant
myocardium (acute) (chronic) — *see* Hypertrophy,
 cardiac
organ or site, congenital NEC — *see* Distortion
pancreatic duct K86.8
pericardium — *see* Pericarditis
pharynx J39.2
prostate N42.89
pulmonary
 artery (idiopathic) I28.8
 valve, congenital Q22.3
pupil H57.04
rectum K59.3
saccule, congenital Q16.5
salivary gland (duct) K11.8
sphincter ani K62.89
stomach K31.89
 acute K31.0
 psychogenic F45.8
submaxillary duct K11.8
trachea, congenital Q32.1
ureter (idiopathic) N28.82
 congenital Q62.2
 due to obstruction N13.4
urethra (acquired) N36.8
vasomotor I73.9
vein I86.8
ventricular, ventricle (acute) (chronic) (*see also* Hypertrophy, cardiac)
 cerebral, congenital Q04.8
venule NEC I86.8
vesical orifice N32.89
Dilated, dilation — *see* Dilatation
Diminished, diminution
hearing (acuity) — *see* Deafness
sense or sensation (cold) (heat) (tactile) (vibratory)
 R20.8
vision NEC H54.7
vital capacity R94.2
Diminuta taenia B71.0

Dimitri-Sturge-Weber disease Q85.8
Dimple
parasacral, pilonidal or postanal — *see* Cyst, pilonidal
Dioctophyme renalis (infection) (infestation) B83.8
Dipetalonemiasis B74.4
Diphallus Q55.69
Diphtheria, diphtheritic (gangrenous) (hemorrhagic)
 A36.9
carrier (suspected) Z22.2
cutaneous A36.3
faucial A36.0
infection of wound A36.3
laryngeal A36.2
myocarditis A36.81
nasal, anterior A36.89
nasopharyngeal A36.1
neurological complication A36.89
pharyngeal A36.0
specified site NEC A36.89
tonsillar A36.0
Diphyllobothriasis (intestine) B70.0
larval B70.1
Diplacusis H93.22- ☑
Diplegia (upper limbs) G83.0
congenital (cerebral) G80.8
facial G51.0
lower limbs G82.20
spastic G80.1
Diplococcus, diplococcal — *see* condition
Diplopia H53.2
Dipsomania F10.20
with
 psychosis — *see* Psychosis, alcoholic
 remission F10.21
Dipylidiasis B71.1
Direction, teeth, abnormal, fully erupted M26.30
Dirofilariasis B74.8
Dirt-eating child F98.3
Disability, disabilities
heart — *see* Disease, heart
intellectual F79
 with
  autistic features F84.9
 mild (I.Q. 50-69) F70
 moderate (I.Q. 35-49) F71
 profound (I.Q. under 20) F73
 severe (I.Q. 20-34) F72
 specified level NEC F78
knowledge acquisition F81.9
learning F81.9
limiting activities Z73.6
spelling, specific F81.81
Disappearance of family member Z63.4
Disarticulation — *see* Amputation
meaning traumatic amputation — *see* Amputation,
 traumatic
Discharge (from)
abnormal finding in — *see* Abnormal, specimen
breast (female) (male) N64.52
diencephalic autonomic idiopathic — *see* Epilepsy,
 specified NEC
ear (*see also* Otorrhea)
 blood — *see* Otorrhagia
excessive urine R35.8
nipple N64.52
penile R36.9
postnasal R09.82
prison, anxiety concerning Z65.2
urethral R36.9
 without blood R36.0
 hematospermia R36.1
vaginal N89.8
Discitis, diskitis M46.40
cervical region M46.42
cervicothoracic region M46.43
lumbar region M46.46
lumbosacral region M46.47
multiple sites M46.49
occipito-atlanto-axial region M46.41
pyogenic — *see* Infection, intervertebral disc, pyogenic
sacrococcygeal region M46.48
thoracic region M46.44
thoracolumbar region M46.45
Discoid
meniscus (congenital) Q68.6
semilunar cartilage (congenital) — *see* Derangement,
 knee, meniscus, specified NEC

Discoloration
nails L60.8
teeth (posteruptive) K03.7
 during formation K00.8
Discomfort
chest R07.89
visual H53.14- ☑
Discontinuity, ossicles, ear H74.2- ☑
Discord (with)
boss Z56.4
classmates Z55.4
counselor Z64.4
employer Z56.4
family Z63.8
fellow employees Z56.4
in-laws Z63.1
landlord Z59.2
lodgers Z59.2
neighbors Z59.2
probation officer Z64.4
social worker Z64.4
teachers Z55.4
workmates Z56.4
Discordant connection
atrioventricular (congenital) Q20.5
ventriculoarterial Q20.3
Discrepancy
centric occlusion maximum intercuspation M26.55
leg length (acquired) — *see* Deformity, limb, unequal
 length
 congenital — *see* Defect, reduction, lower limb
uterine size date O26.84- ☑
Discrimination
ethnic Z60.5
political Z60.5
racial Z60.5
religious Z60.5
sex Z60.5
Disease, diseased (*see also* Syndrome)
absorbent system I87.8
acid-peptic K30
Acosta's T70.29 ☑
Adams-Stokes (-Morgagni) (syncope with heart block)
 I45.9
Addison's anemia (pernicious) D51.0
adenoids (and tonsils) J35.9
adrenal (capsule) (cortex) (gland) (medullary) E27.9
 hyperfunction E27.0
 specified NEC E27.8
ainhum L94.6
airway
 obstructive, chronic J44.9
  due to
   cotton dust J66.0
   specific organic dusts NEC J66.8
 reactive — *see* Asthma
akamushi (scrub typhus) A75.3
Albers-Schönberg (marble bones) Q78.2
Albert's — *see* Tendinitis, Achilles
alimentary canal K63.9
alligator-skin Q80.9
 acquired L85.0
alpha heavy chain C88.3
alpine T70.29 ☑
altitude T70.20 ☑
alveolar ridge
 edentulous K06.9
 specified NEC K06.8
alveoli, teeth K08.9
Alzheimer's G30.9 [F02.80]
 with behavioral disturbance G30.9 [F02.81]
 early onset G30.0 [F02.80]
  with behavioral disturbance G30.0 [F02.81]
 late onset G30.1 [F02.80]
  with behavioral disturbance G30.1 [F02.81]
 specified NEC G30.8 [F02.80]
  with behavioral disturbance G30.8 [F02.81]
amyloid — *see* Amyloidosis
Andersen's (glycogenosis IV) E74.09
Andes T70.29 ☑
Andrews' (bacterid) L08.89
angiospastic I73.9
 cerebral G45.9
 vein I87.8
anterior
 chamber H21.9
 horn cell G12.29

Disease, diseased — *continued*

antiglomerular basement membrane (anti- GBM) antibody M31.0
   tubulo-interstitial nephritis N12
antral — *see* Sinusitis, maxillary
anus K62.9
   specified NEC K62.89
aorta (nonsyphilitic) I77.9
   syphilitic NEC A52.02
aortic (heart) (valve) I35.9
   rheumatic I06.9
Apollo B30.3
aponeuroses — *see* Enthesopathy
appendix K38.9
   specified NEC K38.8
aqueous (chamber) H21.9
Arnold-Chiari — *see* Arnold-Chiari disease
arterial I77.9
   occlusive — *see* Occlusion, by site
   due to stricture or stenosis I77.1
arteriocardiorenal — *see* Hypertension, cardiorenal
arteriolar (generalized) (obliterative) I77.9
arteriorenal — *see* Hypertension, kidney
arteriosclerotic (*see also* Arteriosclerosis)
   cardiovascular — *see* Disease, heart, ischemic, atherosclerotic
   coronary (artery) — *see* Disease, heart, ischemic, atherosclerotic
   heart — *see* Disease, heart, ischemic, atherosclerotic
artery I77.9
   cerebral I67.9
   coronary I25.10
      with angina pectoris — *see* Arteriosclerosis, coronary (artery)
arthropod-borne NOS (viral) A94
   specified type NEC A93.8
atticoantral, chronic H66.20
   left H66.22
      with right H66.23
   right H66.21
      with left H66.23
auditory canal — *see* Disorder, ear, external
auricle, ear NEC — *see* Disorder, pinna
Australian X A83.4
autoimmune (systemic) NOS M35.9
   hemolytic (cold type) (warm type) D59.1
      drug-induced D59.0
   thyroid E06.3
aviator's — *see* Effect, adverse, high altitude
Ayala's Q78.5
Ayerza's (pulmonary artery sclerosis with pulmonary hypertension) I27.0
Babington's (familial hemorrhagic telangiectasia) I78.0
bacterial A49.9
   specified NEC A48.8
   zoonotic A28.9
      specified type NEC A28.8
Baelz's (cheilitis glandularis apostematosa) K13.0
bagasse J67.1
balloon — *see* Effect, adverse, high altitude
Bang's (brucella abortus) A23.1
Bannister's T78.3 ☑
barometer makers' — *see* Poisoning, mercury
Barraquer (-Simons) (progressive lipodystrophy) E88.1
Barrett's — *see* Barrett's, esophagus
Bartholin's gland N75.9
basal ganglia G25.9
   degenerative G23.9
      specified NEC G23.8
   specified NEC G25.89
Basedow's (exophthalmic goiter) — *see* Hyperthyroidism, with, goiter (diffuse)
Bateman's B08.1
Batten-Steinert G71.11
Battey A31.0
Beard's (neurasthenia) F48.8
Becker
   idiopathic mural endomyocardial I42.3
   myotonia congenita G71.12
Begbie's (exophthalmic goiter) — *see* Hyperthyroidism, with, goiter (diffuse)
behavioral, organic F07.9
Beigel's (white piedra) B36.2
Benson's — *see* Deposit, crystalline
Bernard-Soulier (thrombopathy) D69.1
Bernhardt (-Roth) — *see* Mononeuropathy, lower limb, meralgia paresthetica

Disease, diseased — *continued*

Biermer's (pernicious anemia) D51.0
bile duct (common) (hepatic) K83.9
   with calculus, stones — *see* Calculus, bile duct
   specified NEC K83.8
biliary (tract) K83.9
   specified NEC K83.8
Billroth's — *see* Spina bifida
bird fancier's J67.2
black lung J60
bladder N32.9
   in (due to)
      schistosomiasis (bilharziasis) B65.0 [N33]
   specified NEC N32.89
bleeder's D66
blood D75.9
   forming organs D75.9
   vessel I99.9
Bloodgood's — *see* Mastopathy, cystic
Bodechtel-Guttmann (subacute sclerosing panencephalitis) A81.1
bone (*see also* Disorder, bone)
   aluminum M83.4
   fibrocystic NEC
      jaw M27.49
bone-marrow D75.9
Borna A83.9
Bornholm (epidemic pleurodynia) B33.0
Bouchard's (myopathic dilatation of the stomach) K31.0
Bouillaud's (rheumatic heart disease) I01.9
Bourneville (-Brissaud) (tuberous sclerosis) Q85.1
Bouveret (-Hoffmann) (paroxysmal tachycardia) I47.9
bowel K63.9
   functional K59.9
      psychogenic F45.8
brain G93.9
   arterial, artery I67.9
   arteriosclerotic I67.2
   congenital Q04.9
   degenerative — *see* Degeneration, brain
   inflammatory — *see* Encephalitis
   organic G93.9
      arteriosclerotic I67.2
   parasitic NEC B71.9 [G94]
   senile NEC G31.1
   specified NEC G93.89
breast (*see also* Disorder, breast) N64.9
   cystic (chronic) — *see* Mastopathy, cystic
   fibrocystic — *see* Mastopathy, cystic
   Paget's
      female, unspecified side C50.91- ☑
      male, unspecified side C50.92- ☑
   specified NEC N64.89
Breda's — *see* Yaws
Bretonneau's (diphtheritic malignant angina) A36.0
Bright's — *see* Nephritis
   arteriosclerotic — *see* Hypertension, kidney
Brill's (recrudescent typhus) A75.1
Brill-Zinsser (recrudescent typhus) A75.1
Brion-Kayser — *see* Fever, paratyphoid
broad
   beta E78.2
   ligament (noninflammatory) N83.9
      inflammatory — *see* Disease, pelvis, inflammatory
      specified NEC N83.8
Brocq-Duhring (dermatitis herpetiformis) L13.0
Brocq's
   meaning
      dermatitis herpetiformis L13.0
      prurigo L28.2
bronchopulmonary J98.4
bronchus NEC J98.09
bronze Addison's E27.1
   tuberculous A18.7
budgerigar fancier's J67.2
Buerger's (thromboangiitis obliterans) I73.1
bullous L13.9
   chronic of childhood L12.2
   specified NEC L13.8
Bürger-Grütz (essential familial hyperlipemia) E78.3
bursa — *see* Bursopathy
caisson T70.3 ☑
California — *see* Coccidioidomycosis
capillaries I78.9
   specified NEC I78.8
Carapata A68.0

Disease, diseased — *continued*

cardiac — *see* Disease, heart
cardiopulmonary, chronic I27.9
cardiorenal (hepatic) (hypertensive) (vascular) — *see* Hypertension, cardiorenal
cardiovascular (atherosclerotic) I25.10
   with angina pectoris — *see* Arteriosclerosis, coronary (artery),
   congenital Q28.9
   hypertensive — *see* Hypertension, heart
   newborn P29.9
      specified NEC P29.89
   renal (hypertensive) — *see* Hypertension, cardiorenal
   syphilitic (asymptomatic) A52.00
cartilage — *see* Disorder, cartilage
Castellani's A69.8
cat-scratch A28.1
Cavare's (familial periodic paralysis) G72.3
cecum K63.9
celiac (adult) (infantile) K90.0
cellular tissue L98.9
central core G71.2
cerebellar, cerebellum — *see* Disease, brain
cerebral (*see also* Disease, brain)
   degenerative — *see* Degeneration, brain
cerebrospinal G96.9
cerebrovascular I67.9
   acute I67.89
      embolic I63.4- ☑
      thrombotic I63.3- ☑
   arteriosclerotic I67.2
   specified NEC I67.89
cervix (uteri) (noninflammatory) N88.9
   inflammatory — *see* Cervicitis
   specified NEC N88.8
Chabert's A22.9
Chandler's (osteochondritis dissecans, hip) — *see* Osteochondritis, dissecans, hip
Charlouis — *see* Yaws
Chédiak-Steinbrinck (-Higashi) (congenital gigantism of peroxidase granules) E70.330
chest J98.9
Chiari's (hepatic vein thrombosis) I82.0
Chicago B40.9
Chignon B36.8
chigo, chigoe B88.1
childhood granulomatous D71
Chinese liver fluke B66.1
chlamydial A74.9
   specified NEC A74.89
cholecystic K82.9
choroid H31.9
   specified NEC H31.8
Christmas D67
chronic bullous of childhood L12.2
chylomicron retention E78.3
ciliary body H21.9
   specified NEC H21.89
circulatory (system) NEC I99.8
   newborn P29.9
   syphilitic A52.00
      congenital A50.54
coagulation factor deficiency (congenital) — *see* Defect, coagulation
coccidioidal — *see* Coccidioidomycosis
cold
   agglutinin or hemoglobinuria D59.1
      paroxysmal D59.6
   hemagglutinin (chronic) D59.1
collagen NOS (nonvascular) (vascular) M35.9
   specified NEC M35.8
colon K63.9
   functional K59.9
      congenital Q43.2
   ischemic K55.0
combined system — *see* Degeneration, combined
compressed air T70.3 ☑
Concato's (pericardial polyserositis) A19.9
   nontubercular I31.1
   pleural — *see* Pleurisy, with effusion
conjunctiva H11.9
   chlamydial A74.0
   specified NEC H11.89
   viral B30.9
      specified NEC B30.8
connective tissue, systemic (diffuse) M35.9

Disease, diseased — *continued*
connective tissue, systemic — *continued*
  in (due to)
    hypogammaglobulinemia D80.1 [M36.8]
    ochronosis E70.29 [M36.8]
    specified NEC M35.8
Conor and Bruch's (boutonneuse fever) A77.1
Cooper's — *see* Mastopathy, cystic
Cori's (glycogenosis III) E74.03
corkhandler's or corkworker's J67.3
cornea H18.9
  specified NEC H18.89- ☑
coronary (artery) — *see* Disease, heart, ischemic, atherosclerotic
  congenital Q24.5
  ostial, syphilitic (aortic) (mitral) (pulmonary) A52.03
corpus cavernosum N48.9
  specified NEC N48.89
Cotugno's — *see* Sciatica
coxsackie (virus) NEC B34.1
cranial nerve NOS G52.9
Creutzfeldt-Jakob — *see* Creutzfeldt-Jakob disease or syndrome
Crocq's (acrocyanosis) I73.89
Crohn's — *see* Enteritis, regional
Curschmann G71.11
cystic
  breast (chronic) — *see* Mastopathy, cystic
  kidney, congenital Q61.9
  liver, congenital Q44.6
  lung J98.4
    congenital Q33.0
cytomegalic inclusion (generalized) B25.9
  with pneumonia B25.0
  congenital P35.1
cytomegaloviral B25.9
  specified NEC B25.8
Czerny's (periodic hydrarthrosis of the knee) — *see* Effusion, joint, knee
Daae (-Finsen) (epidemic pleurodynia) B33.0
Darling's — *see* Histoplasmosis capsulati
de Quervain's (tendon sheath) M65.4
  thyroid (subacute granulomatous thyroiditis) E06.1
Débove's (splenomegaly) R16.1
deer fly — *see* Tularemia
Degos' I77.89
demyelinating, demyelinizating (nervous system) G37.9
  multiple sclerosis G35
  specified NEC G37.8
dense deposit (*see also* N00-N07 with fourth character .6) N05.6
deposition, hydroxyapatite — *see* Disease, hydroxyapatite deposition
Devergie's (pityriasis rubra pilaris) L44.0
Devic's G36.0
diaphorase deficiency D74.0
diaphragm J98.6
diarrheal, infectious NEC A09
digestive system K92.9
  specified NEC K92.89
disc, degenerative — *see* Degeneration, intervertebral disc
discogenic (*see also* Displacement, intervertebral disc NEC)
  with myelopathy — *see* Disorder, disc, with myelopathy
diverticular — *see* Diverticula
Dubois (thymus) A50.59 [E35]
Duchenne-Griesinger G71.0
Duchenne's
  muscular dystrophy G71.0
  pseudohypertrophy, muscles G71.0
ductless glands E34.9
Duhring's (dermatitis herpetiformis) L13.0
duodenum K31.9
  specified NEC K31.89
Dupré's (meningism) R29.1
Dupuytren's (muscle contracture) M72.0
Durand-Nicholas-Favre (climatic bubo) A55
Duroziez's (congenital mitral stenosis) Q23.2
ear — *see* Disorder, ear
Eberth's — *see* Fever, typhoid
Ebola (virus) A98.4
Ebstein's heart Q22.5
Echinococcus — *see* Echinococcus
echovirus NEC B34.1
Eddowes' (brittle bones and blue sclera) Q78.0

Disease, diseased — *continued*
edentulous (alveolar) ridge K06.9
  specified NEC K06.8
Edsall's T67.2 ☑
Eichstedt's (pityriasis versicolor) B36.0
Ellis-van Creveld (chondroectodermal dysplasia) Q77.6
end stage renal (ESRD) N18.6
  due to hypertension I12.0
endocrine glands or system NEC E34.9
endomyocardial (eosinophilic) I42.3
English (rickets) E55.0
enteroviral, enterovirus NEC B34.1
  central nervous system NEC A88.8
epidemic B99.9
  specified NEC B99.8
epididymis N50.9
Erb (-Landouzy) G71.0
Erdheim-Chester (ECD) E88.89
esophagus K22.9
  functional K22.4
  psychogenic F45.8
  specified NEC K22.8
Eulenburg's (congenital paramyotonia) G71.19
eustachian tube — *see* Disorder, eustachian tube
external
  auditory canal — *see* Disorder, ear, external
  ear — *see* Disorder, ear, external
extrapyramidal G25.9
  specified NEC G25.89
eye H57.9
  anterior chamber H21.9
  inflammatory NEC H57.8
  muscle (external) — *see* Strabismus
  specified NEC H57.8
  syphilitic — *see* Oculopathy, syphilitic
eyeball H44.9
  specified NEC H44.89
eyelid — *see* Disorder, eyelid
  specified NEC — *see* Disorder, eyelid, specified type NEC
eyeworm of Africa B74.3
facial nerve (seventh) G51.9
  newborn (birth injury) P11.3
Fahr (of brain) G23.8
Fahr Volhard (of kidney) I12.- ☑
fallopian tube (noninflammatory) N83.9
  inflammatory — *see* Salpingo-oophoritis
  specified NEC N83.8
familial periodic paralysis G72.3
Fanconi's (congenital pancytopenia) D61.09
fascia NEC (*see also* Disorder, muscle)
  inflammatory — *see* Myositis
  specified NEC M62.89
Fauchard's (periodontitis) — *see* Periodontitis
Favre-Durand-Nicolas (climatic bubo) A55
Fede's K14.0
Feer's — *see* Poisoning, mercury
female pelvic inflammatory (*see also* Disease, pelvis, inflammatory) N73.9
  syphilitic (secondary) A51.42
  tuberculous A18.17
Fernels' (aortic aneurysm) I71.9
fibrocaseous of lung — *see* Tuberculosis, pulmonary
fibrocystic — *see* Fibrocystic disease
Fiedler's (leptospiral jaundice) A27.0
fifth B08.3
file-cutter's — *see* Poisoning, lead
fish-skin Q80.9
  acquired L85.0
Flajani (-Basedow) (exophthalmic goiter) — *see* Hyperthyroidism, with, goiter (diffuse)
flax-dresser's J66.1
fluke — *see* Infestation, fluke
foot and mouth B08.8
foot process N04.9
Forbes' (glycogenosis III) E74.03
Fordyce-Fox (apocrine miliaria) L75.2
Fordyce's (ectopic sebaceous glands) (mouth) Q38.6
Forestier's (rhizomelic pseudopolyarthritis) M35.3
  meaning ankylosing hyperostosis — *see* Hyperostosis, ankylosing
Fothergill's
  neuralgia — *see* Neuralgia, trigeminal
  scarlatina anginosa A38.9
Fournier (gangrene) N49.3
  female N76.89
fourth B08.8
Fox (-Fordyce) (apocrine miliaria) L75.2

Disease, diseased — *continued*
Francis' — *see* Tularemia
Franklin C88.2
Frei's (climatic bubo) A55
Friedreich's
  combined systemic or ataxia G11.1
  myoclonia G25.3
frontal sinus — *see* Sinusitis, frontal
fungus NEC B49
Gaisböck's (polycythemia hypertonica) D75.1
gallbladder K82.9
  calculus — *see* Calculus, gallbladder
  cholecystitis — *see* Cholecystitis
  cholesterolosis K82.4
  fistula — *see* Fistula, gallbladder
  hydrops K82.1
  obstruction — *see* Obstruction, gallbladder
  perforation K82.2
  specified NEC K82.8
gamma heavy chain C88.2
Gamna's (siderotic splenomegaly) D73.2
Gamstorp's (adynamia episodica hereditaria) G72.3
Gandy-Nanta (siderotic splenomegaly) D73.2
ganister J62.8
gastric — *see* Disease, stomach
gastroesophageal reflux (GERD) K21.9
  with esophagitis K21.0
gastrointestinal (tract) K92.9
  amyloid E85.4
  functional K59.9
    psychogenic F45.8
  specified NEC K92.89
Gee (-Herter) (-Heubner) (-Thaysen) (nontropical sprue) K90.0
genital organs
  female N94.9
  male N50.9
Gerhardt's (erythromelalgia) I73.81
Gibert's (pityriasis rosea) L42
Gierke's (glycogenosis I) E74.01
Gilles de la Tourette's (motor-verbal tic) F95.2
gingiva K06.9
  specified NEC K06.8
gland (lymph) I89.9
Glanzmann's (hereditary hemorrhagic thrombasthenia) D69.1
glass-blower's (cataract) — *see* Cataract, specified NEC
  salivary gland hypertrophy K11.1
Glisson's — *see* Rickets
globe H44.9
  specified NEC H44.89
glomerular (*see also* Glomerulonephritis)
  with edema — *see* Nephrosis
  acute — *see* Nephritis, acute
  chronic — *see* Nephritis, chronic
  minimal change N05.0
  rapidly progressive N01.9
glycogen storage E74.00
  Andersen's E74.09
  Cori's E74.03
  Forbes' E74.03
  generalized E74.00
  glucose-6-phosphatase deficiency E74.01
  heart E74.02 [I43]
  hepatorenal E74.09
  Hers' E74.09
  liver and kidney E74.09
  McArdle's E74.04
  muscle phosphofructokinase E74.09
  myocardium E74.02 [I43]
  Pompe's E74.02
  Tauri's E74.09
  type 0 E74.09
  type I E74.01
  type II E74.02
  type III E74.03
  type IV E74.09
  type V E74.04
  type VI-XI E74.09
  Von Gierke's E74.01
Goldstein's (familial hemorrhagic telangiectasia) I78.0
gonococcal NOS A54.9
graft-versus-host (GVH) D89.813
  acute D89.810
  acute on chronic D89.812
  chronic D89.811
grainhandler's J67.8
granulomatous (childhood) (chronic) D71

Index

Disease, diseased — Disease, diseased

Disease, diseased — *continued*
 Graves' (exophthalmic goiter) — *see* Hyperthyroidism,
   with, goiter (diffuse)
 Griesinger's — *see* Ancylostomiasis
 Grisel's M43.6
 Gruby's (tinea tonsurans) B35.0
 Guillain-Barré G61.0
 Guinon's (motor-verbal tic) F95.2
 gum K06.9
 gynecological N94.9
 H (Hartnup's) E72.02
 Haff — *see* Poisoning, mercury
 Hageman (congenital factor XII deficiency) D68.2
 hair (color) (shaft) L67.9
   follicles L73.9
     specified NEC L73.8
 Hamman's (spontaneous mediastinal emphysema)
   J98.2
 hand, foot and mouth B08.4
 Hansen's — *see* Leprosy
 Hantavirus, with pulmonary manifestations B33.4
   with renal manifestations A98.5
 Harada's H30.81- ☑
 Hartnup (pellagra-cerebellar ataxia-renal
   aminoaciduria) E72.02
 Hart's (pellagra-cerebellar ataxia-renal aminoaciduria)
   E72.02
 Hashimoto's (struma lymphomatosa) E06.3
 Hb — *see* Disease, hemoglobin
 heart (organic) I51.9
   with
     pulmonary edema (acute) (*see also* Failure,
       ventricular, left) I50.1
     rheumatic fever (conditions in I00)
       active I01.9
         with chorea I02.0
           specified NEC I01.8
       inactive or quiescent (with chorea) I09.9
         specified NEC I09.89
   amyloid E85.4 [I43]
   aortic (valve) I35.9
   arteriosclerotic or sclerotic (senile) — *see* Disease,
     heart, ischemic, atherosclerotic
   artery, arterial — *see* Disease, heart, ischemic,
     atherosclerotic
   beer drinkers' I42.6
   beriberi (wet) E51.12
   black I27.0
   congenital Q24.9
     cyanotic Q24.9
     specified NEC Q24.8
   coronary — *see* Disease, heart, ischemic
   cryptogenic I51.9
   fibroid — *see* Myocarditis
   functional I51.89
     psychogenic F45.8
   glycogen storage E74.02 [I43]
   gonococcal A54.83
   hypertensive — *see* Hypertension, heart
   hyperthyroid (*see also* Hyperthyroidism)
       E05.90 [I43]
     with thyroid storm E05.91 [I43]
   ischemic (chronic or with a stated duration of over
     4 weeks) I25.9
     atherosclerotic (of) I25.10
       with angina pectoris — *see* Arteriosclerosis,
         coronary (artery)
       coronary artery bypass graft — *see* Arte-
         riosclerosis, coronary (artery),
     cardiomyopathy I25.5
     diagnosed on ECG or other special investiga-
       tion, but currently presenting no symp-
       toms I25.6
     silent I25.6
     specified form NEC I25.89
   kyphoscoliotic I27.1
   meningococcal A39.50
     endocarditis A39.51
     myocarditis A39.52
     pericarditis A39.53
   mitral I05.9
     specified NEC I05.8
   muscular — *see* Degeneration, myocardial
   psychogenic (functional) F45.8
   pulmonary (chronic) I27.9
     in schistosomiasis B65.9 [I52]
     specified NEC I27.89

Disease, diseased — *continued*
 heart — *continued*
   rheumatic (chronic) (inactive) (old) (quiescent)
       (with chorea) I09.9
     active or acute I01.9
       with chorea (acute) (rheumatic) (Syden-
         ham's) I02.0
     specified NEC I09.89
   senile — *see* Myocarditis
   syphilitic A52.06
     aortic A52.03
       aneurysm A52.01
     congenital A50.54 [I52]
   thyrotoxic (*see also* Thyrotoxicosis) E05.90 [I43]
     with thyroid storm E05.91 [I43]
   valve, valvular (obstructive) (regurgitant) (*see also*
       Endocarditis)
     congenital NEC Q24.8
       pulmonary Q22.3
   vascular — *see* Disease, cardiovascular
 heavy chain NEC C88.2
   alpha C88.3
   gamma C88.2
   mu C88.2
 Hebra's
   pityriasis
     maculata et circinata L42
     rubra pilaris L44.0
   prurigo L28.2
 hematopoietic organs D75.9
 hemoglobin or Hb
   abnormal (mixed) NEC D58.2
     with thalassemia D56.9
   AS genotype D57.3
   Bart's D56.0
   C (Hb-C) D58.2
     with other abnormal hemoglobin NEC D58.2
     elliptocytosis D58.1
     Hb-S D57.2- ☑
     sickle-cell D57.2- ☑
     thalassemia D56.8
   Constant Spring D58.2
   D (Hb-D) D58.2
   E (Hb-E) D58.2
   E-beta thalassemia D56.5
   elliptocytosis D58.1
   H (Hb-H) (thalassemia) D56.0
     with other abnormal hemoglobin NEC D56.9
     Constant Spring D56.0
   I thalassemia D56.9
   M D74.0
   S or SS D57.1
   SC D57.2- ☑
   SD D57.8- ☑
   SE D57.8- ☑
   spherocytosis D58.0
   unstable, hemolytic D58.2
 hemolytic (newborn) P55.9
   autoimmune (cold type) (warm type) D59.1
   drug-induced D59.0
   due to or with
     incompatibility
       ABO (blood group) P55.1
       blood (group) (Duffy) (K(ell)) (Kidd) (Lewis)
         (M) (S) NEC P55.8
       Rh (blood group) (factor) P55.0
     Rh negative mother P55.0
   specified type NEC P55.8
   unstable hemoglobin D58.2
 hemorrhagic D69.9
   newborn P53
 Henoch (-Schönlein) (purpura nervosa) D69.0
 hepatic — *see* Disease, liver
 hepatolenticular E83.01
 heredodegenerative NEC
   spinal cord G95.89
 herpesviral, disseminated B00.7
 Hers' (glycogenosis VI) E74.09
 Herter (-Gee) (-Heubner) (nontropical sprue) K90.0
 Heubner-Herter (nontropical sprue) K90.0
 high fetal gene or hemoglobin thalassemia D56.9
 Hildenbrand's — *see* Typhus
 hip (joint) M25.9
   congenital Q65.89
   suppurative M00.9
   tuberculous A18.02
 His (-Werner) (trench fever) A79.0
 Hodgson's I71.2

Disease, diseased — *continued*
 Hodgson's — *continued*
   ruptured I71.1
 Holla — *see* Spherocytosis
 hookworm B76.9
   specified NEC B76.8
 host-versus-graft D89.813
   acute D89.810
   acute on chronic D89.812
   chronic D89.811
 human immunodeficiency virus (HIV) B20
 Huntington's G10
 Hutchinson's (cheiropompholyx) — *see* Hutchinson's
   disease
 hyaline (diffuse) (generalized)
   membrane (lung) (newborn) P22.0
     adult J80
 hydatid — *see* Echinococcus
 hydroxyapatite deposition M11.00
   ankle M11.07- ☑
   elbow M11.02- ☑
   foot joint M11.07- ☑
   hand joint M11.04- ☑
   hip M11.05- ☑
   knee M11.06- ☑
   multiple site M11.09
   shoulder M11.01- ☑
   vertebra M11.08
   wrist M11.03- ☑
 hyperkinetic — *see* Hyperkinesia
 hypertensive — *see* Hypertension
 hypophysis E23.7
 Iceland G93.3
 I-cell E77.0
 immune D89.9
 immunoproliferative (malignant) C88.9
   small intestinal C88.3
   specified NEC C88.8
 inclusion B25.9
   salivary gland B25.9
 infectious, infective B99.9
   congenital P37.9
     specified NEC P37.8
     viral P35.9
       specified type NEC P35.8
   specified NEC B99.8
 inflammatory
   penis N48.29
     abscess N48.21
     cellulitis N48.22
   prepuce N47.7
     balanoposthitis N47.6
   tubo-ovarian — *see* Salpingo-oophoritis
 intervertebral disc (*see also* Disorder, disc)
   with myelopathy — *see* Disorder, disc, with,
     myelopathy
   cervical, cervicothoracic — *see* Disorder, disc, cer-
     vical
     with
       myelopathy — *see* Disorder, disc, cervical,
         with myelopathy
       neuritis, radiculitis or radiculopathy — *see*
         Disorder, disc, cervical, with neuritis
       specified NEC — *see* Disorder, disc, cervical,
         specified type NEC
   lumbar (with)
     myelopathy M51.06
     neuritis, radiculitis, radiculopathy or sciatica
       M51.16
     specified NEC M51.86
   lumbosacral (with)
     neuritis, radiculitis, radiculopathy or sciatica
       M51.17
     specified NEC M51.87
   specified NEC — *see* Disorder, disc, specified NEC
   thoracic (with)
     myelopathy M51.04
     neuritis, radiculitis or radiculopathy M51.14
     specified NEC M51.84
   thoracolumbar (with)
     myelopathy M51.05
     neuritis, radiculitis or radiculopathy M51.15
     specified NEC M51.85
 intestine K63.9
   functional K59.9
     psychogenic F45.8
     specified NEC K59.8
   organic K63.9

Disease, diseased — *continued*
- intestine — *continued*
  - protozoal A07.9
  - specified NEC K63.89
- iris H21.9
  - specified NEC H21.89
- iron metabolism or storage E83.10
- island (scrub typhus) A75.3
- itai-itai — *see* Poisoning, cadmium
- Jakob-Creutzfeldt — *see* Creutzfeldt-Jakob disease or syndrome
- jaw M27.9
  - fibrocystic M27.49
  - specified NEC M27.8
- jigger B88.1
- joint (*see also* Disorder, joint)
  - Charcot's — *see* Arthropathy, neuropathic (Charcot)
  - degenerative — *see* Osteoarthritis
    - multiple M15.9
    - spine — *see* Spondylosis
  - hypertrophic — *see* Osteoarthritis
  - sacroiliac M53.3
  - specified NEC — *see* Disorder, joint, specified type NEC
  - spine NEC — *see* Dorsopathy
  - suppurative — *see* Arthritis, pyogenic or pyemic
- Jourdain's (acute gingivitis) K05.00
  - nonplaque induced K05.01
  - plaque induced K05.00
- Kaschin-Beck (endemic polyarthritis) M12.10
  - ankle M12.17- ☑
  - elbow M12.12- ☑
  - foot joint M12.17- ☑
  - hand joint M12.14- ☑
  - hip M12.15- ☑
  - knee M12.16- ☑
  - multiple site M12.19
  - shoulder M12.11- ☑
  - vertebra M12.18
  - wrist M12.13- ☑
- Katayama B65.2
- Kedani (scrub typhus) A75.3
- Keshan E59
- kidney (functional) (pelvis) N28.9
  - chronic N18.9
    - hypertensive — *see* Hypertension, kidney
    - stage 1 N18.1
    - stage 2 (mild) N18.2
    - stage 3 (moderate) N18.3
    - stage 4 (severe) N18.4
    - stage 5 N18.5
  - complicating pregnancy — *see* Pregnancy, complicated by, renal disease
  - cystic (congenital) Q61.9
  - fibrocystic (congenital) Q61.8
  - hypertensive — *see* Hypertension, kidney
  - in (due to)
    - schistosomiasis (bilharziasis) B65.9 [N29]
  - multicystic Q61.4
  - polycystic Q61.3
    - adult type Q61.2
    - childhood type NEC Q61.19
      - collecting duct dilatation Q61.11
- Kimmelstiel (-Wilson) (intercapillary polycystic (congenital) glomerulosclerosis) — *see* E08-E13 with .21
- Kinnier Wilson's (hepatolenticular degeneration) E83.01
- kissing — *see* Mononucleosis, infectious
- Klebs' (*see also* Glomerulonephritis) N05- ☑
- Klippel-Feil (brevicollis) Q76.1
- Köhler-Pellegrini-Stieda (calcification, knee joint) — *see* Bursitis, tibial collateral
- Kok Q89.8
- König's (osteochondritis dissecans) — *see* Osteochondritis, dissecans
- Korsakoff's (nonalcoholic) F04
  - alcoholic F10.96
    - with dependence F10.26
- Kostmann's (infantile genetic agranulocytosis) D70.0
- kuru A81.81
- Kyasanur Forest A98.2
- labyrinth, ear — *see* Disorder, ear, inner
- lacrimal system — *see* Disorder, lacrimal system
- Lafora's — *see* Epilepsy, generalized, idiopathic
- Lancereaux-Mathieu (leptospiral jaundice) A27.0
- Landry's G61.0

Disease, diseased — *continued*
- Larrey-Weil (leptospiral jaundice) A27.0
- larynx J38.7
- legionnaires' A48.1
  - nonpneumonic A48.2
- Lenegre's I44.2
- lens H27.9
  - specified NEC H27.8
- Lev's (acquired complete heart block) I44.2
- Lewy body (dementia) G31.83 [F02.80]
  - with behavioral disturbance G31.83 [F02.81]
- Lichtheim's (subacute combined sclerosis with pernicious anemia) D51.0
- Lightwood's (renal tubular acidosis) N25.89
- Lignac's (cystinosis) E72.04
- lip K13.0
- lipid-storage E75.6
  - specified NEC E75.5
- Lipschütz's N76.6
- liver (chronic) (organic) K76.9
  - alcoholic (chronic) K70.9
    - acute — *see* Disease, liver, alcoholic, hepatitis
    - cirrhosis K70.30
      - with ascites K70.31
    - failure K70.40
      - with coma K70.41
    - fatty liver K70.0
    - fibrosis K70.2
    - hepatitis K70.10
      - with ascites K70.11
    - sclerosis K70.2
  - cystic, congenital Q44.6
  - drug-induced (idiosyncratic) (toxic) (predictable) (unpredictable) — *see* Disease, liver, toxic
  - end stage K72.90
    - due to hepatitis — *see* Hepatitis
  - fatty, nonalcoholic (NAFLD) K76.0
    - alcoholic K70.0
  - fibrocystic (congenital) Q44.6
  - fluke
    - Chinese B66.1
    - oriental B66.1
    - sheep B66.3
  - glycogen storage E74.09 [K77]
  - in (due to)
    - schistosomiasis (bilharziasis) B65.9 [K77]
  - inflammatory K75.9
    - alcoholic K70.1 ☑
    - specified NEC K75.89
  - polycystic (congenital) Q44.6
  - toxic K71.9
    - with
      - cholestasis K71.0
      - cirrhosis (liver) K71.7
      - fibrosis (liver) K71.7
      - focal nodular hyperplasia K71.8
      - hepatic granuloma K71.8
      - hepatic necrosis K71.10
        - with coma K71.11
      - hepatitis NEC K71.6
        - acute K71.2
        - chronic
          - active K71.50
            - with ascites K71.51
          - lobular K71.4
          - persistent K71.3
        - lupoid K71.50
          - with ascites K71.51
      - peliosis hepatis K71.8
    - veno-occlusive disease (VOD) of liver K71.8
  - veno-occlusive K76.5
- Lobo's (keloid blastomycosis) B48.0
- Lobstein's (brittle bones and blue sclera) Q78.0
- Ludwig's (submaxillary cellulitis) K12.2
- lumbosacral region M53.87
- lung J98.4
  - black J60
  - congenital Q33.9
  - cystic J98.4
    - congenital Q33.0
  - fibroid (chronic) — *see* Fibrosis, lung
  - fluke B66.4
    - oriental B66.4
  - in
    - amyloidosis E85.4 [J99]
    - sarcoidosis D86.0
    - Sjögren's syndrome M35.02

Disease, diseased — *continued*
- lung — *continued*
  - in — *continued*
    - systemic
      - lupus erythematosus M32.13
      - sclerosis M34.81
    - interstitial J84.9
      - of childhood, specified NEC J84.848
      - respiratory bronchiolitis J84.115
      - specified NEC J84.89
    - obstructive (chronic) J44.9
      - with
        - acute
          - bronchitis J44.0
            - exacerbation NEC J44.1
          - lower respiratory infection J44.0
        - alveolitis, allergic J67.9
        - asthma J44.9
        - bronchiectasis J47.9
          - with
            - exacerbation (acute) J47.1
            - lower respiratory infection J47.0
        - bronchitis J44.9
          - with
            - exacerbation (acute) J44.1
            - lower respiratory infection J44.0
        - emphysema J44.9
        - hypersensitivity pneumonitis J67.9
      - decompensated J44.1
        - with
          - exacerbation (acute) J44.1
    - polycystic J98.4
      - congenital Q33.0
    - rheumatoid (diffuse) (interstitial) — *see* Rheumatoid, lung
- Lutembacher's (atrial septal defect with mitral stenosis) Q21.1
- Lyme A69.20
- lymphatic (gland) (system) (channel) (vessel) I89.9
- lymphoproliferative D47.9
  - specified NEC D47.Z9 (*following* D47.4)
  - T-gamma D47.Z9 (*following* D47.4)
  - X-linked D82.3
- Magitot's M27.2
- malarial — *see* Malaria
- malignant (*see also* Neoplasm, malignant, by site)
- Manson's B65.1
- maple bark J67.6
- maple-syrup-urine E71.0
- Marburg (virus) A98.3
- Marion's (bladder neck obstruction) N32.0
- Marsh's (exophthalmic goiter) — *see* Hyperthyroidism, with, goiter (diffuse)
- mastoid (process) — *see* Disorder, ear, middle
- Mathieu's (leptospiral jaundice) A27.0
- Maxcy's A75.2
- McArdle (-Schmid-Pearson) (glycogenosis V) E74.04
- mediastinum J98.5
- medullary center (idiopathic) (respiratory) G93.89
- Meige's (chronic hereditary edema) Q82.0
- meningococcal — *see* Infection, meningococcal
- mental F99
  - organic F09
- mesenchymal M35.9
- mesenteric embolic K55.0
- metabolic, metabolism E88.9
  - bilirubin E80.7
- metal-polisher's J62.8
- metastatic (*see also* Neoplasm, secondary, by site) C79.9
- microvascular - code to condition
- microvillus
  - atrophy Q43.8
  - inclusion (MVD) Q43.8
- middle ear — *see* Disorder, ear, middle
- Mikulicz' (dryness of mouth, absent or decreased lacrimation) K11.8
- Milroy's (chronic hereditary edema) Q82.0
- Minamata — *see* Poisoning, mercury
- minicore G71.2
- Minor's G95.19
- Minot's (hemorrhagic disease, newborn) P53
- Minot-von Willebrand-Jürgens (angiohemophilia) D68.0
- Mitchell's (erythromelalgia) I73.81
- mitral (valve) I05.9
  - nonrheumatic I34.9
- mixed connective tissue M35.1

Disease, diseased — *continued*
moldy hay J67.0
Monge's T70.29 ☑
Morgagni-Adams-Stokes (syncope with heart block) I45.9
Morgagni's (syndrome) (hyperostosis frontalis interna) M85.2
Morton's (with metatarsalgia) — *see* Lesion, nerve, plantar
Morvan's G60.8
motor neuron (bulbar) (familial) (mixed type) (spinal) G12.20
    amyotrophic lateral sclerosis G12.21
    progressive bulbar palsy G12.22
    specified NEC G12.29
moyamoya I67.5
mu heavy chain disease C88.2
multicore G71.2
muscle (*see also* Disorder, muscle)
    inflammatory — *see* Myositis
    ocular (external) — *see* Strabismus
musculoskeletal system, soft tissue — *see also* Disorder, soft tissue
    specified NEC — *see* Disorder, soft tissue, specified type NEC
mushroom workers' J67.5
mycotic B49
myelodysplastic, not classified C94.6
myeloproliferative, not classified C94.6
    chronic D47.1
myocardium, myocardial (*see also* Degeneration, myocardial) I51.5
    primary (idiopathic) I42.9
myoneural G70.9
Naegeli's D69.1
nails L60.9
    specified NEC L60.8
Nairobi (sheep virus) A93.8
nasal J34.9
nemaline body G71.2
nerve — *see* Disorder, nerve
nervous system G98.8
    autonomic G90.9
    central G96.9
        specified NEC G96.8
    congenital Q07.9
    parasympathetic G90.9
    specified NEC G98.8
    sympathetic G90.9
    vegetative G90.9
neuromuscular system G70.9
Newcastle B30.8
Nicolas (-Durand)-Favre (climatic bubo) A55
nipple N64.9
    Paget's C50.01- ☑
        female C50.01- ☑
        male C50.02- ☑
Nishimoto (-Takeuchi) I67.5
nonarthropod-borne NOS (viral) B34.9
    enterovirus NEC B34.1
nonautoimmune hemolytic D59.4
    drug-induced D59.2
Nonne-Milroy-Meige (chronic hereditary edema) Q82.0
nose J34.9
nucleus pulposus — *see* Disorder, disc
nutritional E63.9
oast-house-urine E72.19
    ocular
        herpesviral B00.50
        zoster B02.30
    obliterative vascular I77.1
Ohara's — *see* Tularemia
Opitz's (congestive splenomegaly) D73.2
Oppenheim-Urbach (necrobiosis lipoidica diabeticorum) — *see* E08-E13 with .620
optic nerve NEC — *see* Disorder, nerve, optic
orbit — *see* Disorder, orbit
Oriental liver fluke B66.1
Oriental lung fluke B66.4
Ormond's N13.5
Oropouche virus A93.0
Osler-Rendu (familial hemorrhagic telangiectasia) I78.0
osteofibrocystic E21.0
Otto's M24.7
outer ear — *see* Disorder, ear, external
ovary (noninflammatory) N83.9
    cystic N83.20
    inflammatory — *see* Salpingo-oophoritis

Disease, diseased — *continued*
ovary — *continued*
    polycystic E28.2
    specified NEC N83.8
Owren's (congenital) — *see* Defect, coagulation
pancreas K86.9
    cystic K86.2
    fibrocystic E84.9
    specified NEC K86.8
panvalvular I08.9
    specified NEC I08.8
parametrium (noninflammatory) N83.9
parasitic B89
    cerebral NEC B71.9 [G94]
    intestinal NOS B82.9
    mouth B37.0
    skin NOS B88.9
    specified type — *see* Infestation
    tongue B37.0
parathyroid (gland) E21.5
    specified NEC E21.4
Parkinson's G20
parodontal K05.6
Parrot's (syphilitic osteochondritis) A50.02
Parry's (exophthalmic goiter) — *see* Hyperthyroidism, with, goiter (diffuse)
Parson's (exophthalmic goiter) — *see* Hyperthyroidism, with, goiter (diffuse)
Paxton's (white piedra) B36.2
pearl-worker's — *see* Osteomyelitis, specified type NEC
Pellegrini-Stieda (calcification, knee joint) — *see* Bursitis, tibial collateral
pelvis, pelvic
    female NOS N94.9
        specified NEC N94.89
    gonococcal (acute) (chronic) A54.24
    inflammatory (female) N73.9
        acute N73.0
        chronic N73.1
        specified NEC N73.8
        syphilitic (secondary) A51.42
            late A52.76
        tuberculous A18.17
    organ, female N94.9
    peritoneum, female NEC N94.89
penis N48.9
    inflammatory N48.29
        abscess N48.21
        cellulitis N48.22
    specified NEC N48.89
periapical tissues NOS K04.90
periodontal K05.6
    specified NEC K05.5
periosteum — *see* Disorder, bone, specified type NEC
peripheral
    arterial I73.9
    autonomic nervous system G90.9
    nerves — *see* Polyneuropathy
    vascular NOS I73.9
peritoneum K66.9
    pelvic, female NEC N94.89
    specified NEC K66.8
persistent mucosal (middle ear) H66.20
    left H66.22
        with right H66.23
    right H66.21
        with left H66.23
Petit's — *see* Hernia, abdomen, specified site NEC
pharynx J39.2
    specified NEC J39.2
Phocas' — *see* Mastopathy, cystic
photochromogenic (acid-fast bacilli) (pulmonary) A31.0
    nonpulmonary A31.9
Pick's G31.01 [F02.80]
    with behavioral disturbance G31.01 [F02.81]
pigeon fancier's J67.2
pineal gland E34.8
pink — *see* Poisoning, mercury
Pinkus' (lichen nitidus) L44.1
pinworm B80
Piry virus A93.8
pituitary (gland) E23.7
pituitary-snuff-taker's J67.8
pleura (cavity) J94.9
    specified NEC J94.8
pneumatic drill (hammer) T75.21 ☑

Disease, diseased — *continued*
Pollitzer's (hidradenitis suppurativa) L73.2
polycystic
    kidney or renal Q61.3
        adult type Q61.2
        childhood type NEC Q61.19
            collecting duct dilatation Q61.11
    liver or hepatic Q44.6
    lung or pulmonary J98.4
        congenital Q33.0
    ovary, ovaries E28.2
    spleen Q89.09
polyethylene T84.05- ☑
Pompe's (glycogenosis II) E74.02
Posadas-Wernicke B38.9
Potain's (pulmonary edema) — *see* Edema, lung
prepuce N47.8
    inflammatory N47.7
        balanoposthitis N47.6
Pringle's (tuberous sclerosis) Q85.1
prion, central nervous system A81.9
    specified NEC A81.89
prostate N42.9
    specified NEC N42.89
protozoal B64
    acanthamebiasis — *see* Acanthamebiasis
    African trypanosomiasis — *see* African trypanosomiasis
    babesiosis B60.0
    Chagas disease — *see* Chagas disease
    intestine, intestinal A07.9
    leishmaniasis — *see* Leishmaniasis
    malaria — *see* Malaria
    naegleriasis B60.2
    pneumocystosis B59
    specified organism NEC B60.8
    toxoplasmosis — *see* Toxoplasmosis
pseudo-Hurler's E77.0
psychiatric F99
psychotic — *see* Psychosis
Puente's (simple glandular cheilitis) K13.0
puerperal (*see also* Puerperal) O90.89
pulmonary (*see also* Disease, lung)
    artery I28.9
    chronic obstructive J44.9
        with
            acute bronchitis J44.0
            exacerbation (acute) J44.1
            lower respiratory infection (acute) J44.0
        decompensated J44.1
            with
                exacerbation (acute) J44.1
    heart I27.9
        specified NEC I27.89
    hypertensive (vascular) I27.0
    valve I37.9
        rheumatic I09.89
pulp (dental) NOS K04.90
pulseless M31.4
Putnam's (subacute combined sclerosis with pernicious anemia) D51.0
Pyle (-Cohn) (craniometaphyseal dysplasia) Q78.5
ragpicker's or ragsorter's A22.1
Raynaud's — *see* Raynaud's disease
reactive airway — *see* Asthma
Reclus' (cystic) — *see* Mastopathy, cystic
rectum K62.9
    specified NEC K62.89
Refsum's (heredopathia atactica polyneuritiformis) G60.1
renal (functional) (pelvis) (*see also* Disease, kidney) N28.9
    with
        edema — *see* Nephrosis
        glomerular lesion — *see* Glomerulonephritis
            with edema — *see* Nephrosis
        interstitial nephritis N12
    acute N28.9
    chronic (*see also* Disease, kidney, chronic) N18.9
    cystic, congenital Q61.9
    diabetic — *see* E08-E13 with .22
    end-stage (failure) N18.6
        due to hypertension I12.0
    fibrocystic (congenital) Q61.8
    hypertensive — *see* Hypertension, kidney
    lupus M32.14
    phosphate-losing (tubular) N25.0
    polycystic (congenital) Q61.3

Disease, diseased — continued
renal (see also Disease, kidney) — continued
  polycystic — continued
    adult type Q61.2
    childhood type NEC Q61.19
      collecting duct dilatation Q61.11
  rapidly progressive N01.9
  subacute N01.9
Rendu-Osler-Weber (familial hemorrhagic telangiectasia) I78.0
renovascular (arteriosclerotic) — see Hypertension, kidney
respiratory (tract) J98.9
  acute or subacute NOS J06.9
    due to
      chemicals, gases, fumes or vapors (inhalation) J68.3
      external agent J70.9
        specified NEC J70.8
      radiation J70.0
      smoke inhalation J70.5
  noninfectious J39.8
  chronic NOS J98.9
    due to
      chemicals, gases, fumes or vapors J68.4
      external agent J70.9
        specified NEC J70.8
      radiation J70.1
  newborn P27.9
    specified NEC P27.8
  due to
    chemicals, gases, fumes or vapors J68.9
      acute or subacute NEC J68.3
      chronic J68.4
    external agent J70.9
      specified NEC J70.8
  newborn P28.9
    specified type NEC P28.89
  upper J39.9
    acute or subacute J06.9
    noninfectious NEC J39.8
    specified NEC J39.8
    streptococcal J06.9
retina, retinal H35.9
  Batten's or Batten-Mayou E75.4 [H36]
  specified NEC H35.89
rheumatoid — see Arthritis, rheumatoid
rickettsial NOS A79.9
  specified type NEC A79.89
Riga (-Fede) (cachectic aphthae) K14.0
Riggs' (compound periodontitis) — see Periodontitis
Ritter's L00
Rivalta's (cervicofacial actinomycosis) A42.2
Robles' (onchocerciasis) B73.01
Roger's (congenital interventricular septal defect) Q21.0
Rosenthal's (factor XI deficiency) D68.1
Ross River B33.1
Rossbach's (hyperchlorhydria) K30
Rotes Quérol — see Hyperostosis, ankylosing
Roth (-Bernhardt) — see Mononeuropathy, lower limb, meralgia paresthetica
Runeberg's (progressive pernicious anemia) D51.0
sacroiliac NEC M53.3
salivary gland or duct K11.9
  inclusion B25.9
  specified NEC K11.8
  virus B25.9
sandworm B76.9
Schimmelbusch's — see Mastopathy, cystic
Schmorl's — see Schmorl's disease or nodes
Schönlein (-Henoch) (purpura rheumatica) D69.0
Schottmüller's — see Fever, paratyphoid
Schultz's (agranulocytosis) — see Agranulocytosis
Schwalbe-Ziehen-Oppenheim G24.1
Schwartz-Jampel G71.13
sclera H15.9
  specified NEC H15.89
scrofulous (tuberculous) A18.2
scrotum N50.9
sebaceous glands L73.9
semilunar cartilage, cystic (see also Derangement, knee, meniscus, cystic)
seminal vesicle N50.9
serum NEC (see also Reaction, serum) T80.69 ☑
sexually transmitted A64
  anogenital
    herpesviral infection — see Herpes, anogenital

Disease, diseased — continued
sexually transmitted — continued
  anogenital — continued
    warts A63.0
  chancroid A57
  chlamydial infection — see Chlamydia
  gonorrhea — see Gonorrhea
  granuloma inguinale A58
  specified organism NEC A63.8
  syphilis — see Syphilis
  trichomoniasis — see Trichomoniasis
Sézary C84.1- ☑
shimamushi (scrub typhus) A75.3
shipyard B30.0
sickle-cell D57.1
  with crisis (vasoocclusive pain) D57.00
    with
      acute chest syndrome D57.01
      splenic sequestration D57.02
  elliptocytosis D57.8- ☑
  Hb-C D57.20
    with crisis (vasoocclusive pain) D57.219
      with
        acute chest syndrome D57.211
        splenic sequestration D57.212
    without crisis D57.20
  Hb-SD D57.80
    with crisis D57.819
      with
        acute chest syndrome D57.811
        splenic sequestration D57.812
  Hb-SE D57.80
    with crisis D57.819
      with
        acute chest syndrome D57.811
        splenic sequestration D57.812
  specified NEC D57.80
    with crisis D57.819
      with
        acute chest syndrome D57.811
        splenic sequestration D57.812
  spherocytosis D57.80
    with crisis D57.819
      with
        acute chest syndrome D57.811
        splenic sequestration D57.812
  thalassemia D57.40
    with crisis (vasoocclusive pain) D57.419
      with
        acute chest syndrome D57.411
        splenic sequestration D57.412
    without crisis D57.40
silo-filler's J68.8
  bronchitis J68.0
  pneumonitis J68.0
  pulmonary edema J68.1
simian B B00.4
Simons' (progressive lipodystrophy) E88.1
sin nombre virus B33.4
sinus — see Sinusitis
Sirkari's B55.0
sixth B08.20
  due to human herpesvirus 6 B08.21
  due to human herpesvirus 7 B08.22
skin L98.9
  due to metabolic disorder NEC E88.9 [L99]
  specified NEC L98.8
slim (HIV) B20
small vessel I73.9
Sneddon-Wilkinson (subcorneal pustular dermatosis) L13.1
South African creeping B88.0
spinal (cord) G95.9
  congenital Q06.9
  specified NEC G95.89
spine (see also Spondylopathy)
  joint — see Dorsopathy
  tuberculous A18.01
spinocerebellar (hereditary) G11.9
  specified NEC G11.8
spleen D73.9
  amyloid E85.4 [D77]
  organic D73.9
  polycystic Q89.09
  postinfectional D73.89
sponge-diver's — see Toxicity, venom, marine animal, sea anemone
Startle Q89.8

Disease, diseased — continued
Steinert's G71.11
Sticker's (erythema infectiosum) B08.3
Stieda's (calcification, knee joint) — see Bursitis, tibial collateral
Stokes' (exophthalmic goiter) — see Hyperthyroidism, with, goiter (diffuse)
Stokes-Adams (syncope with heart block) I45.9
stomach K31.9
  functional, psychogenic F45.8
  specified NEC K31.89
stonemason's J62.8
storage
  glycogen — see Disease, glycogen storage
  mucopolysaccharide — see Mucopolysaccharidosis
striatopallidal system NEC G25.89
Stuart-Prower (congenital factor X deficiency) D68.2
Stuart's (congenital factor X deficiency) D68.2
subcutaneous tissue — see Disease, skin
supporting structures of teeth K08.9
  specified NEC K08.8
suprarenal (capsule) (gland) E27.9
  hyperfunction E27.0
  specified NEC E27.8
sweat glands L74.9
  specified NEC L74.8
Sweeley-Klionsky E75.21
Swift (-Feer) — see Poisoning, mercury
swimming-pool granuloma A31.1
Sylvest's (epidemic pleurodynia) B33.0
sympathetic nervous system G90.9
synovium — see Disorder, synovium
syphilitic — see Syphilis
systemic tissue mast cell C96.2
tanapox (virus) B08.71
Tangier E78.6
Tarral-Besnier (pityriasis rubra pilaris) L44.0
Tauri's E74.09
tear duct — see Disorder, lacrimal system
tendon, tendinous (see also Disorder, tendon)
  nodular — see Trigger finger
terminal vessel I73.9
testis N50.9
thalassemia Hb-S — see Disease, sickle-cell, thalassemia
Thaysen-Gee (nontropical sprue) K90.0
Thomsen G71.12
throat J39.2
  septic J02.0
thromboembolic — see Embolism
thymus (gland) E32.9
  specified NEC E32.8
thyroid (gland) E07.9
  heart (see also Hyperthyroidism) E05.90 [I43]
    with thyroid storm E05.91 [I43]
  specified NEC E07.89
Tietze's M94.0
tongue K14.9
  specified NEC K14.8
tonsils, tonsillar (and adenoids) J35.9
tooth, teeth K08.9
  hard tissues K03.9
    specified NEC K03.89
  pulp NEC K04.99
  specified NEC K08.8
Tourette's F95.2
trachea NEC J39.8
tricuspid I07.9
  nonrheumatic I36.9
triglyceride-storage E75.5
trophoblastic — see Mole, hydatidiform
tsutsugamushi A75.3
tube (fallopian) (noninflammatory) N83.9
  inflammatory — see Salpingitis
  specified NEC N83.8
tuberculous NEC — see Tuberculosis
tubo-ovarian (noninflammatory) N83.9
  inflammatory — see Salpingo-oophoritis
  specified NEC N83.8
tubotympanic, chronic — see Otitis, media, suppurative, chronic, tubotympanic
tubulo-interstitial N15.9
  specified NEC N15.8
tympanum — see Disorder, tympanic membrane
Uhl's Q24.8
Underwood's (sclerema neonatorum) P83.0
Unverricht (-Lundborg) — see Epilepsy, generalized, idiopathic

Index

Disease, diseased — Dislocation

Disease, diseased — *continued*
  Urbach-Oppenheim (necrobiosis lipoidica diabetico-
      rum) — *see* E08-E13 with .620
  ureter N28.9
    in (due to)
      schistosomiasis (bilharziasis) B65.0 [N29]
  urethra N36.9
    specified NEC N36.8
  urinary (tract) N39.9
    bladder N32.9
      specified NEC N32.89
    specified NEC N39.8
  uterus (noninflammatory) N85.9
    infective — *see* Endometritis
    inflammatory — *see* Endometritis
    specified NEC N85.8
  uveal tract (anterior) H21.9
    posterior H31.9
  vagabond's B85.1
  vagina, vaginal (noninflammatory) N89.9
    inflammatory NEC N76.89
    specified NEC N89.8
  valve, valvular I38
    multiple I08.9
    specified NEC I08.8
  van Creveld-von Gierke (glycogenosis I) E74.01
  vas deferens N50.9
  vascular I99.9
    arteriosclerotic — *see* Arteriosclerosis
    ciliary body NEC — *see* Disorder, iris, vascular
    hypertensive — *see* Hypertension
    iris NEC — *see* Disorder, iris, vascular
    obliterative I77.1
      peripheral I73.9
    occlusive I99.8
    peripheral (occlusive) I73.9
      in diabetes mellitus — *see* E08-E13 with .51
  vasomotor I73.9
  vasospastic I73.9
  vein I87.9
  venereal (*see also* Disease, sexually transmitted) A64
    chlamydial NEC A56.8
      anus A56.3
      genitourinary NOS A56.2
      pharynx A56.4
      rectum A56.3
    fifth A55
    sixth A55
    specified nature or type NEC A63.8
  vertebra, vertebral (*see also* Spondylopathy)
    disc — *see* Disorder, disc
  vibration — *see* Vibration, adverse effects
  viral, virus (*see also* Disease, by type of virus) B34.9
    arbovirus NOS A94
    arthropod-borne NOS A94
    congenital P35.9
      specified NEC P35.8
    Hanta (with renal manifestations) (Dobrava) (Pu-
        umala) (Seoul) A98.5
      with pulmonary manifestations (Andes) (Bayou)
          (Bermejo) (Black Creek Canal) (Choclo)
          (Juquitiba) (Laguna negra) (Lechiguanas)
          (New York) (Oran) (Sin nombre) B33.4
    Hantaan (Korean hemorrhagic fever) A98.5
    human immunodeficiency (HIV) B20
    Kunjin A83.4
    nonarthropod-borne NOS B34.9
    Powassan A84.8
    Rocio (encephalitis) A83.6
    Sin nombre (Hantavirus) (cardio)-pulmonary syn-
        drome) B33.4
    Tahyna B33.8
    vesicular stomatitis A93.8
  vitreous H43.9
    specified NEC H43.89
  vocal cord J38.3
  Volkmann's, acquired T79.6 ☑
  von Eulenburg's (congenital paramyotonia) G71.19
  von Gierke's (glycogenosis I) E74.01
  von Graefe's — *see* Strabismus, paralytic, ophthalmo-
      plegia, progressive
  von Willebrand (-Jürgens) (angiohemophilia) D68.0
  Vrolik's (osteogenesis imperfecta) Q78.0
  vulva (noninflammatory) N90.9
    inflammatory NEC N76.89
    specified NEC N90.89
  Wallgren's (obstruction of splenic vein with collateral
      circulation) I87.8

Disease, diseased — *continued*
  Wassilieff's (leptospiral jaundice) A27.0
  wasting NEC R64
    due to malnutrition E41
  Waterhouse-Friderichsen A39.1
  Wegner's (syphilitic osteochondritis) A50.02
  Weil's (leptospiral jaundice of lung) A27.0
  Weir Mitchell's (erythromelalgia) I73.81
  Werdnig-Hoffmann G12.0
  Wermer's E31.21
  Werner-His (trench fever) A79.0
  Werner-Schultz (neutropenic splenomegaly) D73.81
  Wernicke-Posadas B38.9
  whipworm B79
  white blood cells D72.9
    specified NEC D72.89
  white matter R90.82
  white-spot, meaning lichen sclerosus et atrophicus
      L90.0
    penis N48.0
    vulva N90.4
  Wilkie's K55.1
  Wilkinson-Sneddon (subcorneal pustular dermatosis)
      L13.1
  Willis' — *see* Diabetes
  Wilson's (hepatolenticular degeneration) E83.01
  woolsorter's A22.1
  yaba monkey tumor B08.72
  yaba pox (virus) B08.72
  zoonotic, bacterial A28.9
    specified type NEC A28.8
Disfigurement (due to scar) L90.5
Disgerminoma — *see* Dysgerminoma
DISH (diffuse idiopathic skeletal hyperostosis) — *see*
      Hyperostosis, ankylosing
Disinsertion, retina — *see* Detachment, retina
Dislocatable hip, congenital Q65.6
Dislocation (articular)
  with fracture — *see* Fracture
  acromioclavicular (joint) S43.10- ☑
    with displacement
      100%-200% S43.12- ☑
      more than 200% S43.13- ☑
    inferior S43.14- ☑
    posterior S43.15- ☑
  ankle S93.0- ☑
  astragalus — *see* Dislocation, ankle
  atlantoaxial S13.121 ☑
  atlantooccipital S13.111 ☑
  atloidooccipital S13.111 ☑
  breast bone S23.29 ☑
  capsule, joint — *code by* site under Dislocation
  carpal (bone) — *see* Dislocation, wrist
  carpometacarpal (joint) NEC S63.05- ☑
    thumb S63.04- ☑
  cartilage (joint) — *code by* site under Dislocation
  cervical spine (vertebra) — *see* Dislocation, vertebra,
      cervical
  chronic — *see* Dislocation, recurrent
  clavicle — *see* Dislocation, acromioclavicular joint
  coccyx S33.2
  congenital NEC Q68.8
  coracoid — *see* Dislocation, shoulder
  costal cartilage S23.29 ☑
  costochondral S23.29 ☑
  cricoarytenoid articulation S13.29 ☑
  cricothyroid articulation S13.29 ☑
  dorsal vertebra — *see* Dislocation, vertebra, thoracic
  ear ossicle — *see* Discontinuity, ossicles, ear
  elbow S53.10- ☑
    congenital Q68.8
    pathological — *see* Dislocation, pathological NEC,
        elbow
    radial head alone — *see* Dislocation, radial head
    recurrent — *see* Dislocation, recurrent, elbow
    traumatic S53.10- ☑
      anterior S53.11- ☑
      lateral S53.14- ☑
      medial S53.13- ☑
      posterior S53.12- ☑
      specified type NEC S53.19- ☑
  eye, nontraumatic — *see* Luxation, globe
  eyeball, nontraumatic — *see* Luxation, globe
  femur
    distal end — *see* Dislocation, knee
    proximal end — *see* Dislocation, hip

Dislocation — *continued*
  fibula
    distal end — *see* Dislocation, ankle
    proximal end — *see* Dislocation, knee
  finger S63.25- ☑
    index S63.25- ☑
    interphalangeal S63.27- ☑
      distal S63.29- ☑
        index S63.29- ☑
        little S63.29- ☑
        middle S63.29- ☑
        ring S63.29- ☑
      index S63.27- ☑
      little S63.27- ☑
      middle S63.27- ☑
      proximal S63.28- ☑
        index S63.28- ☑
        little S63.28- ☑
        middle S63.28- ☑
        ring S63.28- ☑
      ring S63.27- ☑
    little S63.25- ☑
    metacarpophalangeal S63.26- ☑
      index S63.26- ☑
      little S63.26- ☑
      middle S63.26- ☑
      ring S63.26- ☑
    middle S63.25- ☑
    recurrent — *see* Dislocation, recurrent, finger
    ring S63.25- ☑
    thumb — *see* Dislocation, thumb
  foot S93.30- ☑
    recurrent — *see* Dislocation, recurrent, foot
    specified site NEC S93.33- ☑
    tarsal joint S93.31- ☑
    tarsometatarsal joint S93.32- ☑
    toe — *see* Dislocation, toe
  fracture — *see* Fracture
  glenohumeral (joint) — *see* Dislocation, shoulder
  glenoid — *see* Dislocation, shoulder
  habitual — *see* Dislocation, recurrent
  hip S73.00- ☑
    anterior S73.03- ☑
      obturator S73.02- ☑
    central S73.04- ☑
    congenital (total) Q65.2
      bilateral Q65.1
      partial Q65.5
        bilateral Q65.4
        unilateral Q65.3- ☑
      unilateral Q65.0- ☑
    developmental M24.85- ☑
    pathological — *see* Dislocation, pathological NEC,
        hip
    posterior S73.01- ☑
    recurrent — *see* Dislocation, recurrent, hip
  humerus, proximal end — *see* Dislocation, shoulder
  incomplete — *see* Subluxation, by site
  incus — *see* Discontinuity, ossicles, ear
  infracoracoid — *see* Dislocation, shoulder
  innominate (pubic junction) (sacral junction) S33.39 ☑
    acetabulum — *see* Dislocation, hip
  interphalangeal (joint(s))
    finger S63.279 ☑
      distal S63.29- ☑
        index S63.29- ☑
        little S63.29- ☑
        middle S63.29- ☑
        ring S63.29- ☑
      index S63.27- ☑
      little S63.27- ☑
      middle S63.27- ☑
      proximal S63.28- ☑
        index S63.28- ☑
        little S63.28- ☑
        middle S63.28- ☑
        ring S63.28- ☑
      ring S63.27- ☑
    foot or toe — *see* Dislocation, toe
    thumb S63.12- ☑
      distal joint S63.14- ☑
      proximal joint S63.13- ☑
  jaw (cartilage) (meniscus) S03.0 ☑
  joint prosthesis — *see* Complications, joint prosthesis,
      mechanical, displacement, by site
  knee S83.106 ☑

Dislocation — *continued*
- knee — *continued*
  - cap — *see* Dislocation, patella
  - congenital Q68.2
  - old M23.8X-
  - patella — *see* Dislocation, patella
  - pathological — *see* Dislocation, pathological NEC, knee
  - proximal tibia
    - anteriorly S83.11- ☑
    - laterally S83.14- ☑
    - medially S83.13- ☑
    - posteriorly S83.12- ☑
  - recurrent (*see also* Derangement, knee, specified NEC)
  - specified type NEC S83.19- ☑
- lacrimal gland H04.16- ☑
- lens (complete) H27.10
  - anterior H27.12- ☑
  - congenital Q12.1
  - ocular implant — *see* Complications, intraocular lens
  - partial H27.11- ☑
  - posterior H27.13- ☑
  - traumatic S05.8X- ☑
- ligament — *code by* site under Dislocation
- lumbar (vertebra) — *see* Dislocation, vertebra, lumbar
- lumbosacral (vertebra) (*see also* Dislocation, vertebra, lumbar)
  - congenital Q76.49
- mandible S03.0 ☑
- meniscus (knee) — *see* Tear, meniscus
  - other sites - code by site under Dislocation
- metacarpal (bone)
  - distal end — *see* Dislocation, finger
  - proximal end S63.06- ☑
- metacarpophalangeal (joint)
  - finger S63.26- ☑
    - index S63.26- ☑
    - little S63.26- ☑
    - middle S63.26- ☑
    - ring S63.26- ☑
  - thumb S63.11- ☑
- metatarsal (bone) — *see* Dislocation, foot
- metatarsophalangeal (joint(s)) — *see* Dislocation, toe
- midcarpal (joint) S63.03- ☑
- midtarsal (joint) — *see* Dislocation, foot
- neck S13.20 ☑
  - specified site NEC S13.29 ☑
  - vertebra — *see* Dislocation, vertebra, cervical
- nose (septal cartilage) S03.1 ☑
- occipitoatloid S13.111 ☑
- old — *see* Derangement, joint, specified type NEC
- ossicles, ear — *see* Discontinuity, ossicles, ear
- partial — *see* Subluxation, by site
- patella S83.006 ☑
  - congenital Q74.1
  - lateral S83.01- ☑
  - recurrent (nontraumatic) M22.0- ☑
    - incomplete M22.1- ☑
  - specified type NEC S83.09- ☑
- pathological NEC M24.30
  - ankle M24.37- ☑
  - elbow M24.32- ☑
  - foot joint M24.37- ☑
  - hand joint M24.34- ☑
  - hip M24.35- ☑
  - knee M24.36- ☑
  - lumbosacral joint — *see* subcategory M53.2 ☑
  - pelvic region — *see* Dislocation, pathological, hip
  - sacroiliac — *see* subcategory M53.2 ☑
  - shoulder M24.31- ☑
  - wrist M24.33- ☑
- pelvis NEC S33.30 ☑
  - specified NEC S33.39 ☑
- phalanx
  - finger or hand — *see* Dislocation, finger
  - foot or toe — *see* Dislocation, toe
- prosthesis, internal — *see* Complications, prosthetic device, by site, mechanical
- radial head S53.006 ☑
  - anterior S53.01- ☑
  - posterior S53.02- ☑
  - specified type NEC S53.09- ☑
- radiocarpal (joint) S63.02- ☑
- radiohumeral (joint) — *see* Dislocation, radial head

Dislocation — *continued*
- radioulnar (joint)
  - distal S63.01- ☑
  - proximal — *see* Dislocation, elbow
- radius
  - distal end — *see* Dislocation, wrist
  - proximal end — *see* Dislocation, radial head
- recurrent M24.40
  - ankle M24.47- ☑
  - elbow M24.42- ☑
  - finger M24.44- ☑
  - foot joint M24.47- ☑
  - hand joint M24.44- ☑
  - hip M24.45- ☑
  - knee M24.46- ☑
    - patella — *see* Dislocation, patella, recurrent
  - patella — *see* Dislocation, patella, recurrent
  - sacroiliac — *see* subcategory M53.2 ☑
  - shoulder M24.41- ☑
  - toe M24.47- ☑
  - vertebra (*see also* subcategory) M43.5 ☑
    - atlantoaxial M43.4
      - with myelopathy M43.3
  - wrist M24.43- ☑
- rib (cartilage) S23.29 ☑
- sacrococcygeal S33.2 ☑
- sacroiliac (joint) (ligament) S33.2 ☑
  - congenital Q74.2
  - recurrent — *see* subcategory M53.2 ☑
- sacrum S33.2 ☑
- scaphoid (bone) (hand) (wrist) — *see* Dislocation, wrist
  - foot — *see* Dislocation, foot
- scapula — *see* Dislocation, shoulder, girdle, scapula
- semilunar cartilage, knee — *see* Tear, meniscus
- septal cartilage (nose) S03.1 ☑
- septum (nasal) (old) J34.2
- sesamoid bone — *code by* site under Dislocation
- shoulder (blade) (ligament) (joint) (traumatic) S43.006 ☑
  - acromioclavicular — *see* Dislocation, acromioclavicular
  - chronic — *see* Dislocation, recurrent, shoulder
  - congenital Q68.8
  - girdle S43.30- ☑
    - scapula S43.31- ☑
    - specified site NEC S43.39- ☑
  - humerus S43.00- ☑
    - anterior S43.01- ☑
    - inferior S43.03- ☑
    - posterior S43.02- ☑
  - pathological — *see* Dislocation, pathological NEC, shoulder
  - recurrent — *see* Dislocation, recurrent, shoulder
  - specified type NEC S43.08- ☑
- spine
  - cervical — *see* Dislocation, vertebra, cervical
  - congenital Q76.49
  - due to birth trauma P11.5
  - lumbar — *see* Dislocation, vertebra, lumbar
  - thoracic — *see* Dislocation, vertebra, thoracic
- spontaneous — *see* Dislocation, pathological
- sternoclavicular (joint) S43.206 ☑
  - anterior S43.21- ☑
  - posterior S43.22- ☑
- sternum S23.29 ☑
- subglenoid — *see* Dislocation, shoulder
- symphysis pubis S33.4 ☑
- talus — *see* Dislocation, ankle
- tarsal (bone(s)) (joint(s)) — *see* Dislocation, foot
- tarsometatarsal (joint(s)) — *see* Dislocation, foot
- temporomandibular (joint) S03.0 ☑
- thigh, proximal end — *see* Dislocation, hip
- thorax S23.20 ☑
  - specified site NEC S23.29 ☑
  - vertebra — *see* Dislocation, vertebra
- thumb S63.10- ☑
  - interphalangeal joint — *see* Dislocation, interphalangeal (joint), thumb
  - metacarpophalangeal joint — *see* Dislocation, metacarpophalangeal (joint), thumb
- thyroid cartilage S13.29 ☑
- tibia
  - distal end — *see* Dislocation, ankle
  - proximal end — *see* Dislocation, knee
- tibiofibular (joint)
  - distal — *see* Dislocation, ankle

Dislocation — *continued*
- tibiofibular — *continued*
  - superior — *see* Dislocation, knee
- toe(s) S93.106 ☑
  - great S93.10- ☑
    - interphalangeal joint S93.11- ☑
    - metatarsophalangeal joint S93.12- ☑
  - interphalangeal joint S93.119 ☑
  - lesser S93.106 ☑
    - interphalangeal joint S93.11- ☑
    - metatarsophalangeal joint S93.12- ☑
  - metatarsophalangeal joint S93.12- ☑
- tooth S03.2 ☑
- trachea S23.29 ☑
- ulna
  - distal end S63.07- ☑
  - proximal end — *see* Dislocation, elbow
- ulnohumeral (joint) — *see* Dislocation, elbow
- vertebra (articular process) (body) (traumatic)
  - cervical S13.101 ☑
    - atlantoaxial joint S13.121 ☑
    - atlantooccipital joint S13.111 ☑
    - atloidooccipital joint S13.111 ☑
    - joint between
      - C0 and C1 S13.111 ☑
      - C1 and C2 S13.121 ☑
      - C2 and C3 S13.131 ☑
      - C3 and C4 S13.141 ☑
      - C4 and C5 S13.151 ☑
      - C5 and C6 S13.161 ☑
      - C6 and C7 S13.171 ☑
      - C7 and T1 S13.181 ☑
    - occipitoatloid joint S13.111 ☑
  - congenital Q76.49
  - lumbar S33.101 ☑
    - joint between
      - L1 and L2 S33.111 ☑
      - L2 and L3 S33.121 ☑
      - L3 and L4 S33.131 ☑
      - L4 and L5 S33.141 ☑
    - nontraumatic — *see* Displacement, intervertebral disc
    - partial — *see* Subluxation, by site
    - recurrent NEC — *see* subcategory M43.5 ☑
  - thoracic S23.101 ☑
    - joint between
      - T1 and T2 S23.111 ☑
      - T2 and T3 S23.121 ☑
      - T3 and T4 S23.123 ☑
      - T4 and T5 S23.131 ☑
      - T5 and T6 S23.133 ☑
      - T6 and T7 S23.141 ☑
      - T7 and T8 S23.143 ☑
      - T8 and T9 S23.151 ☑
      - T9 and T10 S23.153 ☑
      - T10 and T11 S23.161 ☑
      - T11 and T12 S23.163 ☑
      - T12 and L1 S23.171 ☑
- wrist (carpal bone) S63.006 ☑
  - carpometacarpal joint — *see* Dislocation, carpometacarpal (joint)
  - distal radioulnar joint — *see* Dislocation, radioulnar (joint), distal
  - metacarpal bone, proximal — *see* Dislocation, metacarpal (bone), proximal end
  - midcarpal — *see* Dislocation, midcarpal (joint)
  - radiocarpal joint — *see* Dislocation, radiocarpal (joint)
  - recurrent — *see* Dislocation, recurrent, wrist
  - specified site NEC S63.09- ☑
  - ulna — *see* Dislocation, ulna, distal end
- xiphoid cartilage S23.29 ☑

Disorder (of) (*see also* Disease)
- acantholytic L11.9
  - specified NEC L11.8
- acute
  - psychotic — *see* Psychosis, acute
  - stress F43.0
- adjustment (grief) F43.20
  - with
    - anxiety F43.22
      - with depressed mood F43.23
    - conduct disturbance F43.24
      - with emotional disturbance F43.25
    - depressed mood F43.21
      - with anxiety F43.23

▽ Subterms under main terms may continue to next column or page   ☑ Additional Character Required — Refer to the Tabular List for Character Selection

Disorder — *continued*
  adjustment — *continued*
    with — *continued*
      other specified symptom F43.29
  adrenal (capsule) (gland) (medullary) E27.9
    specified NEC E27.8
  adrenogenital E25.9
    drug-induced E25.8
    iatrogenic E25.8
    idiopathic E25.8
  adult personality (and behavior) F69
    specified NEC F68.8
  affective (mood) — *see* Disorder, mood
  aggressive, unsocialized F91.1
  alcohol-related F10.99
    with
      amnestic disorder, persisting F10.96
      anxiety disorder F10.980
      dementia, persisting F10.97
      intoxication F10.929
        with delirium F10.921
        uncomplicated F10.920
      mood disorder F10.94
      other specified F10.988
      psychotic disorder F10.959
        with
          delusions F10.950
          hallucinations F10.951
      sexual dysfunction F10.981
      sleep disorder F10.982
  allergic — *see* Allergy
  alveolar NEC J84.09
  amino-acid
    cystathioninuria E72.19
    cystinosis E72.04
    cystinuria E72.01
    glycinuria E72.09
    homocystinuria E72.11
    metabolism — *see* Disturbance, metabolism, amino-acid
    specified NEC E72.8
  neonatal, transitory P74.8
  renal transport NEC E72.09
  transport NEC E72.09
  amnesic, amnestic
    alcohol-induced F10.96
      with dependence F10.26
    due to (secondary to) general medical condition F04
    psychoactive NEC-induced F19.96
      with
        abuse F19.16
        dependence F19.26
    sedative, hypnotic or anxiolytic-induced F13.96
      with dependence F13.26
  anaerobic glycolysis with anemia D55.2
  anxiety F41.9
    due to (secondary to)
      alcohol F10.980
      amphetamine F15.980
        in
          abuse F15.180
          dependence F15.280
      anxiolytic F13.980
        in
          abuse F13.180
          dependence F13.280
      caffeine F15.980
        in
          abuse F15.180
          dependence F15.280
      cannabis F12.980
        in
          abuse F12.180
          dependence F12.280
      cocaine F14.980
        in
          abuse F14.180
          dependence F14.180
      general medical condition F06.4
      hallucinogen F16.980
        in
          abuse F16.180
          dependence F16.280
      hypnotic F13.980
        in
          abuse F13.180
          dependence F13.280

Disorder — *continued*
  anxiety — *continued*
    due to — *continued*
      inhalant F18.980
        in
          abuse F18.180
          dependence F18.280
      phencyclidine F16.980
        in
          abuse F16.180
          dependence F16.280
      psychoactive substance NEC F19.980
        in
          abuse F19.180
          dependence F19.280
      sedative F13.980
        in
          abuse F13.180
          dependence F13.280
      volatile solvents F18.980
        in
          abuse F18.180
          dependence F18.280
    generalized F41.1
    mixed
      with depression (mild) F41.8
      specified NEC F41.3
    organic F06.4
    phobic F40.9
      of childhood F40.8
    specified NEC F41.8
  aortic valve — *see* Endocarditis, aortic
  aromatic amino-acid metabolism E70.9
    specified NEC E70.8
  arteriole NEC I77.89
  artery NEC I77.89
  articulation — *see* Disorder, joint
  attachment (childhood)
    disinhibited F94.2
    reactive F94.1
  attention-deficit hyperactivity (adolescent) (adult) (child) F90.9
    combined type F90.2
    hyperactive type F90.1
    inattentive type F90.0
    specified type NEC F90.8
  attention-deficit without hyperactivity (adolescent) (adult) (child) F90.0
  auditory processing (central) H93.25
  autistic F84.0
  autonomic nervous system G90.9
    specified NEC G90.8
  avoidant, child or adolescent F40.10
  balance
    acid-base E87.8
      mixed E87.4
    electrolyte E87.8
    fluid NEC E87.8
  behavioral (disruptive) — *see* Disorder, conduct
  beta-amino-acid metabolism E72.8
  bile acid and cholesterol metabolism E78.70
    Barth syndrome E78.71
    other specified E78.79
    Smith-Lemli-Opitz syndrome E78.72
  bilirubin excretion E80.6
  binocular
    movement H51.9
      convergence
        excess H51.12
        insufficiency H51.11
      internuclear ophthalmoplegia — *see* Ophthalmoplegia, internuclear
      palsy of conjugate gaze H51.0
      specified type NEC H51.8
    vision NEC — *see* Disorder, vision, binocular
  bipolar (I) F31.9
    current episode
      depressed F31.9
        with psychotic features F31.5
        without psychotic features F31.30
          mild F31.31
          moderate F31.32
          severe (without psychotic features) F31.4
            with psychotic features F31.5
      hypomanic F31.0
      manic F31.9
        with psychotic features F31.2
        without psychotic features F31.10

Disorder — *continued*
  bipolar — *continued*
    current episode — *continued*
      manic — *continued*
        without psychotic features — *continued*
          mild F31.11
          moderate F31.12
          severe (without psychotic features) F31.13
            with psychotic features F31.2
        mixed F31.60
          mild F31.61
          moderate F31.62
          severe (without psychotic features) F31.63
            with psychotic features F31.64
        severe depression (without psychotic features) F31.4
          with psychotic features F31.5
    in remission (currently) F31.70
      in full remission
        most recent episode
          depressed F31.76
          hypomanic F31.72
          manic F31.74
          mixed F31.78
      in partial remission
        most recent episode
          depressed F31.75
          hypomanic F31.71
          manic F31.73
          mixed F31.77
    organic F06.30
    single manic episode F30.9
      mild F30.11
      moderate F30.12
      severe (without psychotic symptoms) F30.13
        with psychotic symptoms F30.2
    specified NEC F31.89
  bipolar II F31.81
  bladder N32.9
    functional NEC N31.9
    in schistosomiasis B65.0 [N33]
    specified NEC N32.89
  bleeding D68.9
  blood D75.9
    in congenital early syphilis A50.09 [D77]
  body dysmorphic F45.22
  bone M89.9
    continuity M84.9
      specified type NEC M84.80
        ankle M84.87- ☑
        fibula M84.86- ☑
        foot M84.87- ☑
        hand M84.84- ☑
        humerus M84.82- ☑
        neck M84.88
        pelvis M84.859
        radius M84.83- ☑
        rib M84.88
        shoulder M84.81- ☑
        skull M84.88
        thigh M84.85- ☑
        tibia M84.86- ☑
        ulna M84.83- ☑
        vertebra M84.88
    density and structure M85.9
      cyst (*see also* Cyst, bone, specified type NEC)
        aneurysmal — *see* Cyst, bone, aneurysmal
        solitary — *see* Cyst, bone, solitary
      diffuse idiopathic skeletal hyperostosis — *see* Hyperostosis, ankylosing
      fibrous dysplasia (monostotic) — *see* Dysplasia, fibrous, bone
      fluorosis — *see* Fluorosis, skeletal
      hyperostosis of skull M85.2
      osteitis condensans — *see* Osteitis, condensans
      specified type NEC M85.8- ☑
        ankle M85.87- ☑
        foot M85.87- ☑
        forearm M85.83- ☑
        hand M85.84- ☑
        lower leg M85.86- ☑
        multiple sites M85.89
        neck M85.88
        rib M85.88
        shoulder M85.81- ☑
        skull M85.88
        thigh M85.85- ☑

☑ Additional Character Required — Refer to the Tabular List for Character Selection ▽ Subterms under main terms may continue to next column or page

Disorder — *continued*
- bone — *continued*
  - density and structure — *continued*
    - specified type — *continued*
      - upper arm M85.82- ☑
      - vertebra M85.88
  - development and growth NEC M89.20
    - carpus M89.24- ☑
    - clavicle M89.21- ☑
    - femur M89.25- ☑
    - fibula M89.26- ☑
    - finger M89.24- ☑
    - humerus M89.22- ☑
    - ilium M89.259
    - ischium M89.259
    - metacarpus M89.24- ☑
    - metatarsus M89.27- ☑
    - multiple sites M89.29
    - neck M89.28
    - radius M89.23- ☑
    - rib M89.28
    - scapula M89.21- ☑
    - skull M89.28
    - tarsus M89.27- ☑
    - tibia M89.26- ☑
    - toe M89.27- ☑
    - ulna M89.23- ☑
    - vertebra M89.28
  - specified type NEC M89.8X- ☑
- brachial plexus G54.0
- branched-chain amino-acid metabolism E71.2
  - specified NEC E71.19
- breast N64.9
  - agalactia — *see* Agalactia
  - associated with
    - lactation O92.70
      - specified NEC O92.79
    - pregnancy O92.20
      - specified NEC O92.29
    - puerperium O92.20
      - specified NEC O92.29
  - cracked nipple — *see* Cracked nipple
  - galactorrhea — *see* Galactorrhea
  - hypogalactia O92.4
  - lactation disorder NEC O92.79
  - mastitis — *see* Mastitis
  - nipple infection — *see* Infection, nipple
  - retracted nipple — *see* Retraction, nipple
  - specified type NEC N64.89
- Briquet's F45.0
- bullous, in diseases classified elsewhere L14
- cannabis use
  - due to drug abuse — *see* Abuse, drug, cannabis
  - due to drug dependence — *see* Dependence, drug, cannabis
- carbohydrate
  - absorption, intestinal NEC E74.39
  - metabolism (congenital) E74.9
    - specified NEC E74.8
- cardiac, functional I51.89
- carnitine metabolism E71.40
- cartilage M94.9
  - articular NEC — *see* Derangement, joint, articular cartilage
  - chondrocalcinosis — *see* Chondrocalcinosis
  - specified type NEC M94.8X- ☑
    - articular — *see* Derangement, joint, articular cartilage
    - multiple sites M94.8X0
- catatonic
  - due to (secondary to) known physiological condition F06.1
  - organic F06.1
- central auditory processing H93.25
- cervical
  - region NEC M53.82
  - root (nerve) NEC G54.2
- character NOS F60.9
- childhood disintegrative NEC F84.3
- cholesterol and bile acid metabolism E78.70
  - Barth syndrome E78.71
  - other specified E78.79
  - Smith-Lemli-Opitz syndrome E78.72
- choroid H31.9
  - atrophy — *see* Atrophy, choroid
  - degeneration — *see* Degeneration, choroid
  - detachment — *see* Detachment, choroid

Disorder — *continued*
- choroid — *continued*
  - dystrophy — *see* Dystrophy, choroid
  - hemorrhage — *see* Hemorrhage, choroid
  - rupture — *see* Rupture, choroid
  - scar — *see* Scar, chorioretinal
  - solar retinopathy — *see* Retinopathy, solar
  - specified type NEC H31.8
- ciliary body — *see* Disorder, iris
  - degeneration — *see* Degeneration, ciliary body
- coagulation (factor) (*see also* Defect, coagulation) D68.9
  - newborn, transient P61.6
- coccyx NEC M53.3
- cognitive F09
  - due to (secondary to) general medical condition F09
  - persisting R41.89
    - due to
      - alcohol F10.97
        - with dependence F10.27
      - anxiolytics F13.97
        - with dependence F13.27
      - hypnotics F13.97
        - with dependence F13.27
      - sedatives F13.97
        - with dependence F13.27
      - specified substance NEC F19.97
        - with
          - abuse F19.17
          - dependence F19.27
- communication F80.9
- conduct (childhood) F91.9
  - adjustment reaction — *see* Disorder, adjustment
  - adolescent onset type F91.2
  - childhood onset type F91.1
  - compulsive F63.9
  - confined to family context F91.0
  - depressive F91.8
  - group type F91.2
  - hyperkinetic — *see* Disorder, attention-deficit hyperactivity
  - oppositional defiance F91.3
  - socialized F91.2
  - solitary aggressive type F91.1
  - specified NEC F91.8
  - unsocialized (aggressive) F91.1
- conduction, heart I45.9
- congenital glycosylation (CDG) E74.8
- conjunctiva H11.9
  - infection — *see* Conjunctivitis
- connective tissue, localized L94.9
  - specified NEC L94.8
- conversion — *see* Disorder, dissociative
- convulsive (secondary) — *see* Convulsions
- cornea H18.9
  - deformity — *see* Deformity, cornea
  - degeneration — *see* Degeneration, cornea
  - deposits — *see* Deposit, cornea
  - due to contact lens H18.82- ☑
    - specified as edema — *see* Edema, cornea
  - edema — *see* Edema, cornea
  - keratitis — *see* Keratitis
  - keratoconjunctivitis — *see* Keratoconjunctivitis
  - membrane change — *see* Change, corneal membrane
  - neovascularization — *see* Neovascularization, cornea
  - scar — *see* Opacity, cornea
  - specified type NEC H18.89- ☑
  - ulcer — *see* Ulcer, cornea
- corpus cavernosum N48.9
- cranial nerve — *see* Disorder, nerve, cranial
- cyclothymic F34.0
- defiant oppositional F91.3
- delusional (persistent) (systematized) F22
  - induced F24
- depersonalization F48.1
- depressive F32.9
  - major F32.9
    - with psychotic symptoms F32.3
    - in remission (full) F32.5
      - partial F32.4
    - recurrent F33.9
    - single episode F32.9
      - mild F32.0
      - moderate F32.1
      - severe (without psychotic symptoms) F32.2

Disorder — *continued*
- depressive — *continued*
  - major — *continued*
    - single episode — *continued*
      - severe — *continued*
        - with psychotic symptoms F32.3
    - organic F06.31
    - recurrent F33.9
      - current episode
        - mild F33.0
        - moderate F33.1
        - severe (without psychotic symptoms) F33.2
          - with psychotic symptoms F33.3
      - in remission F33.40
        - full F33.42
        - partial F33.41
      - specified NEC F33.8
    - single episode — *see* Episode, depressive
- developmental F89
  - arithmetical skills F81.2
  - coordination (motor) F82
  - expressive writing F81.81
  - language F80.9
    - expressive F80.1
    - mixed receptive and expressive F80.2
    - receptive type F80.2
    - specified NEC F80.89
  - learning F81.9
    - arithmetical F81.2
    - reading F81.0
  - mixed F88
  - motor coordination or function F82
  - pervasive F84.9
    - specified NEC F84.8
  - phonological F80.0
  - reading F81.0
  - scholastic skills (*see also* Disorder, learning)
    - mixed F81.89
  - specified NEC F88
  - speech F80.9
    - articulation F80.0
    - specified NEC F80.89
  - written expression F81.81
- diaphragm J98.6
- digestive (system) K92.9
  - newborn P78.9
    - specified NEC P78.89
  - postprocedural — *see* Complication, gastrointestinal
  - psychogenic F45.8
- disc (intervertebral) M51.9
  - with
    - myelopathy
      - cervical region M50.00
      - cervicothoracic region M50.03
      - high cervical region M50.01
      - lumbar region M51.06
      - mid-cervical region M50.02
      - sacrococcygeal region M53.3
      - thoracic region M51.04
      - thoracolumbar region M51.05
    - radiculopathy
      - cervical region M50.10
      - cervicothoracic region M50.13
      - high cervical region M50.11
      - lumbar region M51.16
      - lumbosacral region M51.17
      - mid-cervical region M50.12
      - sacrococcygeal region M53.3
      - thoracic region M51.14
      - thoracolumbar region M51.15
    - cervical M50.90
      - with
        - myelopathy M50.00
          - C2-C3 M50.01
          - C3-C4 M50.01
          - C4-C5 M50.02
          - C5-C6 M50.02
          - C6-C7 M50.02
          - C7-T1 M50.03
          - cervicothoracic region M50.03
          - high cervical region M50.01
          - mid-cervical region M50.02
        - neuritis, radiculitis or radiculopathy M50.10
          - C2-C3 M50.11
          - C3-C4 M50.11
          - C4-C5 M50.12
          - C5-C6 M50.12

Index

Disorder — Disorder

Disorder — *continued*
  disc — *continued*
    cervical — *continued*
      with — *continued*
        neuritis, radiculitis or radiculopathy — *continued*
          C6-C7 M50.12
          C7-T1 M50.13
          cervicothoracic region M50.13
          high cervical region M50.11
          mid-cervical region M50.12
      C2-C3 M50.91
      C3-C4 M50.91
      C4-C5 M50.92
      C5-C6 M50.92
      C6-C7 M50.92
      C7-T1 M50.93
      cervicothoracic region M50.93
      degeneration M50.30
        C2-C3 M50.31
        C3-C4 M50.31
        C4-C5 M50.32
        C5-C6 M50.32
        C6-C7 M50.32
        C7-T1 M50.33
        cervicothoracic region M50.33
        high cervical region M50.31
        mid-cervical region M50.32
      displacement M50.20
        C2-C3 M50.21
        C3-C4 M50.21
        C4-C5 M50.22
        C5-C6 M50.22
        C6-C7 M50.22
        C7-T1 M50.23
        cervicothoracic region M50.23
        high cervical region M50.21
        mid-cervical region M50.22
      high cervical region M50.91
      mid-cervical region M50.92
      specified type NEC M50.80
        C2-C3 M50.81
        C3-C4 M50.81
        C4-C5 M50.82
        C5-C6 M50.82
        C6-C7 M50.82
        C7-T1 M50.83
        cervicothoracic region M50.83
        high cervical region M50.81
        mid-cervical region M50.82
    specified NEC
      lumbar region M51.86
      lumbosacral region M51.87
      sacrococcygeal region M53.3
      thoracic region M51.84
      thoracolumbar region M51.85
  disinhibited attachment (childhood) F94.2
  disintegrative, childhood NEC F84.3
  disruptive behavior F98.9
  dissocial personality F60.2
  dissociative F44.9
    affecting
      motor function F44.4
        and sensation F44.7
      sensation F44.6
        and motor function F44.7
    brief reactive F43.0
    due to (secondary to) general medical condition F06.8
    mixed F44.7
    organic F06.8
    other specified NEC F44.89
  double heterozygous sickling — *see* Disease, sickle-cell
  dream anxiety F51.5
  drug induced hemorrhagic D68.32
  drug related F19.99
    abuse — *see* Abuse, drug
    dependence — *see* Dependence, drug
  dysmorphic body F45.1
  dysthymic F34.1
  ear H93.9- ☑
    bleeding — *see* Otorrhagia
    deafness — *see* Deafness
    degenerative H93.09- ☑
    discharge — *see* Otorrhea
    external H61.9- ☑

Disorder — *continued*
  ear — *continued*
    external — *continued*
      auditory canal stenosis — *see* Stenosis, external auditory canal
      exostosis — *see* Exostosis, external ear canal
      impacted cerumen — *see* Impaction, cerumen
      otitis — *see* Otitis, externa
      perichondritis — *see* Perichondritis, ear
      pinna — *see* Disorder, pinna
      specified type NEC H61.89- ☑
    inner H83.9- ☑
      vestibular dysfunction — *see* Disorder, vestibular function
    middle H74.9- ☑
      adhesive H74.1- ☑
      ossicle — *see* Abnormal, ear ossicles
      polyp — *see* Polyp, ear (middle)
      specified NEC, in diseases classified elsewhere H75.8- ☑
    postprocedural — *see* Complications, ear, procedure
    specified NEC, in diseases classified elsewhere H94.8- ☑
  eating (adult) (psychogenic) F50.9
    anorexia — *see* Anorexia
    bulimia F50.2
    child F98.29
      pica F98.3
      rumination disorder F98.21
    pica F50.8
      childhood F98.3
  electrolyte (balance) NEC E87.8
    with
      abortion — *see* Abortion by type complicated by specified condition NEC
      ectopic pregnancy O08.5
      molar pregnancy O08.5
    acidosis (metabolic) (respiratory) E87.2
    alkalosis (metabolic) (respiratory) E87.3
  elimination, transepidermal L87.9
    specified NEC L87.8
  emotional (persistent) F34.9
    of childhood F93.9
      specified NEC F93.8
  endocrine E34.9
    postprocedural E89.89
    specified NEC E89.89
  erectile (male) (organic) (*see also* Dysfunction, sexual, male, erectile) N52.9
    nonorganic F52.21
  erythematous — *see* Erythema
  esophagus K22.9
    functional K22.4
    psychogenic F45.8
  eustachian tube H69.9- ☑
    infection — *see* Salpingitis, eustachian
    obstruction — *see* Obstruction, eustachian tube
    patulous — *see* Patulous, eustachian tube
    specified NEC H69.8- ☑
  extrapyramidal G25.9
    in deseases classified elsewhere — *see* category G26
    specified type NEC G25.89
  eye H57.9
    postprocedural — *see* Complication, postprocedural, eye
  eyelid H02.9
    cyst — *see* Cyst, eyelid
    degenerative H02.70
      chloasma — *see* Chloasma, eyelid
      madarosis — *see* Madarosis
      specified type NEC H02.79
      vitiligo — *see* Vitiligo, eyelid
      xanthelasma — *see* Xanthelasma
    dermatochalasis — *see* Dermatochalasis
    edema — *see* Edema, eyelid
    elephantiasis — *see* Elephantiasis, eyelid
    foreign body, retained — *see* Foreign body, retained, eyelid
    function H02.59
      abnormal innervation syndrome — *see* Syndrome, abnormal innervation
      blepharochalasis — *see* Blepharochalasis
      blepharoclonus — *see* Blepharoclonus
      blepharophimosis — *see* Blepharophimosis
      blepharoptosis — *see* Blepharoptosis

Disorder — *continued*
  eyelid — *continued*
    function — *continued*
      lagophthalmos — *see* Lagophthalmos
      lid retraction — *see* Retraction, lid
    hypertrichosis — *see* Hypertrichosis, eyelid
    specified type NEC H02.89
    vascular H02.879
      left H02.876
        lower H02.875
        upper H02.874
      right H02.873
        lower H02.872
        upper H02.871
  factitious F68.10
    with predominantly
      physical symptoms F68.12
        with psychological symptoms F68.13
      psychological symptoms F68.11
        with physical symptoms F68.13
  factor, coagulation — *see* Defect, coagulation
  fatty acid
    metabolism E71.30
      specified NEC E71.39
    oxidation
      LCAD E71.310
      MCAD E71.311
      SCAD E71.312
      specified deficiency NEC E71.318
  feeding (infant or child) (*see also* Disorder, eating) R63.3
  feigned (with obvious motivation) Z76.5
    without obvious motivation — *see* Disorder, factitious
  female
    hypoactive sexual desire F52.0
    orgasmic F52.31
    sexual arousal F52.22
  fibroblastic M72.9
    specified NEC M72.8
  fluency
    adult onset F98.5
    childhood onset F80.81
    following
      cerebral infarction I69.323
      cerebrovascular disease I69.923
        specified disease NEC I69.823
      intracerebral hemorrhage I69.123
      nontraumatic intracranial hemorrhage NEC I69.223
      subarachnoid hemorrhage I69.023
    in conditions classified elsewhere R47.82
  fluid balance E87.8
  follicular (skin) L73.9
    specified NEC L73.8
  fructose metabolism E74.10
    essential fructosuria E74.11
    fructokinase deficiency E74.11
    fructose-1, 6-diphosphatase deficiency E74.19
    hereditary fructose intolerance E74.12
    other specified E74.19
  functional polymorphonuclear neutrophils D71
  gallbladder, biliary tract and pancreas in diseases classified elsewhere K87
  gamma-glutamyl cycle E72.8
  gastric (functional) K31.9
    motility K30
    psychogenic F45.8
    secretion K30
  gastrointestinal (functional) NOS K92.9
    newborn P78.9
    psychogenic F45.8
  gender-identity or -role F64.9
    childhood F64.2
    effect on relationship F66
    of adolescence or adulthood (nontranssexual) F64.1
    specified NEC F64.8
    uncertainty F66
  genitourinary system
    female N94.9
    male N50.9
    psychogenic F45.8
  globe H44.9
    degenerated condition H44.50
      absolute glaucoma H44.51- ☑
      atrophy H44.52- ☑
      leucocoria H44.53- ☑
    degenerative H44.30

   ☑ **Additional Character Required** — Refer to the Tabular List for Character Selection   ▽ **Subterms under main terms may continue to next column or page**

Disorder — continued
  globe — continued
    degenerative — continued
      chalcosis H44.31- ☑
      myopia H44.2- ☑
      siderosis H44.32- ☑
      specified type NEC H44.39- ☑
    endophthalmitis — see Endophthalmitis
    foreign body, retained — see Foreign body, intraocular, old, retained
    hemophthalmos — see Hemophthalmos
    hypotony H44.40
      due to
        ocular fistula H44.42- ☑
        specified disorder NEC H44.43- ☑
      flat anterior chamber H44.41- ☑
      primary H44.44- ☑
    luxation — see Luxation, globe
    specified type NEC H44.89
  glomerular (in) N05.9
    amyloidosis E85.4 [N08]
    cryoglobulinemia D89.1 [N08]
    disseminated intravascular coagulation D65 [N08]
    Fabry's disease E75.21 [N08]
    familial lecithin cholesterol acyltransferase deficiency E78.6 [N08]
    Goodpasture's syndrome M31.0
    hemolytic-uremic syndrome D59.3
    Henoch (-Schönlein) purpura D69.0 [N08]
    malariae malaria B52.0
    microscopic polyangiitis M31.7 [N08]
    multiple myeloma C90.0- ☑ [N08]
    mumps B26.83
    schistosomiasis B65.9 [N08]
    sepsis NEC A41.- ☑ [N08]
      streptococcal A40.- ☑ [N08]
    sickle-cell disorders D57.- ☑ [N08]
    strongyloidiasis B78.9 [N08]
    subacute bacterial endocarditis I33.0 [N08]
    syphilis A52.75
    systemic lupus erythematosus M32.14
    thrombotic thrombocytopenic purpura M31.1 [N08]
    Waldenström macroglobulinemia C88.0 [N08]
    Wegener's granulomatosis M31.31
  gluconeogenesis E74.4
  glucosaminoglycan metabolism — see Disorder, metabolism, glucosaminoglycan
  glycine metabolism E72.50
    d-glycericacidemia E72.59
    hyperhydroxyprolinemia E72.59
    hyperoxaluria E72.53
    hyperprolinemia E72.59
    non-ketotic hyperglycinemia E72.51
    oxalosis E72.53
    oxaluria E72.53
    sarcosinemia E72.59
    trimethylaminuria E72.52
  glycoprotein metabolism E77.9
    specified NEC E77.8
  habit (and impulse) F63.9
    involving sexual behavior NEC F65.9
    specified NEC F63.89
  heart action I49.9
  hematological D75.9
    newborn (transient) P61.9
      specified NEC P61.8
  hematopoietic organs D75.9
  hemorrhagic NEC D69.9
    drug-induced D68.32
    due to
      extrinsic circulating anticoagulants D68.32
      increase in
        anti-IIa D68.32
        anti-Xa D68.32
      intrinsic
        circulating anticoagulants D68.318
        increase in
          anti-IXa D68.318
          antithrombin D68.318
          anti-VIIIa D68.318
          anti-XIa D68.318
    following childbirth O72.3
  hemostasis — see Defect, coagulation
  histidine metabolism E70.40
    histidinemia E70.41
    other specified E70.49

Disorder — continued
  hyperkinetic — see Disorder, attention-deficit hyperactivity
  hyperleucine-isoleucinemia E71.19
  hypervalinemia E71.19
  hypoactive sexual desire F52.0
  hypochondriacal F45.20
    body dysmorphic F45.22
    neurosis F45.21
    other specified F45.29
  identity
    dissociative F44.81
    of childhood F93.8
  immune mechanism (immunity) D89.9
    specified type NEC D89.89
  impaired renal tubular function N25.9
    specified NEC N25.89
  impulse (control) F63.9
  inflammatory
    pelvic, in diseases classified elsewhere — see category N74
    penis N48.29
      abscess N48.21
      cellulitis N48.22
  integument, newborn P83.9
    specified NEC P83.8
  intermittent explosive F63.81
  internal secretion pancreas — see Increased, secretion, pancreas, endocrine
  intestine, intestinal
    carbohydrate absorption NEC E74.39
      postoperative K91.2
    functional NEC K59.9
      postoperative K91.89
    psychogenic F45.8
    vascular K55.9
      chronic K55.1
      specified NEC K55.8
  intraoperative (intraprocedural) — see Complications, intraoperative
  involuntary emotional expression (IEED) F07.89
  iris H21.9
    adhesions — see Adhesions, iris
    atrophy — see Atrophy, iris
    chamber angle recession — see Recession, chamber angle
    cyst — see Cyst, iris
    degeneration — see Degeneration, iris
    in diseases classified elsewhere H22
    iridodialysis — see Iridodialysis
    iridoschisis — see Iridoschisis
    miotic pupillary cyst — see Cyst, pupillary
    pupillary
      abnormality — see Abnormality, pupillary
      membrane — see Membrane, pupillary
    specified type NEC H21.89
    vascular NEC H21.1X- ☑
  iron metabolism E83.10
    specified NEC E83.19
  isovaleric acidemia E71.110
  jaw, developmental M27.0
    temporomandibular — see Anomaly, dentofacial, temporomandibular joint
  joint M25.9
    derangement — see Derangement, joint
    effusion — see Effusion, joint
    fistula — see Fistula, joint
    hemarthrosis — see Hemarthrosis
    instability — see Instability, joint
    osteophyte — see Osteophyte
    pain — see Pain, joint
    psychogenic F45.8
    specified type NEC M25.80
      ankle M25.87- ☑
      elbow M25.82- ☑
      foot joint M25.87- ☑
      hand joint M25.84- ☑
      hip M25.85- ☑
      knee M25.86- ☑
      shoulder M25.81- ☑
      wrist M25.83- ☑
    stiffness — see Stiffness, joint
  ketone metabolism E71.32
  kidney N28.9
    functional (tubular) N25.9
    in
      schistosomiasis B65.9 [N29]

Disorder — continued
  kidney — continued
    tubular function N25.9
      specified NEC N25.89
  lacrimal system H04.9
    changes H04.69
      fistula — see Fistula, lacrimal
    gland H04.19
      atrophy — see Atrophy, lacrimal gland
      cyst — see Cyst, lacrimal, gland
      dacryops — see Dacryops
      dislocation — see Dislocation, lacrimal gland
      dry eye syndrome — see Syndrome, dry eye
      infection — see Dacryoadenitis
      granuloma — see Granuloma, lacrimal
      inflammation — see Inflammation, lacrimal
      obstruction — see Obstruction, lacrimal
    specified NEC H04.89
  lactation NEC O92.79
  language (developmental) F80.9
    expressive F80.1
    mixed receptive and expressive F80.2
    receptive F80.2
  late luteal phase dysphoric N94.89
  learning (specific) F81.9
    acalculia R48.8
    alexia R48.0
    mathematics F81.2
    reading F81.0
    specified NEC F81.89
    spelling F81.81
    written expression F81.81
  lens H27.9
    aphakia — see Aphakia
    cataract — see Cataract
    dislocation — see Dislocation, lens
    specified type NEC H27.8
  ligament M24.20
    ankle M24.27- ☑
    attachment, spine — see Enthesopathy, spinal
    elbow M24.22- ☑
    foot joint M24.27- ☑
    hand joint M24.24- ☑
    hip M24.25- ☑
    knee — see Derangement, knee, specified NEC
    shoulder M24.21- ☑
    vertebra M24.28
    wrist M24.23- ☑
  ligamentous attachments (see also Enthesopathy)
    spine — see Enthesopathy, spinal
  lipid
    metabolism, congenital E78.9
    storage E75.6
      specified NEC E75.5
  lipoprotein
    deficiency (familial) E78.6
    metabolism E78.9
      specified NEC E78.89
  liver K76.9
    malarial B54 [K77]
  low back (see also Dorsopathy, specified NEC)
  lumbosacral
    plexus G54.1
    root (nerve) NEC G54.4
  lung, interstitial, drug-induced J70.4
    acute J70.2
    chronic J70.3
  lymphoproliferative, post-transplant (PTLD) D47.Z1 (following D47.4)
  lysine and hydroxylysine metabolism E72.3
  male
    erectile (organic) (see also Dysfunction, sexual, male, erectile) N52.9
      nonorganic F52.21
    hypoactive sexual desire F52.0
    orgasmic F52.32
  manic F30.9
    organic F06.33
  mastoid (see also Disorder, ear, middle)
    postprocedural — see Complications, ear, procedure
  meniscus — see Derangement, knee, meniscus
  menopausal N95.9
    specified NEC N95.8
  menstrual N92.6
    psychogenic F45.8
    specified NEC N92.5
  mental (or behavioral) (nonpsychotic) F99

Disorder — Disorder

Disorder — *continued*
  mental — *continued*
    due to (secondary to)
      amphetamine
        due to drug abuse — *see* Abuse, drug, stimulant
        due to drug dependence — *see* Dependence, drug, stimulant
      brain disease, damage and dysfunction F09
      caffeine use
        due to drug abuse — *see* Abuse, drug, stimulant
        due to drug dependence — *see* Dependence, drug, stimulant
      cannabis use
        due to drug abuse — *see* Abuse, drug, cannabis
        due to drug dependence — *see* Dependence, drug, cannabis
      general medical condition F09
      sedative or hypnotic use
        due to drug abuse — *see* Abuse, drug, sedative
        due to drug dependence — *see* Dependence, drug, sedative
      tobacco (nicotine) use — *see* Dependence, drug, nicotine
    following organic brain damage F07.9
      frontal lobe syndrome F07.0
      personality change F07.0
      postconcussional syndrome F07.81
      specified NEC F07.89
    infancy, childhood or adolescence F98.9
    neurotic — *see* Neurosis
    organic or symptomatic F09
    presenile, psychotic F03 ☑
    problem NEC
    psychoneurotic — *see* Neurosis
    psychotic — *see* Psychosis
    puerperal F53
    senile, psychotic NEC F03 ☑
  metabolic, amino acid, transitory, newborn P74.8
  metabolism NOS E88.9
    amino-acid E72.9
      aromatic E70.9
        albinism — *see* Albinism
        histidine E70.40
          histidinemia E70.41
          other specified E70.49
        hyperphenylalaninemia E70.1
          classical phenylketonuria E70.0
        other specified E70.8
        tryptophan E70.5
        tyrosine E70.20
          hypertyrosinemia E70.21
          other specified E70.29
      branched chain E71.2
        3-methylglutaconic aciduria E71.111
        hyperleucine-isoleucinemia E71.19
        hypervalinemia E71.19
        isovaleric acidemia E71.110
        maple syrup urine disease E71.0
        methylmalonic acidemia E71.120
        organic aciduria NEC E71.118
        other specified E71.19
        proprionate NEC E71.128
        proprionic acidemia E71.121
      glycine E72.50
        d-glycericacidemia E72.59
        hyperhydroxyprolinemia E72.59
        hyperoxaluria E72.53
        hyperprolinemia E72.59
        non-ketotic hyperglycinemia E72.51
        other specified E72.59
        sarcosinemia E72.59
        trimethylaminuria E72.52
      hydroxylysine E72.3
      lysine E72.3
      ornithine E72.4
      other specified E72.8
        beta-amino acid E72.8
        gamma-glutamyl cycle E72.8
      straight-chain E72.8
      sulfur-bearing E72.10
        homocystinuria E72.11
        methylenetetrahydrofolate reductase deficiency E72.12
        other specified E72.19

Disorder — *continued*
  metabolism — *continued*
    bile acid and cholesterol metabolism E78.70
    bilirubin E80.7
      specified NEC E80.6
    calcium E83.50
      hypercalcemia E83.52
      hypocalcemia E83.51
      other specified E83.59
    carbohydrate E74.9
      specified NEC E74.8
    cholesterol and bile acid metabolism E78.70
    congenital E88.9
    copper E83.00
      specified type NEC E83.09
      Wilson's disease E83.01
    cystinuria E72.01
    fructose E74.10
    galactose E74.20
    glucosaminoglycan E76.9
      mucopolysaccharidosis — *see* Mucopolysaccharidosis
      specified NEC E76.8
    glutamine E72.8
    glycine E72.50
    glycogen storage (hepatorenal) E74.09
    glycoprotein E77.9
      specified NEC E77.8
    glycosaminoglycan E76.9
      specified NEC E76.8
    in labor and delivery O75.89
    iron E83.10
    isoleucine E71.19
    leucine E71.19
    lipoid E78.9
    lipoprotein E78.9
      specified NEC E78.89
    magnesium E83.40
      hypermagnesemia E83.41
      hypomagnesemia E83.42
      other specified E83.49
    mineral E83.9
      specified NEC E83.89
    mitochondrial E88.40
      MELAS syndrome E88.41
      MERRF syndrome (myoclonic epilepsy associated with ragged-red fibers) E88.42
      other specified E88.49
    ornithine E72.4
    phosphatases E83.30
    phosphorus E83.30
      acid phosphatase deficiency E83.39
      hypophosphatasia E83.39
      hypophosphatemia E83.39
        familial E83.31
      other specified E83.39
      pseudovitamin D deficiency E83.32
    plasma protein NEC E88.09
    porphyrin — *see* Porphyria
    postprocedural E89.89
      specified NEC E89.89
    purine E79.9
      specified NEC E79.8
    pyrimidine E79.9
      specified NEC E79.8
    pyruvate E74.4
    serine E72.8
    sodium E87.8
    specified NEC E88.89
    threonine E72.8
    valine E71.19
    zinc E83.2
  methylmalonic acidemia E71.120
  micturition NEC R39.19
    feeling of incomplete emptying R39.14
    hesitancy R39.11
    poor stream R39.12
    psychogenic F45.8
    split stream R39.13
    straining R39.16
    urgency R39.15
  mitochondrial metabolism E88.40
  mitral (valve) — *see* Endocarditis, mitral
  mixed
    anxiety and depressive F41.8
    of scholastic skills (developmental) F81.89
    receptive expressive language F80.2
  mood F39

Disorder — *continued*
  mood — *continued*
    bipolar — *see* Disorder, bipolar
    depressive — *see* Disorder, depressive
    due to (secondary to)
      alcohol F10.94
      amphetamine F15.94
        in
          abuse F15.14
          dependence F15.24
      anxiolytic F13.94
        in
          abuse F13.14
          dependence F13.24
      cocaine F14.94
        in
          abuse F14.14
          dependence F14.24
      general medical condition F06.30
      hallucinogen F16.94
        in
          abuse F16.14
          dependence F16.24
      hypnotic F13.94
        in
          abuse F13.14
          dependence F13.24
      inhalant F18.94
        in
          abuse F18.14
          dependence F18.24
      opioid F11.94
        in
          abuse F11.14
          dependence F11.24
      phencyclidine (PCP) F16.94
        in
          abuse F16.14
          dependence F16.24
      physiological condition F06.30
        with
          depressive features F06.31
          major depressive-like episode F06.32
          manic features F06.33
          mixed features F06.34
      psychoactive substance NEC F19.94
        in
          abuse F19.14
          dependence F19.24
      sedative F13.94
        in
          abuse F13.14
          dependence F13.24
      volatile solvents F18.94
        in
          abuse F18.14
          dependence F18.24
    manic episode F30.9
      with psychotic symptoms F30.2
      without psychotic symptoms F30.10
        mild F30.11
        moderate F30.12
        severe F30.13
      in remission (full) F30.4
        partial F30.3
      specified type NEC F30.8
    organic F06.30
      right hemisphere F07.89
    persistent F34.9
      cyclothymia F34.0
      dysthymia F34.1
      specified type NEC F34.8
    recurrent F39
    right hemisphere organic F07.89
  movement G25.9
    drug-induced G25.70
      akathisia G25.71
      specified NEC G25.79
    hysterical F44.4
    in diseases classified elsewhere — *see* category G26
    periodic limb G47.61
      sleep related G47.61
    sleep related NEC G47.69
    specified NEC G25.89
    stereotyped F98.4
    treatment-induced G25.9
  multiple personality F44.81

Disorder — *continued*

muscle M62.9
  attachment, spine — *see* Enthesopathy, spinal
  in trichinellosis — *see* Trichinellosis, with muscle disorder
  psychogenic F45.8
  specified type NEC M62.89
  tone, newborn P94.9
    specified NEC P94.8
muscular
  attachments (*see also* Enthesopathy)
    spine — *see* Enthesopathy, spinal
  urethra N36.44
musculoskeletal system, soft tissue — *see* Disorder, soft tissue
  postprocedural M96.89
  psychogenic F45.8
myoneural G70.9
  due to lead G70.1
  specified NEC G70.89
  toxic G70.1
myotonic NEC G71.19
nail, in diseases classified elsewhere L62
neck region NEC — *see* Dorsopathy, specified NEC
nerve G58.9
  abducent NEC — *see* Strabismus, paralytic, sixth nerve
  accessory G52.8
  acoustic — *see* subcategory H93.3 ☑
  auditory — *see* subcategory H93.3 ☑
  auriculotemporal G50.8
  axillary G54.0
  cerebral — *see* Disorder, nerve, cranial
  cranial G52.9
    eighth — *see* subcategory H93.3 ☑
    eleventh G52.8
    fifth G50.9
    first G52.0
    fourth NEC — *see* Strabismus, paralytic, fourth nerve
    multiple G52.7
    ninth G52.1
    second NEC — *see* Disorder, nerve, optic
    seventh NEC G51.8
    sixth NEC — *see* Strabismus, paralytic, sixth nerve
    specified NEC G52.8
    tenth G52.2
    third NEC — *see* Strabismus, paralytic, third nerve
    twelfth G52.3
  entrapment — *see* Neuropathy, entrapment
  facial G51.9
    specified NEC G51.8
  femoral — *see* Lesion, nerve, femoral
  glossopharyngeal NEC G52.1
  hypoglossal G52.3
  intercostal G58.0
  lateral
    cutaneous of thigh — *see* Mononeuropathy, lower limb, meralgia paresthetica
    popliteal — *see* Lesion, nerve, popliteal
  lower limb — *see* Mononeuropathy, lower limb
  medial popliteal — *see* Lesion, nerve, popliteal, medial
  median NEC — *see* Lesion, nerve, median
  multiple G58.7
  oculomotor NEC — *see* Strabismus, paralytic, third nerve
  olfactory G52.0
  optic NEC H47.09- ☑
    hemorrhage into sheath — *see* Hemorrhage, optic nerve
    ischemic H47.01- ☑
  peroneal — *see* Lesion, nerve, popliteal
  phrenic G58.8
  plantar — *see* Lesion, nerve, plantar
  pneumogastric G52.2
  posterior tibial — *see* Syndrome, tarsal tunnel
  radial — *see* Lesion, nerve, radial
  recurrent laryngeal G52.2
  root G54.9
    cervical G54.2
    lumbosacral G54.1
    specified NEC G54.8
    thoracic G54.3
  sciatic NEC — *see* Lesion, nerve, sciatic

Disorder — *continued*

nerve — *continued*
  specified NEC G58.8
    lower limb — *see* Mononeuropathy, lower limb, specified NEC
    upper limb — *see* Mononeuropathy, upper limb, specified NEC
  sympathetic NEC G90.8
  tibial — *see* Lesion, nerve, popliteal, medial
  trigeminal G50.9
    specified NEC G50.8
  trochlear NEC — *see* Strabismus, paralytic, fourth nerve
  ulnar — *see* Lesion, nerve, ulnar
  upper limb — *see* Mononeuropathy, upper limb
  vagus G52.2
nervous system G98.8
  autonomic (peripheral) G90.9
    specified NEC G90.8
  central G96.9
    specified NEC G96.8
  parasympathetic G90.9
  specified NEC G98.8
  sympathetic G90.9
  vegetative G90.9
neurohypophysis NEC E23.3
neurological NEC R29.818
neuromuscular G70.9
  hereditary NEC G71.9
  specified NEC G70.89
  toxic G70.1
neurotic F48.9
  specified NEC F48.8
neutrophil, polymorphonuclear D71
nicotine use — *see* Dependence, drug, nicotine
nightmare F51.5
nose J34.9
  specified NEC J34.89
obsessive-compulsive F42
odontogenesis NOS K00.9
opioid use
  with
    opioid-induced psychotic disorder F11.959
      with
        delusions F11.950
        hallucinations F11.951
  due to drug abuse — *see* Abuse, drug, opioid
  due to drug dependence — *see* Dependence, drug, opioid
oppositional defiant F91.3
optic
  chiasm H47.49
    due to
      inflammatory disorder H47.41
      neoplasm H47.42
      vascular disorder H47.43
  disc H47.39- ☑
    coloboma — *see* Coloboma, optic disc
    drusen — *see* Drusen, optic disc
    pseudopapilledema — *see* Pseudopapilledema
  radiations — *see* Disorder, visual, pathway
  tracts — *see* Disorder, visual, pathway
orbit H05.9
  cyst — *see* Cyst, orbit
  deformity — *see* Deformity, orbit
  edema — *see* Edema, orbit
  enophthalmos — *see* Enophthalmos
  exophthalmos — *see* Exophthalmos
  hemorrhage — *see* Hemorrhage, orbit
  inflammation — *see* Inflammation, orbit
  myopathy — *see* Myopathy, extraocular muscles
  retained foreign body — *see* Foreign body, orbit, old
  specified type NEC H05.89
organic
  anxiety F06.4
  catatonic F06.1
  delusional F06.2
  dissociative F06.8
  emotionally labile (asthenic) F06.8
  mood (affective) F06.30
  schizophrenia-like F06.2
orgasmic (female) F52.31
  male F52.32
ornithine metabolism E72.4
overanxious F41.1
  of childhood F93.8

Disorder — *continued*

pain
  with related psychological factors F45.42
  exclusively related to psychological factors F45.41
pancreatic internal secretion E16.9
  specified NEC E16.8
panic F41.0
  with agoraphobia F40.01
papulosquamous L44.9
  in diseases classified elsewhere L45
  specified NEC L44.8
paranoid F22
  induced F24
  shared F24
parathyroid (gland) E21.5
  specified NEC E21.4
parietoalveolar NEC J84.09
paroxysmal, mixed R56.9
patella M22.9- ☑
  chondromalacia — *see* Chondromalacia, patella
  derangement NEC M22.3X- ☑
  recurrent
    dislocation — *see* Dislocation, patella, recurrent
    subluxation — *see* Dislocation, patella, recurrent, incomplete
  specified NEC M22.8X- ☑
patellofemoral M22.2X- ☑
pentose phosphate pathway with anemia D55.1
perception, due to hallucinogens F16.983
  in
    abuse F16.183
    dependence F16.283
peripheral nervous system NEC G64
peroxisomal E71.50
  biogenesis
    neonatal adrenoleukodystrophy E71.511
    specified disorder NEC E71.518
    Zellweger syndrome E71.510
  rhizomelic chondrodysplasia punctata E71.540
  specified form NEC E71.548
    group 1 E71.518
    group 2 E71.53
    group 3 E71.542
  X-linked adrenoleukodystrophy E71.529
    adolescent E71.521
    adrenomyeloneuropathy E71.522
    childhood E71.520
    specified form NEC E71.528
  Zellweger-like syndrome E71.541
persistent
  (somatoform) pain F45.41
  affective (mood) F34.9
personality (*see also* Personality) F60.9
  affective F34.0
  aggressive F60.3
  amoral F60.2
  anankastic F60.5
  antisocial F60.2
  anxious F60.6
  asocial F60.2
  asthenic F60.7
  avoidant F60.6
  borderline F60.3
  change (secondary) due to general medical condition F07.0
  compulsive F60.5
  cyclothymic F34.0
  dependent (passive) F60.7
  depressive F34.1
  dissocial F60.2
  emotional instability F60.3
  expansive paranoid F60.0
  explosive F60.3
  following organic brain damage F07.9
  histrionic F60.4
  hyperthymic F34.0
  hypothymic F34.1
  hysterical F60.4
  immature F60.89
  inadequate F60.7
  labile F60.3
  mixed (nonspecific) F60.89
  moral deficiency F60.2
  narcissistic F60.81
  negativistic F60.89
  obsessional F60.5
  obsessive (-compulsive) F60.5
  organic F07.9

Disorder — continued

personality (see also Personality) — continued
  overconscientious F60.5
  paranoid F60.0
  passive (-dependent) F60.7
  passive-aggressive F60.89
  pathological NEC F60.9
  pseudosocial F60.2
  psychopathic F60.2
  schizoid F60.1
  schizotypal F21
  self-defeating F60.7
  specified NEC F60.89
  type A F60.5
  unstable (emotional) F60.3
pervasive, developmental F84.9
phobic anxiety, childhood F40.8
phosphate-losing tubular N25.0
pigmentation L81.9
  choroid, congenital Q14.3
  diminished melanin formation L81.6
  iron L81.8
  specified NEC L81.8
pinna (noninfective) H61.10- ☑
  deformity, acquired H61.11- ☑
  hematoma H61.12- ☑
  perichondritis — see Perichondritis, ear
  specified type NEC H61.19- ☑
pituitary gland E23.7
  iatrogenic (postprocedural) E89.3
  specified NEC E23.6
platelets D69.1
plexus G54.9
  specified NEC G54.8
polymorphonuclear neutrophils D71
porphyrin metabolism — see Porphyria
postconcussional F07.81
posthallucinogen perception F16.983
  in
    abuse F16.183
    dependence F16.283
postmenopausal N95.9
  specified NEC N95.8
postprocedural (postoperative) — see Complications, postprocedural
post-transplant lymphoproliferative D47.Z1 (following D47.4)
post-traumatic stress (PTSD) F43.10
  acute F43.11
  chronic F43.12
premenstrual dysphoric (PMDD) N94.3
prepuce N47.8
propionic acidemia E71.121
prostate N42.9
  specified NEC N42.89
psychogenic NOS (see also condition) F45.9
  anxiety F41.8
  appetite F50.9
  asthenic F48.8
  cardiovascular (system) F45.8
  compulsive F42
  cutaneous F54
  depressive F32.9
  digestive (system) F45.8
  dysmenorrheic F45.8
  dyspneic F45.8
  endocrine (system) F54
  eye NEC F45.8
  feeding — see Disorder, eating
  functional NEC F45.8
  gastric F45.8
  gastrointestinal (system) F45.8
  genitourinary (system) F45.8
  heart (function) (rhythm) F45.8
  hyperventilatory F45.8
  hypochondriacal — see Disorder, hypochondriacal
  intestinal F45.8
  joint F45.8
  learning F81.9
  limb F45.8
  lymphatic (system) F45.8
  menstrual F45.8
  micturition F45.8
  monoplegic NEC F44.4
  motor F44.4
  muscle F45.8
  musculoskeletal F45.8
  neurocirculatory F45.8

psychogenic (see also condition) — continued
  obsessive F42
  occupational F48.8
  organ or part of body NEC F45.8
  paralytic NEC F44.4
  phobic F40.9
  physical NEC F45.8
  rectal F45.8
  respiratory (system) F45.8
  rheumatic F45.8
  sexual (function) F52.9
  skin (allergic) (eczematous) F54
  sleep F51.9
  specified part of body NEC F45.8
  stomach F45.8
psychological F99
  associated with
    disease classified elsewhere F54
    sexual
      development F66
      relationship F66
      uncertainty about gender identity F66
psychomotor NEC F44.4
  hysterical F44.4
psychoneurotic (see also Neurosis)
  mixed NEC F48.8
psychophysiologic — see Disorder, somatoform
psychosexual F65.9
  development F66
  identity of childhood F64.2
psychosomatic NOS — see Disorder, somatoform
  multiple F45.0
  undifferentiated F45.1
psychotic — see Psychosis
  transient (acute) F23
puberty E30.9
  specified NEC E30.8
pulmonary (valve) — see Endocarditis, pulmonary
purine metabolism E79.9
pyrimidine metabolism E79.9
pyruvate metabolism E74.4
reactive attachment (childhood) F94.1
reading R48.0
  developmental (specific) F81.0
receptive language F80.2
receptor, hormonal, peripheral (see also Syndrome, androgen insensitivity) E34.50
recurrent brief depressive F33.8
reflex R29.2
refraction H52.7
  aniseikonia H52.32
  anisometropia H52.31
  astigmatism — see Astigmatism
  hypermetropia — see Hypermetropia
  myopia — see Myopia
  presbyopia H52.4
  specified NEC H52.6
relationship F68.8
  due to sexual orientation F66
REM sleep behavior G47.52
renal function, impaired (tubular) N25.9
resonance R49.9
  specified NEC R49.8
respiratory function, impaired (see also Failure, respiration)
  postprocedural — see Complication, postoperative, respiratory system
  psychogenic F45.8
retina H35.9
  angioid streaks H35.33
  changes in vascular appearance H35.01- ☑
  degeneration — see Degeneration, retina
  dystrophy (hereditary) — see Dystrophy, retina
  edema H35.81
  hemorrhage — see Hemorrhage, retina
  ischemia H35.82
  macular degeneration — see Degeneration, macula
  microaneurysms H35.04- ☑
  microvascular abnormality NEC H35.09
  neovascularization — see Neovascularization, retina
  retinopathy — see Retinopathy
  separation of layers H35.70
    central serous chorioretinopathy H35.71- ☑
    pigment epithelium detachment (serous) H35.72- ☑
    hemorrhagic H35.73- ☑

retina — continued
  specified type NEC H35.89
  telangiectasis — see Telangiectasis, retina
  vasculitis — see Vasculitis, retina
retroperitoneal K68.9
right hemisphere organic affective F07.89
rumination (infant or child) F98.21
sacrum, sacrococcygeal NEC M53.3
schizoaffective F25.9
  bipolar type F25.0
  depressive type F25.1
  manic type F25.0
  mixed type F25.0
  specified NEC F25.8
schizoid of childhood F84.5
schizophreniform F20.81
  brief F23
schizotypal (personality) F21
secretion, thyrocalcitonin E07.0
seizure (see also Epilepsy) G40.909
  intractable G40.919
    with status epilepticus G40.911
semantic pragmatic F80.89
  with autism F84.0
sense of smell R43.1
  psychogenic F45.8
separation anxiety, of childhood F93.0
sexual
  arousal, female F52.22
  aversion F52.1
  function, psychogenic F52.9
  maturation F66
  nonorganic F52.9
  preference (see also Deviation, sexual) F65.9
    fetishistic transvestism F65.1
  relationship F66
shyness, of childhood and adolescence F40.10
sibling rivalry F93.8
sickle-cell (sickling) (homozygous) — see Disease, sickle-cell
  heterozygous D57.3
  specified type NEC D57.8- ☑
  trait D57.3
sinus (nasal) J34.9
  specified NEC J34.89
skin L98.9
  atrophic L90.9
    specified NEC L90.8
  granulomatous L92.9
    specified NEC L92.8
  hypertrophic L91.9
    specified NEC L91.8
  infiltrative NEC L98.6
  newborn P83.9
    specified NEC P83.8
  psychogenic (allergic) (eczematous) F54
sleep G47.9
  breathing-related — see Apnea, sleep
  circadian rhythm G47.20
    advance sleep phase type G47.22
    delayed sleep phase type G47.21
    due to
      alcohol
        abuse F10.182
        dependence F10.282
        use F10.982
      amphetamines
        abuse F15.182
        dependence F15.282
        use F15.982
      caffeine
        abuse F15.182
        dependence F15.282
        use F15.982
      cocaine
        abuse F14.182
        dependence F14.282
        use F14.982
      drug NEC
        abuse F19.182
        dependence F19.282
        use F19.982
      opioid
        abuse F11.182
        dependence F11.282
        use F11.982

Disorder — *continued*
  sleep — *continued*
    circadian rhythm — *continued*
      due to — *continued*
        psychoactive substance
          abuse F19.182
          dependence F19.282
          use F19.982
        sedative, hypnotic, or anxiolytic
          abuse F13.182
          dependence F13.282
          use F13.982
        stimulant NEC
          abuse F15.182
          dependence F15.282
          use F15.982
      free running type G47.24
      in conditions classified elsewhere G47.27
      irregular sleep wake type G47.23
      jet lag type G47.25
      shift work type G47.26
      specified NEC G47.29
    due to
      alcohol
        abuse F10.182
        dependence F10.282
        use F10.982
      amphetamine
        abuse F15.182
        dependence F15.282
        use F15.982
      anxiolytic
        abuse F13.182
        dependence F13.282
        use F13.982
      caffeine
        abuse F15.182
        dependence F15.282
        use F15.982
      cocaine
        abuse F14.182
        dependence F14.282
        use F14.982
      drug NEC
        abuse F19.182
        dependence F19.282
        use F19.982
      hypnotic
        abuse F13.182
        dependence F13.282
        use F13.982
      opioid
        abuse F11.182
        dependence F11.282
        use F11.982
      psychoactive substance NEC
        abuse F19.182
        dependence F19.282
        use F19.982
      sedative
        abuse F13.182
        dependence F13.282
        use F13.982
      stimulant NEC
        abuse F15.182
        dependence F15.282
        use F15.982
    emotional F51.9
    excessive somnolence — *see* Hypersomnia
    hypersomnia type — *see* Hypersomnia
    initiating or maintaining — *see* Insomnia
    nightmares F51.5
    nonorganic F51.9
      specified NEC F51.8
    parasomnia type G47.50
    specified NEC G47.8
    terrors F51.4
    walking F51.3
  sleep-wake pattern or schedule — *see* Disorder, sleep, circadian rhythm
  social
    anxiety of childhood F40.10
    functioning in childhood F94.9
      specified NEC F94.8
  soft tissue M79.9
    ankle M79.9
    due to use, overuse and pressure M70.90
      ankle M70.97- ☑

Disorder — *continued*
  soft tissue — *continued*
    due to use, overuse and pressure — *continued*
      bursitis — *see* Bursitis
      foot M70.97- ☑
      forearm M70.93- ☑
      hand M70.94- ☑
      lower leg M70.96- ☑
      multiple sites M70.99
      pelvic region M70.95- ☑
      shoulder region M70.91- ☑
      specified site NEC M70.98
      specified type NEC M70.80
        ankle M70.87- ☑
        foot M70.87- ☑
        forearm M70.83- ☑
        hand M70.84- ☑
        lower leg M70.86- ☑
        multiple sites M70.89
        pelvic region M70.85- ☑
        shoulder region M70.81- ☑
        specified site NEC M70.88
        thigh M70.85- ☑
        upper arm M70.82- ☑
      thigh M70.95- ☑
      upper arm M70.92- ☑
    foot M79.9
    forearm M79.9
    hand M79.9
    lower leg M79.9
    multiple sites M79.9
    occupational — *see* Disorder, soft tissue, due to use, overuse and pressure
    pelvic region M79.9
    shoulder region M79.9
    specified type NEC M79.89
    thigh M79.9
    upper arm M79.9
  somatization F45.0
  somatoform F45.9
    pain (persistent) F45.41
    somatization (multiple) (long-lasting) F45.0
    specified NEC F45.8
    undifferentiated F45.1
  somnolence, excessive — *see* Hypersomnia
  specific
    arithmetical F81.2
    developmental, of motor F82
    reading F81.0
    speech and language F80.9
    spelling F81.81
    written expression F81.81
  speech R47.9
    articulation (functional) (specific) F80.0
    developmental F80.9
    specified NEC R47.89
  spelling (specific) F81.81
  spine (*see also* Dorsopathy)
    ligamentous or muscular attachments, peripheral — *see* Enthesopathy, spinal
    specified NEC — *see* Dorsopathy, specified NEC
  stereotyped, habit or movement F98.4
  stomach (functional) — *see* Disorder, gastric
  stress F43.9
    post-traumatic F43.10
      acute F43.11
      chronic F43.12
  sulfur-bearing amino-acid metabolism E72.10
  sweat gland (eccrine) L74.9
    apocrine L75.9
      specified NEC L75.8
    specified NEC L74.8
  synovium M67.90
    acromioclavicular M67.91- ☑
    ankle M67.97- ☑
    elbow M67.92- ☑
    foot M67.97- ☑
    forearm M67.93- ☑
    hand M67.94- ☑
    hip M67.95- ☑
    knee M67.96- ☑
    multiple sites M67.99
    rupture — *see* Rupture, synovium
    shoulder M67.91- ☑
    specified type NEC M67.80
      acromioclavicular M67.81- ☑
      ankle M67.87- ☑

Disorder — *continued*
  synovium — *continued*
    specified type — *continued*
      elbow M67.82- ☑
      foot M67.87- ☑
      hand M67.84- ☑
      hip M67.85- ☑
      knee M67.86- ☑
      multiple sites M67.89
      wrist M67.83- ☑
    synovitis — *see* Synovitis
    upper arm M67.92- ☑
    wrist M67.93- ☑
  temperature regulation, newborn P81.9
    specified NEC P81.8
  temporomandibular joint — *see* Anomaly, dentofacial, temporomandibular joint
  tendon M67.90
    acromioclavicular M67.91- ☑
    ankle M67.97- ☑
    contracture — *see* Contracture, tendon
    elbow M67.92- ☑
    foot M67.97- ☑
    forearm M67.93- ☑
    hand M67.94- ☑
    hip M67.95- ☑
    knee M67.96- ☑
    multiple sites M67.99
    rupture — *see* Rupture, tendon
    shoulder M67.91- ☑
    specified type NEC M67.80
      acromioclavicular M67.81- ☑
      ankle M67.87- ☑
      elbow M67.82- ☑
      foot M67.87- ☑
      hand M67.84- ☑
      hip M67.85- ☑
      knee M67.86- ☑
      multiple sites M67.89
      trunk M67.88
      wrist M67.83- ☑
    synovitis — *see* Synovitis
    tendinitis — *see* Tendinitis
    tenosynovitis — *see* Tenosynovitis
    trunk M67.98
    upper arm M67.92- ☑
    wrist M67.93- ☑
  thoracic root (nerve) NEC G54.3
  thyrocalcitonin hypersecretion E07.0
  thyroid (gland) E07.9
    function NEC, neonatal, transitory P72.2
    iodine-deficiency related E01.8
    specified NEC E07.89
  tic — *see* Tic
  tooth K08.9
    development K00.9
      specified NEC K00.8
    eruption K00.6
  Tourette's F95.2
  trance and possession F44.89
  tricuspid (valve) — *see* Endocarditis, tricuspid
  tryptophan metabolism E70.5
  tubular, phosphate-losing N25.0
  tubulo-interstitial (in)
    brucellosis A23.9 [N16]
    cystinosis E72.04
    diphtheria A36.84
    glycogen storage disease E74.00 [N16]
    leukemia NEC C95.9- ☑ [N16]
    lymphoma NEC C85.9- ☑ [N16]
    mixed cryoglobulinemia D89.1 [N16]
    multiple myeloma C90.0- ☑ [N16]
    Salmonella infection A02.25
    sarcoidosis D86.84
    sepsis A41.9 [N16]
      streptococcal A40.9 [N16]
    systemic lupus erythematosus M32.15
    toxoplasmosis B58.83
    transplant rejection T86.91 [N16]
    Wilson's disease E83.01 [N16]
  tubulo-renal function, impaired N25.9
    specified NEC N25.89
  tympanic membrane H73.9- ☑
    atrophy — *see* Atrophy, tympanic membrane
    infection — *see* Myringitis
    perforation — *see* Perforation, tympanum
    specified NEC H73.89- ☑

Disorder — continued
  unsocialized aggressive F91.1
  urea cycle metabolism E72.20
    argininemia E72.21
    argininosuccinic aciduria E72.22
    citrullinemia E72.23
    ornithine transcarbamylase deficiency E72.4
    other specified E72.29
  ureter (in) N28.9
    schistosomiasis B65.0 [N29]
    tuberculosis A18.11
  urethra N36.9
    specified NEC N36.8
  urinary system N39.9
    specified NEC N39.8
  valve, heart
    aortic — see Endocarditis, aortic
    mitral — see Endocarditis, mitral
    pulmonary — see Endocarditis, pulmonary
    rheumatic
      aortic — see Endocarditis, aortic, rheumatic
      mitral — see Endocarditis, mitral
      pulmonary — see Endocarditis, pulmonary,
        rheumatic
      tricuspid — see Endocarditis, tricuspid
    tricuspid — see Endocarditis, tricuspid
  vestibular function H81.9- ✓
    specified NEC — see subcategory H81.8 ✓
      in diseases classified elsewhere H82.- ✓
    vertigo — see Vertigo
  vision, binocular H53.30
    abnormal retinal correspondence H53.31
    diplopia H53.2
    fusion with defective stereopsis H53.32
    simultaneous perception H53.33
    suppression H53.34
  visual
    cortex
      blindness H47.619
        left brain H47.612
        right brain H47.611
      due to
        inflammatory disorder H47.629
          left brain H47.622
          right brain H47.621
        neoplasm H47.639
          left brain H47.632
          right brain H47.631
        vascular disorder H47.649
          left brain H47.642
          right brain H47.641
    pathway H47.9
      due to
        inflammatory disorder H47.51- ✓
        neoplasm H47.52- ✓
        vascular disorder H47.53- ✓
      optic chiasm — see Disorder, optic, chiasm
  vitreous body H43.9
    crystalline deposits — see Deposit, crystalline
    degeneration — see Degeneration, vitreous
    hemorrhage — see Hemorrhage, vitreous
    opacities — see Opacity, vitreous
    prolapse — see Prolapse, vitreous
    specified type NEC H43.89
  voice R49.9
    specified type NEC R49.8
  volatile solvent use
    due to drug abuse — see Abuse, drug, inhalant
    due to drug dependence — see Dependence, drug,
      inhalant
  white blood cells D72.9
    specified NEC D72.89
  withdrawing, child or adolescent F40.10
Disorientation R41.0
Displacement, displaced
  acquired traumatic of bone, cartilage, joint, tendon
    NEC — see Dislocation
  adrenal gland (congenital) Q89.1
  appendix, retrocecal (congenital) Q43.8
  auricle (congenital) Q17.4
  bladder (acquired) N32.89
    congenital Q64.19
  brachial plexus (congenital) Q07.8
  brain stem, caudal (congenital) Q04.8
  canaliculus (lacrimalis), congenital Q10.6
  cardia through esophageal hiatus (congenital) Q40.1
  cerebellum, caudal (congenital) Q04.8
  cervix — see Malposition, uterus

Displacement, displaced — continued
  colon (congenital) Q43.3
  device, implant or graft (see also Complications, by
    site and type, mechanical) T85.628 ✓
    arterial graft NEC — see Complication, cardiovas-
      cular device, mechanical, vascular
    breast (implant) T85.42 ✓
    catheter NEC T85.628 ✓
      dialysis (renal) T82.42 ✓
        intraperitoneal T85.621 ✓
      infusion NEC T82.524 ✓
        spinal (epidural) (subdural) T85.620 ✓
      urinary (indwelling) T83.028 ✓
        cystostomy T83.020 ✓
    electronic (electrode) (pulse generator) (stimulator)
      — see Complication, electronic stimulator
    fixation, internal (orthopedic) NEC — see Compli-
      cation, fixation device, mechanical
    gastrointestinal — see Complications, prosthetic
      device, mechanical, gastrointestinal device
    genital NEC T83.428 ✓
      intrauterine contraceptive device T83.32 ✓
      penile prosthesis T83.420 ✓
    heart NEC — see Complication, cardiovascular de-
      vice, mechanical
    joint prosthesis — see Complications, joint prosthe-
      sis, mechanical
    ocular — see Complications, prosthetic device,
      mechanical, ocular device
    orthopedic NEC — see Complication, orthopedic,
      device or graft, mechanical
    specified NEC T85.628 ✓
    urinary NEC (see also Complication, genitourinary,
      device, urinary, mechanical)
      graft T83.22 ✓
    vascular NEC — see Complication, cardiovascular
      device, mechanical
    ventricular intracranial shunt T85.02 ✓
  electronic stimulator
    bone T84.320 ✓
    cardiac — see Complications, cardiac device, elec-
      tronic
    nervous system — see Complication, prosthetic
      device, mechanical, electronic nervous sys-
      tem stimulator
    urinary — see Complications, electronic stimulator,
      urinary
  esophageal mucosa into cardia of stomach, congenital
    Q39.8
  esophagus (acquired) K22.8
    congenital Q39.8
  eyeball (acquired) (lateral) (old) — see Displacement,
    globe
    congenital Q15.8
    current — see Avulsion, eye
  fallopian tube (acquired) N83.4
    congenital Q50.6
    opening (congenital) Q50.6
  gallbladder (congenital) Q44.1
  gastric mucosa (congenital) Q40.2
  globe (acquired) (old) (lateral) H05.21- ✓
    current — see Avulsion, eye
  heart (congenital) Q24.8
    acquired I51.89
  hymen (upward) (congenital) Q52.4
  intervertebral disc NEC
    with myelopathy — see Disorder, disc, with,
      myelopathy
    cervical, cervicothoracic (with) M50.20
      myelopathy — see Disorder, disc, cervical, with
        myelopathy
      neuritis, radiculitis or radiculopathy — see Dis-
        order, disc, cervical, with neuritis
    due to trauma — see Dislocation, vertebra
    lumbar region M51.26
      with
        myelopathy M51.06
        neuritis, radiculitis, radiculopathy or sciatica
          M51.16
    lumbosacral region M51.27
      with
        neuritis, radiculitis, radiculopathy or sciatica
          M51.17
    sacrococcygeal region M53.3
    thoracic region M51.24
      with
        myelopathy M51.04

Displacement, displaced — continued
  intervertebral disc — continued
    thoracic region — continued
      with — continued
        neuritis, radiculitis, radiculopathy M51.14
    thoracolumbar region M51.25
      with
        myelopathy M51.05
        neuritis, radiculitis, radiculopathy M51.15
  intrauterine device T83.32 ✓
  kidney (acquired) N28.83
    congenital Q63.2
  lachrymal, lacrimal apparatus or duct (congenital)
    Q10.6
  lens, congenital Q12.1
  macula (congenital) Q14.1
  Meckel's diverticulum Q43.0
    malignant — see Table of Neoplasms, small intes-
      tine, malignant
  nail (congenital) Q84.6
    acquired L60.8
  opening of Wharton's duct in mouth Q38.4
  organ or site, congenital NEC — see Malposition,
    congenital
  ovary (acquired) N83.4
    congenital Q50.39
    free in peritoneal cavity (congenital) Q50.39
    into hernial sac N83.4
  oviduct (acquired) N83.4
    congenital Q50.6
  parathyroid (gland) E21.4
  parotid gland (congenital) Q38.4
  punctum lacrimale (congenital) Q10.6
  sacro-iliac (joint) (congenital) Q74.2
    current injury S33.2 ✓
    old — see subcategory M53.2 ✓
  salivary gland (any) (congenital) Q38.4
  spleen (congenital) Q89.09
  stomach, congenital Q40.2
  sublingual duct Q38.4
  tongue (downward) (congenital) Q38.3
  tooth, teeth, fully erupted M26.30
    horizontal M26.33
    vertical M26.34
  trachea (congenital) Q32.1
  ureter or ureteric opening or orifice (congenital)
    Q62.62
  uterine opening of oviducts or fallopian tubes Q50.6
  uterus, uterine — see Malposition, uterus
  ventricular septum Q21.0
    with rudimentary ventricle Q20.4
Disproportion
  between native and reconstructed breast N65.1
  fiber-type G71.2
Disruptio uteri — see Rupture, uterus
Disruption (of)
  ciliary body NEC H21.89
  closure of
    cornea T81.31 ✓
    craniotomy T81.32 ✓
    fascia (muscular) (superficial) T81.32 ✓
    internal organ or tissue T81.32 ✓
    laceration (external) (internal) T81.33 ✓
    ligament T81.32 ✓
    mucosa T81.31 ✓
    muscle or muscle flap T81.32 ✓
    ribs or rib cage T81.32 ✓
    skin and subcutaneous tissue (full-thickness) (su-
      perficial) T81.31 ✓
    skull T81.32 ✓
    sternum (sternotomy) T81.32 ✓
    tendon T81.32 ✓
    traumatic laceration (external) (internal) T81.33 ✓
  family Z63.8
    due to
      absence of family member due to military de-
        ployment Z63.31
      absence of family member NEC Z63.32
      alcoholism and drug addiction in family Z63.72
      bereavement Z63.4
      death (assumed) or disappearance of family
        member Z63.4
      divorce or separation Z63.5
      drug addiction in family Z63.72
      return of family member from military deploy-
        ment (current or past conflict) Z63.71
      stressful life events NEC Z63.79
  iris NEC H21.89

Disruption — continued
  ligament(s) (see also Sprain)
    knee
      current injury — see Dislocation, knee
      old (chronic) — see Derangement, knee, instability
      spontaneous NEC — see Derangement, knee, disruption ligament
  ossicular chain — see Discontinuity, ossicles, ear
  pelvic ring (stable) S32.810 ☑
    unstable S32.811 ☑
  traumatic injury wound repair T81.33 ☑
  wound T81.30 ☑
    episiotomy O90.1
    operation T81.31 ☑
      cesarean O90.0
      external operation wound (superficial) T81.31 ☑
      internal operation wound (deep) T81.32 ☑
    perineal (obstetric) O90.1
    traumatic injury repair T81.33 ☑
Dissatisfaction with
  employment Z56.9
  school environment Z55.4
Dissecting — see condition
Dissection
  aorta I71.00
    abdominal I71.02
    thoracic I71.01
    thoracoabdominal I71.03
  artery
    carotid I77.71
    cerebral (nonruptured) I67.0
      ruptured — see Hemorrhage, intracranial, subarachnoid
    coronary I25.42
    iliac I77.72
    renal I77.73
    specified NEC I77.79
    vertebral I77.74
  traumatic — see Wound, open, by site
  vascular I99.8
  wound — see Wound, open
Disseminated — see condition
Dissociation
  auriculoventricular or atrioventricular (AV) (any degree) (isorhythmic) I45.89
    with heart block I44.2
  interference I45.89
Dissociative reaction, state F44.9
Dissolution, vertebra — see Osteoporosis
Distension, distention
  abdomen R14.0
  bladder N32.89
  cecum K63.89
  colon K63.89
  gallbladder K82.8
  intestine K63.89
  kidney N28.89
  liver K76.89
  seminal vesicle N50.8
  stomach K31.89
    acute K31.0
    psychogenic F45.8
  ureter — see Dilatation, ureter
  uterus N85.8
Distoma hepaticum infestation B66.3
Distomiasis B66.9
  bile passages B66.3
  hemic B65.9
  hepatic B66.3
    due to Clonorchis sinensis B66.1
  intestinal B66.5
  liver B66.3
    due to Clonorchis sinensis B66.1
  lung B66.4
  pulmonary B66.4
Distomolar (fourth molar) K00.1
Disto-occlusion (Division I) (Division II) M26.212
Distortion(s) (congenital)
  adrenal (gland) Q89.1
  arm NEC Q68.8
  bile duct or passage Q44.5
  bladder Q64.79
  brain Q04.9
  cervix (uteri) Q51.9
  chest (wall) Q67.8

Distortion(s) — continued
  chest — continued
    bones Q76.8
  clavicle Q74.0
  clitoris Q52.6
  coccyx Q76.49
  common duct Q44.5
  coronary Q24.5
  cystic duct Q44.5
  ear (auricle) (external) Q17.3
    inner Q16.5
    middle Q16.4
      ossicles Q16.3
  endocrine NEC Q89.2
  eustachian tube Q17.8
  eye (adnexa) Q15.8
  face bone(s) NEC Q75.8
  fallopian tube Q50.6
  femur NEC Q68.8
  fibula NEC Q68.8
  finger(s) Q68.1
  foot Q66.9
  genitalia, genital organ(s)
    female Q52.8
      external Q52.79
      internal NEC Q52.8
  gyri Q04.8
  hand bone(s) NEC Q68.1
  heart (auricle) (ventricle) Q24.8
    valve (cusp) Q24.8
  hepatic duct Q44.5
  humerus NEC Q68.8
  hymen Q52.4
  intrafamilial communications Z63.8
  jaw NEC M26.89
  labium (majus) (minus) Q52.79
  leg NEC Q68.8
  lens Q12.8
  liver Q44.7
  lumbar spine Q76.49
    with disproportion O33.8
      causing obstructed labor O65.0
  lumbosacral (joint) (region) Q76.49
    kyphosis — see Kyphosis, congenital
    lordosis — see Lordosis, congenital
  nerve Q07.8
  nose Q30.8
  organ
    of Corti Q16.5
    or site not listed — see Anomaly, by site
  ossicles, ear Q16.3
  oviduct Q50.6
  pancreas Q45.3
  parathyroid (gland) Q89.2
  pituitary (gland) Q89.2
  radius NEC Q68.8
  sacroiliac joint Q74.2
  sacrum Q76.49
  scapula Q74.0
  shoulder girdle Q74.0
  skull bone(s) NEC Q75.8
    with
      anencephalus Q00.0
      encephalocele — see Encephalocele
      hydrocephalus Q03.9
        with spina bifida — see Spina bifida, with hydrocephalus
      microcephaly Q02
  spinal cord Q06.8
  spine Q76.49
    kyphosis — see Kyphosis, congenital
    lordosis — see Lordosis, congenital
  spleen Q89.09
  sternum NEC Q76.7
  thorax (wall) Q67.8
    bony Q76.8
  thymus (gland) Q89.2
  thyroid (gland) Q89.2
  tibia NEC Q68.8
  toe(s) Q66.9
  tongue Q38.3
  trachea (cartilage) Q32.1
  ulna NEC Q68.8
  ureter Q62.8
  urethra Q64.79
    causing obstruction Q64.39
  uterus Q51.9
  vagina Q52.4

Distortion(s) — continued
  vertebra Q76.49
    kyphosis — see Kyphosis, congenital
    lordosis — see Lordosis, congenital
  visual (see also Disturbance, vision)
    shape and size H53.15
  vulva Q52.79
  wrist (bones) (joint) Q68.8
Distress
  abdomen — see Pain, abdominal
  acute respiratory (adult) (child) J80
  epigastric R10.13
  fetal P84
    complicating pregnancy — see Stress, fetal
  gastrointestinal (functional) K30
    psychogenic F45.8
  intestinal (functional) NOS K59.9
    psychogenic F45.8
  maternal, during labor and delivery O75.0
  respiratory R06.00
    adult J80
    child J80
    newborn P22.9
      specified NEC P22.8
    orthopnea R06.01
    psychogenic F45.8
    shortness of breath R06.02
    specified type NEC R06.09
Distribution vessel, atypical Q27.9
  coronary artery Q24.5
  precerebral Q28.1
Districhiasis L68.8
Disturbance(s) (see also Disease)
  absorption K90.9
    calcium E58
    carbohydrate K90.4
    fat K90.4
      pancreatic K90.3
    protein K90.4
    starch K90.4
    vitamin — see Deficiency, vitamin
  acid-base equilibrium E87.8
    mixed E87.4
  activity and attention (with hyperkinesis) — see Disorder, attention-deficit hyperactivity
  amino acid transport E72.00
  assimilation, food K90.9
  auditory nerve, except deafness — see subcategory H93.3 ☑
  behavior — see Disorder, conduct
  blood clotting (mechanism) (see also Defect, coagulation) D68.9
  cerebral
    nerve — see Disorder, nerve, cranial
    status, newborn P91.9
      specified NEC P91.8
  circulatory I99.9
  conduct (see also Disorder, conduct) F91.9
    adjustment reaction — see Disorder, adjustment
    compulsive F63.9
    disruptive F91.9
    hyperkinetic — see Disorder, attention-deficit hyperactivity
    socialized F91.2
    specified NEC F91.8
    unsocialized F91.1
  coordination R27.8
  cranial nerve — see Disorder, nerve, cranial
  deep sensibility — see Disturbance, sensation
  digestive K30
    psychogenic F45.8
  electrolyte (see also Imbalance, electrolyte)
    newborn, transitory P74.4
      hyperammonemia P74.6
      potassium balance P74.3
      sodium balance P74.2
      specified type NEC P74.4
  emotions specific to childhood and adolescence F93.9
    with
      anxiety and fearfulness NEC F93.8
      elective mutism F94.0
      oppositional disorder F91.3
      sensitivity (withdrawal) F40.10
      shyness F40.10
      social withdrawal F40.10
    involving relationship problems F93.8
    mixed F93.8
    specified NEC F93.8

Disturbance(s) — *continued*
　endocrine (gland) E34.9
　　neonatal, transitory P72.9
　　　specified NEC P72.8
　equilibrium R42
　fructose metabolism E74.10
　gait — *see* Gait
　　hysterical F44.4
　　psychogenic F44.4
　gastrointestinal (functional) K30
　　psychogenic F45.8
　habit, child F98.9
　hearing, except deafness and tinnitus — *see* Abnormal, auditory perception
　heart, functional (conditions in I44-I50)
　　due to presence of (cardiac) prosthesis I97.19- ☑
　　postoperative I97.89
　　　cardiac surgery I97.19- ☑
　hormones E34.9
　innervation uterus (parasympathetic) (sympathetic) N85.8
　keratinization NEC
　　gingiva K05.10
　　　nonplaque induced K05.11
　　　plaque induced K05.10
　　lip K13.0
　　oral (mucosa) (soft tissue) K13.29
　　tongue K13.29
　learning (specific) — *see* Disorder, learning
　memory — *see* Amnesia
　　mild, following organic brain damage F06.8
　mental F99
　　associated with diseases classified elsewhere F54
　metabolism E88.9
　　with
　　　abortion — *see* Abortion, by type with other specified complication
　　　ectopic pregnancy O08.5
　　　molar pregnancy O08.5
　　amino-acid E72.9
　　　aromatic E70.9
　　　branched-chain E71.2
　　　straight-chain E72.8
　　　sulfur-bearing E72.10
　　ammonia E72.20
　　arginine E72.21
　　arginosuccinic acid E72.22
　　carbohydrate E74.9
　　cholesterol E78.9
　　citrulline E72.23
　　cystathionine E72.19
　　general E88.9
　　glutamine E72.8
　　histidine E70.40
　　homocystine E72.19
　　hydroxylysine E72.3
　　in labor or delivery O75.89
　　iron E83.10
　　lipoid E78.9
　　lysine E72.3
　　methionine E72.19
　　neonatal, transitory P74.9
　　　calcium and magnesium P71.9
　　　　specified type NEC P71.8
　　　carbohydrate metabolism P70.9
　　　　specified type NEC P70.8
　　　specified NEC P74.8
　　ornithine E72.4
　　phosphate E83.39
　　sodium NEC E87.8
　　threonine E72.8
　　tryptophan E70.5
　　tyrosine E70.20
　　urea cycle E72.20
　motor R29.2
　nervous, functional R45.0
　neuromuscular mechanism (eye), due to syphilis A52.15
　nutritional E63.9
　　nail L60.3
　ocular motion H51.9
　　psychogenic F45.8
　oculogyric H51.8
　　psychogenic F45.8
　oculomotor H51.9
　　psychogenic F45.8
　olfactory nerve R43.1
　optic nerve NEC — *see* Disorder, nerve, optic

Disturbance(s) — *continued*
　oral epithelium, including tongue NEC K13.29
　perceptual due to
　　alcohol withdrawal F10.232
　　amphetamine intoxication F15.922
　　　in
　　　　abuse F15.122
　　　　dependence F15.222
　　anxiolytic withdrawal F13.232
　　cannabis intoxication (acute) F12.922
　　　in
　　　　abuse F12.122
　　　　dependence F12.222
　　cocaine intoxication (acute) F14.922
　　　in
　　　　abuse F14.122
　　　　dependence F14.222
　　hypnotic withdrawal F13.232
　　opioid intoxication (acute) F11.922
　　　in
　　　　abuse F11.122
　　　　dependence F11.222
　　phencyclidine intoxication (acute) F19.922
　　　in
　　　　abuse F19.122
　　　　dependence F19.222
　　sedative withdrawal F13.232
　personality (pattern) (trait) (*see also* Disorder, personality) F60.9
　　following organic brain damage F07.9
　polyglandular E31.9
　　specified NEC E31.8
　potassium balance, newborn P74.3
　psychogenic F45.9
　psychomotor F44.4
　psychophysical visual H53.16
　pupillary — *see* Anomaly, pupil, function
　reflex R29.2
　rhythm, heart I49.9
　salivary secretion K11.7
　sensation (cold) (heat) (localization) (tactile discrimination) (texture) (vibratory) NEC R20.9
　　hysterical F44.6
　　skin R20.9
　　　anesthesia R20.0
　　　hyperesthesia R20.3
　　　hypoesthesia R20.1
　　　paresthesia R20.2
　　　specified type NEC R20.8
　　smell R43.9
　　　and taste (mixed) R43.8
　　　anosmia R43.0
　　　parosmia R43.1
　　　specified NEC R43.8
　　taste R43.9
　　　and smell (mixed) R43.8
　　　parageusia R43.2
　　　specified NEC R43.8
　sensory — *see* Disturbance, sensation
　situational (transient) (*see also* Disorder, adjustment)
　　acute F43.0
　sleep G47.9
　　nonorganic origin F51.9
　smell — *see* Disturbance, sensation, smell
　sociopathic F60.2
　sodium balance, newborn P74.2
　speech R47.9
　　developmental F80.9
　　specified NEC R47.89
　stomach (functional) K31.9
　sympathetic (nerve) G90.9
　taste — *see* Disturbance, sensation, taste
　temperature
　　regulation, newborn P81.9
　　　specified NEC P81.8
　　sense R20.8
　　　hysterical F44.6
　tooth
　　eruption K00.6
　　formation K00.4
　　structure, hereditary NEC K00.5
　touch — *see* Disturbance, sensation
　vascular I99.9
　　arteriosclerotic — *see* Arteriosclerosis
　vasomotor I73.9
　vasospastic I73.9
　vision, visual H53.9

Disturbance(s) — *continued*
　vision, visual — *continued*
　　following
　　　cerebral infarction I69.398
　　　cerebrovascular disease I69.998
　　　　specified NEC I69.898
　　　intracerebral hemorrhage I69.198
　　　nontraumatic intracranial hemorrhage NEC I69.298
　　　specified disease NEC I69.898
　　　subarachnoid hemorrhage I69.098
　　psychophysical H53.16
　　specified NEC H53.8
　　subjective H53.10
　　　day blindness H53.11
　　　discomfort H53.14- ☑
　　　distortions of shape and size H53.15
　　　loss
　　　　sudden H53.13- ☑
　　　　transient H53.12- ☑
　　　specified type NEC H53.19
　voice R49.9
　　psychogenic F44.4
　　specified NEC R49.8
Diuresis R35.8
Diver's palsy, paralysis or squeeze T70.3 ☑
Diverticulitis (acute) K57.92
　bladder — *see* Cystitis
　ileum — *see* Diverticulitis, intestine, small
　intestine K57.92
　　with
　　　abscess, perforation or peritonitis K57.80
　　　　with bleeding K57.81
　　　bleeding K57.93
　　congenital Q43.8
　　large K57.32
　　　with
　　　　abscess, perforation or peritonitis K57.20
　　　　　with bleeding K57.21
　　　　bleeding K57.33
　　　　small intestine K57.52
　　　　　with
　　　　　　abscess, perforation or peritonitis K57.40
　　　　　　　with bleeding K57.41
　　　　　　bleeding K57.53
　　small K57.12
　　　with
　　　　abscess, perforation or peritonitis K57.00
　　　　　with bleeding K57.01
　　　　bleeding K57.13
　　　　large intestine K57.52
　　　　　with
　　　　　　abscess, perforation or peritonitis K57.40
　　　　　　　with bleeding K57.41
　　　　　　bleeding K57.53
Diverticulosis K57.90
　with bleeding K57.91
　large intestine K57.30
　　with
　　　bleeding K57.31
　　　small intestine K57.50
　　　　with bleeding K57.51
　small intestine K57.10
　　with
　　　bleeding K57.11
　　　large intestine K57.50
　　　　with bleeding K57.51
Diverticulum, diverticula (multiple) K57.90
　appendix (noninflammatory) K38.2
　bladder (sphincter) N32.3
　　congenital Q64.6
　bronchus (congenital) Q32.4
　　acquired J98.09
　calyx, calyceal (kidney) N28.89
　cardia (stomach) K31.4
　cecum — *see* Diverticulosis, intestine, large
　　congenital Q43.8
　colon — *see* Diverticulosis, intestine, large
　　congenital Q43.8
　duodenum — *see* Diverticulosis, intestine, small
　　congenital Q43.8
　epiphrenic (esophagus) K22.5
　esophagus (congenital) Q39.6
　　acquired (epiphrenic) (pulsion) (traction) K22.5
　eustachian tube — *see* Disorder, eustachian tube, specified NEC

Diverticulum, diverticula — *continued*
  fallopian tube N83.8
  gastric K31.4
  heart (congenital) Q24.8
  ileum — *see* Diverticulosis, intestine, small
  jejunum — *see* Diverticulosis, intestine, small
  kidney (pelvis) (calyces) N28.89
    with calculus — *see* Calculus, kidney
  Meckel's (displaced) (hypertrophic) Q43.0
    malignant — *see* Table of Neoplasms, small intestine, malignant
  midthoracic K22.5
  organ or site, congenital NEC — *see* Distortion
  pericardium (congenital) (cyst) Q24.8
    acquired I31.8
  pharyngoesophageal (congenital) Q39.6
    acquired K22.5
  pharynx (congenital) Q38.7
  rectosigmoid — *see* Diverticulosis, intestine, large
    congenital Q43.8
  rectum — *see* Diverticulosis, intestine, large
  Rokitansky's K22.5
  seminal vesicle N50.8
  sigmoid — *see* Diverticulosis, intestine, large
    congenital Q43.8
  stomach (acquired) K31.4
    congenital Q40.2
  trachea (acquired) J39.8
  ureter (acquired) N28.89
    congenital Q62.8
  ureterovesical orifice N28.89
  urethra (acquired) N36.1
    congenital Q64.79
  ventricle, left (congenital) Q24.8
  vesical N32.3
    congenital Q64.6
  Zenker's (esophagus) K22.5
Division
  cervix uteri (acquired) N88.8
  glans penis S55.69
  labia minora (congenital) Q52.79
  ligament (partial or complete) (current) (*see also* Sprain)
    with open wound — *see* Wound, open
  muscle (partial or complete) (current) (*see also* Injury, muscle)
    with open wound — *see* Wound, open
  nerve (traumatic) — *see* Injury, nerve
  spinal cord — *see* Injury, spinal cord, by region
  vein I87.8
Divorce, causing family disruption Z63.5
Dix-Hallpike neurolabyrinthitis — *see* Neuronitis, vestibular
Dizziness R42
  hysterical F44.89
  psychogenic F45.8
DMAC (disseminated mycobacterium avium- intracellulare complex) A31.2
DNR (do not resuscitate) Z66
Doan-Wiseman syndrome (primary splenic neutropenia) — *see* Agranulocytosis
Doehle-Heller aortitis A52.02
Dog bite — *see* Bite
Dohle body panmyelopathic syndrome D72.0
Dolichocephaly Q67.2
Dolichocolon Q43.8
Dolichostenomelia — *see* Syndrome, Marfan's
Donohue's syndrome E34.8
Donor (organ or tissue) Z52.9
  blood (whole) Z52.000
    autologous Z52.010
    specified component (lymphocytes) (platelets) NEC Z52.008
      autologous Z52.018
      specified donor NEC Z52.098
    specified donor NEC Z52.090
    stem cells Z52.001
      autologous Z52.011
      specified donor NEC Z52.091
  bone Z52.20
    autologous Z52.21
    marrow Z52.3
    specified type NEC Z52.29
  cornea Z52.5
  egg (Oocyte) Z52.819
    age 35 and over Z52.812
      anonymous recipient Z52.812
      designated recipient Z52.813

Donor — *continued*
  egg — *continued*
    under age 35 Z52.810
      anonymous recipient Z52.810
      designated recipient Z52.811
  kidney Z52.4
  liver Z52.6
  lung Z52.89
  lymphocyte — *see* Donor, blood, specified components NEC
  Oocyte — *see* Donor, egg
  platelets Z52.008
  potential, examination of Z00.5
  semen Z52.89
  skin Z52.10
    autologous Z52.11
    specified type NEC Z52.19
  specified organ or tissue NEC Z52.89
  sperm Z52.89
Donovanosis A58
Dorsalgia M54.9
  psychogenic F45.41
  specified NEC M54.89
Dorsopathy M53.9
  deforming M43.9
    specified NEC — *see* subcategory M43.8 ☑
  specified NEC M53.80
    cervical region M53.82
    cervicothoracic region M53.83
    lumbar region M53.86
    lumbosacral region M53.87
    occipito-atlanto-axial region M53.81
    sacrococcygeal region M53.88
    thoracic region M53.84
    thoracolumbar region M53.85
Double
  albumin E88.09
  aortic arch Q25.4
  auditory canal Q17.8
  auricle (heart) Q20.8
  bladder Q64.79
  cervix Q51.820
    with doubling of uterus (and vagina) Q51.10
      with obstruction Q51.11
  inlet ventricle Q20.4
  kidney with double pelvis (renal) Q63.0
  meatus urinarius Q64.75
  monster Q89.4
  outlet
    left ventricle Q20.2
    right ventricle Q20.1
  pelvis (renal) with double ureter Q62.5
  tongue Q38.3
  ureter (one or both sides) Q62.5
    with double pelvis (renal) Q62.5
  urethra Q64.74
  urinary meatus Q64.75
  uterus Q51.2
    with
      doubling of cervix (and vagina) Q51.10
        with obstruction Q51.11
      in pregnancy or childbirth O34.59- ☑
        causing obstructed labor O65.5
  vagina Q52.10
    with doubling of uterus (and cervix) Q51.10
      with obstruction Q51.11
  vision H53.2
  vulva Q52.79
Douglas' pouch, cul-de-sac — *see* condition
Down syndrome Q90.9
  meiotic nondisjunction Q90.0
  mitotic nondisjunction Q90.1
  mosaicism Q90.1
  translocation Q90.2
DPD (dihydropyrimidine dehydrogenase deficiency) E88.89
Dracontiasis B72
Dracunculiasis, dracunculosis B72
Dream state, hysterical F44.89
Drepanocytic anemia — *see* Disease, sickle-cell
Dresbach's syndrome (elliptocytosis) D58.1
Dreschlera (hawaiiensis) (infection) B43.8
Dressler's syndrome I24.1
Drift, ulnar — *see* Deformity, limb, specified type NEC, forearm
Drinking (alcohol)
  excessive, to excess NEC (without dependence) F10.10
    habitual (continual) (without remission) F10.20

Drinking — *continued*
  excessive, to excess — *continued*
    habitual — *continued*
      with remission F10.21
Drip, postnasal (chronic) R09.82
  due to
    allergic rhinitis — *see* Rhinitis, allergic
    common cold J00
    gastroesophageal reflux — *see* Reflux, gastroesophageal
    nasopharyngitis — *see* Nasopharyngitis
    other known condition — *code to* condition
    sinusitis — *see* Sinusitis
Droop
  facial R29.810
    cerebrovascular disease I69.992
      cerebral infarction I69.392
      intracerebral hemorrhage I69.192
      nontraumatic intracranial hemorrhage NEC I69.292
      specified disease NEC I69.892
      subarachnoid hemorrhage I69.092
Drop (in)
  attack NEC R55
  finger — *see* Deformity, finger
  foot — *see* Deformity, limb, foot, drop
  hematocrit (precipitous) R71.0
  hemoglobin R71.0
  toe — *see* Deformity, toe, specified NEC
  wrist — *see* Deformity, limb, wrist drop
Dropped heart beats I45.9
Dropsy, dropsical (*see also* Hydrops)
  abdomen R18.8
  brain — *see* Hydrocephalus
  cardiac, heart — *see* Failure, heart, congestive
  gangrenous — *see* Gangrene
  heart — *see* Failure, heart, congestive
  kidney — *see* Nephrosis
  lung — *see* Edema, lung
  newborn due to isoimmunization P56.0
  pericardium — *see* Pericarditis
Drowned, drowning (near) T75.1 ☑
Drowsiness R40.0
Drug
  abuse counseling and surveillance Z71.51
  addiction — *see* Dependence
  dependence — *see* Dependence
  habit — *see* Dependence
  harmful use — *see* Abuse, drug
  induced fever R50.2
  overdose — *see* Table of Drugs and Chemicals, by drug, poisoning
  poisoning — *see* Table of Drugs and Chemicals, by drug, poisoning
  resistant organism infection (*see also* Resistant, organism, to, drug) Z16.30
  therapy
    long term (current) (prophylactic) — *see* Therapy, drug long-term (current) (prophylactic)
    short term — *omit code*
  wrong substance given or taken in error — *see* Table of Drugs and Chemicals, by drug, poisoning
Drunkenness (without dependence) F10.129
  acute in alcoholism F10.229
  chronic (without remission) F10.20
    with remission F10.21
  pathological (without dependence) F10.129
    with dependence F10.229
  sleep F51.9
Drusen
  macula (degenerative) (retina) — *see* Degeneration, macula, drusen
  optic disc H47.32- ☑
Dry, dryness (*see also* condition)
  larynx J38.7
  mouth R68.2
    due to dehydration E86.0
  nose J34.89
  socket (teeth) M27.3
  throat J39.2
DSAP L56.5
Duane's syndrome H50.81- ☑
Dubin-Johnson disease or syndrome E80.6
Dubois' disease (thymus gland) A50.59 [E35]
Dubowitz' syndrome Q87.1
Duchenne-Aran muscular atrophy G12.21
Duchenne-Griesinger disease G71.0

Duchenne's
disease or syndrome
motor neuron disease G12.22
muscular dystrophy G71.0
locomotor ataxia (syphilitic) A52.11
paralysis
birth injury P14.0
due to or associated with
motor neuron disease G12.22
muscular dystrophy G71.0
Ducrey's chancre A57
Duct, ductus — see condition
Duhring's disease (dermatitis herpetiformis) L13.0
Dullness, cardiac (decreased) (increased) R01.2
Dumb ague — see Malaria
Dumbness — see Aphasia
Dumdum fever B55.0
Dumping syndrome (postgastrectomy) K91.1
Duodenitis (nonspecific) (peptic) K29.80
with bleeding K29.81
Duodenocholangitis — see Cholangitis
Duodenum, duodenal — see condition
Duplay's bursitis or periarthritis — see Tendinitis, calcific, shoulder
Duplication, duplex (see also Accessory)
alimentary tract Q45.8
anus Q43.4
appendix (and cecum) Q43.4
biliary duct (any) Q44.5
bladder Q64.79
cecum (and appendix) Q43.4
cervix Q51.820
chromosome NEC
with complex rearrangements NEC Q92.5
seen only at prometaphase Q92.8
cystic duct Q44.5
digestive organs Q45.8
esophagus Q39.8
frontonasal process Q75.8
intestine (large) (small) Q43.4
kidney Q63.0
liver Q44.7
pancreas Q45.3
penis Q55.69
respiratory organs NEC Q34.8
salivary duct Q38.4
spinal cord (incomplete) Q06.2
stomach Q40.2
Dupré's disease (meningism) R29.1
Dupuytren's contraction or disease M72.0
Durand-Nicolas-Favre disease A55
Durotomy (inadvertent) (incidental) G97.41
Duroziez's disease (congenital mitral stenosis) Q23.2
Dutton's relapsing fever (West African) A68.1
Dwarfism E34.3
achondroplastic Q77.4
congenital E34.3
constitutional E34.3
hypochondroplastic Q77.4
hypophyseal E23.0
infantile E34.3
Laron-type E34.3
Lorain (-Levi) type E23.0
metatropic Q77.8
nephrotic-glycosuric (with hypophosphatemic rickets) E72.09
nutritional E45
pancreatic K86.8
pituitary E23.0
renal N25.0
thanatophoric Q77.1
Dyke-Young anemia (secondary) (symptomatic) D59.1
Dysacusis — see Abnormal, auditory perception
Dysadrenocortism E27.9
hyperfunction E27.0
Dysarthria R47.1
following
cerebral infarction I69.322
cerebrovascular disease I69.922
specified disease NEC I69.822
intracerebral hemorrhage I69.122
nontraumatic intracranial hemorrhage NEC I69.222
subarachnoid hemorrhage I69.022
Dysautonomia (familial) G90.1
Dysbarism T70.3 ☑
Dysbasia R26.2
angiosclerotica intermittens I73.9
hysterical F44.4

Dysbasia — continued
lordotica (progressiva) G24.1
nonorganic origin F44.4
psychogenic F44.4
Dysbetalipoproteinemia (familial) E78.2
Dyscalculia R48.8
developmental F81.2
Dyschezia K59.00
Dyschondroplasia (with hemangiomata) Q78.4
Dyschromia (skin) L81.9
Dyscollagenosis M35.9
Dyscranio-pygo-phalangy Q87.0
Dyscrasia
blood (with) D75.9
antepartum hemorrhage — see Hemorrhage, antepartum, with coagulation defect
intrapartum hemorrhage O67.0
newborn P61.9
specified type NEC P61.8
puerperal, postpartum O72.3
polyglandular, pluriglandular E31.9
Dysendocrinism E34.9
Dysentery, dysenteric (catarrhal) (diarrhea) (epidemic) (hemorrhagic) (infectious) (sporadic) (tropical) A09
abscess, liver A06.4
amebic (see also Amebiasis) A06.0
with abscess — see Abscess, amebic
acute A06.0
chronic A06.1
arthritis (see also category M01) A09
bacillary (see also category M01) A03.9
bacillary A03.9
arthritis (see also category M01) A03.9
Boyd A03.2
Flexner A03.1
Schmitz (-Stutzer) A03.0
Shiga (-Kruse) A03.0
Shigella A03.9
boydii A03.2
dysenteriae A03.0
flexneri A03.1
group A A03.0
group B A03.1
group C A03.2
group D A03.3
sonnei A03.3
specified type NEC A03.8
Sonne A03.3
specified type NEC A03.8
balantidial A07.0
Balantidium coli A07.0
Boyd's A03.2
candidal B37.82
Chilomastix A07.8
Chinese A03.9
coccidial A07.3
Dientamoeba (fragilis) A07.8
Embadomonas A07.8
Entamoeba, entambic — see Dysentery, amebic
Flexner-Boyd A03.2
Flexner's A03.1
Giardia lamblia A07.1
Hiss-Russell A03.1
Lamblia A07.1
leishmanial B55.0
malarial — see Malaria
metazoal B82.0
monilial B37.82
protozoal A07.9
Salmonella A02.0
schistosomal B65.1
Schmitz (-Stutzer) A03.0
Shiga (-Kruse) A03.0
Shigella NOS — see Dysentery, bacillary
Sonne A03.3
strongyloidiasis B78.0
trichomonal A07.8
viral (see also Enteritis, viral) A08.4
Dysequilibrium R42
Dysesthesia R20.8
hysterical F44.6
Dysfibrinogenemia (congenital) D68.2
Dysfunction
adrenal E27.9
hyperfunction E27.0
autonomic
due to alcohol G31.2
somatoform F45.8

Dysfunction — continued
bladder N31.9
neurogenic NOS — see Dysfunction, bladder, neuromuscular
neuromuscular NOS N31.9
atonic (motor) (sensory) N31.2
autonomous N31.2
flaccid N31.2
nonreflex N31.2
reflex N31.1
specified NEC N31.8
uninhibited N31.0
bleeding, uterus N93.8
cerebral G93.89
colon K59.9
psychogenic F45.8
colostomy K94.03
cystic duct K82.8
cystostomy (stoma) — see Complications, cystostomy
ejaculatory N53.19
anejaculatory orgasm N53.13
painful N53.12
premature F52.4
retarded N53.11
endocrine NOS E34.9
endometrium N85.8
enterostomy K94.13
gallbladder K82.8
gastrostomy (stoma) K94.23
gland, glandular NOS E34.9
heart I51.89
hemoglobin D75.89
hepatic K76.89
hypophysis E23.7
hypothalamic NEC E23.3
ileostomy (stoma) K94.13
jejunostomy (stoma) K94.13
kidney — see Disease, renal
labyrinthine — see subcategory H83.2 ☑
left ventricular, following sudden emotional stress I51.81
liver K76.89
male — see Dysfunction, sexual, male
orgasmic (female) F52.31
male F52.32
ovary E28.9
specified NEC E28.8
papillary muscle I51.89
parathyroid E21.4
physiological NEC R68.89
psychogenic F59
pineal gland E34.8
pituitary (gland) E23.3
platelets D69.1
polyglandular E31.9
specified NEC E31.8
psychophysiologic F59
psychosexual F52.9
with
dyspareunia F52.6
premature ejaculation F52.4
vaginismus F52.5
pylorus K31.9
rectum K59.9
psychogenic F45.8
reflex (sympathetic) — see Syndrome, pain, complex regional I
segmental — see Dysfunction, somatic
senile R54
sexual (due to) R37
alcohol F10.981
amphetamine F15.981
in
abuse F15.181
dependence F15.281
anxiolytic F13.981
in
abuse F13.181
dependence F13.281
cocaine F14.981
in
abuse F14.181
dependence F14.281
excessive sexual drive F52.8
failure of genital response (male) F52.21
female F52.22
female N94.9
aversion F52.1

Dysfunction — continued
  sexual — continued
    female — continued
      dyspareunia N94.1
        psychogenic F52.6
      frigidity F52.22
      nymphomania F52.8
      orgasmic F52.31
      psychogenic F52.9
        aversion F52.1
        dyspareunia F52.6
        frigidity F52.22
        nymphomania F52.8
        orgasmic F52.31
        vaginismus F52.5
      vaginismus N94.2
        psychogenic F52.5
    hypnotic F13.981
      in
        abuse F13.181
        dependence F13.281
    inhibited orgasm (female) F52.31
      male F52.32
    lack
      of sexual enjoyment F52.1
      or loss of sexual desire F52.0
    male N53.9
      anejaculatory orgasm N53.13
      ejaculatory N53.19
        painful N53.12
        premature F52.4
        retarded N53.11
      erectile N52.9
        drug induced N52.2
        due to
          disease classified elsewhere N52.1
          drug N52.2
        postoperative (postprocedural) N52.39
          following
            prostatectomy N52.34
              radical N52.31
            radical cystectomy N52.32
            urethral surgery N52.33
        psychogenic F52.21
        specified cause NEC N52.8
        vasculogenic
          arterial insufficiency N52.01
            with corporo-venous occlusive N52.03
          corporo-venous occlusive N52.02
            with arterial insufficiency N52.03
      impotence — see Dysfunction, sexual, male, erectile
      psychogenic F52.9
        aversion F52.1
        erectile F52.21
        orgasmic F52.32
        premature ejaculation F52.4
        satyriasis F52.8
        specified type NEC F52.8
      specified type NEC N53.8
    nonorganic F52.9
      specified NEC F52.8
    opioid F11.981
      in
        abuse F11.181
        dependence F11.281
    orgasmic dysfunction (female) F52.31
      male F52.32
    premature ejaculation F52.4
    psychoactive substances NEC F19.981
      in
        abuse F19.181
        dependence F19.281
    psychogenic F52.9
    sedative F13.981
      in
        abuse F13.181
        dependence F13.281
    sexual aversion F52.1
    vaginismus (nonorganic) (psychogenic) F52.5
  sinoatrial node I49.5
  somatic M99.09
    abdomen M99.09
    acromioclavicular M99.07
    cervical region M99.01
    cervicothoracic M99.01
    costochondral M99.08

Dysfunction — continued
  somatic — continued
    costovertebral M99.08
    head region M99.00
    hip M99.05
    lower extremity M99.06
    lumbar region M99.03
    lumbosacral M99.03
    occipitocervical M99.00
    pelvic region M99.05
    pubic M99.05
    rib cage M99.08
    sacral region M99.04
    sacrococcygeal M99.04
    sacroiliac M99.04
    specified NEC M99.09
    sternochondral M99.08
    sternoclavicular M99.07
    thoracic region M99.02
    thoracolumbar M99.02
    upper extremity M99.07
  somatoform autonomic F45.8
  stomach K31.89
    psychogenic F45.8
  suprarenal E27.9
    hyperfunction E27.0
  symbolic R48.9
    specified type NEC R48.8
  temporomandibular (joint) M26.69
    joint-pain syndrome M26.62
  testicular (endocrine) E29.9
    specified NEC E29.8
  thymus E32.9
  thyroid E07.9
  ureterostomy (stoma) — see Complications, stoma, urinary tract
  urethrostomy (stoma) — see Complications, stoma, urinary tract
  uterus, complicating delivery O62.9
    hypertonic O62.4
    hypotonic O62.2
      primary O62.0
      secondary O62.1
  ventricular I51.9
    with congestive heart failure I50.9
    left, reversible, following sudden emotional stress I51.81

Dysgenesis
  gonadal (due to chromosomal anomaly) Q96.9
    pure Q99.1
  renal Q60.5
    bilateral Q60.4
    unilateral Q60.3
  reticular D72.0
  tidal platelet D69.3

Dysgerminoma
  specified site — see Neoplasm, malignant, by site
  unspecified site
    female C56.9
    male C62.90

Dysgeusia R43.2

Dysgraphia R27.8

Dyshidrosis, dysidrosis L30.1

Dyskaryotic cervical smear R87.619

Dyskeratosis L85.8
  cervix — see Dysplasia, cervix
  congenital Q82.8
  uterus NEC N85.8

Dyskinesia G24.9
  biliary (cystic duct or gallbladder) K82.8
  drug induced
    orofacial G24.01
  esophagus K22.4
  hysterical F44.4
  intestinal K59.8
  nonorganic origin F44.4
  orofacial (idiopathic) G24.4
    drug induced G24.01
  psychogenic F44.4
  subacute, drug induced G24.01
  tardive G24.01
    neuroleptic induced G24.01
  trachea J39.8
  tracheobronchial J98.09

Dyslalia (developmental) F80.0

Dyslexia R48.0
  developmental F81.0

Dyslipidemia E78.5
  depressed HDL cholesterol E78.6
  elevated fasting triglycerides E78.1

Dysmaturity (see also Light for dates)
  pulmonary (newborn) (Wilson-Mikity) P27.0

Dysmenorrhea (essential) (exfoliative) N94.6
  congestive (syndrome) N94.6
  primary N94.4
  psychogenic F45.8
  secondary N94.5

Dysmetabolic syndrome X E88.81

Dysmetria R27.8

Dysmorphism (due to)
  alcohol Q86.0
  exogenous cause NEC Q86.8
  hydantoin Q86.1
  warfarin Q86.2

Dysmorphophobia (nondelusional) F45.22
  delusional F22

Dysnomia R47.01

Dysorexia R63.0
  psychogenic F50.8

Dysostosis
  cleidocranial, cleidocranialis Q74.0
  craniofacial Q75.1
  Fairbank's (idiopathic familial generalized osteophytosis) Q78.9
  mandibulofacial (incomplete) Q75.4
  multiplex E76.01
  oculomandibular Q75.5

Dyspareunia (female) N94.1
  male N53.12
  nonorganic F52.6
  psychogenic F52.6
  secondary N94.1

Dyspepsia R10.13
  atonic K30
  functional (allergic) (congenital) (gastrointestinal) (occupational) (reflex) K30
  intestinal K59.8
  nervous F45.8
  neurotic F45.8
  psychogenic F45.8

Dysphagia R13.10
  cervical R13.19
  following
    cerebral infarction I69.391
    cerebrovascular disease I69.991
      specified NEC I69.891
    intracerebral hemorrhage I69.191
    nontraumatic intracranial hemorrhage NEC I69.291
    specified disease NEC I69.891
    subarachnoid hemorrhage I69.091
  functional (hysterical) F45.8
  hysterical F45.8
  nervous (hysterical) F45.8
  neurogenic R13.19
  oral phase R13.11
  oropharyngeal phase R13.12
  pharyneal phase R13.13
  pharyngoesophageal phase R13.14
  psychogenic F45.8
  sideropenic D50.1
  spastica K22.4
  specified NEC R13.19

Dysphagocytosis, congenital D71

Dysphasia R47.02
  developmental
    expressive type F80.1
    receptive type F80.2
  following
    cerebrovascular disease I69.921
      cerebral infarction I69.321
      intracerebral hemorrhage I69.121
      nontraumatic intracranial hemorrhage NEC I69.221
      specified disease NEC I69.821
      subarachnoid hemorrhage I69.021

Dysphonia R49.0
  functional F44.4
  hysterical F44.4
  psychogenic F44.4
  spastica J38.3

Dysphoria, postpartal O90.6

Dyspituitarism E23.3

Dysplasia (see also Anomaly)
  acetabular, congenital Q65.89
  alveolar capillary, with vein misalignment J84.843

Dysplasia — *continued*
  anus (histologically confirmed) (mild) (moderate) K62.82
    severe D01.3
  arrhythmogenic right ventricular I42.8
  arterial, fibromuscular I77.3
  asphyxiating thoracic (congenital) Q77.2
  brain Q07.9
  bronchopulmonary, perinatal P27.1
  cervix (uteri) N87.9
    mild N87.0
    moderate N87.1
    severe D06.9
  chondroectodermal Q77.6
  colon D12.6
  craniometaphyseal Q78.5
  dentinal K00.5
  diaphyseal, progressive Q78.3
  dystrophic Q77.5
  ectodermal (anhidrotic) (congenital) (hereditary) Q82.4
    hydrotic Q82.8
  epithelial, uterine cervix — *see* Dysplasia, cervix
  eye (congenital) Q11.2
  fibrous
    bone NEC (monostotic) M85.00
      ankle M85.07- ☑
      foot M85.07- ☑
      forearm M85.03- ☑
      hand M85.04- ☑
      lower leg M85.06- ☑
      multiple site M85.09
      neck M85.08
      rib M85.08
      shoulder M85.01- ☑
      skull M85.08
      specified site NEC M85.08
      thigh M85.05- ☑
      toe M85.07- ☑
      upper arm M85.02- ☑
      vertebra M85.08
    diaphyseal, progressive Q78.3
    jaw M27.8
    polyostotic Q78.1
  florid osseous (*see also* Cyst, calcifying odontogenic)
  high grade, focal D12.6
  hip, congenital Q65.89
  joint, congenital Q74.8
  kidney Q61.4
    multicystic Q61.4
  leg Q74.2
  lung, congenital (not associated with short gestation) Q33.6
  mammary (gland) (benign) N60.9- ☑
    cyst (solitary) — *see* Cyst, breast
    cystic — *see* Mastopathy, cystic
    duct ectasia — *see* Ectasia, mammary duct
    fibroadenosis — *see* Fibroadenosis, breast
    fibrosclerosis — *see* Fibrosclerosis, breast
    specified type NEC N60.8- ☑
  metaphyseal (Jansen's) (McKusick's) (Schmid's) Q78.5
  muscle Q79.8
  oculodentodigital Q87.0
  periapical (cemental) (cemento-osseous) — *see* Cyst, calcifying odontogenic
  periosteum — *see* Disorder, bone, specified type NEC
  polyostotic fibrous Q78.1
  prostate (*see also* Neoplasia, intraepithelial, prostate) N42.3
    severe D07.5
  renal Q61.4
    multicystic Q61.4
  retinal, congenital Q14.1
  right ventricular, arrhythmogenic I42.8
  septo-optic Q04.4
  skin L98.8
  spinal cord Q06.1
  spondyloepiphyseal Q77.7
  thymic, with immunodeficiency D82.1
  vagina N89.3
    mild N89.0
    moderate N89.1
    severe NEC D07.2
  vulva N90.3
    mild N90.0
    moderate N90.1
    severe NEC D07.1

Dyspnea (nocturnal) (paroxysmal) R06.00
  asthmatic (bronchial) J45.909
    with
      bronchitis J45.909
        with
          exacerbation (acute) J45.901
          status asthmaticus J45.902
        chronic J44.9
      exacerbation (acute) J45.901
      status asthmaticus J45.902
    cardiac — *see* Failure, ventricular, left
  cardiac — *see* Failure, ventricular, left
  functional F45.8
  hyperventilation R06.4
  hysterical F45.8
  newborn P28.89
  orthopnea R06.01
  psychogenic F45.8
  shortness of breath R06.02
  specified type NEC R06.09
Dyspraxia R27.8
  developmental (syndrome) F82
Dysproteinemia E88.09
Dysreflexia, autonomic G90.4
Dysrhythmia
  cardiac I49.9
    newborn
      bradycardia P29.12
      occurring before birth P03.819
        before onset of labor P03.810
        during labor P03.811
      tachycardia P29.11
    postoperative I97.89
  cerebral or cortical — *see* Epilepsy
Dyssomnia — *see* Disorder, sleep
Dyssynergia
  biliary K83.8
  bladder sphincter N36.44
  cerebellaris myoclonica (Hunt's ataxia) G11.1
Dysthymia F34.1
Dysthyroidism E07.9
Dystocia O66.9
  affecting newborn P03.1
  cervical (hypotonic) O62.2
    affecting newborn P03.6
    primary O62.0
    secondary O62.1
  contraction ring O62.4
  fetal O66.9
    abnormality NEC O66.3
    conjoined twins O66.3
    oversize O66.2
  maternal O66.9
  positional O64.9 ☑
  shoulder (girdle) O66.0
    causing obstructed labor O66.0
  uterine NEC O62.4
Dystonia G24.9
  deformans progressiva G24.1
  drug induced NEC G24.09
    acute G24.02
    specified NEC G24.09
  familial G24.1
  idiopathic G24.1
    familial G24.1
    nonfamilial G24.2
    orofacial G24.4
  lenticularis G24.8
  musculorum deformans G24.1
  neuroleptic induced (acute) G24.02
  orofacial (idiopathic) G24.4
  oromandibular G24.4
    due to drug G24.01
  specified NEC G24.8
  torsion (familial) (idiopathic) G24.1
    acquired G24.8
    genetic G24.1
    symptomatic (nonfamilial) G24.2
Dystonic movements R25.8
Dystrophy, dystrophia
  adiposogenital E23.6
  Becker's type G71.0
  cervical sympathetic G90.2
  choroid (hereditary) H31.20
    central areolar H31.22
    choroideremia H31.21
    gyrate atrophy H31.23
    specified type NEC H31.29

Dystrophy, dystrophia — *continued*
  cornea (hereditary) H18.50
    endothelial H18.51
    epithelial H18.52
    granular H18.53
    lattice H18.54
    macular H18.55
    specified type NEC H18.59
  Duchenne's type G71.0
  due to malnutrition E45
  Erb's G71.0
  Fuchs' H18.51
  Gower's muscular G71.0
  hair L67.8
  infantile neuraxonal G31.89
  Landouzy-Déjérine G71.0
  Leyden-Möbius G71.0
  muscular G71.0
    benign (Becker type) G71.0
    congenital (hereditary) (progressive) (with specific morphological abnormalities of the muscle fiber) G71.0
      myotonic G71.11
    distal G71.0
    Duchenne type G71.0
    Emery-Dreifuss G71.0
    Erb type G71.0
    facioscapulohumeral G71.0
    Gower's G71.0
    hereditary (progressive) G71.0
    Landouzy-Déjérine type G71.0
    limb-girdle G71.0
    myotonic G71.11
    progressive (hereditary) G71.0
      Charcot-Marie (-Tooth) type G60.0
    pseudohypertrophic (infantile) G71.0
    severe (Duchenne type) G71.0
  myocardium, myocardial — *see* Degeneration, myocardial
  nail L60.3
    congenital Q84.6
  nutritional E45
  ocular G71.0
  oculocerebrorenal E72.03
  oculopharyngeal G71.0
  ovarian N83.8
  polyglandular E31.8
  reflex (neuromuscular) (sympathetic) — *see* Syndrome, pain, complex regional I
  retinal (hereditary) H35.50
    in
      lipid storage disorders E75.6 [H36]
      systemic lipidoses E75.6 [H36]
    involving
      pigment epithelium H35.54
      sensory area H35.53
    pigmentary H35.52
    vitreoretinal H35.51
  Salzmann's nodular — *see* Degeneration, cornea, nodular
  scapuloperoneal G71.0
  skin NEC L98.8
  sympathetic (reflex) — *see* Syndrome, pain, complex regional I
    cervical G90.2
  tapetoretinal H35.54
  thoracic, asphyxiating Q77.2
  unguium L60.3
    congenital Q84.6
  vitreoretinal H35.51
  vulva N90.4
  yellow (liver) — *see* Failure, hepatic
Dysuria R30.0
  psychogenic F45.8

E

Eales' disease H35.06- ☑
Ear (*see also* condition)
  piercing Z41.3
  tropical B36.8
  wax (impacted) H61.20
    left H61.22
      with right H61.23
    right H61.21
      with left H61.23
Earache — *see* subcategory H92.0 ☑
Early satiety R68.81

Eaton-Lambert syndrome — *see* Syndrome, Lambert-Eaton
Eberth's disease (typhoid fever) A01.00
Ebola virus disease A98.4
Ebstein's anomaly or syndrome (heart) Q22.5
Eccentro-osteochondrodysplasia E76.29
Ecchondroma — *see* Neoplasm, bone, benign
Ecchondrosis D48.0
Ecchymosis R58
  conjunctiva — *see* Hemorrhage, conjunctiva
  eye (traumatic) — *see* Contusion, eyeball
  eyelid (traumatic) — *see* Contusion, eyelid
  newborn P54.5
  spontaneous R23.3
  traumatic — *see* Contusion
Echinococciasis — *see* Echinococcus
Echinococcosis — *see* Echinococcus
Echinococcus (infection) B67.90
  granulosus B67.4
    bone B67.2
    liver B67.0
    lung B67.1
    multiple sites B67.32
    specified site NEC B67.39
    thyroid B67.31 [E35]
  liver NOS B67.8
    granulosus B67.0
    multilocularis B67.5
  lung NEC B67.99
    granulosus B67.1
    multilocularis B67.69
  multilocularis B67.7
    liver B67.5
    multiple sites B67.61
    specified site NEC B67.69
  specified site NEC B67.99
    granulosus B67.39
    multilocularis B67.69
  thyroid NEC B67.99
    granulosus B67.31 [E35]
    multilocularis B67.69 [E35]
Echinorhynchiasis B83.8
Echinostomiasis B66.8
Echolalia R48.8
Echovirus, as cause of disease classified elsewhere B97.12
Eclampsia, eclamptic (coma) (convulsions) (delirium) (with hypertension) NEC O15.9
  during labor and delivery O15.1
  postpartum O15.2
  pregnancy O15.0- ☑
  puerperal O15.2
Economic circumstances affecting care Z59.9
Economo's disease A85.8
Ectasia, ectasis
  annuloaortic I35.8
  aorta I77.819
    with aneurysm — *see* Aneurysm, aorta
    abdominal I77.811
    thoracic I77.810
    thoracoabdominal I77.812
  breast — *see* Ectasia, mammary duct
  capillary I78.8
  cornea H18.71- ☑
  gastric antral vascular (GAVE) K31.819
    with hemorrhage K31.811
    without hemorrhage K31.819
  mammary duct N60.4- ☑
  salivary gland (duct) K11.8
  sclera — *see* Sclerectasia
Ecthyma L08.0
  contagiosum B08.02
  gangrenosum L08.0
  infectiosum B08.02
Ectocardia Q24.8
Ectodermal dysplasia (anhidrotic) Q82.4
Ectodermosis erosiva pluriorificialis L51.1
Ectopic, ectopia (congenital)
  abdominal viscera Q45.8
    due to defect in anterior abdominal wall Q79.59
  ACTH syndrome E24.3
  adrenal gland Q89.1
  anus Q43.5
  atrial beats I49.1
  beats I49.49
    atrial I49.1
    ventricular I49.3

Ectopic, ectopia — *continued*
  bladder Q64.10
  bone and cartilage in lung Q33.5
  brain Q04.8
  breast tissue Q83.8
  cardiac Q24.8
  cerebral Q04.8
  cordis Q24.8
  endometrium — *see* Endometriosis
  gastric mucosa Q40.2
  gestation — *see* Pregnancy, by site
  heart Q24.8
  hormone secretion NEC E34.2
  kidney (crossed) (pelvis) Q63.2
  lens, lentis Q12.1
  mole — *see* Pregnancy, by site
  organ or site NEC — *see* Malposition, congenital
  pancreas Q45.3
  pregnancy — *see* Pregnancy, ectopic
  pupil — *see* Abnormality, pupillary
  renal Q63.2
  sebaceous glands of mouth Q38.6
  spleen Q89.09
  testis Q53.00
    bilateral Q53.02
    unilateral Q53.01
  thyroid Q89.2
  tissue in lung Q33.5
  ureter Q62.63
  ventricular beats I49.3
  vesicae Q64.10
Ectromelia Q73.8
  lower limb — *see* Defect, reduction, limb, lower, specified type NEC
  upper limb — *see* Defect, reduction, limb, upper, specified type NEC
Ectropion H02.109
  cervix N86
    with cervicitis N72
  congenital Q10.1
  eyelid (paralytic) H02.109
    cicatricial H02.119
      left H02.116
        lower H02.115
        upper H02.114
      right H02.113
        lower H02.112
        upper H02.111
    congenital Q10.1
    left H02.106
      lower H02.105
      upper H02.104
    mechanical H02.129
      left H02.126
        lower H02.125
        upper H02.124
      right H02.123
        lower H02.122
        upper H02.121
    right H02.103
      lower H02.102
      upper H02.101
    senile H02.139
      left H02.136
        lower H02.135
        upper H02.134
      right H02.133
        lower H02.132
        upper H02.131
    spastic H02.149
      left H02.146
        lower H02.145
        upper H02.144
      right H02.143
        lower H02.142
        upper H02.141
  iris H21.89
  lip (acquired) K13.0
    congenital Q38.0
  urethra N36.8
  uvea H21.89
Eczema (acute) (chronic) (erythematous) (fissum) (rubrum) (squamous) (*see also* Dermatitis) L30.9
  contact — *see* Dermatitis, contact
  dyshydrotic L30.1
  external ear — *see* Otitis, externa, acute, eczematoid
  flexural L20.82
  herpeticum B00.0

Eczema — *continued*
  hypertrophicum L28.0
  hypostatic — *see* Varix, leg, with, inflammation
  impetiginous L01.1
  infantile (due to any substance) L20.83
    intertriginous L21.1
    seborrheic L21.1
  intertriginous NEC L30.4
    infantile L21.1
  intrinsic (allergic) L20.84
  lichenified NEC L28.0
  marginatum (hebrae) B35.6
  pustular L30.3
  stasis — *see* Varix, leg, with, inflammation
  vaccination, vaccinatum T88.1 ☑
  varicose — *see* Varix, leg, with, inflammation
Eczematid L30.2
Eddowes (-Spurway) **syndrome** Q78.0
Edema, edematous (infectious) (pitting) (toxic) R60.9
  with nephritis — *see* Nephrosis
  allergic T78.3 ☑
  amputation stump (surgical) (sequelae (late effect)) T87.89
  angioneurotic (allergic) (any site) (with urticaria) T78.3 ☑
    hereditary D84.1
  angiospastic I73.9
  Berlin's (traumatic) S05.8X- ☑
  brain (cytotoxic) (vasogenic) G93.6
    due to birth injury P11.0
    newborn (anoxia or hypoxia) P52.4
      birth injury P11.0
    traumatic — *see* Injury, intracranial, cerebral edema
  cardiac — *see* Failure, heart, congestive
  cardiovascular — *see* Failure, heart, congestive
  cerebral — *see* Edema, brain
  cerebrospinal — *see* Edema, brain
  cervix (uteri) (acute) N88.8
    puerperal, postpartum O90.89
  chronic hereditary Q82.0
  circumscribed, acute T78.3 ☑
    hereditary D84.1
  conjunctiva H11.42- ☑
  cornea H18.2- ☑
    idiopathic H18.22- ☑
    secondary H18.23- ☑
      due to contact lens H18.21- ☑
  due to
    lymphatic obstruction I89.0
    salt retention E87.0
  epiglottis — *see* Edema, glottis
  essential, acute T78.3 ☑
    hereditary D84.1
  extremities, lower — *see* Edema, legs
  eyelid NEC H02.849
    left H02.846
      lower H02.845
      upper H02.844
    right H02.843
      lower H02.842
      upper H02.841
  familial, hereditary Q82.0
  famine — *see* Malnutrition, severe
  generalized R60.1
  glottis, glottic, glottidis (obstructive) (passive) J38.4
    allergic T78.3 ☑
      hereditary D84.1
  heart — *see* Failure, heart, congestive
  heat T67.7 ☑
  hereditary Q82.0
  inanition — *see* Malnutrition, severe
  intracranial G93.6
  iris H21.89
  joint — *see* Effusion, joint
  larynx — *see* Edema, glottis
  legs R60.0
    due to venous obstruction I87.1
    hereditary Q82.0
  localized R60.0
    due to venous obstruction I87.1
  lower limbs — *see* Edema, legs
  lung J81.1
    with heart condition or failure — *see* Failure, ventricular, left
    acute J81.0
    chemical (acute) J68.1
      chronic J68.1

Edema, edematous — *continued*
- lung — *continued*
  - chronic J81.1
    - due to
      - chemicals, gases, fumes or vapors (inhalation) J68.1
      - external agent J70.9
        - specified NEC J70.8
      - radiation J70.1
    - due to
      - chemicals, fumes or vapors (inhalation) J68.1
      - external agent J70.9
        - specified NEC J70.8
      - high altitude T70.29 ✓
      - near drowning T75.1 ✓
      - radiation J70.0
    - meaning failure, left ventricle I50.1
- lymphatic I89.0
  - due to mastectomy I97.2
- macula H35.81
  - cystoid, following cataract surgery — *see* Complications, postprocedural, following cataract surgery
  - diabetic — *see* Diabetes, by type, with, retinopathy, with macular edema
- malignant — *see* Gangrene, gas
- Milroy's Q82.0
- nasopharynx J39.2
- newborn P83.30
  - hydrops fetalis — *see* Hydrops, fetalis
  - specified NEC P83.39
- nutritional (*see also* Malnutrition, severe)
  - with dyspigmentation, skin and hair E40
- optic disc or nerve — *see* Papilledema
- orbit H05.22- ✓
- pancreas K86.8
- papilla, optic — *see* Papilledema
- penis N48.89
- periodic T78.3 ✓
  - hereditary D84.1
- pharynx J39.2
- pulmonary — *see* Edema, lung
- Quincke's T78.3 ✓
  - hereditary D84.1
- renal — *see* Nephrosis
- retina H35.81
  - diabetic — *see* Diabetes, by type, with, retinopathy, with macular edema
- salt E87.0
- scrotum N50.8
- seminal vesicle N50.8
- spermatic cord N50.8
- spinal (cord) (vascular) (nontraumatic) G95.19
- starvation — *see* Malnutrition, severe
- stasis — *see* Hypertension, venous, (chronic)
- subglottic — *see* Edema, glottis
- supraglottic — *see* Edema, glottis
- testis N44.8
- tunica vaginalis N50.8
- vas deferens N50.8
- vulva (acute) N90.89

Edentulism — *see* Absence, teeth, acquired

Edsall's disease T67.2 ✓

Educational handicap Z55.9
- specified NEC Z55.8

Edward's syndrome — *see* Trisomy, 18

Effect(s) (of) (from) — *see* Effect, adverse NEC

Effect, adverse
- abnormal gravitational (G) forces or states T75.81 ✓
- abuse — *see* Maltreatment
- air pressure T70.9 ✓
  - specified NEC T70.8 ✓
- altitude (high) — *see* Effect, adverse, high altitude
- anesthesia (*see also* Anesthesia) T88.59 ✓
  - in labor and delivery O74.9
  - in pregnancy NEC O29.3- ✓
  - local, toxic
    - in labor and delivery O74.4
    - postpartum, puerperal O89.3
  - postpartum, puerperal O89.9
  - specified NEC T88.59 ✓
    - in labor and delivery O74.8
    - postpartum, puerperal O89.8
  - spinal and epidural T88.59 ✓
    - headache T88.59 ✓
      - in labor and delivery O74.5
      - postpartum, puerperal O89.4

Effect, adverse — *continued*
- anesthesia (*see also* Anesthesia) — *continued*
  - spinal and epidural — *continued*
    - specified NEC
      - in labor and delivery O74.6
      - postpartum, puerperal O89.5
- antitoxin — *see* Complications, vaccination
- atmospheric pressure T70.9 ✓
  - due to explosion T70.8 ✓
  - high T70.3 ✓
  - low — *see* Effect, adverse, high altitude
  - specified effect NEC T70.8 ✓
- biological, correct substance properly administered — *see* Effect, adverse, drug
- blood (derivatives) (serum) (transfusion) — *see* Complications, transfusion
- chemical substance — *see* Table of Drugs and Chemicals
- cold (temperature) (weather) T69.9 ✓
  - chilblains T69.1 ✓
  - frostbite — *see* Frostbite
  - specified effect NEC T69.8 ✓
- drugs and medicaments T88.7 ✓
  - specified drug — *see* Table of Drugs and Chemicals, by drug, adverse effect
  - specified effect — *code to* condition
- electric current, electricity (shock) T75.4 ✓
  - burn — *see* Burn
- exertion (excessive) T73.3 ✓
- exposure — *see* Exposure
- external cause NEC T75.89 ✓
- foodstuffs T78.1 ✓
  - allergic reaction — *see* Allergy, food
    - causing anaphylaxis — *see* Shock, anaphylactic, due to food
  - chylous — *see* Effusion, pleura
  - noxious — *see* Poisoning, food, noxious
- gases, fumes, or vapors T59.9- ✓
  - specified agent — *see* Table of Drugs and Chemicals
- glue (airplane) sniffing
  - due to drug abuse — *see* Abuse, drug, inhalant
  - due to drug dependence — *see* Dependence, drug, inhalant
- heat — *see* Heat
- high altitude NEC T70.29 ✓
  - anoxia T70.29 ✓
  - on
    - ears T70.0 ✓
    - sinuses T70.1 ✓
  - polycythemia D75.1
- high pressure fluids T70.4 ✓
- hot weather — *see* Heat
- hunger T73.0 ✓
- immersion, foot — *see* Immersion
- immunization — *see* Complications, vaccination
- immunological agents — *see* Complications, vaccination
- infrared (radiation) (rays) NOS T66 ✓
  - dermatitis or eczema L59.8
- infusion — *see* Complications, infusion
- lack of care of infants — *see* Maltreatment, child
- lightning — *see* Lightning
- medical care T88.9 ✓
  - specified NEC T88.8 ✓
- medicinal substance, correct, properly administered — *see* Effect, adverse, drug
- motion T75.3 ✓
- noise, on inner ear — *see* subcategory H83.3 ✓
- overheated places — *see* Heat
- psychosocial, of work environment Z56.5
- radiation (diagnostic) (infrared) (natural source) (therapeutic) (ultraviolet) (X-ray) NOS T66 ✓
  - dermatitis or eczema — *see* Dermatitis, due to, radiation
  - fibrosis of lung J70.1
  - pneumonitis J70.0
  - pulmonary manifestations
    - acute J70.0
    - chronic J70.1
  - skin L59.9
- radioactive substance NOS
  - dermatitis or eczema — *see* Radiodermatitis
- reduced temperature T69.9 ✓
  - immersion foot or hand — *see* Immersion
  - specified effect NEC T69.8 ✓
- serum NEC (*see also* Reaction, serum) T80.69 ✓

Effect, adverse — *continued*
- specified NEC T78.8 ✓
  - external cause NEC T75.89 ✓
- strangulation — *see* Asphyxia, traumatic
- submersion T75.1 ✓
- thirst T73.1 ✓
- toxic — *see* Toxicity
- transfusion — *see* Complications, transfusion
- ultraviolet (radiation) (rays) NOS T66 ✓
  - burn — *see* Burn
  - dermatitis or eczema — *see* Dermatitis, due to, ultraviolet rays
    - acute L56.8
- vaccine (any) — *see* Complications, vaccination
- vibration — *see* Vibration, adverse effects
- water pressure NEC T70.9 ✓
  - specified NEC T70.8 ✓
- weightlessness T75.82 ✓
- whole blood — *see* Complications, transfusion
- work environment Z56.5

Effects, late — *see* Sequelae

Effluvium
- anagen L65.1
- telogen L65.0

Effort syndrome (psychogenic) F45.8

Effusion
- amniotic fluid — *see* Pregnancy, complicated by, premature rupture of membranes
- brain (serous) G93.6
- bronchial — *see* Bronchitis
- cerebral G93.6
- cerebrospinal (*see also* Meningitis)
  - vessel G93.6
- chest — *see* Effusion, pleura
- chylous, chyliform (pleura) J94.0
- intracranial G93.6
- joint M25.40
  - ankle M25.47- ✓
  - elbow M25.42- ✓
  - foot joint M25.47- ✓
  - hand joint M25.44- ✓
  - hip M25.45- ✓
  - knee M25.46- ✓
  - shoulder M25.41- ✓
  - specified joint NEC M25.48
  - wrist M25.43- ✓
- malignant pleural J91.0
- meninges — *see* Meningitis
- pericardium, pericardial (noninflammatory) I31.3
  - acute — *see* Pericarditis, acute
- peritoneal (chronic) R18.8
- pleura, pleurisy, pleuritic, pleuropericardial J90
  - chylous, chyliform J94.0
  - due to systemic lupus erythematosis M32.13
  - influenzal — *see* Influenza, with, respiratory manifestations NEC
  - malignant J91.0
  - newborn P28.89
  - tuberculous NEC A15.6
    - primary (progressive) A15.7
- spinal — *see* Meningitis
- thorax, thoracic — *see* Effusion, pleura

Egg shell nails L60.3
- congenital Q84.6

Egyptian splenomegaly B65.1

Ehlers-Danlos syndrome Q79.6

Ehrlichiosis A77.40
- due to
  - E. chafeensis A77.41
  - E. sennetsu A79.81
  - specified organism NEC A77.49

Eichstedt's disease B36.0

Eisenmenger's
- complex or syndrome I27.89
- defect Q21.8

Ejaculation
- painful N53.12
- premature F52.4
- retarded N53.11
- retrograde N53.14
- semen, painful N53.12
  - psychogenic F52.6

Ekbom's syndrome (restless legs) G25.81

Ekman's syndrome (brittle bones and blue sclera) Q78.0

Elastic skin Q82.8
- acquired L57.4

Elastofibroma — *see* Neoplasm, connective tissue, benign
Elastoma (juvenile) Q82.8
　Miescher's L87.2
Elastomyofibrosis I42.4
Elastosis
　actinic, solar L57.8
　atrophicans (senile) L57.4
　perforans serpiginosa L87.2
　senilis L57.4
Elbow — *see* condition
Electric current, electricity, effects (concussion) (fatal) (nonfatal) (shock) T75.4 ☑
　burn — *see* Burn
Electric feet syndrome E53.8
Electrocution T75.4 ☑
　from electroshock gun (taser) T75.4 ☑
Electrolyte imbalance E87.8
　with
　　abortion — *see* Abortion by type, complicated by, electrolyte imbalance
　　ectopic pregnancy O08.5
　　molar pregnancy O08.5
Elephantiasis (nonfilarial) I89.0
　arabicum — *see* Infestation, filarial
　bancroftian B74.0
　congenital (any site) (hereditary) Q82.0
　due to
　　Brugia (malayi) B74.1
　　　timori B74.2
　　mastectomy I97.2
　　Wuchereria (bancrofti) B74.0
　eyelid H02.859
　　left H02.856
　　　lower H02.855
　　　upper H02.854
　　right H02.853
　　　lower H02.852
　　　upper H02.851
　filarial, filariensis — *see* Infestation, filarial
　glandular I89.0
　graecorum A30.9
　lymphangiectatic I89.0
　lymphatic vessel I89.0
　　due to mastectomy I97.2
　scrotum (nonfilarial) I89.0
　streptococcal I89.0
　surgical I97.89
　　postmastectomy I97.2
　telangiectodes I89.0
　vulva (nonfilarial) N90.89
Elevated, elevation
　antibody titer R76.0
　basal metabolic rate R94.8
　blood pressure (*see also* Hypertension)
　　reading (incidental) (isolated) (nonspecific), no diagnosis of hypertension R03.0
　blood sugar R73.9
　body temperature (of unknown origin) R50.9
　cancer antigen 125 [CA 125] R97.1
　carcinoembryonic antigen [CEA] R97.0
　cholesterol E78.0
　　with high triglycerides E78.2
　conjugate, eye H51.0
　C-reactive protein (CRP) R79.82
　diaphragm, congenital Q79.1
　erythrocyte sedimentation rate R70.0
　fasting glucose R73.01
　fasting triglycerides E78.1
　finding on laboratory examination — *see* Findings, abnormal, inconclusive, without diagnosis, by type of exam
　GFR (glomerular filtration rate) — *see* Findings, abnormal, inconclusive, without diagnosis, by type of exam
　glucose tolerance (oral) R73.02
　immunoglobulin level R76.8
　indoleacetic acid R82.5
　lactic acid dehydrogenase (LDH) level R74.0
　leukocytes D72.829
　lipoprotein a level E78.8 ☑
　liver function
　　study R94.5
　　test R79.89
　　　alkaline phosphatase R74.8
　　　aminotransferase R74.0
　　　bilirubin R17
　　　hepatic enzyme R74.8

Elevated, elevation — *continued*
　liver function — *continued*
　　test — *continued*
　　　lactate dehydrogenase R74.0
　lymphocytes D72.820
　prostate specific antigen [PSA] R97.2
　Rh titer — *see* Complication(s), transfusion, incompatibility reaction, Rh (factor)
　scapula, congenital Q74.0
　sedimentation rate R70.0
　SGOT R74.0
　SGPT R74.0
　transaminase level R74.0
　triglycerides E78.1
　　with high cholesterol E78.2
　tumor associated antigens [TAA] NEC R97.8
　tumor specific antigens [TSA] NEC R97.8
　urine level of
　　17-ketosteroids R82.5
　　catecholamine R82.5
　　indoleacetic acid R82.5
　　steroids R82.5
　　vanillylmandelic acid (VMA) R82.5
　venous pressure I87.8
　white blood cell count D72.829
　　specified NEC D72.828
Elliptocytosis (congenital) (hereditary) D58.1
　Hb C (disease) D58.1
　hemoglobin disease D58.1
　sickle-cell (disease) D57.8- ☑
　　trait D57.3
Ellison-Zollinger syndrome E16.4
Ellis-van Creveld syndrome (chondroectodermal dysplasia) Q77.6
Elongated, elongation (congenital) (*see also* Distortion)
　bone Q79.9
　cervix (uteri) Q51.828
　　acquired N88.4
　　hypertrophic N88.4
　colon Q43.8
　common bile duct Q44.5
　cystic duct Q44.5
　frenulum, penis Q55.69
　labia minora (acquired) N90.6
　ligamentum patellae Q74.1
　petiolus (epiglottidis) Q31.8
　tooth, teeth K00.2
　uvula Q38.6
Eltor cholera A00.1
Emaciation (due to malnutrition) E41
Embadomoniasis A07.8
Embedded tooth, teeth K01.0
　root only K08.3
Embolic — *see* condition
Embolism (multiple) (paradoxical) I74.9
　air (any site) (traumatic) T79.0 ☑
　　following
　　　abortion — *see* Abortion by type complicated by embolism
　　　ectopic pregnancy O08.2
　　　infusion, therapeutic injection or transfusion T80.0 ☑
　　　molar pregnancy O08.2
　　　procedure NEC
　　　　artery T81.719 ☑
　　　　　mesenteric T81.710 ☑
　　　　　renal T81.711 ☑
　　　　　specified NEC T81.718 ☑
　　　　vein T81.72 ☑
　　in pregnancy, childbirth or puerperium — *see* Embolism, obstetric
　amniotic fluid (pulmonary) (*see also* Embolism, obstetric)
　　following
　　　abortion — *see* Abortion by type complicated by embolism
　　　ectopic pregnancy O08.2
　　　molar pregnancy O08.2
　aorta, aortic I74.10
　　abdominal I74.09
　　　saddle I74.01
　　bifurcation I74.09
　　　saddle I74.01
　　thoracic I74.11
　artery I74.9
　　auditory, internal I65.8
　　basilar — *see* Occlusion, artery, basilar

Embolism — *continued*
　artery — *continued*
　　carotid (common) (internal) — *see* Occlusion, artery, carotid
　　cerebellar (anterior inferior) (posterior inferior) (superior) I66.3
　　cerebral — *see* Occlusion, artery, cerebral
　　choroidal (anterior) I66.8
　　communicating posterior I66.8
　　coronary (*see also* Infarct, myocardium)
　　　not resulting in infarction I24.0
　　extremity I74.4
　　　lower I74.3
　　　upper I74.2
　　hypophyseal I66.8
　　iliac I74.5
　　limb I74.4
　　　lower I74.3
　　　upper I74.2
　　mesenteric (with gangrene) K55.0
　　ophthalmic — *see* Occlusion, artery, retina
　　peripheral I74.4
　　pontine I66.8
　　precerebral — *see* Occlusion, artery, precerebral
　　pulmonary — *see* Embolism, pulmonary
　　renal N28.0
　　retinal — *see* Occlusion, artery, retina
　　septic I76
　　specified NEC I74.8
　　vertebral — *see* Occlusion, artery, vertebral
　basilar (artery) I65.1
　blood clot
　　following
　　　abortion — *see* Abortion by type complicated by embolism
　　　ectopic or molar pregnancy O08.2
　　　in pregnancy, childbirth or puerperium — *see* Embolism, obstetric
　brain (*see also* Occlusion, artery, cerebral)
　　following
　　　abortion — *see* Abortion by type complicated by embolism
　　　ectopic or molar pregnancy O08.2
　　puerperal, postpartum, childbirth — *see* Embolism, obstetric
　capillary I78.8
　cardiac (*see also* Infarct, myocardium)
　　not resulting in infarction I24.0
　carotid (artery) (common) (internal) — *see* Occlusion, artery, carotid
　cavernous sinus (venous) — *see* Embolism, intracranial venous sinus
　cerebral — *see* Occlusion, artery, cerebral
　cholesterol — *see* Atheroembolism
　coronary (artery or vein) (systemic) — *see* Occlusion, coronary
　due to device, implant or graft (*see also* Complications, by site and type, specified NEC)
　　arterial graft NEC T82.818 ☑
　　breast (implant) T85.81 ☑
　　catheter NEC T85.81 ☑
　　　dialysis (renal) T82.818 ☑
　　　　intraperitoneal T85.81 ☑
　　　infusion NEC T82.818 ☑
　　　　spinal (epidural) (subdural) T85.81 ☑
　　　urinary (indwelling) T83.81 ☑
　　electronic (electrode) (pulse generator) (stimulator)
　　　bone T84.81 ☑
　　　cardiac T82.817 ☑
　　　nervous system (brain) (peripheral nerve) (spinal) T85.81 ☑
　　　urinary T83.81 ☑
　　fixation, internal (orthopedic) NEC T84.81 ☑
　　gastrointestinal (bile duct) (esophagus) T85.81 ☑
　　genital NEC T83.81 ☑
　　heart (graft) (valve) T82.817 ☑
　　joint prosthesis T84.81 ☑
　　ocular (corneal graft) (orbital implant) T85.81 ☑
　　orthopedic (bone graft) NEC T86.838
　　specified NEC T85.81 ☑
　　urinary (graft) NEC T83.81 ☑
　　vascular NEC T82.818 ☑
　　ventricular intracranial shunt T85.81 ☑
　extremities
　　lower — *see* Embolism, vein, lower extremity
　　　arterial I74.3
　　upper I74.2

Embolism — *continued*
  eye H34.9
  fat (cerebral) (pulmonary) (systemic) T79.1 ☑
    complicating delivery — *see* Embolism, obstetric
    following
      abortion — *see* Abortion by type complicated
        by embolism
      ectopic or molar pregnancy O08.2
  following
    abortion — *see* Abortion by type complicated by
      embolism
    ectopic or molar pregnancy O08.2
    infusion, therapeutic injection or transfusion
      air T80.0 ☑
  heart (fatty) (*see also* Infarct, myocardium)
    not resulting in infarction I24.0
  hepatic (vein) I82.0
  in pregnancy, childbirth or puerperium — *see* Embolism, obstetric
  intestine (artery) (vein) (with gangrene) K55.0
  intracranial (*see also* Occlusion, artery, cerebral)
    venous sinus (any) G08
      nonpyogenic I67.6
  intraspinal venous sinuses or veins G08
    nonpyogenic G95.19
  kidney (artery) N28.0
  lateral sinus (venous) — *see* Embolism, intracranial, venous sinus
  leg — *see* Embolism, vein, lower extremity
    arterial I74.3
  longitudinal sinus (venous) — *see* Embolism, intracranial, venous sinus
  lung (massive) — *see* Embolism, pulmonary
  meninges I66.8
  mesenteric (artery) (vein) (with gangrene) K55.0
  obstetric (in) (pulmonary)
    childbirth O88.82
      air O88.02
      amniotic fluid O88.12
      blood clot O88.22
      fat O88.82
      pyemic O88.32
      septic O88.32
      specified type NEC O88.82
    pregnancy O88.81- ☑
      air O88.01- ☑
      amniotic fluid O88.11- ☑
      blood clot O88.21- ☑
      fat O88.81- ☑
      pyemic O88.31- ☑
      septic O88.31- ☑
      specified type NEC O88.81- ☑
    puerperal O88.83
      air O88.03
      amniotic fluid O88.13
      blood clot O88.23
      fat O88.83
      pyemic O88.33
      septic O88.33
      specified type NEC O88.83
  ophthalmic — *see* Occlusion, artery, retina
  penis N48.81
  peripheral artery NOS I74.4
  pituitary E23.6
  popliteal (artery) I74.3
  portal (vein) I81
  postoperative, postrpocedural
    artery T81.719 ☑
      mesenteric T81.710 ☑
      renal T81.711 ☑
      specified NEC T81.718 ☑
    vein T81.72 ☑
  precerebral artery — *see* Occlusion, artery, precerebral
  puerperal — *see* Embolism, obstetric
  pulmonary (acute) (artery) (vein) I26.99
    with acute cor pulmonale I26.09
    chronic I27.82
    following
      abortion — *see* Abortion by type complicated
        by embolism
      ectopic or molar pregnancy O08.2
    healed or old Z86.711
    in pregnancy, childbirth or puerperium — *see*
      Embolism, obstetric
    personal history of Z86.711
    saddle I26.92
      with acute cor pulmonale I26.02

Embolism — *continued*
  pulmonary — *continued*
    septic I26.90
      with acute cor pulmonale I26.01
  pyemic (multiple) I76
    following
      abortion — *see* Abortion by type complicated
        by embolism
      ectopic or molar pregnancy O08.2
    Hemophilus influenzae A41.3
    pneumococcal A40.3
      with pneumonia J13
    puerperal, postpartum, childbirth (any organism)
      — *see* Embolism, obstetric
    specified organism NEC A41.89
    staphylococcal A41.2
    streptococcal A40.9
  renal (artery) N28.0
    vein I82.3
  retina, retinal — *see* Occlusion, artery, retina
  saddle
    abdominal aorta I74.01
    pulmonary artery I26.92
      with acute cor pulmonale I26.02
  septic (arterial) I76
    complicating abortion — *see* Abortion, by type,
      complicated by, embolism
  sinus — *see* Embolism, intracranial, venous sinus
  soap complicating abortion — *see* Abortion, by type,
    complicated by, embolism
  spinal cord G95.19
    pyogenic origin G06.1
  spleen, splenic (artery) I74.8
  upper extremity I74.2
  vein (acute) I82.90
    antecubital I82.61- ☑
      chronic I82.71- ☑
    axillary I82.A1- ☑ (*following* I82.7)
      chronic I82.A2- ☑ (*following* I82.7)
    basilic I82.61-
      chronic I82.71-
    brachial I82.62- ☑
      chronic I82.72- ☑
    brachiocephalic (innominate) I82.290
      chronic I82.291
    cephalic I82.61- ☑
      chronic I82.71- ☑
    chronic I82.91
    deep (DVT) I82.40- ☑
      calf I82.4Z- ☑
        chronic I82.5Z- ☑
      lower leg I82.4Z- ☑
        chronic I82.5Z- ☑
      thigh I82.4Y- ☑
        chronic I82.5Y- ☑
      upper leg I82.4Y ☑
        chronic I82.5Y-
    femoral I82.41- ☑
      chronic I82.51- ☑
    iliac (iliofemoral) I82.42- ☑
      chronic I82.52- ☑
    innominate I82.290
      chronic I82.291
    internal jugular I82.C1- ☑ (*following* I82.7)
      chronic I82.C2- ☑ (*following* I82.7)
    lower extremity
      deep I82.40- ☑
        chronic I82.50- ☑
        specified NEC I82.49- ☑
          chronic NEC I82.59- ☑
      distal
        deep I82.4Z- ☑
      proximal
        deep I82.4Y- ☑
          chronic I82.5Y- ☑
      superficial I82.81- ☑
    popliteal I82.43- ☑
      chronic I82.53- ☑
    radial I82.62- ☑
      chronic I82.72- ☑
    renal I82.3
    saphenous (greater) (lesser) I82.81- ☑
    specified NEC I82.890
      chronic NEC I82.891
    subclavian I82.B1- ☑ (*following* I82.7)
      chronic I82.B2- ☑ (*following* I82.7)
    thoracic NEC I82.290

Embolism — *continued*
  vein — *continued*
    thoracic — *continued*
      chronic I82.291
    tibial I82.44- ☑
      chronic I82.54- ☑
    ulnar I82.62- ☑
      chronic I82.72- ☑
    upper extremity I82.60- ☑
      chronic I82.70- ☑
      deep I82.62- ☑
        chronic I82.72- ☑
      superficial I82.61- ☑
        chronic I82.71- ☑
  vena cava
    inferior (acute) I82.220
      chronic I82.221
    superior (acute) I82.210
      chronic I82.211
  venous sinus G08
  vessels of brain — *see* Occlusion, artery, cerebral
Embolus — *see* Embolism
Embryoma (*see also* Neoplasm, uncertain behavior, by
  site)
  benign — *see* Neoplasm, benign, by site
  kidney C64.- ☑
  liver C22.0
  malignant (*see also* Neoplasm, malignant, by site)
    kidney C64.- ☑
    liver C22.0
    testis C62.9- ☑
      descended (scrotal) C62.1- ☑
      undescended C62.0- ☑
  testis C62.9- ☑
    descended (scrotal) C62.1- ☑
    undescended C62.0- ☑
Embryonic
  circulation Q28.9
  heart Q28.9
  vas deferens Q55.4
Embryopathia NOS Q89.9
Embryotoxon Q13.4
Emesis — *see* Vomiting
Emotional lability R45.86
Emotionality, pathological F60.3
Emotogenic disease — *see* Disorder, psychogenic
Emphysema (atrophic) (bullous) (chronic) (interlobular)
  (lung) (obstructive) (pulmonary) (senile) (vesicular)
  J43.9
  cellular tissue (traumatic) T79.7 ☑
    surgical T81.82 ☑
  centrilobular J43.2
  compensatory J98.3
  congenital (interstitial) P25.0
  conjunctiva H11.89
  connective tissue (traumatic) T79.7 ☑
    surgical T81.82 ☑
  due to chemicals, gases, fumes or vapors J68.4
  eyelid(s) — *see* Disorder, eyelid, specified type NEC
    surgical T81.82 ☑
    traumatic T79.7 ☑
  interstitial J98.2
    congenital P25.0
    perinatal period P25.0
  laminated tissue T79.7 ☑
    surgical T81.82 ☑
  mediastinal J98.2
    newborn P25.2
  orbit, orbital — *see* Disorder, orbit, specified type NEC
  panacinar J43.1
  panlobular J43.1
  specified NEC J43.8
  subcutaneous (traumatic) T79.7 ☑
    nontraumatic J98.2
    postprocedural T81.82 ☑
    surgical T81.82 ☑
  surgical T81.82 ☑
  thymus (gland) (congenital) E32.8
  traumatic (subcutaneous) T79.7 ☑
  unilateral J43.0
Empty nest syndrome Z60.0
Empyema (acute) (chest) (double) (pleura) (supradi-
  aphragmatic) (thorax) J86.9
  with fistula J86.0
  accessory sinus (chronic) — *see* Sinusitis
  antrum (chronic) — *see* Sinusitis, maxillary
  brain (any part) — *see* Abscess, brain

Empyema — *continued*
  ethmoidal (chronic) (sinus) — *see* Sinusitis, ethmoidal
  extradural — *see* Abscess, extradural
  frontal (chronic) (sinus) — *see* Sinusitis, frontal
  gallbladder K81.0
  mastoid (process) (acute) — *see* Mastoiditis, acute
  maxilla, maxillary M27.2
    sinus (chronic) — *see* Sinusitis, maxillary
  nasal sinus (chronic) — *see* Sinusitis
  sinus (accessory) (chronic) (nasal) — *see* Sinusitis
  sphenoidal (sinus) (chronic) — *see* Sinusitis, sphe-
    noidal
  subarachnoid — *see* Abscess, extradural
  subdural — *see* Abscess, subdural
  tuberculous A15.6
  ureter — *see* Ureteritis
  ventricular — *see* Abscess, brain
En coup de sabre lesion L94.1
Enamel pearls K00.2
Enameloma K00.2
Enanthema, viral B09
Encephalitis (chronic) (hemorrhagic) (idiopathic)
  (nonepidemic) (spurious) (subacute) G04.90
  acute (*see also* Encephalitis, viral) A86
    disseminated G04.00
      infectious G04.01
      noninfectious G04.81
      postimmunization (postvaccination) G04.02
      postinfectious G04.01
    inclusion body A85.8
    necrotizing hemorrhagic G04.30
      postimmunization G04.32
      postinfectious G04.31
      specified NEC G04.39
  arboviral, arbovirus NEC A85.2
  arthropod-borne NEC (viral) A85.2
  Australian A83.4
  California (virus) A83.5
  Central European (tick-borne) A84.1
  Czechoslovakian A84.1
  Dawson's (inclusion body) A81.1
  diffuse sclerosing A81.1
  disseminated, acute G04.00
  due to
    cat scratch disease A28.1
    human immunodeficiency virus (HIV) disease
      B20 [G05.3]
    malaria — *see* Malaria
    rickettsiosis — *see* Rickettsiosis
    smallpox inoculation G04.02
    typhus — *see* Typhus
  Eastern equine A83.2
  endemic (viral) A86
  epidemic NEC (viral) A86
  equine (acute) (infectious) (viral) A83.9
    Eastern A83.2
    Venezuelan A92.2
    Western A83.1
  Far Eastern (tick-borne) A84.0
  following vaccination or other immunization proce-
    dure G04.02
  herpes zoster B02.0
  herpesviral B00.4
    due to herpesvirus 6 B10.01
    due to herpesvirus 7 B10.09
    specified NEC B10.09
  Ilheus (virus) A83.8
  in (due to)
    actinomycosis A42.82
    adenovirus A85.1
    African trypanosomiasis B56.9 [G05.3]
    Chagas' disease (chronic) B57.42
    cytomegalovirus B25.8
    enterovirus A85.0
    herpes (simplex) virus B00.4
      due to herpesvirus 6 B10.01
      due to herpesvirus 7 B10.09
      specified NEC B10.09
    infectious disease NEC B99 ☑ [G05.3]
    influenza — *see* Influenza, with, encephalopathy
    listeriosis A32.12
    measles B05.0
    mumps B26.2
    naegleriasis B60.2
    parasitic disease NEC B89 [G05.3]
    poliovirus A80.9 [G05.3]
    rubella B06.01

Encephalitis — *continued*
  in — *continued*
    syphilis
      congenital A50.42
      late A52.14
    systemic lupus erythematosus M32.19
    toxoplasmosis (acquired) B58.2
      congenital P37.1
    tuberculosis A17.82
    zoster B02.0
  inclusion body A81.1
  infectious (acute) (virus) NEC A86
  Japanese (B type) A83.0
  La Crosse A83.5
  lead — *see* Poisoning, lead
  lethargica (acute) (infectious) A85.8
  louping ill A84.8
  lupus erythematosus, systemic M32.19
  lymphatica A87.2
  Mengo A85.8
  meningococcal A39.81
  Murray Valley A83.4
  otitic NEC H66.40 [G05.3]
  parasitic NOS B71.9
  periaxial G37.0
  periaxialis (concentrica) (diffuse) G37.5
  postchickenpox B01.11
  postexanthematous NEC B09
  postimmunization G04.02
  postinfectious NEC G04.01
  postmeasles B05.0
  postvaccinal G04.02
  postvaricella B01.11
  postviral NEC A86
  Powassan A84.8
  Rasmussen G04.81
  Rio Bravo A85.8
  Russian
    autumnal A83.0
    spring-summer (taiga) A84.0
  saturnine — *see* Poisoning, lead
  specified NEC G04.81
  St. Louis A83.3
  subacute sclerosing A81.1
  summer A83.0
  suppurative G04.81
  tick-borne A84.9
  Torula, torular (cryptococcal) B45.1
  toxic NEC G92
  trichinosis B75 [G05.3]
  type
    B A83.0
    C A83.3
  van Bogaert's A81.1
  Venezuelan equine A92.2
  Vienna A85.8
  viral, virus A86
    arthropod-borne NEC A85.2
      mosquito-borne A83.9
        Australian X disease A83.4
        California virus A83.5
        Eastern equine A83.2
        Japanese (B type) A83.0
        Murray Valley A83.4
        specified NEC A83.8
        St. Louis A83.3
        type B A83.0
        type C A83.3
        Western equine A83.1
      tick-borne A84.9
        biundulant A84.1
        central European A84.1
        Czechoslovakian A84.1
        diphasic meningoencephalitis A84.1
        Far Eastern A84.0
        Russian spring-summer (taiga) A84.0
        specified NEC A84.8
    specified type NEC A85.8
  Western equine A83.1
Encephalocele Q01.9
  frontal Q01.0
  nasofrontal Q01.1
  occipital Q01.2
  specified NEC Q01.8
Encephalocystocele — *see* Encephalocele
Encephaloduroarteriomyosynangiosis (EDAMS) I67.5
Encephalomalacia (brain) (cerebellar) (cerebral) —
  Softening, brain

Encephalomeningitis — *see* Meningoencephalitis
Encephalomeningocele — *see* Encephalocele
Encephalomeningomyelitis — *see* Meningoencephalitis
Encephalomyelitis (*see also* Encephalitis) G04.90
  acute disseminated G04.00
    infectious G04.01
    noninfectious G04.81
    postimmunization G04.02
    postinfectious G04.01
  acute necrotizing hemorrhagic G04.30
    postimmunization G04.32
    postinfectious G04.31
    specified NEC G04.39
  benign myalgic G93.3
  equine A83.9
    Eastern A83.2
    Venezuelan A92.2
    Western A83.1
  in diseases classified elsewhere G05.3
  myalgic, benign G93.3
  postchickenpox B01.11
  postinfectious NEC G04.01
  postmeasles B05.0
  postvaccinal G04.02
  postvaricella B01.11
  rubella B06.01
  specified NEC G04.81
  Venezuelan equine A92.2
Encephalomyelocele — *see* Encephalocele
Encephalomyelomeningitis — *see* Meningoencephalitis
Encephalomyelopathy G96.9
Encephalomyeloradiculitis (acute) G61.0
Encephalomyeloradiculoneuritis (acute) (Guillain-
  Barré) G61.0
Encephalomyeloradiculopathy G96.9
Encephalopathia hyperbilirubinemica, newborn
  P57.9
  due to isoimmunization (conditions in P55) P57.0
Encephalopathy (acute) G93.40
  acute necrotizing hemorrhagic G04.30
    postimmunization G04.32
    postinfectious G04.31
    specified NEC G04.39
  alcoholic G31.2
  anoxic — *see* Damage, brain, anoxic
  arteriosclerotic I67.2
  centrolobar progressive (Schilder) G37.0
  congenital Q07.9
  degenerative, in specified disease NEC G32.89
  demyelinating callosal G37.1
  due to
    drugs (*see also* Table of Drugs and Chemicals) G92
  hepatic — *see* Failure, hepatic
  hyperbilirubinemic, newborn P57.9
    due to isoimmunization (conditions in P55) P57.0
  hypertensive I67.4
  hypoglycemic E16.2
  hypoxic — *see* Damage, brain, anoxic
  hypoxic ischemic P91.60
    mild P91.61
    moderate P91.62
    severe P91.63
  in (due to) (with)
    birth injury P11.1
    hyperinsulinism E16.1 [G94]
    influenza — *see* Influenza, with, encephalopathy
    lack of vitamin (*see also* Deficiency, vitamin)
      E56.9 [G32.89]
    neoplastic disease (*see also* Neoplasm)
      D49.9 [G13.1]
    serum (*see also* Reaction, serum) T80.69 ☑
    syphilis A52.17
    trauma (postconcussional) F07.81
      current injury — *see* Injury, intracranial
    vaccination G04.02
  lead — *see* Poisoning, lead
  metabolic G93.41
    drug induced G92
    toxic G92
  myoclonic, early, symptomatic — *see* Epilepsy, gener-
    alized, specified NEC
  necrotizing, subacute (Leigh) G31.82
  pellagrous E52 [G32.89]
  portosystemic — *see* Failure, hepatic
  postcontusional F07.81
    current injury — *see* Injury, intracranial, diffuse

Encephalopathy — *continued*
posthypoglycemic (coma) E16.1 [G94]
postradiation G93.89
saturnine — *see* Poisoning, lead
septic G93.41
specified NEC G93.49
spongioform, subacute (viral) A81.09
toxic G92
metabolic G92
traumatic (postconcussional) F07.81
current injury — *see* Injury, intracranial
vitamin B deficiency NEC E53.9 [G32.89]
vitamin B1 E51.2
Wernicke's E51.2
Encephalorrhagia — *see* Hemorrhage, intracranial, intracerebral
Encephalosis, posttraumatic F07.81
Enchondroma (*see also* Neoplasm, bone, benign)
Enchondromatosis (cartilaginous) (multiple) Q78.4
Encopresis R15.9
functional F98.1
nonorganic origin F98.1
psychogenic F98.1
Encounter (with health service) (for) Z76.89
adjustment and management (of)
breast implant Z45.81 ☑
implanted device NEC Z45.89
myringotomy device (stent) (tube) Z45.82
administrative purpose only Z02.9
examination for
adoption Z02.82
armed forces Z02.3
disability determination Z02.71
driving license Z02.4
employment Z02.1
insurance Z02.6
medical certificate NEC Z02.79
paternity testing Z02.81
residential institution admission Z02.2
school admission Z02.0
sports Z02.5
specified reason NEC Z02.89
aftercare — *see* Aftercare
antenatal screening Z36
assisted reproductive fertility procedure cycle Z31.83
blood typing Z01.83
Rh typing Z01.83
breast augmentation or reduction Z41.1
breast implant exchange (different material) (different size) Z45.81 ☑
breast reconstruction following mastectomy Z42.1
check-up — *see* Examination
chemotherapy for neoplasm Z51.11
colonoscopy, screening Z12.11
counseling — *see* Counseling
delivery, full-term, uncomplicated O80
cesarean, without indication O82
ear piercing Z41.3
examination — *see* Examination
expectant parent(s) (adoptive) pre-birth pediatrician visit Z76.81
fertility preservation procedure (prior to cancer therapy) (prior to removal of gonads) Z31.84
fitting (of) — *see* Fitting (and adjustment) (of)
genetic
counseling Z31.5
testing — *see* Test, genetic
hearing conservation and treatment Z01.12
immunotherapy for neoplasm Z51.12
in vitro fertilization cycle Z31.83
instruction (in)
child care (postpartal) (prenatal) Z32.3
childbirth Z32.2
natural family planning
procreative Z31.61
to avoid pregnancy Z30.02
insulin pump titration Z46.81
joint prosthesis insertion following prior explantation of joint prosthesis (staged procedure)
hip Z47.32
knee Z47.33
shoulder Z47.31
laboratory (as part of a general medical examination) Z00.00
with abnormal findings Z00.01
mental health services (for)
abuse NEC
perpetrator Z69.82

Encounter — *continued*
mental health services — *continued*
abuse — *continued*
victim Z69.81
child abuse
nonparental
perpetrator Z69.021
victim Z69.020
parental
perpetrator Z69.011
victim Z69.010
spousal or partner abuse
perpetrator Z69.12
victim Z69.11
observation (for) (ruled out)
exposure to (suspected)
anthrax Z03.810
biological agent NEC Z03.818
pediatrician visit, by expectant parent(s) (adoptive) Z76.81
plastic and reconstructive surgery following medical procedure or healed injury NEC Z42.8
pregnancy
supervision of — *see* Pregnancy, supervision of
test Z32.00
result negative Z32.02
result positive Z32.01
radiation therapy (antineoplastic) Z51.0
radiological (as part of a general medical examination) Z00.00
with abnormal findings Z00.01
reconstructive surgery following medical procedure or healed injury NEC Z42.8
removal (of) (*see also* Removal)
artificial
arm Z44.00- ☑
complete Z44.01- ☑
partial Z44.02- ☑
eye Z44.2- ☑
leg Z44.10- ☑
complete Z44.11- ☑
partial Z44.12- ☑
breast implant Z45.81 ☑
tissue expander (without synchronous insertion of permanent implant) Z45.81 ☑
device Z46.9
specified NEC Z46.89
external
fixation device — *code to* fracture with seventh character D
prosthesis, prosthetic device Z44.9
breast Z44.3- ☑
specified NEC Z44.8
implanted device NEC Z45.89
insulin pump Z46.81
internal fixation device Z47.2
myringotomy device (stent) (tube) Z45.82
nervous system device NEC Z46.2
brain neuropacemaker Z46.2
visual substitution device Z46.2
implanted Z45.31
non-vascular catheter Z46.82
orthodontic device Z46.4
stent
ureteral Z46.6
urinary device Z46.6
repeat cervical smear to confirm findings of recent normal smear following initial abnormal smear Z01.42
respirator [ventilator] use during power failure Z99.12
Rh typing Z01.83
screening — *see* Screening
specified NEC Z76.89
sterilization Z30.2
suspected condition, ruled out
amniotic cavity and membrane Z03.71
cervical shortening Z03.75
fetal anomaly Z03.73
fetal growth Z03.74
maternal and fetal conditions NEC Z03.79
oligohydramnios Z03.71
placental problem Z03.72
polyhydramnios Z03.71
suspected exposure (to), ruled out
anthrax Z03.810
biological agents NEC Z03.818
termination of pregnancy, elective Z33.2
testing — *see* Test

Encounter — *continued*
therapeutic drug level monitoring Z51.81
titration, insulin pump Z46.81
to determine fetal viability of pregnancy O36.80 ☑
training
insulin pump Z46.81
X-ray of chest (as part of a general medical examination) Z00.00
with abnormal findings Z00.01
Encystment — *see* Cyst
Endarteritis (bacterial, subacute) (infective) I77.6
brain I67.7
cerebral or cerebrospinal I67.7
deformans — *see* Arteriosclerosis
embolic — *see* Embolism
obliterans (*see also* Arteriosclerosis)
pulmonary I28.8
pulmonary I28.8
retina — *see* Vasculitis, retina
senile — *see* Arteriosclerosis
syphilitic A52.09
brain or cerebral A52.04
congenital A50.54 [I79.8]
tuberculous A18.89
Endemic — *see* condition
Endocarditis (chronic) (marantic) (nonbacterial) (thrombotic) (valvular) I38
with rheumatic fever (conditions in I00)
active — *see* Endocarditis, acute, rheumatic
inactive or quiescent (with chorea) I09.1
acute or subacute I33.9
infective I33.0
rheumatic (aortic) (mitral) (pulmonary) (tricuspid) I01.1
with chorea (acute) (rheumatic) (Sydenham's) I02.0
aortic (heart) (nonrheumatic) (valve) I35.8
with
mitral disease I08.0
with tricuspid (valve) disease I08.3
active or acute I01.1
with chorea (acute) (rheumatic) (Sydenham's) I02.0
rheumatic fever (conditions in I00)
active — *see* Endocarditis, acute, rheumatic
inactive or quiescent (with chorea) I06.9
tricuspid (valve) disease I08.2
with mitral (valve) disease I08.3
acute or subacute I33.9
arteriosclerotic I35.8
rheumatic I06.9
with mitral disease I08.0
with tricuspid (valve) disease I08.3
active or acute I01.1
with chorea (acute) (rheumatic) (Sydenham's) I02.0
active or acute I01.1
with chorea (acute) (rheumatic) (Sydenham's) I02.0
specified NEC I06.8
specified cause NEC I35.8
syphilitic A52.03
arteriosclerotic I38
atypical verrucous (Libman-Sacks) M32.11
bacterial (acute) (any valve) (subacute) I33.0
candidal B37.6
congenital Q24.8
constrictive I33.0
Coxiella burnetii A78 [I39]
Coxsackie B33.21
due to
prosthetic cardiac valve T82.6 ☑
Q fever A78 [I39]
Serratia marcescens I33.0
typhoid (fever) A01.02
gonococcal A54.83
infectious or infective (acute) (any valve) (subacute) I33.0
lenta (acute) (any valve) (subacute) I33.0
Libman-Sacks M32.11
listerial A32.82
Löffler's I42.3
malignant (acute) (any valve) (subacute) I33.0
meningococcal A39.51
mitral (chronic) (double) (fibroid) (heart) (inactive) (valve) (with chorea) I05.9
with
aortic (valve) disease I08.0

☑ **Additional Character Required — Refer to the Tabular List for Character Selection**   ▽ **Subterms under main terms may continue to next column or page**

Endocarditis — *continued*
 mitral — *continued*
  with — *continued*
   aortic disease — *continued*
    with tricuspid (valve) disease I08.3
    active or acute I01.1
     with chorea (acute) (rheumatic) (Sydenham's) I02.0
   rheumatic fever (conditions in I00)
    active — *see* Endocarditis, acute, rheumatic
    inactive or quiescent (with chorea) I05.9
   tricuspid (valve) disease I08.1
    with aortic (valve) disease I08.3
   active or acute I01.1
    with chorea (acute) (rheumatic) (Sydenham's) I02.0
   bacterial I33.0
   arteriosclerotic I34.8
   nonrheumatic I34.8
    acute or subacute I33.9
   specified NEC I05.8
  monilial B37.6
  multiple valves I08.9
   specified disorders I08.8
  mycotic (acute) (any valve) (subacute) I33.0
  pneumococcal (acute) (any valve) (subacute) I33.0
  pulmonary (chronic) (heart) (valve) I37.8
   with rheumatic fever (conditions in I00)
    active — *see* Endocarditis, acute, rheumatic
    inactive or quiescent (with chorea) I09.89
     with aortic, mitral or tricuspid disease I08.8
   acute or subacute I33.9
    rheumatic I01.1
     with chorea (acute) (rheumatic) (Sydenham's) I02.0
   arteriosclerotic I37.8
   congenital Q22.2
   rheumatic (chronic) (inactive) (with chorea) I09.89
    active or acute I01.1
     with chorea (acute) (rheumatic) (Sydenham's) I02.0
   syphilitic A52.03
  purulent (acute) (any valve) (subacute) I33.0
  Q fever A78 [I39]
  rheumatic (chronic) (inactive) (with chorea) I09.1
   active or acute (aortic) (mitral) (pulmonary) (tricuspid) I01.1
    with chorea (acute) (rheumatic) (Sydenham's) I02.0
  rheumatoid — *see* Rheumatoid, carditis
  septic (acute) (any valve) (subacute) I33.0
  streptococcal (acute) (any valve) (subacute) I33.0
  subacute — *see* Endocarditis, acute
  suppurative (acute) (any valve) (subacute) I33.0
  syphilitic A52.03
  toxic I33.9
  tricuspid (chronic) (heart) (inactive) (rheumatic) (valve) (with chorea) I07.9
   with
    aortic (valve) disease I08.2
     mitral (valve) disease I08.3
    mitral (valve) disease I08.1
     aortic (valve) disease I08.3
    rheumatic fever (conditions in I00)
     active — *see* Endocarditis, acute, rheumatic
     inactive or quiescent (with chorea) I07.8
   active or acute I01.1
    with chorea (acute) (rheumatic) (Sydenham's) I02.0
   arteriosclerotic I36.8
   nonrheumatic I36.8
    acute or subacute I33.9
   specified cause, except rheumatic I36.8
  tuberculous — *see* Tuberculosis, endocarditis
  typhoid A01.02
  ulcerative (acute) (any valve) (subacute) I33.0
  vegetative (acute) (any valve) (subacute) I33.0
  verrucous (atypical) (nonbacterial) (nonrheumatic) M32.11
Endocardium, endocardial (*see also* condition)
 cushion defect Q21.2
Endocervicitis (*see also* Cervicitis)
 due to intrauterine (contraceptive) device T83.6 ☑
 hyperplastic N72
Endocrine — *see* condition
Endocrinopathy, pluriglandular E31.9
Endodontic
 overfill M27.52

Endodontic — *continued*
 underfill M27.53
Endodontitis K04.0
Endomastoiditis — *see* Mastoiditis
Endometrioma N80.9
Endometriosis N80.9
 appendix N80.5
 bladder N80.8
 bowel N80.5
 broad ligament N80.3
 cervix N80.0
 colon N80.5
 cul-de-sac (Douglas') N80.3
 exocervix N80.0
 fallopian tube N80.2
 female genital organ NEC N80.8
 gallbladder N80.8
 in scar of skin N80.6
 internal N80.0
 intestine N80.5
 lung N80.8
 myometrium N80.0
 ovary N80.1
 parametrium N80.3
 pelvic peritoneum N80.3
 peritoneal (pelvic) N80.3
 rectovaginal septum N80.4
 rectum N80.5
 round ligament N80.3
 skin (scar) N80.6
 specified site NEC N80.8
 stromal D39.0
 umbilicus N80.8
 uterus (internal) N80.0
 vagina N80.4
 vulva N80.8
Endometritis (decidual) (nonspecific) (purulent) (senile) (atrophic) (suppurative) N71.9
 with ectopic pregnancy O08.0
 acute N71.0
 blenorrhagic (gonococcal) (acute) (chronic) A54.24
 cervix, cervical (with erosion or ectropion) (*see also* Cervicitis)
  hyperplastic N72
 chlamydial A56.11
 chronic N71.1
 following
  abortion — *see* Abortion by type complicated by genital infection
  ectopic or molar pregnancy O08.0
 gonococcal, gonorrheal (acute) (chronic) A54.24
 hyperplastic (*see also* Hyperplasia, endometrial) N85.00
  cervix N72
 puerperal, postpartum, childbirth O86.12
 subacute N71.0
 tuberculous A18.17
Endometrium — *see* condition
Endomyocardiopathy, South African I42.3
Endomyocarditis — *see* Endocarditis
Endomyofibrosis I42.3
Endomyometritis — *see* Endometritis
Endopericarditis — *see* Endocarditis
Endoperineuritis — *see* Disorder, nerve
Endophlebitis — *see* Phlebitis
Endophthalmia — *see* Endophthalmitis, purulent
Endophthalmitis (acute) (infective) (metastatic) (subacute) H44.009
 bleb associated (*see also* Bleb, inflamed (infected), postprocedural H59.4 ☑
 gonorrheal A54.39
 in (due to)
  cysticercosis B69.1
  onchocerciasis B73.01
  toxocariasis B83.0
 panuveitis — *see* Panuveitis
 parasitic H44.12- ☑
 purulent H44.00- ☑
  panophthalmitis — *see* Panophthalmitis
  vitreous abscess H44.02- ☑
 specified NEC H44.19
 sympathetic — *see* Uveitis, sympathetic
Endosalpingioma D28.2
Endosalpingiosis N94.89
Endosteitis — *see* Osteomyelitis
Endothelioma, bone — *see* Neoplasm, bone, malignant
Endotheliosis (hemorrhagic infectional) D69.8
Endotoxemia — *code to* condition

Endotrachelitis — *see* Cervicitis
Engelmann (-Camurati) **syndrome** Q78.3
English disease — *see* Rickets
Engman's disease L30.3
Engorgement
 breast N64.59
  newborn P83.4
  puerperal, postpartum O92.79
 lung (passive) — *see* Edema, lung
 pulmonary (passive) — *see* Edema, lung
 stomach K31.89
 venous — *see* Occlusion, retina, vein, engorgement
Enlargement, enlarged (*see also* Hypertrophy)
 adenoids J35.2
  with tonsils J35.3
 alveolar ridge K08.8
  congenital — *see* Anomaly, alveolar
 apertures of diaphragm (congenital) Q79.1
 gingival K06.1
 heart, cardiac — *see* Hypertrophy, cardiac
 lacrimal gland, chronic H04.03- ☑
 liver — *see* Hypertrophy, liver
 lymph gland or node R59.9
  generalized R59.1
  localized R59.0
 orbit H05.34- ☑
 organ or site, congenital NEC — *see* Anomaly, by site
 parathyroid (gland) E21.0
 pituitary fossa R93.0
 prostate N40.0
  with lower urinary tract symptoms (LUTS) N40.1
  without lower urinary tract symtpoms (LUTS) N40.0
 sella turcica R93.0
 spleen — *see* Splenomegaly
 thymus (gland) (congenital) E32.0
 thyroid (gland) — *see* Goiter
 tongue K14.8
 tonsils J35.1
  with adenoids J35.3
 uterus N85.2
Enophthalmos H05.40- ☑
 due to
  orbital tissue atrophy H05.41- ☑
  trauma or surgery H05.42- ☑
Enostosis M27.8
Entamebic, entamebiasis — *see* Amebiasis
Entanglement
 umbilical cord(s) O69.2 ☑
  with compression O69.2 ☑
   without compression O69.82 ☑
  around neck (with compression) O69.1 ☑
   without compression O69.81 ☑
  of twins in monoamniotic sac O69.2 ☑
Enteralgia — *see* Pain, abdominal
Enteric — *see* condition
Enteritis (acute) (diarrheal) (hemorrhagic) (noninfective) (septic) K52.9
 adenovirus A08.2
 aertrycke infection A02.0
 allergic K52.2
 amebic (acute) A06.0
  with abscess — *see* Abscess, amebic
  chronic A06.1
   with abscess — *see* Abscess, amebic
   nondysenteric A06.2
  nondysenteric A06.2
 astrovirus A08.32
 bacillary NOS A03.9
 bacterial A04.9
  specified NEC A04.8
 calicivirus A08.31
 candidal B37.82
 Chilomastix A07.8
 choleriformis A00.1
 chronic (noninfectious) K52.9
  ulcerative — *see* Colitis, ulcerative
 cicatrizing (chronic) — *see* Enteritis, regional, small intestine
 Clostridium
  botulinum (food poisoning) A05.1
  difficile A04.7
 coccidial A07.3
 coxsackie virus A08.39
 dietetic K52.2
 drug-induced K52.1

Enteritis — *continued*
 due to
  astrovirus A08.32
  calicivirus A08.31
  coxsackie virus A08.39
  drugs K52.1
  echovirus A08.39
  enterovirus NEC A08.39
  food hypersensitivity K52.2
  infectious organism (bacterial) (viral) — *see* Enteritis, infectious
  torovirus A08.39
  Yersinia enterocolitica A04.6
 echovirus A08.39
 eltor A00.1
 enterovirus NEC A08.39
 eosinophilic K52.81
 epidemic (infectious) A09
 fulminant K55.0
 gangrenous — *see* Enteritis, infectious
 giardial A07.1
 infectious NOS A09
  due to
   adenovirus A08.2
   Aerobacter aerogenes A04.8
   Arizona (bacillus) A02.0
   bacteria NOS A04.9
    specified NEC A04.8
   Campylobacter A04.5
   Clostridium difficile A04.7
   Clostridium perfringens A04.8
   Enterobacter aerogenes A04.8
   enterovirus A08.39
   Escherichia coli A04.4
    enteroaggregative A04.4
    enterohemorrhagic A04.3
    enteroinvasive A04.2
    enteropathogenic A04.0
    enterotoxigenic A04.1
    specified NEC A04.4
   specified
    bacteria NEC A04.8
    virus NEC A08.39
   Staphylococcus A04.8
   virus NEC A08.4
    specified type NEC A08.39
   Yersinia enterocolitica A04.6
  specified organism NEC A08.8
 influenzal — *see* Influenza, with, digestive manifestations
 ischemic K55.9
  acute K55.0
  chronic K55.1
 microsporidial A07.8
 mucomembranous, myxomembranous — *see* Syndrome, irritable bowel
 mucous — *see* Syndrome, irritable bowel
 necroticans A05.2
 necrotizing of newborn — *see* Enterocolitis, necrotizing, in newborn
 neurogenic — *see* Syndrome, irritable bowel
 newborn necrotizing — *see* Enterocolitis, necrotizing, in newborn
 noninfectious K52.9
 norovirus A08.11
 parasitic NEC B82.9
 paratyphoid (fever) — *see* Fever, paratyphoid
 protozoal A07.9
  specified NEC A07.8
 radiation K52.0
 regional (of) K50.90
  with
   complication K50.919
    abscess K50.914
    fistula K50.913
    intestinal obstruction K50.912
    rectal bleeding K50.911
    specified complication NEC K50.918
  colon — *see* Enteritis, regional, large intestine
  duodenum — *see* Enteritis, regional, small intestine
  ileum — *see* Enteritis, regional, small intestine
  jejunum — *see* Enteritis, regional, small intestine
  large bowel — *see* Enteritis, regional, large intestine
  large intestine (colon) (rectum) K50.10
   with
    complication K50.119
     abscess K50.114

Enteritis — *continued*
 regional — *continued*
  large intestine — *continued*
   with — *continued*
    complication — *continued*
     fistula K50.113
     intestinal obstruction K50.112
     rectal bleeding K50.111
     small intestine (duodenum) (ileum) (jejunum) involvement K50.80
      with
       complication K50.819
        abscess K50.814
        fistula K50.813
        intestinal obstruction K50.812
        rectal bleeding K50.811
        specified complication NEC K50.818
     specified complication NEC K50.118
  rectum — *see* Enteritis, regional, large intestine
  small intestine (duodenum) (ileum) (jejunum) K50.00
   with
    complication K50.019
     abscess K50.014
     fistula K50.013
     intestinal obstruction K50.012
     large intestine (colon) (rectum) involvement K50.80
      with
       complication K50.819
        abscess K50.814
        fistula K50.813
        intestinal obstruction K50.812
        rectal bleeding K50.811
        specified complication NEC K50.818
     rectal bleeding K50.011
     specified complication NEC K50.018
 rotaviral A08.0
 Salmonella, salmonellosis (arizonae) (cholerae-suis) (enteritidis) (typhimurium) A02.0
 segmental — *see* Enteritis, regional
 septic A09
 Shigella — *see* Infection, Shigella
 small round structured NEC A08.19
 spasmodic, spastic — *see* Syndrome, irritable bowel
 staphylococcal A04.8
  due to food A05.0
 torovirus A08.39
 toxic NEC K52.1
  due to Clostridium difficile A04.7
 trichomonal A07.8
 tuberculous A18.32
 typhosa A01.00
 ulcerative (chronic) — *see* Colitis, ulcerative
 viral A08.4
  adenovirus A08.2
  enterovirus A08.39
  Rotavirus A08.0
  small round structured NEC A08.19
  specified NEC A08.39
  virus specified NEC A08.39

Enterobiasis B80
Enterobius vermicularis (infection) (infestation) B80
Enterocele (*see also* Hernia, abdomen)
 pelvic, pelvis (acquired) (congenital) N81.5
 vagina, vaginal (acquired) (congenital) NEC N81.5
Enterocolitis (*see also* Enteritis) K52.9
 due to Clostridium difficile A04.7
 fulminant ischemic K55.0
 granulomatous — *see* Enteritis, regional
 hemorrhagic (acute) K55.0
  chronic K55.1
 infectious NEC A09
 ischemic K55.9
 necrotizing
  due to Clostridium difficile A04.7
  in newborn P77.9
   stage 1 (without pneumatosis, without perforation) P77.1
   stage 2 (with pneumatosis, without perforation) P77.2
   stage 3 (with pneumatosis, with perforation) P77.3
 noninfectious K52.9
 newborn — *see* Enterocolitis, necrotizing, in newborn

Enterocolitis — *continued*
 pseudomembranous (newborn) A04.7
 radiation K52.0
  newborn — *see* Enterocolitis, necrotizing, in newborn
 ulcerative (chronic) — *see* Pancolitis, ulcerative (chronic)
Enterogastritis — *see* Enteritis
Enteropathy K63.9
 gluten-sensitive K90.0
 hemorrhagic, terminal K55.0
 protein-losing K90.4
Enteroperitonitis — *see* Peritonitis
Enteroptosis K63.4
Enterorrhagia K92.2
Enterospasm (*see also* Syndrome, irritable, bowel)
 psychogenic F45.8
Enterostenosis (*see also* Obstruction, intestine) K56.69
Enterostomy
 complication — *see* Complication, enterostomy
 status Z93.4
Enterovirus, as cause of disease classified elsewhere B97.10
 coxsackievirus B97.11
 echovirus B97.12
 other specified B97.19
Enthesopathy (peripheral) M77.9
 Achilles tendinitis — *see* Tendinitis, Achilles
 ankle and tarsus M77.9
  specified type NEC — *see* Enthesopathy, foot, specified type NEC
 anterior tibial syndrome M76.81- ☑
 calcaneal spur — *see* Spur, bone, calcaneal
 elbow region M77.8
  lateral epicondylitis — *see* Epicondylitis, lateral
  medial epicondylitis — *see* Epicondylitis, medial
 foot NEC M77.9
  metatarsalgia — *see* Metatarsalgia
  specified type NEC M77.5- ☑
 forearm M77.9
 gluteal tendinitis — *see* Tendinitis, gluteal
 hand M77.9
 hip — *see* Enthesopathy, lower limb, specified type NEC
 iliac crest spur — *see* Spur, bone, iliac crest
 iliotibial band syndrome — *see* Syndrome, iliotibial band
 knee — *see* Enthesopathy, lower limb, lower leg, specified type NEC
 lateral epicondylitis — *see* Epicondylitis, lateral
 lower limb (excluding foot) M76.9
  Achilles tendinitis — *see* Tendinitis, Achilles
  anterior tibial syndrome M76.81- ☑
  gluteal tendinitis — *see* Tendinitis, gluteal
  iliac crest spur — *see* Spur, bone, iliac crest
  iliotibial band syndrome — *see* Syndrome, iliotibial band
  patellar tendinitis — *see* Tendinitis, patellar
  pelvic region — *see* Enthesopathy, lower limb, specified type NEC
  peroneal tendinitis — *see* Tendinitis, peroneal
  posterior tibial syndrome M76.82- ☑
  psoas tendinitis — *see* Tendinitis, psoas
  shoulder M77.9
  specified type NEC M76.89- ☑
  tibial collateral bursitis — *see* Bursitis, tibial collateral
 medial epicondylitis — *see* Epicondylitis, medial
 metatarsalgia — *see* Metatarsalgia
 multiple sites M77.9
 patellar tendinitis — *see* Tendinitis, patellar
 pelvis M77.9
 periarthritis of wrist — *see* Periarthritis, wrist
 peroneal tendinitis — *see* Tendinitis, peroneal
 posterior tibial syndrome M76.82- ☑
 psoas tendinitis — *see* Tendinitis, psoas
 shoulder region — *see* Lesion, shoulder
 specified site NEC M77.9
 specified type NEC M77.8
 spinal M46.00
  cervical region M46.02
  cervicothoracic region M46.03
  lumbar region M46.06
  lumbosacral region M46.07
  multiple sites M46.09
  occipito-atlanto-axial region M46.01
  sacrococcygeal region M46.08

Enthesopathy — *continued*
　spinal — *continued*
　　thoracic region M46.04
　　thoracolumbar region M46.05
　tibial collateral bursitis — *see* Bursitis, tibial collateral
　upper arm M77.9
　wrist and carpus NEC M77.8
　　calcaneal spur — *see* Spur, bone, calcaneal
　　periarthritis of wrist — *see* Periarthritis, wrist
Entomophobia F40.218
Entomophthoromycosis B46.8
Entrance, air into vein — *see* Embolism, air
Entrapment, nerve — *see* Neuropathy, entrapment
Entropion (eyelid) (paralytic) H02.009
　cicatricial H02.019
　　left H02.016
　　　lower H02.015
　　　upper H02.014
　　right H02.013
　　　lower H02.012
　　　upper H02.011
　congenital Q10.2
　　left H02.006
　　　lower H02.005
　　　upper H02.004
　mechanical H02.029
　　left H02.026
　　　lower H02.025
　　　upper H02.024
　　right H02.023
　　　lower H02.022
　　　upper H02.021
　right H02.003
　　lower H02.002
　　upper H02.001
　senile H02.039
　　left H02.036
　　　lower H02.035
　　　upper H02.034
　　right H02.033
　　　lower H02.032
　　　upper H02.031
　spastic H02.049
　　left H02.046
　　　lower H02.045
　　　upper H02.044
　　right H02.043
　　　lower H02.042
　　　upper H02.041
Enucleated eye (traumatic, current) S05.7- ☑
Enuresis R32
　functional F98.0
　habit disturbance F98.0
　nocturnal N39.44
　　psychogenic F98.0
　nonorganic origin F98.0
　psychogenic F98.0
Eosinopenia — *see* Agranulocytosis
Eosinophilia (allergic) (hereditary) (idiopathic) (secondary) D72.1
　with
　　angiolymphoid hyperplasia (ALHE) D18.01
　infiltrative J82
　Löffler's J82
　peritoneal — *see* Peritonitis, eosinophilic
　pulmonary NEC J82
　tropical (pulmonary) J82
Eosinophilia-myalgia syndrome M35.8
Ependymitis (acute) (cerebral) (chronic) (granular) — *see* Encephalomyelitis
Ependymoblastoma
　specified site — *see* Neoplasm, malignant, by site
　unspecified site C71.9
Ependymoma (epithelial) (malignant)
　anaplastic
　　specified site — *see* Neoplasm, malignant, by site
　　unspecified site C71.9
　benign
　　specified site — *see* Neoplasm, benign, by site
　　unspecified site D33.2
　myxopapillary D43.2
　　specified site — *see* Neoplasm, uncertain behavior, by site
　　unspecified site D43.2
　papillary D43.2
　　specified site — *see* Neoplasm, uncertain behavior, by site
　　unspecified site D43.2

Ependymoma — *continued*
　specified site — *see* Neoplasm, malignant, by site
　unspecified site C71.9
Ependymopathy G93.89
Ephelis, ephelides L81.2
Epiblepharon (congenital) Q10.3
Epicanthus, epicanthic fold (eyelid) (congenital) Q10.3
Epicondylitis (elbow)
　lateral M77.1- ☑
　medial M77.0- ☑
Epicystitis — *see* Cystitis
Epidemic — *see* condition
Epidermidalization, cervix — *see* Dysplasia, cervix
Epidermis, epidermal — *see* condition
Epidermodysplasia verruciformis B07.8
Epidermolysis
　bullosa (congenital) Q81.9
　　acquired L12.30
　　　drug-induced L12.31
　　　specified cause NEC L12.35
　　dystrophica Q81.2
　　letalis Q81.1
　　simplex Q81.0
　　specified NEC Q81.8
　necroticans combustiformis L51.2
　　due to drug — *see* Table of Drugs and Chemicals, by drug
Epidermophytid — *see* Dermatophytosis
Epidermophytosis (infected) — *see* Dermatophytosis
Epididymis — *see* condition
Epididymitis (acute) (nonvenereal) (recurrent) (residual) N45.1
　with orchitis N45.3
　blennorrhagic (gonococcal) A54.23
　caseous (tuberculous) A18.15
　chlamydial A56.19
　filarial (*see also* Infestation, filarial) B74.9 [N51]
　gonococcal A54.23
　syphilitic A52.76
　tuberculous A18.15
Epididymo-orchitis (*see also* Epididymitis) N45.3
Epidural — *see* condition
Epigastrium, epigastric — *see* condition
Epigastrocele — *see* Hernia, ventral
Epiglottis — *see* condition
Epiglottitis, epiglottiditis (acute) J05.10
　with obstruction J05.11
　chronic J37.0
Epignathus Q89.4
Epilepsia partialis continua (*see also* Kozhevnikof's epilepsy) G40.1- ☑
Epilepsy, epileptic, epilepsia (attack) (cerebral) (convulsion) (fit) (seizure) G40.909

> *Note: the following terms are to be considered equivalent to intractable: pharmacoresistant (pharmacologically resistant), treatment resistant, refractory (medically) and poorly controlled*

　with
　　complex partial seizures — *see* Epilepsy, localization-related, symptomatic, with complex partial seizures
　　grand mal seizures on awakening — *see* Epilepsy, generalized, specified NEC
　　myoclonic absences — *see* Epilepsy, generalized, specified NEC
　　myoclonic-astatic seizures — *see* Epilepsy, generalized, specified NEC
　　simple partial seizures — *see* Epilepsy, localization-related, symptomatic, with simple partial seizures
　akinetic — *see* Epilepsy, generalized, specified NEC
　benign childhood with centrotemporal EEG spikes — *see* Epilepsy, localization-related, idiopathic
　benign myoclonic in infancy G40.80- ☑
　Bravais-jacksonian — *see* Epilepsy, localization-related, symptomatic, with simple partial seizures
　childhood
　　with occipital EEG paroxysms — *see* Epilepsy, localization-related, idiopathic
　　absence G40.A09 (*following* G40.3)
　　　intractable G40.A19 (*following* G40.3)
　　　　with status epilepticus G40.A11 (*following* G40.3)
　　　　without status epilepticus G40.A19 (*following* G40.3)
　　　not intractable G40.A09 (*following* G40.3)

Epilepsy, epileptic, epilepsia — *continued*
　childhood — *continued*
　　absence — *continued*
　　　not intractable — *continued*
　　　　with status epilepticus G40.A01 (*following* G40.3)
　　　　without status epilepticus G40.A09 (*following* G40.3)
　climacteric — *see* Epilepsy, specified NEC
　cysticercosis B69.0
　deterioration (mental) F06.8
　due to syphilis A52.19
　focal — *see* Epilepsy, localization-related, symptomatic, with simple partial seizures
　generalized
　　idiopathic G40.309
　　　intractable G40.319
　　　　with status epilepticus G40.311
　　　　without status epilepticus G40.319
　　　not intractable G40.309
　　　　with status epilepticus G40.301
　　　　without status epilepticus G40.309
　　specified NEC G40.409
　　　intractable G40.419
　　　　with status epilepticus G40.411
　　　　without status epilepticus G40.419
　　　not intractable G40.409
　　　　with status epilepticus G40.401
　　　　without status epilepticus G40.409
　impulsive petit mal — *see* Epilepsy, juvenile myoclonic
　intractable G40.919
　　with status epilepticus G40.911
　　without status epilepticus G40.919
　juvenile absence G40.A09 (*following* G40.3)
　　intractable G40.A19 (*following* G40.3)
　　　with status epilepticus G40.A11 (*following* G40.3)
　　　without status epilepticus G40.A19 (*following* G40.3)
　　not intractable G40.A09 (*following* G40.3)
　　　with status epilepticus G40.A01 (*following* G40.3)
　　　without status epilepticus G40.A09 (*following* G40.3)
　juvenile myoclonic G40.B09 (*following* G40.3)
　　intractable G40.B19 (*following* G40.3)
　　　with status epilepticus G40.B11 (*following* G40.3)
　　　without status epilepticus G40.B19 (*following* G40.3)
　　not intractable G40.B09 (*following* G40.3)
　　　with status epilepticus G40.B01 (*following* G40.3)
　　　without status epilepticus G40.B09 (*following* G40.3)
　localization-related (focal) (partial)
　　idiopathic G40.009
　　　with seizures of localized onset G40.009
　　　　intractable G40.019
　　　　　with status epilepticus G40.011
　　　　　without status epilepticus G40.019
　　　　not intractable G40.009
　　　　　with status epilepticus G40.001
　　　　　without status epilepticus G40.009
　　symptomatic
　　　with complex partial seizures G40.209
　　　　intractable G40.219
　　　　　with status epilepticus G40.211
　　　　　without status epilepticus G40.219
　　　　not intractable G40.209
　　　　　with status epilepticus G40.201
　　　　　without status epilepticus G40.209
　　　with simple partial seizures G40.109
　　　　intractable G40.119
　　　　　with status epilepticus G40.111
　　　　　without status epilepticus G40.119
　　　　not intractable G40.109
　　　　　with status epilepticus G40.101
　　　　　without status epilepticus G40.109
　myoclonus, myoclonic (progressive) — *see* Epilepsy, generalized, specified NEC
　not intractable G40.909
　　with status epilepticus G40.901
　　without status epilepticus G40.909
　on awakening — *see* Epilepsy, generalized, specified NEC
　parasitic NOS B71.9 [G94]

Epilepsy, epileptic, epilepsia — *continued*
  partialis continua (*see also* Kozhevnikof's epilepsy)
    G40.1- ☑
  peripheral — *see* Epilepsy, specified NEC
  procursiva — *see* Epilepsy, localization-related,
    symptomatic, with simple partial seizures
  progressive (familial) myoclonic — *see* Epilepsy, gen-
    eralized, idiopathic
  reflex — *see* Epilepsy, specified NEC
  related to
    alcohol G40.509
      not intractable G40.509
        with status epilepticus G40.501
        without status epilepticus G40.509
    drugs G40.509
      not intractable G40.509
        with status epilepticus G40.501
        without status epilepticus G40.509
    external causes G40.509
      not intractable G40.509
        with status epilepticus G40.501
        without status epilepticus G40.509
    hormonal changes G40.509
      not intractable G40.509
        with status epilepticus G40.501
        without status epilepticus G40.509
    sleep deprivation G40.509
      not intractable G40.509
        with status epilepticus G40.501
        without status epilepticus G40.509
    stress G40.509
      not intractable G40.509
        with status epilepticus G40.501
        without status epilepticus G40.509
  somatomotor — *see* Epilepsy, localization-related,
    symptomatic, with simple partial seizures
  somatosensory — *see* Epilepsy, localization-related,
    symptomatic, with simple partial seizures
  spasms G40.822
    intractable G40.824
      with status epilepticus G40.823
      without status epilepticus G40.824
    not intractable G40.822
      with status epilepticus G40.821
      without status epilepticus G40.822
  specified NEC G40.802
    intractable G40.804
      with status epilepticus G40.803
      without status epilepticus G40.804
    not intractable G40.802
      with status epilepticus G40.801
      without status epilepticus G40.802
  syndromes
    generalized
      idiopathic G40.309
        intractable G40.319
          with status epilepticus G40.311
          without status epilepticus G40.319
        not intractable G40.309
          with status epilepticus G40.301
          without status epilepticus G40.309
      specified NEC G40.409
        intractable G40.419
          with status epilepticus G40.411
          without status epilepticus G40.419
        not intractable G40.409
          with status epilepticus G40.401
          without status epilepticus G40.409
    localization-related (focal) (partial)
      idiopathic G40.009
        with seizures of localized onset G40.009
          intractable G40.019
            with status epilepticus G40.011
            without status epilepticus G40.019
          not intractable G40.009
            with status epilepticus G40.001
            without status epilepticus G40.009
      symptomatic
        with complex partial seizures G40.209
          intractable G40.219
            with status epilepticus G40.211
            without status epilepticus G40.219
          not intractable G40.209
            with status epilepticus G40.201
            without status epilepticus G40.209
        with simple partial seizures G40.109
          intractable G40.119
            with status epilepticus G40.111

Epilepsy, epileptic, epilepsia — *continued*
  syndromes — *continued*
    localization-related — *continued*
      symptomatic — *continued*
        with simple partial seizures — *continued*
          intractable — *continued*
            without status epilepticus G40.119
          not intractable G40.109
            with status epilepticus G40.101
            without status epilepticus G40.109
      specified NEC G40.802
        intractable G40.804
          with status epilepticus G40.803
          without status epilepticus G40.804
        not intractable G40.802
          with status epilepticus G40.801
          without status epilepticus G40.802
    tonic (-clonic) — *see* Epilepsy, generalized, specified
      NEC
    twilight F05
    uncinate (gyrus) — *see* Epilepsy, localization-related,
      symptomatic, with complex partial seizures
    Unverricht (-Lundborg) (familial myoclonic) — *see*
      Epilepsy, generalized, idiopathic
    visceral — *see* Epilepsy, specified NEC
    visual — *see* Epilepsy, specified NEC
Epiloia Q85.1
Epimenorrhea N92.0
Epipharyngitis — *see* Nasopharyngitis
Epiphora H04.20- ☑
  due to
    excess lacrimation H04.21- ☑
    insufficient drainage H04.22- ☑
Epiphyseal arrest — *see* Arrest, epiphyseal
Epiphyseolysis, epiphysiolysis — *see* Osteochondropa-
  thy
Epiphysitis (*see also* Osteochondropathy)
  juvenile M92.9
  syphilitic (congenital) A50.02
Epiplocele — *see* Hernia, abdomen
Epiploitis — *see* Peritonitis
Epiplosarcomphalocele — *see* Hernia, umbilicus
Episcleritis (suppurative) H15.10- ☑
  in (due to)
    syphilis A52.71
    tuberculosis A18.51
  nodular H15.12- ☑
  periodica fugax H15.11- ☑
    angioneurotic — *see* Edema, angioneurotic
  syphilitic (late) A52.71
  tuberculous A18.51
Episode
  affective, mixed F39
  depersonalization (in neurotic state) F48.1
  depressive F32.9
    major F32.9
      mild F32.0
      moderate F32.1
      severe (without psychotic symptoms) F32.2
        with psychotic symptoms F32.3
    recurrent F33.9
      brief F33.8
    specified NEC F32.8
  hypomanic F30.8
  manic F30.9
    with
      psychotic symptoms F30.2
      remission (full) F30.4
        partial F30.3
    without psychotic symptoms F30.10
      mild F30.11
      moderate F30.12
      severe (without psychotic symptoms) F30.13
        with psychotic symptoms F30.2
    other specified F30.8
  recurrent F31.89
  psychotic F23
    organic F06.8
  schizophrenic (acute) NEC, brief F23
Epispadias (female) (male) Q64.0
Episplenitis D73.89
Epistaxis (multiple) R04.0
  hereditary I78.0
  vicarious menstruation N94.89
Epithelioma (malignant) (*see also* Neoplasm, malignant,
  by site)
  adenoides cysticum — *see* Neoplasm, skin, benign
  basal cell — *see* Neoplasm, skin, malignant

Epithelioma — *continued*
  benign — *see* Neoplasm, benign, by site
  Bowen's — *see* Neoplasm, skin, in situ
  calcifying, of Malherbe — *see* Neoplasm, skin, benign
  external site — *see* Neoplasm, skin, malignant
  intraepidermal, Jadassohn — *see* Neoplasm, skin, be-
    nign
  squamous cell — *see* Neoplasm, malignant, by site
Epitheliomatosis pigmented Q82.1
Epitheliopathy, multifocal placoid pigment
  H30.14- ☑
Epithelium, epithelial — *see* condition
Epituberculosis (with atelectasis) (allergic) A15.7
Eponychia Q84.6
Epstein's
  nephrosis or syndrome — *see* Nephrosis
  pearl K09.8
Epulis (gingiva) (fibrous) (giant cell) K06.8
Equinia A24.0
Equinovarus (congenital) (talipes) Q66.0
  acquired — *see* Deformity, limb, clubfoot
Equivalent
  convulsive (abdominal) — *see* Epilepsy, specified NEC
  epileptic (psychic) — *see* Epilepsy, localization-related,
    symptomatic, with complex partial seizures
Erb (-Duchenne) **paralysis** (birth injury) (newborn) P14.0
Erb-Goldflam disease or syndrome G70.00
  with exacerbation (acute) G70.01
  in crisis G70.01
Erb's
  disease G71.0
  palsy, paralysis (brachial) (birth) (newborn) P14.0
    spinal (spastic) syphilitic A52.17
  pseudohypertrophic muscular dystrophy G71.0
Erdheim's syndrome (acromegalic macrospondylitis)
  E22.0
Erection, painful (persistent) — *see* Priapism
Ergosterol deficiency (vitamin D) E55.9
  with
    adult osteomalacia M83.8
    rickets — *see* Rickets
Ergotism (*see also* Poisoning, food, noxious, plant)
  from ergot used as drug (migraine therapy) — *see*
    Table of Drugs and Chemicals
Erosio interdigitalis blastomycetica B37.2
Erosion
  artery I77.2
    without rupture I77.89
  bone — *see* Disorder, bone, density and structure,
    specified NEC
  bronchus J98.09
  cartilage (joint) — *see* Disorder, cartilage, specified
    type NEC
  cervix (uteri) (acquired) (chronic) (congenital) N86
    with cervicitis N72
  cornea (nontraumatic) — *see* Ulcer, cornea
    recurrent H18.83- ☑
    traumatic — *see* Abrasion, cornea
  dental (idiopathic) (occupational) (due to diet, drugs
    or vomiting) K03.2
  duodenum, postpyloric — *see* Ulcer, duodenum
  esophagus K22.10
    with bleeding K22.11
  gastric — *see* Ulcer, stomach
  gastrojejunal — *see* Ulcer, gastrojejunal
  implanted mesh — *see* Complications, mesh
  intestine K63.3
  lymphatic vessel I89.8
  pylorus, pyloric (ulcer) — *see* Ulcer, stomach
  spine, aneurysmal A52.09
  stomach — *see* Ulcer, stomach
  teeth (idiopathic) (occupational) (due to diet, drugs
    or vomiting) K03.2
  urethra N36.8
  uterus N85.8
Erotomania F52.8
Error
  metabolism, inborn — *see* Disorder, metabolism
  refractive — *see* Disorder, refraction
Eructation R14.2
  nervous or psychogenic F45.8
Eruption
  creeping B76.9
  drug (generalized) (taken internally) L27.0
    fixed L27.1
    in contact with skin — *see* Dermatitis, due to drugs
    localized L27.1

Eruption — *continued*
  Hutchinson, summer L56.4
  Kaposi's varicelliform B00.0
  napkin L22
  polymorphous light (sun) L56.4
  recalcitrant pustular L13.8
  ringed R23.8
  skin (nonspecific) R21
    creeping (meaning hookworm) B76.9
    due to inoculation/vaccination (generalized) (*see
        also* Dermatitis, due to, vaccine) L27.0
      localized L27.1
    erysipeloid A26.0
    feigned L98.1
    Kaposi's varicelliform B00.0
    lichenoid L28.0
    meaning dermatitis — *see* Dermatitis
    toxic NEC L53.0
  tooth, teeth, abnormal (incomplete) (late) (premature)
    (sequence) K00.6
  vesicular R23.8
Erysipelas (gangrenous) (infantile) (newborn) (phleg-
    monous) (suppurative) A46
  external ear A46 [H62.40]
  puerperal, postpartum O86.89
Erysipeloid A26.9
  cutaneous (Rosenbach's) A26.0
  disseminated A26.8
  sepsis A26.7
  specified NEC A26.8
Erythema, erythematous (infectional) (inflammation)
    L53.9
  ab igne L59.0
  annulare (centrifugum) (rheumaticum) L53.1
  arthriticum epidemicum A25.1
  brucellum — *see* Brucellosis
  chronic figurate NEC L53.3
  chronicum migrans (Borrelia burgdorferi) A69.20
  diaper L22
  due to
    chemical NEC L53.0
      in contact with skin L24.5
    drug (internal use) — *see* Dermatitis, due to, drugs
  elevatum diutinum L95.1
  endemic E52
  epidemic, arthritic A25.1
  figuratum perstans L53.3
  gluteal L22
  heat — *code by site under* Burn, first degree
  ichthyosiforme congenitum bullous Q80.3
  in diseases classified elsewhere L54
  induratum (nontuberculous) L52
    tuberculous A18.4
  infectiosum B08.3
  intertrigo L30.4
  iris L51.9
  marginatum L53.2
    in (due to) acute rheumatic fever I00
  medicamentosum — *see* Dermatitis, due to, drugs
  migrans A26.0
    chronicum A69.20
    tongue K14.1
  multiforme (major) (minor) L51.9
    bullous, bullosum L51.1
    conjunctiva L51.1
    nonbullous L51.0
    pemphigoides L12.0
    specified NEC L51.8
  napkin L22
  neonatorum P83.8
    toxic P83.1
  nodosum L52
    tuberculous A18.4
  palmar L53.8
  pernio T69.1 ☑
  rash, newborn P83.8
  scarlatiniform (recurrent) (exfoliative) L53.8
  solare L55.0
  specified NEC L53.8
  toxic, toxicum NEC L53.0
    newborn P83.1
  tuberculous (primary) A18.4
Erythematous, erythematosus — *see* condition
Erythermalgia (primary) I73.81
Erythralgia I73.81
Erythrasma L08.1
Erythredema (polyneuropathy) — *see* Poisoning, mer-
    cury

Erythremia (acute) C94.0- ☑
  chronic D45
  secondary D75.1
Erythroblastopenia (*see also* Aplasia, red cell) D60.9
  congenital D61.01
Erythroblastophthisis D61.09
Erythroblastosis (fetalis) (newborn) P55.9
  due to
    ABO (antibodies) (incompatibility) (isoimmuniza-
        tion) P55.1
    Rh (antibodies) (incompatibility) (isoimmunization)
        P55.0
Erythrocyanosis (crurum) I73.89
Erythrocythemia — *see* Erythremia
Erythrocytosis (megalosplenic) (secondary) D75.1
  familial D75.0
  oval, hereditary — *see* Elliptocytosis
  secondary D75.1
  stress D75.1
Erythroderma (secondary) (*see also* Erythema) L53.9
  bullous ichthyosiform, congenital Q80.3
  desquamativum L21.1
  ichthyosiform, congenital (bullous) Q80.3
  neonatorum P83.8
  psoriaticum L40.8
Erythrodysesthesia, palmar plantar (PPE) L27.1
Erythrogenesis imperfecta D61.09
Erythroleukemia C94.0- ☑
Erythromelalgia I73.81
Erythrophagocytosis D75.89
Erythrophobia F40.298
Erythroplakia, oral epithelium, and tongue K13.29
Erythroplasia (Queyrat) D07.4
  specified site — *see* Neoplasm, skin, in situ
  unspecified site D07.4
**Escherichia coli (E. coli), as cause of disease classified
    elsewhere** B96.20
  non-O157 Shiga toxin-producing (with known O
      group) B96.22
  non-Shiga toxin-producing B96.29
  O157 B96.21
  O157 with confirmation of Shiga toxin when H antigen
      is unknown, or is not H7 B96.21
  O157:H- (nonmotile) with confirmation of Shiga toxin
      B96.21
  O157:H7 with or without confirmation of Shiga toxin-
      production B96.21
    specified NEC B96.22
  Shiga toxin-producing (with unspecified O group)
      (STEC) B96.23
  specified NEC B96.29
Esophagismus K22.4
Esophagitis (acute) (alkaline) (chemical) (chronic) (infec-
    tional) (necrotic) (peptic) (postoperative) K20.9
  candidal B37.81
  due to gastrointestinal reflux disease K21.0
  eosinophilic K20.0
  reflux K21.0
  specified NEC K20.8
  tuberculous A18.83
  ulcerative K22.10
    with bleeding K22.11
Esophagocele K22.5
Esophagomalacia K22.8
Esophagospasm K22.4
Esophagostenosis K22.2
Esophagostomiasis B81.8
Esophagotracheal — *see* condition
Esophagus — *see* condition
Esophoria H50.51
  convergence, excess H51.12
  divergence, insufficiency H51.8
Esotropia — *see* Strabismus, convergent concomitant
Espundia B55.2
Essential — *see* condition
Esthesioneuroblastoma C30.0
Esthesioneurocytoma C30.0
Esthesioneuroepithelioma C30.0
Esthiomene A55
Estivo-autumnal malaria (fever) B50.9
Estrangement (marital) Z63.5
  parent-child NEC Z62.890
Estriasis — *see* Myiasis
Ethanolism — *see* Alcoholism
Etherism — *see* Dependence, drug, inhalant
Ethmoid, ethmoidal — *see* condition

Ethmoiditis (chronic) (nonpurulent) (purulent) (*see also*
    Sinusitis, ethmoidal)
  influenzal — *see* Influenza, with, respiratory manifes-
      tations NEC
  Woakes' J33.1
Ethylism — *see* Alcoholism
Eulenburg's disease (congenital paramyotonia) G71.19
Eumycetoma B47.0
Eunuchoidism E29.1
  hypogonadotropic E23.0
European blastomycosis — *see* Cryptococcosis
Eustachian — *see* condition
Evaluation (for) (of)
  development state
    adolescent Z00.3
    period of
      delayed growth in childhood Z00.70
        with abnormal findings Z00.71
      rapid growth in childhood Z00.2
    puberty Z00.3
  growth and developmental state (period of rapid
      growth) Z00.2
    delayed growth Z00.70
      with abnormal findings Z00.71
  mental health (status) Z00.8
    requested by authority Z04.6
  period of
    delayed growth in childhood Z00.70
      with abnormal findings Z00.71
    rapid growth in childhood Z00.2
  suspected condition — *see* Observation
Evans syndrome D69.41
**Event, apparent life threatening in newborn and
    infant** (ALTE) R68.13
Eventration (*see also* Hernia, ventral)
  colon into chest — *see* Hernia, diaphragm
  diaphragm (congenital) Q79.1
Eversion
  bladder N32.89
  cervix (uteri) N86
    with cervicitis N72
  foot NEC (*see also* Deformity, valgus, ankle)
    congenital Q66.6
  punctum lacrimale (postinfectional) (senile) H04.52- ☑
  ureter (meatus) N28.89
  urethra (meatus) N36.8
  uterus N81.4
Evidence
  cytologic
    of malignancy on anal smear R85.614
    of malignancy on cervical smear R87.614
    of malignancy on vaginal smear R87.624
Evisceration
  birth injury P15.8
  traumatic NEC
    eye — *see* Enucleated eye
Evulsion — *see* Avulsion
Ewing's sarcoma or tumor — *see* Neoplasm, bone,
    malignant
Examination (for) (following) (general) (of) (routine)
    Z00.00
  with abnormal findings Z00.01
  abuse, physical (alleged), ruled out
    adult Z04.71
    child Z04.72
  adolescent (development state) Z00.3
  alleged rape or sexual assault (victim), ruled out
    adult Z04.41
    child Z04.42
  allergy Z01.82
  annual (adult) (periodic) (physical) Z00.00
    with abnormal findings Z00.01
    gynecological Z01.419
      with abnormal findings Z01.411
  antibody response Z01.84
  blood — *see* Examination, laboratory
  blood pressure Z01.30
    with abnormal findings Z01.31
  cancer staging — *see* Neoplasm, malignant, by site
  cervical Papanicolaou smear Z12.4
    as part of routine gynecological examination
        Z01.419
      with abnormal findings Z01.411
  child (over 28 days old) Z00.129
    with abnormal findings Z00.121
    under 28 days old — *see* Newborn, examination
  clinical research control or normal comparison (con-
      trol) (participant) Z00.6

Examination — *continued*
contraceptive (drug) maintenance (routine) Z30.8
  device (intrauterine) Z30.431
dental Z01.20
  with abnormal findings Z01.21
developmental — *see* Examination, child
donor (potential) Z00.5
ear Z01.10
  with abnormal findings NEC Z01.118
eye Z01.00
  with abnormal findings Z01.01
following
  accident NEC Z04.3
    transport Z04.1
    work Z04.2
  assault, alleged, ruled out
    adult Z04.71
    child Z04.72
  motor vehicle accident Z04.1
  treatment (for) Z09
    combined NEC Z09
      fracture Z09
        malignant neoplasm Z08
      malignant neoplasm Z08
      mental disorder Z09
      specified condition NEC Z09
follow-up (routine) (following) Z09
  chemotherapy NEC Z09
    malignant neoplasm Z08
  fracture Z09
  malignant neoplasm Z08
  postpartum Z39.2
  psychotherapy Z09
  radiotherapy NEC Z09
    malignant neoplasm Z08
  surgery NEC Z09
    malignant neoplasm Z08
gynecological Z01.419
  with abnormal findings Z01.411
  for contraceptive maintenance Z30.8
health — *see* Examination, medical
hearing Z01.10
  with abnormal findings NEC Z01.118
  following failed hearing screening Z01.110
immunity status testing Z01.84
laboratory (as part of a general medical examination) Z00.00
  with abnormal findings Z00.01
  preprocedural Z01.812
lactating mother Z39.1
medical (adult) (for) (of) Z00.00
  with abnormal findings Z00.01
  administrative purpose only Z02.9
    specified NEC Z02.89
  admission to
    armed forces Z02.3
    old age home Z02.2
    prison Z02.89
    residential institution Z02.2
    school Z02.0
      following illness or medical treatment Z02.0
    summer camp Z02.89
  adoption Z02.82
  blood alcohol or drug level Z02.83
  camp (summer) Z02.89
  clinical research, normal subject (control) (participant) Z00.6
  control subject in clinical research (normal comparison) (participant) Z00.6
  donor (potential) Z00.5
  driving license Z02.4
  general (adult) Z00.00
    with abnormal findings Z00.01
  immigration Z02.89
  insurance purposes Z02.6
  marriage Z02.89
  medicolegal reasons NEC Z04.8
  naturalization Z02.89
  participation in sport Z02.5
  paternity testing Z02.81
  population survey Z00.8
  pre-employment Z02.1
  pre-operative — *see* Examination, pre-procedural
  pre-procedural
    cardiovascular Z01.810
    respiratory Z01.811
    specified NEC Z01.818

Examination — *continued*
medical — *continued*
  preschool children
    for admission to school Z02.0
  prisoners
    for entrance into prison Z02.89
  recruitment for armed forces Z02.3
  specified NEC Z00.8
  sport competition Z02.5
medicolegal reason NEC Z04.8
newborn — *see* Newborn, examination
pelvic (annual) (periodic) Z01.419
  with abnormal findings Z01.411
period of rapid growth in childhood Z00.2
periodic (adult) (annual) (routine) Z00.00
  with abnormal findings Z00.01
physical (adult) (*see also* Examination, medical) Z00.00
  sports Z02.5
postpartum
  immediately after delivery Z39.0
  routine follow-up Z39.2
pre-chemotherapy (antineoplastic) Z01.818
prenatal (normal pregnancy) (*see also* Pregnancy, normal) Z34.9- ☑
pre-procedural (pre-operative)
  cardiovascular Z01.810
  laboratory Z01.812
  respiratory Z01.811
  specified NEC Z01.818
prior to chemotherapy (antineoplastic) Z01.818
psychiatric NEC Z00.8
  follow-up not needing further care Z09
  requested by authority Z04.6
radiological (as part of a general medical examination) Z00.00
  with abnormal findings Z00.01
repeat cervical smear to confirm findings of recent normal smear following initial abnormal smear Z01.42
skin (hypersensitivity) Z01.82
special (*see also* Examination, by type) Z01.89
  specified type NEC Z01.89
specified type or reason NEC Z04.8
teeth Z01.20
  with abnormal findings Z01.21
urine — *see* Examination, laboratory
vision Z01.00
  with abnormal findings Z01.01
Exanthem, exanthema (*see also* Rash)
  with enteroviral vesicular stomatitis B08.4
  Boston A88.0
  epidemic with meningitis A88.0 [G02]
  subitum B08.20
    due to human herpesvirus 6 B08.21
    due to human herpesvirus 7 B08.22
  viral, virus B09
    specified type NEC B08.8
Excess, excessive, excessively
  alcohol level in blood R78.0
  androgen (ovarian) E28.1
  attrition, tooth, teeth K03.0
  carotene, carotin (dietary) E67.1
  cold, effects of T69.9 ☑
    specified effect NEC T69.8 ☑
  convergence H51.12
  crying
    in child, adolescent, or adult R45.83
    in infant R68.11
  development, breast N62
  divergence H51.8
  drinking (alcohol) NEC (without dependence) F10.10
    habitual (continual) (without remission) F10.20
  eating R63.2
  estrogen E28.0
  fat (*see also* Obesity)
    in heart — *see* Degeneration, myocardial
    localized E65
  foreskin N47.8
  gas R14.0
  glucagon E16.3
  heat — *see* Heat
  intermaxillary vertical dimension of fully erupted teeth M26.37
  interocclusal distance of fully erupted teeth M26.37
  kalium E87.5
  large
    colon K59.3
      congenital Q43.8

Excess, excessive, excessively — *continued*
  large — *continued*
    infant P08.0
    organ or site, congenital NEC — *see* Anomaly, by site
  long
    organ or site, congenital NEC — *see* Anomaly, by site
  menstruation (with regular cycle) N92.0
    with irregular cycle N92.1
  napping Z72.821
  natrium E87.0
  number of teeth K00.1
  nutrient (dietary) NEC R63.2
  potassium (K) E87.5
  salivation K11.7
  secretion (*see also* Hypersecretion)
    milk O92.6
    sputum R09.3
    sweat R61
  sexual drive F52.8
  short
    organ or site, congenital NEC — *see* Anomaly, by site
    umbilical cord in labor or delivery O69.3 ☑
  skin, eyelid (acquired) — *see* Blepharochalasis
    congenital Q10.3
  sodium (Na) E87.0
  spacing of fully erupted teeth M26.32
  sputum R09.3
  sweating R61
  thirst R63.1
    due to deprivation of water T73.1 ☑
  tuberosity of jaw M26.07
  vitamin
    A (dietary) E67.0
      administered as drug (prolonged intake) — *see* Table of Drugs and Chemicals, vitamins, adverse effect
      overdose or wrong substance given or taken — *see* Table of Drugs and Chemicals, vitamins, poisoning
    D (dietary) E67.3
      administered as drug (prolonged intake) — *see* Table of Drugs and Chemicals, vitamins, adverse effect
      overdose or wrong substance given or taken — *see* Table of Drugs and Chemicals, vitamins, poisoning
  weight
    gain R63.5
    loss R63.4
Excitability, abnormal, under minor stress (personality disorder) F60.3
Excitation
  anomalous atrioventricular I45.6
  psychogenic F30.8
  reactive (from emotional stress, psychological trauma) F30.8
Excitement
  hypomanic F30.8
  manic F30.9
  mental, reactive (from emotional stress, psychological trauma) F30.8
  state, reactive (from emotional stress, psychological trauma) F30.8
Excoriation (traumatic) (*see also* Abrasion)
  neurotic L98.1
Exfoliation
  due to erythematous conditions according to extent of body surface involved L49.0
    less than 10 percent of body surface L49.0
    10-19 percent of body surface L49.1
    20-29 percent of body surface L49.2
    30-39 percent of body surface L49.3
    40-49 percent of body surface L49.4
    50-59 percent of body surface L49.5
    60-69 percent of body surface L49.6
    70-79 percent of body surface L49.7
    80-89 percent of body surface L49.8
    90-99 percent of body surface L49.9
  teeth, due to systemic causes K08.0
Exfoliative — *see* condition
Exhaustion, exhaustive (physical NEC) R53.83
  battle F43.0
  cardiac — *see* Failure, heart
  delirium F43.0

Index

Examination — Exhaustion, exhaustive

Exhaustion, exhaustive — *continued*
  due to
    cold T69.8 ☑
    excessive exertion T73.3 ☑
    exposure T73.2 ☑
    neurasthenia F48.8
  heart — *see* Failure, heart
  heat (*see also* Heat, exhaustion) T67.5 ☑
    due to
      salt depletion T67.4 ☑
      water depletion T67.3 ☑
  maternal, complicating delivery O75.81
  mental F48.8
  myocardium, myocardial — *see* Failure, heart
  nervous F48.8
  old age R54
  psychogenic F48.8
  psychosis F43.0
  senile R54
  vital NEC Z73.0
Exhibitionism F65.2
Exocervicitis — *see* Cervicitis
Exomphalos Q79.2
  meaning hernia — *see* Hernia, umbilicus
Exophoria H50.52
  convergence, insufficiency H51.11
  divergence, excess H51.8
Exophthalmos H05.2- ☑
  congenital Q15.8
  constant NEC H05.24- ☑
  displacement, globe — *see* Displacement, globe
  due to thyrotoxicosis (hyperthyroidism) — *see* Hyperthyroidism, with, goiter (diffuse)
  dysthyroid — *see* Hyperthyroidism, with, goiter (diffuse)
  goiter — *see* Hyperthyroidism, with, goiter (diffuse)
  intermittent NEC H05.25- ☑
  malignant — *see* Hyperthyroidism, with, goiter (diffuse)
  orbital
    edema — *see* Edema, orbit
    hemorrhage — *see* Hemorrhage, orbit
  pulsating NEC H05.26- ☑
  thyrotoxic, thyrotropic — *see* Hyperthyroidism, with, goiter (diffuse)
Exostosis (*see also* Disorder, bone)
  cartilaginous — *see* Neoplasm, bone, benign
  congenital (multiple) Q78.6
  external ear canal H61.81- ☑
  gonococcal A54.49
  jaw (bone) M27.8
  multiple, congenital Q78.6
  orbit H05.35- ☑
  osteocartilaginous — *see* Neoplasm, bone, benign
  syphilitic A52.77
Exotropia — *see* Strabismus, divergent concomitant
Explanation of
  investigation finding Z71.2
  medication Z71.89
Exposure (to) (*see also* Contact, with) T75.89 ☑
  acariasis Z20.7
  AIDS virus Z20.6
  air pollution Z77.110
  algae and algae toxins Z77.121
  algae bloom Z77.121
  anthrax Z20.810
  aromatic amines Z77.020
  aromatic (hazardous) compounds NEC Z77.028
  aromatic dyes NOS Z77.028
  arsenic Z77.010
  asbestos Z77.090
  bacterial disease NEC Z20.818
  benzene Z77.021
  blue-green algae bloom Z77.121
  body fluids (potentially hazardous) Z77.21
  brown tide Z77.121
  chemicals (chiefly nonmedicinal) (hazardous) NEC Z77.098
  cholera Z20.09
  chromium compounds Z77.018
  cold, effects of T69.9 ☑
    specified effect NEC T69.8 ☑
  communicable disease Z20.9
    bacterial NEC Z20.818
    specified NEC Z20.89
    viral NEC Z20.828
  cyanobacteria bloom Z77.121

Exposure — *continued*
  disaster Z65.5
  discrimination Z60.5
  dyes Z77.098
  effects of T73.9 ☑
  environmental tobacco smoke (acute) (chronic) Z77.22
  Escherichia coli (E. coli) Z20.01
  exhaustion due to T73.2 ☑
  fiberglass — *see* Table of Drugs and Chemicals, fiberglass
  German measles Z20.4
  gonorrhea Z20.2
  hazardous metals NEC Z77.018
  hazardous substances NEC Z77.29
  hazards in the physical environment NEC Z77.128
  hazards to health NEC Z77.9
  human immunodeficiency virus (HIV) Z20.6
  human T-lymphotropic virus type-1 (HTLV-1) Z20.89
  implanted
    mesh — *see* Complications, mesh
    prosthetic materials NEC — *see* Complications, prosthetic materials NEC
  infestation (parasitic) NEC Z20.7
  intestinal infectious disease NEC Z20.09
    Escherichia coli (E. coli) Z20.01
  lead Z77.011
  meningococcus Z20.811
  mold (toxic) Z77.120
  nickel dust Z77.018
  noise Z77.122
  occupational
    air contaminants NEC Z57.39
    dust Z57.2
    environmental tobacco smoke Z57.31
    extreme temperature Z57.6
    noise Z57.0
    radiation Z57.1
    risk factors Z57.9
      specified NEC Z57.8
    toxic agents (gases) (liquids) (solids) (vapors) in agriculture Z57.4
    toxic agents (gases) (liquids) (solids) (vapors) in industry NEC Z57.5
    vibration Z57.7
  parasitic disease NEC Z20.7
  pediculosis Z20.7
  persecution Z60.5
  pfiesteria piscicida Z77.121
  poliomyelitis Z20.89
  pollution
    air Z77.110
    environmental NEC Z77.118
    soil Z77.112
    water Z77.111
  polycyclic aromatic hydrocarbons Z77.028
  prenatal (drugs) (toxic chemicals) — *see* Newborn, affected by (suspected to be), noxious substances transmitted via placenta or breast milk
  rabies Z20.3
  radiation, naturally occurring NEC Z77.123
  radon Z77.123
  red tide (Florida) Z77.121
  rubella Z20.4
  second hand tobacco smoke (acute) (chronic) Z77.22
    in the perinatal period P96.81
  sexually-transmitted disease Z20.2
  smallpox (laboratory) Z20.89
  syphilis Z20.2
  terrorism Z65.4
  torture Z65.4
  tuberculosis Z20.1
  uranium Z77.012
  varicella Z20.820
  venereal disease Z20.2
  viral disease NEC Z20.828
  war Z65.5
  water pollution Z77.111
Exsanguination — *see* Hemorrhage
Exstrophy
  abdominal contents Q45.8
  bladder Q64.10
    cloacal Q64.12
    specified type NEC Q64.19
    supravesical fissure Q64.11
Extensive — *see* condition
Extra (*see also* Accessory)
  marker chromosomes (normal individual) Q92.61
    in abnormal individual Q92.62

Extra — *continued*
  rib Q76.6
    cervical Q76.5
Extrasystoles (supraventricular) I49.49
  atrial I49.1
  auricular I49.1
  junctional I49.2
  ventricular I49.3
Extrauterine gestation or pregnancy — *see* Pregnancy, by site
Extravasation
  blood R58
  chyle into mesentery I89.8
  pelvicalyceal N13.8
  pyelosinus N13.8
  urine (from ureter) R39.0
  vesicant agent
    antineoplastic chemotherapy T80.810 ☑
    other agent NEC T80.818 ☑
Extremity — *see* condition, limb
Extrophy — *see* Exstrophy
Extroversion
  bladder Q64.19
  uterus N81.4
    complicating delivery O71.2
    postpartal (old) N81.4
Extruded tooth (teeth) M26.34
Extrusion
  breast implant (prosthetic) T85.42 ☑
  eye implant (globe) (ball) T85.328 ☑
  intervertebral disc — *see* Displacement, intervertebral disc
  ocular lens implant (prosthetic) — *see* Complications, intraocular lens
  vitreous — *see* Prolapse, vitreous
Exudate
  pleural — *see* Effusion, pleura
  retina H35.89
Exudative — *see* condition
Eye, eyeball, eyelid — *see* condition
Eyestrain — *see* Disturbance, vision, subjective
Eyeworm disease of Africa B74.3

F

Faber's syndrome (achlorhydric anemia) D50.9
Fabry (-Anderson) **disease** E75.21
Faciocephalalgia, autonomic (*see also* Neuropathy, peripheral, autonomic) G90.09
Factor(s)
  psychic, associated with diseases classified elsewhere F54
  psychological
    affecting physical conditions F54
    or behavioral
      affecting general medical condition F54
      associated with disorders or diseases classified elsewhere F54
Fahr disease (of brain) G23.8
Fahr Volhard disease (of kidney) I12.- ☑
Failure, failed
  abortion — *see* Abortion, attempted
  aortic (valve) I35.8
    rheumatic I06.8
  attempted abortion — *see* Abortion, attempted
  biventricular I50.9
  bone marrow — *see* Anemia, aplastic
  cardiac — *see* Failure, heart
  cardiorenal (chronic) I50.9
    hypertensive I13.2
  cardiorespiratory (*see also* Failure, heart) R09.2
  cardiovascular (chronic) — *see* Failure, heart
  cerebrovascular I67.9
  cervical dilatation in labor O62.0
  circulation, circulatory (peripheral) R57.9
    newborn P29.89
  compensation — *see* Disease, heart
  compliance with medical treatment or regimen — *see* Noncompliance
  congestive — *see* Failure, heart, congestive
  dental implant (endosseous) M27.69
    due to
      failure of dental prosthesis M27.63
      lack of attached gingiva M27.62
      occlusal trauma (poor prosthetic design) M27.62
      parafunctional habits M27.62

Failure, failed — *continued*
- dental implant — *continued*
  - due to — *continued*
    - periodontal infection (peri-implantitis) M27.62
    - poor oral hygiene M27.62
    - osseointegration M27.61
      - due to
        - complications of systemic disease M27.61
        - poor bone quality M27.61
      - iatrogenic M27.61
    - post-osseointegration
      - biological M27.62
        - due to complications of systemic disease M27.62
      - iatrogenic M27.62
      - mechanical M27.63
    - pre-integration M27.61
    - pre-osseointegration M27.61
    - specified NEC M27.69
- descent of head (at term) of pregnancy (mother) O32.4 ☑
- endosseous dental implant — *see* Failure, dental implant
- engagement of head (term of pregnancy) (mother) O32.4 ☑
- erection (penile) (*see also* Dysfunction, sexual, male, erectile) N52.9
  - nonorgqanic F52.21
- examination(s), anxiety concerning Z55.2
- expansion terminal respiratory units (newborn) (primary) P28.0
- forceps NOS (with subsequent cesarean delivery) O66.5
- gain weight (child over 28 days old) R62.51
  - adult R62.7
  - newborn P92.6
- genital response (male) F52.21
  - female F52.22
- heart (acute) (senile) (sudden) I50.9
  - with
    - acute pulmonary edema — *see* Failure, ventricular, left
    - decompensation — *see* Failure, heart, congestive
    - dilatation — *see* Disease, heart
  - arteriosclerotic I70.90
  - biventricular I50.9
  - combined left-right sided I50.9
  - compensated I50.9
  - complicating
    - anesthesia (general) (local) or other sedation
      - in labor and delivery O74.2
      - in pregnancy O29.12- ☑
      - postpartum, puerperal O89.1
    - delivery (cesarean) (instrumental) O75.4
  - congestive (compensated) (decompensated) I50.9
    - with rheumatic fever (conditions in I00)
      - active I01.8
      - inactive or quiescent (with chorea) I09.81
    - newborn P29.0
    - rheumatic (chronic) (inactive) (with chorea) I09.81
      - active or acute I01.8
        - with chorea I02.0
  - decompensated I50.9
  - degenerative — *see* Degeneration, myocardial
  - diastolic (congestive) I50.30
    - acute (congestive) I50.31
      - and (on) chronic (congestive) I50.33
    - chronic (congestive) I50.32
      - and (on) acute (congestive) I50.33
    - combined with systolic (congestive) I50.40
      - acute (congestive) I50.41
        - and (on) chronic (congestive) I50.43
      - chronic (congestive) I50.42
        - and (on) acute (congestive) I50.43
  - due to presence of cardiac prosthesis I97.13- ☑
  - following cardiac surgery I97.13- ☑
  - high output NOS I50.9
  - hypertensive — *see* Hypertension, heart
  - left (ventricular) — *see* Failure, ventricular, left
  - low output (syndrome) NOS I50.9
  - newborn P29.0
  - organic — *see* Disease, heart
  - peripartum O90.3
  - postprocedural I97.13- ☑
  - rheumatic (chronic) (inactive) I09.9
  - right (ventricular) (secondary to left heart failure) — *see* Failure, heart, congestive

Failure, failed — *continued*
- heart — *continued*
  - systolic (congestive) I50.20
    - acute (congestive) I50.21
      - and (on) chronic (congestive) I50.23
    - chronic (congestive) I50.22
      - and (on) acute (congestive) I50.23
    - combined with diastolic (congestive) I50.40
      - acute (congestive) I50.41
        - and (on) chronic (congestive) I50.43
      - chronic (congestive) I50.42
        - and (on) acute (congestive) I50.43
  - thyrotoxic (*see also* Thyrotoxicosis) E05.90 [I43]
    - with thyroid storm E05.91 [I43]
  - valvular — *see* Endocarditis
- hepatic K72.90
  - with coma K72.91
  - acute or subacute K72.00
    - with coma K72.01
    - due to drugs K71.10
      - with coma K71.11
  - alcoholic (acute) (chronic) (subacute) K70.40
    - with coma K70.41
  - chronic K72.10
    - with coma K72.11
    - due to drugs (acute) (subacute) (chronic) K71.10
      - with coma K71.11
  - due to drugs (acute) (subacute) (chronic) K71.10
    - with coma K71.11
  - postprocedural K91.82
- hepatorenal K76.7
- induction (of labor) O61.9
  - abortion — *see* Abortion, attempted
  - by
    - oxytocic drugs O61.0
    - prostaglandins O61.0
  - instrumental O61.1
  - mechanical O61.1
  - medical O61.0
  - specified NEC O61.8
  - surgical O61.1
- intubation during anesthesia T88.4 ☑
  - in pregnancy O29.6- ☑
  - labor and delivery O74.7
  - postpartum, puerperal O89.6
- involution, thymus (gland) E32.0
- kidney (*see also* Disease, kidney, chronic) N19
  - acute (*see also* Failure, renal, acute) N17.9
- lactation (complete) O92.3
  - partial O92.4
- Leydig's cell, adult E29.1
- liver — *see* Failure, hepatic
- menstruation at puberty N91.0
- mitral I05.8
- myocardial, myocardium (*see also* Failure, heart) I50.9
  - chronic (*see also* Failure, heart, congestive) I50.9
  - congestive (*see also* Failure, heart, congestive) I50.9
- orgasm (female) (psychogenic) F52.31
  - male F52.32
- ovarian (primary) E28.39
  - iatrogenic E89.40
    - asymptomatic E89.40
    - symptomatic E89.41
  - postprocedural (postablative) (postirradiation) (postsurgical) E89.40
    - asymptomatic E89.40
    - symptomatic E89.41
- ovulation causing infertility N97.0
- polyglandular, autoimmune E31.0
- prosthetic joint implant — *see* Complications, joint prosthesis, mechanical, breakdown, by site
- renal N19
  - with
    - tubular necrosis (acute) N17.0
  - acute N17.9
    - with
      - cortical necrosis N17.1
      - medullary necrosis N17.2
      - tubular necrosis N17.0
    - specified NEC N17.8
  - chronic N18.9
    - hypertensive — *see* Hypertension, kidney
  - congenital P96.0
  - end stage (chronic) N18.6
    - due to hypertension I12.0
  - following
    - abortion — *see* Abortion by type complicated by specified condition NEC

Failure, failed — *continued*
- renal — *continued*
  - following — *continued*
    - crushing T79.5 ☑
    - ectopic or molar pregnancy O08.4
    - labor and delivery (acute) O90.4
  - hypertensive — *see* Hypertension, kidney
  - postprocedural N99.0
- respiration, respiratory J96.90
  - with
    - hypercapnia J96.92
    - hypoxia J96.91
  - acute J96.00
    - with
      - hypercapnia J96.02
      - hypoxia J96.01
  - acute and (on) chronic J96.20
    - with
      - hypercapnia J96.22
      - hypoxia J96.21
  - center G93.89
  - chronic J96.10
    - with
      - hypercapnia J96.12
      - hypoxia J96.11
  - newborn P28.5
  - postprocedural (acute) J95.821
    - acute and chronic J95.822
- rotation
  - cecum Q43.3
  - colon Q43.3
  - intestine Q43.3
  - kidney Q63.2
- sedation (conscious) (moderate) during procedure T88.52 ☑
  - history of Z92.83
- segmentation (*see also* Fusion)
  - fingers — *see* Syndactylism, complex, fingers
  - vertebra Q76.49
    - with scoliosis Q76.3
- seminiferous tubule, adult E29.1
- senile (general) R54
- sexual arousal (male) F52.21
  - female F52.22
- testicular endocrine function E29.1
- to thrive (child over 28 days old) R62.51
  - adult R62.7
  - newborn P92.6
- transplant T86.92
  - bone T86.831
    - marrow T86.02
  - cornea T86.841
  - heart T86.22
    - with lung(s) T86.32
  - intestine T86.851
  - kidney T86.12
  - liver T86.42
  - lung(s) T86.811
    - with heart T86.32
  - pancreas T86.891
  - skin (allograft) (autograft) T86.821
  - specified organ or tissue NEC T86.891
  - stem cell (peripheral blood) (umbilical cord) T86.5
- trial of labor (with subsequent cesarean delivery) O66.40
  - following previous cesarean delivery O66.41
- tubal ligation N99.89
- urinary — *see* Disease, kidney, chronic
- vacuum extraction NOS (with subsequent cesarean delivery) O66.5
- vasectomy N99.89
- ventouse NOS (with subsequent cesarean delivery) O66.5
- ventricular (*see also* Failure, heart) I50.9
  - left I50.1
    - with rheumatic fever (conditions in I00)
      - active I01.8
        - with chorea I02.0
      - inactive or quiescent (with chorea) I09.81
    - rheumatic (chronic) (inactive) (with chorea) I09.81
      - active or acute I01.8
        - with chorea I02.0
  - right (*see also* Failure, heart, congestive) I50.9
- vital centers, newborn P91.8

Fainting (fit) R55
Fallen arches — *see* Deformity, limb, flat foot
Falling, falls (repeated) R29.6

Falling, falls — *continued*
  any organ or part — *see* Prolapse
Fallopian
  insufflation Z31.41
  tube — *see* condition
Fallot's
  pentalogy Q21.8
  tetrad or tetralogy Q21.3
  triad or trilogy Q22.3
False (*see also* condition)
  croup J38.5
  joint — *see* Nonunion, fracture
  labor (pains) O47.9
    at or after 37 completed weeks of gestation O47.1
    before 37 completed weeks of gestation O47.0- ☑
  passage, urethra (prostatic) N36.5
  pregnancy F45.8
Family, familial (*see also* condition)
  disruption Z63.8
    involving divorce or separation Z63.5
  Li-Fraumeni (syndrome) Z15.01
  planning advice Z30.09
  problem Z63.9
    specified NEC Z63.8
  retinoblastoma C69.2- ☑
Famine (effects of) T73.0 ☑
  edema — *see* Malnutrition, severe
Fanconi (-de Toni)(-Debré) **syndrome** E72.09
  with cystinosis E72.04
Fanconi's anemia (congenital pancytopenia) D61.09
Farber's disease or syndrome E75.29
Farcy A24.0
Farmer's
  lung J67.0
  skin L57.8
Farsightedness — *see* Hypermetropia
Fascia — *see* condition
Fasciculation R25.3
Fasciitis M72.9
  diffuse (eosinophilic) M35.4
  infective M72.8
    necrotizing M72.6
  necrotizing M72.6
  nodular M72.4
  perirenal (with ureteral obstruction) N13.5
    with infection N13.6
  plantar M72.2
  specified NEC M72.8
  traumatic (old) M72.8
    current — *code by* site under Sprain
Fascioliasis B66.3
Fasciolopsis, fasciolopsiasis (intestinal) B66.5
Fascioscapulohumeral myopathy G71.0
Fast pulse R00.0
Fat
  embolism — *see* Embolism, fat
  excessive (*see also* Obesity)
    in heart — *see* Degeneration, myocardial
  in stool R19.5
  localized (pad) E65
    heart — *see* Degeneration, myocardial
    knee M79.4
    retropatellar M79.4
  necrosis
    breast N64.1
    mesentery K65.4
    omentum K65.4
  pad E65
    knee M79.4
Fatigue R53.83
  auditory deafness — *see* Deafness
  chronic R53.82
  combat F43.0
  general R53.83
    psychogenic F48.8
  heat (transient) T67.6 ☑
  muscle M62.89
  myocardium — *see* Failure, heart
  neoplasm-related R53.0
  nervous, neurosis F48.8
  operational F48.8
  psychogenic (general) F48.8
  senile R54
  voice R49.8
Fatness — *see* Obesity
Fatty (*see also* condition)
  apron E65

Fatty — *continued*
  degeneration — *see* Degeneration, fatty
  heart (enlarged) — *see* Degeneration, myocardial
  liver NEC K76.0
    alcoholic K70.0
    nonalcoholic K76.0
  necrosis — *see* Degeneration, fatty
Fauces — *see* condition
Fauchard's disease (periodontitis) — *see* Periodontitis
Faucitis J02.9
Favism (anemia) D55.0
Favus — *see* Dermatophytosis
Fazio-Londe disease or syndrome G12.1
Fear complex or reaction F40.9
Fear of — *see* Phobia
Feared complaint unfounded Z71.1
Febris, febrile (*see also* Fever)
  flava (*see also* Fever, yellow) A95.9
  melitensis A23.0
  pestis — *see* Plague
  recurrens — *see* Fever, relapsing
  rubra A38.9
Fecal
  incontinence R15.9
  smearing R15.1
  soiling R15.1
  urgency R15.2
Fecalith (impaction) K56.41
  appendix K38.1
  congenital P76.8
Fede's disease K14.0
Feeble rapid pulse due to shock following injury
  T79.4 ☑
Feeble-minded F70
Feeding
  difficulties R63.3
  problem R63.3
    newborn P92.9
      specified NEC P92.8
    nonorganic (adult) — *see* Disorder, eating
Feeling (of)
  foreign body in throat R09.89
Feer's disease — *see* Poisoning, mercury
Feet — *see* condition
Feigned illness Z76.5
Feil-Klippel syndrome (brevicollis) Q76.1
Feinmesser's (hidrotic) **ectodermal dysplasia** Q82.4
Felinophobia F40.218
Felon (*see also* Cellulitis, digit)
  with lymphangitis — *see* Lymphangitis, acute, digit
Felty's syndrome M05.00
  ankle M05.07- ☑
  elbow M05.02- ☑
  foot joint M05.07- ☑
  hand joint M05.04- ☑
  hip M05.05- ☑
  knee M05.06- ☑
  multiple site M05.09
  shoulder M05.01- ☑
  vertebra — *see* Spondylitis, ankylosing
  wrist M05.03- ☑
Female genital cutting status — *see* Female genital mutilation status (FGM)
Female genital mutilation status (FGM) N90.810
  specified NEC N90.818
  type I (clitorectomy status) N90.811
  type II (clitorectomy with excision of labia minora status) N90.812
  type III (infibulation status) N90.813
  type IV N90.818
Femur, femoral — *see* condition
Fenestration, fenestrated (*see also* Imperfect, closure)
  aortico-pulmonary Q21.4
  cusps, heart valve NEC Q24.8
    pulmonary Q22.3
  pulmonic cusps Q22.3
Fernell's disease (aortic aneurysm) I71.9
Fertile eunuch syndrome E23.0
Fetid
  breath R19.6
  sweat L75.0
Fetishism F65.0
  transvestic F65.1
Fetus, fetal (*see also* condition)
  alcohol syndrome (dysmorphic) Q86.0
  compressus O31.0- ☑
  hydantoin syndrome Q86.1

Fetus, fetal — *continued*
  lung tissue P28.0
  papyraceous O31.0- ☑
Fever (inanition) (of unknown origin) (persistent) (with chills) (with rigor) R50.9
  abortus A23.1
  Aden (dengue) A90
  African tick-borne A68.1
  American
    mountain (tick) A93.2
    spotted A77.0
  aphthous B08.8
  arbovirus, arboviral A94
    hemorrhagic A94
    specified NEC A93.8
  Argentinian hemorrhagic A96.0
  Assam B55.0
  Australian Q A78
  Bangkok hemorrhagic A91
  Barmah forest A92.8
  Bartonella A44.0
  bilious, hemoglobinuric B50.8
  blackwater B50.8
  blister B00.1
  Bolivian hemorrhagic A96.1
  Bonvale dam T73.3 ☑
  boutonneuse A77.1
  brain — *see* Encephalitis
  Brazilian purpuric A48.4
  breakbone A90
  Bullis A77.0
  Bunyamwera A92.8
  Burdwan B55.0
  Bwamba A92.8
  Cameroon — *see* Malaria
  Canton A75.9
  catarrhal (acute) J00
    chronic J31.0
  cat-scratch A28.1
  Central Asian hemorrhagic A98.0
  cerebral — *see* Encephalitis
  cerebrospinal meningococcal A39.0
  Chagres B50.9
  Chandipura A92.8
  Changuinola A93.1
  Charcot's (biliary) (hepatic) (intermittent) — *see* Calculus, bile duct
  Chikungunya (viral) (hemorrhagic) A92.0
  Chitral A93.1
  Colombo — *see* Fever, paratyphoid
  Colorado tick (virus) A93.2
  congestive (remittent) — *see* Malaria
  Congo virus A98.0
  continued malarial B50.9
  Corsican — *see* Malaria
  Crimean-Congo hemorrhagic A98.0
  Cyprus — *see* Brucellosis
  dandy A90
  deer fly — *see* Tularemia
  dengue (virus) A90
    hemorrhagic A91
    sandfly A93.1
  desert B38.0
  drug induced R50.2
  due to
    conditions classified elsewhere R50.81
    heat T67.0 ☑
  enteric A01.00
  enteroviral exanthematous (Boston exanthem) A88.0
  ephemeral (of unknown origin) R50.9
  epidemic hemorrhagic A98.5
  erysipelatous — *see* Erysipelas
  estivo-autumnal (malarial) B50.9
  famine A75.0
  five day A79.0
  following delivery O86.4
  Fort Bragg A27.89
  gastroenteric A01.00
  gastromalarial — *see* Malaria
  Gibraltar — *see* Brucellosis
  glandular — *see* Mononucleosis, infectious
  Guama (viral) A92.8
  Haverhill A25.1
  hay (allergic) J30.1
    with asthma (bronchial) J45.909
      with
        exacerbation (acute) J45.901
        status asthmaticus J45.902

Fever — *continued*
hay — *continued*
  due to
    allergen other than pollen J30.89
    pollen, any plant or tree J30.1
heat (effects) T67.0 ☑
hematuric, bilious B50.8
hemoglobinuric (malarial) (bilious) B50.8
hemorrhagic (arthropod-borne) NOS A94
  with renal syndrome A98.5
  arenaviral A96.9
    specified NEC A96.8
  Argentinian A96.0
  Bangkok A91
  Bolivian A96.1
  Central Asian A98.0
  Chikungunya A92.0
  Crimean-Congo A98.0
  dengue (virus) A91
  epidemic A98.5
  Junin (virus) A96.0
  Korean A98.5
  Kyasanur forest A98.2
  Machupo (virus) A96.1
  mite-borne A93.8
  mosquito-borne A92.8
  Omsk A98.1
  Philippine A91
  Russian A98.5
  Singapore A91
  Southeast Asia A91
  Thailand A91
  tick-borne NEC A93.8
  viral A99
    specified NEC A98.8
hepatic — *see* Cholecystitis
herpetic — *see* Herpes
icterohemorrhagic A27.0
Indiana A93.8
infective B99.9
  specified NEC B99.8
intermittent (bilious) (*see also* Malaria)
  of unknown origin R50.9
  pernicious B50.9
iodide R50.2
Japanese river A75.3
jungle (*see also* Malaria)
  yellow A95.0
Junin (virus) hemorrhagic A96.0
Katayama B65.2
kedani A75.3
Kenya (tick) A77.1
Kew Garden A79.1
Korean hemorrhagic A98.5
Lassa A96.2
Lone Star A77.0
Machupo (virus) hemorrhagic A96.1
malaria, malarial — *see* Malaria
Malta A23.9
Marseilles A77.1
marsh — *see* Malaria
Mayaro (viral) A92.8
Mediterranean (*see also* Brucellosis) A23.9
  familial E85.0
  tick A77.1
meningeal — *see* Meningitis
Meuse A79.0
Mexican A75.2
mianeh A68.1
miasmatic — *see* Malaria
mosquito-borne (viral) A92.9
  hemorrhagic A92.8
mountain (*see also* Brucellosis)
  meaning Rocky Mountain spotted fever A77.0
  tick (American) (Colorado) (viral) A93.2
Mucambo (viral) A92.8
mud A27.9
Neapolitan — *see* Brucellosis
neutropenic D70.9
newborn P81.9
  environmental P81.0
Nine-Mile A78
non-exanthematous tick A93.2
North Asian tick-borne A77.2
Omsk hemorrhagic A98.1
O'nyong-nyong (viral) A92.1
Oropouche (viral) A93.0
Oroya A44.0

Fever — *continued*
paludal — *see* Malaria
Panama (malarial) B50.9
Pappataci A93.1
paratyphoid A01.4
  A A01.1
  B A01.2
  C A01.3
parrot A70
periodic (Mediterranean) E85.0
persistent (of unknown origin) R50.9
petechial A39.0
pharyngoconjunctival B30.2
Philippine hemorrhagic A91
phlebotomus A93.1
Piry (virus) A93.8
Pixuna (viral) A92.8
Plasmodium ovale B53.0
polioviral (nonparalytic) A80.4
Pontiac A48.2
postimmunization R50.83
postoperative R50.82
  due to infection T81.4 ☑
posttransfusion R50.84
postvaccination R50.83
presenting with conditions classified elsewhere R50.81
pretibial A27.89
puerperal O86.4
Q A78
quadrilateral A78
quartan (malaria) B52.9
Queensland (coastal) (tick) A77.3
quintan A79.0
rabbit — *see* Tularemia
rat-bite A25.9
  due to
    Spirillum A25.0
    Streptobacillus moniliformis A25.1
recurrent — *see* Fever, relapsing
relapsing (Borrelia) A68.9
  Carter's (Asiatic) A68.1
  Dutton's (West African) A68.1
  Koch's A68.9
  louse-borne A68.0
  Novy's
    louse-borne A68.0
    tick-borne A68.1
  Obermeyer's (European) A68.0
  tick-borne A68.1
remittent (bilious) (congestive) (gastric) — *see* Malaria
rheumatic (active) (acute) (chronic) (subacute) I00
  with central nervous system involvement I02.9
  active with heart involvement — *see* category
    I01 ☑
  inactive or quiescent with
    cardiac hypertrophy I09.89
    carditis I09.9
    endocarditis I09.1
      aortic (valve) I06.9
        with mitral (valve) disease I08.0
      mitral (valve) I05.9
        with aortic (valve) disease I08.0
      pulmonary (valve) I09.89
      tricuspid (valve) I07.8
    heart disease NEC I09.89
    heart failure (congestive) (conditions in I50.9)
      I09.81
    left ventricular failure (conditions in I50.1)
      I09.81
    myocarditis, myocardial degeneration (conditions in I51.4) I09.0
    pancarditis I09.9
    pericarditis I09.2
Rift Valley (viral) A92.4
Rocky Mountain spotted A77.0
rose J30.1
Ross River B33.1
Russian hemorrhagic A98.5
San Joaquin (Valley) B38.0
sandfly A93.1
Sao Paulo A77.0
scarlet A38.9
seven day (leptospirosis) (autumnal) (Japanese) A27.89
  dengue A90
shin-bone A79.0
Singapore hemorrhagic A91
solar A90
Songo A98.5

Fever — *continued*
sore B00.1
South African tick-bite A68.1
Southeast Asia hemorrhagic A91
spinal — *see* Meningitis
spirillary A25.0
splenic — *see* Anthrax
spotted A77.9
  American A77.0
  Brazilian A77.0
  cerebrospinal meningitis A39.0
  Colombian A77.0
  due to Rickettsia
    australis A77.3
    conorii A77.1
    rickettsii A77.0
    sibirica A77.2
    specified type NEC A77.8
  Ehrlichiosis A77.40
    due to
      E. chafeensis A77.41
      specified organism NEC A77.49
  Rocky Mountain A77.0
steroid R50.2
streptobacillary A25.1
subtertian B50.9
Sumatran mite A75.3
sun A90
swamp A27.9
swine A02.8
sylvatic, yellow A95.0
Tahyna B33.8
tertian — *see* Malaria, tertian
Thailand hemorrhagic A91
thermic T67.0 ☑
three-day A93.1
tick
  American mountain A93.2
  Colorado A93.2
  Kemerovo A93.8
  Mediterranean A77.1
  mountain A93.2
  nonexanthematous A93.2
  Quaranfil A93.8
tick-bite NEC A93.8
tick-borne (hemorrhagic) NEC A93.8
trench A79.0
tsutsugamushi A75.3
typhogastric A01.00
typhoid (abortive) (hemorrhagic) (intermittent) (malignant) A01.00
  complicated by
    arthritis A01.04
    heart involvement A01.02
    meningitis A01.01
    osteomyelitis A01.05
    pneumonia A01.03
    specified NEC A01.09
typhomalarial — *see* Malaria
typhus — *see* Typhus (fever)
undulant — *see* Brucellosis
unknown origin R50.9
uveoparotid D86.89
valley B38.0
Venezuelan equine A92.2
vesicular stomatitis A93.8
viral hemorrhagic — *see* Fever, hemorrhagic, by type
  of virus
Volhynian A79.0
Wesselsbron (viral) A92.8
West
  African B50.8
  Nile (viral) A92.30
    with
      complications NEC A92.39
      cranial nerve disorders A92.32
      encephalitis A92.31
      encephalomyelitis A92.31
      neurologic manifestation NEC A92.32
      optic neuritis A92.32
      polyradiculitis A92.32
Whitmore's — *see* Melioidosis
Wolhynian A79.0
worm B83.9
yellow A95.9
  jungle A95.0
  sylvatic A95.0
  urban A95.1

136

☑ Additional Character Required — Refer to the Tabular List for Character Selection   ▼ Subterms under main terms may continue to next column or page

Fever — *continued*
Zika (viral) A92.8

Fibrillation
atrial or auricular (established) I48.91
  chronic I48.2
  paroxysmal I48.0
  permanent I48.2
  persistent I48.1
cardiac I49.8
heart I49.8
muscular M62.89
ventricular I49.01

Fibrin
ball or bodies, pleural (sac) J94.1
chamber, anterior (eye) (gelatinous exudate) — *see* Iridocyclitis, acute

Fibrinogenolysis — *see* Fibrinolysis

Fibrinogenopenia D68.8
acquired D65
congenital D68.2

Fibrinolysis (hemorrhagic) (acquired) D65
antepartum hemorrhage — *see* Hemorrhage, antepartum, with coagulation defect
following
  abortion — *see* Abortion by type complicated by hemorrhage
  ectopic or molar pregnancy O08.1
intrapartum O67.0
newborn, transient P60
postpartum O72.3

Fibrinopenia (hereditary) D68.2
acquired D68.4

Fibrinopurulent — *see* condition

Fibrinous — *see* condition

Fibroadenoma
cellular intracanalicular D24- ☑
giant D24- ☑
intracanalicular
  cellular D24- ☑
  giant D24- ☑
  specified site — *see* Neoplasm, benign, by site
  unspecified site D24- ☑
juvenile D24- ☑
pericanalicular
  specified site — *see* Neoplasm, benign, by site
  unspecified site D24- ☑
phyllodes D24- ☑
prostate D29.1
specified site NEC — *see* Neoplasm, benign, by site
unspecified site D24- ☑

Fibroadenosis, breast (chronic) (cystic) (diffuse) (periodic) (segmental) N60.2- ☑

Fibroangioma (*see also* Neoplasm, benign, by site)
juvenile
  specified site — *see* Neoplasm, benign, by site
  unspecified site D10.6

Fibrochondrosarcoma — *see* Neoplasm, cartilage, malignant

Fibrocystic
disease (*see also* Fibrosis, cystic)
  breast — *see* Mastopathy, cystic
  jaw M27.49
  kidney (congenital) Q61.8
  liver Q44.6
  pancreas E84.9
kidney (congenital) Q61.8

Fibrodysplasia ossificans progressiva — *see* Myositis, ossificans, progressiva

Fibroelastosis (cordis) (endocardial) (endomyocardial) I42.4

Fibroid (tumor) (*see also* Neoplasm, connective tissue, benign)
disease, lung (chronic) — *see* Fibrosis, lung
heart (disease) — *see* Myocarditis
in pregnancy or childbirth O34.1- ☑
  causing obstructed labor O65.5
induration, lung (chronic) — *see* Fibrosis, lung
lung — *see* Fibrosis, lung
pneumonia (chronic) — *see* Fibrosis, lung
uterus D25.9

Fibrolipoma — *see* Lipoma

Fibroliposarcoma — *see* Neoplasm, connective tissue, malignant

Fibroma (*see also* Neoplasm, connective tissue, benign)
ameloblastic — *see* Cyst, calcifying odontogenic
bone (nonossifying) — *see* Disorder, bone, specified type NEC

Fibroma — *continued*
bone — *see* Disorder, bone, specified type — *continued*
  ossifying — *see* Neoplasm, bone, benign
cementifying — *see* Neoplasm, bone, benign
chondromyxoid — *see* Neoplasm, bone, benign
desmoplastic — *see* Neoplasm, connective tissue, uncertain behavior
durum — *see* Neoplasm, connective tissue, benign
fascial — *see* Neoplasm, connective tissue, benign
invasive — *see* Neoplasm, connective tissue, uncertain behavior
molle — *see* Lipoma
myxoid — *see* Neoplasm, connective tissue, benign
nasopharynx, nasopharyngeal (juvenile) D10.6
nonosteogenic (nonossifying) — *see* Dysplasia, fibrous
odontogenic (central) — *see* Cyst, calcifying odontogenic
ossifying — *see* Neoplasm, bone, benign
periosteal — *see* Neoplasm, bone, benign
soft — *see* Lipoma

Fibromatosis M72.9
abdominal — *see* Neoplasm, connective tissue, uncertain behavior
aggressive — *see* Neoplasm, connective tissue, uncertain behavior
congenital generalized — *see* Neoplasm, connective tissue, uncertain behavior
Dupuytren's M72.0
gingival K06.1
palmar (fascial) M72.0
plantar (fascial) M72.2
pseudosarcomatous (proliferative) (subcutaneous) M72.4
retroperitoneal D48.3
specified NEC M72.8

Fibromyalgia M79.7

Fibromyoma (*see also* Neoplasm, connective tissue, benign)
uterus (corpus) (*see also* Leiomyoma, uterus)
  in pregnancy or childbirth — *see* Fibroid, in pregnancy or childbirth
    causing obstructed labor O65.5

Fibromyositis M79.7

Fibromyxolipoma D17.9

Fibromyxoma — *see* Neoplasm, connective tissue, benign

Fibromyxosarcoma — *see* Neoplasm, connective tissue, malignant

Fibro-odontoma, ameloblastic — *see* Cyst, calcifying odontogenic

Fibro-osteoma — *see* Neoplasm, bone, benign

Fibroplasia, retrolental H35.17- ☑

Fibropurulent — *see* condition

Fibrosarcoma (*see also* Neoplasm, connective tissue, malignant)
ameloblastic C41.1
  upper jaw (bone) C41.0
congenital — *see* Neoplasm, connective tissue, malignant
fascial — *see* Neoplasm, connective tissue, malignant
infantile — *see* Neoplasm, connective tissue, malignant
odontogenic C41.1
  upper jaw (bone) C41.0
periosteal — *see* Neoplasm, bone, malignant

Fibrosclerosis
breast N60.3- ☑
multifocal M35.5
penis (corpora cavernosa) N48.6

Fibrosis, fibrotic
adrenal (gland) E27.8
amnion O41.8X- ☑
anal papillae K62.89
arteriocapillary — *see* Arteriosclerosis
bladder N32.89
  interstitial — *see* Cystitis, chronic, interstitial
  localized submucosal — *see* Cystitis, chronic, interstitial
  panmural — *see* Cystitis, chronic, interstitial
breast — *see* Fibrosclerosis, breast
capillary (*see also* Arteriosclerosis) I70.90
  lung (chronic) — *see* Fibrosis, lung
cardiac — *see* Myocarditis
cervix N88.8
chorion O41.8X- ☑
corpus cavernosum (sclerosing) N48.6

Fibrosis, fibrotic — *continued*
cystic (of pancreas) E84.9
  with
    distal intestinal obstruction syndrome E84.19
    fecal impaction E84.19
    intestinal manifestations NEC E84.19
    pulmonary manifestations E84.0
    specified manifestations NEC E84.8
due to device, implant or graft (*see also* Complications, by site and type, specified NEC) T85.82 ☑
  arterial graft NEC T82.828 ☑
  breast (implant) T85.82 ☑
  catheter NEC T85.82 ☑
    dialysis (renal) T82.828 ☑
      intraperitoneal T85.82 ☑
    infusion NEC T82.828 ☑
      spinal (epidural) (subdural) T85.82 ☑
    urinary (indwelling) T83.82 ☑
  electronic (electrode) (pulse generator) (stimulator)
    bone T84.82 ☑
    cardiac T82.827 ☑
    nervous system (brain) (peripheral nerve) (spinal) T85.82 ☑
    urinary T83.82 ☑
  fixation, internal (orthopedic) NEC T84.82 ☑
  gastrointestinal (bile duct) (esophagus) T85.82 ☑
  genital NEC T83.82 ☑
  heart NEC T82.827 ☑
  joint prosthesis T84.82 ☑
  ocular (corneal graft) (orbital implant) NEC T85.82 ☑
  orthopedic NEC T84.82 ☑
  specified NEC T85.82 ☑
  urinary NEC T83.82 ☑
  vascular NEC T82.828 ☑
  ventricular intracranial shunt T85.82 ☑
ejaculatory duct N50.8
endocardium — *see* Endocarditis
endomyocardial (tropical) I42.3
epididymis N50.8
eye muscle — *see* Strabismus, mechanical
heart — *see* Myocarditis
hepatic — *see* Fibrosis, liver
hepatolienal (portal hypertension) K76.6
hepatosplenic (portal hypertension) K76.6
infrapatellar fat pad M79.4
intrascrotal N50.8
kidney N26.9
liver K74.0
  with sclerosis K74.2
    alcoholic K70.2
lung (atrophic) (chronic) (confluent) (massive) (perialveolar) (peribronchial) J84.10
  with
    anthracosilicosis J60
    anthracosis J60
    asbestosis J61
    bagassosis J67.1
    bauxite J63.1
    berylliosis J63.2
    byssinosis J66.0
    calcicosis J62.8
    chalicosis J62.8
    dust reticulation J64
    farmer's lung J67.0
    ganister disease J62.8
    graphite J63.3
    pneumoconiosis NOS J64
    siderosis J63.4
    silicosis J62.8
  capillary J84.10
  congenital P27.8
  diffuse (idiopathic) J84.10
    chemicals, gases, fumes or vapors (inhalation) J68.4
    interstitial J84.10
      acute J84.114
    talc J62.0
  following radiation J70.1
  idiopathic J84.112
  postinflammatory J84.10
  silicotic J62.8
  tuberculous — *see* Tuberculosis, pulmonary
lymphatic gland I89.8
median bar — *see* Hyperplasia, prostate
mediastinum (idiopathic) J98.5
meninges G96.19

Index

Fever — Fibrosis, fibrotic

Fibrosis, fibrotic — continued
  myocardium, myocardial — see Myocarditis
  ovary N83.8
  oviduct N83.8
  pancreas K86.8
  penis NEC N48.6
  pericardium I31.0
  perineum, in pregnancy or childbirth O34.7- ☑
    causing obstructed labor O65.5
  pleura J94.1
  popliteal fat pad M79.4
  prostate (chronic) — see Hyperplasia, prostate
  pulmonary (see also Fibrosis, lung) J84.10
    congenital P27.8
    idiopathic J84.112
  rectal sphincter K62.89
  retroperitoneal, idiopathic (with ureteral obstruction)
    N13.5
    with infection N13.6
  sclerosing mesenteric (idiopathic) K65.4
  scrotum N50.8
  seminal vesicle N50.8
  senile R54
  skin L90.5
  spermatic cord N50.8
  spleen D73.89
    in schistosomiasis (bilharziasis) B65.9 [D77]
  subepidermal nodular — see Neoplasm, skin, benign
  submucous (oral) (tongue) K13.5
  testis N44.8
    chronic, due to syphilis A52.76
  thymus (gland) E32.8
  tongue, submucous K13.5
  tunica vaginalis N50.8
  uterus (non-neoplastic) N85.8
  vagina N89.8
  valve, heart — see Endocarditis
  vas deferens N50.8
  vein I87.8
Fibrositis (periarticular) M79.7
  nodular, chronic (Jaccoud's) (rheumatoid) — see
    Arthropathy, postrheumatic, chronic
Fibrothorax J94.1
Fibrotic — see Fibrosis
Fibrous — see condition
Fibroxanthoma (see also Neoplasm, connective tissue,
  benign)
  atypical — see Neoplasm, connective tissue, uncertain
    behavior
  malignant — see Neoplasm, connective tissue, malig-
    nant
Fibroxanthosarcoma — see Neoplasm, connective tissue, malignant
Fiedler's
  disease (icterohemorrhagic leptospirosis) A27.0
  myocarditis (acute) I40.1
Fifth disease B08.3
  venereal A55
Filaria, filarial, filariasis — see Infestation, filarial
Filatov's disease — see Mononucleosis, infectious
File-cutter's disease — see Poisoning, lead
Filling defect
  biliary tract R93.2
  bladder R93.4
  duodenum R93.3
  gallbladder R93.2
  gastrointestinal tract R93.3
  intestine R93.3
  kidney R93.4
  stomach R93.3
  ureter R93.4
Fimbrial cyst Q50.4
Financial problem affecting care NOS Z59.9
  bankruptcy Z59.8
  foreclosure on loan Z59.8
Findings, abnormal, inconclusive, without diagnosis
  (see also Abnormal)
  17-ketosteroids, elevated R82.5
  acetonuria R82.4
  alcohol in blood R78.0
  anisocytosis R71.8
  antenatal screening of mother O28.9
    biochemical O28.1
    chromosomal O28.5
    cytological O28.2
    genetic O28.5
    hematological O28.0
    radiological O28.4

Findings, abnormal, inconclusive, without diagnosis
  — continued
  antenatal screening of mother — continued
    specified NEC O28.8
    ultrasonic O28.3
  antibody titer, elevated R76.0
  anticardiolipin antibody R76.0
  antiphosphatidylglycerol antibody R76.0
  antiphosphatidylinositol antibody R76.0
  antiphosphatidylserine antibody R76.0
  antiphospholipid antibody R76.0
  bacteriuria N39.0
  bicarbonate E87.8
  bile in urine R82.2
  blood sugar R73.09
    high R73.9
    low (transient) E16.2
  body fluid or substance, specified NEC R88.8
  casts, urine R82.99
  catecholamines R82.5
  cells, urine R82.99
  chloride E87.8
  cholesterol E78.9
    high E78.0
      with high triglycerides E78.2
  chyluria R82.0
  cloudy
    dialysis effluent R88.0
    urine R82.90
  creatinine clearance R94.4
  crystals, urine R82.99
  culture
    blood R78.81
    positive — see Positive, culture
  echocardiogram R93.1
  electrolyte level, urinary R82.99
  function study NEC R94.8
    bladder R94.8
    endocrine NEC R94.7
      thyroid R94.6
    kidney R94.4
    liver R94.5
    pancreas R94.8
    placenta R94.8
    pulmonary R94.2
    spleen R94.8
  gallbladder, nonvisualization R93.2
  glucose (tolerance test) (non-fasting) R73.09
  glycosuria R81
  heart
    shadow R93.1
    sounds R01.2
  hematinuria R82.3
  hematocrit drop (precipitous) R71.0
  hemoglobinuria R82.3
  human papillomavirus (HPV) DNA test positive
    cervix
      high risk R87.810
      low risk R87.820
    vagina
      high risk R87.811
      low risk R87.821
  in blood (of substance not normally found in blood)
    R78.9
    addictive drug NEC R78.4
    alcohol (excessive level) R78.0
    cocaine R78.2
    hallucinogen R78.3
    heavy metals (abnormal level) R78.79
    lead R78.71
    lithium (abnormal level) R78.89
    opiate drug R78.1
    psychotropic drug R78.5
    specified substance NEC R78.89
    steroid agent R78.6
  indoleacetic acid, elevated R82.5
  ketonuria R82.4
  lactic acid dehydrogenase (LDH) R74.0
  liver function test R79.89
  mammogram NEC R92.8
    calcification (calculus) R92.1
    inconclusive result (due to dense breasts) R92.2
    microcalcification R92.0
  mediastinal shift R93.8
  melanin, urine R82.99
  myoglobinuria R82.1
  neonatal screening P09
  nonvisualization of gallbladder R93.2

Findings, abnormal, inconclusive, without diagnosis
  — continued
  odor of urine NOS R82.90
  Papanicolaou cervix R87.619
    non-atypical endometrial cells R87.618
  pneumoencephalogram R93.0
  poikilocytosis R71.8
  potassium (deficiency) E87.6
    excess E87.5
  PPD R76.11
  radiologic (X-ray) R93.8
    abdomen R93.5
    biliary tract R93.2
    breast R92.8
    gastrointestinal tract R93.3
    genitourinary organs R93.8
    head R93.0
    inconclusive due to excess body fat of patient R93.9
    intrathoracic organs NEC R93.1
    placenta R93.8
    retroperitoneum R93.5
    skin R93.8
    skull R93.0
    subcutaneous tissue R93.8
  red blood cell (count) (morphology) (sickling) (volume)
    R71.8
  scan NEC R94.8
    bladder R94.8
    bone R94.8
    kidney R94.4
    liver R93.2
    lung R94.2
    pancreas R94.8
    placental R94.8
    spleen R94.8
    thyroid R94.6
  sedimentation rate, elevated R70.0
  SGOT R74.0
  SGPT R74.0
  sodium (deficiency) E87.1
    excess E87.0
  specified body fluid NEC R88.8
  stress test R94.39
  thyroid (function) (metabolic rate) (scan) (uptake)
    R94.6
  transaminase (level) R74.0
  triglycerides E78.9
    high E78.1
      with high cholesterol E78.2
  tuberculin skin test (without active tuberculosis)
    R76.11
  urine R82.90
    acetone R82.4
    bacteria N39.0
    bile R82.2
    casts or cells R82.99
    chyle R82.0
    culture positive R82.7
    glucose R81
    hemoglobin R82.3
    ketone R82.4
    sugar R81
  vanillylmandelic acid (VMA), elevated R82.5
  vectorcardiogram (VCG) R94.39
  ventriculogram R93.0
  white blood cell (count) (differential) (morphology)
    D72.9
  xerography R92.8
Finger — see condition
Fire, Saint Anthony's — see Erysipelas
Fire-setting
  pathological (compulsive) F63.1
Fish hook stomach K31.89
Fishmeal-worker's lung J67.8
Fissure, fissured
  anus, anal K60.2
    acute K60.0
    chronic K60.1
    congenital Q43.8
  ear, lobule, congenital Q17.8
  epiglottis (congenital) Q31.8
  larynx J38.7
    congenital Q31.8
  lip K13.0
    congenital — see Cleft, lip
  nipple N64.0
    associated with
      lactation O92.13

Fissure, fissured — *continued*
- nipple — *continued*
  - associated with — *continued*
    - pregnancy O92.11- ☑
    - puerperium O92.12
  - nose Q30.2
  - palate (congenital) — *see* Cleft, palate
  - skin R23.4
  - spine (congenital) (*see also* Spina bifida)
    - with hydrocephalus — *see* Spina bifida, by site, with hydrocephalus
  - tongue (acquired) K14.5
    - congenital Q38.3

Fistula (cutaneous) L98.8
- abdomen (wall) K63.2
  - bladder N32.2
  - intestine NEC K63.2
  - ureter N28.89
  - uterus N82.5
- abdominorectal K63.2
- abdominosigmoidal K63.2
- abdominothoracic J86.0
- abdominouterine N82.5
  - congenital Q51.7
- abdominovesical N32.2
- accessory sinuses — *see* Sinusitis
- actinomycotic — *see* Actinomycosis
- alveolar antrum — *see* Sinusitis, maxillary
- alveolar process K04.6
- anorectal K60.5
- antrobuccal — *see* Sinusitis, maxillary
- antrum — *see* Sinusitis, maxillary
- anus, anal (recurrent) (infectional) K60.3
  - congenital Q43.6
    - with absence, atresia and stenosis Q42.2
  - tuberculous A18.32
- aorta-duodenal I77.2
- appendix, appendicular K38.3
- arteriovenous (acquired) (nonruptured) I77.0
  - brain I67.1
    - congenital Q28.2
      - ruptured I60.8
    - ruptured I60.8
  - cerebral — *see* Fistula, arteriovenous, brain
  - congenital (peripheral) (*see also* Malformation, arteriovenous)
    - brain Q28.2
      - ruptured I60.8
    - coronary Q24.5
    - pulmonary Q25.72
  - coronary I25.41
    - congenital Q24.5
  - pulmonary I28.0
    - congenital Q25.72
  - surgically created (for dialysis) Z99.2
    - complication — *see* Complication, arteriovenous, fistula, surgically created
  - traumatic — *see* Injury, blood vessel
- artery I77.2
- aural (mastoid) — *see* Mastoiditis, chronic
- auricle (*see also* Disorder, pinna, specified type NEC)
  - congenital Q18.1
- Bartholin's gland N82.8
- bile duct (common) (hepatic) K83.3
  - with calculus, stones — *see* Calculus, bile duct
- biliary (tract) — *see* Fistula, bile duct
- bladder (sphincter) NEC (*see also* Fistula, vesico-) N32.2
  - into seminal vesicle N32.2
- bone (*see also* Disorder, bone, specified type NEC)
  - with osteomyelitis, chronic — *see* Osteomyelitis, chronic, with draining sinus
- brain G93.89
  - arteriovenous (acquired) I67.1
    - congenital Q28.2
- branchial (cleft) Q18.0
- branchiogenous Q18.0
- breast N61
  - puerperal, postpartum or gestational, due to mastitis (purulent) — *see* Mastitis, obstetric, purulent
- bronchial J86.0
- bronchocutaneous, bronchomediastinal, bronchopleural, bronchopleuromediastinal (infective) J86.0
  - tuberculous NEC A15.5
- bronchoesophageal J86.0
  - congenital Q39.2
    - with atresia of esophagus Q39.1
- bronchovisceral J86.0

Fistula — *continued*
- buccal cavity (infective) K12.2
- cecosigmoidal K63.2
- cecum K63.2
- cerebrospinal (fluid) G96.0
- cervical, lateral Q18.1
- cervicoaural Q18.1
- cervicosigmoidal N82.4
- cervicovesical N82.1
- cervix N82.8
- chest (wall) J86.0
- cholecystenteric — *see* Fistula, gallbladder
- cholecystocolic — *see* Fistula, gallbladder
- cholecystocolonic — *see* Fistula, gallbladder
- cholecystoduodenal — *see* Fistula, gallbladder
- cholecystogastric — *see* Fistula, gallbladder
- cholecystointestinal — *see* Fistula, gallbladder
- choledochoduodenal — *see* Fistula, bile duct
- cholocolic K82.3
- coccyx — *see* Sinus, pilonidal
- colon K63.2
- colostomy K94.09
- common duct — *see* Fistula, bile duct
- congenital, site not listed — *see* Anomaly, by site
- coronary, arteriovenous I25.41
  - congenital Q24.5
- costal region J86.0
- cul-de-sac, Douglas' N82.8
- cystic duct (*see also* Fistula, gallbladder)
  - congenital Q44.5
- dental K04.6
- diaphragm J86.0
- duodenum K31.6
- ear (external) (canal) — *see* Disorder, ear, external, specified type NEC
- enterocolic K63.2
- enterocutaneous K63.2
- enterouterine N82.4
  - congenital Q51.7
- enterovaginal N82.4
  - congenital Q52.2
  - large intestine N82.3
  - small intestine N82.2
- enterovesical N32.1
- epididymis N50.8
  - tuberculous A18.15
- esophagobronchial J86.0
  - congenital Q39.2
    - with atresia of esophagus Q39.1
- esophagocutaneous K22.8
- esophagopleural-cutaneous J86.0
- esophagotracheal J86.0
  - congenital Q39.2
    - with atresia of esophagus Q39.1
- esophagus K22.8
  - congenital Q39.2
    - with atresia of esophagus Q39.1
- ethmoid — *see* Sinusitis, ethmoidal
- eyeball (cornea) (sclera) — *see* Disorder, globe, hypotony
- eyelid H01.8
- fallopian tube, external N82.5
- fecal K63.2
  - congenital Q43.6
- from periapical abscess K04.6
- frontal sinus — *see* Sinusitis, frontal
- gallbladder K82.3
  - with calculus, cholelithiasis, stones — *see* Calculus, gallbladder
- gastric K31.6
- gastrocolic K31.6
  - congenital Q40.2
  - tuberculous A18.32
- gastroenterocolic K31.6
- gastroesophageal K31.6
- gastrojejunal K31.6
- gastrojejunocolic K31.6
- genital tract (female) N82.9
  - specified NEC N82.8
  - to intestine NEC N82.4
  - to skin N82.5
- hepatic artery-portal vein, congenital Q26.6
- hepatopleural J86.0
- hepatopulmonary J86.0
- ileorectal or ileosigmoidal K63.2
- ileovaginal N82.2
- ileovesical N32.1
- ileum K63.2

Fistula — *continued*
- in ano K60.3
  - tuberculous A18.32
- inner ear (labyrinth) — *see* subcategory H83.1 ☑
- intestine NEC K63.2
- intestinocolonic (abdominal) K63.2
- intestinoureteral N28.89
- intestinouterine N82.4
- intestinovaginal N82.4
  - large intestine N82.3
  - small intestine N82.2
- intestinovesical N32.1
- ischiorectal (fossa) K61.3
- jejunum K63.2
- joint M25.10
  - ankle M25.17- ☑
  - elbow M25.12- ☑
  - foot joint M25.17- ☑
  - hand joint M25.14- ☑
  - hip M25.15- ☑
  - knee M25.16- ☑
  - shoulder M25.11- ☑
  - specified joint NEC M25.18
  - tuberculous — *see* Tuberculosis, joint
  - vertebrae M25.18
  - wrist M25.13- ☑
- kidney N28.89
- labium (majus) (minus) N82.8
- labyrinth — *see* subcategory H83.1 ☑
- lacrimal (gland) (sac) H04.61- ☑
- lacrimonasal duct — *see* Fistula, lacrimal
- laryngotracheal, congenital Q34.8
- larynx J38.7
- lip K13.0
  - congenital Q38.0
- lumbar, tuberculous A18.01
- lung J86.0
- lymphatic I89.8
- mammary (gland) N61
- mastoid (process) (region) — *see* Mastoiditis, chronic
- maxillary J32.0
- medial, face and neck Q18.8
- mediastinal J86.0
- mediastinobronchial J86.0
- mediastinocutaneous J86.0
- middle ear — *see* subcategory H74.8 ☑
- mouth K12.2
- nasal J34.89
  - sinus — *see* Sinusitis
- nasopharynx J39.2
- nipple N64.0
- nose J34.89
- oral (cutaneous) K12.2
  - maxillary J32.0
  - nasal (with cleft palate) — *see* Cleft, palate
- orbit, orbital — *see* Disorder, orbit, specified type NEC
- oroantral J32.0
- oviduct, external N82.5
- palate (hard) M27.8
- pancreatic K86.8
- pancreaticoduodenal K86.8
- parotid (gland) K11.4
  - region K12.2
- penis N48.89
- perianal K60.3
- pericardium (pleura) (sac) — *see* Pericarditis
- pericecal K63.2
- perineorectal K60.4
- perineosigmoidal K63.2
- perineum, perineal (with urethral involvement) NEC N36.0
  - tuberculous A18.13
  - ureter N28.89
- perirectal K60.4
  - tuberculous A18.32
- peritoneum K65.9
- pharyngoesophageal J39.2
- pharynx J39.2
  - branchial cleft (congenital) Q18.0
- pilonidal (infected) (rectum) — *see* Sinus, pilonidal
- pleura, pleural, pleurocutaneous, pleuroperitoneal J86.0
  - tuberculous NEC A15.6
- pleuropericardial I31.8
- portal vein-hepatic artery, congenital Q26.6
- postauricular H70.81- ☑
- postoperative, persistent T81.83 ☑
  - specified site — *see* Fistula, by site

Fistula — *continued*
preauricular (congenital) Q18.1
prostate N42.89
pulmonary J86.0
  arteriovenous I28.0
    congenital Q25.72
  tuberculous — *see* Tuberculosis, pulmonary
pulmonoperitoneal J86.0
rectolabial N82.4
rectosigmoid (intercommunicating) K63.2
rectoureteral N28.89
rectourethral N36.0
  congenital Q64.73
rectouterine N82.4
  congenital Q51.7
rectovaginal N82.3
  congenital Q52.2
  tuberculous A18.18
rectovesical N32.1
  congenital Q64.79
rectovesicovaginal N82.3
rectovulval N82.4
  congenital Q52.79
rectum (to skin) K60.4
  congenital Q43.6
    with absence, atresia and stenosis Q42.0
  tuberculous A18.32
renal N28.89
retroauricular — *see* Fistula, postauricular
salivary duct or gland (any) K11.4
  congenital Q38.4
scrotum (urinary) N50.8
  tuberculous A18.15
semicircular canals — *see* subcategory H83.1 ☑
sigmoid K63.2
  to bladder N32.1
sinus — *see* Sinusitis
skin L98.8
  to genital tract (female) N82.5
splenocolic D73.89
stercoral K63.2
stomach K31.6
sublingual gland K11.4
submandibular gland K11.4
submaxillary (gland) K11.4
  region K12.2
thoracic J86.0
  duct I89.8
thoracoabdominal J86.0
thoracogastric J86.0
thoracointestinal J86.0
thorax J86.0
thyroglossal duct Q89.2
thyroid E07.89
trachea, congenital (external) (internal) Q32.1
tracheoesophageal J86.0
  congenital Q39.2
    with atresia of esophagus Q39.1
  following tracheostomy J95.04
traumatic arteriovenous — *see* Injury, blood vessel, by site
tuberculous — *code by* site under Tuberculosis
typhoid A01.09
umbilicourinary Q64.8
urachus, congenital Q64.4
ureter (persistent) N28.89
ureteroabdominal N28.89
ureterorectal N28.89
ureterosigmoido-abdominal N28.89
ureterovaginal N82.1
ureterovesical N32.2
urethra N36.0
  congenital Q64.79
  tuberculous A18.13
urethroperineal N36.0
urethroperineovesical N32.2
urethrorectal N36.0
  congenital Q64.73
urethroscrotal N50.8
urethrovaginal N82.1
urethrovesical N32.2
urinary (tract) (persistent) (recurrent) N36.0
uteroabdominal N82.5
  congenital Q51.7
uteroenteric, uterointestinal N82.4
  congenital Q51.7
uterorectal N82.4
  congenital Q51.7

Fistula — *continued*
uteroureteric N82.1
uterourethral Q51.7
uterovaginal N82.8
uterovesical N82.1
  congenital Q51.7
uterus N82.8
vagina (postpartal) (wall) N82.8
vaginocutaneous (postpartal) N82.5
vaginointestinal NEC N82.4
  large intestine N82.3
  small intestine N82.2
vaginoperineal N82.5
vasocutaneous, congenital Q55.7
vesical NEC N32.2
vesicoabdominal N32.2
vesicocervicovaginal N82.1
vesicocolic N32.1
vesicocutaneous N32.2
vesicoenteric N32.1
vesicointestinal N32.1
vesicometrorectal N82.4
vesicoperineal N32.2
vesicorectal N32.1
  congenital Q64.79
vesicosigmoidal N32.1
vesicosigmoidovaginal N82.3
vesicoureteral N32.2
vesicoureterovaginal N82.1
vesicourethral N32.2
vesicourethrorectal N32.1
vesicouterine N82.1
  congenital Q51.7
vesicovaginal N82.0
vulvorectal N82.4
  congenital Q52.79

Fit R56.9
epileptic — *see* Epilepsy
fainting R55
hysterical F44.5
newborn P90
Fitting (and adjustment) (of)
artificial
  arm — *see* Admission, adjustment, artificial, arm
  breast Z44.3 ☑
  eye Z44.2 ☑
  leg — *see* Admission, adjustment, artificial, leg
automatic implantable cardiac defibrillator (with synchronous cardiac pacemaker) Z45.02
brain neuropacemaker Z46.2
  implanted Z45.42
cardiac defibrillator — *see* Fitting (and adjustment) (of), automatic implantable cardiac defibrillator
catheter, non-vascular Z46.82
colostomy belt Z46.89
contact lenses Z46.0
cystostomy device Z46.6
defibrillator, cardiac — *see* Fitting (and adjustment) (of), automatic implantable cardiac defibrillator
dentures Z46.3
device NOS Z46.9
  abdominal Z46.89
  gastrointestinal NEC Z46.59
  implanted NEC Z45.89
  nervous system Z46.2
    implanted — *see* Admission, adjustment, device, implanted, nervous system
  orthodontic Z46.4
  orthoptic Z46.0
  orthotic Z46.89
  prosthetic (external) Z44.9
    breast Z44.3 ☑
    dental Z46.3
    eye Z44.2 ☑
    specified NEC Z44.8
  specified NEC Z46.89
  substitution
    auditory Z46.2
      implanted — *see* Admission, adjustment, device, implanted, hearing device
    nervous system Z46.2
      implanted — *see* Admission, adjustment, device, implanted, nervous system
    visual Z46.2
      implanted Z45.31
  urinary Z46.6
gastric lap band Z46.51
gastrointestinal appliance NEC Z46.59

Fitting — *continued*
glasses (reading) Z46.0
hearing aid Z46.1
ileostomy device Z46.89
insulin pump Z46.81
intestinal appliance NEC Z46.89
myringotomy device (stent) (tube) Z45.82
neuropacemaker Z46.2
  implanted Z45.42
non-vascular catheter Z46.82
orthodontic device Z46.4
orthopedic device (brace) (cast) (corset) (shoes) Z46.89
pacemaker (cardiac) Z45.018
  nervous system (brain) (peripheral nerve) (spinal cord) Z46.2
    implanted Z45.42
  pulse generator Z45.010
portacath (port-a-cath) Z45.2
prosthesis (external) Z44.9
  arm — *see* Admission, adjustment, artificial, arm
  breast Z44.3 ☑
  dental Z46.3
  eye Z44.2 ☑
  leg — *see* Admission, adjustment, artificial, leg
  specified NEC Z44.8
spectacles Z46.0
wheelchair Z46.89
Fitzhugh-Curtis syndrome
due to
  Chlamydia trachomatis A74.81
  Neisseria gonorrhorea (gonococcal peritonitis) A54.85
Fitz's syndrome (acute hemorrhagic pancreatitis) K85.8
Fixation
joint — *see* Ankylosis
larynx J38.7
stapes — *see* Ankylosis, ear ossicles
  deafness — *see* Deafness, conductive
uterus (acquired) — *see* Malposition, uterus
vocal cord J38.3
Flabby ridge K06.8
Flaccid (*see also* condition)
palate, congenital Q38.5
Flail
chest S22.5 ☑
  newborn (birth injury) P13.8
joint (paralytic) M25.20
  ankle M25.27- ☑
  elbow M25.22- ☑
  foot joint M25.27- ☑
  hand joint M25.24- ☑
  hip M25.25- ☑
  knee M25.26- ☑
  shoulder M25.21- ☑
  specified joint NEC M25.28
  wrist M25.23- ☑
Flajani's disease — *see* Hyperthyroidism, with, goiter (diffuse)
Flap, liver K71.3
Flashbacks (residual to hallucinogen use) F16.283
Flat
chamber (eye) — *see* Disorder, globe, hypotony, flat anterior chamber
chest, congenital Q67.8
foot (acquired) (fixed type) (painful) (postural) (*see also* Deformity, limb, flat foot)
  congenital (rigid) (spastic (everted)) Q66.5- ☑
  rachitic sequelae (late effect) E64.3
organ or site, congenital NEC — *see* Anomaly, by site
pelvis M95.5
  with disproportion (fetopelvic) O33.0
    causing obstructed labor O65.0
  congenital Q74.2
Flatau-Schilder disease G37.0
Flatback syndrome M40.30
lumbar region M40.36
lumbosacral region M40.37
thoracolumbar region M40.35
Flattening
head, femur M89.8X5
hip — *see* Coxa, plana
lip (congenital) Q18.8
nose (congenital) Q67.4
  acquired M95.0
Flatulence R14.3
psychogenic F45.8

Flatus R14.3
 vaginalis N89.8
Flax-dresser's disease J66.1
Flea bite — *see* Injury, bite, by site, superficial, insect
Flecks, glaucomatous (subcapsular) — *see* Cataract, complicated
Fleischer (-Kayser) **ring** (cornea) H18.04- ☑
Fleshy mole O02.0
Flexibilitas cerea — *see* Catalepsy
Flexion
 amputation stump (surgical) T87.89
 cervix — *see* Malposition, uterus
 contracture, joint — *see* Contraction, joint
 deformity, joint (*see also* Deformity, limb, flexion) M21.20
  hip, congenital Q65.89
 uterus (*see also* Malposition, uterus)
  lateral — *see* Lateroversion, uterus
Flexner-Boyd dysentery A03.2
Flexner's dysentery A03.1
Flexure — *see* Flexion
Flint murmur (aortic insufficiency) I35.1
Floater, vitreous — *see* Opacity, vitreous
Floating
 cartilage (joint) (*see also* Loose, body, joint)
  knee — *see* Derangement, knee, loose body
 gallbladder, congenital Q44.1
 kidney N28.89
  congenital Q63.8
 spleen D73.89
Flooding N92.0
Floor — *see* condition
Floppy
 baby syndrome (nonspecific) P94.2
 iris syndrome (intraoperative) (IFIS) H21.81
 nonrheumatic mitral valve syndrome I34.1
Flu (*see also* Influenza)
 avian (*see also* Influenza, due to, identified novel influenza A virus) J09.X2
 bird (*see also* Influenza, due to, identified novel influenza A virus) J09.X2
 intestinal NEC A08.4
 swine (viruses that normally cause infections in pigs) (*see also* Influenza, due to, identified novel influenza A virus) J09.X2
Fluctuating blood pressure I99.8
Fluid
 abdomen R18.8
 chest J94.8
 heart — *see* Failure, heart, congestive
 joint — *see* Effusion, joint
 loss (acute) E86.9
  with
   hypernatremia E87.0
   hyponatremia E87.1
 lung — *see* Edema, lung
 overload E87.70
  specified NEC E87.79
 peritoneal cavity R18.8
 pleural cavity J94.8
 retention R60.9
Flukes NEC (*see also* Infestation, fluke)
 blood NEC — *see* Schistosomiasis
 liver B66.3
Fluor (vaginalis) N89.8
 trichomonal or due to Trichomonas (vaginalis) A59.00
Fluorosis
 dental K00.3
 skeletal M85.10
  ankle M85.17- ☑
  foot M85.17- ☑
  forearm M85.13- ☑
  hand M85.14- ☑
  lower leg M85.16- ☑
  multiple site M85.19
  neck M85.18
  rib M85.18
  shoulder M85.11- ☑
  skull M85.18
  specified site NEC M85.18
  thigh M85.15- ☑
  toe M85.17- ☑
  upper arm M85.12- ☑
  vertebra M85.18
Flush syndrome E34.0
Flushing R23.2
 menopausal N95.1

Flutter
 atrial or auricular I48.92
  atypical I48.4
  type I I48.3
  type II I48.4
  typical I48.3
 heart I49.8
  atrial or auricular I48.92
   atypical I48.4
   type I I48.3
   type II I48.4
   typical I48.3
  ventricular I49.02
 ventricular I49.02
FNHTR (febrile nonhemolytic transfusion reaction) R50.84
Fochier's abscess — *code by* site under Abscess
Focus, Assmann's — *see* Tuberculosis, pulmonary
Fogo selvagem L10.3
Foix-Alajouanine syndrome G95.19
Fold, folds (anomalous) (*see also* Anomaly, by site)
 Descemet's membrane — *see* Change, corneal membrane, Descemet's, fold
 epicanthic Q10.3
 heart Q24.8
Folie à deux F24
Follicle
 cervix (nabothian) (ruptured) N88.8
 graafian, ruptured, with hemorrhage N83.0
 nabothian N88.8
Follicular — *see* condition
Folliculitis (superficial) L73.9
 abscedens et suffodiens L66.3
 cyst N83.0
 decalvans L66.2
 deep — *see* Furuncle, by site
 gonococcal (acute) (chronic) A54.01
 keloid, keloidalis L73.0
 pustular L01.02
 ulerythematosa reticulata L66.4
Folliculome lipidique
 specified site — *see* Neoplasm, benign, by site
 unspecified site
  female D27.9
  male D29.20
Følling's disease E70.0
Follow-up — *see* Examination, follow-up
Fong's syndrome (hereditary osteo-onychodysplasia) Q78.5
Food
 allergy L27.2
 asphyxia (from aspiration or inhalation) — *see* Foreign body, by site
 choked on — *see* Foreign body, by site
 deprivation T73.0 ☑
  specified kind of food NEC E63.8
 intoxication — *see* Poisoning, food
 lack of T73.0 ☑
 poisoning — *see* Poisoning, food
 rejection NEC — *see* Disorder, eating
 strangulation or suffocation — *see* Foreign body, by site
 toxemia — *see* Poisoning, food
Foot — *see* condition
Foramen ovale (nonclosure) (patent) (persistent) Q21.1
Forbes' glycogen storage disease E74.03
Fordyce-Fox disease L75.2
Fordyce's disease (mouth) Q38.6
Forearm — *see* condition
Foreign body
 with
  laceration — *see* Laceration, by site, with foreign body
  puncture wound — *see* Puncture, by site, with foreign body
 accidentally left following a procedure T81.509 ☑
  aspiration T81.506 ☑
   resulting in
    adhesions T81.516 ☑
    obstruction T81.526 ☑
    perforation T81.536 ☑
    specified complication NEC T81.596 ☑
  cardiac catheterization T81.505 ☑
   resulting in
    acute reaction T81.60 ☑
     aseptic peritonitis T81.61 ☑
     specified NEC T81.69 ☑
    adhesions T81.515 ☑

Foreign body — *continued*
 accidentally left following a procedure — *continued*
  cardiac catheterization — *continued*
   resulting in — *continued*
    obstruction T81.525 ☑
    perforation T81.535 ☑
    specified complication NEC T81.595 ☑
   causing
    acute reaction T81.60 ☑
     aseptic peritonitis T81.61 ☑
     specified complication NEC T81.69 ☑
    adhesions T81.519 ☑
    aseptic peritonitis T81.61 ☑
    obstruction T81.529 ☑
    perforation T81.539 ☑
    specified complication NEC T81.599 ☑
  endoscopy T81.504 ☑
   resulting in
    adhesions T81.514 ☑
    obstruction T81.524 ☑
    perforation T81.534 ☑
    specified complication NEC T81.594 ☑
  immunization T81.503 ☑
   resulting in
    adhesions T81.513 ☑
    obstruction T81.523 ☑
    perforation T81.533 ☑
    specified complication NEC T81.593 ☑
  infusion T81.501 ☑
   resulting in
    adhesions T81.511 ☑
    obstruction T81.521 ☑
    perforation T81.531 ☑
    specified complication NEC T81.591 ☑
  injection T81.503 ☑
   resulting in
    adhesions T81.513 ☑
    obstruction T81.523 ☑
    perforation T81.533 ☑
    specified complication NEC T81.593 ☑
  kidney dialysis T81.502 ☑
   resulting in
    adhesions T81.512 ☑
    obstruction T81.522 ☑
    perforation T81.532 ☑
    specified complication NEC T81.592 ☑
  packing removal T81.507 ☑
   resulting in
    acute reaction T81.60 ☑
     aseptic peritonitis T81.61 ☑
     specified NEC T81.69 ☑
    adhesions T81.517 ☑
    obstruction T81.527 ☑
    perforation T81.537 ☑
    specified complication NEC T81.597 ☑
  puncture T81.506 ☑
   resulting in
    adhesions T81.516 ☑
    obstruction T81.526 ☑
    perforation T81.536 ☑
    specified complication NEC T81.596 ☑
  specified procedure NEC T81.508 ☑
   resulting in
    acute reaction T81.60 ☑
     aseptic peritonitis T81.61 ☑
     specified NEC T81.69 ☑
    adhesions T81.518 ☑
    obstruction T81.528 ☑
    perforation T81.538 ☑
    specified complication NEC T81.598 ☑
  surgical operation T81.500 ☑
   resulting in
    acute reaction T81.60 ☑
     aseptic peritonitis T81.61 ☑
     specified NEC T81.69 ☑
    adhesions T81.510 ☑
    obstruction T81.520 ☑
    perforation T81.530 ☑
    specified complication NEC T81.590 ☑
  transfusion T81.501 ☑
   resulting in
    adhesions T81.511 ☑
    obstruction T81.521 ☑
    perforation T81.531 ☑
    specified complication NEC T81.591 ☑

Foreign body — *continued*
- alimentary tract T18.9 ☑
  - anus T18.5 ☑
  - colon T18.4 ☑
  - esophagus — *see* Foreign body, esophagus
  - mouth T18.0 ☑
  - multiple sites T18.8 ☑
  - rectosigmoid (junction) T18.5 ☑
  - rectum T18.5 ☑
  - small intestine T18.3 ☑
  - specified site NEC T18.8 ☑
  - stomach T18.2 ☑
- anterior chamber (eye) S05.5- ☑
- auditory canal — *see* Foreign body, entering through orifice, ear
- bronchus T17.508 ☑
  - causing
    - asphyxiation T17.500 ☑
      - food (bone) (seed) T17.520 ☑
      - gastric contents (vomitus) T17.510 ☑
      - specified type NEC T17.590 ☑
    - injury NEC T17.508 ☑
      - food (bone) (seed) T17.528 ☑
      - gastric contents (vomitus) T17.518 ☑
      - specified type NEC T17.598 ☑
- canthus — *see* Foreign body, conjunctival sac
- ciliary body (eye) S05.5- ☑
- conjunctival sac T15.1- ☑
- cornea T15.0- ☑
- entering through orifice
  - accessory sinus T17.0 ☑
  - alimentary canal T18.9 ☑
    - multiple parts T18.8 ☑
    - specified part NEC T18.8 ☑
  - alveolar process T18.0 ☑
  - antrum (Highmore's) T17.0 ☑
  - anus T18.5 ☑
  - appendix T18.4 ☑
  - auditory canal — *see* Foreign body, entering through orifice, ear
  - auricle — *see* Foreign body, entering through orifice, ear
  - bladder T19.1 ☑
  - bronchioles — *see* Foreign body, respiratory tract, specified site NEC
  - bronchus (main) — *see* Foreign body, bronchus
  - buccal cavity T18.0 ☑
  - canthus (inner) — *see* Foreign body, conjunctival sac
  - cecum T18.4 ☑
  - cervix (canal) (uteri) T19.3 ☑
  - colon T18.4 ☑
  - conjunctival sac — *see* Foreign body, conjunctival sac
  - cornea — *see* Foreign body, cornea
  - digestive organ or tract NOS T18.9 ☑
    - multiple parts T18.8 ☑
    - specified part NEC T18.8 ☑
  - duodenum T18.3 ☑
  - ear (external) T16.- ☑
  - esophagus — *see* Foreign body, esophagus
  - eye (external) NOS T15.9- ☑
    - conjunctival sac — *see* Foreign body, conjunctival sac
    - cornea — *see* Foreign body, cornea
    - specified part NEC T15.8- ☑
  - eyeball (*see also* Foreign body, entering through orifice, eye, specified part NEC)
    - with penetrating wound — *see* Puncture, eyeball
  - eyelid (*see also* Foreign body, conjunctival sac) with
    - laceration — *see* Laceration, eyelid, with foreign body
    - puncture — *see* Puncture, eyelid, with foreign body
    - superficial injury — *see* Foreign body, superficial, eyelid
  - gastrointestinal tract T18.9 ☑
    - multiple parts T18.8 ☑
    - specified part NEC T18.8 ☑
  - genitourinary tract T19.9 ☑
    - multiple parts T19.8 ☑
    - specified part NEC T19.8 ☑
  - globe — *see* Foreign body, entering through orifice, eyeball

Foreign body — *continued*
- entering through orifice — *continued*
  - gum T18.0 ☑
  - Highmore's antrum T17.0 ☑
  - hypopharynx — *see* Foreign body, pharynx
  - ileum T18.3 ☑
  - intestine (small) T18.3 ☑
    - large T18.4 ☑
  - lacrimal apparatus (punctum) — *see* Foreign body, entering through orifice, eye, specified part NEC
  - large intestine T18.4 ☑
  - larynx — *see* Foreign body, larynx
  - lung — *see* Foreign body, respiratory tract, specified site NEC
  - maxillary sinus T17.0 ☑
  - mouth T18.0 ☑
  - nasal sinus T17.0 ☑
  - nasopharynx — *see* Foreign body, pharynx
  - nose (passage) T17.1 ☑
  - nostril T17.1 ☑
  - oral cavity T18.0 ☑
  - palate T18.0 ☑
  - penis T19.4 ☑
  - pharynx — *see* Foreign body, pharynx
  - piriform sinus — *see* Foreign body, pharynx
  - rectosigmoid (junction) T18.5 ☑
  - rectum T18.5 ☑
  - respiratory tract — *see* Foreign body, respiratory tract
  - sinus (accessory) (frontal) (maxillary) (nasal) T17.0 ☑
    - piriform — *see* Foreign body, pharynx
  - small intestine T18.3 ☑
  - stomach T18.2 ☑
  - suffocation by — *see* Foreign body, by site
  - tear ducts or glands — *see* Foreign body, entering through orifice, eye, specified part NEC
  - throat — *see* Foreign body, pharynx
  - tongue T18.0 ☑
  - tonsil, tonsillar (fossa) — *see* Foreign body, pharynx
  - trachea — *see* Foreign body, trachea
  - ureter T19.8 ☑
  - urethra T19.0 ☑
  - uterus (any part) T19.3 ☑
  - vagina T19.2 ☑
  - vulva T19.2 ☑
- esophagus T18.108 ☑
  - causing
    - injury NEC T18.108 ☑
      - food (bone) (seed) T18.128 ☑
      - gastric contents (vomitus) T18.118 ☑
      - specified type NEC T18.198 ☑
    - tracheal compression T18.100 ☑
      - food (bone) (seed) T18.120 ☑
      - gastric contents (vomitus) T18.110 ☑
      - specified type NEC T18.190 ☑
- felling of, in throat R09.89
- fragment — *see* Retained, foreign body fragments (type of)
- genitourinary tract T19.9 ☑
  - bladder T19.1 ☑
  - multiple parts T19.8 ☑
  - penis T19.4 ☑
  - specified site NEC T19.8 ☑
  - urethra T19.0 ☑
  - uterus T19.3 ☑
    - IUD Z97.5
  - vagina T19.2 ☑
    - contraceptive device Z97.5
  - vulva T19.2 ☑
- granuloma (old) (soft tissue) (*see also* Granuloma, foreign body)
  - skin L92.3
- in
  - laceration — *see* Laceration, by site, with foreign body
  - puncture wound — *see* Puncture, by site, with foreign body
  - soft tissue (residual) M79.5
- inadvertently left in operation wound — *see* Foreign body, accidentally left during a procedure
- ingestion, ingested NOS T18.9 ☑
- inhalation or inspiration — *see* Foreign body, by site
- internal organ, not entering through a natural orifice — code as specific injury with foreign body

Foreign body — *continued*
- intraocular S05.5- ☑
  - old, retained (nonmagnetic) H44.70- ☑
    - anterior chamber H44.71- ☑
    - ciliary body H44.72- ☑
    - iris H44.72- ☑
    - lens H44.73- ☑
    - magnetic H44.60- ☑
      - anterior chamber H44.61- ☑
      - ciliary body H44.62- ☑
      - iris H44.62- ☑
      - lens H44.63- ☑
      - posterior wall H44.64- ☑
      - specified site NEC H44.69- ☑
      - vitreous body H44.65- ☑
    - posterior wall H44.74- ☑
    - specified site NEC H44.79- ☑
    - vitreous body H44.75- ☑
- iris — *see* Foreign body, intraocular
- lacrimal punctum — *see* Foreign body, entering through orifice, eye, specified part NEC
- larynx T17.308 ☑
  - causing
    - asphyxiation T17.300 ☑
      - food (bone) (seed) T17.320 ☑
      - gastric contents (vomitus) T17.310 ☑
      - specified type NEC T17.390 ☑
    - injury NEC T17.308 ☑
      - food (bone) (seed) T17.328 ☑
      - gastric contents (vomitus) T17.318 ☑
      - specified type NEC T17.398 ☑
- lens — *see* Foreign body, intraocular
- ocular muscle S05.4- ☑
  - old, retained — *see* Foreign body, orbit, old
- old or residual
  - soft tissue (residual) M79.5
- operation wound, left accidentally — *see* Foreign body, accidentally left during a procedure
- orbit S05.4- ☑
  - old, retained H05.5- ☑
- pharynx T17.208 ☑
  - causing
    - asphyxiation T17.200 ☑
      - food (bone) (seed) T17.220 ☑
      - gastric contents (vomitus) T17.210 ☑
      - specified type NEC T17.290 ☑
    - injury NEC T17.208 ☑
      - food (bone) (seed) T17.228 ☑
      - gastric contents (vomitus) T17.218 ☑
      - specified type NEC T17.298 ☑
- respiratory tract T17.908 ☑
  - bronchioles — *see* Foreign body, respiratory tract, specified site NEC
  - bronchus — *see* Foreign body, bronchus
  - causing
    - asphyxiation T17.900 ☑
      - food (bone) (seed) T17.920 ☑
      - gastric contents (vomitus) T17.910 ☑
      - specified type NEC T17.990 ☑
    - injury NEC T17.908 ☑
      - food (bone) (seed) T17.928 ☑
      - gastric contents (vomitus) T17.918 ☑
      - specified type NEC T17.998 ☑
  - larynx — *see* Foreign body, larynx
  - lung — *see* Foreign body, respiratory tract, specified site NEC
  - multiple parts — *see* Foreign body, respiratory tract, specified site NEC
  - nasal sinus T17.0 ☑
  - nasopharynx — *see* Foreign body, pharynx
  - nose T17.1 ☑
  - nostril T17.1 ☑
  - pharynx — *see* Foreign body, pharynx
  - specified site NEC T17.808 ☑
    - causing
      - asphyxiation T17.800 ☑
        - food (bone) (seed) T17.820 ☑
        - gastric contents (vomitus) T17.810 ☑
        - specified type NEC T17.890 ☑
      - injury NEC T17.808 ☑
        - food (bone) (seed) T17.828 ☑
        - gastric contents (vomitus) T17.818 ☑
        - specified type NEC T17.898 ☑
  - throat — *see* Foreign body, pharynx
  - trachea — *see* Foreign body, trachea
- retained (old) (nonmagnetic) (in)

Foreign body — *continued*
  retained — *continued*
    anterior chamber (eye) — *see* Foreign body, intraocular, old, retained, anterior chamber
      magnetic — *see* Foreign body, intraocular, old, retained, magnetic, anterior chamber
    ciliary body — *see* Foreign body, intraocular, old, retained, ciliary body
      magnetic — *see* Foreign body, intraocular, old, retained, magnetic, ciliary body
    eyelid H02.819
      left H02.816
        lower H02.815
        upper H02.814
      right H02.813
        lower H02.812
        upper H02.811
    fragments — *see* Retained, foreign body fragments (type of)
    globe — *see* Foreign body, intraocular, old, retained
      magnetic — *see* Foreign body, intraocular, old, retained, magnetic
    intraocular — *see* Foreign body, intraocular, old, retained
      magnetic — *see* Foreign body, intraocular, old, retained, magnetic
    iris — *see* Foreign body, intraocular, old, retained, iris
      magnetic — *see* Foreign body, intraocular, old, retained, magnetic, iris
    lens — *see* Foreign body, intraocular, old, retained, lens
      magnetic — *see* Foreign body, intraocular, old, retained, magnetic, lens
    muscle — *see* Foreign body, retained, soft tissue
    orbit — *see* Foreign body, orbit, old
    posterior wall of globe — *see* Foreign body, intraocular, old, retained, posterior wall
      magnetic — *see* Foreign body, intraocular, old, retained, magnetic, posterior wall
    retrobulbar — *see* Foreign body, orbit, old, retrobulbar
    soft tissue M79.5
    vitreous — *see* Foreign body, intraocular, old, retained, vitreous body
      magnetic — *see* Foreign body, intraocular, old, retained, magnetic, vitreous body
  retina S05.5- ☑
  superficial, without open wound
    abdomen, abdominal (wall) S30.851 ☑
    alveolar process S00.552 ☑
    ankle S90.55- ☑
    antecubital space — *see* Foreign body, superficial, forearm
    anus S30.857 ☑
    arm (upper) S40.85- ☑
    auditory canal — *see* Foreign body, superficial, ear
    auricle — *see* Foreign body, superficial, ear
    axilla — *see* Foreign body, superficial, arm
    back, lower S30.850 ☑
    breast S20.15- ☑
    brow S00.85 ☑
    buttock S30.850 ☑
    calf — *see* Foreign body, superficial, leg
    canthus — *see* Foreign body, superficial, eyelid
    cheek S00.85 ☑
      internal S00.552 ☑
    chest wall — *see* Foreign body, superficial, thorax
    chin S00.85 ☑
    clitoris S30.854 ☑
    costal region — *see* Foreign body, superficial, thorax
    digit(s)
      foot — *see* Foreign body, superficial, toe
      hand — *see* Foreign body, superficial, finger
    ear S00.45- ☑
    elbow S50.35- ☑
    epididymis S30.853 ☑
    epigastric region S30.851 ☑
    epiglottis S10.15 ☑
    esophagus, cervical S10.15 ☑
    eyebrow — *see* Foreign body, superficial, eyelid
    eyelid S00.25- ☑
    face S00.85 ☑
    finger(s) S60.459 ☑
      index S60.45- ☑

Foreign body — *continued*
  superficial, without open wound — *continued*
    finger(s) — *continued*
      little S60.45- ☑
      middle S60.45- ☑
      ring S60.45- ☑
    flank S30.851 ☑
    foot (except toe(s) alone) S90.85- ☑
      toe — *see* Foreign body, superficial, toe
    forearm S50.85- ☑
      elbow only — *see* Foreign body, superficial, elbow
    forehead S00.85 ☑
    genital organs, external
      female S30.856 ☑
      male S30.855 ☑
    groin S30.851 ☑
    gum S00.552 ☑
    hand S60.55- ☑
    head S00.95 ☑
      ear — *see* Foreign body, superficial, ear
      eyelid — *see* Foreign body, superficial, eyelid
      lip S00.551 ☑
      nose S00.35 ☑
      oral cavity S00.552 ☑
      scalp S00.05 ☑
      specified site NEC S00.85 ☑
    heel — *see* Foreign body, superficial, foot
    hip S70.25- ☑
    inguinal region S30.851 ☑
    interscapular region S20.459 ☑
    jaw S00.85 ☑
    knee S80.25- ☑
    labium (majus) (minus) S30.854 ☑
    larynx S10.15 ☑
    leg (lower) S80.85- ☑
      knee — *see* Foreign body, superficial, knee
      upper — *see* Foreign body, superficial, thigh
    lip S00.551 ☑
    lower back S30.850 ☑
    lumbar region S30.850 ☑
    malar region S00.85 ☑
    mammary — *see* Foreign body, superficial, breast
    mastoid region S00.85 ☑
    mouth S00.552 ☑
    nail
      finger — *see* Foreign body, superficial, finger
      toe — *see* Foreign body, superficial, toe
    nape S10.85 ☑
    nasal S00.35 ☑
    neck S10.95 ☑
      specified site NEC S10.85 ☑
      throat S10.15 ☑
    nose S00.35 ☑
    occipital region S00.05 ☑
    oral cavity S00.552 ☑
    orbital region — *see* Foreign body, superficial, eyelid
    palate S00.552 ☑
    palm — *see* Foreign body, superficial, hand
    parietal region S00.05 ☑
    pelvis S30.850 ☑
    penis S30.852 ☑
    perineum
      female S30.854 ☑
      male S30.850 ☑
    periocular area — *see* Foreign body, superficial, eyelid
    phalanges
      finger — *see* Foreign body, superficial, finger
      toe — *see* Foreign body, superficial, toe
    pharynx S10.15 ☑
    pinna — *see* Foreign body, superficial, ear
    popliteal space — *see* Foreign body, superficial, knee
    prepuce S30.852 ☑
    pubic region S30.850 ☑
    pudendum
      female S30.856 ☑
      male S30.855 ☑
    sacral region S30.850 ☑
    scalp S00.05 ☑
    scapular region — *see* Foreign body, superficial, shoulder
    scrotum S30.853 ☑
    shin — *see* Foreign body, superficial, leg

Foreign body — *continued*
  superficial, without open wound — *continued*
    shoulder S40.25- ☑
    sternal region S20.359 ☑
    submaxillary region S00.85 ☑
    submental region S00.85 ☑
    subungual
      finger(s) — *see* Foreign body, superficial, finger
      toe(s) — *see* Foreign body, superficial, toe
    supraclavicular fossa S10.85 ☑
    supraorbital S00.85 ☑
    temple S00.85 ☑
    temporal region S00.85 ☑
    testis S30.853 ☑
    thigh S70.35- ☑
    thorax, thoracic (wall) S20.95 ☑
      back S20.45- ☑
      front S20.35- ☑
    throat S10.15 ☑
    thumb S60.35- ☑
    toe(s) (lesser) S90.456 ☑
      great S90.45- ☑
    tongue S00.552 ☑
    trachea S10.15 ☑
    tunica vaginalis S30.853 ☑
    tympanum, tympanic membrane — *see* Foreign body, superficial, ear
    uvula S00.552 ☑
    vagina S30.854 ☑
    vocal cords S10.15 ☑
    vulva S30.854 ☑
    wrist S60.85- ☑
  swallowed T18.9 ☑
  trachea T17.408 ☑
    causing
      asphyxiation T17.400 ☑
        food (bone) (seed) T17.420 ☑
        gastric contents (vomitus) T17.410 ☑
        specified type NEC T17.490 ☑
      injury NEC T17.408 ☑
        food (bone) (seed) T17.428 ☑
        gastric contents (vomitus) T17.418 ☑
        specified type NEC T17.498 ☑
  type of fragment — *see* Retained, foreign body fragments (type of)
  vitreous (humor) S05.5- ☑
Forestier's disease (rhizomelic pseudopolyarthritis) M35.3
  meaning ankylosing hyperostosis — *see* Hyperostosis, ankylosing
Formation
  hyalin in cornea — *see* Degeneration, cornea
  sequestrum in bone (due to infection) — *see* Osteomyelitis, chronic
  valve
    colon, congenital Q43.8
    ureter (congenital) Q62.39
Formication R20.2
Fort Bragg fever A27.89
Fossa (*see also* condition)
  pyriform — *see* condition
Foster-Kennedy syndrome H47.14- ☑
Fothergill's
  disease (trigeminal neuralgia) (*see also* Neuralgia, trigeminal)
  scarlatina anginosa A38.9
Foul breath R19.6
Foundling Z76.1
Fournier disease or gangrene N49.3
  female N76.89
Fourth
  cranial nerve — *see* condition
  molar K00.1
Foville's (peduncular) **disease or syndrome** G46.3
Fox (-Fordyce) disease (apocrine miliaria) L75.2
Fracture, burst — *see* Fracture, traumatic, by site
Fracture, chronic — *see* Fracture, pathological
Fracture, insufficiency — *see* Fracture, pathologic, by site
Fracture, pathological (pathologic) (*see also* Fracture, traumatic) M84.40 ☑
  ankle M84.47- ☑
  carpus M84.44- ☑
  clavicle M84.41- ☑
  dental implant M27.63
  dental restorative material K08.539

Fracture, pathological — *continued*
- dental restorative material — *continued*
  - with loss of material K08.531
  - without loss of material K08.530
- due to
  - neoplastic disease NEC (*see also* Neoplasm) M84.50
    - ankle M84.57- ☑
    - carpus M84.54- ☑
    - clavicle M84.51- ☑
    - femur M84.55- ☑
    - fibula M84.56- ☑
    - finger M84.54- ☑
    - hip M84.559 ☑
    - humerus M84.52- ☑
    - ilium M84.550 ☑
    - ischium M84.550 ☑
    - metacarpus M84.54- ☑
    - metatarsus M84.57- ☑
    - neck M84.58 ☑
    - pelvis M84.550 ☑
    - radius M84.53- ☑
    - rib M84.58 ☑
    - scapula M84.51- ☑
    - skull M84.58 ☑
    - specified site NEC M84.58 ☑
    - tarsus M84.57- ☑
    - tibia M84.56- ☑
    - toe M84.57- ☑
    - ulna M84.53- ☑
    - vertebra M84.58 ☑
  - osteoporosis M80.80 ☑
    - disuse — *see* Osteoporosis, specified type NEC, with pathological fracture
    - drug-induced — *see* Osteoporosis, drug induced, with pathological fracture
    - idiopathic — *see* Osteoporosis, specified type NEC, with pathological fracture
    - postmenopausal — *see* Osteoporosis, postmenopausal, with pathological fracture
    - postoophorectomy — *see* Osteoporosis, postoophorectomy, with pathological fracture
    - postsurgical malabsorption — *see* Osteoporosis, specified type NEC, with pathological fracture
    - specified cause NEC — *see* Osteoporosis, specified type NEC, with pathological fracture
  - specified disease NEC M84.60 ☑
    - ankle M84.67- ☑
    - carpus M84.64- ☑
    - clavicle M84.61- ☑
    - femur M84.65- ☑
    - fibula M84.66- ☑
    - finger M84.64- ☑
    - hip M84.65- ☑
    - humerus M84.62- ☑
    - ilium M84.650 ☑
    - ischium M84.650 ☑
    - metacarpus M84.64- ☑
    - metatarsus M84.67- ☑
    - neck M84.68 ☑
    - radius M84.63- ☑
    - rib M84.68 ☑
    - scapula M84.61- ☑
    - skull M84.68 ☑
    - tarsus M84.67- ☑
    - tibia M84.66- ☑
    - toe M84.67- ☑
    - ulna M84.63- ☑
    - vertebra M84.68 ☑
- femur M84.45- ☑
- fibula M84.46- ☑
- finger M84.44- ☑
- hip M84.459 ☑
- humerus M84.42- ☑
- ilium M84.454 ☑
- ischium M84.454 ☑
- joint prosthesis — *see* Complications, joint prosthesis, mechanical, breakdown, by site
  - periprosthetic — *see* Complications, joint prosthesis, mechanical, periprosthesis, fracture, by site
- metacarpus M84.44- ☑
- metatarsus M84.47- ☑
- neck M84.48 ☑

Fracture, pathological — *continued*
- pelvis M84.454 ☑
- radius M84.43- ☑
- restorative material (dental) K08.539
  - with loss of material K08.531
  - without loss of material K08.530
- rib M84.48 ☑
- scapula M84.41- ☑
- skull M84.48 ☑
- tarsus M84.47- ☑
- tibia M84.46- ☑
- toe M84.47- ☑
- ulna M84.43- ☑
- vertebra M84.48 ☑

Fracture, traumatic (abduction) (adduction) (separation) (*see also* Fracture, pathological) T14.8
- acetabulum S32.40- ☑
  - column
    - anterior (displaced) (iliopubic) S32.43- ☑
      - nondisplaced S32.436 ☑
    - posterior (displaced) (ilioischial) S32.443 ☑
      - nondisplaced S32.44- ☑
  - dome (displaced) S32.48- ☑
    - nondisplaced S32.48 ☑
  - specified NEC S32.49- ☑
  - transverse (displaced) S32.45- ☑
    - with associated posterior wall fracture (displaced) S32.46- ☑
      - nondisplaced S32.46- ☑
    - nondisplaced S32.45- ☑
  - wall
    - anterior (displaced) S32.41- ☑
      - nondisplaced S32.41- ☑
    - medial (displaced) S32.47- ☑
      - nondisplaced S32.47- ☑
    - posterior (displaced) S32.42- ☑
      - with associated transverse fracture (displaced) S32.46- ☑
        - nondisplaced S32.46- ☑
      - nondisplaced S32.42- ☑
- acromion — *see* Fracture, scapula, acromial process
- ankle S82.899 ☑
  - bimalleolar (displaced) S82.84- ☑
    - nondisplaced S82.84- ☑
  - lateral malleolus only (displaced) S82.6- ☑
    - nondisplaced S82.6- ☑
  - medial malleolus (displaced) S82.5- ☑
    - associated with Maisonneuve's fracture — *see* Fracture, Maisonneuve's
    - nondisplaced S82.5- ☑
  - talus — *see* Fracture, tarsal, talus
  - trimalleolar (displaced) S82.85- ☑
    - nondisplaced S82.85- ☑
- arm (upper) (*see also* Fracture, humerus, shaft)
  - humerus — *see* Fracture, humerus
  - radius — *see* Fracture, radius
  - ulna — *see* Fracture, ulna
- astragalus — *see* Fracture, tarsal, talus
- atlas — *see* Fracture, neck, cervical vertebra, first
- axis — *see* Fracture, neck, cervical vertebra, second
- back — *see* Fracture, vertebra
- Barton's — *see* Barton's fracture
- base of skull — *see* Fracture, skull, base
- basicervical (basal) (femoral) S72.0 ☑
- Bennett's — *see* Bennett's fracture
- bimalleolar — *see* Fracture, ankle, bimalleolar
- blow-out S02.3 ☑
- bone NEC T14.8
  - birth injury P13.9
  - following insertion of orthopedic implant, joint prosthesis or bone plate — *see* Fracture, following insertion of orthopedic implant, joint prosthesis or bone plate
  - in (due to) neoplastic disease NEC — *see* Fracture, pathological, due to, neoplastic disease
  - pathological (cause unknown) — *see* Fracture, pathological
- breast bone — *see* Fracture, sternum
- bucket handle (semilunar cartilage) — *see* Tear, meniscus
- burst — *see* Fracture, traumatic, by site
- calcaneus — *see* Fracture, tarsal, calcaneus
- carpal bone(s) S62.10- ☑
  - capitate (displaced) S62.13- ☑
    - nondisplaced S62.13- ☑
  - cuneiform — *see* Fracture, carpal bone, triquetrum

Fracture, traumatic — *continued*
- carpal bone(s) — *continued*
  - hamate (body) (displaced) S62.143 ☑
    - hook process (displaced) S62.15- ☑
      - nondisplaced S62.15- ☑
    - nondisplaced S62.14- ☑
  - larger multangular — *see* Fracture, carpal bones, trapezium
  - lunate (displaced) S62.12- ☑
    - nondisplaced S62.12- ☑
  - navicular S62.00- ☑
    - distal pole (displaced) S62.01- ☑
      - nondisplaced S62.01- ☑
    - middle third (displaced) S62.02- ☑
      - nondisplaced S62.02- ☑
    - proximal third (displaced) S62.03- ☑
      - nondisplaced S62.03- ☑
    - volar tuberosity — *see* Fracture, carpal bones, navicular, distal pole
  - os magnum — *see* Fracture, carpal bones, capitate
  - pisiform (displaced) S62.16- ☑
    - nondisplaced S62.16- ☑
  - semilunar — *see* Fracture, carpal bones, lunate
  - smaller multangular — *see* Fracture, carpal bones, trapezoid
  - trapezium (displaced) S62.17- ☑
    - nondisplaced S62.17- ☑
  - trapezoid (displaced) S62.18- ☑
    - nondisplaced S62.18- ☑
  - triquetrum (displaced) S62.11- ☑
    - nondisplaced S62.11- ☑
  - unciform — *see* Fracture, carpal bones, hamate
- cervical — *see* Fracture, vertebra, cervical
- clavicle S42.00- ☑
  - acromial end (displaced) S42.03- ☑
    - nondisplaced S42.03- ☑
  - birth injury P13.4
  - lateral end — *see* Fracture, clavicle, acromial end
  - shaft (displaced) S42.02- ☑
    - nondisplaced S42.02- ☑
  - sternal end (anterior) (displaced) S42.01- ☑
    - nondisplaced S42.01- ☑
    - posterior S42.01- ☑
- coccyx S32.2 ☑
- collapsed — *see* Collapse, vertebra
- collar bone — *see* Fracture, clavicle
- Colles' — *see* Colles' fracture
- compression, not due to trauma — *see* Collapse, vertebra
- coronoid process — *see* Fracture, ulna, upper end, coronoid process
- corpus cavernosum penis S39.840 ☑
- costochondral cartilage S23.41 ☑
- costochondral, costosternal junction — *see* Fracture, rib
- cranium — *see* Fracture, skull
- cricoid cartilage S12.8 ☑
- cuboid (ankle) — *see* Fracture, tarsal, cuboid
- cuneiform
  - foot — *see* Fracture, tarsal, cuneiform
  - wrist — *see* Fracture, carpal, triquetrum
- delayed union — *see* Delay, union, fracture
- dental restorative material K08.539
  - with loss of material K08.531
  - without loss of material K08.530
- due to
  - birth injury — *see* Birth, injury, fracture
  - osteoporosis — *see* Osteoporosis, with fracture
- Dupuytren's — *see* Fracture, ankle, lateral malleolus
- elbow S42.40- ☑
- ethmoid (bone) (sinus) — *see* Fracture, skull, base
- face bone S02.92 ☑
- fatigue (*see also* Fracture, stress)
  - vertebra M48.40 ☑
    - cervical region M48.42 ☑
    - cervicothoracic region M48.43 ☑
    - lumbar region M48.46 ☑
    - lumbosacral region M48.47 ☑
    - occipito-atlanto-axial region M48.41 ☑
    - sacrococcygeal region M48.48 ☑
    - thoracic region M48.44 ☑
    - thoracolumbar region M48.45 ☑
- femur, femoral S72.9- ☑
  - basicervical (basal) S72.0 ☑
  - birth injury P13.2
  - capital epiphyseal S79.01- ☑

Fracture, traumatic — *continued*
  femur, femoral — *continued*
    condyles, epicondyles — *see* Fracture, femur, lower end
    distal end — *see* Fracture, femur, lower end
    epiphysis
      head — *see* Fracture, femur, upper end, epiphysis
      lower — *see* Fracture, femur, lower end, epiphysis
      upper — *see* Fracture, femur, upper end, epiphysis
    following insertion of implant, prosthesis or plate M96.66- ☑
    head — *see* Fracture, femur, upper end, head
    intertrochanteric — *see* Fracture, femur, trochanteric
    intratrochanteric — *see* Fracture, femur, trochanteric
    lower end S72.40- ☑
      condyle (displaced) S72.41- ☑
        lateral (displaced) S72.42- ☑
          nondisplaced S72.42- ☑
        medial (displaced) S72.43- ☑
          nondisplaced S72.43- ☑
        nondisplaced S72.41- ☑
      epiphysis (displaced) S72.44- ☑
        nondisplaced S72.44- ☑
      physeal S79.10- ☑
        Salter-Harris
          Type I S79.11- ☑
          Type II S79.12- ☑
          Type III S79.13- ☑
          Type IV S79.14- ☑
        specified NEC S79.19- ☑
      specified NEC S72.49- ☑
      supracondylar (displaced) S72.45- ☑
        with intracondylar extension (displaced) S72.46- ☑
          nondisplaced S72.46- ☑
        nondisplaced S72.45- ☑
      torus S72.47- ☑
    neck — *see* Fracture, femur, upper end, neck
    pertrochanteric — *see* Fracture, femur, trochanteric
    shaft (lower third) (middle third) (upper third) S72.30- ☑
      comminuted (displaced) S72.35- ☑
        nondisplaced S72.35- ☑
      oblique (displaced) S72.33- ☑
        nondisplaced S72.33- ☑
      segmental (displaced) S72.36- ☑
        nondisplaced S72.36- ☑
      specified NEC S72.39- ☑
      spiral (displaced) S72.34- ☑
        nondisplaced S72.34- ☑
      transverse (displaced) S72.32- ☑
        nondisplaced S72.32- ☑
    specified site NEC — *see* subcategory S72.8 ☑
    subcapital (displaced) S72.01- ☑
    subtrochanteric (region) (section) (displaced) S72.2- ☑
      nondisplaced S72.2- ☑
    transcervical — *see* Fracture, femur, upper end, neck
    transtrochanteric — *see* Fracture, femur, trochanteric
    trochanteric S72.10- ☑
      apophyseal (displaced) S72.14- ☑
        nondisplaced S72.14- ☑
      greater trochanter (displaced) S72.11- ☑
        nondisplaced S72.11- ☑
      intertrochanteric (displaced) S72.13- ☑
        nondisplaced S72.13- ☑
      lesser trochanter (displaced) S72.12- ☑
        nondisplaced S72.12- ☑
    upper end S72.00- ☑
      apophyseal (displaced) S72.13- ☑
        nondisplaced S72.13- ☑
      cervicotrochanteric — *see* Fracture, femur, upper end, neck, base
      epiphysis (displaced) S72.02- ☑
        nondisplaced S72.02- ☑
      head S72.05- ☑
        articular (displaced) S72.06- ☑
          nondisplaced S72.06- ☑

Fracture, traumatic — *continued*
  femur, femoral — *continued*
    upper end — *continued*
      head — *continued*
        specified NEC S72.09- ☑
      intertrochanteric (displaced) S72.14- ☑
        nondisplaced S72.14- ☑
      intracapsular S72.01- ☑
      midcervical (displaced) S72.03- ☑
        nondisplaced S72.03- ☑
      neck S72.00- ☑
        base (displaced) S72.04- ☑
          nondisplaced S72.04- ☑
        specified NEC S72.09- ☑
      pertrochanteric — *see* Fracture, femur, upper end, trochanteric
      physeal S79.00- ☑
        Salter-Harris type I S79.01- ☑
        specified NEC S79.09- ☑
      subcapital (displaced) S72.01- ☑
      subtrochanteric (displaced) S72.2- ☑
        nondisplaced S72.2- ☑
      transcervical — *see* Fracture, femur, upper end, midcervical
      trochanteric S72.10- ☑
        greater (displaced) S72.11- ☑
          nondisplaced S72.11- ☑
        lesser (displaced) S72.12- ☑
          nondisplaced S72.12- ☑
  fibula (shaft) (styloid) S82.40- ☑
    comminuted (displaced) S82.45- ☑
      nondisplaced S82.45- ☑
    following insertion of implant, prosthesis or plate M96.67- ☑
    involving ankle or malleolus — *see* Fracture, fibula, lateral malleolus
    lateral malleolus (displaced) S82.6- ☑
      nondisplaced S82.6- ☑
    lower end
      physeal S89.30- ☑
        Salter-Harris
          Type I S89.31- ☑
          Type II S89.32- ☑
        specified NEC S89.39- ☑
      specified NEC S82.83- ☑
      torus S82.82- ☑
    oblique (displaced) S82.43- ☑
      nondisplaced S82.43- ☑
    segmental (displaced) S82.46- ☑
      nondisplaced S82.46- ☑
    specified NEC S82.49- ☑
    spiral (displaced) S82.44- ☑
      nondisplaced S82.44- ☑
    transverse (displaced) S82.42- ☑
      nondisplaced S82.42- ☑
    upper end
      physeal S89.20- ☑
        Salter-Harris
          Type I S89.21- ☑
          Type II S89.22- ☑
        specified NEC S89.29- ☑
      specified NEC S82.83- ☑
      torus S82.81- ☑
  finger (except thumb) S62.60- ☑
    distal phalanx (displaced) S62.63- ☑
      nondisplaced S62.66- ☑
    index S62.60- ☑
      distal phalanx (displaced) S62.63- ☑
        nondisplaced S62.66- ☑
      medial phalanx (displaced) S62.62- ☑
        nondisplaced S62.65- ☑
      proximal phalanx (displaced) S62.61- ☑
        nondisplaced S62.64- ☑
    little S62.60- ☑
      distal phalanx (displaced) S62.63- ☑
        nondisplaced S62.66- ☑
      medial phalanx (displaced) S62.62- ☑
        nondisplaced S62.65- ☑
      proximal phalanx (displaced) S62.61- ☑
        nondisplaced S62.64- ☑
    medial phalanx (displaced) S62.62- ☑
      nondisplaced S62.65- ☑
    middle S62.60- ☑
      distal phalanx (displaced) S62.63- ☑
        nondisplaced S62.66- ☑
      medial phalanx (displaced) S62.62-

Fracture, traumatic — *continued*
  finger — *continued*
    middle — *continued*
      medial phalanx — *continued*
        nondisplaced S62.65- ☑
        proximal phalanx (displaced) S62.61- ☑
      proximal phalanx (displaced) S62.61- ☑
        nondisplaced S62.64- ☑
    ring S62.60- ☑
      distal phalanx (displaced) S62.63- ☑
        nondisplaced S62.66- ☑
      medial phalanx (displaced) S62.62- ☑
        nondisplaced S62.65- ☑
      proximal phalanx (displaced) S62.61- ☑
        nondisplaced S62.64- ☑
    thumb — *see* Fracture, thumb
  following insertion (intraoperative) (postoperative) of orthopedic implant, joint prosthesis or bone plate M96.69
    femur M96.66- ☑
    fibula M96.67- ☑
    humerus M96.62- ☑
    pelvis M96.65
    radius M96.63- ☑
    specified bone NEC M96.69
    tibia M96.67- ☑
    ulna M96.63- ☑
  foot S92.90- ☑
    astragalus — *see* Fracture, tarsal, talus
    calcaneus — *see* Fracture, tarsal, calcaneus
    cuboid — *see* Fracture, tarsal, cuboid
    cuneiform — *see* Fracture, tarsal, cuneiform
    metatarsal — *see* Fracture, metatarsal
    navicular — *see* Fracture, tarsal, navicular
    talus — *see* Fracture, tarsal, talus
    tarsal — *see* Fracture, tarsal
    toe — *see* Fracture, toe
  forearm S52.9- ☑
    radius — *see* Fracture, radius
    ulna — *see* Fracture, ulna
  fossa (anterior) (middle) (posterior) S02.19 ☑
  frontal (bone) (skull) S02.0 ☑
    sinus S02.19 ☑
  glenoid (cavity) (scapula) — *see* Fracture, scapula, glenoid cavity
  greenstick — *see* Fracture, by site
  hallux — *see* Fracture, toe, great
  hand S62.9- ☑
    carpal — *see* Fracture, carpal bone
    finger (except thumb) — *see* Fracture, finger
    metacarpal — *see* Fracture, metacarpal
    navicular (scaphoid) (hand) — *see* Fracture, carpal bone, navicular
    thumb — *see* Fracture, thumb
  healed or old
    with complications — *code by* Nature of the complication
  heel bone — *see* Fracture, tarsal, calcaneus
  Hill-Sachs S42.29- ☑
  hip — *see* Fracture, femur, neck
  humerus S42.30- ☑
    anatomical neck — *see* Fracture, humerus, upper end
    articular process — *see* Fracture, humerus, lower end
    capitellum — *see* Fracture, humerus, lower end, condyle, lateral
    distal end — *see* Fracture, humerus, lower end
    epiphysis
      lower — *see* Fracture, humerus, lower end, physeal
      upper — *see* Fracture, humerus, upper end, physeal
    external condyle — *see* Fracture, humerus, lower end, condyle, lateral
    following insertion of implant, prosthesis or plate M96.62- ☑
    great tuberosity — *see* Fracture, humerus, upper end, greater tuberosity
    intercondylar — *see* Fracture, humerus, lower end
    internal epicondyle — *see* Fracture, humerus, lower end, epicondyle, medial
    lesser tuberosity — *see* Fracture, humerus, upper end, lesser tuberosity
    lower end S42.40- ☑

Fracture, traumatic — *continued*
  humerus — *continued*
    lower end — *continued*
      condyle
        lateral (displaced) S42.45- ☑
          nondisplaced S42.45- ☑
        medial (displaced) S42.46- ☑
          nondisplaced S42.46- ☑
      epicondyle
        lateral (displaced) S42.43- ☑
          nondisplaced S42.43- ☑
        medial (displaced) S42.44- ☑
          incarcerated S42.44- ☑
          nondisplaced S42.44- ☑
      physeal S49.10- ☑
        Salter-Harris
          Type I S49.11- ☑
          Type II S49.12- ☑
          Type III S49.13- ☑
          Type IV S49.14- ☑
          specified NEC S49.19- ☑
      specified NEC (displaced) S42.49- ☑
        nondisplaced S42.49- ☑
      supracondylar (simple) (displaced) S42.41- ☑
        comminuted (displaced) S42.42- ☑
          nondisplaced S42.42- ☑
        nondisplaced S42.41- ☑
      torus S42.48- ☑
      transcondylar (displaced) S42.47- ☑
        nondisplaced S42.47- ☑
    proximal end — *see* Fracture, humerus, upper end
    shaft S42.30- ☑
      comminuted (displaced) S42.35- ☑
        nondisplaced S42.35- ☑
      greenstick S42.31- ☑
      oblique (displaced) S42.33- ☑
        nondisplaced S42.33- ☑
      segmental (displaced) S42.36- ☑
        nondisplaced S42.36- ☑
      specified NEC S42.39- ☑
      spiral (displaced) S42.34- ☑
        nondisplaced S42.34- ☑
      transverse (displaced) S42.32- ☑
        nondisplaced S42.32- ☑
    supracondylar — *see* Fracture, humerus, lower end
    surgical neck — *see* Fracture, humerus, upper end, surgical neck
    trochlea — *see* Fracture, humerus, lower end, condyle, medial
    tuberosity — *see* Fracture, humerus, upper end
    upper end S42.20- ☑
      anatomical neck — *see* Fracture, humerus, upper end, specified NEC
      articular head — *see* Fracture, humerus, upper end, specified NEC
      epiphysis — *see* Fracture, humerus, upper end, physeal
      greater tuberosity (displaced) S42.25- ☑
        nondisplaced S42.25- ☑
      lesser tuberosity (displaced) S42.26- ☑
        nondisplaced S42.26- ☑
      physeal S49.00- ☑
        Salter-Harris
          Type I S49.01- ☑
          Type II S49.02- ☑
          Type III S49.03- ☑
          Type IV S49.04- ☑
          specified NEC S49.09- ☑
      specified NEC (displaced) S42.29- ☑
        nondisplaced S42.29- ☑
      surgical neck (displaced) S42.21- ☑
        four-part S42.24- ☑
        nondisplaced S42.21- ☑
        three-part S42.23- ☑
        two-part (displaced) S42.22- ☑
          nondisplaced S42.22- ☑
      torus S42.27- ☑
      transepiphyseal — *see* Fracture, humerus, upper end, physeal
  hyoid bone S12.8 ☑
  ilium S32.30- ☑
    with disruption of pelvic ring — *see* Disruption, pelvic ring
    avulsion (displaced) S32.31- ☑
      nondisplaced S32.31- ☑
    specified NEC S32.39- ☑

Fracture, traumatic — *continued*
  impaction, impacted — *code as* Fracture, by site
  innominate bone — *see* Fracture, ilium
  instep — *see* Fracture, foot
  ischium S32.60- ☑
    with disruption of pelvic ring — *see* Disruption, pelvic ring
    avulsion (displaced) S32.61- ☑
      nondisplaced S32.61- ☑
    specified NEC S32.69- ☑
  jaw (bone) (lower) — *see* Fracture, mandible
    upper — *see* Fracture, maxilla
  joint prosthesis — *see* Complications, joint prosthesis, mechanical, breakdown, by site
    periprosthetic — *see* Complications, joint prosthesis, mechanical, periprosthesis, fracture, by site
  knee cap — *see* Fracture, patella
  larynx S12.8 ☑
  late effects — *see* Sequelae, fracture
  leg (lower) S82.9- ☑
    ankle — *see* Fracture, ankle
    femur — *see* Fracture, femur
    fibula — *see* Fracture, fibula
    malleolus — *see* Fracture, ankle
    patella — *see* Fracture, patella
    specified site NEC S82.89- ☑
    tibia — *see* Fracture, tibia
  lumbar spine — *see* Fracture, vertebra, lumbar
  lumbosacral spine S32.9 ☑
  Maisonneuve's (displaced) S82.86- ☑
    nondisplaced S82.86- ☑
  malar bone (*see also* Fracture, maxilla) S02.400 ☑
  malleolus — *see* Fracture, ankle
  malunion — *see* Fracture, by site
  mandible (lower jaw (bone)) S02.609 ☑
    alveolus S02.67 ☑
    angle (of jaw) S02.65 ☑
    body, unspecified S02.600 ☑
    condylar process S02.61 ☑
    coronoid process S02.63 ☑
    ramus, unspecified S02.64 ☑
    specified site NEC S02.69 ☑
    subcondylar process S02.62 ☑
    symphysis S02.66 ☑
  manubrium (sterni) S22.21 ☑
    dissociation from sternum S22.23 ☑
  march — *see* Fracture, traumatic, stress, by site
  maxilla, maxillary (bone) (sinus) (superior) (upper jaw) S02.401 ☑
    alveolus S02.42 ☑
    inferior — *see* Fracture, mandible
    LeFort I S02.411 ☑
    LeFort II S02.412 ☑
    LeFort III S02.413 ☑
  metacarpal S62.309 ☑
    base (displaced) S62.319 ☑
      nondisplaced S62.349 ☑
    fifth S62.30- ☑
      base (displaced) S62.31- ☑
        nondisplaced S62.34- ☑
      neck (displaced) S62.33- ☑
        nondisplaced S62.36- ☑
      shaft (displaced) S62.32- ☑
        nondisplaced S62.35- ☑
      specified NEC S62.398 ☑
    first S62.20- ☑
      base NEC (displaced) S62.23- ☑
        nondisplaced S62.23- ☑
      Bennett's — *see* Bennett's fracture
      neck (displaced) S62.25- ☑
        nondisplaced S62.25- ☑
      shaft (displaced) S62.24- ☑
        nondisplaced S62.24- ☑
      specified NEC S62.29- ☑
    fourth S62.30- ☑
      base (displaced) S62.31- ☑
        nondisplaced S62.34- ☑
      neck (displaced) S62.33- ☑
        nondisplaced S62.36- ☑
      shaft (displaced) S62.32- ☑
        nondisplaced S62.35- ☑
      specified NEC S62.39- ☑
    neck (displaced) S62.33- ☑
      nondisplaced S62.36- ☑
    Rolando's — *see* Rolando's fracture

Fracture, traumatic — *continued*
  metacarpal — *continued*
    second S62.30- ☑
      base (displaced) S62.31- ☑
        nondisplaced S62.34- ☑
      neck (displaced) S62.33- ☑
        nondisplaced S62.36- ☑
      shaft (displaced) S62.32- ☑
        nondisplaced S62.35- ☑
      specified NEC S62.39- ☑
    shaft (displaced) S62.32- ☑
      nondisplaced S62.35- ☑
    specified NEC S62.399 ☑
    third S62.30- ☑
      base (displaced) S62.31- ☑
        nondisplaced S62.34- ☑
      neck (displaced) S62.33- ☑
        nondisplaced S62.36- ☑
      shaft (displaced) S62.32- ☑
        nondisplaced S62.35- ☑
      specified NEC S62.39- ☑
  metastatic — *see* Fracture, pathological, due to, neoplastic disease (*see also* Neoplasm)
  metatarsal bone S92.30- ☑
    fifth (displaced) S92.35- ☑
      nondisplaced S92.35- ☑
    first (displaced) S92.31- ☑
      nondisplaced S92.31- ☑
    fourth (displaced) S92.34- ☑
      nondisplaced S92.34- ☑
    second (displaced) S92.32- ☑
      nondisplaced S92.32- ☑
    third (displaced) S92.33- ☑
      nondisplaced S92.33- ☑
  Monteggia's — *see* Monteggia's fracture
  multiple
    hand (and wrist) NEC — *see* Fracture, by site
    ribs — *see* Fracture, rib, multiple
  nasal (bone(s)) S02.2 ☑
  navicular (scaphoid) (foot) (*see also* Fracture, tarsal, navicular)
    hand — *see* Fracture, carpal, navicular
  neck S12.9 ☑
    cervical vertebra S12.9 ☑
      fifth (displaced) S12.400 ☑
        nondisplaced S12.401 ☑
        specified type NEC (displaced) S12.490 ☑
          nondisplaced S12.491 ☑
      first (displaced) S12.000 ☑
        burst (stable) S12.01 ☑
          unstable S12.02 ☑
        lateral mass (displaced) S12.040 ☑
          nondisplaced S12.041 ☑
        nondisplaced S12.001 ☑
        posterior arch (displaced) S12.030 ☑
          nondisplaced S12.031 ☑
        specified type NEC (displaced) S12.090 ☑
          nondisplaced S12.091 ☑
      fourth (displaced) S12.300 ☑
        nondisplaced S12.301 ☑
        specified type NEC (displaced) S12.390 ☑
          nondisplaced S12.391 ☑
      second (displaced) S12.100 ☑
        dens (anterior) (displaced) (type II) S12.110 ☑
          nondisplaced S12.112 ☑
          posterior S12.111 ☑
          specified type NEC (displaced) S12.120 ☑
            nondisplaced S12.121 ☑
        nondisplaced S12.101 ☑
        specified type NEC (displaced) S12.190 ☑
          nondisplaced S12.191 ☑
      seventh (displaced) S12.600 ☑
        nondisplaced S12.601 ☑
        specified type NEC (displaced) S12.690 ☑
          displaced S12.691 ☑
      sixth (displaced) S12.500 ☑
        nondisplaced S12.501 ☑
        specified type NEC (displaced) S12.590 ☑
          displaced S12.591 ☑
      third (displaced) S12.200 ☑
        nondisplaced S12.201 ☑
        specified type NEC (displaced) S12.290 ☑
          displaced S12.291 ☑

☑ Additional Character Required — Refer to the Tabular List for Character Selection   ▽ Subterms under main terms may continue to next column or page

Fracture, traumatic — *continued*
neck — *continued*
　hyoid bone S12.8 ☑
　larynx S12.8 ☑
　specified site NEC S12.8 ☑
　thyroid cartilage S12.8 ☑
　trachea S12.8 ☑
neoplastic NEC — *see* Fracture, pathological, due to, neoplastic disease
neural arch — *see* Fracture, vertebra
newborn — *see* Birth, injury, fracture
nontraumatic — *see* Fracture, pathological
nonunion — *see* Nonunion, fracture
nose, nasal (bone) (septum) S02.2
occiput — *see* Fracture, skull, base, occiput
odontoid process — *see* Fracture, neck, cervical vertebra, second
olecranon (process) (ulna) — *see* Fracture, ulna, upper end, olecranon process
orbit, orbital (bone) (region) S02.8 ☑
　floor (blow-out) S02.3 ☑
　roof S02.19 ☑
os
　calcis — *see* Fracture, tarsal, calcaneus
　magnum — *see* Fracture, carpal, capitate
　pubis — *see* Fracture, pubis
palate S02.8 ☑
parietal bone (skull) S02.0 ☑
patella S82.00- ☑
　comminuted (displaced) S82.04- ☑
　　nondisplaced S82.04- ☑
　longitudinal (displaced) S82.02- ☑
　　nondisplaced S82.02- ☑
　osteochondral (displaced) S82.01- ☑
　　nondisplaced S82.01- ☑
　specified NEC S82.09- ☑
　transverse (displaced) S82.03- ☑
　　nondisplaced S82.03- ☑
pedicle (of vertebral arch) — *see* Fracture, vertebra
pelvis, pelvic (bone) S32.9 ☑
　acetabulum — *see* Fracture, acetabulum
　circle — *see* Disruption, pelvic ring
　following insertion of implant, prosthesis or plate M96.65
　ilium — *see* Fracture, ilium
　ischium — *see* Fracture, ischium
　multiple
　　with disruption of pelvic ring (circle) — *see* Disruption, pelvic ring
　　without disruption of pelvic ring (circle) S32.82 ☑
　pubis — *see* Fracture, pubis
　sacrum — *see* Fracture, sacrum
　specified site NEC S32.89 ☑
phalanx
　foot — *see* Fracture, toe
　hand — *see* Fracture, finger
pisiform — *see* Fracture, carpal, pisiform
pond — *see* Fracture, skull
prosthetic device, internal — *see* Complications, prosthetic device, by site, mechanical
pubis S32.50- ☑
　with disruption of pelvic ring — *see* Disruption, pelvic ring
　specified site NEC S32.59- ☑
　superior rim S32.51- ☑
radius S52.9- ☑
　distal end — *see* Fracture, radius, lower end
　following insertion of implant, prosthesis or plate M96.63- ☑
　head — *see* Fracture, radius, upper end, head
　lower end S52.50- ☑
　　Barton's — *see* Barton's fracture
　　Colles' — *see* Colles' fracture
　　extraarticular NEC S52.55- ☑
　　intraarticular NEC S52.57- ☑
　　physeal S59.20- ☑
　　　Salter-Harris
　　　　Type I S59.21- ☑
　　　　Type II S59.22- ☑
　　　　Type III S59.23- ☑
　　　　Type IV S59.24- ☑
　　　specified NEC S59.29- ☑
　　Smith's — *see* Smith's fracture
　　specified NEC S52.59- ☑
　　styloid process (displaced) S52.51- ☑

Fracture, traumatic — *continued*
radius — *continued*
　lower end — *continued*
　　styloid process — *continued*
　　　nondisplaced S52.51- ☑
　　torus S52.52- ☑
　neck — *see* Fracture, radius, upper end
　proximal end — *see* Fracture, radius, upper end
　shaft S52.30- ☑
　　bent bone S52.38- ☑
　　comminuted (displaced) S52.35- ☑
　　　nondisplaced S52.35- ☑
　　Galeazzi's — *see* Galeazzi's fracture
　　greenstick S52.31- ☑
　　oblique (displaced) S52.33- ☑
　　　nondisplaced S52.33- ☑
　　segmental (displaced) S52.36- ☑
　　　nondisplaced S52.36- ☑
　　specified NEC S52.39- ☑
　　spiral (displaced) S52.34- ☑
　　　nondisplaced S52.34- ☑
　　transverse (displaced) S52.32- ☑
　　　nondisplaced S52.32- ☑
　upper end S52.10- ☑
　　head (displaced) S52.12- ☑
　　　nondisplaced S52.12- ☑
　　neck (displaced) S52.13- ☑
　　　nondisplaced S52.13- ☑
　　physeal S59.10- ☑
　　　Salter-Harris
　　　　Type I S59.11- ☑
　　　　Type II S59.12- ☑
　　　　Type III S59.13- ☑
　　　　Type IV S59.14- ☑
　　　specified NEC S59.19- ☑
　　specified NEC S52.18- ☑
　　torus S52.11- ☑
ramus
　inferior or superior, pubis — *see* Fracture, pubis
　mandible — *see* Fracture, mandible
restorative material (dental) K08.539
　with loss of material K08.531
　without loss of material K08.530
rib S22.3- ☑
　with flail chest — *see* Flail, chest
　multiple S22.4- ☑
　　with flail chest — *see* Flail, chest
root, tooth — *see* Fracture, tooth
sacrum S32.10 ☑
　specified NEC S32.19 ☑
　Type
　　1 S32.14 ☑
　　2 S32.15 ☑
　　3 S32.16 ☑
　　4 S32.17 ☑
　Zone
　　I S32.119 ☑
　　　displaced (minimally) S32.111 ☑
　　　　severely S32.112 ☑
　　　nondisplaced S32.110 ☑
　　II S32.129 ☑
　　　displaced (minimally) S32.121 ☑
　　　　severely S32.122 ☑
　　　nondisplaced S32.120 ☑
　　III S32.139 ☑
　　　displaced (minimally) S32.131 ☑
　　　　severely S32.132 ☑
　　　nondisplaced S32.130 ☑
scaphoid (hand) (*see also* Fracture, carpal, navicular)
　foot — *see* Fracture, tarsal, navicular
scapula S42.10- ☑
　acromial process (displaced) S42.12- ☑
　　nondisplaced S42.12- ☑
　body (displaced) S42.11- ☑
　　nondisplaced S42.11- ☑
　coracoid process (displaced) S42.13- ☑
　　nondisplaced S42.13- ☑
　glenoid cavity (displaced) S42.14- ☑
　　nondisplaced S42.14- ☑
　neck (displaced) S42.15- ☑
　　nondisplaced S42.15- ☑
　specified NEC S42.19- ☑
semilunar bone, wrist — *see* Fracture, carpal, lunate
sequelae — *see* Sequelae, fracture
sesamoid bone
　hand — *see* Fracture, carpal

Fracture, traumatic — *continued*
sesamoid bone — *continued*
　other — *code by* site under Fracture
shepherd's — *see* Fracture, tarsal, talus
shoulder (girdle) S42.9- ☑
　blade — *see* Fracture, scapula
sinus (ethmoid) (frontal) S02.19 ☑
skull S02.91 ☑
　base S02.10 ☑
　　occiput S02.119 ☑
　　　condyle S02.113 ☑
　　　　type I S02.110 ☑
　　　　type II S02.111 ☑
　　　　type III S02.112 ☑
　　　　specified NEC S02.118 ☑
　　specified NEC S02.19 ☑
　birth injury P13.0
　frontal bone S02.0 ☑
　parietal bone S02.0 ☑
　specified site NEC S02.8 ☑
　temporal bone S02.19 ☑
　vault S02.0 ☑
Smith's — *see* Smith's fracture
sphenoid (bone) (sinus) S02.19 ☑
spine — *see* Fracture, vertebra
spinous process — *see* Fracture, vertebra
spontaneous (cause unknown) — *see* Fracture, pathological
stave (of thumb) — *see* Fracture, metacarpal, first
sternum S22.20 ☑
　with flail chest — *see* Flail, chest
　body S22.22 ☑
　manubrium S22.21 ☑
　xiphoid (process) S22.24 ☑
stress M84.30 ☑
　ankle M84.37- ☑
　carpus M84.34- ☑
　clavicle M84.31- ☑
　femoral neck M84.359 ☑
　femur M84.35- ☑
　fibula M84.36- ☑
　finger M84.34- ☑
　hip M84.359 ☑
　humerus M84.32- ☑
　ilium M84.350 ☑
　ischium M84.350 ☑
　metacarpus M84.34- ☑
　metatarsus M84.37- ☑
　neck — *see* Fracture, fatigue, vertebra
　pelvis M84.350 ☑
　radius M84.33- ☑
　rib M84.38 ☑
　scapula M84.31- ☑
　skull M84.38 ☑
　tarsus M84.37- ☑
　tibia M84.36- ☑
　toe M84.37- ☑
　ulna M84.33- ☑
　vertebra — *see* Fracture, fatigue, vertebra
supracondylar, elbow — *see* Fracture, humerus, lower end, supracondylar
symphysis pubis — *see* Fracture, pubis
talus (ankle bone) — *see* Fracture, tarsal, talus
tarsal bone(s) S92.20- ☑
　astragalus — *see* Fracture, tarsal, talus
　calcaneus S92.00- ☑
　　anterior process (displaced) S92.02- ☑
　　　nondisplaced S92.02- ☑
　　body (displaced) S92.01- ☑
　　　nondisplaced S92.01- ☑
　　extraarticular NEC (displaced) S92.05- ☑
　　　nondisplaced S92.05- ☑
　　intraarticular (displaced) S92.06- ☑
　　　nondisplaced S92.06- ☑
　　tuberosity (displaced) S92.04- ☑
　　　avulsion (displaced) S92.03- ☑
　　　　nondisplaced S92.03- ☑
　　　nondisplaced S92.04- ☑
　cuboid (displaced) S92.21- ☑
　　nondisplaced S92.21- ☑
　cuneiform
　　intermediate (displaced) S92.23- ☑
　　　nondisplaced S92.23- ☑
　　lateral (displaced) S92.22- ☑
　　　nondisplaced S92.22- ☑
　　medial (displaced) S92.24- ☑

Index

Fracture, traumatic — Fracture, traumatic

Fracture, traumatic — *continued*
  tarsal bone(s) — *continued*
    cuneiform — *continued*
      medial — *continued*
        nondisplaced S92.24- ☑
    navicular (displaced) S92.25- ☑
      nondisplaced S92.25- ☑
    scaphoid — *see* Fracture, tarsal, navicular
    talus S92.10- ☑
      avulsion (displaced) S92.15- ☑
        nondisplaced S92.15- ☑
      body (displaced) S92.12- ☑
        nondisplaced S92.12- ☑
      dome (displaced) S92.14- ☑
        nondisplaced S92.14- ☑
      head (displaced) S92.12- ☑
        nondisplaced S92.12- ☑
      lateral process (displaced) S92.14- ☑
        nondisplaced S92.14- ☑
      neck (displaced) S92.11- ☑
        nondisplaced S92.11- ☑
      posterior process (displaced) S92.13- ☑
        nondisplaced S92.13- ☑
      specified NEC S92.19- ☑
  temporal bone (styloid) S02.19 ☑
  thorax (bony) S22.9 ☑
    with flail chest — *see* Flail, chest
    rib S22.3- ☑
      multiple S22.4- ☑
        with flail chest — *see* Flail, chest
    sternum S22.20 ☑
      body S22.22 ☑
      manubrium S22.21 ☑
      xiphoid process S22.24 ☑
    vertebra (displaced) S22.009 ☑
      burst (stable) S22.001 ☑
        unstable S22.002 ☑
      eighth S22.069 ☑
        burst (stable) S22.061 ☑
          unstable S22.062 ☑
        specified type NEC S22.068 ☑
        wedge compression S22.060 ☑
      eleventh S22.089 ☑
        burst (stable) S22.081 ☑
          unstable S22.082 ☑
        specified type NEC S22.088 ☑
        wedge compression S22.080 ☑
      fifth S22.059 ☑
        burst (stable) S22.051 ☑
          unstable S22.052 ☑
        specified type NEC S22.058 ☑
        wedge compression S22.050 ☑
      first S22.019 ☑
        burst (stable) S22.011 ☑
          unstable S22.012 ☑
        specified type NEC S22.018 ☑
        wedge compression S22.010 ☑
      fourth S22.049 ☑
        burst (stable) S22.041 ☑
          unstable S22.042 ☑
        specified type NEC S22.048 ☑
        wedge compression S22.040 ☑
      ninth S22.079 ☑
        burst (stable) S22.071 ☑
          unstable S22.072 ☑
        specified type NEC S22.078 ☑
        wedge compression S22.070 ☑
      nondisplaced S22.001 ☑
      second S22.029 ☑
        burst (stable) S22.021 ☑
          unstable S22.022 ☑
        specified type NEC S22.028 ☑
        wedge compression S22.020 ☑
      seventh S22.069 ☑
        burst (stable) S22.061 ☑
          unstable S22.062 ☑
        specified type NEC S22.068 ☑
        wedge compression S22.060 ☑
      sixth S22.059 ☑
        burst (stable) S22.051 ☑
          unstable S22.052 ☑
        specified type NEC S22.058 ☑
        wedge compression S22.050 ☑
      specified type NEC S22.008 ☑
      tenth S22.079 ☑

Fracture, traumatic — *continued*
  thorax — *continued*
    vertebra — *continued*
      tenth — *continued*
        burst (stable) S22.071 ☑
          unstable S22.072 ☑
        specified type NEC S22.078 ☑
        wedge compression S22.070 ☑
      third S22.039 ☑
        burst (stable) S22.031 ☑
          unstable S22.032 ☑
        specified type NEC S22.038 ☑
        wedge compression S22.030 ☑
      twelfth S22.089 ☑
        burst (stable) S22.081 ☑
          unstable S22.082 ☑
        specified type NEC S22.088 ☑
        wedge compression S22.080 ☑
      wedge compression S22.000 ☑
  thumb S62.50- ☑
    distal phalanx (displaced) S62.52- ☑
      nondisplaced S62.52- ☑
    proximal phalanx (displaced) S62.51- ☑
      nondisplaced S62.51- ☑
  thyroid cartilage S12.8 ☑
  tibia (shaft) S82.20- ☑
    comminuted (displaced) S82.25- ☑
      nondisplaced S82.25- ☑
    condyles — *see* Fracture, tibia, upper end
    distal end — *see* Fracture, tibia, lower end
    epiphysis
      lower — *see* Fracture, tibia, lower end
      upper — *see* Fracture, tibia, upper end
    following insertion of implant, prosthesis or plate
      M96.67- ☑
    head (involving knee joint) — *see* Fracture, tibia,
      upper end
    intercondyloid eminence — *see* Fracture, tibia,
      upper end
    involving ankle or malleolus — *see* Fracture, ankle,
      medial malleolus
    lower end S82.30- ☑
      physeal S89.10- ☑
        Salter-Harris
          Type I S89.11- ☑
          Type II S89.12- ☑
          Type III S89.13- ☑
          Type IV S89.14- ☑
          specified NEC S89.19- ☑
      pilon (displaced) S82.87- ☑
        nondisplaced S82.87- ☑
      specified NEC S82.39- ☑
      torus S82.31- ☑
    malleolus — *see* Fracture, ankle, medial malleolus
    oblique (displaced) S82.23- ☑
      nondisplaced S82.23- ☑
    pilon — *see* Fracture, tibia, lower end, pilon
    proximal end — *see* Fracture, tibia, upper end
    segmental (displaced) S82.26- ☑
      nondisplaced S82.26- ☑
    specified NEC S82.29- ☑
    spine — *see* Fracture, upper end, spine
    spiral (displaced) S82.24- ☑
      nondisplaced S82.24- ☑
    transverse (displaced) S82.22- ☑
      nondisplaced S82.22- ☑
    tuberosity — *see* Fracture, tibia, upper end,
      tuberosity
    upper end S82.10- ☑
      bicondylar (displaced) S82.14- ☑
        nondisplaced S82.14- ☑
      lateral condyle (displaced) S82.12- ☑
        nondisplaced S82.12- ☑
      medial condyle (displaced) S82.13- ☑
        nondisplaced S82.13- ☑
      physeal S89.00- ☑
        Salter-Harris
          Type I S89.01- ☑
          Type II S89.02- ☑
          Type III S89.03- ☑
          Type IV S89.04- ☑
          specified NEC S89.09- ☑
      plateau — *see* Fracture, tibia, upper end, bi-
        condylar
      specified NEC S82.19- ☑
      spine (displaced) S82.11- ☑

Fracture, traumatic — *continued*
  tibia — *continued*
    upper end — *continued*
      spine — *continued*
        nondisplaced S82.11- ☑
      torus S82.16- ☑
      tuberosity (displaced) S82.15- ☑
        nondisplaced S82.15- ☑
  toe S92.91- ☑
    great (displaced) S92.40- ☑
      distal phalanx (displaced) S92.42- ☑
        nondisplaced S92.42- ☑
      nondisplaced S92.40- ☑
      proximal phalanx (displaced) S92.41- ☑
        nondisplaced S92.41- ☑
      specified NEC S92.49- ☑
    lesser (displaced) S92.50- ☑
      distal phalanx (displaced) S92.53- ☑
        nondisplaced S92.53- ☑
      medial phalanx (displaced) S92.52- ☑
        nondisplaced S92.52- ☑
      nondisplaced S92.50- ☑
      proximal phalanx (displaced) S92.51- ☑
        nondisplaced S92.51- ☑
      specified NEC S92.59- ☑
  tooth (root) S02.5 ☑
  trachea (cartilage) S12.8 ☑
  transverse process — *see* Fracture, vertebra
  trapezium or trapezoid bone — *see* Fracture, carpal
  trimalleolar — *see* Fracture, ankle, trimalleolar
  triquetrum (cuneiform of carpus) — *see* Fracture,
    carpal, triquetrum
  trochanter — *see* Fracture, femur, trochanteric
  tuberosity (external) — *code by* site under Fracture
  ulna (shaft) S52.20- ☑
    bent bone S52.28- ☑
    coronoid process — *see* Fracture, ulna, upper end,
      coronoid process
    distal end — *see* Fracture, ulna, lower end
    following insertion of implant, prosthesis or plate
      M96.63- ☑
    head S52.00- ☑
    lower end S52.60- ☑
      physeal S59.00- ☑
        Salter-Harris
          Type I S59.01- ☑
          Type II S59.02- ☑
          Type III S59.03- ☑
          Type IV S59.04- ☑
          specified NEC S59.09- ☑
      specified NEC S52.69- ☑
      styloid process (displaced) S52.61- ☑
        nondisplaced S52.61- ☑
      torus S52.62- ☑
    proximal end — *see* Fracture, ulna, upper end
    shaft S52.20- ☑
      comminuted (displaced) S52.25- ☑
        nondisplaced S52.25- ☑
      greenstick S52.21- ☑
      Monteggia's — *see* Monteggia's fracture
      oblique (displaced) S52.23- ☑
        nondisplaced S52.23- ☑
      segmental (displaced) S52.26- ☑
        nondisplaced S52.26- ☑
      specified NEC S52.29- ☑
      spiral (displaced) S52.24- ☑
        nondisplaced S52.24- ☑
      transverse (displaced) S52.22- ☑
        nondisplaced S52.22- ☑
    upper end S52.00- ☑
      coronoid process (displaced) S52.04- ☑
        nondisplaced S52.04- ☑
      olecranon process (displaced) S52.02- ☑
        with intraarticular extension S52.03- ☑
        nondisplaced S52.02- ☑
          with intraarticular extension S52.03- ☑
      specified NEC S52.09- ☑
      torus S52.01- ☑
  unciform — *see* Fracture, carpal, hamate
  vault of skull S02.0 ☑
  vertebra, vertebral (arch) (body) (column) (neural arch)
    (pedicle) (spinous process) (transverse process)
    atlas — *see* Fracture, neck, cervical vertebra, first
    axis — *see* Fracture, neck, cervical vertebra, second
    cervical (teardrop) S12.9 ☑

Fracture, traumatic — *continued*
  vertebra, vertebral — *continued*
    cervical — *continued*
      axis — *see* Fracture, neck, cervical vertebra, second
      first (atlas) — *see* Fracture, neck, cervical vertebra, first
      second (axis) — *see* Fracture, neck, cervical vertebra, second
    chronic M84.48 ☑
    coccyx S32.2 ☑
    dorsal — *see* Fracture, thorax, vertebra
    lumbar S32.009 ☑
      burst (stable) S32.001 ☑
        unstable S32.002 ☑
      fifth S32.059 ☑
        burst (stable) S32.051 ☑
          unstable S32.052 ☑
        specified type NEC S32.058 ☑
        wedge compression S32.050 ☑
      first S32.019 ☑
        burst (stable) S32.011 ☑
          unstable S32.012 ☑
        specified type NEC S32.018 ☑
        wedge compression S32.010 ☑
      fourth S32.049 ☑
        burst (stable) S32.041 ☑
          unstable S32.042 ☑
        specified type NEC S32.048 ☑
        wedge compression S32.040 ☑
      second S32.029 ☑
        burst (stable) S32.021 ☑
          unstable S32.022 ☑
        specified type NEC S32.028 ☑
        wedge compression S32.020 ☑
      specified type NEC S32.008 ☑
      third S32.039 ☑
        burst (stable) S32.031 ☑
          unstable S32.032 ☑
        specified type NEC S32.038 ☑
        wedge compression S32.030 ☑
      wedge compression S32.000 ☑
    metastatic — *see* Collapse, vertebra, in, specified disease NEC (*see also* Neoplasm)
    newborn (birth injury) P11.5
    sacrum S32.10 ☑
      specified NEC S32.19 ☑
      Type
        1 S32.14 ☑
        2 S32.15 ☑
        3 S32.16 ☑
        4 S32.17 ☑
      Zone
        I S32.119 ☑
          displaced (minimally) S32.111 ☑
            severely S32.112 ☑
          nondisplaced S32.110 ☑
        II S32.129 ☑
          displaced (minimally) S32.121 ☑
            severely S32.122 ☑
          nondisplaced S32.120 ☑
        III S32.139 ☑
          displaced (minimally) S32.131 ☑
            severely S32.132 ☑
          nondisplaced S32.130 ☑
    thoracic — *see* Fracture, thorax, vertebra
  vertex S02.0 ☑
  vomer (bone) S02.2 ☑
  wrist S62.10- ☑
    carpal — *see* Fracture, carpal bone
    navicular (scaphoid) (hand) — *see* Fracture, carpal, navicular
  xiphisternum, xiphoid (process) S22.24 ☑
  zygoma S02.402 ☑
Fragile, fragility
  autosomal site Q95.5
  bone, congenital (with blue sclera) Q78.0
  capillary (hereditary) D69.8
  hair L67.8
  nails L60.3
  non-sex chromosome site Q95.5
  X chromosome Q99.2
Fragilitas
  crinium L67.8
  ossium (with blue sclerae) (hereditary) Q78.0
  unguium L60.3

Fragilitas — *continued*
  unguium — *continued*
    congenital Q84.6
Fragments, cataract (lens), **following cataract surgery** H59.02- ☑
  retained foreign body — *see* Retained, foreign body fragments (type of)
Frailty (frail) R54
  mental R41.81
Frambesia, frambesial (tropica) (*see also* Yaws)
  initial lesion or ulcer A66.0
  primary A66.0
Frambeside
  gummatous A66.4
  of early yaws A66.2
Frambesioma A66.1
Franceschetti-Klein (-Wildervanck) **disease or syndrome** Q75.4
Francis' disease — *see* Tularemia
Franklin disease C88.2
Frank's essential thrombocytopenia D69.3
Fraser's syndrome Q87.0
Freckle(s) L81.2
  malignant melanoma in — *see* Melanoma
  melanotic (Hutchinson's) — *see* Melanoma, in situ
  retinal D49.81
Frederickson's hyperlipoproteinemia, type
  I and V E78.3
  IIA E78.0
  IIB and III E78.2
  IV E78.1
Freeman Sheldon syndrome Q87.0
Freezing (*see also* Effect, adverse, cold) T69.9 ☑
Freiberg's disease (infraction of metatarsal head or osteochondrosis) — *see* Osteochondrosis, juvenile, metatarsus
Frei's disease A55
Fremitus, friction, cardiac R01.2
Frenum, frenulum
  external os Q51.828
  tongue (shortening) (congenital) Q38.1
Frequency micturition (nocturnal) R35.0
  psychogenic F45.8
Frey's syndrome
  auriculotemporal G50.8
  hyperhidrosis L74.52
Friction
  burn — *see* Burn, by site
  fremitus, cardiac R01.2
  precordial R01.2
  sounds, chest R09.89
Friderichsen-Waterhouse syndrome or disease A39.1
Friedländer's B (bacillus) **NEC** (*see also* condition) A49.8
Friedreich's
  ataxia G11.1
  combined systemic disease G11.1
  facial hemihypertrophy Q67.4
  sclerosis (cerebellum) (spinal cord) G11.1
Frigidity F52.22
Fröhlich's syndrome E23.6
Frontal (*see also* condition)
  lobe syndrome F07.0
Frostbite (superficial) T33.90 ☑
  with
    partial thickness skin loss — *see* Frostbite (superficial), by site
    tissue necrosis T34.90 ☑
  abdominal wall T33.3 ☑
    with tissue necrosis T34.3 ☑
  ankle T33.81- ☑
    with tissue necrosis T34.81- ☑
  arm T33.4- ☑
    with tissue necrosis T34.4- ☑
    finger(s) — *see* Frostbite, finger
    hand — *see* Frostbite, hand
    wrist — *see* Frostbite, wrist
  ear T33.01- ☑
    with tissue necrosis T34.01- ☑
  face T33.09 ☑
    with tissue necrosis T34.09 ☑
  finger T33.53- ☑
    with tissue necrosis T34.53- ☑
  foot T33.82- ☑
    with tissue necrosis T34.82- ☑
  hand T33.52- ☑
    with tissue necrosis T34.52- ☑
  head T33.09 ☑

Frostbite — *continued*
  head — *continued*
    with tissue necrosis T34.09 ☑
    ear — *see* Frostbite, ear
    nose — *see* Frostbite, nose
  hip (and thigh) T33.6- ☑
    with tissue necrosis T34.6- ☑
  knee T33.7- ☑
    with tissue necrosis T34.7- ☑
  leg T33.9- ☑
    with tissue necrosis T34.9- ☑
    ankle — *see* Frostbite, ankle
    foot — *see* Frostbite, foot
    knee — *see* Frostbite, knee
    lower T33.7- ☑
      with tissue necrosis T34.7- ☑
    thigh — *see* Frostbite, hip
    toe — *see* Frostbite, toe
  limb
    lower T33.99 ☑
      with tissue necrosis T34.99 ☑
    upper — *see* Frostbite, arm
  neck T33.1 ☑
    with tissue necrosis T34.1 ☑
  nose T33.02 ☑
    with tissue necrosis T34.02 ☑
  pelvis T33.3 ☑
    with tissue necrosis T34.3 ☑
  specified site NEC T33.99 ☑
    with tissue necrosis T34.99 ☑
  thigh — *see* Frostbite, hip
  thorax T33.2 ☑
    with tissue necrosis T34.2 ☑
  toes T33.83- ☑
    with tissue necrosis T34.83- ☑
  trunk T33.99 ☑
    with tissue necrosis T34.99 ☑
  wrist T33.51- ☑
    with tissue necrosis T34.51- ☑
Frotteurism F65.81
Frozen (*see also* Effect, adverse, cold) T69.9 ☑
  pelvis (female) N94.89
    male K66.8
  shoulder — *see* Capsulitis, adhesive
Fructokinase deficiency E74.11
Fructose 1,6 diphosphatase deficiency E74.19
Fructosemia (benign) (essential) E74.12
Fructosuria (benign) (essential) E74.11
Fuchs'
  black spot (myopic) H44.2- ☑
  dystrophy (corneal endothelium) H18.51
  heterochromic cyclitis — *see* Cyclitis, Fuchs' heterochromic
Fucosidosis E77.1
Fugue R68.89
  dissociative F44.1
  hysterical (dissociative) F44.1
  postictal in epilepsy — *see* Epilepsy
  reaction to exceptional stress (transient) F43.0
Fulminant, fulminating — *see* condition
Functional (*see also* condition)
  bleeding (uterus) N93.8
Functioning, intellectual, borderline R41.83
Fundus — *see* condition
Fungemia NOS B49
Fungus, fungous
  cerebral G93.89
  disease NOS B49
  infection — *see* Infection, fungus
Funiculitis (acute) (chronic) (endemic) N49.1
  gonococcal (acute) (chronic) A54.23
  tuberculous A18.15
Funnel
  breast (acquired) M95.4
    congenital Q67.6
    sequelae (late effect) of rickets E64.3
  chest (acquired) M95.4
    congenital Q67.6
    sequelae (late effect) of rickets E64.3
  pelvis (acquired) M95.5
    with disproportion (fetopelvic) O33.3 ☑
      causing obstructed labor O65.3
    congenital Q74.2
FUO (fever of unknown origin) R50.9
Furfur L21.0
  microsporon B36.0

Furrier's lung J67.8
Furrowed K14.5
  nail(s) (transverse) L60.4
    congenital Q84.6
  tongue K14.5
    congenital Q38.3
Furuncle L02.92
  abdominal wall L02.221
  ankle — *see* Furuncle, lower limb
  antecubital space — *see* Furuncle, upper limb
  anus K61.0
  arm — *see* Furuncle, upper limb
  auditory canal, external — *see* Abscess, ear, external
  auricle (ear) — *see* Abscess, ear, external
  axilla (region) L02.42- ☑
  back (any part) L02.222
  breast N61
  buttock L02.32
  cheek (external) L02.02
  chest wall L02.223
  chin L02.02
  corpus cavernosum N48.21
  ear, external — *see* Abscess, ear, external
  external auditory canal — *see* Abscess, ear, external
  eyelid — *see* Abscess, eyelid
  face L02.02
  femoral (region) — *see* Furuncle, lower limb
  finger — *see* Furuncle, hand
  flank L02.221
  foot L02.62- ☑
  forehead L02.02
  gluteal (region) L02.32
  groin L02.224
  hand L02.52- ☑
  head L02.821
    face L02.02
  hip — *see* Furuncle, lower limb
  kidney — *see* Abscess, kidney
  knee — *see* Furuncle, lower limb
  labium (majus) (minus) N76.4
  lacrimal
    gland — *see* Dacryoadenitis
    passages (duct) (sac) — *see* Inflammation, lacrimal, passages, acute
  leg (any part) — *see* Furuncle, lower limb
  lower limb L02.42- ☑
  malignant A22.0
  mouth K12.2
  navel L02.226

Furuncle — *continued*
  neck L02.12
  nose J34.0
  orbit, orbital — *see* Abscess, orbit
  palmar (space) — *see* Furuncle, hand
  partes posteriores L02.32
  pectoral region L02.223
  penis N48.21
  perineum L02.225
  pinna — *see* Abscess, ear, external
  popliteal — *see* Furuncle, lower limb
  prepatellar — *see* Furuncle, lower limb
  scalp L02.821
  seminal vesicle N49.0
  shoulder — *see* Furuncle, upper limb
  specified site NEC L02.828
  submandibular K12.2
  temple (region) L02.02
  thumb — *see* Furuncle, hand
  toe — *see* Furuncle, foot
  trunk L02.229
    abdominal wall L02.221
    back L02.222
    chest wall L02.223
    groin L02.224
    perineum L02.225
    umbilicus L02.226
  umbilicus L02.226
  upper limb L02.42- ☑
  vulva N76.4
Furunculosis — *see* Furuncle
Fused — *see* Fusion, fused
Fusion, fused (congenital)
  astragaloscaphoid Q74.2
  atria Q21.1
  auditory canal Q16.1
  auricles, heart Q21.1
  binocular with defective stereopsis H53.32
  bone Q79.8
  cervical spine M43.22
  choanal Q30.0
  commissure, mitral valve Q23.2
  cusps, heart valve NEC Q24.8
    mitral Q23.2
    pulmonary Q22.1
    tricuspid Q22.4
  ear ossicles Q16.3
  fingers Q70.0 ☑
  hymen Q52.3

Fusion, fused — *continued*
  joint (acquired) (*see also* Ankylosis)
    congenital Q74.8
  kidneys (incomplete) Q63.1
  labium (majus) (minus) Q52.5
  larynx and trachea Q34.8
  limb, congenital Q74.8
    lower Q74.2
    upper Q74.0
  lobes, lung Q33.8
  lumbosacral (acquired) M43.27
    arthrodesis status Z98.1
    congenital Q76.49
    postprocedural status Z98.1
  nares, nose, nasal, nostril(s) Q30.0
  organ or site not listed — *see* Anomaly, by site
  ossicles Q79.9
    auditory Q16.3
  pulmonic cusps Q22.1
  ribs Q76.6
  sacroiliac (joint) (acquired) M43.28
    arthrodesis status Z98.1
    congenital Q74.2
    postprocedural status Z98.1
  spine (acquired) NEC M43.20
    arthrodesis status Z98.1
    cervical region M43.22
    cervicothoracic region M43.23
    congenital Q76.49
    lumbar M43.26
    lumbosacral region M43.27
    occipito-atlanto-axial region M43.21
    postoperative status Z98.1
    sacrococcygeal region M43.28
    thoracic region M43.24
    thoracolumbar region M43.25
  sublingual duct with submaxillary duct at opening in mouth Q38.4
  testes Q55.1
  toes Q70.2- ☑
  tooth, teeth K00.2
  trachea and esophagus Q39.8
  twins Q89.4
  vagina Q52.4
  ventricles, heart Q21.0
  vertebra (arch) — *see* Fusion, spine
  vulva Q52.5
Fusospirillosis (mouth) (tongue) (tonsil) A69.1
Fussy baby R68.12

  ☑ **Additional Character Required — Refer to the Tabular List for Character Selection**   ▼ Subterms under main terms may continue to next column or page

G

Gain in weight (abnormal) (excessive) (see also Weight, gain)
Gaisböck's disease (polycythemia hypertonica) D75.1
Gait abnormality R26.9
  ataxic R26.0
  falling R29.6
  hysterical (ataxic) (staggering) F44.4
  paralytic R26.1
  spastic R26.1
  specified type NEC R26.89
  staggering R26.0
  unsteadiness R26.81
  walking difficulty NEC R26.2
Galactocele (breast) N64.89
  puerperal, postpartum O92.79
Galactokinase deficiency E74.29
Galactophoritis N61
  gestational, puerperal, postpartum O91.2- ☑
Galactorrhea O92.6
  not associated with childbirth N64.3
Galactosemia (classic) (congenital) E74.21
Galactosuria E74.29
Galacturia R82.0
  schistosomiasis (bilharziasis) B65.0
Galeazzi's fracture S52.37- ☑
Galen's vein — see condition
Galeophobia F40.218
Gall duct — see condition
Gallbladder (see also condition)
  acute K81.0
Gallop rhythm R00.8
Gallstone (colic) (cystic duct) (gallbladder) (impacted) (multiple) (see also Calculus, gallbladder)
  with
    cholecystitis — see Calculus, gallbladder, with cholecystitis
  bile duct (common) (hepatic) — see Calculus, bile duct
  causing intestinal obstruction K56.3
  specified NEC K80.80
    with obstruction K80.81
Gambling Z72.6
  pathological (compulsive) F63.0
Gammopathy (of undetermined significance [MGUS]) D47.2
  associated with lymphoplasmacytic dyscrasia D47.2
  monoclonal D47.2
  polyclonal D89.0
Gamna's disease (siderotic splenomegaly) D73.1
Gamophobia F40.298
Gampsodactylia (congenital) Q66.7
Gamstorp's disease (adynamia episodica hereditaria) G72.3
Gandy-Nanta disease (siderotic splenomegaly) D73.1
Gang
  membership offenses Z72.810
Gangliocytoma D36.10
Ganglioglioma — see Neoplasm, uncertain behavior, by site
Ganglion (compound) (diffuse) (joint) (tendon (sheath)) M67.40
  ankle M67.47- ☑
  foot M67.47- ☑
  forearm M67.43- ☑
  hand M67.44- ☑
  lower leg M67.46- ☑
  multiple sites M67.49
  of yaws (early) (late) A66.6
  pelvic region M67.45- ☑
  periosteal — see Periostitis
  shoulder region M67.41- ☑
  specified site NEC M67.48
  thigh region M67.45- ☑
  tuberculous A18.09
  upper arm M67.42- ☑
  wrist M67.43- ☑
Ganglioneuroblastoma — see Neoplasm, nerve, malignant
Ganglioneuroma D36.10

Ganglioneuroma — continued
  malignant — see Neoplasm, nerve, malignant
Ganglioneuromatosis D36.10
Ganglionitis
  fifth nerve — see Neuralgia, trigeminal
  gasserian (postherpetic) (postzoster) B02.21
  geniculate G51.1
    newborn (birth injury) P11.3
    postherpetic, postzoster B02.21
  herpes zoster B02.21
  postherpetic geniculate B02.21
Gangliosidosis E75.10
  GM1 E75.19
  GM2 E75.00
    other specified E75.09
    Sandhoff disease E75.01
    Tay-Sachs disease E75.02
  GM3 E75.19
  mucolipidosis IV E75.11
Gangosa A66.5
Gangrene, gangrenous (connective tissue) (dropsical) (dry) (moist) (skin) (ulcer) (see also Necrosis) I96
  with diabetes (mellitus) — see Diabetes, gangrene
  abdomen (wall) I96
  alveolar M27.3
  appendix K35.80
    with
      perforation or rupture K35.2
      peritoneal abscess K35.3
      peritonitis NEC K35.3
        generalized (with perforation or rupture) K35.2
        localized (with perforation or rupture) K35.3
  arteriosclerotic (general) (senile) — see Arteriosclerosis, extremities, with, gangrene
  auricle I96
  Bacillus welchii A48.0
  bladder (infectious) — see Cystitis, specified type NEC
  bowel, cecum, or colon — see Gangrene, intestine
  Clostridium perfringens or welchii A48.0
  cornea H18.89- ☑
  corpora cavernosa N48.29
    noninfective N48.89
  cutaneous, spreading I96
  decubital — see Ulcer, pressure, by site
  diabetic (any site) — see Diabetes, gangrene
  emphysematous — see Gangrene, gas
  epidemic — see Poisoning, food, noxious, plant
  epididymis (infectional) N45.1
  erysipelas — see Erysipelas
  extremity (lower) (upper) I96
  Fournier N49.3
    female N76.89
  fusospirochetal A69.0
  gallbladder — see Cholecystitis, acute
  gas (bacillus) A48.0
    following
      abortion — see Abortion by type complicated by infection
      ectopic or molar pregnancy O08.0
  glossitis K14.0
  hernia — see Hernia, by site, with gangrene
  intestine, intestinal (hemorrhagic) (massive) K55.0
    with
      mesenteric embolism K55.0
      obstruction — see Obstruction, intestine
  laryngitis J04.0
  limb (lower) (upper) I96
  lung J85.0
    spirochetal A69.8
  lymphangitis I89.1
  Meleney's (synergistic) — see Ulcer, skin
  mesentery K55.0
    with
      embolism K55.0
      intestinal obstruction — see Obstruction, intestine
  mouth A69.0
  ovary — see Oophoritis
  pancreas K85.9
  penis N48.29
    noninfective N48.89

Gangrene, gangrenous — continued
  perineum I96
  pharynx (see also Pharyngitis)
    Vincent's A69.1
  presenile I73.1
  progressive synergistic — see Ulcer, skin
  pulmonary J85.0
  pulpal (dental) K04.1
  quinsy J36
  Raynaud's (symmetric gangrene) I73.01
  retropharyngeal J39.2
  scrotum N49.3
    noninfective N50.8
  senile (atherosclerotic) — see Arteriosclerosis, extremities, with, gangrene
  spermatic cord N49.1
    noninfective N50.8
  spine I96
  spirochetal NEC A69.8
  spreading cutaneous I96
  stomatitis A69.0
  symmetrical I73.01
  testis (infectional) N45.2
    noninfective N44.8
  throat (see also Pharyngitis)
    diphtheritic A36.0
    Vincent's A69.1
  thyroid (gland) E07.89
  tooth (pulp) K04.1
  tuberculous NEC — see Tuberculosis
  tunica vaginalis N49.1
    noninfective N50.8
  umbilicus I96
  uterus — see Endometritis
  uvulitis K12.2
  vas deferens N49.1
    noninfective N50.8
  vulva N76.89
Ganister disease J62.8
Ganser's syndrome (hysterical) F44.89
Gardner-Diamond syndrome (autoerythrocyte sensitization) D69.2
Gargoylism E76.01
Garré's disease, osteitis (sclerosing), osteomyelitis — see Osteomyelitis, specified type NEC
Garrod's pad, knuckle M72.1
Gartner's duct
  cyst Q52.4
  persistent Q50.6
Gas R14.3
  asphyxiation, inhalation, poisoning, suffocation NEC — see Table of Drugs and Chemicals
  excessive R14.0
  gangrene A48.0
    following
      abortion — see Abortion by type complicated by infection
      ectopic or molar pregnancy O08.0
  on stomach R14.0
  pains R14.1
Gastralgia (see also Pain, abdominal)
Gastrectasis K31.0
  psychogenic F45.8
Gastric — see condition
Gastrinoma
  malignant
    pancreas C25.4
    specified site NEC — see Neoplasm, malignant, by site
    unspecified site C25.4
  specified site — see Neoplasm, uncertain behavior
  unspecified site D37.9
Gastritis (simple) K29.70
  with bleeding K29.71
  acute (erosive) K29.00
    with bleeding K29.01
  alcoholic K29.20
    with bleeding K29.21
  allergic K29.60
    with bleeding K29.61
  atrophic (chronic) K29.40
    with bleeding K29.41

Gastritis — *continued*
  chronic (antral) (fundal) K29.50
    with bleeding K29.51
    atrophic K29.40
      with bleeding K29.41
    superficial K29.30
      with bleeding K29.31
  dietary counseling and surveillance Z71.3
  due to diet deficiency E63.9
  eosinophilic K52.81
  giant hypertrophic K29.60
    with bleeding K29.61
  granulomatous K29.60
    with bleeding K29.61
  hypertrophic (mucosa) K29.60
    with bleeding K29.61
  nervous F54
  spastic K29.60
    with bleeding K29.61
  specified NEC K29.60
    with bleeding K29.61
  superficial chronic K29.30
    with bleeding K29.31
  tuberculous A18.83
  viral NEC A08.4
Gastrocarcinoma — *see* Neoplasm, malignant, stomach
Gastrocolic — *see* condition
Gastrodisciasis, gastrodiscoidiasis B66.8
Gastroduodenitis K29.90
  with bleeding K29.91
  virus, viral A08.4
    specified type NEC A08.39
Gastrodynia — *see* Pain, abdominal
Gastroenteritis (acute) (chronic) (noninfectious) (*see also* Enteritis) K52.9
  allergic K52.2
  dietetic K52.2
  drug-induced K52.1
  due to
    Cryptosporidium A07.2
    drugs K52.1
    food poisoning — *see* Intoxication, foodborne
    radiation K52.0
  eosinophilic K52.81
  epidemic (infectious) A09
  food hypersensitivity K52.2
  infectious — *see* Enteritis, infectious
  influenzal — *see* Influenza, with gastroenteritis
  noninfectious K52.9
    specified NEC K52.89
  rotaviral A08.0
  Salmonella A02.0
  toxic K52.1
  viral NEC A08.4
    acute infectious A08.39
      type Norwalk A08.11
    infantile (acute) A08.39
    Norwalk agent A08.11
    rotaviral A08.0
    severe of infants A08.39
    specified type NEC A08.39
Gastroenteropathy (*see also* Gastroenteritis) K52.9
  acute, due to Norovirus A08.11
  acute, due to Norwalk agent A08.11
  infectious A09
Gastroenteroptosis K63.4
Gastroesophageal laceration- hemorrhage syndrome K22.6
Gastrointestinal — *see* condition
Gastrojejunal — *see* condition
Gastrojejunitis (*see also* Enteritis) K52.9
Gastrojejunocolic — *see* condition
Gastroliths K31.89
Gastromalacia K31.89
Gastroparalysis K31.84
  diabetic — *see* Diabetes, gastroparalysis
Gastroparesis K31.84
  diabetic — *see* Diabetes, by type, with gastroparesis
Gastropathy K31.9
  congestive portal K31.89
  erythematous K29.70
  exudative K90.89
  portal hypertensive K31.89
Gastroptosis K31.89
Gastrorrhagia K92.2
  psychogenic F45.8
Gastroschisis (congenital) Q79.3
Gastrospasm (neurogenic) (reflex) K31.89

Gastrospasm — *continued*
  neurotic F45.8
  psychogenic F45.8
Gastrostaxis — *see* Gastritis, with bleeding
Gastrostenosis K31.89
Gastrostomy
  attention to Z43.1
  status Z93.1
Gastrosuccorrhea (continuous) (intermittent) K31.89
  neurotic F45.8
  psychogenic F45.8
Gatophobia F40.218
Gaucher's disease or splenomegaly (adult) (infantile) E75.22
Gee (-Herter)(-Thaysen) **disease** (nontropical sprue) K90.0
Gélineau's syndrome G47.419
  with cataplexy G47.411
Gemination, tooth, teeth K00.2
Gemistocytoma
  specified site — *see* Neoplasm, malignant, by site
  unspecified site C71.9
General, generalized — *see* condition
Genetic
  carrier (status)
    cystic fibrosis Z14.1
    hemophilia A (asymptomatic) Z14.01
      symptomatic Z14.02
    specified NEC Z14.8
  susceptibility to disease NEC Z15.89
    malignant neoplasm Z15.09
      breast Z15.01
      endometrium Z15.04
      ovary Z15.02
      prostate Z15.03
      specified NEC Z15.09
    multiple endocrine neoplasia Z15.81
Genital — *see* condition
Genito-anorectal syndrome A55
Genitourinary system — *see* condition
Genu
  congenital Q74.1
  extrorsum (acquired) (*see also* Deformity, varus, knee)
    congenital Q74.1
    sequelae (late effect) of rickets E64.3
  introrsum (acquired) (*see also* Deformity, valgus, knee)
    congenital Q74.1
    sequelae (late effect) of rickets E64.3
  rachitic (old) E64.3
  recurvatum (acquired) (*see also* Deformity, limb, specified type NEC, lower leg)
    congenital Q68.2
    sequelae (late effect) of rickets E64.3
  valgum (acquired) (knock-knee) M21.06- ☑
    congenital Q74.1
    sequelae (late effect) of rickets E64.3
  varum (acquired) (bowleg) M21.16- ☑
    congenital Q74.1
    sequelae (late effect) of rickets E64.3
Geographic tongue K14.1
Geophagia — *see* Pica
Geotrichosis B48.3
  stomatitis B48.3
Gephyrophobia F40.242
Gerbode defect Q21.0
GERD (gastroesophageal reflux disease) K21.9
Gerhardt's
  disease (erythromelalgia) I73.81
  syndrome (vocal cord paralysis) J38.00
    bilateral J38.02
    unilateral J38.01
German measles (*see also* Rubella)
  exposure to Z20.4
Germinoblastoma (diffuse) C85.9- ☑
  follicular C82.9- ☑
Germinoma — *see* Neoplasm, malignant, by site
Gerontoxon — *see* Degeneration, cornea, senile
Gerstmann's syndrome R48.8
  developmental F81.2
Gerstmann-Sträussler-Scheinker syndrome (GSS) A81.82
Gestation (period) (*see also* Pregnancy)
  ectopic — *see* Pregnancy, by site
  multiple O30.9- ☑
    greater than quadruplets — *see* Pregnancy, multiple (gestation), specified NEC
    specified NEC — *see* Pregnancy, multiple (gestation), specified NEC

Gestational
  mammary abscess O91.11- ☑
  purulent mastitis O91.11- ☑
  subareolar abscess O91.11- ☑
Ghon tubercle, primary infection A15.7
Ghost
  teeth K00.4
  vessels (cornea) H16.41- ☑
Ghoul hand A66.3
Gianotti-Crosti disease L44.4
Giant
  cell
    epulis K06.8
    peripheral granuloma K06.8
  esophagus, congenital Q39.5
  kidney, congenital Q63.3
  urticaria T78.3 ☑
    hereditary D84.1
Giardiasis A07.1
Gibert's disease or pityriasis L42
Giddiness R42
  hysterical F44.89
  psychogenic F45.8
Gierke's disease (glycogenosis I) E74.01
Gigantism (cerebral) (hypophyseal) (pituitary) E22.0
  constitutional E34.4
Gilbert's disease or syndrome E80.4
Gilchrist's disease B40.9
Gilford-Hutchinson disease E34.8
Gilles de la Tourette's disease or syndrome (motor-verbal tic) F95.2
Gingivitis K05.10
  acute (catarrhal) K05.00
    necrotizing A69.1
    nonplaque induced K05.01
    plaque induced K05.00
  chronic (desquamative) (hyperplastic) (simple marginal) (ulcerative) K05.10
    nonplaque induced K05.11
    plaque induced K05.10
  expulsiva — *see* Periodontitis
  necrotizing ulcerative (acute) A69.1
  pellagrous E52
    acute necrotizing A69.1
  Vincent's A69.1
Gingivoglossitis K14.0
Gingivopericementitis — *see* Periodontitis
Gingivosis — *see* Gingivitis, chronic
Gingivostomatitis K05.10
  herpesviral B00.2
  necrotizing ulcerative (acute) A69.1
Gland, glandular — *see* condition
Glanders A24.0
Glanzmann (-Naegeli) **disease or thrombasthenia** D69.1
Glasgow coma scale
  total score
    3-8 R40.243
    9-12 R40.242
    13-15 R40.241
Glass-blower's disease (cataract) — *see* Cataract, specified NEC
Glaucoma H40.9
  with
    increased episcleral venous pressure H40.81- ☑
    pseudoexfoliation of lens — *see* Glaucoma, open angle, primary, capsular
  absolute H44.51- ☑
  angle-closure (primary) H40.20- ☑
    acute (attack) (crisis) H40.21- ☑
    chronic H40.22- ☑
    intermittent H40.23- ☑
    residual stage H40.24- ☑
  borderline H40.00- ☑
  capsular (with pseudoexfoliation of lens) — *see* Glaucoma, open angle, primary, capsular
  childhood Q15.0
  closed angle — *see* Glaucoma, angle-closure
  congenital Q15.0
  corticosteroid-induced — *see* Glaucoma, secondary, drugs
  hypersecretion H40.82- ☑
  in (due to)
    amyloidosis E85.4 [H42]
    aniridia Q13.1 [H42]
    concussion of globe — *see* Glaucoma, secondary, trauma

☑ **Additional Character Required** — **Refer to the Tabular List for Character Selection**   🔺 **Subterms under main terms may continue to next column or page**

Glaucoma — *continued*
  in — *continued*
    dislocation of lens — *see* Glaucoma, secondary
    disorder of lens NEC — *see* Glaucoma, secondary
    drugs — *see* Glaucoma, secondary, drugs
    endocrine disease NOS E34.9 [H42]
    eye
      inflammation — *see* Glaucoma, secondary, in-
        flammation
      trauma — *see* Glaucoma, secondary, trauma
    hypermature cataract — *see* Glaucoma, secondary
    iridocyclitis — *see* Glaucoma, secondary, inflamma-
      tion
    lens disorder — *see* Glaucoma, secondary
    Lowe's syndrome E72.03 [H42]
    metabolic disease NOS E88.9 [H42]
    ocular disorders NEC — *see* Glaucoma, secondary
    onchocerciasis B73.02
    pupillary block — *see* Glaucoma, secondary
    retinal vein occlusion — *see* Glaucoma, secondary
    Rieger's anomaly Q13.81 [H42]
    rubeosis of iris — *see* Glaucoma, secondary
    tumor of globe — *see* Glaucoma, secondary
  infantile Q15.0
  low tension — *see* Glaucoma, open angle, primary,
    low-tension
  malignant H40.83- ☑
  narrow angle — *see* Glaucoma, angle-closure
  newborn Q15.0
  noncongestive (chronic) — *see* Glaucoma, open angle
  nonobstructive — *see* Glaucoma, open angle
  obstructive (*see also* Glaucoma, angle-closure)
    due to lens changes — *see* Glaucoma, secondary
  open angle H40.10- ☑
    primary H40.11- ☑
      capsular (with pseudoexfoliation of lens)
        H40.14- ☑
      low-tension H40.12- ☑
      pigmentary H40.13- ☑
      residual stage H40.15- ☑
  phacolytic — *see* Glaucoma, secondary
  pigmentary — *see* Glaucoma, open angle, primary,
    pigmentary
  postinfectious — *see* Glaucoma, secondary, inflamma-
    tion
  secondary (to) H40.5- ☑
    drugs H40.6- ☑
    inflammation H40.4- ☑
    trauma H40.3- ☑
  simple (chronic) H40.11 ☑
  simplex H40.11 ☑
  specified type NEC H40.89
  suspect H40.00- ☑
  syphilitic A52.71
  traumatic (*see also* Glaucoma, secondary, trauma)
    newborn (birth injury) P15.3
  tuberculous A18.59
Glaucomatous flecks (subcapsular) — *see* Cataract,
  complicated
Glazed tongue K14.4
Gleet (gonococcal) A54.01
Glénard's disease K63.4
Glioblastoma (multiforme)
  with sarcomatous component
    specified site — *see* Neoplasm, malignant, by site
    unspecified site C71.9
  giant cell
    specified site — *see* Neoplasm, malignant, by site
    unspecified site C71.9
  specified site — *see* Neoplasm, malignant, by site
  unspecified site C71.9
Glioma (malignant)
  astrocytic
    specified site — *see* Neoplasm, malignant, by site
    unspecified site C71.9
  mixed
    specified site — *see* Neoplasm, malignant, by site
    unspecified site C71.9
  nose Q30.8
  specified site NEC — *see* Neoplasm, malignant, by site
  subependymal D43.2
    specified site — *see* Neoplasm, uncertain behavior,
      by site
    unspecified site D43.2
  unspecified site C71.9
Gliomatosis cerebri C71.0

Glioneuroma — *see* Neoplasm, uncertain behavior, by
  site
Gliosarcoma
  specified site — *see* Neoplasm, malignant, by site
  unspecified site C71.9
Gliosis (cerebral) G93.89
  spinal G95.89
Glisson's disease — *see* Rickets
Globinuria R82.3
Globus (hystericus) F45.8
Glomangioma D18.00
  intra-abdominal D18.03
  intracranial D18.02
  skin D18.01
  specified site NEC D18.09
Glomangiomyoma D18.00
  intra-abdominal D18.03
  intracranial D18.02
  skin D18.01
  specified site NEC D18.09
Glomangiosarcoma — *see* Neoplasm, connective tissue,
  malignant
Glomerular
  disease in syphilis A52.75
  nephritis — *see* Glomerulonephritis
Glomerulitis — *see* Glomerulonephritis
Glomerulonephritis (*see also* Nephritis) N05.9
  with
    edema — *see* Nephrosis
    minimal change N05.0
    minor glomerular abnormality N05.0
  acute N00.9
  chronic N03.9
  crescentic (diffuse) NEC (*see also* N00-N07 with fourth
    character .7) N05.7
  dense deposit (*see also* N00-N07 with fourth character
    .6) N05.6
  diffuse
    crescentic (*see also* N00-N07 with fourth character
      .7) N05.7
    endocapillary proliferative (*see also* N00-N07 with
      fourth character .4) N05.4
    membranous (*see also* N00-N07 with fourth char-
      acter .2) N05.2
    mesangial proliferative (*see also* N00-N07 with
      fourth character .3) N05.3
    mesangiocapillary (*see also* N00-N07 with
      character .5) N05.5
    sclerosing N05.8
  endocapillary proliferative (diffuse) NEC (*see also* N00-
    N07 with fourth character .4) N05.4
  extracapillary NEC (*see also* N00-N07 with fourth
    character .7) N05.7
  focal (and segmental) (*see also* N00-N07 with fourth
    character .1) N05.1
  hypocomplementemic — *see* Glomerulonephritis,
    membranoproliferative
  IgA — *see* Nephropathy, IgA
  immune complex (circulating) NEC N05.8
  in (due to)
    amyloidosis E85.4 [N08]
    bilharziasis B65.9 [N08]
    cryoglobulinemia D89.1 [N08]
    defibrination syndrome D65 [N08]
    diabetes mellitus — *see* Diabetes, glomeruloscle-
      rosis
    disseminated intravascular coagulation D65 [N08]
    Fabry (-Anderson) disease E75.21 [N08]
    Goodpasture's syndrome M31.0
    hemolytic-uremic syndrome D59.3
    Henoch (-Schönlein) purpura D69.0 [N08]
    lecithin cholesterol acyltransferase deficiency
      E78.6 [N08]
    microscopic polyangiitis M31.7 [N08]
    multiple myeloma C90.0- ☑ [N08]
    Plasmodium malariae B52.0
    schistosomiasis B65.9 [N08]
    sepsis A41.9 [N08]
      streptococcal A40- ☑ [N08]
    sickle-cell disorders D57.- ☑ [N08]
    strongyloidiasis B78.9 [N08]
    subacute bacterial endocarditis I33.0 [N08]
    syphilis (late) congenital A50.59 [N08]
    systemic lupus erythematosus M32.14
    thrombotic thrombocytopenic purpura
      M31.1 [N08]
    typhoid fever A01.09
    Waldenström macroglobulinemia C88.0 [N08]

Glomerulonephritis — *continued*
  in — *continued*
    Wegener's granulomatosis M31.31
  latent or quiescent N03.9
  lobular, lobulonodular — *see* Glomerulonephritis,
    membranoproliferative
  membranoproliferative (diffuse)(type 1 or 3) (*see also*
    N00-N07 with fourth character .5) N05.5
    dense deposit (type 2) NEC (*see also* N00-N07 with
      fourth character .6) N05.6
  membranous (diffuse) NEC (*see also* N00-N07 with
    fourth character .2) N05.2
  mesangial
    IgA/IgG — *see* Nephropathy, IgA
    proliferative (diffuse) NEC (*see also* N00-N07 with
      fourth character .3) N05.3
  mesangiocapillary (diffuse) NEC (*see also* N00-N07
    with fourth character .5) N05.5
  necrotic, necrotizing NEC (*see also* N00- N07 with
    fourth character .8) N05.8
  nodular — *see* Glomerulonephritis, membranoprolif-
    erative
  poststreptococcal NEC N05.9
    acute N00.9
    chronic N03.9
    rapidly progressive N01.9
  proliferative NEC (*see also* N00-N07 with fourth char-
    acter .8) N05.8
    diffuse (lupus) M32.14
  rapidly progressive N01.9
  sclerosing, diffuse N05.8
  specified pathology NEC (*see also* N00- N07 with fourth
    character .8) N05.8
  subacute N01.9
Glomerulopathy — *see* Glomerulonephritis
Glomerulosclerosis (*see also* Sclerosis, renal)
  intercapillary (nodular) (with diabetes) — *see* Diabetes,
    glomerulosclerosis
  intracapillary — *see* Diabetes, glomerulosclerosis
Glossagra K14.6
Glossalgia K14.6
Glossitis (chronic superficial) (gangrenous) (Moeller's)
  K14.0
  areata exfoliativa K14.1
  atrophic K14.4
  benign migratory K14.1
  cortical superficial, sclerotic K14.0
  Hunter's D51.0
  interstitial, sclerous K14.0
  median rhomboid K14.2
  pellagrous E52
  superficial, chronic K14.0
Glossocele K14.8
Glossodynia K14.6
  exfoliativa K14.4
Glossoncus K14.8
Glossopathy K14.9
Glossophytia K14.3
Glossoplegia K14.8
Glossoptosis K14.8
Glossopyrosis K14.6
Glossotrichia K14.3
Glossy skin L90.8
Glottis — *see* condition
Glottitis (*see also* Laryngitis) J04.0
Glucagonoma
  pancreas
    benign D13.7
    malignant C25.4
    uncertain behavior D37.8
  specified site NEC
    benign — *see* Neoplasm, benign, by site
    malignant — *see* Neoplasm, malignant, by site
    uncertain behavior — *see* Neoplasm, uncertain
      behavior, by site
  unspecified site
    benign D13.7
    malignant C25.4
    uncertain behavior D37.8
Glucoglycinuria E72.51
Glucose-galactose malabsorption E74.39
Glue
  ear — *see* Otitis, media, nonsuppurative, chronic,
    mucoid
  sniffing (airplane) — *see* Abuse, drug, inhalant
    dependence — *see* Dependence, drug, inhalant
Glutaric aciduria E72.3

Glycinemia E72.51
Glycinuria (renal) (with ketosis) E72.09
Glycogen
  infiltration — see Disease, glycogen storage
  storage disease — see Disease, glycogen storage
Glycogenosis (diffuse) (generalized) (see also Disease, glycogen storage)
  cardiac E74.02 [I43]
  diabetic, secondary — see Diabetes, glycogenosis, secondary
  pulmonary interstitial J84.842
Glycopenia E16.2
Glycosuria R81
  renal E74.8
Gnathostoma spinigerum (infection) (infestation), **gnathostomiasis** (wandering swelling) B83.1
Goiter (plunging) (substernal) E04.9
  with
    hyperthyroidism (recurrent) — see Hyperthyroidism, with, goiter
    thyrotoxicosis — see Hyperthyroidism, with, goiter
  adenomatous — see Goiter, nodular
  cancerous C73
  congenital (nontoxic) E03.0
    diffuse E03.0
    parenchymatous E03.0
    transitory, with normal functioning P72.0
  cystic E04.2
    due to iodine-deficiency E01.1
  due to
    enzyme defect in synthesis of thyroid hormone E07.1
    iodine-deficiency (endemic) E01.2
  dyshormonogenetic (familial) E07.1
  endemic (iodine-deficiency) E01.2
    diffuse E01.0
    multinodular E01.1
  exophthalmic — see Hyperthyroidism, with, goiter
  iodine-deficiency (endemic) E01.2
    diffuse E01.0
    multinodular E01.1
    nodular E01.1
  lingual Q89.2
  lymphadenoid E06.3
  malignant C73
  multinodular (cystic) (nontoxic) E04.2
    toxic or with hyperthyroidism E05.20
      with thyroid storm E05.21
  neonatal NEC P72.0
  nodular (nontoxic) (due to) E04.9
    with
      hyperthyroidism E05.20
        with thyroid storm E05.21
      thyrotoxicosis E05.20
        with thyroid storm E05.21
    endemic E01.1
    iodine-deficiency E01.1
    sporadic E04.9
    toxic E05.20
      with thyroid storm E05.21
  nontoxic E04.9
    diffuse (colloid) E04.0
    multinodular E04.2
    simple E04.0
    specified NEC E04.8
    uninodular E04.1
  simple E04.0
  toxic — see Hyperthyroidism, with, goiter
  uninodular (nontoxic) E04.1
    toxic or with hyperthyroidism E05.10
      with thyroid storm E05.11
Goiter-deafness syndrome E07.1
Goldberg syndrome Q89.8
Goldberg-Maxwell syndrome E34.51
Goldblatt's hypertension or kidney I70.1
Goldenhar (-Gorlin) **syndrome** Q87.0
Goldflam-Erb disease or syndrome G70.00
  with exacerbation (acute) G70.01
  in crisis G70.01
Goldscheider's disease Q81.8
Goldstein's disease (familial hemorrhagic telangiectasia) I78.0
Golfer's elbow — see Epicondylitis, medial
Gonadoblastoma
  specified site — see Neoplasm, uncertain behavior, by site
  unspecified site
    female D39.10

Gonadoblastoma — continued
  unspecified site — continued
    male D40.10
Gonecystitis — see Vesiculitis
Gongylonemiasis B83.8
Goniosynechiae — see Adhesions, iris, goniosynechiae
Gonococcemia A54.86
Gonococcus, gonococcal (disease) (infection) (see also condition) A54.9
  anus A54.6
  bursa, bursitis A54.49
  conjunctiva, conjunctivitis (neonatorum) A54.31
  endocardium A54.83
  eye A54.30
    conjunctivitis A54.31
    iridocyclitis A54.32
    keratitis A54.33
    newborn A54.31
    other specified A54.39
  fallopian tubes (acute) (chronic) A54.24
  genitourinary (organ) (system) (tract) (acute)
    lower A54.00
      with abscess (accessory gland) (periurethral) A54.1
    upper (see also condition) A54.29
  heart A54.83
  iridocyclitis A54.32
  joint A54.42
  lymphatic (gland) (node) A54.89
  meninges, meningitis A54.81
  musculoskeletal A54.40
    arthritis A54.42
    osteomyelitis A54.43
    other specified A54.49
    spondylopathy A54.41
  pelviperitonitis A54.24
  pelvis (acute) (chronic) A54.24
  pharynx A54.5
  proctitis A54.6
  pyosalpinx (acute) (chronic) A54.24
  rectum A54.6
  skin A54.89
  specified site NEC A54.89
  tendon sheath A54.49
  throat A54.5
  urethra (acute) (chronic) A54.01
    with abscess (accessory gland) (periurethral) A54.1
  vulva (acute) (chronic) A54.02
Gonocytoma
  specified site — see Neoplasm, uncertain behavior, by site
  unspecified site
    female D39.10
    male D40.10
Gonorrhea (acute) (chronic) A54.9
  Bartholin's gland (acute) (chronic) (purulent) A54.02
    with abscess (accessory gland) (periurethral) A54.1
  bladder A54.01
  cervix A54.03
  conjunctiva, conjunctivitis (neonatorum) A54.31
  contact Z20.2
  Cowper's gland (with abscess) A54.1
  exposure to Z20.2
  fallopian tube (acute) (chronic) A54.24
  kidney (acute) (chronic) A54.21
  lower genitourinary tract A54.00
    with abscess (accessory gland) (periurethral) A54.1
  ovary (acute) (chronic) A54.24
  pelvis (acute) (chronic) A54.24
    female pelvic inflammatory disease A54.24
  penis A54.09
  prostate (acute) (chronic) A54.22
  seminal vesicle (acute) (chronic) A54.23
  specified site not listed (see also Gonococcus) A54.89
  spermatic cord (acute) (chronic) A54.23
  urethra A54.01
    with abscess (accessory gland) (periurethral) A54.1
  vagina A54.02
  vas deferens (acute) (chronic) A54.23
  vulva A54.02
Goodall's disease A08.19
Goodpasture's syndrome M31.0
Gopalan's syndrome (burning feet) E53.0
Gorlin-Chaudry-Moss syndrome Q87.0
Gottron's papules L94.4
Gougerot-Blum syndrome (pigmented purpuric lichenoid dermatitis) L81.7

Gougerot-Carteaud disease or syndrome (confluent reticulate papillomatosis) L83
Gougerot's syndrome (trisymptomatic) L81.7
Gouley's syndrome (constrictive pericarditis) I31.1
Goundou A66.6
Gout, chronic (see also Gout, gouty) M1A.9 ☑ (following M08)
  drug-induced M1A.20 ☑ (following M08)
    ankle M1A.27- ☑ (following M08)
    elbow M1A.22- ☑ (following M08)
    foot joint M1A.27- ☑ (following M08)
    hand joint M1A.24- ☑ (following M08)
    hip M1A.25- ☑ (following M08)
    knee M1A.26- ☑ (following M08)
    multiple site M1A.29- ☑ (following M08)
    shoulder M1A.21- ☑ (following M08)
    vertebrae M1A.28 ☑ (following M08)
    wrist M1A.23- ☑ (following M08)
  idiopathic M1A.00 ☑ (following M08)
    ankle M1A.07- ☑ (following M08)
    elbow M1A.02- ☑ (following M08)
    foot joint M1A.07- ☑ (following M08)
    hand joint M1A.04- ☑ (following M08)
    hip M1A.05- ☑ (following M08)
    knee M1A.06- ☑ (following M08)
    multiple site M1A.09 ☑ (following M08)
    shoulder M1A.01- ☑ (following M08)
    vertebrae M1A.08 ☑ (following M08)
    wrist M1A.03- ☑ (following M08)
  in (due to) renal impairment M1A.30 ☑ (following M08)
    ankle M1A.37- ☑ (following M08)
    elbow M1A.32- ☑ (following M08)
    foot joint M1A.37- ☑ (following M08)
    hand joint M1A.34- ☑ (following M08)
    hip M1A.35- ☑ (following M08)
    knee M1A.36- ☑ (following M08)
    multiple site M1A.39 ☑ (following M08)
    shoulder M1A.31- ☑ (following M08)
    vertebrae M1A.38 ☑ (following M08)
    wrist M1A.33- ☑ (following M08)
  lead-induced M1A.10 ☑ (following M08)
    ankle M1A.17- ☑ (following M08)
    elbow M1A.12- ☑ (following M08)
    foot joint M1A.17- ☑ (following M08)
    hand joint M1A.14- ☑ (following M08)
    hip M1A.15- ☑ (following M08)
    knee M1A.16- ☑ (following M08)
    multiple site M1A.19 ☑ (following M08)
    shoulder M1A.11- ☑ (following M08)
    vertebrae M1A.18 ☑ (following M08)
    wrist M1A.13- ☑ (following M08)
  primary — see Gout, chronic, idiopathic
  saturnine — see Gout, chronic, lead-induced
  secondary NEC M1A.40 ☑ (following M08)
    ankle M1A.47- ☑ (following M08)
    elbow M1A.42- ☑ (following M08)
    foot joint M1A.47- ☑ (following M08)
    hand joint M1A.44- ☑ (following M08)
    hip M1A.45- ☑ (following M08)
    knee M1A.46- ☑ (following M08)
    multiple site M1A.49 ☑ (following M08)
    shoulder M1A.41- ☑ (following M08)
    vertebrae M1A.48 ☑ (following M08)
    wrist M1A.43- ☑ (following M08)
  syphilitic (see also subcategory M14.8-) A52.77
  tophi M1A.9 ☑ (following M08)
Gout, gouty (acute) (attack) (flare) (see also Gout, chronic) M10.9
  drug-induced M10.20
    ankle M10.27- ☑
    elbow M10.22- ☑
    foot joint M10.27- ☑
    hand joint M10.24- ☑
    hip M10.25- ☑
    knee M10.26- ☑
    multiple site M10.29
    shoulder M10.21- ☑
    vertebrae M10.28
    wrist M10.23- ☑
  idiopathic M10.00
    ankle M10.07- ☑
    elbow M10.02- ☑
    foot joint M10.07- ☑
    hand joint M10.04- ☑
    hip M10.05- ☑

☑ **Additional Character Required** — Refer to the Tabular List for Character Selection   ᵂᴷ **Subterms under main terms may continue to next column or page**

Gout, gouty — *continued*
idiopathic — *continued*
knee M10.06- ☑
multiple site M10.09
shoulder M10.01- ☑
vertebrae M10.08
wrist M10.03- ☑
in (due to) renal impairment M10.30
ankle M10.37- ☑
elbow M10.32- ☑
foot joint M10.37- ☑
hand joint M10.34- ☑
hip M10.35- ☑
knee M10.36- ☑
multiple site M10.39
shoulder M10.31- ☑
vertebrae M10.38
wrist M10.33- ☑
lead-induced M10.10
ankle M10.17- ☑
elbow M10.12- ☑
foot joint M10.17- ☑
hand joint M10.14- ☑
hip M10.15- ☑
knee M10.16- ☑
multiple site M10.19
shoulder M10.11- ☑
vertebrae M10.18
wrist M10.13- ☑
primary — *see* Gout, idiopathic
saturnine — *see* Gout, lead-induced
secondary NEC M10.40
ankle M10.47- ☑
elbow M10.42- ☑
foot joint M10.47- ☑
hand joint M10.44- ☑
hip M10.45- ☑
knee M10.46- ☑
multiple site M10.49
shoulder M10.41- ☑
vertebrae M10.48
wrist M10.43- ☑
syphilitic (*see also* subcategory M14.8-) A52.77
tophi — *see* Gout, chronic
Gower's
muscular dystrophy G71.0
syndrome (vasovagal attack) R55
Gradenigo's syndrome — *see* Otitis, media, suppurative, acute
Graefe's disease — *see* Strabismus, paralytic, ophthalmoplegia, progressive
Graft-versus-host disease D89.813
acute D89.810
acute on chronic D89.812
chronic D89.811
Grain mite (itch) B88.0
Grainhandler's disease or lung J67.8
Grand mal — *see* Epilepsy, generalized, specified NEC
Grand multipara status only (not pregnant) Z64.1
pregnant — *see* Pregnancy, complicated by, grand multiparity
Granite worker's lung J62.8
Granular (*see also* condition)
inflammation, pharynx J31.2
kidney (contracting) — *see* Sclerosis, renal
liver K74.69
Granulation tissue (abnormal) (excessive) L92.9
postmastoidectomy cavity — *see* Complications, postmastoidectomy, granulation
Granulocytopenia (primary) (malignant) — *see* Agranulocytosis
Granuloma L92.9
abdomen K66.8
from residual foreign body L92.3
pyogenicum L98.0
actinic L57.5
annulare (perforating) L92.0
apical K04.5
aural — *see* Otitis, externa, specified NEC
beryllium (skin) L92.3
bone
eosinophilic C96.6
from residual foreign body — *see* Osteomyelitis, specified type NEC
lung C96.6
brain (any site) G06.0
schistosomiasis B65.9 [G07]

Granuloma — *continued*
canaliculus lacrimalis — *see* Granuloma, lacrimal
candidal (cutaneous) B37.2
cerebral (any site) G06.0
coccidioidal (primary) (progressive) B38.7
lung B38.1
meninges B38.4
colon K63.89
conjunctiva H11.22- ☑
dental K04.5
ear, middle — *see* Cholesteatoma
eosinophilic C96.6
bone C96.6
lung C96.6
oral mucosa K13.4
skin L92.2
eyelid H01.8
facial (e) L92.2
foreign body (in soft tissue) NEC M60.20
ankle M60.27- ☑
foot M60.27- ☑
forearm M60.23- ☑
hand M60.24- ☑
in operation wound — *see* Foreign body, accidentally left during a procedure
lower leg M60.26- ☑
pelvic region M60.25- ☑
shoulder region M60.21- ☑
skin L92.3
specified site NEC M60.28
subcutaneous tissue L92.3
thigh M60.25- ☑
upper arm M60.22- ☑
gangraenescens M31.2
genito-inguinale A58
giant cell (central) (reparative) (jaw) M27.1
gingiva (peripheral) K06.8
gland (lymph) I88.8
hepatic NEC K75.3
in (due to)
berylliosis J63.2 [K77]
sarcoidosis D86.89
Hodgkin C81.9 ☑
ileum K63.89
infectious B99.9
specified NEC B99.8
inguinale (Donovan) (venereal) A58
intestine NEC K63.89
intracranial (any site) G06.0
intraspinal (any part) G06.1
iridocyclitis — *see* Iridocyclitis, chronic
jaw (bone) (central) M27.1
reparative giant cell M27.1
kidney (*see also* Infection, kidney) N15.8
lacrimal H04.81- ☑
larynx J38.7
lethal midline (faciale(e)) M31.2
liver NEC — *see* Granuloma, hepatic
lung (infectious) (*see also* Fibrosis, lung)
coccidioidal B38.1
eosinophilic C96.6
Majocchi's B35.8
malignant (facial(e)) M31.2
mandible (central) M27.1
midline (lethal) M31.2
monilial (cutaneous) B37.2
nasal sinus — *see* Sinusitis
operation wound T81.89 ☑
foreign body — *see* Foreign body, accidentally left during a procedure
stitch T81.89 ☑
talc — *see* Foreign body, accidentally left during a procedure
oral mucosa K13.4
orbit, orbital H05.11- ☑
paracoccidioidal B41.8
penis, venereal A58
periapical K04.5
peritoneum K66.8
due to ova of helminths NOS (*see also* Helminthiasis) B83.9 [K67]
postmastoidectomy cavity — *see* Complications, postmastoidectomy, recurrent cholesteatoma
prostate N42.89
pudendi (ulcerating) A58
pulp, internal (tooth) K03.3
pyogenic, pyogenicum (of) (skin) L98.0
gingiva K06.8

Granuloma — *continued*
pyogenic, pyogenicum — *continued*
maxillary alveolar ridge K04.5
oral mucosa K13.4
rectum K62.89
reticulohistiocytic D76.3
rubrum nasi L74.8
Schistosoma — *see* Schistosomiasis
septic (skin) L98.0
silica (skin) L92.3
sinus (accessory) (infective) (nasal) — *see* Sinusitis
skin L92.9
from residual foreign body L92.3
pyogenicum L98.0
spine
syphilitic (epidural) A52.19
tuberculous A18.01
stitch (postoperative) T81.89 ☑
suppurative (skin) L98.0
swimming pool A31.1
talc (*see also* Granuloma, foreign body)
in operation wound — *see* Foreign body, accidentally left during a procedure
telangiectaticum (skin) L98.0
tracheostomy J95.09
trichophyticum B35.8
tropicum A66.4
umbilicus L92.9
urethra N36.8
uveitis — *see* Iridocyclitis, chronic
vagina A58
venereum A58
vocal cord J38.3
Granulomatosis L92.9
lymphoid C83.8- ☑
miliary (listerial) A32.89
necrotizing, respiratory M31.30
progressive septic D71
specified NEC L92.8
Wegener's M31.30
with renal involvement M31.31
Granulomatous tissue (abnormal) (excessive) L92.9
Granulosis rubra nasi L74.8
Graphite fibrosis (of lung) J63.3
Graphospasm F48.8
organic G25.89
Grating scapula M89.8X1
Gravel (urinary) — *see* Calculus, urinary
Graves' disease — *see* Hyperthyroidism, with, goiter
Gravis — *see* condition
Grawitz tumor C64.-
Gray syndrome (newborn) P93.0
Grayness, hair (premature) L67.1
congenital Q84.2
Green sickness D50.8
Greenfield's disease
meaning
concentric sclerosis (encephalitis periaxialis concentrica) G37.5
metachromatic leukodystrophy E75.25
Greenstick fracture — *code as* Fracture, by site
Grey syndrome (newborn) P93.0
Grief F43.21
prolonged F43.29
reaction (*see also* Disorder, adjustment) F43.20
Griesinger's disease B76.9
Grinder's lung or pneumoconiosis J62.8
Grinding, teeth
psychogenic F45.8
sleep related G47.63
Grip
Dabney's B33.0
devil's B33.0
Grippe, grippal (*see also* Influenza)
Balkan A78
summer, of Italy A93.1
Grisel's disease M43.6
Groin — *see* condition
Grooved tongue K14.5
Ground itch B76.9
Grover's disease or syndrome L11.1
Growing pains, children R29.898
Growth (fungoid) (neoplastic) (new) (*see also* Neoplasm)
adenoid (vegetative) J35.8
benign — *see* Neoplasm, benign, by site
malignant — *see* Neoplasm, malignant, by site
rapid, childhood Z00.2

Index

Growth — Headache

Growth — *continued*
secondary — *see* Neoplasm, secondary, by site
Gruby's disease B35.0
Gubler-Millard paralysis or syndrome G46.3
Guerin-Stern syndrome Q74.3
Guidance, insufficient anterior (occlusal) M26.54
Guillain-Barré disease or syndrome G61.0
sequelae G65.0
Guinea worms (infection) (infestation) B72
Guinon's disease (motor-verbal tic) F95.2
Gull's disease E03.4
Gum — *see* condition
Gumboil K04.7
with sinus K04.6
Gumma (syphilitic) A52.79
artery A52.09
cerebral A52.04
bone A52.77
of yaws (late) A66.6
brain A52.19
cauda equina A52.19
central nervous system A52.3
ciliary body A52.71
congenital A50.59
eyelid A52.71
heart A52.06
intracranial A52.19
iris A52.71
kidney A52.75
larynx A52.73
leptomeninges A52.19
liver A52.74
meninges A52.19
myocardium A52.06
nasopharynx A52.73
neurosyphilitic A52.3
nose A52.73
orbit A52.71
palate (soft) A52.79
penis A52.76
pericardium A52.06
pharynx A52.73
pituitary A52.79
scrofulous (tuberculous) A18.4
skin A52.79
specified site NEC A52.79
spinal cord A52.19
tongue A52.79
tonsil A52.73
trachea A52.73
tuberculous A18.4
ulcerative due to yaws A66.4
ureter A52.75
yaws A66.4
bone A66.6
Gunn's syndrome Q07.8
Gunshot wound (*see also* Wound, open)
fracture — *code as* Fracture, by site
internal organs — *see* Injury, by site
Gynandrism Q56.0
Gynandroblastoma
specified site — *see* Neoplasm, uncertain behavior, by site
unspecified site
female D39.10
male D40.10
Gynecological examination (periodic) (routine) Z01.419
with abnormal findings Z01.411
Gynecomastia N62
Gynephobia F40.291
Gyrate scalp Q82.8

H

H (Hartnup's) **disease** E72.02
Haas' disease or osteochondrosis (juvenile) (head of humerus) — *see* Osteochondrosis, juvenile, humerus
Habit, habituation
bad sleep Z72.821
chorea F95.8
disturbance, child F98.9
drug — *see* Dependence, drug
irregular sleep Z72.821
laxative F55.2
spasm — *see* Tic
tic — *see* Tic

Haemophilus (H.) **influenzae, as cause of disease classified elsewhere** B96.3
Haff disease — *see* Poisoning, mercury
Hageman's factor defect, deficiency or disease D68.2
Haglund's disease or osteochondrosis (juvenile) (os tibiale externum) — *see* Osteochondrosis, juvenile, tarsus
Hailey-Hailey disease Q82.8
Hair (*see also* condition)
plucking F63.3
in stereotyped movement disorder F98.4
tourniquet syndrome (*see also* Constriction, external, by site)
finger S60.44- ☑
penis S30.842 ☑
thumb S60.34- ☑
toe S90.44- ☑
Hairball in stomach T18.2 ☑
Hair-pulling, pathological (compulsive) F63.3
Hairy black tongue K14.3
Half vertebra Q76.49
Halitosis R19.6
Hallerman-Streiff syndrome Q87.0
Hallervorden-Spatz disease G23.0
Hallopeau's acrodermatitis or disease L40.2
Hallucination R44.3
auditory R44.0
gustatory R44.2
olfactory R44.2
specified NEC R44.2
tactile R44.2
visual R44.1
Hallucinosis (chronic) F28
alcoholic (acute) F10.951
in
abuse F10.151
dependence F10.251
drug-induced F19.951
cannabis F12.951
cocaine F14.951
hallucinogen F16.151
in
abuse F19.151
cannabis F12.151
cocaine F14.151
hallucinogen F16.151
inhalant F18.151
opioid F11.151
sedative, anxiolytic or hypnotic F13.151
stimulant NEC F15.151
dependence F19.251
cannabis F12.251
cocaine F14.251
hallucinogen F16.251
inhalant F18.251
opioid F11.251
sedative, anxiolytic or hypnotic F13.251
stimulant NEC F15.251
inhalant F18.951
opioid F11.951
sedative, anxiolytic or hypnotic F13.951
stimulant NEC F15.951
organic F06.0
Hallux
deformity (acquired) NEC M20.5X- ☑
limitus M20.5X- ☑
malleus (acquired) NEC M20.3- ☑
rigidus (acquired) M20.2- ☑
congenital Q74.2
sequelae (late effect) of rickets E64.3
valgus (acquired) M20.1- ☑
congenital Q66.6
varus (acquired) M20.3- ☑
congenital Q66.3
Halo, visual H53.19
Hamartoma, hamartoblastoma Q85.9
epithelial (gingival), odontogenic, central or peripheral — *see* Cyst, calcifying odontogenic
Hamartosis Q85.9
Hamman-Rich syndrome J84.114
Hammer toe (acquired) NEC (*see also* Deformity, toe, hammer toe)
congenital Q66.89
sequelae (late effect) of rickets E64.3
Hand — *see* condition
Hand-foot syndrome L27.1

Handicap, handicapped
educational Z55.9
specified NEC Z55.8
Hand-Schüller-Christian disease or syndrome C96.5
Hanging (asphyxia) (strangulation) (suffocation) — *see* Asphyxia, traumatic, due to mechanical threat
Hangnail (*see also* Cellulitis, digit)
with lymphangitis — *see* Lymphangitis, acute, digit
Hangover (alcohol) F10.129
Hanhart's syndrome Q87.0
Hanot-Chauffard (-Troisier) **syndrome** E83.19
Hanot's cirrhosis or disease K74.3
Hansen's disease — *see* Leprosy
Hantaan virus disease (Korean hemorrhagic fever) A98.5
Hantavirus disease (with renal manifestations) (Dobrava) (Puumala) (Seoul) A98.5
with pulmonary manifestations (Andes) (Bayou) (Bermejo) (Black Creek Canal) (Choclo) (Juquitiba) (Laguna negra) (Lechiguanas) (New York) (Oran) (Sin nombre) B33.4
Happy puppet syndrome Q93.5
Harada's disease or syndrome H30.81- ☑
Hardening
artery — *see* Arteriosclerosis
brain G93.89
Harelip (complete) (incomplete) — *see* Cleft, lip
Harlequin (newborn) Q80.4
Harley's disease D59.6
Harmful use (of)
alcohol F10.10
anxiolytics — *see* Abuse, drug, sedative
cannabinoids — *see* Abuse, drug, cannabis
cocaine — *see* Abuse, drug, cocaine
drug — *see* Abuse, drug
hallucinogens — *see* Abuse, drug, hallucinogen
hypnotics — *see* Abuse, drug, sedative
opioids — *see* Abuse, drug, opioid
PCP (phencyclidine) — *see* Abuse, drug, hallucinogen
sedatives — *see* Abuse, drug, sedative
stimulants NEC — *see* Abuse, drug, stimulant
Harris' lines — *see* Arrest, epiphyseal
Hartnup's disease E72.02
Harvester's lung J67.0
Harvesting ovum for in vitro fertilization Z31.83
Hashimoto's disease or thyroiditis E06.3
Hashitoxicosis (transient) E06.3
Hassal-Henle bodies or warts (cornea) H18.49
Haut mal — *see* Epilepsy, generalized, specified NEC
Haverhill fever A25.1
Hay fever (*see also* Fever, hay) J30.1
Hayem-Widal syndrome D59.8
Haygarth's nodes M15.8
Haymaker's lung J67.0
Hb (abnormal)
Bart's disease D56.0
disease — *see* Disease, hemoglobin
trait — *see* Trait
Head — *see* condition
Headache R51
allergic NEC G44.89
associated with sexual activity G44.82
chronic daily R51
cluster G44.009
chronic G44.029
intractable G44.021
not intractable G44.029
episodic G44.019
intractable G44.011
not intractable G44.019
intractable G44.001
not intractable G44.009
cough (primary) G44.83
daily chronic R51
drug-induced NEC G44.40
intractable G44.41
not intractable G44.40
exertional (primary) G44.84
histamine G44.009
intractable G44.001
not intractable G44.009
hypnic G44.81
lumbar puncture G97.1
medication overuse G44.40
intractable G44.41
not intractable G44.40
menstrual — *see* Migraine, menstrual
migraine (type) (*see also* Migraine) G43.909

☑ **Additional Character Required** — **Refer to the Tabular List for Character Selection**   ▽ **Subterms under main terms may continue to next column or page**

Headache — *continued*
  nasal septum R51
  neuralgiform, short lasting unilateral, with conjunctival
    injection and tearing (SUNCT) G44.059
    intractable G44.051
    not intractable G44.059
  new daily persistent (NDPH) G44.52
  orgasmic G44.82
  periodic syndromes in adults and children G43.C0
    (*following* G43.7)
    with refractory migraine G43.C1 (*following* G43.7)
    without refractory migraine G43.C0 (*following*
      G43.7)
    intractable G43.C1 (*following* G43.7)
    not intractable G43.C0 (*following* G43.7)
  postspinal puncture G97.1
  post-traumatic G44.309
    acute G44.319
      intractable G44.311
      not intractable G44.319
    chronic G44.329
      intractable G44.321
      not intractable G44.329
    intractable G44.301
    not intractable G44.309
  pre-menstrual — *see* Migraine, menstrual
  preorgasmic G44.82
  primary
    cough G44.83
    exertional G44.84
    stabbing G44.85
    thunderclap G44.53
  rebound G44.40
    intractable G44.41
    not intractable G44.40
  short lasting unilateral neuralgiform, with conjunctival
    injection and tearing (SUNCT) G44.059
    intractable G44.051
    not intractable G44.059
  specified syndrome NEC G44.89
  spinal and epidural anesthesia - induced T88.59 ☑
    in labor and delivery O74.5
    in pregnancy O29.4- ☑
    postpartum, puerperal O89.4
  spinal fluid loss (from puncture) G97.1
  stabbing (primary) G44.85
  tension (-type) G44.209
    chronic G44.229
      intractable G44.221
      not intractable G44.229
    episodic G44.219
      intractable G44.211
      not intractable G44.219
    intractable G44.201
    not intractable G44.209
  thunderclap (primary) G44.53
  vascular NEC G44.1
Healthy
  infant
    accompanying sick mother Z76.3
    receiving care Z76.2
  person accompanying sick person Z76.3
Hearing examination Z01.10
  with abnormal findings NEC Z01.118
  following failed hearing screening Z01.110
  for hearing conservation and treatment Z01.12
Heart — *see* condition
Heart beat
  abnormality R00.9
    specified NEC R00.8
  awareness R00.2
  rapid R00.0
  slow R00.1
Heartburn R12
  psychogenic F45.8
Heat (effects) T67.9 ☑
  apoplexy T67.0 ☑
  burn (*see also* Burn) L55.9
  collapse T67.1 ☑
  cramps T67.2 ☑
  dermatitis or eczema L59.0
  edema T67.7 ☑
  erythema — *code by site under* Burn, first degree
  excessive T67.9 ☑
    specified effect NEC T67.8 ☑
  exhaustion T67.5 ☑
    anhydrotic T67.3 ☑

Heat — *continued*
  exhaustion — *continued*
    due to
      salt (and water) depletion T67.4 ☑
      water depletion T67.3 ☑
        with salt depletion T67.4 ☑
  fatigue (transient) T67.6 ☑
  fever T67.0 ☑
  hyperpyrexia T67.0 ☑
  prickly L74.0
  prostration — *see* Heat, exhaustion
  pyrexia T67.0 ☑
  rash L74.0
  specified effect NEC T67.8 ☑
  stroke T67.0 ☑
  sunburn — *see* Sunburn
  syncope T67.1 ☑
Heavy-for-dates NEC (infant) (4000g to 4499g) P08.1
  exceptionally (4500g or more) P08.0
Hebephrenia, hebephrenic (schizophrenia) F20.1
Heberden's disease or nodes (with arthropathy) M15.1
Hebra's
  pityriasis L26
  prurigo L28.2
Heel — *see* condition
Heerfordt's disease D86.89
Hegglin's anomaly or syndrome D72.0
Heilmeyer-Schoner disease D45
Heine-Medin disease A80.9
Heinz body anemia, congenital D58.2
Heliophobia F40.228
Heller's disease or syndrome F84.3
HELLP syndrome (hemolysis, elevated liver enzymes
  and low platelet count) O14.2- ☑
Helminthiasis (*see also* Infestation, helminth)
  Ancylostoma B76.0
  intestinal B82.0
    mixed types (types classifiable to more than one
      of the titles B65.0-B81.3 and B81.8) B81.4
    specified type NEC B81.8
  mixed types (intestinal) (types classifiable to more
    than one of the titles B65.0-B81.3 and B81.8)
    B81.4
  Necator (americanus) B76.1
  specified type NEC B83.8
Heloma L84
Hemangioblastoma — *see* Neoplasm, connective tissue,
  uncertain behavior
  malignant — *see* Neoplasm, connective tissue, malig-
    nant
Hemangioendothelioma (*see also* Neoplasm, uncertain
  behavior, by site)
  benign D18.00
    intra-abdominal D18.03
    intracranial D18.02
    skin D18.01
    specified site NEC D18.09
  bone (diffuse) — *see* Neoplasm, bone, malignant
  epithelioid (*see also* Neoplasm, uncertain behavior,
    by site)
    malignant — *see* Neoplasm, malignant, by site
  malignant — *see* Neoplasm, connective tissue, malig-
    nant
Hemangiofibroma — *see* Neoplasm, benign, by site
Hemangiolipoma — *see* Lipoma
Hemangioma D18.00
  arteriovenous D18.00
    intra-abdominal D18.03
    intracranial D18.02
    skin D18.01
    specified site NEC D18.09
  capillary D18.00
    intra-abdominal D18.03
    intracranial D18.02
    skin D18.01
    specified site NEC D18.09
  cavernous D18.00
    intra-abdominal D18.03
    intracranial D18.02
    skin D18.01
    specified site NEC D18.09
  epithelioid D18.00
    intra-abdominal D18.03
    intracranial D18.02
    skin D18.01
    specified site NEC D18.09
  histiocytoid D18.00

Hemangioma — *continued*
  histiocytoid — *continued*
    intra-abdominal D18.03
    intracranial D18.02
    skin D18.01
    specified site NEC D18.09
  infantile D18.00
    intra-abdominal D18.03
    intracranial D18.02
    skin D18.01
    specified site NEC D18.09
  intra-abdominal D18.03
  intracranial D18.02
  intramuscular D18.00
    intra-abdominal D18.03
    intracranial D18.02
    skin D18.01
    specified site NEC D18.09
  juvenile D18.00
  malignant — *see* Neoplasm,connective tissue, malig-
    nant
  plexiform D18.00
    intra-abdominal D18.03
    intracranial D18.02
    skin D18.01
    specified site NEC D18.09
  racemose D18.00
    intra-abdominal D18.03
    intracranial D18.02
    skin D18.01
    specified site NEC D18.09
  sclerosing — *see* Neoplasm, skin, benign
  simplex D18.00
    intra-abdominal D18.03
    intracranial D18.02
    skin D18.01
    specified site NEC D18.09
  skin D18.01
  specified site NEC D18.09
  venous D18.00
    intra-abdominal D18.03
    intracranial D18.02
    skin D18.01
    specified site NEC D18.09
  verrucous keratotic D18.00
    intra-abdominal D18.03
    intracranial D18.02
    skin D18.01
    specified site NEC D18.09
Hemangiomatosis (systemic) I78.8
  involving single site — *see* Hemangioma
Hemangiopericytoma (*see also* Neoplasm, connective
  tissue, uncertain behavior)
  benign — *see* Neoplasm, connective tissue, benign
  malignant — *see* Neoplasm, connective tissue, malig-
    nant
Hemangiosarcoma — *see* Neoplasm, connective tissue,
  malignant
Hemarthrosis (nontraumatic) M25.00
  ankle M25.07- ☑
  elbow M25.02- ☑
  foot joint M25.07- ☑
  hand joint M25.04- ☑
  hip M25.05- ☑
  in hemophilic arthropathy — *see* Arthropathy,
    hemophilic
  knee M25.06- ☑
  shoulder M25.01- ☑
  specified joint NEC M25.08
  traumatic — *see* Sprain, by site
  vertebrae M25.08
  wrist M25.03- ☑
Hematemesis K92.0
  with ulcer — *code by site under* Ulcer, with hemor-
    rhage K27.4
  newborn, neonatal P54.0
    due to swallowed maternal blood P78.2
Hematidrosis L74.8
Hematinuria (*see also* Hemoglobinuria)
  malarial B50.8
Hematobilia K83.8
Hematocele
  female NEC N94.89
    with ectopic pregnancy O00.9
    ovary N83.8
  male N50.1
Hematochezia (*see also* Melena) K92.1

Hematochyluria (see also Infestation, filarial)
  schistosomiasis (bilharziasis) B65.0
Hematocolpos (with hematometra or hematosalpinx)
  N89.7
Hematocornea — see Pigmentation, cornea, stromal
Hematogenous — see condition
Hematoma (traumatic) (skin surface intact) (see also
  Contusion)
  with
    injury of internal organs — see Injury, by site
    open wound — see Wound, open
  amputation stump (surgical) (late) T87.89
  aorta, dissecting I71.00
    abdominal I71.02
    thoracic I71.01
    thoracoabdominal I71.03
  aortic intramural — see Dissection, aorta
  arterial (complicating trauma) — see Injury, blood
    vessel, by site
  auricle — see Contusion, ear
    nontraumatic — see Disorder, pinna, hematoma
  birth injury NEC P15.8
  brain (traumatic)
    with
      cerebral laceration or contusion (diffuse) — see
        Injury, intracranial, diffuse
        focal — see Injury, intracranial, focal
    cerebellar, traumatic S06.37- ☑
    intracerebral, traumatic — see Injury, intracranial,
      intracerebral hemorrhage
    newborn NEC P52.4
      birth injury P10.1
    nontraumatic — see Hemorrhage, intracranial
    subarachnoid, arachnoid, traumatic — see Injury,
      intracranial, subarachnoid hemorrhage
    subdural, traumatic — see Injury, intracranial,
      subdural hemorrhage
  breast (nontraumatic) N64.89
  broad ligament (nontraumatic) N83.7
    traumatic S37.892 ☑
  cerebellar, traumatic S06.37- ☑
  cerebral — see Hematoma, brain
  cerebrum S06.36- ☑
    left S06.35- ☑
    right S06.34- ☑
  cesarean delivery wound O90.2
  complicating delivery (perineal) (pelvic) (vagina) (vulva) O71.7
  corpus cavernosum (nontraumatic) N48.89
  epididymis (nontraumatic) N50.1
  epidural (traumatic) — see Injury, intracranial, epidural
    hemorrhage
    spinal — see Injury, spinal cord, by region
  episiotomy O90.2
  face, birth injury P15.4
  genital organ NEC (nontraumatic)
    female (nonobstetric) N94.89
      traumatic S30.202 ☑
    male N50.1
      traumatic S30.201 ☑
  internal organs — see Injury, by site
  intracerebral, traumatic — see Injury, intracranial, intracerebral hemorrhage
  intraoperative — see Complications, intraoperative, hemorrhage
  labia (nontraumatic) (nonobstetric) N90.89
  liver (subcapsular) (nontraumatic) K76.89
    birth injury P15.0
  mediastinum — see Injury, intrathoracic
  mesosalpinx (nontraumatic) N83.7
    traumatic S37.898 ☑
  muscle — code by site under Contusion
  nontraumatic
    muscle M79.81
    soft tissue M79.81
  obstetrical surgical wound O90.2
  orbit, orbital (nontraumatic) (see also Hemorrhage,
    orbit)
    traumatic — see Contusion, orbit
  pelvis (female) (nontraumatic) (nonobstetric) N94.89
    obstetric O71.7
    traumatic — see Injury, by site
  penis (nontraumatic) N48.89
    birth injury P15.5
  perianal (nontraumatic) K64.5
  perineal S30.23 ☑
    complicating delivery O71.7

Hematoma — continued
  perirenal — see Injury, kidney
  pinna — see Contusion, ear
    nontraumatic — see Disorder, pinna, hematoma
  placenta O43.89- ☑
  postoperative (postprocedural) — see Complication,
    postprocedural, hemorrhage
  retroperitoneal (nontraumatic) K66.1
    traumatic S36.892 ☑
  scrotum, superficial S30.22 ☑
    birth injury P15.5
  seminal vesicle (nontraumatic) N50.1
    traumatic S37.892 ☑
  spermatic cord (traumatic) S37.892 ☑
    nontraumatic N50.1
  spinal (cord) (meninges) (see also Injury, spinal cord,
    by region)
    newborn (birth injury) P11.5
  spleen D73.5
    intraoperative — see Complications, intraoperative,
      hemorrhage, spleen
    postprocedural (postoperative) — see Complications, postprocedural, hemorrhage, spleen
  sternocleidomastoid, birth injury P15.2
  sternomastoid, birth injury P15.2
  subarachnoid (traumatic) — see Injury, intracranial,
    subarachnoid hemorrhage
    newborn (nontraumatic) P52.5
      due to birth injury P10.3
    nontraumatic — see Hemorrhage, intracranial,
      subarachnoid
  subdural (traumatic) — see Injury, intracranial, subdural hemorrhage
    newborn (localized) P52.8
      birth injury P10.0
    nontraumatic — see Hemorrhage, intracranial,
      subdural
  superficial, newborn P54.5
  testis (nontraumatic) N50.1
    birth injury P15.5
  tunica vaginalis (nontraumatic) N50.1
  umbilical cord, complicating delivery O69.5 ☑
  uterine ligament (broad) (nontraumatic) N83.7
    traumatic S37.892 ☑
  vagina (ruptured) (nontraumatic) N89.8
    complicating delivery O71.7
  vas deferens (nontraumatic) N50.1
    traumatic S37.892 ☑
  vitreous — see Hemorrhage, vitreous
  vulva (nontraumatic) (nonobstetric) N90.89
    complicating delivery O71.7
    newborn (birth injury) P15.5
Hematometra N85.7
  with hematocolpos N89.7
Hematomyelia (central) G95.19
  newborn (birth injury) P11.5
  traumatic T14.8
Hematomyelitis G04.90
Hematoperitoneum — see Hemoperitoneum
Hematophobia F40.230
Hematopneumothorax (see Hemothorax)
Hematopoiesis, cyclic D70.4
Hematoporphyria — see Porphyria
Hematorachis, hematorrhachis G95.19
  newborn (birth injury) P11.5
Hematosalpinx N83.6
  with
    hematocolpos N89.7
    hematometra N85.7
      with hematocolpos N89.7
  infectional — see Salpingitis
Hematospermia R36.1
Hematothorax (see Hemothorax)
Hematuria R31.9
  benign (familial) (of childhood) (see also Hematuria,
    idiopathic)
    essential microscopic R31.1
  due to sulphonamide, sulfonamide — see Table of
    Drugs and Chemicals, by drug
  endemic (see also Schistosomiasis) B65.0
  gross R31.0
  idiopathic N02.9
    with glomerular lesion
      crescentic (diffuse) glomerulonephritis N02.7
      dense deposit disease N02.6
      endocapillary proliferative glomerulonephritis
        N02.4

Hematuria — continued
  idiopathic — continued
    with glomerular lesion — continued
      focal and segmental hyalinosis or sclerosis
        N02.1
      membranoproliferative (diffuse) N02.5
      membranous (diffuse) N02.2
      mesangial proliferative (diffuse) N02.3
      mesangiocapillary (diffuse) N02.5
      minor abnormality N02.0
      proliferative NEC N02.8
      specified pathology NEC N02.8
  intermittent — see Hematuria, idiopathic
  malarial B50.8
  microscopic NEC R31.2
    benign essential R31.1
  paroxysmal (see also Hematuria, idiopathic)
    nocturnal D59.5
  persistent — see Hematuria, idiopathic
  recurrent — see Hematuria, idiopathic
  tropical (see also Schistosomiasis) B65.0
  tuberculous A18.13
Hemeralopia (day blindness) H53.11
  vitamin A deficiency E50.5
Hemi-akinesia R41.4
Hemianalgesia R20.0
Hemianencephaly Q00.0
Hemianesthesia R20.0
Hemianopia, hemianopsia (heteronymous) H53.47
  homonymous H53.46- ☑
  syphilitic A52.71
Hemiathetosis R25.8
Hemiatrophy R68.89
  cerebellar G31.9
  face, facial, progressive (Romberg) G51.8
  tongue K14.8
Hemiballism (us) G25.5
Hemicardia Q24.8
Hemicephalus, hemicephaly Q00.0
Hemichorea G25.5
Hemicolitis, left — see Colitis, left sided
Hemicrania
  congenital malformation Q00.0
  continua G44.51
  meaning migraine (see also Migraine) G43.909
  paroxysmal G44.039
    chronic G44.049
      intractable G44.041
      not intractable G44.049
    episodic G44.039
      intractable G44.031
      not intractable G44.039
    intractable G44.031
    not intractable G44.039
Hemidystrophy — see Hemiatrophy
Hemiectromelia Q73.8
Hemihypalgesia R20.8
Hemihypesthesia R20.1
Hemi-inattention R41.4
Hemimelia Q73.8
  lower limb — see Defect, reduction, lower limb, specified type NEC
  upper limb — see Defect, reduction, upper limb,
    specified type NEC
Hemiparalysis — see Hemiplegia
Hemiparesis — see Hemiplegia
Hemiparesthesia R20.2
Hemiparkinsonism G20
Hemiplegia G81.9- ☑
  alternans facialis G83.89
  ascending NEC G81.90
    spinal G95.89
  congenital (cerebral) G80.8
    spastic G80.2
  embolic (current episode) I63.4- ☑
  flaccid G81.0- ☑
  following
    cerebrovascular disease I69.959
      cerebral infarction I69.35- ☑
      intracerebral hemorrhage I69.15- ☑
      nontraumatic intracranial hemorrhage NEC
        I69.25- ☑
      specified disease NEC I69.85- ☑
      stroke NOS I69.35- ☑
      subarachnoid hemorrhage I69.05- ☑
  hysterical F44.4
  newborn NEC P91.8

Hemiplegia — continued
  newborn — continued
    birth injury P11.9
    spastic G81.1- ☑
      congenital G80.2
    thrombotic (current episode) I63.3 ☑
Hemisection, spinal cord — see Injury, spinal cord, by region
Hemispasm (facial) R25.2
Hemisporosis B48.8
Hemitremor R25.1
Hemivertebra Q76.49
  failure of segmentation with scoliosis Q76.3
  fusion with scoliosis Q76.3
Hemochromatosis E83.119
  with refractory anemia D46.1
  due to repeated red blood cell transfusion E83.111
  hereditary (primary) E83.110
  primary E83.110
  specified NEC E83.118
Hemoglobin (see also condition)
  abnormal (disease) — see Disease, hemoglobin
  AS genotype D57.3
  Constant Spring D58.2
  E-beta thalassemia D56.5
  fetal, hereditary persistence (HPFH) D56.4
  H Constant Spring D56.0
  low NOS D64.9
  S (Hb S), heterozygous D57.3
Hemoglobinemia D59.9
  due to blood transfusion T80.89 ☑
  paroxysmal D59.6
    nocturnal D59.5
Hemoglobinopathy (mixed) D58.2
  with thalassemia D56.8
  sickle-cell D57.1
    with thalassemia D57.40
      with crisis (vasoocclusive pain) D57.419
        with
          acute chest syndrome D57.411
          splenic sequestration D57.412
      without crisis D57.40
Hemoglobinuria R82.3
  with anemia, hemolytic, acquired (chronic) NEC D59.6
  cold (agglutinin) (paroxysmal) (with Raynaud's syndrome) D59.6
  due to exertion or hemolysis NEC D59.6
  intermittent D59.6
  malarial B50.8
  march D59.6
  nocturnal (paroxysmal) D59.5
  paroxysmal (cold) D59.6
    nocturnal D59.5
Hemolymphangioma D18.1
Hemolysis
  intravascular
    with
      abortion — see Abortion, by type, complicated by, hemorrhage
      ectopic or molar pregnancy O08.1
      hemorrhage
        antepartum — see Hemorrhage, antepartum, with coagulation defect
        intrapartum (see also Hemorrhage, complicating, delivery) O67.0
        postpartum O72.3
    neonatal (excessive) P58.9
    specified NEC P58.8
Hemolytic — see condition
Hemopericardium I31.2
  following acute myocardial infarction (current complication) I23.0
  newborn P54.8
  traumatic — see Injury, heart, with hemopericardium
Hemoperitoneum K66.1
  infectional K65.9
  traumatic S36.899 ☑
    with open wound — see Wound, open, with penetration into peritoneal cavity
Hemophilia (classical) (familial) (hereditary) D66
  A D66
  acquired D68.311
  autoimmune D68.311
  B D67
  C D68.1
  calcipriva (see also Defect, coagulation) D68.4
  nonfamilial (see also Defect, coagulation) D68.4
  secondary D68.311

Hemophilia — continued
  vascular D68.0
Hemophthalmos H44.81- ☑
Hemopneumothorax (see also Hemothorax)
  traumatic S27.2 ☑
Hemoptysis R04.2
  newborn P26.9
  tuberculous — see Tuberculosis, pulmonary
Hemorrhage, hemorrhagic (concealed) R58
  abdomen R58
  accidental antepartum — see Hemorrhage, antepartum
  acute idiopathic pulmonary, in infants R04.81
  adenoid J35.8
  adrenal (capsule) (gland) E27.49
    medulla E27.8
    newborn P54.4
  after delivery — see Hemorrhage, postpartum
  alveolar
    lung, newborn P26.8
    process K08.8
  alveolus K08.8
  amputation stump (surgical) T87.89
  anemia (chronic) D50.0
    acute D62
  antepartum (with) O46.90
    with coagulation defect O46.00- ☑
      afibrinogenemia O46.01- ☑
      disseminated intravascular coagulation O46.02- ☑
      hypofibrinogenemia O46.01- ☑
      specified defect NEC O46.09- ☑
    before 20 weeks gestation O20.9
      specified type NEC O20.8
      threatened abortion O20.0
    due to
      abruptio placenta (see also Abruptio placentae) O45.9- ☑
      leiomyoma, uterus — see Hemorrhage, antepartum, specified cause NEC
      placenta previa O44.1- ☑
    specified cause NEC — see subcategory O46.8X- ☑
  anus (sphincter) K62.5
  apoplexy (stroke) — see Hemorrhage, intracranial, intracerebral
  arachnoid — see Hemorrhage, intracranial, subarachnoid
  artery R58
    brain — see Hemorrhage, intracranial, intracerebral
  basilar (ganglion) I61.0
  bladder N32.89
  bowel K92.2
    newborn P54.3
  brain (miliary) (nontraumatic) — see Hemorrhage, intracranial, intracerebral
    due to
      birth injury P10.1
      syphilis A52.05
    epidural or extradural (traumatic) — see Injury, intracranial, epidural hemorrhage
    newborn P52.4
      birth injury P10.1
    subarachnoid — see Hemorrhage, intracranial, subarachnoid
    subdural — see Hemorrhage, intracranial, subdural
  brainstem (nontraumatic) I61.3
    traumatic S06.38- ☑
  breast N64.59
  bronchial tube — see Hemorrhage, lung
  bronchopulmonary — see Hemorrhage, lung
  bronchus — see Hemorrhage, lung
  bulbar I61.5
  capillary I78.8
    primary D69.8
  cecum K92.2
  cerebellar, cerebellum (nontraumatic) I61.4
    newborn P52.6
    traumatic S06.37- ☑
  cerebral, cerebrum (see also Hemorrhage, intracranial, intracerebral)
    lobe I61.1
    newborn (anoxic) P52.4
      birth injury P10.1
  cerebromeningeal I61.8
  cerebrospinal — see Hemorrhage, intracranial, intracerebral
  cervix (uteri) (stump) NEC N88.8

Hemorrhage, hemorrhagic — continued
  chamber, anterior (eye) — see Hyphema
  childbirth — see Hemorrhage, complicating, delivery
  choroid H31.30- ☑
    expulsive H31.31- ☑
  ciliary body — see Hyphema
  cochlea — see subcategory H83.8 ☑
  colon K92.2
  complicating
    abortion — see Abortion, by type, complicated by, hemorrhage
    delivery O67.9
      associated with coagulation defect (afibrinogenemia) (DIC) (hyperfibrinolysis) O67.0
      specified cause NEC O67.8
    surgical procedure — see Hemorrhage, intraoperative
  conjunctiva H11.3- ☑
    newborn P54.8
  cord, newborn (stump) P51.9
  corpus luteum (ruptured) cyst N83.1
  cortical (brain) I61.1
  cranial — see Hemorrhage, intracranial
  cutaneous R23.3
    due to autosensitivity, erythrocyte D69.2
    newborn P54.5
  delayed
    following ectopic or molar pregnancy O08.1
    postpartum O72.2
  diathesis (familial) D69.9
  disease D69.9
    newborn P53
    specified type NEC D69.8
  due to or associated with
    afibrinogenemia or other coagulation defect (conditions in categories D65- D69)
      antepartum — see Hemorrhage, antepartum, with coagulation defect
      intrapartum O67.0
  dental implant M27.61
  device, implant or graft (see also Complications, by site and type, specified NEC) T85.83 ☑
    arterial graft NEC T82.838 ☑
    breast T85.83 ☑
    catheter NEC T85.83 ☑
      dialysis (renal) T82.838 ☑
        intraperitoneal T85.83 ☑
      infusion NEC T82.838 ☑
        spinal (epidural) (subdural) T85.83 ☑
      urinary (indwelling) T83.83 ☑
    electronic (electrode) (pulse generator) (stimulator)
      bone T84.83 ☑
      cardiac T82.837 ☑
      nervous system (brain) (peripheral nerve) (spinal) T85.83 ☑
      urinary T83.83 ☑
    fixation, internal (orthopedic) NEC T84.83 ☑
    gastrointestinal (bile duct) (esophagus) T85.83 ☑
    genital NEC T83.83 ☑
    heart NEC T82.837 ☑
    joint prosthesis T84.83 ☑
    ocular (corneal graft) (orbital implant) NEC T85.83 ☑
    orthopedic NEC T84.83 ☑
      bone graft T86.838
    specified NEC T85.83 ☑
    urinary NEC T83.83 ☑
    vascular NEC T82.838 ☑
    ventricular intracranial shunt T85.83 ☑
  duodenum, duodenal K92.2
    ulcer — see Ulcer, duodenum, with hemorrhage
  dura mater — see Hemorrhage, intracranial, subdural
  endotracheal — see Hemorrhage, lung
  epicranial subaponeurotic (massive), birth injury P12.2
  epidural (traumatic) (see also Injury, intracranial, epidural hemorrhage)
    nontraumatic I62.1
  esophagus K22.8
    varix I85.01
      secondary I85.11
  excessive, following ectopic gestation (subsequent episode) O08.1
  extradural (traumatic) — see Injury, intracranial, epidural hemorrhage
    birth injury P10.8

Hemorrhage, hemorrhagic — *continued*
  extradural — *see* Injury, intracranial, epidural hemorrhage — *continued*
    newborn (anoxic) (nontraumatic) P52.8
    nontraumatic I62.1
  eye NEC H57.8
    fundus — *see* Hemorrhage, retina
    lid — *see* Disorder, eyelid, specified type NEC
  fallopian tube N83.6
  fibrinogenolysis — *see* Fibrinolysis
  fibrinolytic (acquired) — *see* Fibrinolysis
  from
    ear (nontraumatic) — *see* Otorrhagia
    tracheostomy stoma J95.01
  fundus, eye — *see* Hemorrhage, retina
  funis — *see* Hemorrhage, umbilicus, cord
  gastric — *see* Hemorrhage, stomach
  gastroenteric K92.2
    newborn P54.3
  gastrointestinal (tract) K92.2
    newborn P54.3
  genital organ, male N50.1
  genitourinary (tract) NOS R31.9
  gingiva K06.8
  globe (eye) — *see* Hemophthalmos
  graafian follicle cyst (ruptured) N83.0
  gum K06.8
  heart I51.89
  hypopharyngeal (throat) R04.1
  intermenstrual (regular) N92.3
    irregular N92.1
  internal (organs) NEC R58
    capsule I61.0
    ear — *see* subcategory H83.8 ☑
    newborn P54.8
  intestine K92.2
    newborn P54.3
  intra-abdominal R58
  intra-alveolar (lung), newborn P26.8
  intracerebral (nontraumatic) — *see* Hemorrhage, intracranial, intracerebral
  intracranial (nontraumatic) I62.9
    birth injury P10.9
    epidural, nontraumatic I62.1
    extradural, nontraumatic I62.1
    intracerebral (nontraumatic) (in) I61.9
      brain stem I61.3
      cerebellum I61.4
      hemisphere I61.2
        cortical (superficial) I61.1
        subcortical (deep) I61.0
      intraoperative
        during a nervous system procedure G97.31
        during other procedure G97.32
      intraventricular I61.5
      multiple localized I61.6
      newborn P52.4
        birth injury P10.1
      postprocedural
        following a nervous system procedure G97.51
        following other procedure G97.52
      specified NEC I61.8
      superficial I61.1
      traumatic (diffuse) — *see* Injury, intracranial, diffuse
        focal — *see* Injury, intracranial, focal
    newborn P52.9
      specified NEC P52.8
    subarachnoid (nontraumatic) (from) I60.9
      intracranial (cerebral) artery I60.7
        anterior communicating I60.2- ☑
        basilar I60.4
        carotid siphon and bifurcation I60.0- ☑
        communicating I60.7
          anterior I60.2- ☑
          posterior I60.3- ☑
        middle cerebral I60.1- ☑
        posterior communicating I60.3- ☑
        specified artery NEC I60.6
        vertebral I60.5- ☑
      newborn P52.5
        birth injury P10.3
      specified NEC I60.8
      traumatic S06.6X- ☑
    subdural (nontraumatic) I62.00
      acute I62.01
        birth injury P10.0

Hemorrhage, hemorrhagic — *continued*
  intracranial — *continued*
    subdural — *continued*
      chronic I62.03
      newborn (anoxic) (hypoxic) P52.8
        birth injury P10.0
      spinal G95.19
      subacute I62.02
      traumatic — *see* Injury, intracranial, subdural hemorrhage
    traumatic — *see* Injury, intracranial, focal brain injury
  intramedullary NEC G95.19
  intraocular — *see* Hemophthalmos
  intraoperative, intraprocedural — *see* Complication, hemorrhage (hematoma), intraoperative (intraprocedural), by site
  intrapartum — *see* Hemorrhage, complicating, delivery
  intrapelvic
    female N94.89
    male K66.1
  intraperitoneal K66.1
  intrapontine I61.3
  intraprocedural — *see* Complication, hemorrhage (hematoma), intraoperative (intraprocedural), by site
  intrauterine N85.7
    complicating delivery (*see also* Hemorrhage, complicating, delivery) O67.9
    postpartum — *see* Hemorrhage, postpartum
  intraventricular I61.5
    newborn (nontraumatic) (*see also* Newborn, affected by, hemorrhage) P52.3
      due to birth injury P10.2
      grade
        1 P52.0
        2 P52.1
        3 P52.21
        4 P52.22
  intravesical N32.89
  iris (postinfectional) (postinflammatory) (toxic) — *see* Hyphema
  joint (nontraumatic) — *see* Hemarthrosis
  kidney N28.89
  knee (joint) (nontraumatic) — *see* Hemarthrosis, knee
  labyrinth — *see* subcategory H83.8 ☑
  lenticular striate artery I61.0
  ligature, vessel — *see* Hemorrhage, postoperative
  liver K76.89
  lung R04.89
    newborn P26.9
      massive P26.1
      specified NEC P26.8
    tuberculous — *see* Tuberculosis, pulmonary
  massive umbilical, newborn P51.0
  mediastinum — *see* Hemorrhage, lung
  medulla I61.3
  membrane (brain) I60.8
    spinal cord — *see* Hemorrhage, spinal cord
  meninges, meningeal (brain) (middle) I60.8
    spinal cord — *see* Hemorrhage, spinal cord
  mesentery K66.1
  metritis — *see* Endometritis
  mouth K13.79
  mucous membrane NEC R58
    newborn P54.8
  muscle M62.89
  nail (subungual) L60.8
  nasal turbinate R04.0
    newborn P54.8
  navel, newborn P51.9
  newborn P54.9
    specified NEC P54.8
  nipple N64.59
  nose R04.0
    newborn P54.8
  omentum K66.1
  optic nerve (sheath) H47.02- ☑
  orbit, orbital H05.23- ☑
  ovary NEC N83.8
  oviduct N83.6
  pancreas K86.8
  parathyroid (gland) (spontaneous) E21.4
  parturition — *see* Hemorrhage, complicating, delivery
  penis N48.89
  pericardium, pericarditis I31.2
  peritoneum, peritoneal K66.1

Hemorrhage, hemorrhagic — *continued*
  peritonsillar tissue J35.8
    due to infection J36
  petechial R23.3
    due to autosensitivity, erythrocyte D69.2
  pituitary (gland) E23.6
  pleura — *see* Hemorrhage, lung
  polioencephalitis, superior E51.2
  polymyositis — *see* Polymyositis
  pons, pontine I61.3
  posterior fossa (nontraumatic) I61.8
    newborn P52.6
  postmenopausal N95.0
  postnasal R04.0
  postoperative — *see* Complications, postprocedural, hemorrhage, by site
  postpartum NEC (following delivery of placenta) O72.1
    delayed or secondary O72.2
    retained placenta O72.0
    third stage O72.0
  pregnancy — *see* Hemorrhage, antepartum
  preretinal — *see* Hemorrhage, retina
  prostate N42.1
  puerperal — *see* Hemorrhage, postpartum
    delayed or secondary O72.2
  pulmonary R04.89
    newborn P26.9
      massive P26.1
      specified NEC P26.8
    tuberculous — *see* Tuberculosis, pulmonary
  purpura (primary) D69.3
  rectum (sphincter) K62.5
    newborn P54.2
  recurring, following initial hemorrhage at time of injury T79.2 ☑
  renal N28.89
  respiratory passage or tract R04.9
    specified NEC R04.89
  retina, retinal (vessels) H35.6- ☑
    diabetic — *see* Diabetes, retinal, hemorrhage
  retroperitoneal R58
  scalp R58
  scrotum N50.1
  secondary (nontraumatic) R58
    following initial hemorrhage at time of injury T79.2 ☑
  seminal vesicle N50.1
  skin R23.3
    newborn P54.5
  slipped umbilical ligature P51.8
  spermatic cord N50.1
  spinal (cord) G95.19
    newborn (birth injury) P11.5
  spleen D73.5
    intraoperative — *see* Complications, intraoperative, hemorrhage, spleen
    postprocedural — *see* Complications, postprocedural, hemorrhage, spleen
  stomach K92.2
    newborn P54.3
    ulcer — *see* Ulcer, stomach, with hemorrhage
  subarachnoid (nontraumatic) — *see* Hemorrhage, intracranial, subarachnoid
  subconjunctival (*see also* Hemorrhage, conjunctiva)
    birth injury P15.3
  subcortical (brain) I61.0
  subcutaneous R23.3
  subdiaphragmatic R58
  subdural (acute) (nontraumatic) — *see* Hemorrhage, intracranial, subdural
  subependymal
    newborn P52.0
      with intraventricular extension P52.1
        and intracerebral extension P52.22
  subgaleal P12.1
  subhyaloid — *see* Hemorrhage, retina
  subperiosteal — *see* Disorder, bone, specified type NEC
  subretinal — *see* Hemorrhage, retina
  subtentorial — *see* Hemorrhage, intracranial, subdural
  subungual L60.8
  suprarenal (capsule) (gland) E27.49
    newborn P54.4
  tentorium (traumatic) NEC — *see* Hemorrhage, brain
    newborn (birth injury) P10.4
  testis N50.1
  third stage (postpartum) O72.0
  thorax — *see* Hemorrhage, lung

Hemorrhage, hemorrhagic — *continued*
  throat R04.1
  thymus (gland) E32.8
  thyroid (cyst) (gland) E07.89
  tongue K14.8
  tonsil J35.8
  trachea — *see* Hemorrhage, lung
  tracheobronchial R04.89
    newborn P26.0
  traumatic — *code to* specific injury
    cerebellar — *see* Hemorrhage, brain
    intracranial — *see* Hemorrhage, brain
    recurring or secondary (following initial hemor-
      rhage at time of injury) T79.2 ☑
  tuberculous NEC (*see also* Tuberculosis, pulmonary)
    A15.0
  tunica vaginalis N50.1
  ulcer — *code by* site under Ulcer, with hemorrhage
    K27.4
  umbilicus, umbilical
    cord
      after birth, newborn P51.9
      complicating delivery O69.5 ☑
    newborn P51.9
      massive P51.0
      slipped ligature P51.8
    stump P51.9
  urethra (idiopathic) N36.8
  uterus, uterine (abnormal) N93.9
    climacteric N92.4
    complicating delivery — *see* Hemorrhage, compli-
      cating, delivery
    dysfunctional or functional N93.8
    intermenstrual (regular) N92.3
      irregular N92.1
    postmenopausal N95.0
    postpartum — *see* Hemorrhage, postpartum
    preclimacteric or premenopausal N92.4
    prepubertal N93.8
    pubertal N92.2
  vagina (abnormal) N93.9
    newborn P54.6
  vas deferens N50.1
  vasa previa O69.4 ☑
  ventricular I61.5
  vesical N32.89
  viscera NEC R58
    newborn P54.8
  vitreous (humor) (intraocular) H43.1- ☑
  vulva N90.89
Hemorrhoids (bleeding) (without mention of degree)
  K64.9
  1st degree (grade/stage I) (without prolapse outside
    of anal canal) K64.0
  2nd degree (grade/stage II) (that prolapse with
    straining but retract spontaneously) K64.1
  3rd degree (grade/stage III) (that prolapse with
    straining and require manual replacement back
    inside anal canal) K64.2
  4th degree (grade/stage IV) (with prolapsed tissue that
    cannot be manually replaced) K64.3
  complicating
    pregnancy O22.4 ☑
    puerperium O87.2
  external K64.4
    with
      thrombosis K64.5
  internal (without mention of degree) K64.8
  prolapsed K64.8
  skin tags
    anus K64.4
    residual K64.4
  specified NEC K64.8
  strangulated (*see also* Hemorrhoids, by degree) K64.8
  thrombosed (*see also* Hemorrhoids, by degree) K64.5
  ulcerated (*see also* Hemorrhoids, by degree) K64.8
Hemosalpinx N83.6
  with
    hematocolpos N89.7
    hematometra N85.7
      with hematocolpos N89.7
Hemosiderosis (dietary) E83.19
  pulmonary, idiopathic E83.1- ☑ [J84.03]
  transfusion T80.89 ☑
Hemothorax (bacterial) (nontuberculous) J94.2
  newborn P54.8
  traumatic S27.1 ☑
    with pneumothorax S27.2 ☑

Hemothorax — *continued*
  tuberculous NEC A15.6
Henoch (-Schönlein) **disease or syndrome** (purpura)
  D69.0
Henpue, henpuye A66.6
Hepar lobatum (syphilitic) A52.74
Hepatalgia K76.89
Hepatitis K75.9
  acute B17.9
    with coma K72.01
    with hepatic failure — *see* Failure, hepatic
    alcoholic — *see* Hepatitis, alcoholic
    infectious B15.9
      with hepatic coma B15.0
    viral B17.9
  alcoholic (acute) (chronic) K70.10
    with ascites K70.11
  amebic — *see* Abscess, liver, amebic
  anicteric, (viral) — *see* Hepatitis, viral
  antigen-associated (HAA) — *see* Hepatitis, B
  Australia-antigen (positive) — *see* Hepatitis, B
  autoimmune K75.4
  B B19.10
    with hepatic coma B19.11
    acute B16.9
      with
        delta-agent (coinfection) (without hepatic
          coma) B16.1
          with hepatic coma B16.0
        hepatic coma (without delta-agent coinfec-
          tion) B16.2
    chronic B18.1
      with delta-agent B18.0
  bacterial NEC K75.89
  C (viral) B19.20
    with hepatic coma B19.21
    acute B17.10
      with hepatic coma B17.11
    chronic B18.2
  catarrhal (acute) B15.9
    with hepatic coma B15.0
  cholangiolitic K75.89
  cholestatic K75.89
  chronic K73.9
    active NEC K73.2
    lobular NEC K73.1
    persistent NEC K73.0
    specified NEC K73.8
  cytomegaloviral B25.1
  due to ethanol (acute) (chronic) — *see* Hepatitis, alco-
    holic
  epidemic B15.9
    with hepatic coma B15.0
  fulminant NEC (viral) — *see* Hepatitis, viral
  granulomatous NEC K75.3
  herpesviral B00.81
  history of
    B Z86.19
    C Z86.19
  homologous serum — *see* Hepatitis, viral, type B
  in (due to)
    mumps B26.81
    toxoplasmosis (acquired) B58.1
      congenital (active) P37.1 [K77]
  infectious, infective (acute) (chronic) (subacute) B15.9
    with hepatic coma B15.0
  inoculation — *see* Hepatitis, viral, type B
  interstitial (chronic) K74.69
  lupoid NEC K75.4
  malignant NEC (with hepatic failure) K72.90
    with coma K72.91
  neonatal (idiopathic) (toxic) P59.29
  neonatal giant cell P59.29
  newborn P59.29
  postimmunization — *see* Hepatitis, viral, type B
  post-transfusion — *see* Hepatitis, viral, type B
  reactive, nonspecific K75.2
  serum — *see* Hepatitis, viral, type B
  specified type NEC
    with hepatic failure — *see* Failure, hepatic
  syphilitic (late) A52.74
    congenital (early) A50.08 [K77]
      late A50.59 [K77]
    secondary A51.45
  toxic (*see also* Disease, liver, toxic) K71.6
  tuberculous A18.83
  viral, virus B19.9
    with hepatic coma B19.0

Hepatitis — *continued*
  viral, virus — *continued*
    acute B17.9
    chronic B18.9
      specified NEC B18.8
    type
      B B18.1
        with delta-agent B18.0
      C B18.2
    congenital P35.3
    coxsackie B33.8 [K77]
    cytomegalic inclusion B25.1
    in remission, any type — *code to* Hepatitis, chronic,
      by type
    non-A, non-B B17.8
    specified type NEC (with or without coma) B17.8
    type
      A B15.9
        with hepatic coma B15.0
      B B19.10
        with hepatic coma B19.11
        acute B16.9
          with
            delta-agent (coinfection) (without
              hepatic coma) B16.1
              with hepatic coma B16.0
            hepatic coma (without delta-agent
              coinfection) B16.2
        chronic B18.1
          with delta-agent B18.0
      C B19.20
        with hepatic coma B19.21
        acute B17.10
          with hepatic coma B17.11
        chronic B18.2
      E B17.2
    non-A, non-B B17.8
Hepatization lung (acute) — *see* Pneumonia, lobar
Hepatoblastoma C22.2
Hepatocarcinoma C22.0
Hepatocholangiocarcinoma C22.0
Hepatocholangioma, benign D13.4
Hepatocholangitis K75.89
Hepatolenticular degeneration E83.01
Hepatoma (malignant) C22.0
  benign D13.4
  embryonal C22.0
Hepatomegaly (*see also* Hypertrophy, liver)
  with splenomegaly R16.2
  congenital Q44.7
  in mononucleosis
    gammaherpesviral B27.09
    infectious specified NEC B27.89
Hepatoptosis K76.89
Hepatorenal syndrome following labor and delivery
  O90.4
Hepatosis K76.89
Hepatosplenomegaly R16.2
  hyperlipemic (Bürger-Grütz type) E78.3 [K77]
Hereditary — *see* condition
Heredodegeneration, macular — *see* Dystrophy, retina
Heredopathia atactica polyneuritiformis G60.1
Heredosyphilis — *see* Syphilis, congenital
Herlitz' syndrome Q81.1
Hermansky-Pudlak syndrome E70.331
Hermaphrodite, hermaphroditism (true) Q56.0
  46,XX with streak gonads Q99.1
  46,XX/46,XY Q99.0
  46,XY with streak gonads Q99.1
  chimera 46,XX/46,XY Q99.0
Hernia, hernial (acquired) (recurrent) K46.9
  with
    gangrene — *see* Hernia, by site, with, gangrene
    incarceration — *see* Hernia, by site, with, obstruc-
      tion
    irreducible — *see* Hernia, by site, with, obstruction
    obstruction — *see* Hernia, by site, with, obstruction
    strangulation — *see* Hernia, by site, with, obstruc-
      tion
  abdomen, abdominal K46.9
    with
      gangrene (and obstruction) K46.1
      obstruction K46.0
    femoral — *see* Hernia, femoral
    incisional — *see* Hernia, incisional
    inguinal — *see* Hernia, inguinal
    specified site NEC K45.8

Hernia, hernial — *continued*
  abdomen, abdominal — *continued*
    specified site — *continued*
      with
        gangrene (and obstruction) K45.1
        obstruction K45.0
      umbilical — *see* Hernia, umbilical
      wall — *see* Hernia, ventral
  appendix — *see* Hernia, abdomen
  bladder (mucosa) (sphincter)
    congenital (female) (male) Q79.51
    female — *see* Cystocele
    male N32.89
  brain, congenital — *see* Encephalocele
  cartilage, vertebra — *see* Displacement, intervertebral
      disc
  cerebral, congenital (*see also* Encephalocele)
    endaural Q01.8
  ciliary body (traumatic) S05.2- ☑
  colon — *see* Hernia, abdomen
  Cooper's — *see* Hernia, abdomen, specified site NEC
  crural — *see* Hernia, femoral
  diaphragm, diaphragmatic K44.9
    with
      gangrene (and obstruction) K44.1
      obstruction K44.0
    congenital Q79.0
  direct (inguinal) — *see* Hernia, inguinal
  diverticulum, intestine — *see* Hernia, abdomen
  double (inguinal) — *see* Hernia, inguinal, bilateral
  due to adhesions (with obstruction) K56.5
  epigastric (*see also* Hernia, ventral) K43.9
  esophageal hiatus — *see* Hernia, hiatal
  external (inguinal) — *see* Hernia, inguinal
  fallopian tube N83.4
  fascia M62.89
  femoral K41.90
    with
      gangrene (and obstruction) K41.40
        not specified as recurrent K41.40
        recurrent K41.41
      obstruction K41.30
        not specified as recurrent K41.30
        recurrent K41.31
    bilateral K41.20
      with
        gangrene (and obstruction) K41.10
          not specified as recurrent K41.10
          recurrent K41.11
        obstruction K41.00
          not specified as recurrent K41.00
          recurrent K41.01
      not specified as recurrent K41.20
      recurrent K41.21
    not specified as recurrent K41.90
    recurrent K41.91
    unilateral K41.90
      with
        gangrene (and obstruction) K41.40
          not specified as recurrent K41.40
          recurrent K41.41
        obstruction K41.30
          not specified as recurrent K41.30
          recurrent K41.31
      not specified as recurrent K41.90
      recurrent K41.91
  foramen magnum G93.5
    congenital Q01.8
  funicular (umbilical) (*see also* Hernia, umbilicus)
    spermatic (cord) — *see* Hernia, inguinal
  gastrointestinal tract — *see* Hernia, abdomen
  Hesselbach's — *see* Hernia, femoral, specified site NEC
  hiatal (esophageal) (sliding) K44.9
    with
      gangrene (and obstruction) K44.1
      obstruction K44.0
    congenital Q40.1
  hypogastric — *see* Hernia, ventral
  incarcerated (*see also* Hernia, by site, with obstruction)
    with gangrene — *see* Hernia, by site, with gan-
        grene
  incisional K43.2
    with
      gangrene (and obstruction) K43.1
      obstruction K43.0
  indirect (inguinal) — *see* Hernia, inguinal
  inguinal (direct) (external) (funicular) (indirect) (inter-
      nal) (oblique) (scrotal) (sliding) K40.90

Hernia, hernial — *continued*
  inguinal — *continued*
    with
      gangrene (and obstruction) K40.40
        not specified as recurrent K40.40
        recurrent K40.41
      obstruction K40.30
        not specified as recurrent K40.30
        recurrent K40.31
    bilateral K40.20
      with
        gangrene (and obstruction) K40.10
          not specified as recurrent K40.10
          recurrent K40.11
        obstruction K40.00
          not specified as recurrent K40.00
          recurrent K40.01
      not specified as recurrent K40.20
      recurrent K40.21
    not specified as recurrent K40.90
    recurrent K40.91
    unilateral K40.90
      with
        gangrene (and obstruction) K40.40
          not specified as recurrent K40.40
          recurrent K40.41
        obstruction K40.30
          not specified as recurrent K40.30
          recurrent K40.31
      not specified as recurrent K40.90
      recurrent K40.91
  internal (*see also* Hernia, abdomen)
    inguinal — *see* Hernia, inguinal
  interstitial — *see* Hernia, abdomen
  intervertebral cartilage or disc — *see* Displacement,
      intervertebral disc
  intestine, intestinal — *see* Hernia, by site
  intra-abdominal — *see* Hernia, abdomen
  iris (traumatic) S05.2- ☑
  irreducible (*see also* Hernia, by site, with obstruction)
    with gangrene — *see* Hernia, by site, with gan-
        grene
  ischiatic — *see* Hernia, abdomen, specified site NEC
  ischiorectal — *see* Hernia, abdomen, specified site
      NEC
  lens (traumatic) S05.2- ☑
  linea (alba) (semilunaris) — *see* Hernia, ventral
  Littre's — *see* Hernia, abdomen
  lumbar — *see* Hernia, abdomen, specified site NEC
  lung (subcutaneous) J98.4
  mediastinum J98.5
  mesenteric (internal) — *see* Hernia, abdomen
  midline — *see* Hernia, ventral
  muscle (sheath) M62.89
  nucleus pulposus — *see* Displacement, intervertebral
      disc
  oblique (inguinal) — *see* Hernia, inguinal
  obstructive (*see also* Hernia, by site, with obstruction)
    with gangrene — *see* Hernia, by site, with gan-
        grene
  obturator — *see* Hernia, abdomen, specified site NEC
  omental — *see* Hernia, abdomen
  ovary N83.4
  oviduct N83.4
  paraesophageal (*see also* Hernia, diaphragm)
    congenital Q40.1
  parastomal K43.5
    with
      gangrene (and obstruction) K43.4
      obstruction K43.3
  paraumbilical — *see* Hernia, umbilicus
  perineal — *see* Hernia, abdomen, specified site NEC
  Petit's — *see* Hernia, abdomen, specified site NEC
  postoperative — *see* Hernia, incisional
  pregnant uterus — *see* Abnormal, uterus in pregnancy
      or childbirth
  prevesical N32.89
  properitoneal — *see* Hernia, abdomen, specified site
      NEC
  pudendal — *see* Hernia, abdomen, specified site NEC
  rectovaginal N81.6
  retroperitoneal — *see* Hernia, abdomen, specified site
      NEC
  Richter's — *see* Hernia, abdomen, with obstruction
  Rieux's, Riex's — *see* Hernia, abdomen, specified site
      NEC

Hernia, hernial — *continued*
  sac condition (adhesion) (dropsy) (inflammation)
      (laceration) (suppuration) — *code by site under*
      Hernia
  sciatic — *see* Hernia, abdomen, specified site NEC
  scrotum, scrotal — *see* Hernia, inguinal
  sliding (inguinal) (*see also* Hernia, inguinal)
    hiatus — *see* Hernia, hiatal
  spigelian — *see* Hernia, ventral
  spinal — *see* Spina bifida
  strangulated (*see also* Hernia, by site, with obstruction)
    with gangrene — *see* Hernia, by site, with gan-
        grene
  subxiphoid — *see* Hernia, ventral
  supra-umbilicus — *see* Hernia, ventral
  tendon — *see* Disorder, tendon, specified type NEC
  Treitz's (fossa) — *see* Hernia, abdomen, specified site
      NEC
  tunica vaginalis Q55.29
  umbilicus, umbilical K42.9
    with
      gangrene (and obstruction) K42.1
      obstruction K42.0
  ureter N28.89
  urethra, congenital Q64.79
  urinary meatus, congenital Q64.79
  uterus N81.4
    pregnant — *see* Abnormal, uterus in pregnancy or
        childbirth
  vaginal (anterior) (wall) — *see* Cystocele
  Velpeau's — *see* Hernia, femoral
  ventral K43.9
    with
      gangrene (and obstruction) K43.7
      obstruction K43.6
    incisional K43.2
      with
        gangrene (and obstruction) K43.1
        obstruction K43.0
    recurrent — *see* Hernia, incisional
    specified NEC K43.9
      with
        gangrene (and obstruction) K43.7
        obstruction K43.6
  vesical
    congenital (female) (male) Q79.51
    female — *see* Cystocele
    male N32.89
  vitreous (into wound) S05.2- ☑
    into anterior chamber — *see* Prolapse, vitreous
Herniation (*see also* Hernia)
  brain (stem) G93.5
  cerebral G93.5
  mediastinum J98.5
  nucleus pulposus — *see* Displacement, intervertebral
      disc
Herpangina B08.5
Herpes, herpesvirus, herpetic B00.9
  anogenital A60.9
    perianal skin A60.1
    rectum A60.1
    urogenital tract A60.00
      cervix A60.03
      male genital organ NEC A60.02
      penis A60.01
      specified site NEC A60.09
      vagina A60.04
      vulva A60.04
  blepharitis (zoster) B02.39
    simplex B00.59
  circinatus B35.4
    bullosus L12.0
  conjunctivitis (simplex) B00.53
    zoster B02.31
  cornea B02.33
  encephalitis B00.4
    due to herpesvirus 6 B10.01
    due to herpesvirus 7 B10.09
    specified NEC B10.09
  eye (zoster) B02.30
    simplex B00.50
  eyelid (zoster) B02.39
    simplex B00.59
  facialis B00.1
  febrilis B00.1
  geniculate ganglionitis B02.21
  genital, genitalis A60.00
    female A60.09

Herpes, herpesvirus, herpetic — *continued*
  genital, genitalis — *continued*
    male A60.02
  gestational, gestationis O26.4- ☑
  gingivostomatitis B00.2
  human B00.9
    1 — *see* Herpes, simplex
    2 — *see* Herpes, simplex
    3 — *see* Varicella
    4 — *see* Mononucleosis, Epstein-Barr (virus)
    5 — *see* Disease, cytomegalic inclusion (generalized)
    6
      encephalitis B10.01
      specified NEC B10.81
    7
      encephalitis B10.09
      specified NEC B10.82
    8 B10.89
  infection NEC B10.89
    Kaposi's sarcoma associated B10.89
  iridocyclitis (simplex) B00.51
    zoster B02.32
  iris (vesicular erythema multiforme) L51.9
  iritis (simplex) B00.51
  Kaposi's sarcoma associated B10.89
  keratitis (simplex) (dendritic) (disciform) (interstitial) B00.52
    zoster (interstitial) B02.33
  keratoconjunctivitis (simplex) B00.52
    zoster B02.33
  labialis B00.1
  lip B00.1
  meningitis (simplex) B00.3
    zoster B02.1
  ophthalmicus (zoster) NEC B02.30
    simplex B00.50
  penis A60.01
  perianal skin A60.1
  pharyngitis, pharyngotonsillitis B00.2
  rectum A60.1
  scrotum A60.02
  sepsis B00.7
  simplex B00.9
    complicated NEC B00.89
    congenital P35.2
    conjunctivitis B00.53
    external ear B00.1
    eyelid B00.59
    hepatitis B00.81
    keratitis (interstitial) B00.52
    myeitis B00.82
    specified complication NEC B00.89
    visceral B00.89
  stomatitis B00.2
  tonsurans B35.0
  visceral B00.89
  vulva A60.04
  whitlow B00.89
  zoster (*see also* condition) B02.9
    auricularis B02.21
    complicated NEC B02.8
    conjunctivitis B02.31
    disseminated B02.7
    encephalitis B02.0
    eye (lid) B02.39
    geniculate ganglionitis B02.21
    keratitis (interstitial) B02.33
    meningitis B02.1
    myelitis B02.24
    neuritis, neuralgia B02.29
    ophthalmicus NEC B02.30
    oticus B02.21
    polyneuropathy B02.23
    specified complication NEC B02.8
    trigeminal neuralgia B02.22
Herpesvirus (human) — *see* Herpes
Herpetophobia F40.218
Herrick's anemia — *see* Disease, sickle-cell
Hers' disease E74.09
Herter-Gee syndrome K90.0
Herxheimer's reaction R68.89
Hesitancy
  of micturition R39.11
  urinary R39.11
Hesselbach's hernia — *see* Hernia, femoral, specified site NEC
Heterochromia (congenital) Q13.2

Heterochromia — *continued*
  cataract — *see* Cataract, complicated
  cyclitis (Fuchs) — *see* Cyclitis, Fuchs' heterochromic
  hair L67.1
  iritis — *see* Cyclitis, Fuchs' heterochromic
  retained metallic foreign body (nonmagnetic) — *see* Foreign body, intraocular, old, retained
    magnetic — *see* Foreign body, intraocular, old, retained, magnetic
  uveitis — *see* Cyclitis, Fuchs' heterochromic
Heterophoria — *see* Strabismus, heterophoria
Heterophyes, heterophyiasis (small intestine) B66.8
Heterotopia, heterotopic (*see also* Malposition, congenital)
  cerebralis Q04.8
Heterotropia — *see* Strabismus
Heubner-Herter disease K90.0
Hexadactylism Q69.9
HGSIL (cytology finding) (high grade squamous intraepithelial lesion on cytologic smear) (Pap smear finding)
  anus R85.613
  cervix R87.613
    biopsy (histology) finding — *code to* CIN II or CIN III
  vagina R87.623
    biopsy (histology) finding — *code to* VAIN II or VAIN III
Hibernoma — *see* Lipoma
Hiccup, hiccough R06.6
  epidemic B33.0
  psychogenic F45.8
Hidden penis (congenital) Q55.64
  acquired N48.83
Hidradenitis (axillaris) (suppurative) L73.2
Hidradenoma (nodular) (*see also* Neoplasm, skin, benign)
  clear cell — *see* Neoplasm, skin, benign
  papillary — *see* Neoplasm, skin, benign
Hidrocystoma — *see* Neoplasm, skin, benign
High
  altitude effects T70.20 ☑
    anoxia T70.29 ☑
    on
      ears T70.0 ☑
      sinuses T70.1 ☑
    polycythemia D75.1
  arch
    foot Q66.7
    palate, congenital Q38.5
  arterial tension — *see* Hypertension
  basal metabolic rate R94.8
  blood pressure (*see also* Hypertension)
    borderline R03.0
    reading (incidental) (isolated) (nonspecific), without diagnosis of hypertension R03.0
  cholesterol E78.0
    with high triglycerides E78.2
  diaphragm (congenital) Q79.1
  expressed emotional level within family Z63.8
  head at term O32.4 ☑
  palate, congenital Q38.5
  risk
    infant NEC Z76.2
    sexual behavior (heterosexual) Z72.51
      bisexual Z72.53
      homosexual Z72.52
  temperature (of unknown origin) R50.9
  thoracic rib Q76.6
  triglycerides E78.1
    with high cholesterol E78.2
Hildenbrand's disease A75.0
Hilum — *see* condition
Hip — *see* condition
Hippel's disease Q85.8
Hippophobia F40.218
Hippus H57.09
Hirschsprung's disease or megacolon Q43.1
Hirsutism, hirsuties L68.0
Hirudiniasis
  external B88.3
  internal B83.4
Hiss-Russell dysentery A03.1
Histidinemia, histidinuria E70.41
Histiocytoma (*see also* Neoplasm, skin, benign)
  fibrous (*see also* Neoplasm, skin, benign)
    atypical — *see* Neoplasm, connective tissue, uncertain behavior

Histiocytoma — *continued*
  fibrous (*see also* Neoplasm, skin, benign) — *continued*
    malignant — *see* Neoplasm, connective tissue, malignant
Histiocytosis D76.3
  acute differentiated progressive C96.0
  Langerhans' cell NEC C96.6
    multifocal X
      multisystemic (disseminated) C96.0
      unisystemic C96.5
    pulmonary, adult (adult PLCH) J84.82
    unifocal (X) C96.6
  lipid, lipoid D76.3
    essential E75.29
  malignant C96.A (*following* C96.6)
  mononuclear phagocytes NEC D76.1
    Langerhans' cells C96.6
  non-Langerhans cell D76.3
  polyostotic sclerosing D76.3
  sinus, with massive lymphadenopathy D76.3
  syndrome NEC D76.3
  X NEC C96.6
    acute (progressive) C96.0
    chronic C96.6
    multifocal C96.5
    multisystemic C96.0
    unifocal C96.6
Histoplasmosis B39.9
  with pneumonia NEC B39.2
  African B39.5
  American — *see* Histoplasmosis, capsulati
  capsulati B39.4
    disseminated B39.3
    generalized B39.3
    pulmonary B39.2
      acute B39.0
      chronic B39.1
  Darling's B39.4
  duboisii B39.5
  lung NEC B39.2
History
  family (of) (*see also* History, personal (of))
    alcohol abuse Z81.1
    allergy NEC Z84.89
    anemia Z83.2
    arthritis Z82.61
    asthma Z82.5
    blindness Z82.1
    cardiac death (sudden) Z82.41
    carrier of genetic disease Z84.81
    chromosomal anomaly Z82.79
    chronic
      disabling disease NEC Z82.8
      lower respiratory disease Z82.5
    colonic polyps Z83.71
    congenital malformations and deformations Z82.79
      polycystic kidney Z82.71
    consanguinity Z84.3
    deafness Z82.2
    diabetes mellitus Z83.3
    disability NEC Z82.8
    disease or disorder (of)
      allergic NEC Z84.89
      behavioral NEC Z81.8
      blood and blood-forming organs Z83.2
      cardiovascular NEC Z82.49
      chronic disabling NEC Z82.8
      digestive Z83.79
      ear NEC Z83.52
      endocrine NEC Z83.49
      eye NEC Z83.518
        glaucoma Z83.511
      genitourinary NEC Z84.2
      glaucoma Z83.511
      hematological Z83.2
      immune mechanism Z83.2
      infectious NEC Z83.1
      ischemic heart Z82.49
      kidney Z84.1
      mental NEC Z81.8
      metabolic Z83.49
      musculoskeletal NEC Z82.69
      neurological NEC Z82.0
      nutritional Z83.49
      parasitic NEC Z83.1
      psychiatric NEC Z81.8
      respiratory NEC Z83.6

- **History** — *continued*
  - family (*see also* History, personal) — *continued*
    - disease or disorder — *continued*
      - skin and subcutaneous tissue NEC Z84.Ø
      - specified NEC Z84.89
    - drug abuse NEC Z81.3
    - epilepsy Z82.Ø
    - genetic disease carrier Z84.81
    - glaucoma Z83.511
    - hearing loss Z82.2
    - human immunodeficiency virus (HIV) infection Z83.Ø
    - Huntington's chorea Z82.Ø
    - intellectual disability Z81.Ø
    - leukemia Z8Ø.6
    - malignant neoplasm (of) NOS Z8Ø.9
      - bladder Z8Ø.52
      - breast Z8Ø.3
      - bronchus Z8Ø.1
      - digestive organ Z8Ø.Ø
      - gastrointestinal tract Z8Ø.Ø
      - genital organ Z8Ø.49
        - ovary Z8Ø.41
        - prostate Z8Ø.42
        - specified organ NEC Z8Ø.49
        - testis Z8Ø.43
      - hematopoietic NEC Z8Ø.7
      - intrathoracic organ NEC Z8Ø.2
      - kidney Z8Ø.51
      - lung Z8Ø.1
      - lymphatic NEC Z8Ø.7
      - ovary Z8Ø.41
      - prostate Z8Ø.42
      - respiratory organ NEC Z8Ø.2
      - specified site NEC Z8Ø.8
      - testis Z8Ø.43
      - trachea Z8Ø.1
      - urinary organ or tract Z8Ø.59
        - bladder Z8Ø.52
        - kidney Z8Ø.51
    - mental
      - disorder NEC Z81.8
    - multiple endocrine neoplasia (MEN) syndrome Z83.41
    - osteoporosis Z82.62
    - polycystic kidney Z82.71
    - polyps (colon) Z83.71
    - psychiatric disorder Z81.8
    - psychoactive substance abuse NEC Z81.3
    - respiratory condition NEC Z83.6
      - asthma and other lower respiratory conditions Z82.5
    - self-harmful behavior Z81.8
    - skin condition Z84.Ø
    - specified condition NEC Z84.89
    - stroke (cerebrovascular) Z82.3
    - substance abuse NEC Z81.4
      - alcohol Z81.1
      - drug NEC Z81.3
      - psychoactive NEC Z81.3
      - tobacco Z81.2
    - sudden cardiac death Z82.41
    - tobacco abuse Z81.2
    - violence, violent behavior Z81.8
    - visual loss Z82.1
  - personal (of) (*see also* History, family (of))
    - abuse
      - adult Z91.419
        - physical and sexual Z91.41Ø
        - psychological Z91.411
      - childhood Z62.819
        - physical Z62.81Ø
        - psychological Z62.811
        - sexual Z62.81Ø
    - alcohol dependence F1Ø.21
    - allergy (to) Z88.9
      - analgesic agent NEC Z88.6
      - anesthetic Z88.4
      - antibiotic agent NEC Z88.1
      - anti-infective agent NEC Z88.3
      - contrast media Z91.Ø41
      - drugs, medicaments and biological substances Z88.9
        - specified NEC Z88.8
      - food Z91.Ø18
        - additives Z91.Ø2
        - eggs Z91.Ø12
        - milk products Z91.Ø11

- **History** — *continued*
  - personal (*see also* History, family) — *continued*
    - allergy — *continued*
      - food — *continued*
        - peanuts Z91.Ø1Ø
        - seafood Z91.Ø13
        - specified food NEC Z91.Ø18
      - insect Z91.Ø38
        - bee Z91.Ø3Ø
      - latex Z91.Ø4Ø
      - medicinal agents Z88.9
        - specified NEC Z88.8
      - narcotic agent NEC Z88.5
      - nonmedicinal agents Z91.Ø48
      - penicillin Z88.Ø
      - serum Z88.7
      - specified NEC Z91.Ø9
      - sulfonamides Z88.2
      - vaccine Z88.7
    - anaphylactic shock Z87.892
    - anaphylaxis Z87.892
    - behavioral disorders Z86.59
    - benign carcinoid tumor Z86.Ø12
    - benign neoplasm Z86.Ø18
      - brain Z86.Ø11
      - carcinoid Z86.Ø12
      - colonic polyps Z86.Ø1Ø
    - brain injury (traumatic) Z87.82Ø
    - breast implant removal Z98.86
    - calculi, renal Z87.442
    - cancer — *see* History, personal (of), malignant neoplasm (of)
    - cardiac arrest (death), successfully resuscitated Z86.74
    - cerebral infarction without residual deficit Z86.73
    - cervical dysplasia Z87.41Ø
    - chemotherapy for neoplastic condition Z92.21
    - childhood abuse — *see* History, personal (of), abuse
    - cleft lip (corrected) Z87.73Ø
    - cleft palate (corrected) Z87.73Ø
    - collapsed vertebra (healed) Z87.311
      - due to osteoporosis Z87.31Ø
    - combat and operational stress reaction Z86.51
    - congenital malformation (corrected) Z87.798
      - circulatory system (corrected) Z87.74
      - digestive system (corrected) NEC Z87.738
      - ear (corrected) Z87.72Ø
      - eye (corrected) Z87.721
      - face and neck (corrected) Z87.79Ø
      - genitourinary system (corrected) NEC Z87.718
      - heart (corrected) Z87.74
      - integument (corrected) Z87.76
      - limb(s) (corrected) Z87.76
      - musculoskeletal system (corrected) Z87.76
      - neck (corrected) Z87.79Ø
      - nervous system (corrected) NEC Z87.728
      - respiratory system (corrected) Z87.75
      - sense organs (corrected) NEC Z87.728
      - specified NEC Z87.798
    - contraception Z92.Ø
    - deployment (military) Z91.82
    - diabetic foot ulcer Z86.31
    - disease or disorder (of) Z87.898
      - anaphylaxis Z87.892
      - blood and blood-forming organs Z86.2
      - circulatory system Z86.79
        - specified condition NEC Z86.79
      - connective tissue Z87.39
      - digestive system Z87.19
        - colonic polyp Z86.Ø1Ø
        - peptic ulcer disease Z87.11
        - specified condition NEC Z87.19
      - ear Z86.69
      - endocrine Z86.39
        - diabetic foot ulcer Z86.31
        - gestational diabetes Z86.32
        - specified type NEC Z86.39
      - eye Z86.69
      - genital (track) system NEC
        - female Z87.42
        - male Z87.438
      - hematological Z86.2
      - Hodgkin Z85.71
      - immune mechanism Z86.2
      - infectious Z86.19
        - malaria Z86.13

- **History** — *continued*
  - personal (*see also* History, family) — *continued*
    - disease or disorder — *continued*
      - infectious — *continued*
        - Methicillin resistant Staphylococcus aureus (MRSA) Z86.14
        - poliomyelitis Z86.12
        - specified NEC Z86.19
        - tuberculosis Z86.11
      - mental NEC Z86.59
      - metabolic Z86.39
        - diabetic foot ulcer Z86.31
        - gestational diabetes Z86.32
        - specified type NEC Z86.39
      - musculoskeletal NEC Z87.39
      - nervous system Z86.69
      - nutritional Z86.39
      - parasitic Z86.19
      - respiratory system NEC Z87.Ø9
      - sense organs Z86.69
      - skin Z87.2
      - specified site or type NEC Z87.898
      - subcutaneous tissue Z87.2
      - trophoblastic Z87.59
      - urinary system NEC Z87.448
    - drug dependence — *see* Dependence, drug, by type, in remission
    - drug therapy
      - antineoplastic chemotherapy Z92.21
      - estrogen Z92.23
      - immunosupression Z92.25
      - inhaled steroids Z92.24Ø
      - monoclonal drug Z92.22
      - specified NEC Z92.29
      - steroid Z92.241
      - systemic steroids Z92.241
    - dysplasia
      - cervical Z87.41Ø
      - prostatic Z87.43Ø
      - vaginal Z87.411
      - vulvar Z87.412
    - embolism (venous) Z86.718
      - pulmonary Z86.711
    - encephalitis Z86.61
    - estrogen therapy Z92.23
    - extracorporeal membrane oxygenation (ECMO) Z92.81
    - failed conscious sedation Z92.83
    - failed moderate sedation Z92.83
    - fall, falling Z91.81
    - fracture (healed)
      - fatigue Z87.312
      - fragility Z87.31Ø
      - osteoporosis Z87.31Ø
      - pathological NEC Z87.311
      - stress Z87.312
      - traumatic Z87.81
    - gestational diabetes Z86.32
    - hepatitis
      - B Z86.19
      - C Z86.19
    - Hodgkin disease Z85.71
    - hyperthermia, malignant Z88.4
    - hypospadias (corrected) Z87.71Ø
    - hysterectomy Z9Ø.71Ø
    - immunosupression therapy Z92.25
    - in situ neoplasm
      - breast Z86.ØØØ
      - cervix uteri Z86.ØØ1
      - specified NEC Z86.ØØ8
    - in utero procedure during pregnancy Z98.87Ø
    - in utero procedure while a fetus Z98.871
    - infection NEC Z86.19
      - central nervous system Z86.61
      - Methicillin resistant Staphylococcus aureus (MRSA) Z86.14
      - urinary (recurrent) (tract) Z87.44Ø
    - injury NEC Z87.828
    - irradiation Z92.3
    - kidney stones Z87.442
    - leukemia Z85.6
    - lymphoma (non-Hodgkin) Z85.72
    - malignant melanoma (skin) Z85.82Ø
    - malignant neoplasm (of) Z85.9
      - accessory sinuses Z85.22
      - anus NEC Z85.Ø48
        - carcinoid Z85.Ø4Ø
      - bladder Z85.51

History — *continued*
  personal (*see also* History, family) — *continued*
    malignant neoplasm — *continued*
      bone Z85.830
      brain Z85.841
      breast Z85.3
      bronchus NEC Z85.118
        carcinoid Z85.110
      carcinoid — *see* History, personal (of), malig-
        nant neoplasm, by site, carcinioid
      cervix Z85.41
      colon NEC Z85.038
        carcinoid Z85.030
      digestive organ Z85.00
        specified NEC Z85.09
      endocrine gland NEC Z85.858
      epididymis Z85.48
      esophagus Z85.01
      eye Z85.840
      gastrointestinal tract — *see* History, malignant
        neoplasm, digestive organ
      genital organ
        female Z85.40
          specified NEC Z85.44
        male Z85.45
          specified NEC Z85.49
      hematopoietic NEC Z85.79
      intrathoracic organ Z85.20
      kidney NEC Z85.528
        carcinoid Z85.520
      large intestine NEC Z85.038
        carcinoid Z85.030
      larynx Z85.21
      liver Z85.05
      lung NEC Z85.118
        carcinoid Z85.110
      mediastinum Z85.29
      Merkel cell Z85.821
      middle ear Z85.22
      nasal cavities Z85.22
      nervous system NEC Z85.848
      oral cavity Z85.819
        specified site NEC Z85.818
      ovary Z85.43
      pancreas Z85.07
      pelvis Z85.53
      pharynx Z85.819
        specified site NEC Z85.818
      pleura Z85.29
      prostate Z85.46
      rectosigmoid junction NEC Z85.048
        carcinoid Z85.040
      rectum NEC Z85.048
        carcinoid Z85.040
      respiratory organ Z85.20
      sinuses, accessory Z85.22
      skin NEC Z85.828
        melanoma Z85.820
        Merkel cell Z85.821
      small intestine NEC Z85.068
        carcinoid Z85.060
      soft tissue Z85.831
      specified site NEC Z85.89
      stomach NEC Z85.028
        carcinoid Z85.020
      testis Z85.47
      thymus NEC Z85.238
        carcinoid Z85.230
      thyroid Z85.850
      tongue Z85.810
      trachea Z85.12
      urinary organ or tract Z85.50
        specified NEC Z85.59
      uterus Z85.42
    maltreatment Z91.89
    medical treatment NEC Z92.89
    melanoma (malignant) (skin) Z85.820
    meningitis Z86.61
    mental disorder Z86.59
    Merkel cell carcinoma (skin) Z85.821
    Methicillin resistant Staphylococcus aureus (MRSA)
      Z86.14
    military deployment Z91.82
    military war, peacekeeping and humanitarian de-
      ployment (current or past conflict) Z91.82
    myocardial infarction (old) I25.2
    neglect (in)
      adult Z91.412

History — *continued*
  personal (*see also* History, family) — *continued*
    neglect — *continued*
      childhood Z62.812
    neoplasm
      benign Z86.018
        brain Z86.011
        colon polyp Z86.010
      in situ
        breast Z86.000
        cervix uteri Z86.001
        specified NEC Z86.008
      malignant — *see* History of, malignant neo-
        plasm
      uncertain behavior Z86.03
    nephrotic syndrome Z87.441
    nicotine dependence Z87.891
    noncompliance with medical treatment or regimen
      — *see* Noncompliance
    nutritional deficiency Z86.39
    obstetric complications Z87.59
      childbirth Z87.59
      pregnancy Z87.59
      pre-term labor Z87.51
      puerperium Z87.59
    osteoporosis fractures Z87.31 ☑
    parasuicide (attempt) Z91.5
    physical trauma NEC Z87.828
      self-harm or suicide attempt Z91.5
    pneumonia (recurrent) Z87.01
    poisoning NEC Z91.89
      self-harm or suicide attempt Z91.5
    poor personal hygiene Z91.89
    preterm labor Z87.51
    procedure during pregnancy Z98.870
    procedure while a fetus Z98.871
    prolonged reversible ischemic neurologic deficit
      (PRIND) Z86.73
    prostatic dysplasia Z87.430
    psychological
      abuse
        adult Z91.411
        child Z62.811
      trauma, specified NEC Z91.49
    radiation therapy Z92.3
    removal
      implant
        breast Z98.86
      renal calculi Z87.442
    respiratory condition NEC Z87.09
    retained foreign body fully removed Z87.821
    risk factors NEC Z91.89
    self-harm Z91.5
    self-poisoning attempt Z91.5
    sex reassignment Z87.890
    sleep-wake cycle problem Z72.821
    specified NEC Z87.898
    steroid therapy (systemic) Z92.241
      inhaled Z92.240
    stroke without residual deficits Z86.73
    substance abuse NEC F10-F19 with fifth character
      1
    sudden cardiac arrest Z86.74
    sudden cardiac death successfully resuscitated
      Z86.74
    suicide attempt Z91.5
    surgery NEC Z98.89
      sex reassignment Z87.890
      transplant — *see* Transplant
    thrombophlebitis Z86.72
    thrombosis (venous) Z86.718
      pulmonary Z86.711
    tobacco dependence Z87.891
    transient ischemic attack (TIA) without residual
      deficits Z86.73
    trauma (physical) NEC Z87.828
      psychological NEC Z91.49
      self-harm Z91.5
    traumatic brain injury Z87.820
    unhealthy sleep-wake cycle Z72.821
    urinary calculi Z87.442
    urinary (recurrent) (tract) infection(s) Z87.440
    vaginal dysplasia Z87.411
    venous thrombosis or embolism Z86.718
      pulmonary Z86.711
    vulvar dysplasia Z87.412
His-Werner disease A79.0
HIV (*see also* Human, immunodeficiency virus) B20

HIV — *continued*
  laboratory evidence (nonconclusive) R75
  nonconclusive test (in infants) R75
  positive, seropositive Z21
Hives (bold) — *see* Urticaria
Hoarseness R49.0
Hobo Z59.0
Hodgkin disease — *see* Lymphoma, Hodgkin
Hodgson's disease I71.2
  ruptured I71.1
Hoffa-Kastert disease E88.89
Hoffa's disease E88.89
Hoffmann-Bouveret syndrome I47.9
Hoffmann's syndrome E03.9 [G73.7]
Hole (round)
  macula H35.34- ☑
  retina (without detachment) — *see* Break, retina,
    round hole
    with detachment — *see* Detachment, retina, with
      retinal, break
Holiday relief care Z75.5
Hollenhorst's plaque — *see* Occlusion, artery, retina
Hollow foot (congenital) Q66.7
  acquired — *see* Deformity, limb, foot, specified NEC
Holoprosencephaly Q04.2
Holt-Oram syndrome Q87.2
Homelessness Z59.0
Homesickness — *see* Disorder, adjustment
Homocystinemia, homocystinuria E72.11
Homogentisate 1,2-dioxygenase deficiency E70.29
Homologous serum hepatitis (prophylactic) (therapeu-
  tic) — *see* Hepatitis, viral, type B
Honeycomb lung J98.4
  congenital Q33.0
Hooded
  clitoris Q52.6
  penis Q55.69
Hookworm (anemia) (disease) (infection) (infestation)
  B76.9
  specified NEC B76.8
Hordeolum (eyelid) (externum) (recurrent) H00.019
  internum H00.029
    left H00.026
      lower H00.025
      upper H00.024
    right H00.023
      lower H00.022
      upper H00.021
  left H00.016
    lower H00.015
    upper H00.014
  right H00.013
    lower H00.012
    upper H00.011
Horn
  cutaneous L85.8
  nail L60.2
    congenital Q84.6
Horner (-Claude Bernard) **syndrome** G90.2
  traumatic — *see* Injury, nerve, cervical sympathetic
Horseshoe kidney (congenital) Q63.1
Horton's headache or neuralgia G44.099
  intractable G44.091
  not intractable G44.099
Hospital hopper syndrome — *see* Disorder, factitious
Hospitalism in children — *see* Disorder, adjustment
Hostility R45.5
  towards child Z62.3
Hot flashes
  menopausal N95.1
Hourglass (contracture) (*see also* Contraction, hourglass)
  stomach K31.89
    congenital Q40.2
    stricture K31.2
Household, housing circumstance affecting care
  Z59.9
  specified NEC Z59.8
Housemaid's knee — *see* Bursitis, prepatellar
Hudson (-Stähli) **line** (cornea) — *see* Pigmentation,
  cornea, anterior
Human
  bite (open wound) (*see also* Bite)
    intact skin surface — *see* Bite, superficial
  herpesvirus — *see* Herpes
  immunodeficiency virus (HIV) disease (infection) B20
    asymptomatic status Z21
    contact Z20.6

Human — *continued*
  immunodeficiency virus disease — *continued*
    counseling Z71.7
    dementia B20 [F02.80]
      with behavioral disturbance B20 [F02.81]
    exposure to Z20.6
    laboratory evidence R75
    type-2 (HIV 2) as cause of disease classified elsewhere B97.35
  papillomavirus (HPV)
    DNA test positive
      high risk
        cervix R87.810
        vagina R87.811
      low risk
        cervix R87.820
        vagina R87.821
    screening for Z11.51
  T-cell lymphotropic virus
    type-1 (HTLV-I) infection B33.3
      as cause of disease classified elsewhere B97.33
      carrier Z22.6
    type-2 (HTLV-II) as cause of disease classified elsewhere B97.34
Humidifier lung or pneumonitis J67.7
Humiliation (experience) **in childhood** Z62.898
Humpback (acquired) — *see* Kyphosis
Hunchback (acquired) — *see* Kyphosis
Hunger T73.0 ☑
  air, psychogenic F45.8
Hungry bone syndrome E83.81
Hunner's ulcer — *see* Cystitis, chronic, interstitial
Hunter's
  glossitis D51.0
  syndrome E76.1
Huntington's disease or chorea G10
  with dementia G10 [F02.80]
    with behavioral disturbance G10 [F02.81]
Hunt's
  disease or syndrome (herpetic geniculate ganglionitis) B02.21
    dyssynergia cerebellaris myoclonica G11.1
  neuralgia B02.21
Hurler (-Scheie) **disease or syndrome** E76.02
Hurst's disease G36.1
Hurthle cell
  adenocarcinoma C73
  adenoma D34
  carcinoma C73
  tumor D34
Hutchinson-Boeck disease or syndrome — *see* Sarcoidosis
Hutchinson-Gilford disease or syndrome E34.8
Hutchinson's
  disease, meaning
    angioma serpiginosum L81.7
    pompholyx (cheiropompholyx) L30.1
    prurigo estivalis L56.4
    summer eruption or summer prurigo L56.4
  melanotic freckle — *see* Melanoma, in situ
    malignant melanoma in — *see* Melanoma
  teeth or incisors (congenital syphilis) A50.52
  triad (congenital syphilis) A50.53
Hyalin plaque, sclera, senile H15.89
Hyaline membrane (disease) (lung) (pulmonary) (newborn) P22.0
Hyalinosis
  cutis (et mucosae) E78.89
  focal and segmental (glomerular) (*see also* N00-N07 with fourth character .1) N05.1
Hyalitis, hyalosis, asteroid (*see also* Deposit, crystalline)
  syphilitic (late) A52.71
Hydatid
  cyst or tumor — *see* Echinococcus
  mole — *see* Hydatidiform mole
  Morgagni
    female Q50.5
    male (epididymal) Q55.4
    testicular Q55.29
Hydatidiform mole (benign) (complicating pregnancy) (delivered) (undelivered) O01.9
  classical O01.0
  complete O01.0
  incomplete O01.1
  invasive D39.2
  malignant D39.2
  partial O01.1
Hydatidosis — *see* Echinococcus

Hydradenitis (axillaris) (suppurative) L73.2
Hydradenoma — *see* Hidradenoma
Hydramnios O40.- ☑
Hydrancephaly, hydranencephaly Q04.3
  with spina bifida — *see* Spina bifida, with hydrocephalus
Hydrargyrism NEC — *see* Poisoning, mercury
Hydrarthrosis (*see also* Effusion, joint)
  gonococcal A54.42
  intermittent M12.40
    ankle M12.47- ☑
    elbow M12.42- ☑
    foot joint M12.47- ☑
    hand joint M12.44- ☑
    hip M12.45- ☑
    knee M12.46- ☑
    multiple site M12.49
    shoulder M12.41- ☑
    specified joint NEC M12.48
    wrist M12.43- ☑
  of yaws (early) (late) (*see also* subcategory M14.8-) A66.6
  syphilitic (late) A52.77
    congenital A50.55 [M12.80]
Hydremia D64.89
Hydrencephalocele (congenital) — *see* Encephalocele
Hydrencephalomeningocele (congenital) — *see* Encephalocele
Hydroa R23.8
  aestivale L56.4
  vacciniforme L56.4
Hydroadenitis (axillaris) (suppurative) L73.2
Hydrocalycosis — *see* Hydronephrosis
Hydrocele (spermatic cord) (testis) (tunica vaginalis) N43.3
  canal of Nuck N94.89
  communicating N43.2
    congenital P83.5
  congenital P83.5
  encysted N43.0
  female NEC N94.89
  infected N43.1
  newborn P83.5
  round ligament N94.89
  specified NEC N43.2
  spinalis — *see* Spina bifida
  vulva N90.89
Hydrocephalus (acquired) (external) (internal) (malignant) (recurrent) G91.9
  aqueduct Sylvius stricture Q03.0
  causing disproportion O33.6 ☑
    with obstructed labor O66.3
  communicating G91.0
  congenital (external) (internal) Q03.9
    with spina bifida Q05.4
      cervical Q05.0
      dorsal Q05.1
      lumbar Q05.2
      lumbosacral Q05.2
      sacral Q05.3
      thoracic Q05.1
      thoracolumbar Q05.1
    specified NEC Q03.8
  due to toxoplasmosis (congenital) P37.1
  foramen Magendie block (acquired) G91.1
    congenital (*see also* Hydrocephalus, congenital) Q03.1
  in (due to)
    infectious disease NEC B89 [G91.4]
    neoplastic disease NEC (*see also* Neoplasm) G91.4
    parasitic disease B89 [G91.4]
  newborn Q03.9
    with spina bifida — *see* Spina bifida, with hydrocephalus
  noncommunicating G91.1
  normal pressure G91.2
    secondary G91.0
  obstructive G91.1
  otitic G93.2
  post-traumatic NEC G91.3
  secondary G91.4
    post-traumatic G91.3
  specified NEC G91.8
  syphilitic, congenital A50.49
Hydrocolpos (congenital) N89.8
Hydrocystoma — *see* Neoplasm, skin, benign
Hydroencephalocele (congenital) — *see* Encephalocele

Hydroencephalomeningocele (congenital) — *see* Encephalocele
Hydrohematopneumothorax — *see* Hemothorax
Hydromeningitis — *see* Meningitis
Hydromeningocele (spinal) (*see also* Spina bifida)
  cranial — *see* Encephalocele
Hydrometra N85.8
Hydrometrocolpos N89.8
Hydromicrocephaly Q02
Hydromphalos (since birth) Q45.8
Hydromyelia Q06.4
Hydromyelocele — *see* Spina bifida
Hydronephrosis (atrophic) (early) (functionless) (intermittent) (primary) (secondary) NEC N13.30
  with
    infection N13.6
    obstruction (by) (of)
      renal calculus N13.2
        with infection N13.6
      ureteral NEC N13.1
        with infection N13.6
        calculus N13.2
          with infection N13.6
      ureteropelvic junction (congenital) Q62.0
        with infection N13.6
    ureteral stricture NEC N13.1
      with infection N13.6
  congenital Q62.0
  specified type NEC N13.39
  tuberculous A18.11
Hydropericarditis — *see* Pericarditis
Hydropericardium — *see* Pericarditis
Hydroperitoneum R18.8
Hydrophobia — *see* Rabies
Hydrophthalmos Q15.0
Hydropneumohemothorax — *see* Hemothorax
Hydropneumopericarditis — *see* Pericarditis
Hydropneumopericardium — *see* Pericarditis
Hydropneumothorax J94.8
  traumatic — *see* Injury, intrathoracic, lung
  tuberculous NEC A15.6
Hydrops R60.9
  abdominis R18.8
  articulorum intermittens — *see* Hydrarthrosis, intermittent
  cardiac — *see* Failure, heart, congestive
  causing obstructed labor (mother) O66.3
  endolymphatic H81.0- ☑
  fetal — *see* Pregnancy, complicated by, hydrops, fetalis
  fetalis P83.2
    due to
      ABO isoimmunization P56.0
      alpha thalassemia D56.0
      hemolytic disease P56.90
        specified NEC P56.99
      isoimmunization (ABO) (Rh) P56.0
      other specified nonhemolytic disease NEC P83.2
      Rh incompatibility P56.0
    during pregnancy — *see* Pregnancy, complicated by, hydrops, fetalis
  gallbladder K82.1
  joint — *see* Effusion, joint
  labyrinth H81.0- ☑
  newborn (idiopathic) P83.2
    due to
      ABO isoimmunization P56.0
      alpha thalassemia D56.0
      hemolytic disease P56.90
        specified NEC P56.99
      isoimmunization (ABO) (Rh) P56.0
      Rh incompatibility P56.0
  nutritional — *see* Malnutrition, severe
  pericardium — *see* Pericarditis
  pleura — *see* Hydrothorax
  spermatic cord — *see* Hydrocele
Hydropyonephrosis N13.6
Hydrorachis Q06.4
Hydrorrhea (nasal) J34.89
  pregnancy — *see* Rupture, membranes, premature
Hydrosadenitis (axillaris) (suppurative) L73.2
Hydrosalpinx (fallopian tube) (follicularis) N70.11
Hydrothorax (double) (pleura) J94.8
  chylous (nonfilarial) I89.8
    filarial (*see also* Infestation, filarial) B74.9 [J91.8]
  traumatic — *see* Injury, intrathoracic
  tuberculous NEC (non primary) A15.6
Hydroureter (*see also* Hydronephrosis) N13.4

Hydroureter — *continued*
  with infection N13.6
  congenital Q62.39
Hydroureteronephrosis — *see* Hydronephrosis
Hydrourethra N36.8
Hydroxykynureninuria E70.8
Hydroxylysinemia E72.3
Hydroxyprolinemia E72.59
Hygiene, sleep
  abuse Z72.821
  inadequate Z72.821
  poor Z72.821
Hygroma (congenital) (cystic) D18.1
  praepatellare, prepatellar — *see* Bursitis, prepatellar
Hymen — *see* condition
Hymenolepis, hymenolepiasis (diminuta) (infection)
    (infestation) (nana) B71.0
Hypalgesia R20.8
Hyperacidity (gastric) K31.89
  psychogenic F45.8
Hyperactive, hyperactivity F90.9
  basal cell, uterine cervix — *see* Dysplasia, cervix
  bowel sounds R19.12
  cervix epithelial (basal) — *see* Dysplasia, cervix
  child F90.9
    attention deficit — *see* Disorder, attention-deficit
      hyperactivity
  detrusor muscle N32.81
  gastrointestinal K31.89
    psychogenic F45.8
  nasal mucous membrane J34.3
  stomach K31.89
  thyroid (gland) — *see* Hyperthyroidism
Hyperacusis H93.23- ☑
Hyperadrenalism E27.5
Hyperadrenocorticism E24.9
  congenital E25.0
  iatrogenic E24.2
    correct substance properly administered — *see*
      Table of Drugs and Chemicals, by drug, adverse effect
    overdose or wrong substance given or taken —
      see Table of Drugs and Chemicals, by drug, poisoning
  not associated with Cushing's syndrome E27.0
  pituitary-dependent E24.0
Hyperaldosteronism E26.9
  familial (type I) E26.02
  glucocorticoid-remediable E26.02
  primary (due to (bilateral) adrenal hyperplasia) E26.09
  primary NEC E26.09
  secondary E26.1
  specified NEC E26.89
Hyperalgesia R20.8
Hyperalimentation R63.2
  carotene, carotin E67.1
  specified NEC E67.8
  vitamin
    A E67.0
    D E67.3
Hyperaminoaciduria
  arginine E72.21
  cystine E72.01
  lysine E72.3
  ornithine E72.4
Hyperammonemia (congenital) E72.20
Hyperazotemia — *see* Uremia
Hyperbetalipoproteinemia (familial) E78.0
  with prebetalipoproteinemia E78.2
Hyperbilirubinemia
  constitutional E80.6
  familial conjugated E80.6
  neonatal (transient) — *see* Jaundice, newborn
Hypercalcemia, hypocalciuric, familial E83.52
Hypercalciuria, idiopathic E83.52
Hypercapnia R06.89
  newborn P84
Hypercarotenemia, hypercarotinemia (dietary) E67.1
Hypercementosis K03.4
Hyperchloremia E87.8
Hyperchlorhydria K31.89
  neurotic F45.8
  psychogenic F45.8
Hypercholesterinemia — *see* Hypercholesterolemia
Hypercholesterolemia (essential) (familial) (hereditary)
    (primary) (pure) E78.0
  with hyperglyceridemia, endogenous E78.2

Hypercholesterolemia — *continued*
  dietary counseling and surveillance Z71.3
Hyperchylia gastrica, psychogenic F45.8
Hyperchylomicronemia (familial) (primary) E78.3
  with hyperbetalipoproteinemia E78.3
Hypercoagulable (state) D68.59
  activated protein C resistance D68.51
  antithrombin (III) deficiency D68.59
  factor V Leiden mutation D68.51
  primary NEC D68.59
  protein C deficiency D68.59
  protein S deficiency D68.59
  prothrombin gene mutation D68.52
  secondary D68.69
  specified NEC D68.69
Hypercoagulation (state) D68.59
Hypercorticalism, pituitary-dependent E24.0
Hypercorticosolism — *see* Cushing's, syndrome
Hypercorticosteronism E24.2
  correct substance properly administered — *see* Table
    of Drugs and Chemicals, by drug, adverse effect
  overdose or wrong substance given or taken — *see*
    Table of Drugs and Chemicals, by drug, poisoning
Hypercortisonism E24.2
  correct substance properly administered — *see* Table
    of Drugs and Chemicals, by drug, adverse effect
  overdose or wrong substance given or taken — *see*
    Table of Drugs and Chemicals, by drug, poisoning
Hyperekplexia Q89.8
Hyperelectrolytemia E87.8
Hyperemesis R11.10
  with nausea R11.2
  gravidarum (mild) O21.0
    with
      carbohydrate depletion O21.1
      dehydration O21.1
      electrolyte imbalance O21.1
      metabolic disturbance O21.1
      severe (with metabolic disturbance) O21.1
  projectile R11.12
  psychogenic F45.8
Hyperemia (acute) (passive) R68.89
  anal mucosa K62.89
  bladder N32.89
  cerebral I67.89
  conjunctiva H11.43- ☑
  ear internal, acute — *see* subcategory H83.0 ☑
  enteric K59.8
  eye — *see* Hyperemia, conjunctiva
  eyelid (active) (passive) — *see* Disorder, eyelid, specified type NEC
  intestine K59.8
  iris — *see* Disorder, iris, vascular
  kidney N28.89
  labyrinth — *see* subcategory H83.0 ☑
  liver (active) K76.89
  lung (passive) — *see* Edema, lung
  pulmonary (passive) — *see* Edema, lung
  renal N28.89
  retina H35.89
  stomach K31.89
Hyperesthesia (body surface) R20.3
  larynx (reflex) J38.7
    hysterical F44.89
  pharynx (reflex) J39.2
    hysterical F44.89
Hyperestrogenism (drug-induced) (iatrogenic) E28.0
Hyperexplexia Q89.8
Hyperfibrinolysis — *see* Fibrinolysis
Hyperfructosemia E74.19
Hyperfunction
  adrenal cortex, not associated with Cushing's syndrome E27.0
  medulla E27.5
    adrenomedullary E27.5
    virilism E25.9
      congenital E25.0
  ovarian E28.8
  pancreas K86.8
  parathyroid (gland) E21.3
  pituitary (gland) (anterior) E22.9
    specified NEC E22.8
  polyglandular E31.1
  testicular E29.0

Hypergammaglobulinemia D89.2
  polyclonal D89.0
  Waldenström D89.0
Hypergastrinemia E16.4
Hyperglobulinemia R77.1
Hyperglycemia, hyperglycemic (transient) R73.9
  coma — *see* Diabetes, by type, with coma
  postpancreatectomy E89.1
Hyperglyceridemia (endogenous) (essential) (familial)
    (hereditary) (pure) E78.1
  mixed E78.3
Hyperglycinemia (non-ketotic) E72.51
Hypergonadism
  ovarian E28.8
  testicular (primary) (infantile) E29.0
Hyperheparinemia D68.32
Hyperhidrosis, hyperidrosis R61
  focal
    primary L74.519
      axilla L74.510
      face L74.511
      palms L74.512
      soles L74.513
    secondary L74.52
  generalized R61
  localized
    primary L74.519
      axilla L74.510
      face L74.511
      palms L74.512
      soles L74.513
    secondary L74.52
  psychogenic F45.8
  secondary R61
    focal L74.52
Hyperhistidinemia E70.41
Hyperhomocysteinemia E72.11
Hyperhydroxyprolinemia E72.59
Hyperinsulinism (functional) E16.1
  with
    coma (hypoglycemic) E15
    encephalopathy E16.1 [G94]
  ectopic E16.1
  therapeutic misadventure (from administration of insulin) — *see* subcategory T38.3 ☑
Hyperkalemia E87.5
Hyperkeratosis (*see also* Keratosis) L85.9
  cervix N88.0
  due to yaws (early) (late) (palmar or plantar) A66.3
  follicularis Q82.8
    penetrans (in cutem) L87.0
  palmoplantaris climacterica L85.1
  pinta A67.1
  senile (with pruritus) L57.0
  universalis congenita Q80.8
  vocal cord J38.3
  vulva N90.4
Hyperkinesia, hyperkinetic (disease) (reaction) (syndrome) (childhood) (adolescence) (*see also* Disorder, attention-deficit hyperactivity)
  heart I51.89
Hyperleucine-isoleucinemia E71.19
Hyperlipemia, hyperlipidemia E78.5
  combined E78.2
    familial E78.4
  group
    A E78.0
    B E78.1
    C E78.2
    D E78.3
  mixed E78.2
  specified NEC E78.4
Hyperlipidosis E75.6
  hereditary NEC E75.5
Hyperlipoproteinemia E78.5
  Fredrickson's type
    I E78.3
    IIa E78.0
    IIb E78.2
    III E78.2
    IV E78.1
    V E78.3
  low-density-lipoprotein-type (LDL) E78.0
  very-low-density-lipoprotein-type (VLDL) E78.1
Hyperlucent lung, unilateral J43.0
Hyperlysinemia E72.3
Hypermagnesemia E83.41
  neonatal P71.8

Hypermenorrhea N92.0
Hypermethioninemia E72.19
Hypermetropia (congenital) H52.0- ☑
Hypermobility, hypermotility
  cecum — *see* Syndrome, irritable bowel
  coccyx — *see* subcategory M53.2 ☑
  colon — *see* Syndrome, irritable bowel
    psychogenic F45.8
  ileum K58.9
  intestine (*see also* Syndrome, irritable bowel) K58.9
    psychogenic F45.8
  meniscus (knee) — *see* Derangement, knee, meniscus
  scapula — *see* Instability, joint, shoulder
  stomach K31.89
    psychogenic F45.8
  syndrome M35.7
  urethra N36.41
    with intrinsic sphincter deficiency N36.43
Hypernasality R49.21
Hypernatremia E87.0
Hypernephroma C64.- ☑
Hyperopia — *see* Hypermetropia
Hyperorexia nervosa F50.2
Hyperornithinemia E72.4
Hyperosmia R43.1
Hyperosmolality E87.0
Hyperostosis (monomelic) (*see also* Disorder, bone, density and structure, specified NEC)
  ankylosing (spine) M48.10
    cervical region M48.12
    cervicothoracic region M48.13
    lumbar region M48.16
    lumbosacral region M48.17
    multiple sites M48.19
    occipito-atlanto-axial region M48.11
    sacrococcygeal region M48.18
    thoracic region M48.14
    thoracolumbar region M48.15
  cortical (skull) M85.2
    infantile M89.8X- ☑
  frontal, internal of skull M85.2
  interna frontalis M85.2
  skeletal, diffuse idiopathic — *see* Hyperostosis, ankylosing
  skull M85.2
    congenital Q75.8
  vertebral, ankylosing — *see* Hyperostosis, ankylosing
Hyperovarism E28.8
Hyperoxaluria (primary) E72.53
Hyperparathyroidism E21.3
  primary E21.0
  secondary (renal) N25.81
    non-renal E21.1
  specified NEC E21.2
  tertiary E21.2
Hyperpathia R20.8
Hyperperistalsis R19.2
  psychogenic F45.8
Hyperpermeability, capillary I78.8
Hyperphagia R63.2
Hyperphenylalaninemia NEC E70.1
Hyperphoria (alternating) H50.53
Hyperphosphatemia E83.39
Hyperpiesis, hyperpiesia — *see* Hypertension
Hyperpigmentation (*see also* Pigmentation)
  melanin NEC L81.4
  postinflammatory L81.0
Hyperpinealism E34.8
Hyperpituitarism E22.9
Hyperplasia, hyperplastic
  adenoids J35.2
  adrenal (capsule) (cortex) (gland) E27.8
    with
      sexual precocity (male) E25.9
        congenital E25.0
      virilism, adrenal E25.9
        congenital E25.0
      virilization (female) E25.9
        congenital E25.0
    congenital E25.0
    salt-losing E25.0
  adrenomedullary E27.5
  angiolymphoid, eosinophilia (ALHE) D18.01
  appendix (lymphoid) K38.0
  artery, fibromuscular I77.3
  bone (*see also* Hypertrophy, bone)
    marrow D75.89

Hyperplasia, hyperplastic — *continued*
  breast (*see also* Hypertrophy, breast)
    ductal (atypical) N60.9- ☑
  C-cell, thyroid E07.0
  cementation (tooth) (teeth) K03.4
  cervical gland R59.0
  cervix (uteri) (basal cell) (endometrium) (polypoid) (*see also* Dysplasia, cervix)
    congenital Q51.828
  clitoris, congenital Q52.6
  denture K06.2
  endocervicitis N72
  endometrium, endometrial (adenomatous) (benign) (cystic) (glandular) (glandular-cystic) (polypoid) N85.00
    with atypia N85.02
    cervix — *see* Dysplasia, cervix
    complex (without atypia) N85.01
    simple (without atypia) N85.01
  epithelial L85.9
    focal, oral, including tongue K13.29
    nipple N62
    skin L85.9
    tongue K13.29
    vaginal wall N89.3
  erythroid D75.89
  fibromuscular of artery (carotid) (renal) I77.3
  genital
    female NEC N94.89
    male N50.8
  gingiva K06.1
  glandularis cystica uteri (interstitialis) (*see also* Hyperplasia, endometrial) N85.00
  gum K06.1
  hymen, congenital Q52.4
  irritative, edentulous (alveolar) K06.2
  jaw M26.09
    alveolar M26.79
    lower M26.03
      alveolar M26.72
    upper M26.01
      alveolar M26.71
  kidney (congenital) Q63.3
  labia N90.6
    epithelial N90.3
  liver (congenital) Q44.7
    nodular, focal K76.89
  lymph gland or node R59.9
  mandible, mandibular M26.03
    alveolar M26.72
    unilateral condylar M27.8
  maxilla, maxillary M26.01
    alveolar M26.71
  myometrium, myometrial N85.2
  neuroendocrine cell, of infancy J84.841
  nose
    lymphoid J34.89
    polypoid J33.9
  oral mucosa (irritative) K13.6
  organ or site, congenital NEC — *see* Anomaly, by site
  ovary N83.8
  palate, papillary (irritative) K13.6
  pancreatic islet cells E16.9
    alpha E16.8
      with excess
        gastrin E16.4
        glucagon E16.3
    beta E16.1
  parathyroid (gland) E21.0
  pharynx (lymphoid) J39.2
  prostate (adenofibromatous) (nodular) N40.0
    with lower urinary tract symptoms (LUTS) N40.1
    without lower urinary tract symtpoms (LUTS) N40.0
  renal artery I77.89
  reticulo-endothelial (cell) D75.89
  salivary gland (any) K11.1
  Schimmelbusch's — *see* Mastopathy, cystic
  suprarenal capsule (gland) E27.8
  thymus (gland) (persistent) E32.0
  thyroid (gland) — *see* Goiter
  tonsils (faucial) (infective) (lingual) (lymphoid) J35.1
    with adenoids J35.3
  unilateral condylar M27.8
  uterus, uterine N85.2
    endometrium (glandular) (*see also* Hyperplasia, endometrial) N85.00
  vulva N90.6
    epithelial N90.3

Hyperpnea — *see* Hyperventilation
Hyperpotassemia E87.5
Hyperprebetalipoproteinemia (familial) E78.1
Hyperprolactinemia E22.1
Hyperprolinemia (type I) (type II) E72.59
Hyperproteinemia E88.09
Hyperprothrombinemia, causing coagulation factor deficiency D68.4
Hyperpyrexia R50.9
  heat (effects) T67.0 ☑
  malignant, due to anesthetic T88.3 ☑
  rheumatic — *see* Fever, rheumatic
  unknown origin R50.9
Hyper-reflexia R29.2
Hypersalivation K11.7
Hypersecretion
  ACTH (not associated with Cushing's syndrome) E27.0
    pituitary E24.0
  adrenaline E27.5
  adrenomedullary E27.5
  androgen (testicular) E29.0
    ovarian (drug-induced) (iatrogenic) E28.1
  calcitonin E07.0
  catecholamine E27.5
  corticoadrenal E24.9
  cortisol E24.9
  epinephrine E27.5
  estrogen E28.0
  gastric K31.89
    psychogenic F45.8
  gastrin E16.4
  glucagon E16.3
  hormone(s)
    ACTH (not associated with Cushing's syndrome) E27.0
      pituitary E24.0
    antidiuretic E22.2
    growth E22.0
    intestinal NEC E34.1
    ovarian androgen E28.1
    pituitary E22.9
    testicular E29.0
    thyroid stimulating E05.80
      with thyroid storm E05.81
  insulin — *see* Hyperinsulinism
  lacrimal glands — *see* Epiphora
  medulloadrenal E27.5
  milk O92.6
  ovarian androgens E28.1
  salivary gland (any) K11.7
  thyrocalcitonin E07.0
  upper respiratory J39.8
Hypersegmentation, leukocytic, hereditary D72.0
Hypersensitive, hypersensitiveness, hypersensitivity (*see also* Allergy)
  carotid sinus G90.01
  colon — *see* Irritable, colon
  drug T88.7 ☑
  gastrointestinal K52.2
    psychogenic F45.8
  labyrinth — *see* subcategory H83.2 ☑
  pain R20.8
  pneumonitis — *see* Pneumonitis, allergic
  reaction T78.40 ☑
    upper respiratory tract NEC J39.3
Hypersomnia (organic) G47.10
  due to
    alcohol
      abuse F10.182
      dependence F10.282
      use F10.982
    amphetamines
      abuse F15.182
      dependence F15.282
      use F15.982
    caffeine
      abuse F15.182
      dependence F15.282
      use F15.982
    cocaine
      abuse F14.182
      dependence F14.282
      use F14.982
    drug NEC
      abuse F19.182
      dependence F19.282
      use F19.982
    medical condition G47.14

Hypersomnia — *continued*
  due to — *continued*
    mental disorder F51.13
    opioid
      abuse F11.182
      dependence F11.282
      use F11.982
    psychoactive substance NEC
      abuse F19.182
      dependence F19.282
      use F19.982
    sedative, hypnotic, or anxiolytic
      abuse F13.182
      dependence F13.282
      use F13.982
    stimulant NEC
      abuse F15.182
      dependence F15.282
      use F15.982
  idiopathic G47.11
    with long sleep time G47.11
    without long sleep time G47.12
  menstrual related G47.13
  nonorganic origin F51.11
    specified NEC F51.19
  not due to a substance or known physiological condition F51.11
    specified NEC F51.19
  primary F51.11
  recurrent G47.13
  specified NEC G47.19
Hypersplenia, hypersplenism D73.1
Hyperstimulation, ovaries (associated with induced ovulation) N98.1
Hypersusceptibility — *see* Allergy
Hypertelorism (ocular) (orbital) Q75.2
Hypertension, hypertensive (accelerated) (benign) (essential) (idiopathic) (malignant) (systemic) I10
  with
    heart involvement (conditions in I51.4 - I51.9 due to hypertension) — *see* Hypertension, heart
    kidney involvement — *see* Hypertension, kidney
  benign, intracranial G93.2
  borderline R03.0
  cardiorenal (disease) I13.10
    with heart failure I13.0
      with stage 1 through stage 4 chronic kidney disease I13.0
      with stage 5 or end stage renal disease I13.2
    without heart failure I13.10
      with stage 1 through stage 4 chronic kidney disease I13.10
      with stage 5 or end stage renal disease I13.11
  cardiovascular
    disease (arteriosclerotic) (sclerotic) — *see* Hypertension, heart
    renal (disease) — *see* Hypertension, cardiorenal
  chronic venous — *see* Hypertension, venous (chronic)
  complicating
    childbirth (labor) O10.92
      with
        heart disease O10.12
          with renal disease O10.32
        renal disease O10.22
          with heart disease O10.32
      essential O10.02
      secondary O10.42
    pregnancy O16.- ☑
      with edema (*see also* Pre-eclampsia) O14.9- ☑
      gestational (pregnancy induced) (transient) (without proteinuria) O13.- ☑
        with proteinuria O14.9- ☑
          mild pre-eclampsia O14.0- ☑
          moderate pre-eclampsia O14.0- ☑
          severe pre-eclampsia O14.1- ☑
            with hemolysis, elevated liver enzymes and low platelet count (HELLP) O14.2- ☑
      pre-existing O10.91- ☑
        with
          heart disease O10.11- ☑
            with renal disease O10.31- ☑
          pre-eclampsia O11.- ☑
          renal disease O10.21- ☑
            with heart disease O10.31- ☑
        essential O10.01- ☑
        secondary O10.41- ☑
      puerperium, pre-existing O10.93

Hypertension, hypertensive — *continued*
  complicating — *continued*
    puerperium, pre-existing — *continued*
      with
        heart disease O10.13
          with renal disease O10.33
        renal disease O10.23
          with heart disease O10.33
      essential O10.03
      pregnancy-induced O13.9
      secondary O10.43
  due to
    endocrine disorders I15.2
    pheochromocytoma I15.2
    renal disorders NEC I15.1
      arterial I15.0
    renovascular disorders I15.0
    specified disease NEC I15.8
  encephalopathy I67.4
  gestational (without significant proteinuria) (pregnancy-induced) (transient) O13.- ☑
    with significant proteinuria — *see* Pre-eclampsia
  Goldblatt's I70.1
  heart (disease) (conditions in I51.4-I51.9 due to hypertension) I11.9
    with
      heart failure (congestive) I11.0
      kidney disease (chronic) — *see* Hypertension, cardiorenal
  intracranial (benign) G93.2
  kidney I12.9
    with
      heart disease — *see* Hypertension, cardiorenal
      stage 1 through stage 4 chronic kidney disease I12.9
      stage 5 chronic kidney disease (CKD) or end stage renal disease (ESRD) I12.0
  lesser circulation I27.0
  newborn P29.2
    pulmonary (persistent) P29.3
  ocular H40.05- ☑
  pancreatic duct — *code to* underlying condition
    with chronic pancreatitis K86.1
  portal (due to chronic liver disease) (idiopathic) K76.6
    gastropathy K31.89
    in (due to) schistosomiasis (bilharziasis) B65.9 [K77]
  postoperative I97.3
  psychogenic F45.8
  pulmonary (artery) (secondary) NEC I27.2
    with
      cor pulmonale (chronic) I27.2
        acute I26.09
      right heart ventricular strain/failure I27.2
        acute I26.09
    of newborn (persistent) P29.3
    primary (idiopathic) I27.0
  renal — *see* Hypertension, kidney
  renovascular I15.0
  secondary NEC I15.9
    due to
      endocrine disorders I15.2
      pheochromocytoma I15.2
      renal disorders NEC I15.1
        arterial I15.0
      renovascular disorders I15.0
      specified NEC I15.8
  venous (chronic)
    due to
      deep vein thrombosis — *see* Syndrome, post-thrombotic
    idiopathic I87.309
      with
        inflammation I87.32- ☑
          with ulcer I87.33- ☑
        specified complication NEC I87.39- ☑
        ulcer I87.31- ☑
          with inflammation I87.33- ☑
      asymptomatic I87.30- ☑
Hypertensive urgency — *see* Hypertension
Hyperthecosis ovary E28.8
Hyperthermia (of unknown origin) (*see also* Hyperpyrexia)
  malignant, due to anesthesia T88.3 ☑
  newborn P81.9
    environmental P81.0
Hyperthyroid (recurrent) — *see* Hyperthyroidism
Hyperthyroidism (latent) (pre-adult) (recurrent) E05.90

Hyperthyroidism — *continued*
  with
    goiter (diffuse) E05.00
      with thyroid storm E05.01
      nodular (multinodular) E05.20
        with thyroid storm E05.21
        uninodular E05.10
          with thyroid storm E05.11
    storm E05.91
  due to ectopic thyroid tissue E05.30
    with thyroid storm E05.31
  neonatal, transitory P72.1
  specified NEC E05.80
    with thyroid storm E05.81
Hypertony, hypertonia, hypertonicity
  bladder N31.8
  congenital P94.1
  stomach K31.89
    psychogenic F45.8
  uterus, uterine (contractions) (complicating delivery) O62.4
Hypertrichosis L68.9
  congenital Q84.2
  eyelid H02.869
    left H02.866
      lower H02.865
      upper H02.864
    right H02.863
      lower H02.862
      upper H02.861
  lanuginosa Q84.2
    acquired L68.1
  localized L68.2
  specified NEC L68.8
Hypertriglyceridemia, essential E78.1
Hypertrophy, hypertrophic
  adenofibromatous, prostate — *see* Enlargement, enlarged, prostate
  adenoids (infective) J35.2
    with tonsils J35.3
  adrenal cortex E27.8
  alveolar process or ridge — *see* Anomaly, alveolar
  anal papillae K62.89
  artery I77.89
    congenital NEC Q27.8
      digestive system Q27.8
      lower limb Q27.8
      specified site NEC Q27.8
      upper limb Q27.8
  auricular — *see* Hypertrophy, cardiac
  Bartholin's gland N75.8
  bile duct (common) (hepatic) K83.8
  bladder (sphincter) (trigone) N32.89
  bone M89.30
    carpus M89.34- ☑
    clavicle M89.31- ☑
    femur M89.35- ☑
    fibula M89.36- ☑
    finger M89.34- ☑
    humerus M89.32- ☑
    ilium M89.359
    ischium M89.359
    metacarpus M89.34- ☑
    metatarsus M89.37- ☑
    multiple sites M89.39
    neck M89.38
    radius M89.33- ☑
    rib M89.38
    scapula M89.31- ☑
    skull M89.38
    tarsus M89.37- ☑
    tibia M89.36- ☑
    toe M89.37- ☑
    ulna M89.33- ☑
    vertebra M89.38
  brain G93.89
  breast N62
    cystic — *see* Mastopathy, cystic
    newborn P83.4
    pubertal, massive N62
    puerperal, postpartum — *see* Disorder, breast, specified type NEC
    senile (parenchymatous) N62
  cardiac (chronic) (idiopathic) I51.7
    with rheumatic fever (conditions in I00)
      active I01.8
      inactive or quiescent (with chorea) I09.89
    congenital NEC Q24.8

Hypertrophy, hypertrophic — *continued*
- cardiac — *continued*
  - fatty — *see* Degeneration, myocardial
  - hypertensive — *see* Hypertension, heart
  - rheumatic (with chorea) I09.89
    - active or acute I01.8
      - with chorea I02.0
  - valve — *see* Endocarditis
- cartilage — *see* Disorder, cartilage, specified type NEC
- cecum — *see* Megacolon
- cervix (uteri) N88.8
  - congenital Q51.828
  - elongation N88.4
- clitoris (cirrhotic) N90.89
  - congenital Q52.6
- colon (*see also* Megacolon)
  - congenital Q43.2
- conjunctiva, lymphoid H11.89
- corpora cavernosa N48.89
- cystic duct K82.8
- duodenum K31.89
- endometrium (glandular) (*see also* Hyperplasia, endometrial) N85.00
  - cervix N88.8
- epididymis N50.8
- esophageal hiatus (congenital) Q79.1
  - with hernia — *see* Hernia, hiatal
- eyelid — *see* Disorder, eyelid, specified type NEC
- fat pad E65
  - knee (infrapatellar) (popliteal) (prepatellar) (retropatellar) M79.4
- foot (congenital) Q74.2
- frenulum, frenum (tongue) K14.8
  - lip K13.0
- gallbladder K82.8
- gastric mucosa K29.60
  - with bleeding K29.61
- gland, glandular R59.9
  - generalized R59.1
  - localized R59.0
- gum (mucous membrane) K06.1
- heart (idiopathic) (*see also* Hypertrophy, cardiac)
  - valve (*see also* Endocarditis) I38
- hemifacial Q67.4
- hepatic — *see* Hypertrophy, liver
- hiatus (esophageal) Q79.1
- hilus gland R59.0
- hymen, congenital Q52.4
- ileum K63.89
- intestine NEC K63.89
- jejunum K63.89
- kidney (compensatory) N28.81
  - congenital Q63.3
- labium (majus) (minus) N90.6
- ligament — *see* Disorder, ligament
- lingual tonsil (infective) J35.1
  - with adenoids J35.3
- lip K13.0
  - congenital Q18.6
- liver R16.0
  - acute K76.89
  - cirrhotic — *see* Cirrhosis, liver
  - congenital Q44.7
  - fatty — *see* Fatty, liver
- lymph, lymphatic gland R59.9
  - generalized R59.1
  - localized R59.0
  - tuberculous — *see* Tuberculosis, lymph gland
- mammary gland — *see* Hypertrophy, breast
- Meckel's diverticulum (congenital) Q43.0
  - malignant — *see* Table of Neoplasms, small intestine, malignant
- median bar — *see* Hyperplasia, prostate
- meibomian gland — *see* Chalazion
- meniscus, knee, congenital Q74.1
- metatarsal head — *see* Hypertrophy, bone, metatarsus
- metatarsus — *see* Hypertrophy, bone, metatarsus
- mucous membrane
  - alveolar ridge K06.2
  - gum K06.1
  - nose (turbinate) J34.3
- muscle M62.89
- muscular coat, artery I77.89
- myocardium (*see also* Hypertrophy, cardiac)
  - idiopathic I42.2
- myometrium N85.2
- nail L60.2
  - congenital Q84.5

Hypertrophy, hypertrophic — *continued*
- nasal J34.89
  - alae J34.89
  - bone J34.89
  - cartilage J34.89
  - mucous membrane (septum) J34.3
  - sinus J34.89
  - turbinate J34.3
- nasopharynx, lymphoid (infectional) (tissue) (wall) J35.2
- nipple N62
- organ or site, congenital NEC — *see* Anomaly, by site
- ovary N83.8
- palate (hard) M27.8
  - soft K13.79
- pancreas, congenital Q45.3
- parathyroid (gland) E21.0
- parotid gland K11.1
- penis N48.89
- pharyngeal tonsil J35.2
- pharynx J39.2
  - lymphoid (infectional) (tissue) (wall) J35.2
- pituitary (anterior) (fossa) (gland) E23.6
- prepuce (congenital) N47.8
  - female N90.89
- prostate — *see* Enlargement, enlarged, prostate
  - congenital Q55.4
- pseudomuscular G71.0
- pylorus (adult) (muscle) (sphincter) K31.1
  - congenital or infantile Q40.0
- rectal, rectum (sphincter) K62.89
- rhinitis (turbinate) J31.0
- salivary gland (any) K11.1
  - congenital Q38.4
- scaphoid (tarsal) — *see* Hypertrophy, bone, tarsus
- scar L91.0
- scrotum N50.8
- seminal vesicle N50.8
- sigmoid — *see* Megacolon
- skin L91.9
  - specified NEC L91.8
- spermatic cord N50.8
- spleen — *see* Splenomegaly
- spondylitis — *see* Spondylosis
- stomach K31.89
- sublingual gland K11.1
- submandibular gland K11.1
- suprarenal cortex (gland) E27.8
- synovial NEC M67.20
  - acromioclavicular M67.21- ☑
  - ankle M67.27- ☑
  - elbow M67.22- ☑
  - foot M67.27- ☑
  - hand M67.24- ☑
  - hip M67.25- ☑
  - knee M67.26- ☑
  - multiple sites M67.29
  - specified site NEC M67.28
  - wrist M67.23- ☑
- tendon — *see* Disorder, tendon, specified type NEC
- testis N44.8
  - congenital Q55.29
- thymic, thymus (gland) (congenital) E32.0
- thyroid (gland) — *see* Goiter
- toe (congenital) Q74.2
  - acquired (*see also* Deformity, toe, specified NEC)
- tongue K14.8
  - congenital Q38.2
  - papillae (foliate) K14.3
- tonsils (faucial) (infective) (lingual) (lymphoid) J35.1
  - with adenoids J35.3
- tunica vaginalis N50.8
- ureter N28.89
- urethra N36.8
- uterus N85.2
  - neck (with elongation) N88.4
  - puerperal O90.89
- uvula K13.79
- vagina N89.8
- vas deferens N50.8
- vein I87.8
- ventricle, ventricular (heart) (*see also* Hypertrophy, cardiac)
  - congenital Q24.8
  - in tetralogy of Fallot Q21.3
- verumontanum N36.8
- vocal cord J38.3
- vulva N90.6

Hypertrophy, hypertrophic — *continued*
- vulva — *continued*
  - stasis (nonfilarial) N90.6

Hypertropia H50.2- ☑
Hypertyrosinemia E70.21
Hyperuricemia (asymptomatic) E79.0
Hypervalinemia E71.19
Hyperventilation (tetany) R06.4
- hysterical F45.8
- psychogenic F45.8
- syndrome F45.8
Hypervitaminosis (dietary) NEC E67.8
- A E67.0
  - administered as drug (prolonged intake) — *see* Table of Drugs and Chemicals, vitamins, adverse effect
  - overdose or wrong substance given or taken — *see* Table of Drugs and Chemicals, vitamins, poisoning
- B6 E67.2
- D E67.3
  - administered as drug (prolonged intake) — *see* Table of Drugs and Chemicals, vitamins, adverse effect
  - overdose or wrong substance given or taken — *see* Table of Drugs and Chemicals, vitamins, poisoning
- K E67.8
  - administered as drug (prolonged intake) — *see* Table of Drugs and Chemicals, vitamins, adverse effect
  - overdose or wrong substance given or taken — *see* Table of Drugs and Chemicals, vitamins, poisoning
Hypervolemia E87.70
- specified NEC E87.79
Hypesthesia R20.1
- cornea — *see* Anesthesia, cornea
Hyphema H21.0- ☑
- traumatic S05.1- ☑
Hypoacidity, gastric K31.89
- psychogenic F45.8
Hypoadrenalism, hypoadrenia E27.40
- primary E27.1
- tuberculous A18.7
Hypoadrenocorticism E27.40
- pituitary E23.0
- primary E27.1
Hypoalbuminemia E88.09
Hypoaldosteronism E27.40
Hypoalphalipoproteinemia E78.6
Hypobarism T70.29 ☑
Hypobaropathy T70.29 ☑
Hypobetalipoproteinemia (familial) E78.6
Hypocalcemia E83.51
- dietary E58
- neonatal P71.1
  - due to cow's milk P71.0
- phosphate-loading (newborn) P71.1
Hypochloremia E87.8
Hypochlorhydria K31.89
- neurotic F45.8
- psychogenic F45.8
Hypochondria, hypochondriac, hypochondriasis (reaction) F45.21
- sleep F51.03
Hypochondrogenesis Q77.0
Hypochondroplasia Q77.4
Hypochromasia, blood cells D50.8
Hypodontia — *see* Anodontia
Hypoeosinophilia D72.89
Hypoesthesia R20.1
Hypofibrinogenemia D68.8
- acquired D65
- congenital (hereditary) D68.2
Hypofunction
- adrenocortical E27.40
  - drug-induced E27.3
  - postprocedural E89.6
  - primary E27.1
- adrenomedullary, postprocedural E89.6
- cerebral R29.818
- corticoadrenal NEC E27.40
- intestinal K59.8
- labyrinth — *see* subcategory H83.2 ☑
- ovary E28.39
- pituitary (gland) (anterior) E23.0

Hypofunction — *continued*
　testicular E29.1
　　postprocedural (postsurgical) (postirradiation) (iatrogenic) E89.5
Hypogalactia O92.4
Hypogammaglobulinemia (*see also* Agammaglobulinemia) D80.1
　hereditary D80.0
　nonfamilial D80.1
　transient, of infancy D80.7
Hypogenitalism (congenital) — *see* Hypogonadism
Hypoglossia Q38.3
Hypoglycemia (spontaneous) E16.2
　coma E15
　　diabetic — *see* Diabetes, coma
　diabetic — *see* Diabetes, hypoglycemia
　dietary counseling and surveillance Z71.3
　drug-induced E16.0
　　with coma (nondiabetic) E15
　due to insulin E16.0
　　with coma (nondiabetic) E15
　　therapeutic misadventure — *see* subcategory T38.3 ☑
　functional, nonhyperinsulinemic E16.1
　iatrogenic E16.0
　　with coma (nondiabetic) E15
　in infant of diabetic mother P70.1
　　gestational diabetes P70.0
　infantile E16.1
　leucine-induced E71.19
　neonatal (transitory) P70.4
　　iatrogenic P70.3
　reactive (not drug-induced) E16.1
　transitory neonatal P70.4
Hypogonadism
　female E28.39
　hypogonadotropic E23.0
　male E29.1
　ovarian (primary) E28.39
　pituitary E23.0
　testicular (primary) E29.1
Hypohidrosis, hypoidrosis L74.4
Hypoinsulinemia, postprocedural E89.1
Hypokalemia E87.6
Hypoleukocytosis — *see* Agranulocytosis
Hypolipoproteinemia (alpha) (beta) E78.6
Hypomagnesemia E83.42
　neonatal P71.2
Hypomania, hypomanic reaction F30.8
Hypomenorrhea — *see* Oligomenorrhea
Hypometabolism R63.8
Hypomotility
　gastrointestinal (tract) K31.89
　　psychogenic F45.8
　intestine K59.8
　　psychogenic F45.8
　stomach K31.89
　　psychogenic F45.8
Hyponasality R49.22
Hyponatremia E87.1
Hypo-osmolality E87.1
Hypo-ovarianism, hypo-ovarism E28.39
Hypoparathyroidism E20.9
　familial E20.8
　idiopathic E20.0
　neonatal, transitory P71.4
　postprocedural E89.2
　specified NEC E20.8
Hypoperfusion (in)
　newborn P96.89
Hypopharyngitis — *see* Laryngopharyngitis
Hypophoria H50.53
Hypophosphatemia, hypophosphatasia (acquired) (congenital) (renal) E83.39
　familial E83.31
Hypophyseal, hypophysis (*see also* condition)
　dwarfism E23.0
　gigantism E22.0
Hypopiesis — *see* Hypotension
Hypopinealism E34.8
Hypopituitarism (juvenile) E23.0
　drug-induced E23.1
　due to
　　hypophysectomy E89.3
　　radiotherapy E89.3
　iatrogenic NEC E23.1
　postirradiation E89.3

Hypopituitarism — *continued*
　postpartum E23.0
　postprocedural E89.3
Hypoplasia, hypoplastic
　adrenal (gland), congenital Q89.1
　alimentary tract, congenital Q45.8
　　upper Q40.8
　anus, anal (canal) Q42.3
　　with fistula Q42.2
　aorta, aortic Q25.4
　　ascending, in hypoplastic left heart syndrome Q23.4
　　valve Q23.1
　　　in hypoplastic left heart syndrome Q23.4
　areola, congenital Q83.8
　arm (congenital) — *see* Defect, reduction, upper limb
　artery (peripheral) Q27.8
　　brain (congenital) Q28.3
　　coronary Q24.5
　　digestive system Q27.8
　　lower limb Q27.8
　　pulmonary Q25.79
　　　functional, unilateral J43.0
　　retinal (congenital) Q14.1
　　specified site NEC Q27.8
　　umbilical Q27.0
　　upper limb Q27.8
　auditory canal Q17.8
　　causing impairment of hearing Q16.9
　biliary duct or passage Q44.5
　bone NOS Q79.9
　　face Q75.8
　　marrow D61.9
　　　megakaryocytic D69.49
　　skull — *see* Hypoplasia, skull
　brain Q02
　　gyri Q04.3
　　part of Q04.3
　breast (areola) N64.82
　bronchus Q32.4
　cardiac Q24.8
　carpus — *see* Defect, reduction, upper limb, specified type NEC
　cartilage hair Q78.5
　cecum Q42.8
　cementum K00.4
　cephalic Q02
　cerebellum Q04.3
　cervix (uteri), congenital Q51.821
　clavicle (congenital) Q74.0
　coccyx Q76.49
　colon Q42.9
　　specified NEC Q42.8
　corpus callosum Q04.0
　cricoid cartilage Q31.2
　digestive organ(s) or tract NEC Q45.8
　　upper (congenital) Q40.8
　ear (auricle) (lobe) Q17.2
　　middle Q16.4
　enamel of teeth (neonatal) (postnatal) (prenatal) K00.4
　endocrine (gland) NEC Q89.2
　endometrium N85.8
　epididymis (congenital) Q55.4
　epiglottis Q31.2
　erythroid, congenital D61.01
　esophagus (congenital) Q39.8
　eustachian tube Q17.8
　eye Q11.2
　eyelid (congenital) Q10.3
　face Q18.8
　　bone(s) Q75.8
　femur (congenital) — *see* Defect, reduction, lower limb, specified type NEC
　fibula (congenital) — *see* Defect, reduction, lower limb, specified type NEC
　finger (congenital) — *see* Defect, reduction, upper limb, specified type NEC
　focal dermal Q82.8
　foot — *see* Defect, reduction, lower limb, specified type NEC
　gallbladder Q44.0
　genitalia, genital organ(s)
　　female, congenital Q52.8
　　　external Q52.79
　　　internal NEC Q52.8
　　in adiposogenital dystrophy E23.6
　glottis Q31.2
　hair Q84.2

Hypoplasia, hypoplastic — *continued*
　hand (congenital) — *see* Defect, reduction, upper limb, specified type NEC
　heart Q24.8
　humerus (congenital) — *see* Defect, reduction, upper limb, specified type NEC
　intestine (small) Q41.9
　　large Q42.9
　　　specified NEC Q42.8
　jaw M26.09
　　alveolar M26.79
　　lower M26.04
　　　alveolar M26.74
　　upper M26.02
　　　alveolar M26.73
　kidney(s) Q60.5
　　bilateral Q60.4
　　unilateral Q60.3
　labium (majus) (minus), congenital Q52.79
　larynx Q31.2
　left heart syndrome Q23.4
　leg (congenital) — *see* Defect, reduction, lower limb
　limb Q73.8
　　lower (congenital) — *see* Defect, reduction, lower limb
　　upper (congenital) — *see* Defect, reduction, upper limb
　liver Q44.7
　lung (lobe) (not associated with short gestation) Q33.6
　　associated with immaturity, low birth weight, prematurity, or short gestation P28.0
　mammary (areola), congenital Q83.8
　mandible, mandibular M26.04
　　alveolar M26.74
　　unilateral condylar M27.8
　maxillary M26.02
　　alveolar M26.73
　medullary D61.9
　megakaryocytic D69.49
　metacarpus — *see* Defect, reduction, upper limb, specified type NEC
　metatarsus — *see* Defect, reduction, lower limb, specified type NEC
　muscle Q79.8
　nail(s) Q84.6
　nose, nasal Q30.1
　optic nerve H47.03- ☑
　osseous meatus (ear) Q17.8
　ovary, congenital Q50.39
　pancreas Q45.0
　parathyroid (gland) Q89.2
　parotid gland Q38.4
　patella Q74.1
　pelvis, pelvic girdle Q74.2
　penis (congenital) Q55.62
　peripheral vascular system Q27.8
　　digestive system Q27.8
　　lower limb Q27.8
　　specified site NEC Q27.8
　　upper limb Q27.8
　pituitary (gland) (congenital) Q89.2
　pulmonary (not associated with short gestation) Q33.6
　　artery, functional J43.0
　　associated with short gestation P28.0
　radioulnar — *see* Defect, reduction, upper limb, specified type NEC
　radius — *see* Defect, reduction, upper limb
　rectum Q42.1
　　with fistula Q42.0
　respiratory system NEC Q34.8
　rib Q76.6
　right heart syndrome Q22.6
　sacrum Q76.49
　scapula Q74.0
　scrotum Q55.1
　shoulder girdle Q74.0
　skin Q82.8
　skull (bone) Q75.8
　　with
　　　anencephaly Q00.0
　　　encephalocele — *see* Encephalocele
　　　hydrocephalus Q03.9
　　　　with spina bifida — *see* Spina bifida, by site, with hydrocephalus
　　　microcephaly Q02
　spinal (cord) (ventral horn cell) Q06.1
　spine Q76.49
　sternum Q76.7

Hypoplasia, hypoplastic — continued
  tarsus — see Defect, reduction, lower limb, specified type NEC
  testis Q55.1
  thymic, with immunodeficiency D82.1
  thymus (gland) Q89.2
    with immunodeficiency D82.1
  thyroid (gland) E03.1
    cartilage Q31.2
  tibiofibular (congenital) — see Defect, reduction, lower limb, specified type NEC
  toe — see Defect, reduction, lower limb, specified type NEC
  tongue Q38.3
  Turner's K00.4
  ulna (congenital) — see Defect, reduction, upper limb
  umbilical artery Q27.0
  unilateral condylar M27.8
  ureter Q62.8
  uterus, congenital Q51.811
  vagina Q52.4
  vascular NEC peripheral Q27.8
    brain Q28.3
    digestive system Q27.8
    lower limb Q27.8
    specified site NEC Q27.8
    upper limb Q27.8
  vein(s) (peripheral) Q27.8
    brain Q28.3
    digestive system Q27.8
    great Q26.8
    lower limb Q27.8
    specified site NEC Q27.8
    upper limb Q27.8
  vena cava (inferior) (superior) Q26.8
  vertebra Q76.49
  vulva, congenital Q52.79
  zonule (ciliary) Q12.8
Hypopotassemia E87.6
Hypoproconvertinemia, congenital (hereditary) D68.2
Hypoproteinemia E77.8
Hypoprothrombinemia (congenital) (hereditary) (idiopathic) D68.2
  acquired D68.4
  newborn, transient P61.6
Hypoptyalism K11.7
Hypopyon (eye) (anterior chamber) — see Iridocyclitis, acute, hypopyon
Hypopyrexia R68.0
Hyporeflexia R29.2
Hyposecretion
  ACTH E23.0
  antidiuretic hormone E23.2
  ovary E28.39
  salivary gland (any) K11.7
  vasopressin E23.2
Hyposegmentation, leukocytic, hereditary D72.0
Hyposiderinemia D50.9
Hypospadias Q54.9
  balanic Q54.0
  coronal Q54.0
  glandular Q54.0
  penile Q54.1
  penoscrotal Q54.2
  perineal Q54.3
  specified NEC Q54.8
Hypospermatogenesis — see Oligospermia
Hyposplenism D73.0
Hypostasis pulmonary, passive — see Edema, lung
Hypostatic — see condition
Hyposthenuria N28.89
Hypotension (arterial) (constitutional) I95.9
  chronic I95.89
  drug-induced I95.2
  due to (of) hemodialysis I95.3
  iatrogenic I95.89
  idiopathic (permanent) I95.0
  intracranial, following ventricular shunting (ventriculostomy) G97.2
  intra-dialytic I95.3
  maternal, syndrome (following labor and delivery) O26.5-
  neurogenic, orthostatic G90.3
  orthostatic (chronic) I95.1
    due to drugs I95.2
    neurogenic G90.3
  postoperative I95.81
  postural I95.1

Hypotension — continued
  specified NEC I95.89
Hypothermia (accidental) T68 ☑
  due to anesthesia, anesthetic T88.51 ☑
  low environmental temperature T68 ☑
  neonatal P80.9
    environmental (mild) NEC P80.8
    mild P80.8
    severe (chronic) (cold injury syndrome) P80.0
    specified NEC P80.8
  not associated with low environmental temperature R68.0
Hypothyroidism (acquired) E03.9
  congenital (without goiter) E03.1
    with goiter (diffuse) E03.0
  due to
    exogenous substance NEC E03.2
    iodine-deficiency, acquired E01.8
      subclinical E02
    irradiation therapy E89.0
    medicament NEC E03.2
    P-aminosalicylic acid (PAS) E03.2
    phenylbutazone E03.2
    resorcinol E03.2
    sulfonamide E03.2
    surgery E89.0
    thiourea group drugs E03.2
  iatrogenic NEC E03.2
  iodine-deficiency (acquired) E01.8
    congenital — see Syndrome, iodine- deficiency, congenital
    subclinical E02
  neonatal, transitory P72.2
  postinfectious E03.3
  postirradiation E89.0
  postprocedural E89.0
  postsurgical E89.0
  specified NEC E03.8
  subclinical, iodine-deficiency related E02
Hypotonia, hypotonicity, hypotony
  bladder N31.2
  congenital (benign) P94.2
  eye — see Disorder, globe, hypotony
Hypotrichosis — see Alopecia
Hypotropia H50.2- ☑
Hypoventilation R06.89
  congenital central alveolar G47.35
  sleep related
    idiopathic nonobstructive alveolar G47.34
    in conditions classified elsewhere G47.36
Hypovitaminosis — see Deficiency, vitamin
Hypovolemia E86.1
  surgical shock T81.19 ☑
  traumatic (shock) T79.4 ☑
Hypoxemia R09.02
  newborn P84
  sleep related, in conditions classified elsewhere G47.36
Hypoxia (see also Anoxia) R09.02
  cerebral, during a procedure NEC G97.81
    postprocedural NEC G97.82
  intrauterine P84
  myocardial — see Insufficiency, coronary
  newborn P84
  sleep-related G47.34
Hypsarhythmia — see Epilepsy, generalized, specified NEC
Hysteralgia, pregnant uterus O26.89- ☑
Hysteria, hysterical (conversion) (dissociative state) F44.9
  anxiety F41.8
  convulsions F44.5
  psychosis, acute F44.9
Hysteroepilepsy F44.5

I

Ichthyoparasitism due to Vandellia cirrhosa B88.8
Ichthyosis (congenital) Q80.9
  acquired L85.0
  fetalis Q80.4
  hystrix Q80.8
  lamellar Q80.2
  lingual K13.29
  palmaris and plantaris Q82.8
  simplex Q80.0
  vera Q80.8
  vulgaris Q80.0

Ichthyosis — continued
  X-linked Q80.1
Ichthyotoxism — see Poisoning, fish
  bacterial — see Intoxication, foodborne
Icteroanemia, hemolytic (acquired) D59.9
  congenital — see Spherocytosis
Icterus (see also Jaundice)
  conjunctiva R17
  gravis, newborn P55.0
  hematogenous (acquired) D59.9
  hemolytic (acquired) D59.9
    congenital — see Spherocytosis
  hemorrhagic (acute) (leptospiral) (spirochetal) A27.0
    newborn P53
  infectious B15.9
    with hepatic coma B15.0
    leptospiral A27.0
    spirochetal A27.0
  neonatorum — see Jaundice, newborn
  newborn P59.9
  spirochetal A27.0
Ictus solaris, solis T67.0 ☑
Id reaction (due to bacteria) L30.2
Ideation
  homicidal R45.850
  suicidal R45.851
Identity disorder (child) F64.9
  gender role F64.2
  psychosexual F64.2
Idioglossia F80.0
Idiopathic — see condition
Idiot, idiocy (congenital) F73
  amaurotic (Bielschowsky(-Jansky)) (family) (infantile (late)) (juvenile (late)) (Vogt-Spielmeyer) E75.4
  microcephalic Q02
IgE asthma J45.909
IIAC (idiopathic infantile arterial calcification) Q28.8
Ileitis (chronic) (noninfectious) (see also Enteritis) K52.9
  backwash — see Pancolitis, ulcerative (chronic)
  infectious A09
  regional (ulcerative) — see Enteritis, regional, small intestine
  segmental — see Enteritis, regional
  terminal (ulcerative) — see Enteritis, regional, small intestine
Ileocolitis (see also Enteritis) K52.9
  infectious A09
  regional — see Enteritis, regional
Ileostomy
  attention to Z43.2
  malfunctioning K94.13
  status Z93.2
    with complication — see Complications, enterostomy
Ileotyphus — see Typhoid
Ileum — see condition
Ileus (bowel) (colon) (inhibitory) (intestine) K56.7
  adynamic K56.0
  due to gallstone (in intestine) K56.3
  duodenal (chronic) K31.5
  gallstone K56.3
  mechanical NEC K56.69
  meconium P76.0
    in cystic fibrosis E84.11
    meaning meconium plug (without cystic fibrosis) P76.0
  myxedema K59.8
  neurogenic K56.0
    Hirschsprung's disease or megacolon Q43.1
  newborn
    due to meconium P76.0
      in cystic fibrosis E84.11
      meaning meconium plug (without cystic fibrosis) P76.0
    transitory P76.1
  obstructive K56.69
  paralytic K56.0
Iliac — see condition
Iliotibial band syndrome M76.3- ☑
Illiteracy Z55.0
Illness (see also Disease) R69
  manic-depressive — see Disorder, bipolar
Imbalance R26.89
  autonomic G90.8
  constituents of food intake E63.1
  electrolyte E87.8

☑ Additional Character Required — Refer to the Tabular List for Character Selection   ▽ Subterms under main terms may continue to next column or page

Imbalance — *continued*
  electrolyte — *continued*
    with
      abortion — *see* Abortion by type, complicated by, electrolyte imbalance
      molar pregnancy O08.5
      due to hyperemesis gravidarum O21.1
      following ectopic or molar pregnancy O08.5
      neonatal, transitory NEC P74.4
        potassium P74.3
        sodium P74.2
  endocrine E34.9
  eye muscle NOS H50.9
  hormone E34.9
  hysterical F44.4
  labyrinth — *see* subcategory H83.2 ☑
  posture R29.3
  protein-energy — *see* Malnutrition
  sympathetic G90.8
Imbecile, imbecility (I.Q. 35-49) F71
Imbedding, intrauterine device T83.39 ☑
Imbibition, cholesterol (gallbladder) K82.4
Imbrication, teeth,, fully erupted M26.30
Imerslund (-Gräsbeck) **syndrome** D51.1
Immature (*see also* Immaturity)
  birth (less than 37 completed weeks) — *see* Preterm, newborn
    extremely (less than 28 completed weeks) — *see* Immaturity, extreme
  personality F60.89
Immaturity (less than 37 completed weeks) (*see also* Preterm, newborn)
  extreme of newborn (less than 28 completed weeks of gestation) (less than 196 completed days of gestation) (unspecified weeks of gestation) P07.20
    gestational age
      less than 23 completed weeks P07.21
      23 completed weeks (23 weeks, 0 days through 23 weeks, 6 days) P07.22
      24 completed weeks (24 weeks, 0 days through 24 weeks, 6 days) P07.23
      25 completed weeks (25 weeks, 0 days through 25 weeks, 6 days) P07.24
      26 completed weeks (26 weeks, 0 days through 26 weeks, 6 days) P07.25
      27 completed weeks (27 weeks, 0 days through 27 weeks, 6 days) P07.26
  fetus or infant light-for-dates — *see* Light-for-dates
  lung, newborn P28.0
  organ or site NEC — *see* Hypoplasia
  pulmonary, newborn P28.0
  reaction F60.89
  sexual (female) (male), after puberty E30.0
Immersion T75.1 ☑
  foot T69.02- ☑
  hand T69.01- ☑
Immobile, immobility
  complete, due to severe physical disability or frailty R53.2
  intestine K59.8
  syndrome (paraplegic) M62.3
Immune reconstitution (inflammatory) syndrome [IRIS] D89.3
Immunization (*see also* Vaccination)
  ABO — *see* Incompatibility, ABO
    in newborn P55.1
  complication — *see* Complications, vaccination
  encounter for Z23
  not done (not carried out) Z28.9
    because (of)
      acute illness of patient Z28.01
      allergy to vaccine (or component) Z28.04
      caregiver refusal Z28.82
      chronic illness of patient Z28.02
      contraindication NEC Z28.09
      group pressure Z28.1
      guardian refusal Z28.82
      immune compromised state of patient Z28.03
      parent refusal Z28.82
      patient had disease being vaccinated against Z28.81
      patient refusal Z28.21
      patient's belief Z28.1
      religious beliefs of patient Z28.1
      specified reason NEC Z28.89
        of patient Z28.29
      unspecified patient reason Z28.20

Immunization — *continued*
  Rh factor
    affecting management of pregnancy NEC O36.09- ☑
      anti-D antibody O36.01- ☑
    from transfusion — *see* Complication(s), transfusion, incompatibility reaction, Rh (factor)
Immunocytoma C83.0- ☑
Immunodeficiency D84.9
  with
    adenosine-deaminase deficiency D81.3
    antibody defects D80.9
      specified type NEC D80.8
    hyperimmunoglobulinemia D80.6
    increased immunoglobulin M (IgM) D80.5
    major defect D82.9
      specified type NEC D82.8
    partial albinism D82.8
    short-limbed stature D82.2
    thrombocytopenia and eczema D82.0
  antibody with
    hyperimmunoglobulinemia D80.6
    near-normal immunoglobulins D80.6
  autosomal recessive, Swiss type D80.0
  combined D81.9
    biotin-dependent carboxylase D81.819
      biotinidase D81.810
      holocarboxylase synthetase D81.818
      specified type NEC D81.818
    severe (SCID) D81.9
      with
        low or normal B-cell numbers D81.2
        low T- and B-cell numbers D81.1
        reticular dysgenesis D81.0
    specified type NEC D81.89
  common variable D83.9
    with
      abnormalities of B-cell numbers and function D83.0
      autoantibodies to B- or T-cells D83.2
      immunoregulatory T-cell disorders D83.1
    specified type NEC D83.8
  following hereditary defective response to Epstein-Barr virus (EBV) D82.3
  selective, immunoglobulin
    A (IgA) D80.2
    G (IgG) (subclasses) D80.3
    M (IgM) D80.4
  severe combined (SCID) D81.9
  specified type NEC D84.8
  X-linked, with increased IgM D80.5
Immunotherapy (encounter for)
  antineoplastic Z51.12
Impaction, impacted
  bowel, colon, rectum (*see also* Impaction, fecal) K56.49
    by gallstone K56.3
  calculus — *see* Calculus
  cerumen (ear) (external) H61.2- ☑
  cuspid — *see* Impaction, tooth
  dental (same or adjacent tooth) K01.1
  fecal, feces K56.41
  fracture — *see* Fracture, by site
  gallbladder — *see* Calculus, gallbladder
  gallstone(s) — *see* Calculus, gallbladder
    bile duct (common) (hepatic) — *see* Calculus, bile duct
    cystic duct — *see* Calculus, gallbladder
    in intestine, with obstruction (any part) K56.3
  intestine (calculous) NEC (*see also* Impaction, fecal) K56.49
    gallstone, with ileus K56.3
  intrauterine device (IUD) T83.39 ☑
  molar — *see* Impaction, tooth
  shoulder, causing obstructed labor O66.0
  tooth, teeth K01.1
  turbinate J34.89
Impaired, impairment (function)
  auditory discrimination — *see* Abnormal, auditory perception
  cognitive, mild, so stated G31.84
  dual sensory Z73.82
  fasting glucose R73.01
  glucose tolerance (oral) R73.02
  hearing — *see* Deafness
  heart — *see* Disease, heart
  kidney N28.9
    disorder resulting from N25.9
      specified NEC N25.89

Impaired, impairment — *continued*
  liver K72.90
    with coma K72.91
  mastication K08.8
  mild cognitive, so stated G31.84
  mobility
    ear ossicles — *see* Ankylosis, ear ossicles
    requiring care provider Z74.09
  myocardium, myocardial — *see* Insufficiency, myocardial
  rectal sphincter R19.8
  renal (acute) (chronic) N28.9
    disorder resulting from N25.9
      specified NEC N25.89
  vision NEC H54.7
    both eyes H54.3
Impediment, speech R47.9
  psychogenic (childhood) F98.8
  slurring R47.81
  specified NEC R47.89
Impending
  coronary syndrome I20.0
  delirium tremens F10.239
  myocardial infarction I20.0
Imperception auditory (acquired) (*see also* Deafness)
  congenital H93.25
Imperfect
  aeration, lung (newborn) NEC — *see* Atelectasis
  closure (congenital)
    alimentary tract NEC Q45.8
      lower Q43.8
      upper Q40.8
    atrioventricular ostium Q21.2
    atrium (secundum) Q21.1
    branchial cleft or sinus Q18.0
    choroid Q14.3
    cricoid cartilage Q31.8
    cusps, heart valve NEC Q24.8
      pulmonary Q22.3
    ductus
      arteriosus Q25.0
      Botalli Q25.0
    ear drum (causing impairment of hearing) Q16.4
    esophagus with communication to bronchus or trachea Q39.1
    eyelid Q10.3
    foramen
      botalli Q21.1
      ovale Q21.1
    genitalia, genital organ(s) or system
      female Q52.8
        external Q52.79
        internal NEC Q52.8
      male Q55.8
    glottis Q31.8
    interatrial ostium or septum Q21.1
    interauricular ostium or septum Q21.1
    interventricular ostium or septum Q21.0
    larynx Q31.8
    lip — *see* Cleft, lip
    nasal septum Q30.3
    nose Q30.2
    omphalomesenteric duct Q43.0
    optic nerve entry Q14.2
    organ or site not listed — *see* Anomaly, by site
    ostium
      interatrial Q21.1
      interauricular Q21.1
      interventricular Q21.0
    palate — *see* Cleft, palate
    preauricular sinus Q18.1
    retina Q14.1
    roof of orbit Q75.8
    sclera Q13.5
    septum
      aorticopulmonary Q21.4
      atrial (secundum) Q21.1
      between aorta and pulmonary artery Q21.4
      heart Q21.9
      interatrial (secundum) Q21.1
      interauricular (secundum) Q21.1
      interventricular Q21.0
        in tetralogy of Fallot Q21.3
      nasal Q30.3
      ventricular Q21.0
        with pulmonary stenosis or atresia, dextraposition of aorta, and hypertrophy of right ventricle Q21.3

Imperfect — continued
  closure — continued
    septum — continued
      ventricular — continued
        in tetralogy of Fallot Q21.3
      skull Q75.0
        with
          anencephaly Q00.0
          encephalocele — see Encephalocele
          hydrocephalus Q03.9
            with spina bifida — see Spina bifida, by
              site, with hydrocephalus
          microcephaly Q02
      spine (with meningocele) — see Spina bifida
      trachea Q32.1
      tympanic membrane (causing impairment of
        hearing) Q16.4
      uterus Q51.818
      vitelline duct Q43.0
  erection — see Dysfunction, sexual, male, erectile
  fusion — see Imperfect, closure
  inflation, lung (newborn) — see Atelectasis
  posture R29.3
  rotation, intestine Q43.3
  septum, ventricular Q21.0
Imperfectly descended testis — see Cryptorchid
Imperforate (congenital) (see also Atresia)
  anus Q42.3
    with fistula Q42.2
  cervix (uteri) Q51.828
  esophagus Q39.0
    with tracheoesophageal fistula Q39.1
  hymen Q52.3
  jejunum Q41.1
  pharynx Q38.8
  rectum Q42.1
    with fistula Q42.0
  urethra Q64.39
  vagina Q52.4
Impervious (congenital) (see also Atresia)
  anus Q42.3
    with fistula Q42.2
  bile duct Q44.2
  esophagus Q39.0
    with tracheoesophageal fistula Q39.1
  intestine (small) Q41.9
    large Q42.9
      specified NEC Q42.8
  rectum Q42.1
    with fistula Q42.0
  ureter — see Atresia, ureter
  urethra Q64.39
Impetiginization of dermatoses L01.1
Impetigo (any organism) (any site) (circinate) (conta-
    giosa) (simplex) (vulgaris) L01.00
  Bockhart's L01.02
  bullous, bullosa L01.03
  external ear L01.00 [H62.40]
  follicularis L01.02
  furfuracea L30.5
  herpetiformis L40.1
    nonobstetrical L40.1
  neonatorum L01.03
  nonbullous L01.01
  specified type NEC L01.09
  ulcerative L01.09
Impingement (on teeth)
  soft tissue
    anterior M26.81
    posterior M26.82
Implant, endometrial N80.9
Implantation
  anomalous — see Anomaly, by site
    ureter Q62.63
  cyst
    external area or site (skin) NEC L72.0
    iris — see Cyst, iris, implantation
    vagina N89.8
    vulva N90.7
  dermoid (cyst) — see Implantation, cyst
Impotence (sexual) N52.9
  counseling Z70.1
  organic origin (see also Dysfunction, sexual, male,
    erectile) N52.9
  psychogenic F52.21
Impression, basilar Q75.8
Imprisonment, anxiety concerning Z65.1
Improper care (child) (newborn) — see Maltreatment

Improperly tied umbilical cord (causing hemorrhage)
  P51.8
Impulsiveness (impulsive) R45.87
Inability to swallow — see Aphagia
Inaccessible, inaccessibility
  health care NEC Z75.3
    due to
      waiting period Z75.2
        for admission to facility elsewhere Z75.1
    other helping agencies Z75.4
Inactive — see condition
Inadequate, inadequacy
  aesthetics of dental restoration K08.56
  biologic, constitutional, functional, or social F60.7
  development
    child R62.50
    genitalia
      after puberty NEC E30.0
      congenital
        female Q52.8
          external Q52.79
          internal Q52.8
        male Q55.8
    lungs Q33.6
      associated with short gestation P28.0
    organ or site not listed — see Anomaly, by site
  diet (causing nutritional deficiency) E63.9
  eating habits Z72.4
  environment, household Z59.1
  family support Z63.8
  food (supply) NEC Z59.4
    hunger effects T73.0 ☑
  functional F60.7
  household care, due to
    family member
      handicapped or ill Z74.2
      on vacation Z75.5
      temporarily away from home Z74.2
    technical defects in home Z59.1
    temporary absence from home of person rendering
      care Z74.2
  housing (heating) (space) Z59.1
  income (financial) Z59.6
  intrafamilial communication Z63.8
  material resources Z59.9
  mental — see Disability, intellectual
  parental supervision or control of child Z62.0
  personality F60.7
  pulmonary
    function R06.89
      newborn P28.5
    ventilation, newborn P28.5
  sample of cytologic smear
    anus R85.615
    cervix R87.615
    vagina R87.625
  social F60.7
    insurance Z59.7
    skills NEC Z73.4
  supervision of child by parent Z62.0
  teaching affecting education Z55.8
  welfare support Z59.7
Inanition R64
  with edema — see Malnutrition, severe
  due to
    deprivation of food T73.0 ☑
    malnutrition — see Malnutrition
  fever R50.9
Inappropriate
  change in quantitative human chorionic gonadotropin
    (hCG) in early pregnancy O02.81
  diet or eating habits Z72.4
  level of quantitative human chorionic gonadotropin
    (hCG) for gestational age in early pregnancy
    O02.81
  secretion
    antidiuretic hormone (ADH) (excessive) E22.2
      deficiency E23.2
    pituitary (posterior) E22.2
Inattention at or after birth — see Neglect
Incarceration, incarcerated
  enterocele K46.0
    gangrenous K46.1
  epiplocele K46.0
    gangrenous K46.1
  exophthalmos K42.0
    gangrenous K42.1
  hernia (see also Hernia, by site, with obstruction)

Incarceration, incarcerated — continued
  hernia (see also Hernia, by site, with obstruction) —
    continued
    with gangrene — see Hernia, by site, with gan-
      grene
    iris, in wound — see Injury, eye, laceration, with pro-
      lapse
    lens, in wound — see Injury, eye, laceration, with
      prolapse
    omphalocele K42.0
    prison, anxiety concerning Z65.1
    rupture — see Hernia, by site
    sarcoepiplocele K46.0
      gangrenous K46.1
    sarcoepiplomphalocele K42.0
      with gangrene K42.1
    uterus N85.8
      gravid O34.51- ☑
        causing obstructed labor O65.5
Incised wound
  external — see Laceration
  internal organs — see Injury, by site
Incision, incisional
  hernia K43.2
    with
      gangrene (and obstruction) K43.1
      obstruction K43.0
    surgical, complication — see Complications, surgical
      procedure
    traumatic
      external — see Laceration
      internal organs — see Injury, by site
Inclusion
  azurophilic leukocytic D72.0
  blennorrhea (neonatal) (newborn) P39.1
  gallbladder in liver (congenital) Q44.1
Incompatibility
  ABO
    affecting management of pregnancy O36.11- ☑
      anti-A sensitization O36.11- ☑
      anti-B sensitization O36.19- ☑
      specified NEC O36.19- ☑
    infusion or transfusion reaction — see Complica-
      tion(s), transfusion, incompatibility reaction,
      ABO
    newborn P55.1
  blood (group) (Duffy) (K(ell)) (Kidd) (Lewis) (M) (S) NEC
    affecting management of pregnancy O36.11- ☑
      anti-A sensitization O36.11- ☑
      anti-B sensitization O36.19- ☑
    infusion or transfusion reaction T80.89 ☑
    newborn P55.8
  divorce or estrangement Z63.5
  Rh (blood group) (factor) Z31.82
    affecting management of pregnancy NEC
      O36.09- ☑
      anti-D antibody O36.01- ☑
    infusion or transfusion reaction — see Complica-
      tion(s), transfusion, incompatibility reaction,
      Rh (factor)
    newborn P55.0
  rhesus — see Incompatibility, Rh
Incompetency, incompetent, incompetence
  annular
    aortic (valve) — see Insufficiency, aortic
    mitral (valve) I34.0
    pulmonary valve (heart) I37.1
  aortic (valve) — see Insufficiency, aortic
  cardiac valve — see Endocarditis
  cervix, cervical (os) N88.3
    in pregnancy O34.3- ☑
  chronotropic I45.89
    with
      autonomic dysfunction G90.8
      ischemic heart disease I25.89
      left ventricular dysfunction I51.89
      sinus node dysfunction I49.8
  esophagogastric (junction) (sphincter) K22.0
  mitral (valve) — see Insufficiency, mitral
  pelvic fundus N81.89
  pubocervical tissue N81.82
  pulmonary valve (heart) I37.1
    congenital Q22.3
  rectovaginal tissue N81.83
  tricuspid (annular) (valve) — see Insufficiency, tricuspid
  valvular — see Endocarditis
    congenital Q24.8

☑ Additional Character Required — Refer to the Tabular List for Character Selection ▼ Subterms under main terms may continue to next column or page

Incompetency, incompetent, incompetence — *continued*
  vein, venous (saphenous) (varicose) — *see* Varix, leg
Incomplete (*see also* condition)
  bladder, emptying R33.9
  defecation R15.0
  expansion lungs (newborn) NEC — *see* Atelectasis
  rotation, intestine Q43.3
Inconclusive
  diagnostic imaging due to excess body fat of patient R93.9
  findings on diagnostic imaging of breast NEC R92.8
  mammogram (due to dense breasts) R92.2
Incontinence R32
  anal sphincter R15.9
  feces R15.9
    nonorganic origin F98.1
  overflow N39.490
  psychogenic F45.8
  rectal R15.9
  reflex N39.498
  stress (female) (male) N39.3
    and urge N39.46
  urethral sphincter R32
  urge N39.41
    and stress (female) (male) N39.46
  urine (urinary) R32
    continuous N39.45
    due to cognitive impairment, or severe physical disability or immobility R39.81
    functional R39.81
    mixed (stress and urge) N39.46
    nocturnal N39.44
    nonorganic origin F98.0
    overflow N39.490
    post dribbling N39.43
    reflex N39.498
    specified NEC N39.498
    stress (female) (male) N39.3
      and urge N39.46
    total N39.498
    unaware N39.42
    urge N39.41
      and stress (female) (male) N39.46
Incontinentia pigmenti Q82.3
Incoordinate, incoordination
  esophageal-pharyngeal (newborn) — *see* Dysphagia
  muscular R27.8
  uterus (action) (contractions) (complicating delivery) O62.4
Increase, increased
  abnormal, in development R63.8
  androgens (ovarian) E28.1
  anticoagulants (antithrombin) (anti-VIIIa) (anti-IXa) (anti-Xa) (anti-XIa) — *see* Circulating anticoagulants
  cold sense R20.8
  estrogen E28.0
  function
    adrenal
      cortex — *see* Cushing's, syndrome
      medulla E27.5
    pituitary (gland) (anterior) (lobe) E22.9
      posterior E22.2
  heat sense R20.8
  intracranial pressure (benign) G93.2
  permeability, capillaries I78.8
  pressure, intracranial G93.2
  secretion
    gastrin E16.4
    glucagon E16.3
    pancreas, endocrine E16.9
      growth hormone-releasing hormone E16.8
      pancreatic polypeptide E16.8
      somatostatin E16.8
      vasoactive-intestinal polypeptide E16.8
  sphericity, lens Q12.4
  splenic activity D73.1
  venous pressure I87.8
    portal K76.6
Increta placenta O43.22- ☑
Incrustation, cornea, foreign body (lead)(zinc) — *see* Foreign body, cornea
Incyclophoria H50.54
Incyclotropia — *see* Cyclotropia
Indeterminate sex Q56.4
India rubber skin Q82.8
Indigestion (acid) (bilious) (functional) K30

Indigestion — *continued*
  catarrhal K31.89
  due to decomposed food NOS A05.9
  nervous F45.8
  psychogenic F45.8
Indirect — *see* condition
Induratio penis plastica N48.6
Induration, indurated
  brain G93.89
  breast (fibrous) N64.51
    puerperal, postpartum O92.29
  broad ligament N83.8
  chancre
    anus A51.1
    congenital A50.07
    extragenital NEC A51.2
  corpora cavernosa (penis) (plastic) N48.6
  liver (chronic) K76.89
  lung (black) (chronic) (fibroid) (*see also* Fibrosis, lung) J84.10
    essential brown J84.03
  penile (plastic) N48.6
  phlebitic — *see* Phlebitis
  skin R23.4
Inebriety (without dependence) — *see* Alcohol, intoxication
Inefficiency, kidney N28.9
Inelasticity, skin R23.4
Inequality, leg (length) (acquired) (*see also* Deformity, limb, unequal length)
  congenital — *see* Defect, reduction, lower limb
  lower leg — *see* Deformity, limb, unequal length
Inertia
  bladder (neurogenic) N31.2
  stomach K31.89
    psychogenic F45.8
  uterus, uterine during labor O62.2
    during latent phase of labor O62.0
    primary O62.0
    secondary O62.1
  vesical (neurogenic) N31.2
Infancy, infantile, infantilism (*see also* condition)
  celiac K90.0
  genitalia, genitals (after puberty) E30.0
  Herter's (nontropical sprue) K90.0
  intestinal K90.0
  Lorain E23.0
  pancreatic K86.8
  pelvis M95.5
    with disproportion (fetopelvic) O33.1
      causing obstructed labor O65.1
  pituitary E23.0
  renal N25.0
  uterus — *see* Infantile, genitalia
Infant(s) (*see also* Infancy)
  excessive crying R68.11
  irritable child R68.12
  lack of care — *see* Neglect
  liveborn (singleton) Z38.2
    born in hospital Z38.00
      by cesarean Z38.01
    born outside hospital Z38.1
    multiple NEC Z38.8
      born in hospital Z38.68
        by cesarean Z38.69
      born outside hospital Z38.7
    quadruplet Z38.8
      born in hospital Z38.63
        by cesarean Z38.64
      born outside hospital Z38.7
    quintuplet Z38.8
      born in hospital Z38.65
        by cesarean Z38.66
      born outside hospital Z38.7
    triplet Z38.8
      born in hospital Z38.61
        by cesarean Z38.62
      born outside hospital Z38.7
    twin Z38.5
      born in hospital Z38.30
        by cesarean Z38.31
      born outside hospital Z38.4
  of diabetic mother (syndrome of) P70.1
    gestational diabetes P70.0
Infantile (*see also* condition)
  genitalia, genitals E30.0
  os, uterine E30.0
  penis E30.0

Infantile — *continued*
  testis E29.1
  uterus E30.0
Infantilism — *see* Infancy
Infarct, infarction
  adrenal (capsule) (gland) E27.49
  appendices epiploicae K55.0
  bowel K55.0
  brain (stem) — *see* Infarct, cerebral
  breast N64.89
  brewer's (kidney) N28.0
  cardiac — *see* Infarct, myocardium
  cerebellar — *see* Infarct, cerebral
  cerebral (*see also* Occlusion, artery cerebral or precerebral, with infarction) I63.9
    aborted I63.9
    cortical I63.9
    due to
      cerebral venous thrombosis, nonpyogenic I63.6
      embolism
        cerebral arteries I63.4- ☑
        precerebral arteries I63.1- ☑
      occlusion NEC
        cerebral arteries I63.5- ☑
        precerebral arteries I63.2- ☑
      stenosis NEC
        cerebral arteries I63.5- ☑
        precerebral arteries I63.2- ☑
      thrombosis
        cerebral artery I63.3- ☑
        precerebral artery I63.0- ☑
    intraoperative
      during cardiac surgery I97.810
      during other surgery I97.811
    postprocedural
      following cardiac surgery I97.820
      following other surgery I97.821
    specified NEC I63.8
  colon (acute) (agnogenic) (embolic) (hemorrhagic) (nonocclusive) (nonthrombotic) (occlusive) (segmental) (thrombotic) (with gangrene) K55.0
  coronary artery — *see* Infarct, myocardium
  embolic — *see* Embolism
  fallopian tube N83.8
  gallbladder K82.8
  heart — *see* Infarct, myocardium
  hepatic K76.3
  hypophysis (anterior lobe) E23.6
  impending (myocardium) I20.0
  intestine (acute) (agnogenic) (embolic) (hemorrhagic) (nonocclusive) (nonthrombotic) (occlusive) (thrombotic) (with gangrene) K55.0
  kidney N28.0
  liver K76.3
  lung (embolic) (thrombotic) — *see* Embolism, pulmonary
  lymph node I89.8
  mesentery, mesenteric (embolic) (thrombotic) (with gangrene) K55.0
  muscle (ischemic) M62.20
    ankle M62.27- ☑
    foot M62.27- ☑
    forearm M62.23- ☑
    hand M62.24- ☑
    lower leg M62.26- ☑
    pelvic region M62.25- ☑
    shoulder region M62.21- ☑
    specified site NEC M62.28
    thigh M62.25- ☑
    upper arm M62.22- ☑
  myocardium, myocardial (acute) (with stated duration of 4 weeks or less) I21.3
    diagnosed on ECG, but presenting no symptoms I25.2
    healed or old I25.2
    intraoperative
      during cardiac surgery I97.790
      during other surgery I97.791
    non-Q wave I21.4
    non-ST elevation (NSTEMI) I21.4
      subsequent I22.2
    nontransmural I21.4
    past (diagnosed on ECG or other investigation, but currently presenting no symptoms) I25.2
    postprocedural
      following cardiac surgery I97.190
      following other surgery I97.191
    Q wave (*see also*, Infarct, myocardium, by site) I21.3

Infarct, infarction — continued
  myocardium, myocardial — continued
    ST elevation (STEMI) I21.3
      anterior (anteroapical) (anterolateral) (anteroseptal) (Q wave) (wall) I21.09
        subsequent I22.0
      inferior (diaphragmatic) (inferolateral) (inferoposterior) (wall) NEC I21.19
        subsequent I22.1
      inferoposterior transmural (Q wave) I21.11
      involving
        coronary artery of anterior wall NEC I21.09
        coronary artery of inferior wall NEC I21.19
        diagonal coronary artery I21.02
        left anterior descending coronary artery I21.02
        left circumflex coronary artery I21.21
        left main coronary artery I21.01
        oblique marginal coronary artery I21.21
        right coronary artery I21.11
      lateral (apical-lateral) (basal-lateral) (high) I21.29
        subsequent I22.8
      posterior (posterobasal) (posterolateral) (posteroseptal) (true) I21.29
        subsequent I22.8
      septal I21.29
        subsequent I22.8
      specified NEC I21.29
        subsequent I22.8
      subsequent I22.9
    subsequent (recurrent) (reinfarction) I22.9
      anterior (anteroapical) (anterolateral) (anteroseptal) (wall) I22.0
      diaphragmatic (wall) I22.1
      inferior (diaphragmatic) (inferolateral) (inferoposterior) (wall) I22.1
      lateral (apical-lateral) (basal-lateral) (high) I22.8
      non-ST elevation (NSTEMI) I22.2
      posterior (posterobasal) (posterolateral) (posteroseptal) (true) I22.8
      septal I22.8
      specified NEC I22.8
      ST elevation I22.9
        anterior (anteroapical) (anterolateral) (anteroseptal) (wall) I22.0
        inferior (diaphragmatic) (inferolateral) (inferoposterior) (wall) I22.1
        specified NEC I22.8
      subendocardial I22.2
      transmural I22.9
        anterior (anteroapical) (anterolateral) (anteroseptal) (wall) I22.0
        diaphragmatic (wall) I22.1
        inferior (diaphragmatic) (inferolateral) (inferoposterior) (wall) I22.1
        lateral (apical-lateral) (basal-lateral) (high) I22.8
        posterior (posterobasal) (posterolateral) (posteroseptal) (true) I22.8
        specified NEC I22.8
    syphilitic A52.06
    transmural I21.3
      anterior (anteroapical) (anterolateral) (anteroseptal) (Q wave) (wall) NEC I21.09
      inferior (diaphragmatic) (inferolateral) (inferoposterior) (Q wave) (wall) NEC I21.19
      inferoposterior (Q wave) I21.11
      lateral (apical-lateral) (basal-lateral) (high) NEC I21.29
      posterior (posterobasal) (posterolateral) (posteroseptal) (true) NEC I21.29
      septal NEC I21.29
      specified NEC I21.29
  nontransmural I21.4
  omentum K55.0
  ovary N83.8
  pancreas K86.8
  papillary muscle — see Infarct, myocardium
  parathyroid gland E21.4
  pituitary (gland) E23.6
  placenta O43.81- ☑
  prostate N42.89
  pulmonary (artery) (vein) (hemorrhagic) — see Embolism, pulmonary
  renal (embolic) (thrombotic) N28.0
  retina, retinal (artery) — see Occlusion, artery, retina
  spinal (cord) (acute) (embolic) (nonembolic) G95.11

Infarct, infarction — continued
  spleen D73.5
    embolic or thrombotic I74.8
  subendocardial (acute) (nontransmural) I21.4
  suprarenal (capsule) (gland) E27.49
  testis N50.1
  thrombotic (see also Thrombosis)
    artery, arterial — see Embolism
  thyroid (gland) E07.89
  ventricle (heart) — see Infarct, myocardium
Infecting — see condition
Infection, infected, infective (opportunistic) B99.9
  with
    drug resistant organism — see Resistance (to), drug (see also specific organism)
    lymphangitis — see Lymphangitis
    organ dysfunction (acute) R65.20
      with septic shock R65.21
  abscess (skin) — code by site under Abscess
  Absidia — see Mucormycosis
  Acanthamoeba — see Acanthamebiasis
  Acanthocheilonema (perstans) (streptocerca) B74.4
  accessory sinus (chronic) — see Sinusitis
  achorion — see Dermatophytosis
  acromioclavicular M00.9
  Acremonium falciforme B47.0
  Actinobacillus (actinomycetem-comitans) A28.8
    mallei A24.0
    muris A25.1
  Actinomadura B47.1
  Actinomyces (israelii) (see also Actinomycosis) A42.9
  Actinomycetales — see Actinomycosis
  actinomycotic NOS — see Actinomycosis
  adenoid (and tonsil) J03.90
    chronic J35.02
  adenovirus NEC
    as cause of disease classified elsewhere B97.0
    unspecified nature or site B34.0
  aerogenes capsulatus A48.0
  aertrycke — see Infection, salmonella
  alimentary canal NOS — see Enteritis, infectious
  Allescheria boydii B48.2
  Alternaria B48.8
  alveolus, alveolar (process) K04.7
  Ameba, amebic (histolytica) — see Amebiasis
  amniotic fluid, sac or cavity O41.10- ☑
    chorioamnionitis O41.12- ☑
      placentitis O41.14- ☑
  amputation stump (surgical) — see Complication, amputation stump, infection
  Ancylostoma (duodenalis) B76.0
  Anisakiasis, Anisakis larvae B81.0
  anthrax — see Anthrax
  antrum (chronic) — see Sinusitis, maxillary
  anus, anal (papillae) (sphincter) K62.89
  arbovirus (arbor virus) A94
    specified type NEC A93.8
  artificial insemination N98.0
  Ascaris lumbricoides — see Ascariasis
  Ascomycetes B47.0
  Aspergillus (flavus) (fumigatus) (terreus) — see Aspergillosis
  atypical
    acid-fast (bacilli) — see Mycobacterium, atypical
    mycobacteria — see Mycobacterium, atypical
    virus A81.9
      specified type NEC A81.89
  auditory meatus (external) — see Otitis, externa, infective
  auricle (ear) — see Otitis, externa, infective
  axillary gland (lymph) L04.2
  Bacillus A49.9
    abortus A23.1
    anthracis — see Anthrax
    Ducrey's (any location) A57
    Flexner's A03.1
    Friedländer's NEC A49.8
    gas (gangrene) A48.0
    mallei A24.0
    melitensis A23.0
    paratyphoid, paratyphosus A01.4
      A A01.1
      B A01.2
      C A01.3
    Shiga (-Kruse) A03.0
    suipestifer — see Infection, salmonella
    swimming pool A31.1

Infection, infected, infective — continued
  Bacillus — continued
    typhosa A01.00
    welchii — see Gangrene, gas
  bacterial NOS A49.9
    as cause of disease classified elsewhere B96.89
      Bacteroides fragilis [B. fragilis] B96.6
      Clostridium perfringens [C. perfringens] B96.7
      Enterobacter sakazakii B96.89
      Enterococcus B95.2
      Escherichia coli [E. coli] (see also Escherichia coli) B96.20
      Helicobacter pylori [H.pylori] B96.81
      Hemophilus influenzae [H. influenzae] B96.3
      Klebsiella pneumoniae [K. pneumoniae] B96.1
      Mycoplasma pneumoniae [M. pneumoniae] B96.0
      Proteus (mirabilis) (morganii) B96.4
      Pseudomonas (aeruginosa) (mallei) (pseudomallei) B96.5
      Staphylococcus B95.8
        aureus (methicillin susceptible) (MSSA) B95.61
        methicillin resistant (MRSA) B95.62
        specified NEC B95.7
      Streptococcus B95.5
        group A B95.0
        group B B95.1
        pneumoniae B95.3
        specified NEC B95.4
      Vibrio vulnificus B96.82
    specified NEC A48.8
  Bacterium
    paratyphosum A01.4
      A A01.1
      B A01.2
      C A01.3
    typhosum A01.00
  Bacteroides NEC A49.8
    fragilis, as cause of disease classified elsewhere B96.6
  Balantidium coli A07.0
  Bartholin's gland N75.8
  Basidiobolus B46.8
  bile duct (common) (hepatic) — see Cholangitis
  bladder — see Cystitis
  Blastomyces, blastomycotic (see also Blastomycosis)
    brasiliensis — see Paracoccidioidomycosis
    dermatitidis — see Blastomycosis
    European — see Cryptococcosis
    Loboi B48.0
    North American B40.9
    South American — see Paracoccidioidomycosis
  bleb, postprocedure — see Blebitis
  bone — see Osteomyelitis
  Bordetella — see Whooping cough
  Borrelia bergdorfi A69.20
  brain (see also Encephalitis) G04.90
    membranes — see Meningitis
    septic G06.0
      meninges — see Meningitis, bacterial
  branchial cyst Q18.0
  breast — see Mastitis
  bronchus — see Bronchitis
  Brucella A23.9
    abortus A23.1
    canis A23.3
    melitensis A23.0
    mixed A23.8
    specified NEC A23.8
    suis A23.2
  Brugia (malayi) B74.1
    timori B74.2
  bursa — see Bursitis, infective
  buttocks (skin) L08.9
  Campylobacter, intestinal A04.5
    as cause of disease classified elsewhere B96.81
  Candida (albicans) (tropicalis) — see Candidiasis
  candiru B88.8
  Capillaria (intestinal) B81.1
    hepatica B83.8
    philippinensis B81.1
  cartilage — see Disorder, cartilage, specified type NEC
  cat liver fluke B66.0
  catheter-related bloodstream (CRBSI) T80.211 ☑
  cellulitis — code by site under Cellulitis
  central line-associated T80.219 ☑
    bloodstream (CLABSI) T80.211 ☑

Infection, infected, infective — *continued*
- central line-associated — *continued*
  - specified NEC B80.218 ☑
- Cephalosporium falciforme B47.0
- cerebrospinal — *see* Meningitis
- cervical gland (lymph) L04.0
- cervix — *see* Cervicitis
- cesarean delivery wound (puerperal) O86.0
- cestodes — *see* Infestation, cestodes
- chest J22
- Chilomastix (intestinal) A07.8
- Chlamydia, chlamydial A74.9
  - anus A56.3
  - genitourinary tract A56.2
    - lower A56.00
      - specified NEC A56.19
  - lymphogranuloma A55
  - pharynx A56.4
  - psittaci A70
  - rectum A56.3
  - sexually transmitted NEC A56.8
- cholera — *see* Cholera
- Cladosporium
  - bantianum (brain abscess) B43.1
  - carrionii B43.0
  - castellanii B36.1
  - trichoides (brain abscess) B43.1
  - werneckii B36.1
- Clonorchis (sinensis) (liver) B66.1
- Clostridium NEC
  - bifermentans A48.0
  - botulinum (food poisoning) A05.1
    - infant A48.51
    - wound A48.52
  - difficile
    - as cause of disease classified elsewhere B96.89
    - foodborne (disease) A04.7
    - gas gangrene A48.0
    - necrotizing enterocolitis A04.7
    - sepsis A41.4
  - gas-forming NEC A48.0
  - histolyticum A48.0
  - novyi, causing gas gangrene A48.0
  - oedematiens A48.0
  - perfringens
    - as cause of disease classified elsewhere B96.7
    - due to food A05.2
    - foodborne (disease) A05.2
    - gas gangrene A48.0
    - sepsis A41.4
  - septicum, causing gas gangrene A48.0
  - sordellii, causing gas gangrene A48.0
  - welchii
    - as cause of disease classified elsewhere B96.7
    - foodborne (disease) A05.2
    - gas gangrene A48.0 ☑
    - necrotizing enteritis A05.2
    - sepsis A41.4
- Coccidioides (immitis) — *see* Coccidioidomycosis
- colon — *see* Enteritis, infectious
- colostomy K94.02
- common duct — *see* Cholangitis
- congenital P39.9
  - Candida (albicans) P37.5
  - cytomegalovirus P35.1
  - hepatitis, viral P35.3
  - herpes simplex P35.2
  - infectious or parasitic disease P37.9
    - specified NEC P37.8
  - listeriosis (disseminated) P37.2
  - malaria NEC P37.4
    - falciparum P37.3
  - Plasmodium falciparum P37.3
  - poliomyelitis P35.8
  - rubella P35.0
  - skin P39.4
  - toxoplasmosis (acute) (subacute) (chronic) P37.1
  - tuberculosis P37.0
  - urinary (tract) P39.3
  - vaccinia P35.8
  - virus P35.9
    - specified type NEC P35.8
- Conidiobolus B46.8
- coronavirus NEC B34.2
  - as cause of disease classified elsewhere B97.29
  - severe acute respiratory syndrome (SARS associated) B97.21
- corpus luteum — *see* Salpingo-oophoritis

Infection, infected, infective — *continued*
- Corynebacterium diphtheriae — *see* Diphtheria
- cotia virus B08.8
- Coxiella burnetii A78
- coxsackie — *see* Coxsackie
- Cryptococcus neoformans — *see* Cryptococcosis
- Cryptosporidium A07.2
- Cunninghamella — *see* Mucormycosis
- cyst — *see* Cyst
- cystic duct (*see also* Cholecystitis) K81.9
- Cysticercus cellulosae — *see* Cysticercosis
- cytomegalovirus, cytomegaloviral B25.9
  - congenital P35.1
  - maternal, maternal care for (suspected) damage to fetus O35.3 ☑
  - mononucleosis B27.10
    - with
      - complication NEC B27.19
      - meningitis B27.12
      - polyneuropathy B27.11
- delta-agent (acute), in hepatitis B carrier B17.0
- dental (pulpal origin) K04.7
- Deuteromycetes B47.0
- Dicrocoelium dendriticum B66.2
- Dipetalonema (perstans) (streptocerca) B74.4
- diphtherial — *see* Diphtheria
- Diphyllobothrium (adult) (latum) (pacificum) B70.0
  - larval B70.1
- Diplogonoporus (grandis) B71.8
- Dipylidium caninum B67.4
- Dirofilaria B74.8
- Dracunculus medinensis B72
- Drechslera (hawaiiensis) B43.8
- Ducrey Haemophilus (any location) A57
- due to or resulting from
  - artificial insemination N98.0
  - central venous catheter T80.219 ☑
    - bloodstream T80.211 ☑
    - exit or insertion site T80.212 ☑
    - localized T80.212 ☑
    - port or reservoir T80.212 ☑
    - specified NEC T80.218 ☑
    - tunnel T80.212 ☑
  - device, implant or graft (*see also* Complications, by site and type, infection or inflammation) T85.79 ☑
    - arterial graft NEC T82.7 ☑
    - breast (implant) T85.79 ☑
    - catheter NEC T85.79 ☑
      - dialysis (renal) T82.7 ☑
        - intraperitoneal T85.71 ☑
      - infusion NEC T82.7 ☑
        - spinal (epidural) (subdural) T85.79 ☑
      - urinary (indwelling) T83.51 ☑
    - electronic (electrode) (pulse generator) (stimulator)
      - bone T84.7 ☑
      - cardiac T82.7 ☑
      - nervous system (brain) (peripheral nerve) (spinal) T85.79 ☑
      - urinary T83.59 ☑
    - fixation, internal (orthopedic) NEC — *see* Complication, fixation device, infection
    - gastrointestinal (bile duct) (esophagus) T85.79 ☑
    - genital NEC T83.6 ☑
    - heart NEC T82.7 ☑
      - valve (prosthesis) T82.6 ☑
        - graft T82.7 ☑
    - joint prosthesis — *see* Complication, joint prosthesis, infection
    - ocular (corneal graft) (orbital implant) NEC T85.79 ☑
    - orthopedic NEC T84.7 ☑
    - specified NEC T85.79 ☑
    - urinary NEC T83.59 ☑
    - vascular NEC T82.7 ☑
    - ventricular intracranial shunt T85.79 ☑
  - Hickman catheter T80.219 ☑
    - bloodstream T80.211 ☑
    - localized T80.212 ☑
    - specified NEC T80.218 ☑
  - immunization or vaccination T88.0 ☑
  - infusion, injection or transfusion NEC T80.29 ☑
  - injury NEC — *code by* site under Wound, open
  - peripherally inserted central catheter (PICC) T80.219 ☑

Infection, infected, infective — *continued*
- due to or resulting from — *continued*
  - peripherally inserted central catheter — *continued*
    - bloodstream T80.211 ☑
    - localized T80.212 ☑
    - specified NEC T80.218 ☑
  - portacath (port-a-cath) T80.219 ☑
    - bloodstream T80.211 ☑
    - localized T80.212 ☑
    - specified NEC T80.218 ☑
  - surgery T81.4 ☑
  - triple lumen catheter T80.219 ☑
    - bloodstream T80.211 ☑
    - localized T80.212 ☑
    - specified NEC T80.218 ☑
  - umbilical venous catheter T80.219 ☑
    - bloodstream T80.211 ☑
    - localized T80.212 ☑
    - specified NEC T80.218 ☑
- during labor NEC O75.3
- ear (middle) (*see also* Otitis media)
  - external — *see* Otitis, externa, infective
  - inner — *see* subcategory H83.0 ☑
- Eberthella typhosa A01.00
- Echinococcus — *see* Echinococcus
- echovirus
  - as cause of disease classified elsewhere B97.12
  - unspecified nature or site B34.1
- endocardium I33.0
- endocervix — *see* Cervicitis
- Entamoeba — *see* Amebiasis
- enteric — *see* Enteritis, infectious
- Enterobacter sakazakii B96.89
- Enterobius vermicularis B80
- enterostomy K94.12
- enterovirus B34.1
  - as cause of disease classified elsewhere B97.10
    - coxsackievirus B97.11
    - echovirus B97.12
    - specified NEC B97.19
- Entomophthora B46.8
- Epidermophyton — *see* Dermatophytosis
- epididymis — *see* Epididymitis
- episiotomy (puerperal) O86.0
- Erysipelothrix (insidiosa) (rhusiopathiae) — *see* Erysipeloid
- erythema infectiosum B08.3
- Escherichia (E.) coli NEC A49.8
  - as cause of disease classified elsewhere (*see also* Escherichia coli) B96.20
    - congenital P39.8
    - sepsis P36.4
  - generalized A41.51
  - intestinal — *see* Enteritis, infectious, due to, Escherichia coli
- ethmoidal (chronic) (sinus) — *see* Sinusitis, ethmoidal
- eustachian tube (ear) — *see* Salpingitis, eustachian
- external auditory canal (meatus) NEC — *see* Otitis, externa, infective
- eye (purulent) — *see* Endophthalmitis, purulent
- eyelid — *see* Inflammation, eyelid
- fallopian tube — *see* Salpingo-oophoritis
- Fasciola (gigantica) (hepatica) (indica) B66.3
- Fasciolopsis (buski) B66.5
- filarial — *see* Infestation, filarial
- finger (skin) L08.9
  - nail L03.01- ☑
    - fungus B35.1
- fish tapeworm B70.0
  - larval B70.1
- flagellate, intestinal A07.9
- fluke — *see* Infestation, fluke
- focal
  - teeth (pulpal origin) K04.7
  - tonsils J35.01
- Fonsecaea (compactum) (pedrosoi) B43.0
- food — *see* Intoxication, foodborne
- foot (skin) L08.9
  - dermatophytic fungus B35.3
- Francisella tularensis — *see* Tularemia
- frontal (sinus) (chronic) — *see* Sinusitis, frontal
- fungus NOS B49
  - beard B35.0
  - dermatophytic — *see* Dermatophytosis
  - foot B35.3
  - groin B35.6

Infection, infected, infective — *continued*
- fungus — *continued*
  - hand B35.2
  - nail B35.1
  - pathogenic to compromised host only B48.8
  - perianal (area) B35.6
  - scalp B35.0
  - skin B36.9
    - foot B35.3
    - hand B35.2
    - toenails B35.1
- Fusarium B48.8
- gallbladder — *see* Cholecystitis
- gas bacillus — *see* Gangrene, gas
- gastrointestinal — *see* Enteritis, infectious
- generalized NEC — *see* Sepsis
- genital organ or tract
  - female — *see* Disease, pelvis, inflammatory
  - male N49.9
    - multiple sites N49.8
    - specified NEC N49.8
- Ghon tubercle, primary A15.7
- Giardia lamblia A07.1
- gingiva (chronic) K05.10
  - acute K05.00
    - nonplaque induced K05.01
    - plaque induced K05.00
  - nonplaque induced K05.11
  - plaque induced K05.10
- glanders A24.0
- glenosporopsis B48.0
- Gnathostoma (spinigerum) B83.1
- Gongylonema B83.8
- gonococcal — *see* Gonococcus
- gram-negative bacilli NOS A49.9
- guinea worm B72
- gum (chronic) K05.10
  - acute K05.00
    - nonplaque induced K05.01
    - plaque induced K05.00
  - nonplaque induced K05.11
  - plaque induced K05.10
- Haemophilus — *see* Infection, Hemophilus
- heart — *see* Carditis
- Helicobacter pylori A04.8
  - as cause of disease classified elsewhere B96.81
- helminths B83.9
  - intestinal B82.0
    - mixed (types classifiable to more than one of the titles B65.0-B81.3 and B81.8) B81.4
    - specified type NEC B81.8
  - specified type NEC B83.8
- Hemophilus
  - aegyptius, systemic A48.4
  - ducrey (any location) A57
  - generalized A41.3
  - influenzae NEC A49.2
    - as cause of disease classified elsewhere B96.3
- herpes (simplex) (*see also* Herpes)
  - congenital P35.2
  - disseminated B00.7
  - zoster B02.9
- herpesvirus, herpesviral — *see* Herpes
- Heterophyes (heterophyes) B66.8
- hip (joint) NEC M00.9
  - due to internal joint prosthesis
    - left T84.52 ☑
    - right T84.51 ☑
  - skin NEC L08.9
- Histoplasma — *see* Histoplasmosis
  - American B39.4
  - capsulatum B39.4
- hookworm B76.9
- human
  - papilloma virus A63.0
  - T-cell lymphotropic virus type-1 (HTLV-1) B33.3
- hydrocele N43.0
- Hymenolepis B71.0
- hypopharynx — *see* Pharyngitis
- inguinal (lymph) glands L04.1
  - due to soft chancre A57
- intervertebral disc, pyogenic M46.30
  - cervical region M46.32
  - cervicothoracic region M46.33
  - lumbar region M46.36
  - lumbosacral region M46.37
  - multiple sites M46.39
  - occipito-atlanto-axial region M46.31

Infection, infected, infective — *continued*
- intervertebral disc, pyogenic — *continued*
  - sacrococcygeal region M46.38
  - thoracic region M46.34
  - thoracolumbar region M46.35
- intestine, intestinal — *see* Enteritis, infectious
  - specified NEC A08.8
- intra-amniotic affecting newborn NEC P39.2
- Isospora belli or hominis A07.3
- Japanese B encephalitis A83.0
- jaw (bone) (lower) (upper) M27.2
- joint NEC M00.9
  - due to internal joint prosthesis T84.50 ☑
- kidney (cortex) (hematogenous) N15.9
  - with calculus N20.0
    - with hydronephrosis N13.6
  - following ectopic gestation O08.83
  - pelvis and ureter (cystic) N28.85
  - puerperal (postpartum) O86.21
  - specified NEC N15.8
- Klebsiella (K.) pneumoniae NEC A49.8
  - as cause of disease classified elsewhere B96.1
- knee (joint) NEC M00.9
  - due to internal joint prosthesis
    - left T84.54 ☑
    - right T84.53 ☑
  - joint M00.9
  - skin L08.9
- Koch's — *see* Tuberculosis
- labia (majora) (minora) (acute) — *see* Vulvitis
- lacrimal
  - gland — *see* Dacryoadenitis
  - passages (duct) (sac) — *see* Inflammation, lacrimal, passages
- lancet fluke B66.2
- larynx NEC J38.7
- leg (skin) NOS L08.9
- Legionella pneumophila A48.1
  - nonpneumonic A48.2
- Leishmania (*see also* Leishmaniasis)
  - aethiopica B55.1
  - braziliensis B55.2
  - chagasi B55.0
  - donovani B55.0
  - infantum B55.0
  - major B55.1
  - mexicana B55.1
  - tropica B55.1
- lentivirus, as cause of disease classified elsewhere B97.31
- Leptosphaeria senegalensis B47.0
- Leptospira interrogans A27.9
  - autumnalis A27.89
  - canicola A27.89
  - hebdomadis A27.89
  - icterohaemorrhagiae A27.0
  - pomona A27.89
  - specified type NEC A27.89
- leptospirochetal NEC — *see* Leptospirosis
- Listeria monocytogenes (*see also* Listeriosis)
  - congenital P37.2
- Loa loa B74.3
  - with conjunctival infestation B74.3
  - eyelid B74.3
- Loboa loboi B48.0
- local, skin (staphylococcal) (streptococcal) L08.9
  - abscess — *code by* site under Abscess
  - cellulitis — *code by* site under Cellulitis
  - specified NEC L08.89
  - ulcer — *see* Ulcer, skin
- Loefflerella mallei A24.0
- lung (*see also* Pneumonia) J18.9
  - atypical Mycobacterium A31.0
  - spirochetal A69.8
  - tuberculous — *see* Tuberculosis, pulmonary
  - virus — *see* Pneumonia, viral
- lymph gland (*see also* Lymphadenitis, acute)
  - mesenteric I88.0
- lymphoid tissue, base of tongue or posterior pharynx, NEC (chronic) J35.03
- Madurella (grisea) (mycetomii) B47.0
- major
  - following ectopic or molar pregnancy O08.0
  - puerperal, postpartum, childbirth O85
- Malassezia furfur B36.0
- Malleomyces
  - mallei A24.0
  - pseudomallei (whitmori) — *see* Melioidosis

Infection, infected, infective — *continued*
- mammary gland N61
- Mansonella (ozzardi) (perstans) (streptocerca) B74.4
- mastoid — *see* Mastoiditis
- maxilla, maxillary M27.2
  - sinus (chronic) — *see* Sinusitis, maxillary
- mediastinum J98.5
- Medina (worm) B72
- meibomian cyst or gland — *see* Hordeolum
- meninges — *see* Meningitis, bacterial
- meningococcal (*see also* condition) A39.9
  - adrenals A39.1
  - brain A39.81
  - cerebrospinal A39.0
  - conjunctiva A39.89
  - endocardium A39.51
  - heart A39.50
    - endocardium A39.51
    - myocardium A39.52
    - pericardium A39.53
  - joint A39.83
  - meninges A39.0
  - meningococcemia A39.4
    - acute A39.2
    - chronic A39.3
  - myocardium A39.52
  - pericardium A39.53
  - retrobulbar neuritis A39.82
  - specified site NEC A39.89
- mesenteric lymph nodes or glands NEC I88.0
- Metagonimus B66.8
- metatarsophalangeal M00.9
- methicillin
  - resistant Staphylococcus aureus (MRSA) A49.02
  - susceptible Staphylococcus aureus (MSSA) A49.01
- Microsporum, microsporic — *see* Dermatophytosis
- mixed flora (bacterial) NEC A49.8
- Monilia — *see* Candidiasis
- Monosporium apiospermum B48.2
- mouth, parasitic B37.0
- Mucor — *see* Mucormycosis
- muscle NEC — *see* Myositis, infective
- mycelium NOS B49
- mycetoma B47.9
  - actinomycotic NEC B47.1
  - mycotic NEC B47.0
- Mycobacterium, mycobacterial — *see* Mycobacterium
- Mycoplasma NEC A49.3
  - pneumoniae, as cause of disease classified elsewhere B96.0
- mycotic NOS B49
  - pathogenic to compromised host only B48.8
  - skin NOS B36.9
- myocardium NEC I40.0
- nail (chronic)
  - with lymphangitis — *see* Lymphangitis, acute, digit
  - finger L03.01- ☑
    - fungus B35.1
  - ingrowing L60.0
  - toe L03.03- ☑
    - fungus B35.1
- nasal sinus (chronic) — *see* Sinusitis
- nasopharynx — *see* Nasopharyngitis
- navel L08.82
- Necator americanus B76.1
- Neisseria — *see* Gonococcus
- Neotestudina rosatii B47.0
- newborn P39.9
  - intra-amniotic NEC P39.2
  - skin P39.4
  - specified type NEC P39.8
- nipple N61
  - associated with
    - lactation O91.03
    - pregnancy O91.01- ☑
    - puerperium O91.02
- Nocardia — *see* Nocardiosis
- obstetrical surgical wound (puerperal) O86.0
- Oesophagostomum (apiostomum) B81.8
- Oestrus ovis — *see* Myiasis
- Oidium albicans B37.9
- Onchocerca (volvulus) — *see* Onchocerciasis
- oncovirus, as cause of disease classified elsewhere B97.32
- operation wound T81.4 ☑
- Opisthorchis (felineus) (viverrini) B66.0
- orbit, orbital — *see* Inflammation, orbit

Infection, infected, infective — *continued*
orthopoxvirus NEC B08.09
ovary — *see* Salpingo-oophoritis
Oxyuris vermicularis B80
pancreas (acute) K85.9
  abscess — *see* Pancreatitis, acute
  specified NEC K85.8
papillomavirus, as cause of disease classified elsewhere
  B97.7
papovavirus NEC B34.4
Paracoccidioides brasiliensis — *see* Paracoccidioidomycosis
Paragonimus (westermani) B66.4
parainfluenza virus B34.8
paramΕningococcus NOS A39.9
parapoxvirus B08.60
  specified NEC B08.69
parasitic B89
Parastrongylus
  cantonensis B83.2
  costaricensis B81.3
  paratyphoid A01.4
    Type A A01.1
    Type B A01.2
    Type C A01.3
paraurethral ducts N34.2
parotid gland — *see* Sialoadenitis
parvovirus NEC B34.3
  as cause of disease classified elsewhere B97.6
Pasteurella NEC A28.0
  multocida A28.0
  pestis — *see* Plague
  pseudotuberculosis A28.0
  septica (cat bite) (dog bite) A28.0
  tularensis — *see* Tularemia
pelvic, female — *see* Disease, pelvis, inflammatory
Penicillium (marneffei) B48.4
penis (glans) (retention) NEC N48.29
periapical K04.5
peridental, periodontal K05.20
  generalized K05.22
  localized K05.21
perinatal period P39.9
  specified type NEC P39.8
perineal repair (puerperal) O86.0
periorbital — *see* Inflammation, orbit
perirectal K62.89
perirenal — *see* Infection, kidney
peritoneal — *see* Peritonitis
periureteral N28.89
Petriellidium boydii B48.2
pharynx (*see also* Pharyngitis)
  coxsackievirus B08.5
  posterior, lymphoid (chronic) J35.03
Phialophora
  gougerotii (subcutaneous abscess or cyst) B43.2
  jeanselmei (subcutaneous abscess or cyst) B43.2
  verrucosa (skin) B43.0
Piedraia hortae B36.3
pinta A67.9
  intermediate A67.1
  late A67.2
  mixed A67.3
  primary A67.0
pinworm B80
pityrosporum furfur B36.0
pleuro-pneumonia-like organism (PPLO) NEC A49.3
  as cause of disease classified elsewhere B96.0
pneumococcus, pneumococcal NEC A49.1
  as cause of disease classified elsewhere B95.3
  generalized (purulent) A40.3
    with pneumonia J13
Pneumocystis carinii (pneumonia) B59
Pneumocystis jiroveci (pneumonia) B59
port or reservoir T80.212 ☑
postoperative T81.4 ☑
postoperative wound T81.4 ☑
postprocedural T81.4 ☑
postvaccinal T88.0 ☑
prepuce NEC N47.7
  with penile inflammation N47.6
prion — *see* Disease, prion, central nervous system
prostate (capsule) — *see* Prostatitis
Proteus (mirabilis) (morganii) (vulgaris) NEC A49.8
  as cause of disease classified elsewhere B96.4
protozoal NEC B64
  intestinal A07.9
    specified NEC A07.8

Infection, infected, infective — *continued*
protozoal — *continued*
  specified NEC B60.8
Pseudoallescheria boydii B48.2
Pseudomonas NEC A49.8
  as cause of disease classified elsewhere B96.5
  mallei A24.0
  pneumonia J15.1
  pseudomallei — *see* Melioidosis
puerperal O86.4
  genitourinary tract NEC O86.89
  major or generalized O85
  minor O86.4
  specified NEC O86.89
pulmonary — *see* Infection, lung
purulent — *see* Abscess
Pyrenochaeta romeroi B47.0
Q fever A78
rectum (sphincter) K62.89
renal (*see also* Infection, kidney)
  pelvis and ureter (cystic) N28.85
reovirus, as cause of disease classified elsewhere B97.5
respiratory (tract) NEC J98.8
  acute J22
  chronic J98.8
  influenzal (upper) (acute) — *see* Influenza, with,
    respiratory manifestations NEC
  lower (acute) J22
    chronic — *see* Bronchitis, chronic
  rhinovirus J00
  syncytial virus, as cause of disease classified else-
    where B97.4
  upper (acute) NOS J06.9
    chronic J39.8
    streptococcal J06.9
    viral NOS J06.9
resulting from
  presence of internal prosthesis, implant, graft —
    see Complications, by site and type, infection
retortamoniasis A07.8
retroperitoneal NEC K68.9
retrovirus B33.3
  as cause of disease classified elsewhere B97.30
    human
      immunodeficiency, type 2 (HIV 2) B97.35
      T-cell lymphotropic
        type I (HTLV-I) B97.33
        type II (HTLV-II) B97.34
    lentivirus B97.31
    oncovirus B97.32
    specified NEC B97.39
Rhinosporidium (seeberi) B48.1
rhinovirus
  as cause of disease classified elsewhere B97.89
  unspecified nature or site B34.8
Rhizopus — *see* Mucormycosis
rickettsial NOS A79.9
roundworm (large) NEC B82.0
  Ascariasis (*see also* Ascariasis) B77.9
rubella — *see* Rubella
Saccharomyces — *see* Candidiasis
salivary duct or gland (any) — *see* Sialoadenitis
Salmonella (aertrycke) (arizonae) (callinarum)
  (cholerae-suis) (enteritidis) (suipestifer) (typhimurium) A02.9
  with
    (gastro)enteritis A02.0
    sepsis A02.1
    specified manifestation NEC A02.8
  due to food (poisoning) A02.9
  hirschfeldii A01.3
  localized A02.20
    arthritis A02.23
    meningitis A02.21
    osteomyelitis A02.24
    pneumonia A02.22
    pyelonephritis A02.25
    specified NEC A02.29
  paratyphi A01.4
    A A01.1
    B A01.2
    C A01.3
  schottmuelleri A01.2
  typhi, typhosa — *see* Typhoid
Sarcocystis A07.8
scabies B86
Schistosoma — *see* Infestation, Schistosoma
scrotum (acute) NEC N49.2

Infection, infected, infective — *continued*
seminal vesicle — *see* Vesiculitis
septic
  localized, skin — *see* Abscess
sheep liver fluke B66.3
Shigella A03.9
  boydii A03.2
  dysenteriae A03.0
  flexneri A03.1
  group
    A A03.0
    B A03.1
    C A03.2
    D A03.3
  Schmitz (-Stutzer) A03.0
  schmitzii A03.0
  shigae A03.0
  sonnei A03.3
  specified NEC A03.8
shoulder (joint) NEC M00.9
  due to internal joint prosthesis T84.59 ☑
skin NEC L08.9
sinus (accessory) (chronic) (nasal) (*see also* Sinusitis)
  pilonidal — *see* Sinus, pilonidal
  skin NEC L08.89
Skene's duct or gland — *see* Urethritis
skin (local) (staphylococcal) (streptococcal) L08.9
  abscess — *code by* site under Abscess
  cellulitis — *code by* site under Cellulitis
  due to fungus B36.9
    specified type NEC B36.8
  mycotic B36.9
    specified NEC B36.8
  newborn P39.4
  ulcer — *see* Ulcer, skin
slow virus A81.9
  specified NEC A81.89
Sparganum (mansoni) (proliferum) (baxteri) B70.1
specific (*see also* Syphilis)
  to perinatal period — *see* Infection, congenital
specified NEC B99.8
spermatic cord NEC N49.1
sphenoidal (sinus) — *see* Sinusitis, sphenoidal
spinal cord NOS (*see also* Myelitis) G04.91
  abscess G06.1
  meninges — *see* Meningitis
  streptococcal G04.89
Spirillum A25.0
spirochetal NOS A69.9
  lung A69.8
  specified NEC A69.8
Spirometra larvae B70.1
spleen D73.89
Sporotrichum, Sporothrix (schenckii) — *see* Sporotrichosis
staphylococcal, unspecified site
  as cause of disease classified elsewhere B95.8
    aureus (methicillin susceptible) (MSSA) B95.61
      methicillin resistant (MRSA) B95.62
    specified NEC B95.7
  aureus (methicillin susceptible) (MSSA) A49.01
    methicillin resistant (MRSA) A49.02
  food poisoning A05.0
  generalized (purulent) A41.2
  pneumonia — *see* Pneumonia, staphylococcal
Stellantchasmus falcatus B66.8
streptobacillus moniliformis A25.1
streptococcal NEC A49.1
  as cause of disease classified elsewhere B95.5
  B genitourinary complicating
    childbirth O98.82
    pregnancy O98.81- ☑
    puerperium O98.83
  congenital
    sepsis P36.10
      group B P36.0
      specified NEC P36.19
  generalized (purulent) A40.9
Streptomyces B47.1
Strongyloides (stercoralis) — *see* Strongyloidiasis
stump (amputation) (surgical) — *see* Complication,
  amputation stump, infection
subcutaneous tissue, local L08.9
suipestifer — *see* Infection, salmonella
swimming pool bacillus A31.1
Taenia — *see* Infestation, Taenia
Taeniarhynchus saginatus B68.1
tapeworm — *see* Infestation, tapeworm

Infection, infected, infective — continued
tendon (sheath) — see Tenosynovitis, infective NEC
Ternidens diminutus B81.8
testis — see Orchitis
threadworm B80
throat — see Pharyngitis
thyroglossal duct K14.8
toe (skin) L08.9
  cellulitis L03.03- ☑
    fungus B35.1
  nail L03.03- ☑
    fungus B35.1
tongue NEC K14.0
  parasitic B37.0
tonsil (and adenoid) (faucial) (lingual) (pharyngeal) —
  see Tonsillitis
tooth, teeth K04.7
  periapical K04.7
  peridental, periodontal K05.20
    generalized K05.22
    localized K05.21
  pulp K04.0
  socket M27.3
TORCH — see Infection, congenital
  without active infection P00.2
Torula histolytica — see Cryptococcosis
Toxocara (canis) (cati) (felis) B83.0
Toxoplasma gondii — see Toxoplasma
trachea, chronic J42
trematode NEC — see Infestation, fluke
trench fever A79.0
Treponema pallidum — see Syphilis
Trichinella (spiralis) B75
Trichomonas A59.9
  cervix A59.09
  intestine A07.8
  prostate A59.02
  specified site NEC A59.8
  urethra A59.03
  urogenitalis A59.00
  vagina A59.01
  vulva A59.01
Trichophyton, trichophytic — see Dermatophytosis
Trichosporon (beigelii) cutaneum B36.2
Trichostrongylus B81.2
Trichuris (trichiura) B79
Trombicula (irritans) B88.0
Trypanosoma
  brucei
    gambiense B56.0
    rhodesiense B56.1
  cruzi — see Chagas' disease
tubal — see Salpingo-oophoritis
tuberculous NEC — see Tuberculosis
tubo-ovarian — see Salpingo-oophoritis
tunica vaginalis N49.1
tunnel T80.212 ☑
tympanic membrane NEC — see Myringitis
typhoid (abortive) (ambulant) (bacillus) — see Typhoid
typhus A75.9
  flea-borne A75.2
  mite-borne A75.3
  recrudescent A75.1
  tick-borne A77.9
    African A77.1
    North Asian A77.2
umbilicus L08.82
ureter N28.86
urethra — see Urethritis
urinary (tract) N39.0
  bladder — see Cystitis
  complicating
    pregnancy O23.4- ☑
      specified type NEC O23.3- ☑
  kidney — see Infection, kidney
  newborn P39.3
  puerperal (postpartum) O86.20
  tuberculous A18.13
  urethra — see Urethritis
uterus, uterine — see Endometritis
vaccination T88.0 ☑
vaccinia not from vaccination B08.011
vagina (acute) — see Vaginitis
varicella B01.9
varicose veins — see Varix
vas deferens NEC N49.1
vesical — see Cystitis

Infection, infected, infective — continued
Vibrio
  cholerae A00.0
    El Tor A00.1
  parahaemolyticus (food poisoning) A05.3
  vulnificus
    as cause of disease classified elsewhere B96.82
    foodborne intoxication A05.5
Vincent's (gum) (mouth) (tonsil) A69.1
virus, viral NOS B34.9
  adenovirus
    as cause of disease classified elsewhere B97.0
    unspecified nature or site B34.0
  arbovirus, arbovirus arthropod-borne A94
  as cause of disease classified elsewhere B97.89
    adenovirus B97.0
    coronavirus B97.29
      SARS-associated B97.21
    coxsackievirus B97.11
    echovirus B97.12
    enterovirus B97.10
      coxsackievirus B97.11
      echovirus B97.12
      specified NEC B97.19
    human
      immunodeficiency, type 2 (HIV 2) B97.35
      metapneumovirus B97.81
      T-cell lymphotropic,
        type I (HTLV-I) B97.33
        type II (HTLV-II) B97.34
    papillomavirus B97.7
    parvovirus B97.6
    reovirus B97.5
    respiratory syncytial B97.4
    retrovirus B97.30
      human
        immunodeficiency, type 2 (HIV 2) B97.35
        T-cell lymphotropic,
          type I (HTLV-I) B97.33
          type II (HTLV-II) B97.34
      lentivirus B97.31
      oncovirus B97.32
      specified NEC B97.39
    specified NEC B97.89
  central nervous system A89
    atypical A81.9
      specified NEC A81.89
    enterovirus NEC A88.8
      meningitis A87.0
    slow virus A81.9
      specified NEC A81.89
    specified NEC A88.8
  chest J98.8
  cotia B08.8
  coxsackie (see also Infection, coxsackie) B34.1
    as cause of disease classified elsewhere B97.11
  ECHO
    as cause of disease classified elsewhere B97.12
    unspecified nature or site B34.1
  encephalitis, tick-borne A84.9
  enterovirus, as cause of disease classified elsewhere
    B97.10
    coxsackievirus B97.11
    echovirus B97.12
    specified NEC B97.19
  exanthem NOS B09
  human metapneumovirus as cause of disease
    classified elsewhere B97.81
  human papilloma as cause of disease classified
    elsewhere B97.7
  intestine — see Enteritis, viral
  respiratory syncytial
    as cause of disease classified elsewhere B97.4
    bronchopneumonia J12.1
    common cold syndrome J00
    nasopharyngitis (acute) J00
  rhinovirus
    as cause of disease classified elsewhere B97.89
    unspecified nature or site B34.8
  slow A81.9
    specified NEC A81.89
  specified type NEC B33.8
    as cause of disease classified elsewhere B97.89
    unspecified nature or site B34.8
  unspecified nature or site B34.9
  West Nile — see Virus, West Nile
vulva (acute) — see Vulvitis
West Nile — see Virus, West Nile

Infection, infected, infective — continued
whipworm B79
worms B83.9
  specified type NEC B83.8
Wuchereria (bancrofti) B74.0
  malayi B74.1
yatapoxvirus B08.70
  specified NEC B08.79
yeast (see also Candidiasis) B37.9
yellow fever — see Fever, yellow
Yersinia
  enterocolitica (intestinal) A04.6
  pestis — see Plague
  pseudotuberculosis A28.2
Zeis' gland — see Hordeolum
zoonotic bacterial NOS A28.9
Zopfia senegalensis B47.0
Infective, infectious — see condition
Infertility N97.9
  female N97.9
    age-related N97.8
    associated with
      anovulation N97.0
      cervical (mucus) disease or anomaly N88.3
      congenital anomaly
        cervix N88.3
        fallopian tube N97.1
        uterus N97.2
        vagina N97.8
      dysmucorrhea N88.3
      fallopian tube disease or anomaly N97.1
      pituitary-hypothalamic origin E23.0
      specified origin NEC N97.8
      Stein-Leventhal syndrome E28.2
      uterine disease or anomaly N97.2
      vaginal disease or anomaly N97.8
    due to
      cervical anomaly N88.3
      fallopian tube anomaly N97.1
      ovarian failure E28.39
      Stein-Leventhal syndrome E28.2
      uterine anomaly N97.2
      vaginal anomaly N97.8
    nonimplantation N97.2
    origin
      cervical N88.3
      tubal (block) (occlusion) (stenosis) N97.1
      uterine N97.2
      vaginal N97.8
  male N46.9
    azoospermia N46.01
      extratesticular cause N46.029
        drug therapy N46.021
        efferent duct obstruction N46.023
        infection N46.022
        radiation N46.024
        specified cause NEC N46.029
        systemic disease N46.025
    oligospermia N46.11
      extratesticular cause N46.129
        drug therapy N46.121
        efferent duct obstruction N46.123
        infection N46.122
        radiation N46.124
        specified cause NEC N46.129
        systemic disease N46.125
    specified type NEC N46.8
Infestation B88.9
  Acanthocheilonema (perstans) (streptocerca) B74.4
  Acariasis B88.0
    demodex folliculorum B88.0
    sarcoptes scabiei B86
    trombiculae B88.0
  Agamofilaria streptocerca B74.4
  Ancylostoma, ankylostoma (braziliense) (caninum)
    (ceylanicum) (duodenale) B76.0
    americanum B76.1
    new world B76.1
  Anisakis larvae, anisakiasis B81.0
  arthropod NEC B88.2
  Ascaris lumbricoides — see Ascariasis
  Balantidium coli A07.0
  beef tapeworm B68.1
  Bothriocephalus (latus) B70.0
    larval B70.1
  broad tapeworm B70.0
    larval B70.1
  Brugia (malayi) B74.1

☑ **Additional Character Required** — Refer to the Tabular List for Character Selection   🔄 **Subterms under main terms may continue to next column or page**

Infestation — *continued*
- Brugia — *continued*
  - timori B74.2
- candiru B88.8
- Capillaria
  - hepatica B83.8
  - philippinensis B81.1
- cat liver fluke B66.0
- cestodes B71.9
  - diphyllobothrium — *see* Infestation, diphyllobothrium
  - dipylidiasis B71.1
  - hymenolepiasis B71.0
  - specified type NEC B71.8
- chigger B88.0
- chigo, chigoe B88.1
- Clonorchis (sinensis) (liver) B66.1
- coccidial A07.3
- crab-lice B85.3
- Cysticercus cellulosae — *see* Cysticercosis
- Demodex (folliculorum) B88.0
- Dermanyssus gallinae B88.0
- Dermatobia (hominis) — *see* Myiasis
- Dibothriocephalus (latus) B70.0
  - larval B70.1
- Dicrocoelium dendriticum B66.2
- Diphyllobothrium (adult) (latum) (intestinal) (pacificum) B70.0
  - larval B70.1
- Diplogonoporus (grandis) B71.8
- Dipylidium caninum B67.4
- Distoma hepaticum B66.3
- dog tapeworm B67.4
- Dracunculus medinensis B72
- dragon worm B72
- dwarf tapeworm B71.0
- Echinococcus — *see* Echinococcus
- Echinostomum ilocanum B66.8
- Entamoeba (histolytica) — *see* Infection, Ameba
- Enterobius vermicularis B80
- eyelid
  - in (due to)
    - leishmaniasis B55.1
    - loiasis B74.3
    - onchocerciasis B73.09
    - phthiriasis B85.3
    - parasitic NOS B89
- eyeworm B74.3
- Fasciola (gigantica) (hepatica) (indica) B66.3
- Fasciolopsis (buski) (intestine) B66.5
- filarial B74.9
  - bancroftian B74.0
  - conjunctiva B74.9
  - due to
    - Acanthocheilonema (perstans) (streptocerca) B74.4
    - Brugia (malayi) B74.1
      - timori B74.2
    - Dracunculus medinensis B72
    - guinea worm B72
    - loa loa B74.3
    - Mansonella (ozzardi) (perstans) (streptocerca) B74.4
    - Onchocerca volvulus B73.00
      - eye B73.00
      - eyelid B73.09
    - Wuchereria (bancrofti) B74.0
  - Malayan B74.1
  - ozzardi B74.4
  - specified type NEC B74.8
- fish tapeworm B70.0
  - larval B70.1
- fluke B66.9
  - blood NOS — *see* Schistosomiasis
  - cat liver B66.0
  - intestinal B66.5
  - lancet B66.2
  - liver (sheep) B66.3
    - cat B66.0
    - Chinese B66.1
    - due to clonorchiasis B66.1
    - oriental B66.1
  - lung (oriental) B66.4
  - sheep liver B66.3
  - specified type NEC B66.8
- fly larvae — *see* Myiasis
- Gasterophilus (intestinalis) — *see* Myiasis
- Gastrodiscoides hominis B66.8

Infestation — *continued*
- Giardia lamblia A07.1
- Gnathostoma (spinigerum) B83.1
- Gongylonema B83.8
- guinea worm B72
- helminth B83.9
  - angiostrongyliasis B83.2
    - intestinal B81.3
  - gnathostomiasis B83.1
  - hirudiniasis, internal B83.4
  - intestinal B82.0
    - angiostrongyliasis B81.3
    - anisakiasis B81.0
    - ascariasis — *see* Ascariasis
    - capillariasis B81.1
    - cysticercosis — *see* Cysticercosis
    - diphyllobothriasis — *see* Infestation, diphyllobothriasis
    - dracunculiasis B72
    - echinococcus — *see* Echinococcosis
    - enterobiasis B80
    - filariasis — *see* Infestation, filarial
    - fluke — *see* Infestation, fluke
    - hookworm — *see* Infestation, hookworm
    - mixed (types classifiable to more than one of the titles B65.0-B81.3 and B81.8) B81.4
    - onchocerciasis — *see* Onchocerciasis
    - schistosomiasis — *see* Infestation, schistosoma
    - specified
      - cestode NEC — *see* Infestation, cestode type NEC B81.8
    - strongyloidiasis — *see* Strongyloidiasis
    - taenia — *see* Infestation, taenia
    - trichinellosis B75
    - trichostrongyliasis B81.2
    - trichuriasis B79
  - specified type NEC B83.8
  - syngamiasis B83.3
  - visceral larva migrans B83.0
- Heterophyes (heterophyes) B66.8
- hookworm B76.9
  - ancylostomiasis B76.0
  - necatoriasis B76.1
  - specified type NEC B76.8
- Hymenolepis (diminuta) (nana) B71.0
- intestinal NEC B82.9
- leeches (aquatic) (land) — *see* Hirudiniasis
- Leishmania — *see* Leishmaniasis
- lice, louse — *see* Infestation, Pediculus
- Linguatula B88.8
- Liponyssoides sanguineus B88.0
- Loa loa B74.3
  - conjunctival B74.3
  - eyelid B74.3
- louse — *see* Infestation, Pediculus
- maggots — *see* Myiasis
- Mansonella (ozzardi) (perstans) (streptocerca) B74.4
- Medina (worm) B72
- Metagonimus (yokogawai) B66.8
- microfilaria streptocerca — *see* Onchocerciasis
  - eye B73.00
  - eyelid B73.09
- mites B88.9
  - scabic B86
- Monilia (albicans) — *see* Candidiasis
- mouth B37.0
- Necator americanus B76.1
- nematode NEC (intestinal) B82.0
  - Ancylostoma B76.0
  - conjunctiva NEC B83.9
  - Enterobius vermicularis B80
  - Gnathostoma spinigerum B83.1
  - physaloptera B80
  - specified NEC B81.8
  - trichostrongylus B81.2
  - trichuris (trichuria) B79
- Oesophagostomum (apiostomum) B81.8
- Oestrus ovis (*see also* Myiasis) B87.9
- Onchocerca (volvulus) — *see* Onchocerciasis
- Opisthorchis (felineus) (viverrini) B66.0
- orbit, parasitic NOS B89
- Oxyuris vermicularis B80
- Paragonimus (westermani) B66.4
- parasite, parasitic B89
  - eyelid B89
  - intestinal NOS B82.9
  - mouth B37.0
  - skin B88.9

Infestation — *continued*
- parasite, parasitic — *continued*
  - tongue B37.0
- Parastrongylus
  - cantonensis B83.2
  - costaricensis B81.3
- Pediculus B85.2
  - body B85.1
  - capitis (humanus) (any site) B85.0
  - corporis (humanus) (any site) B85.1
  - head B85.0
  - mixed (classifiable to more than one of the titles B85.0 - B85.3) B85.4
  - pubis (any site) B85.3
- Pentastoma B88.8
- Phthirus (pubis) (any site) B85.3
  - with any infestation classifiable to B85.0 - B85.2 B85.4
- pinworm B80
- pork tapeworm (adult) B68.0
- protozoal NEC B64
  - intestinal A07.9
    - specified NEC A07.8
  - specified NEC B60.8
- pubic, louse B85.3
- rat tapeworm B71.0
- red bug B88.0
- roundworm (large) NEC B82.0
  - Ascariasis (*see also* Ascariasis) B77.9
- sandflea B88.1
- Sarcoptes scabiei B86
- scabies B86
- Schistosoma B65.9
  - bovis B65.8
  - cercariae B65.3
  - haematobium B65.0
  - intercalatum B65.8
  - japonicum B65.2
  - mansoni B65.1
  - mattheei B65.8
  - mekongi B65.8
  - specified type NEC B65.8
  - spindale B65.8
- screw worms — *see* Myiasis
- skin NOS B88.9
- Sparganum (mansoni) (proliferum) (baxteri) B70.1
  - larval B70.1
- specified type NEC B88.8
- Spirometra larvae B70.1
- Stellantchasmus falcatus B66.8
- Strongyloides stercoralis — *see* Strongyloidiasis
- Taenia B68.9
  - diminuta B71.0
  - echinococcus — *see* Echinococcus
  - mediocanellata B68.1
  - nana B71.0
  - saginata B68.1
  - solium (intestinal form) B68.0
    - larval form — *see* Cysticercosis
- Taeniarhynchus saginatus B68.1
- tapeworm B71.9
  - beef B68.1
  - broad B70.0
    - larval B70.1
  - dog B67.4
  - dwarf B71.0
  - fish B70.0
    - larval B70.1
  - pork B68.0
  - rat B71.0
- Ternidens diminutus B81.8
- Tetranychus molestissimus B88.0
- threadworm B80
- tongue B37.0
- Toxocara (canis) (cati) (felis) B83.0
- trematode(s) NEC — *see* Infestation, fluke
- Trichinella (spiralis) B75
- Trichocephalus B79
- Trichomonas — *see* Trichomoniasis
- Trichostrongylus B81.2
- Trichuris (trichiura) B79
- Trombicula (irritans) B88.0
- Tunga penetrans B88.1
- Uncinaria americana B76.1
- Vandellia cirrhosa B88.8
- whipworm B79
- worms B83.9
  - intestinal B82.0

Infestation — *continued*
  Wuchereria (bancrofti) B74.Ø

Infiltrate, infiltration
  amyloid (generalized) (localized) — *see* Amyloidosis
  calcareous NEC R89.7
    localized — *see* Degeneration, by site
  calcium salt R89.7
  cardiac
    fatty — *see* Degeneration, myocardial
    glycogenic E74.02 [I43]
  corneal — *see* Edema, cornea
  eyelid — *see* Inflammation, eyelid
  glycogen, glycogenic — *see* Disease, glycogen storage
  heart, cardiac
    fatty — *see* Degeneration, myocardial
    glycogenic E74.02 [I43]
  inflammatory in vitreous H43.89
  kidney N28.89
  leukemic — *see* Leukemia
  liver K76.89
    fatty — *see* Fatty, liver NEC
    glycogen (*see also* Disease, glycogen storage)
      E74.03 [K77]
  lung R91.8
    eosinophilic J82
  lymphatic (*see also* Leukemia, lymphatic) C91.9- ☑
    gland I88.9
  muscle, fatty M62.89
  myocardium, myocardial
    fatty — *see* Degeneration, myocardial
    glycogenic E74.02 [I43]
  on chest x-ray R91.8
  pulmonary R91.8
    with eosinophilia J82
  skin (lymphocytic) L98.6
  thymus (gland) (fatty) E32.8
  urine R39.0
  vesicant agent
    antineoplastic chemotherapy T80.81Ø ☑
    other agent NEC T80.818 ☑
  vitreous body H43.89

Infirmity R68.89
  senile R54

Inflammation, inflamed, inflammatory (with exudation)
  abducent (nerve) — *see* Strabismus, paralytic, sixth nerve
  accessory sinus (chronic) — *see* Sinusitis
  adrenal (gland) E27.8
  alveoli, teeth M27.3
    scorbutic E54
  anal canal, anus K62.89
  antrum (chronic) — *see* Sinusitis, maxillary
  appendix — *see* Appendicitis
  arachnoid — *see* Meningitis
  areola N61
    puerperal, postpartum or gestational — *see* Infection, nipple
  areolar tissue NOS L08.9
  artery — *see* Arteritis
  auditory meatus (external) — *see* Otitis, externa
  Bartholin's gland N75.8
  bile duct (common) (hepatic) or passage — *see* Cholangitis
  bladder — *see* Cystitis
  bone — *see* Osteomyelitis
  brain (*see also* Encephalitis)
    membrane — *see* Meningitis
  breast N61
    puerperal, postpartum, gestational — *see* Mastitis, obstetric
  broad ligament — *see* Disease, pelvis, inflammatory
  bronchi — *see* Bronchitis
  catarrhal J00
  cecum — *see* Appendicitis
  cerebral (*see also* Encephalitis)
    membrane — *see* Meningitis
  cerebrospinal
    meningococcal A39.0
  cervix (uteri) — *see* Cervicitis
  chest J98.8
  chorioretinal H30.9- ☑
    cyclitis — *see* Cyclitis
    disseminated H30.10- ☑
      generalized H30.13- ☑
      peripheral H30.12- ☑
      posterior pole H30.11- ☑

Inflammation, inflamed, inflammatory — *continued*
  chorioretinal — *continued*
    epitheliopathy — *see* Epitheliopathy
    focal H30.00- ☑
      juxtapapillary H30.01- ☑
      macular H30.04- ☑
      paramacular — *see* Inflammation, chorioretinal, focal, macular
      peripheral H30.03- ☑
      posterior pole H30.02- ☑
    specified type NEC H30.89- ☑
  choroid — *see* Inflammation, chorioretinal
  chronic, postmastoidectomy cavity — *see* Complications, postmastoidectomy, inflammation
  colon — *see* Enteritis
  connective tissue (diffuse) NEC — *see* Disorder, soft tissue, specified type NEC
  cornea — *see* Keratitis
  corpora cavernosa N48.29
  cranial nerve — *see* Disorder, nerve, cranial
  Douglas' cul-de-sac or pouch (chronic) N73.0
  due to device, implant or graft (*see also* Complications, by site and type, infection or inflammation)
    arterial graft T82.7 ☑
    breast (implant) T85.79 ☑
    catheter T85.79 ☑
      dialysis (renal) T82.7 ☑
        intraperitoneal T85.71 ☑
      infusion T82.7 ☑
        spinal (epidural) (subdural) T85.79 ☑
      urinary (indwelling) T83.51 ☑
    electronic (electrode) (pulse generator) (stimulator)
      bone T84.7 ☑
      cardiac T82.7 ☑
      nervous system (brain) (peripheral nerve) (spinal) T85.79 ☑
      urinary T83.59 ☑
    fixation, internal (orthopedic) NEC — *see* Complication, fixation device, infection
    gastrointestinal (bile duct) (esophagus) T85.79 ☑
    genital NEC T83.6 ☑
    heart NEC T82.7 ☑
      valve (prosthesis) T82.6 ☑
        graft T82.7 ☑
    joint prosthesis — *see* Complication, joint prosthesis, infection
    ocular (corneal graft) (orbital implant) NEC T85.79 ☑
    orthopedic NEC T84.7 ☑
    specified NEC T85.79 ☑
    urinary NEC T83.59 ☑
    vascular NEC T82.7 ☑
    ventricular intracranial shunt T85.79 ☑
  duodenum K29.80
    with bleeding K29.81
  dura mater — *see* Meningitis
  ear (middle) (*see also* Otitis, media)
    external — *see* Otitis, externa
    inner — *see* subcategory H83.0 ☑
  epididymis — *see* Epididymitis
  esophagus K20.9
  ethmoidal (sinus) (chronic) — *see* Sinusitis, ethmoidal
  eustachian tube (catarrhal) — *see* Salpingitis, eustachian
  eyelid H01.9
    abscess — *see* Abscess, eyelid
    blepharitis — *see* Blepharitis
    chalazion — *see* Chalazion
    dermatosis (noninfectious) — *see* Dermatosis, eyelid
    hordeolum — *see* Hordeolum
    specified NEC H01.8
  fallopian tube — *see* Salpingo-oophoritis
  fascia — *see* Myositis
  follicular, pharynx J31.2
  frontal (sinus) (chronic) — *see* Sinusitis, frontal
  gallbladder — *see* Cholecystitis
  gastric — *see* Gastritis
  gastrointestinal — *see* Enteritis
  genital organ (internal) (diffuse)
    female — *see* Disease, pelvis, inflammatory
    male N49.9
      multiple sites N49.8
      specified NEC N49.8
  gland (lymph) — *see* Lymphadenitis

Inflammation, inflamed, inflammatory — *continued*
  glottis — *see* Laryngitis
  granular, pharynx J31.2
  gum K05.10
    nonplaque induced K05.11
    plaque induced K05.10
  heart — *see* Carditis
  hepatic duct — *see* Cholangitis
  ileoanal (internal) pouch K91.850
  ileum (*see also* Enteritis)
    regional or terminal — *see* Enteritis, regional
  intestinal pouch K91.850
  intestine (any part) — *see* Enteritis
  jaw (acute) (bone) (chronic) (lower) (suppurative) (upper) M27.2
  joint NEC — *see* Arthritis
    sacroiliac M46.1
  kidney — *see* Nephritis
  knee (joint) M13.169
    tuberculous A18.02
  labium (majus) (minus) — *see* Vulvitis
  lacrimal
    gland — *see* Dacryoadenitis
    passages (duct) (sac) (*see also* Dacryocystitis)
      canaliculitis — *see* Canaliculitis, lacrimal
  larynx — *see* Laryngitis
  leg NOS L08.9
  lip K13.0
  liver (capsule) (*see also* Hepatitis)
    chronic K73.9
    suppurative K75.0
  lung (acute) (*see also* Pneumonia)
    chronic J98.4
  lymph gland or node — *see* Lymphadenitis
  lymphatic vessel — *see* Lymphangitis
  maxilla, maxillary M27.2
    sinus (chronic) — *see* Sinusitis, maxillary
  membranes of brain or spinal cord — *see* Meningitis
  meninges — *see* Meningitis
  mouth K12.1
  muscle — *see* Myositis
  myocardium — *see* Myocarditis
  nasal sinus (chronic) — *see* Sinusitis
  nasopharynx — *see* Nasopharyngitis
  navel L08.82
  nerve NEC — *see* Neuralgia
  nipple N61
    puerperal, postpartum or gestational — *see* Infection, nipple
  nose — *see* Rhinitis
  oculomotor (nerve) — *see* Strabismus, paralytic, third nerve
  optic nerve — *see* Neuritis, optic
  orbit (chronic) H05.10
    acute H05.00
      abscess — *see* Abscess, orbit
      cellulitis — *see* Cellulitis, orbit
      osteomyelitis — *see* Osteomyelitis, orbit
      periostitis — *see* Periostitis, orbital
      tenonitis — *see* Tenonitis, eye
    granuloma — *see* Granuloma, orbit
    myositis — *see* Myositis, orbital
  ovary — *see* Salpingo-oophoritis
  oviduct — *see* Salpingo-oophoritis
  pancreas (acute) — *see* Pancreatitis
  parametrium N73.0
  parotid region L08.9
  pelvis, female — *see* Disease, pelvis, inflammatory
  penis (corpora cavernosa) N48.29
  perianal K62.89
  pericardium — *see* Pericarditis
  perineum (female) (male) L08.9
  perirectal K62.89
  peritoneum — *see* Peritonitis
  periuterine — *see* Disease, pelvis, inflammatory
  perivesical — *see* Cystitis
  petrous bone (acute) (chronic) — *see* Petrositis
  pharynx (acute) — *see* Pharyngitis
  pia mater — *see* Meningitis
  pleura — *see* Pleurisy
  polyp, colon (*see also* Polyp, colon, inflammatory) K51.40
  prostate (*see also* Prostatitis)
    specified type NEC N41.8
  rectosigmoid — *see* Rectosigmoiditis
  rectum (*see also* Proctitis) K62.89

Inflammation, inflamed, inflammatory —
    continued
  respiratory, upper (*see also* Infection, respiratory, up-
    per) J06.9
    acute, due to radiation J70.0
    chronic, due to external agent — *see* condition,
      respiratory, chronic, due to
    due to
      chemicals, gases, fumes or vapors (inhalation)
        J68.2
      radiation J70.1
  retina — *see* Chorioretinitis
  retrocecal — *see* Appendicitis
  retroperitoneal — *see* Peritonitis
  salivary duct or gland (any) (suppurative) — *see*
    Sialoadenitis
  scorbutic, alveoli, teeth E54
  scrotum N49.2
  seminal vesicle — *see* Vesiculitis
  sigmoid — *see* Enteritis
  sinus — *see* Sinusitis
  Skene's duct or gland — *see* Urethritis
  skin L08.9
  spermatic cord N49.1
  sphenoidal (sinus) — *see* Sinusitis, sphenoidal
  spinal
    cord — *see* Encephalitis
    membrane — *see* Meningitis
    nerve — *see* Disorder, nerve
  spine — *see* Spondylopathy, inflammatory
  spleen (capsule) D73.89
  stomach — *see* Gastritis
  subcutaneous tissue L08.9
  suprarenal (gland) E27.8
  synovial — *see* Tenosynovitis
  tendon (sheath) NEC — *see* Tenosynovitis
  testis — *see* Orchitis
  throat (acute) — *see* Pharyngitis
  thymus (gland) E32.8
  thyroid (gland) — *see* Thyroiditis
  tongue K14.0
  tonsil — *see* Tonsillitis
  trachea — *see* Tracheitis
  trochlear (nerve) — *see* Strabismus, paralytic, fourth
    nerve
  tubal — *see* Salpingo-oophoritis
  tuberculous NEC — *see* Tuberculosis
  tubo-ovarian — *see* Salpingo-oophoritis
  tunica vaginalis N49.1
  tympanic membrane — *see* Tympanitis
  umbilicus, umbilical L08.82
  uterine ligament — *see* Disease, pelvis, inflammatory
  uterus (catarrhal) — *see* Endometritis
  uveal tract (anterior) NOS (*see also* Iridocyclitis)
    posterior — *see* Chorioretinitis
  vagina — *see* Vaginitis
  vas deferens N49.1
  vein (*see also* Phlebitis)
    intracranial or intraspinal (septic) G08
    thrombotic I80.9
      leg — *see* Phlebitis, leg
      lower extremity — *see* Phlebitis, leg
  vocal cord J38.3
  vulva — *see* Vulvitis
  Wharton's duct (suppurative) — *see* Sialoadenitis
Inflation, lung, imperfect (newborn) — *see* Atelectasis
Influenza (bronchial) (epidemic) (respiratory (upper))
    (unidentified influenza virus) J11.1
  with
    digestive manifestations J11.2
    encephalopathy J11.81
    enteritis J11.2
    gastroenteritis J11.2
    gastrointestinal manifestations J11.2
    laryngitis J11.1
    myocarditis J11.82
    otitis media J11.83
    pharyngitis J11.1
    pneumonia J11.00
      specified type J11.08
    respiratory manifestations NEC J11.1
    specified manifestation NEC J11.89
  A/H5N1 (*see also* Influenza, due to, identified novel
    influenza A virus) J09.X2
  avian (*see also* Influenza, due to, identified novel in-
    fluenza A virus) J09.X2

Influenza — *continued*
  bird (*see also* Influenza, due to, identified novel influen-
    za A virus) J09.X2
  due to
    avian (*see also* Influenza, due to, identified novel
      influenza A virus) J09.X2
    identified influenza virus NEC J10.1
      with
        digestive manifestations J10.2
        encephalopathy J10.81
        enteritis J10.2
        gastroenteritis J10.2
        gastrointestinal manifestations J10.2
        laryngitis J10.1
        myocarditis J10.82
        otitis media J10.83
        pharyngitis J10.1
        pneumonia (unspecified type) J10.00
          with same identified influenza virus
            J10.01
          specified type NEC J10.08
        respiratory manifestations NEC J10.1
        specified manifestation NEC J10.89
    identified novel influenza A virus J09.X2
      with
        digestive manifestations J09.X3
        encephalopathy J09.X9
        enteritis J09.X3
        gastroenteritis J09.X3
        gastrointestinal manifestations J09.X3
        laryngitis J09.X2
        myocarditis J09.X9
        otitis media J09.X9
        pharyngitis J09.X2
        pneumonia J09.X1
        respiratory manifestations NEC J09.X2
        specified manifestation NEC J09.X9
        upper respiratory symptoms J09.X2
  novel (2009) H1N1 influenza (*see also* Influenza, due
    to, identified influenza virus NEC) J10.1
  novel influenza A/H1N1 (*see also* Influenza, due to,
    identified influenza virus NEC) J10.1
  of other animal origin, not bird or swine (*see also* In-
    fluenza, due to, identified novel influenza A
    virus) J09.X2
  swine (viruses that normally cause infections in pigs)
    (*see also* Influenza, due to, identified novel in-
    fluenza A virus) J09.X2
Influenzal — *see* Influenza
Influenza-like disease — *see* Influenza
Infraction, Freiberg's (metatarsal head) — *see* Osteo-
    chondrosis, juvenile, metatarsus
Infraeruption of tooth (teeth) M26.34
Infusion complication, misadventure, or reaction
    — *see* Complications, infusion
Ingestion
  chemical — *see* Table of Drugs and Chemicals, by
    substance, poisoning
  drug or medicament
    correct substance properly administered — *see*
      Table of Drugs and Chemicals, by drug, ad-
      verse effect
    overdose or wrong substance given or taken —
      see Table of Drugs and Chemicals, by drug,
      poisoning
  foreign body — *see* Foreign body, alimentary tract
  tularemia A21.3
Ingrowing
  hair (beard) L73.1
  nail (finger) (toe) L60.0
Inguinal (*see also* condition)
  testicle Q53.9
    bilateral Q53.21
    unilateral Q53.11
Inhalation
  anthrax A22.1
  flame T27.3 ☑
  food or foreign body — *see* Foreign body, by site
  gases, fumes, or vapors NEC T59.9- ☑
    specified agent — *see* Table of Drugs and Chemi-
      cals, by substance
  liquid or vomitus — *see* Asphyxia
  meconium (newborn) P24.00
    with
      with respiratory symptoms P24.01
      pneumonia (pneumonitis) P24.01
  mucus — *see* Asphyxia, mucus

Inhalation — *continued*
  oil or gasoline (causing suffocation) — *see* Foreign
    body, by site
  smoke J70.5
    due to chemicals, gases, fumes and vapors J68.9
  steam — *see* Toxicity, vapors
  stomach contents or secretions — *see* Foreign body,
    by site
    due to anesthesia (general) (local) or other sedation
      T88.59 ☑
      in labor and delivery O74.0
      in pregnancy O29.01- ☑
      postpartum, puerperal O89.01
Inhibition, orgasm
  female F52.31
  male F52.32
Inhibitor, systemic lupus erythematosus (presence
    of) D68.62
Iniencephalus, iniencephaly Q00.2
Injection, traumatic jet (air) (industrial) (water) (paint
    or dye) T70.4 ☑
Injury (*see also* specified injury type) T14.90
  abdomen, abdominal S39.91 ☑
    blood vessel — *see* Injury, blood vessel, abdomen
    cavity — *see* Injury, intra-abdominal
    contusion S30.1 ☑
    internal — *see* Injury, intra-abdominal
    intra-abdominal organ — *see* Injury, intra-abdom-
      inal
    nerve — *see* Injury, nerve, abdomen
    open — *see* Wound, open, abdomen
    specified NEC S39.81 ☑
    superficial — *see* Injury, superficial, abdomen
  Achilles tendon S86.00- ☑
    laceration S86.02- ☑
    specified type NEC S86.09- ☑
    strain S86.01- ☑
  acoustic, resulting in deafness — *see* Injury, nerve,
    acoustic
  adrenal (gland) S37.819 ☑
    contusion S37.812 ☑
    laceration S37.813 ☑
    specified type NEC S37.818 ☑
  alveolar (process) S09.93 ☑
  ankle S99.91- ☑
    contusion — *see* Contusion, ankle
    dislocation — *see* Dislocation, ankle
    fracture — *see* Fracture, ankle
    nerve — *see* Injury, nerve, ankle
    open — *see* Wound, open, ankle
    specified type NEC S99.81- ☑
    sprain — *see* Sprain, ankle
    superficial — *see* Injury, superficial, ankle
  anterior chamber, eye — *see* Injury, eye, specified site
    NEC
  anus — *see* Injury, abdomen
  aorta (thoracic) S25.00 ☑
    abdominal S35.00 ☑
      laceration (minor) (superficial) S35.01 ☑
        major S35.02 ☑
      specified type NEC S35.09 ☑
    laceration (minor) (superficial) S25.01 ☑
      major S25.02 ☑
    specified type NEC S25.09 ☑
  arm (upper) S49.9- ☑
    blood vessel — *see* Injury, blood vessel, arm
    contusion — *see* Contusion, arm, upper
    fracture — *see* Fracture, humerus
    lower — *see* Injury, forearm
    muscle — *see* Injury, muscle, shoulder
    nerve — *see* Injury, nerve, arm
    open — *see* Wound, open, arm
    specified type NEC S49.8- ☑
    superficial — *see* Injury, superficial, arm
  artery (complicating trauma) (*see also* Injury, blood
    vessel, by site)
    cerebral or meningeal — *see* Injury, intracranial
  auditory canal (external) (meatus) S09.91 ☑
  auricle, auris, ear S09.91 ☑
  axilla — *see* Injury, shoulder
  back — *see* Injury, back, lower
  bile duct S36.13 ☑
  birth (*see also* Birth, injury) P15.9
  bladder (sphincter) S37.20 ☑
    at delivery O71.5
    contusion S37.22 ☑

Injury — *continued*
  bladder — *continued*
    laceration S37.23 ☑
    obstetrical trauma O71.5
    specified type NEC S37.29 ☑
  blast (air) (hydraulic) (immersion) (underwater) NEC
    T14.8
    acoustic nerve trauma — *see* Injury, nerve, acoustic
    bladder — *see* Injury, bladder
    brain — *see* Concussion
    colon — *see* Injury, intestine, large
    ear (primary) S09.31- ☑
      secondary S09.39- ☑
    generalized T70.8 ☑
    lung — *see* Injury, intrathoracic, lung
    multiple body organs T70.8 ☑
    peritoneum S36.81 ☑
    rectum S36.61 ☑
    retroperitoneum S36.898 ☑
    small intestine S36.419 ☑
      duodenum S36.410 ☑
      specified site NEC S36.418 ☑
    specified
      intra-abdominal organ NEC S36.898 ☑
      pelvic organ NEC S37.899 ☑
  blood vessel NEC T14.8
    abdomen S35.9 ☑
      aorta — *see* Injury, aorta, abdominal
      celiac artery — *see* Injury, blood vessel, celiac
        artery
      iliac vessel — *see* Injury, blood vessel, iliac
      laceration S35.91 ☑
      mesenteric vessel — *see* Injury, mesenteric
      portal vein — *see* Injury, blood vessel, portal
        vein
      renal vessel — *see* Injury, blood vessel, renal
      specified vessel NEC S35.8X- ☑
      splenic vessel — *see* Injury, blood vessel,
        splenic
      vena cava — *see* Injury, vena cava, inferior
    ankle — *see* Injury, blood vessel, foot
    aorta (abdominal) (thoracic) — *see* Injury, aorta
    arm (upper) NEC S45.90- ☑
      forearm — *see* Injury, blood vessel, forearm
      laceration S45.91- ☑
      specified
        site NEC S45.80- ☑
          laceration S45.81- ☑
          specified type NEC S45.89- ☑
        type NEC S45.99- ☑
      superficial vein S45.30- ☑
        laceration S45.31- ☑
        specified type NEC S45.39- ☑
    axillary
      artery S45.00- ☑
        laceration S45.01- ☑
        specified type NEC S45.09- ☑
      vein S45.20- ☑
        laceration S45.21- ☑
        specified type NEC S45.29- ☑
    azygos vein — *see* Injury, blood vessel, thoracic,
      specified site NEC
    brachial
      artery S45.10- ☑
        laceration S45.11- ☑
        specified type NEC S45.19- ☑
      vein S45.20- ☑
        laceration S45.219 ☑
        specified type NEC S45.29- ☑
    carotid artery (common) (external) (internal, ex-
      tracranial) S15.00- ☑
      internal, intracranial S06.8- ☑
      laceration (minor) (superficial) S15.01- ☑
        major S15.02- ☑
      specified type NEC S15.09- ☑
    celiac artery S35.219 ☑
      branch S35.299 ☑
        laceration (minor) (superficial) S35.291 ☑
          major S35.292 ☑
        specified NEC S35.298 ☑
      laceration (minor) (superficial) S35.211 ☑
        major S35.212 ☑
      specified type NEC S35.218 ☑
    cerebral — *see* Injury, intracranial
    deep plantar — *see* Injury, blood vessel, plantar
      artery

Injury — *continued*
  blood vessel — *continued*
    digital (hand) — *see* Injury, blood vessel, finger
    dorsal
      artery (foot) S95.00- ☑
        laceration S95.01- ☑
        specified type NEC S95.09- ☑
      vein (foot) S95.20- ☑
        laceration S95.21- ☑
        specified type NEC S95.29- ☑
    due to accidental laceration during procedure —
      see Laceration, accidental complicating
      surgery
    extremity — *see* Injury, blood vessel, limb
    femoral
      artery (common) (superficial) S75.00- ☑
        laceration (minor) (superficial) S75.01- ☑
          major S75.02- ☑
        specified type NEC S75.09- ☑
      vein (hip level) (thigh level) S75.10- ☑
        laceration (minor) (superficial) S75.11- ☑
          major S75.12- ☑
        specified type NEC S75.19- ☑
    finger S65.50- ☑
      index S65.50- ☑
        laceration S65.51- ☑
        specified type NEC S65.59- ☑
      laceration S65.51- ☑
      little S65.50- ☑
        laceration S65.51- ☑
        specified type NEC S65.59- ☑
      middle S65.50- ☑
        laceration S65.51- ☑
        specified type NEC S65.59- ☑
      specified type NEC S65.59- ☑
      thumb — *see* Injury, blood vessel, thumb
    foot S95.90- ☑
      dorsal
        artery — *see* Injury, blood vessel, dorsal,
          artery
        vein — *see* Injury, blood vessel, dorsal, vein
      laceration S95.91- ☑
      plantar artery — *see* Injury, blood vessel, plan-
        tar artery
      specified
        site NEC S95.80- ☑
          laceration S95.81- ☑
          specified type NEC S95.89- ☑
        specified type NEC S95.99- ☑
    forearm S55.90- ☑
      laceration S55.91- ☑
      radial artery — *see* Injury, blood vessel, radial
        artery
      specified
        site NEC S55.80- ☑
          laceration S55.81- ☑
          specified type NEC S55.89- ☑
        type NEC S55.99- ☑
      ulnar artery — *see* Injury, blood vessel, ulnar
        artery
      vein S55.20- ☑
        laceration S55.21- ☑
        specified type NEC S55.29- ☑
    gastric
      artery — *see* Injury, mesenteric, artery, branch
      vein — *see* Injury, blood vessel, abdomen
    gastroduodenal artery — *see* Injury, mesenteric,
      artery, branch
    greater saphenous vein (lower leg level) S85.30- ☑
      hip (and thigh) level S75.20- ☑
        laceration (minor) (superficial) S75.21- ☑
          major S75.22- ☑
        specified type NEC S75.29- ☑
      laceration S85.31- ☑
      specified type NEC S85.39- ☑
    hand (level) S65.90- ☑
      finger — *see* Injury, blood vessel, finger
      laceration S65.91- ☑
      palmar arch — *see* Injury, blood vessel, palmar
        arch
      radial artery — *see* Injury, blood vessel, radial
        artery, hand
      specified
        site NEC S65.80- ☑
          laceration S65.81- ☑
          specified type NEC S65.89- ☑

Injury — *continued*
  blood vessel — *continued*
    hand — *continued*
      specified — *continued*
        type NEC S65.99- ☑
      thumb — *see* Injury, blood vessel, thumb
      ulnar artery — *see* Injury, blood vessel, ulnar
        artery, hand
    head S09.0 ☑
      intracranial — *see* Injury, intracranial
      multiple S09.0 ☑
    hepatic
      artery — *see* Injury, mesenteric, artery
      vein — *see* Injury, vena cava, inferior
    hip S75.90- ☑
      femoral artery — *see* Injury, blood vessel,
        femoral, artery
      femoral vein — *see* Injury, blood vessel,
        femoral, vein
      greater saphenous vein — *see* Injury, blood
        vessel, greater saphenous, hip level
      laceration S75.91- ☑
      specified
        site NEC S75.80- ☑
          laceration S75.81- ☑
          specified type NEC S75.89- ☑
        type NEC S75.99- ☑
    hypogastric (artery) (vein) — *see* Injury, blood
      vessel, iliac
    iliac S35.5- ☑
      artery S35.51- ☑
      specified vessel NEC S35.5- ☑
      uterine vessel — *see* Injury, blood vessel, uter-
        ine
      vein S35.51- ☑
    innominate — *see* Injury, blood vessel, thoracic,
      innominate
    intercostal (artery) (vein) — *see* Injury, blood vessel,
      thoracic, intercostal
    jugular vein (external) S15.20- ☑
      internal S15.30- ☑
        laceration (minor) (superficial) S15.31- ☑
          major S15.32- ☑
        specified type NEC S15.39- ☑
      laceration (minor) (superficial) S15.21- ☑
        major S15.22- ☑
      specified type NEC S15.29- ☑
    leg (level) (lower) S85.90- ☑
      greater saphenous — *see* Injury, blood vessel,
        greater saphenous
      laceration S85.91- ☑
      lesser saphenous — *see* Injury, blood vessel,
        lesser saphenous
      peroneal artery — *see* Injury, blood vessel,
        peroneal artery
      popliteal
        artery — *see* Injury, blood vessel, popliteal,
          artery
        vein — *see* Injury, blood vessel, popliteal,
          vein
      specified
        site NEC S85.80- ☑
          laceration S85.81- ☑
          specified type NEC S85.89- ☑
        type NEC S85.99- ☑
      thigh — *see* Injury, blood vessel, hip
      tibial artery — *see* Injury, blood vessel, tibial
        artery
    lesser saphenous vein (lower leg level) S85.40- ☑
      laceration S85.41- ☑
      specified type NEC S85.49- ☑
    limb
      lower — *see* Injury, blood vessel, leg
      upper — *see* Injury, blood vessel, arm
    lower back — *see* Injury, blood vessel, abdomen
      specified NEC — *see* Injury, blood vessel, ab-
        domen, specified, site NEC
    mammary (artery) (vein) — *see* Injury, blood vessel,
      thoracic, specified site NEC
    mesenteric (inferior) (superior)
      artery — *see* Injury, mesenteric, artery
      vein — *see* Injury, blood vessel, mesenteric,
        vein
    neck S15.9
      specified site NEC S15.8
    ovarian (artery) (vein) — *see* subcategory S35.8 ☑

☑ Additional Character Required — Refer to the Tabular List for Character Selection   ▼ Subterms under main terms may continue to next column or page

Injury — *continued*
blood vessel — *continued*
palmar arch (superficial) S65.20- ☑
deep S65.30- ☑
laceration S65.31- ☑
specified type NEC S65.39- ☑
laceration S65.21- ☑
specified type NEC S65.29- ☑
pelvis — *see* Injury, blood vessel, abdomen
specified NEC — *see* Injury, blood vessel, abdomen, specified, site NEC
peroneal artery S85.20- ☑
laceration S85.21- ☑
specified type NEC S85.29- ☑
plantar artery (deep) (foot) S95.10- ☑
laceration S95.11- ☑
specified type NEC S95.19- ☑
popliteal
artery S85.00- ☑
laceration S85.01- ☑
specified type NEC S85.09- ☑
vein S85.50- ☑
laceration S85.51- ☑
specified type NEC S85.59- ☑
portal vein S35.319 ☑
laceration S35.311 ☑
specified type NEC S35.318 ☑
precerebral — *see* Injury, blood vessel, neck
pulmonary (artery) (vein) — *see* Injury, blood vessel, thoracic, pulmonary
radial artery (forearm level) S55.10- ☑
hand and wrist (level) S65.10- ☑
laceration S65.11- ☑
specified type NEC S65.19- ☑
laceration S55.11- ☑
specified type NEC S55.19- ☑
renal
artery S35.40- ☑
laceration S35.41- ☑
specified NEC S35.49- ☑
vein S35.40- ☑
laceration S35.41- ☑
specified NEC S35.49- ☑
saphenous vein (greater) (lower leg level) — *see* Injury, blood vessel, greater saphenous
hip and thigh level — *see* Injury, blood vessel, greater saphenous, hip level
lesser — *see* Injury, blood vessel, lesser saphenous
shoulder
specified NEC — *see* Injury, blood vessel, arm, specified site NEC
superficial vein — *see* Injury, blood vessel, arm, superficial vein
specified NEC T14.8
splenic
artery — *see* Injury, blood vessel, celiac artery, branch
vein S35.329 ☑
laceration S35.321 ☑
specified NEC S35.328 ☑
subclavian — *see* Injury, blood vessel, thoracic, innominate
thigh — *see* Injury, blood vessel, hip
thoracic S25.90 ☑
aorta S25.00 ☑
laceration (minor) (superficial) S25.01 ☑
major S25.02 ☑
specified type NEC S25.09 ☑
azygos vein — *see* Injury, blood vessel, thoracic, specified, site NEC
innominate
artery S25.10- ☑
laceration (minor) (superficial) S25.11- ☑
major S25.12- ☑
specified type NEC S25.19- ☑
vein S25.30- ☑
laceration (minor) (superficial) S25.31- ☑
major S25.32- ☑
specified type NEC S25.39- ☑
intercostal S25.50- ☑
laceration S25.51- ☑
specified type NEC S25.59- ☑
laceration S25.91 ☑

Injury — *continued*
blood vessel — *continued*
thoracic — *continued*
mammary vessel — *see* Injury, blood vessel, thoracic, specified, site NEC
pulmonary S25.40- ☑
laceration (minor) (superficial) S25.41- ☑
major S25.42- ☑
specified type NEC S25.49- ☑
specified
site NEC S25.80- ☑
laceration S25.81 ☑
specified type NEC S25.89 ☑
type NEC S25.99 ☑
subclavian — *see* Injury, blood vessel, thoracic, innominate
vena cava (superior) S25.20 ☑
laceration (minor) (superficial) S25.21 ☑
major S25.22 ☑
specified type NEC S25.29 ☑
thumb S65.40- ☑
laceration S65.41- ☑
specified type NEC S65.49- ☑
tibial artery S85.10- ☑
anterior S85.13- ☑
laceration S85.14- ☑
specified injury NEC S85.15- ☑
laceration S85.11- ☑
posterior S85.16- ☑
laceration S85.17- ☑
specified injury NEC S85.18- ☑
specified injury NEC S85.12- ☑
ulnar artery (forearm level) S55.00- ☑
hand and wrist (level) S65.00- ☑
laceration S65.01- ☑
specified type NEC S65.09- ☑
laceration S55.01- ☑
specified type NEC S55.09- ☑
upper arm (level) — *see* Injury, blood vessel, arm
superficial vein — *see* Injury, blood vessel, arm, superficial vein
uterine S35.5- ☑
artery S35.53- ☑
vein S35.53- ☑
vena cava — *see* Injury, vena cava
vertebral artery S15.10- ☑
laceration (minor) (superficial) S15.11- ☑
major S15.12- ☑
specified type NEC S15.19- ☑
wrist (level) — *see* Injury, blood vessel, hand
brachial plexus S14.3 ☑
newborn P14.3
brain (traumatic) S06.9- ☑
diffuse (axonal) S06.2X- ☑
focal S06.30- ☑
traumatic — *see* category S06
brainstem S06.38- ☑
breast NOS S29.9
broad ligament — *see* Injury, pelvic organ, specified site NEC
bronchus, bronchi — *see* Injury, intrathoracic, bronchus
brow S09.90 ☑
buttock S39.92 ☑
canthus, eye S05.90 ☑
cardiac plexus — *see* Injury, nerve, thorax, sympathetic
cauda equina S34.3 ☑
cavernous sinus — *see* Injury, intracranial
cecum — *see* Injury, colon
celiac ganglion or plexus — *see* Injury, nerve, lumbosacral, sympathetic
cerebellum — *see* Injury, intracranial
cerebral — *see* Injury, intracranial
cervix (uteri) — *see* Injury, uterus
cheek (wall) S09.93 ☑
chest — *see* Injury, thorax
childbirth (newborn) (*see also* Birth, injury)
maternal NEC O71.9
chin S09.93 ☑
choroid (eye) — *see* Injury, eye, specified site NEC
clitoris S39.94 ☑
coccyx (*see also* Injury, back, lower)
complicating delivery O71.6
colon — *see* Injury, intestine, large
common bile duct — *see* Injury, liver
conjunctiva (superficial) — *see* Injury, eye, conjunctiva

Injury — *continued*
conus medullaris — *see* Injury, spinal, sacral cord
spermatic (pelvic region) S37.898 ☑
scrotal region S39.848 ☑
spinal — *see* Injury, spinal cord, by region
cornea — *see* Injury, eye, specified site NEC
abrasion — *see* Injury, eye, cornea, abrasion
cortex (cerebral) (*see also* Injury, intracranial)
visual — *see* Injury, nerve, optic
costal region NEC S29.9 ☑
costochondral NEC S29.9 ☑
cranial
cavity — *see* Injury, intracranial
nerve — *see* Injury, nerve, cranial
crushing — *see* Crush
cutaneous sensory nerve
cystic duct — *see* Injury, liver
deep tissue — *see* Contusion, by site
meaning pressure ulcer — *see* Ulcer, pressure, unstageable, by site
delivery (newborn) P15.9
maternal NEC O71.9
Descemet's membrane — *see* Injury, eyeball, penetrating
diaphragm — *see* Injury, intrathoracic, diaphragm
duodenum — *see* Injury, intestine, small, duodenum
ear (auricle) (external) (canal) S09.91 ☑
abrasion — *see* Abrasion, ear
bite — *see* Bite, ear
blister — *see* Blister, ear
bruise — *see* Contusion, ear
contusion — *see* Contusion, ear
external constriction — *see* Constriction, external, ear
hematoma — *see* Hematoma, ear
inner — *see* Injury, ear, middle
laceration — *see* Laceration, ear
middle S09.30- ☑
blast — *see* Injury, blast, ear
specified NEC S09.39- ☑
puncture — *see* Puncture, ear
superficial — *see* Injury, superficial, ear
eighth cranial nerve (acoustic or auditory) — *see* Injury, nerve, acoustic
elbow S59.90- ☑
contusion — *see* Contusion, elbow
dislocation — *see* Dislocation, elbow
fracture — *see* Fracture, ulna, upper end
open — *see* Wound, open, elbow
specified NEC S59.80- ☑
sprain — *see* Sprain, elbow
superficial — *see* Injury, superficial, elbow
eleventh cranial nerve (accessory) — *see* Injury, nerve, accessory
epididymis S39.94 ☑
epigastric region S39.91 ☑
epiglottis NEC S19.89 ☑
esophageal plexus — *see* Injury, nerve, thorax, sympathetic
esophagus (thoracic part) (*see also* Injury, intrathoracic, esophagus)
cervical NEC S19.85 ☑
eustachian tube S09.30 ☑
eye S05.9- ☑
avulsion S05.7- ☑
ball — *see* Injury, eyeball
conjunctiva S05.0- ☑
cornea
abrasion S05.0- ☑
laceration S05.3- ☑
with prolapse S05.2- ☑
lacrimal apparatus S05.8X- ☑
orbit penetration S05.4- ☑
specified site NEC S05.8X- ☑
eyeball S05.8X- ☑
contusion S05.1- ☑
penetrating S05.6- ☑
with
foreign body S05.5- ☑
prolapse or loss of intraocular tissue S05.2- ☑
without prolapse or loss of intraocular tissue S05.3- ☑
specified type NEC S05.8- ☑
eyebrow S09.93 ☑

Injury — *continued*
- eyelid S09.93 ☑
  - abrasion — *see* Abrasion, eyelid
  - contusion — *see* Contusion, eyelid
  - open — *see* Wound, open, eyelid
- face S09.93 ☑
- fallopian tube S37.509 ☑
  - bilateral S37.502 ☑
    - blast injury S37.512 ☑
    - contusion S37.522 ☑
    - laceration S37.532 ☑
    - specified type NEC S37.592 ☑
  - blast injury (primary) S37.519 ☑
    - bilateral S37.512 ☑
    - secondary — *see* Injury, fallopian tube, specified type NEC
    - unilateral S37.511 ☑
  - contusion S37.529 ☑
    - bilateral S37.522 ☑
    - unilateral S37.521 ☑
  - laceration S37.539 ☑
    - bilateral S37.532 ☑
    - unilateral S37.531 ☑
  - specified type NEC S37.599 ☑
    - bilateral S37.592 ☑
    - unilateral S37.591 ☑
  - unilateral S37.501 ☑
    - blast injury S37.511 ☑
    - contusion S37.521 ☑
    - laceration S37.531 ☑
    - specified type NEC S37.591 ☑
- fascia — *see* Injury, muscle
- fifth cranial nerve (trigeminal) — *see* Injury, nerve, trigeminal
- finger (nail) S69.9- ☑
  - blood vessel — *see* Injury, blood vessel, finger
  - contusion — *see* Contusion, finger
  - dislocation — *see* Dislocation, finger
  - fracture — *see* Fracture, finger
  - muscle — *see* Injury, muscle, finger
  - nerve — *see* Injury, nerve, digital, finger
  - open — *see* Wound, open, finger
  - specified NEC S69.8- ☑
  - sprain — *see* Sprain, finger
  - superficial — *see* Injury, superficial, finger
- first cranial nerve (olfactory) — *see* Injury, nerve, olfactory
- flank — *see* Injury, abdomen
- foot S99.92- ☑
  - blood vessel — *see* Injury, blood vessel, foot
  - contusion — *see* Contusion, foot
  - dislocation — *see* Dislocation, foot
  - fracture — *see* Fracture, foot
  - muscle — *see* Injury, muscle, foot
  - open — *see* Wound, open, foot
  - specified type NEC S99.82- ☑
  - sprain — *see* Sprain, foot
  - superficial — *see* Injury, superficial, foot
- forceps NOS P15.9
- forearm S59.91- ☑
  - blood vessel — *see* Injury, blood vessel, forearm
  - contusion — *see* Contusion, forearm
  - fracture — *see* Fracture, forearm
  - muscle — *see* Injury, muscle, forearm
  - nerve — *see* Injury, nerve, forearm
  - open — *see* Wound, open, forearm
  - specified NEC S59.81- ☑
  - superficial — *see* Injury, superficial, forearm
- forehead S09.90 ☑
- fourth cranial nerve (trochlear) — *see* Injury, nerve, trochlear
- gallbladder S36.129 ☑
  - contusion S36.122 ☑
  - laceration S36.123 ☑
  - specified NEC S36.128 ☑
- ganglion
  - celiac, coeliac — *see* Injury, nerve, lumbosacral, sympathetic
  - gasserian — *see* Injury, nerve, trigeminal
  - stellate — *see* Injury, nerve, thorax, sympathetic
  - thoracic sympathetic — *see* Injury, nerve, thorax, sympathetic
- gasserian ganglion — *see* Injury, nerve, trigeminal
- gastric artery — *see* Injury, blood vessel, celiac artery, branch

Injury — *continued*
- gastroduodenal artery — *see* Injury, blood vessel, celiac artery, branch
- gastrointestinal tract — *see* Injury, intra-abdominal
  - with open wound into abdominal cavity — *see* Wound, open, with penetration into peritoneal cavity
  - colon — *see* Injury, intestine, large
  - rectum — *see* Injury, intestine, large, rectum
    - with open wound into abdominal cavity S36.61
  - small intestine — *see* Injury, intestine, small
  - specified site NEC — *see* Injury, intra-abdominal, specified, site NEC
  - stomach — *see* Injury, stomach
- genital organ(s)
  - external S39.94 ☑
    - specified NEC S39.848 ☑
  - internal S37.90 ☑
    - fallopian tube — *see* Injury, fallopian tube
    - ovary — *see* Injury, ovary
    - prostate — *see* Injury, prostate
    - seminal vesicle — *see* Injury, pelvis, organ, specified site NEC
    - uterus — *see* Injury, uterus
    - vas deferens — *see* Injury, pelvis, organ, specified site NEC
  - obstetrical trauma O71.9
- gland
  - lacrimal laceration — *see* Injury, eye, specified site NEC
  - salivary S09.90 ☑
  - thyroid NEC S19.84 ☑
- globe (eye) S05.90 ☑
  - specified NEC S05.8X- ☑
- groin — *see* Injury, abdomen
- gum S09.90 ☑
- hand S69.9- ☑
  - blood vessel — *see* Injury, blood vessel, hand
  - contusion — *see* Contusion, hand
  - fracture — *see* Fracture, hand
  - muscle — *see* Injury, muscle, hand
  - nerve — *see* Injury, nerve, hand
  - open — *see* Wound, open, hand
  - specified NEC S69.8- ☑
  - sprain — *see* Sprain, hand
  - superficial — *see* Injury, superficial, hand
- head S09.90 ☑
  - with loss of consciousness S06.9- ☑
  - specified NEC S09.8 ☑
- heart S26.90 ☑
  - with hemopericardium S26.00 ☑
    - contusion S26.01 ☑
    - laceration (mild) S26.020 ☑
      - major S26.022 ☑
      - moderate S26.021 ☑
    - specified type NEC S26.09 ☑
  - without hemopericardium S26.10 ☑
    - contusion S26.11 ☑
    - laceration S26.12 ☑
    - specified type NEC S26.19 ☑
  - contusion S26.91 ☑
  - laceration S26.92 ☑
  - specified type NEC S26.99 ☑
- heel — *see* Injury, foot
- hepatic
  - artery — *see* Injury, blood vessel, celiac artery, branch
  - duct — *see* Injury, liver
  - vein — *see* Injury, vena cava, inferior
- hip S79.91- ☑
  - blood vessel — *see* Injury, blood vessel, hip
  - contusion — *see* Contusion, hip
  - dislocation — *see* Dislocation, hip
  - fracture — *see* Fracture, femur, neck
  - muscle — *see* Injury, muscle, hip
  - nerve — *see* Injury, nerve, hip
  - open — *see* Wound, open, hip
  - specified NEC S79.81- ☑
  - sprain — *see* Sprain, hip
  - superficial — *see* Injury, superficial, hip
- hymen S39.94 ☑
- hypogastric
  - blood vessel — *see* Injury, blood vessel, iliac
  - plexus — *see* Injury, nerve, lumbosacral, sympathetic

Injury — *continued*
- ileum — *see* Injury, intestine, small
- iliac region S39.91 ☑
- instrumental (during surgery) — *see* Laceration, accidental complicating surgery
  - birth injury — *see* Birth, injury
  - nonsurgical — *see* Injury, by site
  - obstetrical O71.9
    - bladder O71.5
    - cervix O71.3
    - high vaginal O71.4
    - perineal NOS O70.9
    - urethra O71.5
    - uterus O71.5
      - with rupture or perforation O71.1
- internal T14.8
  - aorta — *see* Injury, aorta
  - bladder (sphincter) — *see* Injury, bladder
    - with
      - ectopic or molar pregnancy O08.6
      - following ectopic or molar pregnancy O08.6
      - obstetrical trauma O71.5
  - bronchus, bronchi — *see* Injury, intrathoracic, bronchus
  - cecum — *see* Injury, intestine, large
  - cervix (uteri) (*see also* Injury, uterus)
    - with ectopic or molar pregnancy O08.6
    - following ectopic or molar pregnancy O08.6
    - obstetrical trauma O71.3
  - chest — *see* Injury, intrathoracic
  - gastrointestinal tract — *see* Injury, intra-abdominal
  - heart — *see* Injury, heart
  - intestine NEC — *see* Injury, intestine
  - intrauterine — *see* Injury, uterus
  - mesentery — *see* Injury, intra-abdominal, specified, site NEC
  - pelvis, pelvic (organ) S37.90 ☑
    - following ectopic or molar pregnancy (subsequent episode) O08.6
    - obstetrical trauma NEC O71.5
      - rupture or perforation O71.1
    - specified NEC S39.83 ☑
  - rectum — *see* Injury, intestine, large, rectum
  - stomach — *see* Injury, stomach
  - ureter — *see* Injury, ureter
  - urethra (sphincter) following ectopic or molar pregnancy O08.6
  - uterus — *see* Injury, uterus
- interscapular area — *see* Injury, thorax
- intestine
  - large S36.509 ☑
    - ascending (right) S36.500 ☑
      - blast injury (primary) S36.510 ☑
        - secondary S36.590 ☑
      - contusion S36.520 ☑
      - laceration S36.530 ☑
      - specified type NEC S36.590 ☑
    - blast injury (primary) S36.519 ☑
      - ascending (right) S36.510 ☑
      - descending (left) S36.512 ☑
      - rectum S36.61 ☑
      - sigmoid S36.513 ☑
      - specified site NEC S36.518 ☑
      - transverse S36.511 ☑
    - contusion S36.529 ☑
      - ascending (right) S36.520 ☑
      - descending (left) S36.522 ☑
      - rectum S36.62 ☑
      - sigmoid S36.523 ☑
      - specified site NEC S36.528 ☑
      - transverse S36.521 ☑
    - descending (left) S36.502 ☑
      - blast injury (primary) S36.512 ☑
        - secondary S36.592 ☑
      - contusion S36.522 ☑
      - laceration S36.532 ☑
      - specified type NEC S36.592 ☑
    - laceration S36.539 ☑
      - ascending (right) S36.530 ☑
      - descending (left) S36.532 ☑
      - rectum S36.63 ☑
      - sigmoid S36.533 ☑
      - specified site NEC S36.538 ☑
      - transverse S36.531 ☑
    - rectum S36.60 ☑
      - blast injury (primary) S36.61 ☑

☑ Additional Character Required — Refer to the Tabular List for Character Selection

▽ Subterms under main terms may continue to next column or page

Injury — *continued*
  intestine — *continued*
    large — *continued*
      rectum — *continued*
        blast injury — *continued*
          secondary S36.69 ☑
        contusion S36.62 ☑
        laceration S36.63 ☑
        specified type NEC S36.69 ☑
      sigmoid S36.503 ☑
        blast injury (primary) S36.513 ☑
          secondary S36.593 ☑
        contusion S36.523 ☑
        laceration S36.533 ☑
        specified type NEC S36.593 ☑
      specified
        site NEC S36.508 ☑
          blast injury (primary) S36.518 ☑
            secondary S36.598 ☑
          contusion S36.528 ☑
          laceration S36.538 ☑
          specified type NEC S36.598 ☑
        type NEC S36.599 ☑
          ascending (right) S36.590 ☑
          descending (left) S36.592 ☑
          rectum S36.69 ☑
          sigmoid S36.593 ☑
          specified site NEC S36.598 ☑
          transverse S36.591 ☑
      transverse S36.501 ☑
        blast injury (primary) S36.511 ☑
          secondary S36.591 ☑
        contusion S36.521 ☑
        laceration S36.531 ☑
        specified type NEC S36.591 ☑
    small S36.409 ☑
      blast injury (primary) S36.419 ☑
        duodenum S36.410 ☑
        secondary S36.499 ☑
          duodenum S36.490 ☑
          specified site NEC S36.498 ☑
        specified site NEC S36.418 ☑
      contusion S36.429 ☑
        duodenum S36.420 ☑
        specified site NEC S36.428 ☑
      duodenum S36.400 ☑
        blast injury (primary) S36.410 ☑
          secondary S36.490 ☑
        contusion S36.420 ☑
        laceration S36.430 ☑
        specified NEC S36.490 ☑
      laceration S36.439 ☑
        duodenum S36.430 ☑
        specified site NEC S36.438 ☑
      specified
        site NEC S36.408 ☑
        type NEC S36.499 ☑
          duodenum S36.490 ☑
          specified site NEC S36.498 ☑
  intra-abdominal S36.90 ☑
    adrenal gland — *see* Injury, adrenal gland
    bladder — *see* Injury, bladder
    colon — *see* Injury, intestine, large
    contusion S36.92 ☑
    fallopian tube — *see* Injury, fallopian tube
    gallbladder — *see* Injury, gallbladder
    intestine — *see* Injury, intestine
    kidney — *see* Injury, kidney
    laceration S36.93 ☑
    liver — *see* Injury, liver
    ovary — *see* Injury, ovary
    pancreas — *see* Injury, pancreas
    pelvic NOS S37.90 ☑
    peritoneum — *see* Injury, intra-abdominal, speci-
      fied, site NEC
    prostate — *see* Injury, prostate
    rectum — *see* Injury, intestine, large, rectum
    retroperitoneum — *see* Injury, intra-abdominal,
      specified, site NEC
    seminal vesicle — *see* Injury, pelvis, organ, speci-
      fied site NEC
    small intestine — *see* Injury, intestine, small
    specified
      pelvic S37.90 ☑
        specified
          site NEC S37.899 ☑

Injury — *continued*
  intra-abdominal — *continued*
    specified — *continued*
      pelvic — *continued*
        specified — *continued*
          site — *continued*
            specified type NEC S37.898 ☑
          type NEC S37.99 ☑
        site NEC S36.899 ☑
          contusion S36.892 ☑
          laceration S36.893 ☑
          specified type NEC S36.898 ☑
        type NEC S36.99 ☑
    spleen — *see* Injury, spleen
    stomach — *see* Injury, stomach
    ureter — *see* Injury, ureter
    urethra — *see* Injury, urethra
    uterus — *see* Injury, uterus
    vas deferens — *see* Injury, pelvis, organ, specified
      site NEC
  intracranial (traumatic) S06.9- ☑
    cerebellar hemorrhage, traumatic — *see* Injury,
      intracranial, focal
    cerebral edema, traumatic S06.1X- ☑
      diffuse S06.1X- ☑
      focal S06.1X- ☑
    diffuse (axonal) S06.2X- ☑
    epidural hemorrhage (traumatic) S06.4X- ☑
    focal brain injury S06.30- ☑
      contusion — *see* Contusion, cerebral
      laceration — *see* Laceration, cerebral
      intracerebral hemorrhage, traumatic S06.36- ☑
        left side S06.35- ☑
        right side S06.34- ☑
    subarachnoid hemorrhage, traumatic S06.6X- ☑
    subdural hemorrhage, traumatic S06.5X- ☑
  intraocular — *see* Injury, eyeball, penetrating
  intrathoracic S27.9 ☑
    bronchus S27.409 ☑
      bilateral S27.402 ☑
      blast injury (primary) S27.419 ☑
        bilateral S27.412 ☑
        secondary — *see* Injury, intrathoracic,
          bronchus, specified type NEC
        unilateral S27.411 ☑
      contusion S27.429 ☑
        bilateral S27.422 ☑
        unilateral S27.421 ☑
      laceration S27.439 ☑
        bilateral S27.432 ☑
        unilateral S27.431 ☑
      specified type NEC S27.499 ☑
        bilateral S27.492 ☑
        unilateral S27.491 ☑
      unilateral S27.401 ☑
    diaphragm S27.809 ☑
      contusion S27.802 ☑
      laceration S27.803 ☑
      specified type NEC S27.808 ☑
    esophagus (thoracic) S27.819 ☑
      contusion S27.812 ☑
      laceration S27.813 ☑
      specified type NEC S27.818 ☑
    heart — *see* Injury, heart
    hemopneumothorax S27.2 ☑
    hemothorax S27.1 ☑
    lung S27.309 ☑
      aspiration J69.0
      bilateral S27.302 ☑
      blast injury (primary) S27.319 ☑
        bilateral S27.312 ☑
        secondary — *see* Injury, intrathoracic, lung,
          specified type NEC
        unilateral S27.311 ☑
      contusion S27.329 ☑
        bilateral S27.322 ☑
        unilateral S27.321 ☑
      laceration S27.339 ☑
        bilateral S27.332 ☑
        unilateral S27.331 ☑
      specified type NEC S27.399 ☑
        bilateral S27.392 ☑
        unilateral S27.391 ☑
      unilateral S27.301 ☑
    pleura S27.60 ☑
      laceration S27.63 ☑

Injury — *continued*
  intrathoracic — *continued*
    pleura — *continued*
      specified type NEC S27.69 ☑
    pneumothorax S27.0 ☑
    specified organ NEC S27.899 ☑
      contusion S27.892 ☑
      laceration S27.893 ☑
      specified type NEC S27.898 ☑
    thoracic duct — *see* Injury, intrathoracic, specified
      organ NEC
    thymus gland — *see* Injury, intrathoracic, specified
      organ NEC
    trachea, thoracic S27.50 ☑
      blast (primary) S27.51 ☑
      contusion S27.52 ☑
      laceration S27.53 ☑
      specified type NEC S27.59 ☑
  iris — *see* Injury, eye, specified site NEC
    penetrating — *see* Injury, eyeball, penetrating
  jaw S09.93 ☑
  jejunum — *see* Injury, intestine, small
  joint NOS T14.8
    old or residual — *see* Disorder, joint, specified type
      NEC
  kidney S37.00- ☑
    acute (nontraumatic) N17.9
    contusion — *see* Contusion, kidney
    laceration — *see* Laceration, kidney
    specified NEC S37.09- ☑
  knee S89.9- ☑
    contusion — *see* Contusion, knee
    dislocation — *see* Dislocation, knee
    meniscus (lateral) (medial) — *see* Sprain, knee,
      specified site NEC
      old injury or tear — *see* Derangement, knee,
        meniscus, due to old injury
    open — *see* Wound, open, knee
    specified NEC S89.8- ☑
    sprain — *see* Sprain, knee
    superficial — *see* Injury, superficial, knee
  labium (majus) (minus) S39.94 ☑
  labyrinth, ear S09.30- ☑
  lacrimal apparatus, duct, gland, or sac — *see* Injury,
    eye, specified site NEC
  larynx NEC S19.81 ☑
  leg (lower) S89.9- ☑
    blood vessel — *see* Injury, blood vessel, leg
    contusion — *see* Contusion, leg
    fracture — *see* Fracture, leg
    muscle — *see* Injury, muscle, leg
    nerve — *see* Injury, nerve, leg
    open — *see* Wound, open, leg
    specified NEC S89.8- ☑
    superficial — *see* Injury, superficial, leg
  lens, eye — *see* Injury, eye, specified site NEC
    penetrating — *see* Injury, eyeball, penetrating
  limb NEC T14.8
  lip S09.93 ☑
  liver S36.119 ☑
    contusion S36.112 ☑
    laceration S36.113 ☑
      major (stellate) S36.116 ☑
      minor S36.114 ☑
      moderate S36.115 ☑
    specified NEC S36.118 ☑
  lower back S39.92 ☑
    specified NEC S39.82 ☑
  lumbar, lumbosacral (region) S39.92 ☑
    plexus — *see* Injury, lumbosacral plexus
  lumbosacral plexus S34.4 ☑
  lung (*see also* Injury, intrathoracic, lung)
    aspiration J69.0
    transfusion-related (TRALI) J95.84
  lymphatic thoracic duct — *see* Injury, intrathoracic,
    specified organ NEC
  malar region S09.93 ☑
  mastoid region S09.90 ☑
  maxilla S09.93 ☑
  mediastinum — *see* Injury, intrathoracic, specified
    organ NEC
  membrane, brain — *see* Injury, intracranial
  meningeal artery — *see* Injury, intracranial, subdural
    hemorrhage
  meninges (cerebral) — *see* Injury, intracranial

Injury — continued
  mesenteric
    artery
      branch S35.299 ☑
        laceration (minor) (superficial) S35.291 ☑
          major S35.292 ☑
        specified NEC S35.298 ☑
      inferior S35.239 ☑
        laceration (minor) (superficial) S35.231 ☑
          major S35.232 ☑
        specified NEC S35.238 ☑
      superior S35.229 ☑
        laceration (minor) (superficial) S35.221 ☑
          major S35.222 ☑
        specified NEC S35.228 ☑
    plexus (inferior) (superior) — see Injury, nerve, lumbosacral, sympathetic
    vein
      inferior S35.349 ☑
        laceration S35.341 ☑
        specified NEC S35.348 ☑
      superior S35.339 ☑
        laceration S35.331 ☑
        specified NEC S35.338 ☑
  mesentery — see Injury, intra-abdominal, specified site NEC
  mesosalpinx — see Injury, pelvic organ, specified site NEC
  middle ear S09.30- ☑
  midthoracic region NOS S29.9 ☑
  mouth S09.93 ☑
  multiple NOS T07
  muscle (and fascia) (and tendon)
    abdomen S39.001 ☑
      laceration S39.021 ☑
      specified type NEC S39.091 ☑
      strain S39.011 ☑
    abductor
      thumb, forearm level — see Injury, muscle, thumb, abductor
    adductor
      thigh S76.20- ☑
        laceration S76.22- ☑
        specified type NEC S76.29- ☑
        strain S76.21- ☑
    ankle — see Injury, muscle, foot
    anterior muscle group, at leg level (lower) S86.20- ☑
      laceration S86.22- ☑
      specified type NEC S86.29- ☑
      strain S86.21- ☑
    arm (upper) — see Injury, muscle, shoulder
    biceps (parts NEC) S46.20- ☑
      laceration S46.22- ☑
      long head S46.10- ☑
        laceration S46.12- ☑
        specified type NEC S46.19- ☑
        strain S46.11- ☑
      specified type NEC S46.29- ☑
      strain S46.21- ☑
    extensor
      finger(s) (other than thumb) — see Injury, muscle, finger by site, extensor
      forearm level, specified NEC — see Injury, muscle, forearm, extensor
      thumb — see Injury, muscle, thumb, extensor
      toe (large) (ankle level) (foot level) — see Injury, muscle, toe, extensor
    finger
      extensor (forearm level) S56.40- ☑
        hand level S66.309 ☑
          laceration S66.329 ☑
          specified type NEC S66.399 ☑
          strain S66.319 ☑
        laceration S56.429 ☑
        specified type NEC S56.499 ☑
        strain S56.419 ☑
      flexor (forearm level) S56.10- ☑
        hand level S66.109 ☑
          laceration S66.129 ☑
          specified type NEC S66.199 ☑
          strain S66.119 ☑
        laceration S56.129 ☑
        specified type NEC S56.199 ☑
        strain S56.119 ☑
      index

Injury — continued
  muscle — continued
    finger — continued
      index — continued
        extensor (forearm level)
          hand level S66.308 ☑
            laceration S66.32- ☑
            specified type NEC S66.39- ☑
            strain S66.31- ☑
          specified type NEC S56.492- ☑
        flexor (forearm level)
          hand level S66.108 ☑
            laceration S66.12- ☑
            specified type NEC S66.19- ☑
            strain S66.11- ☑
          specified type NEC S56.19- ☑
          strain S56.11- ☑
        intrinsic S66.50- ☑
          laceration S66.52- ☑
          specified type NEC S66.59- ☑
          strain S66.51- ☑
      intrinsic S66.509 ☑
        laceration S66.529 ☑
        specified type NEC S66.599 ☑
        strain S66.519 ☑
      little
        extensor (forearm level)
          hand level S66.30- ☑
            laceration S66.32- ☑
            specified type NEC S66.39- ☑
            strain S66.31- ☑
          laceration S56.42- ☑
          specified type NEC S56.49- ☑
          strain S56.41- ☑
        flexor (forearm level)
          hand level S66.10- ☑
            laceration S66.12- ☑
            specified type NEC S66.19- ☑
            strain S66.11- ☑
          laceration S56.12- ☑
          specified type NEC S56.19- ☑
          strain S56.11- ☑
        intrinsic S66.50- ☑
          laceration S66.52- ☑
          specified type NEC S66.59- ☑
          strain S66.51- ☑
      middle
        extensor (forearm level)
          hand level S66.30- ☑
            laceration S66.32- ☑
            specified type NEC S66.39- ☑
            strain S66.31- ☑
          laceration S56.42- ☑
          specified type NEC S56.49- ☑
          strain S56.41- ☑
        flexor (forearm level)
          hand level S66.10- ☑
            laceration S66.12- ☑
            specified type NEC S66.19- ☑
            strain S66.11- ☑
          laceration S56.12- ☑
          specified type NEC S56.19- ☑
          strain S56.11- ☑
        intrinsic S66.50- ☑
          laceration S66.52- ☑
          specified type NEC S66.59- ☑
          strain S66.51- ☑
      ring
        extensor (forearm level)
          hand level S66.30- ☑
            laceration S66.32- ☑
            specified type NEC S66.39- ☑
            strain S66.31- ☑
          laceration S56.42- ☑
          specified type NEC S56.49- ☑
          strain S56.41- ☑
        flexor (forearm level)
          hand level S66.10- ☑
            laceration S66.12- ☑
            specified type NEC S66.19- ☑
            strain S66.11- ☑
          laceration S56.12- ☑
          specified type NEC S56.19- ☑
          strain S56.11- ☑
        intrinsic S66.50- ☑
          laceration S66.52- ☑

Injury — continued
  muscle — continued
    finger — continued
      ring — continued
        intrinsic — continued
          specified type NEC S66.59- ☑
          strain S66.51- ☑
    flexor
      finger(s) (other than thumb) — see Injury, muscle, finger
      forearm level, specified NEC — see Injury, muscle, forearm, flexor
      thumb — see Injury, muscle, thumb, flexor
      toe (long) (ankle level) (foot level) — see Injury, muscle, toe, flexor
    foot S96.90- ☑
      intrinsic S96.20- ☑
        laceration S96.22- ☑
        specified type NEC S96.29- ☑
        strain S96.21- ☑
      laceration S96.92- ☑
      long extensor, toe — see Injury, muscle, toe, extensor
      long flexor, toe — see Injury, muscle, toe, flexor
      specified
        site NEC S96.80- ☑
          laceration S96.82- ☑
          specified type NEC S96.89- ☑
          strain S96.81- ☑
        type S96.99- ☑
      strain S96.91- ☑
    forearm (level) S56.90- ☑
      extensor S56.50- ☑
        laceration S56.52- ☑
        specified type NEC S56.59- ☑
        strain S56.51- ☑
      flexor S56.20- ☑
        laceration S56.22- ☑
        specified type NEC S56.29- ☑
        strain S56.21- ☑
      laceration S56.92- ☑
      specified S56.99- ☑
        site NEC S56.80- ☑
          laceration S56.82- ☑
          strain S56.81- ☑
          type NEC S56.89- ☑
      strain S56.91- ☑
    hand (level) S66.90- ☑
      laceration S66.92- ☑
      specified
        site NEC S66.80- ☑
          laceration S66.82- ☑
          specified type NEC S66.89- ☑
          strain S66.81- ☑
          type NEC S66.99- ☑
      strain S66.91- ☑
    head S09.10 ☑
      laceration S09.12 ☑
      specified type NEC S09.19 ☑
      strain S09.11 ☑
    hip NEC S76.00- ☑
      laceration S76.02- ☑
      specified type NEC S76.09- ☑
      strain S76.01- ☑
    intrinsic
      ankle and foot level — see Injury, muscle, foot, intrinsic
      finger (other than thumb) — see Injury, muscle, finger by site, intrinsic
      foot (level) — see Injury, muscle, foot, intrinsic
      thumb — see Injury, muscle, thumb, intrinsic
    leg (level) (lower) S86.90- ☑
      Achilles tendon — see Injury, Achilles tendon
      anterior muscle group — see Injury, muscle, anterior muscle group
      laceration S86.92- ☑
      peroneal muscle group — see Injury, muscle, peroneal muscle group
      posterior muscle group — see Injury, muscle, posterior muscle group, leg level
      specified
        site NEC S86.80- ☑
          laceration S86.82- ☑
          specified type NEC S86.89- ☑
          strain S86.81- ☑
          type NEC S86.99- ☑

Injury — *continued*
  muscle — *continued*
    leg — *continued*
      strain S86.91- ☑
    long
      extensor toe, at ankle and foot level — *see* Injury, muscle, toe, extensor
      flexor, toe, at ankle and foot level — *see* Injury, muscle, toe, flexor
      head, biceps — *see* Injury, muscle, biceps, long head
    lower back S39.002 ☑
      laceration S39.022 ☑
      specified type NEC S39.092 ☑
      strain S39.012 ☑
    neck (level) S16.9 ☑
      laceration S16.2 ☑
      specified type NEC S16.8 ☑
      strain S16.1 ☑
    pelvis S39.003 ☑
      laceration S39.023 ☑
      specified type NEC S39.093 ☑
      strain S39.013 ☑
    peroneal muscle group, at leg level (lower) S86.30- ☑
      laceration S86.32- ☑
      specified type NEC S86.39- ☑
      strain S86.31- ☑
    posterior muscle (group)
      leg level (lower) S86.10- ☑
        laceration S86.12- ☑
        specified type NEC S86.19- ☑
        strain S86.11- ☑
      thigh level S76.30- ☑
        laceration S76.32- ☑
        specified type NEC S76.39- ☑
        strain S76.31- ☑
    quadriceps (thigh) S76.10- ☑
      laceration S76.12- ☑
      specified type NEC S76.19- ☑
      strain S76.11- ☑
    shoulder S46.90- ☑
      laceration S46.92- ☑
      rotator cuff — *see* Injury, rotator cuff
      specified site NEC S46.80- ☑
        laceration S46.82- ☑
        specified type NEC S46.89- ☑
        strain S46.81- ☑
      specified type NEC S46.99- ☑
      strain S46.91- ☑
    thigh NEC (level) S76.90- ☑
      adductor — *see* Injury, muscle, adductor, thigh
      laceration S76.92- ☑
      posterior muscle (group) — *see* Injury, muscle, posterior muscle, thigh level
      quadriceps — *see* Injury, muscle, quadriceps
      specified
        site NEC S76.80- ☑
          laceration S76.82- ☑
          specified type NEC S76.89- ☑
          strain S76.81- ☑
        type NEC S76.99- ☑
      strain S76.91- ☑
    thorax (level) S29.009 ☑
      back wall S29.002 ☑
      front wall S29.001 ☑
      laceration S29.029 ☑
        back wall S29.022 ☑
        front wall S29.021 ☑
      specified type NEC S29.099 ☑
        back wall S29.092 ☑
        front wall S29.091 ☑
      strain S29.019 ☑
        back wall S29.012 ☑
        front wall S29.011 ☑
    thumb
      abductor (forearm level) S56.30- ☑
        laceration S56.32- ☑
        specified type NEC S56.39- ☑
        strain S56.31- ☑
      extensor (forearm level) S56.30- ☑
        hand level S66.20- ☑
          laceration S66.22- ☑
          specified type NEC S66.29- ☑
          strain S66.21- ☑
        laceration S56.32- ☑

Injury — *continued*
  muscle — *continued*
    thumb — *continued*
      extensor — *continued*
        specified type NEC S56.39- ☑
        strain S56.31- ☑
      flexor (forearm level) S56.00- ☑
        hand level S66.00- ☑
          laceration S66.02- ☑
          specified type NEC S66.09- ☑
          strain S66.01- ☑
        laceration S56.02- ☑
        specified type NEC S56.09- ☑
        strain S56.01- ☑
        wrist level — *see* Injury, muscle, thumb, flexor, hand level
      intrinsic S66.40- ☑
        laceration S66.42- ☑
        specified type NEC S66.49- ☑
        strain S66.41- ☑
    toe (*see also* Injury, muscle, foot)
      extensor, long S96.10- ☑
        laceration S96.12- ☑
        specified type NEC S96.19- ☑
        strain S96.11- ☑
      flexor, long S96.00- ☑
        laceration S96.02- ☑
        specified type NEC S96.09- ☑
        strain S96.01- ☑
    triceps S46.30- ☑
      laceration S46.32- ☑
      specified type NEC S46.39- ☑
      strain S46.31- ☑
    wrist (and hand) level — *see* Injury, muscle, hand
  musculocutaneous nerve — *see* Injury, nerve, musculocutaneous
  myocardium — *see* Injury, heart
  nape — *see* Injury, neck
  nasal (septum) (sinus) S09.92 ☑
  nasopharynx S09.92 ☑
  neck S19.9 ☑
    specified NEC S19.80 ☑
    specified site NEC S19.89 ☑
  nerve NEC T14.8
    abdomen S34.9 ☑
      peripheral S34.6 ☑
      specified site NEC S34.8 ☑
    abducens S04.4- ☑
      contusion S04.4- ☑
      laceration S04.4- ☑
      specified type NEC S04.4- ☑
    abducent — *see* Injury, nerve, abducens
    accessory S04.7- ☑
      contusion S04.7- ☑
      laceration S04.7- ☑
      specified type NEC S04.7- ☑
    acoustic S04.6- ☑
      contusion S04.6- ☑
      laceration S04.6- ☑
      specified type NEC S04.6- ☑
    ankle S94.9- ☑
      cutaneous sensory S94.3- ☑
      specified site NEC — *see* subcategory S94.8 ☑
    anterior crural, femoral — *see* Injury, nerve, femoral
    arm (upper) S44.9- ☑
      axillary — *see* Injury, nerve, axillary
      cutaneous — *see* Injury, nerve, cutaneous, arm
      median — *see* Injury, nerve, median, upper arm
      musculocutaneous — *see* Injury, nerve, musculocutaneous
      radial — *see* Injury, nerve, radial, upper arm
      specified site NEC — *see* subcategory S44.8 ☑
      ulnar — *see* Injury, nerve, ulnar, arm
    auditory — *see* Injury, nerve, acoustic
    axillary S44.3- ☑
    brachial plexus — *see* Injury, brachial plexus
    cervical sympathetic S14.5 ☑
    cranial S04.9 ☑
      contusion S04.9 ☑
      eighth (acoustic or auditory) — *see* Injury, nerve, acoustic
      eleventh (accessory) — *see* Injury, nerve, accessory
      fifth (trigeminal) — *see* Injury, nerve, trigeminal
      first (olfactory) — *see* Injury, nerve, olfactory
      fourth (trochlear) — *see* Injury, nerve, trochlear

Injury — *continued*
  nerve — *continued*
    cranial — *continued*
      laceration S04.9 ☑
      ninth (glossopharyngeal) — *see* Injury, nerve, glossopharyngeal
      second (optic) — *see* Injury, nerve, optic
      seventh (facial) — *see* Injury, nerve, facial
      sixth (abducent) — *see* Injury, nerve, abducens
      specified
        nerve NEC S04.89- ☑
          contusion S04.89- ☑
          laceration S04.89- ☑
          specified type NEC S04.89- ☑
        type NEC S04.9 ☑
      tenth (pneumogastric or vagus) — *see* Injury, nerve, vagus
      third (oculomotor) — *see* Injury, nerve, oculomotor
      twelfth (hypoglossal) — *see* Injury, nerve, hypoglossal
    cutaneous sensory
      ankle (level) S94.3- ☑
      arm (upper) (level) S44.5- ☑
      foot (level) — *see* Injury, nerve, cutaneous sensory, ankle
      forearm (level) S54.3- ☑
      hip (level) S74.2- ☑
      leg (lower level) S84.2- ☑
      shoulder (level) — *see* Injury, nerve, cutaneous sensory, arm
      thigh (level) — *see* Injury, nerve, cutaneous sensory, hip
    deep peroneal — *see* Injury, nerve, peroneal, foot
    digital
      finger S64.4- ☑
        index S64.49- ☑
        little S64.49- ☑
        middle S64.49- ☑
        ring S64.49- ☑
        thumb S64.3- ☑
      toe — *see* Injury, nerve, ankle, specified site NEC
    eighth cranial (acoustic or auditory) — *see* Injury, nerve, acoustic
    eleventh cranial (accessory) — *see* Injury, nerve, accessory
    facial S04.5- ☑
      contusion S04.5- ☑
      laceration S04.5- ☑
      newborn P11.3
      specified type NEC S04.5- ☑
    femoral (hip level) (thigh level) S74.1- ☑
    fifth cranial (trigeminal) — *see* Injury, nerve, trigeminal
    finger (digital) — *see* Injury, nerve, digital, finger
    first cranial (olfactory) — *see* Injury, nerve, olfactory
    foot S94.9- ☑
      cutaneous sensory S94.3- ☑
      deep peroneal S94.2- ☑
      lateral plantar S94.0- ☑
      medial plantar S94.1- ☑
      specified site NEC — *see* subcategory S94.8 ☑
    forearm (level) S54.9- ☑
      cutaneous sensory — *see* Injury, nerve, cutaneous sensory, forearm
      median — *see* Injury, nerve, median
      radial — *see* Injury, nerve, radial
      specified site NEC — *see* subcategory S54.8 ☑
      ulnar — *see* Injury, nerve, ulnar
    fourth cranial (trochlear) — *see* Injury, nerve, trochlear
    glossopharyngeal S04.89- ☑
      specified type NEC S04.89- ☑
    hand S64.9- ☑
      median — *see* Injury, nerve, median, hand
      radial — *see* Injury, nerve, radial, hand
      specified NEC — *see* subcategory S64.8 ☑
      ulnar — *see* Injury, nerve, ulnar, hand
    hip (level) S74.9- ☑
      cutaneous sensory — *see* Injury, nerve, cutaneous sensory, hip
      femoral — *see* Injury, nerve, femoral
      sciatic — *see* Injury, nerve, sciatic
      specified site NEC — *see* subcategory S74.8 ☑
    hypoglossal S04.89- ☑

Injury — *continued*
  nerve — *continued*
    hypoglossal — *continued*
      specified type NEC S04.89- ☑
    lateral plantar S94.0- ☑
    leg (lower) S84.9- ☑
      cutaneous sensory — *see* Injury, nerve, cutaneous sensory, leg
      peroneal — *see* Injury, nerve, peroneal
      specified site NEC — *see* subcategory S84.8 ☑
      tibial — *see* Injury, nerve, tibial
      upper — *see* Injury, nerve, thigh
    lower
      back — *see* Injury, nerve, abdomen, specified site NEC
        peripheral — *see* Injury, nerve, abdomen, peripheral
      limb — *see* Injury, nerve, leg
    lumbar plexus — *see* Injury, nerve, lumbosacral, sympathetic
    lumbar spinal — *see* Injury, nerve, spinal, lumbar
    lumbosacral
      plexus — *see* Injury, nerve, lumbosacral, sympathetic
      sympathetic S34.5 ☑
    medial plantar S94.1- ☑
    median (forearm level) S54.1- ☑
      hand (level) S64.1- ☑
      upper arm (level) S44.1- ☑
      wrist (level) — *see* Injury, nerve, median, hand
    musculocutaneous S44.4- ☑
    musculospiral (upper arm level) — *see* Injury, nerve, radial, upper arm
    neck S14.9 ☑
      peripheral S14.4 ☑
      specified site NEC S14.8 ☑
      sympathetic S14.5 ☑
    ninth cranial (glossopharyngeal) — *see* Injury, nerve, glossopharyngeal
    oculomotor S04.1- ☑
      contusion S04.1- ☑
      laceration S04.1- ☑
      specified type NEC S04.1- ☑
    olfactory S04.81- ☑
      specified type NEC S04.81- ☑
    optic S04.01- ☑
      contusion S04.01- ☑
      laceration S04.01- ☑
      specified type NEC S04.01- ☑
    pelvic girdle — *see* Injury, nerve, hip
    pelvis — *see* Injury, nerve, abdomen, specified site NEC
      peripheral — *see* Injury, nerve, abdomen, peripheral
    peripheral NEC T14.8
      abdomen — *see* Injury, nerve, abdomen, peripheral
      lower back — *see* Injury, nerve, abdomen, peripheral
      neck — *see* Injury, nerve, neck, peripheral
      pelvis — *see* Injury, nerve, abdomen, peripheral
      specified NEC T14.8
    peroneal (lower leg level) S84.1- ☑
      foot S94.2- ☑
    plexus
      brachial — *see* Injury, brachial plexus
      celiac, coeliac — *see* Injury, nerve, lumbosacral, sympathetic
      mesenteric, inferior — *see* Injury, nerve, lumbosacral, sympathetic
      sacral — *see* Injury, lumbosacral plexus
      spinal
        brachial — *see* Injury, brachial plexus
        lumbosacral — *see* Injury, lumbosacral plexus
    pneumogastric — *see* Injury, nerve, vagus
    radial (forearm level) S54.2- ☑
      hand (level) S64.2- ☑
      upper arm (level) S44.2- ☑
      wrist (level) — *see* Injury, nerve, radial, hand
    root — *see* Injury, nerve, spinal, root
    sacral plexus — *see* Injury, lumbosacral plexus
    sacral spinal — *see* Injury, nerve, spinal, sacral
    sciatic (hip level) (thigh level) S74.0- ☑
    second cranial (optic) — *see* Injury, nerve, optic
    seventh cranial (facial) — *see* Injury, nerve, facial

Injury — *continued*
  nerve — *continued*
    shoulder — *see* Injury, nerve, arm
    sixth cranial (abducent) — *see* Injury, nerve, abducens
    spinal
      plexus — *see* Injury, nerve, plexus, spinal
      root
        cervical S14.2 ☑
        dorsal S24.2 ☑
        lumbar S34.21 ☑
        sacral S34.22 ☑
        thoracic — *see* Injury, nerve, spinal, root, dorsal
    splanchnic — *see* Injury, nerve, lumbosacral, sympathetic
    sympathetic NEC — *see* Injury, nerve, lumbosacral, sympathetic
      cervical — *see* Injury, nerve, cervical sympathetic
    tenth cranial (pneumogastric or vagus) — *see* Injury, nerve, vagus
    thigh (level) — *see* Injury, nerve, hip
      cutaneous sensory — *see* Injury, nerve, cutaneous sensory, hip
      femoral — *see* Injury, nerve, femoral
      sciatic — *see* Injury, nerve, sciatic
      specified NEC — *see* Injury, nerve, hip
    third cranial (oculomotor) — *see* Injury, nerve, oculomotor
    thorax S24.9 ☑
      peripheral S24.3 ☑
      specified site NEC S24.8 ☑
      sympathetic S24.4 ☑
    thumb, digital — *see* Injury, nerve, digital, thumb
    tibial (lower leg level) (posterior) S84.0- ☑
    toe — *see* Injury, nerve, ankle
    trigeminal S04.3- ☑
      contusion S04.3- ☑
      laceration S04.3- ☑
      specified type NEC S04.3- ☑
    trochlear S04.2- ☑
      contusion S04.2- ☑
      laceration S04.2- ☑
      specified type NEC S04.2- ☑
    twelfth cranial (hypoglossal) — *see* Injury, nerve, hypoglossal
    ulnar (forearm level) S54.0- ☑
      arm (upper) (level) S44.0- ☑
      hand (level) S64.0- ☑
      wrist (level) — *see* Injury, nerve, ulnar, hand
    vagus S04.89- ☑
      specified type NEC S04.89- ☑
    wrist (level) — *see* Injury, nerve, hand
  ninth cranial nerve (glossopharyngeal) — *see* Injury, nerve, glossopharyngeal
  nose (septum) S09.92 ☑
  obstetrical O71.9
    specified NEC O71.89
  occipital (region) (scalp) S09.90 ☑
    lobe — *see* Injury, intracranial
  optic chiasm S04.02 ☑
  optic radiation S04.03- ☑
  optic tract and pathways S04.03- ☑
  orbit, orbital (region) — *see* Injury, eye
    penetrating (with foreign body) — *see* Injury, eye, orbit, penetrating
    specified NEC — *see* Injury, eye, specified site NEC
  ovary, ovarian S37.409 ☑
    bilateral S37.402 ☑
      contusion S37.422 ☑
      laceration S37.432 ☑
      specified type NEC S37.492 ☑
    blood vessel — *see* Injury, blood vessel, ovarian
    contusion S37.429 ☑
      bilateral S37.422 ☑
      unilateral S37.421 ☑
    laceration S37.439 ☑
      bilateral S37.432 ☑
      unilateral S37.431 ☑
    specified type NEC S37.499 ☑
      bilateral S37.492 ☑
      unilateral S37.491 ☑
    unilateral S37.401 ☑
      contusion S37.421 ☑
      laceration S37.431 ☑

Injury — *continued*
  ovary, ovarian — *continued*
    unilateral — *continued*
      specified type NEC S37.491 ☑
  palate (hard) (soft) S09.93 ☑
  pancreas S36.209 ☑
    body S36.201 ☑
      contusion S36.221 ☑
      laceration S36.231 ☑
        major S36.261 ☑
        minor S36.241 ☑
        moderate S36.251 ☑
      specified type NEC S36.291 ☑
    contusion S36.229 ☑
    head S36.200 ☑
      contusion S36.220 ☑
      laceration S36.230 ☑
        major S36.260 ☑
        minor S36.240 ☑
        moderate S36.250 ☑
      specified type NEC S36.290 ☑
    laceration S36.239 ☑
      major S36.269 ☑
      minor S36.249 ☑
      moderate S36.259 ☑
    specified type NEC S36.299 ☑
    tail S36.202 ☑
      contusion S36.222 ☑
      laceration S36.232 ☑
        major S36.262 ☑
        minor S36.242 ☑
        moderate S36.252 ☑
      specified type NEC S36.292 ☑
  parietal (region) (scalp) S09.90 ☑
    lobe — *see* Injury, intracranial
  patellar ligament (tendon) S76.10- ☑
    laceration S76.12- ☑
    specified NEC S76.19- ☑
    strain S76.11- ☑
  pelvis, pelvic (floor) S39.93 ☑
    complicating delivery O70.1
    joint or ligament, complicating delivery O71.6
    organ S37.90 ☑
      with ectopic or molar pregnancy O08.6
      complication of abortion — *see* Abortion
      contusion S37.92 ☑
      following ectopic or molar pregnancy O08.6
      laceration S37.93 ☑
      obstetrical trauma NEC O71.5
      specified
        site NEC S37.899 ☑
          contusion S37.892 ☑
          laceration S37.893 ☑
          specified type NEC S37.898 ☑
        type NEC S37.99 ☑
    specified NEC S39.83 ☑
  penis S39.94 ☑
  perineum S39.94 ☑
  peritoneum S36.81 ☑
    laceration S36.893 ☑
  periurethral tissue — *see* Injury, urethra
    complicating delivery O71.82
  phalanges
    foot — *see* Injury, foot
    hand — *see* Injury, hand
  pharynx NEC S19.85 ☑
  pleura — *see* Injury, intrathoracic, pleura
  plexus
    brachial — *see* Injury, brachial plexus
    cardiac — *see* Injury, nerve, thorax, sympathetic
    celiac, coeliac — *see* Injury, nerve, lumbosacral, sympathetic
    esophageal — *see* Injury, nerve, thorax, sympathetic
    hypogastric — *see* Injury, nerve, lumbosacral, sympathetic
    lumbar, lumbosacral — *see* Injury, lumbosacral plexus
    mesenteric — *see* Injury, nerve, lumbosacral, sympathetic
    pulmonary — *see* Injury, nerve, thorax, sympathetic
  postcardiac surgery (syndrome) I97.0
  prepuce S39.94 ☑
  prostate S37.829 ☑
    contusion S37.822 ☑

Injury — *continued*
  prostate — *continued*
    laceration S37.823 ☑
    specified type NEC S37.828 ☑
  pubic region S39.94 ☑
  pudendum S39.94 ☑
  pulmonary plexus — *see* Injury, nerve, thorax, sympathetic
  rectovaginal septum NEC S39.83 ☑
  rectum — *see* Injury, intestine, large, rectum
  retina — *see* Injury, eye, specified site NEC
    penetrating — *see* Injury, eyeball, penetrating
  retroperitoneal — *see* Injury, intra-abdominal, specified site NEC
  rotator cuff (muscle(s)) (tendon(s)) S46.00- ☑
    laceration S46.02- ☑
    specified type NEC S46.09- ☑
    strain S46.01- ☑
  round ligament — *see* Injury, pelvic organ, specified site NEC
  sacral plexus — *see* Injury, lumbosacral plexus
  salivary duct or gland S09.93 ☑
  scalp S09.90 ☑
    newborn (birth injury) P12.9
      due to monitoring (electrode) (sampling incision) P12.4
      specified NEC P12.89
        caput succedaneum P12.81
  scapular region — *see* Injury, shoulder
  sclera — *see* Injury, eye, specified site NEC
    penetrating — *see* Injury, eyeball, penetrating
  scrotum S39.94 ☑
  second cranial nerve (optic) — *see* Injury, nerve, optic
  seminal vesicle — *see* Injury, pelvic organ, specified site NEC
  seventh cranial nerve (facial) — *see* Injury, nerve, facial
  shoulder S49.9- ☑
    blood vessel — *see* Injury, blood vessel, arm
    contusion — *see* Contusion, shoulder
    dislocation — *see* Dislocation, shoulder
    fracture — *see* Fracture, shoulder
    muscle — *see* Injury, muscle, shoulder
    nerve — *see* Injury, nerve, shoulder
    open — *see* Wound, open, shoulder
    specified type NEC S49.8- ☑
    sprain — *see* Sprain, shoulder girdle
    superficial — *see* Injury, superficial, shoulder
  sinus
    cavernous — *see* Injury, intracranial
    nasal S09.92 ☑
  sixth cranial nerve (abducent) — *see* Injury, nerve, abducens
  skeleton, birth injury P13.9
    specified part NEC P13.8
  skin NEC T14.8
    surface intact — *see* Injury, superficial
  skull NEC S09.90 ☑
  specified NEC T14.8
  spermatic cord (pelvic region) S37.898 ☑
    scrotal region S39.848 ☑
  spinal (cord)
    cervical (neck) S14.109 ☑
      anterior cord syndrome S14.139 ☑
        C1 level S14.131 ☑
        C2 level S14.132 ☑
        C3 level S14.133 ☑
        C4 level S14.134 ☑
        C5 level S14.135 ☑
        C6 level S14.136 ☑
        C7 level S14.137 ☑
        C8 level S14.138 ☑
      Brown-Séquard syndrome S14.149 ☑
        C1 level S14.141 ☑
        C2 level S14.142 ☑
        C3 level S14.143 ☑
        C4 level S14.144 ☑
        C5 level S14.145 ☑
        C6 level S14.146 ☑
        C7 level S14.147 ☑
        C8 level S14.148 ☑
      C1 level S14.101 ☑
      C2 level S14.102 ☑
      C3 level S14.103 ☑
      C4 level S14.104 ☑
      C5 level S14.105 ☑
      C6 level S14.106 ☑

Injury — *continued*
  spinal — *continued*
    cervical — *continued*
      C7 level S14.107 ☑
      C8 level S14.108 ☑
      central cord syndrome S14.129 ☑
        C1 level S14.121 ☑
        C2 level S14.122 ☑
        C3 level S14.123 ☑
        C4 level S14.124 ☑
        C5 level S14.125 ☑
        C6 level S14.126 ☑
        C7 level S14.127 ☑
        C8 level S14.128 ☑
      complete lesion S14.119 ☑
        C1 level S14.111 ☑
        C2 level S14.112 ☑
        C3 level S14.113 ☑
        C4 level S14.114 ☑
        C5 level S14.115 ☑
        C6 level S14.116 ☑
        C7 level S14.117 ☑
        C8 level S14.118 ☑
      concussion S14.0 ☑
      edema S14.0 ☑
      incomplete lesion specified NEC S14.159 ☑
        C1 level S14.151 ☑
        C2 level S14.152 ☑
        C3 level S14.153 ☑
        C4 level S14.154 ☑
        C5 level S14.155 ☑
        C6 level S14.156 ☑
        C7 level S14.157 ☑
        C8 level S14.158 ☑
      posterior cord syndrome S14.159 ☑
        C1 level S14.151 ☑
        C2 level S14.152 ☑
        C3 level S14.153 ☑
        C4 level S14.154 ☑
        C5 level S14.155 ☑
        C6 level S14.156 ☑
        C7 level S14.157 ☑
        C8 level S14.158 ☑
    dorsal — *see* Injury, spinal, thoracic
    lumbar S34.109 ☑
      complete lesion S34.119 ☑
        L1 level S34.111 ☑
        L2 level S34.112 ☑
        L3 level S34.113 ☑
        L4 level S34.114 ☑
        L5 level S34.115 ☑
      concussion S34.01 ☑
      edema S34.01 ☑
      incomplete lesion S34.129 ☑
        L1 level S34.121 ☑
        L2 level S34.122 ☑
        L3 level S34.123 ☑
        L4 level S34.124 ☑
        L5 level S34.125 ☑
      L1 level S34.101 ☑
      L2 level S34.102 ☑
      L3 level S34.103 ☑
      L4 level S34.104 ☑
      L5 level S34.105 ☑
    nerve root NEC
      cervical — *see* Injury, nerve, spinal, root, cervical
      dorsal — *see* Injury, nerve, spinal, root, dorsal
      lumbar S34.21 ☑
      sacral S34.22 ☑
      thoracic — *see* Injury, nerve, spinal, root, dorsal
    plexus
      brachial — *see* Injury, brachial plexus
      lumbosacral — *see* Injury, lumbosacral plexus
    sacral S34.139 ☑
      complete lesion S34.131 ☑
      incomplete lesion S34.132 ☑
    thoracic S24.109 ☑
      anterior cord syndrome S24.139 ☑
        T1 level S24.131 ☑
        T2-T6 level S24.132 ☑
        T7-T10 level S24.133 ☑
        T11-T12 level S24.134 ☑
      Brown-Séquard syndrome S24.149 ☑
        T1 level S24.141 ☑

Injury — *continued*
  spinal — *continued*
    thoracic — *continued*
      Brown-Séquard syndrome — *continued*
        T2-T6 level S24.142 ☑
        T7-T10 level S24.143 ☑
        T11-T12 level S24.144 ☑
      complete lesion S24.119 ☑
        T1 level S24.111 ☑
        T2-T6 level S24.112 ☑
        T7-T10 level S24.113 ☑
        T11-T12 level S24.114 ☑
      concussion S24.0 ☑
      edema S24.0 ☑
      incomplete lesion specified NEC S24.159 ☑
        T1 level S24.151 ☑
        T2-T6 level S24.152 ☑
        T7-T10 level S24.153 ☑
        T11-T12 level S24.154 ☑
      posterior cord syndrome S24.159 ☑
        T1 level S24.151 ☑
        T2-T6 level S24.152 ☑
        T7-T10 level S24.153 ☑
        T11-T12 level S24.154 ☑
      T1 level S24.101 ☑
      T2-T6 level S24.102 ☑
      T7-T10 level S24.103 ☑
      T11-T12 level S24.104 ☑
  splanchnic nerve — *see* Injury, nerve, lumbosacral, sympathetic
  spleen S36.00 ☑
    contusion S36.029 ☑
      major S36.021 ☑
      minor S36.020 ☑
    laceration S36.039 ☑
      major (massive) (stellate) S36.032 ☑
      moderate S36.031 ☑
      superficial (capsular) (minor) S36.030 ☑
    specified type NEC S36.09 ☑
  splenic artery — *see* Injury, blood vessel, celiac artery, branch
  stellate ganglion — *see* Injury, nerve, thorax, sympathetic
  sternal region S29.9 ☑
  stomach S36.30 ☑
    contusion S36.32 ☑
    laceration S36.33 ☑
    specified type NEC S36.39 ☑
  subconjunctival — *see* Injury, eye, conjunctiva
  subcutaneous NEC T14.8
  submaxillary region S09.93 ☑
  submental region S09.93 ☑
  subungual
    fingers — *see* Injury, hand
    toes — *see* Injury, foot
  superficial NEC T14.8
    abdomen, abdominal (wall) S30.92 ☑
      abrasion S30.811 ☑
      bite S30.871 ☑
        insect S30.861 ☑
      contusion S30.1 ☑
      external constriction S30.841 ☑
      foreign body S30.851 ☑
    abrasion — *see* Abrasion, by site
    adnexa, eye NEC — *see* Injury, eye, specified site NEC
    alveolar process — *see* Injury, superficial, oral cavity
    ankle S90.91- ☑
      abrasion — *see* Abrasion, ankle
      bite — *see* Bite, ankle
      blister — *see* Blister, ankle
      contusion — *see* Contusion, ankle
      external constriction — *see* Constriction, external, ankle
      foreign body — *see* Foreign body, superficial, ankle
    anus S30.98 ☑
    arm (upper) S40.92- ☑
      abrasion — *see* Abrasion, arm
      bite — *see* Bite, superficial, arm
      blister — *see* Blister, arm (upper)
      contusion — *see* Contusion, arm
      external constriction — *see* Constriction, external, arm

Injury — *continued*
  superficial — *continued*
    arm — *continued*
      foreign body — *see* Foreign body, superficial, arm
    auditory canal (external) (meatus) — *see* Injury, superficial, ear
    auricle — *see* Injury, superficial, ear
    axilla — *see* Injury, superficial, arm
    back (*see also* Injury, superficial, thorax, back)
      lower S30.91
        abrasion S30.810 ☑
        contusion S30.0 ☑
        external constriction S30.840 ☑
        superficial
          bite NEC S30.870 ☑
            insect S30.860 ☑
          foreign body S30.850 ☑
    bite NEC — *see* Bite, superficial NEC, by site
    blister — *see* Blister, by site
    breast S20.10- ☑
      abrasion — *see* Abrasion, breast
      bite — *see* Bite, superficial, breast
      contusion — *see* Contusion, breast
      external constriction — *see* Constriction, external, breast
      foreign body — *see* Foreign body, superficial, breast
    brow — *see* Injury, superficial, head, specified NEC
    buttock S30.91 ☑
    calf — *see* Injury, superficial, leg
    canthus, eye — *see* Injury, superficial, periocular area
    cheek (external) — *see* Injury, superficial, head, specified NEC
      internal — *see* Injury, superficial, oral cavity
    chest wall — *see* Injury, superficial, thorax
    chin — *see* Injury, superficial, head NEC
    clitoris S30.95 ☑
    conjunctiva — *see* Injury, eye, conjunctiva
      with foreign body (in conjunctival sac) — *see* Foreign body, conjunctival sac
    contusion — *see* Contusion, by site
    costal region — *see* Injury, superficial, thorax
    digit(s)
      hand — *see* Injury, superficial, finger
    ear (auricle) (canal) (external) S00.40- ☑
      abrasion — *see* Abrasion, ear
      bite — *see* Bite, superficial, ear
      contusion — *see* Contusion, ear
      external constriction — *see* Constriction, external, ear
      foreign body — *see* Foreign body, superficial, ear
    elbow S50.90- ☑
      abrasion — *see* Abrasion, elbow
      bite — *see* Bite, superficial, elbow
      blister — *see* Blister, elbow
      contusion — *see* Contusion, elbow
      external constriction — *see* Constriction, external, elbow
      foreign body — *see* Foreign body, superficial, elbow
    epididymis S30.94 ☑
    epigastric region S30.92 ☑
    epiglottis — *see* Injury, superficial, throat
    esophagus
      cervical — *see* Injury, superficial, throat
    external constriction — *see* Constriction, external, by site
    extremity NEC T14.8
    eyeball NEC — *see* Injury, eye, specified site NEC
    eyebrow — *see* Injury, superficial, periocular area
    eyelid S00.20- ☑
      abrasion — *see* Abrasion, eyelid
      bite — *see* Bite, superficial, eyelid
      contusion — *see* Contusion, eyelid
      external constriction — *see* Constriction, external, eyelid
      foreign body — *see* Foreign body, superficial, eyelid
    face NEC — *see* Injury, superficial, head, specified NEC
    finger(s) S60.949 ☑
      abrasion — *see* Abrasion, finger
      bite — *see* Bite, superficial, finger

Injury — *continued*
  superficial — *continued*
    finger(s) — *continued*
      blister — *see* Blister, finger
      contusion — *see* Contusion, finger
      external constriction — *see* Constriction, external, finger
      foreign body — *see* Foreign body, superficial, finger
      index S60.94- ☑
      insect bite — *see* Bite, by site, superficial, insect
      little S60.94- ☑
      middle S60.94- ☑
      ring S60.94- ☑
    flank S30.92 ☑
    foot S90.92- ☑
      abrasion — *see* Abrasion, foot
      bite — *see* Bite, foot
      blister — *see* Blister, foot
      contusion — *see* Contusion, foot
      external constriction — *see* Constriction, external, foot
      foreign body — *see* Foreign body, superficial, foot
    forearm S50.91- ☑
      abrasion — *see* Abrasion, forearm
      bite — *see* Bite, forearm, superficial
      blister — *see* Blister, forearm
      contusion — *see* Contusion, forearm
      elbow only — *see* Injury, superficial, elbow
      external constriction — *see* Constriction, external, forearm
      foreign body — *see* Foreign body, superficial, forearm
    forehead — *see* Injury, superficial, head NEC
    foreign body — *see* Foreign body, superficial
    genital organs, external
      female S30.97 ☑
      male S30.96 ☑
    globe (eye) — *see* Injury, eye, specified site NEC
    groin S30.92 ☑
    gum — *see* Injury, superficial, oral cavity
    hand S60.92- ☑
      abrasion — *see* Abrasion, hand
      bite — *see* Bite, superficial, hand
      contusion — *see* Contusion, hand
      external constriction — *see* Constriction, external, hand
      foreign body — *see* Foreign body, superficial, hand
    head S00.90 ☑
      ear — *see* Injury, superficial, ear
      eyelid — *see* Injury, superficial, eyelid
      nose S00.30 ☑
      oral cavity S00.502 ☑
      scalp S00.00 ☑
      specified site NEC S00.80 ☑
    heel — *see* Injury, superficial, foot
    hip S70.91- ☑
      abrasion — *see* Abrasion, hip
      bite — *see* Bite, superficial, hip
      blister — *see* Blister, hip
      contusion — *see* Contusion, hip
      external constriction — *see* Constriction, external, hip
      foreign body — *see* Foreign body, superficial, hip
    iliac region — *see* Injury, superficial, abdomen
    inguinal region — *see* Injury, superficial, abdomen
    insect bite — *see* Bite, by site, superficial, insect
    interscapular region — *see* Injury, superficial, thorax, back
    jaw — *see* Injury, superficial, head, specified NEC
    knee S80.91- ☑
      abrasion — *see* Abrasion, knee
      bite — *see* Bite, superficial, knee
      blister — *see* Blister, knee
      contusion — *see* Contusion, knee
      external constriction — *see* Constriction, external, knee
      foreign body — *see* Foreign body, superficial, knee
    labium (majus) (minus) S30.95 ☑
    lacrimal (apparatus) (gland) (sac) — *see* Injury, eye, specified site NEC
    larynx — *see* Injury, superficial, throat

Injury — *continued*
  superficial — *continued*
    leg (lower) S80.92- ☑
      abrasion — *see* Abrasion, leg
      bite — *see* Bite, superficial, leg
      contusion — *see* Contusion, leg
      external constriction — *see* Constriction, external, leg
      foreign body — *see* Foreign body, superficial, leg
      knee — *see* Injury, superficial, knee
    limb NEC T14.8
    lip S00.501 ☑
    lower back S30.91 ☑
    lumbar region S30.91 ☑
    malar region — *see* Injury, superficial, head, specified NEC
    mammary — *see* Injury, superficial, breast
    mastoid region — *see* Injury, superficial, head, specified NEC
    mouth — *see* Injury, superficial, oral cavity
    muscle NEC T14.8
    nail NEC T14.8
      finger — *see* Injury, superficial, finger
      toe — *see* Injury, superficial, toe
    nasal (septum) — *see* Injury, superficial, nose
    neck S10.90 ☑
      specified site NEC S10.80 ☑
    nose (septum) S00.30 ☑
    occipital region — *see* Injury, superficial, scalp
    oral cavity S00.502 ☑
    orbital region — *see* Injury, superficial, periocular area
    palate — *see* Injury, superficial, oral cavity
    palm — *see* Injury, superficial, hand
    parietal region — *see* Injury, superficial, scalp
    pelvis S30.91 ☑
      girdle — *see* Injury, superficial, hip
    penis S30.93 ☑
    perineum
      female S30.95 ☑
      male S30.91 ☑
    periocular area S00.20- ☑
      abrasion — *see* Abrasion, eyelid
      bite — *see* Bite, superficial, eyelid
      contusion — *see* Contusion, eyelid
      external constriction — *see* Constriction, external, eyelid
      foreign body — *see* Foreign body, superficial, eyelid
    phalanges
      finger — *see* Injury, superficial, finger
      toe — *see* Injury, superficial, toe
    pharynx — *see* Injury, superficial, throat
    pinna — *see* Injury, superficial, ear
    popliteal space — *see* Injury, superficial, knee
    prepuce S30.93 ☑
    pubic region S30.91 ☑
    pudendum
      female S30.97 ☑
      male S30.96 ☑
    sacral region S30.91 ☑
    scalp S00.00 ☑
    scapular region — *see* Injury, superficial, shoulder
    sclera — *see* Injury, eye, specified site NEC
    scrotum S30.94 ☑
    shin — *see* Injury, superficial, leg
    shoulder S40.91- ☑
      abrasion — *see* Abrasion, shoulder
      bite — *see* Bite, superficial, shoulder
      blister — *see* Blister, shoulder
      contusion — *see* Contusion, shoulder
      external constriction — *see* Constriction, external, shoulder
      foreign body — *see* Foreign body, superficial, shoulder
    skin NEC T14.8
    sternal region — *see* Injury, superficial, thorax, front
    subconjunctival — *see* Injury, eye, specified site NEC
    subcutaneous NEC T14.8
    submaxillary region — *see* Injury, superficial, head, specified NEC
    submental region — *see* Injury, superficial, head, specified NEC

Injury — *continued*
  superficial — *continued*
    subungual
      finger(s) — *see* Injury, superficial, finger
      toe(s) — *see* Injury, superficial, toe
    supraclavicular fossa — *see* Injury, superficial, neck
    supraorbital — *see* Injury, superficial, head, specified NEC
    temple — *see* Injury, superficial, head, specified NEC
    temporal region — *see* Injury, superficial, head, specified NEC
    testis S30.94 ☑
    thigh S70.92- ☑
      abrasion — *see* Abrasion, thigh
      bite — *see* Bite, superficial, thigh
      blister — *see* Blister, thigh
      contusion — *see* Contusion, thigh
      external constriction — *see* Constriction, external, thigh
      foreign body — *see* Foreign body, superficial, thigh
    thorax, thoracic (wall) S20.90 ☑
      abrasion — *see* Abrasion, thorax
      back S20.40- ☑
      bite — *see* Bite, thorax, superficial
      blister — *see* Blister, thorax
      contusion — *see* Contusion, thorax
      external constriction — *see* Constriction, external, thorax
      foreign body — *see* Foreign body, superficial, thorax
      front S20.30- ☑
    throat S10.10 ☑
      abrasion S10.11 ☑
      bite S10.17 ☑
        insect S10.16 ☑
      blister S10.12 ☑
      contusion S10.0 ☑
      external constriction S10.14 ☑
      foreign body S10.15 ☑
    thumb S60.93- ☑
      abrasion — *see* Abrasion, thumb
      bite — *see* Bite, superficial, thumb
      blister — *see* Blister, thumb
      contusion — *see* Contusion, thumb
      external constriction — *see* Constriction, external, thumb
      foreign body — *see* Foreign body, superficial, thumb
      insect bite — *see* Bite, by site, superficial, insect
      specified type NEC S60.39 ☑
    toe(s) S90.93- ☑
      abrasion — *see* Abrasion, toe
      bite — *see* Bite, toe
      blister — *see* Blister, toe
      contusion — *see* Contusion, toe
      external constriction — *see* Constriction, external, toe
      foreign body — *see* Foreign body, superficial, toe
      great S90.93- ☑
    tongue — *see* Injury, superficial, oral cavity
    tooth, teeth — *see* Injury, superficial, oral cavity
    trachea S10.10 ☑
    tunica vaginalis S30.94 ☑
    tympanum, tympanic membrane — *see* Injury, superficial, ear
    uvula — *see* Injury, superficial, oral cavity
    vagina S30.95 ☑
    vocal cords — *see* Injury, superficial, throat
    vulva S30.95 ☑
    wrist S60.91- ☑
  supraclavicular region — *see* Injury, neck
  supraorbital S09.93 ☑
  suprarenal gland (multiple) — *see* Injury, adrenal
  surgical complication (external or internal site) — *see* Laceration, accidental complicating surgery
  temple S09.90 ☑
  temporal region S09.90 ☑
  tendon (*see also* Injury, muscle, by site)
    abdomen — *see* Injury, muscle, abdomen
    Achilles — *see* Injury, Achilles tendon
    lower back — *see* Injury, muscle, lower back
    pelvic organs — *see* Injury, muscle, pelvis

Injury — *continued*
  tenth cranial nerve (pneumogastric or vagus) — *see* Injury, nerve, vagus
  testis S39.94 ☑
  thigh S79.92- ☑
    blood vessel — *see* Injury, blood vessel, hip
    contusion — *see* Contusion, thigh
    fracture — *see* Fracture, femur
    muscle — *see* Injury, muscle, thigh
    nerve — *see* Injury, nerve, thigh
    open — *see* Wound, open, thigh
    specified NEC S79.82- ☑
    superficial — *see* Injury, superficial, thigh
  third cranial nerve (oculomotor) — *see* Injury, nerve, oculomotor
  thorax, thoracic S29.9 ☑
    blood vessel — *see* Injury, blood vessel, thorax
    cavity — *see* Injury, intrathoracic
    dislocation — *see* Dislocation, thorax
    external (wall) S29.9 ☑
      contusion — *see* Contusion, thorax
      nerve — *see* Injury, nerve, thorax
      open — *see* Wound, open, thorax
      specified NEC S29.8 ☑
      sprain — *see* Sprain, thorax
      superficial — *see* Injury, superficial, thorax
    fracture — *see* Fracture, thorax
    internal — *see* Injury, intrathoracic
    intrathoracic organ — *see* Injury, intrathoracic
    sympathetic ganglion — *see* Injury, nerve, thorax, sympathetic
  throat (*see also* Injury, neck) S19.9 ☑
  thumb S69.9- ☑
    blood vessel — *see* Injury, blood vessel, thumb
    contusion — *see* Contusion, thumb
    dislocation — *see* Dislocation, thumb
    fracture — *see* Fracture, thumb
    muscle — *see* Injury, muscle, thumb
    nerve — *see* Injury, nerve, digital, thumb
    open — *see* Wound, open, thumb
    specified NEC S69.8- ☑
    sprain — *see* Sprain, thumb
    superficial — *see* Injury, superficial, thumb
  thymus (gland) — *see* Injury, intrathoracic, specified organ NEC
  thyroid (gland) NEC S19.84 ☑
  toe S99.92- ☑
    contusion — *see* Contusion, toe
    dislocation — *see* Dislocation, toe
    fracture — *see* Fracture, toe
    muscle — *see* Injury, muscle, toe
    open — *see* Wound, open, toe
    specified type NEC S99.82- ☑
    sprain — *see* Sprain, toe
    superficial — *see* Injury, superficial, toe
  tongue S09.93 ☑
  tonsil S09.93 ☑
  tooth S09.93 ☑
  trachea (cervical) NEC S19.82 ☑
    thoracic — *see* Injury, intrathoracic, trachea, thoracic
  transfusion-related acute lung (TRALI) J95.84
  tunica vaginalis S39.94 ☑
  twelfth cranial nerve (hypoglossal) — *see* Injury, nerve, hypoglossal
  ureter S37.10 ☑
    contusion S37.12 ☑
    laceration S37.13 ☑
    specified type NEC S37.19 ☑
  urethra (sphincter) S37.30 ☑
    at delivery O71.5
    contusion S37.32 ☑
    laceration S37.33 ☑
    specified type NEC S37.39 ☑
  urinary organ S37.90 ☑
    contusion S37.92 ☑
    laceration S37.93 ☑
    specified
      site NEC S37.899 ☑
        contusion S37.892 ☑
        laceration S37.893 ☑
        specified type NEC S37.898 ☑
      type NEC S37.99 ☑
  uterus, uterine S37.60 ☑
    with ectopic or molar pregnancy O08.6
    blood vessel — *see* Injury, blood vessel, iliac

Injury — *continued*
  uterus, uterine — *continued*
    contusion S37.62 ☑
    laceration S37.63 ☑
      cervix at delivery O71.3
    rupture associated with obstetrics — *see* Rupture, uterus
    specified type NEC S37.69 ☑
  uvula S09.93 ☑
  vagina S39.93 ☑
    abrasion S30.814 ☑
    bite S31.45 ☑
      insect S30.864 ☑
      superficial NEC S30.874 ☑
    contusion S30.23 ☑
    crush S38.03 ☑
    during delivery — *see* Laceration, vagina, during delivery
    external constriction S30.844 ☑
    insect bite S30.864 ☑
    laceration S31.41 ☑
      with foreign body S31.42 ☑
    open wound S31.40 ☑
    puncture S31.43 ☑
      with foreign body S31.44 ☑
    superficial S30.95 ☑
      foreign body S30.854 ☑
  vas deferens — *see* Injury, pelvic organ, specified site NEC
  vascular NEC T14.8
  vein — *see* Injury, blood vessel
  vena cava (superior) S25.20 ☑
    inferior S35.10 ☑
      laceration (minor) (superficial) S35.11 ☑
        major S35.12 ☑
      specified type NEC S35.19 ☑
    laceration (minor) (superficial) S25.21 ☑
      major S25.22 ☑
    specified type NEC S25.29 ☑
  vesical (sphincter) — *see* Injury, bladder
  visual cortex S04.04- ☑
  vitreous (humor) S05.90 ☑
    specified NEC S05.8X- ☑
  vocal cord NEC S19.83 ☑
  vulva S39.94 ☑
    abrasion S30.814 ☑
    bite S31.45 ☑
      insect S30.864 ☑
      superficial NEC S30.874 ☑
    contusion S30.23 ☑
    crush S38.03 ☑
    during delivery — *see* Laceration, perineum, female, during delivery
    external constriction S30.844 ☑
    insect bite S30.864 ☑
    laceration S31.41 ☑
      with foreign body S31.42 ☑
    open wound S31.40 ☑
    puncture S31.43 ☑
      with foreign body S31.44 ☑
    superficial S30.95 ☑
      foreign body S30.854 ☑
  whiplash (cervical spine) S13.4 ☑
  wrist S69.9- ☑
    blood vessel — *see* Injury, blood vessel, hand
    contusion — *see* Contusion, wrist
    dislocation — *see* Dislocation, wrist
    fracture — *see* Fracture, wrist
    muscle — *see* Injury, muscle, hand
    nerve — *see* Injury, nerve, hand
    open — *see* Wound, open, wrist
    specified NEC S69.8- ☑
    sprain — *see* Sprain, wrist
    superficial — *see* Injury, superficial, wrist
Inoculation (*see also* Vaccination)
  complication or reaction — *see* Complications, vaccination
Insanity, insane (*see also* Psychosis)
  adolescent — *see* Schizophrenia
  confusional F28
    acute or subacute F05
  delusional F22
  senile F03 ☑
Insect
  bite — *see* Bite, by site, superficial, insect

Insect — *continued*
  venomous, poisoning NEC (by) — *see* Venom, arthropod

Insensitivity
  adrenocorticotropin hormone (ACTH) E27.49
  androgen E34.50
    complete E34.51
    partial E34.52

Insertion
  cord (umbilical) lateral or velamentous O43.12- ☑
  intrauterine contraceptive device (encounter for) — *see* Intrauterine contraceptive device

Insolation (sunstroke) T67.0 ☑

Insomnia (organic) G47.00
  without objective findings F51.02
  adjustment F51.02
  adjustment disorder F51.02
  behavioral, of childhood Z73.819
    combined type Z73.812
    limit setting type Z73.811
    sleep-onset association type Z73.810
  childhood Z73.819
  chronic F51.04
    somatized tension F51.04
  conditioned F51.04
  due to
    alcohol
      abuse F10.182
      dependence F10.282
      use F10.982
    amphetamines
      abuse F15.182
      dependence F15.282
      use F15.982
    anxiety disorder F51.05
    caffeine
      abuse F15.182
      dependence F15.282
      use F15.982
    cocaine
      abuse F14.182
      dependence F14.282
      use F14.982
    depression F51.05
    drug NEC
      abuse F19.182
      dependence F19.282
      use F19.982
    medical condition G47.01
    mental disorder NEC F51.05
    opioid
      abuse F11.182
      dependence F11.282
      use F11.982
    psychoactive substance NEC
      abuse F19.182
      dependence F19.182
      use F19.982
    sedative, hypnotic, or anxiolytic
      abuse F13.182
      dependence F13.282
      use F13.982
    stimulant NEC
      abuse F15.182
      dependence F15.282
      use F15.982
  fatal familial (FFI) A81.83 ☑
  idiopathic F51.01
  learned F51.3
  nonorganic origin F51.01
  not due to a substance or known physiological condition F51.01
    specified NEC F51.09
  paradoxical F51.03
  primary F51.01
  psychiatric F51.05
  psychophysiologic F51.04
  related to psychopathology F51.05
  short-term F51.02
  specified NEC G47.09
  stress-related F51.02
  transient F51.02

Inspiration
  food or foreign body — *see* Foreign body, by site
  mucus — *see* Asphyxia, mucus

Inspissated bile syndrome (newborn) P59.1

Instability
  emotional (excessive) F60.3

Instability — *continued*
  joint (post-traumatic) M25.30
    ankle M25.37- ☑
    due to old ligament injury — *see* Disorder, ligament
    elbow M25.32- ☑
    flail — *see* Flail, joint
    foot M25.37- ☑
    hand M25.34- ☑
    hip M25.35- ☑
    knee M25.36- ☑
    lumbosacral — *see* subcategory M53.2 ☑
    prosthesis — *see* Complications, joint prosthesis, mechanical, displacement, by site
    sacroiliac — *see* subcategory M53.2 ☑
    secondary to
      old ligament injury — *see* Disorder, ligament
      removal of joint prosthesis M96.89
    shoulder (region) M25.31- ☑
    spine — *see* subcategory M53.2 ☑
    wrist M25.33- ☑
  knee (chronic) M23.5- ☑
  lumbosacral — *see* subcategory M53.2 ☑
  nervous F48.8
  personality (emotional) F60.3
  spine — *see* Instability, joint, spine
  vasomotor R55

Institutional syndrome (childhood) F94.2

Institutionalization, affecting child Z62.22
  disinhibited attachment F94.2

Insufficiency, insufficient
  accommodation, old age H52.4
  adrenal (gland) E27.40
    primary E27.1
  adrenocortical E27.40
    drug-induced E27.3
    iatrogenic E27.3
    primary E27.1
  anterior (occlusal) guidance M26.54
  anus K62.89
  aortic (valve) I35.1
    with
      mitral (valve) disease I08.0
        with tricuspid (valve) disease I08.3
      stenosis I35.2
      tricuspid (valve) disease I08.2
        with mitral (valve) disease I08.3
    congenital Q23.1
    rheumatic I06.1
      with
        mitral (valve) disease I08.0
          with tricuspid (valve) disease I08.3
        stenosis I06.2
          with mitral (valve) disease I08.0
            with tricuspid (valve) disease I08.3
        tricuspid (valve) disease I08.2
          with mitral (valve) disease I08.3
    specified cause NEC I35.1
    syphilitic A52.03
  arterial I77.1
    basilar G45.0
    carotid (hemispheric) G45.1
    cerebral I67.81
    coronary (acute or subacute) I24.8
    mesenteric K55.1
    peripheral I73.9
    precerebral (multiple) (bilateral) G45.2
    vertebral G45.0
  arteriovenous I99.8
  biliary K83.8
  cardiac (*see also* Insufficiency, myocardial)
    due to presence of (cardiac) prosthesis I97.11- ☑
    postprocedural I97.11- ☑
  cardiorenal, hypertensive I13.2
  cardiovascular — *see* Disease, cardiovascular
  cerebrovascular (acute) I67.81
    with transient focal neurological signs and symptoms G45.8
  circulatory NEC I99.8
    newborn P29.89
  convergence H51.11
  coronary (acute or subacute) I24.8
    chronic or with a stated duration of over 4 weeks I25.89
  corticoadrenal E27.40
    primary E27.1
  dietary E63.9
  divergence H51.8

Insufficiency, insufficient — *continued*
  food T73.0 ☑
  gastroesophageal K22.8
  gonadal
    ovary E28.39
    testis E29.1
  heart (*see also* Insufficiency, myocardial)
    newborn P29.0
    valve — *see* Endocarditis
  hepatic — *see* Failure, hepatic
  idiopathic autonomic G90.09
  interocclusal distance of fully erupted teeth (ridge) M26.36
  kidney N28.9
    acute N28.9
    chronic N18.9
  lacrimal (secretion) H04.12- ☑
    passages — *see* Stenosis, lacrimal
  liver — *see* Failure, hepatic
  lung — *see* Insufficiency, pulmonary
  mental (congenital) — *see* Disability, intellectual
  mesenteric K55.1
  mitral (valve) I34.0
    with
      aortic valve disease I08.0
        with tricuspid (valve) disease I08.3
      obstruction or stenosis I05.2
        with aortic valve disease I08.0
      tricuspid (valve) disease I08.1
        with aortic (valve) disease I08.3
    congenital Q23.3
    rheumatic I05.1
      with
        aortic valve disease I08.0
          with tricuspid (valve) disease I08.3
        obstruction or stenosis I05.2
          with aortic valve disease I08.0
            with tricuspid (valve) disease I08.3
        tricuspid (valve) disease I08.1
          with aortic (valve) disease I08.3
      active or acute I01.1
        with chorea, rheumatic (Sydenham's) I02.0
    specified cause, except rheumatic I34.0
  muscle (*see also* Disease, muscle)
    heart — *see* Insufficiency, myocardial
    ocular NEC H50.9
  myocardial, myocardium (with arteriosclerosis) I50.9
    with
      rheumatic fever (conditions in I00) I09.0
        active, acute or subacute I01.2
          with chorea I02.0
        inactive or quiescent (with chorea) I09.0
    congenital Q24.8
    hypertensive — *see* Hypertension, heart
    newborn P29.0
    rheumatic I09.0
      active, acute, or subacute I01.2
    syphilitic A52.06
  nourishment T73.0 ☑
  pancreatic K86.8
  parathyroid (gland) E20.9
  peripheral vascular (arterial) I73.9
  pituitary E23.0
  placental (mother) O36.51- ☑
  platelets D69.6
  prenatal care affecting management of pregnancy O09.3- ☑
  progressive pluriglandular E31.0
  pulmonary J98.4
    acute, following surgery (nonthoracic) J95.2
      thoracic J95.1
    chronic, following surgery J95.3
    following
      shock J98.4
      trauma J98.4
    newborn P28.5
    valve I37.1
      with stenosis I37.2
      congenital Q22.2
      rheumatic I09.89
        with aortic, mitral or tricuspid (valve) disease I08.8
  pyloric K31.89
  renal (acute) N28.9
    chronic N18.9
  respiratory R06.89
    newborn P28.5
  rotation — *see* Malrotation

☑ Additional Character Required — Refer to the Tabular List for Character Selection   ▽ Subterms under main terms may continue to next column or page

Insufficiency, insufficient — *continued*
 sleep syndrome F51.12
 social insurance Z59.7
 suprarenal E27.40
  primary E27.1
 tarso-orbital fascia, congenital Q10.3
 testis E29.1
 thyroid (gland) (acquired) E03.9
  congenital E03.1
 tricuspid (valve) (rheumatic) I07.1
  with
   aortic (valve) disease I08.2
    with mitral (valve) disease I08.3
   mitral (valve) disease I08.1
    with aortic (valve) disease I08.3
   obstruction or stenosis I07.2
    with aortic (valve) disease I08.2
     with mitral (valve) disease I08.3
  congenital Q22.8
  nonrheumatic I36.1
   with stenosis I36.2
 urethral sphincter R32
 valve, valvular (heart) — *see* Endocarditis
  congenital Q24.8
 vascular I99.8
  intestine K55.9
   acute K55.0
  mesenteric K55.1
  peripheral I73.9
  renal — *see* Hypertension, kidney
 velopharyngeal
  acquired K13.79
  congenital Q38.8
 venous (chronic) (peripheral) I87.2
 ventricular — *see* Insufficiency, myocardial
 welfare support Z59.7
Insufflation, fallopian Z31.41
Insular — *see* condition
Insulinoma
 pancreas
  benign D13.7
  malignant C25.4
  uncertain behavior D37.8
 specified site
  benign — *see* Neoplasm, by site, benign
  malignant — *see* Neoplasm, by site, malignant
  uncertain behavior — *see* Neoplasm, by site, uncertain behavior
 unspecified site
  benign D13.7
  malignant C25.4
  uncertain behavior D37.8
Insuloma — *see* Insulinoma
Interference
 balancing side M26.56
 non-working side M26.56
Intermenstrual — *see* condition
Intermittent — *see* condition
Internal — *see* condition
Interrogation
 cardiac defibrillator (automatic) (implantable) Z45.02
 cardiac pacemaker Z45.018
 cardiac (event) (loop) recorder Z45.09
 infusion pump (implanted) (intrathecal) Z45.1
 neurostimulator Z46.2
Interruption
 bundle of His I44.30
 phase-shift, sleep cycle — *see* Disorder, sleep, circadian rhythm
 sleep phase-shift, or 24 hour sleep-wake cycle — *see* Disorder, sleep, circadian rhythm
Interstitial — *see* condition
Intertrigo L30.4
 labialis K13.0
Intervertebral disc — *see* condition
Intestine, intestinal — *see* condition
Intolerance
 carbohydrate K90.4
 disaccharide, hereditary E73.0
 fat NEC K90.4
  pancreatic K90.3
 food K90.4
  dietary counseling and surveillance Z71.3
 fructose E74.10
  hereditary E74.12
 glucose (-galactose) E74.39
 gluten K90.0
 lactose E73.9

Intolerance — *continued*
 lactose — *continued*
  specified NEC E73.8
 lysine E72.3
 milk NEC K90.4
  lactose E73.9
 protein K90.4
 starch NEC K90.4
 sucrose (-isomaltose) E74.31
Intoxicated NEC (without dependence) — *see* Alcohol, intoxication
Intoxication
 acid E87.2
 alcoholic (acute) (without dependence) — *see* Alcohol, intoxication
 alimentary canal K52.1
 amphetamine (without dependence) — *see* Abuse, drug, stimulant, with intoxication
  with dependence — *see* Dependence, drug, stimulant, with intoxication
 anxiolytic (acute) (without dependence) — *see* Abuse, drug, sedative, with intoxication
  with dependence — *see* Dependence, drug, sedative, with intoxication
 caffeine (acute) (without dependence) — *see* Abuse, drug, stimulant, with intoxication
  with dependence — *see* Dependence, drug, stimulant, with intoxication
 cannabinoids (acute) (without dependence) — *see* Abuse, drug, cannabis, with intoxication
  with dependence — *see* Dependence, drug, cannabis, with intoxication
 chemical — *see* Table of Drugs and Chemicals
  via placenta or breast milk — *see* - Absorption, chemical, through placenta
 cocaine (acute) (without dependence) — *see* Abuse, drug, cocaine, with intoxication
  with dependence — *see* Dependence, drug, cocaine, with intoxication
 drug
  acute (without dependence) — *see* Abuse, drug, by type with intoxication
   with dependence — *see* Dependence, drug, by type with intoxication
  addictive
   via placenta or breast milk — *see* Absorption, drug, addictive, through placenta
  newborn P93.8
   gray baby syndrome P93.0
  overdose or wrong substance given or taken — *see* Table of Drugs and Chemicals, by drug, poisoning
 enteric K52.1
 foodborne A05.9
  bacterial A05.9
  classical (Clostridium botulinum) A05.1
  due to
   Bacillus cereus A05.4
   bacterium A05.9
    specified NEC A05.8
   Clostridium
    botulinum A05.1
    perfringens A05.2
    welchii A05.2
   Salmonella A02.9
    with
     (gastro)enteritis A02.0
     localized infection(s) A02.20
      arthritis A02.23
      meningitis A02.21
      osteomyelitis A02.24
      pneumonia A02.22
      pyelonephritis A02.25
      specified NEC A02.29
     sepsis A02.1
     specified manifestation NEC A02.8
   Staphylococcus A05.0
   Vibrio
    parahaemolyticus A05.3
    vulnificus A05.5
  enterotoxin, staphylococcal A05.0
  noxious — *see* Poisoning, food, noxious
 gastrointestinal K52.1
 hallucinogenic (without dependence) — *see* Abuse, drug, hallucinogen, with intoxication
  with dependence — *see* Dependence, drug, hallucinogen, with intoxication

Intoxication — *continued*
 hypnotic (acute) (without dependence) — *see* Abuse, drug, sedative, with intoxication
  with dependence — *see* Dependence, drug, sedative, with intoxication
 inhalant (acute) (without dependence) — *see* Abuse, drug, inhalant, with intoxication
  with dependence — *see* Dependence, drug, inhalant, with intoxication
 meaning
  inebriation — *see* category F10 ☑
  poisoning — *see* Table of Drugs and Chemicals
 methyl alcohol (acute) (without dependence) — *see* Alcohol, intoxication
 opioid (acute) (without dependence) — *see* Abuse, drug, opioid, with intoxication
  with dependence — *see* Dependence, drug, opioid, with intoxication
 pathologic NEC (without dependence) — *see* Alcohol, intoxication
 phencyclidine (without dependence) — *see* Abuse, drug, psychoactive NEC, with intoxication
  with dependence — *see* Dependence, drug, psychoactive NEC, with intoxication
 potassium (K) E87.5
 psychoactive substance NEC (without dependence) — *see* Abuse, drug, psychoactive NEC, with intoxication
  with dependence — *see* Dependence, drug, psychoactive NEC, with intoxication
 sedative (acute) (without dependence) — *see* Abuse, drug, sedative, with intoxication
  with dependence — *see* Dependence, drug, sedative, with intoxication
 serum (*see also* Reaction, serum) T80.69 ☑
 uremic — *see* Uremia
 volatile solvents (acute) (without dependence) — *see* Abuse, drug, inhalant, with intoxication
  with dependence — *see* Dependence, drug, inhalant, with intoxication
 water E87.79
Intracranial — *see* condition
Intrahepatic gallbladder Q44.1
Intraligamentous — *see* condition
Intrathoracic (*see also* condition)
 kidney Q63.2
Intrauterine contraceptive device
 checking Z30.431
 in situ Z97.5
 insertion Z30.430
  immediately following removal Z30.433
 management Z30.431
 reinsertion Z30.433
 removal Z30.432
 replacement Z30.433
 retention in pregnancy O26.3- ☑
Intraventricular — *see* condition
Intrinsic deformity — *see* Deformity
Intubation, difficult or failed T88.4 ☑
Intumescence, lens (eye) (cataract) — *see* Cataract
Intussusception (bowel) (colon) (enteric) (ileocecal) (ileocolic) (intestine) (rectum) K56.1
 appendix K38.8
 congenital Q43.8
 ureter (with obstruction) N13.5
Invagination (bowel, colon, intestine or rectum) K56.1
Inversion
 albumin-globulin (A-G) ratio E88.09
 bladder N32.89
 cecum — *see* Intussusception
 cervix N88.8
 chromosome in normal individual Q95.1
 circadian rhythm — *see* Disorder, sleep, circadian rhythm
 nipple N64.59
  congenital Q83.8
  gestational — *see* Retraction, nipple
  puerperal, postpartum — *see* Retraction, nipple
 nyctohemeral rhythm — *see* Disorder, sleep, circadian rhythm
 optic papilla Q14.2
 organ or site, congenital NEC — *see* Anomaly, by site
 sleep rhythm — *see* Disorder, sleep, circadian rhythm
 testis (congenital) Q55.29
 uterus (chronic) (postinfectional) (postpartal, old) N85.5
  postpartum O71.2

Inversion — *continued*
  vagina (posthysterectomy) N99.3
  ventricular Q20.5
Investigation (*see also* Examination) Z04.9
  clinical research subject (control) (normal comparison) (participant) Z00.6
Involuntary movement, abnormal R25.9
Involution, involutional (*see also* condition)
  breast, cystic — *see* Dysplasia, mammary, specified type NEC
  depression (single episode) F32.8
    recurrent episode F33.9
  melancholia (recurrent episode) (single episode) F32.8
  ovary, senile — *see* Atrophy, ovary
  thymus failure E32.8
I.Q.
  under 20 F73
  20-34 F72
  35-49 F71
  50-69 F70
IRDS (type I) P22.0
  type II P22.1
Irideremia Q13.1
Iridis rubeosis — *see* Disorder, iris, vascular
Iridochoroiditis (panuveitis) — *see* Panuveitis
Iridocyclitis H20.9
  acute H20.0- ☑
    hypopyon H20.05- ☑
    primary H20.01- ☑
    recurrent H20.02- ☑
    secondary (noninfectious) H20.04- ☑
      infectious H20.03- ☑
  chronic H20.1- ☑
  due to allergy — *see* Iridocyclitis, acute, secondary
  endogenous — *see* Iridocyclitis, acute, primary
  Fuchs' — *see* Cyclitis, Fuchs' heterochromic
  gonococcal A54.32
  granulomatous — *see* Iridocyclitis, chronic
  herpes, herpetic (simplex) B00.51
    zoster B02.32
  hypopyon — *see* Iridocyclitis, acute, hypopyon
  in (due to)
    ankylosing spondylitis M45.9
    gonococcal infection A54.32
    herpes (simplex) virus B00.51
      zoster B02.32
    infectious disease NOS B99 ☑
    parasitic disease NOS B89 [H22]
    sarcoidosis D86.83
    syphilis A51.43
    tuberculosis A18.54
    zoster B02.32
  lens-induced H20.2- ☑
  nongranulomatous — *see* Iridocyclitis, acute
  recurrent — *see* Iridocyclitis, acute, recurrent
  rheumatic — *see* Iridocyclitis, chronic
  subacute — *see* Iridocyclitis, acute
  sympathetic — *see* Uveitis, sympathetic
  syphilitic (secondary) A51.43
  tuberculous (chronic) A18.54
  Vogt-Koyanagi H20.82- ☑
Iridocyclochoroiditis (panuveitis) — *see* Panuveitis
Iridodialysis H21.53- ☑
Iridodonesis H21.89
Iridoplegia (complete) (partial) (reflex) H57.09
Iridoschisis H21.25- ☑
Iris (*see also* condition)
  bombé — *see* Membrane, pupillary
Iritis (*see also* Iridocyclitis)
  chronic — *see* Iridocyclitis, chronic
  diabetic — *see* E08-E13 with .39
  due to
    herpes simplex B00.51
    leprosy A30.9 [H22]
  gonococcal A54.32
  gouty M10.9
  granulomatous — *see* Iridocyclitis, chronic
  lens induced — *see* Iridocyclitis, lens-induced
  papulosa (syphilitic) A52.71
  rheumatic — *see* Iridocyclitis, chronic
  syphilitic (secondary) A51.43
    congenital (early) A50.01
    late A52.71
  tuberculous A18.54
Iron — *see* condition
Iron-miner's lung J63.4
Irradiated enamel (tooth, teeth) K03.89

Irradiation effects, adverse T66 ☑
Irreducible, irreducibility — *see* condition
Irregular, irregularity
  action, heart I49.9
  alveolar process K08.8
  bleeding N92.6
  breathing R06.89
  contour of cornea (acquired) — *see* Deformity, cornea
    congenital Q13.4
  contour, reconstructed breast N65.0
  dentin (in pulp) K04.3
  eye movements H55.89
    nystagmus — *see* Nystagmus
    saccadic H55.81
  labor O62.2
  menstruation (cause unknown) N92.6
  periods N92.6
  prostate N42.9
  pupil — *see* Abnormality, pupillary
  reconstructed breast N65.0
  respiratory R06.89
  septum (nasal) J34.2
  shape, organ or site, congenital NEC — *see* Distortion
  sleep-wake pattern (rhythm) G47.23
Irritable, irritability R45.4
  bladder N32.89
  bowel (syndrome) K58.9
    with diarrhea K58.0
    psychogenic F45.8
  bronchial — *see* Bronchitis
  cerebral, in newborn P91.3
  colon K58.9
    with diarrhea K58.0
    psychogenic F45.8
  duodenum K59.8
  heart (psychogenic) F45.8
  hip — *see* Derangement, joint, specified type NEC, hip
  ileum K59.8
  infant R68.12
  jejunum K59.8
  rectum K59.8
  stomach K31.89
    psychogenic F45.8
  sympathetic G90.8
  urethra N36.8
Irritation
  anus K62.89
  axillary nerve G54.0
  bladder N32.89
  brachial plexus G54.0
  bronchial — *see* Bronchitis
  cervical plexus G54.2
  cervix — *see* Cervicitis
  choroid, sympathetic — *see* Endophthalmitis
  cranial nerve — *see* Disorder, nerve, cranial
  gastric K31.89
    psychogenic F45.8
  globe, sympathetic — *see* Uveitis, sympathetic
  labyrinth — *see* subcategory H83.2 ☑
  lumbosacral plexus G54.1
  meninges (traumatic) — *see* Injury, intracranial
    nontraumatic — *see* Meningismus
  nerve — *see* Disorder, nerve
  nervous R45.0
  penis N48.89
  perineum NEC L29.3
  peripheral autonomic nervous system G90.8
  peritoneum — *see* Peritonitis
  pharynx J39.2
  plantar nerve — *see* Lesion, nerve, plantar
  spinal (cord) (traumatic) (*see also* Injury, spinal cord, by region)
    nerve G58.9
      root NEC — *see* Radiculopathy
    nontraumatic — *see* Myelopathy
  stomach K31.89
    psychogenic F45.8
  sympathetic nerve NEC G90.8
  ulnar nerve — *see* Lesion, nerve, ulnar
  vagina N89.8
Ischemia, ischemic I99.8
  bowel (transient)
    acute K55.0
    chronic K55.1
    due to mesenteric artery insufficiency K55.1
  brain — *see* Ischemia, cerebral
  cardiac (see Disease, heart, ischemic)
  cardiomyopathy I25.5

Ischemia, ischemic — *continued*
  cerebral (chronic) (generalized) I67.82
    arteriosclerotic I67.2
    intermittent G45.9
    newborn P91.0
    recurrent focal G45.8
    transient G45.9
  colon chronic (due to mesenteric artery insufficiency) K55.1
  coronary — *see* Disease, heart, ischemic
  demand (coronary) (*see also* Angina) I24.8
  heart (chronic or with a stated duration of over 4 weeks) I25.9
    acute or with a stated duration of 4 weeks or less I24.9
    subacute I24.9
  infarction, muscle — *see* Infarct, muscle
  intestine (large) (small) (transient) K55.9
    acute K55.0
    chronic K55.1
    due to mesenteric artery insufficiency K55.1
  kidney N28.0
  mesenteric, acute K55.0
  muscle, traumatic T79.6 ☑
  myocardium, myocardial (chronic or with a stated duration of over 4 weeks) I25.9
    acute, without myocardial infarction I24.0
    silent (asymptomatic) I25.6
    transient of newborn P29.4
  renal N28.0
  retina, retinal — *see* Occlusion, artery, retina
  small bowel
    acute K55.0
    chronic K55.1
    due to mesenteric artery insufficiency K55.1
  spinal cord G95.11
  subendocardial — *see* Insufficiency, coronary
  supply (coronary) (*see also* Angina) I25.9
    due to vasospasm I20.1
Ischial spine — *see* condition
Ischialgia — *see* Sciatica
Ischiopagus Q89.4
Ischium, ischial — *see* condition
Ischuria R34
Iselin's disease or osteochondrosis — *see* Osteochondrosis, juvenile, metatarsus
Islands of
  parotid tissue in
    lymph nodes Q38.6
    neck structures Q38.6
  submaxillary glands in
    fascia Q38.6
    lymph nodes Q38.6
    neck muscles Q38.6
Islet cell tumor, pancreas D13.7
Isoimmunization NEC (*see also* Incompatibility)
  affecting management of pregnancy (ABO) (with hydrops fetalis) O36.11- ☑
    anti-A sensitization O36.11- ☑
    anti-B sensitization O36.19- ☑
    anti-c sensitization O36.09- ☑
    anti-C sensitization O36.09- ☑
    anti-E sensitization O36.09- ☑
    anti-e sensitization O36.09- ☑
    Rh NEC O36.09- ☑
      anti-D antibody O36.01- ☑
    specified NEC O36.19- ☑
  newborn P55.9
    with
      hydrops fetalis P56.0
      kernicterus P57.0
    ABO (blood groups) P55.1
    Rhesus (Rh) factor P55.0
    specified type NEC P55.8
Isolation, isolated
  dwelling Z59.8
  family Z63.79
  social Z60.4
Isoleucinosis E71.19
Isomerism atrial appendages (with asplenia or polysplenia) Q20.6
Isosporiasis, isosporosis A07.3
Isovaleric acidemia E71.110
Issue of
  medical certificate Z02.79
    for disability determination Z02.71

Issue of — *continued*
  repeat prescription (appliance) (glasses) (medicinal substance, medicament, medicine) Z76.0
    contraception — *see* Contraception
Itch, itching (*see also* Pruritus)
  baker's L23.6
  barber's B35.0
  bricklayer's L24.5
  cheese B88.0
  clam digger's B65.3
  coolie B76.9
  copra B88.0
  dew B76.9
  dhobi B35.6
  filarial — *see* Infestation, filarial
  grain B88.0
  grocer's B88.0
  ground B76.9
  harvest B88.0
  jock B35.6
  Malabar B35.5
    beard B35.0
    foot B35.3
    scalp B35.0
  meaning scabies B86
  Norwegian B86
  perianal L29.0
  poultrymen's B88.0
  sarcoptic B86
  scabies B86
  scrub B88.0
  straw B88.0
  swimmer's B65.3
  water B76.9
  winter L29.8
Ivemark's syndrome (asplenia with congenital heart disease) Q89.01
Ivory bones Q78.2
Ixodiasis NEC B88.8

J

Jaccoud's syndrome — *see* Arthropathy, postrheumatic, chronic
Jackson's
  membrane Q43.3
  paralysis or syndrome G83.89
  veil Q43.3
Jacquet's dermatitis (diaper dermatitis) L22
Jadassohn-Pellizari's disease or anetoderma L90.2
Jadassohn's
  blue nevus — *see* Nevus
  intraepidermal epithelioma — *see* Neoplasm, skin, benign
Jaffe-Lichtenstein (-Uehlinger) **syndrome** — *see* Dysplasia, fibrous, bone NEC
Jakob-Creutzfeldt disease or syndrome — *see* Creutzfeldt-Jakob disease or syndrome
Jaksch-Luzet disease D64.89
Jamaican
  neuropathy G92
  paraplegic tropical ataxic-spastic syndrome G92
Janet's disease F48.8
Janiceps Q89.4
Jansky-Bielschowsky amaurotic idiocy E75.4
Japanese
  B-type encephalitis A83.0
  river fever A75.3
Jaundice (yellow) R17
  acholuric (familial) (splenomegalic) (*see also* Spherocytosis)
    acquired D59.8
  breast-milk (inhibitor) P59.3
  catarrhal (acute) B15.9
    with hepatic coma B15.0
  cholestatic (benign) R17
  due to or associated with
    delayed conjugation P59.8
      associated with (due to) preterm delivery P59.0
    preterm delivery P59.0
  epidemic (catarrhal) B15.9
    with hepatic coma B15.0
    leptospiral A27.0
    spirochetal A27.0
  familial nonhemolytic (congenital) (Gilbert) E80.4
    Crigler-Najjar E80.5
  febrile (acute) B15.9
    with hepatic coma B15.0

Jaundice — *continued*
  febrile — *continued*
    leptospiral A27.0
    spirochetal A27.0
  hematogenous D59.9
  hemolytic (acquired) D59.9
    congenital — *see* Spherocytosis
  hemorrhagic (acute) (leptospiral) (spirochetal) A27.0
  infectious (acute) (subacute) B15.9
    with hepatic coma B15.0
    leptospiral A27.0
    spirochetal A27.0
  leptospiral (hemorrhagic) A27.0
  malignant (without coma) K72.90
    with coma K72.91
  neonatal — *see* Jaundice, newborn
  newborn P59.9
    due to or associated with
      ABO
        antibodies P55.1
        incompatibility, maternal/fetal P55.1
        isoimmunization P55.1
      absence or deficiency of enzyme system for bilirubin conjugation (congenital) P59.8
      bleeding P58.1
      breast milk inhibitors to conjugation P59.3
        associated with preterm delivery P59.0
      bruising P58.0
      Crigler-Najjar syndrome E80.5
      delayed conjugation P59.8
        associated with preterm delivery P59.0
      drugs or toxins
        given to newborn P58.42
        transmitted from mother P58.41
      excessive hemolysis P58.9
        due to
          bleeding P58.1
          bruising P58.0
          drugs or toxins
            given to newborn P58.42
            transmitted from mother P58.41
          infection P58.2
          polycythemia P58.3
          swallowed maternal blood P58.5
        specified type NEC P58.8
      galactosemia E74.21
      Gilbert syndrome E80.4
      hemolytic disease P55.9
        ABO isoimmunization P55.1
        Rh isoimmunization P55.0
        specified NEC P55.8
      hepatocellular damage P59.20
        specified NEC P59.29
      hereditary hemolytic anemia P58.8
      hypothyroidism, congenital E03.1
      incompatibility, maternal/fetal NOS P55.9
      infection P58.2
      inspissated bile syndrome P59.1
      isoimmunization NOS P55.9
      mucoviscidosis E84.9
      polycythemia P58.3
      preterm delivery P59.0
      Rh
        antibodies P55.0
        incompatibility, maternal/fetal P55.0
        isoimmunization P55.0
      specified cause NEC P59.8
      swallowed maternal blood P58.5
    spherocytosis (congenital) D58.0
  nonhemolytic congenital familial (Gilbert) E80.4
  nuclear, newborn (*see also* Kernicterus of newborn) P57.9
  obstructive (*see also* Obstruction, bile duct) K83.1
  post-immunization — *see* Hepatitis, viral, type, B
  post-transfusion — *see* Hepatitis, viral, type, B
  regurgitation (*see also* Obstruction, bile duct) K83.1
  serum (homologous) (prophylactic) (therapeutic) — *see* Hepatitis, viral, type, B
  spirochetal (hemorrhagic) A27.0
  symptomatic R17
    newborn P59.9
Jaw — *see* condition
Jaw-winking phenomenon or syndrome Q07.8
Jealousy
  alcoholic F10.988
  childhood F93.8
  sibling F93.8
Jejunitis — *see* Enteritis

Jejunostomy status Z93.4
Jejunum, jejunal — *see* condition
Jensen's disease — *see* Inflammation, chorioretinal, focal, juxtapapillary
Jerks, myoclonic G25.3
Jervell-Lange-Nielsen syndrome I45.81
Jeune's disease Q77.2
Jigger disease B88.1
Job's syndrome (chronic granulomatous disease) D71
Joint (*see also* condition)
  mice — *see* Loose, body, joint
    knee M23.4- ☑
Jordan's anomaly or syndrome D72.0
Joseph-Diamond-Blackfan anemia (congenital hypoplastic) D61.01
Jungle yellow fever A95.0
Jüngling's disease — *see* Sarcoidosis
Juvenile — *see* condition

K

Kahler's disease C90.0- ☑
Kakke E51.11
Kala-azar B55.0
Kallmann's syndrome E23.0
Kanner's syndrome (autism) — *see* Psychosis, childhood
Kaposi's
  dermatosis (xeroderma pigmentosum) Q82.1
  lichen ruber L44.0
    acuminatus L44.0
  sarcoma
    colon C46.4
    connective tissue C46.1
    gastrointestinal organ C46.4
    lung C46.5- ☑
    lymph node (multiple) C46.3
    palate (hard) (soft) C46.2
    rectum C46.4
    skin (multiple sites) C46.0
    specified site NEC C46.7
    stomach C46.4
    unspecified site C46.9
  varicelliform eruption B00.0
    vaccinia T88.1 ☑
Kartagener's syndrome or triad (sinusitis, bronchiectasis, situs inversus) Q89.3
Karyotype
  with abnormality except iso (Xq) Q96.2
  45,X Q96.0
  46,X
    iso (Xq) Q96.1
  46,XX Q98.3
    with streak gonads Q50.32
    hermaphrodite (true) Q99.1
    male Q98.3
  46,XY
    with streak gonads Q56.1
    female Q97.3
    hermaphrodite (true) Q99.1
  47,XXX Q97.0
  47,XXY Q98.0
  47,XYY Q98.5
Kaschin-Beck disease — *see* Disease, Kaschin-Beck
Katayama's disease or fever B65.2
Kawasaki's syndrome M30.3
Kayser-Fleischer ring (cornea) (pseudosclerosis) H18.04- ☑
Kaznelson's syndrome (congenital hypoplastic anemia) D61.01
Kearns-Sayre syndrome H49.81- ☑
Kedani fever A75.3
Kelis L91.0
Kelly (-Patterson) **syndrome** (sideropenic dysphagia) D50.1
Keloid, cheloid L91.0
  acne L73.0
  Addison's L94.0
  cornea — *see* Opacity, cornea
  Hawkin's L91.0
  scar L91.0
Keloma L91.0
Kenya fever A77.1
Keratectasia (*see also* Ectasia, cornea)
  congenital Q13.4
Keratinization of alveolar ridge mucosa
  excessive K13.23
  minimal K13.22

Keratinized residual ridge mucosa
  excessive K13.23
  minimal K13.22
Keratitis (nodular) (nonulcerative) (simple) (zonular) H16.9
  with ulceration (central) (marginal) (perforated) (ring) — see Ulcer, cornea
  actinic — see Photokeratitis
  arborescens (herpes simplex) B00.52
  areolar H16.11- ☑
  bullosa H16.8
  deep H16.309
    specified type NEC H16.399
  dendritic (a) (herpes simplex) B00.52
  disciform (is) (herpes simplex) B00.52
    varicella B01.81
  filamentary H16.12- ☑
  gonococcal (congenital or prenatal) A54.33
  herpes, herpetic (simplex) B00.52
    zoster B02.33
  in (due to)
    acanthamebiasis B60.13
    adenovirus B30.0
    exanthema (see also Exanthem) B09
    herpes (simplex) virus B00.52
    measles B05.81
    syphilis A50.31
    tuberculosis A18.52
    zoster B02.33
  interstitial (nonsyphilitic) H16.30- ☑
    diffuse H16.32- ☑
    herpes, herpetic (simplex) B00.52
      zoster B02.33
    sclerosing H16.33- ☑
    specified type NEC H16.39- ☑
    syphilitic (congenital) (late) A50.31
    tuberculous A18.52
  macular H16.11- ☑
  nummular H16.11- ☑
  oyster shuckers' H16.8
  parenchymatous — see Keratitis, interstitial
  petrificans H16.8
  postmeasles B05.81
  punctata
    leprosa A30.9 [H16.14-] ☑
    syphilitic (profunda) A50.31
  punctate H16.14- ☑
  purulent H16.8
  rosacea L71.8
  sclerosing H16.33- ☑
  specified type NEC H16.8
  stellate H16.11- ☑
  striate H16.11- ☑
  superficial H16.10- ☑
    with conjunctivitis — see Keratoconjunctivitis
    due to light — see Photokeratitis
  suppurative H16.8
  syphilitic (congenital) (prenatal) A50.31
  trachomatous A71.1
    sequelae B94.0
  tuberculous A18.52
  vesicular H16.8
  xerotic (see also Keratomalacia) H16.8
    vitamin A deficiency E50.4
Keratoacanthoma L85.8
Keratocele — see Descemetocele
Keratoconjunctivitis H16.20- ☑
  Acanthamoeba B60.13
  adenoviral B30.0
  epidemic B30.0
  exposure H16.21- ☑
  herpes, herpetic (simplex) B00.52
    zoster B02.33
  in exanthema (see also Exanthem) B09
  infectious B30.0
  lagophthalmic — see Keratoconjunctivitis, specified type NEC
  neurotrophic H16.23- ☑
  phlyctenular H16.25- ☑
  postmeasles B05.81
  shipyard B30.0
  sicca (Sjogren's) M35.0- ☑
    not Sjogren's H16.22- ☑
  specified type NEC H16.29- ☑
  tuberculous (phlyctenular) A18.52
  vernal H16.26- ☑
Keratoconus H18.60- ☑

Keratoconus — continued
  congenital Q13.4
  stable H18.61- ☑
  unstable H18.62- ☑
Keratocyst (dental) (odontogenic) — see Cyst, calcifying odontogenic
Keratoderma, keratodermia (congenital) (palmaris et plantaris) (symmetrical) Q82.8
  acquired L85.1
    in diseases classified elsewhere L86
  climactericum L85.1
  gonococcal A54.89
  gonorrheal A54.89
  punctata L85.2
  Reiter's — see Reiter's disease
Keratodermatocele — see Descemetocele
Keratoglobus H18.79 ☑
  congenital Q15.8
    with glaucoma Q15.0
Keratohemia — see Pigmentation, cornea, stromal
Keratoiritis (see also Iridocyclitis)
  syphilitic A50.39
  tuberculous A18.54
Keratoma L57.0
  palmaris and plantaris hereditarium Q82.8
  senile L57.0
Keratomalacia H18.44- ☑
  vitamin A deficiency E50.4
Keratomegaly Q13.4
Keratomycosis B49
  nigrans, nigricans (palmaris) B36.1
Keratopathy H18.9
  band H18.42- ☑
  bullous (aphakic), following cataract surgery H59.01- ☑
  bullous H18.1- ☑
Keratoscleritis, tuberculous A18.52
Keratosis L57.0
  actinic L57.0
  arsenical L85.8
  congenital, specified NEC Q80.8
  female genital NEC N94.89
  follicularis Q82.8
    acquired L11.0
    congenita Q82.8
    et parafollicularis in cutem penetrans L87.0
    spinulosa (decalvans) Q82.8
    vitamin A deficiency E50.8
  gonococcal A54.89
  male genital (external) N50.8
  nigricans L83
  obturans, external ear (canal) — see Cholesteatoma, external ear
  palmaris et plantaris (inherited) (symmetrical) Q82.8
    acquired L85.1
  penile N48.89
  pharynx J39.2
  pilaris, acquired L85.8
  punctata (palmaris et plantaris) L85.2
  scrotal N50.8
  seborrheic L82.1
    inflamed L82.0
  senile L57.0
  solar L57.0
  tonsillaris J35.8
  vagina N89.4
  vegetans Q82.8
  vitamin A deficiency E50.8
  vocal cord J38.3
Kerato-uveitis — see Iridocyclitis
Kerion (celsi) B35.0
Kernicterus of newborn (not due to isoimmunization) P57.9
  due to isoimmunization (conditions in P55.0-P55.9) P57.0
  specified type NEC P57.8
Kerunoparalysis T75.09 ☑
Keshan disease E59
Ketoacidosis E87.2
  diabetic — see Diabetes, by type, with ketoacidosis
Ketonuria R82.4
Ketosis NEC E88.89
  diabetic — see Diabetes, by type, with with ketoacidosis
Kew Garden fever A79.1
Kidney — see condition

Kienböck's disease (see also Osteochondrosis, juvenile, hand, carpal lunate)
  adult M93.1
Kimmelstiel (-Wilson) **disease** — see Diabetes, Kimmelstiel (-Wilson) disease
Kink, kinking
  artery I77.1
  hair (acquired) L67.8
  ileum or intestine — see Obstruction, intestine
  Lane's — see Obstruction, intestine
  organ or site, congenital NEC — see Anomaly, by site
  ureter (pelvic junction) N13.5
    with
      hydronephrosis N13.1
        with infection N13.6
      pyelonephritis (chronic) N11.1
    congenital Q62.39
  vein(s) I87.8
    caval I87.1
    peripheral I87.1
Kinnier Wilson's disease (hepatolenticular degeneration) E83.01
Kissing spine M48.20
  cervical region M48.22
  cervicothoracic region M48.23
  lumbar region M48.26
  lumbosacral region M48.27
  occipito-atlanto-axial region M48.21
  thoracic region M48.24
  thoracolumbar region M48.25
Klatskin's tumor C22.1
Klauder's disease A26.8
Klebs' disease (see also Glomerulonephritis) N05- ☑
Klebsiella (K.) **pneumoniae, as cause of disease classified elsewhere** B96.1
Klein (e)-**Levin syndrome** G47.13
Kleptomania F63.2
Klinefelter's syndrome Q98.4
  karyotype 47,XXY Q98.0
  male with more than two X chromosomes Q98.1
Klippel-Feil deficiency, disease, or syndrome (brevicollis) Q76.1
Klippel's disease I67.2
Klippel-Trenaunay (-Weber) **syndrome** Q87.2
Klumpke (-Déjerine) **palsy, paralysis** (birth) (newborn) P14.1
Knee — see condition
Knock knee (acquired) M21.06- ☑
  congenital Q74.1
Knot(s)
  intestinal, syndrome (volvulus) K56.2
  surfer S89.8- ☑
  umbilical cord (true) O69.2 ☑
Knotting (of)
  hair L67.8
  intestine K56.2
Knuckle pad (Garrod's) M72.1
Koch's
  infection — see Tuberculosis
  relapsing fever A68.9
Koch-Weeks' conjunctivitis — see Conjunctivitis, acute, mucopurulent
Köebner's syndrome Q81.8
Köenig's disease (osteochondritis dissecans) — see Osteochondritis, dissecans
Köhler-Pellegrini-Steida disease or syndrome (calcification, knee joint) — see Bursitis, tibial collateral
Köhler's disease
  patellar — see Osteochondrosis, juvenile, patella
  tarsal navicular — see Osteochondrosis, juvenile, tarsus
Koilonychia L60.3
  congenital Q84.6
Kojevnikov's, epilepsy — see Kozhevnikof's epilepsy
Koplik's spots B05.9
Kopp's asthma E32.8
Korsakoff's (Wernicke) **disease, psychosis or syndrome** (alcoholic) F10.96
  with dependence F10.26
  drug-induced
    due to drug abuse — see Abuse, drug, by type, with amnestic disorder
    due to drug dependence — see Dependence, drug, by type, with amnestic disorder
  nonalcoholic F04
Korsakov's disease, psychosis or syndrome — see Korsakoff's disease

☑ Additional Character Required — Refer to the Tabular List for Character Selection   ☑ Subterms under main terms may continue to next column or page

Korsakow's disease, psychosis or syndrome — *see* Korsakoff's disease
Kostmann's disease or syndrome (infantile genetic agranulocytosis) — *see* Agranulocytosis
Kozhevnikof's epilepsy G40.109
　intractable G40.119
　　with status epilepticus G40.111
　　without status epilepticus G40.119
　not intractable G40.109
　　with status epilepticus G40.101
　　without status epilepticus G40.109
Krabbe's
　disease E75.23
　syndrome, congenital muscle hypoplasia Q79.8
Kraepelin-Morel disease — *see* Schizophrenia
Kraft-Weber-Dimitri disease Q85.8
Kraurosis
　ani K62.89
　penis N48.0
　vagina N89.8
　vulva N90.4
Kreotoxism A05.9
Krukenberg's
　spindle — *see* Pigmentation, cornea, posterior
　tumor C79.6- ☑
Kufs' disease E75.4
Kugelberg-Welander disease G12.1
Kuhnt-Junius degeneration (*see also* Degeneration, macula) H35.32
Kümmell's disease or spondylitis — *see* Spondylopathy, traumatic
Kupffer cell sarcoma C22.3
Kuru A81.81
Kussmaul's
　disease M30.0
　respiration E87.2
　　in diabetic acidosis — *see* Diabetes, by type, with ketoacidosis
Kwashiorkor E40
　marasmic, marasmus type E42
Kyasanur Forest disease A98.2
Kyphoscoliosis, kyphoscoliotic (acquired) (*see also* Scoliosis) M41.9
　congenital Q67.5
　heart (disease) I27.1
　sequelae of rickets E64.3
　tuberculous A18.01
Kyphosis, kyphotic (acquired) M40.209
　cervical region M40.202
　cervicothoracic region M40.203
　congenital Q76.419
　　cervical region Q76.412
　　cervicothoracic region Q76.413
　　occipito-atlanto-axial region Q76.411
　　thoracic region Q76.414
　　thoracolumbar region Q76.415
　Morquio-Brailsford type (spinal) (*see also* subcategory M49.8) E76.219
　postlaminectomy M96.3
　postradiation therapy M96.2
　postural (adolescent) M40.00
　　cervicothoracic region M40.03
　　thoracic region M40.04
　　thoracolumbar region M40.05
　secondary NEC M40.10
　　cervical region M40.12
　　cervicothoracic region M40.13
　　thoracic region M40.14
　　thoracolumbar region M40.15
　sequelae of rickets E64.3
　specified type NEC M40.299
　　cervical region M40.292
　　cervicothoracic region M40.293
　　thoracic region M40.294
　　thoracolumbar region M40.295
　syphilitic, congenital A50.56
　thoracic region M40.204
　thoracolumbar region M40.205
　tuberculous A18.01
Kyrle disease L87.0

L

Labia, labium — *see* condition
Labile
　blood pressure R09.89
　vasomotor system I73.9

Labioglossal paralysis G12.29
Labium leporinum — *see* Cleft, lip
Labor — *see* Delivery
Labored breathing — *see* Hyperventilation
Labyrinthitis (circumscribed) (destructive) (diffuse) (inner ear) (latent) (purulent) (suppurative) (*see also* subcategory) H83.0 ☑
　syphilitic A52.79
Laceration
　with abortion — *see* Abortion, by type, complicated by laceration of pelvic organs
　abdomen, abdominal
　　wall S31.119 ☑
　　　with
　　　　foreign body S31.129 ☑
　　　　penetration into peritoneal cavity S31.619 ☑
　　　　　with foreign body S31.629 ☑
　　　epigastric region S31.112 ☑
　　　　with
　　　　　foreign body S31.122 ☑
　　　　　penetration into peritoneal cavity S31.612 ☑
　　　　　　with foreign body S31.622 ☑
　　　left
　　　　lower quadrant S31.114 ☑
　　　　　with
　　　　　　foreign body S31.124 ☑
　　　　　　penetration into peritoneal cavity S31.614 ☑
　　　　　　　with foreign body S31.624 ☑
　　　　upper quadrant S31.111 ☑
　　　　　with
　　　　　　foreign body S31.121 ☑
　　　　　　penetration into peritoneal cavity S31.611 ☑
　　　　　　　with foreign body S31.621 ☑
　　　periumbilic region S31.115 ☑
　　　　with
　　　　　foreign body S31.125 ☑
　　　　　penetration into peritoneal cavity S31.615 ☑
　　　　　　with foreign body S31.625 ☑
　　　right
　　　　lower quadrant S31.113 ☑
　　　　　with
　　　　　　foreign body S31.123 ☑
　　　　　　penetration into peritoneal cavity S31.613 ☑
　　　　　　　with foreign body S31.623 ☑
　　　　upper quadrant S31.110 ☑
　　　　　with
　　　　　　foreign body S31.120 ☑
　　　　　　penetration into peritoneal cavity S31.610 ☑
　　　　　　　with foreign body S31.620 ☑
　　accidental, complicating surgery — *see* Complications, surgical, accidental puncture or laceration
　　Achilles tendon S86.02- ☑
　　adrenal gland S37.813 ☑
　　alveolar (process) — *see* Laceration, oral cavity
　　ankle S91.01- ☑
　　　with
　　　　foreign body S91.02- ☑
　　antecubital space — *see* Laceration, elbow
　　anus (sphincter) S31.831 ☑
　　　with
　　　　ectopic or molar pregnancy O08.6
　　　　foreign body S31.832 ☑
　　　complicating delivery — *see* Delivery, complicated, by, laceration, anus (sphincter)
　　　following ectopic or molar pregnancy O08.6
　　　nontraumatic, nonpuerperal — *see* Fissure, anus
　　arm (upper) S41.11- ☑
　　　with foreign body S41.12- ☑
　　　lower — *see* Laceration, forearm
　　auditory canal (external) (meatus) — *see* Laceration, ear
　　auricle, ear — *see* Laceration, ear
　　axilla — *see* Laceration, arm
　　back (*see also* Laceration, thorax, back)
　　　lower S31.010 ☑
　　　　with
　　　　　foreign body S31.020 ☑
　　　　　with penetration into retroperitoneal space S31.021 ☑

Laceration — *continued*
　back (*see also* Laceration, thorax, back) — *continued*
　　lower — *continued*
　　　with — *continued*
　　　　penetration into retroperitoneal space S31.011 ☑
　bile duct S36.13 ☑
　bladder S37.23 ☑
　　with ectopic or molar pregnancy O08.6
　　following ectopic or molar pregnancy O08.6
　　obstetrical trauma O71.5
　blood vessel — *see* Injury, blood vessel
　bowel (*see also* Laceration, intestine)
　　with ectopic or molar pregnancy O08.6
　　complicating abortion — *see* Abortion, by type, complicated by, specified condition NEC
　　following ectopic or molar pregnancy O08.6
　　obstetrical trauma O71.5
　brain (any part) (cortex) (diffuse) (membrane) (*see also* Injury, intracranial, diffuse)
　　during birth P10.8
　　　with hemorrhage P10.1
　　focal — *see* Injury, intracranial, focal brain injury
　brainstem S06.38- ☑
　breast S21.01- ☑
　　with foreign body S21.02- ☑
　broad ligament S37.893 ☑
　　with ectopic or molar pregnancy O08.6
　　following ectopic or molar pregnancy O08.6
　　laceration syndrome N83.8
　　obstetrical trauma O71.6
　　syndrome (laceration) N83.8
　buttock S31.801 ☑
　　with foreign body S31.802 ☑
　　left S31.821 ☑
　　　with foreign body S31.822 ☑
　　right S31.811 ☑
　　　with foreign body S31.812 ☑
　calf — *see* Laceration, leg
　canaliculus lacrimalis — *see* Laceration, eyelid
　canthus, eye — *see* Laceration, eyelid
　capsule, joint — *see* Sprain
　causing eversion of cervix uteri (old) N86
　central (perineal), complicating delivery O70.9
　cerebellum, traumatic S06.37- ☑
　cerebral S06.33- ☑
　　during birth P10.8
　　　with hemorrhage P10.1
　　left side S06.32- ☑
　　right side S06.31- ☑
　cervix (uteri)
　　with ectopic or molar pregnancy O08.6
　　following ectopic or molar pregnancy O08.6
　　nonpuerperal, nontraumatic N88.1
　　obstetrical trauma (current) O71.3
　　old (postpartal) N88.1
　　traumatic S37.63 ☑
　cheek (external) S01.41- ☑
　　with foreign body S01.42- ☑
　　internal — *see* Laceration, oral cavity
　chest wall — *see* Laceration, thorax
　chin — *see* Laceration, head, specified site NEC
　chordae tendinae NEC I51.1
　　concurrent with acute myocardial infarction — *see* Infarct, myocardium
　　following acute myocardial infarction (current complication) I23.4
　clitoris — *see* Laceration, vulva
　colon — *see* Laceration, intestine, large, colon
　common bile duct S36.13 ☑
　cortex (cerebral) — *see* Injury, intracranial, diffuse
　costal region — *see* Laceration, thorax
　cystic duct S36.13 ☑
　diaphragm S27.803 ☑
　digit(s)
　　foot — *see* Laceration, toe
　　hand — *see* Laceration, finger
　duodenum S36.430 ☑
　ear (canal) (external) S01.31- ☑
　　with foreign body S01.32- ☑
　　drum S09.2- ☑
　elbow S51.01- ☑
　　with
　　　foreign body S51.02- ☑
　epididymis — *see* Laceration, testis

Laceration — *continued*
- epigastric region — *see* Laceration, abdomen, wall, epigastric region
- esophagus K22.8
  - traumatic
    - cervical S11.21 ☑
      - with foreign body S11.22 ☑
    - thoracic S27.813 ☑
- eye (ball) S05.3- ☑
  - with prolapse or loss of intraocular tissue S05.2- ☑
  - penetrating S05.6- ☑
- eyebrow — *see* Laceration, eyelid
- eyelid S01.11- ☑
  - with foreign body S01.12- ☑
- face NEC — *see* Laceration, head, specified site NEC
- fallopian tube S37.539 ☑
  - bilateral S37.532 ☑
  - unilateral S37.531 ☑
- finger(s) S61.219 ☑
  - with
    - damage to nail S61.319 ☑
      - with
        - foreign body S61.329 ☑
    - foreign body S61.229 ☑
  - index S61.218 ☑
    - with
      - damage to nail S61.318 ☑
        - with
          - foreign body S61.328 ☑
      - foreign body S61.228 ☑
    - left S61.211 ☑
      - with
        - damage to nail S61.311 ☑
          - with
            - foreign body S61.321 ☑
        - foreign body S61.221 ☑
    - right S61.210 ☑
      - with
        - damage to nail S61.310 ☑
          - with
            - foreign body S61.320 ☑
        - foreign body S61.220 ☑
  - little S61.218 ☑
    - with
      - damage to nail S61.318 ☑
        - with
          - foreign body S61.328 ☑
      - foreign body S61.228 ☑
    - left S61.217 ☑
      - with
        - damage to nail S61.317 ☑
          - with
            - foreign body S61.327 ☑
        - foreign body S61.227 ☑
    - right S61.216 ☑
      - with
        - damage to nail S61.316 ☑
          - with
            - foreign body S61.326 ☑
        - foreign body S61.226 ☑
  - middle S61.218 ☑
    - with
      - damage to nail S61.318 ☑
        - with
          - foreign body S61.328 ☑
      - foreign body S61.228 ☑
    - left S61.213 ☑
      - with
        - damage to nail S61.313 ☑
          - with
            - foreign body S61.323 ☑
        - foreign body S61.223 ☑
    - right S61.212 ☑
      - with
        - damage to nail S61.312 ☑
          - with
            - foreign body S61.322 ☑
        - foreign body S61.222 ☑
  - ring S61.218 ☑
    - with
      - damage to nail S61.318 ☑
        - with
          - foreign body S61.328 ☑
      - foreign body S61.228 ☑
    - left S61.215 ☑

Laceration — *continued*
- finger(s) — *continued*
  - ring — *continued*
    - left — *continued*
      - with
        - damage to nail S61.315 ☑
          - with
            - foreign body S61.325 ☑
        - foreign body S61.225 ☑
    - right S61.214 ☑
      - with
        - damage to nail S61.314 ☑
          - with
            - foreign body S61.324 ☑
        - foreign body S61.224 ☑
- flank S31.119 ☑
  - with foreign body S31.129 ☑
- foot (except toe(s) alone) S91.319 ☑
  - with foreign body S91.329 ☑
  - left S91.312 ☑
    - with foreign body S91.322 ☑
  - right S91.311 ☑
    - with foreign body S91.321 ☑
  - toe — *see* Laceration, toe
- forearm S51.819 ☑
  - with
    - foreign body S51.829 ☑
  - elbow only — *see* Laceration, elbow
  - left S51.812 ☑
    - with
      - foreign body S51.822 ☑
  - right S51.811 ☑
    - with
      - foreign body S51.821 ☑
- forehead S01.81 ☑
  - with foreign body S01.82 ☑
- fourchette O70.0
  - with ectopic or molar pregnancy O08.6
  - complicating delivery O70.0
  - following ectopic or molar pregnancy O08.6
- gallbladder S36.123 ☑
- genital organs, external
  - female S31.512 ☑
    - with foreign body S31.522 ☑
    - vagina — *see* Laceration, vagina
    - vulva — *see* Laceration, vulva
  - male S31.511 ☑
    - with foreign body S31.521 ☑
    - penis — *see* Laceration, penis
    - scrotum — *see* Laceration, scrotum
    - testis — *see* Laceration, testis
- groin — *see* Laceration, abdomen, wall
- gum — *see* Laceration, oral cavity
- hand S61.419 ☑
  - with
    - foreign body S61.429 ☑
  - finger — *see* Laceration, finger
  - left S61.412 ☑
    - with
      - foreign body S61.422 ☑
  - right S61.411 ☑
    - with
      - foreign body S61.421 ☑
  - thumb — *see* Laceration, thumb
- head S01.91 ☑
  - with foreign body S01.92 ☑
  - cheek — *see* Laceration, cheek
  - ear — *see* Laceration, ear
  - eyelid — *see* Laceration, eyelid
  - lip — *see* Laceration, lip
  - nose — *see* Laceration, nose
  - oral cavity — *see* Laceration, oral cavity
  - scalp S01.01 ☑
    - with foreign body S01.02 ☑
  - specified site NEC S01.81 ☑
    - with foreign body S01.82 ☑
  - temporomandibular area — *see* Laceration, cheek
- heart — *see* Injury, heart, laceration
- heel — *see* Laceration, foot
- hepatic duct S36.13 ☑
- hip S71.019 ☑
  - with foreign body S71.029 ☑
  - left S71.012 ☑
    - with foreign body S71.022 ☑
  - right S71.011 ☑
    - with foreign body S71.021 ☑

Laceration — *continued*
- hymen — *see* Laceration, vagina
- hypochondrium — *see* Laceration, abdomen, wall
- hypogastric region — *see* Laceration, abdomen, wall
- ileum S36.438 ☑
- inguinal region — *see* Laceration, abdomen, wall
- instep — *see* Laceration, foot
- internal organ — *see* Injury, by site
- interscapular region — *see* Laceration, thorax, back
- intestine
  - large
    - colon S36.539 ☑
      - ascending S36.530 ☑
      - descending S36.532 ☑
      - sigmoid S36.533 ☑
      - specified site NEC S36.538 ☑
    - rectum S36.63 ☑
    - transverse S36.531 ☑
  - small S36.439 ☑
    - duodenum S36.430 ☑
    - specified site NEC S36.438 ☑
- intra-abdominal organ S36.93 ☑
  - intestine — *see* Laceration, intestine
  - liver — *see* Laceration, liver
  - pancreas — *see* Laceration, pancreas
  - peritoneum S36.81 ☑
  - specified site NEC S36.893 ☑
  - spleen — *see* Laceration, spleen
  - stomach — *see* Laceration, stomach
- intracranial NEC (*see also* Injury, intracranial, diffuse)
  - birth injury P10.9
- jaw — *see* Laceration, head, specified site NEC
- jejunum S36.438 ☑
- joint capsule — *see* Sprain, by site
- kidney S37.03- ☑
  - major (greater than 3 cm) (massive) (stellate) S37.06- ☑
  - minor (less than 1 cm) S37.04- ☑
  - moderate (1 to 3 cm) S37.05- ☑
    - multiple S37.06- ☑
- knee S81.01- ☑
  - with foreign body S81.02- ☑
- labium (majus) (minus) — *see* Laceration, vulva
- lacrimal duct — *see* Laceration, eyelid
- large intestine — *see* Laceration, intestine, large
- larynx S11.011 ☑
  - with foreign body S11.012 ☑
- leg (lower) S81.819 ☑
  - with foreign body S81.829 ☑
  - foot — *see* Laceration, foot
  - knee — *see* Laceration, knee
  - left S81.812 ☑
    - with foreign body S81.822 ☑
  - right S81.811 ☑
    - with foreign body S81.821 ☑
  - upper — *see* Laceration, thigh
- ligament — *see* Sprain
- lip S01.511 ☑
  - with foreign body S01.521 ☑
- liver S36.113 ☑
  - major (stellate) S36.116 ☑
  - minor S36.114 ☑
  - moderate S36.115 ☑
- loin — *see* Laceration, abdomen, wall
- lower back — *see* Laceration, back, lower
- lumbar region — *see* Laceration, back, lower
- lung S27.339 ☑
  - bilateral S27.332 ☑
  - unilateral S27.331 ☑
- malar region — *see* Laceration, head, specified site NEC
- mammary — *see* Laceration, breast
- mastoid region — *see* Laceration, head, specified site NEC
- meninges — *see* Injury, intracranial, diffuse
- meniscus — *see* Tear, meniscus
- mesentery S36.893 ☑
- mesosalpinx S37.893 ☑
- mouth — *see* Laceration, oral cavity
- muscle — *see* Injury, muscle, by site, laceration
- nail
  - finger — *see* Laceration, finger, with damage to nail
  - toe — *see* Laceration, toe, with damage to nail
- nasal (septum) (sinus) — *see* Laceration, nose

200

☑ **Additional Character Required** — **Refer to the Tabular List for Character Selection**   ▽ Subterms under main terms may continue to next column or page

Laceration — *continued*
- nasopharynx — *see* Laceration, head, specified site NEC
- neck S11.91 ☑
  - with foreign body S11.92 ☑
  - involving
    - cervical esophagus S11.21 ☑
      - with foreign body S11.22 ☑
    - larynx — *see* Laceration, larynx
    - pharynx — *see* Laceration, pharynx
    - thyroid gland — *see* Laceration, thyroid gland
    - trachea — *see* Laceration, trachea
    - specified site NEC S11.81 ☑
      - with foreign body S11.82 ☑
- nerve — *see* Injury, nerve
- nose (septum) (sinus) S01.21 ☑
  - with foreign body S01.22 ☑
- ocular NOS S05.3- ☑
  - adnexa NOS S01.11- ☑
- oral cavity S01.512 ☑
  - with foreign body S01.522 ☑
- orbit (eye) — *see* Wound, open, ocular, orbit
- ovary S37.439 ☑
  - bilateral S37.432 ☑
  - unilateral S37.431 ☑
- palate — *see* Laceration, oral cavity
- palm — *see* Laceration, hand
- pancreas S36.239 ☑
- pelvic S31.010 ☑
  - with
    - foreign body S31.020 ☑
      - penetration into retroperitoneal cavity S31.021 ☑
    - penetration into retroperitoneal cavity S31.011 ☑
  - floor (*see also* Laceration, back, lower)
    - with ectopic or molar pregnancy O08.6
    - complicating delivery O70.1
    - following ectopic or molar pregnancy O08.6
    - old (postpartal) N81.89
  - organ S37.93 ☑
- penis S31.21 ☑
  - with foreign body S31.22 ☑
- perineum
  - female S31.41 ☑
    - with
      - ectopic or molar pregnancy O08.6
      - foreign body S31.42 ☑
    - during delivery O70.9
      - first degree O70.0
      - fourth degree O70.3
      - second degree O70.1
      - third degree O70.2
    - old (postpartal) N81.89
    - postpartal N81.89
    - secondary (postpartal) O90.1
  - male S31.119 ☑
    - with foreign body S31.129 ☑
- periocular area (with or without lacrimal passages) — *see* Laceration, eyelid
- peritoneum S36.893 ☑
- periumbilic region — *see* Laceration, abdomen, wall, periumbilic
- periurethral tissue — *see* Laceration, urethra
- phalanges
  - finger — *see* Laceration, finger
  - toe — *see* Laceration, toe
- pharynx S11.21 ☑
  - with foreign body S11.22 ☑
- pinna — *see* Laceration, ear
- popliteal space — *see* Laceration, knee
- prepuce — *see* Laceration, penis
- prostate S37.823 ☑
- pubic region S31.119 ☑
  - with foreign body S31.129 ☑
- pudendum — *see* Laceration, genital organs, external
- rectovaginal septum — *see* Laceration, vagina
- rectum S36.63 ☑
- retroperitoneum S36.893 ☑
- round ligament S37.893 ☑
- sacral region — *see* Laceration, back, lower
- sacroiliac region — *see* Laceration, back, lower
- salivary gland — *see* Laceration, oral cavity
- scalp S01.01 ☑
  - with foreign body S01.02 ☑
- scapular region — *see* Laceration, shoulder

Laceration — *continued*
- scrotum S31.31 ☑
  - with foreign body S31.32 ☑
- seminal vesicle S37.893 ☑
- shin — *see* Laceration, leg
- shoulder S41.019 ☑
  - with foreign body S41.029 ☑
  - left S41.012 ☑
    - with foreign body S41.022 ☑
  - right S41.011 ☑
    - with foreign body S41.021 ☑
- small intestine — *see* Laceration, intestine, small
- spermatic cord — *see* Laceration, testis
- spinal cord (meninges) (*see also* Injury, spinal cord, by region)
  - due to injury at birth P11.5
  - newborn (birth injury) P11.5
- spleen S36.039 ☑
  - major (massive) (stellate) S36.032 ☑
  - moderate S36.031 ☑
  - superficial (minor) S36.030 ☑
- sternal region — *see* Laceration, thorax, front
- stomach S36.33 ☑
- submaxillary region — *see* Laceration, head, specified site NEC
- submental region — *see* Laceration, head, specified site NEC
- subungual
  - finger(s) — *see* Laceration, finger, with damage to nail
  - toe(s) — *see* Laceration, toe, with damage to nail
- suprarenal gland — *see* Laceration, adrenal gland
- temple, temporal region — *see* Laceration, head, specified site NEC
- temporomandibular area — *see* Laceration, cheek
- tendon — *see* Injury, muscle, by site, laceration
  - Achilles S86.02- ☑
- tentorium cerebelli — *see* Injury, intracranial, diffuse
- testis S31.31 ☑
  - with foreign body S31.32 ☑
- thigh S71.11- ☑
  - with foreign body S71.12- ☑
- thorax, thoracic (wall) S21.91 ☑
  - with foreign body S21.92 ☑
    - back S21.22- ☑
      - with penetration into thoracic cavity S21.42- ☑
    - front S21.12- ☑
      - with penetration into thoracic cavity S21.32- ☑
  - back S21.21- ☑
    - with
      - foreign body S21.22- ☑
        - with penetration into thoracic cavity S21.42- ☑
      - penetration into thoracic cavity S21.41- ☑
  - breast — *see* Laceration, breast
  - front S21.11- ☑
    - with
      - foreign body S21.12- ☑
        - with penetration into thoracic cavity S21.32- ☑
      - penetration into thoracic cavity S21.31- ☑
- thumb S61.019 ☑
  - with
    - damage to nail S61.119 ☑
      - with
        - foreign body S61.129 ☑
    - foreign body S61.029 ☑
  - left S61.012 ☑
    - with
      - damage to nail S61.112 ☑
        - with
          - foreign body S61.122 ☑
      - foreign body S61.022 ☑
  - right S61.011 ☑
    - with
      - damage to nail S61.111 ☑
        - with
          - foreign body S61.121 ☑
      - foreign body S61.021 ☑
- thyroid gland S11.11 ☑
  - with foreign body S11.12 ☑
- toe(s) S91.119 ☑
  - with
    - damage to nail S91.219 ☑

Laceration — *continued*
- toe(s) — *continued*
  - with — *continued*
    - damage to nail — *continued*
      - with
        - foreign body S91.229 ☑
      - foreign body S91.129 ☑
    - great S91.113 ☑
      - with
        - damage to nail S91.213 ☑
          - with
            - foreign body S91.223 ☑
        - foreign body S91.123 ☑
      - left S91.112 ☑
        - with
          - damage to nail S91.212 ☑
            - with
              - foreign body S91.222 ☑
          - foreign body S91.122 ☑
      - right S91.111 ☑
        - with
          - damage to nail S91.211 ☑
            - with
              - foreign body S91.221 ☑
          - foreign body S91.121 ☑
    - lesser S91.116 ☑
      - with
        - damage to nail S91.216 ☑
          - with
            - foreign body S91.226 ☑
        - foreign body S91.126 ☑
      - left S91.115 ☑
        - with
          - damage to nail S91.215 ☑
            - with
              - foreign body S91.225 ☑
          - foreign body S91.125 ☑
      - right S91.114 ☑
        - with
          - damage to nail S91.214 ☑
            - with
              - foreign body S91.224 ☑
          - foreign body S91.124 ☑
- tongue — *see* Laceration, oral cavity
- trachea S11.021 ☑
  - with foreign body S11.022 ☑
- tunica vaginalis — *see* Laceration, testis
- tympanum, tympanic membrane — *see* Laceration, ear, drum
- umbilical region S31.115 ☑
  - with foreign body S31.125 ☑
- ureter S37.13 ☑
- urethra S37.33 ☑
  - with or following ectopic or molar pregnancy O08.6
  - obstetrical trauma O71.5
- urinary organ NEC S37.893 ☑
- uterus S37.63 ☑
  - with ectopic or molar pregnancy O08.6
  - following ectopic or molar pregnancy O08.6
  - nonpuerperal, nontraumatic N85.8
  - obstetrical trauma NEC O71.81
  - old (postpartal) N85.8
- uvula — *see* Laceration, oral cavity
- vagina S31.41 ☑
  - with
    - ectopic or molar pregnancy O08.6
    - foreign body S31.42 ☑
  - during delivery O71.4
    - with perineal laceration — *see* Laceration, perineum, female, during delivery
  - following ectopic or molar pregnancy O08.6
  - nonpuerperal, nontraumatic N89.8
  - old (postpartal) N89.8
- vas deferens S37.893 ☑
- vesical — *see* Laceration, bladder
- vocal cords S11.031 ☑
  - with foreign body S11.032 ☑
- vulva S31.41 ☑
  - with
    - ectopic or molar pregnancy O08.6
    - foreign body S31.42 ☑
  - complicating delivery O70.0
  - following ectopic or molar pregnancy O08.6
  - nonpuerperal, nontraumatic N90.89
  - old (postpartal) N90.89
- wrist S61.519 ☑

Laceration — continued
 wrist — continued
  with
   foreign body S61.529 ☑
  left S61.512 ☑
   with
    foreign body S61.522 ☑
  right S61.511 ☑
   with
    foreign body S61.521 ☑
Lack of
 achievement in school Z55.3
 adequate
  food Z59.4
  intermaxillary vertical dimension of fully erupted teeth M26.36
  sleep Z72.820
 appetite (see Anorexia) R63.0
 awareness R41.9
 care
  in home Z74.2
  of infant (at or after birth) T76.02 ☑
   confirmed T74.02 ☑
 cognitive functions R41.9
 coordination R27.9
  ataxia R27.0
  specified type NEC R27.8
 development (physiological) R62.50
  failure to thrive (child over 28 days old) R62.51
   adult R62.7
   newborn P92.6
  short stature R62.52
  specified type NEC R62.59
 energy R53.83
 financial resources Z59.6
 food T73.0 ☑
 growth R62.52
 heating Z59.1
 housing (permanent) (temporary) Z59.0
  adequate Z59.1
 learning experiences in childhood Z62.898
 leisure time (affecting life-style) Z73.2
 material resources Z59.9
 memory (see also Amnesia)
  mild, following organic brain damage F06.8
 ovulation N97.0
 parental supervision or control of child Z62.0
 person able to render necessary care Z74.2
 physical exercise Z72.3
 play experience in childhood Z62.898
 posterior occlusal support M26.57
 relaxation (affecting life-style) Z73.2
 sexual
  desire F52.0
  enjoyment F52.1
 shelter Z59.0
 sleep (adequate) Z72.820
 supervision of child by parent Z62.0
 support, posterior occlusal M26.57
 water T73.1 ☑
Lacrimal — see condition
Lacrimation, abnormal — see Epiphora
Lacrimonasal duct — see condition
Lactation, lactating (breast) (puerperal, postpartum)
 associated
  cracked nipple O92.13
  retracted nipple O92.03
 defective O92.4
 disorder NEC O92.79
 excessive O92.6
 failed (complete) O92.3
  partial O92.4
 mastitis NEC — see Mastitis, obstetric
 mother (care and/or examination) Z39.1
 nonpuerperal N64.3
Lacticemia, excessive E87.2
Lacunar skull Q75.8
Laennec's cirrhosis K74.69
 alcoholic K70.30
  with ascites K70.31
Lafora's disease — see Epilepsy, generalized, idiopathic
Lag, lid (nervous) — see Retraction, lid
Lagophthalmos (eyelid) (nervous) H02.209
 cicatricial H02.219
  left H02.216
   lower H02.215
   upper H02.214
  right H02.213

Lagophthalmos — continued
 cicatricial — continued
  right — continued
   lower H02.212
   upper H02.211
 keratoconjunctivitis — see Keratoconjunctivitis
 left H02.206
  lower H02.205
  upper H02.204
 mechanical H02.229
  left H02.226
   lower H02.225
   upper H02.224
  right H02.223
   lower H02.222
   upper H02.221
 paralytic H02.239
  left H02.236
   lower H02.235
   upper H02.234
  right H02.233
   lower H02.232
   upper H02.231
 right H02.203
  lower H02.202
  upper H02.201
Laki-Lorand factor deficiency — see Defect, coagulation, specified type NEC
Lalling F80.0
Lambert-Eaton syndrome — see Syndrome, Lambert-Eaton
Lambliasis, lambliosis A07.1
Landau-Kleffner syndrome — see Epilepsy, specified NEC
Landouzy-Déjérine dystrophy or facioscapulohumeral atrophy G71.0
Landouzy's disease (icterohemorrhagic leptospirosis) A27.0
Landry-Guillain-Barré, syndrome or paralysis G61.0
Landry's disease or paralysis G61.0
Lane's
 band Q43.3
 kink — see Obstruction, intestine
 syndrome K90.2
Langdon Down syndrome — see Trisomy, 21
Lapsed immunization schedule status Z28.3
Large
 baby (regardless of gestational age) (4000g to 4499g) P08.1
 ear, congenital Q17.1
 physiological cup Q14.2
 stature R68.89
Large-for-dates NEC (infant) (4000g to 4499g) P08.1
 affecting management of pregnancy O36.6- ☑
 exceptionally (4500g or more) P08.0
Larsen-Johansson disease orosteochondrosis — see Osteochondrosis, juvenile, patella
Larsen's syndrome (flattened facies and multiple congenital dislocations) Q74.8
Larva migrans
 cutaneous B76.9
  Ancylostoma B76.0
 visceral B83.0
Laryngeal — see condition
Laryngismus (stridulus) J38.5
 congenital P28.89
 diphtheritic A36.2
Laryngitis (acute) (edematous) (fibrinous) (infective) (infiltrative) (malignant) (membranous) (phlegmonous) (pneumococcal) (pseudomembranous) (septic) (subglottic) (suppurative) (ulcerative) J04.0
 with
  influenza, flu, or grippe — see Influenza, with, laryngitis
  tracheitis (acute) — see Laryngotracheitis
 atrophic J37.0
 catarrhal J37.0
 chronic J37.0
  with tracheitis (chronic) J37.1
 diphtheritic A36.2
 due to external agent — see Inflammation, respiratory, upper, due to
 H. influenzae J04.0
 Hemophilus influenzae J04.0
 hypertrophic J37.0
 influenzal — see Influenza, with, respiratory manifestations NEC
 obstructive J05.0

Laryngitis — continued
 sicca J37.0
 spasmodic J05.0
  acute J04.0
 streptococcal J04.0
 stridulous J05.0
 syphilitic (late) A52.73
  congenital A50.59 [J99]
   early A50.03 [J99]
 tuberculous A15.5
 Vincent's A69.1
Laryngocele (congenital) (ventricular) Q31.3
Laryngofissure J38.7
 congenital Q31.8
Laryngomalacia (congenital) Q31.5
Laryngopharyngitis (acute) J06.0
 chronic J37.0
 due to external agent — see Inflammation, respiratory, upper, due to
Laryngoplegia J38.00
 bilateral J38.02
 unilateral J38.01
Laryngoptosis J38.7
Laryngospasm J38.5
Laryngostenosis J38.6
Laryngotracheitis (acute) (Infectional) (infective) (viral) J04.2
 atrophic J37.1
 catarrhal J37.1
 chronic J37.1
 diphtheritic A36.2
 due to external agent — see Inflammation, respiratory, upper, due to
 Hemophilus influenzae J04.2
 hypertrophic J37.1
 influenzal -— see Influenza, with, respiratory manifestations NEC
 pachydermic J38.7
 sicca J37.1
 spasmodic J38.5
  acute J05.0
 streptococcal J04.2
 stridulous J38.5
 syphilitic (late) A52.73
  congenital A50.59 [J99]
   early A50.03 [J99]
 tuberculous A15.5
 Vincent's A69.1
Laryngotracheobronchitis — see Bronchitis
Larynx, laryngeal — see condition
Lassa fever A96.2
Lassitude — see Weakness
Late
 talker R62.0
 walker R62.0
Late effect(s) — see Sequelae
Latent — see condition
Laterocession — see Lateroversion
Lateroflexion — see Lateroversion
Lateroversion
 cervix — see Lateroversion, uterus
 uterus, uterine (cervix) (postinfectional) (postpartal, old) N85.4
  congenital Q51.818
  in pregnancy or childbirth O34.59- ☑
Lathyrism — see Poisoning, food, noxious, plant
Launois' syndrome (pituitary gigantism) E22.0
Launois-Bensaude adenolipomatosis E88.89
Laurence-Moon (-Bardet)-**Biedl syndrome** Q87.89
Lax, laxity (see also Relaxation)
 ligament (ous) (see also Disorder, ligament)
  familial M35.7
  knee — see Derangement, knee
 skin (acquired) L57.4
  congenital Q82.8
Laxative habit F55.2
Lazy leukocyte syndrome D70.8
Lead miner's lung J63.6
Leak, leakage
 air NEC J93.82
  postprocedural J95.812
 amniotic fluid — see Rupture, membranes, premature
 blood (microscopic), fetal, into maternal circulation
  affecting management of pregnancy — see Pregnancy, complicated by
 cerebrospinal fluid G96.0
  from spinal (lumbar) puncture G97.0

Leak, leakage — *continued*
  device, implant or graft (*see also* Complications, by site and type, mechanical)
    arterial graft NEC — *see* Complication, cardiovascular device, mechanical, vascular
    breast (implant) T85.43 ☑
    catheter NEC T85.638 ☑
      dialysis (renal) T82.43 ☑
        intraperitoneal T85.631 ☑
      infusion NEC T82.534 ☑
        spinal (epidural) (subdural) T85.630 ☑
      urinary, indwelling T83.038 ☑
        cystostomy T83.030 ☑
    gastrointestinal — *see* Complications, prosthetic device, mechanical, gastrointestinal device
    genital NEC T83.498 ☑
      penile prosthesis T83.490 ☑
    heart NEC — *see* Complication, cardiovascular device, mechanical
    joint prosthesis — *see* Complications, joint prosthesis, mechanical, specified NEC, by site
    ocular NEC — *see* Complications, prosthetic device, mechanical, ocular device
    orthopedic NEC — *see* Complication, orthopedic, device, mechanical
    persistent air J93.82
    specified NEC T85.638 ☑
    urinary NEC (*see also* Complication, genitourinary, device, urinary, mechanical)
      graft T83.23 ☑
    vascular NEC — *see* Complication, cardiovascular device, mechanical
    ventricular intracranial shunt T85.03 ☑
  urine — *see* Incontinence
Leaky heart — *see* Endocarditis
Learning defect (specific) F81.9
Leather bottle stomach C16.9
Leber's
  congenital amaurosis H35.50
  optic atrophy (hereditary) H47.22
Lederer's anemia D59.1
Leeches (external) — *see* Hirudiniasis
Leg — *see* condition
Legg (-Calvé)-**Perthes disease, syndrome or osteochondrosis** M91.1- ☑
Legionellosis A48.1
  nonpneumonic A48.2
Legionnaires'
  disease A48.1
    nonpneumonic A48.2
  pneumonia A48.1
Leigh's disease G31.82
Leiner's disease L21.1
Leiofibromyoma — *see* Leiomyoma
Leiomyoblastoma — *see* Neoplasm, connective tissue, benign
Leiomyofibroma (*see also* Neoplasm, connective tissue, benign)
  uterus (cervix) (corpus) D25.9
Leiomyoma (*see also* Neoplasm, connective tissue, benign)
  bizarre — *see* Neoplasm, connective tissue, benign
  cellular — *see* Neoplasm, connective tissue, benign
  epithelioid — *see* Neoplasm, connective tissue, benign
  uterus (cervix) (corpus) D25.9
    intramural D25.1
    submucous D25.0
    subserosal D25.2
  vascular — *see* Neoplasm, connective tissue, benign
Leiomyoma, leiomyomatosis (intravascular) — *see* Neoplasm, connective tissue, uncertain behavior
Leiomyosarcoma (*see also* Neoplasm, connective tissue, malignant)
  epithelioid — *see* Neoplasm, connective tissue, malignant
  myxoid — *see* Neoplasm, connective tissue, malignant
Leishmaniasis B55.9
  American (mucocutaneous) B55.2
    cutaneous B55.1
  Asian Desert B55.1
  Brazilian B55.2
  cutaneous (any type) B55.1
  dermal (*see also* Leishmaniasis, cutaneous)
    post-kala-azar B55.0
  eyelid B55.1
  infantile B55.0
  Mediterranean B55.0

Leishmaniasis — *continued*
  mucocutaneous (American) (New World) B55.2
  naso-oral B55.2
  nasopharyngeal B55.2
  old world B55.1
  tegumentaria diffusa B55.1
  visceral B55.0
Leishmanoid, dermal (*see also* Leishmaniasis, cutaneous)
  post-kala-azar B55.0
Lenegre's disease I44.2
Lengthening, leg — *see* Deformity, limb, unequal length
Lennert's lymphoma — *see* Lymphoma, Lennert's
Lennox-Gastaut syndrome G40.812
  intractable G40.814
    with status epilepticus G40.813
    without status epilepticus G40.814
  not intractable G40.812
    with status epilepticus G40.811
    without status epilepticus G40.812
Lens — *see* condition
Lenticonus (anterior) (posterior) (congenital) Q12.8
Lenticular degeneration, progressive E83.01
Lentiglobus (posterior) (congenital) Q12.8
Lentigo (congenital) L81.4
  maligna (*see also* Melanoma, in situ)
    melanoma — *see* Melanoma
Lentivirus, as cause of disease classified elsewhere B97.31
Leontiasis
  ossium M85.2
  syphilitic (late) A52.78
    congenital A50.59
Lepothrix A48.8
Lepra — *see* Leprosy
Leprechaunism E34.8
Leprosy A30.- ☑
  with muscle disorder A30.9 [M63.80]
    ankle A30.9 [M63.87-] ☑
    foot A30.9 [M63.87-] ☑
    forearm A30.9 [M63.83-] ☑
    hand A30.9 [M63.84-] ☑
    lower leg A30.9 [M63.86-] ☑
    multiple sites A30.9 [M63.89]
    pelvic region A30.9 [M63.85-] ☑
    shoulder region A30.9 [M63.81-] ☑
    specified site NEC A30.9 [M63.88]
    thigh A30.9 [M63.85-] ☑
    upper arm A30.9 [M63.82-] ☑
  anesthetic A30.9
  BB A30.3
  BL A30.4
  borderline (infiltrated) (neuritic) A30.3
    lepromatous A30.4
    tuberculoid A30.2
  BT A30.2
  dimorphous (infiltrated) (neuritic) A30.3
  I A30.0
  indeterminate (macular) (neuritic) A30.0
  lepromatous (diffuse) (infiltrated) (macular) (neuritic) (nodular) A30.5
  LL A30.5
  macular (early) (neuritic) (simple) A30.9
  maculoanesthetic A30.9
  mixed A30.3
  neural A30.9
  nodular A30.5
  primary neuritic A30.3
  specified type NEC A30.8
  TT A30.1
  tuberculoid (major) (minor) A30.1
Leptocytosis, hereditary D56.9
Leptomeningitis (chronic) (circumscribed) (hemorrhagic) (nonsuppurative) — *see* Meningitis
Leptomeningopathy G96.19
Leptospiral — *see* condition
Leptospirochetal — *see* condition
Leptospirosis A27.9
  canicola A27.89
  due to Leptospira interrogans serovar icterohaemorrhagiae A27.0
  icterohemorrhagica A27.0
  pomona A27.89
  Weil's disease A27.0
Leptus dermatitis B88.0
Leriche's syndrome (aortic bifurcation occlusion) I74.09
Leri's pleonosteosis Q78.8

Leri-Weill syndrome Q77.8
Lermoyez' syndrome — *see* Vertigo, peripheral NEC
Lesch-Nyhan syndrome E79.1
Leser-Trélat disease L82.1
  inflamed L82.0
Lesion(s) (nontraumatic)
  abducens nerve — *see* Strabismus, paralytic, sixth nerve
  alveolar process K08.9
  angiocentric immunoproliferative D47.Z9 (*following* D47.4)
  anorectal K62.9
  aortic (valve) I35.9
  auditory nerve — *see* subcategory H93.3 ☑
  basal ganglion G25.9
  bile duct — *see* Disease, bile duct
  biomechanical M99.9
    specified type NEC M99.89
      abdomen M99.89
      acromioclavicular M99.87
      cervical region M99.81
      cervicothoracic M99.81
      costochondral M99.88
      costovertebral M99.88
      head region M99.80
      hip M99.85
      lower extremity M99.86
      lumbar region M99.83
      lumbosacral M99.83
      occipitocervical M99.80
      pelvic region M99.85
      pubic M99.85
      rib cage M99.88
      sacral region M99.84
      sacrococcygeal M99.84
      sacroiliac M99.84
      specified NEC M99.89
      sternochondral M99.88
      sternoclavicular M99.87
      thoracic region M99.82
      thoracolumbar M99.82
      upper extremity M99.87
  bladder N32.9
  bone — *see* Disorder, bone
  brachial plexus G54.0
  brain G93.9
    congenital Q04.9
    vascular I67.9
      degenerative I67.9
      hypertensive I67.4
  buccal cavity K13.79
  calcified — *see* Calcification
  canthus — *see* Disorder, eyelid
  carate — *see* Pinta, lesions
  cardia K22.9
  cardiac (*see also* Disease, heart) I51.9
    congenital Q24.9
    valvular — *see* Endocarditis
  cauda equina G83.4
  cecum K63.9
  cerebral — *see* Lesion, brain
  cerebrovascular I67.9
    degenerative I67.9
    hypertensive I67.4
  cervical (nerve) root NEC G54.2
  chiasmal — *see* Disorder, optic, chiasm
  chorda tympani G51.8
  coin, lung R91.1
  colon K63.9
  congenital — *see* Anomaly, by site
  conjunctiva H11.9
  conus medullaris — *see* Injury, conus medullaris
  coronary artery — *see* Ischemia, heart
  cranial nerve G52.9
    eighth — *see* Disorder, ear
    eleventh G52.9
    fifth G50.9
    first G52.0
    fourth — *see* Strabismus, paralytic, fourth nerve
    seventh G51.9
    sixth — *see* Strabismus, paralytic, sixth nerve
    tenth G52.2
    twelfth G52.3
  cystic — *see* Cyst
  degenerative — *see* Degeneration
  duodenum K31.9
  edentulous (alveolar) ridge, associated with trauma, due to traumatic occlusion K06.2

Lesion(s) — continued
en coup de sabre L94.1
eyelid — see Disorder, eyelid
gasserian ganglion G50.8
gastric K31.9
gastroduodenal K31.9
gastrointestinal K63.9
gingiva, associated with trauma K06.2
glomerular
  focal and segmental (see also N00-N07 with fourth
    character .1) N05.1
  minimal change (see also N00-N07 with fourth
    character .0) N05.0
heart (organic) — see Disease, heart
hyperchromic, due to pinta (carate) A67.1
hyperkeratotic — see Hyperkeratosis
hypothalamic E23.7
ileocecal K63.9
ileum K63.9
iliohypogastric nerve G57.8- ☑
inflammatory — see Inflammation
intestine K63.9
intracerebral — see Lesion, brain
intrachiasmal (optic) — see Disorder, optic, chiasm
intracranial, space-occupying R90.0
joint — see Disorder, joint
  sacroiliac (old) M53.3
keratotic — see Keratosis
kidney — see Disease, renal
laryngeal nerve (recurrent) G52.2
lip K13.0
liver K76.9
lumbosacral
  plexus G54.1
  root (nerve) NEC G54.4
lung (coin) R91.1
maxillary sinus J32.0
mitral I05.9
Morel-Lavallée — see Hematoma, by site
motor cortex NEC G93.89
mouth K13.79
nerve G58.9
  femoral G57.2- ☑
  median G56.1- ☑
    carpal tunnel syndrome — see Syndrome,
      carpal tunnel
  plantar G57.6- ☑
  popliteal (lateral) G57.3- ☑
    medial G57.4- ☑
  radial G56.3- ☑
  sciatic G57.0- ☑
  spinal — see Injury, nerve, spinal
  ulnar G56.2- ☑
nervous system, congenital Q07.9
nonallopathic — see Lesion, biomechanical
nose (internal) J34.89
obstructive — see Obstruction
obturator nerve G57.8- ☑
oral mucosa K13.70
organ or site NEC — see Disease, by site
osteolytic — see Osteolysis
peptic K27.9
periodontal, due to traumatic occlusion K05.5
pharynx J39.2
pigment, pigmented (skin) L81.9
pinta — see Pinta, lesions
polypoid — see Polyp
prechiasmal (optic) — see Disorder, optic, chiasm
primary (see also Syphilis, primary) A51.0
  carate A67.0
  pinta A67.0
  yaws A66.0
pulmonary J98.4
  valve I37.9
pylorus K31.9
rectosigmoid K63.9
retina, retinal H35.9
sacroiliac (joint) (old) M53.3
salivary gland K11.9
  benign lymphoepithelial K11.8
saphenous nerve G57.8- ☑
sciatic nerve G57.0- ☑
secondary — see Syphilis, secondary
shoulder (region) M75.9- ☑
  specified NEC M75.8- ☑
sigmoid K63.9
sinus (accessory) (nasal) J34.89

Lesion(s) — continued
skin L98.9
  suppurative L08.0
SLAP S43.43- ☑
spinal cord G95.9
  congenital Q06.9
spleen D73.89
stomach K31.9
superior glenoid labrum S43.43- ☑
syphilitic — see Syphilis
tertiary — see Syphilis, tertiary
thoracic root (nerve) NEC G54.3
tonsillar fossa J35.9
tooth, teeth K08.9
  white spot
    chewing surface K02.51
    pit and fissure surface K02.51
    smooth surface K02.61
traumatic — see specific type of injury by site
tricuspid (valve) I07.9
  nonrheumatic I36.9
trigeminal nerve G50.9
ulcerated or ulcerative — see Ulcer, skin
uterus N85.9
vagus nerve G52.2
valvular — see Endocarditis
vascular I99.9
  affecting central nervous system I67.9
  following trauma NEC T14.8
  umbilical cord, complicating delivery O69.5 ☑
warty — see Verruca
white spot (tooth)
  chewing surface K02.51
  pit and fissure surface K02.51
  smooth surface K02.61
Lethargic — see condition
Lethargy R53.83
Letterer-Siwe's disease C96.0
Leukemia, leukemic C95.9- ☑
acute basophilic C94.8- ☑
acute bilineal C95.0- ☑
acute erythroid C94.0- ☑
acute lymphoblastic C91.0- ☑
acute megakaryoblastic C94.2- ☑
acute megakaryocytic C94.2- ☑
acute mixed lineage C95.0- ☑
acute monoblastic (monoblastic/monocytic) C93.0- ☑
acute monocytic (monoblastic/monocytic) C93.0- ☑
acute myeloblastic (minimal differentiation) (with
  maturation) C92.0- ☑
acute myeloid
  with
    11q23-abnormality C92.6- ☑
    dysplasia of remaining hematopoesis and/or
      myelodysplastic disease in its history
      C92.A- ☑ (following C92.6)
    multilineage dysplasia C92.A- ☑ (following
      C92.6)
    variation of MLL-gene C92.6- ☑
  M6 (a)(b) C94.0- ☑
  M7 C94.2- ☑
acute myelomonocytic C92.5- ☑
acute promyelocytic C92.4- ☑
adult T-cell (HTLV-1-associated) (acute variant)
  (chronic variant) (lymphomatoid variant)
  (smouldering variant) C91.5- ☑
aggressive NK-cell C94.8- ☑
AML (1/ETO) (M0) (M1) (M2) (without a FAB classification) C92.0- ☑
AML M3 C92.4- ☑
AML M4 (Eo with inv(16) or t(16;16)) C92.5- ☑
AML M5 C93.0- ☑
AML M5a C93.0- ☑
AML M5b C93.0- ☑
AML Me with t (15;17) and variants C92.4- ☑
atypical chronic myeloid, BCR/ABL-negative C92.2- ☑
biphenotypic acute C95.0- ☑
blast cell C95.0- ☑
Burkitt-type, mature B-cell C91.A- ☑ (following C91.6)
chronic lymphocytic, of B-cell type C91.1- ☑
chronic monocytic C93.1- ☑
chronic myelogenous (Philadelphia chromosome (Ph1)
  positive) (t(9;22)) (q34;q11) (with crisis of blast
  cells) C92.1- ☑
chronic myeloid, BCR/ABL-positive C92.1- ☑
  atypical, BCR/ABL-negative C92.2- ☑
chronic myelomonocytic C93.1- ☑

Leukemia, leukemic — continued
chronic neutrophilic D47.1
CMML (-1) (-2) (with eosinophilia) C93.1- ☑
granulocytic (see also Category C92) C92.9- ☑
hairy cell C91.4- ☑
juvenile myelomonocytic C93.3- ☑
lymphoid C91.9- ☑
  specified NEC C91.Z- ☑ (following C91.6)
mast cell C94.3- ☑
mature B-cell, Burkitt-type C91.A- ☑ (following C91.6)
monocytic (subacute) C93.9- ☑
  specified NEC C93.Z- ☑ (following C93.3)
myelogenous (see also Category C92) C92.9- ☑
myeloid C92.9- ☑
  specified NEC C92.Z- ☑ (following C92.6)
plasma cell C90.1- ☑
plasmacytic C90.1- ☑
prolymphocytic
  of B-cell type C91.3- ☑
  of T-cell type C91.6- ☑
specified NEC C94.8- ☑
stem cell, of unclear lineage C95.0- ☑
subacute lymphocytic C91.9- ☑
T-cell large granular lymphocytic C91.Z- ☑ (following
  C91.6)
unspecified cell type C95.9- ☑
  acute C95.0- ☑
  chronic C95.1- ☑
Leukemoid reaction (see also Reaction, leukemoid)
  D72.823
Leukoaraiosis (hypertensive) I67.81
Leukoariosis — see Leukoaraiosis
Leukocoria — see Disorder, globe, degenerated condition, leucocoria
Leukocytopenia D72.819
Leukocytosis D72.829
eosinophilic D72.1
Leukoderma, leukodermia NEC L81.5
syphilitic A51.39
  late A52.79
Leukodystrophy E75.29
Leukoedema, oral epithelium K13.29
Leukoencephalitis G04.81
acute (subacute) hemorrhagic G36.1
  postimmunization or postvaccinal G04.02
postinfectious G04.01
subacute sclerosing A81.1
van Bogaert's (sclerosing) A81.1
Leukoencephalopathy (see also Encephalopathy)
  G93.49
Binswanger's I67.3
heroin vapor G92
metachromatic E75.25
multifocal (progressive) A81.2
postimmunization and postvaccinal G04.02
progressive multifocal A81.2
reversible, posterior G93.6
van Bogaert's (sclerosing) A81.1
vascular, progressive I67.3
Leukoerythroblastosis D75.9
Leukokeratosis (see also Leukoplakia)
mouth K13.21
nicotina palati K13.24
oral mucosa K13.21
tongue K13.21
vocal cord J38.3
Leukokraurosis vulva (e) N90.4
Leukoma (cornea) (see also Opacity, cornea)
adherent H17.0- ☑
interfering with central vision — see Opacity, cornea,
  central
Leukomalacia, cerebral, newborn P91.2
periventricular P91.2
Leukomelanopathy, hereditary D72.0
Leukonychia (punctata) (striata) L60.8
congenital Q84.4
Leukopathia unguium L60.8
congenital Q84.4
Leukopenia D72.819
basophilic D72.818
chemotherapy (cancer) induced D70.1
congenital D70.0
cyclic D70.0
drug induced NEC D70.2
  due to cytoreductive cancer chemotherapy D70.1
eosinophilic D72.818
familial D70.0

Leukopenia — continued
  infantile genetic D70.0
  malignant D70.9
  periodic D70.0
  transitory neonatal P61.5
Leukopenic — see condition
Leukoplakia
  anus K62.89
  bladder (postinfectional) N32.89
  buccal K13.21
  cervix (uteri) N88.0
  esophagus K22.8
  gingiva K13.21
  hairy (oral mucosa) (tongue) K13.3
  kidney (pelvis) N28.89
  larynx J38.7
  lip K13.21
  mouth K13.21
  oral epithelium, including tongue (mucosa) K13.21
  palate K13.21
  pelvis (kidney) N28.89
  penis (infectional) N48.0
  rectum K62.89
  syphilitic (late) A52.79
  tongue K13.21
  ureter (postinfectional) N28.89
  urethra (postinfectional) N36.8
  uterus N85.8
  vagina N89.4
  vocal cord J38.3
  vulva N90.4
Leukorrhea N89.8
  due to Trichomonas (vaginalis) A59.00
  trichomonal A59.00
Leukosarcoma C85.9- ☑
Levocardia (isolated) Q24.1
  with situs inversus Q89.3
Levotransposition Q20.5
Lev's disease or syndrome (acquired complete heart
    block) I44.2
Levulosuria — see Fructosuria
Levurid L30.2
Lewy body (ies) (dementia) (disease) G31.83
Leyden-Moebius dystrophy G71.0
Leydig cell
  carcinoma
    specified site — see Neoplasm, malignant, by site
    unspecified site
      female C56.9
      male C62.9- ☑
  tumor
    benign
      specified site — see Neoplasm, benign, by site
      unspecified site
        female D27.- ☑
        male D29.2- ☑
    malignant
      specified site — see Neoplasm, malignant, by
        site
      unspecified site
        female C56.- ☑
        male C62.9- ☑
    specified site — see Neoplasm, uncertain behavior,
      by site
    unspecified site
      female D39.1- ☑
      male D40.1- ☑
Leydig-Sertoli cell tumor
  specified site — see Neoplasm, benign, by site
  unspecified site
    female D27.- ☑
    male D29.2- ☑
LGSIL (Low grade squamous intraepithelial lesion on cy-
    tologic smear of)
  anus R85.612
  cervix R87.612
  vagina R87.622
Liar, pathologic F60.2
Libido
  decreased R68.82
Libman-Sacks disease M32.11
Lice (infestation) B85.2
  body (Pediculus corporis) B85.1
  crab B85.3
  head (Pediculus capitis) B85.0
  mixed (classifiable to more than one of the titles B85.0-
    B85.3) B85.4

Lice — continued
  pubic (Phthirus pubis) B85.3
Lichen L28.0
  albus L90.0
    penis N48.0
    vulva N90.4
  amyloidosis E85.4 [L99]
  atrophicus L90.0
    penis N48.0
    vulva N90.4
  congenital Q82.8
  myxedematosus L98.5
  nitidus L44.1
  pilaris Q82.8
    acquired L85.8
  planopilaris L66.1
  planus (chronicus) L43.9
    annularis L43.8
    bullous L43.1
    follicular L66.1
    hypertrophic L43.0
    moniliformis L44.3
    of Wilson L43.9
    specified NEC L43.8
    subacute (active) L43.3
    tropicus L43.3
  ruber
    acuminatus L44.0
    moniliformis L44.3
    planus L43.9
  sclerosus (et atrophicus) L90.0
    penis N48.0
    vulva N90.4
  scrofulosus (primary) (tuberculous) A18.4
  simplex (chronicus) (circumscriptus) L28.0
  striatus L44.2
  urticatus L28.2
Lichenification L28.0
Lichenoides tuberculosis (primary) A18.4
Lichtheim's disease or syndrome — see Degeneration,
    combined
Lien migrans D73.89
Ligament — see condition
Light
  for gestational age — see Light for dates
  headedness R42
Light-for-dates (infant) P05.00
  with weight of
    1000-1249 grams P05.04
    1250-1499 grams P05.05
    1500-1749 grams P05.06
    1750-1999 grams P05.07
    2000-2499 grams P05.08
    499 grams or less P05.01
    500-749 grams P05.02
    750-999 grams P05.03
  affecting management of pregnancy O36.59- ☑
  and small-for-dates — see Small for dates
Lightning (effects) (stroke) (struck by) T75.00 ☑
  burn — see Burn
  foot E53.8
  shock T75.01 ☑
  specified effect NEC T75.09 ☑
Lightwood-Albright syndrome N25.89
Lightwood's disease or syndrome (renal tubular acido-
    sis) N25.89
Lignac (-de Toni) (-Fanconi) (-Debré) **disease or syn-
    drome** E72.09
  with cystinosis E72.04
Ligneous thyroiditis E06.5
Likoff's syndrome I20.8
Limb — see condition
Limbic epilepsy personality syndrome F07.0
Limitation, limited
  activities due to disability Z73.6
  cardiac reserve — see Disease, heart
  eye muscle duction, traumatic — see Strabismus,
    mechanical
  mandibular range of motion M26.52
Lindau (-von Hippel) **disease** Q85.8
Line(s)
  Beau's L60.4
  Harris' — see Arrest, epiphyseal
  Hudson's (cornea) — see Pigmentation, cornea, ante-
    rior
  Stähli's (cornea) — see Pigmentation, cornea, anterior
Linea corneae senilis — see Change, cornea, senile

Lingua
  geographica K14.1
  nigra (villosa) K14.3
  plicata K14.5
  tylosis K13.29
Lingual — see condition
Linguatulosis B88.8
Linitis (gastric) **plastica** C16.9
Lip — see condition
Lipedema — see Edema
Lipemia (see also Hyperlipidemia)
  retina, retinalis E78.3
Lipidosis E75.6
  cerebral (infantile) (juvenile) (late) E75.4
  cerebroretinal E75.4
  cerebroside E75.22
  cholesterol (cerebral) E75.5
  glycolipid E75.21
  hepatosplenomegalic E78.3
  sphingomyelin — see Niemann-Pick disease or syn-
    drome
  sulfatide E75.29
Lipoadenoma — see Neoplasm, benign, by site
Lipoblastoma — see Lipoma
Lipoblastomatosis — see Lipoma
Lipochondrodystrophy E76.01
Lipochrome histiocytosis (familial) D71
Lipodermatosclerosis — see Varix, leg, with, inflamma-
    tion
  ulcerated — see Varix, leg, with, ulcer, with inflamma-
    tion by site
Lipodystrophia progressiva E88.1
Lipodystrophy (progressive) E88.1
  insulin E88.1
  intestinal K90.81
  mesenteric K65.4
Lipofibroma — see Lipoma
Lipofuscinosis, neuronal (with ceroidosis) E75.4
Lipogranuloma, sclerosing L92.8
Lipogranulomatosis E78.89
Lipoid (see also condition)
  histiocytosis D76.3
    essential E75.29
  nephrosis N04.9
  proteinosis of Urbach E78.89
Lipoidemia — see Hyperlipidemia
Lipoidosis — see Lipidosis
Lipoma D17.9
  fetal D17.9
    fat cell D17.9
  infiltrating D17.9
  intramuscular D17.9
  pleomorphic D17.9
  site classification
    arms (skin) (subcutaneous) D17.2- ☑
    connective tissue D17.30
      intra-abdominal D17.5
      intrathoracic D17.4
      peritoneum D17.79
      retroperitoneum D17.79
      specified site NEC D17.39
      spermatic cord D17.6
    face (skin) (subcutaneous) D17.0
    genitourinary organ NEC D17.72
    head (skin) (subcutaneous) D17.0
    intra-abdominal D17.5
    intrathoracic D17.4
    kidney D17.71
    legs (skin) (subcutaneous) D17.2- ☑
    neck (skin) (subcutaneous) D17.0
    peritoneum D17.79
    retroperitoneum D17.79
    skin D17.30
      specified site NEC D17.39
    specified site NEC D17.79
    spermatic cord D17.6
    subcutaneous D17.30
      specified site NEC D17.39
    trunk (skin) (subcutaneous) D17.1
    unspecified D17.9
  spindle cell D17.9
Lipomatosis E88.2
  dolorosa (Dercum) E88.2
  fetal — see Lipoma
  Launois-Bensaude E88.89
Lipomyoma — see Lipoma
Lipomyxoma — see Lipoma

Lipomyxosarcoma — see Neoplasm, connective tissue, malignant
Lipoprotein metabolism disorder E78.9
Lipoproteinemia E78.5
  broad-beta E78.2
  floating-beta E78.2
  hyper-pre-beta E78.1
Liposarcoma (see also Neoplasm, connective tissue, malignant)
  dedifferentiated — see Neoplasm, connective tissue, malignant
  differentiated type — see Neoplasm, connective tissue, malignant
  embryonal — see Neoplasm, connective tissue, malignant
  mixed type — see Neoplasm, connective tissue, malignant
  myxoid — see Neoplasm, connective tissue, malignant
  pleomorphic — see Neoplasm, connective tissue, malignant
  round cell — see Neoplasm, connective tissue, malignant
  well differentiated type — see Neoplasm, connective tissue, malignant
Liposynovitis prepatellaris E88.89
Lipping, cervix N86
Lipschütz disease or ulcer N76.6
Lipuria R82.0
  schistosomiasis (bilharziasis) B65.0
Lisping F80.0
Lissauer's paralysis A52.17
Lissencephalia, lissencephaly Q04.3
Listeriosis, listerellosis A32.9
  congenital (disseminated) P37.2
  cutaneous A32.0
  neonatal, newborn (disseminated) P37.2
  oculoglandular A32.81
  specified NEC A32.89
Lithemia E79.0
Lithiasis — see Calculus
Lithosis J62.8
Lithuria R82.99
Litigation, anxiety concerning Z65.3
Little leaguer's elbow — see Epicondylitis, medial
Little's disease G80.9
Littre's
  gland — see condition
  hernia — see Hernia, abdomen
Littritis — see Urethritis
Livedo (annularis) (racemosa) (reticularis) R23.1
Liver — see condition
Living alone (problems with) Z60.2
  with handicapped person Z74.2
Lloyd's syndrome — see Adenomatosis, endocrine
Loa loa, loaiasis, loasis B74.3
Lobar — see condition
Lobomycosis B48.0
Lobo's disease B48.0
Lobotomy syndrome F07.0
Lobstein (-Ekman) **disease or syndrome** Q78.0
Lobster-claw hand Q71.6- ☑
Lobulation (congenital) (see also Anomaly, by site)
  kidney, Q63.1
  liver, abnormal Q44.7
  spleen Q89.09
Lobule, lobular — see condition
Local, localized — see condition
Locked twins causing obstructed labor O66.1
Locked-in state G83.5
Locking
  joint — see Derangement, joint, specified type NEC
  knee — see Derangement, knee
Lockjaw — see Tetanus
Löffler's
  endocarditis I42.3
  eosinophilia J82
  pneumonia J82
  syndrome (eosinophilic pneumonitis) J82
Loiasis (with conjunctival infestation) (eyelid) B74.3
Lone Star fever A77.0
Long
  labor O63.9
    first stage O63.0
    second stage O63.1
  QT syndrome I45.81
Longitudinal stripes or grooves, nails L60.8
  congenital Q84.6

Long-term (current) (prophylactic) **drug therapy** (use of)
  agents affecting estrogen receptors and estrogen levels NEC Z79.818
  anastrozole (Arimidex) Z79.811
  antibiotics Z79.2
    short-term use — omit code
  anticoagulants Z79.01
  anti-inflammatory, non-steroidal (NSAID) Z79.1
  antiplatelet Z79.02
  antithrombotics Z79.02
  aromatase inhibitors Z79.811
  aspirin Z79.82
  birth control pill or patch Z79.3
  bisphosphonates Z79.83
  contraceptive, oral Z79.3
  drug, specified NEC Z79.899
  estrogen receptor downregulators Z79.818
  Evista Z79.810
  exemestane (Aromasin) Z79.811
  Fareston Z79.810
  fulvestrant (Faslodex) Z79.818
  gonadotropin-releasing hormone (GnRH) agonist Z79.818
  goserelin acetate (Zoladex) Z79.818
  hormone replacement (postmenopausal) Z79.890
  insulin Z79.4
  letrozole (Femara) Z79.811
  leuprolide acetate (leuprorelin) (Lupron) Z79.818
  megestrol acetate (Megace) Z79.818
  methadone for pain management Z79.891
  Nolvadex Z79.810
  non-steroidal anti-inflammatories (NSAID) Z79.1
  opiate analgesic Z79.891
  oral contraceptive Z79.3
  raloxifene (Evista) Z79.810
  selective estrogen receptor modulators (SERMs) Z79.810
  steroids
    inhaled Z79.51
    systemic Z79.52
  tamoxifen (Nolvadex) Z79.810
  toremifene (Fareston) Z79.810
Loop
  intestine — see Volvulus
  vascular on papilla (optic) Q14.2
Loose (see also condition)
  body
    joint M24.00
      ankle M24.07- ☑
      elbow M24.02- ☑
      hand M24.04- ☑
      hip M24.05- ☑
      knee M23.4- ☑
      shoulder (region) M24.01- ☑
      specified site NEC M24.08
      toe M24.07- ☑
      vertebra M24.08
      wrist M24.03- ☑
    knee M23.4-
    sheath, tendon — see Disorder, tendon, specified type NEC
  cartilage — see Loose, body, joint
  tooth, teeth K08.8
Loosening
  aseptic
    joint prosthesis — see Complications, joint prosthesis, mechanical, loosening, by site
    epiphysis — see Osteochondropathy
  mechanical
    joint prosthesis — see Complications, joint prosthesis, mechanical, loosening, by site
Looser-Milkman (-Debray) **syndrome** M83.8
Lop ear (deformity) Q17.3
Lorain (-Levi) **short stature syndrome** E23.0
Lordosis M40.50
  acquired — see Lordosis, specified type NEC
  congenital Q76.429
    lumbar region Q76.426
    lumbosacral region Q76.427
    sacral region Q76.428
    sacrococcygeal region Q76.428
    thoracolumbar region Q76.425
  lumbar region M40.56
  lumbosacral region M40.57
  postsurgical M96.4
  postural — see Lordosis, specified type NEC
  rachitic (late effect) (sequelae) E64.3

Lordosis — continued
  sequelae of rickets E64.3
  specified type NEC M40.40
    lumbar region M40.46
    lumbosacral region M40.47
    thoracolumbar region M40.45
  thoracolumbar region M40.55
  tuberculous A18.01
Loss (of)
  appetite (see Anorexia) R63.0
    hysterical F50.8
    nonorganic origin F50.8
    psychogenic F50.8
  blood — see Hemorrhage
  consciousness, transient R55
    traumatic — see Injury, intracranial
  control, sphincter, rectum R15.9
    nonorganic origin F98.1
  elasticity, skin R23.4
  family (member) in childhood Z62.898
  fluid (acute) E86.9
    with
      hypernatremia E87.0
      hyponatremia E87.1
  function of labyrinth — see subcategory H83.2 ☑
  hair, nonscarring — see Alopecia
  hearing (see also Deafness)
    central NOS H90.5
    neural NOS H90.5
    perceptive NOS H90.5
    sensorineural NOS H90.5
    sensory NOS H90.5
  height R29.890
  limb or member, traumatic, current — see Amputation, traumatic
  love relationship in childhood Z62.898
  memory (see also Amnesia)
    mild, following organic brain damage F06.8
  mind — see Psychosis
  occlusal vertical dimension of fully erupted teeth M26.37
  organ or part — see Absence, by site, acquired
  ossicles, ear (partial) H74.32- ☑
  parent in childhood Z63.4
  pregnancy, recurrent N96
    without current pregnancy N96
    care in current pregnancy O26.2- ☑
  recurrent pregnancy — see Loss, pregnancy, recurrent
  self-esteem, in childhood Z62.898
  sense of
    smell — see Disturbance, sensation, smell
    taste — see Disturbance, sensation, taste
    touch R20.8
  sensory R44.9
    dissociative F44.6
  sexual desire F52.0
  sight (acquired) (complete) (congenital) — see Blindness
  substance of
    bone — see Disorder, bone, density and structure, specified NEC
    cartilage — see Disorder, cartilage, specified type NEC
    auricle (ear) — see Disorder, pinna, specified type NEC
    vitreous (humor) H15.89
  tooth, teeth — see Absence, teeth, acquired
  vision, visual H54.7
    both eyes H54.3
    one eye H54.60
      left (normal vision on right) H54.62
      right (normal vision on left) H54.61
    specified as blindness — see Blindness
    subjective
      sudden H53.13- ☑
      transient H53.12- ☑
  vitreous — see Prolapse, vitreous
  voice — see Aphonia
  weight (abnormal) (cause unknown) R63.4
Louis-Bar syndrome (ataxia-telangiectasia) G11.3
Louping ill (encephalitis) A84.8
Louse, lousiness — see Lice
Low
  achiever, school Z55.3
  back syndrome M54.5
  basal metabolic rate R94.8
  birthweight (2499 grams or less) P07.10

Low — *continued*
  birthweight — *continued*
    with weight of
      1000-1249 grams P07.14
      1250-1499 grams P07.15
      1500-1749 grams P07.16
      1750-1999 grams P07.17
      2000-2499 grams P07.18
    extreme (999 grams or less) P07.00
      with weight of
        499 grams or less P07.01
        500-749 grams P07.02
        750-999 grams P07.03
    for gestational age — *see* Light for dates
  blood pressure (*see also* Hypotension)
    reading (incidental) (isolated) (nonspecific) R03.1
  cardiac reserve — *see* Disease, heart
  function (*see also* Hypofunction)
    kidney N28.9
  hematocrit D64.9
  hemoglobin D64.9
  income Z59.6
  level of literacy Z55.0
  lying
    kidney N28.89
    organ or site, congenital — *see* Malposition, congenital
  output syndrome (cardiac) — *see* Failure, heart
  platelets (blood) — *see* Thrombocytopenia
  reserve, kidney N28.89
  salt syndrome E87.1
  self esteem R45.81
  set ears Q17.4
  vision H54.2
    one eye (other eye normal) H54.50
      left (normal vision on right) H54.52
        other eye blind — *see* Blindness
      right (normal vision on left) H54.51
Low-density-lipoprotein-type (LDL) **hyperlipoproteinemia** E78.0
Lowe's syndrome E72.03
Lown-Ganong-Levine syndrome I45.6
LSD reaction (acute) (without dependence) F16.90
  with dependence F16.20
L-shaped kidney Q63.8
Ludwig's angina or disease K12.2
Lues (venerea), **luetic** — *see* Syphilis
Luetscher's syndrome (dehydration) E86.0
Lumbago, lumbalgia M54.5
  with sciatica M54.4- ☑
    due to intervertebral disc disorder M51.17
  due to displacement, intervertebral disc M51.27
    with sciatica M51.17
Lumbar — *see* condition
Lumbarization, vertebra, congenital Q76.49
Lumbermen's itch B88.0
Lump — *see* Mass
Lunacy — *see* Psychosis
Lung — *see* condition
Lupoid (miliary) **of Boeck** D86.3
Lupus
  anticoagulant D68.62
    with
      hemorrhagic disorder D68.312
      hypercoagulable state D68.62
      finding without diagnosis R76.0
  discoid (local) L93.0
  erythematosus (discoid) (local) L93.0
    disseminated — *see* Lupus, erythematosus, systemic
    eyelid H01.129
      left H01.126
        lower H01.125
        upper H01.124
      right H01.123
        lower H01.122
        upper H01.121
    profundus L93.2
    specified NEC L93.2
    subacute cutaneous L93.1
    systemic M32.9
      with organ or system involvement M32.10
        endocarditis M32.11
        lung M32.13
        pericarditis M32.12
        renal (glomerular) M32.14
          tubulo-interstitial M32.15
        specified organ or system NEC M32.19

Lupus — *continued*
  erythematosus — *continued*
    systemic — *continued*
      drug-induced M32.0
      inhibitor (presence of) D68.62
        with
          hemorrhagic disorder D68.312
          hypercoagulable state D68.62
        finding without diagnosis R76.0
      specified NEC M32.8
  exedens A18.4
  hydralazine M32.0
    correct substance properly administered — *see* Table of Drugs and Chemicals, by drug, adverse effect
    overdose or wrong substance given or taken — *see* Table of Drugs and Chemicals, by drug, poisoning
  nephritis (chronic) M32.14
  nontuberculous, not disseminated L93.0
  panniculitis L93.2
  pernio (Besnier) D86.3
  systemic — *see* Lupus, erythematosus, systemic
  tuberculous A18.4
    eyelid A18.4
  vulgaris A18.4
    eyelid A18.4
Luteinoma D27.- ☑
Lutembacher's disease or syndrome (atrial septal defect with mitral stenosis) Q21.1
Luteoma D27.- ☑
Lutz (-Splendore-de Almeida) **disease** — *see* Paracoccidioidomycosis
Luxation (*see also* Dislocation)
  eyeball (nontraumatic) — *see* Luxation, globe
    birth injury P15.3
  globe, nontraumatic H44.82- ☑
  lacrimal gland — *see* Dislocation, lacrimal gland
  lens (old) (partial) (spontaneous)
    congenital Q12.1
    syphilitic A50.39
Lycanthropy F22
Lyell's syndrome L51.2
  due to drug L51.2
    correct substance properly administered — *see* Table of Drugs and Chemicals, by drug, adverse effect
    overdose or wrong substance given or taken — *see* Table of Drugs and Chemicals, by drug, poisoning
Lyme disease A69.20
Lymph
  gland or node — *see* condition
  scrotum — *see* Infestation, filarial
Lymphadenitis I88.9
  with ectopic or molar pregnancy O08.0
  acute L04.9
    axilla L04.2
    face L04.0
    head L04.0
    hip L04.3
    limb
      lower L04.3
      upper L04.2
    neck L04.0
    shoulder L04.2
    specified site NEC L04.8
    trunk L04.1
  anthracosis (occupational) J60
  any site, except mesenteric I88.9
    chronic I88.1
    subacute I88.1
  breast
    gestational — *see* Mastitis, obstetric
    puerperal, postpartum (nonpurulent) O91.22
  chancroidal (congenital) A57
  chronic I88.1
    mesenteric I88.0
  due to
    Brugia (malayi) B74.1
      timori B74.2
    chlamydial lymphogranuloma A55
    diphtheria (toxin) A36.89
    lymphogranuloma venereum A55
    Wuchereria bancrofti B74.0
  following ectopic or molar pregnancy O08.0
  gonorrheal A54.89
  infective — *see* Lymphadenitis, acute

Lymphadenitis — *continued*
  mesenteric (acute) (chronic) (nonspecific) (subacute) I88.0
    due to Salmonella typhi A01.09
    tuberculous A18.39
  mycobacterial A31.8
  purulent — *see* Lymphadenitis, acute
  pyogenic — *see* Lymphadenitis, acute
  regional, nonbacterial I88.8
  septic — *see* Lymphadenitis, acute
  subacute, unspecified site I88.1
  suppurative — *see* Lymphadenitis, acute
  syphilitic (early) (secondary) A51.49
    late A52.79
  tuberculous — *see* Tuberculosis, lymph gland
  venereal (chlamydial) A55
Lymphadenoid goiter E06.3
Lymphadenopathy (generalized) R59.1
  angioimmunoblastic, with dysproteinemia (AILD) C86.5
  due to toxoplasmosis (acquired) B58.89
    congenital (acute) (subacute) (chronic) P37.1
  localized R59.0
  syphilitic (early) (secondary) A51.49
Lymphadenosis R59.1
Lymphangiectasis I89.0
  conjunctiva H11.89
  postinfectional I89.0
  scrotum I89.0
Lymphangiectatic elephantiasis, nonfilarial I89.0
Lymphangioendothelioma D18.1
  malignant — *see* Neoplasm, connective tissue, malignant
Lymphangioleiomyomatosis J84.81
Lymphangioma D18.1
  capillary D18.1
  cavernous D18.1
  cystic D18.1
  malignant — *see* Neoplasm, connective tissue, malignant
Lymphangiomyoma D18.1
Lymphangiomyomatosis J84.81
Lymphangiosarcoma — *see* Neoplasm, connective tissue, malignant
Lymphangitis I89.1
  with
    abscess — *code by* site under Abscess
    cellulitis — *code by* site under Cellulitis
    ectopic or molar pregnancy O08.0
  acute L03.91
    abdominal wall L03.321
    ankle — *see* Lymphangitis, acute, lower limb
    arm — *see* Lymphangitis, acute, upper limb
    auricle (ear) — *see* Lymphangitis, acute, ear
    axilla L03.12- ☑
    back (any part) L03.322
    buttock L03.327
    cervical (meaning neck) L03.222
    cheek (external) L03.212
    chest wall L03.323
    digit
      finger — *see* Lymphangitis, acute, finger
      toe — *see* Lymphangitis, acute, toe
    ear (external) H60.1- ☑
    external auditory canal — *see* Lymphangitis, acute, ear
    eyelid — *see* Abscess, eyelid
    face NEC L03.212
    finger (intrathecal) (periosteal) (subcutaneous) (subcuticular) L03.02- ☑
    foot — *see* Lymphangitis, acute, lower limb
    gluteal (region) L03.327
    groin L03.324
    hand — *see* Lymphangitis, acute, upper limb
    head NEC L03.891
      face (any part, except ear, eye and nose) L03.212
    heel — *see* Lymphangitis, acute, lower limb
    hip — *see* Lymphangitis, acute, lower limb
    jaw (region) L03.212
    knee — *see* Lymphangitis, acute, lower limb
    leg — *see* Lymphangitis, acute, lower limb
    lower limb L03.12- ☑
      toe — *see* Lymphangitis, acute, toe
    navel L03.326
    neck (region) L03.222
    orbit, orbital — *see* Cellulitis, orbit

Lymphangitis — continued
  acute — continued
    pectoral (region) LØ3.323
    perineal, perineum LØ3.325
    scalp (any part) LØ3.891
    shoulder — see Lymphangitis, acute, upper limb
    specified site NEC LØ3.898
    thigh — see Lymphangitis, acute, lower limb
    thumb (intrathecal) (periosteal) (subcutaneous)
      (subcuticular) — see Lymphangitis, acute,
      finger
    toe (intrathecal) (periosteal) (subcutaneous) (sub-
      cuticular) LØ3.Ø4- ☑
    trunk LØ3.329
      abdominal wall LØ3.321
      back (any part) LØ3.322
      buttock LØ3.327
      chest wall LØ3.323
      groin LØ3.324
      perineal, perineum LØ3.325
      umbilicus LØ3.326
    umbilicus LØ3.326
    upper limb LØ3.12- ☑
      axilla — see Lymphangitis, acute, axilla
      finger — see Lymphangitis, acute, finger
      thumb — see Lymphangitis, acute, finger
      wrist — see Lymphangitis, acute, upper limb
  breast
    gestational — see Mastitis, obstetric
  chancroidal A57
  chronic (any site) I89.1
  due to
    Brugia (malayi) B74.1
      timori B74.2
    Wuchereria bancrofti B74.Ø
  following ectopic or molar pregnancy OØ8.89
  penis
    acute N48.29
    gonococcal (acute) (chronic) A54.Ø9
  puerperal, postpartum, childbirth O86.89
  strumous, tuberculous A18.2
  subacute (any site) I89.1
  tuberculous — see Tuberculosis, lymph gland
Lymphatic (vessel) — see condition
Lymphatism E32.8
Lymphectasia I89.Ø
Lymphedema (acquired) (see also Elephantiasis)
  congenital Q82.Ø
  hereditary (chronic) (idiopathic) Q82.Ø
  postmastectomy I97.2
  praecox I89.Ø
  secondary I89.Ø
  surgical NEC I97.89
    postmastectomy (syndrome) I97.2
Lymphoblastic — see condition
Lymphoblastoma (diffuse) — see Lymphoma, lymphoblastic (diffuse)
  giant follicular — see Lymphoma, lymphoblastic (dif-
    fuse)
  macrofollicular — see Lymphoma, lymphoblastic
    (diffuse)
Lymphocele I89.8
Lymphocytic
  chorioencephalitis (acute) (serous) A87.2
  choriomeningitis (acute) (serous) A87.2
  meningoencephalitis A87.2
Lymphocytoma, benign cutis L98.8
Lymphocytopenia D72.81Ø
Lymphocytosis (symptomatic) D72.82Ø
  infectious (acute) B33.8
Lymphoepithelioma — see Neoplasm, malignant, by
  site
Lymphogranuloma (malignant) (see also Lymphoma,
  Hodgkin)
  chlamydial A55
  inguinale A55
  venereum (any site) (chlamydial) (with stricture of
    rectum) A55
Lymphogranulomatosis (malignant) (see also Lymphoma, Hodgkin)
  benign (Boeck's sarcoid) (Schaumann's) D86.1
Lymphohistiocytosis, hemophagocytic (familial) D76.1
Lymphoid — see condition
Lymphoma (of) (malignant) C85.9Ø
  adult T-cell (HTLV-1-associated) (acute variant)
    (chronic variant) (lymphomatoid variant)
    (smouldering variant) C91.5- ☑

Lymphoma — continued
  anaplastic large cell
    ALK-negative C84.7- ☑
    ALK-positive C84.6- ☑
    CD3Ø-positive C84.6- ☑
    primary cutaneous C86.6
  angioimmunoblastic T-cell C86.5
  BALT C88.4
  B-cell C85.1- ☑
  blastic NK-cell C86.4
  B-precursor C83.5- ☑
  bronchial-associated lymphoid tissue [BALT-lym-
    phoma] C88.4
  Burkitt C83.7- ☑
  Burkitt-like C83.7- ☑
  centrocytic C83.1- ☑
  cutaneous follicle center C82.6- ☑
  cutaneous T-cell C84.A- ☑ (following C84.7)
  diffuse follicle center C82.5- ☑
  diffuse large cell C83.3- ☑
    anaplastic C83.3- ☑
    B-cell C83.3- ☑
    CD3Ø-positive C83.3- ☑
    centroblastic C83.3- ☑
    immunoblastic C83.3- ☑
    plasmablastic C83.3- ☑
    subtype not specified C83.3- ☑
    T-cell rich C83.3- ☑
  enteropathy-type (associated) (intestinal) T-cell C86.2
  extranodal marginal zone B-cell lymphoma of mucosa-
    associated lymphoid tissue [MALT-lymphoma]
    C88.4
  extranodal NK/T-cell, nasal type C86.Ø
  follicular C82.9- ☑
    grade
      I C82.Ø- ☑
      II C82.1- ☑
      III C82.2- ☑
      IIIa C82.3- ☑
      IIIb C82.4- ☑
    specified NEC C82.8- ☑
  hepatosplenic T-cell (alpha-beta) (gamma-delta) C86.1
  histiocytic C85.9- ☑
    true C96.A (following C96.6)
  Hodgkin C81.9 ☑
    classical C81.7- ☑
      lymphocyte depleted C81.3- ☑
      lymphocyte-rich C81.4- ☑
      mixed cellularity C81.2- ☑
      nodular sclerosis C81.1- ☑
      specified NEC C81.7- ☑
    lymphocyte depleted classical C81.3- ☑
    lymphocyte-rich classical C81.4- ☑
    mixed cellularity classical C81.2- ☑
    nodular
      lymphocyte predominant C81.Ø- ☑
      sclerosis classical C81.1- ☑
  intravascular large B-cell C83.8- ☑
  Lennert's C84.4- ☑
  lymphoblastic (diffuse) C83.5- ☑
  lymphoblastic B-cell C83.5- ☑
  lymphoblastic T-cell C83.5- ☑
  lymphoepithelioid C84.4- ☑
  lymphoplasmacytic C83.Ø- ☑
    with IgM-production C88.Ø
  MALT C88.4
  mantle cell C83.1- ☑
  mature T-cell NEC C84.4- ☑
  mature T/NK-cell C84.9- ☑
    specified NEC C84.Z- ☑ (following C84.7)
  mediastinal (thymic) large B-cell C85.2- ☑
  Mediterranean C88.3
  mucosa-associated lymphoid tissue [MALT-lymphoma]
    C88.4
  NK/T cell C84.9- ☑
  nodal marginal zone C83.Ø- ☑
  non-follicular (diffuse) C83.9- ☑
    specified NEC C83.8- ☑
  non-Hodgkin (see also Lymphoma, by type) C85.9- ☑
    specified NEC C85.8- ☑
  non-leukemic variant of B-CLL C83.Ø- ☑
  peripheral T-cell, not classified C84.4- ☑
  primary cutaneous
    anaplastic large cell C86.6
    CD3Ø-positive large T-cell C86.6
  primary effusion B-cell C83.8- ☑

Lymphoma — continued
  SALT C88.4
  skin-associated lymphoid tissue [SALT-lymphoma]
    C88.4
  small cell B-cell C83.Ø- ☑
  splenic marginal zone C83.Ø- ☑
  subcutaneous panniculitis-like T-cell C86.3
  T-precursor C83.5- ☑
  true histiocytic C96.A (following C96.6)
Lymphomatosis — see Lymphoma
Lymphopathia venereum, veneris A55
Lymphopenia D72.81Ø
Lymphoplasmacytic leukemia — see Leukemia,
  chronic lymphocytic, B-cell type
Lymphoproliferation, X-linked disease D82.3
Lymphoreticulosis, benign (of inoculation) A28.1
Lymphorrhea I89.8
Lymphosarcoma (diffuse) (see also Lymphoma)
  C85.9- ☑
Lymphostasis I89.8
Lypemania — see Melancholia
Lysine and hydroxylysine metabolism disorder E72.3
Lyssa — see Rabies

M

Macacus ear Q17.3
Maceration, wet feet, tropical (syndrome) T69.Ø2- ☑
MacLeod's syndrome J43.Ø
Macrocephalia, macrocephaly Q75.3
Macrocheilia, macrochilia (congenital) Q18.6
Macrocolon (see also Megacolon) Q43.1
Macrocornea Q15.8
  with glaucoma Q15.Ø
Macrocytic — see condition
Macrocytosis D75.89
Macrodactylia, macrodactylism (fingers) (thumbs)
  Q74.Ø
  toes Q74.2
Macrodontia KØØ.2
Macrogenia M26.Ø5
Macrogenitosomia (adrenal) (male) (praecox) E25.9
  congenital E25.Ø
Macroglobulinemia (idiopathic) (primary) C88.Ø
  monoclonal (essential) D47.2
  Waldenström C88.Ø
Macroglossia (congenital) Q38.2
  acquired K14.8
Macrognathia, macrognathism (congenital)
  (mandibular) (maxillary) M26.Ø9
Macrogyria (congenital) QØ4.8
Macrohydrocephalus — see Hydrocephalus
Macromastia — see Hypertrophy, breast
Macrophthalmos Q11.3
  in congenital glaucoma Q15.Ø
Macropsia H53.15
Macrosigmoid K59.3
  congenital Q43.2
Macrospondylitis, acromegalic E22.Ø
Macrostomia (congenital) Q18.4
Macrotia (external ear) (congenital) Q17.1
Macula
  cornea, corneal — see Opacity, cornea
  degeneration (atrophic) (exudative) (senile) (see also
    Degeneration, macula)
    hereditary — see Dystrophy, retina
Maculae ceruleae B85.1
Maculopathy, toxic — see Degeneration, macula, toxic
Madarosis (eyelid) HØ2.729
  left HØ2.726
    lower HØ2.725
    upper HØ2.724
  right HØ2.723
    lower HØ2.722
    upper HØ2.721
Madelung's
  deformity (radius) Q74.Ø
  disease
    radial deformity Q74.Ø
    symmetrical lipomas, neck E88.89
Madness — see Psychosis
Madura
  foot B47.9
    actinomycotic B47.1
    mycotic B47.Ø
Maduromycosis B47.Ø
Maffucci's syndrome Q78.4

Magnesium metabolism disorder — *see* Disorder, metabolism, magnesium
Main en griffe (acquired) (*see also* Deformity, limb, clawhand)
   congenital Q74.0
Maintenance (encounter for)
   antineoplastic chemotherapy Z51.11
   antineoplastic radiation therapy Z51.0
   methadone F11.20
Majocchi's
   disease L81.7
   granuloma B35.8
Major — *see* condition
Mal de los pintos — *see* Pinta
Mal de mer T75.3 ☑
Malabar itch (any site) B35.5
Malabsorption K90.9
   calcium K90.89
   carbohydrate K90.4
   disaccharide E73.9
   fat K90.4
   galactose E74.20
   glucose (-galactose) E74.39
   intestinal K90.9
     specified NEC K90.89
   isomaltose E74.31
   lactose E73.9
   methionine E72.19
   monosaccharide E74.39
   postgastrectomy K91.2
   postsurgical K91.2
   protein K90.4
   starch K90.4
   sucrose E74.39
   syndrome K90.9
     postsurgical K91.2
Malacia, bone (adult) M83.9
   juvenile — *see* Rickets
Malacoplakia
   bladder N32.89
   pelvis (kidney) N28.89
   ureter N28.89
   urethra N36.8
Malacosteon, juvenile — *see* Rickets
Maladaptation — *see* Maladjustment
Maladie de Roger Q21.0
Maladjustment
   conjugal Z63.0
     involving divorce or estrangement Z63.5
   educational Z55.4
   family Z63.9
   marital Z63.0
     involving divorce or estrangement Z63.5
   occupational NEC Z56.89
   simple, adult — *see* Disorder, adjustment
   situational — *see* Disorder, adjustment
   social Z60.9
     due to
       acculturation difficulty Z60.3
       discrimination and persecution (perceived) Z60.5
       exclusion and isolation Z60.4
       life-cycle (phase of life) transition Z60.0
       rejection Z60.4
       specified reason NEC Z60.8
Malaise R53.81
Malakoplakia — *see* Malacoplakia
Malaria, malarial (fever) B54
   with
     blackwater fever B50.8
       hemoglobinuric (bilious) B50.8
     hemoglobinuria B50.8
   accidentally induced (therapeutically) — *code by* type under Malaria
   algid B50.9
   cerebral B50.0 [G94]
   clinically diagnosed (without parasitological confirmation) B54
   congenital NEC P37.4
     falciparum P37.3
   congestion, congestive B54
   continued (fever) B50.9
   estivo-autumnal B50.9
   falciparum B50.9
     with complications NEC B50.8
       cerebral B50.0 [G94]
     severe B50.8
   hemorrhagic B54

Malaria, malarial — *continued*
   malariae B52.9
     with
       complications NEC B52.8
       glomerular disorder B52.0
   malignant (tertian) — *see* Malaria, falciparum
   mixed infections — *code to* first listed type in B50-B53
   ovale B53.0
   parasitologically confirmed NEC B53.8
   pernicious, acute — *see* Malaria, falciparum
   Plasmodium (P.)
     falciparum NEC — *see* Malaria, falciparum
     malariae NEC B52.9
       with Plasmodium
         falciparum (and or vivax) — *see* Malaria, falciparum
         vivax (*see also* Malaria, vivax)
           and falciparum — *see* Malaria, falciparum
     ovale B53.0
       with Plasmodium malariae (*see also* Malaria, malariae)
       and vivax (*see also* Malaria, vivax)
         and falciparum — *see* Malaria, falciparum
     simian B53.1
       with Plasmodium malariae (*see also* Malaria, malariae)
       and vivax (*see also* Malaria, vivax)
         and falciparum — *see* Malaria, falciparum
     vivax NEC B51.9
       with Plasmodium falciparum — *see* Malaria, falciparum
   quartan — *see* Malaria, malariae
   quotidian — *see* Malaria, falciparum
   recurrent B54
   remittent B54
   specified type NEC (parasitologically confirmed) B53.8
   spleen B54
   subtertian (fever) — *see* Malaria, falciparum
   tertian (benign) (*see also* Malaria, vivax)
     malignant B50.9
   tropical B50.9
   typhoid B54
   vivax B51.9
     with
       complications NEC B51.8
       ruptured spleen B51.0
Malassez's disease (cystic) N50.8
Malassimilation K90.9
Maldescent, testis Q53.9
   bilateral Q53.20
     abdominal Q53.21
     perineal Q53.22
   unilateral Q53.10
     abdominal Q53.11
     perineal Q53.12
Maldevelopment (*see also* Anomaly)
   brain Q07.9
   colon Q43.9
   hip Q74.2
     congenital dislocation Q65.2
       bilateral Q65.1
       unilateral Q65.0- ☑
   mastoid process Q75.8
   middle ear Q16.4
     except ossicles Q16.4
     ossicles Q16.3
   ossicles Q16.3
   spine Q76.49
   toe Q74.2
Male type pelvis Q74.2
   with disproportion (fetopelvic) O33.3 ☑
     causing obstructed labor O65.3
Malformation (congenital) (*see also* Anomaly)
   adrenal gland Q89.1
   affecting multiple systems with skeletal changes NEC Q87.5
   alimentary tract Q45.9
     specified type NEC Q45.8
     upper Q40.9
       specified type NEC Q40.8
   aorta Q25.9
     atresia Q25.2
     coarctation (preductal) (postductal) Q25.1
     patent ductus arteriosus Q25.0
     specified type NEC Q25.4

Malformation — *continued*
   aorta — *continued*
     stenosis (supravalvular) Q25.3
   aortic valve Q23.9
     specified NEC Q23.8
   arteriovenous, aneurysmatic (congenital) Q27.30
     brain Q28.2
     cerebral Q28.2
     peripheral Q27.30
       digestive system Q27.33
       lower limb Q27.32
       other specified site Q27.39
       renal vessel Q27.34
       upper limb Q27.31
     precerebral vessels (nonruptured) Q28.0
   auricle
     ear (congenital) Q17.3
       acquired H61.119
         left H61.112
           with right H61.113
         right H61.111
           with left H61.113
   bile duct Q44.5
   bladder Q64.79
     aplasia Q64.5
     diverticulum Q64.6
     exstrophy — *see* Exstrophy, bladder
     neck obstruction Q64.31
   bone Q79.9
     face Q75.9
       specified type NEC Q75.8
     skull Q75.9
       specified type NEC Q75.8
   brain (multiple) Q04.9
     arteriovenous Q28.2
     specified type NEC Q04.8
   branchial cleft Q18.2
   breast Q83.9
     specified type NEC Q83.8
   broad ligament Q50.6
   bronchus Q32.4
   bursa Q79.9
   cardiac
     chambers Q20.9
       specified type NEC Q20.8
     septum Q21.9
       specified type NEC Q21.8
   cerebral Q04.9
     vessels Q28.3
   cervix uteri Q51.9
     specified type NEC Q51.828
   Chiari
     Type I G93.5
     Type II Q07.01
   choroid (congenital) Q14.3
     plexus Q07.8
   circulatory system Q28.9
   cochlea Q16.5
   cornea Q13.4
   coronary vessels Q24.5
   corpus callosum (congenital) Q04.0
   diaphragm Q79.1
   digestive system NEC, specified type NEC Q45.8
   dura Q07.9
     brain Q04.9
     spinal Q06.9
   ear Q17.9
     causing impairment of hearing Q16.9
     external Q17.9
       accessory auricle Q17.0
       causing impairment of hearing Q16.9
         absence of
           auditory canal Q16.1
           auricle Q16.0
       macrotia Q17.1
       microtia Q17.2
       misplacement Q17.4
       misshapen NEC Q17.3
       prominence Q17.5
       specified type NEC Q17.8
     inner Q16.5
     middle Q16.4
       absence of eustachian tube Q16.2
       ossicles (fusion) Q16.3
     ossicles Q16.3
     specified type NEC Q17.8
   epididymis Q55.4
   esophagus Q39.9

▼ Subterms under main terms may continue to next column or page   ☑ Additional Character Required — Refer to the Tabular List for Character Selection   209

Index

Magnesium metabolism disorder — Malformation

Malformation — *continued*
  esophagus — *continued*
    specified type NEC Q39.8
  eye Q15.9
    lid Q10.3
    specified NEC Q15.8
  fallopian tube Q50.6
  genital organ — *see* Anomaly, genitalia
  great
    artery Q25.9
      aorta — *see* Malformation, aorta
      pulmonary artery — *see* Malformation, pulmonary, artery
      specified type NEC Q25.8
    vein Q26.9
      anomalous
        portal venous connection Q26.5
        pulmonary venous connection Q26.4
          partial Q26.3
          total Q26.2
      persistent left superior vena cava Q26.1
      portal vein-hepatic artery fistula Q26.6
      specified type NEC Q26.8
      vena cava stenosis, congenital Q26.0
  gum Q38.6
  hair Q84.2
  heart Q24.9
    specified type NEC Q24.8
  integument Q84.9
    specified type NEC Q84.8
  internal ear Q16.5
  intestine Q43.9
    specified type NEC Q43.8
  iris Q13.2
  joint Q74.9
    ankle Q74.2
    lumbosacral Q76.49
    sacroiliac Q74.2
    specified type NEC Q74.8
  kidney Q63.9
    accessory Q63.0
    giant Q63.3
    horseshoe Q63.1
    hydronephrosis Q62.0
    malposition Q63.2
    specified type NEC Q63.8
  lacrimal apparatus Q10.6
  lingual Q38.3
  lip Q38.0
  liver Q44.7
  lung Q33.9
  meninges or membrane (congenital) Q07.9
    cerebral Q04.8
    spinal (cord) Q06.9
  middle ear Q16.4
    ossicles Q16.3
  mitral valve Q23.9
    specified NEC Q23.8
  Mondini's (congenital) (malformation, cochlea) Q16.5
  mouth (congenital) Q38.6
  multiple types NEC Q89.7
  musculoskeletal system Q79.9
  myocardium Q24.8
  nail Q84.6
  nervous system (central) Q07.9
  nose Q30.9
    specified type NEC Q30.8
  optic disc Q14.2
  orbit Q10.7
  ovary Q50.39
  palate Q38.5
  parathyroid gland Q89.2
  pelvic organs or tissues NEC
    in pregnancy or childbirth O34.8- ☑
      causing obstructed labor O65.5
  penis Q55.69
    aplasia Q55.5
    curvature (lateral) Q55.61
    hypoplasia Q55.62
  pericardium Q24.8
  peripheral vascular system Q27.9
    specified type NEC Q27.8
  pharynx Q38.8
  precerebral vessels Q28.1
  prostate Q55.4
  pulmonary
    arteriovenous Q25.72
    artery Q25.9

Malformation — *continued*
  pulmonary — *continued*
    artery — *continued*
      atresia Q25.5
      specified type NEC Q25.79
      stenosis Q25.6
    valve Q22.3
  renal artery Q27.2
  respiratory system Q34.9
  retina Q14.1
  scrotum — *see* Malformation, testis and scrotum
  seminal vesicles Q55.4
  sense organs NEC Q07.9
  skin Q82.9
  specified NEC Q89.8
  spinal
    cord Q06.9
    nerve root Q07.8
  spine Q76.49
    kyphosis — *see* Kyphosis, congenital
    lordosis — *see* Lordosis, congenital
  spleen Q89.09
  stomach Q40.3
    specified type NEC Q40.2
  teeth, tooth K00.9
  tendon Q79.9
  testis and scrotum Q55.20
    aplasia Q55.0
    hypoplasia Q55.1
    polyorchism Q55.21
    retractile testis Q55.22
    scrotal transposition Q55.23
    specified NEC Q55.29
  thorax, bony Q76.9
  throat Q38.8
  thyroid gland Q89.2
  tongue (congenital) Q38.3
    hypertrophy Q38.2
    tie Q38.1
  trachea Q32.1
  tricuspid valve Q22.9
    specified type NEC Q22.8
  umbilical cord NEC (complicating delivery) O69.89 ☑
  umbilicus Q89.9
  ureter Q62.8
    agenesis Q62.4
    duplication Q62.5
    malposition — *see* Malposition, congenital, ureter
    obstructive defect — *see* Defect, obstructive, ureter
    vesico-uretero-renal reflux Q62.7
  urethra Q64.79
    aplasia Q64.5
    duplication Q64.74
    posterior valves Q64.2
    prolapse Q64.71
    stricture Q64.32
  urinary system Q64.9
  uterus Q51.9
    specified type NEC Q51.818
  vagina Q52.4
  vas deferens Q55.4
    atresia Q55.3
  vascular system, peripheral Q27.9
  venous — *see* Anomaly, vein(s)
  vulva Q52.70

Malfunction (*see also* Dysfunction)
  cardiac electronic device T82.119 ☑
    electrode T82.110 ☑
    pulse generator T82.111 ☑
    specified type NEC T82.118 ☑
  catheter device NEC T85.618 ☑
    cystostomy T83.010 ☑
    dialysis (renal) (vascular) T82.41 ☑
      intraperitoneal T85.611 ☑
    infusion NEC T82.514 ☑
      spinal (epidural) (subdural) T85.610 ☑
    urinary, indwelling T83.018 ☑
  colostomy K94.03
    valve K94.03
  cystostomy (stoma) N99.512
    catheter T83.010 ☑
  enteric stoma K94.13
  enterostomy K94.13
  esophagostomy K94.33
  gastroenteric K31.89
  gastrostomy K94.23
  ileostomy K94.13
    valve K94.13

Malfunction — *continued*
  jejunostomy K94.13
  pacemaker — *see* Malfunction, cardiac electronic device
  prosthetic device, internal — *see* Complications, prosthetic device, by site, mechanical
  tracheostomy J95.03
  urinary device NEC — *see* Complication, genitourinary, device, urinary, mechanical
  valve
    colostomy K94.03
    heart T82.09 ☑
    ileostomy K94.13
  vascular graft or shunt NEC — *see* Complication, cardiovascular device, mechanical, vascular
  ventricular (communicating shunt) T85.01 ☑
Malherbe's tumor — *see* Neoplasm, skin, benign
Malibu disease L98.8
Malignancy (*see also* Neoplasm, malignant, by site)
  unspecified site (primary) C80.1
Malignant — *see* condition
Malingerer, malingering Z76.5
Mallet finger (acquired) — *see* Deformity, finger, mallet finger
  congenital Q74.0
  sequelae of rickets E64.3
Malleus A24.0
Mallory's bodies R89.7
Mallory-Weiss syndrome K22.6
Malnutrition E46
  degree
    first E44.1
    mild (protein) E44.1
    moderate (protein) E44.0
    second E44.0
    severe (protein-energy) E43
      intermediate form E42
        with
          kwashiorkor (and marasmus) E42
          marasmus E41
    third E43
  following gastrointestinal surgery K91.2
  intrauterine
    light-for-dates — *see* Light for dates
    small-for-dates — *see* Small for dates
  lack of care, or neglect (child) (infant) T76.02 ☑
    confirmed T74.02 ☑
  malignant E40
  protein E46
    calorie E46
      mild E44.1
      moderate E44.0
      severe E43
        intermediate form E42
          with
            kwashiorkor (and marasmus) E42
            marasmus E41
    energy E46
      mild E44.1
      moderate E44.0
      severe E43
        intermediate form E42
          with
            kwashiorkor (and marasmus) E42
            marasmus E41
  severe (protein-energy) E43
    with
      kwashiorkor (and marasmus) E42
      marasmus E41
Malocclusion (teeth) M26.4
  Angle's M26.219
    class I M26.211
    class II M26.212
    class III M26.213
  due to
    abnormal swallowing M26.59
    mouth breathing M26.59
    tongue, lip or finger habits M26.59
  temporomandibular (joint) M26.69
Malposition
  cervix — *see* Malposition, uterus
  congenital
    adrenal (gland) Q89.1
    alimentary tract Q45.8
      lower Q43.8
      upper Q40.8
    aorta Q25.4
    appendix Q43.8

Malposition — *continued*
  congenital — *continued*
    arterial trunk Q20.0
    artery (peripheral) Q27.8
      coronary Q24.5
      digestive system Q27.8
      lower limb Q27.8
      pulmonary Q25.79
      specified site NEC Q27.8
      upper limb Q27.8
    auditory canal Q17.8
      causing impairment of hearing Q16.9
    auricle (ear) Q17.4
      causing impairment of hearing Q16.9
      cervical Q18.2
    biliary duct or passage Q44.5
    bladder (mucosa) — *see* Exstrophy, bladder
    brachial plexus Q07.8
    brain tissue Q04.8
    breast Q83.8
    bronchus Q32.4
    cecum Q43.8
    clavicle Q74.0
    colon Q43.8
    digestive organ or tract NEC Q45.8
      lower Q43.8
      upper Q40.8
    ear (auricle) (external) Q17.4
      ossicles Q16.3
    endocrine (gland) NEC Q89.2
    epiglottis Q31.8
    eustachian tube Q17.8
    eye Q15.8
    facial features Q18.8
    fallopian tube Q50.6
    finger(s) Q68.1
      supernumerary Q69.0
    foot Q66.9
    gallbladder Q44.1
    gastrointestinal tract Q45.8
    genitalia, genital organ(s) or tract
      female Q52.8
        external Q52.79
        internal NEC Q52.8
      male Q55.8
    glottis Q31.8
    hand Q68.1
    heart Q24.8
      dextrocardia Q24.0
        with complete transposition of viscera Q89.3
    hepatic duct Q44.5
    hip (joint) Q65.89
    intestine (large) (small) Q43.8
      with anomalous adhesions, fixation or malrotation Q43.3
    joint NEC Q68.8
    kidney Q63.2
    larynx Q31.8
    limb Q68.8
      lower Q68.8
      upper Q68.8
    liver Q44.7
    lung (lobe) Q33.8
    nail(s) Q84.6
    nerve Q07.8
    nervous system NEC Q07.8
    nose, nasal (septum) Q30.8
    organ or site not listed — *see* Anomaly, by site
    ovary Q50.39
    pancreas Q45.3
    parathyroid (gland) Q89.2
    patella Q74.1
    peripheral vascular system Q27.8
    pituitary (gland) Q89.2
    respiratory organ or system NEC Q34.8
    rib (cage) Q76.6
      supernumerary in cervical region Q76.5
    scapula Q74.0
    shoulder Q74.0
    spinal cord Q06.8
    spleen Q89.09
    sternum NEC Q76.7
    stomach Q40.2
    symphysis pubis Q74.2
    thymus (gland) Q89.2
    thyroid (gland) (tissue) Q89.2
      cartilage Q31.8
    toe(s) Q66.9

Malposition — *continued*
  congenital — *continued*
    toe(s) — *continued*
      supernumerary Q69.2
    tongue Q38.3
    trachea Q32.1
    ureter Q62.60
      deviation Q62.61
      displacement Q62.62
      ectopia Q62.63
      specified type NEC Q62.69
    uterus Q51.818
    vein(s) (peripheral) Q27.8
      great Q26.8
    vena cava (inferior) (superior) Q26.8
  device, implant or graft (*see also* Complications, by site and type, mechanical) T85.628 ☑
    arterial graft NEC — *see* Complication, cardiovascular device, mechanical, vascular
    breast (implant) T85.42 ☑
    catheter NEC T85.628 ☑
      cystostomy T83.020 ☑
      dialysis (renal) T82.42 ☑
        intraperitoneal T85.621 ☑
      infusion NEC T82.524 ☑
        spinal (epidural) (subdural) T85.620 ☑
      urinary, indwelling T83.028 ☑
    electronic (electrode) (pulse generator) (stimulator)
      bone T84.320 ☑
      cardiac T82.129 ☑
        electrode T82.120 ☑
        pulse generator T82.121 ☑
        specified type NEC T82.128 ☑
      nervous system — *see* Complication, prosthetic device, mechanical, electronic nervous system stimulator
      urinary — *see* Complication, genitourinary, device, urinary, mechanical
    fixation, internal (orthopedic) NEC — *see* Complication, fixation device, mechanical
    gastrointestinal — *see* Complications, prosthetic device, mechanical, gastrointestinal device
    genital NEC T83.428 ☑
      intrauterine contraceptive device T83.32 ☑
      penile prosthesis T83.420 ☑
    heart NEC — *see* Complication, cardiovascular device, mechanical
    joint prosthesis — *see* Complication, joint prosthesis, mechanical
    ocular NEC — *see* Complications, prosthetic device, mechanical, ocular device
    orthopedic NEC — *see* Complication, orthopedic, device, mechanical
    specified NEC T85.628 ☑
    urinary NEC (*see also* Complication, genitourinary, device, urinary, mechanical)
      graft T83.22 ☑
    vascular NEC — *see* Complication, cardiovascular device, mechanical
    ventricular intracranial shunt T85.02 ☑
  fetus — *see* Pregnancy, complicated by (management affected by), presentation, fetal
  gallbladder K82.8
  gastrointestinal tract, congenital Q45.8
  heart, congenital NEC Q24.8
  joint prosthesis — *see* Complications, joint prosthesis, mechanical, displacement, by site
  stomach K31.89
    congenital Q40.2
  tooth, teeth, fully erupted M26.30
  uterus (acute) (acquired) (adherent) (asymptomatic) (postinfectional) (postpartal, old) N85.4
    anteflexion or anteversion N85.4
      congenital Q51.818
    flexion N85.4
      lateral — *see* Lateroversion, uterus
    inversion N85.5
    lateral (flexion) (version) — *see* Lateroversion, uterus
      in pregnancy or childbirth — *see* subcategory O34.5 ☑
    retroflexion or retroversion — *see* Retroversion, uterus

Malposture R29.3
Malrotation
  cecum Q43.3
  colon Q43.3

Malrotation — *continued*
  intestine Q43.3
  kidney Q63.2
Malta fever — *see* Brucellosis
Maltreatment
  adult
    abandonment
      confirmed T74.01 ☑
      suspected T76.01 ☑
    confirmed T74.91 ☑
    history of Z91.419
    neglect
      confirmed T74.01 ☑
      suspected T76.01 ☑
    physical abuse
      confirmed T74.11 ☑
      suspected T76.11 ☑
    psychological abuse
      confirmed T74.31 ☑
      history of Z91.411
      suspected T76.31 ☑
    sexual abuse
      confirmed T74.21 ☑
      suspected T76.21 ☑
    suspected T76.91 ☑
  child
    abandonment
      confirmed T74.02 ☑
      suspected T76.02 ☑
    confirmed T74.92 ☑
    history of — *see* History, personal (of), abuse
    neglect
      confirmed T74.02 ☑
      history of — *see* History, personal (of), abuse
      suspected T76.02 ☑
    physical abuse
      confirmed T74.12 ☑
      history of — *see* History, personal (of), abuse
      suspected T76.12 ☑
    psychological abuse
      confirmed T74.32 ☑
      history of — *see* History, personal (of), abuse
      suspected T76.32 ☑
    sexual abuse
      confirmed T74.22 ☑
      history of — *see* History, personal (of), abuse
      suspected T76.22 ☑
    suspected T76.92 ☑
  personal history of Z91.89
Maltworker's lung J67.4
Malunion, fracture — *see* Fracture, by site
Mammillitis N61
  puerperal, postpartum O91.02
Mammitis — *see* Mastitis
Mammogram (examination) Z12.39
  routine Z12.31
Mammoplasia N62
Management (of)
  bone conduction hearing device (implanted) Z45.320
  cardiac pacemaker NEC Z45.018
  cerebrospinal fluid drainage device Z45.41
  cochlear device (implanted) Z45.321
  contraceptive Z30.9
    specified NEC Z30.8
  implanted device Z45.9
    specified NEC Z45.89
  infusion pump Z45.1
  procreative Z31.9
    male factor infertility in female Z31.81
    specified NEC Z31.89
  prosthesis (external) (*see also* Fitting) Z44.9
    implanted Z45.9
      specified NEC Z45.89
  renal dialysis catheter Z49.01
  vascular access device Z45.2
Mangled — *see* specified injury by site
Mania (monopolar) (*see also* Disorder, mood, manic episode)
  with psychotic symptoms F30.2
  without psychotic symptoms F30.10
    mild F30.11
    moderate F30.12
    severe F30.13
  Bell's F30.8
  chronic (recurrent) F31.89
  hysterical F44.89
  puerperal F30.8

Index

Mania — Megacolon

Mania — *continued*
  recurrent F31.89
Manic-depressive insanity, psychosis, or syndrome — *see* Disorder, bipolar
Mannosidosis E77.1
Mansonelliasis, mansonellosis B74.4
Manson's
  disease B65.1
  schistosomiasis B65.1
Manual — *see* condition
Maple-bark-stripper's lung (disease) J67.6
Maple-syrup-urine disease E71.0
Marable's syndrome (celiac artery compression) I77.4
Marasmus E41
  due to malnutrition E41
  intestinal E41
  nutritional E41
  senile R54
  tuberculous NEC — *see* Tuberculosis
Marble
  bones Q78.2
  skin R23.8
Marburg virus disease A98.3
March
  fracture — *see* Fracture, traumatic, stress, by site
  hemoglobinuria D59.6
Marchesani (-Weill) **syndrome** Q87.0
Marchiafava (-Bignami) **syndrome or disease** G37.1
Marchiafava-Micheli syndrome D59.5
Marcus Gunn's syndrome Q07.8
Marfan's syndrome — *see* Syndrome, Marfan's
Marie-Bamberger disease — *see* Osteoarthropathy, hypertrophic, specified NEC
Marie-Charcot-Tooth neuropathic muscular atrophy G60.0
Marie's
  cerebellar ataxia (late-onset) G11.2
  disease or syndrome (acromegaly) E22.0
Marie-Strümpell arthritis, disease or spondylitis — *see* Spondylitis, ankylosing
Marion's disease (bladder neck obstruction) N32.0
Marital conflict Z63.0
Mark
  port wine Q82.5
  raspberry Q82.5
  strawberry Q82.5
  stretch L90.6
  tattoo L81.8
Marker heterochromatin — *see* Extra, marker chromosomes
Maroteaux-Lamy syndrome (mild) (severe) E76.29
Marrow (bone)
  arrest D61.9
  poor function D75.89
Marseilles fever A77.1
Marsh fever — *see* Malaria
Marshall's (hidrotic) **ectodermal dysplasia** Q82.4
Marsh's disease (exophthalmic goiter) E05.00
  with storm E05.01
Masculinization (female) **with adrenal hyperplasia** E25.9
  congenital E25.0
Masculinovoblastoma D27.- ☑
Masochism (sexual) F65.51
Mason's lung J62.8
Mass
  abdominal R19.00
    epigastric R19.06
    generalized R19.07
    left lower quadrant R19.04
    left upper quadrant R19.02
    periumbilic R19.05
    right lower quadrant R19.03
    right upper quadrant R19.01
    specified site NEC R19.09
  breast N63
  chest R22.2
  cystic — *see* Cyst
  ear H93.8- ☑
  head R22.0
  intra-abdominal (diffuse) (generalized) — *see* Mass, abdominal
  kidney N28.89
  liver R16.0
  localized (skin) R22.9
    chest R22.2
    head R22.0

Mass — *continued*
  localized — *continued*
    limb
      lower R22.4- ☑
      upper R22.3- ☑
    neck R22.1
    trunk R22.2
  lung R91.8
  malignant — *see* Neoplasm, malignant, by site
  neck R22.1
  pelvic (diffuse) (generalized) — *see* Mass, abdominal
  specified organ NEC — *see* Disease, by site
  splenic R16.1
  substernal thyroid — *see* Goiter
  superficial (localized) R22.9
  umbilical (diffuse) (generalized) R19.09
Massive — *see* condition
Mast cell
  disease, systemic tissue D47.0
  leukemia C94.3- ☑
  sarcoma C96.2
  tumor D47.0
    malignant C96.2
Mastalgia N64.4
Masters-Allen syndrome N83.8
Mastitis (acute) (diffuse) (nonpuerperal) (subacute) N61
  chronic (cystic) — *see* Mastopathy, cystic
  cystic (Schimmelbusch's type) — *see* Mastopathy, cystic
  fibrocystic — *see* Mastopathy, cystic
  infective N61
    newborn P39.0
  interstitial, gestational or puerperal — *see* Mastitis, obstetric
  neonatal (noninfective) P83.4
    infective P39.0
  obstetric (interstitial) (nonpurulent)
    associated with
      lactation O91.23
      pregnancy O91.21- ☑
      puerperium O91.22
    purulent
      associated with
        lactation O91.13
        pregnancy O91.11- ☑
        puerperium O91.12
  periductal — *see* Ectasia, mammary duct
  phlegmonous — *see* Mastopathy, cystic
  plasma cell — *see* Ectasia, mammary duct
Mastocytoma D47.0
  malignant C96.2
Mastocytosis Q82.2
  aggressive systemic C96.2
  indolent systemic D47.0
  malignant C96.2
  systemic, associated with clonal hematopoetic non-mast-cell disease (SM-AHNMD) D47.0
Mastodynia N64.4
Mastoid — *see* condition
Mastoidalgia — *see* subcategory H92.0 ☑
Mastoiditis (coalescent) (hemorrhagic) (suppurative) H70.9- ☑
  acute, subacute H70.00- ☑
    complicated NEC H70.09- ☑
    subperiosteal H70.01- ☑
  chronic (necrotic) (recurrent) H70.1- ☑
  in (due to)
    infectious disease NEC B99 ☑ [H75.0-] ☑
    parasitic disease NEC B89 [H75.0-] ☑
    tuberculosis A18.03
  petrositis — *see* Petrositis
  postauricular fistula — *see* Fistula, postauricular
  specified NEC H70.89- ☑
  tuberculous A18.03
Mastopathy, mastopathia N64.9
  chronica cystica — *see* Mastopathy, cystic
  cystic (chronic) (diffuse) N60.1- ☑
    with epithelial proliferation N60.3- ☑
  diffuse cystic — *see* Mastopathy, cystic
  estrogenic, oestrogenica N64.89
  ovarian origin N64.89
Mastoplasia, mastoplastia N62
Masturbation (excessive) F98.8
Maternal care (for) — *see* Pregnancy (complicated by) (management affected by)
Matheiu's disease (leptospiral jaundice) A27.0

Mauclaire's disease or osteochondrosis — *see* Osteochondrosis, juvenile, hand, metacarpal
Maxcy's disease A75.2
Maxilla, maxillary — *see* condition
May (-Hegglin) **anomaly or syndrome** D72.0
McArdle (-Schmid)(-Pearson) **disease** (glycogen storage) E74.04
McCune-Albright syndrome Q78.1
McQuarrie's syndrome (idiopathic familial hypoglycemia) E16.2
Meadow's syndrome Q86.1
Measles (black) (hemorrhagic) (suppressed) B05.9
  with
    complications NEC B05.89
    encephalitis B05.0
    intestinal complications B05.4
    keratitis (keratoconjunctivitis) B05.81
    meningitis B05.1
    otitis media B05.3
    pneumonia B05.2
  French — *see* Rubella
  German — *see* Rubella
  Liberty — *see* Rubella
Meatitis, urethral — *see* Urethritis
Meatus, meatal — *see* condition
Meat-wrappers' asthma J68.9
Meckel-Gruber syndrome Q61.9
Meckel's diverticulitis, diverticulum (displaced) (hypertrophic) Q43.0
  malignant — *see* Table of Neoplasms, small intestine, malignant
Meconium
  ileus, newborn P76.0
    in cystic fibrosis E84.11
    meaning meconium plug (without cystic fibrosis) P76.0
  obstruction, newborn P76.0
    due to fecaliths P76.0
    in mucoviscidosis E84.11
  peritonitis P78.0
  plug syndrome (newborn) NEC P76.0
Median (*see also* condition)
  arcuate ligament syndrome I77.4
  bar (prostate) (vesical orifice) — *see* Hyperplasia, prostate
  rhomboid glossitis K14.2
Mediastinal shift R93.8
Mediastinitis (acute) (chronic) J98.5
  syphilitic A52.73
  tuberculous A15.8
Mediastinopericarditis (*see also* Pericarditis)
  acute I30.9
  adhesive I31.0
  chronic I31.8
  rheumatic I09.2
Mediastinum, mediastinal — *see* condition
Medicine poisoning — *see* Table of Drugs and Chemicals, by drug, poisoning
Mediterranean
  fever — *see* Brucellosis
    familial E85.0
    tick A77.1
  kala-azar B55.0
  leishmaniasis B55.0
  tick fever A77.1
Medulla — *see* condition
Medullary cystic kidney Q61.5
Medullated fibers
  optic (nerve) Q14.8
  retina Q14.1
Medulloblastoma
  desmoplastic C71.6
  specified site — *see* Neoplasm, malignant, by site
  unspecified site C71.6
Medulloepithelioma (*see also* Neoplasm, malignant, by site)
  teratoid — *see* Neoplasm, malignant, by site
Medullomyoblastoma
  specified site — *see* Neoplasm, malignant, by site
  unspecified site C71.6
Meekeren-Ehlers-Danlos syndrome Q79.6
Megacolon (acquired) (functional) (not Hirschsprung's disease) (in) K59.3
  Chagas' disease B57.32
  congenital, congenitum (aganglionic) Q43.1
  Hirschsprung's (disease) Q43.1
  toxic NEC K59.3

☑ **Additional Character Required — Refer to the Tabular List for Character Selection**   ▽ Subterms under main terms may continue to next column or page

Megacolon — *continued*
  toxic — *continued*
    due to Clostridium difficile A04.7
Megaesophagus (functional) K22.0
  congenital Q39.5
  in (due to) Chagas' disease B57.31
Megalencephaly Q04.5
Megalerythema (epidemic) B08.3
Megaloappendix Q43.8
Megalocephalus, megalocephaly NEC Q75.3
Megalocornea Q15.8
  with glaucoma Q15.0
Megalocytic anemia D53.1
Megalodactylia (fingers) (thumbs) (congenital) Q74.0
  toes Q74.2
Megaloduodenum Q43.8
Megaloesophagus (functional) K22.0
  congenital Q39.5
Megalogastria (acquired) K31.89
  congenital Q40.2
Megalophthalmos Q11.3
Megalopsia H53.15
Megalosplenia — *see* Splenomegaly
Megaloureter N28.82
  congenital Q62.2
Megarectum K62.89
Megasigmoid K59.3
  congenital Q43.2
Megaureter N28.82
  congenital Q62.2
Megavitamin-B6 syndrome E67.2
Megrim — *see* Migraine
Meibomian
  cyst, infected — *see* Hordeolum
  gland — *see* condition
  sty, stye — *see* Hordeolum
Meibomitis — *see* Hordeolum
Meige-Milroy disease (chronic hereditary edema) Q82.0
Meige's syndrome Q82.0
Melalgia, nutritional E53.8
Melancholia F32.9
  climacteric (single episode) F32.8
    recurrent episode F33.9
  hypochondriac F45.29
  intermittent (single episode) F32.8
    recurrent episode F33.9
  involutional (single episode) F32.8
    recurrent episode F33.9
  menopausal (single episode) F32.8
    recurrent episode F33.9
  puerperal F32.8
  reactive (emotional stress or trauma) F32.3
  recurrent F33.9
  senile F03 ☑
  stuporous (single episode) F32.8
    recurrent episode F33.9
Melanemia R79.89
Melanoameloblastoma — *see* Neoplasm, bone, benign
Melanoblastoma — *see* Melanoma
Melanocarcinoma — *see* Melanoma
Melanocytoma, eyeball D31.4- ☑
Melanocytosis, neurocutaneous Q82.8
Melanoderma, melanodermia L81.4
Melanodontia, infantile K03.89
Melanodontoclasia K03.89
Melanoepithelioma — *see* Melanoma
Melanoma (malignant) C43.9
  acral lentiginous, malignant — *see* Melanoma, skin, by site
  amelanotic — *see* Melanoma, skin, by site
  balloon cell — *see* Melanoma, skin, by site
  benign — *see* Nevus
  desmoplastic, malignant — *see* Melanoma, skin, by site
  epithelioid cell — *see* Melanoma, skin, by site
    with spindle cell, mixed — *see* Melanoma, skin, by site
  in
    giant pigmented nevus — *see* Melanoma, skin, by site
    Hutchinson's melanotic freckle — *see* Melanoma, skin, by site
    junctional nevus — *see* Melanoma, skin, by site
    precancerous melanosis — *see* Melanoma, skin, by site
  in situ D03.9
    abdominal wall D03.59

Melanoma — *continued*
  in situ — *continued*
    ala nasi D03.39
    ankle D03.7- ☑
    anus, anal (margin) (skin) D03.51
    arm D03.6- ☑
    auditory canal D03.2- ☑
    auricle (ear) D03.2- ☑
    auricular canal (external) D03.2- ☑
    axilla, axillary fold D03.59
    back D03.59
    breast D03.52
    brow D03.39
    buttock D03.59
    canthus (eye) D03.1- ☑
    cheek (external) D03.39
    chest wall D03.59
    chin D03.39
    choroid D03.8
    conjunctiva D03.8
    ear (external) D03.2- ☑
    external meatus (ear) D03.2- ☑
    eye D03.8
    eyebrow D03.39
    eyelid (lower) (upper) D03.1- ☑
    face D03.30
      specified NEC D03.39
    female genital organ (external) NEC D03.8
    finger D03.6- ☑
    flank D03.59
    foot D03.7- ☑
    forearm D03.6- ☑
    forehead D03.39
    foreskin D03.8
    gluteal region D03.59
    groin D03.59
    hand D03.6- ☑
    heel D03.7- ☑
    helix D03.2- ☑
    hip D03.7- ☑
    interscapular region D03.59
    iris D03.8
    jaw D03.39
    knee D03.7- ☑
    labium (majus) (minus) D03.8
    lacrimal gland D03.8
    leg D03.7- ☑
    lip (lower) (upper) D03.0
    lower limb NEC D03.7- ☑
    male genital organ (external) NEC D03.8
    nail D03.9
      finger D03.6- ☑
      toe D03.7- ☑
    neck D03.4
    nose (external) D03.39
    orbit D03.8
    penis D03.8
    perianal skin D03.51
    perineum D03.51
    pinna D03.2- ☑
    popliteal fossa or space D03.7- ☑
    prepuce D03.8
    pudendum D03.8
    retina D03.8
    retrobulbar D03.8
    scalp D03.4
    scrotum D03.8
    shoulder D03.6- ☑
    specified site NEC D03.8
    submammary fold D03.52
    temple D03.39
    thigh D03.7- ☑
    toe D03.7- ☑
    trunk NEC D03.59
    umbilicus D03.59
    upper limb NEC D03.6- ☑
    vulva D03.8
  juvenile — *see* Nevus
  malignant, of soft parts except skin — *see* Neoplasm, connective tissue, malignant
  metastatic
    breast C79.81
    genital organ C79.82
    specified site NEC C79.89
  neurotropic, malignant — *see* Melanoma, skin, by site
  nodular — *see* Melanoma, skin, by site
  regressing, malignant — *see* Melanoma, skin, by site

Melanoma — *continued*
  skin C43.9
    abdominal wall C43.59
    ala nasi C43.31
    ankle C43.7- ☑
    anus, anal (skin) C43.51
    arm C43.6- ☑
    auditory canal (external) C43.2- ☑
    auricle (ear) C43.2- ☑
    auricular canal (external) C43.2- ☑
    axilla, axillary fold C43.59
    back C43.59
    breast (female) (male) C43.52
    brow C43.39
    buttock C43.59
    canthus (eye) C43.1- ☑
    cheek (external) C43.39
    chest wall C43.59
    chin C43.39
    ear (external) C43.2- ☑
    elbow C43.6- ☑
    external meatus (ear) C43.2- ☑
    eyebrow C43.39
    eyelid (lower) (upper) C43.1- ☑
    face C43.30
      specified NEC C43.39
    female genital organ (external) NEC C51.9
    finger C43.6- ☑
    flank C43.59
    foot C43.7- ☑
    forearm C43.6- ☑
    forehead C43.39
    foreskin C60.0
    glabella C43.39
    gluteal region C43.59
    groin C43.59
    hand C43.6- ☑
    heel C43.7- ☑
    helix C43.2- ☑
    hip C43.7- ☑
    interscapular region C43.59
    jaw (external) C43.39
    knee C43.7- ☑
    labium C51.9
      majus C51.0
      minus C51.1
    leg C43.7- ☑
    lip (lower) (upper) C43.0
    lower limb NEC C43.7- ☑
    male genital organ (external) NEC C63.9
    nail
      finger C43.6- ☑
      toe C43.7- ☑
    nasolabial groove C43.39
    nates C43.59
    neck C43.4
    nose (external) C43.31
    overlapping site C43.8
    palpebra C43.1- ☑
    penis C60.9
    perianal skin C43.51
    perineum C43.51
    pinna C43.2- ☑
    popliteal fossa or space C43.7- ☑
    prepuce C60.0
    pudendum C51.9
    scalp C43.4
    scrotum C63.2
    shoulder C43.6- ☑
    skin NEC C43.9
    submammary fold C43.52
    temple C43.39
    thigh C43.7- ☑
    toe C43.7- ☑
    trunk NEC C43.59
    umbilicus C43.59
    upper limb NEC C43.6- ☑
    vulva C51.9
      overlapping sites C51.8
  spindle cell
    with epithelioid, mixed — *see* Melanoma, skin, by site
    type A C69.4- ☑
    type B C69.4- ☑
  superficial spreading — *see* Melanoma, skin, by site
Melanosarcoma (*see also* Melanoma)
  epithelioid cell — *see* Melanoma

▽ Subterms under main terms may continue to next column or page   ☑ Additional Character Required — Refer to the Tabular List for Character Selection   **213**

Megacolon — Melanosarcoma

Melanosis L81.4
  addisonian E27.1
    tuberculous A18.7
  adrenal E27.1
  colon K63.89
  conjunctiva — *see* Pigmentation, conjunctiva
    congenital Q13.89
  cornea (presenile) (senile) (*see also* Pigmentation, cornea)
    congenital Q13.4
  eye NEC H57.8
    congenital Q15.8
  lenticularis progressiva Q82.1
  liver K76.89
  precancerous (*see also* Melanoma, in situ)
    malignant melanoma in — *see* Melanoma
  Riehl's L81.4
  sclera H15.89
    congenital Q13.89
  suprarenal E27.1
  tar L81.4
  toxic L81.4
Melanuria R82.99
MELAS syndrome E88.41
Melasma L81.1
  adrenal (gland) E27.1
  suprarenal (gland) E27.1
Melena K92.1
  with ulcer — *code by* site under Ulcer, with hemorrhage K27.4
  due to swallowed maternal blood P78.2
  newborn, neonatal P54.1
    due to swallowed maternal blood P78.2
Meleney's
  gangrene (cutaneous) — *see* Ulcer, skin
  ulcer (chronic undermining) — *see* Ulcer, skin
Melioidosis A24.9
  acute A24.1
  chronic A24.2
  fulminating A24.1
  pneumonia A24.1
  pulmonary (chronic) A24.2
    acute A24.1
    subacute A24.2
  sepsis A24.1
  specified NEC A24.3
  subacute A24.2
Melitensis, febris A23.0
Melkersson (-Rosenthal) **syndrome** G51.2
Mellitus, diabetes — *see* Diabetes
Melorheostosis (bone) — *see* Disorder, bone, density and structure, specified NEC
Meloschisis Q18.4
Melotia Q17.4
Membrana
  capsularis lentis posterior Q13.89
  epipapillaris Q14.2
Membranacea placenta O43.19- ☑
Membranaceous uterus N85.8
Membrane(s), membranous (*see also* condition)
  cyclitic — *see* Membrane, pupillary
  folds, congenital — *see* Web
  Jackson's Q43.3
  over face of newborn P28.9
  premature rupture — *see* Rupture, membranes, premature
  pupillary H21.4- ☑
    persistent Q13.89
  retained (with hemorrhage) (complicating delivery) O72.2
    without hemorrhage O73.1
  secondary cataract — *see* Cataract, secondary
  unruptured (causing asphyxia) — *see* Asphyxia, newborn
  vitreous — *see* Opacity, vitreous, membranes and strands
Membranitis — *see* Chorioamnionitis
Memory disturbance, lack or loss (*see also* Amnesia)
  mild, following organic brain damage F06.8
Menadione deficiency E56.1
Menarche
  delayed E30.0
  precocious E30.1
Mendacity, pathologic F60.2
Mendelson's syndrome (due to anesthesia) J95.4
  in labor and delivery O74.0
  in pregnancy O29.01- ☑

Mendelson's syndrome — *continued*
  obstetric O74.0
  postpartum, puerperal O89.01
Ménétrier's disease or syndrome K29.60
  with bleeding K29.61
Ménière's disease, syndrome or vertigo H81.0- ☑
Meninges, meningeal — *see* condition
Meningioma (*see also* Neoplasm, meninges, benign)
  angioblastic — *see* Neoplasm, meninges, benign
  angiomatous — *see* Neoplasm, meninges, benign
  endotheliomatous — *see* Neoplasm, meninges, benign
  fibroblastic — *see* Neoplasm, meninges, benign
  fibrous — *see* Neoplasm, meninges, benign
  hemangioblastic — *see* Neoplasm, meninges, benign
  hemangiopericytic — *see* Neoplasm, meninges, benign
  malignant — *see* Neoplasm, meninges, malignant
  meningiothelial — *see* Neoplasm, meninges, benign
  meningotheliomatous — *see* Neoplasm, meninges, benign
  mixed — *see* Neoplasm, meninges, benign
  multiple — *see* Neoplasm, meninges, uncertain behavior
  papillary — *see* Neoplasm, meninges, uncertain behavior
  psammomatous — *see* Neoplasm, meninges, benign
  syncytial — *see* Neoplasm, meninges, benign
  transitional — *see* Neoplasm, meninges, benign
Meningiomatosis (diffuse) — *see* Neoplasm, meninges, uncertain behavior
Meningism — *see* Meningismus
Meningismus (infectional) (pneumococcal) R29.1
  due to serum or vaccine R29.1
  influenzal — *see* Influenza, with, manifestations NEC
Meningitis (basal) (basic) (brain) (cerebral) (cervical) (congestive) (diffuse) (hemorrhagic) (infantile) (membranous) (metastatic) (nonspecific) (pontine) (progressive) (simple) (spinal) (subacute) (sympathetic) (toxic) G03.9
  abacterial G03.0
  actinomycotic A42.81
  adenoviral A87.1
  arbovirus A87.8
  aseptic (acute) G03.0
  bacterial G00.9
    Escherichia coli (E. coli) G00.8
    Friedländer (bacillus) G00.8
    gram-negative G00.9
    H. influenzae G00.0
    Klebsiella G00.8
    pneumococcal G00.1
    specified organism NEC G00.8
    staphylococcal G00.3
    streptococcal (acute) G00.2
  benign recurrent (Mollaret) G03.2
  candidal B37.5
  caseous (tuberculous) A17.0
  cerebrospinal A39.0
  chronic NEC G03.1
  clear cerebrospinal fluid NEC G03.0
  coxsackievirus A87.0
  cryptococcal B45.1
  diplococcal (gram positive) A39.0
  echovirus A87.0
  enteroviral A87.0
  eosinophilic B83.2
  epidemic NEC A39.0
  Escherichia coli (E. coli) G00.8
  fibrinopurulent G00.9
    specified organism NEC G00.8
  Friedländer (bacillus) G00.8
  gonococcal A54.81
  gram-negative cocci G00.9
  gram-positive cocci G00.9
  H. influenzae G00.0
  Haemophilus (influenzae) G00.0
  in (due to)
    adenovirus A87.1
    African trypanosomiasis B56.9 [G02]
    anthrax A22.8
    bacterial disease NEC A48.8 [G01]
    Chagas' disease (chronic) B57.41
    chickenpox B01.0
    coccidioidomycosis B38.4
    Diplococcus pneumoniae G00.1
    enterovirus A87.0
    herpes (simplex) virus B00.3
      zoster B02.1

Meningitis — *continued*
  in — *continued*
    infectious mononucleosis B27.92
    leptospirosis A27.81
    Listeria monocytogenes A32.11
    Lyme disease A69.21
    measles B05.1
    mumps (virus) B26.1
    neurosyphilis (late) A52.13
    parasitic disease NEC B89 [G02]
    poliovirus A80.9 [G02]
    preventive immunization, inoculation or vaccination G03.8
    rubella B06.02
    Salmonella infection A02.21
    specified cause NEC G03.8
    typhoid fever A01.01
    varicella B01.0
    viral disease NEC A87.8
    whooping cough A37.90
    zoster B02.1
  infectious G00.9
  influenzal (H. influenzae) G00.0
  Klebsiella G00.8
  leptospiral (aseptic) A27.81
  lymphocytic (acute) (benign) (serous) A87.2
  meningococcal A39.0
  Mima polymorpha G00.8
  Mollaret (benign recurrent) G03.2
  monilial B37.5
  mycotic NEC B49 [G02]
  Neisseria A39.0
  nonbacterial G03.0
  nonpyogenic NEC G03.0
  ossificans G96.19
  pneumococcal G00.1
  poliovirus A80.9 [G02]
  postmeasles B05.1
  purulent G00.9
    specified organism NEC G00.8
  pyogenic G00.9
    specified organism NEC G00.8
  Salmonella (arizonae) (Cholerae-Suis) (enteritidis) (typhimurium) A02.21
  septic G00.9
    specified organism NEC G00.8
  serosa circumscripta NEC G03.0
  serous NEC G93.2
  specified organism NEC G00.8
  sporotrichosis B42.81
  staphylococcal G00.3
  sterile G03.0
  streptococcal (acute) G00.2
  suppurative G00.9
    specified organism NEC G00.8
  syphilitic (late) (tertiary) A52.13
    acute A51.41
    congenital A50.41
    secondary A51.41
  Torula histolytica (cryptococcal) B45.1
  traumatic (complication of injury) T79.8 ☑
  tuberculous A17.0
  typhoid A01.01
  viral NEC A87.9
  Yersinia pestis A20.3
Meningocele (spinal) (*see also* Spina bifida)
  with hydrocephalus — *see* Spina bifida, by site, with hydrocephalus
  acquired (traumatic) G96.19
  cerebral — *see* Encephalocele
Meningocerebritis — *see* Meningoencephalitis
Meningococcemia A39.4
  acute A39.2
  chronic A39.3
Meningococcus, meningococcal (*see also* condition) A39.9
  adrenalitis, hemorrhagic A39.1
  carrier (suspected) of Z22.31
  meningitis (cerebrospinal) A39.0
Meningoencephalitis (*see also* Encephalitis) G04.90
  acute NEC (*see also* Encephalitis, viral) A86
  bacterial NEC G04.2
  California A83.5
  diphasic A84.1
  eosinophilic B83.2
  epidemic A39.81
  herpesviral, herpetic B00.4
    due to herpesvirus 6 B10.01

Meningoencephalitis — *continued*
  herpesviral, herpetic — *continued*
    due to herpesvirus 7 B10.09
    specified NEC B10.09
  in (due to)
    blastomycosis NEC B40.81
    diseases classified elsewhere G05.3
    free-living amebae B60.2
    H. influenzae G00.0
    Hemophilus influenzae (H .influenzae) G04.2
    herpes B00.4
      due to herpesvirus 6 B10.01
      due to herpesvirus 7 B10.09
      specified NEC B10.09
    Lyme disease A69.22
    mercury — *see* subcategory T56.1 ☑
    mumps B26.2
    Naegleria (amebae) (organisms) (fowleri) B60.2
    Parastrongylus cantonensis B83.2
    toxoplasmosis (acquired) B58.2
      congenital P37.1
  infectious (acute) (viral) A86
  influenzal (H. influenzae) G04.2
  Listeria monocytogenes A32.12
  lymphocytic (serous) A87.2
  mumps B26.2
  parasitic NEC B89 [G05.3]
  pneumococcal G00.1
  primary amebic B60.2
  specific (syphilitic) A52.14
  specified organism NEC G04.81
  staphylococcal G04.2
  streptococcal G04.2
  syphilitic A52.14
  toxic NEC G92
    due to mercury — *see* subcategory T56.1 ☑
  tuberculous A17.82
  virus NEC A86
Meningoencephalocele (*see also* Encephalocele)
  syphilitic A52.19
    congenital A50.49
Meningoencephalomyelitis (*see also* Meningoencephalitis)
  acute NEC (viral) A86
    disseminated G04.00
      postimmunization or postvaccination G04.02
      postinfectious G04.01
  due to
    actinomycosis A42.82
    Torula B45.1
    Toxoplasma or toxoplasmosis (acquired) B58.2
      congenital P37.1
  postimmunization or postvaccination G04.02
Meningoencephalomyelopathy G96.9
Meningoencephalopathy G96.9
Meningomyelitis (*see also* Meningoencephalitis)
  bacterial NEC G04.2
  blastomycotic NEC B40.81
  cryptococcal B45.1
  in diseases classified elsewhere G05.4
  meningococcal A39.81
  syphilitic A52.14
  tuberculous A17.82
Meningomyelocele (*see also* Spina bifida)
  syphilitic A52.19
Meningomyeloneuritis — *see* Meningoencephalitis
Meningoradiculitis — *see* Meningitis
Meningovascular — *see* condition
Menkes' disease or syndrome E83.09
  meaning maple-syrup-urine disease E71.0
Menometrorrhagia N92.1
Menopause, menopausal (asymptomatic) (state) Z78.0
  arthritis (any site) NEC — *see* Arthritis, specified form NEC
  bleeding N92.4
  depression (single episode) F32.8
    agitated (single episode) F32.2
      recurrent episode F33.9
    psychotic (single episode) F32.8
      recurrent episode F33.9
    recurrent episode F33.9
  melancholia (single episode) F32.8
    recurrent episode F33.9
  paranoid state F22
  premature E28.319
    asymptomatic E28.319
      postirradiation E89.40
      postsurgical E89.40

Menopause, menopausal — *continued*
  premature — *continued*
    symptomatic E28.310
      postirradiation E89.41
      postsurgical E89.41
  psychosis NEC F28
  symptomatic N95.1
  toxic polyarthritis NEC — *see* Arthritis, specified form NEC
Menorrhagia (primary) N92.0
  climacteric N92.4
    menopausal N92.4
  menopausal N92.4
  postclimacteric N95.0
  postmenopausal N95.0
  preclimacteric or premenopausal N92.4
  pubertal (menses retained) N92.2
Menostaxis N92.0
Menses, retention N94.89
Menstrual — *see* Menstruation
Menstruation
  absent — *see* Amenorrhea
  anovulatory N97.0
  cycle, irregular N92.6
  delayed N91.0
  disorder N93.9
    psychogenic F45.8
  during pregnancy O20.8
  excessive (with regular cycle) N92.0
    with irregular cycle N92.1
    at puberty N92.2
  frequent N92.0
  infrequent — *see* Oligomenorrhea
  irregular N92.6
    specified NEC N92.5
  latent N92.5
  membranous N92.5
  painful (*see also* Dysmenorrhea) N94.6
    primary N94.4
    psychogenic F45.8
    secondary N94.5
  passage of clots N92.0
  precocious E30.1
  protracted N92.5
  rare — *see* Oligomenorrhea
  retained N94.89
  retrograde N92.5
  scanty — *see* Oligomenorrhea
  suppression N94.89
  vicarious (nasal) N94.89
Mental (*see also* condition)
  deficiency — *see* Disability, intellectual
  deterioration — *see* Psychosis
  disorder — *see* Disorder, mental
  exhaustion F48.8
  insufficiency (congenital) — *see* Disability, intellectual
  observation without need for further medical care Z03.89
  retardation — *see* Disability, intellectual
  subnormality — *see* Disability, intellectuall
  upset — *see* Disorder, mental
Meralgia paresthetica G57.1- ☑
Mercurial — *see* condition
Mercurialism — *see* subcategory T56.1 ☑
Merkel cell tumor — *see* Carcinoma, Merkel cell
Merocele — *see* Hernia, femoral
Meromelia
  lower limb — *see* Defect, reduction, lower limb
    intercalary
      femur — *see* Defect, reduction, lower limb, specified type NEC
        tibiofibular (complete) (incomplete) — *see* Defect, reduction, lower limb
  upper limb — *see* Defect, reduction, upper limb
    intercalary, humeral, radioulnar — *see* Agenesis, arm, with hand present
MERRF syndrome (myoclonic epilepsy associated with ragged-red fiber) E88.42
Merzbacher-Pelizaeus disease E75.29
Mesaortitis — *see* Aortitis
Mesarteritis — *see* Arteritis
Mesencephalitis — *see* Encephalitis
Mesenchymoma (*see also* Neoplasm, connective tissue, uncertain behavior)
  benign — *see* Neoplasm, connective tissue, benign
  malignant — *see* Neoplasm, connective tissue, malignant

Mesenteritis
  retractile K65.4
  sclerosing K65.4
Mesentery, mesenteric — *see* condition
Mesiodens, mesiodentes K00.1
Mesio-occlusion M26.213
Mesocolon — *see* condition
Mesonephroma (malignant) — *see* Neoplasm, malignant, by site
  benign — *see* Neoplasm, benign, by site
Mesophlebitis — *see* Phlebitis
Mesostromal dysgenesia Q13.89
Mesothelioma (malignant) C45.9
  benign
    mesentery D19.1
    mesocolon D19.1
    omentum D19.1
    peritoneum D19.1
    pleura D19.0
    specified site NEC D19.7
    unspecified site D19.9
  biphasic C45.9
    benign
      mesentery D19.1
      mesocolon D19.1
      omentum D19.1
      peritoneum D19.1
      pleura D19.0
      specified site NEC D19.7
      unspecified site D19.9
  cystic D48.4
  epithelioid C45.9
    benign
      mesentery D19.1
      mesocolon D19.1
      omentum D19.1
      peritoneum D19.1
      pleura D19.0
      specified site NEC D19.7
      unspecified site D19.9
  fibrous C45.9
    benign
      mesentery D19.1
      mesocolon D19.1
      omentum D19.1
      peritoneum D19.1
      pleura D19.0
      specified site NEC D19.7
      unspecified site D19.9
  site classification
    liver C45.7
    lung C45.7
    mediastinum C45.7
    mesentery C45.1
    mesocolon C45.1
    omentum C45.1
    pericardium C45.2
    peritoneum C45.1
    pleura C45.0
      parietal C45.0
    retroperitoneum C45.7
    specified site NEC C45.7
    unspecified C45.9
Metabolic syndrome E88.81
Metagonimiasis B66.8
Metagonimus infestation (intestine) B66.8
Metal
  pigmentation L81.8
  polisher's disease J62.8
Metamorphopsia H53.15
Metaplasia
  apocrine (breast) — *see* Dysplasia, mammary, specified type NEC
  cervix (squamous) — *see* Dysplasia, cervix
  endometrium (squamous) (uterus) N85.8
  esophagus
  kidney (pelvis) (squamous) N28.89
  myelogenous D73.1
  myeloid (agnogenic) (megakaryocytic) D73.1
  spleen D73.1
  squamous cell, bladder N32.89
Metastasis, metastatic
  abscess — *see* Abscess
  calcification E83.59
  cancer
    from specified site — *see* Neoplasm, malignant, by site

Metastasis, metastatic — *continued*
  cancer — *continued*
    to specified site — *see* Neoplasm, secondary, by site
    deposits (in) — *see* Neoplasm, secondary, by site
    disease (*see also* Neoplasm, secondary, by site) C79.9
    spread (to) — *see* Neoplasm, secondary, by site
Metastrongyliasis B83.8
Metatarsalgia M77.4- ☑
  anterior G57.6- ☑
  Morton's G57.6- ☑
Metatarsus, metatarsal (*see also* condition)
  valgus (abductus), congenital Q66.6
  varus (adductus) (congenital) Q66.2
Methadone use F11.20
Methemoglobinemia D74.9
  acquired (with sulfhemoglobinemia) D74.8
  congenital D74.0
  enzymatic (congenital) D74.0
  Hb M disease D74.0
  hereditary D74.0
  toxic D74.8
Methemoglobinuria — *see* Hemoglobinuria
Methioninemia E72.19
Methylmalonic acidemia E71.120
Metritis (catarrhal) (hemorrhagic) (septic) (suppurative) (*see also* Endometritis)
  cervical — *see* Cervicitis
Metropathia hemorrhagica N93.8
Metroperitonitis — *see* Peritonitis, pelvic, female
Metrorrhagia N92.1
  climacteric N92.4
  menopausal N92.4
  postpartum NEC (atonic) (following delivery of placenta) O72.1
    delayed or secondary O72.2
  preclimacteric or premenopausal N92.4
  psychogenic F45.8
Metrorrhexis — *see* Rupture, uterus
Metrosalpingitis N70.91
Metrostaxis N93.8
Metrovaginitis — *see* Endometritis
Meyer-Schwickerath and Weyers syndrome Q87.0
Meynert's amentia (nonalcoholic) F04
  alcoholic F10.96
    with dependence F10.26
Mibelli's disease (porokeratosis) Q82.8
Mice, joint — *see* Loose, body, joint
  knee M23.4- ☑
Micrencephalon, micrencephaly Q02
Microalbuminuria R80.9
Microaneurysm, retinal (*see also* Disorder, retina, microaneurysms)
  diabetic — *see* E08-E13 with .31
Microangiopathy (peripheral) I73.9
  thrombotic M31.1
Microcalcifications, breast R92.0
Microcephalus, microcephalic, microcephaly Q02
  due to toxoplasmosis (congenital) P37.1
Microcheilia Q18.7
Microcolon (congenital) Q43.8
Microcornea (congenital) Q13.4
Microcytic — *see* condition
Microdeletions NEC Q93.88
Microdontia K00.2
Microdrepanocytosis D57.40
  with crisis (vasoocclusive pain) D57.419
    with
      acute chest syndrome D57.411
      splenic sequestration D57.412
Microembolism
  atherothrombotic — *see* Atheroembolism
  retinal — *see* Occlusion, artery, retina
Microencephalon Q02
Microfilaria streptocerca infestation — *see* Onchocerciasis
Microgastria (congenital) Q40.2
Microgenia M26.06
Microgenitalia, congenital
  female Q52.8
  male Q55.8
Microglioma — *see* Lymphoma, non-Hodgkin, specified NEC
Microglossia (congenital) Q38.3
Micrognathia, micrognathism (congenital) (mandibular) (maxillary) M26.09
Microgyria (congenital) Q04.3

Microinfarct of heart — *see* Insufficiency, coronary
Microlentia (congenital) Q12.8
Microlithiasis, alveolar, pulmonary J84.02
Micromastia N64.82
Micromyelia (congenital) Q06.8
Micropenis Q55.62
Microphakia (congenital) Q12.8
Microphthalmos, microphthalmia (congenital) Q11.2
  due to toxoplasmosis P37.1
Micropsia H53.15
Microscopic polyangiitis (polyarteritis) M31.7
Microsporidiosis B60.8
  intestinal A07.8
Microsporon furfur infestation B36.0
Microsporosis (*see also* Dermatophytosis)
  nigra B36.1
Microstomia (congenital) Q18.5
Microtia (congenital) (external ear) Q17.2
Microtropia H50.40
Microvillus inclusion disease (MVD) (MVID) Q43.8
Micturition
  disorder NEC R39.19
    psychogenic F45.8
  frequency R35.0
    psychogenic F45.8
  hesitancy R39.11
  incomplete emptying R39.14
  nocturnal R35.1
  painful R30.9
    dysuria R30.0
    psychogenic F45.8
    tenesmus R30.1
  poor stream R39.12
  split stream R39.13
  straining R39.16
  urgency R39.15
Mid plane — *see* condition
Middle
  ear — *see* condition
  lobe (right) syndrome J98.19
Miescher's elastoma L87.2
Mietens' syndrome Q87.2
Migraine (idiopathic) G43.909
  with aura (acute-onset) (prolonged) (typical) (without headache) G43.109
    with refractory migraine G43.119
      with status migrainosus G43.111
      without status migrainosus G43.119
    without mention of refractory migraine G43.109
      with status migrainosus G43.101
      without status migrainosus G43.109
    intractable G43.119
      with status migrainosus G43.111
      without status migrainosus G43.119
    not intractable G43.109
      with status migrainosus G43.101
      without status migrainosus G43.109
    persistent G43.509
      with cerebral infarction G43.609
        with refractory migraine G43.619
          with status migrainosus G43.611
          without status migrainosus G43.619
        without refractory migraine G43.609
          with status migrainosus G43.601
          without status migrainosus G43.609
        intractable G43.619
          with status migrainosus G43.611
          without status migrainosus G43.619
        not intractable G43.609
          with status migrainosus G43.601
          without status migrainosus G43.609
      without cerebral infarction G43.509
        with refractory migraine G43.519
          with status migrainosus G43.511
          without status migrainosus G43.519
        without refractory migraine G43.509
          with status migrainosus G43.501
          without status migrainosus G43.509
        intractable G43.519
          with status migrainosus G43.511
          without status migrainosus G43.519
        not intractable G43.509
          with status migrainosus G43.501
          without status migrainosus G43.509
    with refractory migraine G43.911
      with status migrainosus G43.911
      without status migrainosus G43.919
  without aura G43.009

Migraine — *continued*
  without aura — *continued*
    with refractory migraine G43.019
      with status migrainosus G43.011
      without status migrainosus G43.019
    without mention of refractory migraine G43.009
      with status migrainosus G43.001
      without status migrainosus G43.009
    chronic G43.709
      with refractory migraine G43.719
        with status migrainosus G43.711
        without status migrainosus G43.719
      without refractory migraine G43.709
        with status migrainosus G43.701
        without status migrainosus G43.709
      intractable
        with status migrainosus G43.711
        without status migrainosus G43.719
      not intractable
        with status migrainosus G43.701
        without status migrainosus G43.709
    intractable
      with status migrainosus G43.011
      without status migrainosus G43.019
    not intractable
      with status migrainosus G43.001
      without status migrainosus G43.009
  without refractory migraine G43.909
    with status migrainosus G43.901
    without status migrainosus G43.919
  abdominal G43.D0 (*following* G43.7)
    with refractory migraine G43.D1 (*following* G43.7)
    without refractory migraine G43.D0 (*following* G43.7)
    intractable G43.D1 (*following* G43.7)
    not intractable G43.D0 (*following* G43.7)
  basilar — *see* Migraine, with aura
  classical — *see* Migraine, with aura
  common — *see* Migraine, without aura
  complicated G43.109
  equivalents — *see* Migraine, with aura
  familiar — *see* Migraine, hemiplegic
  hemiplegic G43.409
    with refractory migraine G43.419
      with status migrainosus G43.411
      without status migrainosus G43.419
    without refractory migraine G43.409
      with status migrainosus G43.401
      without status migrainosus G43.409
    intractable G43.419
      with status migrainosus G43.411
      without status migrainosus G43.419
    not intractable G43.409
      with status migrainosus G43.401
      without status migrainosus G43.409
  intractable G43.919
    with status migrainosus G43.911
    without status migrainosus G43.919
  menstrual G43.829
    with refractory migraine G43.839
      with status migrainosus G43.831
      without status migrainosus G43.839
    without refractory migraine G43.829
      with status migrainosus G43.821
      without status migrainosus G43.829
    intractable G43.839
      with status migrainosus G43.831
      without status migrainosus G43.839
    not intractable G43.829
      with status migrainosus G43.821
      without status migrainosus G43.829
  menstrually related — *see* Migraine, menstrual
  not intractable G43.909
    with status migrainosus G43.901
    without status migrainosus G43.919
  ophthalmoplegic G43.B0 (*following* G43.7)
    with refractory migraine G43.B1 (*following* G43.7)
    without refractory migraine G43.B0 (*following* G43.7)
    intractable G43.B1 (*following* G43.7)
    not intractable G43.B0 (*following* G43.7)
  persistent aura (with, without) cerebral infarction — *see* Migraine, with aura, persistent
  preceded or accompanied by transient focal neurological phenomena — *see* Migraine, with aura
  pre-menstrual — *see* Migraine, menstrual
  pure menstrual — *see* Migraine, menstrual
  retinal — *see* Migraine, with aura

Migraine — *continued*
 specified NEC G43.809
  intractable G43.819
   with status migrainosus G43.811
   without status migrainosus G43.819
  not intractable G43.809
   with status migrainosus G43.801
   without status migrainosus G43.809
 sporadic — *see* Migraine, hemiplegic
 transformed — *see* Migraine, without aura, chronic
 triggered seizures — *see* Migraine, with aura
Migrant, social Z59.0
Migration, anxiety concerning Z60.3
Migratory, migrating (*see also* condition)
 person Z59.0
 testis Q55.29
Mikity-Wilson disease or syndrome P27.0
Mikulicz' disease or syndrome K11.8
Miliaria L74.3
 alba L74.1
 apocrine L75.2
 crystallina L74.1
 profunda L74.2
 rubra L74.0
 tropicalis L74.2
Miliary — *see* condition
Milium L72.0
 colloid L57.8
Milk
 crust L21.0
 excessive secretion O92.6
 poisoning — *see* Poisoning, food, noxious
 retention O92.79
 sickness — *see* Poisoning, food, noxious
 spots I31.0
Milk-alkali disease or syndrome E83.52
Milk-leg (deep vessels) (nonpuerperal) — *see* Embolism, vein, lower extremity
 complicating pregnancy O22.3- ☑
 puerperal, postpartum, childbirth O87.1
Milky urine — *see* Chyluria
Millard-Gubler (-Foville) **paralysis or syndrome** G46.3
Millar's asthma J38.5
Miller Fisher syndrome G61.0
Mills' disease — *see* Hemiplegia
Millstone maker's pneumoconiosis J62.8
Milroy's disease (chronic hereditary edema) Q82.0
Minamata disease T26.1- ☑
Miners' asthma or lung J60
Minkowski-Chauffard syndrome — *see* Spherocytosis
Minor — *see* condition
Minor's disease (hematomyelia) G95.19
Minot's disease (hemorrhagic disease), newborn P53
Minot-von Willebrand-Jurgens disease or syndrome (angiohemophilia) D68.0
Minus (and plus) **hand** (intrinsic) — *see* Deformity, limb, specified type NEC, forearm
Miosis (pupil) H57.03
Mirizzi's syndrome (hepatic duct stenosis) K83.1
Mirror writing F81.0
Misadventure (of) (prophylactic) (therapeutic) (*see also* Complications) T88.9 ☑
 administration of insulin (by accident) — *see* subcategory T38.3
 infusion — *see* Complications, infusion
 local applications (of fomentations, plasters, etc.) T88.9 ☑
  burn or scald — *see* Burn
  specified NEC T88.8 ☑
 medical care (early) (late) T88.9 ☑
  adverse effect of drugs or chemicals — *see* Table of Drugs and Chemicals
  burn or scald — *see* Burn
  specified NEC T88.8 ☑
 specified NEC T88.8 ☑
 surgical procedure (early) (late) — *see* Complications, surgical procedure
 transfusion — *see* Complications, transfusion
 vaccination or other immunological procedure — *see* Complications, vaccination
Miscarriage O03.9
Misdirection, aqueous H40.83- ☑
Misperception, sleep state F51.02
Misplaced, misplacement
 ear Q17.4
 kidney (acquired) N28.89

Misplaced, misplacement — *continued*
 kidney — *continued*
  congenital Q63.2
 organ or site, congenital NEC — *see* Malposition, congenital
Missed
 abortion O02.1
 delivery O36.4 ☑
Missing — *see* Absence
Misuse of drugs F19.99
Mitchell's disease (erythromelalgia) I73.81
Mite(s) (infestation) B88.9
 diarrhea B88.0
 grain (itch) B88.0
 hair follicle (itch) B88.0
 in sputum B88.0
Mitral — *see* condition
Mittelschmerz N94.0
Mixed — *see* condition
MNGIE (Mitochondrial Neurogastrointestinal Encephalopathy) **syndrome** E88.49
Mobile, mobility
 cecum Q43.3
 excessive — *see* Hypermobility
 gallbladder, congenital Q44.1
 kidney N28.89
 organ or site, congenital NEC — *see* Malposition, congenital
Mobitz heart block (atrioventricular) I44.1
Moebius, Möbius
 disease (ophthalmoplegic migraine) — *see* Migraine, ophthalmoplegic
 syndrome Q87.0
  congenital oculofacial paralysis (with other anomalies) Q87.0
  ophthalmoplegic migraine — *see* Migraine, ophthalmoplegic
Moeller's glossitis K14.0
Mohr's syndrome (Types I and II) Q87.0
Mola destruens D39.2
Molar pregnancy O02.0
Molarization of premolars K00.2
Molding, head (during birth) — *omit code*
Mole (pigmented) (*see also* Nevus)
 blood O02.0
 Breus' O02.0
 cancerous — *see* Melanoma
 carneous O02.0
 destructive D39.2
 fleshy O02.0
 hydatid, hydatidiform (benign) (complicating pregnancy) (delivered) (undelivered) O01.9
  classical O01.0
  complete O01.0
  incomplete O01.1
  invasive D39.2
  malignant D39.2
  partial O01.1
 intrauterine O02.0
 invasive (hydatidiform) D39.2
 malignant
  meaning
   malignant hydatidiform mole D39.2
   melanoma — *see* Melanoma
 nonhydatidiform O02.0
 nonpigmented — *see* Nevus
 pregnancy NEC O02.0
 skin — *see* Nevus
 tubal O00.1
 vesicular — *see* Mole, hydatidiform
Molimen, molimina (menstrual) N94.3
Molluscum contagiosum (epitheliale) B08.1
Mönckeberg's arteriosclerosis, disease, or sclerosis — *see* Arteriosclerosis, extremities
Mondini's malformation (cochlea) Q16.5
Mondor's disease I80.8
Monge's disease T70.29 ☑
Monilethrix (congenital) Q84.1
Moniliasis (*see also* Candidiasis) B37.9
 neonatal P37.5
Monitoring (encounter for)
 therapeutic drug level Z51.81
Monkey malaria B53.1
Monkeypox B04
Monoarthritis M13.10
 ankle M13.17- ☑
 elbow M13.12- ☑

Monoarthritis — *continued*
 foot joint M13.17- ☑
 hand joint M13.14- ☑
 hip M13.15- ☑
 knee M13.16- ☑
 shoulder M13.11- ☑
 wrist M13.13- ☑
Monoblastic — *see* condition
Monochromat (ism), monochromatopsia (acquired) (congenital) H53.51
Monocytic — *see* condition
Monocytopenia D72.818
Monocytosis (symptomatic) D72.821
Monomania — *see* Psychosis
Mononeuritis G58.9
 cranial nerve — *see* Disorder, nerve, cranial
 femoral nerve G57.2- ☑
 lateral
  cutaneous nerve of thigh G57.1- ☑
  popliteal nerve G57.3- ☑
 lower limb G57.9- ☑
  specified nerve NEC G57.8- ☑
 medial popliteal nerve G57.4- ☑
 median nerve G56.1- ☑
 multiplex G58.7
 plantar nerve G57.6- ☑
 posterior tibial nerve G57.5- ☑
 radial nerve G56.3- ☑
 sciatic nerve G57.0- ☑
 specified NEC G58.8
 tibial nerve G57.4- ☑
 ulnar nerve G56.2- ☑
 upper limb G56.9- ☑
  specified nerve NEC G56.8- ☑
 vestibular — *see* subcategory H93.3 ☑
Mononeuropathy G58.9
 carpal tunnel syndrome — *see* Syndrome, carpal tunnel
 diabetic NEC — *see* E08-E13 with .41
 femoral nerve — *see* Lesion, nerve, femoral
 ilioinguinal nerve G57.8- ☑
 in diseases classified elsewhere — *see* category G59
 intercostal G58.0
 lower limb G57.9- ☑
  causalgia — *see* Causalgia, lower limb
  femoral nerve — *see* Lesion, nerve, femoral
  meralgia paresthetica G57.1- ☑
  plantar nerve — *see* Lesion, nerve, plantar
  popliteal nerve — *see* Lesion, nerve, popliteal
  sciatic nerve — *see* Lesion, nerve, sciatic
  specified NEC G57.8- ☑
  tarsal tunnel syndrome — *see* Syndrome, tarsal tunnel
 median nerve — *see* Lesion, nerve, median
 multiplex G58.7
 obturator nerve G57.8- ☑
 popliteal nerve — *see* Lesion, nerve, popliteal
 radial nerve — *see* Lesion, nerve, radial
 saphenous nerve G57.8- ☑
 specified NEC G58.8
 tarsal tunnel syndrome — *see* Syndrome, tarsal tunnel
 tuberculous A17.83
 ulnar nerve — *see* Lesion, nerve, ulnar
 upper limb G56.9- ☑
  carpal tunnel syndrome — *see* Syndrome, carpal tunnel
  causalgia — *see* Causalgia
  median nerve — *see* Lesion, nerve, median
  radial nerve — *see* Lesion, nerve, radial
  specified site NEC G56.8- ☑
  ulnar nerve — *see* Lesion, nerve, ulnar
Mononucleosis, infectious B27.90
 with
  complication NEC B27.99
  meningitis B27.92
  polyneuropathy B27.91
 cytomegaloviral B27.10
  with
   complication NEC B27.19
   meningitis B27.12
   polyneuropathy B27.11
 Epstein-Barr (virus) B27.00
  with
   complication NEC B27.09
   meningitis B27.02
   polyneuropathy B27.01

Mononucleosis, infectious — continued
  gammaherpesviral B27.00
    with
      complication NEC B27.09
      meningitis B27.02
      polyneuropathy B27.01
  specified NEC B27.80
    with
      complication NEC B27.89
      meningitis B27.82
      polyneuropathy B27.81
Monoplegia G83.3- ☑
  congenital (cerebral) G80.8
    spastic G80.1
  embolic (current episode) I63.4 ☑
  following
    cerebrovascular disease
      cerebral infarction
        lower limb I69.34- ☑
        upper limb I69.33- ☑
      intracerebral hemorrhage
        lower limb I69.14- ☑
        upper limb I69.13- ☑
      lower limb I69.94- ☑
      nontraumatic intracranial hemorrhage NEC
        lower limb I69.24- ☑
        upper limb I69.23- ☑
      specified disease NEC
        lower limb I69.84- ☑
        upper limb I69.83- ☑
      stroke NOS
        lower limb I69.34- ☑
        upper limb I69.33- ☑
      subarachnoid hemorrhage
        lower limb I69.04- ☑
        upper limb I69.03- ☑
      upper limb I69.93- ☑
  hysterical (transient) F44.4
  lower limb G83.1- ☑
  psychogenic (conversion reaction) F44.4
  thrombotic (current episode) I63.3 ☑
  transient R29.818
  upper limb G83.2- ☑
Monorchism, monorchidism Q55.0
Monosomy (see also Deletion, chromosome) Q93.9
  specified NEC Q93.89
  whole chromosome
    meiotic nondisjunction Q93.0
    mitotic nondisjunction Q93.1
    mosaicism Q93.1
  X Q96.9
Monster, monstrosity (single) Q89.7
  acephalic Q00.0
  twin Q89.4
Monteggia's fracture (-dislocation) S52.27- ☑
Mooren's ulcer (cornea) — see Ulcer, cornea, Mooren's
Moore's syndrome — see Epilepsy, specified NEC
Mooser-Neill reaction A75.2
Mooser's bodies A75.2
Morbidity not stated or unknown R69
Morbilli — see Measles
Morbus (see also Disease)
  angelicus, anglorum E55.0
  Beigel B36.2
  caducus — see Epilepsy
  celiacus K90.0
  comitialis — see Epilepsy
  cordis (see also Disease, heart) I51.9
    valvulorum — see Endocarditis
  coxae senilis M16.9
    tuberculous A18.02
  hemorrhagicus neonatorum P53
  maculosus neonatorum P54.5
Morel (-Stewart)(-Morgagni) **syndrome** M85.2
Morel-Kraepelin disease — see Schizophrenia
Morel-Moore syndrome M85.2
Morgagni's
  cyst, organ, hydatid, or appendage
    female Q50.5
    male (epididymal) Q55.4
      testicular Q55.29
  syndrome M85.2
Morgagni-Stewart-Morel syndrome M85.2
Morgagni-Stokes-Adams syndrome I45.9
Morgagni-Turner (-Albright) **syndrome** Q96.9
Moria F07.0
Moron (I.Q. 50-69) F70

Morphea L94.0
Morphinism (without remission) F11.20
  with remission F11.21
Morphinomania (without remission) F11.20
  with remission F11.21
Morquio (-Ullrich)(-Brailsford) **disease or syndrome** —
  see Mucopolysaccharidosis
Mortification (dry) (moist) — see Gangrene
Morton's metatarsalgia (neuralgia)(neuroma) (syn-
  drome) G57.6-
Morvan's disease or syndrome G60.8
Mosaicism, mosaic (autosomal) (chromosomal)
  45,X/46,XX Q96.3
  45,X/other cell lines NEC with abnormal sex chromo-
    some Q96.4
  sex chromosome
    female Q97.8
    lines with various numbers of X chromosomes
      Q97.2
    male Q98.7
  XY Q96.3
Moschowitz' disease M31.1
Mother yaw A66.0
Motion sickness (from travel, any vehicle) (from round-
  abouts or swings) T75.3 ☑
Mottled, mottling, teeth (enamel) (endemic) (nonen-
  demic) K00.3
Mounier-Kuhn syndrome Q32.4
  with bronchiectasis J47.9
    exacerbation (acute) J47.1
    lower respiratory infection J47.0
  acquired J98.09
    with bronchiectasis J47.9
      with
        exacerbation (acute) J47.1
        lower respiratory infection J47.0
Mountain
  sickness T70.29 ☑
    with polycythemia , acquired (acute) D75.1
  tick fever A93.2
Mouse, joint — see Loose, body, joint
  knee M23.4- ☑
Mouth — see condition
Movable
  coccyx — see subcategory M53.2 ☑
  kidney N28.89
    congenital Q63.8
  spleen D73.89
Movements, dystonic R25.8
Moyamoya disease I67.5
MRSA (Methicillin resistant Staphylococcus aureus)
  infection A49.02
    as the cause of diseases classified elsewhere B95.62
  sepsis A41.02
MSSA (Methicillin susceptible Staphylococcus aureus)
  infection A49.01
    as the cause of diseases classified elsewhere B95.61
  sepsis A41.01
Mucha-Habermann disease L41.0
Mucinosis (cutaneous) (focal) (papular) (skin) L98.5
  oral K13.79
Mucocele
  appendix K38.8
  buccal cavity K13.79
  gallbladder K82.1
  lacrimal sac, chronic H04.43- ☑
  nasal sinus J34.1
  nose J34.1
  salivary gland (any) K11.6
  sinus (accessory) (nasal) J34.1
  turbinate (bone) (middle) (nasal) J34.1
  uterus N85.8
Mucolipidosis
  I E77.1
  II, III E77.0
  IV E75.11
Mucopolysaccharidosis E76.3
  beta-gluduronidase deficiency E76.29
  cardiopathy E76.3 [I52]
  Hunter's syndrome E76.1
  Hurler's syndrome E76.01
  Hurler-Scheie syndrome E76.02
  Maroteaux-Lamy syndrome E76.29
  Morquio syndrome E76.219
    A E76.210
    B E76.211
    classic E76.210

Mucopolysaccharidosis — continued
  Sanfilippo syndrome E76.22
  Scheie's syndrome E76.03
  specified NEC E76.29
  type
    I
      Hurler's syndrome E76.01
      Hurler-Scheie syndrome E76.02
      Scheie's syndrome E76.03
    II E76.1
    III E76.22
    IV E76.219
    IVA E76.210
    IVB E76.211
    VI E76.29
    VII E76.29
Mucormycosis B46.5
  cutaneous B46.3
  disseminated B46.4
  gastrointestinal B46.2
  generalized B46.4
  pulmonary B46.0
  rhinocerebral B46.1
  skin B46.3
  subcutaneous B46.3
Mucositis (ulcerative) K12.30
  due to drugs NEC K12.32
  gastrointestinal K92.81
  mouth (oral) (oropharyngeal) K12.30
    due to antineoplastic therapy K12.31
    due to drugs NEC K12.32
    due to radiation K12.33
    specified NEC K12.39
    viral K12.39
  nasal J34.81
  oral cavity — see Mucositis, mouth
  oral soft tissues — see Mucositis, mouth
  vagina and vulva N76.81
Mucositis necroticans agranulocytica — see Agranulocytosis
Mucous (see also condition)
  patches (syphilitic) A51.39
    congenital A50.07
Mucoviscidosis E84.9
  with meconium obstruction E84.11
Mucus
  asphyxia or suffocation — see Asphyxia, mucus
  in stool R19.5
  plug — see Asphyxia, mucus
Muguet B37.0
Mulberry molars (congenital syphilis) A50.52
Müllerian mixed tumor
  specified site — see Neoplasm, malignant, by site
  unspecified site C54.9
Multicystic kidney (development) Q61.4
Multiparity (grand) Z64.1
  affecting management of pregnancy, labor and deliv-
    ery (supervision only) O09.4- ☑
  requiring contraceptive management — see Contra-
    ception
Multipartita placenta O43.19- ☑
Multiple, multiplex (see also condition)
  digits (congenital) Q69.9
  endocrine neoplasia — see Neoplasia, endocrine,
    multiple (MEN)
  personality F44.81
Mumps B26.9
  arthritis B26.85
  complication NEC B26.89
  encephalitis B26.2
  hepatitis B26.81
  meningitis (aseptic) B26.1
  meningoencephalitis B26.2
  myocarditis B26.82
  oophoritis B26.89
  orchitis B26.0
  pancreatitis B26.3
  polyneuropathy B26.84
Mumu (see also Infestation, filarial) B74.9 [N51]
Münchhausen's syndrome — see Disorder, factitious
Münchmeyer's syndrome — see Myositis, ossificans,
  progressiva
Mural — see condition
Murmur (cardiac) (heart) (organic) R01.1
  abdominal R19.15
  aortic (valve) — see Endocarditis, aortic
  benign R01.0
  diastolic — see Endocarditis

Murmur — *continued*
Flint I35.1
functional R01.0
Graham Steell I37.1
innocent R01.0
mitral (valve) — *see* Insufficiency, mitral
nonorganic R01.0
presystolic, mitral — *see* Insufficiency, mitral
pulmonic (valve) I37.8
systolic (valvular) — *see* Endocarditis
tricuspid (valve) I07.9
valvular — *see* Endocarditis
Murri's disease (intermittent hemoglobinuria) D59.6
Muscle, muscular (*see also* condition)
carnitine (palmityltransferase) deficiency E71.314
Musculoneuralgia — *see* Neuralgia
Mushrooming hip — *see* Derangement, joint, specified NEC, hip
Mushroom-workers' (pickers') **disease or lung** J67.5
Mutation(s)
factor V Leiden D68.51
prothrombin gene D68.52
surfactant, of lung J84.83
Mutism (*see also* Aphasia)
deaf (acquired) (congenital) NEC H91.3
elective (adjustment reaction) (childhood) F94.0
hysterical F44.4
selective (childhood) F94.0
MVD (microvillus inclusion disease) Q43.8
MVID (microvillus inclusion disease) Q43.8
Myalgia M79.1
epidemic (cervical) B33.0
traumatic NEC T14.8
Myasthenia G70.9
congenital G70.2
cordis — *see* Failure, heart
developmental G70.2
gravis G70.00
with exacerbation (acute) G70.01
in crisis G70.01
neonatal, transient P94.0
pseudoparalytica G70.00
with exacerbation (acute) G70.01
in crisis G70.01
stomach, psychogenic F45.8
syndrome
in
diabetes mellitus — *see* E08-E13 with .44
neoplastic disease (*see also* Neoplasm)
D49.9 [G73.3]
pernicious anemia D51.0 [G73.3]
thyrotoxicosis E05.90 [G73.3]
with thyroid storm E05.91 [G73.3]
Myasthenic M62.81
Mycelium infection B49
Mycetismus — *see* Poisoning, food, noxious, mushroom
Mycetoma B47.9
actinomycotic B47.1
bone (mycotic) B47.9 [M90.80]
eumycotic B47.0
foot B47.9
actinomycotic B47.1
mycotic B47.0
madurae NEC B47.9
mycotic B47.0
maduromycotic B47.0
mycotic B47.0
nocardial B47.1
Mycobacteriosis — *see* Mycobacterium
Mycobacterium, mycobacterial (infection) A31.9
anonymous A31.9
atypical A31.9
cutaneous A31.1
pulmonary A31.0
tuberculous — *see* Tuberculosis, pulmonary
specified site NEC A31.8
avium (intracellulare complex) A31.0
balnei A31.1
Battey A31.0
chelonei A31.8
cutaneous A31.1
extrapulmonary systemic A31.8
fortuitum A31.8
intracellulare (Battey bacillus) A31.0
kakaferifu A31.8
kansasii (yellow bacillus) A31.0
kasongo A31.8
leprae (*see also* Leprosy) A30.9

Mycobacterium, mycobacterial — *continued*
luciflavum A31.1
marinum (M. balnei) A31.1
nonspecific — *see* Mycobacterium, atypical
pulmonary (atypical) A31.0
tuberculous — *see* Tuberculosis, pulmonary
scrofulaceum A31.8
simiae A31.8
systemic, extrapulmonary A31.8
szulgai A31.8
terrae A31.8
triviale A31.8
tuberculosis (human, bovine) — *see* Tuberculosis
ulcerans A31.1
xenopi A31.8
Mycoplasma (M.) **pneumoniae, as cause of disease classified elsewhere** B96.0
Mycosis, mycotic B49
cutaneous NEC B36.9
ear B36.8
fungoides (extranodal) (solid organ) C84.0- ☑
mouth B37.0
nails B35.1
opportunistic B48.8
skin NEC B36.9
specified NEC B48.8
stomatitis B37.0
vagina, vaginitis (candidal) B37.3
Mydriasis (pupil) H57.04
Myelatelia Q06.1
Myelinolysis, pontine, central G37.2
Myelitis (acute) (ascending) (childhood) (chronic) (descending) (diffuse) (disseminated) (idiopathic) (pressure) (progressive) (spinal cord) (subacute) (*see also* Encephalitis) G04.91
herpes simplex B00.82
herpes zoster B02.24
in diseases classified elsewhere G05.4
necrotizing, subacute G37.4
optic neuritis in G36.0
postchickenpox B01.12
postherpetic B02.24
postimmunization G04.02
postinfectious NEC G04.89
postvaccinal G04.02
specified NEC G04.89
syphilitic (transverse) A52.14
toxic G92
transverse (in demyelinating diseases of central nervous system) G37.3
tuberculous A17.82
varicella B01.12
Myeloblastic — *see* condition
Myeloblastoma
granular cell (*see also* Neoplasm, connective tissue)
malignant — *see* Neoplasm, connective tissue, malignant
tongue D10.1
Myelocele — *see* Spina bifida
Myelocystocele — *see* Spina bifida
Myelocytic — *see* condition
Myelodysplasia D46.9
specified NEC D46.Z (*following* D46.4)
spinal cord (congenital) Q06.1
Myelodysplastic syndrome D46.9
with
5q deletion D46.C (*following* D46.2)
isolated del (5q) chromosomal abnormality D46.C (*following* D46.2)
specified NEC D46.Z (*following* D46.4)
Myeloencephalitis — *see* Encephalitis
Myelofibrosis D75.81
with myeloid metaplasia D47.4
acute C94.4- ☑
idiopathic (chronic) D47.4
primary D47.1
secondary D75.81
in myeloproliferative disease D47.4
Myelogenous — *see* condition
Myeloid — *see* condition
Myelokathexis D70.9
Myeloleukodystrophy E75.29
Myelolipoma — *see* Lipoma
Myeloma (multiple) C90.0- ☑
monostotic C90.3 ☑
plasma cell C90.0- ☑
plasma cell C90.0- ☑

Myeloma — *continued*
solitary (*see also* Plasmacytoma, solitary) C90.3- ☑
Myelomalacia G95.89
Myelomatosis C90.0- ☑
Myelomeningitis — *see* Meningoencephalitis
Myelomeningocele (spinal cord) — *see* Spina bifida
Myelo-osteo-musculodysplasia hereditaria Q79.8
Myelopathic
anemia D64.89
muscle atrophy — *see* Atrophy, muscle, spinal
pain syndrome G89.0
Myelopathy (spinal cord) G95.9
drug-induced G95.89
in (due to)
degeneration or displacement, intervertebral disc NEC — *see* Disorder, disc, with, myelopathy
infection — *see* Encephalitis
intervertebral disc disorder (*see also* Disorder, disc, with, myelopathy)
mercury — *see* subcategory T56.1 ☑
neoplastic disease (*see also* Neoplasm) D49.9 [G99.2]
pernicious anemia D51.0 [G99.2]
spondylosis — *see* Spondylosis, with myelopathy NEC
necrotic (subacute) (vascular) G95.19
radiation-induced G95.89
spondylogenic NEC — *see* Spondylosis, with myelopathy NEC
toxic G95.89
transverse, acute G37.3
vascular G95.19
vitamin B12 E53.8 [G32.0]
Myelophthisis D61.82
Myeloradiculitis G04.91
Myeloradiculodysplasia (spinal) Q06.1
Myelosarcoma C92.3- ☑
Myelosclerosis D75.89
with myeloid metaplasia D47.4
disseminated, of nervous system G35
megakaryocytic D47.4
with myeloid metaplasia D47.4
Myelosis
acute C92.0- ☑
aleukemic C92.9- ☑
chronic D47.1
erythremic (acute) C94.0- ☑
megakaryocytic C94.2- ☑
nonleukemic D72.828
subacute C92.9- ☑
Myiasis (cavernous) B87.9
aural B87.4
creeping B87.0
cutaneous B87.0
dermal B87.0
ear (external) (middle) B87.4
eye B87.2
genitourinary B87.81
intestinal B87.82
laryngeal B87.3
nasopharyngeal B87.3
ocular B87.2
orbit B87.2
skin B87.0
specified site NEC B87.89
traumatic B87.1
wound B87.1
Myoadenoma, prostate — *see* Hyperplasia, prostate
Myoblastoma
granular cell (*see also* Neoplasm, connective tissue, benign)
malignant — *see* Neoplasm, connective tissue, malignant
tongue D10.1
Myocardial — *see* condition
Myocardiopathy (congestive) (constrictive) (familial) (hypertrophic nonobstructive) (idiopathic) (infiltrative) (obstructive) (primary) (restrictive) (sporadic) (*see also* Cardiomyopathy) I42.9
alcoholic I42.6
cobalt-beer I42.6
glycogen storage E74.02 [I43]
hypertrophic obstructive I42.1
in (due to)
beriberi E51.12
cardiac glycogenosis E74.02 [I43]
Friedreich's ataxia G11.1 [I43]

Myocardiopathy — continued
  in — continued
    myotonia atrophica G71.11 [I43]
    progressive muscular dystrophy G71.0 [I43]
  obscure (African) I42.8
  secondary I42.9
  thyrotoxic E05.90 [I43]
    with storm E05.91 [I43]
  toxic NEC I42.7
Myocarditis (with arteriosclerosis)(chronic)(fibroid) (interstitial) (old) (progressive) (senile) I51.4
  with
    rheumatic fever (conditions in I00) I09.0
      active — see Myocarditis, acute, rheumatic
      inactive or quiescent (with chorea) I09.0
  active I40.9
    rheumatic I01.2
      with chorea (acute) (rheumatic) (Sydenham's) I02.0
  acute or subacute (interstitial) I40.9
    due to
      streptococcus (beta-hemolytic) I01.2
    idiopathic I40.1
    rheumatic I01.2
      with chorea (acute) (rheumatic) (Sydenham's) I02.0
    specified NEC I40.8
  aseptic of newborn B33.22
  bacterial (acute) I40.0
  Coxsackie (virus) B33.22
  diphtheritic A36.81
  eosinophilic I40.1
  epidemic of newborn (Coxsackie) B33.22
  Fiedler's (acute) (isolated) I40.1
  giant cell (acute) (subacute) I40.1
  gonococcal A54.83
  granulomatous (idiopathic) (isolated) (nonspecific) I40.1
  hypertensive — see Hypertension, heart
  idiopathic (granulomatous) I40.1
  in (due to)
    diphtheria A36.81
    epidemic louse-borne typhus A75.0 [I41]
    Lyme disease A69.29
    sarcoidosis D86.85
    scarlet fever A38.1
    toxoplasmosis (acquired) B58.81
    typhoid A01.02
    typhus NEC A75.9 [I41]
  infective I40.0
  influenzal — see Influenza, with, myocarditis
  isolated (acute) I40.1
  meningococcal A39.52
  mumps B26.82
  nonrheumatic, active I40.9
  parenchymatous I40.9
  pneumococcal I40.0
  rheumatic (chronic) (inactive) (with chorea) I09.0
    active or acute I01.2
      with chorea (acute) (rheumatic) (Sydenham's) I02.0
  rheumatoid — see Rheumatoid, carditis
  septic I40.0
  staphylococcal I40.0
  suppurative I40.0
  syphilitic (chronic) A52.06
  toxic I40.8
    rheumatic — see Myocarditis, acute, rheumatic
  tuberculous A18.84
  typhoid A01.02
  valvular — see Endocarditis
  virus, viral I40.0
    of newborn (Coxsackie) B33.22
Myocardium, myocardial — see condition
Myocardosis — see Cardiomyopathy
Myoclonus, myoclonic, myoclonia (familial) (essential) (multifocal) (simplex) G25.3
  drug-induced G25.3
  epilepsy (see also Epilepsy, generalized, specified NEC) G40.4- ☑
    familial (progressive) G25.3
  epileptica G40.409
    with status epilepticus G40.401
  facial G51.3
  familial progressive G25.3
  Friedreich's G25.3
  jerks G25.3
  massive G25.3

Myoclonus, myoclonic, myoclonia — continued
  palatal G25.3
  pharyngeal G25.3
Myocytolysis I51.5
Myodiastasis — see Diastasis, muscle
Myoendocarditis — see Endocarditis
Myoepithelioma — see Neoplasm, benign, by site
Myofasciitis (acute) — see Myositis
Myofibroma (see also Neoplasm, connective tissue, benign)
  uterus (cervix) (corpus) — see Leiomyoma
Myofibromatosis D48.1
  infantile Q89.8
Myofibrosis M62.89
  heart — see Myocarditis
  scapulohumeral — see Lesion, shoulder, specified NEC
Myofibrositis M79.7
  scapulohumeral — see Lesion, shoulder, specified NEC
Myoglobulinuria, myoglobinuria (primary) R82.1
Myokymia, facial G51.4
Myolipoma — see Lipoma
Myoma (see also Neoplasm, connective tissue, benign)
  malignant — see Neoplasm, connective tissue, malignant
  prostate D29.1
  uterus (cervix) (corpus) — see Leiomyoma
Myomalacia M62.89
Myometritis — see Endometritis
Myometrium — see condition
Myonecrosis, clostridial A48.0
Myopathy G72.9
  acute
    necrotizing G72.81
    quadriplegic G72.81
  alcoholic G72.1
  benign congenital G71.2
  central core G71.2
  centronuclear G71.2
  congenital (benign) G71.2
  critical illness G72.81
  distal G71.0
  drug-induced G72.0
  endocrine NEC E34.9 [G73.7]
  extraocular muscles H05.82- ☑
  facioscapulohumeral G71.0
  hereditary G71.9
    specified NEC G71.8
  immune NEC G72.49
  in (due to)
    Addison's disease E27.1 [G73.7]
    alcohol G72.1
    amyloidosis E85.0 [G73.7]
    cretinism E00.9 [G73.7]
    Cushing's syndrome E24.9 [G73.7]
    drugs G72.0
    endocrine disease NEC E34.9 [G73.7]
    giant cell arteritis M31.6 [G73.7]
    glycogen storage disease E74.00 [G73.7]
    hyperadrenocorticism E24.9 [G73.7]
    hyperparathyroidism NEC E21.3 [G73.7]
    hypoparathyroidism E20.9 [G73.7]
    hypopituitarism E23.0 [G73.7]
    hypothyroidism E03.9 [G73.7]
    infectious disease NEC B99 ☑ [G73.7]
    lipid storage disease E75.6 [G73.7]
    metabolic disease NEC E88.9 [G73.7]
    myxedema E03.9 [G73.7]
    parasitic disease NEC B89 [G73.7]
    polyarteritis nodosa M30.0 [G73.7]
    rheumatoid arthritis — see Rheumatoid, myopathy
    sarcoidosis D86.87
    scleroderma M34.82
    sicca syndrome M35.03
    Sjögren's syndrome M35.03
    systemic lupus erythematosus M32.19
    thyrotoxicosis (hyperthyroidism) E05.90 [G73.7]
      with thyroid storm E05.91 [G73.7]
    toxic agent NEC G72.2
  inflammatory NEC G72.49
  intensive care (ICU) G72.81
  limb-girdle G71.0
  mitochondrial NEC G71.3
  myotubular G71.2
  mytonic, proximal (PROMM) G71.11
  nemaline G71.2
  ocular G71.0
  oculopharyngeal G71.0
  of critical illness G72.81

Myopathy — continued
  primary G71.9
    specified NEC G71.8
  progressive NEC G72.89
  proximal myotonic (PROMM) G71.11
  rod G71.2
  scapulohumeral G71.0
  specified NEC G72.89
  toxic G72.2
Myopericarditis (see also Pericarditis)
  chronic rheumatic I09.2
Myopia (axial) (congenital) H52.1- ☑
  degenerative (malignant) H44.2- ☑
  malignant H44.2- ☑
  pernicious H44.2- ☑
  progressive high (degenerative) H44.2- ☑
Myosarcoma — see Neoplasm, connective tissue, malignant
Myosis (pupil) H57.03
  stromal (endolymphatic) D39.0
Myositis M60.9
  clostridial A48.0
  due to posture — see Myositis, specified type NEC
  epidemic B33.0
  fibrosa or fibrous (chronic), Volkmann's T79.6 ☑
  foreign body granuloma — see Granuloma, foreign body
  in (due to)
    bilharziasis B65.9 [M63.8-] ☑
    cysticercosis B69.81
    leprosy A30.9 [M63.8-] ☑
    mycosis B49 [M63.8-] ☑
    sarcoidosis D86.87
    schistosomiasis B65.9 [M63.8-] ☑
    syphilis
      late A52.78
      secondary A51.49
    toxoplasmosis (acquired) B58.82
    trichinellosis B75 [M63.8-] ☑
    tuberculosis A18.09
  inclusion body [IBM] G72.41
  infective M60.009
    arm M60.002
      left M60.001
      right M60.000
    leg M60.005
      left M60.004
      right M60.003
    lower limb M60.005
      ankle M60.07- ☑
      foot M60.07- ☑
      lower leg M60.06- ☑
      thigh M60.05- ☑
      toe M60.07- ☑
    multiple sites M60.09
    specified site NEC M60.08
    upper limb M60.002
      finger M60.04- ☑
      forearm M60.03- ☑
      hand M60.04- ☑
      shoulder region M60.01- ☑
      upper arm M60.02- ☑
  interstitial M60.10
    ankle M60.17- ☑
    foot M60.17- ☑
    forearm M60.13- ☑
    hand M60.14- ☑
    lower leg M60.16- ☑
    multiple sites M60.19
    shoulder region M60.11- ☑
    specified site NEC M60.18
    thigh M60.15- ☑
    upper arm M60.12- ☑
  mycotic B49 [M63.8-] ☑
  orbital, chronic H05.12- ☑
  ossificans or ossifying (circumscripta) (see also Ossification, muscle, specified NEC)
    in (due to)
      burns M61.30
        ankle M61.37- ☑
        foot M61.37- ☑
        forearm M61.33- ☑
        hand M61.34- ☑
        lower leg M61.36- ☑
        multiple sites M61.39
        pelvic region M61.35- ☑
        shoulder region M61.31- ☑

Myositis — *continued*
ossificans or ossifying (*see also* Ossification, muscle, specified) — *continued*
in — *continued*
burns — *continued*
specified site NEC M61.38
thigh M61.35- ☑
upper arm M61.32- ☑
quadriplegia or paraplegia M61.20
ankle M61.27- ☑
foot M61.27- ☑
forearm M61.23- ☑
hand M61.24- ☑
lower leg M61.26- ☑
multiple sites M61.29
pelvic region M61.25- ☑
shoulder region M61.21- ☑
specified site NEC M61.28
thigh M61.25- ☑
upper arm M61.22- ☑
progressiva M61.10
ankle M61.17- ☑
finger M61.14- ☑
foot M61.17- ☑
forearm M61.13- ☑
hand M61.14- ☑
lower leg M61.16- ☑
multiple sites M61.19
pelvic region M61.15- ☑
shoulder region M61.11- ☑
specified site NEC M61.18
thigh M61.15- ☑
toe M61.17- ☑
upper arm M61.12- ☑
traumatica M61.00
ankle M61.07- ☑
foot M61.07- ☑
forearm M61.03- ☑
hand M61.04- ☑

Myositis — *continued*
ossificans or ossifying (*see also* Ossification, muscle, specified) — *continued*
traumatica — *continued*
lower leg M61.06- ☑
multiple sites M61.09
pelvic region M61.05- ☑
shoulder region M61.01- ☑
specified site NEC M61.08
thigh M61.05- ☑
upper arm M61.02- ☑
purulent — *see* Myositis, infective
specified type NEC M60.80
ankle M60.87- ☑
foot M60.87- ☑
forearm M60.83- ☑
hand M60.84- ☑
lower leg M60.86- ☑
multiple sites M60.89
pelvic region M60.85- ☑
shoulder region M60.81- ☑
specified site NEC M60.88
thigh M60.85- ☑
upper arm M60.82- ☑
suppurative — *see* Myositis, infective
traumatic (old) — *see* Myositis, specified type NEC
Myospasia impulsiva F95.2
Myotonia (acquisita) (intermittens) M62.89
atrophica G71.11
chondrodystrophic G71.13
congenita (acetazolamide responsive) (dominant) (recessive) G71.12
drug-induced G71.14
dystrophica G71.11
fluctuans G71.19
levior G71.12
permanens G71.19
symptomatic G71.19

Myotonic pupil — *see* Anomaly, pupil, function, tonic pupil
Myriapodiasis B88.2
Myringitis H73.2- ☑
with otitis media — *see* Otitis, media
acute H73.00- ☑
bullous H73.01- ☑
specified NEC H73.09- ☑
bullous — *see* Myringitis, acute, bullous
chronic H73.1- ☑
Mysophobia F40.228
Mytilotoxism — *see* Poisoning, fish
Myxadenitis labialis K13.0
Myxedema (adult) (idiocy) (infantile) (juvenile) (*see also* Hypothyroidism) E03.9
circumscribed E05.90
with storm E05.91
coma E03.5
congenital E00.1
cutis L98.5
localized (pretibial) E05.90
with storm E05.91
papular L98.5
Myxochondrosarcoma — *see* Neoplasm, cartilage, malignant
Myxofibroma — *see* Neoplasm, connective tissue, benign
odontogenic — *see* Cyst, calcifying odontogenic
Myxofibrosarcoma — *see* Neoplasm, connective tissue, malignant
Myxolipoma D17.9
Myxoliposarcoma — *see* Neoplasm, connective tissue, malignant
Myxoma (*see also* Neoplasm, connective tissue, benign)
nerve sheath — *see* Neoplasm, nerve, benign
odontogenic — *see* Cyst, calcifying odontogenic
Myxosarcoma — *see* Neoplasm, connective tissue, malignant

N

Naegeli's
 disease Q82.8
 leukemia, monocytic C93.1- ☑
Naegleriasis (with meningoencephalitis) B60.2
Naffziger's syndrome G54.0
Naga sore — *see* Ulcer, skin
Nägele's pelvis M95.5
 with disproportion (fetopelvic) O33.0
  causing obstructed labor O65.0
Nail (*see also* condition)
 biting F98.8
 patella syndrome Q87.2
Nanism, nanosomia — *see* Dwarfism
Nanophyetiasis B66.8
Nanukayami A27.89
Napkin rash L22
Narcolepsy G47.419
 with cataplexy G47.411
 in conditions classified elsewhere G47.429
  with cataplexy G47.421
Narcosis R06.89
Narcotism — *see* Dependence
NARP (Neuropathy, Ataxia and Retinitis pigmentosa)
 syndrome E88.49
Narrow
 anterior chamber angle H40.03- ☑
 pelvis — *see* Contraction, pelvis
Narrowing (*see also* Stenosis)
 artery I77.1
  auditory, internal I65.8
  basilar — *see* Occlusion, artery, basilar
  carotid — *see* Occlusion, artery, carotid
  cerebellar — *see* Occlusion, artery, cerebellar
  cerebral — *see* Occlusion artery, cerebral
  choroidal — *see* Occlusion, artery, cerebral, specified NEC
  communicating posterior — *see* Occlusion, artery, cerebral, specified NEC
  coronary (*see also* Disease, heart, ischemic, atherosclerotic)
   congenital Q24.5
    syphilitic A50.54 [I52]
   due to syphilis NEC A52.06
  hypophyseal — *see* Occlusion, artery, cerebral, specified NEC
  pontine — *see* Occlusion, artery, cerebral, specified NEC
  precerebral — *see* Occlusion, artery, precerebral
  vertebral — *see* Occlusion, artery, vertebral
 auditory canal (external) — *see* Stenosis, external ear canal
 eustachian tube — *see* Obstruction, eustachian tube
 eyelid — *see* Disorder, eyelid function
 larynx J38.6
 mesenteric artery K55.0
 palate M26.89
 palpebral fissure — *see* Disorder, eyelid function
 ureter N13.5
  with infection N13.6
 urethra — *see* Stricture, urethra
Narrowness, abnormal, eyelid Q10.3
Nasal — *see* condition
Nasolachrymal, nasolacrimal — *see* condition
Nasopharyngeal (*see also* condition)
 pituitary gland Q89.2
 torticollis M43.6
Nasopharyngitis (acute) (infective) (streptococcal) (subacute) J00
 chronic (suppurative) (ulcerative) J31.1
Nasopharynx, nasopharyngeal — *see* condition
Natal tooth, teeth K00.6
Nausea (without vomiting) R11.0
 with vomiting R11.2
 gravidarum — *see* Hyperemesis, gravidarum
 marina T75.3 ☑
 navalis T75.3 ☑
Navel — *see* condition
Neapolitan fever — *see* Brucellosis

Near drowning T75.1 ☑
Nearsightedness — *see* Myopia
Near-syncope R55
Nebula, cornea — *see* Opacity, cornea
Necator americanus infestation B76.1
Necatoriasis B76.1
Neck — *see* condition
Necrobiosis R68.89
 lipoidica NEC L92.1
  with diabetes — *see* E08-E13 with .620
Necrolysis, toxic epidermal L51.2
 due to drug
  correct substance properly administered — *see* Table of Drugs and Chemicals, by drug, adverse effect
  overdose or wrong substance given or taken — *see* Table of Drugs and Chemicals, by drug, poisoning
Necrophilia F65.89
Necrosis, necrotic (ischemic) (*see also* Gangrene)
 adrenal (capsule) (gland) E27.49
 amputation stump (surgical) (late) T87.50
  arm T87.5- ☑
  leg T87.5- ☑
 antrum J32.0
 aorta (hyaline) (*see also* Aneurysm, aorta)
  cystic medial — *see* Dissection, aorta
 artery I77.5
 bladder (aseptic) (sphincter) N32.89
 bone (*see also* Osteonecrosis) M87.9
  aseptic or avascular — *see* Osteonecrosis
   idiopathic M87.00
  ethmoid J32.2
  jaw M27.2
  tuberculous — *see* Tuberculosis, bone
 brain I67.89
 breast (aseptic) (fat) (segmental) N64.1
 bronchus J98.09
 central nervous system NEC I67.89
 cerebellar I67.89
 cerebral I67.89
 colon K55.0
 cornea H18.40
 cortical (acute) (renal) N17.1
 cystic medial (aorta) — *see* Dissection, aorta
 dental pulp K04.1
 esophagus K22.8
 ethmoid (bone) J32.2
 eyelid — *see* Disorder, eyelid, degenerative
 fat, fatty (generalized) (*see also* Disorder, soft tissue, specified type NEC)
  abdominal wall K65.4
  breast (aseptic) (segmental) N64.1
  localized — *see* Degeneration, by site, fatty
  mesentery K65.4
  omentum K65.4
  pancreas K86.8
  peritoneum K65.4
  skin (subcutaneous), newborn P83.0
  subcutaneous, due to birth injury P15.6
 gallbladder — *see* Cholecystitis, acute
 heart — *see* Infarct, myocardium
 hip, aseptic or avascular — *see* Osteonecrosis, by type, femur
 intestine (acute) (hemorrhagic) (massive) K55.0
 jaw M27.2
 kidney (bilateral) N28.0
  acute N17.9
  cortical (acute) (bilateral) N17.1
   with ectopic or molar pregnancy O08.4
  medullary (bilateral) (in acute renal failure) (papillary) N17.2
  papillary (bilateral) (in acute renal failure) N17.2
  tubular N17.0
   with ectopic or molar pregnancy O08.4
   complicating
    abortion — *see* Abortion, by type, complicated by, tubular necrosis
    ectopic or molar pregnancy O08.4
    pregnancy — *see* Pregnancy, complicated by, diseases of, specified type or system NEC

Necrosis, necrotic — *continued*
 kidney — *continued*
  tubular — *continued*
   following ectopic or molar pregnancy O08.4
   traumatic T79.5 ☑
 larynx J38.7
 liver (with hepatic failure) (cell) — *see* Failure, hepatic
  hemorrhagic, central K76.2
 lung J85.0
 lymphatic gland — *see* Lymphadenitis, acute
 mammary gland (fat) (segmental) N64.1
 mastoid (chronic) — *see* Mastoiditis, chronic
 medullary (acute) (renal) N17.2
 mesentery K55.0
  fat K65.4
 mitral valve — *see* Insufficiency, mitral
 myocardium, myocardial — *see* Infarct, myocardium
 nose J34.0
 omentum (with mesenteric infarction) K55.0
  fat K65.4
 orbit, orbital — *see* Osteomyelitis, orbit
 ossicles, ear — *see* Abnormal, ear ossicles
 ovary N70.92
 pancreas (aseptic) (duct) (fat) K86.8
  acute (infective) — *see* Pancreatitis, acute
  infective — *see* Pancreatitis, acute
 papillary (acute) (renal) N17.2
 perineum N90.89
 peritoneum (with mesenteric infarction) K55.0
  fat K65.4
 pharynx J02.9
  in granulocytopenia — *see* Neutropenia
  Vincent's A69.1
 phosphorus — *see* subcategory T54.2 ☑
 pituitary (gland) (postpartum) (Sheehan) E23.0
 pressure — *see* Ulcer, pressure, by site
 pulmonary J85.0
 pulp (dental) K04.1
 radiation — *see* Necrosis, by site
 radium — *see* Necrosis, by site
 renal — *see* Necrosis, kidney
 sclera H15.89
 scrotum N50.8
 skin or subcutaneous tissue NEC I96
 spine, spinal (column) (*see also* Osteonecrosis, by type, vertebra)
  cord G95.19
 spleen D73.5
 stomach K31.89
 stomatitis (ulcerative) A69.0
 subcutaneous fat, newborn P83.8
 subendocardial (acute) I21.4
  chronic I25.89
 suprarenal (capsule) (gland) E27.49
 testis N50.8
 thymus (gland) E32.8
 tonsil J35.8
 trachea J39.8
 tuberculous NEC — *see* Tuberculosis
 tubular (acute) (anoxic) (renal) (toxic) N17.0
  postprocedural N99.0
 vagina N89.8
 vertebra (*see also* Osteonecrosis, by type, vertebra)
  tuberculous A18.01
 vulva N90.89
 X-ray — *see* Necrosis, by site
Necrospermia — *see* Infertility, male
Need (for)
 care provider because (of)
  assistance with personal care Z74.1
  continuous supervision required Z74.3
  impaired mobility Z74.09
  no other household member able to render care Z74.2
  specified reason NEC Z74.8
 immunization — *see* Vaccination
 vaccination — *see* Vaccination
Neglect
 adult
  confirmed T74.01 ☑
  history of Z91.412
  suspected T76.01 ☑

Neglect — continued
  child (childhood)
    confirmed T74.02 ☑
    history of Z62.812
    suspected T76.02 ☑
  emotional, in childhood Z62.898
  hemispatial R41.4
  left-sided R41.4
  sensory R41.4
  visuospatial R41.4
Neisserian infection NEC — see Gonococcus
Nelaton's syndrome G60.8
Nelson's syndrome E24.1
Nematodiasis (intestinal) B82.0
  Ancylostoma B76.0
Neonatal (see also Newborn)
  acne L70.4
  bradycardia P29.12
  screening, abnormal findings on P09
  tachycardia P29.11
  tooth, teeth K00.6
Neonatorum — see condition
Neoplasia
  endocrine, multiple (MEN) E31.20
    type I E31.21
    type IIA E31.22
    type IIB E31.23
  intraepithelial (histologically confirmed)
    anal (AIN) (histologically confirmed) K62.82
      grade I K62.82
      grade II K62.82
      severe D01.3
    cervical glandular (histologically confirmed) D06.9
    cervix (uteri) (CIN) (histologically confirmed) N87.9
      glandular D06.9
      grade I N87.0
      grade II N87.1
      grade III (severe dysplasia) (see also Carcinoma, cervix uteri, in situ) D06.9
    prostate (histologically confirmed) (PIN I) (PIN II) N42.3
      grade I N42.3
      grade II N42.3
      severe D07.5
    vagina (histologically confirmed) (VAIN) N89.3
      grade I N89.0
      grade II N89.1
      grade III (severe dysplasia) D07.2
    vulva (histologically confirmed) (VIN) N90.3
      grade I N90.0
      grade II N90.1
      grade III (severe dysplasia) D07.1
Neoplasm, neoplastic (see also Table of Neoplasms)
  lipomatous, benign — see Lipoma
Neovascularization
  ciliary body — see Disorder, iris, vascular
  cornea H16.40- ☑
    deep H16.44- ☑
    ghost vessels — see Ghost, vessels
    localized H16.43- ☑
    pannus — see Pannus
  iris — see Disorder, iris, vascular
  retina H35.05- ☑
Nephralgia N23
Nephritis, nephritic (albuminuric) (azotemic) (congenital) (disseminated) (epithelial) (familial) (focal) (granulomatous) (hemorrhagic) (infantile) (nonsuppurative, excretory) (uremic) N05.9
  with
    dense deposit disease N05.6
    diffuse
      crescentic glomerulonephritis N05.7
      endocapillary proliferative glomerulonephritis N05.4
      membranous glomerulonephritis N05.2
      mesangial proliferative glomerulonephritis N05.3
      mesangiocapillary glomerulonephritis N05.5
    edema — see Nephrosis
    focal and segmental glomerular lesions N05.1
    foot process disease N04.9
    glomerular lesion
      diffuse sclerosing N05.8
      hypocomplementemic — see Nephritis, membranoproliferative
      IgA — see Nephropathy, IgA
      lobular, lobulonodular — see Nephritis, membranoproliferative

Nephritis, nephritic — continued
  with — continued
    glomerular lesion — continued
      nodular — see Nephritis, membranoproliferative
    lesion of
      glomerulonephritis, proliferative N05.8
      renal necrosis N05.9
    minor glomerular abnormality N05.0
    specified morphological changes NEC N05.8
  acute N00.9
    with
      dense deposit disease N00.6
      diffuse
        crescentic glomerulonephritis N00.7
        endocapillary proliferative glomerulonephritis N00.4
        membranous glomerulonephritis N00.2
        mesangial proliferative glomerulonephritis N00.3
        mesangiocapillary glomerulonephritis N00.5
      focal and segmental glomerular lesions N00.1
      minor glomerular abnormality N00.0
      specified morphological changes NEC N00.8
  amyloid E85.4 [N08]
  antiglomerular basement membrane (anti-GBM) antibody NEC
    in Goodpasture's syndrome M31.0
  antitubular basement membrane (tubulo-interstitial) NEC N12
    toxic — see Nephropathy, toxic
  arteriolar — see Hypertension, kidney
  arteriosclerotic — see Hypertension, kidney
  ascending — see Nephritis, tubulo-interstitial
  atrophic N03.9
  Balkan (endemic) N15.0
  calculous, calculus — see Calculus, kidney
  cardiac — see Hypertension, kidney
  cardiovascular — see Hypertension, kidney
  chronic N03.9
    with
      dense deposit disease N03.6
      diffuse
        crescentic glomerulonephritis N03.7
        endocapillary proliferative glomerulonephritis N03.4
        membranous glomerulonephritis N03.2
        mesangial proliferative glomerulonephritis N03.3
        mesangiocapillary glomerulonephritis N03.5
      focal and segmental glomerular lesions N03.1
      minor glomerular abnormality N03.0
      specified morphological changes NEC N03.8
    arteriosclerotic — see Hypertension, kidney
  cirrhotic N26.9
  complicating pregnancy O26.83- ☑
  croupous N00.9
  degenerative — see Nephrosis
  diffuse sclerosing N05.8
  due to
    diabetes mellitus — see E08-E13 with .21
    subacute bacterial endocarditis I33.0
    systemic lupus erythematosus (chronic) M32.14
    typhoid fever A01.09
  gonococcal (acute) (chronic) A54.21
  hypocomplementemic — see Nephritis, membranoproliferative
  IgA — see Nephropathy, IgA
  immune complex (circulating) NEC N05.8
  infective — see Nephritis, tubulo-interstitial
  interstitial — see Nephritis, tubulo-interstitial
  lead N14.3
  membranoproliferative (diffuse) (type 1 or 3) (see also N00-N07 with fourth character .5) N05.5
    type 2 (see also N00-N07 with fourth character .6) N05.6
  minimal change N05.0
  necrotic, necrotizing NEC (see also N00-N07 with fourth character .8) N05.8
  nephrotic — see Nephrosis
  nodular — see Nephritis, membranoproliferative
  polycystic Q61.3
    adult type Q61.2
    autosomal
      dominant Q61.2
      recessive NEC Q61.19
    childhood type NEC Q61.19
    infantile type NEC Q61.19

Nephritis, nephritic — continued
  poststreptococcal N05.9
    acute N00.9
    chronic N03.9
    rapidly progressive N01.9
  proliferative NEC (see also N00-N07 with fourth character .8) N05.8
  purulent — see Nephritis, tubulo-interstitial
  rapidly progressive N01.9
    with
      dense deposit disease N01.6
      diffuse
        crescentic glomerulonephritis N01.7
        endocapillary proliferative glomerulonephritis N01.4
        membranous glomerulonephritis N01.2
        mesangial proliferative glomerulonephritis N01.3
        mesangiocapillary glomerulonephritis N01.5
      focal and segmental glomerular lesions N01.1
      minor glomerular abnormality N01.0
      specified morphological changes NEC N01.8
  salt losing or wasting NEC N28.89
  saturnine N14.3
  sclerosing, diffuse N05.8
  septic — see Nephritis, tubulo-interstitial
  specified pathology NEC (see also N00-N07 with fourth character .8) N05.8
  subacute N01.9
  suppurative — see Nephritis, tubulo-interstitial
  syphilitic (late) A52.75
    congenital A50.59 [N08]
    early (secondary) A51.44
  toxic — see Nephropathy, toxic
  tubal, tubular — see Nephritis, tubulo-interstitial
  tuberculous A18.11
  tubulo-interstitial (in) N12
    acute (infectious) N10
    chronic (infectious) N11.9
      nonobstructive N11.8
        reflux-associated N11.0
      obstructive N11.1
      specified NEC N11.8
    due to
      brucellosis A23.9 [N16]
      cryoglobulinemia D89.1 [N16]
      glycogen storage disease E74.00 [N16]
      Sjögren's syndrome M35.04
  vascular — see Hypertension, kidney
  war N00.9
Nephroblastoma (epithelial) (mesenchymal) C64- ☑
Nephrocalcinosis E83.59 [N29]
Nephrocystitis, pustular — see Nephritis, tubulo-interstitial
Nephrolithiasis (congenital) (pelvis) (recurrent) (see also Calculus, kidney)
Nephroma C64- ☑
  mesoblastic D41.0- ☑
Nephronephritis — see Nephrosis
Nephronophthisis Q61.5
Nephropathia epidemica A98.5
Nephropathy (see also Nephritis) N28.9
  with
    edema — see Nephrosis
    glomerular lesion — see Glomerulonephritis
  amyloid, hereditary E85.0
  analgesic N14.0
    with medullary necrosis, acute N17.2
  Balkan (endemic) N15.0
  chemical — see Nephropathy, toxic
  diabetic — see E08-E13 with .21
  drug-induced N14.2
    specified NEC N14.1
  focal and segmental hyalinosis or sclerosis N02.1
  heavy metal-induced N14.3
  hereditary NEC N07.9
    with
      dense deposit disease N07.6
      diffuse
        crescentic glomerulonephritis N07.7
        endocapillary proliferative glomerulonephritis N07.4
        membranous glomerulonephritis N07.2
        mesangial proliferative glomerulonephritis N07.3
        mesangiocapillary glomerulonephritis N07.5
      focal and segmental glomerular lesions N07.1
      minor glomerular abnormality N07.0

Nephropathy — continued
  hereditary — continued
    with — continued
      specified morphological changes NEC N07.8
  hypercalcemic N25.89
  hypertensive — see Hypertension, kidney
  hypokalemic (vacuolar) N25.89
  IgA N02.8
    with glomerular lesion N02.9
      focal and segmental hyalinosis or sclerosis
        N02.1
      membranoproliferative (diffuse) N02.5
      membranous (diffuse) N02.2
      mesangial proliferative (diffuse) N02.3
      mesangiocapillary (diffuse) N02.5
      proliferative NEC N02.8
      specified pathology NEC N02.8
  lead N14.3
  membranoproliferative (diffuse) N02.5
  membranous (diffuse) N02.2
  mesangial (IgA/IgG) — see Nephropathy, IgA
    proliferative (diffuse) N02.3
  mesangiocapillary (diffuse) N02.5
  obstructive N13.8
  phenacetin N17.2
  phosphate-losing N25.0
  potassium depletion N25.89
  pregnancy-related O26.83- ☑
  proliferative NEC (see also N00-N07 with fourth character .8) N05.8
  protein-losing N25.89
  saturnine N14.3
  sickle-cell D57.- ☑ [N08]
  toxic NEC N14.4
    due to
      drugs N14.2
        analgesic N14.0
        specified NEC N14.1
      heavy metals N14.3
  vasomotor N17.0
  water-losing N25.89
Nephroptosis N28.83
Nephropyosis — see Abscess, kidney
Nephrorrhagia N28.89
Nephrosclerosis (arteriolar)(arteriosclerotic) (chronic) (hyaline) (see also Hypertension, kidney)
  hyperplastic — see Hypertension, kidney
  senile N26.9
Nephrosis, nephrotic (Epstein's) (syndrome) (congenital) N04.9
  with
    foot process disease N04.9
    glomerular lesion N04.1
    hypocomplementemic N04.5
  acute N04.9
  anoxic — see Nephrosis, tubular
  chemical — see Nephrosis, tubular
  cholemic K76.7
  diabetic — see E08-E13 with .21
  Finnish type (congenital) Q89.8
  hemoglobin N10
  hemoglobinuric — see Nephrosis, tubular
  in
    amyloidosis E85.4 [N08]
    diabetes mellitus — see E08-E13 with .21
    epidemic hemorrhagic fever A98.5
    malaria (malariae) B52.0
  ischemic — see Nephrosis, tubular
  lipoid N04.9
  lower nephron — see Nephrosis, tubular
  malarial (malariae) B52.0
  minimal change N04.0
  myoglobin N10
  necrotizing — see Nephrosis, tubular
  osmotic (sucrose) N25.89
  radiation N04.9
  syphilitic (late) A52.75
  toxic — see Nephrosis, tubular
  tubular (acute) N17.0
    postprocedural N99.0
    radiation N04.9
Nephrosonephritis, hemorrhagic (endemic) A98.5
Nephrostomy
  attention to Z43.6
  status Z93.6
Nerve (see also condition)
  injury — see Injury, nerve, by body site
Nerves R45.0

Nervous (see also condition) R45.0
  heart F45.8
  stomach F45.8
  tension R45.0
Nervousness R45.0
Nesidioblastoma
  pancreas D13.7
  specified site NEC — see Neoplasm, benign, by site
  unspecified site D13.7
Nettleship's syndrome Q82.2
Neumann's disease or syndrome L10.1
Neuralgia, neuralgic (acute) M79.2
  accessory (nerve) G52.8
  acoustic (nerve) — see subcategory H93.3 ☑
  auditory (nerve) — see subcategory H93.3 ☑
  ciliary G44.009
    intractable G44.001
    not intractable G44.009
  cranial
    nerve (see also Disorder, nerve, cranial)
      fifth or trigeminal — see Neuralgia, trigeminal
    postherpetic, postzoster B02.29
  ear — see subcategory H92.0 ☑
  facialis vera G51.1
  Fothergill's — see Neuralgia, trigeminal
  glossopharyngeal (nerve) G52.1
  Horton's G44.099
    intractable G44.091
    not intractable G44.099
  Hunt's B02.21
  hypoglossal (nerve) G52.3
  infraorbital — see Neuralgia, trigeminal
  malarial — see Malaria
  migrainous G44.009
    intractable G44.001
    not intractable G44.009
  Morton's G57.6- ☑
  nerve, cranial — see Disorder, nerve, cranial
  nose G52.0
  occipital M54.81
  olfactory G52.0
  penis N48.9
  perineum R10.2
  postherpetic NEC B02.29
    trigeminal B02.22
  pubic region R10.2
  scrotum R10.2
  Sluder's G44.89
  specified nerve NEC G58.8
  spermatic cord R10.2
  sphenopalatine (ganglion) G90.09
  trifacial — see Neuralgia, trigeminal
  trigeminal G50.0
    postherpetic, postzoster B02.22
  vagus (nerve) G52.2
  writer's F48.8
    organic G25.89
Neurapraxia — see Injury, nerve
Neurasthenia F48.8
  cardiac F45.8
  gastric F45.8
  heart F45.8
Neurilemmoma (see also Neoplasm, nerve, benign)
  acoustic (nerve) D33.3
  malignant (see also Neoplasm, nerve, malignant)
    acoustic (nerve) C72.4- ☑
Neurilemmosarcoma — see Neoplasm, nerve, malignant
Neurinoma — see Neoplasm, nerve, benign
Neurinomatosis — see Neoplasm, nerve, uncertain behavior
Neuritis (rheumatoid) M79.2
  abducens (nerve) — see Strabismus, paralytic, sixth nerve
  accessory (nerve) G52.8
  acoustic (nerve) (see also subcategory) H93.3 ☑
    in (due to)
      infectious disease NEC B99 [H94.0-] ☑
      parasitic disease NEC B89 [H94.0-] ☑
      syphilitic A52.15
  alcoholic G62.1
    with psychosis — see Psychosis, alcoholic
  amyloid, any site E85.4 [G63]
  auditory (nerve) — see subcategory H93.3 ☑
  brachial — see Radiculopathy
    due to displacement, intervertebral disc — see Disorder, disc, cervical, with neuritis

Neuritis — continued
  cranial nerve
    due to Lyme disease A69.22
    eighth or acoustic or auditory — see subcategory H93.3 ☑
    eleventh or accessory G52.8
    fifth or trigeminal G51.0
    first or olfactory G52.0
    fourth or trochlear — see Strabismus, paralytic, fourth nerve
    second or optic — see Neuritis, optic
    seventh or facial G51.8
      newborn (birth injury) P11.3
    sixth or abducent — see Strabismus, paralytic, sixth nerve
    tenth or vagus G52.2
    third or oculomotor — see Strabismus, paralytic, third nerve
    twelfth or hypoglossal G52.3
  Déjérine-Sottas G60.0
  diabetic (mononeuropathy) — see E08-E13 with .41
    polyneuropathy — see E08-E13 with .42
  due to
    beriberi E51.11
    displacement, prolapse or rupture, intervertebral disc — see Disorder, disc, with, radiculopathy
    herniation, nucleus pulposus M51.9 [G55]
  endemic E51.11
  facial G51.8
    newborn (birth injury) P11.3
  general — see Polyneuropathy
  geniculate ganglion G51.1
    due to herpes (zoster) B02.21
  gouty M10.00 [G63]
  hypoglossal (nerve) G52.3
  ilioinguinal (nerve) G57.9- ☑
  infectious (multiple) NEC G61.0
  interstitial hypertrophic progressive G60.0
  lumbar M54.16
  lumbosacral M54.17
  multiple (see also Polyneuropathy)
    endemic E51.11
    infective, acute G61.0
  multiplex endemica E51.11
  nerve root — see Radiculopathy
  oculomotor (nerve) — see Strabismus, paralytic, third nerve
  olfactory nerve G52.0
  optic (nerve) (hereditary) (sympathetic) H46.9
    with demyelination G36.0
    in myelitis G36.0
    nutritional H46.2
    papillitis — see Papillitis, optic
    retrobulbar H46.1- ☑
    specified type NEC H46.8
    toxic H46.3
  peripheral (nerve) G62.9
    multiple — see Polyneuropathy
    single — see Mononeuritis
  pneumogastric (nerve) G52.2
  postherpetic, postzoster B02.29
  progressive hypertrophic interstitial G60.0
  retrobulbar (see also Neuritis, optic, retrobulbar)
    in (due to)
      late syphilis A52.15
      meningococcal infection A39.82
    meningococcal A39.82
    syphilitic A52.15
  sciatic (nerve) (see also Sciatica)
    due to displacement of intervertebral disc — see Disorder, disc, with, radiculopathy
  serum (see also Reaction, serum) T80.69 ☑
  shoulder-girdle G54.5
  specified nerve NEC G58.8
  spinal (nerve) root — see Radiculopathy
  syphilitic A52.15
  thenar (median) G56.1- ☑
  thoracic M54.14
  toxic NEC G62.2
  trochlear (nerve) — see Strabismus, paralytic, fourth nerve
  vagus (nerve) G52.2
Neuroastrocytoma — see Neoplasm, uncertain behavior, by site
Neuroavitaminosis E56.9 [G99.8]
Neuroblastoma
  olfactory C30.0
  specified site — see Neoplasm, malignant, by site

Neuroblastoma — *continued*
  unspecified site C74.90
Neurochorioretinitis — *see* Chorioretinitis
Neurocirculatory asthenia F45.8
Neurocysticercosis B69.0
Neurocytoma — *see* Neoplasm, benign, by site
Neurodermatitis (circumscribed) (circumscripta) (local) L28.0
  atopic L20.81
  diffuse (Brocq) L20.81
  disseminated L20.81
Neuroencephalomyelopathy, optic G36.0
Neuroepithelioma (*see also* Neoplasm, malignant, by site)
  olfactory C30.0
Neurofibroma (*see also* Neoplasm, nerve, benign)
  melanotic — *see* Neoplasm, nerve, benign
  multiple — *see* Neurofibromatosis
  plexiform — *see* Neoplasm, nerve, benign
Neurofibromatosis (multiple) (nonmalignant) Q85.00
  acoustic Q85.02
  malignant — *see* Neoplasm, nerve, malignant
  specified NEC Q85.09
  type 1 (von Recklinghausen) Q85.01
  type 2 Q85.02
Neurofibrosarcoma — *see* Neoplasm, nerve, malignant
Neurogenic (*see also* condition)
  bladder (*see also* Dysfunction, bladder, neuromuscular) N31.9
    cauda equina syndrome G83.4
  bowel NEC K59.2
  heart F45.8
Neuroglioma — *see* Neoplasm, uncertain behavior, by site
Neurolabyrinthitis (of Dix and Hallpike) — *see* Neuronitis, vestibular
Neurolathyrism — *see* Poisoning, food, noxious, plant
Neuroleprosy A30.9
Neuroma (*see also* Neoplasm, nerve, benign)
  acoustic (nerve) D33.3
  amputation (stump) (traumatic) (surgical complication) (late) T87.3- ☑
    arm T87.3- ☑
    leg T87.3- ☑
  digital (toe) G57.6- ☑
  interdigital (toe) G58.8
    lower limb G57.8- ☑
    upper limb G56.8- ☑
  intermetatarsal G57.8- ☑
  Morton's G57.6- ☑
  nonneoplastic
    arm G56.9- ☑
    leg G57.9- ☑
    lower extremity G57.9- ☑
    upper extremity G56.9- ☑
  optic (nerve) D33.3
  plantar G57.6- ☑
  plexiform — *see* Neoplasm, nerve, benign
  surgical (nonneoplastic)
    arm G56.9- ☑
    leg G57.9- ☑
    lower extremity G57.9- ☑
    upper extremity G56.9- ☑
Neuromyalgia — *see* Neuralgia
Neuromyasthenia (epidemic) (postinfectious) G93.3
Neuromyelitis G36.9
  ascending G61.0
  optica G36.0
Neuromyopathy G70.9
  paraneoplastic D49.9 [G13.0]
Neuromyotonia (Isaacs) G71.19
Neuronevus — *see* Nevus
Neuronitis G58.9
  ascending (acute) G57.2- ☑
  vestibular H81.2- ☑
Neuroparalytic — *see* condition
Neuropathy, neuropathic G62.9
  acute motor G62.81
  alcoholic G62.1
    with psychosis — *see* Psychosis, alcoholic
  arm G56.9- ☑
  autonomic, peripheral — *see* Neuropathy, peripheral, autonomic
  axillary G56.9- ☑
  bladder N31.9
    atonic (motor) (sensory) N31.2
    autonomous N31.2

Neuropathy, neuropathic — *continued*
  bladder — *continued*
    flaccid N31.2
    nonreflex N31.2
    reflex N31.1
    uninhibited N31.0
  brachial plexus G54.0
  cervical plexus G54.2
  chronic
    progressive segmentally demyelinating G62.89
    relapsing demyelinating G62.89
  Déjérine-Sottas G60.0
  diabetic — *see* E08-E13 with .40
    mononeuropathy — *see* E08-E13 with .41
    polyneuropathy — *see* E08-E13 with .42
  entrapment G58.9
    iliohypogastric nerve G57.8- ☑
    ilioinguinal nerve G57.8- ☑
    lateral cutaneous nerve of thigh G57.1- ☑
    median nerve G56.0- ☑
    obturator nerve G57.8- ☑
    peroneal nerve G57.3- ☑
    posterior tibial nerve G57.5- ☑
    saphenous nerve G57.8- ☑
    ulnar nerve G56.2- ☑
  facial nerve G51.9
  hereditary G60.9
    motor and sensory (types I-IV) G60.0
    sensory G60.8
    specified NEC G60.8
  hypertrophic G60.0
    Charcot-Marie-Tooth G60.0
    Déjérine-Sottas G60.0
    interstitial progressive G60.0
    of infancy G60.0
    Refsum G60.1
  idiopathic G60.9
    progressive G60.3
    specified NEC G60.8
  in association with hereditary ataxia G60.2
  intercostal G58.0
  ischemic — *see* Disorder, nerve
  Jamaica (ginger) G62.2
  leg NEC G57.9- ☑
  lower extremity G57.9- ☑
  lumbar plexus G54.1
  median nerve G56.1- ☑
  motor and sensory (*see also* Polyneuropathy)
    hereditary (types I-IV) G60.0
  multiple (acute) (chronic) — *see* Polyneuropathy
  optic (nerve) (*see also* Neuritis, optic)
    ischemic H47.01- ☑
  paraneoplastic (sensorial) (Denny Brown) D49.9 [G13.0]
  peripheral (nerve) (*see also* Polyneuropathy) G62.9
    autonomic G90.9
      idiopathic G90.09
      in (due to)
        amyloidosis E85.4 [G99.0]
        diabetes mellitus — *see* E08-E13 with .43
        endocrine disease NEC E34.9 [G99.0]
        gout M10.00 [G99.0]
        hyperthyroidism E05.90 [G99.0]
          with thyroid storm E05.91 [G99.0]
        metabolic disease NEC E88.9 [G99.0]
    idiopathic G60.9
      progressive G60.3
    in (due to)
      antitetanus serum G62.0
      arsenic G62.2
      drugs NEC G62.0
      lead G62.2
      organophosphate compounds G62.2
      toxic agent NEC G62.2
  plantar nerves G57.6- ☑
  progressive
    hypertrophic interstitial G60.0
    inflammatory G62.81
  radicular NEC — *see* Radiculopathy
  sacral plexus G54.1
  sciatic G57.0- ☑
  serum G61.1
  toxic NEC G62.2
  trigeminal sensory G50.8
  ulnar nerve G56.2- ☑
  uremic N18.9 [G63]
  vitamin B12 E53.8 [G63]
    with anemia (pernicious) D51.0 [G63]
      due to dietary deficiency D51.3 [G63]

Neurophthisis (*see also* Disorder, nerve)
  peripheral, diabetic — *see* E08-E13 with .42
Neuroretinitis — *see* Chorioretinitis
Neuroretinopathy, hereditary optic H47.22
Neurosarcoma — *see* Neoplasm, nerve, malignant
Neurosclerosis — *see* Disorder, nerve
Neurosis, neurotic F48.9
  anankastic F42
  anxiety (state) F41.1
    panic type F41.0
  asthenic F48.8
  bladder F45.8
  cardiac (reflex) F45.8
  cardiovascular F45.8
  character F60.9
  colon F45.8
  compensation F68.1 ☑
  compulsive, compulsion F42
  conversion F44.9
  craft F48.8
  cutaneous F45.8
  depersonalization F48.1
  depressive (reaction) (type) F34.1
  environmental F48.8
  excoriation L98.1
  fatigue F48.8
  functional — *see* Disorder, somatoform
  gastric F45.8
  gastrointestinal F45.8
  heart F45.8
  hypochondriacal F45.21
  hysterical F44.9
  incoordination F45.8
    larynx F45.8
    vocal cord F45.8
  intestine F45.8
  larynx (sensory) F45.8
    hysterical F44.4
  mixed NEC F48.8
  musculoskeletal F45.8
  obsessional F42
  obsessive-compulsive F42
  occupational F48.8
  ocular NEC F45.8
  organ — *see* Disorder, somatoform
  pharynx F45.8
  phobic F40.9
  posttraumatic (situational) F43.10
    acute F43.11
    chronic F43.12
  psychasthenic (type) F48.8
  railroad F48.8
  rectum F45.8
  respiratory F45.8
  rumination F45.8
  sexual F65.9
  situational F48.8
  social F40.10
    generalized F40.11
  specified type NEC F48.8
  state F48.9
    with depersonalization episode F48.1
  stomach F45.8
  traumatic F43.10
    acute F43.11
    chronic F43.12
  vasomotor F45.8
  visceral F45.8
  war F48.8
Neurospongioblastosis diffusa Q85.1
Neurosyphilis (arrested) (early) (gumma) (late) (latent) (recurrent) (relapse) A52.3
  with ataxia (cerebellar) (locomotor) (spastic) (spinal) A52.19
  aneurysm (cerebral) A52.05
  arachnoid (adhesive) A52.13
  arteritis (any artery) (cerebral) A52.04
  asymptomatic A52.2
  congenital A50.40
  dura (mater) A52.13
  general paresis A52.17
  hemorrhagic A52.05
  juvenile (asymptomatic) (meningeal) A50.40
  leptomeninges (aseptic) A52.13
  meningeal, meninges (adhesive) A52.13
  meningitis A52.13
  meningovascular (diffuse) A52.13
  optic atrophy A52.15

Neurosyphilis — *continued*
  parenchymatous (degenerative) A52.19
  paresis, paretic A52.17
    juvenile A50.45
  remission in (sustained) A52.3
  serological (without symptoms) A52.2
  specified nature or site NEC A52.19
  tabes, tabetic (dorsalis) A52.11
    juvenile A50.45
  taboparesis A52.17
    juvenile A50.45
  thrombosis (cerebral) A52.05
  vascular (cerebral) NEC A52.05
Neurothekeoma — *see* Neoplasm, nerve, benign
Neurotic — *see* Neurosis
Neurotoxemia — *see* Toxemia
Neutroclusion M26.211
Neutropenia, neutropenic (chronic) (genetic) (idiopathic) (immune) (infantile) (malignant) (pernicious) (splenic) D70.9
  congenital (primary) D70.0
  cyclic D70.4
  cytoreductive cancer chemotherapy sequela D70.1
  drug-induced D70.2
    due to cytoreductive cancer chemotherapy D70.1
  due to infection D70.3
  fever D70.9
  neonatal, transitory (isoimmune) (maternal transfer) P61.5
  periodic D70.4
  secondary (cyclic) (periodic) (splenic) D70.4
    drug-induced D70.2
      due to cytoreductive cancer chemotherapy D70.1
  toxic D70.8
Neutrophilia, hereditary giant D72.0
Nevocarcinoma — *see* Melanoma
Nevus D22.9
  achromic — *see* Neoplasm, skin, benign
  amelanotic — *see* Neoplasm, skin, benign
  angiomatous D18.00
    intra-abdominal D18.03
    intracranial D18.02
    skin D18.01
    specified site NEC D18.09
  araneus I78.1
  balloon cell — *see* Neoplasm, skin, benign
  bathing trunk D48.5
  blue — *see* Neoplasm, skin, benign
    cellular — *see* Neoplasm, skin, benign
    giant — *see* Neoplasm, skin, benign
    Jadassohn's — *see* Neoplasm, skin, benign
    malignant — *see* Melanoma
  capillary D18.00
    intra-abdominal D18.03
    intracranial D18.02
    skin D18.01
    specified site NEC D18.09
  cavernous D18.00
    intra-abdominal D18.03
    intracranial D18.02
    skin D18.01
    specified site NEC D18.09
  cellular — *see* Neoplasm, skin, benign
    blue — *see* Neoplasm, skin, benign
  choroid D31.3- ☑
  comedonicus Q82.5
  conjunctiva D31.0- ☑
  dermal — *see* Neoplasm, skin, benign
    with epidermal nevus — *see* Neoplasm, skin, benign
  dysplastic — *see* Neoplasm, skin, benign
  eye D31.9- ☑
  flammeus Q82.5
  hemangiomatous D18.00
    intra-abdominal D18.03
    intracranial D18.02
    skin D18.01
    specified site NEC D18.09
  iris D31.4- ☑
  lacrimal gland D31.5- ☑
  lymphatic D18.1
  magnocellular
    specified site — *see* Neoplasm, benign, by site
    unspecified site D31.40
  malignant — *see* Melanoma
  meaning hemangioma D18.00
    intra-abdominal D18.03

Nevus — *continued*
  meaning hemangioma — *continued*
    intracranial D18.02
    skin D18.01
    specified site NEC D18.09
  mouth (mucosa) D10.30
    specified site NEC D10.39
    white sponge Q38.6
  multiplex Q85.1
  non-neoplastic I78.1
  oral mucosa D10.30
    specified site NEC D10.39
    white sponge Q38.6
  orbit D31.6- ☑
  pigmented
    giant (*see also* Neoplasm, skin, uncertain behavior) D48.5
      malignant melanoma in — *see* Melanoma
  portwine Q82.5
  retina D31.2- ☑
  retrobulbar D31.6- ☑
  sanguineous Q82.5
  senile I78.1
  skin D22.9
    abdominal wall D22.5
    ala nasi D22.39
    ankle D22.7- ☑
    anus, anal D22.5
    arm D22.6- ☑
    auditory canal (external) D22.2- ☑
    auricle (ear) D22.2- ☑
    auricular canal (external) D22.2- ☑
    axilla, axillary fold D22.5
    back D22.5
    breast D22.5
    brow D22.39
    buttock D22.5
    canthus (eye) D22.1- ☑
    cheek (external) D22.39
    chest wall D22.5
    chin D22.39
    ear (external) D22.2- ☑
    external meatus (ear) D22.2- ☑
    eyebrow D22.39
    eyelid (lower) (upper) D22.1- ☑
    face D22.30
      specified NEC D22.39
    female genital organ (external) NEC D28.0
    finger D22.6- ☑
    flank D22.5
    foot D22.7- ☑
    forearm D22.6- ☑
    forehead D22.39
    foreskin D29.0
    genital organ (external) NEC
      female D28.0
      male D29.9
    gluteal region D22.5
    groin D22.5
    hand D22.6- ☑
    heel D22.7- ☑
    helix D22.2- ☑
    hip D22.7- ☑
    interscapular region D22.5
    jaw D22.39
    knee D22.7- ☑
    labium (majus) (minus) D28.0
    leg D22.7- ☑
    lip (lower) (upper) D22.0
    lower limb D22.7- ☑
    male genital organ (external) D29.9
    nail D22.9
      finger D22.6- ☑
      toe D22.7- ☑
    nasolabial groove D22.39
    nates D22.5
    neck D22.4
    nose (external) D22.39
    palpebra D22.1- ☑
    penis D29.0
    perianal skin D22.5
    perineum D22.5
    pinna D22.2- ☑
    popliteal fossa or space D22.7- ☑
    prepuce D29.0
    pudendum D28.0
    scalp D22.4

Nevus — *continued*
  skin — *continued*
    scrotum D29.4
    shoulder D22.6- ☑
    submammary fold D22.5
    temple D22.39
    thigh D22.7- ☑
    toe D22.7- ☑
    trunk NEC D22.5
    umbilicus D22.5
    upper limb D22.6- ☑
    vulva D28.0
  specified site NEC — *see* Neoplasm, by site, benign
  spider I78.1
  stellar I78.1
  strawberry Q82.5
  Sutton's — *see* Neoplasm, skin, benign
  unius lateris Q82.5
  Unna's Q82.5
  vascular Q82.5
  verrucous Q82.5
Newborn (infant) (liveborn) (singleton) Z38.2
  abstinence syndrome P96.1
  acne L70.4
  affected by (suspected to be)
    abnormalities of membranes P02.9
      specified NEC P02.8
    abruptio placenta P02.1
    amino-acid metabolic disorder, transitory P74.8
    amniocentesis (while in utero) P00.6
    amnionitis P02.7
    apparent life threatening event (ALTE) R68.13
    bleeding (into)
      cerebral cortex P52.22
      germinal matrix P52.0
      ventricles P52.1
    breech delivery P03.0
    cardiac arrest P29.81
    cardiomyopathy I42.8
      congenital I42.4
    cerebral ischemia P91.0
    Cesarean delivery P03.4
    chemotherapy agents P04.1
    chorioamnionitis P02.7
    cocaine (crack) P04.41
    complications of labor and delivery P03.9
      specified NEC P03.89
    compression of umbilical cord NEC P02.5
    contracted pelvis P03.1
    delivery P03.9
      Cesarean P03.4
      forceps P03.2
      vacuum extractor P03.3
    entanglement (knot) in umbilical cord P02.5
    environmental chemicals P04.6
    fetal (intrauterine)
      growth retardation P05.9
      malnutrition not light or small for gestational age P05.2
    forceps delivery P03.2
    heart rate abnormalities
      bradycardia P29.12
      intrauterine P03.819
        before onset of labor P03.810
        during labor P03.811
      tachycardia P29.11
    hemorrhage (antepartum) P02.1
      cerebellar (nontraumatic) P52.6
      intracerebral (nontraumatic) P52.4
      intracranial (nontraumatic) P52.9
        specified NEC P52.8
      intraventricular (nontraumatic) P52.3
        grade 1 P52.0
        grade 2 P52.1
        grade 3 P52.21
        grade 4 P52.22
      posterior fossa (nontraumatic) P52.6
      subarachnoid (nontraumatic) P52.5
      subependymal P52.0
        with intracerebral extension P52.22
        with intraventricular extension P52.1
          with enlargment of ventricles P52.21
        without intraventricular extension P52.0
    hypoxic ischemic encephalopathy [HIE] P91.60
      mild P91.61
      moderate P91.62
      severe P91.63
    induction of labor P03.89

226

☑ Additional Character Required — Refer to the Tabular List for Character Selection   ▽ Subterms under main terms may continue to next column or page

Newborn — continued
  affected by — continued
    intestinal perforation P78.0
    intrauterine (fetal) blood loss P50.9
      due to (from)
        cut end of co-twin cord P50.5
        hemorrhage into
          co-twin P50.3
            maternal circulation P50.4
        placenta P50.2
        ruptured cord blood P50.1
        vasa previa P50.0
      specified NEC P50.8
    intrauterine (fetal) hemorrhage P50.9
    intrauterine (in utero) procedure P96.5
    malpresentation (malposition) NEC P03.1
    maternal (complication of) (use of)
      alcohol P04.3
      analgesia (maternal) P04.0
      anesthesia (maternal) P04.0
      blood loss P02.1
      circulatory disease P00.3
      condition P00.9
        specified NEC P00.89
      delivery P03.9
        Cesarean P03.4
        forceps P03.2
        vacuum extractor P03.3
      diabetes mellitus (pre-existing) P70.1
      disorder P00.9
        specified NEC P00.89
      drugs (addictive) (illegal) NEC P04.49
      ectopic pregnancy P01.4
      gestational diabetes P70.0
      hemorrhage P02.1
      hypertensive disorder P00.0
      incompetent cervix P01.0
      infectious disease P00.2
      injury P00.5
      labor and delivery P03.9
      malpresentation before labor P01.7
      maternal death P01.6
      medical procedure P00.7
      medication P04.1
      multiple pregnancy P01.5
      nutritional disorder P00.4
      oligohydramnios P01.2
      parasitic disease P00.2
      periodontal disease P00.81
      placenta previa P02.0
      polyhydramnios P01.3
      precipitate delivery P03.5
      pregnancy P01.9
        specified P01.8
      premature rupture of membranes P01.1
      renal disease P00.1
      respiratory disease P00.3
      surgical procedure P00.6
      urinary tract disease P00.1
      uterine contraction (abnormal) P03.6
    meconium peritonitis P78.0
    medication (legal) (maternal use) (prescribed) P04.1
    membrane abnormalities P02.9
      specified NEC P02.8
    membranitis P02.7
    methamphetamine(s) P04.49
    mixed metabolic and respiratory acidosis P84
    neonatal abstinence syndrome P96.1
    noxious substances transmitted via placenta or
      breast milk P04.9
      specified NEC P04.8
    nutritional supplements P04.5
    placenta previa P02.0
    placental
      abnormality (functional) (morphological)
        P02.20
        specified NEC P02.29
      dysfunction P02.29
      infarction P02.29
      insufficiency P02.29
      separation NEC P02.1
      transfusion syndromes P02.3
    placentitis P02.7
    precipitate delivery P03.5
    prolapsed cord P02.4
    respiratory arrest P28.81
    slow intrauterine growth P05.9
    tobacco P04.2

Newborn — continued
  affected by — continued
    twin to twin transplacental transfusion P02.3
    umbilical cord (tightly) around neck P02.5
    umbilical cord condition P02.60
      short cord P02.69
      specified NEC P02.69
    uterine contractions (abnormal) P03.6
    vasa previa P02.69
      from intrauterine blood loss P50.0
  apnea P28.3
    obstructive P28.4
    primary P28.3
    specified NEC P28.4
  born in hospital Z38.00
    by cesarean Z38.01
  born outside hospital Z38.1
  breast buds P96.89
  breast engorgement P83.4
  check-up — see Newborn, examination
  convulsion P90
  dehydration P74.1
  examination
    8 to 28 days old Z00.111
    under 8 days old Z00.110
  fever P81.9
    environmentally-induced P81.0
  hyperbilirubinemia P59.9
    of prematurity P59.0
  hypernatremia P74.2
  hyponatremia P74.2
  infection P39.9
    candidal P37.5
    specified NEC P39.8
    urinary tract P39.3
  jaundice P59.8
    due to
      breast milk inhibitor P59.3
      hepatocellular damage P59.20
        specified NEC P59.29
      preterm delivery P59.0
    of prematurity P59.0
    specified NEC P59.8
  late metabolic acidosis P74.0
  mastitis P39.0
    infective P39.0
    noninfective P83.4
  multiple born NEC Z38.8
    born in hospital Z38.68
      by cesarean Z38.69
    born outside hospital Z38.7
  omphalitis P38.9
    with mild hemorrhage P38.1
    without hemorrhage P38.9
  post-term P08.21
  prolonged gestation (over 42 completed weeks)
    P08.22
  quadruplet Z38.8
    born in hospital Z38.63
      by cesarean Z38.64
    born outside hospital Z38.7
  quintuplet Z38.8
    born in hospital Z38.65
      by cesarean Z38.66
    born outside hospital Z38.7
  seizure P90
  sepsis (congenital) P36.9
    due to
      anaerobes NEC P36.5
      Escherichia coli P36.4
      Staphylococcus P36.30
        aureus P36.2
        specified NEC P36.39
      Streptococcus P36.10
        group B P36.0
        specified NEC P36.19
      specified NEC P36.8
  triplet Z38.8
    born in hospital Z38.61
      by cesarean Z38.62
    born outside hospital Z38.7
  twin Z38.5
    born in hospital Z38.30
      by cesarean Z38.31
    born outside hospital Z38.4
  vomiting P92.09
    bilious P92.01
  weight check Z00.111

Newcastle conjunctivitis or disease B30.8
Nezelof's syndrome (pure alymphocytosis) D81.4
Niacin (amide) **deficiency** E52
Nicolas (-Durand)-**Favre disease** A55
Nicotine — see Tobacco
Nicotinic acid deficiency E52
Niemann-Pick disease or syndrome E75.249
  specified NEC E75.248
  type
    A E75.240
    B E75.241
    C E75.242
    D E75.243
Night
  blindness — see Blindness, night
  sweats R61
  terrors (child) F51.4
Nightmares (REM sleep type) F51.5
Nipple — see condition
Nisbet's chancre A57
Nishimoto (-Takeuchi) **disease** I67.5
Nitritoid crisis or reaction — see Crisis, nitritoid
Nitrosohemoglobinemia D74.8
Njovera A65
Nocardiosis, nocardiasis A43.9
  cutaneous A43.1
  lung A43.0
  pneumonia A43.0
  pulmonary A43.0
  specified site NEC A43.8
Nocturia R35.1
  psychogenic F45.8
Nocturnal — see condition
Nodal rhythm I49.8
Node(s) (see also Nodule)
  Bouchard's (with arthropathy) M15.2
  Haygarth's M15.8
  Heberden's (with arthropathy) M15.1
  larynx J38.7
  lymph — see condition
  milker's B08.03
  Osler's I33.0
  Schmorl's — see Schmorl's disease
  singer's J38.2
  teacher's J38.2
  tuberculous — see Tuberculosis, lymph gland
  vocal cord J38.2
Nodule(s), nodular
  actinomycotic — see Actinomycosis
  breast NEC N63
  colloid (cystic), thyroid E04.1
  cutaneous — see Swelling, localized
  endometrial (stromal) D26.1
  Haygarth's M15.8
  inflammatory — see Inflammation
  juxta-articular
    syphilitic A52.77
    yaws A66.7
  larynx J38.7
  lung, solitary (subsegmental branch of the bronchial
    tree) R91.1
    multiple R91.8
  milker's B08.03
  prostate N40.2
    with lower urinary tract symptoms (LUTS) N40.3
    without lower urinary tract symtpoms (LUTS) N40.2
  pulmonary, solitary (subsegmental branch of the
    bronchial tree) R91.1
  retrocardiac R09.89
  rheumatoid M06.30
    ankle M06.37- ☑
    elbow M06.32- ☑
    foot joint M06.37- ☑
    hand joint M06.34- ☑
    hip M06.35- ☑
    knee M06.36- ☑
    multiple site M06.39
    shoulder M06.31- ☑
    vertebra M06.38
    wrist M06.33- ☑
  scrotum (inflammatory) N49.2
  singer's J38.2
  solitary, lung (subsegmental branch of the bronchial
    tree) R91.1
    multiple R91.8
  subcutaneous — see Swelling, localized
  teacher's J38.2

Nodule(s), nodular — *continued*
  thyroid (cold) (gland) (nontoxic) E04.1
    with thyrotoxicosis E05.20
      with thyroid storm E05.21
      toxic or with hyperthyroidism E05.20
        with thyroid storm E05.21
  vocal cord J38.2
Noma (gangrenous) (hospital) (infective) A69.0
  auricle I96
  mouth A69.0
  pudendi N76.89
  vulvae N76.89
Nomad, nomadism Z59.0
Nonautoimmune hemolytic anemia D59.4
  drug-induced D59.2
Nonclosure (*see also* Imperfect, closure)
  ductus arteriosus (Botallo's) Q25.0
  foramen
    botalli Q21.1
    ovale Q21.1
Noncompliance Z91.19
  with
    dialysis Z91.15
    dietary regimen Z91.11
    medical treatment Z91.19
    medication regimen NEC Z91.14
      underdosing (*see also* Table of Drugs and
        Chemicals, categories T36-T50, with final
        character 6) Z91.14
      intentional NEC Z91.128
        due to financial hardship of patient
          Z91.120
      unintentional NEC Z91.138
        due to patient's age related debility
          Z91.130
    renal dialysis Z91.15
Nondescent (congenital) (*see also* Malposition, congen-
    ital)
  cecum Q43.3
  colon Q43.3
  testicle Q53.9
    bilateral Q53.20
      abdominal Q53.21
      perineal Q53.22
    unilateral Q53.10
      abdominal Q53.11
      perineal Q53.12
Nondevelopment
  brain Q02
    part of Q04.3
  heart Q24.8
  organ or site, congenital NEC — *see* Hypoplasia
Nonengagement
  head NEC O32.4 ☑
    in labor, causing obstructed labor O64.8 ☑
Nonexanthematous tick fever A93.2
Nonexpansion, lung (newborn) P28.0
Nonfunctioning
  cystic duct (*see also* Disease, gallbladder) K82.8
  gallbladder (*see also* Disease, gallbladder) K82.8
  kidney N28.9
  labyrinth — *see* subcategory H83.2 ☑
Non-Hodgkin lymphoma NEC — *see* Lymphoma, non-
  Hodgkin
Nonimplantation, ovum N97.2
Noninsufflation, fallopian tube N97.1
Non-ketotic hyperglycinemia E72.51
Nonne-Milroy syndrome Q82.0
Nonovulation N97.0
Nonpatent fallopian tube N97.1
Nonpneumatization, lung NEC P28.0
Nonrotation — *see* Malrotation
Nonsecretion, urine — *see* Anuria
Nonunion
  fracture — *see* Fracture, by site
  organ or site, congenital NEC — *see* Imperfect, closure
  symphysis pubis, congenital Q74.2
Nonvisualization, gallbladder R93.2
Nonvital, nonvitalized tooth K04.99
Non-working side interference M26.56
Noonan's syndrome Q87.1
Normocytic anemia (infectional) due to blood loss
  (chronic) D50.0
  acute D62
Norrie's disease (congenital) Q15.8
North American blastomycosis B40.9
Norwegian itch B86

Nose, nasal — *see* condition
Nosebleed R04.0
Nose-picking F98.8
Nosomania F45.21
Nosophobia F45.22
Nostalgia F43.20
Notch of iris Q13.2
Notching nose, congenital (tip) Q30.2
Nothnagel's
  syndrome — *see* Strabismus, paralytic, third nerve
  vasomotor acroparesthesia I73.89
Novy's relapsing fever A68.9
  louse-borne A68.0
  tick-borne A68.1
Noxious
  foodstuffs, poisoning by — *see* Poisoning, food, nox-
    ious, plant
  substances transmitted through placenta or breast
    milk P04.9
Nucleus pulposus — *see* condition
Numbness R20.0
Nuns' knee — *see* Bursitis, prepatellar
Nursemaid's elbow S53.03- ☑
Nutcracker esophagus K22.4
Nutmeg liver K76.1
Nutrient element deficiency E61.9
  specified NEC E61.8
Nutrition deficient or insufficient (*see also* Malnutri-
    tion) E46
  due to
    insufficient food T73.0 ☑
    lack of
      care (child) T76.02 ☑
        adult T76.01 ☑
      food T73.0 ☑
Nutritional stunting E45
Nyctalopia (night blindness) — *see* Blindness, night
Nycturia R35.1
  psychogenic F45.8
Nymphomania F52.8
Nystagmus H55.00
  benign paroxysmal — *see* Vertigo, benign paroxysmal
  central positional H81.4- ☑
  congenital H55.01
  dissociated H55.04
  latent H55.02
  miners' H55.09
  positional
    benign paroxysmal H81.4- ☑
    central H81.4- ☑
  specified form NEC H55.09
  visual deprivation H55.03

O

Obermeyer's relapsing fever (European) A68.0
Obesity E66.9
  with alveolar hyperventilation E66.2
  adrenal E27.8
  complicating
    childbirth O99.214
    pregnancy O99.21- ☑
    puerperium O99.215
  constitutional E66.8
  dietary counseling and surveillance Z71.3
  drug-induced E66.1
  due to
    drug E66.1
    excess calories E66.09
      morbid E66.01
      severe E66.01
  endocrine E66.8
  endogenous E66.8
  familial E66.8
  glandular E66.8
  hypothyroid — *see* Hypothyroidism
  morbid E66.01
    with alveolar hypoventilation E66.2
    due to excess calories E66.01
  nutritional E66.09
  pituitary E23.6
  severe E66.01
  specified type NEC E66.8
Oblique — *see* condition
Obliteration
  appendix (lumen) K38.8
  artery I77.1

Obliteration — *continued*
  bile duct (noncalculous) K83.1
  common duct (noncalculous) K83.1
  cystic duct — *see* Obstruction, gallbladder
  disease, arteriolar I77.1
  endometrium N85.8
  eye, anterior chamber — *see* Disorder, globe, hy-
    potony
  fallopian tube N97.1
  lymphatic vessel I89.0
    due to mastectomy I97.2
  organ or site, congenital NEC — *see* Atresia, by site
  ureter N13.5
    with infection N13.6
  urethra — *see* Stricture, urethra
  vein I87.8
  vestibule (oral) K08.8
Observation (following) (for) (without need for further
    medical care) Z04.9
  accident NEC Z04.3
    at work Z04.2
    transport Z04.1
  adverse effect of drug Z03.6
  alleged rape or sexual assault (victim), ruled out
    adult Z04.41
    child Z04.42
  criminal assault Z04.8
  development state
    adolescent Z00.3
    period of rapid growth in childhood Z00.2
    puberty Z00.3
  disease, specified NEC Z03.89
  following work accident Z04.2
  growth and development state — *see* Observation,
    development state
  injuries (accidental) NEC (*see also* Observation, acci-
    dent)
  newborn (for suspected condition, ruled out) — *see* -
    Newborn, affected by (suspected to be), mater-
    nal (complication of) (use of)
  postpartum
    immediately after delivery Z39.0
    routine follow-up Z39.2
  pregnancy (normal) (without complication) Z34.9- ☑
    high risk O09.9- ☑
  suicide attempt, alleged NEC Z03.89
    self-poisoning Z03.6
  suspected, ruled out (*see also* Suspected condition,
    ruled out)
    abuse, physical
      adult Z04.71
      child Z04.72
    accident at work Z04.2
    adult battering victim Z04.71
    child battering victim Z04.72
    condition NEC Z03.89
      newborn — *see* Newborn, affected by (suspect-
        ed to be), maternal (complication of) (use
        of)
    drug poisoning or adverse effect Z03.6
    exposure (to)
      anthrax Z03.810
      biological agent NEC Z03.818
    inflicted injury NEC Z04.8
    suicide attempt, alleged Z03.89
      self-poisoning Z03.6
    toxic effects from ingested substance (drug) (poi-
      son) Z03.6
  toxic effects from ingested substance (drug) (poison)
    Z03.6
Obsession, obsessional state F42
Obsessive-compulsive neurosis or reaction F42
Obstetric embolism, septic — *see* Embolism, obstetric,
  septic
Obstetrical trauma (complicating delivery) O71.9
  with or following ectopic or molar pregnancy O08.6
  specified type NEC O71.89
Obstipation — *see* Constipation
Obstruction, obstructed, obstructive
  airway J98.8
    with
      allergic alveolitis J67.9
      asthma J45.909
        with
          exacerbation (acute) J45.901
          status asthmaticus J45.902
      bronchiectasis J47.9

Obstruction, obstructed, obstructive — *continued*
  airway — *continued*
    with — *continued*
      bronchiectasis — *continued*
        with
          exacerbation (acute) J47.1
          lower respiratory infection J47.0
      bronchitis (chronic) J44.9
      emphysema J43.9
    chronic J44.9
      with
        allergic alveolitis — *see* Pneumonitis, hypersensitivity
        bronchiectasis J47.9
          with
            exacerbation (acute) J47.1
            lower respiratory infection J47.0
    due to
      foreign body — *see* Foreign body, by site, causing asphyxia
      inhalation of fumes or vapors J68.9
      laryngospasm J38.5
  ampulla of Vater K83.1
  aortic (heart) (valve) — *see* Stenosis, aortic
  aortoiliac I74.09
  aqueduct of Sylvius G91.1
    congenital Q03.0
      with spina bifida — *see* Spina bifida, by site, with hydrocephalus
  Arnold-Chiari — *see* Arnold-Chiari disease
  artery (*see also* Embolism, artery) I74.9
    basilar (complete) (partial) — *see* Occlusion, artery, basilar
    carotid (complete) (partial) — *see* Occlusion, artery, carotid
    cerebellar — *see* Occlusion, artery, cerebellar
    cerebral (anterior) (middle) (posterior) — *see* Occlusion, artery, cerebral
    precerebral — *see* Occlusion, artery, precerebral
    renal N28.0
    retinal NEC — *see* Occlusion, artery, retina
    vertebral (complete) (partial) — *see* Occlusion, artery, vertebral
  band (intestinal) K56.69
  bile duct or passage (common) (hepatic) (noncalculous) K83.1
    with calculus K80.51
    congenital (causing jaundice) Q44.3
  biliary (duct) (tract) K83.1
    gallbladder K82.0
  bladder-neck (acquired) N32.0
    congenital Q64.31
    due to hyperplasia (hypertrophy) of prostate — *see* Hyperplasia, prostate
  bowel — *see* Obstruction, intestine
  bronchus J98.09
  canal, ear — *see* Stenosis, external ear canal
  cardia K22.2
  caval veins (inferior) (superior) I87.1
  cecum — *see* Obstruction, intestine
  circulatory I99.8
  colon — *see* Obstruction, intestine
  common duct (noncalculous) K83.1
  coronary (artery) — *see* Occlusion, coronary
  cystic duct (*see also* Obstruction, gallbladder)
    with calculus K80.21
  device, implant or graft (*see also* Complications, by site and type, mechanical) T85.698 ☑
    arterial graft NEC — *see* Complication, cardiovascular device, mechanical, vascular
    catheter NEC T85.628 ☑
      cystostomy T83.090 ☑
      dialysis (renal) T82.49 ☑
        intraperitoneal T85.691 ☑
      infusion NEC T82.594 ☑
        spinal (epidural) (subdural) T85.690 ☑
      urinary, indwelling T83.098 ☑
    due to infection T85.79 ☑
    gastrointestinal — *see* Complications, prosthetic device, mechanical, gastrointestinal device
    genital NEC T83.498 ☑
      intrauterine contraceptive device T83.39 ☑
      penile prosthesis T83.490 ☑
    heart NEC — *see* Complication, cardiovascular device, mechanical
    joint prosthesis — *see* Complications, joint prosthesis, mechanical, specified NEC, by site

Obstruction, obstructed, obstructive — *continued*
  device, implant or graft (*see also* Complications, by site and type, mechanical) — *continued*
    orthopedic NEC — *see* Complication, orthopedic, device, mechanical
    specified NEC T85.628 ☑
    urinary NEC (*see also* Complication, genitourinary, device, urinary, mechanical)
      graft T83.29 ☑
    vascular NEC — *see* Complication, cardiovascular device, mechanical
    ventricular intracranial shunt T85.09 ☑
  due to foreign body accidentally left in operative wound T81.529 ☑
  duodenum K31.5
  ejaculatory duct N50.8
  esophagus K22.2
  eustachian tube (complete) (partial) H68.10- ☑
    cartilagenous (extrinsic) H68.13- ☑
      intrinsic H68.12- ☑
    osseous H68.11- ☑
  fallopian tube (bilateral) N97.1
  fecal K56.41
    with hernia — *see* Hernia, by site, with obstruction
  foramen of Monro (congenital) Q03.8
    with spina bifida — *see* Spina bifida, by site, with hydrocephalus
  foreign body — *see* Foreign body
  gallbladder K82.0
    with calculus, stones K80.21
    congenital Q44.1
  gastric outlet K31.1
  gastrointestinal — *see* Obstruction, intestine
  hepatic K76.89
    duct (noncalculous) K83.1
  ileum — *see* Obstruction, intestine
  iliofemoral (artery) I74.5
  intestine K56.60
    with
      adhesions (intestinal) (peritoneal) K56.5
    adynamic K56.0
    by gallstone K56.3
    congenital (small) Q41.9
      large Q42.9
        specified part NEC Q42.8
    neurogenic K56.0
      Hirschsprung's disease or megacolon Q43.1
    newborn P76.9
      due to
        fecaliths P76.8
        inspissated milk P76.2
        meconium (plug) P76.0
          in mucoviscidosis E84.11
      specified NEC P76.8
    postoperative K91.3
    reflex K56.0
    specified NEC K56.69
    volvulus K56.2
  intracardiac ball valve prosthesis T82.09 ☑
  jejunum — *see* Obstruction, intestine
  joint prosthesis — *see* Complications, joint prosthesis, mechanical, specified NEC, by site
  kidney (calices) N28.89
  labor — *see* Delivery
  lacrimal (passages) (duct)
    by
      dacryolith — *see* Dacryolith
      stenosis — *see* Stenosis, lacrimal
    congenital Q10.5
    neonatal H04.53- ☑
  lacrimonasal duct — *see* Obstruction, lacrimal
  lacteal, with steatorrhea K90.2
  laryngitis — *see* Laryngitis
  larynx NEC J38.6
    congenital Q31.8
  lung J98.4
    disease, chronic J44.9
  lymphatic I89.0
  meconium (plug)
    newborn P76.0
      due to fecaliths P76.0
    in mucoviscidosis E84.11
  mitral — *see* Stenosis, mitral
  nasal J34.89
  nasolacrimal duct (*see also* Obstruction, lacrimal)
    congenital Q10.5
  nasopharynx J39.2
  nose J34.89

Obstruction, obstructed, obstructive — *continued*
  organ or site, congenital NEC — *see* Atresia, by site
  pancreatic duct K86.8
  parotid duct or gland K11.8
  pelviureteral junction N13.5
    congenital Q62.39
  pharynx J39.2
  portal (circulation) (vein) I81
  prostate (*see also* Hyperplasia, prostate)
    valve (urinary) N32.0
  pulmonary valve (heart) I37.0
  pyelonephritis (chronic) N11.1
  pylorus
    adult K31.1
    congenital or infantile Q40.0
  rectosigmoid — *see* Obstruction, intestine
  rectum K62.4
  renal N28.89
    outflow N13.8
    pelvis, congenital Q62.39
  respiratory J98.8
    chronic J44.9
  retinal (vessels) H34.9
  salivary duct (any) K11.8
    with calculus K11.5
  sigmoid — *see* Obstruction, intestine
  sinus (accessory) (nasal) J34.89
  Stensen's duct K11.8
  stomach NEC K31.89
    acute K31.0
    congenital Q40.2
    due to pylorospasm K31.3
  submandibular duct K11.8
  submaxillary gland K11.8
    with calculus K11.5
  thoracic duct I89.0
  thrombotic — *see* Thrombosis
  trachea J39.8
  tracheostomy airway J95.03
  tricuspid (valve) — *see* Stenosis, tricuspid
  upper respiratory, congenital Q34.8
  ureter (functional) (pelvic junction) NEC N13.5
    with
      hydronephrosis N13.1
        with infection N13.6
      pyelonephritis (chronic) N11.1
    congenital Q62.39
    due to calculus — *see* Calculus, ureter
  urethra NEC N36.8
    congenital Q64.39
  urinary (moderate) N13.9
    due to hyperplasia (hypertrophy) of prostate — *see* Hyperplasia, prostate
    organ or tract (lower) N13.9
    prostatic valve N32.0
    specified NEC N13.8
  uropathy N13.9
  uterus N85.8
  vagina N89.5
  valvular — *see* Endocarditis
  vein, venous I87.1
    caval (inferior) (superior) I87.1
    thrombotic — *see* Thrombosis
  vena cava (inferior) (superior) I87.1
  vesical NEC N32.0
  vesicourethral orifice N32.0
    congenital Q64.31
  vessel NEC I99.8
Obturator — *see* condition
Occlusal wear, teeth K03.0
Occlusio pupillae — *see* Membrane, pupillary
Occlusion, occluded
  anus K62.4
    congenital Q42.3
      with fistula Q42.2
  aortoiliac (chronic) I74.09
  aqueduct of Sylvius G91.1
    congenital Q03.0
      with spina bifida — *see* Spina bifida, by site, with hydrocephalus
  artery (*see also* Embolism, artery) I74.9
    auditory, internal I65.8
    basilar I65.1
      with
        infarction I63.22
          due to
            embolism I63.12
            thrombosis I63.02

Occlusion, occluded — *continued*
  artery (*see also* Embolism, artery) — *continued*
    brain or cerebral I66.9
      with infarction (due to) I63.5 ☑
        embolism I63.4 ☑
        thrombosis I63.3 ☑
    carotid I65.2- ☑
      with
        infarction I63.23- ☑
          due to
            embolism I63.13- ☑
            thrombosis I63.03- ☑
    cerebellar (anterior inferior) (posterior inferior) (superior) I66.3
      with infarction I63.54- ☑
        due to
          embolism I63.44- ☑
          thrombosis I63.34- ☑
    cerebral I66.9
      with infarction I63.50
        due to
          embolism I63.40
            specified NEC I63.49
          thrombosis I63.30
            specified NEC I63.39
      anterior I66.1- ☑
        with infarction I63.52- ☑
          due to
            embolism I63.42- ☑
            thrombosis I63.32- ☑
      middle I66.0- ☑
        with infarction I63.51- ☑
          due to
            embolism I63.41- ☑
            thrombosis I63.31- ☑
      posterior I66.2- ☑
        with infarction I63.53- ☑
          due to
            embolism I63.43- ☑
            thrombosis I63.33- ☑
      specified NEC I66.8
        with infarction I63.59
          due to
            embolism I63.4 ☑
            thrombosis I63.3 ☑
    choroidal (anterior) — *see* Occlusion, artery, precerebral, specified NEC
    communicating posterior — *see* Occlusion, artery, cerebral, specified NEC
    complete
      coronary I25.82
      extremities I70.92
    coronary (acute) (thrombotic) (without myocardial infarction) I24.0
      with myocardial infarction — *see* Infarction, myocardium
      chronic total I25.82
      complete I25.82
      healed or old I25.2
      total (chronic) I25.82
    hypophyseal — *see* Occlusion, artery, precerebral, specified NEC
    iliac I74.5
    lower extremities due to stenosis or stricture I77.1
    mesenteric (embolic) (thrombotic) K55.0
    perforating — *see* Occlusion, artery, cerebral, specified NEC
    peripheral I77.9
      thrombotic or embolic I74.4
    pontine — *see* Occlusion, artery, cerebral, specified NEC
    precerebral I65.9
      with infarction I63.20
        due to
          embolism I63.10
            specified NEC I63.19
          thrombosis I63.00
            specified NEC I63.09
        specified NEC I63.29
      basilar — *see* Occlusion, artery, basilar
      carotid — *see* Occlusion, artery, carotid
      puerperal O88.23
      specified NEC I65.8
        with infarction I63.29
          due to
            embolism I63.19
            thrombosis I63.00

Occlusion, occluded — *continued*
  artery (*see also* Embolism, artery) — *continued*
    precerebral — *continued*
      vertebral — *see* Occlusion, artery, vertebral
    renal N28.0
    retinal
      branch H34.23- ☑
      central H34.1- ☑
      partial H34.21- ☑
      transient H34.0- ☑
    spinal — *see* Occlusion, artery, precerebral, vertebral
    total (chronic)
      coronary I25.82
      extremities I70.92
    vertebral I65.0- ☑
      with
        infarction I63.21- ☑
          due to
            embolism I63.11- ☑
            thrombosis I63.01- ☑
  basilar artery — *see* Occlusion, artery, basilar
  bile duct (common) (hepatic) (noncalculous) K83.1
  bowel — *see* Obstruction, intestine
  carotid (artery) (common) (internal) — *see* Occlusion, artery, carotid
  centric (of teeth) M26.59
    maximum intercuspation discrepancy M26.55
  cerebellar (artery) — *see* Occlusion, artery, cerebellar
  cerebral (artery) — *see* Occlusion, artery, cerebral
  cerebrovascular (*see also* Occlusion, artery, cerebral)
    with infarction I63.5 ☑
  cervical canal — *see* Stricture, cervix
  cervix (uteri) — *see* Stricture, cervix
  choanal Q30.0
  choroidal (artery) — *see* Occlusion, artery, precerebral, specified NEC
  colon — *see* Obstruction, intestine
  communicating posterior artery — *see* Occlusion, artery, precerebral, specified NEC
  coronary (artery) (vein) (thrombotic) (*see also* Infarct, myocardium)
    chronic total I25.82
    healed or old I25.2
    not resulting in infarction I24.0
    total (chronic) I25.82
  cystic duct — *see* Obstruction, gallbladder
  embolic — *see* Embolism
  fallopian tube N97.1
    congenital Q50.6
  gallbladder (*see also* Obstruction, gallbladder)
    congenital (causing jaundice) Q44.1
  gingiva, traumatic K06.2
  hymen N89.6
    congenital Q52.3
  hypophyseal (artery) — *see* Occlusion, artery, precerebral, specified NEC
  iliac artery I74.5
  intestine — *see* Obstruction, intestine
  lacrimal passages — *see* Obstruction, lacrimal
  lung J98.4
  lymph or lymphatic channel I89.0
  mammary duct N64.89
  mesenteric artery (embolic) (thrombotic) K55.0
  nose J34.89
    congenital Q30.0
  organ or site, congenital NEC — *see* Atresia, by site
  oviduct N97.1
    congenital Q50.6
  peripheral arteries
    due to stricture or stenosis I77.1
    upper extremity I74.2
  pontine (artery) — *see* Occlusion, artery, precerebral, specified NEC
  posterior lingual, of mandibular teeth M26.29
  precerebral artery — *see* Occlusion, artery, precerebral
  punctum lacrimale — *see* Obstruction, lacrimal
  pupil — *see* Membrane, pupillary
  pylorus, adult (*see also* Stricture, pylorus) K31.1
  renal artery N28.0
  retina, retinal
    artery — *see* Occlusion, artery, retinal
    vein (central) H34.81- ☑
      engorgement H34.82- ☑
      tributary H34.83- ☑
    vessels H34.9

Occlusion, occluded — *continued*
  spinal artery — *see* Occlusion, artery, precerebral, vertebral
  teeth (mandibular) (posterior lingual) M26.29
  thoracic duct I89.0
  thrombotic — *see* Thrombosis, artery
  traumatic
    edentulous (alveolar) ridge K06.2
    gingiva K06.2
    periodontal K05.5
  tubal N97.1
  ureter (complete) (partial) N13.5
    congenital Q62.10
  ureteropelvic junction N13.5
    congenital Q62.11
  ureterovesical orifice N13.5
    congenital Q62.12
  urethra — *see* Stricture, urethra
  uterus N85.8
  vagina N89.5
  vascular NEC I99.8
  vein — *see* Thrombosis
    retinal — *see* Occlusion, retinal, vein
  vena cava (inferior) (superior) — *see* Embolism, vena cava
  ventricle (brain) NEC G91.1
  vertebral (artery) — *see* Occlusion, artery, vertebral
  vessel (blood) I99.8
  vulva N90.5

Occult
  blood in feces (stools) R19.5

Occupational
  problems NEC Z56.89

Ochlophobia — *see* Agoraphobia

Ochronosis (endogenous) E70.29

Ocular muscle — *see* condition

Oculogyric crisis or disturbance H51.8
  psychogenic F45.8

Oculomotor syndrome H51.9

Oculopathy
  syphilitic NEC A52.71
    congenital
      early A50.01
      late A50.30
    early (secondary) A51.43
    late A52.71

Oddi's sphincter spasm K83.4

Odontalgia K08.8

Odontoameloblastoma — *see* Cyst, calcifying odontogenic

Odontoclasia K03.89

Odontodysplasia, regional K00.4

Odontogenesis imperfecta K00.5

Odontoma (ameloblastic) (complex) (compound) (fibroameloblastic) — *see* Cyst, calcifying odontogenic

Odontomyelitis (closed) (open) K04.0

Odontorrhagia K08.8

Odontosarcoma, ameloblastic C41.1
  upper jaw (bone) C41.0

Oestriasis — *see* Myiasis

Oguchi's disease H53.63

Ohara's disease — *see* Tularemia

Oidiomycosis — *see* Candidiasis

Oidium albicans infection — *see* Candidiasis

Old age (without mention of debility) R54
  dementia F03 ☑

Old (previous) **myocardial infarction** I25.2

Olfactory — *see* condition

Oligemia — *see* Anemia

Oligoastrocytoma
  specified site — *see* Neoplasm, malignant, by site
  unspecified site C71.9

Oligocythemia D64.9

Oligodendroblastoma
  specified site — *see* Neoplasm, malignant
  unspecified site C71.9

Oligodendroglioma
  anaplastic type
    specified site — *see* Neoplasm, malignant, by site
    unspecified site C71.9
  specified site — *see* Neoplasm, malignant, by site
  unspecified site C71.9

Oligodontia — *see* Anodontia

Oligoencephalon Q02

Oligohidrosis L74.4

Oligohydramnios O41.0- ☑

Oligohydrosis L74.4

Oligomenorrhea N91.5
  primary N91.3
  secondary N91.4
Oligophrenia (see also Disability, intellectual)
  phenylpyruvic E70.0
Oligospermia N46.11
  due to
    drug therapy N46.121
    efferent duct obstruction N46.123
    infection N46.122
    radiation N46.124
    specified cause NEC N46.129
    systemic disease N46.125
Oligotrichia — see Alopecia
Oliguria R34
  postprocedural N99.0
  with, complicating or following ectopic or molar
    pregnancy O08.4
Ollier's disease Q78.4
Omenotocele — see Hernia, abdomen, specified site
  NEC
Omentitis — see Peritonitis
Omentum, omental — see condition
Omphalitis (congenital) (newborn) P38.9
  with mild hemorrhage P38.1
  without hemorrhage P38.9
  not of newborn L08.82
  tetanus A33
Omphalocele Q79.2
Omphalomesenteric duct, persistent Q43.0
Omphalorrhagia, newborn P51.9
Omsk hemorrhagic fever A98.1
Onanism (excessive) F98.8
Onchocerciasis, onchocercosis B73.1
  with
    eye disease B73.00
      endophthalmitis B73.01
      eyelid B73.09
      glaucoma B73.02
      specified NEC B73.09
    eyelid B73.09
    eye NEC B73.00
Oncocytoma — see Neoplasm, benign, by site
Oncovirus, as cause of disease classified elsewhere
  B97.32
Ondine's curse — see Apnea, sleep
Oneirophrenia F23
Onychauxis L60.2
  congenital Q84.5
Onychia (see also Cellulitis, digit)
  with lymphangitis — see Lymphangitis, acute, digit
  candidal B37.2
  dermatophytic B35.1
Onychitis (see also Cellulitis, digit)
  with lymphangitis — see Lymphangitis, acute, digit
Onychocryptosis L60.0
Onychodystrophy L60.3
  congenital Q84.6
Onychogryphosis, onychogryposis L60.2
Onycholysis L60.1
Onychomadesis L60.8
Onychomalacia L60.3
Onychomycosis (finger) (toe) B35.1
Onycho-osteodysplasia Q79.8
Onychophagia F98.8
Onychophosis L60.8
Onychoptosis L60.8
Onychorrhexis L60.3
  congenital Q84.6
Onychoschizia L60.3
Onyxis (finger) (toe) L60.0
Onyxitis (see also Cellulitis, digit)
  with lymphangitis — see Lymphangitis, acute, digit
Oophoritis (cystic) (infectional) (interstitial) N70.92
  with salpingitis N70.93
  acute N70.02
    with salpingitis N70.03
  chronic N70.12
    with salpingitis N70.13
  complicating abortion — see Abortion, by type, com-
    plicated by, oophoritis
Oophorocele N83.4
Opacity, opacities
  cornea H17.- ☑
    central H17.1- ☑
    congenital Q13.3
    degenerative — see Degeneration, cornea

Opacity, opacities — continued
  cornea — continued
    hereditary — see Dystrophy, cornea
    inflammatory — see Keratitis
    minor H17.81- ☑
    peripheral H17.82- ☑
    sequelae of trachoma (healed) B94.0
    specified NEC H17.89
  enamel (teeth) (fluoride) (nonfluoride) K00.3
  lens — see Cataract
  snowball — see Deposit, crystalline
  vitreous (humor) NEC H43.39- ☑
    congenital Q14.0
    membranes and strands H43.31- ☑
Opalescent dentin (hereditary) K00.5
Open, opening
  abnormal, organ or site, congenital — see Imperfect,
    closure
  angle with
    borderline
      findings
        high risk H40.02- ☑
        low risk H40.01- ☑
      intraocular pressure H40.00- ☑
    cupping of discs H40.01- ☑
    glaucoma (primary) — see Glaucoma, open angle
  bite
    anterior M26.220
    posterior M26.221
  false — see Imperfect, closure
  margin on tooth restoration K08.51
  restoration margins of tooth K08.51
  wound — see Wound, open
Operational fatigue F48.8
Operative — see condition
Operculitis — see Periodontitis
Operculum — see Break, retina
Ophiasis L63.2
Ophthalmia (see also Conjunctivitis) H10.9
  actinic rays — see Photokeratitis
  allergic (acute) — see Conjunctivitis, acute, atopic
  blennorrhagic (gonococcal) (neonatorum) A54.31
  diphtheritic A36.86
  Egyptian A71.1
  electrica — see Photokeratitis
  gonococcal (neonatorum) A54.31
  metastatic — see Endophthalmitis, purulent
  migraine — see Migraine, ophthalmoplegic
  neonatorum, newborn P39.1
    gonococcal A54.31
  nodosa H16.24- ☑
  purulent — see Conjunctivitis, acute, mucopurulent
  spring — see Conjunctivitis, acute, atopic
  sympathetic — see Uveitis, sympathetic
Ophthalmitis — see Ophthalmia
Ophthalmocele (congenital) Q15.8
Ophthalmoneuromyelitis G36.0
Ophthalmoplegia (see also Strabismus, paralytic)
  anterior internuclear — see Ophthalmoplegia, inter-
    nuclear
  ataxia-areflexia G61.0
  diabetic — see E08-E13 with .39
  exophthalmic E05.00
    with thyroid storm E05.01
  external H49.88- ☑
    progressive H49.4- ☑
      with pigmentary retinopathy — see Kearns-
        Sayre syndrome
    total H49.3- ☑
  internal (complete) (total) H52.51- ☑
  internuclear H51.2- ☑
  migraine — see Migraine, ophthalmoplegic
  Parinaud's H49.88- ☑
  progressive external — see Ophthalmoplegia, external,
    progressive
  supranuclear, progressive G23.1
  total (external) — see Ophthalmoplegia, external, total
Opioid(s)
  abuse — see Abuse, drug, opioids
  dependence — see Dependence, drug, opioids
Opisthognathism M26.09
Opisthorchiasis (felineus) (viverrini) B66.0
Opitz' disease D73.2
Opiumism — see Dependence, drug, opioid
Oppenheim's disease G70.2
Oppenheim-Urbach disease (necrobiosis lipoidica dia-
  beticorum) — see E08-E13 with .620

Optic nerve — see condition
Orbit — see condition
Orchioblastoma C62.9- ☑
Orchitis (gangrenous) (nonspecific) (septic) (suppurative)
  N45.2
  blennorrhagic (gonococcal) (acute) (chronic) A54.23
  chlamydial A56.19
  filarial (see also Infestation, filarial) B74.9 [N51]
  gonococcal (acute) (chronic) A54.23
  mumps B26.0
  syphilitic A52.76
  tuberculous A18.15
Orf (virus disease) B08.02
Organic (see also condition)
  brain syndrome F09
  heart — see Disease, heart
  mental disorder F09
  psychosis F09
Orgasm
  anejaculatory N53.13
Oriental
  bilharziasis B65.2
  schistosomiasis B65.2
Orifice — see condition
Origin of both great vessels from right ventricle
  Q20.1
Ormond's disease (with ureteral obstruction) N13.5
  with infection N13.6
Ornithine metabolism disorder E72.4
Ornithinemia (Type I) (Type II) E72.4
Ornithosis A70
Orotaciduria, oroticaciduria (congenital) (hereditary)
  (pyrimidine deficiency) E79.8
  anemia D53.0
Orthodontics
  adjustment Z46.4
  fitting Z46.4
Orthopnea R06.01
Orthopoxvirus B08.09
  specified NEC B08.09
Os, uterus — see condition
Osgood-Schlatter disease or osteochondrosis — see
  Osteochondrosis, juvenile, tibia
Osler (-Weber)-**Rendu disease** I78.0
Osler's nodes I33.0
Osmidrosis L75.0
Osseous — see condition
Ossification
  artery — see Arteriosclerosis
  auricle (ear) — see Disorder, pinna, specified type NEC
  bronchial J98.09
  cardiac — see Degeneration, myocardial
  cartilage (senile) — see Disorder, cartilage, specified
    type NEC
  coronary (artery) — see Disease, heart, ischemic,
    atherosclerotic
  diaphragm J98.6
  ear, middle — see Otosclerosis
  falx cerebri G96.19
  fontanel, premature Q75.0
  heart (see also Degeneration, myocardial)
    valve — see Endocarditis
  larynx J38.7
  ligament — see Disorder, tendon, specified type NEC
    posterior longitudinal — see Spondylopathy,
      specified NEC
  meninges (cerebral) (spinal) G96.19
  multiple, eccentric centers — see Disorder, bone, de-
    velopment or growth
  muscle (see also Calcification, muscle)
    due to burns — see Myositis, ossificans, in, burns
    paralytic — see Myositis, ossificans, in, quadriplegia
    progressive — see Myositis, ossificans, progressiva
    specified NEC M61.50
      ankle M61.57- ☑
      foot M61.57- ☑
      forearm M61.53- ☑
      hand M61.54- ☑
      lower leg M61.56- ☑
      multiple sites M61.59
      pelvic region M61.55- ☑
      shoulder region M61.51- ☑
      specified site NEC M61.58
      thigh M61.55- ☑
      upper arm M61.52- ☑
    traumatic — see Myositis, ossificans, traumatica

Index

Ossification — Osteochondropathy

Ossification — *continued*
myocardium, myocardial — *see* Degeneration, myocardial
penis N48.89
periarticular — *see* Disorder, joint, specified type NEC
pinna — *see* Disorder, pinna, specified type NEC
rider's bone — *see* Ossification, muscle, specified NEC
sclera H15.89
subperiosteal, post-traumatic M89.8X- ☑
tendon — *see* Disorder, tendon, specified type NEC
trachea J39.8
tympanic membrane — *see* Disorder, tympanic membrane, specified NEC
vitreous (humor) — *see* Deposit, crystalline
Osteitis (*see also* Osteomyelitis)
alveolar M27.3
condensans M85.30
ankle M85.37- ☑
foot M85.37- ☑
forearm M85.33- ☑
hand M85.34- ☑
lower leg M85.36- ☑
multiple site M85.39
neck M85.38
rib M85.38
shoulder M85.31- ☑
skull M85.38
specified site NEC M85.38
thigh M85.35- ☑
toe M85.37- ☑
upper arm M85.32- ☑
vertebra M85.38
deformans M88.9
in (due to)
malignant neoplasm of bone C41.9 [M90.60]
neoplastic disease (*see also* Neoplasm) D49.9 [M90.60]
carpus D49.9 [M90.64-] ☑
clavicle D49.9 [M90.61-] ☑
femur D49.9 [M90.65-] ☑
fibula D49.9 [M90.66-] ☑
finger D49.9 [M90.64-] ☑
humerus D49.9 [M90.62-] ☑
ilium D49.9 [M90.65-] ☑
ischium D49.9 [M90.65-] ☑
metacarpus D49.9 [M90.64-] ☑
metatarsus D49.9 [M90.67-] ☑
multiple sites D49.9 [M90.69]
neck D49.9 [M90.68]
radius D49.9 [M90.63-] ☑
rib D49.9 [M90.68]
scapula D49.9 [M90.61-] ☑
skull D49.9 [M90.68]
tarsus D49.9 [M90.67-] ☑
tibia D49.9 [M90.66-] ☑
toe D49.9 [M90.67-] ☑
ulna D49.9 [M90.63-] ☑
vertebra D49.9 [M90.68]
skull M88.0
specified NEC — *see* Paget's disease, bone, by site
vertebra M88.1
due to yaws A66.6
fibrosa NEC — *see* Cyst, bone, by site
circumscripta — *see* Dysplasia, fibrous, bone NEC
cystica (generalisata) E21.0
disseminata Q78.1
osteoplastica E21.0
fragilitans Q78.0
Garr's (sclerosing) — *see* Osteomyelitis, specified type NEC
jaw (acute) (chronic) (lower) (suppurative) (upper) M27.2
parathyroid E21.0
petrous bone (acute) (chronic) — *see* Petrositis
sclerotic, nonsuppurative — *see* Osteomyelitis, specified type NEC
tuberculosa A18.09
cystica D86.89
multiplex cystoides D86.89
Osteoarthritis M19.90
ankle M19.07- ☑
elbow M19.02- ☑
foot joint M19.07- ☑
generalized M15.9
erosive M15.4
primary M15.0
specified NEC M15.8

Osteoarthritis — *continued*
hand joint M19.04- ☑
first carpometacarpal joint M18.9
hip M16.1- ☑
bilateral M16.0
due to hip dysplasia (unilateral) M16.3- ☑
bilateral M16.2
interphalangeal
distal (Heberden) M15.1
proximal (Bouchard) M15.2
knee M17.9
bilateral M17.0
post-traumatic NEC M19.92
ankle M19.17- ☑
elbow M19.12- ☑
foot joint M19.17- ☑
hand joint M19.14- ☑
first carpometacarpal joint M18.3- ☑
bilateral M18.2
hip M16.5- ☑
bilateral M16.4
knee M17.3- ☑
bilateral M17.2
shoulder M19.11- ☑
wrist M19.13- ☑
primary M19.91
ankle M19.07- ☑
elbow M19.02- ☑
foot joint M19.07- ☑
hand joint M19.04- ☑
first carpometacarpal joint M18.1- ☑
bilateral M18.0
hip M16.1- ☑
bilateral M16.0
knee M17.1- ☑
bilateral M17.0
shoulder M19.01- ☑
spine — *see* Spondylosis
wrist M19.03- ☑
secondary M19.93
ankle M19.27- ☑
elbow M19.22- ☑
foot joint M19.27- ☑
hand joint M19.24- ☑
first carpometacarpal joint M18.5- ☑
bilateral M18.4
hip M16.7
bilateral M16.6
knee M17.5
bilateral M17.4
multiple M15.3
shoulder M19.21- ☑
spine — *see* Spondylosis
wrist M19.23- ☑
shoulder M19.01- ☑
spine — *see* Spondylosis
wrist M19.03- ☑
Osteoarthropathy (hypertrophic) M19.90
ankle — *see* Osteoarthritis, primary, ankle
elbow — *see* Osteoarthritis, primary, elbow
foot joint — *see* Osteoarthritis, primary, foot
hand joint — *see* Osteoarthritis, primary, hand joint
knee joint — *see* Osteoarthritis, primary, knee
multiple site — *see* Osteoarthritis, primary, multiple joint
pulmonary (*see also* Osteoarthropathy, specified type NEC)
hypertrophic — *see* Osteoarthropathy, hypertrophic, specified type NEC
secondary — *see* Osteoarthropathy, specified type NEC
secondary hypertrophic — *see* Osteoarthropathy, specified type NEC
shoulder — *see* Osteoarthritis, primary, shoulder
specified joint NEC — *see* Osteoarthritis, primary, specified joint NEC
specified type NEC M89.40
carpus M89.44- ☑
clavicle M89.41- ☑
femur M89.45- ☑
fibula M89.46- ☑
finger M89.44- ☑
humerus M89.42- ☑
ilium M89.459
ischium M89.459
metacarpus M89.44- ☑

Osteoarthropathy — *continued*
specified type — *continued*
metatarsus M89.47- ☑
multiple sites M89.49
neck M89.48
radius M89.43- ☑
rib M89.48
scapula M89.41- ☑
skull M89.48
tarsus M89.47- ☑
tibia M89.46- ☑
toe M89.47- ☑
ulna M89.43- ☑
vertebra M89.48
spine — *see* Spondylosis
wrist — *see* Osteoarthritis, primary, wrist
Osteoarthrosis (degenerative) (hypertrophic) (joint) (*see also* Osteoarthritis)
deformans alkaptonurica E70.29 [M36.8]
erosive M15.4
generalized M15.9
primary M15.0
polyarticular M15.9
spine — *see* Spondylosis
Osteoblastoma — *see* Neoplasm, bone, benign
aggressive — *see* Neoplasm, bone, uncertain behavior
Osteochondritis (*see also* Osteochondropathy, by site)
Brailsford's — *see* Osteochondrosis, juvenile, radius
dissecans M93.20
ankle M93.27- ☑
elbow M93.22- ☑
foot M93.27- ☑
hand M93.24- ☑
hip M93.25- ☑
knee M93.26- ☑
multiple sites M93.29
shoulder joint M93.21- ☑
specified site NEC M93.28
wrist M93.23- ☑
juvenile M92.9
patellar — *see* Osteochondrosis, juvenile, patella
syphilitic (congenital) (early) A50.02 [M90.80]
ankle A50.02 [M90.87-] ☑
elbow A50.02 [M90.82-] ☑
foot A50.02 [M90.87-] ☑
forearm A50.02 [M90.83-] ☑
hand A50.02 [M90.84-] ☑
hip A50.02 [M90.85-] ☑
knee A50.02 [M90.86-] ☑
multiple sites A50.02 [M90.89]
shoulder joint A50.02 [M90.81-] ☑
specified site NEC A50.02 [M90.88]
Osteochondroarthrosis deformans endemica — *see* Disease, Kaschin-Beck
Osteochondrodysplasia Q78.9
with defects of growth of tubular bones and spine Q77.9
specified NEC Q77.8
specified NEC Q78.8
Osteochondrodystrophy E78.9
Osteochondrolysis — *see* Osteochondritis, dissecans
Osteochondroma — *see* Neoplasm, bone, benign
Osteochondromatosis D48.0
syndrome Q78.4
Osteochondromyxosarcoma — *see* Neoplasm, bone, malignant
Osteochondropathy M93.90
ankle M93.97- ☑
elbow M93.92- ☑
foot M93.97- ☑
hand M93.94- ☑
hip M93.95- ☑
Kienböck's disease of adults M93.1
knee M93.96- ☑
multiple joints M93.99
osteochondritis dissecans — *see* Osteochondritis, dissecans
osteochondrosis — *see* Osteochondrosis
shoulder region M93.91- ☑
slipped upper femoral epiphysis — *see* Slipped, epiphysis, upper femoral
specified joint NEC M93.98
specified type NEC M93.80
ankle M93.87- ☑
elbow M93.82- ☑
foot M93.87- ☑

Osteochondropathy — *continued*
  specified type — *continued*
    hand M93.84- ☑
    hip M93.85- ☑
    knee M93.86- ☑
    multiple joints M93.89
    shoulder region M93.81- ☑
    specified joint NEC M93.88
    wrist M93.83- ☑
  syphilitic, congenital
    early A50.02 [M90.80]
    late A50.56 [M90.80]
  wrist M93.93- ☑
Osteochondrosarcoma — *see* Neoplasm, bone, malignant
Osteochondrosis (*see also* Osteochondropathy, by site)
  acetabulum (juvenile) M91.0
  adult — *see* Osteochondropathy, specified type NEC, by site
  astragalus (juvenile) — *see* Osteochondrosis, juvenile, tarsus
  Blount's — *see* Osteochondrosis, juvenile, tibia
  Buchanan's M91.0
  Burns' — *see* Osteochondrosis, juvenile, ulna
  calcaneus (juvenile) — *see* Osteochondrosis, juvenile, tarsus
  capitular epiphysis (femur) (juvenile) — *see* Legg-Calvé-Perthes disease
  carpal (juvenile) (lunate) (scaphoid) — *see* Osteochondrosis, juvenile, hand, carpal lunate
    adult M93.1
  coxae juvenilis — *see* Legg-Calvé-Perthes disease
  deformans juvenilis, coxae — *see* Legg-Calvé-Perthes disease
  Diaz's — *see* Osteochondrosis, juvenile, tarsus
  dissecans (knee) (shoulder) — *see* Osteochondritis, dissecans
  femoral capital epiphysis (juvenile) — *see* Legg-Calvé-Perthes disease
  femur (head), juvenile — *see* Legg-Calvé-Perthes disease
  fibula (juvenile) — *see* Osteochondrosis, juvenile, fibula
  foot NEC (juvenile) M92.8
  Freiberg's — *see* Osteochondrosis, juvenile, metatarsus
  Haas' (juvenile) — *see* Osteochondrosis, juvenile, humerus
  Haglund's — *see* Osteochondrosis, juvenile, tarsus
  hip (juvenile) — *see* Legg-Calvé-Perthes disease
  humerus (capitulum) (head) (juvenile) — *see* Osteochondrosis, juvenile, humerus
  ilium, iliac crest (juvenile) M91.0
  ischiopubic synchondrosis M91.0
  Iselin's — *see* Osteochondrosis, juvenile, metatarsus
  juvenile, juvenilis M92.9
    after congenital dislocation of hip reduction — *see* Osteochondrosis, juvenile, hip, specified NEC
    arm — *see* Osteochondrosis, juvenile, upper limb NEC
    capitular epiphysis (femur) — *see* Legg-Calvé-Perthes disease
    clavicle, sternal epiphysis — *see* Osteochondrosis, juvenile, upper limb NEC
    coxae — *see* Legg-Calvé-Perthes disease
    deformans M92.9
    fibula M92.5- ☑
    foot NEC M92.8
    hand M92.20- ☑
      carpal lunate M92.21- ☑
      metacarpal head M92.22- ☑
      specified site NEC M92.29- ☑
    head of femur — *see* Legg-Calvé-Perthes disease
    hip and pelvis M91.9-
      coxa plana — *see* Coxa, plana
      femoral head — *see* Legg-Calvé-Perthes disease
      pelvis M91.0
      pseudocoxalgia — *see* Pseudocoxalgia
      specified NEC M91.8- ☑
    humerus M92.0- ☑
    limb
      lower NEC M92.8
      upper NEC — *see* Osteochondrosis, juvenile, upper limb NEC
    medial cuneiform bone — *see* Osteochondrosis, juvenile, tarsus
    metatarsus M92.7- ☑
    patella M92.4- ☑

Osteochondrosis — *continued*
  juvenile, juvenilis — *continued*
    radius M92.1- ☑
    specified site NEC M92.8
    spine M42.00
      cervical region M42.02
      cervicothoracic region M42.03
      lumbar region M42.06
      lumbosacral region M42.07
      multiple sites M42.09
      occipito-atlanto-axial region M42.01
      sacrococcygeal region M42.08
      thoracic region M42.04
      thoracolumbar region M42.05
    tarsus M92.6- ☑
    tibia M92.5- ☑
    ulna M92.1- ☑
    upper limb NEC M92.3- ☑
    vertebra (body) (epiphyseal plates) (Calvé's) (Scheuermann's) — *see* Osteochondrosis, juvenile, spine
  Kienböck's — *see* Osteochondrosis, juvenile, hand, carpal lunate
    adult M93.1
  Köhler's
    patellar — *see* Osteochondrosis, juvenile, patella
    tarsal navicular — *see* Osteochondrosis, juvenile, tarsus
  Legg-Perthes (-Calvé)(-Waldenström) — *see* Legg-Calvé-Perthes disease
  limb
    lower NEC (juvenile) M92.8
    upper NEC (juvenile) — *see* Osteochondrosis, juvenile, upper limb NEC
  lunate bone (carpal) (juvenile) (*see also* Osteochondrosis, juvenile, hand, carpal lunate)
    adult M93.1
  Mauclaire's — *see* Osteochondrosis, juvenile, hand, metacarpal
  metacarpal (head) (juvenile) — *see* Osteochondrosis, juvenile, hand, metacarpal
  metatarsus (fifth) (head) (juvenile) (second) — *see* Osteochondrosis, juvenile, metatarsus
  navicular (juvenile) — *see* Osteochondrosis, juvenile, tarsus
  os
    calcis (juvenile) — *see* Osteochondrosis, juvenile, tarsus
    tibiale externum (juvenile) — *see* Osteochondrosis, juvenile, tarsus
  Osgood-Schlatter — *see* Osteochondrosis, juvenile, tibia
  Panner's — *see* Osteochondrosis, juvenile, humerus
  patellar center (juvenile) (primary) (secondary) — *see* Osteochondrosis, juvenile, patella
  pelvis (juvenile) M91.0
  Pierson's M91.0
  radius (head) (juvenile) — *see* Osteochondrosis, juvenile, radius
  Scheuermann's — *see* Osteochondrosis, juvenile, spine
  Sever's — *see* Osteochondrosis, juvenile, tarsus
  Sinding-Larsen — *see* Osteochondrosis, juvenile, patella
  spine M42.9
    adult M42.10
      cervical region M42.12
      cervicothoracic region M42.13
      lumbar region M42.16
      lumbosacral region M42.17
      multiple sites M42.19
      occipito-atlanto-axial region M42.11
      sacrococcygeal region M42.18
      thoracic region M42.14
      thoracolumbar region M42.15
    juvenile — *see* Osteochondrosis, juvenile, spine
  symphysis pubis (juvenile) M91.0
  syphilitic (congenital) A50.02
  talus (juvenile) — *see* Osteochondrosis, juvenile, tarsus
  tarsus (navicular) (juvenile) — *see* Osteochondrosis, juvenile, tarsus
  tibia (proximal) (tubercle) (juvenile) — *see* Osteochondrosis, juvenile, tibia
  tuberculous — *see* Tuberculosis, bone
  ulna (lower) (juvenile) — *see* Osteochondrosis, juvenile, ulna
  van Neck's M91.0
  vertebral — *see* Osteochondrosis, spine

Osteoclastoma D48.0
  malignant — *see* Neoplasm, bone, malignant
Osteodynia — *see* Disorder, bone, specified type NEC
Osteodystrophy Q78.9
  azotemic N25.0
  congenital Q78.9
  parathyroid, secondary E21.1
  renal N25.0
Osteofibroma — *see* Neoplasm, bone, benign
Osteofibrosarcoma — *see* Neoplasm, bone, malignant
Osteogenesis imperfecta Q78.0
Osteogenic — *see* condition
Osteolysis M89.50
  carpus M89.54- ☑
  clavicle M89.51- ☑
  femur M89.55- ☑
  fibula M89.56- ☑
  finger M89.54- ☑
  humerus M89.52- ☑
  ilium M89.559
  ischium M89.559
  joint prosthesis (periprosthetic) — *see* Complications, joint prosthesis, mechanical, periprosthetic, osteolysis, by site
  metacarpus M89.54- ☑
  metatarsus M89.57- ☑
  multiple sites M89.59
  neck M89.58
  periprosthetic — *see* Complications, joint prosthesis, mechanical, periprosthetic, osteolysis, by site
  radius M89.53- ☑
  rib M89.58
  scapula M89.51- ☑
  skull M89.58
  tarsus M89.57- ☑
  tibia M89.56- ☑
  toe M89.57- ☑
  ulna M89.53- ☑
  vertebra M89.58
Osteoma (*see also* Neoplasm, bone, benign)
  osteoid (*see also* Neoplasm, bone, benign)
    giant — *see* Neoplasm, bone, benign
Osteomalacia M83.9
  adult M83.9
    drug-induced NEC M83.5
    due to
      malabsorption (postsurgical) M83.2
      malnutrition M83.3
    specified NEC M83.8
  aluminium-induced M83.4
  infantile — *see* Rickets
  juvenile — *see* Rickets
  oncogenic E83.89
  pelvis M83.8
  puerperal M83.0
  senile M83.1
  vitamin-D-resistant in adults E83.31 [M90.8-] ☑
    carpus E83.31 [M90.84-] ☑
    clavicle E83.31 [M90.81-] ☑
    femur E83.31 [M90.85-] ☑
    fibula E83.31 [M90.86-] ☑
    finger E83.31 [M90.84-] ☑
    humerus E83.31 [M90.82-] ☑
    ilium E83.31 [M90.859]
    ischium E83.31 [M90.859]
    metacarpus E83.31 [M90.84-] ☑
    metatarsus E83.31 [M90.87-] ☑
    multiple sites E83.31 [M90.89]
    neck E83.31 [M90.88]
    radius E83.31 [M90.83-] ☑
    rib E83.31 [M90.88]
    scapula E83.31 [M90.819]
    skull E83.31 [M90.88]
    tarsus E83.31 [M90.879]
    tibia E83.31 [M90.869]
    toe E83.31 [M90.879]
    ulna E83.31 [M90.839]
    vertebra E83.31 [M90.88]
Osteomyelitis (general) (infective) (localized) (neonatal) (purulent) (septic) (staphylococcal) (streptococcal) (suppurative) (with periostitis) M86.9
  acute M86.10
    carpus M86.14- ☑
    clavicle M86.11- ☑
    femur M86.15- ☑
    fibula M86.16- ☑
    finger M86.14- ☑

Osteomyelitis — *continued*
- acute — *continued*
  - hematogenous M86.00
    - carpus M86.04- ☑
    - clavicle M86.01- ☑
    - femur M86.05- ☑
    - fibula M86.06- ☑
    - finger M86.04- ☑
    - humerus M86.02- ☑
    - ilium M86.059
    - ischium M86.059
    - mandible M27.2
    - metacarpus M86.04- ☑
    - metatarsus M86.07- ☑
    - multiple sites M86.09
    - neck M86.08
    - orbit H05.02- ☑
    - petrous bone — *see* Petrositis
    - radius M86.03- ☑
    - rib M86.08
    - scapula M86.01- ☑
    - skull M86.08
    - tarsus M86.07- ☑
    - tibia M86.06- ☑
    - toe M86.07- ☑
    - ulna M86.03- ☑
    - vertebra — *see* Osteomyelitis, vertebra
  - humerus M86.12- ☑
  - ilium M86.159
  - ischium M86.159
  - mandible M27.2
  - metacarpus M86.14- ☑
  - metatarsus M86.17- ☑
  - multiple sites M86.19
  - neck M86.18
  - orbit H05.02- ☑
  - petrous bone — *see* Petrositis
  - radius M86.13- ☑
  - rib M86.18
  - scapula M86.11- ☑
  - skull M86.18
  - tarsus M86.17- ☑
  - tibia M86.16- ☑
  - toe M86.17- ☑
  - ulna M86.13- ☑
  - vertebra — *see* Osteomyelitis, vertebra
- chronic (or old) M86.60
  - with draining sinus M86.40
    - carpus M86.44- ☑
    - clavicle M86.41- ☑
    - femur M86.45- ☑
    - fibula M86.46- ☑
    - finger M86.44- ☑
    - humerus M86.42- ☑
    - ilium M86.459
    - ischium M86.459
    - mandible M27.2
    - metacarpus M86.44- ☑
    - metatarsus M86.47- ☑
    - multiple sites M86.49
    - neck M86.48
    - orbit H05.02- ☑
    - petrous bone — *see* Petrositis
    - radius M86.43- ☑
    - rib M86.48
    - scapula M86.41- ☑
    - skull M86.48
    - tarsus M86.47- ☑
    - tibia M86.46- ☑
    - toe M86.47- ☑
    - ulna M86.43- ☑
    - vertebra — *see* Osteomyelitis, vertebra
  - carpus M86.64- ☑
  - clavicle M86.61- ☑
  - femur M86.65- ☑
  - fibula M86.66- ☑
  - finger M86.64- ☑
  - hematogenous NEC M86.50
    - carpus M86.54- ☑
    - clavicle M86.51- ☑
    - femur M86.55- ☑
    - fibula M86.56- ☑
    - finger M86.54- ☑
    - humerus M86.52- ☑
    - ilium M86.559
    - ischium M86.559

Osteomyelitis — *continued*
- chronic — *continued*
  - hematogenous — *continued*
    - mandible M27.2
    - metacarpus M86.54- ☑
    - metatarsus M86.57- ☑
    - multifocal M86.30
      - carpus M86.34- ☑
      - clavicle M86.31- ☑
      - femur M86.35- ☑
      - fibula M86.36- ☑
      - finger M86.34- ☑
      - humerus M86.32- ☑
      - ilium M86.359
      - ischium M86.359
      - metacarpus M86.34- ☑
      - metatarsus M86.37- ☑
      - multiple sites M86.39
      - neck M86.38
      - radius M86.33- ☑
      - rib M86.38
      - scapula M86.31- ☑
      - skull M86.38
      - tarsus M86.37- ☑
      - tibia M86.36- ☑
      - toe M86.37- ☑
      - ulna M86.33- ☑
      - vertebra — *see* Osteomyelitis, vertebra
    - multiple sites M86.59
    - neck M86.58
    - orbit H05.02- ☑
    - petrous bone — *see* Petrositis
    - radius M86.53- ☑
    - rib M86.58
    - scapula M86.51- ☑
    - skull M86.58
    - tarsus M86.57- ☑
    - tibia M86.56- ☑
    - toe M86.57- ☑
    - ulna M86.53- ☑
    - vertebra — *see* Osteomyelitis, vertebra
  - humerus M86.62- ☑
  - ilium M86.659
  - ischium M86.659
  - mandible M27.2
  - metacarpus M86.64- ☑
  - metatarsus M86.67- ☑
  - multifocal — *see* Osteomyelitis, chronic, hematogenous, multifocal
  - multiple sites M86.69
  - neck M86.68
  - orbit H05.02- ☑
  - petrous bone — *see* Petrositis
  - radius M86.63- ☑
  - rib M86.68
  - scapula M86.61- ☑
  - skull M86.68
  - tarsus M86.67- ☑
  - tibia M86.66- ☑
  - toe M86.67- ☑
  - ulna M86.63- ☑
  - vertebra — *see* Osteomyelitis, vertebra
- echinococcal B67.2
- Garr's — *see* Osteomyelitis, specified type NEC
- jaw (acute) (chronic) (lower) (neonatal) (suppurative) (upper) M27.2
- nonsuppurating — *see* Osteomyelitis, specified type NEC
- orbit H05.02- ☑
- petrous bone — *see* Petrositis
- Salmonella (arizonae) (cholerae-suis) (enteritidis) (typhimurium) A02.24
- sclerosing, nonsuppurative — *see* Osteomyelitis, specified type NEC
- specified type NEC (*see also* subcategory) M86.8X- ☑
  - mandible M27.2
  - orbit H05.02- ☑
  - petrous bone — *see* Petrositis
  - vertebra — *see* Osteomyelitis, vertebra
- subacute M86.20
  - carpus M86.24- ☑
  - clavicle M86.21- ☑
  - femur M86.25- ☑
  - fibula M86.26- ☑
  - finger M86.24- ☑
  - humerus M86.22- ☑

Osteomyelitis — *continued*
- subacute — *continued*
  - mandible M27.2
  - metacarpus M86.24- ☑
  - metatarsus M86.27- ☑
  - multiple sites M86.29
  - neck M86.28
  - orbit H05.02- ☑
  - petrous bone — *see* Petrositis
  - radius M86.23- ☑
  - rib M86.28
  - scapula M86.21- ☑
  - skull M86.28
  - tarsus M86.27- ☑
  - tibia M86.26- ☑
  - toe M86.27- ☑
  - ulna M86.23- ☑
  - vertebra — *see* Osteomyelitis, vertebra
- syphilitic A52.77
  - congenital (early) A50.02 [M90.80]
- tuberculous — *see* Tuberculosis, bone
- typhoid A01.05
- vertebra M46.20
  - cervical region M46.22
  - cervicothoracic region M46.23
  - lumbar region M46.26
  - lumbosacral region M46.27
  - occipito-atlanto-axial region M46.21
  - sacrococcygeal region M46.28
  - thoracic region M46.24
  - thoracolumbar region M46.25

Osteomyelofibrosis D75.89
Osteomyelosclerosis D75.89
Osteonecrosis M87.9
- due to
  - drugs — *see* Osteonecrosis, secondary, due to, drugs
  - trauma — *see* Osteonecrosis, secondary, due to, trauma
- idiopathic aseptic M87.00
  - ankle M87.07- ☑
  - carpus M87.03- ☑
  - clavicle M87.01- ☑
  - femur M87.05- ☑
  - fibula M87.06- ☑
  - finger M87.04- ☑
  - humerus M87.02- ☑
  - ilium M87.050
  - ischium M87.050
  - metacarpus M87.04- ☑
  - metatarsus M87.07- ☑
  - multiple sites M87.09
  - neck M87.08
  - pelvis M87.050
  - radius M87.03- ☑
  - rib M87.08
  - scapula M87.01- ☑
  - skull M87.08
  - tarsus M87.07- ☑
  - tibia M87.06- ☑
  - toe M87.07- ☑
  - ulna M87.03- ☑
  - vertebra M87.08
- secondary NEC M87.30
  - carpus M87.33- ☑
  - clavicle M87.31- ☑
  - due to
    - drugs M87.10
      - carpus M87.13- ☑
      - clavicle M87.11- ☑
      - femur M87.15- ☑
      - fibula M87.16- ☑
      - finger M87.14- ☑
      - humerus M87.12- ☑
      - ilium M87.159
      - ischium M87.159
      - jaw M87.180
      - metacarpus M87.14- ☑
      - metatarsus M87.17- ☑
      - multiple sites M87.19
      - neck M87.18
      - radius M87.13- ☑
      - rib M87.18
      - scapula M87.11- ☑
      - skull M87.18
      - tarsus M87.17- ☑
      - tibia M87.16- ☑

☑ **Additional Character Required** — Refer to the Tabular List for Character Selection   ▽ **Subterms under main terms may continue to next column or page**

Osteonecrosis — *continued*
  secondary — *continued*
    due to — *continued*
      drugs — *continued*
        toe M87.17- ☑
        ulna M87.13- ☑
        vertebra M87.18 ☑
      hemoglobinopathy NEC D58.2 [M90.50]
        carpus D58.2 [M90.54-] ☑
        clavicle D58.2 [M90.51-] ☑
        femur D58.2 [M90.55-] ☑
        fibula D58.2 [M90.56-] ☑
        finger D58.2 [M90.54-] ☑
        humerus D58.2 [M90.52-] ☑
        ilium D58.2 [M90.55-] ☑
        ischium D58.2 [M90.55-] ☑
        metacarpus D58.2 [M90.54-] ☑
        metatarsus D58.2 [M90.57-] ☑
        multiple sites D58.2 [M90.58]
        neck D58.2 [M90.58]
        radius D58.2 [M90.53-] ☑
        rib D58.2 [M90.58]
        scapula D58.2 [M90.51-] ☑
        skull D58.2 [M90.58]
        tarsus D58.2 [M90.57-] ☑
        tibia D58.2 [M90.56-] ☑
        toe D58.2 [M90.57-] ☑
        ulna D58.2 [M90.53-] ☑
        vertebra D58.2 [M90.58]
      trauma (previous) M87.20
        carpus M87.23- ☑
        clavicle M87.21- ☑
        femur M87.25- ☑
        fibula M87.26- ☑
        finger M87.24- ☑
        humerus M87.22- ☑
        ilium M87.25- ☑
        ischium M87.25- ☑
        metacarpus M87.24- ☑
        metatarsus M87.27- ☑
        multiple sites M87.29
        neck M87.28
        radius M87.23- ☑
        rib M87.28
        scapula M87.21- ☑
        skull M87.28
        tarsus M87.27- ☑
        tibia M87.26- ☑
        toe M87.27- ☑
        ulna M87.23- ☑
        vertebra M87.28
  femur M87.35- ☑
  fibula M87.36- ☑
  finger M87.34- ☑
  humerus M87.32- ☑
  ilium M87.350
  in
    caisson disease T70.3 [M90.50]
      carpus T70.3 ☑ [M90.54-]
      clavicle T70.3 ☑ [M90.51-] ☑
      femur T70.3 ☑ [M90.55-] ☑
      fibula T70.3 ☑ [M90.56-] ☑
      finger T70.3 ☑ [M90.54-] ☑
      humerus T70.3 ☑ [M90.52-] ☑
      ilium T70.3 ☑ [M90.55-] ☑
      ischium T70.3 ☑ [M90.55-] ☑
      metacarpus T70.3 ☑ [M90.54-] ☑
      metatarsus T70.3 ☑ [M90.57-] ☑
      multiple sites T70.3 ☑ [M90.59]
      neck T70.3 ☑ [M90.58]
      radius T70.3 ☑ [M90.53-] ☑
      rib T70.3 ☑ [M90.58]
      scapula T70.3 ☑ [M90.51-] ☑
      skull T70.3 ☑ [M90.58]
      tarsus T70.3 ☑ [M90.57-] ☑
      tibia T70.3 ☑ [M90.56-] ☑
      toe T70.3 ☑ [M90.57-] ☑
      ulna T70.3 ☑ [M90.53-] ☑
      vertebra T70.3 ☑ [M90.58]
  ischium M87.350
  metacarpus M87.34- ☑
  metatarsus M87.37- ☑
  multiple site M87.39
  neck M87.38
  radius M87.33- ☑
  rib M87.38

Osteonecrosis — *continued*
  secondary — *continued*
    scapula M87.319
    skull M87.38
    tarsus M87.379
    tibia M87.366
    toe M87.379
    ulna M87.33- ☑
    vertebra M87.38
  specified type NEC M87.80
    carpus M87.83- ☑
    clavicle M87.81- ☑
    femur M87.85- ☑
    fibula M87.86- ☑
    finger M87.84- ☑
    humerus M87.82- ☑
    ilium M87.85- ☑
    ischium M87.85- ☑
    metacarpus M87.84- ☑
    metatarsus M87.87- ☑
    multiple sites M87.89
    neck M87.88
    radius M87.83- ☑
    rib M87.88
    scapula M87.81- ☑
    skull M87.88
    tarsus M87.87- ☑
    tibia M87.86- ☑
    toe M87.87- ☑
    ulna M87.83- ☑
    vertebra M87.88

Osteo-onycho-arthro-dysplasia Q79.8
Osteo-onychodysplasia, hereditary Q79.8
Osteopathia condensans disseminata Q78.8
Osteopathy (*see also* Osteomyelitis, Osteonecrosis, Osteoporosis)
  after poliomyelitis M89.60
    carpus M89.64- ☑
    clavicle M89.61- ☑
    femur M89.65- ☑
    fibula M89.66- ☑
    finger M89.64- ☑
    humerus M89.62- ☑
    ilium M89.659
    ischium M89.659
    metacarpus M89.64- ☑
    metatarsus M89.67- ☑
    multiple sites M89.69
    neck M89.68
    radius M89.63- ☑
    rib M89.68
    scapula M89.61- ☑
    skull M89.68
    tarsus M89.67- ☑
    tibia M89.66- ☑
    toe M89.67- ☑
    ulna M89.63- ☑
    vertebra M89.68
  in (due to)
    renal osteodystrophy N25.0
    specified diseases classified elsewhere — *see* subcategory M90.8
Osteopenia M85.8- ☑
  borderline M85.8- ☑
Osteoperiostitis — *see* Osteomyelitis, specified type NEC
Osteopetrosis (familial) Q78.2
Osteophyte M25.70
  ankle M25.77- ☑
  elbow M25.72- ☑
  foot joint M25.77- ☑
  hand joint M25.74- ☑
  hip M25.75- ☑
  knee M25.76- ☑
  shoulder M25.71- ☑
  spine M25.78
  vertebrae M25.78
  wrist M25.73- ☑
Osteopoikilosis Q78.8
Osteoporosis (female) (male) M81.0
  with current pathological fracture M80.00 ☑
  age-related M81.0
    with current pathologic fracture M80.00 ☑
      carpus M80.04- ☑
      clavicle M80.01- ☑
      fibula M80.06- ☑

Osteoporosis — *continued*
  age-related — *continued*
    with current pathologic fracture — *continued*
      finger M80.04- ☑
      humerus M80.02- ☑
      ilium M80.05- ☑
      ischium M80.05- ☑
      metacarpus M80.04- ☑
      metatarsus M80.07- ☑
      pelvis M80.05- ☑
      radius M80.03- ☑
      scapula M80.01- ☑
      tarsus M80.07- ☑
      tibia M80.06- ☑
      toe M80.07- ☑
      ulna M80.03- ☑
      vertebra M80.08 ☑
  disuse M81.8
    with current pathological fracture M80.80 ☑
      carpus M80.84- ☑
      clavicle M80.81- ☑
      fibula M80.86- ☑
      finger M80.84- ☑
      humerus M80.82- ☑
      ilium M80.85- ☑
      ischium M80.85- ☑
      metacarpus M80.84- ☑
      metatarsus M80.87- ☑
      pelvis M80.85- ☑
      radius M80.83- ☑
      scapula M80.81- ☑
      tarsus M80.87- ☑
      tibia M80.86- ☑
      toe M80.87- ☑
      ulna M80.83- ☑
      vertebra M80.88 ☑
  drug-induced — *see* Osteoporosis, specified type NEC
  idiopathic — *see* Osteoporosis, specified type NEC
  involutional — *see* Osteoporosis, age-related
  Lequesne M81.6
  localized M81.6
  postmenopausal M81.0
    with pathological fracture M80.00 ☑
      carpus M80.04- ☑
      clavicle M80.01- ☑
      fibula M80.06- ☑
      finger M80.04- ☑
      humerus M80.02- ☑
      ilium M80.05- ☑
      ischium M80.05- ☑
      metacarpus M80.04- ☑
      metatarsus M80.07- ☑
      pelvis M80.05- ☑
      radius M80.03- ☑
      scapula M80.01- ☑
      tarsus M80.07- ☑
      tibia M80.06- ☑
      toe M80.07- ☑
      ulna M80.03- ☑
      vertebra M80.08 ☑
  postoophorectomy — *see* Osteoporosis, specified type NEC
  postsurgical malabsorption — *see* Osteoporosis, specified type NEC
  post-traumatic — *see* Osteoporosis, specified type NEC
  senile — *see* Osteoporosis, age-related
  specified type NEC M81.8
    with pathological fracture M80.80 ☑
      carpus M80.84- ☑
      clavicle M80.81- ☑
      fibula M80.86- ☑
      finger M80.84- ☑
      humerus M80.82- ☑
      ilium M80.85- ☑
      ischium M80.85- ☑
      metacarpus M80.84- ☑
      metatarsus M80.87- ☑
      pelvis M80.85- ☑
      radius M80.83- ☑
      scapula M80.81- ☑
      tarsus M80.87- ☑
      tibia M80.86- ☑
      toe M80.87- ☑
      ulna M80.83- ☑
      vertebra M80.88 ☑

Index

Osteonecrosis — Osteoporosis

Osteopsathyrosis (idiopathica) Q78.Ø
Osteoradionecrosis, jaw (acute) (chronic) (lower) (suppurative) (upper) M27.2
Osteosarcoma (any form) — see Neoplasm, bone, malignant
Osteosclerosis Q78.2
  acquired M85.8- ☑
  congenita Q77.4
  fragilitas (generalisata) Q78.2
  myelofibrosis D75.81
Osteosclerotic anemia D64.89
Osteosis
  cutis L94.2
  renal fibrocystic N25.Ø
Österreicher-Turner syndrome Q87.2
Ostium
  atrioventriculare commune Q21.2
  primum (arteriosum) (defect) (persistent) Q21.2
  secundum (arteriosum) (defect) (patent) (persistent) Q21.1
Ostrum-Furst syndrome Q75.8
Otalgia H92.Ø ☑
Otitis (acute) H66.9Ø
  with effusion (see also Otitis, media, nonsuppurative)
    purulent — see Otitis, media, suppurative
  adhesive — see subcategory H74.1
  chronic (see also Otitis, media, chronic)
    with effusion (see also Otitis, media, nonsuppurative, chronic)
  externa H6Ø.9- ☑
    abscess — see Abscess, ear, external
    acute (noninfective) H6Ø.5Ø- ☑
      actinic H6Ø.51- ☑
      chemical H6Ø.52- ☑
      contact H6Ø.53- ☑
      eczematoid H6Ø.54- ☑
      infective — see Otitis, externa, infective
      reactive H6Ø.55- ☑
      specified NEC H6Ø.59- ☑
    cellulitis — see Cellulitis, ear
    chronic H6Ø.6- ☑
    diffuse — see Otitis, externa, infective, diffuse
    hemorrhagic — see Otitis, externa, infective, hemorrhagic
    in (due to)
      aspergillosis B44.89
      candidiasis B37.84
      erysipelas A46 [H62.4Ø]
      herpes (simplex) virus infection BØØ.1
        zoster BØ2.8
      impetigo LØ1.ØØ [H62.4Ø]
      infectious disease NEC B99 ☑ [H62.4-] ☑
      mycosis NEC B36.9 [H62.4Ø]
      parasitic disease NEC B89 [H62.4Ø]
      viral disease NEC B34.9 [H62.4Ø]
      zoster BØ2.8
    infective NEC H6Ø.39- ☑
      abscess — see Abscess, ear, external
      cellulitis — see Cellulitis, ear
      diffuse H6Ø.31- ☑
      hemorrhagic H6Ø.32- ☑
      swimmer's ear — see Swimmer's, ear
    malignant H6Ø.2- ☑
    mycotic B36.9 [H62.4Ø]
    necrotizing — see Otitis, externa, malignant
    Pseudomonas aeruginosa — see Otitis, externa, malignant
    reactive — see Otitis, externa, acute, reactive
    specified NEC — see subcategory H6Ø.8 ☑
    tropical B36.8
  insidiosa — see Otosclerosis
  interna H83.Ø ☑
  media (hemorrhagic) (staphylococcal) (streptococcal) H66.9- ☑
    with effusion (nonpurulent) — see Otitis, media, nonsuppurative
    acute, subacute H66.9Ø
      allergic — see Otitis, media, nonsuppurative, acute, allergic
      exudative — see Otitis, media, nonsuppurative, acute
      mucoid — see Otitis, media, nonsuppurative, acute
      necrotizing (see also Otitis, media, suppurative, acute)
        in
          measles BØ5.3

Otitis — continued
  media — continued
    acute, subacute — continued
      necrotizing (see also Otitis, media, suppurative, acute) — continued
        in — continued
          scarlet fever A38.Ø
      nonsuppurative NEC — see Otitis, media, nonsuppurative, acute
      purulent — see Otitis, media, suppurative, acute
      sanguinous — see Otitis, media, nonsuppurative, acute
      secretory — see Otitis, media, nonsuppurative, acute, serous
      seromucinous — see Otitis, media, nonsuppurative, acute
      serous — see Otitis, media, nonsuppurative, acute, serous
      suppurative — see Otitis, media, suppurative, acute
    allergic — see Otitis, media, nonsuppurative
    catarrhal — see Otitis, media, nonsuppurative
    chronic H66.9Ø
      with effusion (nonpurulent) — see Otitis, media, nonsuppurative, chronic
      allergic — see Otitis, media, nonsuppurative, chronic, allergic
      benign suppurative — see Otitis, media, suppurative, chronic, tubotympanic
      catarrhal — see Otitis, media, nonsuppurative, chronic, serous
      exudative — see Otitis, media, nonsuppurative, chronic
      mucinous — see Otitis, media, nonsuppurative, chronic, mucoid
      mucoid — see Otitis, media, nonsuppurative, chronic, mucoid
      nonsuppurative NEC — see Otitis, media, nonsuppurative, chronic
      purulent — see Otitis, media, suppurative, chronic
      secretory — see Otitis, media, nonsuppurative, chronic, mucoid
      seromucinous — see Otitis, media, nonsuppurative, chronic
      serous — see Otitis, media, nonsuppurative, chronic, serous
      suppurative — see Otitis, media, suppurative, chronic
      transudative — see Otitis, media, nonsuppurative, chronic, mucoid
    exudative — see Otitis, media, nonsuppurative
    in (due to) (with)
      influenza — see Influenza, with, otitis media
      measles BØ5.3
      scarlet fever A38.Ø
      tuberculosis A18.6
      viral disease NEC B34.- ☑ [H67.-] ☑
    mucoid — see Otitis, media, nonsuppurative
    nonsuppurative H65.9- ☑
      acute or subacute NEC H65.19- ☑
        allergic H65.11- ☑
          recurrent H65.11- ☑
        recurrent H65.19- ☑
        secretory — see Otitis, media, nonsuppurative, serous
        serous H65.Ø- ☑
          recurrent H65.Ø- ☑
      chronic H65.49- ☑
        allergic H65.41- ☑
        mucoid H65.3- ☑
        serous H65.2- ☑
    postmeasles BØ5.3
    purulent — see Otitis, media, suppurative
    secretory — see Otitis, media, nonsuppurative
    seromucinous — see Otitis, media, nonsuppurative
    serous — see Otitis, media, nonsuppurative
    suppurative H66.4- ☑
      acute H66.ØØ- ☑
        with rupture of ear drum H66.Ø1- ☑
        recurrent H66.ØØ- ☑
          with rupture of ear drum H66.Ø1- ☑
      chronic (see also subcategory) H66.3 ☑
        atticoantral H66.2- ☑
        benign — see Otitis, media, suppurative, chronic, tubotympanic

Otitis — continued
  media — continued
    suppurative — continued
      chronic (see also subcategory) — continued
        tubotympanic H66.1- ☑
      transudative — see Otitis, media, nonsuppurative
      tuberculous A18.6
Otocephaly Q18.2
Otolith syndrome — see subcategory H81.8 ☑
Otomycosis (diffuse) **NEC** B36.9 [H62.4Ø]
  in
    aspergillosis B44.89
    candidiasis B37.84
    moniliasis B37.84
Otoporosis — see Otosclerosis
Otorrhagia (nontraumatic) H92.2- ☑
  traumatic — code by Type of injury
Otorrhea H92.1- ☑
  cerebrospinal G96.Ø
Otosclerosis (general) H8Ø.9- ☑
  cochlear (endosteal) H8Ø.2- ☑
  involving
    otic capsule — see Otosclerosis, cochlear
    oval window
      nonobliterative H8Ø.Ø- ☑
      obliterative H8Ø.1- ☑
    round window — see Otosclerosis, cochlear
  nonobliterative — see Otosclerosis, involving, oval window, nonobliterative
  obliterative — see Otosclerosis, involving, oval window, obliterative
  specified NEC H8Ø.8- ☑
Otospongiosis — see Otosclerosis
Otto's disease or pelvis M24.7
Outcome of delivery Z37.9
  multiple births Z37.9
    all liveborn Z37.5Ø
      quadruplets Z37.52
      quintuplets Z37.53
      sextuplets Z37.54
      specified number NEC Z37.59
      triplets Z37.51
    all stillborn Z37.7
    some liveborn Z37.6Ø
      quadruplets Z37.62
      quintuplets Z37.63
      sextuplets Z37.64
      specified number NEC Z37.69
      triplets Z37.61
  single NEC Z37.9
    liveborn Z37.Ø
    stillborn Z37.1
  twins NEC Z37.9
    both liveborn Z37.2
    both stillborn Z37.4
    one liveborn, one stillborn Z37.3
Outlet — see condition
Ovalocytosis (congenital) (hereditary) — see Elliptocytosis
Ovarian — see Condition
Ovariocele N83.4
Ovaritis (cystic) — see Oophoritis
Ovary, ovarian (see also condition)
  resistant syndrome E28.39
  vein syndrome N13.8
Overactive (see also Hyperfunction)
  adrenal cortex NEC E27.Ø
  bladder N32.81
  hypothalamus E23.3
  thyroid — see Hyperthyroidism
Overactivity R46.3
  child — see Disorder, attention-deficit hyperactivity
Overbite (deep) (excessive) (horizontal) (vertical) M26.29
Overbreathing — see Hyperventilation
Overconscientious personality F6Ø.5
Overdevelopment — see Hypertrophy
Overdistension — see Distension
Overdose, overdosage (drug) — see Table of Drugs and Chemicals, by drug, poisoning
Overeating R63.2
  nonorganic origin F5Ø.8
  psychogenic F5Ø.8
Overexertion (effects) (exhaustion) T73.3 ☑
Overexposure (effects) T73.9 ☑
  exhaustion T73.2 ☑
Overfeeding — see Overeating
  newborn P92.4

☑ **Additional Character Required** — **Refer to the Tabular List for Character Selection**   ▽ **Subterms under main terms may continue to next column or page**

Overfill, endodontic M27.52
Overgrowth, bone — *see* Hypertrophy, bone
Overhanging of dental restorative material (unrepairable) K08.52
Overheated (places) (effects) — *see* Heat
Overjet (excessive horizontal) M26.23
Overlaid, overlying (suffocation) — *see* Asphyxia, traumatic, due to mechanical threat
Overlap, excessive horizontal (teeth) M26.23
Overlapping toe (acquired) (*see also* Deformity, toe, specified NEC)
  congenital (fifth toe) Q66.89
Overload
  circulatory, due to transfusion (blood) (blood components) (TACO) E87.71
  fluid E87.70
    due to transfusion (blood) (blood components) E87.71
    specified NEC E87.79
  iron, due to repeated red blood cell transfusions E83.111
  potassium (K) E87.5
  sodium (Na) E87.0
Overnutrition — *see* Hyperalimentation
Overproduction (*see also* Hypersecretion)
  ACTH E27.0
  catecholamine E27.5
  growth hormone E22.0
Overprotection, child by parent Z62.1
Overriding
  aorta Q25.4
  finger (acquired) — *see* Deformity, finger
    congenital Q68.1
  toe (acquired) (*see also* Deformity, toe, specified NEC)
    congenital Q66.89
Overstrained R53.83
  heart — *see* Hypertrophy, cardiac
Overuse, muscle NEC M70.8- ☑
Overweight E66.3
Overworked R53.83
Oviduct — *see* condition
Ovotestis Q56.0
Ovulation (cycle)
  failure or lack of N97.0
  pain N94.0
Ovum — *see* condition
Owren's disease or syndrome (parahemophilia) D68.2
Ox heart — *see* Hypertrophy, cardiac
Oxalosis E72.53
Oxaluria E72.53
Oxycephaly, oxycephalic Q75.0
  syphilitic, congenital A50.02
Oxyuriasis B80
Oxyuris vermicularis (infestation) B80
Ozena J31.0

P

Pachyderma, pachydermia L85.9
  larynx (verrucosa) J38.7
Pachydermatocele (congenital) Q82.8
Pachydermoperiostosis (*see also* Osteoarthropathy, hypertrophic, specified type NEC)
  clubbed nail M89.40 [L62]
Pachygyria Q04.3
Pachymeningitis (adhesive) (basal) (brain) (cervical) (chronic)(circumscribed) (external) (fibrous) (hemorrhagic) (hypertrophic) (internal) (purulent) (spinal) (suppurative) — *see* Meningitis
Pachyonychia (congenital) Q84.5
Pacinian tumor — *see* Neoplasm, skin, benign
Pad, knuckle or Garrod's M72.1
Paget's disease
  with infiltrating duct carcinoma — *see* Neoplasm, breast, malignant
  bone M88.9
    carpus M88.84- ☑
    clavicle M88.81- ☑
    femur M88.85- ☑
    fibula M88.86- ☑
    finger M88.84- ☑
    humerus M88.82- ☑
    ilium M88.85- ☑
    in neoplastic disease — *see* Osteitis, deformans, in neoplastic disease
    ischium M88.85- ☑
    metacarpus M88.84- ☑

Paget's disease — *continued*
  bone — *continued*
    metatarsus M88.87- ☑
    multiple sites M88.89
    neck M88.88
    radius M88.83- ☑
    rib M88.88
    scapula M88.81- ☑
    skull M88.0
    tarsus M88.87- ☑
    tibia M88.86- ☑
    toe M88.87- ☑
    ulna M88.83- ☑
    vertebra M88.88
  breast (female) C50.01- ☑
    male C50.02- ☑
  extramammary (*see also* Neoplasm, skin, malignant)
    anus C21.0
      margin C44.590
      skin C44.590
  intraductal carcinoma — *see* Neoplasm, breast, malignant
  malignant — *see* Neoplasm, skin, malignant
    breast (female) C50.01- ☑
      male C50.02- ☑
    unspecified site (female) C50.01- ☑
      male C50.02- ☑
  mammary — *see* Paget's disease, breast
  nipple — *see* Paget's disease, breast
  osteitis deformans — *see* Paget's disease, bone
Paget-Schroetter syndrome I82.890
Pain(s) (*see also* Painful) R52
  abdominal R10.9
    colic R10.83
    generalized R10.84
      with acute abdomen R10.0
    lower R10.30
      left quadrant R10.32
      pelvic or perineal R10.2
      periumbilical R10.33
      right quadrant R10.31
    rebound — *see* Tenderness, abdominal, rebound
    severe with abdominal rigidity R10.0
    tenderness — *see* Tenderness, abdominal
    upper R10.10
      epigastric R10.13
      left quadrant R10.12
      right quadrant R10.11
  acute R52
    due to trauma G89.11
    neoplasm related G89.3
    postprocedural NEC G89.18
    post-thoracotomy G89.12
    specified by site — *code to* Pain, by site
  adnexa (uteri) R10.2
  anginoid — *see* Pain, precordial
  anus K62.89
  arm — *see* Pain, limb, upper
  axillary (axilla) M79.62- ☑
  back (postural) M54.9
  bladder R39.89
    associated with micturition — *see* Micturition, painful
  bone — *see* Disorder, bone, specified type NEC
  breast N64.4
  broad ligament R10.2
  cancer associated (acute) (chronic) G89.3
  cecum — *see* Pain, abdominal
  cervicobrachial M53.1
  chest (central) R07.9
    anterior wall R07.89
    atypical R07.89
    ischemic I20.9
    musculoskeletal R07.89
    non-cardiac R07.89
    on breathing R07.1
    pleurodynia R07.81
    precordial R07.2
    wall (anterior) R07.89
  chronic G89.29
    associated with significant psychosocial dysfunction G89.4
    due to trauma G89.21
    neoplasm related G89.3
    postoperative NEC G89.28
    postprocedural NEC G89.28
    post-thoracotomy G89.22

Pain(s) — *continued*
  chronic — *continued*
    specified NEC G89.29
  coccyx M53.3
  colon — *see* Pain, abdominal
  coronary — *see* Angina
  costochondral R07.1
  diaphragm R07.1
  due to cancer G89.3
  due to device, implant or graft (*see also* Complications, by site and type, specified NEC) T85.84 ☑
    arterial graft NEC T82.848 ☑
    breast (implant) T85.84 ☑
    catheter NEC T85.84 ☑
      dialysis (renal) T82.848 ☑
        intraperitoneal T85.84 ☑
      infusion NEC T82.848 ☑
        spinal (epidural) (subdural) T85.84 ☑
      urinary (indwelling) T83.84 ☑
    electronic (electrode) (pulse generator) (stimulator)
      bone T84.84 ☑
      cardiac T82.847 ☑
      nervous system (brain) (peripheral nerve) (spinal) T85.84 ☑
      urinary T83.84 ☑
    fixation, internal (orthopedic) NEC T84.84 ☑
    gastrointestinal (bile duct) (esophagus) T85.84 ☑
    genital NEC T83.84 ☑
    heart NEC T82.847 ☑
    infusion NEC T85.84 ☑
    joint prosthesis T84.84 ☑
    ocular (corneal graft) (orbital implant) NEC T85.84 ☑
    orthopedic NEC T84.84 ☑
    specified NEC T85.84 ☑
    urinary NEC T83.84 ☑
    vascular NEC T82.848 ☑
    ventricular intracranial shunt T85.84 ☑
  due to malignancy (primary) (secondary) G89.3
  ear — *see* subcategory H92.0 ☑
  epigastric, epigastrium R10.13
  eye — *see* Pain, ocular
  face, facial R51
    atypical G50.1
  female genital organs NEC N94.89
  finger — *see* Pain, limb, upper
  flank — *see* Pain, abdominal
  foot — *see* Pain, limb, lower
  gallbladder K82.9
  gas (intestinal) R14.1
  gastric — *see* Pain, abdominal
  generalized NOS R52
  genital organ
    female N94.89
    male N50.8
  groin — *see* Pain, abdominal, lower
  hand — *see* Pain, limb, upper
  head — *see* Headache
  heart — *see* Pain, precordial
  infra-orbital — *see* Neuralgia, trigeminal
  intercostal R07.82
  intermenstrual N94.0
  jaw R68.84
  joint M25.50
    ankle M25.57- ☑
    elbow M25.52- ☑
    finger M79.64- ☑
    foot M25.57- ☑
    hand M79.64- ☑
    hip M25.55- ☑
    knee M25.56- ☑
    shoulder M25.51- ☑
    toe M25.57- ☑
    wrist M25.53- ☑
  kidney N23
  laryngeal R07.0
  leg — *see* Pain, limb, lower
  limb M79.609
    lower M79.60- ☑
      foot M79.67- ☑
      lower leg M79.66- ☑
      thigh M79.65- ☑
      toe M79.67- ☑
    upper M79.60- ☑
      axilla M79.62- ☑
      finger M79.64- ☑

Pain(s) — continued
  limb — continued
    upper — continued
      forearm M79.63- ☑
      hand M79.64- ☑
      upper arm M79.62- ☑
  loin M54.5
  low back M54.5
  lumbar region M54.5
  mandibular R68.84
  mastoid — see subcategory H92.0 ☑
  maxilla R68.84
  menstrual (see also Dysmenorrhea) N94.6
  metacarpophalangeal (joint) — see Pain, joint, hand
  metatarsophalangeal (joint) — see Pain, joint, foot
  mouth K13.79
  muscle — see Myalgia
  musculoskeletal (see also Pain, by site) M79.1
  myofascial M79.1
  nasal J34.89
  nasopharynx J39.2
  neck NEC M54.2
  nerve NEC — see Neuralgia
  neuromuscular — see Neuralgia
  nose J34.89
  ocular H57.1- ☑
  ophthalmic — see Pain, ocular
  orbital region — see Pain, ocular
  ovary N94.89
  over heart — see Pain, precordial
  ovulation N94.0
  pelvic (female) R10.2
  penis N48.89
  pericardial — see Pain, precordial
  perineal, perineum R10.2
  pharynx J39.2
  pleura, pleural, pleuritic R07.81
  postoperative NOS G89.18
  postprocedural NOS G89.18
  post-thoracotomy G89.12
  precordial (region) R07.2
  premenstrual N94.3
  psychogenic (persistent) (any site) F45.41
  radicular (spinal) — see Radiculopathy
  rectum K62.89
  respiration R07.1
  retrosternal R07.2
  rheumatoid, muscular — see Myalgia
  rib R07.81
  root (spinal) — see Radiculopathy
  round ligament (stretch) R10.2
  sacroiliac M53.3
  sciatic — see Sciatica
  scrotum N50.8
  seminal vesicle N50.8
  shoulder M25.51- ☑
  spermatic cord N50.8
  spinal root — see Radiculopathy
  spine M54.9
    cervical M54.2
    low back M54.5
      with sciatica M54.4- ☑
    thoracic M54.6
  stomach — see Pain, abdominal
  substernal R07.2
  temporomandibular (joint) M26.62
  testis N50.8
  thoracic spine M54.6
    with radicular and visceral pain M54.14
  throat R07.0
  tibia — see Pain, limb, lower
  toe — see Pain, limb, lower
  tongue K14.6
  tooth K08.8
  trigeminal — see Neuralgia, trigeminal
  tumor associated G89.3
  ureter N23
  urinary (organ) (system) N23
  uterus NEC N94.89
  vagina R10.2
  vertebrogenic (syndrome) M54.89
  vesical R39.89
    associated with micturition — see Micturition, painful
  vulva R10.2
Painful (see also Pain)
  coitus
    female N94.1

Painful — continued
  coitus — continued
    male N53.12
    psychogenic F52.6
  ejaculation (semen) N53.12
    psychogenic F52.6
  erection — see Priapism
  feet syndrome E53.8
  joint replacement (hip) (knee) T84.84 ☑
  menstruation — see Dysmenorrhea
    psychogenic F45.8
  micturition — see Micturition, painful
  respiration R07.1
  scar NEC L90.5
  wire sutures T81.89 ☑
Painter's colic — see subcategory T56.0 ☑
Palate — see condition
Palatoplegia K13.79
Palatoschisis — see Cleft, palate
Palilalia R48.8
Palliative care Z51.5
Pallor R23.1
  optic disc, temporal — see Atrophy, optic
Palmar (see also condition)
  fascia — see condition
Palpable
  cecum K63.89
  kidney N28.89
  ovary N83.8
  prostate N42.9
  spleen — see Splenomegaly
Palpitations (heart) R00.2
  psychogenic F45.8
Palsy (see also Paralysis) G83.9
  atrophic diffuse (progressive) G12.22
  Bell's (see also Palsy, facial)
    newborn P11.3
  brachial plexus NEC G54.0
    newborn (birth injury) P14.3
  brain — see Palsy, cerebral
  bulbar (progressive) (chronic) G12.22
    of childhood (Fazio-Londe) G12.1
    pseudo NEC G12.29
    supranuclear (progressive) G23.1
  cerebral (congenital) G80.9
    ataxic G80.4
    athetoid G80.3
    choreathetoid G80.3
    diplegic G80.8
      spastic G80.1
    dyskinetic G80.3
      athetoid G80.3
      choreathetoid G80.3
      distonic G80.3
    dystonic G80.3
    hemiplegic G80.8
      spastic G80.2
    mixed G80.8
    monoplegic G80.8
      spastic G80.1
    paraplegic G80.8
      spastic G80.1
    quadriplegic G80.8
      spastic G80.0
    spastic G80.1
      diplegic G80.1
      hemiplegic G80.2
      monoplegic G80.1
      quadriplegic G80.0
      specified NEC G80.1
      tetrapelgic G80.0
    specified NEC G80.8
    syphilitic A52.12
      congenital A50.49
    tetraplegic G80.8
      spastic G80.0
  cranial nerve (see also Disorder, nerve, cranial)
    multiple G52.7
      in
        infectious disease B99 ☑ [G53]
        neoplastic disease (see also Neoplasm) D49.9 [G53]
        parasitic disease B89 [G53]
        sarcoidosis D86.82
  creeping G12.22
  diver's T70.3 ☑
  Erb's P14.0
  facial G51.0

Palsy — continued
  facial — continued
    newborn (birth injury) P11.3
  glossopharyngeal G52.1
  Klumpke (-Déjérine) P14.1
  lead — see subcategory T56.0 ☑
  median nerve (tardy) G56.1- ☑
  nerve G58.9
    specified NEC G58.8
  peroneal nerve (acute) (tardy) G57.3- ☑
  progressive supranuclear G23.1
  pseudobulbar NEC G12.29
  radial nerve (acute) G56.3- ☑
  seventh nerve (see also Palsy, facial)
    newborn P11.3
  shaking — see Parkinsonism
  spastic (cerebral) (spinal) G80.1
  ulnar nerve (tardy) G56.2- ☑
  wasting G12.29
Paludism — see Malaria
Panangiitis M30.0
Panaris, panaritium (see also Cellulitis, digit)
  with lymphangitis — see Lymphangitis, acute, digit
Panarteritis nodosa M30.0
  brain or cerebral I67.7
Pancake heart R93.1
  with cor pulmonale (chronic) I27.81
Pancarditis (acute) (chronic) I51.89
  rheumatic I09.89
    active or acute I01.8
Pancoast's syndrome or tumor C34.1- ☑
Pancolitis, ulcerative (chronic) K51.00
  with
    abscess K51.014
    complication K51.019
    fistula K51.013
    obstruction K51.012
    rectal bleeding K51.011
    specified complication NEC K51.018
Pancreas, pancreatic — see condition
Pancreatitis (annular) (apoplectic) (calcareous) (edematous) (hemorrhagic) (malignant) (recurrent) (subacute) (suppurative) K85.9
  acute K85.9
    alcohol induced K85.2
    biliary K85.1
    drug induced K85.3
    gallstone K85.1
    idiopathic K85.0
    specified NEC K85.8
  chronic (infectious) K86.1
    alcohol-induced K86.0
    recurrent K86.1
    relapsing K86.1
  cystic (chronic) K86.1
  cytomegaloviral B25.2
  fibrous (chronic) K86.1
  gallstone K85.1
  gangrenous K85.8
  interstitial (chronic) K86.1
    acute K85.8
  mumps B26.3
  recurrent (chronic) K86.1
  relapsing, chronic K86.1
  syphilitic A52.74
Pancreatoblastoma — see Neoplasm, pancreas, malignant
Pancreolithiasis K86.8
Pancytolysis D75.89
Pancytopenia (acquired) D61.818
  with
    malformations D61.09
    myelodysplastic syndrome — see Syndrome, myelodysplastic
  antineoplastic chemotherapy induced D61.810
  congenital D61.09
  drug-induced NEC D61.811
Panencephalitis, subacute, sclerosing A81.1
Panhematopenia D61.9
  congenital D61.09
  constitutional D61.09
  splenic, primary D73.1
Panhemocytopenia D61.9
  congenital D61.09
  constitutional D61.09
Panhypogonadism E29.1
Panhypopituitarism E23.0
  prepubertal E23.0

Panic (attack) (state) F41.Ø
  reaction to exceptional stress (transient) F43.Ø
Panmyelopathy, familial, constitutional D61.Ø9
Panmyelophthisis D61.82
  congenital D61.Ø9
Panmyelosis (acute) (with myelofibrosis) C94.4- ☑
Panner's disease — *see* Osteochondrosis, juvenile, humerus
Panneuritis endemica E51.11
Panniculitis (nodular) (nonsuppurative) M79.3
  back M54.ØØ
    cervical region M54.Ø2
    cervicothoracic region M54.Ø3
    lumbar region M54.Ø6
    lumbosacral region M54.Ø7
    multiple sites M54.Ø9
    occipito-atlanto-axial region M54.Ø1
    sacrococcygeal region M54.Ø8
    thoracic region M54.Ø4
    thoracolumbar region M54.Ø5
  lupus L93.2
  mesenteric K65.4
  neck M54.Ø2
    cervicothoracic region M54.Ø3
    occipito-atlanto-axial region M54.Ø1
  relapsing M35.6
Panniculus adiposus (abdominal) E65
Pannus (allergic) (cornea) (degenerativus) (keratic) H16.42- ☑
  abdominal (symptomatic) E65
  trachomatosus, trachomatous (active) A71.1
Panophthalmitis H44.Ø1- ☑
Pansinusitis (chronic) (hyperplastic) (nonpurulent) (purulent) J32.4
  acute JØ1.4Ø
    recurrent JØ1.41
  tuberculous A15.8
Panuveitis (sympathetic) H44.11- ☑
Panvalvular disease IØ8.9
  specified NEC IØ8.8
Papanicolaou smear, cervix Z12.4
  as part of routine gynecological examination ZØ1.419
    with abnormal findings ZØ1.411
  for suspected neoplasm Z12.4
  nonspecific abnormal finding R87.619
  routine ZØ1.419
    with abnormal findings ZØ1.411
Papilledema (choked disc) H47.1Ø
  associated with
    decreased ocular pressure H47.12
    increased intracranial pressure H47.11
    retinal disorder H47.13
  Foster-Kennedy syndrome H47.14- ☑
Papillitis H46.ØØ
  anus K62.89
  chronic lingual K14.4
  necrotizing, kidney N17.2
  optic H46.Ø- ☑
  rectum K62.89
  renal, necrotizing N17.2
  tongue K14.Ø
Papilloma (*see also* Neoplasm, benign, by site)
  acuminatum (female) (male) (anogenital) A63.Ø
  benign pinta (primary) A67.Ø
  bladder (urinary) (transitional cell) D41.4
  choroid plexus (lateral ventricle) (third ventricle) D33.Ø
    anaplastic C71.5
    fourth ventricle D33.1
    malignant C71.5
  renal pelvis (transitional cell) D41.1- ☑
    benign D3Ø.1- ☑
  Schneiderian
    specified site — *see* Neoplasm, benign, by site
    unspecified site D14.Ø
  serous surface
    borderline malignancy
      specified site — *see* Neoplasm, uncertain behavior, by site
      unspecified site D39.1Ø
    specified site — *see* Neoplasm, benign, by site
    unspecified site D27.9
  transitional (cell)
    bladder (urinary) D41.4
    inverted type — *see* Neoplasm, uncertain behavior, by site
    renal pelvis D41.1- ☑
    ureter D41.2- ☑

Papilloma — *continued*
  ureter (transitional cell) D41.2- ☑
    benign D3Ø.2- ☑
  urothelial — *see* Neoplasm, uncertain behavior, by site
  villous — *see* Neoplasm, uncertain behavior, by site
    adenocarcinoma in — *see* Neoplasm, malignant, by site
    in situ — *see* Neoplasm, in situ
  yaws, plantar or palmar A66.1
Papillomata, multiple, of yaws A66.1
Papillomatosis (*see also* Neoplasm, benign, by site)
  confluent and reticulated L83
  cystic, breast — *see* Mastopathy, cystic
  ductal, breast — *see* Mastopathy, cystic
  intraductal (diffuse) — *see* Neoplasm, benign, by site
  subareolar duct D24- ☑
Papillomavirus, as cause of disease classified elsewhere B97.7
Papillon-Léage and Psaume syndrome Q87.Ø
Papule(s) R23.8
  carate (primary) A67.Ø
  fibrous, of nose D22.39
  Gottron's L94.4
  pinta (primary) A67.Ø
Papulosis
  lymphomatoid C86.6
  malignant I77.89
Papyraceous fetus O31.Ø- ☑
Para-albuminemia E88.Ø9
Paracephalus Q89.7
Parachute mitral valve Q23.2
Paracoccidioidomycosis B41.9
  disseminated B41.7
  generalized B41.7
  mucocutaneous-lymphangitic B41.8
  pulmonary B41.Ø
  specified NEC B41.8
  visceral B41.8
Paradentosis KØ5.4
Paraffinoma T88.8 ☑
Paraganglioma D44.7
  adrenal D35.Ø- ☑
    malignant C74.1- ☑
  aortic body D44.7
    malignant C75.5
  carotid body D44.6
    malignant C75.4
  chromaffin (*see also* Neoplasm, benign, by site)
    malignant — *see* Neoplasm, malignant, by site
  extra-adrenal D44.7
    malignant C75.5
      specified site — *see* Neoplasm, malignant, by site
      unspecified site C75.5
    specified site — *see* Neoplasm, uncertain behavior, by site
    unspecified site D44.7
  gangliocytic D13.2
    specified site — *see* Neoplasm, benign, by site
    unspecified site D13.2
  glomus jugulare D44.7
    malignant C75.5
  jugular D44.7
  malignant C75.5
    specified site — *see* Neoplasm, malignant, by site
    unspecified site C75.5
  nonchromaffin D44.7
    malignant C75.5
      specified site — *see* Neoplasm, malignant, by site
      unspecified site C75.5
    specified site — *see* Neoplasm, uncertain behavior, by site
    unspecified site D44.7
  parasympathetic D44.7
    specified site — *see* Neoplasm, uncertain behavior, by site
    unspecified site D44.7
  specified site — *see* Neoplasm, uncertain behavior, by site
  sympathetic D44.7
    specified site — *see* Neoplasm, uncertain behavior, by site
    unspecified site D44.7
  unspecified site D44.7
Parageusia R43.2

Parageusia — *continued*
  psychogenic F45.8
Paragonimiasis B66.4
Paragranuloma, Hodgkin — *see* Lymphoma, Hodgkin, classical, specified NEC
Parahemophilia (*see also* Defect, coagulation) D68.2
Parakeratosis R23.4
  variegata L41.Ø
Paralysis, paralytic (complete) (incomplete) G83.9
  with
    syphilis A52.17
  abducens, abducent (nerve) — *see* Strabismus, paralytic, sixth nerve
  abductor, lower extremity G57.9- ☑
  accessory nerve G52.8
  accommodation (*see also* Paresis, of accommodation)
    hysterical F44.89
  acoustic nerve (except Deafness) H93.3 ☑
  agitans (*see also* Parkinsonism) G2Ø
    arteriosclerotic G21.4
  alternating (oculomotor) G83.89
  amyotrophic G12.21
  ankle G57.9- ☑
  anus (sphincter) K62.89
  arm — *see* Monoplegia, upper limb
  ascending (spinal), acute G61.Ø
  association G12.29
  asthenic bulbar G7Ø.ØØ
    with exacerbation (acute) G7Ø.Ø1
    in crisis G7Ø.Ø1
  ataxic (hereditary) G11.9
    general (syphilitic) A52.17
  atrophic G58.9
    infantile, acute — *see* Poliomyelitis, paralytic
    progressive G12.22
    spinal (acute) — *see* Poliomyelitis, paralytic
  axillary G54.Ø
  Babinski-Nageotte's G83.89
  Bell's G51.Ø
    newborn P11.3
  Benedikt's G46.3
  birth injury P14.9
    spinal cord P11.5
  bladder (neurogenic) (sphincter) N31.2
  bowel, colon or intestine K56.Ø
  brachial plexus G54.Ø
    birth injury P14.3
    newborn (birth injury) P14.3
  brain G83.9
    diplegia G83.Ø
    triplegia G83.89
  bronchial J98.Ø9
  Brown-Séquard G83.81
  bulbar (chronic) (progressive) G12.22
    infantile — *see* Poliomyelitis, paralytic
    poliomyelitic — *see* Poliomyelitis, paralytic
    pseudo G12.29
  bulbospinal G7Ø.ØØ
    with exacerbation (acute) G7Ø.Ø1
    in crisis G7Ø.Ø1
  cardiac (*see also* Failure, heart) I5Ø.9
  cerebrocerebellar, diplegic G8Ø.1
  cervical
    plexus G54.2
    sympathetic G9Ø.Ø9
  Céstan-Chenais G46.3
  Charcot-Marie-Tooth type G6Ø.Ø
  Clark's G8Ø.9
  colon K56.Ø
  compressed air T7Ø.3 ☑
  compression
    arm G56.9- ☑
    leg G57.9- ☑
    lower extremity G57.9- ☑
    upper extremity G56.9- ☑
  congenital (cerebral) — *see* Palsy, cerebral
  conjugate movement (gaze) (of eye) H51.Ø
    cortical (nuclear) (supranuclear) H51.Ø
  cordis — *see* Failure, heart
  cranial or cerebral nerve G52.9
  creeping G12.22
  crossed leg G83.89
  crutch — *see* Injury, brachial plexus
  deglutition R13.Ø
    hysterical F44.4
  dementia A52.17
  descending (spinal) NEC G12.29
  diaphragm (flaccid) J98.6

Paralysis, paralytic — *continued*
- diaphragm — *continued*
  - due to accidental dissection of phrenic nerve during procedure — *see* Puncture, accidental complicating surgery
- digestive organs NEC K59.8
- diplegic — *see* Diplegia
- divergence (nuclear) H51.8
- diver's T70.3 ☑
- Duchenne's
  - birth injury P14.0
  - due to or associated with
    - motor neuron disease G12.22
    - muscular dystrophy G71.0
- due to intracranial or spinal birth injury — *see* Palsy, cerebral
- embolic (current episode) I63.4 ☑
- Erb (-Duchenne) (birth) (newborn) P14.0
- Erb's syphilitic spastic spinal A52.17
- esophagus K22.8
- eye muscle (extrinsic) H49.9
  - intrinsic (*see also* Paresis, of accommodation)
- facial (nerve) G51.0
  - birth injury P11.3
  - congenital P11.3
  - following operation NEC — *see* Puncture, accidental complicating surgery
  - newborn (birth injury) P11.3
- familial (recurrent) (periodic) G72.3
  - spastic G11.4
- fauces J39.2
- finger G56.9- ☑
- gait R26.1
- gastric nerve (nondiabetic) G52.2
- gaze, conjugate H51.0
- general (progressive) (syphilitic) A52.17
  - juvenile A50.45
- glottis J38.00
  - bilateral J38.02
  - unilateral J38.01
- gluteal G54.1
- Gubler (-Millard) G46.3
- hand — *see* Monoplegia, upper limb
- heart — *see* Arrest, cardiac
- hemiplegic — *see* Hemiplegia
- hyperkalemic periodic (familial) G72.3
- hypoglossal (nerve) G52.3
- hypokalemic periodic G72.3
- hysterical F44.4
- ileus K56.0
- infantile (*see also* Poliomyelitis, paralytic) A80.30
  - bulbar — *see* Poliomyelitis, paralytic
  - cerebral — *see* Palsy, cerebral
  - spastic — *see* Palsy, cerebral, spastic
- infective — *see* Poliomyelitis, paralytic
- inferior nuclear G83.9
- internuclear — *see* Ophthalmoplegia, internuclear
- intestine K56.0
- iris H57.09
  - due to diphtheria (toxin) A36.89
- ischemic, Volkmann's (complicating trauma) T79.6 ☑
- Jackson's G83.89
- jake — *see* Poisoning, food, noxious, plant
- Jamaica ginger (jake) G62.2
- juvenile general A50.45
- Klumpke (-Déjérine) (birth) (newborn) P14.1
- labioglossal (laryngeal) (pharyngeal) G12.29
- Landry's G61.0
- laryngeal nerve (recurrent) (superior) (unilateral) J38.00
  - bilateral J38.02
  - unilateral J38.01
- larynx J38.00
  - bilateral J38.02
  - due to diphtheria (toxin) A36.2
  - unilateral J38.01
- lateral G12.21
- lead T56.0 ☑
- left side — *see* Hemiplegia
- leg G83.1- ☑
  - both — *see* Paraplegia
  - crossed G83.89
  - hysterical F44.4
  - psychogenic F44.4
  - transient or transitory R29.818
    - traumatic NEC — *see* Injury, nerve, leg
- levator palpebrae superioris — *see* Blepharoptosis, paralytic
- limb — *see* Monoplegia

Paralysis, paralytic — *continued*
- lip K13.0
- Lissauer's A52.17
- lower limb — *see* Monoplegia, lower limb
  - both — *see* Paraplegia
- lung J98.4
- median nerve G56.1- ☑
- medullary (tegmental) G83.89
- mesencephalic NEC G83.89
  - tegmental G83.89
- middle alternating G83.89
- Millard-Gubler-Foville G46.3
- monoplegic — *see* Monoplegia
- motor G83.9
- muscle, muscular NEC G72.89
  - due to nerve lesion G58.9
  - eye (extrinsic) H49.9
    - intrinsic — *see* Paresis, of accommodation
    - oblique — *see* Strabismus, paralytic, fourth nerve
  - iris sphincter H21.9
  - ischemic (Volkmann's) (complicating trauma) T79.6 ☑
  - progressive G12.21
  - pseudohypertrophic G71.0
- musculocutaneous nerve G56.9- ☑
- musculospiral G56.9- ☑
- nerve (*see also* Disorder, nerve)
  - abducent — *see* Strabismus, paralytic, sixth nerve
  - accessory G52.8
  - auditory (except Deafness) H93.3 ☑
  - birth injury P14.9
  - cranial or cerebral G52.9
  - facial G51.0
    - birth injury P11.3
    - congenital P11.3
    - newborn (birth injury) P11.3
  - fourth or trochlear — *see* Strabismus, paralytic, fourth nerve
  - newborn (birth injury) P14.9
  - oculomotor — *see* Strabismus, paralytic, third nerve
  - phrenic (birth injury) P14.2
  - radial G56.3- ☑
  - seventh or facial G51.0
    - newborn (birth injury) P11.3
  - sixth or abducent — *see* Strabismus, paralytic, sixth nerve
  - syphilitic A52.15
  - third or oculomotor — *see* Strabismus, paralytic, third nerve
  - trigeminal G50.9
  - trochlear — *see* Strabismus, paralytic, fourth nerve
  - ulnar G56.2- ☑
- normokalemic periodic G72.3
- ocular H49.9
  - alternating G83.89
- oculofacial, congenital (Moebius) Q87.0
- oculomotor (external bilateral) (nerve) — *see* Strabismus, paralytic, third nerve
- palate (soft) K13.79
- paratrigeminal G50.9
- periodic (familial) (hyperkalemic) (hypokalemic) (myotonic) (normokalemic) (potassium sensitive) (secondary) G72.3
- peripheral autonomic nervous system — *see* Neuropathy, peripheral, autonomic
- peroneal (nerve) G57.3- ☑
- pharynx J39.2
- phrenic nerve G56.8- ☑
- plantar nerve(s) G57.6- ☑
- pneumogastric nerve G52.2
- poliomyelitis (current) — *see* Poliomyelitis, paralytic
- popliteal nerve G57.3- ☑
- postepileptic transitory G83.84
- progressive (atrophic) (bulbar) (spinal) G12.22
  - general A52.17
  - infantile acute — *see* Poliomyelitis, paralytic
  - supranuclear G23.1
- pseudobulbar G12.29
- pseudohypertrophic (muscle) G71.0
- psychogenic F44.4
- quadriceps G57.9- ☑
- quadriplegic — *see* Tetraplegia
- radial nerve G56.3- ☑
- rectus muscle (eye) H49.9
- recurrent isolated sleep G47.53

Paralysis, paralytic — *continued*
- respiratory (muscle) (system) (tract) R06.81
  - center NEC G93.89
  - congenital P28.89
  - newborn P28.89
- right side — *see* Hemiplegia
- saturnine T56.0 ☑
- sciatic nerve G57.0- ☑
- senile G83.9
- shaking — *see* Parkinsonism
- shoulder G56.9- ☑
- sleep, recurrent isolated G47.53
- spastic G83.9
  - cerebral — *see* Palsy, cerebral, spastic
  - congenital (cerebral) — *see* Palsy, cerebral, spastic
  - familial G11.4
  - hereditary G11.4
  - quadriplegic G80.0
  - syphilitic (spinal) A52.17
- sphincter, bladder — *see* Paralysis, bladder
- spinal (cord) G83.9
  - accessory nerve G52.8
  - acute — *see* Poliomyelitis, paralytic
  - ascending acute G61.0
  - atrophic (acute) (*see also* Poliomyelitis, paralytic) spastic, syphilitic A52.17
  - congenital NEC — *see* Palsy, cerebral
  - hereditary G95.89
  - infantile — *see* Poliomyelitis, paralytic
  - progressive G12.21
  - sequelae NEC G83.89
- sternomastoid G52.8
- stomach K31.84
  - diabetic — *see* Diabetes, by type, with gastroparesis
  - nerve G52.2
    - diabetic — *see* Diabetes, by type, with gastroparesis
- stroke — *see* Infarct, brain
- subcapsularis G56.8- ☑
- supranuclear (progressive) G23.1
- sympathetic G90.8
  - cervical G90.09
  - nervous system — *see* Neuropathy, peripheral, autonomic
- syndrome G83.9
  - specified NEC G83.89
- syphilitic spastic spinal (Erb's) A52.17
- thigh G57.9- ☑
- throat J39.2
  - diphtheritic A36.0
  - muscle J39.2
- thrombotic (current episode) I63.3 ☑
- thumb G56.9- ☑
- tick — *see* Toxicity, venom, arthropod, specified NEC
- Todd's (postepileptic transitory paralysis) G83.84
- toe G57.6- ☑
- tongue K14.8
- transient R29.5
  - arm or leg NEC R29.818
  - traumatic NEC — *see* Injury, nerve
- trapezius G52.8
- traumatic, transient NEC — *see* Injury, nerve
- trembling — *see* Parkinsonism
- triceps brachii G56.9- ☑
- trigeminal nerve G50.9
- trochlear (nerve) — *see* Strabismus, paralytic, fourth nerve
- ulnar nerve G56.2- ☑
- upper limb — *see* Monoplegia, upper limb
- uremic N18.9 [G99.8]
- uveoparotitic D86.89
- uvula K13.79
  - postdiphtheritic A36.0
- vagus nerve G52.2
- vasomotor NEC G90.8
- velum palati K13.79
- vesical — *see* Paralysis, bladder
- vestibular nerve (except Vertigo) H93.3 ☑
- vocal cords J38.00
  - bilateral J38.02
  - unilateral J38.01
- Volkmann's (complicating trauma) T79.6 ☑
- wasting G12.29
- Weber's G46.3
- wrist G56.9- ☑

Paramedial urethrovesical orifice Q64.79

Paramenia N92.6
Parametritis (*see also* Disease, pelvis, inflammatory) N73.2
  acute N73.0
  complicating abortion — *see* Abortion, by type, complicated by, parametritis
Parametrium, parametric — *see* condition
Paramnesia — *see* Amnesia
Paramolar K00.1
Paramyloidosis E85.8
Paramyoclonus multiplex G25.3
Paramyotonia (congenita) G71.19
Parangi — *see* Yaws
Paranoia (querulans) F22
  senile F03 ☑
Paranoid
  dementia (senile) F03 ☑
    praecox — *see* Schizophrenia
  personality F60.0
  psychosis (climacteric) (involutional) (menopausal) F22
    psychogenic (acute) F23
    senile F03 ☑
  reaction (acute) F23
    chronic F22
  schizophrenia F20.0
  state (climacteric) (involutional) (menopausal) (simple) F22
    senile F03 ☑
  tendencies F60.0
  traits F60.0
  trends F60.0
  type, psychopathic personality F60.0
Paraparesis — *see* Paraplegia
Paraphasia R47.02
Paraphilia F65.9
Paraphimosis (congenital) N47.2
  chancroidal A57
Paraphrenia, paraphrenic (late) F22
  schizophrenia F20.0
Paraplegia (lower) G82.20
  ataxic — *see* Degeneration, combined, spinal cord
  complete G82.21
  congenital (cerebral) G80.8
    spastic G80.1
  familial spastic G11.4
  functional (hysterical) F44.4
  hereditary, spastic G11.4
  hysterical F44.4
  incomplete G82.22
  Pott's A18.01
  psychogenic F44.4
  spastic
    Erb's spinal, syphilitic A52.17
    hereditary G11.4
    tropical G04.1
  syphilitic (spastic) A52.17
  tropical spastic G04.1
Parapoxvirus B08.60
  specified NEC B08.69
Paraproteinemia D89.2
  benign (familial) D89.2
  monoclonal D47.2
  secondary to malignant disease D47.2
Parapsoriasis L41.9
  en plaques L41.4
  guttata L41.1
  large plaque L41.4
  retiform, retiformis L41.5
  small plaque L41.3
  specified NEC L41.8
  varioliformis (acuta) L41.0
Parasitic (*see also* condition)
  disease NEC B89
  stomatitis B37.0
  sycosis (beard) (scalp) B35.0
  twin Q89.4
Parasitism B89
  intestinal B82.9
  skin B88.9
  specified — *see* Infestation
Parasitophobia F40.218
Parasomnia G47.50
  due to
    alcohol
      abuse F10.182
      dependence F10.282

Parasomnia — *continued*
  due to — *continued*
    alcohol — *continued*
      use F10.982
    amphetamines
      abuse F15.182
      dependence F15.282
      use F15.982
    caffeine
      abuse F15.182
      dependence F15.282
      use F15.982
    cocaine
      abuse F14.182
      dependence F14.282
      use F14.982
    drug NEC
      abuse F19.182
      dependence F19.282
      use F19.982
    opioid
      abuse F11.182
      dependence F11.282
      use F11.982
    psychoactive substance NEC
      abuse F19.182
      dependence F19.282
      use F19.982
    sedative, hypnotic, or anxiolytic
      abuse F13.182
      dependence F13.282
      use F13.982
    stimulant NEC
      abuse F15.182
      dependence F15.282
      use F15.982
  in conditions classified elsewhere G47.54
  nonorganic origin F51.8
  organic G47.50
  specified NEC G47.59
Paraspadias Q54.9
Paraspasmus facialis G51.8
Parasuicide (attempt)
  history of (personal) Z91.5
    in family Z81.8
Parathyroid gland — *see* condition
Parathyroid tetany E20.9
Paratrachoma A74.0
Paratyphilitis — *see* Appendicitis
Paratyphoid (fever) — *see* Fever, paratyphoid
Paratyphus — *see* Fever, paratyphoid
Paraurethral duct Q64.79
  nonorganic origin F51.5
Paraurethritis (*see also* Urethritis)
  gonococcal (acute) (chronic) (with abscess) A54.1
Paravaccinia NEC B08.04
Paravaginitis — *see* Vaginitis
Parencephalitis (*see also* Encephalitis)
  sequelae G09
Parent-child conflict — *see* Conflict, parent-child
  estrangement NEC Z62.890
Paresis (*see also* Paralysis)
  accommodation — *see* Paresis, of accommodation
  Bernhardt's G57.1- ☑
  bladder (sphincter) (*see also* Paralysis, bladder)
    tabetic A52.17
  bowel, colon or intestine K56.0
  extrinsic muscle, eye H49.9
  general (progressive) (syphilitic) A52.17
    juvenile A50.45
  heart — *see* Failure, heart
  insane (syphilitic) A52.17
  juvenile (general) A50.45
  of accommodation H52.52- ☑
  peripheral progressive (idiopathic) G60.3
  pseudohypertrophic G71.0
  senile G83.9
  syphilitic (general) A52.17
    congenital A50.45
  vesical NEC N31.2
Paresthesia (*see also* Disturbance, sensation)
  Bernhardt G57.1- ☑
Paretic — *see* condition
Parinaud's
  conjunctivitis H10.89
  oculoglandular syndrome H10.89
  ophthalmoplegia H49.88- ☑
Parkinsonism (idiopathic) (primary) G20

Parkinsonism — *continued*
  with neurogenic orthostatic hypotension (symptomatic) G90.3
  arteriosclerotic G21.4
  dementia G31.83 [F02.80]
    with behavioral disturbance G31.83 [F02.81]
  due to
    drugs NEC G21.19
      neuroleptic G21.11
  neuroleptic induced G21.11
  postencephalitic G21.3
  secondary G21.9
    due to
      arteriosclerosis G21.4
      drugs NEC G21.19
        neuroleptic G21.11
      encephalitis G21.3
      external agents NEC G21.2
      syphilis A52.19
    specified NEC G21.8
  syphilitic A52.19
  treatment-induced NEC G21.19
  vascular G21.4
Parkinson's disease, syndrome or tremor — *see* Parkinsonism
Parodontitis — *see* Periodontitis
Parodontosis K05.4
Paronychia (*see also* Cellulitis, digit)
  with lymphangitis — *see* Lymphangitis, acute, digit
  candidal (chronic) B37.2
  tuberculous (primary) A18.4
Parorexia (psychogenic) F50.8
Parosmia R43.1
  psychogenic F45.8
Parotid gland — *see* condition
Parotitis, parotiditis (allergic)(nonspecific toxic) (purulent) (septic) (suppurative) (*see also* Sialoadenitis)
  epidemic — *see* Mumps
  infectious — *see* Mumps
  postoperative K91.89
  surgical K91.89
Parrot fever A70
Parrot's disease (early congenital syphilitic pseudoparalysis) A50.02
Parry-Romberg syndrome G51.8
Parry's disease or syndrome E05.00
  with thyroid storm E05.01
Pars planitis — *see* Cyclitis
Parsonage (-Aldren)-**Turner syndrome** G54.5
Parson's disease (exophthalmic goiter) E05.00
  with thyroid storm E05.01
Particolored infant Q82.8
Parturition — *see* Delivery
Parulis K04.7
  with sinus K04.6
Parvovirus, as cause of disease classified elsewhere B97.6
Pasini and Pierini's atrophoderma L90.3
Passage
  false, urethra N36.5
  meconium (newborn) during delivery P03.82
  of sounds or bougies — *see* Attention to, artificial, opening
Passive — *see* condition
  smoking Z77.22
Pasteurella septica A28.0
Pasteurellosis — *see* Infection, Pasteurella
PAT (paroxysmal atrial tachycardia) I47.1
Patau's syndrome — *see* Trisomy, 13
Patches
  mucous (syphilitic) A51.39
    congenital A50.07
  smokers' (mouth) K13.24
Patellar — *see* condition
Patent (*see also* Imperfect, closure)
  canal of Nuck Q52.4
  cervix N88.3
  ductus arteriosus or Botallo's Q25.0
  foramen
    botalli Q21.1
    ovale Q21.1
  interauricular septum Q21.1
  interventricular septum Q21.0
  omphalomesenteric duct Q43.0
  os (uteri) — *see* Patent, cervix
  ostium secundum Q21.1
  urachus Q64.4

Patent — *continued*
  vitelline duct Q43.0
Paterson (-Brown)(-Kelly) **syndrome or web** D50.1
Pathologic, pathological (*see also* condition)
  asphyxia R09.01
  fire-setting F63.1
  gambling F63.0
  ovum O02.0
  resorption, tooth K03.3
  stealing F63.2
Pathology (of) — *see* Disease
  periradicular, associated with previous endodontic
    treatment NEC M27.59
Pattern, sleep-wake, irregular G47.23
Patulous (*see also* Imperfect, closure (congenital))
  alimentary tract Q45.8
    lower Q43.8
    upper Q40.8
  eustachian tube H69.0- ☑
Pause, sinoatrial I49.5
Paxton's disease B36.2
Pearl(s)
  enamel K00.2
  Epstein's K09.8
Pearl-worker's disease — *see* Osteomyelitis, specified
    type NEC
Pectenosis K62.4
Pectoral — *see* condition
Pectus
  carinatum (congenital) Q67.7
    acquired M95.4
    rachitic sequelae (late effect) E64.3
  excavatum (congenital) Q67.6
    acquired M95.4
    rachitic sequelae (late effect) E64.3
  recurvatum (congenital) Q67.6
Pedatrophia E41
Pederosis F65.4
Pediculosis (infestation) B85.2
  capitis (head-louse) (any site) B85.0
  corporis (body-louse) (any site) B85.1
  eyelid B85.0
  mixed (classifiable to more than one of the titles B85.0-
    B85.3) B85.4
  pubis (pubic louse) (any site) B85.3
  vestimenti B85.1
  vulvae B85.3
Pediculus (infestation) — *see* Pediculosis
Pedophilia F65.4
Peg-shaped teeth K00.2
Pelade — *see* Alopecia, areata
Pelger-Huët anomaly or syndrome D72.0
Peliosis (rheumatica) D69.0
  hepatis K76.4
    with toxic liver disease K71.8
Pelizaeus-Merzbacher disease E75.29
Pellagra (alcoholic) (with polyneuropathy) E52
Pellagra-cerebellar-ataxia-renal aminoaciduria
  syndrome E72.02
Pellegrini (-Stieda) **disease or syndrome** — *see* Bursitis,
  tibial collateral
Pellizzi's syndrome E34.8
Pel's crisis A52.11
Pelvic (*see also* condition)
  examination (periodic) (routine) Z01.419
    with abnormal findings Z01.411
  kidney, congenital Q63.2
Pelviolithiasis — *see* Calculus, kidney
Pelviperitonitis (*see also* Peritonitis, pelvic)
  gonococcal A54.24
  puerperal O85
Pelvis — *see* condition or type
Pemphigoid L12.9
  benign, mucous membrane L12.1
  bullous L12.0
  cicatricial L12.1
  juvenile L12.2
  ocular L12.1
  specified NEC L12.8
Pemphigus L10.9
  benign familial (chronic) Q82.8
  Brazilian L10.3
  circinatus L13.0
  conjunctiva L12.1
  drug-induced L10.5
  erythematosus L10.4
  foliaceous L10.2

Pemphigus — *continued*
  gangrenous — *see* Gangrene
  neonatorum L01.03
  ocular L12.1
  paraneoplastic L10.81
  specified NEC L10.89
  syphilitic (congenital) A50.06
  vegetans L10.1
  vulgaris L10.0
  wildfire L10.3
Pendred's syndrome E07.1
Pendulous
  abdomen, in pregnancy — *see* Pregnancy, complicat-
    ed by, abnormal, pelvic organs or tissues NEC
  breast N64.89
Penetrating wound (*see also* Puncture)
  with internal injury — *see* Injury, by site
  eyeball — *see* Puncture, eyeball
  orbit (with or without foreign body) — *see* Puncture,
    orbit
  uterus by instrument with or following ectopic or
    molar pregnancy O08.6
Penicillosis B48.4
Penis — *see* condition
Penitis N48.29
Pentalogy of Fallot Q21.8
Pentasomy X syndrome Q97.1
Pentosuria (essential) E74.8
Percreta placenta - O43.23 ☑
Peregrinating patient — *see* Disorder, factitious
Perforation, perforated (nontraumatic) (of)
  accidental during procedure (blood vessel) (nerve)
    (organ) — *see* Complication, accidental punc-
    ture or laceration
  antrum — *see* Sinusitis, maxillary
  appendix K35.2
  atrial septum, multiple Q21.1
  attic, ear — *see* Perforation, tympanum, attic
  bile duct (common) (hepatic) K83.2
    cystic K82.2
  bladder (urinary)
    with or following ectopic or molar pregnancy O08.6
    obstetrical trauma O71.5
    traumatic S37.29 ☑
      at delivery O71.5
  bowel K63.1
    with or following ectopic or molar pregnancy O08.6
    newborn P78.0
    obstetrical trauma O71.5
    traumatic — *see* Laceration, intestine
  broad ligament N83.8
    with or following ectopic or molar pregnancy O08.6
    obstetrical trauma O71.6
  by
    device, implant or graft (*see also* Complications,
      by site and type, mechanical) T85.628 ☑
      arterial graft NEC — *see* Complication, cardio-
        vascular device, mechanical, vascular
      breast (implant) T85.49 ☑
      catheter NEC T85.698 ☑
        cystostomy T83.090 ☑
        dialysis (renal) T82.49 ☑
          intraperitoneal T85.691 ☑
        infusion NEC T82.594 ☑
          spinal (epidural) (subdural) T85.690 ☑
      electronic (electrode) (pulse generator) (stimu-
        lator)
        bone T84.390 ☑
        cardiac T82.199 ☑
          electrode T82.190 ☑
          pulse generator T82.191 ☑
          specified type NEC T82.198 ☑
        nervous system — *see* Complication, pros-
          thetic device, mechanical, electronic
          nervous system stimulator
        urinary — *see* Complication, genitourinary,
          device, urinary, mechanical
      fixation, internal (orthopedic) NEC — *see*
        Complication, fixation device, mechanical
      gastrointestinal — *see* Complications, prosthet-
        ic device, mechanical, gastrointestinal
        device
      genital NEC T83.498 ☑
        intrauterine contraceptive device T83.39 ☑
        penile prosthesis T83.490 ☑
      heart NEC — *see* Complication, cardiovascular
        device, mechanical

Perforation, perforated — *continued*
  by — *continued*
    device, implant or graft (*see also* Complications, by
      site and type, mechanical) — *continued*
      joint prosthesis — *see* Complications, joint
        prosthesis, mechanical, specified NEC, by
        site
      ocular NEC — *see* Complications, prosthetic
        device, mechanical, ocular device
      orthopedic NEC — *see* Complication, orthope-
        dic, device, mechanical
      specified NEC T85.628 ☑
      urinary, indwelling T83.098 ☑
      urinary NEC (*see also* Complication, genitouri-
        nary, device, urinary, mechanical)
        graft T83.29 ☑
      vascular NEC — *see* Complication, cardiovascu-
        lar device, mechanical
      ventricular intracranial shunt T85.09 ☑
    foreign body left accidentally in operative wound
      T81.539 ☑
    instrument (any) during a procedure, accidental
      — *see* Puncture, accidental complicating
      surgery
  cecum K35.2
  cervix (uteri) N88.8
    with or following ectopic or molar pregnancy O08.6
    obstetrical trauma O71.3
  colon K63.1
    newborn P78.0
    obstetrical trauma O71.5
    traumatic — *see* Laceration, intestine, large
  common duct (bile) K83.2
  cornea (due to ulceration) — *see* Ulcer, cornea, perfo-
    rated
  cystic duct K82.2
  diverticulum (intestine) K57.80
    with bleeding K57.81
    large intestine K57.20
      with
        bleeding K57.21
        small intestine K57.40
          with bleeding K57.41
      small intestine K57.00
      with
        bleeding K57.01
        large intestine K57.40
          with bleeding K57.41
  ear drum — *see* Perforation, tympanum
  esophagus K22.3
  ethmoidal sinus — *see* Sinusitis, ethmoidal
  frontal sinus — *see* Sinusitis, frontal
  gallbladder K82.2
  heart valve — *see* Endocarditis
  ileum K63.1
    newborn P78.0
    obstetrical trauma O71.5
    traumatic — *see* Laceration, intestine, small
  instrumental, surgical (accidental) (blood vessel)
    (nerve) (organ) — *see* Puncture, accidental
    complicating surgery
  intestine NEC K63.1
    with ectopic or molar pregnancy O08.6
    newborn P78.0
    obstetrical trauma O71.5
    traumatic — *see* Laceration, intestine
    ulcerative NEC K63.1
      newborn P78.0
  jejunum, jejunal K63.1
    obstetrical trauma O71.5
    traumatic — *see* Laceration, intestine, small
    ulcer — *see* Ulcer, gastrojejunal, with perforation
  joint prosthesis — *see* Complications, joint prosthesis,
    mechanical, specified NEC, by site
  mastoid (antrum) (cell) — *see* Disorder, mastoid,
    specified NEC
  maxillary sinus — *see* Sinusitis, maxillary
  membrana tympani — *see* Perforation, tympanum
  nasal
    septum J34.89
      congenital Q30.3
      syphilitic A52.73
    sinus J34.89
      congenital Q30.8
      due to sinusitis — *see* Sinusitis
  palate (*see also* Cleft, palate) Q35.9
    syphilitic A52.79

Perforation, perforated — continued
  palatine vault (see also Cleft, palate, hard) Q35.1
    syphilitic A52.79
      congenital A50.59
  pars flaccida (ear drum) — see Perforation, tympanum, attic
  pelvic
    floor S31.030 ☑
      with
        ectopic or molar pregnancy O08.6
        penetration into retroperitoneal space S31.031 ☑
          retained foreign body S31.040 ☑
            with penetration into retroperitoneal space S31.041 ☑
        following ectopic or molar pregnancy O08.6
      obstetrical trauma O70.1
    organ S37.99 ☑
      adrenal gland S37.818 ☑
      bladder — see Perforation, bladder
      fallopian tube S37.599 ☑
        bilateral S37.592 ☑
        unilateral S37.591 ☑
      kidney S37.09-
      obstetrical trauma O71.5
      ovary S37.499 ☑
        bilateral S37.492 ☑
        unilateral S37.491 ☑
      prostate S37.828 ☑
      specified organ NEC S37.898 ☑
      ureter — see Perforation, ureter
      urethra — see Perforation, urethra
      uterus — see Perforation, uterus
  perineum — see Laceration, perineum
  pharynx J39.2
  rectum K63.1
    newborn P78.0
    obstetrical trauma O71.5
    traumatic S36.63 ☑
  root canal space due to endodontic treatment M27.51
  sigmoid K63.1
    newborn P78.0
    obstetrical trauma O71.5
    traumatic S36.533 ☑
  sinus (accessory) (chronic) (nasal) J34.89
  sphenoidal sinus — see Sinusitis, sphenoidal
  surgical (accidental) (by instrument) (blood vessel) (nerve) (organ) — see Puncture, accidental complicating surgery
  traumatic
    external — see Puncture
    eye — see Puncture, eyeball
    internal organ — see Injury, by site
  tympanum, tympanic (membrane) (persistent post-traumatic) (postinflammatory) H72.9- ☑
    attic H72.1- ☑
      multiple — see Perforation, tympanum, multiple
      total — see Perforation, tympanum, total
    central H72.0- ☑
      multiple — see Perforation, tympanum, multiple
      total — see Perforation, tympanum, total
    marginal NEC — see subcategory H72.2 ☑
    multiple H72.81- ☑
    pars flaccida — see Perforation, tympanum, attic
    total H72.82- ☑
    traumatic, current episode S09.2- ☑
  typhoid, gastrointestinal — see Typhoid
  ulcer — see Ulcer, by site, with perforation
  ureter N28.89
    traumatic S37.19 ☑
  urethra N36.8
    with ectopic or molar pregnancy O08.6
    following ectopic or molar pregnancy O08.6
    obstetrical trauma O71.5
    traumatic S37.39 ☑
      at delivery O71.5
  uterus
    with ectopic or molar pregnancy O08.6
    by intrauterine contraceptive device T83.39 ☑
    following ectopic or molar pregnancy O08.6
    obstetrical trauma O71.1
    traumatic S37.69 ☑
      obstetric O71.1
  uvula K13.79
    syphilitic A52.79

Perforation, perforated — continued
  vagina O71.4
    obstetrical trauma O71.4
    other trauma — see Puncture, vagina
Periadenitis mucosa necrotica recurrens K12.0
Periappendicitis (acute) — see Appendicitis
Periarteritis nodosa (disseminated) (infectious) (necrotizing) M30.0
Periarthritis (joint) (see also Enthesopathy)
  Duplay's M75.0- ☑
  gonococcal A54.42
  humeroscapularis — see Capsulitis, adhesive
  scapulohumeral — see Capsulitis, adhesive
  shoulder — see Capsulitis, adhesive
  wrist M77.2-
Periarthrosis (angioneural) — see Enthesopathy
Pericapsulitis, adhesive (shoulder) — see Capsulitis, adhesive
Pericarditis (with decompensation) (with effusion) I31.9
  with rheumatic fever (conditions in I00)
    active — see Pericarditis, rheumatic
    inactive or quiescent I09.2
  acute (hemorrhagic) (nonrheumatic) (Sicca) I30.9
    with chorea (acute) (rheumatic) (Sydenham's) I02.0
    benign I30.8
    nonspecific I30.0
    rheumatic I01.0
      with chorea (acute) (Sydenham's) I02.0
  adhesive or adherent (chronic) (external) (internal) I31.0
    acute — see Pericarditis, acute
    rheumatic I09.2
  bacterial (acute) (subacute) (with serous or seropurulent effusion) I30.1
  calcareous I31.1
  cholesterol (chronic) I31.8
    acute I30.9
  chronic (nonrheumatic) I31.9
    rheumatic I09.2
  constrictive (chronic) I31.1
  coxsackie B33.23
  fibrinocaseous (tuberculous) A18.84
  fibrinopurulent I30.1
  fibrinous I30.8
  fibrous I31.0
  gonococcal A54.83
  idiopathic I30.0
  in systemic lupus erythematosus M32.12
  infective I30.1
  meningococcal A39.53
  neoplastic (chronic) I31.8
    acute I30.9
  obliterans, obliterating I31.0
  plastic I31.0
  pneumococcal I30.1
  postinfarction I24.1
  purulent I30.1
  rheumatic (active) (acute) (with effusion) (with pneumonia) I01.0
    with chorea (acute) (rheumatic) (Sydenham's) I02.0
    chronic or inactive (with chorea) I09.2
  rheumatoid — see Rheumatoid, carditis
  septic I30.1
  serofibrinous I30.8
  staphylococcal I30.1
  streptococcal I30.1
  suppurative I30.1
  syphilitic A52.06
  tuberculous A18.84
  uremic N18.9 [I32]
  viral I30.1
Pericardium, pericardial — see condition
Pericellulitis — see Cellulitis
Pericementitis (chronic) (suppurative) (see also Periodontitis)
  acute K05.20
    generalized K05.22
    localized K05.21
Perichondritis
  auricle — see Perichondritis, ear
  bronchus J98.09
  ear (external) H61.00- ☑
    acute H61.01- ☑
    chronic H61.02- ☑
  external auditory canal — see Perichondritis, ear
  larynx J38.7
    syphilitic A52.73
    typhoid A01.09

Perichondritis — continued
  nose J34.89
  pinna — see Perichondritis, ear
  trachea J39.8
Periclasia K05.4
Pericoronitis — see Periodontitis
Pericystitis N30.90
  with hematuria N30.91
Peridiverticulitis (intestine) K57.92
  cecum — see Diverticulitis, intestine, large
  colon — see Diverticulitis, intestine, large
  duodenum — see Diverticulitis, intestine, small
  intestine — see Diverticulitis, intestine
  jejunum — see Diverticulitis, intestine, small
  rectosigmoid — see Diverticulitis, intestine, large
  rectum — see Diverticulitis, intestine, large
  sigmoid — see Diverticulitis, intestine, large
Periendocarditis — see Endocarditis
Periepididymitis N45.1
Perifolliculitis L01.02
  abscedens, caput, scalp L66.3
  capitis, abscedens (et suffodiens) L66.3
  superficial pustular L01.02
Perihepatitis K65.8
Perilabyrinthitis (acute) — see subcategory H83.0 ☑
Perimeningitis — see Meningitis
Perimetritis — see Endometritis
Perimetrosalpingitis — see Salpingo-oophoritis
Perineocele N81.81
Perinephric, perinephritic — see condition
Perinephritis (see also Infection, kidney)
  purulent — see Abscess, kidney
Perineum, perineal — see condition
Perineuritis NEC — see Neuralgia
Periodic — see condition
Periodontitis (chronic) (complex) (compound) (local) (simplex) K05.30
  acute K05.20
    generalized K05.22
    localized K05.21
  apical K04.5
    acute (pulpal origin) K04.4
  generalized K05.32
  localized K05.31
Periodontoclasia K05.4
Periodontosis (juvenile) K05.4
Periods (see also Menstruation)
  heavy N92.0
  irregular N92.6
  shortened intervals (irregular) N92.1
Perionychia (see also Cellulitis, digit)
  with lymphangitis — see Lymphangitis, acute, digit
Perioophoritis — see Salpingo-oophoritis
Periorchitis N45.2
Periosteum, periosteal — see condition
Periostitis (albuminosa) (circumscribed) (diffuse) (infective) (monomelic) (see also Osteomyelitis)
  alveolar M27.3
  alveolodental M27.3
  dental M27.3
  gonorrheal A54.43
  jaw (lower) (upper) M27.2
  orbit H05.03- ☑
  syphilitic A52.77
    congenital (early) A50.02 [M90.80]
    secondary A51.46
  tuberculous — see Tuberculosis, bone
  yaws (hypertrophic) (early) (late) A66.6 [M90.80]
Periostosis (hyperplastic) (see also Disorder, bone, specified type NEC)
  with osteomyelitis — see Osteomyelitis, specified type NEC
Peripartum
  cardiomyopathy O90.3
Periphlebitis — see Phlebitis
Periproctitis K62.89
Periprostatitis — see Prostatitis
Perirectal — see condition
Perirenal — see condition
Perisalpingitis — see Salpingo-oophoritis
Perisplenitis (infectional) D73.89
Peristalsis, visible or reversed R19.2
Peritendinitis — see Enthesopathy
Peritoneum, peritoneal — see condition
Peritonitis (adhesive) (bacterial) (fibrinous) (hemorrhagic) (idiopathic) (localized) (perforative) (primary) (with adhesions) (with effusion) K65.9

Peritonitis — *continued*
　with or following
　　abscess K65.1
　　appendicitis K35.2
　　　with perforation or rupture K35.2
　　　　generalized K35.2
　　　　localized K35.3
　　diverticular disease (intestine) K57.80
　　　with bleeding K57.81
　　　ectopic or molar pregnancy O08.0
　　　large intestine K57.20
　　　　with
　　　　　bleeding K57.21
　　　　　small intestine K57.40
　　　　　　with bleeding K57.41
　　　　small intestine K57.00
　　　　　with
　　　　　　bleeding K57.01
　　　　　　large intestine K57.40
　　　　　　　with bleeding K57.41
　acute (generalized) K65.0
　aseptic T81.61 ☑
　bile, biliary K65.3
　chemical T81.61 ☑
　chlamydial A74.81
　chronic proliferative K65.8
　complicating abortion — *see* Abortion, by type, complicated by, pelvic peritonitis
　congenital P78.1
　diaphragmatic K65.0
　diffuse K65.0
　diphtheritic A36.89
　disseminated K65.0
　due to
　　bile K65.3
　　foreign
　　　body or object accidentally left during a procedure (instrument) (sponge) (swab) T81.599 ☑
　　　substance accidentally left during a procedure (chemical) (powder) (talc) T81.61 ☑
　　talc T81.61 ☑
　　urine K65.8
　eosinophilic K65.8
　　acute K65.0
　fibrocaseous (tuberculous) A18.31
　fibropurulent K65.0
　following ectopic or molar pregnancy O08.0
　general (ized) K65.0
　gonococcal A54.85
　meconium (newborn) P78.0
　neonatal P78.1
　　meconium P78.0
　pancreatic K65.0
　paroxysmal, familial E85.0
　　benign E85.0
　pelvic
　　female N73.5
　　　acute N73.3
　　　chronic N73.4
　　　　with adhesions N73.6
　　male K65.0
　periodic, familial E85.0
　proliferative, chronic K65.8
　puerperal, postpartum, childbirth O85
　purulent K65.0
　septic K65.0
　specified NEC K65.8
　spontaneous bacterial K65.2
　subdiaphragmatic K65.0
　subphrenic K65.0
　suppurative K65.0
　syphilitic A52.74
　　congenital (early) A50.08 [K67]
　talc T81.61 ☑
　tuberculous A18.31
　urine K65.8
Peritonsillar — *see* condition
Peritonsillitis J36
Periphlitis K37
Periureteritis N28.89
Periurethral — *see* condition
Periurethritis (gangrenous) — *see* Urethritis
Periuterine — *see* condition
Perivaginitis — *see* Vaginitis
Perivasculitis, retinal H35.06- ☑
Perivasitis (chronic) N49.1
Perivesiculitis (seminal) — *see* Vesiculitis

Perlèche NEC K13.0
　due to
　　candidiasis B37.83
　　moniliasis B37.83
　　riboflavin deficiency E53.0
　　vitamin B2 (riboflavin) deficiency E53.0
Pernicious — *see* condition
Pernio, perniosis T69.1 ☑
Perpetrator (of abuse) — *see* Index to External Causes of Injury, Perpetrator
Persecution
　delusion F22
　social Z60.5
Perseveration (tonic) R48.8
Persistence, persistent (congenital)
　anal membrane Q42.3
　　with fistula Q42.2
　arteria stapedia Q16.3
　atrioventricular canal Q21.2
　branchial cleft Q18.0
　bulbus cordis in left ventricle Q21.8
　canal of Cloquet Q14.0
　capsule (opaque) Q12.8
　cilioretinal artery or vein Q14.8
　cloaca Q43.7
　communication — *see* Fistula, congenital
　convolutions
　　aortic arch Q25.4
　　fallopian tube Q50.6
　　oviduct Q50.6
　　uterine tube Q50.6
　double aortic arch Q25.4
　ductus arteriosus (Botalli) Q25.0
　fetal
　　circulation P29.3
　　form of cervix (uteri) Q51.828
　　hemoglobin, hereditary (HPFH) D56.4
　foramen
　　Botalli Q21.1
　　ovale Q21.1
　Gartner's duct Q52.4
　hemoglobin, fetal (hereditary) (HPFH) D56.4
　hyaloid
　　artery (generally incomplete) Q14.0
　　system Q14.8
　hymen, in pregnancy or childbirth — *see* Pregnancy, complicated by, abnormal, vulva
　lanugo Q84.2
　left
　　posterior cardinal vein Q26.8
　　root with right arch of aorta Q25.4
　　superior vena cava Q26.1
　Meckel's diverticulum Q43.0
　　malignant — *see* Table of Neoplasms, small intestine, malignant
　mucosal disease (middle ear) — *see* Otitis, media, suppurative, chronic, tubotympanic
　nail(s), anomalous Q84.6
　omphalomesenteric duct Q43.0
　organ or site not listed — *see* Anomaly, by site
　ostium
　　atrioventriculare commune Q21.2
　　primum Q21.2
　　secundum Q21.1
　ovarian rests in fallopian tube Q50.6
　pancreatic tissue in intestinal tract Q43.8
　primary (deciduous)
　　teeth K00.6
　　vitreous hyperplasia Q14.0
　pupillary membrane Q13.89
　rhesus (Rh) titer — *see* Complication(s), transfusion, incompatibility reaction, Rh (factor)
　right aortic arch Q25.4
　sinus
　　urogenitalis
　　　female Q52.8
　　　male Q55.8
　　venosus with imperfect incorporation in right auricle Q26.8
　thymus (gland) (hyperplasia) E32.0
　thyroglossal duct Q89.2
　thyrolingual duct Q89.2
　truncus arteriosus or communis Q20.0
　tunica vasculosa lentis Q12.2
　umbilical sinus Q64.4
　urachus Q64.4
　vitelline duct Q43.0

Person (with)
　admitted for clinical research, as a control subject (normal comparison) (participant) Z00.6
　awaiting admission to adequate facility elsewhere Z75.1
　concern (normal) about sick person in family Z63.6
　consulting on behalf of another Z71.0
　feigning illness Z76.5
　living (in)
　　without
　　　adequate housing (heating) (space) Z59.1
　　　housing (permanent) (temporary) Z59.0
　　　person able to render necessary care Z74.2
　　　shelter Z59.0
　　alone Z60.2
　　boarding school Z59.3
　　residential institution Z59.3
　on waiting list Z75.1
　sick or handicapped in family Z63.6
Personality (disorder) F60.9
　accentuation of traits (type A pattern) Z73.1
　affective F34.0
　aggressive F60.3
　amoral F60.2
　anacastic, anankastic F60.5
　antisocial F60.2
　anxious F60.6
　asocial F60.2
　asthenic F60.7
　avoidant F60.6
　borderline F60.3
　change due to organic condition (enduring) F07.0
　compulsive F60.5
　cycloid F34.0
　cyclothymic F34.0
　dependent F60.7
　depressive F34.1
　dissocial F60.2
　dual F44.81
　eccentric F60.89
　emotionally unstable F60.3
　expansive paranoid F60.0
　explosive F60.3
　fanatic F60.0
　haltlose type F60.89
　histrionic F60.4
　hyperthymic F34.0
　hypothymic F34.1
　hysterical F60.4
　immature F60.89
　inadequate F60.7
　labile (emotional) F60.3
　mixed (nonspecific) F60.81
　morally defective F60.2
　multiple F44.81
　narcissistic F60.81
　obsessional F60.5
　obsessive (-compulsive) F60.5
　organic F07.0
　overconscientious F60.5
　paranoid F60.0
　passive (-dependent) F60.7
　passive-aggressive F60.89
　pathologic F60.9
　pattern defect or disturbance F60.9
　pseudopsychopathic (organic) F07.0
　pseudoretarded (organic) F07.0
　psychoinfantile F60.4
　psychoneurotic NEC F60.89
　psychopathic F60.2
　querulant F60.0
　sadistic F60.89
　schizoid F60.1
　self-defeating F60.7
　sensitive paranoid F60.0
　sociopathic (amoral) (antisocial) (asocial) (dissocial) F60.2
　specified NEC F60.89
　type A Z73.1
　unstable (emotional) F60.3
Perthes' disease — *see* Legg-Calvé-Perthes disease
Pertussis (*see also* Whooping cough) A37.90
Perversion, perverted
　appetite F50.8
　　psychogenic F50.8
　function
　　pituitary gland E23.2
　　　posterior lobe E22.2

Perversion, perverted — *continued*
  sense of smell and taste R43.8
    psychogenic F45.8
  sexual — *see* Deviation, sexual
Pervious, congenital (*see also* Imperfect, closure)
  ductus arteriosus Q25.0
Pes (congenital) (*see also* Talipes)
  acquired (*see also* Deformity, limb, foot, specified NEC)
    planus — *see* Deformity, limb, flat foot
  adductus Q66.89
  cavus Q66.7
  deformity NEC, acquired — *see* Deformity, limb, foot, specified NEC
  planus (acquired) (any degree) (*see also* Deformity, limb, flat foot)
    rachitic sequelae (late effect) E64.3
  valgus Q66.6
Pest, pestis — *see* Plague
Petechia, petechiae R23.3
  newborn P54.5
Petechial typhus A75.9
Peter's anomaly Q13.4
Petit mal seizure — *see* Epilepsy, generalized, specified NEC
Petit's hernia — *see* Hernia, abdomen, specified site NEC
Petrellidosis B48.2
Petrositis H70.20- ☑
  acute H70.21- ☑
  chronic H70.22- ☑
Peutz-Jeghers disease or syndrome Q85.8
Peyronie's disease N48.6
Pfeiffer's disease — *see* Mononucleosis, infectious
Phagedena (dry) (moist) (sloughing) (*see also* Gangrene)
  geometric L88
  penis N48.29
  tropical — *see* Ulcer, skin
  vulva N76.6
Phagedenic — *see* condition
Phakoma H35.89
Phakomatosis (*see also* specific eponymous syndromes) Q85.9
  Bourneville's Q85.1
  specified NEC Q85.8
Phantom limb syndrome (without pain) G54.7
  with pain G54.6
Pharyngeal pouch syndrome D82.1
Pharyngitis (acute) (catarrhal)(gangrenous) (infective) (malignant) (membranous) (phlegmonous) (pseudomembranous) (simple) (subacute) (suppurative) (ulcerative) (viral) J02.9
  with influenza, flu, or grippe — *see* Influenza, with, pharyngitis
  aphthous B08.5
  atrophic J31.2
  chlamydial A56.4
  chronic (atrophic) (granular) (hypertrophic) J31.2
  coxsackievirus B08.5
  diphtheritic A36.0
  enteroviral vesicular B08.5
  follicular (chronic) J31.2
  fusospirochetal A69.1
  gonococcal A54.5
  granular (chronic) J31.2
  herpesviral B00.2
  hypertrophic J31.2
  infectional, chronic J31.2
  influenzal — *see* Influenza, with, respiratory manifestations NEC
  lymphonodular, acute (enteroviral) B08.8
  pneumococcal J02.8
  purulent J02.9
  putrid J02.9
  septic J02.0
  sicca J31.2
  specified organism NEC J02.8
  staphylococcal J02.8
  streptococcal J02.0
  syphilitic, congenital (early) A50.03
  tuberculous A15.8
  vesicular, enteroviral B08.5
  viral NEC J02.8
Pharyngoconjunctivitis, viral B30.2
Pharyngolaryngitis (acute) J06.0
  chronic J37.0
Pharyngoplegia J39.2
Pharyngotonsillitis, herpesviral B00.2

Pharyngotracheitis, chronic J42
Pharynx, pharyngeal — *see* condition
Phenomenon
  Arthus' — *see* Arthus' phenomenon
  jaw-winking Q07.8
  lupus erythematosus (LE) cell M32.9
  Raynaud's (secondary) I73.00
    with gangrene I73.01
  vasomotor R55
  vasospastic I73.9
  vasovagal R55
  Wenckebach's I44.1
Phenylketonuria E70.1
  classical E70.0
  maternal E70.1
Pheochromoblastoma
  specified site — *see* Neoplasm, malignant, by site
  unspecified site C74.10
Pheochromocytoma
  malignant
    specified site — *see* Neoplasm, malignant, by site
    unspecified site C74.10
  specified site — *see* Neoplasm, benign, by site
  unspecified site D35.00
Pheohyphomycosis — *see* Chromomycosis
Pheomycosis — *see* Chromomycosis
Phimosis (congenital) (due to infection) N47.1
  chancroidal A57
Phlebectasia (*see also* Varix)
  congenital Q27.4
Phlebitis (infective) (pyemic) (septic) (suppurative) I80.9
  antepartum — *see* Thrombophlebitis, antepartum
  blue — *see* Phlebitis, leg, deep
  breast, superficial I80.8
  cavernous (venous) sinus — *see* Phlebitis, intracranial (venous) sinus
  cerebral (venous) sinus — *see* Phlebitis, intracranial (venous) sinus
  chest wall, superficial I80.8
  cranial (venous) sinus — *see* Phlebitis, intracranial (venous) sinus
  deep (vessels) — *see* Phlebitis, leg, deep
  due to implanted device — *see* Complications, by site and type, specified NEC
  during or resulting from a procedure T81.72 ☑
  femoral vein (superficial) I80.1- ☑
  femoropopliteal vein I80.0- ☑
  gestational — *see* Phlebopathy, gestational
  hepatic veins I80.8
  iliofemoral — *see* Phlebitis, femoral vein
  intracranial (venous) sinus (any) G08
    nonpyogenic I67.6
  intraspinal venous sinuses and veins G08
    nonpyogenic G95.19
  lateral (venous) sinus — *see* Phlebitis, intracranial (venous) sinus
  leg I80.3
    antepartum — *see* Thrombophlebitis, antepartum
    deep (vessels) NEC I80.20- ☑
      iliac I80.21- ☑
      popliteal vein I80.22- ☑
      specified vessel NEC I80.29- ☑
      tibial vein I80.23- ☑
    femoral vein (superficial) I80.1- ☑
    superficial (vessels) I80.0- ☑
  longitudinal sinus — *see* Phlebitis, intracranial (venous) sinus
  lower limb — *see* Phlebitis, leg
  migrans, migrating (superficial) I82.1
  pelvic
    with ectopic or molar pregnancy O08.0
    following ectopic or molar pregnancy O08.0
    puerperal, postpartum O87.1
  popliteal vein — *see* Phlebitis, leg, deep, popliteal
  portal (vein) K75.1
  postoperative T81.72 ☑
  pregnancy — *see* Thrombophlebitis, antepartum
  puerperal, postpartum, childbirth O87.0
    deep O87.1
    pelvic O87.1
    superficial O87.0
  retina — *see* Vasculitis, retina
  saphenous (accessory) (great) (long) (small) — *see* Phlebitis, leg, superficial
  sinus (meninges) — *see* Phlebitis, intracranial (venous) sinus
  specified site NEC I80.8

Phlebitis — *continued*
  syphilitic A52.09
  tibial vein — *see* Phlebitis, leg, deep, tibial
  ulcerative I80.9
    leg — *see* Phlebitis, leg
  umbilicus I80.8
  uterus (septic) — *see* Endometritis
  varicose (leg) (lower limb) — *see* Varix, leg, with, inflammation
Phlebofibrosis I87.8
Phleboliths I87.8
Phlebopathy,
  gestational O22.9- ☑
  puerperal O87.9
Phlebosclerosis I87.8
Phlebothrombosis (*see also* Thrombosis)
  antepartum — *see* Thrombophlebitis, antepartum
  pregnancy — *see* Thrombophlebitis, antepartum
  puerperal — *see* Thrombophlebitis, puerperal
Phlebotomus fever A93.1
Phlegmasia
  alba dolens O87.1
    nonpuerperal — *see* Phlebitis, femoral vein
  cerulea dolens — *see* Phlebitis, leg, deep
Phlegmon — *see* Abscess
Phlegmonous — *see* condition
Phlyctenulosis (allergic) (keratoconjunctivitis) (nontuberculous) (*see also* Keratoconjunctivitis)
  cornea — *see* Keratoconjunctivitis
  tuberculous A18.52
Phobia, phobic F40.9
  animal F40.218
    spiders F40.210
  examination F40.298
  reaction F40.9
  simple F40.298
  social F40.10
    generalized F40.11
  specific (isolated) F40.298
    animal F40.218
      spiders F40.210
    blood F40.230
    injection F40.231
    injury F40.233
    men F40.290
    natural environment F40.228
      thunderstorms F40.220
    situational F40.248
      bridges F40.242
      closed in spaces F40.240
      flying F40.243
      heights F40.241
    specified focus NEC F40.298
    transfusion F40.231
    women F40.291
  specified NEC F40.8
    medical care NEC F40.232
  state F40.9
Phocas' disease — *see* Mastopathy, cystic
Phocomelia Q73.1
  lower limb — *see* Agenesis, leg, with foot present
  upper limb — *see* Agenesis, arm, with hand present
Phoria H50.50
Phosphate-losing tubular disorder N25.0
Phosphatemia E83.39
Phosphaturia E83.39
Photodermatitis (sun) L56.8
  chronic L57.8
  due to drug L56.8
  light other than sun L59.8
Photokeratitis H16.13- ☑
Photophobia H53.14- ☑
Photophthalmia — *see* Photokeratitis
Photopsia H53.19
Photoretinitis — *see* Retinopathy, solar
Photosensitivity, photosensitization (sun) skin L56.8
  light other than sun L59.8
Phrenitis — *see* Encephalitis
Phrynoderma (vitamin A deficiency) E50.8
Phthiriasis (pubis) B85.3
  with any infestation classifiable to B85.0-B85.2 B85.4
Phthirus infestation — *see* Phthiriasis
Phthisis (*see also* Tuberculosis)
  bulbi (infectional) — *see* Disorder, globe, degenerated condition, atrophy
  eyeball (due to infection) — *see* Disorder, globe, degenerated condition, atrophy

Index

Phycomycosis — Pneumocephalus

Phycomycosis — *see* Zygomycosis
Physalopteriasis B81.8
Physical restraint status Z78.1
Phytobezoar T18.9 ☑
  intestine T18.3 ☑
  stomach T18.2 ☑
Pian — *see* Yaws
Pianoma A66.1
Pica F50.8
  in adults F50.8
  infant or child F98.3
Picking, nose F98.8
Pick-Niemann disease — *see* Niemann-Pick disease or syndrome
Pick's
  cerebral atrophy G31.01 [F02.80]
    with behavioral disturbance G31.01 [F02.81]
  disease or syndrome (brain) G31.01 [F02.80]
    with behavioral disturbance G31.01 [F02.81]
Pickwickian syndrome E66.2
Piebaldism E70.39
Piedra (beard) (scalp) B36.8
  black B36.3
  white B36.2
Pierre Robin deformity or syndrome Q87.0
Pierson's disease or osteochondrosis M91.0
Pig-bel A05.2
Pigeon
  breast or chest (acquired) M95.4
    congenital Q67.7
    rachitic sequelae (late effect) E64.3
  breeder's disease or lung J67.2
  fancier's disease or lung J67.2
  toe — *see* Deformity, toe, specified NEC
Pigmentation (abnormal) (anomaly) L81.9
  conjunctiva H11.13- ☑
  cornea (anterior) H18.01- ☑
    posterior H18.05- ☑
    stromal H18.06- ☑
  diminished melanin formation NEC L81.6
  iron L81.8
  lids, congenital Q82.8
  limbus corneae — *see* Pigmentation, cornea
  metals L81.8
  optic papilla, congenital Q14.2
  retina, congenital (grouped) (nevoid) Q14.1
  scrotum, congenital Q82.8
  tattoo L81.8
Piles (*see also* Hemorrhoids) K64.9
Pili
  annulati or torti (congenital) Q84.1
  incarnati L73.1
Pill roller hand (intrinsic) — *see* Parkinsonism
Pilomatrixoma — *see* Neoplasm, skin, benign
  malignant — *see* Neoplasm, skin, malignant
Pilonidal — *see* condition
Pimple R23.8
Pinched nerve — *see* Neuropathy, entrapment
Pindborg tumor — *see* Cyst, calcifying odontogenic
Pineal body or gland — *see* condition
Pinealoblastoma C75.3
Pinealoma D44.5
  malignant C75.3
Pineoblastoma C75.3
Pineocytoma D44.5
Pinguecula H11.15- ☑
Pingueculitis H10.81- ☑
Pinhole meatus (*see also* Stricture, urethra) N35.9
Pink
  disease — *see* subcategory T56.1 ☑
  eye — *see* Conjunctivitis, acute, mucopurulent
Pinkus' disease (lichen nitidus) L44.1
Pinpoint
  meatus — *see* Stricture, urethra
  os (uteri) — *see* Stricture, cervix
Pins and needles R20.2
Pinta A67.9
  cardiovascular lesions A67.2
  chancre (primary) A67.0
  erythematous plaques A67.1
  hyperchromic lesions A67.1
  hyperkeratosis A67.1
  lesions A67.9
    cardiovascular A67.2
    hyperchromic A67.1
    intermediate A67.1
    late A67.2

Pinta — *continued*
  lesions — *continued*
    mixed A67.3
    primary A67.0
    skin (achromic) (cicatricial) (dyschromic) A67.2
      hyperchromic A67.1
      mixed (achromic and hyperchromic) A67.3
    papule (primary) A67.0
    skin lesions (achromic) (cicatricial) (dyschromic) A67.2
      hyperchromic A67.1
      mixed (achromic and hyperchromic) A67.3
    vitiligo A67.2
Pintids A67.1
Pinworm (disease) (infection) (infestation) B80
Piroplasmosis B60.0
Pistol wound — *see* Gunshot wound
Pitchers' elbow — *see* Derangement, joint, specified type NEC, elbow
Pithecoid pelvis Q74.2
  with disproportion (fetopelvic) O33.0
    causing obstructed labor O65.0
Pithiatism F48.8
Pitted — *see* Pitting
Pitting (*see also* Edema) R60.9
  lip R60.0
  nail L60.8
  teeth K00.4
Pituitary gland — *see* condition
Pituitary-snuff-taker's disease J67.8
Pityriasis (capitis) L21.0
  alba L30.5
  circinata (et maculata) L42
  furfuracea L21.0
  Hebra's L26
  lichenoides L41.0
    chronica L41.1
    et varioliformis (acuta) L41.0
  maculata (et circinata) L30.5
  nigra B36.1
  pilaris, Hebra's L44.0
  rosea L42
  rotunda L44.8
  rubra (Hebra) pilaris L44.0
  simplex L30.5
  specified type NEC L30.5
  streptogenes L30.5
  versicolor (scrotal) B36.0
Placenta, placental — *see* Pregnancy, complicated by (care of) (management affected by), specified condition
Placentitis O41.14- ☑
Plagiocephaly Q67.3
Plague A20.9
  abortive A20.8
  ambulatory A20.8
  asymptomatic A20.8
  bubonic A20.0
  cellulocutaneous A20.1
  cutaneobubonic A20.1
  lymphatic gland A20.0
  meningitis A20.3
  pharyngeal A20.8
  pneumonic (primary) (secondary) A20.2
  pulmonary, pulmonic A20.2
  septicemic A20.7
  tonsillar A20.8
    septicemic A20.7
Planning, family
  contraception Z30.9
  procreation Z31.69
Plaque(s)
  artery, arterial — *see* Arteriosclerosis
  calcareous — *see* Calcification
  coronary, lipid rich I25.83
  epicardial I31.8
  erythematous, of pinta A67.1
  Hollenhorst's — *see* Occlusion, artery, retina
  lipid rich, coronary I25.83
  pleural (without asbestos) J92.9
    with asbestos J92.0
  tongue K13.29
Plasmacytoma C90.3- ☑
  extramedullary C90.2- ☑
  medullary C90.0- ☑
  solitary C90.3- ☑
Plasmacytopenia D72.818
Plasmacytosis D72.822
Plaster ulcer — *see* Ulcer, pressure, by site

Plateau iris syndrome (post-iridectomy) (postprocedural) (without glaucoma) H21.82
  with glaucoma H40.22- ☑
Platybasia Q75.8
Platyonychia (congenital) Q84.6
  acquired L60.8
Platypelloid pelvis M95.5
  with disproportion (fetopelvic) O33.0
    causing obstructed labor O65.0
  congenital Q74.2
Platyspondylisis Q76.49
Plaut (-Vincent) **disease** (*see also* Vincent's) A69.1
Plethora R23.2
  newborn P61.1
Pleura, pleural — *see* condition
Pleuralgia R07.81
Pleurisy (acute) (adhesive) (chronic) (costal) (diaphragmatic) (double) (dry) (fibrinous) (fibrous) (interlobar) (latent) (plastic) (primary) (residual) (sicca) (sterile) (subacute) (unresolved) R09.1
  with
    adherent pleura J86.0
    effusion J90
      chylous, chyliform J94.0
      tuberculous (non primary) A15.6
        primary (progressive) A15.7
    tuberculosis — *see* Pleurisy, tuberculous (non primary)
  encysted — *see* Pleurisy, with effusion
  exudative — *see* Pleurisy, with effusion
  fibrinopurulent, fibropurulent — *see* Pyothorax
  hemorrhagic — *see* Hemothorax
  pneumococcal J90
  purulent — *see* Pyothorax
  septic — *see* Pyothorax
  serofibrinous — *see* Pleurisy, with effusion
  seropurulent — *see* Pyothorax
  serous — *see* Pleurisy, with effusion
  staphylococcal J86.9
  streptococcal J90
  suppurative — *see* Pyothorax
  traumatic (post) (current) — *see* Injury, intrathoracic, pleura
  tuberculous (with effusion) (non primary) A15.6
    primary (progressive) A15.7
Pleuritis sicca — *see* Pleurisy
Pleurobronchopneumonia — *see* Pneumonia, broncho-
Pleurodynia R07.81
  epidemic B33.0
  viral B33.0
Pleuropericarditis (*see also* Pericarditis)
  acute I30.9
Pleuropneumonia (acute) (bilateral) (double) (septic) (*see also* Pneumonia) J18.8
  chronic — *see* Fibrosis, lung
Pleuro-pneumonia-like-organism (PPLO), as cause of disease classified elsewhere B96.0
Pleurorrhea — *see* Pleurisy, with effusion
Plexitis, brachial G54.0
Plica
  polonica B85.0
  syndrome, knee M67.5- ☑
  tonsil J35.8
Plicated tongue K14.5
Plug
  bronchus NEC J98.09
  meconium (newborn) NEC syndrome P76.0
  mucus — *see* Asphyxia, mucus
Plumbism — *see* subcategory T56.0 ☑
Plummer's disease E05.20
  with thyroid storm E05.21
Plummer-Vinson syndrome D50.1
Pluricarential syndrome of infancy E40
Plus (and minus) **hand** (intrinsic) — *see* Deformity, limb, specified type NEC, forearm
Pneumathemia — *see* Air, embolism
Pneumatic hammer (drill) syndrome T75.21 ☑
Pneumatocele (lung) J98.4
  intracranial G93.89
  tension J44.9
Pneumatosis
  cystoides intestinalis K63.89
  intestinalis K63.89
  peritonei K66.8
Pneumaturia R39.89
Pneumoblastoma — *see* Neoplasm, lung, malignant
Pneumocephalus G93.89

Pneumococcemia A40.3
Pneumococcus, pneumococcal — *see* condition
Pneumoconiosis (due to) (inhalation of) J64
   with tuberculosis (any type in A15) J65
   aluminum J63.0
   asbestos J61
   bagasse, bagassosis J67.1
   bauxite J63.1
   beryllium J63.2
   coal miners' (simple) J60
   coalworkers' (simple) J60
   collier's J60
   cotton dust J66.0
   diatomite (diatomaceous earth) J62.8
   dust
      inorganic NEC J63.6
      lime J62.8
      marble J62.8
      organic NEC J66.8
   fumes or vapors (from silo) J68.9
   graphite J63.3
   grinder's J62.8
   kaolin J62.8
   mica J62.8
   millstone maker's J62.8
   mineral fibers NEC J61
   miner's J60
   moldy hay J67.0
   potter's J62.8
   rheumatoid — *see* Rheumatoid, lung
   sandblaster's J62.8
   silica, silicate NEC J62.8
      with carbon J60
   stonemason's J62.8
   talc (dust) J62.0
Pneumocystis carinii pneumonia B59
Pneumocystis jiroveci (pneumonia) B59
Pneumocystosis (with pneumonia) B59
Pneumohemopericardium I31.2
Pneumohemothorax J94.2
   traumatic S27.2 ☑
Pneumohydropericardium — *see* Pericarditis
Pneumohydrothorax — *see* Hydrothorax
Pneumomediastinum J98.2
   congenital or perinatal P25.2
Pneumomycosis B49 [J99]
Pneumonia (acute) (double) (migratory) (purulent)
      (septic) (unresolved) J18.9
   with
      influenza — *see* Influenza, with, pneumonia
      lung abscess J85.1
      due to specified organism — *see* Pneumonia,
            in (due to)
   adenoviral J12.0
   adynamic J18.2
   alba A50.04
   allergic (eosinophilic) J82
   alveolar — *see* Pneumonia, lobar
   anaerobes J15.8
   anthrax A22.1
   apex, apical — *see* Pneumonia, lobar
   Ascaris B77.81
   aspiration J69.0
      due to
         aspiration of microorganisms
            bacterial J15.9
            viral J12.9
         food (regurgitated) J69.0
         gastric secretions J69.0
         milk (regurgitated) J69.0
         oils, essences J69.1
         solids, liquids NEC J69.8
         vomitus J69.0
      newborn P24.81
         amniotic fluid (clear) P24.11
         blood P24.21
         food (regurgitated) P24.31
         liquor (amnii) P24.11
         meconium P24.01
         milk P24.31
         mucus P24.11
         specified NEC P24.81
         stomach contents P24.31
      postprocedural J95.4
   atypical NEC J18.9
   bacillus J15.9
      specified NEC J15.8
   bacterial J15.9

Pneumonia — *continued*
   bacterial — *continued*
      specified NEC J15.8
   Bacteroides (fragilis) (oralis) (melaninogenicus) J15.8
   basal, basic, basilar — *see* Pneumonia, by type
   bronchiolitis obliterans organized (BOOP) J84.89
   broncho-, bronchial (confluent) (croupous) (diffuse)
         (disseminated) (hemorrhagic) (involving lobes)
         (lobar) (terminal) J18.0
      allergic (eosinophilic) J82
      aspiration — *see* Pneumonia, aspiration
      bacterial J15.9
         specified NEC J15.8
      chronic — *see* Fibrosis, lung
      diplococcal J13
      Eaton's agent J15.7
      Escherichia coli (E. coli) J15.5
      Friedländer's bacillus J15.0
      Hemophilus influenzae J14
      hypostatic J18.2
      inhalation (*see also* Pneumonia, aspiration)
         due to fumes or vapors (chemical) J68.0
         of oils or essences J69.1
      Klebsiella (pneumoniae) J15.0
      lipid, lipoid J69.1
         endogenous J84.89
      Mycoplasma (pneumoniae) J15.7
      pleuro-pneumonia-like-organisms (PPLO) J15.7
      pneumococcal J13
      Proteus J15.6
      Pseudomonas J15.1
      Serratia marcescens J15.6
      specified organism NEC J16.8
      staphylococcal — *see* Pneumonia, staphylococcal
      streptococcal NEC J15.4
         group B J15.3
         pneumoniae J13
      viral, virus — *see* Pneumonia, viral
   Butyrivibrio (fibriosolvens) J15.8
   Candida B37.1
   caseous — *see* Tuberculosis, pulmonary
   catarrhal — *see* Pneumonia, broncho
   chlamydial J16.0
      congenital P23.1
   cholesterol J84.89
   cirrhotic (chronic) — *see* Fibrosis, lung
   Clostridium (haemolyticum) (novyi) J15.8
   confluent — *see* Pneumonia, broncho
   congenital (infective) P23.9
      due to
         bacterium NEC P23.6
         Chlamydia P23.1
         Escherichia coli P23.4
         Haemophilus influenzae P23.6
         infective organism NEC P23.8
         Klebsiella pneumoniae P23.6
         Mycoplasma P23.6
         Pseudomonas P23.5
         Staphylococcus P23.2
         Streptococcus (except group B) P23.6
            group B P23.3
         viral agent P23.0
      specified NEC P23.8
   croupous — *see* Pneumonia, lobar
   cryptogenic organizing J84.116
   cytomegalic inclusion B25.0
   cytomegaloviral B25.0
   deglutition — *see* Pneumonia, aspiration
   desquamative interstitial J84.117
   diffuse — *see* Pneumonia, broncho
   diplococcal, diplococcus (broncho-) (lobar) J13
   disseminated (focal) — *see* Pneumonia, broncho
   Eaton's agent J15.7
   embolic, embolism — *see* Embolism, pulmonary
   Enterobacter J15.6
   eosinophilic J82
   Escherichia coli (E. coli) J15.5
   Eubacterium J15.8
   fibrinous — *see* Pneumonia, lobar
   fibroid, fibrous (chronic) — *see* Fibrosis, lung
   Friedländer's bacillus J15.0
   Fusobacterium (nucleatum) J15.8
   gangrenous J85.0
   giant cell (measles) B05.2
   gonococcal A54.84
   gram-negative bacteria NEC J15.6
      anaerobic J15.8
   Hemophilus influenzae (broncho) (lobar) J14

Pneumonia — *continued*
   human metapneumovirus J12.3
   hypostatic (broncho) (lobar) J18.2
   in (due to)
      actinomycosis A42.0
      adenovirus J12.0
      anthrax A22.1
      ascariasis B77.81
      aspergillosis B44.9
      Bacillus anthracis A22.1
      Bacterium anitratum J15.6
      candidiasis B37.1
      chickenpox B01.2
      Chlamydia J16.0
         neonatal P23.1
      coccidioidomycosis B38.2
         acute B38.0
         chronic B38.1
      cytomegalovirus disease B25.0
      Diplococcus (pneumoniae) J13
      Eaton's agent J15.7
      Enterobacter J15.6
      Escherichia coli (E. coli) J15.5
      Friedländer's bacillus J15.0
      fumes and vapors (chemical) (inhalation) J68.0
      gonorrhea A54.84
      Hemophilus influenzae (H. influenzae) J14
      Herellea J15.6
      histoplasmosis B39.2
         acute B39.0
         chronic B39.1
      human metapneumovirus J12.3
      Klebsiella (pneumoniae) J15.0
      measles B05.2
      Mycoplasma (pneumoniae) J15.7
      nocardiosis, nocardiasis A43.0
      ornithosis A70
      parainfluenza virus J12.2
      pleuro-pneumonia-like-organism (PPLO) J15.7
      pneumococcus J13
      pneumocystosis (Pneumocystis carinii) (Pneumo-
            cystis jiroveci) B59
      Proteus J15.6
      Pseudomonas NEC J15.1
         pseudomallei A24.1
      psittacosis A70
      Q fever A78
      respiratory syncytial virus J12.1
      rheumatic fever I00 [J17]
      rubella B06.81
      Salmonella (infection) A02.22
         typhi A01.03
      schistosomiasis B65.9 [J17]
      Serratia marcescens J15.6
      specified
         bacterium NEC J15.8
         organism NEC J16.8
      spirochetal NEC A69.8
      Staphylococcus J15.20
         aureus (methicillin susceptible) (MSSA) J15.211
            methicillin resistant (MRSA) J15.212
         specified NEC J15.29
      Streptococcus J15.4
         group B J15.3
         pneumoniae J13
         specified NEC J15.4
      toxoplasmosis B58.3
      tularemia A21.2
      typhoid (fever) A01.03
      varicella B01.2
      virus — *see* Pneumonia, viral
      whooping cough A37.91
         due to
            Bordetella parapertussis A37.11
            Bordetella pertussis A37.01
            specified NEC A37.81
      Yersinia pestis A20.2
   inhalation of food or vomit — *see* Pneumonia, aspira-
         tion
   interstitial J84.9
      chronic J84.111
      desquamative J84.117
      due to
         collagen vascular disease J84.17
         known underlying cause J84.17
      idiopathic NOS J84.111
      in disease classified elsewhere J84.17

Pneumonia — *continued*
  interstitial — *continued*
    lymphocytic (due to collagen vascular disease) (in diseases classified elsewhere) J84.17
    lymphoid J84.2
    non-specific J84.89
      due to
        collagen vascular disease J84.17
          known underlying cause J84.17
      idiopathic J84.113
      in diseases classified elsewhere J84.17
    plasma cell B59
    pseudomonas J15.1
    usual J84.112
      due to collagen vascular disease J84.17
      idiopathic J84.112
      in diseases classified elsewhere J84.17
  Klebsiella (pneumoniae) J15.0
  lipid, lipoid (exogenous) J69.1
    endogenous J84.89
  lobar (disseminated) (double) (interstitial) J18.1
    bacterial J15.9
      specified NEC J15.8
    chronic — *see* Fibrosis, lung
    Escherichia coli (E. coli) J15.5
    Friedländer's bacillus J15.0
    Hemophilus influenzae J14
    hypostatic J18.2
    Klebsiella (pneumoniae) J15.0
    pneumococcal J13
    Proteus J15.6
    Pseudomonas J15.1
    specified organism NEC J16.8
    staphylococcal — *see* Pneumonia, staphylococcal
    streptococcal NEC J15.4
    Streptococcus pneumoniae J13
    viral, virus — *see* Pneumonia, viral
  lobular — *see* Pneumonia, broncho
  Löffler's J82
  lymphoid interstitial J84.2
  massive — *see* Pneumonia, lobar
  meconium P24.01
  MSSA (methicillin susceptible Staphylococcus aureus) J15.211
  multilobar — *see* Pneumonia, by type
  Mycoplasma (pneumoniae) J15.7
  necrotic J85.0
  neonatal P23.9
    aspiration — *see* Aspiration, by substance, with pneumonia
  nitrogen dioxide J68.9
  organizing J84.89
    due to
      collagen vascular disease J84.17
      known underlying cause J84.17
    in diseases classified elsewhere J84.17
  orthostatic J18.2
  parainfluenza virus J12.2
  parenchymatous — *see* Fibrosis, lung
  passive J18.2
  patchy — *see* Pneumonia, broncho
  Peptococcus J15.8
  Peptostreptococcus J15.8
  plasma cell (of infants) B59
  pleurolobar — *see* Pneumonia, lobar
  pleuro-pneumonia-like organism (PPLO) J15.7
  pneumococcal (broncho) (lobar) J13
  Pneumocystis (carinii) (jiroveci) B59
  postinfectional NEC B99 ☑ [J17]
  postmeasles B05.2
  Proteus J15.6
  Pseudomonas J15.1
  psittacosis A70
  radiation J70.0
  respiratory syncytial virus J12.1
  resulting from a procedure J95.89
  rheumatic I00 [J17]
  Salmonella (arizonae) (cholerae-suis) (enteritidis) (typhimurium) A02.22
    typhi A01.03
    typhoid fever A01.03
  SARS-associated coronavirus J12.81
  segmented, segmental — *see* Pneumonia, broncho-
  Serratia marcescens J15.6
  specified NEC J18.8
    bacterium NEC J15.8
    organism NEC J16.8
    virus NEC J12.89

Pneumonia — *continued*
  spirochetal NEC A69.8
  staphylococcal (broncho) (lobar) J15.20
    aureus (methicillin susceptible) (MSSA) J15.211
      methicillin resistant (MRSA) J15.212
    specified NEC J15.29
  static, stasis J18.2
  streptococcal NEC (broncho) (lobar) J15.4
    group
      A J15.4
      B J15.3
    specified NEC J15.4
  Streptococcus pneumoniae J13
  syphilitic, congenital (early) A50.04
  traumatic (complication) (early) (secondary) T79.8 ☑
  tuberculous (any) — *see* Tuberculosis, pulmonary
  tularemic A21.2
  varicella B01.2
  Veillonella J15.8
  ventilator associated J95.851
  viral, virus (broncho) (interstitial) (lobar) J12.9
    adenoviral J12.0
    congenital P23.0
    human metapneumovirus J12.3
    parainfluenza J12.2
    respiratory syncytial J12.1
    SARS-associated coronavirus J12.81
    specified NEC J12.89
  white (congenital) A50.04
Pneumonic — *see* condition
Pneumonitis (acute) (primary) (*see also* Pneumonia)
  air-conditioner J67.7
  allergic (due to) J67.9
    organic dust NEC J67.8
    red cedar dust J67.8
    sequoiosis J67.8
    wood dust J67.8
  aspiration J69.0
    due to
      anesthesia J95.4
        during
          labor and delivery O74.0
          pregnancy O29.01- ☑
          puerperium O89.01
      fumes or gases J68.0
    obstetric O74.0
  chemical (due to gases, fumes or vapors) (inhalation) J68.0
    due to anesthesia J95.4
  cholesterol J84.89
  chronic — *see* Fibrosis, lung
  congenital rubella P35.0
  crack (cocaine) J68.0
  due to
    beryllium J68.0
    cadmium J68.0
    crack (cocaine) J68.0
    detergent J69.8
    fluorocarbon-polymer J68.0
    food, vomit (aspiration) J69.0
    fumes or vapors J68.0
    gases, fumes or vapors (inhalation) J68.0
    inhalation
      blood J69.8
      essences J69.1
      food (regurgitated), milk, vomit J69.0
      oils, essences J69.1
      saliva J69.0
      solids, liquids NEC J69.8
    manganese J68.0
    nitrogen dioxide J68.0
    oils, essences J69.1
    solids, liquids NEC J69.8
    toxoplasmosis (acquired) B58.3
      congenital P37.1
    vanadium J68.0
    ventilator J95.851
  eosinophilic J82
  hypersensitivity J67.9
    air conditioner lung J67.7
    bagassosis J67.1
    bird fancier's lung J67.2
    farmer's lung J67.0
    maltworker's lung J67.4
    maple bark-stripper's lung J67.6
    mushroom worker's lung J67.5
    specified organic dust NEC J67.8
    suberosis J67.3

Pneumonitis — *continued*
  interstitial (chronic) J84.89
    acute J84.114
    lymphoid J84.2
    non-specific J84.89
      idiopathic J84.113
  lymphoid, interstitial J84.2
  meconium P24.01
  postanesthetic J95.4
    correct substance properly administered — *see* Table of Drugs and Chemicals, by drug, adverse effect
    in labor and delivery O74.0
    in pregnancy O29.01- ☑
    obstetric O74.0
    overdose or wrong substance given or taken (by accident) — *see* Table of Drugs and Chemicals, by drug, poisoning
    postpartum, puerperal O89.01
  postoperative J95.4
    obstetric O74.0
  radiation J70.0
  rubella, congenital P35.0
  ventilation (air-conditioning) J67.7
  ventilator associated J95.851
  wood-dust J67.8
Pneumoconiosis — *see* Pneumoconiosis
Pneumoparotid K11.8
Pneumopathy NEC J98.4
  alveolar J84.09
  due to organic dust NEC J66.8
  parietoalveolar J84.09
Pneumopericarditis (*see also* Pericarditis)
  acute I30.1
Pneumopericardium (*see also* Pericarditis)
  congenital P25.3
  newborn P25.3
  traumatic (post) — *see* Injury, heart
Pneumophagia (psychogenic) F45.8
Pneumopleurisy, pneumopleuritis (*see also* Pneumonia) J18.8
Pneumopyopericardium I30.1
Pneumopyothorax — *see* Pyopneumothorax
  with fistula J86.0
Pneumorrhagia (*see also* Hemorrhage, lung)
  tuberculous — *see* Tuberculosis, pulmonary
Pneumothorax NOS J93.9
  acute J93.83
  chronic J93.81
  congenital P25.1
  perinatal period P25.1
  postprocedural J95.811
  specified NEC J93.83
  spontaneous NOS J93.83
    newborn P25.1
    primary J93.11
    secondary J93.12
    tension J93.0
  tense valvular, infectional J93.0
  tension (spontaneous) J93.0
  traumatic S27.0 ☑
    with hemothorax S27.2 ☑
  tuberculous — *see* Tuberculosis, pulmonary
Podagra (*see also* Gout) M10.9
Podencephalus Q01.9
Poikilocytosis R71.8
Poikiloderma L81.6
  Civatte's L57.3
  congenital Q82.8
  vasculare atrophicans L94.5
Poikilodermatomyositis M33.10
  with
    myopathy M33.12
    respiratory involvement M33.11
    specified organ involvement NEC M33.19
Pointed ear (congenital) Q17.3
Poison ivy, oak, sumac or other plant dermatitis (allergic) (contact) L23.7
Poisoning (acute) (*see also* Table of Drugs and Chemicals)
  algae and toxins T65.82- ☑
  Bacillus B (aertrycke) (cholerae (suis)) (paratyphosus) (suipestifer) A02.9
    botulinus A05.1
  bacterial toxins A05.9
  berries, noxious — *see* Poisoning, food, noxious, berries
  botulism A05.1
  ciguatera fish T61.0- ☑

☑ **Additional Character Required** — Refer to the Tabular List for Character Selection

⬇ **Subterms under main terms may continue to next column or page**

Poisoning — *continued*
  Clostridium botulinum A05.1
  death-cap (Amanita phalloides) (Amanita verna) —
    see Poisoning, food, noxious, mushrooms
  drug — *see* Table of Drugs and Chemicals, by drug,
    poisoning
  epidemic, fish (noxious) — *see* Poisoning, seafood
    bacterial A05.9
  fava bean D55.0
  fish (noxious) T61.9- ☑
    bacterial — *see* Intoxication, foodborne, by agent
    ciguatera fish — *see* Poisoning, ciguatera fish
    scombroid fish — *see* Poisoning, scombroid fish
    specified type NEC T61.77- ☑
  food (acute) (diseased) (infected) (noxious) NEC
    T62.9- ☑
    bacterial — *see* Intoxication, foodborne, by agent
    due to
      Bacillus (aertrycke) (choleraesuis) (paratypho-
        sus) (suipestifer) A02.9
        botulinus A05.1
      Clostridium (perfringens) (Welchii) A05.2
      salmonella (aertrycke) (callinarum) (choleraesu-
        is) (enteritidis) (paratyphi) (suipestifer)
        A02.9
        with
          gastroenteritis A02.0
          sepsis A02.1
      staphylococcus A05.0
      Vibrio
        parahaemolyticus A05.3
        vulnificus A05.5
    noxious or naturally toxic T62.9- ☑
      berries — *see* subcategory T62.1 ☑
      fish — *see* Poisoning, seafood
      mushrooms — *see* subcategory T62.0X ☑
      plants NEC — *see* subcategory T62.2X ☑
      seafood — *see* Poisoning, seafood
      specified NEC — *see* subcategory T62.8X ☑
  ichthyotoxism — *see* Poisoning, seafood
  kreotoxism, food A05.9
  latex T65.81- ☑
  lead T56.0- ☑
  mushroom — *see* Poisoning, food, noxious, mushroom
  mussels (*see also* Poisoning, shellfish)
    bacterial — *see* Intoxication, foodborne, by agent
  nicotine (tobacco) T65.2- ☑
  noxious foodstuffs — *see* Poisoning, food, noxious
  plants, noxious — *see* Poisoning, food, noxious, plants
    NEC
  ptomaine — *see* Poisoning, food
  radiation J70.0
  Salmonella (arizonae) (cholerae-suis) (enteritidis) (ty-
    phimurium) A02.9
  scombroid fish T61.1- ☑
  seafood (noxious) T61.9- ☑
    bacterial — *see* Intoxication, foodborne, by agent
    fish — *see* Poisoning, fish
    shellfish — *see* Poisoning, shellfish
    specified NEC — *see* subcategory T61.8X ☑
  shellfish (amnesic) (azaspiracid) (diarrheic) (neurotoxic)
    (noxious) (paralytic) T61.78- ☑
    bacterial — *see* Intoxication, foodborne, by agent
    ciguatera mollusk — *see* Poisoning, ciguatera fish
  specified substance NEC T65.891 ☑
  Staphylococcus, food A05.0
  tobacco (nicotine) T65.2- ☑
  water E87.79
Poker spine — *see* Spondylitis, ankylosing
Poland syndrome Q79.8
Polioencephalitis (acute) (bulbar) A80.9
  inferior G12.22
  influenzal — *see* Influenza, with, encephalopathy
  superior hemorrhagic (acute) (Wernicke's) E51.2
  Wernicke's E51.2
Polioencephalomyelitis (acute) (anterior) A80.9
  with beriberi E51.2
Polioencephalopathy, superior hemorrhagic E51.2
  with
    beriberi E51.11
    pellagra E52
Poliomeningoencephalitis — *see* Meningoencephalitis
Poliomyelitis (acute) (anterior) (epidemic) A80.9
  with paralysis (bulbar) — *see* Poliomyelitis, paralytic
  abortive A80.4
  ascending (progressive) — *see* Poliomyelitis, paralytic
  bulbar (paralytic) — *see* Poliomyelitis, paralytic

Poliomyelitis — *continued*
  congenital P35.8
  nonepidemic A80.9
  nonparalytic A80.4
  paralytic A80.30
    specified NEC A80.39
    vaccine-associated A80.0
    wild virus
      imported A80.1
      indigenous A80.2
  spinal, acute A80.9
Poliosis (eyebrow) (eyelashes) L67.1
  circumscripta, acquired L67.1
Pollakiuria R35.0
  psychogenic F45.8
Pollinosis J30.1
Pollitzer's disease L73.2
Polyadenitis (*see also* Lymphadenitis)
  malignant A20.0
Polyalgia M79.89
Polyangiitis M30.0
  microscopic M31.7
  overlap syndrome M30.8
Polyarteritis
  microscopic M31.7
  nodosa M30.0
    with lung involvement M30.1
    juvenile M30.2
    related condition NEC M30.8
Polyarthralgia — *see* Pain, joint
Polyarthritis, polyarthropathy (*see also* Arthritis) M13.0
  due to or associated with other specified conditions
    — *see* Arthritis
  epidemic (Australian) (with exanthema) B33.1
  infective — *see* Arthritis, pyogenic or pyemic
  inflammatory M06.4
  juvenile (chronic) (seronegative) M08.3
  migratory — *see* Fever, rheumatic
  rheumatic, acute — *see* Fever, rheumatic
Polyarthrosis M15.9
  post-traumatic M15.3
  primary M15.0
  specified NEC M15.8
Polycarential syndrome of infancy E40
Polychondritis (atrophic) (chronic) (*see also* Disorder,
  cartilage, specified type NEC)
  relapsing M94.1
Polycoria Q13.2
Polycystic (disease)
  degeneration, kidney Q61.3
    autosomal dominant (adult type) Q61.2
    autosomal recessive (infantile type) NEC Q61.19
  kidney Q61.3
    autosomal
      dominant Q61.2
      recessive NEC Q61.19
    autosomal dominant (adult type) Q61.2
    autosomal recessive (childhood type) NEC Q61.19
    infantile type NEC Q61.19
  liver Q44.6
  lung J98.4
    congenital Q33.0
  ovary, ovaries E28.2
  spleen Q89.09
Polycythemia (secondary) D75.1
  acquired D75.1
  benign (familial) D75.0
  due to
    donor twin P61.1
    erythropoietin D75.1
    fall in plasma volume D75.1
    high altitude D75.1
    maternal-fetal transfusion P61.1
    stress D75.1
  emotional D75.1
  erythropoietin D75.1
  familial (benign) D75.0
  Gaisböck's (hypertonica) D75.1
  high altitude D75.1
  hypertonica D75.1
  hypoxemic D75.1
  neonatorum P61.1
  nephrogenous D75.1
  relative D75.1
  secondary D75.1
  spurious D75.1
  stress D75.1
  vera D45

Polycytosis cryptogenica D75.1
Polydactylism, polydactyly Q69.9
  toes Q69.2
Polydipsia R63.1
Polydystrophy, pseudo-Hurler E77.0
Polyembryoma — *see* Neoplasm, malignant, by site
Polyglandular
  deficiency E31.0
  dyscrasia E31.9
  dysfunction E31.9
  syndrome E31.8
Polyhydramnios O40.- ☑
Polymastia Q83.1
Polymenorrhea N92.0
Polymyalgia M35.3
  arteritica, giant cell M31.5
  rheumatica M35.3
    with giant cell arteritis M31.5
Polymyositis (acute) (chronic) (hemorrhagic) M33.20
  with
    myopathy M33.22
    respiratory involvement M33.21
    skin involvement — *see* Dermatopolymyositis
    specified organ involvement NEC M33.29
  ossificans (generalisata) (progressiva) — *see* Myositis,
    ossificans, progressiva
Polyneuritis, polyneuritic (*see also* Polyneuropathy)
  acute (post-)infective G61.0
  alcoholic G62.1
  cranialis G52.7
  demyelinating, chronic inflammatory (CIDP) G61.81
  diabetic — *see* Diabetes, polyneuropathy
  diphtheritic A36.83
  due to lack of vitamin NEC E56.9 [G63]
  endemic E51.11
  erythredema — *see* subcategory T56.1 ☑
  febrile, acute G61.0
  hereditary ataxic G60.1
  idiopathic, acute G61.0
  infective (acute) G61.0
  inflammatory, chronic demyelinating (CIDP) G61.81
  nutritional E63.9 [G63]
  postinfective (acute) G61.0
  specified NEC G62.89
Polyneuropathy (peripheral) G62.9
  alcoholic G62.1
  amyloid (Portuguese) E85.1 [G63]
  arsenical G62.2
  critical illness G62.81
  demyelinating, chronic inflammatory (CIDP) G61.81
  diabetic — *see* Diabetes, polyneuropathy
  drug-induced G62.0
  hereditary G60.9
    specified NEC G60.8
  idiopathic G60.9
    progressive G60.3
  in (due to)
    alcohol G62.1
      sequelae G65.2
    amyloidosis, familial (Portuguese) E85.1 [G63]
    antitetanus serum G61.1
    arsenic G62.2
      sequelae G65.2
    avitaminosis NEC E56.9 [G63]
    beriberi E51.11
    collagen vascular disease NEC M35.9 [G63]
    deficiency (of)
      B (-complex) vitamins E53.9 [G63]
      vitamin B6 E53.1 [G63]
    diabetes — *see* Diabetes, polyneuropathy
    diphtheria A36.83
    drug or medicament G62.0
      correct substance properly administered — *see*
        Table of Drugs and Chemicals, by drug,
        adverse effect
      overdose or wrong substance given or taken
        — *see* Table of Drugs and Chemicals, by
        drug, poisoning
    endocrine disease NEC E34.9 [G63]
    herpes zoster B02.23
    hypoglycemia E16.2 [G63]
    infectious
      disease NEC B99 ☑ [G63]
      mononucleosis B27.91
    lack of vitamin NEC E56.9 [G63]
    lead G62.2
      sequelae G65.2
    leprosy A30.9 [G63]

Polyneuropathy — *continued*
  in — *continued*
    Lyme disease A69.22
    metabolic disease NEC E88.9 [G63]
    microscopic polyangiitis M31.7 [G63]
    mumps B26.84
    neoplastic disease (*see also* Neoplasm) D49.9 [G63]
    nutritional deficiency NEC E63.9 [G63]
    organophosphate compounds G62.2
      sequelae G65.2
    parasitic disease NEC B89 [G63]
    pellagra E52 [G63]
    polyarteritis nodosa M30.0
    porphyria E80.20 [G63]
    radiation G62.82
    rheumatoid arthritis — *see* Rheumatoid, polyneu-
      ropathy
    sarcoidosis D86.89
    serum G61.1
    syphilis (late) A52.15
      congenital A50.43
    systemic
      connective tissue disorder M35.9 [G63]
      lupus erythematosus M32.19
    toxic agent NEC G62.2
      sequelae G65.2
    triorthocresyl phosphate G62.2
      sequelae G65.2
    tuberculosis A17.89
    uremia N18.9 [G63]
    vitamin B12 deficiency E53.8 [G63]
      with anemia (pernicious) D51.0 [G63]
        due to dietary deficiency D51.3 [G63]
    zoster B02.23
  inflammatory G61.9
    chronic demyelinating (CIDP) G61.81
    sequelae G65.1
    specified NEC G61.89
  lead G62.2
    sequelae G65.2
  nutritional NEC E63.9 [G63]
  postherpetic (zoster) B02.23
  progressive G60.3
  radiation-induced G62.82
  sensory (hereditary) (idiopathic) G60.8
  specified NEC G62.89
  syphilitic (late) A52.15
    congenital A50.43
Polyopia H53.8
Polyorchism, polyorchidism Q55.21
Polyosteoarthritis (*see also* Osteoarthritis, generalized)
  M15.9
  post-traumatic M15.3
  specified NEC M15.8
Polyostotic fibrous dysplasia Q78.1
Polyotia Q17.0
Polyp, polypus
  accessory sinus J33.8
  adenocarcinoma in — *see* Neoplasm, malignant, by
    site
  adenocarcinoma in situ in — *see* Neoplasm, in situ, by
    site
  adenoid tissue J33.0
  adenomatous (*see also* Neoplasm, benign, by site)
    adenocarcinoma in — *see* Neoplasm, malignant,
      by site
    adenocarcinoma in situ in — *see* Neoplasm, in situ,
      by site
    carcinoma in — *see* Neoplasm, malignant, by site
    carcinoma in situ in — *see* Neoplasm, in situ, by
      site
    multiple — *see* Neoplasm, benign
      adenocarcinoma in — *see* Neoplasm, malig-
        nant, by site
      adenocarcinoma in situ in — *see* Neoplasm, in
        situ, by site
  antrum J33.8
  anus, anal (canal) K62.0
  Bartholin's gland N84.3
  bladder D41.4
  carcinoma in — *see* Neoplasm, malignant, by site
  carcinoma in situ in — *see* Neoplasm, in situ, by site
  cecum D12.0
  cervix (uteri) N84.1
    in pregnancy or childbirth — *see* Pregnancy,
      complicated by, abnormal, cervix
    mucous N84.1
    nonneoplastic N84.1

Polyp, polypus — *continued*
  choanal J33.0
  cholesterol K82.4
  clitoris N84.3
  colon K63.5
    adenomatous D12.6
    ascending D12.2
    cecum D12.0
    descending D12.4
    inflammatory K51.40
      with
        abscess K51.414
        complication K51.419
          specified NEC K51.418
        fistula K51.413
        intestinal obstruction K51.412
        rectal bleeding K51.411
    sigmoid D12.5
    transverse D12.3
  corpus uteri N84.0
  dental K04.0
  duodenum K31.7
  ear (middle) H74.4- ☑
  endometrium N84.0
  ethmoidal (sinus) J33.8
  fallopian tube N84.8
  female genital tract N84.9
    specified NEC N84.8
  frontal (sinus) J33.8
  gallbladder K82.4
  gingiva, gum K06.8
  labia, labium (majus) (minus) N84.3
  larynx (mucous) J38.1
    adenomatous D14.1
  malignant — *see* Neoplasm, malignant, by site
  maxillary (sinus) J33.8
  middle ear — *see* Polyp, ear (middle)
  myometrium N84.0
  nares
    anterior J33.9
    posterior J33.0
  nasal (mucous) J33.9
    cavity J33.0
    septum J33.0
  nasopharyngeal J33.0
  nose (mucous) J33.9
  oviduct N84.8
  pharynx J39.2
  placenta O90.89
  prostate — *see* Enlargement, enlarged, prostate
  pudenda, pudendum N84.3
  pulpal (dental) K04.0
  rectum (nonadenomatous) K62.1
    adenomatous — *see* Polyp, adenomatous
  septum (nasal) J33.0
  sinus (accessory) (ethmoidal) (frontal) (maxillary)
    (sphenoidal) J33.8
  sphenoidal (sinus) J33.8
  stomach K31.7
    adenomatous D13.1
  tube, fallopian N84.8
  turbinate, mucous membrane J33.8
  umbilical, newborn P83.6
  ureter N28.89
  urethra N36.2
  uterus (body) (corpus) (mucous) N84.0
    cervix N84.1
    in pregnancy or childbirth — *see* Pregnancy,
      complicated by, tumor, uterus
  vagina N84.2
  vocal cord (mucous) J38.1
  vulva N84.3
Polyphagia R63.2
Polyploidy Q92.7
Polypoid — *see* condition
Polyposis (*see also* Polyp)
  coli (adenomatous) D12.6
    adenocarcinoma in C18.9
    adenocarcinoma in situ in — *see* Neoplasm, in situ,
      by site
    carcinoma in C18.9
  colon (adenomatous) D12.6
  familial D12.6
    adenocarcinoma in situ in — *see* Neoplasm, in situ,
      by site
  intestinal (adenomatous) D12.6
  malignant lymphomatous C83.1- ☑

Polyposis — *continued*
  multiple, adenomatous (*see also* Neoplasm, benign)
    D36.9
Polyradiculitis — *see* Polyneuropathy
Polyradiculoneuropathy (acute) (postinfective) (seg-
  mentally demyelinating) G61.0
Polyserositis
  due to pericarditis I31.1
  pericardial I31.1
  periodic, familial E85.0
  tuberculous A19.9
    acute A19.1
    chronic A19.8
Polysplenia syndrome Q89.09
Polysyndactyly (*see also* Syndactylism, syndactyly) Q70.4
Polytrichia L68.3
Polyunguia Q84.6
Polyuria R35.8
  nocturnal R35.1
  psychogenic F45.8
Pompe's disease (glycogen storage) E74.02
Pompholyx L30.1
Poncet's disease (tuberculous rheumatism) A18.09
Pond fracture — *see* Fracture, skull
Ponos B55.0
Pons, pontine — *see* condition
Poor
  aesthetic of existing restoration of tooth K08.56
  contractions, labor O62.2
  gingival margin to tooth restoration K08.51
  personal hygiene R46.0
  prenatal care, affecting management of pregnancy
    — *see* Pregnancy, complicated by, insufficient,
    prenatal care
  sucking reflex (newborn) R29.2
  urinary stream R39.12
  vision NEC H54.7
Poradenitis, nostras inguinalis or venerea A55
Porencephaly (congenital) (developmental) (true) Q04.6
  acquired G93.0
  nondevelopmental G93.0
  traumatic (post) F07.89
Porocephaliasis B88.8
Porokeratosis Q82.8
Poroma, eccrine — *see* Neoplasm, skin, benign
Porphyria (South African) E80.20
  acquired E80.20
  acute intermittent (hepatic) (Swedish) E80.21
  cutanea tarda (hereditary) (symptomatic) E80.1
  due to drugs E80.20
    correct substance properly administered — *see*
      Table of Drugs and Chemicals, by drug, ad-
      verse effect
    overdose or wrong substance given or taken —
      see Table of Drugs and Chemicals, by drug,
      poisoning
  erythropoietic (congenital) (hereditary) E80.0
  hepatocutaneous type E80.1
  secondary E80.20
  toxic NEC E80.20
  variegata E80.20
Porphyrinuria — *see* Porphyria
Porphyruria — *see* Porphyria
Port wine nevus, mark, or stain Q82.5
Portal — *see* condition
Posadas-Wernicke disease B38.9
Positive
  culture (nonspecific)
    blood R78.81
    bronchial washings R84.5
    cerebrospinal fluid R83.5
    cervix uteri R87.5
    nasal secretions R84.5
    nipple discharge R89.5
    nose R84.5
      staphylococcus (Methicillin susceptible) Z22.321
        Methicillin resistant Z22.322
    peritoneal fluid R85.5
    pleural fluid R84.5
    prostatic secretions R86.5
    saliva R85.5
    seminal fluid R86.5
    sputum R84.5
    synovial fluid R89.5
    throat scrapings R84.5
    urine R82.7
    vagina R87.5
    vulva R87.5

Positive — *continued*
  culture — *continued*
    wound secretions R89.5
  PPD (skin test) R76.11
  serology for syphilis A53.0
    with signs or symptoms — *code as* Syphilis, by site and stage
    false R76.8
  skin test, tuberculin (without active tuberculosis) R76.11
  test, human immunodeficiency virus (HIV) R75
  VDRL A53.0
    with signs or symptoms — *code by* site and stage under Syphilis A53.9
  Wassermann reaction A53.0
Postcardiotomy syndrome I97.0
Postcaval ureter Q62.62
Postcholecystectomy syndrome K91.5
Postclimacteric bleeding N95.0
Postcommissurotomy syndrome I97.0
Postconcussional syndrome F07.81
Postcontusional syndrome F07.81
Postcricoid region — *see* condition
Post-dates (40-42 weeks) (pregnancy) (mother) O48.0
  more than 42 weeks gestation O48.1
Postencephalitic syndrome F07.89
Posterior — *see* condition
Posterolateral sclerosis (spinal cord) — *see* Degeneration, combined
Postexanthematous — *see* condition
Postfebrile — *see* condition
Postgastrectomy dumping syndrome K91.1
Posthemiplegic chorea — *see* Monoplegia
Posthemorrhagic anemia (chronic) D50.0
  acute D62
  newborn P61.3
Postherpetic neuralgia (zoster) B02.29
  trigeminal B02.22
Posthitis N47.7
Postimmunization complication or reaction — *see* Complications, vaccination
Postinfectious — *see* condition
Postlaminectomy syndrome NEC M96.1
Postleukotomy syndrome F07.0
Postmastectomy lymphedema (syndrome) I97.2
Postmaturity, postmature (over 42 weeks)
  maternal (over 42 weeks gestation) O48.1
  newborn P08.22
Postmeasles complication NEC (*see also* condition) B05.89
Postmenopausal
  endometrium (atrophic) N95.8
    suppurative (*see also* Endometritis) N71.9
  osteoporosis — *see* Osteoporosis, postmenopausal
Postnasal drip R09.82
  due to
    allergic rhinitis — *see* Rhinitis, allergic
    common cold J00
    gastroesophageal reflux — *see* Reflux, gastroesophageal
    nasopharyngitis — *see* Nasopharyngitis
    other known condition — *code to* condition
    sinusitis — *see* Sinusitis
Postnatal — *see* condition
Postoperative (postprocedural) — *see* Complication, postoperative
  pneumothorax, therapeutic Z98.3
  state NEC Z98.89
Postpancreatectomy hyperglycemia E89.1
Postpartum — *see* Puerperal
Postphlebitic syndrome — *see* Syndrome, postthrombotic
Postpolio (myelitic) **syndrome** G14
Postpoliomyelitic (*see also* condition)
  osteopathy — *see* Osteopathy, after poliomyelitis
Postprocedural (*see also* Postoperative)
  hypoinsulinemia E89.1
Postschizophrenic depression F32.8
Postsurgery status (*see also* Status (post))
  pneumothorax, therapeutic Z98.3
Post-term (40-42 weeks) (pregnancy) (mother) O48.0
  infant P08.21
  more than 42 weeks gestation (mother) O48.1
Post-traumatic brain syndrome, nonpsychotic F07.81
Post-typhoid abscess A01.09
Postures, hysterical F44.2

Postvaccinal reaction or complication — *see* Complications, vaccination
Postvalvulotomy syndrome I97.0
Potain's
  disease (pulmonary edema) — *see* Edema, lung
  syndrome (gastrectasis with dyspepsia) K31.0
Potter's
  asthma J62.8
  facies Q60.6
  lung J62.8
  syndrome (with renal agenesis) Q60.6
Pott's
  curvature (spinal) A18.01
  disease or paraplegia A18.01
  spinal curvature A18.01
  tumor, puffy — *see* Osteomyelitis, specified type NEC
Pouch
  bronchus Q32.4
  Douglas' — *see* condition
  esophagus, esophageal, congenital Q39.6
    acquired K22.5
  gastric K31.4
  Hartmann's K82.8
  pharynx, pharyngeal (congenital) Q38.7
Pouchitis K91.850
Poultrymen's itch B88.0
Poverty NEC Z59.6
  extreme Z59.5
Poxvirus NEC B08.8
Prader-Willi syndrome Q87.1
Preauricular appendage or tag Q17.0
Prebetalipoproteinemia (acquired) (essential) (familial) (hereditary) (primary) (secondary) E78.1
  with chylomicronemia E78.3
Precipitate labor or delivery O62.3
Preclimacteric bleeding (menorrhagia) N92.4
Precocious
  adrenarche E30.1
  menarche E30.1
  menstruation E30.1
  pubarche E30.1
  puberty E30.1
    central E22.8
  sexual development NEC E30.1
  thelarche E30.8
Precocity, sexual (constitutional) (cryptogenic) (female) (idiopathic) (male) E30.1
  with adrenal hyperplasia E25.9
    congenital E25.0
Precordial pain R07.2
Predeciduous teeth K00.2
Prediabetes, prediabetic R73.09
  complicating
    pregnancy — *see* Pregnancy, complicated by, diseases of, specified type or system NEC
    puerperium O99.89
Predislocation status of hip at birth Q65.6
Pre-eclampsia O14.9- ☑
  with pre-existing hypertension — *see* Hypertension, complicating pregnancy, pre-existing, with, pre-eclampsia
  mild O14.0- ☑
  moderate O14.0- ☑
  severe O14.1- ☑
    with hemolysis, elevated liver enzymes and low platelet count (HELLP) O14.2- ☑
Pre-eruptive color change, teeth, tooth K00.8
Pre-excitation atrioventricular conduction I45.6
Preglaucoma H40.00- ☑
Pregnancy (single) (uterine) (*see also* Delivery and Puerperal)

> *Note: The Tabular must be reviewed for assignment of appropriate seventh character for multiple gestation codes in Chapter 15*

> *Note: The Tabular must be reviewed for assignment of the appropriate character indicating the trimester of the pregnancy*

  abdominal (ectopic) O00.0
    with viable fetus O36.7- ☑
  ampullar O00.1
  biochemical O02.81
  broad ligament O00.8
  cervical O00.8
  chemical O02.81

Pregnancy — *continued*
  complicated by (care of) (management affected by)
    abnormal, abnormality
      cervix O34.4- ☑
        causing obstructed labor O65.5
      cord (umbilical) O69.9 ☑
      findings on antenatal screening of mother O28.9
        biochemical O28.1
        chromosomal O28.5
        cytological O28.2
        genetic O28.5
        hematological O28.0
        radiological O28.4
        specified NEC O28.8
        ultrasonic O28.3
      glucose (tolerance) NEC O99.810
      pelvic organs O34.9- ☑
        specified NEC O34.8- ☑
          causing obstructed labor O65.5
      pelvis (bony) (major) NEC O33.0
      perineum O34.7- ☑
      position
        placenta O44.1- ☑
          without hemorrhage O44.0- ☑
        uterus O34.59- ☑
      uterus O34.59- ☑
        causing obstructed labor O65.5
        congenital O34.0- ☑
      vagina O34.6- ☑
        causing obstructed labor O65.5
      vulva O34.7- ☑
        causing obstructed labor O65.5
    abruptio placentae — *see* Abruptio placentae
    abscess or cellulitis
      bladder O23.1- ☑
      breast O91.11- ☑
      genital organ or tract O23.9- ☑
    abuse
      physical O9A.31 ☑ (*following* O99)
      psychological O9A.51 ☑ (*following* O99)
      sexual O9A.41 ☑ (*following* O99)
    adverse effect anesthesia O29.9- ☑
      aspiration pneumonitis O29.01- ☑
      cardiac arrest O29.11- ☑
      cardiac complication NEC O29.19- ☑
      cardiac failure O29.12- ☑
      central nervous system complication NEC O29.29- ☑
      cerebral anoxia O29.21- ☑
      failed or difficult intubation O29.6- ☑
      inhalation of stomach contents or secretions NOS O29.01- ☑
      local, toxic reaction O29.3X- ☑
      Mendelson's syndrome O29.01- ☑
      pressure collapse of lung O29.02- ☑
      pulmonary complications NEC O29.09- ☑
      specified NEC O29.8X- ☑
      spinal and epidural type NEC O29.5X- ☑
        induced headache O29.4- ☑
    albuminuria O12.1- ☑
    alcohol use O99.31- ☑
    amnionitis O41.12- ☑
    anaphylactoid syndrome of pregnancy O88.01- ☑
    anemia (conditions in D50-D64) (pre-existing) O99.01- ☑
      complicating the puerperium O99.03
    antepartum hemorrhage O46.9- ☑
      with coagulation defect — *see* Hemorrhage, antepartum, with coagulation defect
      specified NEC O46.8X- ☑
    appendicitis O99.61- ☑
    atrophy (yellow) (acute) liver (subacute) O26.61- ☑
    bariatric surgery status O99.84- ☑
    bicornis or bicornuate uterus O34.59- ☑
    biliary tract problems O26.61- ☑
    breech presentation O32.1 ☑
    cardiovascular diseases (conditions in I00-I09, I20-I52, I70-I99) O99.41- ☑
    cerebrovascular disorders (conditions in I60-I69) O99.41- ☑
    cervical shortening O26.87- ☑
    cervicitis O23.51- ☑
    chloasma (gravidarum) O26.89- ☑
    cholecystitis O99.61- ☑
    cholestasis (intrahepatic) O26.61- ☑

Pregnancy — *continued*
  complicated by — *continued*
    chorioamnionitis O41.12- ☑
    circulatory system disorder (conditions in I00-I09, I20-I99, O99.41-)
    compound presentation O32.6 ☑
    conjoined twins O30.02- ☑
    connective system disorders (conditions in M00-M99) O99.89
    contracted pelvis (general) O33.1
      inlet O33.2
      outlet O33.3 ☑
    convulsions (eclamptic) (uremic) (*see also* Eclampsia) O15.9
    cracked nipple O92.11- ☑
    cystitis O23.1- ☑
    cystocele O34.8- ☑
    death of fetus (near term) O36.4 ☑
      early pregnancy O02.1
      of one fetus or more in multiple gestation O31.2- ☑
    deciduitis O41.14- ☑
    decreased fetal movement O36.81- ☑
    dental problems O99.61- ☑
    diabetes (mellitus) O24.91- ☑
      gestational (pregnancy induced) — *see* Diabetes, gestational
      pre-existing O24.31- ☑
        specified NEC O24.81- ☑
        type 1 O24.01- ☑
        type 2 O24.11- ☑
    digestive system disorders (conditions in K00-K93) O99.61- ☑
    diseases of — *see* Pregnancy, complicated by, specified body system disease
      biliary tract O26.61- ☑
      blood NEC (conditions in D65-D77) O99.11- ☑
      liver O26.61- ☑
      specified NEC O99.89
    disorders of — *see* Pregnancy, complicated by, specified body system disorder
      amniotic fluid and membranes O41.9- ☑
        specified NEC O41.8X- ☑
      biliary tract O26.61- ☑
      ear and mastoid process (conditions in H60-H95) O99.89
      eye and adnexa (conditions in H00-H59) O99.89
      liver O26.61- ☑
      skin (conditions in L00-L99) O99.71- ☑
      specified NEC O99.89
    displacement, uterus NEC O34.59- ☑
      causing obstructed labor O65.5
    disproportion (due to) O33.9
      fetal deformities NEC O33.7
      generally contracted pelvis O33.1
      hydrocephalic fetus O33.6 ☑
      inlet contraction of pelvis O33.2
      mixed maternal and fetal origin O33.4 ☑
      specified NEC O33.8
    double uterus O34.59- ☑
      causing obstructed labor O65.5
    drug use (conditions in F11-F19) O99.32- ☑
    eclampsia, eclamptic (coma) (convulsions) (delirium) (nephritis) (uremia) (*see also* Eclampsia) O15.- ☑
    ectopic pregnancy — *see* Pregnancy, ectopic
    edema O12.0- ☑
      with
        gestational hypertension, mild (*see also* Pre-eclampsia) O14.0- ☑
        proteinuria O12.2- ☑
    effusion, amniotic fluid — *see* Pregnancy, complicated by, premature rupture of membranes
    elderly
      multigravida O09.52- ☑
      primigravida O09.51- ☑
    embolism (*see also* Embolism, obstetric, pregnancy) O88.- ☑
    endocrine diseases NEC O99.28- ☑
    endometritis O86.12
    excessive weight gain O26.0- ☑
    exhaustion O26.81- ☑
      during labor and delivery O75.81
    face presentation O32.3 ☑
    failed induction of labor O61.9
      instrumental O61.1
      mechanical O61.1

Pregnancy — *continued*
  complicated by — *continued*
    failed induction of labor — *continued*
      medical O61.0
      specified NEC O61.8
      surgical O61.1
    failed or difficult intubation for anesthesia O29.6- ☑
    false labor (pains) O47.9
      at or after 37 completed weeks of pregnancy O47.1
      before 37 completed weeks of pregnancy O47.0- ☑
    fatigue O26.81- ☑
      during labor and delivery O75.81
    fatty metamorphosis of liver O26.61- ☑
    female genital mutilation O34.8- ☑ [N90.81-] ☑
    fetal (maternal care for)
      abnormality or damage O35.9 ☑
        acid-base balance O68
        specified type NEC O35.8 ☑
      acidemia O68
      acidosis O68
      alkalosis O68
      anemia and thrombocytopenia O36.82- ☑
      anencephaly O35.0
      chromosomal abnormality (conditions in Q90-Q99) O35.1 ☑
      conjoined twins O30.02- ☑
      damage from
        amniocentesis O35.7 ☑
        biopsy procedures O35.7 ☑
        drug addiction O35.5
        hematological investigation O35.7 ☑
        intrauterine contraceptive device O35.7 ☑
        maternal
          alcohol addiction O35.4 ☑
          cytomegalovirus infection O35.3 ☑
          disease NEC O35.8 ☑
          drug addiction O35.5 ☑
          listeriosis O35.8 ☑
          rubella O35.3 ☑
          toxoplasmosis O35.8 ☑
          viral infection O35.3 ☑
        medical procedure NEC O35.7 ☑
        radiation O35.6 ☑
      death (near term) O36.4 ☑
        early pregnancy O02.1
      decreased movement O36.81- ☑
      disproportion due to deformity (fetal) O33.7
      excessive growth (large for dates) O36.6- ☑
      growth retardation O36.59- ☑
        light for dates O36.59- ☑
        small for dates O36.59- ☑
      heart rate irregularity (bradycardia) (decelerations) (tachycardia) O76
      hereditary disease O35.2 ☑
      hydrocephalus O35.0 ☑
      intrauterine death O36.4 ☑
      poor growth O36.59- ☑
        light for dates O36.59- ☑
        small for dates O36.59- ☑
      problem O36.9- ☑
        specified NEC O36.89- ☑
      reduction (elective) O31.3- ☑
      selective termination O31.3- ☑
      spina bifida O35.0 ☑
      thrombocytopenia O36.82- ☑
    fibroid (tumor) (uterus) O34.1- ☑
    fissure of nipple O92.11- ☑
    gallstones O99.61- ☑
    gastric banding status O99.84- ☑
    gastric bypass status O99.84- ☑
    genital herpes (asymptomatic) (history of) (inactive) O98.51- ☑
    genital tract infection O23.9- ☑
    glomerular diseases (conditions in N00-N07) O26.83- ☑
      with hypertension, pre-existing — *see* Hypertension, complicating, pregnancy, pre-existing, with, renal disease
    gonorrhea O98.21- ☑
    grand multiparity O09.4 ☑
    habitual aborter — *see* Pregnancy, complicated by, recurrent pregnancy loss

Pregnancy — *continued*
  complicated by — *continued*
    HELLP syndrome (hemolysis, elevated liver enzymes and low platelet count) O14.2- ☑
    hemorrhage
      antepartum — *see* Hemorrhage, antepartum
      before 20 completed weeks gestation O20.9
        specified NEC O20.8
      due to premature separation, placenta (*see also* Abruptio placentae) O45.9- ☑
      early O20.9
        specified NEC O20.8
      threatened abortion O20.0
    hemorrhoids O22.4- ☑
    hepatitis (viral) O98.41- ☑
    herniation of uterus O34.59- ☑
    high
      head at term O32.4 ☑
      risk — *see* Supervision (of) (for), high-risk
    history of in utero procedure during previous pregnancy O09.82- ☑
    HIV O98.71- ☑
    human immunodeficiency virus (HIV) disease O98.71- ☑
    hydatidiform mole (*see also* Mole, hydatidiform) O01.9
    hydramnios O40.- ☑
    hydrocephalic fetus (disproportion) O33.6 ☑
    hydrops
      amnii O40.- ☑
      fetalis O36.2- ☑
        associated with isoimmunization (*see also* Pregnancy, complicated by, isoimmunization) O36.11- ☑
    hydrorrhea O42.90
    hyperemesis (gravidarum) (mild) (*see also* Hyperemesis, gravidarum) O21.0
    hypertension — *see* Hypertension, complicating pregnancy
    hypertensive
      heart and renal disease, pre-existing — *see* Hypertension, complicating, pregnancy, pre-existing, with, heart disease, with renal disease
      heart disease, pre-existing — *see* Hypertension, complicating, pregnancy, pre-existing, with, heart disease
      renal disease, pre-existing — *see* Hypertension, complicating, pregnancy, pre-existing, with, renal disease
    hypotension O26.5- ☑
    immune disorders NEC (conditions in D80-D89) O99.11- ☑
    incarceration, uterus O34.51- ☑
    incompetent cervix O34.3- ☑
    inconclusive fetal viability O36.80 ☑
    infection(s) O98.91- ☑
      amniotic fluid or sac O41.10- ☑
      bladder O23.1- ☑
      carrier state NEC O99.830
        streptococcus B O99.820
      genital organ or tract O23.9- ☑
        specified NEC O23.59- ☑
      genitourinary tract O23.9- ☑
      gonorrhea O98.21- ☑
      hepatitis (viral) O98.41- ☑
      HIV O98.71- ☑
      human immunodeficiency virus (HIV) O98.71- ☑
      kidney O23.0- ☑
      nipple O91.01- ☑
      parasitic disease O98.91- ☑
        specified NEC O98.81- ☑
      protozoal disease O98.61- ☑
      sexually transmitted NEC O98.31- ☑
      specified type NEC O98.81- ☑
      syphilis O98.11- ☑
      tuberculosis O98.01- ☑
      urethra O23.2- ☑
      urinary (tract) O23.4- ☑
        specified NEC O23.3- ☑
      viral disease O98.51- ☑
    injury or poisoning (conditions in S00-T88) O9A.21- ☑ (*following* O99)
      due to abuse
        physical O9A.31- ☑ (*following* O99)

Pregnancy — *continued*
  complicated by — *continued*
    injury or poisoning — *continued*
      due to abuse — *continued*
        psychological O9A.51- ☑ (*following* O99)
        sexual O9A.41- ☑ (*following* O99)
    insufficient
      prenatal care O09.3- ☑
      weight gain O26.1- ☑
    insulin resistance O26.89 ☑
    intrauterine fetal death (near term) O36.4 ☑
      early pregnancy O02.1
      multiple gestation (one fetus or more) O31.2- ☑
    isoimmunization O36.11- ☑
      anti-A sensitization O36.11- ☑
      anti-B sensitization O36.19- ☑
      Rh O36.09- ☑
        anti-D antibody O36.01- ☑
      specified NEC O36.19- ☑
    laceration of uterus NEC O71.81
    malformation
      placenta, placental (vessel) O43.10- ☑
        specified NEC O43.19- ☑
      uterus (congenital) O34.0- ☑
    malnutrition (conditions in E40-E46) O25.1- ☑
    maternal hypotension syndrome O26.5- ☑
    mental disorders (conditions in F01-F09, F20-F99) O99.34- ☑
      alcohol use O99.31- ☑
      drug use O99.32- ☑
      smoking O99.33- ☑
    mentum presentation O32.3 ☑
    metabolic disorders O99.28- ☑
    missed
      abortion O02.1
      delivery O36.4 ☑
    multiple gestations O30.9- ☑
      conjoined twins O30.02- ☑
      quadruplet — *see* Pregnancy, quadruplet
      specified complication NEC O31.8X- ☑
      specified number of multiples NEC — *see* Pregnancy, multiple (gestation), specified NEC
      triplet — *see* Pregnancy, triplet
      twin — *see* Pregnancy, twin
    musculoskeletal condition (conditions is M00-M99) O99.89
    necrosis, liver (conditions in K72) O26.61- ☑
    neoplasm
      benign
        cervix O34.4- ☑
        corpus uteri O34.1- ☑
        uterus O34.1- ☑
      malignant O9A.11- ☑ (*following* O99)
    nephropathy NEC O26.83- ☑
    nervous system condition (conditions in G00-G99) O99.35- ☑
    nutritional diseases NEC O99.28- ☑
    obesity (pre-existing) O99.21- ☑
    obesity surgery status O99.84- ☑
    oblique lie or presentation O32.2 ☑
    older mother — *see* Pregnancy, complicated by, elderly
    oligohydramnios O41.0- ☑
      with premature rupture of membranes (*see also* Pregnancy, complicated by, premature rupture of membranes) O42.- ☑
    onset (spontaneous) of labor after 37 completed weeks of gestation but before 39 completed weeks gestation, with delivery by (planned) cesarean section O75.82
    oophoritis O23.52- ☑
    overdose, drug (*see also* Table of Drugs and Chemicals, by drug, poisoning) O9A.21- ☑ (*following* O99)
    oversize fetus O33.5 ☑
    papyraceous fetus O31.0- ☑
    pelvic inflammatory disease O99.89
    periodontal disease O99.61- ☑
    peripheral neuritis O26.82- ☑
    peritoneal (pelvic) adhesions O99.89
    phlebitis O22.9- ☑
    phlebopathy O22.9- ☑
    phlebothrombosis (superficial) O22.2- ☑
      deep O22.3- ☑

Pregnancy — *continued*
  complicated by — *continued*
    placenta accreta O43.21- ☑
    placenta increta O43.22- ☑
    placenta percreta O43.23- ☑
    placenta previa O44.1- ☑
      without hemorrhage O44.0- ☑
    placental disorder O43.9- ☑
      specified NEC O43.89- ☑
    placental dysfunction O43.89- ☑
    placental infarction O43.81- ☑
    placental insufficiency O36.51- ☑
    placental transfusion syndromes
      fetomaternal O43.01- ☑
      fetus to fetus O43.02- ☑
      maternofetal O43.01- ☑
    placentitis O41.14- ☑
    pneumonia O99.51- ☑
    poisoning (*see also* Table of Drugs and Chemicals) O9A.21 (*following* O99)
    polyhydramnios O40- ☑
    polymorphic eruption of pregnancy O26.86
    poor obstetric history NEC O09.29- ☑
    postmaturity (post-term) (40 to 42 weeks) O48.0
      more than 42 completed weeks gestation (prolonged) O48.1
    pre-eclampsia O14.9- ☑
      mild O14.0- ☑
      moderate O14.0- ☑
      severe O14.1- ☑
        with hemolysis, elevated liver enzymes and low platelet count (HELLP) O14.2- ☑
    premature labor — *see* Pregnancy, complicated by, preterm labor
    premature rupture of membranes O42.90
      with onset of labor
        after 24 hours O42.10
          after 37 weeks gestation O42.12
          pre-term (before 37 completed weeks of gestation) O42.11- ☑
        within 24 hours O42.00
          after 37 weeks gestation O42.02
          pre-term (before 37 completed weeks of gestation) O42.01- ☑
      after 37 weeks gestation O42.92
      full-term O42.92
      pre-term (before 37 completed weeks of gestation) O42.91- ☑
    premature separation of placenta (*see also* Abruptio placentae) O45.9- ☑
    presentation, fetal — *see* Delivery, complicated by, malposition
    preterm delivery O60.10 ☑
    preterm labor
      with delivery O60.10 ☑
        preterm O60.10 ☑
        term O60.20 ☑
      without delivery O60.00 ☑
        second trimester O60.02
        third trimester O60.03
      second trimester
        with preterm delivery
          second trimester O60.12 ☑
          third trimester O60.13 ☑
        with term delivery O60.22 ☑
        without delivery O60.02
      third trimester
        with term delivery O60.23 ☑
        with third trimester preterm delivery O60.14 ☑
        without delivery O60.03
    previous history of — *see* Pregnancy, supervision of, high-risk
    prolapse, uterus O34.52- ☑
    proteinuria (gestational) O12.1- ☑
      with edema O12.2- ☑
    pruritic urticarial papules and plaques of pregnancy (PUPPP) O26.86
    pruritus (neurogenic) O26.89- ☑
    psychosis or psychoneurosis (puerperal) F53
    ptyalism O26.89- ☑
    PUPPP (pruritic urticarial papules and plaques of pregnancy) O26.86
    pyelitis O23.0- ☑
    recurrent pregnancy loss O26.2- ☑
    renal disease or failure NEC O26.83- ☑

Pregnancy — *continued*
  complicated by — *continued*
    renal disease or failure — *continued*
      with secondary hypertension, pre-existing — *see* Hypertension, complicating, pregnancy, pre-existing, secondary
      hypertensive, pre-existing — *see* Hypertension, complicating, pregnancy, pre-existing, with, renal disease
    respiratory condition (conditions in J00-J99) O99.51- ☑
    retained, retention
      dead ovum O02.0
      intrauterine contraceptive device O26.3- ☑
    retroversion, uterus O34.53- ☑
    Rh immunization, incompatibility or sensitization NEC O36.09- ☑
      anti-D antibody O36.01- ☑
    rupture
      amnion (premature) (*see also* Pregnancy, complicated by, premature rupture of membranes) O42- ☑
      membranes (premature) (*see also* Pregnancy, complicated by, premature rupture of membranes) O42- ☑
      uterus (during labor) O71.1
        before onset of labor O71.0- ☑
    salivation (excessive) O26.89- ☑
    salpingitis O23.52- ☑
    salpingo-oophoritis O23.52- ☑
    sepsis (conditions in A40, A41) O98.81- ☑
    size date discrepancy (uterine) O26.84- ☑
    skin condition (conditions in L00-L99) O99.71- ☑
    smoking (tobacco) O99.33- ☑
    social problem O09.7- ☑
    specified condition NEC O26.89- ☑
    spotting O26.85- ☑
    streptococcus B carrier state O99.820
    subluxation of symphysis (pubis) O26.71- ☑
    syphilis (conditions in A50-A53) O98.11- ☑
    threatened
      abortion O20.0
      labor O47.9
        at or after 37 completed weeks of gestation O47.1
        before 37 completed weeks of gestation O47.0- ☑
    thrombophlebitis (superficial) O22.2- ☑
    thrombosis O22.9- ☑
      cerebral venous O22.5- ☑
      cerebrovenous sinus O22.5- ☑
      deep O22.3- ☑
    torsion of uterus O34.59- ☑
    toxemia O14.9- ☑
    transverse lie or presentation O32.2 ☑
    tuberculosis (conditions in A15-A19) O98.01- ☑
    tumor (benign)
      cervix O34.4- ☑
      malignant O9A.11- ☑ (*following* O99)
      uterus O34.1- ☑
    unstable lie O32.0 ☑
    upper respiratory infection O99.51- ☑
    urethritis O23.2- ☑
    uterine size date discrepancy O26.84- ☑
    vaginitis or vulvitis O23.59- ☑
    varicose veins (lower extremities) O22.0- ☑
      genitals O22.1- ☑
      legs O22.0- ☑
      perineal O22.1- ☑
      vaginal or vulval O22.1- ☑
    venereal disease NEC (conditions in A63.8) O98.31- ☑
    venous disorders O22.9- ☑
      specified NEC O22.8X- ☑
    very young mother — *see* Pregnancy, complicated by, young mother
    viral diseases (conditions in A80-B09, B25-B34) O98.51- ☑
    vomiting O21.9
      due to diseases classified elsewhere O21.8
      hyperemesis gravidarum (mild) (*see also* Hyperemesis, gravidarum) O21.0
      late (occurring after 20 weeks of gestation) O21.2
    young mother
      multigravida O09.62- ☑

Pregnancy — *continued*
  complicated by — *continued*
    young mother — *continued*
      primigravida O09.61- ☑
  complicated NOS O26.9- ☑
  concealed O09.3- ☑
  continuing following
    elective fetal reduction of one or more fetus
      O31.3- ☑
    intrauterine death of one or more fetus O31.2- ☑
    spontaneous abortion of one or more fetus
      O31.1- ☑
  cornual O00.8
  ectopic (ruptured) O00.9
    abdominal O00.0
      with viable fetus O36.7- ☑
    cervical O00.8
    complicated (by) O08.9
      afibrinogenemia O08.1
      cardiac arrest O08.81
      chemical damage of pelvic organ(s) O08.6
      circulatory collapse O08.3
      defibrination syndrome O08.1
      electrolyte imbalance O08.5
      embolism (amniotic fluid) (blood clot) (pul-
        monary) (septic) O08.2
      endometritis O08.0
      genital tract and pelvic infection O08.0
      hemorrhage (delayed) (excessive) O08.1
      infection
        genital tract or pelvic O08.0
          kidney O08.83
          urinary tract O08.3
      intravascular coagulation O08.1
      laceration of pelvic organ(s) O08.6
      metabolic disorder O08.5
      oliguria O08.4
      oophoritis O08.0
      parametritis O08.0
      pelvic peritonitis O08.0
      perforation of pelvic organ(s) O08.6
      renal failure or shutdown O08.4
      salpingitis or salpingo-oophoritis O08.0
      sepsis O08.82
      shock O08.83
        septic O08.82
      specified condition NEC O08.89
      tubular necrosis (renal) O08.4
      uremia O08.4
      urinary infection O08.83
      venous complication NEC O08.7
        embolism O08.2
    cornual O00.8
    intraligamentous O00.8
    mural O00.8
    ovarian O00.2
    specified site NEC O00.8
    tubal (ruptured) O00.1
  examination (normal) Z34.9- ☑
    first Z34.0- ☑
    high-risk — *see* Pregnancy, supervision of, high-risk
    specified Z34.8- ☑
  extrauterine — *see* Pregnancy, ectopic
  fallopian O00.1
  false F45.8
  hidden O09.3- ☑
  high-risk — *see* Pregnancy, supervision of, high-risk
  incidental finding Z33.1
  interstitial O00.8
  intraligamentous O00.8
  intramural O00.8
  intraperitoneal O00.0
  isthmian O00.1
  mesometric (mural) O00.8
  molar NEC O02.0
    complicated (by) O08.9
      afibrinogenemia O08.1
      cardiac arrest O08.81
      chemical damage of pelvic organ(s) O08.6
      circulatory collapse O08.3
      defibrination syndrome O08.1
      electrolyte imbalance O08.5
      embolism (amniotic fluid) (blood clot) (pul-
        monary) (septic) O08.2
      endometritis O08.0
      genital tract and pelvic infection O08.0
      hemorrhage (delayed) (excessive) O08.1

Pregnancy — *continued*
  molar — *continued*
    complicated — *continued*
      infection
        genital tract or pelvic O08.0
          kidney O08.83
          urinary tract O08.83
      intravascular coagulation O08.1
      laceration of pelvic organ(s) O08.6
      metabolic disorder O08.5
      oliguria O08.4
      oophoritis O08.0
      parametritis O08.0
      pelvic peritonitis O08.0
      perforation of pelvic organ(s) O08.6
      renal failure or shutdown O08.4
      salpingitis or salpingo-oophoritis O08.0
      sepsis O08.82
      shock O08.3
        septic O08.82
      specified condition NEC O08.89
      tubular necrosis (renal) O08.4
      uremia O08.4
      urinary infection O08.83
      venous complication NEC O08.7
        embolism O08.2
    hydatidiform (*see also* Mole, hydatidiform) O01.9
  multiple (gestation) O30.9- ☑
    greater than quadruplets — *see* Pregnancy, multiple (gestation), specified NEC
    specified NEC O30.80- ☑
      with
        two or more monoamniotic fetuses
          O30.82- ☑
        two or more monochorionic fetuses
          O30.81- ☑
      two or more monoamniotic fetuses O30.82- ☑
      two or more monochorionic fetuses O30.81- ☑
      unable to determine number of placenta and
        number of amniotic sacs O30.89- ☑
      unspecified number of placenta and unspeci-
        fied number of amniotic sacs O30.80- ☑
  mural O00.8
  normal (supervision of) Z34.9- ☑
    first Z34.0- ☑
    high-risk — *see* Pregnancy, supervision of, high-risk
    specified Z34.8- ☑
  ovarian O00.2
  postmature (40 to 42 weeks) O48.0
    more than 42 weeks gestation O48.1
  post-term (40 to 42 weeks) O48.0
  prenatal care only Z34.9- ☑
    first Z34.0- ☑
    high-risk — *see* Pregnancy, supervision of, high-risk
    specified Z34.8- ☑
  prolonged (more than 42 weeks gestation) O48.1
  quadruplet O30.20- ☑
    with
      two or more monoamniotic fetuses O30.22- ☑
      two or more monochorionic fetuses O30.21- ☑
    two or more monoamniotic fetuses O30.22- ☑
    two or more monochorionic fetuses O30.21- ☑
    unable to determine number of placenta and
      number of amniotic sacs O30.29- ☑
    unspecified number of placenta and unspecified
      number of amniotic sacs O30.20- ☑
  quintuplet — *see* Pregnancy, multiple (gestation),
    specified NEC
  sextuplet — *see* Pregnancy, multiple (gestation),
    specified NEC
  supervision of
    concealed pregnancy O09.3- ☑
    elderly mother
      multigravida O09.52- ☑
      primigravida O09.51- ☑
    hidden pregnancy O09.3- ☑
    high-risk O09.9- ☑
      due to (history of)
        ectopic pregnancy O09.1- ☑
        elderly — *see* Pregnancy, supervision, elder-
          ly mother
        grand multiparity O09.4 ☑
        in utero procedure during previous pregnan-
          cy O09.82- ☑
        in vitro fertilization O09.81- ☑

Pregnancy — *continued*
  supervision of — *continued*
    high-risk — *continued*
      due to — *continued*
        infertility O09.0- ☑
        insufficient prenatal care O09.3- ☑
        molar pregnancy O09.1- ☑
        multiple previous pregnancies O09.4- ☑
        older mother — *see* Pregnancy, supervision
          of, elderly mother
        poor reproductive or obstetric history NEC
          O09.29- ☑
        pre-term labor O09.21- ☑
        previous
          neonatal death O09.29- ☑
        social problems O09.7- ☑
        specified NEC O09.89- ☑
        very young mother — *see* Pregnancy, super-
          vision, young mother
      resulting from in vitro fertilization O09.81- ☑
    normal Z34.9- ☑
      first Z34.0- ☑
      specified NEC Z34.8- ☑
    young mother
      multigravida O09.62- ☑
      primigravida O09.61- ☑
  triplet O30.10- ☑
    with
      two or more monoamniotic fetuses O30.12- ☑
      two or more monochrorionic fetuses O30.11- ☑
    two or more monoamniotic fetuses O30.12- ☑
    two or more monochrorionic fetuses O30.11- ☑
    unable to determine number of placenta and
      number of amniotic sacs O30.19- ☑
    unspecified number of placenta and unspecified
      number of amniotic sacs O30.10- ☑
  tubal (with abortion) (with rupture) O00.1
  twin O30.00- ☑
    conjoined O30.02- ☑
    dichorionic/diamniotic (two placenta, two amniotic
      sacs) O30.04- ☑
    monochorionic/diamniotic (one placenta, two
      amniotic sacs) O30.03- ☑
    monochorionic/monoamniotic (one placenta, one
      amniotic sac) O30.01- ☑
    unable to determine number of placenta and
      number of amniotic sacs O30.09- ☑
    unspecified number of placenta and unspecified
      number of amniotic sacs O30.00- ☑
  unwanted Z64.0
  weeks of gestation
    less than 8 weeks Z3A.01 (*following* Z36)
    8 weeks Z3A.08 (*following* Z36)
    9 weeks Z3A.09 (*following* Z36)
    10 weeks Z3A.10 (*following* Z36)
    11 weeks Z3A.11 (*following* Z36)
    12 weeks Z3A.12 (*following* Z36)
    13 weeks Z3A.13 (*following* Z36)
    14 weeks Z3A.14 (*following* Z36)
    15 weeks Z3A.15 (*following* Z36)
    16 weeks Z3A.16 (*following* Z36)
    17 weeks Z3A.17 (*following* Z36)
    18 weeks Z3A.18 (*following* Z36)
    19 weeks Z3A.19 (*following* Z36)
    20 weeks Z3A.20 (*following* Z36)
    21 weeks Z3A.21 (*following* Z36)
    22 weeks Z3A.22 (*following* Z36)
    23 weeks Z3A.23 (*following* Z36)
    24 weeks Z3A.24 (*following* Z36)
    25 weeks Z3A.25 (*following* Z36)
    26 weeks Z3A.26 (*following* Z36)
    27 weeks Z3A.27 (*following* Z36)
    28 weeks Z3A.28 (*following* Z36)
    29 weeks Z3A.29 (*following* Z36)
    30 weeks Z3A.30 (*following* Z36)
    31 weeks Z3A.31 (*following* Z36)
    32 weeks Z3A.32 (*following* Z36)
    33 weeks Z3A.33 (*following* Z36)
    34 weeks Z3A.34 (*following* Z36)
    35 weeks Z3A.35 (*following* Z36)
    36 weeks Z3A.36 (*following* Z36)
    37 weeks Z3A.37 (*following* Z36)
    38 weeks Z3A.38 (*following* Z36)
    39 weeks Z3A.39 (*following* Z36)
    40 weeks Z3A.40 (*following* Z36)
    41 weeks Z3A.41 (*following* Z36)
    42 weeks Z3A.42 (*following* Z36)

Pregnancy — *continued*
  weeks of gestation — *continued*
    greater than 42 weeks Z3A.49 (*following* Z36)
    not specified Z3A.00 (*following* Z36)
Preiser's disease — *see* Osteonecrosis, secondary, due
  to, trauma, metacarpus
Pre-kwashiorkor — *see* Malnutrition, severe
Preleukemia (syndrome) D46.9
Preluxation, hip, congenital Q65.6
Premature (*see also* condition)
  adrenarche E27.0
  aging E34.8
  beats I49.40
    atrial I49.1
    auricular I49.1
    supraventricular I49.1
  birth NEC — *see* Preterm, newborn
  closure, foramen ovale Q21.8
  contraction
    atrial I49.1
    atrioventricular I49.2
    auricular I49.1
    auriculoventricular I49.49
    heart (extrasystole) I49.49
    junctional I49.2
    ventricular I49.3
  delivery (*see also* Pregnancy, complicated by, preterm
    labor) O60.10 ☑
  ejaculation F52.4
  infant NEC — *see* Preterm, newborn
    light-for-dates — *see* Light for dates
  labor — *see* Pregnancy, complicated by, preterm labor
  lungs P28.0
  menopause E28.319
    asymptomatic E28.319
    symptomatic E28.310
  newborn
    less than 37 completed weeks — *see* Preterm,
      newborn
    extreme (less than 28 completed weeks) — *see*
      Immaturity, extreme
  puberty E30.1
  rupture membranes or amnion — *see* Pregnancy,
    complicated by, premature rupture of mem-
    branes
  senility E34.8
  thelarche E30.8
  ventricular systole I49.3
Prematurity NEC (less than 37 completed weeks) — *see*
  Preterm, newborn
  extreme (less than 28 completed weeks) — *see* Imma-
    turity, extreme
Premenstrual
  dysphoric disorder (PMDD) N94.3
  tension (syndrome) N94.3
Premolarization, cuspids K00.2
Prenatal
  care, normal pregnancy — *see* Pregnancy, normal
  screening of mother Z36
  teeth K00.6
Preparatory care for subsequent treatment NEC
  for dialysis Z49.01
    peritoneal Z49.02
Prepartum — *see* condition
Preponderance, left or right ventricular I51.7
Prepuce — *see* condition
PRES (posterior reversible encephalopathy syndrome)
  I67.83
Presbycardia R54
Presbycusis, presbyacusia H91.1- ☑
Presbyesophagus K22.8
Presbyophrenia F03 ☑
Presbyopia H52.4
Prescription of contraceptives (initial) Z30.019
  emergency (postcoital) Z30.012
  implantable subdermal Z30.019
  injectable Z30.013
  intrauterine contraceptive device Z30.014
  pills Z30.011
  postcoital (emergency) Z30.012
  repeat Z30.40
    implantable subdermal Z30.49
    injectable Z30.42
    pills Z30.41
    specified type NEC Z30.49
  specified type NEC Z30.018

Presence (of)
  ankle-joint implant (functional) (prosthesis) Z96.66- ☑
  aortocoronary (bypass) graft Z95.1
  arterial-venous shunt (dialysis) Z99.2
  artificial
    eye (globe) Z97.0
    heart (fully implantable) (mechanical) Z95.812
      valve Z95.2
    larynx Z96.3
    lens (intraocular) Z96.1
    limb (complete) (partial) Z97.1- ☑
      arm Z97.1- ☑
        bilateral Z97.15
      leg Z97.1- ☑
        bilateral Z97.16
  audiological implant (functional) Z96.29
  bladder implant (functional) Z96.0
  bone
    conduction hearing device Z96.29
    implant (functional) NEC Z96.7
    joint (prosthesis) — *see* Presence, joint implant
  cardiac
    defibrillator (functional) (with synchronous cardiac
      pacemaker) Z95.810
    implant or graft Z95.9
      specified type NEC Z95.818
    pacemaker Z95.0
  cerebrospinal fluid drainage device Z98.2
  cochlear implant (functional) Z96.21
  contact lens (es) Z97.3
  coronary artery graft or prosthesis Z95.5
  CSF shunt Z98.2
  dental prosthesis device Z97.2
  dentures Z97.2
  device (external) NEC Z97.8
    cardiac NEC Z95.818
    heart assist Z95.811
    implanted (functional) Z96.9
      specified NEC Z96.89
    prosthetic Z97.8
  ear implant Z96.20
    cochlear implant Z96.21
    myringotomy tube Z96.22
    specified type NEC Z96.29
  elbow-joint implant (functional) (prosthesis)
    Z96.62- ☑
  endocrine implant (functional) NEC Z96.49
  eustachian tube stent or device (functional) Z96.29
  external hearing-aid or device Z97.4
  finger-joint implant (functional) (prosthetic) Z96.69- ☑
  functional implant Z96.9
    specified NEC Z96.89
  graft
    cardiac NEC Z95.818
    vascular NEC Z95.828
  hearing-aid or device (external) Z97.4
    implant (bone) (cochlear) (functional) Z96.21
  heart assist device Z95.811
  heart valve implant (functional) Z95.2
    prosthetic Z95.2
    specified type NEC Z95.4
    xenogenic Z95.3
  hip-joint implant (functional) (prosthesis) Z96.64- ☑
  implanted device (artificial) (functional) (prosthetic)
    Z96.9
    automatic cardiac defibrillator (with synchronous
      cardiac pacemaker) Z95.810
    cardiac pacemaker Z95.0
    cochlear Z96.21
    dental Z96.5
    heart Z95.812
    heart valve Z95.2
      prosthetic Z95.2
      specified NEC Z95.4
      xenogenic Z95.3
    insulin pump Z96.41
    intraocular lens Z96.1
    joint Z96.60
      ankle Z96.66- ☑
      elbow Z96.62- ☑
      finger Z96.69- ☑
      hip Z96.64- ☑
      knee Z96.65- ☑
      shoulder Z96.61- ☑
      specified NEC Z96.698
      wrist Z96.63- ☑
    larynx Z96.3
    myringotomy tube Z96.22

Presence — *continued*
  implanted device — *continued*
    otological Z96.20
      cochlear Z96.21
      eustachian stent Z96.29
      myringotomy Z96.22
      specified NEC Z96.29
      stapes Z96.29
    skin Z96.81
    skull plate Z96.7
    specified NEC Z96.89
    urogenital Z96.0
  insulin pump (functional) Z96.41
  intestinal bypass or anastomosis Z98.0
  intraocular lens (functional) Z96.1
  intrauterine contraceptive device (IUD) Z97.5
  intravascular implant (functional) (prosthetic) NEC
    Z95.9
    coronary artery Z95.5
    defibrillator (with synchronous cardiac pacemaker)
      Z95.810
    peripheral vessel (with angioplasty) Z95.820
  joint implant (prosthetic) (any) Z96.60
    ankle — *see* Presence, ankle joint implant
    elbow — *see* Presence, elbow joint implant
    finger — *see* Presence, finger joint implant
    hip — *see* Presence, hip joint implant
    knee — *see* Presence, knee joint implant
    shoulder — *see* Presence, shoulder joint implant
    specified joint NEC Z96.698
    wrist — *see* Presence, wrist joint implant
  knee-joint implant (functional) (prosthesis) Z96.65- ☑
  laryngeal implant (functional) Z96.3
  mandibular implant (dental) Z96.5
  myringotomy tube(s) Z96.22
  orthopedic-joint implant (prosthetic) (any) — *see*
    Presence, joint implant
  otological implant (functional) Z96.29
  shoulder-joint implant (functional) (prosthesis)
    Z96.61- ☑
  skull-plate implant Z96.7
  spectacles Z97.3
  stapes implant (functional) Z96.29
  systemic lupus erythematosus [SLE] inhibitor D68.62
  tendon implant (functional) (graft) Z96.7
  tooth root(s) implant Z96.5
  ureteral stent Z96.0
  urethral stent Z96.0
  urogenital implant (functional) Z96.0
  vascular implant or device Z95.9
    access port device Z95.828
    specified type NEC Z95.828
  wrist-joint implant (functional) (prosthesis) Z96.63- ☑
Presenile (*see also* condition)
  dementia F03 ☑
  premature aging E34.8
Presentation, fetal — *see* Delivery, complicated by,
  malposition
Prespondylolisthesis (congenital) Q76.2
Pressure
  area, skin — *see* Ulcer, pressure, by site
  brachial plexus G54.0
  brain G93.5
    injury at birth NEC P11.1
  cerebral — *see* Pressure, brain
  chest R07.89
  cone, tentorial G93.5
  hyposystolic (*see also* Hypotension)
    incidental reading, without diagnosis of hypoten-
      sion R03.1
  increased
    intracranial (benign) G93.2
      injury at birth P11.0
    intraocular H40.05- ☑
  lumbosacral plexus G54.1
  mediastinum J98.5
  necrosis (chronic) — *see* Ulcer, pressure, by site
  parental, inappropriate (excessive) Z62.6
  sore (chronic) — *see* Ulcer, pressure, by site
  spinal cord G95.20
  ulcer (chronic) — *see* Ulcer, pressure, by site
  venous, increased I87.8
Pre-syncope R55
Preterm
  delivery (*see also* Pregnancy, complicated by, preterm
    labor) O60.10 ☑
  labor — *see* Pregnancy, complicated by, preterm labor
  newborn (infant) P07.30

Preterm — *continued*
  newborn — *continued*
    gestational age
      28 completed weeks (28 weeks, Ø days through
        28 weeks, 6 days) PØ7.31
      29 completed weeks (29 weeks, Ø days through
        29 weeks, 6 days) PØ7.32
      30 completed weeks (30 weeks, Ø days through
        30 weeks, 6 days) PØ7.33
      31 completed weeks (31 weeks, Ø days through
        31 weeks, 6 days) PØ7.34
      32 completed weeks (32 weeks, Ø days through
        32 weeks, 6 days) PØ7.35
      33 completed weeks (33 weeks, Ø days through
        33 weeks, 6 days) PØ7.36
      34 completed weeks (34 weeks, Ø days through
        34 weeks, 6 days) PØ7.37
      35 completed weeks (35 weeks, Ø days through
        35 weeks, 6 days) PØ7.38
      36 completed weeks (36 weeks, Ø days through
        36 weeks, 6 days) PØ7.39
Previa
  placenta (low) (marginal) (partial) (total) (with hemorrhage) O44.1- ☑
    without hemorrhage O44.Ø- ☑
  vasa O69.4 ☑
Priapism N48.3Ø
  due to
    disease classified elsewhere N48.32
    drug N48.33
    specified cause NEC N48.39
    trauma N48.31
Prickling sensation (skin) R2Ø.2
Prickly heat L74.Ø
Primary — *see* condition
Primigravida
  elderly, affecting management of pregnancy, labor and delivery (supervision only) — *see* Pregnancy, complicated by, elderly, primigravida
  older, affecting management of pregnancy, labor and delivery (supervision only) — *see* Pregnancy, complicated by, elderly, primigravida
  very young, affecting management of pregnancy, labor and delivery (supervision only) — *see* Pregnancy, complicated by, young mother, primigravida
Primipara
  elderly, affecting management of pregnancy, labor and delivery (supervision only) — *see* Pregnancy, complicated by, elderly, primigravida
  older, affecting management of pregnancy, labor and delivery (supervision only) — *see* Pregnancy, complicated by, elderly, primigravida
  very young, affecting management of pregnancy, labor and delivery (supervision only) — *see* Pregnancy, complicated by, young mother, primigravida
Primus varus (bilateral) Q66.2
PRIND (Prolonged reversible ischemic neurologic deficit) I63.9
Pringle's disease (tuberous sclerosis) Q85.1
Prinzmetal angina I2Ø.1
Prizefighter ear — *see* Cauliflower ear
Problem (with) (related to)
  academic Z55.8
  acculturation Z6Ø.3
  adjustment (to)
    change of job Z56.1
    life-cycle transition Z6Ø.Ø
    pension Z6Ø.Ø
    retirement Z6Ø.Ø
  adopted child Z62.821
  alcoholism in family Z63.72
  atypical parenting situation Z62.9
  bankruptcy Z59.8
  behavioral (adult) F69
    drug seeking Z72.89
  birth of sibling affecting child Z62.898
  care (of)
    provider dependency Z74.9
      specified NEC Z74.8
    sick or handicapped person in family or household Z63.6
  child
    abuse (affecting the child) — *see* Maltreatment, child
    custody or support proceedings Z65.3
    in care of non-parental family member Z62.21
    in foster care Z62.21
    in welfare custody Z62.21

Problem — *continued*
  child — *continued*
    living in orphanage or group home Z62.22
  child-rearing Z62.9
    specified NEC Z62.898
  communication (developmental) F8Ø.9
  conflict or discord (with)
    boss Z56.4
    classmates Z55.4
    counselor Z64.4
    employer Z56.4
    family Z63.9
      specified NEC Z63.8
    probation officer Z64.4
    social worker Z64.4
    teachers Z55.4
    workmates Z56.4
  conviction in legal proceedings Z65.Ø
    with imprisonment Z65.1
  counselor Z64.4
  creditors Z59.8
  digestive K92.9
  drug addict in family Z63.72
  ear — *see* Disorder, ear
  economic Z59.9
    affecting care Z59.9
    specified NEC Z59.8
  education Z55.9
    specified NEC Z55.8
  employment Z56.9
    change of job Z56.1
    discord Z56.4
    environment Z56.5
    sexual harassment Z56.81
    specified NEC Z56.89
    stressful schedule Z56.3
    stress NEC Z56.6
    threat of job loss Z56.2
    unemployment Z56.Ø
  enuresis, child F98.Ø
  eye H57.9
  failed examinations (school) Z55.2
  falling Z91.81
  family (*see also* Disruption, family) Z63.9
    specified NEC Z63.8
  feeding (elderly) (infant) R63.3
    newborn P92.9
      breast P92.5
      overfeeding P92.4
      slow P92.2
      specified NEC P92.8
      underfeeding P92.3
    nonorganic F5Ø.8
  finance Z59.9
    specified NEC Z59.8
  foreclosure on loan Z59.8
  foster child Z62.822
  frightening experience(s) in childhood Z62.898
  genital NEC
    female N94.9
    male N5Ø.9
  health care Z75.9
    specified NEC Z75.8
  hearing — *see* Deafness
  homelessness Z59.Ø
  housing Z59.9
    inadequate Z59.1
    isolated Z59.8
    specified NEC Z59.8
  identity (of childhood) F93.8
  illegitimate pregnancy (unwanted) Z64.Ø
  illiteracy Z55.9
  impaired mobility Z74.Ø9
  imprisonment or incarceration Z65.1
  inadequate teaching affecting education Z55.8
  inappropriate (excessive) parental pressure Z62.6
  influencing health status NEC Z78.9
  in-law Z63.1
  institutionalization, affecting child Z62.22
  intrafamilial communication Z63.8
  jealousy, child F93.8
  landlord Z59.2
  language (developmental) F8Ø.9
  learning (developmental) F81.9
  legal Z65.3
    conviction without imprisonment Z65.Ø
    imprisonment Z65.1
    release from prison Z65.2

Problem — *continued*
  life-management Z73.9
    specified NEC Z73.89
  life-style Z72.9
    gambling Z72.6
    high-risk sexual behavior (heterosexual) Z72.51
      bisexual Z72.53
      homosexual Z72.52
    inappropriate eating habits Z72.4
    self-damaging behavior NEC Z72.89
    specified NEC Z72.89
    tobacco use Z72.Ø
  literacy Z55.9
    low level Z55.Ø
    specified NEC Z55.8
  living alone Z6Ø.2
  lodgers Z59.2
  loss of love relationship in childhood Z62.898
  marital Z63.Ø
    involving
      divorce Z63.5
      estrangement Z63.5
      gender identity F66
  mastication KØ8.8
  medical
    care, within family Z63.6
    facilities Z75.9
      specified NEC Z75.8
  mental F48.9
  multiparity Z64.1
  negative life events in childhood Z62.9
    altered pattern of family relationships Z62.898
    frightening experience Z62.898
    loss of
      love relationship Z62.898
      self-esteem Z62.898
    physical abuse (alleged) — *see* Maltreatment, child
    removal from home Z62.29
    specified event NEC Z62.898
  neighbor Z59.2
  neurological NEC R29.818
  new step-parent affecting child Z62.898
  none (feared complaint unfounded) Z71.1
  occupational NEC Z56.89
  parent-child — *see* Conflict, parent-child
  personal hygiene Z91.89
  personality F69
  phase-of-life transition, adjustment Z6Ø.Ø
  presence of sick or disabled person in family or household Z63.79
    needing care Z63.6
  primary support group (family) Z63.9
    specified NEC Z63.8
  probation officer Z64.4
  psychiatric F99
  psychosexual (development) F66
  psychosocial Z65.9
    specified NEC Z65.8
  relationship Z63.9
    childhood F93.8
  release from prison Z65.2
  removal from home affecting child Z62.29
  seeking and accepting known hazardous and harmful behavioral or psychological interventions Z65.8
    chemical, nutritional or physical interventions Z65.8
  sexual function (nonorganic) F52.9
  sight H54.7
  sleep disorder, child F51.9
  smell — *see* Disturbance, sensation, smell
  social
    environment Z6Ø.9
      specified NEC Z6Ø.8
    exclusion and rejection Z6Ø.4
    worker Z64.4
  speech R47.9
    developmental F8Ø.9
    specified NEC R47.89
  swallowing — *see* Dysphagia
  taste — *see* Disturbance, sensation, taste
  tic, child F95.Ø
  underachievement in school Z55.3
  unemployment Z56.Ø
    threatened Z56.2
  unwanted pregnancy Z64.Ø
  upbringing Z62.9
    specified NEC Z62.898
  urinary N39.9
  voice production R47.89

☑ Additional Character Required — Refer to the Tabular List for Character Selection   ▧ Subterms under main terms may continue to next column or page

Problem — *continued*
 work schedule (stressful) Z56.3
Procedure (surgical)
 for purpose other than remedying health state Z41.9
  specified NEC Z41.8
 not done Z53.9
  because of
   administrative reasons Z53.8
   contraindication Z53.09
    smoking Z53.01
   patient's decision Z53.20
    for reasons of belief or group pressure Z53.1
    left against medical advice (AMA) Z53.21
    specified reason NEC Z53.29
   specified reason NEC Z53.8
Procidentia (uteri) N81.3
Proctalgia K62.89
 fugax K59.4
 spasmodic K59.4
Proctitis K62.89
 amebic (acute) A06.0
 chlamydial A56.3
 gonococcal A54.6
 granulomatous — *see* Enteritis, regional, large intestine
 herpetic A60.1
 radiation K62.7
 tuberculous A18.32
 ulcerative (chronic) K51.20
  with
   complication K51.219
    abscess K51.214
    fistula K51.213
    obstruction K51.212
    rectal bleeding K51.211
    specified NEC K51.218
Proctocele
 female (without uterine prolapse) N81.6
  with uterine prolapse N81.2
   complete N81.3
 male K62.3
Proctocolitis, mucosal — *see* Rectosigmoiditis, ulcerative
Proctoptosis K62.3
Proctorrhagia K62.5
Proctosigmoiditis K63.89
 ulcerative (chronic) — *see* Rectosigmoiditis, ulcerative
Proctospasm K59.4
 psychogenic F45.8
Profichet's disease — *see* Disorder, soft tissue, specified type NEC
Progeria E34.8
Prognathism (mandibular) (maxillary) M26.19
Progonoma (melanotic) — *see* Neoplasm, benign, by site
Progressive — *see* condition
Prolactinoma
 specified site — *see* Neoplasm, benign, by site
 unspecified site D35.2
Prolapse, prolapsed
 anus, anal (canal) (sphincter) K62.2
 arm or hand O32.2 ☑
  causing obstructed labor O64.4 ☑
 bladder (mucosa) (sphincter) (acquired)
  congenital Q79.4
  female — *see* Cystocele
  male N32.89
 breast implant (prosthetic) T85.49 ☑
 cecostomy K94.09
 cecum K63.4
 cervix, cervical (hypertrophied) N81.2
  anterior lip, obstructing labor O65.5
  congenital Q51.828
  postpartal, old N81.2
  stump N81.85
 ciliary body (traumatic) — *see* Laceration, eye(ball), with prolapse or loss of interocular tissue
 colon (pedunculated) K63.4
 colostomy K94.09
 disc (intervertebral) — *see* Displacement, intervertebral disc
 eye implant (orbital) T85.398 ☑
  lens (ocular) — *see* Complications, intraocular lens
 fallopian tube N83.4
 gastric (mucosa) K31.89
 genital, female N81.9
  specified NEC N81.89
 globe, nontraumatic — *see* Luxation, globe

Prolapse, prolapsed — *continued*
 ileostomy bud K94.19
 intervertebral disc — *see* Displacement, intervertebral disc
 intestine (small) K63.4
 iris (traumatic) — *see* Laceration, eye(ball), with prolapse or loss of interocular tissue
  nontraumatic H21.89
 kidney N28.83
  congenital Q63.2
 laryngeal muscles or ventricle J38.7
 liver K76.89
 meatus urinarius N36.8
 mitral (valve) I34.1
 ocular lens implant — *see* Complications, intraocular lens
 organ or site, congenital NEC — *see* Malposition, congenital
 ovary N83.4
 pelvic floor, female N81.89
 perineum, female N81.89
 rectum (mucosa) (sphincter) K62.3
  due to trichuris trichuria B79
 spleen D73.89
 stomach K31.89
 umbilical cord
  complicating delivery O69.0 ☑
 urachus, congenital Q64.4
 ureter N28.89
  with obstruction N13.5
   with infection N13.6
 ureterovesical orifice N28.89
 urethra (acquired) (infected) (mucosa) N36.8
  congenital Q64.71
 urinary meatus N36.8
  congenital Q64.72
 uterovaginal N81.4
  complete N81.3
  incomplete N81.2
 uterus (with prolapse of vagina) N81.4
  complete N81.3
  congenital Q51.818
  first degree N81.2
  in pregnancy or childbirth — *see* Pregnancy, complicated by, abnormal, uterus
  incomplete N81.2
  postpartal (old) N81.4
  second degree N81.2
  third degree N81.3
 uveal (traumatic) — *see* Laceration, eye(ball), with prolapse or loss of interocular tissue
 vagina (anterior) (wall) — *see* Cystocele
  with prolapse of uterus N81.4
   complete N81.3
   incomplete N81.2
  posterior wall N81.6
  posthysterectomy N99.3
 vitreous (humor) H43.0- ☑
  in wound — *see* Laceration, eye(ball), with prolapse or loss of interocular tissue
 womb — *see* Prolapse, uterus
Prolapsus, female N81.9
 specified NEC N81.89
Proliferation(s)
 primary cutaneous CD30-positive large T-cell C86.6
Proliferative — *see* condition
Prolonged, prolongation (of)
 bleeding (time) (idiopathic) R79.1
 coagulation (time) R79.1
 gestation (over 42 completed weeks)
  mother O48.1
  newborn P08.22
 interval I44.0
 labor O63.9
  first stage O63.0
  second stage O63.1
 partial thromboplastin time (PTT) R79.1
 pregnancy (more than 42 weeks gestation) O48.1
 prothrombin time R79.1
 QT interval I45.81
 uterine contractions in labor O62.4
Prominence, prominent
 auricle (congenital) (ear) Q17.5
 ischial spine or sacral promontory
  with disproportion (fetopelvic) O33.0
   causing obstructed labor O65.0
 nose (congenital) acquired M95.0
Promiscuity — *see* High, risk, sexual behavior

Pronation
 ankle — *see* Deformity, limb, foot, specified NEC
 foot (*see also* Deformity, limb, foot, specified NEC)
  congenital Q74.2
Prophylactic
 administration of
  antibiotics, long-term Z79.2
   short-term use — *omit code*
  drug (*see also* Long-term (current) drug therapy (use of)) Z79.899
 medication Z79.899
 organ removal (for neoplasia management) Z40.00
  breast Z40.01
  ovary Z40.02
  specified site NEC Z40.09
 surgery Z40.9
  for risk factors related to malignant neoplasm — *see* Prophylactic, organ removal
  specified NEC Z40.8
 vaccination Z23
Propionic acidemia E71.121
Proptosis (ocular) (*see also* Exophthalmos)
 thyroid — *see* Hyperthyroidism, with goiter
Prosecution, anxiety concerning Z65.3
Prosopagnosia R48.3
Prostadynia N42.81
Prostate, prostatic — *see* condition
Prostatism — *see* Hyperplasia, prostate
Prostatitis (congestive) (suppurative) (with cystitis) N41.9
 acute N41.0
 cavitary N41.8
 chronic N41.1
 diverticular N41.8
 due to Trichomonas (vaginalis) A59.02
 fibrous N41.1
 gonococcal (acute) (chronic) A54.22
 granulomatous N41.4
 hypertrophic N41.1
 subacute N41.1
 trichomonal A59.02
 tuberculous A18.14
Prostatocystitis N41.3
Prostatorrhea N42.89
Prostatosis N42.82
Prostration R53.83
 heat (*see also* Heat, exhaustion)
  anhydrotic T67.3 ☑
  due to
   salt (and water) depletion T67.4 ☑
   water depletion T67.3 ☑
 nervous F48.8
 senile R54
Protanomaly (anomalous trichromat) H53.54
Protanopia (complete) (incomplete) H53.54
Protection (against) (from) — *see* Prophylactic
Protein
 deficiency NEC — *see* Malnutrition
 malnutrition — *see* Malnutrition
 sickness (*see also* Reaction, serum) T80.69 ☑
Proteinemia R77.9
Proteinosis
 alveolar (pulmonary) J84.01
 lipid or lipoid (of Urbach) E78.89
Proteinuria R80.9
 Bence Jones R80.3
 complicating pregnancy — *see* Proteinuria, gestational
 gestational O12.1- ☑
  with edema O12.2- ☑
 idiopathic R80.0
 isolated R80.0
  with glomerular lesion N06.9
   dense deposit disease N06.6
   diffuse
    crescentic glomerulonephritis N06.7
    endocapillary proliferative glomerulonephritis N06.4
    mesangiocapillary glomerulonephritis N06.5
   focal and segmental hyalinosis or sclerosis N06.1
   membranous (diffuse) N06.2
   mesangial proliferative (diffuse) N06.3
   minimal change N06.0
   specified pathology NEC N06.8
 orthostatic R80.2
  with glomerular lesion — *see* Proteinuria, isolated, with glomerular lesion
 persistent R80.1

Proteinuria — continued
  persistent — continued
    with glomerular lesion — see Proteinuria, isolated, with glomerular lesion
  postural R80.2
    with glomerular lesion — see Proteinuria, isolated, with glomerular lesion
  pre-eclamptic — see Pre-eclampsia
  specified type NEC R80.8
Proteolysis, pathologic D65
Proteus (mirabilis) (morganii), **as cause of disease classified elsewhere** B96.4
Prothrombin gene mutation D68.52
Protoporphyria, erythropoietic E80.0
Protozoal (see also condition)
  disease B64
    specified NEC B60.8
Protrusion, protrusio
  acetabuli M24.7
  acetabulum (into pelvis) M24.7
  device, implant or graft (see also Complications, by site and type, mechanical) T85.698 ☑
    arterial graft NEC — see Complication, cardiovascular device, mechanical, vascular
    breast (implant) T85.49 ☑
    catheter NEC T85.698 ☑
      cystostomy T83.090 ☑
      dialysis (renal) T82.49 ☑
        intraperitoneal T85.691 ☑
      infusion NEC T82.594 ☑
        spinal (epidural) (subdural) T85.690 ☑
      urinary, indwelling T83.098 ☑
    electronic (electrode) (pulse generator) (stimulator) bone T84.390 ☑
      nervous system — see Complication, prosthetic device, mechanical, electronic nervous system stimulator
    fixation, internal (orthopedic) NEC — see Complication, fixation device, mechanical
    gastrointestinal — see Complications, prosthetic device, mechanical, gastrointestinal device
    genital NEC T83.498 ☑
      intrauterine contraceptive device T83.39 ☑
      penile prosthesis T83.490 ☑
    heart NEC — see Complication, cardiovascular device, mechanical
    joint prosthesis — see Complications, joint prosthesis, mechanical, specified NEC, by site
    ocular NEC — see Complications, prosthetic device, mechanical, ocular device
    orthopedic NEC — see Complication, orthopedic, device, mechanical
    specified NEC T85.628 ☑
    urinary NEC (see also Complication, genitourinary, device, urinary, mechanical)
      graft T83.29 ☑
    vascular NEC — see Complication, cardiovascular device, mechanical
    ventricular intracranial shunt T85.09 ☑
  intervertebral disc — see Displacement, intervertebral disc
  joint prosthesis — see Complications, joint prosthesis, mechanical, specified NEC, by site
  nucleus pulposus — see Displacement, intervertebral disc
Prune belly (syndrome) Q79.4
Prurigo (ferox) (gravis) (Hebrae) (Hebra's) (mitis) (simplex) L28.2
  Besnier's L20.0
  estivalis L56.4
  nodularis L28.1
  psychogenic F45.8
Pruritus, pruritic (essential) L29.9
  ani, anus L29.0
    psychogenic F45.8
  anogenital L29.3
    psychogenic F45.8
  due to onchocerca volvulus B73.1
  gravidarum — see Pregnancy, complicated by, specified pregnancy-related condition NEC
  hiemalis L29.8
  neurogenic (any site) F45.8
  perianal L29.0
  psychogenic (any site) F45.8
  scroti, scrotum L29.1
    psychogenic F45.8
  senile, senilis L29.8

Pruritus, pruritic — continued
  specified NEC L29.8
    psychogenic F45.8
  Trichomonas A59.9
  vulva, vulvae L29.2
    psychogenic F45.8
Pseudarthrosis, pseudoarthrosis (bone) — see Nonunion, fracture
  clavicle, congenital Q74.0
  joint, following fusion or arthrodesis M96.0
Pseudoaneurysm — see Aneurysm
Pseudoangina (pectoris) — see Angina
Pseudoangioma I81
Pseudoarteriosus Q28.8
Pseudoarthrosis — see Pseudarthrosis
Pseudobulbar affect (PBA) F48.8
Pseudochromhidrosis L67.8
Pseudocirrhosis, liver, pericardial I31.1
Pseudocowpox B08.03
Pseudocoxalgia M91.3- ☑
Pseudocroup J38.5
Pseudo-Cushing's syndrome, alcohol-induced E24.4
Pseudocyesis F45.8
Pseudocyst
  lung J98.4
  pancreas K86.3
  retina — see Cyst, retina
Pseudoelephantiasis neuroarthritica Q82.0
Pseudoexfoliation, capsule (lens) — see Cataract, specified NEC
Pseudofolliculitis barbae L73.1
Pseudoglioma H44.89
Pseudohemophilia (Bernuth's) (hereditary) (type B) D68.0
  Type A D69.8
  vascular D69.8
Pseudohermaphroditism Q56.3
  adrenal E25.8
  female Q56.2
    with adrenocortical disorder E25.8
    without adrenocortical disorder Q56.2
    adrenal, congenital E25.0
  male Q56.1
    with
      5-alpha-reductase deficiency E29.1
      adrenocortical disorder E25.8
      androgen resistance E34.51
      cleft scrotum Q56.1
      feminizing testis E34.51
    without gonadal disorder Q56.1
    adrenal E25.8
Pseudo-Hurler's polydystrophy E77.0
Pseudohydrocephalus G93.2
Pseudohypertrophic muscular dystrophy (Erb's) G71.0
Pseudohypertrophy, muscle G71.0
Pseudohypoparathyroidism E20.1
Pseudoinsomnia F51.03
Pseudoleukemia, infantile D64.89
Pseudomembranous — see condition
Pseudomeningocele (cerebral) (infective) (post-traumatic) G96.19
  postprocedural (spinal) G97.82
Pseudomenses (newborn) P54.6
Pseudomenstruation (newborn) P54.6
Pseudomonas
  aeruginosa, as cause of disease classified elsewhere B96.5
  mallei infection A24.0
    as cause of disease classified elsewhere B96.5
  pseudomallei, as cause of disease classified elsewhere B96.5
Pseudomyotonia G71.19
Pseudomyxoma peritonei C78.6
Pseudoneuritis, optic (nerve) (disc) (papilla), **congenital** Q14.2
Pseudo-obstruction intestine (acute) (chronic) (idiopathic) (intermittent secondary) (primary) K59.8
Pseudopapilledema H47.33- ☑
  congenital Q14.2
Pseudoparalysis
  arm or leg R29.818
  atonic, congenital P94.2
Pseudopelade L66.0
Pseudophakia Z96.1
Pseudopolyarthritis, rhizomelic M35.3
Pseudopolycythemia D75.1
Pseudopseudohypoparathyroidism E20.1

Pseudopterygium H11.81- ☑
Pseudoptosis (eyelid) — see Blepharochalasis
Pseudopuberty, precocious
  female heterosexual E25.8
  male isosexual E25.8
Pseudorickets (renal) N25.0
Pseudorubella B08.20
Pseudosclerema, newborn P83.8
Pseudosclerosis (brain)
  Jakob's — see Creutzfeldt-Jakob disease or syndrome
  of Westphal (Strümpell) E83.01
  spastic — see Creutzfeldt-Jakob disease or syndrome
Pseudotetanus — see Convulsions
Pseudotetany R29.0
  hysterical F44.5
Pseudotruncus arteriosus Q25.4
Pseudotuberculosis A28.2
  enterocolitis A04.8
  pasteurella (infection) A28.0
Pseudotumor
  cerebri G93.2
  orbital H05.11 ☑
Pseudoxanthoma elasticum Q82.8
Psilosis (sprue) (tropical) K90.1
  nontropical K90.0
Psittacosis A70
Psoitis M60.88
Psoriasis L40.9
  arthropathic L40.50
    arthritis mutilans L40.52
    distal interphalangeal L40.51
    juvenile L40.54
    other specified L40.59
    spondylitis L40.53
  buccal K13.29
  flexural L40.8
  guttate L40.4
  mouth K13.29
  nummular L40.0
  plaque L40.0
  psychogenic F54
  pustular (generalized) L40.1
    palmaris et plantaris L40.3
  specified NEC L40.8
  vulgaris L40.0
Psychasthenia F48.8
Psychiatric disorder or problem F99
Psychogenic (see also condition)
  factors associated with physical conditions F54
Psychological and behavioral factors affecting medical condition F59
Psychoneurosis, psychoneurotic (see also Neurosis)
  anxiety (state) F41.1
  depersonalization F48.1
  hypochondriacal F45.21
  hysteria F44.9
  neurasthenic F48.8
  personality NEC F60.89
Psychopathy, psychopathic
  affectionless F94.2
  autistic F84.5
  constitution, post-traumatic F07.81
  personality — see Disorder, personality
  sexual — see Deviation, sexual
  state F60.2
Psychosexual identity disorder of childhood F64.2
Psychosis, psychotic F29
  acute (transient) F23
    hysterical F44.9
  affective — see Disorder, mood
  alcoholic F10.959
    with
      abuse F10.159
      anxiety disorder F10.980
        with
          abuse F10.180
          dependence F10.280
      delirium tremens F10.231
      delusions F10.950
        with
          abuse F10.150
          dependence F10.250
      dementia F10.97
        with dependence F10.27
      dependence F10.259
      hallucinosis F10.951

☑ **Additional Character Required** — Refer to the Tabular List for Character Selection   ▼ Subterms under main terms may continue to next column or page

Psychosis, psychotic — *continued*
  alcoholic — *continued*
    with
      hallucinosis — *continued*
        with
          abuse F10.151
          dependence F10.251
      mood disorder F10.94
        with
          abuse F10.14
          dependence F10.24
      paranoia F10.950
        with
          abuse F10.150
          dependence F10.250
      persisting amnesia F10.96
        with dependence F10.26
    amnestic confabulatory F10.96
      with dependence F10.26
    delirium tremens F10.231
    Korsakoff's, Korsakov's, Korsakow's F10.26
    paranoid type F10.950
      with
        abuse F10.150
        dependence F10.250
  anergastic — *see* Psychosis, organic
  arteriosclerotic (simple type) (uncomplicated) F01.50
    with behavioral disturbance F01.51
  childhood F84.0
    atypical F84.8
  climacteric — *see* Psychosis, involutional
  confusional F29
    acute or subacute F05
    reactive F23
  cycloid F23
  depressive — *see* Disorder, depressive
  disintegrative (childhood) F84.3
  drug-induced — *see* F11-F19 with .X59
    paranoid and hallucinatory states — *see* F11-F19
      with .X50 or .X51
  due to or associated with
    addiction, drug — *see* F11-F19 with .X59
    dependence
      alcohol F10.259
      drug — *see* F11-F19 with .X59
    epilepsy F06.8
    Huntington's chorea F06.8
    ischemia, cerebrovascular (generalized) F06.8
    multiple sclerosis F06.8
    physical disease F06.8
    presenile dementia F03 ☑
    senile dementia F03 ☑
    vascular disease (arteriosclerotic) (cerebral) F01.50
      with behavioral disturbance F01.51
  epileptic F06.8
  episode F23
    due to or associated with physical condition F06.8
  exhaustive F43.0
  hallucinatory, chronic F28
  hypomanic F30.8
  hysterical (acute) F44.9
  induced F24
  infantile F84.0
    atypical F84.8
  infective (acute) (subacute) F05
  involutional F28
    depressive — *see* Disorder, depressive
    melancholic — *see* Disorder, depressive
    paranoid (state) F22
  Korsakoff's, Korsakov's, Korsakow's (nonalcoholic) F04
    alcoholic F10.96
      in dependence F10.26
    induced by other psychoactive substance — *see*
      categories F11-F19 with .X5X
  mania, manic (single episode) F30.2
    recurrent type F31.89
  manic-depressive — *see* Disorder, mood
  menopausal — *see* Psychosis, involutional
  mixed schizophrenic and affective F25.8
  multi-infarct (cerebrovascular) F01.50
    with behavioral disturbance F01.51
  nonorganic F29
    specified NEC F28
  organic F09
    due to or associated with
      arteriosclerosis (cerebral) — *see* Psychosis, ar-
        teriosclerotic

Psychosis, psychotic — *continued*
  organic — *continued*
    due to or associated with — *continued*
      cerebrovascular disease, arteriosclerotic — *see*
        Psychosis, arteriosclerotic
      childbirth — *see* Psychosis, puerperal
      Creutzfeldt-Jakob disease or syndrome — *see*
        Creutzfeldt-Jakob disease or syndrome
      dependence, alcohol F10.259
      disease
        alcoholic liver F10.259
        brain, arteriosclerotic — *see* Psychosis, arte-
          riosclerotic
        cerebrovascular F01.50
          with behavioral disturbance F01.51
        Creutzfeldt-Jakob — *see* Creutzfeldt-Jakob
          disease or syndrome
        endocrine or metabolic F06.8
          acute or subacute F05
        liver, alcoholic F10.259
      epilepsy transient (acute) F05
      infection
        brain (intracranial) F06.8
          acute or subacute F05
      intoxication
        alcoholic (acute) F10.259
        drug F11-F19 with .X59
      ischemia, cerebrovascular (generalized) — *see*
        Psychosis, arteriosclerotic
      puerperium — *see* Psychosis, puerperal
      trauma, brain (birth) (from electric current)
        (surgical) F06.8
        acute or subacute F05
    infective F06.8
      acute or subacute F05
    post-traumatic F06.8
      acute or subacute F05
  paranoiac F22
  paranoid (climacteric) (involutional) (menopausal) F22
    psychogenic (acute) F23
    schizophrenic F20.0
    senile F03 ☑
  postpartum F53
  presbyophrenic (type) F03 ☑
  presenile F03 ☑
  psychogenic (paranoid) F23
    depressive F32.3
  puerperal F53
    specified type — *see* Psychosis, by type
  reactive (brief) (transient) (emotional stress) (psycho-
    logical trauma) F23
    depressive F32.3
      recurrent F33.3
    excitative type F30.8
  schizoaffective F25.9
    depressive type F25.1
    manic type F25.0
  schizophrenia, schizophrenic — *see* Schizophrenia
  schizophrenia-like, in epilepsy F06.2
  schizophreniform F20.81
    affective type F25.9
    brief F23
    confusional type F23
    depressive type F25.1
    manic type F25.0
    mixed type F25.0
  senile NEC F03 ☑
    depressed or paranoid type F03 ☑
    simple deterioration F03 ☑
    specified type — *code to* condition
  shared F24
  situational (reactive) F23
  symbiotic (childhood) F84.3
  symptomatic F09
Psychosomatic — *see* Disorder, psychosomatic
Psychosyndrome, organic F07.9
Psychotic episode due to or associated with physical
  condition F06.8
Pterygium (eye) H11.00- ☑
  amyloid H11.01- ☑
  central H11.02- ☑
  colli Q18.3
  double H11.03- ☑
  peripheral
    progressive H11.05- ☑
    stationary H11.04- ☑
  recurrent H11.06- ☑

Ptilosis (eyelid) — *see* Madarosis
Ptomaine (poisoning) — *see* Poisoning, food
Ptosis (*see also* Blepharoptosis)
  adiposa (false) — *see* Blepharoptosis
  breast N64.81
  cecum K63.4
  colon K63.4
  congenital (eyelid) Q10.0
    specified site NEC — *see* Anomaly, by site
  eyelid — *see* Blepharoptosis
    congenital Q10.0
  gastric K31.89
  intestine K63.4
  kidney N28.83
  liver K76.89
  renal N28.83
  splanchnic K63.4
  spleen D73.89
  stomach K31.89
  viscera K63.4
PTP D69.51
Ptyalism (periodic) K11.7
  hysterical F45.8
  pregnancy — *see* Pregnancy, complicated by, specified
    pregnancy-related condition NEC
  psychogenic F45.8
Ptyalolithiasis K11.5
Pubarche, precocious E30.1
Pubertas praecox E30.1
Puberty (development state) Z00.3
  bleeding (excessive) N92.2
  delayed E30.0
  precocious (constitutional) (cryptogenic) (idiopathic)
    E30.1
    central E22.8
    due to
      ovarian hyperfunction E28.1
        estrogen E28.0
      testicular hyperfunction E29.0
    premature E30.1
    due to
      adrenal cortical hyperfunction E25.8
      pineal tumor E34.8
      pituitary (anterior) hyperfunction E22.8
Puckering, macula — *see* Degeneration, macula, puckering
Pudenda, pudendum — *see* condition
Puente's disease (simple glandular cheilitis) K13.0
Puerperal, puerperium (complicated by, complications)
  abnormal glucose (tolerance test) O99.815
  abscess
    areola O91.02
      associated with lactation O91.03
    Bartholin's gland O86.19
    breast O91.12
      associated with lactation O91.13
    cervix (uteri) O86.11
    genital organ NEC O86.19
    kidney O86.21
    mammary O91.12
      associated with lactation O91.13
    nipple O91.02
      associated with lactation O91.03
    peritoneum O85
    subareolar O91.12
      associated with lactation O91.13
    urinary tract — *see* Puerperal, infection, urinary
    uterus O86.12
    vagina (wall) O86.13
    vaginorectal O86.13
    vulvovaginal gland O86.13
  adnexitis O86.19
  afibrinogenemia, or other coagulation defect O72.3
  albuminuria (acute) (subacute) — *see* Proteinuria,
    gestational
  alcohol use O99.315
  anemia O90.81
    pre-existing (pre-pregnancy) O99.03
  anesthetic death O89.8
  apoplexy O99.43
  bariatric surgery status O99.845
  blood disorder NEC O99.13
  blood dyscrasia O72.3
  cardiomyopathy O90.3
  cerebrovascular disorder (conditions in I60-I69) O99.43
  cervicitis O86.11
  circulatory system disorder O99.43
  coagulopathy (any) O72.3

Index

Psychosis, psychotic — Puerperal, puerperium

Puerperal, puerperium — *continued*
- complications O90.9
  - specified NEC O90.89
- convulsions — *see* Eclampsia
- cystitis O86.22
- cystopyelitis O86.29
- delirium NEC F05
- diabetes O24.93
  - gestational — *see* Puerperal, gestational diabetes
  - pre-existing O24.33
    - specified NEC O24.83
      - type 1 O24.03
      - type 2 O24.13
- digestive system disorder O99.63
- disease O90.9
  - breast NEC O92.29
  - cerebrovascular (acute) O99.43
  - nonobstetric NEC O99.89
  - tubo-ovarian O86.19
  - Valsuani's O99.03
- disorder O90.9
  - biliary tract O26.63
  - lactation O92.70
  - liver O26.63
  - nonobstetric NEC O99.89
- disruption
  - cesarean wound O90.0
  - episiotomy wound O90.1
  - perineal laceration wound O90.1
- drug use O99.325
- eclampsia (with pre-existing hypertension) O15.2
- embolism (pulmonary) (blood clot) — *see* Embolism, obstetric, puerperal
- endocrine, nutritional or metabolic disease NEC O99.285
- endophlebitis — *see* Puerperal, phlebitis
- endotrachelitis O86.11
- failure
  - lactation (complete) O92.3
    - partial O92.4
  - renal, acute O90.4
- fever (of unknown origin) O86.4
  - septic O85
- fissure, nipple O92.12
  - associated with lactation O92.13
- fistula
  - breast (due to mastitis) O91.12
    - associated with lactation O91.13
  - nipple O91.02
    - associated with lactation O91.03
- galactophoritis O91.22
  - associated with lactation O91.23
- galactorrhea O92.6
- gastric banding status O99.845
- gastric bypass status O99.845
- gastrointestinal disease NEC O99.63
- gestational diabetes O24.439
  - diet controlled O24.430
  - insulin (and diet) controlled O24.434
- gonorrhea O98.23
- hematoma, subdural O99.43
- hemiplegia, cerebral O99.355
  - due to cerbrovascular disorder O99.43
- hemorrhage O72.1
  - brain O99.43
  - bulbar O99.43
  - cerebellar O99.43
  - cerebral O99.43
  - cortical O99.43
  - delayed or secondary O72.2
  - extradural O99.43
  - internal capsule O99.43
  - intracranial O99.43
  - intrapontine O99.43
  - meningeal O99.43
  - pontine O99.43
  - retained placenta O72.0
  - subarachnoid O99.43
  - subcortical O99.43
  - subdural O99.43
  - third stage O72.0
  - uterine, delayed O72.2
  - ventricular O99.43
- hemorrhoids O87.2
- hepatorenal syndrome O90.4
- hypertension — *see* Hypertension, complicating, puerperium
- hypertrophy, breast O92.29

Puerperal, puerperium — *continued*
- induration breast (fibrous) O92.29
- infection O86.4
  - cervix O86.11
  - generalized O85
  - genital tract NEC O86.19
    - obstetric surgical wound O86.0
  - kidney (bacillus coli) O86.21
  - maternal O98.93
    - carrier state NEC O99.835
    - gonorrhea O98.23
    - human immunodeficiency virus (HIV) O98.73
    - protozoal O98.63
    - sexually transmitted NEC O98.33
    - specified NEC O98.83
    - streptococcus B carrier state O99.825
    - syphilis O98.13
    - tuberculosis O98.03
    - viral hepatitis O98.43
    - viral NEC O98.53
  - nipple O91.02
    - associated with lactation O91.03
  - peritoneum O85
  - renal O86.21
  - specified NEC O86.89
  - urinary (asymptomatic) (tract) NEC O86.20
    - bladder O86.22
    - kidney O86.21
    - specified site NEC O86.29
    - urethra O86.22
  - vagina O86.13
  - vein — *see* Puerperal, phlebitis
- ischemia, cerebral O99.43
- lymphangitis O86.89
  - breast O91.22
    - associated with lactation O91.23
- malignancy O9A.13 (*following* O99)
- malnutrition O25.3
- mammillitis O91.02
  - associated with lactation O91.03
- mammitis O91.22
  - associated with lactation O91.23
- mania F30.8
- mastitis O91.22
  - associated with lactation O91.23
  - purulent O91.12
    - associated with lactation O91.13
- melancholia — *see* Disorder, depressive
- mental disorder NEC O99.345
- metroperitonitis O85
- metrorrhagia — *see* Hemorrhage, postpartum
- metrosalpingitis O86.19
- metrovaginitis O86.13
- milk leg O87.1
- monoplegia, cerebral O99.43
- mood disturbance O90.6
- necrosis, liver (acute) (subacute) (conditions in subcategory K72.0) O26.63
  - with renal failure O90.4
- nervous system disorder O99.355
- obesity (pre-existing prior to pregnancy) O99.215
- obesity surgery status O99.845
- occlusion, precerebral artery O99.43
- paralysis
  - bladder (sphincter) O90.89
  - cerebral O99.43
- paralytic stroke O99.43
- parametritis O85
- paravaginitis O86.13
- pelviperitonitis O85
- perimetritis O86.12
- perimetrosalpingitis O86.19
- perinephritis O86.21
- periphlebitis — *see* Puerperal phlebitis
- peritoneal infection O85
- peritonitis (pelvic) O85
- perivaginitis O86.13
- phlebitis O87.0
  - deep O87.1
  - pelvic O87.1
  - superficial O87.0
- phlebothrombosis, deep O87.1
- phlegmasia alba dolens O87.1
- placental polyp O90.89
- pneumonia, embolic — *see* Embolism, obstetric, puerperal
- pre-eclampsia — *see* Pre-eclampsia
- psychosis F53

Puerperal, puerperium — *continued*
- pyelitis O86.21
- pyelocystitis O86.29
- pyelonephritis O86.21
- pyelonephrosis O86.21
- pyemia O85
- pyocystitis O86.29
- pyohemia O85
- pyometra O86.12
- pyonephritis O86.21
- pyosalpingitis O86.19
- pyrexia (of unknown origin) O86.4
- renal
  - disease NEC O90.89
  - failure O90.4
- respiratory disease NEC O99.53
- retention
  - decidua — *see* Retention, decidua
  - placenta O72.0
  - secundines — *see* Retention, secundines
- retrated nipple O92.02
- salpingo-ovaritis O86.19
- salpingoperitonitis O85
- secondary perineal tear O90.1
- sepsis (pelvic) O85
- sepsis O85
- septic thrombophlebitis O86.81
- skin disorder NEC O99.73
- specified condition NEC O99.89
- stroke O99.43
- subinvolution (uterus) O90.89
- subluxation of symphysis (pubis) O26.73
- suppuration — *see* Puerperal, abscess
- tetanus A34
- thelitis O91.02
  - associated with lactation O91.03
- thrombocytopenia O72.3
- thrombophlebitis (superficial) O87.0
  - deep O87.1
  - pelvic O87.1
  - septic O86.81
- thrombosis (venous) — *see* Thrombosis, puerperal
- thyroiditis O90.5
- toxemia (eclamptic) (pre-eclamptic) (with convulsions) O15.2
- trauma, non-obstetric O9A.23 (*following* O99)
  - caused by abuse (physical) (suspected) O9A.33 (*following* O99)
    - confirmed O9A.33 (*following* O99)
    - psychological (suspected) O9A.53 (*following* O99)
      - confirmed O9A.53 (*following* O99)
    - sexual (suspected) O9A.43 (*following* O99)
      - confirmed O9A.43 (*following* O99)
- uremia (due to renal failure) O90.4
- urethritis O86.22
- vaginitis O86.13
- varicose veins (legs) O87.4
  - vulva or perineum O87.8
- venous O87.9
- vulvitis O86.13
- vulvovaginitis O86.13
- white leg O87.1

Puerperium — *see* Puerperal

Pulmolithiasis J98.4

Pulmonary — *see* condition

Pulpitis (acute) (anachoretic) (chronic) (hyperplastic) (irreversible) (putrescent) (reversible) (suppurative) (ulcerative) K04.0

Pulpless tooth K04.99

Pulse
- alternating R00.8
- bigeminal R00.8
- fast R00.0
- feeble, rapid due to shock following injury T79.4 ☑
- rapid R00.0
- weak R09.89

Pulsus alternans or trigeminus R00.8

Punch drunk F07.81

Punctum lacrimale occlusion — *see* Obstruction, lacrimal

Puncture
- abdomen, abdominal
  - wall S31.139 ☑
    - with
      - foreign body S31.149 ☑
      - penetration into peritoneal cavity S31.639 ☑

☑ Additional Character Required — Refer to the Tabular List for Character Selection   ▼ Subterms under main terms may continue to next column or page

Puncture — *continued*
  abdomen, abdominal — *continued*
    wall — *continued*
      with — *continued*
        penetration into peritoneal cavity — *continued*
          with foreign body S31.649 ☑
      epigastric region S31.132 ☑
        with
          foreign body S31.142 ☑
          penetration into peritoneal cavity S31.632 ☑
            with foreign body S31.642 ☑
        left
          lower quadrant S31.134 ☑
            with
              foreign body S31.144 ☑
              penetration into peritoneal cavity S31.634 ☑
                with foreign body S31.644 ☑
          upper quadrant S31.131 ☑
            with
              foreign body S31.141 ☑
              penetration into peritoneal cavity S31.631 ☑
                with foreign body S31.641 ☑
      periumbilic region S31.135 ☑
        with
          foreign body S31.145 ☑
          penetration into peritoneal cavity S31.635 ☑
            with foreign body S31.645 ☑
      right
        lower quadrant S31.133 ☑
          with
            foreign body S31.143 ☑
            penetration into peritoneal cavity S31.633 ☑
              with foreign body S31.643 ☑
        upper quadrant S31.130 ☑
          with
            foreign body S31.140 ☑
            penetration into peritoneal cavity S31.630 ☑
              with foreign body S31.640 ☑
  accidental, complicating surgery — *see* Complication, accidental puncture or laceration
  alveolar (process) — *see* Puncture, oral cavity
  ankle S91.039 ☑
    with
      foreign body S91.049 ☑
    left S91.032 ☑
      with
        foreign body S91.042 ☑
    right S91.031 ☑
      with
        foreign body S91.041 ☑
  anus S31.833 ☑
    with foreign body S31.834 ☑
  arm (upper) S41.139 ☑
    with foreign body S41.149 ☑
    left S41.132 ☑
      with foreign body S41.142 ☑
    lower — *see* Puncture, forearm
    right S41.131 ☑
      with foreign body S41.141 ☑
  auditory canal (external) (meatus) — *see* Puncture, ear
  auricle, ear — *see* Puncture, ear
  axilla — *see* Puncture, arm
  back (*see also* Puncture, thorax, back)
    lower S31.030 ☑
      with
        foreign body S31.040 ☑
          with penetration into retroperitoneal space S31.041 ☑
        penetration into retroperitoneal space S31.031 ☑
  bladder (traumatic) S37.29 ☑
    nontraumatic N32.89
  breast S21.039 ☑
    with foreign body S21.049 ☑
    left S21.032 ☑
      with foreign body S21.042 ☑
    right S21.031 ☑
      with foreign body S21.041 ☑

Puncture — *continued*
  buttock S31.803 ☑
    with foreign body S31.804 ☑
    left S31.823 ☑
      with foreign body S31.824 ☑
    right S31.813 ☑
      with foreign body S31.814 ☑
  by
    device, implant or graft — *see* Complications, by site and type, mechanical
    foreign body left accidentally in operative wound T81.539 ☑
    instrument (any) during a procedure, accidental — *see* Puncture, accidental complicating surgery
  calf — *see* Puncture, leg
  canaliculus lacrimalis — *see* Puncture, eyelid
  canthus, eye — *see* Puncture, eyelid
  cervical esophagus S11.23 ☑
    with foreign body S11.24 ☑
  cheek (external) S01.439 ☑
    with foreign body S01.449 ☑
    internal — *see* Puncture, oral cavity
    left S01.432 ☑
      with foreign body S01.442 ☑
    right S01.431 ☑
      with foreign body S01.441 ☑
  chest wall — *see* Puncture, thorax
  chin — *see* Puncture, head, specified site NEC
  clitoris — *see* Puncture, vulva
  costal region — *see* Puncture, thorax
  digit(s)
    foot — *see* Puncture, toe
    hand — *see* Puncture, finger
  ear (canal) (external) S01.339 ☑
    with foreign body S01.349 ☑
    drum S09.2- ☑
    left S01.332 ☑
      with foreign body S01.342 ☑
    right S01.331 ☑
      with foreign body S01.341 ☑
  elbow S51.039 ☑
    with
      foreign body S51.049 ☑
    left S51.032 ☑
      with
        foreign body S51.042 ☑
    right S51.031 ☑
      with
        foreign body S51.041 ☑
  epididymis — *see* Puncture, testis
  epigastric region — *see* Puncture, abdomen, wall, epigastric
  epiglottis S11.83 ☑
    with foreign body S11.84 ☑
  esophagus
    cervical S11.23 ☑
      with foreign body S11.24 ☑
    thoracic S27.818 ☑
  eyeball S05.6- ☑
    with foreign body S05.5- ☑
  eyebrow — *see* Puncture, eyelid
  eyelid S01.13- ☑
    with foreign body S01.14- ☑
    left S01.132 ☑
      with foreign body S01.142 ☑
    right S01.131 ☑
      with foreign body S01.141 ☑
  face NEC — *see* Puncture, head, specified site NEC
  finger(s) S61.239 ☑
    with
      damage to nail S61.339 ☑
        with
          foreign body S61.349 ☑
      foreign body S61.249 ☑
    index S61.238 ☑
      with
        damage to nail S61.338 ☑
          with
            foreign body S61.348 ☑
        foreign body S61.248 ☑
      left S61.231 ☑
        with
          damage to nail S61.331 ☑
            with
              foreign body S61.341 ☑

Puncture — *continued*
  finger(s) — *continued*
    index — *continued*
      left — *continued*
        with — *continued*
          foreign body S61.241 ☑
      right S61.230 ☑
        with
          damage to nail S61.330 ☑
            with
              foreign body S61.340 ☑
          foreign body S61.240 ☑
    little S61.238 ☑
      with
        damage to nail S61.338 ☑
          with
            foreign body S61.348 ☑
        foreign body S61.248 ☑
      left S61.237 ☑
        with
          damage to nail S61.337 ☑
            with
              foreign body S61.347 ☑
          foreign body S61.247 ☑
      right S61.236 ☑
        with
          damage to nail S61.336 ☑
            with
              foreign body S61.346 ☑
          foreign body S61.246 ☑
    middle S61.238 ☑
      with
        damage to nail S61.338 ☑
          with
            foreign body S61.348 ☑
        foreign body S61.248 ☑
      left S61.233 ☑
        with
          damage to nail S61.333 ☑
            with
              foreign body S61.343 ☑
          foreign body S61.243 ☑
      right S61.232 ☑
        with
          damage to nail S61.332 ☑
            with
              foreign body S61.342 ☑
          foreign body S61.242 ☑
    ring S61.238 ☑
      with
        damage to nail S61.338 ☑
          with
            foreign body S61.348 ☑
        foreign body S61.248 ☑
      left S61.235 ☑
        with
          damage to nail S61.335 ☑
            with
              foreign body S61.345 ☑
          foreign body S61.245 ☑
      right S61.234 ☑
        with
          damage to nail S61.334 ☑
            with
              foreign body S61.344 ☑
          foreign body S61.244 ☑
  flank S31.139 ☑
    with foreign body S31.149 ☑
  foot (except toe(s) alone) S91.339 ☑
    with foreign body S91.349 ☑
    left S91.332 ☑
      with foreign body S91.342 ☑
    right S91.331 ☑
      with foreign body S91.341 ☑
    toe — *see* Puncture, toe
  forearm S51.839 ☑
    with
      foreign body S51.849 ☑
    elbow only — *see* Puncture, elbow
    left S51.832 ☑
      with
        foreign body S51.842 ☑
    right S51.831 ☑
      with
        foreign body S51.841 ☑
  forehead — *see* Puncture, head, specified site NEC

Puncture — *continued*
genital organs, external
    female S31.532 ☑
      with foreign body S31.542 ☑
      vagina — *see* Puncture, vagina
      vulva — *see* Puncture, vulva
    male S31.531 ☑
      with foreign body S31.541 ☑
      penis — *see* Puncture, penis
      scrotum — *see* Puncture, scrotum
      testis — *see* Puncture, testis
groin — *see* Puncture, abdomen, wall
gum — *see* Puncture, oral cavity
hand S61.439 ☑
  with
    foreign body S61.449 ☑
  finger — *see* Puncture, finger
  left S61.432 ☑
    with
      foreign body S61.442 ☑
  right S61.431 ☑
    with
      foreign body S61.441 ☑
  thumb — *see* Puncture, thumb
head S01.93 ☑
  with foreign body S01.94 ☑
  cheek — *see* Puncture, cheek
  ear — *see* Puncture, ear
  eyelid — *see* Puncture, eyelid
  lip — *see* Puncture, oral cavity
  nose — *see* Puncture, nose
  oral cavity — *see* Puncture, oral cavity
  scalp S01.03 ☑
    with foreign body S01.04 ☑
  specified site NEC S01.83 ☑
    with foreign body S01.84 ☑
  temporomandibular area — *see* Puncture, cheek
heart S26.99 ☑
  with hemopericardium S26.09 ☑
  without hemopericardium S26.19 ☑
heel — *see* Puncture, foot
hip S71.039 ☑
  with foreign body S71.049 ☑
  left S71.032 ☑
    with foreign body S71.042 ☑
  right S71.031 ☑
    with foreign body S71.041 ☑
hymen — *see* Puncture, vagina
hypochondrium — *see* Puncture, abdomen, wall
hypogastric region — *see* Puncture, abdomen, wall
inguinal region — *see* Puncture, abdomen, wall
instep — *see* Puncture, foot
internal organs — *see* Injury, by site
interscapular region — *see* Puncture, thorax, back
intestine
  large
    colon S36.599 ☑
      ascending S36.590 ☑
      descending S36.592 ☑
      sigmoid S36.593 ☑
      specified site NEC S36.598 ☑
      transverse S36.591 ☑
    rectum S36.69 ☑
  small S36.499 ☑
    duodenum S36.490 ☑
    specified site NEC S36.498 ☑
intra-abdominal organ S36.99 ☑
  gallbladder S36.128 ☑
  intestine — *see* Puncture, intestine
  liver S36.118 ☑
  pancreas — *see* Puncture, pancreas
  peritoneum S36.81 ☑
  specified site NEC S36.898 ☑
  spleen S36.09 ☑
  stomach S36.39 ☑
jaw — *see* Puncture, head, specified site NEC
knee S81.039 ☑
  with foreign body S81.049 ☑
  left S81.032 ☑
    with foreign body S81.042 ☑
  right S81.031 ☑
    with foreign body S81.041 ☑
labium (majus) (minus) — *see* Puncture, vulva
lacrimal duct — *see* Puncture, eyelid
larynx S11.013 ☑
  with foreign body S11.014 ☑

Puncture — *continued*
leg (lower) S81.839 ☑
  with foreign body S81.849 ☑
  foot — *see* Puncture, foot
  knee — *see* Puncture, knee
  left S81.832 ☑
    with foreign body S81.842 ☑
  right S81.831 ☑
    with foreign body S81.841 ☑
  upper — *see* Puncture, thigh
lip S01.531 ☑
  with foreign body S01.541 ☑
loin — *see* Puncture, abdomen, wall
lower back — *see* Puncture, back, lower
lumbar region — *see* Puncture, back, lower
malar region — *see* Puncture, head, specified site NEC
mammary — *see* Puncture, breast
mastoid region — *see* Puncture, head, specified site NEC
mouth — *see* Puncture, oral cavity
nail
  finger — *see* Puncture, finger, with damage to nail
  toe — *see* Puncture, toe, with damage to nail
nasal (septum) (sinus) — *see* Puncture, nose
nasopharynx — *see* Puncture, head, specified site NEC
neck S11.93 ☑
  with foreign body S11.94 ☑
  involving
    cervical esophagus — *see* Puncture, cervical esophagus
    larynx — *see* Puncture, larynx
    pharynx — *see* Puncture, pharynx
    thyroid gland — *see* Puncture, thyroid gland
    trachea — *see* Puncture, trachea
  specified site NEC S11.83 ☑
    with foreign body S11.84 ☑
nose (septum) (sinus) S01.23 ☑
  with foreign body S01.24 ☑
ocular — *see* Puncture, eyeball
oral cavity S01.532 ☑
  with foreign body S01.542 ☑
orbit S05.4- ☑
palate — *see* Puncture, oral cavity
palm — *see* Puncture, hand
pancreas S36.299 ☑
  body S36.291 ☑
  head S36.290 ☑
  tail S36.292 ☑
pelvis — *see* Puncture, back, lower
penis S31.23 ☑
  with foreign body S31.24 ☑
perineum
  female S31.43 ☑
    with foreign body S31.44 ☑
  male S31.139 ☑
    with foreign body S31.149 ☑
periocular area (with or without lacrimal passages) — *see* Puncture, eyelid
phalanges
  finger — *see* Puncture, finger
  toe — *see* Puncture, toe
pharynx S11.23 ☑
  with foreign body S11.24 ☑
pinna — *see* Puncture, ear
popliteal space — *see* Puncture, knee
prepuce — *see* Puncture, penis
pubic region S31.139 ☑
  with foreign body S31.149 ☑
pudendum — *see* Puncture, genital organs, external
rectovaginal septum — *see* Puncture, vagina
sacral region — *see* Puncture, back, lower
sacroiliac region — *see* Puncture, back, lower
salivary gland — *see* Puncture, oral cavity
scalp S01.03 ☑
  with foreign body S01.04 ☑
scapular region — *see* Puncture, shoulder
scrotum S31.33 ☑
  with foreign body S31.34 ☑
shin — *see* Puncture, leg
shoulder S41.039 ☑
  with foreign body S41.049 ☑
  left S41.032 ☑
    with foreign body S41.042 ☑
  right S41.031 ☑
    with foreign body S41.041 ☑
spermatic cord — *see* Puncture, testis

Puncture — *continued*
sternal region — *see* Puncture, thorax, front
submaxillary region — *see* Puncture, head, specified site NEC
submental region — *see* Puncture, head, specified site NEC
subungual
  finger(s) — *see* Puncture, finger, with damage to nail
  toe — *see* Puncture, toe, with damage to nail
supraclavicular fossa — *see* Puncture, neck, specified site NEC
temple, temporal region — *see* Puncture, head, specified site NEC
temporomandibular area — *see* Puncture, cheek
testis S31.33 ☑
  with foreign body S31.34 ☑
thigh S71.139 ☑
  with foreign body S71.149 ☑
  left S71.132 ☑
    with foreign body S71.142 ☑
  right S71.131 ☑
    with foreign body S71.141 ☑
thorax, thoracic (wall) S21.93 ☑
  with foreign body S21.94 ☑
  back S21.23- ☑
    with
      foreign body S21.24- ☑
        with penetration S21.44 ☑
      penetration S21.43 ☑
  breast — *see* Puncture, breast
  front S21.13- ☑
    with
      foreign body S21.14- ☑
        with penetration S21.34 ☑
      penetration S21.33 ☑
throat — *see* Puncture, neck
thumb S61.039 ☑
  with
    damage to nail S61.139 ☑
      with
        foreign body S61.149 ☑
    foreign body S61.049 ☑
  left S61.032 ☑
    with
      damage to nail S61.132 ☑
        with
          foreign body S61.142 ☑
      foreign body S61.042 ☑
  right S61.031 ☑
    with
      damage to nail S61.131 ☑
        with
          foreign body S61.141 ☑
      foreign body S61.041 ☑
thyroid gland S11.13 ☑
  with foreign body S11.14 ☑
toe(s) S91.139 ☑
  with
    damage to nail S91.239 ☑
      with
        foreign body S91.249 ☑
    foreign body S91.149 ☑
  great S91.133 ☑
    with
      damage to nail S91.233 ☑
        with
          foreign body S91.243 ☑
      foreign body S91.143 ☑
    left S91.132 ☑
      with
        damage to nail S91.232 ☑
          with
            foreign body S91.242 ☑
        foreign body S91.142 ☑
    right S91.131 ☑
      with
        damage to nail S91.231 ☑
          with
            foreign body S91.241 ☑
        foreign body S91.141 ☑
  lesser S91.136 ☑
    with
      damage to nail S91.236 ☑
        with
          foreign body S91.246 ☑

☑ Additional Character Required — Refer to the Tabular List for Character Selection   ▽ Subterms under main terms may continue to next column or page

Puncture — *continued*
  toe(s) — *continued*
    lesser — *continued*
      with — *continued*
        foreign body S91.146 ☑
      left S91.135 ☑
        with
          damage to nail S91.235 ☑
            with
              foreign body S91.245 ☑
          foreign body S91.145 ☑
      right S91.134 ☑
        with
          damage to nail S91.234 ☑
            with
              foreign body S91.244 ☑
          foreign body S91.144 ☑
  tongue — *see* Puncture, oral cavity
  trachea S11.023 ☑
    with foreign body S11.024 ☑
  tunica vaginalis — *see* Puncture, testis
  tympanum, tympanic membrane S09.2- ☑
  umbilical region S31.135 ☑
    with foreign body S31.145 ☑
  uvula — *see* Puncture, oral cavity
  vagina S31.43 ☑
    with foreign body S31.44 ☑
  vocal cords S11.033 ☑
    with foreign body S11.034 ☑
  vulva S31.43 ☑
    with foreign body S31.44 ☑
  wrist S61.539 ☑
    with
      foreign body S61.549 ☑
    left S61.532 ☑
      with
        foreign body S61.542 ☑
    right S61.531 ☑
      with
        foreign body S61.541 ☑
PUO (pyrexia of unknown origin) R50.9
Pupillary membrane (persistent) Q13.89
Pupillotonia — *see* Anomaly, pupil, function, tonic pupil
Purpura D69.2
  abdominal D69.0
  allergic D69.0
  anaphylactoid D69.0
  annularis telangiectodes L81.7
  arthritic D69.0
  autoerythrocyte sensitization D69.2
  autoimmune D69.0
  bacterial D69.0
  Bateman's (senile) D69.2
  capillary fragility (hereditary) (idiopathic) D69.8
  cryoglobulinemic D89.1
  Devil's pinches D69.2
  fibrinolytic — *see* Fibrinolysis
  fulminans, fulminous D65
  gangrenous D65
  hemorrhagic, hemorrhagica D69.3
    not due to thrombocytopenia D69.0
  Henoch (-Schönlein) (allergic) D69.0
  hypergammaglobulinemic (benign) (Waldenström) D89.0
  idiopathic (thrombocytopenic) D69.3
    nonthrombocytopenic D69.0
  immune thrombocytopenic D69.3
  infectious D69.0
  malignant D69.0
  neonatorum P54.5
  nervosa D69.0
  newborn P54.5
  nonthrombocytopenic D69.2
    hemorrhagic D69.0
    idiopathic D69.0
  nonthrombopenic D69.2
  peliosis rheumatica D69.0
  posttransfusion (post-transfusion) (from (fresh) whole blood or blood products) D69.51
  primary D69.49
  red cell membrane sensitivity D69.2
  rheumatica D69.0
  Schönlein (-Henoch) (allergic) D69.0
  scorbutic E54 [D77]
  senile D69.2
  simplex D69.2
  symptomatica D69.0

Purpura — *continued*
  telangiectasia annularis L81.7
  thrombocytopenic D69.49
    congenital D69.42
    hemorrhagic D69.3
    hereditary D69.42
    idiopathic D69.3
    immune D69.3
    neonatal, transitory P61.0
    thrombotic M31.1
  thrombohemolytic — *see* Fibrinolysis
  thrombolytic — *see* Fibrinolysis
  thrombopenic D69.49
  thrombotic, thrombocytopenic M31.1
  toxic D69.0
  vascular D69.0
  visceral symptoms D69.0
Purpuric spots R23.3
Purulent — *see* condition
Pus
  in
    stool R19.5
    urine N39.0
  tube (rupture) — *see* Salpingo-oophoritis
Pustular rash L08.0
Pustule (nonmalignant) L08.9
  malignant A22.0
Pustulosis palmaris et plantaris L40.3
Putnam (-Dana) **disease or syndrome** — *see* Degeneration, combined
Putrescent pulp (dental) K04.1
Pyarthritis, pyarthrosis — *see* Arthritis, pyogenic or pyemic
  tuberculous — *see* Tuberculosis, joint
Pyelectasis — *see* Hydronephrosis
Pyelitis (congenital) (uremic) (*see also* Pyelonephritis)
  with
    calculus — *see* category N20 ☑
      with hydronephrosis N13.2
    contracted kidney N11.9
  acute N10
  chronic N11.9
    with calculus — *see* category N20 ☑
      with hydronephrosis N13.2
  cystica N28.84
  puerperal (postpartum) O86.21
  tuberculous A18.11
Pyelocystitis — *see* Pyelonephritis
Pyelonephritis (*see also* Nephritis, tubulo-interstitial)
  with
    calculus — *see* category N20 ☑
      with hydronephrosis N13.2
    contracted kidney N11.9
  acute N10
  calculous — *see* category N20 ☑
    with hydronephrosis N13.2
  chronic N11.9
    with calculus — *see* category N20 ☑
      with hydronephrosis N13.2
    associated with ureteral obstruction or stricture N11.1
    nonobstructive N11.8
      with reflux (vesicoureteral) N11.0
    obstructive N11.1
    specified NEC N11.8
  in (due to)
    brucellosis A23.9 [N16]
    cryoglobulinemia (mixed) D89.1 [N16]
    cystinosis E72.04
    diphtheria A36.84
    glycogen storage disease E74.09 [N16]
    leukemia NEC C95.9- ☑ [N16]
    lymphoma NEC C85.90 [N16]
    multiple myeloma C90.0- ☑ [N16]
    obstruction N11.1
    Salmonella infection A02.25
    sarcoidosis D86.84
    sepsis A41.9 [N16]
    Sjögren's disease M35.04
    toxoplasmosis B58.83
    transplant rejection T86.91 [N16]
    Wilson's disease E83.01 [N16]
  nonobstructive N12
    with reflux (vesicoureteral) N11.0
    chronic N11.8
  syphilitic A52.75
Pyelonephrosis (obstructive) N11.1
  chronic N11.9

Pyelophlebitis I80.8
Pyeloureteritis cystica N28.85
Pyemia, pyemic (fever) (infection) (purulent) (*see also* Sepsis)
  joint — *see* Arthritis, pyogenic or pyemic
  liver K75.1
  pneumococcal A40.3
  portal K75.1
  postvaccinal T88.0 ☑
  puerperal, postpartum, childbirth O85
  specified organism NEC A41.89
  tuberculous — *see* Tuberculosis, miliary
Pygopagus Q89.4
Pyknoepilepsy (idiopathic) — *see* Pyknolepsy
Pyknolepsy G40.A09 (*following* G40.3)
  intractable G40.A19 (*following* G40.3)
    with status epilepticus G40.A11 (*following* G40.3)
    without status epilepticus G40.A19 (*following* G40.3)
  not intractable G40.A09 (*following* G40.3)
    with status epilepticus G40.A01 (*following* G40.3)
    without status epilepticus G40.A09 (*following* G40.3)
Pylephlebitis K75.1
Pyle's syndrome Q78.5
Pylethrombophlebitis K75.1
Pylethrombosis K75.1
Pyloritis K29.90
  with bleeding K29.91
Pylorospasm (reflex) **NEC** K31.3
  congenital or infantile Q40.0
  neurotic F45.8
  newborn Q40.0
  psychogenic F45.8
Pylorus, pyloric — *see* condition
Pyoarthrosis — *see* Arthritis, pyogenic or pyemic
Pyocele
  mastoid — *see* Mastoiditis, acute
  sinus (accessory) — *see* Sinusitis
  turbinate (bone) J32.9
  urethra (*see also* Urethritis) N34.0
Pyocolpos — *see* Vaginitis
Pyocystitis N30.80
  with hematuria N30.81
Pyoderma, pyodermia L08.0
  gangrenosum L88
  newborn P39.4
  phagedenic L88
  vegetans L08.81
Pyodermatitis L08.0
  vegetans L08.81
Pyogenic — *see* condition
Pyohydronephrosis N13.6
Pyometra, pyometrium, pyometritis — *see* Endometritis
Pyomyositis (tropical) — *see* Myositis, infective
Pyonephritis N12
Pyonephrosis N13.6
  tuberculous A18.11
Pyo-oophoritis — *see* Salpingo-oophoritis
Pyo-ovarium — *see* Salpingo-oophoritis
Pyopericarditis, pyopericardium I30.1
Pyophlebitis — *see* Phlebitis
Pyopneumopericardium I30.1
Pyopneumothorax (infective) J86.9
  with fistula J86.0
  tuberculous NEC A15.6
Pyosalpinx, pyosalpingitis (*see also* Salpingo-oophoritis)
Pyothorax J86.9
  with fistula J86.0
  tuberculous NEC A15.6
Pyoureter N28.89
  tuberculous A18.11
Pyramidopallidonigral syndrome G20
Pyrexia (of unknown origin) R50.9
  atmospheric T67.0 ☑
  during labor NEC O75.2
  heat T67.0 ☑
  newborn P81.9
    environmentally-induced P81.0
  persistent R50.9
  puerperal O86.4
Pyroglobulinemia NEC E88.09
Pyromania F63.1
Pyrosis R12
Pyuria (bacterial) N39.0

Q

Q fever A78
  with pneumonia A78
Quadricuspid aortic valve Q23.8
Quadrilateral fever A78
Quadriparesis — *see* Quadriplegia
  meaning muscle weakness M62.81
Quadriplegia G82.50
  complete
    C1-C4 level G82.51
    C5-C7 level G82.53
  congenital (cerebral) (spinal) G80.8
    spastic G80.0
  embolic (current episode) I63.4 ☑
  functional R53.2
  incomplete
    C1-C4 level G82.52
    C5-C7 level G82.54
  thrombotic (current episode) I63.3 ☑
  traumatic — *code to* injury with seventh character S
    current episode — *see* Injury, spinal (cord), cervical
Quadruplet, pregnancy — *see* Pregnancy, quadruplet
Quarrelsomeness F60.3
Queensland fever A77.3
Quervain's disease M65.4
  thyroid E06.1
Queyrat's erythroplasia D07.4
  penis D07.4
  specified site — *see* Neoplasm, skin, in situ
  unspecified site D07.4
Quincke's disease or edema T78.3 ☑
  hereditary D84.1
Quinsy (gangrenous) J36
Quintan fever A79.0
Quintuplet, pregnancy — *see* Pregnancy, quintuplet

R

Rabbit fever — *see* Tularemia
Rabies A82.9
  contact Z20.3
  exposure to Z20.3
  inoculation reaction — *see* Complications, vaccination
  sylvatic A82.0
  urban A82.1
Rachischisis — *see* Spina bifida
Rachitic (*see also* condition)
  deformities of spine (late effect) (sequelae) E64.3
  pelvis (late effect) (sequelae) E64.3
    with disproportion (fetopelvic) O33.0
      causing obstructed labor O65.0
Rachitis, rachitism (acute) (tarda) (*see also* Rickets)
  renalis N25.0
  sequelae E64.3
Radial nerve — *see* condition
Radiation
  burn — *see* Burn
  effects NOS T66 ☑
  sickness NOS T66 ☑
  therapy, encounter for Z51.0
Radiculitis (pressure) (vertebrogenic) — *see* Radiculopathy
Radiculomyelitis (*see also* Encephalitis)
  toxic, due to
    Clostridium tetani A35
    Corynebacterium diphtheriae A36.82
Radiculopathy M54.10
  cervical region M54.12
  cervicothoracic region M54.13
  due to
    disc disorder
      C3 M50.11
      C4 M50.11
      C5 M50.12
      C6 M50.12
      C7 M50.12
      C8 M50.13
    displacement of intervertebral disc — *see* Disorder, disc, with, radiculopathy
  leg M54.1- ☑
  lumbar region M54.16
  lumbosacral region M54.17
  occipito-atlanto-axial region M54.11
  postherpetic B02.29
  sacrococcygeal region M54.18

Radiculopathy — *continued*
  syphilitic A52.11
  thoracic region (with visceral pain) M54.14
  thoracolumbar region M54.15
Radiodermal burns (acute, chronic, or occupational) — *see* Burn
Radiodermatitis L58.9
  acute L58.0
  chronic L58.1
Radiotherapy session Z51.0
Rage, meaning rabies — *see* Rabies
Ragpicker's disease A22.1
Ragsorter's disease A22.1
Raillietiniasis B71.8
Railroad neurosis F48.8
Railway spine F48.8
Raised (*see also* Elevated)
  antibody titer R76.0
Rake teeth, tooth M26.39
Rales R09.89
Ramifying renal pelvis Q63.8
Ramsay-Hunt disease or syndrome (*see also* Hunt's disease) B02.21
  meaning dyssynergia cerebellaris myoclonica G11.1
Ranula K11.6
  congenital Q38.4
Rape
  adult
    confirmed T74.21 ☑
    suspected T76.21 ☑
  alleged, observation or examination, ruled out
    adult Z04.41
    child Z04.42
  child
    confirmed T74.22 ☑
    suspected T76.22 ☑
Rapid
  feeble pulse, due to shock, following injury T79.4 ☑
  heart (beat) R00.0
    psychogenic F45.8
  second stage (delivery) O62.3
  time-zone change syndrome — *see* Disorder, sleep, circadian rhythm, psychogenic
Rarefaction, bone — *see* Disorder, bone, density and structure, specified NEC
Rash (toxic) R21
  canker A38.9
  diaper L22
  drug (internal use) L27.0
    contact (*see also* Dermatitis, due to, drugs, external) L25.1
  following immunization T88.1 ☑
  food — *see* Dermatitis, due to, food
  heat L74.0
  napkin (psoriasiform) L22
  nettle — *see* Urticaria
  pustular L08.0
  rose R21
    epidemic B06.9
  scarlet A38.9
  serum (*see also* Reaction, serum) T80.69 ☑
  wandering tongue K14.1
Rasmussen aneurysm — *see* Tuberculosis, pulmonary
Rasmussen encephalitis G04.81
Rat-bite fever A25.9
  due to Streptobacillus moniliformis A25.1
  spirochetal (morsus muris) A25.0
Rathke's pouch tumor D44.3
Raymond (-Céstan) **syndrome** I65.8
Raynaud's disease, phenomenon or syndrome (secondary) I73.00
  with gangrene (symmetric) I73.01
RDS (newborn) (type I) P22.0
  type II P22.1
Reaction (*see also* Disorder)
  adaptation — *see* Disorder, adjustment
  adjustment (anxiety) (conduct disorder) (depressiveness) (distress) — *see* Disorder, adjustment
    with
      mutism, elective (child) (adolescent) F94.0
  adverse
    food (any) (ingested) NEC T78.1 ☑
      anaphylactic — *see* Shock, anaphylactic, due to food
  affective — *see* Disorder, mood
  allergic — *see* Allergy
  anaphylactic — *see* Shock, anaphylactic

Reaction — *continued*
  anaphylactoid — *see* Shock, anaphylactic
  anesthesia — *see* Anesthesia, complication
  antitoxin (prophylactic) (therapeutic) — *see* Complications, vaccination
  anxiety F41.1
  Arthus — *see* Arthus' phenomenon
  asthenic F48.8
  combat and operational stress F43.0
  compulsive F42
  conversion F44.9
  crisis, acute F43.0
  deoxyribonuclease (DNA) (DNase) hypersensitivity D69.2
  depressive (single episode) F32.9
    affective (single episode) F31.4
      recurrent episode F33.9
    neurotic F34.1
    psychoneurotic F34.1
    psychotic F32.3
    recurrent — *see* Disorder, depressive, recurrent
  dissociative F44.9
  drug NEC T88.7 ☑
    addictive — *see* Dependence, drug
      transmitted via placenta or breast milk — *see* Absorption, drug, addictive, through placenta
    allergic — *see* Allergy, drug
    lichenoid L43.2
    newborn P93.8
      gray baby syndrome P93.0
    overdose or poisoning (by accident) — *see* Table of Drugs and Chemicals, by drug, poisoning
    photoallergic L56.1
    phototoxic L56.0
    withdrawal — *see* Dependence, by drug, with, withdrawal
      infant of dependent mother P96.1
      newborn P96.1
    wrong substance given or taken (by accident) — *see* Table of Drugs and Chemicals, by drug, poisoning
  fear F40.9
    child (abnormal) F93.8
  febrile nonhemolytic transfusion (FNHTR) R50.84
  fluid loss, cerebrospinal G97.1
  foreign
    body NEC — *see* Granuloma, foreign body
      in operative wound (inadvertently left) — *see* Foreign body, accidentally left during a procedure
    substance accidentally left during a procedure (chemical) (powder) (talc) T81.60 ☑
      aseptic peritonitis T81.61 ☑
      body or object (instrument) (sponge) (swab) — *see* Foreign body, accidentally left during a procedure
      specified reaction NEC T81.69 ☑
  grief — *see* Disorder, adjustment
  Herxheimer's R68.89
  hyperkinetic — *see* Hyperkinesia
  hypochondriacal F45.20
  hypoglycemic, due to insulin E16.0
    with coma (diabetic) — *see* Diabetes, coma
      nondiabetic E15
    therapeutic misadventure — *see* subcategory T38.3 ☑
  hypomanic F30.8
  hysterical F44.9
  immunization — *see* Complications, vaccination
  incompatibility
    ABO blood group (infusion) (transfusion) — *see* Complication(s), transfusion, incompatibility reaction, ABO
      delayed serologic T80.39 ☑
    minor blood group (Duffy) (E) (K(ell)) (Kidd) (Lewis) (M) (N) (P) (S) T80.89 ☑
    Rh (factor) (infusion) (transfusion) — *see* Complication(s), transfusion, incompatibility reaction, Rh (factor)
  inflammatory — *see* Infection
  infusion — *see* Complications, infusion
  inoculation (immune serum) — *see* Complications, vaccination
  insulin T38.3- ☑
  involutional psychotic — *see* Disorder, depressive
  leukemoid D72.823

☑ Additional Character Required — Refer to the Tabular List for Character Selection   ▽ Subterms under main terms may continue to next column or page

Reaction — *continued*
- leukemoid — *continued*
  - basophilic D72.823
  - lymphocytic D72.823
  - monocytic D72.823
  - myelocytic D72.823
  - neutrophilic D72.823
- LSD (acute)
  - due to drug abuse — *see* Abuse, drug, hallucinogen
  - due to drug dependence — *see* Dependence, drug, hallucinogen
- lumbar puncture G97.1
- manic-depressive — *see* Disorder, bipolar
- neurasthenic F48.8
- neurogenic — *see* Neurosis
- neurotic F48.9
- neurotic-depressive F34.1
- nitritoid — *see* Crisis, nitritoid
- nonspecific
  - to
    - cell mediated immunity measurement of gamma interferon antigen response without active tuberculosis R76.12
    - QuantiFERON-TB test (QFT) without active tuberculosis R76.12
    - tuberculin test (*see also* Reaction, tuberculin skin test) R76.11
- obsessive-compulsive F42
- organic, acute or subacute — *see* Delirium
- paranoid (acute) F23
  - chronic F22
  - senile F03 ☑
- passive dependency F60.7
- phobic F40.9
- post-traumatic stress, uncomplicated Z73.3
- psychogenic F99
- psychoneurotic (*see also* Neurosis)
  - compulsive F42
  - depersonalization F48.1
  - depressive F34.1
  - hypochondriacal F45.20
  - neurasthenic F48.8
  - obsessive F42
- psychophysiologic — *see* Disorder, somatoform
- psychosomatic — *see* Disorder, somatoform
- psychotic — *see* Psychosis
- scarlet fever toxin — *see* Complications, vaccination
- schizophrenic F23
  - acute (brief) (undifferentiated) F23
  - latent F21
  - undifferentiated (acute) (brief) F23
- serological for syphilis — *see* Serology for syphilis
- serum T80.69 ☑
  - anaphylactic (immediate) (*see also* Shock, anaphylactic) T80.59 ☑
  - specified reaction NEC
    - due to
      - administration of blood and blood products T80.61 ☑
      - immunization T80.62 ☑
      - serum specified NEC T80.69 ☑
      - vaccination T80.62 ☑
- situational — *see* Disorder, adjustment
- somatization — *see* Disorder, somatoform
- spinal puncture G97.1
- stress (severe) F43.9
  - acute (agitation) ("daze") (disorientation) (disturbance of consciousness) (flight reaction) (fugue) F43.0
  - specified NEC F43.8
- surgical procedure — *see* Complications, surgical procedure
- tetanus antitoxin — *see* Complications, vaccination
- toxic, to local anesthesia T81.89 ☑
  - in labor and delivery O74.4
  - in pregnancy O29.3X- ☑
  - postpartum, puerperal O89.3
- toxin-antitoxin — *see* Complications, vaccination
- transfusion (blood) (bone marrow) (lymphocytes) (allergic) — *see* Complications, transfusion
- tuberculin skin test, abnormal R76.11
- vaccination (any) — *see* Complications, vaccination
- withdrawing, child or adolescent F93.8

Reactive airway disease — *see* Asthma
Reactive depression — *see* Reaction, depressive

Rearrangement
- chromosomal
  - balanced (in) Q95.9
    - abnormal individual (autosomal) Q95.2
      - non-sex (autosomal) chromosomes Q95.2
      - sex/non-sex chromosomes Q95.3
    - specified NEC Q95.8

Recalcitrant patient — *see* Noncompliance
Recanalization, thrombus — *see* Thrombosis
Recession, receding
- chamber angle (eye) H21.55- ☑
- chin M26.09
- gingival (generalized) (localized) (postinfective) (postoperative) K06.0

Recklinghausen disease Q85.01
- bones E21.0

Reclus' disease (cystic) — *see* Mastopathy, cystic
Recrudescent typhus (fever) A75.1
Recruitment, auditory H93.21- ☑
Rectalgia K62.89
Rectitis K62.89
Rectocele
- female (without uterine prolapse) N81.6
  - with uterine prolapse N81.4
    - incomplete N81.2
- in pregnancy — *see* Pregnancy, complicated by, abnormal, pelvic organs or tissues NEC
- male K62.3

Rectosigmoid junction — *see* condition
Rectosigmoiditis K63.89
- ulcerative (chronic) K51.30
  - with
    - complication K51.319
      - abscess K51.314
      - fistula K51.313
      - obstruction K51.312
      - rectal bleeding K51.311
      - specified NEC K51.318

Rectourethral — *see* condition
Rectovaginal — *see* condition
Rectovesical — *see* condition
Rectum, rectal — *see* condition
Recurrent — *see* condition
- pregnancy loss — *see* Loss (of), pregnancy, recurrent

Red bugs B88.0
Red tide (*see also* Table of Drugs and Chemicals) T65.82- ☑
Red-cedar lung or pneumonitis J67.8
Reduced
- mobility Z74.09
- ventilatory or vital capacity R94.2

Redundant, redundancy
- anus (congenital) Q43.8
- clitoris N90.89
- colon (congenital) Q43.8
- foreskin (congenital) N47.8
- intestine (congenital) Q43.8
- labia N90.6
- organ or site, congenital NEC — *see* Accessory
- panniculus (abdominal) E65
- prepuce (congenital) N47.8
- pylorus K31.89
- rectum (congenital) Q43.8
- scrotum N50.8
- sigmoid (congenital) Q43.8
- skin (of face) L57.4
  - eyelids — *see* Blepharochalasis
- stomach K31.89

Reduplication — *see* Duplication
Reflex R29.2
- hyperactive gag J39.2
- pupillary, abnormal — *see* Anomaly, pupil, function
- vasoconstriction I73.9
- vasovagal R55

Reflux K21.9
- acid K21.9
- esophageal K21.9
  - with esophagitis K21.0
  - newborn P78.83
- gastroesophageal K21.9
  - with esophagitis K21.0
- mitral — *see* Insufficiency, mitral
- ureteral — *see* Reflux, vesicoureteral
- vesicoureteral (with scarring) N13.70
  - with
    - nephropathy N13.729
      - with hydroureter N13.739

Reflux — *continued*
- vesicoureteral — *continued*
  - with — *continued*
    - nephropathy — *continued*
      - with hydroureter — *continued*
        - bilateral N13.732
        - unilateral N13.731
      - without hydroureter N13.729
        - bilateral N13.722
        - unilateral N13.721
      - bilateral N13.722
      - unilateral N13.721
  - pyelonephritis (chronic) N11.0
  - without nephropathy N13.71
  - congenital Q62.7

Reforming, artificial openings — *see* Attention to, artificial, opening
Refractive error — *see* Disorder, refraction
Refsum's disease or syndrome G60.1
Refusal of
- food, psychogenic F50.8
- treatment (because of) Z53.20
  - left against medical advice (AMA) Z53.21
  - patient's decision NEC Z53.29
  - reasons of belief or group pressure Z53.1

Regional — *see* condition
Regurgitation R11.10
- aortic (valve) — *see* Insufficiency, aortic
- food (*see also* Vomiting)
  - with reswallowing — *see* Rumination
  - newborn P92.1
- gastric contents — *see* Vomiting
- heart — *see* Endocarditis
- mitral (valve) — *see* Insufficiency, mitral
  - congenital Q23.3
- myocardial — *see* Endocarditis
- pulmonary (valve) (heart) I37.1
  - congenital Q22.2
  - syphilitic A52.03
- tricuspid — *see* Insufficiency, tricuspid
- valve, valvular — *see* Endocarditis
  - congenital Q24.8
- vesicoureteral — *see* Reflux, vesicoureteral

Reichmann's disease or syndrome K31.89
Reifenstein syndrome E34.52
Reinsertion, contraceptive device Z30.433
Reiter's disease, syndrome, or urethritis M02.30
- ankle M02.37- ☑
- elbow M02.32- ☑
- foot joint M02.37- ☑
- hand joint M02.34- ☑
- hip M02.35- ☑
- knee M02.36- ☑
- multiple site M02.39
- shoulder M02.31- ☑
- vertebra M02.38
- wrist M02.33- ☑

Rejection
- food, psychogenic F50.8
- transplant T86.91
  - bone T86.830
    - marrow T86.01
  - cornea T86.840
  - heart T86.21
    - with lung(s) T86.31
  - intestine T86.850
  - kidney T86.11
  - liver T86.41
  - lung(s) T86.810
    - with heart T86.31
  - organ (immune or nonimmune cause) T86.91
  - pancreas T86.890
  - skin (allograft) (autograft) T86.820
  - specified NEC T86.890
  - stem cell (peripheral blood) (umbilical cord) T86.5

Relapsing fever A68.9
- Carter's (Asiatic) A68.1
- Dutton's (West African) A68.1
- Koch's A68.9
- louse-borne (epidemic) A68.0
- Novy's (American) A68.1
- Obermeyers's (European) A68.0
- Spirillum A68.9
- tick-borne (endemic) A68.1

Relationship
- occlusal
  - open anterior M26.220

Relationship — *continued*
  occlusal — *continued*
    open posterior M26.221
Relaxation
  anus (sphincter) K62.89
    psychogenic F45.8
  arch (foot) (*see also* Deformity, limb, flat foot)
  back ligaments — *see* Instability, joint, spine
  bladder (sphincter) N31.2
  cardioesophageal K21.9
  cervix — *see* Incompetency, cervix
  diaphragm J98.6
  joint (capsule) (ligament) (paralytic) — *see* Flail, joint
    congenital NEC Q74.8
  lumbosacral (joint) — *see* subcategory M53.2 ☑
  pelvic floor N81.89
  perineum N81.89
  posture R29.3
  rectum (sphincter) K62.89
  sacroiliac (joint) — *see* subcategory M53.2 ☑
  scrotum N50.8
  urethra (sphincter) N36.44
  vesical N31.2
Release from prison, anxiety concerning Z65.2
Remains
  canal of Cloquet Q14.0
  capsule (opaque) Q14.8
Remittent fever (malarial) B54
Remnant
  canal of Cloquet Q14.0
  capsule (opaque) Q14.8
  cervix, cervical stump (acquired) (postoperative) N88.8
  cystic duct, postcholecystectomy K91.5
  fingernail L60.8
    congenital Q84.6
  meniscus, knee — *see* Derangement, knee, meniscus,
    specified NEC
  thyroglossal duct Q89.2
  tonsil J35.8
    infected (chronic) J35.01
  urachus Q64.4
Removal (from) (of)
  artificial
    arm Z44.00- ☑
      complete Z44.01- ☑
      partial Z44.02- ☑
    eye Z44.2- ☑
    leg Z44.10- ☑
      complete Z44.11- ☑
      partial Z44.12- ☑
  breast implant Z45.81 ☑
  cardiac pulse generator (battery) (end-of-life) Z45.010
  catheter (urinary) (indwelling) Z46.6
    from artificial opening — *see* Attention to, artificial,
      opening
    non-vascular Z46.82
    vascular NEC Z45.2
  device Z46.9
    contraceptive Z30.432
    implanted NEC Z45.89
    specified NEC Z46.89
  drains Z48.03
  dressing (nonsurgical) Z48.00
    surgical Z48.01
  external
    fixation device — *code to* fracture with seventh
      character D
    prosthesis, prosthetic device Z44.9
      breast Z44.3- ☑
      specified NEC Z44.8
  home in childhood (to foster home or institution)
    Z62.29
  ileostomy Z43.2
  insulin pump Z46.81
  myringotomy device (stent) (tube) Z45.82
  nervous system device NEC Z46.2
    brain neuropacemaker Z46.2
    visual substitution device Z46.2
      implanted Z45.31
  non-vascular catheter Z46.82
  organ, prophylactic (for neoplasia management) —
    see Prophylactic, organ removal
  orthodontic device Z46.4
  staples Z48.02
  stent
    ureteral Z46.6
  suture Z48.02
  urinary device Z46.6

Removal — *continued*
  vascular access device or catheter Z45.2
Ren
  arcuatus Q63.1
  mobile, mobilis N28.89
    congenital Q63.8
  unguliformis Q63.1
Renal — *see* condition
Rendu-Osler-Weber disease or syndrome I78.0
Reninoma D41.0- ☑
Renon-Delille syndrome E23.3
Reovirus, as cause of disease classified elsewhere
  B97.5
Repeated falls NEC R29.6
Replaced chromosome by dicentric ring Q93.2
Replacement by artificial or mechanical device or
     prosthesis of
  bladder Z96.0
  blood vessel NEC Z95.828
  bone NEC Z96.7
  cochlea Z96.21
  coronary artery Z95.5
  eustachian tube Z96.29
  eye globe Z97.0
  heart Z95.812
    valve Z95.2
      prosthetic Z95.2
      specified NEC Z95.4
      xenogenic Z95.3
  intestine Z96.89
  joint Z96.60
    hip — *see* Presence, hip joint implant
    knee — *see* Presence, knee joint implant
    specified site NEC Z96.698
  larynx Z96.3
  lens Z96.1
  limb(s) — *see* Presence, artificial, limb
  mandible NEC (for tooth root implant(s)) Z96.5
  organ NEC Z96.89
  peripheral vessel NEC Z95.828
  stapes Z96.29
  teeth Z97.2
  tendon Z96.7
  tissue NEC Z96.89
  tooth root(s) Z96.5
  vessel NEC Z95.828
    coronary (artery) Z95.5
Request for expert evidence Z04.8
Reserve, decreased or low
  cardiac — *see* Disease, heart
  kidney N28.89
Residual (*see also* condition)
  ovary syndrome N99.83
  state, schizophrenic F20.5
  urine R39.19
Resistance, resistant (to)
  activated protein C D68.51
  complicating pregnancy O26.89 ☑
  insulin E88.81
  organism(s)
    to
      drug
        aminoglycosides Z16.29
        amoxicillin Z16.11
        ampicillin Z16.11
        antibiotic(s) Z16.20
          multiple Z16.24
          specified NEC Z16.29
        antifungal Z16.32
        antimicrobial (single) Z16.30
          multiple Z16.35
          specified NEC Z16.39
        antimycbacterial (single) Z16.341
          multiple Z16.342
        antiparasitic Z16.31
        antiviral Z16.33
        beta lactam antibiotics Z16.10
          specified NEC Z16.19
        cephalosporins Z16.19
        extended beta lactamase (ESBL) Z16.12
        fluoroquinolones Z16.23
        macrolides Z16.29
        methicillin — *see* MRSA
        multiple drugs (MDRO)
          antibiotics Z16.24
        penicillins Z16.11
        quinine (and related compounds) Z16.31
        quinolones Z16.23

Resistance, resistant — *continued*
  organism(s) — *continued*
    to — *continued*
      drug — *continued*
        sulfonamides Z16.29
        tetracyclines Z16.29
        tuberculostatics (single) Z16.341
          multiple Z16.342
        vancomycin Z16.21
          related antibiotics Z16.22
  thyroid hormone E07.89
Resorption
  dental (roots) K03.3
    alveoli M26.79
  teeth (external) (internal) (pathological) (roots) K03.3
Respiration
  Cheyne-Stokes R06.3
  decreased due to shock, following injury T79.4 ☑
  disorder of, psychogenic F45.8
  insufficient, or poor R06.89
    newborn P28.5
  painful R07.1
  sighing, psychogenic F45.8
Respiratory (*see also* condition)
  distress syndrome (newborn) (type I) P22.0
    type II P22.1
  syncytial virus, as cause of disease classified elsewhere
    B97.4
Respite care Z75.5
Response (drug)
  photoallergic L56.1
  phototoxic L56.0
Restless legs (syndrome) G25.81
Restlessness R45.1
Restoration (of)
  dental
    aesthetically inadequate or displeasing K08.56
    defective K08.50
      specified NEC K08.59
    failure of marginal integrity K08.51
    failure of periodontal anatomical intergrity K08.54
  organ continuity from previous sterilization (tuboplas-
    ty) (vasoplasty) Z31.0
    aftercare Z31.42
  tooth (existing)
    contours biologically incompatible with oral health
      K08.54
    open margins K08.51
    overhanging K08.52
    poor aesthetic K08.56
    poor gingival margins K08.51
    unsatisfactory, of tooth K08.50
      specified NEC K08.59
Restorative material (dental)
  allergy to K08.55
  fractured K08.539
    with loss of material K08.531
    without loss of material K08.530
  unrepairable overhanging of K08.52
Restriction of housing space Z59.1
Rests, ovarian, in fallopian tube Q50.6
Restzustand (schizophrenic) F20.5
Retained (*see also* Retention)
  cholelithiasis following cholecystectomy K91.86
  foreign body fragments (type of) Z18.9
    acrylics Z18.2
    animal quill(s) or spines Z18.31
    cement Z18.83
    concrete Z18.83
    crystalline Z18.83
    depleted isotope Z18.09
    depleted uranium Z18.01
    diethylhexylphthalates Z18.2
    glass Z18.81
    isocyanate Z18.2
    magnetic metal Z18.11
    metal Z18.10
    nonmagnetic metal Z18.12
    nontherapeutic radioactive Z18.09
    organic NEC Z18.39
    plastic Z18.2
    quill(s) (animal) Z18.31
    radioactive (nontherapeutic) NEC Z18.09
    specified NEC Z18.89
    spine(s) (animal) Z18.31
    stone Z18.83
    tooth (teeth) Z18.32
    wood Z18.33

Retained — *continued*
  fragments (type of) Z18.9
    acrylics Z18.2
    animal quill(s) or spines Z18.31
    cement Z18.83
    concrete Z18.83
    crystalline Z18.83
    depleted isotope Z18.09
    depleted uranium Z18.01
    diethylhexylphthalates Z18.2
    glass Z18.81
    isocyanate Z18.2
    magnetic metal Z18.11
    metal Z18.10
    nonmagnectic metal Z18.12
    nontherapeutic radioactive Z18.09
    organic NEC Z18.39
    plastic Z18.2
    quill(s) (animal) Z18.31
    radioactive (nontherapeutic) NEC Z18.09
    specified NEC Z18.89
    spine(s) (animal) Z18.31
    stone Z18.83
    tooth (teeth) Z18.32
    wood Z18.33
  gallstones, following cholecystectomy K91.86
Retardation
  development, developmental, specific — *see* Disorder, developmental
  endochondral bone growth — *see* Disorder, bone, development or growth
  growth R62.50
    due to malnutrition E45
  mental — *see* Disability, intellectual
  motor function, specific F82
  physical (child) R62.52
    due to malnutrition E45
  reading (specific) F81.0
  spelling (specific) (without reading disorder) F81.81
Retching — *see* Vomiting
Retention (*see also* Retained)
  bladder — *see* Retention, urine
  carbon dioxide E87.2
  cholelithiasis following cholecystectomy K91.86
  cyst — *see* Cyst
  dead
    fetus (at or near term) (mother) O36.4 ☑
      early fetal death O02.1
    ovum O02.0
  decidua (fragments) (following delivery) (with hemorrhage) O72.2
    without hemorrhage O73.1
  deciduous tooth K00.6
  dental root K08.3
  fecal — *see* Constipation
  fetus
    dead O36.4 ☑
      early O02.1
  fluid R60.9
  foreign body (*see also* Foreign body, retained)
    current trauma — *code as* Foreign body, by site or type
  gallstones, following cholecystectomy K91.86
  gastric K31.89
  intrauterine contraceptive device, in pregnancy — *see* Pregnancy, complicated by, retention, intrauterine device
  membranes (complicating delivery) (with hemorrhage) O72.2
    with abortion — *see* Abortion, by type
    without hemorrhage O73.1
  meniscus — *see* Derangement, meniscus
  menses N94.89
  milk (puerperal, postpartum) O92.79
  nitrogen, extrarenal R39.2
  ovary syndrome N99.83
  placenta (total) (with hemorrhage) O72.0
    without hemorrhage O73.0
    portions or fragments (with hemorrhage) O72.2
      without hemorrhage O73.1
  products of conception
    early pregnancy (dead fetus) O02.1
    following
      delivery (with hemorrhage) O72.2
        without hemorrhage O73.1
  secundines (following delivery) (with hemorrhage) O72.0
    without hemorrhage O73.0

Retention — *continued*
  secundines — *continued*
    complicating puerperium (delayed hemorrhage) O72.2
    partial O72.2
      without hemorrhage O73.1
  smegma, clitoris N90.89
  urine R33.9
    drug-induced R33.0
    due to hyperplasia (hypertrophy) of prostate — *see* Hyperplasia, prostate
    organic R33.8
      drug-induced R33.0
    psychogenic F45.8
    specified NEC R33.8
  water (in tissues) — *see* Edema
Reticulation, dust — *see* Pneumoconiosis
Reticulocytosis R70.1
Reticuloendotheliosis
  acute infantile C96.0
  leukemic C91.4- ☑
  malignant C96.9
  nonlipid C96.0
Reticulohistiocytoma (giant-cell) D76.3
Reticuloid, actinic L57.1
Reticulosis (skin)
  acute of infancy C96.0
  hemophagocytic, familial D76.1
  histiocytic medullary C96.9
  lipomelanotic I89.8
  malignant (midline) C86.0
  nonlipid C96.0
  polymorphic C83.8- ☑
  Sézary — *see* Sézary disease
Retina, retinal (*see also* condition)
  dark area D49.81
Retinitis (*see also* Inflammation, chorioretinal)
  albuminurica N18.9 [H32]
  diabetic — *see* Diabetes, retinitis
  disciformis — *see* Degeneration, macula
  focal — *see* Inflammation, chorioretinal, focal
  gravidarum — *see* Pregnancy, complicated by, specified pregnancy-related condition NEC
  juxtapapillaris — *see* Inflammation, chorioretinal, focal, juxtapapillary
  luetic — *see* Retinitis, syphilitic
  pigmentosa H35.52
  proliferans — *see* Disorder, globe, degenerative, specified type NEC
  proliferating — *see* Disorder, globe, degenerative, specified type NEC
  renal N18.9 [H32]
  syphilitic (early) (secondary) A51.43
    central, recurrent A52.71
    congenital (early) A50.01 [H32]
    late A52.71
  tuberculous A18.53
Retinoblastoma C69.2- ☑
  differentiated C69.2- ☑
  undifferentiated C69.2- ☑
Retinochoroiditis (*see also* Inflammation, chorioretinal)
  disseminated — *see* Inflammation, chorioretinal, disseminated
    syphilitic A52.71
  focal — *see* Inflammation, chorioretinal
  juxtapapillaris — *see* Inflammation, chorioretinal, focal, juxtapapillary
Retinopathy (background) H35.00
  arteriosclerotic I70.8 [H35.0-] ☑
  atherosclerotic I70.8 [H35.0-] ☑
  central serous — *see* Chorioretinopathy, central serous
  Coats H35.02- ☑
  diabetic — *see* Diabetes, retinopathy
  exudative H35.02- ☑
  hypertensive H35.03- ☑
  in (due to)
    diabetes — *see* Diabetes, retinopathy
    sickle-cell disorders D57.- ☑ [H36]
  of prematurity H35.10- ☑
    stage 0 H35.11- ☑
    stage 1 H35.12- ☑
    stage 2 H35.13- ☑
    stage 3 H35.14- ☑
    stage 4 H35.15- ☑
    stage 5 H35.16- ☑
  pigmentary, congenital — *see* Dystrophy, retina
  proliferative NEC H35.2- ☑

Retinopathy — *continued*
  proliferative — *continued*
    diabetic — *see* Diabetes, retinopathy, proliferative
    sickle-cell D57.- ☑ [H36]
  solar H31.02- ☑
Retinoschisis H33.10- ☑
  congenital Q14.1
  specified type NEC H33.19- ☑
Retortamoniasis A07.8
Retractile testis Q55.22
Retraction
  cervix — *see* Retroversion, uterus
  drum (membrane) — *see* Disorder, tympanic membrane, specified NEC
  finger — *see* Deformity, finger
  lid H02.539
    left H02.536
      lower H02.535
      upper H02.534
    right H02.533
      lower H02.532
      upper H02.531
  lung J98.4
  mediastinum J98.5
  nipple N64.53
    associated with
      lactation O92.03
      pregnancy O92.01- ☑
      puerperium O92.02
    congenital Q83.8
  palmar fascia M72.0
  pleura — *see* Pleurisy
  ring, uterus (Bandl's) (pathological) O62.4
  sternum (congenital) Q76.7
    acquired M95.4
  uterus — *see* Retroversion, uterus
  valve (heart) — *see* Endocarditis
Retrobulbar — *see* condition
Retrocecal — *see* condition
Retrocession — *see* Retroversion
Retrodisplacement — *see* Retroversion
Retroflection, retroflexion — *see* Retroversion
Retrognathia, retrognathism (mandibular) (maxillary) M26.19
Retrograde menstruation N92.5
Retroperineal — *see* condition
Retroperitoneal — *see* condition
Retroperitonitis K68.9
Retropharyngeal — *see* condition
Retroplacental — *see* condition
Retroposition — *see* Retroversion
Retroprosthetic membrane T85.398 ☑
Retrosternal thyroid (congenital) Q89.2
Retroversion, retroverted
  cervix — *see* Retroversion, uterus
  female NEC — *see* Retroversion, uterus
  iris H21.89
  testis (congenital) Q55.29
  uterus (acquired) (acute) (any degree) (asymptomatic) (cervix) (postinfectional) (postpartal, old) N85.4
    congenital Q51.818
    in pregnancy O34.53- ☑
Retrovirus, as cause of disease classified elsewhere B97.30
  human
    immunodeficiency, type 2 (HIV 2) B97.35
    T-cell lymphotropic
      type I (HTLV-I) B97.33
      type II (HTLV-II) B97.34
  lentivirus B97.31
  oncovirus B97.32
  specified NEC B97.39
Retrusion, premaxilla (developmental) M26.09
Rett's disease or syndrome F84.2
Reverse peristalsis R19.2
Reye's syndrome G93.7
Rh (factor)
  hemolytic disease (newborn) P55.0
  incompatibility, immunization or sensitization
    affecting management of pregnancy NEC O36.09- ☑
      anti-D antibody O36.01- ☑
    newborn P55.0
    transfusion reaction — *see* Complication(s), transfusion, incompatibility reaction, Rh (factor)
  negative mother affecting newborn P55.0

Rh — *continued*
  titer elevated — *see* Complication(s), transfusion, incompatibility reaction, Rh (factor)
  transfusion reaction — *see* Complication(s), transfusion, incompatibility reaction, Rh (factor)
Rhabdomyolysis (idiopathic) NEC M62.82
  traumatic T79.6 ☑
Rhabdomyoma (*see also* Neoplasm, connective tissue, benign)
  adult — *see* Neoplasm, connective tissue, benign
  fetal — *see* Neoplasm, connective tissue, benign
  glycogenic — *see* Neoplasm, connective tissue, benign
Rhabdomyosarcoma (any type) — *see* Neoplasm, connective tissue, malignant
Rhabdosarcoma — *see* Rhabdomyosarcoma
Rhesus (factor) **incompatibility** — *see* Rh, incompatibility
Rheumatic (acute) (subacute) (chronic)
  adherent pericardium I09.2
  coronary arteritis I01.9
  degeneration, myocardium I09.0
  fever (acute) — *see* Fever, rheumatic
  heart — *see* Disease, heart, rheumatic
  myocardial degeneration — *see* Degeneration, myocardium
  myocarditis (chronic) (inactive) (with chorea) I09.0
    with chorea (acute) (rheumatic) (Sydenham's) I02.0
    active or acute I01.2
  pancarditis, acute I01.8
    with chorea (acute) (rheumatic) Sydenham's) I02.0
  pericarditis (active) (acute) (with effusion) (with pneumonia) I01.0
    with chorea (acute) (rheumatic) (Sydenham's) I02.0
    chronic or inactive I09.2
  pneumonia I00 [J17]
  torticollis M43.6
  typhoid fever A01.09
Rheumatism (articular) (neuralgic) (nonarticular) M79.0
  gout — *see* Arthritis, rheumatoid
  intercostal, meaning Tietze's disease M94.0
  palindromic (any site) M12.30
    ankle M12.37- ☑
    elbow M12.32- ☑
    foot joint M12.37- ☑
    hand joint M12.34- ☑
    hip M12.35- ☑
    knee M12.36- ☑
    multiple site M12.39
    shoulder M12.31- ☑
    specified joint NEC M12.38
    vertebrae M12.38
    wrist M12.33- ☑
  sciatic M54.4- ☑
Rheumatoid (*see also* condition)
  arthritis (*see also* Arthritis, rheumatoid)
    with involvement of organs NEC M05.60
      ankle M05.67- ☑
      elbow M05.62- ☑
      foot joint M05.67- ☑
      hand joint M05.64- ☑
      hip M05.65- ☑
      knee M05.66- ☑
      multiple site M05.69
      shoulder M05.61- ☑
      vertebra — *see* Spondylitis, ankylosing
      wrist M05.63- ☑
    seronegative — *see* Arthritis, rheumatoid, seronegative
    seropositive — *see* Arthritis, rheumatoid, seropositive
  carditis M05.30
    ankle M05.37- ☑
    elbow M05.32- ☑
    foot joint M05.37- ☑
    hand joint M05.34- ☑
    hip M05.35- ☑
    knee M05.36- ☑
    multiple site M05.39
    shoulder M05.31- ☑
    vertebra — *see* Spondylitis, ankylosing
    wrist M05.33- ☑
  endocarditis — *see* Rheumatoid, carditis
  lung (disease) M05.10
    ankle M05.17- ☑
    elbow M05.12- ☑
    foot joint M05.17- ☑
    hand joint M05.14- ☑

Rheumatoid — *continued*
  lung — *continued*
    hip M05.15- ☑
    knee M05.16- ☑
    multiple site M05.19
    shoulder M05.11- ☑
    vertebra — *see* Spondylitis, ankylosing
    wrist M05.13- ☑
  myocarditis — *see* Rheumatoid, carditis
  myopathy M05.40
    ankle M05.47- ☑
    elbow M05.42- ☑
    foot joint M05.47- ☑
    hand joint M05.44- ☑
    hip M05.45- ☑
    knee M05.46- ☑
    multiple site M05.49
    shoulder M05.41- ☑
    vertebra — *see* Spondylitis, ankylosing
    wrist M05.43- ☑
  pericarditis — *see* Rheumatoid, carditis
  polyarthritis — *see* Arthritis, rheumatoid
  polyneuropathy M05.50
    ankle M05.57- ☑
    elbow M05.52- ☑
    foot joint M05.57- ☑
    hand joint M05.54- ☑
    hip M05.55- ☑
    knee M05.56- ☑
    multiple site M05.59
    shoulder M05.51- ☑
    vertebra — *see* Spondylitis, ankylosing
    wrist M05.53- ☑
  vasculitis M05.20
    ankle M05.27- ☑
    elbow M05.22- ☑
    foot joint M05.27- ☑
    hand joint M05.24- ☑
    hip M05.25- ☑
    knee M05.26- ☑
    multiple site M05.29
    shoulder M05.21- ☑
    vertebra — *see* Spondylitis, ankylosing
    wrist M05.23- ☑
Rhinitis (atrophic) (catarrhal) (chronic) (croupous) (fibrinous) (granulomatous) (hyperplastic) (hypertrophic) (membranous) (obstructive) (purulent) (suppurative) (ulcerative) J31.0
  with
    sore throat — *see* Nasopharyngitis
  acute J00
  allergic J30.9
    with asthma J45.909
      with
        exacerbation (acute) J45.901
        status asthmaticus J45.902
    due to
      food J30.5
      pollen J30.1
    nonseasonal J30.89
    perennial J30.89
    seasonal NEC J30.2
    specified NEC J30.89
  infective J00
  pneumococcal J00
  syphilitic A52.73
    congenital A50.05 [J99]
  tuberculous A15.8
  vasomotor J30.0
Rhinoantritis (chronic) — *see* Sinusitis, maxillary
Rhinodacryolith — *see* Dacryolith
Rhinolith (nasal sinus) J34.89
Rhinomegaly J34.89
Rhinopharyngitis (acute) (subacute) (*see also* Nasopharyngitis)
  chronic J31.1
  destructive ulcerating A66.5
  mutilans A66.5
Rhinophyma L71.1
Rhinorrhea J34.89
  cerebrospinal (fluid) G96.0
  paroxysmal — *see* Rhinitis, allergic
  spasmodic — *see* Rhinitis, allergic
Rhinosalpingitis — *see* Salpingitis, eustachian
Rhinoscleroma A48.8
Rhinosporidiosis B48.1
Rhinovirus infection NEC B34.8

Rhizomelic chondrodysplasia punctata E71.540
Rhythm
  atrioventricular nodal I49.8
  disorder I49.9
    coronary sinus I49.8
    ectopic I49.8
    nodal I49.8
  escape I49.9
  heart, abnormal I49.9
  idioventricular I44.2
  nodal I49.8
  sleep, inversion G47.2- ☑
    nonorganic origin — *see* Disorder, sleep, circadian rhythm, psychogenic
Rhytidosis facialis L98.8
Rib (*see also* condition)
  cervical Q76.5
Riboflavin deficiency E53.0
Rice bodies (*see also* Loose, body, joint)
  knee M23.4- ☑
Richter syndrome — *see* Leukemia, chronic lymphocytic, B-cell type
Richter's hernia — *see* Hernia, abdomen, with obstruction
Ricinism — *see* Poisoning, food, noxious, plant
Rickets (active) (acute) (adolescent) (chest wall) (congenital) (current) (infantile) (intestinal) E55.0
  adult — *see* Osteomalacia
  celiac K90.0
  hypophosphatemic with nephrotic-glycosuric dwarfism E72.09
  inactive E64.3
  kidney N25.0
  renal N25.0
  sequelae, any E64.3
  vitamin-D-resistant E83.31 [M90.80]
Rickettsial disease A79.9
  specified type NEC A79.89
Rickettsialpox (Rickettsia akari) A79.1
Rickettsiosis A79.9
  due to
    Ehrlichia sennetsu A79.81
    Rickettsia akari (rickettsialpox) A79.1
  specified type NEC A79.89
  tick-borne A77.9
  vesicular A79.1
Rider's bone — *see* Ossification, muscle, specified NEC
Ridge, aiveolus (*see also* condition)
  flabby K06.8
Ridged ear, congenital Q17.3
Riedel's
  lobe, liver Q44.7
  struma, thyroiditis or disease E06.5
Rieger's anomaly or syndrome Q13.81
Riehl's melanosis L81.4
Rietti-Greppi-Micheli anemia D56.9
Rieux's hernia — *see* Hernia, abdomen, specified site NEC
Riga (-Fede) **disease** K14.0
Riggs' disease — *see* Periodontitis
Right middle lobe syndrome J98.11
Rigid, rigidity (*see also* condition)
  abdominal R19.30
    with severe abdominal pain R10.0
    epigastric R19.36
    generalized R19.37
    left lower quadrant R19.34
    left upper quadrant R19.32
    periumbilic R19.35
    right lower quadrant R19.33
    right upper quadrant R19.31
  articular, multiple, congenital Q68.8
  cervix (uteri) in pregnancy — *see* Pregnancy, complicated by, abnormal, cervix
  hymen (acquired) (congenital) N89.6
  nuchal R29.1
  pelvic floor in pregnancy — *see* Pregnancy, complicated by, abnormal, pelvic organs or tissues NEC
  perineum or vulva in pregnancy — *see* Pregnancy, complicated by, abnormal, vulva
  spine — *see* Dorsopathy, specified NEC
  vagina in pregnancy — *see* Pregnancy, complicated by, abnormal, vagina
Rigors R68.89
  with fever R50.9
Riley-Day syndrome G90.1
RIND (reversible ischemic neurologic deficit) I63.9

☑ **Additional Character Required** — **Refer to the Tabular List for Character Selection**   ▽ **Subterms under main terms may continue to next column or page**

Ring(s)
aorta (vascular) Q25.4
Bandl's O62.4
contraction, complicating delivery O62.4
esophageal, lower (muscular) K22.2
Fleischer's (cornea) H18.04- ☑
hymenal, tight (acquired) (congenital) N89.6
Kayser-Fleischer (cornea) H18.04- ☑
retraction, uterus, pathological O62.4
Schatzki's (esophagus) (lower) K22.2
congenital Q39.3
Soemmerring's — see Cataract, secondary
vascular (congenital) Q25.8
aorta Q25.4
Ringed hair (congenital) Q84.1
Ringworm B35.9
beard B35.0
black dot B35.0
body B35.4
Burmese B35.5
corporeal B35.4
foot B35.3
groin B35.6
hand B35.2
honeycomb B35.0
nails B35.1
perianal (area) B35.6
scalp B35.0
specified NEC B35.8
Tokelau B35.5
Rise, venous pressure I87.8
Risk, suicidal
meaning personal history of attempted suicide Z91.5
meaning suicidal ideation — see Ideation, suicidal
Ritter's disease L00
Rivalry, sibling Z62.891
Rivalta's disease A42.2
River blindness B73.01
Robert's pelvis Q74.2
with disproportion (fetopelvic) O33.0
causing obstructed labor O65.0
Robin (-Pierre) **syndrome** Q87.0
Robinow-Silvermann-Smith syndrome Q87.1
Robinson's (hidrotic) **ectodermal dysplasia or syndrome** Q82.4
Robles' disease B73.01
Rocky Mountain (spotted) **fever** A77.0
Roetheln — see Rubella
Roger's disease Q21.0
Rokitansky-Aschoff sinuses (gallbladder) K82.8
Rolando's fracture (displaced) S62.22- ☑
nondisplaced S62.22- ☑
Romano-Ward (prolonged QT interval) **syndrome** I45.81
Romberg's disease or syndrome G51.8
Roof, mouth — see condition
Rosacea L71.9
acne L71.9
keratitis L71.8
specified NEC L71.8
Rosary, rachitic E55.0
Rose
cold J30.1
fever J30.1
rash R21
epidemic B06.9
Rosenbach's erysipeloid A26.0
Rosenthal's disease or syndrome D68.1
Roseola B09
infantum B08.20
due to human herpesvirus 6 B08.21
due to human herpesvirus 7 B08.22
Ross River disease or fever B33.1
Rossbach's disease K31.89
psychogenic F45.8
Rostan's asthma (cardiac) — see Failure, ventricular, left
Rotation
anomalous, incomplete or insufficient, intestine Q43.3
cecum (congenital) Q43.3
colon (congenital) Q43.3
spine, incomplete or insufficient — see Dorsopathy, deforming, specified NEC
tooth, teeth, fully erupted M26.35
vertebra, incomplete or insufficient — see Dorsopathy, deforming, specified NEC
Rotes Quérol disease or syndrome — see Hyperostosis, ankylosing

Roth (-Bernhardt) **disease or syndrome** — see Meralgia paraesthetica
Rothmund (-Thomson) **syndrome** Q82.8
Rotor's disease or syndrome E80.6
Round
back (with wedging of vertebrae) — see Kyphosis
sequelae (late effect) of rickets E64.3
worms (large) (infestation) NEC B82.0
Ascariasis (see also Ascariasis) B77.9
Roussy-Lévy syndrome G60.0
Rubella (German measles) B06.9
complication NEC B06.09
neurological B06.00
congenital P35.0
contact Z20.4
exposure to Z20.4
maternal
care for (suspected) damage to fetus O35.3 ☑
manifest rubella in infant P35.0
suspected damage to fetus affecting management of pregnancy O35.3 ☑
specified complications NEC B06.89
Rubeola (meaning measles) — see Measles
meaning rubella — see Rubella
Rubeosis, iris — see Disorder, iris, vascular
Rubinstein-Taybi syndrome Q87.2
Rudimentary (congenital) (see also Agenesis)
arm — see Defect, reduction, upper limb
bone Q79.9
cervix uteri Q51.828
eye Q11.2
lobule of ear Q17.3
patella Q74.1
respiratory organs in thoracopagus Q89.4
tracheal bronchus Q32.4
uterus Q51.818
in male Q56.1
vagina Q52.0
Ruled out condition — see Observation, suspected
Rumination R11.10
with nausea R11.2
disorder of infancy F98.21
neurotic F42
newborn P92.1
obsessional F42
psychogenic F42
Runeberg's disease D51.0
Runny nose R09.89
Rupia (syphilitic) A51.39
congenital A50.06
tertiary A52.79
Rupture, ruptured
abscess (spontaneous) — code by site under Abscess
aneurysm — see Aneurysm
anus (sphincter) — see Laceration, anus
aorta, aortic I71.8
abdominal I71.3
arch I71.1
ascending I71.1
descending I71.8
abdominal I71.3
thoracic I71.1
syphilitic A52.01
thoracoabdominal I71.5
thorax, thoracic I71.1
transverse I71.1
traumatic — see Injury, aorta, laceration, major
valve or cusp (see also Endocarditis, aortic) I35.8
appendix (with peritonitis) K35.2
arteriovenous fistula, brain I60.8
artery I77.2
brain — see Hemorrhage, intracranial, intracerebral
coronary — see Infarct, myocardium
heart — see Infarct, myocardium
pulmonary I28.8
traumatic (complication) — see Injury, blood vessel
bile duct (common) (hepatic) K83.2
cystic K82.2
bladder (sphincter) (nontraumatic) (spontaneous) N32.89
following ectopic or molar pregnancy O08.6
obstetrical trauma O71.5
traumatic S37.29 ☑
blood vessel (see also Hemorrhage)
brain — see Hemorrhage, intracranial, intracerebral
heart — see Infarct, myocardium

Rupture, ruptured — continued
blood vessel (see also Hemorrhage) — continued
traumatic (complication) — see Injury, blood vessel, laceration, major, by site
bone — see Fracture
bowel (nontraumatic) K63.1
brain
aneurysm (congenital) (see also Hemorrhage, intracranial, subarachnoid)
syphilitic A52.05
hemorrhagic — see Hemorrhage, intracranial, intracerebral
capillaries I78.8
cardiac (auricle) (ventricle) (wall) I23.3
with hemopericardium I23.0
infectional I40.9
traumatic — see Injury, heart
cartilage (articular) (current) (see also Sprain)
knee S83.3- ☑
semilunar — see Tear, meniscus
cecum (with peritonitis) K65.0
with peritoneal abscess K35.3
traumatic S36.598 ☑
celiac artery, traumatic — see Injury, blood vessel, celiac artery, laceration, major
cerebral aneurysm (congenital) (see Hemorrhage, intracranial, subarachnoid)
cervix (uteri)
with ectopic or molar pregnancy O08.6
following ectopic or molar pregnancy O08.6
obstetrical trauma O71.3
traumatic S37.69 ☑
chordae tendineae NEC I51.1
concurrent with acute myocardial infarction — see Infarct, myocardium
following acute myocardial infarction (current complication) I23.4
choroid (direct) (indirect) (traumatic) H31.32- ☑
circle of Willis I60.6
colon (nontraumatic) K63.1
traumatic — see Injury, intestine, large
cornea (traumatic) — see Injury, eye, laceration
coronary (artery) (thrombotic) — see Infarct, myocardium
corpus luteum (infected) (ovary) N83.1
cyst — see Cyst
cystic duct K82.2
Descemet's membrane — see Change, corneal membrane, Descemet's, rupture
traumatic — see Injury, eye, laceration
diaphragm, traumatic — see Injury, intrathoracic, diaphragm
disc — see Rupture, intervertebral disc
diverticulum (intestine) K57.80
with bleeding K57.81
bladder N32.3
large intestine K57.20
with
bleeding K57.21
small intestine K57.40
with bleeding K57.41
small intestine K57.00
with
bleeding K57.01
large intestine K57.40
with bleeding K57.41
duodenal stump K31.89
ear drum (nontraumatic) (see also Perforation, tympanum)
traumatic S09.2- ☑
due to blast injury — see Injury, blast, ear
esophagus K22.3
eye (without prolapse or loss of intraocular tissue) — see Injury, eye, laceration
fallopian tube NEC (nonobstetric) (nontraumatic) N83.8
due to pregnancy O00.1
fontanel P13.1
gallbladder K82.2
traumatic S36.128 ☑
gastric (see also Rupture, stomach)
vessel K92.2
globe (eye) (traumatic) — see Injury, eye, laceration
graafian follicle (hematoma) N83.0
heart — see Rupture, cardiac
hymen (nontraumatic) (nonintentional) N89.8
internal organ, traumatic — see Injury, by site

Rupture, ruptured — *continued*
  intervertebral disc — *see* Displacement, intervertebral disc
    traumatic — *see* Rupture, traumatic, intervertebral disc
  intestine NEC (nontraumatic) K63.1
    traumatic — *see* Injury, intestine
  iris (*see also* Abnormality, pupillary)
    traumatic — *see* Injury, eye, laceration
  joint capsule, traumatic — *see* Sprain
  kidney (traumatic) S37.06- ☑
    birth injury P15.8
    nontraumatic N28.89
  lacrimal duct (traumatic) — *see* Injury, eye, specified site NEC
  lens (cataract) (traumatic) — *see* Cataract, traumatic
  ligament, traumatic — *see* Rupture, traumatic, ligament, by site
  liver S36.116 ☑
    birth injury P15.0
  lymphatic vessel I89.8
  marginal sinus (placental) (with hemorrhage) — *see* Hemorrhage, antepartum, specified cause NEC
  membrana tympani (nontraumatic) — *see* Perforation, tympanum
  membranes (spontaneous)
    artificial
      delayed delivery following O75.5
    delayed delivery following — *see* Pregnancy, complicated by, premature rupture of membranes
  meningeal artery I60.8
  meniscus (knee) (*see also* Tear, meniscus)
    old — *see* Derangement, meniscus
    site other than knee — *code as* Sprain
  mesenteric artery, traumatic — *see* Injury, mesenteric, artery, laceration, major
  mesentery (nontraumatic) K66.8
    traumatic — *see* Injury, intra-abdominal, specified, site NEC
  mitral (valve) I34.8
  muscle (traumatic) (*see also* Strain)
    diastasis — *see* Diastasis, muscle
    nontraumatic M62.10
      ankle M62.17- ☑
      foot M62.17- ☑
      forearm M62.13- ☑
      hand M62.14- ☑
      lower leg M62.16- ☑
      pelvic region M62.15- ☑
      shoulder region M62.11- ☑
      specified site NEC M62.18
      thigh M62.15- ☑
      upper arm M62.12- ☑
    traumatic — *see* Strain, by site
  musculotendinous junction NEC, nontraumatic — *see* Rupture, tendon, spontaneous
  mycotic aneurysm causing cerebral hemorrhage — *see* Hemorrhage, intracranial, subarachnoid
  myocardium, myocardial — *see* Rupture, cardiac
    traumatic — *see* Injury, heart
  nontraumatic, meaning hernia — *see* Hernia
  obstructed — *see* Hernia, by site, obstructed
  operation wound — *see* Disruption, wound, operation
  ovary, ovarian N83.0
    corpus luteum cyst N83.1
    follicle (graafian) N83.0
  oviduct (nonobstetric) (nontraumatic) N83.8
    due to pregnancy O00.1
  pancreas (nontraumatic) K86.8
    traumatic S36.299 ☑
  papillary muscle NEC I51.2
    following acute myocardial infarction (current complication) I23.5
  pelvic
    floor, complicating delivery O70.1
    organ NEC, obstetrical trauma O71.5
  perineum (nonobstetric) (nontraumatic) N90.89
    complicating delivery — *see* Delivery, complicated, by, laceration, anus (sphincter)
  postoperative wound — *see* Disruption, wound, operation
  prostate (traumatic) S37.828 ☑
  pulmonary
    artery I28.8
    valve (heart) I37.8
    vein I28.8

Rupture, ruptured — *continued*
  pulmonary — *continued*
    vessel I28.8
  pus tube — *see* Salpingitis
  pyosalpinx — *see* Salpingitis
  rectum (nontraumatic) K63.1
    traumatic S36.69 ☑
  retina, retinal (traumatic) (without detachment) (*see also* Break, retina)
    with detachment — *see* Detachment, retina, with retinal, break
  rotator cuff (nontraumatic) M75.10- ☑
    complete M75.12- ☑
    incomplete M75.11- ☑
  sclera — *see* Injury, eye, laceration
  sigmoid (nontraumatic) K63.1
    traumatic S36.593 ☑
  spinal cord (*see also* Injury, spinal cord, by region)
    due to injury at birth P11.5
    newborn (birth injury) P11.5
  spleen S36.09 ☑
    birth injury P15.1
    congenital (birth injury) P15.1
    due to P. vivax malaria B51.0
    nontraumatic D73.5
    spontaneous D73.5
  splenic vein R58
    traumatic — *see* Injury, blood vessel, splenic vein
  stomach (nontraumatic) (spontaneous) K31.89
    traumatic S36.39 ☑
  supraspinatus (complete) (incomplete) (nontraumatic) — *see* Tear, rotator cuff
  symphysis pubis
    obstetric O71.6
    traumatic S33.4 ☑
  synovium (cyst) M66.10
    ankle M66.17- ☑
    elbow M66.12- ☑
    finger M66.14- ☑
    foot M66.17- ☑
    forearm M66.13- ☑
    hand M66.14- ☑
    pelvic region M66.15- ☑
    shoulder region M66.11- ☑
    specified site NEC M66.18
    thigh M66.15- ☑
    toe M66.17- ☑
    upper arm M66.12- ☑
    wrist M66.13- ☑
  tendon (traumatic) — *see* Strain
    nontraumatic (spontaneous) M66.9
      ankle M66.87- ☑
      extensor M66.20
        ankle M66.27- ☑
        foot M66.27- ☑
        forearm M66.23- ☑
        hand M66.24- ☑
        lower leg M66.26- ☑
        multiple sites M66.29
        pelvic region M66.25- ☑
        shoulder region M66.21- ☑
        specified site NEC M66.28
        thigh M66.25- ☑
        upper arm M66.22- ☑
      flexor M66.30
        ankle M66.37- ☑
        foot M66.37- ☑
        forearm M66.33- ☑
        hand M66.34- ☑
        lower leg M66.36- ☑
        multiple sites M66.39
        pelvic region M66.35- ☑
        shoulder region M66.31- ☑
        specified site NEC M66.38
        thigh M66.35- ☑
        upper arm M66.32- ☑
      foot M66.87- ☑
      forearm M66.83- ☑
      hand M66.84- ☑
      lower leg M66.86- ☑
      multiple sites M66.89
      pelvic region M66.85- ☑
      shoulder region M66.81- ☑
      specified
        site NEC M66.88
        tendon M66.80

Rupture, ruptured — *continued*
  tendon — *see* Strain — *continued*
    nontraumatic — *continued*
      thigh M66.85- ☑
      upper arm M66.82- ☑
  thoracic duct I89.8
  tonsil J35.8
  traumatic
    aorta — *see* Injury, aorta, laceration, major
    diaphragm — *see* Injury, intrathoracic, diaphragm
    external site — *see* Wound, open, by site
    eye — *see* Injury, eye, laceration
    internal organ — *see* Injury, by site
    intervertebral disc
      cervical S13.0 ☑
      lumbar S33.0 ☑
      thoracic S23.0 ☑
    kidney S37.06- ☑
    ligament (*see also* Sprain)
      ankle — *see* Sprain, ankle
      carpus — *see* Rupture, traumatic, ligament, wrist
      collateral (hand) — *see* Rupture, traumatic, ligament, finger, collateral
      finger (metacarpophalangeal) (interphalangeal) S63.40- ☑
        collateral S63.41- ☑
          index S63.41- ☑
          little S63.41- ☑
          middle S63.41- ☑
          ring S63.41- ☑
        index S63.40- ☑
        little S63.40- ☑
        middle S63.40- ☑
        palmar S63.42- ☑
          index S63.42- ☑
          little S63.42- ☑
          middle S63.42- ☑
          ring S63.42- ☑
        ring S63.40- ☑
        specified site NEC S63.499 ☑
          index S63.49- ☑
          little S63.49- ☑
          middle S63.49- ☑
          ring S63.49- ☑
        volar plate S63.43- ☑
          index S63.43- ☑
          little S63.43- ☑
          middle S63.43- ☑
          ring S63.43- ☑
      foot — *see* Sprain, foot
      radial collateral S53.2- ☑
      radiocarpal — *see* Rupture, traumatic, ligament, wrist, radiocarpal
      ulnar collateral S53.3- ☑
      ulnocarpal — *see* Rupture, traumatic, ligament, wrist, ulnocarpal
      wrist S63.30- ☑
        collateral S63.31- ☑
        radiocarpal S63.32- ☑
        specified site NEC S63.39- ☑
        ulnocarpal (palmar) S63.33- ☑
    liver S36.116 ☑
    membrana tympani — *see* Rupture, ear drum, traumatic
    muscle or tendon — *see* Strain
    myocardium — *see* Injury, heart
    pancreas S36.299 ☑
    rectum S36.69 ☑
    sigmoid S36.593 ☑
    spleen S36.09 ☑
    stomach S36.39 ☑
    symphysis pubis S33.4 ☑
    tympanum, tympanic (membrane) — *see* Rupture, ear drum, traumatic
    ureter S37.19 ☑
    uterus S37.69 ☑
    vagina — *see* Injury, vagina
    vena cava — *see* Injury, vena cava, laceration, major
  tricuspid (heart) (valve) I07.8
  tube, tubal (nonobstetric) (nontraumatic) N83.8
    abscess — *see* Salpingitis
    due to pregnancy O00.1

    ☑ **Additional Character Required** — Refer to the Tabular List for Character Selection   ▽ Subterms under main terms may continue to next column or page

Rupture, ruptured — *continued*
- tympanum, tympanic (membrane) (nontraumatic) (*see also* Perforation, tympanic membrane) H72.9- ☑
  - traumatic — *see* Rupture, ear drum, traumatic
- umbilical cord, complicating delivery O69.89 ☑
- ureter (traumatic) S37.19 ☑
  - nontraumatic N28.89
- urethra (nontraumatic) N36.8
  - with ectopic or molar pregnancy O08.6
  - following ectopic or molar pregnancy O08.6
  - obstetrical trauma O71.5
  - traumatic S37.39 ☑
- uterosacral ligament (nonobstetric) (nontraumatic) N83.8
- uterus (traumatic) S37.69 ☑
  - before labor O71.0- ☑
  - during or after labor O71.1
  - nonpuerperal, nontraumatic N85.8
  - pregnant (during labor) O71.1
    - before labor O71.0- ☑
- vagina — *see* Injury, vagina
- valve, valvular (heart) — *see* Endocarditis
- varicose vein — *see* Varix
- varix — *see* Varix
- vena cava R58
  - traumatic — *see* Injury, vena cava, laceration, major
- vesical (urinary) N32.89
- vessel (blood) R58
  - pulmonary I28.8
  - traumatic — *see* Injury, blood vessel
- viscus R19.8
- vulva complicating delivery O70.0

Russell-Silver syndrome Q87.1
Russian spring-summer type encephalitis A84.0
Rust's disease (tuberculous cervical spondylitis) A18.01
Ruvalcaba-Myhre-Smith syndrome E71.440
Rytand-Lipsitch syndrome I44.2

S

Saber, sabre shin or tibia (syphilitic) A50.56 [M90.8-] ☑
Sac lacrimal — *see* condition
Saccharomyces infection B37.9
Saccharopinuria E72.3
Saccular — *see* condition
Sacculation
- aorta (nonsyphilitic) — *see* Aneurysm, aorta
- bladder N32.3
- intralaryngeal (congenital) (ventricular) Q31.3
- larynx (ventricular) Q31.3
- organ or site, congenital — *see* Distortion
- pregnant uterus — *see* Pregnancy, complicated by, abnormal, uterus
- ureter N28.89
- urethra N36.1
- vesical N32.3

Sachs' amaurotic familial idiocy or disease E75.02
Sachs-Tay disease E75.02
Sacks-Libman disease M32.11
Sacralgia M53.3
Sacralization Q76.49
Sacrodynia M53.3
Sacroiliac joint — *see* condition
Sacroiliitis NEC M46.1
Sacrum — *see* condition
Saddle
- back — *see* Lordosis
- embolus
  - abdominal aorta I74.01
  - pulmonary artery I26.92
    - with acute cor pulmonale I26.02
  - injury — *code to* condition
- nose M95.0
  - due to syphilis A50.57

Sadism (sexual) F65.52
Sadness, postpartal O90.6
Sadomasochism F65.50
Saemisch's ulcer (cornea) — *see* Ulcer, cornea, central
Sahib disease B55.0
Sailors' skin L57.8
Saint
- Anthony's fire — *see* Erysipelas
- triad — *see* Hernia, diaphragm
- Vitus' dance — *see* Chorea, Sydenham's

Salaam
- attack(s) — *see* Epilepsy, spasms

Salaam — *continued*
- tic R25.8

Salicylism
- abuse F55.8
- overdose or wrong substance given — *see* Table of Drugs and Chemicals, by drug, poisoning

Salivary duct or gland — *see* condition
Salivation, excessive K11.7
Salmonella — *see* Infection, Salmonella
Salmonellosis A02.0
Salpingitis (catarrhal) (fallopian tube) (nodular) (pseudofollicular) (purulent) (septic) N70.91
- with oophoritis N70.93
- acute N70.01
  - with oophoritis N70.03
- chlamydial A56.11
- chronic N70.11
  - with oophoritis N70.13
- complicating abortion — *see* Abortion, by type, complicated by, salpingitis
- ear — *see* Salpingitis, eustachian
- eustachian (tube) H68.00- ☑
  - acute H68.01- ☑
  - chronic H68.02- ☑
- follicularis N70.11
  - with oophoritis N70.13
- gonococcal (acute) (chronic) A54.24
- interstitial, chronic N70.11
  - with oophoritis N70.13
- isthmica nodosa N70.11
  - with oophoritis N70.13
- specific (gonococcal) (acute) (chronic) A54.24
- tuberculous (acute) (chronic) A18.17
- venereal (gonococcal) (acute) (chronic) A54.24

Salpingocele N83.4
Salpingo-oophoritis (catarrhal) (purulent) (ruptured) (septic) (suppurative) N70.93
- acute N70.03
  - with ectopic or molar pregnancy O08.0
  - following ectopic or molar pregnancy O08.0
  - gonococcal A54.24
- chronic N70.13
- following ectopic or molar pregnancy O08.0
- gonococcal (acute) (chronic) A54.24
- puerperal O86.19
- specific (gonococcal) (acute) (chronic) A54.24
- subacute N70.03
- tuberculous (acute) (chronic) A18.17
- venereal (gonococcal) (acute) (chronic) A54.24

Salpingo-ovaritis — *see* Salpingo-oophoritis
Salpingoperitonitis — *see* Salpingo-oophoritis
Salzmann's nodular dystrophy — *see* Degeneration, cornea, nodular
Sampson's cyst or tumor N80.1
San Joaquin (Valley) **fever** B38.0
Sandblaster's asthma, lung or pneumoconiosis J62.8
Sander's disease (paranoia) F22
Sandfly fever A93.1
Sandhoff's disease E75.01
Sanfilippo (Type B) (Type C) (Type D) **syndrome** E76.22
Sanger-Brown ataxia G11.2
Sao Paulo fever or typhus A77.0
Saponification, mesenteric K65.8
Sarcocele (benign)
- syphilitic A52.76
  - congenital A50.59

Sarcocystosis A07.8
Sarcoepiplocele — *see* Hernia
Sarcoepiplomphalocele Q79.2
Sarcoid (*see also* Sarcoidosis)
- arthropathy D86.86
- Boeck's D86.9
- Darier-Roussy D86.3
- iridocyclitis D86.83
- meningitis D86.81
- myocarditis D86.85
- myositis D86.87
- pyelonephritis D86.84
- Spiegler-Fendt L08.89

Sarcoidosis D86.9
- with
  - cranial nerve palsies D86.82
  - hepatic granuloma D86.89
  - polyarthritis D86.86
  - tubulo-interstitial nephropathy D86.84
- combined sites NEC D86.89
- lung D86.0

Sarcoidosis — *continued*
- lung — *continued*
  - and lymph nodes D86.2
- lymph nodes D86.1
  - and lung D86.2
- meninges D86.81
- skin D86.3
- specified type NEC D86.89

Sarcoma (of) (*see also* Neoplasm, connective tissue, malignant)
- alveolar soft part — *see* Neoplasm, connective tissue, malignant
- ameloblastic C41.1
  - upper jaw (bone) C41.0
- botryoid — *see* Neoplasm, connective tissue, malignant
- botryoides — *see* Neoplasm, connective tissue, malignant
- cerebellar C71.6
  - circumscribed (arachnoidal) C71.6
- circumscribed (arachnoidal) cerebellar C71.6
- clear cell (*see also* Neoplasm, connective tissue, malignant)
  - kidney C64.- ☑
- dendritic cells (accessory cells) C96.4
- embryonal — *see* Neoplasm, connective tissue, malignant
- endometrial (stromal) C54.1
  - isthmus C54.0
- epithelioid (cell) — *see* Neoplasm, connective tissue, malignant
- Ewing's — *see* Neoplasm, bone, malignant
- follicular dendritic cell C96.4
- germinoblastic (diffuse) — *see* Lymphoma, diffuse large cell
- follicular — *see* Lymphoma, follicular, specified NEC
- giant cell (except of bone) (*see also* Neoplasm, connective tissue, malignant)
  - bone — *see* Neoplasm, bone, malignant
- glomoid — *see* Neoplasm, connective tissue, malignant
- granulocytic C92.3- ☑
- hemangioendothelial — *see* Neoplasm, connective tissue, malignant
- hemorrhagic, multiple — *see* Sarcoma, Kaposi's
- histiocytic C96.A (*following* C96.6)
- Hodgkin — *see* Lymphoma, Hodgkin
- immunoblastic (diffuse) — *see* Lymphoma, diffuse large cell
- interdigitating dendritic cell C96.4
- Kaposi's
  - colon C46.4
  - connective tissue C46.1
  - gastrointestinal organ C46.4
  - lung C46.5- ☑
  - lymph node(s) C46.3
  - palate (hard) (soft) C46.2
  - rectum C46.4
  - skin C46.0
  - specified site NEC C46.7
  - stomach C46.4
  - unspecified site C46.9
- Kupffer cell C22.3
- Langerhans cell C96.4
- leptomeningeal — *see* Neoplasm, meninges, malignant
- liver NEC C22.4
- lymphangioendothelial — *see* Neoplasm, connective tissue, malignant
- lymphoblastic — *see* Lymphoma, lymphoblastic (diffuse)
- lymphocytic — *see* Lymphoma, small cell B-cell
- mast cell C96.2
- melanotic — *see* Melanoma
- meningeal — *see* Neoplasm, meninges, malignant
- meningothelial — *see* Neoplasm, meninges, malignant
- mesenchymal (*see also* Neoplasm, connective tissue, malignant)
  - mixed — *see* Neoplasm, connective tissue, malignant
- mesothelial — *see* Mesothelioma
- monstrocellular
  - specified site — *see* Neoplasm, malignant, by site
  - unspecified site C71.9
- myeloid C92.3- ☑
- neurogenic — *see* Neoplasm, nerve, malignant

Sarcoma — *continued*
  odontogenic C41.1
    upper jaw (bone) C41.0
  osteoblastic — *see* Neoplasm, bone, malignant
  osteogenic (*see also* Neoplasm, bone, malignant)
    juxtacortical — *see* Neoplasm, bone, malignant
    periosteal — *see* Neoplasm, bone, malignant
  periosteal (*see also* Neoplasm, bone, malignant)
    osteogenic — *see* Neoplasm, bone, malignant
  pleomorphic cell — *see* Neoplasm, connective tissue, malignant
  reticulum cell (diffuse) — *see* Lymphoma, diffuse large cell
    nodular — *see* Lymphoma, follicular
    pleomorphic cell type — *see* Lymphoma, diffuse large cell
  rhabdoid — *see* Neoplasm, malignant, by site
  round cell — *see* Neoplasm, connective tissue, malignant
  small cell — *see* Neoplasm, connective tissue, malignant
  soft tissue — *see* Neoplasm, connective tissue, malignant
  spindle cell — *see* Neoplasm, connective tissue, malignant
  stromal (endometrial) C54.1
    isthmus C54.0
  synovial (*see also* Neoplasm, connective tissue, malignant)
    biphasic — *see* Neoplasm, connective tissue, malignant
    epithelioid cell — *see* Neoplasm, connective tissue, malignant
    spindle cell — *see* Neoplasm, connective tissue, malignant
Sarcomatosis
  meningeal — *see* Neoplasm, meninges, malignant
  specified site NEC — *see* Neoplasm, connective tissue, malignant
  unspecified site C80.1
Sarcosinemia E72.59
Sarcosporidiosis (intestinal) A07.8
Satiety, early R68.81
Saturnine — *see* condition
Saturnism
  overdose or wrong substance given or taken — *see* Table of Drugs and Chemicals, by drug, poisoning
Satyriasis F52.8
Sauriasis — *see* Ichthyosis
SBE (subacute bacterial endocarditis) I33.0
Scabies (any site) B86
Scabs R23.4
Scaglietti-Dagnini syndrome E22.0
Scald — *see* Burn
Scalenus anticus (anterior) **syndrome** G54.0
Scales R23.4
Scaling, skin R23.4
Scalp — *see* condition
Scapegoating affecting child Z62.3
Scaphocephaly Q75.0
Scapulalgia M89.8X1
Scapulohumeral myopathy G71.0
Scar, scarring (*see also* Cicatrix) L90.5
  adherent L90.5
  atrophic L90.5
  cervix
    in pregnancy or childbirth — *see* Pregnancy, complicated by, abnormal cervix
  cheloid L91.0
  chorioretinal H31.00- ☑
    posterior pole macula H31.01- ☑
    postsurgical H59.81- ☑
    solar retinopathy H31.02- ☑
    specified type NEC H31.09- ☑
  choroid — *see* Scar, chorioretinal
  conjunctiva H11.24- ☑
  cornea H17.9
    xerophthalmic (*see also* Opacity, cornea)
      vitamin A deficiency E50.6
  duodenum, obstructive K31.5
  hypertrophic L91.0
  keloid L91.0
  labia N90.89
  lung (base) J98.4
  macula — *see* Scar, chorioretinal, posterior pole
  muscle M62.89

Scar, scarring — *continued*
  myocardium, myocardial I25.2
  painful L90.5
  posterior pole (eye) — *see* Scar, chorioretinal, posterior pole
  retina — *see* Scar, chorioretinal
  trachea J39.8
  uterus N85.8
    in pregnancy O34.29
  vagina N89.8
    postoperative N99.2
  vulva N90.89
Scarabiasis B88.2
Scarlatina (anginosa) (maligna) (ulcerosa) A38.9
  myocarditis (acute) A38.1
    old — *see* Myocarditis
  otitis media A38.0
Scarlet fever (albuminuria) (angina) A38.9
Schamberg's disease (progressive pigmentary dermatosis) L81.7
Schatzki's ring (acquired) (esophagus) (lower) K22.2
  congenital Q39.3
Schaufenster krankheit I20.8
Schaumann's
  benign lymphogranulomatosis D86.1
  disease or syndrome — *see* Sarcoidosis
Scheie's syndrome E76.03
Schenck's disease B42.1
Scheuermann's disease or osteochondrosis — *see* Osteochondrosis, juvenile, spine
Schilder (-Flatau) **disease** G37.0
Schilling-type monocytic leukemia C93.0- ☑
Schimmelbusch's disease, cystic mastitis, or hyperplasia — *see* Mastopathy, cystic
Schistosoma infestation — *see* Infestation, Schistosoma
Schistosomiasis B65.9
  with muscle disorder B65.9 [M63.80]
    ankle B65.9 [M63.87-] ☑
    foot B65.9 [M63.87-] ☑
    forearm B65.9 [M63.83-] ☑
    hand B65.9 [M63.84-] ☑
    lower leg B65.9 [M63.86-] ☑
    multiple sites B65.9 [M63.89]
    pelvic region B65.9 [M63.85-] ☑
    shoulder region B65.9 [M63.81-] ☑
    specified site NEC B65.9 [M63.88]
    thigh B65.9 [M63.85-] ☑
    upper arm B65.9 [M63.82-] ☑
  Asiatic B65.2
  bladder B65.0
  chestermani B65.8
  colon B65.1
  cutaneous B65.3
  due to
    S. haematobium B65.0
    S. japonicum B65.2
    S. mansoni B65.1
    S. mattheii B65.8
  Eastern B65.2
  genitourinary tract B65.0
  intestinal B65.1
  lung NEC B65.9 [J99]
    pneumonia B65.9 [J17]
  Manson's (intestinal) B65.1
  oriental B65.2
  pulmonary NEC B65.9 [J99]
    pneumonia B65.9
  Schistosoma
    haematobium B65.0
    japonicum B65.2
    mansoni B65.1
  specified type NEC B65.8
  urinary B65.0
  vesical B65.0
Schizencephaly Q04.6
Schizoaffective psychosis F25.9
Schizodontia K00.2
Schizoid personality F60.1
Schizophrenia, schizophrenic F20.9
  acute (brief) (undifferentiated) F23
  atypical (form) F20.3
  borderline F21
  catalepsy F20.2
  catatonic (type) (excited) (withdrawn) F20.2
  cenesthopathic, cenesthesiopathic F20.89
  childhood type F84.5
  chronic undifferentiated F20.5

Schizophrenia, schizophrenic — *continued*
  cyclic F25.0
  disorganized (type) F20.1
  flexibilitas cerea F20.2
  hebephrenic (type) F20.1
  incipient F21
  latent F21
  negative type F20.5
  paranoid (type) F20.0
  paraphrenic F20.0
  post-psychotic depression F32.8
  prepsychotic F21
  prodromal F21
  pseudoneurotic F21
  pseudopsychopathic F21
  reaction F23
  residual (state) (type) F20.5
  restzustand F20.5
  schizoaffective (type) — *see* Psychosis, schizoaffective
  simple (type) F20.89
  simplex F20.89
  specified type NEC F20.89
  stupor F20.2
  syndrome of childhood F84.5
  undifferentiated (type) F20.3
    chronic F20.5
Schizothymia (persistent) F60.1
Schlatter-Osgood disease or osteochondrosis — *see* Osteochondrosis, juvenile, tibia
Schlatter's tibia — *see* Osteochondrosis, juvenile, tibia
Schmidt's syndrome (polyglandular, autoimmune) E31.0
Schmincke's carcinoma or tumor — *see* Neoplasm, nasopharynx, malignant
Schmitz (-Stutzer) **dysentery** A03.0
Schmorl's disease or nodes
  lumbar region M51.46
  lumbosacral region M51.47
  sacrococcygeal region M53.3
  thoracic region M51.44
  thoracolumbar region M51.45
Schneiderian
  papilloma — *see* Neoplasm, nasopharynx, benign
    specified site — *see* Neoplasm, benign, by site
    unspecified site D14.0
  specified site — *see* Neoplasm, malignant, by site
    unspecified site C30.0
Scholte's syndrome (malignant carcinoid) E34.0
Scholz (-Bielchowsky-Henneberg) **disease or syndrome** E75.25
Schönlein (-Henoch) disease or purpura (primary) (rheumatic) D69.0
Schottmuller's disease A01.4
Schroeder's syndrome (endocrine hypertensive) E27.0
Schüller-Christian disease or syndrome C96.5
Schultze's type acroparesthesia, simple I73.89
Schultz's disease or syndrome — *see* Agranulocytosis
Schwalbe-Ziehen-Oppenheim disease G24.1
Schwannoma (*see also* Neoplasm, nerve, benign)
  malignant (*see also* Neoplasm, nerve, malignant)
    with rhabdomyoblastic differentiation — *see* Neoplasm, nerve, malignant
    melanocytic — *see* Neoplasm, nerve, benign
    pigmented — *see* Neoplasm, nerve, benign
Schwannomatosis Q85.03
Schwartz (-Jampel) **syndrome** G71.13
Schwartz-Bartter syndrome E22.2
Schweniger-Buzzi anetoderma L90.1
Sciatic — *see* condition
Sciatica (infective)
  with lumbago M54.4- ☑
    due to intervertebral disc disorder — *see* Disorder, disc, with, radiculopathy
  due to displacement of intervertebral disc (with lumbago) — *see* Disorder, disc, with, radiculopathy
  wallet M54.3- ☑
Scimitar syndrome Q26.8
Sclera — *see* condition
Sclerectasia H15.84- ☑
Scleredema
  adultorum — *see* Sclerosis, systemic
  Buschke's — *see* Sclerosis, systemic
  newborn P83.0
Sclerema (adiposum) (edematosum) (neonatorum) (newborn) P83.0
  adultorum — *see* Sclerosis, systemic
Scleriasis — *see* Scleroderma
Scleritis H15.00- ☑

Scleritis — *continued*
  with corneal involvement H15.04- ☑
    anterior H15.01- ☑
    brawny H15.02- ☑
    in (due to) zoster B02.34
    posterior H15.03- ☑
    specified type NEC H15.09- ☑
    syphilitic A52.71
    tuberculous (nodular) A18.51
Sclerochoroiditis H31.8
Scleroconjunctivitis — *see* Scleritis
Sclerocystic ovary syndrome E28.2
Sclerodactyly, sclerodactylia L94.3
Scleroderma, sclerodermia (acrosclerotic) (diffuse) (generalized) (progressive) (pulmonary) (*see also* Sclerosis, systemic) M34.9
  circumscribed L94.0
  linear L94.1
  localized L94.0
  newborn P83.8
  systemic M34.9
Sclerokeratitis H16.8
  tuberculous A18.52
Scleroma nasi A48.8
Scleromalacia (perforans) H15.05- ☑
Scleromyxedema L98.5
Sclérose en plaques G35
Sclerosis, sclerotic
  adrenal (gland) E27.8
  Alzheimer's — *see* Disease, Alzheimer's
  amyotrophic (lateral) G12.21
  aorta, aortic I70.0
    valve — *see* Endocarditis, aortic
  artery, arterial, arteriolar, arteriovascular — *see* Arteriosclerosis
  ascending multiple G35
  brain (generalized) (lobular) G37.9
    artery, arterial I67.2
    diffuse G37.0
    disseminated G35
    insular G35
    Krabbe's E75.23
    miliary G35
    multiple G35
    presenile (Alzheimer's) — *see* Disease, Alzheimer's, early onset
    senile (arteriosclerotic) I67.2
    stem, multiple G35
    tuberous Q85.1
  bulbar, multiple G35
  bundle of His I44.39
  cardiac — *see* Disease, heart, ischemic, atherosclerotic
  cardiorenal — *see* Hypertension, cardiorenal
  cardiovascular (*see also* Disease, cardiovascular)
    renal — *see* Hypertension, cardiorenal
  cerebellar — *see* Sclerosis, brain
  cerebral — *see* Sclerosis, brain
  cerebrospinal (disseminated) (multiple) G35
  cerebrovascular I67.2
  choroid — *see* Degeneration, choroid
  combined (spinal cord) (*see also* Degeneration, combined)
    multiple G35
  concentric (Balo) G37.5
  cornea — *see* Opacity, cornea
  coronary (artery) I25.10
    with angina pectoris — *see* Arteriosclerosis, coronary (artery),
  corpus cavernosum
    female N90.89
    male N48.6
  diffuse (brain) (spinal cord) G37.0
  disseminated G35
  dorsal G35
  dorsolateral (spinal cord) — *see* Degeneration, combined
  endometrium N85.5
  extrapyramidal G25.9
  eye, nuclear (senile) — *see* Cataract, senile, nuclear
  focal and segmental (glomerular) (*see also* N00-N07 with fourth character .1) N05.1
  Friedreich's (spinal cord) G11.1
  funicular (spermatic cord) N50.8
  general (vascular) — *see* Arteriosclerosis
  gland (lymphatic) I89.8
  hepatic K74.1
    alcoholic K70.2

Sclerosis, sclerotic — *continued*
  hereditary
    cerebellar G11.9
    spinal (Friedreich's ataxia) G11.1
  hippocampal G93.81
  insular G35
  kidney — *see* Sclerosis, renal
  larynx J38.7
  lateral (amyotrophic) (descending) (primary) (spinal) G12.21
  lens, senile nuclear — *see* Cataract, senile, nuclear
  liver K74.1
    with fibrosis K74.2
      alcoholic K70.2
    alcoholic K70.2
    cardiac K76.1
  lung — *see* Fibrosis, lung
  mastoid — *see* Mastoiditis, chronic
  mesial temporal G93.81
  mitral I05.8
  Mönckeberg's (medial) — *see* Arteriosclerosis, extremities
  multiple (brain stem) (cerebral) (generalized) (spinal cord) G35
  myocardium, myocardial — *see* Disease, heart, ischemic, atherosclerotic
  nuclear (senile), eye — *see* Cataract, senile, nuclear
  ovary N83.8
  pancreas K86.8
  penis N48.6
  peripheral arteries — *see* Arteriosclerosis, extremities
  plaques G35
  pluriglandular E31.8
  polyglandular E31.8
  posterolateral (spinal cord) — *see* Degeneration, combined
  presenile (Alzheimer's) — *see* Disease, Alzheimer's, early onset
  primary, lateral G12.29
  progressive, systemic M34.0
  pulmonary — *see* Fibrosis, lung
    artery I27.0
    valve (heart) — *see* Endocarditis, pulmonary
  renal N26.9
    with
      cystine storage disease E72.09
      hypertensive heart disease (conditions in I11) — *see* Hypertension, cardiorenal
    arteriolar (hyaline) (hyperplastic) — *see* Hypertension, kidney
  retina (senile) (vascular) H35.00
  senile (vascular) — *see* Arteriosclerosis
  spinal (cord) (progressive) G95.89
    ascending G61.0
    combined (*see also* Degeneration, combined)
      multiple G35
      syphilitic A52.11
    disseminated G35
    dorsolateral — *see* Degeneration, combined
    hereditary (Friedreich's) (mixed form) G11.1
    lateral (amyotrophic) G12.21
    multiple G35
    posterior (syphilitic) A52.11
  stomach K31.89
  subendocardial, congenital I42.4
  systemic M34.9
    with
      lung involvement M34.81
      myopathy M34.82
      polyneuropathy M34.83
    drug-induced M34.2
    due to chemicals NEC M34.2
    progressive M34.0
    specified NEC M34.89
  temporal (mesial) G93.81
  tricuspid (heart) (valve) I07.8
  tuberous (brain) Q85.1
  tympanic membrane — *see* Disorder, tympanic membrane, specified NEC
  valve, valvular (heart) — *see* Endocarditis
  vascular — *see* Arteriosclerosis
  vein I87.8
Scoliosis (acquired) (postural) M41.9
  adolescent (idiopathic) — *see* Scoliosis, idiopathic, juvenile
  congenital Q67.5
    due to bony malformation Q76.3
    failure of segmentation (hemivertebra) Q76.3

Scoliosis — *continued*
  congenital — *continued*
    hemivertebra fusion Q76.3
    postural Q67.5
  idiopathic M41.20
    adolescent M41.129
      cervical region M41.122
      cervicothoracic region M41.123
      lumbar region M41.126
      lumbosacral region M41.127
      thoracic region M41.124
      thoracolumbar region M41.125
    cervical region M41.22
    cervicothoracic region M41.23
    infantile M41.00
      cervical region M41.02
      cervicothoracic region M41.03
      lumbar region M41.06
      lumbosacral region M41.07
      sacrococcygeal region M41.08
      thoracic region M41.04
      thoracolumbar region M41.05
    juvenile M41.119
      cervical region M41.112
      cervicothoracic region M41.113
      lumbar region M41.116
      lumbosacral region M41.117
      thoracic region M41.114
      thoracolumbar region M41.115
    lumbar region M41.26
    lumbosacral region M41.27
    thoracic region M41.24
    thoracolumbar region M41.25
  neuromuscular M41.40
    cervical region M41.42
    cervicothoracic region M41.43
    lumbar region M41.46
    lumbosacral region M41.47
    occipito-atlanto-axial region M41.41
    thoracic region M41.44
    thoracolumbar region M41.45
  paralytic — *see* Scoliosis, neuromuscular
  postradiation therapy M96.5
  rachitic (late effect or sequelae) E64.3 [M49.80]
    cervical region E64.3 [M49.82]
    cervicothoracic region E64.3 [M49.83]
    lumbar region E64.3 [M49.86]
    lumbosacral region E64.3 [M49.87]
    multiple sites E64.3 [M49.89]
    occipito-atlanto-axial region E64.3 [M49.81]
    sacrococcygeal region E64.3 [M49.88]
    thoracic region E64.3 [M49.84]
    thoracolumbar region E64.3 [M49.85]
  sciatic M54.4- ☑
  secondary (to) NEC M41.50
    cerebral palsy, Friedreich's ataxia, poliomyelitis, neuromuscular disorders — *see* Scoliosis, neuromuscular
    cervical region M41.52
    cervicothoracic region M41.53
    lumbar region M41.56
    lumbosacral region M41.57
    thoracic region M41.54
    thoracolumbar region M41.55
  specified form NEC M41.80
    cervical region M41.82
    cervicothoracic region M41.83
    lumbar region M41.86
    lumbosacral region M41.87
    thoracic region M41.84
    thoracolumbar region M41.85
  thoracogenic M41.30
    thoracic region M41.34
    thoracolumbar region M41.35
  tuberculous A18.01
Scoliotic pelvis
  with disproportion (fetopelvic) O33.0
    causing obstructed labor O65.0
Scorbutus, scorbutic (*see also* Scurvy)
  anemia D53.2
Scotoma (arcuate) (Bjerrum) (central) (ring) (*see also* Defect, visual field, localized, scotoma)
  scintillating H53.19
Scratch — *see* Abrasion
Scratchy throat R09.89
Screening (for) Z13.9
  alcoholism Z13.89
  anemia Z13.0

Screening — *continued*
anomaly, congenital Z13.89
antenatal, of mother Z36
arterial hypertension Z13.6
arthropod-borne viral disease NEC Z11.59
bacteriuria, asymptomatic Z13.89
behavioral disorder Z13.89
brain injury, traumatic Z13.850
bronchitis, chronic Z13.83
brucellosis Z11.2
cardiovascular disorder Z13.6
cataract Z13.5
chlamydial diseases Z11.8
cholera Z11.0
chromosomal abnormalities (nonprocreative) NEC
    Z13.79
colonoscopy Z12.11
congenital
    dislocation of hip Z13.89
    eye disorder Z13.5
    malformation or deformation Z13.89
contamination NEC Z13.88
cystic fibrosis Z13.228
dengue fever Z11.59
dental disorder Z13.84
depression Z13.89
developmental handicap Z13.4
    in early childhood Z13.4
diabetes mellitus Z13.1
diphtheria Z11.2
disability, intellectual Z13.4
disease or disorder Z13.9
    bacterial NEC Z11.2
        intestinal infectious Z11.0
        respiratory tuberculosis Z11.1
    blood or blood-forming organ Z13.0
    cardiovascular Z13.6
    Chagas' Z11.6
    chlamydial Z11.8
    dental Z13.89
    developmental Z13.4
    digestive tract NEC Z13.818
        lower GI Z13.811
        upper GI Z13.810
    ear Z13.5
    endocrine Z13.29
    eye Z13.5
    genitourinary Z13.89
    heart Z13.6
    human immunodeficiency virus (HIV) infection
        Z11.4
    immunity Z13.0
    infection
        intestinal Z11.0
        specified NEC Z11.6
    infectious Z11.9
    mental Z13.89
    metabolic Z13.228
    neurological Z13.89
    nutritional Z13.21
        metabolic Z13.228
        lipoid disorders Z13.220
    protozoal Z11.6
        intestinal Z11.0
    respiratory Z13.83
    rheumatic Z13.828
    rickettsial Z11.8
    sexually-transmitted NEC Z11.3
        human immunodeficiency virus (HIV) Z11.4
    sickle-cell (trait) Z13.0
    skin Z13.89
    specified NEC Z13.89
    spirochetal Z11.8
    thyroid Z13.29
    vascular Z13.6
    venereal Z11.3
    viral NEC Z11.59
        human immunodeficiency virus (HIV) Z11.4
        intestinal Z11.0
elevated titer Z13.89
emphysema Z13.83
encephalitis, viral (mosquito- or tick-borne) Z11.59
exposure to contaminants (toxic) Z13.88
fever
    dengue Z11.59
    hemorrhagic Z11.59
    yellow Z11.59
filariasis Z11.6

Screening — *continued*
galactosemia Z13.228
gastrointestinal condition Z13.818
genetic (nonprocreative) - for procreative manage-
    ment — *see* Testing, genetic, for procreative
    management
    disease carrier status (nonprocreative) Z13.71
    specified NEC (nonprocreative) Z13.79
genitourinary condition Z13.89
glaucoma Z13.5
gonorrhea Z11.3
gout Z13.89
helminthiasis (intestinal) Z11.6
hematopoietic malignancy Z12.89
hemoglobinopathies NEC Z13.0
hemorrhagic fever Z11.59
Hodgkin disease Z12.89
human immunodeficiency virus (HIV) Z11.4
human papillomavirus Z11.51
hypertension Z13.6
immunity disorders Z13.0
infection
    mycotic Z11.8
    parasitic Z11.6
ingestion of radioactive substance Z13.88
intellectual disability Z13.4
intestinal
    helminthiasis Z11.6
    infectious disease Z11.0
leishmaniasis Z11.6
leprosy Z11.2
leptospirosis Z11.8
leukemia Z12.89
lymphoma Z12.89
malaria Z11.6
malnutrition Z13.29
    metabolic Z13.228
    nutritional Z13.21
measles Z11.59
mental disorder Z13.89
metabolic errors, inborn Z13.228
multiphasic Z13.89
musculoskeletal disorder Z13.828
    osteoporosis Z13.820
mycoses Z11.8
myocardial infarction (acute) Z13.6
neoplasm (malignant) (of) Z12.9
    bladder Z12.6
    blood Z12.89
    breast Z12.39
        routine mammogram Z12.31
    cervix Z12.4
    colon Z12.11
    genitourinary organs NEC Z12.79
        bladder Z12.6
        cervix Z12.4
        ovary Z12.73
        prostate Z12.5
        testis Z12.71
        vagina Z12.72
    hematopoietic system Z12.89
    intestinal tract Z12.10
        colon Z12.11
        rectum Z12.12
        small intestine Z12.13
    lung Z12.2
    lymph (glands) Z12.89
    nervous system Z12.82
    oral cavity Z12.81
    prostate Z12.5
    rectum Z12.12
    respiratory organs Z12.2
    skin Z12.83
    small intestine Z12.13
    specified site NEC Z12.89
    stomach Z12.0
nephropathy Z13.89
nervous system disorders NEC Z13.858
neurological condition Z13.89
osteoporosis Z13.820
parasitic infestation Z11.9
    specified NEC Z11.8
phenylketonuria Z13.228
plague Z11.2
poisoning (chemical) (heavy metal) Z13.88
poliomyelitis Z11.59
postnatal, chromosomal abnormalities Z13.89
prenatal, of mother Z36

Screening — *continued*
protozoal disease Z11.6
    intestinal Z11.0
pulmonary tuberculosis Z11.1
radiation exposure Z13.88
respiratory condition Z13.83
respiratory tuberculosis Z11.1
rheumatoid arthritis Z13.828
rubella Z11.59
schistosomiasis Z11.6
sexually-transmitted disease NEC Z11.3
    human immunodeficiency virus (HIV) Z11.4
sickle-cell disease or trait Z13.0
skin condition Z13.89
sleeping sickness Z11.6
special Z13.9
    specified NEC Z13.89
syphilis Z11.3
tetanus Z11.2
trachoma Z11.8
traumatic brain injury Z13.850
trypanosomiasis Z11.6
tuberculosis, respiratory Z11.1
venereal disease Z11.3
viral encephalitis (mosquito- or tick-borne) Z11.59
whooping cough Z11.2
worms, intestinal Z11.6
yaws Z11.8
yellow fever Z11.59
Scrofula, scrofulosis (tuberculosis of cervical lymph
    glands) A18.2
Scrofulide (primary) (tuberculous) A18.4
Scrofuloderma, scrofulodermia (any site) (primary)
    A18.4
Scrofulosus lichen (primary) (tuberculous) A18.4
Scrofulous — *see* condition
Scrotal tongue K14.5
Scrotum — *see* condition
Scurvy, scorbutic E54
    anemia D53.2
    gum E54
    infantile E54
    rickets E55.0 [M90.80]
Sealpox B08.62
Seasickness T75.3 ☑
Seatworm (infection) (infestation) B80
Sebaceous (*see also* condition)
    cyst — *see* Cyst, sebaceous
Seborrhea, seborrheic L21.9
    capillitii R23.8
    capitis L21.0
    dermatitis L21.9
        infantile L21.1
    eczema L21.9
        infantile L21.1
    sicca L21.0
Seckel's syndrome Q87.1
Seclusion, pupil — *see* Membrane, pupillary
Second hand tobacco smoke exposure (acute)
    (chronic) Z77.22
    in the perinatal period P96.81
Secondary
    dentin (in pulp) K04.3
    neoplasm, secondaries — *see* Table of Neoplasms,
        secondary
Secretion
    antidiuretic hormone, inappropriate E22.2
    catecholamine, by pheochromocytoma E27.5
    hormone
        antidiuretic, inappropriate (syndrome) E22.2
        by
            carcinoid tumor E34.0
            pheochromocytoma E27.5
        ectopic NEC E34.2
    urinary
        excessive R35.8
        suppression R34
Section
    nerve, traumatic — *see* Injury, nerve
Segmentation, incomplete (congenital) (*see also* Fu-
    sion)
    bone NEC Q78.8
    lumbosacral (joint) (vertebra) Q76.49
Seitelberger's syndrome (infantile neuraxonal dystro-
    phy) G31.89
Seizure(s) (*see also* Convulsions) R56.9
    akinetic — *see* Epilepsy, generalized, specified NEC
    atonic — *see* Epilepsy, generalized, specified NEC

Index

Seizure(s) — *continued*
  autonomic (hysterical) F44.5
  convulsive — *see* Convulsions
  cortical (focal) (motor) — *see* Epilepsy, localization-related, symptomatic, with simple partial seizures
  disorder (*see also* Epilepsy) G40.909
  due to stroke — *see* Sequelae (of), disease, cerebrovascular, by type, specified NEC
  epileptic — *see* Epilepsy
  febrile (simple) R56.00
    with status epilepticus G40.901
    complex (atypical) (complicated) R56.01
      with status epilepticus G40.901
  grand mal G40.409
    intractable G40.419
      with status epilepticus G40.411
      without status epilepticus G40.419
    not intractable G40.409
      with status epilepticus G40.401
      without status epilepticus G40.409
  heart — *see* Disease, heart
  hysterical F44.5
  intractable G40.919
    with status epilepticus G40.911
  Jacksonian (focal) (motor type) (sensory type) — *see* Epilepsy, localization-related, symptomatic, with simple partial seizures
  newborn P90
  nonspecific epileptic
    atonic — *see* Epilepsy, generalized, specified NEC
    clonic — *see* Epilepsy, generalized, specified NEC
    myoclonic — *see* Epilepsy, generalized, specified NEC
    tonic — *see* Epilepsy, generalized, specified NEC
    tonic-clonic — *see* Epilepsy, generalized, specified NEC
  partial, developing into secondarily generalized seizures
    complex — *see* Epilepsy, localization-related, symptomatic, with complex partial seizures
    simple — *see* Epilepsy, localization-related, symptomatic, with simple partial seizures
  petit mal G40.409
    intractable G40.419
      with status epilepticus G40.411
      without status epilepticus G40.419
    not intractable G40.409
      with status epilepticus G40.401
      without status epilepticus G40.409
  post traumatic R56.1
  recurrent G40.909
  specified NEC G40.89
  uncinate — *see* Epilepsy, localization-related, symptomatic, with complex partial seizures
Selenium deficiency, dietary E59
Self-damaging behavior (life-style) Z72.89
Self-harm (attempted)
  history (personal) Z91.5
    in family Z81.8
Self-mutilation (attempted)
  history (personal) Z91.5
    in family Z81.8
Self-poisoning
  history (personal) Z91.5
    in family Z81.8
  observation following (alleged) attempt Z03.6
Semicoma R40.1
Seminal vesiculitis N49.0
Seminoma C62.9-
  specified site — *see* Neoplasm, malignant, by site
Senear-Usher disease or syndrome L10.4
Senectus R54
Senescence (without mention of psychosis) R54
Senile, senility (*see also* condition) R41.81
  with
    acute confusional state F05
    mental changes NOS F03
    psychosis NEC — *see* Psychosis, senile
  asthenia R54
  cervix (atrophic) N88.8
  debility R54
  endometrium (atrophic) N85.8
  fallopian tube (atrophic) — *see* Atrophy, fallopian tube
  heart (failure) R54
  ovary (atrophic) — *see* Atrophy, ovary
  premature E34.8

Senile, senility — *continued*
  vagina, vaginitis (atrophic) N95.2
  wart L82.1
Sensation
  burning (skin) R20.8
    tongue K14.6
  loss of R20.8
  prickling (skin) R20.2
  tingling (skin) R20.2
Sense loss
  smell — *see* Disturbance, sensation, smell
  taste — *see* Disturbance, sensation, taste
  touch R20.8
Sensibility disturbance (cortical) (deep) (vibratory) R20.9
Sensitive, sensitivity (*see also* Allergy)
  carotid sinus G90.01
  child (excessive) F93.8
  cold, autoimmune D59.1
  dentin K03.89
  latex Z91.040
  methemoglobin D74.8
  tuberculin, without clinical or radiological symptoms R76.11
  visual
    glare H53.71
    impaired contrast H53.72
Sensitiver Beziehungswahn F22
Sensitization, auto-erythrocytic D69.2
Separation
  anxiety, abnormal (of childhood) F93.0
  apophysis, traumatic — *code as* Fracture, by site
  choroid — *see* Detachment, choroid
  epiphysis, epiphyseal
    nontraumatic (*see also* Osteochondropathy, specified type NEC)
      upper femoral — *see* Slipped, epiphysis, upper femoral
    traumatic — *code as* Fracture, by site
  fracture — *see* Fracture
  infundibulum cardiac from right ventricle by a partition Q24.3
  joint (traumatic) (current) — *code by* site under Dislocation
  pubic bone, obstetrical trauma O71.6
  retina, retinal — *see* Detachment, retina
  symphysis pubis, obstetrical trauma O71.6
  tracheal ring, incomplete, congenital Q32.1
Sepsis (generalized) (unspecified organism) A41.9
  with
    organ dysfunction (acute) (multiple) R65.20
      with septic shock R65.21
  actinomycotic A42.7
  adrenal hemorrhage syndrome (meningococcal) A39.1
  anaerobic A41.4
  Bacillus anthracis A22.7
  Brucella (*see also* Brucellosis) A23.9
  candidal B37.7
  cryptogenic A41.9
  due to device, implant or graft T85.79 ☑
    arterial graft NEC T82.7 ☑
    breast (implant) T85.79 ☑
    catheter NEC T85.79 ☑
      dialysis (renal) T82.7 ☑
        intraperitoneal T85.71 ☑
      infusion NEC T82.7 ☑
        spinal (epidural) (subdural) T85.79 ☑
      urinary (indwelling) T83.51 ☑
    ectopic or molar pregnancy O08.82
    electronic (electrode) (pulse generator) (stimulator)
      bone T84.7 ☑
      cardiac T82.7 ☑
      nervous system (brain) (peripheral nerve) (spinal) T85.79 ☑
      urinary T83.59 ☑
    fixation, internal (orthopedic) — *see* Complication, fixation device, infection
    gastrointestinal (bile duct) (esophagus) T85.79 ☑
    genital T83.6 ☑
    heart NEC T82.7 ☑
      valve (prosthesis) T82.6 ☑
        graft T82.7 ☑
    joint prosthesis — *see* Complication, joint prosthesis, infection
    ocular (corneal graft) (orbital implant) T85.79 ☑
    orthopedic NEC T84.7 ☑

Sepsis — *continued*
  due to device, implant or graft — *continued*
    orthopedic — *continued*
      fixation device, internal — *see* Complication, fixation device, infection
    specified NEC T85.79 ☑
    vascular T82.7 ☑
    ventricular intracranial shunt T85.79 ☑
  during labor O75.3
  Enterococcus A41.81
  Erysipelothrix (rhusiopathiae) (erysipeloid) A26.7
  Escherichia coli (E. coli) A41.5 ☑
  extraintestinal yersiniosis A28.2
  following
    abortion (subsequent episode) O08.0
      current episode — *see* Abortion
    ectopic or molar pregnancy O08.82
    immunization T88.0 ☑
    infusion, therapeutic injection or transfusion NEC T80.29 ☑
  gangrenous A41.9
  gonococcal A54.86
  Gram-negative (organism) A41.5 ☑
    anaerobic A41.4
  Haemophilus influenzae A41.3
  herpesviral B00.7
  intra-abdominal K65.1
  intraocular — *see* Endophthalmitis, purulent
  Listeria monocytogenes A32.7
  localized — *code to* specific localized infection
    in operation wound T81.4 ☑
    skin — *see* Abscess
  malleus A24.0
  melioidosis A24.1
  meningeal — *see* Meningitis
  meningococcal A39.4
    acute A39.2
    chronic A39.3
  MSSA (Methicillin susceptible Staphylococcus aureus) A41.01
  newborn P36.9
    due to
      anaerobes NEC P36.5
      Escherichia coli P36.4
      Staphylococcus P36.30
        aureus P36.2
        specified NEC P36.39
      Streptococcus P36.10
        group B P36.0
        specified NEC P36.19
    specified NEC P36.8
  Pasteurella multocida A28.0
  pelvic, puerperal, postpartum, childbirth O85
  pneumococcal A40.3
  postprocedural T81.4 ☑
  puerperal, postpartum, childbirth (pelvic) O85
  Salmonella (arizonae) (cholerae-suis) (enteritidis) (typhimurium) A02.1
  severe R65.20
    with septic shock R65.21
  Shigella (*see also* Dysentery, bacillary) A03.9
  skin, localized — *see* Abscess
  specified organism NEC A41.89
  Staphylococcus, staphylococcal A41.2
    aureus (methicillin susceptible) (MSSA) A41.01
      methicillin resistant (MRSA) A41.02
    coagulase-negative A41.1
    specified NEC A41.1
  Streptococcus, streptococcal A40.9
    agalactiae A40.1
    group
      A A40.0
      B A40.1
      D A41.81
    neonatal P36.10
      group B P36.0
      specified NEC P36.19
    pneumoniae A40.3
    pyogenes A40.0
    specified NEC A40.8
  tracheostomy stoma J95.02
  tularemic A21.7
  umbilical, umbilical cord (newborn) — *see* Sepsis, newborn
  Yersinia pestis A20.7
Septate — *see* Septum
Septic — *see* condition
  arm — *see* Cellulitis, upper limb

Seizure(s) — Septic

Index

Septic — Sequelae

Septic — *continued*
  arm — *see* Cellulitis, upper limb — *continued*
    with lymphangitis — *see* Lymphangitis, acute,
      upper limb
  embolus — *see* Embolism
  finger — *see* Cellulitis, digit
    with lymphangitis — *see* Lymphangitis, acute,
      digit
  foot — *see* Cellulitis, lower limb
    with lymphangitis — *see* Lymphangitis, acute,
      lower limb
  gallbladder (acute) K81.0
  hand — *see* Cellulitis, upper limb
    with lymphangitis — *see* Lymphangitis, acute,
      upper limb
  joint — *see* Arthritis, pyogenic or pyemic
  leg — *see* Cellulitis, lower limb
    with lymphangitis — *see* Lymphangitis, acute,
      lower limb
  nail (*see also* Cellulitis, digit)
    with lymphangitis — *see* Lymphangitis, acute,
      digit
  sore (*see also* Abscess)
    throat J02.0
      streptococcal J02.0
  spleen (acute) D73.89
  teeth, tooth (pulpal origin) K04.4
  throat — *see* Pharyngitis
  thrombus — *see* Thrombosis
  toe — *see* Cellulitis, digit
    with lymphangitis — *see* Lymphangitis, acute,
      digit
  tonsils, chronic J35.01
    with adenoiditis J35.03
  uterus — *see* Endometritis
Septicemia A41.9
  meaning sepsis — *see* Sepsis
Septum, septate (congenital) (*see also* Anomaly, by site)
  anal Q42.3
    with fistula Q42.2
  aqueduct of Sylvius Q03.0
    with spina bifida — *see* Spina bifida, by site, with
      hydrocephalus
  uterus (complete) (partial) Q51.2
  vagina Q52.10
    in pregnancy — *see* Pregnancy, complicated by,
      abnormal vagina
      causing obstructed labor O65.5
    longitudinal (with or without obstruction) Q52.12
    transverse Q52.11
Sequelae (of) (*see also* condition)
  abscess, intracranial or intraspinal (conditions in G06)
    G09
  amputation — *code to* injury with seventh character
    S
  burn and corrosion — *code to* injury with seventh
    character S
  calcium deficiency E64.8
  cerebrovascular disease — *see* Sequelae, disease,
    cerebrovascular
  childbirth O94
  contusion — *code to* injury with seventh character S
  corrosion — *see* Sequelae, burn and corrosion
  crushing injury — *code to* injury with seventh charac-
    ter S
  disease
    cerebrovascular I69.90
      alteration of sensation I69.998
      aphasia I69.920
      apraxia I69.990
      ataxia I69.993
      cognitive deficits I69.91
      disturbance of vision I69.998
      dysarthria I69.922
      dysphagia I69.991
      dysphasia I69.921
      facial droop I69.992
      facial weakness I69.992
      fluency disorder I69.923
      hemiplegia I69.95- ☑
      hemorrhage
        intracerebral — *see* Sequelae, hemorrhage,
          intracerebral
        intracranial, nontraumatic NEC — *see* Seque-
          lae, hemorrhage, intracranial, nontrau-
          matic

Sequelae — *continued*
  disease — *continued*
    cerebrovascular — *continued*
      hemorrhage — *continued*
        subarachnoid — *see* Sequelae, hemorrhage,
          subarachnoid
      language deficit I69.928
      monoplegia
        lower limb I69.84- ☑
        upper limb I69.93- ☑
      paralytic syndrome I69.96- ☑
      specified effect NEC I69.998
      specified type NEC I69.80
        alteration of sensation I69.898
        aphasia I69.820
        apraxia I69.890
        ataxia I69.893
        cognitive deficits I69.81
        disturbance of vision I69.898
        dysarthria I69.822
        dysphagia I69.891
        dysphasia I69.821
        facial droop I69.892
        facial weakness I69.892
        fluency disorder I69.823
        hemiplegia I69.85- ☑
        language deficit I69.828
        monoplegia
          lower limb I69.84- ☑
          upper limb I69.83- ☑
        paralytic syndrome I69.86- ☑
        specified effect NEC I69.898
      speech deficit I69.928
        speech deficit I69.828
      stroke NOS — *see* Sequelae, stroke NOS
  dislocation — *code to* injury with seventh character S
  encephalitis or encephalomyelitis (conditions in G04)
    G09
    in infectious disease NEC B94.8
    viral B94.1
  external cause — *code to* injury with seventh character
    S
  foreign body entering natural orifice — *code to* injury
    with seventh character S
  fracture — *code to* injury with seventh character S
  frostbite — *code to* injury with seventh character S
  Hansen's disease B92
  hemorrhage
    intracerebral I69.10
      alteration of sensation I69.198
      aphasia I69.120
      apraxia I69.190
      ataxia I69.193
      cognitive deficits I69.11
      disturbance of vision I69.198
      dysarthria I69.122
      dysphagia I69.191
      dysphasia I69.121
      facial droop I69.192
      facial weakness I69.192
      fluency disorder I69.123
      hemiplegia I69.15- ☑
      language deficit NEC I69.128
      monoplegia
        lower limb I69.14- ☑
        upper limb I69.13- ☑
      paralytic syndrome I69.16- ☑
      specified effect NEC I69.198
      speech deficit NEC I69.128
    intracranial, nontraumatic NEC I69.20
      alteration of sensation I69.298
      aphasia I69.220
      apraxia I69.290
      ataxia I69.293
      cognitive deficits I69.21
      disturbance of vision I69.298
      dysarthria I69.222
      dysphagia I69.291
      dysphasia I69.221
      facial droop I69.292
      facial weakness I69.292
      fluency disorder I69.223
      hemiplegia I69.25- ☑
      language deficit NEC I69.228
      monoplegia
        lower limb I69.24- ☑
        upper limb I69.23- ☑
      paralytic syndrome I69.26- ☑

Sequelae — *continued*
  hemorrhage — *continued*
    intracranial, nontraumatic — *continued*
      specified effect NEC I69.298
      speech deficit NEC I69.228
    subarachnoid I69.00
      alteration of sensation I69.098
      aphasia I69.020
      apraxia I69.090
      ataxia I69.093
      cognitive deficits I69.01
      disturbance of vision I69.098
      dysarthria I69.022
      dysphagia I69.091
      dysphasia I69.021
      facial droop I69.092
      facial weakness I69.092
      fluency disorder I69.023
      hemiplegia I69.05- ☑
      language deficit NEC I69.028
      monoplegia
        lower limb I69.04- ☑
        upper limb I69.03- ☑
      paralytic syndrome I69.06- ☑
      specified effect NEC I69.098
      speech deficit NEC I69.028
  hepatitis, viral B94.2
  hyperalimentation E68
  infarction
    cerebral I69.30
      alteration of sensation I69.398
      aphasia I69.320
      apraxia I69.390
      ataxia I69.393
      cognitive deficits I69.31
      disturbance of vision I69.398
      dysarthria I69.322
      dysphagia I69.391
      dysphasia I69.321
      facial droop I69.392
      facial weakness I69.392
      fluency disorder I69.323
      hemiplegia I69.35- ☑
      language deficit NEC I69.328
      monoplegia
        lower limb I69.34- ☑
        upper limb I69.33- ☑
      paralytic syndrome I69.36- ☑
      specified effect NEC I69.398
      speech deficit NEC I69.328
  infection, pyogenic, intracranial or intraspinal G09
  infectious disease B94.9
    specified NEC B94.8
  injury — *code to* injury with seventh character S
  leprosy B92
  meningitis
    bacterial (conditions in G00) G09
    other or unspecified cause (conditions in G03) G09
  muscle (and tendon) injury — *code to* injury with
    seventh character S
  myelitis — *see* Sequelae, encephalitis
  niacin deficiency E64.8
  nutritional deficiency E64.9
    specified NEC E64.8
  obstetrical condition O94
  parasitic disease B94.9
  phlebitis or thrombophlebitis of intracranial or in-
    traspinal venous sinuses and veins (conditions
    in G08) G09
  poisoning — *code to* poisoning with seventh character
    S
    nonmedicinal substance — *see* Sequelae, toxic ef-
      fect, nonmedicinal substance
  poliomyelitis (acute) B91
  pregnancy O94
  protein-energy malnutrition E64.0
  puerperium O94
  rickets E64.3
  selenium deficiency E64.8
  sprain and strain — *code to* injury with seventh char-
    acter S
  stroke NOS I69.30
    alteration in sensation I69.398
    aphasia I69.320
    apraxia I69.390
    ataxia I69.393
    cognitive deficits I69.31
    disturbance of vision I69.398

Sequelae — *continued*
  stroke — *continued*
    dysarthria I69.322
    dysphagia I69.391
    dysphasia I69.321
    facial droop I69.392
    facial weakness I69.392
    hemiplegia I69.35- ☑
    language deficit NEC I69.328
    monoplegia
      lower limb I69.34- ☑
      upper limb I69.33- ☑
    paralytic syndrome I69.36- ☑
    specified effect NEC I69.398
    speech deficit NEC I69.328
  tendon and muscle injury — *code to* injury with seventh character S
  thiamine deficiency E64.8
  trachoma B94.0
  tuberculosis B90.9
    bones and joints B90.2
    central nervous system B90.0
    genitourinary B90.1
    pulmonary (respiratory) B90.9
    specified organs NEC B90.8
  viral
    encephalitis B94.1
    hepatitis B94.2
  vitamin deficiency NEC E64.8
    A E64.1
    B E64.8
    C E64.2
  wound, open — *code to* injury with seventh character S

Sequestration (*see also* Sequestrum)
  lung, congenital Q33.2
Sequestrum
  bone — *see* Osteomyelitis, chronic
  dental M27.2
  jaw bone M27.2
  orbit — *see* Osteomyelitis, orbit
  sinus (accessory) (nasal) — *see* Sinusitis
Sequoiosis lung or pneumonitis J67.8
Serology for syphilis
  doubtful
    with signs or symptoms — *code by* site and stage under Syphilis
    follow-up of latent syphilis — *see* Syphilis, latent
  negative, with signs or symptoms — *code by* site and stage under Syphilis
  positive A53.0
    with signs or symptoms — *code by* site and stage under Syphilis
  reactivated A53.0
Seroma (*see also* Hematoma)
  traumatic, secondary and recurrent T79.2 ☑
Seropurulent — *see* condition
Serositis, multiple K65.8
  pericardial I31.1
  peritoneal K65.8
Serous — *see* condition
Sertoli cell
  adenoma
    specified site — *see* Neoplasm, benign, by site
    unspecified site
      female D27.9
      male D29.20
  carcinoma
    specified site — *see* Neoplasm, malignant, by site
    unspecified site (male) C62.9- ☑
      female C56.9
  tumor
    with lipid storage
      specified site — *see* Neoplasm, benign, by site
      unspecified site
        female D27.9
        male D29.20
    specified site — *see* Neoplasm, benign, by site
    unspecified site
      female D27.9
      male D29.20
Sertoli-Leydig cell tumor — *see* Neoplasm, benign, by site
  specified site — *see* Neoplasm, benign, by site
  unspecified site
    female D27.9
    male D29.20

Serum
  allergy, allergic reaction (*see also* Reaction, serum) T80.69 ☑
    shock (*see also* Shock, anaphylactic) T80.59 ☑
  arthritis (*see also* Reaction, serum) T80.69 ☑
  complication or reaction NEC (*see also* Reaction, serum) T80.69 ☑
  disease NEC (*see also* Reaction, serum) T80.69 ☑
  hepatitis (*see also* Hepatitis, viral, type B)
    carrier (suspected) of Z22.51
  intoxication (*see also* Reaction, serum) T80.69 ☑
  neuritis (*see also* Reaction, serum) T80.69 ☑
  neuropathy G61.1
  poisoning NEC (*see also* Reaction, serum) T80.69 ☑
  rash NEC (*see also* Reaction, serum) T80.69 ☑
  reaction NEC (*see also* Reaction, serum) T80.69 ☑
  sickness NEC (*see also* Reaction, serum) T80.69 ☑
  urticaria (*see also* Reaction, serum) T80.69 ☑
Sesamoiditis M25.8- ☑
Severe sepsis R65.20
  with septic shock R65.21
Sever's disease or osteochondrosis — *see* Osteochondrosis, juvenile, tarsus
Sex
  chromosome mosaics Q97.8
    lines with various numbers of X chromosomes Q97.2
  education Z70.8
  reassignment surgery status Z87.890
Sextuplet pregnancy — *see* Pregnancy, sextuplet
Sexual
  function, disorder of (psychogenic) F52.9
  immaturity (female) (male) E30.0
  impotence (psychogenic) organic origin NEC — *see* Dysfunction, sexual, male
  precocity (constitutional) (cryptogenic)(female) (idiopathic) (male) E30.1
Sexuality, pathologic — *see* Deviation, sexual
Sézary disease C84.1- ☑
Shadow, lung R91.8
Shaking palsy or paralysis — *see* Parkinsonism
Shallowness, acetabulum — *see* Derangement, joint, specified type NEC, hip
Shaver's disease J63.1
Sheath (tendon) — *see* condition
Sheathing, retinal vessels H35.01- ☑
Shedding
  nail L60.8
  premature, primary (deciduous) teeth K00.6
Sheehan's disease or syndrome E23.0
Shelf, rectal K62.89
Shell teeth K00.5
Shellshock (current) F43.0
  lasting state — *see* Disorder, post-traumatic stress
Shield kidney Q63.1
Shift
  auditory threshold (temporary) H93.24- ☑
  mediastinal R93.8
Shifting sleep-work schedule (affecting sleep) G47.26
Shiga (-Kruse) **dysentery** A03.0
Shiga's bacillus A03.0
Shigella (dysentery) — *see* Dysentery, bacillary
Shigellosis A03.9
  Group A A03.0
  Group B A03.1
  Group C A03.2
  Group D A03.3
Shin splints S86.89- ☑
Shingles — *see* Herpes, zoster
Shipyard disease or eye B30.0
Shirodkar suture, in pregnancy — *see* Pregnancy, complicated by, incompetent cervix
Shock R57.9
  with ectopic or molar pregnancy O08.3
  adrenal (cortical) (Addisonian) E27.2
  adverse food reaction (anaphylactic) — *see* Shock, anaphylactic, due to food
  allergic — *see* Shock, anaphylactic
  anaphylactic T78.2 ☑
    chemical — *see* Table of Drugs and Chemicals
    due to drug or medicinal substance
      correct substance properly administered T88.6 ☑
      overdose or wrong substance given or taken (by accident) — *see* Table of Drugs and Chemicals, by drug, poisoning

Shock — *continued*
  anaphylactic — *continued*
    due to food (nonpoisonous) T78.00 ☑
      additives T78.06 ☑
      dairy products T78.07 ☑
      eggs T78.08 ☑
      fish T78.03 ☑
        shellfish T78.02 ☑
      fruit T78.04 ☑
      milk T78.07 ☑
      nuts T78.05 ☑
        peanuts T78.01 ☑
      peanuts T78.01 ☑
      seeds T78.05 ☑
      specified type NEC T78.09 ☑
      vegetable T78.04 ☑
    following sting(s) — *see* Venom
    immunization T80.52 ☑
    serum T80.59 ☑
      blood and blood products T80.51 ☑
      immunization T80.52 ☑
      specified NEC T80.59 ☑
      vaccination T80.52 ☑
  anaphylactoid — *see* Shock, anaphylactic
  anesthetic
    correct substance properly administered T88.2 ☑
    overdose or wrong substance given or taken — *see* Table of Drugs and Chemicals, by drug, poisoning
    specified anesthetic — *see* Table of Drugs and Chemicals, by drug, poisoning
  cardiogenic R57.0
  chemical substance — *see* Table of Drugs and Chemicals
  complicating ectopic or molar pregnancy O08.3
  culture — *see* Disorder, adjustment
  drug
    due to correct substance properly administered T88.6 ☑
    overdose or wrong substance given or taken (by accident) — *see* Table of Drugs and Chemicals, by drug, poisoning
  during or after labor and delivery O75.1
  electric T75.4 ☑
    (taser) T75.4 ☑
  endotoxic R65.21
    postprocedural (during or resulting from a procedure, not elsewhere classified) T81.12 ☑
  following
    ectopic or molar pregnancy O08.3
    injury (immediate) (delayed) T79.4 ☑
    labor and delivery O75.1
  food (anaphylactic) — *see* Shock, anaphylactic, due to food
  from electroshock gun (taser) T75.4 ☑
  gram-negative R65.21
    postprocedural (during or resulting from a procedure, not elsewhere classified) T81.12 ☑
  hematologic R57.8
  hemorrhagic
    surgery (intraoperative) (postoperative) T81.19 ☑
    trauma T79.4 ☑
  hypovolemic R57.1
    surgical T81.19 ☑
    traumatic T79.4 ☑
  insulin E15
    therapeutic misadventure — *see* subcategory T38.3 ☑
  kidney N17.0
    traumatic (following crushing) T79.5 ☑
  lightning T75.01 ☑
  lung J80
  obstetric O75.1
    with ectopic or molar pregnancy O08.3
    following ectopic or molar pregnancy O08.3
  pleural (surgical) T81.19 ☑
    due to trauma T79.4 ☑
  postprocedural (postoperative) T81.10 ☑
    with ectopic or molar pregnancy O08.3
    cardiogenic T81.11 ☑
    endotoxic T81.12 ☑
    following ectopic or molar pregnancy O08.3
    gram-negative T81.12 ☑
    hypovolemic T81.19 ☑
    septic T81.12 ☑
    specified type NEC T81.19 ☑

Shock — *continued*
 psychic F43.Ø
 septic (due to severe sepsis) R65.21
 specified NEC R57.8
 surgical T81.1Ø ☑
 taser gun (taser) T75.4 ☑
 therapeutic misadventure NEC T81.1Ø ☑
 thyroxin
  overdose or wrong substance given or taken —
   see Table of Drugs and Chemicals, by drug,
   poisoning
 toxic, syndrome A48.3
 transfusion — *see* Complications, transfusion
 traumatic (immediate) (delayed) T79.4 ☑
Shoemaker's chest M95.4
Short, shortening, shortness
 arm (acquired) (*see also* Deformity, limb, unequal
  length)
  congenital Q71.81- ☑
  forearm — *see* Deformity, limb, unequal length
 bowel syndrome K91.2
 breath RØ6.Ø2
 cervical (complicating pregnancy) O26.87- ☑
  non-gravid uterus N88.3
 common bile duct, congenital Q44.5
 cord (umbilical), complicating delivery O69.3 ☑
 cystic duct, congenital Q44.5
 esophagus (congenital) Q39.8
 femur (acquired) — *see* Deformity, limb, unequal
  length, femur
  congenital — *see* Defect, reduction, lower limb,
   longitudinal, femur
 frenum, frenulum, linguae (congenital) Q38.1
 hip (acquired) (*see also* Deformity, limb, unequal
  length)
  congenital Q65.89
 leg (acquired) (*see also* Deformity, limb, unequal
  length)
  congenital Q72.81- ☑
  lower leg (*see also* Deformity, limb, unequal length)
 limbed stature, with immunodeficiency D82.2
 lower limb (acquired) (*see also* Deformity, limb, unequal length)
  congenital Q72.81- ☑
 organ or site, congenital NEC — *see* Distortion
 palate, congenital Q38.5
 radius (acquired) (*see also* Deformity, limb, unequal
  length)
  congenital — *see* Defect, reduction, upper limb,
   longitudinal, radius
 rib syndrome Q77.2
 stature (child) (hereditary) (idiopathic) NEC R62.52
  constitutional E34.3
  due to endocrine disorder E34.3
  Laron-type E34.3
 tendon (*see also* Contraction, tendon)
  with contracture of joint — *see* Contraction, joint
  Achilles (acquired) M67.Ø- ☑
   congenital Q66.89
  congenital Q79.8
 thigh (acquired) (*see also* Deformity, limb, unequal
  length, femur)
  congenital — *see* Defect, reduction, lower limb,
   longitudinal, femur
 tibialis anterior (tendon) — *see* Contraction, tendon
 umbilical cord
  complicating delivery O69.3 ☑
 upper limb, congenital — *see* Defect, reduction, upper
  limb, specified type NEC
 urethra N36.8
 uvula, congenital Q38.5
 vagina (congenital) Q52.4
Shortsightedness — *see* Myopia
Shoshin (acute fulminating beriberi) E51.11
Shoulder — *see* condition
Shovel-shaped incisors KØØ.2
Shower, thromboembolic — *see* Embolism
Shunt
 arterial-venous (dialysis) Z99.2
 arteriovenous, pulmonary (acquired) I28.Ø
  congenital Q25.72
 cerebral ventricle (communicating) in situ Z98.2
 surgical, prosthetic, with complications — *see* Complications, cardiovascular, device or implant
Shutdown, renal N28.9
Shy-Drager syndrome G9Ø.3

Sialadenitis, sialadenosis (any gland) (chronic) (period-
 ic) (suppurative) — *see* Sialoadenitis
Sialectasia K11.8
Sialidosis E77.1
Sialitis, silitis (any gland) (chronic) (suppurative) — *see*
 Sialoadenitis
Sialoadenitis (any gland) (periodic) (suppurative) K11.2Ø
 acute K11.21
  recurrent K11.22
 chronic K11.23
Sialoadenopathy K11.9
Sialoangitis — *see* Sialoadenitis
Sialodochitis (fibrinosa) — *see* Sialoadenitis
Sialodocholithiasis K11.5
Sialolithiasis K11.5
Sialometaplasia, necrotizing K11.8
Sialorrhea (*see also* Ptyalism)
 periodic — *see* Sialoadenitis
Sialosis K11.7
Siamese twin Q89.4
Sibling rivalry Z62.891
Sicard's syndrome G52.7
Sicca syndrome M35.ØØ
 with
  keratoconjunctivitis M35.Ø1
  lung involvement M35.Ø2
  myopathy M35.Ø3
  renal tubulo-interstitial disorders M35.Ø4
 specified organ involvement NEC M35.Ø9
Sick R69
 or handicapped person in family Z63.79
  needing care at home Z63.6
 sinus (syndrome) I49.5
Sick-euthyroid syndrome EØ7.81
Sickle-cell
 anemia — *see* Disease, sickle-cell
 trait D57.3
Sicklemia (*see also* Disease, sickle-cell)
 trait D57.3
Sickness
 air (travel) T75.3 ☑
 airplane T75.3 ☑
 alpine T7Ø.29 ☑
 altitude T7Ø.2Ø ☑
 Andes T7Ø.29 ☑
 aviator's T7Ø.29 ☑
 balloon T7Ø.29 ☑
 car T75.3 ☑
 compressed air T7Ø.3 ☑
 decompression T7Ø.3 ☑
 green D5Ø.8
 milk — *see* Poisoning, food, noxious
 motion T75.3 ☑
 mountain T7Ø.29 ☑
  acute D75.1
 protein (*see also* Reaction, serum) T8Ø.69 ☑
 radiation T66 ☑
 roundabout (motion) T75.3 ☑
 sea T75.3 ☑
 serum NEC (*see also* Reaction, serum) T8Ø.69 ☑
 sleeping (African) B56.9
  by Trypanosoma B56.9
   brucei
    gambiense B56.Ø
    rhodesiense B56.1
  East African B56.1
  Gambian B56.Ø
  Rhodesian B56.1
  West African B56.Ø
 swing (motion) T75.3 ☑
 train (railway) (travel) T75.3 ☑
 travel (any vehicle) T75.3 ☑
Sideropenia — *see* Anemia, iron deficiency
Siderosilicosis J62.8
Siderosis (lung) J63.4
 eye (globe) — *see* Disorder, globe, degenerative,
  siderosis
Siemens' syndrome (ectodermal dysplasia) Q82.8
Sighing RØ6.89
 psychogenic F45.8
Sigmoid (*see also* condition)
 flexure — *see* condition
 kidney Q63.1
Sigmoiditis (*see also* Enteritis) K52.9
 infectious AØ9
 noninfectious K52.9
Silfversköld's syndrome Q78.9

Silicosiderosis J62.8
Silicosis, silicotic (simple) (complicated) J62.8
 with tuberculosis J65
Silicotuberculosis J65
Silo-fillers' disease J68.8
 bronchitis J68.Ø
 pneumonitis J68.Ø
 pulmonary edema J68.1
Silver's syndrome Q87.1
Simian malaria B53.1
Simmonds' cachexia or disease E23.Ø
Simons' disease or syndrome (progressive lipodystro-
 phy) E88.1
Simple, simplex — *see* condition
Simulation, conscious (of illness) Z76.5
Simultanagnosia (asimultagnosia) R48.3
Sin Nombre virus disease (Hantavirus) (cardio)-pul-
 monary syndrome) B33.4
Sinding-Larsen disease or osteochondrosis — *see*
 Osteochondrosis, juvenile, patella
Singapore hemorrhagic fever A91
Singer's node or nodule J38.2
Single
 atrium Q21.2
 coronary artery Q24.5
 umbilical artery Q27.Ø
 ventricle Q2Ø.4
Singultus RØ6.6
 epidemicus B33.Ø
Sinus (*see also* Fistula)
 abdominal K63.89
 arrest I45.5
 arrhythmia I49.8
 bradycardia RØØ.1
 branchial cleft (internal) (external) Q18.Ø
 coccygeal — *see* Sinus, pilonidal
 dental KØ4.6
 dermal (congenital) QØ6.8
  with abscess QØ6.8
  coccygeal, pilonidal — *see* Sinus, coccygeal
 infected, skin NEC LØ8.89
 marginal, ruptured or bleeding — *see* Hemorrhage,
  antepartum, specified cause NEC
 medial, face and neck Q18.8
 pause I45.5
 pericranii QØ1.9
 pilonidal (infected) (rectum) LØ5.92
  with abscess LØ5.Ø2
 preauricular Q18.1
 rectovaginal N82.3
 Rokitansky-Aschoff (gallbladder) K82.8
 sacrococcygeal (dermoid) (infected) — *see* Sinus, pilonidal
 tachycardia RØØ.Ø
  paroxysmal I47.1
 tarsi syndrome M25.57- ☑
 testis N5Ø.8
 tract (postinfective) — *see* Fistula
 urachus Q64.4
Sinusitis (accessory) (chronic) (hyperplastic) (nasal)
 (nonpurulent) (purulent) J32.9
 acute JØ1.9Ø
  ethmoidal JØ1.2Ø
   recurrent JØ1.21
  frontal JØ1.1Ø
   recurrent JØ1.11
  involving more than one sinus, other than pansinusitis JØ1.8Ø
   recurrent JØ1.81
  maxillary JØ1.ØØ
   recurrent JØ1.Ø1
  pansinusitis JØ1.4Ø
   recurrent JØ1.41
  recurrent JØ1.91
  specified NEC JØ1.8Ø
   recurrent JØ1.81
  sphenoidal JØ1.3Ø
   recurrent JØ1.31
 allergic — *see* Rhinitis, allergic
 due to high altitude T7Ø.1 ☑
 ethmoidal J32.2
  acute JØ1.2Ø
   recurrent JØ1.21
 frontal J32.1
  acute JØ1.1Ø
   recurrent JØ1.11
 influenzal — *see* Influenza, with, respiratory manifestations NEC

  ☑ **Additional Character Required** — Refer to the Tabular List for Character Selection   ▼ **Subterms under main terms may continue to next column or page**

Sinusitis — *continued*
  involving more than one sinus but not pansinusitis
      J32.8
    acute J01.80
      recurrent J01.81
  maxillary J32.0
    acute J01.00
      recurrent J01.01
  sphenoidal J32.3
    acute J01.30
      recurrent J01.31
  tuberculous, any sinus A15.8
Sinusitis-bronchiectasis-situs inversus (syndrome) (triad) Q89.3
Sipple's syndrome E31.22
Sirenomelia (syndrome) Q87.2
Siriasis T67.0 ☑
Sirkari's disease B55.0
Siti A65
Situation, psychiatric F99
Situational
  disturbance (transient) — *see* Disorder, adjustment
    acute F43.0
  maladjustment — *see* Disorder, adjustment
  reaction — *see* Disorder, adjustment
    acute F43.0
Situs inversus or transversus (abdominalis) (thoracis) Q89.3
Sixth disease B08.20
  due to human herpesvirus 6 B08.21
  due to human herpesvirus 7 B08.22
Sjögren-Larsson syndrome Q87.1
Sjögren's syndrome or disease — *see* Sicca syndrome
Skeletal — *see* condition
Skene's gland — *see* condition
Skenitis — *see* Urethritis
Skerljevo A65
Skevas-Zerfus disease — *see* Toxicity, venom, marine animal, sea anemone
Skin (*see also* condition)
  clammy R23.1
  donor — *see* Donor, skin
  hidebound M35.9
Slate-dressers' or slate-miners' lung J62.8
Sleep
  apnea — *see* Apnea, sleep
  deprivation Z72.820
  disorder or disturbance G47.9
    child F51.9
    nonorganic origin F51.9
    specified NEC G47.8
  disturbance G47.9
    nonorganic origin F51.9
  drunkenness F51.9
  rhythm inversion G47.2- ☑
  terrors F51.4
  walking F51.3
    hysterical F44.89
Sleep hygiene
  abuse Z72.821
  inadequate Z72.821
  poor Z72.821
Sleeping sickness — *see* Sickness, sleeping
Sleeplessness — *see* Insomnia
  menopausal N95.1
Sleep-wake schedule disorder G47.20
Slim disease (in HIV infection) B20
Slipped, slipping
  epiphysis (traumatic) (*see also* Osteochondropathy, specified type NEC)
    capital femoral (traumatic)
      acute (on chronic) S79.01- ☑
    current traumatic — *code as* Fracture, by site
    upper femoral (nontraumatic) M93.00- ☑
      acute M93.01- ☑
        on chronic M93.03- ☑
      chronic M93.02- ☑
  intervertebral disc — *see* Displacement, intervertebral disc
  ligature, umbilical P51.8
  patella — *see* Disorder, patella, derangement NEC
  rib M89.8X8
  sacroiliac joint — *see* subcategory M53.2 ☑
  tendon — *see* Disorder, tendon
  ulnar nerve, nontraumatic — *see* Lesion, nerve, ulnar
  vertebra NEC — *see* Spondylolisthesis
Slocumb's syndrome E27.0

Sloughing (multiple) (phagedena) (skin) (*see also* Gangrene)
  abscess — *see* Abscess
  appendix K38.8
  fascia — *see* Disorder, soft tissue, specified type NEC
  scrotum N50.8
  tendon — *see* Disorder, tendon
  transplanted organ — *see* Rejection, transplant
  ulcer — *see* Ulcer, skin
Slow
  feeding, newborn P92.2
  flow syndrome, coronary I20.8
  heart (beat) R00.1
Slowing, urinary stream R39.19
Sluder's neuralgia (syndrome) G44.89
Slurred, slurring speech R47.81
Small (ness)
  for gestational age — *see* Small for dates
  introitus, vagina N89.6
  kidney (unknown cause) N27.9
    bilateral N27.1
    unilateral N27.0
  ovary (congenital) Q50.39
  pelvis
    with disproportion (fetopelvic) O33.1
      causing obstructed labor O65.1
  uterus N85.8
  white kidney N03.9
Small-and-light-for-dates — *see* Small for dates
Small-for-dates (infant) P05.10
  with weight of
    1000-1249 grams P05.14
    1250-1499 grams P05.15
    1500-1749 grams P05.16
    1750-1999 grams P05.17
    2000-2499 grams P05.18
    499 grams or less P05.11
    500-749 grams P05.12
    750-999 grams P05.13
Smallpox B03
Smearing, fecal R15.1
Smith-Lemli-Opitz syndrome E78.72
Smith's fracture S52.54- ☑
Smoker — *see* Dependence, drug, nicotine
Smoker's
  bronchitis J41.0
  cough J41.0
  palate K13.24
  throat J31.2
  tongue K13.24
Smoking
  passive Z77.22
Smothering spells R06.81
Snaggle teeth, tooth M26.39
Snapping
  finger — *see* Trigger finger
  hip — *see* Derangement, joint, specified type NEC, hip
    involving the iliotibial band M76.3- ☑
  knee — *see* Derangement, knee
    involving the iliotibial band M76.3- ☑
Sneddon-Wilkinson disease or syndrome (sub-corneal pustular dermatosis) L13.1
Sneezing (intractable) R06.7
Sniffing
  cocaine
    abuse — *see* Abuse, drug, cocaine
    dependence — *see* Dependence, drug, cocaine
  gasoline
    abuse — *see* Abuse, drug, inhalant
    dependence — *see* Dependence, drug, inhalant
  glue (airplane)
    abuse — *see* Abuse, drug, inhalant
    drug dependence — *see* Dependence, drug, inhalant
Sniffles
  newborn P28.89
Snoring R06.83
Snow blindness — *see* Photokeratitis
Snuffles (non-syphilitic) R06.5
  newborn P28.89
  syphilitic (infant) A50.05 [J99]
Social
  exclusion Z60.4
    due to discrimination or persecution (perceived) Z60.5
  migrant Z59.0
    acculturation difficulty Z60.3

Social — *continued*
  rejection Z60.4
    due to discrimination or persecution Z60.5
  role conflict NEC Z73.5
  skills inadequacy NEC Z73.4
  transplantation Z60.3
Sodoku A25.0
Soemmerring's ring — *see* Cataract, secondary
Soft (*see also* condition)
  nails L60.3
Softening
  bone — *see* Osteomalacia
  brain (necrotic) (progressive) G93.89
    congenital Q04.8
    embolic I63.4 ☑
    hemorrhagic — *see* Hemorrhage, intracranial, intracerebral
      occlusive I63.5 ☑
      thrombotic I63.3 ☑
  cartilage M94.2- ☑
    patella M22.4- ☑
  cerebellar — *see* Softening, brain
  cerebral — *see* Softening, brain
  cerebrospinal — *see* Softening, brain
  myocardial, heart — *see* Degeneration, myocardial
  spinal cord G95.89
  stomach K31.89
Soldier's
  heart F45.8
  patches I31.0
Solitary
  cyst, kidney N28.1
  kidney, congenital Q60.0
Solvent abuse — *see* Abuse, drug, inhalant
  dependence — *see* Dependence, drug, inhalant
Somatization reaction, somatic reaction — *see* Disorder, somatoform
Somnambulism F51.3
  hysterical F44.89
Somnolence R40.0
  nonorganic origin F51.11
Sonne dysentery A03.3
Soor B37.0
Sore
  bed — *see* Ulcer, pressure, by site
  chiclero B55.1
  Delhi B55.1
  desert — *see* Ulcer, skin
  eye H57.1- ☑
  Lahore B55.1
  mouth K13.79
    canker K12.0
  muscle M79.1
  Naga — *see* Ulcer, skin
  of skin — *see* Ulcer, skin
  oriental B55.1
  pressure — *see* Ulcer, pressure, by site
  skin L98.9
  soft A57
  throat (acute) (*see also* Pharyngitis)
    with influenza, flu, or grippe — *see* Influenza, with, respiratory manifestations NEC
    chronic J31.2
    coxsackie (virus) B08.5
    diphtheritic A36.0
    herpesviral B00.2
    influenzal — *see* Influenza, with, respiratory manifestations NEC
    septic J02.0
    streptococcal (ulcerative) J02.0
    viral NEC J02.8
      coxsackie B08.5
    tropical — *see* Ulcer, skin
    veldt — *see* Ulcer, skin
Soto's syndrome (cerebral gigantism) Q87.3
South African cardiomyopathy syndrome I42.8
Southeast Asian hemorrhagic fever A91
Spacing
  abnormal, tooth, teeth, fully erupted M26.30
  excessive, tooth, fully erupted M26.32
Spade-like hand (congenital) Q68.1
Spading nail L60.8
  congenital Q84.6
Spanish collar N47.1
Sparganosis B70.1
Spasm(s), **spastic, spasticity** (*see also* condition) R25.2
  accommodation — *see* Spasm, of accommodation

Spasm(s), spastic, spasticity — *continued*
ampulla of Vater K83.4
anus, ani (sphincter) (reflex) K59.4
 psychogenic F45.8
artery I73.9
 cerebral G45.9
Bell's G51.3
bladder (sphincter, external or internal) N32.89
 psychogenic F45.8
bronchus, bronchiole J98.01
cardia K22.0
cardiac I20.1
carpopedal — *see* Tetany
cerebral (arteries) (vascular) G45.9
cervix, complicating delivery O62.4
ciliary body (of accommodation) — *see* Spasm, of accommodation
colon K58.9
 with diarrhea K58.0
 psychogenic F45.8
common duct K83.8
compulsive — *see* Tic
conjugate H51.8
coronary (artery) I20.1
diaphragm (reflex) R06.6
 epidemic B33.0
 psychogenic F45.8
duodenum K59.8
epidemic diaphragmatic (transient) B33.0
esophagus (diffuse) K22.4
 psychogenic F45.8
facial G51.3
fallopian tube N83.8
gastrointestinal (tract) K31.89
 psychogenic F45.8
glottis J38.5
 hysterical F44.4
 psychogenic F45.8
 conversion reaction F44.4
 reflex through recurrent laryngeal nerve J38.5
habit — *see* Tic
heart I20.1
hemifacial (clonic) G51.3
hourglass — *see* Contraction, hourglass
hysterical F44.4
infantile — *see* Epilepsy, spasms
inferior oblique, eye H51.8
intestinal (*see also* Syndrome, irritable bowel) K58.9
 psychogenic F45.8
larynx, laryngeal J38.5
 hysterical F44.4
 psychogenic F45.8
 conversion reaction F44.4
levator palpebrae superioris — *see* Disorder, eyelid function
muscle NEC M62.838
 back M62.830
nerve, trigeminal G51.0
nervous F45.8
nodding F98.4
occupational F48.8
oculogyric H51.8
 psychogenic F45.8
of accommodation H52.53- ☑
ophthalmic artery — *see* Occlusion, artery, retina
perineal, female N94.89
peroneo-extensor (*see also* Deformity, limb, flat foot)
pharynx (reflex) J39.2
 hysterical F45.8
 psychogenic F45.8
psychogenic F45.8
pylorus NEC K31.3
 adult hypertrophic K31.89
 congenital or infantile Q40.0
 psychogenic F45.8
rectum (sphincter) K59.4
 psychogenic F45.8
retinal (artery) — *see* Occlusion, artery, retina
sigmoid (*see also* Syndrome, irritable bowel) K58.9
 psychogenic F45.8
sphincter of Oddi K83.4
stomach K31.89
 neurotic F45.8
throat J39.2
 hysterical F45.8
 psychogenic F45.8
tic F95.9
 chronic F95.1

Spasm(s), spastic, spasticity — *continued*
tic — *continued*
 transient of childhood F95.0
tongue K14.8
torsion (progressive) G24.1
trigeminal nerve — *see* Neuralgia, trigeminal
ureter N13.5
urethra (sphincter) N35.9
uterus N85.8
 complicating labor O62.4
vagina N94.2
 psychogenic F52.5
vascular I73.9
vasomotor I73.9
vein NEC I87.8
viscera — *see* Pain, abdominal
Spasmodic — *see* condition
Spasmophilia — *see* Tetany
Spasmus nutans F98.4
Spastic, spasticity (*see also* Spasm)
 child (cerebral) (congenital) (paralysis) G80.1
Speaker's throat R49.8
Specific, specified — *see* condition
Speech
 defect, disorder, disturbance, impediment R47.9
 psychogenic, in childhood and adolescence F98.8
 slurring R47.81
 specified NEC R47.89
Spencer's disease A08.19
Spens' syndrome (syncope with heart block) I45.9
Sperm counts (fertility testing) Z31.41
 postvasectomy Z30.8
 reversal Z31.42
Spermatic cord — *see* condition
Spermatocele N43.40
 congenital Q55.4
 multiple N43.42
 single N43.41
Spermatocystitis N49.0
Spermatocytoma C62.9- ☑
 specified site — *see* Neoplasm, malignant, by site
Spermatorrhea N50.8
Sphacelus — *see* Gangrene
Sphenoidal — *see* condition
Sphenoiditis (chronic) — *see* Sinusitis, sphenoidal
Sphenopalatine ganglion neuralgia G90.09
Sphericity, increased, lens (congenital) Q12.4
Spherocytosis (congenital) (familial) (hereditary) D58.0
 hemoglobin disease D58.0
 sickle-cell (disease) D57.8- ☑
Spherophakia Q12.4
Sphincter — *see* condition
Sphincteritis, sphincter of Oddi — *see* Cholangitis
Sphingolipidosis E75.3
 specified NEC E75.29
Sphingomyelinosis E75.3
Spicule tooth K00.2
Spider
 bite — *see* Toxicity, venom, spider
 fingers — *see* Syndrome, Marfan's
 nevus I78.1
 toes — *see* Syndrome, Marfan's
 vascular I78.1
Spiegler-Fendt
 benign lymphocytoma L98.8
 sarcoid L08.89
Spielmeyer-Vogt disease E75.4
Spina bifida (aperta) Q05.9
 with hydrocephalus NEC Q05.4
 cervical Q05.5
 with hydrocephalus Q05.0
 dorsal Q05.6
 with hydrocephalus Q05.1
 lumbar Q05.7
 with hydrocephalus Q05.2
 lumbosacral Q05.7
 with hydrocephalus Q05.2
 occulta Q76.0
 sacral Q05.8
 with hydrocephalus Q05.3
 thoracic Q05.6
 with hydrocephalus Q05.1
 thoracolumbar Q05.6
 with hydrocephalus Q05.1
Spindle, Krukenberg's — *see* Pigmentation, cornea, posterior
Spine, spinal — *see* condition

Spiradenoma (eccrine) — *see* Neoplasm, skin, benign
Spirillosis A25.0
Spirillum
 minus A25.0
 obermeieri infection A68.0
Spirochetal — *see* condition
Spirochetosis A69.9
 arthritic, arthritica A69.9
 bronchopulmonary A69.8
 icterohemorrhagic A27.0
 lung A69.8
Spirometrosis B70.1
Spitting blood — *see* Hemoptysis
Splanchnoptosis K63.4
Spleen, splenic — *see* condition
Splenectasis — *see* Splenomegaly
Splenitis (interstitial) (malignant) (nonspecific) D73.89
 malarial (*see also* Malaria) B54 [D77]
 tuberculous A18.85
Splenocele D73.89
Splenomegaly, splenomegalia (Bengal) (cryptogenic) (idiopathic) (tropical) R16.1
 with hepatomegaly R16.2
 cirrhotic D73.2
 congenital Q89.09
 congestive, chronic D73.2
 Egyptian B65.1
 Gaucher's E75.22
 malarial (*see also* Malaria) B54 [D77]
 neutropenic D73.81
 Niemann-Pick — *see* Niemann-Pick disease or syndrome
 siderotic D73.2
 syphilitic A52.79
 congenital (early) A50.08 [D77]
Splenopathy D73.9
Splenoptosis D73.89
Splenosis D73.89
Splinter — *see* Foreign body, superficial, by site
Split, splitting
 foot Q72.7- ☑
 heart sounds R01.2
 lip, congenital — *see* Cleft, lip
 nails L60.3
 urinary stream R39.13
Spondylarthrosis — *see* Spondylosis
Spondylitis (chronic) (*see also* Spondylopathy, inflammatory)
 ankylopoietica — *see* Spondylitis, ankylosing
 ankylosing (chronic) M45.9
 with lung involvement M45.9 [J99]
 cervical region M45.2
 cervicothoracic region M45.3
 juvenile M08.1
 lumbar region M45.6
 lumbosacral region M45.7
 multiple sites M45.0
 occipito-atlanto-axial region M45.1
 sacrococcygeal region M45.8
 thoracic region M45.4
 thoracolumbar region M45.5
 atrophic (ligamentous) — *see* Spondylitis, ankylosing
 deformans (chronic) — *see* Spondylosis
 gonococcal A54.41
 gouty M10.08
 in (due to)
 brucellosis A23.9 [M49.80]
 cervical region A23.9 [M49.82]
 cervicothoracic region A23.9 [M49.83]
 lumbar region A23.9 [M49.86]
 lumbosacral region A23.9 [M49.87]
 multiple sites A23.9 [M49.89]
 occipito-atlanto-axial region A23.9 [M49.81]
 sacrococcygeal region A23.9 [M49.88]
 thoracic region A23.9 [M49.84]
 thoracolumbar region A23.9 [M49.85]
 enterobacteria (*see also* subcategory M49.8) A04.9
 tuberculosis A18.01
 infectious NEC — *see* Spondylopathy, infective
 juvenile ankylosing (chronic) M08.1
 Kümmell's — *see* Spondylopathy, traumatic
 Marie-Strümpell — *see* Spondylitis, ankylosing
 muscularis — *see* Spondylopathy, specified NEC
 psoriatic L40.53
 rheumatoid — *see* Spondylitis, ankylosing
 rhizomelica — *see* Spondylitis, ankylosing
 sacroiliac NEC M46.1

☑ **Additional Character Required** — Refer to the Tabular List for Character Selection   ▽ Subterms under main terms may continue to next column or page

Spondylitis — *continued*
  senescent, senile — *see* Spondylosis
  traumatic (chronic) or post-traumatic — *see* Spondylopathy, traumatic
  tuberculous A18.01
  typhosa A01.05
Spondylolisthesis (acquired) (degenerative) M43.10
  with disproportion (fetopelvic) O33.0
    causing obstructed labor O65.0
  cervical region M43.12
  cervicothoracic region M43.13
  congenital Q76.2
  lumbar region M43.16
  lumbosacral region M43.17
  multiple sites M43.19
  occipito-atlanto-axial region M43.11
  sacrococcygeal region M43.18
  thoracic region M43.14
  thoracolumbar region M43.15
  traumatic (old) M43.10
    acute
      fifth cervical (displaced) S12.430 ☑
        nondisplaced S12.431 ☑
        specified type NEC (displaced) S12.450 ☑
          nondisplaced S12.451 ☑
        type III S12.44 ☑
      fourth cervical (displaced) S12.330 ☑
        nondisplaced S12.331 ☑
        specified type NEC (displaced) S12.350 ☑
          nondisplaced S12.351 ☑
        type III S12.34 ☑
      second cervical (displaced) S12.130 ☑
        nondisplaced S12.131 ☑
        specified type NEC (displaced) S12.150 ☑
          nondisplaced S12.151 ☑
        type III S12.14 ☑
      seventh cervical (displaced) S12.630 ☑
        nondisplaced S12.631 ☑
        specified type NEC (displaced) S12.650 ☑
          nondisplaced S12.651 ☑
        type III S12.64 ☑
      sixth cervical (displaced) S12.530 ☑
        nondisplaced S12.531 ☑
        specified type NEC (displaced) S12.550 ☑
          nondisplaced S12.551 ☑
        type III S12.54 ☑
      third cervical (displaced) S12.230 ☑
        nondisplaced S12.231 ☑
        specified type NEC (displaced) S12.250 ☑
          nondisplaced S12.251 ☑
        type III S12.24 ☑
Spondylolysis (acquired) M43.00
  cervical region M43.02
  cervicothoracic region M43.03
  congenital Q76.2
  lumbar region M43.06
  lumbosacral region M43.07
    with disproportion (fetopelvic) O33.0
      causing obstructed labor O65.8
  multiple sites M43.09
  occipito-atlanto-axial region M43.01
  sacrococcygeal region M43.08
  thoracic region M43.04
  thoracolumbar region M43.05
Spondylopathy M48.9
  infective NEC M46.50
    cervical region M46.52
    cervicothoracic region M46.53
    lumbar region M46.56
    lumbosacral region M46.57
    multiple sites M46.59
    occipito-atlanto-axial region M46.51
    sacrococcygeal region M46.58
    thoracic region M46.54
    thoracolumbar region M46.55
  inflammatory M46.90
    cervical region M46.92
    cervicothoracic region M46.93
    lumbar region M46.96
    lumbosacral region M46.97
    multiple sites M46.99
    occipito-atlanto-axial region M46.91
    sacrococcygeal region M46.98
    specified type NEC M46.80
      cervical region M46.82
      cervicothoracic region M46.83
      lumbar region M46.86

Spondylopathy — *continued*
  inflammatory — *continued*
    specified type — *continued*
      lumbosacral region M46.87
      multiple sites M46.89
      occipito-atlanto-axial region M46.81
      sacrococcygeal region M46.88
      thoracic region M46.84
      thoracolumbar region M46.85
    thoracic region M46.94
    thoracolumbar region M46.95
  neuropathic, in
    syringomyelia and syringobulbia G95.0
    tabes dorsalis A52.11
  specified NEC — *see* subcategory M48.8 ☑
  traumatic M48.30
    cervical region M48.32
    cervicothoracic region M48.33
    lumbar region M48.36
    lumbosacral region M48.37
    occipito-atlanto-axial region M48.31
    sacrococcygeal region M48.38
    thoracic region M48.34
    thoracolumbar region M48.35
Spondylosis M47.9
  with
    disproportion (fetopelvic) O33.0
      causing obstructed labor O65.0
    myelopathy NEC M47.10
      cervical region M47.12
      cervicothoracic region M47.13
      lumbar region M47.16
      occipito-atlanto-axial region M47.11
      thoracic region M47.14
      thoracolumbar region M47.15
    radiculopathy M47.20
      cervical region M47.22
      cervicothoracic region M47.23
      lumbar region M47.26
      lumbosacral region M47.27
      occipito-atlanto-axial region M47.21
      sacrococcygeal region M47.28
      thoracic region M47.24
      thoracolumbar region M47.25
  without myelopathy or radiculopathy M47.819
    cervical region M47.812
    cervicothoracic region M47.813
    lumbar region M47.816
    lumbosacral region M47.817
    occipito-atlanto-axial region M47.811
    sacrococcygeal region M47.818
    thoracic region M47.814
    thoracolumbar region M47.815
    specified NEC M47.899
      cervical region M47.892
      cervicothoracic region M47.893
      lumbar region M47.896
      lumbosacral region M47.897
      occipito-atlanto-axial region M47.891
      sacrococcygeal region M47.898
      thoracic region M47.894
      thoracolumbar region M47.895
  traumatic — *see* Spondylopathy, traumatic
Sponge
  inadvertently left in operation wound — *see* Foreign body, accidentally left during a procedure
  kidney (medullary) Q61.5
Sponge-diver's disease — *see* Toxicity, venom, marine animal, sea anemone
Spongioblastoma (any type) — *see* Neoplasm, malignant, by site
  specified site — *see* Neoplasm, malignant, by site
  unspecified site C71.9
Spongioneuroblastoma — *see* Neoplasm, malignant, by site
Spontaneous (*see also* condition)
  fracture (cause unknown) — *see* Fracture, pathological
Spoon nail L60.3
  congenital Q84.6
Sporadic — *see* condition
Sporothrix schenckii infection — *see* Sporotrichosis
Sporotrichosis B42.9
  arthritis B42.82
  disseminated B42.7
  generalized B42.7
  lymphocutaneous (fixed) (progressive) B42.1
  pulmonary B42.0
  specified NEC B42.89

Spots, spotting (in) (of)
  Bitot's (*see also* Pigmentation, conjunctiva)
    in the young child E50.1
    vitamin A deficiency E50.1
  café, au lait L81.3
  Cayenne pepper I78.1
  cotton wool, retina — *see* Occlusion, artery, retina
  de Morgan's (senile angiomas) I78.1
  Fuchs' black (myopic) H44.2-
  intermenstrual (regular) N92.0
    irregular N92.1
  Koplik's B05.9
  liver L81.4
  pregnancy O26.85- ☑
  purpuric R23.3
  ruby I78.1
Spotted fever — *see* Fever, spotted N92.3
Sprain (joint) (ligament)
  acromioclavicular joint or ligament S43.5- ☑
  ankle S93.40- ☑
    calcaneofibular ligament S93.41- ☑
    deltoid ligament S93.42- ☑
    internal collateral ligament — *see* Sprain, ankle, specified ligament NEC
    specified ligament NEC S93.49- ☑
    talofibular ligament — *see* Sprain, ankle, specified ligament NEC
    tibiofibular ligament S93.43- ☑
  anterior longitudinal, cervical S13.4 ☑
  atlas, atlanto-axial, atlanto-occipital S13.4 ☑
  breast bone — *see* Sprain, sternum
  calcaneofibular — *see* Sprain, ankle
  carpal — *see* Sprain, wrist
  carpometacarpal — *see* Sprain, hand, specified site NEC
  cartilage
    costal S23.41 ☑
    semilunar (knee) — *see* Sprain, knee, specified site NEC
      with current tear — *see* Tear, meniscus
    thyroid region S13.5 ☑
    xiphoid — *see* Sprain, sternum
  cervical, cervicodorsal, cervicothoracic S13.4 ☑
  chondrosternal S23.421 ☑
  coracoclavicular S43.8- ☑
  coracohumeral S43.41- ☑
  coronary, knee — *see* Sprain, knee, specified site NEC
  costal cartilage S23.41 ☑
  cricoarytenoid articulation or ligament S13.5 ☑
  cricothyroid articulation S13.5 ☑
  cruciate, knee — *see* Sprain, knee, cruciate
  deltoid, ankle — *see* Sprain, ankle
  dorsal (spine) S23.3 ☑
  elbow S53.40- ☑
    radial collateral ligament S53.43- ☑
    radiohumeral S53.41- ☑
    rupture
      radial collateral ligament — *see* Rupture, traumatic, ligament, radial collateral
      ulnar collateral ligament — *see* Rupture, traumatic, ligament, ulnar collateral
    specified type NEC S53.49- ☑
    ulnar collateral ligament S53.44- ☑
    ulnohumeral S53.42- ☑
  femur, head — *see* Sprain, hip
  fibular collateral, knee — *see* Sprain, knee, collateral
  fibulocalcaneal — *see* Sprain, ankle
  finger(s) S63.61- ☑
    index S63.61- ☑
    interphalangeal (joint) S63.63- ☑
      index S63.63- ☑
      little S63.63- ☑
      middle S63.63- ☑
      ring S63.63- ☑
    little S63.61- ☑
    metacarpophalangeal (joint) S63.65- ☑
    middle S63.61- ☑
    ring S63.61- ☑
    specified site NEC S63.69- ☑
      index S63.69- ☑
      little S63.69- ☑
      middle S63.69- ☑
      ring S63.69- ☑
  foot S93.60- ☑
    specified ligament NEC S93.69- ☑
    tarsal ligament S93.61- ☑

Sprain — *continued*
  foot — *continued*
    tarsometatarsal ligament S93.62- ☑
    toe — *see* Sprain, toe
  hand S63.9- ☑
    finger — *see* Sprain, finger
    specified site NEC — *see* subcategory S63.8 ☑
    thumb — *see* Sprain, thumb
  head S03.9 ☑
  hip S73.10- ☑
    iliofemoral ligament S73.11- ☑
    ischiocapsular (ligament) S73.12- ☑
    specified NEC S73.19- ☑
  iliofemoral — *see* Sprain, hip
  innominate
    acetabulum — *see* Sprain, hip
    sacral junction S33.6 ☑
  internal
    collateral, ankle — *see* Sprain, ankle
    semilunar cartilage — *see* Sprain, knee, specified
        site NEC
  interphalangeal
    finger — *see* Sprain, finger, interphalangeal (joint)
    toe — *see* Sprain, toe, interphalangeal joint
  ischiocapsular — *see* Sprain, hip
  ischiofemoral — *see* Sprain, hip
  jaw (articular disc) (cartilage) (meniscus) S03.4 ☑
    old M26.69
  knee S83.9- ☑
    collateral ligament S83.40- ☑
      lateral (fibular) S83.42- ☑
      medial (tibial) S83.41- ☑
    cruciate ligament S83.50- ☑
      anterior S83.51- ☑
      posterior S83.52- ☑
    lateral (fibular) collateral ligament S83.42- ☑
    medial (tibial) collateral ligament S83.41- ☑
    patellar ligament S76.11- ☑
    specified site NEC S83.8X- ☑
    superior tibiofibular joint (ligament) S83.6- ☑
  lateral collateral, knee — *see* Sprain, knee, collateral
  lumbar (spine) S33.5 ☑
  lumbosacral S33.9 ☑
  mandible (articular disc) S03.4 ☑
    old M26.69
  medial collateral, knee — *see* Sprain, knee, collateral
  meniscus
    jaw S03.4 ☑
      old M26.69
    knee — *see* Sprain, knee, specified site NEC
      with current tear — *see* Tear, meniscus
        old — *see* Derangement, knee, meniscus,
            due to old tear
    mandible S03.4 ☑
      old M26.69
  metacarpal (distal) (proximal) — *see* Sprain, hand,
      specified site NEC
  metacarpophalangeal — *see* Sprain, finger, metacar-
      pophalangeal (joint)
  metatarsophalangeal — *see* Sprain, toe, metatarsopha-
      langeal joint
  midcarpal — *see* Sprain, hand, specified site NEC
  midtarsal — *see* Sprain, foot, specified site NEC
  neck S13.9 ☑
    anterior longitudinal cervical ligament S13.4 ☑
    atlanto-axial joint S13.4 ☑
    atlanto-occipital joint S13.4 ☑
    cervical spine S13.4 ☑
    cricoarytenoid ligament S13.5 ☑
    cricothyroid ligament S13.5 ☑
    specified site NEC S13.8 ☑
    thyroid region (cartilage) S13.5 ☑
  nose S03.8 ☑
  orbicular, hip — *see* Sprain, hip
  patella — *see* Sprain, knee, specified site NEC
  patellar ligament S76.11- ☑
  pelvis NEC S33.8 ☑
  phalanx
    finger — *see* Sprain, finger
    toe — *see* Sprain, toe
  pubofemoral — *see* Sprain, hip
  radiocarpal — *see* Sprain, wrist
  radiohumeral — *see* Sprain, elbow
  radius, collateral — *see* Rupture, traumatic, ligament,
      radial collateral
  rib (cage) S23.41 ☑

Sprain — *continued*
  rotator cuff (capsule) S43.42- ☑
  sacroiliac (region)
    chronic or old — *see* subcategory M53.2 ☑
    joint S33.6 ☑
  scaphoid (hand) — *see* Sprain, hand, specified site
      NEC
  scapula (r) — *see* Sprain, shoulder girdle, specified site
      NEC
  semilunar cartilage (knee) — *see* Sprain, knee, speci-
      fied site NEC
    with current tear — *see* Tear, meniscus
      old — *see* Derangement, knee, meniscus, due
          to old tear
  shoulder joint S43.40- ☑
    acromioclavicular joint (ligament) — *see* Sprain,
        acromioclavicular joint
    blade — *see* Sprain, shoulder, girdle, specified site
        NEC
    coracoclavicular joint (ligament) — *see* Sprain,
        coracoclavicular joint
    coracohumeral ligament — *see* Sprain, coraco-
        humeral joint
    girdle S43.9- ☑
      specified site NEC S43.8- ☑
    rotator cuff — *see* Sprain, rotator cuff
    specified site NEC S43.49- ☑
    sternoclavicular joint (ligament) — *see* Sprain,
        sternoclavicular joint
  spine
    cervical S13.4 ☑
    lumbar S33.5 ☑
    thoracic S23.3 ☑
  sternoclavicular joint S43.6- ☑
  sternum S23.429 ☑
    chondrosternal joint S23.421 ☑
    specified site NEC S23.428 ☑
    sternoclavicular (joint) (ligament) S23.420 ☑
  symphysis
    jaw S03.4 ☑
      old M26.69
    mandibular S03.4 ☑
      old M26.69
  talofibular — *see* Sprain, ankle
  tarsal — *see* Sprain, foot, specified site NEC
  tarsometatarsal — *see* Sprain, foot, specified site NEC
  temporomandibular S03.4 ☑
    old M26.69
  thorax S23.9 ☑
    ribs S23.41 ☑
    specified site NEC S23.8 ☑
    spine S23.3 ☑
    sternum — *see* Sprain, sternum
  thumb S63.60- ☑
    interphalangeal (joint) S63.62- ☑
    metacarpophalangeal (joint) S63.64- ☑
    specified site NEC S63.68- ☑
  thyroid cartilage or region S13.5 ☑
  tibia (proximal end) — *see* Sprain, knee, specified site
      NEC
  tibial collateral, knee — *see* Sprain, knee, collateral
  tibiofibular
    distal — *see* Sprain, ankle
    superior — *see* Sprain, knee, specified site NEC
  toe(s) S93.50- ☑
    great S93.50- ☑
    interphalangeal joint S93.51- ☑
      great S93.51- ☑
      lesser S93.51- ☑
    lesser S93.50- ☑
    metatarsophalangeal joint S93.52- ☑
      great S93.52- ☑
      lesser S93.52- ☑
  ulna, collateral — *see* Rupture, traumatic, ligament,
      ulnar collateral
  ulnohumeral — *see* Sprain, elbow
  wrist S63.50- ☑
    carpal S63.51- ☑
    radiocarpal S63.52- ☑
    specified site NEC S63.59- ☑
  xiphoid cartilage — *see* Sprain, sternum
Sprengel's deformity (congenital) Q74.0
Sprue (tropical) K90.1
  celiac K90.0
  idiopathic K90.0
  meaning thrush B37.0

Sprue — *continued*
  nontropical K90.0
Spur, bone (*see also* Enthesopathy)
  calcaneal M77.3- ☑
  iliac crest M76.2- ☑
  nose (septum) J34.89
Spurway's syndrome Q78.0
Sputum
  abnormal (amount) (color) (odor) (purulent) R09.3
  blood-stained R04.2
  excessive (cause unknown) R09.3
Squamous (*see also* condition)
  epithelium in
    cervical canal (congenital) Q51.828
    uterine mucosa (congenital) Q51.818
Squashed nose M95.0
  congenital Q67.4
Squeeze, diver's T70.3 ☑
Squint (*see also* Strabismus)
  accommodative — *see* Strabismus, convergent con-
      comitant
St. Hubert's disease A82.9
Stab (*see also* Laceration)
  internal organs — *see* Injury, by site
Stafne's cyst or cavity M27.0
Staggering gait R26.0
  hysterical F44.4
Staghorn calculus — *see* Calculus, kidney
Stähli's line (cornea) (pigment) — *see* Pigmentation,
    cornea, anterior
Stain, staining
  meconium (newborn) P96.83
  port wine Q82.5
  tooth, teeth (hard tissues) (extrinsic) K03.6
    due to
      accretions K03.6
      deposits (betel) (black) (green) (materia alba)
          (orange) (soft) (tobacco) K03.6
      metals (copper) (silver) K03.7
      nicotine K03.6
      pulpal bleeding K03.7
      tobacco K03.6
    intrinsic K00.8
Stammering (*see also* Disorder, fluency) F80.81
Standstill
  auricular I45.5
  cardiac — *see* Arrest, cardiac
  sinoatrial I45.5
  ventricular — *see* Arrest, cardiac
Stannosis J63.5
Stanton's disease — *see* Melioidosis
Staphylitis (acute) (catarrhal) (chronic) (gangrenous)
    (membranous) (suppurative) (ulcerative) K12.2
Staphylococcal scalded skin syndrome L00
Staphylococcemia A41.2
Staphylococcus, staphylococcal (*see also* condition)
  as cause of disease classified elsewhere B95.8
    aureus (methicillin susceptible) (MSSA) B95.61
      methicillin resistant (MRSA) B95.62
  specified NEC, as cause of disease classified elsewhere
      B95.7
Staphyloma (sclera)
  cornea H18.72- ☑
  equatorial H15.81- ☑
  localized (anterior) H15.82- ☑
  posticum H15.83- ☑
  ring H15.85- ☑
Stargardt's disease — *see* Dystrophy, retina
Starvation (inanition) (due to lack of food) T73.0 ☑
  edema — *see* Malnutrition, severe
Stasis
  bile (noncalculous) K83.1
  bronchus J98.09
    with infection — *see* Bronchitis
  cardiac — *see* Failure, heart, congestive
  cecum K59.8
  colon K59.8
  dermatitis — *see* Varix, leg, with, inflammation
  duodenal K31.5
  eczema — *see* Varix, leg, with, inflammation
  edema — *see* Hypertension, venous (chronic), idiopath-
      ic
  foot T69.0- ☑
  ileocecal coil K59.8
  ileum K59.8
  intestinal K59.8
  jejunum K59.8

Stasis— *continued*
kidney N19
liver (cirrhotic) K76.1
lymphatic I89.8
pneumonia J18.2
pulmonary — *see* Edema, lung
rectal K59.8
renal N19
    tubular N17.0
ulcer — *see* Varix, leg, with, ulcer
    without varicose veins I87.2
urine — *see* Retention, urine
venous I87.8
State (of)
affective and paranoid, mixed, organic psychotic F06.8
agitated R45.1
    acute reaction to stress F43.0
anxiety (neurotic) F41.1
apprehension F41.1
burn-out Z73.0
climacteric, female Z78.0
    symptomatic N95.1
compulsive F42
    mixed with obsessional thoughts F42
confusional (psychogenic) F44.89
    acute (*see also* Delirium)
        with
            arteriosclerotic dementia F01.50
                with behavioral disturbance F01.51
            senility or dementia F05
        alcoholic F10.231
        epileptic F05
    reactive (from emotional stress, psychological
        trauma) F44.89
    subacute — *see* Delirium
convulsive — *see* Convulsions
crisis F43.0
depressive F32.9
    neurotic F34.1
dissociative F44.9
emotional shock (stress) R45.7
hypercoagulation — *see* Hypercoagulable
locked-in G83.5
menopausal Z78.0
    symptomatic N95.1
neurotic F48.9
    with depersonalization F48.1
obsessional F42
oneiroid (schizophrenia-like) F23
organic
    hallucinatory (nonalcoholic) F06.0
    paranoid (hallucinatory) F06.2
panic F41.0
paranoid F22
    climacteric F22
    involutional F22
    menopausal F22
    organic F06.2
    senile F03 ☑
    simple F22
persistent vegetative R40.3
phobic F40.9
postleukotomy F07.0
pregnant, incidental Z33.1
psychogenic, twilight F44.89
psychopathic (constitutional) F60.2
psychotic, organic (*see also* Psychosis, organic)
    mixed paranoid and affective F06.8
    senile or presenile F03 ☑
    transient NEC F06.8
        with
            depression F06.31
            hallucinations F06.0
residual schizophrenic F20.5
restlessness R45.1
stress (emotional) R45.7
tension (mental) F48.9
    specified NEC F48.8
transient organic psychotic NEC F06.8
    depressive type F06.31
    hallucinatory type F06.30
twilight
    epileptic F05
    psychogenic F44.89
vegetative, persistent R40.3
vital exhaustion Z73.0
withdrawal, — *see* Withdrawal, state

Status (post) (*see also* Presence (of))
absence, epileptic — *see* Epilepsy, by type, with status
    epilepticus
administration of tPA (rtPA) in a different facility
    within the last 24 hours prior to admission to
    current facility Z92.82
adrenalectomy (unilateral) (bilateral) E89.6
anastomosis Z98.0
anginosus I20.9
angioplasty (peripheral) Z98.62
    with implant Z95.820
    coronary artery Z98.61
        with implant Z95.5
aortocoronary bypass Z95.1
arthrodesis Z98.1
artificial opening (of) Z93.9
    gastrointestinal tract Z93.4
    specified NEC Z93.8
    urinary tract Z93.6
    vagina Z93.8
asthmaticus — *see* Asthma, by type, with status asth-
    maticus
awaiting organ transplant Z76.82
bariatric surgery Z98.84
bed confinement Z74.01
bleb, filtering (vitreous), after glaucoma surgery Z98.83
breast implant Z98.82
    removal Z98.86
cataract extraction Z98.4- ☑
cholecystectomy Z90.49
clitorectomy N90.811
    with excision of labia minora N90.812
colectomy (complete) (partial) Z90.49
colonization — *see* Carrier (suspected) of
colostomy Z93.3
convulsivus idiopathicus — *see* Epilepsy, by type, with
    status epilepticus
coronary artery angioplasty — *see* Status, angioplasty,
    coronary artery
cystectomy (urinary bladder) Z90.6
cystostomy Z93.50
    appendico-vesicostomy Z93.52
    cutaneous Z93.51
    specified NEC Z93.59
delinquent immunization Z28.3
dental Z98.818
    crown Z98.811
    fillings Z98.811
    restoration Z98.811
    sealant Z98.810
    specified NEC Z98.818
deployment (current) (military) Z56.82
dialysis (hemodialysis) (peritoneal) Z99.2
do not resuscitate (DNR) Z66
donor — *see* Donor
embedded fragments — *see* Retained, foreign body
    fragments (type of)
embedded splinter — *see* Retained, foreign body
    fragments (type of)
enterostomy Z93.4
epileptic, epilepticus (*see also* Epilepsy, by type, with
    status epilepticus) G40.901
estrogen receptor
    negative Z17.1
    positive Z17.0
female genital cutting — *see* Female genital mutilation
    status
female genital mutilation — *see* Female genital muti-
    lation status
filtering (vitreous) bleb after glaucoma surgery Z98.83
gastrectomy (complete) (partial) Z90.3
gastric banding Z98.84
gastric bypass for obesity Z98.84
gastrostomy Z93.1
human immunodeficiency virus (HIV) infection,
    asymptomatic Z21
hysterectomy (complete) (total) Z90.710
    partial (with remaining cervial stump) Z90.711
ileostomy Z93.2
implant
    breast Z98.82
infibulation N90.813
intestinal bypass Z98.0
jejunostomy Z93.4
lapsed immunization schedule Z28.3
laryngectomy Z90.02
lymphaticus E32.8
marmoratus G80.3

Status — *continued*
mastectomy (unilateral) (bilateral) Z90.1- ☑
military deployment status (current) Z56.82
    in theater or in support of military war, peacekeep-
        ing and humanitarian operations Z56.82
nephrectomy (unilateral) (bilateral) Z90.5
nephrostomy Z93.6
obesity surgery Z98.84
oophorectomy
    bilateral Z90.722
    unilateral Z90.721
organ replacement
    by artificial or mechanical device or prosthesis of
        artery Z95.828
        bladder Z96.0
        blood vessel Z95.828
        breast Z97.8
        eye globe Z97.0
        heart Z95.812
            valve Z95.2
        intestine Z97.8
        joint Z96.60
            hip — *see* Presence, hip joint implant
            knee — *see* Presence, knee joint implant
            specified site NEC Z96.698
        kidney Z97.8
        larynx Z96.3
        lens Z96.1
        limbs — *see* Presence, artificial, limb
        liver Z97.8
        lung Z97.8
        pancreas Z97.8
    by organ transplant (heterologous)(homologous)
        — *see* Transplant
pacemaker
    brain Z96.89
    cardiac Z95.0
    specified NEC Z96.89
pancreatectomy Z90.410
    complete Z90.410
    partial Z90.411
    total Z90.410
physical restraint Z78.1
pneumonectomy (complete) (partial) Z90.2
pneumothorax, therapeutic Z98.3
postcommotio cerebri F07.81
postoperative (postprocedural) NEC Z98.89
    breast implant Z98.82
    dental Z98.818
        crown Z98.811
        fillings Z98.811
        restoration Z98.811
        sealant Z98.810
        specified NEC Z98.818
    pneumothorax, therapeutic Z98.3
postpartum (routine follow-up) Z39.2
    care immediately after delivery Z39.0
postsurgical (postprocedural) NEC Z98.89
    pneumothorax, therapeutic Z98.3
pregnancy, incidental Z33.1
prosthesis coronary angioplasty Z95.5
pseudophakia Z96.1
renal dialysis (hemodialysis) (peritoneal) Z99.2
retained foreign body — *see* Retained, foreign body
    fragments (type of)
reversed jejunal transposition (for bypass) Z98.0
salpingo-oophorectomy
    bilateral Z90.722
    unilateral Z90.721
sex reassignment surgery status Z87.890
shunt
    arteriovenous (for dialysis) Z99.2
    cerebrospinal fluid Z98.2
    ventricular (communicating) (for drainage) Z98.2
splenectomy Z90.81
thymicolymphaticus E32.8
thymicus E32.8
thymolymphaticus E32.8
thyroidectomy (hypothyroidism) E89.0
tooth (teeth) extraction (*see also* Absence, teeth, ac-
    quired) K08.409
tPA (rtPA) administration in a different facility within
    the last 24 hours prior to admission to current
    facility Z92.82
tracheostomy Z93.0
transplant — *see* Transplant
    organ removed Z98.85
tubal ligation Z98.51

Status — *continued*
underimmunization Z28.3
ureterostomy Z93.6
urethrostomy Z93.6
vagina, artificial Z93.8
vasectomy Z98.52
wheelchair confinement Z99.3
Stealing
child problem F91.8
in company with others Z72.810
pathological (compulsive) F63.2
Steam burn — *see* Burn
Steatocystoma multiplex L72.2
Steatohepatitis (nonalcoholic) (NASH) K75.81
Steatoma L72.3
eyelid (cystic) — *see* Dermatosis, eyelid
infected — *see* Hordeolum
Steatorrhea (chronic) K90.4
with lacteal obstruction K90.2
idiopathic (adult) (infantile) K90.0
pancreatic K90.3
primary K90.0
tropical K90.1
Steatosis E88.89
heart — *see* Degeneration, myocardial
kidney N28.89
liver NEC K76.0
Steele-Richardson-Olszewski disease or syndrome
G23.1
Steinbrocker's syndrome G90.8
Steinert's disease G71.11
Stein-Leventhal syndrome E28.2
Stein's syndrome E28.2
STEMI (*see also* Infarct, myocardium, ST elevation) I21.3
Stenocardia I20.8
Stenocephaly Q75.8
Stenosis, stenotic (cicatricial) (*see also* Stricture)
ampulla of Vater K83.1
anus, anal (canal) (sphincter) K62.4
and rectum K62.4
congenital Q42.3
with fistula Q42.2
aorta (ascending) (supraventricular) (congenital) Q25.3
arteriosclerotic I70.0
calcified I70.0
aortic (valve) I35.0
with insufficiency I35.2
congenital Q23.0
rheumatic I06.0
with
incompetency, insufficiency or regurgitation
I06.2
with mitral (valve) disease I08.0
with tricuspid (valve) disease I08.3
mitral (valve) disease I08.0
with tricuspid (valve) disease I08.3
tricuspid (valve) disease I08.2
with mitral (valve) disease I08.3
specified cause NEC I35.0
syphilitic A52.03
aqueduct of Sylvius (congenital) Q03.0
with spina bifida — *see* Spina bifida, by site, with
hydrocephalus
acquired G91.1
artery NEC (*see also* Arteriosclerosis) I77.1
celiac I77.4
cerebral — *see* Occlusion, artery, cerebral
extremities — *see* Arteriosclerosis, extremities
precerebral — *see* Occlusion, artery, precerebral
pulmonary (congenital) Q25.6
acquired I28.8
renal I70.1
bile duct (common) (hepatic) K83.1
congenital Q44.3
bladder-neck (acquired) N32.0
congenital Q64.31
brain G93.89
bronchus J98.09
congenital Q32.3
syphilitic A52.72
cardia (stomach) K22.2
congenital Q39.3
cardiovascular — *see* Disease, cardiovascular
caudal M48.08
cervix, cervical (canal) N88.2
congenital Q51.828
in pregnancy or childbirth — *see* Pregnancy,
complicated by, abnormal cervix

Stenosis, stenotic — *continued*
colon (*see also* Obstruction, intestine)
congenital Q42.9
specified NEC Q42.8
colostomy K94.03
common (bile) duct K83.1
congenital Q44.3
coronary (artery) — *see* Disease, heart, ischemic,
atherosclerotic
cystic duct — *see* Obstruction, gallbladder
due to presence of device, implant or graft (*see also*
Complications, by site and type, specified NEC)
T85.85 ☑
arterial graft NEC T82.858 ☑
breast (implant) T85.85 ☑
catheter T85.85 ☑
dialysis (renal) T82.858 ☑
intraperitoneal T85.85 ☑
infusion NEC T82.858 ☑
spinal (epidural) (subdural) T85.85 ☑
urinary (indwelling) T83.85 ☑
fixation, internal (orthopedic) NEC T84.85 ☑
gastrointestinal (bile duct) (esophagus) T85.85 ☑
genital NEC T83.85 ☑
heart NEC T82.857 ☑
joint prosthesis T84.85 ☑
ocular (corneal graft) (orbital implant) NEC
T85.85 ☑
orthopedic NEC T84.85 ☑
specified NEC T85.85 ☑
urinary NEC T83.85 ☑
vascular NEC T82.858 ☑
ventricular intracranial shunt T85.85 ☑
duodenum K31.5
congenital Q41.0
ejaculatory duct NEC N50.8
endocervical os — *see* Stenosis, cervix
enterostomy K94.13
esophagus K22.2
congenital Q39.3
syphilitic A52.79
congenital A50.59 [K23]
eustachian tube — *see* Obstruction, eustachian tube
external ear canal (acquired) H61.30- ☑
congenital Q16.1
due to
inflammation H61.32- ☑
trauma H61.31- ☑
postprocedural H95.81- ☑
specified cause NEC H61.39- ☑
gallbladder — *see* Obstruction, gallbladder
glottis J38.6
heart valve (congenital) Q24.8
aortic Q23.0
mitral Q23.2
pulmonary Q22.1
tricuspid Q22.4
hepatic duct K83.1
hymen N89.6
hypertrophic subaortic (idiopathic) I42.1
ileum K56.69
congenital Q41.2
infundibulum cardia Q24.3
intervertebral foramina (*see also* Lesion, biomechanical, specified NEC)
connective tissue M99.79
abdomen M99.79
cervical region M99.71
cervicothoracic M99.71
head region M99.70
lumbar region M99.73
lumbosacral M99.73
occipitocervical M99.70
sacral region M99.74
sacrococcygeal M99.74
sacroiliac M99.74
specified NEC M99.79
thoracic region M99.72
thoracolumbar M99.72
disc M99.79
abdomen M99.79
cervical region M99.71
cervicothoracic M99.71
head region M99.70
lower extremity M99.76
lumbar region M99.73
lumbosacral M99.73

Stenosis, stenotic — *continued*
intervertebral foramina (*see also* Lesion, biomechanical,
specified) — *continued*
disc — *continued*
occipitocervical M99.70
pelvic M99.75
rib cage M99.78
sacral region M99.74
sacrococcygeal M99.74
sacroiliac M99.74
specified NEC M99.79
thoracic region M99.72
thoracolumbar M99.72
upper extremity M99.77
osseous M99.69
abdomen M99.69
cervical region M99.61
cervicothoracic M99.61
head region M99.60
lower extremity M99.66
lumbar region M99.63
lumbosacral M99.63
occipitocervical M99.60
pelvic M99.65
rib cage M99.68
sacral region M99.64
sacrococcygeal M99.64
sacroiliac M99.64
specified NEC M99.69
thoracic region M99.62
thoracolumbar M99.62
upper extremity M99.67
subluxation — *see* Stenosis, intervertebral foramina, osseous
intestine (*see also* Obstruction, intestine)
congenital (small) Q41.9
large Q42.9
specified NEC Q42.8
specified NEC Q41.8
jejunum K56.69
congenital Q41.1
lacrimal (passage)
canaliculi H04.54- ☑
congenital Q10.5
duct H04.55- ☑
punctum H04.56- ☑
sac H04.57- ☑
lacrimonasal duct — *see* Stenosis, lacrimal, duct
congenital Q10.5
larynx J38.6
congenital NEC Q31.8
subglottic Q31.1
syphilitic A52.73
congenital A50.59 [J99]
mitral (chronic) (inactive) (valve) I05.0
with
aortic valve disease I08.0
incompetency, insufficiency or regurgitation
I05.2
active or acute I01.1
with rheumatic or Sydenham's chorea I02.0
congenital Q23.2
specified cause, except rheumatic I34.2
syphilitic A52.03
myocardium, myocardial (*see also* Degeneration, myocardial)
hypertrophic subaortic (idiopathic) I42.1
nares (anterior) (posterior) J34.89
congenital Q30.0
nasal duct (*see also* Stenosis, lacrimal, duct)
congenital Q10.5
nasolacrimal duct (*see also* Stenosis, lacrimal, duct)
congenital Q10.5
neural canal (*see also* Lesion, biomechanical, specified
NEC)
connective tissue M99.49
abdomen M99.49
cervical region M99.41
cervicothoracic M99.41
head region M99.40
lower extremity M99.46
lumbar region M99.43
lumbosacral M99.43
occipitocervical M99.40
pelvic M99.45
rib cage M99.48
sacral region M99.44
sacrococcygeal M99.44

☑ **Additional Character Required** — **Refer to the Tabular List for Character Selection**   ▽ **Subterms under main terms may continue to next column or page**

Stenosis, stenotic — *continued*
  neural canal (*see also* Lesion, biomechanical, specified)
      — *continued*
    connective tissue — *continued*
      sacroiliac M99.44
      specified NEC M99.49
      thoracic region M99.42
      thoracolumbar M99.42
      upper extremity M99.47
    intervertebral disc M99.59
      abdomen M99.59
      cervical region M99.51
      cervicothoracic M99.51
      head region M99.50
      lower extremity M99.56
      lumbar region M99.53
      lumbosacral M99.53
      occipitocervical M99.50
      pelvic M99.55
      rib cage M99.58
      sacral region M99.54
      sacrococcygeal M99.54
      sacroiliac M99.54
      specified NEC M99.59
      thoracic region M99.52
      thoracolumbar M99.52
      upper extremity M99.57
    osseous M99.39
      abdomen M99.39
      cervical region M99.31
      cervicothoracic M99.31
      head region M99.30
      lower extremity M99.36
      lumbar region M99.33
      lumbosacral M99.33
      occipitocervical M99.30
      pelvic M99.35
      rib cage M99.38
      sacral region M99.34
      sacrococcygeal M99.34
      sacroiliac M99.34
      specified NEC M99.39
      thoracic region M99.32
      thoracolumbar M99.32
      upper extremity M99.37
    subluxation M99.29
      cervical region M99.21
      cervicothoracic M99.21
      head region M99.20
      lower extremity M99.26
      lumbar region M99.23
      lumbosacral M99.23
      occipitocervical M99.20
      pelvic M99.25
      rib cage M99.28
      sacral region M99.24
      sacrococcygeal M99.24
      sacroiliac M99.24
      specified NEC M99.29
      thoracic region M99.22
      thoracolumbar M99.22
      upper extremity M99.27
  organ or site, congenital NEC — *see* Atresia, by site
  papilla of Vater K83.1
  pulmonary (artery) (congenital) Q25.6
    with ventricular septal defect, transposition of
        aorta, and hypertrophy of right ventricle
        Q21.3
    acquired I28.8
    in tetralogy of Fallot Q21.3
    infundibular Q24.3
    subvalvular Q24.3
    supravalvular Q25.6
    valve I37.0
      with insufficiency I37.2
      congenital Q22.1
      rheumatic I09.89
        with aortic, mitral or tricuspid (valve) disease
            I08.8
    vein, acquired I28.8
    vessel NEC I28.8
  pulmonic (congenital) Q22.1
    infundibular Q24.3
    subvalvular Q24.3
  pylorus (hypertrophic) (acquired) K31.1
    adult K31.1
    congenital Q40.0
    infantile Q40.0

Stenosis, stenotic — *continued*
  rectum (sphincter) — *see* Stricture, rectum
  renal artery I70.1
    congenital Q27.1
  salivary duct (any) K11.8
  sphincter of Oddi K83.1
  spinal M48.00
    cervical region M48.02
    cervicothoracic region M48.03
    lumbar region M48.06
    lumbosacral region M48.07
    occipito-atlanto-axial region M48.01
    sacrococcygeal region M48.08
    thoracic region M48.04
    thoracolumbar region M48.05
  stomach, hourglass K31.2
  subaortic (congenital) Q24.4
    hypertrophic (idiopathic) I42.1
  subglottic J38.6
    congenital Q31.1
    postprocedural J95.5
  trachea J39.8
    congenital Q32.1
    syphilitic A52.73
    tuberculous NEC A15.5
  tracheostomy J95.03
  tricuspid (valve) I07.0
    with
      aortic (valve) disease I08.2
      incompetency, insufficiency or regurgitation
          I07.2
        with aortic (valve) disease I08.2
          with mitral (valve) disease I08.3
        mitral (valve) disease I08.1
          with aortic (valve) disease I08.3
    congenital Q22.4
    nonrheumatic I36.0
      with insufficiency I36.2
  tubal N97.1
  ureter — *see* Atresia, ureter
  ureteropelvic junction, congenital Q62.11
  ureterovesical orifice, congenital Q62.12
  urethra (valve) (*see also* Stricture, urethra)
    congenital Q64.32
  urinary meatus, congenital Q64.33
  vagina N89.5
    congenital Q52.4
    in pregnancy — *see* Pregnancy, complicated by,
        abnormal vagina
    causing obstructed labor O65.5
  valve (cardiac) (heart) (*see also* Endocarditis) I38
    congenital Q24.8
      aortic Q23.0
      mitral Q23.2
      pulmonary Q22.1
      tricuspid Q22.4
  vena cava (inferior) (superior) I87.1
    congenital Q26.0
  vesicourethral orifice Q64.31
  vulva N90.5
Stent jail T82.897 ☑
Stercolith (impaction) K56.41
  appendix K38.1
Stercoraceous, stercoral ulcer K63.3
  anus or rectum K62.6
Stereotypies NEC F98.4
Sterility — *see* Infertility
Sterilization — *see* Encounter (for), sterilization
Sternalgia — *see* Angina
Sternopagus Q89.4
Sternum bifidum Q76.7
Steroid
  effects (adverse) (adrenocortical) (iatrogenic)
    cushingoid E24.2
      correct substance properly administered — *see*
          Table of Drugs and Chemicals, by drug,
          adverse effect
      overdose or wrong substance given or taken
          — *see* Table of Drugs and Chemicals, by
          drug, poisoning
    diabetes — *see* subcategory E09 ☑
      correct substance properly administered — *see*
          Table of Drugs and Chemicals, by drug,
          adverse effect
      overdose or wrong substance given or taken
          — *see* Table of Drugs and Chemicals, by
          drug, poisoning
    fever R50.2

Steroid — *continued*
  effects — *continued*
    insufficiency E27.3
      correct substance properly administered — *see*
          Table of Drugs and Chemicals, by drug,
          adverse effect
      overdose or wrong substance given or taken
          — *see* Table of Drugs and Chemicals, by
          drug, poisoning
  responder H40.04- ☑
Stevens-Johnson disease or syndrome L51.1
  toxic epidermal necrolysis overlap L51.3
Stewart-Morel syndrome M85.2
Sticker's disease B08.3
Sticky eye — *see* Conjunctivitis, acute, mucopurulent
Stieda's disease — *see* Bursitis, tibial collateral
Stiff neck — *see* Torticollis
Stiff-man syndrome G25.82
Stiffness, joint NEC M25.60
  ankle M25.67- ☑
  ankylosis — *see* Ankylosis, joint
  contracture — *see* Contraction, joint
  elbow M25.62- ☑
  foot M25.67- ☑
  hand M25.64- ☑
  hip M25.65- ☑
  knee M25.66- ☑
  shoulder M25.61- ☑
  wrist M25.63- ☑
Stigmata congenital syphilis A50.59
Stillbirth P95
Still-Felty syndrome — *see* Felty's syndrome
Still's disease or syndrome (juvenile) M08.20
  adult-onset M06.1
  ankle M08.27- ☑
  elbow M08.22- ☑
  foot joint M08.27- ☑
  hand joint M08.24- ☑
  hip M08.25- ☑
  knee M08.26- ☑
  multiple site M08.29
  shoulder M08.21- ☑
  vertebra M08.28
  wrist M08.23- ☑
Stimulation, ovary E28.1
Sting (venomous) (with allergic or anaphylactic shock)
    — *see* Table of Drugs and Chemicals, by animal or
    substance, poisoning
Stippled epiphyses Q78.8
Stitch
  abscess T81.4 ☑
  burst (in operation wound) — *see* Disruption, wound,
      operation
Stokes' disease E05.00
  with thyroid storm E05.01
Stokes-Adams disease or syndrome I45.9
Stokvis (-Talma) **disease** D74.8
Stoma malfunction
  colostomy K94.03
  enterostomy K94.13
  gastrostomy K94.23
  ileostomy K94.13
  tracheostomy J95.03
Stomach — *see* condition
Stomatitis (denture) (ulcerative) K12.1
  angular K13.0
    due to dietary or vitamin deficiency E53.0
  aphthous K12.0
  bovine B08.61
  candidal B37.0
  catarrhal K12.1
  diphtheritic A36.89
  due to
    dietary deficiency E53.0
    thrush B37.0
    vitamin deficiency
      B group NEC E53.9
      B2 (riboflavin) E53.0
  epidemic B08.8
  epizootic B08.8
  follicular K12.1
  gangrenous A69.0
  Geotrichum B48.3
  herpesviral, herpetic B00.2
  herpetiformis K12.0
  malignant K12.1
  membranous acute K12.1

Stomatitis — *continued*
  monilial B37.Ø
  mycotic B37.Ø
  necrotizing ulcerative A69.Ø
  parasitic B37.Ø
  septic K12.1
  spirochetal A69.1
  suppurative (acute) K12.2
  ulceromembranous A69.1
  vesicular K12.1
    with exanthem (enteroviral) BØ8.4
    virus disease A93.8
  Vincent's A69.1
Stomatocytosis D58.8
Stomatomycosis B37.Ø
Stomatorrhagia K13.79
Stone(s) (*see also* Calculus)
  bladder (diverticulum) N21.Ø
  cystine E72.Ø9
  heart syndrome I5Ø.1
  kidney N2Ø.Ø
  prostate N42.Ø
  pulpal (dental) KØ4.2
  renal N2Ø.Ø
  salivary gland or duct (any) K11.5
  urethra (impacted) N21.1
  urinary (duct) (impacted) (passage) N2Ø.9
    bladder (diverticulum) N21.Ø
    lower tract N21.9
    specified NEC N21.8
  xanthine E79.8 [N22]
Stonecutter's lung J62.8
Stonemason's asthma, disease, lung or pneumoconiosis J62.8
Stoppage
  heart — *see* Arrest, cardiac
  urine — *see* Retention, urine
Storm, thyroid — *see* Thyrotoxicosis
Strabismus (congenital) (nonparalytic) H5Ø.9
  concomitant H5Ø.4Ø
    convergent — *see* Strabismus, convergent concomitant
    divergent — *see* Strabismus, divergent concomitant
  convergent concomitant H5Ø.ØØ
    accommodative component H5Ø.43
    alternating H5Ø.Ø5
      with
        A pattern H5Ø.Ø6
        specified nonconcomitances NEC H5Ø.Ø8
        V pattern H5Ø.Ø7
    monocular H5Ø.Ø1- ☑
      with
        A pattern H5Ø.Ø2- ☑
        specified nonconcomitances NEC H5Ø.Ø4- ☑
        V pattern H5Ø.Ø3- ☑
      intermittent H5Ø.31- ☑
        alternating H5Ø.32
  cyclotropia H5Ø.1- ☑
  divergent concomitant H5Ø.1Ø
    alternating H5Ø.15
      with
        A pattern H5Ø.16
        specified nonconcomitances NEC H5Ø.18
        V pattern H5Ø.17
    monocular H5Ø.11- ☑
      with
        A pattern H5Ø.12- ☑
        specified nonconcomitances NEC H5Ø.14- ☑
        V pattern H5Ø.13- ☑
      intermittent H5Ø.33 ☑
        alternating H5Ø.34
  Duane's syndrome H5Ø.81- ☑
  due to adhesions, scars H5Ø.69
  heterophoria H5Ø.5Ø
    alternating H5Ø.55
    cyclophoria H5Ø.54
    esophoria H5Ø.51
    exophoria H5Ø.52
    vertical H5Ø.53
  heterotropia H5Ø.4Ø
    intermittent H5Ø.3Ø
  hypertropia H5Ø.2- ☑
  hypotropia — *see* Hypertropia
  latent H5Ø.5Ø
  mechanical H5Ø.6Ø
    Brown's sheath syndrome H5Ø.61- ☑

Strabismus — *continued*
  mechanical — *continued*
    specified type NEC H5Ø.69
  monofixation syndrome H5Ø.42
  paralytic H49.9
    abducens nerve H49.2- ☑
    fourth nerve H49.1- ☑
    Kearns-Sayre syndrome H49.81- ☑
    ophthalmoplegia (external)
      progressive H49.4- ☑
        with pigmentary retinopathy H49.81- ☑
      total H49.3- ☑
    sixth nerve H49.2- ☑
    specified type NEC H49.88- ☑
    third nerve H49.Ø- ☑
    trochlear nerve H49.1- ☑
  specified type NEC H5Ø.89
  vertical H5Ø.2- ☑
Strain
  back S39.Ø12 ☑
  cervical S16.1 ☑
  eye NEC — *see* Disturbance, vision, subjective
  heart — *see* Disease, heart
  low back S39.Ø12 ☑
  mental NOS Z73.3
    work-related Z56.6
  muscle (tendon) — *see* Injury, muscle, by site, strain
  neck S16.1 ☑
  physical NOS Z73.3
    work-related Z56.6
  postural (*see also* Disorder, soft tissue, due to use)
  psychological NEC Z73.3
  tendon — *see* Injury, muscle, by site, strain
Straining, on urination R39.16
Strand, vitreous — *see* Opacity, vitreous, membranes and strands
Strangulation, strangulated (*see also* Asphyxia, traumatic)
  appendix K38.8
  bladder-neck N32.Ø
  bowel or colon K56.2
  food or foreign body — *see* Foreign body, by site
  hemorrhoids — *see* Hemorrhoids, with complication
  hernia (*see also* Hernia, by site, with obstruction)
    with gangrene — *see* Hernia, by site, with gangrene
  intestine (large) (small) K56.2
    with hernia (*see also* Hernia, by site, with obstruction)
      with gangrene — *see* Hernia, by site, with gangrene
  mesentery K56.2
  mucus — *see* Asphyxia, mucus
  omentum K56.2
  organ or site, congenital NEC — *see* Atresia, by site
  ovary — *see* Torsion, ovary
  penis N48.89
    foreign body T19.4 ☑
  rupture — *see* Hernia, by site, with obstruction
  stomach due to hernia (*see also* Hernia, by site, with obstruction)
    with gangrene — *see* Hernia, by site, with gangrene
  vesicourethral orifice N32.Ø
Strangury R3Ø.Ø
Straw itch B88.Ø
Strawberry
  gallbladder K82.4
  mark Q82.5
  tongue (red) (white) K14.3
Streak(s)
  macula, angioid H35.33
  ovarian Q5Ø.32
Strephosymbolia F81.Ø
  secondary to organic lesion R48.8
Streptobacillary fever A25.1
Streptobacillosis A25.1
Streptobacillus moniliformis A25.1
Streptococcus, streptococcal (*see also* condition)
  as cause of disease classified elsewhere B95.5
  group
    A, as cause of disease classified elsewhere B95.Ø
    B, as cause of disease classified elsewhere B95.1
    D, as cause of disease classified elsewhere B95.2
    pneumoniae, as cause of disease classified elsewhere B95.3

Streptococcus, streptococcal — *continued*
  specified NEC, as cause of disease classified elsewhere B95.4
Streptomycosis B47.1
Streptotrichosis A48.8
Stress F43.9
  family — *see* Disruption, family
  fetal P84
    complicating pregnancy O77.9
      due to drug administration O77.1
  mental NEC Z73.3
    work-related Z56.6
  physical NEC Z73.3
    work-related Z56.6
  polycythemia D75.1
  reaction (*see also* Reaction, stress) F43.9
  work schedule Z56.3
Stretching, nerve — *see* Injury, nerve
Striae albicantes, atrophicae or distensae (cutis) L9Ø.6
Stricture (*see also* Stenosis)
  ampulla of Vater K83.1
  anus (sphincter) K62.4
    congenital Q42.3
      with fistula Q42.2
    infantile Q42.3
      with fistula Q42.2
  aorta (ascending) (congenital) Q25.3
    arteriosclerotic I7Ø.Ø
    calcified I7Ø.Ø
    supravalvular, congenital Q25.3
  aortic (valve) — *see* Stenosis, aortic
  aqueduct of Sylvius (congenital) QØ3.Ø
    with spina bifida — *see* Spina bifida, by site, with hydrocephalus
    acquired G91.1
  artery I77.1
    basilar — *see* Occlusion, artery, basilar
    carotid — *see* Occlusion, artery, carotid
    celiac I77.4
    congenital (peripheral) Q27.8
      cerebral Q28.3
      coronary Q24.5
      digestive system Q27.8
      lower limb Q27.8
      retinal Q14.1
      specified site NEC Q27.8
      umbilical Q27.Ø
      upper limb Q27.8
    coronary — *see* Disease, heart, ischemic, atherosclerotic
      congenital Q24.5
    precerebral — *see* Occlusion, artery, precerebral
    pulmonary (congenital) Q25.6
      acquired I28.8
    renal I7Ø.1
    vertebral — *see* Occlusion, artery, vertebral
  auditory canal (external) (congenital)
    acquired — *see* Stenosis, external ear canal
  bile duct (common) (hepatic) K83.1
    congenital Q44.3
    postoperative K91.89
  bladder N32.89
    neck N32.Ø
  bowel — *see* Obstruction, intestine
  brain G93.89
  bronchus J98.Ø9
    congenital Q32.3
    syphilitic A52.72
  cardia (stomach) K22.2
    congenital Q39.3
  cardiac (*see also* Disease, heart)
    orifice (stomach) K22.2
  cecum — *see* Obstruction, intestine
  cervix, cervical (canal) N88.2
    congenital Q51.828
    in pregnancy — *see* Pregnancy, complicated by, abnormal cervix
      causing obstructed labor O65.5
  colon (*see also* Obstruction, intestine)
    congenital Q42.9
      specified NEC Q42.8
  colostomy K94.Ø3
  common (bile) duct K83.1
  coronary (artery) — *see* Disease, heart, ischemic, atherosclerotic
  cystic duct — *see* Obstruction, gallbladder
  digestive organs NEC, congenital Q45.8
  duodenum K31.5

Stricture — *continued*
- duodenum — *continued*
  - congenital Q41.0
- ear canal (external) (congenital) Q16.1
  - acquired — *see* Stricture, auditory canal, acquired
- ejaculatory duct N50.8
- enterostomy K94.13
- esophagus K22.2
  - congenital Q39.3
  - syphilitic A52.79
    - congenital A50.59 [K23]
- eustachian tube (*see also* Obstruction, eustachian tube)
  - congenital Q17.8
- fallopian tube N97.1
  - gonococcal A54.24
  - tuberculous A18.17
- gallbladder — *see* Obstruction, gallbladder
- glottis J38.6
- heart (*see also* Disease, heart)
  - valve (*see also* Endocarditis) I38
    - aortic Q23.0
    - mitral Q23.4
    - pulmonary Q22.1
    - tricuspid Q22.4
- hepatic duct K83.1
- hourglass, of stomach K31.2
- hymen N89.6
- hypopharynx J39.2
- ileum K56.69
  - congenital Q41.2
- intestine (*see also* Obstruction, intestine)
  - congenital (small) Q41.9
    - large Q42.9
      - specified NEC Q42.8
    - specified NEC Q41.8
  - ischemic K55.1
- jejunum K56.69
  - congenital Q41.1
- lacrimal passages (*see also* Stenosis, lacrimal)
  - congenital Q10.5
- larynx J38.6
  - congenital NEC Q31.8
    - subglottic Q31.1
  - syphilitic A52.73
    - congenital A50.59 [J99]
- meatus
  - ear (congenital) Q16.1
    - acquired — *see* Stricture, auditory canal, acquired
  - osseous (ear) (congenital) Q16.1
    - acquired — *see* Stricture, auditory canal, acquired
  - urinarius (*see also* Stricture, urethra)
    - congenital Q64.33
- mitral (valve) — *see* Stenosis, mitral
- myocardium, myocardial I51.5
  - hypertrophic subaortic (idiopathic) I42.1
- nares (anterior) (posterior) J34.89
  - congenital Q30.0
- nasal duct (*see also* Stenosis, lacrimal, duct)
  - congenital Q10.5
- nasolacrimal duct (*see also* Stenosis, lacrimal, duct)
  - congenital Q10.5
- nasopharynx J39.2
  - syphilitic A52.73
- nose J34.89
  - congenital Q30.0
- nostril (anterior) (posterior) J34.89
  - congenital Q30.0
  - syphilitic A52.73
    - congenital A50.59 [J99]
- organ or site, congenital NEC — *see* Atresia, by site
- os uteri — *see* Stricture, cervix
- osseous meatus (ear) (congenital) Q16.1
  - acquired — *see* Stricture, auditory canal, acquired
- oviduct — *see* Stricture, fallopian tube
- pelviureteric junction (congenital) Q62.11
- penis, by foreign body T19.4 ☑
- pharynx J39.2
- prostate N42.89
- pulmonary, pulmonic
  - artery (congenital) Q25.6
    - acquired I28.8
    - noncongenital I28.8
  - infundibulum (congenital) Q24.3
  - valve I37.0
    - congenital Q22.1
  - vein, acquired I28.8

Stricture — *continued*
- pulmonary, pulmonic — *continued*
  - vessel NEC I28.8
- punctum lacrimale (*see also* Stenosis, lacrimal, punctum)
  - congenital Q10.5
- pylorus (hypertrophic) K31.1
  - adult K31.1
  - congenital Q40.0
  - infantile Q40.0
- rectosigmoid K56.69
- rectum (sphincter) K62.4
  - congenital Q42.1
    - with fistula Q42.0
  - due to
    - chlamydial lymphogranuloma A55
    - irradiation K91.89
    - lymphogranuloma venereum A55
  - gonococcal A54.6
  - inflammatory (chlamydial) A55
  - syphilitic A52.74
  - tuberculous A18.32
- renal artery I70.1
  - congenital Q27.1
- salivary duct or gland (any) K11.8
- sigmoid (flexure) — *see* Obstruction, intestine
- spermatic cord N50.8
- stoma (following) (of)
  - colostomy K94.03
  - enterostomy K94.13
  - gastrostomy K94.23
  - ileostomy K94.13
  - tracheostomy J95.03
- stomach K31.89
  - congenital Q40.2
  - hourglass K31.2
- subaortic Q24.4
  - hypertrophic (acquired) (idiopathic) I42.1
- subglottic J38.6
- syphilitic NEC A52.79
- trachea J39.8
  - congenital Q32.1
  - syphilitic A52.73
  - tuberculous NEC A15.5
- tracheostomy J95.03
- tricuspid (valve) — *see* Stenosis, tricuspid
- tunica vaginalis N50.8
- ureter (postoperative) N13.5
  - with
    - hydronephrosis N13.1
      - with infection N13.6
    - pyelonephritis (chronic) N11.1
  - congenital — *see* Atresia, ureter
  - tuberculous A18.11
- ureteropelvic junction (congenital) Q62.11
- ureterovesical orifice N13.5
  - with infection N13.6
- urethra (organic) (spasmodic) N35.9
  - associated with schistosomiasis B65.0 [N37]
  - congenital Q64.39
    - valvular (posterior) Q64.2
  - due to
    - infection — *see* Stricture, urethra, postinfective
    - trauma — *see* Stricture, urethra, post-traumatic
  - gonococcal, gonorrheal A54.01
  - infective NEC — *see* Stricture, urethra, postinfective
  - late effect (sequelae) of injury — *see* Stricture, urethra, post-traumatic
  - postcatheterization — *see* Stricture, urethra, postprocedural
  - postinfective NEC
    - female N35.12
    - male N35.119
      - anterior urethra N35.114
      - bulbous urethra N35.112
      - meatal N35.111
      - membranous urethra N35.113
  - postobstetric N35.021
  - postoperative — *see* Stricture, urethra, postprocedural
  - postprocedural
    - female N99.12
    - male N99.114
      - anterior urethra N99.113
      - bulbous urethra N99.111
      - meatal N99.110
      - membranous urethra N99.112

Stricture — *continued*
- urethra — *continued*
  - post-traumatic
    - female N35.028
      - due to childbirth N35.021
    - male N35.014
      - anterior urethra N35.013
      - bulbous urethra N35.011
      - meatal N35.010
      - membranous urethra N35.012
  - sequela (late effect) of
    - childbirth N35.021
    - injury — *see* Stricture, urethra, post-traumatic
  - specified cause NEC N35.8
  - syphilitic A52.76
  - traumatic — *see* Stricture, urethra, post-traumatic
  - valvular (posterior), congenital Q64.2
- urinary meatus — *see* Stricture, urethra
- uterus, uterine (synechiae) N85.6
  - os (external) (internal) — *see* Stricture, cervix
- vagina (outlet) — *see* Stenosis, vagina
- valve (cardiac) (heart) (*see also* Endocarditis)
  - congenital
    - aortic Q23.0
    - mitral Q23.4
    - pulmonary Q22.1
    - tricuspid Q22.4
- vas deferens N50.8
  - congenital Q55.4
- vein I87.1
- vena cava (inferior) (superior) NEC I87.1
  - congenital Q26.0
- vesicourethral orifice N32.0
  - congenital Q64.31
- vulva (acquired) N90.5

Stridor R06.1
- congenital (larynx) P28.89

Stridulous — *see* condition

Stroke (apoplectic) (brain) (embolic) (ischemic) (paralytic) (thrombotic) I63.9
- epileptic — *see* Epilepsy
- heat T67.0 ☑
- in evolution I63.9
- intraoperative
  - during cardiac surgery I97.810
  - during other surgery I97.811
- lightning — *see* Lightning
- meaning
  - cerebral hemorrhage — *code to* Hemorrhage, intracranial
  - cerebral infarction — *code to* Infarction, cerebral
- postprocedural
  - following cardiac surgery I97.820
  - following other surgery I97.821
- unspecified (NOS) I63.9

Stromatosis, endometrial D39.0

Strongyloidiasis, strongyloidosis B78.9
- cutaneous B78.1
- disseminated B78.7
- intestinal B78.0

Strophulus pruriginosus L28.2

Struck by lightning — *see* Lightning

Struma (*see also* Goiter)
- Hashimoto E06.3
- lymphomatosa E06.3
- nodosa (simplex) E04.9
  - endemic E01.2
    - multinodular E01.1
  - multinodular E04.2
    - iodine-deficiency related E01.1
  - toxic or with hyperthyroidism E05.20
    - with thyroid storm E05.21
    - multinodular E05.20
      - with thyroid storm E05.21
    - uninodular E05.10
      - with thyroid storm E05.11
  - toxicosa E05.20
    - with thyroid storm E05.21
    - multinodular E05.20
      - with thyroid storm E05.21
    - uninodular E05.10
      - with thyroid storm E05.11
  - uninodular E04.1
- ovarii D27.- ☑
- Riedel's E06.5

Strumipriva cachexia E03.4

Strümpell-Marie spine — *see* Spondylitis, ankylosing

Strümpell-Westphal pseudosclerosis E83.01

Stuart deficiency disease (factor X) D68.2
Stuart-Prower factor deficiency (factor X) D68.2
Student's elbow — *see* Bursitis, elbow, olecranon
Stump — *see* Amputation
Stunting, nutritional E45
Stupor (catatonic) R40.1
  depressive F32.8
  dissociative F44.2
  manic F30.2
  manic-depressive F31.89
  psychogenic (anergic) F44.2
  reaction to exceptional stress (transient) F43.0
Sturge (-Weber) (-Dimitri) (-Kalischer) **disease or syndrome** Q85.8
Stuttering F80.81
  adult onset F98.5
  childhood onset F80.81
  following cerebrovascular disease — *see* Disorder, fluency. following cerebrovascular disease
  in conditions classified elsewhere R47.82
Sty, stye (external) (internal) (meibomian) (zeisian) — *see* Hordeolum
Subacidity, gastric K31.89
  psychogenic F45.8
Subacute — *see* condition
Subarachnoid — *see* condition
Subcortical — *see* condition
Subcostal syndrome, nerve compression — *see* Mononeuropathy, upper limb, specified site NEC
Subcutaneous, subcuticular — *see* condition
Subdural — *see* condition
Subendocardium — *see* condition
Subependymoma
  specified site — *see* Neoplasm, uncertain behavior, by site
  unspecified site D43.2
Suberosis J67.3
Subglossitis — *see* Glossitis
Subhemophilia D66
Subinvolution
  breast (postlactational) (postpuerperal) N64.89
  puerperal O90.89
  uterus (chronic) (nonpuerperal) N85.3
    puerperal O90.89
Sublingual — *see* condition
Sublinguitis — *see* Sialoadenitis
Subluxatable hip Q65.6
Subluxation (*see also* Dislocation)
  acromioclavicular S43.11- ☑
  ankle S93.0- ☑
  atlantoaxial, recurrent M43.4
    with myelopathy M43.3
  carpometacarpal (joint) NEC S63.05- ☑
    thumb S63.04- ☑
  complex, vertebral — *see* Complex, subluxation
  congenital (*see also* Malposition, congenital)
    hip — *see* Dislocation, hip, congenital, partial
    joint (excluding hip)
      lower limb Q68.8
      shoulder Q68.8
      upper limb Q68.8
  elbow (traumatic) S53.10- ☑
    anterior S53.11- ☑
    lateral S53.14- ☑
    medial S53.13- ☑
    posterior S53.12- ☑
    specified type NEC S53.19- ☑
  finger S63.20- ☑
    index S63.20- ☑
    interphalangeal S63.22- ☑
      distal S63.24- ☑
        index S63.24- ☑
        little S63.24- ☑
        middle S63.24- ☑
        ring S63.24- ☑
      index S63.22- ☑
      little S63.22- ☑
      middle S63.22- ☑
      proximal S63.23- ☑
        index S63.23- ☑
        little S63.23- ☑
        middle S63.23- ☑
        ring S63.23- ☑
      ring S63.22- ☑
    little S63.20- ☑
    metacarpophalangeal S63.21- ☑

Subluxation — *continued*
  finger — *continued*
    metacarpophalangeal — *continued*
      index S63.21- ☑
      little S63.21- ☑
      middle S63.21- ☑
      ring S63.21- ☑
    middle S63.20- ☑
    ring S63.20- ☑
  foot S93.30- ☑
    specified site NEC S93.33- ☑
    tarsal joint S93.31- ☑
    tarsometatarsal joint S93.32- ☑
    toe — *see* Subluxation, toe
  hip S73.00- ☑
    anterior S73.03- ☑
      obturator S73.02- ☑
    central S73.04- ☑
    posterior S73.01- ☑
  interphalangeal (joint)
    finger S63.22- ☑
      distal joint S63.24- ☑
        index S63.24- ☑
        little S63.24- ☑
        middle S63.24- ☑
        ring S63.24- ☑
      index S63.22- ☑
      little S63.22- ☑
      middle S63.22- ☑
      proximal joint S63.23- ☑
        index S63.23- ☑
        little S63.23- ☑
        middle S63.23- ☑
        ring S63.23- ☑
      ring S63.22- ☑
    thumb S63.12- ☑
      distal joint S63.14- ☑
      proximal joint S63.13- ☑
    toe S93.13- ☑
      great S93.13- ☑
      lesser S93.13- ☑
  joint prosthesis — *see* Complications, joint prosthesis, mechanical, displacement, by site
  knee S83.10- ☑
    cap — *see* Subluxation, patella
    patella — *see* Subluxation, patella
    proximal tibia
      anteriorly S83.11- ☑
      laterally S83.14- ☑
      medially S83.13- ☑
      posteriorly S83.12- ☑
    specified type NEC S83.19- ☑
  lens — *see* Dislocation, lens, partial
  ligament, traumatic — *see* Sprain, by site
  metacarpal (bone)
    proximal end S63.06- ☑
  metacarpophalangeal (joint)
    finger S63.21- ☑
      index S63.21- ☑
      little S63.21- ☑
      middle S63.21- ☑
      ring S63.21- ☑
    thumb S63.11- ☑
  metatarsophalangeal joint S93.14- ☑
    great toe S93.14- ☑
    lesser toe S93.14- ☑
  midcarpal (joint) S63.03- ☑
  patella S83.00- ☑
    lateral S83.01- ☑
    recurrent (nontraumatic) — *see* Dislocation, patella, recurrent, incomplete
    specified type NEC S83.09- ☑
  pathological — *see* Dislocation, pathological
  radial head S53.00- ☑
    anterior S53.01- ☑
    nursemaid's elbow S53.03- ☑
    posterior S53.02- ☑
    specified type NEC S53.09- ☑
  radiocarpal (joint) S63.02- ☑
  radioulnar (joint)
    distal S63.01- ☑
    proximal — *see* Subluxation, elbow
  shoulder
    congenital Q68.8
    girdle S43.30- ☑
      scapula S43.31- ☑

Subluxation — *continued*
  shoulder — *continued*
    girdle — *continued*
      specified site NEC S43.39- ☑
    traumatic S43.00- ☑
      anterior S43.01- ☑
      inferior S43.03- ☑
      posterior S43.02- ☑
      specified type NEC S43.08- ☑
  sternoclavicular (joint) S43.20- ☑
    anterior S43.21- ☑
    posterior S43.22- ☑
  symphysis (pubis)
  thumb S63.103
    interphalangeal joint — *see* Subluxation, interphalangeal (joint), thumb
    metacarpophalangeal joint — *see* Subluxation, metacarpophalangeal (joint), thumb
  toe(s) S93.10- ☑
    great S93.10- ☑
      interphalangeal joint S93.13- ☑
      metatarsophalangeal joint S93.14- ☑
    interphalangeal joint S93.13- ☑
    lesser S93.10- ☑
      interphalangeal joint S93.13- ☑
      metatarsophalangeal joint S93.14- ☑
    metatarsophalangeal joint S93.149 ☑
  ulna
    distal end S63.07- ☑
    proximal end — *see* Subluxation, elbow
  ulnohumeral joint — *see* Subluxation, elbow
  vertebral
    recurrent NEC — *see* subcategory M43.5 ☑
    traumatic
      cervical S13.100 ☑
        atlantoaxial joint S13.120 ☑
        atlantooccipital joint S13.110 ☑
        atloidooccipital joint S13.110 ☑
        joint between
          C0 and C1 S13.110 ☑
          C1 and C2 S13.120 ☑
          C2 and C3 S13.130 ☑
          C3 and C4 S13.140 ☑
          C4 and C5 S13.150 ☑
          C5 and C6 S13.160 ☑
          C6 and C7 S13.170 ☑
          C7 and T1 S13.180 ☑
        occipitoatloid joint S13.110 ☑
      lumbar S33.100 ☑
        joint between
          L1 and L2 S33.110 ☑
          L2 and L3 S33.120 ☑
          L3 and L4 S33.130 ☑
          L4 and L5 S33.140 ☑
      thoracic S23.100 ☑
        joint between
          T1 and T2 S23.110 ☑
          T2 and T3 S23.120 ☑
          T3 and T4 S23.122 ☑
          T4 and T5 S23.130 ☑
          T5 and T6 S23.132 ☑
          T6 and T7 S23.140 ☑
          T7 and T8 S23.142 ☑
          T8 and T9 S23.150 ☑
          T9 and T10 S23.152 ☑
          T10 and T11 S23.160 ☑
          T11 and T12 S23.162 ☑
          T12 and L1 S23.170 ☑
  wrist (carpal bone) S63.00- ☑
    carpometacarpal joint — *see* Subluxation, carpometacarpal (joint)
    distal radioulnar joint — *see* Subluxation, radioulnar (joint), distal
    metacarpal bone, proximal — *see* Subluxation, metacarpal (bone), proximal end
    midcarpal — *see* Subluxation, midcarpal (joint)
    radiocarpal joint — *see* Subluxation, radiocarpal (joint)
    recurrent — *see* Dislocation, recurrent, wrist
    specified site NEC S63.09- ☑
    ulna — *see* Subluxation, ulna, distal end
Submaxillary — *see* condition
Submersion (fatal) (nonfatal) T75.1 ☑
Submucous — *see* condition
Subnormal, subnormality
  accommodation (old age) H52.4

☑ Additional Character Required — Refer to the Tabular List for Character Selection   ▽ Subterms under main terms may continue to next column or page

Subnormal, subnormality — *continued*
  mental — *see* Disability, intellectual
  temperature (accidental) T68 ☑
Subphrenic — *see* condition
Subscapular nerve — *see* condition
Subseptus uterus Q51.2
Subsiding appendicitis K36
Substernal thyroid E04.9
  congenital Q89.2
Substitution disorder F44.9
Subtentorial — *see* condition
Subthyroidism (acquired) (*see also* Hypothyroidism)
  congenital E03.1
Succenturiate placenta O43.19- ☑
Sucking thumb, child (excessive) F98.8
Sudamen, sudamina L74.1
Sudanese kala-azar B55.0
Sudden
  hearing loss — *see* Deafness, sudden
  heart failure — *see* Failure, heart
Sudeck's atrophy, disease, or syndrome — *see* Algo-
  neurodystrophy
Suffocation — *see* Asphyxia, traumatic
Sugar
  blood
    high (transient) R73.9
    low (transient) E16.2
  in urine R81
Suicide, suicidal (attempted) T14.91
  by poisoning — *see* Table of Drugs and Chemicals
  history of (personal) Z91.5
    in family Z81.8
  ideation — *see* Ideation, suicidal
  risk
    meaning personal history of attempted suicide
      Z91.5
    meaning suicidal ideation — *see* Ideation, suicidal
  tendencies
    meaning personal history of attempted suicide
      Z91.5
    meaning suicidal ideation — *see* Ideation, suicidal
  trauma — *see* nature of injury by site
Suipestifer infection — *see* Infection, salmonella
Sulfhemoglobinemia, sulphemoglobinemia (acquired) (with methemoglobinemia) D74.8
Sumatran mite fever A75.3
Summer — *see* condition
Sunburn L55.9
  first degree L55.0
  second degree L55.1
  third degree L55.2
SUNCT (short lasting unilateral neuralgiform headache
  with conjunctival injection and tearing) G44.059
  intractable G44.051
  not intractable G44.059
Sunken acetabulum — *see* Derangement, joint, specified type NEC, hip
Sunstroke T67.0 ☑
Superfecundation — *see* Pregnancy, multiple
Superfetation — *see* Pregnancy, multiple
Superinvolution (uterus) N85.8
Supernumerary (congenital)
  aortic cusps Q23.8
  auditory ossicles Q16.3
  bone Q79.8
  breast Q83.1
  carpal bones Q74.0
  cusps, heart valve NEC Q24.8
    aortic Q23.8
    mitral Q23.2
    pulmonary Q22.3
  digit(s) Q69.9
  ear (lobule) Q17.0
  fallopian tube Q50.6
  finger Q69.0
  hymen Q52.4
  kidney Q63.0
  lacrimonasal duct Q10.6
  lobule (ear) Q17.0
  mitral cusps Q23.2
  muscle Q79.8
  nipple(s) Q83.3
  organ or site not listed — *see* Accessory
  ossicles, auditory Q16.3
  ovary Q50.31
  oviduct Q50.6
  pulmonary, pulmonic cusps Q22.3

Supernumerary — *continued*
  rib Q76.6
    cervical or first (syndrome) Q76.5
  roots (of teeth) K00.2
  spleen Q89.09
  tarsal bones Q74.2
  teeth K00.1
  testis Q55.29
  thumb Q69.1
  toe Q69.2
  uterus Q51.2
  vagina Q52.1 ☑
  vertebra Q76.49
Supervision (of)
  contraceptive — *see* Prescription, contraceptives
  dietary (for) Z71.3
    allergy (food) Z71.3
    colitis Z71.3
    diabetes mellitus Z71.3
    food allergy or intolerance Z71.3
    gastritis Z71.3
    hypercholesterolemia Z71.3
    hypoglycemia Z71.3
    intolerance (food) Z71.3
    obesity Z71.3
    specified NEC Z71.3
  healthy infant or child Z76.2
    foundling Z76.1
  high-risk pregnancy — *see* Pregnancy, complicated
    by, high, risk
  lactation Z39.1
  pregnancy — *see* Pregnancy, supervision of
Supplemental teeth K00.1
Suppression
  binocular vision H53.34
  lactation O92.5
  menstruation N94.89
  ovarian secretion E28.39
  renal N28.9
  urine, urinary secretion R34
Suppuration, suppurative (*see also* condition)
  accessory sinus (chronic) — *see* Sinusitis
  adrenal gland
  antrum (chronic) — *see* Sinusitis, maxillary
  bladder — *see* Cystitis
  brain G06.0
    sequelae G09
  breast N61
    puerperal, postpartum or gestational — *see* Masti-
      tis, obstetric, purulent
  dental periosteum M27.3
  ear (middle) (*see also* Otitis, media)
    external NEC — *see* Otitis, externa, infective
    internal — *see* subcategory H83.0 ☑
  ethmoidal (chronic) (sinus) — *see* Sinusitis, ethmoidal
  fallopian tube — *see* Salpingo-oophoritis
  frontal (chronic) (sinus) — *see* Sinusitis, frontal
  gallbladder (acute) K81.0
  gum K05.20
    generalized K05.22
    localized K05.21
  intracranial G06.0
  joint — *see* Arthritis, pyogenic or pyemic
  labyrinthine — *see* subcategory H83.0 ☑
  lung — *see* Abscess, lung
  mammary gland N61
    puerperal, postpartum O91.12
      associated with lactation O91.13
  maxilla, maxillary M27.2
    sinus (chronic) — *see* Sinusitis, maxillary
  muscle — *see* Myositis, infective
  nasal sinus (chronic) — *see* Sinusitis
  pancreas, acute K85.8
  parotid gland — *see* Sialoadenitis
  pelvis, pelvic
    female — *see* Disease, pelvis, inflammatory
    male K65.0
  pericranial — *see* Osteomyelitis
  salivary duct or gland (any) — *see* Sialoadenitis
  sinus (accessory) (chronic) (nasal) — *see* Sinusitis
  sphenoidal sinus (chronic) — *see* Sinusitis, sphenoidal
  thymus (gland) E32.1
  thyroid (gland) E06.0
  tonsil — *see* Tonsillitis
  uterus — *see* Endometritis
Supraeruption of tooth (teeth) M26.34
Supraglottitis J04.30

Supraglottitis — *continued*
  with obstruction J04.31
Suprarenal (gland) — *see* condition
Suprascapular nerve — *see* condition
Suprasellar — *see* condition
Surfer's knots or nodules S89.8- ☑
Surgical
  emphysema T81.82 ☑
  procedures, complication or misadventure — *see*
    Complications, surgical procedures
  shock T81.10 ☑
Surveillance (of) (for) (*see also* Observation)
  alcohol abuse Z71.41
  contraceptive — *see* Prescription, contraceptives
  dietary Z71.3
  drug abuse Z71.51
Susceptibility to disease, genetic Z15.89
  malignant neoplasm Z15.09
    breast Z15.01
    endometrium Z15.04
    ovary Z15.02
    prostate Z15.03
    specified NEC Z15.09
  multiple endocrine neoplasia Z15.81
Suspected condition, ruled out (*see also* Observation,
  suspected)
  amniotic cavity and membrane Z03.71
  cervical shortening Z03.75
  fetal anomaly Z03.73
  fetal growth Z03.74
  maternal and fetal conditions NEC Z03.79
  oligohydramnios Z03.71
  placental problem Z03.72
  polyhydramnios Z03.71
Suspended uterus
  in pregnancy or childbirth — *see* Pregnancy, compli-
    cated by, abnormal uterus
Sutton's nevus D22.9
Suture
  burst (in operation wound) T81.31 ☑
    external operation wound T81.31 ☑
    internal operation wound T81.32 ☑
  inadvertently left in operation wound — *see* Foreign
    body, accidentally left during a procedure
  removal Z48.02
Swab inadvertently left in operation wound — *see*
  Foreign body, accidentally left during a procedure
Swallowed, swallowing
  difficulty — *see* Dysphagia
  foreign body — *see* Foreign body, alimentary tract
Swan-neck deformity (finger) — *see* Deformity, finger,
  swan-neck
Swearing, compulsive F42
  in Gilles de la Tourette's syndrome F95.2
Sweat, sweats
  fetid L75.0
  night R61
Sweating, excessive R61
Sweeley-Klionsky disease E75.21
Sweet's disease or dermatosis L98.2
Swelling (of) R60.9
  abdomen, abdominal (not referable to any particular
    organ) — *see* Mass, abdominal
  ankle — *see* Effusion, joint, ankle
  arm M79.89
    forearm M79.89
  breast N63
  Calabar B74.3
  cervical gland R59.0
  chest, localized R22.2
  ear H93.8- ☑
  extremity (lower) (upper) — *see* Disorder, soft tissue,
    specified type NEC
  finger M79.89
  foot M79.89
  glands R59.9
    generalized R59.1
    localized R59.0
  hand M79.89
  head (localized) R22.0
  inflammatory — *see* Inflammation
  intra-abdominal — *see* Mass, abdominal
  joint — *see* Effusion, joint
  leg M79.89
    lower M79.89
  limb — *see* Disorder, soft tissue, specified type NEC

Swelling — continued
  localized (skin) R22.9
    chest R22.2
    head R22.0
    limb
      lower — see Mass, localized, limb, lower
      upper — see Mass, localized, limb, upper
    neck R22.1
    trunk R22.2
  neck (localized) R22.1
  pelvic — see Mass, abdominal
  scrotum N50.8
  splenic — see Splenomegaly
  testis N50.8
  toe M79.89
  umbilical R19.09
  wandering, due to Gnathostoma (spinigerum) B83.1
  white — see Tuberculosis, arthritis
Swift (-Feer) disease
  overdose or wrong substance given or taken — see Table of Drugs and Chemicals, by drug, poisoning
Swimmer's
  cramp T75.1 ☑
  ear H60.33- ☑
  itch B65.3
Swimming in the head R42
Swollen — see Swelling
Swyer syndrome Q99.1
Sycosis L73.8
  barbae (not parasitic) L73.8
  contagiosa (mycotic) B35.0
  lupoides L73.8
  mycotic B35.0
  parasitic B35.0
  vulgaris L73.8
Sydenham's chorea — see Chorea, Sydenham's
Sylvatic yellow fever A95.0
Sylvest's disease B33.0
Symblepharon H11.23- ☑
  congenital Q10.3
Symond's syndrome G93.2
Sympathetic — see condition
Sympatheticotonia G90.8
Sympathicoblastoma
  specified site — see Neoplasm, malignant, by site
  unspecified site C74.90
Sympathogonioma — see Sympathicoblastoma
Symphalangy (fingers) (toes) Q70.9
Symptoms NEC R68.89
  breast NEC N64.59
  development NEC R63.8
  factitious, self-induced — see Disorder, factitious
  genital organs, female R10.2
  involving
    abdomen NEC R19.8
    appearance NEC R46.89
    awareness R41.9
      altered mental status R41.82
      amnesia — see Amnesia
      borderline intellectual functioning R41.83
      coma — see Coma
      disorientation R41.0
      neurologic neglect syndrome R41.4
      senile cognitive decline R41.81
      specified symptom NEC R41.89
    behavior NEC R46.89
    cardiovascular system NEC R09.89
    chest NEC R09.89
    circulatory system NEC R09.89
    cognitive functions R41.9
      altered mental status R41.82
      amnesia — see Amnesia
      borderline intellectual functioning R41.83
      coma — see Coma
      disorientation R41.0
      neurologic neglect syndrome R41.4
      senile cognitive decline R41.81
      specified symptom NEC R41.89
    development NEC R62.50
    digestive system NEC R19.8
    emotional state NEC R45.89
      emotional lability R45.86
    food and fluid intake R63.8
    general perceptions and sensations R44.9
      specified NEC R44.8
    musculoskeletal system R29.91

Symptoms — continued
  involving — continued
    musculoskeletal system — continued
      specified NEC R29.898
    nervous system R29.90
      specified NEC R29.818
    pelvis NEC R19.8
    respiratory system NEC R09.89
    skin and integument R23.9
    urinary system R39.9
  menopausal N95.1
  metabolism NEC R63.8
  neurotic F48.8
  of infancy R68.19
  pelvis NEC, female R10.2
  skin and integument NEC R23.9
  subcutaneous tissue NEC R23.9
Sympus Q74.2
Syncephalus Q89.4
Synchondrosis
  abnormal (congenital) Q78.8
  ischiopubic M91.0
Synchysis (scintillans) (senile) (vitreous body) H43.89
Syncope (near) (pre-) R55
  anginosa I20.8
  bradycardia R00.1
  cardiac R55
  carotid sinus G90.01
  due to spinal (lumbar) puncture G97.1
  heart R55
  heat T67.1 ☑
  laryngeal R05
  psychogenic F48.8
  tussive R05
  vasoconstriction R55
  vasodepressor R55
  vasomotor R55
  vasovagal R55
Syndactylism, syndactyly Q70.9
  complex (with synostosis)
    fingers Q70.0- ☑
    toes Q70.2- ☑
  simple (without synostosis)
    fingers Q70.1- ☑
    toes Q70.3- ☑
Syndrome (see also Disease)
  48,XXXX Q97.1
  49,XXXXX Q97.1
  5q minus NOS D46.C (following D46.2)
  abdominal
    acute R10.0
    muscle deficiency Q79.4
  abnormal innervation H02.519
    left H02.516
      lower H02.515
      upper H02.514
    right H02.513
      lower H02.512
      upper H02.511
  abstinence, neonatal P96.1
  acid pulmonary aspiration, obstetric O74.0
  acquired immunodeficiency — see Human, immunodeficiency virus (HIV) disease
  acute abdominal R10.0
  acute respiratory distress (adult) (child) J80
  Adair-Dighton Q78.0
  Adams-Stokes (-Morgagni) I45.9
  adiposogenital E23.6
  adrenal
    hemorrhage (meningococcal) A39.1
    meningococcic A39.1
  adrenocortical — see Cushing's, syndrome
  adrenogenital E25.9
    congenital, associated with enzyme deficiency E25.0
  afferent loop NEC K91.89
  Alagille's Q44.7
  alcohol withdrawal (without convulsions) — see Dependence, alcohol, with, withdrawal
  Alder's D72.0
  Aldrich (-Wiskott) D82.0
  alien hand R41.4
  Alport Q87.81
  alveolar hypoventilation E66.2
  alveolocapillary block J84.10
  amnesic, amnestic (confabulatory) (due to) — see Disorder, amnesic
  amyostatic (Wilson's disease) E83.01

Syndrome — continued
  androgen insensitivity E34.50
    complete E34.51
    partial E34.52
  androgen resistance (see also Syndrome, androgen insensitivity) E34.50
  Angelman Q93.5
  anginal — see Angina
  ankyloglossia superior Q38.1
  anterior
    chest wall R07.89
    cord G83.82
    spinal artery G95.19
      compression M47.019
        cervical region M47.012
        cervicothoracic region M47.013
        lumbar region M47.016
        occipito-atlanto-axial region M47.011
        thoracic region M47.014
        thoracolumbar region M47.015
    tibial M76.81- ☑
  antibody deficiency D80.9
    agammaglobulinemic D80.1
      hereditary D80.0
    congenital D80.0
    hypogammaglobulinemic D80.1
      hereditary D80.0
  anticardiolipin (-antibody) D68.61
  antiphospholipid (-antibody) D68.61
  aortic
    arch M31.4
    bifurcation I74.09
  aortomesenteric duodenum occlusion K31.5
  apical ballooning (transient left ventricular) I51.81
  arcuate ligament I77.4
  argentaffin, argintaffinoma E34.0
  Arnold-Chiari — see Arnold-Chiari disease
  Arrillaga-Ayerza I27.0
  Asherman's N85.6
  aspiration, of newborn — see Aspiration, by substance, with pneumonia
    meconium P24.01
  ataxia-telangiectasia G11.3
  auriculotemporal G50.8
  autoerythrocyte sensitization (Gardner-Diamond) D69.2
  autoimmune lymphoproliferative [ALPS] D89.82
  autoimmune polyglandular E31.0
  autosomal — see Abnormal, autosomes
  Avellis' G46.8
  Ayerza (-Arrillaga) I27.0
  Babinski-Nageotte G83.89
  Bakwin-Krida Q79.8
  bare lymphocyte D81.6
  Barré-Guillain G61.0
  Barré-Liéou M53.0
  Barrett's — see Barrett's, esophagus
  Barsony-Polgar K22.4
  Bársony-Teschendorf K22.4
  Barth E78.71
  Bartter's E26.81
  basal cell nevus Q87.89
  Basedow's E05.00
    with thyroid storm E05.01
  basilar artery G45.0
  Batten-Steinert G71.11
  battered
    baby or child — see Maltreatment, child, physical abuse
    spouse — see Maltreatment, adult, physical abuse
  Beals Q87.40
  Beau's I51.5
  Beck's I65.8
  Benedikt's G46.3
  Béquez César (-Steinbrinck-Chédiak-Higashi) E70.330
  Bernhardt-Roth — see Meralgia paresthetica
  Bernheim's I50.9
  big spleen D73.1
  bilateral polycystic ovarian E28.2
  Bing-Horton's — see Horton's headache
  Birt-Hogg-Dube syndrome Q87.89
  Björck (-Thorsen) E34.0
  black
    lung J60
    widow spider bite — see Toxicity, venom, spider, black widow
  Blackfan-Diamond D61.01

☑ Additional Character Required — Refer to the Tabular List for Character Selection   ▽ Subterms under main terms may continue to next column or page

Syndrome — *continued*
- blind loop K90.2
  - congenital Q43.8
  - postsurgical K91.2
- blue sclera Q78.0
- blue toe I75.02- ✓
- Boder-Sedgewick G11.3
- Boerhaave's K22.3
- Borjeson Forssman Lehmann Q89.8
- Bouillaud's I01.9
- Bourneville (-Pringle) Q85.1
- Bouveret (-Hoffman) I47.9
- brachial plexus G54.0
- bradycardia-tachycardia I49.5
- brain (nonpsychotic) F09
  - with psychosis, psychotic reaction F09
  - acute or subacute — *see* Delirium
  - congenital — *see* Disability, intellectual
  - organic F09
    - post-traumatic (nonpsychotic) F07.81
      - psychotic F09
    - personality change F07.0
    - postcontusional F07.81
    - post-traumatic, nonpsychotic F07.81
    - psycho-organic F09
    - psychotic F06.8
- brain stem stroke G46.3
- Brandt's (acrodermatitis enteropathica) E83.2
- broad ligament laceration N83.8
- Brock's J98.11
- bronze baby P83.8
- Brown-Sequard G83.81
- bubbly lung P27.0
- Buchem's M85.2
- Budd-Chiari I82.0
- bulbar (progressive) G12.22
- Bürger-Grütz E78.3
- Burke's K86.8
- Burnett's (milk-alkali) E83.52
- burning feet E53.9
- Bywaters' T79.5 ✓
- Call-Fleming I67.841
- carbohydrate-deficient glycoprotein (CDGS) E77.8
- carcinogenic thrombophlebitis I82.1
- carcinoid E34.0
- cardiac asthma I50.1
- cardiacos negros I27.0
- cardiofaciocutaneous Q87.89
- cardiopulmonary-obesity E66.2
- cardiorenal — *see* Hypertension, cardiorenal
- cardiorespiratory distress (idiopathic), newborn P22.0
- cardiovascular renal — *see* Hypertension, cardiorenal
- carotid
  - artery (hemispheric) (internal) G45.1
  - body G90.01
  - sinus G90.01
- carpal tunnel G56.0- ✓
- Cassidy (-Scholte) E34.0
- cat cry Q93.4
- cat eye Q92.8
- cauda equina G83.4
- causalgia — *see* Causalgia
- celiac K90.0
  - artery compression I77.4
  - axis I77.4
- central pain G89.0
- cerebellar
  - hereditary G11.9
  - stroke G46.4
- cerebellomedullary malformation — *see* Spina bifida
- cerebral
  - artery
    - anterior G46.1
    - middle G46.0
    - posterior G46.2
  - gigantism E22.0
- cervical (root) M53.1
  - disc — *see* Disorder, disc, cervical, with neuritis
  - fusion Q76.1
  - posterior, sympathicus M53.0
  - rib Q76.5
  - sympathetic paralysis G90.2
- cervicobrachial (diffuse) M53.1
- cervicocranial M53.0
- cervicodorsal outlet G54.2
- cervicothoracic outlet G54.0
- Céstan (-Raymond) I65.8

Syndrome — *continued*
- Charcot's (angina cruris) (intermittent claudication) I73.9
- Charcot-Weiss-Baker G90.09
- CHARGE Q89.8
- Chédiak-Higashi (-Steinbrinck) E70.330
- chest wall R07.1
- Chiari's (hepatic vein thrombosis) I82.0
- Chilaiditi's Q43.3
- child maltreatment — *see* Maltreatment, child
- chondrocostal junction M94.0
- chondroectodermal dysplasia Q77.6
- chromosome 4 short arm deletion Q93.3
- chromosome 5 short arm deletion Q93.4
- chronic
  - pain G89.4
    - personality F68.8
- Clarke-Hadfield K86.8
- Clerambault's automatism G93.89
- Clouston's (hidrotic ectodermal dysplasia) Q82.4
- clumsiness, clumsy child F82
- cluster headache G44.009
  - intractable G44.001
  - not intractable G44.009
- Coffin-Lowry Q89.8
- cold injury (newborn) P80.0
- combined immunity deficiency D81.9
- compartment (deep) (posterior) (traumatic) T79.A0 ✓ (*following* T79.7)
  - abdomen T79.A3 ✓ (*following* T79.7)
  - lower extremity (hip, buttock, thigh, leg, foot, toes) T79.A2 ✓ (*following* T79.7)
  - nontraumatic
    - abdomen M79.A3 (*following* M79.7)
    - lower extremity (hip, buttock, thigh, leg, foot, toes) M79.A2- ✓ (*following* M79.7)
    - specified site NEC M79.A9 (*following* M79.7)
    - upper extremity (shoulder, arm, forearm, wrist, hand, fingers) M79.A1- ✓ (*following* M79.7)
  - postprocedural — *see* Syndrome, compartment, nontraumatic
  - specified site NEC T79.A9 ✓ (*following* T79.7)
  - upper extremity (shoulder, arm, forearm, wrist, hand, fingers) T79.A1 ✓ (*following* T79.7)
- complex regional pain — *see* Syndrome, pain, complex regional
- compression T79.5 ✓
  - anterior spinal — *see* Syndrome, anterior, spinal artery, compression
  - cauda equina G83.4
  - celiac artery I77.4
  - vertebral artery M47.029
    - cervical region M47.022
    - occipito-atlanto-axial region M47.021
- concussion F07.81
- congenital
  - affecting multiple systems NEC Q87.89
  - central alveolar hypoventilation G47.35
  - facial diplegia Q87.0
  - muscular hypertrophy-cerebral Q87.89
  - oculo-auriculovertebral Q87.0
  - oculofacial diplegia (Moebius) Q87.0
  - rubella (manifest) P35.0
- congestion-fibrosis (pelvic), female N94.89
- congestive dysmenorrhea N94.6
- connective tissue M35.9
  - overlap NEC M35.1
- Conn's E26.01
- conus medullaris G95.81
- cord
  - anterior G83.82
  - posterior G83.83
- coronary
  - acute NEC I24.9
  - insufficiency or intermediate I20.0
  - slow flow I20.8
- Costen's (complex) M26.69
- costochondral junction M94.0
- costoclavicular G54.0
- costovertebral E22.0
- Cowden Q85.8
- craniovertebral M53.0
- Creutzfeldt-Jakob — *see* Creutzfeldt-Jakob disease or syndrome
- crib death R99
- cricopharyngeal — *see* Dysphagia
- cri-du-chat Q93.4

Syndrome — *continued*
- croup J05.0
- CRPS I — *see* Syndrome, pain, complex regional I
- crush T79.5 ✓
- cryptophthalmos Q87.0
- cubital tunnel — *see* Lesion, nerve, ulnar
- Curschmann (-Batten) (-Steinert) G71.11
- Cushing's E24.9
  - alcohol-induced E24.4
  - drug-induced E24.2
  - due to
    - alcohol
      - drugs E24.2
      - ectopic ACTH E24.3
      - overproduction of pituitary ACTH E24.0
    - overdose or wrong substance given or taken — *see* Table of Drugs and Chemicals, by drug, poisoning
  - pituitary-dependent E24.0
  - specified type NEC E24.8
- cystic duct stump K91.5
- Dana-Putnam D51.0
- Danbolt (-Cross) (acrodermatitis enteropathica) E83.2
- Dandy-Walker Q03.1
  - with spina bifida Q07.01
- Danlos' Q79.8
- De Quervain E34.51
- de Toni-Fanconi (-Debré) E72.09
  - with cystinosis E72.04
- defibrination (*see also* Fibrinolysis)
  - with
    - antepartum hemorrhage — *see* Hemorrhage, antepartum, with coagulation defect
    - intrapartum hemorrhage — *see* Hemorrhage, complicating, delivery
  - newborn P60
  - postpartum O72.3
- Degos' I77.89
- Déjérine-Roussy G89.0
- delayed sleep phase G47.21
- demyelinating G37.9
- dependence — *see* F10-F19 with fourth character .2
- depersonalization (-derealization) F48.1
- di George's D82.1
- diabetes mellitus in newborn infant P70.2
- diabetes mellitus-hypertension-nephrosis — *see* Diabetes, nephrosis
- diabetes-nephrosis — *see* Diabetes, nephrosis
- diabetic amyotrophy — *see* Diabetes, amyotrophy
- Diamond-Blackfan D61.01
- Diamond-Gardener D69.2
- DIC (diffuse or disseminated intravascular coagulopathy) D65
- Dighton's Q78.0
- disequilibrium E87.8
- Döhle body-panmyelopathic D72.0
- dorsolateral medullary G46.4
- double athetosis G80.3
- Down (*see also* Down syndrome) Q90.9
- Dresbach's (elliptocytosis) D58.1
- Dressler's (postmyocardial infarction) I24.1
  - postcardiotomy I97.0
- drug withdrawal, infant of dependent mother P96.1
- dry eye H04.12- ✓
- due to abnormality
  - chromosomal Q99.9
    - sex
      - female phenotype Q97.9
      - male phenotype Q98.9
    - specified NEC Q99.8
- dumping (postgastrectomy) K91.1
  - nonsurgical K31.89
- Dupré's (meningism) R29.1
- dysmetabolic X E88.81
- dyspraxia, developmental F82
- Eagle-Barrett Q79.4
- Eaton-Lambert — *see* Syndrome, Lambert-Eaton
- Ebstein's Q22.5
- ectopic ACTH E24.3
- eczema-thrombocytopenia D82.0
- Eddowes' Q78.0
- effort (psychogenic) F45.8
- Ehlers-Danlos Q79.6
- Eisenmenger's I27.89
- Ekman's Q78.0
- electric feet E53.8
- Ellis-van Creveld Q77.6
- empty nest Z60.0

Index

Syndrome — Syndrome

Syndrome — *continued*
  endocrine-hypertensive E27.0
  entrapment — *see* Neuropathy, entrapment
  eosinophilia-myalgia M35.8
  epileptic (*see also* Epilepsy, by type)
    absence G40.A09 (*following* G40.3)
      intractable G40.A19 (*following* G40.3)
        with status epilepticus G40.A11 (*following* G40.3)
        without status epilepticus G40.A19 (*following* G40.3)
      not intractable G40.A09 (*following* G40.3)
        with status epilepticus G40.A01 (*following* G40.3)
        without status epilepticus G40.A09 (*following* G40.3)
  Erdheim-Chester (ECD) E88.89
  Erdheim's E22.0
  erythrocyte fragmentation D59.4
  Evans D69.41
  exhaustion F48.8
  extrapyramidal G25.9
    specified NEC G25.89
  eye retraction — *see* Strabismus
  eyelid-malar-mandible Q87.0
  Faber's D50.9
  facial pain, paroxysmal G50.0
  Fallot's Q21.3
  familial eczema-thrombocytopenia (Wiskott-Aldrich) D82.0
  Fanconi (-de Toni) (-Debré) E72.09
    with cystinosis E72.04
  Fanconi's (anemia) (congenital pancytopenia) D61.09
  fatigue
    chronic R53.82
    psychogenic F48.8
  faulty bowel habit K59.3
  Feil-Klippel (brevicollis) Q76.1
  Felty's — *see* Felty's syndrome
  fertile eunuch E23.0
  fetal
    alcohol (dysmorphic) Q86.0
    hydantoin Q86.1
  Fiedler's I40.1
  first arch Q87.0
  fish odor E72.8
  Fisher's G61.0
  Fitzhugh-Curtis
    due to
      Chlamydia trachomatis A74.81
      Neisseria gonorrhorea (gonococcal peritonitis) A54.85
  Fitz's K85.8
  Flajani (-Basedow) E05.00
    with thyroid storm E05.01
  flatback — *see* Flatback syndrome
  floppy
    baby P94.2
    iris (intraoperative) (IFIS) H21.81
    mitral valve I34.1
  flush E34.0
  Foix-Alajouanine G95.19
  Fong's Q79.8
  foramen magnum G93.5
  Foster-Kennedy H47.14- ☑
  Foville's (peduncular) G46.3
  fragile X Q99.2
  Franceschetti Q75.4
  Frey's
    auriculotemporal G50.8
    hyperhidrosis L74.52
  Friderichsen-Waterhouse A39.1
  Froin's G95.89
  frontal lobe F07.0
  Fukuhara E88.49
  functional
    bowel K59.9
    prepubertal castrate E29.1
  Gaisböck's D75.1
  ganglion (basal ganglia brain) G25.9
    geniculi G51.1
  Gardner-Diamond D69.2
  gastroesophageal
    junction K22.0
    laceration-hemorrhage K22.6
  gastrojejunal loop obstruction K91.89
  Gee-Herter-Heubner K90.0
  Gelineau's G47.419

Syndrome — *continued*
  Gelineau's — *continued*
    with cataplexy G47.411
  genito-anorectal A55
  Gerstmann-Sträussler-Scheinker (GSS) A81.82
  Gianotti-Crosti L44.4
  giant platelet (Bernard-Soulier) D69.1
  Gilles de la Tourette's F95.2
  goiter-deafness E07.1
  Goldberg Q89.8
  Goldberg-Maxwell E34.51
  Good's D83.8
  Gopalan' (burning feet) E53.8
  Gorlin's Q87.89
  Gougerot-Blum L81.7
  Gouley's I31.1
  Gower's R55
  gray or grey (newborn) P93.0
    platelet D69.1
  Gubler-Millard G46.3
  Guillain-Barré (-Strohl) G61.0
  gustatory sweating G50.8
  Hadfield-Clarke K86.8
  hair tourniquet — *see* Constriction, external, by site
  Hamman's J98.19
  hand-foot L27.1
  hand-shoulder G90.8
  hantavirus (cardio)-pulmonary (HPS) (HCPS) B33.4
  happy puppet Q93.5
  Harada's H30.81- ☑
  Hayem-Faber D50.9
  headache NEC G44.89
    complicated NEC G44.59
  Heberden's I20.8
  Hedinger's E34.0
  Hegglin's D72.0
  HELLP (hemolysis, elevated liver enzymes and low platelet count) O14.2- ☑
  hemolytic-uremic D59.3
  hemophagocytic, infection-associated D76.2
  Henoch-Schönlein D69.0
  hepatic flexure K59.8
  hepatopulmonary K76.81
  hepatorenal K76.7
    following delivery O90.4
    postoperative or postprocedural K91.83
    postpartum, puerperal O90.4
  hepatourologic K76.7
  Herter (-Gee) (nontropical sprue) K90.0
  Heubner-Herter K90.0
  Heyd's K76.7
  Hilger's G90.09
  histamine-like (fish poisoning) — *see* Poisoning, fish
  histiocytic D76.3
  histiocytosis NEC D76.3
  HIV infection, acute B20
  Hoffmann-Werdnig G12.0
  Hollander-Simons E88.1
  Hoppe-Goldflam G70.00
    with exacerbation (acute) G70.01
    in crisis G70.01
  Horner's G90.2
  hungry bone E83.81
  hunterian glossitis D51.0
  Hutchinson's triad A50.53
  hyperabduction G54.0
  hyperammonemia-hyperornithinemia-homocitrullinemia E72.4
  hypereosinophilic (idiopathic) D72.1
  hyperimmunoglobulin E (IgE) D82.4
  hyperkalemic E87.5
  hyperkinetic — *see* Hyperkinesia
  hypermobility M35.7
  hypernatremia E87.0
  hyperosmolarity E87.0
  hyperperfusion G97.82
  hypersplenic D73.1
  hypertransfusion, newborn P61.1
  hyperventilation F45.8
  hyperviscosity (of serum)
    polycythemic D75.1
    sclerothymic D58.8
  hypoglycemic (familial) (neonatal) E16.2
  hypokalemic E87.6
  hyponatremic E87.1
  hypopituitarism E23.0
  hypoplastic left-heart Q23.4
  hypopotassemia E87.6

Syndrome — *continued*
  hyposmolality E87.1
  hypotension, maternal O26.5- ☑
  hypothenar hammer I73.89
  ICF (intravascular coagulation-fibrinolysis) D65
  idiopathic
    cardiorespiratory distress, newborn P22.0
    nephrotic (infantile) N04.9
  iliotibial band M76.3- ☑
  immobility, immobilization (paraplegic) M62.3
  immune reconstitution D89.3
  immune reconstitution inflammatory [IRIS] D89.3
  immunity deficiency, combined D81.9
  immunodeficiency
    acquired — *see* Human, immunodeficiency virus (HIV) disease
    combined D81.9
  impending coronary I20.0
  impingement, shoulder M75.4- ☑
  inappropriate secretion of antidiuretic hormone E22.2
  infant
    gestational diabetes P70.0
    of diabetic mother P70.1
  infantilism (pituitary) E23.0
  inferior vena cava I87.1
  inspissated bile (newborn) P59.1
  institutional (childhood) F94.2
  insufficient sleep F51.12
  intermediate coronary (artery) I20.0
  interspinous ligament — *see* Spondylopathy, specified NEC
  intestinal
    carcinoid E34.0
    knot K56.2
  intravascular coagulation-fibrinolysis (ICF) D65
  iodine-deficiency, congenital E00.9
    type
      mixed E00.2
      myxedematous E00.1
      neurological E00.0
  IRDS (idiopathic respiratory distress, newborn) P22.0
  irritable
    bowel K58.9
      with diarrhea K58.0
      psychogenic F45.8
    heart (psychogenic) F45.8
    weakness F48.8
  ischemic bowel (transient) K55.9
    chronic K55.1
    due to mesenteric artery insufficiency K55.1
  IVC (intravascular coagulopathy) D65
  Ivemark's Q89.01
  Jaccoud's — *see* Arthropathy, postrheumatic, chronic
  Jackson's G83.89
  Jakob-Creutzfeldt — *see* Creutzfeldt-Jakob disease or syndrome
  jaw-winking Q07.8
  Jervell-Lange-Nielsen I45.81
  jet lag G47.25
  Job's D71
  Joseph-Diamond-Blackfan D61.01
  jugular foramen G52.7
  Kabuki Q89.8
  Kanner's (autism) F84.0
  Kartagener's Q89.3
  Kelly's D50.1
  Kimmelstiel-Wilson — *see* Diabetes, specified type, with Kimmelstiel-Wilson disease
  Klein (e)-Levine G47.13
  Klippel-Feil (brevicollis) Q76.1
  Köhler-Pellegrini-Steida — *see* Bursitis, tibial collateral
  König's K59.8
  Korsakoff (-Wernicke) (nonalcoholic) F04
    alcoholic F10.26
  Kostmann's D70.0
  Krabbe's congenital muscle hypoplasia Q79.8
  labyrinthine — *see* subcategory H83.2 ☑
  lacunar NEC G46.7
  Lambert-Eaton G70.80
    in
      neoplastic disease G73.1
      specified disease NEC G70.81
  Landau-Kleffner — *see* Epilepsy, specified NEC
  Larsen's Q74.8
  lateral
    cutaneous nerve of thigh G57.1- ☑
    medullary G46.4
  Launois' E22.0

Syndrome — continued
- lazy
  - leukocyte D70.8
  - posture M62.3
- Lemiere I80.8
- Lennox-Gastaut G40.812
  - intractable G40.814
    - with status epilepticus G40.813
    - without status epilepticus G40.814
  - not intractable G40.812
    - with status epilepticus G40.811
    - without status epilepticus G40.812
- lenticular, progressive E83.01
- Leopold-Levi's E05.90
- Lev's I44.2
- Lichtheim's D51.0
- Li-Fraumeni Z15.01
- Lightwood's N25.89
- Lignac (de Toni) (-Fanconi) (-Debré) E72.09
  - with cystinosis E72.04
- Likoff's I20.8
- limbic epilepsy personality F07.0
- liver-kidney K76.7
- lobotomy F07.0
- Loffler's J82
- long arm 18 or 21 deletion Q93.89
- long QT I45.81
- Louis-Barré G11.3
- low
  - atmospheric pressure T70.29 ☑
  - back M54.5
  - output (cardiac) I50.9
- lower radicular, newborn (birth injury) P14.8
- Luetscher's (dehydration) E86.0
- Lupus anticoagulant D68.62
- Lutembacher's Q21.1
- macrophage activation D76.1
  - due to infection D76.2
- magnesium-deficiency R29.0
- Mal de Debarquement R42
- malabsorption K90.9
  - postsurgical K91.2
- malformation, congenital, due to
  - alcohol Q86.0
  - exogenous cause NEC Q86.8
  - hydantoin Q86.1
  - warfarin Q86.2
- malignant
  - carcinoid E34.0
  - neuroleptic G21.0
- Mallory-Weiss K22.6
- mandibulofacial dysostosis Q75.4
- manic-depressive — see Disorder, bipolar, affective
- maple-syrup-urine E71.0
- Marable's I77.4
- Marfan's Q87.40
  - with
    - cardiovascular manifestations Q87.418
      - aortic dilation Q87.410
    - ocular manifestations Q87.42
    - skeletal manifestations Q87.43
- Marie's (acromegaly) E22.0
- maternal hypotension — see Syndrome, hypotension, maternal
- May (-Hegglin) D72.0
- McArdle (-Schmidt) (-Pearson) E74.04
- McQuarrie's E16.2
- meconium plug (newborn) P76.0
- median arcuate ligament I77.4
- Meekeren-Ehlers-Danlos Q79.6
- megavitamin-B6 E67.2
- Meige G24.4
- MELAS E88.41
- Mendelson's O74.0
- MERRF (myoclonic epilepsy associated with ragged-red fibers) E88.42
- mesenteric
  - artery (superior) K55.1
  - vascular insufficiency K55.1
- metabolic E88.81
- metastatic carcinoid E34.0
- micrognathia-glossoptosis Q87.0
- midbrain NEC G93.89
- middle lobe (lung) J98.19
- middle radicular G54.0
- migraine (see also Migraine) G43.909
- Mikulicz' K11.8
- milk-alkali E83.52

Syndrome — continued
- Millard-Gubler G46.3
- Miller-Dieker Q93.88
- Miller-Fisher G61.0
- Minkowski-Chauffard D58.0
- Mirizzi's K83.1
- MNGIE (Mitochondrial Neurogastrointestinal Encephalopathy) E88.49
- Möbius, ophthalmoplegic migraine — see Migraine, ophthalmoplegic
- monofixation H50.42
- Morel-Moore M85.2
- Morel-Morgagni M85.2
- Morgagni (-Morel) (-Stewart) M85.2
- Morgagni-Adams-Stokes I45.9
- Mounier-Kuhn Q32.4
  - with bronchiectasis J47.9
    - with
      - exacerbation (acute) J47.1
      - lower respiratory infection J47.0
  - acquired J98.09
    - with bronchiectasis J47.9
      - with
        - exacerbation (acute) J47.1
        - lower respiratory infection J47.0
- mucocutaneous lymph node (acute febrile) (MCLS) M30.3
- multiple endocrine neoplasia (MEN) — see Neoplasia, endocrine, multiple (MEN)
- multiple operations — see Disorder, factitious
- myasthenic G70.9
  - in
    - diabetes mellitus — see Diabetes, amyotrophy
    - endocrine disease NEC E34.9 [G73.3]
    - neoplastic disease (see also Neoplasm) D49.9 [G73.3]
    - thyrotoxicosis (hyperthyroidism) E05.90 [G73.3]
      - with thyroid storm E05.91 [G73.3]
- myelodysplastic D46.9
  - with
    - 5q deletion D46.C (following D46.2)
    - isolated del (5q) chromosomal abnormality D46.C (following D46.2)
  - lesions, low grade D46.20
  - specified NEC D46.Z (following D46.4)
- myelopathic pain G89.0
- myeloproliferative (chronic) D47.1
- myofascial pain M79.1
- Naffziger's G54.0
- nail patella Q87.2
- NARP (Neuropathy, Ataxia and Retinitis pigmentosa) E88.49
- neonatal abstinence P96.1
- nephritic (see also Nephritis)
  - with edema — see Nephrosis
  - acute N00.9
  - chronic N03.9
  - rapidly progressive N01.9
- nephrotic (congenital) (see also Nephrosis) N04.9
  - with
    - dense deposit disease N04.6
    - diffuse
      - crescentic glomerulonephritis N04.7
      - endocapillary proliferative glomerulonephritis N04.4
      - membranous glomerulonephritis N04.2
      - mesangial proliferative glomerulonephritis N04.3
      - mesangiocapillary glomerulonephritis N04.5
    - focal and segmental glomerular lesions N04.1
    - minor glomerular abnormality N04.0
    - specified morphological changes NEC N04.8
  - diabetic — see Diabetes, nephrosis
- neurologic neglect R41.4
- Nezelof's D81.4
- Nonne-Milroy-Meige Q82.0
- Nothnagel's vasomotor acroparesthesia I73.89
- oculomotor H51.9
- ophthalmoplegia-cerebellar ataxia — see Strabismus, paralytic, third nerve
- oral-facial-digital Q87.0
- organic
  - affective F06.30
  - amnesic (not alcohol- or drug-induced) F04
  - brain F09
  - depressive F06.31
  - hallucinosis F06.0
  - personality F07.0

Syndrome — continued
- Ormond's N13.5
- oro-facial-digital Q87.0
- os trigonum Q68.8
- Osler-Weber-Rendu I78.0
- osteoporosis-osteomalacia M83.8
- Osterreicher-Turner Q79.8
- otolith — see subcategory H81.8 ☑
- oto-palatal-digital Q87.0
- outlet (thoracic) G54.0
- ovary
  - polycystic E28.2
  - resistant E28.39
  - sclerocystic E28.2
- Owren's D68.2
- Paget-Schroetter I82.890
- pain (see also Pain)
  - complex regional I G90.50
    - lower limb G90.52- ☑
    - specified site NEC G90.59
    - upper limb G90.51- ☑
  - complex regional II — see Causalgia
- painful
  - bruising D69.2
  - feet E53.8
  - prostate N42.81
- paralysis agitans — see Parkinsonism
- paralytic G83.9
  - specified NEC G83.89
- Parinaud's H51.0
- parkinsonian — see Parkinsonism
- Parkinson's — see Parkinsonism
- paroxysmal facial pain G50.0
- Parry's E05.00
  - with thyroid storm E05.01
- Parsonage (-Aldren)-Turner G54.5
- patella clunk M25.86- ☑
- Paterson (-Brown) (-Kelly) D50.1
- pectoral girdle I77.89
- pectoralis minor I77.89
- Pelger-Huet D72.0
- pellagra-cerebellar ataxia-renal aminoaciduria E72.02
- pellagroid E52
- Pellegrini-Stieda — see Bursitis, tibial collateral
- pelvic congestion-fibrosis, female N94.89
- penta X Q97.1
- peptic ulcer — see Ulcer, peptic
- perabduction I77.89
- periodic headache, in adults and children — see Headache, periodic syndromes in adults and children
- periurethral fibrosis N13.5
- phantom limb (without pain) G54.7
  - with pain G54.6
- pharyngeal pouch D82.1
- Pick's (heart) (liver) I31.1
- Pickwickian E66.2
- PIE (pulmonary infiltration with eosinophilia) J82
- pigmentary pallidal degeneration (progressive) G23.0
- pineal E34.8
- pituitary E22.0
- placental transfusion — see Pregnancy, complicated by, placental transfusion syndromes
- plantar fascia M72.2
- plateau iris (post-iridectomy) (postprocedural) H21.82
- Plummer-Vinson D50.1
- pluricarential of infancy E40
- plurideficiency E40
- pluriglandular (compensatory) E31.8
  - autoimmune E31.0
- pneumatic hammer T75.21 ☑
- polyangiitis overlap M30.8
- polycarential of infancy E40
- polyglandular E31.8
  - autoimmune E31.0
- polysplenia Q89.09
- pontine NEC G93.89
- popliteal
  - artery entrapment I77.89
  - web Q87.89
- post chemoembolization — code to associated conditions
- postcardiac injury
  - postcardiotomy I97.0
  - postmyocardial infarction I24.1
- postcardiotomy I97.0
- postcholecystectomy K91.5
- postcommissurotomy I97.0

Syndrome — continued
  postconcussional F07.81
  postcontusional F07.81
  postencephalitic F07.89
  posterior
    cervical sympathetic M53.0
    cord G83.83
    fossa compression G93.5
    reversible encephalopathy (PRES) I67.83
  postgastrectomy (dumping) K91.1
  postgastric surgery K91.1
  postinfarction I24.1
  postlaminectomy NEC M96.1
  postleukotomy F07.0
  postmastectomy lymphedema I97.2
  postmyocardial infarction I24.1
  postoperative NEC T81.9 ☑
    blind loop K90.2
  postpartum panhypopituitary (Sheehan) E23.0
  postpolio (myelitic) G14
  postthrombotic I87.009
    with
      inflammation I87.02- ☑
        with ulcer I87.03- ☑
      specified complication NEC I87.09- ☑
      ulcer I87.01- ☑
        with inflammation I87.03- ☑
    asymptomatic I87.00- ☑
  postvagotomy K91.1
  postvalvulotomy I97.0
  postviral NEC G93.3
    fatigue G93.3
  Potain's K31.0
  potassium intoxication E87.5
  precerebral artery (multiple) (bilateral) G45.2
  preinfarction I20.0
  preleukemic D46.9
  premature senility E34.8
  premenstrual dysphoric N94.3
  premenstrual tension N94.3
  Prinzmetal-Massumi R07.1
  prune belly Q79.4
  pseudo -Turner's Q87.1
  pseudocarpal tunnel (sublimis) — see Syndrome,
    carpal tunnel
  pseudoparalytica G70.00
    with exacerbation (acute) G70.01
    in crisis G70.01
  psycho-organic (nonpsychotic severity) F07.9
    acute or subacute F05
    depressive type F06.31
    hallucinatory type F06.0
    nonpsychotic severity F07.0
    specified NEC F07.89
  pulmonary
    arteriosclerosis I27.0
    dysmaturity (Wilson-Mikity) P27.0
    hypoperfusion (idiopathic) P22.0
    renal (hemorrhagic) (Goodpasture's) M31.0
  pure
    motor lacunar G46.5
    sensory lacunar G46.6
  Putnam-Dana D51.0
  pyramidopallidonigral G20
  pyriformis — see Lesion, nerve, sciatic
  QT interval prolongation I45.81
  radicular NEC — see Radiculopathy
    upper limbs, newborn (birth injury) P14.3
  rapid time-zone change G47.25
  Rasmussen G04.81
  Raymond (-Céstan) I65.8
  Raynaud's I73.00
    with gangrene I73.01
  RDS (respiratory distress syndrome, newborn) P22.0
  reactive airways dysfunction J68.3
  Refsum's G60.1
  Reifenstein E34.52
  renal glomerulohyalinosis-diabetic — see Diabetes,
    nephrosis
  Rendu-Osler-Weber I78.0
  residual ovary N99.83
  resistant ovary E28.39
  respiratory
    distress
      acute J80
        adult J80
        child J80
      newborn (idiopathic) (type I) P22.0

Syndrome — continued
  respiratory — continued
    distress — continued
      newborn — continued
        type II P22.1
  restless legs G25.81
  retinoblastoma (familial) C69.2 ☑
  retroperitoneal fibrosis N13.5
  retroviral seroconversion (acute) Z21
  Reye's G93.7
  Richter — see Leukemia, chronic lymphocytic, B-cell
    type
  Ridley's I50.1
  right
    heart, hypoplastic Q22.6
    ventricular obstruction — see Failure, heart, con-
      gestive
  Romano-Ward (prolonged QT interval) I45.81
  rotator cuff, shoulder (see also Tear, rotator cuff)
    M75.10- ☑
  Rotes Quérol — see Hyperostosis, ankylosing
  Roth — see Meralgia paresthetica
  rubella (congenital) P35.0
  Ruvalcaba-Myhre-Smith E71.440
  Rytand-Lipsitch I44.2
  salt
    depletion E87.1
      due to heat NEC T67.8 ☑
        causing heat exhaustion or prostration
          T67.4 ☑
    low E87.1
  salt-losing N28.89
  Scaglietti-Dagnini E22.0
  scalenus anticus (anterior) G54.0
  scapulocostal — see Mononeuropathy, upper limb,
    specified site NEC
  scapuloperoneal G71.0
  schizophrenic, of childhood NEC F84.5
  Schnitzler D47.2
  Scholte's E34.0
  Schroeder's E27.0
  Schüller-Christian C96.5
  Schwachman's — see Syndrome, Shwachman's
  Schwartz (-Jampel) G71.13
  Schwartz-Bartter E22.2
  scimitar Q26.8
  sclerocystic ovary E28.2
  Seitelberger's G31.89
  septicemic adrenal hemorrhage A39.1
  seroconversion, retroviral (acute) Z21
  serous meningitis G93.2
  severe acute respiratory (SARS) J12.81
  shaken infant T74.4 ☑
  shock (traumatic) T79.4 ☑
    kidney N17.0
      following crush injury T79.5 ☑
    toxic A48.3
  shock-lung J80
  Shone's — code to specific anomalies
  short
    bowel K91.2
    rib Q77.2
  shoulder-hand — see Algoneurodystrophy
  Shwachman's D70.4
  sicca — see Sicca syndrome
  sick
    cell E87.1
    sinus I49.5
  sick-euthyroid E07.81
  sideropenic D50.1
  Siemens' ectodermal dysplasia Q82.4
  Silfversköld's Q78.9
  Simons' E88.1
  sinus tarsi M25.57- ☑
  sinusitis-bronchiectasis-situs inversus Q89.3
  Sipple's E31.22
  sirenomelia Q87.2
  Slocumb's E27.0
  slow flow, coronary I20.8
  Sluder's G44.89
  Smith-Magenis Q93.88
  Sneddon-Wilkinson L13.1
  Sotos' Q22.0
  South African cardiomyopathy I42.8
  spasmodic
    upward movement, eyes H51.8
    winking F95.8
  Spen's I45.9

Syndrome — continued
  splenic
    agenesis Q89.01
    flexure K59.8
    neutropenia D73.81
  Spurway's Q78.0
  staphylococcal scalded skin L00
  Stein-Leventhal E28.2
  Stein's E28.2
  Stevens-Johnson syndrome L51.1
    toxic epidermal necrolysis overlap L51.3
  Stewart-Morel M85.2
  Stickler Q89.8
  stiff baby Q89.8
  stiff man G25.82
  Still-Felty — see Felty's syndrome
  Stokes (-Adams) I45.9
  stone heart I50.1
  straight back, congenital Q76.49
  subclavian steal G45.8
  subcoracoid-pectoralis minor G54.0
  subcostal nerve compression I77.89
  subphrenic interposition Q43.3
  superior
    cerebellar artery I63.8
    mesenteric artery K55.1
    semi-circular canal dehiscence H83.8X- ☑
    vena cava I87.1
  supine hypotensive (maternal) — see Syndrome, hy-
    potension, maternal
  suprarenal cortical E27.0
  supraspinatus (see also Tear, rotator cuff) M75.10- ☑
  Susac G93.49
  swallowed blood P78.2
  sweat retention L74.0
  Swyer Q99.1
  Symond's G93.2
  sympathetic
    cervical paralysis G90.2
    pelvic, female N94.89
  systemic inflammatory response (SIRS), of non-infec-
    tious origin (without organ dysfunction) R65.10
    with acute organ dysfunction R65.11
  tachycardia-bradycardia I49.5
  takotsubo I51.81
  TAR (thrombocytopenia with absent radius) Q87.2
  tarsal tunnel G57.5- ☑
  teething K00.7
  tegmental G93.89
  telangiectasic-pigmentation-cataract Q82.8
  temporal pyramidal apex — see Otitis, media, suppu-
    rative, acute
  temporomandibular joint-pain-dysfunction M26.62
  Terry's H44.2- ☑
  testicular feminization (see also Syndrome, androgen
    insensitivity) E34.51
  thalamic pain (hyperesthetic) G89.0
  thoracic outlet (compression) G54.0
  Thorson-Björck E34.0
  thrombocytopenia with absent radius (TAR) Q87.2
  thyroid-adrenocortical insufficiency E31.0
  tibial
    anterior M76.81- ☑
    posterior M76.82- ☑
  Tietze's M94.0
  time-zone (rapid) G47.25
  Toni-Fanconi E72.09
    with cystinosis E72.04
  Touraine's Q79.8
  tourniquet — see Constriction, external, by site
  toxic shock A48.3
  transient left ventricular apical ballooning I51.81
  traumatic vasospastic T75.22 ☑
  Treacher Collins Q75.4
  triple X, female Q97.0
  trisomy Q92.9
    13 Q91.7
      meiotic nondisjunction Q91.4
      mitotic nondisjunction Q91.5
      mosaicism Q91.5
      translocation Q91.6
    18 Q91.3
      meiotic nondisjunction Q91.0
      mitotic nondisjunction Q91.1
      mosaicism Q91.1
      translocation Q91.2
    20 (q)(p) Q92.8
    21 Q90.9

Syndrome — *continued*
- trisomy — *continued*
  - 21 — *continued*
    - meiotic nondisjunction Q90.0
    - mitotic nondisjunction Q90.1
    - mosaicism Q90.1
    - translocation Q90.2
  - 22 Q92.8
- tropical wet feet T69.0- ☑
- Trousseau's I82.1
- tumor lysis (following antineoplastic chemotherapy) (spontaneous) NEC E88.3
- Twiddler's (due to)
  - automatic implantable defibrillator T82.198 ☑
  - cardiac pacemaker T82.198 ☑
- Unverricht (-Lundborg) — *see* Epilepsy, generalized, idiopathic
- upward gaze H51.8
- uremia, chronic (*see also* Disease, kidney, chronic) N18.9
- urethral N34.3
- urethro-oculo-articular — *see* Reiter's disease
- urohepatic K76.7
- vago-hypoglossal G52.7
- van Buchem's M85.2
- van der Hoeve's Q78.0
- vascular NEC in cerebrovascular disease G46.8
- vasoconstriction, reversible cerebrovascular I67.841
- vasomotor I73.9
- vasospastic (traumatic) T75.22 ☑
- vasovagal R55
- VATER Q87.2
- velo-cardio-facial Q93.81
- vena cava (inferior) (superior) (obstruction) I87.1
- vertebral
  - artery G45.0
    - compression — *see* Syndrome, anterior, spinal artery, compression
  - steal G45.0
- vertebro-basilar artery G45.0
- vertebrogenic (pain) M54.89
- vertiginous — *see* Disorder, vestibular function
- Vinson-Plummer D50.1
- virus B34.9
- visceral larva migrans B83.0
- visual disorientation H53.8
- vitamin B6 deficiency E53.1
- vitreal corneal H59.01- ☑
- vitreous (touch) H59.01- ☑
- Vogt-Koyanagi H20.82- ☑
- Volkmann's T79.6
- von Schroetter's I82.890
- von Willebrand (-Jürgen) D68.0
- Waldenström-Kjellberg D50.1
- Wallenberg's G46.3
- water retention E87.79
- Waterhouse (-Friderichsen) A39.1
- Weber-Gubler G46.3
- Weber-Leyden G46.3
- Weber's G46.3
- Wegener's M31.30
  - with
    - kidney involvement M31.31
    - lung involvement M31.30
      - with kidney involvement M31.31
- Weingarten's (tropical eosinophilia) J82
- Weiss-Baker G90.09
- Werdnig-Hoffman G12.0
- Wermer's E31.21
- Werner's E34.8
- Wernicke-Korsakoff (nonalcoholic) F04
  - alcoholic F10.26
- Westphal-Strümpell E83.01
- West's — *see* Epilepsy, spasms
- wet
  - feet (maceration) (tropical) T69.0- ☑
  - lung, newborn P22.1
- whiplash S13.4 ☑
- whistling face Q87.0
- Wilkie's K55.1
- Wilkinson-Sneddon L13.1
- Willebrand (-Jürgens) D68.0
- Wilson's (hepatolenticular degeneration) E83.01
- Wiskott-Aldrich D82.0
- withdrawal — *see* Withdrawal, state
  - drug
    - infant of dependent mother P96.1
    - therapeutic use, newborn P96.2

Syndrome — *continued*
- Woakes' (ethmoiditis) J33.1
- Wright's (hyperabduction) I77.89
- X I20.9
- XXXX Q97.1
- XXXXX Q97.1
- XXXXY Q98.1
- XXY Q98.0
- yellow nail L60.5
- Zahorsky's B08.5
- Zellweger syndrome E71.510
- Zellweger-like syndrome E71.541

Synechia (anterior) (iris) (posterior) (pupil) (*see also* Adhesions, iris)
- intra-uterine (traumatic) N85.6

Synesthesia R20.8

Syngamiasis, syngamosis B83.3

Synodontia K00.2

Synorchidism, synorchism Q55.1

Synostosis (congenital) Q78.8
- astragalo-scaphoid Q74.2
- radioulnar Q74.0

Synovial sarcoma — *see* Neoplasm, connective tissue, malignant

Synovioma (malignant) (*see also* Neoplasm, connective tissue, malignant)
- benign — *see* Neoplasm, connective tissue, benign

Synoviosarcoma — *see* Neoplasm, connective tissue, malignant

Synovitis (*see also* Tenosynovitis)
- crepitant
  - hand M70.0- ☑
  - wrist M70.03- ☑
- gonococcal A54.49
- gouty — *see* Gout, idiopathic
- in (due to)
  - crystals M65.8- ☑
  - gonorrhea A54.49
  - syphilis (late) A52.78
  - use, overuse, pressure — *see* Disorder, soft tissue, due to use
- infective NEC — *see* Tenosynovitis, infective NEC
- specified NEC — *see* Tenosynovitis, specified type NEC
- syphilitic A52.78
  - congenital (early) A50.02
- toxic — *see* Synovitis, transient
- transient M67.3- ☑
  - ankle M67.37- ☑
  - elbow M67.32- ☑
  - foot joint M67.37- ☑
  - hand joint M67.34- ☑
  - hip M67.35- ☑
  - knee M67.36- ☑
  - multiple site M67.39
  - pelvic region M67.35- ☑
  - shoulder M67.31- ☑
  - specified joint NEC M67.38
  - wrist M67.33- ☑
- traumatic, current — *see* Sprain
- tuberculous — *see* Tuberculosis, synovitis
- villonodular (pigmented) M12.2- ☑
  - ankle M12.27- ☑
  - elbow M12.22- ☑
  - foot joint M12.27- ☑
  - hand joint M12.24- ☑
  - hip M12.25- ☑
  - knee M12.26- ☑
  - multiple site M12.29
  - pelvic region M12.25- ☑
  - shoulder M12.21- ☑
  - specified joint NEC M12.28
  - vertebrae M12.28
  - wrist M12.23- ☑

Syphilid A51.39
- congenital A50.06
- newborn A50.06
- tubercular (late) A52.79

Syphilis, syphilitic (acquired) A53.9
- abdomen (late) A52.79
- acoustic nerve A52.15
- adenopathy (secondary) A51.49
- adrenal (gland) (with cortical hypofunction) A52.79
- age under 2 years NOS (*see also* Syphilis, congenital, early)
  - acquired A51.9
- alopecia (secondary) A51.32
- anemia (late) A52.79 [D63.8]

Syphilis, syphilitic — *continued*
- aneurysm (aorta) (ruptured) A52.01
  - central nervous system A52.05
  - congenital A50.54 [I79.0]
- anus (late) A52.74
  - primary A51.1
  - secondary A51.39
- aorta (arch) (abdominal) (thoracic) A52.02
  - aneurysm A52.01
- aortic (insufficiency) (regurgitation) (stenosis) A52.03
  - aneurysm A52.01
- arachnoid (adhesive) (cerebral) (spinal) A52.13
- asymptomatic — *see* Syphilis, latent
- ataxia (locomotor) A52.11
- atrophoderma maculatum A51.39
- auricular fibrillation A52.06
- bladder (late) A52.76
- bone A52.77
  - secondary A51.46
- brain A52.17
- breast (late) A52.79
- bronchus (late) A52.72
- bubo (primary) A51.0
- bulbar palsy A52.19
- bursa (late) A52.78
- cardiac decompensation A52.06
- cardiovascular A52.00
- central nervous system (late) (recurrent) (relapse) (tertiary) A52.3
  - with
    - ataxia A52.11
    - general paralysis A52.17
      - juvenile A50.45
    - paresis (general) A52.17
      - juvenile A50.45
    - tabes (dorsalis) A52.11
      - juvenile A50.45
    - taboparesis A52.17
      - juvenile A50.45
  - aneurysm A52.05
  - congenital A50.40
    - juvenile A50.40
  - remission in (sustained) A52.3
  - serology doubtful, negative, or positive A52.3
  - specified nature or site NEC A52.19
  - vascular A52.05
- cerebral A52.17
  - meningovascular A52.13
  - nerves (multiple palsies) A52.15
  - sclerosis A52.17
  - thrombosis A52.05
- cerebrospinal (tabetic type) A52.12
- cerebrovascular A52.05
- cervix (late) A52.76
- chancre (multiple) A51.0
  - extragenital A51.2
  - Rollet's A51.0
- Charcot's joint A52.16
- chorioretinitis A51.43
  - congenital A50.01
  - late A52.71
  - prenatal A50.01
- choroiditis — *see* Syphilitic chorioretinitis
- choroidoretinitis — *see* Syphilitic chorioretinitis
- ciliary body (secondary) A51.43
  - late A52.71
- colon A52.74
- combined spinal sclerosis A52.11
- condyloma (latum) A51.31
- congenital A50.9
  - with
    - paresis (general) A50.45
    - tabes (dorsalis) A50.45
    - taboparesis A50.45
  - early, or less than 2 years after birth NEC A50.2
    - with manifestations — *see* Syphilis, congenital, early, symptomatic
    - latent (without manifestations) A50.1
      - negative spinal fluid test A50.1
      - serology positive A50.1
    - symptomatic A50.09
      - cutaneous A50.06
      - mucocutaneous A50.07
      - oculopathy A50.01
      - osteochondropathy A50.02
      - pharyngitis A50.03
      - pneumonia A50.04
      - rhinitis A50.05

Syphilis, syphilitic — *continued*
  congenital — *continued*
    early, or less than 2 years after birth — *continued*
      symptomatic — *continued*
        visceral A50.08
      chorioretinitis, choroiditis A50.01 [H32]
      interstitial keratitis A50.31
      juvenile neurosyphilis A50.45
      late, or 2 years or more after birth NEC A50.7
        chorioretinitis, choroiditis A50.32
        interstitial keratitis A50.31
        juvenile neurosyphilis A50.45
        latent (without manifestations) A50.6
          negative spinal fluid test A50.6
          serology positive A50.6
        symptomatic or with manifestations NEC A50.59
          arthropathy A50.55
          cardiovascular A50.54
          Clutton's joints A50.51
          Hutchinson's teeth A50.52
          Hutchinson's triad A50.53
          osteochondropathy A50.56
          saddle nose A50.57
  conjugal A53.9
    tabes A52.11
  conjunctiva (late) A52.71
  contact Z20.2
  cord bladder A52.19
  cornea, late A52.71
  coronary (artery) (sclerosis) A52.06
  coryza, congenital A50.05
  cranial nerve A52.15
    multiple palsies A52.15
  cutaneous — *see* Syphilis, skin
  dacryocystitis (late) A52.71
  degeneration, spinal cord A52.12
  dementia paralytica A52.17
    juvenilis A50.45
  destruction of bone A52.77
  dilatation, aorta A52.01
  due to blood transfusion A53.9
  dura mater A52.13
  ear A52.79
    inner A52.79
      nerve (eighth) A52.15
      neurorecurrence A52.15
  early A51.9
    cardiovascular A52.00
    central nervous system A52.3
    latent (without manifestations) (less than 2 years after infection) A51.5
      negative spinal fluid test A51.5
      serological relapse after treatment A51.5
      serology positive A51.5
    relapse (treated, untreated) A51.9
    skin A51.39
    symptomatic A51.9
      extragenital chancre A51.2
      primary, except extragenital chancre A51.0
      secondary (*see also* Syphilis, secondary) A51.39
        relapse (treated, untreated) A51.49
    ulcer A51.39
  eighth nerve (neuritis) A52.15
  endemic A65
  endocarditis A52.03
    aortic A52.03
    pulmonary A52.03
  epididymis (late) A52.76
  epiglottis (late) A52.73
  epiphysitis (congenital) (early) A50.02
  episcleritis (late) A52.71
  esophagus A52.79
  eustachian tube A52.73
  exposure to Z20.2
  eye A52.71
  eyelid (late) (with gumma) A52.71
  fallopian tube (late) A52.76
  fracture A52.77
  gallbladder (late) A52.74
  gastric (polyposis) (late) A52.74
  general A53.9
    paralysis A52.17
      juvenile A50.45
  genital (primary) A51.0
  glaucoma A52.71
  gumma NEC A52.79

Syphilis, syphilitic — *continued*
  gumma — *continued*
    cardiovascular system A52.00
    central nervous system A52.3
    congenital A50.59
  heart (block) (decompensation) (disease) (failure) A52.06 [I52]
    valve NEC A52.03
  hemianesthesia A52.19
  hemianopsia A52.71
  hemiparesis A52.17
  hemiplegia A52.17
  hepatic artery A52.09
  hepatis A52.74
  hepatomegaly, congenital A50.08
  hereditaria tarda — *see* Syphilis, congenital, late
  hereditary — *see* Syphilis, congenital
  Hutchinson's teeth A50.52
  hyalitis A52.71
  inactive — *see* Syphilis, latent
  infantum — *see* Syphilis, congenital
  inherited — *see* Syphilis, congenital
  internal ear A52.79
  intestine (late) A52.74
  iris, iritis (secondary) A51.43
    late A52.71
  joint (late) A52.77
  keratitis (congenital) (interstitial) (late) A50.31
  kidney A52.75
  lacrimal passages (late) A52.71
  larynx (late) A52.73
  late A52.9
    cardiovascular A52.00
    central nervous system A52.3
    kidney A52.75
    latent or 2 years or more after infection (without manifestations) A52.8
      negative spinal fluid test A52.8
      serology positive A52.8
    paresis A52.17
    specified site NEC A52.79
    symptomatic or with manifestations A52.79
    tabes A52.11
  latent A53.0
    with signs or symptoms — *code by* site and stage under Syphilis
    early, or less than 2 years after infection A51.5
    central nervous system A52.2
    date of infection unspecified A53.0
    follow-up of latent syphilis A53.0
      date of infection unspecified A53.0
      late, or 2 years or more after infection A52.8
    late, or 2 years or more after infection A52.8
    positive serology (only finding) A53.0
      early, or less than 2 years after infection A51.5
      date of infection unspecified A53.0
      late, or 2 years or more after infection A52.8
  lens (late) A52.71
  leukoderma A51.39
    late A52.79
  lienitis A52.79
  lip A51.39
    chancre (primary) A51.2
    late A52.79
  Lissauer's paralysis A52.17
  liver A52.74
  locomotor ataxia A52.11
  lung A52.72
  lymph gland (early) (secondary) A51.49
    late A52.79
  lymphadenitis (secondary) A51.49
  macular atrophy of skin A51.39
    striated A52.79
  mediastinum (late) A52.73
  meninges (adhesive) (brain) (spinal cord) A52.13
  meningitis A52.13
    acute (secondary) A51.41
    congenital A50.41
  meningoencephalitis A52.14
  meningovascular A52.13
    congenital A50.41
  mesarteritis A52.09
    brain A52.04
  middle ear A52.77
  mitral stenosis A52.03
  monoplegia A52.17
  mouth (secondary) A51.39
    late A52.79

Syphilis, syphilitic — *continued*
  mucocutaneous (secondary) A51.39
    late A52.79
  mucous
    membrane (secondary) A51.39
      late A52.79
    patches A51.39
      congenital A50.07
  mulberry molars A50.52
  muscle A52.78
  myocardium A52.06
  nasal sinus (late) A52.73
  neonatorum — *see* Syphilis, congenital
  nephrotic syndrome (secondary) A51.44
  nerve palsy (any cranial nerve) A52.15
    multiple A52.15
  nervous system, central A52.3
  neuritis A52.15
    acoustic A52.15
  neurorecidive of retina A52.19
  neuroretinitis A52.19
  newborn — *see* Syphilis, congenital
  nodular superficial (late) A52.79
  nonvenereal A65
  nose (late) A52.73
    saddle back deformity A50.57
  occlusive arterial disease A52.09
  oculopathy A52.71
  ophthalmic (late) A52.71
  optic nerve (atrophy) (neuritis) (papilla) A52.15
  orbit (late) A52.71
  organic A53.9
  osseous (late) A52.77
  osteochondritis (congenital) (early) A50.02 [M90.80]
  osteoporosis A52.77
  ovary (late) A52.76
  oviduct (late) A52.76
  palate (late) A52.79
  pancreas (late) A52.74
  paralysis A52.17
    general A52.17
      juvenile A50.45
  paresis (general) A52.17
    juvenile A50.45
  paresthesia A52.19
  Parkinson's disease or syndrome A52.19
  paroxysmal tachycardia A52.06
  pemphigus (congenital) A50.06
  penis (chancre) A51.0
    late A52.76
  pericardium A52.06
  perichondritis, larynx (late) A52.73
  periosteum (late) A52.77
    congenital (early) A50.02 [M90.80]
    early (secondary) A51.46
  peripheral nerve A52.79
  petrous bone (late) A52.77
  pharynx A52.73
    secondary A51.39
  pituitary (gland) A52.79
  pleura (late) A52.73
  pneumonia, white A50.04
  pontine lesion A52.17
  portal vein A52.09
  primary A51.0
    anal A51.1
    and secondary — *see* Syphilis, secondary
    central nervous system A52.3
    extragenital chancre NEC A51.2
    fingers A51.2
    genital A51.0
    lip A51.2
    specified site NEC A51.2
    tonsils A51.2
  prostate (late) A52.76
  ptosis (eyelid) A52.71
  pulmonary (late) A52.72
    artery A52.09
  pyelonephritis (late) A52.75
  recently acquired, symptomatic A51.9
  rectum (late) A52.74
  respiratory tract (late) A52.73
  retina, late A52.71
  retrobulbar neuritis A52.15
  salpingitis A52.76
  sclera (late) A52.71
  sclerosis
    cerebral A52.17

☑ Additional Character Required — Refer to the Tabular List for Character Selection   ▽ Subterms under main terms may continue to next column or page

Syphilis, syphilitic — *continued*
  sclerosis — *continued*
    coronary A52.06
    multiple A52.11
  scotoma (central) A52.71
  scrotum (late) A52.76
  secondary (and primary) A51.49
    adenopathy A51.49
    anus A51.39
    bone A51.46
    chorioretinitis, choroiditis A51.43
    hepatitis A51.45
    liver A51.45
    lymphadenitis A51.49
    meningitis (acute) A51.41
    mouth A51.39
    mucous membranes A51.39
    periosteum, periostitis A51.46
    pharynx A51.39
    relapse (treated, untreated) A51.49
    skin A51.39
    specified form NEC A51.49
    tonsil A51.39
    ulcer A51.39
    viscera NEC A51.49
    vulva A51.39
  seminal vesicle (late) A52.76
  seronegative with signs or symptoms — *code by* site and stage under Syphilis
  seropositive
    with signs or symptoms — *code by* site and stage under Syphilis
    follow-up of latent syphilis — *see* Syphilis, latent
    only finding — *see* Syphilis, latent
  seventh nerve (paralysis) A52.15
  sinus, sinusitis (late) A52.73
  skeletal system A52.77
  skin (with ulceration) (early) (secondary) A51.39
    late or tertiary A52.79
  small intestine A52.74
  spastic spinal paralysis A52.17
  spermatic cord (late) A52.76
  spinal (cord) A52.12

Syphilis, syphilitic — *continued*
  spleen A52.79
  splenomegaly A52.79
  spondylitis A52.77
  staphyloma A52.71
  stigmata (congenital) A50.59
  stomach A52.74
  synovium A52.78
  tabes dorsalis (late) A52.11
    juvenile A50.45
  tabetic type A52.11
    juvenile A50.45
  taboparesis A52.17
    juvenile A50.45
  tachycardia A52.06
  tendon (late) A52.78
  tertiary A52.9
    with symptoms NEC A52.79
    cardiovascular A52.00
    central nervous system A52.3
    multiple NEC A52.79
    specified site NEC A52.79
  testis A52.76
  thorax A52.73
  throat A52.73
  thymus (gland) (late) A52.79
  thyroid (late) A52.79
  tongue (late) A52.79
  tonsil (lingual) (late) A52.73
    primary A51.2
    secondary A51.39
  trachea (late) A52.73
  tunica vaginalis (late) A52.76
  ulcer (any site) (early) (secondary) A51.39
    late A52.79
    perforating A52.79
      foot A52.11
  urethra (late) A52.76
  urogenital (late) A52.76
  uterus (late) A52.76
  uveal tract (secondary) A51.43
    late A52.71
  uveitis (secondary) A51.43

Syphilis, syphilitic — *continued*
  uveitis — *continued*
    late A52.71
  uvula (late) (perforated) A52.79
  vagina A51.0
    late A52.76
  valvulitis NEC A52.03
  vascular A52.00
    brain (cerebral) A52.05
  ventriculi A52.74
  vesicae urinariae (late) A52.76
  viscera (abdominal) (late) A52.74
    secondary A51.49
  vitreous (opacities) (late) A52.71
    hemorrhage A52.71
  vulva A51.0
    late A52.76
    secondary A51.39
Syphiloma A52.79
  cardiovascular system A52.00
  central nervous system A52.3
  circulatory system A52.00
  congenital A50.59
Syphilophobia F45.29
Syringadenoma (*see also* Neoplasm, skin, benign)
  papillary — *see* Neoplasm, skin, benign
Syringobulbia G95.0
Syringocystadenoma — *see* Neoplasm, skin, benign
  papillary — *see* Neoplasm, skin, benign
Syringoma (*see also* Neoplasm, skin, benign)
  chondroid — *see* Neoplasm, skin, benign
Syringomyelia G95.0
Syringomyelitis — *see* Encephalitis
Syringomyelocele — *see* Spina bifida
Syringopontia G95.0
System, systemic (*see also* condition)
  disease, combined — *see* Degeneration, combined
  inflammatory response syndrome (SIRS) of non-infectious origin (without organ dysfunction) R65.10
    with acute organ dysfunction R65.11
  lupus erythematosus M32.9
    inhibitor present D68.62

T

Tabacism, tabacosis, tabagism (*see also* Poisoning, tobacco)
  meaning dependence (without remission) F17.200
    with
      disorder F17.299
        remission F17.211
        specified disorder NEC F17.298
        withdrawal F17.203
Tabardillo A75.9
  flea-borne A75.2
  louse-borne A75.0
Tabes, tabetic A52.10
  with
    central nervous system syphilis A52.10
    Charcot's joint A52.16
    cord bladder A52.19
    crisis, viscera (any) A52.19
    paralysis, general A52.17
    paresis (general) A52.17
    perforating ulcer (foot) A52.19
  arthropathy (Charcot) A52.16
  bladder A52.19
  bone A52.11
  cerebrospinal A52.12
  congenital A50.45
  conjugal A52.10
  dorsalis A52.11
    juvenile A50.49
  juvenile A50.49
  latent A52.19
  mesenterica A18.39
  paralysis, insane, general A52.17
  spasmodic A52.17
  syphilis (cerebrospinal) A52.12
Taboparalysis A52.17
Taboparesis (remission) A52.17
  juvenile A50.45
TAC (trigeminal autonomic cephalgia) **NEC** G44.099
  intractable G44.091
  not intractable G44.099
Tache noir S60.22- ☑
Tachyalimentation K91.2
Tachyarrhythmia, tachyrhythmia — *see* Tachycardia
Tachycardia R00.0
  atrial (paroxysmal) I47.1
  auricular I47.1
  AV nodal re-entry (re-entrant) I47.1
  junctional (paroxysmal) I47.1
  newborn P29.11
  nodal (paroxysmal) I47.1
  non-paroxysmal AV nodal I45.89
  paroxysmal (sustained) (nonsustained) I47.9
    with sinus bradycardia I49.5
    atrial (PAT) I47.1
    atrioventricular (AV) (re-entrant) I47.1
      psychogenic F54
    junctional I47.1
      ectopic I47.1
    nodal I47.1
    psychogenic (atrial) (supraventricular) (ventricular) F54
    supraventricular (sustained) I47.1
      psychogenic F54
    ventricular I47.2
      psychogenic F54
  psychogenic F45.8
  sick sinus I49.5
  sinoauricular NOS R00.0
    paroxysmal I47.1
  sinus [sinusal] NOS R00.0
    paroxysmal I47.1
  supraventricular I47.1
  ventricular (paroxysmal) (sustained) I47.2
    psychogenic F54
Tachygastria K31.89
Tachypnea R06.82
  hysterical F45.8
  newborn (idiopathic) (transitory) P22.1
  psychogenic F45.8
  transitory, of newborn P22.1

TACO (transfusion associated circulatory overload) E87.71
Taenia (infection) (infestation) B68.9
  diminuta B71.0
  echinococcal infestation B67.90
  mediocanellata B68.1
  nana B71.0
  saginata B68.1
  solium (intestinal form) B68.0
    larval form — *see* Cysticercosis
Taeniasis (intestine) — *see* Taenia
Tag (hypertrophied skin) (infected) L91.8
  adenoid J35.8
  anus K64.4
  hemorrhoidal K64.4
  hymen N89.8
  perineal N90.89
  preauricular Q17.0
  sentinel K64.4
  skin L91.8
    accessory (congenital) Q82.8
    anus K64.4
    congenital Q82.8
    preauricular Q17.0
  tonsil J35.8
  urethra, urethral N36.8
  vulva N90.89
Tahyna fever B33.8
Takahara's disease E80.3
Takayasu's disease or syndrome M31.4
Talcosis (pulmonary) J62.0
Talipes (congenital) Q66.89
  acquired, planus — *see* Deformity, limb, flat foot
  asymmetric Q66.89
  calcaneovalgus Q66.4
  calcaneovarus Q66.1
  calcaneus Q66.89
  cavus Q66.7
  equinovalgus Q66.6
  equinovarus Q66.0
  equinus Q66.89
  percavus Q66.7
  planovalgus Q66.6
  planus (acquired) (any degree) (*see also* Deformity, limb, flat foot)
    congenital Q66.5- ☑
    due to rickets (sequelae) E64.3
  valgus Q66.6
  varus Q66.3
Tall stature, constitutional E34.4
Talma's disease M62.89
Talon noir S90.3- ☑
  hand S60.22- ☑
  heel S90.3- ☑
  toe S90.1- ☑
Tamponade, heart I31.4
Tanapox (virus disease) B08.71
Tangier disease E78.6
Tantrum, child problem F91.8
Tapeworm (infection) (infestation) — *see* Infestation, tapeworm
Tapia's syndrome G52.7
TAR (thrombocytopenia with absent radius) **syndrome** Q87.2
Tarral-Besnier disease L44.0
Tarsal tunnel syndrome — *see* Syndrome, tarsal tunnel
Tarsalgia — *see* Pain, limb, lower
Tarsitis (eyelid) H01.8
  syphilitic A52.71
  tuberculous A18.4
Tartar (teeth) (dental calculus) K03.6
Tattoo (mark) L81.8
Tauri's disease E74.09
Taurodontism K00.2
Taussig-Bing syndrome Q20.1
Taybi's syndrome Q87.2
Tay-Sachs amaurotic familial idiocy or disease E75.02
TBI (traumatic brain injury) — *see* category S06 ☑
Teacher's node or nodule J38.2
Tear, torn (traumatic) (*see also* Laceration)
  with abortion — *see* Abortion
  annular fibrosis M51.35
  anus, anal (sphincter) S31.831 ☑

Tear, torn — *continued*
  anus, anal — *continued*
    complicating delivery
      with third degree perineal laceration O70.2
        with mucosa O70.3
      without third degree perineal laceration O70.4
    nontraumatic (healed) (old) K62.81
  articular cartilage, old — *see* Derangement, joint, articular cartilage, by site
  bladder
    with ectopic or molar pregnancy O08.6
    following ectopic or molar pregnancy O08.6
    obstetrical O71.5
    traumatic — *see* Injury, bladder
  bowel
    with ectopic or molar pregnancy O08.6
    following ectopic or molar pregnancy O08.6
    obstetrical trauma O71.5
  broad ligament
    with ectopic or molar pregnancy O08.6
    following ectopic or molar pregnancy O08.6
    obstetrical trauma O71.6
  bucket handle (knee) (meniscus) — *see* Tear, meniscus
  capsule, joint — *see* Sprain
  cartilage (*see also* Sprain)
    articular, old — *see* Derangement, joint, articular cartilage, by site
  cervix
    with ectopic or molar pregnancy O08.6
    following ectopic or molar pregnancy O08.6
    obstetrical trauma (current) O71.3
    old N88.1
    traumatic — *see* Injury, uterus
  dural G97.41
    nontraumatic G96.11
  internal organ — *see* Injury, by site
  knee cartilage
    articular (current) S83.3- ☑
    old — *see* Derangement, knee, meniscus, due to old tear
  ligament — *see* Sprain
  meniscus (knee) (current injury) S83.209 ☑
    bucket-handle S83.20- ☑
    lateral
      bucket-handle S83.25- ☑
      complex S83.27- ☑
      peripheral S83.26- ☑
      specified type NEC S83.28- ☑
    medial
      bucket-handle S83.21- ☑
      complex S83.23- ☑
      peripheral S83.22- ☑
      specified type NEC S83.24- ☑
    old — *see* Derangement, knee, meniscus, due to old tear
    site other than knee — *code as* Sprain
    specified type NEC S83.20- ☑
  muscle — *see* Strain
  pelvic
    floor, complicating delivery O70.1
    organ NEC, obstetrical trauma O71.5
      with ectopic or molar pregnancy O08.6
      following ectopic or molar pregnancy O08.6
  perineal, secondary O90.1
  periurethral tissue, obstetrical trauma O71.82
    with ectopic or molar pregnancy O08.6
    following ectopic or molar pregnancy O08.6
  rectovaginal septum — *see* Laceration, vagina
  retina, retinal (without detachment) (horseshoe) (*see also* Break, retina, horseshoe)
    with detachment — *see* Detachment, retina, with retinal, break
  rotator cuff (nontraumatic) M75.10- ☑
    complete M75.12- ☑
    incomplete M75.11- ☑
    traumatic S46.01- ☑
      capsule S43.42- ☑
  semilunar cartilage, knee — *see* Tear, meniscus
  supraspinatus (complete) (incomplete) (nontraumatic) (*see also* Tear, rotator cuff) M75.10- ☑
  tendon — *see* Strain
  tentorial, at birth P10.4

Tear, torn — *continued*
umbilical cord
complicating delivery O69.89 ☑
urethra
with ectopic or molar pregnancy O08.6
following ectopic or molar pregnancy O08.6
obstetrical trauma O71.5
uterus — *see* Injury, uterus
vagina — *see* Laceration, vagina
vessel, from catheter — *see* Puncture, accidental
complicating surgery
vulva, complicating delivery O70.0
Tear-stone — *see* Dacryolith
Teeth (*see also* condition)
grinding
psychogenic F45.8
sleep related G47.63
Teething (syndrome) K00.7
Telangiectasia, telangiectasis (verrucous) I78.1
ataxic (cerebellar) (Louis-Bar) G11.3
familial I78.0
hemorrhagic, hereditary (congenital) (senile) I78.0
hereditary, hemorrhagic (congenital) (senile) I78.0
juxtafoveal H35.07- ☑
macular H35.07- ☑
parafoveal H35.07- ☑
retinal (idiopathic) (juxtafoveal) (macular) (parafoveal) H35.07- ☑
spider I78.1
Telephone scatologia F65.89
Telescoped bowel or intestine K56.1
congenital Q43.8
Temperature
body, high (of unknown origin) R50.9
cold, trauma from T69.9
newborn P80.0
specified effect NEC T69.8 ☑
Temple — *see* condition
Temporal — *see* condition
Temporomandibular joint pain-dysfunction syndrome M26.62
Temporosphenoidal — *see* condition
Tendency
bleeding — *see* Defect, coagulation
suicide
meaning personal history of attempted suicide Z91.5
meaning suicidal ideation — *see* Ideation, suicidal
to fall R29.6
Tenderness, abdominal R10.819
epigastric R10.816
generalized R10.817
left lower quadrant R10.814
left upper quadrant R10.812
periumbilic R10.815
rebound R10.829
epigastric R10.826
generalized R10.827
left lower quadrant R10.824
left upper quadrant R10.822
periumbilic R10.825
right lower quadrant R10.823
right upper quadrant R10.821
right lower quadrant R10.813
right upper quadrant R10.811
Tendinitis, tendonitis (*see also* Enthesopathy)
Achilles M76.6- ☑
adhesive — *see* Tenosynovitis, specified type NEC
shoulder — *see* Capsulitis, adhesive
bicipital M75.2- ☑
calcific M65.2- ☑
ankle M65.27- ☑
foot M65.27- ☑
forearm M65.23- ☑
hand M65.24- ☑
lower leg M65.26- ☑
multiple sites M65.29
pelvic region M65.25- ☑
shoulder M75.3- ☑
specified site NEC M65.28
thigh M65.25- ☑
upper arm M65.22- ☑
due to use, overuse, pressure (*see also* Disorder, soft tissue, due to use)
specified NEC — *see* Disorder, soft tissue, due to use, specified NEC
gluteal M76.0- ☑

Tendinitis, tendonitis — *continued*
patellar M76.5- ☑
peroneal M76.7- ☑
psoas M76.1- ☑
tibial (posterior) M76.82- ☑
anterior M76.81- ☑
trochanteric — *see* Bursitis, hip, trochanteric
Tendon — *see* condition
Tendosynovitis — *see* Tenosynovitis
Tenesmus (rectal) R19.8
vesical R30.1
Tennis elbow — *see* Epicondylitis, lateral
Tenonitis (*see also* Tenosynovitis)
eye (capsule) H05.04- ☑
Tenontosynovitis — *see* Tenosynovitis
Tenontothecitis — *see* Tenosynovitis
Tenophyte — *see* Disorder, synovium, specified type NEC
Tenosynovitis (*see also* Synovitis) M65.9
adhesive — *see* Tenosynovitis, specified type NEC
shoulder — *see* Capsulitis, adhesive
bicipital (calcifying) — *see* Tendinitis, bicipital
gonococcal A54.49
in (due to)
crystals M65.8- ☑
gonorrhea A54.49
syphilis (late) A52.78
use, overuse, pressure (*see also* Disorder, soft tissue, due to use)
specified NEC — *see* Disorder, soft tissue, due to use, specified NEC
infective NEC M65.1- ☑
ankle M65.17- ☑
foot M65.17- ☑
forearm M65.13- ☑
hand M65.14- ☑
lower leg M65.16- ☑
multiple sites M65.19
pelvic region M65.15- ☑
shoulder region M65.11- ☑
specified site NEC M65.18
thigh M65.15- ☑
upper arm M65.12- ☑
radial styloid M65.4
shoulder region M65.81- ☑
adhesive — *see* Capsulitis, adhesive
specified type NEC M65.88
ankle M65.87- ☑
foot M65.87- ☑
forearm M65.83- ☑
hand M65.84- ☑
lower leg M65.86- ☑
multiple sites M65.89
pelvic region M65.85- ☑
shoulder region M65.81- ☑
specified site NEC M65.88
thigh M65.85- ☑
upper arm M65.82- ☑
tuberculous — *see* Tuberculosis, tenosynovitis
Tenovaginitis — *see* Tenosynovitis
Tension
arterial, high (*see also* Hypertension)
without diagnosis of hypertension R03.0
headache G44.209
intractable G44.201
not intractable G44.209
nervous R45.0
pneumothorax J93.0
premenstrual N94.3
state (mental) F48.9
Tentorium — *see* condition
Teratencephalus Q89.8
Teratism Q89.7
Teratoblastoma (malignant) — *see* Neoplasm, malignant, by site
Teratocarcinoma (*see also* Neoplasm, malignant, by site)
liver C22.7
Teratoma (solid) (*see also* Neoplasm, uncertain behavior, by site)
with embryonal carcinoma, mixed — *see* Neoplasm, malignant, by site
with malignant transformation — *see* Neoplasm, malignant, by site
adult (cystic) — *see* Neoplasm, benign, by site
benign — *see* Neoplasm, benign, by site

Teratoma — *continued*
combined with choriocarcinoma — *see* Neoplasm, malignant, by site
cystic (adult) — *see* Neoplasm, benign, by site
differentiated — *see* Neoplasm, benign, by site
embryonal (*see also* Neoplasm, malignant, by site)
liver C22.7
immature — *see* Neoplasm, malignant, by site
liver C22.7
adult, benign, cystic, differentiated type or mature D13.4
malignant (*see also* Neoplasm, malignant, by site)
anaplastic — *see* Neoplasm, malignant, by site
intermediate — *see* Neoplasm, malignant, by site
specified site — *see* Neoplasm, malignant, by site
unspecified site C62.90
undifferentiated — *see* Neoplasm, malignant, by site
mature — *see* Neoplasm, uncertain behavior, by site
malignant — *see* Neoplasm, by site, malignant, by site
ovary D27.- ☑
embryonal, immature or malignant C56- ☑
solid — *see* Neoplasm, uncertain behavior, by site
testis C62.9- ☑
adult, benign, cystic, differentiated type or mature D29.2- ☑
scrotal C62.1- ☑
undescended C62.0- ☑
Termination
anomalous (*see also* Malposition, congenital)
right pulmonary vein Q26.3
pregnancy, elective Z33.2
Ternidens diminutus infestation B81.8
Ternidensiasis B81.8
Terror(s) night (child) F51.4
Terrorism, victim of Z65.4
Terry's syndrome H44.2- ☑
Tertiary — *see* condition
Test, tests, testing (for)
adequacy (for dialysis)
hemodialysis Z49.31
peritoneal Z49.32
blood pressure Z01.30
abnormal reading — *see* Blood, pressure
blood typing Z01.83
Rh typing Z01.83
blood-alcohol Z04.8
positive — *see* Findings, abnormal, in blood
blood-drug Z04.8
positive — *see* Findings, abnormal, in blood
cardiac pulse generator (battery) Z45.010
fertility Z31.41
genetic
disease carrier status for procreative management
female Z31.430
male Z31.440
male partner of patient with recurrent pregnancy loss Z31.441
procreative management NEC
female Z31.438
male Z31.448
hearing Z01.10
with abnormal findings NEC Z01.118
HIV (human immunodeficiency virus)
nonconclusive (in infants) R75
positive Z21
seropositive Z21
immunity status Z01.84
intelligence NEC Z01.89
laboratory (as part of a general medical examination) Z00.00
with abnormal finding Z00.01
for medicolegal reason NEC Z04.8
male partner of patient with recurrent pregnancy loss Z31.441
Mantoux (for tuberculosis) Z11.1
abnormal result R76.11
pregnancy, positive first pregnancy — *see* Pregnancy, normal, first
procreative Z31.49
fertility Z31.41
skin, diagnostic
allergy Z01.82
special screening examination — *see* Screening, by name of disease

Test, tests, testing — *continued*
  skin, diagnostic — *continued*
    Mantoux Z11.1
    tuberculin Z11.1
  specified NEC Z01.89
  tuberculin Z11.1
    abnormal result R76.11
  vision Z01.00
    with abnormal findings Z01.01
  Wassermann Z11.3
    positive — *see* Serology for syphilis, positive
Testicle, testicular, testis (*see also* condition)
  feminization syndrome (*see also* Syndrome, androgen insensitivity) E34.51
  migrans Q55.29
Tetanus, tetanic (cephalic) (convulsions) A35
  with
    abortion A34
    ectopic or molar pregnancy O08.0
  following ectopic or molar pregnancy O08.0
  inoculation reaction (due to serum) — *see* Complications, vaccination
  neonatorum A33
  obstetrical A34
  puerperal, postpartum, childbirth A34
Tetany (due to) R29.0
  alkalosis E87.3
  associated with rickets E55.0
  convulsions R29.0
    hysterical F44.5
  functional (hysterical) F44.5
  hyperkinetic R29.0
    hysterical F44.5
  hyperpnea R06.4
    hysterical F44.5
    psychogenic F45.8
  hyperventilation (*see also* Hyperventilation) R06.4
    hysterical F44.5
  neonatal (without calcium or magnesium deficiency) P71.3
  parathyroid (gland) E20.9
  parathyroprival E89.2
  post- (para)thyroidectomy E89.2
  postoperative E89.2
  pseudotetany R29.0
  psychogenic (conversion reaction) F44.5
Tetralogy of Fallot Q21.3
Tetraplegia (chronic) (*see also* Quadriplegia) G82.50
Thailand hemorrhagic fever A91
Thalassanemia — *see* Thalassemia
Thalassemia (anemia) (disease) D56.9
  with other hemoglobinopathy D56.8
  alpha (major) (severe) (triple gene defect) D56.0
    minor D56.3
    silent carrier D56.3
    trait D56.3
  beta (severe) D56.1
    homozygous D56.1
    major D56.1
    minor D56.3
    trait D56.3
  delta-beta (homozygous) D56.2
    minor D56.3
    trait D56.3
  dominant D56.8
  hemoglobin
    C D56.8
    E-beta D56.5
  intermedia D56.1
  major D56.1
  minor D56.3
  mixed D56.8
  sickle-cell — *see* Disease, sickle-cell, thalassemia
  specified type NEC D56.8
  trait D56.3
  variants D56.8
Thanatophoric dwarfism or short stature Q77.1
Thaysen-Gee disease (nontropical sprue) K90.0
Thaysen's disease K90.0
Thecoma D27- ☑
  luteinized D27- ☑
  malignant C56- ☑
Thelarche, premature E30.8
Thelaziasis B83.8
Thelitis N61
  puerperal, postpartum or gestational — *see* Infection, nipple
Therapeutic — *see* condition

Therapy
  drug, long-term (current) (prophylactic)
    agents affecting estrogen receptors and estrogen levels NEC Z79.818
    anastrozole (Arimidex) Z79.811
    antibiotics Z79.2
      short-term use — *omit code*
    anticoagulants Z79.01
    anti-inflammatory Z79.1
    antiplatelet Z79.02
    antithrombotics Z79.02
    aromatase inhibitors Z79.811
    aspirin Z79.82
    birth control pill or patch Z79.3
    bisphosphonates Z79.83
    contraceptive, oral Z79.3
    drug, specified NEC Z79.899
    estrogen receptor downregulators Z79.818
    Evista Z79.810
    exemestane (Aromasin) Z79.811
    Fareston Z79.810
    fulvestrant (Faslodex) Z79.818
    gonadotropin-releasing hormone (GnRH) agonist Z79.818
    goserelin acetate (Zoladex) Z79.818
    hormone replacement (postmenopausal) Z79.890
    insulin Z79.4
    letrozole (Femara) Z79.811
    leuprolide acetate (leuprorelin) (Lupron) Z79.818
    megestrol acetate (Megace) Z79.818
    methadone
      for pain management Z79.891
      maintenance therapy F11.20
    Nolvadex Z79.810
    opiate analgesic Z79.891
    oral contraceptive Z79.3
    raloxifene (Evista) Z79.810
    selective estrogen receptor modulators (SERMs) Z79.810
    short term — *omit code*
    steroids
      inhaled Z79.51
      systemic Z79.52
    tamoxifen (Nolvadex) Z79.810
    toremifene (Fareston) Z79.810
Thermic — *see* condition
Thermography (abnormal) (*see also* Abnormal, diagnostic imaging) R93.8
  breast R92.8
Thermoplegia T67.0 ☑
Thesaurismosis, glycogen — *see* Disease, glycogen storage
Thiamin deficiency E51.9
  specified NEC E51.8
Thiaminic deficiency with beriberi E51.11
Thibierge-Weissenbach syndrome — *see* Sclerosis, systemic
Thickening
  bone — *see* Hypertrophy, bone
  breast N64.59
  endometrium R93.8
  epidermal L85.9
    specified NEC L85.8
  hymen N89.6
  larynx J38.7
  nail L60.2
    congenital Q84.5
  periosteal — *see* Hypertrophy, bone
  pleura J92.9
    with asbestos J92.0
  skin R23.4
  subepiglottic J38.7
  tongue K14.8
  valve, heart — *see* Endocarditis
Thigh — *see* condition
Thinning vertebra — *see* Spondylopathy, specified NEC
Thirst, excessive R63.1
  due to deprivation of water T73.1 ☑
Thomsen disease G71.12
Thoracic (*see also* condition)
  kidney Q63.2
  outlet syndrome G54.0
Thoracogastroschisis (congenital) Q79.8
Thoracopagus Q89.4
Thorax — *see* condition
Thorn's syndrome N28.89
Thorson-Björck syndrome E34.0
Threadworm (infection) (infestation) B80

Threatened
  abortion O20.0
    with subsequent abortion O03.9
  job loss, anxiety concerning Z56.2
  labor (without delivery) O47.9
    after 37 completed weeks of gestation O47.1
    before 37 completed weeks of gestation O47.0- ☑
  loss of job, anxiety concerning Z56.2
  miscarriage O20.0
  unemployment, anxiety concerning Z56.2
Three-day fever A93.1
Threshers' lung J67.0
Thrix annulata (congenital) Q84.1
Throat — *see* condition
Thrombasthenia (Glanzmann) (hemorrhagic) (hereditary) D69.1
Thromboangiitis I73.1
  obliterans (general) I73.1
    cerebral I67.89
    vessels
      brain I67.89
      spinal cord I67.89
Thromboarteritis — *see* Arteritis
Thromboasthenia (Glanzmann) (hemorrhagic) (hereditary) D69.1
Thrombocytasthenia (Glanzmann) D69.1
Thrombocythemia (essential) (hemorrhagic) (idiopathic) (primary) D47.3
Thrombocytopathy (dystrophic) (granulopenic) D69.1
Thrombocytopenia, thrombocytopenic D69.6
  with absent radius (TAR) Q87.2
  congenital D69.42
  dilutional D69.59
  due to
    (massive) blood transfusion D69.59
    drugs D69.59
    extracorporeal circulation of blood D69.59
    platelet alloimmunization D69.59
  essential D69.3
  heparin induced (HIT) D75.82
  hereditary D69.42
  idiopathic D69.3
  neonatal, transitory P61.0
    due to
      exchange transfusion P61.0
      idiopathic maternal thrombocytopenia P61.0
      isoimmunization P61.0
  primary NEC D69.49
    idiopathic D69.3
  puerperal, postpartum O72.3
  secondary D69.59
  transient neonatal P61.0
Thrombocytosis, essential D47.3
  primary D47.3
Thromboembolism — *see* Embolism
Thrombopathy (Bernard-Soulier) D69.1
  constitutional D68.0
  Willebrand-Jurgens D68.0
Thrombopenia — *see* Thrombocytopenia
Thrombophilia D68.59
  primary NEC D68.59
  secondary NEC D68.69
  specified NEC D68.69
Thrombophlebitis I80.9
  antepartum O22.2- ☑
    deep O22.3- ☑
    superficial O22.2- ☑
  cavernous (venous) sinus G08
    complicating pregnancy O22.5- ☑
    nonpyogenic I67.6
  cerebral (sinus) (vein) G08
    nonpyogenic I67.6
    sequelae G09
  due to implanted device — *see* Complications, by site and type, specified NEC
  during or resulting from a procedure NEC T81.72 ☑
  femoral vein (superficial) I80.1- ☑
  femoropopliteal vein I80.0- ☑
  hepatic (vein) I80.8
  idiopathic, recurrent I82.1
  iliofemoral I80.1- ☑
  intracranial venous sinus (any) G08
    nonpyogenic I67.6
    sequelae G09
  intraspinal venous sinuses and veins G08
    nonpyogenic G95.19
  lateral (venous) sinus G08
    nonpyogenic I67.6

☑ **Additional Character Required** — Refer to the Tabular List for Character Selection   ▽ **Subterms under main terms may continue to next column or page**

Thrombophlebitis — *continued*
leg I80.299
  superficial I80.0- ☑
longitudinal (venous) sinus G08
  nonpyogenic I67.6
lower extremity I80.299
migrans, migrating I82.1
pelvic
  with ectopic or molar pregnancy O08.0
  following ectopic or molar pregnancy O08.0
  puerperal O87.1
popliteal vein — *see* Phlebitis, leg, deep, popliteal
portal (vein) K75.1
postoperative T81.72 ☑
pregnancy — *see* Thrombophlebitis, antepartum
puerperal, postpartum, childbirth O87.0
  deep O87.1
  pelvic O87.1
  septic O86.81
  superficial O87.0
saphenous (greater) (lesser) I80.0- ☑
sinus (intracranial) G08
  nonpyogenic I67.6
specified site NEC I80.8
tibial vein I80.23-

Thrombosis, thrombotic (bland) (multiple) (progressive)
  (silent) (vessel) I82.90
anal K64.5
antepartum — *see* Thrombophlebitis, antepartum
aorta, aortic I74.10
  abdominal I74.09
    saddle I74.01
  bifurcation I74.09
  saddle I74.01
  specified site NEC I74.19
  terminal I74.09
  thoracic I74.11
  valve — *see* Endocarditis, aortic
apoplexy I63.3 ☑
artery, arteries (postinfectional) I74.9
  auditory, internal — *see* Occlusion, artery, precerebral, specified NEC
  basilar — *see* Occlusion, artery, basilar
  carotid (common) (internal) — *see* Occlusion, artery, carotid
  cerebellar (anterior inferior) (posterior inferior) (superior) — *see* Occlusion, artery, cerebellar
  cerebral — *see* Occlusion, artery, cerebral
  choroidal (anterior) — *see* Occlusion, artery, cerebral, specified NEC
  communicating, posterior — *see* Occlusion, artery, cerebral, specified NEC
  coronary (*see also* Infarct, myocardium)
    not resulting in infarction I24.0
  hepatic I74.8
  hypophyseal — *see* Occlusion, artery, cerebral, specified NEC
  iliac I74.5
  limb I74.4
    lower I74.3
    upper I74.2
  meningeal, anterior or posterior — *see* Occlusion, artery, cerebral, specified NEC
  mesenteric (with gangrene) K55.0
  ophthalmic — *see* Occlusion, artery, retina
  pontine — *see* Occlusion, artery, cerebral, specified NEC
  precerebral — *see* Occlusion, artery, precerebral
  pulmonary (iatrogenic) — *see* Embolism, pulmonary
  renal N28.0
  retinal — *see* Occlusion, artery, retina
  spinal, anterior or posterior G95.11
  traumatic NEC T14.8
  vertebral — *see* Occlusion, artery, vertebral
atrium, auricular (*see also* Infarct, myocardium)
  following acute myocardial infarction (current complication) I23.6
  not resulting in infarction I24.0
basilar (artery) — *see* Occlusion, artery, basilar
brain (artery) (stem) (*see also* Occlusion, artery, cerebral)
  due to syphilis A52.05
  puerperal O99.43
  sinus — *see* Thrombosis, intracranial venous sinus
capillary I78.8

Thrombosis, thrombotic — *continued*
cardiac (*see also* Infarct, myocardium)
  not resulting in infarction I24.0
  valve — *see* Endocarditis
carotid (artery) (common) (internal) — *see* Occlusion, artery, carotid
cavernous (venous) sinus — *see* Thrombosis, intracranial venous sinus
cerebellar artery (anterior inferior) (posterior inferior) (superior) I66.3
cerebral (artery) — *see* Occlusion, artery, cerebral
cerebrovenous sinus (*see also* Thrombosis, intracranial venous sinus)
  puerperium O87.3
chronic I82.91
coronary (artery) (vein) (*see also* Infarct, myocardium)
  not resulting in infarction I24.0
corpus cavernosum N48.89
cortical I66.9
deep — *see* Embolism, vein, lower extremity
due to device, implant or graft (*see also* Complications, by site and type, specified NEC) T85.86 ☑
  arterial graft NEC T82.868 ☑
  breast (implant) T85.86 ☑
  catheter NEC T85.86 ☑
    dialysis (renal) T82.868 ☑
      intraperitoneal T85.86 ☑
    infusion NEC T82.868 ☑
      spinal (epidural) (subdural) T85.86 ☑
    urinary (indwelling) T83.86 ☑
  electronic (electrode) (pulse generator) (stimulator)
    bone T84.86 ☑
    cardiac T82.867 ☑
    nervous system (brain) (peripheral nerve) (spinal) T85.86 ☑
    urinary T83.86 ☑
  fixation, internal (orthopedic) NEC T84.86 ☑
  gastrointestinal (bile duct) (esophagus) T85.86 ☑
  genital NEC T83.86 ☑
  heart T82.867 ☑
  joint prosthesis T84.86 ☑
  ocular (corneal graft) (orbital implant) NEC T85.86 ☑
  orthopedic NEC T84.86 ☑
  specified NEC T85.86 ☑
  urinary NEC T83.86 ☑
  vascular NEC T82.868 ☑
  ventricular intracranial shunt T85.86 ☑
during the puerperium — *see* Thrombosis, puerperal
endocardial (*see also* Infarct, myocardium)
  not resulting in infarction I24.0
eye — *see* Occlusion, retina
genital organ
  female NEC N94.89
    pregnancy — *see* Thrombophlebitis, antepartum
  male N50.1
gestational — *see* Phlebopathy, gestational
heart (chamber) (*see also* Infarct, myocardium)
  not resulting in infarction I24.0
hepatic (vein) I82.0
  artery I74.8
history (of) Z86.718
intestine (with gangrene) K55.0
intracardiac NEC (apical) (atrial) (auricular) (ventricular) (old) I51.3
intracranial (arterial) I66.9
  venous sinus (any) G08
    nonpyogenic origin I67.6
    puerperium O87.3
intramural (*see also* Infarct, myocardium)
  not resulting in infarction I24.0
intraspinal venous sinuses and veins G08
  nonpyogenic G95.19
kidney (artery) N28.0
lateral (venous) sinus — *see* Thrombosis, intracranial venous sinus
leg — *see* Thrombosis, vein, lower extremity
  arterial I74.3
liver (venous) I82.0
  artery I74.8
  portal vein I81
longitudinal (venous) sinus — *see* Thrombosis, intracranial venous sinus
lower limb — *see* Thrombosis, vein, lower extremity
lung (iatrogenic) (postoperative) — *see* Embolism, pulmonary

Thrombosis, thrombotic — *continued*
meninges (brain) (arterial) I66.8
mesenteric (artery) (with gangrene) K55.0
  vein (inferior) (superior) I81
mitral I34.8
mural (*see also* Infarct, myocardium)
  due to syphilis A52.06
  not resulting in infarction I24.0
omentum (with gangrene) K55.0
ophthalmic — *see* Occlusion, retina
pampiniform plexus (male) N50.1
parietal (*see also* Infarct, myocardium)
  not resulting in infarction I24.0
penis, superficial vein N48.81
perianal venous K64.5
peripheral arteries I74.4
  upper I74.2
personal history (of) Z86.718
portal I81
  due to syphilis A52.09
precerebral artery — *see* Occlusion, artery, precerebral
puerperal, postpartum O87.0
  brain (artery) O99.43
    venous (sinus) O87.3
  cardiac O99.43
  cerebral (artery) O99.43
    venous (sinus) O87.3
  superficial O87.0
pulmonary (artery) (iatrogenic) (postoperative) (vein) — *see* Embolism, pulmonary
renal (artery) N28.0
  vein I82.3
resulting from presence of device, implant or graft — *see* Complications, by site and type, specified NEC
retina, retinal — *see* Occlusion, retina
scrotum N50.1
seminal vesicle N50.1
sigmoid (venous) sinus — *see* Thrombosis, intracranial venous sinus
sinus, intracranial (any) — *see* Thrombosis, intracranial venous sinus
specified site NEC I82.890
  chronic I82.891
spermatic cord N50.1
spinal cord (arterial) G95.11
  due to syphilis A52.09
  pyogenic origin G06.1
spleen, splenic D73.5
  artery I74.8
testis N50.1
traumatic NEC T14.8
tricuspid I07.8
tumor — *see* Neoplasm, unspecified behavior, by site
tunica vaginalis N50.1
umbilical cord (vessels), complicating delivery O69.5 ☑
vas deferens N50.1
vein (acute) I82.90
  antecubital I82.61- ☑
    chronic I82.71- ☑
  axillary I82.A1- ☑ (*following* I82.7)
    chronic I82.A2- ☑ (*following* I82.7)
  basilic I82.61- ☑
    chronic I82.71- ☑
  brachial I82.62- ☑
    chronic I82.72- ☑
  brachiocephalic (innominate) I82.290
    chronic I82.291
  cephalic I82.61- ☑
    chronic I82.71- ☑
  cerebral, nonpyogenic I67.6
  chronic I82.91
  deep (DVT) I82.40- ☑
    calf I82.4Z- ☑
      chronic I82.5Z- ☑
    lower leg I82.4Z- ☑
      chronic I82.5Z- ☑
    thigh I82.4Y- ☑
      chronic I82.5Y- ☑
    upper leg I82.4Y ☑
      chronic I82.5y-
  femoral I82.41- ☑
    chronic I82.51- ☑
  iliac (iliofemoral) I82.42- ☑
    chronic I82.52- ☑
  innominate I82.290
    chronic I82.291

Thrombosis, thrombotic — continued
  vein — continued
    internal jugular I82.C1- ☑ (following I82.7)
      chronic I82.C2- ☑ (following I82.7)
    lower extremity
      deep I82.40- ☑
        chronic I82.50- ☑
          specified NEC I82.49- ☑
            chronic NEC I82.59- ☑
      distal
        deep I82.4Z- ☑
      proximal
        deep I82.4Y- ☑
          chronic I82.5Y- ☑
      superficial I82.81- ☑
    perianal K64.5
    popliteal I82.43- ☑
      chronic I82.53- ☑
    radial I82.62- ☑
      chronic I82.72- ☑
    renal I82.3
    saphenous (greater) (lesser) I82.81- ☑
    specified NEC I82.890
      chronic NEC I82.891
    subclavian I82.B1- ☑ (following I82.7)
      chronic I82.B2- ☑ (following I82.7)
    thoracic NEC I82.290
      chronic I82.291
    tibial I82.44- ☑
      chronic I82.54- ☑
    ulnar I82.62- ☑
      chronic I82.72- ☑
    upper extremity I82.60- ☑
      chronic I82.70- ☑
      deep I82.62- ☑
        chronic I82.72- ☑
      superficial I82.61- ☑
        chronic I82.71- ☑
  vena cava
    inferior I82.220
      chronic I82.221
    superior I82.210
      chronic I82.211
  venous, perianal K64.5
  ventricle (see also Infarct, myocardium)
    following acute myocardial infarction (current complication) I23.6
    not resulting in infarction I24.0
Thrombus — see Thrombosis
Thrush (see also Candidiasis)
  newborn P37.5
  oral B37.0
  vaginal B37.3
Thumb (see also condition)
  sucking (child problem) F98.8
Thymitis E32.8
Thymoma (benign) D15.0
  malignant C37
Thymus, thymic (gland) — see condition
Thyrocele — see Goiter
Thyroglossal (see also condition)
  cyst Q89.2
  duct, persistent Q89.2
Thyroid (gland) (body) (see also condition)
  hormone resistance E07.89
  lingual Q89.2
  nodule (cystic) (nontoxic) (single) E04.1
Thyroiditis E06.9
  acute (nonsuppurative) (pyogenic) (suppurative) E06.0
  autoimmune E06.3
  chronic (nonspecific) (sclerosing) E06.5
    with thyrotoxicosis, transient E06.2
    fibrous E06.5
    lymphadenoid E06.3
    lymphocytic E06.3
    lymphoid E06.3
  de Quervain's E06.1
  drug-induced E06.4
  fibrous (chronic) E06.5
  giant-cell (follicular) E06.1
  granulomatous (de Quervain) (subacute) E06.1
  Hashimoto's (struma lymphomatosa) E06.3
  iatrogenic E06.4
  ligneous E06.5
  lymphocytic (chronic) E06.3
  lymphoid E06.3
  lymphomatous E06.3

Thyroiditis — continued
  nonsuppurative E06.1
  postpartum, puerperal O90.5
  pseudotuberculous E06.1
  pyogenic E06.0
  radiation E06.4
  Riedel's E06.5
  subacute (granulomatous) E06.1
  suppurative E06.0
  tuberculous A18.81
  viral E06.1
  woody E06.5
Thyrolingual duct, persistent Q89.2
Thyromegaly E01.0
Thyrotoxic
  crisis — see Thyrotoxicosis
  heart disease or failure (see also Thyrotoxicosis) E05.90 [I43]
    with thyroid storm E05.91 [I43]
  storm — see Thyrotoxicosis
Thyrotoxicosis (recurrent) E05.90
  with
    goiter (diffuse) E05.00
      with thyroid storm E05.01
      adenomatous uninodular E05.10
        with thyroid storm E05.11
      multinodular E05.20
        with thyroid storm E05.21
      nodular E05.20
        with thyroid storm E05.21
      uninodular E05.10
        with thyroid storm E05.11
    infiltrative
      dermopathy E05.00
        with thyroid storm E05.01
      ophthalmopathy E05.00
        with thyroid storm E05.01
    single thyroid nodule E05.10
      with thyroid storm E05.11
    thyroid storm E05.91
  due to
    ectopic thyroid nodule or tissue E05.30
      with thyroid storm E05.31
    ingestion of (excessive) thyroid material E05.40
      with thyroid storm E05.41
    overproduction of thyroid-stimulating hormone E05.80
      with thyroid storm E05.81
    specified cause NEC E05.80
      with thyroid storm E05.81
  factitia E05.40
    with thyroid storm E05.41
  heart E05.90 [I43]
    with thyroid storm E05.91 [I43]
  failure E05.90 [I43]
  neonatal (transient) P72.1
  transient with chronic thyroiditis E06.2
Tibia vara — see Osteochondrosis, juvenile, tibia
Tic (disorder) F95.9
  breathing F95.8
  child problem F95.0
  compulsive F95.1
  de la Tourette F95.2
  degenerative (generalized) (localized) G25.69
    facial G25.69
  disorder
    chronic
      motor F95.1
      vocal F95.1
    combined vocal and multiple motor F95.2
    transient F95.0
  douloureux G50.0
    atypical G50.1
    postherpetic, postzoster B02.22
  drug-induced G25.61
  eyelid F95.8
  habit F95.9
    chronic F95.1
    transient of childhood F95.0
  lid, transient of childhood F95.0
  motor-verbal F95.2
  occupational F48.8
  orbicularis F95.8
    transient of childhood F95.0
  organic origin G25.69
  postchoreic G25.69
  psychogenic, compulsive F95.1
  salaam R25.8

Tic — continued
  spasm (motor or vocal) F95.9
    chronic F95.1
    transient of childhood F95.0
  specified NEC F95.8
Tick-borne — see condition
Tietze's disease or syndrome M94.0
Tight, tightness
  anus K62.89
  chest R07.89
  fascia (lata) M62.89
  foreskin (congenital) N47.1
  hymen, hymenal ring N89.6
  introitus (acquired) (congenital) N89.6
  rectal sphincter K62.89
  tendon — see Short, tendon
  urethral sphincter N35.9
Tilting vertebra — see Dorsopathy, deforming, specified NEC
Timidity, child F93.8
Tinea (intersecta) (tarsi) B35.9
  amiantacea L44.8
  asbestina B35.0
  barbae B35.0
  beard B35.0
  black dot B35.0
  blanca B36.2
  capitis B35.0
  corporis B35.4
  cruris B35.6
  flava B36.0
  foot B35.3
  furfuracea B36.0
  imbricata (Tokelau) B35.5
  kerion B35.0
  manuum B35.2
  microsporic — see Dermatophytosis
  nigra B36.1
  nodosa — see Piedra
  pedis B35.3
  scalp B35.0
  specified site NEC B35.8
  sycosis B35.0
  tonsurans B35.0
  trichophytic — see Dermatophytosis
  unguium B35.1
  versicolor B36.0
Tingling sensation (skin) R20.2
Tin-miner's lung J63.5
Tinnitus (audible) (aurium) (subjective) — see subcategory H93.1 ☑
Tipped tooth (teeth) M26.33
Tipping
  pelvis M95.5
    with disproportion (fetopelvic) O33.0
      causing obstructed labor O65.0
  tooth (teeth), fully erupted M26.33
Tiredness R53.83
Tissue — see condition
Tobacco (nicotine)
  dependence — see Dependence, drug, nicotine
  harmful use Z72.0
  heart — see Tobacco, toxic effect
  maternal use, affecting newborn P04.2
  toxic effect — see Table of Drugs and Chemicals, by substance, poisoning
    chewing tobacco — see Table of Drugs and Chemicals, by substance, poisoning
    cigarettes — see Table of Drugs and Chemicals, by substance, poisoning
  use Z72.0
    complicating
      childbirth O99.334
      pregnancy O99.33- ☑
      puerperium O99.335
    counseling and surveillance Z71.6
  withdrawal state — see Dependence, drug, nicotine
Tocopherol deficiency E56.0
Todd's
  cirrhosis K74.3
  paralysis (postepileptic) (transitory) G83.84
Toe — see condition
Toilet, artificial opening — see Attention to, artificial, opening
Tokelau (ringworm) B35.5
Tollwut — see Rabies

Tommaselli's disease R31.9
   correct substance properly administered — *see* Table of Drugs and Chemicals, by drug, adverse effect
   overdose or wrong substance given or taken — *see* Table of Drugs and Chemicals, by drug, poisoning
Tongue (*see also* condition)
   tie Q38.1
Tonic pupil — *see* Anomaly, pupil, function, tonic pupil
Toni-Fanconi syndrome (cystinosis) E72.09
   with cystinosis E72.04
Tonsil — *see* condition
Tonsillitis (acute) (catarrhal) (croupous) (follicular) (gangrenous) (infective) (lacunar) (lingual) (malignant) (membranous) (parenchymatous) (phlegmonous) (pseudomembranous) (purulent) (septic) (subacute) (suppurative) (toxic) (ulcerative) (vesicular) (viral) J03.90
   chronic J35.01
     with adenoiditis J35.03
   diphtheritic A36.0
   hypertrophic J35.01
     with adenoiditis J35.03
   recurrent J03.91
   specified organism NEC J03.80
     recurrent J03.81
   staphylococcal J03.80
     recurrent J03.81
   streptococcal J03.00
     recurrent J03.01
   tuberculous A15.8
   Vincent's A69.1
Tooth, teeth — *see* condition
Toothache K08.8
Topagnosis R20.8
Tophi — *see* Gout, chronic
TORCH infection — *see* Infection, congenital
   without active infection P00.2
Torn — *see* Tear
Tornwaldt's cyst or disease J39.2
Torsion
   accessory tube — *see* Torsion, fallopian tube
   adnexa (female) — *see* Torsion, fallopian tube
   aorta, acquired I77.1
   appendix epididymis N44.04
   appendix testis N44.03
   bile duct (common) (hepatic) K83.8
     congenital Q44.5
   bowel, colon or intestine K56.2
   cervix — *see* Malposition, uterus
   cystic duct K82.8
   dystonia — *see* Dystonia, torsion
   epididymis (appendix) N44.04
   fallopian tube N83.52
     with ovary N83.53
   gallbladder K82.8
     congenital Q44.1
   hydatid of Morgagni
     female N83.52
     male N44.03
   kidney (pedicle) (leading to infarction) N28.0
   Meckel's diverticulum (congenital) Q43.0
     malignant — *see* Table of Neoplasms, small intestine, malignant
   mesentery K56.2
   omentum K56.2
   organ or site, congenital NEC — *see* Anomaly, by site
   ovary (pedicle) N83.51
     with fallopian tube N83.53
     congenital Q50.2
   oviduct — *see* Torsion, fallopian tube
   penis (acquired) N48.82
     congenital Q55.63
   spasm — *see* Dystonia, torsion
   spermatic cord N44.02
     extravaginal N44.01
     intravaginal N44.02
   spleen D73.5
   testis, testicle N44.00
     appendix N44.03
   tibia — *see* Deformity, limb, specified type NEC, lower leg
   uterus — *see* Malposition, uterus
Torticollis (intermittent) (spastic) M43.6
   congenital (sternomastoid) Q68.0
   due to birth injury P15.8
   hysterical F44.4
   ocular R29.891

Torticollis — *continued*
   psychogenic F45.8
     conversion reaction F44.4
   rheumatic M43.6
   rheumatoid M06.88
   spasmodic G24.3
   traumatic, current S13.4 ☑
Tortipelvis G24.1
Tortuous
   artery I77.1
   organ or site, congenital NEC — *see* Distortion
   retinal vessel, congenital Q14.1
   ureter N13.8
   urethra N36.8
   vein — *see* Varix
Torture, victim of Z65.4
Torula, torular (histolytica) (infection) — *see* Cryptococcosis
Torulosis — *see* Cryptococcosis
Torus (mandibularis) (palatinus) M27.0
   fracture — *see* Fracture, by site, torus
Touraine's syndrome Q79.8
Tourette's syndrome F95.2
Tourniquet syndrome — *see* Constriction, external, by site
Tower skull Q75.0
   with exophthalmos Q87.0
Toxemia R68.89
   bacterial — *see* Sepsis
   burn — *see* Burn
   eclamptic (with pre-existing hypertension) — *see* Eclampsia
   erysipelatous — *see* Erysipelas
   fatigue R68.89
   food — *see* Poisoning, food
   gastrointestinal K52.1
   intestinal K52.1
   kidney — *see* Uremia
   malarial — *see* Malaria
   myocardial — *see* Myocarditis, toxic
   of pregnancy — *see* Pre-eclampsia
   pre-eclamptic — *see* Pre-eclampsia
   small intestine K52.1
   staphylococcal, due to food A05.0
   stasis R68.89
   uremic — *see* Uremia
   urinary — *see* Uremia
Toxemica cerebropathia psychica (nonalcoholic) F04
   alcoholic — *see* Alcohol, amnestic disorder
Toxic (poisoning) (*see also* condition) T65.91 ☑
   effect — *see* Table of Drugs and Chemicals, by substance, poisoning
   shock syndrome A48.3
   thyroid (gland) — *see* Thyrotoxicosis
Toxicemia — *see* Toxemia
Toxicity — *see* Table of Drugs and Chemicals, by substance, poisoning
   fava bean D55.0
   food, noxious — *see* Poisoning, food
   from drug or nonmedicinal substance — *see* Table of Drugs and Chemicals, by drug
Toxicosis (*see also* Toxemia)
   capillary, hemorrhagic D69.0
Toxinfection, gastrointestinal K52.1
Toxocariasis B83.0
Toxoplasma, toxoplasmosis (acquired) B58.9
   with
     hepatitis B58.1
     meningoencephalitis B58.2
     ocular involvement B58.00
     other organ involvement B58.89
     pneumonia, pneumonitis B58.3
   congenital (acute) (subacute) (chronic) P37.1
   maternal, manifest toxoplasmosis in infant (acute) (subacute) (chronic) P37.1
tPA (rtPA) **administration in a different facility within the last 24 hours prior to admission to current facility** Z92.82
Trabeculation, bladder N32.89
Trachea — *see* condition
Tracheitis (catarrhal) (infantile) (membranous) (plastic) (septal) (suppurative) (viral) J04.10
   with
     bronchitis (15 years of age and above) J40
       acute or subacute — *see* Bronchitis, acute
       chronic J42
       tuberculous NEC A15.5

Tracheitis — *continued*
   with — *continued*
     bronchitis — *continued*
       under 15 years of age J20.9
     laryngitis (acute) J04.2
       chronic J37.1
       tuberculous NEC A15.5
   acute J04.10
     with obstruction J04.11
   chronic J42
     with
       bronchitis (chronic) J42
       laryngitis (chronic) J37.1
   diphtheritic (membranous) A36.89
   due to external agent — *see* Inflammation, respiratory, upper, due to
   syphilitic A52.73
   tuberculous A15.5
Trachelitis (nonvenereal) — *see* Cervicitis
Tracheobronchial — *see* condition
Tracheobronchitis (15 years of age and above) (*see also* Bronchitis)
   due to
     Bordetella bronchiseptica A37.80
       with pneumonia A37.81
     Francisella tularensis A21.8
Tracheobronchomegaly Q32.4
   with bronchiectasis J47.9
     with
       exacerbation (acute) J47.1
       lower respiratory infection J47.0
   acquired J98.09
     with bronchiectasis J47.9
       with
         exacerbation (acute) J47.1
         lower respiratory infection J47.0
Tracheobronchopneumonitis — *see* Pneumonia, broncho-
Tracheocele (external) (internal) J39.8
   congenital Q32.1
Tracheomalacia J39.8
   congenital Q32.0
Tracheopharyngitis (acute) J06.9
   chronic J42
   due to external agent — *see* Inflammation, respiratory, upper, due to
Tracheostenosis J39.8
Tracheostomy
   complication — *see* Complication, tracheostomy
   status Z93.0
     attention to Z43.0
     malfunctioning J95.03
Trachoma, trachomatous A71.9
   active (stage) A71.1
   contraction of conjunctiva A71.1
   dubium A71.0
   healed or sequelae B94.0
   initial (stage) A71.0
   pannus A71.1
   Türck's J37.0
Traction, vitreomacular H43.82- ☑
Train sickness T75.3 ☑
Trait(s)
   Hb-S D57.3
   hemoglobin
     abnormal NEC D58.2
       with thalassemia D56.3
     C — *see* Disease, hemoglobin C
     S (Hb-S) D57.3
   Lepore D56.3
   personality, accentuated Z73.1
   sickle-cell D57.3
     with elliptocytosis or spherocytosis D57.3
   type A personality Z73.1
Tramp Z59.0
Trance R41.89
   hysterical F44.89
Transaminasemia R74.0
Transection
   abdomen (partial) S38.3 ☑
   aorta (incomplete) (*see also* Injury, aorta)
     complete — *see* Injury, aorta, laceration, major
   carotid artery (incomplete) (*see also* Injury, blood vessel, carotid, laceration)
     complete — *see* Injury, blood vessel, carotid, laceration, major
   celiac artery (incomplete) S35.211 ☑
     branch (incomplete) S35.291 ☑

Transection — *continued*
celiac artery — *continued*
  branch — *continued*
    complete S35.292 ☑
  complete S35.212 ☑
innominate
  artery (incomplete) (*see also* Injury, blood vessel, thoracic, innominate, artery, laceration)
    complete — *see* Injury, blood vessel, thoracic, innominate, artery, laceration, major
  vein (incomplete) (*see also* Injury, blood vessel, thoracic, innominate, vein, laceration)
    complete — *see* Injury, blood vessel, thoracic, innominate, vein, laceration, major
jugular vein (external) (incomplete) (*see also* Injury, blood vessel, jugular vein, laceration)
  complete — *see* Injury, blood vessel, jugular vein, laceration, major
  internal (incomplete) (*see also* Injury, blood vessel, jugular vein, internal, laceration)
    complete — *see* Injury, blood vessel, jugular vein, internal, laceration, major
mesenteric artery (incomplete) (*see also* Injury, mesenteric, artery, laceration)
  complete — *see* Injury, mesenteric artery, laceration, major
pulmonary vessel (incomplete) (*see also* Injury, blood vessel, thoracic, pulmonary, laceration)
  complete — *see* Injury, blood vessel, thoracic, pulmonary, laceration, major
subclavian — *see* Transection, innominate
vena cava (incomplete) (*see also* Injury, vena cava)
  complete — *see* Injury, vena cava, laceration, major
vertebral artery (incomplete) (*see also* Injury, blood vessel, vertebral, laceration)
  complete — *see* Injury, blood vessel, vertebral, laceration, major
Transfusion
associated (red blood cell) hemochromatosis E83.111
blood
  ABO incompatible — *see* Complication(s), transfusion, incompatibility reaction, ABO
  minor blood group (Duffy) (E) (K(ell)) (Kidd) (Lewis) (M) (N) (P) (S) T80.89 ☑
  reaction or complication — *see* Complications, transfusion
fetomaternal (mother) — *see* Pregnancy, complicated by, placenta, transfusion syndrome
maternofetal (mother) — *see* Pregnancy, complicated by, placenta, transfusion syndrome
placental (syndrome) (mother) — *see* Pregnancy, complicated by, placenta, transfusion syndrome
reaction (adverse) — *see* Complications, transfusion
related acute lung injury (TRALI) J95.84
twin-to-twin — *see* Pregnancy, complicated by, placenta, transfusion syndrome, fetus to fetus
Transient (meaning homeless) (*see also* condition) Z59.0
Translocation
balanced autosomal Q95.9
  in normal individual Q95.0
chromosomes NEC Q99.8
  balanced and insertion in normal individual Q95.0
Down syndrome Q90.2
trisomy
  13 Q91.6
  18 Q91.2
  21 Q90.2
Translucency, iris — *see* Degeneration, iris
Transmission of chemical substances through the placenta — *see* Absorption, chemical, through placenta
Transparency, lung, unilateral J43.0
Transplant (ed) (status) Z94.9
awaiting organ Z76.82
bone Z94.6
  marrow Z94.81
candidate Z76.82
complication — *see* Complication, transplant
cornea Z94.7
heart Z94.1
  and lung(s) Z94.3
  valve Z95.2
    prosthetic Z95.2
    specified NEC Z95.4
    xenogenic Z95.3
intestine Z94.82
kidney Z94.0

Transplant — *continued*
liver Z94.4
lung(s) Z94.2
  and heart Z94.3
organ (failure) (infection) (rejection) Z94.9
  removal status Z98.85
pancreas Z94.83
skin Z94.5
social Z60.3
specified organ or tissue NEC Z94.89
stem cells Z94.84
tissue Z94.9
Transplants, ovarian, endometrial N80.1
Transposed — *see* Transposition
Transposition (congenital) (*see also* Malposition, congenital)
abdominal viscera Q89.3
aorta (dextra) Q20.3
appendix Q43.8
colon Q43.8
corrected Q20.5
great vessels (complete) (partial) Q20.3
heart Q24.0
  with complete transposition of viscera Q89.3
intestine (large) (small) Q43.8
reversed jejunal (for bypass) (status) Z98.0
scrotum Q55.23
stomach Q40.2
  with general transposition of viscera Q89.3
tooth, teeth, fully erupted M26.30
vessels, great (complete) (partial) Q20.3
viscera (abdominal) (thoracic) Q89.3
Transsexualism F64.1
Transverse (*see also* condition)
arrest (deep), in labor O64.0 ☑
lie (mother) O32.2 ☑
  causing obstructed labor O64.8 ☑
Transvestism, transvestitism (dual-role) F64.1
fetishistic F65.1
Trapped placenta (with hemorrhage) O72.0
without hemorrhage O73.0
Trauma, traumatism (*see also* Injury)
acoustic — *see* subcategory H83.3 ☑
birth — *see* Birth, injury
complicating ectopic or molar pregnancy O08.6
during delivery O71.9
following ectopic or molar pregnancy O08.6
obstetric O71.9
  specified NEC O71.89
Traumatic (*see also* condition)
brain injury — *see* category S06 ☑
Treacher Collins syndrome Q75.4
Treitz's hernia — *see* Hernia, abdomen, specified site NEC
Trematode infestation — *see* Infestation, fluke
Trematodiasis — *see* Infestation, fluke
Trembling paralysis — *see* Parkinsonism
Tremor(s) R25.1
drug induced G25.1
essential (benign) G25.0
familial G25.0
hereditary G25.0
hysterical F44.4
intention G25.2
medication induced postural G25.1
mercurial — *see* subcategory T56.1 ☑
Parkinson's — *see* Parkinsonism
psychogenic (conversion reaction) F44.4
senilis R54
specified type NEC G25.2
Trench
fever A79.0
foot — *see* Immersion, foot
mouth A69.1
Treponema pallidum infection — *see* Syphilis
Treponematosis
due to
  T. pallidum — *see* Syphilis
  T. pertenue — *see* Yaws
Triad
Hutchinson's (congenital syphilis) A50.53
Kartagener's Q89.3
Saint's — *see* Hernia, diaphragm
Trichiasis (eyelid) H02.059
with entropion — *see* Entropion
left H02.056
  lower H02.055

Trichiasis — *continued*
left — *continued*
  upper H02.054
right H02.053
  lower H02.052
  upper H02.051
Trichinella spiralis (infection) (infestation) B75
Trichinellosis, trichiniasis, trichinelliasis, trichinosis B75
with muscle disorder B75 [M63.80]
  ankle B75 [M63.87-] ☑
  foot B75 [M63.87-] ☑
  forearm B75 [M63.83-] ☑
  hand B75 [M63.84-] ☑
  lower leg B75 [M63.86-] ☑
  multiple sites B75 [M63.89]
  pelvic region B75 [M63.85-] ☑
  shoulder region B75 [M63.81-] ☑
  specified site NEC B75 [M63.88]
  thigh B75 [M63.85-] ☑
  upper arm B75 [M63.82-] ☑
Trichobezoar T18.9 ☑
intestine T18.3 ☑
stomach T18.2 ☑
Trichocephaliasis, trichocephalosis B79
Trichocephalus infestation B79
Trichoclasis L67.8
Trichoepithelioma (*see also* Neoplasm, skin, benign)
malignant — *see* Neoplasm, skin, malignant
Trichofolliculoma — *see* Neoplasm, skin, benign
Tricholemmoma — *see* Neoplasm, skin, benign
Trichomoniasis A59.9
bladder A59.03
cervix A59.09
intestinal A07.8
prostate A59.02
seminal vesicles A59.09
specified site NEC A59.8
urethra A59.03
urogenitalis A59.00
vagina A59.01
vulva A59.01
Trichomycosis
axillaris A48.8
nodosa, nodularis B36.8
Trichonodosis L67.8
Trichophytid, trichophyton infection — *see* Dermatophytosis
Trichophytobezoar T18.9 ☑
intestine T18.3 ☑
stomach T18.2 ☑
Trichophytosis — *see* Dermatophytosis
Trichoptilosis L67.8
Trichorrhexis (nodosa) (invaginata) L67.0
Trichosis axillaris A48.8
Trichosporosis nodosa B36.2
Trichostasis spinulosa (congenital) Q84.1
Trichostrongyliasis, trichostrongylosis (small intestine) B81.2
Trichostrongylus infection B81.2
Trichotillomania F63.3
Trichromat, trichromatopsia, anomalous (congenital) H53.55
Trichuriasis B79
Trichuris trichiura (infection) (infestation) (any site) B79
Tricuspid (valve) — *see* condition
Trifid (*see also* Accessory)
kidney (pelvis) Q63.8
tongue Q38.3
Trigeminal neuralgia — *see* Neuralgia, trigeminal
Trigeminy R00.8
Trigger finger (acquired) M65.30
congenital Q74.0
index finger M65.32- ☑
little finger M65.35- ☑
middle finger M65.33- ☑
ring finger M65.34- ☑
thumb M65.31- ☑
Trigonitis (bladder) (chronic) (pseudomembranous) N30.30
with hematuria N30.31
Trigonocephaly Q75.0
Trilocular heart — *see* Cor triloculare
Trimethylaminuria E72.52
Tripartite placenta O43.19- ☑
Triphalangeal thumb Q74.0

Triple (*see also* Accessory)
  kidneys Q63.0
  uteri Q51.818
  X, female Q97.0
Triplegia G83.89
  congenital G80.8
Triplet (newborn) (*see also* Newborn, triplet)
  complicating pregnancy — *see* Pregnancy, triplet
Triplication — *see* Accessory
Triploidy Q92.7
Trismus R25.2
  neonatorum A33
  newborn A33
Trisomy (syndrome) Q92.9
  13 (partial) Q91.7
    meiotic nondisjunction Q91.4
    mitotic nondisjunction Q91.5
    mosaicism Q91.5
    translocation Q91.6
  18 (partial) Q91.3
    meiotic nondisjunction Q91.0
    mitotic nondisjunction Q91.1
    mosaicism Q91.1
    translocation Q91.2
  20 Q92.8
  21 (partial) Q90.9
    meiotic nondisjunction Q90.0
    mitotic nondisjunction Q90.1
    mosaicism Q90.1
    translocation Q90.2
  22 Q92.8
  autosomes Q92.9
  chromosome specified NEC Q92.8
    partial Q92.2
      due to unbalanced translocation Q92.5
    specified NEC Q92.8
    whole (nonsex chromosome)
      meiotic nondisjunction Q92.0
      mitotic nondisjunction Q92.1
      mosaicism Q92.1
  due to
    dicentrics — *see* Extra, marker chromosomes
    extra rings — *see* Extra, marker chromosomes
    isochromosomes — *see* Extra, marker chromo-
      somes
  specified NEC Q92.8
  whole chromosome Q92.9
    meiotic nondisjunction Q92.0
    mitotic nondisjunction Q92.1
    mosaicism Q92.1
    partial Q92.9
    specified NEC Q92.8
Tritanomaly, tritanopia H53.55
Trombiculosis, trombiculiasis, trombidiosis B88.0
Trophedema (congenital) (hereditary) Q82.0
Trophoblastic disease (*see also* Mole, hydatidiform)
  O01.9
Tropholymphedema Q82.0
Trophoneurosis NEC G96.8
  disseminated M34.9
Tropical — *see* condition
Trouble (*see also* Disease)
  heart — *see* Disease, heart
  kidney — *see* Disease, renal
  nervous R45.0
  sinus — *see* Sinusitis
Trousseau's syndrome (thrombophlebitis migrans) I82.1
Truancy, childhood
  from school Z72.810
Truncus
  arteriosus (persistent) Q20.0
  communis Q20.0
Trunk — *see* condition
Trypanosomiasis
  African B56.9
    by Trypanosoma brucei
      gambiense B56.0
      rhodesiense B56.1
  American — *see* Chagas' disease
  Brazilian — *see* Chagas' disease
  by Trypanosoma
    brucei gambiense B56.0
    brucei rhodesiense B56.1
    cruzi — *see* Chagas' disease
  gambiensis, Gambian B56.0
  rhodesiensis, Rhodesian B56.1
  South American — *see* Chagas' disease

Trypanosomiasis — *continued*
  where
    African trypanosomiasis is prevalent B56.9
    Chagas' disease is prevalent B57.2
T-shaped incisors K00.2
Tsutsugamushi (disease) (fever) A75.3
Tube, tubal, tubular — *see* condition
Tubercle (*see also* Tuberculosis)
  brain, solitary A17.81
  Darwin's Q17.8
  Ghon, primary infection A15.7
Tuberculid, tuberculide (indurating, subcutaneous)
  (lichenoid) (miliary) (papulonecrotic) (primary) (skin)
  A18.4
Tuberculoma (*see also* Tuberculosis)
  brain A17.81
  meninges (cerebral) (spinal) A17.1
  spinal cord A17.81
Tuberculosis, tubercular, tuberculous (calcification)
  (calcified) (caseous) (chromogenic acid-fast bacilli)
  (degeneration) (fibrocaseous) (fistula) (interstitial)
  (isolated circumscribed lesions) (necrosis)
  (parenchymatous) (ulcerative) A15.9
  with pneumoconiosis (any condition in J60-J64) J65
  abdomen (lymph gland) A18.39
  abscess (respiratory) A15.9
    bone A18.03
      hip A18.02
      knee A18.02
      sacrum A18.01
      specified site NEC A18.03
      spinal A18.01
      vertebra A18.01
    brain A17.81
    breast A18.89
    Cowper's gland A18.15
    dura (mater) (cerebral) (spinal) A17.81
    epidural (cerebral) (spinal) A17.81
    female pelvis A18.17
    frontal sinus A15.8
    genital organs NEC A18.10
    genitourinary A18.10
    gland (lymphatic) — *see* Tuberculosis, lymph gland
    hip A18.02
    intestine A18.32
    ischiorectal A18.32
    joint NEC A18.02
      hip A18.02
      knee A18.02
      specified NEC A18.02
      vertebral A18.01
    kidney A18.11
    knee A18.02
    latent R76.11
    lumbar (spine) A18.01
    lung — *see* Tuberculosis, pulmonary
    meninges (cerebral) (spinal) A17.0
    muscle A18.09
    perianal (fistula) A18.32
    perinephric A18.11
    perirectal A18.32
    rectum A18.32
    retropharyngeal A15.8
    sacrum A18.01
    scrofulous A18.2
    scrotum A18.15
    skin (primary) A18.4
    spinal cord A17.81
    spine or vertebra (column) A18.01
    subdiaphragmatic A18.31
    testis A18.15
    urinary A18.13
    uterus A18.17
  accessory sinus — *see* Tuberculosis, sinus
  Addison's disease A18.7
  adenitis — *see* Tuberculosis, lymph gland
  adenoids A15.8
  adenopathy — *see* Tuberculosis, lymph gland
  adherent pericardium A18.84
  adnexa (uteri) A18.17
  adrenal (capsule) (gland) A18.7
  alimentary canal A18.32
  anemia A18.89
  ankle (joint) (bone) A18.02
  anus A18.32
  apex, apical — *see* Tuberculosis, pulmonary
  appendicitis, appendix A18.32
  arachnoid A17.0

Tuberculosis, tubercular, tuberculous — *continued*
  artery, arteritis A18.89
    cerebral A18.89
  arthritis (chronic) (synovial) A18.02
    spine or vertebra (column) A18.01
  articular — *see* Tuberculosis, joint
  ascites A18.31
  asthma — *see* Tuberculosis, pulmonary
  axilla, axillary (gland) A18.2
  bladder A18.12
  bone A18.03
    hip A18.02
    knee A18.02
    limb NEC A18.03
    sacrum A18.01
    spine or vertebral column A18.01
  bowel (miliary) A18.32
  brain A17.81
  breast A18.89
  broad ligament A18.17
  bronchi, bronchial, bronchus A15.5
    ectasia, ectasis (bronchiectasis) — *see* Tuberculosis,
      pulmonary
    fistula A15.5
      primary (progressive) A15.7
    gland or node A15.4
      primary (progressive) A15.7
    lymph gland or node A15.4
      primary (progressive) A15.7
  bronchiectasis — *see* Tuberculosis, pulmonary
  bronchitis A15.5
  bronchopleural A15.6
  bronchopneumonia, bronchopneumonic — *see* Tuber-
    culosis, pulmonary
  bronchorrhagia A15.5
  bronchotracheal A15.5
  bronze disease A18.7
  buccal cavity A18.83
  bulbourethral gland A18.15
  bursa A18.09
  cachexia A15.9
  cardiomyopathy A18.84
  caries — *see* Tuberculosis, bone
  cartilage A18.02
    intervertebral A18.01
  catarrhal — *see* Tuberculosis, respiratory
  cecum A18.32
  cellulitis (primary) A18.4
  cerebellum A17.81
  cerebral, cerebrum A17.81
  cerebrospinal A17.81
    meninges A17.0
  cervical (lymph gland or node) A18.2
  cervicitis, cervix (uteri) A18.16
  chest — *see* Tuberculosis, respiratory
  chorioretinitis A18.53
  choroid, choroiditis A18.53
  ciliary body A18.54
  colitis A18.32
  collier's J65
  colliquativa (primary) A18.4
  colon A18.32
  complex, primary A15.7
  congenital P37.0
  conjunctiva A18.59
  connective tissue (systemic) A18.89
  contact Z20.1
  cornea (ulcer) A18.52
  Cowper's gland A18.15
  coxae A18.02
  coxalgia A18.02
  cul-de-sac of Douglas A18.17
  curvature, spine A18.01
  cutis (colliquativa) (primary) A18.4
  cyst, ovary A18.18
  cystitis A18.12
  dactylitis A18.03
  diarrhea A18.32
  diffuse — *see* Tuberculosis, miliary
  digestive tract A18.32
  disseminated — *see* Tuberculosis, miliary
  duodenum A18.32
  dura (mater) (cerebral) (spinal) A17.0
    abscess (cerebral) (spinal) A17.81
  dysentery A18.32
  ear (inner) (middle) A18.6
    bone A18.03
    external (primary) A18.4

Tuberculosis, tubercular, tuberculous — *continued*
- ear — *continued*
  - skin (primary) A18.4
- elbow A18.02
- emphysema — *see* Tuberculosis, pulmonary
- empyema A15.6
- encephalitis A17.82
- endarteritis A18.89
- endocarditis A18.84
  - aortic A18.84
  - mitral A18.84
  - pulmonary A18.84
  - tricuspid A18.84
- endocrine glands NEC A18.82
- endometrium A18.17
- enteric, enterica, enteritis A18.32
- enterocolitis A18.32
- epididymis, epididymitis A18.15
- epidural abscess (cerebral) (spinal) A17.81
- epiglottis A15.5
- episcleritis A18.51
- erythema (induratum) (nodosum) (primary) A18.4
- esophagus A18.83
- eustachian tube A18.6
- exposure (to) Z20.1
- exudative — *see* Tuberculosis, pulmonary
- eye A18.50
- eyelid (primary) (lupus) A18.4
- fallopian tube (acute) (chronic) A18.17
- fascia A18.09
- fauces A15.8
- female pelvic inflammatory disease A18.17
- finger A18.03
- first infection A15.7
- gallbladder A18.83
- ganglion A18.09
- gastritis A18.83
- gastrocolic fistula A18.32
- gastroenteritis A18.32
- gastrointestinal tract A18.32
- general, generalized — *see* Tuberculosis, miliary
- genital organs A18.10
- genitourinary A18.10
- genu A18.02
- glandula suprarenalis A18.7
- glandular, general A18.2
- glottis A15.5
- grinder's J65
- gum A18.83
- hand A18.03
- heart A18.84
- hematogenous — *see* Tuberculosis, miliary
- hemoptysis — *see* Tuberculosis, pulmonary
- hemorrhage NEC — *see* Tuberculosis, pulmonary
- hemothorax A15.6
- hepatitis A18.83
- hilar lymph nodes A15.4
  - primary (progressive) A15.7
- hip (joint) (disease) (bone) A18.02
- hydropneumothorax A15.6
- hydrothorax A15.6
- hypoadrenalism A18.7
- hypopharynx A15.8
- ileocecal (hyperplastic) A18.32
- ileocolitis A18.32
- ileum A18.32
- iliac spine (superior) A18.03
- immunological findings only A15.7
- indurativa (primary) A18.4
- infantile A15.7
- infection A15.9
  - without clinical manifestations A15.7
- infraclavicular gland A18.2
- inguinal gland A18.2
- inguinalis A18.2
- intestine (any part) A18.32
- iridocyclitis A18.54
- iris, iritis A18.54
- ischiorectal A18.32
- jaw A18.03
- jejunum A18.32
- joint A18.02
  - vertebral A18.01
- keratitis (interstitial) A18.52
- keratoconjunctivitis A18.52
- kidney A18.11
- knee (joint) A18.02
- kyphosis, kyphoscoliosis A18.01

Tuberculosis, tubercular, tuberculous — *continued*
- laryngitis A15.5
- larynx A15.5
- leptomeninges, leptomeningitis (cerebral) (spinal) A17.0
- lichenoides (primary) A18.4
- linguae A18.83
- lip A18.83
- liver A18.83
- lordosis A18.01
- lung — *see* Tuberculosis, pulmonary
- lupus vulgaris A18.4
- lymph gland or node (peripheral) A18.2
  - abdomen A18.39
  - bronchial A15.4
    - primary (progressive) A15.7
  - cervical A18.2
  - hilar A15.4
    - primary (progressive) A15.7
  - intrathoracic A15.4
    - primary (progressive) A15.7
  - mediastinal A15.4
    - primary (progressive) A15.7
  - mesenteric A18.39
  - retroperitoneal A18.39
  - tracheobronchial A15.4
    - primary (progressive) A15.7
- lymphadenitis — *see* Tuberculosis, lymph gland
- lymphangitis — *see* Tuberculosis, lymph gland
- lymphatic (gland) (vessel) — *see* Tuberculosis, lymph gland
- mammary gland A18.89
- marasmus A15.9
- mastoiditis A18.03
- mediastinal lymph gland or node A15.4
  - primary (progressive) A15.7
- mediastinitis A15.8
  - primary (progressive) A15.7
- mediastinum A15.8
  - primary (progressive) A15.7
- medulla A17.81
- melanosis, Addisonian A18.7
- meninges, meningitis (basilar) (cerebral) (cerebrospinal) (spinal) A17.0
- meningoencephalitis A17.82
- mesentery, mesenteric (gland or node) A18.39
- miliary A19.9
  - acute A19.2
    - multiple sites A19.1
    - single specified site A19.0
  - chronic A19.8
  - specified NEC A19.8
- millstone makers' J65
- miner's J65
- molder's J65
- mouth A18.83
- multiple A19.9
  - acute A19.1
  - chronic A19.8
- muscle A18.09
- myelitis A17.82
- myocardium, myocarditis A18.84
- nasal (passage) (sinus) A15.8
- nasopharynx A15.8
- neck gland A18.2
- nephritis A18.11
- nerve (mononeuropathy) A17.83
- nervous system A17.9
- nose (septum) A15.8
- ocular A18.50
- omentum A18.31
- oophoritis (acute) (chronic) A18.17
- optic (nerve trunk) (papilla) A18.59
- orbit A18.59
- orchitis A18.15
- organ, specified NEC A18.89
- osseous — *see* Tuberculosis, bone
- osteitis — *see* Tuberculosis, bone
- osteomyelitis — *see* Tuberculosis, bone
- otitis media A18.6
- ovary, ovaritis (acute) (chronic) A18.17
- oviduct (acute) (chronic) A18.17
- pachymeningitis A17.0
- palate (soft) A18.83
- pancreas A18.83
- papulonecrotic (a) (primary) A18.4
- parathyroid glands A18.82
- paronychia (primary) A18.4

Tuberculosis, tubercular, tuberculous — *continued*
- parotid gland or region A18.83
- pelvis (bony) A18.03
- penis A18.15
- peribronchitis A15.5
- pericardium, pericarditis A18.84
- perichondritis, larynx A15.5
- periostitis — *see* Tuberculosis, bone
- perirectal fistula A18.32
- peritoneum NEC A18.31
- peritonitis A18.31
- pharynx, pharyngitis A15.8
- phlyctenulosis (keratoconjunctivitis) A18.52
- phthisis NEC — *see* Tuberculosis, pulmonary
- pituitary gland A18.82
- pleura, pleural, pleurisy, pleuritis (fibrinous) (obliterative) (purulent) (simple plastic) (with effusion) A15.6
  - primary (progressive) A15.7
- pneumonia, pneumonic — *see* Tuberculosis, pulmonary
- pneumothorax (spontaneous) (tense valvular) — *see* Tuberculosis, pulmonary
- polyneuropathy A17.89
- polyserositis A19.9
  - acute A19.1
  - chronic A19.8
- potter's J65
- prepuce A18.15
- primary (complex) A15.7
- proctitis A18.32
- prostate, prostatitis A18.14
- pulmonalis — *see* Tuberculosis, pulmonary
- pulmonary (cavitated) (fibrotic) (infiltrative) (nodular) A15.0
  - childhood type or first infection A15.7
  - primary (complex) A15.7
- pyelitis A18.11
- pyelonephritis A18.11
- pyemia — *see* Tuberculosis, miliary
- pyonephrosis A18.11
- pyopneumothorax A15.6
- pyothorax A15.6
- rectum (fistula) (with abscess) A18.32
- reinfection stage — *see* Tuberculosis, pulmonary
- renal A18.11
- renis A18.11
- respiratory A15.9
  - primary A15.7
  - specified site NEC A15.8
- retina, retinitis A18.53
- retroperitoneal (lymph gland or node) A18.39
- rheumatism NEC A18.09
- rhinitis A15.8
- sacroiliac (joint) A18.01
- sacrum A18.01
- salivary gland A18.83
- salpingitis (acute) (chronic) A18.17
- sandblaster's J65
- sclera A18.51
- scoliosis A18.01
- scrofulous A18.2
- scrotum A18.15
- seminal tract or vesicle A18.15
- senile A15.9
- septic — *see* Tuberculosis, miliary
- shoulder (joint) A18.02
  - blade A18.03
- sigmoid A18.32
- sinus (any nasal) A15.8
  - bone A18.03
  - epididymis A18.15
- skeletal NEC A18.03
- skin (any site) (primary) A18.4
- small intestine A18.32
- soft palate A18.83
- spermatic cord A18.15
- spine, spinal (column) A18.01
  - cord A17.81
  - medulla A17.81
  - membrane A17.0
  - meninges A17.0
- spleen, splenitis A18.85
- spondylitis A18.01
- sternoclavicular joint A18.02
- stomach A18.83
- stonemason's J65
- subcutaneous tissue (cellular) (primary) A18.4

☑ **Additional Character Required** — Refer to the Tabular List for Character Selection ▽ **Subterms under main terms may continue to next column or page**

Tuberculosis, tubercular, tuberculous — *continued*
  subcutis (primary) A18.4
  subdeltoid bursa A18.83
  submaxillary (region) A18.83
  supraclavicular gland A18.2
  suprarenal (capsule) (gland) A18.7
  swelling, joint (*see also* category M01) (*see also* Tuberculosis, joint) A18.02
  symphysis pubis A18.02
  synovitis A18.09
   articular A18.02
   spine or vertebra A18.01
  systemic — *see* Tuberculosis, miliary
  tarsitis A18.4
  tendon (sheath) — *see* Tuberculosis, tenosynovitis
  tenosynovitis A18.09
   spine or vertebra A18.01
  testis A18.15
  throat A15.8
  thymus gland A18.82
  thyroid gland A18.81
  tongue A18.83
  tonsil, tonsillitis A15.8
  trachea, tracheal A15.5
   lymph gland or node A15.4
    primary (progressive) A15.7
  tracheobronchial A15.5
   lymph gland or node A15.4
    primary (progressive) A15.7
  tubal (acute) (chronic) A18.17
  tunica vaginalis A18.15
  ulcer (skin) (primary) A18.4
   bowel or intestine A18.32
   specified NEC — *see* Tuberculosis, by site
  unspecified site A15.9
  ureter A18.11
  urethra, urethral (gland) A18.13
  urinary organ or tract A18.13
  uterus A18.17
  uveal tract A18.54
  uvula A18.83
  vagina A18.18
  vas deferens A18.15
  verruca, verrucosa (cutis) (primary) A18.4
  vertebra (column) A18.01
  vesiculitis A18.15
  vulva A18.18
  wrist (joint) A18.02

Tuberculum
  Carabelli — *see* Excludes Note at K00.2
  occlusal — *see* Excludes Note at K00.2
  paramolare K00.2

Tuberosity, enitre maxillary M26.07
Tuberous sclerosis (brain) Q85.1
Tubo-ovarian — *see* condition
Tuboplasty, after previous sterilization Z31.0
  aftercare Z31.42
Tubotympanitis, catarrhal (chronic) — *see* Otitis, media, nonsuppurative, chronic, serous
Tularemia A21.9
  with
   conjunctivitis A21.1
   pneumonia A21.2
  abdominal A21.3
  bronchopneumonic A21.2
  conjunctivitis A21.1
  cryptogenic A21.3
  enteric A21.3
  gastrointestinal A21.3
  generalized A21.7
  ingestion A21.3
  intestinal A21.3
  oculoglandular A21.1
  ophthalmic A21.1
  pneumonia (any), pneumonic A21.2
  pulmonary A21.2
  sepsis A21.7
  specified NEC A21.8
  typhoidal A21.7
  ulceroglandular A21.0
Tularensis conjunctivitis A21.1
Tumefaction (*see also* Swelling)
  liver — *see* Hypertrophy, liver
Tumor (*see also* Neoplasm, unspecified behavior, by site)
  acinar cell — *see* Neoplasm, uncertain behavior, by site
  acinic cell — *see* Neoplasm, uncertain behavior, by site

Tumor — *continued*
  adenocarcinoid — *see* Neoplasm, malignant, by site
  adenomatoid (*see also* Neoplasm, benign, by site)
   odontogenic — *see* Cyst, calcifying odontogenic
  adnexal (skin) — *see* Neoplasm, skin, benign, by site
  adrenal
   cortical (benign) D35.0- ☑
    malignant C74.0- ☑
   rest — *see* Neoplasm, benign, by site
  alpha-cell
   malignant
    pancreas C25.4
    specified site NEC — *see* Neoplasm, malignant, by site
    unspecified site C25.4
   pancreas D13.7
   specified site NEC — *see* Neoplasm, benign, by site
   unspecified site D13.7
  aneurysmal — *see* Aneurysm
  aortic body D44.7
   malignant C75.5
  Askin's — *see* Neoplasm, connective tissue, malignant
  basal cell (*see also* Neoplasm, skin, uncertain behavior) D48.5
  Bednar — *see* Neoplasm, skin, malignant
  benign (unclassified) — *see* Neoplasm, benign, by site
  beta-cell
   malignant
    pancreas C25.4
    specified site NEC — *see* Neoplasm, malignant, by site
    unspecified site C25.4
   pancreas D13.7
   specified site NEC — *see* Neoplasm, benign, by site
   unspecified site D13.7
  Brenner D27.9
   borderline malignancy D39.1- ☑
   malignant C56- ☑
   proliferating D39.1- ☑
  bronchial alveolar, intravascular D38.1
  Brooke's — *see* Neoplasm, skin, benign
  brown fat — *see* Lipoma
  Burkitt — *see* Lymphoma, Burkitt
  calcifying epithelial odontogenic — *see* Cyst, calcifying odontogenic
  carcinoid
   benign D3A.00 (*following* D36)
    appendix D3A.020 (*following* D36)
    ascending colon D3A.022 (*following* D36)
    bronchus (lung) D3A.090 (*following* D36)
    cecum D3A.021 (*following* D36)
    colon D3A.029 (*following* D36)
    descending colon D3A.024 (*following* D36)
    duodenum D3A.010 (*following* D36)
    foregut NOS D3A.094 (*following* D36)
    hindgut NOS D3A.096 (*following* D36)
    ileum D3A.012 (*following* D36)
    jejunum D3A.011 (*following* D36)
    kidney D3A.093 (*following* D36)
    large intestine D3A.029 (*following* D36)
    lung (bronchus) D3A.090 (*following* D36)
    midgut NOS D3A.095 (*following* D36)
    rectum D3A.026 (*following* D36)
    sigmoid colon D3A.025 (*following* D36)
    small intestine D3A.019 (*following* D36)
    specified NEC D3A.098 (*following* D36)
    stomach D3A.092 (*following* D36)
    thymus D3A.091 (*following* D36)
    transverse colon D3A.023 (*following* D36)
   malignant C7A.00 (*following* C75)
    appendix C7A.020 (*following* C75)
    ascending colon C7A.022 (*following* C75)
    bronchus (lung) C7A.090 (*following* C75)
    cecum C7A.021 (*following* C75)
    colon C7A.029 (*following* C75)
    descending colon C7A.024 (*following* C75)
    duodenum C7A.010 (*following* C75)
    foregut NOS C7A.094 (*following* C75)
    hindgut NOS C7A.096 (*following* C75)
    ileum C7A.012 (*following* C75)
    jejunum C7A.011 (*following* C75)
    kidney C7A.093 (*following* C75)
    large intestine C7A.029 (*following* C75)
    lung (bronchus) C7A.090 (*following* C75)
    midgut NOS C7A.095 (*following* C75)
    rectum C7A.026 (*following* C75)
    sigmoid colon C7A.025 (*following* C75)
    small intestine C7A.019 (*following* C75)

Tumor — *continued*
  carcinoid — *continued*
   malignant — *continued*
    specified NEC C7A.098 (*following* C75)
    stomach C7A.092 (*following* C75)
    thymus C7A.091 (*following* C75)
    transverse colon C7A.023 (*following* C75)
    mesentery metastasis C7B.04 (*following* C75)
    secondary C7B.00 (*following* C75)
     bone C7B.03 (*following* C75)
     distant lymph nodes C7B.01 (*following* C75)
     liver C7B.02 (*following* C75)
     peritoneum C7B.04 (*following* C75)
     specified NEC C7B.09 (*following* C75)
  carotid body D44.6
   malignant C75.4
  cells (*see also* Neoplasm, unspecified behavior, by site)
   benign — *see* Neoplasm, benign, by site
   malignant — *see* Neoplasm, malignant, by site
   uncertain whether benign or malignant — *see* Neoplasm, uncertain behavior, by site
  cervix, in pregnancy or childbirth — *see* Pregnancy, complicated by, tumor, cervix
  chondromatous giant cell — *see* Neoplasm, bone, benign
  chromaffin (*see also* Neoplasm, benign, by site)
   malignant — *see* Neoplasm, malignant, by site
  Cock's peculiar L72.3
  Codman's — *see* Neoplasm, bone, benign
  dentigerous, mixed — *see* Cyst, calcifying odontogenic
  dermoid — *see* Neoplasm, benign, by site
   with malignant transformation C56- ☑
  desmoid (extra-abdominal) (*see also* Neoplasm, connective tissue, uncertain behavior)
   abdominal — *see* Neoplasm, connective tissue, uncertain behavior
  embolus — *see* Neoplasm, secondary, by site
  embryonal (mixed) (*see also* Neoplasm, uncertain behavior, by site)
   liver C22.7
  endodermal sinus
   specified site — *see* Neoplasm, malignant, by site
   unspecified site
    female C56.- ☑
    male C62.90
  epithelial
   benign — *see* Neoplasm, benign, by site
   malignant — *see* Neoplasm, malignant, by site
  Ewing's — *see* Neoplasm, bone, malignant, by site
  fatty — *see* Lipoma
  fibroid — *see* Leiomyoma
  G cell
   malignant
    pancreas C25.4
    specified site NEC — *see* Neoplasm, malignant, by site
    unspecified site C25.4
   specified site — *see* Neoplasm, uncertain behavior, by site
   unspecified site D37.8
  germ cell (*see also* Neoplasm, malignant, by site)
   mixed — *see* Neoplasm, malignant, by site
  ghost cell, odontogenic — *see* Cyst, calcifying odontogenic
  giant cell (*see also* Neoplasm, uncertain behavior, by site)
   bone D48.0
    malignant — *see* Neoplasm, bone, malignant
   chondromatous — *see* Neoplasm, bone, benign
   malignant — *see* Neoplasm, malignant, by site
   soft parts — *see* Neoplasm, connective tissue, uncertain behavior
    malignant — *see* Neoplasm, connective tissue, malignant
  glomus D18.00
   intra-abdominal D18.03
   intracranial D18.02
   jugulare D44.7
    malignant C75.5
   skin D18.01
   specified site NEC D18.09
  gonadal stromal — *see* Neoplasm, uncertain behavior, by site
  granular cell (*see also* Neoplasm, connective tissue, benign)
   malignant — *see* Neoplasm, connective tissue, malignant

Tumor — *continued*
  granulosa cell D39.1- ☑
    juvenile D39.1- ☑
    malignant C56- ☑
  granulosa cell-theca cell D39.1- ☑
    malignant C56- ☑
  Grawitz's C64- ☑
  hemorrhoidal — *see* Hemorrhoids
  hilar cell D27- ☑
  hilus cell D27- ☑
  Hurthle cell (benign) D34
    malignant C73
  hydatid — *see* Echinococcus
  hypernephroid (*see also* Neoplasm, uncertain behavior, by site)
  interstitial cell (*see also* Neoplasm, uncertain behavior, by site)
    benign — *see* Neoplasm, benign, by site
    malignant — *see* Neoplasm, malignant, by site
  intravascular bronchial alveolar D38.1
  islet cell — *see* Neoplasm, benign, by site
    malignant — *see* Neoplasm, malignant, by site
      pancreas C25.4
      specified site NEC — *see* Neoplasm, malignant, by site
      unspecified site C25.4
    pancreas D13.7
    specified site NEC — *see* Neoplasm, benign, by site
    unspecified site D13.7
  juxtaglomerular D41.0- ☑
  Klatskin's C22.1
  Krukenberg's C79.6- ☑
  Leydig cell — *see* Neoplasm, uncertain behavior, by site
    benign — *see* Neoplasm, benign, by site
      specified site — *see* Neoplasm, benign, by site
      unspecified site
        female D27.9
        male D29.20
    malignant — *see* Neoplasm, malignant, by site
      specified site — *see* Neoplasm, malignant, by site
      unspecified site
        female C56.9
        male C62.90
    specified site — *see* Neoplasm, uncertain behavior, by site
    unspecified site
      female D39.10
      male D40.10
  lipid cell, ovary D27- ☑
  lipoid cell, ovary D27- ☑
  malignant (*see also* Neoplasm, malignant, by site) C80.1
    fusiform cell (type) C80.1
    giant cell (type) C80.1
    localized, plasma cell — *see* Plasmacytoma, solitary
    mixed NEC C80.1
    small cell (type) C80.1
    spindle cell (type) C80.1
    unclassified C80.1
  mast cell D47.0
    malignant C96.2
  melanotic, neuroectodermal — *see* Neoplasm, benign, by site
  Merkel cell — *see* Carcinoma, Merkel cell
  mesenchymal
    malignant — *see* Neoplasm, connective tissue, malignant
    mixed — *see* Neoplasm, connective tissue, uncertain behavior
  mesodermal, mixed (*see also* Neoplasm, malignant, by site)
    liver C22.4
  mesonephric (*see also* Neoplasm, uncertain behavior, by site)
    malignant — *see* Neoplasm, malignant, by site
  metastatic
    from specified site — *see* Neoplasm, malignant, by site
    of specified site — *see* Neoplasm, malignant, by site
    to specified site — *see* Neoplasm, secondary, by site
  mixed NEC (*see also* Neoplasm, benign, by site)
    malignant — *see* Neoplasm, malignant, by site

Tumor — *continued*
  mucinous of low malignant potential
    specified site — *see* Neoplasm, malignant, by site
    unspecified site C56.9
  mucocarcinoid
    specified site — *see* Neoplasm, malignant, by site
    unspecified site C18.1
  mucoepidermoid — *see* Neoplasm, uncertain behavior, by site
  Müllerian, mixed
    specified site — *see* Neoplasm, malignant, by site
    unspecified site C54.9
  myoepithelial — *see* Neoplasm, benign, by site
  neuroectodermal (peripheral) — *see* Neoplasm, malignant, by site
    primitive
      specified site — *see* Neoplasm, malignant, by site
      unspecified site C71.9
  neuroendocrine D3A.8 (*following* D36)
    malignant poorly differentiated C7A.1 (*following* C75)
    secondary NEC C7B.8 (*following* C75)
    specified NEC C7A.8 (*following* C75)
  neurogenic olfactory C30.0
  nonencapsulated sclerosing C73
  odontogenic (adenomatoid) (benign) (calcifying epithelial) (keratocystic) (squamous) — *see* Cyst, calcifying odontogenic
    malignant C41.1
      upper jaw (bone) C41.0
  ovarian stromal D39.1- ☑
  ovary, in pregnancy — *see* Pregnancy, complicated by
  pacinian — *see* Neoplasm, skin, benign
  Pancoast's — *see* Pancoast's syndrome
  papillary (*see also* Papilloma)
    cystic D37.9
    mucinous of low malignant potential C56- ☑
      specified site — *see* Neoplasm, malignant, by site
      unspecified site C56.9
    serous of low malignant potential
      specified site — *see* Neoplasm, malignant, by site
      unspecified site C56.9
  pelvic, in pregnancy or childbirth — *see* Pregnancy, complicated by
  phantom F45.8
  phyllodes D48.6- ☑
    benign D24- ☑
    malignant — *see* Neoplasm, breast, malignant
  Pindborg — *see* Cyst, calcifying odontogenic
  placental site trophoblastic D39.2
  plasma cell (malignant) (localized) — *see* Plasmacytoma, solitary
  polyvesicular vitelline
    specified site — *see* Neoplasm, malignant, by site
    unspecified site
      female C56.9
      male C62.90
  Pott's puffy — *see* Osteomyelitis, specified NEC
  Rathke's pouch D44.3
  retinal anlage — *see* Neoplasm, benign, by site
  salivary gland type, mixed — *see* Neoplasm, salivary gland, benign
    malignant — *see* Neoplasm, salivary gland, malignant
  Sampson's N80.1
  Schmincke's — *see* Neoplasm, nasopharynx, malignant
  sclerosing stromal D27- ☑
  sebaceous — *see* Cyst, sebaceous
  secondary — *see* Neoplasm, secondary, by site
    carcinoid C7B.00 (*following* C75)
      bone C7B.03 (*following* C75)
      distant lymph nodes C7B.01 (*following* C75)
      liver C7B.02 (*following* C75)
      peritoneum C7B.04 (*following* C75)
      specified NEC C7B.09 (*following* C75)
    neuroendocrine NEC C7B.8 (*following* C75)
  serous of low malignant potential
    specified site — *see* Neoplasm, malignant, by site
    unspecified site C56.9
  Sertoli cell — *see* Neoplasm, benign, by site
    with lipid storage
      specified site — *see* Neoplasm, benign, by site
      unspecified site

Tumor — *continued*
  Sertoli cell — *see* Neoplasm, benign, by site — *continued*
    with lipid storage — *continued*
      unspecified site — *continued*
        female D27.9
        male D29.20
      specified site — *see* Neoplasm, benign, by site
      unspecified site
        female D27.9
        male D29.20
  Sertoli-Leydig cell — *see* Neoplasm, benign, by site
    specified site — *see* Neoplasm, benign, by site
    unspecified site
      female D27.9
      male D29.20
  sex cord (-stromal) — *see* Neoplasm, uncertain behavior, by site
    with annular tubules D39.1- ☑
  skin appendage — *see* Neoplasm, skin, benign
  smooth muscle — *see* Neoplasm, connective tissue, uncertain behavior
  soft tissue
    benign — *see* Neoplasm, connective tissue, benign
    malignant — *see* Neoplasm, connective tissue, malignant
  sternomastoid (congenital) Q68.0
  stromal
    endometrial D39.0
    gastric D48.1
      benign D21.4
      malignant C16.9
      uncertain behavior D48.1
    gastrointestinal
      benign D21.4
      malignant C49.4
      uncertain behavior D48.1
    intestine
      benign D21.4
      malignant C49.4
      uncertain behavior D48.1
    ovarian D39.1- ☑
    stomach
      benign D21.4
      malignant C16.9
      uncertain behavior D48.1
  sweat gland (*see also* Neoplasm, skin, uncertain behavior)
    benign — *see* Neoplasm, skin, benign
    malignant — *see* Neoplasm, skin, malignant
  syphilitic, brain A52.17
  testicular D40.10
  testicular stromal D40.1- ☑
  theca cell D27.- ☑
  theca cell-granulosa cell D39.1- ☑
  Triton, malignant — *see* Neoplasm, nerve, malignant
  trophoblastic, placental site D39.2
  turban D23.4
  uterus (body), in pregnancy or childbirth — *see* Pregnancy, complicated by, tumor, uterus
  vagina, in pregnancy or childbirth — *see* Pregnancy, complicated by
  varicose — *see* Varix
  von Recklinghausen's — *see* Neurofibromatosis
  vulva or perineum, in pregnancy or childbirth — *see* Pregnancy, complicated by
    causing obstructed labor O65.5
  Warthin's — *see* Neoplasm, salivary gland, benign
  Wilms' C64- ☑
  yolk sac — *see* Neoplasm, malignant, by site
    specified site — *see* Neoplasm, malignant, by site
    unspecified site
      female C56.9
      male C62.90
Tumor lysis syndrome (following antineoplastic chemotherapy) (spontaneous) NEC E88.3
Tumorlet — *see* Neoplasm, uncertain behavior, by site
Tungiasis B88.1
Tunica vasculosa lentis Q12.2
Turban tumor D23.4
Türck's trachoma J37.0
Turner-Kieser syndrome Q79.8
Turner-like syndrome Q87.1
Turner's
  hypoplasia (tooth) K00.4
  syndrome Q96.9
    specified NEC Q96.8

308
☑ Additional Character Required — Refer to the Tabular List for Character Selection
▽ Subterms under main terms may continue to next column or page

Turner's — *continued*
  tooth K00.4
Turner-Ullrich syndrome Q96.9
Tussis convulsiva — *see* Whooping cough
Twiddler's syndrome (due to)
  automatic implantable defibrillatorT82.198
  cardiac pacemaker T82.198 ☑
Twilight state
  epileptic F05
  psychogenic F44.89
Twin (newborn) (*see also* Newborn, twin)
  conjoined Q89.4
  pregnancy — *see* Pregnancy, twin, conjoined
Twinning, teeth K00.2
Twist, twisted
  bowel, colon or intestine K56.2
  hair (congenital) Q84.1
  mesentery K56.2
  omentum K56.2
  organ or site, congenital NEC — *see* Anomaly, by site
  ovarian pedicle — *see* Torsion, ovary
Twitching R25.3
Tylosis (acquired) L84
  buccalis K13.29
  linguae K13.29
  palmaris et plantaris (congenital) (inherited) Q82.8
    acquired L85.1
Tympanism R14.0
Tympanites (abdominal) (intestinal) R14.0
Tympanitis — *see* Myringitis
Tympanosclerosis H74.0 ☑
Tympanum — *see* condition
Tympany
  abdomen R14.0
  chest R09.89
Type A behavior pattern Z73.1
Typhlitis — *see* Appendicitis
Typhoenteritis — *see* Typhoid
Typhoid (abortive) (ambulant) (any site) (clinical) (fever) (hemorrhagic) (infection) (intermittent) (malignant) (rheumatic) (Widal negative) A01.00
  with pneumonia A01.03
  abdominal A01.09
  arthritis A01.04
  carrier (suspected) of Z22.0
  cholecystitis (current) A01.09
  endocarditis A01.02
  heart involvement A01.02
  inoculation reaction — *see* Complications, vaccination
  meningitis A01.01
  mesenteric lymph nodes A01.09
  myocarditis A01.02
  osteomyelitis A01.05
  perichondritis, larynx A01.09
  pneumonia A01.03
  specified NEC A01.09
  spine A01.05
  ulcer (perforating) A01.09
Typhomalaria (fever) — *see* Malaria
Typhomania A01.00
Typhoperitonitis A01.09
Typhus (fever) A75.9
  abdominal, abdominalis — *see* Typhoid
  African tick A77.1
  amarillic A95.9
  brain A75.9 [G94]
  cerebral A75.9 [G94]
  classical A75.0
  due to Rickettsia
    prowazekii A75.0
      recrudescent A75.1
    tsutsugamushi A75.3
    typhi A75.2
  endemic (flea-borne) A75.2
  epidemic (louse-borne) A75.0
  exanthematicus SAI A75.0
    brillii SAI A75.1
    mexicanus SAI A75.2
    typhus murinus A75.2
  exanthematic NEC A75.0
  flea-borne A75.2
  India tick A77.1
  Kenya (tick) A77.1
  louse-borne A75.0
  Mexican A75.2
  mite-borne A75.3
  murine A75.2
  North Asian tick-borne A77.2

Typhus — *continued*
  petechial A75.9
  Queensland tick A77.3
  rat A75.2
  recrudescent A75.1
  recurrens — *see* Fever, relapsing
  Sao Paulo A77.0
  scrub (China) (India) (Malaysia) (New Guinea) A75.3
  shop (of Malaysia) A75.2
  Siberian tick A77.2
  tick-borne A77.9
  tropical (mite-borne) A75.3
Tyrosinemia E70.21
  newborn, transitory P74.5
Tyrosinosis E70.21
Tyrosinuria E70.29

U

Uhl's anomaly or disease Q24.8
Ulcer, ulcerated, ulcerating, ulceration, ulcerative
  alveolar process M27.3
  amebic (intestine) A06.1
    skin A06.7
  anastomotic — *see* Ulcer, gastrojejunal
  anorectal K62.6
  antral — *see* Ulcer, stomach
  anus (sphincter) (solitary) K62.6
  aorta — *see* Aneurysm
  aphthous (oral) (recurrent) K12.0
    genital organ(s)
      female N76.6
      male N50.8
  artery I77.2
  atrophic — *see* Ulcer, skin
    decubitus — *see* Ulcer, pressure, by site
  back L98.429
    with
      bone necrosis L98.424
      exposed fat layer L98.422
      muscle necrosis L98.423
      skin breakdown only L98.421
  Barrett's (esophagus) K22.10
    with bleeding K22.11
  bile duct (common) (hepatic) K83.8
  bladder (solitary) (sphincter) NEC N32.89
    bilharzial B65.9 [N33]
    in schistosomiasis (bilharzial) B65.9 [N33]
    submucosal — *see* Cystitis, interstitial
    tuberculous A18.12
  bleeding K27.4
  bone — *see* Osteomyelitis, specified type NEC
  bowel — *see* Ulcer, intestine
  breast N61
  bronchus J98.09
  buccal (cavity) (traumatic) K12.1
  Buruli A31.1
  buttock L98.419
    with
      bone necrosis L98.414
      exposed fat layer L98.412
      muscle necrosis L98.413
      skin breakdown only L98.411
  cancerous — *see* Neoplasm, malignant, by site
  cardia K22.10
    with bleeding K22.11
  cardioesophageal (peptic) K22.10
    with bleeding K22.11
  cecum — *see* Ulcer, intestine
  cervix (uteri) (decubitus) (trophic) N86
    with cervicitis N72
  chancroidal A57
  chiclero B55.1
  chronic (cause unknown) — *see* Ulcer, skin
  Cochin-China B55.1
  colon — *see* Ulcer, intestine
  conjunctiva H10.89
  cornea H16.00- ☑
    with hypopyon H16.03- ☑
    central H16.01- ☑
    dendritic (herpes simplex) B00.52
    marginal H16.04- ☑
    Mooren's H16.05- ☑
    mycotic H16.06- ☑
    perforated H16.07- ☑
    ring H16.02- ☑
    tuberculous (phlyctenular) A18.52

Ulcer, ulcerated, ulcerating, ulceration, ulcerative
  — *continued*
  corpus cavernosum (chronic) N48.5
  crural — *see* Ulcer, lower limb
  Curling's — *see* Ulcer, peptic, acute
  Cushing's — *see* Ulcer, peptic, acute
  cystic duct K82.8
  cystitis (interstitial) — *see* Cystitis, interstitial
  decubitus — *see* Ulcer, pressure, by site
  dendritic, cornea (herpes simplex) B00.52
  diabetes, diabetic — *see* Diabetes, ulcer
  Dieulafoy's K25.0
  due to
    infection NEC — *see* Ulcer, skin
    radiation NEC L59.8
    trophic disturbance (any region) — *see* Ulcer, skin
    X-ray L58.1
  duodenum, duodenal (eroded) (peptic) K26.9
    with
      hemorrhage K26.4
        and perforation K26.6
      perforation K26.5
    acute K26.3
      with
        hemorrhage K26.0
          and perforation K26.2
        perforation K26.1
    chronic K26.7
      with
        hemorrhage K26.4
          and perforation K26.6
        perforation K26.5
  dysenteric A09
  elusive — *see* Cystitis, interstitial
  endocarditis (acute) (chronic) (subacute) I28.8
  epiglottis J38.7
  esophagus (peptic) K22.10
    with bleeding K22.11
    due to
      aspirin K22.10
        with bleeding K22.11
      gastrointestinal reflux disease K21.0
      ingestion of chemical or medicament K22.10
        with bleeding K22.11
      fungal K22.10
        with bleeding K22.11
      infective K22.10
        with bleeding K22.11
    varicose — *see* Varix, esophagus
  eyelid (region) H01.8
  fauces J39.2
  Fenwick (-Hunner) (solitary) — *see* Cystitis, interstitial
  fistulous — *see* Ulcer, skin
  foot (indolent) (trophic) — *see* Ulcer, lower limb
  frambesial, initial A66.0
  frenum (tongue) K14.0
  gallbladder or duct K82.8
  gangrenous — *see* Gangrene
  gastric — *see* Ulcer, stomach
  gastrocolic — *see* Ulcer, gastrojejunal
  gastroduodenal — *see* Ulcer, peptic
  gastroesophageal — *see* Ulcer, stomach
  gastrointestinal — *see* Ulcer, gastrojejunal
  gastrojejunal (peptic) K28.9
    with
      hemorrhage K28.4
        and perforation K28.6
      perforation K28.5
    acute K28.3
      with
        hemorrhage K28.0
          and perforation K28.2
        perforation K28.1
    chronic K28.7
      with
        hemorrhage K28.4
          and perforation K28.6
        perforation K28.5
  gastrojejunocolic — *see* Ulcer, gastrojejunal
  gingiva K06.8
  gingivitis K05.10
    nonplaque induced K05.11
    plaque induced K05.10
  glottis J38.7
  granuloma of pudenda A58
  gum K06.8
  gumma, due to yaws A66.4
  heel — *see* Ulcer, lower limb

Ulcer, ulcerated, ulcerating, ulceration, ulcerative — *continued*

hemorrhoid (*see also* Hemorrhoids, by degree) K64.8
Hunner's — *see* Cystitis, interstitial
hypopharynx J39.2
hypopyon (chronic) (subacute) — *see* Ulcer, cornea, with hypopyon
hypostaticum — *see* Ulcer, varicose
ileum — *see* Ulcer, intestine
intestine, intestinal K63.3
  with perforation K63.1
  amebic A06.1
  duodenal — *see* Ulcer, duodenum
  granulocytopenic (with hemorrhage) — *see* Neutropenia
  marginal — *see* Ulcer, gastrojejunal
  perforating K63.1
    newborn P78.0
  primary, small intestine K63.3
  rectum K62.6
  stercoraceous, stercoral K63.3
  tuberculous A18.32
  typhoid (fever) — *see* Typhoid
  varicose I86.8
jejunum, jejunal — *see* Ulcer, gastrojejunal
keratitis — *see* Ulcer, cornea
knee — *see* Ulcer, lower limb
labium (majus) (minus) N76.6
laryngitis — *see* Laryngitis
larynx (aphthous) (contact) J38.7
  diphtheritic A36.2
leg — *see* Ulcer, lower limb
lip K13.0
Lipschütz's N76.6
lower limb (atrophic) (chronic) (neurogenic) (perforating) (pyogenic) (trophic) (tropical) L97.909
  with
    bone necrosis L97.904
    exposed fat layer L97.902
    muscle necrosis L97.903
    skin breakdown only L97.901
  ankle L97.309
    with
      bone necrosis L97.304
      exposed fat layer L97.302
      muscle necrosis L97.303
      skin breakdown only L97.301
    left L97.329
      with
        bone necrosis L97.324
        exposed fat layer L97.322
        muscle necrosis L97.323
        skin breakdown only L97.321
    right L97.319
      with
        bone necrosis L97.314
        exposed fat layer L97.312
        muscle necrosis L97.313
        skin breakdown only L97.311
  calf L97.209
    with
      bone necrosis L97.204
      exposed fat layer L97.202
      muscle necrosis L97.203
      skin breakdown only L97.201
    left L97.229
      with
        bone necrosis L97.224
        exposed fat layer L97.222
        muscle necrosis L97.223
        skin breakdown only L97.221
    right L97.219
      with
        bone necrosis L97.214
        exposed fat layer L97.212
        muscle necrosis L97.213
        skin breakdown only L97.211
  decubitus — *see* Ulcer, pressure, by site
  foot specified NEC L97.509
    with
      bone necrosis L97.504
      exposed fat layer L97.502
      muscle necrosis L97.503
      skin breakdown only L97.501
    left L97.529
      with
        bone necrosis L97.524
        exposed fat layer L97.522

Ulcer, ulcerated, ulcerating, ulceration, ulcerative — *continued*

lower limb — *continued*
  foot specified — *continued*
    left — *continued*
      with — *continued*
        muscle necrosis L97.523
        skin breakdown only L97.521
    right L97.519
      with
        bone necrosis L97.514
        exposed fat layer L97.512
        muscle necrosis L97.513
        skin breakdown only L97.511
  heel L97.409
    with
      bone necrosis L97.404
      exposed fat layer L97.402
      muscle necrosis L97.403
      skin breakdown only L97.401
    left L97.429
      with
        bone necrosis L97.424
        exposed fat layer L97.422
        muscle necrosis L97.423
        skin breakdown only L97.421
    right L97.419
      with
        bone necrosis L97.414
        exposed fat layer L97.412
        muscle necrosis L97.413
        skin breakdown only L97.411
  left L97.929
    with
      bone necrosis L97.924
      exposed fat layer L97.922
      muscle necrosis L97.923
      skin breakdown only L97.921
  leprous A30.1
  lower leg NOS L97.909
    with
      bone necrosis L97.904
      exposed fat layer L97.902
      muscle necrosis L97.903
      skin breakdown only L97.901
    left L97.929
      with
        bone necrosis L97.924
        exposed fat layer L97.922
        muscle necrosis L97.923
        skin breakdown only L97.921
    right L97.919
      with
        bone necrosis L97.914
        exposed fat layer L97.912
        muscle necrosis L97.913
        skin breakdown only L97.911
  specified site NEC L97.809
    with
      bone necrosis L97.804
      exposed fat layer L97.802
      muscle necrosis L97.803
      skin breakdown only L97.801
    left L97.829
      with
        bone necrosis L97.824
        exposed fat layer L97.822
        muscle necrosis L97.823
        skin breakdown only L97.821
    right L97.819
      with
        bone necrosis L97.814
        exposed fat layer L97.812
        muscle necrosis L97.813
        skin breakdown only L97.811
  midfoot L97.409
    with
      bone necrosis L97.404
      exposed fat layer L97.402
      muscle necrosis L97.403
      skin breakdown only L97.401
    left L97.429
      with
        bone necrosis L97.424
        exposed fat layer L97.422
        muscle necrosis L97.423
        skin breakdown only L97.421

Ulcer, ulcerated, ulcerating, ulceration, ulcerative — *continued*

lower limb — *continued*
  midfoot — *continued*
    right L97.419
      with
        bone necrosis L97.414
        exposed fat layer L97.412
        muscle necrosis L97.413
        skin breakdown only L97.411
  right L97.919
    with
      bone necrosis L97.914
      exposed fat layer L97.912
      muscle necrosis L97.913
      skin breakdown only L97.911
  syphilitic A52.19
  thigh L97.109
    with
      bone necrosis L97.104
      exposed fat layer L97.102
      muscle necrosis L97.103
      skin breakdown only L97.101
    left L97.129
      with
        bone necrosis L97.124
        exposed fat layer L97.122
        muscle necrosis L97.123
        skin breakdown only L97.121
    right L97.119
      with
        bone necrosis L97.114
        exposed fat layer L97.112
        muscle necrosis L97.113
        skin breakdown only L97.111
  toe L97.509
    with
      bone necrosis L97.504
      exposed fat layer L97.502
      muscle necrosis L97.503
      skin breakdown only L97.501
    left L97.529
      with
        bone necrosis L97.524
        exposed fat layer L97.522
        muscle necrosis L97.523
        skin breakdown only L97.521
    right L97.519
      with
        bone necrosis L97.514
        exposed fat layer L97.512
        muscle necrosis L97.513
        skin breakdown only L97.511
  varicose — *see* Varix, leg, with, ulcer
luetic — *see* Ulcer, syphilitic
lung J98.4
  tuberculous — *see* Tuberculosis, pulmonary
malignant — *see* Neoplasm, malignant, by site
marginal NEC — *see* Ulcer, gastrojejunal
meatus (urinarius) N34.2
Meckel's diverticulum Q43.0
  malignant — *see* Table of Neoplasms, small intestine, malignant
Meleney's (chronic undermining) — *see* Ulcer, skin
Mooren's (cornea) — *see* Ulcer, cornea, Mooren's
mycobacterial (skin) A31.1
nasopharynx J39.2
neck, uterus N86
neurogenic NEC — *see* Ulcer, skin
nose, nasal (passage) (infective) (septum) J34.0
  skin — *see* Ulcer, skin
  spirochetal A69.8
  varicose (bleeding) I86.8
oral mucosa (traumatic) K12.1
palate (soft) K12.1
penis (chronic) N48.5
peptic (site unspecified) K27.9
  with
    hemorrhage K27.4
      and perforation K27.6
    perforation K27.5
  acute K27.3
    with
      hemorrhage K27.0
        and perforation K27.2
      perforation K27.1
  chronic K27.7

Ulcer, ulcerated, ulcerating, ulceration, ulcerative
— *continued*
  peptic — *continued*
    chronic — *continued*
      with
        hemorrhage K27.4
          and perforation K27.6
        perforation K27.5
      esophagus K22.10
        with bleeding K22.11
      newborn P78.82
    perforating K27.5
    skin — *see* Ulcer, skin
  peritonsillar J35.8
  phagedenic (tropical) — *see* Ulcer, skin
  pharynx J39.2
  phlebitis — *see* Phlebitis
  plaster — *see* Ulcer, pressure, by site
  popliteal space — *see* Ulcer, lower limb
  postpyloric — *see* Ulcer, duodenum
  prepuce N47.7
  prepyloric — *see* Ulcer, stomach
  pressure (pressure area) L89.9- ☑
    ankle L89.5- ☑
    back L89.1- ☑
    buttock L89.3- ☑
    coccyx L89.15- ☑
    contiguous site of back, buttock, hip L89.4- ☑
    elbow L89.0- ☑
    face L89.81- ☑
    head L89.81- ☑
    heel L89.6- ☑
    hip L89.2- ☑
    sacral region (tailbone) L89.15- ☑
    specified site NEC L89.89- ☑
    stage 1 (healing) (pre-ulcer skin changes limited
      to persistent focal edema)
      ankle L89.5- ☑
      back L89.1- ☑
      buttock L89.3- ☑
      coccyx L89.15- ☑
      contiguous site of back, buttock, hip L89.4- ☑
      elbow L89.0- ☑
      face L89.81- ☑
      head L89.81- ☑
      heel L89.6- ☑
      hip L89.2- ☑
      sacral region (tailbone) L89.15- ☑
      specified site NEC L89.89- ☑
    stage 2 (healing) (abrasion, blister, partial thickness
      skin loss involving epidermis and/or dermis)
      ankle L89.5- ☑
      back L89.1- ☑
      buttock L89.3- ☑
      coccyx L89.15- ☑
      contiguous site of back, buttock, hip L89.4- ☑
      elbow L89.0- ☑
      face L89.81- ☑
      head L89.81- ☑
      heel L89.6- ☑
      hip L89.2- ☑
      sacral region (tailbone) L89.15- ☑
      specified site NEC L89.89- ☑
    stage 3 (healing) (full thickness skin loss involving
      damage or necrosis of subcutaneous tissue)
      ankle L89.5- ☑
      back L89.1- ☑
      buttock L89.3- ☑
      coccyx L89.15- ☑
      contiguous site of back, buttock, hip L89.4- ☑
      elbow L89.0- ☑
      face L89.81- ☑
      head L89.81- ☑
      heel L89.6- ☑
      hip L89.2- ☑
      sacral region (tailbone) L89.15- ☑
      specified site NEC L89.89- ☑
    stage 4 (healing) (necrosis of soft tissues through
      to underlying muscle, tendon, or bone)
      ankle L89.5- ☑
      back L89.1- ☑
      buttock L89.3- ☑
      coccyx L89.15- ☑
      contiguous site of back, buttock, hip L89.4- ☑
      elbow L89.0- ☑
      face L89.81- ☑

Ulcer, ulcerated, ulcerating, ulceration, ulcerative
— *continued*
  pressure — *continued*
    stage 4 — *continued*
      head L89.81- ☑
      heel L89.6- ☑
      hip L89.2- ☑
      sacral region (tailbone) L89.15- ☑
      specified site NEC L89.89- ☑
    unspecified stage
      ankle L89.5- ☑
      back L89.1- ☑
      buttock L89.3- ☑
      coccyx L89.15- ☑
      contiguous site of back, buttock, hip L89.4- ☑
      elbow L89.0- ☑
      face L89.81- ☑
      head L89.81- ☑
      heel L89.6- ☑
      hip L89.2- ☑
      sacral region (tailbone) L89.15- ☑
      specified site NEC L89.89- ☑
    unstageable
      ankle L89.5- ☑
      back L89.1- ☑
      buttock L89.3- ☑
      coccyx L89.15- ☑
      contiguous site of back, buttock, hip L89.4- ☑
      elbow L89.0- ☑
      face L89.81- ☑
      head L89.81- ☑
      heel L89.6- ☑
      hip L89.2- ☑
      sacral region (tailbone) L89.15- ☑
      specified site NEC L89.89- ☑
  primary of intestine K63.3
    with perforation K63.1
  prostate N41.9
  pyloric — *see* Ulcer, stomach
  rectosigmoid K63.3
    with perforation K63.1
  rectum (sphincter) (solitary) K62.6
    stercoraceous, stercoral K62.6
  retina — *see* Inflammation, chorioretinal
  rodent (*see also* Neoplasm, skin, malignant)
  sclera — *see* Scleritis
  scrofulous (tuberculous) A18.2
  scrotum N50.8
    tuberculous A18.15
    varicose I86.1
  seminal vesicle N50.8
  sigmoid — *see* Ulcer, intestine
  skin (atrophic) (chronic) (neurogenic) (non-healing)
    (perforating) (pyogenic) (trophic) (tropical)
    L98.499
    with gangrene — *see* Gangrene
    amebic A06.7
    back — *see* Ulcer, back
    buttock — *see* Ulcer, buttock
    decubitus — *see* Ulcer, pressure
    lower limb — *see* Ulcer, lower limb
    mycobacterial A31.1
    specified site NEC L98.499
      with
        bone necrosis L98.494
        exposed fat layer L98.492
        muscle necrosis L98.493
        skin breakdown only L98.491
    tuberculous (primary) A18.4
    varicose — *see* Ulcer, varicose
  sloughing — *see* Ulcer, skin
  solitary, anus or rectum (sphincter) K62.6
  sore throat J02.9
    streptococcal J02.0
  spermatic cord N50.8
  spine (tuberculous) A18.01
  stasis (venous) — *see* Varix, leg, with, ulcer
    without varicose veins I87.2
  stercoraceous, stercoral K63.3
    with perforation K63.1
    anus or rectum K62.6
  stoma, stomal — *see* Ulcer, gastrojejunal
  stomach (eroded) (peptic) (round) K25.9
    with
      hemorrhage K25.4
        and perforation K25.6
      perforation K25.5

Ulcer, ulcerated, ulcerating, ulceration, ulcerative
— *continued*
  stomach — *continued*
    acute K25.3
      with
        hemorrhage K25.0
          and perforation K25.2
        perforation K25.1
    chronic K25.7
      with
        hemorrhage K25.4
          and perforation K25.6
        perforation K25.5
  stomal — *see* Ulcer, gastrojejunal
  stomatitis K12.1
  stress — *see* Ulcer, peptic
  strumous (tuberculous) A18.2
  submucosal, bladder — *see* Cystitis, interstitial
  syphilitic (any site) (early) (secondary) A51.39
    late A52.79
      perforating A52.79
        foot A52.11
  testis N50.8
  thigh — *see* Ulcer, lower limb
  throat J39.2
    diphtheritic A36.0
  toe — *see* Ulcer, lower limb
  tongue (traumatic) K14.0
  tonsil J35.8
    diphtheritic A36.0
  trachea J39.8
  trophic — *see* Ulcer, skin
  tropical — *see* Ulcer, skin
  tuberculous — *see* Tuberculosis, ulcer
  tunica vaginalis N50.8
  turbinate J34.89
  typhoid (perforating) — *see* Typhoid
  unspecified site — *see* Ulcer, skin
  urethra (meatus) — *see* Urethritis
  uterus N85.8
    cervix N86
      with cervicitis N72
    neck N86
      with cervicitis N72
  vagina N76.5
    in Behçet's disease M35.2 [N77.0]
    pessary N89.8
  valve, heart I33.0
  varicose (lower limb, any part) (*see also* Varix, leg, with,
    ulcer)
    broad ligament I86.2
    esophagus — *see* Varix, esophagus
    inflamed or infected — *see* Varix, leg, with ulcer,
      with inflammation
    nasal septum I86.8
    perineum I86.3
    scrotum I86.1
    specified site NEC I86.8
    sublingual I86.0
    vulva I86.3
  vas deferens N50.8
  vulva (acute) (infectional) N76.6
    in (due to)
      Behçet's disease M35.2 [N77.0]
      herpesviral (herpes simplex) infection A60.04
      tuberculosis A18.18
  vulvobuccal, recurring N76.6
  X-ray L58.1
  yaws A66.4
Ulcerosa scarlatina A38.8
Ulcus (*see also* Ulcer)
  cutis tuberculosum A18.4
  duodeni — *see* Ulcer, duodenum
  durum (syphilitic) A51.0
    extragenital A51.2
  gastrojejunale — *see* Ulcer, gastrojejunal
  hypostaticum — *see* Ulcer, varicose
  molle (cutis) (skin) A57
  serpens corneae — *see* Ulcer, cornea, central
  ventriculi — *see* Ulcer, stomach
Ulegyria Q04.8
Ulerythema
  ophryogenes, congenital Q84.2
  sycosiforme L73.8
Ullrich (-Bonnevie)(-Turner) **syndrome** Q87.1
Ullrich-Feichtiger syndrome Q87.0
Ulnar — *see* condition
Ulorrhagia, ulorrhea K06.8

Umbilicus, umbilical — *see* condition
Unacceptable
 contours of tooth KØ8.54
 morphology of tooth KØ8.54
Unavailability (of)
 bed at medical facility Z75.1
 health service-related agencies Z75.4
 medical facilities (at) Z75.3
  due to
   investigation by social service agency Z75.2
   lack of services at home Z75.Ø
   remoteness from facility Z75.3
   waiting list Z75.1
  home Z75.Ø
  outpatient clinic Z75.3
 schooling Z55.1
 social service agencies Z75.4
Uncinaria americana infestation B76.1
Uncinariasis B76.9
Uncongenial work Z56.5
Unconscious (ness) — *see* Coma
Under observation — *see* Observation
Underachievement in school Z55.3
Underdevelopment (*see also* Undeveloped)
 nose Q3Ø.1
 sexual E3Ø.Ø
Underdosing (*see also* Table of Drugs and Chemicals,
  categories T36-T5Ø, with final character 6) Z91.14
 intentional NEC Z91.128
  due to financial hardship of patient Z91.12Ø
 unintentional NEC Z91.138
  due to patient's age related debility Z91.13Ø
Underfeeding, newborn P92.3
Underfill, endodontic M27.53
Underimmunization status Z28.3
Undernourishment — *see* Malnutrition
Undernutrition — *see* Malnutrition
Underweight R63.6
 for gestational age — *see* Light for dates
Underwood's disease P83.Ø
Undescended (*see also* Malposition, congenital)
 cecum Q43.3
 colon Q43.3
 testicle — *see* Cryptorchid
Undeveloped, undevelopment (*see also* Hypoplasia)
 brain (congenital) QØ2
 cerebral (congenital) QØ2
 heart Q24.8
 lung Q33.6
 testis E29.1
 uterus E3Ø.Ø
Undiagnosed (disease) R69
Undulant fever — *see* Brucellosis
Unemployment, anxiety concerning Z56.Ø
 threatened Z56.2
Unequal length (acquired) (limb) (*see also* Deformity,
  limb, unequal length)
 leg (*see also* Deformity, limb, unequal length)
  congenital Q72.9- ☑
Unextracted dental root KØ8.3
Unguis incarnatus L6Ø.Ø
Unhappiness R45.2
Unicornate uterus Q51.4
Unilateral (*see also* condition)
 development, breast N64.89
 organ or site, congenital NEC — *see* Agenesis, by site
Unilocular heart Q2Ø.8
Union, abnormal (*see also* Fusion)
 larynx and trachea Q34.8
Universal mesentery Q43.3
**Unrepairable overhanging of dental restorative
  materials** KØ8.52
Unsatisfactory
 restoration of tooth KØ8.5Ø
  specified NEC KØ8.59
 sample of cytologic smear
  anus R85.615
  cervix R87.615
  vagina R87.625
 surroundings Z59.1
 work Z56.5
Unsoundness of mind — *see* Psychosis
Unstable
 back NEC — *see* Instability, joint, spine
 hip (congenital) Q65.6
  acquired — *see* Derangement, joint, specified type
   NEC, hip

Unstable — *continued*
 joint — *see* Instability, joint
  secondary to removal of joint prosthesis M96.89
 lie (mother) O32.Ø ☑
 lumbosacral (joint) (congenital)
  acquired — *see* subcategory M53.2 ☑
 sacroiliac — *see* subcategory M53.2 ☑
 spine NEC — *see* Instability, joint, spine
Unsteadiness on feet R26.81
Untruthfulness, child problem F91.8
Unverricht (-Lundborg) **disease or epilepsy** — *see*
  Epilepsy, generalized, idiopathic
Unwanted pregnancy Z64.Ø
Upbringing, institutional Z62.22
 away from parents NEC Z62.29
 in care of non-parental family member Z62.21
 in foster care Z62.21
 in orphanage or group home Z62.22
 in welfare custody Z62.21
Upper respiratory — *see* condition
Upset
 gastric K3Ø
 gastrointestinal K3Ø
  psychogenic F45.8
 intestinal (large) (small) K59.9
  psychogenic F45.8
 menstruation N93.9
 mental F48.9
 stomach K3Ø
  psychogenic F45.8
Urachus (*see also* condition)
 patent or persistent Q64.4
Urbach-Oppenheim disease (necrobiosis lipoidica diabeticorum) — *see* EØ8-E13 with .62Ø
Urbach's lipoid proteinosis E78.89
Urbach-Wiethe disease E78.89
Urban yellow fever A95.1
Urea
 blood, high — *see* Uremia
 cycle metabolism disorder — *see* Disorder, urea cycle
  metabolism
Uremia, uremic N19
 with
  ectopic or molar pregnancy OØ8.4
  polyneuropathy N18.9 [G63]
 chronic (*see also* Disease, kidney, chronic) N18.9
  due to hypertension — *see* Hypertensive, kidney
 complicating
  ectopic or molar pregnancy OØ8.4
 congenital P96.Ø
 extrarenal R39.2
 following ectopic or molar pregnancy OØ8.4
 newborn P96.Ø
 prerenal R39.2
Ureter, ureteral — *see* condition
Ureteralgia N23
Ureterectasis — *see* Hydroureter
Ureteritis N28.89
 cystica N28.86
 due to calculus N2Ø.1
  with calculus, kidney N2Ø.2
   with hydronephrosis N13.2
 gonococcal (acute) (chronic) A54.21
 nonspecific N28.89
Ureterocele N28.89
 congenital (orthotopic) Q62.31
 ectopic Q62.32
Ureterolith, ureterolithiasis — *see* Calculus, ureter
Ureterostomy
 attention to Z43.6
 status Z93.6
Urethra, urethral — *see* condition
Urethralgia R39.89
Urethritis (anterior) (posterior) N34.2
 calculous N21.1
 candidal B37.41
 chlamydial A56.Ø1
 diplococcal (gonococcal) A54.Ø1
  with abscess (accessory gland) (periurethral) A54.1
 gonococcal A54.Ø1
  with abscess (accessory gland) (periurethral) A54.1
 nongonococcal N34.1
  Reiter's — *see* Reiter's disease
 nonspecific N34.1
 nonvenereal N34.1
 postmenopausal N34.2
 puerperal O86.22

Urethritis — *continued*
 Reiter's — *see* Reiter's disease
 specified NEC N34.2
 trichomonal or due to Trichomonas (vaginalis) A59.Ø3
Urethrocele N81.Ø
 with
  cystocele — *see* Cystocele
  prolapse of uterus — *see* Prolapse, uterus
Urethrolithiasis (with colic or infection) N21.1
Urethrorectal — *see* condition
Urethrorrhagia N36.8
Urethrorrhea R36.9
Urethrostomy
 attention to Z43.6
 status Z93.6
Urethrotrigonitis — *see* Trigonitis
Urethrovaginal — *see* condition
Urgency
 fecal R15.2
 hypertensive — *see* Hypertension
 urinary N39.41
Urhidrosis, uridrosis L74.8
Uric acid in blood (increased) E79.Ø
Uricacidemia (asymptomatic) E79.Ø
Uricemia (asymptomatic) E79.Ø
Uricosuria R82.99
Urinary — *see* condition
Urination
 frequent R35.Ø
 painful R3Ø.9
Urine
 blood in — *see* Hematuria
 discharge, excessive R35.8
 enuresis, nonorganic origin F98.Ø
 extravasation R39.Ø
 frequency R35.Ø
 incontinence R32
  nonorganic origin F98.Ø
 intermittent stream R39.19
 pus in N39.Ø
 retention or stasis R33.9
  organic R33.8
   drug-induced R33.Ø
  psychogenic F45.8
 secretion
  deficient R34
  excessive R35.8
  frequency R35.Ø
 stream
  intermittent R39.19
  slowing R39.19
  splitting R39.13
  weak R39.12
Urinemia — *see* Uremia
Urinoma, urethra N36.8
Uroarthritis, infectious (Reiter's) — *see* Reiter's disease
Urodialysis R34
Urolithiasis — *see* Calculus, urinary
Uronephrosis — *see* Hydronephrosis
Uropathy N39.9
 obstructive N13.9
  specified NEC N13.8
 reflux N13.9
  specified NEC N13.8
 vesicoureteral reflux-associated — *see* Reflux, vesicoureteral
Urosepsis — *code to* condition
Urticaria L5Ø.9
 with angioneurotic edema T78.3 ☑
  hereditary D84.1
 allergic L5Ø.Ø
 cholinergic L5Ø.5
 chronic L5Ø.8
 cold, familial L5Ø.2
 contact L5Ø.6
 dermatographic L5Ø.3
 due to
  cold or heat L5Ø.2
  drugs L5Ø.Ø
  food L5Ø.Ø
  inhalants L5Ø.Ø
  plants L5Ø.6
  serum (*see also* Reaction, serum) T8Ø.69 ☑
 factitial L5Ø.8
 giant T78.3 ☑
  hereditary D84.1
 gigantea T78.3 ☑

Urticaria — continued
  idiopathic L50.1
  larynx T78.3 ☑
    hereditary D84.1
  neonatorum P83.8
  nonallergic L50.1
  papulosa (Hebra) L28.2
  pigmentosa Q82.2
  recurrent periodic L50.8
  serum (see also Reaction, serum) T80.69 ☑
  solar L56.3
  specified type NEC L50.8
  thermal (cold) (heat) L50.2
  vibratory L50.4
  xanthelasmoidea Q82.2
Use (of)
  alcohol F10.99
    with sleep disorder F10.982
    harmful — see Abuse, alcohol
  amphetamines — see Use, stimulant NEC
  caffeine — see Use, stimulant NEC
  cannabis F12.90
    with
      anxiety disorder F12.980
      intoxication F12.929
        with
          delirium F12.921
          perceptual disturbance F12.922
        uncomplicated F12.920
      other specified disorder F12.988
      psychosis F12.959
        delusions F12.950
        hallucinations F12.951
      unspecified disorder F12.99
  cocaine F14.90
    with
      anxiety disorder F14.980
      intoxication F14.929
        with
          delirium F14.921
          perceptual disturbance F14.922
        uncomplicated F14.920
      other specified disorder F14.988
      psychosis F14.959
        delusions F14.950
        hallucinations F14.951
      sexual dysfunction F14.981
      sleep disorder F14.982
      unspecified disorder F14.99
    harmful — see Abuse, drug, cocaine
  drug(s) NEC F19.90
    with sleep disorder F19.982
    harmful — see Abuse, drug, by type
  hallucinogen NEC F16.90
    with
      anxiety disorder F16.980
      intoxication F16.929
        with
          delirium F16.921
        uncomplicated F16.920
      mood disorder F16.94
      other specified disorder F16.988
      perception disorder (flashbacks) F16.983
      psychosis F16.959
        delusions F16.950
        hallucinations F16.951
      unspecified disorder F16.99
    harmful — see Abuse, drug, hallucinogen NEC
  inhalants F18.90
    with
      anxiety disorder F18.980
      intoxication F18.929
        with delirium F18.921
        uncomplicated F18.920
      mood disorder F18.94
      other specified disorder F18.988
      persisting dementia F18.97
      psychosis F18.959
        delusions F18.950
        hallucinations F18.951
      unspecified disorder F18.99
    harmful — see Abuse, drug, inhalant
  methadone F11.20
  nonprescribed drugs F19.90
    harmful — see Abuse, non-psychoactive substance
  opioid F11.90

Use — continued
  opioid — continued
    with
      disorder F11.99
        mood F11.94
        sleep F11.982
        specified type NEC F11.988
      intoxication F11.929
        with
          delirium F11.921
          perceptual disturbance F11.922
        uncomplicated F11.920
      withdrawal F11.93
    harmful — see Abuse, drug, opioid
  patent medicines F19.90
    harmful — see Abuse, non-psychoactive substance
  psychoactive drug NEC F19.90
    with
      anxiety disorder F19.980
      intoxication F19.929
        with
          delirium F19.921
          perceptual disturbance F19.922
        uncomplicated F19.920
      mood disorder F19.94
      other specified disorder F19.988
      persisting
        amnestic disorder F19.96
        dementia F19.97
      psychosis F19.959
        delusions F19.950
        hallucinations F19.951
      sexual dysfunction F19.981
      sleep disorder F19.982
      unspecified disorder F19.99
      withdrawal F19.939
        with
          delirium F19.931
          perceptual disturbance F19.932
        uncomplicated F19.930
    harmful — see Abuse, drug NEC, psychoactive NEC
  sedative, hypnotic, or anxiolytic F13.90
    with
      anxiety disorder F13.980
      intoxication F13.929
        with
          delirium F13.921
        uncomplicated F13.920
      other specified disorder F13.988
      persisting
        amnestic disorder F13.96
        dementia F13.97
      psychosis F13.959
        delusions F13.950
        hallucinations F13.951
      sexual dysfunction F13.981
      sleep disorder F13.982
      unspecified disorder F13.99
    harmful — see Abuse, drug, sedative, hypnotic, or anxiolytic
  stimulant NEC F15.90
    with
      anxiety disorder F15.980
      intoxication F15.929
        with
          delirium F15.921
          perceptual disturbance F15.922
        uncomplicated F15.920
      mood disorder F15.94
      other specified disorder F15.988
      psychosis F15.959
        delusions F15.950
        hallucinations F15.951
      sexual dysfunction F15.981
      sleep disorder F15.982
      unspecified disorder F15.99
      withdrawal F15.93
    harmful — see Abuse, drug, stimulant NEC
  tobacco Z72.0
    with dependence — see Dependence, drug, nicotine
  volatile solvents (see also Use, inhalant) F18.90
    harmful — see Abuse, drug, inhalant
Usher-Senear disease or syndrome L10.4
Uta B55.1
Uteromegaly N85.2
Uterovaginal — see condition
Uterovesical — see condition

Uveal — see condition
Uveitis (anterior) (see also Iridocyclitis)
  acute — see Iridocyclitis, acute
  chronic — see Iridocyclitis, chronic
  due to toxoplasmosis (acquired) B58.09
    congenital P37.1
  granulomatous — see Iridocyclitis, chronic
  heterochromic — see Cyclitis, Fuchs' heterochromic
  lens-induced — see Iridocyclitis, lens-induced
  posterior — see Chorioretinitis
  sympathetic H44.13- ☑
  syphilitic (secondary) A51.43
    congenital (early) A50.01
    late A52.71
  tuberculous A18.54
Uveoencephalitis — see Inflammation, chorioretinal
Uveokeratitis — see Iridocyclitis
Uveoparotitis D86.89
Uvula — see condition
Uvulitis (acute) (catarrhal) (chronic) (membranous) (suppurative) (ulcerative) K12.2

V

Vaccination (prophylactic)
  complication or reaction — see Complications, vaccination
  delayed Z28.9
  encounter for Z23
  not done — see Immunization, not done, because (of)
Vaccinia (generalized) (localized) T88.1 ☑
  without vaccination B08.011
  congenital P35.8
Vacuum, in sinus (accessory) (nasal) J34.89
Vagabond, vagabondage Z59.0
Vagabond's disease B85.1
Vagina, vaginal — see condition
Vaginalitis (tunica) (testis) N49.1
Vaginismus (reflex) N94.2
  functional F52.5
  nonorganic F52.5
  psychogenic F52.5
  secondary N94.2
Vaginitis (acute) (circumscribed) (diffuse) (emphysematous) (nonvenereal) (ulcerative) N76.0
  with ectopic or molar pregnancy O08.0
  amebic A06.82
  atrophic, postmenopausal N95.2
  bacterial N76.0
  blennorrhagic (gonococcal) A54.02
  candidal B37.3
  chlamydial A56.02
  chronic N76.1
  due to Trichomonas (vaginalis) A59.01
  following ectopic or molar pregnancy O08.0
  gonococcal A54.02
    with abscess (accessory gland) (periurethral) A54.1
  granuloma A58
  in (due to)
    candidiasis B37.3
    herpesviral (herpes simplex) infection A60.04
    pinworm infection B80 [N77.1]
  monilial B37.3
  mycotic (candidal) B37.3
  postmenopausal atrophic N95.2
  puerperal (postpartum) O86.13
  senile (atrophic) N95.2
  subacute or chronic N76.1
  syphilitic (early) A51.0
    late A52.76
  trichomonal A59.01
  tuberculous A18.18
Vaginosis — see Vaginitis
Vagotonia G52.2
Vagrancy Z59.0
VAIN — see Neoplasia, intraepithelial, vagina
Vallecula — see condition
Valley fever B38.0
Valsuani's disease — see Anemia, obstetric
Valve, valvular (formation) (see also condition)
  cerebral ventricle (communicating) in situ Z98.2
  cervix, internal os Q51.828
  congenital NEC — see Atresia, by site
  ureter (pelvic junction) (vesical orifice) Q62.39
  urethra (congenital) (posterior) Q64.2
Valvulitis (chronic) — see Endocarditis
Valvulopathy — see Endocarditis

Van Bogaert's leukoencephalopathy (sclerosing) (subacute) A81.1
Van Bogaert-Scherer-Epstein disease or syndrome E75.5
Van Buchem's syndrome M85.2
Van Creveld-von Gierke disease E74.01
Van der Hoeve (-de Kleyn) **syndrome** Q78.0
Van der Woude's syndrome Q38.0
Van Neck's disease or osteochondrosis M91.0
Vanishing lung J44.9
Vapor asphyxia or suffocation T59.9 ☑
  specified agent — see Table of Drugs and Chemicals
Variance, lethal ball, prosthetic heart valve T82.09 ☑
Variants, thalassemic D56.8
Variations in hair color L67.1
Varicella B01.9
  with
    complications NEC B01.89
    encephalitis B01.11
    encephalomyelitis B01.11
    meningitis B01.0
    myelitis B01.12
    pneumonia B01.2
  congenital P35.8
Varices — see Varix
Varicocele (scrotum) (thrombosed) I86.1
  ovary I86.2
  perineum I86.3
  spermatic cord (ulcerated) I86.1
Varicose
  aneurysm (ruptured) I77.0
  dermatitis — see Varix, leg, with, inflammation
  eczema — see Varix, leg, with, inflammation
  phlebitis — see Varix, with, inflammation
  tumor — see Varix
  ulcer (lower limb, any part) (see also Varix, leg, with, ulcer)
    anus (see also Hemorrhoids) K64.8
    esophagus — see Varix, esophagus
    inflamed or infected — see Varix, leg, with ulcer, with inflammation
    nasal septum I86.8
    perineum I86.3
    scrotum I86.1
    specified site NEC I86.8
  vein — see Varix
  vessel — see Varix, leg
Varicosis, varicosities, varicosity — see Varix
Variola (major) (minor) B03
Varioloid B03
Varix (lower limb) (ruptured) I83.90
  with
    edema I83.899
    inflammation I83.10
      with ulcer (venous) I83.209
    pain I83.819
    specified complication NEC I83.899
    stasis dermatitis I83.10
      with ulcer (venous) I83.209
    swelling I83.899
    ulcer I83.009
      with inflammation I83.209
  aneurysmal I77.0
  asymptomatic I83.9- ☑
  bladder I86.2
  broad ligament I86.2
  complicating
    childbirth (lower extremity) O87.4
      anus or rectum O87.2
      genital (vagina, vulva or perineum) O87.8
    pregnancy (lower extremity) O22.0- ☑
      anus or rectum O22.4- ☑
      genital (vagina, vulva or perineum) O22.1- ☑
    puerperium (lower extremity) O87.4
      anus or rectum O87.2
      genital (vagina, vulva, perineum) O87.8
  congenital (any site) Q27.8
  esophagus (idiopathic) (primary) (ulcerated) I85.00
    bleeding I85.01
    congenital Q27.8
    in (due to)
      alcoholic liver disease I85.10
        bleeding I85.11
      cirrhosis of liver I85.10
        bleeding I85.11
      portal hypertension I85.10
        bleeding I85.11

Varix — continued
  esophagus — continued
    in — continued
      schistosomiasis I85.10
        bleeding I85.11
      toxic liver disease I85.10
        bleeding I85.11
    secondary I85.10
      bleeding I85.11
  gastric I86.4
  inflamed or infected I83.10
    ulcerated I83.209
  labia (majora) I86.3
  leg (asymptomatic) I83.90
    with
      edema I83.899
      inflammation I83.10
        with ulcer — see Varix, leg, with, ulcer, with inflammation by site
      pain I83.819
      specified complication NEC I83.899
      swelling I83.899
      ulcer I83.009
        with inflammation I83.209
        ankle I83.003
          with inflammation I83.203
        calf I83.002
          with inflammation I83.202
        foot NEC I83.005
          with inflammation I83.205
        heel I83.004
          with inflammation I83.204
        lower leg NEC I83.008
          with inflammation I83.208
        midfoot I83.004
          with inflammation I83.204
        thigh I83.001
          with inflammation I83.201
    bilateral (asymptomatic) I83.93
      with
        edema I83.893
        pain I83.813
        specified complication NEC I83.893
        swelling I83.893
        ulcer I83.009
          with inflammation I83.209
    left (asymptomatic) I83.92
      with
        edema I83.892
        inflammation I83.12
          with ulcer — see Varix, leg, with, ulcer, with inflammation by site
        pain I83.812
        specified complication NEC I83.892
        swelling I83.892
        ulcer I83.029
          with inflammation I83.229
          ankle I83.023
            with inflammation I83.223
          calf I83.022
            with inflammation I83.222
          foot NEC I83.025
            with inflammation I83.225
          heel I83.024
            with inflammation I83.224
          lower leg NEC I83.028
            with inflammation I83.228
          midfoot I83.024
            with inflammation I83.224
          thigh I83.021
            with inflammation I83.221
    right (asymptomatic) I83.91
      with
        edema I83.891
        inflammation I83.11
          with ulcer — see Varix, leg, with, ulcer, with inflammation by site
        pain I83.811
        specified complication NEC I83.891
        swelling I83.891
        ulcer I83.019
          with inflammation I83.219
          ankle I83.013
            with inflammation I83.213
          calf I83.012
            with inflammation I83.212
          foot NEC I83.015
            with inflammation I83.215

Varix — continued
  leg — continued
    right — continued
      with — continued
        ulcer — continued
          heel I83.014
            with inflammation I83.214
          lower leg NEC I83.018
            with inflammation I83.218
          midfoot I83.014
            with inflammation I83.214
          thigh I83.011
            with inflammation I83.211
  nasal septum I86.8
  orbit I86.8
    congenital Q27.8
  ovary I86.2
  papillary I78.1
  pelvis I86.2
  perineum I86.3
  pharynx I86.8
  placenta O43.89- ☑
  renal papilla I86.8
  retina H35.09
  scrotum (ulcerated) I86.1
  sigmoid colon I86.8
  specified site NEC I86.8
  spinal (cord) (vessels) I86.8
  spleen, splenic (vein) (with phlebolith) I86.8
  stomach I86.4
  sublingual I86.0
  ulcerated I83.009
    inflamed or infected I83.209
  uterine ligament I86.2
  vagina I86.8
  vocal cord I86.8
  vulva I86.3
Vas deferens — see condition
Vas deferentitis N49.1
Vasa previa O69.4 ☑
  hemorrhage from, affecting newborn P50.0
Vascular (see also condition)
  loop on optic papilla Q14.2
  spasm I73.9
  spider I78.1
Vascularization, cornea — see Neovascularization, cornea
Vasculitis I77.6
  allergic D69.0
  cryoglobulinemic D89.1
  disseminated I77.6
  hypocomplementemic M31.8
  kidney I77.89
  livedoid L95.0
  nodular L95.8
  retina H35.06- ☑
  rheumatic — see Fever, rheumatic
  rheumatoid — see Rheumatoid, vasculitis
  skin (limited to) L95.9
    specified NEC L95.8
Vasculopathy, necrotizing M31.9
  cardiac allograft T86.290
  specified NEC M31.8
Vasitis (nodosa) N49.1
  tuberculous A18.15
Vasodilation I73.9
Vasomotor — see condition
Vasoplasty, after previous sterilization Z31.0
  aftercare Z31.42
Vasospasm (vasoconstriction) I73.9
  cerebral (cerebrovascular) (artery) I67.848
    reversible I67.841
  coronary I20.1
  nerve
    arm — see Mononeuropathy, upper limb
    brachial plexus G54.0
    cervical plexus G54.2
    leg — see Mononeuropathy, lower limb
    peripheral NOS I73.9
    retina (artery) — see Occlusion, artery, retina
Vasospastic — see condition
Vasovagal attack (paroxysmal) R55
  psychogenic F45.8
VATER syndrome Q87.2
Vater's ampulla — see condition
Vegetation, vegetative
  adenoid (nasal fossa) J35.8
  endocarditis (acute) (any valve) (subacute) I33.0

Vegetation, vegetative — *continued*
  heart (mycotic) (valve) I33.0
Veil
  Jackson's Q43.3
Vein, venous — *see* condition
Veldt sore — *see* Ulcer, skin
Velpeau's hernia — *see* Hernia, femoral
Venereal
  bubo A55
  disease A64
  granuloma inguinale A58
  lymphogranuloma (Durand-Nicolas-Favre) A55
Venofibrosis I87.8
Venom, venomous — *see* Table of Drugs and Chemicals,
    by animal or substance, poisoning
Venous — *see* condition
Ventilator lung, newborn P27.8
Ventral — *see* condition
Ventricle, ventricular (*see also* condition)
  escape I49.3
  inversion Q20.5
Ventriculitis (cerebral) (*see also* Encephalitis) G04.90
Ventriculostomy status Z98.2
Vernet's syndrome G52.7
Verneuil's disease (syphilitic bursitis) A52.78
Verruca (due to HPV) (filiformis) (simplex) (viral) (vulgaris)
    B07.9
  acuminata A63.0
  necrogenica (primary) (tuberculosa) A18.4
  plana B07.8
  plantaris B07.0
  seborrheica L82.1
    inflamed L82.0
  senile (seborrheic) L82.1
    inflamed L82.0
  tuberculosa (primary) A18.4
  venereal A63.0
Verrucosities — *see* Verruca
Verruga peruana, peruviana A44.1
Version
  with extraction
  cervix — *see* Malposition, uterus
  uterus (postinfectional) (postpartal, old) — *see* Malpo-
    sition, uterus
Vertebra, vertebral — *see* condition
Vertical talus (congenital) Q66.80
  left foot Q66.82
  right foot Q66.81
Vertigo R42
  auditory — *see* Vertigo, aural
  aural H81.31- ☑
  benign paroxysmal (positional) H81.1- ☑
  central (origin) H81.4- ☑
  cerebral H81.4- ☑
  Dix and Hallpike (epidemic) — *see* Neuronitis,
    vestibular
  due to infrasound T75.23 ☑
  epidemic A88.1
    Dix and Hallpike — *see* Neuronitis, vestibular
    Pedersen's — *see* Neuronitis, vestibular
    vestibular neuronitis — *see* Neuronitis, vestibular
  hysterical F44.89
  infrasound T75.23 ☑
  labyrinthine — *see* subcategory H81.0 ☑
  laryngeal R05
  malignant positional H81.4- ☑
  Ménière's — *see* subcategory H81.0 ☑
  menopausal N95.1
  otogenic — *see* Vertigo, aural
  paroxysmal positional, benign — *see* Vertigo, benign
    paroxysmal
  Pedersen's (epidemic) — *see* Neuronitis, vestibular
  peripheral NEC H81.39- ☑
  positional
    benign paroxysmal — *see* Vertigo, benign parox-
      ysmal
    malignant H81.4- ☑
Very-low-density-lipoprotein-type (VLDL) **hyper-
    lipoproteinemia** E78.1
Vesania — *see* Psychosis
Vesical — *see* condition
Vesicle
  cutaneous R23.8
  seminal — *see* condition
  skin R23.8
Vesicocolic — *see* condition
Vesicoperineal — *see* condition

Vesicorectal — *see* condition
Vesicourethrorectal — *see* condition
Vesicovaginal — *see* condition
Vesicular — *see* condition
Vesiculitis (seminal) N49.0
  amebic A06.82
  gonorrheal (acute) (chronic) A54.23
  trichomonal A59.09
  tuberculous A18.15
Vestibulitis (ear) (*see also* subcategory) H83.0 ☑
  nose (external) J34.89
  vulvar N94.810
Vestibulopathy , acute peripheral (recurrent) — *see*
    Neuronitis, vestibular
Vestige, vestigial (*see also* Persistence)
  branchial Q18.0
  structures in vitreous Q14.0
Vibration
  adverse effects T75.20 ☑
    pneumatic hammer syndrome T75.21 ☑
    specified effect NEC T75.29 ☑
    vasospastic syndrome T75.22 ☑
    vertigo from infrasound T75.23 ☑
  exposure (occupational) Z57.7
  vertigo T75.23 ☑
Vibriosis A28.9
Victim (of)
  crime Z65.4
  disaster Z65.5
  terrorism Z65.4
  torture Z65.4
  war Z65.5
Vidal's disease L28.0
Villaret's syndrome G52.7
Villous — *see* condition
VIN — *see* Neoplasia, intraepithelial, vulva
Vincent's infection (angina) (gingivitis) A69.1
  stomatitis NEC A69.1
Vinson-Plummer syndrome D50.1
Violence, physical R45.6
Viosterol deficiency — *see* Deficiency, calciferol
Vipoma — *see* Neoplasm, malignant, by site
Viremia B34.9
Virilism (adrenal) E25.9
  congenital E25.0
Virilization (female) (suprarenal) E25.9
  congenital E25.0
  isosexual E28.2
Virulent bubo A57
Virus, viral (*see also* condition)
  as cause of disease classified elsewhere B97.89
  cytomegalovirus B25.9
  human immunodeficiency (HIV) — *see* Human, immun-
    odeficiency virus (HIV) disease
  infection — *see* Infection, virus
  specified NEC B34.8
  swine influenza (viruses that normally cause infections
    in pigs) (*see also* Influenza, due to, identified
    novel influenza A virus) J09.X2
  West Nile (fever) A92.30
    with
      complications NEC A92.39
      cranial nerve disorders A92.32
      encephalitis A92.31
      encephalomyelitis A92.31
      neurologic manifestation NEC A92.32
      optic neuritis A92.32
      polyradiculitis A92.32
Viscera, visceral — *see* condition
Visceroptosis K63.4
Visible peristalsis R19.2
Vision, visual
  binocular, suppression H53.34
  blurred, blurring H53.8
    hysterical F44.6
  defect, defective NEC H54.7
  disorientation (syndrome) H53.8
  disturbance H53.9
    hysterical F44.6
  double H53.2
  examination Z01.00
    with abnormal findings Z01.01
  field, limitation (defect) — *see* Defect, visual field
  hallucinations R44.1
  halos H53.19
  loss — *see* Loss, vision

Vision, visual — *continued*
  loss — *see* Loss, vision — *continued*
    sudden — *see* Disturbance, vision, subjective, loss,
      sudden
    low (both eyes) — *see* Low, vision
  perception, simultaneous without fusion H53.33
Vitality, lack or want of R53.83
  newborn P96.89
Vitamin deficiency — *see* Deficiency, vitamin
Vitelline duct, persistent Q43.0
Vitiligo L80
  eyelid H02.739
    left H02.736
      lower H02.735
      upper H02.734
    right H02.733
      lower H02.732
      upper H02.731
  pinta A67.2
  vulva N90.89
Vitreal corneal syndrome H59.01- ☑
Vitreoretinopathy, proliferative (*see also* Retinopathy,
    proliferative)
  with retinal detachment — *see* Detachment, retina,
    traction
Vitreous (*see also* condition)
  touch syndrome — *see* Complication, postprocedural,
    following cataract surgery
Vocal cord — *see* condition
Vogt-Koyanagi syndrome H20.82- ☑
Vogt's disease or syndrome G80.3
Vogt-Spielmeyer amaurotic idiocy or disease E75.4
Voice
  change R49.9
    specified NEC R49.8
  loss — *see* Aphonia
Volhynian fever A79.0
Volkmann's ischemic contracture or paralysis (com-
    plicating trauma) T79.6 ☑
Volvulus (bowel) (colon) (duodenum) (intestine) K56.2
  with perforation K56.2
  congenital Q43.8
  fallopian tube — *see* Torsion, fallopian tube
  oviduct — *see* Torsion, fallopian tube
  stomach (due to absence of gastrocolic ligament)
    K31.89
Vomiting R11.10
  with nausea R11.2
  without nausea R11.11
  asphyxia — *see* Foreign body, by site, causing asphyx-
    ia, gastric contents
  bilious (cause unknown) R11.14
    following gastro-intestinal surgery K91.0
    in newborn P92.01
  blood — *see* Hematemesis
  causing asphyxia, choking, or suffocation — *see* For-
    eign body, by site
  cyclical G43.A0 (*following* G43.7)
    with refractory migraine G43.A1 (*following* G43.7)
    without refractory migraine G43.A0 (*following*
      G43.7)
    intractable G43.A1 (*following* G43.7)
    not intractable G43.A0 (*following* G43.7)
    psychogenic F50.8
  fecal mater R11.13
  following gastrointestinal surgery K91.0
    psychogenic F50.8
  functional K31.89
  hysterical F50.8
  nervous F50.8
  neurotic F50.8
  newborn NEC P92.09
    bilious P92.01
  periodic R11.10
    psychogenic F50.8
  projectile R11.12
  psychogenic F50.8
  uremic — *see* Uremia
Vomito negro — *see* Fever, yellow
Von Bezold's abscess — *see* Mastoiditis, acute
Von Economo-Cruchet disease A85.8
Von Eulenburg's disease G71.19
Von Gierke's disease E74.01
Von Hippel (-Lindau) **disease or syndrome** Q85.8
Von Jaksch's anemia or disease D64.89
Von Recklinghausen
  disease (neurofibromatosis) Q85.01

Von Recklinghausen — *continued*
  disease — *continued*
    bones E21.0
Von Schroetter's syndrome I82.890
Von Willebrand (-Jurgens)(-Minot) **disease or syndrome** D68.0
Von Zumbusch's disease L40.1
Voyeurism F65.3
Vrolik's disease Q78.0
Vulva — *see* condition
Vulvismus N94.2
Vulvitis (acute) (allergic) (atrophic) (hypertrophic) (intertriginous) (senile) N76.2
  with ectopic or molar pregnancy O08.0
  adhesive, congenital Q52.79
  blennorrhagic (gonococcal) A54.02
  candidal B37.3
  chlamydial A56.02
  due to Haemophilus ducreyi A57
  following ectopic or molar pregnancy O08.0
  gonococcal A54.02
    with abscess (accessory gland) (periurethral) A54.1
  herpesviral A60.04
  leukoplakic N90.4
  monilial B37.3
  puerperal (postpartum) O86.19
  subacute or chronic N76.3
  syphilitic (early) A51.0
    late A52.76
  trichomonal A59.01
  tuberculous A18.18
Vulvodynia N94.819
  specified NEC N94.818
Vulvorectal — *see* condition
Vulvovaginitis (acute) — *see* Vaginitis

W

Waiting list, person on Z75.1
  for organ transplant Z76.82
  undergoing social agency investigation Z75.2
Waldenström
  hypergammaglobulinemia D89.0
  syndrome or macroglobulinemia C88.0
Waldenström-Kjellberg syndrome D50.1
Walking
  difficulty R26.2
    psychogenic F44.4
  sleep F51.3
    hysterical F44.89
Wall, abdominal — *see* condition
Wallenberg's disease or syndrome G46.3
Wallgren's disease I87.8
Wandering
  gallbladder, congenital Q44.1
  in diseases classified elsewhere Z91.83
  kidney, congenital Q63.8
  organ or site, congenital NEC — *see* Malposition, congenital, by site
  pacemaker (heart) I49.8
  spleen D73.89
War neurosis F48.8
Wart (due to HPV) (filiform) (infectious) (viral) B07.9
  anogenital region (venereal) A63.0
  common B07.8
  external genital organs (venereal) A63.0
  flat B07.8
  Hassal-Henle's (of cornea) H18.49
  Peruvian A44.1
  plantar B07.0
  prosector (tuberculous) A18.4
  seborrheic L82.1
    inflamed L82.0
  senile (seborrheic) L82.1
    inflamed L82.0
  tuberculous A18.4
  venereal A63.0
Warthin's tumor — *see* Neoplasm, salivary gland, benign
Wassilieff's disease A27.0
Wasting
  disease R64
    due to malnutrition E41
  extreme (due to malnutrition) E41
  muscle NEC — *see* Atrophy, muscle
Water
  clefts (senile cataract) — *see* Cataract, senile, incipient
  deprivation of T73.1 ☑

Water — *continued*
  intoxication E87.79
  itch B76.9
  lack of T73.1 ☑
  loading E87.70
  on
    brain — *see* Hydrocephalus
    chest J94.8
  poisoning E87.79
Waterbrash R12
Waterhouse (-Friderichsen) **syndrome or disease** (meningococcal) A39.1
Water-losing nephritis N25.89
Watermelon stomach K31.819
  with hemorrhage K31.811
  without hemorrhage K31.819
Watsoniasis B66.8
Wax in ear — *see* Impaction, cerumen
Weak, weakening, weakness (generalized) R53.1
  arches (acquired) (*see also* Deformity, limb, flat foot)
  bladder (sphincter) R32
  facial R29.810
    following
      cerebrovascular disease I69.992
        cerebral infarction I69.392
        intracerebral hemorrhage I69.192
        nontraumatic intracranial hemorrhage NEC I69.292
        specified disease NEC I69.892
        stroke I69.392
        subarachnoid hemorrhage I69.092
  foot (double) — *see* Weak, arches
  heart, cardiac — *see* Failure, heart
  mind F70
  muscle M62.81
  myocardium — *see* Failure, heart
  newborn P96.89
  pelvic fundus N81.89
  pubocervical tissue N81.82
  rectovaginal tissue N81.83
  senile R54
  urinary stream R39.12
  valvular — *see* Endocarditis
Wear, worn (with normal or routine use)
  articular bearing surface of internal joint prosthesis — *see* Complications, joint prosthesis, mechanical, wear of articular bearing surfaces, by site
  device, implant or graft — *see* Complications, by site, mechanical complication
  tooth, teeth (approximal) (hard tissues) (interproximal) (occlusal) K03.0
Weather, weathered
  effects of
    cold T69.9 ☑
      specified effect NEC T69.8 ☑
    hot — *see* Heat
    skin L57.8
Weaver's syndrome Q87.3
Web, webbed (congenital)
  duodenal Q43.8
  esophagus Q39.4
  fingers Q70.1- ☑
  larynx (glottic) (subglottic) Q31.0
  neck (pterygium colli) Q18.3
  Paterson-Kelly D50.1
  popliteal syndrome Q87.89
  toes Q70.3- ☑
Weber-Christian disease M35.6
Weber-Cockayne syndrome (epidermolysis bullosa) Q81.8
Weber-Gubler syndrome G46.3
Weber-Leyden syndrome G46.3
Weber-Osler syndrome I78.0
Weber's paralysis or syndrome G46.3
Wedge-shaped or wedging vertebra — *see* Collapse, vertebra NEC
Wegener's granulomatosis or syndrome M31.30
  with
    kidney involvement M31.31
    lung involvement M31.30
      with kidney involvement M31.31
Wegner's disease A50.02
Weight
  1000-2499 grams at birth (low) — *see* Low, birthweight
  999 grams or less at birth (extremely low) — *see* Low, birthweight, extreme

Weight — *continued*
  gain (abnormal) (excessive) R63.5
    in pregnancy — *see* Pregnancy, complicated by, excessive weight gain
    low — *see* Pregnancy, complicated by, insufficient, weight gain
  loss (abnormal) (cause unknown) R63.4
Weightlessness (effect of) T75.82 ☑
Weil (I)-**Marchesani syndrome** Q87.1
Weil's disease A27.0
Weingarten's syndrome J82
Weir Mitchell's disease I73.81
Weiss-Baker syndrome G90.09
Wells' disease L98.3
Wen — *see* Cyst, sebaceous
Wenckebach's block or phenomenon I44.1
Werdnig-Hoffmann syndrome (muscular atrophy) G12.0
Werlhof's disease D69.3
Wermer's disease or syndrome E31.21
Werner-His disease A79.0
Werner's disease or syndrome E34.8
Wernicke-Korsakoff's syndrome or psychosis (alcoholic) F10.96
  with dependence F10.26
  drug-induced
    due to drug abuse — *see* Abuse, drug, by type, with amnestic disorder
    due to drug dependence — *see* Dependence, drug, by type, with amnestic disorder
  nonalcoholic F04
Wernicke-Posadas disease B38.9
Wernicke's
  developmental aphasia F80.2
  disease or syndrome E51.2
  encephalopathy E51.2
  polioencephalitis, superior E51.2
West African fever B50.8
Westphal-Strümpell syndrome E83.01
West's syndrome — *see* Epilepsy, spasms
Wet
  feet, tropical (maceration) (syndrome) — *see* Immersion, foot
  lung (syndrome), newborn P22.1
Wharton's duct — *see* condition
Wheal — *see* Urticaria
Wheezing R06.2
Whiplash injury S13.4 ☑
Whipple's disease (*see also* subcategory M14.8-) K90.81
Whipworm (disease) (infection) (infestation) B79
Whistling face Q87.0
White (*see also* condition)
  kidney, small N03.9
  leg, puerperal, postpartum, childbirth O87.1
  mouth B37.0
  patches of mouth K13.29
  spot lesions, teeth
    chewing surface K02.51
    pit and fissure surface K02.51
    smooth surface K02.61
Whitehead L70.0
Whitlow (*see also* Cellulitis, digit)
  with lymphangitis — *see* Lymphangitis, acute, digit
  herpesviral B00.89
Whitmore's disease or fever — *see* Melioidosis
Whooping cough A37.90
  with pneumonia A37.91
    due to Bordetella
      bronchiseptica A37.81
      parapertussis A37.11
      pertussis A37.01
    specified organism NEC A37.81
  due to
    Bordetella
      bronchiseptica A37.80
        with pneumonia A37.81
      parapertussis A37.10
        with pneumonia A37.11
      pertussis A37.00
        with pneumonia A37.01
      specified NEC A37.80
        with pneumonia A37.81
Wichman's asthma J38.5
Wide cranial sutures, newborn P96.3
Widening aorta — *see* Ectasia, aorta
  with aneurysm — *see* Aneurysm, aorta
Wilkie's disease or syndrome K55.1

Wilkinson-Sneddon disease or syndrome — Wound, open

Wilkinson-Sneddon disease or syndrome L13.1
Willebrand (-Jürgens) **thrombopathy** D68.0
Willige-Hunt disease or syndrome G23.1
Wilms' tumor C64-
Wilson-Mikity syndrome P27.0
Wilson's
  disease or syndrome E83.01
  hepatolenticular degeneration E83.01
  lichen ruber L43.9
Window (see also Imperfect, closure)
  aorticopulmonary Q21.4
Winter — see condition
Wiskott-Aldrich syndrome D82.0
Withdrawal state (see also Dependence, drug by type, with withdrawal)
  newborn
    correct therapeutic substance properly administered P96.2
    infant of dependent mother P96.1
  therapeutic substance, neonatal P96.2
Witts' anemia D50.8
Witzelsucht F07.0
Woakes' ethmoiditis or syndrome J33.1
Wolff-Hirschorn syndrome Q93.3
Wolff-Parkinson-White syndrome I45.6
Wolhynian fever A79.0
Wolman's disease E75.5
Wood lung or pneumonitis J67.8
Woolly, wooly hair (congenital) (nevus) Q84.1
Woolsorter's disease A22.1
Word
  blindness (congenital) (developmental) F81.0
  deafness (congenital) (developmental) H93.25
Worm(s) (infection) (infestation) (see also Infestation, helminth)
  guinea B72
  in intestine NEC B82.0
Worm-eaten soles A66.3
Worn out — see Exhaustion
  cardiac
    defibrillator (with synchronous cardiace pacemaker) Z45.02
    pacemaker
      battery Z45.010
      lead Z45.018
  device, implant or graft — see Complications, by site, mechanical
Worried well Z71.1
Worries R45.82
Wound, open
  abdomen, abdominal
    wall S31.109
      with penetration into peritoneal cavity S31.609
      bite — see Bite, abdomen, wall
      epigastric region S31.102
        with penetration into peritoneal cavity S31.602
        bite — see Bite, abdomen, wall, epigastric region
        laceration — see Laceration, abdomen, wall, epigastric region
        puncture — see Puncture, abdomen, wall, epigastric region
      laceration — see Laceration, abdomen, wall
      left
        lower quadrant S31.104
          with penetration into peritoneal cavity S31.604
          bite — see Bite, abdomen, wall, left, lower quadrant
          laceration — see Laceration, abdomen, wall, left, lower quadrant
          puncture — see Puncture, abdomen, wall, left, lower quadrant
        upper quadrant S31.101
          with penetration into peritoneal cavity S31.601
          bite — see Bite, abdomen, wall, left, upper quadrant
          laceration — see Laceration, abdomen, wall, left, upper quadrant
          puncture — see Puncture, abdomen, wall, left, upper quadrant
      periumbilic region S31.105
        with penetration into peritoneal cavity S31.605

Wound, open — continued
  abdomen, abdominal — continued
    wall — continued
      periumbilic region — continued
        bite — see Bite, abdomen, wall, periumbilic region
        laceration — see Laceration, abdomen, wall, periumbilic region
        puncture — see Puncture, abdomen, wall, periumbilic region
      puncture — see Puncture, abdomen, wall
      right
        lower quadrant S31.103
          with penetration into peritoneal cavity S31.603
          bite — see Bite, abdomen, wall, right, lower quadrant
          laceration — see Laceration, abdomen, wall, right, lower quadrant
          puncture — see Puncture, abdomen, wall, right, lower quadrant
        upper quadrant S31.100
          with penetration into peritoneal cavity S31.600
          bite — see Bite, abdomen, wall, right, upper quadrant
          laceration — see Laceration, abdomen, wall, right, upper quadrant
          puncture — see Puncture, abdomen, wall, right, upper quadrant
    alveolar (process) — see Wound, open, oral cavity
    ankle S91.00-
      bite — see Bite, ankle
      laceration — see Laceration, ankle
      puncture — see Puncture, ankle
    antecubital space — see Wound, open, elbow
    anterior chamber, eye — see Wound, open, ocular
    anus S31.839
      bite S31.835
      laceration — see Laceration, anus
      puncture — see Puncture, anus
    arm (upper) S41.10-
      with amputation — see Amputation, traumatic, arm
      bite — see Bite, arm
      forearm — see Wound, open, forearm
      laceration — see Laceration, arm
      puncture — see Puncture, arm
    auditory canal (external) (meatus) — see Wound, open, ear
    auricle, ear — see Wound, open, ear
    axilla — see Wound, open, arm
    back (see also Wound, open, thorax, back)
      lower S31.000
        with penetration into retroperitoneal space S31.001
        bite — see Bite, back, lower
        laceration — see Laceration, back, lower
        puncture — see Puncture, back, lower
      bite — see Bite
    blood vessel — see Injury, blood vessel
    breast S21.00-
      with amputation — see Amputation, traumatic, breast
      bite — see Bite, breast
      laceration — see Laceration, breast
      puncture — see Puncture, breast
    buttock S31.809
      bite — see Bite, buttock
      laceration — see Laceration, buttock
      left S31.829
      puncture — see Puncture, buttock
      right S31.819
    calf — see Wound, open, leg
    canaliculus lacrimalis — see Wound, open, eyelid
    canthus, eye — see Wound, open, eyelid
    cervical esophagus S11.20
      bite S11.25
      laceration — see Laceration, esophagus, traumatic, cervical
      puncture — see Puncture, cervical esophagus
    cheek (external) S01.40-
      bite — see Bite, cheek
      internal — see Wound, open, oral cavity
      laceration — see Laceration, cheek
      puncture — see Puncture, cheek

Wound, open — continued
  chest wall — see Wound, open, thorax
  chin — see Wound, open, head, specified site NEC
  choroid — see Wound, open, ocular
  ciliary body (eye) — see Wound, open, ocular
  clitoris S31.40
    with amputation — see Amputation, traumatic, clitoris
    bite S31.45
    laceration — see Laceration, vulva
    puncture — see Puncture, vulva
  conjunctiva — see Wound, open, ocular
  cornea — see Wound, open, ocular
  costal region — see Wound, open, thorax
  Descemet's membrane — see Wound, open, ocular
  digit(s)
    foot — see Wound, open, toe
    hand — see Wound, open, finger
  ear (canal) (external) S01.30-
    with amputation — see Amputation, traumatic, ear
    bite — see Bite, ear
    drum S09.2-
    laceration — see Laceration, ear
    puncture — see Puncture, ear
  elbow S51.00-
    bite — see Bite, elbow
    laceration — see Laceration, elbow
    puncture — see Puncture, elbow
  epididymis — see Wound, open, testis
  epigastric region S31.102
    with penetration into peritoneal cavity S31.602
    bite — see Bite, abdomen, wall, epigastric region
    laceration — see Laceration, abdomen, wall, epigastric region
    puncture — see Puncture, abdomen, wall, epigastric region
  epiglottis — see Wound, open, neck, specified site NEC
  esophagus (thoracic) S27.819
    cervical — see Wound, open, cervical esophagus
    laceration S27.813
    specified type NEC S27.818
  eye — see Wound, open, ocular
  eyeball — see Wound, open, ocular
  eyebrow — see Wound, open, eyelid
  eyelid S01.10-
    bite — see Bite, eyelid
    laceration — see Laceration, eyelid
    puncture — see Puncture, eyelid
  face NEC — see Wound, open, head, specified site NEC
  finger(s) S61.209
    with
      amputation — see Amputation, traumatic, finger
      damage to nail S61.309
    bite — see Bite, finger
    index S61.208
      with
        damage to nail S61.308
      left S61.201
        with
          damage to nail S61.301
      right S61.200
        with
          damage to nail S61.300
    laceration — see Laceration, finger
    little S61.208
      with
        damage to nail S61.308
      left S61.207
        with damage to nail S61.307
      right S61.206
        with damage to nail S61.306
    middle S61.208
      with
        damage to nail S61.308
      left S61.203
        with damage to nail S61.303
      right S61.202
        with damage to nail S61.302
    puncture — see Puncture, finger
    ring S61.208
      with
        damage to nail S61.308
      left S61.205

Wound, open — *continued*
finger(s) — *continued*
  ring — *continued*
    left — *continued*
      with damage to nail S61.305 ☑
    right S61.204 ☑
      with damage to nail S61.304 ☑
flank — *see* Wound, open, abdomen, wall
foot (except toe(s) alone) S91.30- ☑
  with amputation — *see* Amputation, traumatic, foot
  bite — *see* Bite, foot
  laceration — *see* Laceration, foot
  puncture — *see* Puncture, foot
  toe — *see* Wound, open, toe
forearm S51.80- ☑
  with
    amputation — *see* Amputation, traumatic, forearm
  bite — *see* Bite, forearm
  elbow only — *see* Wound, open, elbow
  laceration — *see* Laceration, forearm
  puncture — *see* Puncture, forearm
forehead — *see* Wound, open, head, specified site NEC
genital organs, external
  with amputation — *see* Amputation, traumatic, genital organs
  bite — *see* Bite, genital organ
  female S31.502 ☑
    vagina S31.40 ☑
    vulva S31.40 ☑
  laceration — *see* Laceration, genital organ
  male S31.501 ☑
    penis S31.20 ☑
    scrotum S31.30 ☑
    testes S31.30 ☑
  puncture — *see* Puncture, genital organ
globe (eye) — *see* Wound, open, ocular
groin — *see* Wound, open, abdomen, wall
gum — *see* Wound, open, oral cavity
hand S61.40- ☑
  with
    amputation — *see* Amputation, traumatic, hand
  bite — *see* Bite, hand
  finger(s) — *see* Wound, open, finger
  laceration — *see* Laceration, hand
  puncture — *see* Puncture, hand
  thumb — *see* Wound, open, thumb
head S01.90 ☑
  bite — *see* Bite, head
  cheek — *see* Wound, open, cheek
  ear — *see* Wound, open, ear
  eyelid — *see* Wound, open, eyelid
  laceration — *see* Laceration, head
  lip — *see* Wound, open, lip
  nose S01.20 ☑
  oral cavity — *see* Wound, open, oral cavity
  puncture — *see* Puncture, head
  scalp — *see* Wound, open, scalp
  specified site NEC S01.80 ☑
  temporomandibular area — *see* Wound, open, cheek
heel — *see* Wound, open, foot
hip S71.00- ☑
  with amputation — *see* Amputation, traumatic, hip
  bite — *see* Bite, hip
  laceration — *see* Laceration, hip
  puncture — *see* Puncture, hip
hymen S31.40 ☑
  bite — *see* Bite, vulva
  laceration — *see* Laceration, vagina
  puncture — *see* Puncture, vagina
hypochondrium S31.109 ☑
  bite — *see* Bite, hypochondrium
  laceration — *see* Laceration, hypochondrium
  puncture — *see* Puncture, hypochondrium
hypogastric region S31.109 ☑
  bite — *see* Bite, hypogastric region
  laceration — *see* Laceration, hypogastric region
  puncture — *see* Puncture, hypogastric region
iliac (region) — *see* Wound, open, inguinal region
inguinal region S31.109 ☑
  bite — *see* Bite, abdomen, wall, lower quadrant
  laceration — *see* Laceration, inguinal region

Wound, open — *continued*
inguinal region — *continued*
  puncture — *see* Puncture, inguinal region
instep — *see* Wound, open, foot
interscapular region — *see* Wound, open, thorax, back
intraocular — *see* Wound, open, ocular
iris — *see* Wound, open, ocular
jaw — *see* Wound, open, head, specified site NEC
knee S81.00- ☑
  bite — *see* Bite, knee
  laceration — *see* Laceration, knee
  puncture — *see* Puncture, knee
labium (majus) (minus) — *see* Wound, open, vulva
laceration — *see* Laceration, by site
lacrimal duct — *see* Wound, open, eyelid
larynx S11.019 ☑
  bite — *see* Bite, larynx
  laceration — *see* Laceration, larynx
  puncture — *see* Puncture, larynx
left
  lower quadrant S31.104 ☑
    with penetration into peritoneal cavity S31.604 ☑
    bite — *see* Bite, abdomen, wall, left, lower quadrant
    laceration — *see* Laceration, abdomen, wall, left, lower quadrant
    puncture — *see* Puncture, abdomen, wall, left, lower quadrant
  upper quadrant S31.101 ☑
    with penetration into peritoneal cavity S31.601 ☑
    bite — *see* Bite, abdomen, wall, left, upper quadrant
    laceration — *see* Laceration, abdomen, wall, left, upper quadrant
    puncture — *see* Puncture, abdomen, wall, left, upper quadrant
leg (lower) S81.80- ☑
  with amputation — *see* Amputation, traumatic, leg
  ankle — *see* Wound, open, ankle
  bite — *see* Bite, leg
  foot — *see* Wound, open, foot
  knee — *see* Wound, open, knee
  laceration — *see* Laceration, leg
  puncture — *see* Puncture, leg
  toe — *see* Wound, open, toe
  upper — *see* Wound, open, thigh
lip S01.501 ☑
  bite — *see* Bite, lip
  laceration — *see* Laceration, lip
  puncture — *see* Puncture, lip
loin S31.109 ☑
  bite — *see* Bite, abdomen, wall
  laceration — *see* Laceration, loin
  puncture — *see* Puncture, loin
lower back — *see* Wound, open, back, lower
lumbar region — *see* Wound, open, back, lower
malar region — *see* Wound, open, head, specified site NEC
mammary — *see* Wound, open, breast
mastoid region — *see* Wound, open, head, specified site NEC
mouth — *see* Wound, open, oral cavity
nail
  finger — *see* Wound, open, finger, with damage to nail
  toe — *see* Wound, open, toe, with damage to nail
nape (neck) — *see* Wound, open, neck
nasal (septum) (sinus) — *see* Wound, open, nose
nasopharynx — *see* Wound, open, head, specified site NEC
neck S11.90 ☑
  bite — *see* Bite, neck
  involving
    cervical esophagus S11.20 ☑
    larynx — *see* Wound, open, larynx
    pharynx S11.20 ☑
    thyroid S11.10 ☑
    trachea (cervical) S11.029 ☑
      bite — *see* Bite, trachea
      laceration S11.021 ☑
        with foreign body S11.022 ☑
      puncture S11.023 ☑
        with foreign body S11.024 ☑

Wound, open — *continued*
neck — *continued*
  laceration — *see* Laceration, neck
  puncture — *see* Puncture, neck
  specified site NEC S11.80 ☑
    specified type NEC S11.89 ☑
nose (septum) (sinus) S01.20 ☑
  with amputation — *see* Amputation, traumatic, nose
  bite — *see* Bite, nose
  laceration — *see* Laceration, nose
  puncture — *see* Puncture, nose
ocular S05.90 ☑
  avulsion (traumatic enucleation) S05.7- ☑
  eyeball S05.6- ☑
    with foreign body S05.5- ☑
  eyelid — *see* Wound, open, eyelid
  laceration and rupture S05.3- ☑
    with prolapse or loss of intraocular tissue S05.2- ☑
  orbit (penetrating) (with or without foreign body) S05.4- ☑
  periocular area — *see* Wound, open, eyelid
  specified NEC S05.8X- ☑
oral cavity S01.502 ☑
  bite S01.552 ☑
  laceration — *see* Laceration, oral cavity
  puncture — *see* Puncture, oral cavity
orbit — *see* Wound, open, ocular, orbit
palate — *see* Wound, open, oral cavity
palm — *see* Wound, open, hand
pelvis, pelvic (*see also* Wound, open, back, lower)
  girdle — *see* Wound, open, hip
penetrating — *see* Puncture, by site
penis S31.20 ☑
  with amputation — *see* Amputation, traumatic, penis
  bite S31.25 ☑
  laceration — *see* Laceration, penis
  puncture — *see* Puncture, penis
perineum
  bite — *see* Bite, perineum
  female S31.502 ☑
  laceration — *see* Laceration, perineum
  male S31.501 ☑
  puncture — *see* Puncture, perineum
periocular area (with or without lacrimal passages) — *see* Wound, open, eyelid
periumbilic region S31.105 ☑
  with penetration into peritoneal cavity S31.605 ☑
  bite — *see* Bite, abdomen, wall, periumbilic region
  laceration — *see* Laceration, abdomen, wall, periumbilic region
  puncture — *see* Puncture, abdomen, wall, periumbilic region
phalanges
  finger — *see* Wound, open, finger
  toe — *see* Wound, open, toe
pharynx S11.20 ☑
pinna — *see* Wound, open, ear
popliteal space — *see* Wound, open, knee
prepuce — *see* Wound, open, penis
pubic region — *see* Wound, open, back, lower
pudendum — *see* Wound, open, genital organs, external
puncture wound — *see* Puncture
rectovaginal septum — *see* Wound, open, vagina
right
  lower quadrant S31.103 ☑
    with penetration into peritoneal cavity S31.603 ☑
    bite — *see* Bite, abdomen, wall, right, lower quadrant
    laceration — *see* Laceration, abdomen, wall, right, lower quadrant
    puncture — *see* Puncture, abdomen, wall, right, lower quadrant
  upper quadrant S31.100 ☑
    with penetration into peritoneal cavity S31.600 ☑
    bite — *see* Bite, abdomen, wall, right, upper quadrant
    laceration — *see* Laceration, abdomen, wall, right, upper quadrant
    puncture — *see* Puncture, abdomen, wall, right, upper quadrant

318
☑ Additional Character Required — Refer to the Tabular List for Character Selection
▽ Subterms under main terms may continue to next column or page

Wound, open — *continued*
  sacral region — *see* Wound, open, back, lower
  sacroiliac region — *see* Wound, open, back, lower
  salivary gland — *see* Wound, open, oral cavity
  scalp S01.00 ☑
    bite S01.05 ☑
    laceration — *see* Laceration, scalp
    puncture — *see* Puncture, scalp
  scalpel, newborn (birth injury) P15.8
  scapular region — *see* Wound, open, shoulder
  sclera — *see* Wound, open, ocular
  scrotum S31.30 ☑
    with amputation — *see* Amputation, traumatic, scrotum
    bite S31.35 ☑
    laceration — *see* Laceration, scrotum
    puncture — *see* Puncture, scrotum
  shin — *see* Wound, open, leg
  shoulder S41.00- ☑
    with amputation — *see* Amputation, traumatic, arm
    bite — *see* Bite, shoulder
    laceration — *see* Laceration, shoulder
    puncture — *see* Puncture, shoulder
  skin NOS T14.8
  spermatic cord — *see* Wound, open, testis
  sternal region — *see* Wound, open, thorax, front wall
  submaxillary region — *see* Wound, open, head, specified site NEC
  submental region — *see* Wound, open, head, specified site NEC
  subungual
    finger(s) — *see* Wound, open, finger
    toe(s) — *see* Wound, open, toe
  supraclavicular region — *see* Wound, open, neck, specified site NEC
  temple, temporal region — *see* Wound, open, head, specified site NEC
  temporomandibular area — *see* Wound, open, cheek
  testis S31.30 ☑
    with amputation — *see* Amputation, traumatic, testes
    bite S31.35 ☑
    laceration — *see* Laceration, testis
    puncture — *see* Puncture, testis
  thigh S71.10- ☑
    with amputation — *see* Amputation, traumatic, hip
    bite — *see* Bite, thigh
    laceration — *see* Laceration, thigh
    puncture — *see* Puncture, thigh
  thorax, thoracic (wall) S21.90 ☑
    back S21.20- ☑
      with penetration S21.40 ☑
    bite — *see* Bite, thorax
    breast — *see* Wound, open, breast
    front S21.10- ☑
      with penetration S21.30 ☑
    laceration — *see* Laceration, thorax
    puncture — *see* Puncture, thorax
  throat — *see* Wound, open, neck
  thumb S61.009 ☑
    with
      amputation — *see* Amputation, traumatic, thumb
      damage to nail S61.109 ☑
    bite — *see* Bite, thumb
    laceration — *see* Laceration, thumb
    left S61.002 ☑
      with
        damage to nail S61.102 ☑
    puncture — *see* Puncture, thumb
    right S61.001 ☑
      with
        damage to nail S61.101 ☑
  thyroid (gland) — *see* Wound, open, neck, thyroid
  toe(s) S91.109 ☑
    with
      amputation — *see* Amputation, traumatic, toe
      damage to nail S91.209 ☑
    bite — *see* Bite, toe
    great S91.103 ☑
      with
        damage to nail S91.203 ☑
      left S91.102 ☑

Wound, open — *continued*
  toe(s) — *continued*
    great — *continued*
      left — *continued*
        with
          damage to nail S91.202 ☑
      right S91.101 ☑
        with
          damage to nail S91.201 ☑
      laceration — *see* Laceration, toe
    lesser S91.106 ☑
      with
        damage to nail S91.206 ☑
      left S91.105 ☑
        with
          damage to nail S91.205 ☑
      right S91.104 ☑
        with
          damage to nail S91.204 ☑
    puncture — *see* Puncture, toe
  tongue — *see* Wound, open, oral cavity
  trachea (cervical region) — *see* Wound, open, neck, trachea
  tunica vaginalis — *see* Wound, open, testis
  tympanum, tympanic membrane S09.2- ☑
    laceration — *see* Laceration, ear, drum
    puncture — *see* Puncture, tympanum
  umbilical region — *see* Wound, open, abdomen, wall, periumbilic region
  uvula — *see* Wound, open, oral cavity
  vagina S31.40 ☑
    bite S31.45 ☑
    laceration — *see* Laceration, vagina
    puncture — *see* Puncture, vagina
  vitreous (humor) — *see* Wound, open, ocular
  vocal cord S11.039 ☑
    bite — *see* Bite, vocal cord
    laceration S11.031 ☑
      with foreign body S11.032 ☑
    puncture S11.033 ☑
      with foreign body S11.034 ☑
  vulva S31.40 ☑
    with amputation — *see* Amputation, traumatic, vulva
    bite S31.45 ☑
    laceration — *see* Laceration, vulva
    puncture — *see* Puncture, vulva
  wrist S61.50- ☑
    bite — *see* Bite, wrist
    laceration — *see* Laceration, wrist
    puncture — *see* Puncture, wrist
Wound, superficial — *see* Injury (*see also* specified injury type)
Wright's syndrome G54.0
Wrist — *see* condition
Wrong drug (by accident) (given in error) — *see* Table of Drugs and Chemicals, by drug, poisoning
Wry neck — *see* Torticollis
Wuchereria (bancrofti) **infestation** B74.0
Wuchereriasis B74.0
Wuchernde Struma Langhans C73

X

Xanthelasma (eyelid) (palpebrarum) H02.60
  left H02.66
    lower H02.65
    upper H02.64
  right H02.63
    lower H02.62
    upper H02.61
Xanthelasmatosis (essential) E78.2
Xanthinuria, hereditary E79.8
Xanthoastrocytoma
  specified site — *see* Neoplasm, malignant, by site
  unspecified site C71.9
Xanthofibroma — *see* Neoplasm, connective tissue, benign
Xanthogranuloma D76.3
Xanthoma(s), xanthomatosis (primary) (familial) (hereditary) E75.5
  with
    hyperlipoproteinemia
      Type I E78.3
      Type III E78.2
      Type IV E78.1

Xanthoma(s), xanthomatosis — *continued*
  with — *continued*
    hyperlipoproteinemia — *continued*
      Type V E78.3
  cerebrotendinous E75.5
  cutaneotendinous E75.5
  disseminatum (skin) E78.2
  eruptive E78.2
  hypercholesterinemic E78.0
  hypercholesterolemic E78.0
  hyperlipidemic E78.5
  joint E75.5
  multiple (skin) E78.2
  tendon (sheath) E75.5
  tuberosum E78.2
  tuberous E78.2
  tubo-eruptive E78.2
  verrucous, oral mucosa K13.4
Xanthosis R23.8
Xenophobia F40.10
Xeroderma (*see also* Ichthyosis)
  acquired L85.0
  eyelid H01.149
    left H01.146
      lower H01.145
      upper H01.144
    right H01.143
      lower H01.142
      upper H01.141
  pigmentosum Q82.1
  vitamin A deficiency E50.8
Xerophthalmia (vitamin A deficiency) E50.7
  unrelated to vitamin A deficiency — *see* Keratoconjunctivitis
Xerosis
  conjunctiva H11.14- ☑
    with Bitot's spots (*see also* Pigmentation, conjunctiva)
      vitamin A deficiency E50.1
    vitamin A deficiency E50.0
  cornea H18.89- ☑
    with ulceration — *see* Ulcer, cornea
      vitamin A deficiency E50.3
    vitamin A deficiency E50.2
  cutis L85.3
  skin L85.3
Xerostomia K11.7
Xiphopagus Q89.4
XO syndrome Q96.9
X-ray (of)
  abnormal findings — *see* Abnormal, diagnostic imaging
  breast (mammogram) (routine) Z12.31
  chest
    routine (as part of a general medical examination) Z00.00
      with abnormal findings Z00.01
  routine (as part of a general medical examination) Z00.00
    with abnormal findings Z00.01
XXXXY syndrome Q98.1
XXY syndrome Q98.0

Y

Yaba pox (virus disease) B08.72
Yatapoxvirus B08.70
  specified NEC B08.79
Yawning R06.89
  psychogenic F45.8
Yaws A66.9
  cutaneous, less than five years after infection A66.2
  bone lesions A66.6
  butter A66.1
  chancre A66.0
  early (cutaneous) (macular) (maculopapular) (micropapular) (papular) A66.2
    frambeside A66.2
    skin lesions NEC A66.2
  eyelid A66.2
  ganglion A66.6
  gangosis, gangosa A66.5
  gumma, gummata A66.4
    bone A66.6
  gummatous
    frambeside A66.4
    osteitis A66.6
    periostitis A66.6

Yaws — *continued*
    hydrarthrosis (*see also* subcategory M14.8-) A66.6
    hyperkeratosis (early) (late) A66.3
    initial lesions A66.0
    joint lesions (*see also* subcategory M14.8-) A66.6
    juxta-articular nodules A66.7
    late nodular (ulcerated) A66.4
    latent (without clinical manifestations) (with positive
        serology) A66.8
    mother A66.0
    mucosal A66.7
    multiple papillomata A66.1
    nodular, late (ulcerated) A66.4
    osteitis A66.6
    papilloma, plantar or palmar A66.1
    periostitis (hypertrophic) A66.6
    specified NEC A66.7

Yaws — *continued*
    ulcers A66.4
    wet crab A66.1
Yeast infection (*see also* Candidiasis) B37.9
Yellow
    atrophy (liver) — *see* Failure, hepatic
    fever — *see* Fever, yellow
    jack — *see* Fever, yellow
    jaundice — *see* Jaundice
    nail syndrome L60.5
Yersiniosis (*see also* Infection, Yersinia)
    extraintestinal A28.2
    intestinal A04.6

Z

Zahorsky's syndrome (herpangina) B08.5

Zellweger's syndrome Q87.89
Zenker's diverticulum (esophagus) K22.5
Ziehen-Oppenheim disease G24.1
Zieve's syndrome K70.0
Zinc
    deficiency, dietary E60
    metabolism disorder E83.2
Zollinger-Ellison syndrome E16.4
Zona — *see* Herpes, zoster
Zoophobia F40.218
Zoster (herpes) — *see* Herpes, zoster
Zygomycosis B46.9
    specified NEC B46.8
Zymotic — *see* condition

Yaws — *continued*

☑ **Additional Character Required — Refer to the Tabular List for Character Selection** ▽ **Subterms under main terms may continue to next column or page**

Note: The list below gives the code number for neoplasms by anatomical site. For each site there are six possible code numbers according to whether the neoplasm in question is malignant, benign, in situ, of uncertain behavior, or of unspecified nature. The description of the neoplasm will often indicate which of the six columns is appropriate; e.g., malignant melanoma of skin, benign fibroadenoma of breast, carcinoma in situ of cervix uteri. Where such descriptors are not present, the remainder of the Index should be consulted where guidance is given to the appropriate column for each morphological (histological) variety listed; e.g., Mesonephroma – see Neoplasm, malignant; Embryoma (see also Neoplasm, uncertain behavior); Disease, Bowen's – see Neoplasm, skin, in situ. However, the guidance in the Index can be overridden if one of the descriptors mentioned above is present; e.g., malignant adenoma of colon is coded to C18.9 and not to D12.6 as the adjective "malignant" overrides the Index entry "Adenoma (see also Neoplasm, benign)." Codes listed with a dash -, following the code have a required 5th character for laterality. The tabular list must be reviewed for the complete code.

	Malignant Primary	Malignant Secondary	Ca in situ	Benign	Uncertain	Unspecified Behavior
Neoplasm, neoplastic	C80.1	C79.9	D09.9	D36.9	D48.9	D49.9
abdomen,						
abdominal	C76.2	C79.8-☑	D09.8	D36.7	D48.7	D49.89
cavity	C76.2	C79.8-☑	D09.8	D36.7	D48.7	D49.89
organ	C76.2	C79.8-☑	D09.8	D36.7	D48.7	D49.89
viscera	C76.2	C79.8-☑	D09.8	D36.7	D48.7	D49.89
wall — *see also*						
Neoplasm, abdomen, wall,						
skin	C44.509	C79.2	D04.5	D23.5	D48.5	D49.2
connective						
tissue	C49.4	C79.8-☑	—	D21.4	D48.1	D49.2
skin	C44.509	—	—	—	—	—
basal cell						
carcinoma	C44.519	—	—	—	—	—
specified type						
NEC	C44.599	—	—	—	—	—
squamous cell						
carcinoma	C44.529	—	—	—	—	—
abdominopelvic	C76.8	C79.8-☑	—	D36.7	D48.7	D49.89
accessory sinus — *see*						
Neoplasm, sinus						
acoustic nerve	C72.4-☑	C79.49	—	D33.3	D43.3	D49.7
adenoid (pharynx)						
(tissue)	C11.1	C79.89	D00.08	D10.6	D37.05	D49.0
adipose tissue — *see also*						
Neoplasm, connective						
tissue	C49.4	C79.89	—	D21.9	D48.1	D49.2
adnexa (uterine)	C57.4	C79.89	D07.39	D28.7	D39.8	D49.5
adrenal	C74.9-☑	C79.7-☑	D09.3	D35.0-☑	D44.1-☑	D49.7
capsule	C74.9-☑	C79.7-☑	D09.3	D35.0-☑	D44.1-☑	D49.7
cortex	C74.0-☑	C79.7-☑	D09.3	D35.0-☑	D44.1-☑	D49.7
gland	C74.9-☑	C79.7-☑	D09.3	D35.0-☑	D44.1-☑	D49.7
medulla	C74.1-☑	C79.7-☑	D09.3	D35.0-☑	D44.1-☑	D49.7
ala nasi (external) — *see*						
also Neoplasm, skin,						
nose	C44.301	C79.2	D04.39	D23.39	D48.5	D49.2
alimentary canal or tract						
NEC	C26.9	C78.80	D01.9	D13.9	D37.9	D49.0
alveolar	C03.9	C79.89	D00.03	D10.39	D37.09	D49.0
mucosa	C03.9	C79.89	D00.03	D10.39	D37.09	D49.0
lower	C03.1	C79.89	D00.03	D10.39	D37.09	D49.0
upper	C03.0	C79.89	D00.03	D10.39	D37.09	D49.0
ridge or process	C41.1	C79.51	—	D16.5	D48.0	D49.2
carcinoma	C03.9	C79.8-☑	—	—	—	—
lower	C03.1	C79.8-☑	—	—	—	—
upper	C03.0	C79.8-☑	—	—	—	—
lower	C41.1	C79.51	—	D16.5	D48.0	D49.2
mucosa	C03.9	C79.89	D00.03	D10.39	D37.09	D49.0
lower	C03.1	C79.89	D00.03	D10.39	D37.09	D49.0
upper	C03.0	C79.89	D00.03	D10.39	D37.09	D49.0
upper	C41.0	C79.51	—	D16.4	D48.0	D49.2
sulcus	C06.1	C79.89	D00.02	D10.39	D37.09	D49.0
alveolus	C03.9	C79.89	D00.03	D10.39	D37.09	D49.0
lower	C03.1	C79.89	D00.03	D10.39	D37.09	D49.0
upper	C03.0	C79.89	D00.03	D10.39	D37.09	D49.0
ampulla of Vater	C24.1	C78.89	D01.5	D13.5	D37.6	D49.0
ankle NEC	C76.5-☑	C79.89	D04.7-☑	D36.7	D48.7	D49.89

	Malignant Primary	Malignant Secondary	Ca in situ	Benign	Uncertain	Unspecified Behavior
Neoplasm, neoplastic —						
continued						
anorectum, anorectal						
(junction)	C21.8	C78.5	D01.3	D12.9	D37.8	D49.0
antecubital fossa or						
space	C76.4-☑	C79.89	D04.6-☑	D36.7	D48.7	D49.89
antrum (Highmore)						
(maxillary)	C31.0	C78.39	D02.3	D14.0	D38.5	D49.1
pyloric	C16.3	C78.89	D00.2	D13.1	D37.1	D49.0
tympanicum	C30.1	C78.39	D02.3	D14.0	D38.5	D49.1
anus, anal	C21.0	C78.5	D01.3	D12.9	D37.8	D49.0
canal	C21.1	C78.5	D01.3	D12.9	D37.8	D49.0
cloacogenic zone	C21.2	C78.5	D01.3	D12.9	D37.8	D49.0
margin — *see also*						
Neoplasm, anus,						
skin	C44.500	C79.2	D04.5	D23.5	D48.5	D49.2
overlapping lesion with						
rectosigmoid						
junction or						
rectum	C21.8	—	—	—	—	—
skin	C44.500	C79.2	D04.5	D23.5	D48.5	D49.2
basal cell						
carcinoma	C44.510					
specified type						
NEC	C44.590					
squamous cell						
carcinoma	C44.520		—	—	—	—
sphincter	C21.1	C78.5	D01.3	D12.9	D37.8	D49.0
aorta (thoracic)	C49.3	C79.89	—	D21.3	D48.1	D49.2
abdominal	C49.4	C79.89	—	D21.4	D48.1	D49.2
aortic body	C75.5	C79.89	—	D35.6	D44.7	D49.7
aponeurosis	C49.9	C79.89	—	D21.9	D48.1	D49.2
palmar	C49.1-☑	C79.89	—	D21.1-☑	D48.1	D49.2
plantar	C49.2-☑	C79.89	—	D21.2-☑	D48.1	D49.2
appendix	C18.1	C78.5	D01.0	D12.1	D37.3	D49.0
arachnoid	C70.9	C79.49	—	D32.9	D42.9	D49.7
cerebral	C70.0	C79.32	—	D32.0	D42.0	D49.7
spinal	C70.1	C79.49	—	D32.1	D42.1	D49.7
areola	C50.0-☑	C79.81	D05-☑	D24-☑	D48.6-☑	D49.3
arm NEC	C76.4-☑	C79.89	D04.6-☑	D36.7	D48.7	D49.89
artery — *see* Neoplasm,						
connective tissue						
aryepiglottic fold	C13.1	C79.89	D00.08	D10.7	D37.05	D49.0
hypopharyngeal						
aspect	C13.1	C79.89	D00.08	D10.7	D37.05	D49.0
laryngeal aspect	C32.1	C78.39	D02.0	D14.1	D38.0	D49.1
marginal zone	C13.1	C79.89	D00.08	D10.7	D37.05	D49.0
arytenoid (cartilage)	C32.3	C78.39	D02.0	D14.1	D38.0	D49.1
fold — *see* Neoplasm,						
aryepiglottic						
associated with						
transplanted						
organ	C80.2	—	—	—	—	—
atlas	C41.2	C79.51	—	D16.6	D48.0	D49.2
atrium, cardiac	C38.0	C79.89	—	D15.1	D48.7	D49.89
auditory						
canal (external) (skin)						
A81	C44.20-☑	C79.2	D04.2-☑	D23.2-☑	D48.5	D49.2
internal	C30.1	C78.39	D02.3	D14.0	D38.5	D49.1
nerve	C72.4-☑	C79.49	—	D33.3	D43.3	D49.7
tube	C30.1	C78.39	D02.3	D14.0	D38.5	D49.1
opening	C11.2	C79.89	D00.08	D10.6	D37.05	D49.0
auricle, ear — *see also*						
Neoplasm, skin,						
ear	C44.20-☑	C79.2	D04.2-☑	D23.2-☑	D48.5	D49.2
auricular canal (external)						
— *see also* Neoplasm,						
skin, ear						
internal	C30.1	C78.39	D02.3	D14.0	D38.5	D49.2
autonomic nerve or						
nervous system NEC						
(see Neoplasm, nerve,						
peripheral)						
axilla, axillary	C76.1	C79.89	D09.8	D36.7	D48.7	D49.89
fold — *see also*						
Neoplasm, skin,						
trunk	C44.509	C79.2	D04.5	D23.5	D48.5	D49.2
back NEC	C76.8	C79.89	D04.5	D36.7	D48.7	D49.89

Neoplasm, neoplastic — continued

	Malignant Primary	Malignant Secondary	Ca in situ	Benign	Uncertain	Unspecified Behavior
Bartholin's gland	C51.0	C79.82	D07.1	D28.0	D39.8	D49.5
basal ganglia	C71.0	C79.31	—	D33.0	D43.0	D49.6
basis pedunculi	C71.7	C79.31	—	D33.1	D43.1	D49.6
bile or biliary (tract)	C24.9	C78.89	D01.5	D13.5	D37.6	D49.0
canaliculi (biliferi) (intrahepatic)	C22.1	C78.7	D01.5	D13.4	D37.6	D49.0
canals, interlobular	C22.1	C78.89	D01.5	D13.4	D37.6	D49.0
duct or passage (common) (cystic) (extrahepatic)	C24.0	C78.89	D01.5	D13.5	D37.6	D49.0
interlobular	C22.1	C78.89	D01.5	D13.4	D37.6	D49.0
intrahepatic	C22.1	C78.7	D01.5	D13.4	D37.6	D49.0
and extrahepatic	C24.8	C78.89	D01.5	D13.5	D37.6	D49.0
bladder (urinary)	C67.9	C79.11	D09.0	D30.3	D41.4	D49.4
dome	C67.1	C79.11	D09.0	D30.3	D41.4	D49.4
neck	C67.5	C79.11	D09.0	D30.3	D41.4	D49.4
orifice	C67.9	C79.11	D09.0	D30.3	D41.4	D49.4
ureteric	C67.6	C79.11	D09.0	D30.3	D41.4	D49.4
urethral	C67.5	C79.11	D09.0	D30.3	D41.4	D49.4
overlapping lesion	C67.8	—	—	—	—	—
sphincter	C67.8	C79.11	D09.0	D30.3	D41.4	D49.4
trigone	C67.0	C79.11	D09.0	D30.3	D41.4	D49.4
urachus	C67.7	C79.11	D09.0	D30.3	D41.4	D49.4
wall	C67.9	C79.11	D09.0	D30.3	D41.4	D49.4
anterior	C67.3	C79.11	D09.0	D30.3	D41.4	D49.4
lateral	C67.2	C79.11	D09.0	D30.3	D41.4	D49.4
posterior	C67.4	C79.11	D09.0	D30.3	D41.4	D49.4
blood vessel — see Neoplasm, connective tissue						
bone (periosteum)	C41.9	C79.51	—	D16.9	D48.0	D49.2
acetabulum	C41.4	C79.51	—	D16.8	D48.0	D49.2
ankle	C40.3-✓	C79.51	—	D16.3-✓	—	—
arm NEC	C40.0-✓	C79.51	—	D16.0-✓	—	—
astragalus	C40.3-✓	C79.51	—	D16.3-✓	—	—
atlas	C41.2	C79.51	—	D16.6	D48.0	D49.2
axis	C41.2	C79.51	—	D16.6	D48.0	D49.2
back NEC	C41.2	C79.51	—	D16.6	D48.0	D49.2
calcaneus	C40.3-✓	C79.51	—	D16.3-✓	—	—
calvarium	C41.0	C79.51	—	D16.4	D48.0	D49.2
carpus (any)	C40.1-✓	C79.51	—	D16.1-✓	—	—
cartilage NEC	C41.9	C79.51	—	D16.9	D48.0	D49.2
clavicle	C41.3	C79.51	—	D16.7	D48.0	D49.2
clivus	C41.0	C79.51	—	D16.4	D48.0	D49.2
coccygeal vertebra	C41.4	C79.51	—	D16.8	D48.0	D49.2
coccyx	C41.4	C79.51	—	D16.8	D48.0	D49.2
costal cartilage	C41.3	C79.51	—	D16.7	D48.0	D49.2
costovertebral joint	C41.3	C79.51	—	D16.7	D48.0	D49.2
cranial	C41.0	C79.51	—	D16.4	D48.0	D49.2
cuboid	C40.3-✓	C79.51	—	D16.3-✓	—	—
cuneiform	C41.9	C79.51	—	D16.9	D48.0	D49.2
elbow	C40.0-✓	C79.51	—	D16.0-✓	—	—
ethmoid (labyrinth)	C41.0	C79.51	—	D16.4	D48.0	D49.2
face	C41.0	C79.51	—	D16.4	D48.0	D49.2
femur (any part)	C40.2-✓	C79.51	—	D16.2-✓	—	—
fibula (any part)	C40.2-✓	C79.51	—	D16.2-✓	—	—
finger (any)	C40.1-✓	C79.51	—	D16.1-✓	—	—
foot	C40.3-✓	C79.51	—	D16.3-✓	—	—
forearm	C40.0-✓	C79.51	—	D16.0-✓	—	—
frontal	C41.0	C79.51	—	D16.4	D48.0	D49.2
hand	C40.1-✓	C79.51	—	D16.1-✓	—	—
heel	C40.3-✓	C79.51	—	D16.3-✓	—	—
hip	C41.4	C79.51	—	D16.8	D48.0	D49.2
humerus (any part)	C40.0-✓	C79.51	—	D16.0-✓	—	—
hyoid	C41.0	C79.51	—	D16.4	D48.0	D49.2
ilium	C41.4	C79.51	—	D16.8	D48.0	D49.2
innominate	C41.4	C79.51	—	D16.8	D48.0	D49.2
intervertebral cartilage or disc	C41.2	C79.51	—	D16.6	D48.0	D49.2
ischium	C41.4	C79.51	—	D16.8	D48.0	D49.2
jaw (lower)	C41.1	C79.51	—	D16.5	D48.0	D49.2
knee	C40.2-✓	C79.51	—	D16.2-✓	—	—
leg NEC	C40.2-✓	C79.51	—	D16.2-✓	—	—
limb NEC	C40.9-✓	C79.51	—	D16.9	—	—

Neoplasm, neoplastic — continued

	Malignant Primary	Malignant Secondary	Ca in situ	Benign	Uncertain	Unspecified Behavior
bone — continued						
limb — continued						
lower (long bones)	C40.2-✓	C79.51	—	D16.2-✓	—	—
short bones	C40.3-✓	C79.51	—	D16.3-✓	—	—
upper (long bones)	C40.0-✓	C79.51	—	D16.0-✓	—	—
short bones	C40.1-✓	C79.51	—	D16.1-✓	—	—
malar	C41.0	C79.51	—	D16.4	D48.0	D49.2
mandible	C41.1	C79.51	—	D16.5	D48.0	D49.2
marrow NEC (any bone)	C96.9	C79.52	—	—	D47.9	D49.89
mastoid	C41.0	C79.51	—	D16.4	D48.0	D49.2
maxilla, maxillary (superior)	C41.0	C79.51	—	D16.4	D48.0	D49.2
inferior	C41.1	C79.51	—	D16.5	D48.0	D49.2
metacarpus (any)	C40.1-✓	C79.51	—	D16.1-✓	—	—
metatarsus (any)	C40.3-✓	C79.51	—	D16.3-✓	—	—
navicular						
ankle	C40.3-✓	C79.51	—	—	—	—
hand	C40.1-✓	C79.51	—	—	—	—
nose, nasal	C41.0	C79.51	—	D16.4	D48.0	D49.2
occipital	C41.0	C79.51	—	D16.4	D48.0	D49.2
orbit	C41.0	C79.51	—	D16.4	D48.0	D49.2
overlapping sites	C40.8-✓	—	—	—	—	—
parietal	C41.0	C79.51	—	D16.4	D48.0	D49.2
patella	C40.2-✓	C79.51	—	—	—	—
pelvic	C41.4	C79.51	—	D16.8	D48.0	D49.2
phalanges						
foot	C40.3-✓	C79.51	—	—	—	—
hand	C40.1-✓	C79.51	—	—	—	—
pubic	C41.4	C79.51	—	D16.8	D48.0	D49.2
radius (any part)	C40.0-✓	C79.51	—	D16.0-✓	—	—
rib	C41.3	C79.51	—	D16.7	D48.0	D49.2
sacral vertebra	C41.4	C79.51	—	D16.8	D48.0	D49.2
sacrum	C41.4	C79.51	—	D16.8	D48.0	D49.2
scaphoid						
of ankle	C40.3-✓	C79.51	—	—	—	—
of hand	C40.1-✓	C79.51	—	—	—	—
scapula (any part)	C40.0-✓	C79.51	—	D16.0-✓	—	—
sella turcica	C41.0	C79.51	—	D16.4	D48.0	D49.2
shoulder	C40.0-✓	C79.51	—	D16.0-✓	—	—
skull	C41.0	C79.51	—	D16.4	D48.0	D49.2
sphenoid	C41.0	C79.51	—	D16.4	D48.0	D49.2
spine, spinal (column)	C41.2	C79.51	—	D16.6	D48.0	D49.2
coccyx	C41.4	C79.51	—	D16.8	D48.0	D49.2
sacrum	C41.4	C79.51	—	D16.8	D48.0	D49.2
sternum	C41.3	C79.51	—	D16.7	D48.0	D49.2
tarsus (any)	C40.3-✓	C79.51	—	—	—	—
temporal	C41.0	C79.51	—	D16.4	D48.0	D49.2
thumb	C40.1-✓	C79.51	—	—	—	—
tibia (any part)	C40.2-✓	C79.51	—	—	—	—
toe (any)	C40.3-✓	C79.51	—	—	—	—
trapezium	C40.1-✓	C79.51	—	—	—	—
trapezoid	C40.1-✓	C79.51	—	—	—	—
turbinate	C41.0	C79.51	—	D16.4	D48.0	D49.2
ulna (any part)	C40.0-✓	C79.51	—	D16.0-✓	—	—
unciform	C40.1-✓	C79.51	—	—	—	—
vertebra (column)	C41.2	C79.51	—	D16.6	D48.0	D49.2
coccyx	C41.4	C79.51	—	D16.8	D48.0	D49.2
sacrum	C41.4	C79.51	—	D16.8	D48.0	D49.2
vomer	C41.0	C79.51	—	D16.4	D48.0	D49.2
wrist	C40.1-✓	C79.51	—	—	—	—
xiphoid process	C41.3	C79.51	—	D16.7	D48.0	D49.2
zygomatic	C41.0	C79.51	—	D16.4	D48.0	D49.2
book-leaf (mouth) — ventral surface of tongue and floor of mouth	C06.89	C79.89	D00.00	D10.39	D37.09	D49.0
bowel — see Neoplasm, intestine						
brachial plexus	C47.1-✓	C79.89	—	D36.12	D48.2	D49.2
brain NEC	C71.9	C79.31	—	D33.2	D43.2	D49.6
basal ganglia	C71.0	C79.31	—	D33.0	D43.0	D49.6
cerebellopontine angle	C71.6	C79.31	—	D33.1	D43.1	D49.6
cerebellum NOS	C71.6	C79.31	—	D33.1	D43.1	D49.6
cerebrum	C71.0	C79.31	—	D33.0	D43.0	D49.6

☑ Additional Character Required — Refer to the Tabular List for Character Selection   ▽ Subterms under main terms may continue to next column or page

	Malignant Primary	Malignant Secondary	Ca in situ	Benign	Uncertain	Unspecified Behavior
Neoplasm, neoplastic — *continued*						
brain — *continued*						
choroid plexus	C71.7	C79.31	—	D33.1	D43.1	D49.6
corpus callosum	C71.8	C79.31	—	D33.2	D43.2	D49.6
corpus striatum	C71.0	C79.31	—	D33.0	D43.0	D49.6
cortex (cerebral)	C71.0	C79.31	—	D33.0	D43.0	D49.6
frontal lobe	C71.1	C79.31	—	D33.0	D43.0	D49.6
globus pallidus	C71.0	C79.31	—	D33.0	D43.0	D49.6
hippocampus	C71.2	C79.31	—	D33.0	D43.0	D49.6
hypothalamus	C71.0	C79.31	—	D33.0	D43.0	D49.6
internal capsule	C71.0	C79.31	—	D33.0	D43.0	D49.6
medulla oblongata	C71.7	C79.31	—	D33.1	D43.1	D49.6
meninges	C70.0	C79.32	—	D32.0	D42.0	D49.7
midbrain	C71.7	C79.31	—	D33.1	D43.1	D49.6
occipital lobe	C71.4	C79.31	—	D33.0	D43.0	D49.6
overlapping lesion	C71.8	C79.31	—	—	—	D49.6
parietal lobe	C71.3	C79.31	—	D33.0	D43.0	D49.6
peduncle	C71.7	C79.31	—	D33.1	D43.1	D49.6
pons	C71.7	C79.31	—	D33.1	D43.1	D49.6
stem	C71.7	C79.31	—	D33.1	D43.1	D49.6
tapetum	C71.8	C79.31	—	D33.2	D43.2	D49.6
temporal lobe	C71.2	C79.31	—	D33.0	D43.0	D49.6
thalamus	C71.0	C79.31	—	D33.0	D43.0	D49.6
uncus	C71.2	C79.31	—	D33.0	D43.0	D49.6
ventricle (floor)	C71.5	C79.31	—	D33.0	D43.0	D49.6
fourth	C71.7	C79.31	—	D33.1	D43.1	D49.6
branchial (cleft) (cyst) (vestiges)	C10.4	C79.89	D00.08	D10.5	D37.05	D49.0
breast (connective tissue) (glandular tissue) (soft parts)	C50.9-☑	C79.81	D05.-☑	D24.-☑	D48.6-☑	D49.3
areola	C50.-☑	C79.81	D05.-☑	D24.-☑	D48.6-☑	D49.3
axillary tail	C50.6-☑	C79.81	D05.-☑	D24.-☑	D48.6-☑	D49.3
central portion	C50.1-☑	C79.81	D05.-☑	D24.-☑	D48.6-☑	D49.3
inner	C50.8-☑	C79.81	D05.-☑	D24.-☑	D48.6-☑	D49.3
lower	C50.8-☑	C79.81	D05.-☑	D24.-☑	D48.6-☑	D49.3
lower-inner quadrant	C50.3-☑	C79.81	D05.-☑	D24.-☑	D48.6-☑	D49.3
lower-outer quadrant	C50.5-☑	C79.81	D05.-☑	D24.-☑	D48.6-☑	D49.3
mastectomy site (skin) — *see also* Neoplasm, breast, skin	C44.501	C79.2	—	—	—	—
specified as breast tissue	C50.8-☑	C79.81	—	—	—	—
midline	C50.8-☑	C79.81	D05.-☑	D24.-☑	D48.6-☑	D49.3
nipple	C50.0-☑	C79.81	D05.-☑	D24.-☑	D48.6-☑	D49.3
outer	C50.8-☑	C79.81	D05.-☑	D24.-☑	D48.6-☑	D49.3
overlapping lesion	C50.8-☑	—	—	—	—	—
skin	C44.501	C79.2	D04.5	D23.5	D48.5	D49.2
basal cell carcinoma	C44.511	—	—	—	—	—
specified type NEC	C44.591	—	—	—	—	—
squamous cell carcinoma	C44.521	—	—	—	—	—
tail (axillary)	C50.6-☑	C79.81	D05.-☑	D24.-☑	D48.6-☑	D49.3
upper	C50.8-☑	C79.81	D05.-☑	D24.-☑	D48.6-☑	D49.3
upper-inner quadrant	C50.2-☑	C79.81	D05.-☑	D24.-☑	D48.6-☑	D49.3
upper-outer quadrant	C50.4-☑	C79.81	D05.-☑	D24.-☑	D48.6-☑	D49.3
broad ligament	C57.1-☑	C79.82	D07.39	D28.2	D39.8	D49.5
bronchiogenic, bronchogenic (lung)	C34.9-☑	C78.0-☑	D02.2-☑	D14.3-☑	D38.1	D49.1
bronchiole	C34.9-☑	C78.0-☑	D02.2-☑	D14.3-☑	D38.1	D49.1
bronchus	C34.9-☑	C78.0-☑	D02.2-☑	D14.3-☑	D38.1	D49.1
carina	C34.0-☑	C78.0-☑	D02.2-☑	D14.3-☑	D38.1	D49.1
lower lobe of lung	C34.3-☑	C78.0-☑	D02.2-☑	D14.3-☑	D38.1	D49.1
main	C34.0-☑	C78.0-☑	D02.2-☑	D14.3-☑	D38.1	D49.1
middle lobe of lung	C34.2	C78.0-☑	D02.21	D14.31	D38.1	D49.1
overlapping lesion	C34.8-☑	—	—	—	—	—
upper lobe of lung	C34.1-☑	C78.0-☑	D02.2-☑	D14.3-☑	D38.1	D49.1
brow	C44.309	C79.2	D04.39	D23.39	D48.5	D49.2
basal cell carcinoma	C44.319	—	—	—	—	—
specified type NEC	C44.399	—	—	—	—	—

	Malignant Primary	Malignant Secondary	Ca in situ	Benign	Uncertain	Unspecified Behavior
Neoplasm, neoplastic — *continued*						
brow — *continued*						
squamous cell carcinoma	C44.329	—	—	—	—	—
buccal (cavity)	C06.9	C79.89	D00.00	D10.39	D37.09	D49.0
commissure	C06.0	C79.89	D00.02	D10.39	D37.09	D49.0
groove (lower) (upper)	C06.1	C79.89	D00.02	D10.39	D37.09	D49.0
mucosa	C06.0	C79.89	D00.02	D10.39	D37.09	D49.0
sulcus (lower) (upper)	C06.1	C79.89	D00.02	D10.39	D37.09	D49.0
bulbourethral gland	C68.0	C79.19	D09.19	D30.4	D41.3	D49.5
bursa — *see* Neoplasm, connective tissue						
buttock NEC	C76.3	C79.89	D04.5	D36.7	D48.7	D49.89
calf	C76.5-☑	C79.89	D04.7-☑	D36.7	D48.7	D49.89
calvarium	C41.0	C79.51	—	D16.4	D48.0	D49.2
calyx, renal	C65.-☑	C79.0-☑	D09.19	D30.1-☑	D41.1-☑	D49.5
canal						
anal	C21.1	C78.5	D01.3	D12.9	D37.8	D49.0
auditory (external) — *see also* Neoplasm, skin, ear	C44.20-☑	C79.2	D04.2-☑	D23.2-☑	D48.5	D49.2
auricular (external) — *see also* Neoplasm, skin, ear	C44.20-☑	C79.2	D04.2-☑	D23.2-☑	D48.5	D49.2
canaliculi, biliary (biliferi) (intrahepatic)	C22.1	C78.7	D01.5	D13.4	D37.6	D49.0
canthus (eye) (inner) (outer)	C44.10-☑	C79.2	D04.1-☑	D23.1-☑	D48.5	D49.2
basal cell carcinoma	C44.11-☑	—	—	—	—	—
specified type NEC	C44.19-☑	—	—	—	—	—
squamous cell carcinoma	C44.12-☑	—	—	—	—	—
capillary — *see* Neoplasm, connective tissue						
caput coli	C18.0	C78.5	D01.0	D12.0	D37.4	D49.0
carcinoid — *see* Tumor, carcinoid						
cardia (gastric)	C16.0	C78.89	D00.2	D13.1	D37.1	D49.0
cardiac orifice (stomach)	C16.0	C78.89	D00.2	D13.1	D37.1	D49.0
cardio-esophageal junction	C16.0	C78.89	D00.2	D13.1	D37.1	D49.0
cardio-esophagus	C16.0	C78.89	D00.2	D13.1	D37.1	D49.0
carina (bronchus)	C34.0-☑	C78.0-☑	D02.2-☑	D14.3-☑	D38.1	D49.1
carotid (artery)	C49.0	C79.89	—	D21.0	D48.1	D49.2
body	C75.4	C79.89	—	D35.5	D44.6	D49.7
carpus (any bone)	C40.1-☑	C79.51	—	D16.1-☑	D48.0	D49.2
cartilage (articular) (joint) NEC — *see also* Neoplasm, bone	C41.9	C79.51	—	D16.9	D48.0	D49.2
arytenoid	C32.3	C78.39	D02.0	D14.1	D38.0	D49.1
auricular	C49.0	C79.89	—	D21.0	D48.1	D49.2
bronchi	C34.0-☑	C78.39	—	D14.3-☑	D38.1	D49.1
costal	C41.3	C79.51	—	D16.7	D48.0	D49.2
cricoid	C32.3	C78.39	D02.0	D14.1	D38.0	D49.1
cuneiform	C32.3	C78.39	D02.0	D14.1	D38.0	D49.1
ear (external)	C49.0	C79.89	—	D21.0	D48.1	D49.2
ensiform	C41.3	C79.51	—	D16.7	D48.0	D49.2
epiglottis	C32.1	C78.39	D02.0	D14.1	D38.0	D49.1
anterior surface	C10.1	C79.89	D00.08	D10.5	D37.05	D49.0
eyelid	C49.0	C79.89	—	D21.0	D48.1	D49.2
intervertebral	C41.2	C79.51	—	D16.6	D48.0	D49.2
larynx, laryngeal	C32.3	C78.39	D02.0	D14.1	D38.0	D49.1
nose, nasal	C30.0	C78.39	D02.3	D14.0	D38.5	D49.1
pinna	C49.0	C79.89	—	D21.0	D48.1	D49.2
rib	C41.3	C79.51	—	D16.7	D48.0	D49.2
semilunar (knee)	C40.2-☑	C79.51	—	D16.2-☑	D48.0	D49.2
thyroid	C32.3	C78.39	D02.0	D14.1	D38.0	D49.1
trachea	C33	C78.39	D02.1	D14.2	D38.1	D49.1
cauda equina	C72.1	C79.49	—	D33.4	D43.4	D49.7
cavity						
buccal	C06.9	C79.89	D00.00	D10.30	D37.09	D49.0
nasal	C30.0	C78.39	D02.3	D14.0	D38.5	D49.1
oral	C06.9	C79.89	D00.00	D10.30	D37.09	D49.0
peritoneal	C48.2	C78.6	—	D20.1	D48.4	D49.0
tympanic	C30.1	C78.39	D02.3	D14.0	D38.5	D49.1
cecum	C18.0	C78.5	D01.0	D12.0	D37.4	D49.0

Neoplasm, neoplastic — continued	Malignant Primary	Malignant Secondary	Ca in situ	Benign	Uncertain	Unspecified Behavior
central nervous system	C72.9	C79.40	—	—	—	—
cerebellopontine (angle)	C71.6	C79.31	—	D33.1	D43.1	D49.6
cerebellum, cerebellar	C71.6	C79.31	—	D33.1	D43.1	D49.6
cerebrum, cerebral (cortex) (hemisphere) (white matter)	C71.0	C79.31	—	D33.0	D43.0	D49.6
meninges	C70.0	C79.32	—	D32.0	D42.0	D49.7
peduncle	C71.7	C79.31	—	D33.1	D43.1	D49.6
ventricle	C71.5	C79.31	—	D33.0	D43.0	D49.6
fourth	C71.7	C79.31	—	D33.1	D43.1	D49.6
cervical region	C76.0	C79.89	D09.8	D36.7	D48.7	D49.89
cervix (cervical) (uteri) (uterus)	C53.9	C79.82	D06.9	D26.0	D39.0	D49.5
canal	C53.0	C79.82	D06.0	D26.0	D39.0	D49.5
endocervix (canal) (gland)	C53.0	C79.82	D06.0	D26.0	D39.0	D49.5
exocervix	C53.1	C79.82	D06.1	D26.0	D39.0	D49.5
external os	C53.1	C79.82	D06.1	D26.0	D39.0	D49.5
internal os	C53.0	C79.82	D06.0	D26.0	D39.0	D49.5
nabothian gland	C53.0	C79.82	D06.0	D26.0	D39.0	D49.5
overlapping lesion	C53.8	—	—	—	—	—
squamocolumnar junction	C53.8	C79.82	D06.7	D26.0	D39.0	D49.5
stump	C53.8	C79.82	D06.7	D26.0	D39.0	D49.5
cheek	C76.0	C79.89	D09.8	D36.7	D48.7	D49.89
external	C44.309	C79.2	D04.39	D23.39	D48.5	D49.2
basal cell carcinoma	C44.319	—	—	—	—	—
specified type NEC	C44.399	—	—	—	—	—
squamous cell carcinoma	C44.329	—	—	—	—	—
inner aspect	C06.0	C79.89	D00.02	D10.39	D37.09	D49.0
internal	C06.0	C79.89	D00.02	D10.39	D37.09	D49.0
mucosa	C06.0	C79.89	D00.02	D10.39	D37.09	D49.0
chest (wall) NEC	C76.1	C79.89	D09.8	D36.7	D48.7	D49.89
chiasma opticum	C72.3-☑	C79.49	—	D33.3	D43.3	D49.7
chin	C44.309	C79.2	D04.39	D23.39	D48.5	D49.2
basal cell carcinoma	C44.319	—	—	—	—	—
specified type NEC	C44.399	—	—	—	—	—
squamous cell carcinoma	C44.329	—	—	—	—	—
choana	C11.3	C79.89	D00.08	D10.6	D37.05	D49.0
cholangiole	C22.1	C78.89	D01.5	D13.4	D37.6	D49.0
choledochal duct	C24.0	C78.89	D01.5	D13.5	D37.6	D49.0
choroid	C69.3-☑	C79.49	D09.2-☑	D31.3-☑	D48.7	D49.81
plexus	C71.5	C79.31	—	D33.0	D43.0	D49.6
ciliary body	C69.4-☑	C79.49	D09.2-☑	D31.4-☑	D48.7	D49.89
clavicle	C41.3	C79.51	—	D16.7	D48.0	D49.2
clitoris	C51.2	C79.82	D07.1	D28.0	D39.8	D49.5
clivus	C41.0	C79.51	—	D16.4	D48.0	D49.2
cloacogenic zone	C21.2	C78.5	D01.3	D12.9	D37.8	D49.0
coccygeal body or glomus	C49.5	C79.89	—	D21.5	D48.1	D49.2
vertebra	C41.4	C79.51	—	D16.8	D48.0	D49.2
coccyx	C41.4	C79.51	—	D16.8	D48.0	D49.2
colon — see also Neoplasm, intestine, large	C18.9	C78.5	—	—	—	—
with rectum	C19	C78.5	D01.1	D12.7	D37.5	D49.0
columnella — see also Neoplasm, skin, face	C44.390	C79.2	D04.39	D23.39	D48.5	D49.2
column, spinal — see Neoplasm, spine						
commissure labial, lip	C00.6	C79.89	D00.01	D10.39	D37.01	D49.0
laryngeal	C32.0	C78.39	D02.0	D14.1	D38.0	D49.1
common (bile) duct	C24.0	C78.89	D01.5	D13.5	D37.6	D49.0
concha — see also Neoplasm, skin, ear	C44.20-☑	C79.2	D04.2-☑	D23.2-☑	D48.5	D49.2
nose	C30.0	C78.39	D02.3	D14.0	D38.5	D49.1
conjunctiva	C69.0-☑	C79.49	D09.2-☑	D31.0-☑	D48.7	D49.89

Neoplasm, neoplastic — continued	Malignant Primary	Malignant Secondary	Ca in situ	Benign	Uncertain	Unspecified Behavior
connective tissue NEC	C49.9	C79.89	—	D21.9	D48.1	D49.2

Note: For neoplasms of connective tissue (blood vessel, bursa, fascia, ligament, muscle, peripheral nerves, sympathetic and parasympathetic nerves and ganglia, synovia, tendon, etc.) or of morphological types that indicate connective tissue, code according to the list under "Neoplasm, connective tissue". For sites that do not appear in this list, code to neoplasm of that site; e.g., fibrosarcoma, pancreas (C25.9)

Note: Morphological types that indicate connective tissue appear in their proper place in the alphabetic index with the instruction "see Neoplasm, connective tissue ...."

	Malignant Primary	Malignant Secondary	Ca in situ	Benign	Uncertain	Unspecified Behavior
abdomen	C49.4	C79.89	—	D21.4	D48.1	D49.2
abdominal wall	C49.4	C79.89	—	D21.4	D48.1	D49.2
ankle	C49.2-☑	C79.89	—	D21.2-☑	D48.1	D49.2
antecubital fossa or space	C49.1-☑	C79.89	—	D21.1-☑	D48.1	D49.2
arm	C49.1-☑	C79.89	—	D21.1-☑	D48.1	D49.2
auricle (ear)	C49.0	C79.89	—	D21.0	D48.1	D49.2
axilla	C49.3	C79.89	—	D21.3	D48.1	D49.2
back	C49.6	C79.89	—	D21.6	D48.1	D49.2
breast — see Neoplasm, breast						
buttock	C49.5	C79.89	—	D21.5	D48.1	D49.2
calf	C49.2-☑	C79.89	—	D21.2-☑	D48.1	D49.2
cervical region	C49.0	C79.89	—	D21.0	D48.1	D49.2
cheek	C49.0	C79.89	—	D21.0	D48.1	D49.2
chest (wall)	C49.3	C79.89	—	D21.3	D48.1	D49.2
chin	C49.0	C79.89	—	D21.0	D48.1	D49.2
diaphragm	C49.3	C79.89	—	D21.3	D48.1	D49.2
ear (external)	C49.0	C79.89	—	D21.0	D48.1	D49.2
elbow	C49.1-☑	C79.89	—	D21.1-☑	D48.1	D49.2
extrarectal	C49.5	C79.89	—	D21.5	D48.1	D49.2
extremity	C49.9	C79.89	—	D21.9	D48.1	D49.2
lower	C49.2-☑	C79.89	—	D21.2-☑	D48.1	D49.2
upper	C49.1-☑	C79.89	—	D21.1-☑	D48.1	D49.2
eyelid	C49.0	C79.89	—	D21.0	D48.1	D49.2
face	C49.0	C79.89	—	D21.0	D48.1	D49.2
finger	C49.1-☑	C79.89	—	D21.1-☑	D48.1	D49.2
flank	C49.6	C79.89	—	D21.6	D48.1	D49.2
foot	C49.2-☑	C79.89	—	D21.2-☑	D48.1	D49.2
forearm	C49.1-☑	C79.89	—	D21.1-☑	D48.1	D49.2
forehead	C49.0	C79.89	—	D21.0	D48.1	D49.2
gastric	C49.4	C79.89	—	D21.4	D48.1	D49.2
gastrointestinal	C49.4	C79.89	—	D21.4	D48.1	D49.2
gluteal region	C49.5	C79.89	—	D21.5	D48.1	D49.2
great vessels NEC	C49.3	C79.89	—	D21.3	D48.1	D49.2
groin	C49.5	C79.89	—	D21.5	D48.1	D49.2
hand	C49.1-☑	C79.89	—	D21.1-☑	D48.1	D49.2
head	C49.0	C79.89	—	D21.0	D48.1	D49.2
heel	C49.2-☑	C79.89	—	D21.2-☑	D48.1	D49.2
hip	C49.2-☑	C79.89	—	D21.2-☑	D48.1	D49.2
hypochondrium	C49.4	C79.89	—	D21.4	D48.1	D49.2
iliopsoas muscle	C49.5	C79.89	—	D21.5	D48.1	D49.2
infraclavicular region	C49.3	C79.89	—	D21.3	D48.1	D49.2
inguinal (canal) (region)	C49.5	C79.89	—	D21.5	D48.1	D49.2
intestinal	C49.4	C79.89	—	D21.4	D48.1	D49.2
intrathoracic	C49.3	C79.89	—	D21.3	D48.1	D49.2
ischiorectal fossa	C49.5	C79.89	—	D21.5	D48.1	D49.2
jaw	C03.9	C79.89	D00.03	D10.39	D48.1	D49.0
knee	C49.2-☑	C79.89	—	D21.2-☑	D48.1	D49.2
leg	C49.2-☑	C79.89	—	D21.2-☑	D48.1	D49.2
limb NEC	C49.9	C79.89	—	D21.9	D48.1	D49.2
lower	C49.2-☑	C79.89	—	D21.2-☑	D48.1	D49.2
upper	C49.1-☑	C79.89	—	D21.1-☑	D48.1	D49.2
nates	C49.5	C79.89	—	D21.5	D48.1	D49.2
neck	C49.0	C79.89	—	D21.0	D48.1	D49.2
orbit	C69.6-☑	C79.49	D09.2-☑	D31.6-☑	D48.1	D49.89
overlapping lesion	C49.8	—	—	—	—	—
pararectal	C49.5	C79.89	—	D21.5	D48.1	D49.2
para-urethral	C49.5	C79.89	—	D21.5	D48.1	D49.2
paravaginal	C49.5	C79.89	—	D21.5	D48.1	D49.2
pelvis (floor)	C49.5	C79.89	—	D21.5	D48.1	D49.2
pelvo-abdominal	C49.8			D21.6	D48.1	D49.2
perineum	C49.5	C79.89	—	D21.5	D48.1	D49.2
perirectal (tissue)	C49.5	C79.89	—	D21.5	D48.1	D49.2

Neoplasm, neoplastic — continued	Malignant Primary	Malignant Secondary	Ca in situ	Benign	Uncertain	Unspecified Behavior
connective tissue — continued						
periurethral (tissue)	C49.5	C79.89	—	D21.5	D48.1	D49.2
popliteal fossa or space	C49.2-☑	C79.89	—	D21.2-☑	D48.1	D49.2
presacral	C49.5	C79.89	—	D21.5	D48.1	D49.2
psoas muscle	C49.4	C79.89	—	D21.4	D48.1	D49.2
pterygoid fossa	C49.0	C79.89	—	D21.0	D48.1	D49.2
rectovaginal septum or wall	C49.5	C79.89	—	D21.5	D48.1	D49.2
rectovesical	C49.5	C79.89	—	D21.5	D48.1	D49.2
retroperitoneum	C48.0	C78.6		D20.0	D48.3	D49.0
sacrococcygeal region	C49.5	C79.89	—	D21.5	D48.1	D49.2
scalp	C49.0	C79.89	—	D21.0	D48.1	D49.2
scapular region	C49.3	C79.89	—	D21.3	D48.1	D49.2
shoulder	C49.1-☑	C79.89	—	D21.1-☑	D48.1	D49.2
skin (dermis) NEC — see also Neoplasm, skin, by site	C44.90	C79.2	D04.9	D23.9	D48.5	D49.2
stomach	C49.4	C79.89	—	D21.4	D48.1	D49.2
submental	C49.0	C79.89	—	D21.0	D48.1	D49.2
supraclavicular region	C49.0	C79.89	—	D21.0	D48.1	D49.2
temple	C49.0	C79.89	—	D21.0	D48.1	D49.2
temporal region	C49.0	C79.89	—	D21.0	D48.1	D49.2
thigh	C49.2-☑	C79.89	—	D21.2-☑	D48.1	D49.2
thoracic (duct) (wall)	C49.3	C79.89	—	D21.3	D48.1	D49.2
thorax	C49.3	C79.89	—	D21.3	D48.1	D49.2
thumb	C49.1-☑	C79.89	—	D21.1-☑	D48.1	D49.2
toe	C49.2-☑	C79.89	—	D21.2-☑	D48.1	D49.2
trunk	C49.6	C79.89	—	D21.6	D48.1	D49.2
umbilicus	C49.4	C79.89	—	D21.4	D48.1	D49.2
vesicorectal	C49.5	C79.89	—	D21.5	D48.1	D49.2
wrist	C49.1-☑	C79.89	—	D21.1-☑	D48.1	D49.2
conus medullaris	C72.0	C79.49		D33.4	D43.4	D49.7
cord (true) (vocal)	C32.0	C78.39	D02.0	D14.1	D38.0	D49.1
false	C32.1	C78.39	D02.0	D14.1	D38.0	D49.1
spermatic	C63.1-☑	C79.82	D07.69	D29.8	D40.8	D49.5
spinal (cervical) (lumbar) (thoracic)	C72.0	C79.49	—	D33.4	D43.4	D49.7
cornea (limbus)	C69.1-☑	C79.49	D09.2-☑	D31.1-☑	D48.7	D49.89
corpus						
albicans	C56.-☑	C79.6-☑	D07.39	D27.-☑	D39.1-☑	D49.5
callosum, brain	C71.0	C79.31		D33.2	D43.2	D49.6
cavernosum	C60.2	C79.82	D07.4	D29.0	D40.8	D49.5
gastric	C16.2	C78.89	D00.2	D13.1	D37.1	D49.0
overlapping sites	C54.8	—		—	—	—
penis	C60.2	C79.82	D07.4	D29.0	D40.8	D49.5
striatum, cerebrum	C71.0	C79.31		D33.0	D43.0	D49.6
uteri	C54.9	C79.82	D07.0	D26.1	D39.0	D49.5
isthmus	C54.0	C79.82	D07.0	D26.1	D39.0	D49.5
cortex						
adrenal	C74.0-☑	C79.7-☑	D09.3	D35.0-☑	D44.1-☑	D49.7
cerebral	C71.0	C79.31		D33.0	D43.0	D49.6
costal cartilage	C41.3	C79.51		D16.7	D48.0	D49.2
costovertebral joint	C41.3	C79.51		D16.7	D48.0	D49.2
Cowper's gland	C68.0	C79.19	D09.19	D30.4	D41.3	D49.5
cranial (fossa, any)	C71.9	C79.31		D33.2	D43.2	D49.6
meninges	C70.0	C79.32		D32.0	D42.0	D49.7
nerve	C72.50	C79.49	—	D33.3	D43.3	D49.7
specified NEC	C72.59	C79.49	—	D33.3	D43.3	D49.7
craniobuccal pouch	C75.2	C79.89	D09.3	D35.2	D44.3	D49.7
craniopharyngeal (duct) (pouch)	C75.2	C79.89	D09.3	D35.3	D44.4	D49.7
cricoid	C13.0	C79.89	D00.08	D10.7	D37.05	D49.0
cartilage	C32.3	C78.39	D02.0	D14.1	D38.0	D49.1
cricopharynx	C13.0	C79.89	D00.08	D10.7	D37.05	D49.0
crypt of Morgagni	C21.8	C78.5	D01.3	D12.9	D37.8	D49.0
crystalline lens	C69.4-☑	C79.49	D09.2-☑	D31.4-☑	D48.7	D49.89
cul-de-sac (Douglas')	C48.1	C78.6	—	D20.1	D48.4	D49.0
cuneiform cartilage	C32.3	C78.39	D02.0	D14.1	D38.0	D49.1
cutaneous — see Neoplasm, skin						
cutis — see Neoplasm, skin						

Neoplasm, neoplastic — continued	Malignant Primary	Malignant Secondary	Ca in situ	Benign	Uncertain	Unspecified Behavior
cystic (bile) duct (common)	C24.0	C78.89	D01.5	D13.5	D37.6	D49.0
dermis — see Neoplasm, skin						
diaphragm	C49.3	C79.89	—	D21.3	D48.1	D49.2
digestive organs, system, tube, or tract						
NEC	C26.9	C78.89	D01.9	D13.9	D37.9	D49.0
disc, intervertebral	C41.2	C79.51		D16.6	D48.0	D49.2
disease, generalized	C80.0	—	—	—	—	—
disseminated	C80.0	—	—	—	—	—
Douglas' cul-de-sac or pouch	C48.1	C78.6		D20.1	D48.4	D49.0
duodenojejunal junction	C17.8	C78.4	D01.49	D13.39	D37.2	D49.0
duodenum	C17.0	C78.4	D01.49	D13.2	D37.2	D49.0
dura (cranial) (mater)	C70.9	C79.49		D32.9	D42.9	D49.7
cerebral	C70.0	C79.32		D32.0	D42.0	D49.7
spinal	C70.1	C79.49		D32.1	D42.1	D49.7
ear (external) — see also Neoplasm, skin, ear	C44.20-☑	C79.2	D04.2-☑	D23.2-☑	D48.5	D49.2
auricle or auris — see also Neoplasm, skin, ear	C44.20-☑	C79.2	D04.2-☑	D23.2-☑	D48.5	D49.2
canal, external — see also Neoplasm, skin, ear	C44.20-☑	C79.2	D04.2-☑	D23.2-☑	D48.5	D49.2
cartilage	C49.0	C79.89	—	D21.0	D48.1	D49.2
external meatus — see also Neoplasm, skin, ear	C44.20-☑	C79.2	D04.2-☑	D23.2-☑	D48.5	D49.2
inner	C30.1	C78.39	D02.3	D14.0	D38.5	D49.1
lobule — see also Neoplasm, skin, ear	C44.20-☑	C79.2	D04.2-☑	D23.2-☑	D48.5	D49.2
middle	C30.1	C78.39	D02.3	D14.0	D38.5	D49.1
overlapping lesion with accessory sinuses	C31.8	—	—	—	—	—
skin	C44.20-☑	C79.2	D04.2-☑	D23.2-☑	D48.5	D49.2
basal cell carcinoma	C44.21-☑	—	—	—	—	—
specified type NEC	C44.29-☑	—	—	—	—	—
squamous cell carcinoma	C44.22-☑	—	—	—	—	—
earlobe	C44.20-☑	C79.2	D04.2-☑	D23.2-☑	D48.5	D49.2
basal cell carcinoma	C44.21-☑	—	—	—	—	—
specified type NEC	C44.29-☑	—	—	—	—	—
squamous cell carcinoma	C44.22-☑	—	—	—	—	—
ejaculatory duct	C63.7	C79.82	D07.69	D29.8	D40.8	D49.5
elbow NEC	C76.4-☑	C79.89	D04.6-☑	D36.7	D48.7	D49.89
endocardium	C38.0	C79.89	—	D15.1	D48.7	D49.89
endocervix (canal) (gland)	C53.0	C79.82	D06.0	D26.0	D39.0	D49.5
endocrine gland NEC	C75.9	C79.89	D09.3	D35.9	D44.9	D49.7
pluriglandular	C75.8	C79.89	D09.3	D35.7	D44.9	D49.7
endometrium (gland) (stroma)	C54.1	C79.82	D07.0	D26.1	D39.0	D49.5
ensiform cartilage	C41.3	C79.51	—	D16.7	D48.0	D49.2
enteric — see Neoplasm, intestine						
ependyma (brain)	C71.5	C79.31		D33.0	D43.0	D49.6
fourth ventricle	C71.7	C79.31	—	D33.1	D43.1	D49.6
epicardium	C38.0	C79.89	—	D15.1	D48.7	D49.89
epididymis	C63.0-☑	C79.82	D07.69	D29.3-☑	D40.8	D49.5
epidural	C72.9	C79.49	—	D33.9	D43.9	D49.7
epiglottis	C32.1	C78.39	D02.0	D14.1	D38.0	D49.1
anterior aspect or surface	C10.1	C79.89	D00.08	D10.5	D37.05	D49.0
cartilage	C32.3	C78.39	D02.0	D14.1	D38.0	D49.1
free border (margin)	C10.1	C79.89	D00.08	D10.5	D37.05	D49.0
junctional region	C10.8	C79.89	D00.08	D10.5	D37.05	D49.0
posterior (laryngeal) surface	C32.1	C78.39	D02.0	D14.1	D38.0	D49.1

Neoplasm, neoplastic — *continued*

	Malignant Primary	Malignant Secondary	Ca in situ	Benign	Uncertain	Unspecified Behavior
epiglottis — *continued*						
suprahyoid portion	C32.1	C78.39	D02.0	D14.1	D38.0	D49.1
esophagogastric junction	C16.0	C78.89	D00.2	D13.1	D37.1	D49.0
esophagus	C15.9	C78.89	D00.1	D13.0	D37.8	D49.0
abdominal	C15.5	C78.89	D00.1	D13.0	D37.8	D49.0
cervical	C15.3	C78.89	D00.1	D13.0	D37.8	D49.0
distal (third)	C15.5	C78.89	D00.1	D13.0	D37.8	D49.0
lower (third)	C15.5	C78.89	D00.1	D13.0	D37.8	D49.0
middle (third)	C15.4	C78.89	D00.1	D13.0	D37.8	D49.0
overlapping lesion	C15.8	—	—	—	—	—
proximal (third)	C15.3	C78.89	D00.1	D13.0	D37.8	D49.0
thoracic	C15.4	C78.89	D00.1	D13.0	D37.8	D49.0
upper (third)	C15.3	C78.89	D00.1	D13.0	D37.8	D49.0
ethmoid (sinus)	C31.1	C78.39	D02.3	D14.0	D38.5	D49.1
bone or labyrinth	C41.0	C79.51	—	D16.4	D48.0	D49.2
eustachian tube	C30.1	C78.39	D02.3	D14.0	D38.5	D49.1
exocervix	C53.1	C79.82	D06.1	D26.0	D39.0	D49.5
external						
meatus (ear) — *see also* Neoplasm, skin, ear	C44.20-☑	C79.2	D04.2-☑	D23.2-☑	D48.5	D49.2
os, cervix uteri	C53.1	C79.82	D06.1	D26.0	D39.0	D49.5
extradural	C72.9	C79.49	—	D33.9	D43.9	D49.7
extrahepatic (bile)						
duct	C24.0	C78.89	D01.5	D13.5	D37.6	D49.0
overlapping lesion with gallbladder	C24.8	—	—	—	—	—
extraocular muscle	C69.6-☑	C79.49	D09.2-☑	D31.6-☑	D48.7	D49.89
extrarectal	C76.3	C79.89	D09.8	D36.7	D48.7	D49.89
extremity	C76.8	C79.89	D04.8	D36.7	D48.7	D49.89
lower	C76.5-☑	C79.89	D04.7-☑	D36.7	D48.7	D49.89
upper	C76.4-☑	C79.89	D04.6-☑	D36.7	D48.7	D49.89
eyeball	C69.9-☑	C79.49	D09.2-☑	D31.9-☑	D48.7	D49.89
eyebrow	C44.309	C79.2	D04.39	D23.39	D48.5	D49.2
basal cell carcinoma	C44.319	—	—	—	—	—
specified type NEC	C44.399	—	—	—	—	—
squamous cell carcinoma	C44.329	—	—	—	—	—
eyelid (lower) (skin) (upper)	C44.10-☑	—	—	—	—	—
basal cell carcinoma	C44.11-☑	—	—	—	—	—
cartilage	C49.0	C79.89	—	D21.0	D48.1	D49.2
specified type NEC	C44.19-☑	—	—	—	—	—
squamous cell carcinoma	C44.12-☑	—	—	—	—	—
eye NEC	C69.9-☑	C79.49	D09.2-☑	D31.9-☑	D48.7	D49.89
overlapping sites	C69.8-☑	—	—	—	—	—
face NEC	C76.0	C79.89	D04.39	D36.7	D48.7	D49.89
fallopian tube (accessory)	C57.0-☑	C79.82	D07.39	D28.2	D39.8	D49.5
falx (cerebella) (cerebri)	C70.0	C79.32		D32.0	D42.0	D49.7
fascia — *see also* Neoplasm, connective tissue						
palmar	C49.1-☑	C79.89	—	D21.1-☑	D48.1	D49.2
plantar	C49.2-☑	C79.89	—	D21.2-☑	D48.1	D49.2
fatty tissue — *see* Neoplasm, connective tissue						
fauces, faucial NEC	C10.9	C79.89	D00.08	D10.5	D37.05	D49.0
pillars	C09.1	C79.89	D00.08	D10.5	D37.05	D49.0
tonsil	C09.9	C79.89	D00.08	D10.4	D37.05	D49.0
femur (any part)	C40.2-☑	—	—	D16.2-☑	—	—
fetal membrane	C58	C79.82	D07.0	D26.7	D39.2	D49.5
fibrous tissue — *see* Neoplasm, connective tissue						
fibula (any part)	C40.2-☑	C79.51	—	D16.2-☑	—	—
filum terminale	C72.0	C79.49	—	D33.4	D43.4	D49.7
finger NEC	C76.4-☑	C79.89	D04.6-☑	D36.7	D48.7	D49.89
flank NEC	C76.8	C79.89	D04.5	D36.7	D48.7	D49.89
follicle, nabothian	C53.0	C79.82	D06.0	D26.0	D39.0	D49.5
foot NEC	C76.5-☑	C79.89	D04.7-☑	D36.7	D48.7	D49.89
forearm NEC	C76.4-☑	C79.89	D04.6-☑	D36.7	D48.7	D49.89
forehead (skin)	C44.309	C79.2	D04.39	D23.39	D48.5	D49.2

Neoplasm, neoplastic — *continued*

	Malignant Primary	Malignant Secondary	Ca in situ	Benign	Uncertain	Unspecified Behavior
forehead — *continued*						
basal cell carcinoma	C44.319	—	—	—	—	—
specified type NEC	C44.399	—	—	—	—	—
squamous cell carcinoma	C44.329	—	—	—	—	—
foreskin	C60.0	C79.82	D07.4	D29.0	D40.8	D49.5
fornix						
pharyngeal	C11.3	C79.89	D00.08	D10.6	D37.05	D49.0
vagina	C52	C79.82	D07.2	D28.1	D39.8	D49.5
fossa (of)						
anterior (cranial)	C71.9	C79.31	—	D33.2	D43.2	D49.6
cranial	C71.9	C79.31	—	D33.2	D43.2	D49.6
ischiorectal	C76.3	C79.89	D09.8	D36.7	D48.7	D49.89
middle (cranial)	C71.9	C79.31	—	D33.2	D43.2	D49.6
piriform	C12	C79.89	D00.08	D10.7	D37.05	D49.0
pituitary	C75.1	C79.89	D09.3	D35.2	D44.3	D49.7
posterior (cranial)	C71.9	C79.31	—	D33.2	D43.2	D49.6
pterygoid	C49.0	C79.89	—	D21.0	D48.1	D49.2
pyriform	C12	C79.89	D00.08	D10.7	D37.05	D49.0
Rosenmuller	C11.2	C79.89	D00.08	D10.6	D37.05	D49.0
tonsillar	C09.0	C79.89	D00.08	D10.5	D37.05	D49.0
fourchette	C51.9	C79.82	D07.1	D28.0	D39.8	D49.5
frenulum						
labii — *see* Neoplasm, lip, internal						
linguae	C02.2	C79.89	D00.07	D10.1	D37.02	D49.0
frontal						
bone	C41.0	C79.51	—	D16.4	D48.0	D49.2
lobe, brain	C71.1	C79.31	—	D33.0	D43.0	D49.6
pole	C71.1	C79.31	—	D33.0	D43.0	D49.6
sinus	C31.2	C78.39	D02.3	D14.0	D38.5	D49.1
fundus						
stomach	C16.1	C78.89	D00.2	D13.1	D37.1	D49.0
uterus	C54.3	C79.82	D07.0	D26.1	D39.0	D49.5
gallbladder	C23	C78.89	D01.5	D13.5	D37.6	D49.0
overlapping lesion with extrahepatic bile ducts	C24.8	—	—	—	—	—
gall duct (extrahepatic)	C24.0	C78.89	D01.5	D13.5	D37.6	D49.0
intrahepatic	C22.1	C78.7	D01.5	D13.4	D37.6	D49.0
ganglia — *see also* Neoplasm, nerve, peripheral	C47.9	C79.89	—	D36.10	D48.2	D49.2
basal	C71.0	C79.31	—	D33.0	D43.0	D49.6
cranial nerve	C72.50	C79.49	—	D33.3	D43.3	D49.7
Gartner's duct	C52	C79.82	D07.2	D28.1	D39.8	D49.5
gastric — *see* Neoplasm, stomach						
gastrocolic	C26.9	C78.89	D01.9	D13.9	D37.9	D49.0
gastroesophageal junction	C16.0	C78.89	D00.2	D13.1	D37.1	D49.0
gastrointestinal (tract) NEC	C26.9	C78.89	D01.9	D13.9	D37.9	D49.0
generalized	C80.0	—	—	—	—	—
genital organ or tract						
female NEC	C57.9	C79.82	D07.30	D28.9	D39.9	D49.5
overlapping lesion	C57.8	—	—	—	—	—
specified site NEC	C57.7	C79.82	D07.39	D28.7	D39.8	D49.5
male NEC	C63.9	C79.82	D07.60	D29.9	D40.9	D49.5
overlapping lesion	C63.8	—	—	—	—	—
specified site NEC	C63.7	C79.82	D07.69	D29.8	D40.8	D49.5
genitourinary tract						
female	C57.9	C79.82	D07.30	D28.9	D39.9	D49.5
male	C63.9	C79.82	D07.60	D29.9	D40.9	D49.5
gingiva (alveolar) (marginal)	C03.9	C79.89	D00.03	D10.39	D37.09	D49.0
lower	C03.1	C79.89	D00.03	D10.39	D37.09	D49.0
mandibular	C03.1	C79.89	D00.03	D10.39	D37.09	D49.0
maxillary	C03.0	C79.89	D00.03	D10.39	D37.09	D49.0
upper	C03.0	C79.89	D00.03	D10.39	D37.09	D49.0
gland, glandular (lymphatic) (system) — *see also* Neoplasm, lymph gland						
endocrine NEC	C75.9	C79.89	D09.3	D35.9	D44.9	D49.7

☑ Additional Character Required — Refer to the Tabular List for Character Selection   ▽ Subterms under main terms may continue to next column or page

Neoplasm, neoplastic — continued	Malignant Primary	Malignant Secondary	Ca in situ	Benign	Uncertain	Unspecified Behavior
gland, glandular — see also Neoplasm, lymph gland — continued						
salivary — see Neoplasm, salivary gland						
glans penis	C60.1	C79.82	D07.4	D29.0	D40.8	D49.5
globus pallidus	C71.0	C79.31	—	D33.0	D43.0	D49.6
glomus						
coccygeal	C49.5	C79.89	—	D21.5	D48.1	D49.2
jugularis	C75.5	C79.89	—	D35.6	D44.7	D49.7
glosso-epiglottic fold(s)	C10.1	C79.89	D00.08	D10.5	D37.05	D49.0
glossopalatine fold	C09.1	C79.89	D00.08	D10.5	D37.05	D49.0
glossopharyngeal sulcus	C09.0	C79.89	D00.08	D10.5	D37.05	D49.0
glottis	C32.0	C78.39	D02.0	D14.1	D38.0	D49.1
gluteal region	C76.3	C79.89	D04.5	D36.7	D48.7	D49.89
great vessels NEC	C49.3	C79.89	—	D21.3	D48.1	D49.2
groin NEC	C76.3	C79.89	D04.5	D36.7	D48.7	D49.89
gum	C03.9	C79.89	D00.03	D10.39	D37.09	D49.0
lower	C03.1	C79.89	D00.03	D10.39	D37.09	D49.0
upper	C03.0	C79.89	D00.03	D10.39	D37.09	D49.0
hand NEC	C76.4-✓	C79.89	D04.6-✓	D36.7	D48.7	D49.89
head NEC	C76.0	C79.89	D04.4	D36.7	D48.7	D49.89
heart	C38.0	C79.89	—	D15.1	D48.7	D49.89
heel NEC	C76.5-✓	C79.89	D04.7-✓	D36.7	D48.7	D49.89
helix — see also Neoplasm, skin, ear						
ear	C44.20-✓	C79.2	D04.2-✓	D23.2-✓	D48.5	D49.2
hematopoietic, hemopoietic tissue NEC	C96.9	—	—	—	—	—
specified NEC	C96.Z	—	—	—	—	—
hemisphere, cerebral	C71.0	C79.31	—	D33.0	D43.0	D49.6
hemorrhoidal zone	C21.1	C78.5	D01.3	D12.9	D37.8	D49.0
hepatic — see also Index to disease, by histology	C22.9	C78.7	D01.5	D13.4	D37.6	D49.0
duct (bile)	C24.0	C78.89	D01.5	D13.5	D37.6	D49.0
flexure (colon)	C18.3	C78.5	D01.0	D12.3	D37.4	D49.0
primary	C22.8	C78.7	D01.5	D13.4	D37.6	D49.0
hepatobiliary	C24.9	C78.89	D01.5	D13.5	D37.6	D49.0
hepatoblastoma	C22.2	C78.7	D01.5	D13.4	D37.6	D49.0
hepatoma	C22.0	C78.7	D01.5	D13.4	D37.6	D49.0
hilus of lung	C34.0-✓	C78.0-✓	D02.2-✓	D14.3-✓	D38.1	D49.1
hippocampus, brain	C71.2	C79.31	—	D33.0	D43.0	D49.6
hip NEC	C76.5-✓	C79.89	D04.7-✓	D36.7	D48.7	D49.89
humerus (any part)	C40.0-✓	C79.51	—	D16.0-✓	—	—
hymen	C52	C79.82	D07.2	D28.1	D39.8	D49.5
hypopharynx, hypopharyngeal NEC	C13.9	C79.89	D00.08	D10.7	D37.05	D49.0
overlapping lesion	C13.8	—	—	—	—	—
postcricoid region	C13.0	C79.89	D00.08	D10.7	D37.05	D49.0
posterior wall	C13.2	C79.89	D00.08	D10.7	D37.05	D49.0
pyriform fossa (sinus)	C12	C79.89	D00.08	D10.7	D37.05	D49.0
hypophysis	C75.1	C79.89	D09.3	D35.2	D44.3	D49.7
hypothalamus	C71.0	C79.31	—	D33.0	D43.0	D49.6
ileocecum, ileocecal (coil) (junction) (valve)	C18.0	C78.5	D01.0	D12.0	D37.4	D49.0
ileum	C17.2	C78.4	D01.49	D13.39	D37.2	D49.0
ilium	C41.4	C79.51	—	D16.8	D48.0	D49.2
immunoproliferative NEC	C88.9	—	—	—	—	—
infraclavicular (region)	C76.1	C79.89	D04.5	D36.7	D48.7	D49.89
inguinal (region)	C76.3	C79.89	D04.5	D36.7	D48.7	D49.89
insula	C71.0	C79.31	—	D33.0	D43.0	D49.6
insular tissue (pancreas)	C25.4	C78.89	D01.7	D13.7	D37.8	D49.0
brain	C71.0	C79.31	—	D33.0	D43.0	D49.6
interarytenoid fold	C13.1	C78.39	D00.08	D10.7	D37.05	D49.0
hypopharyngeal aspect	C13.1	C79.89	D00.08	D10.7	D37.05	D49.0
laryngeal aspect	C32.1	C78.39	D02.0	D14.1	D38.0	D49.1
marginal zone	C13.1	C79.89	D00.08	D10.7	D37.05	D49.0
interdental papillae	C03.9	C79.89	D00.03	D10.39	D37.09	D49.0

Neoplasm, neoplastic — continued	Malignant Primary	Malignant Secondary	Ca in situ	Benign	Uncertain	Unspecified Behavior
interdental papillae — continued						
lower	C03.1	C79.89	D00.03	D10.39	D37.09	D49.0
upper	C03.0	C79.89	D00.03	D10.39	D37.09	D49.0
internal						
capsule	C71.0	C79.31	—	D33.0	D43.0	D49.6
os (cervix)	C53.0	C79.82	D06.0	D26.0	D39.0	D49.5
intervertebral cartilage or disc	C41.2	C79.51	—	D16.6	D48.0	D49.2
intestine, intestinal	C26.0	C78.80	D01.40	D13.9	D37.8	D49.0
large	C18.9	C78.5	D01.0	D12.6	D37.4	D49.0
appendix	C18.1	C78.5	D01.0	D12.1	D37.3	D49.0
caput coli	C18.0	C78.5	D01.0	D12.0	D37.4	D49.0
cecum	C18.0	C78.5	D01.0	D12.0	D37.4	D49.0
colon	C18.9	C78.5	D01.0	D12.6	D37.4	D49.0
and rectum	C19	C78.5	D01.1	D12.7	D37.5	D49.0
ascending	C18.2	C78.5	D01.0	D12.2	D37.4	D49.0
caput	C18.0	C78.5	D01.0	D12.0	D37.4	D49.0
descending	C18.6	C78.5	D01.0	D12.4	D37.4	D49.0
distal	C18.6	C78.5	D01.0	D12.4	D37.4	D49.0
left	C18.6	C78.5	D01.0	D12.4	D37.4	D49.0
overlapping lesion	C18.8	—	—	—	—	—
pelvic	C18.7	C78.5	D01.0	D12.5	D37.4	D49.0
right	C18.2	C78.5	D01.0	D12.2	D37.4	D49.0
sigmoid (flexure)	C18.7	C78.5	D01.0	D12.5	D37.4	D49.0
transverse	C18.4	C78.5	D01.0	D12.3	D37.4	D49.0
hepatic flexure	C18.3	C78.5	D01.0	D12.3	D37.4	D49.0
ileocecum, ileocecal (coil) (valve)	C18.0	C78.5	D01.0	D12.0	D37.4	D49.0
overlapping lesion	C18.8					
sigmoid flexure (lower) (upper)	C18.7	C78.5	D01.0	D12.5	D37.4	D49.0
splenic flexure	C18.5	C78.5	D01.0	D12.3	D37.4	D49.0
small	C17.9	C78.4	D01.40	D13.30	D37.2	D49.0
duodenum	C17.0	C78.4	D01.49	D13.2	D37.2	D49.0
ileum	C17.2	C78.4	D01.49	D13.39	D37.2	D49.0
jejunum	C17.1	C78.4	D01.49	D13.39	D37.2	D49.0
overlapping lesion	C17.8	—	—	—	—	—
tract NEC	C26.0	C78.89	D01.40	D13.9	D37.8	D49.0
intra-abdominal	C76.2	C79.89	D09.8	D36.7	D48.7	D49.89
intracranial NEC	C71.9	C79.31	—	D33.2	D43.2	D49.6
intrahepatic (bile) duct	C22.1	C78.7	D01.5	D13.4	D37.6	D49.0
intraocular	C69.9-✓	C79.49	D09.2-✓	D31.9-✓	D48.7	D49.89
intraorbital	C69.6-✓	C79.49	D09.2-✓	D31.6-✓	D48.7	D49.89
intrasellar	C75.1	C79.89	D09.3	D35.2	D44.3	D49.7
intrathoracic (cavity) (organs)	C76.1	C79.89	D09.8	D15.9	D48.7	D49.89
specified NEC	C76.1	C79.89	D09.8	D15.7	—	—
iris	C69.4-✓	C79.49	D09.2-✓	D31.4-✓	D48.7	D49.89
ischiorectal (fossa)	C76.3	C79.89	D09.8	D36.7	D48.7	D49.89
ischium	C41.4	C79.51	—	D16.8	D48.0	D49.2
island of Reil	C71.0	C79.31	—	D33.0	D43.0	D49.6
islands or islets of Langerhans	C25.4	C78.89	D01.7	D13.7	D37.8	D49.0
isthmus uteri	C54.0	C79.82	D07.0	D26.1	D39.0	D49.5
jaw	C76.0	C79.89	D09.8	D36.7	D48.7	D49.89
bone	C41.1	C79.51	—	D16.5	D48.0	D49.2
lower	C41.1	C79.51	—	D16.5	—	—
upper	C41.0	C79.51	—	D16.4	—	—
carcinoma (any type) (lower) (upper)	C76.0	C79.89	—	—	—	—
skin — see also Neoplasm, skin, face	C44.309	C79.2	D04.39	D23.39	D48.5	D49.2
soft tissues	C03.9	C79.89	D00.03	D10.39	D37.09	D49.0
lower	C03.1	C79.89	D00.03	D10.39	D37.09	D49.0
upper	C03.0	C79.89	D00.03	D10.39	D37.09	D49.0
jejunum	C17.1	C78.4	D01.49	D13.39	D37.2	D49.0
joint NEC — see also Neoplasm, bone	C41.9	C79.51	—	D16.9	D48.0	D49.2
acromioclavicular	C40.0-✓	C79.51	—	D16.0-✓	—	—
bursa or synovial membrane — see						

Neoplasm Table

Neoplasm, gland, glandular — Neoplasm, joint NEC

Neoplasm Table

Neoplasm, neoplastic — *continued*	Malignant Primary	Malignant Secondary	Ca in situ	Benign	Uncertain	Unspecified Behavior
joint — *see also* Neoplasm, bone — *continued*						
bursa or synovial membrane — *see* Neoplasm, connective tissue — *continued* Neoplasm, connective tissue						
costovertebral	C41.3	C79.51	—	D16.7	D48.0	D49.2
sternocostal	C41.3	C79.51	—	D16.7	D48.0	D49.2
temporomandibular	C41.1	C79.51	—	D16.5	D48.0	D49.2
junction						
anorectal	C21.8	C78.5	D01.3	D12.9	D37.8	D49.0
cardioesophageal	C16.0	C78.89	D00.2	D13.1	D37.1	D49.0
esophagogastric	C16.0	C78.89	D00.2	D13.1	D37.1	D49.0
gastroesophageal	C16.0	C78.89	D00.2	D13.1	D37.1	D49.0
hard and soft palate	C05.9	C79.89	D00.00	D10.39	D37.09	D49.0
ileocecal	C18.0	C78.5	D01.0	D12.0	D37.4	D49.0
pelvirectal	C19	C78.5	D01.1	D12.7	D37.5	D49.0
pelviureteric	C65.- ☑	C79.0- ☑	D09.19	D30.1- ☑	D41.1- ☑	D49.5
rectosigmoid	C19	C78.5	D01.1	D12.7	D37.5	D49.0
squamocolumnar, of cervix	C53.8	C79.82	D06.7	D26.0	D39.0	D49.5
Kaposi's sarcoma — *see* Kaposi's, sarcoma						
kidney (parenchymal)	C64.- ☑	C79.0- ☑	D09.19	D30.0- ☑	D41.0- ☑	D49.5
calyx	C65.- ☑	C79.0- ☑	D09.19	D30.1- ☑	D41.1- ☑	D49.5
hilus	C65.- ☑	C79.0- ☑	D09.19	D30.1- ☑	D41.1- ☑	D49.5
pelvis	C65.- ☑	C79.0- ☑	D09.19	D30.1- ☑	D41.1- ☑	D49.5
knee NEC	C76.5- ☑	C79.89	D04.7- ☑	D36.7	D48.7	D49.89
labia (skin)	C51.9	C79.82	D07.1	D28.0	D39.8	D49.5
majora	C51.0	C79.82	D07.1	D28.0	D39.8	D49.5
minora	C51.1	C79.82	D07.1	D28.0	D39.8	D49.5
labial — *see also* Neoplasm, lip						
sulcus (lower)	C00.9	C79.89	D00.01	D10.0	D37.01	D49.0
(upper)	C06.1	C79.89	D00.02	D10.39	D37.09	D49.0
labium (skin)	C51.9	C79.82	D07.1	D28.0	D39.8	D49.5
majus	C51.0	C79.82	D07.1	D28.0	D39.8	D49.5
minus	C51.1	C79.82	D07.1	D28.0	D39.8	D49.5
lacrimal						
canaliculi	C69.5- ☑	C79.49	D09.2- ☑	D31.5- ☑	D48.7	D49.89
duct (nasal)	C69.5- ☑	C79.49	D09.2- ☑	D31.5- ☑	D48.7	D49.89
gland	C69.5- ☑	C79.49	D09.2- ☑	D31.5- ☑	D48.7	D49.89
punctum	C69.5- ☑	C79.49	D09.2- ☑	D31.5- ☑	D48.7	D49.89
sac	C69.5- ☑	C79.49	D09.2- ☑	D31.5- ☑	D48.7	D49.89
Langerhans, islands or islets	C25.4	C78.89	D01.7	D13.7	D37.8	D49.0
laryngopharynx	C13.9	C79.89	D00.08	D10.7	D37.05	D49.0
larynx, laryngeal NEC	C32.9	C78.39	D02.0	D14.1	D38.0	D49.1
aryepiglottic fold	C32.1	C78.39	D02.0	D14.1	D38.0	D49.1
cartilage (arytenoid) (cricoid) (cuneiform) (thyroid)	C32.3	C78.39	D02.0	D14.1	D38.0	D49.1
commissure (anterior) (posterior)	C32.0	C78.39	D02.0	D14.1	D38.0	D49.1
extrinsic NEC	C32.1	C78.39	D02.0	D14.1	D38.0	D49.1
meaning hypopharynx	C13.9	C79.89	D00.08	D10.7	D37.05	D49.0
interarytenoid fold	C32.1	C78.39	D02.0	D14.1	D38.0	D49.1
intrinsic	C32.0	C78.39	D02.0	D14.1	D38.0	D49.1
overlapping lesion	C32.8	—	—	—	—	—
ventricular band	C32.1	C78.39	D02.0	D14.1	D38.0	D49.1
leg NEC	C76.5- ☑	C79.89	D04.7- ☑	D36.7	D48.7	D49.89
lens, crystalline	C69.4- ☑	C79.49	D09.2- ☑	D31.4- ☑	D48.7	D49.89
lid (lower) (upper)	C44.10- ☑	C79.2	D04.1- ☑	D23.1- ☑	D48.5	D49.2
basal cell carcinoma	C44.11- ☑	—	—	—	—	—
specified type NEC	C44.19- ☑	—	—	—	—	—
squamous cell carcinoma	C44.12- ☑	—	—	—	—	—
ligament — *see also* Neoplasm, connective tissue						

Neoplasm, neoplastic — *continued*	Malignant Primary	Malignant Secondary	Ca in situ	Benign	Uncertain	Unspecified Behavior
ligament — *see also* Neoplasm, connective tissue — *continued*						
broad	C57.1- ☑	C79.82	D07.39	D28.2	D39.8	D49.5
Mackenrodt's	C57.7	C79.82	D07.39	D28.7	D39.8	D49.5
non-uterine — *see* Neoplasm, connective tissue						
round	C57.2- ☑	C79.82	—	D28.2	D39.8	D49.5
sacro-uterine	C57.3	C79.82	—	D28.2	D39.8	D49.5
uterine	C57.3	C79.82	—	D28.2	D39.8	D49.5
utero-ovarian	C57.7	C79.82	D07.39	D28.2	D39.8	D49.5
uterosacral	C57.3	C79.82	—	D28.2	D39.8	D49.5
limb	C76.8	C79.89	D04.8	D36.7	D48.7	D49.89
lower	C76.5- ☑	C79.89	D04.7- ☑	D36.7	D48.7	D49.89
upper	C76.4- ☑	C79.89	D04.6- ☑	D36.7	D48.7	D49.89
limbus of cornea	C69.1- ☑	C79.49	D09.2- ☑	D31.1- ☑	D48.7	D49.89
lingual NEC — *see also* Neoplasm, tongue	C02.9	C79.89	D00.07	D10.1	D37.02	D49.0
lingula, lung	C34.1- ☑	C78.0- ☑	D02.2- ☑	D14.3- ☑	D38.1	D49.1
lip	C00.9	C79.89	D00.01	D10.0	D37.01	D49.0
buccal aspect — *see* Neoplasm, lip, internal						
commissure	C00.6	C79.89	D00.01	D10.0	D37.01	D49.0
external	C00.2	C79.89	D00.01	D10.0	D37.01	D49.0
lower	C00.1	C79.89	D00.01	D10.0	D37.01	D49.0
upper	C00.0	C79.89	D00.01	D10.0	D37.01	D49.0
frenulum — *see* Neoplasm, lip, internal						
inner aspect — *see* Neoplasm, lip, internal						
internal	C00.5	C79.89	D00.01	D10.0	D37.01	D49.0
lower	C00.4	C79.89	D00.01	D10.0	D37.01	D49.0
upper	C00.3	C79.89	D00.01	D10.0	D37.01	D49.0
lipstick area	C00.2	C79.89	D00.01	D10.0	D37.01	D49.0
lower	C00.1	C79.89	D00.01	D10.0	D37.01	D49.0
upper	C00.0	C79.89	D00.01	D10.0	D37.01	D49.0
lower	C00.1	C79.89	D00.01	D10.0	D37.01	D49.0
internal	C00.4	C79.89	D00.01	D10.0	D37.01	D49.0
mucosa — *see* Neoplasm, lip, internal						
oral aspect — *see* Neoplasm, lip, internal						
overlapping lesion	C00.8	—	—	—	—	—
with oral cavity or pharynx	C14.8	—	—	—	—	—
skin (commissure) (lower) (upper)	C44.00	C79.2	D04.0	D23.0	D48.5	D49.2
basal cell carcinoma	C44.01	—	—	—	—	—
specified type NEC	C44.09	—	—	—	—	—
squamous cell carcinoma	C44.02	—	—	—	—	—
upper	C00.0	C79.89	D00.01	D10.0	D37.01	D49.0
internal	C00.3	C79.89	D00.01	D10.0	D37.01	D49.0
vermilion border	C00.2	C79.89	D00.01	D10.0	D37.01	D49.0
lower	C00.1	C79.89	D00.01	D10.0	D37.01	D49.0
upper	C00.0	C79.89	D00.01	D10.0	D37.01	D49.0
lipomatous — *see* Lipoma, by site						
liver — *see also* Index to disease, by histology	C22.9	C78.7	D01.5	D13.4	D37.6	D49.0
primary	C22.8	C78.7	D01.5	D13.4	D37.6	D49.0
lumbosacral plexus	C47.5	—	—	D36.16	D48.2	D49.2
lung	C34.9- ☑	C78.0- ☑	D02.2- ☑	D14.3- ☑	D38.1	D49.1
azygos lobe	C34.1- ☑	C78.0- ☑	D02.2- ☑	D14.3- ☑	D38.1	D49.1
carina	C34.0- ☑	C78.0- ☑	D02.2- ☑	D14.3- ☑	D38.1	D49.1
hilus	C34.0- ☑	C78.0- ☑	D02.2- ☑	D14.3- ☑	D38.1	D49.1
lingula	C34.1- ☑	C78.0- ☑	D02.2- ☑	D14.3- ☑	D38.1	D49.1
lobe NEC	C34.9- ☑	C78.0- ☑	D02.2- ☑	D14.3- ☑	D38.1	D49.1
lower lobe	C34.3- ☑	C78.0- ☑	D02.2- ☑	D14.3- ☑	D38.1	D49.1

☑ Additional Character Required — Refer to the Tabular List for Character Selection   🔻 Subterms under main terms may continue to next column or page

	Malignant Primary	Malignant Secondary	Ca in situ	Benign	Uncertain	Unspecified Behavior
Neoplasm, neoplastic —						
continued						
lung — *continued*						
main bronchus	C34.0-☑	C78.0-☑	D02.2-☑	D14.3-☑	D38.1	D49.1
mesothelioma — *see*						
Mesothelioma						
middle lobe	C34.2	C78.0-☑	D02.21	D14.31	D38.1	D49.1
overlapping lesion	C34.8-☑					
upper lobe	C34.1-☑	C78.0-☑	D02.2-☑	D14.3-☑	D38.1	D49.1
lymph, lymphatic channel						
NEC	C49.9	C79.89	—	D21.9	D48.1	D49.2
gland (secondary)	—	C77.9	—	D36.0	D48.7	D49.89
abdominal	—	C77.2	—	D36.0	D48.7	D49.89
aortic	—	C77.2	—	D36.0	D48.7	D49.89
arm	—	C77.3	—	D36.0	D48.7	D49.89
auricular (anterior)						
(posterior)	—	C77.0	—	D36.0	D48.7	D49.89
axilla, axillary	—	C77.3	—	D36.0	D48.7	D49.89
brachial	—	C77.3	—	D36.0	D48.7	D49.89
bronchial	—	C77.1	—	D36.0	D48.7	D49.89
bronchopulmonary	—	C77.1	—	D36.0	D48.7	D49.89
celiac	—	C77.2	—	D36.0	D48.7	D49.89
cervical	—	C77.0	—	D36.0	D48.7	D49.89
cervicofacial	—	C77.0	—	D36.0	D48.7	D49.89
Cloquet	—	C77.4	—	D36.0	D48.7	D49.89
colic	—	C77.2	—	D36.0	D48.7	D49.89
common duct	—	C77.2	—	D36.0	D48.7	D49.89
cubital	—	C77.3	—	D36.0	D48.7	D49.89
diaphragmatic	—	C77.1	—	D36.0	D48.7	D49.89
epigastric,						
inferior	—	C77.1	—	D36.0	D48.7	D49.89
epitrochlear	—	C77.3	—	D36.0	D48.7	D49.89
esophageal	—	C77.1	—	D36.0	D48.7	D49.89
face	—	C77.0	—	D36.0	D48.7	D49.89
femoral	—	C77.4	—	D36.0	D48.7	D49.89
gastric	—	C77.2	—	D36.0	D48.7	D49.89
groin	—	C77.4	—	D36.0	D48.7	D49.89
head	—	C77.0	—	D36.0	D48.7	D49.89
hepatic	—	C77.2	—	D36.0	D48.7	D49.89
hilar						
(pulmonary)	—	C77.1	—	D36.0	D48.7	D49.89
splenic	—	C77.2	—	D36.0	D48.7	D49.89
hypogastric	—	C77.5	—	D36.0	D48.7	D49.89
ileocolic	—	C77.2	—	D36.0	D48.7	D49.89
iliac	—	C77.5	—	D36.0	D48.7	D49.89
infraclavicular	—	C77.3	—	D36.0	D48.7	D49.89
inguina, inguinal	—	C77.4	—	D36.0	D48.7	D49.89
innominate	—	C77.1	—	D36.0	D48.7	D49.89
intercostal	—	C77.1	—	D36.0	D48.7	D49.89
intestinal	—	C77.2	—	D36.0	D48.7	D49.89
intrabdominal	—	C77.2	—	D36.0	D48.7	D49.89
intrapelvic	—	C77.5	—	D36.0	D48.7	D49.89
intrathoracic	—	C77.1	—	D36.0	D48.7	D49.89
jugular	—	C77.0	—	D36.0	D48.7	D49.89
leg	—	C77.4	—	D36.0	D48.7	D49.89
limb						
lower	—	C77.4	—	D36.0	D48.7	D49.89
upper	—	C77.3	—	D36.0	D48.7	D49.89
lower limb	—	C77.4	—	D36.0	D48.7	D49.89
lumbar	—	C77.2	—	D36.0	D48.7	D49.89
mandibular	—	C77.0	—	D36.0	D48.7	D49.89
mediastinal	—	C77.1	—	D36.0	D48.7	D49.89
mesenteric (inferior)						
(superior)	—	C77.2	—	D36.0	D48.7	D49.89
midcolic	—	C77.2	—	D36.0	D48.7	D49.89
multiple sites in						
categories C77.0 -						
C77.5	—	C77.8	—	D36.0	D48.7	D49.89
neck	—	C77.0	—	D36.0	D48.7	D49.89
obturator	—	C77.5	—	D36.0	D48.7	D49.89
occipital	—	C77.0	—	D36.0	D48.7	D49.89
pancreatic	—	C77.2	—	D36.0	D48.7	D49.89
para-aortic	—	C77.2	—	D36.0	D48.7	D49.89
paracervical	—	C77.5	—	D36.0	D48.7	D49.89
parametrial	—	C77.5	—	D36.0	D48.7	D49.89
parasternal	—	C77.1	—	D36.0	D48.7	D49.89
parotid	—	C77.0	—	D36.0	D48.7	D49.89
pectoral	—	C77.3	—	D36.0	D48.7	D49.89
pelvic	—	C77.5	—	D36.0	D48.7	D49.89
peri-aortic	—	C77.2	—	D36.0	D48.7	D49.89
peripancreatic	—	C77.2	—	D36.0	D48.7	D49.89
popliteal	—	C77.4	—	D36.0	D48.7	D49.89
porta hepatis	—	C77.2	—	D36.0	D48.7	D49.89

	Malignant Primary	Malignant Secondary	Ca in situ	Benign	Uncertain	Unspecified Behavior
Neoplasm, neoplastic —						
continued						
lymph, lymphatic channel						
— *continued*						
gland — *continued*						
portal	—	C77.2		D36.0	D48.7	D49.89
preauricular	—	C77.0		D36.0	D48.7	D49.89
prelaryngeal	—	C77.0		D36.0	D48.7	D49.89
presymphysial	—	C77.5		D36.0	D48.7	D49.89
pretracheal	—	C77.0		D36.0	D48.7	D49.89
primary (any site)						
NEC	C96.9	—	—	—	—	—
pulmonary						
(hiler)	—	C77.1		D36.0	D48.7	D49.89
pyloric	—	C77.2		D36.0	D48.7	D49.89
retroperitoneal	—	C77.2		D36.0	D48.7	D49.89
retropharyngeal	—	C77.0		D36.0	D48.7	D49.89
Rosenmuller's	—	C77.4		D36.0	D48.7	D49.89
sacral	—	C77.5		D36.0	D48.7	D49.89
scalene	—	C77.0		D36.0	D48.7	D49.89
site NEC	—	C77.9		D36.0	D48.7	D49.89
splenic (hilar)	—	C77.2		D36.0	D48.7	D49.89
subclavicular	—	C77.3		D36.0	D48.7	D49.89
subinguinal	—	C77.4		D36.0	D48.7	D49.89
sublingual	—	C77.0		D36.0	D48.7	D49.89
submandibular	—	C77.0		D36.0	D48.7	D49.89
submaxillary	—	C77.0		D36.0	D48.7	D49.89
submental	—	C77.0		D36.0	D48.7	D49.89
subscapular	—	C77.3		D36.0	D48.7	D49.89
supraclavicular	—	C77.0		D36.0	D48.7	D49.89
thoracic	—	C77.1		D36.0	D48.7	D49.89
tibial	—	C77.4		D36.0	D48.7	D49.89
tracheal	—	C77.1		D36.0	D48.7	D49.89
tracheobronchial	—	C77.1		D36.0	D48.7	D49.89
upper limb	—	C77.3		D36.0	D48.7	D49.89
Virchow's	—	C77.0		D36.0	D48.7	D49.89
node — *see also*						
Neoplasm, lymph						
gland						
primary NEC	C96.9	—				
vessel — *see also*						
Neoplasm,						
connective						
tissue	C49.9	C79.89	—	D21.9	D48.1	D49.2
Mackenrodt's						
ligament	C57.7	C79.82	D07.39	D28.7	D39.8	D49.5
malar	C41.0	C79.51	—	D16.4	D48.0	D49.2
region — *see*						
Neoplasm, cheek						
mammary gland — *see*						
Neoplasm, breast						
mandible	C41.1	C79.51	—	D16.5	D48.0	D49.2
alveolar						
mucosa						
(carcinoma)	C03.1	C79.89	D00.03	D10.39	D37.09	D49.0
ridge or process	C41.1	C79.51	—	D16.5	D48.0	D49.2
marrow (bone) NEC	C96.9	C79.52	—	—	D47.9	D49.89
mastectomy site (skin)						
see also Neoplasm,						
breast, skin	C44.501	C79.2	—	—	—	—
specified as breast						
tissue	C50.8-☑	C79.81	—	—	—	—
mastoid (air cells)						
(antrum) (cavity)	C30.1	C78.39	D02.3	D14.0	D38.5	D49.1
bone or process	C41.0	C79.51	—	D16.4	D48.0	D49.2
maxilla, maxillary						
(superior)	C41.0	C79.51	—	D16.4	D48.0	D49.2
alveolar						
mucosa	C03.0	C79.89	D00.03	D10.39	D37.09	D49.0
ridge or process						
(carcinoma)	C41.0	C79.51	—	D16.4	D48.0	D49.2
antrum	C31.0	C78.39	D02.3	D14.0	D38.5	D49.1
carcinoma	C03.0	C79.51	—	—	—	—
inferior — *see*						
Neoplasm,						
mandible						
sinus	C31.0	C78.39	D02.3	D14.0	D38.5	D49.1
meatus external (ear) —						
see also Neoplasm,						
skin, ear	C44.20-☑	C79.2	D04.2-☑	D23.2-☑	D48.5	D49.2
Meckel diverticulum,						
malignant	C17.3	C78.4	D01.49	D13.39	D37.2	D49.0

Neoplasm, neoplastic — continued

	Malignant Primary	Malignant Secondary	Ca in situ	Benign	Uncertain	Unspecified Behavior
mediastinum, mediastinal	C38.3	C78.1	—	D15.2	D38.3	D49.89
anterior	C38.1	C78.1	—	D15.2	D38.3	D49.89
posterior	C38.2	C78.1	—	D15.2	D38.3	D49.89
medulla						
adrenal	C74.1-✓	C79.7-✓	D09.3	D35.0-✓	D44.1-✓	D49.7
oblongata	C71.7	C79.31	—	D33.1	D43.1	D49.6
meibomian gland	C44.10-✓	C79.2	D04.1-✓	D23.1-✓	D48.5	D49.2
basal cell carcinoma	C44.11-✓	—	—	—	—	—
specified type NEC	C44.19-✓	—	—	—	—	—
squamous cell carcinoma	C44.12-✓	—	—	—	—	—
melanoma — see Melanoma						
meninges	C70.9	C79.49	—	D32.9	D42.9	D49.7
brain	C70.0	C79.32	—	D32.0	D42.0	D49.7
cerebral	C70.0	C79.32	—	D32.0	D42.0	D49.7
crainial	C70.0	C79.32	—	D32.0	D42.0	D49.7
intracranial	C70.0	C79.32	—	D32.0	D42.0	D49.7
spinal (cord)	C70.1	C79.49	—	D32.1	D42.1	D49.7
meniscus, knee joint (lateral) (medial)	C40.2-✓	C79.51	—	D16.2-✓	D48.0	D49.2
Merkel cell — see Carcinoma, Merkel cell						
mesentery, mesenteric	C48.1	C78.6	—	D20.1	D48.4	D49.0
mesoappendix	C48.1	C78.6	—	D20.1	D48.4	D49.0
mesocolon	C48.1	C78.6	—	D20.1	D48.4	D49.0
mesopharynx — see Neoplasm, oropharynx						
mesosalpinx	C57.1-✓	C79.82	D07.39	D28.2	D39.8	D49.5
mesothelial tissue — see Mesothelioma						
mesothelioma — see Mesothelioma						
mesovarium	C57.1-✓	C79.82	D07.39	D28.2	D39.8	D49.5
metacarpus (any bone)	C40.1-✓	C79.51	—	D16.1-✓	—	—
metastatic NEC — see also Neoplasm, by site, secondary	—	C79.9	—	—	—	—
metatarsus (any bone)	C40.3-✓	C79.51	—	D16.3-✓	—	—
midbrain	C71.7	C79.31	—	D33.1	D43.1	D49.6
milk duct — see Neoplasm, breast						
mons						
pubis	C51.9	C79.82	D07.1	D28.0	D39.8	D49.5
veneris	C51.9	C79.82	D07.1	D28.0	D39.8	D49.5
motor tract	C72.9	C79.49	—	D33.9	D43.9	D49.7
brain	C71.9	C79.31	—	D33.2	D43.2	D49.6
cauda equina	C72.1	C79.49	—	D33.4	D43.4	D49.7
spinal	C72.0	C79.49	—	D33.4	D43.4	D49.7
mouth	C06.9	C79.89	D00.00	D10.30	D37.09	D49.0
book-leaf	C06.89	C79.89				
floor	C04.9	C79.89	D00.06	D10.2	D37.09	D49.0
anterior portion	C04.0	C79.89	D00.06	D10.2	D37.09	D49.0
lateral portion	C04.1	C79.89	D00.06	D10.2	D37.09	D49.0
overlapping lesion	C04.8	—	—	—	—	—
overlapping NEC	C06.80	—	—	—	—	—
roof	C05.9	C79.89	D00.00	D10.39	D37.09	D49.0
specified part NEC	C06.89	C79.89	D00.00	D10.39	D37.09	D49.0
vestibule	C06.1	C79.89	D00.00	D10.39	D37.09	D49.0
mucosa						
alveolar (ridge or process)	C03.9	C79.89	D00.03	D10.39	D37.09	D49.0
lower	C03.1	C79.89	D00.03	D10.39	D37.09	D49.0
upper	C03.0	C79.89	D00.03	D10.39	D37.09	D49.0
buccal	C06.0	C79.89	D00.02	D10.39	D37.09	D49.0
cheek	C06.0	C79.89	D00.02	D10.39	D37.09	D49.0
lip — see Neoplasm, lip, internal						
nasal	C30.0	C78.39	D02.3	D14.0	D38.5	D49.1
oral	C06.0	C79.89	D00.02	D10.39	D37.09	D49.0
Mullerian duct						
female	C57.7	C79.82	D07.39	D28.7	D39.8	D49.5
male	C63.7	C79.82	D07.69	D29.8	D40.8	D49.5

Neoplasm, neoplastic — continued

	Malignant Primary	Malignant Secondary	Ca in situ	Benign	Uncertain	Unspecified Behavior
muscle — see also Neoplasm, connective tissue						
extraocular	C69.6-✓	C79.49	D09.2-✓	D31.6-✓	D48.7	D49.89
myocardium	C38.0	C79.89	—	D15.1	D48.7	D49.89
myometrium	C54.2	C79.82	D07.0	D26.1	D39.0	D49.5
myopericardium	C38.0	C79.89	—	D15.1	D48.7	D49.89
nabothian gland (follicle)	C53.0	C79.82	D06.0	D26.0	D39.0	D49.5
nail — see also Neoplasm, skin, limb	C44.90	C79.2	D04.9	D23.9	D48.5	D49.2
finger — see also Neoplasm, skin, limb, upper	C44.60-✓	C79.2	D04.6-✓	D23.6-✓	D48.5	D49.2
toe — see also Neoplasm, skin, limb, lower	C44.70-✓	C79.2	D04.7-✓	D23.7-✓	D48.5	D49.2
nares, naris (anterior) (posterior)	C30.0	C78.39	D02.3	D14.0	D38.5	D49.1
nasal — see Neoplasm, nose						
nasolabial groove — see also Neoplasm, skin, face	C44.309	C79.2	D04.39	D23.39	D48.5	D49.2
nasolacrimal duct	C69.5-✓	C79.49	D09.2-✓	D31.5-✓	D48.7	D49.89
nasopharynx, nasopharyngeal	C11.9	C79.89	D00.08	D10.6	D37.05	D49.0
floor	C11.3	C79.89	D00.08	D10.6	D37.05	D49.0
overlapping lesion	C11.8	—	—	—	—	—
roof	C11.0	C79.89	D00.08	D10.6	D37.05	D49.0
wall	C11.9	C79.89	D00.08	D10.6	D37.05	D49.0
anterior	C11.3	C79.89	D00.08	D10.6	D37.05	D49.0
lateral	C11.2	C79.89	D00.08	D10.6	D37.05	D49.0
posterior	C11.1	C79.89	D00.08	D10.6	D37.05	D49.0
superior	C11.0	C79.89	D00.08	D10.6	D37.05	D49.0
nates — see also Neoplasm, skin, trunk	C44.509	C79.2	D04.5	D23.5	D48.5	D49.2
neck NEC	C76.0	C79.89	D09.8	D36.7	D48.7	D49.89
skin	C44.40					
basal cell carcinoma	C44.41	—	—	—	—	—
specified type NEC	C44.49	—	—	—	—	—
squamous cell carcinoma	C44.42	—	—	—	—	—
nerve (ganglion)	C47.9	C79.89	—	D36.10	D48.2	D49.2
abducens	C72.59	C79.49	—	D33.3	D43.3	D49.7
accessory (spinal)	C72.59	C79.49	—	D33.3	D43.3	D49.7
acoustic	C72.4-✓	C79.49	—	D33.3	D43.3	D49.7
auditory	C72.4-✓	C79.49	—	D33.3	D43.3	D49.7
autonomic NEC — see also Neoplasm, nerve, peripheral	C47.9	C79.89	—	D36.10	D48.2	D49.2
brachial	C47.1-✓	C79.89	—	D36.12	D48.2	D49.2
cranial	C72.50	C79.49	—	D33.3	D43.3	D49.7
specified NEC	C72.59	C79.49	—	D33.3	D43.3	D49.7
facial	C72.59	C79.49	—	D33.3	D43.3	D49.7
femoral	C47.2-✓	C79.89	—	D36.13	D48.2	D49.2
ganglion NEC — see also Neoplasm, nerve, peripheral	C47.9	C79.89	—	D36.10	D48.2	D49.2
glossopharyngeal	C72.59	C79.49	—	D33.3	D43.3	D49.7
hypoglossal	C72.59	C79.49	—	D33.3	D43.3	D49.7
intercostal	C47.3	C79.89	—	D36.14	D48.2	D49.2
lumbar	C47.6	C79.89	—	D36.17	D48.2	D49.2
median	C47.1-✓	C79.89	—	D36.12	D48.2	D49.2
obturator	C47.2-✓	C79.89	—	D36.13	D48.2	D49.2
oculomotor	C72.59	C79.49	—	D33.3	D43.3	D49.7
olfactory	C47.2-✓	C79.49	—	D33.3	D43.3	D49.7
optic	C72.3-✓	C79.49	—	D33.3	D43.3	D49.7
parasympathetic NEC	C47.9	C79.89	—	D36.10	D48.2	D49.2
peripheral NEC	C47.9	C79.89	—	D36.10	D48.2	D49.2
abdomen	C47.4	C79.89	—	D36.15	D48.2	D49.2
abdominal wall	C47.4	C79.89	—	D36.15	D48.2	D49.2
ankle	C47.2-✓	C79.89	—	D36.13	D48.2	D49.2

✓ Additional Character Required — Refer to the Tabular List for Character Selection   ▽ Subterms under main terms may continue to next column or page

Neoplasm, neoplastic — *continued*
nerve — *continued*
  peripheral — *continued*

	Malignant Primary	Malignant Secondary	Ca in situ	Benign	Uncertain	Unspecified Behavior
antecubital fossa or space	C47.1-☑	C79.89	—	D36.12	D48.2	D49.2
arm	C47.1-☑	C79.89	—	D36.12	D48.2	D49.2
auricle (ear)	C47.0	C79.89	—	D36.11	D48.2	D49.2
axilla	C47.3	C79.89	—	D36.12	D48.2	D49.2
back	C47.6	C79.89	—	D36.17	D48.2	D49.2
buttock	C47.5	C79.89	—	D36.16	D48.2	D49.2
calf	C47.2-☑	C79.89	—	D36.13	D48.2	D49.2
cervical region	C47.0	C79.89	—	D36.11	D48.2	D49.2
cheek	C47.0	C79.89	—	D36.11	D48.2	D49.2
chest (wall)	C47.3	C79.89	—	D36.14	D48.2	D49.2
chin	C47.0	C79.89	—	D36.11	D48.2	D49.2
ear (external)	C47.0	C79.89	—	D36.11	D48.2	D49.2
elbow	C47.1-☑	C79.89	—	D36.12	D48.2	D49.2
extrarectal	C47.5	C79.89	—	D36.16	D48.2	D49.2
extremity	C47.9	C79.89	—	D36.10	D48.2	D49.2
lower	C47.2-☑	C79.89	—	D36.13	D48.2	D49.2
upper	C47.1-☑	C79.89	—	D36.12	D48.2	D49.2
eyelid	C47.0	C79.89	—	D36.11	D48.2	D49.2
face	C47.0	C79.89	—	D36.11	D48.2	D49.2
finger	C47.1-☑	C79.89	—	D36.12	D48.2	D49.2
flank	C47.6	C79.89	—	D36.17	D48.2	D49.2
foot	C47.2-☑	C79.89	—	D36.13	D48.2	D49.2
forearm	C47.1-☑	C79.89	—	D36.12	D48.2	D49.2
forehead	C47.0	C79.89	—	D36.11	D48.2	D49.2
gluteal region	C47.5	C79.89	—	D36.16	D48.2	D49.2
groin	C47.5	C79.89	—	D36.16	D48.2	D49.2
hand	C47.1-☑	C79.89	—	D36.12	D48.2	D49.2
head	C47.0	C79.89	—	D36.11	D48.2	D49.2
heel	C47.2-☑	C79.89	—	D36.13	D48.2	D49.2
hip	C47.2-☑	C79.89	—	D36.13	D48.2	D49.2
infraclavicular region	C47.3	C79.89	—	D36.14	D48.2	D49.2
inguinal (canal) (region)	C47.5	C79.89	—	D36.16	D48.2	D49.2
intrathoracic	C47.3	C79.89	—	D36.14	D48.2	D49.2
ischiorectal fossa	C47.5	C79.89	—	D36.16	D48.2	D49.2
knee	C47.2-☑	C79.89	—	D36.13	D48.2	D49.2
leg	C47.2-☑	C79.89	—	D36.13	D48.2	D49.2
limb NEC	C47.9	C79.89	—	D36.10	D48.2	D49.2
lower	C47.2-☑	C79.89	—	D36.13	D48.2	D49.2
upper	C47.1-☑	C79.89	—	D36.12	D48.2	D49.2
nates	C47.5	C79.89	—	D36.16	D48.2	D49.2
neck	C47.0	C79.89	—	D36.11	D48.2	D49.2
orbit	C69.6-☑	C79.49	—	D31.6-☑	D48.7	D49.2
pararectal	C47.5	C79.89	—	D36.16	D48.2	D49.2
paraurethral	C47.5	C79.89	—	D36.16	D48.2	D49.2
paravaginal	C47.5	C79.89	—	D36.16	D48.2	D49.2
pelvis (floor)	C47.5	C79.89	—	D36.16	D48.2	D49.2
pelvoabdominal	C47.8	C79.89	—	D36.17	D48.2	D49.2
perineum	C47.5	C79.89	—	D36.16	D48.2	D49.2
perirectal (tissue)	C47.5	C79.89	—	D36.16	D48.2	D49.2
periurethral (tissue)	C47.5	C79.89	—	D36.16	D48.2	D49.2
popliteal fossa or space	C47.2-☑	C79.89	—	D36.13	D48.2	D49.2
presacral	C47.5	C79.89	—	D36.16	D48.2	D49.2
pterygoid fossa	C47.0	C79.89	—	D36.11	D48.2	D49.2
rectovaginal septum or wall	C47.5	C79.89	—	D36.16	D48.2	D49.2
rectovesical	C47.5	C79.89	—	D36.16	D48.2	D49.2
sacrococcygeal region	C47.5	C79.89	—	D36.16	D48.2	D49.2
scalp	C47.0	C79.89	—	D36.11	D48.2	D49.2
scapular region	C47.3	C79.89	—	D36.14	D48.2	D49.2
shoulder	C47.1-☑	C79.89	—	D36.12	D48.2	D49.2
submental	C47.0	C79.89	—	D36.11	D48.2	D49.2
supraclavicular region	C47.0	C79.89	—	D36.11	D48.2	D49.2
temple	C47.0	C79.89	—	D36.11	D48.2	D49.2
temporal region	C47.0	C79.89	—	D36.11	D48.2	D49.2
thigh	C47.2-☑	C79.89	—	D36.13	D48.2	D49.2
thoracic (duct) (wall)	C47.3	C79.89	—	D36.14	D48.2	D49.2
thorax	C47.3	C79.89	—	D36.14	D48.2	D49.2
thumb	C47.1-☑	C79.89	—	D36.12	D48.2	D49.2

Neoplasm, neoplastic — *continued*
nerve — *continued*
  peripheral — *continued*

	Malignant Primary	Malignant Secondary	Ca in situ	Benign	Uncertain	Unspecified Behavior
toe	C47.2-☑	C79.89	—	D36.13	D48.2	D49.2
trunk	C47.6	C79.89	—	D36.17	D48.2	D49.2
umbilicus	C47.4	C79.89	—	D36.15	D48.2	D49.2
vesicorectal	C47.5	C79.89	—	D36.16	D48.2	D49.2
wrist	C47.1-☑	C79.89	—	D36.12	D48.2	D49.2
radial	C47.1-☑	C79.89	—	D36.12	D48.2	D49.2
sacral	C47.5	C79.89	—	D36.16	D48.2	D49.2
sciatic	C47.2-☑	C79.89	—	D36.13	D48.2	D49.2
spinal NEC	C47.9	C79.89	—	D36.10	D48.2	D49.2
accessory	C72.59	C79.49	—	D33.3	D43.3	D49.7
sympathetic NEC — *see also* Neoplasm, nerve, peripheral	C47.9	C79.89	—	D36.10	D48.2	D49.2
trigeminal	C72.59	C79.49	—	D33.3	D43.3	D49.7
trochlear	C72.59	C79.49	—	D33.3	D43.3	D49.7
ulnar	C47.1-☑	C79.89	—	D36.12	D48.2	D49.2
vagus	C72.59	C79.49	—	D33.3	D43.3	D49.7
nervous system (central)	C72.9	C79.40	—	D33.9	D43.9	D49.7
autonomic — *see* Neoplasm, nerve, peripheral						
parasympathetic — *see* Neoplasm, nerve, peripheral						
specified site NEC	—	C79.49	—	D33.7	D43.8	—
sympathetic — *see* Neoplasm, nerve, peripheral						
nevus — *see* Nevus						
nipple	C50.0-☑	C79.81	D05.-☑	D24.-☑	—	—
nose, nasal	C76.0	C79.89	D09.8	D36.7	D48.7	D49.89
ala (external) (nasi) — see also Neoplasm, nose, skin						
bone	C41.0	C79.51	—	D16.4	D48.0	D49.2
cartilage	C30.0	C78.39	D02.3	D14.0	D38.5	D49.1
cavity	C30.0	C78.39	D02.3	D14.0	D38.5	D49.1
choana	C11.3	C79.89	D00.08	D10.6	D37.05	D49.0
external (skin) — see also Neoplasm, nose, skin	C44.301	C79.2	D04.39	D23.39	D48.5	D49.2
fossa	C30.0	C78.39	D02.3	D14.0	D38.5	D49.1
internal	C30.0	C78.39	D02.3	D14.0	D38.5	D49.1
mucosa	C30.0	C78.39	D02.3	D14.0	D38.5	D49.1
septum	C30.0	C78.39	D02.3	D14.0	D38.5	D49.1
posterior margin	C11.3	C79.89	D00.08	D10.6	D37.05	D49.0
sinus — *see* Neoplasm, sinus						
skin	C44.301	C79.2	D04.39	D23.39	D48.5	D49.2
basal cell carcinoma	C44.311	—	—	—	—	—
specified type NEC	C44.391	—	—	—	—	—
squamous cell carcinoma	C44.321	—	—	—	—	—
turbinate (mucosa)	C30.0	C78.39	D02.3	D14.0	D38.5	D49.1
bone	C41.0	C79.51	—	D16.4	D48.0	D49.2
vestibule	C30.0	C78.39	D02.3	D14.0	D38.5	D49.1
nostril	C30.0	C78.39	D02.3	D14.0	D38.5	D49.1
nucleus pulposus	C41.2	C79.51	—	D16.6	D48.0	D49.2
occipital bone	C41.0	C79.51	—	D16.4	D48.0	D49.2
lobe or pole, brain	C71.4	C79.31	—	D33.0	D43.0	D49.6
odontogenic — *see* Neoplasm, jaw bone						
olfactory nerve or bulb	C72.2-☑	C79.49	—	D33.3	D43.3	D49.7
olive (brain)	C71.7	C79.31	—	D33.1	D43.1	D49.6
omentum	C48.1	C78.6	—	D20.1	D48.4	D49.0
operculum (brain)	C71.0	C79.31	—	D33.0	D43.0	D49.6
optic nerve, chiasm, or tract	C72.3-☑	C79.49	—	D33.3	D43.3	D49.7
oral (cavity)	C06.9	C79.89	D00.00	D10.30	D37.09	D49.0
ill-defined	C14.8	C79.89	D00.00	D10.30	D37.09	D49.0
mucosa	C06.0	C79.89	D00.02	D10.39	D37.09	D49.0
orbit	C69.6-☑	C79.49	D09.2-☑	D31.6-☑	D48.7	D49.89

Neoplasm Table

Neoplasm, orbit — Neoplasm, pole

	Malignant Primary	Malignant Secondary	Ca in situ	Benign	Uncertain	Unspecified Behavior
Neoplasm, neoplastic — continued						
orbit — continued						
autonomic nerve	C69.6-☑	C79.49	—	D31.6-☑	D48.7	D49.2
bone	C41.0	C79.51	—	D16.4	D48.0	D49.2
eye	C69.6-☑	C79.49	D09.2-☑	D31.6-☑	D48.7	D49.89
peripheral nerves	C69.6-☑	C79.49	—	D31.6-☑	D48.7	D49.2
soft parts	C69.6-☑	C79.49	D09.2-☑	D31.6-☑	D48.7	D49.89
organ of Zuckerkandl	C75.5	C79.89	—	D35.6	D44.7	D49.7
oropharynx	C10.9	C79.89	D00.08	D10.5	D37.05	D49.0
branchial cleft (vestige)	C10.4	C79.89	D00.08	D10.5	D37.05	D49.0
junctional region	C10.8	C79.89	D00.08	D10.5	D37.05	D49.0
lateral wall	C10.2	C79.89	D00.08	D10.5	D37.05	D49.0
overlapping lesion	C10.8	—	—	—	—	—
pillars or fauces	C09.1	C79.89	D00.08	D10.5	D37.05	D49.0
posterior wall	C10.3	C79.89	D00.08	D10.5	D37.05	D49.0
vallecula	C10.0	C79.89	D00.08	D10.5	D37.05	D49.0
os						
external	C53.1	C79.82	D06.1	D26.0	D39.0	D49.5
internal	C53.0	C79.82	D06.0	D26.0	D39.0	D49.5
ovary	C56.-☑	C79.6-☑	D07.39	D27.-☑	D39.1-☑	D49.5
oviduct	C57.0-☑	C79.82	D07.39	D28.2	D39.8	D49.5
palate	C05.9	C79.89	D00.00	D10.39	D37.09	D49.0
hard	C05.0	C79.89	D00.05	D10.39	D37.09	D49.0
junction of hard and soft palate	C05.9	C79.89	D00.00	D10.39	D37.09	D49.0
overlapping lesions	C05.8	—	—	—	—	—
soft	C05.1	C79.89	D00.04	D10.39	D37.09	D49.0
nasopharyngeal surface	C11.3	C79.89	D00.08	D10.6	D37.05	D49.0
posterior surface	C11.3	C79.89	D00.08	D10.6	D37.05	D49.0
superior surface	C11.3	C79.89	D00.08	D10.6	D37.05	D49.0
palatoglossal arch	C09.1	C79.89	D00.00	D10.5	D37.09	D49.0
palatopharyngeal arch	C09.1	C79.89	D00.00	D10.5	D37.09	D49.0
pallium	C71.0	C79.31	—	D33.0	D43.0	D49.6
palpebra	C44.10-☑	C79.2	D04.1-☑	D23.1-☑	D48.5	D49.2
basal cell carcinoma	C44.11-☑	—	—	—	—	—
specified type NEC	C44.19-☑	—	—	—	—	—
squamous cell carcinoma	C44.12-☑	—	—	—	—	—
pancreas	C25.9	C78.89	D01.7	D13.6	D37.8	D49.0
body	C25.1	C78.89	D01.7	D13.6	D37.8	D49.0
duct (of Santorini) (of Wirsung)	C25.3	C78.89	D01.7	D13.6	D37.8	D49.0
ectopic tissue	C25.7	C78.89	—	D13.6	D37.8	D49.0
head	C25.0	C78.89	D01.7	D13.6	D37.8	D49.0
islet cells	C25.4	C78.89	D01.7	D13.7	D37.8	D49.0
neck	C25.7	C78.89	D01.7	D13.6	D37.8	D49.0
overlapping lesion	C25.8	—	—	—	—	—
tail	C25.2	C78.89	D01.7	D13.6	D37.8	D49.0
para-aortic body	C75.5	C79.89	—	D35.6	D44.7	D49.7
paraganglion NEC	C75.5	C79.89	—	D35.6	D44.7	D49.7
parametrium	C57.3	C79.82	—	D28.2	D39.8	D49.5
paranephric	C48.0	C78.6	—	D20.0	D48.3	D49.0
pararectal	C76.3	C79.89	—	D36.7	D48.7	D49.89
parasagittal (region)	C76.0	C79.89	D09.8	D36.7	D48.7	D49.89
parasellar	C72.9	C79.49	—	D33.9	D43.8	D49.7
parathyroid (gland)	C75.0	C79.89	D09.3	D35.1	D44.2	D49.7
paraurethral	C76.3	C79.89	—	D36.7	D48.7	D49.89
gland	C68.1	C79.19	D09.19	D30.8	D41.8	D49.5
paravaginal	C76.3	C79.89	—	D36.7	D48.7	D49.89
parenchyma, kidney	C64.-☑	C79.0-☑	D09.19	D30.0-☑	D41.0-☑	D49.5
parietal						
bone	C41.0	C79.51	—	D16.4	D48.0	D49.2
lobe, brain	C71.3	C79.31	—	D33.0	D43.0	D49.6
paroophoron	C57.1-☑	C79.82	D07.39	D28.2	D39.8	D49.5
parotid (duct) (gland)	C07	C79.89	D00.00	D11.0	D37.030	D49.0
parovarium	C57.1-☑	C79.82	D07.39	D28.2	D39.8	D49.5
patella	C40.20	C79.51	—	—	—	—
peduncle, cerebral	C71.7	C79.31	—	D33.1	D43.1	D49.6
pelvirectal junction	C19	C78.5	D01.1	D12.7	D37.5	D49.0
pelvis, pelvic	C76.3	C79.89	D09.8	D36.7	D48.7	D49.89
bone	C41.4	C79.51	—	D16.8	D48.0	D49.2
floor	C76.3	C79.89	D09.8	D36.7	D48.7	D49.89
renal	C65.-☑	C79.0-☑	D09.19	D30.1-☑	D41.1-☑	D49.5
viscera	C76.3	C79.89	D09.8	D36.7	D48.7	D49.89

	Malignant Primary	Malignant Secondary	Ca in situ	Benign	Uncertain	Unspecified Behavior
Neoplasm, neoplastic — continued						
pelvis, pelvic — continued						
wall	C76.3	C79.89	D09.8	D36.7	D48.7	D49.89
pelvo-abdominal	C76.8	C79.89	D09.8	D36.7	D48.7	D49.89
penis	C60.9	C79.82	D07.4	D29.0	D40.8	D49.5
body	C60.2	C79.82	D07.4	D29.0	D40.8	D49.5
corpus (cavernosum)	C60.2	C79.82	D07.4	D29.0	D40.8	D49.5
glans	C60.1	C79.82	D07.4	D29.0	D40.8	D49.5
overlapping sites	C60.8	—	—	—	—	—
skin NEC	C60.9	C79.82	D07.4	D29.0	D40.8	D49.5
periadrenal (tissue)	C48.0	C78.6	—	D20.0	D48.3	D49.0
perianal (skin) — see also Neoplasm, anus, skin	C44.500	C79.2	D04.5	D23.5	D48.5	D49.2
pericardium	C38.0	C79.89	—	D15.1	D48.7	D49.89
perinephric	C48.0	C78.6	—	D20.0	D48.3	D49.0
perineum	C76.3	C79.89	D09.8	D36.7	D48.7	D49.89
periodontal tissue NEC	C03.9	C79.89	D00.03	D10.39	D37.09	D49.0
periosteum — see Neoplasm, bone						
peripancreatic	C48.0	C78.6	—	D20.0	D48.3	D49.0
peripheral nerve NEC	C47.9	C79.89	—	D36.10	D48.2	D49.2
perirectal (tissue)	C76.3	C79.89	—	D36.7	D48.7	D49.89
perirenal (tissue)	C48.0	C78.6	—	D20.0	D48.3	D49.0
peritoneum, peritoneal (cavity)	C48.2	C78.6	—	D20.1	D48.4	D49.0
benign mesothelial tissue — see Mesothelioma, benign						
overlapping lesion with digestive organs	C48.8	—		—	—	—
	C26.9	—		—	—	—
parietal	C48.1	C78.6	—	D20.1	D48.4	D49.0
pelvic	C48.1	C78.6	—	D20.1	D48.4	D49.0
specified part NEC	C48.1	C78.6	—	D20.1	D48.4	D49.0
peritonsillar (tissue)	C76.0	C79.89	D09.8	D36.7	D48.7	D49.89
periurethral tissue	C76.3	C79.89	—	D36.7	D48.7	D49.89
phalanges						
foot	C40.3-☑	C79.51	—	D16.3-☑	—	—
hand	C40.1-☑	C79.51	—	D16.1-☑	—	—
pharynx, pharyngeal	C14.0	C79.89	D00.08	D10.9	D37.05	D49.0
bursa	C11.1	C79.89	D00.08	D10.6	D37.05	D49.0
fornix	C11.3	C79.89	D00.08	D10.6	D37.05	D49.0
recess	C11.2	C79.89	D00.08	D10.6	D37.05	D49.0
region	C14.0	C79.89	D00.08	D10.9	D37.05	D49.0
tonsil	C11.1	C79.89	D00.08	D10.6	D37.05	D49.0
wall (lateral) (posterior)	C14.0	C79.89	D00.08	D10.9	D37.05	D49.0
pia mater	C70.9	C79.40	—	D32.9	D42.9	D49.7
cerebral	C70.0	C79.32	—	D32.0	D42.0	D49.7
cranial	C70.0	C79.32	—	D32.0	D42.0	D49.7
spinal	C70.1	C79.49	—	D32.1	D42.1	D49.7
pillars of fauces	C09.1	C79.89	D00.08	D10.5	D37.05	D49.0
pineal (body) (gland)	C75.3	C79.89	D09.3	D35.4	D44.5	D49.7
pinna (ear) NEC — see also Neoplasm, skin, ear	C44.20-☑	C79.2	D04.2-☑	D23.2-☑	D48.5	D49.2
piriform fossa or sinus	C12	C79.89	D00.08	D10.7	D37.05	D49.0
pituitary (body) (fossa) (gland) (lobe)	C75.1	C79.89	D09.3	D35.2	D44.3	D49.7
placenta	C58	C79.82	D07.0	D26.7	D39.2	D49.5
pleura, pleural (cavity)	C38.4	C78.2	—	D19.0	D38.2	D49.1
overlapping lesion with heart or mediastinum	C38.8	—		—	—	—
parietal	C38.4	C78.2	—	D19.0	D38.2	D49.1
visceral	C38.4	C78.2	—	D19.0	D38.2	D49.1
plexus						
brachial	C47.1-☑	C79.89	—	D36.12	D48.2	D49.2
cervical	C47.0	C79.89	—	D36.11	D48.2	D49.2
choroid	C71.5	C79.31	—	D33.0	D43.0	D49.6
lumbosacral	C47.5	C79.89	—	D36.16	D48.2	D49.2
sacral	C47.5	C79.89	—	D36.16	D48.2	D49.2
pluriendocrine	C75.8	C79.89	D09.3	D35.7	D44.9	D49.7
pole						

☑ Additional Character Required — Refer to the Tabular List for Character Selection   ▼ Subterms under main terms may continue to next column or page

Neoplasm, neoplastic — continued	Malignant Primary	Malignant Secondary	Ca in situ	Benign	Uncertain	Unspecified Behavior
pole — *continued*						
frontal	C71.1	C79.31	—	D33.0	D43.0	D49.6
occipital	C71.4	C79.31	—	D33.0	D43.0	D49.6
pons (varolii)	C71.7	C79.31	—	D33.1	D43.1	D49.6
popliteal fossa or space	C76.5-✓	C79.89	D04.7-✓	D36.7	D48.7	D49.89
postcricoid (region)	C13.0	C79.89	D00.08	D10.7	D37.05	D49.0
posterior fossa (cranial)	C71.9	C79.31	—	D33.2	D43.2	D49.6
postnasal space	C11.9	C79.89	D00.08	D10.6	D37.05	D49.0
prepuce	C60.0	C79.82	D07.4	D29.0	D40.8	D49.5
prepylorus	C16.4	C78.89	D00.2	D13.1	D37.1	D49.0
presacral (region)	C76.3	C79.89	—	D36.7	D48.7	D49.89
prostate (gland)	C61	C79.82	D07.5	D29.1	D40.0	D49.5
utricle	C68.0	C79.19	D09.19	D30.4	D41.3	D49.5
pterygoid fossa	C49.0	C79.89	—	D21.0	D48.1	D49.2
pubic bone	C41.4	C79.51	—	D16.8	D48.0	D49.2
pudenda, pudendum (female)	C51.9	C79.82	D07.1	D28.0	D39.8	D49.5
pulmonary — *see also* Neoplasm, lung	C34.9-✓	C78.0-✓	D02.2-✓	D14.3-✓	D38.1	D49.1
putamen	C71.0	C79.31	—	D33.0	D43.0	D49.6
pyloric						
antrum	C16.3	C78.89	D00.2	D13.1	D37.1	D49.0
canal	C16.4	C78.89	D00.2	D13.1	D37.1	D49.0
pylorus	C16.4	C78.89	D00.2	D13.1	D37.1	D49.0
pyramid (brain)	C71.7	C79.31	—	D33.1	D43.1	D49.6
pyriform fossa or sinus	C12	C79.89	D00.08	D10.7	D37.05	D49.0
radius (any part)	C40.0-✓	C79.51	—	D16.0-✓	—	—
Rathke's pouch	C75.1	C79.89	D09.3	D35.2	D44.3	D49.7
rectosigmoid (junction)	C19	C78.5	D01.1	D12.7	D37.5	D49.0
overlapping lesion with anus or rectum	C21.8	—	—	—	—	—
rectouterine pouch	C48.1	C78.6	—	D20.1	D48.4	D49.0
rectovaginal septum or wall	C76.3	C79.89	D09.8	D36.7	D48.7	D49.89
rectovesical septum	C76.3	C79.89	D09.8	D36.7	D48.7	D49.89
rectum (ampulla)	C20	C78.5	D01.2	D12.8	D37.5	D49.0
and colon	C19	C78.5	D01.1	D12.7	D37.5	D49.0
overlapping lesion with anus or rectosigmoid junction	C21.8	—	—	—	—	—
renal	C64.-✓	C79.0-✓	D09.19	D30.0-✓	D41.0-✓	D49.5
calyx	C65.-✓	C79.0-✓	D09.19	D30.1-✓	D41.1-✓	D49.5
hilus	C65.-✓	C79.0-✓	D09.19	D30.1-✓	D41.1-✓	D49.5
parenchyma	C64.-✓	C79.0-✓	D09.19	D30.0-✓	D41.0-✓	D49.5
pelvis	C65.-✓	C79.0-✓	D09.19	D30.1-✓	D41.1-✓	D49.5
respiratory						
organs or system NEC	C39.9	C78.30	D02.4	D14.4	D38.6	D49.1
tract NEC	C39.9	C78.30	D02.4	D14.4	D38.5	D49.1
upper	C39.0	C78.30	D02.4	D14.4	D38.5	D49.1
retina	C69.2-✓	C79.49	D09.2-✓	D31.2-✓	D48.7	D49.81
retrobulbar	C69.6-✓	C79.49	—	D31.6-✓	D48.7	D49.89
retrocecal	C48.0	C78.6	—	D20.0	D48.3	D49.0
retromolar (area) (triangle) (trigone)	C06.2	C79.89	D00.00	D10.39	D37.09	D49.0
retro-orbital	C76.0	C79.89	D09.8	D36.7	D48.7	D49.89
retroperitoneal (space) (tissue)	C48.0	C78.6	—	D20.0	D48.3	D49.0
retroperitoneum	C48.0	C78.6	—	D20.0	D48.3	D49.0
retropharyngeal	C14.0	C79.89	D00.08	D10.9	D37.05	D49.0
retrovesical (septum)	C76.3	C79.89	D09.8	D36.7	D48.7	D49.89
rhinencephalon	C71.0	C79.31	—	D33.0	D43.0	D49.6
rib	C41.3	C79.51	—	D16.7	D48.0	D49.2
Rosenmuller's fossa	C11.2	C79.89	D00.08	D10.6	D37.05	D49.0
round ligament	C57.2✓	C79.82	—	D28.2	D39.8	D49.5
sacrococcyx, sacrococcygeal	C41.4	C79.51	—	D16.8	D48.0	D49.2
region	C76.3	C79.89	D09.8	D36.7	D48.7	D49.89
sacrouterine ligament	C57.3	C79.82	—	D28.2	D39.8	D49.5
sacrum, sacral (vertebra)	C41.4	C79.51	—	D16.8	D48.0	D49.2

Neoplasm, neoplastic — continued	Malignant Primary	Malignant Secondary	Ca in situ	Benign	Uncertain	Unspecified Behavior
salivary gland or duct (major)	C08.9	C79.89	D00.00	D11.9	D37.039	D49.0
minor NEC	C06.9	C79.89	D00.00	D10.39	D37.04	D49.0
overlapping lesion	C08.9	—	—	—	—	—
parotid	C07	C79.89	D00.00	D11.0	D37.030	D49.0
pluriglandular	C08.9	C79.89	D00.00	D11.9	D37.039	D49.0
sublingual	C08.1	C79.89	D00.00	D11.7	D37.031	D49.0
submandibular	C08.0	C79.89	D00.00	D11.7	D37.032	D49.0
submaxillary	C08.0	C79.89	D00.00	D11.7	D37.032	D49.0
salpinx (uterine)	C57.0-✓	C79.82	D07.39	D28.2	D39.8	D49.5
Santorini's duct	C25.3	C78.89	D01.7	D13.6	D37.8	D49.0
scalp	C44.40	C79.2	D04.4	D23.4	D48.5	D49.2
basal cell carcinoma	C44.41	—	—	—	—	—
specified type NEC	C44.49	—	—	—	—	—
squamous cell carcinoma	C44.42	—	—	—	—	—
scapula (any part)	C40.0-✓	C79.51	—	D16.0-✓	—	—
scapular region	C76.1	C79.89	D09.8	D36.7	D48.7	D49.89
scar NEC — *see also* Neoplasm, skin, by site	C44.90	C79.2	D04.9	D23.9	D48.5	D49.2
sciatic nerve	C47.2-✓	C79.89	—	D36.13	D48.2	D49.2
sclera	C69.4-✓	C79.49	D09.2-✓	D31.4-✓	D48.7	D49.89
scrotum (skin)	C63.2	C79.82	D07.61	D29.4	D40.8	D49.5
sebaceous gland — *see* Neoplasm, skin						
sella turcica	C75.1	C79.89	D09.3	D35.2	D44.3	D49.7
bone	C41.0	C79.51	—	D16.4	D48.0	D49.2
semilunar cartilage (knee)	C40.2-✓	C79.51	—	D16.2-✓	D48.0	D49.2
seminal vesicle	C63.7	C79.82	D07.69	D29.8	D40.8	D49.5
septum						
nasal	C30.0	C78.39	D02.3	D14.0	D38.5	D49.1
posterior margin	C11.3	C79.89	D00.08	D10.6	D37.05	D49.0
rectovaginal	C76.3	C79.89	D09.8	D36.7	D48.7	D49.89
rectovesical	C76.3	C79.89	D09.8	D36.7	D48.7	D49.89
urethrovaginal	C57.9	C79.82	D07.30	D28.9	D39.9	D49.5
vesicovaginal	C57.9	C79.82	D07.30	D28.9	D39.9	D49.5
shoulder NEC	C76.4-✓	C79.89	D04.6-✓	D36.7	D48.7	D49.89
sigmoid flexure (lower) (upper)	C18.7	C78.5	D01.0	D12.5	D37.4	D49.0
sinus (accessory)	C31.9	C78.39	D02.3	D14.0	D38.5	D49.1
bone (any)	C41.0	C79.51	—	D16.4	D48.0	D49.2
ethmoidal	C31.1	C78.39	D02.3	D14.0	D38.5	D49.1
frontal	C31.2	C78.39	D02.3	D14.0	D38.5	D49.1
maxillary	C31.0	C78.39	D02.3	D14.0	D38.5	D49.1
nasal, paranasal NEC	C31.9	C78.39	D02.3	D14.0	D38.5	D49.1
overlapping lesion	C31.8	—	—	—	—	—
pyriform	C12	C79.89	D00.08	D10.7	D37.05	D49.0
sphenoid	C31.3	C78.39	D02.3	D14.0	D38.5	D49.1
skeleton, skeletal NEC	C41.9	C79.51	—	D16.9	D48.0	D49.2
Skene's gland	C68.1	C79.19	D09.19	D30.8	D41.8	D49.5
skin NOS	C44.90	C79.2	D04.9	D23.9	D48.5	D49.2
abdominal wall	C44.509	C79.2	D04.5	D23.5	D48.5	D49.2
basal cell carcinoma	C44.519	—	—	—	—	—
specified type NEC	C44.599	—	—	—	—	—
squamous cell carcinoma	C44.529	—	—	—	—	—
ala nasi — *see also* Neoplasm, nose, skin	C44.301	C79.2	D04.39	D23.39	D48.5	D49.2
ankle — *see also* Neoplasm, skin, limb, lower	C44.70-✓	C79.2	D04.7-✓	D23.7-✓	D48.5	D49.2
antecubital space — *see also* Neoplasm, skin, limb, upper	C44.60-✓	C79.2	D04.6-✓	D23.6-✓	D48.5	D49.2
anus	C44.500	C79.2	D04.5	D23.5	D48.5	D49.2
basal cell carcinoma	C44.510	—	—	—	—	—
specified type NEC	C44.590	—	—	—	—	—
squamous cell carcinoma	C44.520	—	—	—	—	—

Neoplasm Table

Neoplasm, pole — Neoplasm, skin NOS

	Malignant Primary	Malignant Secondary	Ca in situ	Benign	Uncertain	Unspecified Behavior
Neoplasm, neoplastic — continued						
skin — continued						
arm — see also Neoplasm, skin, limb, upper	C44.60-☑	C79.2	D04.6-☑	D23.6-☑	D48.5	D49.2
auditory canal (external) — see also Neoplasm, skin, ear	C44.20-☑	C79.2	D04.2-☑	D23.2-☑	D48.5	D49.2
auricle (ear) — see also Neoplasm, skin, ear	C44.20-☑	C79.2	D04.2-☑	D23.2-☑	D48.5	D49.2
auricular canal (external) — see also Neoplasm, skin, ear	C44.20-☑	C79.2	D04.2-☑	D23.2-☑	D48.5	D49.2
axilla, axillary fold — see also Neoplasm, skin, trunk	C44.509	C79.2	D04.5	D23.5	D48.5	D49.2
back — see also Neoplasm, skin, trunk	C44.509	C79.2	D04.5	D23.5	D48.5	D49.2
basal cell carcinoma	C44.91	—	—	—	—	—
breast	C44.501	C79.2	D04.5	D23.5	D48.5	D49.2
basal cell carcinoma	C44.511	—	—	—	—	—
specified type NEC	C44.591	—	—	—	—	—
squamous cell carcinoma	C44.521	—	—	—	—	—
brow — see also Neoplasm, skin, face	C44.309	C79.2	D04.39	D23.39	D48.5	D49.2
buttock — see also Neoplasm, skin, trunk	C44.509	C79.2	D04.5	D23.5	D48.5	D49.2
calf — see also Neoplasm, skin, limb, lower	C44.70-☑	C79.2	D04.7-☑	D23.7-☑	D48.5	D49.2
canthus (eye) (inner) (outer)	C44.10-☑	C79.2	D04.1-☑	D23.1-☑	D48.5	D49.2
basal cell carcinoma	C44.11-☑	—	—	—	—	—
specified type NEC	C44.19-☑	—	—	—	—	—
squamous cell carcinoma	C44.12-☑	—	—	—	—	—
cervical region — see also Neoplasm, skin, neck	C44.40	C79.2	D04.4	D23.4	D48.5	D49.2
cheek (external) — see also Neoplasm, skin, face	C44.309	C79.2	D04.39	D23.39	D48.5	D49.2
chest (wall) — see also Neoplasm, skin, trunk	C44.509	C79.2	D04.5	D23.5	D48.5	D49.2
chin — see also Neoplasm, skin, face	C44.309	C79.2	D04.39	D23.39	D48.5	D49.2
clavicular area — see also Neoplasm, skin, trunk	C44.509	C79.2	D04.5	D23.5	D48.5	D49.2
clitoris	C51.2	C79.82	D07.1	D28.0	D39.8	D49.5
columnella — see also Neoplasm, skin, face	C44.309	C79.2	D04.39	D23.39	D48.5	D49.2
concha — see also Neoplasm, skin, ear	C44.20-☑	C79.2	D04.2-☑	D23.2-☑	D48.5	D49.2
ear (external)	C44.20-☑	C79.2	D04.2-☑	D23.2-☑	D48.5	D49.2
basal cell carcinoma	C44.21-☑	—	—	—	—	—
specified type NEC	C44.29-☑	—	—	—	—	—
squamous cell carcinoma	C44.22-☑	—	—	—	—	—
elbow — see also Neoplasm, skin, limb, upper	C44.60-☑	C79.2	D04.6-☑	D23.6-☑	D48.5	D49.2

	Malignant Primary	Malignant Secondary	Ca in situ	Benign	Uncertain	Unspecified Behavior
Neoplasm, neoplastic — continued						
skin — continued						
eyebrow — see also Neoplasm, skin, face	C44.309	C79.2	D04.39	D23.39	D48.5	D49.2
eyelid	C44.10-☑	C79.2	D04.1-☑	D23.1-☑	D48.5	D49.2
basal cell carcinoma	C44.11-☑	—	—	—	—	—
specified type NEC	C44.19-☑	—	—	—	—	—
squamous cell carcinoma	C44.12-☑	—	—	—	—	—
face NOS	C44.300	C79.2	D04.30	D23.30	D48.5	D49.2
basal cell carcinoma	C44.310					
specified type NEC	C44.390					
squamous cell carcinoma	C44.320					
female genital organs (external)	C51.9	C79.82	D07.1	D28.0	D39.8	D49.5
clitoris	C51.2	C79.82	D07.1	D28.0	D39.8	D49.5
labium NEC	C51.9	C79.82	D07.1	D28.0	D39.8	D49.5
majus	C51.0	C79.82	D07.1	D28.0	D39.8	D49.5
minus	C51.1	C79.82	D07.1	D28.0	D39.8	D49.5
pudendum	C51.9	C79.82	D07.1	D28.0	D39.8	D49.5
vulva	C51.9	C79.82	D07.1	D28.0	D39.8	D49.5
finger — see also Neoplasm, skin, limb, upper	C44.60-☑	C79.2	D04.6-☑	D23.6-☑	D48.5	D49.2
flank — see also Neoplasm, skin, trunk	C44.509	C79.2	D04.5	D23.5	D48.5	D49.2
foot — see also Neoplasm, skin, limb, lower	C44.70-☑	C79.2	D04.7-☑	D23.7-☑	D48.5	D49.2
forearm — see also Neoplasm, skin, limb, upper	C44.60-☑	C79.2	D04.6-☑	D23.6-☑	D48.5	D49.2
forehead — see also Neoplasm, skin, face	C44.309	C79.2	D04.39	D23.39	D48.5	D49.2
glabella — see also Neoplasm, skin, face	C44.309	C79.2	D04.39	D23.39	D48.5	D49.2
gluteal region — see also Neoplasm, skin, trunk	C44.509	C79.2	D04.5	D23.5	D48.5	D49.2
groin — see also Neoplasm, skin, trunk	C44.509	C79.2	D04.5	D23.5	D48.5	D49.2
hand — see also Neoplasm, skin, limb, upper	C44.60-☑	C79.2	D04.6-☑	D23.6-☑	D48.5	D49.2
head NEC — see also Neoplasm, skin, scalp	C44.40	C79.2	D04.4	D23.4	D48.5	D49.2
heel — see also Neoplasm, skin, limb, lower	C44.70-☑	C79.2	D04.7-☑	D23.7-☑	D48.5	D49.2
helix — see also Neoplasm, skin, ear	C44.20-☑	C79.2	D04.2-☑	D23.2-☑	D48.5	D49.2
hip — see also Neoplasm, skin, limb, lower	C44.70-☑	C79.2	D04.7-☑	D23.7-☑	D48.5	D49.2
infraclavicular region — see also Neoplasm, skin, trunk	C44.509	C79.2	D04.5	D23.5	D48.5	D49.2
inguinal region — see also Neoplasm, skin, trunk	C44.509	C79.2	D04.5	D23.5	D48.5	D49.2
jaw — see also Neoplasm, skin, face	C44.309	C79.2	D04.39	D23.39	D48.5	D49.2
Kaposi's sarcoma — see Kaposi's, sarcoma, skin						
knee — see also Neoplasm, skin, limb, lower	C44.70-☑	C79.2	D04.7-☑	D23.7-☑	D48.5	D49.2
labia						

☑ Additional Character Required — Refer to the Tabular List for Character Selection   ▽ Subterms under main terms may continue to next column or page

Neoplasm Table

Neoplasm, neoplastic — *continued*	Malignant Primary	Malignant Secondary	Ca in situ	Benign	Uncertain	Unspecified Behavior
skin — continued						
labia — continued						
majora	C51.0	C79.82	D07.1	D28.0	D39.8	D49.5
minora	C51.1	C79.82	D07.1	D28.0	D39.8	D49.5
leg — *see also Neoplasm, skin, limb, lower*	C44.70-☑	C79.2	D04.7-☑	D23.7-☑	D48.5	D49.2
lid (lower) (upper)	C44.10-☑	C79.2	D04.1-☑	D23.1-☑	D48.5	D49.2
basal cell carcinoma	C44.11-☑	—	—	—	—	—
specified type NEC	C44.19-☑	—	—	—	—	—
squamous cell carcinoma	C44.12-☑	—	—	—	—	—
limb NEC	C44.90	C79.2	D04.9	D23.9	D48.5	D49.2
basal cell carcinoma	C44.91					
lower	C44.70-☑	C79.2	D04.7-☑	D23.7-☑	D48.5	D49.2
basal cell carcinoma	C44.71-☑	—	—	—		
specified type NEC	C44.79-☑	—	—	—		
squamous cell carcinoma	C44.72-☑	—	—	—		
upper	C44.60-☑	C79.2	D04.6-☑	D23.6-☑	D48.5	D49.2
basal cell carcinoma	C44.61-☑	—	—	—		
specified type NEC	C44.69-☑	—	—	—		
squamous cell carcinoma	C44.62-☑	—	—	—		
lip (lower) (upper)	C44.00	C79.2	D04.0	D23.0	D48.5	D49.2
basal cell carcinoma	C44.01					
specified type NEC	C44.09					
squamous cell carcinoma	C44.02					
male genital organs	C63.9	C79.82	D07.60	D29.9	D40.8	D49.5
penis	C60.9	C79.82	D07.4	D29.0	D40.8	D49.5
prepuce	C60.0	C79.82	D07.4	D29.0	D40.8	D49.5
scrotum	C63.2	C79.82	D07.61	D29.4	D40.8	D49.5
mastectomy site (skin) — *see also Neoplasm, skin, breast*	C44.501	C79.2	—	—	—	—
specified as breast tissue	C50.8-☑	C79.81	—	—	—	—
meatus, acoustic (external) — *see also Neoplasm, skin, ear*	C44.20-☑	C79.2	D04.2-☑	D23.2-☑	D48.5	D49.2
melanotic — *see Melanoma*						
Merkel cell — *see Carcinoma, Merkel cell*						
nates — *see also Neoplasm, skin, trunk*	C44.509	C79.2	D04.5	D23.5	D48.5	D49.2
neck	C44.40	C79.2	D04.4	D23.4	D48.5	D49.2
basal cell carcinoma	C44.41	—	—	—	—	—
specified type NEC	C44.49	—	—	—	—	—
squamous cell carcinoma	C44.42	—	—	—	—	—
nevus — *see Nevus, skin*						
nose (external) — *see also Neoplasm, nose, skin*	C44.301	C79.2	D04.39	D23.39	D48.5	D49.2
overlapping lesion	C44.80					
basal cell carcinoma	C44.81	—	—	—	—	—
specified type NEC	C44.89	—	—	—	—	—
squamous cell carcinoma	C44.82	—	—	—	—	—

Neoplasm, neoplastic — *continued*	Malignant Primary	Malignant Secondary	Ca in situ	Benign	Uncertain	Unspecified Behavior
skin — continued						
palm — *see also Neoplasm, skin, limb, upper*	C44.60-☑	C79.2	D04.6-☑	D23.6-☑	D48.5	D49.2
palpebra	C44.10-☑	C79.2	D04.1-☑	D23.1-☑	D48.5	D49.2
basal cell carcinoma	C44.11-☑	—	—	—	—	—
specified type NEC	C44.19-☑	—	—	—	—	—
squamous cell carcinoma	C44.12-☑	—	—	—	—	—
penis NEC	C60.9	C79.82	D07.4	D29.0	D40.8	D49.5
perianal — *see also Neoplasm, skin, anus*	C44.500	C79.2	D04.5	D23.5	D48.5	D49.2
perineum — *see also Neoplasm, skin, anus*	C44.500	C79.2	D04.5	D23.5	D48.5	D49.2
pinna — *see also Neoplasm, skin, ear*	C44.20-☑	C79.2	D04.2-☑	D23.2-☑	D48.5	D49.2
plantar — *see also Neoplasm, skin, limb, lower*	C44.70-☑	C79.2	D04.7-☑	D23.7-☑	D48.5	D49.2
popliteal fossa or space — *see also Neoplasm, skin, limb, lower*	C44.70-☑	C79.2	D04.7-☑	D23.7-☑	D48.5	D49.2
prepuce	C60.0	C79.82	D07.4	D29.0	D40.8	D49.5
pubes — *see also Neoplasm, skin, trunk*	C44.509	C79.2	D04.5	D23.5	D48.5	D49.2
sacrococcygeal region — *see also Neoplasm, skin, trunk*	C44.509	C79.2	D04.5	D23.5	D48.5	D49.2
scalp	C44.40	C79.2	D04.4	D23.4	D48.5	D49.2
basal cell carcinoma	C44.41	—	—	—	—	—
specified type NEC	C44.49	—	—	—	—	—
squamous cell carcinoma	C44.42	—	—	—	—	—
scapular region — *see also Neoplasm, skin, trunk*	C44.509	C79.2	D04.5	D23.5	D48.5	D49.2
scrotum	C63.2	C79.82	D07.61	D29.4	D40.8	D49.5
shoulder — *see also Neoplasm, skin, limb, upper*	C44.60-☑	C79.2	D04.6-☑	D23.6-☑	D48.5	D49.2
sole (foot) — *see also Neoplasm, skin, limb, lower*	C44.70-☑	C79.2	D04.7-☑	D23.7-☑	D48.5	D49.2
specified sites NEC	C44.80	C79.2	D04.8	D23.9	D48.5	D49.2
basal cell carcinoma	C44.81	—	—	—	—	—
specified type NEC	C44.89	—	—	—	—	—
squamous cell carcinoma	C44.82	—	—	—	—	—
specified type NEC	C44.99	—	—	—	—	—
squamous cell carcinoma	C44.92	—	—	—	—	—
submammary fold — *see also Neoplasm, skin, trunk*	C44.509	C79.2	D04.5	D23.5	D48.5	D49.2
supraclavicular region — *see also Neoplasm, skin, neck*	C44.40	C79.2	D04.4	D23.4	D48.5	D49.2
temple — *see also Neoplasm, skin, face*	C44.309	C79.2	D04.39	D23.39	D48.5	D49.2
thigh — *see also Neoplasm, skin, limb, lower*	C44.70-☑	C79.2	D04.7-☑	D23.7-☑	D48.5	D49.2
thoracic wall — *see also Neoplasm, skin, trunk*	C44.509	C79.2	D04.5	D23.5	D48.5	D49.2

	Malignant Primary	Malignant Secondary	Ca in situ	Benign	Uncertain	Unspecified Behavior
Neoplasm, neoplastic —						
continued						
skin — *continued*						
thumb — *see also*						
Neoplasm, skin, limb, upper	C44.60-☑	C79.2	D04.6-☑	D23.6-☑	D48.5	D49.2
toe — *see also*						
Neoplasm, skin, limb, lower	C44.70-☑	C79.2	D04.7-☑	D23.7-☑	D48.5	D49.2
tragus — *see also*						
Neoplasm, skin, ear	C44.20-☑	C79.2	D04.2-☑	D23.2-☑	D48.5	D49.2
trunk	C44.509	C79.2	D04.5	D23.5	D48.5	D49.2
basal cell carcinoma	C44.519	—	—	—	—	—
specified type NEC	C44.599	—	—	—	—	—
squamous cell carcinoma	C44.529	—	—	—	—	—
umbilicus — *see also*						
Neoplasm, skin, trunk	C44.509	C79.2	D04.5	D23.5	D48.5	D49.2
vulva	C51.9	C79.82	D07.1	D28.0	D39.8	D49.5
overlapping lesion	C51.8	—	—	—	—	—
wrist — *see also*						
Neoplasm, skin, limb, upper	C44.60-☑	C79.2	D04.6-☑	D23.6-☑	D48.5	D49.2
skull	C41.0	C79.51	—	D16.4	D48.0	D49.2
soft parts or tissues — *see* Neoplasm, connective tissue						
specified site NEC	C76.8	C79.89	D09.8	D36.7	D48.7	D49.89
spermatic cord	C63.1-☑	C79.82	D07.69	D29.8	D40.8	D49.5
sphenoid	C31.3	C78.39	D02.3	D14.0	D38.5	D49.1
bone	C41.0	C79.51	—	D16.4	D48.0	D49.2
sinus	C31.3	C78.39	D02.3	D14.0	D38.5	D49.1
sphincter						
anal	C21.1	C78.5	D01.3	D12.9	D37.8	D49.0
of Oddi	C24.0	C78.89	D01.5	D13.5	D37.6	D49.0
spine, spinal (column)	C41.2	C79.51	—	D16.6	D48.0	D49.2
bulb	C71.7	C79.31	—	D33.1	D43.1	D49.6
coccyx	C41.4	C79.51	—	D16.8	D48.0	D49.2
cord (cervical) (lumbar) (sacral) (thoracic)	C72.0	C79.49	—	D33.4	D43.4	D49.7
dura mater	C70.1	C79.49	—	D32.1	D42.1	D49.7
lumbosacral	C41.2	C79.51	—	D16.6	D48.0	D49.2
marrow NEC	C96.9	C79.52	—	—	D47.9	D49.89
membrane	C70.1	C79.49	—	D32.1	D42.1	D49.7
meninges	C70.1	C79.49	—	D32.1	D42.1	D49.7
nerve (root)	C47.9	C79.89	—	D36.10	D48.2	D49.2
pia mater	C70.1	C79.49	—	D32.1	D42.1	D49.7
root	C47.9	C79.89	—	D36.10	D48.2	D49.2
sacrum	C41.4	C79.51	—	D16.8	D48.0	D49.2
spleen, splenic NEC	C26.1	C78.89	D01.7	D13.9	D37.8	D49.0
flexure (colon)	C18.5	C78.5	D01.0	D12.3	D37.4	D49.0
stem, brain	C71.7	C79.31	—	D33.1	D43.1	D49.6
Stensen's duct	C07	C79.89	D00.00	D11.0	D37.030	D49.0
sternum	C41.3	C79.51	—	D16.7	D48.0	D49.2
stomach	C16.9	C78.89	D00.2	D13.1	D37.1	D49.0
antrum (pyloric)	C16.3	C78.89	D00.2	D13.1	D37.1	D49.0
body	C16.2	C78.89	D00.2	D13.1	D37.1	D49.0
cardia	C16.0	C78.89	D00.2	D13.1	D37.1	D49.0
cardiac orifice	C16.0	C78.89	D00.2	D13.1	D37.1	D49.0
corpus	C16.2	C78.89	D00.2	D13.1	D37.1	D49.0
fundus	C16.1	C78.89	D00.2	D13.1	D37.1	D49.0
greater curvature NEC	C16.6	C78.89	D00.2	D13.1	D37.1	D49.0
lesser curvature NEC	C16.5	C78.89	D00.2	D13.1	D37.1	D49.0
overlapping lesion	C16.8	—	—	—	—	—
prepylorus	C16.4	C78.89	D00.2	D13.1	D37.1	D49.0
pylorus	C16.4	C78.89	D00.2	D13.1	D37.1	D49.0
wall NEC	C16.9	C78.89	D00.2	D13.1	D37.1	D49.0
anterior NEC	C16.8	C78.89	D00.2	D13.1	D37.1	D49.0
posterior NEC	C16.8	C78.89	D00.2	D13.1	D37.1	D49.0
stroma, endometrial	C54.1	C79.82	D07.0	D26.1	D39.0	D49.5
stump, cervical	C53.8	C79.82	D06.7	D26.0	D39.0	D49.5
subcutaneous (nodule) (tissue) NEC — *see*						

	Malignant Primary	Malignant Secondary	Ca in situ	Benign	Uncertain	Unspecified Behavior
Neoplasm, neoplastic —						
continued						
subcutaneous — *see* Neoplasm, connective tissue — *continued*						
Neoplasm, connective tissue						
subdural	C70.9	C79.32	—	D32.9	D42.9	D49.7
subglottis, subglottic	C32.2	C78.39	D02.0	D14.1	D38.0	D49.1
sublingual	C04.9	C79.89	D00.06	D10.2	D37.09	D49.0
gland or duct	C08.1	C79.89	D00.00	D11.7	D37.031	D49.0
submandibular gland	C08.0	C79.89	D00.00	D11.7	D37.032	D49.0
submaxillary gland or duct	C08.0	C79.89	D00.00	D11.7	D37.032	D49.0
submental	C76.0	C79.89	D09.8	D36.7	D48.7	D49.89
subpleural	C34.9-☑	C78.0-☑	D02.2-☑	D14.3-☑	D38.1	D49.1
substernal	C38.1	C78.1	—	D15.2	D38.3	D49.89
sudoriferous, sudoriparous gland, site unspecified	C44.90	C79.2	D04.9	D23.9	D48.5	D49.2
specified site — *see* Neoplasm, skin						
supraclavicular region	C76.0	C79.89	D09.8	D36.7	D48.7	D49.89
supraglottis	C32.1	C78.39	D02.0	D14.1	D38.0	D49.1
suprarenal	C74.9-☑	C79.7-☑	D09.3	D35.0-☑	D44.1-☑	D49.7
capsule	C74.9-☑	C79.7-☑	D09.3	D35.0-☑	D44.1-☑	D49.7
cortex	C74.0-☑	C79.7-☑	D09.3	D35.0-☑	D44.1-☑	D49.7
gland	C74.9-☑	C79.7-☑	D09.3	D35.0-☑	D44.1-☑	D49.7
medulla	C74.1-☑	C79.7-☑	D09.3	D35.0-☑	D44.1-☑	D49.7
suprasellar (region)	C71.9	C79.31	—	D33.2	D43.2	D49.6
supratentorial (brain) NEC	C71.0	C79.31	—	D33.0	D43.0	D49.6
sweat gland (apocrine) (eccrine), site unspecified	C44.90	C79.2	D04.9	D23.9	D48.5	D49.2
specified site — *see* Neoplasm, skin						
sympathetic nerve or nervous system NEC	C47.9	C79.89	—	D36.10	D48.2	D49.2
symphysis pubis	C41.4	C79.51	—	D16.8	D48.0	D49.2
synovial membrane — *see* Neoplasm, connective tissue						
tapetum, brain	C71.8	C79.31	—	D33.2	D43.2	D49.6
tarsus (any bone)	C40.3-☑	C79.51	—	D16.3-☑	—	—
temple (skin) — *see also* Neoplasm, skin, face	C44.309	C79.2	D04.39	D23.39	D48.5	D49.2
temporal						
bone	C41.0	C79.51	—	D16.4	D48.0	D49.2
lobe or pole	C71.2	C79.31	—	D33.0	D43.0	D49.6
region	C76.0	C79.89	D09.8	D36.7	D48.7	D49.89
skin — *see also* Neoplasm, skin, face	C44.309	C79.2	D04.39	D23.39	D48.5	D49.2
tendon (sheath) — *see* Neoplasm, connective tissue						
tentorium (cerebelli)	C70.0	C79.32	—	D32.0	D42.0	D49.7
testis, testes	C62.9-☑	C79.82	D07.69	D29.2-☑	D40.1-☑	D49.5
descended	C62.1-☑	C79.82	D07.69	D29.2-☑	D40.1-☑	D49.5
ectopic	C62.0-☑	C79.82	D07.69	D29.2-☑	D40.1-☑	D49.5
retained	C62.0-☑	C79.82	D07.69	D29.2-☑	D40.1-☑	D49.5
scrotal	C62.1-☑	C79.82	D07.69	D29.2-☑	D40.1-☑	D49.5
undescended	C62.0-☑	C79.82	D07.69	D29.2-☑	D40.1-☑	D49.5
unspecified whether descended or undescended	C62.9-☑	C79.82	D07.69	D29.2-☑	D40.1-☑	D49.5
thalamus	C71.0	C79.31	—	D33.0	D43.0	D49.6
thigh NEC	C76.5-☑	C79.89	D04.7-☑	D36.7	D48.7	D49.89
thorax, thoracic (cavity) (organs NEC)	C76.1	C79.89	D09.8	D36.7	D48.7	D49.89
duct	C49.3	C79.89	—	D21.3	D48.1	D49.2
wall NEC	C76.1	C79.89	D09.8	D36.7	D48.7	D49.89
throat	C14.0	C79.89	D00.08	D10.9	D37.05	D49.0
thumb NEC	C76.4-☑	C79.89	D04.6-☑	D36.7	D48.7	D49.89
thymus (gland)	C37	C79.89	D09.3	D15.0	D38.4	D49.89
thyroglossal duct	C73	C79.89	D09.3	D34	D44.0	D49.7

☑ Additional Character Required — Refer to the Tabular List for Character Selection ▽ Subterms under main terms may continue to next column or page

Neoplasm, neoplastic — *continued*	Malignant Primary	Malignant Secondary	Ca in situ	Benign	Uncertain	Unspecified Behavior
thyroid (gland)	C73	C79.89	D09.3	D34	D44.0	D49.7
cartilage	C32.3	C78.39	D02.0	D14.1	D38.0	D49.1
tibia (any part)	C40.2-☑	C79.51	—	D16.2-☑	—	
toe NEC	C76.5-☑	C79.89	D04.7-☑	D36.7	D48.7	D49.89
tongue	C02.9	C79.89	D00.07	D10.1	D37.02	D49.0
anterior (two-thirds) NEC	C02.3	C79.89	D00.07	D10.1	D37.02	D49.0
dorsal surface	C02.0	C79.89	D00.07	D10.1	D37.02	D49.0
ventral surface	C02.2	C79.89	D00.07	D10.1	D37.02	D49.0
base (dorsal surface)	C01	C79.89	D00.07	D10.1	D37.02	D49.0
border (lateral)	C02.1	C79.89	D00.07	D10.1	D37.02	D49.0
dorsal surface NEC	C02.0	C79.89	D00.07	D10.1	D37.02	D49.0
fixed part NEC	C01	C79.89	D00.07	D10.1	D37.02	D49.0
foreamen cecum	C02.0	C79.89	D00.07	D10.1	D37.02	D49.0
frenulum linguae	C02.2	C79.89	D00.07	D10.1	D37.02	D49.0
junctional zone	C02.8	C79.89	D00.07	D10.1	D37.02	D49.0
margin (lateral)	C02.1	C79.89	D00.07	D10.1	D37.02	D49.0
midline NEC	C02.0	C79.89	D00.07	D10.1	D37.02	D49.0
mobile part NEC	C02.3	C79.89	D00.07	D10.1	D37.02	D49.0
overlapping lesion	C02.8	—	—	—	—	—
posterior (third)	C01	C79.89	D00.07	D10.1	D37.02	D49.0
root	C01	C79.89	D00.07	D10.1	D37.02	D49.0
surface (dorsal)	C02.0	C79.89	D00.07	D10.1	D37.02	D49.0
base	C01	C79.89	D00.07	D10.1	D37.02	D49.0
ventral	C02.2	C79.89	D00.07	D10.1	D37.02	D49.0
tip	C02.1	C79.89	D00.07	D10.1	D37.02	D49.0
tonsil	C02.4	C79.89	D00.07	D10.1	D37.02	D49.0
tonsil	C09.9	C79.89	D00.08	D10.4	D37.05	D49.0
fauces, faucial	C09.9	C79.89	D00.08	D10.4	D37.05	D49.0
lingual	C02.4	C79.89	D00.07	D10.1	D37.02	D49.0
overlapping sites	C09.8	—	—	—	—	—
palatine	C09.9	C79.89	D00.08	D10.4	D37.05	D49.0
pharyngeal	C11.1	C79.89	D00.08	D10.6	D37.05	D49.0
pillar (anterior) (posterior)	C09.1	C79.89	D00.08	D10.5	D37.05	D49.0
tonsillar fossa	C09.0	C79.89	D00.08	D10.5	D37.05	D49.0
tooth socket NEC	C03.9	C79.89	D00.03	D10.39	D37.09	D49.0
trachea (cartilage) (mucosa)	C33	C78.39	D02.1	D14.2	D38.1	D49.1
overlapping lesion with bronchus or lung	C34.8-☑	—	—	—	—	
tracheobronchial	C34.8-☑	C78.39	D02.1	D14.2	D38.1	D49.1
overlapping lesion with lung	C34.8-☑	—	—	—	—	
tragus — *see also* Neoplasm, skin, ear	C44.20-☑	C79.2	D04.2-☑	D23.2-☑	D48.5	D49.2
trunk NEC	C76.8	C79.89	D04.5	D36.7	D48.7	D49.89
tubo-ovarian	C57.8	C79.82	D07.39	D28.7	D39.8	D49.5
tunica vaginalis	C63.7	C79.82	D07.69	D29.8	D40.8	D49.5
turbinate (bone)	C41.0	C79.51	—	D16.4	D48.0	D49.2
nasal	C30.0	C78.39	D02.3	D14.0	D38.5	D49.1
tympanic cavity	C30.1	C78.39	D02.3	D14.0	D38.5	D49.1
ulna (any part)	C40.0-☑	C79.51	—	D16.0-☑	—	—
umbilicus, umbilical — *see also* Neoplasm, skin, trunk	C44.509	C79.2	D04.5	D23.5	D48.5	D49.2
uncus, brain	C71.2	C79.31	—	D33.0	D43.0	D49.6
unknown site or unspecified	C80.1	C79.9	D09.9	D36.9	D48.9	D49.9
urachus	C67.7	C79.11	D09.0	D30.3	D41.4	D49.4
ureter-bladder (junction)	C67.6	C79.11	D09.0	D30.3	D41.4	D49.4
ureter, ureteral	C66.-☑	C79.19	D09.19	D30.2-☑	D41.2-☑	D49.5
orifice (bladder)	C67.6	C79.11	D09.0	D30.3	D41.4	D49.4
urethra, urethral (gland)	C68.0	C79.19	D09.19	D30.4	D41.3	D49.5
orifice, internal	C67.5	C79.11	D09.0	D30.3	D41.4	D49.4
urethrovaginal (septum)	C57.9	C79.82	D07.30	D28.9	D39.8	D49.5
urinary organ or system	C68.9	C79.10	D09.10	D30.9	D41.9	D49.5
bladder — *see* Neoplasm, bladder						
overlapping lesion	C68.8	—	—	—	—	—
specified sites NEC	C68.8	C79.19	D09.19	D30.8	D41.8	D49.5
utero-ovarian	C57.8	C79.82	D07.39	D28.7	D39.8	D49.5
ligament	C57.1-☑	C79.82	D07.39	D28.2	D39.8	D49.5
uterosacral ligament	C57.3	C79.82	—	D28.2	D39.8	D49.5

Neoplasm, neoplastic — *continued*	Malignant Primary	Malignant Secondary	Ca in situ	Benign	Uncertain	Unspecified Behavior
uterus, uteri, uterine	C55	C79.82	D07.0	D26.9	D39.0	D49.5
adnexa NEC	C57.4	C79.82	D07.39	D28.7	D39.8	D49.5
body	C54.9	C79.82	D07.0	D26.1	D39.0	D49.5
cervix	C53.9	C79.82	D06.9	D26.0	D39.0	D49.5
cornu	C54.9	C79.82	D07.0	D26.1	D39.0	D49.5
corpus	C54.9	C79.82	D07.0	D26.1	D39.0	D49.5
endocervix (canal) (gland)	C53.0	C79.82	D06.0	D26.0	D39.0	D49.5
endometrium	C54.1	C79.82	D07.0	D26.1	D39.0	D49.5
exocervix	C53.1	C79.82	D06.1	D26.0	D39.0	D49.5
external os	C53.1	C79.82	D06.1	D26.0	D39.0	D49.5
fundus	C54.3	C79.82	D07.0	D26.1	D39.0	D49.5
internal os	C53.0	C79.82	D06.0	D26.0	D39.0	D49.5
isthmus	C54.0	C79.82	D07.0	D26.1	D39.0	D49.5
ligament	C57.3	C79.82	—	D28.2	D39.8	D49.5
broad	C57.1-☑	C79.82	D07.39	D28.2	D39.8	D49.5
round	C57.2-☑	C79.82	—	D28.2	D39.8	D49.5
lower segment	C54.0	C79.82	D07.0	D26.1	D39.0	D49.5
myometrium	C54.2	C79.82	D07.0	D26.1	D39.0	D49.5
overlapping sites	C54.8	—	—	—	—	—
squamocolumnar junction	C53.8	C79.82	D06.7	D26.0	D39.0	D49.5
tube	C57.0-☑	C79.82	D07.39	D28.2	D39.8	D49.5
utricle, prostatic	C68.0	C79.19	D09.19	D30.4	D41.3	D49.5
uveal tract	C69.4-☑	C79.49	D09.2-☑	D31.4-☑	D48.7	D49.89
uvula	C05.2	C79.89	D00.04	D10.39	D37.09	D49.0
vagina, vaginal (fornix) (vault) (wall)	C52	C79.82	D07.2	D28.1	D39.8	D49.5
vaginovesical	C57.9	C79.82	D07.30	D28.9	D39.9	D49.5
septum	C57.9	C79.82	D07.30	D28.9	D39.9	D49.5
valiecula (epiglottis)	C10.0	C79.89	D00.08	D10.5	D37.05	D49.0
vascular — *see* Neoplasm, connective tissue						
vas deferens	C63.1-☑	C79.82	D07.69	D29.8	D40.8	D49.5
Vater's ampulla	C24.1	C78.89	D01.5	D13.5	D37.6	D49.0
vein, venous — *see* Neoplasm, connective tissue						
vena cava (abdominal) (inferior)	C49.4	C79.89	—	D21.4	D48.1	D49.2
superior	C49.3	C79.89	—	D21.3	D48.1	D49.2
ventricle (cerebral) (floor) (lateral) (third)	C71.5	C79.31	—	D33.0	D43.0	D49.6
cardiac (left) (right)	C38.0	C79.89	—	D15.1	D48.7	D49.89
fourth	C71.7	C79.31	—	D33.1	D43.1	D49.6
ventricular band of larynx	C32.1	C78.39	D02.0	D14.1	D38.0	D49.1
ventriculus — *see* Neoplasm, stomach						
vermillion border — *see* Neoplasm, lip						
vermis, cerebellum	C71.6	C79.31	—	D33.1	D43.1	D49.6
vertebra (column)	C41.2	C79.51	—	D16.6	D48.0	D49.2
coccyx	C41.4	C79.51	—	D16.8	D48.0	D49.2
marrow NEC	C96.9	C79.52	—	—	D47.9	D49.89
sacrum	C41.4	C79.51	—	D16.8	D48.0	D49.2
vesical — *see* Neoplasm, bladder						
vesicle, seminal	C63.7	C79.82	D07.69	D29.8	D40.8	D49.5
vesicocervical tissue	C57.9	C79.82	D07.30	D28.9	D39.9	D49.5
vesicorectal	C76.3	C79.82	D09.8	D36.7	D48.7	D49.89
vesicovaginal	C57.9	C79.82	D07.30	D28.9	D39.8	D49.5
septum	C57.9	C79.82	D07.30	D28.9	D39.8	D49.5
vessel (blood) — *see* Neoplasm, connective tissue						
vestibular gland, greater	C51.0	C79.82	D07.1	D28.0	D39.8	D49.5
vestibule						
mouth	C06.1	C79.89	D00.00	D10.39	D37.09	D49.0
nose	C30.0	C78.39	D02.3	D14.0	D38.5	D49.1
Virchow's gland	C77.0	C77.0		D36.0	D48.7	D49.89
viscera NEC	C76.8	C79.89	D09.8	D36.7	D48.7	D49.89
vocal cords (true)	C32.0	C78.39	D02.0	D14.1	D38.0	D49.1
false	C32.1	C78.39	D02.0	D14.1	D38.0	D49.1
vomer	C41.0	C79.51	—	D16.4	D48.0	D49.2
vulva	C51.9	C79.82	D07.1	D28.0	D39.8	D49.5
vulvovaginal gland	C51.0	C79.82	D07.1	D28.0	D39.8	D49.5
Waldeyer's ring	C14.2	C79.89	D00.08	D10.9	D37.05	D49.0
Wharton's duct	C08.0	C79.89	D00.00	D11.7	D37.032	D49.0

Neoplasm Table

Neoplasm, white matter — Neoplasm, Zuckerkandl organ

	Malignant Primary	Malignant Secondary	Ca in situ	Benign	Uncertain	Unspecified Behavior
Neoplasm, neoplastic — *continued*						
white matter (central) (cerebral)	C71.0	C79.31	—	D33.0	D43.0	D49.6
windpipe	C33	C78.39	D02.1	D14.2	D38.1	D49.1
Wirsung's duct	C25.3	C78.89	D01.7	D13.6	D37.8	D49.0
wolffian (body) (duct)						
female	C57.7	C79.82	D07.39	D28.7	D39.8	D49.5
male	C63.7	C79.82	D07.69	D29.8	D40.8	D49.5
womb — *see* Neoplasm, uterus						
wrist NEC	C76.4-☑	C79.89	D04.6-☑	D36.7	D48.7	D49.89
xiphoid process	C41.3	C79.51		D16.7	D48.0	D49.2
Zuckerkandl organ	C75.5	C79.89	—	D35.6	D44.7	D49.7

☑ Additional Character Required — Refer to the Tabular List for Character Selection   ▽ Subterms under main terms may continue to next column or page

ICD-10-CM Table of Drugs and Chemicals

Substance	Poisoning, Accidental (unintentional)	Poisoning, Intentional Self-harm	Poisoning, Assault	Poisoning, Undetermined	Adverse Effect	Under-dosing
14-Hydroxydihydromorphinone	T40.2X1	T40.2X2	T40.2X3	T40.2X4	T40.2X5	T40.2X6
1-Propanol	T51.3X1	T51.3X2	T51.3X3	T51.3X4	—	—
2,3,7,8-Tetrachlorodibenzo-p-dioxin	T53.7X1	T53.7X2	T53.7X3	T53.7X4	—	—
2,4,5-T (trichlorophenoxyacetic acid)	T60.1X1	T60.1X2	T60.1X3	T60.1X4	—	—
2,4,5-Trichlorophenoxyacetic acid	T60.3X1	T60.3X2	T60.3X3	T60.3X4	—	—
2,4-D (dichlorophenoxyacetic acid)	T60.3X1	T60.3X2	T60.3X3	T60.3X4	—	—
2,4-Toluene diisocyanate	T65.0X1	T65.0X2	T65.0X3	T65.0X4	—	—
2-Deoxy-5-fluorouridine	T45.1X1	T45.1X2	T45.1X3	T45.1X4	T45.1X5	T45.1X6
2-Ethoxyethanol	T52.3X1	T52.3X2	T52.3X3	T52.3X4	—	—
2-Methoxyethanol	T52.3X1	T52.3X2	T52.3X3	T52.3X4	—	—
2-Propanol	T51.2X1	T51.2X2	T51.2X3	T51.2X4	—	—
4-Aminobutyric acid	T43.8X1	T43.8X2	T43.8X3	T43.8X4	T43.8X5	T43.8X6
4-Aminophenol derivatives	T39.1X1	T39.1X2	T39.1X3	T39.1X4	T39.1X5	T39.1X6
5-Deoxy-5-fluorouridine	T45.1X1	T45.1X2	T45.1X3	T45.1X4	T45.1X5	T45.1X6
5-Methoxypsoralen (5-MOP)	T50.991	T50.992	T50.993	T50.994	T50.995	T50.996
8-Aminoquinoline drugs	T37.2X1	T37.2X2	T37.2X3	T37.2X4	T37.2X5	T37.2X6
8-Methoxypsoralen (8-MOP)	T50.991	T50.992	T50.993	T50.994	T50.995	T50.996
ABOB	T37.5X1	T37.5X2	T37.5X3	T37.5X4	T37.5X5	T37.5X6
Abrine	T62.2X1	T62.2X2	T62.2X3	T62.2X4	—	—
Abrus (seed)	T62.2X1	T62.2X2	T62.2X3	T62.2X4	—	—
Absinthe	T51.0X1	T51.0X2	T51.0X3	T51.0X4	—	—
beverage	T51.0X1	T51.0X2	T51.0X3	T51.0X4	—	—
Acaricide	T60.8X1	T60.8X2	T60.8X3	T60.8X4	—	—
Acebutolol	T44.7X1	T44.7X2	T44.7X3	T44.7X4	T44.7X5	T44.7X6
Acecarbromal	T42.6X1	T42.6X2	T42.6X3	T42.6X4	T42.6X5	T42.6X6
Aceclidine	T44.1X1	T44.1X2	T44.1X3	T44.1X4	T44.1X5	T44.1X6
Acedapsone	T37.0X1	T37.0X2	T37.0X3	T37.0X4	T37.0X5	T37.0X6
Acefylline piperazine	T48.6X1	T48.6X2	T48.6X3	T48.6X4	T48.6X5	T48.6X6
Acemorphan	T40.2X1	T40.2X2	T40.2X3	T40.2X4	T40.2X5	T40.2X6
Acenocoumarin	T45.511	T45.512	T45.513	T45.514	T45.515	T45.516
Acenocoumarol	T45.511	T45.512	T45.513	T45.514	T45.515	T45.516
Acepifylline	T48.6X1	T48.6X2	T48.6X3	T48.6X4	T48.6X5	T48.6X6
Acepromazine	T43.3X1	T43.3X2	T43.3X3	T43.3X4	T43.3X5	T43.3X6
Acesulfamethoxypyridazine	T37.0X1	T37.0X2	T37.0X3	T37.0X4	T37.0X5	T37.0X6
Acetal	T52.8X1	T52.8X2	T52.8X3	T52.8X4	—	—
Acetaldehyde (vapor)	T52.8X1	T52.8X2	T52.8X3	T52.8X4	—	—
liquid	T65.891	T65.892	T65.893	T65.894	—	—
Acetaminophen	T39.1X1	T39.1X2	T39.1X3	T39.1X4	T39.1X5	T39.1X6
Acetaminosalol	T39.1X1	T39.1X2	T39.1X3	T39.1X4	T39.1X5	T39.1X6
Acetanilide	T39.1X1	T39.1X2	T39.1X3	T39.1X4	T39.1X5	T39.1X6
Acetarsol	T37.3X1	T37.3X2	T37.3X3	T37.3X4	T37.3X5	T37.3X6
Acetazolamide	T50.2X1	T50.2X2	T50.2X3	T50.2X4	T50.2X5	T50.2X6
Acetiamine	T45.2X1	T45.2X2	T45.2X3	T45.2X4	T45.2X5	T45.2X6
Acetic						
acid	T54.2X1	T54.2X2	T54.2X3	T54.2X4	—	—
with sodium acetate (ointment)	T49.3X1	T49.3X2	T49.3X3	T49.3X4	T49.3X5	T49.3X6
ester (solvent)(vapor)	T52.8X1	T52.8X2	T52.8X3	T52.8X4	—	—
irrigating solution	T50.3X1	T50.3X2	T50.3X3	T50.3X4	T50.3X5	T50.3X6
medicinal (lotion)	T49.2X1	T49.2X2	T49.2X3	T49.2X4	T49.2X5	T49.2X6
anhydride	T65.891	T65.892	T65.893	T65.894	—	—
ether (vapor)	T52.8X1	T52.8X2	T52.8X3	T52.8X4	—	—
Acetohexamide	T38.3X1	T38.3X2	T38.3X3	T38.3X4	T38.3X5	T38.3X6
Acetohydroxamic acid	T50.991	T50.992	T50.993	T50.994	T50.995	T50.996
Acetomenaphthone	T45.7X1	T45.7X2	T45.7X3	T45.7X4	T45.7X5	T45.7X6
Acetomorphine	T40.1X1	T40.1X2	T40.1X3	T40.1X4	—	—
Acetone (oils)	T52.4X1	T52.4X2	T52.4X3	T52.4X4	—	—
chlorinated	T52.4X1	T52.4X2	T52.4X3	T52.4X4	—	—
vapor	T52.4X1	T52.4X2	T52.4X3	T52.4X4	—	—
Acetonitrile	T52.8X1	T52.8X2	T52.8X3	T52.8X4	—	—
Acetophenazine	T43.3X1	T43.3X2	T43.3X3	T43.3X4	T43.3X5	T43.3X6
Acetophenetedin	T39.1X1	T39.1X2	T39.1X3	T39.1X4	T39.1X5	T39.1X6
Acetophenone	T52.4X1	T52.4X2	T52.4X3	T52.4X4	—	—
Acetorphine	T40.2X1	T40.2X2	T40.2X3	T40.2X4	—	—
Acetosulfone (sodium)	T37.1X1	T37.1X2	T37.1X3	T37.1X4	T37.1X5	T37.1X6
Acetrizoate (sodium)	T50.8X1	T50.8X2	T50.8X3	T50.8X4	T50.8X5	T50.8X6
Acetrizoic acid	T50.8X1	T50.8X2	T50.8X3	T50.8X4	T50.8X5	T50.8X6
Acetyl						
bromide	T53.6X1	T53.6X2	T53.6X3	T53.6X4	—	—
chloride	T53.6X1	T53.6X2	T53.6X3	T53.6X4	—	—
Acetylcarbromal	T42.6X1	T42.6X2	T42.6X3	T42.6X4	T42.6X5	T42.6X6

Substance	Poisoning, Accidental (unintentional)	Poisoning, Intentional Self-harm	Poisoning, Assault	Poisoning, Undetermined	Adverse Effect	Under-dosing
Acetylcholine						
chloride	T44.1X1	T44.1X2	T44.1X3	T44.1X4	T44.1X5	T44.1X6
derivative	T44.1X1	T44.1X2	T44.1X3	T44.1X4	T44.1X5	T44.1X6
Acetylcysteine	T48.4X1	T48.4X2	T48.4X3	T48.4X4	T48.4X5	T48.4X6
Acetyldigitoxin	T46.0X1	T46.0X2	T46.0X3	T46.0X4	T46.0X5	T46.0X6
Acetyldigoxin	T46.0X1	T46.0X2	T46.0X3	T46.0X4	T46.0X5	T46.0X6
Acetyldihydrocodeine	T40.2X1	T40.2X2	T40.2X3	T40.2X4	—	—
Acetyldihydrocodeinone	T40.2X1	T40.2X2	T40.2X3	T40.2X4	—	—
Acetylene (gas)	T59.891	T59.892	T59.893	T59.894	—	—
dichloride	T53.6X1	T53.6X2	T53.6X3	T53.6X4	—	—
incomplete combustion of	T58.11	T58.12	T58.13	T58.14	—	—
industrial	T59.891	T59.892	T59.893	T59.894	—	—
tetrachloride	T53.6X1	T53.6X2	T53.6X3	T53.6X4	—	—
vapor	T53.6X1	T53.6X2	T53.6X3	T53.6X4	—	—
Acetylpheneturide	T42.6X1	T42.6X2	T42.6X3	T42.6X4	T42.6X5	T42.6X6
Acetylphenylhydrazine	T39.8X1	T39.8X2	T39.8X3	T39.8X4	T39.8X5	T39.8X6
Acetylsalicylic acid (salts)	T39.011	T39.012	T39.013	T39.014	T39.015	T39.016
enteric coated	T39.011	T39.012	T39.013	T39.014	T39.015	T39.016
Acetylsulfamethoxypyridazine	T37.0X1	T37.0X2	T37.0X3	T37.0X4	T37.0X5	T37.0X6
Achromycin	T36.4X1	T36.4X2	T36.4X3	T36.4X4	T36.4X5	T36.4X6
ophthalmic preparation	T49.5X1	T49.5X2	T49.5X3	T49.5X4	T49.5X5	T49.5X6
topical NEC	T49.0X1	T49.0X2	T49.0X3	T49.0X4	T49.0X5	T49.0X6
Aciclovir	T37.5X1	T37.5X2	T37.5X3	T37.5X4	T37.5X5	T37.5X6
Acidifying agent NEC	T50.901	T50.902	T50.903	T50.904	T50.905	T50.906
Acid (corrosive) NEC	T54.2X1	T54.2X2	T54.2X3	T54.2X4	—	—
Acipimox	T46.6X1	T46.6X2	T46.6X3	T46.6X4	T46.6X5	T46.6X6
Acitretin	T50.991	T50.992	T50.993	T50.994	T50.995	T50.996
Aclarubicin	T45.1X1	T45.1X2	T45.1X3	T45.1X4	T45.1X5	T45.1X6
Aclatonium napadisilate	T48.1X1	T48.1X2	T48.1X3	T48.1X4	T48.1X5	T48.1X6
Aconite (wild)	T46.991	T46.992	T46.993	T46.994	T46.995	T46.996
Aconitine	T46.991	T46.992	T46.993	T46.994	T46.995	T46.996
Aconitum ferox	T46.991	T46.992	T46.993	T46.994	T46.995	T46.996
Acridine	T65.6X1	T65.6X2	T65.6X3	T65.6X4	—	—
vapor	T59.891	T59.892	T59.893	T59.894	—	—
Acriflavine	T37.91	T37.92	T37.93	T37.94	T37.95	T37.96
Acriflavinium chloride	T49.0X1	T49.0X2	T49.0X3	T49.0X4	T49.0X5	T49.0X6
Acrinol	T49.0X1	T49.0X2	T49.0X3	T49.0X4	T49.0X5	T49.0X6
Acrisorcin	T49.0X1	T49.0X2	T49.0X3	T49.0X4	T49.0X5	T49.0X6
Acrivastine	T45.0X1	T45.0X2	T45.0X3	T45.0X4	T45.0X5	T45.0X6
Acrolein (gas)	T59.891	T59.892	T59.893	T59.894	—	—
liquid	T54.1X1	T54.1X2	T54.1X3	T54.1X4	—	—
Acrylamide	T65.891	T65.892	T65.893	T65.894	—	—
Acrylic resin	T49.3X1	T49.3X2	T49.3X3	T49.3X4	T49.3X5	T49.3X6
Acrylonitrile	T65.891	T65.892	T65.893	T65.894	—	—
Actaea spicata	T62.2X1	T62.2X2	T62.2X3	T62.2X4	—	—
berry	T62.1X1	T62.1X2	T62.1X3	T62.1X4	—	—
Acterol	T37.3X1	T37.3X2	T37.3X3	T37.3X4	T37.3X5	T37.3X6
ACTH	T38.811	T38.812	T38.813	T38.814	T38.815	T38.816
Actinomycin C	T45.1X1	T45.1X2	T45.1X3	T45.1X4	T45.1X5	T45.1X6
Actinomycin D	T45.1X1	T45.1X2	T45.1X3	T45.1X4	T45.1X5	T45.1X6
Activated charcoal — see also Charcoal, medicinal	T47.6X1	T47.6X2	T47.6X3	T47.6X4	T47.6X5	T47.6X6
Acyclovir	T37.5X1	T37.5X2	T37.5X3	T37.5X4	T37.5X5	T37.5X6
Adenine	T45.2X1	T45.2X2	T45.2X3	T45.2X4	T45.2X5	T45.2X6
arabinoside	T37.5X1	T37.5X2	T37.5X3	T37.5X4	T37.5X5	T37.5X6
Adenosine (phosphate)	T46.2X1	T46.2X2	T46.2X3	T46.2X4	T46.2X5	T46.2X6
ADH	T38.891	T38.892	T38.893	T38.894	T38.895	T38.896
Adhesive NEC	T65.891	T65.892	T65.893	T65.894	—	—
Adicillin	T36.0X1	T36.0X2	T36.0X3	T36.0X4	T36.0X5	T36.0X6
Adiphenine	T44.3X1	T44.3X2	T44.3X3	T44.3X4	T44.3X5	T44.3X6
Adipiodone	T50.8X1	T50.8X2	T50.8X3	T50.8X4	T50.8X5	T50.8X6
Adjunct, pharmaceutical	T50.901	T50.902	T50.903	T50.904	T50.905	T50.906
Adrenal (extract, cortex or medulla) (glucocorticoids) (hormones) (mineralocorticoids)	T38.0X1	T38.0X2	T38.0X3	T38.0X4	T38.0X5	T38.0X6
ENT agent	T49.6X1	T49.6X2	T49.6X3	T49.6X4	T49.6X5	T49.6X6
ophthalmic preparation	T49.5X1	T49.5X2	T49.5X3	T49.5X4	T49.5X5	T49.5X6
topical NEC	T49.0X1	T49.0X2	T49.0X3	T49.0X4	T49.0X5	T49.0X6
Adrenalin — see Adrenaline						
Adrenaline	T44.5X1	T44.5X2	T44.5X3	T44.5X4	T44.5X5	T44.5X6
Adrenergic NEC	T44.901	T44.902	T44.903	T44.904	T44.905	T44.906
blocking agent NEC	T44.8X1	T44.8X2	T44.8X3	T44.8X4	T44.8X5	T44.8X6
beta, heart	T44.7X1	T44.7X2	T44.7X3	T44.7X4	T44.7X5	T44.7X6
specified NEC	T44.991	T44.992	T44.993	T44.994	T44.995	T44.996
Adrenochrome						
derivative	T46.991	T46.992	T46.993	T46.994	T46.995	T46.996

Substance	Poisoning, Accidental (unintentional)	Poisoning, Intentional Self-harm	Poisoning, Assault	Poisoning, Undetermined	Adverse Effect	Under-dosing
Adrenochrome — continued						
(mono) semicarbazone	T46.991	T46.992	T46.993	T46.994	T46.995	T46.996
Adrenocorticotrophic hormone	T38.811	T38.812	T38.813	T38.814	T38.815	T38.816
Adrenocorticotrophin	T38.811	T38.812	T38.813	T38.814	T38.815	T38.816
Adriamycin	T45.1X1	T45.1X2	T45.1X3	T45.1X4	T45.1X5	T45.1X6
Aerosol spray NEC	T65.91	T65.92	T65.93	T65.94	—	—
Aerosporin	T36.8X1	T36.8X2	T36.8X3	T36.8X4	T36.8X5	T36.8X6
ENT agent	T49.6X1	T49.6X2	T49.6X3	T49.6X4	T49.6X5	T49.6X6
ophthalmic preparation	T49.5X1	T49.5X2	T49.5X3	T49.5X4	T49.5X5	T49.5X6
topical NEC	T49.0X1	T49.0X2	T49.0X3	T49.0X4	T49.0X5	T49.0X6
Aethusa cynapium	T62.2X1	T62.2X2	T62.2X3	T62.2X4		
Afghanistan black	T40.7X1	T40.7X2	T40.7X3	T40.7X4	T40.7X5	T40.7X6
Aflatoxin	T64.01	T64.02	T64.03	T64.04	—	—
Afloqualone	T42.8X1	T42.8X2	T42.8X3	T42.8X4	T42.8X5	T42.8X6
African boxwood	T62.2X1	T62.2X2	T62.2X3	T62.2X4		
Agar	T47.4X1	T47.4X2	T47.4X3	T47.4X4	T47.4X5	T47.4X6
Agonist						
predominantly						
alpha-adrenoreceptor	T44.4X1	T44.4X2	T44.4X3	T44.4X4	T44.4X5	T44.4X6
beta-adrenoreceptor	T44.5X1	T44.5X2	T44.5X3	T44.5X4	T44.5X5	T44.5X6
Agricultural agent NEC	T65.91	T65.92	T65.93	T65.94	—	—
Agrypnal	T42.3X1	T42.3X2	T42.3X3	T42.3X4	T42.3X5	T42.3X6
AHLG	T50.Z11	T50.Z12	T50.Z13	T50.Z14	T50.Z15	T50.Z16
Air contaminant(s), source/type NOS	T65.91	T65.92	T65.93	T65.94	—	—
Ajmaline	T46.2X1	T46.2X2	T46.2X3	T46.2X4	T46.2X5	T46.2X6
Akee	T62.1X1	T62.1X2	T62.1X3	T62.1X4		
Akrinol	T49.0X1	T49.0X2	T49.0X3	T49.0X4	T49.0X5	T49.0X6
Akritoin	T37.8X1	T37.8X2	T37.8X3	T37.8X4	T37.8X5	T37.8X6
Alacepril	T46.4X1	T46.4X2	T46.4X3	T46.4X4	T46.4X5	T46.4X6
Alantolactone	T37.4X1	T37.4X2	T37.4X3	T37.4X4	T37.4X5	T37.4X6
Albamycin	T36.8X1	T36.8X2	T36.8X3	T36.8X4	T36.8X5	T36.8X6
Albendazole	T37.4X1	T37.4X2	T37.4X3	T37.4X4	T37.4X5	T37.4X6
Albumin						
bovine	T45.8X1	T45.8X2	T45.8X3	T45.8X4	T45.8X5	T45.8X6
human serum	T45.8X1	T45.8X2	T45.8X3	T45.8X4	T45.8X5	T45.8X6
salt-poor	T45.8X1	T45.8X2	T45.8X3	T45.8X4	T45.8X5	T45.8X6
normal human serum	T45.8X1	T45.8X2	T45.8X3	T45.8X4	T45.8X5	T45.8X6
Albuterol	T48.6X1	T48.6X2	T48.6X3	T48.6X4	T48.6X5	T48.6X6
Albutoin	T42.0X1	T42.0X2	T42.0X3	T42.0X4	T42.0X5	T42.0X6
Alclometasone	T49.0X1	T49.0X2	T49.0X3	T49.0X4	T49.0X5	T49.0X6
Alcohol	T51.91	T51.92	T51.93	T51.94	—	—
absolute	T51.0X1	T51.0X2	T51.0X3	T51.0X4	—	—
beverage	T51.0X1	T51.0X2	T51.0X3	T51.0X4	—	—
allyl	T51.8X1	T51.8X2	T51.8X3	T51.8X4	—	—
amyl	T51.3X1	T51.3X2	T51.3X3	T51.3X4	—	—
antifreeze	T51.1X1	T51.1X2	T51.1X3	T51.1X4	—	—
beverage	T51.0X1	T51.0X2	T51.0X3	T51.0X4	—	—
butyl	T51.3X1	T51.3X2	T51.3X3	T51.3X4	—	—
dehydrated	T51.0X1	T51.0X2	T51.0X3	T51.0X4	—	—
beverage	T51.0X1	T51.0X2	T51.0X3	T51.0X4	—	—
denatured	T51.0X1	T51.0X2	T51.0X3	T51.0X4	—	—
deterrent NEC	T50.6X1	T50.6X2	T50.6X3	T50.6X4	T50.6X5	T50.6X6
diagnostic (gastric function)	T50.8X1	T50.8X2	T50.8X3	T50.8X4	T50.8X5	T50.8X6
ethyl	T51.0X1	T51.0X2	T51.0X3	T51.0X4	—	—
beverage	T51.0X1	T51.0X2	T51.0X3	T51.0X4	—	—
grain	T51.0X1	T51.0X2	T51.0X3	T51.0X4	—	—
beverage	T51.0X1	T51.0X2	T51.0X3	T51.0X4	—	—
industrial	T51.0X1	T51.0X2	T51.0X3	T51.0X4	—	—
isopropyl	T51.2X1	T51.2X2	T51.2X3	T51.2X4	—	—
methyl	T51.1X1	T51.1X2	T51.1X3	T51.1X4	—	—
preparation for consumption	T51.0X1	T51.0X2	T51.0X3	T51.0X4	—	—
propyl	T51.3X1	T51.3X2	T51.3X3	T51.3X4	—	—
secondary	T51.2X1	T51.2X2	T51.2X3	T51.2X4	—	—
radiator	T51.1X1	T51.1X2	T51.1X3	T51.1X4	—	—
rubbing	T51.2X1	T51.2X2	T51.2X3	T51.2X4	—	—
specified type NEC	T51.8X1	T51.8X2	T51.8X3	T51.8X4	—	—
surgical	T51.0X1	T51.0X2	T51.0X3	T51.0X4	—	—
vapor (from any type of Alcohol)	T59.891	T59.892	T59.893	T59.894	—	—
wood	T51.1X1	T51.1X2	T51.1X3	T51.1X4	—	—
Alcuronium (chloride)	T48.1X1	T48.1X2	T48.1X3	T48.1X4	T48.1X5	T48.1X6
Aldactone	T50.0X1	T50.0X2	T50.0X3	T50.0X4	T50.0X5	T50.0X6
Aldesulfone sodium	T37.1X1	T37.1X2	T37.1X3	T37.1X4	T37.1X5	T37.1X6
Aldicarb	T60.0X1	T60.0X2	T60.0X3	T60.0X4	—	—
Aldomet	T46.5X1	T46.5X2	T46.5X3	T46.5X4	T46.5X5	T46.5X6
Aldosterone	T50.0X1	T50.0X2	T50.0X3	T50.0X4	T50.0X5	T50.0X6
Aldrin (dust)	T60.1X1	T60.1X2	T60.1X3	T60.1X4	—	—
Aleve — see Naproxen						
Alexitol sodium	T47.1X1	T47.1X2	T47.1X3	T47.1X4	T47.1X5	T47.1X6

Substance	Poisoning, Accidental (unintentional)	Poisoning, Intentional Self-harm	Poisoning, Assault	Poisoning, Undetermined	Adverse Effect	Under-dosing
Alfacalcidol	T45.2X1	T45.2X2	T45.2X3	T45.2X4	T45.2X5	T45.2X6
Alfadolone	T41.1X1	T41.1X2	T41.1X3	T41.1X4	T41.1X5	T41.1X6
Alfaxalone	T41.1X1	T41.1X2	T41.1X3	T41.1X4	T41.1X5	T41.1X6
Alfentanil	T40.4X1	T40.4X2	T40.4X3	T40.4X4	T40.4X5	T40.4X6
Alfuzosin (hydrochloride)	T44.8X1	T44.8X2	T44.8X3	T44.8X4	T44.8X5	T44.8X6
Algae (harmful) (toxin)	T65.821	T65.822	T65.823	T65.824	—	—
Algeldrate	T47.1X1	T47.1X2	T47.1X3	T47.1X4	T47.1X5	T47.1X6
Algin	T47.8X1	T47.8X2	T47.8X3	T47.8X4	T47.8X5	T47.8X6
Alglucerase	T45.3X1	T45.3X2	T45.3X3	T45.3X4	T45.3X5	T45.3X6
Alidase	T45.3X1	T45.3X2	T45.3X3	T45.3X4	T45.3X5	T45.3X6
Alimemazine	T43.3X1	T43.3X2	T43.3X3	T43.3X4	T43.3X5	T43.3X6
Aliphatic thiocyanates	T65.0X1	T65.0X2	T65.0X3	T65.0X4	—	—
Alizapride	T45.0X1	T45.0X2	T45.0X3	T45.0X4	T45.0X5	T45.0X6
Alkali (caustic)	T54.3X1	T54.3X2	T54.3X3	T54.3X4	—	—
Alkaline antiseptic solution (aromatic)	T49.6X1	T49.6X2	T49.6X3	T49.6X4	T49.6X5	T49.6X6
Alkalinizing agents (medicinal)	T50.901	T50.902	T50.903	T50.904	T50.905	T50.906
Alkalizing agent NEC	T50.901	T50.902	T50.903	T50.904	T50.905	T50.906
Alka-seltzer	T39.011	T39.012	T39.013	T39.014	T39.015	T39.016
Alkavervir	T46.5X1	T46.5X2	T46.5X3	T46.5X4	T46.5X5	T46.5X6
Alkonium (bromide)	T49.0X1	T49.0X2	T49.0X3	T49.0X4	T49.0X5	T49.0X6
Alkylating drug NEC	T45.1X1	T45.1X2	T45.1X3	T45.1X4	T45.1X5	T45.1X6
antimyeloproliferative	T45.1X1	T45.1X2	T45.1X3	T45.1X4	T45.1X5	T45.1X6
lymphatic	T45.1X1	T45.1X2	T45.1X3	T45.1X4	T45.1X5	T45.1X6
Alkylisocyanate	T65.0X1	T65.0X2	T65.0X3	T65.0X4	—	—
Allantoin	T49.4X1	T49.4X2	T49.4X3	T49.4X4	T49.4X5	T49.4X6
Allegron	T43.011	T43.012	T43.013	T43.014	T43.015	T43.016
Allethrin	T49.0X1	T49.0X2	T49.0X3	T49.0X4	T49.0X5	T49.0X6
Allobarbital	T42.3X1	T42.3X2	T42.3X3	T42.3X4	T42.3X5	T42.3X6
Allopurinol	T50.4X1	T50.4X2	T50.4X3	T50.4X4	T50.4X5	T50.4X6
Allyl						
alcohol	T51.8X1	T51.8X2	T51.8X3	T51.8X4	—	—
disulfide	T46.6X1	T46.6X2	T46.6X3	T46.6X4	T46.6X5	T46.6X6
Allylestrenol	T38.5X1	T38.5X2	T38.5X3	T38.5X4	T38.5X5	T38.5X6
Allylisopropylacetylurea	T42.6X1	T42.6X2	T42.6X3	T42.6X4	T42.6X5	T42.6X6
Allylisopropylmalonylurea	T42.3X1	T42.3X2	T42.3X3	T42.3X4	T42.3X5	T42.3X6
Allylthiourea	T49.3X1	T49.3X2	T49.3X3	T49.3X4	T49.3X5	T49.3X6
Allyltribromide	T42.6X1	T42.6X2	T42.6X3	T42.6X4	T42.6X5	T42.6X6
Allypropymal	T42.3X1	T42.3X2	T42.3X3	T42.3X4	T42.3X5	T42.3X6
Almagate	T47.1X1	T47.1X2	T47.1X3	T47.1X4	T47.1X5	T47.1X6
Almasilate	T47.1X1	T47.1X2	T47.1X3	T47.1X4	T47.1X5	T47.1X6
Almitrine	T50.7X1	T50.7X2	T50.7X3	T50.7X4	T50.7X5	T50.7X6
Aloes	T47.2X1	T47.2X2	T47.2X3	T47.2X4	T47.2X5	T47.2X6
Aloglutamol	T47.1X1	T47.1X2	T47.1X3	T47.1X4	T47.1X5	T47.1X6
Aloin	T47.2X1	T47.2X2	T47.2X3	T47.2X4	T47.2X5	T47.2X6
Aloxidone	T42.2X1	T42.2X2	T42.2X3	T42.2X4	T42.2X5	T42.2X6
Alpha						
acetyldigoxin	T46.0X1	T46.0X2	T46.0X3	T46.0X4	T46.0X5	T46.0X6
adrenergic blocking drug	T44.6X1	T44.6X2	T44.6X3	T44.6X4	T44.6X5	T44.6X6
amylase	T45.3X1	T45.3X2	T45.3X3	T45.3X4	T45.3X5	T45.3X6
tocoferol (acetate)	T45.2X1	T45.2X2	T45.2X3	T45.2X4	T45.2X5	T45.2X6
tocopherol	T45.2X1	T45.2X2	T45.2X3	T45.2X4	T45.2X5	T45.2X6
Alphadolone	T41.1X1	T41.1X2	T41.1X3	T41.1X4	T41.1X5	T41.1X6
Alphaprodine	T40.4X1	T40.4X2	T40.4X3	T40.4X4	T40.4X5	T40.4X6
Alphaxalone	T41.1X1	T41.1X2	T41.1X3	T41.1X4	T41.1X5	T41.1X6
Alprazolam	T42.4X1	T42.4X2	T42.4X3	T42.4X4	T42.4X5	T42.4X6
Alprenolol	T44.7X1	T44.7X2	T44.7X3	T44.7X4	T44.7X5	T44.7X6
Alprostadil	T46.7X1	T46.7X2	T46.7X3	T46.7X4	T46.7X5	T46.7X6
Alsactide	T38.811	T38.812	T38.813	T38.814	T38.815	T38.816
Alseroxylon	T46.5X1	T46.5X2	T46.5X3	T46.5X4	T46.5X5	T46.5X6
Alteplase	T45.611	T45.612	T45.613	T45.614	T45.615	T45.616
Altizide	T50.2X1	T50.2X2	T50.2X3	T50.2X4	T50.2X5	T50.2X6
Altretamine	T45.1X1	T45.1X2	T45.1X3	T45.1X4	T45.1X5	T45.1X6
Alum (medicinal)	T49.4X1	T49.4X2	T49.4X3	T49.4X4	T49.4X5	T49.4X6
nonmedicinal (ammonium) (potassium)	T56.891	T56.892	T56.893	T56.894		
Aluminium, aluminum						
acetate	T49.2X1	T49.2X2	T49.2X3	T49.2X4	T49.2X5	T49.2X6
solution	T49.0X1	T49.0X2	T49.0X3	T49.0X4	T49.0X5	T49.0X6
aspirin	T39.011	T39.012	T39.013	T39.014	T39.015	T39.016
bis (acetylsalicylate)	T39.011	T39.012	T39.013	T39.014	T39.015	T39.016
carbonate (gel, basic)	T47.1X1	T47.1X2	T47.1X3	T47.1X4	T47.1X5	T47.1X6
chlorhydroxide-complex	T47.1X1	T47.1X2	T47.1X3	T47.1X4	T47.1X5	T47.1X6
chloride	T49.2X1	T49.2X2	T49.2X3	T49.2X4	T49.2X5	T49.2X6
clofibrate	T46.6X1	T46.6X2	T46.6X3	T46.6X4	T46.6X5	T46.6X6
diacetate	T49.2X1	T49.2X2	T49.2X3	T49.2X4	T49.2X5	T49.2X6
glycinate	T47.1X1	T47.1X2	T47.1X3	T47.1X4	T47.1X5	T47.1X6
hydroxide (gel)	T47.1X1	T47.1X2	T47.1X3	T47.1X4	T47.1X5	T47.1X6
hydroxide-magnesium carb. gel	T47.1X1	T47.1X2	T47.1X3	T47.1X4	T47.1X5	T47.1X6
magnesium silicate	T47.1X1	T47.1X2	T47.1X3	T47.1X4	T47.1X5	T47.1X6
nicotinate	T46.7X1	T46.7X2	T46.7X3	T46.7X4	T46.7X5	T46.7X6

Substance	Poisoning, Accidental (unintentional)	Poisoning, Intentional Self-harm	Poisoning, Assault	Poisoning, Undetermined	Adverse Effect	Under-dosing
Aluminium, aluminum — *continued*						
ointment (surgical) (topical)	T49.3X1	T49.3X2	T49.3X3	T49.3X4	T49.3X5	T49.3X6
phosphate	T47.1X1	T47.1X2	T47.1X3	T47.1X4	T47.1X5	T47.1X6
salicylate	T39.091	T39.092	T39.093	T39.094	T39.095	T39.096
silicate	T47.1X1	T47.1X2	T47.1X3	T47.1X4	T47.1X5	T47.1X6
sodium silicate	T47.1X1	T47.1X2	T47.1X3	T47.1X4	T47.1X5	T47.1X6
subacetate	T49.2X1	T49.2X2	T49.2X3	T49.2X4	T49.2X5	T49.2X6
sulfate	T49.0X1	T49.0X2	T49.0X3	T49.0X4	T49.0X5	T49.0X6
tannate	T47.6X1	T47.6X2	T47.6X3	T47.6X4	T47.6X5	T47.6X6
topical NEC	T49.3X1	T49.3X2	T49.3X3	T49.3X4	T49.3X5	T49.3X6
Alurate	T42.3X1	T42.3X2	T42.3X3	T42.3X4	T42.3X5	T42.3X6
Alverine	T44.3X1	T44.3X2	T44.3X3	T44.3X4	T44.3X5	T44.3X6
Alvodine	T40.2X1	T40.2X2	T40.2X3	T40.2X4	T40.2X5	T40.2X6
Amanita phalloides	T62.0X1	T62.0X2	T62.0X3	T62.0X4	—	—
Amanitine	T62.0X1	T62.0X2	T62.0X3	T62.0X4	—	—
Amantadine	T42.8X1	T42.8X2	T42.8X3	T42.8X4	T42.8X5	T42.8X6
Ambazone	T49.6X1	T49.6X2	T49.6X3	T49.6X4	T49.6X5	T49.6X6
Ambenonium (chloride)	T44.0X1	T44.0X2	T44.0X3	T44.0X4	T44.0X5	T44.0X6
Ambroxol	T48.4X1	T48.4X2	T48.4X3	T48.4X4	T48.4X5	T48.4X6
Ambuphylline	T48.6X1	T48.6X2	T48.6X3	T48.6X4	T48.6X5	T48.6X6
Ambutonium bromide	T44.3X1	T44.3X2	T44.3X3	T44.3X4	T44.3X5	T44.3X6
Amcinonide	T49.0X1	T49.0X2	T49.0X3	T49.0X4	T49.0X5	T49.0X6
Amdinocilline	T36.0X1	T36.0X2	T36.0X3	T36.0X4	T36.0X5	T36.0X6
Ametazole	T50.8X1	T50.8X2	T50.8X3	T50.8X4	T50.8X5	T50.8X6
Amethocaine	T41.3X1	T41.3X2	T41.3X3	T41.3X4	T41.3X5	T41.3X6
regional	T41.3X1	T41.3X2	T41.3X3	T41.3X4	T41.3X5	T41.3X6
spinal	T41.3X1	T41.3X2	T41.3X3	T41.3X4	T41.3X5	T41.3X6
Amethopterin	T45.1X1	T45.1X2	T45.1X3	T45.1X4	T45.1X5	T45.1X6
Amezinium metilsulfate	T44.991	T44.992	T44.993	T44.994	T44.995	T44.996
Amfebutamone	T43.291	T43.292	T43.293	T43.294	T43.295	T43.296
Amfepramone	T50.5X1	T50.5X2	T50.5X3	T50.5X4	T50.5X5	T50.5X6
Amfetamine	T43.621	T43.622	T43.623	T43.624	T43.625	T43.626
Amfetaminil	T43.621	T43.622	T43.623	T43.624	T43.625	T43.626
Amfomycin	T36.8X1	T36.8X2	T36.8X3	T36.8X4	T36.8X5	T36.8X6
Amidefrine mesilate	T48.5X1	T48.5X2	T48.5X3	T48.5X4	T48.5X5	T48.5X6
Amidone	T40.3X1	T40.3X2	T40.3X3	T40.3X4	T40.3X5	T40.3X6
Amidopyrine	T39.2X1	T39.2X2	T39.2X3	T39.2X4	T39.2X5	T39.2X6
Amidotrizoate	T50.8X1	T50.8X2	T50.8X3	T50.8X4	T50.8X5	T50.8X6
Amiflamine	T43.1X1	T43.1X2	T43.1X3	T43.1X4	T43.1X5	T43.1X6
Amikacin	T36.5X1	T36.5X2	T36.5X3	T36.5X4	T36.5X5	T36.5X6
Amikhelline	T46.3X1	T46.3X2	T46.3X3	T46.3X4	T46.3X5	T46.3X6
Amiloride	T50.2X1	T50.2X2	T50.2X3	T50.2X4	T50.2X5	T50.2X6
Aminacrine	T49.0X1	T49.0X2	T49.0X3	T49.0X4	T49.0X5	T49.0X6
Amineptine	T43.011	T43.012	T43.013	T43.014	T43.015	T43.016
Aminitrozole	T37.3X1	T37.3X2	T37.3X3	T37.3X4	T37.3X5	T37.3X6
Aminoacetic acid (derivatives)	T50.3X1	T50.3X2	T50.3X3	T50.3X4	T50.3X5	T50.3X6
Amino acids	T50.3X1	T50.3X2	T50.3X3	T50.3X4	T50.3X5	T50.3X6
Aminoacridine	T49.0X1	T49.0X2	T49.0X3	T49.0X4	T49.0X5	T49.0X6
Aminobenzoic acid (-p)	T49.3X1	T49.3X2	T49.3X3	T49.3X4	T49.3X5	T49.3X6
Aminocaproic acid	T45.621	T45.622	T45.623	T45.624	T45.625	T45.626
Aminoethylisothiourium	T45.8X1	T45.8X2	T45.8X3	T45.8X4	T45.8X5	T45.8X6
Aminofenazone	T39.2X1	T39.2X2	T39.2X3	T39.2X4	T39.2X5	T39.2X6
Aminoglutethimide	T45.1X1	T45.1X2	T45.1X3	T45.1X4	T45.1X5	T45.1X6
Aminohippuric acid	T50.8X1	T50.8X2	T50.8X3	T50.8X4	T50.8X5	T50.8X6
Aminomethylbenzoic acid	T45.691	T45.692	T45.693	T45.694	T45.695	T45.696
Aminometradine	T50.2X1	T50.2X2	T50.2X3	T50.2X4	T50.2X5	T50.2X6
Aminopentamide	T44.3X1	T44.3X2	T44.3X3	T44.3X4	T44.3X5	T44.3X6
Aminophenazone	T39.2X1	T39.2X2	T39.2X3	T39.2X4	T39.2X5	T39.2X6
Aminophenol	T54.0X1	T54.0X2	T54.0X3	T54.0X4	—	—
Aminophenylpyridone	T43.591	T43.592	T43.593	T43.594	T43.595	T43.596
Aminophylline	T48.6X1	T48.6X2	T48.6X3	T48.6X4	T48.6X5	T48.6X6
Aminopterin sodium	T45.1X1	T45.1X2	T45.1X3	T45.1X4	T45.1X5	T45.1X6
Aminopyrine	T39.2X1	T39.2X2	T39.2X3	T39.2X4	T39.2X5	T39.2X6
Aminorex	T50.5X1	T50.5X2	T50.5X3	T50.5X4	T50.5X5	T50.5X6
Aminosalicylic acid	T37.1X1	T37.1X2	T37.1X3	T37.1X4	T37.1X5	T37.1X6
Aminosalylum	T37.1X1	T37.1X2	T37.1X3	T37.1X4	T37.1X5	T37.1X6
Amiodarone	T46.2X1	T46.2X2	T46.2X3	T46.2X4	T46.2X5	T46.2X6
Amiphenazole	T50.7X1	T50.7X2	T50.7X3	T50.7X4	T50.7X5	T50.7X6
Amiquinsin	T46.5X1	T46.5X2	T46.5X3	T46.5X4	T46.5X5	T46.5X6
Amisometradine	T50.2X1	T50.2X2	T50.2X3	T50.2X4	T50.2X5	T50.2X6
Amisulpride	T43.591	T43.592	T43.593	T43.594	T43.595	T43.596
Amitriptyline	T43.011	T43.012	T43.013	T43.014	T43.015	T43.016
Amitriptylinoxide	T43.011	T43.012	T43.013	T43.014	T43.015	T43.016
Amlexanox	T48.6X1	T48.6X2	T48.6X3	T48.6X4	T48.6X5	T48.6X6
Ammonia (fumes) (gas) (vapor)	T59.891	T59.892	T59.893	T59.894	—	—
aromatic spirit	T48.991	T48.992	T48.993	T48.994	T48.995	T48.996
liquid (household)	T54.3X1	T54.3X2	T54.3X3	T54.3X4	—	—
Ammoniated mercury	T49.0X1	T49.0X2	T49.0X3	T49.0X4	T49.0X5	T49.0X6
Ammonium						
acid tartrate	T49.5X1	T49.5X2	T49.5X3	T49.5X4	T49.5X5	T49.5X6
Ammonium — *continued*						
bromide	T42.6X1	T42.6X2	T42.6X3	T42.6X4	T42.6X5	T42.6X6
carbonate	T54.3X1	T54.3X2	T54.3X3	T54.3X4	—	—
chloride	T50.991	T50.992	T50.993	T50.994	T50.995	T50.996
expectorant	T48.4X1	T48.4X2	T48.4X3	T48.4X4	T48.4X5	T48.4X6
compounds (household) NEC	T54.3X1	T54.3X2	T54.3X3	T54.3X4	—	—
fumes (any usage)	T59.891	T59.892	T59.893	T59.894	—	—
industrial	T54.3X1	T54.3X2	T54.3X3	T54.3X4	—	—
ichthyosulronate	T49.4X1	T49.4X2	T49.4X3	T49.4X4	T49.4X5	T49.4X6
mandelate	T37.91	T37.92	T37.93	T37.94	T37.95	T37.96
sulfamate	T60.3X1	T60.3X2	T60.3X3	T60.3X4	—	—
sulfonate resin	T47.8X1	T47.8X2	T47.8X3	T47.8X4	T47.8X5	T47.8X6
Amobarbital (sodium)	T42.3X1	T42.3X2	T42.3X3	T42.3X4	T42.3X5	T42.3X6
Amodiaquine	T37.2X1	T37.2X2	T37.2X3	T37.2X4	T37.2X5	T37.2X6
Amopyroquin (e)	T37.2X1	T37.2X2	T37.2X3	T37.2X4	T37.2X5	T37.2X6
Amoxapine	T43.011	T43.012	T43.013	T43.014	T43.015	T43.016
Amoxicillin	T36.0X1	T36.0X2	T36.0X3	T36.0X4	T36.0X5	T36.0X6
Amperozide	T43.591	T43.592	T43.593	T43.594	T43.595	T43.596
Amphenidone	T43.591	T43.592	T43.593	T43.594	T43.595	T43.596
Amphetamine NEC	T43.621	T43.622	T43.623	T43.624	T43.625	T43.626
Amphomycin	T36.8X1	T36.8X2	T36.8X3	T36.8X4	T36.8X5	T36.8X6
Amphotalide	T37.4X1	T37.4X2	T37.4X3	T37.4X4	T37.4X5	T37.4X6
Amphotericin B	T36.7X1	T36.7X2	T36.7X3	T36.7X4	T36.7X5	T36.7X6
topical	T49.0X1	T49.0X2	T49.0X3	T49.0X4	T49.0X5	T49.0X6
Ampicillin	T36.0X1	T36.0X2	T36.0X3	T36.0X4	T36.0X5	T36.0X6
Amprotropine	T44.3X1	T44.3X2	T44.3X3	T44.3X4	T44.3X5	T44.3X6
Amsacrine	T45.1X1	T45.1X2	T45.1X3	T45.1X4	T45.1X5	T45.1X6
Amygdaline	T62.2X1	T62.2X2	T62.2X3	T62.2X4	—	—
Amyl						
acetate	T52.8X1	T52.8X2	T52.8X3	T52.8X4	—	—
vapor	T59.891	T59.892	T59.893	T59.894	—	—
alcohol	T51.3X1	T51.3X2	T51.3X3	T51.3X4	—	—
chloride	T53.6X1	T53.6X2	T53.6X3	T53.6X4	—	—
formate	T52.8X1	T52.8X2	T52.8X3	T52.8X4	—	—
nitrite	T46.3X1	T46.3X2	T46.3X3	T46.3X4	T46.3X5	T46.3X6
propionate	T65.891	T65.892	T65.893	T65.894	—	—
Amylase	T47.5X1	T47.5X2	T47.5X3	T47.5X4	T47.5X5	T47.5X6
Amyleine, regional	T41.3X1	T41.3X2	T41.3X3	T41.3X4	T41.3X5	T41.3X6
Amylene						
dichloride	T53.6X1	T53.6X2	T53.6X3	T53.6X4	—	—
hydrate	T51.3X1	T51.3X2	T51.3X3	T51.3X4	—	—
Amylmetacresol	T49.6X1	T49.6X2	T49.6X3	T49.6X4	T49.6X5	T49.6X6
Amylobarbitone	T42.3X1	T42.3X2	T42.3X3	T42.3X4	T42.3X5	T42.3X6
Amylocaine, regional	T41.3X1	T41.3X2	T41.3X3	T41.3X4	T41.3X5	T41.3X6
infiltration (subcutaneous)	T41.3X1	T41.3X2	T41.3X3	T41.3X4	T41.3X5	T41.3X6
nerve block (peripheral) (plexus)	T41.3X1	T41.3X2	T41.3X3	T41.3X4	T41.3X5	T41.3X6
spinal	T41.3X1	T41.3X2	T41.3X3	T41.3X4	T41.3X5	T41.3X6
topical (surface)	T41.3X1	T41.3X2	T41.3X3	T41.3X4	T41.3X5	T41.3X6
Amylopectin	T47.6X1	T47.6X2	T47.6X3	T47.6X4	T47.6X5	T47.6X6
Amytal (sodium)	T42.3X1	T42.3X2	T42.3X3	T42.3X4	T42.3X5	T42.3X6
Anabolic steroid	T38.7X1	T38.7X2	T38.7X3	T38.7X4	T38.7X5	T38.7X6
Analeptic NEC	T50.7X1	T50.7X2	T50.7X3	T50.7X4	T50.7X5	T50.7X6
Analgesic	T39.91	T39.92	T39.93	T39.94	T39.95	T39.96
anti-inflammatory NEC	T39.91	T39.92	T39.93	T39.94	T39.95	T39.96
propionic acid derivative	T39.311	T39.312	T39.313	T39.314	T39.315	T39.316
antirheumatic NEC	T39.4X1	T39.4X2	T39.4X3	T39.4X4	T39.4X5	T39.4X6
aromatic NEC	T39.1X1	T39.1X2	T39.1X3	T39.1X4	T39.1X5	T39.1X6
narcotic NEC	T40.601	T40.602	T40.603	T40.604	T40.605	T40.606
combination	T40.601	T40.602	T40.603	T40.604	T40.605	T40.606
obstetric	T40.601	T40.602	T40.603	T40.604	T40.605	T40.606
non-narcotic NEC	T39.91	T39.92	T39.93	T39.94	T39.95	T39.96
combination	T39.91	T39.92	T39.93	T39.94	T39.95	T39.96
pyrazole	T39.2X1	T39.2X2	T39.2X3	T39.2X4	T39.2X5	T39.2X6
specified NEC	T39.8X1	T39.8X2	T39.8X3	T39.8X4	T39.8X5	T39.8X6
Analgin	T39.2X1	T39.2X2	T39.2X3	T39.2X4	T39.2X5	T39.2X6
Anamirta cocculus	T62.1X1	T62.1X2	T62.1X3	T62.1X4	—	—
Ancillin	T36.0X1	T36.0X2	T36.0X3	T36.0X4	T36.0X5	T36.0X6
Ancrod	T45.691	T45.692	T45.693	T45.694	T45.695	T45.696
Androgen	T38.7X1	T38.7X2	T38.7X3	T38.7X4	T38.7X5	T38.7X6
Androgen-estrogen mixture	T38.7X1	T38.7X2	T38.7X3	T38.7X4	T38.7X5	T38.7X6
Androstalone	T38.7X1	T38.7X2	T38.7X3	T38.7X4	T38.7X5	T38.7X6
Androstanolone	T38.7X1	T38.7X2	T38.7X3	T38.7X4	T38.7X5	T38.7X6
Androsterone	T38.7X1	T38.7X2	T38.7X3	T38.7X4	T38.7X5	T38.7X6
Anemone pulsatilla	T62.2X1	T62.2X2	T62.2X3	T62.2X4	—	—
Anesthesia						
caudal	T41.3X1	T41.3X2	T41.3X3	T41.3X4	T41.3X5	T41.3X6
endotracheal	T41.0X1	T41.0X2	T41.0X3	T41.0X4	T41.0X5	T41.0X6
epidural	T41.3X1	T41.3X2	T41.3X3	T41.3X4	T41.3X5	T41.3X6
inhalation	T41.0X1	T41.0X2	T41.0X3	T41.0X4	T41.0X5	T41.0X6
local	T41.3X1	T41.3X2	T41.3X3	T41.3X4	T41.3X5	T41.3X6

Substance	Poisoning, Accidental (unintentional)	Poisoning, Intentional Self-harm	Poisoning, Assault	Poisoning, Undetermined	Adverse Effect	Under-dosing
Anesthesia — continued						
mucosal	T41.3X1	T41.3X2	T41.3X3	T41.3X4	T41.3X5	T41.3X6
muscle relaxation	T48.1X1	T48.1X2	T48.1X3	T48.1X4	T48.1X5	T48.1X6
nerve blocking	T41.3X1	T41.3X2	T41.3X3	T41.3X4	T41.3X5	T41.3X6
plexus blocking	T41.3X1	T41.3X2	T41.3X3	T41.3X4	T41.3X5	T41.3X6
potentiated	T41.201	T41.202	T41.203	T41.204	T41.205	T41.206
rectal	T41.201	T41.202	T41.203	T41.204	T41.205	T41.206
general	T41.201	T41.202	T41.203	T41.204	T41.205	T41.206
local	T41.3X1	T41.3X2	T41.3X3	T41.3X4	T41.3X5	T41.3X6
regional	T41.3X1	T41.3X2	T41.3X3	T41.3X4	T41.3X5	T41.3X6
surface	T41.3X1	T41.3X2	T41.3X3	T41.3X4	T41.3X5	T41.3X6
Anesthetic NEC — see also Anesthesia	T41.41	T41.42	T41.43	T41.44	T41.45	T41.46
with muscle relaxant	T41.201	T41.202	T41.203	T41.204	T41.205	T41.206
general	T41.201	T41.202	T41.203	T41.204	T41.205	T41.206
local	T41.3X1	T41.3X2	T41.3X3	T41.3X4	T41.3X5	T41.3X6
gaseous NEC	T41.0X1	T41.0X2	T41.0X3	T41.0X4	T41.0X5	T41.0X6
general NEC	T41.201	T41.202	T41.203	T41.204	T41.205	T41.206
halogenated hydrocarbon derivatives NEC	T41.0X1	T41.0X2	T41.0X3	T41.0X4	T41.0X5	T41.0X6
infiltration NEC	T41.3X1	T41.3X2	T41.3X3	T41.3X4	T41.3X5	T41.3X6
intravenous NEC	T41.1X1	T41.1X2	T41.1X3	T41.1X4	T41.1X5	T41.1X6
local NEC	T41.3X1	T41.3X2	T41.3X3	T41.3X4	T41.3X5	T41.3X6
rectal	T41.201	T41.202	T41.203	T41.204	T41.205	T41.206
general	T41.201	T41.202	T41.203	T41.204	T41.205	T41.206
local	T41.3X1	T41.3X2	T41.3X3	T41.3X4	T41.3X5	T41.3X6
regional NEC	T41.3X1	T41.3X2	T41.3X3	T41.3X4	T41.3X5	T41.3X6
spinal NEC	T41.3X1	T41.3X2	T41.3X3	T41.3X4	T41.3X5	T41.3X6
thiobarbiturate	T41.1X1	T41.1X2	T41.1X3	T41.1X4	T41.1X5	T41.1X6
topical	T41.3X1	T41.3X2	T41.3X3	T41.3X4	T41.3X5	T41.3X6
Aneurine	T45.2X1	T45.2X2	T45.2X3	T45.2X4	T45.2X5	T45.2X6
Angio-Conray	T50.8X1	T50.8X2	T50.8X3	T50.8X4	T50.8X5	T50.8X6
Angiotensin	T44.5X1	T44.5X2	T44.5X3	T44.5X4	T44.5X5	T44.5X6
Angiotensinamide	T44.991	T44.992	T44.993	T44.994	T44.995	T44.996
Anhydrohydroxy-progesterone	T38.5X1	T38.5X2	T38.5X3	T38.5X4	T38.5X5	T38.5X6
Anhydron	T50.2X1	T50.2X2	T50.2X3	T50.2X4	T50.2X5	T50.2X6
Anileridine	T40.4X1	T40.4X2	T40.4X3	T40.4X4	T40.4X5	T40.4X6
Aniline (dye) (liquid)	T65.3X1	T65.3X2	T65.3X3	T65.3X4		
analgesic	T39.1X1	T39.1X2	T39.1X3	T39.1X4	T39.1X5	T39.1X6
derivatives, therapeutic NEC	T39.1X1	T39.1X2	T39.1X3	T39.1X4	T39.1X5	T39.1X6
vapor	T65.3X1	T65.3X2	T65.3X3	T65.3X4	—	—
Aniscoropine	T44.3X1	T44.3X2	T44.3X3	T44.3X4	T44.3X5	T44.3X6
Anise oil	T47.5X1	T47.5X2	T47.5X3	T47.5X4	T47.5X5	T47.5X6
Anisidine	T65.3X1	T65.3X2	T65.3X3	T65.3X4	—	—
Anisindione	T45.511	T45.512	T45.513	T45.514	T45.515	T45.516
Anisotropine methyl-bromide	T44.3X1	T44.3X2	T44.3X3	T44.3X4	T44.3X5	T44.3X6
Anistreplase	T45.611	T45.612	T45.613	T45.614	T45.615	T45.616
Anorexiant (central)	T50.5X1	T50.5X2	T50.5X3	T50.5X4	T50.5X5	T50.5X6
Anorexic agents	T50.5X1	T50.5X2	T50.5X3	T50.5X4	T50.5X5	T50.5X6
Ansamycin	T36.6X1	T36.6X2	T36.6X3	T36.6X4	T36.6X5	T36.6X6
Ant (bite) (sting)	T63.421	T63.422	T63.423	T63.424	—	—
Antabuse	T50.6X1	T50.6X2	T50.6X3	T50.6X4	T50.6X5	T50.6X6
Antacid NEC	T47.1X1	T47.1X2	T47.1X3	T47.1X4	T47.1X5	T47.1X6
Antagonist						
Aldosterone	T50.0X1	T50.0X2	T50.0X3	T50.0X4	T50.0X5	T50.0X6
alpha-adrenoreceptor	T44.6X1	T44.6X2	T44.6X3	T44.6X4	T44.6X5	T44.6X6
anticoagulant	T45.7X1	T45.7X2	T45.7X3	T45.7X4	T45.7X5	T45.7X6
beta-adrenoreceptor	T44.7X1	T44.7X2	T44.7X3	T44.7X4	T44.7X5	T44.7X6
extrapyramidal NEC	T44.3X1	T44.3X2	T44.3X3	T44.3X4	T44.3X5	T44.3X6
folic acid	T45.1X1	T45.1X2	T45.1X3	T45.1X4	T45.1X5	T45.1X6
H2 receptor	T47.0X1	T47.0X2	T47.0X3	T47.0X4	T47.0X5	T47.0X6
heavy metal	T45.8X1	T45.8X2	T45.8X3	T45.8X4	T45.8X5	T45.8X6
narcotic analgesic	T50.7X1	T50.7X2	T50.7X3	T50.7X4	T50.7X5	T50.7X6
opiate	T50.7X1	T50.7X2	T50.7X3	T50.7X4	T50.7X5	T50.7X6
pyrimidine	T45.1X1	T45.1X2	T45.1X3	T45.1X4	T45.1X5	T45.1X6
serotonin	T46.5X1	T46.5X2	T46.5X3	T46.5X4	T46.5X5	T46.5X6
Antazolin (e)	T45.0X1	T45.0X2	T45.0X3	T45.0X4	T45.0X5	T45.0X6
Anterior pituitary hormone NEC	T38.811	T38.812	T38.813	T38.814	T38.815	T38.816
Anthelmintic NEC	T37.4X1	T37.4X2	T37.4X3	T37.4X4	T37.4X5	T37.4X6
Anthiolimine	T37.4X1	T37.4X2	T37.4X3	T37.4X4	T37.4X5	T37.4X6
Anthralin	T49.4X1	T49.4X2	T49.4X3	T49.4X4	T49.4X5	T49.4X6
Anthramycin	T45.1X1	T45.1X2	T45.1X3	T45.1X4	T45.1X5	T45.1X6
Antiadrenergic NEC	T44.8X1	T44.8X2	T44.8X3	T44.8X4	T44.8X5	T44.8X6
Antiallergic NEC	T45.0X1	T45.0X2	T45.0X3	T45.0X4	T45.0X5	T45.0X6
Antiandrogen NEC	T38.6X1	T38.6X2	T38.6X3	T38.6X4	T38.6X5	T38.6X6
Anti-anemic (drug) (preparation)	T45.8X1	T45.8X2	T45.8X3	T45.8X4	T45.8X5	T45.8X6
Antianxiety drug NEC	T43.501	T43.502	T43.503	T43.504	T43.505	T43.506
Antiaris toxicaria	T65.891	T65.892	T65.893	T65.894	—	—
Antiarteriosclerotic drug	T46.6X1	T46.6X2	T46.6X3	T46.6X4	T46.6X5	T46.6X6

Substance	Poisoning, Accidental (unintentional)	Poisoning, Intentional Self-harm	Poisoning, Assault	Poisoning, Undetermined	Adverse Effect	Under-dosing
Antiasthmatic drug NEC	T48.6X1	T48.6X2	T48.6X3	T48.6X4	T48.6X5	T48.6X6
Antibiotic NEC	T36.91	T36.92	T36.93	T36.94	T36.95	T36.96
aminoglycoside	T36.5X1	T36.5X2	T36.5X3	T36.5X4	T36.5X5	T36.5X6
anticancer	T45.1X1	T45.1X2	T45.1X3	T45.1X4	T45.1X5	T45.1X6
antifungal	T36.7X1	T36.7X2	T36.7X3	T36.7X4	T36.7X5	T36.7X6
antimycobacterial	T36.5X1	T36.5X2	T36.5X3	T36.5X4	T36.5X5	T36.5X6
antineoplastic	T45.1X1	T45.1X2	T45.1X3	T45.1X4	T45.1X5	T45.1X6
b-lactam NEC	T36.1X1	T36.1X2	T36.1X3	T36.1X4	T36.1X5	T36.1X6
cephalosporin (group)	T36.1X1	T36.1X2	T36.1X3	T36.1X4	T36.1X5	T36.1X6
chloramphenicol (group)	T36.2X1	T36.2X2	T36.2X3	T36.2X4	T36.2X5	T36.2X6
ENT	T49.6X1	T49.6X2	T49.6X3	T49.6X4	T49.6X5	T49.6X6
eye	T49.5X1	T49.5X2	T49.5X3	T49.5X4	T49.5X5	T49.5X6
fungicidal (local)	T49.0X1	T49.0X2	T49.0X3	T49.0X4	T49.0X5	T49.0X6
intestinal	T36.8X1	T36.8X2	T36.8X3	T36.8X4	T36.8X5	T36.8X6
local	T49.0X1	T49.0X2	T49.0X3	T49.0X4	T49.0X5	T49.0X6
macrolides	T36.3X1	T36.3X2	T36.3X3	T36.3X4	T36.3X5	T36.3X6
polypeptide	T36.8X1	T36.8X2	T36.8X3	T36.8X4	T36.8X5	T36.8X6
specified NEC	T36.8X1	T36.8X2	T36.8X3	T36.8X4	T36.8X5	T36.8X6
tetracycline (group)	T36.4X1	T36.4X2	T36.4X3	T36.4X4	T36.4X5	T36.4X6
throat	T49.6X1	T49.6X2	T49.6X3	T49.6X4	T49.6X5	T49.6X6
Anticancer agents NEC	T45.1X1	T45.1X2	T45.1X3	T45.1X4	T45.1X5	T45.1X6
Anticholesterolemic drug NEC	T46.6X1	T46.6X2	T46.6X3	T46.6X4	T46.6X5	T46.6X6
Anticholinergic NEC	T44.3X1	T44.3X2	T44.3X3	T44.3X4	T44.3X5	T44.3X6
Anticholinesterase	T44.0X1	T44.0X2	T44.0X3	T44.0X4	T44.0X5	T44.0X6
organophosphorus	T44.0X1	T44.0X2	T44.0X3	T44.0X4	T44.0X5	T44.0X6
insecticide	T60.0X1	T60.0X2	T60.0X3	T60.0X4	—	—
nerve gas	T59.891	T59.892	T59.893	T59.894	—	—
reversible	T44.0X1	T44.0X2	T44.0X3	T44.0X4	T44.0X5	T44.0X6
ophthalmological	T49.5X1	T49.5X2	T49.5X3	T49.5X4	T49.5X5	T49.5X6
Anticoagulant NEC	T45.511	T45.512	T45.513	T45.514	T45.515	T45.516
Antagonist	T45.7X1	T45.7X2	T45.7X3	T45.7X4	T45.7X5	T45.7X6
Anti-common-cold drug NEC	T48.5X1	T48.5X2	T48.5X3	T48.5X4	T48.5X5	T48.5X6
Anticonvulsant	T42.71	T42.72	T42.73	T42.74	T42.75	T42.76
barbiturate	T42.3X1	T42.3X2	T42.3X3	T42.3X4	T42.3X5	T42.3X6
combination (with barbiturate)	T42.3X1	T42.3X2	T42.3X3	T42.3X4	T42.3X5	T42.3X6
hydantoin	T42.0X1	T42.0X2	T42.0X3	T42.0X4	T42.0X5	T42.0X6
hypnotic NEC	T42.6X1	T42.6X2	T42.6X3	T42.6X4	T42.6X5	T42.6X6
oxazolidinedione	T42.2X1	T42.2X2	T42.2X3	T42.2X4	T42.2X5	T42.2X6
pyrimidinedione	T42.6X1	T42.6X2	T42.6X3	T42.6X4	T42.6X5	T42.6X6
specified NEC	T42.6X1	T42.6X2	T42.6X3	T42.6X4	T42.6X5	T42.6X6
succinimide	T42.2X1	T42.2X2	T42.2X3	T42.2X4	T42.2X5	T42.2X6
Antidepressant	T43.201	T43.202	T43.203	T43.204	T43.205	T43.206
monoamine oxidase inhibitor	T43.1X1	T43.1X2	T43.1X3	T43.1X4	T43.1X5	T43.1X6
selective serotonin norepinephrine reuptake inhibitor	T43.211	T43.212	T43.213	T43.214	T43.215	T43.216
selective serotonin reuptake inhibitor	T43.221	T43.222	T43.223	T43.224	T43.225	T43.226
specified NEC	T43.291	T43.292	T43.293	T43.294	T43.295	T43.296
tetracyclic	T43.021	T43.022	T43.023	T43.024	T43.025	T43.026
triazolopyridine	T43.211	T43.212	T43.213	T43.214	T43.215	T43.216
tricyclic	T43.011	T43.012	T43.013	T43.014	T43.015	T43.016
Antidiabetic NEC	T38.3X1	T38.3X2	T38.3X3	T38.3X4	T38.3X5	T38.3X6
biguanide	T38.3X1	T38.3X2	T38.3X3	T38.3X4	T38.3X5	T38.3X6
and sulfonyl combined	T38.3X1	T38.3X2	T38.3X3	T38.3X4	T38.3X5	T38.3X6
combined	T38.3X1	T38.3X2	T38.3X3	T38.3X4	T38.3X5	T38.3X6
sulfonylurea	T38.3X1	T38.3X2	T38.3X3	T38.3X4	T38.3X5	T38.3X6
Antidiarrheal drug NEC	T47.6X1	T47.6X2	T47.6X3	T47.6X4	T47.6X5	T47.6X6
absorbent	T47.6X1	T47.6X2	T47.6X3	T47.6X4	T47.6X5	T47.6X6
Anti-D immunoglobulin (human)	T50.Z11	T50.Z12	T50.Z13	T50.Z14	T50.Z15	T50.Z16
Antidiphtheria serum	T50.Z11	T50.Z12	T50.Z13	T50.Z14	T50.Z15	T50.Z16
Antidiuretic hormone	T38.891	T38.892	T38.893	T38.894	T38.895	T38.896
Antidote NEC	T50.6X1	T50.6X2	T50.6X3	T50.6X4	T50.6X5	T50.6X6
heavy metal	T45.8X1	T45.8X2	T45.8X3	T45.8X4	T45.8X5	T45.8X6
Antidysrhythmic NEC	T46.2X1	T46.2X2	T46.2X3	T46.2X4	T46.2X5	T46.2X6
Antiemetic drug	T45.0X1	T45.0X2	T45.0X3	T45.0X4	T45.0X5	T45.0X6
Antiepilepsy agent	T42.71	T42.72	T42.73	T42.74	T42.75	T42.76
combination	T42.5X1	T42.5X2	T42.5X3	T42.5X4	T42.5X5	T42.5X6
mixed	T42.5X1	T42.5X2	T42.5X3	T42.5X4	T42.5X5	T42.5X6
specified, NEC	T42.6X1	T42.6X2	T42.6X3	T42.6X4	T42.6X5	T42.6X6
Antiestrogen NEC	T38.6X1	T38.6X2	T38.6X3	T38.6X4	T38.6X5	T38.6X6
Antifertility pill	T38.4X1	T38.4X2	T38.4X3	T38.4X4	T38.4X5	T38.4X6
Antifibrinolytic drug	T45.621	T45.622	T45.623	T45.624	T45.625	T45.626
Antifilarial drug	T37.4X1	T37.4X2	T37.4X3	T37.4X4	T37.4X5	T37.4X6
Antiflatulent	T47.5X1	T47.5X2	T47.5X3	T47.5X4	T47.5X5	T47.5X6
Antifreeze	T65.91	T65.92	T65.93	T65.94		
alcohol	T51.1X1	T51.1X2	T51.1X3	T51.1X4	—	—
ethylene glycol	T51.8X1	T51.8X2	T51.8X3	T51.8X4	—	—

Additional Character May Be Required — Refer to the Tabular List for Character Selection   ▽ Subterms under main terms may continue to next column or page

Table of Drugs and Chemicals

Antifungal — Argyrol

Substance	Poisoning, Accidental (unintentional)	Poisoning, Intentional Self-harm	Poisoning, Assault	Poisoning, Undetermined	Adverse Effect	Under-dosing
Antifungal						
antibiotic (systemic)	T36.7X1	T36.7X2	T36.7X3	T36.7X4	T36.7X5	T36.7X6
anti-infective NEC	T37.91	T37.92	T37.93	T37.94	T37.95	T37.96
disinfectant, local	T49.0X1	T49.0X2	T49.0X3	T49.0X4	T49.0X5	T49.0X6
nonmedicinal (spray)	T60.3X1	T60.3X2	T60.3X3	T60.3X4	—	—
topical	T49.0X1	T49.0X2	T49.0X3	T49.0X4	T49.0X5	T49.0X6
Anti-gastric-secretion drug NEC	T47.1X1	T47.1X2	T47.1X3	T47.1X4	T47.1X5	T47.1X6
Antigonadotrophin NEC	T38.6X1	T38.6X2	T38.6X3	T38.6X4	T38.6X5	T38.6X6
Antihallucinogen	T43.501	T43.502	T43.503	T43.504	T43.505	T43.506
Antihelmintics	T37.4X1	T37.4X2	T37.4X3	T37.4X4	T37.4X5	T37.4X6
Antihemophilic						
factor	T45.8X1	T45.8X2	T45.8X3	T45.8X4	T45.8X5	T45.8X6
fraction	T45.8X1	T45.8X2	T45.8X3	T45.8X4	T45.8X5	T45.8X6
globulin concentrate	T45.7X1	T45.7X2	T45.7X3	T45.7X4	T45.7X5	T45.7X6
human plasma	T45.8X1	T45.8X2	T45.8X3	T45.8X4	T45.8X5	T45.8X6
plasma, dried	T45.7X1	T45.7X2	T45.7X3	T45.7X4	T45.7X5	T45.7X6
Antihemorrhoidal preparation	T49.2X1	T49.2X2	T49.2X3	T49.2X4	T49.2X5	T49.2X6
Antiheparin drug	T45.7X1	T45.7X2	T45.7X3	T45.7X4	T45.7X5	T45.7X6
Antihistamine	T45.0X1	T45.0X2	T45.0X3	T45.0X4	T45.0X5	T45.0X6
Antihookworm drug	T37.4X1	T37.4X2	T37.4X3	T37.4X4	T37.4X5	T37.4X6
Anti-human lymphocytic globulin	T50.Z11	T50.Z12	T50.Z13	T50.Z14	T50.Z15	T50.Z16
Antihyperlipidemic drug	T46.6X1	T46.6X2	T46.6X3	T46.6X4	T46.6X5	T46.6X6
Antihypertensive drug NEC	T46.5X1	T46.5X2	T46.5X3	T46.5X4	T46.5X5	T46.5X6
Anti-infective NEC	T37.91	T37.92	T37.93	T37.94	T37.95	T37.96
anthelmintic	T37.4X1	T37.4X2	T37.4X3	T37.4X4	T37.4X5	T37.4X6
antibiotics	T36.91	T36.92	T36.93	T36.94	T36.95	T36.96
specified NEC	T36.8X1	T36.8X2	T36.8X3	T36.8X4	T36.8X5	T36.8X6
antimalarial	T37.2X1	T37.2X2	T37.2X3	T37.2X4	T37.2X5	T37.2X6
antimycobacterial NEC	T37.1X1	T37.1X2	T37.1X3	T37.1X4	T37.1X5	T37.1X6
antibiotics	T36.5X1	T36.5X2	T36.5X3	T36.5X4	T36.5X5	T36.5X6
antiprotozoal NEC	T37.3X1	T37.3X2	T37.3X3	T37.3X4	T37.3X5	T37.3X6
blood	T37.2X1	T37.2X2	T37.2X3	T37.2X4	T37.2X5	T37.2X6
antiviral	T37.5X1	T37.5X2	T37.5X3	T37.5X4	T37.5X5	T37.5X6
arsenical	T37.8X1	T37.8X2	T37.8X3	T37.8X4	T37.8X5	T37.8X6
bismuth, local	T49.0X1	T49.0X2	T49.0X3	T49.0X4	T49.0X5	T49.0X6
ENT	T49.6X1	T49.6X2	T49.6X3	T49.6X4	T49.6X5	T49.6X6
eye NEC	T49.5X1	T49.5X2	T49.5X3	T49.5X4	T49.5X5	T49.5X6
heavy metals NEC	T37.8X1	T37.8X2	T37.8X3	T37.8X4	T37.8X5	T37.8X6
local NEC	T49.0X1	T49.0X2	T49.0X3	T49.0X4	T49.0X5	T49.0X6
specified NEC	T49.0X1	T49.0X2	T49.0X3	T49.0X4	T49.0X5	T49.0X6
mixed	T37.91	T37.92	T37.93	T37.94	T37.95	T37.96
ophthalmic preparation	T49.5X1	T49.5X2	T49.5X3	T49.5X4	T49.5X5	T49.5X6
topical NEC	T49.0X1	T49.0X2	T49.0X3	T49.0X4	T49.0X5	T49.0X6
Anti-inflammatory drug NEC	T39.391	T39.392	T39.393	T39.394	T39.395	T39.396
local	T49.0X1	T49.0X2	T49.0X3	T49.0X4	T49.0X5	T49.0X6
nonsteroidal NEC	T39.391	T39.392	T39.393	T39.394	T39.395	T39.396
propionic acid derivative	T39.311	T39.312	T39.313	T39.314	T39.315	T39.316
specified NEC	T39.391	T39.392	T39.393	T39.394	T39.395	T39.396
Antikaluretic	T50.3X1	T50.3X2	T50.3X3	T50.3X4	T50.3X5	T50.3X6
Antiknock (tetraethyl lead)	T56.0X1	T56.0X2	T56.0X3	T56.0X4	—	—
Antilipemic drug NEC	T46.6X1	T46.6X2	T46.6X3	T46.6X4	T46.6X5	T46.6X6
Antimalarial	T37.2X1	T37.2X2	T37.2X3	T37.2X4	T37.2X5	T37.2X6
prophylactic NEC	T37.2X1	T37.2X2	T37.2X3	T37.2X4	T37.2X5	T37.2X6
pyrimidine derivative	T37.2X1	T37.2X2	T37.2X3	T37.2X4	T37.2X5	T37.2X6
Antimetabolite	T45.1X1	T45.1X2	T45.1X3	T45.1X4	T45.1X5	T45.1X6
Antimitotic agent	T45.1X1	T45.1X2	T45.1X3	T45.1X4	T45.1X5	T45.1X6
Antimony (compounds) (vapor) NEC	T56.891	T56.892	T56.893	T56.894	—	—
anti-infectives	T37.8X1	T37.8X2	T37.8X3	T37.8X4	T37.8X5	T37.8X6
dimercaptosuccinate	T37.3X1	T37.3X2	T37.3X3	T37.3X4	T37.3X5	T37.3X6
hydride	T56.891	T56.892	T56.893	T56.894	—	—
pesticide (vapor)	T60.8X1	T60.8X2	T60.8X3	T60.8X4	—	—
potassium (sodium) tartrate	T37.8X1	T37.8X2	T37.8X3	T37.8X4	T37.8X5	T37.8X6
sodium	T37.3X1	T37.3X2	T37.3X3	T37.3X4	T37.3X5	T37.3X6
dimercaptosuccinate						
tartrated	T37.8X1	T37.8X2	T37.8X3	T37.8X4	T37.8X5	T37.8X6
Antimuscarinic NEC	T44.3X1	T44.3X2	T44.3X3	T44.3X4	T44.3X5	T44.3X6
Antimycobacterial drug NEC	T37.1X1	T37.1X2	T37.1X3	T37.1X4	T37.1X5	T37.1X6
antibiotics	T36.5X1	T36.5X2	T36.5X3	T36.5X4	T36.5X5	T36.5X6
combination	T37.1X1	T37.1X2	T37.1X3	T37.1X4	T37.1X5	T37.1X6
Antinausea drug	T45.0X1	T45.0X2	T45.0X3	T45.0X4	T45.0X5	T45.0X6
Antinematode drug	T37.4X1	T37.4X2	T37.4X3	T37.4X4	T37.4X5	T37.4X6
Antineoplastic NEC	T45.1X1	T45.1X2	T45.1X3	T45.1X4	T45.1X5	T45.1X6
alkaloidal	T45.1X1	T45.1X2	T45.1X3	T45.1X4	T45.1X5	T45.1X6
antibiotics	T45.1X1	T45.1X2	T45.1X3	T45.1X4	T45.1X5	T45.1X6
combination	T45.1X1	T45.1X2	T45.1X3	T45.1X4	T45.1X5	T45.1X6
estrogen	T38.5X1	T38.5X2	T38.5X3	T38.5X4	T38.5X5	T38.5X6

Substance	Poisoning, Accidental (unintentional)	Poisoning, Intentional Self-harm	Poisoning, Assault	Poisoning, Undetermined	Adverse Effect	Under-dosing
Antineoplastic — continued						
steroid	T38.7X1	T38.7X2	T38.7X3	T38.7X4	T38.7X5	T38.7X6
Antiparasitic drug (systemic)	T37.91	T37.92	T37.93	T37.94	T37.95	T37.96
local	T49.0X1	T49.0X2	T49.0X3	T49.0X4	T49.0X5	T49.0X6
specified NEC	T37.8X1	T37.8X2	T37.8X3	T37.8X4	T37.8X5	T37.8X6
Antiparkinsonism drug NEC	T42.8X1	T42.8X2	T42.8X3	T42.8X4	T42.8X5	T42.8X6
Antiperspirant NEC	T49.2X1	T49.2X2	T49.2X3	T49.2X4	T49.2X5	T49.2X6
Antiphlogistic NEC	T39.4X1	T39.4X2	T39.4X3	T39.4X4	T39.4X5	T39.4X6
Antiplatyhelmintic drug	T37.4X1	T37.4X2	T37.4X3	T37.4X4	T37.4X5	T37.4X6
Antiprotozoal drug NEC	T37.3X1	T37.3X2	T37.3X3	T37.3X4	T37.3X5	T37.3X6
blood	T37.2X1	T37.2X2	T37.2X3	T37.2X4	T37.2X5	T37.2X6
local	T49.0X1	T49.0X2	T49.0X3	T49.0X4	T49.0X5	T49.0X6
Antipruritic drug NEC	T49.1X1	T49.1X2	T49.1X3	T49.1X4	T49.1X5	T49.1X6
Antipsychotic drug	T43.501	T43.502	T43.503	T43.504	T43.505	T43.506
specified NEC	T43.591	T43.592	T43.593	T43.594	T43.595	T43.596
Antipyretic	T39.91	T39.92	T39.93	T39.94	T39.95	T39.96
specified NEC	T39.8X1	T39.8X2	T39.8X3	T39.8X4	T39.8X5	T39.8X6
Antipyrine	T39.2X1	T39.2X2	T39.2X3	T39.2X4	T39.2X5	T39.2X6
Antirabies hyperimmune serum	T50.Z11	T50.Z12	T50.Z13	T50.Z14	T50.Z15	T50.Z16
Antirheumatic NEC	T39.4X1	T39.4X2	T39.4X3	T39.4X4	T39.4X5	T39.4X6
Antirigidity drug NEC	T42.8X1	T42.8X2	T42.8X3	T42.8X4	T42.8X5	T42.8X6
Antischistosomal drug	T37.4X1	T37.4X2	T37.4X3	T37.4X4	T37.4X5	T37.4X6
Antiscorpion sera	T50.Z11	T50.Z12	T50.Z13	T50.Z14	T50.Z15	T50.Z16
Antiseborrheics	T49.4X1	T49.4X2	T49.4X3	T49.4X4	T49.4X5	T49.4X6
Antiseptics (external) (medicinal)	T49.0X1	T49.0X2	T49.0X3	T49.0X4	T49.0X5	T49.0X6
Antistine	T45.0X1	T45.0X2	T45.0X3	T45.0X4	T45.0X5	T45.0X6
Antitapeworm drug	T37.4X1	T37.4X2	T37.4X3	T37.4X4	T37.4X5	T37.4X6
Antitetanus immunoglobulin	T50.Z11	T50.Z12	T50.Z13	T50.Z14	T50.Z15	T50.Z16
Antithyroid drug NEC	T38.2X1	T38.2X2	T38.2X3	T38.2X4	T38.2X5	T38.2X6
Antitoxin	T50.Z11	T50.Z12	T50.Z13	T50.Z14	T50.Z15	T50.Z16
diphtheria	T50.Z11	T50.Z12	T50.Z13	T50.Z14	T50.Z15	T50.Z16
gas gangrene	T50.Z11	T50.Z12	T50.Z13	T50.Z14	T50.Z15	T50.Z16
tetanus	T50.Z11	T50.Z12	T50.Z13	T50.Z14	T50.Z15	T50.Z16
Antitrichomonal drug	T37.3X1	T37.3X2	T37.3X3	T37.3X4	T37.3X5	T37.3X6
Antituberculars	T37.1X1	T37.1X2	T37.1X3	T37.1X4	T37.1X5	T37.1X6
antibiotics	T36.5X1	T36.5X2	T36.5X3	T36.5X4	T36.5X5	T36.5X6
Antitussive NEC	T48.3X1	T48.3X2	T48.3X3	T48.3X4	T48.3X5	T48.3X6
codeine mixture	T40.2X1	T40.2X2	T40.2X3	T40.2X4	T40.2X5	T40.2X6
opiate	T40.2X1	T40.2X2	T40.2X3	T40.2X4	T40.2X5	T40.2X6
Antivaricose drug	T46.8X1	T46.8X2	T46.8X3	T46.8X4	T46.8X5	T46.8X6
Antivenin, antivenom (sera)	T50.Z11	T50.Z12	T50.Z13	T50.Z14	T50.Z15	T50.Z16
crotaline	T50.Z11	T50.Z12	T50.Z13	T50.Z14	T50.Z15	T50.Z16
spider bite	T50.Z11	T50.Z12	T50.Z13	T50.Z14	T50.Z15	T50.Z16
Antivertigo drug	T45.0X1	T45.0X2	T45.0X3	T45.0X4	T45.0X5	T45.0X6
Antiviral drug NEC	T37.5X1	T37.5X2	T37.5X3	T37.5X4	T37.5X5	T37.5X6
eye	T49.5X1	T49.5X2	T49.5X3	T49.5X4	T49.5X5	T49.5X6
Antiwhipworm drug	T37.4X1	T37.4X2	T37.4X3	T37.4X4	T37.4X5	T37.4X6
Ant poison — see Insecticide						
Antrol — see also by specific chemical substance	T60.91	T60.92	T60.93	T60.94	—	—
fungicide	T60.91	T60.92	T60.93	T60.94	—	—
ANTU (alpha naphthylthiourea)	T60.4X1	T60.4X2	T60.4X3	T60.4X4	—	—
Apalcillin	T36.0X1	T36.0X2	T36.0X3	T36.0X4	T36.0X5	T36.0X6
APC	T48.5X1	T48.5X2	T48.5X3	T48.5X4	T48.5X5	T48.5X6
Aplonidine	T44.4X1	T44.4X2	T44.4X3	T44.4X4	T44.4X5	T44.4X6
Apomorphine	T47.7X1	T47.7X2	T47.7X3	T47.7X4	T47.7X5	T47.7X6
Appetite depressants, central	T50.5X1	T50.5X2	T50.5X3	T50.5X4	T50.5X5	T50.5X6
Apraclonidine (hydrochloride)	T44.4X1	T44.4X2	T44.4X3	T44.4X4	T44.4X5	T44.4X6
Apresoline	T46.5X1	T46.5X2	T46.5X3	T46.5X4	T46.5X5	T46.5X6
Aprindine	T46.2X1	T46.2X2	T46.2X3	T46.2X4	T46.2X5	T46.2X6
Aprobarbital	T42.3X1	T42.3X2	T42.3X3	T42.3X4	T42.3X5	T42.3X6
Apronalide	T42.6X1	T42.6X2	T42.6X3	T42.6X4	T42.6X5	T42.6X6
Aprotinin	T45.621	T45.622	T45.623	T45.624	T45.625	T45.626
Aptocaine	T41.3X1	T41.3X2	T41.3X3	T41.3X4	T41.3X5	T41.3X6
Aqua fortis	T54.2X1	T54.2X2	T54.2X3	T54.2X4	—	—
Ara-A	T37.5X1	T37.5X2	T37.5X3	T37.5X4	T37.5X5	T37.5X6
Ara-C	T45.1X1	T45.1X2	T45.1X3	T45.1X4	T45.1X5	T45.1X6
Arachis oil	T49.3X1	T49.3X2	T49.3X3	T49.3X4	T49.3X5	T49.3X6
cathartic	T47.4X1	T47.4X2	T47.4X3	T47.4X4	T47.4X5	T47.4X6
Aralen	T37.2X1	T37.2X2	T37.2X3	T37.2X4	T37.2X5	T37.2X6
Arecoline	T44.1X1	T44.1X2	T44.1X3	T44.1X4	T44.1X5	T44.1X6
Arginine	T50.991	T50.992	T50.993	T50.994	T50.995	T50.996
glutamate	T50.991	T50.992	T50.993	T50.994	T50.995	T50.996
Argyrol	T49.0X1	T49.0X2	T49.0X3	T49.0X4	T49.0X5	T49.0X6
ENT agent	T49.6X1	T49.6X2	T49.6X3	T49.6X4	T49.6X5	T49.6X6

Table of Drugs and Chemicals

Argyrol — Benzalkonium

Substance	Poisoning, Accidental (unintentional)	Poisoning, Intentional Self-harm	Poisoning, Assault	Poisoning, Undetermined	Adverse Effect	Under-dosing
Argyrol — continued						
ophthalmic preparation	T49.5X1	T49.5X2	T49.5X3	T49.5X4	T49.5X5	T49.5X6
Aristocort	T38.0X1	T38.0X2	T38.0X3	T38.0X4	T38.0X5	T38.0X6
ENT agent	T49.6X1	T49.6X2	T49.6X3	T49.6X4	T49.6X5	T49.6X6
ophthalmic preparation	T49.5X1	T49.5X2	T49.5X3	T49.5X4	T49.5X5	T49.5X6
topical NEC	T49.0X1	T49.0X2	T49.0X3	T49.0X4	T49.0X5	T49.0X6
Aromatics, corrosive	T54.1X1	T54.1X2	T54.1X3	T54.1X4	—	—
disinfectants	T54.1X1	T54.1X2	T54.1X3	T54.1X4	—	—
Arsenate of lead	T57.0X1	T57.0X2	T57.0X3	T57.0X4	—	—
herbicide	T57.0X1	T57.0X2	T57.0X3	T57.0X4	—	—
Arsenic, arsenicals (compounds) (dust) (vapor) **NEC**	T57.0X1	T57.0X2	T57.0X3	T57.0X4	—	—
anti-infectives	T37.8X1	T37.8X2	T37.8X3	T37.8X4	T37.8X5	T37.8X6
pesticide (dust) (fumes)	T57.0X1	T57.0X2	T57.0X3	T57.0X4	—	—
Arsine (gas)	T57.0X1	T57.0X2	T57.0X3	T57.0X4	—	—
Arsphenamine (silver)	T37.8X1	T37.8X2	T37.8X3	T37.8X4	T37.8X5	T37.8X6
Arsthinol	T37.3X1	T37.3X2	T37.3X3	T37.3X4	T37.3X5	T37.3X6
Artane	T44.3X1	T44.3X2	T44.3X3	T44.3X4	T44.3X5	T44.3X6
Arthropod (venomous) **NEC**	T63.481	T63.482	T63.483	T63.484	—	—
Articaine	T41.3X1	T41.3X2	T41.3X3	T41.3X4	T41.3X5	T41.3X6
Asbestos	T57.8X1	T57.8X2	T57.8X3	T57.8X4	—	—
Ascaridole	T37.4X1	T37.4X2	T37.4X3	T37.4X4	T37.4X5	T37.4X6
Ascorbic acid	T45.2X1	T45.2X2	T45.2X3	T45.2X4	T45.2X5	T45.2X6
Asiaticoside	T49.0X1	T49.0X2	T49.0X3	T49.0X4	T49.0X5	T49.0X6
Asparaginase	T45.1X1	T45.1X2	T45.1X3	T45.1X4	T45.1X5	T45.1X6
Aspidium (oleoresin)	T37.4X1	T37.4X2	T37.4X3	T37.4X4	T37.4X5	T37.4X6
Aspirin (aluminum) (soluble)	T39.011	T39.012	T39.013	T39.014	T39.015	T39.016
Aspoxicillin	T36.0X1	T36.0X2	T36.0X3	T36.0X4	T36.0X5	T36.0X6
Astemizole	T45.0X1	T45.0X2	T45.0X3	T45.0X4	T45.0X5	T45.0X6
Astringent (local)	T49.2X1	T49.2X2	T49.2X3	T49.2X4	T49.2X5	T49.2X6
specified NEC	T49.2X1	T49.2X2	T49.2X3	T49.2X4	T49.2X5	T49.2X6
Astromicin	T36.5X1	T36.5X2	T36.5X3	T36.5X4	T36.5X5	T36.5X6
Ataractic drug NEC	T43.501	T43.502	T43.503	T43.504	T43.505	T43.506
Atenolol	T44.7X1	T44.7X2	T44.7X3	T44.7X4	T44.7X5	T44.7X6
Atonia drug, intestinal	T47.4X1	T47.4X2	T47.4X3	T47.4X4	T47.4X5	T47.4X6
Atophan	T50.4X1	T50.4X2	T50.4X3	T50.4X4	T50.4X5	T50.4X6
Atracurium besilate	T48.1X1	T48.1X2	T48.1X3	T48.1X4	T48.1X5	T48.1X6
Atropine	T44.3X1	T44.3X2	T44.3X3	T44.3X4	T44.3X5	T44.3X6
derivative	T44.3X1	T44.3X2	T44.3X3	T44.3X4	T44.3X5	T44.3X6
methonitrate	T44.3X1	T44.3X2	T44.3X3	T44.3X4	T44.3X5	T44.3X6
Attapulgite	T47.6X1	T47.6X2	T47.6X3	T47.6X4	T47.6X5	T47.6X6
Auramine	T65.891	T65.892	T65.893	T65.894	—	—
dye	T65.6X1	T65.6X2	T65.6X3	T65.6X4	—	—
fungicide	T60.3X1	T60.3X2	T60.3X3	T60.3X4	—	—
Auranofin	T39.4X1	T39.4X2	T39.4X3	T39.4X4	T39.4X5	T39.4X6
Aurantiin	T46.991	T46.992	T46.993	T46.994	T46.995	T46.996
Aureomycin	T36.4X1	T36.4X2	T36.4X3	T36.4X4	T36.4X5	T36.4X6
ophthalmic preparation	T49.5X1	T49.5X2	T49.5X3	T49.5X4	T49.5X5	T49.5X6
topical NEC	T49.0X1	T49.0X2	T49.0X3	T49.0X4	T49.0X5	T49.0X6
Aurothioglucose	T39.4X1	T39.4X2	T39.4X3	T39.4X4	T39.4X5	T39.4X6
Aurothioglycanide	T39.4X1	T39.4X2	T39.4X3	T39.4X4	T39.4X5	T39.4X6
Aurothiomalate sodium	T39.4X1	T39.4X2	T39.4X3	T39.4X4	T39.4X5	T39.4X6
Aurotioprol	T39.4X1	T39.4X2	T39.4X3	T39.4X4	T39.4X5	T39.4X6
Automobile fuel	T52.0X1	T52.0X2	T52.0X3	T52.0X4	—	—
Autonomic nervous system agent NEC	T44.901	T44.902	T44.903	T44.904	T44.905	T44.906
Avlosulfon	T37.1X1	T37.1X2	T37.1X3	T37.1X4	T37.1X5	T37.1X6
Avomine	T42.6X1	T42.6X2	T42.6X3	T42.6X4	T42.6X5	T42.6X6
Axerophthol	T45.2X1	T45.2X2	T45.2X3	T45.2X4	T45.2X5	T45.2X6
Azacitidine	T45.1X1	T45.1X2	T45.1X3	T45.1X4	T45.1X5	T45.1X6
Azacyclonol	T43.591	T43.592	T43.593	T43.594	T43.595	T43.596
Azadirachta	T60.2X1	T60.2X2	T60.2X3	T60.2X4	—	—
Azanidazole	T37.3X1	T37.3X2	T37.3X3	T37.3X4	T37.3X5	T37.3X6
Azapetine	T46.7X1	T46.7X2	T46.7X3	T46.7X4	T46.7X5	T46.7X6
Azapropazone	T39.2X1	T39.2X2	T39.2X3	T39.2X4	T39.2X5	T39.2X6
Azaribine	T45.1X1	T45.1X2	T45.1X3	T45.1X4	T45.1X5	T45.1X6
Azaserine	T45.1X1	T45.1X2	T45.1X3	T45.1X4	T45.1X5	T45.1X6
Azatadine	T45.0X1	T45.0X2	T45.0X3	T45.0X4	T45.0X5	T45.0X6
Azatepa	T45.1X1	T45.1X2	T45.1X3	T45.1X4	T45.1X5	T45.1X6
Azathioprine	T45.1X1	T45.1X2	T45.1X3	T45.1X4	T45.1X5	T45.1X6
Azelaic acid	T49.0X1	T49.0X2	T49.0X3	T49.0X4	T49.0X5	T49.0X6
Azelastine	T45.0X1	T45.0X2	T45.0X3	T45.0X4	T45.0X5	T45.0X6
Azidocillin	T36.0X1	T36.0X2	T36.0X3	T36.0X4	T36.0X5	T36.0X6
Azidothymidine	T37.5X1	T37.5X2	T37.5X3	T37.5X4	T37.5X5	T37.5X6
Azinphos (ethyl) (methyl)	T60.0X1	T60.0X2	T60.0X3	T60.0X4	—	—
Aziridine (chelating)	T54.1X1	T54.1X2	T54.1X3	T54.1X4	—	—
Azithromycin	T36.3X1	T36.3X2	T36.3X3	T36.3X4	T36.3X5	T36.3X6
Azlocillin	T36.0X1	T36.0X2	T36.0X3	T36.0X4	T36.0X5	T36.0X6
Azobenzene smoke	T65.3X1	T65.3X2	T65.3X3	T65.3X4	—	—
acaricide	T60.8X1	T60.8X2	T60.8X3	T60.8X4	—	—
Azosulfamide	T37.0X1	T37.0X2	T37.0X3	T37.0X4	T37.0X5	T37.0X6
AZT	T37.5X1	T37.5X2	T37.5X3	T37.5X4	T37.5X5	T37.5X6
Aztreonam	T36.1X1	T36.1X2	T36.1X3	T36.1X4	T36.1X5	T36.1X6

Substance	Poisoning, Accidental (unintentional)	Poisoning, Intentional Self-harm	Poisoning, Assault	Poisoning, Undetermined	Adverse Effect	Under-dosing
Azulfidine	T37.0X1	T37.0X2	T37.0X3	T37.0X4	T37.0X5	T37.0X6
Azuresin	T50.8X1	T50.8X2	T50.8X3	T50.8X4	T50.8X5	T50.8X6
b-acetyldigoxin	T46.0X1	T46.0X2	T46.0X3	T46.0X4	T46.0X5	T46.0X6
P-Acetamidophenol	T39.1X1	T39.1X2	T39.1X3	T39.1X4	T39.1X5	T39.1X6
Bacampicillin	T36.0X1	T36.0X2	T36.0X3	T36.0X4	T36.0X5	T36.0X6
Bacillus						
lactobacillus	T47.8X1	T47.8X2	T47.8X3	T47.8X4	T47.8X5	T47.8X6
subtilis	T47.6X1	T47.6X2	T47.6X3	T47.6X4	T47.6X5	T47.6X6
Bacimycin	T49.0X1	T49.0X2	T49.0X3	T49.0X4	T49.0X5	T49.0X6
ophthalmic preparation	T49.5X1	T49.5X2	T49.5X3	T49.5X4	T49.5X5	T49.5X6
Bacitracin zinc	T49.0X1	T49.0X2	T49.0X3	T49.0X4	T49.0X5	T49.0X6
with neomycin	T49.0X1	T49.0X2	T49.0X3	T49.0X4	T49.0X5	T49.0X6
ENT agent	T49.6X1	T49.6X2	T49.6X3	T49.6X4	T49.6X5	T49.6X6
ophthalmic preparation	T49.5X1	T49.5X2	T49.5X3	T49.5X4	T49.5X5	T49.5X6
topical NEC	T49.0X1	T49.0X2	T49.0X3	T49.0X4	T49.0X5	T49.0X6
Baclofen	T42.8X1	T42.8X2	T42.8X3	T42.8X4	T42.8X5	T42.8X6
Baking soda	T50.991	T50.992	T50.993	T50.994	T50.995	T50.996
BAL	T45.8X1	T45.8X2	T45.8X3	T45.8X4	T45.8X5	T45.8X6
Bambuterol	T48.6X1	T48.6X2	T48.6X3	T48.6X4	T48.6X5	T48.6X6
Bamethan (sulfate)	T46.7X1	T46.7X2	T46.7X3	T46.7X4	T46.7X5	T46.7X6
Bamifylline	T48.6X1	T48.6X2	T48.6X3	T48.6X4	T48.6X5	T48.6X6
Bamipine	T45.0X1	T45.0X2	T45.0X3	T45.0X4	T45.0X5	T45.0X6
Baneberry — see Actaea spicata						
Banewort — see Belladonna						
Barbenyl	T42.3X1	T42.3X2	T42.3X3	T42.3X4	T42.3X5	T42.3X6
Barbexaclone	T42.6X1	T42.6X2	T42.6X3	T42.6X4	T42.6X5	T42.6X6
Barbital	T42.3X1	T42.3X2	T42.3X3	T42.3X4	T42.3X5	T42.3X6
sodium	T42.3X1	T42.3X2	T42.3X3	T42.3X4	T42.3X5	T42.3X6
Barbitone	T42.3X1	T42.3X2	T42.3X3	T42.3X4	T42.3X5	T42.3X6
Barbiturate NEC	T42.3X1	T42.3X2	T42.3X3	T42.3X4	T42.3X5	T42.3X6
with tranquilizer	T42.3X1	T42.3X2	T42.3X3	T42.3X4	T42.3X5	T42.3X6
anesthetic (intravenous)	T41.1X1	T41.1X2	T41.1X3	T41.1X4	T41.1X5	T41.1X6
Barium (carbonate) (chloride) (sulfite)	T57.8X1	T57.8X2	T57.8X3	T57.8X4	—	—
diagnostic agent	T50.8X1	T50.8X2	T50.8X3	T50.8X4	T50.8X5	T50.8X6
pesticide	T60.4X1	T60.4X2	T60.4X3	T60.4X4	—	—
rodenticide	T60.4X1	T60.4X2	T60.4X3	T60.4X4	—	—
sulfate (medicinal)	T50.8X1	T50.8X2	T50.8X3	T50.8X4	T50.8X5	T50.8X6
Barrier cream	T49.3X1	T49.3X2	T49.3X3	T49.3X4	T49.3X5	T49.3X6
Basic fuchsin	T49.0X1	T49.0X2	T49.0X3	T49.0X4	T49.0X5	T49.0X6
Battery acid or fluid	T54.2X1	T54.2X2	T54.2X3	T54.2X4	—	—
Bay rum	T51.8X1	T51.8X2	T51.8X3	T51.8X4	—	—
b-benzalbutyramide	T46.6X1	T46.6X2	T46.6X3	T46.6X4	T46.6X5	T46.6X6
BCG (vaccine)	T50.A91	T50.A92	T50.A93	T50.A94	T50.A95	T50.A96
BCNU	T45.1X1	T45.1X2	T45.1X3	T45.1X4	T45.1X5	T45.1X6
Bearsfoot	T62.2X1	T62.2X2	T62.2X3	T62.2X4	—	—
Beclamide	T42.6X1	T42.6X2	T42.6X3	T42.6X4	T42.6X5	T42.6X6
Beclomethasone	T44.5X1	T44.5X2	T44.5X3	T44.5X4	T44.5X5	T44.5X6
Bee (sting) (venom)	T63.441	T63.442	T63.443	T63.444	—	—
Befunolol	T49.5X1	T49.5X2	T49.5X3	T49.5X4	T49.5X5	T49.5X6
Bekanamycin	T36.5X1	T36.5X2	T36.5X3	T36.5X4	T36.5X5	T36.5X6
Belladonna — see also Nightshade						
alkaloids	T44.3X1	T44.3X2	T44.3X3	T44.3X4	T44.3X5	T44.3X6
extract	T44.3X1	T44.3X2	T44.3X3	T44.3X4	T44.3X5	T44.3X6
herb	T44.3X1	T44.3X2	T44.3X3	T44.3X4	T44.3X5	T44.3X6
Bemegride	T50.7X1	T50.7X2	T50.7X3	T50.7X4	T50.7X5	T50.7X6
Benactyzine	T44.3X1	T44.3X2	T44.3X3	T44.3X4	T44.3X5	T44.3X6
Benadryl	T45.0X1	T45.0X2	T45.0X3	T45.0X4	T45.0X5	T45.0X6
Benaprizine	T44.3X1	T44.3X2	T44.3X3	T44.3X4	T44.3X5	T44.3X6
Benazepril	T46.4X1	T46.4X2	T46.4X3	T46.4X4	T46.4X5	T46.4X6
Bencyclane	T46.7X1	T46.7X2	T46.7X3	T46.7X4	T46.7X5	T46.7X6
Bendazol	T46.3X1	T46.3X2	T46.3X3	T46.3X4	T46.3X5	T46.3X6
Bendrofluazide	T50.2X1	T50.2X2	T50.2X3	T50.2X4	T50.2X5	T50.2X6
Bendroflumethiazide	T50.2X1	T50.2X2	T50.2X3	T50.2X4	T50.2X5	T50.2X6
Benemid	T50.4X1	T50.4X2	T50.4X3	T50.4X4	T50.4X5	T50.4X6
Benethamine penicillin	T36.0X1	T36.0X2	T36.0X3	T36.0X4	T36.0X5	T36.0X6
Benexate	T47.1X1	T47.1X2	T47.1X3	T47.1X4	T47.1X5	T47.1X6
Benfluorex	T46.6X1	T46.6X2	T46.6X3	T46.6X4	T46.6X5	T46.6X6
Benfotiamine	T45.2X1	T45.2X2	T45.2X3	T45.2X4	T45.2X5	T45.2X6
Benisone	T49.0X1	T49.0X2	T49.0X3	T49.0X4	T49.0X5	T49.0X6
Benomyl	T60.0X1	T60.0X2	T60.0X3	T60.0X4	—	—
Benoquin	T49.8X1	T49.8X2	T49.8X3	T49.8X4	T49.8X5	T49.8X6
Benoxinate	T41.3X1	T41.3X2	T41.3X3	T41.3X4	T41.3X5	T41.3X6
Benperidol	T43.4X1	T43.4X2	T43.4X3	T43.4X4	T43.4X5	T43.4X6
Benproperine	T48.3X1	T48.3X2	T48.3X3	T48.3X4	T48.3X5	T48.3X6
Benserazide	T42.8X1	T42.8X2	T42.8X3	T42.8X4	T42.8X5	T42.8X6
Bentazepam	T42.4X1	T42.4X2	T42.4X3	T42.4X4	T42.4X5	T42.4X6
Bentiromide	T50.8X1	T50.8X2	T50.8X3	T50.8X4	T50.8X5	T50.8X6
Bentonite	T49.3X1	T49.3X2	T49.3X3	T49.3X4	T49.3X5	T49.3X6
Benzalbutyramide	T46.6X1	T46.6X2	T46.6X3	T46.6X4	T46.6X5	T46.6X6
Benzalkonium (chloride)	T49.0X1	T49.0X2	T49.0X3	T49.0X4	T49.0X5	T49.0X6
ophthalmic preparation	T49.5X1	T49.5X2	T49.5X3	T49.5X4	T49.5X5	T49.5X6

Substance	Poisoning, Accidental (unintentional)	Poisoning, Intentional Self-harm	Poisoning, Assault	Poisoning, Undetermined	Adverse Effect	Under-dosing
Benzamidosalicylate (calcium)	T37.1X1	T37.1X2	T37.1X3	T37.1X4	T37.1X5	T37.1X6
Benzamine	T41.3X1	T41.3X2	T41.3X3	T41.3X4	T41.3X5	T41.3X6
lactate	T49.1X1	T49.1X2	T49.1X3	T49.1X4	T49.1X5	T49.1X6
Benzamphetamine	T50.5X1	T50.5X2	T50.5X3	T50.5X4	T50.5X5	T50.5X6
Benzapril hydrochloride	T46.5X1	T46.5X2	T46.5X3	T46.5X4	T46.5X5	T46.5X6
Benzathine benzylpenicillin	T36.0X1	T36.0X2	T36.0X3	T36.0X4	T36.0X5	T36.0X6
Benzathine penicillin	T36.0X1	T36.0X2	T36.0X3	T36.0X4	T36.0X5	T36.0X6
Benzatropine	T42.8X1	T42.8X2	T42.8X3	T42.8X4	T42.8X5	T42.8X6
Benzbromarone	T50.4X1	T50.4X2	T50.4X3	T50.4X4	T50.4X5	T50.4X6
Benzcarbimine	T45.1X1	T45.1X2	T45.1X3	T45.1X4	T45.1X5	T45.1X6
Benzedrex	T44.991	T44.992	T44.993	T44.994	T44.995	T44.996
Benzedrine (amphetamine)	T43.621	T43.622	T43.623	T43.624	T43.625	T43.626
Benzenamine	T65.3X1	T65.3X2	T65.3X3	T65.3X4	—	—
Benzene	T52.1X1	T52.1X2	T52.1X3	T52.1X4	—	—
homologues (acetyl) (dimethyl) (methyl) (solvent)	T52.2X1	T52.2X2	T52.2X3	T52.2X4	—	—
Benzethonium (chloride)	T49.0X1	T49.0X2	T49.0X3	T49.0X4	T49.0X5	T49.0X6
Benzfetamine	T50.5X1	T50.5X2	T50.5X3	T50.5X4	T50.5X5	T50.5X6
Benzhexol	T44.3X1	T44.3X2	T44.3X3	T44.3X4	T44.3X5	T44.3X6
Benzhydramine (chloride)	T45.0X1	T45.0X2	T45.0X3	T45.0X4	T45.0X5	T45.0X6
Benzidine	T65.891	T65.892	T65.893	T65.894	—	—
Benzilonium bromide	T44.3X1	T44.3X2	T44.3X3	T44.3X4	T44.3X5	T44.3X6
Benzimidazole	T60.3X1	T60.3X2	T60.3X3	T60.3X4	—	—
Benzin (e) — see Ligroin						
Benziodarone	T46.3X1	T46.3X2	T46.3X3	T46.3X4	T46.3X5	T46.3X6
Benznidazole	T37.3X1	T37.3X2	T37.3X3	T37.3X4	T37.3X5	T37.3X6
Benzocaine	T41.3X1	T41.3X2	T41.3X3	T41.3X4	T41.3X5	T41.3X6
Benzodiapin	T42.4X1	T42.4X2	T42.4X3	T42.4X4	T42.4X5	T42.4X6
Benzodiazepine NEC	T42.4X1	T42.4X2	T42.4X3	T42.4X4	T42.4X5	T42.4X6
Benzoic acid	T49.0X1	T49.0X2	T49.0X3	T49.0X4	T49.0X5	T49.0X6
with salicylic acid	T49.0X1	T49.0X2	T49.0X3	T49.0X4	T49.0X5	T49.0X6
Benzoin (tincture)	T48.5X1	T48.5X2	T48.5X3	T48.5X4	T48.5X5	T48.5X6
Benzol (benzene)	T52.1X1	T52.1X2	T52.1X3	T52.1X4	—	—
vapor	T52.0X1	T52.0X2	T52.0X3	T52.0X4	—	—
Benzomorphan	T40.2X1	T40.2X2	T40.2X3	T40.2X4	T40.2X5	T40.2X6
Benzonatate	T48.3X1	T48.3X2	T48.3X3	T48.3X4	T48.3X5	T48.3X6
Benzophenones	T49.3X1	T49.3X2	T49.3X3	T49.3X4	T49.3X5	T49.3X6
Benzopyrone	T46.991	T46.992	T46.993	T46.994	T46.995	T46.996
Benzothiadiazides	T50.2X1	T50.2X2	T50.2X3	T50.2X4	T50.2X5	T50.2X6
Benzoxonium chloride	T49.0X1	T49.0X2	T49.0X3	T49.0X4	T49.0X5	T49.0X6
Benzoylpas calcium	T37.1X1	T37.1X2	T37.1X3	T37.1X4	T37.1X5	T37.1X6
Benzoyl peroxide	T49.0X1	T49.0X2	T49.0X3	T49.0X4	T49.0X5	T49.0X6
Benzperidin	T43.591	T43.592	T43.593	T43.594	T43.595	T43.596
Benzperidol	T43.591	T43.592	T43.593	T43.594	T43.595	T43.596
Benzphetamine	T50.5X1	T50.5X2	T50.5X3	T50.5X4	T50.5X5	T50.5X6
Benzpyrinium bromide	T44.1X1	T44.1X2	T44.1X3	T44.1X4	T44.1X5	T44.1X6
Benzquinamide	T45.0X1	T45.0X2	T45.0X3	T45.0X4	T45.0X5	T45.0X6
Benzthiazide	T50.2X1	T50.2X2	T50.2X3	T50.2X4	T50.2X5	T50.2X6
Benztropine						
anticholinergic	T44.3X1	T44.3X2	T44.3X3	T44.3X4	T44.3X5	T44.3X6
antiparkinson	T42.8X1	T42.8X2	T42.8X3	T42.8X4	T42.8X5	T42.8X6
Benzydamine	T49.0X1	T49.0X2	T49.0X3	T49.0X4	T49.0X5	T49.0X6
Benzyl						
acetate	T52.8X1	T52.8X2	T52.8X3	T52.8X4	—	—
alcohol	T49.0X1	T49.0X2	T49.0X3	T49.0X4	T49.0X5	T49.0X6
benzoate	T49.0X1	T49.0X2	T49.0X3	T49.0X4	T49.0X5	T49.0X6
Benzoic acid	T49.0X1	T49.0X2	T49.0X3	T49.0X4	T49.0X5	T49.0X6
morphine	T40.2X1	T40.2X2	T40.2X3	T40.2X4	—	—
nicotinate	T46.6X1	T46.6X2	T46.6X3	T46.6X4	T46.6X5	T46.6X6
penicillin	T36.0X1	T36.0X2	T36.0X3	T36.0X4	T36.0X5	T36.0X6
Benzylhydrochlorthiazide	T50.2X1	T50.2X2	T50.2X3	T50.2X4	T50.2X5	T50.2X6
Benzylpenicillin	T36.0X1	T36.0X2	T36.0X3	T36.0X4	T36.0X5	T36.0X6
Benzylthiouracil	T38.2X1	T38.2X2	T38.2X3	T38.2X4	T38.2X5	T38.2X6
Bephenium hydroxynaphthoate	T37.4X1	T37.4X2	T37.4X3	T37.4X4	T37.4X5	T37.4X6
Bepridil	T46.1X1	T46.1X2	T46.1X3	T46.1X4	T46.1X5	T46.1X6
Bergamot oil	T65.891	T65.892	T65.893	T65.894	—	—
Bergapten	T50.991	T50.992	T50.993	T50.994	T50.995	T50.996
Berries, poisonous	T62.1X1	T62.1X2	T62.1X3	T62.1X4	—	—
Beryllium (compounds)	T56.7X1	T56.7X2	T56.7X3	T56.7X4	—	—
beta adrenergic blocking agent, heart	T44.7X1	T44.7X2	T44.7X3	T44.7X4	T44.7X5	T44.7X6
Betacarotene	T45.2X1	T45.2X2	T45.2X3	T45.2X4	T45.2X5	T45.2X6
Beta-Chlor	T42.6X1	T42.6X2	T42.6X3	T42.6X4	T42.6X5	T42.6X6
Betahistine	T46.7X1	T46.7X2	T46.7X3	T46.7X4	T46.7X5	T46.7X6
Betaine	T47.5X1	T47.5X2	T47.5X3	T47.5X4	T47.5X5	T47.5X6
Betamethasone	T49.0X1	T49.0X2	T49.0X3	T49.0X4	T49.0X5	T49.0X6
topical	T49.0X1	T49.0X2	T49.0X3	T49.0X4	T49.0X5	T49.0X6
Betamicin	T36.8X1	T36.8X2	T36.8X3	T36.8X4	T36.8X5	T36.8X6
Betanidine	T46.5X1	T46.5X2	T46.5X3	T46.5X4	T46.5X5	T46.5X6
Betaxolol	T44.7X1	T44.7X2	T44.7X3	T44.7X4	T44.7X5	T44.7X6

Substance	Poisoning, Accidental (unintentional)	Poisoning, Intentional Self-harm	Poisoning, Assault	Poisoning, Undetermined	Adverse Effect	Under-dosing
Betazole	T50.8X1	T50.8X2	T50.8X3	T50.8X4	T50.8X5	T50.8X6
Bethanechol	T44.1X1	T44.1X2	T44.1X3	T44.1X4	T44.1X5	T44.1X6
chloride	T44.1X1	T44.1X2	T44.1X3	T44.1X4	T44.1X5	T44.1X6
Bethanidine	T46.5X1	T46.5X2	T46.5X3	T46.5X4	T46.5X5	T46.5X6
Betoxycaine	T41.3X1	T41.3X2	T41.3X3	T41.3X4	T41.3X5	T41.3X6
Betula oil	T49.3X1	T49.3X2	T49.3X3	T49.3X4	T49.3X5	T49.3X6
Bevantolol	T44.7X1	T44.7X2	T44.7X3	T44.7X4	T44.7X5	T44.7X6
Bevonium metilsulfate	T44.3X1	T44.3X2	T44.3X3	T44.3X4	T44.3X5	T44.3X6
Bezafibrate	T46.6X1	T46.6X2	T46.6X3	T46.6X4	T46.6X5	T46.6X6
Bezitramide	T40.4X1	T40.4X2	T40.4X3	T40.4X4	T40.4X5	T40.4X6
BHA	T50.991	T50.992	T50.993	T50.994	T50.995	T50.996
Bhang	T40.7X1	T40.7X2	T40.7X3	T40.7X4	T40.7X5	T40.7X6
BHC (medicinal)	T49.0X1	T49.0X2	T49.0X3	T49.0X4	T49.0X5	T49.0X6
nonmedicinal (vapor)	T53.6X1	T53.6X2	T53.6X3	T53.6X4	—	—
Bialamicol	T37.3X1	T37.3X2	T37.3X3	T37.3X4	T37.3X5	T37.3X6
Bibenzonium bromide	T48.3X1	T48.3X2	T48.3X3	T48.3X4	T48.3X5	T48.3X6
Bibrocathol	T49.5X1	T49.5X2	T49.5X3	T49.5X4	T49.5X5	T49.5X6
Bichloride of mercury — see Mercury, chloride						
Bichromates (calcium) (potassium)(sodium) (crystals)	T57.8X1	T57.8X2	T57.8X3	T57.8X4		
fumes	T56.2X1	T56.2X2	T56.2X3	T56.2X4		
Biclotymol	T49.6X1	T49.6X2	T49.6X3	T49.6X4	T49.6X5	T49.6X6
Bicucculine	T50.7X1	T50.7X2	T50.7X3	T50.7X4	T50.7X5	T50.7X6
Bifemelane	T43.291	T43.292	T43.293	T43.294	T43.295	T43.296
Biguanide derivatives, oral	T38.3X1	T38.3X2	T38.3X3	T38.3X4	T38.3X5	T38.3X6
Bile salts	T47.5X1	T47.5X2	T47.5X3	T47.5X4	T47.5X5	T47.5X6
Biligrafin	T50.8X1	T50.8X2	T50.8X3	T50.8X4	T50.8X5	T50.8X6
Bilopaque	T50.8X1	T50.8X2	T50.8X3	T50.8X4	T50.8X5	T50.8X6
Binifibrate	T46.6X1	T46.6X2	T46.6X3	T46.6X4	T46.6X5	T46.6X6
Binitrobenzol	T65.3X1	T65.3X2	T65.3X3	T65.3X4	—	—
Bioflavonoid(s)	T46.991	T46.992	T46.993	T46.994	T46.995	T46.996
Biological substance NEC	T50.901	T50.902	T50.903	T50.904	T50.905	T50.906
Biotin	T45.2X1	T45.2X2	T45.2X3	T45.2X4	T45.2X5	T45.2X6
Biperiden	T44.3X1	T44.3X2	T44.3X3	T44.3X4	T44.3X5	T44.3X6
Bisacodyl	T47.2X1	T47.2X2	T47.2X3	T47.2X4	T47.2X5	T47.2X6
Bisbentiamine	T45.2X1	T45.2X2	T45.2X3	T45.2X4	T45.2X5	T45.2X6
Bisbutiamine	T45.2X1	T45.2X2	T45.2X3	T45.2X4	T45.2X5	T45.2X6
Bisdequalinium (salts) (diacetate)	T49.6X1	T49.6X2	T49.6X3	T49.6X4	T49.6X5	T49.6X6
Bishydroxycoumarin	T45.511	T45.512	T45.513	T45.514	T45.515	T45.516
Bismarsen	T37.8X1	T37.8X2	T37.8X3	T37.8X4	T37.8X5	T37.8X6
Bismuth salts	T47.6X1	T47.6X2	T47.6X3	T47.6X4	T47.6X5	T47.6X6
aluminate	T47.1X1	T47.1X2	T47.1X3	T47.1X4	T47.1X5	T47.1X6
anti-infectives	T37.8X1	T37.8X2	T37.8X3	T37.8X4	T37.8X5	T37.8X6
formic iodide	T49.0X1	T49.0X2	T49.0X3	T49.0X4	T49.0X5	T49.0X6
glycolylarsenate	T49.0X1	T49.0X2	T49.0X3	T49.0X4	T49.0X5	T49.0X6
nonmedicinal (compounds) NEC	T65.91	T65.92	T65.93	T65.94	—	—
subcarbonate	T47.6X1	T47.6X2	T47.6X3	T47.6X4	T47.6X5	T47.6X6
subsalicylate	T37.8X1	T37.8X2	T37.8X3	T37.8X4	T37.8X5	T37.8X6
sulfarsphenamine	T37.8X1	T37.8X2	T37.8X3	T37.8X4	T37.8X5	T37.8X6
Bisoprolol	T44.7X1	T44.7X2	T44.7X3	T44.7X4	T44.7X5	T44.7X6
Bisoxatin	T47.2X1	T47.2X2	T47.2X3	T47.2X4	T47.2X5	T47.2X6
Bisulepin (hydrochloride)	T45.0X1	T45.0X2	T45.0X3	T45.0X4	T45.0X5	T45.0X6
Bithionol	T37.8X1	T37.8X2	T37.8X3	T37.8X4	T37.8X5	T37.8X6
anthelminthic	T37.4X1	T37.4X2	T37.4X3	T37.4X4	T37.4X5	T37.4X6
Bitolterol	T48.6X1	T48.6X2	T48.6X3	T48.6X4	T48.6X5	T48.6X6
Bitoscanate	T37.4X1	T37.4X2	T37.4X3	T37.4X4	T37.4X5	T37.4X6
Bitter almond oil	T62.8X1	T62.8X2	T62.8X3	T62.8X4	—	—
Bittersweet	T62.2X1	T62.2X2	T62.2X3	T62.2X4	—	—
Black						
flag	T60.91	T60.92	T60.93	T60.94	—	—
henbane	T62.2X1	T62.2X2	T62.2X3	T62.2X4	—	—
leaf (40)	T60.91	T60.92	T60.93	T60.94	—	—
widow spider (bite)	T63.311	T63.312	T63.313	T63.314	—	—
antivenin	T50.Z11	T50.Z12	T50.Z13	T50.Z14	T50.Z15	T50.Z16
Blast furnace gas (carbon monoxide from)	T58.8X1	T58.8X2	T58.8X3	T58.8X4	—	—
Bleach	T54.91	T54.92	T54.93	T54.94	—	—
Bleaching agent (medicinal)	T49.4X1	T49.4X2	T49.4X3	T49.4X4	T49.4X5	T49.4X6
Bleomycin	T45.1X1	T45.1X2	T45.1X3	T45.1X4	T45.1X5	T45.1X6
Blockain	T41.3X1	T41.3X2	T41.3X3	T41.3X4	T41.3X5	T41.3X6
infiltration (subcutaneous)	T41.3X1	T41.3X2	T41.3X3	T41.3X4	T41.3X5	T41.3X6
nerve block (peripheral) (plexus)	T41.3X1	T41.3X2	T41.3X3	T41.3X4	T41.3X5	T41.3X6
topical (surface)	T41.3X1	T41.3X2	T41.3X3	T41.3X4	T41.3X5	T41.3X6
Blockers, calcium channel	T46.1X1	T46.1X2	T46.1X3	T46.1X4	T46.1X5	T46.1X6
Blood (derivatives) (natural) (plasma) (whole)	T45.8X1	T45.8X2	T45.8X3	T45.8X4	T45.8X5	T45.8X6
dried	T45.8X1	T45.8X2	T45.8X3	T45.8X4	T45.8X5	T45.8X6
drug affecting NEC	T45.91	T45.92	T45.93	T45.94	T45.95	T45.96

Table of Drugs and Chemicals

Blood — Butyl

Substance	Poisoning, Accidental (unintentional)	Poisoning, Intentional Self-harm	Poisoning, Assault	Poisoning, Undetermined	Adverse Effect	Under-dosing
Blood — continued						
expander NEC	T45.8X1	T45.8X2	T45.8X3	T45.8X4	T45.8X5	T45.8X6
fraction NEC	T45.8X1	T45.8X2	T45.8X3	T45.8X4	T45.8X5	T45.8X6
substitute (macromolecular)	T45.8X1	T45.8X2	T45.8X3	T45.8X4	T45.8X5	T45.8X6
Blue velvet	T40.2X1	T40.2X2	T40.2X3	T40.2X4	—	—
Bone meal	T62.8X1	T62.8X2	T62.8X3	T62.8X4	—	—
Bonine	T45.0X1	T45.0X2	T45.0X3	T45.0X4	T45.0X5	T45.0X6
Bopindolol	T44.7X1	T44.7X2	T44.7X3	T44.7X4	T44.7X5	T44.7X6
Boracic acid	T49.0X1	T49.0X2	T49.0X3	T49.0X4	T49.0X5	T49.0X6
ENT agent	T49.6X1	T49.6X2	T49.6X3	T49.6X4	T49.6X5	T49.6X6
ophthalmic preparation	T49.5X1	T49.5X2	T49.5X3	T49.5X4	T49.5X5	T49.5X6
Borane complex	T57.8X1	T57.8X2	T57.8X3	T57.8X4	—	—
Borate(s)	T57.8X1	T57.8X2	T57.8X3	T57.8X4	—	—
buffer	T50.991	T50.992	T50.993	T50.994	T50.995	T50.996
cleanser	T54.91	T54.92	T54.93	T54.94	—	—
sodium	T57.8X1	T57.8X2	T57.8X3	T57.8X4	—	—
Borax (cleanser)	T54.91	T54.92	T54.93	T54.94	—	—
Bordeaux mixture	T60.3X1	T60.3X2	T60.3X3	T60.3X4	—	—
Boric acid	T49.0X1	T49.0X2	T49.0X3	T49.0X4	T49.0X5	T49.0X6
ENT agent	T49.6X1	T49.6X2	T49.6X3	T49.6X4	T49.6X5	T49.6X6
ophthalmic preparation	T49.5X1	T49.5X2	T49.5X3	T49.5X4	T49.5X5	T49.5X6
Bornaprine	T44.3X1	T44.3X2	T44.3X3	T44.3X4	T44.3X5	T44.3X6
Boron	T57.8X1	T57.8X2	T57.8X3	T57.8X4	—	—
hydride NEC	T57.8X1	T57.8X2	T57.8X3	T57.8X4	—	—
fumes or gas	T57.8X1	T57.8X2	T57.8X3	T57.8X4	—	—
trifluoride	T59.891	T59.892	T59.893	T59.894	—	—
Botox	T48.291	T48.292	T48.293	T48.294	T48.295	T48.296
Botulinus anti-toxin (type A, B)	T50.Z11	T50.Z12	T50.Z13	T50.Z14	T50.Z15	T50.Z16
Brake fluid vapor	T59.891	T59.892	T59.893	T59.894	—	—
Brallobarbital	T42.3X1	T42.3X2	T42.3X3	T42.3X4	T42.3X5	T42.3X6
Bran (wheat)	T47.4X1	T47.4X2	T47.4X3	T47.4X4	T47.4X5	T47.4X6
Brass (fumes)	T56.891	T56.892	T56.893	T56.894	—	—
Brasso	T52.0X1	T52.0X2	T52.0X3	T52.0X4	—	—
Bretylium tosilate	T46.2X1	T46.2X2	T46.2X3	T46.2X4	T46.2X5	T46.2X6
Brevital (sodium)	T41.1X1	T41.1X2	T41.1X3	T41.1X4	T41.1X5	T41.1X6
Brinase	T45.3X1	T45.3X2	T45.3X3	T45.3X4	T45.3X5	T45.3X6
British antilewisite	T45.8X1	T45.8X2	T45.8X3	T45.8X4	T45.8X5	T45.8X6
Brodifacoum	T60.4X1	T60.4X2	T60.4X3	T60.4X4	—	—
Bromal (hydrate)	T42.6X1	T42.6X2	T42.6X3	T42.6X4	T42.6X5	T42.6X6
Bromazepam	T42.4X1	T42.4X2	T42.4X3	T42.4X4	T42.4X5	T42.4X6
Bromazine	T45.0X1	T45.0X2	T45.0X3	T45.0X4	T45.0X5	T45.0X6
Brombenzylcyanide	T59.3X1	T59.3X2	T59.3X3	T59.3X4	—	—
Bromelains	T45.3X1	T45.3X2	T45.3X3	T45.3X4	T45.3X5	T45.3X6
Bromethalin	T60.4X1	T60.4X2	T60.4X3	T60.4X4	—	—
Bromhexine	T48.4X1	T48.4X2	T48.4X3	T48.4X4	T48.4X5	T48.4X6
Bromide salts	T42.6X1	T42.6X2	T42.6X3	T42.6X4	T42.6X5	T42.6X6
Bromindione	T45.511	T45.512	T45.513	T45.514	T45.515	T45.516
Bromine						
compounds (medicinal)	T42.6X1	T42.6X2	T42.6X3	T42.6X4	T42.6X5	T42.6X6
sedative	T42.6X1	T42.6X2	T42.6X3	T42.6X4	T42.6X5	T42.6X6
vapor	T59.891	T59.892	T59.893	T59.894	—	—
Bromisoval	T42.6X1	T42.6X2	T42.6X3	T42.6X4	T42.6X5	T42.6X6
Bromisovalum	T42.6X1	T42.6X2	T42.6X3	T42.6X4	T42.6X5	T42.6X6
Bromobenzylcyanide	T59.3X1	T59.3X2	T59.3X3	T59.3X4	—	—
Bromochlorosalicylani-lide	T49.0X1	T49.0X2	T49.0X3	T49.0X4	T49.0X5	T49.0X6
Bromocriptine	T42.8X1	T42.8X2	T42.8X3	T42.8X4	T42.8X5	T42.8X6
Bromodiphenhydramine	T45.0X1	T45.0X2	T45.0X3	T45.0X4	T45.0X5	T45.0X6
Bromoform	T42.6X1	T42.6X2	T42.6X3	T42.6X4	T42.6X5	T42.6X6
Bromophenol blue reagent	T50.991	T50.992	T50.993	T50.994	T50.995	T50.996
Bromopride	T47.8X1	T47.8X2	T47.8X3	T47.8X4	T47.8X5	T47.8X6
Bromosalicylchloranitide	T49.0X1	T49.0X2	T49.0X3	T49.0X4	T49.0X5	T49.0X6
Bromosalicylhydroxamic acid	T37.1X1	T37.1X2	T37.1X3	T37.1X4	T37.1X5	T37.1X6
Bromo-seltzer	T39.1X1	T39.1X2	T39.1X3	T39.1X4	T39.1X5	T39.1X6
Bromoxynil	T60.3X1	T60.3X2	T60.3X3	T60.3X4	—	—
Bromperidol	T43.4X1	T43.4X2	T43.4X3	T43.4X4	T43.4X5	T43.4X6
Brompheniramine	T45.0X1	T45.0X2	T45.0X3	T45.0X4	T45.0X5	T45.0X6
Bromsulfophthalein	T50.8X1	T50.8X2	T50.8X3	T50.8X4	T50.8X5	T50.8X6
Bromural	T42.6X1	T42.6X2	T42.6X3	T42.6X4	T42.6X5	T42.6X6
Bromvaletone	T42.6X1	T42.6X2	T42.6X3	T42.6X4	T42.6X5	T42.6X6
Bronchodilator NEC	T48.6X1	T48.6X2	T48.6X3	T48.6X4	T48.6X5	T48.6X6
Brotizolam	T42.4X1	T42.4X2	T42.4X3	T42.4X4	T42.4X5	T42.4X6
Brovincamine	T46.7X1	T46.7X2	T46.7X3	T46.7X4	T46.7X5	T46.7X6
Brown recluse spider (bite) (venom)	T63.331	T63.332	T63.333	T63.334	—	—
Brown spider (bite) (venom)	T63.391	T63.392	T63.393	T63.394	—	—
Broxaterol	T48.6X1	T48.6X2	T48.6X3	T48.6X4	T48.6X5	T48.6X6
Broxuridine	T45.1X1	T45.1X2	T45.1X3	T45.1X4	T45.1X5	T45.1X6
Broxyquinoline	T37.8X1	T37.8X2	T37.8X3	T37.8X4	T37.8X5	T37.8X6
Bruceine	T48.291	T48.292	T48.293	T48.294	T48.295	T48.296
Brucia	T62.2X1	T62.2X2	T62.2X3	T62.2X4	—	—
Brucine	T65.1X1	T65.1X2	T65.1X3	T65.1X4	—	—
Brunswick green — see Copper						
Bruten — see Ibuprofen						
Bryonia	T47.2X1	T47.2X2	T47.2X3	T47.2X4	T47.2X5	T47.2X6
Buclizine	T45.0X1	T45.0X2	T45.0X3	T45.0X4	T45.0X5	T45.0X6
Buclosamide	T49.0X1	T49.0X2	T49.0X3	T49.0X4	T49.0X5	T49.0X6
Budesonide	T44.5X1	T44.5X2	T44.5X3	T44.5X4	T44.5X5	T44.5X6
Budralazine	T46.5X1	T46.5X2	T46.5X3	T46.5X4	T46.5X5	T46.5X6
Bufferin	T39.011	T39.012	T39.013	T39.014	T39.015	T39.016
Buflomedil	T46.7X1	T46.7X2	T46.7X3	T46.7X4	T46.7X5	T46.7X6
Buformin	T38.3X1	T38.3X2	T38.3X3	T38.3X4	T38.3X5	T38.3X6
Bufotenine	T40.991	T40.992	T40.993	T40.994	—	—
Bufrolin	T48.6X1	T48.6X2	T48.6X3	T48.6X4	T48.6X5	T48.6X6
Bufylline	T48.6X1	T48.6X2	T48.6X3	T48.6X4	T48.6X5	T48.6X6
Bulk filler	T50.5X1	T50.5X2	T50.5X3	T50.5X4	T50.5X5	T50.5X6
cathartic	T47.4X1	T47.4X2	T47.4X3	T47.4X4	T47.4X5	T47.4X6
Bumetanide	T50.1X1	T50.1X2	T50.1X3	T50.1X4	T50.1X5	T50.1X6
Bunaftine	T46.2X1	T46.2X2	T46.2X3	T46.2X4	T46.2X5	T46.2X6
Bunamiodyl	T50.8X1	T50.8X2	T50.8X3	T50.8X4	T50.8X5	T50.8X6
Bunazosin	T44.6X1	T44.6X2	T44.6X3	T44.6X4	T44.6X5	T44.6X6
Bunitrolol	T44.7X1	T44.7X2	T44.7X3	T44.7X4	T44.7X5	T44.7X6
Buphenine	T46.7X1	T46.7X2	T46.7X3	T46.7X4	T46.7X5	T46.7X6
Bupivacaine	T41.3X1	T41.3X2	T41.3X3	T41.3X4	T41.3X5	T41.3X6
infiltration (subcutaneous)	T41.3X1	T41.3X2	T41.3X3	T41.3X4	T41.3X5	T41.3X6
nerve block (peripheral) (plexus)	T41.3X1	T41.3X2	T41.3X3	T41.3X4	T41.3X5	T41.3X6
spinal	T41.3X1	T41.3X2	T41.3X3	T41.3X4	T41.3X5	T41.3X6
Bupranolol	T44.7X1	T44.7X2	T44.7X3	T44.7X4	T44.7X5	T44.7X6
Buprenorphine	T40.4X1	T40.4X2	T40.4X3	T40.4X4	T40.4X5	T40.4X6
Bupropion	T43.291	T43.292	T43.293	T43.294	T43.295	T43.296
Burimamide	T47.1X1	T47.1X2	T47.1X3	T47.1X4	T47.1X5	T47.1X6
Buserelin	T38.891	T38.892	T38.893	T38.894	T38.895	T38.896
Buspirone	T43.591	T43.592	T43.593	T43.594	T43.595	T43.596
Busulfan, busulphan	T45.1X1	T45.1X2	T45.1X3	T45.1X4	T45.1X5	T45.1X6
Butabarbital (sodium)	T42.3X1	T42.3X2	T42.3X3	T42.3X4	T42.3X5	T42.3X6
Butabarbitone	T42.3X1	T42.3X2	T42.3X3	T42.3X4	T42.3X5	T42.3X6
Butabarpal	T42.3X1	T42.3X2	T42.3X3	T42.3X4	T42.3X5	T42.3X6
Butacaine	T41.3X1	T41.3X2	T41.3X3	T41.3X4	T41.3X5	T41.3X6
Butalamine	T46.7X1	T46.7X2	T46.7X3	T46.7X4	T46.7X5	T46.7X6
Butalbital	T42.3X1	T42.3X2	T42.3X3	T42.3X4	T42.3X5	T42.3X6
Butallylonal	T42.3X1	T42.3X2	T42.3X3	T42.3X4	T42.3X5	T42.3X6
Butamben	T41.3X1	T41.3X2	T41.3X3	T41.3X4	T41.3X5	T41.3X6
Butamirate	T48.3X1	T48.3X2	T48.3X3	T48.3X4	T48.3X5	T48.3X6
Butane (distributed in mobile container)	T59.891	T59.892	T59.893	T59.894	—	—
distributed through pipes	T59.891	T59.892	T59.893	T59.894	—	—
incomplete combustion	T58.11	T58.12	T58.13	T58.14	—	—
Butanilicaine	T41.3X1	T41.3X2	T41.3X3	T41.3X4	T41.3X5	T41.3X6
Butanol	T51.3X1	T51.3X2	T51.3X3	T51.3X4	—	—
Butanone, 2-butanone	T52.4X1	T52.4X2	T52.4X3	T52.4X4	—	—
Butantrone	T49.4X1	T49.4X2	T49.4X3	T49.4X4	T49.4X5	T49.4X6
Butaperazine	T43.3X1	T43.3X2	T43.3X3	T43.3X4	T43.3X5	T43.3X6
Butazolidin	T39.2X1	T39.2X2	T39.2X3	T39.2X4	T39.2X5	T39.2X6
Butetamate	T48.6X1	T48.6X2	T48.6X3	T48.6X4	T48.6X5	T48.6X6
Butethal	T42.3X1	T42.3X2	T42.3X3	T42.3X4	T42.3X5	T42.3X6
Butethamate	T44.3X1	T44.3X2	T44.3X3	T44.3X4	T44.3X5	T44.3X6
Buthalitone (sodium)	T41.1X1	T41.1X2	T41.1X3	T41.1X4	T41.1X5	T41.1X6
Butisol (sodium)	T42.3X1	T42.3X2	T42.3X3	T42.3X4	T42.3X5	T42.3X6
Butizide	T50.2X1	T50.2X2	T50.2X3	T50.2X4	T50.2X5	T50.2X6
Butobarbital	T42.3X1	T42.3X2	T42.3X3	T42.3X4	T42.3X5	T42.3X6
sodium	T42.3X1	T42.3X2	T42.3X3	T42.3X4	T42.3X5	T42.3X6
Butobarbitone	T42.3X1	T42.3X2	T42.3X3	T42.3X4	T42.3X5	T42.3X6
Butoconazole (nitrate)	T49.0X1	T49.0X2	T49.0X3	T49.0X4	T49.0X5	T49.0X6
Butorphanol	T40.4X1	T40.4X2	T40.4X3	T40.4X4	T40.4X5	T40.4X6
Butriptyline	T43.011	T43.012	T43.013	T43.014	T43.015	T43.016
Butropium bromide	T44.3X1	T44.3X2	T44.3X3	T44.3X4	T44.3X5	T44.3X6
Buttercups	T62.2X1	T62.2X2	T62.2X3	T62.2X4	—	—
Butter of antimony — see Antimony						
Butyl						
acetate (secondary)	T52.8X1	T52.8X2	T52.8X3	T52.8X4	—	—
alcohol	T51.3X1	T51.3X2	T51.3X3	T51.3X4	—	—
aminobenzoate	T41.3X1	T41.3X2	T41.3X3	T41.3X4	T41.3X5	T41.3X6
butyrate	T52.8X1	T52.8X2	T52.8X3	T52.8X4	—	—
carbinol	T51.3X1	T51.3X2	T51.3X3	T51.3X4	—	—
carbitol	T52.3X1	T52.3X2	T52.3X3	T52.3X4	—	—
cellosolve	T52.3X1	T52.3X2	T52.3X3	T52.3X4	—	—
chloral (hydrate)	T42.6X1	T42.6X2	T42.6X3	T42.6X4	T42.6X5	T42.6X6
formate	T52.8X1	T52.8X2	T52.8X3	T52.8X4	—	—
lactate	T52.8X1	T52.8X2	T52.8X3	T52.8X4	—	—
propionate	T52.8X1	T52.8X2	T52.8X3	T52.8X4	—	—
scopolamine bromide	T44.3X1	T44.3X2	T44.3X3	T44.3X4	T44.3X5	T44.3X6
thiobarbital sodium	T41.1X1	T41.1X2	T41.1X3	T41.1X4	T41.1X5	T41.1X6

Substance	Poisoning, Accidental (unintentional)	Poisoning, Intentional Self-harm	Poisoning, Assault	Poisoning, Undetermined	Adverse Effect	Under-dosing
Butylated hydroxyanisole	T50.991	T50.992	T50.993	T50.994	T50.995	T50.996
Butylchloral hydrate	T42.6X1	T42.6X2	T42.6X3	T42.6X4	T42.6X5	T42.6X6
Butyltoluene	T52.2X1	T52.2X2	T52.2X3	T52.2X4	—	—
Butyn	T41.3X1	T41.3X2	T41.3X3	T41.3X4	T41.3X5	T41.3X6
Butyrophenone (-based tranquilizers)	T43.4X1	T43.4X2	T43.4X3	T43.4X4	T43.4X5	T43.4X6
Cabergoline	T42.8X1	T42.8X2	T42.8X3	T42.8X4	T42.8X5	T42.8X6
Cacodyl, cacodylic acid	T57.0X1	T57.0X2	T57.0X3	T57.0X4	—	—
Cactinomycin	T45.1X1	T45.1X2	T45.1X3	T45.1X4	T45.1X5	T45.1X6
Cade oil	T49.4X1	T49.4X2	T49.4X3	T49.4X4	T49.4X5	T49.4X6
Cadexomer iodine	T49.0X1	T49.0X2	T49.0X3	T49.0X4	T49.0X5	T49.0X6
Cadmium (chloride) (fumes) (oxide)	T56.3X1	T56.3X2	T56.3X3	T56.3X4	—	—
sulfide (medicinal) NEC	T49.4X1	T49.4X2	T49.4X3	T49.4X4	T49.4X5	T49.4X6
Cadralazine	T46.5X1	T46.5X2	T46.5X3	T46.5X4	T46.5X5	T46.5X6
Caffeine	T43.611	T43.612	T43.613	T43.614	T43.615	T43.616
Calabar bean	T62.2X1	T62.2X2	T62.2X3	T62.2X4	—	—
Caladium seguinum	T62.2X1	T62.2X2	T62.2X3	T62.2X4	—	—
Calamine (lotion)	T49.3X1	T49.3X2	T49.3X3	T49.3X4	T49.3X5	T49.3X6
Calcifediol	T45.2X1	T45.2X2	T45.2X3	T45.2X4	T45.2X5	T45.2X6
Calciferol	T45.2X1	T45.2X2	T45.2X3	T45.2X4	T45.2X5	T45.2X6
Calcitonin	T50.991	T50.992	T50.993	T50.994	T50.995	T50.996
Calcitriol	T45.2X1	T45.2X2	T45.2X3	T45.2X4	T45.2X5	T45.2X6
Calcium	T50.3X1	T50.3X2	T50.3X3	T50.3X4	T50.3X5	T50.3X6
actylsalicylate	T39.011	T39.012	T39.013	T39.014	T39.015	T39.016
benzamidosalicylate	T37.1X1	T37.1X2	T37.1X3	T37.1X4	T37.1X5	T37.1X6
bromide	T42.6X1	T42.6X2	T42.6X3	T42.6X4	T42.6X5	T42.6X6
bromolactobionate	T42.6X1	T42.6X2	T42.6X3	T42.6X4	T42.6X5	T42.6X6
carbaspirin	T39.011	T39.012	T39.013	T39.014	T39.015	T39.016
carbimide	T50.6X1	T50.6X2	T50.6X3	T50.6X4	T50.6X5	T50.6X6
carbonate	T47.1X1	T47.1X2	T47.1X3	T47.1X4	T47.1X5	T47.1X6
chloride	T50.991	T50.992	T50.993	T50.994	T50.995	T50.996
anhydrous	T50.991	T50.992	T50.993	T50.994	T50.995	T50.996
cyanide	T57.8X1	T57.8X2	T57.8X3	T57.8X4	—	—
dioctyl sulfosuccinate	T47.4X1	T47.4X2	T47.4X3	T47.4X4	T47.4X5	T47.4X6
disodium edathamil	T45.8X1	T45.8X2	T45.8X3	T45.8X4	T45.8X5	T45.8X6
disodium edetate	T45.8X1	T45.8X2	T45.8X3	T45.8X4	T45.8X5	T45.8X6
dobesilate	T46.991	T46.992	T46.993	T46.994	T46.995	T46.996
EDTA	T45.8X1	T45.8X2	T45.8X3	T45.8X4	T45.8X5	T45.8X6
ferrous citrate	T45.4X1	T45.4X2	T45.4X3	T45.4X4	T45.4X5	T45.4X6
folinate	T45.8X1	T45.8X2	T45.8X3	T45.8X4	T45.8X5	T45.8X6
glubionate	T50.3X1	T50.3X2	T50.3X3	T50.3X4	T50.3X5	T50.3X6
gluconate	T50.3X1	T50.3X2	T50.3X3	T50.3X4	T50.3X5	T50.3X6
gluconogalactogluconate	T50.3X1	T50.3X2	T50.3X3	T50.3X4	T50.3X5	T50.3X6
hydrate, hydroxide	T54.3X1	T54.3X2	T54.3X3	T54.3X4	—	—
hypochlorite	T54.3X1	T54.3X2	T54.3X3	T54.3X4	—	—
iodide	T48.4X1	T48.4X2	T48.4X3	T48.4X4	T48.4X5	T48.4X6
ipodate	T50.8X1	T50.8X2	T50.8X3	T50.8X4	T50.8X5	T50.8X6
lactate	T50.3X1	T50.3X2	T50.3X3	T50.3X4	T50.3X5	T50.3X6
leucovorin	T45.8X1	T45.8X2	T45.8X3	T45.8X4	T45.8X5	T45.8X6
mandelate	T37.91	T37.92	T37.93	T37.94	T37.95	T37.96
oxide	T54.3X1	T54.3X2	T54.3X3	T54.3X4	—	—
pantothenate	T45.2X1	T45.2X2	T45.2X3	T45.2X4	T45.2X5	T45.2X6
phosphate	T50.3X1	T50.3X2	T50.3X3	T50.3X4	T50.3X5	T50.3X6
salicylate	T39.091	T39.092	T39.093	T39.094	T39.095	T39.096
salts	T50.3X1	T50.3X2	T50.3X3	T50.3X4	T50.3X5	T50.3X6
Calculus-dissolving drug	T50.991	T50.992	T50.993	T50.994	T50.995	T50.996
Calomel	T49.0X1	T49.0X2	T49.0X3	T49.0X4	T49.0X5	T49.0X6
Caloric agent	T50.3X1	T50.3X2	T50.3X3	T50.3X4	T50.3X5	T50.3X6
Calusterone	T38.7X1	T38.7X2	T38.7X3	T38.7X4	T38.7X5	T38.7X6
Camazepam	T42.4X1	T42.4X2	T42.4X3	T42.4X4	T42.4X5	T42.4X6
Camomile	T49.0X1	T49.0X2	T49.0X3	T49.0X4	T49.0X5	T49.0X6
Camoquin	T37.2X1	T37.2X2	T37.2X3	T37.2X4	T37.2X5	T37.2X6
Camphor						
insecticide	T60.2X1	T60.2X2	T60.2X3	T60.2X4	—	—
medicinal	T49.8X1	T49.8X2	T49.8X3	T49.8X4	T49.8X5	T49.8X6
Camylofin	T44.3X1	T44.3X2	T44.3X3	T44.3X4	T44.3X5	T44.3X6
Cancer chemotherapy drug regimen	T45.1X1	T45.1X2	T45.1X3	T45.1X4	T45.1X5	T45.1X6
Candeptin	T49.0X1	T49.0X2	T49.0X3	T49.0X4	T49.0X5	T49.0X6
Candicidin	T49.0X1	T49.0X2	T49.0X3	T49.0X4	T49.0X5	T49.0X6
Cannabinol	T40.7X1	T40.7X2	T40.7X3	T40.7X4	T40.7X5	T40.7X6
Cannabis (derivatives)	T40.7X1	T40.7X2	T40.7X3	T40.7X4	T40.7X5	T40.7X6
Canned heat	T51.1X1	T51.1X2	T51.1X3	T51.1X4	—	—
Canrenoic acid	T50.0X1	T50.0X2	T50.0X3	T50.0X4	T50.0X5	T50.0X6
Canrenone	T50.0X1	T50.0X2	T50.0X3	T50.0X4	T50.0X5	T50.0X6
Cantharides, cantharidin, cantharis	T49.8X1	T49.8X2	T49.8X3	T49.8X4	T49.8X5	T49.8X6
Canthaxanthin	T50.991	T50.992	T50.993	T50.994	T50.995	T50.996
Capillary-active drug NEC	T46.901	T46.902	T46.903	T46.904	T46.905	T46.906
Capreomycin	T36.8X1	T36.8X2	T36.8X3	T36.8X4	T36.8X5	T36.8X6
Capsicum	T49.4X1	T49.4X2	T49.4X3	T49.4X4	T49.4X5	T49.4X6
Captafol	T60.3X1	T60.3X2	T60.3X3	T60.3X4	—	—

Substance	Poisoning, Accidental (unintentional)	Poisoning, Intentional Self-harm	Poisoning, Assault	Poisoning, Undetermined	Adverse Effect	Under-dosing
Captan	T60.3X1	T60.3X2	T60.3X3	T60.3X4	—	—
Captodiame, captodiamine	T43.591	T43.592	T43.593	T43.594	T43.595	T43.596
Captopril	T46.4X1	T46.4X2	T46.4X3	T46.4X4	T46.4X5	T46.4X6
Caramiphen	T44.3X1	T44.3X2	T44.3X3	T44.3X4	T44.3X5	T44.3X6
Carazolol	T44.7X1	T44.7X2	T44.7X3	T44.7X4	T44.7X5	T44.7X6
Carbachol	T44.1X1	T44.1X2	T44.1X3	T44.1X4	T44.1X5	T44.1X6
Carbacrylamine (resin)	T50.3X1	T50.3X2	T50.3X3	T50.3X4	T50.3X5	T50.3X6
Carbamate (insecticide)	T60.0X1	T60.0X2	T60.0X3	T60.0X4	—	—
Carbamate (sedative)	T42.6X1	T42.6X2	T42.6X3	T42.6X4	T42.6X5	T42.6X6
herbicide	T60.0X1	T60.0X2	T60.0X3	T60.0X4	—	—
insecticide	T60.0X1	T60.0X2	T60.0X3	T60.0X4	—	—
Carbamazepine	T42.1X1	T42.1X2	T42.1X3	T42.1X4	T42.1X5	T42.1X6
Carbamide	T47.3X1	T47.3X2	T47.3X3	T47.3X4	T47.3X5	T47.3X6
peroxide	T49.0X1	T49.0X2	T49.0X3	T49.0X4	T49.0X5	T49.0X6
topical	T49.8X1	T49.8X2	T49.8X3	T49.8X4	T49.8X5	T49.8X6
Carbamylcholine chloride	T44.1X1	T44.1X2	T44.1X3	T44.1X4	T44.1X5	T44.1X6
Carbaril	T60.0X1	T60.0X2	T60.0X3	T60.0X4	—	—
Carbarsone	T37.3X1	T37.3X2	T37.3X3	T37.3X4	T37.3X5	T37.3X6
Carbaryl	T60.0X1	T60.0X2	T60.0X3	T60.0X4	—	—
Carbaspirin	T39.011	T39.012	T39.013	T39.014	T39.015	T39.016
Carbazochrome (salicylate) (sodium sulfonate)	T49.4X1	T49.4X2	T49.4X3	T49.4X4	T49.4X5	T49.4X6
Carbenicillin	T36.0X1	T36.0X2	T36.0X3	T36.0X4	T36.0X5	T36.0X6
Carbenoxolone	T47.1X1	T47.1X2	T47.1X3	T47.1X4	T47.1X5	T47.1X6
Carbetapentane	T48.3X1	T48.3X2	T48.3X3	T48.3X4	T48.3X5	T48.3X6
Carbethyl salicylate	T39.091	T39.092	T39.093	T39.094	T39.095	T39.096
Carbidopa (with levodopa)	T42.8X1	T42.8X2	T42.8X3	T42.8X4	T42.8X5	T42.8X6
Carbimazole	T38.2X1	T38.2X2	T38.2X3	T38.2X4	T38.2X5	T38.2X6
Carbinol	T51.1X1	T51.1X2	T51.1X3	T51.1X4	—	—
Carbinoxamine	T45.0X1	T45.0X2	T45.0X3	T45.0X4	T45.0X5	T45.0X6
Carbiphene	T39.8X1	T39.8X2	T39.8X3	T39.8X4	T39.8X5	T39.8X6
Carbitol	T52.3X1	T52.3X2	T52.3X3	T52.3X4	—	—
Carbocaine	T41.3X1	T41.3X2	T41.3X3	T41.3X4	T41.3X5	T41.3X6
infiltration (subcutaneous)	T41.3X1	T41.3X2	T41.3X3	T41.3X4	T41.3X5	T41.3X6
nerve block (peripheral) (plexus)	T41.3X1	T41.3X2	T41.3X3	T41.3X4	T41.3X5	T41.3X6
topical (surface)	T41.3X1	T41.3X2	T41.3X3	T41.3X4	T41.3X5	T41.3X6
Carbocisteine	T48.4X1	T48.4X2	T48.4X3	T48.4X4	T48.4X5	T48.4X6
Carbocromen	T46.3X1	T46.3X2	T46.3X3	T46.3X4	T46.3X5	T46.3X6
Carbol fuchsin	T49.0X1	T49.0X2	T49.0X3	T49.0X4	T49.0X5	T49.0X6
Carbolic acid — see also Phenol	T54.0X1	T54.0X2	T54.0X3	T54.0X4	—	—
Carbolonium (bromide)	T48.1X1	T48.1X2	T48.1X3	T48.1X4	T48.1X5	T48.1X6
Carbo medicinalis	T47.6X1	T47.6X2	T47.6X3	T47.6X4	T47.6X5	T47.6X6
Carbomycin	T36.8X1	T36.8X2	T36.8X3	T36.8X4	T36.8X5	T36.8X6
Carbon						
bisulfide (liquid)	T65.4X1	T65.4X2	T65.4X3	T65.4X4	—	—
vapor	T65.4X1	T65.4X2	T65.4X3	T65.4X4	—	—
dioxide (gas)	T59.7X1	T59.7X2	T59.7X3	T59.7X4	—	—
medicinal	T41.5X1	T41.5X2	T41.5X3	T41.5X4	T41.5X5	T41.5X6
nonmedicinal	T59.7X1	T59.7X2	T59.7X3	T59.7X4	—	—
snow	T49.4X1	T49.4X2	T49.4X3	T49.4X4	T49.4X5	T49.4X6
disulfide (liquid)	T65.4X1	T65.4X2	T65.4X3	T65.4X4	—	—
vapor	T65.4X1	T65.4X2	T65.4X3	T65.4X4	—	—
monoxide (from incomplete combustion)	T58.91	T58.92	T58.93	T58.94	—	—
blast furnace gas	T58.8X1	T58.8X2	T58.8X3	T58.8X4	—	—
butane (distributed in mobile container)	T58.11	T58.12	T58.13	T58.14	—	—
distributed through pipes	T58.11	T58.12	T58.13	T58.14	—	—
charcoal fumes	T58.2X1	T58.2X2	T58.2X3	T58.2X4	—	—
coal	T58.2X1	T58.2X2	T58.2X3	T58.2X4	—	—
coke (in domestic stoves, fireplaces)	T58.2X1	T58.2X2	T58.2X3	T58.2X4	—	—
exhaust gas (motor) not in transit	T58.01	T58.02	T58.03	T58.04	—	—
combustion engine, any not in watercraft	T58.01	T58.02	T58.03	T58.04	—	—
farm tractor, not in transit	T58.01	T58.02	T58.03	T58.04	—	—
gas engine	T58.01	T58.02	T58.03	T58.04	—	—
motor pump	T58.01	T58.02	T58.03	T58.04	—	—
motor vehicle, not in transit	T58.01	T58.02	T58.03	T58.04	—	—
fuel (in domestic use)	T58.2X1	T58.2X2	T58.2X3	T58.2X4	—	—
gas (piped)	T58.11	T58.12	T58.13	T58.14	—	—
in mobile container	T58.11	T58.12	T58.13	T58.14	—	—
piped (natural)	T58.11	T58.12	T58.13	T58.14	—	—
utility	T58.11	T58.12	T58.13	T58.14	—	—
in mobile container	T58.11	T58.12	T58.13	T58.14	—	—
gas (piped)	T58.11	T58.12	T58.13	T58.14	—	—
illuminating gas	T58.11	T58.12	T58.13	T58.14	—	—

Substance	Poisoning, Accidental (unintentional)	Poisoning, Intentional Self-harm	Poisoning, Assault	Poisoning, Undetermined	Adverse Effect	Under-dosing
Carbon — continued						
monoxide — continued						
industrial fuels or gases, any	T58.8X1	T58.8X2	T58.8X3	T58.8X4	—	—
kerosene (in domestic stoves, fireplaces)	T58.2X1	T58.2X2	T58.2X3	T58.2X4	—	—
kiln gas or vapor	T58.8X1	T58.8X2	T58.8X3	T58.8X4	—	—
motor exhaust gas, not in transit	T58.Ø1	T58.Ø2	T58.Ø3	T58.Ø4	—	—
piped gas (manufactured) (natural)	T58.11	T58.12	T58.13	T58.14	—	—
producer gas	T58.8X1	T58.8X2	T58.8X3	T58.8X4	—	—
propane (distributed in mobile container)	T58.11	T58.12	T58.13	T58.14	—	—
distributed through pipes	T58.11	T58.12	T58.13	T58.14	—	—
solid (in domestic stoves, fireplaces)	T58.2X1	T58.2X2	T58.2X3	T58.2X4	—	—
specified source NEC	T58.8X1	T58.8X2	T58.8X3	T58.8X4	—	—
stove gas	T58.11	T58.12	T58.13	T58.14	—	—
piped	T58.11	T58.12	T58.13	T58.14	—	—
utility gas	T58.11	T58.12	T58.13	T58.14	—	—
piped	T58.11	T58.12	T58.13	T58.14	—	—
water gas	T58.11	T58.12	T58.13	T58.14	—	—
wood (in domestic stoves, fireplaces)	T58.2X1	T58.2X2	T58.2X3	T58.2X4	—	—
tetrachloride (vapor) NEC	T53.ØX1	T53.ØX2	T53.ØX3	T53.ØX4	—	—
liquid (cleansing agent) NEC	T53.ØX1	T53.ØX2	T53.ØX3	T53.ØX4	—	—
solvent	T53.ØX1	T53.ØX2	T53.ØX3	T53.ØX4	—	—
Carbonic acid gas	T59.7X1	T59.7X2	T59.7X3	T59.7X4	—	—
anhydrase inhibitor NEC	T5Ø.2X1	T5Ø.2X2	T5Ø.2X3	T5Ø.2X4	T5Ø.2X5	T5Ø.2X6
Carbophenothion	T6Ø.ØX1	T6Ø.ØX2	T6Ø.ØX3	T6Ø.ØX4	—	—
Carboplatin	T45.1X1	T45.1X2	T45.1X3	T45.1X4	T45.1X5	T45.1X6
Carboprost	T48.ØX1	T48.ØX2	T48.ØX3	T48.ØX4	T48.ØX5	T48.ØX6
Carboquone	T45.1X1	T45.1X2	T45.1X3	T45.1X4	T45.1X5	T45.1X6
Carbowax	T49.3X1	T49.3X2	T49.3X3	T49.3X4	T49.3X5	T49.3X6
Carboxymethylcellulose	T47.4X1	T47.4X2	T47.4X3	T47.4X4	T47.4X5	T47.4X6
Carbrital	T42.3X1	T42.3X2	T42.3X3	T42.3X4	T42.3X5	T42.3X6
Carbromal	T42.6X1	T42.6X2	T42.6X3	T42.6X4	T42.6X5	T42.6X6
Carbutamide	T38.3X1	T38.3X2	T38.3X3	T38.3X4	T38.3X5	T38.3X6
Carbuterol	T48.6X1	T48.6X2	T48.6X3	T48.6X4	T48.6X5	T48.6X6
Cardiac						
depressants	T46.2X1	T46.2X2	T46.2X3	T46.2X4	T46.2X5	T46.2X6
rhythm regulator	T46.2X1	T46.2X2	T46.2X3	T46.2X4	T46.2X5	T46.2X6
specified NEC	T46.2X1	T46.2X2	T46.2X3	T46.2X4	T46.2X5	T46.2X6
Cardiografin	T5Ø.8X1	T5Ø.8X2	T5Ø.8X3	T5Ø.8X4	T5Ø.8X5	T5Ø.8X6
Cardiogreen	T5Ø.8X1	T5Ø.8X2	T5Ø.8X3	T5Ø.8X4	T5Ø.8X5	T5Ø.8X6
Cardiotonic (glycoside) **NEC**	T46.ØX1	T46.ØX2	T46.ØX3	T46.ØX4	T46.ØX5	T46.ØX6
Cardiovascular drug NEC	T46.9Ø1	T46.9Ø2	T46.9Ø3	T46.9Ø4	T46.9Ø5	T46.9Ø6
Cardrase	T5Ø.2X1	T5Ø.2X2	T5Ø.2X3	T5Ø.2X4	T5Ø.2X5	T5Ø.2X6
Carfecillin	T36.ØX1	T36.ØX2	T36.ØX3	T36.ØX4	T36.ØX5	T36.ØX6
Carfenazine	T43.3X1	T43.3X2	T43.3X3	T43.3X4	T43.3X5	T43.3X6
Carfusin	T49.ØX1	T49.ØX2	T49.ØX3	T49.ØX4	T49.ØX5	T49.ØX6
Carindacillin	T36.ØX1	T36.ØX2	T36.ØX3	T36.ØX4	T36.ØX5	T36.ØX6
Carisoprodol	T42.8X1	T42.8X2	T42.8X3	T42.8X4	T42.8X5	T42.8X6
Carmellose	T47.4X1	T47.4X2	T47.4X3	T47.4X4	T47.4X5	T47.4X6
Carminative	T47.5X1	T47.5X2	T47.5X3	T47.5X4	T47.5X5	T47.5X6
Carmofur	T45.1X1	T45.1X2	T45.1X3	T45.1X4	T45.1X5	T45.1X6
Carmustine	T45.1X1	T45.1X2	T45.1X3	T45.1X4	T45.1X5	T45.1X6
Carotene	T45.2X1	T45.2X2	T45.2X3	T45.2X4	T45.2X5	T45.2X6
Carphenazine	T43.3X1	T43.3X2	T43.3X3	T43.3X4	T43.3X5	T43.3X6
Carpipramine	T42.4X1	T42.4X2	T42.4X3	T42.4X4	T42.4X5	T42.4X6
Carprofen	T39.311	T39.312	T39.313	T39.314	T39.315	T39.316
Carpronium chloride	T44.3X1	T44.3X2	T44.3X3	T44.3X4	T44.3X5	T44.3X6
Carrageenan	T47.8X1	T47.8X2	T47.8X3	T47.8X4	T47.8X5	T47.8X6
Carteolol	T44.7X1	T44.7X2	T44.7X3	T44.7X4	T44.7X5	T44.7X6
Carter's Little Pills	T47.2X1	T47.2X2	T47.2X3	T47.2X4	T47.2X5	T47.2X6
Cascara (sagrada)	T47.2X1	T47.2X2	T47.2X3	T47.2X4	T47.2X5	T47.2X6
Cassava	T62.2X1	T62.2X2	T62.2X3	T62.2X4	—	—
Castellani's paint	T49.ØX1	T49.ØX2	T49.ØX3	T49.ØX4	T49.ØX5	T49.ØX6
Castor						
bean	T62.2X1	T62.2X2	T62.2X3	T62.2X4	—	—
oil	T47.2X1	T47.2X2	T47.2X3	T47.2X4	T47.2X5	T47.2X6
Catalase	T45.3X1	T45.3X2	T45.3X3	T45.3X4	T45.3X5	T45.3X6
Caterpillar (sting)	T63.431	T63.432	T63.433	T63.434	—	—
Catha (edulis) (tea)	T43.691	T43.692	T43.693	T43.694	—	—
Cathartic NEC	T47.4X1	T47.4X2	T47.4X3	T47.4X4	T47.4X5	T47.4X6
anthacene derivative	T47.2X1	T47.2X2	T47.2X3	T47.2X4	T47.2X5	T47.2X6
bulk	T47.4X1	T47.4X2	T47.4X3	T47.4X4	T47.4X5	T47.4X6
contact	T47.2X1	T47.2X2	T47.2X3	T47.2X4	T47.2X5	T47.2X6
emollient NEC	T47.4X1	T47.4X2	T47.4X3	T47.4X4	T47.4X5	T47.4X6
irritant NEC	T47.2X1	T47.2X2	T47.2X3	T47.2X4	T47.2X5	T47.2X6

Substance	Poisoning, Accidental (unintentional)	Poisoning, Intentional Self-harm	Poisoning, Assault	Poisoning, Undetermined	Adverse Effect	Under-dosing
Cathartic — continued						
mucilage	T47.4X1	T47.4X2	T47.4X3	T47.4X4	T47.4X5	T47.4X6
saline	T47.3X1	T47.3X2	T47.3X3	T47.3X4	T47.3X5	T47.3X6
vegetable	T47.2X1	T47.2X2	T47.2X3	T47.2X4	T47.2X5	T47.2X6
Cathine	T5Ø.5X1	T5Ø.5X2	T5Ø.5X3	T5Ø.5X4	T5Ø.5X5	T5Ø.5X6
Cathomycin	T36.8X1	T36.8X2	T36.8X3	T36.8X4	T36.8X5	T36.8X6
Cation exchange resin	T5Ø.3X1	T5Ø.3X2	T5Ø.3X3	T5Ø.3X4	T5Ø.3X5	T5Ø.3X6
Caustic(s) NEC	T54.91	T54.92	T54.93	T54.94	—	—
alkali	T54.3X1	T54.3X2	T54.3X3	T54.3X4	—	—
hydroxide	T54.3X1	T54.3X2	T54.3X3	T54.3X4	—	—
potash	T54.3X1	T54.3X2	T54.3X3	T54.3X4	—	—
soda	T54.3X1	T54.3X2	T54.3X3	T54.3X4	—	—
specified NEC	T54.91	T54.92	T54.93	T54.94	—	—
Ceepryn	T49.ØX1	T49.ØX2	T49.ØX3	T49.ØX4	T49.ØX5	T49.ØX6
ENT agent	T49.6X1	T49.6X2	T49.6X3	T49.6X4	T49.6X5	T49.6X6
lozenges	T49.6X1	T49.6X2	T49.6X3	T49.6X4	T49.6X5	T49.6X6
Cefacetrile	T36.1X1	T36.1X2	T36.1X3	T36.1X4	T36.1X5	T36.1X6
Cefaclor	T36.1X1	T36.1X2	T36.1X3	T36.1X4	T36.1X5	T36.1X6
Cefadroxil	T36.1X1	T36.1X2	T36.1X3	T36.1X4	T36.1X5	T36.1X6
Cefalexin	T36.1X1	T36.1X2	T36.1X3	T36.1X4	T36.1X5	T36.1X6
Cefaloglycin	T36.1X1	T36.1X2	T36.1X3	T36.1X4	T36.1X5	T36.1X6
Cefaloridine	T36.1X1	T36.1X2	T36.1X3	T36.1X4	T36.1X5	T36.1X6
Cefalosporins	T36.1X1	T36.1X2	T36.1X3	T36.1X4	T36.1X5	T36.1X6
Cefalotin	T36.1X1	T36.1X2	T36.1X3	T36.1X4	T36.1X5	T36.1X6
Cefamandole	T36.1X1	T36.1X2	T36.1X3	T36.1X4	T36.1X5	T36.1X6
Cefamycin antibiotic	T36.1X1	T36.1X2	T36.1X3	T36.1X4	T36.1X5	T36.1X6
Cefapirin	T36.1X1	T36.1X2	T36.1X3	T36.1X4	T36.1X5	T36.1X6
Cefatrizine	T36.1X1	T36.1X2	T36.1X3	T36.1X4	T36.1X5	T36.1X6
Cefazedone	T36.1X1	T36.1X2	T36.1X3	T36.1X4	T36.1X5	T36.1X6
Cefazolin	T36.1X1	T36.1X2	T36.1X3	T36.1X4	T36.1X5	T36.1X6
Cefbuperazone	T36.1X1	T36.1X2	T36.1X3	T36.1X4	T36.1X5	T36.1X6
Cefetamet	T36.1X1	T36.1X2	T36.1X3	T36.1X4	T36.1X5	T36.1X6
Cefixime	T36.1X1	T36.1X2	T36.1X3	T36.1X4	T36.1X5	T36.1X6
Cefmenoxime	T36.1X1	T36.1X2	T36.1X3	T36.1X4	T36.1X5	T36.1X6
Cefmetazole	T36.1X1	T36.1X2	T36.1X3	T36.1X4	T36.1X5	T36.1X6
Cefminox	T36.1X1	T36.1X2	T36.1X3	T36.1X4	T36.1X5	T36.1X6
Cefonicid	T36.1X1	T36.1X2	T36.1X3	T36.1X4	T36.1X5	T36.1X6
Cefoperazone	T36.1X1	T36.1X2	T36.1X3	T36.1X4	T36.1X5	T36.1X6
Ceforanide	T36.1X1	T36.1X2	T36.1X3	T36.1X4	T36.1X5	T36.1X6
Cefotaxime	T36.1X1	T36.1X2	T36.1X3	T36.1X4	T36.1X5	T36.1X6
Cefotetan	T36.1X1	T36.1X2	T36.1X3	T36.1X4	T36.1X5	T36.1X6
Cefotiam	T36.1X1	T36.1X2	T36.1X3	T36.1X4	T36.1X5	T36.1X6
Cefoxitin	T36.1X1	T36.1X2	T36.1X3	T36.1X4	T36.1X5	T36.1X6
Cefpimizole	T36.1X1	T36.1X2	T36.1X3	T36.1X4	T36.1X5	T36.1X6
Cefpiramide	T36.1X1	T36.1X2	T36.1X3	T36.1X4	T36.1X5	T36.1X6
Cefradine	T36.1X1	T36.1X2	T36.1X3	T36.1X4	T36.1X5	T36.1X6
Cefroxadine	T36.1X1	T36.1X2	T36.1X3	T36.1X4	T36.1X5	T36.1X6
Cefsulodin	T36.1X1	T36.1X2	T36.1X3	T36.1X4	T36.1X5	T36.1X6
Ceftazidime	T36.1X1	T36.1X2	T36.1X3	T36.1X4	T36.1X5	T36.1X6
Cefteram	T36.1X1	T36.1X2	T36.1X3	T36.1X4	T36.1X5	T36.1X6
Ceftezole	T36.1X1	T36.1X2	T36.1X3	T36.1X4	T36.1X5	T36.1X6
Ceftizoxime	T36.1X1	T36.1X2	T36.1X3	T36.1X4	T36.1X5	T36.1X6
Ceftriaxone	T36.1X1	T36.1X2	T36.1X3	T36.1X4	T36.1X5	T36.1X6
Cefuroxime	T36.1X1	T36.1X2	T36.1X3	T36.1X4	T36.1X5	T36.1X6
Cefuzonam	T36.1X1	T36.1X2	T36.1X3	T36.1X4	T36.1X5	T36.1X6
Celestone	T38.ØX1	T38.ØX2	T38.ØX3	T38.ØX4	T38.ØX5	T38.ØX6
topical	T49.ØX1	T49.ØX2	T49.ØX3	T49.ØX4	T49.ØX5	T49.ØX6
Celiprolol	T44.7X1	T44.7X2	T44.7X3	T44.7X4	T44.7X5	T44.7X6
Cell stimulants and proliferants	T49.8X1	T49.8X2	T49.8X3	T49.8X4	T49.8X5	T49.8X6
Cellosolve	T52.91	T52.92	T52.93	T52.94	—	—
Cellulose						
cathartic	T47.4X1	T47.4X2	T47.4X3	T47.4X4	T47.4X5	T47.4X6
hydroxyethyl	T47.4X1	T47.4X2	T47.4X3	T47.4X4	T47.4X5	T47.4X6
nitrates (topical)	T49.3X1	T49.3X2	T49.3X3	T49.3X4	T49.3X5	T49.3X6
oxidized	T49.4X1	T49.4X2	T49.4X3	T49.4X4	T49.4X5	T49.4X6
Centipede (bite)	T63.411	T63.412	T63.413	T63.414	—	—
Central nervous system						
depressants	T42.71	T42.72	T42.73	T42.74	T42.75	T42.76
anesthetic (general) NEC	T41.2Ø1	T41.2Ø2	T41.2Ø3	T41.2Ø4	T41.2Ø5	T41.2Ø6
gases NEC	T41.ØX1	T41.ØX2	T41.ØX3	T41.ØX4	T41.ØX5	T41.ØX6
intravenous	T41.1X1	T41.1X2	T41.1X3	T41.1X4	T41.1X5	T41.1X6
barbiturates	T42.3X1	T42.3X2	T42.3X3	T42.3X4	T42.3X5	T42.3X6
benzodiazepines	T42.4X1	T42.4X2	T42.4X3	T42.4X4	T42.4X5	T42.4X6
bromides	T42.6X1	T42.6X2	T42.6X3	T42.6X4	T42.6X5	T42.6X6
cannabis sativa	T4Ø.7X1	T4Ø.7X2	T4Ø.7X3	T4Ø.7X4	T4Ø.7X5	T4Ø.7X6
chloral hydrate	T42.6X1	T42.6X2	T42.6X3	T42.6X4	T42.6X5	T42.6X6
ethanol	T51.ØX1	T51.ØX2	T51.ØX3	T51.ØX4	—	—
hallucinogenics	T4Ø.9Ø1	T4Ø.9Ø2	T4Ø.9Ø3	T4Ø.9Ø4	T4Ø.9Ø5	T4Ø.9Ø6
hypnotics	T42.71	T42.72	T42.73	T42.74	T42.75	T42.76
specified NEC	T42.6X1	T42.6X2	T42.6X3	T42.6X4	T42.6X5	T42.6X6
muscle relaxants	T42.8X1	T42.8X2	T42.8X3	T42.8X4	T42.8X5	T42.8X6
paraldehyde	T42.6X1	T42.6X2	T42.6X3	T42.6X4	T42.6X5	T42.6X6

Additional Character May Be Required — Refer to the Tabular List for Character Selection   ▽ Subterms under main terms may continue to next column or page

Substance	Poisoning, Accidental (unintentional)	Poisoning, Intentional Self-harm	Poisoning, Assault	Poisoning, Undetermined	Adverse Effect	Under-dosing
Central nervous system — *continued*						
depressants — *continued*						
sedatives; sedative-hypnotics	T42.71	T42.72	T42.73	T42.74	T42.75	T42.76
mixed NEC	T42.6X1	T42.6X2	T42.6X3	T42.6X4	T42.6X5	T42.6X6
specified NEC	T42.6X1	T42.6X2	T42.6X3	T42.6X4	T42.6X5	T42.6X6
muscle-tone depressants	T42.8X1	T42.8X2	T42.8X3	T42.8X4	T42.8X5	T42.8X6
stimulants	T43.601	T43.602	T43.603	T43.604	T43.605	T43.606
amphetamines	T43.621	T43.622	T43.623	T43.624	T43.625	T43.626
analeptics	T50.7X1	T50.7X2	T50.7X3	T50.7X4	T50.7X5	T50.7X6
antidepressants	T43.201	T43.202	T43.203	T43.204	T43.205	T43.206
opiate antagonists	T50.7X1	T50.7X2	T50.7X3	T50.7X4	T50.7X5	T50.7X6
specified NEC	T43.691	T43.692	T43.693	T43.694	T43.695	T43.696
Cephalexin	T36.1X1	T36.1X2	T36.1X3	T36.1X4	T36.1X5	T36.1X6
Cephaloglycin	T36.1X1	T36.1X2	T36.1X3	T36.1X4	T36.1X5	T36.1X6
Cephaloridine	T36.1X1	T36.1X2	T36.1X3	T36.1X4	T36.1X5	T36.1X6
Cephalosporins	T36.1X1	T36.1X2	T36.1X3	T36.1X4	T36.1X5	T36.1X6
N (adicillin)	T36.0X1	T36.0X2	T36.0X3	T36.0X4	T36.0X5	T36.0X6
Cephalothin	T36.1X1	T36.1X2	T36.1X3	T36.1X4	T36.1X5	T36.1X6
Cephalotin	T36.1X1	T36.1X2	T36.1X3	T36.1X4	T36.1X5	T36.1X6
Cephradine	T36.1X1	T36.1X2	T36.1X3	T36.1X4	T36.1X5	T36.1X6
Cerbera (odallam)	T62.2X1	T62.2X2	T62.2X3	T62.2X4	—	—
Cerberin	T46.0X1	T46.0X2	T46.0X3	T46.0X4	T46.0X5	T46.0X6
Cerebral stimulants	T43.601	T43.602	T43.603	T43.604	T43.605	T43.606
psychotherapeutic	T43.601	T43.602	T43.603	T43.604	T43.605	T43.606
specified NEC	T43.691	T43.692	T43.693	T43.694	T43.695	T43.696
Cerium oxalate	T45.0X1	T45.0X2	T45.0X3	T45.0X4	T45.0X5	T45.0X6
Cerous oxalate	T45.0X1	T45.0X2	T45.0X3	T45.0X4	T45.0X5	T45.0X6
Ceruletide	T50.8X1	T50.8X2	T50.8X3	T50.8X4	T50.8X5	T50.8X6
Cetalkonium (chloride)	T49.0X1	T49.0X2	T49.0X3	T49.0X4	T49.0X5	T49.0X6
Cethexonium chloride	T49.0X1	T49.0X2	T49.0X3	T49.0X4	T49.0X5	T49.0X6
Cetiedil	T46.7X1	T46.7X2	T46.7X3	T46.7X4	T46.7X5	T46.7X6
Cetirizine	T45.0X1	T45.0X2	T45.0X3	T45.0X4	T45.0X5	T45.0X6
Cetomacrogol	T50.991	T50.992	T50.993	T50.994	T50.995	T50.996
Cetotiamine	T45.2X1	T45.2X2	T45.2X3	T45.2X4	T45.2X5	T45.2X6
Cetoxime	T45.0X1	T45.0X2	T45.0X3	T45.0X4	T45.0X5	T45.0X6
Cetraxate	T47.1X1	T47.1X2	T47.1X3	T47.1X4	T47.1X5	T47.1X6
Cetrimide	T49.0X1	T49.0X2	T49.0X3	T49.0X4	T49.0X5	T49.0X6
Cetrimonium (bromide)	T49.0X1	T49.0X2	T49.0X3	T49.0X4	T49.0X5	T49.0X6
Cetylpyridinium chloride	T49.0X1	T49.0X2	T49.0X3	T49.0X4	T49.0X5	T49.0X6
ENT agent	T49.6X1	T49.6X2	T49.6X3	T49.6X4	T49.6X5	T49.6X6
lozenges	T49.6X1	T49.6X2	T49.6X3	T49.6X4	T49.6X5	T49.6X6
Cevadilla — *see* Sabadilla						
Cevitamic acid	T45.2X1	T45.2X2	T45.2X3	T45.2X4	T45.2X5	T45.2X6
Chalk, precipitated	T47.1X1	T47.1X2	T47.1X3	T47.1X4	T47.1X5	T47.1X6
Chamomile	T49.0X1	T49.0X2	T49.0X3	T49.0X4	T49.0X5	T49.0X6
Ch'an su	T46.0X1	T46.0X2	T46.0X3	T46.0X4	T46.0X5	T46.0X6
Charcoal	T47.6X1	T47.6X2	T47.6X3	T47.6X4	T47.6X5	T47.6X6
activated — *see also* Charcoal, medicinal	T47.6X1	T47.6X2	T47.6X3	T47.6X4	T47.6X5	T47.6X6
fumes (Carbon monoxide)	T58.2X1	T58.2X2	T58.2X3	T58.2X4	—	—
industrial	T58.8X1	T58.8X2	T58.8X3	T58.8X4	—	—
medicinal (activated)	T47.6X1	T47.6X2	T47.6X3	T47.6X4	T47.6X5	T47.6X6
antidiarrheal	T47.6X1	T47.6X2	T47.6X3	T47.6X4	T47.6X5	T47.6X6
poison control	T47.8X1	T47.8X2	T47.8X3	T47.8X4	T47.8X5	T47.8X6
specified use other than for diarrhea	T47.8X1	T47.8X2	T47.8X3	T47.8X4	T47.8X5	T47.8X6
topical	T49.8X1	T49.8X2	T49.8X3	T49.8X4	T49.8X5	T49.8X6
Chaulmosulfone	T37.1X1	T37.1X2	T37.1X3	T37.1X4	T37.1X5	T37.1X6
Chelating agent NEC	T50.6X1	T50.6X2	T50.6X3	T50.6X4	T50.6X5	T50.6X6
Chelidonium majus	T62.2X1	T62.2X2	T62.2X3	T62.2X4	—	—
Chemical substance NEC	T65.91	T65.92	T65.93	T65.94	—	—
Chenodeoxycholic acid	T47.5X1	T47.5X2	T47.5X3	T47.5X4	T47.5X5	T47.5X6
Chenodiol	T47.5X1	T47.5X2	T47.5X3	T47.5X4	T47.5X5	T47.5X6
Chenopodium	T37.4X1	T37.4X2	T37.4X3	T37.4X4	T37.4X5	T37.4X6
Cherry laurel	T62.2X1	T62.2X2	T62.2X3	T62.2X4	—	—
Chinidin (e)	T46.2X1	T46.2X2	T46.2X3	T46.2X4	T46.2X5	T46.2X6
Chiniofon	T37.8X1	T37.8X2	T37.8X3	T37.8X4	T37.8X5	T37.8X6
Chlophedianol	T48.3X1	T48.3X2	T48.3X3	T48.3X4	T48.3X5	T48.3X6
Chloral	T42.6X1	T42.6X2	T42.6X3	T42.6X4	T42.6X5	T42.6X6
derivative	T42.6X1	T42.6X2	T42.6X3	T42.6X4	T42.6X5	T42.6X6
hydrate	T42.6X1	T42.6X2	T42.6X3	T42.6X4	T42.6X5	T42.6X6
Chloralamide	T42.6X1	T42.6X2	T42.6X3	T42.6X4	T42.6X5	T42.6X6
Chloralodol	T42.6X1	T42.6X2	T42.6X3	T42.6X4	T42.6X5	T42.6X6
Chloraiose	T60.4X1	T60.4X2	T60.4X3	T60.4X4	—	—
Chlorambucil	T45.1X1	T45.1X2	T45.1X3	T45.1X4	T45.1X5	T45.1X6
Chloramine	T57.8X1	T57.8X2	T57.8X3	T57.8X4	—	—
T	T49.0X1	T49.0X2	T49.0X3	T49.0X4	T49.0X5	T49.0X6
topical	T49.0X1	T49.0X2	T49.0X3	T49.0X4	T49.0X5	T49.0X6
Chloramphenicol	T36.2X1	T36.2X2	T36.2X3	T36.2X4	T36.2X5	T36.2X6
ENT agent	T49.6X1	T49.6X2	T49.6X3	T49.6X4	T49.6X5	T49.6X6
ophthalmic preparation	T49.5X1	T49.5X2	T49.5X3	T49.5X4	T49.5X5	T49.5X6

Substance	Poisoning, Accidental (unintentional)	Poisoning, Intentional Self-harm	Poisoning, Assault	Poisoning, Undetermined	Adverse Effect	Under-dosing
Chloramphenicol — *continued*						
topical NEC	T49.0X1	T49.0X2	T49.0X3	T49.0X4	T49.0X5	T49.0X6
Chlorate (potassium) (sodium) NEC	T60.3X1	T60.3X2	T60.3X3	T60.3X4		
herbicide	T60.3X1	T60.3X2	T60.3X3	T60.3X4	—	—
Chlorazanil	T50.2X1	T50.2X2	T50.2X3	T50.2X4	T50.2X5	T50.2X6
Chlorbenzene, chlorbenzol	T53.7X1	T53.7X2	T53.7X3	T53.7X4		
Chlorbenzoxamine	T44.3X1	T44.3X2	T44.3X3	T44.3X4	T44.3X5	T44.3X6
Chlorbutol	T42.6X1	T42.6X2	T42.6X3	T42.6X4	T42.6X5	T42.6X6
Chlorcyclizine	T45.0X1	T45.0X2	T45.0X3	T45.0X4	T45.0X5	T45.0X6
Chlordan (e) (dust)	T60.1X1	T60.1X2	T60.1X3	T60.1X4	—	—
Chlordantoin	T49.0X1	T49.0X2	T49.0X3	T49.0X4	T49.0X5	T49.0X6
Chlordiazepoxide	T42.4X1	T42.4X2	T42.4X3	T42.4X4	T42.4X5	T42.4X6
Chlordiethyl benzamide	T49.3X1	T49.3X2	T49.3X3	T49.3X4	T49.3X5	T49.3X6
Chloresium	T49.8X1	T49.8X2	T49.8X3	T49.8X4	T49.8X5	T49.8X6
Chlorethiazol	T42.6X1	T42.6X2	T42.6X3	T42.6X4	T42.6X5	T42.6X6
Chlorethyl — *see* Ethyl chloride						
Chloretone	T42.6X1	T42.6X2	T42.6X3	T42.6X4	T42.6X5	T42.6X6
Chlorex	T53.6X1	T53.6X2	T53.6X3	T53.6X4	—	—
insecticide	T60.1X1	T60.1X2	T60.1X3	T60.1X4	—	—
Chlorfenvinphos	T60.0X1	T60.0X2	T60.0X3	T60.0X4	—	—
Chlorhexadol	T42.6X1	T42.6X2	T42.6X3	T42.6X4	T42.6X5	T42.6X6
Chlorhexamide	T45.1X1	T45.1X2	T45.1X3	T45.1X4	T45.1X5	T45.1X6
Chlorhexidine	T49.0X1	T49.0X2	T49.0X3	T49.0X4	T49.0X5	T49.0X6
Chlorhydroxyquinolin	T49.0X1	T49.0X2	T49.0X3	T49.0X4	T49.0X5	T49.0X6
Chloride of lime (bleach)	T54.3X1	T54.3X2	T54.3X3	T54.3X4		
Chlorimipramine	T43.011	T43.012	T43.013	T43.014	T43.015	T43.016
Chlorinated						
camphene	T53.6X1	T53.6X2	T53.6X3	T53.6X4		
diphenyl	T53.7X1	T53.7X2	T53.7X3	T53.7X4		
hydrocarbons NEC	T53.91	T53.92	T53.93	T53.94		
solvents	T53.91	T53.92	T53.93	T53.94		
lime (bleach)	T54.3X1	T54.3X2	T54.3X3	T54.3X4		
and boric acid solution	T49.0X1	T49.0X2	T49.0X3	T49.0X4	T49.0X5	T49.0X6
naphthalene (insecticide)	T60.1X1	T60.1X2	T60.1X3	T60.1X4	—	—
industrial (non-pesticide)	T53.7X1	T53.7X2	T53.7X3	T53.7X4		
pesticide NEC	T60.8X1	T60.8X2	T60.8X3	T60.8X4		
soda — *see also* sodium hypochlorite						
solution	T49.0X1	T49.0X2	T49.0X3	T49.0X4	T49.0X5	T49.0X6
Chlorine (fumes) (gas)	T59.4X1	T59.4X2	T59.4X3	T59.4X4		
bleach	T54.3X1	T54.3X2	T54.3X3	T54.3X4		
compound gas NEC	T59.4X1	T59.4X2	T59.4X3	T59.4X4		
disinfectant	T59.4X1	T59.4X2	T59.4X3	T59.4X4		
releasing agents NEC	T59.4X1	T59.4X2	T59.4X3	T59.4X4		
Chlorisondamine chloride	T46.991	T46.992	T46.993	T46.994	T46.995	T46.996
Chlormadinone	T38.5X1	T38.5X2	T38.5X3	T38.5X4	T38.5X5	T38.5X6
Chlormephos	T60.0X1	T60.0X2	T60.0X3	T60.0X4	—	—
Chlormerodrin	T50.2X1	T50.2X2	T50.2X3	T50.2X4	T50.2X5	T50.2X6
Chlormethiazole	T42.6X1	T42.6X2	T42.6X3	T42.6X4	T42.6X5	T42.6X6
Chlormethine	T45.1X1	T45.1X2	T45.1X3	T45.1X4	T45.1X5	T45.1X6
Chlormethylenecycline	T36.4X1	T36.4X2	T36.4X3	T36.4X4	T36.4X5	T36.4X6
Chlormezanone	T42.6X1	T42.6X2	T42.6X3	T42.6X4	T42.6X5	T42.6X6
Chloroacetic acid	T60.3X1	T60.3X2	T60.3X3	T60.3X4	—	—
Chloroacetone	T59.3X1	T59.3X2	T59.3X3	T59.3X4		
Chloroacetophenone	T59.3X1	T59.3X2	T59.3X3	T59.3X4		
Chloroaniline	T53.7X1	T53.7X2	T53.7X3	T53.7X4		
Chlorobenzene, chlorobenzol	T53.7X1	T53.7X2	T53.7X3	T53.7X4		
Chlorobromomethane (fire extinguisher)	T53.6X1	T53.6X2	T53.6X3	T53.6X4		
Chlorobutanol	T49.0X1	T49.0X2	T49.0X3	T49.0X4	T49.0X5	T49.0X6
Chlorocresol	T49.0X1	T49.0X2	T49.0X3	T49.0X4	T49.0X5	T49.0X6
Chlorodehydromethyltestosterone	T38.7X1	T38.7X2	T38.7X3	T38.7X4	T38.7X5	T38.7X6
Chlorodinitrobenzene	T53.7X1	T53.7X2	T53.7X3	T53.7X4		
dust or vapor	T53.7X1	T53.7X2	T53.7X3	T53.7X4		
Chlorodiphenyl	T53.7X1	T53.7X2	T53.7X3	T53.7X4		
Chloroethane — *see* Ethyl chloride						
Chloroethylene	T53.6X1	T53.6X2	T53.6X3	T53.6X4	—	—
Chlorofluorocarbons	T53.5X1	T53.5X2	T53.5X3	T53.5X4	—	—
Chloroform (fumes) (vapor)	T53.1X1	T53.1X2	T53.1X3	T53.1X4		
anesthetic	T41.0X1	T41.0X2	T41.0X3	T41.0X4	T41.0X5	T41.0X6
solvent	T53.1X1	T53.1X2	T53.1X3	T53.1X4		
water, concentrated	T41.0X1	T41.0X2	T41.0X3	T41.0X4	T41.0X5	T41.0X6
Chloroguanide	T37.2X1	T37.2X2	T37.2X3	T37.2X4	T37.2X5	T37.2X6
Chloromycetin	T36.2X1	T36.2X2	T36.2X3	T36.2X4	T36.2X5	T36.2X6
ENT agent	T49.6X1	T49.6X2	T49.6X3	T49.6X4	T49.6X5	T49.6X6
ophthalmic preparation	T49.5X1	T49.5X2	T49.5X3	T49.5X4	T49.5X5	T49.5X6
otic solution	T49.6X1	T49.6X2	T49.6X3	T49.6X4	T49.6X5	T49.6X6
topical NEC	T49.0X1	T49.0X2	T49.0X3	T49.0X4	T49.0X5	T49.0X6
Chloronitrobenzene	T53.7X1	T53.7X2	T53.7X3	T53.7X4	—	—
dust or vapor	T53.7X1	T53.7X2	T53.7X3	T53.7X4	—	—

Substance	Poisoning, Accidental (unintentional)	Poisoning, Intentional Self-harm	Poisoning, Assault	Poisoning, Undetermined	Adverse Effect	Under-dosing
Chlorophacinone	T60.4X1	T60.4X2	T60.4X3	T60.4X4	—	—
Chlorophenol	T53.7X1	T53.7X2	T53.7X3	T53.7X4	—	—
Chlorophenothane	T60.1X1	T60.1X2	T60.1X3	T60.1X4	—	—
Chlorophyll	T50.991	T50.992	T50.993	T50.994	T50.995	T50.996
Chloropicrin (fumes)	T53.6X1	T53.6X2	T53.6X3	T53.6X4	—	—
fumigant	T60.8X1	T60.8X2	T60.8X3	T60.8X4	—	—
fungicide	T60.3X1	T60.3X2	T60.3X3	T60.3X4	—	—
pesticide	T60.8X1	T60.8X2	T60.8X3	T60.8X4	—	—
Chloroprocaine	T41.3X1	T41.3X2	T41.3X3	T41.3X4	T41.3X5	T41.3X6
infiltration (subcutaneous)	T41.3X1	T41.3X2	T41.3X3	T41.3X4	T41.3X5	T41.3X6
nerve block (peripheral) (plexus)	T41.3X1	T41.3X2	T41.3X3	T41.3X4	T41.3X5	T41.3X6
spinal	T41.3X1	T41.3X2	T41.3X3	T41.3X4	T41.3X5	T41.3X6
Chloroptic	T49.5X1	T49.5X2	T49.5X3	T49.5X4	T49.5X5	T49.5X6
Chloropurine	T45.1X1	T45.1X2	T45.1X3	T45.1X4	T45.1X5	T45.1X6
Chloropyramine	T45.0X1	T45.0X2	T45.0X3	T45.0X4	T45.0X5	T45.0X6
Chloropyrifos	T60.0X1	T60.0X2	T60.0X3	T60.0X4	—	—
Chloropyrilene	T45.0X1	T45.0X2	T45.0X3	T45.0X4	T45.0X5	T45.0X6
Chloroquine	T37.2X1	T37.2X2	T37.2X3	T37.2X4	T37.2X5	T37.2X6
Chlorothalonil	T60.3X1	T60.3X2	T60.3X3	T60.3X4	—	—
Chlorothen	T45.0X1	T45.0X2	T45.0X3	T45.0X4	T45.0X5	T45.0X6
Chlorothiazide	T50.2X1	T50.2X2	T50.2X3	T50.2X4	T50.2X5	T50.2X6
Chlorothymol	T49.4X1	T49.4X2	T49.4X3	T49.4X4	T49.4X5	T49.4X6
Chlorotrianisene	T38.5X1	T38.5X2	T38.5X3	T38.5X4	T38.5X5	T38.5X6
Chlorovinyldichloroarsine, not in war	T57.0X1	T57.0X2	T57.0X3	T57.0X4	—	—
Chloroxine	T49.4X1	T49.4X2	T49.4X3	T49.4X4	T49.4X5	T49.4X6
Chloroxylenol	T49.0X1	T49.0X2	T49.0X3	T49.0X4	T49.0X5	T49.0X6
Chlorphenamine	T45.0X1	T45.0X2	T45.0X3	T45.0X4	T45.0X5	T45.0X6
Chlorphenesin	T42.8X1	T42.8X2	T42.8X3	T42.8X4	T42.8X5	T42.8X6
topical (antifungal)	T49.0X1	T49.0X2	T49.0X3	T49.0X4	T49.0X5	T49.0X6
Chlorpheniramine	T45.0X1	T45.0X2	T45.0X3	T45.0X4	T45.0X5	T45.0X6
Chlorphenoxamine	T45.0X1	T45.0X2	T45.0X3	T45.0X4	T45.0X5	T45.0X6
Chlorphentermine	T50.5X1	T50.5X2	T50.5X3	T50.5X4	T50.5X5	T50.5X6
Chlorprocaine — see Chloroprocaine						
Chlorproguanil	T37.2X1	T37.2X2	T37.2X3	T37.2X4	T37.2X5	T37.2X6
Chlorpromazine	T43.3X1	T43.3X2	T43.3X3	T43.3X4	T43.3X5	T43.3X6
Chlorpropamide	T38.3X1	T38.3X2	T38.3X3	T38.3X4	T38.3X5	T38.3X6
Chlorprothixene	T43.4X1	T43.4X2	T43.4X3	T43.4X4	T43.4X5	T43.4X6
Chlorquinaldol	T49.0X1	T49.0X2	T49.0X3	T49.0X4	T49.0X5	T49.0X6
Chlorquinol	T49.0X1	T49.0X2	T49.0X3	T49.0X4	T49.0X5	T49.0X6
Chlortalidone	T50.2X1	T50.2X2	T50.2X3	T50.2X4	T50.2X5	T50.2X6
Chlortetracycline	T36.4X1	T36.4X2	T36.4X3	T36.4X4	T36.4X5	T36.4X6
Chlorthalidone	T50.2X1	T50.2X2	T50.2X3	T50.2X4	T50.2X5	T50.2X6
Chlorthion	T60.0X1	T60.0X2	T60.0X3	T60.0X4	—	—
Chlorthiophos	T60.0X1	T60.0X2	T60.0X3	T60.0X4	—	—
Chlortrianisene	T38.5X1	T38.5X2	T38.5X3	T38.5X4	T38.5X5	T38.5X6
Chlor-Trimeton	T45.0X1	T45.0X2	T45.0X3	T45.0X4	T45.0X5	T45.0X6
Chlorzoxazone	T42.8X1	T42.8X2	T42.8X3	T42.8X4	T42.8X5	T42.8X6
Choke damp	T59.7X1	T59.7X2	T59.7X3	T59.7X4	—	—
Cholagogues	T47.5X1	T47.5X2	T47.5X3	T47.5X4	T47.5X5	T47.5X6
Cholebrine	T50.8X1	T50.8X2	T50.8X3	T50.8X4	T50.8X5	T50.8X6
Cholecalciferol	T45.2X1	T45.2X2	T45.2X3	T45.2X4	T45.2X5	T45.2X6
Cholecystokinin	T50.8X1	T50.8X2	T50.8X3	T50.8X4	T50.8X5	T50.8X6
Cholera vaccine	T50.A91	T50.A92	T50.A93	T50.A94	T50.A95	T50.A96
Choleretic	T47.5X1	T47.5X2	T47.5X3	T47.5X4	T47.5X5	T47.5X6
Cholesterol-lowering agents	T46.6X1	T46.6X2	T46.6X3	T46.6X4	T46.6X5	T46.6X6
Cholestyramine (resin)	T46.6X1	T46.6X2	T46.6X3	T46.6X4	T46.6X5	T46.6X6
Cholic acid	T47.5X1	T47.5X2	T47.5X3	T47.5X4	T47.5X5	T47.5X6
Choline	T48.6X1	T48.6X2	T48.6X3	T48.6X4	T48.6X5	T48.6X6
chloride	T50.991	T50.992	T50.993	T50.994	T50.995	T50.996
dihydrogen citrate	T50.991	T50.992	T50.993	T50.994	T50.995	T50.996
salicylate	T39.091	T39.092	T39.093	T39.094	T39.095	T39.096
theophyllinate	T48.6X1	T48.6X2	T48.6X3	T48.6X4	T48.6X5	T48.6X6
Cholinergic (drug) NEC	T44.1X1	T44.1X2	T44.1X3	T44.1X4	T44.1X5	T44.1X6
muscle tone enhancer	T44.1X1	T44.1X2	T44.1X3	T44.1X4	T44.1X5	T44.1X6
organophosphorus	T44.0X1	T44.0X2	T44.0X3	T44.0X4	T44.0X5	T44.0X6
insecticide	T60.0X1	T60.0X2	T60.0X3	T60.0X4	—	—
nerve gas	T59.891	T59.892	T59.893	T59.894	—	—
trimethyl ammonium propanediol	T44.1X1	T44.1X2	T44.1X3	T44.1X4	T44.1X5	T44.1X6
Cholinesterase reactivator	T50.6X1	T50.6X2	T50.6X3	T50.6X4	T50.6X5	T50.6X6
Cholografin	T50.8X1	T50.8X2	T50.8X3	T50.8X4	T50.8X5	T50.8X6
Chorionic gonadotropin	T38.891	T38.892	T38.893	T38.894	T38.895	T38.896
Chromate	T56.2X1	T56.2X2	T56.2X3	T56.2X4	—	—
dust or mist	T56.2X1	T56.2X2	T56.2X3	T56.2X4	—	—
lead — see also lead	T56.0X1	T56.0X2	T56.0X3	T56.0X4	—	—
paint	T56.0X1	T56.0X2	T56.0X3	T56.0X4	—	—
Chromic						
acid	T56.2X1	T56.2X2	T56.2X3	T56.2X4	—	—
dust or mist	T56.2X1	T56.2X2	T56.2X3	T56.2X4	—	—

Substance	Poisoning, Accidental (unintentional)	Poisoning, Intentional Self-harm	Poisoning, Assault	Poisoning, Undetermined	Adverse Effect	Under-dosing
Chromic — continued						
phosphate 32P	T45.1X1	T45.1X2	T45.1X3	T45.1X4	T45.1X5	T45.1X6
Chromium	T56.2X1	T56.2X2	T56.2X3	T56.2X4	—	—
compounds — see Chromate						
sesquioxide	T50.8X1	T50.8X2	T50.8X3	T50.8X4	T50.8X5	T50.8X6
Chromomycin A3	T45.1X1	T45.1X2	T45.1X3	T45.1X4	T45.1X5	T45.1X6
Chromonar	T46.3X1	T46.3X2	T46.3X3	T46.3X4	T46.3X5	T46.3X6
Chromyl chloride	T56.2X1	T56.2X2	T56.2X3	T56.2X4	—	—
Chrysarobin	T49.4X1	T49.4X2	T49.4X3	T49.4X4	T49.4X5	T49.4X6
Chrysazin	T47.2X1	T47.2X2	T47.2X3	T47.2X4	T47.2X5	T47.2X6
Chymar	T45.3X1	T45.3X2	T45.3X3	T45.3X4	T45.3X5	T45.3X6
ophthalmic preparation	T49.5X1	T49.5X2	T49.5X3	T49.5X4	T49.5X5	T49.5X6
Chymopapain	T45.3X1	T45.3X2	T45.3X3	T45.3X4	T45.3X5	T45.3X6
Chymotrypsin	T45.3X1	T45.3X2	T45.3X3	T45.3X4	T45.3X5	T45.3X6
ophthalmic preparation	T49.5X1	T49.5X2	T49.5X3	T49.5X4	T49.5X5	T49.5X6
Cianidanol	T50.991	T50.992	T50.993	T50.994	T50.995	T50.996
Cianopramine	T43.011	T43.012	T43.013	T43.014	T43.015	T43.016
Cibenzoline	T46.2X1	T46.2X2	T46.2X3	T46.2X4	T46.2X5	T46.2X6
Ciclacillin	T36.0X1	T36.0X2	T36.0X3	T36.0X4	T36.0X5	T36.0X6
Ciclobarbital — see Hexobarbital						
Ciclonicate	T46.7X1	T46.7X2	T46.7X3	T46.7X4	T46.7X5	T46.7X6
Ciclopirox (olamine)	T49.0X1	T49.0X2	T49.0X3	T49.0X4	T49.0X5	T49.0X6
Ciclosporin	T45.1X1	T45.1X2	T45.1X3	T45.1X4	T45.1X5	T45.1X6
Cicuta maculata or virosa	T62.2X1	T62.2X2	T62.2X3	T62.2X4	—	—
Cicutoxin	T62.2X1	T62.2X2	T62.2X3	T62.2X4	—	—
Cigarette lighter fluid	T52.0X1	T52.0X2	T52.0X3	T52.0X4	—	—
Cigarettes (tobacco)	T65.221	T65.222	T65.223	T65.224	—	—
Ciguatoxin	T61.01	T61.02	T61.03	T61.04	—	—
Cilazapril	T46.4X1	T46.4X2	T46.4X3	T46.4X4	T46.4X5	T46.4X6
Cimetidine	T47.0X1	T47.0X2	T47.0X3	T47.0X4	T47.0X5	T47.0X6
Cimetropium bromide	T44.3X1	T44.3X2	T44.3X3	T44.3X4	T44.3X5	T44.3X6
Cinchocaine	T41.3X1	T41.3X2	T41.3X3	T41.3X4	T41.3X5	T41.3X6
topical (surface)	T41.3X1	T41.3X2	T41.3X3	T41.3X4	T41.3X5	T41.3X6
Cinchona	T37.2X1	T37.2X2	T37.2X3	T37.2X4	T37.2X5	T37.2X6
Cinchonine alkaloids	T37.2X1	T37.2X2	T37.2X3	T37.2X4	T37.2X5	T37.2X6
Cinchophen	T50.4X1	T50.4X2	T50.4X3	T50.4X4	T50.4X5	T50.4X6
Cinepazide	T46.7X1	T46.7X2	T46.7X3	T46.7X4	T46.7X5	T46.7X6
Cinnamedrine	T48.5X1	T48.5X2	T48.5X3	T48.5X4	T48.5X5	T48.5X6
Cinnarizine	T45.0X1	T45.0X2	T45.0X3	T45.0X4	T45.0X5	T45.0X6
Cinoxacin	T37.8X1	T37.8X2	T37.8X3	T37.8X4	T37.8X5	T37.8X6
Ciprofibrate	T46.6X1	T46.6X2	T46.6X3	T46.6X4	T46.6X5	T46.6X6
Ciprofloxacin	T36.8X1	T36.8X2	T36.8X3	T36.8X4	T36.8X5	T36.8X6
Cisapride	T47.8X1	T47.8X2	T47.8X3	T47.8X4	T47.8X5	T47.8X6
Cisplatin	T45.1X1	T45.1X2	T45.1X3	T45.1X4	T45.1X5	T45.1X6
Citalopram	T43.221	T43.222	T43.223	T43.224	T43.225	T43.226
Citanest	T41.3X1	T41.3X2	T41.3X3	T41.3X4	T41.3X5	T41.3X6
infiltration (subcutaneous)	T41.3X1	T41.3X2	T41.3X3	T41.3X4	T41.3X5	T41.3X6
nerve block (peripheral) (plexus)	T41.3X1	T41.3X2	T41.3X3	T41.3X4	T41.3X5	T41.3X6
Citric acid	T47.5X1	T47.5X2	T47.5X3	T47.5X4	T47.5X5	T47.5X6
Citrovorum (factor)	T45.8X1	T45.8X2	T45.8X3	T45.8X4	T45.8X5	T45.8X6
Claviceps purpurea	T62.2X1	T62.2X2	T62.2X3	T62.2X4	—	—
Clavulanic acid	T36.1X1	T36.1X2	T36.1X3	T36.1X4	T36.1X5	T36.1X6
Cleaner, cleansing agent, type not specified	T65.891	T65.892	T65.893	T65.894	—	—
of paint or varnish	T52.91	T52.92	T52.93	T52.94	—	—
specified type NEC	T65.891	T65.892	T65.893	T65.894	—	—
Clebopride	T47.8X1	T47.8X2	T47.8X3	T47.8X4	T47.8X5	T47.8X6
Clefamide	T37.3X1	T37.3X2	T37.3X3	T37.3X4	T37.3X5	T37.3X6
Clemastine	T45.0X1	T45.0X2	T45.0X3	T45.0X4	T45.0X5	T45.0X6
Clematis vitalba	T62.2X1	T62.2X2	T62.2X3	T62.2X4	—	—
Clemizole	T45.0X1	T45.0X2	T45.0X3	T45.0X4	T45.0X5	T45.0X6
penicillin	T36.0X1	T36.0X2	T36.0X3	T36.0X4	T36.0X5	T36.0X6
Clenbuterol	T48.6X1	T48.6X2	T48.6X3	T48.6X4	T48.6X5	T48.6X6
Clidinium bromide	T44.3X1	T44.3X2	T44.3X3	T44.3X4	T44.3X5	T44.3X6
Clindamycin	T36.8X1	T36.8X2	T36.8X3	T36.8X4	T36.8X5	T36.8X6
Clinofibrate	T46.6X1	T46.6X2	T46.6X3	T46.6X4	T46.6X5	T46.6X6
Clioquinol	T37.8X1	T37.8X2	T37.8X3	T37.8X4	T37.8X5	T37.8X6
Cliradon	T40.2X1	T40.2X2	T40.2X3	T40.2X4		
Clobazam	T42.4X1	T42.4X2	T42.4X3	T42.4X4	T42.4X5	T42.4X6
Clobenzorex	T50.5X1	T50.5X2	T50.5X3	T50.5X4	T50.5X5	T50.5X6
Clobetasol	T49.0X1	T49.0X2	T49.0X3	T49.0X4	T49.0X5	T49.0X6
Clobetasone	T49.0X1	T49.0X2	T49.0X3	T49.0X4	T49.0X5	T49.0X6
Clobutinol	T48.3X1	T48.3X2	T48.3X3	T48.3X4	T48.3X5	T48.3X6
Clocortolone	T38.0X1	T38.0X2	T38.0X3	T38.0X4	T38.0X5	T38.0X6
Clodantoin	T49.0X1	T49.0X2	T49.0X3	T49.0X4	T49.0X5	T49.0X6
Clodronic acid	T50.991	T50.992	T50.993	T50.994	T50.995	T50.996
Clofazimine	T37.1X1	T37.1X2	T37.1X3	T37.1X4	T37.1X5	T37.1X6
Clofedanol	T48.3X1	T48.3X2	T48.3X3	T48.3X4	T48.3X5	T48.3X6
Clofenamide	T50.2X1	T50.2X2	T50.2X3	T50.2X4	T50.2X5	T50.2X6
Clofenotane	T49.0X1	T49.0X2	T49.0X3	T49.0X4	T49.0X5	T49.0X6
Clofezone	T39.2X1	T39.2X2	T39.2X3	T39.2X4	T39.2X5	T39.2X6
Clofibrate	T46.6X1	T46.6X2	T46.6X3	T46.6X4	T46.6X5	T46.6X6

Substance	Poisoning, Accidental (unintentional)	Poisoning, Intentional Self-harm	Poisoning, Assault	Poisoning, Undetermined	Adverse Effect	Under-dosing
Clofibride	T46.6X1	T46.6X2	T46.6X3	T46.6X4	T46.6X5	T46.6X6
Cloforex	T50.5X1	T50.5X2	T50.5X3	T50.5X4	T50.5X5	T50.5X6
Clomethiazole	T42.6X1	T42.6X2	T42.6X3	T42.6X4	T42.6X5	T42.6X6
Clometocillin	T36.0X1	T36.0X2	T36.0X3	T36.0X4	T36.0X5	T36.0X6
Clomifene	T38.5X1	T38.5X2	T38.5X3	T38.5X4	T38.5X5	T38.5X6
Clomiphene	T38.5X1	T38.5X2	T38.5X3	T38.5X4	T38.5X5	T38.5X6
Clomipramine	T43.011	T43.012	T43.013	T43.014	T43.015	T43.016
Clomocycline	T36.4X1	T36.4X2	T36.4X3	T36.4X4	T36.4X5	T36.4X6
Clonazepam	T42.4X1	T42.4X2	T42.4X3	T42.4X4	T42.4X5	T42.4X6
Clonidine	T46.5X1	T46.5X2	T46.5X3	T46.5X4	T46.5X5	T46.5X6
Clonixin	T39.8X1	T39.8X2	T39.8X3	T39.8X4	T39.8X5	T39.8X6
Clopamide	T50.2X1	T50.2X2	T50.2X3	T50.2X4	T50.2X5	T50.2X6
Clopenthixol	T43.4X1	T43.4X2	T43.4X3	T43.4X4	T43.4X5	T43.4X6
Cloperastine	T48.3X1	T48.3X2	T48.3X3	T48.3X4	T48.3X5	T48.3X6
Clophedianol	T48.3X1	T48.3X2	T48.3X3	T48.3X4	T48.3X5	T48.3X6
Cloponone	T36.2X1	T36.2X2	T36.2X3	T36.2X4	T36.2X5	T36.2X6
Cloprednol	T38.0X1	T38.0X2	T38.0X3	T38.0X4	T38.0X5	T38.0X6
Cloral betaine	T42.6X1	T42.6X2	T42.6X3	T42.6X4	T42.6X5	T42.6X6
Cloramfenicol	T36.2X1	T36.2X2	T36.2X3	T36.2X4	T36.2X5	T36.2X6
Clorazepate (dipotassium)	T42.4X1	T42.4X2	T42.4X3	T42.4X4	T42.4X5	T42.4X6
Clorexolone	T50.2X1	T50.2X2	T50.2X3	T50.2X4	T50.2X5	T50.2X6
Clorfenamine	T45.0X1	T45.0X2	T45.0X3	T45.0X4	T45.0X5	T45.0X6
Clorgiline	T43.1X1	T43.1X2	T43.1X3	T43.1X4	T43.1X5	T43.1X6
Clorotepine	T44.3X1	T44.3X2	T44.3X3	T44.3X4	T44.3X5	T44.3X6
Clorox (bleach)	T54.91	T54.92	T54.93	T54.94		
Clorprenaline	T48.6X1	T48.6X2	T48.6X3	T48.6X4	T48.6X5	T48.6X6
Clortermine	T50.5X1	T50.5X2	T50.5X3	T50.5X4	T50.5X5	T50.5X6
Clotiapine	T43.591	T43.592	T43.593	T43.594	T43.595	T43.596
Clotiazepam	T42.4X1	T42.4X2	T42.4X3	T42.4X4	T42.4X5	T42.4X6
Clotibric acid	T46.6X1	T46.6X2	T46.6X3	T46.6X4	T46.6X5	T46.6X6
Clotrimazole	T49.0X1	T49.0X2	T49.0X3	T49.0X4	T49.0X5	T49.0X6
Cloxacillin	T36.0X1	T36.0X2	T36.0X3	T36.0X4	T36.0X5	T36.0X6
Cloxazolam	T42.4X1	T42.4X2	T42.4X3	T42.4X4	T42.4X5	T42.4X6
Cloxiquine	T49.0X1	T49.0X2	T49.0X3	T49.0X4	T49.0X5	T49.0X6
Clozapine	T42.4X1	T42.4X2	T42.4X3	T42.4X4	T42.4X5	T42.4X6
Coagulant NEC	T45.7X1	T45.7X2	T45.7X3	T45.7X4	T45.7X5	T45.7X6
Coal (carbon monoxide from) — see also Carbon, monoxide, coal	T58.2X1	T58.2X2	T58.2X3	T58.2X4	—	—
oil — see Kerosene						
tar	T49.1X1	T49.1X2	T49.1X3	T49.1X4	T49.1X5	T49.1X6
fumes	T59.891	T59.892	T59.893	T59.894		
medicinal (ointment)	T49.4X1	T49.4X2	T49.4X3	T49.4X4	T49.4X5	T49.4X6
analgesics NEC	T39.2X1	T39.2X2	T39.2X3	T39.2X4	T39.2X5	T39.2X6
naphtha (solvent)	T52.0X1	T52.0X2	T52.0X3	T52.0X4		
Cobalamine	T45.2X1	T45.2X2	T45.2X3	T45.2X4	T45.2X5	T45.2X6
Cobalt (nonmedicinal) (fumes) (industrial)	T56.891	T56.892	T56.893	T56.894		
medicinal (trace) (chloride)	T45.8X1	T45.8X2	T45.8X3	T45.8X4	T45.8X5	T45.8X6
Cobra (venom)	T63.041	T63.042	T63.043	T63.044		
Coca (leaf)	T40.5X1	T40.5X2	T40.5X3	T40.5X4	T40.5X5	T40.5X6
Cocaine	T40.5X1	T40.5X2	T40.5X3	T40.5X4	T40.5X5	T40.5X6
topical anesthetic	T41.3X1	T41.3X2	T41.3X3	T41.3X4	T41.3X5	T41.3X6
Cocarboxylase	T45.3X1	T45.3X2	T45.3X3	T45.3X4	T45.3X5	T45.3X6
Coccidioidin	T50.8X1	T50.8X2	T50.8X3	T50.8X4	T50.8X5	T50.8X6
Cocculus indicus	T62.1X1	T62.1X2	T62.1X3	T62.1X4	—	—
Cochineal	T65.6X1	T65.6X2	T65.6X3	T65.6X4	—	—
medicinal products	T50.991	T50.992	T50.993	T50.994	T50.995	T50.996
Codeine	T40.2X1	T40.2X2	T40.2X3	T40.2X4	T40.2X5	T40.2X6
Cod-liver oil	T45.2X1	T45.2X2	T45.2X3	T45.2X4	T45.2X5	T45.2X6
Coenzyme A	T50.991	T50.992	T50.993	T50.994	T50.995	T50.996
Coffee	T62.8X1	T62.8X2	T62.8X3	T62.8X4	—	—
Cogalactoisomerase	T50.991	T50.992	T50.993	T50.994	T50.995	T50.996
Cogentin	T44.3X1	T44.3X2	T44.3X3	T44.3X4	T44.3X5	T44.3X6
Coke fumes or gas (carbon monoxide)	T58.2X1	T58.2X2	T58.2X3	T58.2X4		
industrial use	T58.8X1	T58.8X2	T58.8X3	T58.8X4	—	—
Colace	T47.4X1	T47.4X2	T47.4X3	T47.4X4	T47.4X5	T47.4X6
Colaspase	T45.1X1	T45.1X2	T45.1X3	T45.1X4	T45.1X5	T45.1X6
Colchicine	T50.4X1	T50.4X2	T50.4X3	T50.4X4	T50.4X5	T50.4X6
Colchicum	T62.2X1	T62.2X2	T62.2X3	T62.2X4	—	—
Cold cream	T49.3X1	T49.3X2	T49.3X3	T49.3X4	T49.3X5	T49.3X6
Colecalciferol	T45.2X1	T45.2X2	T45.2X3	T45.2X4	T45.2X5	T45.2X6
Colestipol	T46.6X1	T46.6X2	T46.6X3	T46.6X4	T46.6X5	T46.6X6
Colestyramine	T46.6X1	T46.6X2	T46.6X3	T46.6X4	T46.6X5	T46.6X6
Colimycin	T36.8X1	T36.8X2	T36.8X3	T36.8X4	T36.8X5	T36.8X6
Colistimethate	T36.8X1	T36.8X2	T36.8X3	T36.8X4	T36.8X5	T36.8X6
Colistin	T36.8X1	T36.8X2	T36.8X3	T36.8X4	T36.8X5	T36.8X6
sulfate (eye preparation)	T49.5X1	T49.5X2	T49.5X3	T49.5X4	T49.5X5	T49.5X6
Collagen	T50.991	T50.992	T50.993	T50.994	T50.995	T50.996
Collagenase	T49.4X1	T49.4X2	T49.4X3	T49.4X4	T49.4X5	T49.4X6
Collodion	T49.3X1	T49.3X2	T49.3X3	T49.3X4	T49.3X5	T49.3X6
Colocynth	T47.2X1	T47.2X2	T47.2X3	T47.2X4	T47.2X5	T47.2X6

Substance	Poisoning, Accidental (unintentional)	Poisoning, Intentional Self-harm	Poisoning, Assault	Poisoning, Undetermined	Adverse Effect	Under-dosing
Colophony adhesive	T49.3X1	T49.3X2	T49.3X3	T49.3X4	T49.3X5	T49.3X6
Colorant — see also Dye	T50.991	T50.992	T50.993	T50.994	T50.995	T50.996
Coloring matter — see Dye(s)						
Combustion gas (after combustion) — see Carbon, monoxide						
prior to combustion	T59.891	T59.892	T59.893	T59.894		
Compazine	T43.3X1	T43.3X2	T43.3X3	T43.3X4	T43.3X5	T43.3X6
Compound						
42 (warfarin)	T60.4X1	T60.4X2	T60.4X3	T60.4X4	—	—
269 (endrin)	T60.1X1	T60.1X2	T60.1X3	T60.1X4	—	—
497 (dieldrin)	T60.1X1	T60.1X2	T60.1X3	T60.1X4	—	—
1080 (sodium fluoroacetate)	T60.4X1	T60.4X2	T60.4X3	T60.4X4		
3422 (parathion)	T60.0X1	T60.0X2	T60.0X3	T60.0X4	—	—
3911 (phorate)	T60.0X1	T60.0X2	T60.0X3	T60.0X4	—	—
3956 (toxaphene)	T60.1X1	T60.1X2	T60.1X3	T60.1X4	—	—
4049 (malathion)	T60.0X1	T60.0X2	T60.0X3	T60.0X4		
4069 (malathion)	T60.0X1	T60.0X2	T60.0X3	T60.0X4		
4124 (dicapthon)	T60.0X1	T60.0X2	T60.0X3	T60.0X4		
E (cortisone)	T38.0X1	T38.0X2	T38.0X3	T38.0X4	T38.0X5	T38.0X6
F (hydrocortisone)	T38.0X1	T38.0X2	T38.0X3	T38.0X4	T38.0X5	T38.0X6
Congener, anabolic	T38.7X1	T38.7X2	T38.7X3	T38.7X4	T38.7X5	T38.7X6
Congo red	T50.8X1	T50.8X2	T50.8X3	T50.8X4	T50.8X5	T50.8X6
Coniine, conine	T62.2X1	T62.2X2	T62.2X3	T62.2X4		
Conium (maculatum)	T62.2X1	T62.2X2	T62.2X3	T62.2X4		
Conjugated estrogenic substances	T38.5X1	T38.5X2	T38.5X3	T38.5X4	T38.5X5	T38.5X6
Contac	T48.5X1	T48.5X2	T48.5X3	T48.5X4	T48.5X5	T48.5X6
Contact lens solution	T49.5X1	T49.5X2	T49.5X3	T49.5X4	T49.5X5	T49.5X6
Contraceptive (oral)	T38.4X1	T38.4X2	T38.4X3	T38.4X4	T38.4X5	T38.4X6
vaginal	T49.8X1	T49.8X2	T49.8X3	T49.8X4	T49.8X5	T49.8X6
Contrast medium, radiography	T50.8X1	T50.8X2	T50.8X3	T50.8X4	T50.8X5	T50.8X6
Convallaria glycosides	T46.0X1	T46.0X2	T46.0X3	T46.0X4	T46.0X5	T46.0X6
Convallaria majalis	T62.2X1	T62.2X2	T62.2X3	T62.2X4	—	—
berry	T62.1X1	T62.1X2	T62.1X3	T62.1X4	—	—
Copperhead snake (bite) (venom)	T63.061	T63.062	T63.063	T63.064		
Copper (dust) (fumes) (nonmedicinal) NEC	T56.4X1	T56.4X2	T56.4X3	T56.4X4		
arsenate, arsenite	T57.0X1	T57.0X2	T57.0X3	T57.0X4		
insecticide	T60.2X1	T60.2X2	T60.2X3	T60.2X4		
emetic	T47.7X1	T47.7X2	T47.7X3	T47.7X4	T47.7X5	T47.7X6
fungicide	T60.3X1	T60.3X2	T60.3X3	T60.3X4		
gluconate	T49.0X1	T49.0X2	T49.0X3	T49.0X4	T49.0X5	T49.0X6
insecticide	T60.2X1	T60.2X2	T60.2X3	T60.2X4		
medicinal (trace)	T45.8X1	T45.8X2	T45.8X3	T45.8X4	T45.8X5	T45.8X6
oleate	T49.0X1	T49.0X2	T49.0X3	T49.0X4	T49.0X5	T49.0X6
sulfate	T56.4X1	T56.4X2	T56.4X3	T56.4X4		
cupric	T56.4X1	T56.4X2	T56.4X3	T56.4X4		
fungicide	T60.3X1	T60.3X2	T60.3X3	T60.3X4		
medicinal						
ear	T49.6X1	T49.6X2	T49.6X3	T49.6X4	T49.6X5	T49.6X6
emetic	T47.7X1	T47.7X2	T47.7X3	T47.7X4	T47.7X5	T47.7X6
eye	T49.5X1	T49.5X2	T49.5X3	T49.5X4	T49.5X5	T49.5X6
cuprous	T56.4X1	T56.4X2	T56.4X3	T56.4X4		
fungicide	T60.3X1	T60.3X2	T60.3X3	T60.3X4		
medicinal						
ear	T49.6X1	T49.6X2	T49.6X3	T49.6X4	T49.6X5	T49.6X6
emetic	T47.7X1	T47.7X2	T47.7X3	T47.7X4	T47.7X5	T47.7X6
eye	T49.5X1	T49.5X2	T49.5X3	T49.5X4	T49.5X5	T49.5X6
Coral (sting)	T63.691	T63.692	T63.693	T63.694	—	—
snake (bite) (venom)	T63.021	T63.022	T63.023	T63.024	—	—
Corbadrine	T49.6X1	T49.6X2	T49.6X3	T49.6X4	T49.6X5	T49.6X6
Cordite	T65.891	T65.892	T65.893	T65.894		
vapor	T59.891	T59.892	T59.893	T59.894	—	—
Cordran	T49.0X1	T49.0X2	T49.0X3	T49.0X4	T49.0X5	T49.0X6
Corn cures	T49.4X1	T49.4X2	T49.4X3	T49.4X4	T49.4X5	T49.4X6
Cornhusker's lotion	T49.3X1	T49.3X2	T49.3X3	T49.3X4	T49.3X5	T49.3X6
Corn starch	T49.3X1	T49.3X2	T49.3X3	T49.3X4	T49.3X5	T49.3X6
Coronary vasodilator NEC	T46.3X1	T46.3X2	T46.3X3	T46.3X4	T46.3X5	T46.3X6
Corrosive NEC	T54.91	T54.92	T54.93	T54.94	—	—
acid NEC	T54.2X1	T54.2X2	T54.2X3	T54.2X4	—	—
aromatics	T54.1X1	T54.1X2	T54.1X3	T54.1X4	—	—
disinfectant	T54.1X1	T54.1X2	T54.1X3	T54.1X4	—	—
fumes NEC	T54.91	T54.92	T54.93	T54.94		
specified NEC	T54.91	T54.92	T54.93	T54.94	—	—
sublimate	T56.1X1	T56.1X2	T56.1X3	T56.1X4	—	—
Cortate	T38.0X1	T38.0X2	T38.0X3	T38.0X4	T38.0X5	T38.0X6
Cort-Dome	T38.0X1	T38.0X2	T38.0X3	T38.0X4	T38.0X5	T38.0X6
ENT agent	T49.6X1	T49.6X2	T49.6X3	T49.6X4	T49.6X5	T49.6X6
ophthalmic preparation	T49.5X1	T49.5X2	T49.5X3	T49.5X4	T49.5X5	T49.5X6

Substance	Poisoning, Accidental (unintentional)	Poisoning, Intentional Self-harm	Poisoning, Assault	Poisoning, Undetermined	Adverse Effect	Under-dosing
Cort-Dome — *continued*						
topical NEC	T49.0X1	T49.0X2	T49.0X3	T49.0X4	T49.0X5	T49.0X6
Cortef	T38.0X1	T38.0X2	T38.0X3	T38.0X4	T38.0X5	T38.0X6
ENT agent	T49.6X1	T49.6X2	T49.6X3	T49.6X4	T49.6X5	T49.6X6
ophthalmic preparation	T49.5X1	T49.5X2	T49.5X3	T49.5X4	T49.5X5	T49.5X6
topical NEC	T49.0X1	T49.0X2	T49.0X3	T49.0X4	T49.0X5	T49.0X6
Corticosteroid	T38.0X1	T38.0X2	T38.0X3	T38.0X4	T38.0X5	T38.0X6
ENT agent	T49.6X1	T49.6X2	T49.6X3	T49.6X4	T49.6X5	T49.6X6
mineral	T50.0X1	T50.0X2	T50.0X3	T50.0X4	T50.0X5	T50.0X6
ophthalmic	T49.5X1	T49.5X2	T49.5X3	T49.5X4	T49.5X5	T49.5X6
topical NEC	T49.0X1	T49.0X2	T49.0X3	T49.0X4	T49.0X5	T49.0X6
Corticotropin	T38.811	T38.812	T38.813	T38.814	T38.815	T38.816
Cortisol	T49.0X1	T49.0X2	T49.0X3	T49.0X4	T49.0X5	T49.0X6
ENT agent	T49.6X1	T49.6X2	T49.6X3	T49.6X4	T49.6X5	T49.6X6
ophthalmic preparation	T49.5X1	T49.5X2	T49.5X3	T49.5X4	T49.5X5	T49.5X6
topical NEC	T49.0X1	T49.0X2	T49.0X3	T49.0X4	T49.0X5	T49.0X6
Cortisone (acetate)	T38.0X1	T38.0X2	T38.0X3	T38.0X4	T38.0X5	T38.0X6
ENT agent	T49.6X1	T49.6X2	T49.6X3	T49.6X4	T49.6X5	T49.6X6
ophthalmic preparation	T49.5X1	T49.5X2	T49.5X3	T49.5X4	T49.5X5	T49.5X6
topical NEC	T49.0X1	T49.0X2	T49.0X3	T49.0X4	T49.0X5	T49.0X6
Cortivazol	T38.0X1	T38.0X2	T38.0X3	T38.0X4	T38.0X5	T38.0X6
Cortogen	T38.0X1	T38.0X2	T38.0X3	T38.0X4	T38.0X5	T38.0X6
ENT agent	T49.6X1	T49.6X2	T49.6X3	T49.6X4	T49.6X5	T49.6X6
ophthalmic preparation	T49.5X1	T49.5X2	T49.5X3	T49.5X4	T49.5X5	T49.5X6
Cortone	T38.0X1	T38.0X2	T38.0X3	T38.0X4	T38.0X5	T38.0X6
ENT agent	T49.6X1	T49.6X2	T49.6X3	T49.6X4	T49.6X5	T49.6X6
ophthalmic preparation	T49.5X1	T49.5X2	T49.5X3	T49.5X4	T49.5X5	T49.5X6
Cortril	T38.0X1	T38.0X2	T38.0X3	T38.0X4	T38.0X5	T38.0X6
ENT agent	T49.6X1	T49.6X2	T49.6X3	T49.6X4	T49.6X5	T49.6X6
ophthalmic preparation	T49.5X1	T49.5X2	T49.5X3	T49.5X4	T49.5X5	T49.5X6
topical NEC	T49.0X1	T49.0X2	T49.0X3	T49.0X4	T49.0X5	T49.0X6
Corynebacterium parvum	T45.1X1	T45.1X2	T45.1X3	T45.1X4	T45.1X5	T45.1X6
Cosmetic preparation	T49.8X1	T49.8X2	T49.8X3	T49.8X4	T49.8X5	T49.8X6
Cosmetics	T49.8X1	T49.8X2	T49.8X3	T49.8X4	T49.8X5	T49.8X6
Cosyntropin	T38.811	T38.812	T38.813	T38.814	T38.815	T38.816
Cotarnine	T45.7X1	T45.7X2	T45.7X3	T45.7X4	T45.7X5	T45.7X6
Co-trimoxazole	T36.8X1	T36.8X2	T36.8X3	T36.8X4	T36.8X5	T36.8X6
Cottonseed oil	T49.3X1	T49.3X2	T49.3X3	T49.3X4	T49.3X5	T49.3X6
Cough mixture (syrup)	T48.4X1	T48.4X2	T48.4X3	T48.4X4	T48.4X5	T48.4X6
containing opiates	T40.2X1	T40.2X2	T40.2X3	T40.2X4	T40.2X5	T40.2X6
expectorants	T48.4X1	T48.4X2	T48.4X3	T48.4X4	T48.4X5	T48.4X6
Coumadin	T45.511	T45.512	T45.513	T45.514	T45.515	T45.516
rodenticide	T60.4X1	T60.4X2	T60.4X3	T60.4X4	—	—
Coumaphos	T60.0X1	T60.0X2	T60.0X3	T60.0X4	—	—
Coumarin	T45.511	T45.512	T45.513	T45.514	T45.515	T45.516
Coumetarol	T45.511	T45.512	T45.513	T45.514	T45.515	T45.516
Cowbane	T62.2X1	T62.2X2	T62.2X3	T62.2X4	—	—
Cozyme	T45.2X1	T45.2X2	T45.2X3	T45.2X4	T45.2X5	T45.2X6
Crack	T40.5X1	T40.5X2	T40.5X3	T40.5X4	—	—
Crataegus extract	T46.0X1	T46.0X2	T46.0X3	T46.0X4	T46.0X5	T46.0X6
Creolin	T54.1X1	T54.1X2	T54.1X3	T54.1X4	—	—
disinfectant	T54.1X1	T54.1X2	T54.1X3	T54.1X4	—	—
Creosol (compound)	T49.0X1	T49.0X2	T49.0X3	T49.0X4	T49.0X5	T49.0X6
Creosote (coal tar) (beechwood)	T49.0X1	T49.0X2	T49.0X3	T49.0X4	T49.0X5	T49.0X6
medicinal (expectorant)	T48.4X1	T48.4X2	T48.4X3	T48.4X4	T48.4X5	T48.4X6
syrup	T48.4X1	T48.4X2	T48.4X3	T48.4X4	T48.4X5	T48.4X6
Cresol(s)	T49.0X1	T49.0X2	T49.0X3	T49.0X4	T49.0X5	T49.0X6
and soap solution	T49.0X1	T49.0X2	T49.0X3	T49.0X4	T49.0X5	T49.0X6
Cresyl acetate	T49.0X1	T49.0X2	T49.0X3	T49.0X4	T49.0X5	T49.0X6
Cresylic acid	T49.0X1	T49.0X2	T49.0X3	T49.0X4	T49.0X5	T49.0X6
Crimidine	T60.4X1	T60.4X2	T60.4X3	T60.4X4	—	—
Croconazole	T37.8X1	T37.8X2	T37.8X3	T37.8X4	T37.8X5	T37.8X6
Cromoglicic acid	T48.6X1	T48.6X2	T48.6X3	T48.6X4	T48.6X5	T48.6X6
Cromolyn	T48.6X1	T48.6X2	T48.6X3	T48.6X4	T48.6X5	T48.6X6
Cromonar	T46.3X1	T46.3X2	T46.3X3	T46.3X4	T46.3X5	T46.3X6
Cropropamide	T39.8X1	T39.8X2	T39.8X3	T39.8X4	T39.8X5	T39.8X6
with crotethamide	T50.7X1	T50.7X2	T50.7X3	T50.7X4	T50.7X5	T50.7X6
Crotamiton	T49.0X1	T49.0X2	T49.0X3	T49.0X4	T49.0X5	T49.0X6
Crotethamide	T39.8X1	T39.8X2	T39.8X3	T39.8X4	T39.8X5	T39.8X6
with cropropamide	T50.7X1	T50.7X2	T50.7X3	T50.7X4	T50.7X5	T50.7X6
Croton (oil)	T47.2X1	T47.2X2	T47.2X3	T47.2X4	T47.2X5	T47.2X6
chloral	T42.6X1	T42.6X2	T42.6X3	T42.6X4	T42.6X5	T42.6X6
Crude oil	T52.0X1	T52.0X2	T52.0X3	T52.0X4	—	—
Cryogenine	T39.8X1	T39.8X2	T39.8X3	T39.8X4	T39.8X5	T39.8X6
Cryolite (vapor)	T60.1X1	T60.1X2	T60.1X3	T60.1X4	—	—
insecticide	T60.1X1	T60.1X2	T60.1X3	T60.1X4	—	—
Cryptenamine (tannates)	T46.5X1	T46.5X2	T46.5X3	T46.5X4	T46.5X5	T46.5X6
Crystal violet	T49.0X1	T49.0X2	T49.0X3	T49.0X4	T49.0X5	T49.0X6
Cuckoopint	T62.2X1	T62.2X2	T62.2X3	T62.2X4	—	—
Cumetharol	T45.511	T45.512	T45.513	T45.514	T45.515	T45.516
Cupric						
acetate	T60.3X1	T60.3X2	T60.3X3	T60.3X4	—	—

Substance	Poisoning, Accidental (unintentional)	Poisoning, Intentional Self-harm	Poisoning, Assault	Poisoning, Undetermined	Adverse Effect	Under-dosing
Cupric — *continued*						
acetoarsenite	T57.0X1	T57.0X2	T57.0X3	T57.0X4	—	—
arsenate	T57.0X1	T57.0X2	T57.0X3	T57.0X4	—	—
gluconate	T49.0X1	T49.0X2	T49.0X3	T49.0X4	T49.0X5	T49.0X6
oleate	T49.0X1	T49.0X2	T49.0X3	T49.0X4	T49.0X5	T49.0X6
sulfate	T56.4X1	T56.4X2	T56.4X3	T56.4X4	—	—
Cuprous sulfate — *see also* Copper sulfate	T56.4X1	T56.4X2	T56.4X3	T56.4X4	—	—
Curare, curarine	T48.1X1	T48.1X2	T48.1X3	T48.1X4	T48.1X5	T48.1X6
Cyamemazine	T43.3X1	T43.3X2	T43.3X3	T43.3X4	T43.3X5	T43.3X6
Cyamopsis tetragonoloba	T46.6X1	T46.6X2	T46.6X3	T46.6X4	T46.6X5	T46.6X6
Cyanacetyl hydrazide	T37.1X1	T37.1X2	T37.1X3	T37.1X4	T37.1X5	T37.1X6
Cyanic acid (gas)	T59.891	T59.892	T59.893	T59.894	—	—
Cyanide(s) (compounds) (potassium) (sodium) NEC	T65.0X1	T65.0X2	T65.0X3	T65.0X4	—	—
dust or gas (inhalation) NEC	T57.3X1	T57.3X2	T57.3X3	T57.3X4	—	—
fumigant	T65.0X1	T65.0X2	T65.0X3	T65.0X4	—	—
hydrogen	T57.3X1	T57.3X2	T57.3X3	T57.3X4	—	—
mercuric — *see* Mercury						
pesticide (dust) (fumes)	T65.0X1	T65.0X2	T65.0X3	T65.0X4	—	—
Cyanoacrylate adhesive	T49.3X1	T49.3X2	T49.3X3	T49.3X4	T49.3X5	T49.3X6
Cyanocobalamin	T45.8X1	T45.8X2	T45.8X3	T45.8X4	T45.8X5	T45.8X6
Cyanogen (chloride) (gas) NEC	T59.891	T59.892	T59.893	T59.894	—	—
Cyclacillin	T36.0X1	T36.0X2	T36.0X3	T36.0X4	T36.0X5	T36.0X6
Cyclaine	T41.3X1	T41.3X2	T41.3X3	T41.3X4	T41.3X5	T41.3X6
Cyclamate	T50.991	T50.992	T50.993	T50.994	T50.995	T50.996
Cyclamen europaeum	T62.2X1	T62.2X2	T62.2X3	T62.2X4	—	—
Cyclandelate	T46.7X1	T46.7X2	T46.7X3	T46.7X4	T46.7X5	T46.7X6
Cyclazocine	T50.7X1	T50.7X2	T50.7X3	T50.7X4	T50.7X5	T50.7X6
Cyclizine	T45.0X1	T45.0X2	T45.0X3	T45.0X4	T45.0X5	T45.0X6
Cyclobarbital	T42.3X1	T42.3X2	T42.3X3	T42.3X4	T42.3X5	T42.3X6
Cyclobarbitone	T42.3X1	T42.3X2	T42.3X3	T42.3X4	T42.3X5	T42.3X6
Cyclobenzaprine	T48.1X1	T48.1X2	T48.1X3	T48.1X4	T48.1X5	T48.1X6
Cyclodrine	T44.3X1	T44.3X2	T44.3X3	T44.3X4	T44.3X5	T44.3X6
Cycloguanil embonate	T37.2X1	T37.2X2	T37.2X3	T37.2X4	T37.2X5	T37.2X6
Cyclohexane	T52.8X1	T52.8X2	T52.8X3	T52.8X4	—	—
Cyclohexanol	T51.8X1	T51.8X2	T51.8X3	T51.8X4	—	—
Cyclohexanone	T52.4X1	T52.4X2	T52.4X3	T52.4X4	—	—
Cycloheximide	T60.3X1	T60.3X2	T60.3X3	T60.3X4	—	—
Cyclohexyl acetate	T52.8X1	T52.8X2	T52.8X3	T52.8X4	—	—
Cycloleucin	T45.1X1	T45.1X2	T45.1X3	T45.1X4	T45.1X5	T45.1X6
Cyclomethycaine	T41.3X1	T41.3X2	T41.3X3	T41.3X4	T41.3X5	T41.3X6
Cyclopentamine	T44.4X1	T44.4X2	T44.4X3	T44.4X4	T44.4X5	T44.4X6
Cyclopenthiazide	T50.2X1	T50.2X2	T50.2X3	T50.2X4	T50.2X5	T50.2X6
Cyclopentolate	T44.3X1	T44.3X2	T44.3X3	T44.3X4	T44.3X5	T44.3X6
Cyclophosphamide	T45.1X1	T45.1X2	T45.1X3	T45.1X4	T45.1X5	T45.1X6
Cycloplegic drug	T49.5X1	T49.5X2	T49.5X3	T49.5X4	T49.5X5	T49.5X6
Cyclopropane	T41.291	T41.292	T41.293	T41.294	T41.295	T41.296
Cyclopyrabital	T39.8X1	T39.8X2	T39.8X3	T39.8X4	T39.8X5	T39.8X6
Cycloserine	T37.1X1	T37.1X2	T37.1X3	T37.1X4	T37.1X5	T37.1X6
Cyclosporin	T45.1X1	T45.1X2	T45.1X3	T45.1X4	T45.1X5	T45.1X6
Cyclothiazide	T50.2X1	T50.2X2	T50.2X3	T50.2X4	T50.2X5	T50.2X6
Cycrimine	T44.3X1	T44.3X2	T44.3X3	T44.3X4	T44.3X5	T44.3X6
Cyhalothrin	T60.1X1	T60.1X2	T60.1X3	T60.1X4	—	—
Cymarin	T46.0X1	T46.0X2	T46.0X3	T46.0X4	T46.0X5	T46.0X6
Cypermethrin	T60.1X1	T60.1X2	T60.1X3	T60.1X4	—	—
Cyphenothrin	T60.2X1	T60.2X2	T60.2X3	T60.2X4	—	—
Cyproheptadine	T45.0X1	T45.0X2	T45.0X3	T45.0X4	T45.0X5	T45.0X6
Cyproterone	T38.6X1	T38.6X2	T38.6X3	T38.6X4	T38.6X5	T38.6X6
Cysteamine	T50.6X1	T50.6X2	T50.6X3	T50.6X4	T50.6X5	T50.6X6
Cytarabine	T45.1X1	T45.1X2	T45.1X3	T45.1X4	T45.1X5	T45.1X6
Cytisus						
laburnum	T62.2X1	T62.2X2	T62.2X3	T62.2X4	—	—
scoparius	T62.2X1	T62.2X2	T62.2X3	T62.2X4	—	—
Cytochrome C	T47.5X1	T47.5X2	T47.5X3	T47.5X4	T47.5X5	T47.5X6
Cytomel	T38.1X1	T38.1X2	T38.1X3	T38.1X4	T38.1X5	T38.1X6
Cytosine arabinoside	T45.1X1	T45.1X2	T45.1X3	T45.1X4	T45.1X5	T45.1X6
Cytoxan	T45.1X1	T45.1X2	T45.1X3	T45.1X4	T45.1X5	T45.1X6
Cytozyme	T45.7X1	T45.7X2	T45.7X3	T45.7X4	T45.7X5	T45.7X6
S-Carboxymethylcysteine	T48.4X1	T48.4X2	T48.4X3	T48.4X4	T48.4X5	T48.4X6
Dacarbazine	T45.1X1	T45.1X2	T45.1X3	T45.1X4	T45.1X5	T45.1X6
Dactinomycin	T45.1X1	T45.1X2	T45.1X3	T45.1X4	T45.1X5	T45.1X6
DADPS	T37.1X1	T37.1X2	T37.1X3	T37.1X4	T37.1X5	T37.1X6
Dakin's solution	T49.0X1	T49.0X2	T49.0X3	T49.0X4	T49.0X5	T49.0X6
Dalapon (sodium)	T60.3X1	T60.3X2	T60.3X3	T60.3X4	—	—
Dalmane	T42.4X1	T42.4X2	T42.4X3	T42.4X4	T42.4X5	T42.4X6
Danazol	T38.6X1	T38.6X2	T38.6X3	T38.6X4	T38.6X5	T38.6X6
Danilone	T45.511	T45.512	T45.513	T45.514	T45.515	T45.516
Danthron	T47.2X1	T47.2X2	T47.2X3	T47.2X4	T47.2X5	T47.2X6
Dantrolene	T42.8X1	T42.8X2	T42.8X3	T42.8X4	T42.8X5	T42.8X6
Dantron	T47.2X1	T47.2X2	T47.2X3	T47.2X4	T47.2X5	T47.2X6

Substance	Poisoning, Accidental (unintentional)	Poisoning, Intentional Self-harm	Poisoning, Assault	Poisoning, Undetermined	Adverse Effect	Underdosing
Daphne (gnidium) (mezereum)	T62.2X1	T62.2X2	T62.2X3	T62.2X4	—	—
berry	T62.1X1	T62.1X2	T62.1X3	T62.1X4	—	—
Dapsone	T37.1X1	T37.1X2	T37.1X3	T37.1X4	T37.1X5	T37.1X6
Daraprim	T37.2X1	T37.2X2	T37.2X3	T37.2X4	T37.2X5	T37.2X6
Darnel	T62.2X1	T62.2X2	T62.2X3	T62.2X4		
Darvon	T39.8X1	T39.8X2	T39.8X3	T39.8X4	T39.8X5	T39.8X6
Daunomycin	T45.1X1	T45.1X2	T45.1X3	T45.1X4	T45.1X5	T45.1X6
Daunorubicin	T45.1X1	T45.1X2	T45.1X3	T45.1X4	T45.1X5	T45.1X6
DBI	T38.3X1	T38.3X2	T38.3X3	T38.3X4	T38.3X5	T38.3X6
D-Con	T60.91	T60.92	T60.93	T60.94	—	—
insecticide	T60.2X1	T60.2X2	T60.2X3	T60.2X4		
rodenticide	T60.4X1	T60.4X2	T60.4X3	T60.4X4		
DDAVP	T38.891	T38.892	T38.893	T38.894	T38.895	T38.896
DDE (bis(chlorophenyl)-dichloroethylene)	T60.2X1	T60.2X2	T60.2X3	T60.2X4		
DDS	T37.1X1	T37.1X2	T37.1X3	T37.1X4	T37.1X5	T37.1X6
DDT (dust)	T60.1X1	T60.1X2	T60.1X3	T60.1X4		
Deadly nightshade — see also Belladonna	T62.2X1	T62.2X2	T62.2X3	T62.2X4		
berry	T62.1X1	T62.1X2	T62.1X3	T62.1X4		
Deamino-D-arginine vasopressin	T38.891	T38.892	T38.893	T38.894	T38.895	T38.896
Deanol (aceglumate)	T50.991	T50.992	T50.993	T50.994	T50.995	T50.996
Debrisoquine	T46.5X1	T46.5X2	T46.5X3	T46.5X4	T46.5X5	T46.5X6
Decaborane	T57.8X1	T57.8X2	T57.8X3	T57.8X4	—	—
fumes	T59.891	T59.892	T59.893	T59.894	—	—
Decadron	T38.0X1	T38.0X2	T38.0X3	T38.0X4	T38.0X5	T38.0X6
ENT agent	T49.6X1	T49.6X2	T49.6X3	T49.6X4	T49.6X5	T49.6X6
ophthalmic preparation	T49.5X1	T49.5X2	T49.5X3	T49.5X4	T49.5X5	T49.5X6
topical NEC	T49.0X1	T49.0X2	T49.0X3	T49.0X4	T49.0X5	T49.0X6
Decahydronaphthalene	T52.8X1	T52.8X2	T52.8X3	T52.8X4		
Decalin	T52.8X1	T52.8X2	T52.8X3	T52.8X4	—	—
Decamethonium (bromide)	T48.1X1	T48.1X2	T48.1X3	T48.1X4	T48.1X5	T48.1X6
Decholin	T47.5X1	T47.5X2	T47.5X3	T47.5X4	T47.5X5	T47.5X6
Declomycin	T36.4X1	T36.4X2	T36.4X3	T36.4X4	T36.4X5	T36.4X6
Decongestant, nasal (mucosa)	T48.5X1	T48.5X2	T48.5X3	T48.5X4	T48.5X5	T48.5X6
combination	T48.5X1	T48.5X2	T48.5X3	T48.5X4	T48.5X5	T48.5X6
Deet	T60.8X1	T60.8X2	T60.8X3	T60.8X4	—	—
Deferoxamine	T45.8X1	T45.8X2	T45.8X3	T45.8X4	T45.8X5	T45.8X6
Deflazacort	T38.0X1	T38.0X2	T38.0X3	T38.0X4	T38.0X5	T38.0X6
Deglycyrrhizinized extract of licorice	T48.4X1	T48.4X2	T48.4X3	T48.4X4	T48.4X5	T48.4X6
Dehydrocholic acid	T47.5X1	T47.5X2	T47.5X3	T47.5X4	T47.5X5	T47.5X6
Dehydroemetine	T37.3X1	T37.3X2	T37.3X3	T37.3X4	T37.3X5	T37.3X6
Dekalin	T52.8X1	T52.8X2	T52.8X3	T52.8X4	—	—
Delalutin	T38.5X1	T38.5X2	T38.5X3	T38.5X4	T38.5X5	T38.5X6
Delorazepam	T42.4X1	T42.4X2	T42.4X3	T42.4X4	T42.4X5	T42.4X6
Delphinium	T62.2X1	T62.2X2	T62.2X3	T62.2X4	—	—
Deltamethrin	T60.1X1	T60.1X2	T60.1X3	T60.1X4	—	—
Deltasone	T38.0X1	T38.0X2	T38.0X3	T38.0X4	T38.0X5	T38.0X6
Deltra	T38.0X1	T38.0X2	T38.0X3	T38.0X4	T38.0X5	T38.0X6
Delvinal	T42.3X1	T42.3X2	T42.3X3	T42.3X4	T42.3X5	T42.3X6
Demecarium (bromide)	T49.5X1	T49.5X2	T49.5X3	T49.5X4	T49.5X5	T49.5X6
Demeclocycline	T36.4X1	T36.4X2	T36.4X3	T36.4X4	T36.4X5	T36.4X6
Demecolcine	T45.1X1	T45.1X2	T45.1X3	T45.1X4	T45.1X5	T45.1X6
Demegestone	T38.5X1	T38.5X2	T38.5X3	T38.5X4	T38.5X5	T38.5X6
Demelanizing agents	T49.8X1	T49.8X2	T49.8X3	T49.8X4	T49.8X5	T49.8X6
Demephion -O and -S	T60.0X1	T60.0X2	T60.0X3	T60.0X4	—	—
Demerol	T40.2X1	T40.2X2	T40.2X3	T40.2X4	T40.2X5	T40.2X6
Demethylchlortetracycline	T36.4X1	T36.4X2	T36.4X3	T36.4X4	T36.4X5	T36.4X6
Demethyltetracycline	T36.4X1	T36.4X2	T36.4X3	T36.4X4	T36.4X5	T36.4X6
Demeton -O and -S	T60.0X1	T60.0X2	T60.0X3	T60.0X4	—	—
Demulcent (external)	T49.3X1	T49.3X2	T49.3X3	T49.3X4	T49.3X5	T49.3X6
specified NEC	T49.3X1	T49.3X2	T49.3X3	T49.3X4	T49.3X5	T49.3X6
Demulen	T38.4X1	T38.4X2	T38.4X3	T38.4X4	T38.4X5	T38.4X6
Denatured alcohol	T51.0X1	T51.0X2	T51.0X3	T51.0X4	—	—
Dendrid	T49.5X1	T49.5X2	T49.5X3	T49.5X4	T49.5X5	T49.5X6
Dental drug, topical application NEC	T49.7X1	T49.7X2	T49.7X3	T49.7X4	T49.7X5	T49.7X6
Dentifrice	T49.7X1	T49.7X2	T49.7X3	T49.7X4	T49.7X5	T49.7X6
Deodorant spray (feminine hygiene)	T49.8X1	T49.8X2	T49.8X3	T49.8X4	T49.8X5	T49.8X6
Deoxycortone	T50.0X1	T50.0X2	T50.0X3	T50.0X4	T50.0X5	T50.0X6
Deoxyribonuclease (pancreatic)	T45.3X1	T45.3X2	T45.3X3	T45.3X4	T45.3X5	T45.3X6
Depilatory	T49.4X1	T49.4X2	T49.4X3	T49.4X4	T49.4X5	T49.4X6
Deprenalin	T42.8X1	T42.8X2	T42.8X3	T42.8X4	T42.8X5	T42.8X6
Deprenyl	T42.8X1	T42.8X2	T42.8X3	T42.8X4	T42.8X5	T42.8X6
Depressant						
appetite (central)	T50.5X1	T50.5X2	T50.5X3	T50.5X4	T50.5X5	T50.5X6
cardiac	T46.2X1	T46.2X2	T46.2X3	T46.2X4	T46.2X5	T46.2X6

Substance	Poisoning, Accidental (unintentional)	Poisoning, Intentional Self-harm	Poisoning, Assault	Poisoning, Undetermined	Adverse Effect	Underdosing
Depressant — continued						
central nervous system (anesthetic) — see also Central nervous system, depressants	T42.71	T42.72	T42.73	T42.74	T42.75	T42.76
general anesthetic	T41.201	T41.202	T41.203	T41.204	T41.205	T41.206
muscle tone	T42.8X1	T42.8X2	T42.8X3	T42.8X4	T42.8X5	T42.8X6
muscle tone, central	T42.8X1	T42.8X2	T42.8X3	T42.8X4	T42.8X5	T42.8X6
psychotherapeutic	T43.501	T43.502	T43.503	T43.504	T43.505	T43.506
Depressant, appetite	T50.5X1	T50.5X2	T50.5X3	T50.5X4	T50.5X5	T50.5X6
Deptropine	T45.0X1	T45.0X2	T45.0X3	T45.0X4	T45.0X5	T45.0X6
Dequalinium (chloride)	T49.0X1	T49.0X2	T49.0X3	T49.0X4	T49.0X5	T49.0X6
Derris root	T60.2X1	T60.2X2	T60.2X3	T60.2X4	—	—
Deserpidine	T46.5X1	T46.5X2	T46.5X3	T46.5X4	T46.5X5	T46.5X6
Desferrioxamine	T45.8X1	T45.8X2	T45.8X3	T45.8X4	T45.8X5	T45.8X6
Desipramine	T43.011	T43.012	T43.013	T43.014	T43.015	T43.016
Deslanoside	T46.0X1	T46.0X2	T46.0X3	T46.0X4	T46.0X5	T46.0X6
Desloughing agent	T49.4X1	T49.4X2	T49.4X3	T49.4X4	T49.4X5	T49.4X6
Desmethylimipramine	T43.011	T43.012	T43.013	T43.014	T43.015	T43.016
Desmopressin	T38.891	T38.892	T38.893	T38.894	T38.895	T38.896
Desocodeine	T40.2X1	T40.2X2	T40.2X3	T40.2X4	T40.2X5	T40.2X6
Desogestrel	T38.5X1	T38.5X2	T38.5X3	T38.5X4	T38.5X5	T38.5X6
Desomorphine	T40.2X1	T40.2X2	T40.2X3	T40.2X4	—	—
Desonide	T49.0X1	T49.0X2	T49.0X3	T49.0X4	T49.0X5	T49.0X6
Desoximetasone	T49.0X1	T49.0X2	T49.0X3	T49.0X4	T49.0X5	T49.0X6
Desoxycorticosteroid	T50.0X1	T50.0X2	T50.0X3	T50.0X4	T50.0X5	T50.0X6
Desoxycortone	T50.0X1	T50.0X2	T50.0X3	T50.0X4	T50.0X5	T50.0X6
Desoxyephedrine	T43.621	T43.622	T43.623	T43.624	T43.625	T43.626
Detaxtran	T46.6X1	T46.6X2	T46.6X3	T46.6X4	T46.6X5	T46.6X6
Detergent	T49.2X1	T49.2X2	T49.2X3	T49.2X4	T49.2X5	T49.2X6
external medication	T49.2X1	T49.2X2	T49.2X3	T49.2X4	T49.2X5	T49.2X6
local	T49.2X1	T49.2X2	T49.2X3	T49.2X4	T49.2X5	T49.2X6
medicinal	T49.2X1	T49.2X2	T49.2X3	T49.2X4	T49.2X5	T49.2X6
nonmedicinal	T55.1X2	T55.1X2	T55.1X3	T55.1X4	—	—
specified NEC	T55.1X1	T55.1X2	T55.1X3	T55.1X4	—	—
Deterrent, alcohol	T50.6X1	T50.6X2	T50.6X3	T50.6X4	T50.6X5	T50.6X6
Detoxifying agent	T50.6X1	T50.6X2	T50.6X3	T50.6X4	T50.6X5	T50.6X6
Detrothyronine	T38.1X1	T38.1X2	T38.1X3	T38.1X4	T38.1X5	T38.1X6
Dettol (external medication)	T49.0X1	T49.0X2	T49.0X3	T49.0X4	T49.0X5	T49.0X6
Dexamethasone	T38.0X1	T38.0X2	T38.0X3	T38.0X4	T38.0X5	T38.0X6
ENT agent	T49.6X1	T49.6X2	T49.6X3	T49.6X4	T49.6X5	T49.6X6
ophthalmic preparation	T49.5X1	T49.5X2	T49.5X3	T49.5X4	T49.5X5	T49.5X6
topical NEC	T49.0X1	T49.0X2	T49.0X3	T49.0X4	T49.0X5	T49.0X6
Dexamfetamine	T43.621	T43.622	T43.623	T43.624	T43.625	T43.626
Dexamphetamine	T43.621	T43.622	T43.623	T43.624	T43.625	T43.626
Dexbrompheniramine	T45.0X1	T45.0X2	T45.0X3	T45.0X4	T45.0X5	T45.0X6
Dexchlorpheniramine	T45.0X1	T45.0X2	T45.0X3	T45.0X4	T45.0X5	T45.0X6
Dexedrine	T43.621	T43.622	T43.623	T43.624	T43.625	T43.626
Dexetimide	T44.3X1	T44.3X2	T44.3X3	T44.3X4	T44.3X5	T44.3X6
Dexfenfluramine	T50.5X1	T50.5X2	T50.5X3	T50.5X4	T50.5X5	T50.5X6
Dexpanthenol	T45.2X1	T45.2X2	T45.2X3	T45.2X4	T45.2X5	T45.2X6
Dextran (40) (70) (150)	T45.8X1	T45.8X2	T45.8X3	T45.8X4	T45.8X5	T45.8X6
Dextriferron	T45.4X1	T45.4X2	T45.4X3	T45.4X4	T45.4X5	T45.4X6
Dextroamphetamine	T43.621	T43.622	T43.623	T43.624	T43.625	T43.626
Dextro calcium pantothenate	T45.2X1	T45.2X2	T45.2X3	T45.2X4	T45.2X5	T45.2X6
Dextromethorphan	T48.3X1	T48.3X2	T48.3X3	T48.3X4	T48.3X5	T48.3X6
Dextromoramide	T40.4X1	T40.4X2	T40.4X3	T40.4X4	—	—
topical	T49.8X1	T49.8X2	T49.8X3	T49.8X4	T49.8X5	T49.8X6
Dextro pantothenyl alcohol	T45.2X1	T45.2X2	T45.2X3	T45.2X4	T45.2X5	T45.2X6
Dextropropoxyphene	T40.4X1	T40.4X2	T40.4X3	T40.4X4	T40.4X5	T40.4X6
Dextrorphan	T40.2X1	T40.2X2	T40.2X3	T40.2X4	T40.2X5	T40.2X6
Dextrose	T50.3X1	T50.3X2	T50.3X3	T50.3X4	T50.3X5	T50.3X6
concentrated solution, intravenous	T46.8X1	T46.8X2	T46.8X3	T46.8X4	T46.8X5	T46.8X6
Dextrothyroxin	T38.1X1	T38.1X2	T38.1X3	T38.1X4	T38.1X5	T38.1X6
Dextrothyroxine sodium	T38.1X1	T38.1X2	T38.1X3	T38.1X4	T38.1X5	T38.1X6
DFP	T44.0X1	T44.0X2	T44.0X3	T44.0X4	T44.0X5	T44.0X6
DHE	T37.3X1	T37.3X2	T37.3X3	T37.3X4	T37.3X5	T37.3X6
45	T46.5X1	T46.5X2	T46.5X3	T46.5X4	T46.5X5	T46.5X6
Diabinese	T38.3X1	T38.3X2	T38.3X3	T38.3X4	T38.3X5	T38.3X6
Diacetone alcohol	T52.4X1	T52.4X2	T52.4X3	T52.4X4	—	—
Diacetyl monoxime	T50.991	T50.992	T50.993	T50.994	—	—
Diacetylmorphine	T40.1X1	T40.1X2	T40.1X3	T40.1X4	—	—
Diachylon plaster	T49.4X1	T49.4X2	T49.4X3	T49.4X4	T49.4X5	T49.4X6
Diaethylstilboestrolum	T38.5X1	T38.5X2	T38.5X3	T38.5X4	T38.5X5	T38.5X6
Diagnostic agent NEC	T50.8X1	T50.8X2	T50.8X3	T50.8X4	T50.8X5	T50.8X6
Dial (soap)	T49.2X1	T49.2X2	T49.2X3	T49.2X4	T49.2X5	T49.2X6
sedative	T42.3X1	T42.3X2	T42.3X3	T42.3X4	T42.3X5	T42.3X6
Dialkyl carbonate	T52.91	T52.92	T52.93	T52.94	—	—
Diallylbarbituric acid	T42.3X1	T42.3X2	T42.3X3	T42.3X4	T42.3X5	T42.3X6
Diallymal	T42.3X1	T42.3X2	T42.3X3	T42.3X4	T42.3X5	T42.3X6

Substance	Poisoning, Accidental (unintentional)	Poisoning, Intentional Self-harm	Poisoning, Assault	Poisoning, Undetermined	Adverse Effect	Under-dosing
Dialysis solution (intraperitoneal)	T50.3X1	T50.3X2	T50.3X3	T50.3X4	T50.3X5	T50.3X6
Diaminodiphenylsulfone	T37.1X1	T37.1X2	T37.1X3	T37.1X4	T37.1X5	T37.1X6
Diamorphine	T40.1X1	T40.1X2	T40.1X3	T40.1X4	—	—
Diamox	T50.2X1	T50.2X2	T50.2X3	T50.2X4	T50.2X5	T50.2X6
Diamthazole	T49.0X1	T49.0X2	T49.0X3	T49.0X4	T49.0X5	T49.0X6
Dianthone	T47.2X1	T47.2X2	T47.2X3	T47.2X4	T47.2X5	T47.2X6
Diaphenylsulfone	T37.0X1	T37.0X2	T37.0X3	T37.0X4	T37.0X5	T37.0X6
Diasone (sodium)	T37.1X1	T37.1X2	T37.1X3	T37.1X4	T37.1X5	T37.1X6
Diastase	T47.5X1	T47.5X2	T47.5X3	T47.5X4	T47.5X5	T47.5X6
Diatrizoate	T50.8X1	T50.8X2	T50.8X3	T50.8X4	T50.8X5	T50.8X6
Diazepam	T42.4X1	T42.4X2	T42.4X3	T42.4X4	T42.4X5	T42.4X6
Diazinon	T60.0X1	T60.0X2	T60.0X3	T60.0X4	—	—
Diazomethane (gas)	T59.891	T59.892	T59.893	T59.894	—	—
Diazoxide	T46.5X1	T46.5X2	T46.5X3	T46.5X4	T46.5X5	T46.5X6
Dibekacin	T36.5X1	T36.5X2	T36.5X3	T36.5X4	T36.5X5	T36.5X6
Dibenamine	T44.6X1	T44.6X2	T44.6X3	T44.6X4	T44.6X5	T44.6X6
Dibenzepin	T43.011	T43.012	T43.013	T43.014	T43.015	T43.016
Dibenzheptropine	T45.0X1	T45.0X2	T45.0X3	T45.0X4	T45.0X5	T45.0X6
Dibenzyline	T44.6X1	T44.6X2	T44.6X3	T44.6X4	T44.6X5	T44.6X6
Diborane (gas)	T59.891	T59.892	T59.893	T59.894	—	—
Dibromochloropropane	T60.8X1	T60.8X2	T60.8X3	T60.8X4	—	—
Dibromodulcitol	T45.1X1	T45.1X2	T45.1X3	T45.1X4	T45.1X5	T45.1X6
Dibromoethane	T53.6X1	T53.6X2	T53.6X3	T53.6X4	—	—
Dibromomannitol	T45.1X1	T45.1X2	T45.1X3	T45.1X4	T45.1X5	T45.1X6
Dibromopropamidine isethionate	T49.0X1	T49.0X2	T49.0X3	T49.0X4	T49.0X5	T49.0X6
Dibrompropamidine	T49.0X1	T49.0X2	T49.0X3	T49.0X4	T49.0X5	T49.0X6
Dibucaine	T41.3X1	T41.3X2	T41.3X3	T41.3X4	T41.3X5	T41.3X6
topical (surface)	T41.3X1	T41.3X2	T41.3X3	T41.3X4	T41.3X5	T41.3X6
Dibunate sodium	T48.3X1	T48.3X2	T48.3X3	T48.3X4	T48.3X5	T48.3X6
Dibutoline sulfate	T44.3X1	T44.3X2	T44.3X3	T44.3X4	T44.3X5	T44.3X6
Dicamba	T60.3X1	T60.3X2	T60.3X3	T60.3X4	—	—
Dicapthon	T60.0X1	T60.0X2	T60.0X3	T60.0X4	—	—
Dichlobenil	T60.3X1	T60.3X2	T60.3X3	T60.3X4	—	—
Dichlone	T60.3X1	T60.3X2	T60.3X3	T60.3X4	—	—
Dichloralphenozone	T42.6X1	T42.6X2	T42.6X3	T42.6X4	T42.6X5	T42.6X6
Dichlorbenzidine	T65.3X1	T65.3X2	T65.3X3	T65.3X4	—	—
Dichlorhydrin	T52.8X1	T52.8X2	T52.8X3	T52.8X4	—	—
Dichlorhydroxyquinoline	T37.8X1	T37.8X2	T37.8X3	T37.8X4	T37.8X5	T37.8X6
Dichlorobenzene	T53.7X1	T53.7X2	T53.7X3	T53.7X4	—	—
Dichlorobenzyl alcohol	T49.6X1	T49.6X2	T49.6X3	T49.6X4	T49.6X5	T49.6X6
Dichlorodifluoromethane	T53.5X1	T53.5X2	T53.5X3	T53.5X4	—	—
Dichloroethane	T52.8X1	T52.8X2	T52.8X3	T52.8X4	—	—
Dichloroethylene	T53.6X1	T53.6X2	T53.6X3	T53.6X4	—	—
Dichloroethyl sulfide, not in war	T59.891	T59.892	T59.893	T59.894	—	—
Dichloroformoxine, not in war	T59.891	T59.892	T59.893	T59.894	—	—
Dichlorohydrin, alpha-dichlorohydrin	T52.8X1	T52.8X2	T52.8X3	T52.8X4	—	—
Dichloromethane (solvent)	T53.4X1	T53.4X2	T53.4X3	T53.4X4	—	—
vapor	T53.4X1	T53.4X2	T53.4X3	T53.4X4	—	—
Dichloronaphthoquinone	T60.3X1	T60.3X2	T60.3X3	T60.3X4	—	—
Dichlorophen	T37.4X1	T37.4X2	T37.4X3	T37.4X4	T37.4X5	T37.4X6
Dichloropropene	T60.3X1	T60.3X2	T60.3X3	T60.3X4	—	—
Dichloropropionic acid	T60.3X1	T60.3X2	T60.3X3	T60.3X4	—	—
Dichlorphenamide	T50.2X1	T50.2X2	T50.2X3	T50.2X4	T50.2X5	T50.2X6
Dichlorvos	T60.0X1	T60.0X2	T60.0X3	T60.0X4	—	—
Diclofenac	T39.391	T39.392	T39.393	T39.394	T39.395	T39.396
Diclofenamide	T50.2X1	T50.2X2	T50.2X3	T50.2X4	T50.2X5	T50.2X6
Diclofensine	T43.291	T43.292	T43.293	T43.294	T43.295	T43.296
Diclonixine	T39.8X1	T39.8X2	T39.8X3	T39.8X4	T39.8X5	T39.8X6
Dicloxacillin	T36.0X1	T36.0X2	T36.0X3	T36.0X4	T36.0X5	T36.0X6
Dicophane	T49.0X1	T49.0X2	T49.0X3	T49.0X4	T49.0X5	T49.0X6
Dicoumarol, dicoumarin, dicumarol	T45.511	T45.512	T45.513	T45.514	T45.515	T45.516
Dicrotophos	T60.0X1	T60.0X2	T60.0X3	T60.0X4	—	—
Dicyanogen (gas)	T65.0X1	T65.0X2	T65.0X3	T65.0X4	—	—
Dicyclomine	T44.3X1	T44.3X2	T44.3X3	T44.3X4	T44.3X5	T44.3X6
Dicycloverine	T44.3X1	T44.3X2	T44.3X3	T44.3X4	T44.3X5	T44.3X6
Dideoxycytidine	T37.5X1	T37.5X2	T37.5X3	T37.5X4	T37.5X5	T37.5X6
Dideoxyinosine	T37.5X1	T37.5X2	T37.5X3	T37.5X4	T37.5X5	T37.5X6
Dieldrin (vapor)	T60.1X1	T60.1X2	T60.1X3	T60.1X4	—	—
Diemal	T42.3X1	T42.3X2	T42.3X3	T42.3X4	T42.3X5	T42.3X6
Dienestrol	T38.5X1	T38.5X2	T38.5X3	T38.5X4	T38.5X5	T38.5X6
Dienoestrol	T38.5X1	T38.5X2	T38.5X3	T38.5X4	T38.5X5	T38.5X6
Dietetic drug NEC	T50.901	T50.902	T50.903	T50.904	T50.905	T50.906
Diethazine	T42.8X1	T42.8X2	T42.8X3	T42.8X4	T42.8X5	T42.8X6
Diethyl						
barbituric acid	T42.3X1	T42.3X2	T42.3X3	T42.3X4	T42.3X5	T42.3X6
carbamazine	T37.4X1	T37.4X2	T37.4X3	T37.4X4	T37.4X5	T37.4X6
carbinol	T51.3X1	T51.3X2	T51.3X3	T51.3X4	—	—

Substance	Poisoning, Accidental (unintentional)	Poisoning, Intentional Self-harm	Poisoning, Assault	Poisoning, Undetermined	Adverse Effect	Under-dosing
Diethyl — continued						
carbonate	T52.8X1	T52.8X2	T52.8X3	T52.8X4	—	—
ether (vapor) — see also ether	T41.0X1	T41.0X2	T41.0X3	T41.0X4	T41.0X5	T41.0X6
oxide	T52.8X1	T52.8X2	T52.8X3	T52.8X4	—	—
propion	T50.5X1	T50.5X2	T50.5X3	T50.5X4	T50.5X5	T50.5X6
stilbestrol	T38.5X1	T38.5X2	T38.5X3	T38.5X4	T38.5X5	T38.5X6
toluamide (nonmedicinal)	T60.8X1	T60.8X2	T60.8X3	T60.8X4	—	—
medicinal	T49.3X1	T49.3X2	T49.3X3	T49.3X4	T49.3X5	T49.3X6
Diethylcarbamazine	T37.4X1	T37.4X2	T37.4X3	T37.4X4	T37.4X5	T37.4X6
Diethylene						
dioxide	T52.8X1	T52.8X2	T52.8X3	T52.8X4	—	—
glycol (monoacetate) (monobutyl ether) (monoethyl ether)	T52.3X1	T52.3X2	T52.3X3	T52.3X4	—	—
Diethylhexylphthalate	T65.891	T65.892	T65.893	T65.894	—	—
Diethylpropion	T50.5X1	T50.5X2	T50.5X3	T50.5X4	T50.5X5	T50.5X6
Diethylstilbestrol	T38.5X1	T38.5X2	T38.5X3	T38.5X4	T38.5X5	T38.5X6
Diethylstilboestrol	T38.5X1	T38.5X2	T38.5X3	T38.5X4	T38.5X5	T38.5X6
Diethylsulfone-diethylmethane	T42.6X1	T42.6X2	T42.6X3	T42.6X4	T42.6X5	T42.6X6
Diethyltoluamide	T49.0X1	T49.0X2	T49.0X3	T49.0X4	T49.0X5	T49.0X6
Diethyltryptamine (DET)	T40.991	T40.992	T40.993	T40.994	—	—
Difebarbamate	T42.3X1	T42.3X2	T42.3X3	T42.3X4	T42.3X5	T42.3X6
Difencloxazine	T40.2X1	T40.2X2	T40.2X3	T40.2X4	T40.2X5	T40.2X6
Difenidol	T45.0X1	T45.0X2	T45.0X3	T45.0X4	T45.0X5	T45.0X6
Difenoxin	T47.6X1	T47.6X2	T47.6X3	T47.6X4	T47.6X5	T47.6X6
Difetarsone	T37.3X1	T37.3X2	T37.3X3	T37.3X4	T37.3X5	T37.3X6
Diffusin	T45.3X1	T45.3X2	T45.3X3	T45.3X4	T45.3X5	T45.3X6
Diflorasone	T49.0X1	T49.0X2	T49.0X3	T49.0X4	T49.0X5	T49.0X6
Diflos	T44.0X1	T44.0X2	T44.0X3	T44.0X4	T44.0X5	T44.0X6
Diflubenzuron	T60.1X1	T60.1X2	T60.1X3	T60.1X4	—	—
Diflucortolone	T49.0X1	T49.0X2	T49.0X3	T49.0X4	T49.0X5	T49.0X6
Diflunisal	T39.091	T39.092	T39.093	T39.094	T39.095	T39.096
Difluoromethyldopa	T42.8X1	T42.8X2	T42.8X3	T42.8X4	T42.8X5	T42.8X6
Difluorophate	T44.0X1	T44.0X2	T44.0X3	T44.0X4	T44.0X5	T44.0X6
Digestant NEC	T47.5X1	T47.5X2	T47.5X3	T47.5X4	T47.5X5	T47.5X6
Digitalin (e)	T46.0X1	T46.0X2	T46.0X3	T46.0X4	T46.0X5	T46.0X6
Digitalis (leaf)(glycoside)	T46.0X1	T46.0X2	T46.0X3	T46.0X4	T46.0X5	T46.0X6
lanata	T46.0X1	T46.0X2	T46.0X3	T46.0X4	T46.0X5	T46.0X6
purpurea	T46.0X1	T46.0X2	T46.0X3	T46.0X4	T46.0X5	T46.0X6
Digitoxin	T46.0X1	T46.0X2	T46.0X3	T46.0X4	T46.0X5	T46.0X6
Digitoxose	T46.0X1	T46.0X2	T46.0X3	T46.0X4	T46.0X5	T46.0X6
Digoxin	T46.0X1	T46.0X2	T46.0X3	T46.0X4	T46.0X5	T46.0X6
Digoxine	T46.0X1	T46.0X2	T46.0X3	T46.0X4	T46.0X5	T46.0X6
Dihydralazine	T46.5X1	T46.5X2	T46.5X3	T46.5X4	T46.5X5	T46.5X6
Dihydrazine	T46.5X1	T46.5X2	T46.5X3	T46.5X4	T46.5X5	T46.5X6
Dihydrocodeine	T40.2X1	T40.2X2	T40.2X3	T40.2X4	T40.2X5	T40.2X6
Dihydrocodeinone	T40.2X1	T40.2X2	T40.2X3	T40.2X4	T40.2X5	T40.2X6
Dihydroergocornine	T46.7X1	T46.7X2	T46.7X3	T46.7X4	T46.7X5	T46.7X6
Dihydroergocristine (mesilate)	T46.7X1	T46.7X2	T46.7X3	T46.7X4	T46.7X5	T46.7X6
Dihydroergokryptine	T46.7X1	T46.7X2	T46.7X3	T46.7X4	T46.7X5	T46.7X6
Dihydroergotamine	T46.5X1	T46.5X2	T46.5X3	T46.5X4	T46.5X5	T46.5X6
Dihydroergotoxine	T46.7X1	T46.7X2	T46.7X3	T46.7X4	T46.7X5	T46.7X6
mesilate	T46.7X1	T46.7X2	T46.7X3	T46.7X4	T46.7X5	T46.7X6
Dihydrohydroxycodeinone	T40.2X1	T40.2X2	T40.2X3	T40.2X4	T40.2X5	T40.2X6
Dihydrohydroxymorphinone	T40.2X1	T40.2X2	T40.2X3	T40.2X4	T40.2X5	T40.2X6
Dihydroisocodeine	T40.2X1	T40.2X2	T40.2X3	T40.2X4	T40.2X5	T40.2X6
Dihydromorphine	T40.2X1	T40.2X2	T40.2X3	T40.2X4	—	T40.2X6
Dihydromorphinone	T40.2X1	T40.2X2	T40.2X3	T40.2X4	—	T40.2X6
Dihydrostreptomycin	T36.5X1	T36.5X2	T36.5X3	T36.5X4	T36.5X5	T36.5X6
Dihydrotachysterol	T45.2X1	T45.2X2	T45.2X3	T45.2X4	T45.2X5	T45.2X6
Dihydroxyaluminum aminoacetate	T47.1X1	T47.1X2	T47.1X3	T47.1X4	T47.1X5	T47.1X6
Dihydroxyaluminum sodium carbonate	T47.1X1	T47.1X2	T47.1X3	T47.1X4	T47.1X5	T47.1X6
Dihydroxyanthraquinone	T47.2X1	T47.2X2	T47.2X3	T47.2X4	T47.2X5	T47.2X6
Dihydroxycodeinone	T40.2X1	T40.2X2	T40.2X3	T40.2X4	T40.2X5	T40.2X6
Dihydroxypropyl theophylline	T50.2X1	T50.2X2	T50.2X3	T50.2X4	T50.2X5	T50.2X6
Diiodohydroxyquin	T37.8X1	T37.8X2	T37.8X3	T37.8X4	T37.8X5	T37.8X6
topical	T49.0X1	T49.0X2	T49.0X3	T49.0X4	T49.0X5	T49.0X6
Diiodohydroxyquinoline	T37.8X1	T37.8X2	T37.8X3	T37.8X4	T37.8X5	T37.8X6
Diiodotyrosine	T38.2X1	T38.2X2	T38.2X3	T38.2X4	T38.2X5	T38.2X6
Diisopromine	T44.3X1	T44.3X2	T44.3X3	T44.3X4	T44.3X5	T44.3X6
Diisopropylamine	T46.3X1	T46.3X2	T46.3X3	T46.3X4	T46.3X5	T46.3X6
Diisopropylfluorophosphonate	T44.0X1	T44.0X2	T44.0X3	T44.0X4	T44.0X5	T44.0X6
Dilantin	T42.0X1	T42.0X2	T42.0X3	T42.0X4	T42.0X5	T42.0X6
Dilaudid	T40.2X1	T40.2X2	T40.2X3	T40.2X4	T40.2X5	T40.2X6
Dilazep	T46.3X1	T46.3X2	T46.3X3	T46.3X4	T46.3X5	T46.3X6
Dill	T47.5X1	T47.5X2	T47.5X3	T47.5X4	T47.5X5	T47.5X6
Diloxanide	T37.3X1	T37.3X2	T37.3X3	T37.3X4	T37.3X5	T37.3X6
Diltiazem	T46.1X1	T46.1X2	T46.1X3	T46.1X4	T46.1X5	T46.1X6

Additional Character May Be Required — Refer to the Tabular List for Character Selection ▽ Subterms under main terms may continue to next column or page

Substance	Poisoning, Accidental (unintentional)	Poisoning, Intentional Self-harm	Poisoning, Assault	Poisoning, Undetermined	Adverse Effect	Under-dosing
Dimazole	T49.0X1	T49.0X2	T49.0X3	T49.0X4	T49.0X5	T49.0X6
Dimefline	T50.7X1	T50.7X2	T50.7X3	T50.7X4	T50.7X5	T50.7X6
Dimefox	T60.0X1	T60.0X2	T60.0X3	T60.0X4	—	—
Dimemorfan	T48.3X1	T48.3X2	T48.3X3	T48.3X4	T48.3X5	T48.3X6
Dimenhydrinate	T45.0X1	T45.0X2	T45.0X3	T45.0X4	T45.0X5	T45.0X6
Dimercaprol (British anti-lewisite)	T45.8X1	T45.8X2	T45.8X3	T45.8X4	T45.8X5	T45.8X6
Dimercaptopropanol	T45.8X1	T45.8X2	T45.8X3	T45.8X4	T45.8X5	T45.8X6
Dimestrol	T38.5X1	T38.5X2	T38.5X3	T38.5X4	T38.5X5	T38.5X6
Dimetane	T45.0X1	T45.0X2	T45.0X3	T45.0X4	T45.0X5	T45.0X6
Dimethicone	T47.1X1	T47.1X2	T47.1X3	T47.1X4	T47.1X5	T47.1X6
Dimethindene	T45.0X1	T45.0X2	T45.0X3	T45.0X4	T45.0X5	T45.0X6
Dimethisoquin	T49.1X1	T49.1X2	T49.1X3	T49.1X4	T49.1X5	T49.1X6
Dimethisterone	T38.5X1	T38.5X2	T38.5X3	T38.5X4	T38.5X5	T38.5X6
Dimethoate	T60.0X1	T60.0X2	T60.0X3	T60.0X4	—	—
Dimethocaine	T41.3X1	T41.3X2	T41.3X3	T41.3X4	T41.3X5	T41.3X6
Dimethoxanate	T48.3X1	T48.3X2	T48.3X3	T48.3X4	T48.3X5	T48.3X6
Dimethyl						
arsine, arsinic acid	T57.0X1	T57.0X2	T57.0X3	T57.0X4	—	—
carbinol	T51.2X1	T51.2X2	T51.2X3	T51.2X4	—	—
carbonate	T52.8X1	T52.8X2	T52.8X3	T52.8X4	—	—
diguanide	T38.3X1	T38.3X2	T38.3X3	T38.3X4	T38.3X5	T38.3X6
ketone	T52.4X1	T52.4X2	T52.4X3	T52.4X4	—	—
vapor	T52.4X1	T52.4X2	T52.4X3	T52.4X4	—	—
meperidine	T40.2X1	T40.2X2	T40.2X3	T40.2X4	T40.2X5	T40.2X6
parathion	T60.0X1	T60.0X2	T60.0X3	T60.0X4	—	—
phthlate	T49.3X1	T49.3X2	T49.3X3	T49.3X4	T49.3X5	T49.3X6
polysiloxane	T47.8X1	T47.8X2	T47.8X3	T47.8X4	T47.8X5	T47.8X6
sulfate (fumes)	T59.891	T59.892	T59.893	T59.894	—	—
liquid	T65.891	T65.892	T65.893	T65.894	—	—
sulfoxide (nonmedicinal)	T52.8X1	T52.8X2	T52.8X3	T52.8X4	—	—
medicinal	T49.4X1	T49.4X2	T49.4X3	T49.4X4	T49.4X5	T49.4X6
tryptamine	T40.991	T40.992	T40.993	T40.994	—	—
tubocurarine	T48.1X1	T48.1X2	T48.1X3	T48.1X4	T48.1X5	T48.1X6
Dimethylamine sulfate	T49.4X1	T49.4X2	T49.4X3	T49.4X4	T49.4X5	T49.4X6
Dimethylformamide	T52.8X1	T52.8X2	T52.8X3	T52.8X4	—	—
Dimethyltubocurarinium chloride	T48.1X1	T48.1X2	T48.1X3	T48.1X4	T48.1X5	T48.1X6
Dimeticone	T47.1X1	T47.1X2	T47.1X3	T47.1X4	T47.1X5	T47.1X6
Dimetilan	T60.0X1	T60.0X2	T60.0X3	T60.0X4	—	—
Dimetindene	T45.0X1	T45.0X2	T45.0X3	T45.0X4	T45.0X5	T45.0X6
Dimetotiazine	T43.3X1	T43.3X2	T43.3X3	T43.3X4	T43.3X5	T43.3X6
Dimorpholamine	T50.7X1	T50.7X2	T50.7X3	T50.7X4	T50.7X5	T50.7X6
Dimoxyline	T46.3X1	T46.3X2	T46.3X3	T46.3X4	T46.3X5	T46.3X6
Dinitrobenzene	T65.3X1	T65.3X2	T65.3X3	T65.3X4	—	—
vapor	T59.891	T59.892	T59.893	T59.894	—	—
Dinitrobenzol	T65.3X1	T65.3X2	T65.3X3	T65.3X4	—	—
vapor	T59.891	T59.892	T59.893	T59.894	—	—
Dinitrobutylphenol	T65.3X1	T65.3X2	T65.3X3	T65.3X4	—	—
Dinitro (-ortho-)cresol (pesticide) (spray)	T65.3X1	T65.3X2	T65.3X3	T65.3X4	—	—
Dinitrocyclohexylphenol	T65.3X1	T65.3X2	T65.3X3	T65.3X4	—	—
Dinitrophenol	T65.3X1	T65.3X2	T65.3X3	T65.3X4	—	—
Dinoprost	T48.0X1	T48.0X2	T48.0X3	T48.0X4	T48.0X5	T48.0X6
Dinoprostone	T48.0X1	T48.0X2	T48.0X3	T48.0X4	T48.0X5	T48.0X6
Dinoseb	T60.3X1	T60.3X2	T60.3X3	T60.3X4	—	—
Dioctyl sulfosuccinate (calcium) (sodium)	T47.4X1	T47.4X2	T47.4X3	T47.4X4	T47.4X5	T47.4X6
Diodone	T50.8X1	T50.8X2	T50.8X3	T50.8X4	T50.8X5	T50.8X6
Diodoquin	T37.8X1	T37.8X2	T37.8X3	T37.8X4	T37.8X5	T37.8X6
Dionin	T40.2X1	T40.2X2	T40.2X3	T40.2X4	T40.2X5	T40.2X6
Diosmin	T46.991	T46.992	T46.993	T46.994	T46.995	T46.996
Dioxane	T52.8X1	T52.8X2	T52.8X3	T52.8X4	—	—
Dioxathion	T60.0X1	T60.0X2	T60.0X3	T60.0X4	—	—
Dioxin	T53.7X1	T53.7X2	T53.7X3	T53.7X4	—	—
Dioxopromethazine	T43.3X1	T43.3X2	T43.3X3	T43.3X4	T43.3X5	T43.3X6
Dioxyline	T46.3X1	T46.3X2	T46.3X3	T46.3X4	T46.3X5	T46.3X6
Dipentene	T52.8X1	T52.8X2	T52.8X3	T52.8X4	—	—
Diperodon	T41.3X1	T41.3X2	T41.3X3	T41.3X4	T41.3X5	T41.3X6
Diphacinone	T60.4X1	T60.4X2	T60.4X3	T60.4X4	—	—
Diphemanil	T44.3X1	T44.3X2	T44.3X3	T44.3X4	T44.3X5	T44.3X6
metilsulfate	T44.3X1	T44.3X2	T44.3X3	T44.3X4	T44.3X5	T44.3X6
Diphenadione	T45.511	T45.512	T45.513	T45.514	T45.515	T45.516
rodenticide	T60.4X1	T60.4X2	T60.4X3	T60.4X4	—	—
Diphenhydramine	T45.0X1	T45.0X2	T45.0X3	T45.0X4	T45.0X5	T45.0X6
Diphenidol	T45.0X1	T45.0X2	T45.0X3	T45.0X4	T45.0X5	T45.0X6
Diphenoxylate	T47.6X1	T47.6X2	T47.6X3	T47.6X4	T47.6X5	T47.6X6
Diphenylamine	T65.3X1	T65.3X2	T65.3X3	T65.3X4	—	—
Diphenylbutazone	T39.2X1	T39.2X2	T39.2X3	T39.2X4	T39.2X5	T39.2X6
Diphenylchloroarsine, not in war	T57.0X1	T57.0X2	T57.0X3	T57.0X4	—	—
Diphenylhydantoin	T42.0X1	T42.0X2	T42.0X3	T42.0X4	T42.0X5	T42.0X6
Diphenylmethane dye	T52.1X1	T52.1X2	T52.1X3	T52.1X4	—	—
Diphenylpyraline	T45.0X1	T45.0X2	T45.0X3	T45.0X4	T45.0X5	T45.0X6
Diphtheria						
antitoxin	T50.Z11	T50.Z12	T50.Z13	T50.Z14	T50.Z15	T50.Z16
toxoid	T50.A91	T50.A92	T50.A93	T50.A94	T50.A95	T50.A96
with tetanus toxoid	T50.A21	T50.A22	T50.A23	T50.A24	T50.A25	T50.A26
with pertussis component	T50.A11	T50.A12	T50.A13	T50.A14	T50.A15	T50.A16
vaccine	T50.A91	T50.A92	T50.A93	T50.A94	T50.A95	T50.A96
combination						
without pertussis	T50.A21	T50.A22	T50.A23	T50.A24	T50.A25	T50.A26
including pertussis	T50.A11	T50.A12	T50.A13	T50.A14	T50.A15	T50.A16
Diphylline	T50.2X1	T50.2X2	T50.2X3	T50.2X4	T50.2X5	T50.2X6
Dipipanone	T40.4X1	T40.4X2	T40.4X3	T40.4X4	—	—
Dipivefrine	T49.5X1	T49.5X2	T49.5X3	T49.5X4	T49.5X5	T49.5X6
Diplovax	T50.B91	T50.B92	T50.B93	T50.B94	T50.B95	T50.B96
Diprophylline	T50.2X1	T50.2X2	T50.2X3	T50.2X4	T50.2X5	T50.2X6
Dipropyline	T48.291	T48.292	T48.293	T48.294	T48.295	T48.296
Dipyridamole	T46.3X1	T46.3X2	T46.3X3	T46.3X4	T46.3X5	T46.3X6
Dipyrone	T39.2X1	T39.2X2	T39.2X3	T39.2X4	T39.2X5	T39.2X6
Diquat (dibromide)	T60.3X1	T60.3X2	T60.3X3	T60.3X4	—	—
Disinfectant	T65.891	T65.892	T65.893	T65.894	—	—
alkaline	T54.3X1	T54.3X2	T54.3X3	T54.3X4	—	—
aromatic	T54.1X1	T54.1X2	T54.1X3	T54.1X4	—	—
intestinal	T37.8X1	T37.8X2	T37.8X3	T37.8X4	T37.8X5	T37.8X6
Disipal	T42.8X1	T42.8X2	T42.8X3	T42.8X4	T42.8X5	T42.8X6
Disodium edetate	T50.6X1	T50.6X2	T50.6X3	T50.6X4	T50.6X5	T50.6X6
Disoprofol	T41.291	T41.292	T41.293	T41.294	T41.295	T41.296
Disopyramide	T46.2X1	T46.2X2	T46.2X3	T46.2X4	T46.2X5	T46.2X6
Distigmine (bromide)	T44.0X1	T44.0X2	T44.0X3	T44.0X4	T44.0X5	T44.0X6
Disulfamide	T50.2X1	T50.2X2	T50.2X3	T50.2X4	T50.2X5	T50.2X6
Disulfanilamide	T37.0X1	T37.0X2	T37.0X3	T37.0X4	T37.0X5	T37.0X6
Disulfiram	T50.6X1	T50.6X2	T50.6X3	T50.6X4	T50.6X5	T50.6X6
Disulfoton	T60.0X1	T60.0X2	T60.0X3	T60.0X4	—	—
Dithiazanine iodide	T37.4X1	T37.4X2	T37.4X3	T37.4X4	T37.4X5	T37.4X6
Dithiocarbamate	T60.0X1	T60.0X2	T60.0X3	T60.0X4	—	—
Dithranol	T49.4X1	T49.4X2	T49.4X3	T49.4X4	T49.4X5	T49.4X6
Diucardin	T50.2X1	T50.2X2	T50.2X3	T50.2X4	T50.2X5	T50.2X6
Diupres	T50.2X1	T50.2X2	T50.2X3	T50.2X4	T50.2X5	T50.2X6
Diuretic NEC	T50.2X1	T50.2X2	T50.2X3	T50.2X4	T50.2X5	T50.2X6
benzothiadiazine	T50.2X1	T50.2X2	T50.2X3	T50.2X4	T50.2X5	T50.2X6
carbonic acid anhydrase inhibitors	T50.2X1	T50.2X2	T50.2X3	T50.2X4	T50.2X5	T50.2X6
furfuryl NEC	T50.2X1	T50.2X2	T50.2X3	T50.2X4	T50.2X5	T50.2X6
loop (high-ceiling)	T50.1X1	T50.1X2	T50.1X3	T50.1X4	T50.1X5	T50.1X6
mercurial NEC	T50.2X1	T50.2X2	T50.2X3	T50.2X4	T50.2X5	T50.2X6
osmotic	T50.2X1	T50.2X2	T50.2X3	T50.2X4	T50.2X5	T50.2X6
purine NEC	T50.2X1	T50.2X2	T50.2X3	T50.2X4	T50.2X5	T50.2X6
saluretic NEC	T50.2X1	T50.2X2	T50.2X3	T50.2X4	T50.2X5	T50.2X6
sulfonamide	T50.2X1	T50.2X2	T50.2X3	T50.2X4	T50.2X5	T50.2X6
thiazide NEC	T50.2X1	T50.2X2	T50.2X3	T50.2X4	T50.2X5	T50.2X6
xanthine	T50.2X1	T50.2X2	T50.2X3	T50.2X4	T50.2X5	T50.2X6
Diurgin	T50.2X1	T50.2X2	T50.2X3	T50.2X4	T50.2X5	T50.2X6
Diuril	T50.2X1	T50.2X2	T50.2X3	T50.2X4	T50.2X5	T50.2X6
Diuron	T60.3X1	T60.3X2	T60.3X3	T60.3X4	—	—
Divalproex	T42.6X1	T42.6X2	T42.6X3	T42.6X4	T42.6X5	T42.6X6
Divinyl ether	T41.0X1	T41.0X2	T41.0X3	T41.0X4	T41.0X5	T41.0X6
Dixanthogen	T49.0X1	T49.0X2	T49.0X3	T49.0X4	T49.0X5	T49.0X6
Dixyrazine	T43.3X1	T43.3X2	T43.3X3	T43.3X4	T43.3X5	T43.3X6
D-lysergic acid diethylamide	T40.8X1	T40.8X2	T40.8X3	T40.8X4	—	—
DMCT	T36.4X1	T36.4X2	T36.4X3	T36.4X4	T36.4X5	T36.4X6
DMSO — see Dimethyl sulfoxide						
DNBP	T60.3X1	T60.3X2	T60.3X3	T60.3X4	—	—
DNOC	T65.3X1	T65.3X2	T65.3X3	T65.3X4	—	—
Dobutamine	T44.5X1	T44.5X2	T44.5X3	T44.5X4	T44.5X5	T44.5X6
DOCA	T38.0X1	T38.0X2	T38.0X3	T38.0X4	T38.0X5	T38.0X6
Docusate sodium	T47.4X1	T47.4X2	T47.4X3	T47.4X4	T47.4X5	T47.4X6
Dodicin	T49.0X1	T49.0X2	T49.0X3	T49.0X4	T49.0X5	T49.0X6
Dofamium chloride	T49.0X1	T49.0X2	T49.0X3	T49.0X4	T49.0X5	T49.0X6
Dolophine	T40.3X1	T40.3X2	T40.3X3	T40.3X4	T40.3X5	T40.3X6
Doloxene	T39.8X1	T39.8X2	T39.8X3	T39.8X4	T39.8X5	T39.8X6
Domestic gas (after combustion) — see Gas, utility						
prior to combustion	T59.891	T59.892	T59.893	T59.894	—	—
Domiodol	T48.4X1	T48.4X2	T48.4X3	T48.4X4	T48.4X5	T48.4X6
Domiphen (bromide)	T49.0X1	T49.0X2	T49.0X3	T49.0X4	T49.0X5	T49.0X6
Domperidone	T45.0X1	T45.0X2	T45.0X3	T45.0X4	T45.0X5	T45.0X6
Dopa	T42.8X1	T42.8X2	T42.8X3	T42.8X4	T42.8X5	T42.8X6
Dopamine	T44.991	T44.992	T44.993	T44.994	T44.995	T44.996
Doriden	T42.6X1	T42.6X2	T42.6X3	T42.6X4	T42.6X5	T42.6X6
Dormiral	T42.3X1	T42.3X2	T42.3X3	T42.3X4	T42.3X5	T42.3X6
Dormison	T42.6X1	T42.6X2	T42.6X3	T42.6X4	T42.6X5	T42.6X6
Dornase	T48.4X1	T48.4X2	T48.4X3	T48.4X4	T48.4X5	T48.4X6

Substance	Poisoning, Accidental (unintentional)	Poisoning, Intentional Self-harm	Poisoning, Assault	Poisoning, Undetermined	Adverse Effect	Under-dosing
Dorsacaine	T41.3X1	T41.3X2	T41.3X3	T41.3X4	T41.3X5	T41.3X6
Dosulepin	T43.011	T43.012	T43.013	T43.014	T43.015	T43.016
Dothiepin	T43.011	T43.012	T43.013	T43.014	T43.015	T43.016
Doxantrazole	T48.6X1	T48.6X2	T48.6X3	T48.6X4	T48.6X5	T48.6X6
Doxapram	T50.7X1	T50.7X2	T50.7X3	T50.7X4	T50.7X5	T50.7X6
Doxazosin	T44.6X1	T44.6X2	T44.6X3	T44.6X4	T44.6X5	T44.6X6
Doxepin	T43.011	T43.012	T43.013	T43.014	T43.015	T43.016
Doxifluridine	T45.1X1	T45.1X2	T45.1X3	T45.1X4	T45.1X5	T45.1X6
Doxorubicin	T45.1X1	T45.1X2	T45.1X3	T45.1X4	T45.1X5	T45.1X6
Doxycycline	T36.4X1	T36.4X2	T36.4X3	T36.4X4	T36.4X5	T36.4X6
Doxylamine	T45.0X1	T45.0X2	T45.0X3	T45.0X4	T45.0X5	T45.0X6
Dramamine	T45.0X1	T45.0X2	T45.0X3	T45.0X4	T45.0X5	T45.0X6
Drano (drain cleaner)	T54.3X1	T54.3X2	T54.3X3	T54.3X4	—	—
Dressing, live pulp	T49.7X1	T49.7X2	T49.7X3	T49.7X4	T49.7X5	T49.7X6
Drocode	T40.2X1	T40.2X2	T40.2X3	T40.2X4	T40.2X5	T40.2X6
Dromoran	T40.2X1	T40.2X2	T40.2X3	T40.2X4	T40.2X5	T40.2X6
Dromostanolone	T38.7X1	T38.7X2	T38.7X3	T38.7X4	T38.7X5	T38.7X6
Dronabinol	T40.7X1	T40.7X2	T40.7X3	T40.7X4	T40.7X5	T40.7X6
Droperidol	T43.591	T43.592	T43.593	T43.594	T43.595	T43.596
Dropropizine	T48.3X1	T48.3X2	T48.3X3	T48.3X4	T48.3X5	T48.3X6
Drostanolone	T38.7X1	T38.7X2	T38.7X3	T38.7X4	T38.7X5	T38.7X6
Drotaverine	T44.3X1	T44.3X2	T44.3X3	T44.3X4	T44.3X5	T44.3X6
Drotrecogin alfa	T45.511	T45.512	T45.513	T45.514	T45.515	T45.516
Drug NEC	T50.901	T50.902	T50.903	T50.904	T50.905	T50.906
specified NEC	T50.991	T50.992	T50.993	T50.994	T50.995	T50.996
DTIC	T45.1X1	T45.1X2	T45.1X3	T45.1X4	T45.1X5	T45.1X6
Duboisine	T44.3X1	T44.3X2	T44.3X3	T44.3X4	T44.3X5	T44.3X6
Dulcolax	T47.2X1	T47.2X2	T47.2X3	T47.2X4	T47.2X5	T47.2X6
Duponol (C) (EP)	T49.2X1	T49.2X2	T49.2X3	T49.2X4	T49.2X5	T49.2X6
Durabolin	T38.7X1	T38.7X2	T38.7X3	T38.7X4	T38.7X5	T38.7X6
Dyclone	T41.3X1	T41.3X2	T41.3X3	T41.3X4	T41.3X5	T41.3X6
Dyclonine	T41.3X1	T41.3X2	T41.3X3	T41.3X4	T41.3X5	T41.3X6
Dydrogesterone	T38.5X1	T38.5X2	T38.5X3	T38.5X4	T38.5X5	T38.5X6
Dye NEC	T65.6X1	T65.6X2	T65.6X3	T65.6X4	—	—
antiseptic	T49.0X1	T49.0X2	T49.0X3	T49.0X4	T49.0X5	T49.0X6
diagnostic agents	T50.8X1	T50.8X2	T50.8X3	T50.8X4	T50.8X5	T50.8X6
pharmaceutical NEC	T50.901	T50.902	T50.903	T50.904	T50.905	T50.906
Dyflos	T44.0X1	T44.0X2	T44.0X3	T44.0X4	T44.0X5	T44.0X6
Dymelor	T38.3X1	T38.3X2	T38.3X3	T38.3X4	T38.3X5	T38.3X6
Dynamite	T65.3X1	T65.3X2	T65.3X3	T65.3X4	—	—
fumes	T59.891	T59.892	T59.893	T59.894	—	—
Dyphylline	T44.3X1	T44.3X2	T44.3X3	T44.3X4	T44.3X5	T44.3X6
b-eucaine	T49.1X1	T49.1X2	T49.1X3	T49.1X4	T49.1X5	T49.1X6
Ear drug NEC	T49.6X1	T49.6X2	T49.6X3	T49.6X4	T49.6X5	T49.6X6
Ear preparations	T49.6X1	T49.6X2	T49.6X3	T49.6X4	T49.6X5	T49.6X6
Echothiophate, echothiopate, ecothiopate	T49.5X1	T49.5X2	T49.5X3	T49.5X4	T49.5X5	T49.5X6
Econazole	T49.0X1	T49.0X2	T49.0X3	T49.0X4	T49.0X5	T49.0X6
Ecothiopate iodide	T49.5X1	T49.5X2	T49.5X3	T49.5X4	T49.5X5	T49.5X6
Ecstasy	T43.621	T43.622	T43.623	T43.624	T43.625	T43.626
Ectylurea	T42.6X1	T42.6X2	T42.6X3	T42.6X4	T42.6X5	T42.6X6
Edathamil disodium	T45.8X1	T45.8X2	T45.8X3	T45.8X4	T45.8X5	T45.8X6
Edecrin	T50.1X1	T50.1X2	T50.1X3	T50.1X4	T50.1X5	T50.1X6
Edetate, disodium (calcium)	T45.8X1	T45.8X2	T45.8X3	T45.8X4	T45.8X5	T45.8X6
Edoxudine	T49.5X1	T49.5X2	T49.5X3	T49.5X4	T49.5X5	T49.5X6
Edrophonium	T44.0X1	T44.0X2	T44.0X3	T44.0X4	T44.0X5	T44.0X6
chloride	T44.0X1	T44.0X2	T44.0X3	T44.0X4	T44.0X5	T44.0X6
EDTA	T50.6X1	T50.6X2	T50.6X3	T50.6X4	T50.6X5	T50.6X6
Eflornithine	T37.2X1	T37.2X2	T37.2X3	T37.2X4	T37.2X5	T37.2X6
Efloxate	T46.3X1	T46.3X2	T46.3X3	T46.3X4	T46.3X5	T46.3X6
Elase	T49.8X1	T49.8X2	T49.8X3	T49.8X4	T49.8X5	T49.8X6
Elastase	T47.5X1	T47.5X2	T47.5X3	T47.5X4	T47.5X5	T47.5X6
Elaterium	T47.2X1	T47.2X2	T47.2X3	T47.2X4	T47.2X5	T47.2X6
Elcatonin	T50.991	T50.992	T50.993	T50.994	T50.995	T50.996
Elder	T62.2X1	T62.2X2	T62.2X3	T62.2X4	—	—
berry, (unripe)	T62.1X1	T62.1X2	T62.1X3	T62.1X4	—	—
Electrolyte balance drug	T50.3X1	T50.3X2	T50.3X3	T50.3X4	T50.3X5	T50.3X6
Electrolytes NEC	T50.3X1	T50.3X2	T50.3X3	T50.3X4	T50.3X5	T50.3X6
Electrolytic agent NEC	T50.3X1	T50.3X2	T50.3X3	T50.3X4	T50.3X5	T50.3X6
Elemental diet	T50.901	T50.902	T50.903	T50.904	T50.905	T50.906
Elliptinium acetate	T45.1X1	T45.1X2	T45.1X3	T45.1X4	T45.1X5	T45.1X6
Embramine	T45.0X1	T45.0X2	T45.0X3	T45.0X4	T45.0X5	T45.0X6
Emepronium (salts)	T44.3X1	T44.3X2	T44.3X3	T44.3X4	T44.3X5	T44.3X6
bromide	T44.3X1	T44.3X2	T44.3X3	T44.3X4	T44.3X5	T44.3X6
Emetic NEC	T47.7X1	T47.7X2	T47.7X3	T47.7X4	T47.7X5	T47.7X6
Emetine	T37.3X1	T37.3X2	T37.3X3	T37.3X4	T37.3X5	T37.3X6
Emollient NEC	T49.3X1	T49.3X2	T49.3X3	T49.3X4	T49.3X5	T49.3X6
Emorfazone	T39.8X1	T39.8X2	T39.8X3	T39.8X4	T39.8X5	T39.8X6
Emylcamate	T43.591	T43.592	T43.593	T43.594	T43.595	T43.596
Enalapril	T46.4X1	T46.4X2	T46.4X3	T46.4X4	T46.4X5	T46.4X6
Enalaprilat	T46.4X1	T46.4X2	T46.4X3	T46.4X4	T46.4X5	T46.4X6
Encainide	T46.2X1	T46.2X2	T46.2X3	T46.2X4	T46.2X5	T46.2X6
Endocaine	T41.3X1	T41.3X2	T41.3X3	T41.3X4	T41.3X5	T41.3X6

Substance	Poisoning, Accidental (unintentional)	Poisoning, Intentional Self-harm	Poisoning, Assault	Poisoning, Undetermined	Adverse Effect	Under-dosing
Endosulfan	T60.2X1	T60.2X2	T60.2X3	T60.2X4	—	—
Endothall	T60.3X1	T60.3X2	T60.3X3	T60.3X4	—	—
Endralazine	T46.5X1	T46.5X2	T46.5X3	T46.5X4	T46.5X5	T46.5X6
Endrin	T60.1X1	T60.1X2	T60.1X3	T60.1X4	—	—
Enflurane	T41.0X1	T41.0X2	T41.0X3	T41.0X4	T41.0X5	T41.0X6
Enhexymal	T42.3X1	T42.3X2	T42.3X3	T42.3X4	T42.3X5	T42.3X6
Enocitabine	T45.1X1	T45.1X2	T45.1X3	T45.1X4	T45.1X5	T45.1X6
Enovid	T38.4X1	T38.4X2	T38.4X3	T38.4X4	T38.4X5	T38.4X6
Enoxacin	T36.8X1	T36.8X2	T36.8X3	T36.8X4	T36.8X5	T36.8X6
Enoxaparin (sodium)	T45.511	T45.512	T45.513	T45.514	T45.515	T45.516
Enpiprazole	T43.591	T43.592	T43.593	T43.594	T43.595	T43.596
Enprofylline	T48.6X1	T48.6X2	T48.6X3	T48.6X4	T48.6X5	T48.6X6
Enprostil	T47.1X1	T47.1X2	T47.1X3	T47.1X4	T47.1X5	T47.1X6
Enterogastrone	T38.891	T38.892	T38.893	T38.894	T38.895	T38.896
ENT preparations (anti-infectives)	T49.6X1	T49.6X2	T49.6X3	T49.6X4	T49.6X5	T49.6X6
Enviomycin	T36.8X1	T36.8X2	T36.8X3	T36.8X4	T36.8X5	T36.8X6
Enzodase	T45.3X1	T45.3X2	T45.3X3	T45.3X4	T45.3X5	T45.3X6
Enzyme NEC	T45.3X1	T45.3X2	T45.3X3	T45.3X4	T45.3X5	T45.3X6
depolymerizing	T49.8X1	T49.8X2	T49.8X3	T49.8X4	T49.8X5	T49.8X6
fibrolytic	T45.3X1	T45.3X2	T45.3X3	T45.3X4	T45.3X5	T45.3X6
gastric	T47.5X1	T47.5X2	T47.5X3	T47.5X4	T47.5X5	T47.5X6
intestinal	T47.5X1	T47.5X2	T47.5X3	T47.5X4	T47.5X5	T47.5X6
local action	T49.4X1	T49.4X2	T49.4X3	T49.4X4	T49.4X5	T49.4X6
proteolytic	T49.4X1	T49.4X2	T49.4X3	T49.4X4	T49.4X5	T49.4X6
thrombolytic	T45.3X1	T45.3X2	T45.3X3	T45.3X4	T45.3X5	T45.3X6
EPAB	T41.3X1	T41.3X2	T41.3X3	T41.3X4	T41.3X5	T41.3X6
Epanutin	T42.0X1	T42.0X2	T42.0X3	T42.0X4	T42.0X5	T42.0X6
Ephedra	T44.991	T44.992	T44.993	T44.994	T44.995	T44.996
Ephedrine	T44.991	T44.992	T44.993	T44.994	T44.995	T44.996
Epichlorhydrin, epichlorohydrin	T52.8X1	T52.8X2	T52.8X3	T52.8X4	—	—
Epicillin	T36.0X1	T36.0X2	T36.0X3	T36.0X4	T36.0X5	T36.0X6
Epiestriol	T38.5X1	T38.5X2	T38.5X3	T38.5X4	T38.5X5	T38.5X6
Epilim — see Sodium valproate						
Epimestrol	T38.5X1	T38.5X2	T38.5X3	T38.5X4	T38.5X5	T38.5X6
Epinephrine	T44.5X1	T44.5X2	T44.5X3	T44.5X4	T44.5X5	T44.5X6
Epirubicin	T45.1X1	T45.1X2	T45.1X3	T45.1X4	T45.1X5	T45.1X6
Epitiostanol	T38.7X1	T38.7X2	T38.7X3	T38.7X4	T38.7X5	T38.7X6
Epitizide	T50.2X1	T50.2X2	T50.2X3	T50.2X4	T50.2X5	T50.2X6
EPN	T60.0X1	T60.0X2	T60.0X3	T60.0X4	—	—
EPO	T45.8X1	T45.8X2	T45.8X3	T45.8X4	T45.8X5	T45.8X6
Epoetin alpha	T45.8X1	T45.8X2	T45.8X3	T45.8X4	T45.8X5	T45.8X6
Epomediol	T50.991	T50.992	T50.993	T50.994	T50.995	T50.996
Epoprostenol	T45.521	T45.522	T45.523	T45.524	T45.525	T45.526
Epoxy resin	T65.891	T65.892	T65.893	T65.894	—	—
Eprazinone	T48.4X1	T48.4X2	T48.4X3	T48.4X4	T48.4X5	T48.4X6
Epsilon aminocaproic acid	T45.621	T45.622	T45.623	T45.624	T45.625	T45.626
Epsom salt	T47.3X1	T47.3X2	T47.3X3	T47.3X4	T47.3X5	T47.3X6
Eptazocine	T40.4X1	T40.4X2	T40.4X3	T40.4X4	T40.4X5	T40.4X6
Equanil	T43.591	T43.592	T43.593	T43.594	T43.595	T43.596
Equisetum	T62.2X1	T62.2X2	T62.2X3	T62.2X4	—	—
diuretic	T50.2X1	T50.2X2	T50.2X3	T50.2X4	T50.2X5	T50.2X6
Ergobasine	T48.0X1	T48.0X2	T48.0X3	T48.0X4	T48.0X5	T48.0X6
Ergocalciferol	T45.2X1	T45.2X2	T45.2X3	T45.2X4	T45.2X5	T45.2X6
Ergoloid mesylates	T46.7X1	T46.7X2	T46.7X3	T46.7X4	T46.7X5	T46.7X6
Ergometrine	T48.0X1	T48.0X2	T48.0X3	T48.0X4	T48.0X5	T48.0X6
Ergonovine	T48.0X1	T48.0X2	T48.0X3	T48.0X4	T48.0X5	T48.0X6
Ergotamine	T46.5X1	T46.5X2	T46.5X3	T46.5X4	T46.5X5	T46.5X6
Ergotocine	T48.0X1	T48.0X2	T48.0X3	T48.0X4	T48.0X5	T48.0X6
Ergotrate	T48.0X1	T48.0X2	T48.0X3	T48.0X4	T48.0X5	T48.0X6
Ergot NEC	T64.81	T64.82	T64.83	T64.84	—	—
derivative	T48.0X1	T48.0X2	T48.0X3	T48.0X4	T48.0X5	T48.0X6
medicinal (alkaloids)	T48.0X1	T48.0X2	T48.0X3	T48.0X4	T48.0X5	T48.0X6
prepared	T48.0X1	T48.0X2	T48.0X3	T48.0X4	T48.0X5	T48.0X6
Eritrityl tetranitrate	T46.3X1	T46.3X2	T46.3X3	T46.3X4	T46.3X5	T46.3X6
Erythrityl tetranitrate	T46.3X1	T46.3X2	T46.3X3	T46.3X4	T46.3X5	T46.3X6
Erythrol tetranitrate	T46.3X1	T46.3X2	T46.3X3	T46.3X4	T46.3X5	T46.3X6
Erythromycin (salts)	T36.3X1	T36.3X2	T36.3X3	T36.3X4	T36.3X5	T36.3X6
ophthalmic preparation	T49.5X1	T49.5X2	T49.5X3	T49.5X4	T49.5X5	T49.5X6
topical NEC	T49.0X1	T49.0X2	T49.0X3	T49.0X4	T49.0X5	T49.0X6
Erythropoietin	T45.8X1	T45.8X2	T45.8X3	T45.8X4	T45.8X5	T45.8X6
human	T45.8X1	T45.8X2	T45.8X3	T45.8X4	T45.8X5	T45.8X6
Escin	T46.991	T46.992	T46.993	T46.994	T46.995	T46.996
Esculin	T45.2X1	T45.2X2	T45.2X3	T45.2X4	T45.2X5	T45.2X6
Esculoside	T45.2X1	T45.2X2	T45.2X3	T45.2X4	T45.2X5	T45.2X6
ESDT (ether-soluble tar distillate)	T49.1X1	T49.1X2	T49.1X3	T49.1X4	T49.1X5	T49.1X6
Eserine	T49.5X1	T49.5X2	T49.5X3	T49.5X4	T49.5X5	T49.5X6
Esflurbiprofen	T39.311	T39.312	T39.313	T39.314	T39.315	T39.316
Eskabarb	T42.3X1	T42.3X2	T42.3X3	T42.3X4	T42.3X5	T42.3X6
Eskalith	T43.8X1	T43.8X2	T43.8X3	T43.8X4	T43.8X5	T43.8X6
Esmolol	T44.7X1	T44.7X2	T44.7X3	T44.7X4	T44.7X5	T44.7X6

Additional Character May Be Required — Refer to the Tabular List for Character Selection ▽ Subterms under main terms may continue to next column or page

Substance	Poisoning, Accidental (unintentional)	Poisoning, Intentional Self-harm	Poisoning, Assault	Poisoning, Undetermined	Adverse Effect	Under-dosing
Estanozolol	T38.7X1	T38.7X2	T38.7X3	T38.7X4	T38.7X5	T38.7X6
Estazolam	T42.4X1	T42.4X2	T42.4X3	T42.4X4	T42.4X5	T42.4X6
Estradiol	T38.5X1	T38.5X2	T38.5X3	T38.5X4	T38.5X5	T38.5X6
with testosterone	T38.7X1	T38.7X2	T38.7X3	T38.7X4	T38.7X5	T38.7X6
benzoate	T38.5X1	T38.5X2	T38.5X3	T38.5X4	T38.5X5	T38.5X6
Estramustine	T45.1X1	T45.1X2	T45.1X3	T45.1X4	T45.1X5	T45.1X6
Estriol	T38.5X1	T38.5X2	T38.5X3	T38.5X4	T38.5X5	T38.5X6
Estrogen	T38.5X1	T38.5X2	T38.5X3	T38.5X4	T38.5X5	T38.5X6
with progesterone	T38.5X1	T38.5X2	T38.5X3	T38.5X4	T38.5X5	T38.5X6
conjugated	T38.5X1	T38.5X2	T38.5X3	T38.5X4	T38.5X5	T38.5X6
Estrone	T38.5X1	T38.5X2	T38.5X3	T38.5X4	T38.5X5	T38.5X6
Estropipate	T38.5X1	T38.5X2	T38.5X3	T38.5X4	T38.5X5	T38.5X6
Etacrynate sodium	T50.1X1	T50.1X2	T50.1X3	T50.1X4	T50.1X5	T50.1X6
Etacrynic acid	T50.1X1	T50.1X2	T50.1X3	T50.1X4	T50.1X5	T50.1X6
Etafedrine	T48.6X1	T48.6X2	T48.6X3	T48.6X4	T48.6X5	T48.6X6
Etafenone	T46.3X1	T46.3X2	T46.3X3	T46.3X4	T46.3X5	T46.3X6
Etambutol	T37.1X1	T37.1X2	T37.1X3	T37.1X4	T37.1X5	T37.1X6
Etamiphyllin	T48.6X1	T48.6X2	T48.6X3	T48.6X4	T48.6X5	T48.6X6
Etamivan	T50.7X1	T50.7X2	T50.7X3	T50.7X4	T50.7X5	T50.7X6
Etamsylate	T45.7X1	T45.7X2	T45.7X3	T45.7X4	T45.7X5	T45.7X6
Etebenecid	T50.4X1	T50.4X2	T50.4X3	T50.4X4	T50.4X5	T50.4X6
Ethacridine	T49.0X1	T49.0X2	T49.0X3	T49.0X4	T49.0X5	T49.0X6
Ethacrynic acid	T50.1X1	T50.1X2	T50.1X3	T50.1X4	T50.1X5	T50.1X6
Ethadione	T42.2X1	T42.2X2	T42.2X3	T42.2X4	T42.2X5	T42.2X6
Ethambutol	T37.1X1	T37.1X2	T37.1X3	T37.1X4	T37.1X5	T37.1X6
Ethamide	T50.2X1	T50.2X2	T50.2X3	T50.2X5	T50.2X6	
Ethamivan	T50.7X1	T50.7X2	T50.7X3	T50.7X4	T50.7X5	T50.7X6
Ethamsylate	T45.7X1	T45.7X2	T45.7X3	T45.7X4	T45.7X5	T45.7X6
Ethanol	T51.0X1	T51.0X2	T51.0X3	T51.0X4	—	—
beverage	T51.0X1	T51.0X2	T51.0X3	T51.0X4	—	—
Ethanolamine oleate	T46.8X1	T46.8X2	T46.8X3	T46.8X4	T46.8X5	T46.8X6
Ethaverine	T44.3X1	T44.3X2	T44.3X3	T44.3X4	T44.3X5	T44.3X6
Ethchlorvynol	T42.6X1	T42.6X2	T42.6X3	T42.6X4	T42.6X5	T42.6X6
Ethebenecid	T50.4X1	T50.4X2	T50.4X3	T50.4X4	T50.4X5	T50.4X6
Ether (vapor)	T41.0X1	T41.0X2	T41.0X3	T41.0X4	T41.0X5	T41.0X6
anesthetic	T41.0X1	T41.0X2	T41.0X3	T41.0X4	T41.0X5	T41.0X6
divinyl	T41.0X1	T41.0X2	T41.0X3	T41.0X4	T41.0X5	T41.0X6
ethyl (medicinal)	T41.0X1	T41.0X2	T41.0X3	T41.0X4	T41.0X5	T41.0X6
nonmedicinal	T52.8X1	T52.8X2	T52.8X3	T52.8X4	—	—
petroleum — see Ligroin						
solvent	T52.8X1	T52.8X2	T52.8X3	T52.8X4	—	—
Ethiazide	T50.2X1	T50.2X2	T50.2X3	T50.2X4	T50.2X5	T50.2X6
Ethidium chloride (vapor)	T59.891	T59.892	T59.893	T59.894		
Ethinamate	T42.6X1	T42.6X2	T42.6X3	T42.6X4	T42.6X5	T42.6X6
Ethinylestradiol, ethinyloestradiol	T38.5X1	T38.5X2	T38.5X3	T38.5X4	T38.5X5	T38.5X6
with						
levonorgestrel	T38.4X1	T38.4X2	T38.4X3	T38.4X4	T38.4X5	T38.4X6
norethisterone	T38.4X1	T38.4X2	T38.4X3	T38.4X4	T38.4X5	T38.4X6
Ethiodized oil (131 I)	T50.8X1	T50.8X2	T50.8X3	T50.8X4	T50.8X5	T50.8X6
Ethion	T60.0X1	T60.0X2	T60.0X3	T60.0X4		
Ethionamide	T37.1X1	T37.1X2	T37.1X3	T37.1X4	T37.1X5	T37.1X6
Ethioniamide	T37.1X1	T37.1X2	T37.1X3	T37.1X4	T37.1X5	T37.1X6
Ethisterone	T38.5X1	T38.5X2	T38.5X3	T38.5X4	T38.5X5	T38.5X6
Ethobral	T42.3X1	T42.3X2	T42.3X3	T42.3X4	T42.3X5	T42.3X6
Ethocaine (infiltration) (topical)	T41.3X1	T41.3X2	T41.3X3	T41.3X4	T41.3X5	T41.3X6
nerve block (peripheral) (plexus)	T41.3X1	T41.3X2	T41.3X3	T41.3X4	T41.3X5	T41.3X6
spinal	T41.3X1	T41.3X2	T41.3X3	T41.3X4	T41.3X5	T41.3X6
Ethoheptazine	T40.4X1	T40.4X2	T40.4X3	T40.4X4	T40.4X5	T40.4X6
Ethopropazine	T44.3X1	T44.3X2	T44.3X3	T44.3X4	T44.3X5	T44.3X6
Ethosuximide	T42.2X1	T42.2X2	T42.2X3	T42.2X4	T42.2X5	T42.2X6
Ethotoin	T42.0X1	T42.0X2	T42.0X3	T42.0X4	T42.0X5	T42.0X6
Ethoxazene	T37.91	T37.92	T37.93	T37.94	T37.95	T37.96
Ethoxazorutoside	T46.991	T46.992	T46.993	T46.994	T46.995	T46.996
Ethoxzolamide	T50.2X1	T50.2X2	T50.2X3	T50.2X4	T50.2X5	T50.2X6
Ethyl						
acetate	T52.8X1	T52.8X2	T52.8X3	T52.8X4	—	—
alcohol	T51.0X1	T51.0X2	T51.0X3	T51.0X4	—	—
beverage	T51.0X1	T51.0X2	T51.0X3	T51.0X4	—	—
aldehyde (vapor)	T59.891	T59.892	T59.893	T59.894	—	—
liquid	T52.8X1	T52.8X2	T52.8X3	T52.8X4	—	—
aminobenzoate	T41.3X1	T41.3X2	T41.3X3	T41.3X4	T41.3X5	T41.3X6
aminophenothiazine	T43.3X1	T43.3X2	T43.3X3	T43.3X4	T43.3X5	T43.3X6
benzoate	T52.8X1	T52.8X2	T52.8X3	T52.8X4	—	—
biscoumacetate	T45.511	T45.512	T45.513	T45.514	T45.515	T45.516
bromide (anesthetic)	T41.0X1	T41.0X2	T41.0X3	T41.0X4	T41.0X5	T41.0X6
carbamate	T45.1X1	T45.1X2	T45.1X3	T45.1X4	T45.1X5	T45.1X6
carbinol	T51.3X1	T51.3X2	T51.3X3	T51.3X4	—	—
carbonate	T52.8X1	T52.8X2	T52.8X3	T52.8X4	—	—
chaulmoograte	T37.1X1	T37.1X2	T37.1X3	T37.1X4	T37.1X5	T37.1X6
chloride (anesthetic)	T41.0X1	T41.0X2	T41.0X3	T41.0X4	T41.0X5	T41.0X6

Substance	Poisoning, Accidental (unintentional)	Poisoning, Intentional Self-harm	Poisoning, Assault	Poisoning, Undetermined	Adverse Effect	Under-dosing
Ethyl — continued						
chloride — continued						
anesthetic (local)	T41.3X1	T41.3X2	T41.3X3	T41.3X4	T41.3X5	T41.3X6
inhaled	T41.0X1	T41.0X2	T41.0X3	T41.0X4	T41.0X5	T41.0X6
local	T49.4X1	T49.4X2	T49.4X3	T49.4X4	T49.4X5	T49.4X6
solvent	T53.6X1	T53.6X2	T53.6X3	T53.6X4		
dibunate	T48.3X1	T48.3X2	T48.3X3	T48.3X4	T48.3X5	T48.3X6
dichloroarsine (vapor)	T57.0X1	T57.0X2	T57.0X3	T57.0X4		
estranol	T38.7X1	T38.7X2	T38.7X3	T38.7X4	T38.7X5	T38.7X6
ether — see also ether	T52.8X1	T52.8X2	T52.8X3	T52.8X4		
formate NEC (solvent)	T52.0X1	T52.0X2	T52.0X3	T52.0X4		
fumarate	T49.4X1	T49.4X2	T49.4X3	T49.4X4	T49.4X5	T49.4X6
hydroxyisobutyrate NEC (solvent)	T52.8X1	T52.8X2	T52.8X3	T52.8X4		
iodoacetate	T59.3X1	T59.3X2	T59.3X3	T59.3X4		
lactate NEC (solvent)	T52.8X1	T52.8X2	T52.8X3	T52.8X4		
loflazepate	T42.4X1	T42.4X2	T42.4X3	T42.4X4	T42.4X5	T42.4X6
mercuric chloride	T56.1X1	T56.1X2	T56.1X3	T56.1X4		
methylcarbinol	T51.8X1	T51.8X2	T51.8X3	T51.8X4		
morphine	T40.2X1	T40.2X2	T40.2X3	T40.2X4	T40.2X5	T40.2X6
noradrenaline	T48.6X1	T48.6X2	T48.6X3	T48.6X4	T48.6X5	T48.6X6
oxybutyrate NEC (solvent)	T52.8X1	T52.8X2	T52.8X3	T52.8X4		
Ethylene (gas)	T59.891	T59.892	T59.893	T59.894		
anesthetic (general)	T41.0X1	T41.0X2	T41.0X3	T41.0X4	T41.0X5	T41.0X6
chlorohydrin	T52.8X1	T52.8X2	T52.8X3	T52.8X4		
vapor	T53.6X1	T53.6X2	T53.6X3	T53.6X4		
dichloride	T52.8X1	T52.8X2	T52.8X3	T52.8X4		
vapor	T53.6X1	T53.6X2	T53.6X3	T53.6X4		
dinitrate	T52.3X1	T52.3X2	T52.3X3	T52.3X4		
glycol(s)	T52.8X1	T52.8X2	T52.8X3	T52.8X4		
dinitrate	T52.3X1	T52.3X2	T52.3X3	T52.3X4		
monobutyl ether	T52.3X1	T52.3X2	T52.3X3	T52.3X4		
imine	T54.1X1	T54.1X2	T54.1X3	T54.1X4		
oxide (fumigant) (nonmedicinal)	T59.891	T59.892	T59.893	T59.894		
medicinal	T49.0X1	T49.0X2	T49.0X3	T49.0X4	T49.0X5	T49.0X6
Ethylenediaminetetra-acetic acid	T50.6X1	T50.6X2	T50.6X3	T50.6X4	T50.6X5	T50.6X6
Ethylenediamine theophylline	T48.6X1	T48.6X2	T48.6X3	T48.6X4	T48.6X5	T48.6X6
Ethylenedinitrilotetra-acetate	T50.6X1	T50.6X2	T50.6X3	T50.6X4	T50.6X5	T50.6X6
Ethylestrenol	T38.7X1	T38.7X2	T38.7X3	T38.7X4	T38.7X5	T38.7X6
Ethylhydrocellulose	T47.4X1	T47.4X2	T47.4X3	T47.4X4	T47.4X5	T47.4X6
Ethylidene						
chloride NEC	T53.6X1	T53.6X2	T53.6X3	T53.6X4	—	—
diacetate	T60.3X1	T60.3X2	T60.3X3	T60.3X4	—	—
dicoumarin	T45.511	T45.512	T45.513	T45.514	T45.515	T45.516
dicoumarol	T45.511	T45.512	T45.513	T45.514	T45.515	T45.516
diethyl ether	T52.0X1	T52.0X2	T52.0X3	T52.0X4		
Ethylmorphine	T40.2X1	T40.2X2	T40.2X3	T40.2X4	T40.2X5	T40.2X6
Ethylnorepinephrine	T48.6X1	T48.6X2	T48.6X3	T48.6X4	T48.6X5	T48.6X6
Ethylparachlorophen-oxyisobutyrate	T46.6X1	T46.6X2	T46.6X3	T46.6X4	T46.6X5	T46.6X6
Ethynodiol	T38.4X1	T38.4X2	T38.4X3	T38.4X4	T38.4X5	T38.4X6
with mestranol diacetate	T38.4X1	T38.4X2	T38.4X3	T38.4X4	T38.4X5	T38.4X6
Etidocaine	T41.3X1	T41.3X2	T41.3X3	T41.3X4	T41.3X5	T41.3X6
infiltration (subcutaneous)	T41.3X1	T41.3X2	T41.3X3	T41.3X4	T41.3X5	T41.3X6
nerve (peripheral) (plexus)	T41.3X1	T41.3X2	T41.3X3	T41.3X4	T41.3X5	T41.3X6
Etidronate	T50.991	T50.992	T50.993	T50.994	T50.995	T50.996
Etidronic acid (disodium salt)	T50.991	T50.992	T50.993	T50.994	T50.995	T50.996
Etifoxine	T42.6X1	T42.6X2	T42.6X3	T42.6X4	T42.6X5	T42.6X6
Etilefrine	T44.4X1	T44.4X2	T44.4X3	T44.4X4	T44.4X5	T44.4X6
Etilfen	T42.3X1	T42.3X2	T42.3X3	T42.3X4	T42.3X5	T42.3X6
Etinodiol	T38.4X1	T38.4X2	T38.4X3	T38.4X4	T38.4X5	T38.4X6
Etiroxate	T46.6X1	T46.6X2	T46.6X3	T46.6X4	T46.6X5	T46.6X6
Etizolam	T42.4X1	T42.4X2	T42.4X3	T42.4X4	T42.4X5	T42.4X6
Etodolac	T39.391	T39.392	T39.393	T39.394	T39.395	T39.396
Etofamide	T37.3X1	T37.3X2	T37.3X3	T37.3X4	T37.3X5	T37.3X6
Etofibrate	T46.6X1	T46.6X2	T46.6X3	T46.6X4	T46.6X5	T46.6X6
Etofylline	T46.7X1	T46.7X2	T46.7X3	T46.7X4	T46.7X5	T46.7X6
clofibrate	T46.6X1	T46.6X2	T46.6X3	T46.6X4	T46.6X5	T46.6X6
Etoglucid	T45.1X1	T45.1X2	T45.1X3	T45.1X4	T45.1X5	T45.1X6
Etomidate	T41.1X1	T41.1X2	T41.1X3	T41.1X4	T41.1X5	T41.1X6
Etomide	T39.8X1	T39.8X2	T39.8X3	T39.8X4	T39.8X5	T39.8X6
Etomidoline	T44.3X1	T44.3X2	T44.3X3	T44.3X4	T44.3X5	T44.3X6
Etoposide	T45.1X1	T45.1X2	T45.1X3	T45.1X4	T45.1X5	T45.1X6
Etorphine	T40.2X1	T40.2X2	T40.2X3	T40.2X4	T40.2X5	T40.2X6
Etoval	T42.3X1	T42.3X2	T42.3X3	T42.3X4	T42.3X5	T42.3X6
Etozolin	T50.1X1	T50.1X2	T50.1X3	T50.1X4	T50.1X5	T50.1X6
Etretinate	T50.991	T50.992	T50.993	T50.994	T50.995	T50.996
Etryptamine	T43.691	T43.692	T43.693	T43.694	T43.695	T43.696
Etybenzatropine	T44.3X1	T44.3X2	T44.3X3	T44.3X4	T44.3X5	T44.3X6

Substance	Poisoning, Accidental (unintentional)	Poisoning, Intentional Self-harm	Poisoning, Assault	Poisoning, Undetermined	Adverse Effect	Under-dosing
Etynodiol	T38.4X1	T38.4X2	T38.4X3	T38.4X4	T38.4X5	T38.4X6
Eucaine	T41.3X1	T41.3X2	T41.3X3	T41.3X4	T41.3X5	T41.3X6
Eucalyptus oil	T49.7X1	T49.7X2	T49.7X3	T49.7X4	T49.7X5	T49.7X6
Eucatropine	T49.5X1	T49.5X2	T49.5X3	T49.5X4	T49.5X5	T49.5X6
Eucodal	T40.2X1	T40.2X2	T40.2X3	T40.2X4	T40.2X5	T40.2X6
Euneryl	T42.3X1	T42.3X2	T42.3X3	T42.3X4	T42.3X5	T42.3X6
Euphthalmine	T44.3X1	T44.3X2	T44.3X3	T44.3X4	T44.3X5	T44.3X6
Eurax	T49.0X1	T49.0X2	T49.0X3	T49.0X4	T49.0X5	T49.0X6
Euresol	T49.4X1	T49.4X2	T49.4X3	T49.4X4	T49.4X5	T49.4X6
Euthroid	T38.1X1	T38.1X2	T38.1X3	T38.1X4	T38.1X5	T38.1X6
Evans blue	T50.8X1	T50.8X2	T50.8X3	T50.8X4	T50.8X5	T50.8X6
Evipal	T42.3X1	T42.3X2	T42.3X3	T42.3X4	T42.3X5	T42.3X6
sodium	T41.1X1	T41.1X2	T41.1X3	T41.1X4	T41.1X5	T41.1X6
Evipan	T42.3X1	T42.3X2	T42.3X3	T42.3X4	T42.3X5	T42.3X6
sodium	T41.1X1	T41.1X2	T41.1X3	T41.1X4	T41.1X5	T41.1X6
Exalamide	T49.0X1	T49.0X2	T49.0X3	T49.0X4	T49.0X5	T49.0X6
Exalgin	T39.1X1	T39.1X2	T39.1X3	T39.1X4	T39.1X5	T39.1X6
Excipients, pharmaceutical	T50.901	T50.902	T50.903	T50.904	T50.905	T50.906
Exhaust gas (engine) (motor vehicle)	T58.01	T58.02	T58.03	T58.04	—	—
Ex-Lax (phenolphthalein)	T47.2X1	T47.2X2	T47.2X3	T47.2X4	T47.2X5	T47.2X6
Expectorant NEC	T48.4X1	T48.4X2	T48.4X3	T48.4X4	T48.4X5	T48.4X6
Extended insulin zinc suspension	T38.3X1	T38.3X2	T38.3X3	T38.3X4	T38.3X5	T38.3X6
External medications (skin) (mucous membrane)	T49.91	T49.92	T49.93	T49.94	T49.95	T49.96
dental agent	T49.7X1	T49.7X2	T49.7X3	T49.7X4	T49.7X5	T49.7X6
ENT agent	T49.6X1	T49.6X2	T49.6X3	T49.6X4	T49.6X5	T49.6X6
ophthalmic preparation	T49.5X1	T49.5X2	T49.5X3	T49.5X4	T49.5X5	T49.5X6
specified NEC	T49.8X1	T49.8X2	T49.8X3	T49.8X4	T49.8X5	T49.8X6
Extrapyramidal antagonist NEC	T44.3X1	T44.3X2	T44.3X3	T44.3X4	T44.3X5	T44.3X6
Eye agents (anti-infective)	T49.5X1	T49.5X2	T49.5X3	T49.5X4	T49.5X5	T49.5X6
Eye drug NEC	T49.5X1	T49.5X2	T49.5X3	T49.5X4	T49.5X5	T49.5X6
FAC (fluorouracil + doxorubicin + cyclophosphamide)	T45.1X1	T45.1X2	T45.1X3	T45.1X4	T45.1X5	T45.1X6
Factor						
I (fibrinogen)	T45.8X1	T45.8X2	T45.8X3	T45.8X4	T45.8X5	T45.8X6
III (thromboplastin)	T45.8X1	T45.8X2	T45.8X3	T45.8X4	T45.8X5	T45.8X6
IX complex	T45.7X1	T45.7X2	T45.7X3	T45.7X4	T45.7X5	T45.7X6
human	T45.8X1	T45.8X2	T45.8X3	T45.8X4	T45.8X5	T45.8X6
VIII (antihemophilic Factor) (concentrate)	T45.8X1	T45.8X2	T45.8X3	T45.8X4	T45.8X5	T45.8X6
Famotidine	T47.0X1	T47.0X2	T47.0X3	T47.0X4	T47.0X5	T47.0X6
Fat suspension, intravenous	T50.991	T50.992	T50.993	T50.994	T50.995	T50.996
Fazadinium bromide	T48.1X1	T48.1X2	T48.1X3	T48.1X4	T48.1X5	T48.1X6
Febarbamate	T42.3X1	T42.3X2	T42.3X3	T42.3X4	T42.3X5	T42.3X6
Fecal softener	T47.4X1	T47.4X2	T47.4X3	T47.4X4	T47.4X5	T47.4X6
Fedrilate	T48.3X1	T48.3X2	T48.3X3	T48.3X4	T48.3X5	T48.3X6
Felodipine	T46.1X1	T46.1X2	T46.1X3	T46.1X4	T46.1X5	T46.1X6
Felypressin	T38.891	T38.892	T38.893	T38.894	T38.895	T38.896
Femoxetine	T43.221	T43.222	T43.223	T43.224	T43.225	T43.226
Fenalcomine	T46.3X1	T46.3X2	T46.3X3	T46.3X4	T46.3X5	T46.3X6
Fenamisal	T37.1X1	T37.1X2	T37.1X3	T37.1X4	T37.1X5	T37.1X6
Fenazone	T39.2X1	T39.2X2	T39.2X3	T39.2X4	T39.2X5	T39.2X6
Fenbendazole	T37.4X1	T37.4X2	T37.4X3	T37.4X4	T37.4X5	T37.4X6
Fenbutrazate	T50.5X1	T50.5X2	T50.5X3	T50.5X4	T50.5X5	T50.5X6
Fencamfamine	T43.691	T43.692	T43.693	T43.694	T43.695	T43.696
Fendiline	T46.1X1	T46.1X2	T46.1X3	T46.1X4	T46.1X5	T46.1X6
Fenetylline	T43.691	T43.692	T43.693	T43.694	T43.695	T43.696
Fenflumizole	T39.391	T39.392	T39.393	T39.394	T39.395	T39.396
Fenfluramine	T50.5X1	T50.5X2	T50.5X3	T50.5X4	T50.5X5	T50.5X6
Fenobarbital	T42.3X1	T42.3X2	T42.3X3	T42.3X4	T42.3X5	T42.3X6
Fenofibrate	T46.6X1	T46.6X2	T46.6X3	T46.6X4	T46.6X5	T46.6X6
Fenoprofen	T39.311	T39.312	T39.313	T39.314	T39.315	T39.316
Fenoterol	T48.6X1	T48.6X2	T48.6X3	T48.6X4	T48.6X5	T48.6X6
Fenoverine	T44.3X1	T44.3X2	T44.3X3	T44.3X4	T44.3X5	T44.3X6
Fenoxazoline	T48.5X1	T48.5X2	T48.5X3	T48.5X4	T48.5X5	T48.5X6
Fenproporex	T50.5X1	T50.5X2	T50.5X3	T50.5X4	T50.5X5	T50.5X6
Fenquizone	T50.2X1	T50.2X2	T50.2X3	T50.2X4	T50.2X5	T50.2X6
Fentanyl	T40.4X1	T40.4X2	T40.4X3	T40.4X4	T40.4X5	T40.4X6
Fentazin	T43.3X1	T43.3X2	T43.3X3	T43.3X4	T43.3X5	T43.3X6
Fenthion	T60.0X1	T60.0X2	T60.0X3	T60.0X4	—	—
Fenticlor	T49.0X1	T49.0X2	T49.0X3	T49.0X4	T49.0X5	T49.0X6
Fenylbutazone	T39.2X1	T39.2X2	T39.2X3	T39.2X4	T39.2X5	T39.2X6
Feprazone	T39.2X1	T39.2X2	T39.2X3	T39.2X4	T39.2X5	T39.2X6
Fer de lance (bite) (venom)	T63.061	T63.062	T63.063	T63.064	—	—
Ferric — see also Iron						
chloride	T45.4X1	T45.4X2	T45.4X3	T45.4X4	T45.4X5	T45.4X6
citrate	T45.4X1	T45.4X2	T45.4X3	T45.4X4	T45.4X5	T45.4X6
hydroxide						
colloidal	T45.4X1	T45.4X2	T45.4X3	T45.4X4	T45.4X5	T45.4X6
Ferric — see also Iron — continued						
hydroxide — continued						
polymaltose	T45.4X1	T45.4X2	T45.4X3	T45.4X4	T45.4X5	T45.4X6
pyrophosphate	T45.4X1	T45.4X2	T45.4X3	T45.4X4	T45.4X5	T45.4X6
Ferritin	T45.4X1	T45.4X2	T45.4X3	T45.4X4	T45.4X5	T45.4X6
Ferrocholinate	T45.4X1	T45.4X2	T45.4X3	T45.4X4	T45.4X5	T45.4X6
Ferrodextrane	T45.4X1	T45.4X2	T45.4X3	T45.4X4	T45.4X5	T45.4X6
Ferropolimaler	T45.4X1	T45.4X2	T45.4X3	T45.4X4	T45.4X5	T45.4X6
Ferrous — see also Iron						
phosphate	T45.4X1	T45.4X2	T45.4X3	T45.4X4	T45.4X5	T45.4X6
salt	T45.4X1	T45.4X2	T45.4X3	T45.4X4	T45.4X5	T45.4X6
with folic acid	T45.4X1	T45.4X2	T45.4X3	T45.4X4	T45.4X5	T45.4X6
Ferrous fumerate, gluconate, lactate, salt NEC, sulfate (medicinal)	T45.4X1	T45.4X2	T45.4X3	T45.4X4	T45.4X5	T45.4X6
Ferrovanadium (fumes)	T59.891	T59.892	T59.893	T59.894	—	—
Ferrum — see Iron						
Fertilizers NEC	T65.891	T65.892	T65.893	T65.894	—	—
with herbicide mixture	T60.3X1	T60.3X2	T60.3X3	T60.3X4	—	—
Fetoxilate	T47.6X1	T47.6X2	T47.6X3	T47.6X4	T47.6X5	T47.6X6
Fiber, dietary	T47.4X1	T47.4X2	T47.4X3	T47.4X4	T47.4X5	T47.4X6
Fiberglass	T65.831	T65.832	T65.833	T65.834	—	—
Fibrinogen (human)	T45.8X1	T45.8X2	T45.8X3	T45.8X4	T45.8X5	T45.8X6
Fibrinolysin (human)	T45.691	T45.692	T45.693	T45.694	T45.695	T45.696
Fibrinolysis						
affecting drug	T45.601	T45.602	T45.603	T45.604	T45.605	T45.606
inhibitor NEC	T45.621	T45.622	T45.623	T45.624	T45.625	T45.626
Fibrinolytic drug	T45.611	T45.612	T45.613	T45.614	T45.615	T45.616
Filix mas	T37.4X1	T37.4X2	T37.4X3	T37.4X4	T37.4X5	T37.4X6
Filtering cream	T49.3X1	T49.3X2	T49.3X3	T49.3X4	T49.3X5	T49.3X6
Fiorinal	T39.011	T39.012	T39.013	T39.014	T39.015	T39.016
Firedamp	T59.891	T59.892	T59.893	T59.894	—	—
Fish, noxious, nonbacterial	T61.91	T61.92	T61.93	T61.94	—	—
ciguatera	T61.01	T61.02	T61.03	T61.04	—	—
scombroid	T61.11	T61.12	T61.13	T61.14	—	—
shell	T61.781	T61.782	T61.783	T61.784	—	—
specified NEC	T61.771	T61.772	T61.773	T61.774	—	—
Flagyl	T37.3X1	T37.3X2	T37.3X3	T37.3X4	T37.3X5	T37.3X6
Flavine adenine dinucleotide	T45.2X1	T45.2X2	T45.2X3	T45.2X4	T45.2X5	T45.2X6
Flavodic acid	T46.991	T46.992	T46.993	T46.994	T46.995	T46.996
Flavoxate	T44.3X1	T44.3X2	T44.3X3	T44.3X4	T44.3X5	T44.3X6
Flaxedil	T48.1X1	T48.1X2	T48.1X3	T48.1X4	T48.1X5	T48.1X6
Flaxseed (medicinal)	T49.3X1	T49.3X2	T49.3X3	T49.3X4	T49.3X5	T49.3X6
Flecainide	T46.2X1	T46.2X2	T46.2X3	T46.2X4	T46.2X5	T46.2X6
Fleroxacin	T36.8X1	T36.8X2	T36.8X3	T36.8X4	T36.8X5	T36.8X6
Floctafenine	T39.8X1	T39.8X2	T39.8X3	T39.8X4	T39.8X5	T39.8X6
Flomax	T44.6X1	T44.6X2	T44.6X3	T44.6X4	T44.6X5	T44.6X6
Flomoxef	T36.1X1	T36.1X2	T36.1X3	T36.1X4	T36.1X5	T36.1X6
Flopropione	T44.3X1	T44.3X2	T44.3X3	T44.3X4	T44.3X5	T44.3X6
Florantyrone	T47.5X1	T47.5X2	T47.5X3	T47.5X4	T47.5X5	T47.5X6
Floraquin	T37.8X1	T37.8X2	T37.8X3	T37.8X4	T37.8X5	T37.8X6
Florinef	T38.0X1	T38.0X2	T38.0X3	T38.0X4	T38.0X5	T38.0X6
ENT agent	T49.6X1	T49.6X2	T49.6X3	T49.6X4	T49.6X5	T49.6X6
ophthalmic preparation	T49.5X1	T49.5X2	T49.5X3	T49.5X4	T49.5X5	T49.5X6
topical NEC	T49.0X1	T49.0X2	T49.0X3	T49.0X4	T49.0X5	T49.0X6
Flowers of sulfur	T49.4X1	T49.4X2	T49.4X3	T49.4X4	T49.4X5	T49.4X6
Floxuridine	T45.1X1	T45.1X2	T45.1X3	T45.1X4	T45.1X5	T45.1X6
Fluanisone	T43.4X1	T43.4X2	T43.4X3	T43.4X4	T43.4X5	T43.4X6
Flubendazole	T37.4X1	T37.4X2	T37.4X3	T37.4X4	T37.4X5	T37.4X6
Fluclorolone acetonide	T49.0X1	T49.0X2	T49.0X3	T49.0X4	T49.0X5	T49.0X6
Flucloxacillin	T36.0X1	T36.0X2	T36.0X3	T36.0X4	T36.0X5	T36.0X6
Fluconazole	T37.8X1	T37.8X2	T37.8X3	T37.8X4	T37.8X5	T37.8X6
Flucytosine	T37.8X1	T37.8X2	T37.8X3	T37.8X4	T37.8X5	T37.8X6
Fludeoxyglucose (18F)	T50.8X1	T50.8X2	T50.8X3	T50.8X4	T50.8X5	T50.8X6
Fludiazepam	T42.4X1	T42.4X2	T42.4X3	T42.4X4	T42.4X5	T42.4X6
Fludrocortisone	T50.0X1	T50.0X2	T50.0X3	T50.0X4	T50.0X5	T50.0X6
ENT agent	T49.6X1	T49.6X2	T49.6X3	T49.6X4	T49.6X5	T49.6X6
ophthalmic preparation	T49.5X1	T49.5X2	T49.5X3	T49.5X4	T49.5X5	T49.5X6
topical NEC	T49.0X1	T49.0X2	T49.0X3	T49.0X4	T49.0X5	T49.0X6
Fludroxycortide	T49.0X1	T49.0X2	T49.0X3	T49.0X4	T49.0X5	T49.0X6
Flufenamic acid	T39.391	T39.392	T39.393	T39.394	T39.395	T39.396
Fluindione	T45.511	T45.512	T45.513	T45.514	T45.515	T45.516
Flumequine	T37.8X1	T37.8X2	T37.8X3	T37.8X4	T37.8X5	T37.8X6
Flumethasone	T49.0X1	T49.0X2	T49.0X3	T49.0X4	T49.0X5	T49.0X6
Flumethiazide	T50.2X1	T50.2X2	T50.2X3	T50.2X4	T50.2X5	T50.2X6
Flumidin	T37.5X1	T37.5X2	T37.5X3	T37.5X4	T37.5X5	T37.5X6
Flunarizine	T46.7X1	T46.7X2	T46.7X3	T46.7X4	T46.7X5	T46.7X6
Flunidazole	T37.8X1	T37.8X2	T37.8X3	T37.8X4	T37.8X5	T37.8X6
Flunisolide	T48.6X1	T48.6X2	T48.6X3	T48.6X4	T48.6X5	T48.6X6
Flunitrazepam	T42.4X1	T42.4X2	T42.4X3	T42.4X4	T42.4X5	T42.4X6
Fluocinolone (acetonide)	T49.0X1	T49.0X2	T49.0X3	T49.0X4	T49.0X5	T49.0X6
Fluocinonide	T49.0X1	T49.0X2	T49.0X3	T49.0X4	T49.0X5	T49.0X6

Substance	Poisoning, Accidental (unintentional)	Poisoning, Intentional Self-harm	Poisoning, Assault	Poisoning, Undetermined	Adverse Effect	Under-dosing
Fluocortin (butyl)	T49.0X1	T49.0X2	T49.0X3	T49.0X4	T49.0X5	T49.0X6
Fluocortolone	T49.0X1	T49.0X2	T49.0X3	T49.0X4	T49.0X5	T49.0X6
Fluohydrocortisone	T38.0X1	T38.0X2	T38.0X3	T38.0X4	T38.0X5	T38.0X6
ENT agent	T49.6X1	T49.6X2	T49.6X3	T49.6X4	T49.6X5	T49.6X6
ophthalmic preparation	T49.5X1	T49.5X2	T49.5X3	T49.5X4	T49.5X5	T49.5X6
topical NEC	T49.0X1	T49.0X2	T49.0X3	T49.0X4	T49.0X5	T49.0X6
Fluonid	T49.0X1	T49.0X2	T49.0X3	T49.0X4	T49.0X5	T49.0X6
Fluopromazine	T43.3X1	T43.3X2	T43.3X3	T43.3X4	T43.3X5	T43.3X6
Fluoracetate	T60.8X1	T60.8X2	T60.8X3	T60.8X4	—	—
Fluorescein	T50.8X1	T50.8X2	T50.8X3	T50.8X4	T50.8X5	T50.8X6
Fluorhydrocortisone	T50.0X1	T50.0X2	T50.0X3	T50.0X4	T50.0X5	T50.0X6
Fluoride (nonmedicinal) (pesticide) (sodium) NEC	T60.8X1	T60.8X2	T60.8X3	T60.8X4		
hydrogen — see Hydrofluoric acid						
medicinal NEC	T50.991	T50.992	T50.993	T50.994	T50.995	T50.996
dental use	T49.7X1	T49.7X2	T49.7X3	T49.7X4	T49.7X5	T49.7X6
not pesticide NEC	T54.91	T54.92	T54.93	T54.94	—	—
stannous	T49.7X1	T49.7X2	T49.7X3	T49.7X4	T49.7X5	T49.7X6
Fluorinated corticosteroids	T38.0X1	T38.0X2	T38.0X3	T38.0X4	T38.0X5	T38.0X6
Fluorine (gas)	T59.5X1	T59.5X2	T59.5X3	T59.5X4	—	—
salt — see Fluoride(s)						
Fluoristan	T49.7X1	T49.7X2	T49.7X3	T49.7X4	T49.7X5	T49.7X6
Fluormetholone	T49.0X1	T49.0X2	T49.0X3	T49.0X4	T49.0X5	T49.0X6
Fluoroacetate	T60.8X1	T60.8X2	T60.8X3	T60.8X4	—	—
Fluorocarbon monomer	T53.6X1	T53.6X2	T53.6X3	T53.6X4	—	—
Fluorocytosine	T37.8X1	T37.8X2	T37.8X3	T37.8X4	T37.8X5	T37.8X6
Fluorodeoxyuridine	T45.1X1	T45.1X2	T45.1X3	T45.1X4	T45.1X5	T45.1X6
Fluorometholone	T49.0X1	T49.0X2	T49.0X3	T49.0X4	T49.0X5	T49.0X6
ophthalmic preparation	T49.5X1	T49.5X2	T49.5X3	T49.5X4	T49.5X5	T49.5X6
Fluorophosphate insecticide	T60.0X1	T60.0X2	T60.0X3	T60.0X4	—	—
Fluorosol	T46.3X1	T46.3X2	T46.3X3	T46.3X4	T46.3X5	T46.3X6
Fluorouracil	T45.1X1	T45.1X2	T45.1X3	T45.1X4	T45.1X5	T45.1X6
Fluorphenylalanine	T49.5X1	T49.5X2	T49.5X3	T49.5X4	T49.5X5	T49.5X6
Fluothane	T41.0X1	T41.0X2	T41.0X3	T41.0X4	T41.0X5	T41.0X6
Fluoxetine	T43.221	T43.222	T43.223	T43.224	T43.225	T43.226
Fluoxymesterone	T38.7X1	T38.7X2	T38.7X3	T38.7X4	T38.7X5	T38.7X6
Flupenthixol	T43.4X1	T43.4X2	T43.4X3	T43.4X4	T43.4X5	T43.4X6
Flupentixol	T43.4X1	T43.4X2	T43.4X3	T43.4X4	T43.4X5	T43.4X6
Fluphenazine	T43.3X1	T43.3X2	T43.3X3	T43.3X4	T43.3X5	T43.3X6
Fluprednidene	T49.0X1	T49.0X2	T49.0X3	T49.0X4	T49.0X5	T49.0X6
Fluprednisolone	T38.0X1	T38.0X2	T38.0X3	T38.0X4	T38.0X5	T38.0X6
Fluradoline	T39.8X1	T39.8X2	T39.8X3	T39.8X4	T39.8X5	T39.8X6
Flurandrenolide	T49.0X1	T49.0X2	T49.0X3	T49.0X4	T49.0X5	T49.0X6
Flurandrenolone	T49.0X1	T49.0X2	T49.0X3	T49.0X4	T49.0X5	T49.0X6
Flurazepam	T42.4X1	T42.4X2	T42.4X3	T42.4X4	T42.4X5	T42.4X6
Flurbiprofen	T39.311	T39.312	T39.313	T39.314	T39.315	T39.316
Flurobate	T49.0X1	T49.0X2	T49.0X3	T49.0X4	T49.0X5	T49.0X6
Fluroxene	T41.0X1	T41.0X2	T41.0X3	T41.0X4	T41.0X5	T41.0X6
Fluspirilene	T43.591	T43.592	T43.593	T43.594	T43.595	T43.596
Flutamide	T38.6X1	T38.6X2	T38.6X3	T38.6X4	T38.6X5	T38.6X6
Flutazolam	T42.4X1	T42.4X2	T42.4X3	T42.4X4	T42.4X5	T42.4X6
Fluticasone propionate	T49.1X1	T49.1X2	T49.1X3	T49.1X4	T49.1X5	T49.1X6
Flutoprazepam	T42.4X1	T42.4X2	T42.4X3	T42.4X4	T42.4X5	T42.4X6
Flutropium bromide	T48.6X1	T48.6X2	T48.6X3	T48.6X4	T48.6X5	T48.6X6
Fluvoxamine	T43.221	T43.222	T43.223	T43.224	T43.225	T43.226
Folacin	T45.8X1	T45.8X2	T45.8X3	T45.8X4	T45.8X5	T45.8X6
Folic acid	T45.8X1	T45.8X2	T45.8X3	T45.8X4	T45.8X5	T45.8X6
with ferrous salt	T45.2X1	T45.2X2	T45.2X3	T45.2X4	T45.2X5	T45.2X6
antagonist	T45.1X1	T45.1X2	T45.1X3	T45.1X4	T45.1X5	T45.1X6
Folinic acid	T45.8X1	T45.8X2	T45.8X3	T45.8X4	T45.8X5	T45.8X6
Folium stramoniae	T48.6X1	T48.6X2	T48.6X3	T48.6X4	T48.6X5	T48.6X6
Follicle-stimulating hormone, human	T38.811	T38.812	T38.813	T38.814	T38.815	T38.816
Folpet	T60.3X1	T60.3X2	T60.3X3	T60.3X4	—	—
Fominoben	T48.3X1	T48.3X2	T48.3X3	T48.3X4	T48.3X5	T48.3X6
Food, foodstuffs, noxious, nonbacterial, NEC	T62.91	T62.92	T62.93	T62.94	—	—
berries	T62.1X1	T62.1X2	T62.1X3	T62.1X4	—	—
fish — see also Fish	T61.91	T61.92	T61.93	T61.94	—	—
mushrooms	T62.0X1	T62.0X2	T62.0X3	T62.0X4	—	—
plants	T62.2X1	T62.2X2	T62.2X3	T62.2X4	—	—
seafood	T61.91	T61.92	T61.93	T61.94	—	—
specified NEC	T61.8X1	T61.8X2	T61.8X3	T61.8X4	—	—
seeds	T62.2X1	T62.2X2	T62.2X3	T62.2X4	—	—
shellfish	T61.781	T61.782	T61.783	T61.784	—	—
specified NEC	T62.8X1	T62.8X2	T62.8X3	T62.8X4	—	—
Fool's parsley	T62.2X1	T62.2X2	T62.2X3	T62.2X4	—	—
Formaldehyde (solution), gas or vapor	T59.2X1	T59.2X2	T59.2X3	T59.2X4	—	—
fungicide	T60.3X1	T60.3X2	T60.3X3	T60.3X4	—	—
Formalin	T59.2X1	T59.2X2	T59.2X3	T59.2X4	—	—
Formalin — continued						
fungicide	T60.3X1	T60.3X2	T60.3X3	T60.3X4	—	—
vapor	T59.2X1	T59.2X2	T59.2X3	T59.2X4	—	—
Formic acid	T54.2X1	T54.2X2	T54.2X3	T54.2X4	—	—
vapor	T59.891	T59.892	T59.893	T59.894	—	—
Foscarnet sodium	T37.5X1	T37.5X2	T37.5X3	T37.5X4	T37.5X5	T37.5X6
Fosfestrol	T38.5X1	T38.5X2	T38.5X3	T38.5X4	T38.5X5	T38.5X6
Fosfomycin	T36.8X1	T36.8X2	T36.8X3	T36.8X4	T36.8X5	T36.8X6
Fosfonet sodium	T37.5X1	T37.5X2	T37.5X3	T37.5X4	T37.5X5	T37.5X6
Fosinopril	T46.4X1	T46.4X2	T46.4X3	T46.4X4	T46.4X5	T46.4X6
sodium	T46.4X1	T46.4X2	T46.4X3	T46.4X4	T46.4X5	T46.4X6
Fowler's solution	T57.0X1	T57.0X2	T57.0X3	T57.0X4	—	—
Foxglove	T62.2X1	T62.2X2	T62.2X3	T62.2X4	—	—
Framycetin	T36.5X1	T36.5X2	T36.5X3	T36.5X4	T36.5X5	T36.5X6
Frangula	T47.2X1	T47.2X2	T47.2X3	T47.2X4	T47.2X5	T47.2X6
extract	T47.2X1	T47.2X2	T47.2X3	T47.2X4	T47.2X5	T47.2X6
Frei antigen	T50.8X1	T50.8X2	T50.8X3	T50.8X4	T50.8X5	T50.8X6
Freon	T53.5X1	T53.5X2	T53.5X3	T53.5X4	—	—
Fructose	T50.3X1	T50.3X2	T50.3X3	T50.3X4	T50.3X5	T50.3X6
Frusemide	T50.1X1	T50.1X2	T50.1X3	T50.1X4	T50.1X5	T50.1X6
FSH	T38.811	T38.812	T38.813	T38.814	T38.815	T38.816
Ftorafur	T45.1X1	T45.1X2	T45.1X3	T45.1X4	T45.1X5	T45.1X6
Fuel						
automobile	T52.0X1	T52.0X2	T52.0X3	T52.0X4	—	—
exhaust gas, not in transit	T58.01	T58.02	T58.03	T58.04	—	—
vapor NEC	T52.0X1	T52.0X2	T52.0X3	T52.0X4	—	—
gas (domestic use) — see also Carbon, monoxide, fuel, utility						
utility	T59.891	T59.892	T59.893	T59.894	—	—
incomplete combustion of — see Carbon, monoxide, fuel, utility						
in mobile container	T59.891	T59.892	T59.893	T59.894	—	—
piped (natural)	T59.891	T59.892	T59.893	T59.894	—	—
industrial, incomplete combustion	T58.8X1	T58.8X2	T58.8X3	T58.8X4	—	—
Fugillin	T36.8X1	T36.8X2	T36.8X3	T36.8X4	T36.8X5	T36.8X6
Fulminate of mercury	T56.1X1	T56.1X2	T56.1X3	T56.1X4	—	—
Fulvicin	T36.7X1	T36.7X2	T36.7X3	T36.7X4	T36.7X5	T36.7X6
Fumadil	T36.8X1	T36.8X2	T36.8X3	T36.8X4	T36.8X5	T36.8X6
Fumagillin	T36.8X1	T36.8X2	T36.8X3	T36.8X4	T36.8X5	T36.8X6
Fumaric acid	T49.4X1	T49.4X2	T49.4X3	T49.4X4	T49.4X5	T49.4X6
Fumes (from)	T59.91	T59.92	T59.93	T59.94		
carbon monoxide — see Carbon, monoxide						
charcoal (domestic use) — see Charcoal, fumes						
chloroform — see Chloroform						
coke (in domestic stoves, fireplaces) — see Coke fumes						
corrosive NEC	T54.91	T54.92	T54.93	T54.94	—	—
ether — see ether						
freons	T53.5X1	T53.5X2	T53.5X3	T53.5X4	—	—
hydrocarbons	T59.891	T59.892	T59.893	T59.894	—	—
petroleum (liquefied)	T59.891	T59.892	T59.893	T59.894	—	—
distributed through pipes (pure or mixed with air)	T59.891	T59.892	T59.893	T59.894		
lead — see lead						
metal — see Metals, or the specified metal						
nitrogen dioxide	T59.0X1	T59.0X2	T59.0X3	T59.0X4		
pesticides — see Pesticides						
petroleum (liquefied)	T59.891	T59.892	T59.893	T59.894	—	—
distributed through pipes (pure or mixed with air)	T59.891	T59.892	T59.893	T59.894		
polyester	T59.891	T59.892	T59.893	T59.894	—	—
specified source NEC — see also substance specified	T59.891	T59.892	T59.893	T59.894	—	—
sulfur dioxide	T59.1X1	T59.1X2	T59.1X3	T59.1X4	—	—
Fumigant NEC	T60.91	T60.92	T60.93	T60.94	—	—
Fungicide NEC (nonmedicinal)	T60.3X1	T60.3X2	T60.3X3	T60.3X4	—	—
Fungi, noxious, used as food	T62.0X1	T62.0X2	T62.0X3	T62.0X4	—	—
Fungizone	T36.7X1	T36.7X2	T36.7X3	T36.7X4	T36.7X5	T36.7X6
topical	T49.0X1	T49.0X2	T49.0X3	T49.0X4	T49.0X5	T49.0X6
Furacin	T49.0X1	T49.0X2	T49.0X3	T49.0X4	T49.0X5	T49.0X6
Furadantin	T37.91	T37.92	T37.93	T37.94	T37.95	T37.96
Furazolidone	T37.8X1	T37.8X2	T37.8X3	T37.8X4	T37.8X5	T37.8X6

Substance	Poisoning, Accidental (unintentional)	Poisoning, Intentional Self-harm	Poisoning, Assault	Poisoning, Undetermined	Adverse Effect	Under-dosing
Furazolium chloride	T49.0X1	T49.0X2	T49.0X3	T49.0X4	T49.0X5	T49.0X6
Furfural	T52.8X1	T52.8X2	T52.8X3	T52.8X4	—	—
Furnace (coal burning) (domestic), gas from	T58.2X1	T58.2X2	T58.2X3	T58.2X4	—	—
industrial	T58.8X1	T58.8X2	T58.8X3	T58.8X4	—	—
Furniture polish	T65.891	T65.892	T65.893	T65.894	—	—
Furosemide	T50.1X1	T50.1X2	T50.1X3	T50.1X4	T50.1X5	T50.1X6
Furoxone	T37.91	T37.92	T37.93	T37.94	T37.95	T37.96
Fursultiamine	T45.2X1	T45.2X2	T45.2X3	T45.2X4	T45.2X5	T45.2X6
Fusafungine	T36.8X1	T36.8X2	T36.8X3	T36.8X4	T36.8X5	T36.8X6
Fusel oil (any) (amyl) (butyl) (propyl), vapor	T51.3X1	T51.3X2	T51.3X3	T51.3X4	—	—
Fusidate (ethanolamine) (sodium)	T36.8X1	T36.8X2	T36.8X3	T36.8X4	T36.8X5	T36.8X6
Fusidic acid	T36.8X1	T36.8X2	T36.8X3	T36.8X4	T36.8X5	T36.8X6
Fytic acid, nonasodium	T50.6X1	T50.6X2	T50.6X3	T50.6X4	T50.6X5	T50.6X6
b-Galactosidase	T47.5X1	T47.5X2	T47.5X3	T47.5X4	T47.5X5	T47.5X6
GABA	T43.8X1	T43.8X2	T43.8X3	T43.8X4	T43.8X5	T43.8X6
Gadopentetic acid	T50.8X1	T50.8X2	T50.8X3	T50.8X4	T50.8X5	T50.8X6
Galactose	T50.3X1	T50.3X2	T50.3X3	T50.3X4	T50.3X5	T50.3X6
Galantamine	T44.0X1	T44.0X2	T44.0X3	T44.0X4	T44.0X5	T44.0X6
Gallamine (triethiodide)	T48.1X1	T48.1X2	T48.1X3	T48.1X4	T48.1X5	T48.1X6
Gallium citrate	T50.991	T50.992	T50.993	T50.994	T50.995	T50.996
Gallopamil	T46.1X1	T46.1X2	T46.1X3	T46.1X4	T46.1X5	T46.1X6
Gamboge	T47.2X1	T47.2X2	T47.2X3	T47.2X4	T47.2X5	T47.2X6
Gamimune	T50.Z11	T50.Z12	T50.Z13	T50.Z14	T50.Z15	T50.Z16
Gamma-aminobutyric acid	T43.8X1	T43.8X2	T43.8X3	T43.8X4	T43.8X5	T43.8X6
Gamma-benzene hexachloride (medicinal)	T49.0X1	T49.0X2	T49.0X3	T49.0X4	T49.0X5	T49.0X6
nonmedicinal, vapor	T53.6X1	T53.6X2	T53.6X3	T53.6X4	—	—
Gamma-BHC (medicinal) — *see also* Gamma-benzene hexachloride	T49.0X1	T49.0X2	T49.0X3	T49.0X4	T49.0X5	T49.0X6
Gamma globulin	T50.Z11	T50.Z12	T50.Z13	T50.Z14	T50.Z15	T50.Z16
Gamulin	T50.Z11	T50.Z12	T50.Z13	T50.Z14	T50.Z15	T50.Z16
Ganciclovir (sodium)	T37.5X1	T37.5X2	T37.5X3	T37.5X4	T37.5X5	T37.5X6
Ganglionic blocking drug NEC	T44.2X1	T44.2X2	T44.2X3	T44.2X4	T44.2X5	T44.2X6
specified NEC	T44.2X1	T44.2X2	T44.2X3	T44.2X4	T44.2X5	T44.2X6
Ganja	T40.7X1	T40.7X2	T40.7X3	T40.7X4	T40.7X5	T40.7X6
Garamycin	T36.5X1	T36.5X2	T36.5X3	T36.5X4	T36.5X5	T36.5X6
ophthalmic preparation	T49.5X1	T49.5X2	T49.5X3	T49.5X4	T49.5X5	T49.5X6
topical NEC	T49.0X1	T49.0X2	T49.0X3	T49.0X4	T49.0X5	T49.0X6
Gardenal	T42.3X1	T42.3X2	T42.3X3	T42.3X4	T42.3X5	T42.3X6
Gardepanyl	T42.3X1	T42.3X2	T42.3X3	T42.3X4	T42.3X5	T42.3X6
Gas	T59.91	T59.92	T59.93	T59.94	—	—
acetylene	T59.891	T59.892	T59.893	T59.894	—	—
incomplete combustion of	T58.11	T58.12	T58.13	T58.14	—	—
air contaminants, source or type not specified	T59.91	T59.92	T59.93	T59.94	—	—
anesthetic	T41.0X1	T41.0X2	T41.0X3	T41.0X4	T41.0X5	T41.0X6
blast furnace	T58.8X1	T58.8X2	T58.8X3	T58.8X4	—	—
butane — *see* butane						
carbon monoxide — *see* Carbon, monoxide						
chlorine	T59.4X1	T59.4X2	T59.4X3	T59.4X4	—	—
coal	T58.2X1	T58.2X2	T58.2X3	T58.2X4	—	—
cyanide	T57.3X1	T57.3X2	T57.3X3	T57.3X4	—	—
dicyanogen	T65.0X1	T65.0X2	T65.0X3	T65.0X4	—	—
domestic — *see* Domestic gas						
exhaust	T58.01	T58.02	T58.03	T58.04	—	—
from utility (for cooking, heating, or lighting) (after combustion) — *see* Carbon, monoxide, fuel, utility						
prior to combustion	T59.891	T59.892	T59.893	T59.894	—	—
from wood- or coal-burning stove or fireplace	T58.2X1	T58.2X2	T58.2X3	T58.2X4	—	—
fuel (domestic use) (after combustion) — *see also* Carbon, monoxide, fuel						
industrial use	T58.8X1	T58.8X2	T58.8X3	T58.8X4	—	—
prior to combustion	T59.891	T59.892	T59.893	T59.894	—	—
utility	T59.891	T59.892	T59.893	T59.894	—	—
incomplete combustion of — *see* Carbon, monoxide, fuel, utility						
in mobile container	T59.891	T59.892	T59.893	T59.894	—	—
piped (natural)	T59.891	T59.892	T59.893	T59.894	—	—
garage	T58.01	T58.02	T58.03	T58.04	—	—
hydrocarbon NEC	T59.891	T59.892	T59.893	T59.894	—	—

Substance	Poisoning, Accidental (unintentional)	Poisoning, Intentional Self-harm	Poisoning, Assault	Poisoning, Undetermined	Adverse Effect	Under-dosing
Gas — *continued*						
hydrocarbon — *continued*						
incomplete combustion of — *see* Carbon, monoxide, fuel, utility						
liquefied — *see* butane						
piped	T59.891	T59.892	T59.893	T59.894	—	—
hydrocyanic acid	T65.0X1	T65.0X2	T65.0X3	T65.0X4	—	—
illuminating (after combustion)	T58.11	T58.12	T58.13	T58.14	—	—
prior to combustion	T59.891	T59.892	T59.893	T59.894	—	—
incomplete combustion, any — *see* Carbon, monoxide						
kiln	T58.8X1	T58.8X2	T58.8X3	T58.8X4	—	—
lacrimogenic	T59.3X1	T59.3X2	T59.3X3	T59.3X4	—	—
liquefied petroleum — *see* butane						
marsh	T59.891	T59.892	T59.893	T59.894	—	—
motor exhaust, not in transit	T58.01	T58.02	T58.03	T58.04	—	—
mustard, not in war	T59.891	T59.892	T59.893	T59.894	—	—
natural	T59.891	T59.892	T59.893	T59.894	—	—
nerve, not in war	T59.91	T59.92	T59.93	T59.94	—	—
oil	T52.0X1	T52.0X2	T52.0X3	T52.0X4	—	—
petroleum (liquefied) (distributed in mobile containers)	T59.891	T59.892	T59.893	T59.894	—	—
piped (pure or mixed with air)	T59.891	T59.892	T59.893	T59.894	—	—
piped (manufactured) (natural) NEC	T59.891	T59.892	T59.893	T59.894	—	—
producer	T58.8X1	T58.8X2	T58.8X3	T58.8X4	—	—
propane — *see* propane						
refrigerant (chlorofluoro-carbon)	T53.5X1	T53.5X2	T53.5X3	T53.5X4	—	—
not chlorofluoro-carbon	T59.891	T59.892	T59.893	T59.894	—	—
sewer	T59.91	T59.92	T59.93	T59.94	—	—
specified source NEC	T59.91	T59.92	T59.93	T59.94	—	—
stove (after combustion)	T58.11	T58.12	T58.13	T58.14	—	—
prior to combustion	T59.891	T59.892	T59.893	T59.894	—	—
tear	T59.3X1	T59.3X2	T59.3X3	T59.3X4	—	—
therapeutic	T41.5X1	T41.5X2	T41.5X3	T41.5X4	T41.5X5	T41.5X6
utility (for cooking, heating, or lighting) (piped) NEC	T59.891	T59.892	T59.893	T59.894	—	—
incomplete combustion of — *see* Carbon, monoxide, fuel, utilty						
in mobile container	T59.891	T59.892	T59.893	T59.894	—	—
piped (natural)	T59.891	T59.892	T59.893	T59.894	—	—
water	T58.11	T58.12	T58.13	T58.14	—	—
incomplete combustion of — *see* Carbon, monoxide, fuel, utility						
Gaseous substance — *see* Gas						
Gasoline	T52.0X1	T52.0X2	T52.0X3	T52.0X4	—	—
vapor	T52.0X1	T52.0X2	T52.0X3	T52.0X4	—	—
Gastric enzymes	T47.5X1	T47.5X2	T47.5X3	T47.5X4	T47.5X5	T47.5X6
Gastrografin	T50.8X1	T50.8X2	T50.8X3	T50.8X4	T50.8X5	T50.8X6
Gastrointestinal drug	T47.91	T47.92	T47.93	T47.94	T47.95	T47.96
biological	T47.8X1	T47.8X2	T47.8X3	T47.8X4	T47.8X5	T47.8X6
specified NEC	T47.8X1	T47.8X2	T47.8X3	T47.8X4	T47.8X5	T47.8X6
Gaultheria procumbens	T62.2X1	T62.2X2	T62.2X3	T62.2X4	—	—
Gefarnate	T44.3X1	T44.3X2	T44.3X3	T44.3X4	T44.3X5	T44.3X6
Gelatin (intravenous)	T45.8X1	T45.8X2	T45.8X3	T45.8X4	T45.8X5	T45.8X6
absorbable (sponge)	T45.7X1	T45.7X2	T45.7X3	T45.7X4	T45.7X5	T45.7X6
Gelfilm	T49.8X1	T49.8X2	T49.8X3	T49.8X4	T49.8X5	T49.8X6
Gelfoam	T45.7X1	T45.7X2	T45.7X3	T45.7X4	T45.7X5	T45.7X6
Gelsemine	T50.991	T50.992	T50.993	T50.994	T50.995	T50.996
Gelsemium (sempervirens)	T62.2X1	T62.2X2	T62.2X3	T62.2X4	—	—
Gemeprost	T48.0X1	T48.0X2	T48.0X3	T48.0X4	T48.0X5	T48.0X6
Gemfibrozil	T46.6X1	T46.6X2	T46.6X3	T46.6X4	T46.6X5	T46.6X6
Gemonil	T42.3X1	T42.3X2	T42.3X3	T42.3X4	T42.3X5	T42.3X6
Gentamicin	T36.5X1	T36.5X2	T36.5X3	T36.5X4	T36.5X5	T36.5X6
ophthalmic preparation	T49.5X1	T49.5X2	T49.5X3	T49.5X4	T49.5X5	T49.5X6
topical NEC	T49.0X1	T49.0X2	T49.0X3	T49.0X4	T49.0X5	T49.0X6
Gentian	T47.5X1	T47.5X2	T47.5X3	T47.5X4	T47.5X5	T47.5X6
violet	T49.0X1	T49.0X2	T49.0X3	T49.0X4	T49.0X5	T49.0X6
Gepefrine	T44.4X1	T44.4X2	T44.4X3	T44.4X4	T44.4X5	T44.4X6
Gestonorone caproate	T38.5X1	T38.5X2	T38.5X3	T38.5X4	T38.5X5	T38.5X6
Gexane	T49.0X1	T49.0X2	T49.0X3	T49.0X4	T49.0X5	T49.0X6
Gila monster (venom)	T63.111	T63.112	T63.113	T63.114	—	—
Ginger	T47.5X1	T47.5X2	T47.5X3	T47.5X4	T47.5X5	T47.5X6
Jamaica — *see* Jamaica, ginger						

Additional Character May Be Required — Refer to the Tabular List for Character Selection ▽ Subterms under main terms may continue to next column or page

Substance	Poisoning, Accidental (unintentional)	Poisoning, Intentional Self-harm	Poisoning, Assault	Poisoning, Undetermined	Adverse Effect	Under-dosing
Gitalin	T46.0X1	T46.0X2	T46.0X3	T46.0X4	T46.0X5	T46.0X6
amorphous	T46.0X1	T46.0X2	T46.0X3	T46.0X4	T46.0X5	T46.0X6
Gitaloxin	T46.0X1	T46.0X2	T46.0X3	T46.0X4	T46.0X5	T46.0X6
Gitoxin	T46.0X1	T46.0X2	T46.0X3	T46.0X4	T46.0X5	T46.0X6
Glafenine	T39.8X1	T39.8X2	T39.8X3	T39.8X4	T39.8X5	T39.8X6
Glandular extract (medicinal) NEC	T50.Z91	T50.Z92	T50.Z93	T50.Z94	T50.Z95	T50.Z96
Glaucarubin	T37.3X1	T37.3X2	T37.3X3	T37.3X4	T37.3X5	T37.3X6
Glibenclamide	T38.3X1	T38.3X2	T38.3X3	T38.3X4	T38.3X5	T38.3X6
Glibornuride	T38.3X1	T38.3X2	T38.3X3	T38.3X4	T38.3X5	T38.3X6
Gliclazide	T38.3X1	T38.3X2	T38.3X3	T38.3X4	T38.3X5	T38.3X6
Glimidine	T38.3X1	T38.3X2	T38.3X3	T38.3X4	T38.3X5	T38.3X6
Glipizide	T38.3X1	T38.3X2	T38.3X3	T38.3X4	T38.3X5	T38.3X6
Gliquidone	T38.3X1	T38.3X2	T38.3X3	T38.3X4	T38.3X5	T38.3X6
Glisolamide	T38.3X1	T38.3X2	T38.3X3	T38.3X4	T38.3X5	T38.3X6
Glisoxepide	T38.3X1	T38.3X2	T38.3X3	T38.3X4	T38.3X5	T38.3X6
Globin zinc insulin	T38.3X1	T38.3X2	T38.3X3	T38.3X4	T38.3X5	T38.3X6
Globulin						
antilymphocytic	T50.Z11	T50.Z12	T50.Z13	T50.Z14	T50.Z15	T50.Z16
antirhesus	T50.Z11	T50.Z12	T50.Z13	T50.Z14	T50.Z15	T50.Z16
antivenin	T50.Z11	T50.Z12	T50.Z13	T50.Z14	T50.Z15	T50.Z16
antiviral	T50.Z11	T50.Z12	T50.Z13	T50.Z14	T50.Z15	T50.Z16
Glucagon	T38.3X1	T38.3X2	T38.3X3	T38.3X4	T38.3X5	T38.3X6
Glucocorticoids	T38.0X1	T38.0X2	T38.0X3	T38.0X4	T38.0X5	T38.0X6
Glucocorticosteroid	T38.0X1	T38.0X2	T38.0X3	T38.0X4	T38.0X5	T38.0X6
Gluconic acid	T50.991	T50.992	T50.993	T50.994	T50.995	T50.996
Glucosamine sulfate	T39.4X1	T39.4X2	T39.4X3	T39.4X4	T39.4X5	T39.4X6
Glucose	T50.3X1	T50.3X2	T50.3X3	T50.3X4	T50.3X5	T50.3X6
with sodium chloride	T50.3X1	T50.3X2	T50.3X3	T50.3X4	T50.3X5	T50.3X6
Glucosulfone sodium	T37.1X1	T37.1X2	T37.1X3	T37.1X4	T37.1X5	T37.1X6
Glucurolactone	T47.8X1	T47.8X2	T47.8X3	T47.8X4	T47.8X5	T47.8X6
Glue NEC	T52.8X1	T52.8X2	T52.8X3	T52.8X4	—	—
Glutamic acid	T47.5X1	T47.5X2	T47.5X3	T47.5X4	T47.5X5	T47.5X6
Glutaral (medicinal)	T49.0X1	T49.0X2	T49.0X3	T49.0X4	T49.0X5	T49.0X6
nonmedicinal	T65.891	T65.892	T65.893	T65.894	—	—
Glutaraldehyde (nonmedicinal)	T65.891	T65.892	T65.893	T65.894	—	—
medicinal	T49.0X1	T49.0X2	T49.0X3	T49.0X4	T49.0X5	T49.0X6
Glutathione	T50.6X1	T50.6X2	T50.6X3	T50.6X4	T50.6X5	T50.6X6
Glutethimide	T42.6X1	T42.6X2	T42.6X3	T42.6X4	T42.6X5	T42.6X6
Glyburide	T38.3X1	T38.3X2	T38.3X3	T38.3X4	T38.3X5	T38.3X6
Glycerin	T47.4X1	T47.4X2	T47.4X3	T47.4X4	T47.4X5	T47.4X6
Glycerol	T47.4X1	T47.4X2	T47.4X3	T47.4X4	T47.4X5	T47.4X6
borax	T49.6X1	T49.6X2	T49.6X3	T49.6X4	T49.6X5	T49.6X6
intravenous	T50.3X1	T50.3X2	T50.3X3	T50.3X4	T50.3X5	T50.3X6
iodinated	T48.4X1	T48.4X2	T48.4X3	T48.4X4	T48.4X5	T48.4X6
Glycerophosphate	T50.991	T50.992	T50.993	T50.994	T50.995	T50.996
Glyceryl						
gualacolate	T48.4X1	T48.4X2	T48.4X3	T48.4X4	T48.4X5	T48.4X6
nitrate	T46.3X1	T46.3X2	T46.3X3	T46.3X4	T46.3X5	T46.3X6
triacetate (topical)	T49.0X1	T49.0X2	T49.0X3	T49.0X4	T49.0X5	T49.0X6
trinitrate	T46.3X1	T46.3X2	T46.3X3	T46.3X4	T46.3X5	T46.3X6
Glycine	T50.3X1	T50.3X2	T50.3X3	T50.3X4	T50.3X5	T50.3X6
Glyclopyramide	T38.3X1	T38.3X2	T38.3X3	T38.3X4	T38.3X5	T38.3X6
Glycobiarsol	T37.3X1	T37.3X2	T37.3X3	T37.3X4	T37.3X5	T37.3X6
Glycols (ether)	T52.3X1	T52.3X2	T52.3X3	T52.3X4	—	—
Glyconiazide	T37.1X1	T37.1X2	T37.1X3	T37.1X4	T37.1X5	T37.1X6
Glycopyrrolate	T44.3X1	T44.3X2	T44.3X3	T44.3X4	T44.3X5	T44.3X6
Glycopyrronium	T44.3X1	T44.3X2	T44.3X3	T44.3X4	T44.3X5	T44.3X6
bromide	T44.3X1	T44.3X2	T44.3X3	T44.3X4	T44.3X5	T44.3X6
Glycoside, cardiac (stimulant)	T46.0X1	T46.0X2	T46.0X3	T46.0X4	T46.0X5	T46.0X6
Glycyclamide	T38.3X1	T38.3X2	T38.3X3	T38.3X4	T38.3X5	T38.3X6
Glycyrrhiza extract	T48.4X1	T48.4X2	T48.4X3	T48.4X4	T48.4X5	T48.4X6
Glycyrrhizic acid	T48.4X1	T48.4X2	T48.4X3	T48.4X4	T48.4X5	T48.4X6
Glycyrrhizinate potassium	T48.4X1	T48.4X2	T48.4X3	T48.4X4	T48.4X5	T48.4X6
Glymidine sodium	T38.3X1	T38.3X2	T38.3X3	T38.3X4	T38.3X5	T38.3X6
Glyphosate	T60.3X1	T60.3X2	T60.3X3	T60.3X4	—	—
Glyphylline	T48.6X1	T48.6X2	T48.6X3	T48.6X4	T48.6X5	T48.6X6
Gold						
colloidal (l98Au)	T45.1X1	T45.1X2	T45.1X3	T45.1X4	T45.1X5	T45.1X6
salts	T39.4X1	T39.4X2	T39.4X3	T39.4X4	T39.4X5	T39.4X6
Golden sulfide of antimony	T56.891	T56.892	T56.893	T56.894	—	—
Goldylocks	T62.2X1	T62.2X2	T62.2X3	T62.2X4	—	—
Gonadal tissue extract	T38.901	T38.902	T38.903	T38.904	T38.905	T38.906
female	T38.5X1	T38.5X2	T38.5X3	T38.5X4	T38.5X5	T38.5X6
male	T38.7X1	T38.7X2	T38.7X3	T38.7X4	T38.7X5	T38.7X6
Gonadorelin	T38.891	T38.892	T38.893	T38.894	T38.895	T38.896
Gonadotropin	T38.891	T38.892	T38.893	T38.894	T38.895	T38.896
chorionic	T38.891	T38.892	T38.893	T38.894	T38.895	T38.896
pituitary	T38.811	T38.812	T38.813	T38.814	T38.815	T38.816
Goserelin	T45.1X1	T45.1X2	T45.1X3	T45.1X4	T45.1X5	T45.1X6
Grain alcohol	T51.0X1	T51.0X2	T51.0X3	T51.0X4	—	—

Substance	Poisoning, Accidental (unintentional)	Poisoning, Intentional Self-harm	Poisoning, Assault	Poisoning, Undetermined	Adverse Effect	Under-dosing
Gramicidin	T49.0X1	T49.0X2	T49.0X3	T49.0X4	T49.0X5	T49.0X6
Granisetron	T45.0X1	T45.0X2	T45.0X3	T45.0X4	T45.0X5	T45.0X6
Gratiola officinalis	T62.2X1	T62.2X2	T62.2X3	T62.2X4	—	—
Grease	T65.891	T65.892	T65.893	T65.894	—	—
Green hellebore	T62.2X1	T62.2X2	T62.2X3	T62.2X4	—	—
Green soap	T49.2X1	T49.2X2	T49.2X3	T49.2X4	T49.2X5	T49.2X6
Grifulvin	T36.7X1	T36.7X2	T36.7X3	T36.7X4	T36.7X5	T36.7X6
Griseofulvin	T36.7X1	T36.7X2	T36.7X3	T36.7X4	T36.7X5	T36.7X6
Growth hormone	T38.811	T38.812	T38.813	T38.814	T38.815	T38.816
Guaiacol derivatives	T48.4X1	T48.4X2	T48.4X3	T48.4X4	T48.4X5	T48.4X6
Guaiac reagent	T50.991	T50.992	T50.993	T50.994	T50.995	T50.996
Guaifenesin	T48.4X1	T48.4X2	T48.4X3	T48.4X4	T48.4X5	T48.4X6
Guaimesal	T48.4X1	T48.4X2	T48.4X3	T48.4X4	T48.4X5	T48.4X6
Guaiphenesin	T48.4X1	T48.4X2	T48.4X3	T48.4X4	T48.4X5	T48.4X6
Guamecycline	T36.4X1	T36.4X2	T36.4X3	T36.4X4	T36.4X5	T36.4X6
Guanabenz	T46.5X1	T46.5X2	T46.5X3	T46.5X4	T46.5X5	T46.5X6
Guanacline	T46.5X1	T46.5X2	T46.5X3	T46.5X4	T46.5X5	T46.5X6
Guanadrel	T46.5X1	T46.5X2	T46.5X3	T46.5X4	T46.5X5	T46.5X6
Guanatol	T37.2X1	T37.2X2	T37.2X3	T37.2X4	T37.2X5	T37.2X6
Guanethidine	T46.5X1	T46.5X2	T46.5X3	T46.5X4	T46.5X5	T46.5X6
Guanfacine	T46.5X1	T46.5X2	T46.5X3	T46.5X4	T46.5X5	T46.5X6
Guano	T65.891	T65.892	T65.893	T65.894	—	—
Guanochlor	T46.5X1	T46.5X2	T46.5X3	T46.5X4	T46.5X5	T46.5X6
Guanoclor	T46.5X1	T46.5X2	T46.5X3	T46.5X4	T46.5X5	T46.5X6
Guanoctine	T46.5X1	T46.5X2	T46.5X3	T46.5X4	T46.5X5	T46.5X6
Guanoxabenz	T46.5X1	T46.5X2	T46.5X3	T46.5X4	T46.5X5	T46.5X6
Guanoxan	T46.5X1	T46.5X2	T46.5X3	T46.5X4	T46.5X5	T46.5X6
Guar gum (medicinal)	T46.6X1	T46.6X2	T46.6X3	T46.6X4	T46.6X5	T46.6X6
Hachimycin	T36.7X1	T36.7X2	T36.7X3	T36.7X4	T36.7X5	T36.7X6
Hair						
dye	T49.4X1	T49.4X2	T49.4X3	T49.4X4	T49.4X5	T49.4X6
preparation NEC	T49.4X1	T49.4X2	T49.4X3	T49.4X4	T49.4X5	T49.4X6
Halazepam	T42.4X1	T42.4X2	T42.4X3	T42.4X4	T42.4X5	T42.4X6
Halcinolone	T49.0X1	T49.0X2	T49.0X3	T49.0X4	T49.0X5	T49.0X6
Halcinonide	T49.0X1	T49.0X2	T49.0X3	T49.0X4	T49.0X5	T49.0X6
Halethazole	T49.0X1	T49.0X2	T49.0X3	T49.0X4	T49.0X5	T49.0X6
Hallucinogen NEC	T40.901	T40.902	T40.903	T40.904	T40.905	T40.906
Halofantrine	T37.2X1	T37.2X2	T37.2X3	T37.2X4	T37.2X5	T37.2X6
Halofenate	T46.6X1	T46.6X2	T46.6X3	T46.6X4	T46.6X5	T46.6X6
Halometasone	T49.0X1	T49.0X2	T49.0X3	T49.0X4	T49.0X5	T49.0X6
Haloperidol	T43.4X1	T43.4X2	T43.4X3	T43.4X4	T43.4X5	T43.4X6
Haloprogin	T49.0X1	T49.0X2	T49.0X3	T49.0X4	T49.0X5	T49.0X6
Halotex	T49.0X1	T49.0X2	T49.0X3	T49.0X4	T49.0X5	T49.0X6
Halothane	T41.0X1	T41.0X2	T41.0X3	T41.0X4	T41.0X5	T41.0X6
Haloxazolam	T42.4X1	T42.4X2	T42.4X3	T42.4X4	T42.4X5	T42.4X6
Halquinols	T49.0X1	T49.0X2	T49.0X3	T49.0X4	T49.0X5	T49.0X6
Hamamelis	T49.2X1	T49.2X2	T49.2X3	T49.2X4	T49.2X5	T49.2X6
Haptendextran	T45.8X1	T45.8X2	T45.8X3	T45.8X4	T45.8X5	T45.8X6
Harmonyl	T46.5X1	T46.5X2	T46.5X3	T46.5X4	T46.5X5	T46.5X6
Hartmann's solution	T50.3X1	T50.3X2	T50.3X3	T50.3X4	T50.3X5	T50.3X6
Hashish	T40.7X1	T40.7X2	T40.7X3	T40.7X4	T40.7X5	T40.7X6
Hawaiian Woodrose seeds	T40.991	T40.992	T40.993	T40.994	—	—
HCB	T60.3X1	T60.3X2	T60.3X3	T60.3X4	—	—
HCH	T53.6X1	T53.6X2	T53.6X3	T53.6X4	—	—
medicinal	T49.0X1	T49.0X2	T49.0X3	T49.0X4	T49.0X5	T49.0X6
HCN	T57.3X1	T57.3X2	T57.3X3	T57.3X4	—	—
Headache cures, drugs, powders NEC	T50.901	T50.902	T50.903	T50.904	T50.905	T50.906
Heavenly Blue (morning glory)	T40.991	T40.992	T40.993	T40.994	—	—
Heavy metal antidote	T45.8X1	T45.8X2	T45.8X3	T45.8X4	T45.8X5	T45.8X6
Hedaquinium	T49.0X1	T49.0X2	T49.0X3	T49.0X4	T49.0X5	T49.0X6
Hedge hyssop	T62.2X1	T62.2X2	T62.2X3	T62.2X4	—	—
Heet	T49.8X1	T49.8X2	T49.8X3	T49.8X4	T49.8X5	T49.8X6
Helenin	T37.4X1	T37.4X2	T37.4X3	T37.4X4	T37.4X5	T37.4X6
Helium (nonmedicinal) NEC	T59.891	T59.892	T59.893	T59.894	—	—
medicinal	T48.991	T48.992	T48.993	T48.994	T48.995	T48.996
Hellebore (black) (green) (white)	T62.2X1	T62.2X2	T62.2X3	T62.2X4	—	—
Hematin	T45.8X1	T45.8X2	T45.8X3	T45.8X4	T45.8X5	T45.8X6
Hematinic preparation	T45.8X1	T45.8X2	T45.8X3	T45.8X4	T45.8X5	T45.8X6
Hematological agent	T45.91	T45.92	T45.93	T45.94	T45.95	T45.96
specified NEC	T45.8X1	T45.8X2	T45.8X3	T45.8X4	T45.8X5	T45.8X6
Hemlock	T62.2X1	T62.2X2	T62.2X3	T62.2X4	—	—
Hemostatic	T45.621	T45.622	T45.623	T45.624	T45.625	T45.626
drug, systemic	T45.621	T45.622	T45.623	T45.624	T45.625	T45.626
Hemostyptic	T49.4X1	T49.4X2	T49.4X3	T49.4X4	T49.4X5	T49.4X6
Henbane	T62.2X1	T62.2X2	T62.2X3	T62.2X4	—	—
Heparin (sodium)	T45.511	T45.512	T45.513	T45.514	T45.515	T45.516
action reverser	T45.7X1	T45.7X2	T45.7X3	T45.7X4	T45.7X5	T45.7X6
Heparin-fraction	T45.511	T45.512	T45.513	T45.514	T45.515	T45.516
Heparinoid (systemic)	T45.511	T45.512	T45.513	T45.514	T45.515	T45.516

Substance	Poisoning, Accidental (unintentional)	Poisoning, Intentional Self-harm	Poisoning, Assault	Poisoning, Undetermined	Adverse Effect	Under-dosing
Hepatic secretion stimulant	T47.8X1	T47.8X2	T47.8X3	T47.8X4	T47.8X5	T47.8X6
Hepatitis B						
immune globulin	T50.Z11	T50.Z12	T50.Z13	T50.Z14	T50.Z15	T50.Z16
vaccine	T50.B91	T50.B92	T50.B93	T50.B94	T50.B95	T50.B96
Hepronicate	T46.7X1	T46.7X2	T46.7X3	T46.7X4	T46.7X5	T46.7X6
Heptabarb	T42.3X1	T42.3X2	T42.3X3	T42.3X4	T42.3X5	T42.3X6
Heptabarbital	T42.3X1	T42.3X2	T42.3X3	T42.3X4	T42.3X5	T42.3X6
Heptabarbitone	T42.3X1	T42.3X2	T42.3X3	T42.3X4	T42.3X5	T42.3X6
Heptachlor	T60.1X1	T60.1X2	T60.1X3	T60.1X4	—	—
Heptalgin	T40.2X1	T40.2X2	T40.2X3	T40.2X4	T40.2X5	T40.2X6
Heptaminol	T46.3X1	T46.3X2	T46.3X3	T46.3X4	T46.3X5	T46.3X6
Herbicide NEC	T60.3X1	T60.3X2	T60.3X3	T60.3X4	—	—
Heroin	T40.1X1	T40.1X2	T40.1X3	T40.1X4	—	—
Herplex	T49.5X1	T49.5X2	T49.5X3	T49.5X4	T49.5X5	T49.5X6
HES	T45.8X1	T45.8X2	T45.8X3	T45.8X4	T45.8X5	T45.8X6
Hesperidin	T46.991	T46.992	T46.993	T46.994	T46.995	T46.996
Hetacillin	T36.0X1	T36.0X2	T36.0X3	T36.0X4	T36.0X5	T36.0X6
Hetastarch	T45.8X1	T45.8X2	T45.8X3	T45.8X4	T45.8X5	T45.8X6
HETP	T60.0X1	T60.0X2	T60.0X3	T60.0X4	—	—
Hexachlorobenzene (vapor)	T60.3X1	T60.3X2	T60.3X3	T60.3X4	—	—
Hexachlorocyclohexane	T53.6X1	T53.6X2	T53.6X3	T53.6X4		
Hexachlorophene	T49.0X1	T49.0X2	T49.0X3	T49.0X4	T49.0X5	T49.0X6
Hexadiline	T46.3X1	T46.3X2	T46.3X3	T46.3X4	T46.3X5	T46.3X6
Hexadimethrine (bromide)	T45.7X1	T45.7X2	T45.7X3	T45.7X4	T45.7X5	T45.7X6
Hexadylamine	T46.3X1	T46.3X2	T46.3X3	T46.3X4	T46.3X5	T46.3X6
Hexaethyl tetraphosphate	T60.0X1	T60.0X2	T60.0X3	T60.0X4	—	—
Hexafluorenium bromide	T48.1X1	T48.1X2	T48.1X3	T48.1X4	T48.1X5	T48.1X6
Hexafluronium (bromide)	T48.1X1	T48.1X2	T48.1X3	T48.1X4	T48.1X5	T48.1X6
Hexa-germ	T49.2X1	T49.2X2	T49.2X3	T49.2X4	T49.2X5	T49.2X6
Hexahydrobenzol	T52.8X1	T52.8X2	T52.8X3	T52.8X4	—	—
Hexahydrocresol(s)	T51.8X1	T51.8X2	T51.8X3	T51.8X4	—	—
arsenide	T57.0X1	T57.0X2	T57.0X3	T57.0X4		
arseniurated	T57.0X1	T57.0X2	T57.0X3	T57.0X4		
cyanide	T57.3X1	T57.3X2	T57.3X3	T57.3X4		
gas	T59.891	T59.892	T59.893	T59.894		
Fluoride (liquid)	T57.8X1	T57.8X2	T57.8X3	T57.8X4	—	—
vapor	T59.891	T59.892	T59.893	T59.894		—
phophorated	T60.0X1	T60.0X2	T60.0X3	T60.0X4		
sulfate	T57.8X1	T57.8X2	T57.8X3	T57.8X4		
sulfide (gas)	T59.6X1	T59.6X2	T59.6X3	T59.6X4	—	—
arseniurated	T57.0X1	T57.0X2	T57.0X3	T57.0X4		
sulfurated	T57.8X1	T57.8X2	T57.8X3	T57.8X4		
Hexahydrophenol	T51.8X1	T51.8X2	T51.8X3	T51.8X4	—	—
Hexalen	T51.8X1	T51.8X2	T51.8X3	T51.8X4	—	—
Hexamethonium bromide	T44.2X1	T44.2X2	T44.2X3	T44.2X4	T44.2X5	T44.2X6
Hexamethylene	T52.8X1	T52.8X2	T52.8X3	T52.8X4	—	—
Hexamethylmelamine	T45.1X1	T45.1X2	T45.1X3	T45.1X4	T45.1X5	T45.1X6
Hexamidine	T49.0X1	T49.0X2	T49.0X3	T49.0X4	T49.0X5	T49.0X6
Hexamine (mandelate)	T37.8X1	T37.8X2	T37.8X3	T37.8X4	T37.8X5	T37.8X6
Hexanone, 2-hexanone	T52.4X1	T52.4X2	T52.4X3	T52.4X4	—	—
Hexanuorenium	T48.1X1	T48.1X2	T48.1X3	T48.1X4	T48.1X5	T48.1X6
Hexapropymate	T42.6X1	T42.6X2	T42.6X3	T42.6X4	T42.6X5	T42.6X6
Hexasonium iodide	T44.3X1	T44.3X2	T44.3X3	T44.3X4	T44.3X5	T44.3X6
Hexcarbacholine bromide	T48.1X1	T48.1X2	T48.1X3	T48.1X4	T48.1X5	T48.1X6
Hexemal	T42.3X1	T42.3X2	T42.3X3	T42.3X4	T42.3X5	T42.3X6
Hexestrol	T38.5X1	T38.5X2	T38.5X3	T38.5X4	T38.5X5	T38.5X6
Hexethal (sodium)	T42.3X1	T42.3X2	T42.3X3	T42.3X4	T42.3X5	T42.3X6
Hexetidine	T37.8X1	T37.8X2	T37.8X3	T37.8X4	T37.8X5	T37.8X6
Hexobarbital	T42.3X1	T42.3X2	T42.3X3	T42.3X4	T42.3X5	T42.3X6
rectal	T41.291	T41.292	T41.293	T41.294	T41.295	T41.296
sodium	T41.1X1	T41.1X2	T41.1X3	T41.1X4	T41.1X5	T41.1X6
Hexobendine	T46.3X1	T46.3X2	T46.3X3	T46.3X4	T46.3X5	T46.3X6
Hexocyclium	T44.3X1	T44.3X2	T44.3X3	T44.3X4	T44.3X5	T44.3X6
metilsulfate	T44.3X1	T44.3X2	T44.3X3	T44.3X4	T44.3X5	T44.3X6
Hexoestrol	T38.5X1	T38.5X2	T38.5X3	T38.5X4	T38.5X5	T38.5X6
Hexone	T52.4X1	T52.4X2	T52.4X3	T52.4X4	—	—
Hexoprenaline	T48.6X1	T48.6X2	T48.6X3	T48.6X4	T48.6X5	T48.6X6
Hexylcaine	T41.3X1	T41.3X2	T41.3X3	T41.3X4	T41.3X5	T41.3X6
Hexylresorcinol	T52.2X1	T52.2X2	T52.2X3	T52.2X4	—	—
HGH (human growth hormone)	T38.811	T38.812	T38.813	T38.814	T38.815	T38.816
Hinkle's pills	T47.2X1	T47.2X2	T47.2X3	T47.2X4	T47.2X5	T47.2X6
Histalog	T50.8X1	T50.8X2	T50.8X3	T50.8X4	T50.8X5	T50.8X6
Histamine (phosphate)	T50.8X1	T50.8X2	T50.8X3	T50.8X4	T50.8X5	T50.8X6
Histoplasmin	T50.8X1	T50.8X2	T50.8X3	T50.8X4	T50.8X5	T50.8X6
Holly berries	T62.2X1	T62.2X2	T62.2X3	T62.2X4	—	—
Homatropine	T44.3X1	T44.3X2	T44.3X3	T44.3X4	T44.3X5	T44.3X6
methylbromide	T44.3X1	T44.3X2	T44.3X3	T44.3X4	T44.3X5	T44.3X6
Homochlorcyclizine	T45.0X1	T45.0X2	T45.0X3	T45.0X4	T45.0X5	T45.0X6
Homosalate	T49.3X1	T49.3X2	T49.3X3	T49.3X4	T49.3X5	T49.3X6
Homo-tet	T50.Z11	T50.Z12	T50.Z13	T50.Z14	T50.Z15	T50.Z16
Hormone	T38.801	T38.802	T38.803	T38.804	T38.805	T38.806
Hormone — continued						
adrenal cortical steroids	T38.0X1	T38.0X2	T38.0X3	T38.0X4	T38.0X5	T38.0X6
androgenic	T38.7X1	T38.7X2	T38.7X3	T38.7X4	T38.7X5	T38.7X6
anterior pituitary NEC	T38.811	T38.812	T38.813	T38.814	T38.815	T38.816
antidiabetic agents	T38.3X1	T38.3X2	T38.3X3	T38.3X4	T38.3X5	T38.3X6
antidiuretic	T38.891	T38.892	T38.893	T38.894	T38.895	T38.896
cancer therapy	T45.1X1	T45.1X2	T45.1X3	T45.1X4	T45.1X5	T45.1X6
follicle stimulating	T38.811	T38.812	T38.813	T38.814	T38.815	T38.816
gonadotropic	T38.891	T38.892	T38.893	T38.894	T38.895	T38.896
pituitary	T38.811	T38.812	T38.813	T38.814	T38.815	T38.816
growth	T38.811	T38.812	T38.813	T38.814	T38.815	T38.816
luteinizing	T38.811	T38.812	T38.813	T38.814	T38.815	T38.816
ovarian	T38.5X1	T38.5X2	T38.5X3	T38.5X4	T38.5X5	T38.5X6
oxytocic	T48.0X1	T48.0X2	T48.0X3	T48.0X4	T48.0X5	T48.0X6
parathyroid (derivatives)	T50.991	T50.992	T50.993	T50.994	T50.995	T50.996
pituitary (posterior) NEC	T38.891	T38.892	T38.893	T38.894	T38.895	T38.896
anterior	T38.811	T38.812	T38.813	T38.814	T38.815	T38.816
specified, NEC	T38.891	T38.892	T38.893	T38.894	T38.895	T38.896
thyroid	T38.1X1	T38.1X2	T38.1X3	T38.1X4	T38.1X5	T38.1X6
Hornet (sting)	T63.451	T63.452	T63.453	T63.454		
Horse anti-human lymphocytic serum	T50.Z11	T50.Z12	T50.Z13	T50.Z14	T50.Z15	T50.Z16
Horticulture agent NEC	T65.91	T65.92	T65.93	T65.94	—	—
with pesticide	T60.91	T60.92	T60.93	T60.94	—	—
Human						
albumin	T45.8X1	T45.8X2	T45.8X3	T45.8X4	T45.8X5	T45.8X6
growth hormone (HGH)	T38.811	T38.812	T38.813	T38.814	T38.815	T38.816
immune serum	T50.Z11	T50.Z12	T50.Z13	T50.Z14	T50.Z15	T50.Z16
Hyaluronidase	T45.3X1	T45.3X2	T45.3X3	T45.3X4	T45.3X5	T45.3X6
Hyazyme	T45.3X1	T45.3X2	T45.3X3	T45.3X4	T45.3X5	T45.3X6
Hycodan	T40.2X1	T40.2X2	T40.2X3	T40.2X4	T40.2X5	T40.2X6
Hydantoin derivative NEC	T42.0X1	T42.0X2	T42.0X3	T42.0X4	T42.0X5	T42.0X6
Hydeltra	T38.0X1	T38.0X2	T38.0X3	T38.0X4	T38.0X5	T38.0X6
Hydergine	T44.6X1	T44.6X2	T44.6X3	T44.6X4	T44.6X5	T44.6X6
Hydrabamine penicillin	T36.0X1	T36.0X2	T36.0X3	T36.0X4	T36.0X5	T36.0X6
Hydralazine	T46.5X1	T46.5X2	T46.5X3	T46.5X4	T46.5X5	T46.5X6
Hydrargaphen	T49.0X1	T49.0X2	T49.0X3	T49.0X4	T49.0X5	T49.0X6
Hydrargyri aminochloridum	T49.0X1	T49.0X2	T49.0X3	T49.0X4	T49.0X5	T49.0X6
Hydrastine	T48.291	T48.292	T48.293	T48.294	T48.295	T48.296
Hydrazine	T54.1X1	T54.1X2	T54.1X3	T54.1X4		
monoamine oxidase inhibitors	T43.1X1	T43.1X2	T43.1X3	T43.1X4	T43.1X5	T43.1X6
Hydrazoic acid, azides	T54.2X1	T54.2X2	T54.2X3	T54.2X4		
Hydriodic acid	T48.4X1	T48.4X2	T48.4X3	T48.4X4	T48.4X5	T48.4X6
Hydrocarbon gas	T59.891	T59.892	T59.893	T59.894		
incomplete combustion of — see Carbon, monoxide, fuel, utility						
liquefied (mobile container)	T59.891	T59.892	T59.893	T59.894		
piped (natural)	T59.891	T59.892	T59.893	T59.894		
Hydrochloric acid (liquid)	T54.2X1	T54.2X2	T54.2X3	T54.2X4		
medicinal (digestant)	T47.5X1	T47.5X2	T47.5X3	T47.5X4	T47.5X5	T47.5X6
vapor	T59.891	T59.892	T59.893	T59.894		
Hydrochlorothiazide	T50.2X1	T50.2X2	T50.2X3	T50.2X4	T50.2X5	T50.2X6
Hydrocodone	T40.2X1	T40.2X2	T40.2X3	T40.2X4	T40.2X5	T40.2X6
Hydrocortisone (derivatives)	T49.0X1	T49.0X2	T49.0X3	T49.0X4	T49.0X5	T49.0X6
aceponate	T49.0X1	T49.0X2	T49.0X3	T49.0X4	T49.0X5	T49.0X6
ENT agent	T49.6X1	T49.6X2	T49.6X3	T49.6X4	T49.6X5	T49.6X6
ophthalmic preparation	T49.5X1	T49.5X2	T49.5X3	T49.5X4	T49.5X5	T49.5X6
topical NEC	T49.0X1	T49.0X2	T49.0X3	T49.0X4	T49.0X5	T49.0X6
Hydrocortone	T38.0X1	T38.0X2	T38.0X3	T38.0X4	T38.0X5	T38.0X6
ENT agent	T49.6X1	T49.6X2	T49.6X3	T49.6X4	T49.6X5	T49.6X6
ophthalmic preparation	T49.5X1	T49.5X2	T49.5X3	T49.5X4	T49.5X5	T49.5X6
topical NEC	T49.0X1	T49.0X2	T49.0X3	T49.0X4	T49.0X5	T49.0X6
Hydrocyanic acid (liquid)	T57.3X1	T57.3X2	T57.3X3	T57.3X4	—	—
gas	T65.0X1	T65.0X2	T65.0X3	T65.0X4	—	—
Hydroflumethiazide	T50.2X1	T50.2X2	T50.2X3	T50.2X4	T50.2X5	T50.2X6
Hydrofluoric acid (liquid)	T54.2X1	T54.2X2	T54.2X3	T54.2X4	—	—
vapor	T59.891	T59.892	T59.893	T59.894		
Hydrogen	T59.891	T59.892	T59.893	T59.894		
arsenide	T57.0X1	T57.0X2	T57.0X3	T57.0X4		
arseniureted	T57.0X1	T57.0X2	T57.0X3	T57.0X4		
chloride	T57.8X1	T57.8X2	T57.8X3	T57.8X4		
cyanide (salts)	T57.3X1	T57.3X2	T57.3X3	T57.3X4		
gas	T57.3X1	T57.3X2	T57.3X3	T57.3X4		
Fluoride	T59.5X1	T59.5X2	T59.5X3	T59.5X4		
vapor	T59.5X1	T59.5X2	T59.5X3	T59.5X4		
peroxide	T49.0X1	T49.0X2	T49.0X3	T49.0X4	T49.0X5	T49.0X6
phosphureted	T57.1X1	T57.1X2	T57.1X3	T57.1X4		
sulfide	T59.6X1	T59.6X2	T59.6X3	T59.6X4		
arseniureted	T57.0X1	T57.0X2	T57.0X3	T57.0X4		
sulfureted	T59.6X1	T59.6X2	T59.6X3	T59.6X4		

Substance	Poisoning, Accidental (unintentional)	Poisoning, Intentional Self-harm	Poisoning, Assault	Poisoning, Undetermined	Adverse Effect	Under-dosing
Hydromethylpyridine	T46.7X1	T46.7X2	T46.7X3	T46.7X4	T46.7X5	T46.7X6
Hydromorphinol	T40.2X1	T40.2X2	T40.2X3	T40.2X4	—	—
Hydromorphinone	T40.2X1	T40.2X2	T40.2X3	T40.2X4	T40.2X5	T40.2X6
Hydromorphone	T40.2X1	T40.2X2	T40.2X3	T40.2X4	T40.2X5	T40.2X6
Hydromox	T50.2X1	T50.2X2	T50.2X3	T50.2X4	T50.2X5	T50.2X6
Hydrophilic lotion	T49.3X1	T49.3X2	T49.3X3	T49.3X4	T49.3X5	T49.3X6
Hydroquinidine	T46.2X1	T46.2X2	T46.2X3	T46.2X4	T46.2X5	T46.2X6
Hydroquinone	T52.2X1	T52.2X2	T52.2X3	T52.2X4	—	—
vapor	T59.891	T59.892	T59.893	T59.894	—	—
Hydrosulfuric acid (gas)	T59.6X1	T59.6X2	T59.6X3	T59.6X4	—	—
Hydrotalcite	T47.1X1	T47.1X2	T47.1X3	T47.1X4	T47.1X5	T47.1X6
Hydrous wool fat	T49.3X1	T49.3X2	T49.3X3	T49.3X4	T49.3X5	T49.3X6
Hydroxide, caustic	T54.3X1	T54.3X2	T54.3X3	T54.3X4	—	—
Hydroxocobalamin	T45.8X1	T45.8X2	T45.8X3	T45.8X4	T45.8X5	T45.8X6
Hydroxyamphetamine	T49.5X1	T49.5X2	T49.5X3	T49.5X4	T49.5X5	T49.5X6
Hydroxycarbamide	T45.1X1	T45.1X2	T45.1X3	T45.1X4	T45.1X5	T45.1X6
Hydroxychloroquine	T37.8X1	T37.8X2	T37.8X3	T37.8X4	T37.8X5	T37.8X6
Hydroxydihydrocodeinone	T40.2X1	T40.2X2	T40.2X3	T40.2X4	T40.2X5	T40.2X6
Hydroxyestrone	T38.5X1	T38.5X2	T38.5X3	T38.5X4	T38.5X5	T38.5X6
Hydroxyethyl starch	T45.8X1	T45.8X2	T45.8X3	T45.8X4	T45.8X5	T45.8X6
Hydroxymethylpentanone	T52.4X1	T52.4X2	T52.4X3	T52.4X4	—	—
Hydroxyphenamate	T43.591	T43.592	T43.593	T43.594	T43.595	T43.596
Hydroxyphenylbutazone	T39.2X1	T39.2X2	T39.2X3	T39.2X4	T39.2X5	T39.2X6
Hydroxyprogesterone	T38.5X1	T38.5X2	T38.5X3	T38.5X4	T38.5X5	T38.5X6
caproate	T38.5X1	T38.5X2	T38.5X3	T38.5X4	T38.5X5	T38.5X6
Hydroxyquinoline (derivatives) NEC	T37.8X1	T37.8X2	T37.8X3	T37.8X4	T37.8X5	T37.8X6
Hydroxystilbamidine	T37.3X1	T37.3X2	T37.3X3	T37.3X4	T37.3X5	T37.3X6
Hydroxytoluene (nonmedicinal)	T54.0X1	T54.0X2	T54.0X3	T54.0X4	—	—
medicinal	T49.0X1	T49.0X2	T49.0X3	T49.0X4	T49.0X5	T49.0X6
Hydroxyurea	T45.1X1	T45.1X2	T45.1X3	T45.1X4	T45.1X5	T45.1X6
Hydroxyzine	T43.591	T43.592	T43.593	T43.594	T43.595	T43.596
Hyoscine	T44.3X1	T44.3X2	T44.3X3	T44.3X4	T44.3X5	T44.3X6
Hyoscyamine	T44.3X1	T44.3X2	T44.3X3	T44.3X4	T44.3X5	T44.3X6
Hyoscyamus	T44.3X1	T44.3X2	T44.3X3	T44.3X4	T44.3X5	T44.3X6
dry extract	T44.3X1	T44.3X2	T44.3X3	T44.3X4	T44.3X5	T44.3X6
Hypaque	T50.8X1	T50.8X2	T50.8X3	T50.8X4	T50.8X5	T50.8X6
Hypertussis	T50.Z11	T50.Z12	T50.Z13	T50.Z14	T50.Z15	T50.Z16
Hypnotic	T42.71	T42.72	T42.73	T42.74	T42.75	T42.76
anticonvulsant	T42.71	T42.72	T42.73	T42.74	T42.75	T42.76
specified NEC	T42.6X1	T42.6X2	T42.6X3	T42.6X4	T42.6X5	T42.6X6
Hypochlorite	T49.0X1	T49.0X2	T49.0X3	T49.0X4	T49.0X5	T49.0X6
Hypophysis, posterior	T38.891	T38.892	T38.893	T38.894	T38.895	T38.896
Hypotensive NEC	T46.5X1	T46.5X2	T46.5X3	T46.5X4	T46.5X5	T46.5X6
Hypromellose	T49.5X1	T49.5X2	T49.5X3	T49.5X4	T49.5X5	T49.5X6
Ibacitabine	T37.5X1	T37.5X2	T37.5X3	T37.5X4	T37.5X5	T37.5X6
Ibopamine	T44.991	T44.992	T44.993	T44.994	T44.995	T44.996
Ibufenac	T39.311	T39.312	T39.313	T39.314	T39.315	T39.316
Ibuprofen	T39.311	T39.312	T39.313	T39.314	T39.315	T39.316
Ibuproxam	T39.311	T39.312	T39.313	T39.314	T39.315	T39.316
Ibuterol	T48.6X1	T48.6X2	T48.6X3	T48.6X4	T48.6X5	T48.6X6
Ichthammol	T49.0X1	T49.0X2	T49.0X3	T49.0X4	T49.0X5	T49.0X6
Ichthyol	T49.4X1	T49.4X2	T49.4X3	T49.4X4	T49.4X5	T49.4X6
Idarubicin	T45.1X1	T45.1X2	T45.1X3	T45.1X4	T45.1X5	T45.1X6
Idrocilamide	T42.8X1	T42.8X2	T42.8X3	T42.8X4	T42.8X5	T42.8X6
Ifenprodil	T46.7X1	T46.7X2	T46.7X3	T46.7X4	T46.7X5	T46.7X6
Ifosfamide	T45.1X1	T45.1X2	T45.1X3	T45.1X4	T45.1X5	T45.1X6
Iletin	T38.3X1	T38.3X2	T38.3X3	T38.3X4	T38.3X5	T38.3X6
Ilex	T62.2X1	T62.2X2	T62.2X3	T62.2X4	—	—
Illuminating gas (after combustion)	T58.11	T58.12	T58.13	T58.14	—	—
prior to combustion	T59.891	T59.892	T59.893	T59.894	—	—
Ilopan	T45.2X1	T45.2X2	T45.2X3	T45.2X4	T45.2X5	T45.2X6
Iloprost	T46.7X1	T46.7X2	T46.7X3	T46.7X4	T46.7X5	T46.7X6
Ilotycin	T36.3X1	T36.3X2	T36.3X3	T36.3X4	T36.3X5	T36.3X6
ophthalmic preparation	T49.5X1	T49.5X2	T49.5X3	T49.5X4	T49.5X5	T49.5X6
topical NEC	T49.0X1	T49.0X2	T49.0X3	T49.0X4	T49.0X5	T49.0X6
Imidazole-4-carboxamide	T45.1X1	T45.1X2	T45.1X3	T45.1X4	T45.1X5	T45.1X6
Iminostilbene	T42.1X1	T42.1X2	T42.1X3	T42.1X4	T42.1X5	T42.1X6
Imipenem	T36.0X1	T36.0X2	T36.0X3	T36.0X4	T36.0X5	T36.0X6
Imipramine	T43.011	T43.012	T43.013	T43.014	T43.015	T43.016
Immu-G	T50.Z11	T50.Z12	T50.Z13	T50.Z14	T50.Z15	T50.Z16
Immuglobin	T50.Z11	T50.Z12	T50.Z13	T50.Z14	T50.Z15	T50.Z16
Immune						
globulin	T50.Z11	T50.Z12	T50.Z13	T50.Z14	T50.Z15	T50.Z16
serum globulin	T50.Z11	T50.Z12	T50.Z13	T50.Z14	T50.Z15	T50.Z16
Immunoglobin human (intravenous) (normal)	T50.Z11	T50.Z12	T50.Z13	T50.Z14	T50.Z15	T50.Z16
unmodified	T50.Z11	T50.Z12	T50.Z13	T50.Z14	T50.Z15	T50.Z16
Immunosuppressive drug	T45.1X1	T45.1X2	T45.1X3	T45.1X4	T45.1X5	T45.1X6
Immu-tetanus	T50.Z11	T50.Z12	T50.Z13	T50.Z14	T50.Z15	T50.Z16
Indalpine	T43.221	T43.222	T43.223	T43.224	T43.225	T43.226
Indanazoline	T48.5X1	T48.5X2	T48.5X3	T48.5X4	T48.5X5	T48.5X6
Indandione (derivatives)	T45.511	T45.512	T45.513	T45.514	T45.515	T45.516
Indapamide	T46.5X1	T46.5X2	T46.5X3	T46.5X4	T46.5X5	T46.5X6
Indendione (derivatives)	T45.511	T45.512	T45.513	T45.514	T45.515	T45.516
Indenolol	T44.7X1	T44.7X2	T44.7X3	T44.7X4	T44.7X5	T44.7X6
Inderal	T44.7X1	T44.7X2	T44.7X3	T44.7X4	T44.7X5	T44.7X6
Indian						
hemp	T40.7X1	T40.7X2	T40.7X3	T40.7X4	T40.7X5	T40.7X6
tobacco	T62.2X1	T62.2X2	T62.2X3	T62.2X4	—	—
Indigo carmine	T50.8X1	T50.8X2	T50.8X3	T50.8X4	T50.8X5	T50.8X6
Indobufen	T45.521	T45.522	T45.523	T45.524	T45.525	T45.526
Indocin	T39.2X1	T39.2X2	T39.2X3	T39.2X4	T39.2X5	T39.2X6
Indocyanine green	T50.8X1	T50.8X2	T50.8X3	T50.8X4	T50.8X5	T50.8X6
Indometacin	T39.391	T39.392	T39.393	T39.394	T39.395	T39.396
Indomethacin	T39.391	T39.392	T39.393	T39.394	T39.395	T39.396
farnesil	T39.4X1	T39.4X2	T39.4X3	T39.4X4	T39.4X5	T39.4X6
Indoramin	T44.6X1	T44.6X2	T44.6X3	T44.6X4	T44.6X5	T44.6X6
Industrial						
alcohol	T51.0X1	T51.0X2	T51.0X3	T51.0X4	—	—
fumes	T59.891	T59.892	T59.893	T59.894		
solvents (fumes) (vapors)	T52.91	T52.92	T52.93	T52.94	—	—
Influenza vaccine	T50.B91	T50.B92	T50.B93	T50.B94	T50.B95	T50.B96
Ingested substance NEC	T65.91	T65.92	T65.93	T65.94	—	—
INH	T37.1X1	T37.1X2	T37.1X3	T37.1X4	T37.1X5	T37.1X6
Inhalation, gas (noxious) — see Gas						
Inhibitor						
angiotensin-converting enzyme	T46.4X1	T46.4X2	T46.4X3	T46.4X4	T46.4X5	T46.4X6
carbonic anhydrase	T50.2X1	T50.2X2	T50.2X3	T50.2X4	T50.2X5	T50.2X6
fibrinolysis	T45.621	T45.622	T45.623	T45.624	T45.625	T45.626
monoamine oxidase NEC	T43.1X1	T43.1X2	T43.1X3	T43.1X4	T43.1X5	T43.1X6
hydrazine	T43.1X1	T43.1X2	T43.1X3	T43.1X4	T43.1X5	T43.1X6
postsynaptic	T43.8X1	T43.8X2	T43.8X3	T43.8X4	T43.8X5	T43.8X6
prothrombin synthesis	T45.511	T45.512	T45.513	T45.514	T45.515	T45.516
Ink	T65.891	T65.892	T65.893	T65.894	—	—
Inorganic substance NEC	T57.91	T57.92	T57.93	T57.94	—	—
Inosine pranobex	T37.5X1	T37.5X2	T37.5X3	T37.5X4	T37.5X5	T37.5X6
Inositol	T50.991	T50.992	T50.993	T50.994	T50.995	T50.996
nicotinate	T46.7X1	T46.7X2	T46.7X3	T46.7X4	T46.7X5	T46.7X6
Inproquone	T45.1X1	T45.1X2	T45.1X3	T45.1X4	T45.1X5	T45.1X6
Insecticide NEC	T60.91	T60.92	T60.93	T60.94	—	—
carbamate	T60.0X1	T60.0X2	T60.0X3	T60.0X4		
chlorinated	T60.1X1	T60.1X2	T60.1X3	T60.1X4		
mixed	T60.91	T60.92	T60.93	T60.94		
organochlorine	T60.1X1	T60.1X2	T60.1X3	T60.1X4		
organophosphorus	T60.0X1	T60.0X2	T60.0X3	T60.0X4		
Insect (sting), venomous	T63.481	T63.482	T63.483	T63.484		
ant	T63.421	T63.422	T63.423	T63.424		
bee	T63.441	T63.442	T63.443	T63.444		
caterpillar	T63.431	T63.432	T63.433	T63.434		
hornet	T63.451	T63.452	T63.453	T63.454		
wasp	T63.461	T63.462	T63.463	T63.464		
Insular tissue extract	T38.3X1	T38.3X2	T38.3X3	T38.3X4	T38.3X5	T38.3X6
Insulin (amorphous) (globin) (isophane) (Lente) (NPH) (Semilente) (Ultralente)	T38.3X1	T38.3X2	T38.3X3	T38.3X4	T38.3X5	T38.3X6
defalan	T38.3X1	T38.3X2	T38.3X3	T38.3X4	T38.3X5	T38.3X6
human	T38.3X1	T38.3X2	T38.3X3	T38.3X4	T38.3X5	T38.3X6
injection, soluble	T38.3X1	T38.3X2	T38.3X3	T38.3X4	T38.3X5	T38.3X6
biphasic	T38.3X1	T38.3X2	T38.3X3	T38.3X4	T38.3X5	T38.3X6
intermediate acting	T38.3X1	T38.3X2	T38.3X3	T38.3X4	T38.3X5	T38.3X6
protamine zinc	T38.3X1	T38.3X2	T38.3X3	T38.3X4	T38.3X5	T38.3X6
slow acting	T38.3X1	T38.3X2	T38.3X3	T38.3X4	T38.3X5	T38.3X6
zinc						
protamine injection	T38.3X1	T38.3X2	T38.3X3	T38.3X4	T38.3X5	T38.3X6
suspension (amorphous) (crystalline)	T38.3X1	T38.3X2	T38.3X3	T38.3X4	T38.3X5	T38.3X6
Interferon (alpha) (beta) (gamma)	T37.5X1	T37.5X2	T37.5X3	T37.5X4	T37.5X5	T37.5X6
Intestinal motility control drug	T47.6X1	T47.6X2	T47.6X3	T47.6X4	T47.6X5	T47.6X6
biological	T47.8X1	T47.8X2	T47.8X3	T47.8X4	T47.8X5	T47.8X6
Intranarcon	T41.1X1	T41.1X2	T41.1X3	T41.1X4	T41.1X5	T41.1X6
Intravenous						
amino acids	T50.991	T50.992	T50.993	T50.994	T50.995	T50.996
fat suspension	T50.991	T50.992	T50.993	T50.994	T50.995	T50.996
Inulin	T50.8X1	T50.8X2	T50.8X3	T50.8X4	T50.8X5	T50.8X6
Invert sugar	T50.3X1	T50.3X2	T50.3X3	T50.3X4	T50.3X5	T50.3X6
Inza — see Naproxen						
Iobenzamic acid	T50.8X1	T50.8X2	T50.8X3	T50.8X4	T50.8X5	T50.8X6
Iocarmic acid	T50.8X1	T50.8X2	T50.8X3	T50.8X4	T50.8X5	T50.8X6
Iocetamic acid	T50.8X1	T50.8X2	T50.8X3	T50.8X4	T50.8X5	T50.8X6

Substance	Poisoning, Accidental (unintentional)	Poisoning, Intentional Self-harm	Poisoning, Assault	Poisoning, Undetermined	Adverse Effect	Under-dosing
Iodamide	T50.8X1	T50.8X2	T50.8X3	T50.8X4	T50.8X5	T50.8X6
Iodide NEC — see also Iodine	T49.0X1	T49.0X2	T49.0X3	T49.0X4	T49.0X5	T49.0X6
mercury (ointment)	T49.0X1	T49.0X2	T49.0X3	T49.0X4	T49.0X5	T49.0X6
methylate	T49.0X1	T49.0X2	T49.0X3	T49.0X4	T49.0X5	T49.0X6
potassium (expectorant) NEC	T48.4X1	T48.4X2	T48.4X3	T48.4X4	T48.4X5	T48.4X6
Iodinated						
contrast medium	T50.8X1	T50.8X2	T50.8X3	T50.8X4	T50.8X5	T50.8X6
glycerol	T48.4X1	T48.4X2	T48.4X3	T48.4X4	T48.4X5	T48.4X6
human serum albumin (131I)	T50.8X1	T50.8X2	T50.8X3	T50.8X4	T50.8X5	T50.8X6
Iodine (antiseptic, external) (tincture) NEC	T49.0X1	T49.0X2	T49.0X3	T49.0X4	T49.0X5	T49.0X6
125 — see also Radiation sickness, and Exposure to radioactivce isotopes	T50.8X1	T50.8X2	T50.8X3	T50.8X4	T50.8X5	T50.8X6
therapeutic	T50.991	T50.992	T50.993	T50.994	T50.995	T50.996
131 — see also Radiation sickness, and Exposure to radioactivce isotopes	T50.8X1	T50.8X2	T50.8X3	T50.8X4	T50.8X5	T50.8X6
therapeutic	T38.2X1	T38.2X2	T38.2X3	T38.2X4	T38.2X5	T38.2X6
diagnostic	T50.8X1	T50.8X2	T50.8X3	T50.8X4	T50.8X5	T50.8X6
for thyroid conditions (antithyroid)	T38.2X1	T38.2X2	T38.2X3	T38.2X4	T38.2X5	T38.2X6
solution	T49.0X1	T49.0X2	T49.0X3	T49.0X4	T49.0X5	T49.0X6
vapor	T59.891	T59.892	T59.893	T59.894	—	—
Iodipamide	T50.8X1	T50.8X2	T50.8X3	T50.8X4	T50.8X5	T50.8X6
Iodized (poppy seed) oil	T50.8X1	T50.8X2	T50.8X3	T50.8X4	T50.8X5	T50.8X6
Iodobismitol	T37.8X1	T37.8X2	T37.8X3	T37.8X4	T37.8X5	T37.8X6
Iodochlorhydroxyquin	T37.8X1	T37.8X2	T37.8X3	T37.8X4	T37.8X5	T37.8X6
topical	T49.0X1	T49.0X2	T49.0X3	T49.0X4	T49.0X5	T49.0X6
Iodochlorhydroxyquinoline	T37.8X1	T37.8X2	T37.8X3	T37.8X4	T37.8X5	T37.8X6
Iodocholesterol (131I)	T50.8X1	T50.8X2	T50.8X3	T50.8X4	T50.8X5	T50.8X6
Iodoform	T49.0X1	T49.0X2	T49.0X3	T49.0X4	T49.0X5	T49.0X6
Iodohippuric acid	T50.8X1	T50.8X2	T50.8X3	T50.8X4	T50.8X5	T50.8X6
Iodopanoic acid	T50.8X1	T50.8X2	T50.8X3	T50.8X4	T50.8X5	T50.8X6
Iodophthalein (sodium)	T50.8X1	T50.8X2	T50.8X3	T50.8X4	T50.8X5	T50.8X6
Iodopyracet	T50.8X1	T50.8X2	T50.8X3	T50.8X4	T50.8X5	T50.8X6
Iodoquinol	T37.8X1	T37.8X2	T37.8X3	T37.8X4	T37.8X5	T37.8X6
Iodoxamic acid	T50.8X1	T50.8X2	T50.8X3	T50.8X4	T50.8X5	T50.8X6
Iofendylate	T50.8X1	T50.8X2	T50.8X3	T50.8X4	T50.8X5	T50.8X6
Ioglycamic acid	T50.8X1	T50.8X2	T50.8X3	T50.8X4	T50.8X5	T50.8X6
Iohexol	T50.8X1	T50.8X2	T50.8X3	T50.8X4	T50.8X5	T50.8X6
Ion exchange resin						
anion	T47.8X1	T47.8X2	T47.8X3	T47.8X4	T47.8X5	T47.8X6
cation	T50.3X1	T50.3X2	T50.3X3	T50.3X4	T50.3X5	T50.3X6
cholestyramine	T46.6X1	T46.6X2	T46.6X3	T46.6X4	T46.6X5	T46.6X6
intestinal	T47.8X1	T47.8X2	T47.8X3	T47.8X4	T47.8X5	T47.8X6
Iopamidol	T50.8X1	T50.8X2	T50.8X3	T50.8X4	T50.8X5	T50.8X6
Iopanoic acid	T50.8X1	T50.8X2	T50.8X3	T50.8X4	T50.8X5	T50.8X6
Iophenoic acid	T50.8X1	T50.8X2	T50.8X3	T50.8X4	T50.8X5	T50.8X6
Iopodate, sodium	T50.8X1	T50.8X2	T50.8X3	T50.8X4	T50.8X5	T50.8X6
Iopodic acid	T50.8X1	T50.8X2	T50.8X3	T50.8X4	T50.8X5	T50.8X6
Iopromide	T50.8X1	T50.8X2	T50.8X3	T50.8X4	T50.8X5	T50.8X6
Iopydol	T50.8X1	T50.8X2	T50.8X3	T50.8X4	T50.8X5	T50.8X6
Iotalamic acid	T50.8X1	T50.8X2	T50.8X3	T50.8X4	T50.8X5	T50.8X6
Iothalamate	T50.8X1	T50.8X2	T50.8X3	T50.8X4	T50.8X5	T50.8X6
Iothiouracil	T38.2X1	T38.2X2	T38.2X3	T38.2X4	T38.2X5	T38.2X6
Iotrol	T50.8X1	T50.8X2	T50.8X3	T50.8X4	T50.8X5	T50.8X6
Iotrolan	T50.8X1	T50.8X2	T50.8X3	T50.8X4	T50.8X5	T50.8X6
Iotroxate	T50.8X1	T50.8X2	T50.8X3	T50.8X4	T50.8X5	T50.8X6
Iotroxic acid	T50.8X1	T50.8X2	T50.8X3	T50.8X4	T50.8X5	T50.8X6
Ioversol	T50.8X1	T50.8X2	T50.8X3	T50.8X4	T50.8X5	T50.8X6
Ioxaglate	T50.8X1	T50.8X2	T50.8X3	T50.8X4	T50.8X5	T50.8X6
Ioxaglic acid	T50.8X1	T50.8X2	T50.8X3	T50.8X4	T50.8X5	T50.8X6
Ioxitalamic acid	T50.8X1	T50.8X2	T50.8X3	T50.8X4	T50.8X5	T50.8X6
Ipecac	T47.7X1	T47.7X2	T47.7X3	T47.7X4	T47.7X5	T47.7X6
Ipecacuanha	T48.4X1	T48.4X2	T48.4X3	T48.4X4	T48.4X5	T48.4X6
Ipodate, calcium	T50.8X1	T50.8X2	T50.8X3	T50.8X4	T50.8X5	T50.8X6
Ipral	T42.3X1	T42.3X2	T42.3X3	T42.3X4	T42.3X5	T42.3X6
Ipratropium (bromide)	T48.6X1	T48.6X2	T48.6X3	T48.6X4	T48.6X5	T48.6X6
Ipriflavone	T46.3X1	T46.3X2	T46.3X3	T46.3X4	T46.3X5	T46.3X6
Iprindole	T43.011	T43.012	T43.013	T43.014	T43.015	T43.016
Iproclozide	T43.1X1	T43.1X2	T43.1X3	T43.1X4	T43.1X5	T43.1X6
Iprofenin	T50.8X1	T50.8X2	T50.8X3	T50.8X4	T50.8X5	T50.8X6
Iproheptine	T49.2X1	T49.2X2	T49.2X3	T49.2X4	T49.2X5	T49.2X6
Iproniazid	T43.1X1	T43.1X2	T43.1X3	T43.1X4	T43.1X5	T43.1X6
Iproplatin	T45.1X1	T45.1X2	T45.1X3	T45.1X4	T45.1X5	T45.1X6
Iproveratril	T46.1X1	T46.1X2	T46.1X3	T46.1X4	T46.1X5	T46.1X6
Iron (compounds) (medicinal) NEC	T45.4X1	T45.4X2	T45.4X3	T45.4X4	T45.4X5	T45.4X6
ammonium	T45.4X1	T45.4X2	T45.4X3	T45.4X4	T45.4X5	T45.4X6
dextran injection	T45.4X1	T45.4X2	T45.4X3	T45.4X4	T45.4X5	T45.4X6

Substance	Poisoning, Accidental (unintentional)	Poisoning, Intentional Self-harm	Poisoning, Assault	Poisoning, Undetermined	Adverse Effect	Under-dosing
Iron (compounds) (medicinal) NEC — continued						
nonmedicinal	T56.891	T56.892	T56.893	T56.894	—	—
salts	T45.4X1	T45.4X2	T45.4X3	T45.4X4	T45.4X5	T45.4X6
sorbitex	T45.4X1	T45.4X2	T45.4X3	T45.4X4	T45.4X5	T45.4X6
sorbitol citric acid complex	T45.4X1	T45.4X2	T45.4X3	T45.4X4	T45.4X5	T45.4X6
Irrigating fluid (vaginal)	T49.8X1	T49.8X2	T49.8X3	T49.8X4	T49.8X5	T49.8X6
eye	T49.5X1	T49.5X2	T49.5X3	T49.5X4	T49.5X5	T49.5X6
Isepamicin	T36.5X1	T36.5X2	T36.5X3	T36.5X4	T36.5X5	T36.5X6
Isoaminile (citrate)	T48.3X1	T48.3X2	T48.3X3	T48.3X4	T48.3X5	T48.3X6
Isoamyl nitrite	T46.3X1	T46.3X2	T46.3X3	T46.3X4	T46.3X5	T46.3X6
Isobenzan	T60.1X1	T60.1X2	T60.1X3	T60.1X4	—	—
Isobutyl acetate	T52.8X1	T52.8X2	T52.8X3	T52.8X4	—	—
Isocarboxazid	T43.1X1	T43.1X2	T43.1X3	T43.1X4	T43.1X5	T43.1X6
Isoconazole	T49.0X1	T49.0X2	T49.0X3	T49.0X4	T49.0X5	T49.0X6
Isocyanate	T65.0X1	T65.0X2	T65.0X3	T65.0X4	—	—
Isoephedrine	T44.991	T44.992	T44.993	T44.994	T44.995	T44.996
Isoetarine	T48.6X1	T48.6X2	T48.6X3	T48.6X4	T48.6X5	T48.6X6
Isoethadione	T42.2X1	T42.2X2	T42.2X3	T42.2X4	T42.2X5	T42.2X6
Isoetharine	T44.5X1	T44.5X2	T44.5X3	T44.5X4	T44.5X5	T44.5X6
Isoflurane	T41.0X1	T41.0X2	T41.0X3	T41.0X4	T41.0X5	T41.0X6
Isoflurophate	T44.0X1	T44.0X2	T44.0X3	T44.0X4	T44.0X5	T44.0X6
Isomaltose, ferric complex	T45.4X1	T45.4X2	T45.4X3	T45.4X4	T45.4X5	T45.4X6
Isometheptene	T44.3X1	T44.3X2	T44.3X3	T44.3X4	T44.3X5	T44.3X6
Isoniazid	T37.1X1	T37.1X2	T37.1X3	T37.1X4	T37.1X5	T37.1X6
with rifampicin	T36.6X1	T36.6X2	T36.6X3	T36.6X4	T36.6X5	T36.6X6
thioacetazone	T37.1X1	T37.1X2	T37.1X3	T37.1X4	T37.1X5	T37.1X6
Isonicotinic acid hydrazide	T37.1X1	T37.1X2	T37.1X3	T37.1X4	T37.1X5	T37.1X6
Isonipecaine	T40.4X1	T40.4X2	T40.4X3	T40.4X4	T40.4X5	T40.4X6
Isopentaquine	T37.2X1	T37.2X2	T37.2X3	T37.2X4	T37.2X5	T37.2X6
Isophane insulin	T38.3X1	T38.3X2	T38.3X3	T38.3X4	T38.3X5	T38.3X6
Isophorone	T65.891	T65.892	T65.893	T65.894	—	—
Isophosphamide	T45.1X1	T45.1X2	T45.1X3	T45.1X4	T45.1X5	T45.1X6
Isopregnenone	T38.5X1	T38.5X2	T38.5X3	T38.5X4	T38.5X5	T38.5X6
Isoprenaline	T48.6X1	T48.6X2	T48.6X3	T48.6X4	T48.6X5	T48.6X6
Isopromethazine	T43.3X1	T43.3X2	T43.3X3	T43.3X4	T43.3X5	T43.3X6
Isopropamide	T44.3X1	T44.3X2	T44.3X3	T44.3X4	T44.3X5	T44.3X6
iodide	T44.3X1	T44.3X2	T44.3X3	T44.3X4	T44.3X5	T44.3X6
Isopropanol	T51.2X1	T51.2X2	T51.2X3	T51.2X4	—	—
Isopropyl						
acetate	T52.8X1	T52.8X2	T52.8X3	T52.8X4	—	—
alcohol	T51.2X1	T51.2X2	T51.2X3	T51.2X4	—	—
medicinal	T49.4X1	T49.4X2	T49.4X3	T49.4X4	T49.4X5	T49.4X6
ether	T52.8X1	T52.8X2	T52.8X3	T52.8X4	—	—
Isopropylaminophenazone	T39.2X1	T39.2X2	T39.2X3	T39.2X4	T39.2X5	T39.2X6
Isoproterenol	T48.6X1	T48.6X2	T48.6X3	T48.6X4	T48.6X5	T48.6X6
Isosorbide dinitrate	T46.3X1	T46.3X2	T46.3X3	T46.3X4	T46.3X5	T46.3X6
Isothipendyl	T45.0X1	T45.0X2	T45.0X3	T45.0X4	T45.0X5	T45.0X6
Isotretinoin	T50.991	T50.992	T50.993	T50.994	T50.995	T50.996
Isoxazolyl penicillin	T36.0X1	T36.0X2	T36.0X3	T36.0X4	T36.0X5	T36.0X6
Isoxicam	T39.391	T39.392	T39.393	T39.394	T39.395	T39.396
Isoxsuprine	T46.7X1	T46.7X2	T46.7X3	T46.7X4	T46.7X5	T46.7X6
Ispagula	T47.4X1	T47.4X2	T47.4X3	T47.4X4	T47.4X5	T47.4X6
husk	T47.4X1	T47.4X2	T47.4X3	T47.4X4	T47.4X5	T47.4X6
Isradipine	T46.1X1	T46.1X2	T46.1X3	T46.1X4	T46.1X5	T46.1X6
l-thyroxine sodium	T38.1X1	T38.1X2	T38.1X3	T38.1X4	T38.1X5	T38.1X6
Itraconazole	T37.8X1	T37.8X2	T37.8X3	T37.8X4	T37.8X5	T37.8X6
Itramin tosilate	T46.3X1	T46.3X2	T46.3X3	T46.3X4	T46.3X5	T46.3X6
Ivermectin	T37.4X1	T37.4X2	T37.4X3	T37.4X4	T37.4X5	T37.4X6
Izoniazid	T37.1X1	T37.1X2	T37.1X3	T37.1X4	T37.1X5	T37.1X6
with thioacetazone	T37.1X1	T37.1X2	T37.1X3	T37.1X4	T37.1X5	T37.1X6
Jalap	T47.2X1	T47.2X2	T47.2X3	T47.2X4	T47.2X5	T47.2X6
Jamaica						
dogwood (bark)	T39.8X1	T39.8X2	T39.8X3	T39.8X4	T39.8X5	T39.8X6
ginger	T65.891	T65.892	T65.893	T65.894	—	—
root	T62.2X1	T62.2X2	T62.2X3	T62.2X4	—	—
Jatropha	T62.2X1	T62.2X2	T62.2X3	T62.2X4	—	—
curcas	T62.2X1	T62.2X2	T62.2X3	T62.2X4	—	—
Jectofer	T45.4X1	T45.4X2	T45.4X3	T45.4X4	T45.4X5	T45.4X6
Jellyfish (sting)	T63.621	T63.622	T63.623	T63.624	—	—
Jequirity (bean)	T62.2X1	T62.2X2	T62.2X3	T62.2X4	—	—
Jimson weed (stramonium)	T62.2X1	T62.2X2	T62.2X3	T62.2X4	—	—
seeds	T62.2X1	T62.2X2	T62.2X3	T62.2X4	—	—
Josamycin	T36.3X1	T36.3X2	T36.3X3	T36.3X4	T36.3X5	T36.3X6
Juniper tar	T49.1X1	T49.1X2	T49.1X3	T49.1X4	T49.1X5	T49.1X6
Kallidinogenase	T46.7X1	T46.7X2	T46.7X3	T46.7X4	T46.7X5	T46.7X6
Kallikrein	T46.7X1	T46.7X2	T46.7X3	T46.7X4	T46.7X5	T46.7X6
Kanamycin	T36.5X1	T36.5X2	T36.5X3	T36.5X4	T36.5X5	T36.5X6
Kantrex	T36.5X1	T36.5X2	T36.5X3	T36.5X4	T36.5X5	T36.5X6
Kaolin	T47.6X1	T47.6X2	T47.6X3	T47.6X4	T47.6X5	T47.6X6
light	T47.6X1	T47.6X2	T47.6X3	T47.6X4	T47.6X5	T47.6X6
Karaya (gum)	T47.4X1	T47.4X2	T47.4X3	T47.4X4	T47.4X5	T47.4X6

Additional Character May Be Required — Refer to the Tabular List for Character Selection   ▽ Subterms under main terms may continue to next column or page

Substance	Poisoning, Accidental (unintentional)	Poisoning, Intentional Self-harm	Poisoning, Assault	Poisoning, Undetermined	Adverse Effect	Under-dosing
Kebuzone	T39.2X1	T39.2X2	T39.2X3	T39.2X4	T39.2X5	T39.2X6
Kelevan	T60.1X1	T60.1X2	T60.1X3	T60.1X4	—	—
Kemithal	T41.1X1	T41.1X2	T41.1X3	T41.1X4	T41.1X5	T41.1X6
Kenacort	T38.0X1	T38.0X2	T38.0X3	T38.0X4	T38.0X5	T38.0X6
Keratolytic drug NEC	T49.4X1	T49.4X2	T49.4X3	T49.4X4	T49.4X5	T49.4X6
anthracene	T49.4X1	T49.4X2	T49.4X3	T49.4X4	T49.4X5	T49.4X6
Keratoplastic NEC	T49.4X1	T49.4X2	T49.4X3	T49.4X4	T49.4X5	T49.4X6
Kerosene, kerosine (fuel) (solvent) NEC	T52.0X1	T52.0X2	T52.0X3	T52.0X4	—	—
insecticide	T52.0X1	T52.0X2	T52.0X3	T52.0X4	—	—
vapor	T52.0X1	T52.0X2	T52.0X3	T52.0X4	—	—
Ketamine	T41.291	T41.292	T41.293	T41.294	T41.295	T41.296
Ketazolam	T42.4X1	T42.4X2	T42.4X3	T42.4X4	T42.4X5	T42.4X6
Ketazon	T39.2X1	T39.2X2	T39.2X3	T39.2X4	T39.2X5	T39.2X6
Ketobemidone	T40.4X1	T40.4X2	T40.4X3	T40.4X4	—	—
Ketoconazole	T49.0X1	T49.0X2	T49.0X3	T49.0X4	T49.0X5	T49.0X6
Ketols	T52.4X1	T52.4X2	T52.4X3	T52.4X4	—	—
Ketone oils	T52.4X1	T52.4X2	T52.4X3	T52.4X4	—	—
Ketoprofen	T39.311	T39.312	T39.313	T39.314	T39.315	T39.316
Ketorolac	T39.8X1	T39.8X2	T39.8X3	T39.8X4	T39.8X5	T39.8X6
Ketotifen	T45.0X1	T45.0X2	T45.0X3	T45.0X4	T45.0X5	T45.0X6
Khat	T43.691	T43.692	T43.693	T43.694	—	—
Khellin	T46.3X1	T46.3X2	T46.3X3	T46.3X4	T46.3X5	T46.3X6
Khelloside	T46.3X1	T46.3X2	T46.3X3	T46.3X4	T46.3X5	T46.3X6
Kiln gas or vapor (carbon monoxide)	T58.8X1	T58.8X2	T58.8X3	T58.8X4	—	—
Kitasamycin	T36.3X1	T36.3X2	T36.3X3	T36.3X4	T36.3X5	T36.3X6
Konsyl	T47.4X1	T47.4X2	T47.4X3	T47.4X4	T47.4X5	T47.4X6
Kosam seed	T62.2X1	T62.2X2	T62.2X3	T62.2X4	—	—
Krait (venom)	T63.091	T63.092	T63.093	T63.094	—	—
Kwell (insecticide)	T60.1X1	T60.1X2	T60.1X3	T60.1X4	—	—
anti-infective (topical)	T49.0X1	T49.0X2	T49.0X3	T49.0X4	T49.0X5	T49.0X6
Labetalol	T44.8X1	T44.8X2	T44.8X3	T44.8X4	T44.8X5	T44.8X6
Laburnum (seeds)	T62.2X1	T62.2X2	T62.2X3	T62.2X4	—	—
leaves	T62.2X1	T62.2X2	T62.2X3	T62.2X4	—	—
Lachesine	T49.5X1	T49.5X2	T49.5X3	T49.5X4	T49.5X5	T49.5X6
Lacidipine	T46.5X1	T46.5X2	T46.5X3	T46.5X4	T46.5X5	T46.5X6
Lacquer	T65.6X1	T65.6X2	T65.6X3	T65.6X4	—	—
Lacrimogenic gas	T59.3X1	T59.3X2	T59.3X3	T59.3X4	—	—
Lactated potassic saline	T50.3X1	T50.3X2	T50.3X3	T50.3X4	T50.3X5	T50.3X6
Lactic acid	T49.8X1	T49.8X2	T49.8X3	T49.8X4	T49.8X5	T49.8X6
Lactobacillus						
acidophilus	T47.6X1	T47.6X2	T47.6X3	T47.6X4	T47.6X5	T47.6X6
compound	T47.6X1	T47.6X2	T47.6X3	T47.6X4	T47.6X5	T47.6X6
bifidus, lyophilized	T47.6X1	T47.6X2	T47.6X3	T47.6X4	T47.6X5	T47.6X6
bulgaricus	T47.6X1	T47.6X2	T47.6X3	T47.6X4	T47.6X5	T47.6X6
sporogenes	T47.6X1	T47.6X2	T47.6X3	T47.6X4	T47.6X5	T47.6X6
Lactoflavin	T45.2X1	T45.2X2	T45.2X3	T45.2X4	T45.2X5	T45.2X6
Lactose (as excipient)	T50.901	T50.902	T50.903	T50.904	T50.905	T50.906
Lactuca (virosa) (extract)	T42.6X1	T42.6X2	T42.6X3	T42.6X4	T42.6X5	T42.6X6
Lactucarium	T42.6X1	T42.6X2	T42.6X3	T42.6X4	T42.6X5	T42.6X6
Lactulose	T47.3X1	T47.3X2	T47.3X3	T47.3X4	T47.3X5	T47.3X6
Laevo — see Levo-						
Lanatosides	T46.0X1	T46.0X2	T46.0X3	T46.0X4	T46.0X5	T46.0X6
Lanolin	T49.3X1	T49.3X2	T49.3X3	T49.3X4	T49.3X5	T49.3X6
Largactil	T43.3X1	T43.3X2	T43.3X3	T43.3X4	T43.3X5	T43.3X6
Larkspur	T62.2X1	T62.2X2	T62.2X3	T62.2X4	—	—
Laroxyl	T43.011	T43.012	T43.013	T43.015	T43.016	
Lasix	T50.1X1	T50.1X2	T50.1X3	T50.1X4	T50.1X5	T50.1X6
Lassar's paste	T49.4X1	T49.4X2	T49.4X3	T49.4X4	T49.4X5	T49.4X6
Latamoxef	T36.1X1	T36.1X2	T36.1X3	T36.1X4	T36.1X5	T36.1X6
Latex	T65.811	T65.812	T65.813	T65.814	—	—
Lathyrus (seed)	T62.2X1	T62.2X2	T62.2X3	T62.2X4	—	—
Laudanum	T40.0X1	T40.0X2	T40.0X3	T40.0X4	T40.0X5	T40.0X6
Laudexium	T48.1X1	T48.1X2	T48.1X3	T48.1X4	T48.1X5	T48.1X6
Laughing gas	T41.0X1	T41.0X2	T41.0X3	T41.0X4	T41.0X5	T41.0X6
Laurel, black or cherry	T62.2X1	T62.2X2	T62.2X3	T62.2X4	—	—
Laurolinium	T49.0X1	T49.0X2	T49.0X3	T49.0X4	T49.0X5	T49.0X6
Lauryl sulfoacetate	T49.2X1	T49.2X2	T49.2X3	T49.2X4	T49.2X5	T49.2X6
Laxative NEC	T47.4X1	T47.4X2	T47.4X3	T47.4X4	T47.4X5	T47.4X6
osmotic	T47.3X1	T47.3X2	T47.3X3	T47.3X4	T47.3X5	T47.3X6
saline	T47.3X1	T47.3X2	T47.3X3	T47.3X4	T47.3X5	T47.3X6
stimulant	T47.2X1	T47.2X2	T47.2X3	T47.2X4	T47.2X5	T47.2X6
L-dopa	T42.8X1	T42.8X2	T42.8X3	T42.8X4	T42.8X5	T42.8X6
Lead (dust) (fumes) (vapor) NEC	T56.0X1	T56.0X2	T56.0X3	T56.0X4	—	—
acetate	T49.2X1	T49.2X2	T49.2X3	T49.2X4	T49.2X5	T49.2X6
alkyl (fuel additive)	T56.0X1	T56.0X2	T56.0X3	T56.0X4	—	—
anti-infectives	T37.8X1	T37.8X2	T37.8X3	T37.8X4	T37.8X5	T37.8X6
antiknock compound (tetraethyl)	T56.0X1	T56.0X2	T56.0X3	T56.0X4	—	—

Substance	Poisoning, Accidental (unintentional)	Poisoning, Intentional Self-harm	Poisoning, Assault	Poisoning, Undetermined	Adverse Effect	Under-dosing
Lead (dust) (fumes) (vapor) NEC — continued						
arsenate, arsenite (dust)(herbicide) (insecticide) (vapor)	T57.0X1	T57.0X2	T57.0X3	T57.0X4	—	—
carbonate	T56.0X1	T56.0X2	T56.0X3	T56.0X4	—	—
paint	T56.0X1	T56.0X2	T56.0X3	T56.0X4	—	—
chromate	T56.0X1	T56.0X2	T56.0X3	T56.0X4	—	—
paint	T56.0X1	T56.0X2	T56.0X3	T56.0X4	—	—
dioxide	T56.0X1	T56.0X2	T56.0X3	T56.0X4	—	—
inorganic	T56.0X1	T56.0X2	T56.0X3	T56.0X4	—	—
iodide	T56.0X1	T56.0X2	T56.0X3	T56.0X4	—	—
pigment (paint)	T56.0X1	T56.0X2	T56.0X3	T56.0X4	—	—
monoxide (dust)	T56.0X1	T56.0X2	T56.0X3	T56.0X4	—	—
paint	T56.0X1	T56.0X2	T56.0X3	T56.0X4	—	—
organic	T56.0X1	T56.0X2	T56.0X3	T56.0X4	—	—
oxide	T56.0X1	T56.0X2	T56.0X3	T56.0X4	—	—
paint	T56.0X1	T56.0X2	T56.0X3	T56.0X4	—	—
paint	T56.0X1	T56.0X2	T56.0X3	T56.0X4	—	—
salts	T56.0X1	T56.0X2	T56.0X3	T56.0X4	—	—
specified compound NEC	T56.0X1	T56.0X2	T56.0X3	T56.0X4	—	—
tetra-ethyl	T56.0X1	T56.0X2	T56.0X3	T56.0X4	—	—
Lebanese red	T40.7X1	T40.7X2	T40.7X3	T40.7X4	T40.7X5	T40.7X6
Lefetamine	T39.8X1	T39.8X2	T39.8X3	T39.8X4	T39.8X5	T39.8X6
Lenperone	T43.4X1	T43.4X2	T43.4X3	T43.4X4	T43.4X5	T43.4X6
Lente lietin (insulin)	T38.3X1	T38.3X2	T38.3X3	T38.3X4	T38.3X5	T38.3X6
Leptazol	T50.7X1	T50.7X2	T50.7X3	T50.7X4	T50.7X5	T50.7X6
Leptophos	T60.0X1	T60.0X2	T60.0X3	T60.0X4	—	—
Leritine	T40.2X1	T40.2X2	T40.2X3	T40.2X4	T40.2X5	T40.2X6
Letosteine	T48.4X1	T48.4X2	T48.4X3	T48.4X4	T48.4X5	T48.4X6
Letter	T38.1X1	T38.1X2	T38.1X3	T38.1X4	T38.1X5	T38.1X6
Lettuce opium	T42.6X1	T42.6X2	T42.6X3	T42.6X4	T42.6X5	T42.6X6
Leucinocaine	T41.3X1	T41.3X2	T41.3X3	T41.3X4	T41.3X5	T41.3X6
Leucocianidol	T46.991	T46.992	T46.993	T46.994	T46.995	T46.996
Leucovorin (factor)	T45.8X1	T45.8X2	T45.8X3	T45.8X4	T45.8X5	T45.8X6
Leukeran	T45.1X1	T45.1X2	T45.1X3	T45.1X4	T45.1X5	T45.1X6
Leuprolide	T38.891	T38.892	T38.893	T38.894	T38.895	T38.896
Levalbuterol	T48.6X1	T48.6X2	T48.6X3	T48.6X4	T48.6X5	T48.6X6
Levallorphan	T50.7X1	T50.7X2	T50.7X3	T50.7X4	T50.7X5	T50.7X6
Levamisole	T37.4X1	T37.4X2	T37.4X3	T37.4X4	T37.4X5	T37.4X6
Levanil	T42.6X1	T42.6X2	T42.6X3	T42.6X4	T42.6X5	T42.6X6
Levarterenol	T44.4X1	T44.4X2	T44.4X3	T44.4X4	T44.4X5	T44.4X6
Levdropropizine	T48.3X1	T48.3X2	T48.3X3	T48.3X4	T48.3X5	T48.3X6
Levobunolol	T49.5X1	T49.5X2	T49.5X3	T49.5X4	T49.5X5	T49.5X6
Levocabastine (hydrochloride)	T45.0X1	T45.0X2	T45.0X3	T45.0X4	T45.0X5	T45.0X6
Levocarnitine	T50.991	T50.992	T50.993	T50.994	T50.995	T50.996
Levodopa	T42.8X1	T42.8X2	T42.8X3	T42.8X4	T42.8X5	T42.8X6
with carbidopa	T42.8X1	T42.8X2	T42.8X3	T42.8X4	T42.8X5	T42.8X6
Levo-dromoran	T40.2X1	T40.2X2	T40.2X3	T40.2X4	T40.2X5	T40.2X6
Levoglutamide	T50.991	T50.992	T50.993	T50.994	T50.995	T50.996
Levoid	T38.1X1	T38.1X2	T38.1X3	T38.1X4	T38.1X5	T38.1X6
Levo-isomethadone	T40.3X1	T40.3X2	T40.3X3	T40.3X4	T40.3X5	T40.3X6
Levomepromazine	T43.3X1	T43.3X2	T43.3X3	T43.3X4	T43.3X5	T43.3X6
Levonordefrin	T49.6X1	T49.6X2	T49.6X3	T49.6X4	T49.6X5	T49.6X6
Levonorgestrel	T38.4X1	T38.4X2	T38.4X3	T38.4X4	T38.4X5	T38.4X6
with ethinylestradiol	T38.5X1	T38.5X2	T38.5X3	T38.5X4	T38.5X5	T38.5X6
Levopromazine	T43.3X1	T43.3X2	T43.3X3	T43.3X4	T43.3X5	T43.3X6
Levoprome	T42.6X1	T42.6X2	T42.6X3	T42.6X4	T42.6X5	T42.6X6
Levopropoxyphene	T40.4X1	T40.4X2	T40.4X3	T40.4X4	T40.4X5	T40.4X6
Levopropylhexedrine	T50.5X1	T50.5X2	T50.5X3	T50.5X4	T50.5X5	T50.5X6
Levoproxyphylline	T48.6X1	T48.6X2	T48.6X3	T48.6X4	T48.6X5	T48.6X6
Levorphanol	T40.4X1	T40.4X2	T40.4X3	T40.4X4	T40.4X5	T40.4X6
Levothyroxine	T38.1X1	T38.1X2	T38.1X3	T38.1X4	T38.1X5	T38.1X6
sodium	T38.1X1	T38.1X2	T38.1X3	T38.1X4	T38.1X5	T38.1X6
Levsin	T44.3X1	T44.3X2	T44.3X3	T44.3X4	T44.3X5	T44.3X6
Levulose	T50.3X1	T50.3X2	T50.3X3	T50.3X4	T50.3X5	T50.3X6
Lewisite (gas), not in war	T57.0X1	T57.0X2	T57.0X3	T57.0X4	—	—
Librium	T42.4X1	T42.4X2	T42.4X3	T42.4X4	T42.4X5	T42.4X6
Lidex	T49.0X1	T49.0X2	T49.0X3	T49.0X4	T49.0X5	T49.0X6
Lidocaine	T41.3X1	T41.3X2	T41.3X3	T41.3X4	T41.3X5	T41.3X6
regional	T41.3X1	T41.3X2	T41.3X3	T41.3X4	T41.3X5	T41.3X6
spinal	T41.3X1	T41.3X2	T41.3X3	T41.3X4	T41.3X5	T41.3X6
Lidofenin	T50.8X1	T50.8X2	T50.8X3	T50.8X4	T50.8X5	T50.8X6
Lidoflazine	T46.1X1	T46.1X2	T46.1X3	T46.1X4	T46.1X5	T46.1X6
Lighter fluid	T52.0X1	T52.0X2	T52.0X3	T52.0X4	—	—
Lignin hemicellulose	T47.6X1	T47.6X2	T47.6X3	T47.6X4	T47.6X5	T47.6X6
Lignocaine	T41.3X1	T41.3X2	T41.3X3	T41.3X4	T41.3X5	T41.3X6
regional	T41.3X1	T41.3X2	T41.3X3	T41.3X4	T41.3X5	T41.3X6
spinal	T41.3X1	T41.3X2	T41.3X3	T41.3X4	T41.3X5	T41.3X6
Ligroin (e) (solvent)	T52.0X1	T52.0X2	T52.0X3	T52.0X4	—	—
vapor	T59.891	T59.892	T59.893	T59.894	—	—
Ligustrum vulgare	T62.2X1	T62.2X2	T62.2X3	T62.2X4	—	—

Substance	Poisoning, Accidental (unintentional)	Poisoning, Intentional Self-harm	Poisoning, Assault	Poisoning, Undetermined	Adverse Effect	Under-dosing
Lily of the valley	T62.2X1	T62.2X2	T62.2X3	T62.2X4	—	—
Lime (chloride)	T54.3X1	T54.3X2	T54.3X3	T54.3X4	—	—
Limonene	T52.8X1	T52.8X2	T52.8X3	T52.8X4	—	—
Lincomycin	T36.8X1	T36.8X2	T36.8X3	T36.8X4	T36.8X5	T36.8X6
Lindane (insecticide) (nonmedicinal) (vapor)	T53.6X1	T53.6X2	T53.6X3	T53.6X4	—	—
medicinal	T49.0X1	T49.0X2	T49.0X3	T49.0X4	T49.0X5	T49.0X6
Liniments NEC	T49.91	T49.92	T49.93	T49.94	T49.95	T49.96
Linoleic acid	T46.6X1	T46.6X2	T46.6X3	T46.6X4	T46.6X5	T46.6X6
Linolenic acid	T46.6X1	T46.6X2	T46.6X3	T46.6X4	T46.6X5	T46.6X6
Linseed	T47.4X1	T47.4X2	T47.4X3	T47.4X4	T47.4X5	T47.4X6
Liothyronine	T38.1X1	T38.1X2	T38.1X3	T38.1X4	T38.1X5	T38.1X6
Liotrix	T38.1X1	T38.1X2	T38.1X3	T38.1X4	T38.1X5	T38.1X6
Lipancreatin	T47.5X1	T47.5X2	T47.5X3	T47.5X4	T47.5X5	T47.5X6
Lipo-alprostadil	T46.7X1	T46.7X2	T46.7X3	T46.7X4	T46.7X5	T46.7X6
Lipo-Lutin	T38.5X1	T38.5X2	T38.5X3	T38.5X4	T38.5X5	T38.5X6
Lipotropic drug NEC	T50.901	T50.902	T50.903	T50.904	T50.905	T50.906
Liquefied petroleum gases	T59.891	T59.892	T59.893	T59.894	—	—
piped (pure or mixed with air)	T59.891	T59.892	T59.893	T59.894	—	—
Liquid						
paraffin	T47.4X1	T47.4X2	T47.4X3	T47.4X4	T47.4X5	T47.4X6
petrolatum	T47.4X1	T47.4X2	T47.4X3	T47.4X4	T47.4X5	T47.4X6
topical	T49.3X1	T49.3X2	T49.3X3	T49.3X4	T49.3X5	T49.3X6
specified NEC	T65.891	T65.892	T65.893	T65.894	—	—
substance	T65.91	T65.92	T65.93	T65.94	—	—
Liquor creosolis compositus	T65.891	T65.892	T65.893	T65.894	—	—
Liquorice	T48.4X1	T48.4X2	T48.4X3	T48.4X4	T48.4X5	T48.4X6
extract	T47.8X1	T47.8X2	T47.8X3	T47.8X4	T47.8X5	T47.8X6
Lisinopril	T46.4X1	T46.4X2	T46.4X3	T46.4X4	T46.4X5	T46.4X6
Lisuride	T42.8X1	T42.8X2	T42.8X3	T42.8X4	T42.8X5	T42.8X6
Lithane	T43.8X1	T43.8X2	T43.8X3	T43.8X4	T43.8X5	T43.8X6
Lithium	T56.891	T56.892	T56.893	T56.894	—	—
gluconate	T43.591	T43.592	T43.593	T43.594	T43.595	T43.596
salts (carbonate)	T43.591	T43.592	T43.593	T43.594	T43.595	T43.596
Lithonate	T43.8X1	T43.8X2	T43.8X3	T43.8X4	T43.8X5	T43.8X6
Liver						
extract	T45.8X1	T45.8X2	T45.8X3	T45.8X4	T45.8X5	T45.8X6
for parenteral use	T45.8X1	T45.8X2	T45.8X3	T45.8X4	T45.8X5	T45.8X6
fraction 1	T45.8X1	T45.8X2	T45.8X3	T45.8X4	T45.8X5	T45.8X6
hydrolysate	T45.8X1	T45.8X2	T45.8X3	T45.8X4	T45.8X5	T45.8X6
Lizard (bite) (venom)	T63.121	T63.122	T63.123	T63.124	—	—
LMD	T45.8X1	T45.8X2	T45.8X3	T45.8X4	T45.8X5	T45.8X6
Lobelia	T62.2X1	T62.2X2	T62.2X3	T62.2X4	—	—
Lobeline	T50.7X1	T50.7X2	T50.7X3	T50.7X4	T50.7X5	T50.7X6
Local action drug NEC	T49.8X1	T49.8X2	T49.8X3	T49.8X4	T49.8X5	T49.8X6
Locorten	T49.0X1	T49.0X2	T49.0X3	T49.0X4	T49.0X5	T49.0X6
Lofepramine	T43.011	T43.012	T43.013	T43.014	T43.015	T43.016
Lolium temulentum	T62.2X1	T62.2X2	T62.2X3	T62.2X4	—	—
Lomotil	T47.6X1	T47.6X2	T47.6X3	T47.6X4	T47.6X5	T47.6X6
Lomustine	T45.1X1	T45.1X2	T45.1X3	T45.1X4	T45.1X5	T45.1X6
Lonidamine	T45.1X1	T45.1X2	T45.1X3	T45.1X4	T45.1X5	T45.1X6
Loperamide	T47.6X1	T47.6X2	T47.6X3	T47.6X4	T47.6X5	T47.6X6
Loprazolam	T42.4X1	T42.4X2	T42.4X3	T42.4X4	T42.4X5	T42.4X6
Lorajmine	T46.2X1	T46.2X2	T46.2X3	T46.2X4	T46.2X5	T46.2X6
Loratidine	T45.0X1	T45.0X2	T45.0X3	T45.0X4	T45.0X5	T45.0X6
Lorazepam	T42.4X1	T42.4X2	T42.4X3	T42.4X4	T42.4X5	T42.4X6
Lorcainide	T46.2X1	T46.2X2	T46.2X3	T46.2X4	T46.2X5	T46.2X6
Lormetazepam	T42.4X1	T42.4X2	T42.4X3	T42.4X4	T42.4X5	T42.4X6
Lotions NEC	T49.91	T49.92	T49.93	T49.94	T49.95	T49.96
Lotusate	T42.3X1	T42.3X2	T42.3X3	T42.3X4	T42.3X5	T42.3X6
Lovastatin	T46.6X1	T46.6X2	T46.6X3	T46.6X4	T46.6X5	T46.6X6
Lowila	T49.2X1	T49.2X2	T49.2X3	T49.2X4	T49.2X5	T49.2X6
Loxapine	T43.591	T43.592	T43.593	T43.594	T43.595	T43.596
Lozenges (throat)	T49.6X1	T49.6X2	T49.6X3	T49.6X4	T49.6X5	T49.6X6
LSD	T40.8X1	T40.8X2	T40.8X3	T40.8X4	—	—
L-Tryptophan — see amino acid						
Lubricant, eye	T49.5X1	T49.5X2	T49.5X3	T49.5X4	T49.5X5	T49.5X6
Lubricating oil NEC	T52.0X1	T52.0X2	T52.0X3	T52.0X4	—	—
Lucanthone	T37.4X1	T37.4X2	T37.4X3	T37.4X4	T37.4X5	T37.4X6
Luminal	T42.3X1	T42.3X2	T42.3X3	T42.3X4	T42.3X5	T42.3X6
Lung irritant (gas) NEC	T59.91	T59.92	T59.93	T59.94	—	—
Luteinizing hormone	T38.811	T38.812	T38.813	T38.814	T38.815	T38.816
Lutocylol	T38.5X1	T38.5X2	T38.5X3	T38.5X4	T38.5X5	T38.5X6
Lutromone	T38.5X1	T38.5X2	T38.5X3	T38.5X4	T38.5X5	T38.5X6
Lututrin	T48.291	T48.292	T48.293	T48.294	T48.295	T48.296
Lye (concentrated)	T54.3X1	T54.3X2	T54.3X3	T54.3X4	—	—
Lygranum (skin test)	T50.8X1	T50.8X2	T50.8X3	T50.8X4	T50.8X5	T50.8X6
Lymecycline	T36.4X1	T36.4X2	T36.4X3	T36.4X4	T36.4X5	T36.4X6
Lymphogranuloma venereum antigen	T50.8X1	T50.8X2	T50.8X3	T50.8X4	T50.8X5	T50.8X6
Lynestrenol	T38.4X1	T38.4X2	T38.4X3	T38.4X4	T38.4X5	T38.4X6

Substance	Poisoning, Accidental (unintentional)	Poisoning, Intentional Self-harm	Poisoning, Assault	Poisoning, Undetermined	Adverse Effect	Under-dosing
Lyovac Sodium Edecrin	T50.1X1	T50.1X2	T50.1X3	T50.1X4	T50.1X5	T50.1X6
Lypressin	T38.891	T38.892	T38.893	T38.894	T38.895	T38.896
Lysergic acid diethylamide	T40.8X1	T40.8X2	T40.8X3	T40.8X4	—	—
Lysergide	T40.8X1	T40.8X2	T40.8X3	T40.8X4	—	—
Lysine vasopressin	T38.891	T38.892	T38.893	T38.894	T38.895	T38.896
Lysol	T54.1X1	T54.1X2	T54.1X3	T54.1X4	—	—
Lysozyme	T49.0X1	T49.0X2	T49.0X3	T49.0X4	T49.0X5	T49.0X6
Lytta (vitatta)	T49.8X1	T49.8X2	T49.8X3	T49.8X4	T49.8X5	T49.8X6
Mace	T59.3X1	T59.3X2	T59.3X3	T59.3X4	—	—
Macrogol	T50.991	T50.992	T50.993	T50.994	T50.995	T50.996
Macrolide						
anabolic drug	T38.7X1	T38.7X2	T38.7X3	T38.7X4	T38.7X5	T38.7X6
antibiotic	T36.3X1	T36.3X2	T36.3X3	T36.3X4	T36.3X5	T36.3X6
Mafenide	T49.0X1	T49.0X2	T49.0X3	T49.0X4	T49.0X5	T49.0X6
Magaldrate	T47.1X1	T47.1X2	T47.1X3	T47.1X4	T47.1X5	T47.1X6
Magic mushroom	T40.991	T40.992	T40.993	T40.994	—	—
Magnamycin	T36.8X1	T36.8X2	T36.8X3	T36.8X4	T36.8X5	T36.8X6
Magnesia magma	T47.1X1	T47.1X2	T47.1X3	T47.1X4	T47.1X5	T47.1X6
Magnesium NEC	T56.891	T56.892	T56.893	T56.894	—	—
carbonate	T47.1X1	T47.1X2	T47.1X3	T47.1X4	T47.1X5	T47.1X6
citrate	T47.4X1	T47.4X2	T47.4X3	T47.4X4	T47.4X5	T47.4X6
hydroxide	T47.1X1	T47.1X2	T47.1X3	T47.1X4	T47.1X5	T47.1X6
oxide	T47.1X1	T47.1X2	T47.1X3	T47.1X4	T47.1X5	T47.1X6
peroxide	T49.0X1	T49.0X2	T49.0X3	T49.0X4	T49.0X5	T49.0X6
salicylate	T39.091	T39.092	T39.093	T39.094	T39.095	T39.096
silicofluoride	T50.3X1	T50.3X2	T50.3X3	T50.3X4	T50.3X5	T50.3X6
sulfate	T47.4X1	T47.4X2	T47.4X3	T47.4X4	T47.4X5	T47.4X6
thiosulfate	T45.0X1	T45.0X2	T45.0X3	T45.0X4	T45.0X5	T45.0X6
trisilicate	T47.1X1	T47.1X2	T47.1X3	T47.1X4	T47.1X5	T47.1X6
Malathion (medicinal)	T49.0X1	T49.0X2	T49.0X3	T49.0X4	T49.0X5	T49.0X6
insecticide	T60.0X1	T60.0X2	T60.0X3	T60.0X4	—	—
Male fern extract	T37.4X1	T37.4X2	T37.4X3	T37.4X4	T37.4X5	T37.4X6
M-AMSA	T45.1X1	T45.1X2	T45.1X3	T45.1X4	T45.1X5	T45.1X6
Mandelic acid	T37.8X1	T37.8X2	T37.8X3	T37.8X4	T37.8X5	T37.8X6
Manganese (dioxide) (salts)	T57.2X1	T57.2X2	T57.2X3	T57.2X4	—	—
medicinal	T50.991	T50.992	T50.993	T50.994	T50.995	T50.996
Mannitol	T47.3X1	T47.3X2	T47.3X3	T47.3X4	T47.3X5	T47.3X6
hexanitrate	T46.3X1	T46.3X2	T46.3X3	T46.3X4	T46.3X5	T46.3X6
Mannomustine	T45.1X1	T45.1X2	T45.1X3	T45.1X4	T45.1X5	T45.1X6
MAO inhibitors	T43.1X1	T43.1X2	T43.1X3	T43.1X4	T43.1X5	T43.1X6
Mapharsen	T37.8X1	T37.8X2	T37.8X3	T37.8X4	T37.8X5	T37.8X6
Maphenide	T49.0X1	T49.0X2	T49.0X3	T49.0X4	T49.0X5	T49.0X6
Maprotiline	T43.021	T43.022	T43.023	T43.024	T43.025	T43.026
Marcaine	T41.3X1	T41.3X2	T41.3X3	T41.3X4	T41.3X5	T41.3X6
infiltration (subcutaneous)	T41.3X1	T41.3X2	T41.3X3	T41.3X4	T41.3X5	T41.3X6
nerve block (peripheral) (plexus)	T41.3X1	T41.3X2	T41.3X3	T41.3X4	T41.3X5	T41.3X6
Marezine	T45.0X1	T45.0X2	T45.0X3	T45.0X4	T45.0X5	T45.0X6
Marihuana	T40.7X1	T40.7X2	T40.7X3	T40.7X4	T40.7X5	T40.7X6
Marijuana	T40.7X1	T40.7X2	T40.7X3	T40.7X4	T40.7X5	T40.7X6
Marine (sting)	T63.691	T63.692	T63.693	T63.694	—	—
animals (sting)	T63.691	T63.692	T63.693	T63.694	—	—
plants (sting)	T63.711	T63.712	T63.713	T63.714	—	—
Marplan	T43.1X1	T43.1X2	T43.1X3	T43.1X4	T43.1X5	T43.1X6
Marsh gas	T59.891	T59.892	T59.893	T59.894	—	—
Marsilid	T43.1X1	T43.1X2	T43.1X3	T43.1X4	T43.1X5	T43.1X6
Matulane	T45.1X1	T45.1X2	T45.1X3	T45.1X4	T45.1X5	T45.1X6
Mazindol	T50.5X1	T50.5X2	T50.5X3	T50.5X4	T50.5X5	T50.5X6
MCPA	T60.3X1	T60.3X2	T60.3X3	T60.3X4	—	—
MDMA	T43.621	T43.622	T43.623	T43.624	T43.625	T43.626
Meadow saffron	T62.2X1	T62.2X2	T62.2X3	T62.2X4	—	—
Measles virus vaccine (attenuated)	T50.B91	T50.B92	T50.B93	T50.B94	T50.B95	T50.B96
Meat, noxious	T62.8X1	T62.8X2	T62.8X3	T62.8X4	—	—
Meballymal	T42.3X1	T42.3X2	T42.3X3	T42.3X4	T42.3X5	T42.3X6
Mebanazine	T43.1X1	T43.1X2	T43.1X3	T43.1X4	T43.1X5	T43.1X6
Mebaral	T42.3X1	T42.3X2	T42.3X3	T42.3X4	T42.3X5	T42.3X6
Mebendazole	T37.4X1	T37.4X2	T37.4X3	T37.4X4	T37.4X5	T37.4X6
Mebeverine	T44.3X1	T44.3X2	T44.3X3	T44.3X4	T44.3X5	T44.3X6
Mebhydrolin	T45.0X1	T45.0X2	T45.0X3	T45.0X4	T45.0X5	T45.0X6
Mebumal	T42.3X1	T42.3X2	T42.3X3	T42.3X4	T42.3X5	T42.3X6
Mebutamate	T43.591	T43.592	T43.593	T43.594	T43.595	T43.596
Mecamylamine	T44.2X1	T44.2X2	T44.2X3	T44.2X4	T44.2X5	T44.2X6
Mechlorethamine	T45.1X1	T45.1X2	T45.1X3	T45.1X4	T45.1X5	T45.1X6
Mecillinam	T36.0X1	T36.0X2	T36.0X3	T36.0X4	T36.0X5	T36.0X6
Meclizine (hydrochloride)	T45.0X1	T45.0X2	T45.0X3	T45.0X4	T45.0X5	T45.0X6
Meclocycline	T36.4X1	T36.4X2	T36.4X3	T36.4X4	T36.4X5	T36.4X6
Meclofenamate	T39.391	T39.392	T39.393	T39.394	T39.395	T39.396
Meclofenamic acid	T39.391	T39.392	T39.393	T39.394	T39.395	T39.396
Meclofenoxate	T43.691	T43.692	T43.693	T43.694	T43.695	T43.696
Meclozine	T45.0X1	T45.0X2	T45.0X3	T45.0X4	T45.0X5	T45.0X6
Mecobalamin	T45.8X1	T45.8X2	T45.8X3	T45.8X4	T45.8X5	T45.8X6
Mecoprop	T60.3X1	T60.3X2	T60.3X3	T60.3X4	—	—

Substance	Poisoning, Accidental (unintentional)	Poisoning, Intentional Self-harm	Poisoning, Assault	Poisoning, Undetermined	Adverse Effect	Under-dosing
Mecrilate	T49.3X1	T49.3X2	T49.3X3	T49.3X4	T49.3X5	T49.3X6
Mecysteine	T48.4X1	T48.4X2	T48.4X3	T48.4X4	T48.4X5	T48.4X6
Medazepam	T42.4X1	T42.4X2	T42.4X3	T42.4X4	T42.4X5	T42.4X6
Medicament NEC	T50.901	T50.902	T50.903	T50.904	T50.905	T50.906
Medinal	T42.3X1	T42.3X2	T42.3X3	T42.3X4	T42.3X5	T42.3X6
Medomin	T42.3X1	T42.3X2	T42.3X3	T42.3X4	T42.3X5	T42.3X6
Medrogestone	T38.5X1	T38.5X2	T38.5X3	T38.5X4	T38.5X5	T38.5X6
Medroxalol	T44.8X1	T44.8X2	T44.8X3	T44.8X4	T44.8X5	T44.8X6
Medroxyprogesterone acetate (depot)	T38.5X1	T38.5X2	T38.5X3	T38.5X4	T38.5X5	T38.5X6
Medrysone	T49.0X1	T49.0X2	T49.0X3	T49.0X4	T49.0X5	T49.0X6
Mefenamic acid	T39.391	T39.392	T39.393	T39.394	T39.395	T39.396
Mefenorex	T50.5X1	T50.5X2	T50.5X3	T50.5X4	T50.5X5	T50.5X6
Mefloquine	T37.2X1	T37.2X2	T37.2X3	T37.2X4	T37.2X5	T37.2X6
Mefruside	T50.2X1	T50.2X2	T50.2X3	T50.2X4	T50.2X5	T50.2X6
Megahallucinogen	T40.901	T40.902	T40.903	T40.904	T40.905	T40.906
Megestrol	T38.5X1	T38.5X2	T38.5X3	T38.5X4	T38.5X5	T38.5X6
Meglumine						
antimoniate	T37.8X1	T37.8X2	T37.8X3	T37.8X4	T37.8X5	T37.8X6
diatrizoate	T50.8X1	T50.8X2	T50.8X3	T50.8X4	T50.8X5	T50.8X6
iodipamide	T50.8X1	T50.8X2	T50.8X3	T50.8X4	T50.8X5	T50.8X6
iotroxate	T50.8X1	T50.8X2	T50.8X3	T50.8X4	T50.8X5	T50.8X6
MEK (methyl ethyl ketone)	T52.4X1	T52.4X2	T52.4X3	T52.4X4	—	—
Meladinin	T49.3X1	T49.3X2	T49.3X3	T49.3X4	T49.3X5	T49.3X6
Meladrazine	T44.3X1	T44.3X2	T44.3X3	T44.3X4	T44.3X5	T44.3X6
Melaleuca alternifolia oil	T49.0X1	T49.0X2	T49.0X3	T49.0X4	T49.0X5	T49.0X6
Melanizing agents	T49.3X1	T49.3X2	T49.3X3	T49.3X4	T49.3X5	T49.3X6
Melanocyte-stimulating hormone	T38.891	T38.892	T38.893	T38.894	T38.895	T38.896
Melarsonyl potassium	T37.3X1	T37.3X2	T37.3X3	T37.3X4	T37.3X5	T37.3X6
Melarsoprol	T37.3X1	T37.3X2	T37.3X3	T37.3X4	T37.3X5	T37.3X6
Melia azedarach	T62.2X1	T62.2X2	T62.2X3	T62.2X4	—	—
Melitracen	T43.011	T43.012	T43.013	T43.014	T43.015	T43.016
Mellaril	T43.3X1	T43.3X2	T43.3X3	T43.3X4	T43.3X5	T43.3X6
Meloxine	T49.3X1	T49.3X2	T49.3X3	T49.3X4	T49.3X5	T49.3X6
Melperone	T43.4X1	T43.4X2	T43.4X3	T43.4X4	T43.4X5	T43.4X6
Melphalan	T45.1X1	T45.1X2	T45.1X3	T45.1X4	T45.1X5	T45.1X6
Memantine	T43.8X1	T43.8X2	T43.8X3	T43.8X4	T43.8X5	T43.8X6
Menadiol	T45.7X1	T45.7X2	T45.7X3	T45.7X4	T45.7X5	T45.7X6
sodium sulfate	T45.7X1	T45.7X2	T45.7X3	T45.7X4	T45.7X5	T45.7X6
Menadione	T45.7X1	T45.7X2	T45.7X3	T45.7X4	T45.7X5	T45.7X6
sodium bisulfite	T45.7X1	T45.7X2	T45.7X3	T45.7X4	T45.7X5	T45.7X6
Menaphthone	T45.7X1	T45.7X2	T45.7X3	T45.7X4	T45.7X5	T45.7X6
Menaquinone	T45.7X1	T45.7X2	T45.7X3	T45.7X4	T45.7X5	T45.7X6
Menatetrenone	T45.7X1	T45.7X2	T45.7X3	T45.7X4	T45.7X5	T45.7X6
Meningococcal vaccine	T50.A91	T50.A92	T50.A93	T50.A94	T50.A95	T50.A96
Menningovax (-AC) (-C)	T50.A91	T50.A92	T50.A93	T50.A94	T50.A95	T50.A96
Menotropins	T38.811	T38.812	T38.813	T38.814	T38.815	T38.816
Menthol	T48.5X1	T48.5X2	T48.5X3	T48.5X4	T48.5X5	T48.5X6
Mepacrine	T37.2X1	T37.2X2	T37.2X3	T37.2X4	T37.2X5	T37.2X6
Meparfynol	T42.6X1	T42.6X2	T42.6X3	T42.6X4	T42.6X5	T42.6X6
Mepartricin	T36.7X1	T36.7X2	T36.7X3	T36.7X4	T36.7X5	T36.7X6
Mepazine	T43.3X1	T43.3X2	T43.3X3	T43.3X4	T43.3X5	T43.3X6
Mepenzolate	T44.3X1	T44.3X2	T44.3X3	T44.3X4	T44.3X5	T44.3X6
bromide	T44.3X1	T44.3X2	T44.3X3	T44.3X4	T44.3X5	T44.3X6
Meperidine	T40.4X1	T40.4X2	T40.4X3	T40.4X4	T40.4X5	T40.4X6
Mephebarbital	T42.3X1	T42.3X2	T42.3X3	T42.3X4	T42.3X5	T42.3X6
Mephenamin (e)	T42.8X1	T42.8X2	T42.8X3	T42.8X4	T42.8X5	T42.8X6
Mephenesin	T42.8X1	T42.8X2	T42.8X3	T42.8X4	T42.8X5	T42.8X6
Mephenhydramine	T45.0X1	T45.0X2	T45.0X3	T45.0X4	T45.0X5	T45.0X6
Mephenoxalone	T42.8X1	T42.8X2	T42.8X3	T42.8X4	T42.8X5	T42.8X6
Mephentermine	T44.991	T44.992	T44.993	T44.994	T44.995	T44.996
Mephenytoin	T42.0X1	T42.0X2	T42.0X3	T42.0X4	T42.0X5	T42.0X6
with phenobarbital	T42.3X1	T42.3X2	T42.3X3	T42.3X4	T42.3X5	T42.3X6
Mephobarbital	T42.3X1	T42.3X2	T42.3X3	T42.3X4	T42.3X5	T42.3X6
Mephosfolan	T60.0X1	T60.0X2	T60.0X3	T60.0X4	—	—
Mepindolol	T44.7X1	T44.7X2	T44.7X3	T44.7X4	T44.7X5	T44.7X6
Mepiperphenidol	T44.3X1	T44.3X2	T44.3X3	T44.3X4	T44.3X5	T44.3X6
Mepitiostane	T38.7X1	T38.7X2	T38.7X3	T38.7X4	T38.7X5	T38.7X6
Mepivacaine	T41.3X1	T41.3X2	T41.3X3	T41.3X4	T41.3X5	T41.3X6
epidural	T41.3X1	T41.3X2	T41.3X3	T41.3X4	T41.3X5	T41.3X6
Meprednisone	T38.0X1	T38.0X2	T38.0X3	T38.0X4	T38.0X5	T38.0X6
Meprobam	T43.591	T43.592	T43.593	T43.594	T43.595	T43.596
Meprobamate	T43.591	T43.592	T43.593	T43.594	T43.595	T43.596
Meproscillarin	T46.0X1	T46.0X2	T46.0X3	T46.0X4	T46.0X5	T46.0X6
Meprylcaine	T41.3X1	T41.3X2	T41.3X3	T41.3X4	T41.3X5	T41.3X6
Meptazinol	T39.8X1	T39.8X2	T39.8X3	T39.8X4	T39.8X5	T39.8X6
Mepyramine	T45.0X1	T45.0X2	T45.0X3	T45.0X4	T45.0X5	T45.0X6
Mequitazine	T43.3X1	T43.3X2	T43.3X3	T43.3X4	T43.3X5	T43.3X6
Meralluride	T50.2X1	T50.2X2	T50.2X3	T50.2X4	T50.2X5	T50.2X6
Merbaphen	T50.2X1	T50.2X2	T50.2X3	T50.2X4	T50.2X5	T50.2X6
Merbromin	T49.0X1	T49.0X2	T49.0X3	T49.0X4	T49.0X5	T49.0X6

Substance	Poisoning, Accidental (unintentional)	Poisoning, Intentional Self-harm	Poisoning, Assault	Poisoning, Undetermined	Adverse Effect	Under-dosing
Mercaptobenzothiazole salts	T49.0X1	T49.0X2	T49.0X3	T49.0X4	T49.0X5	T49.0X6
Mercaptomerin	T50.2X1	T50.2X2	T50.2X3	T50.2X4	T50.2X5	T50.2X6
Mercaptopurine	T45.1X1	T45.1X2	T45.1X3	T45.1X4	T45.1X5	T45.1X6
Mercumatilin	T50.2X1	T50.2X2	T50.2X3	T50.2X4	T50.2X5	T50.2X6
Mercuramide	T50.2X1	T50.2X2	T50.2X3	T50.2X4	T50.2X5	T50.2X6
Mercurochrome	T49.0X1	T49.0X2	T49.0X3	T49.0X4	T49.0X5	T49.0X6
Mercurophylline	T50.2X1	T50.2X2	T50.2X3	T50.2X4	T50.2X5	T50.2X6
Mercury, mercurial, mercuric, mercurous (compounds) (cyanide) (fumes) (nonmedicinal) (vapor) NEC	T56.1X1	T56.1X2	T56.1X3	T56.1X4	—	—
ammoniated	T49.0X1	T49.0X2	T49.0X3	T49.0X4	T49.0X5	T49.0X6
anti-infective						
local	T49.0X1	T49.0X2	T49.0X3	T49.0X4	T49.0X5	T49.0X6
systemic	T37.8X1	T37.8X2	T37.8X3	T37.8X4	T37.8X5	T37.8X6
topical	T49.0X1	T49.0X2	T49.0X3	T49.0X4	T49.0X5	T49.0X6
chloride (ammoniated)	T49.0X1	T49.0X2	T49.0X3	T49.0X4	T49.0X5	T49.0X6
fungicide	T56.1X1	T56.1X2	T56.1X3	T56.1X4	—	—
diuretic NEC	T50.2X1	T50.2X2	T50.2X3	T50.2X4	T50.2X5	T50.2X6
fungicide	T56.1X1	T56.1X2	T56.1X3	T56.1X4	—	—
organic (fungicide)	T56.1X1	T56.1X2	T56.1X3	T56.1X4	—	—
oxide, yellow	T49.0X1	T49.0X2	T49.0X3	T49.0X4	T49.0X5	T49.0X6
Mersalyl	T50.2X1	T50.2X2	T50.2X3	T50.2X4	T50.2X5	T50.2X6
Merthiolate	T49.0X1	T49.0X2	T49.0X3	T49.0X4	T49.0X5	T49.0X6
ophthalmic preparation	T49.5X1	T49.5X2	T49.5X3	T49.5X4	T49.5X5	T49.5X6
Meruvax	T50.B91	T50.B92	T50.B93	T50.B94	T50.B95	T50.B96
Mesalazine	T47.8X1	T47.8X2	T47.8X3	T47.8X4	T47.8X5	T47.8X6
Mescal buttons	T40.991	T40.992	T40.993	T40.994	—	—
Mescaline	T40.991	T40.992	T40.993	T40.994	—	—
Mesna	T48.4X1	T48.4X2	T48.4X3	T48.4X4	T48.4X5	T48.4X6
Mesoglycan	T46.6X1	T46.6X2	T46.6X3	T46.6X4	T46.6X5	T46.6X6
Mesoridazine	T43.3X1	T43.3X2	T43.3X3	T43.3X4	T43.3X5	T43.3X6
Mestanolone	T38.7X1	T38.7X2	T38.7X3	T38.7X4	T38.7X5	T38.7X6
Mesterolone	T38.7X1	T38.7X2	T38.7X3	T38.7X4	T38.7X5	T38.7X6
Mestranol	T38.5X1	T38.5X2	T38.5X3	T38.5X4	T38.5X5	T38.5X6
Mesulergine	T42.8X1	T42.8X2	T42.8X3	T42.8X4	T42.8X5	T42.8X6
Mesulfen	T49.0X1	T49.0X2	T49.0X3	T49.0X4	T49.0X5	T49.0X6
Mesuximide	T42.2X1	T42.2X2	T42.2X3	T42.2X4	T42.2X5	T42.2X6
Metabutethamine	T41.3X1	T41.3X2	T41.3X3	T41.3X4	T41.3X5	T41.3X6
Metactesylacetate	T49.0X1	T49.0X2	T49.0X3	T49.0X4	T49.0X5	T49.0X6
Metacycline	T36.4X1	T36.4X2	T36.4X3	T36.4X4	T36.4X5	T36.4X6
Metaldehyde (snail killer) NEC	T60.8X1	T60.8X2	T60.8X3	T60.8X4	—	—
Metals (heavy) (nonmedicinal)	T56.91	T56.92	T56.93	T56.94	—	—
dust, fumes, or vapor NEC	T56.91	T56.92	T56.93	T56.94	—	—
light NEC	T56.91	T56.92	T56.93	T56.94	—	—
dust, fumes, or vapor NEC	T56.91	T56.92	T56.93	T56.94	—	—
specified NEC	T56.891	T56.892	T56.893	T56.894	—	—
thallium	T56.811	T56.812	T56.813	T56.814	—	—
Metamfetamine	T43.621	T43.622	T43.623	T43.624	T43.625	T43.626
Metamizole sodium	T39.2X1	T39.2X2	T39.2X3	T39.2X4	T39.2X5	T39.2X6
Metampicillin	T36.0X1	T36.0X2	T36.0X3	T36.0X4	T36.0X5	T36.0X6
Metamucil	T47.4X1	T47.4X2	T47.4X3	T47.4X4	T47.4X5	T47.4X6
Metandienone	T38.7X1	T38.7X2	T38.7X3	T38.7X4	T38.7X5	T38.7X6
Metandrostenolone	T38.7X1	T38.7X2	T38.7X3	T38.7X4	T38.7X5	T38.7X6
Metaphen	T49.0X1	T49.0X2	T49.0X3	T49.0X4	T49.0X5	T49.0X6
Metaphos	T60.0X1	T60.0X2	T60.0X3	T60.0X4	—	—
Metapramine	T43.011	T43.012	T43.013	T43.014	T43.015	T43.016
Metaproterenol	T48.291	T48.292	T48.293	T48.294	T48.295	T48.296
Metaraminol	T44.4X1	T44.4X2	T44.4X3	T44.4X4	T44.4X5	T44.4X6
Metaxalone	T42.8X1	T42.8X2	T42.8X3	T42.8X4	T42.8X5	T42.8X6
Metenolone	T38.7X1	T38.7X2	T38.7X3	T38.7X4	T38.7X5	T38.7X6
Metergoline	T42.8X1	T42.8X2	T42.8X3	T42.8X4	T42.8X5	T42.8X6
Metescufylline	T46.991	T46.992	T46.993	T46.994	T46.995	T46.996
Metetoin	T42.0X1	T42.0X2	T42.0X3	T42.0X4	T42.0X5	T42.0X6
Metformin	T38.3X1	T38.3X2	T38.3X3	T38.3X4	T38.3X5	T38.3X6
Methacholine	T44.1X1	T44.1X2	T44.1X3	T44.1X4	T44.1X5	T44.1X6
Methacycline	T36.4X1	T36.4X2	T36.4X3	T36.4X4	T36.4X5	T36.4X6
Methadone	T40.3X1	T40.3X2	T40.3X3	T40.3X4	T40.3X5	T40.3X6
Methallenestril	T38.5X1	T38.5X2	T38.5X3	T38.5X4	T38.5X5	T38.5X6
Methallenoestril	T38.5X1	T38.5X2	T38.5X3	T38.5X4	T38.5X5	T38.5X6
Methamphetamine	T43.621	T43.622	T43.623	T43.624	T43.625	T43.626
Methampyrone	T39.2X1	T39.2X2	T39.2X3	T39.2X4	T39.2X5	T39.2X6
Methandienone	T38.7X1	T38.7X2	T38.7X3	T38.7X4	T38.7X5	T38.7X6
Methandriol	T38.7X1	T38.7X2	T38.7X3	T38.7X4	T38.7X5	T38.7X6
Methandrostenolone	T38.7X1	T38.7X2	T38.7X3	T38.7X4	T38.7X5	T38.7X6
Methane	T59.891	T59.892	T59.893	T59.894	—	—
Methanethiol	T59.891	T59.892	T59.893	T59.894	—	—
Methaniazide	T37.1X1	T37.1X2	T37.1X3	T37.1X4	T37.1X5	T37.1X6
Methanol (vapor)	T51.1X1	T51.1X2	T51.1X3	T51.1X4	—	—

Table of Drugs and Chemicals

Methantheline — Metrifonate

Substance	Poisoning, Accidental (unintentional)	Poisoning, Intentional Self-harm	Poisoning, Assault	Poisoning, Undetermined	Adverse Effect	Underdosing
Methantheline	T44.3X1	T44.3X2	T44.3X3	T44.3X4	T44.3X5	T44.3X6
Methanthelinium bromide	T44.3X1	T44.3X2	T44.3X3	T44.3X4	T44.3X5	T44.3X6
Methaphenilene	T45.0X1	T45.0X2	T45.0X3	T45.0X4	T45.0X5	T45.0X6
Methapyrilene	T45.0X1	T45.0X2	T45.0X3	T45.0X4	T45.0X5	T45.0X6
Methaqualone (compound)	T42.6X1	T42.6X2	T42.6X3	T42.6X4	T42.6X5	T42.6X6
Metharbital	T42.3X1	T42.3X2	T42.3X3	T42.3X4	T42.3X5	T42.3X6
Methazolamide	T50.2X1	T50.2X2	T50.2X3	T50.2X4	T50.2X5	T50.2X6
Methdilazine	T43.3X1	T43.3X2	T43.3X3	T43.3X4	T43.3X5	T43.3X6
Methedrine	T43.621	T43.622	T43.623	T43.624	T43.625	T43.626
Methenamine (mandelate)	T37.8X1	T37.8X2	T37.8X3	T37.8X4	T37.8X5	T37.8X6
Methenolone	T38.7X1	T38.7X2	T38.7X3	T38.7X4	T38.7X5	T38.7X6
Methergine	T48.0X1	T48.0X2	T48.0X3	T48.0X4	T48.0X5	T48.0X6
Methetoin	T42.0X1	T42.0X2	T42.0X3	T42.0X4	T42.0X5	T42.0X6
Methiacil	T38.2X1	T38.2X2	T38.2X3	T38.2X4	T38.2X5	T38.2X6
Methicillin	T36.0X1	T36.0X2	T36.0X3	T36.0X4	T36.0X5	T36.0X6
Methimazole	T38.2X1	T38.2X2	T38.2X3	T38.2X4	T38.2X5	T38.2X6
Methiodal sodium	T50.8X1	T50.8X2	T50.8X3	T50.8X4	T50.8X5	T50.8X6
Methionine	T50.991	T50.992	T50.993	T50.994	T50.995	T50.996
Methisazone	T37.5X1	T37.5X2	T37.5X3	T37.5X4	T37.5X5	T37.5X6
Methisoprinol	T37.5X1	T37.5X2	T37.5X3	T37.5X4	T37.5X5	T37.5X6
Methitural	T42.3X1	T42.3X2	T42.3X3	T42.3X4	T42.3X5	T42.3X6
Methixene	T44.3X1	T44.3X2	T44.3X3	T44.3X4	T44.3X5	T44.3X6
Methobarbital, methobarbitone	T42.3X1	T42.3X2	T42.3X3	T42.3X4	T42.3X5	T42.3X6
Methocarbamol	T42.8X1	T42.8X2	T42.8X3	T42.8X4	T42.8X5	T42.8X6
skeletal muscle relaxant	T48.1X1	T48.1X2	T48.1X3	T48.1X4	T48.1X5	T48.1X6
Methohexital	T41.1X1	T41.1X2	T41.1X3	T41.1X4	T41.1X5	T41.1X6
Methohexitone	T41.1X1	T41.1X2	T41.1X3	T41.1X4	T41.1X5	T41.1X6
Methoin	T42.0X1	T42.0X2	T42.0X3	T42.0X4	T42.0X5	T42.0X6
Methopholine	T39.8X1	T39.8X2	T39.8X3	T39.8X4	T39.8X5	T39.8X6
Methopromazine	T43.3X1	T43.3X2	T43.3X3	T43.3X4	T43.3X5	T43.3X6
Methorate	T48.3X1	T48.3X2	T48.3X3	T48.3X4	T48.3X5	T48.3X6
Methoserpidine	T46.5X1	T46.5X2	T46.5X3	T46.5X4	T46.5X5	T46.5X6
Methotrexate	T45.1X1	T45.1X2	T45.1X3	T45.1X4	T45.1X5	T45.1X6
Methotrimeprazine	T43.3X1	T43.3X2	T43.3X3	T43.3X4	T43.3X5	T43.3X6
Methoxa-Dome	T49.3X1	T49.3X2	T49.3X3	T49.3X4	T49.3X5	T49.3X6
Methoxamine	T44.4X1	T44.4X2	T44.4X3	T44.4X4	T44.4X5	T44.4X6
Methoxsalen	T50.991	T50.992	T50.993	T50.994	T50.995	T50.996
Methoxyaniline	T65.3X1	T65.3X2	T65.3X3	T65.3X4	—	—
Methoxybenzyl penicillin	T36.0X1	T36.0X2	T36.0X3	T36.0X4	T36.0X5	T36.0X6
Methoxychlor	T53.7X1	T53.7X2	T53.7X3	T53.7X4	—	—
Methoxy-DDT	T53.7X1	T53.7X2	T53.7X3	T53.7X4	—	—
Methoxyflurane	T41.0X1	T41.0X2	T41.0X3	T41.0X4	T41.0X5	T41.0X6
Methoxyphenamine	T48.6X1	T48.6X2	T48.6X3	T48.6X4	T48.6X5	T48.6X6
Methoxypromazine	T43.3X1	T43.3X2	T43.3X3	T43.3X4	T43.3X5	T43.3X6
Methscopolamine bromide	T44.3X1	T44.3X2	T44.3X3	T44.3X4	T44.3X5	T44.3X6
Methsuximide	T42.2X1	T42.2X2	T42.2X3	T42.2X4	T42.2X5	T42.2X6
Methyclothiazide	T50.2X1	T50.2X2	T50.2X3	T50.2X4	T50.2X5	T50.2X6
Methyl						
acetate	T52.4X1	T52.4X2	T52.4X3	T52.4X4	—	—
acetone	T52.4X1	T52.4X2	T52.4X3	T52.4X4	—	—
acrylate	T65.891	T65.892	T65.893	T65.894	—	—
alcohol	T51.1X1	T51.1X2	T51.1X3	T51.1X4	—	—
aminophenol	T65.3X1	T65.3X2	T65.3X3	T65.3X4	—	—
amphetamine	T43.621	T43.622	T43.623	T43.624	T43.625	T43.626
androstanolone	T38.7X1	T38.7X2	T38.7X3	T38.7X4	T38.7X5	T38.7X6
atropine	T44.3X1	T44.3X2	T44.3X3	T44.3X4	T44.3X5	T44.3X6
benzene	T52.2X1	T52.2X2	T52.2X3	T52.2X4	—	—
benzoate	T52.8X1	T52.8X2	T52.8X3	T52.8X4	—	—
benzol	T52.2X1	T52.2X2	T52.2X3	T52.2X4	—	—
bromide (gas)	T59.891	T59.892	T59.893	T59.894	—	—
fumigant	T60.8X1	T60.8X2	T60.8X3	T60.8X4	—	—
butanol	T51.3X1	T51.3X2	T51.3X3	T51.3X4	—	—
carbinol	T51.1X1	T51.1X2	T51.1X3	T51.1X4	—	—
carbonate	T52.8X1	T52.8X2	T52.8X3	T52.8X4	—	—
CCNU	T45.1X1	T45.1X2	T45.1X3	T45.1X4	T45.1X5	T45.1X6
cellosolve	T52.91	T52.92	T52.93	T52.94	—	—
cellulose	T47.4X1	T47.4X2	T47.4X3	T47.4X4	T47.4X5	T47.4X6
chloride (gas)	T59.891	T59.892	T59.893	T59.894	—	—
chloroformate	T59.3X1	T59.3X2	T59.3X3	T59.3X4	—	—
cyclohexane	T52.8X1	T52.8X2	T52.8X3	T52.8X4	—	—
cyclohexanol	T51.8X1	T51.8X2	T51.8X3	T51.8X4	—	—
cyclohexanone	T52.8X1	T52.8X2	T52.8X3	T52.8X4	—	—
cyclohexyl acetate	T52.8X1	T52.8X2	T52.8X3	T52.8X4	—	—
demeton	T60.0X1	T60.0X2	T60.0X3	T60.0X4	—	—
dihydromorphinone	T40.2X1	T40.2X2	T40.2X3	T40.2X4	T40.2X5	T40.2X6
ergometrine	T48.0X1	T48.0X2	T48.0X3	T48.0X4	T48.0X5	T48.0X6
ergonovine	T48.0X1	T48.0X2	T48.0X3	T48.0X4	T48.0X5	T48.0X6
ethyl ketone	T52.4X1	T52.4X2	T52.4X3	T52.4X4	—	—
glucamine antimonate	T37.8X1	T37.8X2	T37.8X3	T37.8X4	T37.8X5	T37.8X6
hydrazine	T65.891	T65.892	T65.893	T65.894	—	—
iodide	T65.891	T65.892	T65.893	T65.894	—	—
isobutyl ketone	T52.4X1	T52.4X2	T52.4X3	T52.4X4	—	—

Substance	Poisoning, Accidental (unintentional)	Poisoning, Intentional Self-harm	Poisoning, Assault	Poisoning, Undetermined	Adverse Effect	Underdosing
Methyl — continued						
isothiocyanate	T60.3X1	T60.3X2	T60.3X3	T60.3X4	—	—
mercaptan	T59.891	T59.892	T59.893	T59.894		
morphine NEC	T40.2X1	T40.2X2	T40.2X3	T40.2X4	T40.2X5	T40.2X6
nicotinate	T49.4X1	T49.4X2	T49.4X3	T49.4X4	T49.4X5	T49.4X6
paraben	T49.0X1	T49.0X2	T49.0X3	T49.0X4	T49.0X5	T49.0X6
parafynol	T42.6X1	T42.6X2	T42.6X3	T42.6X4	T42.6X5	T42.6X6
parathion	T60.0X1	T60.0X2	T60.0X3	T60.0X4	—	—
peridol	T43.4X1	T43.4X2	T43.4X3	T43.4X4	T43.4X5	T43.4X6
phenidate	T43.631	T43.632	T43.633	T43.634	T43.635	T43.636
prednisolone	T38.0X1	T38.0X2	T38.0X3	T38.0X4	T38.0X5	T38.0X6
ENT agent	T49.6X1	T49.6X2	T49.6X3	T49.6X4	T49.6X5	T49.6X6
ophthalmic preparation	T49.5X1	T49.5X2	T49.5X3	T49.5X4	T49.5X5	T49.5X6
topical NEC	T49.0X1	T49.0X2	T49.0X3	T49.0X4	T49.0X5	T49.0X6
propylcarbinol	T51.3X1	T51.3X2	T51.3X3	T51.3X4	—	—
rosaniline NEC	T49.0X1	T49.0X2	T49.0X3	T49.0X4	T49.0X5	T49.0X6
salicylate	T49.2X1	T49.2X2	T49.2X3	T49.2X4	T49.2X5	T49.2X6
sulfate (fumes)	T59.891	T59.892	T59.893	T59.894	—	—
liquid	T52.8X1	T52.8X2	T52.8X3	T52.8X4	—	—
sulfonal	T42.6X1	T42.6X2	T42.6X3	T42.6X4	T42.6X5	T42.6X6
testosterone	T38.7X1	T38.7X2	T38.7X3	T38.7X4	T38.7X5	T38.7X6
thiouracil	T38.2X1	T38.2X2	T38.2X3	T38.2X4	T38.2X5	T38.2X6
Methylamphetamine	T43.621	T43.622	T43.623	T43.624	T43.625	T43.626
Methylated spirit	T51.1X1	T51.1X2	T51.1X3	T51.1X4	—	—
Methylatropine nitrate	T44.3X1	T44.3X2	T44.3X3	T44.3X4	T44.3X5	T44.3X6
Methylbenactyzium bromide	T44.3X1	T44.3X2	T44.3X3	T44.3X4	T44.3X5	T44.3X6
Methylbenzethonium chloride	T49.0X1	T49.0X2	T49.0X3	T49.0X4	T49.0X5	T49.0X6
Methylcellulose	T47.4X1	T47.4X2	T47.4X3	T47.4X4	T47.4X5	T47.4X6
laxative	T47.4X1	T47.4X2	T47.4X3	T47.4X4	T47.4X5	T47.4X6
Methylchlorophenoxyacetic acid	T60.3X1	T60.3X2	T60.3X3	T60.3X4	—	—
Methyldopa	T46.5X1	T46.5X2	T46.5X3	T46.5X4	T46.5X5	T46.5X6
Methyldopate	T46.5X1	T46.5X2	T46.5X3	T46.5X4	T46.5X5	T46.5X6
Methylene						
blue	T50.6X1	T50.6X2	T50.6X3	T50.6X4	T50.6X5	T50.6X6
chloride or dichloride (solvent)	T53.4X1	T53.4X2	T53.4X3	T53.4X4	—	—
NEC						
Methylenedioxyamphetamine	T43.621	T43.622	T43.623	T43.624	T43.625	T43.626
Methylenedioxymethamphetamine	T43.621	T43.622	T43.623	T43.624	T43.625	T43.626
Methylergometrine	T48.0X1	T48.0X2	T48.0X3	T48.0X4	T48.0X5	T48.0X6
Methylergonovine	T48.0X1	T48.0X2	T48.0X3	T48.0X4	T48.0X5	T48.0X6
Methylestrenolone	T38.5X1	T38.5X2	T38.5X3	T38.5X4	T38.5X5	T38.5X6
Methylethyl cellulose	T50.991	T50.992	T50.993	T50.994	T50.995	T50.996
Methylhexabital	T42.3X1	T42.3X2	T42.3X3	T42.3X4	T42.3X5	T42.3X6
Methylmorphine	T40.2X1	T40.2X2	T40.2X3	T40.2X4	T40.2X5	T40.2X6
Methylparaben (ophthalmic)	T49.5X1	T49.5X2	T49.5X3	T49.5X4	T49.5X5	T49.5X6
Methylparafynol	T42.6X1	T42.6X2	T42.6X3	T42.6X4	T42.6X5	T42.6X6
Methylpentynol, methylpenthynol	T42.6X1	T42.6X2	T42.6X3	T42.6X4	T42.6X5	T42.6X6
Methylphenidate	T43.631	T43.632	T43.633	T43.634	T43.635	T43.636
Methylphenobarbital	T42.3X1	T42.3X2	T42.3X3	T42.3X4	T42.3X5	T42.3X6
Methylpolysiloxane	T47.1X1	T47.1X2	T47.1X3	T47.1X4	T47.1X5	T47.1X6
Methylprednisolone — see Methyl, prednisolone						
Methylrosaniline	T49.0X1	T49.0X2	T49.0X3	T49.0X4	T49.0X5	T49.0X6
Methylrosanilinium chloride	T49.0X1	T49.0X2	T49.0X3	T49.0X4	T49.0X5	T49.0X6
Methyltestosterone	T38.7X1	T38.7X2	T38.7X3	T38.7X4	T38.7X5	T38.7X6
Methylthionine chloride	T50.6X1	T50.6X2	T50.6X3	T50.6X4	T50.6X5	T50.6X6
Methylthioninium chloride	T50.6X1	T50.6X2	T50.6X3	T50.6X4	T50.6X5	T50.6X6
Methylthiouracil	T38.2X1	T38.2X2	T38.2X3	T38.2X4	T38.2X5	T38.2X6
Methyprylon	T42.6X1	T42.6X2	T42.6X3	T42.6X4	T42.6X5	T42.6X6
Methysergide	T46.5X1	T46.5X2	T46.5X3	T46.5X4	T46.5X5	T46.5X6
Metiamide	T47.1X1	T47.1X2	T47.1X3	T47.1X4	T47.1X5	T47.1X6
Meticillin	T36.0X1	T36.0X2	T36.0X3	T36.0X4	T36.0X5	T36.0X6
Meticrane	T50.2X1	T50.2X2	T50.2X3	T50.2X4	T50.2X5	T50.2X6
Metildigoxin	T46.0X1	T46.0X2	T46.0X3	T46.0X4	T46.0X5	T46.0X6
Metipranolol	T49.5X1	T49.5X2	T49.5X3	T49.5X4	T49.5X5	T49.5X6
Metirosine	T46.5X1	T46.5X2	T46.5X3	T46.5X4	T46.5X5	T46.5X6
Metisazone	T37.5X1	T37.5X2	T37.5X3	T37.5X4	T37.5X5	T37.5X6
Metixene	T44.3X1	T44.3X2	T44.3X3	T44.3X4	T44.3X5	T44.3X6
Metizoline	T48.5X1	T48.5X2	T48.5X3	T48.5X4	T48.5X5	T48.5X6
Metoclopramide	T45.0X1	T45.0X2	T45.0X3	T45.0X4	T45.0X5	T45.0X6
Metofenazate	T43.3X1	T43.3X2	T43.3X3	T43.3X4	T43.3X5	T43.3X6
Metofoline	T39.8X1	T39.8X2	T39.8X3	T39.8X4	T39.8X5	T39.8X6
Metolazone	T50.2X1	T50.2X2	T50.2X3	T50.2X4	T50.2X5	T50.2X6
Metopon	T40.2X1	T40.2X2	T40.2X3	T40.2X4	T40.2X5	T40.2X6
Metoprine	T45.1X1	T45.1X2	T45.1X3	T45.1X4	T45.1X5	T45.1X6
Metoprolol	T44.7X1	T44.7X2	T44.7X3	T44.7X4	T44.7X5	T44.7X6
Metrifonate	T60.0X1	T60.0X2	T60.0X3	T60.0X4	—	—

Substance	Poisoning, Accidental (unintentional)	Poisoning, Intentional Self-harm	Poisoning, Assault	Poisoning, Undetermined	Adverse Effect	Under-dosing
Metrizamide	T50.8X1	T50.8X2	T50.8X3	T50.8X4	T50.8X5	T50.8X6
Metrizoic acid	T50.8X1	T50.8X2	T50.8X3	T50.8X4	T50.8X5	T50.8X6
Metronidazole	T37.8X1	T37.8X2	T37.8X3	T37.8X4	T37.8X5	T37.8X6
Metycaine	T41.3X1	T41.3X2	T41.3X3	T41.3X4	T41.3X5	T41.3X6
infiltration (subcutaneous)	T41.3X1	T41.3X2	T41.3X3	T41.3X4	T41.3X5	T41.3X6
nerve block (peripheral) (plexus)	T41.3X1	T41.3X2	T41.3X3	T41.3X4	T41.3X5	T41.3X6
topical (surface)	T41.3X1	T41.3X2	T41.3X3	T41.3X4	T41.3X5	T41.3X6
Metyrapone	T50.8X1	T50.8X2	T50.8X3	T50.8X4	T50.8X5	T50.8X6
Mevinphos	T60.0X1	T60.0X2	T60.0X3	T60.0X4	—	—
Mexazolam	T42.4X1	T42.4X2	T42.4X3	T42.4X4	T42.4X5	T42.4X6
Mexenone	T49.3X1	T49.3X2	T49.3X3	T49.3X4	T49.3X5	T49.3X6
Mexiletine	T46.2X1	T46.2X2	T46.2X3	T46.2X4	T46.2X5	T46.2X6
Mezereon	T62.2X1	T62.2X2	T62.2X3	T62.2X4	—	—
berries	T62.1X1	T62.1X2	T62.1X3	T62.1X4	—	—
Mezlocillin	T36.0X1	T36.0X2	T36.0X3	T36.0X4	T36.0X5	T36.0X6
Mianserin	T43.021	T43.022	T43.023	T43.024	T43.025	T43.026
Micatin	T49.0X1	T49.0X2	T49.0X3	T49.0X4	T49.0X5	T49.0X6
Miconazole	T49.0X1	T49.0X2	T49.0X3	T49.0X4	T49.0X5	T49.0X6
Micronomicin	T36.5X1	T36.5X2	T36.5X3	T36.5X4	T36.5X5	T36.5X6
Midazolam	T42.4X1	T42.4X2	T42.4X3	T42.4X4	T42.4X5	T42.4X6
Midecamycin	T36.3X1	T36.3X2	T36.3X3	T36.3X4	T36.3X5	T36.3X6
Mifepristone	T38.6X1	T38.6X2	T38.6X3	T38.6X4	T38.6X5	T38.6X6
Milk of magnesia	T47.1X1	T47.1X2	T47.1X3	T47.1X4	T47.1X5	T47.1X6
Millipede (tropical)	T63.411	T63.412	T63.413	T63.414	—	—
(venomous)						
Miltown	T43.591	T43.592	T43.593	T43.594	T43.595	T43.596
Milverine	T44.3X1	T44.3X2	T44.3X3	T44.3X4	T44.3X5	T44.3X6
Minaprine	T43.291	T43.292	T43.293	T43.294	T43.295	T43.296
Minaxolone	T41.291	T41.292	T41.293	T41.294	T41.295	T41.296
Mineral						
acids	T54.2X1	T54.2X2	T54.2X3	T54.2X4	—	—
oil (laxative)(medicinal)	T47.4X1	T47.4X2	T47.4X3	T47.4X4	T47.4X5	T47.4X6
emulsion	T47.2X1	T47.2X2	T47.2X3	T47.2X4	T47.2X5	T47.2X6
nonmedicinal	T52.0X1	T52.0X2	T52.0X3	T52.0X4	—	—
topical	T49.3X1	T49.3X2	T49.3X3	T49.3X4	T49.3X5	T49.3X6
salt NEC	T50.3X1	T50.3X2	T50.3X3	T50.3X4	T50.3X5	T50.3X6
spirits	T52.0X1	T52.0X2	T52.0X3	T52.0X4	—	—
Mineralocorticosteroid	T50.0X1	T50.0X2	T50.0X3	T50.0X4	T50.0X5	T50.0X6
Minocycline	T36.4X1	T36.4X2	T36.4X3	T36.4X4	T36.4X5	T36.4X6
Minoxidil	T46.7X1	T46.7X2	T46.7X3	T46.7X4	T46.7X5	T46.7X6
Miokamycin	T36.3X1	T36.3X2	T36.3X3	T36.3X4	T36.3X5	T36.3X6
Miotic drug	T49.5X1	T49.5X2	T49.5X3	T49.5X4	T49.5X5	T49.5X6
Mipafox	T60.0X1	T60.0X2	T60.0X3	T60.0X4	—	—
Mirex	T60.1X1	T60.1X2	T60.1X3	T60.1X4	—	—
Mirtazapine	T43.021	T43.022	T43.023	T43.024	T43.025	T43.026
Misonidazole	T37.3X1	T37.3X2	T37.3X3	T37.3X4	T37.3X5	T37.3X6
Misoprostol	T47.1X1	T47.1X2	T47.1X3	T47.1X4	T47.1X5	T47.1X6
Mithramycin	T45.1X1	T45.1X2	T45.1X3	T45.1X4	T45.1X5	T45.1X6
Mitobronitol	T45.1X1	T45.1X2	T45.1X3	T45.1X4	T45.1X5	T45.1X6
Mitoguazone	T45.1X1	T45.1X2	T45.1X3	T45.1X4	T45.1X5	T45.1X6
Mitolactol	T45.1X1	T45.1X2	T45.1X3	T45.1X4	T45.1X5	T45.1X6
Mitomycin	T45.1X1	T45.1X2	T45.1X3	T45.1X4	T45.1X5	T45.1X6
Mitopodozide	T45.1X1	T45.1X2	T45.1X3	T45.1X4	T45.1X5	T45.1X6
Mitotane	T45.1X1	T45.1X2	T45.1X3	T45.1X4	T45.1X5	T45.1X6
Mitoxantrone	T45.1X1	T45.1X2	T45.1X3	T45.1X4	T45.1X5	T45.1X6
Mivacurium chloride	T48.1X1	T48.1X2	T48.1X3	T48.1X4	T48.1X5	T48.1X6
Miyari bacteria	T47.6X1	T47.6X2	T47.6X3	T47.6X4	T47.6X5	T47.6X6
Moclobemide	T43.1X1	T43.1X2	T43.1X3	T43.1X4	T43.1X5	T43.1X6
Moderil	T46.5X1	T46.5X2	T46.5X3	T46.5X4	T46.5X5	T46.5X6
Mofebutazone	T39.2X1	T39.2X2	T39.2X3	T39.2X4	T39.2X5	T39.2X6
Mogadon — see Nitrazepam						
Molindone	T43.591	T43.592	T43.593	T43.594	T43.595	T43.596
Molsidomine	T46.3X1	T46.3X2	T46.3X3	T46.3X4	T46.3X5	T46.3X6
Mometasone	T49.0X1	T49.0X2	T49.0X3	T49.0X4	T49.0X5	T49.0X6
Monistat	T49.0X1	T49.0X2	T49.0X3	T49.0X4	T49.0X5	T49.0X6
Monkshood	T62.2X1	T62.2X2	T62.2X3	T62.2X4	—	—
Monoamine oxidase inhibitor NEC	T43.1X1	T43.1X2	T43.1X3	T43.1X4	T43.1X5	T43.1X6
hydrazine	T43.1X1	T43.1X2	T43.1X3	T43.1X4	T43.1X5	T43.1X6
Monobenzone	T49.4X1	T49.4X2	T49.4X3	T49.4X4	T49.4X5	T49.4X6
Monochloroacetic acid	T60.3X1	T60.3X2	T60.3X3	T60.3X4	—	—
Monochlorobenzene	T53.7X1	T53.7X2	T53.7X3	T53.7X4	—	—
Monoethanolamine	T46.8X1	T46.8X2	T46.8X3	T46.8X4	T46.8X5	T46.8X6
oleate	T46.8X1	T46.8X2	T46.8X3	T46.8X4	T46.8X5	T46.8X6
Monooctanoin	T50.991	T50.992	T50.993	T50.994	T50.995	T50.996
Monophenylbutazone	T39.2X1	T39.2X2	T39.2X3	T39.2X4	T39.2X5	T39.2X6
Monosodium glutamate	T65.891	T65.892	T65.893	T65.894	—	—
Monosulfiram	T49.0X1	T49.0X2	T49.0X3	T49.0X4	T49.0X5	T49.0X6
Monoxide, carbon — see Carbon, monoxide						
Monoxidine hydrochloride	T46.1X1	T46.1X2	T46.1X3	T46.1X4	T46.1X5	T46.1X6
Monuron	T60.3X1	T60.3X2	T60.3X3	T60.3X4	—	—

Substance	Poisoning, Accidental (unintentional)	Poisoning, Intentional Self-harm	Poisoning, Assault	Poisoning, Undetermined	Adverse Effect	Under-dosing
Moperone	T43.4X1	T43.4X2	T43.4X3	T43.4X4	T43.4X5	T43.4X6
Mopidamol	T45.1X1	T45.1X2	T45.1X3	T45.1X4	T45.1X5	T45.1X6
MOPP (mechloreth-amine + vincristine + prednisone + procarba-zine)	T45.1X1	T45.1X2	T45.1X3	T45.1X4	T45.1X5	T45.1X6
Morfin	T40.2X1	T40.2X2	T40.2X3	T40.2X4	T40.2X5	T40.2X6
Morinamide	T37.1X1	T37.1X2	T37.1X3	T37.1X4	T37.1X5	T37.1X6
Morning glory seeds	T40.991	T40.992	T40.993	T40.994	—	—
Moroxydine	T37.5X1	T37.5X2	T37.5X3	T37.5X4	T37.5X5	T37.5X6
Morphazinamide	T37.1X1	T37.1X2	T37.1X3	T37.1X4	T37.1X5	T37.1X6
Morphine	T40.2X1	T40.2X2	T40.2X3	T40.2X4	T40.2X5	T40.2X6
antagonist	T50.7X1	T50.7X2	T50.7X3	T50.7X4	T50.7X5	T50.7X6
Morpholinylethylmorphine	T40.2X1	T40.2X2	T40.2X3	T40.2X4	—	—
Morsuximide	T42.2X1	T42.2X2	T42.2X3	T42.2X4	T42.2X5	T42.2X6
Mosapramine	T43.591	T43.592	T43.593	T43.594	T43.595	T43.596
Moth balls — see also Pesticides	T60.2X1	T60.2X2	T60.2X3	T60.2X4	—	—
naphthalene	T60.2X1	T60.2X2	T60.2X3	T60.2X4	—	—
paradichlorobenzene	T60.1X1	T60.1X2	T60.1X3	T60.1X4	—	—
Motor exhaust gas	T58.01	T58.02	T58.03	T58.04	—	—
Mouthwash (antiseptic) (zinc chloride)	T49.6X1	T49.6X2	T49.6X3	T49.6X4	T49.6X5	T49.6X6
Moxastine	T45.0X1	T45.0X2	T45.0X3	T45.0X4	T45.0X5	T45.0X6
Moxaverine	T44.3X1	T44.3X2	T44.3X3	T44.3X4	T44.3X5	T44.3X6
Moxisylyte	T46.7X1	T46.7X2	T46.7X3	T46.7X4	T46.7X5	T46.7X6
Mucilage, plant	T47.4X1	T47.4X2	T47.4X3	T47.4X4	T47.4X5	T47.4X6
Mucolytic drug	T48.4X1	T48.4X2	T48.4X3	T48.4X4	T48.4X5	T48.4X6
Mucomyst	T48.4X1	T48.4X2	T48.4X3	T48.4X4	T48.4X5	T48.4X6
Mucous membrane agents (external)	T49.91	T49.92	T49.93	T49.94	T49.95	T49.96
specified NEC	T49.8X1	T49.8X2	T49.8X3	T49.8X4	T49.8X5	T49.8X6
Mumps						
immune globulin (human)	T50.Z11	T50.Z12	T50.Z13	T50.Z14	T50.Z15	T50.Z16
skin test antigen	T50.8X1	T50.8X2	T50.8X3	T50.8X4	T50.8X5	T50.8X6
vaccine	T50.B91	T50.B92	T50.B93	T50.B94	T50.B95	T50.B96
Mumpsvax	T50.B91	T50.B92	T50.B93	T50.B94	T50.B95	T50.B96
Mupirocin	T49.0X1	T49.0X2	T49.0X3	T49.0X4	T49.0X5	T49.0X6
Muriatic acid — see Hydrochloric acid						
Muromonab-CD3	T45.1X1	T45.1X2	T45.1X3	T45.1X4	T45.1X5	T45.1X6
Muscle-action drug NEC	T48.201	T48.202	T48.203	T48.204	T48.205	T48.206
Muscle affecting agents NEC	T48.201	T48.202	T48.203	T48.204	T48.205	T48.206
oxytocic	T48.0X1	T48.0X2	T48.0X3	T48.0X4	T48.0X5	T48.0X6
relaxants	T48.201	T48.202	T48.203	T48.204	T48.205	T48.206
central nervous system	T42.8X1	T42.8X2	T42.8X3	T42.8X4	T42.8X5	T42.8X6
skeletal	T48.1X1	T48.1X2	T48.1X3	T48.1X4	T48.1X5	T48.1X6
smooth	T44.3X1	T44.3X2	T44.3X3	T44.3X4	T44.3X5	T44.3X6
Muscle relaxant — see Relaxant, muscle						
Muscle-tone depressant, central NEC	T42.8X1	T42.8X2	T42.8X3	T42.8X4	T42.8X5	T42.8X6
specified NEC	T42.8X1	T42.8X2	T42.8X3	T42.8X4	T42.8X5	T42.8X6
Mushroom, noxious	T62.0X1	T62.0X2	T62.0X3	T62.0X4	—	—
Mussel, noxious	T61.781	T61.782	T61.783	T61.784	—	—
Mustard (emetic)	T47.7X1	T47.7X2	T47.7X3	T47.7X4	T47.7X5	T47.7X6
black	T47.7X1	T47.7X2	T47.7X3	T47.7X4	T47.7X5	T47.7X6
gas, not in war	T59.91	T59.92	T59.93	T59.94	—	—
nitrogen	T45.1X1	T45.1X2	T45.1X3	T45.1X4	T45.1X5	T45.1X6
Mustine	T45.1X1	T45.1X2	T45.1X3	T45.1X4	T45.1X5	T45.1X6
M-vac	T45.1X1	T45.1X2	T45.1X3	T45.1X4	T45.1X5	T45.1X6
Mycifradin	T36.5X1	T36.5X2	T36.5X3	T36.5X4	T36.5X5	T36.5X6
topical	T49.0X1	T49.0X2	T49.0X3	T49.0X4	T49.0X5	T49.0X6
Mycitracin	T36.8X1	T36.8X2	T36.8X3	T36.8X4	T36.8X5	T36.8X6
ophthalmic preparation	T49.5X1	T49.5X2	T49.5X3	T49.5X4	T49.5X5	T49.5X6
Mycostatin	T36.7X1	T36.7X2	T36.7X3	T36.7X4	T36.7X5	T36.7X6
topical	T49.0X1	T49.0X2	T49.0X3	T49.0X4	T49.0X5	T49.0X6
Mycotoxins	T64.81	T64.82	T64.83	T64.84	—	—
aflatoxin	T64.01	T64.02	T64.03	T64.04	—	—
specified NEC	T64.81	T64.82	T64.83	T64.84	—	—
Mydriacyl	T44.3X1	T44.3X2	T44.3X3	T44.3X4	T44.3X5	T44.3X6
Mydriatic drug	T49.5X1	T49.5X2	T49.5X3	T49.5X4	T49.5X5	T49.5X6
Myelobromal	T45.1X1	T45.1X2	T45.1X3	T45.1X4	T45.1X5	T45.1X6
Myleran	T45.1X1	T45.1X2	T45.1X3	T45.1X4	T45.1X5	T45.1X6
Myochrysin (e)	T39.2X1	T39.2X2	T39.2X3	T39.2X4	T39.2X5	T39.2X6
Myoneural blocking agents	T48.1X1	T48.1X2	T48.1X3	T48.1X4	T48.1X5	T48.1X6
Myralact	T49.0X1	T49.0X2	T49.0X3	T49.0X4	T49.0X5	T49.0X6
Myristica fragrans	T62.2X1	T62.2X2	T62.2X3	T62.2X4	—	—
Myristicin	T65.891	T65.892	T65.893	T65.894	—	—
Mysoline	T42.3X1	T42.3X2	T42.3X3	T42.3X4	T42.3X5	T42.3X6
Nabilone	T40.7X1	T40.7X2	T40.7X3	T40.7X4	T40.7X5	T40.7X6
Nabumetone	T39.391	T39.392	T39.393	T39.394	T39.395	T39.396
Nadolol	T44.7X1	T44.7X2	T44.7X3	T44.7X4	T44.7X5	T44.7X6

Substance	Poisoning, Accidental (unintentional)	Poisoning, Intentional Self-harm	Poisoning, Assault	Poisoning, Undetermined	Adverse Effect	Under-dosing
Nafcillin	T36.0X1	T36.0X2	T36.0X3	T36.0X4	T36.0X5	T36.0X6
Nafoxidine	T38.6X1	T38.6X2	T38.6X3	T38.6X4	T38.6X5	T38.6X6
Naftazone	T46.991	T46.992	T46.993	T46.994	T46.995	T46.996
Naftidrofuryl (oxalate)	T46.7X1	T46.7X2	T46.7X3	T46.7X4	T46.7X5	T46.7X6
Naftifine	T49.0X1	T49.0X2	T49.0X3	T49.0X4	T49.0X5	T49.0X6
Nail polish remover	T52.91	T52.92	T52.93	T52.94	—	—
Nalbuphine	T40.4X1	T40.4X2	T40.4X3	T40.4X4	T40.4X5	T40.4X6
Naled	T60.0X1	T60.0X2	T60.0X3	T60.0X4	—	—
Nalidixic acid	T37.8X1	T37.8X2	T37.8X3	T37.8X4	T37.8X5	T37.8X6
Nalorphine	T50.7X1	T50.7X2	T50.7X3	T50.7X4	T50.7X5	T50.7X6
Naloxone	T50.7X1	T50.7X2	T50.7X3	T50.7X4	T50.7X5	T50.7X6
Naltrexone	T50.7X1	T50.7X2	T50.7X3	T50.7X4	T50.7X5	T50.7X6
Namenda	T43.8X1	T43.8X2	T43.8X3	T43.8X4	T43.8X5	T43.8X6
Nandrolone	T38.7X1	T38.7X2	T38.7X3	T38.7X4	T38.7X5	T38.7X6
Naphazoline	T48.5X1	T48.5X2	T48.5X3	T48.5X4	T48.5X5	T48.5X6
Naphtha (painters') (petroleum)	T52.0X1	T52.0X2	T52.0X3	T52.0X4	—	—
solvent	T52.0X1	T52.0X2	T52.0X3	T52.0X4	—	—
vapor	T52.0X1	T52.0X2	T52.0X3	T52.0X4	—	—
Naphthalene (non-chlorinated)	T60.2X1	T60.2X2	T60.2X3	T60.2X4	—	—
chlorinated	T60.1X1	T60.1X2	T60.1X3	T60.1X4	—	—
vapor	T60.1X1	T60.1X2	T60.1X3	T60.1X4	—	—
insecticide or moth repellent	T60.2X1	T60.2X2	T60.2X3	T60.2X4	—	—
chlorinated	T60.1X1	T60.1X2	T60.1X3	T60.1X4	—	—
vapor	T60.2X1	T60.2X2	T60.2X3	T60.2X4	—	—
chlorinated	T60.1X1	T60.1X2	T60.1X3	T60.1X4	—	—
Naphthol	T65.891	T65.892	T65.893	T65.894	—	—
Naphthylamine	T65.891	T65.892	T65.893	T65.894	—	—
Naphthylthiourea (ANTU)	T60.4X1	T60.4X2	T60.4X3	T60.4X4	—	—
Naprosyn — see Naproxen						
Naproxen	T39.311	T39.312	T39.313	T39.314	T39.315	T39.316
Narcotic (drug)	T40.601	T40.602	T40.603	T40.604	T40.605	T40.606
analgesic NEC	T40.601	T40.602	T40.603	T40.604	T40.605	T40.606
antagonist	T50.7X1	T50.7X2	T50.7X3	T50.7X4	T50.7X5	T50.7X6
specified NEC	T40.691	T40.692	T40.693	T40.694	T40.695	T40.696
synthetic	T40.4X1	T40.4X2	T40.4X3	T40.4X4	T40.4X5	T40.4X6
Narcotine	T48.3X1	T48.3X2	T48.3X3	T48.3X4	T48.3X5	T48.3X6
Nardil	T43.1X1	T43.1X2	T43.1X3	T43.1X4	T43.1X5	T43.1X6
Nasal drug NEC	T49.6X1	T49.6X2	T49.6X3	T49.6X4	T49.6X5	T49.6X6
Natamycin	T49.0X1	T49.0X2	T49.0X3	T49.0X4	T49.0X5	T49.0X6
Natrium cyanide — see Cyanide(s)						
Natural						
blood (product)	T45.8X1	T45.8X2	T45.8X3	T45.8X4	T45.8X5	T45.8X6
gas (piped)	T59.891	T59.892	T59.893	T59.894	—	—
incomplete combustion	T58.11	T58.12	T58.13	T58.14	—	—
Nealbarbital	T42.3X1	T42.3X2	T42.3X3	T42.3X4	T42.3X5	T42.3X6
Nectadon	T48.3X1	T48.3X2	T48.3X3	T48.3X4	T48.3X5	T48.3X6
Nedocromil	T48.6X1	T48.6X2	T48.6X3	T48.6X4	T48.6X5	T48.6X6
Nefopam	T39.8X1	T39.8X2	T39.8X3	T39.8X4	T39.8X5	T39.8X6
Nematocyst (sting)	T63.691	T63.692	T63.693	T63.694	—	—
Nembutal	T42.3X1	T42.3X2	T42.3X3	T42.3X4	T42.3X5	T42.3X6
Nemonapride	T43.591	T43.592	T43.593	T43.594	T43.595	T43.596
Neoarsphenamine	T37.8X1	T37.8X2	T37.8X3	T37.8X4	T37.8X5	T37.8X6
Neocinchophen	T50.4X1	T50.4X2	T50.4X3	T50.4X4	T50.4X5	T50.4X6
Neomycin (derivatives)	T36.5X1	T36.5X2	T36.5X3	T36.5X4	T36.5X5	T36.5X6
with						
bacitracin	T49.0X1	T49.0X2	T49.0X3	T49.0X4	T49.0X5	T49.0X6
neostigmine	T44.0X1	T44.0X2	T44.0X3	T44.0X4	T44.0X5	T44.0X6
ENT agent	T49.6X1	T49.6X2	T49.6X3	T49.6X4	T49.6X5	T49.6X6
ophthalmic preparation	T49.5X1	T49.5X2	T49.5X3	T49.5X4	T49.5X5	T49.5X6
topical NEC	T49.0X1	T49.0X2	T49.0X3	T49.0X4	T49.0X5	T49.0X6
Neonal	T42.3X1	T42.3X2	T42.3X3	T42.3X4	T42.3X5	T42.3X6
Neoprontosil	T37.0X1	T37.0X2	T37.0X3	T37.0X4	T37.0X5	T37.0X6
Neosalvarsan	T37.8X1	T37.8X2	T37.8X3	T37.8X4	T37.8X5	T37.8X6
Neosilversalvarsan	T37.8X1	T37.8X2	T37.8X3	T37.8X4	T37.8X5	T37.8X6
Neosporin	T36.8X1	T36.8X2	T36.8X3	T36.8X4	T36.8X5	T36.8X6
ENT agent	T49.6X1	T49.6X2	T49.6X3	T49.6X4	T49.6X5	T49.6X6
opthalmic preparation	T49.5X1	T49.5X2	T49.5X3	T49.5X4	T49.5X5	T49.5X6
topical NEC	T49.0X1	T49.0X2	T49.0X3	T49.0X4	T49.0X5	T49.0X6
Neostigmine bromide	T44.0X1	T44.0X2	T44.0X3	T44.0X4	T44.0X5	T44.0X6
Neraval	T42.3X1	T42.3X2	T42.3X3	T42.3X4	T42.3X5	T42.3X6
Neravan	T42.3X1	T42.3X2	T42.3X3	T42.3X4	T42.3X5	T42.3X6
Nerium oleander	T62.2X1	T62.2X2	T62.2X3	T62.2X4	—	—
Nerve gas, not in war	T59.91	T59.92	T59.93	T59.94	—	—
Nesacaine	T41.3X1	T41.3X2	T41.3X3	T41.3X4	T41.3X5	T41.3X6
infiltration (subcutaneous)	T41.3X1	T41.3X2	T41.3X3	T41.3X4	T41.3X5	T41.3X6
nerve block (peripheral) (plexus)	T41.3X1	T41.3X2	T41.3X3	T41.3X4	T41.3X5	T41.3X6
Netilmicin	T36.5X1	T36.5X2	T36.5X3	T36.5X4	T36.5X5	T36.5X6
Neurobarb	T42.3X1	T42.3X2	T42.3X3	T42.3X4	T42.3X5	T42.3X6

Substance	Poisoning, Accidental (unintentional)	Poisoning, Intentional Self-harm	Poisoning, Assault	Poisoning, Undetermined	Adverse Effect	Under-dosing
Neuroleptic drug NEC	T43.501	T43.502	T43.503	T43.504	T43.505	T43.506
Neuromuscular blocking drug	T48.1X1	T48.1X2	T48.1X3	T48.1X4	T48.1X5	T48.1X6
Neutral insulin injection	T38.3X1	T38.3X2	T38.3X3	T38.3X4	T38.3X5	T38.3X6
Neutral spirits	T51.0X1	T51.0X2	T51.0X3	T51.0X4	—	—
beverage	T51.0X1	T51.0X2	T51.0X3	T51.0X4	—	—
Niacin	T46.7X1	T46.7X2	T46.7X3	T46.7X4	T46.7X5	T46.7X6
Niacinamide	T45.2X1	T45.2X2	T45.2X3	T45.2X4	T45.2X5	T45.2X6
Nialamide	T43.1X1	T43.1X2	T43.1X3	T43.1X4	T43.1X5	T43.1X6
Niaprazine	T42.6X1	T42.6X2	T42.6X3	T42.6X4	T42.6X5	T42.6X6
Nicametate	T46.7X1	T46.7X2	T46.7X3	T46.7X4	T46.7X5	T46.7X6
Nicardipine	T46.1X1	T46.1X2	T46.1X3	T46.1X4	T46.1X5	T46.1X6
Nicergoline	T46.7X1	T46.7X2	T46.7X3	T46.7X4	T46.7X5	T46.7X6
Nickel (carbonyl) (tetra-carbonyl)(fumes) (vapor)	T56.891	T56.892	T56.893	T56.894	—	—
Nickelocene	T56.891	T56.892	T56.893	T56.894	—	—
Niclosamide	T37.4X1	T37.4X2	T37.4X3	T37.4X4	T37.4X5	T37.4X6
Nicofuranose	T46.7X1	T46.7X2	T46.7X3	T46.7X4	T46.7X5	T46.7X6
Nicomorphine	T40.2X1	T40.2X2	T40.2X3	T40.2X4	—	—
Nicorandil	T46.3X1	T46.3X2	T46.3X3	T46.3X4	T46.3X5	T46.3X6
Nicotiana (plant)	T62.2X1	T62.2X2	T62.2X3	T62.2X4	—	—
Nicotinamide	T45.2X1	T45.2X2	T45.2X3	T45.2X4	T45.2X5	T45.2X6
Nicotine (insecticide) (spray) (sulfate) NEC	T60.2X1	T60.2X2	T60.2X3	T60.2X4	—	—
from tobacco	T65.291	T65.292	T65.293	T65.294	—	—
cigarettes	T65.221	T65.222	T65.223	T65.224	—	—
not insecticide	T65.291	T65.292	T65.293	T65.294	—	—
Nicotinic acid	T46.7X1	T46.7X2	T46.7X3	T46.7X4	T46.7X5	T46.7X6
Nicotinyl alcohol	T46.7X1	T46.7X2	T46.7X3	T46.7X4	T46.7X5	T46.7X6
Nicoumalone	T45.511	T45.512	T45.513	T45.514	T45.515	T45.516
Nifedipine	T46.1X1	T46.1X2	T46.1X3	T46.1X4	T46.1X5	T46.1X6
Nifenazone	T39.2X1	T39.2X2	T39.2X3	T39.2X4	T39.2X5	T39.2X6
Nifuraldezone	T37.91	T37.92	T37.93	T37.94	T37.95	T37.96
Nifuratel	T37.8X1	T37.8X2	T37.8X3	T37.8X4	T37.8X5	T37.8X6
Nifurtimox	T37.3X1	T37.3X2	T37.3X3	T37.3X4	T37.3X5	T37.3X6
Nifurtoinol	T37.8X1	T37.8X2	T37.8X3	T37.8X4	T37.8X5	T37.8X6
Nightshade, deadly (solanum) — see also Belladonna	T62.2X1	T62.2X2	T62.2X3	T62.2X4	—	—
berry	T62.1X1	T62.1X2	T62.1X3	T62.1X4	—	—
Nikethamide	T50.7X1	T50.7X2	T50.7X3	T50.7X4	T50.7X5	T50.7X6
Nilstat	T36.7X1	T36.7X2	T36.7X3	T36.7X4	T36.7X5	T36.7X6
topical	T49.0X1	T49.0X2	T49.0X3	T49.0X4	T49.0X5	T49.0X6
Nilutamide	T38.6X1	T38.6X2	T38.6X3	T38.6X4	T38.6X5	T38.6X6
Nimesulide	T39.391	T39.392	T39.393	T39.394	T39.395	T39.396
Nimetazepam	T42.4X1	T42.4X2	T42.4X3	T42.4X4	T42.4X5	T42.4X6
Nimodipine	T46.1X1	T46.1X2	T46.1X3	T46.1X4	T46.1X5	T46.1X6
Nimorazole	T37.3X1	T37.3X2	T37.3X3	T37.3X4	T37.3X5	T37.3X6
Nimustine	T45.1X1	T45.1X2	T45.1X3	T45.1X4	T45.1X5	T45.1X6
Niridazole	T37.4X1	T37.4X2	T37.4X3	T37.4X4	T37.4X5	T37.4X6
Nisentil	T40.2X1	T40.2X2	T40.2X3	T40.2X4	T40.2X5	T40.2X6
Nisoldipine	T46.1X1	T46.1X2	T46.1X3	T46.1X4	T46.1X5	T46.1X6
Nitramine	T65.3X1	T65.3X2	T65.3X3	T65.3X4	—	—
Nitrate, organic	T46.3X1	T46.3X2	T46.3X3	T46.3X4	T46.3X5	T46.3X6
Nitrazepam	T42.4X1	T42.4X2	T42.4X3	T42.4X4	T42.4X5	T42.4X6
Nitrefazole	T50.6X1	T50.6X2	T50.6X3	T50.6X4	T50.6X5	T50.6X6
Nitrendipine	T46.1X1	T46.1X2	T46.1X3	T46.1X4	T46.1X5	T46.1X6
Nitric						
acid (liquid)	T54.2X1	T54.2X2	T54.2X3	T54.2X4	—	—
vapor	T59.891	T59.892	T59.893	T59.894	—	—
oxide (gas)	T59.0X1	T59.0X2	T59.0X3	T59.0X4	—	—
Nitrimidazine	T37.3X1	T37.3X2	T37.3X3	T37.3X4	T37.3X5	T37.3X6
Nitrite, amyl (medicinal) (vapor)	T46.3X1	T46.3X2	T46.3X3	T46.3X4	T46.3X5	T46.3X6
Nitroaniline	T65.3X1	T65.3X2	T65.3X3	T65.3X4	—	—
vapor	T59.891	T59.892	T59.893	T59.894	—	—
Nitrobenzene, nitrobenzol	T65.3X1	T65.3X2	T65.3X3	T65.3X4	—	—
vapor	T65.3X1	T65.3X2	T65.3X3	T65.3X4	—	—
Nitrocellulose	T65.891	T65.892	T65.893	T65.894	—	—
lacquer	T65.891	T65.892	T65.893	T65.894	—	—
Nitrodiphenyl	T65.3X1	T65.3X2	T65.3X3	T65.3X4	—	—
Nitrofural	T49.0X1	T49.0X2	T49.0X3	T49.0X4	T49.0X5	T49.0X6
Nitrofurantoin	T37.8X1	T37.8X2	T37.8X3	T37.8X4	T37.8X5	T37.8X6
Nitrofurazone	T49.0X1	T49.0X2	T49.0X3	T49.0X4	T49.0X5	T49.0X6
Nitrogen	T59.0X1	T59.0X2	T59.0X3	T59.0X4	—	—
mustard	T45.1X1	T45.1X2	T45.1X3	T45.1X4	T45.1X5	T45.1X6
Nitroglycerin, nitroglycerol (medicinal)	T46.3X1	T46.3X2	T46.3X3	T46.3X4	T46.3X5	T46.3X6
nonmedicinal	T65.5X1	T65.5X2	T65.5X3	T65.5X4	—	—
fumes	T65.5X1	T65.5X2	T65.5X3	T65.5X4	—	—
Nitroglycol	T52.3X1	T52.3X2	T52.3X3	T52.3X4	—	—
Nitrohydrochloric acid	T54.2X1	T54.2X2	T54.2X3	T54.2X4	—	—
Nitromersol	T49.0X1	T49.0X2	T49.0X3	T49.0X4	T49.0X5	T49.0X6

Substance	Poisoning, Accidental (unintentional)	Poisoning, Intentional Self-harm	Poisoning, Assault	Poisoning, Undetermined	Adverse Effect	Under-dosing
Nitronaphthalene	T65.891	T65.892	T65.893	T65.894	—	—
Nitrophenol	T54.0X1	T54.0X2	T54.0X3	T54.0X4	—	—
Nitropropane	T52.8X1	T52.8X2	T52.8X3	T52.8X4	—	—
Nitroprusside	T46.5X1	T46.5X2	T46.5X3	T46.5X4	T46.5X5	T46.5X6
Nitrosodimethylamine	T65.3X1	T65.3X2	T65.3X3	T65.3X4	—	—
Nitrothiazol	T37.4X1	T37.4X2	T37.4X3	T37.4X4	T37.4X5	T37.4X6
Nitrotoluene, nitrotoluol	T65.3X1	T65.3X2	T65.3X3	T65.3X4	—	—
vapor	T65.3X1	T65.3X2	T65.3X3	T65.3X4	—	—
Nitrous						
acid (liquid)	T54.2X1	T54.2X2	T54.2X3	T54.2X4	—	—
fumes	T59.891	T59.892	T59.893	T59.894	—	—
ether spirit	T46.3X1	T46.3X2	T46.3X3	T46.3X4	T46.3X5	T46.3X6
oxide	T41.0X1	T41.0X2	T41.0X3	T41.0X4	T41.0X5	T41.0X6
Nitroxoline	T37.8X1	T37.8X2	T37.8X3	T37.8X4	T37.8X5	T37.8X6
Nitrozone	T49.0X1	T49.0X2	T49.0X3	T49.0X4	T49.0X5	T49.0X6
Nizatidine	T47.0X1	T47.0X2	T47.0X3	T47.0X4	T47.0X5	T47.0X6
Nizofenone	T43.8X1	T43.8X2	T43.8X3	T43.8X4	T43.8X5	T43.8X6
Noctec	T42.6X1	T42.6X2	T42.6X3	T42.6X4	T42.6X5	T42.6X6
Noludar	T42.6X1	T42.6X2	T42.6X3	T42.6X4	T42.6X5	T42.6X6
Nomegestrol	T38.5X1	T38.5X2	T38.5X3	T38.5X4	T38.5X5	T38.5X6
Nomifensine	T43.291	T43.292	T43.293	T43.294	T43.295	T43.296
Nonoxinol	T49.8X1	T49.8X2	T49.8X3	T49.8X4	T49.8X5	T49.8X6
Nonylphenoxy	T49.8X1	T49.8X2	T49.8X3	T49.8X4	T49.8X5	T49.8X6
(polyethoxyethanol)						
Noptil	T42.3X1	T42.3X2	T42.3X3	T42.3X4	T42.3X5	T42.3X6
Noradrenaline	T44.4X1	T44.4X2	T44.4X3	T44.4X4	T44.4X5	T44.4X6
Noramidopyrine	T39.2X1	T39.2X2	T39.2X3	T39.2X4	T39.2X5	T39.2X6
methanesulfonate sodium	T39.2X1	T39.2X2	T39.2X3	T39.2X4	T39.2X5	T39.2X6
Norbormide	T60.4X1	T60.4X2	T60.4X3	T60.4X4	—	—
Nordazepam	T42.4X1	T42.4X2	T42.4X3	T42.4X4	T42.4X5	T42.4X6
Norepinephrine	T44.4X1	T44.4X2	T44.4X3	T44.4X4	T44.4X5	T44.4X6
Norethandrolone	T38.7X1	T38.7X2	T38.7X3	T38.7X4	T38.7X5	T38.7X6
Norethindrone	T38.4X1	T38.4X2	T38.4X3	T38.4X4	T38.4X5	T38.4X6
Norethisterone (acetate)	T38.4X1	T38.4X2	T38.4X3	T38.4X4	T38.4X5	T38.4X6
(enantate)						
with ethinylestradiol	T38.5X1	T38.5X2	T38.5X3	T38.5X4	T38.5X5	T38.5X6
Noretynodrel	T38.5X1	T38.5X2	T38.5X3	T38.5X4	T38.5X5	T38.5X6
Norfenefrine	T44.4X1	T44.4X2	T44.4X3	T44.4X4	T44.4X5	T44.4X6
Norfloxacin	T36.8X1	T36.8X2	T36.8X3	T36.8X4	T36.8X5	T36.8X6
Norgestrel	T38.4X1	T38.4X2	T38.4X3	T38.4X4	T38.4X5	T38.4X6
Norgestrienone	T38.4X1	T38.4X2	T38.4X3	T38.4X4	T38.4X5	T38.4X6
Norlestrin	T38.4X1	T38.4X2	T38.4X3	T38.4X4	T38.4X5	T38.4X6
Norlutin	T38.4X1	T38.4X2	T38.4X3	T38.4X4	T38.4X5	T38.4X6
Normal serum albumin (human),	T45.8X1	T45.8X2	T45.8X3	T45.8X4	T45.8X5	T45.8X6
salt-poor						
Normethandrone	T38.5X1	T38.5X2	T38.5X3	T38.5X4	T38.5X5	T38.5X6
Normison — see						
Benzodiazepines						
Normorphine	T40.2X1	T40.2X2	T40.2X3	T40.2X4	—	—
Norpseudoephedrine	T50.5X1	T50.5X2	T50.5X3	T50.5X4	T50.5X5	T50.5X6
Nortestosterone	T38.7X1	T38.7X2	T38.7X3	T38.7X4	T38.7X5	T38.7X6
(furanpropionate)						
Nortriptyline	T43.011	T43.012	T43.013	T43.014	T43.015	T43.016
Noscapine	T48.3X1	T48.3X2	T48.3X3	T48.3X4	T48.3X5	T48.3X6
Nose preparations	T49.6X1	T49.6X2	T49.6X3	T49.6X4	T49.6X5	T49.6X6
Novobiocin	T36.5X1	T36.5X2	T36.5X3	T36.5X4	T36.5X5	T36.5X6
Novocain (infiltration)	T41.3X1	T41.3X2	T41.3X3	T41.3X4	T41.3X5	T41.3X6
(topical)						
nerve block (peripheral)	T41.3X1	T41.3X2	T41.3X3	T41.3X4	T41.3X5	T41.3X6
(plexus)						
spinal	T41.3X1	T41.3X2	T41.3X3	T41.3X4	T41.3X5	T41.3X6
Noxious foodstuff	T62.91	T62.92	T62.93	T62.94	—	—
specified NEC	T62.8X1	T62.8X2	T62.8X3	T62.8X4	—	—
Noxiptiline	T43.011	T43.012	T43.013	T43.014	T43.015	T43.016
Noxytiolin	T49.0X1	T49.0X2	T49.0X3	T49.0X4	T49.0X5	T49.0X6
NPH Iletin (insulin)	T38.3X1	T38.3X2	T38.3X3	T38.3X4	T38.3X5	T38.3X6
Numorphan	T40.2X1	T40.2X2	T40.2X3	T40.2X4	T40.2X5	T40.2X6
Nunol	T42.3X1	T42.3X2	T42.3X3	T42.3X4	T42.3X5	T42.3X6
Nupercaine (spinal	T41.3X1	T41.3X2	T41.3X3	T41.3X4	T41.3X5	T41.3X6
anesthetic)						
topical (surface)	T41.3X1	T41.3X2	T41.3X3	T41.3X4	T41.3X5	T41.3X6
Nutmeg oil (liniment)	T49.3X1	T49.3X2	T49.3X3	T49.3X4	T49.3X5	T49.3X6
Nutritional supplement	T50.901	T50.902	T50.903	T50.904	T50.905	T50.906
Nux vomica	T65.1X1	T65.1X2	T65.1X3	T65.1X4	—	—
Nydrazid	T37.1X1	T37.1X2	T37.1X3	T37.1X4	T37.1X5	T37.1X6
Nylidrin	T46.7X1	T46.7X2	T46.7X3	T46.7X4	T46.7X5	T46.7X6
Nystatin	T36.7X1	T36.7X2	T36.7X3	T36.7X4	T36.7X5	T36.7X6
topical	T49.0X1	T49.0X2	T49.0X3	T49.0X4	T49.0X5	T49.0X6
Nytol	T45.0X1	T45.0X2	T45.0X3	T45.0X4	T45.0X5	T45.0X6
Obidoxime chloride	T50.6X1	T50.6X2	T50.6X3	T50.6X4	T50.6X5	T50.6X6
Octafonium (chloride)	T49.3X1	T49.3X2	T49.3X3	T49.3X4	T49.3X5	T49.3X6
Octamethyl	T60.0X1	T60.0X2	T60.0X3	T60.0X4	—	—
pyrophosphoramide						
Octanoin	T50.991	T50.992	T50.993	T50.994	T50.995	T50.996
Octatropine	T44.3X1	T44.3X2	T44.3X3	T44.3X4	T44.3X5	T44.3X6
methylbromide						
Octotiamine	T45.2X1	T45.2X2	T45.2X3	T45.2X4	T45.2X5	T45.2X6
Octoxinol (9)	T49.8X1	T49.8X2	T49.8X3	T49.8X4	T49.8X5	T49.8X6
Octreotide	T38.991	T38.992	T38.993	T38.994	T38.995	T38.996
Octyl nitrite	T46.3X1	T46.3X2	T46.3X3	T46.3X4	T46.3X5	T46.3X6
Oestradiol	T38.5X1	T38.5X2	T38.5X3	T38.5X4	T38.5X5	T38.5X6
Oestriol	T38.5X1	T38.5X2	T38.5X3	T38.5X4	T38.5X5	T38.5X6
Oestrogen	T38.5X1	T38.5X2	T38.5X3	T38.5X4	T38.5X5	T38.5X6
Oestrone	T38.5X1	T38.5X2	T38.5X3	T38.5X4	T38.5X5	T38.5X6
Ofloxacin	T36.8X1	T36.8X2	T36.8X3	T36.8X4	T36.8X5	T36.8X6
Oil (of)	T65.891	T65.892	T65.893	T65.894	—	—
bitter almond	T62.8X1	T62.8X2	T62.8X3	T62.8X4	—	—
cloves	T49.7X1	T49.7X2	T49.7X3	T49.7X4	T49.7X5	T49.7X6
colors	T65.6X1	T65.6X2	T65.6X3	T65.6X4	—	—
fumes	T59.891	T59.892	T59.893	T59.894	—	—
lubricating	T52.0X1	T52.0X2	T52.0X3	T52.0X4	—	—
Niobe	T52.8X1	T52.8X2	T52.8X3	T52.8X4	—	—
vitriol (liquid)	T54.2X1	T54.2X2	T54.2X3	T54.2X4	—	—
fumes	T54.2X1	T54.2X2	T54.2X3	T54.2X4	—	—
wintergreen (bitter) NEC	T49.3X1	T49.3X2	T49.3X3	T49.3X4	T49.3X5	T49.3X6
Oily preparation (for skin)	T49.3X1	T49.3X2	T49.3X3	T49.3X4	T49.3X5	T49.3X6
Ointment NEC	T49.3X1	T49.3X2	T49.3X3	T49.3X4	T49.3X5	T49.3X6
Olanzapine	T43.591	T43.592	T43.593	T43.594	T43.595	T43.596
Oleander	T62.2X1	T62.2X2	T62.2X3	T62.2X4	—	—
Oleandomycin	T36.3X1	T36.3X2	T36.3X3	T36.3X4	T36.3X5	T36.3X6
Oleandrin	T46.0X1	T46.0X2	T46.0X3	T46.0X4	T46.0X5	T46.0X6
Oleic acid	T46.6X1	T46.6X2	T46.6X3	T46.6X4	T46.6X5	T46.6X6
Oleovitamin A	T45.2X1	T45.2X2	T45.2X3	T45.2X4	T45.2X5	T45.2X6
Oleum ricini	T47.2X1	T47.2X2	T47.2X3	T47.2X4	T47.2X5	T47.2X6
Olive oil (medicinal) NEC	T47.4X1	T47.4X2	T47.4X3	T47.4X4	T47.4X5	T47.4X6
Olivomycin	T45.1X1	T45.1X2	T45.1X3	T45.1X4	T45.1X5	T45.1X6
Olsalazine	T47.8X1	T47.8X2	T47.8X3	T47.8X4	T47.8X5	T47.8X6
Omeprazole	T47.1X1	T47.1X2	T47.1X3	T47.1X4	T47.1X5	T47.1X6
OMPA	T60.0X1	T60.0X2	T60.0X3	T60.0X4	—	—
Oncovin	T45.1X1	T45.1X2	T45.1X3	T45.1X4	T45.1X5	T45.1X6
Ondansetron	T45.0X1	T45.0X2	T45.0X3	T45.0X4	T45.0X5	T45.0X6
Ophthaine	T41.3X1	T41.3X2	T41.3X3	T41.3X4	T41.3X5	T41.3X6
Ophthetic	T41.3X1	T41.3X2	T41.3X3	T41.3X4	T41.3X5	T41.3X6
Opiate NEC	T40.601	T40.602	T40.603	T40.604	T40.605	T40.606
antagonists	T50.7X1	T50.7X2	T50.7X3	T50.7X4	T50.7X5	T50.7X6
Opioid NEC	T40.2X1	T40.2X2	T40.2X3	T40.2X4	T40.2X5	T40.2X6
Opipramol	T43.011	T43.012	T43.013	T43.014	T43.015	T43.016
Opium alkaloids (total)	T40.0X1	T40.0X2	T40.0X3	T40.0X4	T40.0X5	T40.0X6
standardized powdered	T40.0X1	T40.0X2	T40.0X3	T40.0X4	T40.0X5	T40.0X6
tincture (camphorated)	T40.0X1	T40.0X2	T40.0X3	T40.0X4	T40.0X5	T40.0X6
Oracon	T38.4X1	T38.4X2	T38.4X3	T38.4X4	T38.4X5	T38.4X6
Oragrafin	T50.8X1	T50.8X2	T50.8X3	T50.8X4	T50.8X5	T50.8X6
Oral contraceptives	T38.4X1	T38.4X2	T38.4X3	T38.4X4	T38.4X5	T38.4X6
Oral rehydration salts	T50.3X1	T50.3X2	T50.3X3	T50.3X4	T50.3X5	T50.3X6
Orazamide	T50.991	T50.992	T50.993	T50.994	T50.995	T50.996
Orciprenaline	T48.291	T48.292	T48.293	T48.294	T48.295	T48.296
Organidin	T48.4X1	T48.4X2	T48.4X3	T48.4X4	T48.4X5	T48.4X6
Organonitrate NEC	T46.3X1	T46.3X2	T46.3X3	T46.3X4	T46.3X5	T46.3X6
Organophosphates	T60.0X1	T60.0X2	T60.0X3	T60.0X4	—	—
Orimune	T50.B91	T50.B92	T50.B93	T50.B94	T50.B95	T50.B96
Orinase	T38.3X1	T38.3X2	T38.3X3	T38.3X4	T38.3X5	T38.3X6
Ormeloxifene	T38.6X1	T38.6X2	T38.6X3	T38.6X4	T38.6X5	T38.6X6
Ornidazole	T37.3X1	T37.3X2	T37.3X3	T37.3X4	T37.3X5	T37.3X6
Ornithine aspartate	T50.991	T50.992	T50.993	T50.994	T50.995	T50.996
Ornoprostil	T47.1X1	T47.1X2	T47.1X3	T47.1X4	T47.1X5	T47.1X6
Orphenadrine	T42.8X1	T42.8X2	T42.8X3	T42.8X4	T42.8X5	T42.8X6
(hydrochloride)						
Ortal (sodium)	T42.3X1	T42.3X2	T42.3X3	T42.3X4	T42.3X5	T42.3X6
Orthoboric acid	T49.0X1	T49.0X2	T49.0X3	T49.0X4	T49.0X5	T49.0X6
ENT agent	T49.6X1	T49.6X2	T49.6X3	T49.6X4	T49.6X5	T49.6X6
ophthalmic preparation	T49.5X1	T49.5X2	T49.5X3	T49.5X4	T49.5X5	T49.5X6
Orthocaine	T41.3X1	T41.3X2	T41.3X3	T41.3X4	T41.3X5	T41.3X6
Orthodichlorobenzene	T53.7X1	T53.7X2	T53.7X3	T53.7X4	—	—
Ortho-Novum	T38.4X1	T38.4X2	T38.4X3	T38.4X4	T38.4X5	T38.4X6
Orthotolidine (reagent)	T54.2X1	T54.2X2	T54.2X3	T54.2X4	—	—
Osmic acid (liquid)	T54.2X1	T54.2X2	T54.2X3	T54.2X4	—	—
fumes	T54.2X1	T54.2X2	T54.2X3	T54.2X4	—	—
Osmotic diuretics	T50.2X1	T50.2X2	T50.2X3	T50.2X4	T50.2X5	T50.2X6
Otilonium bromide	T44.3X1	T44.3X2	T44.3X3	T44.3X4	T44.3X5	T44.3X6
Otorhinolaryngological drug NEC	T49.6X1	T49.6X2	T49.6X3	T49.6X4	T49.6X5	T49.6X6
Ouabain (e)	T46.0X1	T46.0X2	T46.0X3	T46.0X4	T46.0X5	T46.0X6
Ovarian						
hormone	T38.5X1	T38.5X2	T38.5X3	T38.5X4	T38.5X5	T38.5X6
stimulant	T38.5X1	T38.5X2	T38.5X3	T38.5X4	T38.5X5	T38.5X6
Ovral	T38.4X1	T38.4X2	T38.4X3	T38.4X4	T38.4X5	T38.4X6

Substance	Poisoning, Accidental (unintentional)	Poisoning, Intentional Self-harm	Poisoning, Assault	Poisoning, Undetermined	Adverse Effect	Under-dosing
Ovulen	T38.4X1	T38.4X2	T38.4X3	T38.4X4	T38.4X5	T38.4X6
Oxacillin	T36.0X1	T36.0X2	T36.0X3	T36.0X4	T36.0X5	T36.0X6
Oxalic acid	T54.2X1	T54.2X2	T54.2X3	T54.2X4	—	—
ammonium salt	T50.991	T50.992	T50.993	T50.994	T50.995	T50.996
Oxamniquine	T37.4X1	T37.4X2	T37.4X3	T37.4X4	T37.4X5	T37.4X6
Oxanamide	T43.591	T43.592	T43.593	T43.594	T43.595	T43.596
Oxandrolone	T38.7X1	T38.7X2	T38.7X3	T38.7X4	T38.7X5	T38.7X6
Oxantel	T37.4X1	T37.4X2	T37.4X3	T37.4X4	T37.4X5	T37.4X6
Oxapium iodide	T44.3X1	T44.3X2	T44.3X3	T44.3X4	T44.3X5	T44.3X6
Oxaprotiline	T43.021	T43.022	T43.023	T43.024	T43.025	T43.026
Oxaprozin	T39.311	T39.312	T39.313	T39.314	T39.315	T39.316
Oxatomide	T45.0X1	T45.0X2	T45.0X3	T45.0X4	T45.0X5	T45.0X6
Oxazepam	T42.4X1	T42.4X2	T42.4X3	T42.4X4	T42.4X5	T42.4X6
Oxazimedrine	T50.5X1	T50.5X2	T50.5X3	T50.5X4	T50.5X5	T50.5X6
Oxazolam	T42.4X1	T42.4X2	T42.4X3	T42.4X4	T42.4X5	T42.4X6
Oxazolidine derivatives	T42.2X1	T42.2X2	T42.2X3	T42.2X4	T42.2X5	T42.2X6
Oxazolidinedione (derivative)	T42.2X1	T42.2X2	T42.2X3	T42.2X4	T42.2X5	T42.2X6
Ox bile extract	T47.5X1	T47.5X2	T47.5X3	T47.5X4	T47.5X5	T47.5X6
Oxcarbazepine	T42.1X1	T42.1X2	T42.1X3	T42.1X4	T42.1X5	T42.1X6
Oxedrine	T44.4X1	T44.4X2	T44.4X3	T44.4X4	T44.4X5	T44.4X6
Oxeladin (citrate)	T48.3X1	T48.3X2	T48.3X3	T48.3X4	T48.3X5	T48.3X6
Oxendolone	T38.5X1	T38.5X2	T38.5X3	T38.5X4	T38.5X5	T38.5X6
Oxetacaine	T41.3X1	T41.3X2	T41.3X3	T41.3X4	T41.3X5	T41.3X6
Oxethazine	T41.3X1	T41.3X2	T41.3X3	T41.3X4	T41.3X5	T41.3X6
Oxetorone	T39.8X1	T39.8X2	T39.8X3	T39.8X4	T39.8X5	T39.8X6
Oxiconazole	T49.0X1	T49.0X2	T49.0X3	T49.0X4	T49.0X5	T49.0X6
Oxidizing agent NEC	T54.91	T54.92	T54.93	T54.94	—	—
Oxipurinol	T50.4X1	T50.4X2	T50.4X3	T50.4X4	T50.4X5	T50.4X6
Oxitriptan	T43.291	T43.292	T43.293	T43.294	T43.295	T43.296
Oxitropium bromide	T48.6X1	T48.6X2	T48.6X3	T48.6X4	T48.6X5	T48.6X6
Oxodipine	T46.1X1	T46.1X2	T46.1X3	T46.1X4	T46.1X5	T46.1X6
Oxolamine	T48.3X1	T48.3X2	T48.3X3	T48.3X4	T48.3X5	T48.3X6
Oxolinic acid	T37.8X1	T37.8X2	T37.8X3	T37.8X4	T37.8X5	T37.8X6
Oxomemazine	T43.3X1	T43.3X2	T43.3X3	T43.3X4	T43.3X5	T43.3X6
Oxophenarsine	T37.3X1	T37.3X2	T37.3X3	T37.3X4	T37.3X5	T37.3X6
Oxprenolol	T44.7X1	T44.7X2	T44.7X3	T44.7X4	T44.7X5	T44.7X6
Oxsoralen	T49.3X1	T49.3X2	T49.3X3	T49.3X4	T49.3X5	T49.3X6
Oxtriphylline	T48.6X1	T48.6X2	T48.6X3	T48.6X4	T48.6X5	T48.6X6
Oxybate sodium	T41.291	T41.292	T41.293	T41.294	T41.295	T41.296
Oxybuprocaine	T41.3X1	T41.3X2	T41.3X3	T41.3X4	T41.3X5	T41.3X6
Oxybutynin	T44.3X1	T44.3X2	T44.3X3	T44.3X4	T44.3X5	T44.3X6
Oxychlorosene	T49.0X1	T49.0X2	T49.0X3	T49.0X4	T49.0X5	T49.0X6
Oxycodone	T40.2X1	T40.2X2	T40.2X3	T40.2X4	T40.2X5	T40.2X6
Oxyfedrine	T46.3X1	T46.3X2	T46.3X3	T46.3X4	T46.3X5	T46.3X6
Oxygen	T41.5X1	T41.5X2	T41.5X3	T41.5X4	T41.5X5	T41.5X6
Oxylone	T49.0X1	T49.0X2	T49.0X3	T49.0X4	T49.0X5	T49.0X6
ophthalmic preparation	T49.5X1	T49.5X2	T49.5X3	T49.5X4	T49.5X5	T49.5X6
Oxymesterone	T38.7X1	T38.7X2	T38.7X3	T38.7X4	T38.7X5	T38.7X6
Oxymetazoline	T48.5X1	T48.5X2	T48.5X3	T48.5X4	T48.5X5	T48.5X6
Oxymetholone	T38.7X1	T38.7X2	T38.7X3	T38.7X4	T38.7X5	T38.7X6
Oxymorphone	T40.2X1	T40.2X2	T40.2X3	T40.2X4	T40.2X5	T40.2X6
Oxypertine	T43.591	T43.592	T43.593	T43.594	T43.595	T43.596
Oxyphenbutazone	T39.2X1	T39.2X2	T39.2X3	T39.2X4	T39.2X5	T39.2X6
Oxyphencyclimine	T44.3X1	T44.3X2	T44.3X3	T44.3X4	T44.3X5	T44.3X6
Oxyphenisatine	T47.2X1	T47.2X2	T47.2X3	T47.2X4	T47.2X5	T47.2X6
Oxyphenonium bromide	T44.3X1	T44.3X2	T44.3X3	T44.3X4	T44.3X5	T44.3X6
Oxypolygelatin	T45.8X1	T45.8X2	T45.8X3	T45.8X4	T45.8X5	T45.8X6
Oxyquinoline (derivatives)	T37.8X1	T37.8X2	T37.8X3	T37.8X4	T37.8X5	T37.8X6
Oxytetracycline	T36.4X1	T36.4X2	T36.4X3	T36.4X4	T36.4X5	T36.4X6
Oxytocic drug NEC	T48.0X1	T48.0X2	T48.0X3	T48.0X4	T48.0X5	T48.0X6
Oxytocin (synthetic)	T48.0X1	T48.0X2	T48.0X3	T48.0X4	T48.0X5	T48.0X6
Ozone	T59.891	T59.892	T59.893	T59.894	—	—
PABA	T49.3X1	T49.3X2	T49.3X3	T49.3X4	T49.3X5	T49.3X6
Packed red cells	T45.8X1	T45.8X2	T45.8X3	T45.8X4	T45.8X5	T45.8X6
Padimate	T49.3X1	T49.3X2	T49.3X3	T49.3X4	T49.3X5	T49.3X6
Paint NEC	T65.6X1	T65.6X2	T65.6X3	T65.6X4	—	—
cleaner	T52.91	T52.92	T52.93	T52.94	—	—
fumes NEC	T59.891	T59.892	T59.893	T59.894	—	—
lead (fumes)	T56.0X1	T56.0X2	T56.0X3	T56.0X4	—	—
solvent NEC	T52.8X1	T52.8X2	T52.8X3	T52.8X4	—	—
stripper	T52.8X1	T52.8X2	T52.8X3	T52.8X4	—	—
Palfium	T40.2X1	T40.2X2	T40.2X3	T40.2X4	—	—
Palm kernel oil	T50.991	T50.992	T50.993	T50.994	T50.995	T50.996
Paludrine	T37.2X1	T37.2X2	T37.2X3	T37.2X4	T37.2X5	T37.2X6
PAM (pralidoxime)	T50.6X1	T50.6X2	T50.6X3	T50.6X4	T50.6X5	T50.6X6
Pamaquine (naphthoute)	T37.2X1	T37.2X2	T37.2X3	T37.2X4	T37.2X5	T37.2X6
Panadol	T39.1X1	T39.1X2	T39.1X3	T39.1X4	T39.1X5	T39.1X6
Pancreatic digestive secretion stimulant	T47.8X1	T47.8X2	T47.8X3	T47.8X4	T47.8X5	T47.8X6
dornase	T45.3X1	T45.3X2	T45.3X3	T45.3X4	T45.3X5	T45.3X6
Pancreatin	T47.5X1	T47.5X2	T47.5X3	T47.5X4	T47.5X5	T47.5X6
Pancrelipase	T47.5X1	T47.5X2	T47.5X3	T47.5X4	T47.5X5	T47.5X6
Pancuronium (bromide)	T48.1X1	T48.1X2	T48.1X3	T48.1X4	T48.1X5	T48.1X6
Pangamic acid	T45.2X1	T45.2X2	T45.2X3	T45.2X4	T45.2X5	T45.2X6
Panthenol	T45.2X1	T45.2X2	T45.2X3	T45.2X4	T45.2X5	T45.2X6
topical	T49.8X1	T49.8X2	T49.8X3	T49.8X4	T49.8X5	T49.8X6
Pantopon	T40.0X1	T40.0X2	T40.0X3	T40.0X4	T40.0X5	T40.0X6
Pantothenic acid	T45.2X1	T45.2X2	T45.2X3	T45.2X4	T45.2X5	T45.2X6
Panwarfin	T45.511	T45.512	T45.513	T45.514	T45.515	T45.516
Papain	T47.5X1	T47.5X2	T47.5X3	T47.5X4	T47.5X5	T47.5X6
digestant	T47.5X1	T47.5X2	T47.5X3	T47.5X4	T47.5X5	T47.5X6
Papaveretum	T40.0X1	T40.0X2	T40.0X3	T40.0X4	T40.0X5	T40.0X6
Papaverine	T44.3X1	T44.3X2	T44.3X3	T44.3X4	T44.3X5	T44.3X6
Para-acetamidophenol	T39.1X1	T39.1X2	T39.1X3	T39.1X4	T39.1X5	T39.1X6
Para-aminobenzoic acid	T49.3X1	T49.3X2	T49.3X3	T49.3X4	T49.3X5	T49.3X6
Para-aminophenol derivatives	T39.1X1	T39.1X2	T39.1X3	T39.1X4	T39.1X5	T39.1X6
Para-aminosalicylic acid	T37.1X1	T37.1X2	T37.1X3	T37.1X4	T37.1X5	T37.1X6
Paracetaldehyde	T42.6X1	T42.6X2	T42.6X3	T42.6X4	T42.6X5	T42.6X6
Paracetamol	T39.1X1	T39.1X2	T39.1X3	T39.1X4	T39.1X5	T39.1X6
Parachlorophenol (camphorated)	T49.0X1	T49.0X2	T49.0X3	T49.0X4	T49.0X5	T49.0X6
Paracodin	T40.2X1	T40.2X2	T40.2X3	T40.2X4	T40.2X5	T40.2X6
Paradione	T42.2X1	T42.2X2	T42.2X3	T42.2X4	T42.2X5	T42.2X6
Paraffin(s) (wax)	T52.0X1	T52.0X2	T52.0X3	T52.0X4	—	—
liquid (medicinal)	T47.4X1	T47.4X2	T47.4X3	T47.4X4	T47.4X5	T47.4X6
nonmedicinal	T52.0X1	T52.0X2	T52.0X3	T52.0X4	—	—
Paraformaldehyde	T60.3X1	T60.3X2	T60.3X3	T60.3X4	—	—
Paraldehyde	T42.6X1	T42.6X2	T42.6X3	T42.6X4	T42.6X5	T42.6X6
Paramethadione	T42.2X1	T42.2X2	T42.2X3	T42.2X4	T42.2X5	T42.2X6
Paramethasone	T38.0X1	T38.0X2	T38.0X3	T38.0X4	T38.0X5	T38.0X6
acetate	T49.0X1	T49.0X2	T49.0X3	T49.0X4	T49.0X5	T49.0X6
Paraoxon	T60.0X1	T60.0X2	T60.0X3	T60.0X4	—	—
Paraquat	T60.3X1	T60.3X2	T60.3X3	T60.3X4	—	—
Parasympatholytic NEC	T44.3X1	T44.3X2	T44.3X3	T44.3X4	T44.3X5	T44.3X6
Parasympathomimetic drug NEC	T44.1X1	T44.1X2	T44.1X3	T44.1X4	T44.1X5	T44.1X6
Parathion	T60.0X1	T60.0X2	T60.0X3	T60.0X4	—	—
Parathormone	T50.991	T50.992	T50.993	T50.994	T50.995	T50.996
Parathyroid extract	T50.991	T50.992	T50.993	T50.994	T50.995	T50.996
Paratyphoid vaccine	T50.A91	T50.A92	T50.A93	T50.A94	T50.A95	T50.A96
Paredrine	T44.4X1	T44.4X2	T44.4X3	T44.4X4	T44.4X5	T44.4X6
Paregoric	T40.0X1	T40.0X2	T40.0X3	T40.0X4	T40.0X5	T40.0X6
Pargyline	T46.5X1	T46.5X2	T46.5X3	T46.5X4	T46.5X5	T46.5X6
Paris green	T57.0X1	T57.0X2	T57.0X3	T57.0X4	—	—
insecticide	T57.0X1	T57.0X2	T57.0X3	T57.0X4	—	—
Parnate	T43.1X1	T43.1X2	T43.1X3	T43.1X4	T43.1X5	T43.1X6
Paromomycin	T36.5X1	T36.5X2	T36.5X3	T36.5X4	T36.5X5	T36.5X6
Paroxypropione	T45.1X1	T45.1X2	T45.1X3	T45.1X4	T45.1X5	T45.1X6
Parzone	T40.2X1	T40.2X2	T40.2X3	T40.2X4	T40.2X5	T40.2X6
PAS	T37.1X1	T37.1X2	T37.1X3	T37.1X4	T37.1X5	T37.1X6
Pasiniazid	T37.1X1	T37.1X2	T37.1X3	T37.1X4	T37.1X5	T37.1X6
PBB (polybrominated biphenyls)	T65.891	T65.892	T65.893	T65.894	—	—
PCB	T65.891	T65.892	T65.893	T65.894	—	—
PCP meaning pentachlorophenol	T60.1X1	T60.1X2	T60.1X3	T60.1X4	—	—
fungicide	T60.3X1	T60.3X2	T60.3X3	T60.3X4	—	—
herbicide	T60.3X1	T60.3X2	T60.3X3	T60.3X4	—	—
insecticide	T60.1X1	T60.1X2	T60.1X3	T60.1X4	—	—
meaning phencyclidine	T40.991	T40.992	T40.993	T40.994	—	—
Peach kernel oil (emulsion)	T47.4X1	T47.4X2	T47.4X3	T47.4X4	T47.4X5	T47.4X6
Peanut oil (emulsion) NEC	T47.4X1	T47.4X2	T47.4X3	T47.4X4	T47.4X5	T47.4X6
topical	T49.3X1	T49.3X2	T49.3X3	T49.3X4	T49.3X5	T49.3X6
Pearly Gates (morning glory seeds)	T40.991	T40.992	T40.993	T40.994	—	—
Pecazine	T43.3X1	T43.3X2	T43.3X3	T43.3X4	T43.3X5	T43.3X6
Pectin	T47.6X1	T47.6X2	T47.6X3	T47.6X4	T47.6X5	T47.6X6
Pefloxacin	T37.8X1	T37.8X2	T37.8X3	T37.8X4	T37.8X5	T37.8X6
Pegademase, bovine	T50.Z91	T50.Z92	T50.Z93	T50.Z94	T50.Z95	T50.Z96
Pelletierine tannate	T37.4X1	T37.4X2	T37.4X3	T37.4X4	T37.4X5	T37.4X6
Pemirolast (potassium)	T48.6X1	T48.6X2	T48.6X3	T48.6X4	T48.6X5	T48.6X6
Pemoline	T50.7X1	T50.7X2	T50.7X3	T50.7X4	T50.7X5	T50.7X6
Pempidine	T44.2X1	T44.2X2	T44.2X3	T44.2X4	T44.2X5	T44.2X6
Penamecillin	T36.0X1	T36.0X2	T36.0X3	T36.0X4	T36.0X5	T36.0X6
Penbutolol	T44.7X1	T44.7X2	T44.7X3	T44.7X4	T44.7X5	T44.7X6
Penethamate	T36.0X1	T36.0X2	T36.0X3	T36.0X4	T36.0X5	T36.0X6
Penfluridol	T43.591	T43.592	T43.593	T43.594	T43.595	T43.596
Penflutizide	T50.2X1	T50.2X2	T50.2X3	T50.2X4	T50.2X5	T50.2X6
Pengitoxin	T46.0X1	T46.0X2	T46.0X3	T46.0X4	T46.0X5	T46.0X6
Penicillamine	T50.6X1	T50.6X2	T50.6X3	T50.6X4	T50.6X5	T50.6X6
Penicillin (any)	T36.0X1	T36.0X2	T36.0X3	T36.0X4	T36.0X5	T36.0X6
Penicillinase	T45.3X1	T45.3X2	T45.3X3	T45.3X4	T45.3X5	T45.3X6

Substance	Poisoning, Accidental (unintentional)	Poisoning, Intentional Self-harm	Poisoning, Assault	Poisoning, Undetermined	Adverse Effect	Under-dosing
Penicilloyl polylysine	T50.8X1	T50.8X2	T50.8X3	T50.8X4	T50.8X5	T50.8X6
Penimepicycline	T36.4X1	T36.4X2	T36.4X3	T36.4X4	T36.4X5	T36.4X6
Pentachloroethane	T53.6X1	T53.6X2	T53.6X3	T53.6X4	—	—
Pentachloronaphthalene	T53.7X1	T53.7X2	T53.7X3	T53.7X4	—	—
Pentachlorophenol	T60.1X1	T60.1X2	T60.1X3	T60.1X4	—	—
(pesticide)						
fungicide	T60.3X1	T60.3X2	T60.3X3	T60.3X4	—	—
herbicide	T60.3X1	T60.3X2	T60.3X3	T60.3X4	—	—
insecticide	T60.1X1	T60.1X2	T60.1X3	T60.1X4	—	—
Pentaerythritol	T46.3X1	T46.3X2	T46.3X3	T46.3X4	T46.3X5	T46.3X6
chloral	T42.6X1	T42.6X2	T42.6X3	T42.6X4	T42.6X5	T42.6X6
tetranitrate NEC	T46.3X1	T46.3X2	T46.3X3	T46.3X4	T46.3X5	T46.3X6
Pentaerythrityl tetranitrate	T46.3X1	T46.3X2	T46.3X3	T46.3X4	T46.3X5	T46.3X6
Pentagastrin	T50.8X1	T50.8X2	T50.8X3	T50.8X4	T50.8X5	T50.8X6
Pentalin	T53.6X1	T53.6X2	T53.6X3	T53.6X4	—	—
Pentamethonium bromide	T44.2X1	T44.2X2	T44.2X3	T44.2X4	T44.2X5	T44.2X6
Pentamidine	T37.3X1	T37.3X2	T37.3X3	T37.3X4	T37.3X5	T37.3X6
Pentanol	T51.3X1	T51.3X2	T51.3X3	T51.3X4	—	—
Pentapyrrolinium (bitartrate)	T44.2X1	T44.2X2	T44.2X3	T44.2X4	T44.2X5	T44.2X6
Pentaquine	T37.2X1	T37.2X2	T37.2X3	T37.2X4	T37.2X5	T37.2X6
Pentazocine	T40.4X1	T40.4X2	T40.4X3	T40.4X4	T40.4X5	T40.4X6
Pentetrazole	T50.7X1	T50.7X2	T50.7X3	T50.7X4	T50.7X5	T50.7X6
Penthienate bromide	T44.3X1	T44.3X2	T44.3X3	T44.3X4	T44.3X5	T44.3X6
Pentifylline	T46.7X1	T46.7X2	T46.7X3	T46.7X4	T46.7X5	T46.7X6
Pentobarbital	T42.3X1	T42.3X2	T42.3X3	T42.3X4	T42.3X5	T42.3X6
sodium	T42.3X1	T42.3X2	T42.3X3	T42.3X4	T42.3X5	T42.3X6
Pentobarbitone	T42.3X1	T42.3X2	T42.3X3	T42.3X4	T42.3X5	T42.3X6
Pentolonium tartrate	T44.2X1	T44.2X2	T44.2X3	T44.2X4	T44.2X5	T44.2X6
Pentosan polysulfate (sodium)	T39.8X1	T39.8X2	T39.8X3	T39.8X4	T39.8X5	T39.8X6
Pentostatin	T45.1X1	T45.1X2	T45.1X3	T45.1X4	T45.1X5	T45.1X6
Pentothal	T41.1X1	T41.1X2	T41.1X3	T41.1X4	T41.1X5	T41.1X6
Pentoxifylline	T46.7X1	T46.7X2	T46.7X3	T46.7X4	T46.7X5	T46.7X6
Pentoxyverine	T48.3X1	T48.3X2	T48.3X3	T48.3X4	T48.3X5	T48.3X6
Pentrinat	T46.3X1	T46.3X2	T46.3X3	T46.3X4	T46.3X5	T46.3X6
Pentylenetetrazole	T50.7X1	T50.7X2	T50.7X3	T50.7X4	T50.7X5	T50.7X6
Pentylsalicylamide	T37.1X1	T37.1X2	T37.1X3	T37.1X4	T37.1X5	T37.1X6
Pentymal	T42.3X1	T42.3X2	T42.3X3	T42.3X4	T42.3X5	T42.3X6
Peplomycin	T45.1X1	T45.1X2	T45.1X3	T45.1X4	T45.1X5	T45.1X6
Peppermint (oil)	T47.5X1	T47.5X2	T47.5X3	T47.5X4	T47.5X5	T47.5X6
Pepsin	T47.5X1	T47.5X2	T47.5X3	T47.5X4	T47.5X5	T47.5X6
digestant	T47.5X1	T47.5X2	T47.5X3	T47.5X4	T47.5X5	T47.5X6
Pepstatin	T47.1X1	T47.1X2	T47.1X3	T47.1X4	T47.1X5	T47.1X6
Peptavlon	T50.8X1	T50.8X2	T50.8X3	T50.8X4	T50.8X5	T50.8X6
Perazine	T43.3X1	T43.3X2	T43.3X3	T43.3X4	T43.3X5	T43.3X6
Percaine (spinal)	T41.3X1	T41.3X2	T41.3X3	T41.3X4	T41.3X5	T41.3X6
topical (surface)	T41.3X1	T41.3X2	T41.3X3	T41.3X4	T41.3X5	T41.3X6
Perchloroethylene	T53.3X1	T53.3X2	T53.3X3	T53.3X4	—	—
medicinal	T37.4X1	T37.4X2	T37.4X3	T37.4X4	T37.4X5	T37.4X6
vapor	T53.3X1	T53.3X2	T53.3X3	T53.3X4	—	—
Percodan	T40.2X1	T40.2X2	T40.2X3	T40.2X4	T40.2X5	T40.2X6
Percogesic — see also acetaminophen	T45.0X1	T45.0X2	T45.0X3	T45.0X4	T45.0X5	T45.0X6
Percorten	T38.0X1	T38.0X2	T38.0X3	T38.0X4	T38.0X5	T38.0X6
Pergolide	T42.8X1	T42.8X2	T42.8X3	T42.8X4	T42.8X5	T42.8X6
Pergonal	T38.811	T38.812	T38.813	T38.814	T38.815	T38.816
Perhexilene	T46.3X1	T46.3X2	T46.3X3	T46.3X4	T46.3X5	T46.3X6
Perhexiline (maleate)	T46.3X1	T46.3X2	T46.3X3	T46.3X4	T46.3X5	T46.3X6
Periactin	T45.0X1	T45.0X2	T45.0X3	T45.0X4	T45.0X5	T45.0X6
Periciazine	T43.3X1	T43.3X2	T43.3X3	T43.3X4	T43.3X5	T43.3X6
Periclor	T42.6X1	T42.6X2	T42.6X3	T42.6X4	T42.6X5	T42.6X6
Perindopril	T46.4X1	T46.4X2	T46.4X3	T46.4X4	T46.4X5	T46.4X6
Perisoxal	T39.8X1	T39.8X2	T39.8X3	T39.8X4	T39.8X5	T39.8X6
Peritoneal dialysis solution	T50.3X1	T50.3X2	T50.3X3	T50.3X4	T50.3X5	T50.3X6
Peritrate	T46.3X1	T46.3X2	T46.3X3	T46.3X4	T46.3X5	T46.3X6
Perlapine	T42.4X1	T42.4X2	T42.4X3	T42.4X4	T42.4X5	T42.4X6
Permanganate	T65.891	T65.892	T65.893	T65.894	—	—
Permethrin	T60.1X1	T60.1X2	T60.1X3	T60.1X4	—	—
Pernocton	T42.3X1	T42.3X2	T42.3X3	T42.3X4	T42.3X5	T42.3X6
Pernoston	T42.3X1	T42.3X2	T42.3X3	T42.3X4	T42.3X5	T42.3X6
Peronine	T40.2X1	T40.2X2	T40.2X3	T40.2X4	—	—
Perphenazine	T43.3X1	T43.3X2	T43.3X3	T43.3X4	T43.3X5	T43.3X6
Pertofrane	T43.011	T43.012	T43.013	T43.014	T43.015	T43.016
Pertussis						
immune serum (human)	T50.Z11	T50.Z12	T50.Z13	T50.Z14	T50.Z15	T50.Z16
vaccine (with diphtheria toxoid) (with tetanus toxoid)	T50.A11	T50.A12	T50.A13	T50.A14	T50.A15	T50.A16
Peruvian balsam	T49.0X1	T49.0X2	T49.0X3	T49.0X4	T49.0X5	T49.0X6
Peruvoside	T46.0X1	T46.0X2	T46.0X3	T46.0X4	T46.0X5	T46.0X6
Pesticide (dust) (fumes) (vapor) NEC	T60.91	T60.92	T60.93	T60.94	—	—

Substance	Poisoning, Accidental (unintentional)	Poisoning, Intentional Self-harm	Poisoning, Assault	Poisoning, Undetermined	Adverse Effect	Under-dosing
Pesticide (dust) (fumes) (vapor) NEC — continued						
arsenic	T57.0X1	T57.0X2	T57.0X3	T57.0X4	—	—
chlorinated	T60.1X1	T60.1X2	T60.1X3	T60.1X4	—	—
cyanide	T65.0X1	T65.0X2	T65.0X3	T65.0X4	—	—
kerosene	T52.0X1	T52.0X2	T52.0X3	T52.0X4	—	—
mixture (of compounds)	T60.2X1	T60.2X2	T60.2X3	T60.2X4	—	—
naphthalene	T60.2X1	T60.2X2	T60.2X3	T60.2X4	—	—
organochlorine (compounds)	T60.1X1	T60.1X2	T60.1X3	T60.1X4	—	—
petroleum (distillate) (products) NEC	T60.8X1	T60.8X2	T60.8X3	T60.8X4	—	—
specified ingredient NEC	T60.8X1	T60.8X2	T60.8X3	T60.8X4	—	—
strychnine	T65.1X1	T65.1X2	T65.1X3	T65.1X4	—	—
thallium	T60.4X1	T60.4X2	T60.4X3	T60.4X4	—	—
Pethidine	T40.4X1	T40.4X2	T40.4X3	T40.4X4	T40.4X5	T40.4X6
Petrichloral	T42.6X1	T42.6X2	T42.6X3	T42.6X4	T42.6X5	T42.6X6
Petrol	T52.0X1	T52.0X2	T52.0X3	T52.0X4	—	—
vapor	T52.0X1	T52.0X2	T52.0X3	T52.0X4	—	—
Petrolatum	T49.3X1	T49.3X2	T49.3X3	T49.3X4	T49.3X5	T49.3X6
hydrophilic	T49.3X1	T49.3X2	T49.3X3	T49.3X4	T49.3X5	T49.3X6
liquid	T47.4X1	T47.4X2	T47.4X3	T47.4X4	T47.4X5	T47.4X6
topical	T49.3X1	T49.3X2	T49.3X3	T49.3X4	T49.3X5	T49.3X6
nonmedicinal	T52.0X1	T52.0X2	T52.0X3	T52.0X4	—	—
red veterinary	T49.3X1	T49.3X2	T49.3X3	T49.3X4	T49.3X5	T49.3X6
white	T49.3X1	T49.3X2	T49.3X3	T49.3X4	T49.3X5	T49.3X6
Petroleum (products) NEC	T52.0X1	T52.0X2	T52.0X3	T52.0X4	—	—
benzine(s) — see Ligroin						
ether — see Ligroin						
jelly — see Petrolatum						
naphtha — see Ligroin						
pesticide	T60.8X1	T60.8X2	T60.8X3	T60.8X4	—	—
solids	T52.0X1	T52.0X2	T52.0X3	T52.0X4	—	—
solvents	T52.0X1	T52.0X2	T52.0X3	T52.0X4	—	—
vapor	T52.0X1	T52.0X2	T52.0X3	T52.0X4	—	—
Peyote	T40.991	T40.992	T40.993	T40.994	—	—
Phanodorm, phanodorn	T42.3X1	T42.3X2	T42.3X3	T42.3X4	T42.3X5	T42.3X6
Phanquinone	T37.3X1	T37.3X2	T37.3X3	T37.3X4	T37.3X5	T37.3X6
Phanquone	T37.3X1	T37.3X2	T37.3X3	T37.3X4	T37.3X5	T37.3X6
Pharmaceutical						
adjunct NEC	T50.901	T50.902	T50.903	T50.904	T50.905	T50.906
excipient NEC	T50.901	T50.902	T50.903	T50.904	T50.905	T50.906
sweetener	T50.901	T50.902	T50.903	T50.904	T50.905	T50.906
viscous agent	T50.901	T50.902	T50.903	T50.904	T50.905	T50.906
Phemitone	T42.3X1	T42.3X2	T42.3X3	T42.3X4	T42.3X5	T42.3X6
Phenacaine	T41.3X1	T41.3X2	T41.3X3	T41.3X4	T41.3X5	T41.3X6
Phenacemide	T42.6X1	T42.6X2	T42.6X3	T42.6X4	T42.6X5	T42.6X6
Phenacetin	T39.1X1	T39.1X2	T39.1X3	T39.1X4	T39.1X5	T39.1X6
Phenadoxone	T40.2X1	T40.2X2	T40.2X3	T40.2X4	—	—
Phenaglycodol	T43.591	T43.592	T43.593	T43.594	T43.595	T43.596
Phenantoin	T42.0X1	T42.0X2	T42.0X3	T42.0X4	T42.0X5	T42.0X6
Phenaphthazine reagent	T50.991	T50.992	T50.993	T50.994	T50.995	T50.996
Phenazocine	T40.4X1	T40.4X2	T40.4X3	T40.4X4	T40.4X5	T40.4X6
Phenazone	T39.2X1	T39.2X2	T39.2X3	T39.2X4	T39.2X5	T39.2X6
Phenazopyridine	T39.8X1	T39.8X2	T39.8X3	T39.8X4	T39.8X5	T39.8X6
Phenbenicillin	T36.0X1	T36.0X2	T36.0X3	T36.0X4	T36.0X5	T36.0X6
Phenbutrazate	T50.5X1	T50.5X2	T50.5X3	T50.5X4	T50.5X5	T50.5X6
Phencyclidine	T40.991	T40.992	T40.993	T40.994	T40.995	T40.996
Phendimetrazine	T50.5X1	T50.5X2	T50.5X3	T50.5X4	T50.5X5	T50.5X6
Phenelzine	T43.1X1	T43.1X2	T43.1X3	T43.1X4	T43.1X5	T43.1X6
Phenemal	T42.3X1	T42.3X2	T42.3X3	T42.3X4	T42.3X5	T42.3X6
Phenergan	T42.6X1	T42.6X2	T42.6X3	T42.6X4	T42.6X5	T42.6X6
Pheneticillin	T36.0X1	T36.0X2	T36.0X3	T36.0X4	T36.0X5	T36.0X6
Pheneturide	T42.6X1	T42.6X2	T42.6X3	T42.6X4	T42.6X5	T42.6X6
Phenformin	T38.3X1	T38.3X2	T38.3X3	T38.3X4	T38.3X5	T38.3X6
Phenglutarimide	T44.3X1	T44.3X2	T44.3X3	T44.3X4	T44.3X5	T44.3X6
Phenicarbazide	T39.8X1	T39.8X2	T39.8X3	T39.8X4	T39.8X5	T39.8X6
Phenindamine	T45.0X1	T45.0X2	T45.0X3	T45.0X4	T45.0X5	T45.0X6
Phenindione	T45.511	T45.512	T45.513	T45.514	T45.515	T45.516
Pheniprazine	T43.1X1	T43.1X2	T43.1X3	T43.1X4	T43.1X5	T43.1X6
Pheniramine	T45.0X1	T45.0X2	T45.0X3	T45.0X4	T45.0X5	T45.0X6
Phenisatin	T47.2X1	T47.2X2	T47.2X3	T47.2X4	T47.2X5	T47.2X6
Phenmetrazine	T50.5X1	T50.5X2	T50.5X3	T50.5X4	T50.5X5	T50.5X6
Phenobal	T42.3X1	T42.3X2	T42.3X3	T42.3X4	T42.3X5	T42.3X6
Phenobarbital	T42.3X1	T42.3X2	T42.3X3	T42.3X4	T42.3X5	T42.3X6
with						
mephenytoin	T42.3X1	T42.3X2	T42.3X3	T42.3X4	T42.3X5	T42.3X6
phenytoin	T42.3X1	T42.3X2	T42.3X3	T42.3X4	T42.3X5	T42.3X6
sodium	T42.3X1	T42.3X2	T42.3X3	T42.3X4	T42.3X5	T42.3X6
Phenobarbitone	T42.3X1	T42.3X2	T42.3X3	T42.3X4	T42.3X5	T42.3X6
Phenobutiodil	T50.8X1	T50.8X2	T50.8X3	T50.8X4	T50.8X5	T50.8X6
Phenoctide	T49.0X1	T49.0X2	T49.0X3	T49.0X4	T49.0X5	T49.0X6
Phenol	T49.0X1	T49.0X2	T49.0X3	T49.0X4	T49.0X5	T49.0X6

Table of Drugs and Chemicals

Phenol — Plant

Substance	Poisoning, Accidental (unintentional)	Poisoning, Intentional Self-harm	Poisoning, Assault	Poisoning, Undetermined	Adverse Effect	Under-dosing
Phenol — continued						
disinfectant	T54.0X1	T54.0X2	T54.0X3	T54.0X4	—	—
in oil injection	T46.8X1	T46.8X2	T46.8X3	T46.8X4	T46.8X5	T46.8X6
medicinal	T49.1X1	T49.1X2	T49.1X3	T49.1X4	T49.1X5	T49.1X6
nonmedicinal NEC	T54.0X1	T54.0X2	T54.0X3	T54.0X4	—	—
pesticide	T60.8X1	T60.8X2	T60.8X3	T60.8X4	—	—
red	T50.8X1	T50.8X2	T50.8X3	T50.8X4	T50.8X5	T50.8X6
Phenolic preparation	T49.1X1	T49.1X2	T49.1X3	T49.1X4	T49.1X5	T49.1X6
Phenolphthalein	T47.2X1	T47.2X2	T47.2X3	T47.2X4	T47.2X5	T47.2X6
Phenolsulfonphthalein	T50.8X1	T50.8X2	T50.8X3	T50.8X4	T50.8X5	T50.8X6
Phenomorphan	T40.2X1	T40.2X2	T40.2X3	T40.2X4	—	—
Phenonyl	T42.3X1	T42.3X2	T42.3X3	T42.3X4	T42.3X5	T42.3X6
Phenoperidine	T40.4X1	T40.4X2	T40.4X3	T40.4X4	—	—
Phenopyrazone	T46.991	T46.992	T46.993	T46.994	T46.995	T46.996
Phenoquin	T50.4X1	T50.4X2	T50.4X3	T50.4X4	T50.4X5	T50.4X6
Phenothiazine (psychotropic) NEC	T43.3X1	T43.3X2	T43.3X3	T43.3X4	T43.3X5	T43.3X6
insecticide	T60.2X1	T60.2X2	T60.2X3	T60.2X4	—	—
Phenothrin	T49.0X1	T49.0X2	T49.0X3	T49.0X4	T49.0X5	T49.0X6
Phenoxybenzamine	T46.7X1	T46.7X2	T46.7X3	T46.7X4	T46.7X5	T46.7X6
Phenoxyethanol	T49.0X1	T49.0X2	T49.0X3	T49.0X4	T49.0X5	T49.0X6
Phenoxymethyl penicillin	T36.0X1	T36.0X2	T36.0X3	T36.0X4	T36.0X5	T36.0X6
Phenprobamate	T42.8X1	T42.8X2	T42.8X3	T42.8X4	T42.8X5	T42.8X6
Phenprocoumon	T45.511	T45.512	T45.513	T45.514	T45.515	T45.516
Phensuximide	T42.2X1	T42.2X2	T42.2X3	T42.2X4	T42.2X5	T42.2X6
Phentermine	T50.5X1	T50.5X2	T50.5X3	T50.5X4	T50.5X5	T50.5X6
Phenthicillin	T36.0X1	T36.0X2	T36.0X3	T36.0X4	T36.0X5	T36.0X6
Phentolamine	T46.7X1	T46.7X2	T46.7X3	T46.7X4	T46.7X5	T46.7X6
Phenyl						
butazone	T39.2X1	T39.2X2	T39.2X3	T39.2X4	T39.2X5	T39.2X6
enediamine	T65.3X1	T65.3X2	T65.3X3	T65.3X4	—	—
hydrazine	T65.3X1	T65.3X2	T65.3X3	T65.3X4	—	—
antineoplastic	T45.1X1	T45.1X2	T45.1X3	T45.1X4	T45.1X5	T45.1X6
mercuric compounds — see Mercury						
salicylate	T49.3X1	T49.3X2	T49.3X3	T49.3X4	T49.3X5	T49.3X6
Phenylalanine mustard	T45.1X1	T45.1X2	T45.1X3	T45.1X4	T45.1X5	T45.1X6
Phenylbutazone	T39.2X1	T39.2X2	T39.2X3	T39.2X4	T39.2X5	T39.2X6
Phenylenediamine	T65.3X1	T65.3X2	T65.3X3	T65.3X4	—	—
Phenylephrine	T44.4X1	T44.4X2	T44.4X3	T44.4X4	T44.4X5	T44.4X6
Phenylethylbiguanide	T38.3X1	T38.3X2	T38.3X3	T38.3X4	T38.3X5	T38.3X6
Phenylmercuric						
acetate	T49.0X1	T49.0X2	T49.0X3	T49.0X4	T49.0X5	T49.0X6
borate	T49.0X1	T49.0X2	T49.0X3	T49.0X4	T49.0X5	T49.0X6
nitrate	T49.0X1	T49.0X2	T49.0X3	T49.0X4	T49.0X5	T49.0X6
Phenylmethylbarbitone	T42.3X1	T42.3X2	T42.3X3	T42.3X4	T42.3X5	T42.3X6
Phenylpropanol	T47.5X1	T47.5X2	T47.5X3	T47.5X4	T47.5X5	T47.5X6
Phenylpropanolamine	T44.991	T44.992	T44.993	T44.994	T44.995	T44.996
Phenylsulfthion	T60.0X1	T60.0X2	T60.0X3	T60.0X4	—	—
Phenyltoloxamine	T45.0X1	T45.0X2	T45.0X3	T45.0X4	T45.0X5	T45.0X6
Phenyramidol, phenyramidon	T39.8X1	T39.8X2	T39.8X3	T39.8X4	T39.8X5	T39.8X6
Phenytoin	T42.0X1	T42.0X2	T42.0X3	T42.0X4	T42.0X5	T42.0X6
with Phenobarbital	T42.3X1	T42.3X2	T42.3X3	T42.3X4	T42.3X5	T42.3X6
pHisoHex	T49.2X1	T49.2X2	T49.2X3	T49.2X4	T49.2X5	T49.2X6
Pholcodine	T48.3X1	T48.3X2	T48.3X3	T48.3X4	T48.3X5	T48.3X6
Pholedrine	T46.991	T46.992	T46.993	T46.994	T46.995	T46.996
Phorate	T60.0X1	T60.0X2	T60.0X3	T60.0X4	—	—
Phosdrin	T60.0X1	T60.0X2	T60.0X3	T60.0X4	—	—
Phosfolan	T60.0X1	T60.0X2	T60.0X3	T60.0X4	—	—
Phosgene (gas)	T59.891	T59.892	T59.893	T59.894	—	—
Phosphamidon	T60.0X1	T60.0X2	T60.0X3	T60.0X4	—	—
Phosphate	T65.891	T65.892	T65.893	T65.894	—	—
laxative	T47.4X1	T47.4X2	T47.4X3	T47.4X4	T47.4X5	T47.4X6
organic	T60.0X1	T60.0X2	T60.0X3	T60.0X4	—	—
solvent	T52.91	T52.92	T52.93	T52.94	—	—
tricresyl	T65.891	T65.892	T65.893	T65.894	—	—
Phosphine	T57.1X1	T57.1X2	T57.1X3	T57.1X4	—	—
fumigant	T57.1X1	T57.1X2	T57.1X3	T57.1X4	—	—
Phospholine	T49.5X1	T49.5X2	T49.5X3	T49.5X4	T49.5X5	T49.5X6
Phosphoric acid	T54.2X1	T54.2X2	T54.2X3	T54.2X4	—	—
Phosphorus (compound) NEC	T57.1X1	T57.1X2	T57.1X3	T57.1X4	—	—
pesticide	T60.0X1	T60.0X2	T60.0X3	T60.0X4	—	—
Phthalates	T65.891	T65.892	T65.893	T65.894	—	—
Phthalic anhydride	T65.891	T65.892	T65.893	T65.894	—	—
Phthalimidoglutarimide	T42.6X1	T42.6X2	T42.6X3	T42.6X4	T42.6X5	T42.6X6
Phthalylsulfathiazole	T37.0X1	T37.0X2	T37.0X3	T37.0X4	T37.0X5	T37.0X6
Phylloquinone	T45.7X1	T45.7X2	T45.7X3	T45.7X4	T45.7X5	T45.7X6
Physeptone	T40.3X1	T40.3X2	T40.3X3	T40.3X4	T40.3X5	T40.3X6
Physostigma venenosum	T62.2X1	T62.2X2	T62.2X3	T62.2X4	—	—
Physostigmine	T49.5X1	T49.5X2	T49.5X3	T49.5X4	T49.5X5	T49.5X6
Phytolacca decandra	T62.2X1	T62.2X2	T62.2X3	T62.2X4	—	—

Substance	Poisoning, Accidental (unintentional)	Poisoning, Intentional Self-harm	Poisoning, Assault	Poisoning, Undetermined	Adverse Effect	Under-dosing
Phytolacca decandra — continued						
berries	T62.1X1	T62.1X2	T62.1X3	T62.1X4	—	—
Phytomenadione	T45.7X1	T45.7X2	T45.7X3	T45.7X4	T45.7X5	T45.7X6
Phytonadione	T45.7X1	T45.7X2	T45.7X3	T45.7X4	T45.7X5	T45.7X6
Picoperine	T48.3X1	T48.3X2	T48.3X3	T48.3X4	T48.3X5	T48.3X6
Picosulfate (sodium)	T47.2X1	T47.2X2	T47.2X3	T47.2X4	T47.2X5	T47.2X6
Picric (acid)	T54.2X1	T54.2X2	T54.2X3	T54.2X4	—	—
Picrotoxin	T50.7X1	T50.7X2	T50.7X3	T50.7X4	T50.7X5	T50.7X6
Piketoprofen	T49.0X1	T49.0X2	T49.0X3	T49.0X4	T49.0X5	T49.0X6
Pilocarpine	T44.1X1	T44.1X2	T44.1X3	T44.1X4	T44.1X5	T44.1X6
Pilocarpus (jaborandi) extract	T44.1X1	T44.1X2	T44.1X3	T44.1X4	T44.1X5	T44.1X6
Pilsicainide (hydrochloride)	T46.2X1	T46.2X2	T46.2X3	T46.2X4	T46.2X5	T46.2X6
Pimaricin	T36.7X1	T36.7X2	T36.7X3	T36.7X4	T36.7X5	T36.7X6
Pimeclone	T50.7X1	T50.7X2	T50.7X3	T50.7X4	T50.7X5	T50.7X6
Pimelic ketone	T52.8X1	T52.8X2	T52.8X3	T52.8X4		
Pimethixene	T45.0X1	T45.0X2	T45.0X3	T45.0X4	T45.0X5	T45.0X6
Piminodine	T40.2X1	T40.2X2	T40.2X3	T40.2X4	T40.2X5	T40.2X6
Pimozide	T43.591	T43.592	T43.593	T43.594	T43.595	T43.596
Pinacidil	T46.5X1	T46.5X2	T46.5X3	T46.5X4	T46.5X5	T46.5X6
Pinaverium bromide	T44.3X1	T44.3X2	T44.3X3	T44.3X4	T44.3X5	T44.3X6
Pinazepam	T42.4X1	T42.4X2	T42.4X3	T42.4X4	T42.4X5	T42.4X6
Pindolol	T44.7X1	T44.7X2	T44.7X3	T44.7X4	T44.7X5	T44.7X6
Pindone	T60.4X1	T60.4X2	T60.4X3	T60.4X4	—	—
Pine oil (disinfectant)	T65.891	T65.892	T65.893	T65.894	—	—
Pinkroot	T37.4X1	T37.4X2	T37.4X3	T37.4X4	T37.4X5	T37.4X6
Pipadone	T40.2X1	T40.2X2	T40.2X3	T40.2X4	—	—
Pipamazine	T45.0X1	T45.0X2	T45.0X3	T45.0X4	T45.0X5	T45.0X6
Pipamperone	T43.4X1	T43.4X2	T43.4X3	T43.4X4	T43.4X5	T43.4X6
Pipazetate	T48.3X1	T48.3X2	T48.3X3	T48.3X4	T48.3X5	T48.3X6
Pipemidic acid	T37.8X1	T37.8X2	T37.8X3	T37.8X4	T37.8X5	T37.8X6
Pipenzolate bromide	T44.3X1	T44.3X2	T44.3X3	T44.3X4	T44.3X5	T44.3X6
Piperacetazine	T43.3X1	T43.3X2	T43.3X3	T43.3X4	T43.3X5	T43.3X6
Piperacillin	T36.0X1	T36.0X2	T36.0X3	T36.0X4	T36.0X5	T36.0X6
Piperazine	T37.4X1	T37.4X2	T37.4X3	T37.4X4	T37.4X5	T37.4X6
estrone sulfate	T38.5X1	T38.5X2	T38.5X3	T38.5X4	T38.5X5	T38.5X6
Piper cubeba	T62.2X1	T62.2X2	T62.2X3	T62.2X4	—	—
Piperidione	T48.3X1	T48.3X2	T48.3X3	T48.3X4	T48.3X5	T48.3X6
Piperidolate	T44.3X1	T44.3X2	T44.3X3	T44.3X4	T44.3X5	T44.3X6
Piperocaine	T41.3X1	T41.3X2	T41.3X3	T41.3X4	T41.3X5	T41.3X6
infiltration (subcutaneous)	T41.3X1	T41.3X2	T41.3X3	T41.3X4	T41.3X5	T41.3X6
nerve block (peripheral) (plexus)	T41.3X1	T41.3X2	T41.3X3	T41.3X4	T41.3X5	T41.3X6
topical (surface)	T41.3X1	T41.3X2	T41.3X3	T41.3X4	T41.3X5	T41.3X6
Piperonyl butoxide	T60.8X1	T60.8X2	T60.8X3	T60.8X4	—	—
Pipethanate	T44.3X1	T44.3X2	T44.3X3	T44.3X4	T44.3X5	T44.3X6
Pipobroman	T45.1X1	T45.1X2	T45.1X3	T45.1X4	T45.1X5	T45.1X6
Pipotiazine	T43.3X1	T43.3X2	T43.3X3	T43.3X4	T43.3X5	T43.3X6
Pipoxizine	T45.0X1	T45.0X2	T45.0X3	T45.0X4	T45.0X5	T45.0X6
Pipradrol	T43.691	T43.692	T43.693	T43.694	T43.695	T43.696
Piprinhydrinate	T45.0X1	T45.0X2	T45.0X3	T45.0X4	T45.0X5	T45.0X6
Pirarubicin	T45.1X1	T45.1X2	T45.1X3	T45.1X4	T45.1X5	T45.1X6
Pirazinamide	T37.1X1	T37.1X2	T37.1X3	T37.1X4	T37.1X5	T37.1X6
Pirbuterol	T48.6X1	T48.6X2	T48.6X3	T48.6X4	T48.6X5	T48.6X6
Pirenzepine	T47.1X1	T47.1X2	T47.1X3	T47.1X4	T47.1X5	T47.1X6
Piretanide	T50.1X1	T50.1X2	T50.1X3	T50.1X4	T50.1X5	T50.1X6
Piribedil	T42.8X1	T42.8X2	T42.8X3	T42.8X4	T42.8X5	T42.8X6
Piridoxilate	T46.3X1	T46.3X2	T46.3X3	T46.3X4	T46.3X5	T46.3X6
Piritramide	T40.4X1	T40.4X2	T40.4X3	T40.4X4	—	—
Piromidic acid	T37.8X1	T37.8X2	T37.8X3	T37.8X4	T37.8X5	T37.8X6
Piroxicam	T39.391	T39.392	T39.393	T39.394	T39.395	T39.396
beta-cyclodextrin complex	T39.8X1	T39.8X2	T39.8X3	T39.8X4	T39.8X5	T39.8X6
Pirozadil	T46.6X1	T46.6X2	T46.6X3	T46.6X4	T46.6X5	T46.6X6
Piscidia (bark) (erythrina)	T39.8X1	T39.8X2	T39.8X3	T39.8X4	T39.8X5	T39.8X6
Pitch	T65.891	T65.892	T65.893	T65.894	—	—
Pitkin's solution	T41.3X1	T41.3X2	T41.3X3	T41.3X4	T41.3X5	T41.3X6
Pitocin	T48.0X1	T48.0X2	T48.0X3	T48.0X4	T48.0X5	T48.0X6
Pitressin (tannate)	T38.891	T38.892	T38.893	T38.894	T38.895	T38.896
Pituitary extracts (posterior)	T38.891	T38.892	T38.893	T38.894	T38.895	T38.896
anterior	T38.811	T38.812	T38.813	T38.814	T38.815	T38.816
Pituitrin	T38.891	T38.892	T38.893	T38.894	T38.895	T38.896
Pivampicillin	T36.0X1	T36.0X2	T36.0X3	T36.0X4	T36.0X5	T36.0X6
Pivmecillinam	T36.0X1	T36.0X2	T36.0X3	T36.0X4	T36.0X5	T36.0X6
Placental hormone	T38.891	T38.892	T38.893	T38.894	T38.895	T38.896
Placidyl	T42.6X1	T42.6X2	T42.6X3	T42.6X4	T42.6X5	T42.6X6
Plague vaccine	T50.A91	T50.A92	T50.A93	T50.A94	T50.A95	T50.A96
Plant						
food or fertilizer NEC	T65.891	T65.892	T65.893	T65.894	—	—
containing herbicide	T60.3X1	T60.3X2	T60.3X3	T60.3X4	—	—
noxious, used as food	T62.2X1	T62.2X2	T62.2X3	T62.2X4	—	—
berries	T62.1X1	T62.1X2	T62.1X3	T62.1X4	—	—
seeds	T62.2X1	T62.2X2	T62.2X3	T62.2X4	—	—

Substance	Poisoning, Accidental (unintentional)	Poisoning, Intentional Self-harm	Poisoning, Assault	Poisoning, Undetermined	Adverse Effect	Under-dosing
Plant — *continued*						
noxious, used as food — *continued*						
specified type NEC	T62.2X1	T62.2X2	T62.2X3	T62.2X4	—	—
Plasma	T45.8X1	T45.8X2	T45.8X3	T45.8X4	T45.8X5	T45.8X6
expander NEC	T45.8X1	T45.8X2	T45.8X3	T45.8X4	T45.8X5	T45.8X6
protein fraction (human)	T45.8X1	T45.8X2	T45.8X3	T45.8X4	T45.8X5	T45.8X6
Plasmanate	T45.8X1	T45.8X2	T45.8X3	T45.8X4	T45.8X5	T45.8X6
Plasminogen (tissue)	T45.611	T45.612	T45.613	T45.614	T45.615	T45.616
activator						
Plaster dressing	T49.3X1	T49.3X2	T49.3X3	T49.3X4	T49.3X5	T49.3X6
Plastic dressing	T49.3X1	T49.3X2	T49.3X3	T49.3X4	T49.3X5	T49.3X6
Plegicil	T43.3X1	T43.3X2	T43.3X3	T43.3X4	T43.3X5	T43.3X6
Plicamycin	T45.1X1	T45.1X2	T45.1X3	T45.1X4	T45.1X5	T45.1X6
Podophyllotoxin	T49.8X1	T49.8X2	T49.8X3	T49.8X4	T49.8X5	T49.8X6
Podophyllum (resin)	T49.4X1	T49.4X2	T49.4X3	T49.4X4	T49.4X5	T49.4X6
Poisonous berries	T62.1X1	T62.1X2	T62.1X3	T62.1X4	—	—
Poison NEC	T65.91	T65.92	T65.93	T65.94	—	—
Pokeweed (any part)	T62.2X1	T62.2X2	T62.2X3	T62.2X4	—	—
Poldine metilsulfate	T44.3X1	T44.3X2	T44.3X3	T44.3X4	T44.3X5	T44.3X6
Polidexide (sulfate)	T46.6X1	T46.6X2	T46.6X3	T46.6X4	T46.6X5	T46.6X6
Polidocanol	T46.8X1	T46.8X2	T46.8X3	T46.8X4	T46.8X5	T46.8X6
Poliomyelitis vaccine	T50.B91	T50.B92	T50.B93	T50.B94	T50.B95	T50.B96
Polish (car) (floor) (furni-ture)	T65.891	T65.892	T65.893	T65.894	—	—
(metal) (porcelain) (silver)						
abrasive	T65.891	T65.892	T65.893	T65.894	—	—
porcelain	T65.891	T65.892	T65.893	T65.894	—	—
Poloxalkol	T47.4X1	T47.4X2	T47.4X3	T47.4X4	T47.4X5	T47.4X6
Poloxamer	T47.4X1	T47.4X2	T47.4X3	T47.4X4	T47.4X5	T47.4X6
Polyaminostyrene resins	T50.3X1	T50.3X2	T50.3X3	T50.3X4	T50.3X5	T50.3X6
Polycarbophil	T47.4X1	T47.4X2	T47.4X3	T47.4X4	T47.4X5	T47.4X6
Polychlorinated biphenyl	T65.891	T65.892	T65.893	T65.894	—	—
Polycycline	T36.4X1	T36.4X2	T36.4X3	T36.4X4	T36.4X5	T36.4X6
Polyester fumes	T59.891	T59.892	T59.893	T59.894	—	—
Polyester resin hardener	T52.91	T52.92	T52.93	T52.94	—	—
fumes	T59.891	T59.892	T59.893	T59.894	—	—
Polyestradiol phosphate	T38.5X1	T38.5X2	T38.5X3	T38.5X4	T38.5X5	T38.5X6
Polyethanolamine alkyl sulfate	T49.2X1	T49.2X2	T49.2X3	T49.2X4	T49.2X5	T49.2X6
Polyethylene adhesive	T49.3X1	T49.3X2	T49.3X3	T49.3X4	T49.3X5	T49.3X6
Polyferose	T45.4X1	T45.4X2	T45.4X3	T45.4X4	T45.4X5	T45.4X6
Polygeline	T45.8X1	T45.8X2	T45.8X3	T45.8X4	T45.8X5	T45.8X6
Polymyxin	T36.8X1	T36.8X2	T36.8X3	T36.8X4	T36.8X5	T36.8X6
B	T36.8X1	T36.8X2	T36.8X3	T36.8X4	T36.8X5	T36.8X6
ENT agent	T49.6X1	T49.6X2	T49.6X3	T49.6X4	T49.6X5	T49.6X6
ophthalmic preparation	T49.5X1	T49.5X2	T49.5X3	T49.5X4	T49.5X5	T49.5X6
topical NEC	T49.0X1	T49.0X2	T49.0X3	T49.0X4	T49.0X5	T49.0X6
E sulfate (eye preparation)	T49.5X1	T49.5X2	T49.5X3	T49.5X4	T49.5X5	T49.5X6
Polynoxylin	T49.0X1	T49.0X2	T49.0X3	T49.0X4	T49.0X5	T49.0X6
Polyoestradiol phosphate	T38.5X1	T38.5X2	T38.5X3	T38.5X4	T38.5X5	T38.5X6
Polyoxymethyleneurea	T49.0X1	T49.0X2	T49.0X3	T49.0X4	T49.0X5	T49.0X6
Polysilane	T47.8X1	T47.8X2	T47.8X3	T47.8X4	T47.8X5	T47.8X6
Polytetrafluoroethylene (inhaled)	T59.891	T59.892	T59.893	T59.894	—	—
Polythiazide	T50.2X1	T50.2X2	T50.2X3	T50.2X4	T50.2X5	T50.2X6
Polyvidone	T45.8X1	T45.8X2	T45.8X3	T45.8X4	T45.8X5	T45.8X6
Polyvinylpyrrolidone	T45.8X1	T45.8X2	T45.8X3	T45.8X4	T45.8X5	T45.8X6
Pontocaine (hydrochloride) (infiltration) (topical)	T41.3X1	T41.3X2	T41.3X3	T41.3X4	T41.3X5	T41.3X6
nerve block (peripheral) (plexus)	T41.3X1	T41.3X2	T41.3X3	T41.3X4	T41.3X5	T41.3X6
spinal	T41.3X1	T41.3X2	T41.3X3	T41.3X4	T41.3X5	T41.3X6
Porfiromycin	T45.1X1	T45.1X2	T45.1X3	T45.1X4	T45.1X5	T45.1X6
Posterior pituitary hormone NEC	T38.891	T38.892	T38.893	T38.894	T38.895	T38.896
Pot	T40.7X1	T40.7X2	T40.7X3	T40.7X4	T40.7X5	T40.7X6
Potash (caustic)	T54.3X1	T54.3X2	T54.3X3	T54.3X4	—	—
Potassic saline injection (lactated)	T50.3X1	T50.3X2	T50.3X3	T50.3X4	T50.3X5	T50.3X6
Potassium-removing resin	T50.3X1	T50.3X2	T50.3X3	T50.3X4	T50.3X5	T50.3X6
Potassium-retaining drug	T50.3X1	T50.3X2	T50.3X3	T50.3X4	T50.3X5	T50.3X6
Potassium (salts) NEC	T50.3X1	T50.3X2	T50.3X3	T50.3X4	T50.3X5	T50.3X6
aminobenzoate	T45.8X1	T45.8X2	T45.8X3	T45.8X4	T45.8X5	T45.8X6
aminosalicylate	T37.1X1	T37.1X2	T37.1X3	T37.1X4	T37.1X5	T37.1X6
antimony ' tartrate'	T37.8X1	T37.8X2	T37.8X3	T37.8X4	T37.8X5	T37.8X6
arsenite (solution)	T57.0X1	T57.0X2	T57.0X3	T57.0X4	—	—
bichromate	T56.2X1	T56.2X2	T56.2X3	T56.2X4	—	—
bisulfate	T47.3X1	T47.3X2	T47.3X3	T47.3X4	T47.3X5	T47.3X6
bromide	T42.6X1	T42.6X2	T42.6X4	T42.6X4	T42.6X5	T42.6X6
canrenoate	T50.0X1	T50.0X2	T50.0X3	T50.0X4	T50.0X5	T50.0X6
carbonate	T54.3X1	T54.3X2	T54.3X3	T54.3X4	—	—
chlorate NEC	T65.891	T65.892	T65.893	T65.894	—	—
chloride	T50.3X1	T50.3X2	T50.3X3	T50.3X4	T50.3X5	T50.3X6

Substance	Poisoning, Accidental (unintentional)	Poisoning, Intentional Self-harm	Poisoning, Assault	Poisoning, Undetermined	Adverse Effect	Under-dosing
Potassium (salts) NEC — *continued*						
citrate	T50.991	T50.992	T50.993	T50.994	T50.995	T50.996
cyanide	T65.0X1	T65.0X2	T65.0X3	T65.0X4	—	—
ferric hexacyanoferrate (medicinal)	T50.6X1	T50.6X2	T50.6X3	T50.6X4	T50.6X5	T50.6X6
nonmedicinal	T65.891	T65.892	T65.893	T65.894	—	—
Fluoride	T57.8X1	T57.8X2	T57.8X3	T57.8X4	—	—
glucaldrate	T47.1X1	T47.1X2	T47.1X3	T47.1X4	T47.1X5	T47.1X6
hydroxide	T54.3X1	T54.3X2	T54.3X3	T54.3X4	—	—
iodate	T49.0X1	T49.0X2	T49.0X3	T49.0X4	T49.0X5	T49.0X6
iodide	T48.4X1	T48.4X2	T48.4X3	T48.4X4	T48.4X5	T48.4X6
nitrate	T57.8X1	T57.8X2	T57.8X3	T57.8X4	—	—
oxalate	T65.891	T65.892	T65.893	T65.894	—	—
perchlorate (nonmedicinal) NEC	T65.891	T65.892	T65.893	T65.894	—	—
antithyroid	T38.2X1	T38.2X2	T38.2X3	T38.2X4	T38.2X5	T38.2X6
medicinal	T38.2X1	T38.2X2	T38.2X3	T38.2X4	T38.2X5	T38.2X6
Permanganate (nonmedicinal)	T65.891	T65.892	T65.893	T65.894	—	—
medicinal	T49.0X1	T49.0X2	T49.0X3	T49.0X4	T49.0X5	T49.0X6
sulfate	T47.2X1	T47.2X2	T47.2X3	T47.2X4	T47.2X5	T47.2X6
Povidone	T45.8X1	T45.8X2	T45.8X3	T45.8X4	T45.8X5	T45.8X6
iodine	T49.0X1	T49.0X2	T49.0X3	T49.0X4	T49.0X5	T49.0X6
Practolol	T44.7X1	T44.7X2	T44.7X3	T44.7X4	T44.7X5	T44.7X6
Prajmalium bitartrate	T46.2X1	T46.2X2	T46.2X3	T46.2X4	T46.2X5	T46.2X6
Pralidoxime (iodide)	T50.6X1	T50.6X2	T50.6X3	T50.6X4	T50.6X5	T50.6X6
chloride	T50.6X1	T50.6X2	T50.6X3	T50.6X4	T50.6X5	T50.6X6
Pramiverine	T44.3X1	T44.3X2	T44.3X3	T44.3X4	T44.3X5	T44.3X6
Pramocaine	T49.1X1	T49.1X2	T49.1X3	T49.1X4	T49.1X5	T49.1X6
Pramoxine	T49.1X1	T49.1X2	T49.1X3	T49.1X4	T49.1X5	T49.1X6
Prasterone	T38.7X1	T38.7X2	T38.7X3	T38.7X4	T38.7X5	T38.7X6
Pravastatin	T46.6X1	T46.6X2	T46.6X3	T46.6X4	T46.6X5	T46.6X6
Prazepam	T42.4X1	T42.4X2	T42.4X3	T42.4X4	T42.4X5	T42.4X6
Praziquantel	T37.4X1	T37.4X2	T37.4X3	T37.4X4	T37.4X5	T37.4X6
Prazitone	T43.291	T43.292	T43.293	T43.294	T43.295	T43.296
Prazosin	T44.6X1	T44.6X2	T44.6X3	T44.6X4	T44.6X5	T44.6X6
Prednicarbate	T49.0X1	T49.0X2	T49.0X3	T49.0X4	T49.0X5	T49.0X6
Prednimustine	T45.1X1	T45.1X2	T45.1X3	T45.1X4	T45.1X5	T45.1X6
Prednisolone	T38.0X1	T38.0X2	T38.0X3	T38.0X4	T38.0X5	T38.0X6
ENT agent	T49.6X1	T49.6X2	T49.6X3	T49.6X4	T49.6X5	T49.6X6
ophthalmic preparation	T49.5X1	T49.5X2	T49.5X3	T49.5X4	T49.5X5	T49.5X6
steaglate	T49.0X1	T49.0X2	T49.0X3	T49.0X4	T49.0X5	T49.0X6
topical NEC	T49.0X1	T49.0X2	T49.0X3	T49.0X4	T49.0X5	T49.0X6
Prednisone	T38.0X1	T38.0X2	T38.0X3	T38.0X4	T38.0X5	T38.0X6
Prednylidene	T38.0X1	T38.0X2	T38.0X3	T38.0X4	T38.0X5	T38.0X6
Pregnandiol	T38.5X1	T38.5X2	T38.5X3	T38.5X4	T38.5X5	T38.5X6
Pregneninolone	T38.5X1	T38.5X2	T38.5X3	T38.5X4	T38.5X5	T38.5X6
Preludin	T43.691	T43.692	T43.693	T43.694	T43.695	T43.696
Premarin	T38.5X1	T38.5X2	T38.5X3	T38.5X4	T38.5X5	T38.5X6
Premedication anesthetic	T41.201	T41.202	T41.203	T41.204	T41.205	T41.206
Prenalterol	T44.5X1	T44.5X2	T44.5X3	T44.5X4	T44.5X5	T44.5X6
Prenoxdiazine	T48.3X1	T48.3X2	T48.3X3	T48.3X4	T48.3X5	T48.3X6
Prenylamine	T46.3X1	T46.3X2	T46.3X3	T46.3X4	T46.3X5	T46.3X6
Preparation H	T49.8X1	T49.8X2	T49.8X3	T49.8X4	T49.8X5	T49.8X6
Preparation, local	T49.4X1	T49.4X2	T49.4X3	T49.4X4	T49.4X5	T49.4X6
Preservative (nonmedicinal)	T65.891	T65.892	T65.893	T65.894	—	—
medicinal	T50.901	T50.902	T50.903	T50.904	T50.905	T50.906
wood	T60.91	T60.92	T60.93	T60.94	—	—
Prethcamide	T50.7X1	T50.7X2	T50.7X3	T50.7X4	T50.7X5	T50.7X6
Pride of China	T62.2X1	T62.2X2	T62.2X3	T62.2X4	—	—
Pridinol	T44.3X1	T44.3X2	T44.3X3	T44.3X4	T44.3X5	T44.3X6
Prifinium bromide	T44.3X1	T44.3X2	T44.3X3	T44.3X4	T44.3X5	T44.3X6
Prilocaine	T41.3X1	T41.3X2	T41.3X3	T41.3X4	T41.3X5	T41.3X6
infiltration (subcutaneous)	T41.3X1	T41.3X2	T41.3X3	T41.3X4	T41.3X5	T41.3X6
nerve block (peripheral) (plexus)	T41.3X1	T41.3X2	T41.3X3	T41.3X4	T41.3X5	T41.3X6
regional	T41.3X1	T41.3X2	T41.3X3	T41.3X4	T41.3X5	T41.3X6
Primaquine	T37.2X1	T37.2X2	T37.2X3	T37.2X4	T37.2X5	T37.2X6
Primidone	T42.6X1	T42.6X2	T42.6X3	T42.6X4	T42.6X5	T42.6X6
Primula (veris)	T62.2X1	T62.2X2	T62.2X3	T62.2X4	—	—
Prinadol	T40.2X1	T40.2X2	T40.2X3	T40.2X4	T40.2X5	T40.2X6
Priscol, Priscoline	T44.6X1	T44.6X2	T44.6X3	T44.6X4	T44.6X5	T44.6X6
Pristinamycin	T36.3X1	T36.3X2	T36.3X3	T36.3X4	T36.3X5	T36.3X6
Privet	T62.2X1	T62.2X2	T62.2X3	T62.2X4	—	—
berries	T62.1X1	T62.1X2	T62.1X3	T62.1X4	—	—
Privine	T44.4X1	T44.4X2	T44.4X3	T44.4X4	T44.4X5	T44.4X6
Pro-Banthine	T44.3X1	T44.3X2	T44.3X3	T44.3X4	T44.3X5	T44.3X6
Probarbital	T42.3X1	T42.3X2	T42.3X3	T42.3X4	T42.3X5	T42.3X6
Probenecid	T50.4X1	T50.4X2	T50.4X3	T50.4X4	T50.4X5	T50.4X6
Probucol	T46.6X1	T46.6X2	T46.6X3	T46.6X4	T46.6X5	T46.6X6
Procainamide	T46.2X1	T46.2X2	T46.2X3	T46.2X4	T46.2X5	T46.2X6
Procaine	T41.3X1	T41.3X2	T41.3X3	T41.3X4	T41.3X5	T41.3X6

Table of Drugs and Chemicals

Procaine — Purgative NEC

Substance	Poisoning, Accidental (unintentional)	Poisoning, Intentional Self-harm	Poisoning, Assault	Poisoning, Undetermined	Adverse Effect	Under-dosing
Procaine — continued						
benzylpenicillin	T36.0X1	T36.0X2	T36.0X3	T36.0X4	T36.0X5	T36.0X6
nerve block (periphreal) (plexus)	T41.3X1	T41.3X2	T41.3X3	T41.3X4	T41.3X5	T41.3X6
penicillin G	T36.0X1	T36.0X2	T36.0X3	T36.0X4	T36.0X5	T36.0X6
regional	T41.3X1	T41.3X2	T41.3X3	T41.3X4	T41.3X5	T41.3X6
spinal	T41.3X1	T41.3X2	T41.3X3	T41.3X4	T41.3X5	T41.3X6
Procalmidol	T43.591	T43.592	T43.593	T43.594	T43.595	T43.596
Procarbazine	T45.1X1	T45.1X2	T45.1X3	T45.1X4	T45.1X5	T45.1X6
Procaterol	T44.5X1	T44.5X2	T44.5X3	T44.5X4	T44.5X5	T44.5X6
Prochlorperazine	T43.3X1	T43.3X2	T43.3X3	T43.3X4	T43.3X5	T43.3X6
Procyclidine	T44.3X1	T44.3X2	T44.3X3	T44.3X4	T44.3X5	T44.3X6
Producer gas	T58.8X1	T58.8X2	T58.8X3	T58.8X4	—	—
Profadol	T40.4X1	T40.4X2	T40.4X3	T40.4X4	T40.4X5	T40.4X6
Profenamine	T44.3X1	T44.3X2	T44.3X3	T44.3X4	T44.3X5	T44.3X6
Profenil	T44.3X1	T44.3X2	T44.3X3	T44.3X4	T44.3X5	T44.3X6
Proflavine	T49.0X1	T49.0X2	T49.0X3	T49.0X4	T49.0X5	T49.0X6
Progabide	T42.6X1	T42.6X2	T42.6X3	T42.6X4	T42.6X5	T42.6X6
Progesterone	T38.5X1	T38.5X2	T38.5X3	T38.5X4	T38.5X5	T38.5X6
Progestin	T38.5X1	T38.5X2	T38.5X3	T38.5X4	T38.5X5	T38.5X6
oral contraceptive	T38.4X1	T38.4X2	T38.4X3	T38.4X4	T38.4X5	T38.4X6
Progestogen NEC	T38.5X1	T38.5X2	T38.5X3	T38.5X4	T38.5X5	T38.5X6
Progestone	T38.5X1	T38.5X2	T38.5X3	T38.5X4	T38.5X5	T38.5X6
Proglumide	T47.1X1	T47.1X2	T47.1X3	T47.1X4	T47.1X5	T47.1X6
Proguanil	T37.2X1	T37.2X2	T37.2X3	T37.2X4	T37.2X5	T37.2X6
Prolactin	T38.811	T38.812	T38.813	T38.814	T38.815	T38.816
Prolintane	T43.691	T43.692	T43.693	T43.694	T43.695	T43.696
Proloid	T38.1X1	T38.1X2	T38.1X3	T38.1X4	T38.1X5	T38.1X6
Proluton	T38.5X1	T38.5X2	T38.5X3	T38.5X4	T38.5X5	T38.5X6
Promacetin	T37.1X1	T37.1X2	T37.1X3	T37.1X4	T37.1X5	T37.1X6
Promazine	T43.3X1	T43.3X2	T43.3X3	T43.3X4	T43.3X5	T43.3X6
Promedol	T40.2X1	T40.2X2	T40.2X3	T40.2X4	—	—
Promegestone	T38.5X1	T38.5X2	T38.5X3	T38.5X4	T38.5X5	T38.5X6
Promethazine (teoclate)	T43.3X1	T43.3X2	T43.3X3	T43.3X4	T43.3X5	T43.3X6
Promin	T37.1X1	T37.1X2	T37.1X3	T37.1X4	T37.1X5	T37.1X6
Pronase	T45.3X1	T45.3X2	T45.3X3	T45.3X4	T45.3X5	T45.3X6
Pronestyl (hydrochloride)	T46.2X1	T46.2X2	T46.2X3	T46.2X4	T46.2X5	T46.2X6
Pronetalol	T44.7X1	T44.7X2	T44.7X3	T44.7X4	T44.7X5	T44.7X6
Prontosil	T37.0X1	T37.0X2	T37.0X3	T37.0X4	T37.0X5	T37.0X6
Propachlor	T60.3X1	T60.3X2	T60.3X3	T60.3X4	—	—
Propafenone	T46.2X1	T46.2X2	T46.2X3	T46.2X4	T46.2X5	T46.2X6
Propallylonal	T42.3X1	T42.3X2	T42.3X3	T42.3X4	T42.3X5	T42.3X6
Propamidine	T49.0X1	T49.0X2	T49.0X3	T49.0X4	T49.0X5	T49.0X6
Propane (distributed in mobile container)	T59.891	T59.892	T59.893	T59.894	—	—
distributed through pipes	T59.891	T59.892	T59.893	T59.894	—	—
incomplete combustion	T58.11	T58.12	T58.13	T58.14	—	—
Propanidid	T41.291	T41.292	T41.293	T41.294	T41.295	T41.296
Propanil	T60.3X1	T60.3X2	T60.3X3	T60.3X4	—	—
Propantheline	T44.3X1	T44.3X2	T44.3X3	T44.3X4	T44.3X5	T44.3X6
bromide	T44.3X1	T44.3X2	T44.3X3	T44.3X4	T44.3X5	T44.3X6
Proparacaine	T41.3X1	T41.3X2	T41.3X3	T41.3X4	T41.3X5	T41.3X6
Propatylnitrate	T46.3X1	T46.3X2	T46.3X3	T46.3X4	T46.3X5	T46.3X6
Propicillin	T36.0X1	T36.0X2	T36.0X3	T36.0X4	T36.0X5	T36.0X6
Propiolactone	T49.0X1	T49.0X2	T49.0X3	T49.0X4	T49.0X5	T49.0X6
Propiomazine	T45.0X1	T45.0X2	T45.0X3	T45.0X4	T45.0X5	T45.0X6
Propionaldehyde (medicinal)	T42.6X1	T42.6X2	T42.6X3	T42.6X4	T42.6X5	T42.6X6
Propionate (calcium) (sodium)	T49.0X1	T49.0X2	T49.0X3	T49.0X4	T49.0X5	T49.0X6
Propion gel	T49.0X1	T49.0X2	T49.0X3	T49.0X4	T49.0X5	T49.0X6
Propitocaine	T41.3X1	T41.3X2	T41.3X3	T41.3X4	T41.3X5	T41.3X6
infiltration (subcutaneous)	T41.3X1	T41.3X2	T41.3X3	T41.3X4	T41.3X5	T41.3X6
nerve block (peripheral) (plexus)	T41.3X1	T41.3X2	T41.3X3	T41.3X4	T41.3X5	T41.3X6
Propofol	T41.291	T41.292	T41.293	T41.294	T41.295	T41.296
Propoxur	T60.0X1	T60.0X2	T60.0X3	T60.0X4	—	—
Propoxycaine	T41.3X1	T41.3X2	T41.3X3	T41.3X4	T41.3X5	T41.3X6
infiltration (subcutaneous)	T41.3X1	T41.3X2	T41.3X3	T41.3X4	T41.3X5	T41.3X6
nerve block (peripheral) (plexus)	T41.3X1	T41.3X2	T41.3X3	T41.3X4	T41.3X5	T41.3X6
topical (surface)	T41.3X1	T41.3X2	T41.3X3	T41.3X4	T41.3X5	T41.3X6
Propoxyphene	T40.4X1	T40.4X2	T40.4X3	T40.4X4	T40.4X5	T40.4X6
Propranolol	T44.7X1	T44.7X2	T44.7X3	T44.7X4	T44.7X5	T44.7X6
Propyl						
alcohol	T51.3X1	T51.3X2	T51.3X3	T51.3X4	—	—
carbinol	T51.3X1	T51.3X2	T51.3X3	T51.3X4	—	—
hexadrine	T44.4X1	T44.4X2	T44.4X3	T44.4X4	T44.4X5	T44.4X6
iodone	T50.8X1	T50.8X2	T50.8X3	T50.8X4	T50.8X5	T50.8X6
thiouracil	T38.2X1	T38.2X2	T38.2X3	T38.2X4	T38.2X5	T38.2X6
Propylaminophenothiazine	T43.3X1	T43.3X2	T43.3X3	T43.3X4	T43.3X5	T43.3X6
Propylene	T59.891	T59.892	T59.893	T59.894	—	—
Propylhexedrine	T48.5X1	T48.5X2	T48.5X3	T48.5X4	T48.5X5	T48.5X6

Substance	Poisoning, Accidental (unintentional)	Poisoning, Intentional Self-harm	Poisoning, Assault	Poisoning, Undetermined	Adverse Effect	Under-dosing
Propyliodone	T50.8X1	T50.8X2	T50.8X3	T50.8X4	T50.8X5	T50.8X6
Propylparaben (ophthalmic)	T49.5X1	T49.5X2	T49.5X3	T49.5X4	T49.5X5	T49.5X6
Propylthiouracil	T38.2X1	T38.2X2	T38.2X3	T38.2X4	T38.2X5	T38.2X6
Propyphenazone	T39.2X1	T39.2X2	T39.2X3	T39.2X4	T39.2X5	T39.2X6
Proquazone	T39.391	T39.392	T39.393	T39.394	T39.395	T39.396
Proscillaridin	T46.0X1	T46.0X2	T46.0X3	T46.0X4	T46.0X5	T46.0X6
Prostacyclin	T45.521	T45.522	T45.523	T45.524	T45.525	T45.526
Prostaglandin (I2)	T45.521	T45.522	T45.523	T45.524	T45.525	T45.526
E1	T46.7X1	T46.7X2	T46.7X3	T46.7X4	T46.7X5	T46.7X6
E2	T48.0X1	T48.0X2	T48.0X3	T48.0X4	T48.0X5	T48.0X6
F2 alpha	T48.0X1	T48.0X2	T48.0X3	T48.0X4	T48.0X5	T48.0X6
Prostigmin	T44.0X1	T44.0X2	T44.0X3	T44.0X4	T44.0X5	T44.0X6
Prosultiamine	T45.2X1	T45.2X2	T45.2X3	T45.2X4	T45.2X5	T45.2X6
Protamine sulfate	T45.7X1	T45.7X2	T45.7X3	T45.7X4	T45.7X5	T45.7X6
zinc insulin	T38.3X1	T38.3X2	T38.3X3	T38.3X4	T38.3X5	T38.3X6
Protease	T45.5X1	T45.5X2	T45.5X3	T45.5X4	T45.5X5	T45.5X6
Protectant, skin NEC	T49.3X1	T49.3X2	T49.3X3	T49.3X4	T49.3X5	T49.3X6
Protein hydrolysate	T50.991	T50.992	T50.993	T50.994	T50.995	T50.996
Prothiaden — see Dothiepin hydrochloride						
Prothionamide	T37.1X1	T37.1X2	T37.1X3	T37.1X4	T37.1X5	T37.1X6
Prothipendyl	T43.591	T43.592	T43.593	T43.594	T43.595	T43.596
Prothoate	T60.0X1	T60.0X2	T60.0X3	T60.0X4	—	—
Prothrombin						
activator	T45.7X1	T45.7X2	T45.7X3	T45.7X4	T45.7X5	T45.7X6
synthesis inhibitor	T45.511	T45.512	T45.513	T45.514	T45.515	T45.516
Protionamide	T37.1X1	T37.1X2	T37.1X3	T37.1X4	T37.1X5	T37.1X6
Protirelin	T38.891	T38.892	T38.893	T38.894	T38.895	T38.896
Protokylol	T48.6X1	T48.6X2	T48.6X3	T48.6X4	T48.6X5	T48.6X6
Protopam	T50.6X1	T50.6X2	T50.6X3	T50.6X4	T50.6X5	T50.6X6
Protoveratrine(s) (A) (B)	T46.5X1	T46.5X2	T46.5X3	T46.5X4	T46.5X5	T46.5X6
Protriptyline	T43.011	T43.012	T43.013	T43.014	T43.015	T43.016
Provera	T38.5X1	T38.5X2	T38.5X3	T38.5X4	T38.5X5	T38.5X6
Provitamin A	T45.2X1	T45.2X2	T45.2X3	T45.2X4	T45.2X5	T45.2X6
Proxibarbal	T42.3X1	T42.3X2	T42.3X3	T42.3X4	T42.3X5	T42.3X6
Proxymetacaine	T41.3X1	T41.3X2	T41.3X3	T41.3X4	T41.3X5	T41.3X6
Proxyphylline	T48.6X1	T48.6X2	T48.6X3	T48.6X4	T48.6X5	T48.6X6
Prozac — see Fluoxetine hydrochloride						
Prunus						
laurocerasus	T62.2X1	T62.2X2	T62.2X3	T62.2X4	—	—
virginiana	T62.2X1	T62.2X2	T62.2X3	T62.2X4	—	—
Prussian blue						
commercial	T65.891	T65.892	T65.893	T65.894	—	—
therapeutic	T50.6X1	T50.6X2	T50.6X3	T50.6X4	T50.6X5	T50.6X6
Prussic acid	T65.0X1	T65.0X2	T65.0X3	T65.0X4	—	—
vapor	T57.3X1	T57.3X2	T57.3X3	T57.3X4	—	—
Pseudoephedrine	T44.991	T44.992	T44.993	T44.994	T44.995	T44.996
Psilocin	T40.991	T40.992	T40.993	T40.994		
Psilocybin	T40.991	T40.992	T40.993	T40.994		
Psilocybine	T40.991	T40.992	T40.993	T40.994		
Psoralene (nonmedicinal)	T65.891	T65.892	T65.893	T65.894		
Psoralens (medicinal)	T50.991	T50.992	T50.993	T50.994	T50.995	T50.996
PSP (phenolsulfonphthalein)	T50.8X1	T50.8X2	T50.8X3	T50.8X4	T50.8X5	T50.8X6
Psychodysleptic drug NEC	T40.901	T40.902	T40.903	T40.904	T40.905	T40.906
Psychostimulant	T43.601	T43.602	T43.603	T43.604	T43.605	T43.606
amphetamine	T43.621	T43.622	T43.623	T43.624	T43.625	T43.626
caffeine	T43.611	T43.612	T43.613	T43.614	T43.615	T43.616
methylphenidate	T43.631	T43.632	T43.633	T43.634	T43.635	T43.636
specified NEC	T43.691	T43.692	T43.693	T43.694	T43.695	T43.696
Psychotherapeutic drug NEC	T43.91	T43.92	T43.93	T43.94	T43.95	T43.96
antidepressants — see also Antidepressant	T43.201	T43.202	T43.203	T43.204	T43.205	T43.206
specified NEC	T43.8X1	T43.8X2	T43.8X3	T43.8X4	T43.8X5	T43.8X6
tranquilizers NEC	T43.501	T43.502	T43.503	T43.504	T43.505	T43.506
Psychotomimetic agents	T40.901	T40.902	T40.903	T40.904	T40.905	T40.906
Psychotropic drug NEC	T43.91	T43.92	T43.93	T43.94	T43.95	T43.96
specified NEC	T43.8X1	T43.8X2	T43.8X3	T43.8X4	T43.8X5	T43.8X6
Psyllium hydrophilic mucilloid	T47.4X1	T47.4X2	T47.4X3	T47.4X4	T47.4X5	T47.4X6
Pteroylglutamic acid	T45.8X1	T45.8X2	T45.8X3	T45.8X4	T45.8X5	T45.8X6
Pteroyltriglutamate	T45.1X1	T45.1X2	T45.1X3	T45.1X4	T45.1X5	T45.1X6
PTFE — see Polytetrafluoroethylene						
Pulp						
devitalizing paste	T49.7X1	T49.7X2	T49.7X3	T49.7X4	T49.7X5	T49.7X6
dressing	T49.7X1	T49.7X2	T49.7X3	T49.7X4	T49.7X5	T49.7X6
Pulsatilla	T62.2X1	T62.2X2	T62.2X3	T62.2X4	—	—
Pumpkin seed extract	T37.4X1	T37.4X2	T37.4X3	T37.4X4	T37.4X5	T37.4X6
Purex (bleach)	T54.91	T54.92	T54.93	T54.94	—	—
Purgative NEC — see also Cathartic	T47.4X1	T47.4X2	T47.4X3	T47.4X4	T47.4X5	T47.4X6

Table of Drugs and Chemicals — Purine analogue — Romilar

Substance	Poisoning, Accidental (unintentional)	Poisoning, Intentional Self-harm	Poisoning, Assault	Poisoning, Undetermined	Adverse Effect	Under-dosing
Purine analogue (antineoplastic)	T45.1X1	T45.1X2	T45.1X3	T45.1X4	T45.1X5	T45.1X6
Purine diuretics	T50.2X1	T50.2X2	T50.2X3	T50.2X4	T50.2X5	T50.2X6
Purinethol	T45.1X1	T45.1X2	T45.1X3	T45.1X4	T45.1X5	T45.1X6
PVP	T45.8X1	T45.8X2	T45.8X3	T45.8X4	T45.8X5	T45.8X6
Pyrabital	T39.8X1	T39.8X2	T39.8X3	T39.8X4	T39.8X5	T39.8X6
Pyramidon	T39.2X1	T39.2X2	T39.2X3	T39.2X4	T39.2X5	T39.2X6
Pyrantel	T37.4X1	T37.4X2	T37.4X3	T37.4X4	T37.4X5	T37.4X6
Pyrathiazine	T45.0X1	T45.0X2	T45.0X3	T45.0X4	T45.0X5	T45.0X6
Pyrazinamide	T37.1X1	T37.1X2	T37.1X3	T37.1X4	T37.1X5	T37.1X6
Pyrazinoic acid (amide)	T37.1X1	T37.1X2	T37.1X3	T37.1X4	T37.1X5	T37.1X6
Pyrazole (derivatives)	T39.2X1	T39.2X2	T39.2X3	T39.2X4	T39.2X5	T39.2X6
Pyrazolone analgesic NEC	T39.2X1	T39.2X2	T39.2X3	T39.2X4	T39.2X5	T39.2X6
Pyrethrin, pyrethrum (nonmedicinal)	T60.2X1	T60.2X2	T60.2X3	T60.2X4	—	—
Pyrethrum extract	T49.0X1	T49.0X2	T49.0X3	T49.0X4	T49.0X5	T49.0X6
Pyribenzamine	T45.0X1	T45.0X2	T45.0X3	T45.0X4	T45.0X5	T45.0X6
Pyridine	T52.8X1	T52.8X2	T52.8X3	T52.8X4	—	—
aldoxime methiodide	T50.6X1	T50.6X2	T50.6X3	T50.6X4	T50.6X5	T50.6X6
aldoxime methyl chloride	T50.6X1	T50.6X2	T50.6X3	T50.6X4	T50.6X5	T50.6X6
vapor	T59.891	T59.892	T59.893	T59.894		
Pyridium	T39.8X1	T39.8X2	T39.8X3	T39.8X4	T39.8X5	T39.8X6
Pyridostigmine bromide	T44.0X1	T44.0X2	T44.0X3	T44.0X4	T44.0X5	T44.0X6
Pyridoxal phosphate	T45.2X1	T45.2X2	T45.2X3	T45.2X4	T45.2X5	T45.2X6
Pyridoxine	T45.2X1	T45.2X2	T45.2X3	T45.2X4	T45.2X5	T45.2X6
Pyrilamine	T45.0X1	T45.0X2	T45.0X3	T45.0X4	T45.0X5	T45.0X6
Pyrimethamine	T37.2X1	T37.2X2	T37.2X3	T37.2X4	T37.2X5	T37.2X6
with sulfadoxine	T37.2X1	T37.2X2	T37.2X3	T37.2X4	T37.2X5	T37.2X6
Pyrimidine antagonist	T45.1X1	T45.1X2	T45.1X3	T45.1X4	T45.1X5	T45.1X6
Pyriminil	T60.4X1	T60.4X2	T60.4X3	T60.4X4	—	—
Pyrithione zinc	T49.4X1	T49.4X2	T49.4X3	T49.4X4	T49.4X5	T49.4X6
Pyrithyldione	T42.6X1	T42.6X2	T42.6X3	T42.6X4	T42.6X5	T42.6X6
Pyrogallic acid	T49.0X1	T49.0X2	T49.0X3	T49.0X4	T49.0X5	T49.0X6
Pyrogallol	T49.0X1	T49.0X2	T49.0X3	T49.0X4	T49.0X5	T49.0X6
Pyroxylin	T49.3X1	T49.3X2	T49.3X3	T49.3X4	T49.3X5	T49.3X6
Pyrrobutamine	T45.0X1	T45.0X2	T45.0X3	T45.0X4	T45.0X5	T45.0X6
Pyrrolizidine alkaloids	T62.8X1	T62.8X2	T62.8X3	T62.8X4	—	—
Pyrvinium chloride	T37.4X1	T37.4X2	T37.4X3	T37.4X4	T37.4X5	T37.4X6
PZI	T38.3X1	T38.3X2	T38.3X3	T38.3X4	T38.3X5	T38.3X6
Quaalude	T42.6X1	T42.6X2	T42.6X3	T42.6X4	T42.6X5	T42.6X6
Quarternary ammonium						
anti-infective	T49.0X1	T49.0X2	T49.0X3	T49.0X4	T49.0X5	T49.0X6
ganglion blocking	T44.2X1	T44.2X2	T44.2X3	T44.2X4	T44.2X5	T44.2X6
parasympatholytic	T44.3X1	T44.3X2	T44.3X3	T44.3X4	T44.3X5	T44.3X6
Quazepam	T42.4X1	T42.4X2	T42.4X3	T42.4X4	T42.4X5	T42.4X6
Quicklime	T54.3X1	T54.3X2	T54.3X3	T54.3X4		
Quillaja extract	T48.4X1	T48.4X2	T48.4X3	T48.4X4	T48.4X5	T48.4X6
Quinacrine	T37.2X1	T37.2X2	T37.2X3	T37.2X4	T37.2X5	T37.2X6
Quinaglute	T46.2X1	T46.2X2	T46.2X3	T46.2X4	T46.2X5	T46.2X6
Quinalbarbital	T42.3X1	T42.3X2	T42.3X3	T42.3X4	T42.3X5	T42.3X6
Quinalbarbitone sodium	T42.3X1	T42.3X2	T42.3X3	T42.3X4	T42.3X5	T42.3X6
Quinalphos	T60.0X1	T60.0X2	T60.0X3	T60.0X4		
Quinapril	T46.4X1	T46.4X2	T46.4X3	T46.4X4	T46.4X5	T46.4X6
Quinestradiol	T38.5X1	T38.5X2	T38.5X3	T38.5X4	T38.5X5	T38.5X6
Quinestradol	T38.5X1	T38.5X2	T38.5X3	T38.5X4	T38.5X5	T38.5X6
Quinestrol	T38.5X1	T38.5X2	T38.5X3	T38.5X4	T38.5X5	T38.5X6
Quinethazone	T50.2X1	T50.2X2	T50.2X3	T50.2X4	T50.2X5	T50.2X6
Quingestanol	T38.4X1	T38.4X2	T38.4X3	T38.4X4	T38.4X5	T38.4X6
Quinidine	T46.2X1	T46.2X2	T46.2X3	T46.2X4	T46.2X5	T46.2X6
Quinine	T37.2X1	T37.2X2	T37.2X3	T37.2X4	T37.2X5	T37.2X6
Quiniobine	T37.8X1	T37.8X2	T37.8X3	T37.8X4	T37.8X5	T37.8X6
Quinisocaine	T49.1X1	T49.1X2	T49.1X3	T49.1X4	T49.1X5	T49.1X6
Quinocide	T37.2X1	T37.2X2	T37.2X3	T37.2X4	T37.2X5	T37.2X6
Quinoline (derivatives) NEC	T37.8X1	T37.8X2	T37.8X3	T37.8X4	T37.8X5	T37.8X6
Quinupramine	T43.011	T43.012	T43.013	T43.014	T43.015	T43.016
Quotane	T41.3X1	T41.3X2	T41.3X3	T41.3X4	T41.3X5	T41.3X6
Rabies						
immune globulin (human)	T50.Z11	T50.Z12	T50.Z13	T50.Z14	T50.Z15	T50.Z16
vaccine	T50.B91	T50.B92	T50.B93	T50.B94	T50.B95	T50.B96
Racemoramide	T40.2X1	T40.2X2	T40.2X3	T40.2X4	—	—
Racemorphan	T40.2X1	T40.2X2	T40.2X3	T40.2X4	T40.2X5	T40.2X6
Racepinefrin	T44.5X1	T44.5X2	T44.5X3	T44.5X4	T44.5X5	T44.5X6
Raclopride	T43.591	T43.592	T43.593	T43.594	T43.595	T43.596
Radiator alcohol	T51.1X1	T51.1X2	T51.1X3	T51.1X4		
Radioactive drug NEC	T50.8X1	T50.8X2	T50.8X3	T50.8X4	T50.8X5	T50.8X6
Radio-opaque (drugs) (materials)	T50.8X1	T50.8X2	T50.8X3	T50.8X4	T50.8X5	T50.8X6
Ramifenazone	T39.2X1	T39.2X2	T39.2X3	T39.2X4	T39.2X5	T39.2X6
Ramipril	T46.4X1	T46.4X2	T46.4X3	T46.4X4	T46.4X5	T46.4X6
Ranitidine	T47.0X1	T47.0X2	T47.0X3	T47.0X4	T47.0X5	T47.0X6
Ranunculus	T62.2X1	T62.2X2	T62.2X3	T62.2X4	—	—
Rat poison NEC	T60.4X1	T60.4X2	T60.4X3	T60.4X4	—	—
Rattlesnake (venom)	T63.011	T63.012	T63.013	T63.014	—	—

Substance	Poisoning, Accidental (unintentional)	Poisoning, Intentional Self-harm	Poisoning, Assault	Poisoning, Undetermined	Adverse Effect	Under-dosing
Raubasine	T46.7X1	T46.7X2	T46.7X3	T46.7X4	T46.7X5	T46.7X6
Raudixin	T46.5X1	T46.5X2	T46.5X3	T46.5X4	T46.5X5	T46.5X6
Rautensin	T46.5X1	T46.5X2	T46.5X3	T46.5X4	T46.5X5	T46.5X6
Rautina	T46.5X1	T46.5X2	T46.5X3	T46.5X4	T46.5X5	T46.5X6
Rautotal	T46.5X1	T46.5X2	T46.5X3	T46.5X4	T46.5X5	T46.5X6
Rauwiloid	T46.5X1	T46.5X2	T46.5X3	T46.5X4	T46.5X5	T46.5X6
Rauwoldin	T46.5X1	T46.5X2	T46.5X3	T46.5X4	T46.5X5	T46.5X6
Rauwolfia (alkaloids)	T46.5X1	T46.5X2	T46.5X3	T46.5X4	T46.5X5	T46.5X6
Razoxane	T45.1X1	T45.1X2	T45.1X3	T45.1X4	T45.1X5	T45.1X6
Realgar	T57.0X1	T57.0X2	T57.0X3	T57.0X4	—	—
Recombinant (R) — see specific protein						
Red blood cells, packed	T45.8X1	T45.8X2	T45.8X3	T45.8X4	T45.8X5	T45.8X6
Red squill (scilliroside)	T60.4X1	T60.4X2	T60.4X3	T60.4X4	—	—
Reducing agent, industrial NEC	T65.891	T65.892	T65.893	T65.894	—	—
Refrigerant gas (chlorofluorocarbon)	T53.5X1	T53.5X2	T53.5X3	T53.5X4		
not chlorofluorocarbon	T59.891	T59.892	T59.893	T59.894		
Regroton	T50.2X1	T50.2X2	T50.2X3	T50.2X4	T50.2X5	T50.2X6
Rehydration salts (oral)	T50.3X1	T50.3X2	T50.3X3	T50.3X4	T50.3X5	T50.3X6
Rela	T42.8X1	T42.8X2	T42.8X3	T42.8X4	T42.8X5	T42.8X6
Relaxant, muscle						
anesthetic	T48.1X1	T48.1X2	T48.1X3	T48.1X4	T48.1X5	T48.1X6
central nervous system	T42.8X1	T42.8X2	T42.8X3	T42.8X4	T42.8X5	T42.8X6
skeletal NEC	T48.1X1	T48.1X2	T48.1X3	T48.1X4	T48.1X5	T48.1X6
smooth NEC	T44.3X1	T44.3X2	T44.3X3	T44.3X4	T44.3X5	T44.3X6
Remoxipride	T43.591	T43.592	T43.593	T43.594	T43.595	T43.596
Renese	T50.2X1	T50.2X2	T50.2X3	T50.2X4	T50.2X5	T50.2X6
Renografin	T50.8X1	T50.8X2	T50.8X3	T50.8X4	T50.8X5	T50.8X6
Replacement solution	T50.3X1	T50.3X2	T50.3X3	T50.3X4	T50.3X5	T50.3X6
Reproterol	T48.6X1	T48.6X2	T48.6X3	T48.6X4	T48.6X5	T48.6X6
Rescinnamine	T46.5X1	T46.5X2	T46.5X3	T46.5X4	T46.5X5	T46.5X6
Reserpin (e)	T46.5X1	T46.5X2	T46.5X3	T46.5X4	T46.5X5	T46.5X6
Resorcin, resorcinol (nonmedicinal)	T65.891	T65.892	T65.893	T65.894	—	—
medicinal	T49.4X1	T49.4X2	T49.4X3	T49.4X4	T49.4X5	T49.4X6
Respaire	T48.4X1	T48.4X2	T48.4X3	T48.4X4	T48.4X5	T48.4X6
Respiratory drug NEC	T48.901	T48.902	T48.903	T48.904	T48.905	T48.906
antiasthmatic NEC	T48.6X1	T48.6X2	T48.6X3	T48.6X4	T48.6X5	T48.6X6
anti-common-cold NEC	T48.5X1	T48.5X2	T48.5X3	T48.5X4	T48.5X5	T48.5X6
expectorant NEC	T48.4X1	T48.4X2	T48.4X3	T48.4X4	T48.4X5	T48.4X6
stimulant	T48.901	T48.902	T48.903	T48.904	T48.905	T48.906
Retinoic acid	T49.0X1	T49.0X2	T49.0X3	T49.0X4	T49.0X5	T49.0X6
Retinol	T45.2X1	T45.2X2	T45.2X3	T45.2X4	T45.2X5	T45.2X6
Rh (D) immune globulin (human)	T50.Z11	T50.Z12	T50.Z13	T50.Z14	T50.Z15	T50.Z16
Rhodine	T39.011	T39.012	T39.013	T39.014	T39.015	T39.016
RhoGAM	T50.Z11	T50.Z12	T50.Z13	T50.Z14	T50.Z15	T50.Z16
Rhubarb						
dry extract	T47.2X1	T47.2X2	T47.2X3	T47.2X4	T47.2X5	T47.2X6
tincture, compound	T47.2X1	T47.2X2	T47.2X3	T47.2X4	T47.2X5	T47.2X6
Ribavirin	T37.5X1	T37.5X2	T37.5X3	T37.5X4	T37.5X5	T37.5X6
Riboflavin	T45.2X1	T45.2X2	T45.2X3	T45.2X4	T45.2X5	T45.2X6
Ribostamycin	T36.5X1	T36.5X2	T36.5X3	T36.5X4	T36.5X5	T36.5X6
Ricin	T62.2X1	T62.2X2	T62.2X3	T62.2X4	—	—
Ricinus communis	T62.2X1	T62.2X2	T62.2X3	T62.2X4	—	—
Rickettsial vaccine NEC	T50.A91	T50.A92	T50.A93	T50.A94	T50.A95	T50.A96
Rifabutin	T36.6X1	T36.6X2	T36.6X3	T36.6X4	T36.6X5	T36.6X6
Rifamide	T36.6X1	T36.6X2	T36.6X3	T36.6X4	T36.6X5	T36.6X6
Rifampicin	T36.6X1	T36.6X2	T36.6X3	T36.6X4	T36.6X5	T36.6X6
with isoniazid	T37.1X1	T37.1X2	T37.1X3	T37.1X4	T37.1X5	T37.1X6
Rifampin	T36.6X1	T36.6X2	T36.6X3	T36.6X4	T36.6X5	T36.6X6
Rifamycin	T36.6X1	T36.6X2	T36.6X3	T36.6X4	T36.6X5	T36.6X6
Rifaximin	T36.6X1	T36.6X2	T36.6X3	T36.6X4	T36.6X5	T36.6X6
Rimantadine	T37.5X1	T37.5X2	T37.5X3	T37.5X4	T37.5X5	T37.5X6
Rimazolium metilsulfate	T39.8X1	T39.8X2	T39.8X3	T39.8X4	T39.8X5	T39.8X6
Rimifon	T37.1X1	T37.1X2	T37.1X3	T37.1X4	T37.1X5	T37.1X6
Rimiterol	T48.6X1	T48.6X2	T48.6X3	T48.6X4	T48.6X5	T48.6X6
Ringer (lactate) solution	T50.3X1	T50.3X2	T50.3X3	T50.3X4	T50.3X5	T50.3X6
Ristocetin	T36.8X1	T36.8X2	T36.8X3	T36.8X4	T36.8X5	T36.8X6
Ritalin	T43.631	T43.632	T43.633	T43.634	T43.635	T43.636
Ritodrine	T44.5X1	T44.5X2	T44.5X3	T44.5X4	T44.5X5	T44.5X6
Roach killer — see Insecticide						
Rociverine	T44.3X1	T44.3X2	T44.3X3	T44.3X4	T44.3X5	T44.3X6
Rocky Mountain spotted fever vaccine	T50.A91	T50.A92	T50.A93	T50.A94	T50.A95	T50.A96
Rodenticide NEC	T60.4X1	T60.4X2	T60.4X3	T60.4X4	—	—
Rohypnol	T42.4X1	T42.4X2	T42.4X3	T42.4X4	T42.4X5	T42.4X6
Rokitamycin	T36.3X1	T36.3X2	T36.3X3	T36.3X4	T36.3X5	T36.3X6
Rolaids	T47.1X1	T47.1X2	T47.1X3	T47.1X4	T47.1X5	T47.1X6
Rolitetracycline	T36.4X1	T36.4X2	T36.4X3	T36.4X4	T36.4X5	T36.4X6
Romilar	T48.3X1	T48.3X2	T48.3X3	T48.3X4	T48.3X5	T48.3X6

Table of Drugs and Chemicals

Ronifibrate — Simethicone

Substance	Poisoning, Accidental (unintentional)	Poisoning, Intentional Self-harm	Poisoning, Assault	Poisoning, Undetermined	Adverse Effect	Under-dosing
Ronifibrate	T46.6X1	T46.6X2	T46.6X3	T46.6X4	T46.6X5	T46.6X6
Rosaprostol	T47.1X1	T47.1X2	T47.1X3	T47.1X4	T47.1X5	T47.1X6
Rose bengal sodium (131I)	T50.8X1	T50.8X2	T50.8X3	T50.8X4	T50.8X5	T50.8X6
Rose water ointment	T49.3X1	T49.3X2	T49.3X3	T49.3X4	T49.3X5	T49.3X6
Rosoxacin	T37.8X1	T37.8X2	T37.8X3	T37.8X4	T37.8X5	T37.8X6
Rotenone	T60.2X1	T60.2X2	T60.2X3	T60.2X4	—	—
Rotoxamine	T45.0X1	T45.0X2	T45.0X3	T45.0X4	T45.0X5	T45.0X6
Rough-on-rats	T60.4X1	T60.4X2	T60.4X3	T60.4X4	—	—
Roxatidine	T47.0X1	T47.0X2	T47.0X3	T47.0X4	T47.0X5	T47.0X6
Roxithromycin	T36.3X1	T36.3X2	T36.3X3	T36.3X4	T36.3X5	T36.3X6
Rt-PA	T45.611	T45.612	T45.613	T45.614	T45.615	T45.616
Rubbing alcohol	T51.2X1	T51.2X2	T51.2X3	T51.2X4	—	—
Rubefacient	T49.4X1	T49.4X2	T49.4X3	T49.4X4	T49.4X5	T49.4X6
Rubella vaccine	T50.B91	T50.B92	T50.B93	T50.B94	T50.B95	T50.B96
Rubeola vaccine	T50.B91	T50.B92	T50.B93	T50.B94	T50.B95	T50.B96
Rubidium chloride Rb82	T50.8X1	T50.8X2	T50.8X3	T50.8X4	T50.8X5	T50.8X6
Rubidomycin	T45.1X1	T45.1X2	T45.1X3	T45.1X4	T45.1X5	T45.1X6
Rue	T62.2X1	T62.2X2	T62.2X3	T62.2X4	—	—
Rufocromomycin	T45.1X1	T45.1X2	T45.1X3	T45.1X4	T45.1X5	T45.1X6
Russel's viper venin	T45.7X1	T45.7X2	T45.7X3	T45.7X4	T45.7X5	T45.7X6
Ruta (graveolens)	T62.2X1	T62.2X2	T62.2X3	T62.2X4	—	—
Rutinum	T46.991	T46.992	T46.993	T46.994	T46.995	T46.996
Rutoside	T46.991	T46.992	T46.993	T46.994	T46.995	T46.996
b-sitosterol(s)	T46.6X1	T46.6X2	T46.6X3	T46.6X4	T46.6X5	T46.6X6
Sabadilla (plant)	T62.2X1	T62.2X2	T62.2X3	T62.2X4	—	—
pesticide	T60.2X1	T60.2X2	T60.2X3	T60.2X4	—	—
Saccharated iron oxide	T45.8X1	T45.8X2	T45.8X3	T45.8X4	T45.8X5	T45.8X6
Saccharin	T50.901	T50.902	T50.903	T50.904	T50.905	T50.906
Saccharomyces boulardii	T47.6X1	T47.6X2	T47.6X3	T47.6X4	T47.6X5	T47.6X6
Safflower oil	T46.6X1	T46.6X2	T46.6X3	T46.6X4	T46.6X5	T46.6X6
Safrazine	T43.1X1	T43.1X2	T43.1X3	T43.1X4	T43.1X5	T43.1X6
Salazosulfapyridine	T37.0X1	T37.0X2	T37.0X3	T37.0X4	T37.0X5	T37.0X6
Salbutamol	T48.6X1	T48.6X2	T48.6X3	T48.6X4	T48.6X5	T48.6X6
Salicylamide	T39.091	T39.092	T39.093	T39.094	T39.095	T39.096
Salicylate NEC	T39.091	T39.092	T39.093	T39.094	T39.095	T39.096
methyl	T49.3X1	T49.3X2	T49.3X3	T49.3X4	T49.3X5	T49.3X6
theobromine calcium	T50.2X1	T50.2X2	T50.2X3	T50.2X4	T50.2X5	T50.2X6
Salicylazosulfapyridine	T37.0X1	T37.0X2	T37.0X3	T37.0X4	T37.0X5	T37.0X6
Salicylhydroxamic acid	T49.0X1	T49.0X2	T49.0X3	T49.0X4	T49.0X5	T49.0X6
Salicylic acid	T49.4X1	T49.4X2	T49.4X3	T49.4X4	T49.4X5	T49.4X6
with benzoic acid	T49.4X1	T49.4X2	T49.4X3	T49.4X4	T49.4X5	T49.4X6
congeners	T39.091	T39.092	T39.093	T39.094	T39.095	T39.096
derivative	T39.091	T39.092	T39.093	T39.094	T39.095	T39.096
salts	T39.091	T39.092	T39.093	T39.094	T39.095	T39.096
Salinazid	T37.1X1	T37.1X2	T37.1X3	T37.1X4	T37.1X5	T37.1X6
Salmeterol	T48.6X1	T48.6X2	T48.6X3	T48.6X4	T48.6X5	T48.6X6
Salol	T49.3X1	T49.3X2	T49.3X3	T49.3X4	T49.3X5	T49.3X6
Salsalate	T39.091	T39.092	T39.093	T39.094	T39.095	T39.096
Salt-replacing drug	T50.901	T50.902	T50.903	T50.904	T50.905	T50.906
Salt-retaining mineralocorticoid	T50.0X1	T50.0X2	T50.0X3	T50.0X4	T50.0X5	T50.0X6
Salt substitute	T50.901	T50.902	T50.903	T50.904	T50.905	T50.906
Saluretic NEC	T50.2X1	T50.2X2	T50.2X3	T50.2X4	T50.2X5	T50.2X6
Saluron	T50.2X1	T50.2X2	T50.2X3	T50.2X4	T50.2X5	T50.2X6
Salvarsan 606 (neosilver) (silver)	T37.8X1	T37.8X2	T37.8X3	T37.8X4	T37.8X5	T37.8X6
Sambucus canadensis	T62.2X1	T62.2X2	T62.2X3	T62.2X4	—	—
berry	T62.1X1	T62.1X2	T62.1X3	T62.1X4	—	—
Sandril	T46.5X1	T46.5X2	T46.5X3	T46.5X4	T46.5X5	T46.5X6
Sanguinaria canadensis	T62.2X1	T62.2X2	T62.2X3	T62.2X4	—	—
Saniflush (cleaner)	T54.2X1	T54.2X2	T54.2X3	T54.2X4	—	—
Santonin	T37.4X1	T37.4X2	T37.4X3	T37.4X4	T37.4X5	T37.4X6
Santyl	T49.8X1	T49.8X2	T49.8X3	T49.8X4	T49.8X5	T49.8X6
Saralasin	T46.5X1	T46.5X2	T46.5X3	T46.5X4	T46.5X5	T46.5X6
Sarcolysin	T45.1X1	T45.1X2	T45.1X3	T45.1X4	T45.1X5	T45.1X6
Sarkomycin	T45.1X1	T45.1X2	T45.1X3	T45.1X4	T45.1X5	T45.1X6
Saroten	T43.011	T43.012	T43.013	T43.014	T43.015	T43.016
Saturnine — see Lead						
Savin (oil)	T49.4X1	T49.4X2	T49.4X3	T49.4X4	T49.4X5	T49.4X6
Scammony	T47.2X1	T47.2X2	T47.2X3	T47.2X4	T47.2X5	T47.2X6
Scarlet red	T49.8X1	T49.8X2	T49.8X3	T49.8X4	T49.8X5	T49.8X6
Scheele's green	T57.0X1	T57.0X2	T57.0X3	T57.0X4	—	—
insecticide	T57.0X1	T57.0X2	T57.0X3	T57.0X4	—	—
Schizontozide (blood) (tissue)	T37.2X1	T37.2X2	T37.2X3	T37.2X4	T37.2X5	T37.2X6
Schradan	T60.0X1	T60.0X2	T60.0X3	T60.0X4	—	—
Schweinfurth green	T57.0X1	T57.0X2	T57.0X3	T57.0X4	—	—
insecticide	T57.0X1	T57.0X2	T57.0X3	T57.0X4	—	—
Scilla, rat poison	T60.4X1	T60.4X2	T60.4X3	T60.4X4	—	—
Scillaren	T60.4X1	T60.4X2	T60.4X3	T60.4X4	—	—
Sclerosing agent	T46.8X1	T46.8X2	T46.8X3	T46.8X4	T46.8X5	T46.8X6
Scombrotoxin	T61.11	T61.12	T61.13	T61.14	—	—
Scopolamine	T44.3X1	T44.3X2	T44.3X3	T44.3X4	T44.3X5	T44.3X6

Substance	Poisoning, Accidental (unintentional)	Poisoning, Intentional Self-harm	Poisoning, Assault	Poisoning, Undetermined	Adverse Effect	Under-dosing
Scopolia extract	T44.3X1	T44.3X2	T44.3X3	T44.3X4	T44.3X5	T44.3X6
Scouring powder	T65.891	T65.892	T65.893	T65.894	—	—
Sea						
anemone (sting)	T63.631	T63.632	T63.633	T63.634	—	—
cucumber (sting)	T63.691	T63.692	T63.693	T63.694	—	—
snake (bite) (venom)	T63.091	T63.092	T63.093	T63.094	—	—
urchin spine (puncture)	T63.691	T63.692	T63.693	T63.694	—	—
Seafood	T61.91	T61.92	T61.93	T61.94	—	—
specified NEC	T61.8X1	T61.8X2	T61.8X3	T61.8X4	—	—
Secbutabarbital	T42.3X1	T42.3X2	T42.3X3	T42.3X4	T42.3X5	T42.3X6
Secbutabarbitone	T42.3X1	T42.3X2	T42.3X3	T42.3X4	T42.3X5	T42.3X6
Secnidazole	T37.3X1	T37.3X2	T37.3X3	T37.3X4	T37.3X5	T37.3X6
Secobarbital	T42.3X1	T42.3X2	T42.3X3	T42.3X4	T42.3X5	T42.3X6
Seconal	T42.3X1	T42.3X2	T42.3X3	T42.3X4	T42.3X5	T42.3X6
Secretin	T50.8X1	T50.8X2	T50.8X3	T50.8X4	T50.8X5	T50.8X6
Sedative NEC	T42.71	T42.72	T42.73	T42.74	T42.75	T42.76
mixed NEC	T42.6X1	T42.6X2	T42.6X3	T42.6X4	T42.6X5	T42.6X6
Sedormid	T42.6X1	T42.6X2	T42.6X3	T42.6X4	T42.6X5	T42.6X6
Seed disinfectant or dressing	T60.8X1	T60.8X2	T60.8X3	T60.8X4	—	—
Seeds (poisonous)	T62.2X1	T62.2X2	T62.2X3	T62.2X4	—	—
Selegiline	T42.8X1	T42.8X2	T42.8X3	T42.8X4	T42.8X5	T42.8X6
Selenium NEC	T56.891	T56.892	T56.893	T56.894	—	—
disulfide or sulfide	T49.4X1	T49.4X2	T49.4X3	T49.4X4	T49.4X5	T49.4X6
fumes	T59.891	T59.892	T59.893	T59.894	—	—
sulfide	T49.4X1	T49.4X2	T49.4X3	T49.4X4	T49.4X5	T49.4X6
Selenomethionine (75Se)	T50.8X1	T50.8X2	T50.8X3	T50.8X4	T50.8X5	T50.8X6
Selsun	T49.4X1	T49.4X2	T49.4X3	T49.4X4	T49.4X5	T49.4X6
Semustine	T45.1X1	T45.1X2	T45.1X3	T45.1X4	T45.1X5	T45.1X6
Senega syrup	T48.4X1	T48.4X2	T48.4X3	T48.4X4	T48.4X5	T48.4X6
Senna	T47.2X1	T47.2X2	T47.2X3	T47.2X4	T47.2X5	T47.2X6
Sennoside A+B	T47.2X1	T47.2X2	T47.2X3	T47.2X4	T47.2X5	T47.2X6
Septisol	T49.2X1	T49.2X2	T49.2X3	T49.2X4	T49.2X5	T49.2X6
Seractide	T38.811	T38.812	T38.813	T38.814	T38.815	T38.816
Serax	T42.4X1	T42.4X2	T42.4X3	T42.4X4	T42.4X5	T42.4X6
Serenesil	T42.6X1	T42.6X2	T42.6X3	T42.6X4	T42.6X5	T42.6X6
Serenium (hydrochloride)	T37.91	T37.92	T37.93	T37.94	T37.95	T37.96
Serepax — see Oxazepam						
Sermorelin	T38.891	T38.892	T38.893	T38.894	T38.895	T38.896
Sernyl	T41.1X1	T41.1X2	T41.1X3	T41.1X4	T41.1X5	T41.1X6
Serotonin	T50.991	T50.992	T50.993	T50.994	T50.995	T50.996
Serpasil	T46.5X1	T46.5X2	T46.5X3	T46.5X4	T46.5X5	T46.5X6
Serrapeptase	T45.3X1	T45.3X2	T45.3X3	T45.3X4	T45.3X5	T45.3X6
Serum						
antibotulinus	T50.Z11	T50.Z12	T50.Z13	T50.Z14	T50.Z15	T50.Z16
anticytotoxic	T50.Z11	T50.Z12	T50.Z13	T50.Z14	T50.Z15	T50.Z16
antidiphtheria	T50.Z11	T50.Z12	T50.Z13	T50.Z14	T50.Z15	T50.Z16
antimeningococcus	T50.Z11	T50.Z12	T50.Z13	T50.Z14	T50.Z15	T50.Z16
anti-Rh	T50.Z11	T50.Z12	T50.Z13	T50.Z14	T50.Z15	T50.Z16
anti-snake-bite	T50.Z11	T50.Z12	T50.Z13	T50.Z14	T50.Z15	T50.Z16
antitetanic	T50.Z11	T50.Z12	T50.Z13	T50.Z14	T50.Z15	T50.Z16
antitoxic	T50.Z11	T50.Z12	T50.Z13	T50.Z14	T50.Z15	T50.Z16
complement (inhibitor)	T45.8X1	T45.8X2	T45.8X3	T45.8X4	T45.8X5	T45.8X6
convalescent	T50.Z11	T50.Z12	T50.Z13	T50.Z14	T50.Z15	T50.Z16
hemolytic complement	T45.8X1	T45.8X2	T45.8X3	T45.8X4	T45.8X5	T45.8X6
immune (human)	T50.Z11	T50.Z12	T50.Z13	T50.Z14	T50.Z15	T50.Z16
protective NEC	T50.Z11	T50.Z12	T50.Z13	T50.Z14	T50.Z15	T50.Z16
Setastine	T45.0X1	T45.0X2	T45.0X3	T45.0X4	T45.0X5	T45.0X6
Setoperone	T43.591	T43.592	T43.593	T43.594	T43.595	T43.596
Sewer gas	T59.91	T59.92	T59.93	T59.94	—	—
Shampoo	T55.0X1	T55.0X2	T55.0X3	T55.0X4	—	—
Shellfish, noxious, nonbacterial	T61.781	T61.782	T61.783	T61.784	—	—
Sildenafil	T46.7X1	T46.7X2	T46.7X3	T46.7X4	T46.7X5	T46.7X6
Silibinin	T50.991	T50.992	T50.993	T50.994	T50.995	T50.996
Silicone NEC	T65.891	T65.892	T65.893	T65.894	—	—
medicinal	T49.3X1	T49.3X2	T49.3X3	T49.3X4	T49.3X5	T49.3X6
Silvadene	T49.0X1	T49.0X2	T49.0X3	T49.0X4	T49.0X5	T49.0X6
Silver	T49.0X1	T49.0X2	T49.0X3	T49.0X4	T49.0X5	T49.0X6
anti-infectives	T49.0X1	T49.0X2	T49.0X3	T49.0X4	T49.0X5	T49.0X6
arsphenamine	T37.8X1	T37.8X2	T37.8X3	T37.8X4	T37.8X5	T37.8X6
colloidal	T49.0X1	T49.0X2	T49.0X3	T49.0X4	T49.0X5	T49.0X6
nitrate	T49.0X1	T49.0X2	T49.0X3	T49.0X4	T49.0X5	T49.0X6
ophthalmic preparation	T49.5X1	T49.5X2	T49.5X3	T49.5X4	T49.5X5	T49.5X6
toughened (keratolytic)	T49.4X1	T49.4X2	T49.4X3	T49.4X4	T49.4X5	T49.4X6
nonmedicinal (dust)	T56.891	T56.892	T56.893	T56.894	—	—
protein	T49.5X1	T49.5X2	T49.5X3	T49.5X4	T49.5X5	T49.5X6
salvarsan	T37.8X1	T37.8X2	T37.8X3	T37.8X4	T37.8X5	T37.8X6
sulfadiazine	T49.4X1	T49.4X2	T49.4X3	T49.4X4	T49.4X5	T49.4X6
Silymarin	T50.991	T50.992	T50.993	T50.994	T50.995	T50.996
Simaldrate	T47.1X1	T47.1X2	T47.1X3	T47.1X4	T47.1X5	T47.1X6
Simazine	T60.3X1	T60.3X2	T60.3X3	T60.3X4	—	—
Simethicone	T47.1X1	T47.1X2	T47.1X3	T47.1X4	T47.1X5	T47.1X6

Additional Character May Be Required — Refer to the Tabular List for Character Selection ▽ Subterms under main terms may continue to next column or page

Substance	Poisoning, Accidental (unintentional)	Poisoning, Intentional Self-harm	Poisoning, Assault	Poisoning, Undetermined	Adverse Effect	Under-dosing
Simfibrate	T46.6X1	T46.6X2	T46.6X3	T46.6X4	T46.6X5	T46.6X6
Simvastatin	T46.6X1	T46.6X2	T46.6X3	T46.6X4	T46.6X5	T46.6X6
Sincalide	T50.8X1	T50.8X2	T50.8X3	T50.8X4	T50.8X5	T50.8X6
Sinequan	T43.011	T43.012	T43.013	T43.014	T43.015	T43.016
Singoserp	T46.5X1	T46.5X2	T46.5X3	T46.5X4	T46.5X5	T46.5X6
Sintrom	T45.511	T45.512	T45.513	T45.514	T45.515	T45.516
Sisomicin	T36.5X1	T36.5X2	T36.5X3	T36.5X4	T36.5X5	T36.5X6
Sitosterols	T46.6X1	T46.6X2	T46.6X3	T46.6X4	T46.6X5	T46.6X6
Skeletal muscle relaxants	T48.1X1	T48.1X2	T48.1X3	T48.1X4	T48.1X5	T48.1X6
Skin						
agents (external)	T49.91	T49.92	T49.93	T49.94	T49.95	T49.96
specified NEC	T49.8X1	T49.8X2	T49.8X3	T49.8X4	T49.8X5	T49.8X6
test antigen	T50.8X1	T50.8X2	T50.8X3	T50.8X4	T50.8X5	T50.8X6
Sleep-eze	T45.0X1	T45.0X2	T45.0X3	T45.0X4	T45.0X5	T45.0X6
Sleeping draught, pill	T42.71	T42.72	T42.73	T42.74	T42.75	T42.76
Smallpox vaccine	T50.B11	T50.B12	T50.B13	T50.B14	T50.B15	T50.B16
Smelter fumes NEC	T56.91	T56.92	T56.93	T56.94	—	—
Smog	T59.1X1	T59.1X2	T59.1X3	T59.1X4	—	—
Smoke NEC	T59.811	T59.812	T59.813	T59.814	—	—
Smooth muscle relaxant	T44.3X1	T44.3X2	T44.3X3	T44.3X4	T44.3X5	T44.3X6
Snail killer NEC	T60.8X1	T60.8X2	T60.8X3	T60.8X4	—	—
Snake venom or bite	T63.001	T63.002	T63.003	T63.004	—	—
hemocoagulase	T45.7X1	T45.7X2	T45.7X3	T45.7X4	T45.7X5	T45.7X6
Snuff	T65.211	T65.212	T65.213	T65.214		
Soap (powder) (product)	T55.0X1	T55.0X2	T55.0X3	T55.0X4		
enema	T47.4X1	T47.4X2	T47.4X3	T47.4X4	T47.4X5	T47.4X6
medicinal, soft	T49.2X1	T49.2X2	T49.2X3	T49.2X4	T49.2X5	T49.2X6
superfatted	T49.2X1	T49.2X2	T49.2X3	T49.2X4	T49.2X5	T49.2X6
Sobrerol	T48.4X1	T48.4X2	T48.4X3	T48.4X4	T48.4X5	T48.4X6
Soda (caustic)	T54.3X1	T54.3X2	T54.3X3	T54.3X4		
bicarb	T47.1X1	T47.1X2	T47.1X3	T47.1X4	T47.1X5	T47.1X6
chlorinated — see Sodium, hypochlorite						
Sodium						
acetosulfone	T37.1X1	T37.1X2	T37.1X3	T37.1X4	T37.1X5	T37.1X6
acetrizoate	T50.8X1	T50.8X2	T50.8X3	T50.8X4	T50.8X5	T50.8X6
acid phosphate	T50.3X1	T50.3X2	T50.3X3	T50.3X4	T50.3X5	T50.3X6
alginate	T47.8X1	T47.8X2	T47.8X3	T47.8X4	T47.8X5	T47.8X6
amidotrizoate	T50.8X1	T50.8X2	T50.8X3	T50.8X4	T50.8X5	T50.8X6
aminopterin	T45.1X1	T45.1X2	T45.1X3	T45.1X4	T45.1X5	T45.1X6
amylosulfate	T47.8X1	T47.8X2	T47.8X3	T47.8X4	T47.8X5	T47.8X6
amytal	T42.3X1	T42.3X2	T42.3X3	T42.3X4	T42.3X5	T42.3X6
antimony gluconate	T37.3X1	T37.3X2	T37.3X3	T37.3X4	T37.3X5	T37.3X6
arsenate	T57.0X1	T57.0X2	T57.0X3	T57.0X4	—	—
aurothiomalate	T39.4X1	T39.4X2	T39.4X3	T39.4X4	T39.4X5	T39.4X6
aurothiosulfate	T39.4X1	T39.4X2	T39.4X3	T39.4X4	T39.4X5	T39.4X6
barbiturate	T42.3X1	T42.3X2	T42.3X3	T42.3X4	T42.3X5	T42.3X6
basic phosphate	T47.4X1	T47.4X2	T47.4X3	T47.4X4	T47.4X5	T47.4X6
bicarbonate	T47.1X1	T47.1X2	T47.1X3	T47.1X4	T47.1X5	T47.1X6
bichromate	T57.8X1	T57.8X2	T57.8X3	T57.8X4	—	—
biphosphate	T50.3X1	T50.3X2	T50.3X3	T50.3X4	T50.3X5	T50.3X6
bisulfate	T65.891	T65.892	T65.893	T65.894		
borate						
cleanser	T57.8X1	T57.8X2	T57.8X3	T57.8X4	—	—
eye	T49.5X1	T49.5X2	T49.5X3	T49.5X4	T49.5X5	T49.5X6
therapeutic	T49.8X1	T49.8X2	T49.8X3	T49.8X4	T49.8X5	T49.8X6
bromide	T42.6X1	T42.6X2	T42.6X3	T42.6X4	T42.6X5	T42.6X6
cacodylate (nonmedicinal) NEC	T50.8X1	T50.8X2	T50.8X3	T50.8X4	T50.8X5	T50.8X6
anti-infective	T37.8X1	T37.8X2	T37.8X3	T37.8X4	T37.8X5	T37.8X6
herbicide	T60.3X1	T60.3X2	T60.3X3	T60.3X4	—	—
calcium edetate	T45.8X1	T45.8X2	T45.8X3	T45.8X4	T45.8X5	T45.8X6
carbonate NEC	T54.3X1	T54.3X2	T54.3X3	T54.3X4	—	—
chlorate NEC	T65.891	T65.892	T65.893	T65.894	—	—
herbicide	T54.91	T54.92	T54.93	T54.94	—	—
chloride	T50.3X1	T50.3X2	T50.3X3	T50.3X4	T50.3X5	T50.3X6
with glucose	T50.3X1	T50.3X2	T50.3X3	T50.3X4	T50.3X5	T50.3X6
chromate	T65.891	T65.892	T65.893	T65.894	—	—
citrate	T50.991	T50.992	T50.993	T50.994	T50.995	T50.996
cromoglicate	T48.6X1	T48.6X2	T48.6X3	T48.6X4	T48.6X5	T48.6X6
cyanide	T65.0X1	T65.0X2	T65.0X3	T65.0X4	—	—
cyclamate	T50.3X1	T50.3X2	T50.3X3	T50.3X4	T50.3X5	T50.3X6
dehydrocholate	T45.8X1	T45.8X2	T45.8X3	T45.8X4	T45.8X5	T45.8X6
diatrizoate	T50.8X1	T50.8X2	T50.8X3	T50.8X4	T50.8X5	T50.8X6
dibunate	T48.4X1	T48.4X2	T48.4X3	T48.4X4	T48.4X5	T48.4X6
dioctyl sulfosuccinate	T47.4X1	T47.4X2	T47.4X3	T47.4X4	T47.4X5	T47.4X6
dipantoyl ferrate	T45.8X1	T45.8X2	T45.8X3	T45.8X4	T45.8X5	T45.8X6
edetate	T45.8X1	T45.8X2	T45.8X3	T45.8X4	T45.8X5	T45.8X6
ethacrynate	T50.1X1	T50.1X2	T50.1X3	T50.1X4	T50.1X5	T50.1X6
feredetate	T45.8X1	T45.8X2	T45.8X3	T45.8X4	T45.8X5	T45.8X6
Fluoride — see Fluoride						
fluoroacetate (dust) (pesticide)	T60.4X1	T60.4X2	T60.4X3	T60.4X4	—	—

Substance	Poisoning, Accidental (unintentional)	Poisoning, Intentional Self-harm	Poisoning, Assault	Poisoning, Undetermined	Adverse Effect	Under-dosing
Sodium — continued						
free salt	T50.3X1	T50.3X2	T50.3X3	T50.3X4	T50.3X5	T50.3X6
fusidate	T36.8X1	T36.8X2	T36.8X3	T36.8X4	T36.8X5	T36.8X6
glucaldrate	T47.1X1	T47.1X2	T47.1X3	T47.1X4	T47.1X5	T47.1X6
glucosulfone	T37.1X1	T37.1X2	T37.1X3	T37.1X4	T37.1X5	T37.1X6
glutamate	T45.8X1	T45.8X2	T45.8X3	T45.8X4	T45.8X5	T45.8X6
hydrogen carbonate	T50.3X1	T50.3X2	T50.3X3	T50.3X4	T50.3X5	T50.3X6
hydroxide	T54.3X1	T54.3X2	T54.3X3	T54.3X4	—	—
hypochlorite (bleach) NEC	T54.3X1	T54.3X2	T54.3X3	T54.3X4		
disinfectant	T54.3X1	T54.3X2	T54.3X3	T54.3X4	—	—
medicinal (anti-infective) (external)	T49.0X1	T49.0X2	T49.0X3	T49.0X4	T49.0X5	T49.0X6
vapor	T54.3X1	T54.3X2	T54.3X3	T54.3X4	—	—
hyposulfite	T49.0X1	T49.0X2	T49.0X3	T49.0X4	T49.0X5	T49.0X6
indigotin disulfonate	T50.8X1	T50.8X2	T50.8X3	T50.8X4	T50.8X5	T50.8X6
iodide	T50.991	T50.992	T50.993	T50.994	T50.995	T50.996
I-131	T50.8X1	T50.8X2	T50.8X3	T50.8X4	T50.8X5	T50.8X6
therapeutic	T38.2X1	T38.2X2	T38.2X3	T38.2X4	T38.2X5	T38.2X6
iodohippurate (131I)	T50.8X1	T50.8X2	T50.8X3	T50.8X4	T50.8X5	T50.8X6
iopodate	T50.8X1	T50.8X2	T50.8X3	T50.8X4	T50.8X5	T50.8X6
iothalamate	T50.8X1	T50.8X2	T50.8X3	T50.8X4	T50.8X5	T50.8X6
iron edetate	T45.4X1	T45.4X2	T45.4X3	T45.4X4	T45.4X5	T45.4X6
lactate (compound solution)	T45.8X1	T45.8X2	T45.8X3	T45.8X4	T45.8X5	T45.8X6
lauryl (sulfate)	T49.2X1	T49.2X2	T49.2X3	T49.2X4	T49.2X5	T49.2X6
L-triiodothyronine	T38.1X1	T38.1X2	T38.1X3	T38.1X4	T38.1X5	T38.1X6
magnesium citrate	T50.991	T50.992	T50.993	T50.994	T50.995	T50.996
mersalate	T50.2X1	T50.2X2	T50.2X3	T50.2X4	T50.2X5	T50.2X6
metasilicate	T65.891	T65.892	T65.893	T65.894	—	—
metrizoate	T50.8X1	T50.8X2	T50.8X3	T50.8X4	T50.8X5	T50.8X6
monofluoroacetate (pesticide)	T60.1X1	T60.1X2	T60.1X3	T60.1X4	—	—
morrhuate	T46.8X1	T46.8X2	T46.8X3	T46.8X4	T46.8X5	T46.8X6
nafcillin	T36.0X1	T36.0X2	T36.0X3	T36.0X4	T36.0X5	T36.0X6
nitrate (oxidizing agent)	T65.891	T65.892	T65.893	T65.894	—	—
nitrite	T50.6X1	T50.6X2	T50.6X3	T50.6X4	T50.6X5	T50.6X6
nitroferricyanide	T46.5X1	T46.5X2	T46.5X3	T46.5X4	T46.5X5	T46.5X6
nitroprusside	T46.5X1	T46.5X2	T46.5X3	T46.5X4	T46.5X5	T46.5X6
oxalate	T65.891	T65.892	T65.893	T65.894	—	—
oxide/peroxide	T65.891	T65.892	T65.893	T65.894	—	—
oxybate	T41.291	T41.292	T41.293	T41.294	T41.295	T41.296
para-aminohippurate	T50.8X1	T50.8X2	T50.8X3	T50.8X4	T50.8X5	T50.8X6
perborate (nonmedicinal) NEC	T65.891	T65.892	T65.893	T65.894		
medicinal	T49.0X1	T49.0X2	T49.0X3	T49.0X4	T49.0X5	T49.0X6
soap	T55.0X1	T55.0X2	T55.0X3	T55.0X4	—	—
percarbonate — see Sodium, perborate						
pertechnetate Tc99m	T50.8X1	T50.8X2	T50.8X3	T50.8X4	T50.8X5	T50.8X6
phosphate						
cellulose	T45.8X1	T45.8X2	T45.8X3	T45.8X4	T45.8X5	T45.8X6
dibasic	T47.2X1	T47.2X2	T47.2X3	T47.2X4	T47.2X5	T47.2X6
monobasic	T47.2X1	T47.2X2	T47.2X3	T47.2X4	T47.2X5	T47.2X6
phytate	T50.6X1	T50.6X2	T50.6X3	T50.6X4	T50.6X5	T50.6X6
picosulfate	T47.2X1	T47.2X2	T47.2X3	T47.2X4	T47.2X5	T47.2X6
polyhydroxyaluminium monocarbonate	T47.1X1	T47.1X2	T47.1X3	T47.1X4	T47.1X5	T47.1X6
polystyrene sulfonate	T50.3X1	T50.3X2	T50.3X3	T50.3X4	T50.3X5	T50.3X6
propionate	T49.0X1	T49.0X2	T49.0X3	T49.0X4	T49.0X5	T49.0X6
propyl hydroxybenzoate	T50.991	T50.992	T50.993	T50.994	T50.995	T50.996
psylliate	T46.8X1	T46.8X2	T46.8X3	T46.8X4	T46.8X5	T46.8X6
removing resins	T50.3X1	T50.3X2	T50.3X3	T50.3X4	T50.3X5	T50.3X6
salicylate	T39.091	T39.092	T39.093	T39.094	T39.095	T39.096
salt NEC	T50.3X1	T50.3X2	T50.3X3	T50.3X4	T50.3X5	T50.3X6
selenate	T60.2X1	T60.2X2	T60.2X3	T60.2X4	—	—
stibogluconate	T37.3X1	T37.3X2	T37.3X3	T37.3X4	T37.3X5	T37.3X6
sulfate	T47.4X1	T47.4X2	T47.4X3	T47.4X4	T47.4X5	T47.4X6
sulfoxone	T37.1X1	T37.1X2	T37.1X3	T37.1X4	T37.1X5	T37.1X6
tetradecyl sulfate	T46.8X1	T46.8X2	T46.8X3	T46.8X4	T46.8X5	T46.8X6
thiopental	T41.1X1	T41.1X2	T41.1X3	T41.1X4	T41.1X5	T41.1X6
thiosalicylate	T39.091	T39.092	T39.093	T39.094	T39.095	T39.096
thiosulfate	T50.6X1	T50.6X2	T50.6X3	T50.6X4	T50.6X5	T50.6X6
tolbutamide	T38.3X1	T38.3X2	T38.3X3	T38.3X4	T38.3X5	T38.3X6
(L)-triiodothyronine	T38.1X1	T38.1X2	T38.1X3	T38.1X4	T38.1X5	T38.1X6
tyropanoate	T50.8X1	T50.8X2	T50.8X3	T50.8X4	T50.8X5	T50.8X6
valproate	T42.6X1	T42.6X2	T42.6X3	T42.6X4	T42.6X5	T42.6X6
versenate	T50.6X1	T50.6X2	T50.6X3	T50.6X4	T50.6X5	T50.6X6
Sodium-free salt	T50.901	T50.902	T50.903	T50.904	T50.905	T50.906
Sodium-removing resin	T50.3X1	T50.3X2	T50.3X3	T50.3X4	T50.3X5	T50.3X6
Soft soap	T55.0X1	T55.0X2	T55.0X3	T55.0X4	—	—
Solanine	T62.2X1	T62.2X2	T62.2X3	T62.2X4	—	—
berries	T62.1X1	T62.1X2	T62.1X3	T62.1X4	—	—
Solanum dulcamara	T62.2X1	T62.2X2	T62.2X3	T62.2X4	—	—

Substance	Poisoning, Accidental (unintentional)	Poisoning, Intentional Self-harm	Poisoning, Assault	Poisoning, Undetermined	Adverse Effect	Under-dosing
Solanum dulcamara — *continued*						
berries	T62.1X1	T62.1X2	T62.1X3	T62.1X4	—	—
Solapsone	T37.1X1	T37.1X2	T37.1X3	T37.1X4	T37.1X5	T37.1X6
Solar lotion	T49.3X1	T49.3X2	T49.3X3	T49.3X4	T49.3X5	T49.3X6
Solasulfone	T37.1X1	T37.1X2	T37.1X3	T37.1X4	T37.1X5	T37.1X6
Soldering fluid	T65.891	T65.892	T65.893	T65.894	—	—
Solid substance	T65.91	T65.92	T65.93	T65.94	—	—
specified NEC	T65.891	T65.892	T65.893	T65.894	—	—
Solvent, industrial NEC	T52.91	T52.92	T52.93	T52.94	—	—
naphtha	T52.0X1	T52.0X2	T52.0X3	T52.0X4	—	—
petroleum	T52.0X1	T52.0X2	T52.0X3	T52.0X4	—	—
specified NEC	T52.8X1	T52.8X2	T52.8X3	T52.8X4	—	—
Soma	T42.8X1	T42.8X2	T42.8X3	T42.8X4	T42.8X5	T42.8X6
Somatorelin	T38.891	T38.892	T38.893	T38.894	T38.895	T38.896
Somatostatin	T38.991	T38.992	T38.993	T38.994	T38.995	T38.996
Somatotropin	T38.811	T38.812	T38.813	T38.814	T38.815	T38.816
Somatrem	T38.811	T38.812	T38.813	T38.814	T38.815	T38.816
Somatropin	T38.811	T38.812	T38.813	T38.814	T38.815	T38.816
Sominex	T45.0X1	T45.0X2	T45.0X3	T45.0X4	T45.0X5	T45.0X6
Somnos	T42.6X1	T42.6X2	T42.6X3	T42.6X4	T42.6X5	T42.6X6
Somonal	T42.3X1	T42.3X2	T42.3X3	T42.3X4	T42.3X5	T42.3X6
Soneryl	T42.3X1	T42.3X2	T42.3X3	T42.3X4	T42.3X5	T42.3X6
Soothing syrup	T50.901	T50.902	T50.903	T50.904	T50.905	T50.906
Sopor	T42.6X1	T42.6X2	T42.6X3	T42.6X4	T42.6X5	T42.6X6
Soporific	T42.71	T42.72	T42.73	T42.74	T42.75	T42.76
Soporific drug	T42.71	T42.72	T42.73	T42.74	T42.75	T42.76
specified type NEC	T42.6X1	T42.6X2	T42.6X3	T42.6X4	T42.6X5	T42.6X6
Sorbide nitrate	T46.3X1	T46.3X2	T46.3X3	T46.3X4	T46.3X5	T46.3X6
Sorbitol	T47.4X1	T47.4X2	T47.4X3	T47.4X4	T47.4X5	T47.4X6
Sotalol	T44.7X1	T44.7X2	T44.7X3	T44.7X4	T44.7X5	T44.7X6
Sotradecol	T46.8X1	T46.8X2	T46.8X3	T46.8X4	T46.8X5	T46.8X6
Soysterol	T46.6X1	T46.6X2	T46.6X3	T46.6X4	T46.6X5	T46.6X6
Spacoline	T44.3X1	T44.3X2	T44.3X3	T44.3X4	T44.3X5	T44.3X6
Spanish fly	T49.8X1	T49.8X2	T49.8X3	T49.8X4	T49.8X5	T49.8X6
Sparine	T43.3X1	T43.3X2	T43.3X3	T43.3X4	T43.3X5	T43.3X6
Sparteine	T48.0X1	T48.0X2	T48.0X3	T48.0X4	T48.0X5	T48.0X6
Spasmolytic						
anticholinergics	T44.3X1	T44.3X2	T44.3X3	T44.3X4	T44.3X5	T44.3X6
autonomic	T44.3X1	T44.3X2	T44.3X3	T44.3X4	T44.3X5	T44.3X6
bronchial NEC	T48.6X1	T48.6X2	T48.6X3	T48.6X4	T48.6X5	T48.6X6
quaternary ammonium	T44.3X1	T44.3X2	T44.3X3	T44.3X4	T44.3X5	T44.3X6
skeletal muscle NEC	T48.1X1	T48.1X2	T48.1X3	T48.1X4	T48.1X5	T48.1X6
Spectinomycin	T36.5X1	T36.5X2	T36.5X3	T36.5X4	T36.5X5	T36.5X6
Speed	T43.621	T43.622	T43.623	T43.624	T43.625	T43.626
Spermicide	T49.8X1	T49.8X2	T49.8X3	T49.8X4	T49.8X5	T49.8X6
Spider (bite) (venom)	T63.391	T63.392	T63.393	T63.394	—	—
antivenin	T50.Z11	T50.Z12	T50.Z13	T50.Z14	T50.Z15	T50.Z16
Spigelia (root)	T37.4X1	T37.4X2	T37.4X3	T37.4X4	T37.4X5	T37.4X6
Spindle inactivator	T50.4X1	T50.4X2	T50.4X3	T50.4X4	T50.4X5	T50.4X6
Spiperone	T43.4X1	T43.4X2	T43.4X3	T43.4X4	T43.4X5	T43.4X6
Spiramycin	T36.3X1	T36.3X2	T36.3X3	T36.3X4	T36.3X5	T36.3X6
Spirapril	T46.4X1	T46.4X2	T46.4X3	T46.4X4	T46.4X5	T46.4X6
Spirilene	T43.591	T43.592	T43.593	T43.594	T43.595	T43.596
Spirit(s) (neutral) **NEC**	T51.0X1	T51.0X2	T51.0X3	T51.0X4	—	—
beverage	T51.0X1	T51.0X2	T51.0X3	T51.0X4	—	—
industrial	T51.0X1	T51.0X2	T51.0X3	T51.0X4	—	—
mineral	T52.0X1	T52.0X2	T52.0X3	T52.0X4	—	—
of salt — *see* Hydrochloric acid						
surgical	T51.0X1	T51.0X2	T51.0X3	T51.0X4	—	—
Spironolactone	T50.0X1	T50.0X2	T50.0X3	T50.0X4	T50.0X5	T50.0X6
Spiroperidol	T43.4X1	T43.4X2	T43.4X3	T43.4X4	T43.4X5	T43.4X6
Sponge, absorbable (gelatin)	T45.7X1	T45.7X2	T45.7X3	T45.7X4	T45.7X5	T45.7X6
Sporostacin	T49.0X1	T49.0X2	T49.0X3	T49.0X4	T49.0X5	T49.0X6
Spray (aerosol)	T65.91	T65.92	T65.93	T65.94	—	—
cosmetic	T65.891	T65.892	T65.893	T65.894	—	—
medicinal NEC	T50.901	T50.902	T50.903	T50.904	T50.905	T50.906
pesticides — *see* Pesticides						
specified content — *see* specific substance						
Spurge flax	T62.2X1	T62.2X2	T62.2X3	T62.2X4	—	—
Spurges	T62.2X1	T62.2X2	T62.2X3	T62.2X4	—	—
Sputum viscosity-lowering drug	T48.4X1	T48.4X2	T48.4X3	T48.4X4	T48.4X5	T48.4X6
Squill	T46.0X1	T46.0X2	T46.0X3	T46.0X4	T46.0X5	T46.0X6
rat poison	T60.4X1	T60.4X2	T60.4X3	T60.4X4	—	—
Squirting cucumber (cathartic)	T47.2X1	T47.2X2	T47.2X3	T47.2X4	T47.2X5	T47.2X6
Stains	T65.6X1	T65.6X2	T65.6X3	T65.6X4	—	—
Stannous fluoride	T49.7X1	T49.7X2	T49.7X3	T49.7X4	T49.7X5	T49.7X6
Stanolone	T38.7X1	T38.7X2	T38.7X3	T38.7X4	T38.7X5	T38.7X6
Stanozolol	T38.7X1	T38.7X2	T38.7X3	T38.7X4	T38.7X5	T38.7X6
Staphisagria or stavesacre (pediculicide)	T49.0X1	T49.0X2	T49.0X3	T49.0X4	T49.0X5	T49.0X6
Starch	T50.901	T50.902	T50.903	T50.904	T50.905	T50.906
Stelazine	T43.3X1	T43.3X2	T43.3X3	T43.3X4	T43.3X5	T43.3X6
Stemetil	T43.3X1	T43.3X2	T43.3X3	T43.3X4	T43.3X5	T43.3X6
Stepronin	T48.4X1	T48.4X2	T48.4X3	T48.4X4	T48.4X5	T48.4X6
Sterculia	T47.4X1	T47.4X2	T47.4X3	T47.4X4	T47.4X5	T47.4X6
Sternutator gas	T59.891	T59.892	T59.893	T59.894	—	—
Steroid	T38.0X1	T38.0X2	T38.0X3	T38.0X4	T38.0X5	T38.0X6
anabolic	T38.7X1	T38.7X2	T38.7X3	T38.7X4	T38.7X5	T38.7X6
androgenic	T38.7X1	T38.7X2	T38.7X3	T38.7X4	T38.7X5	T38.7X6
antineoplastic, hormone	T38.7X1	T38.7X2	T38.7X3	T38.7X4	T38.7X5	T38.7X6
estrogen	T38.5X1	T38.5X2	T38.5X3	T38.5X4	T38.5X5	T38.5X6
ENT agent	T49.6X1	T49.6X2	T49.6X3	T49.6X4	T49.6X5	T49.6X6
ophthalmic preparation	T49.5X1	T49.5X2	T49.5X3	T49.5X4	T49.5X5	T49.5X6
topical NEC	T49.0X1	T49.0X2	T49.0X3	T49.0X4	T49.0X5	T49.0X6
Stibine	T56.891	T56.892	T56.893	T56.894	—	—
Stibogluconate	T37.3X1	T37.3X2	T37.3X3	T37.3X4	T37.3X5	T37.3X6
Stibophen	T37.4X1	T37.4X2	T37.4X3	T37.4X4	T37.4X5	T37.4X6
Stilbamidine (isetionate)	T37.3X1	T37.3X2	T37.3X3	T37.3X4	T37.3X5	T37.3X6
Stilbestrol	T38.5X1	T38.5X2	T38.5X3	T38.5X4	T38.5X5	T38.5X6
Stilboestrol	T38.5X1	T38.5X2	T38.5X3	T38.5X4	T38.5X5	T38.5X6
Stimulant						
central nervous system — *see also* Psychostimulant	T43.601	T43.602	T43.603	T43.604	T43.605	T43.606
analeptics	T50.7X1	T50.7X2	T50.7X3	T50.7X4	T50.7X5	T50.7X6
opiate antagonist	T50.7X1	T50.7X2	T50.7X3	T50.7X4	T50.7X5	T50.7X6
psychotherapeutic NEC — *see also* Psychotherapeutic drug	T43.601	T43.602	T43.603	T43.604	T43.605	T43.606
specified NEC	T43.691	T43.692	T43.693	T43.694	T43.695	T43.696
respiratory	T48.901	T48.902	T48.903	T48.904	T48.905	T48.906
Stone-dissolving drug	T50.901	T50.902	T50.903	T50.904	T50.905	T50.906
Storage battery (cells) (acid)	T54.2X1	T54.2X2	T54.2X3	T54.2X4	—	—
Stovaine	T41.3X1	T41.3X2	T41.3X3	T41.3X4	T41.3X5	T41.3X6
infiltration (subcutaneous)	T41.3X1	T41.3X2	T41.3X3	T41.3X4	T41.3X5	T41.3X6
nerve block (peripheral) (plexus)	T41.3X1	T41.3X2	T41.3X3	T41.3X4	T41.3X5	T41.3X6
spinal	T41.3X1	T41.3X2	T41.3X3	T41.3X4	T41.3X5	T41.3X6
topical (surface)	T41.3X1	T41.3X2	T41.3X3	T41.3X4	T41.3X5	T41.3X6
Stovarsal	T37.8X1	T37.8X2	T37.8X3	T37.8X4	T37.8X5	T37.8X6
Stove gas — *see* Gas, stove						
Stoxil	T49.5X1	T49.5X2	T49.5X3	T49.5X4	T49.5X5	T49.5X6
Stramonium	T48.6X1	T48.6X2	T48.6X3	T48.6X4	T48.6X5	T48.6X6
natural state	T62.2X1	T62.2X2	T62.2X3	T62.2X4	—	—
Streptodornase	T45.3X1	T45.3X2	T45.3X3	T45.3X4	T45.3X5	T45.3X6
Streptoduocin	T36.5X1	T36.5X2	T36.5X3	T36.5X4	T36.5X5	T36.5X6
Streptokinase	T45.611	T45.612	T45.613	T45.614	T45.615	T45.616
Streptomycin (derivative)	T36.5X1	T36.5X2	T36.5X3	T36.5X4	T36.5X5	T36.5X6
Streptonivicin	T36.5X1	T36.5X2	T36.5X3	T36.5X4	T36.5X5	T36.5X6
Streptovarycin	T36.5X1	T36.5X2	T36.5X3	T36.5X4	T36.5X5	T36.5X6
Streptozocin	T45.1X1	T45.1X2	T45.1X3	T45.1X4	T45.1X5	T45.1X6
Streptozotocin	T45.1X1	T45.1X2	T45.1X3	T45.1X4	T45.1X5	T45.1X6
Stripper (paint) (solvent)	T52.8X1	T52.8X2	T52.8X3	T52.8X4	—	—
Strobane	T60.1X1	T60.1X2	T60.1X3	T60.1X4	—	—
Strofantina	T46.0X1	T46.0X2	T46.0X3	T46.0X4	T46.0X5	T46.0X6
Strophanthin (g) (k)	T46.0X1	T46.0X2	T46.0X3	T46.0X4	T46.0X5	T46.0X6
Strophanthus	T46.0X1	T46.0X2	T46.0X3	T46.0X4	T46.0X5	T46.0X6
Strophantin	T46.0X1	T46.0X2	T46.0X3	T46.0X4	T46.0X5	T46.0X6
Strophantin-g	T46.0X1	T46.0X2	T46.0X3	T46.0X4	T46.0X5	T46.0X6
Strychnine (nonmedicinal) (pesticide) (salts)	T65.1X1	T65.1X2	T65.1X3	T65.1X4	—	—
medicinal	T48.291	T48.292	T48.293	T48.294	T48.295	T48.296
Strychnos (ignatii) — *see* Strychnine						
Styramate	T42.8X1	T42.8X2	T42.8X3	T42.8X4	T42.8X5	T42.8X6
Styrene	T65.891	T65.892	T65.893	T65.894	—	—
Succinimide, antiepileptic or anticonvulsant	T42.2X1	T42.2X2	T42.2X3	T42.2X4	T42.2X5	T42.2X6
mercuric — *see* Mercury						
Succinylcholine	T48.1X1	T48.1X2	T48.1X3	T48.1X4	T48.1X5	T48.1X6
Succinylsulfathiazole	T37.0X1	T37.0X2	T37.0X3	T37.0X4	T37.0X5	T37.0X6
Sucralfate	T47.1X1	T47.1X2	T47.1X3	T47.1X4	T47.1X5	T47.1X6
Sucrose	T50.3X1	T50.3X2	T50.3X3	T50.3X4	T50.3X5	T50.3X6
Sufentanil	T40.4X1	T40.4X2	T40.4X3	T40.4X4	T40.4X5	T40.4X6
Sulbactam	T36.0X1	T36.0X2	T36.0X3	T36.0X4	T36.0X5	T36.0X6
Sulbenicillin	T36.0X1	T36.0X2	T36.0X3	T36.0X4	T36.0X5	T36.0X6
Sulbentine	T49.0X1	T49.0X2	T49.0X3	T49.0X4	T49.0X5	T49.0X6
Sulfacetamide	T49.0X1	T49.0X2	T49.0X3	T49.0X4	T49.0X5	T49.0X6
ophthalmic preparation	T49.5X1	T49.5X2	T49.5X3	T49.5X4	T49.5X5	T49.5X6
Sulfachlorpyridazine	T37.0X1	T37.0X2	T37.0X3	T37.0X4	T37.0X5	T37.0X6
Sulfacitine	T37.0X1	T37.0X2	T37.0X3	T37.0X4	T37.0X5	T37.0X6
Sulfadiasulfone sodium	T37.0X1	T37.0X2	T37.0X3	T37.0X4	T37.0X5	T37.0X6

Additional Character May Be Required — Refer to the Tabular List for Character Selection ▽ **Subterms under main terms may continue to next column or page**

Substance	Poisoning, Accidental (unintentional)	Poisoning, Intentional Self-harm	Poisoning, Assault	Poisoning, Undetermined	Adverse Effect	Under-dosing
Sulfadiazine	T37.0X1	T37.0X2	T37.0X3	T37.0X4	T37.0X5	T37.0X6
silver (topical)	T49.0X1	T49.0X2	T49.0X3	T49.0X4	T49.0X5	T49.0X6
Sulfadimethoxine	T37.0X1	T37.0X2	T37.0X3	T37.0X4	T37.0X5	T37.0X6
Sulfadimidine	T37.0X1	T37.0X2	T37.0X3	T37.0X4	T37.0X5	T37.0X6
Sulfadoxine	T37.0X1	T37.0X2	T37.0X3	T37.0X4	T37.0X5	T37.0X6
with pyrimethamine	T37.2X1	T37.2X2	T37.2X3	T37.2X4	T37.2X5	T37.2X6
Sulfaethidole	T37.0X1	T37.0X2	T37.0X3	T37.0X4	T37.0X5	T37.0X6
Sulfafurazole	T37.0X1	T37.0X2	T37.0X3	T37.0X4	T37.0X5	T37.0X6
Sulfaguanidine	T37.0X1	T37.0X2	T37.0X3	T37.0X4	T37.0X5	T37.0X6
Sulfalene	T37.0X1	T37.0X2	T37.0X3	T37.0X4	T37.0X5	T37.0X6
Sulfaloxate	T37.0X1	T37.0X2	T37.0X3	T37.0X4	T37.0X5	T37.0X6
Sulfaloxic acid	T37.0X1	T37.0X2	T37.0X3	T37.0X4	T37.0X5	T37.0X6
Sulfamazone	T39.2X1	T39.2X2	T39.2X3	T39.2X4	T39.2X5	T39.2X6
Sulfamerazine	T37.0X1	T37.0X2	T37.0X3	T37.0X4	T37.0X5	T37.0X6
Sulfameter	T37.0X1	T37.0X2	T37.0X3	T37.0X4	T37.0X5	T37.0X6
Sulfamethazine	T37.0X1	T37.0X2	T37.0X3	T37.0X4	T37.0X5	T37.0X6
Sulfamethizole	T37.0X1	T37.0X2	T37.0X3	T37.0X4	T37.0X5	T37.0X6
Sulfamethoxazole	T37.0X1	T37.0X2	T37.0X3	T37.0X4	T37.0X5	T37.0X6
with trimethoprim	T36.8X1	T36.8X2	T36.8X3	T36.8X4	T36.8X5	T36.8X6
Sulfamethoxydiazine	T37.0X1	T37.0X2	T37.0X3	T37.0X4	T37.0X5	T37.0X6
Sulfamethoxypyridazine	T37.0X1	T37.0X2	T37.0X3	T37.0X4	T37.0X5	T37.0X6
Sulfamethylthiazole	T37.0X1	T37.0X2	T37.0X3	T37.0X4	T37.0X5	T37.0X6
Sulfametoxydiazine	T37.0X1	T37.0X2	T37.0X3	T37.0X4	T37.0X5	T37.0X6
Sulfamidopyrine	T39.2X1	T39.2X2	T39.2X3	T39.2X4	T39.2X5	T39.2X6
Sulfamonomethoxine	T37.0X1	T37.0X2	T37.0X3	T37.0X4	T37.0X5	T37.0X6
Sulfamoxole	T37.0X1	T37.0X2	T37.0X3	T37.0X4	T37.0X5	T37.0X6
Sulfamylon	T49.0X1	T49.0X2	T49.0X3	T49.0X4	T49.0X5	T49.0X6
Sulfan blue (diagnostic dye)	T50.8X1	T50.8X2	T50.8X3	T50.8X4	T50.8X5	T50.8X6
Sulfanilamide	T37.0X1	T37.0X2	T37.0X3	T37.0X4	T37.0X5	T37.0X6
Sulfanilylguanidine	T37.0X1	T37.0X2	T37.0X3	T37.0X4	T37.0X5	T37.0X6
Sulfaperin	T37.0X1	T37.0X2	T37.0X3	T37.0X4	T37.0X5	T37.0X6
Sulfaphenazole	T37.0X1	T37.0X2	T37.0X3	T37.0X4	T37.0X5	T37.0X6
Sulfaphenylthiazole	T37.0X1	T37.0X2	T37.0X3	T37.0X4	T37.0X5	T37.0X6
Sulfaproxyline	T37.0X1	T37.0X2	T37.0X3	T37.0X4	T37.0X5	T37.0X6
Sulfapyridine	T37.0X1	T37.0X2	T37.0X3	T37.0X4	T37.0X5	T37.0X6
Sulfapyrimidine	T37.0X1	T37.0X2	T37.0X3	T37.0X4	T37.0X5	T37.0X6
Sulfarsphenamine	T37.8X1	T37.8X2	T37.8X3	T37.8X4	T37.8X5	T37.8X6
Sulfasalazine	T37.0X1	T37.0X2	T37.0X3	T37.0X4	T37.0X5	T37.0X6
Sulfasuxidine	T37.0X1	T37.0X2	T37.0X3	T37.0X4	T37.0X5	T37.0X6
Sulfasymazine	T37.0X1	T37.0X2	T37.0X3	T37.0X4	T37.0X5	T37.0X6
Sulfated amylopectin	T47.8X1	T47.8X2	T47.8X3	T47.8X4	T47.8X5	T47.8X6
Sulfathiazole	T37.0X1	T37.0X2	T37.0X3	T37.0X4	T37.0X5	T37.0X6
Sulfatostearate	T49.2X1	T49.2X2	T49.2X3	T49.2X4	T49.2X5	T49.2X6
Sulfinpyrazone	T50.4X1	T50.4X2	T50.4X3	T50.4X4	T50.4X5	T50.4X6
Sulfiram	T49.0X1	T49.0X2	T49.0X3	T49.0X4	T49.0X5	T49.0X6
Sulfisomidine	T37.0X1	T37.0X2	T37.0X3	T37.0X4	T37.0X5	T37.0X6
Sulfisoxazole	T37.0X1	T37.0X2	T37.0X3	T37.0X4	T37.0X5	T37.0X6
ophthalmic preparation	T49.5X1	T49.5X2	T49.5X3	T49.5X4	T49.5X5	T49.5X6
Sulfobromophthalein (sodium)	T50.8X1	T50.8X2	T50.8X3	T50.8X4	T50.8X5	T50.8X6
Sulfobromphthalein	T50.8X1	T50.8X2	T50.8X3	T50.8X4	T50.8X5	T50.8X6
Sulfogaiacol	T48.4X1	T48.4X2	T48.4X3	T48.4X4	T48.4X5	T48.4X6
Sulfomyxin	T36.8X1	T36.8X2	T36.8X3	T36.8X4	T36.8X5	T36.8X6
Sulfonal	T42.6X1	T42.6X2	T42.6X3	T42.6X4	T42.6X5	T42.6X6
Sulfonamide NEC	T37.0X1	T37.0X2	T37.0X3	T37.0X4	T37.0X5	T37.0X6
eye	T49.5X1	T49.5X2	T49.5X3	T49.5X4	T49.5X5	T49.5X6
Sulfonazide	T37.1X1	T37.1X2	T37.1X3	T37.1X4	T37.1X5	T37.1X6
Sulfones	T37.1X1	T37.1X2	T37.1X3	T37.1X4	T37.1X5	T37.1X6
Sulfonethylmethane	T42.6X1	T42.6X2	T42.6X3	T42.6X4	T42.6X5	T42.6X6
Sulfonmethane	T42.6X1	T42.6X2	T42.6X3	T42.6X4	T42.6X5	T42.6X6
Sulfonphthal, sulfonphthol	T50.8X1	T50.8X2	T50.8X3	T50.8X4	T50.8X5	T50.8X6
Sulfonylurea derivatives, oral	T38.3X1	T38.3X2	T38.3X3	T38.3X4	T38.3X5	T38.3X6
Sulforidazine	T43.3X1	T43.3X2	T43.3X3	T43.3X4	T43.3X5	T43.3X6
Sulfoxone	T37.1X1	T37.1X2	T37.1X3	T37.1X4	T37.1X5	T37.1X6
Sulfuric acid	T54.2X1	T54.2X2	T54.2X3	T54.2X4	—	—
Sulfur, sulfurated, sulfuric, sulfurous, sulfuryl (compounds NEC) (medicinal)	T49.4X1	T49.4X2	T49.4X3	T49.4X4	T49.4X5	T49.4X6
acid	T54.2X1	T54.2X2	T54.2X3	T54.2X4	—	—
dioxide (gas)	T59.1X1	T59.1X2	T59.1X3	T59.1X4	—	—
ether — see Ether(s)						
hydrogen	T59.6X1	T59.6X2	T59.6X3	T59.6X4	—	—
medicinal (keratolytic) (ointment) NEC	T49.4X1	T49.4X2	T49.4X3	T49.4X4	T49.4X5	T49.4X6
ointment	T49.0X1	T49.0X2	T49.0X3	T49.0X4	T49.0X5	T49.0X6
pesticide (vapor)	T60.91	T60.92	T60.93	T60.94	—	—
vapor NEC	T59.891	T59.892	T59.893	T59.894	—	—
Sulglicotide	T47.1X1	T47.1X2	T47.1X3	T47.1X4	T47.1X5	T47.1X6
Sulindac	T39.391	T39.392	T39.393	T39.394	T39.395	T39.396
Sulisatin	T47.2X1	T47.2X2	T47.2X3	T47.2X4	T47.2X5	T47.2X6
Sulisobenzone	T49.3X1	T49.3X2	T49.3X3	T49.3X4	T49.3X5	T49.3X6

Substance	Poisoning, Accidental (unintentional)	Poisoning, Intentional Self-harm	Poisoning, Assault	Poisoning, Undetermined	Adverse Effect	Under-dosing
Sulkowitch's reagent	T50.8X1	T50.8X2	T50.8X3	T50.8X4	T50.8X5	T50.8X6
Sulmetozine	T44.3X1	T44.3X2	T44.3X3	T44.3X4	T44.3X5	T44.3X6
Suloctidil	T46.7X1	T46.7X2	T46.7X3	T46.7X4	T46.7X5	T46.7X6
Sulph- — see also Sulf-						
Sulphadiazine	T37.0X1	T37.0X2	T37.0X3	T37.0X4	T37.0X5	T37.0X6
Sulphadimethoxine	T37.0X1	T37.0X2	T37.0X3	T37.0X4	T37.0X5	T37.0X6
Sulphadimidine	T37.0X1	T37.0X2	T37.0X3	T37.0X4	T37.0X5	T37.0X6
Sulphadione	T37.1X1	T37.1X2	T37.1X3	T37.1X4	T37.1X5	T37.1X6
Sulphafurazole	T37.0X1	T37.0X2	T37.0X3	T37.0X4	T37.0X5	T37.0X6
Sulphamethizole	T37.0X1	T37.0X2	T37.0X3	T37.0X4	T37.0X5	T37.0X6
Sulphamethoxazole	T37.0X1	T37.0X2	T37.0X3	T37.0X4	T37.0X5	T37.0X6
Sulphan blue	T50.8X1	T50.8X2	T50.8X3	T50.8X4	T50.8X5	T50.8X6
Sulphaphenazole	T37.0X1	T37.0X2	T37.0X3	T37.0X4	T37.0X5	T37.0X6
Sulphapyridine	T37.0X1	T37.0X2	T37.0X3	T37.0X4	T37.0X5	T37.0X6
Sulphasalazine	T37.0X1	T37.0X2	T37.0X3	T37.0X4	T37.0X5	T37.0X6
Sulphinpyrazone	T50.4X1	T50.4X2	T50.4X3	T50.4X4	T50.4X5	T50.4X6
Sulpiride	T43.591	T43.592	T43.593	T43.594	T43.595	T43.596
Sulprostone	T48.0X1	T48.0X2	T48.0X3	T48.0X4	T48.0X5	T48.0X6
Sulpyrine	T39.2X1	T39.2X2	T39.2X3	T39.2X4	T39.2X5	T39.2X6
Sultamicillin	T36.0X1	T36.0X2	T36.0X3	T36.0X4	T36.0X5	T36.0X6
Sulthiame	T42.6X1	T42.6X2	T42.6X3	T42.6X4	T42.6X5	T42.6X6
Sultiame	T42.6X1	T42.6X2	T42.6X3	T42.6X4	T42.6X5	T42.6X6
Sultopride	T43.591	T43.592	T43.593	T43.594	T43.595	T43.596
Sumatriptan	T39.8X1	T39.8X2	T39.8X3	T39.8X4	T39.8X5	T39.8X6
Sunflower seed oil	T46.6X1	T46.6X2	T46.6X3	T46.6X4	T46.6X5	T46.6X6
Superinone	T48.4X1	T48.4X2	T48.4X3	T48.4X4	T48.4X5	T48.4X6
Suprofen	T39.311	T39.312	T39.313	T39.314	T39.315	T39.316
Suramin (sodium)	T37.4X1	T37.4X2	T37.4X3	T37.4X4	T37.4X5	T37.4X6
Surfacaine	T41.3X1	T41.3X2	T41.3X3	T41.3X4	T41.3X5	T41.3X6
Surital	T41.1X1	T41.1X2	T41.1X3	T41.1X4	T41.1X5	T41.1X6
Sutilains	T45.3X1	T45.3X2	T45.3X3	T45.3X4	T45.3X5	T45.3X6
Suxamethonium (chloride)	T48.1X1	T48.1X2	T48.1X3	T48.1X4	T48.1X5	T48.1X6
Suxethonium (chloride)	T48.1X1	T48.1X2	T48.1X3	T48.1X4	T48.1X5	T48.1X6
Suxibuzone	T39.2X1	T39.2X2	T39.2X3	T39.2X4	T39.2X5	T39.2X6
Sweetener	T50.901	T50.902	T50.903	T50.904	T50.905	T50.906
Sweet niter spirit	T46.3X1	T46.3X2	T46.3X3	T46.3X4	T46.3X5	T46.3X6
Sweet oil (birch)	T49.3X1	T49.3X2	T49.3X3	T49.3X4	—	T49.3X6
Sym-dichloroethyl ether	T53.6X1	T53.6X2	T53.6X3	T53.6X4		
Sympatholytic NEC	T44.8X1	T44.8X2	T44.8X3	T44.8X4	T44.8X5	T44.8X6
haloalkylamine	T44.8X1	T44.8X2	T44.8X3	T44.8X4	T44.8X5	T44.8X6
Sympathomimetic NEC	T44.901	T44.902	T44.903	T44.904	T44.905	T44.906
anti-common-cold	T48.5X1	T48.5X2	T48.5X3	T48.5X4	T48.5X5	T48.5X6
bronchodilator	T48.6X1	T48.6X2	T48.6X3	T48.6X4	T48.6X5	T48.6X6
specified NEC	T44.991	T44.992	T44.993	T44.994	T44.995	T44.996
Synagis	T50.B91	T50.B92	T50.B93	T50.B94	T50.B95	T50.B96
Synalar	T49.0X1	T49.0X2	T49.0X3	T49.0X4	T49.0X5	T49.0X6
Synthroid	T38.1X1	T38.1X2	T38.1X3	T38.1X4	T38.1X5	T38.1X6
Syntocinon	T48.0X1	T48.0X2	T48.0X3	T48.0X4	T48.0X5	T48.0X6
Syrosingopine	T46.5X1	T46.5X2	T46.5X3	T46.5X4	T46.5X5	T46.5X6
Systemic drug	T45.91	T45.92	T45.93	T45.94	T45.95	T45.96
specified NEC	T45.8X1	T45.8X2	T45.8X3	T45.8X4	T45.8X5	T45.8X6
Tablets — see also specified substance	T50.901	T50.902	T50.903	T50.904	T50.905	T50.906
Tace	T38.5X1	T38.5X2	T38.5X3	T38.5X4	T38.5X5	T38.5X6
Tacrine	T44.0X1	T44.0X2	T44.0X3	T44.0X4	T44.0X5	T44.0X6
Tadalafil	T46.7X1	T46.7X2	T46.7X3	T46.7X4	T46.7X5	T46.7X6
Talampicillin	T36.0X1	T36.0X2	T36.0X3	T36.0X4	T36.0X5	T36.0X6
Talbutal	T42.3X1	T42.3X2	T42.3X3	T42.3X4	T42.3X5	T42.3X6
Talc powder	T49.3X1	T49.3X2	T49.3X3	T49.3X4	T49.3X5	T49.3X6
Talcum	T49.3X1	T49.3X2	T49.3X3	T49.3X4	T49.3X5	T49.3X6
Taleranol	T38.6X1	T38.6X2	T38.6X3	T38.6X4	T38.6X5	T38.6X6
Tamoxifen	T38.6X1	T38.6X2	T38.6X3	T38.6X4	T38.6X5	T38.6X6
Tamsulosin	T44.6X1	T44.6X2	T44.6X3	T44.6X4	T44.6X5	T44.6X6
Tandearil, tanderil	T39.2X1	T39.2X2	T39.2X3	T39.2X4	T39.2X5	T39.2X6
Tannic acid	T49.2X1	T49.2X2	T49.2X3	T49.2X4	T49.2X5	T49.2X6
medicinal (astringent)	T49.2X1	T49.2X2	T49.2X3	T49.2X4	T49.2X5	T49.2X6
Tannin — see Tannic acid						
Tansy	T62.2X1	T62.2X2	T62.2X3	T62.2X4	—	—
TAO	T36.3X1	T36.3X2	T36.3X3	T36.3X4	T36.3X5	T36.3X6
Tapazole	T38.2X1	T38.2X2	T38.2X3	T38.2X4	T38.2X5	T38.2X6
Taractan	T43.591	T43.592	T43.593	T43.594	T43.595	T43.596
Tarantula (venomous)	T63.321	T63.322	T63.323	T63.324	—	—
Tartar emetic	T37.8X1	T37.8X2	T37.8X3	T37.8X4	T37.8X5	T37.8X6
Tartaric acid	T65.891	T65.892	T65.893	T65.894	—	—
Tartrated antimony (anti-infective)	T37.8X1	T37.8X2	T37.8X3	T37.8X4	—	T37.8X6
Tartrate, laxative	T47.4X1	T47.4X2	T47.4X3	T47.4X4	T47.4X5	T47.4X6
Tar NEC	T52.0X1	T52.0X2	T52.0X3	T52.0X4	—	—
camphor	T60.1X1	T60.1X2	T60.1X3	T60.1X4	—	—
distillate	T49.1X1	T49.1X2	T49.1X3	T49.1X4	T49.1X5	T49.1X6
fumes	T59.891	T59.892	T59.893	T59.894	—	—
medicinal	T49.1X1	T49.1X2	T49.1X3	T49.1X4	T49.1X5	T49.1X6
ointment	T49.1X1	T49.1X2	T49.1X3	T49.1X4	T49.1X5	T49.1X6

Table of Drugs and Chemicals

Tauromustine — Thonzylamine

Substance	Poisoning, Accidental (unintentional)	Poisoning, Intentional Self-harm	Poisoning, Assault	Poisoning, Undetermined	Adverse Effect	Under-dosing
Tauromustine	T45.1X1	T45.1X2	T45.1X3	T45.1X4	T45.1X5	T45.1X6
TCA — *see* Trichloroacetic acid						
TCDD	T53.7X1	T53.7X2	T53.7X3	T53.7X4	—	—
TDI (vapor)	T65.0X1	T65.0X2	T65.0X3	T65.0X4	—	—
Tear						
gas	T59.3X1	T59.3X2	T59.3X3	T59.3X4	—	—
solution	T49.5X1	T49.5X2	T49.5X3	T49.5X4	T49.5X5	T49.5X6
Teclothiazide	T50.2X1	T50.2X2	T50.2X3	T50.2X4	T50.2X5	T50.2X6
Teclozan	T37.3X1	T37.3X2	T37.3X3	T37.3X4	T37.3X5	T37.3X6
Tegafur	T45.1X1	T45.1X2	T45.1X3	T45.1X4	T45.1X5	T45.1X6
Tegretol	T42.1X1	T42.1X2	T42.1X3	T42.1X4	T42.1X5	T42.1X6
Teicoplanin	T36.8X1	T36.8X2	T36.8X3	T36.8X4	T36.8X5	T36.8X6
Telepaque	T50.8X1	T50.8X2	T50.8X3	T50.8X4	T50.8X5	T50.8X6
Tellurium	T56.891	T56.892	T56.893	T56.894	—	—
fumes	T56.891	T56.892	T56.893	T56.894	—	—
TEM	T45.1X1	T45.1X2	T45.1X3	T45.1X4	T45.1X5	T45.1X6
Temazepam	T42.4X1	T42.4X2	T42.4X3	T42.4X4	T42.4X5	T42.4X6
Temocillin	T36.0X1	T36.0X2	T36.0X3	T36.0X4	T36.0X5	T36.0X6
Tenamfetamine	T43.621	T43.622	T43.623	T43.624	T43.625	T43.626
Teniposide	T45.1X1	T45.1X2	T45.1X3	T45.1X4	T45.1X5	T45.1X6
Tenitramine	T46.3X1	T46.3X2	T46.3X3	T46.3X4	T46.3X5	T46.3X6
Tenoglicin	T48.4X1	T48.4X2	T48.4X3	T48.4X4	T48.4X5	T48.4X6
Tenonitrozole	T37.3X1	T37.3X2	T37.3X3	T37.3X4	T37.3X5	T37.3X6
Tenoxicam	T39.391	T39.392	T39.393	T39.394	T39.395	T39.396
TEPA	T45.1X1	T45.1X2	T45.1X3	T45.1X4	T45.1X5	T45.1X6
TEPP	T60.0X1	T60.0X2	T60.0X3	T60.0X4		
Teprotide	T46.5X1	T46.5X2	T46.5X3	T46.5X4	T46.5X5	T46.5X6
Terazosin	T44.6X1	T44.6X2	T44.6X3	T44.6X4	T44.6X5	T44.6X6
Terbufos	T60.0X1	T60.0X2	T60.0X3	T60.0X4	—	—
Terbutaline	T48.6X1	T48.6X2	T48.6X3	T48.6X4	T48.6X5	T48.6X6
Terconazole	T49.0X1	T49.0X2	T49.0X3	T49.0X4	T49.0X5	T49.0X6
Terfenadine	T45.0X1	T45.0X2	T45.0X3	T45.0X4	T45.0X5	T45.0X6
Teriparatide (acetate)	T50.991	T50.992	T50.993	T50.994	T50.995	T50.996
Terizidone	T37.1X1	T37.1X2	T37.1X3	T37.1X4	T37.1X5	T37.1X6
Terlipressin	T38.891	T38.892	T38.893	T38.894	T38.895	T38.896
Terodiline	T46.3X1	T46.3X2	T46.3X3	T46.3X4	T46.3X5	T46.3X6
Teroxalene	T37.4X1	T37.4X2	T37.4X3	T37.4X4	T37.4X5	T37.4X6
Terpin (cis) **hydrate**	T48.4X1	T48.4X2	T48.4X3	T48.4X4	T48.4X5	T48.4X6
Terramycin	T36.4X1	T36.4X2	T36.4X3	T36.4X4	T36.4X5	T36.4X6
Tertatolol	T44.7X1	T44.7X2	T44.7X3	T44.7X4	T44.7X5	T44.7X6
Tessalon	T48.3X1	T48.3X2	T48.3X3	T48.3X4	T48.3X5	T48.3X6
Testolactone	T38.7X1	T38.7X2	T38.7X3	T38.7X4	T38.7X5	T38.7X6
Testosterone	T38.7X1	T38.7X2	T38.7X3	T38.7X4	T38.7X5	T38.7X6
Tetanus toxoid or vaccine	T50.A91	T50.A92	T50.A93	T50.A94	T50.A95	T50.A96
antitoxin	T50.Z11	T50.Z12	T50.Z13	T50.Z14	T50.Z15	T50.Z16
immune globulin (human)	T50.Z11	T50.Z12	T50.Z13	T50.Z14	T50.Z15	T50.Z16
toxoid	T50.A91	T50.A92	T50.A93	T50.A94	T50.A95	T50.A96
with diphtheria toxoid	T50.A21	T50.A22	T50.A23	T50.A24	T50.A25	T50.A26
with pertussis	T50.A11	T50.A12	T50.A13	T50.A14	T50.A15	T50.A16
Tetrabenazine	T43.591	T43.592	T43.593	T43.594	T43.595	T43.596
Tetracaine	T41.3X1	T41.3X2	T41.3X3	T41.3X4	T41.3X5	T41.3X6
nerve block (peripheral) (plexus)	T41.3X1	T41.3X2	T41.3X3	T41.3X4	T41.3X5	T41.3X6
regional	T41.3X1	T41.3X2	T41.3X3	T41.3X4	T41.3X5	T41.3X6
spinal	T41.3X1	T41.3X2	T41.3X3	T41.3X4	T41.3X5	T41.3X6
Tetrachlorethylene — *see* Tetrachloroethylene						
Tetrachlormethiazide	T50.2X1	T50.2X2	T50.2X3	T50.2X4	T50.2X5	T50.2X6
Tetrachloroethane	T53.6X1	T53.6X2	T53.6X3	T53.6X4	—	—
vapor	T53.6X1	T53.6X2	T53.6X3	T53.6X4	—	—
paint or varnish	T53.6X1	T53.6X2	T53.6X3	T53.6X4	—	—
Tetrachloroethylene (liquid)	T53.3X1	T53.3X2	T53.3X3	T53.3X4	—	—
medicinal	T37.4X1	T37.4X2	T37.4X3	T37.4X4	T37.4X5	T37.4X6
vapor	T53.3X1	T53.3X2	T53.3X3	T53.3X4	—	—
Tetrachloromethane — *see* Carbon tetrachloride						
Tetracosactide	T38.811	T38.812	T38.813	T38.814	T38.815	T38.816
Tetracosactrin	T38.811	T38.812	T38.813	T38.814	T38.815	T38.816
Tetracycline	T36.4X1	T36.4X2	T36.4X3	T36.4X4	T36.4X5	T36.4X6
ophthalmic preparation	T49.5X1	T49.5X2	T49.5X3	T49.5X4	T49.5X5	T49.5X6
topical NEC	T49.0X1	T49.0X2	T49.0X3	T49.0X4	T49.0X5	T49.0X6
Tetradifon	T60.8X1	T60.8X2	T60.8X3	T60.8X4	—	—
Tetradotoxin	T61.771	T61.772	T61.773	T61.774	—	—
Tetraethyl						
lead	T56.0X1	T56.0X2	T56.0X3	T56.0X4	—	—
pyrophosphate	T60.0X1	T60.0X2	T60.0X3	T60.0X4	—	—
Tetraethylammonium chloride	T44.2X1	T44.2X2	T44.2X3	T44.2X4	T44.2X5	T44.2X6
Tetraethylthiuram disulfide	T50.6X1	T50.6X2	T50.6X3	T50.6X4	T50.6X5	T50.6X6
Tetrahydroaminoacridine	T44.0X1	T44.0X2	T44.0X3	T44.0X4	T44.0X5	T44.0X6
Tetrahydrocannabinol	T40.7X1	T40.7X2	T40.7X3	T40.7X4	T40.7X5	T40.7X6
Tetrahydrofuran	T52.8X1	T52.8X2	T52.8X3	T52.8X4	—	—
Tetrahydronaphthalene	T52.8X1	T52.8X2	T52.8X3	T52.8X4	—	—
Tetrahydrozoline	T49.5X1	T49.5X2	T49.5X3	T49.5X4	T49.5X5	T49.5X6
Tetralin	T52.8X1	T52.8X2	T52.8X3	T52.8X4	—	—
Tetramethrin	T60.2X1	T60.2X2	T60.2X3	T60.2X4	—	—
Tetramethylthiuram (disulfide) **NEC**	T60.3X1	T60.3X2	T60.3X3	T60.3X4	—	—
medicinal	T49.0X1	T49.0X2	T49.0X3	T49.0X4	T49.0X5	T49.0X6
Tetramisole	T37.4X1	T37.4X2	T37.4X3	T37.4X4	T37.4X5	T37.4X6
Tetranicotinoyl fructose	T46.7X1	T46.7X2	T46.7X3	T46.7X4	T46.7X5	T46.7X6
Tetrazepam	T42.4X1	T42.4X2	T42.4X3	T42.4X4	T42.4X5	T42.4X6
Tetronal	T42.6X1	T42.6X2	T42.6X3	T42.6X4	T42.6X5	T42.6X6
Tetryl	T65.3X1	T65.3X2	T65.3X3	T65.3X4	—	—
Tetrylammonium chloride	T44.2X1	T44.2X2	T44.2X3	T44.2X4	T44.2X5	T44.2X6
Tetryzoline	T49.5X1	T49.5X2	T49.5X3	T49.5X4	T49.5X5	T49.5X6
Thalidomide	T45.1X1	T45.1X2	T45.1X3	T45.1X4	T45.1X5	T45.1X6
Thallium (compounds) (dust)	T56.811	T56.812	T56.813	T56.814	—	—
NEC						
pesticide	T60.4X1	T60.4X2	T60.4X3	T60.4X4	—	—
THC	T40.7X1	T40.7X2	T40.7X3	T40.7X4	T40.7X5	T40.7X6
Thebacon	T48.3X1	T48.3X2	T48.3X3	T48.3X4	T48.3X5	T48.3X6
Thebaine	T40.2X1	T40.2X2	T40.2X3	T40.2X4	T40.2X5	T40.2X6
Thenoic acid	T49.6X1	T49.6X2	T49.6X3	T49.6X4	T49.6X5	T49.6X6
Thenyldiamine	T45.0X1	T45.0X2	T45.0X3	T45.0X4	T45.0X5	T45.0X6
Theobromine (calcium salicylate)	T48.6X1	T48.6X2	T48.6X3	T48.6X4	T48.6X5	T48.6X6
sodium salicylate	T48.6X1	T48.6X2	T48.6X3	T48.6X4	T48.6X5	T48.6X6
Theophyllamine	T48.6X1	T48.6X2	T48.6X3	T48.6X4	T48.6X5	T48.6X6
Theophylline	T48.6X1	T48.6X2	T48.6X3	T48.6X4	T48.6X5	T48.6X6
aminobenzoic acid	T48.6X1	T48.6X2	T48.6X3	T48.6X4	T48.6X5	T48.6X6
ethylenediamine	T48.6X1	T48.6X2	T48.6X3	T48.6X4	T48.6X5	T48.6X6
piperazine	T48.6X1	T48.6X2	T48.6X3	T48.6X4	T48.6X5	T48.6X6
p-amino-benzoate						
Thiabendazole	T37.4X1	T37.4X2	T37.4X3	T37.4X4	T37.4X5	T37.4X6
Thialbarbital	T41.1X1	T41.1X2	T41.1X3	T41.1X4	T41.1X5	T41.1X6
Thiamazole	T38.2X1	T38.2X2	T38.2X3	T38.2X4	T38.2X5	T38.2X6
Thiambutosine	T37.1X1	T37.1X2	T37.1X3	T37.1X4	T37.1X5	T37.1X6
Thiamine	T45.2X1	T45.2X2	T45.2X3	T45.2X4	T45.2X5	T45.2X6
Thiamphenicol	T36.2X1	T36.2X2	T36.2X3	T36.2X4	T36.2X5	T36.2X6
Thiamylal	T41.1X1	T41.1X2	T41.1X3	T41.1X4	T41.1X5	T41.1X6
sodium	T41.1X1	T41.1X2	T41.1X3	T41.1X4	T41.1X5	T41.1X6
Thiazesim	T43.291	T43.292	T43.293	T43.294	T43.295	T43.296
Thiazides (diuretics)	T50.2X1	T50.2X2	T50.2X3	T50.2X4	T50.2X5	T50.2X6
Thiazinamium metilsulfate	T43.3X1	T43.3X2	T43.3X3	T43.3X4	T43.3X5	T43.3X6
Thiethylperazine	T43.3X1	T43.3X2	T43.3X3	T43.3X4	T43.3X5	T43.3X6
Thimerosal	T49.0X1	T49.0X2	T49.0X3	T49.0X4	T49.0X5	T49.0X6
ophthalmic preparation	T49.5X1	T49.5X2	T49.5X3	T49.5X4	T49.5X5	T49.5X6
Thioacetazone	T37.1X1	T37.1X2	T37.1X3	T37.1X4	T37.1X5	T37.1X6
with isoniazid	T37.1X1	T37.1X2	T37.1X3	T37.1X4	T37.1X5	T37.1X6
Thiobarbital sodium	T41.1X1	T41.1X2	T41.1X3	T41.1X4	T41.1X5	T41.1X6
Thiobarbiturate anesthetic	T41.1X1	T41.1X2	T41.1X3	T41.1X4	T41.1X5	T41.1X6
Thiobismol	T37.8X1	T37.8X2	T37.8X3	T37.8X4	T37.8X5	T37.8X6
Thiobutabarbital sodium	T41.1X1	T41.1X2	T41.1X3	T41.1X4	T41.1X5	T41.1X6
Thiocarbamate (insecticide)	T60.0X1	T60.0X2	T60.0X3	T60.0X4	—	—
Thiocarbamide	T38.2X1	T38.2X2	T38.2X3	T38.2X4	T38.2X5	T38.2X6
Thiocarbarsone	T37.8X1	T37.8X2	T37.8X3	T37.8X4	T37.8X5	T37.8X6
Thiocarlide	T37.1X1	T37.1X2	T37.1X3	T37.1X4	T37.1X5	T37.1X6
Thioctamide	T50.991	T50.992	T50.993	T50.994	T50.995	T50.996
Thioctic acid	T50.991	T50.992	T50.993	T50.994	T50.995	T50.996
Thiofos	T60.0X1	T60.0X2	T60.0X3	T60.0X4	—	—
Thioglycolate	T49.4X1	T49.4X2	T49.4X3	T49.4X4	T49.4X5	T49.4X6
Thioglycolic acid	T65.891	T65.892	T65.893	T65.894	—	—
Thioguanine	T45.1X1	T45.1X2	T45.1X3	T45.1X4	T45.1X5	T45.1X6
Thiomercaptomerin	T50.2X1	T50.2X2	T50.2X3	T50.2X4	T50.2X5	T50.2X6
Thiomerin	T50.2X1	T50.2X2	T50.2X3	T50.2X4	T50.2X5	T50.2X6
Thiomersal	T49.0X1	T49.0X2	T49.0X3	T49.0X4	T49.0X5	T49.0X6
Thionazin	T60.0X1	T60.0X2	T60.0X3	T60.0X4	—	—
Thiopental (sodium)	T41.1X1	T41.1X2	T41.1X3	T41.1X4	T41.1X5	T41.1X6
Thiopentone (sodium)	T41.1X1	T41.1X2	T41.1X3	T41.1X4	T41.1X5	T41.1X6
Thiopropazate	T43.3X1	T43.3X2	T43.3X3	T43.3X4	T43.3X5	T43.3X6
Thioproperazine	T43.3X1	T43.3X2	T43.3X3	T43.3X4	T43.3X5	T43.3X6
Thioridazine	T43.3X1	T43.3X2	T43.3X3	T43.3X4	T43.3X5	T43.3X6
Thiosinamine	T49.3X1	T49.3X2	T49.3X3	T49.3X4	T49.3X5	T49.3X6
Thiotepa	T45.1X1	T45.1X2	T45.1X3	T45.1X4	T45.1X5	T45.1X6
Thiothixene	T43.4X1	T43.4X2	T43.4X3	T43.4X4	T43.4X5	T43.4X6
Thiouracil (benzyl) (methyl) (propyl)	T38.2X1	T38.2X2	T38.2X3	T38.2X4	T38.2X5	T38.2X6
Thiourea	T38.2X1	T38.2X2	T38.2X3	T38.2X4	T38.2X5	T38.2X6
Thiphenamil	T44.3X1	T44.3X2	T44.3X3	T44.3X4	T44.3X5	T44.3X6
Thiram	T60.3X1	T60.3X2	T60.3X3	T60.3X4	—	—
medicinal	T49.2X1	T49.2X2	T49.2X3	T49.2X4	T49.2X5	T49.2X6
Thonzylamine (systemic)	T45.0X1	T45.0X2	T45.0X3	T45.0X4	T45.0X5	T45.0X6
mucosal decongestant	T48.5X1	T48.5X2	T48.5X3	T48.5X4	T48.5X5	T48.5X6

Additional Character May Be Required — Refer to the Tabular List for Character Selection ▽ Subterms under main terms may continue to next column or page

Substance	Poisoning, Accidental (unintentional)	Poisoning, Intentional Self-harm	Poisoning, Assault	Poisoning, Undetermined	Adverse Effect	Under-dosing
Thorazine	T43.3X1	T43.3X2	T43.3X3	T43.3X4	T43.3X5	T43.3X6
Thorium dioxide suspension	T50.8X1	T50.8X2	T50.8X3	T50.8X4	T50.8X5	T50.8X6
Thornapple	T62.2X1	T62.2X2	T62.2X3	T62.2X4	—	—
Throat drug NEC	T49.6X1	T49.6X2	T49.6X3	T49.6X4	T49.6X5	T49.6X6
Thrombin	T45.7X1	T45.7X2	T45.7X3	T45.7X4	T45.7X5	T45.7X6
Thrombolysin	T45.611	T45.612	T45.613	T45.614	T45.615	T45.616
Thromboplastin	T45.7X1	T45.7X2	T45.7X3	T45.7X4	T45.7X5	T45.7X6
Thurfyl nicotinate	T46.7X1	T46.7X2	T46.7X3	T46.7X4	T46.7X5	T46.7X6
Thymol	T49.0X1	T49.0X2	T49.0X3	T49.0X4	T49.0X5	T49.0X6
Thymopentin	T37.5X1	T37.5X2	T37.5X3	T37.5X4	T37.5X5	T37.5X6
Thymoxamine	T46.7X1	T46.7X2	T46.7X3	T46.7X4	T46.7X5	T46.7X6
Thymus extract	T38.891	T38.892	T38.893	T38.894	T38.895	T38.896
Thyreotrophic hormone	T38.811	T38.812	T38.813	T38.814	T38.815	T38.816
Thyroglobulin	T38.1X1	T38.1X2	T38.1X3	T38.1X4	T38.1X5	T38.1X6
Thyroid (hormone)	T38.1X1	T38.1X2	T38.1X3	T38.1X4	T38.1X5	T38.1X6
Thyrolar	T38.1X1	T38.1X2	T38.1X3	T38.1X4	T38.1X5	T38.1X6
Thyrotrophin	T38.811	T38.812	T38.813	T38.814	T38.815	T38.816
Thyrotropic hormone	T38.811	T38.812	T38.813	T38.814	T38.815	T38.816
Thyroxine	T38.1X1	T38.1X2	T38.1X3	T38.1X4	T38.1X5	T38.1X6
Tiabendazole	T37.4X1	T37.4X2	T37.4X3	T37.4X4	T37.4X5	T37.4X6
Tiamizide	T50.2X1	T50.2X2	T50.2X3	T50.2X4	T50.2X5	T50.2X6
Tianeptine	T43.291	T43.292	T43.293	T43.294	T43.295	T43.296
Tiapamil	T46.1X1	T46.1X2	T46.1X3	T46.1X4	T46.1X5	T46.1X6
Tiapride	T43.591	T43.592	T43.593	T43.594	T43.595	T43.596
Tiaprofenic acid	T39.311	T39.312	T39.313	T39.314	T39.315	T39.316
Tiaramide	T39.8X1	T39.8X2	T39.8X3	T39.8X4	T39.8X5	T39.8X6
Ticarcillin	T36.0X1	T36.0X2	T36.0X3	T36.0X4	T36.0X5	T36.0X6
Ticlatone	T49.0X1	T49.0X2	T49.0X3	T49.0X4	T49.0X5	T49.0X6
Ticlopidine	T45.521	T45.522	T45.523	T45.524	T45.525	T45.526
Ticrynafen	T50.1X1	T50.1X2	T50.1X3	T50.1X4	T50.1X5	T50.1X6
Tidiacic	T50.991	T50.992	T50.993	T50.994	T50.995	T50.996
Tiemonium	T44.3X1	T44.3X2	T44.3X3	T44.3X4	T44.3X5	T44.3X6
iodide	T44.3X1	T44.3X2	T44.3X3	T44.3X4	T44.3X5	T44.3X6
Tienilic acid	T50.1X1	T50.1X2	T50.1X3	T50.1X4	T50.1X5	T50.1X6
Tifenamil	T44.3X1	T44.3X2	T44.3X3	T44.3X4	T44.3X5	T44.3X6
Tigan	T45.0X1	T45.0X2	T45.0X3	T45.0X4	T45.0X5	T45.0X6
Tigloidine	T44.3X1	T44.3X2	T44.3X3	T44.3X4	T44.3X5	T44.3X6
Tilactase	T47.5X1	T47.5X2	T47.5X3	T47.5X4	T47.5X5	T47.5X6
Tiletamine	T41.291	T41.292	T41.293	T41.294	T41.295	T41.296
Tilidine	T40.4X1	T40.4X2	T40.4X3	T40.4X4	—	—
Timepidium bromide	T44.3X1	T44.3X2	T44.3X3	T44.3X4	T44.3X5	T44.3X6
Timiperone	T43.4X1	T43.4X2	T43.4X3	T43.4X4	T43.4X5	T43.4X6
Timolol	T44.7X1	T44.7X2	T44.7X3	T44.7X4	T44.7X5	T44.7X6
Tincture, iodine — see Iodine						
Tindal	T43.3X1	T43.3X2	T43.3X3	T43.3X4	T43.3X5	T43.3X6
Tinidazole	T37.3X1	T37.3X2	T37.3X3	T37.3X4	T37.3X5	T37.3X6
Tinoridine	T39.8X1	T39.8X2	T39.8X3	T39.8X4	T39.8X5	T39.8X6
Tin (chloride) (dust) (oxide)	T56.6X1	T56.6X2	T56.6X3	T56.6X4	—	—
NEC						
anti-infectives	T37.8X1	T37.8X2	T37.8X3	T37.8X4	T37.8X5	T37.8X6
Tiocarlide	T37.1X1	T37.1X2	T37.1X3	T37.1X4	T37.1X5	T37.1X6
Tioclomarol	T45.511	T45.512	T45.513	T45.514	T45.515	T45.516
Tioconazole	T49.0X1	T49.0X2	T49.0X3	T49.0X4	T49.0X5	T49.0X6
Tioguanine	T45.1X1	T45.1X2	T45.1X3	T45.1X4	T45.1X5	T45.1X6
Tiopronin	T50.991	T50.992	T50.993	T50.994	T50.995	T50.996
Tiotixene	T43.4X1	T43.4X2	T43.4X3	T43.4X4	T43.4X5	T43.4X6
Tioxolone	T49.4X1	T49.4X2	T49.4X3	T49.4X4	T49.4X5	T49.4X6
Tipepidine	T48.3X1	T48.3X2	T48.3X3	T48.3X4	T48.3X5	T48.3X6
Tiquizium bromide	T44.3X1	T44.3X2	T44.3X3	T44.3X4	T44.3X5	T44.3X6
Tiratricol	T38.1X1	T38.1X2	T38.1X3	T38.1X4	T38.1X5	T38.1X6
Tisopurine	T50.4X1	T50.4X2	T50.4X3	T50.4X4	T50.4X5	T50.4X6
Titanium (compounds)	T56.891	T56.892	T56.893	T56.894	—	—
(vapor)						
dioxide	T49.3X1	T49.3X2	T49.3X3	T49.3X4	T49.3X5	T49.3X6
ointment	T49.3X1	T49.3X2	T49.3X3	T49.3X4	T49.3X5	T49.3X6
oxide	T49.3X1	T49.3X2	T49.3X3	T49.3X4	T49.3X5	T49.3X6
tetrachloride	T56.891	T56.892	T56.893	T56.894	—	—
Titanocene	T56.891	T56.892	T56.893	T56.894	—	—
Titroid	T38.1X1	T38.1X2	T38.1X3	T38.1X4	T38.1X5	T38.1X6
Tizanidine	T42.8X1	T42.8X2	T42.8X3	T42.8X4	T42.8X5	T42.8X6
TMTD	T60.3X1	T60.3X2	T60.3X3	T60.3X4	—	—
TNT (fumes)	T65.3X1	T65.3X2	T65.3X3	T65.3X4	—	—
Toadstool	T62.0X1	T62.0X2	T62.0X3	T62.0X4	—	—
Tobacco NEC	T65.291	T65.292	T65.293	T65.294	—	—
cigarettes	T65.221	T65.222	T65.223	T65.224	—	—
Indian	T62.2X1	T62.2X2	T62.2X3	T62.2X4	—	—
smoke, second-hand	T65.221	T65.222	T65.223	T65.224	—	—
Tobramycin	T36.5X1	T36.5X2	T36.5X3	T36.5X4	T36.5X5	T36.5X6
Tocainide	T46.2X1	T46.2X2	T46.2X3	T46.2X4	T46.2X5	T46.2X6
Tocoferol	T45.2X1	T45.2X2	T45.2X3	T45.2X4	T45.2X5	T45.2X6
Tocopherol	T45.2X1	T45.2X2	T45.2X3	T45.2X4	T45.2X5	T45.2X6
acetate	T45.2X1	T45.2X2	T45.2X3	T45.2X4	T45.2X5	T45.2X6

Substance	Poisoning, Accidental (unintentional)	Poisoning, Intentional Self-harm	Poisoning, Assault	Poisoning, Undetermined	Adverse Effect	Under-dosing
Tocosamine	T48.0X1	T48.0X2	T48.0X3	T48.0X4	T48.0X5	T48.0X6
Todralazine	T46.5X1	T46.5X2	T46.5X3	T46.5X4	T46.5X5	T46.5X6
Tofisopam	T42.4X1	T42.4X2	T42.4X3	T42.4X4	T42.4X5	T42.4X6
Tofranil	T43.011	T43.012	T43.013	T43.014	T43.015	T43.016
Toilet deodorizer	T65.891	T65.892	T65.893	T65.894		
Tolamolol	T44.7X1	T44.7X2	T44.7X3	T44.7X4	T44.7X5	T44.7X6
Tolazamide	T38.3X1	T38.3X2	T38.3X3	T38.3X4	T38.3X5	T38.3X6
Tolazoline	T46.7X1	T46.7X2	T46.7X3	T46.7X4	T46.7X5	T46.7X6
Tolbutamide (sodium)	T38.3X1	T38.3X2	T38.3X3	T38.3X4	T38.3X5	T38.3X6
Tolciclate	T49.0X1	T49.0X2	T49.0X3	T49.0X4	T49.0X5	T49.0X6
Tolmetin	T39.391	T39.392	T39.393	T39.394	T39.395	T39.396
Tolnaftate	T49.0X1	T49.0X2	T49.0X3	T49.0X4	T49.0X5	T49.0X6
Tolonidine	T46.5X1	T46.5X2	T46.5X3	T46.5X4	T46.5X5	T46.5X6
Toloxatone	T42.6X1	T42.6X2	T42.6X3	T42.6X4	T42.6X5	T42.6X6
Tolperisone	T44.3X1	T44.3X2	T44.3X3	T44.3X4	T44.3X5	T44.3X6
Tolserol	T42.8X1	T42.8X2	T42.8X3	T42.8X4	T42.8X5	T42.8X6
Toluene (liquid)	T52.2X1	T52.2X2	T52.2X3	T52.2X4	—	—
diisocyanate	T65.0X1	T65.0X2	T65.0X3	T65.0X4	—	—
Toluidine	T65.891	T65.892	T65.893	T65.894	—	—
vapor	T59.891	T59.892	T59.893	T59.894	—	—
Toluol (liquid)	T52.2X1	T52.2X2	T52.2X3	T52.2X4	—	—
vapor	T52.2X1	T52.2X2	T52.2X3	T52.2X4	—	—
Toluylenediamine	T65.3X1	T65.3X2	T65.3X3	T65.3X4	—	—
Tolylene-2,4-diisocyanate	T65.0X1	T65.0X2	T65.0X3	T65.0X4	—	—
Tonic NEC	T50.901	T50.902	T50.903	T50.904	T50.905	T50.906
Topical action drug NEC	T49.91	T49.92	T49.93	T49.94	T49.95	T49.96
ear, nose or throat	T49.6X1	T49.6X2	T49.6X3	T49.6X4	T49.6X5	T49.6X6
eye	T49.5X1	T49.5X2	T49.5X3	T49.5X4	T49.5X5	T49.5X6
skin	T49.91	T49.92	T49.93	T49.94	T49.95	T49.96
specified NEC	T49.8X1	T49.8X2	T49.8X3	T49.8X4	T49.8X5	T49.8X6
Toquizine	T44.3X1	T44.3X2	T44.3X3	T44.3X4	T44.3X5	T44.3X6
Toremifene	T38.6X1	T38.6X2	T38.6X3	T38.6X4	T38.6X5	T38.6X6
Tosylchloramide sodium	T49.8X1	T49.8X2	T49.8X3	T49.8X4	T49.8X5	T49.8X6
Toxaphene (dust) (spray)	T60.1X1	T60.1X2	T60.1X3	T60.1X4	—	—
Toxin, diphtheria (Schick Test)	T50.8X1	T50.8X2	T50.8X3	T50.8X4	T50.8X5	T50.8X6
Toxoid						
combined	T50.A21	T50.A22	T50.A23	T50.A24	T50.A25	T50.A26
diphtheria	T50.A91	T50.A92	T50.A93	T50.A94	T50.A95	T50.A96
tetanus	T50.A91	T50.A92	T50.A93	T50.A94	T50.A95	T50.A96
Trace element NEC	T45.8X1	T45.8X2	T45.8X3	T45.8X4	T45.8X5	T45.8X6
Tractor fuel NEC	T52.0X1	T52.0X2	T52.0X3	T52.0X4	—	—
Tragacanth	T50.991	T50.992	T50.993	T50.994	T50.995	T50.996
Tramadol	T40.4X1	T40.4X2	T40.4X3	T40.4X4	T40.4X5	T40.4X6
Tramazoline	T48.5X1	T48.5X2	T48.5X3	T48.5X4	T48.5X5	T48.5X6
Tranexamic acid	T45.621	T45.622	T45.623	T45.624	T45.625	T45.626
Tranilast	T45.0X1	T45.0X2	T45.0X3	T45.0X4	T45.0X5	T45.0X6
Tranquilizer NEC	T43.501	T43.502	T43.503	T43.504	T43.505	T43.506
with hypnotic or sedative	T42.6X1	T42.6X2	T42.6X3	T42.6X4	T42.6X5	T42.6X6
benzodiazepine NEC	T42.4X1	T42.4X2	T42.4X3	T42.4X4	T42.4X5	T42.4X6
butyrophenone NEC	T43.4X1	T43.4X2	T43.4X3	T43.4X4	T43.4X5	T43.4X6
carbamate	T43.591	T43.592	T43.593	T43.594	T43.595	T43.596
dimethylamine	T43.3X1	T43.3X2	T43.3X3	T43.3X4	T43.3X5	T43.3X6
ethylamine	T43.3X1	T43.3X2	T43.3X3	T43.3X4	T43.3X5	T43.3X6
hydroxyzine	T43.591	T43.592	T43.593	T43.594	T43.595	T43.596
major NEC	T43.501	T43.502	T43.503	T43.504	T43.505	T43.506
penothiazine NEC	T43.3X1	T43.3X2	T43.3X3	T43.3X4	T43.3X5	T43.3X6
phenothiazine-based	T43.3X1	T43.3X2	T43.3X3	T43.3X4	T43.3X5	T43.3X6
piperazine NEC	T43.3X1	T43.3X2	T43.3X3	T43.3X4	T43.3X5	T43.3X6
piperidine	T43.3X1	T43.3X2	T43.3X3	T43.3X4	T43.3X5	T43.3X6
propylamine	T43.3X1	T43.3X2	T43.3X3	T43.3X4	T43.3X5	T43.3X6
specified NEC	T43.591	T43.592	T43.593	T43.594	T43.595	T43.596
thioxanthene NEC	T43.591	T43.592	T43.593	T43.594	T43.595	T43.596
Tranxene	T42.4X1	T42.4X2	T42.4X3	T42.4X4	T42.4X5	T42.4X6
Tranylcypromine	T43.1X1	T43.1X2	T43.1X3	T43.1X4	T43.1X5	T43.1X6
Trapidil	T46.3X1	T46.3X2	T46.3X3	T46.3X4	T46.3X5	T46.3X6
Trasentine	T44.3X1	T44.3X2	T44.3X3	T44.3X4	T44.3X5	T44.3X6
Travert	T50.3X1	T50.3X2	T50.3X3	T50.3X4	T50.3X5	T50.3X6
Trazodone	T43.211	T43.212	T43.213	T43.214	T43.215	T43.216
Trecator	T37.1X1	T37.1X2	T37.1X3	T37.1X4	T37.1X5	T37.1X6
Treosulfan	T45.1X1	T45.1X2	T45.1X3	T45.1X4	T45.1X5	T45.1X6
Tretamine	T45.1X1	T45.1X2	T45.1X3	T45.1X4	T45.1X5	T45.1X6
Tretinoin	T49.0X1	T49.0X2	T49.0X3	T49.0X4	T49.0X5	T49.0X6
Tretoquinol	T48.6X1	T48.6X2	T48.6X3	T48.6X4	T48.6X5	T48.6X6
Triacetin	T49.0X1	T49.0X2	T49.0X3	T49.0X4	T49.0X5	T49.0X6
Triacetoxyanthracene	T49.4X1	T49.4X2	T49.4X3	T49.4X4	T49.4X5	T49.4X6
Triacetyloleandomycin	T36.3X1	T36.3X2	T36.3X3	T36.3X4	T36.3X5	T36.3X6
Triamcinolone	T49.0X1	T49.0X2	T49.0X3	T49.0X4	T49.0X5	T49.0X6
ENT agent	T49.6X1	T49.6X2	T49.6X3	T49.6X4	T49.6X5	T49.6X6
hexacetonide	T49.0X1	T49.0X2	T49.0X3	T49.0X4	T49.0X5	T49.0X6
ophthalmic preparation	T49.5X1	T49.5X2	T49.5X3	T49.5X4	T49.5X5	T49.5X6
topical NEC	T49.0X1	T49.0X2	T49.0X3	T49.0X4	T49.0X5	T49.0X6
Triampyzine	T44.3X1	T44.3X2	T44.3X3	T44.3X4	T44.3X5	T44.3X6

Table of Drugs and Chemicals

Triamterene — Urokinase

Substance	Poisoning, Accidental (unintentional)	Poisoning, Intentional Self-harm	Poisoning, Assault	Poisoning, Undetermined	Adverse Effect	Under-dosing
Triamterene	T50.2X1	T50.2X2	T50.2X3	T50.2X4	T50.2X5	T50.2X6
Triazine (herbicide)	T60.3X1	T60.3X2	T60.3X3	T60.3X4	—	—
Triaziquone	T45.1X1	T45.1X2	T45.1X3	T45.1X4	T45.1X5	T45.1X6
Triazolam	T42.4X1	T42.4X2	T42.4X3	T42.4X4	T42.4X5	T42.4X6
Triazole (herbicide)	T60.3X1	T60.3X2	T60.3X3	T60.3X4	—	—
Tribenoside	T46.991	T46.992	T46.993	T46.994	T46.995	T46.996
Tribromacetaldehyde	T42.6X1	T42.6X2	T42.6X3	T42.6X4	T42.6X5	T42.6X6
Tribromoethanol, rectal	T41.291	T41.292	T41.293	T41.294	T41.295	T41.296
Tribromomethane	T42.6X1	T42.6X2	T42.6X3	T42.6X4	T42.6X5	T42.6X6
Trichlorethane	T53.2X1	T53.2X2	T53.2X3	T53.2X4	—	—
Trichlorethylene	T53.2X1	T53.2X2	T53.2X3	T53.2X4	—	—
Trichlorfon	T60.0X1	T60.0X2	T60.0X3	T60.0X4	—	—
Trichlormethiazide	T50.2X1	T50.2X2	T50.2X3	T50.2X4	T50.2X5	T50.2X6
Trichlormethine	T45.1X1	T45.1X2	T45.1X3	T45.1X4	T45.1X5	T45.1X6
Trichloroacetic acid, Trichloracetic acid	T54.2X1	T54.2X2	T54.2X3	T54.2X4	—	—
medicinal	T49.4X1	T49.4X2	T49.4X3	T49.4X4	T49.4X5	T49.4X6
Trichloroethane	T53.2X1	T53.2X2	T53.2X3	T53.2X4	—	—
Trichloroethanol	T42.6X1	T42.6X2	T42.6X3	T42.6X4	T42.6X5	T42.6X6
Trichloroethylene (liquid)	T53.2X1	T53.2X2	T53.2X3	T53.2X4	—	—
(vapor)						
anesthetic (gas)	T41.0X1	T41.0X2	T41.0X3	T41.0X4	T41.0X5	T41.0X6
vapor NEC	T53.2X1	T53.2X2	T53.2X3	T53.2X4	—	—
Trichloroethyl phosphate	T42.6X1	T42.6X2	T42.6X3	T42.6X4	T42.6X5	T42.6X6
Trichlorofluoromethane NEC	T53.5X1	T53.5X2	T53.5X3	T53.5X4	—	—
Trichloronate	T60.0X1	T60.0X2	T60.0X3	T60.0X4	—	—
Trichloropropane	T53.6X1	T53.6X2	T53.6X3	T53.6X4	—	—
Trichlorotriethylamine	T45.1X1	T45.1X2	T45.1X3	T45.1X4	T45.1X5	T45.1X6
Trichomonacides NEC	T37.3X1	T37.3X2	T37.3X3	T37.3X4	T37.3X5	T37.3X6
Trichomycin	T36.7X1	T36.7X2	T36.7X3	T36.7X4	T36.7X5	T36.7X6
Triclobisonium chloride	T49.0X1	T49.0X2	T49.0X3	T49.0X4	T49.0X5	T49.0X6
Triclocarban	T49.0X1	T49.0X2	T49.0X3	T49.0X4	T49.0X5	T49.0X6
Triclofos	T42.6X1	T42.6X2	T42.6X3	T42.6X4	T42.6X5	T42.6X6
Triclosan	T49.0X1	T49.0X2	T49.0X3	T49.0X4	T49.0X5	T49.0X6
Tricresyl phosphate	T65.891	T65.892	T65.893	T65.894	—	—
solvent	T52.91	T52.92	T52.93	T52.94	—	—
Tricyclamol chloride	T44.3X1	T44.3X2	T44.3X3	T44.3X4	T44.3X5	T44.3X6
Tridesilon	T49.0X1	T49.0X2	T49.0X3	T49.0X4	T49.0X5	T49.0X6
Tridihexethyl iodide	T44.3X1	T44.3X2	T44.3X3	T44.3X4	T44.3X5	T44.3X6
Tridione	T42.2X1	T42.2X2	T42.2X3	T42.2X4	T42.2X5	T42.2X6
Trientine	T45.8X1	T45.8X2	T45.8X3	T45.8X4	T45.8X5	T45.8X6
Triethanolamine NEC	T54.3X1	T54.3X2	T54.3X3	T54.3X4	—	—
detergent	T54.3X1	T54.3X2	T54.3X3	T54.3X4	—	—
trinitrate (biphosphate)	T46.3X1	T46.3X2	T46.3X3	T46.3X4	T46.3X5	T46.3X6
Triethanomelamine	T45.1X1	T45.1X2	T45.1X3	T45.1X4	T45.1X5	T45.1X6
Triethylenemelamine	T45.1X1	T45.1X2	T45.1X3	T45.1X4	T45.1X5	T45.1X6
Triethylenephosphoramide	T45.1X1	T45.1X2	T45.1X3	T45.1X4	T45.1X5	T45.1X6
Triethylenethiophosphoramide	T45.1X1	T45.1X2	T45.1X3	T45.1X4	T45.1X5	T45.1X6
Trifluoperazine	T43.3X1	T43.3X2	T43.3X3	T43.3X4	T43.3X5	T43.3X6
Trifluoroethyl vinyl ether	T41.0X1	T41.0X2	T41.0X3	T41.0X4	T41.0X5	T41.0X6
Trifluperidol	T43.4X1	T43.4X2	T43.4X3	T43.4X4	T43.4X5	T43.4X6
Triflupromazine	T43.3X1	T43.3X2	T43.3X3	T43.3X4	T43.3X5	T43.3X6
Trifluridine	T37.5X1	T37.5X2	T37.5X3	T37.5X4	T37.5X5	T37.5X6
Triflusal	T45.521	T45.522	T45.523	T45.524	T45.525	T45.526
Trihexyphenidyl	T44.3X1	T44.3X2	T44.3X3	T44.3X4	T44.3X5	T44.3X6
Triiodothyronine	T38.1X1	T38.1X2	T38.1X3	T38.1X4	T38.1X5	T38.1X6
Trilene	T41.0X1	T41.0X2	T41.0X3	T41.0X4	T41.0X5	T41.0X6
Trilostane	T38.992	T38.992	T38.993	T38.994	T38.995	T38.996
Trimebutine	T44.3X1	T44.3X2	T44.3X3	T44.3X4	T44.3X5	T44.3X6
Trimecaine	T41.3X1	T41.3X2	T41.3X3	T41.3X4	T41.3X5	T41.3X6
Trimeprazine (tartrate)	T44.3X1	T44.3X2	T44.3X3	T44.3X4	T44.3X5	T44.3X6
Trimetaphan camsilate	T44.2X1	T44.2X2	T44.2X3	T44.2X4	T44.2X5	T44.2X6
Trimetazidine	T46.7X1	T46.7X2	T46.7X3	T46.7X4	T46.7X5	T46.7X6
Trimethadione	T42.2X1	T42.2X2	T42.2X3	T42.2X4	T42.2X5	T42.2X6
Trimethaphan	T44.2X1	T44.2X2	T44.2X3	T44.2X4	T44.2X5	T44.2X6
Trimethidinium	T44.2X1	T44.2X2	T44.2X3	T44.2X4	T44.2X5	T44.2X6
Trimethobenzamide	T45.0X1	T45.0X2	T45.0X3	T45.0X4	T45.0X5	T45.0X6
Trimethoprim	T37.8X1	T37.8X2	T37.8X3	T37.8X4	T37.8X5	T37.8X6
with sulfamethoxazole	T36.8X1	T36.8X2	T36.8X3	T36.8X4	T36.8X5	T36.8X6
Trimethylcarbinol	T51.3X1	T51.3X2	T51.3X3	T51.3X4	—	—
Trimethylpsoralen	T49.3X1	T49.3X2	T49.3X3	T49.3X4	T49.3X5	T49.3X6
Trimeton	T45.0X1	T45.0X2	T45.0X3	T45.0X4	T45.0X5	T45.0X6
Trimetrexate	T45.1X1	T45.1X2	T45.1X3	T45.1X4	T45.1X5	T45.1X6
Trimipramine	T43.011	T43.012	T43.013	T43.014	T43.015	T43.016
Trimustine	T45.1X1	T45.1X2	T45.1X3	T45.1X4	T45.1X5	T45.1X6
Trinitrine	T46.3X1	T46.3X2	T46.3X3	T46.3X4	T46.3X5	T46.3X6
Trinitrobenzol	T65.3X1	T65.3X2	T65.3X3	T65.3X4	—	—
Trinitrophenol	T65.3X1	T65.3X2	T65.3X3	T65.3X4	—	—
Trinitrotoluene (fumes)	T65.3X1	T65.3X2	T65.3X3	T65.3X4	—	—
Trional	T42.6X1	T42.6X2	T42.6X3	T42.6X4	T42.6X5	T42.6X6
Triorthocresyl phosphate	T65.891	T65.892	T65.893	T65.894	—	—
Trioxide of arsenic	T57.0X1	T57.0X2	T57.0X3	T57.0X4	—	—

Substance	Poisoning, Accidental (unintentional)	Poisoning, Intentional Self-harm	Poisoning, Assault	Poisoning, Undetermined	Adverse Effect	Under-dosing
Trioxysalen	T49.4X1	T49.4X2	T49.4X3	T49.4X4	T49.4X5	T49.4X6
Tripamide	T50.2X1	T50.2X2	T50.2X3	T50.2X4	T50.2X5	T50.2X6
Triparanol	T46.6X1	T46.6X2	T46.6X3	T46.6X4	T46.6X5	T46.6X6
Tripelennamine	T45.0X1	T45.0X2	T45.0X3	T45.0X4	T45.0X5	T45.0X6
Triperiden	T44.3X1	T44.3X2	T44.3X3	T44.3X4	T44.3X5	T44.3X6
Triperidol	T43.4X1	T43.4X2	T43.4X3	T43.4X4	T43.4X5	T43.4X6
Triphenylphosphate	T65.891	T65.892	T65.893	T65.894	—	—
Triple						
bromides	T42.6X1	T42.6X2	T42.6X3	T42.6X4	T42.6X5	T42.6X6
carbonate	T47.1X1	T47.1X2	T47.1X3	T47.1X4	T47.1X5	T47.1X6
vaccine						
DPT	T50.A11	T50.A12	T50.A13	T50.A14	T50.A15	T50.A16
including pertussis	T50.A11	T50.A12	T50.A13	T50.A14	T50.A15	T50.A16
MMR	T50.B91	T50.B92	T50.B93	T50.B94	T50.B95	T50.B96
Triprolidine	T45.0X1	T45.0X2	T45.0X3	T45.0X4	T45.0X5	T45.0X6
Trisodium hydrogen edetate	T50.6X1	T50.6X2	T50.6X3	T50.6X4	T50.6X5	T50.6X6
Trisoralen	T49.3X1	T49.3X2	T49.3X3	T49.3X4	T49.3X5	T49.3X6
Trisulfapyrimidines	T37.0X1	T37.0X2	T37.0X3	T37.0X4	T37.0X5	T37.0X6
Trithiozine	T44.3X1	T44.3X2	T44.3X3	T44.3X4	T44.3X5	T44.3X6
Tritiozine	T44.3X1	T44.3X2	T44.3X3	T44.3X4	T44.3X5	T44.3X6
Tritoqualine	T45.0X1	T45.0X2	T45.0X3	T45.0X4	T45.0X5	T45.0X6
Trofosfamide	T45.1X1	T45.1X2	T45.1X3	T45.1X4	T45.1X5	T45.1X6
Troleandomycin	T36.3X1	T36.3X2	T36.3X3	T36.3X4	T36.3X5	T36.3X6
Trolnitrate (phosphate)	T46.3X1	T46.3X2	T46.3X3	T46.3X4	T46.3X5	T46.3X6
Tromantadine	T37.5X1	T37.5X2	T37.5X3	T37.5X4	T37.5X5	T37.5X6
Trometamol	T50.2X1	T50.2X2	T50.2X3	T50.2X4	T50.2X5	T50.2X6
Tromethamine	T50.2X1	T50.2X2	T50.2X3	T50.2X4	T50.2X5	T50.2X6
Tronothane	T41.3X1	T41.3X2	T41.3X3	T41.3X4	T41.3X5	T41.3X6
Tropacine	T44.3X1	T44.3X2	T44.3X3	T44.3X4	T44.3X5	T44.3X6
Tropatepine	T44.3X1	T44.3X2	T44.3X3	T44.3X4	T44.3X5	T44.3X6
Tropicamide	T44.3X1	T44.3X2	T44.3X3	T44.3X4	T44.3X5	T44.3X6
Trospium chloride	T44.3X1	T44.3X2	T44.3X3	T44.3X4	T44.3X5	T44.3X6
Troxerutin	T46.991	T46.992	T46.993	T46.994	T46.995	T46.996
Troxidone	T42.2X1	T42.2X2	T42.2X3	T42.2X4	T42.2X5	T42.2X6
Tryparsamide	T37.3X1	T37.3X2	T37.3X3	T37.3X4	T37.3X5	T37.3X6
Trypsin	T45.3X1	T45.3X2	T45.3X3	T45.3X4	T45.3X5	T45.3X6
Tryptizol	T43.011	T43.012	T43.013	T43.014	T43.015	T43.016
TSH	T38.811	T38.812	T38.813	T38.814	T38.815	T38.816
Tuaminoheptane	T48.5X1	T48.5X2	T48.5X3	T48.5X4	T48.5X5	T48.5X6
Tuberculin, purified protein derivative (PPD)	T50.8X1	T50.8X2	T50.8X3	T50.8X4	T50.8X5	T50.8X6
Tubocurare	T48.1X1	T48.1X2	T48.1X3	T48.1X4	T48.1X5	T48.1X6
Tubocurarine (chloride)	T48.1X1	T48.1X2	T48.1X3	T48.1X4	T48.1X5	T48.1X6
Tulobuterol	T48.6X1	T48.6X2	T48.6X3	T48.6X4	T48.6X5	T48.6X6
Turpentine (spirits of)	T52.8X1	T52.8X2	T52.8X3	T52.8X4	—	—
vapor	T52.8X1	T52.8X2	T52.8X3	T52.8X4	—	—
Tybamate	T43.591	T43.592	T43.593	T43.594	T43.595	T43.596
Tyloxapol	T48.4X1	T48.4X2	T48.4X3	T48.4X4	T48.4X5	T48.4X6
Tymazoline	T48.5X1	T48.5X2	T48.5X3	T48.5X4	T48.5X5	T48.5X6
Typhoid-paratyphoid vaccine	T50.A91	T50.A92	T50.A93	T50.A94	T50.A95	T50.A96
Typhus vaccine	T50.A91	T50.A92	T50.A93	T50.A94	T50.A95	T50.A96
Tyropanoate	T50.8X1	T50.8X2	T50.8X3	T50.8X4	T50.8X5	T50.8X6
Tyrothricin	T49.6X1	T49.6X2	T49.6X3	T49.6X4	T49.6X5	T49.6X6
ENT agent	T49.6X1	T49.6X2	T49.6X3	T49.6X4	T49.6X5	T49.6X6
ophthalmic preparation	T49.5X1	T49.5X2	T49.5X3	T49.5X4	T49.5X5	T49.5X6
Ufenamate	T39.391	T39.392	T39.393	T39.394	T39.395	T39.396
Ultraviolet light protectant	T49.3X1	T49.3X2	T49.3X3	T49.3X4	T49.3X5	T49.3X6
Undecenoic acid	T49.0X1	T49.0X2	T49.0X3	T49.0X4	T49.0X5	T49.0X6
Undecoylium	T49.0X1	T49.0X2	T49.0X3	T49.0X4	T49.0X5	T49.0X6
Undecylenic acid (derivatives)	T49.0X1	T49.0X2	T49.0X3	T49.0X4	T49.0X5	T49.0X6
Unna's boot	T49.3X1	T49.3X2	T49.3X3	T49.3X4	T49.3X5	T49.3X6
Unsaturated fatty acid	T46.6X1	T46.6X2	T46.6X3	T46.6X4	T46.6X5	T46.6X6
Uracil mustard	T45.1X1	T45.1X2	T45.1X3	T45.1X4	T45.1X5	T45.1X6
Uramustine	T45.1X1	T45.1X2	T45.1X3	T45.1X4	T45.1X5	T45.1X6
Urapidil	T46.5X1	T46.5X2	T46.5X3	T46.5X4	T46.5X5	T46.5X6
Urari	T48.1X1	T48.1X2	T48.1X3	T48.1X4	T48.1X5	T48.1X6
Urate oxidase	T50.4X1	T50.4X2	T50.4X3	T50.4X4	T50.4X5	T50.4X6
Urea	T47.3X1	T47.3X2	T47.3X3	T47.3X4	T47.3X5	T47.3X6
peroxide	T49.0X1	T49.0X2	T49.0X3	T49.0X4	T49.0X5	T49.0X6
stibamine	T37.4X1	T37.4X2	T37.4X3	T37.4X4	T37.4X5	T37.4X6
topical	T49.8X1	T49.8X2	T49.8X3	T49.8X4	T49.8X5	T49.8X6
Urethane	T45.1X1	T45.1X2	T45.1X3	T45.1X4	T45.1X5	T45.1X6
Urginea (maritima) (scilla) — see Squill						
Uric acid metabolism drug NEC	T50.4X1	T50.4X2	T50.4X3	T50.4X4	T50.4X5	T50.4X6
Uricosuric agent	T50.4X1	T50.4X2	T50.4X3	T50.4X4	T50.4X5	T50.4X6
Urinary anti-infective	T37.8X1	T37.8X2	T37.8X3	T37.8X4	T37.8X5	T37.8X6
Urofollitropin	T38.811	T38.812	T38.813	T38.814	T38.815	T38.816
Urokinase	T45.611	T45.612	T45.613	T45.614	T45.615	T45.616

Additional Character May Be Required — Refer to the Tabular List for Character Selection

▽ Subterms under main terms may continue to next column or page

Substance	Poisoning, Accidental (unintentional)	Poisoning, Intentional Self-harm	Poisoning, Assault	Poisoning, Undetermined	Adverse Effect	Under-dosing
Urokon	T50.8X1	T50.8X2	T50.8X3	T50.8X4	T50.8X5	T50.8X6
Ursodeoxycholic acid	T50.991	T50.992	T50.993	T50.994	T50.995	T50.996
Ursodiol	T50.991	T50.992	T50.993	T50.994	T50.995	T50.996
Urtica	T62.2X1	T62.2X2	T62.2X3	T62.2X4	—	—
Utility gas — *see* Gas, utility						
Vaccine NEC	T50.Z91	T50.Z92	T50.Z93	T50.Z94	T50.Z95	T50.Z96
antineoplastic	T50.Z91	T50.Z92	T50.Z93	T50.Z94	T50.Z95	T50.Z96
bacterial NEC	T50.A91	T50.A92	T50.A93	T50.A94	T50.A95	T50.A96
with						
other bacterial component	T50.A21	T50.A22	T50.A23	T50.A24	T50.A25	T50.A26
pertussis component	T50.A11	T50.A12	T50.A13	T50.A14	T50.A15	T50.A16
viral-rickettsial component	T50.A21	T50.A22	T50.A23	T50.A24	T50.A25	T50.A26
mixed NEC	T50.A21	T50.A22	T50.A23	T50.A24	T50.A25	T50.A26
BCG	T50.A91	T50.A92	T50.A93	T50.A94	T50.A95	T50.A96
cholera	T50.A91	T50.A92	T50.A93	T50.A94	T50.A95	T50.A96
diphtheria	T50.A91	T50.A92	T50.A93	T50.A94	T50.A95	T50.A96
with tetanus	T50.A21	T50.A22	T50.A23	T50.A24	T50.A25	T50.A26
and pertussis	T50.A11	T50.A12	T50.A13	T50.A14	T50.A15	T50.A16
influenza	T50.B91	T50.B92	T50.B93	T50.B94	T50.B95	T50.B96
measles	T50.B91	T50.B92	T50.B93	T50.B94	T50.B95	T50.B96
with mumps and rubella	T50.B91	T50.B92	T50.B93	T50.B94	T50.B95	T50.B96
meningococcal	T50.A91	T50.A92	T50.A93	T50.A94	T50.A95	T50.A96
mumps	T50.B91	T50.B92	T50.B93	T50.B94	T50.B95	T50.B96
paratyphoid	T50.A91	T50.A92	T50.A93	T50.A94	T50.A95	T50.A96
pertussis	T50.A11	T50.A12	T50.A13	T50.A14	T50.A15	T50.A16
with diphtheria	T50.A11	T50.A12	T50.A13	T50.A14	T50.A15	T50.A16
and tetanus	T50.A11	T50.A12	T50.A13	T50.A14	T50.A15	T50.A16
with other component	T50.A11	T50.A12	T50.A13	T50.A14	T50.A15	T50.A16
plague	T50.A91	T50.A92	T50.A93	T50.A94	T50.A95	T50.A96
poliomyelitis	T50.B91	T50.B92	T50.B93	T50.B94	T50.B95	T50.B96
poliovirus	T50.B91	T50.B92	T50.B93	T50.B94	T50.B95	T50.B96
rabies	T50.B91	T50.B92	T50.B93	T50.B94	T50.B95	T50.B96
respiratory syncytial virus	T50.B91	T50.B92	T50.B93	T50.B94	T50.B95	T50.B96
rickettsial NEC	T50.A91	T50.A92	T50.A93	T50.A94	T50.A95	T50.A96
with bacterial component	T50.A21	T50.A22	T50.A23	T50.A24	T50.A25	T50.A26
Rocky Mountain spotted fever	T50.A91	T50.A92	T50.A93	T50.A94	T50.A95	T50.A96
rubella	T50.B91	T50.B92	T50.B93	T50.B94	T50.B95	T50.B96
sabin oral	T50.B91	T50.B92	T50.B93	T50.B94	T50.B95	T50.B96
smallpox	T50.B11	T50.B12	T50.B13	T50.B14	T50.B15	T50.B16
TAB	T50.A91	T50.A92	T50.A93	T50.A94	T50.A95	T50.A96
tetanus	T50.A91	T50.A92	T50.A93	T50.A94	T50.A95	T50.A96
typhoid	T50.A91	T50.A92	T50.A93	T50.A94	T50.A95	T50.A96
typhus	T50.A91	T50.A92	T50.A93	T50.A94	T50.A95	T50.A96
viral NEC	T50.B91	T50.B92	T50.B93	T50.B94	T50.B95	T50.B96
yellow fever	T50.B91	T50.B92	T50.B93	T50.B94	T50.B95	T50.B96
Vaccinia immune globulin	T50.Z11	T50.Z12	T50.Z13	T50.Z14	T50.Z15	T50.Z16
Vaginal contraceptives	T49.8X1	T49.8X2	T49.8X3	T49.8X4	T49.8X5	T49.8X6
Valerian						
root	T42.6X1	T42.6X2	T42.6X3	T42.6X4	T42.6X5	T42.6X6
tincture	T42.6X1	T42.6X2	T42.6X3	T42.6X4	T42.6X5	T42.6X6
Valethamate bromide	T44.3X1	T44.3X2	T44.3X3	T44.3X4	T44.3X5	T44.3X6
Valisone	T49.0X1	T49.0X2	T49.0X3	T49.0X4	T49.0X5	T49.0X6
Valium	T42.4X1	T42.4X2	T42.4X3	T42.4X4	T42.4X5	T42.4X6
Valmid	T42.6X1	T42.6X2	T42.6X3	T42.6X4	T42.6X5	T42.6X6
Valnoctamide	T42.6X1	T42.6X2	T42.6X3	T42.6X4	T42.6X5	T42.6X6
Valproate (sodium)	T42.6X1	T42.6X2	T42.6X3	T42.6X4	T42.6X5	T42.6X6
Valproic acid	T42.6X1	T42.6X2	T42.6X3	T42.6X4	T42.6X5	T42.6X6
Valpromide	T42.6X1	T42.6X2	T42.6X3	T42.6X4	T42.6X5	T42.6X6
Vanadium	T56.891	T56.892	T56.893	T56.894	—	—
Vancomycin	T36.8X1	T36.8X2	T36.8X3	T36.8X4	T36.8X5	T36.8X6
Vapor — *see also* Gas	T59.91	T59.92	T59.93	T59.94	—	—
kiln (carbon monoxide)	T58.8X1	T58.8X2	T58.8X3	T58.8X4	—	—
lead — *see* lead						
specified source NEC	T59.891	T59.892	T59.893	T59.894	—	—
Vardenafil	T46.7X1	T46.7X2	T46.7X3	T46.7X4	T46.7X5	T46.7X6
Varicose reduction drug	T46.8X1	T46.8X2	T46.8X3	T46.8X4	T46.8X5	T46.8X6
Varnish	T65.4X1	T65.4X2	T65.4X3	T65.4X4	—	—
cleaner	T52.91	T52.92	T52.93	T52.94	—	—
Vaseline	T49.3X1	T49.3X2	T49.3X3	T49.3X4	T49.3X5	T49.3X6
Vasodilan	T46.7X1	T46.7X2	T46.7X3	T46.7X4	T46.7X5	T46.7X6
Vasodilator						
coronary NEC	T46.3X1	T46.3X2	T46.3X3	T46.3X4	T46.3X5	T46.3X6
peripheral NEC	T46.7X1	T46.7X2	T46.7X3	T46.7X4	T46.7X5	T46.7X6
Vasopressin	T38.891	T38.892	T38.893	T38.894	T38.895	T38.896
Vasopressor drugs	T38.891	T38.892	T38.893	T38.894	T38.895	T38.896
Vecuronium bromide	T48.1X1	T48.1X2	T48.1X3	T48.1X4	T48.1X5	T48.1X6
Vegetable extract, astringent	T49.2X1	T49.2X2	T49.2X3	T49.2X4	T49.2X5	T49.2X6
Venlafaxine	T43.211	T43.212	T43.213	T43.214	T43.215	T43.216

Substance	Poisoning, Accidental (unintentional)	Poisoning, Intentional Self-harm	Poisoning, Assault	Poisoning, Undetermined	Adverse Effect	Under-dosing
Venom, venomous (bite) (sting)	T63.91	T63.92	T63.93	T63.94	—	—
amphibian NEC	T63.831	T63.832	T63.833	T63.834		
animal NEC	T63.891	T63.892	T63.893	T63.894		
ant	T63.421	T63.422	T63.423	T63.424		
arthropod NEC	T63.481	T63.482	T63.483	T63.484		
bee	T63.441	T63.442	T63.443	T63.444		
centipede	T63.411	T63.412	T63.413	T63.414		
fish	T63.591	T63.592	T63.593	T63.594		
frog	T63.811	T63.812	T63.813	T63.814		
hornet	T63.451	T63.452	T63.453	T63.454		
insect NEC	T63.481	T63.482	T63.483	T63.484		
lizard	T63.121	T63.122	T63.123	T63.124		
marine						
animals	T63.691	T63.692	T63.693	T63.694		
bluebottle	T63.611	T63.612	T63.613	T63.614		
jellyfish NEC	T63.621	T63.622	T63.623	T63.624		
Portugese Man-o-war	T63.611	T63.612	T63.613	T63.614		
sea anemone	T63.631	T63.632	T63.633	T63.634		
specified NEC	T63.691	T63.692	T63.693	T63.694		
fish	T63.591	T63.592	T63.593	T63.594		
plants	T63.711	T63.712	T63.713	T63.714		
sting ray	T63.511	T63.512	T63.513	T63.514		
millipede (tropical)	T63.411	T63.412	T63.413	T63.414		
plant NEC	T63.791	T63.792	T63.793	T63.794		
marine	T63.711	T63.712	T63.713	T63.714		
reptile	T63.191	T63.192	T63.193	T63.194		
gila monster	T63.111	T63.112	T63.113	T63.114		
lizard NEC	T63.121	T63.122	T63.123	T63.124		
scorpion	T63.2X1	T63.2X2	T63.2X3	T63.2X4		
snake	T63.001	T63.002	T63.003	T63.004		
African NEC	T63.081	T63.082	T63.083	T63.084		
American (North) (South) NEC	T63.061	T63.062	T63.063	T63.064		
Asian	T63.081	T63.082	T63.083	T63.084		
Australian	T63.071	T63.072	T63.073	T63.074		
cobra	T63.041	T63.042	T63.043	T63.044		
coral snake	T63.021	T63.022	T63.023	T63.024		
rattlesnake	T63.011	T63.012	T63.013	T63.014		
specified NEC	T63.091	T63.092	T63.093	T63.094		
taipan	T63.031	T63.032	T63.033	T63.034		
specified NEC	T63.891	T63.892	T63.893	T63.894		
spider	T63.301	T63.302	T63.303	T63.304		
black widow	T63.311	T63.312	T63.313	T63.314		
brown recluse	T63.331	T63.332	T63.333	T63.334		
specified NEC	T63.391	T63.392	T63.393	T63.394		
tarantula	T63.321	T63.322	T63.323	T63.324		
sting ray	T63.511	T63.512	T63.513	T63.514		
toad	T63.821	T63.822	T63.823	T63.824		
wasp	T63.461	T63.462	T63.463	T63.464		
Venous sclerosing drug NEC	T46.8X1	T46.8X2	T46.8X3	T46.8X4	T46.8X5	T46.8X6
Ventolin — *see* Albuterol						
Veramon	T42.3X1	T42.3X2	T42.3X3	T42.3X4	T42.3X5	T42.3X6
Verapamil	T46.1X1	T46.1X2	T46.1X3	T46.1X4	T46.1X5	T46.1X6
Veratrine	T46.5X1	T46.5X2	T46.5X3	T46.5X4	T46.5X5	T46.5X6
Veratrum						
album	T62.2X1	T62.2X2	T62.2X3	T62.2X4	—	—
alkaloids	T46.5X1	T46.5X2	T46.5X3	T46.5X4	T46.5X5	T46.5X6
viride	T62.2X1	T62.2X2	T62.2X3	T62.2X4	—	—
Verdigris	T60.3X1	T60.3X2	T60.3X3	T60.3X4	—	—
Veronal	T42.3X1	T42.3X2	T42.3X3	T42.3X4	T42.3X5	T42.3X6
Veroxil	T37.4X1	T37.4X2	T37.4X3	T37.4X4	T37.4X5	T37.4X6
Versenate	T50.6X1	T50.6X2	T50.6X3	T50.6X4	T50.6X5	T50.6X6
Versidyne	T39.8X1	T39.8X2	T39.8X3	T39.8X4	T39.8X5	T39.8X6
Vetrabutine	T48.0X1	T48.0X2	T48.0X3	T48.0X4	T48.0X5	T48.0X6
Vidarabine	T37.5X1	T37.5X2	T37.5X3	T37.5X4	T37.5X5	T37.5X6
Vienna						
green	T57.0X1	T57.0X2	T57.0X3	T57.0X4	—	—
insecticide	T60.2X1	T60.2X2	T60.2X3	T60.2X4	—	—
red	T57.0X1	T57.0X2	T57.0X3	T57.0X4	—	—
pharmaceutical dye	T50.991	T50.992	T50.993	T50.994	T50.995	T50.996
Vigabatrin	T42.6X1	T42.6X2	T42.6X3	T42.6X4	T42.6X5	T42.6X6
Viloxazine	T43.291	T43.292	T43.293	T43.294	T43.295	T43.296
Viminol	T39.8X1	T39.8X2	T39.8X3	T39.8X4	T39.8X5	T39.8X6
Vinbarbital, vinbarbitone	T42.3X1	T42.3X2	T42.3X3	T42.3X4	T42.3X5	T42.3X6
Vinblastine	T45.1X1	T45.1X2	T45.1X3	T45.1X4	T45.1X5	T45.1X6
Vinburnine	T46.7X1	T46.7X2	T46.7X3	T46.7X4	T46.7X5	T46.7X6
Vincamine	T45.1X1	T45.1X2	T45.1X3	T45.1X4	T45.1X5	T45.1X6
Vincristine	T45.1X1	T45.1X2	T45.1X3	T45.1X4	T45.1X5	T45.1X6
Vindesine	T45.1X1	T45.1X2	T45.1X3	T45.1X4	T45.1X5	T45.1X6
Vinesthene, vinethene	T41.0X1	T41.0X2	T41.0X3	T41.0X4	T41.0X5	T41.0X6
Vinorelbine tartrate	T45.1X1	T45.1X2	T45.1X3	T45.1X4	T45.1X5	T45.1X6

Table of Drugs and Chemicals

Vinpocetine — Zyprexa

Substance	Poisoning, Accidental (unintentional)	Poisoning, Intentional Self-harm	Poisoning, Assault	Poisoning, Undetermined	Adverse Effect	Under-dosing
Vinpocetine	T46.7X1	T46.7X2	T46.7X3	T46.7X4	T46.7X5	T46.7X6
Vinyl						
acetate	T65.891	T65.892	T65.893	T65.894	—	—
bital	T42.3X1	T42.3X2	T42.3X3	T42.3X4	T42.3X5	T42.3X6
bromide	T65.891	T65.892	T65.893	T65.894	—	—
chloride	T59.891	T59.892	T59.893	T59.894	—	—
ether	T41.0X1	T41.0X2	T41.0X3	T41.0X4	T41.0X5	T41.0X6
Vinylbital	T42.3X1	T42.3X2	T42.3X3	T42.3X4	T42.3X5	T42.3X6
Vinylidene chloride	T65.891	T65.892	T65.893	T65.894	—	—
Vioform	T37.8X1	T37.8X2	T37.8X3	T37.8X4	T37.8X5	T37.8X6
topical	T49.0X1	T49.0X2	T49.0X3	T49.0X4	T49.0X5	T49.0X6
Viomycin	T36.8X1	T36.8X2	T36.8X3	T36.8X4	T36.8X5	T36.8X6
Viosterol	T45.2X1	T45.2X2	T45.2X3	T45.2X4	T45.2X5	T45.2X6
Viper (venom)	T63.091	T63.092	T63.093	T63.094		
Viprynium	T37.4X1	T37.4X2	T37.4X3	T37.4X4	T37.4X5	T37.4X6
Viquidil	T46.7X1	T46.7X2	T46.7X3	T46.7X4	T46.7X5	T46.7X6
Viral vaccine NEC	T50.B91	T50.B92	T50.B93	T50.B94	T50.B95	T50.B96
Virginiamycin	T36.8X1	T36.8X2	T36.8X3	T36.8X4	T36.8X5	T36.8X6
Virugon	T37.5X1	T37.5X2	T37.5X3	T37.5X4	T37.5X5	T37.5X6
Viscous agent	T50.901	T50.902	T50.903	T50.904	T50.905	T50.906
Visine	T49.5X1	T49.5X2	T49.5X3	T49.5X4	T49.5X5	T49.5X6
Visnadine	T46.3X1	T46.3X2	T46.3X3	T46.3X4	T46.3X5	T46.3X6
Vitamin NEC	T45.2X1	T45.2X2	T45.2X3	T45.2X4	T45.2X5	T45.2X6
A	T45.2X1	T45.2X2	T45.2X3	T45.2X4	T45.2X5	T45.2X6
B1	T45.2X1	T45.2X2	T45.2X3	T45.2X4	T45.2X5	T45.2X6
B2	T45.2X1	T45.2X2	T45.2X3	T45.2X4	T45.2X5	T45.2X6
B6	T45.2X1	T45.2X2	T45.2X3	T45.2X4	T45.2X5	T45.2X6
B12	T45.2X1	T45.2X2	T45.2X3	T45.2X4	T45.2X5	T45.2X6
B15	T45.2X1	T45.2X2	T45.2X3	T45.2X4	T45.2X5	T45.2X6
B NEC	T45.2X1	T45.2X2	T45.2X3	T45.2X4	T45.2X5	T45.2X6
nicotinic acid	T46.7X1	T46.7X2	T46.7X3	T46.7X4	T46.7X5	T46.7X6
C	T45.2X1	T45.2X2	T45.2X3	T45.2X4	T45.2X5	T45.2X6
D	T45.2X1	T45.2X2	T45.2X3	T45.2X4	T45.2X5	T45.2X6
D2	T45.2X1	T45.2X2	T45.2X3	T45.2X4	T45.2X5	T45.2X6
D3	T45.2X1	T45.2X2	T45.2X3	T45.2X4	T45.2X5	T45.2X6
E	T45.2X1	T45.2X2	T45.2X3	T45.2X4	T45.2X5	T45.2X6
E acetate	T45.2X1	T45.2X2	T45.2X3	T45.2X4	T45.2X5	T45.2X6
hematopoietic	T45.8X1	T45.8X2	T45.8X3	T45.8X4	T45.8X5	T45.8X6
K1	T45.7X1	T45.7X2	T45.7X3	T45.7X4	T45.7X5	T45.7X6
K2	T45.7X1	T45.7X2	T45.7X3	T45.7X4	T45.7X5	T45.7X6
K NEC	T45.7X1	T45.7X2	T45.7X3	T45.7X4	T45.7X5	T45.7X6
PP	T45.2X1	T45.2X2	T45.2X3	T45.2X4	T45.2X5	T45.2X6
ulceroprotectant	T47.1X1	T47.1X2	T47.1X3	T47.1X4	T47.1X5	T47.1X6
Vleminckx's solution	T49.4X1	T49.4X2	T49.4X3	T49.4X4	T49.4X5	T49.4X6
Voltaren — see Diclofenac sodium						
Warfarin	T45.511	T45.512	T45.513	T45.514	T45.515	T45.516
rodenticide	T60.4X1	T60.4X2	T60.4X3	T60.4X4	—	—
sodium	T60.4X1	T60.4X2	T60.4X3	T60.4X4	—	—
Wasp (sting)	T63.461	T63.462	T63.463	T63.464	—	—
Water						
balance drug	T50.3X1	T50.3X2	T50.3X3	T50.3X4	T50.3X5	T50.3X6
distilled	T50.3X1	T50.3X2	T50.3X3	T50.3X4	T50.3X5	T50.3X6
gas — see Gas, water						
incomplete combustion of — see Carbon, monoxide, fuel, utility						
hemlock	T62.2X1	T62.2X2	T62.2X3	T62.2X4	—	—
moccasin (venom)	T63.061	T63.062	T63.063	T63.064	—	—
purified	T50.3X1	T50.3X2	T50.3X3	T50.3X4	T50.3X5	T50.3X6
Wax (paraffin) (petroleum)	T52.0X1	T52.0X2	T52.0X3	T52.0X4	—	—
automobile	T65.891	T65.892	T65.893	T65.894	—	—
floor	T52.0X1	T52.0X2	T52.0X3	T52.0X4	—	—
Weed killers NEC	T60.3X1	T60.3X2	T60.3X3	T60.3X4	—	—
Welldorm	T42.6X1	T42.6X2	T42.6X3	T42.6X4	T42.6X5	T42.6X6
White						
arsenic	T57.0X1	T57.0X2	T57.0X3	T57.0X4	—	—
hellebore	T62.2X1	T62.2X2	T62.2X3	T62.2X4	—	—
lotion (keratolytic)	T49.4X1	T49.4X2	T49.4X3	T49.4X4	T49.4X5	T49.4X6
spirit	T52.0X1	T52.0X2	T52.0X3	T52.0X4	—	—
Whitewash	T65.891	T65.892	T65.893	T65.894		
Whole blood (human)	T45.8X1	T45.8X2	T45.8X3	T45.8X4	T45.8X5	T45.8X6
Wild						
black cherry	T62.2X1	T62.2X2	T62.2X3	T62.2X4	—	—
poisonous plants NEC	T62.2X1	T62.2X2	T62.2X3	T62.2X4	—	—
Window cleaning fluid	T65.891	T65.892	T65.893	T65.894		
Wintergreen (oil)	T49.3X1	T49.3X2	T49.3X3	T49.3X4	T49.3X5	T49.3X6
Wisterine	T62.2X1	T62.2X2	T62.2X3	T62.2X4		
Witch hazel	T49.2X1	T49.2X2	T49.2X3	T49.2X4	T49.2X5	T49.2X6
Wood alcohol or spirit	T51.1X1	T51.1X2	T51.1X3	T51.1X4		
Wool fat (hydrous)	T49.3X1	T49.3X2	T49.3X3	T49.3X4	T49.3X5	T49.3X6
Woorali	T48.1X1	T48.1X2	T48.1X3	T48.1X4	T48.1X5	T48.1X6
Wormseed, American	T37.4X1	T37.4X2	T37.4X3	T37.4X4	T37.4X5	T37.4X6

Substance	Poisoning, Accidental (unintentional)	Poisoning, Intentional Self-harm	Poisoning, Assault	Poisoning, Undetermined	Adverse Effect	Under-dosing
Xamoterol	T44.5X1	T44.5X2	T44.5X3	T44.5X4	T44.5X5	T44.5X6
Xanthine diuretics	T50.2X1	T50.2X2	T50.2X3	T50.2X4	T50.2X5	T50.2X6
Xanthinol nicotinate	T46.7X1	T46.7X2	T46.7X3	T46.7X4	T46.7X5	T46.7X6
Xanthotoxin	T49.3X1	T49.3X2	T49.3X3	T49.3X4	T49.3X5	T49.3X6
Xantinol nicotinate	T46.7X1	T46.7X2	T46.7X3	T46.7X4	T46.7X5	T46.7X6
Xantocillin	T36.0X1	T36.0X2	T36.0X3	T36.0X4	T36.0X5	T36.0X6
Xenon (127Xe) (133Xe)	T50.8X1	T50.8X2	T50.8X3	T50.8X4	T50.8X5	T50.8X6
Xenysalate	T49.4X1	T49.4X2	T49.4X3	T49.4X4	T49.4X5	T49.4X6
Xibornol	T37.8X1	T37.8X2	T37.8X3	T37.8X4	T37.8X5	T37.8X6
Xigris	T45.511	T45.512	T45.513	T45.514	T45.515	T45.516
Xipamide	T50.2X1	T50.2X2	T50.2X3	T50.2X4	T50.2X5	T50.2X6
Xylene (vapor)	T52.2X1	T52.2X2	T52.2X3	T52.2X4	—	—
Xylocaine (infiltration) (topical)	T41.3X1	T41.3X2	T41.3X3	T41.3X4	T41.3X5	T41.3X6
nerve block (peripheral) (plexus)	T41.3X1	T41.3X2	T41.3X3	T41.3X4	T41.3X5	T41.3X6
spinal	T41.3X1	T41.3X2	T41.3X3	T41.3X4	T41.3X5	T41.3X6
Xylol (vapor)	T52.2X1	T52.2X2	T52.2X3	T52.2X4	—	—
Xylometazoline	T48.5X1	T48.5X2	T48.5X3	T48.5X4	T48.5X5	T48.5X6
Yeast	T45.2X1	T45.2X2	T45.2X3	T45.2X4	T45.2X5	T45.2X6
dried	T45.2X1	T45.2X2	T45.2X3	T45.2X4	T45.2X5	T45.2X6
Yellow						
fever vaccine	T50.B91	T50.B92	T50.B93	T50.B94	T50.B95	T50.B96
jasmine	T62.2X1	T62.2X2	T62.2X3	T62.2X4		
phenolphthalein	T47.2X1	T47.2X2	T47.2X3	T47.2X4	T47.2X5	T47.2X6
Yew	T62.2X1	T62.2X2	T62.2X3	T62.2X4		
Yohimbic acid	T40.991	T40.992	T40.993	T40.994	T40.995	T40.996
Zactane	T39.8X1	T39.8X2	T39.8X3	T39.8X4	T39.8X5	T39.8X6
Zalcitabine	T37.5X1	T37.5X2	T37.5X3	T37.5X4	T37.5X5	T37.5X6
Zaroxolyn	T50.2X1	T50.2X2	T50.2X3	T50.2X4	T50.2X5	T50.2X6
Zephiran (topical)	T49.0X1	T49.0X2	T49.0X3	T49.0X4	T49.0X5	T49.0X6
ophthalmic preparation	T49.5X1	T49.5X2	T49.5X3	T49.5X4	T49.5X5	T49.5X6
Zeranol	T38.7X1	T38.7X2	T38.7X3	T38.7X4	T38.7X5	T38.7X6
Zerone	T51.1X1	T51.1X2	T51.1X3	T51.1X4		
Zidovudine	T37.5X1	T37.5X2	T37.5X3	T37.5X4	T37.5X5	T37.5X6
Zimeldine	T43.221	T43.222	T43.223	T43.224	T43.225	T43.226
Zinc (compounds) (fumes) (vapor)	T56.5X1	T56.5X2	T56.5X3	T56.5X4	—	—
NEC						
anti-infectives	T49.0X1	T49.0X2	T49.0X3	T49.0X4	T49.0X5	T49.0X6
antivaricose	T46.8X1	T46.8X2	T46.8X3	T46.8X4	T46.8X5	T46.8X6
bacitracin	T49.0X1	T49.0X2	T49.0X3	T49.0X4	T49.0X5	T49.0X6
chloride (mouthwash)	T49.6X1	T49.6X2	T49.6X3	T49.6X4	T49.6X5	T49.6X6
chromate	T56.5X1	T56.5X2	T56.5X3	T56.5X4		
gelatin	T49.3X1	T49.3X2	T49.3X3	T49.3X4	T49.3X5	T49.3X6
oxide	T49.3X1	T49.3X2	T49.3X3	T49.3X4	T49.3X5	T49.3X6
plaster	T49.3X1	T49.3X2	T49.3X3	T49.3X4	T49.3X5	T49.3X6
peroxide	T49.0X1	T49.0X2	T49.0X3	T49.0X4	T49.0X5	T49.0X6
pesticides	T56.5X1	T56.5X2	T56.5X3	T56.5X4		
phosphide	T60.4X1	T60.4X2	T60.4X3	T60.4X4	—	—
pyrithionate	T49.4X1	T49.4X2	T49.4X3	T49.4X4	T49.4X5	T49.4X6
stearate	T49.3X1	T49.3X2	T49.3X3	T49.3X4	T49.3X5	T49.3X6
sulfate	T49.5X1	T49.5X2	T49.5X3	T49.5X4	T49.5X5	T49.5X6
ENT agent	T49.6X1	T49.6X2	T49.6X3	T49.6X4	T49.6X5	T49.6X6
ophthalmic solution	T49.5X1	T49.5X2	T49.5X3	T49.5X4	T49.5X5	T49.5X6
topical NEC	T49.0X1	T49.0X2	T49.0X3	T49.0X4	T49.0X5	T49.0X6
undecylenate	T49.0X1	T49.0X2	T49.0X3	T49.0X4	T49.0X5	T49.0X6
Zineb	T60.0X1	T60.0X2	T60.0X3	T60.0X4		
Zinostatin	T45.1X1	T45.1X2	T45.1X3	T45.1X4	T45.1X5	T45.1X6
Zipeprol	T48.3X1	T48.3X2	T48.3X3	T48.3X4	T48.3X5	T48.3X6
Zofenopril	T46.4X1	T46.4X2	T46.4X3	T46.4X4	T46.4X5	T46.4X6
Zolpidem	T42.6X1	T42.6X2	T42.6X3	T42.6X4	T42.6X5	T42.6X6
Zomepirac	T39.391	T39.392	T39.393	T39.394	T39.395	T39.396
Zopiclone	T42.6X1	T42.6X2	T42.6X3	T42.6X4	T42.6X5	T42.6X6
Zorubicin	T45.1X1	T45.1X2	T45.1X3	T45.1X4	T45.1X5	T45.1X6
Zotepine	T43.591	T43.592	T43.593	T43.594	T43.595	T43.596
Zovant	T45.511	T45.512	T45.513	T45.514	T45.515	T45.516
Zoxazolamine	T42.8X1	T42.8X2	T42.8X3	T42.8X4	T42.8X5	T42.8X6
Zuclopenthixol	T43.4X1	T43.4X2	T43.4X3	T43.4X4	T43.4X5	T43.4X6
Zygadenus (venenosus)	T62.2X1	T62.2X2	T62.2X3	T62.2X4		
Zyprexa	T43.591	T43.592	T43.593	T43.594	T43.595	T43.596

Additional Character May Be Required — Refer to the Tabular List for Character Selection   Subterms under main terms may continue to next column or page

ICD-10-CM Index to External Causes

A

Abandonment (causing exposure to weather conditions) (with intent to injure or kill) NEC X58 ☑
Abuse (adult) (child) (mental) (physical) (sexual) X58 ☑
Accident (to) X58 ☑
aircraft (in transit) (powered) (see also Accident, transport, aircraft)
due to, caused by cataclysm — see Forces of nature, by type
animal-drawn vehicle — see Accident, transport, animal-drawn vehicle occupant
animal-rider — see Accident, transport, animal-rider
automobile — see Accident, transport, car occupant
bare foot water skier V94.4 ☑
boat, boating (see also Accident, watercraft)
striking swimmer
powered V94.11 ☑
unpowered V94.12 ☑
bus — see Accident, transport, bus occupant
<Insert new term here>
cable car, not on rails V98.0 ☑
on rails — see Accident, transport, streetcar occupant
car — see Accident, transport, car occupant
caused by, due to
animal NEC W64 ☑
chain hoist W24.0 ☑
cold (excessive) — see Exposure, cold
corrosive liquid, substance — see Table of Drugs and Chemicals
cutting or piercing instrument — see Contact, with, by type of instrument
drive belt W24.0 ☑
electric
current — see Exposure, electric current
motor (see also Contact, with, by type of machine) W31.3 ☑
current (of) W86.8 ☑
environmental factor NEC X58 ☑
explosive material — see Explosion
fire, flames — see Exposure, fire
firearm missile — see Discharge, firearm by type
heat (excessive) — see Heat
hot — see Contact, with, hot
ignition — see Ignition
lifting device W24.0 ☑
lightning — see subcategory T75.0 ☑
causing fire — see Exposure, fire
machine, machinery — see Contact, with, by type of machine
natural factor NEC X58 ☑
pulley (block) W24.0 ☑
radiation — see Radiation
steam X13.1 ☑
inhalation X13.0 ☑
pipe X16 ☑
thunderbolt — see subcategory T75.0 ☑
causing fire — see Exposure, fire
transmission device W24.1 ☑
coach — see Accident, transport, bus occupant
coal car — see Accident, transport, industrial vehicle occupant
diving (see also Fall, into, water)
with
drowning or submersion — see Drowning
forklift — see Accident, transport, industrial vehicle occupant
heavy transport vehicle NOS — see Accident, transport, truck occupant
ice yacht V98.2 ☑
in
medical, surgical procedure
as, or due to misadventure — see Misadventure
causing an abnormal reaction or later complication without mention of misadventure (see also Complication of or following, by type of procedure) Y84.9
land yacht V98.1 ☑
late effect of — see W00-X58 with 7th character S

logging car — see Accident, transport, industrial vehicle occupant
machine, machinery (see also Contact, with, by type of machine)
on board watercraft V93.69 ☑
explosion — see Explosion, in, watercraft
fire — see Burn, on board watercraft
powered craft V93.63 ☑
ferry boat V93.61 ☑
fishing boat V93.62 ☑
jetskis V93.63 ☑
liner V93.61 ☑
merchant ship V93.60 ☑
passenger ship V93.61 ☑
sailboat V93.64 ☑
mine tram — see Accident, transport, industrial vehicle occupant
mobility scooter (motorized) — see Accident, transport, pedestrian, conveyance, specified type NEC
motor scooter — see Accident, transport, motorcyclist
motor vehicle NOS (traffic) (see also Accident, transport) V89.2 ☑
nontraffic V89.0 ☑
three-wheeled NOS — see Accident, transport, three-wheeled motor vehicle occupant
motorcycle NOS — see Accident, transport, motorcyclist
nonmotor vehicle NOS (nontraffic) (see also Accident, transport) V89.1 ☑
traffic NOS V89.3 ☑
nontraffic (victim's mode of transport NOS) V88.9 ☑
collision (between) V88.7 ☑
bus and truck V88.5 ☑
car and:
bus V88.3 ☑
pickup V88.2 ☑
three-wheeled motor vehicle V88.0 ☑
train V88.6 ☑
truck V88.4 ☑
two-wheeled motor vehicle V88.0 ☑
van V88.2 ☑
specified vehicle NEC and:
three-wheeled motor vehicle V88.1 ☑
two-wheeled motor vehicle V88.1 ☑
known mode of transport — see Accident, transport, by type of vehicle
noncollision V88.8 ☑
on board watercraft V93.89 ☑
powered craft V93.83 ☑
ferry boat V93.81 ☑
fishing boat V93.82 ☑
jetskis V93.83 ☑
liner V93.81 ☑
merchant ship V93.80 ☑
passenger ship V93.81 ☑
unpowered craft V93.88 ☑
canoe V93.85 ☑
inflatable V93.86 ☑
in tow
recreational V94.31 ☑
specified NEC V94.32 ☑
kayak V93.85 ☑
sailboat V93.84 ☑
surf-board V93.88 ☑
water skis V93.87 ☑
windsurfer V93.88 ☑
parachutist V97.29 ☑
entangled in object V97.21 ☑
injured on landing V97.22 ☑
pedal cycle — see Accident, transport, pedal cyclist
pedestrian (on foot)
with
another pedestrian W51 ☑
with fall W03 ☑
due to ice or snow W00.0 ☑
on pedestrian conveyance NEC V00.09 ☑
roller skater (in-line) V00.01 ☑
skate boarder V00.02 ☑
transport vehicle — see Accident, transport

pedestrian — continued
on pedestrian conveyance — see Accident, transport, pedestrian, conveyance
pick-up truck or van — see Accident, transport, pickup truck occupant
quarry truck — see Accident, transport, industrial vehicle occupant
railway vehicle (any) (in motion) — see Accident, transport, railway vehicle occupant
due to cataclysm — see Forces of nature, by type
scooter (non-motorized) — see Accident, transport, pedestrian, conveyance, scooter
sequelae of — see categories W00-X58 with 7th character S
skateboard — see Accident, transport, pedestrian, conveyance, skateboard
ski(ing) — see Accident, transport, pedestrian, conveyance
lift V98.3 ☑
specified cause NEC X58 ☑
streetcar — see Accident, transport, streetcar occupant
traffic (victim's mode of transport NOS) V87.9 ☑
collision (between) V87.7 ☑
bus and truck V87.5 ☑
car and:
bus V87.3 ☑
pickup V87.2 ☑
three-wheeled motor vehicle V87.0 ☑
train V87.6 ☑
truck V87.4 ☑
two-wheeled motor vehicle V87.0 ☑
van V87.2 ☑
specified vehicle NEC and:
three-wheeled motor vehicle V87.1 ☑
two-wheeled motor vehicle V87.1 ☑
known mode of transport — see Accident, transport, by type of vehicle
noncollision V87.8 ☑
transport (involving injury to) V99 ☑
18 wheeler — see Accident, transport, truck occupant
agricultural vehicle occupant (nontraffic) V84.9 ☑
driver V84.5 ☑
hanger-on V84.7 ☑
passenger V84.6 ☑
traffic V84.3 ☑
driver V84.0 ☑
hanger-on V84.2 ☑
passenger V84.1 ☑
while boarding or alighting V84.4 ☑
aircraft NEC V97.89 ☑
military NEC V97.818 ☑
with civilian aircraft V97.810 ☑
civilian injured by V97.811 ☑
occupant injured (in)
nonpowered craft accident V96.9 ☑
balloon V96.00 ☑
collision V96.03 ☑
crash V96.01 ☑
explosion V96.05 ☑
fire V96.04 ☑
forced landing V96.02 ☑
specified type NEC V96.09 ☑
glider V96.20 ☑
collision V96.23 ☑
crash V96.21 ☑
explosion V96.25 ☑
fire V96.24 ☑
forced landing V96.22 ☑
specified type NEC V96.29 ☑
hang glider V96.10 ☑
collision V96.13 ☑
crash V96.11 ☑
explosion V96.15 ☑
fire V96.14 ☑
forced landing V96.12 ☑
specified type NEC V96.19 ☑
specified craft NEC V96.8 ☑
powered craft accident V95.9 ☑

☷ **Subterms under main terms may continue to next column or page**   ☑ **Additional Character Required — Refer to the Tabular List for Character Selection**

Accident — *continued*
  transport — *continued*
   aircraft — *continued*
    occupant injured — *continued*
     powered craft accident — *continued*
      fixed wing
       commercial V95.30 ☑
        collision V95.33 ☑
        crash V95.31 ☑
        explosion V95.35 ☑
        fire V95.34 ☑
        forced landing V95.32 ☑
        specified type NEC V95.39 ☑
       private V95.20 ☑
        collision V95.23 ☑
        crash V95.21 ☑
        explosion V95.25 ☑
        fire V95.24 ☑
        forced landing V95.22 ☑
        specified type NEC V95.29 ☑
      glider V95.10 ☑
       collision V95.13 ☑
       crash V95.11 ☑
       explosion V95.15 ☑
       fire V95.14 ☑
       forced landing V95.12 ☑
       specified type NEC V95.19 ☑
      helicopter V95.00 ☑
       collision V95.03 ☑
       crash V95.01 ☑
       explosion V95.05 ☑
       fire V95.04 ☑
       forced landing V95.02 ☑
       specified type NEC V95.09 ☑
      spacecraft V95.40 ☑
       collision V95.43 ☑
       crash V95.41 ☑
       explosion V95.45 ☑
       fire V95.44 ☑
       forced landing V95.42 ☑
       specified type NEC V95.49 ☑
      specified craft NEC V95.8 ☑
      ultralight V95.10 ☑
       collision V95.13 ☑
       crash V95.11 ☑
       explosion V95.15 ☑
       fire V95.14 ☑
       forced landing V95.12 ☑
       specified type NEC V95.19 ☑
     specified accident NEC V97.0 ☑
     while boarding or alighting V97.1 ☑
    person (injured by)
     falling from, in or on aircraft V97.0 ☑
     machinery on aircraft V97.89 ☑
     on ground with aircraft involvement V97.39 ☑
     rotating propeller V97.32 ☑
     struck by object falling from aircraft V97.31 ☑
     sucked into aircraft jet V97.33 ☑
     while boarding or alighting aircraft V97.1 ☑
   airport (battery-powered) passenger vehicle — *see* Accident, transport, industrial vehicle occupant
   all-terrain vehicle occupant (nontraffic) V86.99 ☑
    driver V86.59 ☑
    dune buggy — *see* Accident, transport, dune buggy occupant
    hanger-on V86.79 ☑
    passenger V86.69 ☑
    snowmobile — *see* Accident, transport, snowmobile occupant
    traffic V86.39 ☑
     driver V86.09 ☑
     hanger-on V86.29 ☑
     passenger V86.19 ☑
    while boarding or alighting V86.49 ☑
   ambulance occupant (traffic) V86.31 ☑
    driver V86.01 ☑
    hanger-on V86.21 ☑
    nontraffic V86.91 ☑
     driver V86.51 ☑
     hanger-on V86.71 ☑
     passenger V86.61 ☑
    passenger V86.11 ☑
    while boarding or alighting V86.41 ☑

Accident — *continued*
  transport — *continued*
   animal-drawn vehicle occupant (in) V80.929 ☑
    collision (with)
     animal V80.12 ☑
      being ridden V80.711 ☑
     animal-drawn vehicle V80.721 ☑
     bus V80.42 ☑
     car V80.42 ☑
     fixed or stationary object V80.82 ☑
     military vehicle V80.920 ☑
     nonmotor vehicle V80.791 ☑
     pedal cycle V80.22 ☑
     pedestrian V80.12 ☑
     pickup V80.42 ☑
     railway train or vehicle V80.62 ☑
     specified motor vehicle NEC V80.52 ☑
     streetcar V80.731 ☑
     truck V80.42 ☑
     two- or three-wheeled motor vehicle V80.32 ☑
     van V80.42 ☑
    noncollision V80.02 ☑
    specified circumstance NEC V80.928 ☑
   animal-rider V80.919 ☑
    collision (with)
     animal V80.11 ☑
      being ridden V80.710 ☑
     animal-drawn vehicle V80.720 ☑
     bus V80.41 ☑
     car V80.41 ☑
     fixed or stationary object V80.81 ☑
     military vehicle V80.910 ☑
     nonmotor vehicle V80.790 ☑
     pedal cycle V80.21 ☑
     pedestrian V80.11 ☑
     pickup V80.41 ☑
     railway train or vehicle V80.61 ☑
     specified motor vehicle NEC V80.51 ☑
     streetcar V80.730 ☑
     truck V80.41 ☑
     two- or three-wheeled motor vehicle V80.31 ☑
     van V80.41 ☑
    noncollision V80.018 ☑
     specified as horse rider V80.010 ☑
    specified circumstance NEC V80.918 ☑
   armored car — *see* Accident, transport, truck occupant
   battery-powered truck (baggage) (mail) — *see* Accident, transport, industrial vehicle occupant
   bus occupant V79.9 ☑
    collision (with)
     animal (traffic) V70.9 ☑
      being ridden (traffic) V76.9 ☑
       nontraffic V76.3 ☑
       while boarding or alighting V76.4 ☑
      nontraffic V70.3 ☑
      while boarding or alighting V70.4 ☑
     animal-drawn vehicle (traffic) V76.9 ☑
      nontraffic V76.3 ☑
      while boarding or alighting V76.4 ☑
     bus (traffic) V74.9 ☑
      nontraffic V74.3 ☑
      while boarding or alighting V74.4 ☑
     car (traffic) V73.9 ☑
      nontraffic V73.3 ☑
      while boarding or alighting V73.4 ☑
     motor vehicle NOS (traffic) V79.60 ☑
      nontraffic V79.20 ☑
      specified type NEC (traffic) V79.69 ☑
       nontraffic V79.29 ☑
     pedal cycle (traffic) V71.9 ☑
      nontraffic V71.3 ☑
      while boarding or alighting V71.4 ☑
     pickup truck (traffic) V73.9 ☑
      nontraffic V73.3 ☑
      while boarding or alighting V73.4 ☑
     railway vehicle (traffic) V75.9 ☑
      nontraffic V75.3 ☑
      while boarding or alighting V75.4 ☑
     specified vehicle NEC (traffic) V76.9 ☑
      nontraffic V76.3 ☑
      while boarding or alighting V76.4 ☑
     stationary object (traffic) V77.9 ☑

Accident — *continued*
  transport — *continued*
   bus occupant — *continued*
    collision — *continued*
     stationary object — *continued*
      nontraffic V77.3 ☑
      while boarding or alighting V77.4 ☑
     streetcar (traffic) V76.9 ☑
      nontraffic V76.3 ☑
      while boarding or alighting V76.4 ☑
     three wheeled motor vehicle (traffic) V72.9 ☑
      nontraffic V72.3 ☑
      while boarding or alighting V72.4 ☑
     truck (traffic) V74.9 ☑
      nontraffic V74.3 ☑
      while boarding or alighting V74.4 ☑
     two wheeled motor vehicle (traffic) V72.9 ☑
      nontraffic V72.3 ☑
      while boarding or alighting V72.4 ☑
     van (traffic) V73.9 ☑
      nontraffic V73.3 ☑
      while boarding or alighting V73.4 ☑
   driver
    collision (with)
     animal (traffic) V70.5 ☑
      being ridden (traffic) V76.5 ☑
       nontraffic V76.0 ☑
      nontraffic V70.0 ☑
     animal-drawn vehicle (traffic) V76.5 ☑
      nontraffic V76.0 ☑
     bus (traffic) V74.5 ☑
      nontraffic V74.0 ☑
     car (traffic) V73.5 ☑
      nontraffic V73.0 ☑
     motor vehicle NOS (traffic) V79.40 ☑
      nontraffic V79.00 ☑
      specified type NEC (traffic) V79.49 ☑
       nontraffic V79.09 ☑
     pedal cycle (traffic) V71.5 ☑
      nontraffic V71.0 ☑
     pickup truck (traffic) V73.5 ☑
      nontraffic V73.0 ☑
     railway vehicle (traffic) V75.5 ☑
      nontraffic V75.0 ☑
     specified vehicle NEC (traffic) V76.5 ☑
      nontraffic V76.0 ☑
     stationary object (traffic) V77.5 ☑
      nontraffic V77.0 ☑
     streetcar (traffic) V76.5 ☑
      nontraffic V76.0 ☑
     three wheeled motor vehicle (traffic) V72.5 ☑
      nontraffic V72.0 ☑
     truck (traffic) V74.5 ☑
      nontraffic V74.0 ☑
     two wheeled motor vehicle (traffic) V72.5 ☑
      nontraffic V72.0 ☑
     van (traffic) V73.5 ☑
      nontraffic V73.0 ☑
    noncollision accident (traffic) V78.5 ☑
     nontraffic V78.0 ☑
   hanger-on
    collision (with)
     animal (traffic) V70.7 ☑
      being ridden (traffic) V76.7 ☑
       nontraffic V76.2 ☑
      nontraffic V70.2 ☑
     animal-drawn vehicle (traffic) V76.7 ☑
      nontraffic V76.2 ☑
     bus (traffic) V74.7 ☑
      nontraffic V74.2 ☑
     car (traffic) V73.7 ☑
      nontraffic V73.2 ☑
     pedal cycle (traffic) V71.7 ☑
      nontraffic V71.2 ☑
     pickup truck (traffic) V73.7 ☑
      nontraffic V73.2 ☑
     railway vehicle (traffic) V75.7 ☑
      nontraffic V75.2 ☑
     specified vehicle NEC (traffic) V76.7 ☑
      nontraffic V76.2 ☑
     stationary object (traffic) V77.7 ☑
      nontraffic V77.2 ☑
     streetcar (traffic) V76.7 ☑

Accident — *continued*
  transport — *continued*
    bus occupant — *continued*
      hanger-on — *continued*
        collision — *continued*
          streetcar — *continued*
            nontraffic V76.2
            three wheeled motor vehicle (traffic)
              V72.7 ☑
              nontraffic V72.2 ☑
            truck (traffic) V74.7 ☑
              nontraffic V74.2 ☑
            two wheeled motor vehicle (traffic)
              V72.7 ☑
              nontraffic V72.2 ☑
            van (traffic) V73.7 ☑
              nontraffic V73.2 ☑
        noncollision accident (traffic) V78.7 ☑
          nontraffic V78.2 ☑
      noncollision accident (traffic) V78.9 ☑
        nontraffic V78.3 ☑
        while boarding or alighting V78.4 ☑
      nontraffic V79.3 ☑
      passenger
        collision (with)
          animal (traffic) V70.6 ☑
            being ridden (traffic) V76.6 ☑
              nontraffic V76.1 ☑
            nontraffic V70.1 ☑
          animal-drawn vehicle (traffic) V76.6 ☑
            nontraffic V76.1 ☑
          bus (traffic) V74.6 ☑
            nontraffic V74.1 ☑
          car (traffic) V73.6 ☑
            nontraffic V73.1 ☑
          motor vehicle NOS (traffic) V79.50 ☑
            nontraffic V79.10 ☑
            specified type NEC (traffic) V79.59 ☑
              nontraffic V79.19 ☑
          pedal cycle (traffic) V71.6 ☑
            nontraffic V71.1 ☑
          pickup truck (traffic) V73.6 ☑
            nontraffic V73.1 ☑
          railway vehicle (traffic) V75.6 ☑
            nontraffic V75.1 ☑
          specified vehicle NEC (traffic) V76.6 ☑
            nontraffic V76.1 ☑
          stationary object (traffic) V77.6 ☑
            nontraffic V77.1 ☑
          streetcar (traffic) V76.6 ☑
            nontraffic V76.1 ☑
          three wheeled motor vehicle (traffic)
            V72.6 ☑
            nontraffic V72.1 ☑
          truck (traffic) V74.6 ☑
            nontraffic V74.1 ☑
          two wheeled motor vehicle (traffic)
            V72.6 ☑
            nontraffic V72.1 ☑
          van (traffic) V73.6 ☑
            nontraffic V73.1 ☑
        noncollision accident (traffic) V78.6 ☑
          nontraffic V78.1 ☑
      specified type NEC V79.88 ☑
        military vehicle V79.81 ☑
    cable car, not on rails V98.0 ☑
      on rails — *see* Accident, transport, streetcar
        occupant
    car occupant V49.9 ☑
      ambulance occupant — *see* Accident, transport,
        ambulance occupant
      collision (with)
        animal (traffic) V40.9 ☑
          being ridden (traffic) V46.9 ☑
            nontraffic V46.3 ☑
            while boarding or alighting V46.4 ☑
          nontraffic V40.3 ☑
          while boarding or alighting V40.4 ☑
        animal-drawn vehicle (traffic) V46.9 ☑
          nontraffic V46.3 ☑
          while boarding or alighting V46.4 ☑
        bus (traffic) V44.9 ☑
          nontraffic V44.3 ☑
          while boarding or alighting V44.4 ☑
        car (traffic) V43.92 ☑
          nontraffic V43.32 ☑

Accident — *continued*
  transport — *continued*
    car occupant — *continued*
      collision — *continued*
        car — *continued*
          while boarding or alighting V43.42 ☑
        motor vehicle NOS (traffic) V49.60 ☑
          nontraffic V49.20 ☑
          specified type NEC (traffic) V49.69 ☑
            nontraffic V49.29 ☑
        pedal cycle (traffic) V41.9 ☑
          nontraffic V41.3 ☑
          while boarding or alighting V41.4 ☑
        pickup truck (traffic) V43.93 ☑
          nontraffic V43.33 ☑
          while boarding or alighting V43.43 ☑
        railway vehicle (traffic) V45.9 ☑
          nontraffic V45.3 ☑
          while boarding or alighting V45.4 ☑
        specified vehicle NEC (traffic) V46.9 ☑
          nontraffic V46.3 ☑
          while boarding or alighting V46.4 ☑
        sport utility vehicle (traffic) V43.91 ☑
          nontraffic V43.31 ☑
          while boarding or alighting V43.41 ☑
        stationary object (traffic) V47.92 ☑
          nontraffic V47.32 ☑
          while boarding or alighting V47.4 ☑
        streetcar (traffic) V46.9 ☑
          nontraffic V46.3 ☑
          while boarding or alighting V46.4 ☑
        three wheeled motor vehicle (traffic)
          V42.9 ☑
          nontraffic V42.3 ☑
          while boarding or alighting V42.4 ☑
        truck (traffic) V44.9 ☑
          nontraffic V44.3 ☑
          while boarding or alighting V44.4 ☑
        two wheeled motor vehicle (traffic) V42.9 ☑
          nontraffic V42.3 ☑
          while boarding or alighting V42.4 ☑
        van (traffic) V43.94 ☑
          nontraffic V43.34 ☑
          while boarding or alighting V43.44 ☑
      driver
        collision (with)
          animal (traffic) V40.5 ☑
            being ridden (traffic) V46.5 ☑
              nontraffic V46.0 ☑
            nontraffic V40.0 ☑
          animal-drawn vehicle (traffic) V46.5 ☑
            nontraffic V46.0 ☑
          bus (traffic) V44.5 ☑
            nontraffic V44.0 ☑
          car (traffic) V43.52 ☑
            nontraffic V43.02 ☑
          motor vehicle NOS (traffic) V49.40 ☑
            nontraffic V49.00 ☑
            specified type NEC (traffic) V49.49 ☑
              nontraffic V49.09 ☑
          pedal cycle (traffic) V41.5 ☑
            nontraffic V41.0 ☑
          pickup truck (traffic) V43.53 ☑
            nontraffic V43.03 ☑
          railway vehicle (traffic) V45.5 ☑
            nontraffic V45.0 ☑
          specified vehicle NEC (traffic) V46.5 ☑
            nontraffic V46.0 ☑
          sport utility vehicle (traffic) V43.51 ☑
            nontraffic V43.01 ☑
          stationary object (traffic) V47.52 ☑
            nontraffic V47.02 ☑
          streetcar (traffic) V46.5 ☑
            nontraffic V46.0 ☑
          three wheeled motor vehicle (traffic)
            V42.5 ☑
            nontraffic V42.0 ☑
          truck (traffic) V44.5 ☑
            nontraffic V44.0 ☑
          two wheeled motor vehicle (traffic)
            V42.5 ☑
            nontraffic V42.0 ☑
          van (traffic) V43.54 ☑
            nontraffic V43.04 ☑
        noncollision accident (traffic) V48.5 ☑
          nontraffic V48.0 ☑

Accident — *continued*
  transport — *continued*
    car occupant — *continued*
      hanger-on
        collision (with)
          animal (traffic) V40.7 ☑
            being ridden (traffic) V46.7 ☑
              nontraffic V46.2 ☑
            nontraffic V40.2 ☑
          animal-drawn vehicle (traffic) V46.7 ☑
            nontraffic V46.2 ☑
          bus (traffic) V44.7 ☑
            nontraffic V44.2 ☑
          car (traffic) V43.72 ☑
            nontraffic V43.22 ☑
          pedal cycle (traffic) V41.7 ☑
            nontraffic V41.2 ☑
          pickup truck (traffic) V43.73 ☑
            nontraffic V43.23 ☑
          railway vehicle (traffic) V45.7 ☑
            nontraffic V45.2 ☑
          specified vehicle NEC (traffic) V46.7 ☑
            nontraffic V46.2 ☑
          sport utility vehicle (traffic) V43.71 ☑
            nontraffic V43.21 ☑
          stationary object (traffic) V47.7 ☑
            nontraffic V47.2 ☑
          streetcar (traffic) V46.7 ☑
            nontraffic V46.2 ☑
          three wheeled motor vehicle (traffic)
            V42.7 ☑
            nontraffic V42.2 ☑
          truck (traffic) V44.7 ☑
            nontraffic V44.2 ☑
          two wheeled motor vehicle (traffic)
            V42.7 ☑
            nontraffic V42.2 ☑
          van (traffic) V43.74 ☑
            nontraffic V43.24 ☑
        noncollision accident (traffic) V48.7 ☑
          nontraffic V48.2 ☑
      noncollision accident (traffic) V48.9 ☑
        nontraffic V48.3 ☑
        while boarding or alighting V48.4 ☑
      nontraffic V49.3 ☑
      passenger
        collision (with)
          animal (traffic) V40.6 ☑
            being ridden (traffic) V46.6 ☑
              nontraffic V46.1 ☑
            nontraffic V40.1 ☑
          animal-drawn vehicle (traffic) V46.6 ☑
            nontraffic V46.1 ☑
          bus (traffic) V44.6 ☑
            nontraffic V44.1 ☑
          car (traffic) V43.62 ☑
            nontraffic V43.12 ☑
          motor vehicle NOS (traffic) V49.50 ☑
            nontraffic V49.10 ☑
            specified type NEC (traffic) V49.59 ☑
              nontraffic V49.19 ☑
          pedal cycle (traffic) V41.6 ☑
            nontraffic V41.1 ☑
          pickup truck (traffic) V43.63 ☑
            nontraffic V43.13 ☑
          railway vehicle (traffic) V45.6 ☑
            nontraffic V45.1 ☑
          specified vehicle NEC (traffic) V46.6 ☑
            nontraffic V46.1 ☑
          sport utility vehicle (traffic) V43.61 ☑
            nontraffic V43.11 ☑
          stationary object (traffic) V47.62 ☑
            nontraffic V47.12 ☑
          streetcar (traffic) V46.6 ☑
            nontraffic V46.1 ☑
          three wheeled motor vehicle (traffic)
            V42.6 ☑
            nontraffic V42.1 ☑
          truck (traffic) V44.6 ☑
            nontraffic V44.1 ☑
          two wheeled motor vehicle (traffic)
            V42.6 ☑
            nontraffic V42.1 ☑
          van (traffic) V43.64 ☑
            nontraffic V43.14 ☑
        noncollision accident (traffic) V48.6 ☑

External Causes Index

Accident — Accident

Accident — *continued*
  transport — *continued*
    car occupant — *continued*
      passenger — *continued*
        noncollision accident — *continued*
          nontraffic V48.1 ☑
        specified type NEC V49.88 ☑
        military vehicle V49.81 ☑
    coal car — *see* Accident, transport, industrial vehicle occupant
    construction vehicle occupant (nontraffic) V85.9 ☑
      driver V85.5 ☑
      hanger-on V85.7 ☑
      passenger V85.6 ☑
      traffic V85.3 ☑
        driver V85.0 ☑
        hanger-on V85.2 ☑
        passenger V85.1 ☑
      while boarding or alighting V85.4 ☑
    dirt bike rider — *see* Accident, transport, all-terrain vehicle occupant
    due to cataclysm — *see* Forces of nature, by type
    dune buggy occupant (nontraffic) V86.93 ☑
      driver V86.53 ☑
      hanger-on V86.73 ☑
      passenger V86.63 ☑
      traffic V86.33 ☑
        driver V86.03 ☑
        hanger-on V86.23 ☑
        passenger V86.13 ☑
      while boarding or alighting V86.43 ☑
    forklift — *see* Accident, transport, industrial vehicle occupant
    go cart — *see* Accident, transport, all-terrain vehicle occupant
    golf cart — *see* Accident, transport, all-terrain vehicle occupant
    heavy transport vehicle occupant — *see* Accident, transport, truck occupant
    ice yacht V98.2 ☑
    industrial vehicle occupant (nontraffic) V83.9 ☑
      driver V83.5 ☑
      hanger-on V83.7 ☑
      passenger V83.6 ☑
      traffic V83.3 ☑
        driver V83.0 ☑
        hanger-on V83.2 ☑
        passenger V83.1 ☑
      while boarding or alighting V83.4 ☑
    interurban electric car — *see* Accident, transport, streetcar
    land yacht V98.1 ☑
    logging car — *see* Accident, transport, industrial vehicle occupant
    military vehicle occupant (traffic) V86.34 ☑
      driver V86.04 ☑
      hanger-on V86.24 ☑
      nontraffic V86.94 ☑
        driver V86.54 ☑
        hanger-on V86.74 ☑
        passenger V86.64 ☑
      passenger V86.14 ☑
      while boarding or alighting V86.44 ☑
    mine tram — *see* Accident, transport, industrial vehicle occupant
    motor vehicle NEC occupant (traffic) V86.39 ☑
      driver V86.09 ☑
      hanger-on V86.29 ☑
      nontraffic V86.99 ☑
        driver V86.59 ☑
        hanger-on V86.79 ☑
        passenger V86.69 ☑
      passenger V86.19 ☑
      while boarding or alighting V86.49 ☑
    motorcoach — *see* Accident, transport, bus occupant
    motorcyclist V29.9 ☑
      collision (with)
        animal (traffic) V20.9 ☑
          being ridden (traffic) V26.9 ☑
            nontraffic V26.2 ☑
              while boarding or alighting V26.3 ☑
          nontraffic V20.2 ☑
          while boarding or alighting V20.3 ☑
        animal-drawn vehicle (traffic) V26.9 ☑
          nontraffic V26.2 ☑

Accident — *continued*
  transport — *continued*
    motorcyclist — *continued*
      collision — *continued*
        animal-drawn vehicle — *continued*
          while boarding or alighting V26.3 ☑
        bus (traffic) V24.9 ☑
          nontraffic V24.2 ☑
          while boarding or alighting V24.3 ☑
        car (traffic) V23.9 ☑
          nontraffic V23.2 ☑
          while boarding or alighting V23.3 ☑
        motor vehicle NOS (traffic) V29.60 ☑
          nontraffic V29.20 ☑
          specified type NEC (traffic) V29.69 ☑
            nontraffic V29.29 ☑
        pedal cycle (traffic) V21.9 ☑
          nontraffic V21.2 ☑
          while boarding or alighting V21.3 ☑
        pickup truck (traffic) V23.9 ☑
          nontraffic V23.2 ☑
          while boarding or alighting V23.3 ☑
        railway vehicle (traffic) V25.9 ☑
          nontraffic V25.2 ☑
          while boarding or alighting V25.3 ☑
        specified vehicle NEC (traffic) V26.9 ☑
          nontraffic V26.2 ☑
          while boarding or alighting V26.3 ☑
        stationary object (traffic) V27.9 ☑
          nontraffic V27.2 ☑
          while boarding or alighting V27.3 ☑
        streetcar (traffic) V26.9 ☑
          nontraffic V26.2 ☑
          while boarding or alighting V26.3 ☑
        three wheeled motor vehicle (traffic) V22.9 ☑
          nontraffic V22.2 ☑
          while boarding or alighting V22.3 ☑
        truck (traffic) V24.9 ☑
          nontraffic V24.2 ☑
          while boarding or alighting V24.3 ☑
        two wheeled motor vehicle (traffic) V22.9 ☑
          nontraffic V22.2 ☑
          while boarding or alighting V22.3 ☑
        van (traffic) V23.9 ☑
          nontraffic V23.2 ☑
          while boarding or alighting V23.3 ☑
      driver
        collision (with)
          animal (traffic) V20.4 ☑
            being ridden (traffic) V26.4 ☑
              nontraffic V26.0 ☑
            nontraffic V20.0 ☑
          animal-drawn vehicle (traffic) V26.4 ☑
            nontraffic V26.0 ☑
          bus (traffic) V24.4 ☑
            nontraffic V24.0 ☑
          car (traffic) V23.4 ☑
            nontraffic V23.0 ☑
          motor vehicle NOS (traffic) V29.40 ☑
            nontraffic V29.00 ☑
            specified type NEC (traffic) V29.49 ☑
              nontraffic V29.09 ☑
          pedal cycle (traffic) V21.4 ☑
            nontraffic V21.0 ☑
          pickup truck (traffic) V23.4 ☑
            nontraffic V23.0 ☑
          railway vehicle (traffic) V25.4 ☑
            nontraffic V25.0 ☑
          specified vehicle NEC (traffic) V26.4 ☑
            nontraffic V26.0 ☑
          stationary object (traffic) V27.4 ☑
            nontraffic V27.0 ☑
          streetcar (traffic) V26.4 ☑
            nontraffic V26.0 ☑
          three wheeled motor vehicle (traffic) V22.4 ☑
            nontraffic V22.0 ☑
          truck (traffic) V24.4 ☑
            nontraffic V24.0 ☑
          two wheeled motor vehicle (traffic) V22.4 ☑
            nontraffic V22.0 ☑
          van (traffic) V23.4 ☑
            nontraffic V23.0 ☑
        noncollision accident (traffic) V28.4 ☑

Accident — *continued*
  transport — *continued*
    motorcyclist — *continued*
      driver — *continued*
        noncollision accident — *continued*
          nontraffic V28.0 ☑
      noncollision accident (traffic) V28.9 ☑
        nontraffic V28.2 ☑
        while boarding or alighting V28.3 ☑
      nontraffic V29.3 ☑
      passenger
        collision (with)
          animal (traffic) V20.5 ☑
            being ridden (traffic) V26.5 ☑
              nontraffic V26.1 ☑
            nontraffic V20.1 ☑
          animal-drawn vehicle (traffic) V26.5 ☑
            nontraffic V26.1 ☑
          bus (traffic) V24.5 ☑
            nontraffic V24.1 ☑
          car (traffic) V23.5 ☑
            nontraffic V23.1 ☑
          motor vehicle NOS (traffic) V29.50 ☑
            nontraffic V29.10 ☑
            specified type NEC (traffic) V29.59 ☑
              nontraffic V29.19 ☑
          pedal cycle (traffic) V21.5 ☑
            nontraffic V21.1 ☑
          pickup truck (traffic) V23.5 ☑
            nontraffic V23.1 ☑
          railway vehicle (traffic) V25.5 ☑
            nontraffic V25.1 ☑
          specified vehicle NEC (traffic) V26.5 ☑
            nontraffic V26.1 ☑
          stationary object (traffic) V27.5 ☑
            nontraffic V27.1 ☑
          streetcar (traffic) V26.5 ☑
            nontraffic V26.1 ☑
          three wheeled motor vehicle (traffic) V22.5 ☑
            nontraffic V22.1 ☑
          truck (traffic) V24.5 ☑
            nontraffic V24.1 ☑
          two wheeled motor vehicle (traffic) V22.5 ☑
            nontraffic V22.1 ☑
          van (traffic) V23.5 ☑
            nontraffic V23.1 ☑
        noncollision accident (traffic) V28.5 ☑
          nontraffic V28.1 ☑
      specified type NEC V29.88 ☑
      military vehicle V29.81 ☑
    occupant (of)
      aircraft (powered) V95.9 ☑
        fixed wing
          commercial — *see* Accident, transport, aircraft, occupant, powered, fixed wing, commercial
          private — *see* Accident, transport, aircraft, occupant, powered, fixed wing, private
        nonpowered V96.9 ☑
        specified NEC V95.8 ☑
      airport battery-powered vehicle — *see* Accident, transport, industrial vehicle occupant
      all-terrain vehicle (ATV) — *see* Accident, transport, all-terrain vehicle occupant
      animal-drawn vehicle — *see* Accident, transport, animal-drawn vehicle occupant
      automobile — *see* Accident, transport, car occupant
      balloon V96.00 ☑
      battery-powered vehicle — *see* Accident, transport, industrial vehicle occupant
      bicycle — *see* Accident, transport, pedal cyclist
        motorized — *see* Accident, transport, motorcycle rider
      boat NEC — *see* Accident, watercraft
      bulldozer — *see* Accident, transport, construction vehicle occupant
      bus — *see* Accident, transport, bus occupant
      cable car (on rails) (*see also* Accident, transport, streetcar occupant)
        not on rails V98.0 ☑
      car (*see also* Accident, transport, car occupant)

Accident — *continued*
  transport — *continued*
    occupant — *continued*
      car (*see also* Accident, transport, car occupant) — *continued*
        cable (on rails) (*see also* Accident, transport, streetcar occupant)
          not on rails V98.0 ☑
        coach — *see* Accident, transport, bus occupant
        coal-car — *see* Accident, transport, industrial vehicle occupant
        digger — *see* Accident, transport, construction vehicle occupant
        dump truck — *see* Accident, transport, construction vehicle occupant
        earth-leveler — *see* Accident, transport, construction vehicle occupant
        farm machinery (self-propelled) — *see* Accident, transport, agricultural vehicle occupant
        forklift — *see* Accident, transport, industrial vehicle occupant
        glider (unpowered) V96.20 ☑
          hang V96.10 ☑
          powered (microlight) (ultralight) — *see* Accident, transport, aircraft, occupant, powered, glider
        glider (unpowered) NEC V96.20 ☑
        hang-glider V96.10 ☑
        harvester — *see* Accident, transport, agricultural vehicle occupant
        heavy (transport) vehicle — *see* Accident, transport, truck occupant
        helicopter — *see* Accident, transport, aircraft, occupant, helicopter
        ice-yacht V98.2 ☑
        kite (carrying person) V96.8 ☑
        land-yacht V98.1 ☑
        logging car — *see* Accident, transport, industrial vehicle occupant
        mechanical shovel — *see* Accident, transport, construction vehicle occupant
        microlight — *see* Accident, transport, aircraft, occupant, powered, glider
        minibus — *see* Accident, transport, car occupant
        minivan — *see* Accident, transport, car occupant
        moped — *see* Accident, transport, motorcycle
        motor scooter — *see* Accident, transport, motorcycle
        motorcycle (with sidecar) — *see* Accident, transport, motorcycle
        pedal cycle (*see also* Accident, transport, pedal cyclist)
        pick-up (truck) — *see* Accident, transport, pickup truck occupant
        railway (train) (vehicle) (subterranean) (elevated) — *see* Accident, transport, railway vehicle occupant
        rickshaw — *see* Accident, transport, pedal cycle
          motorized — *see* Accident, transport, three-wheeled motor vehicle
          pedal driven — *see* Accident, transport, pedal cyclist
        road-roller — *see* Accident, transport, construction vehicle occupant
        ship NOS V94.9 ☑
        ski-lift (chair) (gondola) V98.3 ☑
        snowmobile — *see* Accident, transport, snowmobile occupant
        spacecraft, spaceship — *see* Accident, transport, aircraft, occupant, spacecraft
        sport utility vehicle — *see* Accident, transport, car occupant
        streetcar (interurban) (operating on public street or highway) — *see* Accident, transport, streetcar occupant
        SUV — *see* Accident, transport, car occupant
        téléférique V98.0 ☑
        three-wheeled vehicle (motorized) (*see also* Accident, transport, three-wheeled motor vehicle occupant)
          nonmotorized — *see* Accident, transport, pedal cycle
        tractor (farm) (and trailer) — *see* Accident, transport, agricultural vehicle occupant

Accident — *continued*
  transport — *continued*
    occupant — *continued*
      train — *see* Accident, transport, railway vehicle occupant
      tram — *see* Accident, transport, streetcar occupant
        in mine or quarry — *see* Accident, transport, industrial vehicle occupant
      tricycle — *see* Accident, transport, pedal cycle
        motorized — *see* Accident, transport, three-wheeled motor vehicle
      trolley — *see* Accident, transport, streetcar occupant
        in mine or quarry — *see* Accident, transport, industrial vehicle occupant
      tub, in mine or quarry — *see* Accident, transport, industrial vehicle occupant
      ultralight — *see* Accident, transport, aircraft, occupant, powered, glider
      van — *see* Accident, transport, van occupant
    vehicle NEC V89.9 ☑
      heavy transport — *see* Accident, transport, truck occupant
      motor (traffic) NEC V89.2 ☑
        nontraffic NEC V89.0 ☑
    watercraft NOS V94.9 ☑
      causing drowning B — *see* Drowning, resulting from accident to boat
  parachutist V97.29 ☑
    after accident to aircraft — *see* Accident, transport, aircraft
    entangled in object V97.21 ☑
    injured on landing V97.22 ☑
  pedal cyclist V19.9 ☑
    collision (with)
      animal (traffic) V10.9 ☑
        being ridden (traffic) V16.9 ☑
          nontraffic V16.2 ☑
          while boarding or alighting V16.3 ☑
        nontraffic V10.2 ☑
        while boarding or alighting V10.3 ☑
      animal-drawn vehicle (traffic) V16.9 ☑
        nontraffic V16.2 ☑
        while boarding or alighting V16.3 ☑
      bus (traffic) V14.9 ☑
        nontraffic V14.2 ☑
        while boarding or alighting V14.3 ☑
      car (traffic) V13.9 ☑
        nontraffic V13.2 ☑
        while boarding or alighting V13.3 ☑
      motor vehicle NOS (traffic) V19.60 ☑
        nontraffic V19.20 ☑
        specified type NEC (traffic) V19.69 ☑
          nontraffic V19.29 ☑
      pedal cycle (traffic) V11.9 ☑
        nontraffic V11.2 ☑
        while boarding or alighting V11.3 ☑
      pickup truck (traffic) V13.9 ☑
        nontraffic V13.2 ☑
        while boarding or alighting V13.3 ☑
      railway vehicle (traffic) V15.9 ☑
        nontraffic V15.2 ☑
        while boarding or alighting V15.3 ☑
      specified vehicle NEC (traffic) V16.9 ☑
        nontraffic V16.2 ☑
        while boarding or alighting V16.3 ☑
      stationary object (traffic) V17.9 ☑
        nontraffic V17.2 ☑
        while boarding or alighting V17.3 ☑
      streetcar (traffic) V16.9 ☑
        nontraffic V16.2 ☑
        while boarding or alighting V16.3 ☑
      three wheeled motor vehicle (traffic) V12.9 ☑
        nontraffic V12.2 ☑
        while boarding or alighting V12.3 ☑
      truck (traffic) V14.9 ☑
        nontraffic V14.2 ☑
        while boarding or alighting V14.3 ☑
      two wheeled motor vehicle (traffic) V12.9 ☑
        nontraffic V12.2 ☑
        while boarding or alighting V12.3 ☑
      van (traffic) V13.9 ☑
        nontraffic V13.2 ☑
        while boarding or alighting V13.3 ☑

Accident — *continued*
  transport — *continued*
    pedal cyclist — *continued*
      driver
        collision (with)
          animal (traffic) V10.4 ☑
            being ridden (traffic) V16.4 ☑
              nontraffic V16.0 ☑
            nontraffic V10.0 ☑
          animal-drawn vehicle (traffic) V16.4 ☑
            nontraffic V16.0 ☑
          bus (traffic) V14.4 ☑
            nontraffic V14.0 ☑
          car (traffic) V13.4 ☑
            nontraffic V13.0 ☑
          motor vehicle NOS (traffic) V19.40 ☑
            nontraffic V19.00 ☑
            specified type NEC (traffic) V19.49 ☑
              nontraffic V19.09 ☑
          pedal cycle (traffic) V11.4 ☑
            nontraffic V11.0 ☑
          pickup truck (traffic) V13.4 ☑
            nontraffic V13.0 ☑
          railway vehicle (traffic) V15.4 ☑
            nontraffic V15.0 ☑
          specified vehicle NEC (traffic) V16.4 ☑
            nontraffic V16.0 ☑
          stationary object (traffic) V17.4 ☑
            nontraffic V17.0 ☑
          streetcar (traffic) V16.4 ☑
            nontraffic V16.0 ☑
          three wheeled motor vehicle (traffic) V12.4 ☑
            nontraffic V12.0 ☑
          truck (traffic) V14.4 ☑
            nontraffic V14.0 ☑
          two wheeled motor vehicle (traffic) V12.4 ☑
            nontraffic V12.0 ☑
          van (traffic) V13.4 ☑
            nontraffic V13.0 ☑
        noncollision accident (traffic) V18.4 ☑
          nontraffic V18.0 ☑
      noncollision accident (traffic) V18.9 ☑
        nontraffic V18.2 ☑
        while boarding or alighting V18.3 ☑
      nontraffic V19.3 ☑
      passenger
        collision (with)
          animal (traffic) V10.5 ☑
            being ridden (traffic) V16.5 ☑
              nontraffic V16.1 ☑
            nontraffic V10.1 ☑
          animal-drawn vehicle (traffic) V16.5 ☑
            nontraffic V16.1 ☑
          bus (traffic) V14.5 ☑
            nontraffic V14.1 ☑
          car (traffic) V13.5 ☑
            nontraffic V13.1 ☑
          motor vehicle NOS (traffic) V19.50 ☑
            nontraffic V19.10 ☑
            specified type NEC (traffic) V19.59 ☑
              nontraffic V19.19 ☑
          pedal cycle (traffic) V11.5 ☑
            nontraffic V11.1 ☑
          pickup truck (traffic) V13.5 ☑
            nontraffic V13.1 ☑
          railway vehicle (traffic) V15.5 ☑
            nontraffic V15.1 ☑
          specified vehicle NEC (traffic) V16.5 ☑
            nontraffic V16.1 ☑
          stationary object (traffic) V17.5 ☑
            nontraffic V17.1 ☑
          streetcar (traffic) V16.5 ☑
            nontraffic V16.1 ☑
          three wheeled motor vehicle (traffic) V12.5 ☑
            nontraffic V12.1 ☑
          truck (traffic) V14.5 ☑
            nontraffic V14.1 ☑
          two wheeled motor vehicle (traffic) V12.5 ☑
            nontraffic V12.1 ☑
          van (traffic) V13.5 ☑
            nontraffic V13.1 ☑
        noncollision accident (traffic) V18.5 ☑

Accident — *continued*
  transport — *continued*
    pedal cyclist — *continued*
      passenger — *continued*
        noncollision accident — *continued*
          nontraffic V18.1 ☑
        specified type NEC V19.88 ☑
        military vehicle V19.81 ☑
    pedestrian
      conveyance (occupant) V09.9 ☑
        babystroller V00.828 ☑
          collision (with) V09.9 ☑
            animal being ridden or animal drawn
              vehicle V06.99 ☑
              nontraffic V06.09 ☑
              traffic V06.19 ☑
            bus or heavy transport V04.99 ☑
              nontraffic V04.09 ☑
              traffic V04.19 ☑
            car V03.99 ☑
              nontraffic V03.09 ☑
              traffic V03.19 ☑
            pedal cycle V01.99 ☑
              nontraffic V01.09 ☑
              traffic V01.19 ☑
            pick-up truck or van V03.99 ☑
              nontraffic V03.09 ☑
              traffic V03.19 ☑
            railway (train) (vehicle) V05.99 ☑
              nontraffic V05.09 ☑
              traffic V05.19 ☑
            stationary object V00.822 ☑
            streetcar V06.99 ☑
              nontraffic V06.09 ☑
              traffic V06.19 ☑
            two- or three-wheeled motor vehicle
              V02.99 ☑
              nontraffic V02.09 ☑
              traffic V02.19 ☑
            vehicle V09.9 ☑
              animal-drawn V06.99 ☑
                nontraffic V06.09 ☑
                traffic V06.19 ☑
              motor
                nontraffic V09.00 ☑
                traffic V09.20 ☑
         fall V00.821 ☑
        nontraffic V09.1 ☑
          involving motor vehicle NEC
            V09.00 ☑
        traffic V09.3 ☑
          involving motor vehicle NEC
            V09.20 ☑
        flat-bottomed NEC V00.388 ☑
          collision (with) V09.9 ☑
            animal being ridden or animal drawn
              vehicle V06.99 ☑
              nontraffic V06.09 ☑
              traffic V06.19 ☑
            bus or heavy transport V04.99 ☑
              nontraffic V04.09 ☑
              traffic V04.19 ☑
            car V03.99 ☑
              nontraffic V03.09 ☑
              traffic V03.19 ☑
            pedal cycle V01.99 ☑
              nontraffic V01.09 ☑
              traffic V01.19 ☑
            pick-up truck or van V03.99 ☑
              nontraffic V03.09 ☑
              traffic V03.19 ☑
            railway (train) (vehicle) V05.99 ☑
              nontraffic V05.09 ☑
              traffic V05.19 ☑
            stationary object V00.382 ☑
            streetcar V06.99 ☑
              nontraffic V06.09 ☑
              traffic V06.19 ☑
            two- or three-wheeled motor vehicle
              V02.99 ☑
              nontraffic V02.09 ☑
              traffic V02.19 ☑
            vehicle V09.9 ☑
              animal-drawn V06.99 ☑
                nontraffic V06.09 ☑
                traffic V06.19 ☑

Accident — *continued*
  transport — *continued*
    pedestrian — *continued*
      conveyance — *continued*
        flat-bottomed — *continued*
          collision — *continued*
            vehicle — *continued*
              motor
                nontraffic V09.00 ☑
                traffic V09.20 ☑
        fall V00.381 ☑
        nontraffic V09.1 ☑
          involving motor vehicle NEC
            V09.00 ☑
        snow
          board — *see* Accident, transport,
            pedestrian, conveyance, snow
            board
          ski — *see* Accident, transport,
            pedestrian, conveyance, skis
            (snow)
        traffic V09.3 ☑
          involving motor vehicle NEC
            V09.20 ☑
        gliding type NEC V00.288 ☑
          collision (with) V09.9 ☑
            animal being ridden or animal drawn
              vehicle V06.99 ☑
              nontraffic V06.09 ☑
              traffic V06.19 ☑
            bus or heavy transport V04.99 ☑
              nontraffic V04.09 ☑
              traffic V04.19 ☑
            car V03.99 ☑
              nontraffic V03.09 ☑
              traffic V03.19 ☑
            pedal cycle V01.99 ☑
              nontraffic V01.09 ☑
              traffic V01.19 ☑
            pick-up truck or van V03.99 ☑
              nontraffic V03.09 ☑
              traffic V03.19 ☑
            railway (train) (vehicle) V05.99 ☑
              nontraffic V05.09 ☑
              traffic V05.19 ☑
            stationary object V00.282 ☑
            streetcar V06.99 ☑
              nontraffic V06.09 ☑
              traffic V06.19- ☑
            two- or three-wheeled motor vehicle
              V02.99 ☑
              nontraffic V02.09 ☑
              traffic V02.19 ☑
            vehicle V09.9 ☑
              animal-drawn V06.99 ☑
                nontraffic V06.09 ☑
                traffic V06.19 ☑
              motor
                nontraffic V09.00 ☑
                traffic V09.20 ☑
        fall V00.281 ☑
        heelies — *see* Accident, transport,
          pedestrian, conveyance, heelies
        ice skate — *see* Accident, transport,
          pedestrian, conveyance, ice skate
        nontraffic V09.1 ☑
          involving motor vehicle NEC
            V09.00 ☑
        sled — *see* Accident, transport, pedestri-
          an, conveyance, sled
        traffic V09.3 ☑
          involving motor vehicle NEC
            V09.20 ☑
          wheelies — *see* Accident, transport,
            pedestrian, conveyance, heel-
            ies
        heelies V00.158 ☑
          colliding with stationary object
            V00.152 ☑
          fall V00.151 ☑
        ice skates V00.218 ☑
          collision (with) V09.9 ☑
            animal being ridden or animal drawn
              vehicle V06.99 ☑
              nontraffic V06.09 ☑
              traffic V06.19 ☑

Accident — *continued*
  transport — *continued*
    pedestrian — *continued*
      conveyance — *continued*
        ice skates — *continued*
          collision — *continued*
            bus or heavy transport V04.99 ☑
              nontraffic V04.09 ☑
              traffic V04.19 ☑
            car V03.99 ☑
              nontraffic V03.09 ☑
              traffic V03.19 ☑
            pedal cycle V01.99 ☑
              nontraffic V01.09 ☑
              traffic V01.19 ☑
            pick-up truck or van V03.99 ☑
              nontraffic V03.09 ☑
              traffic V03.19 ☑
            railway (train) (vehicle) V05.99 ☑
              nontraffic V05.09 ☑
              traffic V05.19 ☑
            stationary object V00.212 ☑
            streetcar V06.99 ☑
              nontraffic V06.09 ☑
              traffic V06.19 ☑
            two- or three-wheeled motor vehicle
              V02.99 ☑
              nontraffic V02.09 ☑
              traffic V02.19 ☑
            vehicle V09.9 ☑
              animal-drawn V06.99 ☑
                nontraffic V06.09 ☑
                traffic V06.19 ☑
              motor
                nontraffic V09.00 ☑
                traffic V09.20 ☑
        fall V00.211 ☑
        nontraffic V09.1 ☑
          involving motor vehicle NEC
            V09.00 ☑
        traffic V09.3 ☑
          involving motor vehicle NEC
            V09.20 ☑
        motorized mobility scooter V00.838 ☑
          collision with stationary object
            V00.832 ☑
          fall from V00.831 ☑
        nontraffic V09.1 ☑
          involving motor vehicle V09.00 ☑
           military V09.01 ☑
           specified type NEC V09.09 ☑
        roller skates (non in-line) V00.128 ☑
          collision (with) V09.9 ☑
            animal being ridden or animal drawn
              vehicle V06.91 ☑
              nontraffic V06.01 ☑
              traffic V06.11 ☑
            bus or heavy transport V04.91 ☑
              nontraffic V04.01 ☑
              traffic V04.11 ☑
            car V03.91 ☑
              nontraffic V03.01 ☑
              traffic V03.11 ☑
            pedal cycle V01.91 ☑
              nontraffic V01.01 ☑
              traffic V01.11 ☑
            pick-up truck or van V03.91 ☑
              nontraffic V03.01 ☑
              traffic V03.11 ☑
            railway (train) (vehicle) V05.91 ☑
              nontraffic V05.01 ☑
              traffic V05.11 ☑
            stationary object V00.122 ☑
            streetcar V06.91 ☑
              nontraffic V06.01 ☑
              traffic V06.11 ☑
            two- or three-wheeled motor vehicle
              V02.91 ☑
              nontraffic V02.01 ☑
              traffic V02.11 ☑
            vehicle V09.9 ☑
              animal-drawn V06.91 ☑
                nontraffic V06.01 ☑
                traffic V06.11 ☑
              motor
                nontraffic V09.00 ☑

☑ Additional Character Required — Refer to the Tabular List for Character Selection   ⬇ Subterms under main terms may continue to next column or page

Accident — *continued*
  transport — *continued*
    pedestrian — *continued*
      conveyance — *continued*
        roller skates — *continued*
          collision — *continued*
            vehicle — *continued*
              motor — *continued*
                traffic V09.20 ☑
          fall V00.121 ☑
          in-line V00.118 ☑
            collision — *see also* Accident, transport, pedestrian, conveyance occupant, roller skates, collision
            with stationary object V00.112 ☑
            fall V00.111 ☑
          nontraffic V09.1 ☑
            involving motor vehicle NEC V09.00 ☑
          traffic V09.3 ☑
            involving motor vehicle NEC V09.20 ☑
        rolling shoes V00.158 ☑
          colliding with stationary object V00.152 ☑
          fall V00.151 ☑
        rolling type NEC V00.188 ☑
          collision (with) V09.9 ☑
            animal being ridden or animal drawn vehicle V06.99 ☑
              nontraffic V06.09 ☑
              traffic V06.19 ☑
            bus or heavy transport V04.99 ☑
              nontraffic V04.09 ☑
              traffic V04.19 ☑
            car V03.99 ☑
              nontraffic V03.09 ☑
              traffic V03.19 ☑
            pedal cycle V01.99 ☑
              nontraffic V01.09 ☑
              traffic V01.19 ☑
            pick-up truck or van V03.99 ☑
              nontraffic V03.09 ☑
              traffic V03.19 ☑
            railway (train) (vehicle) V05.99 ☑
              nontraffic V05.09 ☑
              traffic V05.19 ☑
            stationary object V00.182 ☑
            streetcar V06.99 ☑
              nontraffic V06.09 ☑
              traffic V06.19 ☑
            two- or three-wheeled motor vehicle V02.99 ☑
              nontraffic V02.09 ☑
              traffic V02.19 ☑
            vehicle V09.9 ☑
              animal-drawn V06.99 ☑
                nontraffic V06.09 ☑
                traffic V06.19 ☑
              motor
                nontraffic V09.00 ☑
                traffic V09.20 ☑
        fall V00.181 ☑
        in-line roller skate — *see* Accident, transport, pedestrian, conveyance, roller skate, in-line
        nontraffic V09.1 ☑
          involving motor vehicle NEC V09.00 ☑
        roller skate — *see* Accident, transport, pedestrian, conveyance, roller skate
        scooter (non-motorized) — *see* Accident, transport, pedestrian, conveyance, scooter
        skateboard — *see* Accident, transport, pedestrian, conveyance, skateboard
        traffic V09.3 ☑
          involving motor vehicle NEC V09.20 ☑
       scooter (non-motorized) V00.148 ☑
         collision (with) V09.9 ☑
           animal being ridden or animal drawn vehicle V06.99 ☑

Accident — *continued*
  transport — *continued*
    pedestrian — *continued*
      conveyance — *continued*
        scooter — *continued*
          collision — *continued*
            animal being ridden or animal drawn vehicle — *continued*
              nontraffic V06.09 ☑
              traffic V06.19 ☑
            bus or heavy transport V04.99 ☑
              nontraffic V04.09 ☑
              traffic V04.19 ☑
            car V03.99 ☑
              nontraffic V03.09 ☑
              traffic V03.19 ☑
            pedal cycle V01.99 ☑
              nontraffic V01.09 ☑
              traffic V01.19 ☑
            pick-up truck or van V03.99 ☑
              nontraffic V03.09 ☑
              traffic V03.19 ☑
            railway (train) (vehicle) V05.99 ☑
              nontraffic V05.09 ☑
              traffic V05.19 ☑
            stationary object V00.142 ☑
            streetcar V06.99 ☑
              nontraffic V06.09 ☑
              traffic V06.19 ☑
            two- or three-wheeled motor vehicle V02.99 ☑
              nontraffic V02.09 ☑
              traffic V02.19 ☑
            vehicle V09.9 ☑
              animal-drawn V06.99 ☑
                nontraffic V06.09 ☑
                traffic V06.19 ☑
              motor
                nontraffic V09.00 ☑
                traffic V09.20 ☑
        fall V00.141 ☑
        nontraffic V09.1 ☑
          involving motor vehicle NEC V09.00 ☑
        traffic V09.3 ☑
          involving motor vehicle NEC V09.20 ☑
        skate board V00.138 ☑
         collision (with) V09.9 ☑
           animal being ridden or animal drawn vehicle V06.92 ☑
            nontraffic V06.02 ☑
            traffic V06.12 ☑
           bus or heavy transport V04.92 ☑
            nontraffic V04.02 ☑
            traffic V04.12 ☑
           car V03.92 ☑
            nontraffic V03.02 ☑
            traffic V03.12 ☑
           pedal cycle V01.92 ☑
            nontraffic V01.02 ☑
            traffic V01.12 ☑
           pick-up truck or van V03.92 ☑
            nontraffic V03.02 ☑
            traffic V03.12 ☑
           railway (train) (vehicle) V05.92 ☑
            nontraffic V05.02 ☑
            traffic V05.12 ☑
           stationary object V00.132 ☑
           streetcar V06.92 ☑
            nontraffic V06.02 ☑
            traffic V06.12 ☑
           two- or three-wheeled motor vehicle V02.92 ☑
            nontraffic V02.02 ☑
            traffic V02.12 ☑
           vehicle V09.9 ☑
            animal-drawn V06.92 ☑
              nontraffic V06.02 ☑
              traffic V06.12 ☑
            motor
              nontraffic V09.00 ☑
              traffic V09.20 ☑
        fall V00.131 ☑
        nontraffic V09.1 ☑

Accident — *continued*
  transport — *continued*
    pedestrian — *continued*
      conveyance — *continued*
        skate board — *continued*
          nontraffic — *continued*
            involving motor vehicle NEC V09.00 ☑
          traffic V09.3 ☑
            involving motor vehicle NEC V09.20 ☑
        skis (snow) V00.328 ☑
         collision (with) V09.9 ☑
           animal being ridden or animal drawn vehicle V06.99 ☑
            nontraffic V06.09 ☑
            traffic V06.19 ☑
           bus or heavy transport V04.99 ☑
            nontraffic V04.09 ☑
            traffic V04.19 ☑
           car V03.99 ☑
            nontraffic V03.09 ☑
            traffic V03.19 ☑
           pedal cycle V01.99 ☑
            nontraffic V01.09 ☑
            traffic V01.19 ☑
           pick-up truck or van V03.99 ☑
            nontraffic V03.09 ☑
            traffic V03.19 ☑
           railway (train) (vehicle) V05.99 ☑
            nontraffic V05.09 ☑
            traffic V05.19 ☑
           stationary object V00.322 ☑
           streetcar V06.99 ☑
            nontraffic V06.09 ☑
            traffic V06.19 ☑
           two- or three-wheeled motor vehicle V02.99 ☑
            nontraffic V02.09 ☑
            traffic V02.19 ☑
           vehicle V09.9 ☑
            animal-drawn V06.99 ☑
              nontraffic V06.09 ☑
              traffic V06.19 ☑
            motor
              nontraffic V09.00 ☑
              traffic V09.20 ☑
        fall V00.321 ☑
        nontraffic V09.1 ☑
          involving motor vehicle NEC V09.00 ☑
        traffic V09.3 ☑
          involving motor vehicle NEC V09.20 ☑
        sled V00.228 ☑
         collision (with) V09.9 ☑
           animal being ridden or animal drawn vehicle V06.99 ☑
            nontraffic V06.09 ☑
            traffic V06.19 ☑
           bus or heavy transport V04.99 ☑
            nontraffic V04.09 ☑
            traffic V04.19 ☑
           car V03.99 ☑
            nontraffic V03.09 ☑
            traffic V03.19 ☑
           pedal cycle V01.99 ☑
            nontraffic V01.09 ☑
            traffic V01.19 ☑
           pick-up truck or van V03.99 ☑
            nontraffic V03.09 ☑
            traffic V03.19 ☑
           railway (train) (vehicle) V05.99 ☑
            nontraffic V05.09 ☑
            traffic V05.19 ☑
           stationary object V00.222 ☑
           streetcar V06.99 ☑
            nontraffic V06.09 ☑
            traffic V06.19 ☑
           two- or three-wheeled motor vehicle V02.99 ☑
            nontraffic V02.09 ☑
            traffic V02.19 ☑
           vehicle V09.9 ☑
            animal-drawn V06.99 ☑
              nontraffic V06.09 ☑

External Causes Index

Accident — Accident

Accident — *continued*
  transport — *continued*
    pedestrian — *continued*
      conveyance — *continued*
        sled — *continued*
          collision — *continued*
            vehicle — *continued*
              animal-drawn — *continued*
                traffic V06.19 ☑
              motor
                nontraffic V09.00 ☑
                traffic V09.20 ☑
          fall V00.221 ☑
          nontraffic V09.1 ☑
            involving motor vehicle NEC
              V09.00 ☑
          traffic V09.3 ☑
            involving motor vehicle NEC
              V09.20 ☑
        snow board V00.318 ☑
          collision (with) V09.9 ☑
            animal being ridden or animal drawn
              vehicle V06.99 ☑
              nontraffic V06.09 ☑
              traffic V06.19 ☑
            bus or heavy transport V04.99 ☑
              nontraffic V04.09 ☑
              traffic V04.19 ☑
            car V03.99 ☑
              nontraffic V03.09 ☑
              traffic V03.19 ☑
            pedal cycle V01.99 ☑
              nontraffic V01.09 ☑
              traffic V01.19 ☑
            pick-up truck or van V03.99 ☑
              nontraffic V03.09 ☑
              traffic V03.19 ☑
            railway (train) (vehicle) V05.99 ☑
              nontraffic V05.09 ☑
              traffic V05.19 ☑
            stationary object V00.312 ☑
            streetcar V06.99 ☑
              nontraffic V06.09 ☑
              traffic V06.19 ☑
            two- or three-wheeled motor vehicle
              V02.99 ☑
              nontraffic V02.09 ☑
              traffic V02.19 ☑
            vehicle V09.9 ☑
              animal-drawn V06.99 ☑
                nontraffic V06.09 ☑
                traffic V06.19 ☑
              motor
                nontraffic V09.00 ☑
                traffic V09.20 ☑
        fall V00.311 ☑
        nontraffic V09.1 ☑
          involving motor vehicle NEC
            V09.00 ☑
        traffic V09.3 ☑
          involving motor vehicle NEC
            V09.20 ☑
      specified type NEC V00.898 ☑
        collision (with) V09.9 ☑
          animal being ridden or animal drawn
            vehicle V06.99 ☑
            nontraffic V06.09 ☑
            traffic V06.19 ☑
          bus or heavy transport V04.99 ☑
            nontraffic V04.09 ☑
            traffic V04.19 ☑
          car V03.99 ☑
            nontraffic V03.09 ☑
            traffic V03.19 ☑
          pedal cycle V01.99 ☑
            nontraffic V01.09 ☑
            traffic V01.19 ☑
          pick-up truck or van V03.99 ☑
            nontraffic V03.09 ☑
            traffic V03.19 ☑
          railway (train) (vehicle) V05.99 ☑
            nontraffic V05.09 ☑
            traffic V05.19 ☑
          stationary object V00.892 ☑
          streetcar V06.99 ☑
            nontraffic V06.09 ☑

Accident — *continued*
  transport — *continued*
    pedestrian — *continued*
      conveyance — *continued*
        specified type — *continued*
          collision — *continued*
            streetcar — *continued*
              traffic V06.19 ☑
            two- or three-wheeled motor vehicle
              V02.99 ☑
              nontraffic V02.09 ☑
              traffic V02.19 ☑
            vehicle V09.9 ☑
              animal-drawn V06.99 ☑
                nontraffic V06.09 ☑
                traffic V06.19 ☑
              motor
                nontraffic V09.00 ☑
                traffic V09.20 ☑
        fall V00.891 ☑
        nontraffic V09.1 ☑
          involving motor vehicle NEC
            V09.00 ☑
        traffic V09.3 ☑
          involving motor vehicle NEC
            V09.20 ☑
      traffic V09.3 ☑
        involving motor vehicle V09.20 ☑
          military V09.21 ☑
          specified type NEC V09.29 ☑
      wheelchair (powered) V00.818 ☑
        collision (with) V09.9 ☑
          animal being ridden or animal drawn
            vehicle V06.99 ☑
            nontraffic V06.09 ☑
            traffic V06.19 ☑
          bus or heavy transport V04.99 ☑
            nontraffic V04.09 ☑
            traffic V04.19 ☑
          car V03.99 ☑
            nontraffic V03.09 ☑
            traffic V03.19 ☑
          pedal cycle V01.99 ☑
            nontraffic V01.09 ☑
            traffic V01.19 ☑
          pick-up truck or van V03.99 ☑
            nontraffic V03.09 ☑
            traffic V03.19 ☑
          railway (train) (vehicle) V05.99 ☑
            nontraffic V05.09 ☑
            traffic V05.19 ☑
          stationary object V00.812 ☑
          streetcar V06.99 ☑
            nontraffic V06.09 ☑
            traffic V06.19 ☑
          two- or three-wheeled motor vehicle
            V02.99 ☑
            nontraffic V02.09 ☑
            traffic V02.19 ☑
          vehicle V09.9 ☑
            animal-drawn V06.99 ☑
              nontraffic V06.09 ☑
              traffic V06.19 ☑
            motor
              nontraffic V09.00 ☑
              traffic V09.20 ☑
        fall V00.811 ☑
        nontraffic V09.1 ☑
          involving motor vehicle NEC
            V09.00 ☑
        traffic V09.3 ☑
          involving motor vehicle NEC
            V09.20 ☑
      wheeled shoe V00.158 ☑
        colliding with stationary object
          V00.152 ☑
        fall V00.151 ☑
    on foot (*see also* Accident, pedestrian)
      collision (with)
        animal being ridden or animal drawn
          vehicle V06.90 ☑
            nontraffic V06.00 ☑
            traffic V06.10 ☑
        bus or heavy transport V04.90 ☑
          nontraffic V04.00 ☑
          traffic V04.10 ☑

Accident — *continued*
  transport — *continued*
    pedestrian — *continued*
      on foot (*see also* Accident, pedestrian) — *continued*
        collision — *continued*
          car V03.90 ☑
            nontraffic V03.00 ☑
            traffic V03.10 ☑
          pedal cycle V01.90 ☑
            nontraffic V01.00 ☑
            traffic V01.10 ☑
          pick-up truck or van V03.90 ☑
            nontraffic V03.00 ☑
            traffic V03.10 ☑
          railway (train) (vehicle) V05.90 ☑
            nontraffic V05.00 ☑
            traffic V05.10 ☑
          streetcar V06.90 ☑
            nontraffic V06.00 ☑
            traffic V06.10 ☑
          two- or three-wheeled motor vehicle
            V02.90 ☑
            nontraffic V02.00 ☑
            traffic V02.10 ☑
          vehicle V09.9 ☑
            animal-drawn V06.90 ☑
              nontraffic V06.00 ☑
              traffic V06.10 ☑
            motor
        nontraffic V09.1 ☑
          involving motor vehicle V09.00 ☑
           military V09.01 ☑
           specified type NEC V09.09 ☑
        traffic V09.3 ☑
          involving motor vehicle V09.20 ☑
           military V09.21 ☑
           specified type NEC V09.29 ☑
    person NEC (unknown way or transportation)
      V99 ☑
      collision (between)
        bus (with)
          heavy transport vehicle (traffic) V87.5 ☑
            nontraffic V88.5 ☑
        car (with)
          bus (traffic) V87.3 ☑
            nontraffic V88.3 ☑
          heavy transport vehicle (traffic) V87.4 ☑
            nontraffic V88.4 ☑
            nontraffic V88.5 ☑
          pick-up truck or van (traffic) V87.2 ☑
            nontraffic V88.2 ☑
          train or railway vehicle (traffic) V87.6 ☑
            nontraffic V88.6 ☑
          two-or three-wheeled motor vehicle
            (traffic) V87.0 ☑
            nontraffic V88.0 ☑
        motor vehicle (traffic) NEC V87.7 ☑
          nontraffic V88.7 ☑
        two-or three-wheeled vehicle (with) (traffic)
          motor vehicle NEC V87.1 ☑
            nontraffic V88.1 ☑
        nonmotor vehicle (collision) (noncollision)
          (traffic) V87.9 ☑
          nontraffic V88.9 ☑
    pickup truck occupant V59.9 ☑
      collision (with)
        animal (traffic) V50.9 ☑
          being ridden (traffic) V56.9 ☑
            nontraffic V56.3 ☑
            while boarding or alighting V56.4 ☑
          nontraffic V50.3 ☑
          while boarding or alighting V50.4 ☑
        animal-drawn vehicle (traffic) V56.9 ☑
          nontraffic V56.3 ☑
          while boarding or alighting V56.4 ☑
        bus (traffic) V54.9 ☑
          nontraffic V54.3 ☑
          while boarding or alighting V54.4 ☑
        car (traffic) V53.9 ☑
          nontraffic V53.3 ☑
          while boarding or alighting V53.4 ☑
        motor vehicle NOS (traffic) V59.60 ☑
          nontraffic V59.20 ☑
          specified type NEC (traffic) V59.69 ☑
            nontraffic V59.29 ☑

Accident — *continued*
　transport — *continued*
　　pickup truck occupant — *continued*
　　　collision — *continued*
　　　　pedal cycle (traffic) V51.9 ☑
　　　　　nontraffic V51.3 ☑
　　　　　while boarding or alighting V51.4 ☑
　　　　pickup truck (traffic) V53.9 ☑
　　　　　nontraffic V53.3 ☑
　　　　　while boarding or alighting V53.4 ☑
　　　　railway vehicle (traffic) V55.9 ☑
　　　　　nontraffic V55.3 ☑
　　　　　while boarding or alighting V55.4 ☑
　　　　specified vehicle NEC (traffic) V56.9 ☑
　　　　　nontraffic V56.3 ☑
　　　　　while boarding or alighting V56.4 ☑
　　　　stationary object (traffic) V57.9 ☑
　　　　　nontraffic V57.3 ☑
　　　　　while boarding or alighting V57.4 ☑
　　　　streetcar (traffic) V56.9 ☑
　　　　　nontraffic V56.3 ☑
　　　　　while boarding or alighting V56.4 ☑
　　　　three wheeled motor vehicle (traffic)
　　　　　V52.9 ☑
　　　　　nontraffic V52.3 ☑
　　　　　while boarding or alighting V52.4 ☑
　　　　truck (traffic) V54.9 ☑
　　　　　nontraffic V54.3 ☑
　　　　　while boarding or alighting V54.4 ☑
　　　　two wheeled motor vehicle (traffic) V52.9 ☑
　　　　　nontraffic V52.3 ☑
　　　　　while boarding or alighting V52.4 ☑
　　　　van (traffic) V53.9 ☑
　　　　　nontraffic V53.3 ☑
　　　　　while boarding or alighting V53.4 ☑
　　　driver
　　　　collision (with)
　　　　　animal (traffic) V50.5 ☑
　　　　　　being ridden (traffic) V56.5 ☑
　　　　　　　nontraffic V56.0 ☑
　　　　　　nontraffic V50.1 ☑
　　　　　animal-drawn vehicle (traffic) V56.5 ☑
　　　　　　nontraffic V56.0 ☑
　　　　　bus (traffic) V54.5 ☑
　　　　　　nontraffic V54.0 ☑
　　　　　car (traffic) V53.6 ☑
　　　　　　nontraffic V53.0 ☑
　　　　　motor vehicle NOS (traffic) V59.40 ☑
　　　　　　nontraffic V59.00 ☑
　　　　　　specified type NEC (traffic) V59.49 ☑
　　　　　　　nontraffic V59.09 ☑
　　　　　pedal cycle (traffic) V51.5 ☑
　　　　　　nontraffic V51.0 ☑
　　　　　pickup truck (traffic) V53.5 ☑
　　　　　　nontraffic V53.0 ☑
　　　　　railway vehicle (traffic) V55.5 ☑
　　　　　　nontraffic V55.0 ☑
　　　　　specified vehicle NEC (traffic) V56.5 ☑
　　　　　　nontraffic V56.0 ☑
　　　　　stationary object (traffic) V57.5 ☑
　　　　　　nontraffic V57.0 ☑
　　　　　streetcar (traffic) V56.5 ☑
　　　　　　nontraffic V56.0 ☑
　　　　　three wheeled motor vehicle (traffic)
　　　　　　V52.5 ☑
　　　　　　nontraffic V52.0 ☑
　　　　　truck (traffic) V54.5 ☑
　　　　　　nontraffic V54.0 ☑
　　　　　two wheeled motor vehicle (traffic)
　　　　　　V52.5 ☑
　　　　　　nontraffic V52.0 ☑
　　　　　van (traffic) V53.5 ☑
　　　　　　nontraffic V53.0 ☑
　　　　noncollision accident (traffic) V58.5 ☑
　　　　　nontraffic V58.0 ☑
　　　hanger-on
　　　　collision (with)
　　　　　animal (traffic) V50.7 ☑
　　　　　　being ridden (traffic) V56.7 ☑
　　　　　　　nontraffic V56.2 ☑
　　　　　　nontraffic V50.2 ☑
　　　　　animal-drawn vehicle (traffic) V56.7 ☑
　　　　　　nontraffic V56.2 ☑
　　　　　bus (traffic) V54.7 ☑
　　　　　　nontraffic V54.2 ☑
　　　　　car (traffic) V53.7 ☑

Accident — *continued*
　transport — *continued*
　　pickup truck occupant — *continued*
　　　hanger-on — *continued*
　　　　collision — *continued*
　　　　　car — *continued*
　　　　　　nontraffic V53.2 ☑
　　　　　pedal cycle (traffic) V51.7 ☑
　　　　　　nontraffic V51.2 ☑
　　　　　pickup truck (traffic) V53.7 ☑
　　　　　　nontraffic V53.2 ☑
　　　　　railway vehicle (traffic) V55.7 ☑
　　　　　　nontraffic V55.2 ☑
　　　　　specified vehicle NEC (traffic) V56.7 ☑
　　　　　　nontraffic V56.2 ☑
　　　　　stationary object (traffic) V57.7 ☑
　　　　　　nontraffic V57.2 ☑
　　　　　streetcar (traffic) V56.7 ☑
　　　　　　nontraffic V56.2 ☑
　　　　　three wheeled motor vehicle (traffic)
　　　　　　V52.7 ☑
　　　　　　nontraffic V52.2 ☑
　　　　　truck (traffic) V54.7 ☑
　　　　　　nontraffic V54.2 ☑
　　　　　two wheeled motor vehicle (traffic)
　　　　　　V52.7 ☑
　　　　　　nontraffic V52.2 ☑
　　　　　van (traffic) V53.7 ☑
　　　　　　nontraffic V53.2 ☑
　　　　noncollision accident (traffic) V58.7 ☑
　　　　　nontraffic V58.2 ☑
　　　noncollision accident (traffic) V58.9 ☑
　　　　nontraffic V58.3 ☑
　　　　while boarding or alighting V58.4 ☑
　　　nontraffic V59.3 ☑
　　　passenger
　　　　collision (with)
　　　　　animal (traffic) V50.6 ☑
　　　　　　being ridden (traffic) V56.6 ☑
　　　　　　　nontraffic V56.1 ☑
　　　　　　nontraffic V50.1 ☑
　　　　　animal-drawn vehicle (traffic) V56.6 ☑
　　　　　　nontraffic V56.1 ☑
　　　　　bus (traffic) V54.6 ☑
　　　　　　nontraffic V54.1 ☑
　　　　　car (traffic) V53.6 ☑
　　　　　　nontraffic V53.1 ☑
　　　　　motor vehicle NOS (traffic) V59.50 ☑
　　　　　　nontraffic V59.10 ☑
　　　　　　specified type NEC (traffic) V59.59 ☑
　　　　　　　nontraffic V59.19 ☑
　　　　　pedal cycle (traffic) V51.6 ☑
　　　　　　nontraffic V51.1 ☑
　　　　　pickup truck (traffic) V53.6 ☑
　　　　　　nontraffic V53.1 ☑
　　　　　railway vehicle (traffic) V55.6 ☑
　　　　　　nontraffic V55.1 ☑
　　　　　specified vehicle NEC (traffic) V56.6 ☑
　　　　　　nontraffic V56.1 ☑
　　　　　stationary object (traffic) V57.6 ☑
　　　　　　nontraffic V57.1 ☑
　　　　　streetcar (traffic) V56.6 ☑
　　　　　　nontraffic V56.1 ☑
　　　　　three wheeled motor vehicle (traffic)
　　　　　　V52.6 ☑
　　　　　　nontraffic V52.1 ☑
　　　　　truck (traffic) V54.6 ☑
　　　　　　nontraffic V54.1 ☑
　　　　　two wheeled motor vehicle (traffic)
　　　　　　V52.6 ☑
　　　　　　nontraffic V52.1 ☑
　　　　　van (traffic) V53.6 ☑
　　　　　　nontraffic V53.1 ☑
　　　　noncollision accident (traffic) V58.6 ☑
　　　　　nontraffic V58.1 ☑
　　　specified type NEC V59.88 ☑
　　　military vehicle V59.81 ☑
　　quarry truck — *see* Accident, transport, industrial
　　　vehicle occupant
　　race car — *see* Accident, transport, motor vehicle
　　　NEC occupant
　　railway vehicle occupant V81.9 ☑
　　　collision (with) V81.3 ☑
　　　　motor vehicle (non-military) (traffic)
　　　　　V81.1 ☑
　　　　　military V81.83 ☑

Accident — *continued*
　transport — *continued*
　　railway vehicle occupant — *continued*
　　　collision — *continued*
　　　　motor vehicle — *continued*
　　　　　nontraffic V81.0 ☑
　　　　rolling stock V81.2 ☑
　　　　specified object NEC V81.3 ☑
　　　during derailment V81.7 ☑
　　　　with antecedent collision B — *see* Accident,
　　　　　transport, railway vehicle occupant,
　　　　　collision
　　　explosion V81.81 ☑
　　　fall (in railway vehicle) V81.5 ☑
　　　　during derailment V81.7 ☑
　　　　　with antecedent collision B — *see* Acci-
　　　　　　dent, transport, railway vehicle
　　　　　　occupant, collision
　　　　from railway vehicle V81.6 ☑
　　　　　during derailment V81.7 ☑
　　　　　　with antecedent collision B — *see*
　　　　　　　Accident, transport, railway
　　　　　　　vehicle occupant, collision
　　　　while boarding or alighting V81.4 ☑
　　　fire V81.81 ☑
　　　object falling onto train V81.82 ☑
　　　specified type NEC V81.89 ☑
　　　while boarding or alighting V81.4 ☑
　　ski lift V98.3 ☑
　　snowmobile occupant (nontraffic) V86.92 ☑
　　　driver V86.52 ☑
　　　hanger-on V86.72 ☑
　　　passenger V86.62 ☑
　　　traffic V86.32 ☑
　　　　driver V86.02 ☑
　　　　hanger-on V86.22 ☑
　　　　passenger V86.12 ☑
　　　while boarding or alighting V86.42 ☑
　　specified NEC V98.8 ☑
　　sport utility vehicle occupant (*see also* Accident,
　　　transport, car occupant)
　　　collision (with)
　　　　stationary object (traffic) V47.91 ☑
　　　　　nontraffic V47.31 ☑
　　　driver
　　　　collision (with)
　　　　　stationary object (traffic) V47.51 ☑
　　　　　　nontraffic V47.01 ☑
　　　passenger
　　　　collision (with)
　　　　　stationary object (traffic) V47.61 ☑
　　　　　　nontraffic V47.11 ☑
　　streetcar occupant V82.9 ☑
　　　collision (with) V82.3 ☑
　　　　motor vehicle (traffic) V82.1 ☑
　　　　　nontraffic V82.0 ☑
　　　　rolling stock V82.2 ☑
　　　during derailment V82.7 ☑
　　　　with antecedent collision B — *see* Accident,
　　　　　transport, streetcar occupant, collision
　　　fall (in streetcar) V82.5 ☑
　　　　during derailment V82.7 ☑
　　　　　with antecedent collision B — *see* Acci-
　　　　　　dent, transport, streetcar occu-
　　　　　　pant, collision
　　　　from streetcar V82.6 ☑
　　　　　during derailment V82.7 ☑
　　　　　　with antecedent collision B — *see*
　　　　　　　Accident, transport, streetcar
　　　　　　　occupant, collision
　　　　while boarding or alighting V82.4 ☑
　　　　while boarding or alighting V82.4 ☑
　　　specified type NEC V82.8 ☑
　　　while boarding or alighting V82.4 ☑
　　three-wheeled motor vehicle occupant V39.9 ☑
　　　collision (with)
　　　　animal (traffic) V30.9 ☑
　　　　　being ridden (traffic) V36.9 ☑
　　　　　　nontraffic V36.3 ☑
　　　　　　while boarding or alighting V36.4 ☑
　　　　　nontraffic V30.3 ☑
　　　　　while boarding or alighting V30.4 ☑
　　　　animal-drawn vehicle (traffic) V36.9 ☑
　　　　　nontraffic V36.3 ☑
　　　　　while boarding or alighting V36.4 ☑
　　　　bus (traffic) V34.9 ☑

External Causes Index

Accident — *continued*
  transport — *continued*
    three-wheeled motor vehicle occupant — *continued*
      collision — *continued*
        bus — *continued*
          nontraffic V34.3 ☑
          while boarding or alighting V34.4 ☑
        car (traffic) V33.9 ☑
          nontraffic V33.3 ☑
          while boarding or alighting V33.4 ☑
        motor vehicle NOS (traffic) V39.60 ☑
          nontraffic V39.20 ☑
          specified type NEC (traffic) V39.69 ☑
            nontraffic V39.29 ☑
        pedal cycle (traffic) V31.9 ☑
          nontraffic V31.3 ☑
          while boarding or alighting V31.4 ☑
        pickup truck (traffic) V33.9 ☑
          nontraffic V33.3 ☑
          while boarding or alighting V33.4 ☑
        railway vehicle (traffic) V35.9 ☑
          nontraffic V35.3 ☑
          while boarding or alighting V35.4 ☑
        specified vehicle NEC (traffic) V36.9 ☑
          nontraffic V36.3 ☑
          while boarding or alighting V36.4 ☑
        stationary object (traffic) V37.9 ☑
          nontraffic V37.3 ☑
          while boarding or alighting V37.4 ☑
        streetcar (traffic) V36.9 ☑
          nontraffic V36.3 ☑
          while boarding or alighting V36.4 ☑
        three wheeled motor vehicle (traffic) V32.9 ☑
          nontraffic V32.3 ☑
          while boarding or alighting V32.4 ☑
        truck (traffic) V34.9 ☑
          nontraffic V34.3 ☑
          while boarding or alighting V34.4 ☑
        two wheeled motor vehicle (traffic) V32.9 ☑
          nontraffic V32.3 ☑
          while boarding or alighting V32.4 ☑
        van (traffic) V33.9 ☑
          nontraffic V33.3 ☑
          while boarding or alighting V33.4 ☑
    driver
      collision (with)
        animal (traffic) V30.5 ☑
          being ridden (traffic) V36.5 ☑
            nontraffic V36.0 ☑
          nontraffic V30.0 ☑
        animal-drawn vehicle (traffic) V36.5 ☑
          nontraffic V36.0 ☑
        bus (traffic) V34.5 ☑
          nontraffic V34.0 ☑
        car (traffic) V33.5 ☑
          nontraffic V33.0 ☑
        motor vehicle NOS (traffic) V39.40 ☑
          nontraffic V39.00 ☑
          specified type NEC (traffic) V39.49 ☑
            nontraffic V39.09 ☑
        pedal cycle (traffic) V31.5 ☑
          nontraffic V31.0 ☑
        pickup truck (traffic) V33.5 ☑
          nontraffic V33.0 ☑
        railway vehicle (traffic) V35.5 ☑
          nontraffic V35.0 ☑
        specified vehicle NEC (traffic) V36.5 ☑
          nontraffic V36.0 ☑
        stationary object (traffic) V37.5 ☑
          nontraffic V37.0 ☑
        streetcar (traffic) V36.5 ☑
          nontraffic V36.0 ☑
        three wheeled motor vehicle (traffic) V32.5 ☑
          nontraffic V32.0 ☑
        truck (traffic) V34.5 ☑
          nontraffic V34.0 ☑
        two wheeled motor vehicle (traffic) V32.5 ☑
          nontraffic V32.0 ☑
        van (traffic) V33.5 ☑
          nontraffic V33.0 ☑
      noncollision accident (traffic) V38.5 ☑
        nontraffic V38.0 ☑

Accident — *continued*
  transport — *continued*
    three-wheeled motor vehicle occupant — *continued*
      hanger-on
        collision (with)
          animal (traffic) V30.7 ☑
            being ridden (traffic) V36.7 ☑
              nontraffic V36.2 ☑
            nontraffic V30.2 ☑
          animal-drawn vehicle (traffic) V36.7 ☑
            nontraffic V36.2 ☑
          bus (traffic) V34.7 ☑
            nontraffic V34.2 ☑
          car (traffic) V33.7 ☑
            nontraffic V33.2 ☑
          pedal cycle (traffic) V31.7 ☑
            nontraffic V31.2 ☑
          pickup truck (traffic) V33.7 ☑
            nontraffic V33.2 ☑
          railway vehicle (traffic) V35.7 ☑
            nontraffic V35.2 ☑
          specified vehicle NEC (traffic) V36.7 ☑
            nontraffic V36.2 ☑
          stationary object (traffic) V37.7 ☑
            nontraffic V37.2 ☑
          streetcar (traffic) V36.7 ☑
            nontraffic V36.2 ☑
          three wheeled motor vehicle (traffic) V32.7 ☑
            nontraffic V32.2 ☑
          truck (traffic) V34.7 ☑
            nontraffic V34.2 ☑
          two wheeled motor vehicle (traffic) V32.7 ☑
            nontraffic V32.2 ☑
          van (traffic) V33.7 ☑
            nontraffic V33.2 ☑
        noncollision accident (traffic) V38.7 ☑
          nontraffic V38.2 ☑
      noncollision accident (traffic) V38.9 ☑
        nontraffic V38.3 ☑
        while boarding or alighting V38.4 ☑
      nontraffic V39.3 ☑
      passenger
        collision (with)
          animal (traffic) V30.6 ☑
            being ridden (traffic) V36.6 ☑
              nontraffic V36.1 ☑
            nontraffic V30.1 ☑
          animal-drawn vehicle (traffic) V36.6 ☑
          bus (traffic) V34.6 ☑
            nontraffic V34.1 ☑
          car (traffic) V33.6 ☑
            nontraffic V33.1 ☑
          motor vehicle NOS (traffic) V39.50 ☑
            nontraffic V39.10 ☑
            specified type NEC (traffic) V39.59 ☑
              nontraffic V39.19 ☑
          pedal cycle (traffic) V31.6 ☑
            nontraffic V31.1 ☑
          pickup truck (traffic) V33.6 ☑
            nontraffic V33.1 ☑
          railway vehicle (traffic) V35.6 ☑
            nontraffic V35.1 ☑
          specified vehicle NEC (traffic) V36.6 ☑
            nontraffic V36.1 ☑
          stationary object (traffic) V37.6 ☑
            nontraffic V37.1 ☑
          streetcar (traffic) V36.6 ☑
            nontraffic V36.1 ☑
          three wheeled motor vehicle (traffic) V32.6 ☑
            nontraffic V32.1 ☑
          truck (traffic) V34.6 ☑
            nontraffic V34.1 ☑
          two wheeled motor vehicle (traffic) V32.6 ☑
            nontraffic V32.1 ☑
          van (traffic) V33.6 ☑
            nontraffic V33.1 ☑
        noncollision accident (traffic) V38.6 ☑
          nontraffic V38.1 ☑
    specified type NEC V39.89 ☑
    military vehicle V39.81 ☑

Accident — *continued*
  transport — *continued*
    tractor (farm) (and trailer) — *see* Accident, transport, agricultural vehicle occupant
    tram — *see* Accident, transport, streetcar
      in mine or quarry — *see* Accident, transport, industrial vehicle occupant
    trolley — *see* Accident, transport, streetcar
      in mine or quarry — *see* Accident, transport, industrial vehicle occupant
    truck (heavy) occupant V69.9 ☑
      collision (with)
        animal (traffic) V60.9 ☑
          being ridden (traffic) V66.9 ☑
            nontraffic V66.3 ☑
            while boarding or alighting V66.4 ☑
          nontraffic V60.3 ☑
          while boarding or alighting V60.4 ☑
        animal-drawn vehicle (traffic) V66.9 ☑
          nontraffic V66.3 ☑
          while boarding or alighting V66.4 ☑
        bus (traffic) V64.9 ☑
          nontraffic V64.3 ☑
          while boarding or alighting V64.4 ☑
        car (traffic) V63.9 ☑
          nontraffic V63.3 ☑
          while boarding or alighting V63.4 ☑
        motor vehicle NOS (traffic) V69.60 ☑
          nontraffic V69.20 ☑
          specified type NEC (traffic) V69.69 ☑
            nontraffic V69.29 ☑
        pedal cycle (traffic) V61.9 ☑
          nontraffic V61.3 ☑
          while boarding or alighting V61.4 ☑
        pickup truck (traffic) V63.9 ☑
          nontraffic V63.3 ☑
          while boarding or alighting V63.4 ☑
        railway vehicle (traffic) V65.9 ☑
          nontraffic V65.3 ☑
          while boarding or alighting V65.4 ☑
        specified vehicle NEC (traffic) V66.9 ☑
          nontraffic V66.3 ☑
          while boarding or alighting V66.4 ☑
        stationary object (traffic) V67.9 ☑
          nontraffic V67.3 ☑
          while boarding or alighting V67.4 ☑
        streetcar (traffic) V66.9 ☑
          nontraffic V66.3 ☑
          while boarding or alighting V66.4 ☑
        three wheeled motor vehicle (traffic) V62.9 ☑
          nontraffic V62.3 ☑
          while boarding or alighting V62.4 ☑
        truck (traffic) V64.9 ☑
          nontraffic V64.3 ☑
          while boarding or alighting V64.4 ☑
        two wheeled motor vehicle (traffic) V62.9 ☑
          nontraffic V62.3 ☑
          while boarding or alighting V62.4 ☑
        van (traffic) V63.9 ☑
          nontraffic V63.3 ☑
          while boarding or alighting V63.4 ☑
      driver
        collision (with)
          animal (traffic) V60.5 ☑
            being ridden (traffic) V66.5 ☑
              nontraffic V66.0 ☑
            nontraffic V60.0 ☑
          animal-drawn vehicle (traffic) V66.5 ☑
            nontraffic V66.0 ☑
          bus (traffic) V64.5 ☑
            nontraffic V64.0 ☑
          car (traffic) V63.5 ☑
            nontraffic V63.0 ☑
          motor vehicle NOS (traffic) V69.40 ☑
            nontraffic V69.00 ☑
            specified type NEC (traffic) V69.49 ☑
              nontraffic V69.09 ☑
          pedal cycle (traffic) V61.5 ☑
            nontraffic V61.0 ☑
          pickup truck (traffic) V63.5 ☑
            nontraffic V63.0 ☑
          railway vehicle (traffic) V65.5 ☑
            nontraffic V65.0 ☑
          specified vehicle NEC (traffic) V66.5 ☑
            nontraffic V66.0 ☑

  ☑ **Additional Character Required** — Refer to the Tabular List for Character Selection   ▽ **Subterms under main terms may continue to next column or page**

Accident — *continued*
  transport — *continued*
    truck occupant — *continued*
      driver — *continued*
        collision — *continued*
          stationary object (traffic) V67.5 ☑
            nontraffic V67.0 ☑
          streetcar (traffic) V66.5 ☑
            nontraffic V66.0 ☑
          three wheeled motor vehicle (traffic)
            V62.5 ☑
            nontraffic V62.0 ☑
          truck (traffic) V64.5 ☑
            nontraffic V64.0 ☑
          two wheeled motor vehicle (traffic)
            V62.5 ☑
            nontraffic V62.0 ☑
          van (traffic) V63.5 ☑
            nontraffic V63.0 ☑
         noncollision accident (traffic) V68.5 ☑
          nontraffic V68.0 ☑
      dump — *see* Accident, transport, construction
        vehicle occupant
      hanger-on
        collision (with)
          animal (traffic) V60.7 ☑
            being ridden (traffic) V66.7 ☑
              nontraffic V66.2 ☑
            nontraffic V60.2 ☑
          animal-drawn vehicle (traffic) V66.7 ☑
            nontraffic V66.2 ☑
          bus (traffic) V64.7 ☑
            nontraffic V64.2 ☑
          car (traffic) V63.7 ☑
            nontraffic V63.2 ☑
          pedal cycle (traffic) V61.7 ☑
            nontraffic V61.2 ☑
          pickup truck (traffic) V63.7 ☑
            nontraffic V63.2 ☑
          railway vehicle (traffic) V65.7 ☑
            nontraffic V65.2 ☑
          specified vehicle NEC (traffic) V66.7 ☑
            nontraffic V66.2 ☑
          stationary object (traffic) V67.7 ☑
            nontraffic V67.2 ☑
          streetcar (traffic) V66.7 ☑
            nontraffic V66.2 ☑
          three wheeled motor vehicle (traffic)
            V62.7 ☑
            nontraffic V62.2 ☑
          truck (traffic) V64.7 ☑
            nontraffic V64.2 ☑
          two wheeled motor vehicle (traffic)
            V62.7 ☑
            nontraffic V62.2 ☑
          van (traffic) V63.7 ☑
            nontraffic V63.2 ☑
        noncollision accident (traffic) V68.7 ☑
          nontraffic V68.2 ☑
      noncollision accident (traffic) V68.9 ☑
        nontraffic V68.3 ☑
        while boarding or alighting V68.4 ☑
      nontraffic V69.3 ☑
      passenger
        collision (with)
          animal (traffic) V60.6 ☑
            being ridden (traffic) V66.6 ☑
              nontraffic V66.1- ☑
            nontraffic V60.1 ☑
          animal-drawn vehicle (traffic) V66.6 ☑
            nontraffic V66.1 ☑
          bus (traffic) V64.6 ☑
            nontraffic V64.1 ☑
          car (traffic) V63.6 ☑
            nontraffic V63.1 ☑
          motor vehicle NOS (traffic) V69.50 ☑
            nontraffic V69.10 ☑
            specified type NEC (traffic) V69.59 ☑
              nontraffic V69.19 ☑
          pedal cycle (traffic) V61.6 ☑
            nontraffic V61.1 ☑
          pickup truck (traffic) V63.6 ☑
            nontraffic V63.1 ☑
          railway vehicle (traffic) V65.6 ☑
            nontraffic V65.1 ☑
          specified vehicle NEC (traffic) V66.6 ☑

Accident — *continued*
  transport — *continued*
    truck occupant — *continued*
      passenger — *continued*
        collision — *continued*
          specified vehicle — *continued*
            nontraffic V66.1 ☑
          stationary object (traffic) V67.6 ☑
            nontraffic V67.1 ☑
          streetcar (traffic) V66.6 ☑
            nontraffic V66.1 ☑
          three wheeled motor vehicle (traffic)
            V62.6 ☑
            nontraffic V62.1 ☑
          truck (traffic) V64.6 ☑
            nontraffic V64.1 ☑
          two wheeled motor vehicle (traffic)
            V62.6 ☑
            nontraffic V62.1 ☑
          van (traffic) V63.6 ☑
            nontraffic V63.1 ☑
        noncollision accident (traffic) V68.6 ☑
          nontraffic V68.1 ☑
      pickup — *see* Accident, transport, pickup truck
        occupant
      specified type NEC V69.88 ☑
        military vehicle V69.81 ☑
    van occupant V59.9 ☑
      collision (with)
        animal (traffic) V50.9 ☑
          being ridden (traffic) V56.9 ☑
            nontraffic V56.3 ☑
            while boarding or alighting V56.4 ☑
          nontraffic V50.3 ☑
            while boarding or alighting V50.4 ☑
        animal-drawn vehicle (traffic) V56.9 ☑
          nontraffic V56.3 ☑
          while boarding or alighting V56.4 ☑
        bus (traffic) V54.9 ☑
          nontraffic V54.3 ☑
          while boarding or alighting V54.4 ☑
        car (traffic) V53.9 ☑
          nontraffic V53.3 ☑
          while boarding or alighting V53.4 ☑
        motor vehicle NOS (traffic) V59.60 ☑
          nontraffic V59.20 ☑
          specified type NEC (traffic) V59.69 ☑
            nontraffic V59.29 ☑
        pedal cycle (traffic) V51.9 ☑
          nontraffic V51.3 ☑
          while boarding or alighting V51.4 ☑
        pickup truck (traffic) V53.9 ☑
          nontraffic V53.3 ☑
          while boarding or alighting V53.4 ☑
        railway vehicle (traffic) V55.9 ☑
          nontraffic V55.3 ☑
          while boarding or alighting V55.4 ☑
        specified vehicle NEC (traffic) V56.9 ☑
          nontraffic V56.3 ☑
          while boarding or alighting V56.4 ☑
        stationary object (traffic) V57.9 ☑
          nontraffic V57.3 ☑
          while boarding or alighting V57.4 ☑
        streetcar (traffic) V56.9 ☑
          nontraffic V56.3 ☑
          while boarding or alighting V56.4 ☑
        three wheeled motor vehicle (traffic)
          V52.9 ☑
          nontraffic V52.3 ☑
          while boarding or alighting V52.4 ☑
        truck (traffic) V54.9 ☑
          nontraffic V54.3 ☑
          while boarding or alighting V54.4 ☑
        two wheeled motor vehicle (traffic) V52.9 ☑
          nontraffic V52.3 ☑
          while boarding or alighting V52.4 ☑
        van (traffic) V53.9 ☑
          nontraffic V53.3 ☑
          while boarding or alighting V53.4 ☑
      driver
        collision (with)
          animal (traffic) V50.5 ☑
            being ridden (traffic) V56.5 ☑
              nontraffic V56.0 ☑
            nontraffic V50.0 ☑
          animal-drawn vehicle (traffic) V56.5 ☑

Accident — *continued*
  transport — *continued*
    van occupant — *continued*
      driver — *continued*
        collision — *continued*
          animal-drawn vehicle — *continued*
            nontraffic V56.0 ☑
          bus (traffic) V54.5 ☑
            nontraffic V54.0 ☑
          car (traffic) V53.5 ☑
            nontraffic V53.0 ☑
          motor vehicle NOS (traffic) V59.40 ☑
            nontraffic V59.00 ☑
            specified type NEC (traffic) V59.49 ☑
              nontraffic V59.09 ☑
          pedal cycle (traffic) V51.5 ☑
            nontraffic V51.0 ☑
          pickup truck (traffic) V53.5 ☑
            nontraffic V53.0 ☑
          railway vehicle (traffic) V55.5 ☑
            nontraffic V55.0 ☑
          specified vehicle NEC (traffic) V56.5 ☑
            nontraffic V56.0 ☑
          stationary object (traffic) V57.5 ☑
            nontraffic V57.0 ☑
          streetcar (traffic) V56.5 ☑
            nontraffic V56.0 ☑
          three wheeled motor vehicle (traffic)
          V52.5 ☑
          nontraffic V52.0 ☑
          truck (traffic) V54.5 ☑
            nontraffic V54.0 ☑
          two wheeled motor vehicle (traffic)
          V52.5 ☑
          nontraffic V52.0 ☑
          van (traffic) V53.5 ☑
            nontraffic V53.0 ☑
        noncollision accident (traffic) V58.5 ☑
          nontraffic V58.0 ☑
      hanger-on
        collision (with)
          animal (traffic) V50.7 ☑
            being ridden (traffic) V56.7 ☑
              nontraffic V56.2 ☑
            nontraffic V50.2 ☑
          animal-drawn vehicle (traffic) V56.7 ☑
            nontraffic V56.2 ☑
          bus (traffic) V54.7 ☑
            nontraffic V54.2 ☑
          car (traffic) V53.7 ☑
            nontraffic V53.2 ☑
          pedal cycle (traffic) V51.7 ☑
            nontraffic V51.2 ☑
          pickup truck (traffic) V53.7 ☑
            nontraffic V53.2 ☑
          railway vehicle (traffic) V55.7 ☑
            nontraffic V55.2 ☑
          specified vehicle NEC (traffic) V56.7 ☑
            nontraffic V56.2 ☑
          stationary object (traffic) V57.7 ☑
            nontraffic V57.2 ☑
          streetcar (traffic) V56.7 ☑
            nontraffic V56.2 ☑
          three wheeled motor vehicle (traffic)
          V52.7 ☑
          nontraffic V52.2 ☑
          truck (traffic) V54.7 ☑
            nontraffic V54.2 ☑
          two wheeled motor vehicle (traffic)
          V52.7 ☑
          nontraffic V52.2 ☑
          van (traffic) V53.7 ☑
            nontraffic V53.2 ☑
        noncollision accident (traffic) V58.7 ☑
          nontraffic V58.2 ☑
      noncollision accident (traffic) V58.9 ☑
        nontraffic V58.3 ☑
        while boarding or alighting V58.4 ☑
      nontraffic V59.3 ☑
      passenger
        collision (with)
          animal (traffic) V50.6 ☑
            being ridden (traffic) V56.6 ☑
              nontraffic V56.1 ☑
            nontraffic V50.1 ☑
          animal-drawn vehicle (traffic) V56.6 ☑

Accident — *continued*
  transport — *continued*
    van occupant — *continued*
      passenger — *continued*
        collision — *continued*
          animal-drawn vehicle — *continued*
            nontraffic V56.1 ☑
          bus (traffic) V54.6 ☑
            nontraffic V54.1 ☑
          car (traffic) V53.6 ☑
            nontraffic V53.1 ☑
          motor vehicle NOS (traffic) V59.5Ø ☑
            nontraffic V59.1Ø ☑
            specified type NEC (traffic) V59.59 ☑
              nontraffic V59.19 ☑
          pedal cycle (traffic) V51.6 ☑
            nontraffic V51.1 ☑
          pickup truck (traffic) V53.6 ☑
            nontraffic V53.1 ☑
          railway vehicle (traffic) V55.6 ☑
            nontraffic V55.1 ☑
          specified vehicle NEC (traffic) V56.6 ☑
            nontraffic V56.1 ☑
          stationary object (traffic) V57.6 ☑
            nontraffic V57.1 ☑
          streetcar (traffic) V56.6 ☑
            nontraffic V56.1 ☑
          three wheeled motor vehicle (traffic) V52.6 ☑
            nontraffic V52.1 ☑
          truck (traffic) V54.6 ☑
            nontraffic V54.1 ☑
          two wheeled motor vehicle (traffic) V52.6 ☑
            nontraffic V52.1 ☑
          van (traffic) V53.6 ☑
            nontraffic V53.1 ☑
        noncollision accident (traffic) V58.6 ☑
          nontraffic V58.1 ☑
        specified type NEC V59.88 ☑
        military vehicle V59.81 ☑
  watercraft occupant — *see* Accident, watercraft
  vehicle NEC V89.9 ☑
    animal-drawn NEC — *see* Accident, transport, animal-drawn vehicle occupant
    special
      agricultural — *see* Accident, transport, agricultural vehicle occupant
      construction — *see* Accident, transport, construction vehicle occupant
      industrial — *see* Accident, transport, industrial vehicle occupant
      three-wheeled NEC (motorized) — *see* Accident, transport, three-wheeled motor vehicle occupant
  watercraft V94.9 ☑
    causing
      drowning B — *see* Drowning, due to, accident to, watercraft
      injury NEC V91.89 ☑
        crushed between craft and object V91.19 ☑
          powered craft V91.13 ☑
            ferry boat V91.11 ☑
            fishing boat V91.12 ☑
            jetskis V91.13 ☑
            liner V91.11 ☑
            merchant ship V91.10 ☑
            passenger ship V91.11 ☑
          unpowered craft V91.18 ☑
            canoe V91.15 ☑
            inflatable V91.16 ☑
            kayak V91.15 ☑
            sailboat V91.14 ☑
            surf-board V91.18 ☑
            windsurfer V91.18 ☑
        fall on board V91.29 ☑
          powered craft V91.23 ☑
            ferry boat V91.21 ☑
            fishing boat V91.22 ☑
            jetskis V91.23 ☑
            liner V91.21 ☑
            merchant ship V91.20 ☑
            passenger ship V91.21 ☑
          unpowered craft
            canoe V91.25 ☑
            inflatable V91.26 ☑

Accident — *continued*
  watercraft — *continued*
    causing — *continued*
      injury — *continued*
        fall on board — *continued*
          unpowered craft — *continued*
            kayak V91.25 ☑
            sailboat V91.24 ☑
        fire on board causing burn V91.09 ☑
          powered craft V91.03 ☑
            ferry boat V91.01 ☑
            fishing boat V91.02 ☑
            jetskis V91.03 ☑
            liner V91.01 ☑
            merchant ship V91.00 ☑
            passenger ship V91.01 ☑
          unpowered craft V91.08 ☑
            canoe V91.05 ☑
            inflatable V91.06 ☑
            kayak V91.05 ☑
            sailboat V91.04 ☑
            surf-board V91.08 ☑
            water skis V91.07 ☑
            windsurfer V91.08 ☑
        hit by falling object V91.39 ☑
          powered craft V91.33 ☑
            ferry boat V91.31 ☑
            fishing boat V91.32 ☑
            jetskis V91.33 ☑
            liner V91.31 ☑
            merchant ship V91.30 ☑
            passenger ship V91.31 ☑
          unpowered craft V91.38 ☑
            canoe V91.35 ☑
            inflatable V91.36 ☑
            kayak V91.35 ☑
            sailboat V91.34 ☑
            surf-board V91.38 ☑
            water skis V91.37 ☑
            windsurfer V91.38 ☑
        specified type NEC V91.89 ☑
          powered craft V91.83 ☑
            ferry boat V91.81 ☑
            fishing boat V91.82 ☑
            jetskis V91.83 ☑
            liner V91.81 ☑
            merchant ship V91.80 ☑
            passenger ship V91.81 ☑
          unpowered craft V91.88 ☑
            canoe V91.85 ☑
            inflatable V91.86 ☑
            kayak V91.85 ☑
            sailboat V91.84 ☑
            surf-board V91.88 ☑
            water skis V91.87 ☑
            windsurfer V91.88 ☑
      due to, caused by cataclysm — *see* Forces of nature, by type
    military NEC V94.818 ☑
      with civilian watercraft V94.810 ☑
      civilian in water injured by V94.811 ☑
    nonpowered, struck by
      nonpowered vessel V94.22 ☑
      powered vessel V94.21 ☑
    specified type NEC V94.89 ☑
    striking swimmer
      powered V94.11 ☑
      unpowered V94.12 ☑
Acid throwing (assault) Y08.89 ☑
Activity (involving) (of victim at time of event) Y93.9
  aerobic and step exercise (class) Y93.A3 (*following* Y93.7)
  alpine skiing Y93.23
  animal care NEC Y93.K9 (*following* Y93.7)
  arts and handcrafts NEC Y93.D9 (*following* Y93.7)
  athletics played as a team or group NEC Y93.69
  athletics played individually NEC Y93.59
  athletics NEC Y93.79
  baking Y93.G3 (*following* Y93.7)
  ballet Y93.41
  barbells Y93.B3 (*following* Y93.7)
  BASE (Building, Antenna, Span, Earth) jumping Y93.33
  baseball Y93.64
  basketball Y93.67
  bathing (personal) Y93.E1 (*following* Y93.7)
  beach volleyball Y93.68

Activity — *continued*
  bike riding Y93.55
  boogie boarding Y93.18
  bowling Y93.54
  boxing Y93.71
  brass instrument playing Y93.J4 (*following* Y93.7)
  building construction Y93.H3 (*following* Y93.7)
  bungee jumping Y93.34
  calisthenics Y93.A2 (*following* Y93.7)
  canoeing (in calm and turbulent water) Y93.16
  capture the flag Y93.6A
  cardiorespiratory exercise NEC Y93.A9 (*following* Y93.7)
  caregiving (providing) NEC Y93.F9 (*following* Y93.7)
    bathing Y93.F1 (*following* Y93.7)
    lifting Y93.F2 (*following* Y93.7)
  cellular
    communication device Y93.C2 (*following* Y93.7)
    telephone Y93.C2 (*following* Y93.7)
  challenge course Y93.A5 (*following* Y93.7)
  cheerleading Y93.45
  circuit training Y93.A4 (*following* Y93.7)
  cleaning
    floor Y93.E5 (*following* Y93.7)
  climbing NEC Y93.39
    mountain Y93.31
    rock Y93.31
    wall Y93.31
  clothing care and maintenance NEC Y93.E9 (*following* Y93.7)
  combatives Y93.75
  computer
    keyboarding Y93.C1 (*following* Y93.7)
    technology NEC Y93.C9 (*following* Y93.7)
  confidence course Y93.A5 (*following* Y93.7)
  construction (building) Y93.H3 (*following* Y93.7)
  cooking and baking Y93.G3 (*following* Y93.7)
  cool down exercises Y93.A2 (*following* Y93.7)
  cricket Y93.69
  crocheting Y93.D1 (*following* Y93.7)
  cross country skiing Y93.24
  dancing (all types) Y93.41
  digging
    dirt Y93.H1 (*following* Y93.7)
  dirt digging Y93.H1 (*following* Y93.7)
  dishwashing Y93.G1 (*following* Y93.7)
  diving (platform) (springboard) Y93.12
    underwater Y93.15
  dodge ball Y93.6A
  downhill skiing Y93.23
  drum playing Y93.J2 (*following* Y93.7)
  dumbbells Y93.B3 (*following* Y93.7)
  electronic
    devices NEC Y93.C9 (*following* Y93.7)
      hand held interactive Y93.C2 (*following* Y93.7)
    game playing (using) (with)
      interactive device Y93.C2 (*following* Y93.7)
      keyboard or other stationary device Y93.C1 (*following* Y93.7)
  elliptical machine Y93.A1 (*following* Y93.7)
  exercise(s)
    machines ((primarily) for)
      cardiorespiratory conditioning Y93.A1 (*following* Y93.7)
      muscle strengthening Y93.B1 (*following* Y93.7)
    muscle strengthening (non-machine) NEC Y93.B9 (*following* Y93.7)
  external motion NEC Y93.I9 (*following* Y93.7)
    rollercoaster Y93.I1 (*following* Y93.7)
  field hockey Y93.65
  figure skating (pairs) (singles) Y93.21
  flag football Y93.62
  floor mopping and cleaning Y93.E5 (*following* Y93.7)
  food preparation and clean up Y93.G1 (*following* Y93.7)
  football (American) NOS Y93.61
    flag Y93.62
    tackle Y93.61
    touch Y93.62
  four square Y93.6A
  free weights Y93.B3 (*following* Y93.7)
  frisbee (ultimate) Y93.74
  furniture
    building Y93.D3 (*following* Y93.7)
    finishing Y93.D3 (*following* Y93.7)
    repair Y93.D3 (*following* Y93.7)
  game playing (electronic)
    using interactive device Y93.C2 (*following* Y93.7)
    using keyboard or other stationary device Y93.C1 (*following* Y93.7)

Activity — *continued*

gardening Y93.H2 (*following* Y93.7)
golf Y93.53
grass drills Y93.A6 (*following* Y93.7)
grilling and smoking food Y93.G2 (*following* Y93.7)
grooming and shearing an animal Y93.K3 (*following* Y93.7)
guerilla drills Y93.A6 (*following* Y93.7)
gymnastics (rhythmic) Y93.43
hand held interactive electronic device Y93.C2 (*following* Y93.7)
handball Y93.73
handcrafts NEC Y93.D9 (*following* Y93.7)
hang gliding Y93.35
hiking (on level or elevated terrain) Y93.Ø1
hockey (ice) Y93.22
　field Y93.65
horseback riding Y93.52
household (interior) maintenance NEC Y93.E9 (*following* Y93.7)
ice NEC Y93.29
　dancing Y93.21
　hockey Y93.22
　skating Y93.21
inline roller skating Y93.51
ironing Y93.E4 (*following* Y93.7)
judo Y93.75
jumping jacks Y93.A2 (*following* Y93.7)
jumping rope Y93.56
jumping (off) NEC Y93.39
　BASE (Building, Antenna, Span, Earth) Y93.33
　bungee Y93.34
　jacks Y93.A2 (*following* Y93.7)
　rope Y93.56
karate Y93.75
kayaking (in calm and turbulent water) Y93.16
keyboarding (computer) Y93.C1 (*following* Y93.7)
kickball Y93.6A
knitting Y93.D1 (*following* Y93.7)
lacrosse Y93.65
land maintenance NEC Y93.H9 (*following* Y93.7)
landscaping Y93.H2 (*following* Y93.7)
laundry Y93.E2 (*following* Y93.7)
machines (exercise)
　primarily for cardiorespiratory conditioning Y93.A1 (*following* Y93.7)
　primarily for muscle strengthening Y93.B1 (*following* Y93.7)
maintenance
　exterior building NEC Y93.H9 (*following* Y93.7)
　household (interior) NEC Y93.E9 (*following* Y93.7)
　land Y93.H9 (*following* Y93.7)
　property Y93.H9 (*following* Y93.7)
marching (on level or elevated terrain) Y93.Ø1
martial arts Y93.75
microwave oven Y93.G3 (*following* Y93.7)
milking an animal Y93.K2 (*following* Y93.7)
mopping (floor) Y93.E5 (*following* Y93.7)
mountain climbing Y93.31
muscle strengthening
　exercises (non-machine) NEC Y93.B9 (*following* Y93.7)
　machines Y93.B1 (*following* Y93.7)
musical keyboard (electronic) playing Y93.J1 (*following* Y93.7)
nordic skiing Y93.24
obstacle course Y93.A5 (*following* Y93.7)
oven (microwave) Y93.G3 (*following* Y93.7)
packing up and unpacking in moving to a new residence Y93.E6 (*following* Y93.7)
parasailing Y93.19
percussion instrument playing NEC Y93.J2 (*following* Y93.7)
personal
　bathing and showering Y93.E1 (*following* Y93.7)
　hygiene NEC Y93.E8 (*following* Y93.7)
　showering Y93.E1 (*following* Y93.7)
physical games generally associated with school recess, summer camp and children Y93.6A
physical training NEC Y93.A9 (*following* Y93.7)
piano playing Y93.J1 (*following* Y93.7)
pilates Y93.B4 (*following* Y93.7)
platform diving Y93.12
playing musical instrument
　brass instrument Y93.J4 (*following* Y93.7)
　drum Y93.J2 (*following* Y93.7)
　musical keyboard (electronic) Y93.J1 (*following* Y93.7)

Activity — *continued*

playing musical instrument — *continued*
　percussion instrument NEC Y93.J2 (*following* Y93.7)
　piano Y93.J1 (*following* Y93.7)
　string instrument Y93.J3 (*following* Y93.7)
　winds instrument Y93.J4 (*following* Y93.7)
property maintenance
　exterior NEC Y93.H9 (*following* Y93.7)
　interior NEC Y93.E9 (*following* Y93.7)
pruning (garden and lawn) Y93.H2 (*following* Y93.7)
pull-ups Y93.B2 (*following* Y93.7)
push-ups Y93.B2 (*following* Y93.7)
racquetball Y93.73
rafting (in calm and turbulent water) Y93.16
raking (leaves) Y93.H1 (*following* Y93.7)
rappelling Y93.32
refereeing a sports activity Y93.81
residential relocation Y93.E6 (*following* Y93.7)
rhythmic gymnastics Y93.43
rhythmic movement NEC Y93.49
riding
　horseback Y93.52
　rollercoaster Y93.I1 (*following* Y93.7)
rock climbing Y93.31
roller skating (inline) Y93.51
rollercoaster riding Y93.I1 (*following* Y93.7)
rough housing and horseplay Y93.83
rowing (in calm and turbulent water) Y93.16
rugby Y93.63
running Y93.Ø2
SCUBA diving Y93.15
sewing Y93.D2 (*following* Y93.7)
shoveling Y93.H1 (*following* Y93.7)
　dirt Y93.H1 (*following* Y93.7)
　snow Y93.H1 (*following* Y93.7)
showering (personal) Y93.E1 (*following* Y93.7)
sit-ups Y93.B2 (*following* Y93.7)
skateboarding Y93.51
skating (ice) Y93.21
　roller Y93.51
skiing (alpine) (downhill) Y93.23
　cross country Y93.24
　nordic Y93.24
　water Y93.17
sledding (snow) Y93.23
sleeping (sleep) Y93.84
smoking and grilling food Y93.G2 (*following* Y93.7)
snorkeling Y93.15
snow NEC Y93.29
　boarding Y93.23
　shoveling Y93.H1 (*following* Y93.7)
　sledding Y93.23
　tubing Y93.23
soccer Y93.66
softball Y93.64
specified NEC Y93.89
spectator at an event Y93.82
sports NEC Y93.79
　sports played as a team or group NEC Y93.69
　sports played individually NEC Y93.59
springboard diving Y93.12
squash Y93.73
stationary bike Y93.A1 (*following* Y93.7)
step (stepping) exercise (class) Y93.A3 (*following* Y93.7)
stepper machine Y93.A1 (*following* Y93.7)
stove Y93.G3 (*following* Y93.7)
string instrument playing Y93.J3 (*following* Y93.7)
surfing Y93.18
　wind Y93.18
swimming Y93.11
tackle football Y93.61
tap dancing Y93.41
tennis Y93.73
tobogganing Y93.23
touch football Y93.62
track and field events (non-running) Y93.57
　running Y93.Ø2
trampoline Y93.44
treadmill Y93.A1 (*following* Y93.7)
trimming shrubs Y93.H2 (*following* Y93.7)
tubing (in calm and turbulent water) Y93.16
　snow Y93.23
ultimate frisbee Y93.74
underwater diving Y93.15
unpacking in moving to a new residence Y93.E6 (*following* Y93.7)
use of stove, oven and microwave oven Y93.G3 (*following* Y93.7)

Activity — *continued*

vacuuming Y93.E3 (*following* Y93.7)
volleyball (beach) (court) Y93.68
wake boarding Y93.17
walking (on level or elevated terrain) Y93.Ø1
　an animal Y93.K1 (*following* Y93.7)
walking an animal Y93.K1 (*following* Y93.7)
wall climbing Y93.31
warm up and cool down exercises Y93.A2 (*following* Y93.7)
water NEC Y93.19
　aerobics Y93.14
　craft NEC Y93.19
　exercise Y93.14
　polo Y93.13
　skiing Y93.17
　sliding Y93.18
　survival training and testing Y93.19
weeding (garden and lawn) Y93.H2 (*following* Y93.7)
wind instrument playing Y93.J4 (*following* Y93.7)
windsurfing Y93.18
wrestling Y93.72
yoga Y93.42

Adverse effect of drugs — *see* Table of Drugs and Chemicals

Aerosinusitis — *see* Air, pressure

After-effect, late — *see* Sequelae

Air

blast in war operations — *see* War operations, air blast pressure
　change, rapid
　　during
　　　ascent W94.29 ☑
　　　　while (in) (surfacing from)
　　　　　aircraft W94.23 ☑
　　　　　deep water diving W94.21 ☑
　　　　　underground W94.22 ☑
　　　descent W94.39 ☑
　　　　in
　　　　　aircraft W94.31 ☑
　　　　　water W94.32 ☑
　　high, prolonged W94.Ø ☑
　　low, prolonged W94.12 ☑
　　　due to residence or long visit at high altitude W94.11 ☑

Alpine sickness W94.11 ☑

Altitude sickness W94.11 ☑

Anaphylactic shock, anaphylaxis — *see* Table of Drugs and Chemicals

Andes disease W94.11 ☑

Arachnidism, arachnoidism X58 ☑

Arson (with intent to injure or kill) X97 ☑

Asphyxia, asphyxiation

by
　food (bone) (seed) — *see* categories T17 and T18 ☑
　gas (*see also* Table of Drugs and Chemicals)
　　legal
　　　execution — *see* Legal, intervention, gas
　　　intervention — *see* Legal, intervention, gas
from
　fire (*see also* Exposure, fire)
　　in war operations — *see* War operations, fire
　ignition — *see* Ignition
　vomitus T17.81 ☑
in war operations — *see* War operations, restriction of airway

Aspiration

food (any type) (into respiratory tract) (with asphyxia, obstruction respiratory tract, suffocation) — *see* categories T17 and T18 ☑
foreign body — *see* Foreign body, aspiration
vomitus (with asphyxia, obstruction respiratory tract, suffocation) T17.81 ☑

Assassination (attempt) — *see* Assault

Assault (homicidal) (by) (in) YØ9

arson X97 ☑
bite (of human being) YØ4.1 ☑
bodily force YØ4.8 ☑
　bite YØ4.1 ☑
　bumping into YØ4.2 ☑
　sexual — *see* subcategories T74.Ø, T76.Ø ☑
　unarmed fight YØ4.Ø ☑
bomb X96.9 ☑
　antipersonnel X96.Ø ☑
　fertilizer X96.3 ☑
　gasoline X96.1 ☑

Assault — *continued*
- bomb — *continued*
  - letter X96.2 ☑
  - petrol X96.1 ☑
  - pipe X96.3 ☑
  - specified NEC X96.8 ☑
- brawl (hand) (fists) (foot) (unarmed) Y04.0 ☑
- burning, burns (by fire) NEC X97 ☑
  - acid Y08.89 ☑
  - caustic, corrosive substance Y08.89 ☑
  - chemical from swallowing caustic, corrosive substance — *see* Table of Drugs and Chemicals
  - cigarette(s) X97 ☑
  - hot object X98.9 ☑
    - fluid NEC X98.2 ☑
    - household appliance X98.3 ☑
    - specified NEC X98.8 ☑
    - steam X98.0 ☑
    - tap water X98.1 ☑
    - vapors X98.0 ☑
  - scalding — *see* Assault, burning
  - steam X98.0 ☑
  - vitriol Y08.89 ☑
- caustic, corrosive substance (gas) Y08.89 ☑
- crashing of
  - aircraft Y08.81 ☑
  - motor vehicle Y03.8 ☑
    - pushed in front of Y02.0 ☑
    - run over Y03.0 ☑
    - specified NEC Y03.8 ☑
- cutting or piercing instrument X99.9 ☑
  - dagger X99.2 ☑
  - glass X99.0 ☑
  - knife X99.1 ☑
  - specified NEC X99.8 ☑
  - sword X99.2 ☑
- dagger X99.2 ☑
- drowning (in) X92.9 ☑
  - bathtub X92.0 ☑
  - natural water X92.3 ☑
  - specified NEC X92.8 ☑
  - swimming pool X92.1 ☑
    - following fall X92.2 ☑
- dynamite X96.8 ☑
- explosive(s) (material) X96.9 ☑
- fight (hand) (fists) (foot) (unarmed) Y04.0 ☑
  - with weapon — *see* Assault, by type of weapon
- fire X97 ☑
- firearm X95.9 ☑
  - airgun X95.01 ☑
  - handgun X93 ☑
  - hunting rifle X94.1 ☑
  - larger X94.9 ☑
    - specified NEC X94.8 ☑
  - machine gun X94.2 ☑
  - shotgun X94.0 ☑
  - specified NEC X95.8 ☑
- from high place Y01 ☑
- gunshot (wound) NEC — *see* Assault, firearm, by type
- incendiary device X97 ☑
- injury Y09 ☑
  - to child due to criminal abortion attempt NEC Y08.89 ☑
- knife X99.1 ☑
- late effect of — *see* categories X92-Y08 with 7th character S
- placing before moving object NEC Y02.8 ☑
  - motor vehicle Y02.0 ☑
- poisoning — *see* categories T36-T65 with 7th character S
- puncture, any part of body — *see* Assault, cutting or piercing instrument
- pushing
  - before moving object NEC Y02.8 ☑
    - motor vehicle Y02.0 ☑
    - subway train Y02.1 ☑
    - train Y02.1 ☑
  - from high place Y01 ☑
- rape T74.2- ☑
- scalding — *see* Assault, burning
- sequelae of — *see* categories X92-Y08 with 7th character S
- sexual (by bodily force) T74.2- ☑
- shooting — *see* Assault, firearm
- specified means NEC Y08.89 ☑

Assault — *continued*
- stab, any part of body — *see* Assault, cutting or piercing instrument
- steam X98.0 ☑
- striking against
  - other person Y04.2 ☑
  - sports equipment Y08.09 ☑
    - baseball bat Y08.02 ☑
    - hockey stick Y08.01 ☑
- struck by
  - sports equipment Y08.09 ☑
    - baseball bat Y08.02 ☑
    - hockey stick Y08.01 ☑
- submersion — *see* Assault, drowning
- violence Y09
- weapon Y09
  - blunt Y00 ☑
  - cutting or piercing — *see* Assault, cutting or piercing instrument
  - firearm — *see* Assault, firearm
- wound Y09
  - cutting — *see* Assault, cutting or piercing instrument
  - gunshot — *see* Assault, firearm
  - knife X99.1 ☑
  - piercing — *see* Assault, cutting or piercing instrument
  - puncture — *see* Assault, cutting or piercing instrument
  - stab — *see* Assault, cutting or piercing instrument

Attack by mammals NEC W55.89 ☑
Avalanche — *see* Landslide
Aviator's disease — *see* Air, pressure

B

Barotitis, barodontalgia, barosinusitis, barotrauma (otitic) (sinus) — *see* Air, pressure
Battered (baby) (child) (person) (syndrome) X58 ☑
Bayonet wound W26.1 ☑
- in
  - legal intervention — *see* Legal, intervention, sharp object, bayonet
  - war operations — *see* War operations, combat
- stated as undetermined whether accidental or intentional Y28.8 ☑
- suicide (attempt) X78.2 ☑

Bean in nose — *see* categories T17 and T18 ☑
Bed set on fire NEC — *see* Exposure, fire, uncontrolled, building, bed
Beheading (by guillotine)
- homicide X99.9 ☑
- legal execution — *see* Legal, intervention
Bending, injury in — *see* category Y93 ☑
Bends — *see* Air, pressure, change
Bite, bitten by
- alligator W58.01 ☑
- arthropod (nonvenomous) NEC W57 ☑
- bull W55.21 ☑
- cat W55.01 ☑
- cow W55.21 ☑
- crocodile W58.11 ☑
- dog W54.0 ☑
- goat W55.31 ☑
- hoof stock NEC W55.31 ☑
- horse W55.11 ☑
- human being (accidentally) W50.3 ☑
  - with intent to injure or kill Y04.1 ☑
  - as, or caused by, a crowd or human stampede (with fall) W52 ☑
  - assault Y04.1 ☑
  - homicide (attempt) Y04.1 ☑
  - in
    - fight Y04.1 ☑
- insect (nonvenomous) W57 ☑
- lizard (nonvenomous) W59.01 ☑
- mammal NEC W55.81 ☑
- mammal NEC W55.81 ☑
  - marine W56.31 ☑
- marine animal (nonvenomous) W56.81 ☑
- millipede W57 ☑
- moray eel W56.51 ☑
- mouse W53.01 ☑
- person(s) (accidentally) W50.3 ☑
  - with intent to injure or kill Y04.1 ☑

Bite, bitten by — *continued*
- person(s) — *continued*
  - as, or caused by, a crowd or human stampede (with fall) W52 ☑
  - assault Y04.1 ☑
  - homicide (attempt) Y04.1 ☑
  - in
    - fight Y04.1 ☑
- pig W55.41 ☑
- raccoon W55.51 ☑
- rat W53.11 ☑
- reptile W59.81 ☑
  - lizard W59.01 ☑
  - snake W59.11 ☑
  - turtle W59.21 ☑
    - terrestrial W59.81 ☑
- rodent W53.81 ☑
  - mouse W53.01 ☑
  - rat W53.11 ☑
  - specified NEC W53.81 ☑
  - squirrel W53.21 ☑
- shark W56.41 ☑
- sheep W55.31 ☑
- snake (nonvenomous) W59.11 ☑
- spider (nonvenomous) W57 ☑
- squirrel W53.21 ☑

Blast (air) in war operations — *see* War operations, blast
Blizzard X37.2 ☑
Blood alcohol level Y90.9
- less than 20mg/100ml Y90.0
- 20-39mg/100ml Y90.1
- 40-59mg/100ml Y90.2
- 60-79mg/100ml Y90.3
- 80-99mg/100ml Y90.4
- 100-119mg/100ml Y90.5
- 120-199mg/100ml Y90.6
- 200-239mg/100ml Y90.7
- presence in blood, level not specified Y90.9
Blow X58 ☑
- by law-enforcing agent, police (on duty) — *see* Legal, intervention, manhandling
- blunt object — *see* Legal, intervention, blunt object
Blowing up — *see* Explosion
Brawl (hand) (fists) (foot) Y04.0 ☑
Breakage (accidental) (part of)
- ladder (causing fall) W11 ☑
- scaffolding (causing fall) W12 ☑
Broken
- glass, contact with — *see* Contact, with, glass
- power line (causing electric shock) W85 ☑
Bumping against, into (accidentally)
- object NEC W22.8 ☑
  - with fall — *see* Fall, due to, bumping against, object
  - caused by crowd or human stampede (with fall) W52 ☑
  - sports equipment W21.9 ☑
- person(s) W51 ☑
  - with fall W03 ☑
    - due to ice or snow W00.0 ☑
  - assault Y04.2 ☑
  - caused by, a crowd or human stampede (with fall) W52 ☑
  - homicide (attempt) Y04.2 ☑
- sports equipment W21.9 ☑
Burn, burned, burning (accidental) (by) (from) (on)
- acid NEC — *see* Table of Drugs and Chemicals
- bed linen — *see* Exposure, fire, uncontrolled, in building, bed
- blowtorch X08.8 ☑
  - with ignition of clothing NEC X06.2 ☑
    - nightwear X05 ☑
- bonfire, campfire (controlled) (*see also* Exposure, fire, controlled, not in building)
  - uncontrolled — *see* Exposure, fire, uncontrolled, not in building
- candle X08.8 ☑
  - with ignition of clothing NEC X06.2 ☑
    - nightwear X05 ☑
- caustic liquid, substance (external) (internal) NEC — *see* Table of Drugs and Chemicals
- chemical (external) (internal) (*see also* Table of Drugs and Chemicals)
  - in war operations — *see* War operations, fire
- cigar(s) or cigarette(s) X08.8 ☑
  - with ignition of clothing NEC X06.2 ☑

Burn, burned, burning — *continued*
　cigar(s) or cigarette(s) — *continued*
　　with ignition of clothing — *continued*
　　　nightwear X05 ☑
　clothes, clothing NEC (from controlled fire) X06.2 ☑
　　with conflagration — *see* Exposure, fire, uncontrolled, building
　　　not in building or structure — *see* Exposure, fire, uncontrolled, not in building
　cooker (hot) X15.8 ☑
　　stated as undetermined whether accidental or intentional Y27.3 ☑
　　suicide (attempt) X77.3 ☑
　electric blanket X16 ☑
　engine (hot) X17 ☑
　fire, flames — *see* Exposure, fire
　flare, Very pistol — *see* Discharge, firearm NEC
　heat
　　from appliance (electrical) (household) X15.8 ☑
　　　cooker X15.8 ☑
　　　hotplate X15.2 ☑
　　　kettle X15.8 ☑
　　　light bulb X15.8 ☑
　　　saucepan X15.3 ☑
　　　skillet X15.3 ☑
　　　stated as undetermined whether accidental or intentional Y27.3 ☑
　　　stove X15.0 ☑
　　　suicide (attempt) X77.3 ☑
　　　toaster X15.1 ☑
　　in local application or packing during medical or surgical procedure Y63.5
　heating
　　appliance, radiator or pipe X16 ☑
　homicide (attempt) — *see* Assault, burning
　hot
　　air X14.1 ☑
　　cooker X15.8 ☑
　　drink X10.0 ☑
　　engine X17 ☑
　　fat X10.2 ☑
　　fluid NEC X12 ☑
　　food X10.1 ☑
　　gases X14.1 ☑
　　heating appliance X16 ☑
　　household appliance NEC X15.8 ☑
　　kettle X15.8 ☑
　　liquid NEC X12 ☑
　　machinery X17 ☑
　　metal (molten) (liquid) NEC X18 ☑
　　object (not producing fire or flames) NEC X19 ☑
　　oil (cooking) X10.2 ☑
　　pipe(s) X16 ☑
　　radiator X16 ☑
　　saucepan (glass) (metal) X15.3 ☑
　　stove (kitchen) X15.0 ☑
　　substance NEC X19 ☑
　　　caustic or corrosive NEC — *see* Table of Drugs and Chemicals
　　toaster X15.1 ☑
　　tool X17 ☑
　　vapor X13.1 ☑
　　water (tap) — *see* Contact, with, hot, tap water
　hotplate X15.2 ☑
　　suicide (attempt) X77.3 ☑
　ignition — *see* Ignition
　in war operations — *see* War operations, fire
　inflicted by other person X97 ☑
　　by hot objects, hot vapor, and steam — *see* Assault, burning, hot object
　internal, from swallowed caustic, corrosive liquid, substance — *see* Table of Drugs and Chemicals
　iron (hot) X15.8 ☑
　　stated as undetermined whether accidental or intentional Y27.3 ☑
　　suicide (attempt) X77.3 ☑
　kettle (hot) X15.8 ☑
　　stated as undetermined whether accidental or intentional Y27.3 ☑
　　suicide (attempt) X77.3 ☑
　lamp (flame) X08.8 ☑
　　with ignition of clothing NEC X06.2 ☑
　　　nightwear X05 ☑
　lighter (cigar) (cigarette) X08.8 ☑
　　with ignition of clothing NEC X06.2 ☑
　　　nightwear X05 ☑

Burn, burned, burning — *continued*
　lightning — *see* subcategory T75.0 ☑
　　causing fire — *see* Exposure, fire
　liquid (boiling) (hot) NEC X12 ☑
　　stated as undetermined whether accidental or intentional Y27.2 ☑
　　suicide (attempt) X77.2 ☑
　local application of externally applied substance in medical or surgical care Y63.5
　machinery (hot) X17 ☑
　matches X08.8 ☑
　　with ignition of clothing NEC X06.2 ☑
　　　nightwear X05 ☑
　mattress — *see* Exposure, fire, uncontrolled, building, bed
　medicament, externally applied Y63.5
　metal (hot) (liquid) (molten) NEC X18 ☑
　nightwear (nightclothes, nightdress, gown, pajamas, robe) X05 ☑
　object (hot) NEC X19 ☑
　on board watercraft
　　due to
　　　accident to watercraft V91.09 ☑
　　　　powered craft V91.03 ☑
　　　　　ferry boat V91.01 ☑
　　　　　fishing boat V91.02 ☑
　　　　　jetskis V91.03 ☑
　　　　　liner V91.01 ☑
　　　　　merchant ship V91.00 ☑
　　　　　passenger ship V91.01 ☑
　　　　unpowered craft V91.08 ☑
　　　　　canoe V91.05 ☑
　　　　　inflatable V91.06 ☑
　　　　　kayak V91.05 ☑
　　　　　sailboat V91.04 ☑
　　　　　surf-board V91.08 ☑
　　　　　water skis V91.07 ☑
　　　　　windsurfer V91.08 ☑
　　　fire on board V93.09 ☑
　　　　ferry boat V93.01 ☑
　　　　fishing boat V93.02 ☑
　　　　jetskis V93.03 ☑
　　　　liner V93.01 ☑
　　　　merchant ship V93.00 ☑
　　　　passenger ship V93.01 ☑
　　　　powered craft NEC V93.03 ☑
　　　　sailboat V93.04 ☑
　　　specified heat source NEC on board V93.19 ☑
　　　　ferry boat V93.11 ☑
　　　　fishing boat V93.12 ☑
　　　　jetskis V93.13 ☑
　　　　liner V93.11 ☑
　　　　merchant ship V93.10 ☑
　　　　passenger ship V93.11 ☑
　　　　powered craft NEC V93.13 ☑
　　　　sailboat V93.14 ☑
　pipe (hot) X16 ☑
　　smoking X08.8 ☑
　　　with ignition of clothing NEC X06.2 ☑
　　　　nightwear X05 ☑
　powder — *see* Powder burn
　radiator (hot) X16 ☑
　saucepan (hot) (glass) (metal) X15.3 ☑
　　stated as undetermined whether accidental or intentional Y27.3 ☑
　　suicide (attempt) X77.3 ☑
　self-inflicted X76 ☑
　　stated as undetermined whether accidental or intentional Y26 ☑
　stated as undetermined whether accidental or intentional Y27.0 ☑
　steam X13.1 ☑
　　pipe X16 ☑
　　　stated as undetermined whether accidental or intentional Y27.8 ☑
　　stated as undetermined whether accidental or intentional Y27.0 ☑
　　suicide (attempt) X77.0 ☑
　stove (hot) (kitchen) X15.0 ☑
　　stated as undetermined whether accidental or intentional Y27.3 ☑
　　suicide (attempt) X77.3 ☑
　substance (hot) NEC X19 ☑
　　boiling X12 ☑
　　　stated as undetermined whether accidental or intentional Y27.2 ☑

Burn, burned, burning — *continued*
　substance — *continued*
　　boiling — *continued*
　　　suicide (attempt) X77.2 ☑
　　　molten (metal) X18 ☑
　　suicide (attempt) NEC X76 ☑
　　hot
　　　household appliance X77.3 ☑
　　　object X77.9 ☑
　　therapeutic misadventure
　　　heat in local application or packing during medical or surgical procedure Y63.5
　　　overdose of radiation Y63.2
　　toaster (hot) X15.1 ☑
　　　stated as undetermined whether accidental or intentional Y27.3 ☑
　　　suicide (attempt) X77.3 ☑
　　tool (hot) X17 ☑
　　torch, welding X08.8 ☑
　　　with ignition of clothing NEC X06.2 ☑
　　　　nightwear X05 ☑
　　trash fire (controlled) — *see* Exposure, fire, controlled, not in building
　　　uncontrolled — *see* Exposure, fire, uncontrolled, not in building
　　vapor (hot) X13.1 ☑
　　　stated as undetermined whether accidental or intentional Y27.0 ☑
　　　suicide (attempt) X77.0 ☑
　　Very pistol — *see* Discharge, firearm NEC
Butted by animal W55.82 ☑
　bull W55.22 ☑
　cow W55.22 ☑
　goat W55.32 ☑
　horse W55.12 ☑
　pig W55.42 ☑
　sheep W55.32 ☑

C

Caisson disease — *see* Air, pressure, change
Campfire (exposure to) (controlled) (*see also* Exposure, fire, controlled, not in building)
　uncontrolled — *see* Exposure, fire, uncontrolled, not in building
Capital punishment (any means) — *see* Legal, intervention
Car sickness T75.3 ☑
Casualty (not due to war) NEC X58 ☑
　war — *see* War operations
Cat
　bite W55.01 ☑
　scratch W55.03 ☑
Cataclysm, cataclysmic (any injury) NEC — *see* Forces of nature
Catching fire — *see* Exposure, fire
Caught
　between
　　folding object W23.0 ☑
　　objects (moving) (stationary and moving) W23.0 ☑
　　　and machinery — *see* Contact, with, by type of machine
　　stationary W23.1 ☑
　　sliding door and door frame W23.0 ☑
　by, in
　　machinery (moving parts of) — *see* Contact, with, by type of machine
　　washing-machine wringer W23.0 ☑
　under packing crate (due to losing grip) W23.1 ☑
Cave-in caused by cataclysmic earth surface movement or eruption — *see* Landslide
Change(s) in air pressure — *see* Air, pressure, change
Choked, choking (on) (any object except food or vomitus)
　food (bone) (seed) — *see* categories T17 and T18 ☑
　vomitus T17.81- ☑
Civil insurrection — *see* War operations
Cloudburst (any injury) X37.8 ☑
Cold, exposure to (accidental) (excessive) (extreme) (natural) (place) NEC — *see* Exposure, cold
Collapse
　building W20.1 ☑
　　burning (uncontrolled fire) X00.2 ☑
　dam or man-made structure (causing earth movement) X36.0 ☑
　machinery — *see* Contact, with, by type of machine

Collapse — *continued*
  structure W20.1 ☑
    burning (uncontrolled fire) X00.2 ☑
Collision (accidental) NEC (*see also* Accident, transport) V89.9 ☑
  pedestrian W51 ☑
    with fall W03 ☑
      due to ice or snow W00.0 ☑
      involving pedestrian conveyance — *see* Accident, transport, pedestrian, conveyance
    and
      crowd or human stampede (with fall) W52 ☑
      object W22.8 ☑
        with fall — *see* Fall, due to, bumping against, object
  person(s) — *see* Collision, pedestrian
  transport vehicle NEC V89.9 ☑
    and
      avalanche, fallen or not moving — *see* Accident, transport
        falling or moving — *see* Landslide
      landslide, fallen or not moving — *see* Accident, transport
        falling or moving — *see* Landslide
    due to cataclysm — *see* Forces of nature, by type
    intentional, purposeful suicide (attempt) — *see* Suicide, collision
Combustion, spontaneous — *see* Ignition
Complication (delayed) **of or following** (medical or surgical procedure) Y84.9
  with misadventure — *see* Misadventure
  amputation of limb(s) Y83.5
  anastomosis (arteriovenous) (blood vessel) (gastrojejunal) (tendon) (natural or artificial material) Y83.2
  aspiration (of fluid) Y84.4
    tissue Y84.8
  biopsy Y84.8
  blood
    sampling Y84.7
    transfusion
      procedure Y84.8
  bypass Y83.2
  catheterization (urinary) Y84.6
    cardiac Y84.0
  colostomy Y83.3
  cystostomy Y83.3
  dialysis (kidney) Y84.1
  drug — *see* Table of Drugs and Chemicals
  due to misadventure — *see* Misadventure
  duodenostomy Y83.3
  electroshock therapy Y84.3
  external stoma, creation of Y83.3
  formation of external stoma Y83.3
  gastrostomy Y83.3
  graft Y83.2
  hypothermia (medically-induced) Y84.8
  implant, implantation (of)
    artificial
      internal device (cardiac pacemaker) (electrodes in brain) (heart valve prosthesis) (orthopedic) Y83.1
      material or tissue (for anastomosis or bypass) Y83.2
        with creation of external stoma Y83.3
    natural tissues (for anastomosis or bypass) Y83.2
      with creation of external stoma Y83.3
  infusion
    procedure Y84.8
  injection — *see* Table of Drugs and Chemicals
    procedure Y84.8
  insertion of gastric or duodenal sound Y84.5
  insulin-shock therapy Y84.3
  paracentesis (abdominal) (thoracic) (aspirative) Y84.4
  procedures other than surgical operation — *see* Complication of or following, by type of procedure
  radiological procedure or therapy Y84.2
  removal of organ (partial) (total) NEC Y83.6
  sampling
    blood Y84.7
    fluid NEC Y84.4
    tissue Y84.8
  shock therapy Y84.3
  surgical operation NEC (*see also* Complication of or following, by type of operation) Y83.9
    reconstructive NEC Y83.4

Complication (delayed) **of or following** — *continued*
  surgical operation (*see also* Complication of or following, by type of operation) — *continued*
    reconstructive — *continued*
      with
        anastomosis, bypass or graft Y83.2
        formation of external stoma Y83.3
    specified NEC Y83.8
  transfusion (*see also* Table of Drugs and Chemicals)
    procedure Y84.8
  transplant, transplantation (heart) (kidney) (liver) (whole organ, any) Y83.0
    partial organ Y83.4
  ureterostomy Y83.3
  vaccination (*see also* Table of Drugs and Chemicals)
    procedure Y84.8
Compression
  divers' squeeze — *see* Air, pressure, change
  trachea by
    food (lodged in esophagus) — *see* categories T17 and T18 ☑
    vomitus (lodged in esophagus) T17.81- ☑
Conflagration — *see* Exposure, fire, uncontrolled
Constriction (external)
  hair W49.01 ☑
  jewelry W49.04 ☑
  ring W49.04 ☑
  rubber band W49.03 ☑
  specified item NEC W49.09 ☑
  string W49.02 ☑
  thread W49.02 ☑
Contact (accidental)
  with
    abrasive wheel (metalworking) W31.1 ☑
    alligator W58.09 ☑
      bite W58.01 ☑
      crushing W58.03 ☑
      strike W58.02 ☑
    amphibian W62.9 ☑
      frog W62.0 ☑
      toad W62.1 ☑
    animal (nonvenomous) NEC W64 ☑
      marine W56.89 ☑
        bite W56.81 ☑
        dolphin — *see* Contact, with, dolphin
        fish NEC — *see* Contact, with, fish
        mammal — *see* Contact, with, mammal, marine
        orca — *see* Contact, with, orca
        sea lion — *see* Contact, with, sea lion
        shark — *see* Contact, with, shark
        strike W56.82 ☑
    animate mechanical force NEC W64 ☑
    arrow W21.89 ☑
      not thrown, projected or falling W45.8 ☑
    arthropods (nonvenomous) W57 ☑
    axe W27.0 ☑
    band-saw (industrial) W31.2 ☑
    bayonet — *see* Bayonet wound
    bee(s) X58 ☑
    bench-saw (industrial) W31.2 ☑
    bird W61.99 ☑
      bite W61.91 ☑
      chicken — *see* Contact, with, chicken
      duck — *see* Contact, with, duck
      goose — *see* Contact, with, goose
      macaw — *see* Contact, with, macaw
      parrot — *see* Contact, with, parrot
      psittacine — *see* Contact, with, psittacine
      strike W61.92 ☑
      turkey — *see* Contact, with, turkey
    blender W29.0 ☑
    boiling water X12 ☑
      stated as undetermined whether accidental or intentional Y27.2 ☑
      suicide (attempt) X77.2 ☑
    bore, earth-drilling or mining (land) (seabed) W31.0 ☑
    buffalo — *see* Contact, with, hoof stock NEC
    bull W55.29 ☑
      bite W55.21 ☑
      gored W55.22 ☑
      strike W55.22 ☑
    bumper cars W31.81 ☑
    camel — *see* Contact, with, hoof stock NEC

Contact — *continued*
  with — *continued*
    can
      lid W45.2 ☑
      opener W27.4 ☑
        powered W29.0 ☑
    cat W55.09 ☑
      bite W55.01 ☑
      scratch W55.03 ☑
    caterpillar (venomous) X58 ☑
    centipede (venomous) X58 ☑
    chain
      hoist W24.0 ☑
        agricultural operations W30.89 ☑
      saw W29.3 ☑
    chicken W61.39 ☑
      peck W61.33 ☑
      strike W61.32 ☑
    chisel W27.0 ☑
    circular saw W31.2 ☑
    cobra X58 ☑
    combine (harvester) W30.0 ☑
    conveyer belt W24.1 ☑
    cooker (hot) X15.8 ☑
      stated as undetermined whether accidental or intentional Y27.3 ☑
      suicide (attempt) X77.3 ☑
    coral X58 ☑
    cotton gin W31.82 ☑
    cow W55.29 ☑
      bite W55.21 ☑
      strike W55.22 ☑
    crane W24.0 ☑
      agricultural operations W30.89 ☑
    crocodile W58.19 ☑
      bite W58.11 ☑
      crushing W58.13 ☑
      strike W58.12 ☑
    dagger W26.1 ☑
      stated as undetermined whether accidental or intentional Y28.2 ☑
      suicide (attempt) X78.2 ☑
    dairy equipment W31.82 ☑
    dart W21.89 ☑
      not thrown, projected or falling W45.8 ☑
    deer — *see* Contact, with, hoof stock NEC
    derrick W24.0 ☑
      agricultural operations W30.89 ☑
        hay W30.2 ☑
    dog W54.8 ☑
      bite W54.0 ☑
      strike W54.1 ☑
    dolphin W56.09 ☑
      bite W56.01 ☑
      strike W56.02 ☑
    donkey — *see* Contact, with, hoof stock NEC
    drill (powered) W29.8 ☑
      earth (land) (seabed) W31.0 ☑
      nonpowered W27.8 ☑
    drive belt W24.0 ☑
      agricultural operations W30.89 ☑
    dry ice — *see* Exposure, cold, man-made
    dryer (clothes) (powered) (spin) W29.2 ☑
    duck W61.69 ☑
      bite W61.61 ☑
      strike W61.62 ☑
    earth (-)
      drilling machine (industrial) W31.0 ☑
      scraping machine in stationary use W31.83 ☑
    edge of stiff paper W45.1 ☑
    electric
      beater W29.0 ☑
      blanket X16 ☑
      fan W29.2 ☑
        commercial W31.82 ☑
      knife W29.1 ☑
      mixer W29.0 ☑
    elevator (building) W24.0 ☑
      agricultural operations W30.89 ☑
      grain W30.3 ☑
    engine(s), hot NEC X17 ☑
    excavating machine W31.0 ☑
    farm machine W30.9 ☑
    feces — *see* Contact, with, by type of animal
    fer de lance X58 ☑

Contact — *continued*
  with — *continued*
    fish W56.59 ☑
      bite W56.51 ☑
      shark — *see* Contact, with, shark
      strike W56.52 ☑
    flying horses W31.81 ☑
    forging (metalworking) machine W31.1 ☑
    fork W27.4 ☑
    forklift (truck) W24.0 ☑
      agricultural operations W30.89 ☑
    frog W62.0 ☑
    garden
      cultivator (powered) W29.3 ☑
        riding W30.89 ☑
      fork W27.1 ☑
    gas turbine W31.3 ☑
    Gila monster X58 ☑
    giraffe — *see* Contact, with, hoof stock NEC
    glass (sharp) (broken) W25 ☑
      with subsequent fall W18.02 ☑
      assault X99.0 ☑
      due to fall — *see* Fall, by type
      stated as undetermined whether accidental or
        intentional Y28.0 ☑
      suicide (attempt) X78.0 ☑
    goat W55.39 ☑
      bite W55.31 ☑
      strike W55.32 ☑
    goose W61.59 ☑
      bite W61.51 ☑
      strike W61.52 ☑
    hand
      saw W27.0 ☑
      tool (not powered) NEC W27.8 ☑
        powered W29.8 ☑
    harvester W30.0 ☑
    hay-derrick W30.2 ☑
    heating
      appliance (hot) X16 ☑
      pad (electric) X16 ☑
    heat NEC X19 ☑
      from appliance (electrical) (household) — *see*
        Contact, with, hot, household appliance
      heating appliance X16 ☑
    hedge-trimmer (powered) W29.3 ☑
    hoe W27.1 ☑
    hoist (chain) (shaft) NEC W24.0 ☑
      agricultural W30.89 ☑
    hoof stock NEC W55.39 ☑
      bite W55.31 ☑
      strike W55.32 ☑
    hornet(s) X58 ☑
    horse W55.19 ☑
      bite W55.11 ☑
      strike W55.12 ☑
    hot
      air X14.1 ☑
        inhalation X14.0 ☑
      cooker X15.8 ☑
      drinks X10.0 ☑
      engine X17 ☑
      fats X10.2 ☑
      fluids NEC X12 ☑
        assault X98.2 ☑
        suicide (attempt) X77.2 ☑
        undetermined whether accidental or inten-
          tional Y27.2 ☑
      food X10.1 ☑
      gases X14.1 ☑
        inhalation X14.0 ☑
      heating appliance X16 ☑
      household appliance X15.8 ☑
        assault X98.3 ☑
        cooker X15.8 ☑
        hotplate X15.2 ☑
        kettle X15.8 ☑
        light bulb X15.8 ☑
        object NEC X19 ☑
          assault X98.8 ☑
          stated as undetermined whether acciden-
            tal or intentional Y27.9 ☑
          suicide (attempt) X77.8 ☑
        saucepan X15.3 ☑
        skillet X15.3 ☑

Contact — *continued*
  with — *continued*
    hot — *continued*
      household appliance — *continued*
        stated as undetermined whether accidental
          or intentional Y27.3 ☑
        stove X15.0 ☑
        suicide (attempt) X77.3 ☑
        toaster X15.1 ☑
      kettle X15.8 ☑
      light bulb X15.8 ☑
      liquid NEC (*see also* Burn) X12 ☑
        drinks X10.0 ☑
        stated as undetermined whether accidental
          or intentional Y27.2 ☑
        suicide (attempt) X77.2 ☑
        tap water X11.8 ☑
          stated as undetermined whether acciden-
            tal or intentional Y27.1 ☑
          suicide (attempt) X77.1 ☑
      machinery X17 ☑
      metal (molten) (liquid) NEC X18 ☑
      object (not producing fire or flames) NEC X19 ☑
      oil (cooking) X10.2 ☑
      pipe X16 ☑
      plate X15.2 ☑
      radiator X16 ☑
      saucepan (glass) (metal) X15.3 ☑
      skillet X15.3 ☑
      stove (kitchen) X15.0 ☑
      substance NEC X19 ☑
      tap-water X11.8 ☑
        assault X98.1 ☑
        heated on stove X12 ☑
          stated as undetermined whether acciden-
            tal or intentional Y27.2 ☑
          suicide (attempt) X77.2 ☑
        in bathtub X11.0 ☑
        running X11.1 ☑
        stated as undetermined whether accidental
          or intentional Y27.1 ☑
        suicide (attempt) X77.1 ☑
      toaster X15.1 ☑
      tool X17 ☑
      vapors X13.1 ☑
        inhalation X13.0 ☑
      water (tap) X11.8 ☑
        boiling X12 ☑
          stated as undetermined whether acciden-
            tal or intentional Y27.2 ☑
          suicide (attempt) X77.2 ☑
        heated on stove X12 ☑
          stated as undetermined whether acciden-
            tal or intentional Y27.2 ☑
          suicide (attempt) X77.2 ☑
        in bathtub X11.0 ☑
        running X11.1 ☑
        stated as undetermined whether accidental
          or intentional Y27.1 ☑
        suicide (attempt) X77.1 ☑
    hotplate X15.2 ☑
    ice-pick W27.4 ☑
    insect (nonvenomous) NEC W57 ☑
    kettle (hot) X15.8 ☑
    knife W26.0 ☑
      assault X99.1 ☑
      electric W29.1 ☑
      stated as undetermined whether accidental or
        intentional Y28.1 ☑
      suicide (attempt) X78.1 ☑
    lathe (metalworking) W31.1 ☑
      turnings W45.8 ☑
      woodworking W31.2 ☑
    lawnmower (powered) (ridden) W28 ☑
      causing electrocution W86.8 ☑
        suicide (attempt) X83.1 ☑
      unpowered W27.1 ☑
    lift, lifting (devices) W24.0 ☑
      agricultural operations W30.89 ☑
      shaft W24.0 ☑
    liquefied gas — *see* Exposure, cold, man-made
    liquid air, hydrogen, nitrogen — *see* Exposure, cold,
      man-made
    lizard (nonvenomous) W59.09 ☑
      bite W59.01 ☑
      strike W59.02 ☑

Contact — *continued*
  with — *continued*
    llama — *see* Contact, with, hoof stock NEC
    macaw W61.19 ☑
      bite W61.11 ☑
      strike W61.12 ☑
    machine, machinery W31.9 ☑
      abrasive wheel W31.1 ☑
      agricultural including animal-powered
        W30.9 ☑
        combine harvester W30.0 ☑
        grain storage elevator W30.3 ☑
        hay derrick W30.2 ☑
        power take-off device W30.1 ☑
        reaper W30.0 ☑
        specified NEC W30.89 ☑
        thresher W30.0 ☑
        transport vehicle, stationary W30.81 ☑
      band saw W31.2 ☑
      bench saw W31.2 ☑
      circular saw W31.2 ☑
      commercial NEC W31.82 ☑
      drilling, metal (industrial) W31.1 ☑
      earth-drilling W31.0 ☑
      earthmoving or scraping W31.89 ☑
      excavating W31.89 ☑
      forging machine W31.1 ☑
      gas turbine W31.3 ☑
      hot X17 ☑
      internal combustion engine W31.3 ☑
      land drill W31.0 ☑
      lathe W31.1 ☑
      lifting (devices) W24.0 ☑
      metal drill W31.1 ☑
      metalworking (industrial) W31.1 ☑
      milling, metal W31.1 ☑
      mining W31.0 ☑
      molding W31.2 ☑
      overhead plane W31.2 ☑
      power press, metal W31.1 ☑
      prime mover W31.3 ☑
      printing W31.89 ☑
      radial saw W31.2 ☑
      recreational W31.81 ☑
      roller-coaster W31.81 ☑
      rolling mill, metal W31.1 ☑
      sander W31.2 ☑
      seabed drill W31.0 ☑
      shaft
        hoist W31.0 ☑
        lift W31.0 ☑
      specified NEC W31.89 ☑
      spinning W31.89 ☑
      steam engine W31.3 ☑
      transmission W24.1 ☑
      undercutter W31.0 ☑
      water driven turbine W31.3 ☑
      weaving W31.89 ☑
      woodworking or forming (industrial) W31.2 ☑
    mammal (feces) (urine) W55.89 ☑
      bull — *see* Contact, with, bull
      cat — *see* Contact, with, cat
      cow — *see* Contact, with, cow
      goat — *see* Contact, with, goat
      hoof stock — *see* Contact, with, hoof stock
      horse — *see* Contact, with, horse
      marine W56.39 ☑
        dolphin — *see* Contact, with, dolphin
        orca — *see* Contact, with, orca
        sea lion — *see* Contact, with, sea lion
        specified NEC W56.39 ☑
          bite W56.31 ☑
          strike W56.32 ☑
      pig — *see* Contact, with, pig
      raccoon — *see* Contact, with, raccoon
      rodent — *see* Contact, with, rodent
      sheep — *see* Contact, with, sheep
      specified NEC W55.89 ☑
        bite W55.81 ☑
        strike W55.82 ☑
    marine
      animal W56.89 ☑
        bite W56.81 ☑
        dolphin — *see* Contact, with, dolphin
        fish NEC — *see* Contact, with, fish

External Causes Index

Contact — Contact

Contact — *continued*
  with — *continued*
    marine — *continued*
      animal — *continued*
        mammal — *see* Contact, with, mammal, marine
        orca — *see* Contact, with, orca
        sea lion — *see* Contact, with, sea lion
        shark — *see* Contact, with, shark
        strike W56.82 ☑
    meat
      grinder (domestic) W29.0 ☑
        industrial W31.82 ☑
        nonpowered W27.4 ☑
      slicer (domestic) W29.0 ☑
        industrial W31.82 ☑
    merry go round W31.81 ☑
    metal, hot (liquid) (molten) NEC X18 ☑
    millipede W57 ☑
    nail W45.0 ☑
      gun W29.4 ☑
    needle (sewing) W27.3 ☑
      hypodermic W46.0 ☑
        contaminated W46.1 ☑
    object (blunt) NEC
      hot NEC X19 ☑
      legal intervention — *see* Legal, intervention, blunt object
      sharp NEC W45.8 ☑
        inflicted by other person NEC W45.8 ☑
          stated as
            intentional homicide (attempt) — *see* Assault, cutting or piercing instrument
        legal intervention — *see* Legal, intervention, sharp object
        self-inflicted X78.9 ☑
    orca W56.29 ☑
      bite W56.21 ☑
      strike W56.22 ☑
    overhead plane W31.2 ☑
    paper (as sharp object) W45.1 ☑
    paper-cutter W27.5 ☑
    parrot W61.09 ☑
      bite W61.01 ☑
      strike W61.02 ☑
    pig W55.49 ☑
      bite W55.41 ☑
      strike W55.42 ☑
    pipe, hot X16 ☑
    pitchfork W27.1 ☑
    plane (metal) (wood) W27.0 ☑
      overhead W31.2 ☑
    plant thorns, spines, sharp leaves or other mechanisms W60 ☑
    powered
      garden cultivator W29.3 ☑
      household appliance, implement, or machine W29.8 ☑
      saw (industrial) W31.2 ☑
        hand W29.8 ☑
    printing machine W31.89 ☑
    psittacine bird W61.29 ☑
      bite W61.21 ☑
      macaw — *see* Contact, with, macaw
      parrot — *see* Contact, with, parrot
      strike W61.22 ☑
    pulley (block) (transmission) W24.0 ☑
      agricultural operations W30.89 ☑
    raccoon W55.59 ☑
      bite W55.51 ☑
      strike W55.52 ☑
    radial-saw (industrial) W31.2 ☑
    radiator (hot) X16 ☑
    rake W27.1 ☑
    rattlesnake X58 ☑
    reaper W30.0 ☑
    reptile W59.89 ☑
      lizard — *see* Contact, with, lizard
      snake — *see* Contact, with, snake
      specified NEC W59.89 ☑
        bite W59.81 ☑
        crushing W59.83 ☑
        strike W59.82 ☑
      turtle — *see* Contact, with, turtle
    rivet gun (powered) W29.4 ☑

Contact — *continued*
  with — *continued*
    road scraper — *see* Accident, transport, construction vehicle
    rodent (feces) (urine) W53.89 ☑
      bite W53.81 ☑
      mouse W53.09 ☑
        bite W53.01 ☑
      rat W53.19 ☑
        bite W53.11 ☑
      specified NEC W53.89 ☑
        bite W53.81 ☑
      squirrel W53.29 ☑
        bite W53.21 ☑
    roller coaster W31.81 ☑
    rope NEC W24.0 ☑
      agricultural operations W30.89 ☑
    saliva — *see* Contact, with, by type of animal
    sander W29.8 ☑
      industrial W31.2 ☑
    saucepan (hot) (glass) (metal) X15.3 ☑
    saw W27.0 ☑
      band (industrial) W31.2 ☑
      bench (industrial) W31.2 ☑
      chain W29.3 ☑
      hand W27.0 ☑
    sawing machine, metal W31.1 ☑
    scissors W27.2 ☑
    scorpion X58 ☑
    screwdriver W27.0 ☑
      powered W29.8 ☑
    sea
      anemone, cucumber or urchin (spine) X58 ☑
      lion W56.19 ☑
        bite W56.11 ☑
        strike W56.12 ☑
    serpent — *see* Contact, with, snake, by type
    sewing-machine (electric) (powered) W29.2 ☑
      not powered W27.8 ☑
    shaft (hoist) (lift) (transmission) NEC W24.0 ☑
      agricultural W30.89 ☑
    shark W56.49 ☑
      bite W56.41 ☑
      strike W56.42 ☑
    shears (hand) W27.2 ☑
      powered (industrial) W31.1 ☑
        domestic W29.2 ☑
    sheep W55.39 ☑
      bite W55.31 ☑
      strike W55.32 ☑
    shovel W27.8 ☑
      steam — *see* Accident, transport, construction vehicle
    snake (nonvenomous) W59.19 ☑
      bite W59.11 ☑
      crushing W59.13 ☑
      strike W59.12 ☑
    spade W27.1 ☑
    spider (venomous) X58 ☑
    spin-drier W29.2 ☑
    spinning machine W31.89 ☑
    splinter W45.8 ☑
    sports equipment W21.9 ☑
    staple gun (powered) W29.8 ☑
    steam X13.1 ☑
      engine W31.3 ☑
      inhalation X13.0 ☑
      pipe X16 ☑
      shovel W31.89 ☑
    stove (hot) (kitchen) X15.0 ☑
    substance, hot NEC X19 ☑
      molten (metal) X18 ☑
    sword W26.1 ☑
      assault X99.2 ☑
      stated as undetermined whether accidental or intentional Y28.2 ☑
      suicide (attempt) X78.2 ☑
    tarantula X58 ☑
    thresher W30.0 ☑
    tin can lid W45.2 ☑
    toad W62.1 ☑
    toaster (hot) X15.1 ☑
    tool W27.8 ☑
      hand (not powered) W27.8 ☑
        auger W27.0 ☑

Contact — *continued*
  with — *continued*
    tool — *continued*
      hand — *continued*
        axe W27.0 ☑
        can opener W27.4 ☑
        chisel W27.0 ☑
        fork W27.4 ☑
        garden W27.1 ☑
        handsaw W27.0 ☑
        hoe W27.1 ☑
        ice-pick W27.4 ☑
        kitchen utensil W27.4 ☑
        manual
          lawn mower W27.1 ☑
          sewing machine W27.8 ☑
        meat grinder W27.4 ☑
        needle (sewing) W27.3 ☑
          hypodermic W46.0 ☑
            contaminated W46.1 ☑
        paper cutter W27.5 ☑
        pitchfork W27.1 ☑
        rake W27.1 ☑
        scissors W27.2 ☑
        screwdriver W27.0 ☑
        specified NEC W27.8 ☑
        workbench W27.0 ☑
      hot X17 ☑
      powered W29.8 ☑
        blender W29.0 ☑
          commercial W31.82 ☑
        can opener W29.0 ☑
          commercial W31.82 ☑
        chainsaw W29.3 ☑
        clothes dryer W29.2 ☑
          commercial W31.82 ☑
        dishwasher W29.2 ☑
          commercial W31.82 ☑
        edger W29.3 ☑
        electric fan W29.2 ☑
          commercial W31.82 ☑
        electric knife W29.1 ☑
        food processor W29.0 ☑
          commercial W31.82 ☑
        garbage disposal W29.0 ☑
          commercial W31.82 ☑
        garden tool W29.3 ☑
        hedge trimmer W29.3 ☑
        ice maker W29.0 ☑
          commercial W31.82 ☑
        kitchen appliance W29.0 ☑
          commercial W31.82 ☑
        lawn mower W28 ☑
        meat grinder W29.0 ☑
          commercial W31.82 ☑
        mixer W29.0 ☑
          commercial W31.82 ☑
        rototiller W29.3 ☑
        sewing machine W29.2 ☑
          commercial W31.82 ☑
        washing machine W29.2 ☑
          commercial W31.82 ☑
    transmission device (belt, cable, chain, gear, pinion, shaft) W24.1 ☑
      agricultural operations W30.89 ☑
    turbine (gas) (water-driven) W31.3 ☑
    turkey W61.49 ☑
      peck W61.43 ☑
      strike W61.42 ☑
    turtle (nonvenomous) W59.29 ☑
      bite W59.21 ☑
      strike W59.22 ☑
      terrestrial W59.89 ☑
        bite W59.81 ☑
        crushing W59.83 ☑
        strike W59.82 ☑
    under-cutter W31.0 ☑
    urine — *see* Contact, with, by type of animal
    vehicle
      agricultural use (transport) — *see* Accident, transport, agricultural vehicle
        not on public highway W30.81 ☑
      industrial use (transport) — *see* Accident, transport, industrial vehicle
        not on public highway W31.83 ☑

☑ **Additional Character Required — Refer to the Tabular List for Character Selection**   ▽ **Subterms under main terms may continue to next column or page**

Contact — *continued*
  with — *continued*
    vehicle — *continued*
      off-road use (transport) — *see* Accident, transport, all-terrain or off-road vehicle
        not on public highway W31.83 ☑
      special construction use (transport) — *see* Accident, transport, construction vehicle
        not on public highway W31.83 ☑
    venomous
      animal X58 ☑
      arthropods X58 ☑
      lizard X58 ☑
      marine animal NEC X58 ☑
      marine plant NEC X58 ☑
      millipedes (tropical) X58 ☑
      plant(s) X58 ☑
      snake X58 ☑
      spider X58 ☑
      viper X58 ☑
    washing-machine (powered) W29.2 ☑
    wasp X58 ☑
    weaving-machine W31.89 ☑
    winch W24.0 ☑
      agricultural operations W30.89 ☑
    wire NEC W24.0 ☑
      agricultural operations W30.89 ☑
    wood slivers W45.8 ☑
    yellow jacket X58 ☑
    zebra — *see* Contact, with, hoof stock NEC
Coup de soleil X32 ☑
Crash
  aircraft (in transit) (powered) V95.9 ☑
    balloon V96.01 ☑
    fixed wing NEC (private) V95.21 ☑
      commercial V95.31 ☑
    glider V96.21 ☑
      hang V96.11 ☑
      powered V95.11 ☑
    helicopter V95.01 ☑
    in war operations — *see* War operations, destruction of aircraft
    microlight V95.11 ☑
    nonpowered V96.9 ☑
      specified NEC V96.8 ☑
    powered NEC V95.8 ☑
    stated as
      homicide (attempt) Y08.81 ☑
      suicide (attempt) X83.0 ☑
    ultralight V95.11 ☑
  spacecraft V95.41 ☑
  transport vehicle NEC (*see also* Accident, transport) V89.9 ☑
    homicide (attempt) Y03.8 ☑
    motor NEC (traffic) V89.2 ☑
      homicide (attempt) Y03.8 ☑
      suicide (attempt) — *see* Suicide, collision
Cruelty (mental) (physical) (sexual) X58 ☑
Crushed (accidentally) X58 ☑
  between objects (moving) (stationary and moving) W23.0 ☑
  stationary W23.1 ☑
  by
    alligator W58.03 ☑
    avalanche NEC — *see* Landslide
    cave-in W20.0 ☑
      caused by cataclysmic earth surface movement — *see* Landslide
    crocodile W58.13 ☑
    crowd or human stampede W52 ☑
    falling
      aircraft V97.39 ☑
        in war operations — *see* War operations, destruction of aircraft
      earth, material W20.0 ☑
        caused by cataclysmic earth surface movement — *see* Landslide
      object NEC W20.8 ☑
    landslide NEC — *see* Landslide
    lizard (nonvenomous) W59.09 ☑
    machinery — *see* Contact, with, by type of machine
    reptile NEC W59.89 ☑
    snake (nonvenomous) W59.13 ☑
  in
    machinery — *see* Contact, with, by type of machine

Cut, cutting (any part of body) (accidental) (*see also* Contact, with, by object or machine)
  during medical or surgical treatment as misadventure — *see* Index to Diseases and Injuries, Complications
  homicide (attempt) — *see* Assault, cutting or piercing instrument
  inflicted by other person — *see* Assault, cutting or piercing instrument
  legal
    execution — *see* Legal, intervention
    intervention — *see* Legal, intervention, sharp object
  machine NEC (*see also* Contact, with, by type of machine) W31.9 ☑
  self-inflicted — *see* Suicide, cutting or piercing instrument
  suicide (attempt) — *see* Suicide, cutting or piercing instrument
Cyclone (any injury) X37.1 ☑

D

Decapitation (accidental circumstances) NEC X58 ☑
  homicide X99.9 ☑
  legal execution — *see* Legal, intervention
Dehydration from lack of water X58 ☑
Deprivation X58 ☑
Derailment (accidental)
  railway (rolling stock) (train) (vehicle) (without antecedent collision) V81.7 ☑
    with antecedent collision — *see* Accident, transport, railway vehicle occupant
  streetcar (without antecedent collision) V82.7 ☑
    with antecedent collision — *see* Accident, transport, streetcar occupant
Descent
  parachute (voluntary) (without accident to aircraft) V97.29 ☑
    due to accident to aircraft — *see* Accident, transport, aircraft
Desertion X58 ☑
Destitution X58 ☑
Disability, late effect or sequela of injury — *see* Sequelae
Discharge (accidental)
  airgun W34.010 ☑
    assault X95.01 ☑
    homicide (attempt) X95.01 ☑
    stated as undetermined whether accidental or intentional Y24.0 ☑
    suicide (attempt) X74.01 ☑
  BB gun — *see* Discharge, airgun
  firearm (accidental) W34.00 ☑
    assault X95.9 ☑
    handgun (pistol) (revolver) W32.0 ☑
      assault X93 ☑
      homicide (attempt) X93 ☑
      legal intervention — *see* Legal, intervention, firearm, handgun
      stated as undetermined whether accidental or intentional Y22 ☑
      suicide (attempt) X72 ☑
    homicide (attempt) X95.9 ☑
    hunting rifle W33.02 ☑
      assault X94.1 ☑
      homicide (attempt) X94.1 ☑
      legal intervention
        injuring
          bystander Y35.032 ☑
          law enforcement personnel Y35.031 ☑
          suspect Y35.033 ☑
      stated as undetermined whether accidental or intentional Y23.1 ☑
      suicide (attempt) X73.1 ☑
    larger W33.00 ☑
      assault X94.9 ☑
      homicide (attempt) X94.9 ☑
      hunting rifle — *see* Discharge, firearm, hunting rifle
      legal intervention — *see* Legal, intervention, firearm by type of firearm
      machine gun — *see* Discharge, firearm, machine gun
      shotgun — *see* Discharge, firearm, shotgun
      specified NEC W33.09 ☑

Discharge — *continued*
  firearm — *continued*
    larger — *continued*
      specified — *continued*
        assault X94.8 ☑
        homicide (attempt) X94.8 ☑
        legal intervention
          injuring
            bystander Y35.092 ☑
            law enforcement personnel Y35.091 ☑
            suspect Y35.093 ☑
        stated as undetermined whether accidental or intentional Y23.8 ☑
        suicide (attempt) X73.8 ☑
      stated as undetermined whether accidental or intentional Y23.9 ☑
      suicide (attempt) X73.9 ☑
    legal intervention
      injuring
        bystander Y35.002 ☑
        law enforcement personnel Y35.001 ☑
        suspect Y35.03 ☑
      using rubber bullet
        injuring
          bystander Y35.042 ☑
          law enforcement personnel Y35.041 ☑
          suspect Y35.043 ☑
    machine gun W33.03 ☑
      assault X94.2 ☑
      homicide (attempt) X94.2 ☑
      legal intervention — *see* Legal, intervention, firearm, machine gun
      stated as undetermined whether accidental or intentional Y23.3 ☑
      suicide (attempt) X73.2 ☑
    pellet gun — *see* Discharge, airgun
    shotgun W33.01 ☑
      assault X94.0 ☑
      homicide (attempt) X94.0 ☑
      legal intervention — *see* Legal, intervention, firearm, specified NEC
      stated as undetermined whether accidental or intentional Y23.0 ☑
      suicide (attempt) X73.0 ☑
    specified NEC W34.09 ☑
      assault X95.8 ☑
      homicide (attempt) X95.8 ☑
      legal intervention — *see* Legal, intervention, firearm, specified NEC
      stated as undetermined whether accidental or intentional Y24.8 ☑
      suicide (attempt) X74.8 ☑
    stated as undetermined whether accidental or intentional Y24.9 ☑
    suicide (attempt) X74.9 ☑
    Very pistol W34.09 ☑
      assault X95.8 ☑
      homicide (attempt) X95.8 ☑
      stated as undetermined whether accidental or intentional Y24.8 ☑
      suicide (attempt) X74.8 ☑
  firework(s) W39 ☑
    stated as undetermined whether accidental or intentional Y25 ☑
  gas-operated gun NEC W34.018 ☑
    airgun — *see* Discharge, airgun
    assault X95.09 ☑
    homicide (attempt) X95.09 ☑
    paintball gun — *see* Discharge, paintball gun
    stated as undetermined whether accidental or intentional Y24.8 ☑
    suicide (attempt) X74.09 ☑
  gun NEC (*see also* Discharge, firearm NEC)
    air — *see* Discharge, airgun
    BB — *see* Discharge, airgun
    for single hand use — *see* Discharge, firearm, handgun
    hand — *see* Discharge, firearm, handgun
    machine — *see* Discharge, firearm, machine gun
    other specified — *see* Discharge, firearm NEC
    paintball — *see* Discharge, paintball gun
    pellet — *see* Discharge, airgun
  handgun — *see* Discharge, firearm, handgun
  machine gun — *see* Discharge, firearm, machine gun
  paintball gun W34.011 ☑

Discharge — *continued*
  paintball gun — *continued*
    assault X95.02 ☑
    homicide (attempt) X95.02 ☑
    stated as undetermined whether accidental or intentional Y24.8 ☑
    suicide (attempt) X74.02 ☑
  pistol — *see* Discharge, firearm, handgun
    flare — *see* Discharge, firearm, Very pistol
    pellet — *see* Discharge, firearm, airgun
    Very — *see* Discharge, firearm, Very pistol
  revolver — *see* Discharge, firearm, handgun
  rifle (hunting) — *see* Discharge, firearm, hunting rifle
  shotgun — *see* Discharge, firearm, shotgun
  spring-operated gun NEC W34.018 ☑
    assault X95.09 ☑
    homicide (attempt) X95.09 ☑
    stated as undetermined whether accidental or intentional Y24.8 ☑
    suicide (attempt) X74.09 ☑
Disease
  Andes W94.11 ☑
  aviator's — *see* Air, pressure
  range W94.11 ☑
Diver's disease, palsy, paralysis, squeeze — *see* Air, pressure
Diving (into water) — *see* Accident, diving
Dog bite W54.0 ☑
Dragged by transport vehicle NEC (*see also* Accident, transport) V09.9 ☑
Drinking poison (accidental) — *see* Table of Drugs and Chemicals
Dropped (accidentally) **while being carried or supported by other person** W04 ☑
Drowning (accidental) W74 ☑
  assault X92.9 ☑
  due to
    accident (to)
      machinery — *see* Contact, with, by type of machine
      watercraft V90.89 ☑
        burning V90.29 ☑
          powered V90.23 ☑
            fishing boat V90.22 ☑
            jetskis V90.23 ☑
            merchant ship V90.20 ☑
            passenger ship V90.21 ☑
          unpowered V90.28 ☑
            canoe V90.25 ☑
            inflatable V90.26 ☑
            kayak V90.25 ☑
            sailboat V90.24 ☑
            water skis V90.27 ☑
        crushed V90.39 ☑
          powered V90.33 ☑
            fishing boat V90.32 ☑
            jetskis V90.33 ☑
            merchant ship V90.30 ☑
            passenger ship V90.31 ☑
          unpowered V90.38 ☑
            canoe V90.35 ☑
            inflatable V90.36 ☑
            kayak V90.35 ☑
            sailboat V90.34 ☑
            water skis V90.37 ☑
        overturning V90.09 ☑
          powered V90.03 ☑
            fishing boat V90.02 ☑
            jetskis V90.03 ☑
            merchant ship V90.00 ☑
            passenger ship V90.01 ☑
          unpowered V90.08 ☑
            canoe V90.05 ☑
            inflatable V90.06 ☑
            kayak V90.05 ☑
            sailboat V90.04 ☑
        sinking V90.19 ☑
          powered V90.13 ☑
            fishing boat V90.12 ☑
            jetskis V90.13 ☑
            merchant ship V90.10 ☑
            passenger ship V90.11 ☑
          unpowered V90.18 ☑
            canoe V90.15 ☑
            inflatable V90.16 ☑
            kayak V90.15 ☑

Drowning — *continued*
  due to — *continued*
    accident — *continued*
      watercraft — *continued*
        sinking — *continued*
          unpowered — *continued*
            sailboat V90.14 ☑
          specified type NEC V90.89 ☑
          powered V90.83 ☑
            fishing boat V90.82 ☑
            jetskis V90.83 ☑
            merchant ship V90.80 ☑
            passenger ship V90.81 ☑
          unpowered V90.88 ☑
            canoe V90.85 ☑
            inflatable V90.86 ☑
            kayak V90.85 ☑
            sailboat V90.84 ☑
            water skis V90.87 ☑
  avalanche — *see* Landslide
  cataclysmic
    earth surface movement NEC — *see* Forces of nature, earth movement
    storm — *see* Forces of nature, cataclysmic storm
  cloudburst X37.8 ☑
  cyclone X37.1 ☑
  fall overboard (from) V92.09 ☑
    powered craft V92.03 ☑
      ferry boat V92.01 ☑
      fishing boat V92.02 ☑
      jetskis V92.03 ☑
      liner V92.01 ☑
      merchant ship V92.00 ☑
      passenger ship V92.01 ☑
    resulting from
      accident to watercraft — *see* Drowning, due to, accident to, watercraft
      being washed overboard (from) V92.29 ☑
        powered craft V92.23 ☑
          ferry boat V92.21 ☑
          fishing boat V92.22 ☑
          jetskis V92.23 ☑
          liner V92.21 ☑
          merchant ship V92.20 ☑
          passenger ship V92.21 ☑
        unpowered craft V92.28 ☑
          canoe V92.25 ☑
          inflatable V92.26 ☑
          kayak V92.25 ☑
          sailboat V92.24 ☑
          surf-board V92.28 ☑
          water skis V92.27 ☑
          windsurfer V92.28 ☑
      motion of watercraft V92.19 ☑
        powered craft V92.13 ☑
          ferry boat V92.11 ☑
          fishing boat V92.12 ☑
          jetskis V92.13 ☑
          liner V92.11 ☑
          merchant ship V92.10 ☑
          passenger ship V92.11 ☑
        unpowered craft
          canoe V92.15 ☑
          inflatable V92.16 ☑
          kayak V92.15 ☑
          sailboat V92.14 ☑
        unpowered craft V92.08 ☑
          canoe V92.05 ☑
          inflatable V92.06 ☑
          kayak V92.05 ☑
          sailboat V92.04 ☑
          surf-board V92.08 ☑
          water skis V92.07 ☑
          windsurfer V92.08 ☑
  hurricane X37.0 ☑
  jumping into water from watercraft (involved in accident) (*see also* Drowning, due to, accident to, watercraft)
    without accident to or on watercraft W16.711 ☑
  tidal wave NEC — *see* Forces of nature, tidal wave
  torrential rain X37.8 ☑

Drowning — *continued*
  following
    fall
      into
        bathtub W16.211 ☑
        bucket W16.221 ☑
        fountain — *see* Drowning, following, fall, into, water, specified NEC
        quarry — *see* Drowning, following, fall, into, water, specified NEC
        reservoir — *see* Drowning, following, fall, into, water, specified NEC
        swimming-pool W16.011 ☑
          stated as undetermined whether accidental or intentional Y21.3 ☑
          striking
            bottom W16.021 ☑
            wall W16.031 ☑
          suicide (attempt) X71.2 ☑
        water NOS W16.41 ☑
          natural (lake) (open sea) (river) (stream) (pond) W16.111 ☑
            striking
              bottom W16.121 ☑
              side W16.131 ☑
          specified NEC W16.311 ☑
            striking
              bottom W16.321 ☑
              wall W16.331 ☑
      overboard NEC — *see* Drowning, due to, fall overboard
    jump or dive
      from boat W16.711 ☑
        striking bottom W16.721 ☑
      into
        fountain — *see* Drowning, following, jump or dive, into, water, specified NEC
        quarry — *see* Drowning, following, jump or dive, into, water, specified NEC
        reservoir — *see* Drowning, following, jump or dive, into, water, specified NEC
        swimming-pool W16.511 ☑
          striking
            bottom W16.521 ☑
            wall W16.531 ☑
          suicide (attempt) X71.2 ☑
        water NOS W16.91 ☑
          natural (lake) (open sea) (river) (stream) (pond) W16.611 ☑
          specified NEC W16.811 ☑
            bottom W16.821 ☑
            striking
              bottom W16.821 ☑
              wall W16.831 ☑
            striking
              bottom W16.821 ☑
              wall W16.831 ☑
            striking bottom W16.621 ☑
  homicide (attempt) X92.9 ☑
  in
    bathtub (accidental) W65 ☑
      assault X92.0 ☑
      following fall W16.211 ☑
        stated as undetermined whether accidental or intentional Y21.1 ☑
      stated as undetermined whether accidental or intentional Y21.0 ☑
      suicide (attempt) X71.0 ☑
    lake — *see* Drowning, in, natural water
    natural water (lake) (open sea) (river) (stream) (pond) W69 ☑
      assault X92.3 ☑
      following
        dive or jump W16.611 ☑
          striking bottom W16.621 ☑
        fall W16.111 ☑
          striking
            bottom W16.121 ☑
            side W16.131 ☑
      stated as undetermined whether accidental or intentional Y21.4 ☑
      suicide (attempt) X71.3 ☑
    quarry — *see* Drowning, in, specified place NEC
    quenching tank — *see* Drowning, in, specified place NEC
    reservoir — *see* Drowning, in, specified place NEC

☑ Additional Character Required — Refer to the Tabular List for Character Selection   ▽ Subterms under main terms may continue to next column or page

Drowning — *continued*
　in — *continued*
　　river — *see* Drowning, in, natural water
　　sea — *see* Drowning, in, natural water
　　specified place NEC W73 ☑
　　　assault X92.8 ☑
　　　following
　　　　dive or jump W16.811 ☑
　　　　　striking
　　　　　　bottom W16.821 ☑
　　　　　　wall W16.831 ☑
　　　　fall W16.311 ☑
　　　　　striking
　　　　　　bottom W16.321 ☑
　　　　　　wall W16.331 ☑
　　　stated as undetermined whether accidental or
　　　　intentional Y21.8 ☑
　　　suicide (attempt) X71.8 ☑
　　stream — *see* Drowning, in, natural water
　　swimming-pool W67 ☑
　　　assault X92.1 ☑
　　　　following fall X92.2 ☑
　　　following
　　　　dive or jump W16.511 ☑
　　　　　striking
　　　　　　bottom W16.521 ☑
　　　　　　wall W16.531 ☑
　　　　fall W16.011 ☑
　　　　　striking
　　　　　　bottom W16.021 ☑
　　　　　　wall W16.031 ☑
　　　stated as undetermined whether accidental or
　　　　intentional Y21.2 ☑
　　　　following fall Y21.3 ☑
　　　suicide (attempt) X71.1 ☑
　　　　following fall X71.2 ☑
　　war operations — *see* War operations, restriction
　　　of airway
　　resulting from accident to watercraft — *see* Drowning,
　　　due to, accident, watercraft
　self-inflicted X71.9 ☑
　stated as undetermined whether accidental or inten-
　　tional Y21.9 ☑
　suicide (attempt) X71.9 ☑

E

Earth falling (on) W20.0 ☑
　caused by cataclysmic earth surface movement or
　　eruption — *see* Landslide
Earth (surface) movement NEC — *see* Forces of nature,
　earth movement
Earthquake (any injury) X34 ☑
Effect(s) (adverse) of
　air pressure (any) — *see* Air, pressure
　cold, excessive (exposure to) — *see* Exposure, cold
　heat (excessive) — *see* Heat
　hot place (weather) B — *see* Heat
　insolation X30 ☑
　late — *see* Sequelae
　motion — *see* Motion
　nuclear explosion or weapon in war operations — *see*
　　War operations, nuclear weapon
　radiation — *see* Radiation
　travel — *see* Travel
Electric shock (accidental) (by) (in) — *see* Exposure,
　electric current
Electrocution (accidental) — *see* Exposure, electric cur-
　rent
**Endotracheal tube wrongly placed during anesthetic
　procedure**
Entanglement
　in
　　bed linen, causing suffocation T71 ☑
　　wheel of pedal cycle V19.88 ☑
Entry of foreign body or material — *see* Foreign body
Environmental pollution related condition — *see*
　category Z57
Execution, legal (any method) — *see* Legal, intervention
Exhaustion
　cold — *see* Exposure, cold
　due to excessive exertion — *see* category Y93 ☑
　heat — *see* Heat
Explosion (accidental) (of) (with secondary fire) W40.9 ☑
　acetylene W40.1 ☑
　aerosol can W36.1 ☑

Explosion — *continued*
　air tank (compressed) (in machinery) W36.2 ☑
　aircraft (in transit) (powered) NEC V95.9 ☑
　　balloon V96.05 ☑
　　fixed wing NEC (private) V95.25 ☑
　　　commercial V95.35 ☑
　　glider V96.25 ☑
　　　hang V96.15 ☑
　　　powered V95.15 ☑
　　helicopter V95.05 ☑
　　in war operations — *see* War operations, destruc-
　　　tion of aircraft
　　microlight V95.15 ☑
　　nonpowered V96.9 ☑
　　　specified NEC V96.8 ☑
　　powered NEC V95.8 ☑
　　stated as
　　　homicide (attempt) Y03.8 ☑
　　　suicide (attempt) X83.0 ☑
　　ultralight V95.15 ☑
　anesthetic gas in operating room W40.1 ☑
　antipersonnel bomb W40.8 ☑
　　assault X96.0 ☑
　　homicide (attempt) X96.0 ☑
　　suicide (attempt) X75 ☑
　assault X96.9 ☑
　bicycle tire W37.0 ☑
　blasting (cap) (materials) W40.0 ☑
　boiler (machinery), not on transport vehicle W35 ☑
　　on watercraft — *see* Explosion, in, watercraft
　butane W40.1 ☑
　caused by other person X96.9 ☑
　coal gas W40.1 ☑
　detonator W40.0 ☑
　dump (munitions) W40.8 ☑
　dynamite W40.0 ☑
　　in
　　　assault X96.8 ☑
　　　homicide (attempt) X96.8 ☑
　　　legal intervention
　　　　injuring
　　　　　bystander Y35.112 ☑
　　　　　law enforcement personnel Y35.111 ☑
　　　　　suspect Y35.113 ☑
　　　suicide (attempt) X75 ☑
　explosive (material) W40.9 ☑
　　gas W40.1 ☑
　　in blasting operation W40.0 ☑
　　specified NEC W40.8 ☑
　　　in
　　　　assault X96.8 ☑
　　　　homicide (attempt) X96.8 ☑
　　　　legal intervention
　　　　　injuring
　　　　　　bystander Y35.192 ☑
　　　　　　law enforcement personnel
　　　　　　　Y35.191 ☑
　　　　　　suspect Y35.193 ☑
　　　　suicide (attempt) X75 ☑
　factory (munitions) W40.8 ☑
　fertilizer bomb W40.8 ☑
　　assault X96.3 ☑
　　homicide (attempt) X96.3 ☑
　　suicide (attempt) X75 ☑
　firearm (parts) NEC W34.19 ☑
　　airgun W34.110 ☑
　　BB gun W34.110 ☑
　　gas, air or spring-operated gun NEC W34.118 ☑
　　hangun W32.1 ☑
　　hunting rifle W33.12 ☑
　　larger firearm W33.10 ☑
　　　specified NEC W33.19 ☑
　　machine gun W33.13 ☑
　　paintball gun W34.111 ☑
　　pellet gun W34.110 ☑
　　shotgun W33.11 ☑
　　Very pistol [flare] W34.19 ☑
　fire-damp W40.1 ☑
　fireworks W39 ☑
　gas (coal) (explosive) W40.1 ☑
　　cylinder W36.9 ☑
　　　aerosol can W36.1 ☑
　　　air tank W36.2 ☑
　　　pressurized W36.3 ☑
　　　specified NEC W36.8 ☑

Explosion — *continued*
　gasoline (fumes) (tank) not in moving motor vehicle
　　W40.1 ☑
　　bomb W40.8 ☑
　　　assault X96.1 ☑
　　　homicide (attempt) X96.1 ☑
　　　suicide (attempt) X75 ☑
　　in motor vehicle — *see* Accident, transport, by type
　　　of vehicle
　grain store W40.8 ☑
　grenade W40.8 ☑
　　in
　　　assault X96.8 ☑
　　　homicide (attempt) X96.8 ☑
　　　legal intervention
　　　　injuring
　　　　　bystander Y35.192 ☑
　　　　　law enforcement personnel Y35.191 ☑
　　　　　suspect Y35.193 ☑
　　　suicide (attempt) X75 ☑
　handgun (parts) — *see* Explosion, firearm, hangun
　　(parts)
　homicide (attempt) X96.9 ☑
　　antipersonnel bomb — *see* Explosion, antiperson-
　　　nel bomb
　　fertilizer bomb — *see* Explosion, fertilizer bomb
　　gasoline bomb — *see* Explosion, gasoline bomb
　　letter bomb — *see* Explosion, letter bomb
　　pipe bomb — *see* Explosion, pipe bomb
　　specified NEC X96.8 ☑
　hose, pressurized W37.8 ☑
　hot water heater, tank (in machinery) W35 ☑
　　on watercraft — *see* Explosion, in, watercraft
　in, on
　　dump W40.8 ☑
　　factory W40.8 ☑
　　mine (of explosive gases) NEC W40.1 ☑
　　watercraft V93.59 ☑
　　　powered craft V93.53 ☑
　　　　ferry boat V93.51 ☑
　　　　fishing boat V93.52 ☑
　　　　jetskis V93.53 ☑
　　　　liner V93.51 ☑
　　　　merchant ship V93.50 ☑
　　　　passenger ship V93.51 ☑
　　　　sailboat V93.54 ☑
　letter bomb W40.8 ☑
　　assault X96.2 ☑
　　homicide (attempt) X96.2 ☑
　　suicide (attempt) X75 ☑
　machinery (*see also* Contact, with, by type of machine)
　　on board watercraft — *see* Explosion, in, watercraft
　　pressure vessel — *see* Explosion, by type of vessel
　methane W40.1 ☑
　mine W40.1 ☑
　missile NEC W40.8 ☑
　mortar bomb W40.8 ☑
　　in
　　　assault X96.8 ☑
　　　homicide (attempt) X96.8 ☑
　　　legal intervention
　　　　injuring
　　　　　bystander Y35.192 ☑
　　　　　law enforcement personnel Y35.191 ☑
　　　　　suspect Y35.193 ☑
　　　suicide (attempt) X75 ☑
　munitions (dump) (factory) W40.8 ☑
　pipe, pressurized W37.8 ☑
　　bomb W40.8 ☑
　　　assault X96.4 ☑
　　　homicide (attempt) X96.4 ☑
　　　suicide (attempt) X75 ☑
　pressure, pressurized
　　cooker W38 ☑
　　gas tank (in machinery) W36.3 ☑
　　hose W37.8 ☑
　　pipe W37.8 ☑
　　specified device NEC W38 ☑
　　tire W37.8 ☑
　　　bicycle W37.0 ☑
　　vessel (in machinery) W38 ☑
　propane W40.1 ☑
　self-inflicted X75 ☑
　shell (artillery) NEC W40.8 ☑
　　during war operations — *see* War operations, ex-
　　　plosion

▽ **Subterms under main terms may continue to next column or page**　　☑ **Additional Character Required — Refer to the Tabular List for Character Selection**　　**407**

Drowning — Explosion

Explosion — *continued*
  shell — *continued*
    in
      legal intervention
        injuring
          bystander Y35.122 ☑
          law enforcement personnel Y35.121 ☑
          suspect Y35.123 ☑
      war — *see* War operations, explosion
  spacecraft V95.45
  stated as undetermined whether accidental or intentional Y25 ☑
  steam or water lines (in machinery) W37.8 ☑
  stove W40.9 ☑
  suicide (attempt) X75 ☑
  tire, pressurized W37.8 ☑
    bicycle W37.0 ☑
  undetermined whether accidental or intentional Y25 ☑
  vehicle tire NEC W37.8 ☑
    bicycle W37.0 ☑
  war operations — *see* War operations, explosion
Exposure (to) X58 ☑
  air pressure change — *see* Air, pressure
  cold (accidental) (excessive) (extreme) (natural) (place) X31 ☑
    assault Y08.89 ☑
    due to
      man-made conditions W93.8 ☑
        dry ice (contact) W93.01 ☑
          inhalation W93.02 ☑
        liquid air (contact) (hydrogen) (nitrogen) W93.11 ☑
          inhalation W93.12 ☑
        refrigeration unit (deep freeze) W93.2 ☑
          suicide (attempt) X83.2 ☑
      weather (conditions) X31 ☑
    homicide (attempt) Y08.89 ☑
    self-inflicted X83.2 ☑
  due to abandonment or neglect X58 ☑
  electric current W86.8 ☑
    appliance (faulty) W86.8 ☑
      domestic W86.0 ☑
    caused by other person Y08.89 ☑
    conductor (faulty) W86.1 ☑
    control apparatus (faulty) W86.1 ☑
    electric power generating plant, distribution station W86.1 ☑
    electroshock gun — *see* Exposure, electric current, taser
    high-voltage cable W85 ☑
    homicide (attempt) Y08.89 ☑
    legal execution — *see* Legal, intervention, specified means NEC
    lightning — *see* subcategory T75.0 ☑
    live rail W86.8 ☑
    misadventure in medical or surgical procedure in electroshock therapy Y63.4
    motor (electric) (faulty) W86.8 ☑
      domestic W86.0 ☑
    self-inflicted X83.1 ☑
    specified NEC W86.8 ☑
      domestic W86.0 ☑
    stun gun — *see* Exposure, electric current, taser
    suicide (attempt) X83.1 ☑
    taser W86.8 ☑
      assault Y08.89 ☑
      legal intervention — *see* category Y35
      self-harm (intentional) X83.8 ☑
      undetermined intent Y33 ☑
    third rail W86.8 ☑
    transformer (faulty) W86.1 ☑
    transmission lines W85 ☑
  environmental tobacco smoke X58 ☑
  excessive
    cold — *see* Exposure, cold
    heat (natural) NEC X30 ☑
      man-made W92 ☑
  factor(s) NOS X58 ☑
    environmental NEC X58 ☑
      man-made NEC W99 ☑
    natural NEC — *see* Forces of nature
    specified NEC X58 ☑
  fire, flames (accidental) X08.8 ☑
    assault X97 ☑

Exposure — *continued*
  fire, flames — *continued*
    campfire — *see* Exposure, fire, controlled, not in building
    controlled (in)
      with ignition (of) clothing (*see also* Ignition, clothes) X06.2 ☑
        nightwear X05 ☑
      bonfire — *see* Exposure, fire, controlled, not in building
      brazier (in building or structure) (*see also* Exposure, fire, controlled, building)
        not in building or structure — *see* Exposure, fire, controlled, not in building
      building or structure X02.0 ☑
        with
          fall from building X02.3 ☑
          from building X02.5 ☑
          injury due to building collapse X02.2 ☑
          smoke inhalation X02.1 ☑
        hit by object from building X02.4 ☑
        specified mode of injury NEC X02.8 ☑
      fireplace, furnace or stove — *see* Exposure, fire, controlled, building
      not in building or structure X03.0 ☑
        with
          fall X03.3 ☑
          smoke inhalation X03.1 ☑
        hit by object X03.4 ☑
        specified mode of injury NEC X03.8 ☑
      trash — *see* Exposure, fire, controlled, not in building
    fireplace — *see* Exposure, fire, controlled, building
    fittings or furniture (in building or structure) (uncontrolled) — *see* Exposure, fire, uncontrolled, building
    forest (uncontrolled) — *see* Exposure, fire, uncontrolled, not in building
    grass (uncontrolled) — *see* Exposure, fire, uncontrolled, not in building
    hay (uncontrolled) — *see* Exposure, fire, uncontrolled, not in building
    homicide (attempt) X97 ☑
    ignition of highly flammable material X04 ☑
    in, of, on, starting in
      machinery — *see* Contact, with, by type of machine
      motor vehicle (in motion) (*see also* Accident, transport, occupant by type of vehicle) V87.8 ☑
        with collision — *see* Collision
      railway rolling stock, train, vehicle V81.81 ☑
        with collision — *see* Accident, transport, railway vehicle occupant
      street car (in motion) V82.8 ☑
        with collision — *see* Accident, transport, streetcar occupant
      transport vehicle NEC (*see also* Accident, transport)
        with collision — *see* Collision
      war operations (*see also* War operations, fire)
        from nuclear explosion — *see* War operations, nuclear weapons
      watercraft (in transit) (not in transit) V91.09 ☑
        localized — *see* Burn, on board watercraft, due to, fire on board
        powered craft V91.03 ☑
          ferry boat V91.01 ☑
          fishing boat V91.02 ☑
          jet skis V91.03 ☑
          liner V91.01 ☑
          merchant ship V91.00 ☑
          passenger ship V91.01 ☑
        unpowered craft V91.08 ☑
          canoe V91.05 ☑
          inflatable V91.06 ☑
          kayak V91.05 ☑
          sailboat V91.04 ☑
          surf-board V91.08 ☑
          waterskis V91.07 ☑
          windsurfer V91.08 ☑
    lumber (uncontrolled) — *see* Exposure, fire, uncontrolled, not in building
    mine (uncontrolled) — *see* Exposure, fire, uncontrolled, not in building

Exposure — *continued*
  fire, flames — *continued*
    prairie (uncontrolled) — *see* Exposure, fire, uncontrolled, not in building
    resulting from
      explosion — *see* Explosion
      lightning X08.8 ☑
    self-inflicted X76 ☑
    specified NEC X08.8 ☑
    started by other person X97 ☑
    stated as undetermined whether accidental or intentional Y26 ☑
    stove — *see* Exposure, fire, controlled, building
    suicide (attempt) X76 ☑
    tunnel (uncontrolled) — *see* Exposure, fire, uncontrolled, not in building
    uncontrolled
      in building or structure X00.0 ☑
        with
          fall from building X00.3 ☑
          injury due to building collapse X00.2 ☑
          jump from building X00.5 ☑
          smoke inhalation X00.1 ☑
        bed X08.00 ☑
          due to
            cigarette X08.01 ☑
            specified material NEC X08.09 ☑
          furniture NEC X08.20 ☑
            due to
              cigarette X08.21 ☑
              specified material NEC X08.29 ☑
          hit by object from building X00.4 ☑
          sofa X08.10 ☑
            due to
              cigarette X08.11 ☑
              specified material NEC X08.19 ☑
          specified mode of injury NEC X00.8 ☑
      not in building or structure (any) X01.0 ☑
        with
          fall X01.3 ☑
          smoke inhalation X01.1 ☑
        hit by object X01.4 ☑
        specified mode of injury NEC X01.8 ☑
    undetermined whether accidental or intentional Y26 ☑
  forces of nature NEC — *see* Forces of nature
  G-forces (abnormal) W49.9 ☑
  gravitational forces (abnormal) W49.9 ☑
  heat (natural) NEC — *see* Heat
  high-pressure jet (hydraulic) (pneumatic) W49.9 ☑
  hydraulic jet W49.9 ☑
  inanimate mechanical force W49.9 ☑
  jet, high-pressure (hydraulic) (pneumatic) W49.9 ☑
  lightning — *see* subcategory T75.0 ☑
    causing fire — *see* Exposure, fire
  mechanical forces NEC W49.9 ☑
    animate NEC W64 ☑
    inanimate NEC W49.9 ☑
  noise W42.9 ☑
    supersonic W42.0 ☑
  noxious substance — *see* Table of Drugs and Chemicals
  pneumatic jet W49.9 ☑
  prolonged in deep-freeze unit or refrigerator W93.2 ☑
  radiation — *see* Radiation
  smoke (*see also* Exposure, fire)
    tobacco, second hand Z77.22
  specified factors NEC X58 ☑
  sunlight X32 ☑
    man-made (sun lamp) W89.8 ☑
      tanning bed W89.1 ☑
  supersonic waves W42.0 ☑
  transmission line(s), electric W85 ☑
  vibration W49.9 ☑
  waves
    infrasound W49.9 ☑
    sound W42.9 ☑
    supersonic W42.0 ☑
  weather NEC — *see* Forces of nature
External cause status Y99.9
  child assisting in compensated work for family Y99.8
  civilian activity done for financial or other compensation Y99.0
  civilian activity done for income or pay Y99.0
  family member assisting in compensated work for other family member Y99.8

408

☑ **Additional Character Required** — **Refer to the Tabular List for Character Selection**   ▽ **Subterms under main terms may continue to next column or page**

External cause status — *continued*
hobby not done for income Y99.8
leisure activity Y99.8
military activity Y99.1
off-duty activity of military personnel Y99.8
recreation or sport not for income or while a student Y99.8
specified NEC Y99.8
student activity Y99.8
volunteer activity Y99.2

F

Factors, supplemental
alcohol
blood level
less than 20mg/100ml Y90.0
20-39mg/100ml Y90.1
40-59mg/100ml Y90.2
60-79mg/100ml Y90.3
80-99mg/100ml Y90.4
100-119mg/100ml Y90.5
120-199mg/100ml Y90.6
200-239mg/100ml Y90.7
240mg/100ml or more Y90.8
presence in blood, level not specified Y90.9
presence in blood, but level not specified Y90.9
environmental-pollution-related condition- see Z57 ☑
nosocomial condition Y95
work-related condition Y99.0
Failure
in suture or ligature during surgical procedure Y65.2
mechanical, of instrument or apparatus (any) (during any medical or surgical procedure) Y65.8
sterile precautions (during medical and surgical care) — *see* Misadventure, failure, sterile precautions, by type of procedure
to
introduce tube or instrument Y65.4
endotracheal tube during anesthesia Y65.3
make curve (transport vehicle) NEC — *see* Accident, transport
remove tube or instrument Y65.4
Fall, falling (accidental) W19 ☑
building W20.1 ☑
burning (uncontrolled fire) X00.3 ☑
down
embankment W17.81 ☑
escalator W10.0 ☑
hill W17.81 ☑
ladder W11 ☑
ramp W10.2 ☑
stairs, steps W10.9 ☑
due to
bumping against
object W18.00 ☑
sharp glass W18.02 ☑
specified NEC W18.09 ☑
sports equipment W18.01 ☑
person W03 ☑
due to ice or snow W00.0 ☑
on pedestrian conveyance — *see* Accident, transport, pedestrian, conveyance
collision with another person W03 ☑
due to ice or snow W00.0 ☑
involving pedestrian conveyance — *see* Accident, transport, pedestrian, conveyance
grocery cart tipping over W17.82 ☑
ice or snow W00.9 ☑
from one level to another W00.2 ☑
on stairs or steps W00.1 ☑
involving pedestrian conveyance — *see* Accident, transport, pedestrian, conveyance
on same level W00.0 ☑
slipping (on moving sidewalk) W01.0 ☑
with subsequent striking against object W01.10 ☑
furniture W01.190 ☑
sharp object W01.119 ☑
glass W01.110 ☑
power tool or machine W01.111 ☑
specified NEC W01.118 ☑
specified NEC W01.198 ☑
striking against
object W18.00 ☑
sharp glass W18.02 ☑
specified NEC W18.09 ☑

Fall, falling — *continued*
due to — *continued*
striking against — *continued*
object — *continued*
sports equipment W18.01 ☑
person W03 ☑
due to ice or snow W00.0 ☑
on pedestrian conveyance — *see* Accident, transport, pedestrian, conveyance
earth (with asphyxia or suffocation (by pressure)) — *see* Earth, falling
from, off, out of
aircraft NEC (with accident to aircraft NEC) V97.0 ☑
while boarding or alighting V97.1 ☑
balcony W13.0 ☑
bed W06 ☑
boat, ship, watercraft NEC (with drowning or submersion) — *see* Drowning, due to, fall overboard
with hitting bottom or object V94.0 ☑
bridge W13.1 ☑
building W13.9 ☑
burning (uncontrolled fire) X00.3 ☑
cavity W17.2 ☑
chair W07 ☑
cherry picker W17.89 ☑
cliff W15 ☑
dock W17.4 ☑
embankment W17.81 ☑
escalator W10.0 ☑
flagpole W13.8 ☑
furniture NEC W08 ☑
grocery cart W17.82 ☑
haystack W17.89 ☑
high place NEC W17.89 ☑
stated as undetermined whether accidental or intentional Y30 ☑
hole W17.2 ☑
incline W10.2 ☑
ladder W11 ☑
lifting device W17.89 ☑
machine, machinery (*see also* Contact, with, by type of machine)
not in operation W17.89 ☑
manhole W17.1 ☑
mobile elevated work platform [MEWP] W17.89 ☑
motorized mobility scooter W05.2 ☑
one level to another NEC W17.89 ☑
intentional, purposeful, suicide (attempt) X80
stated as undetermined whether accidental or intentional Y30 ☑
pit W17.2 ☑
playground equipment W09.8 ☑
jungle gym W09.2 ☑
slide W09.0 ☑
swing W09.1 ☑
quarry W17.89 ☑
railing W13.9 ☑
ramp W10.2 ☑
roof W13.2 ☑
scaffolding W12 ☑
scooter (nonmotorized) W05.1 ☑
motorized mobility W05.2 ☑
sky lift W17.89 ☑
stairs, steps W10.9 ☑
curb W10.1 ☑
due to ice or snow W00.1 ☑
escalator W10.0 ☑
incline W10.2 ☑
ramp W10.2 ☑
sidewalk curb W10.1 ☑
specified NEC W10.8 ☑
stepladder W11 ☑
storm drain W17.1 ☑
streetcar NEC V82.6 ☑
with antecedent collision — *see* Accident, transport, streetcar occupant
while boarding or alighting V82.4 ☑
structure NEC W13.8 ☑
burning (uncontrolled fire) X00.3 ☑
table W08 ☑
toilet W18.11 ☑
with subsequent striking against object W18.12 ☑
train NEC V81.6 ☑

Fall, falling — *continued*
from, off, out of — *continued*
train — *continued*
during derailment (without antecedent collision) V81.7 ☑
with antecedent collision — *see* Accident, transport, railway vehicle occupant
while boarding or alighting V81.4 ☑
transport vehicle after collision — *see* Accident, transport, by type of vehicle, collision
tree W14 ☑
vehicle (in motion) NEC (*see also* Accident, transport) V89.9 ☑
motor NEC (*see also* Accident, transport, occupant, by type of vehicle) V87.8 ☑
stationary W17.89 ☑
while boarding or alighting B — *see* Accident, transport, by type of vehicle, while boarding or alighting
viaduct W13.8 ☑
wall W13.8 ☑
watercraft (*see also* Drowning, due to, fall overboard)
with hitting bottom or object V94.0 ☑
well W17.0 ☑
wheelchair, non-moving W05.0 ☑
powered — *see* Accident, transport, pedestrian, conveyance occupant, specified type NEC
window W13.4 ☑
in, on
aircraft NEC V97.0 ☑
with accident to aircraft V97.0 ☑
while boarding or alighting V97.1 ☑
bathtub (empty) W18.2 ☑
filled W16.212 ☑
causing drowning W16.211 ☑
escalator W10.0 ☑
incline W10.2 ☑
ladder W11 ☑
machine, machinery — *see* Contact, with, by type of machine
object, edged, pointed or sharp (with cut) — *see* Fall, by type
playground equipment W09.8 ☑
jungle gym W09.2 ☑
slide W09.0 ☑
swing W09.1 ☑
ramp W10.2 ☑
scaffolding W12 ☑
shower W18.2 ☑
causing drowning W16.211 ☑
staircase, stairs, steps W10.9 ☑
curb W10.1 ☑
due to ice or snow W00.1 ☑
escalator W10.0 ☑
incline W10.2 ☑
specified NEC W10.8 ☑
streetcar (without antecedent collision) V82.5 ☑
with antecedent collision — *see* Accident, transport, streetcar occupant
while boarding or alighting V82.4 ☑
train (without antecedent collision) V81.5 ☑
with antecedent collision — *see* Accident, transport, railway vehicle occupant
during derailment (without antecedent collision) V81.7 ☑
with antecedent collision — *see* Accident, transport, railway vehicle occupant
while boarding or alighting V81.4 ☑
transport vehicle after collision — *see* Accident, transport, by type of vehicle, collision
watercraft V93.39 ☑
due to
accident to craft V91.29 ☑
powered craft V91.23 ☑
ferry boat V91.21 ☑
fishing boat V91.22 ☑
jetskis V91.23 ☑
liner V91.21 ☑
merchant ship V91.20 ☑
passenger ship V91.21 ☑
unpowered craft
canoe V91.25 ☑
inflatable V91.26 ☑
kayak V91.25 ☑
sailboat V91.24 ☑

Fall, falling — *continued*
  in, on — *continued*
    watercraft — *continued*
      powered craft V93.33 ☑
        ferry boat V93.31 ☑
        fishing boat V93.32 ☑
        jetskis V93.33 ☑
        liner V93.31 ☑
        merchant ship V93.30 ☑
        passenger ship V93.31 ☑
      unpowered craft V93.38 ☑
        canoe V93.35 ☑
        inflatable V93.36 ☑
        kayak V93.35 ☑
        sailboat V93.34 ☑
        surf-board V93.38 ☑
        windsurfer V93.38 ☑
  into
    cavity W17.2 ☑
    dock W17.4 ☑
    fire — *see* Exposure, fire, by type
    haystack W17.89 ☑
    hole W17.2 ☑
    lake — *see* Fall, into, water
    lake — *see* Fall, into, water
    manhole W17.1 ☑
    moving part of machinery — *see* Contact, with, by type of machine
    ocean — *see* Fall, into, water
    opening in surface NEC W17.89 ☑
    pit W17.2 ☑
    pond — *see* Fall, into, water
    quarry W17.89 ☑
    river — *see* Fall, into, water
    shaft W17.89 ☑
    storm drain W17.1 ☑
    stream — *see* Fall, into, water
    swimming pool (*see also* Fall, into, water, in, swimming pool)
      empty W17.3 ☑
    tank W17.89 ☑
    water W16.42 ☑
      causing drowning W16.41 ☑
      from watercraft — *see* Drowning, due to, fall overboard
      hitting diving board W21.4 ☑
      in
        bathtub W16.212 ☑
          causing drowning W16.211 ☑
        bucket W16.222 ☑
          causing drowning W16.221 ☑
        natural body of water W16.112 ☑
          causing drowning W16.111 ☑
          striking
            bottom W16.122 ☑
              causing drowning W16.121 ☑
            side W16.132 ☑
              causing drowning W16.131 ☑
        specified water NEC W16.312 ☑
          causing drowning W16.311 ☑
          striking
            bottom W16.322 ☑
              causing drowning W16.321 ☑
            wall W16.332 ☑
              causing drowning W16.331 ☑
        swimming pool W16.012 ☑
          causing drowning W16.011 ☑
          striking
            bottom W16.022 ☑
              causing drowning W16.031 ☑
            wall W16.032 ☑
              causing drowning W16.021 ☑
        utility bucket W16.222 ☑
          causing drowning W16.221 ☑
    well W17.0 ☑
  involving
    bed W06 ☑
    chair W07 ☑
    furniture NEC W08 ☑
    glass — *see* Fall, by type
    playground equipment W09.8 ☑
      jungle gym W09.2 ☑
      slide W09.0 ☑
      swing W09.1 ☑
    roller blades — *see* Accident, transport, pedestrian, conveyance

Fall, falling — *continued*
  involving — *continued*
    skateboard(s) — *see* Accident, transport, pedestrian, conveyance
    skates (ice) (in line) (roller) — *see* Accident, transport, pedestrian, conveyance
    skis — *see* Accident, transport, pedestrian, conveyance
    table W08 ☑
    wheelchair, non-moving W05.0 ☑
      powered — *see* Accident, transport, pedestrian, conveyance, specified type NEC
  object — *see* Struck by, object, falling
  off
    toilet W18.11 ☑
      with subsequent striking against object W18.12 ☑
  on same level W18.30 ☑
    due to
      specified NEC W18.39 ☑
      stepping on an object W18.31 ☑
  out of
    bed W06 ☑
    building NEC W13.8 ☑
    chair W07 ☑
    furniture NEC W08 ☑
    wheelchair, non-moving W05.0 ☑
      powered — *see* Accident, transport, pedestrian, conveyance, specified type NEC
    window W13.4 ☑
  over
    animal W01.0 ☑
    cliff W15 ☑
    embankment W17.81 ☑
    small object W01.0 ☑
  rock W20.8 ☑
  same level W18.30 ☑
    from
      being crushed, pushed, or stepped on by a crowd or human stampede W52 ☑
      collision, pushing, shoving, by or with other person W03 ☑
      slipping, stumbling, tripping W01.0 ☑
    involving ice or snow W00.0 ☑
      involving skates (ice) (roller), skateboard, skis — *see* Accident, transport, pedestrian, conveyance
  snowslide (avalanche) — *see* Landslide
  stone W20.8 ☑
  structure W20.1 ☑
    burning (uncontrolled fire) X00.3 ☑
  through
    bridge W13.1 ☑
    floor W13.3 ☑
    roof W13.2 ☑
    wall W13.8 ☑
    window W13.4 ☑
  timber W20.8 ☑
  tree (caused by lightning) W20.8 ☑
  while being carried or supported by other person(s) W04 ☑

Fallen on by
  animal (not being ridden) NEC W55.89 ☑
Felo-de-se — *see* Suicide
Fight (hand) (fists) (foot) — *see* Assault, fight
Fire (accidental) — *see* Exposure, fire
Firearm discharge — *see* Discharge, firearm
Fireball effects from nuclear explosion in war operations — *see* War operations, nuclear weapons
Fireworks (explosion) W39 ☑
Flash burns from explosion — *see* Explosion
Flood (any injury) (caused by) X38 ☑
  collapse of man-made structure causing earth movement X36.0 ☑
  tidal wave — *see* Forces of nature, tidal wave
Food (any type) **in**
  air passages (with asphyxia, obstruction, or suffocation) — *see* categories T17 and T18
  alimentary tract causing asphyxia (due to compression of trachea) — *see* categories T17 and T18
Forces of nature X39.8 ☑
  avalanche X36.1 ☑
    causing transport accident — *see* Accident, transport, by type of vehicle
  blizzard X37.2 ☑
  cataclysmic storm X37.9 ☑

Forces of nature — *continued*
  cataclysmic storm — *continued*
    with flood X38 ☑
    blizzard X37.2 ☑
    cloudburst X37.8 ☑
    cyclone X37.1 ☑
    dust storm X37.3 ☑
    hurricane X37.0 ☑
    specified storm NEC X37.8 ☑
    storm surge X37.0 ☑
    tornado X37.1 ☑
    twister X37.1 ☑
    typhoon X37.0 ☑
  cloudburst X37.8 ☑
  cold (natural) X31 ☑
  cyclone X37.1 ☑
  dam collapse causing earth movement X36.0 ☑
  dust storm X37.3 ☑
  earth movement X36.1 ☑
    caused by dam or structure collapse X36.0 ☑
    earthquake X34 ☑
  earthquake X34 ☑
  flood (caused by) X38 ☑
    dam collapse X36.0 ☑
    tidal wave B — *see* Forces of nature, tidal wave
  heat (natural) X30 ☑
  hurricane X37.0 ☑
  landslide X36.1 ☑
    causing transport accident — *see* Accident, transport, by type of vehicle
  lightning — *see* subcategory T75.0 ☑
    causing fire — *see* Exposure, fire
  mudslide X36.1 ☑
    causing transport accident — *see* Accident, transport, by type of vehicle
  radiation (natural) X39.08 ☑
    radon X39.01 ☑
  radon X39.01 ☑
  specified force NEC X39.8 ☑
  storm surge X37.0 ☑
  structure collapse causing earth movement X36.0 ☑
  sunlight X32 ☑
  tidal wave X37.41 ☑
    due to
      earthquake X37.41 ☑
      landslide X37.43 ☑
      storm X37.42 ☑
      volcanic eruption X37.41 ☑
  tornado X37.1 ☑
  tsunami X37.41 ☑
  twister X37.1 ☑
  typhoon X37.0 ☑
  volcanic eruption X35 ☑
Foreign body
  aspiration — *see* Index to Diseases and Injuries, Foreign body, respiratory tract
  entering through skin W45.8 ☑
    can lid W45.2 ☑
    nail W45.0 ☑
    paper W45.1 ☑
    specified NEC W45.8 ☑
    splinter W45.8 ☑
Forest fire (exposure to) — *see* Exposure, fire, uncontrolled, not in building
Found injured X58 ☑
  from exposure (to) — *see* Exposure
  on
    highway, road(way), street V89.9 ☑
    railway right of way V81.9 ☑
Fracture (circumstances unknown or unspecified) X58 ☑
  due to specified cause NEC X58 ☑
Freezing — *see* Exposure, cold
Frostbite X31 ☑
  due to man-made conditions — *see* Exposure, cold, man-made
Frozen — *see* Exposure, cold

G

Gored by bull W55.22 ☑
Gunshot wound W34.00 ☑

H

Hailstones, injured by X39.8 ☑

Hanged herself or himself — *see* Hanging, self-inflicted
Hanging (accidental) (*see also* category) T71 ☑
  legal execution — *see* Legal, intervention, specified
    means NEC
Heat (effects of) (excessive) X30 ☑
  due to
    man-made conditions W92 ☑
      on board watercraft V93.29 ☑
        fishing boat V93.22 ☑
        merchant ship V93.20 ☑
        passenger ship V93.21 ☑
        sailboat V93.24 ☑
        specified powered craft NEC V93.23 ☑
    weather (conditions) X30 ☑
  from
    electric heating apparatus causing burning X16 ☑
    nuclear explosion in war operations — *see* War
      operations, nuclear weapons
  inappropriate in local application or packing in medical
    or surgical procedure Y63.5
Hemorrhage
  delayed following medical or surgical treatment
    without mention of misadventure — *see* Index
    to Diseases and Injuries, Complication(s)
  during medical or surgical treatment as misadventure
    — *see* Index to Diseases and Injuries, Complica-
    tion(s)
High
  altitude (effects) — *see* Air, pressure, low
  level of radioactivity, effects — *see* Radiation
  pressure (effects) — *see* Air, pressure, high
  temperature, effects — *see* Heat
Hit, hitting (accidental) by — *see* Struck by
Hitting against — *see* Striking against
Homicide (attempt) (justifiable) — *see* Assault
Hot
  place, effects (*see also* Heat)
  weather, effects X30 ☑
House fire (uncontrolled) — *see* Exposure, fire, uncon-
  trolled, building
Humidity, causing problem X39.8 ☑
Hunger X58 ☑
Hurricane (any injury) X37.0 ☑
Hypobarism, hypobaropathy — *see* Air, pressure, low

I

Ictus
  caloris (*see also* Heat)
  solaris X30 ☑
Ignition (accidental) (*see also* Exposure, fire) X08.8 ☑
  anesthetic gas in operating room W40.1 ☑
  apparel X06.2 ☑
    from highly flammable material X04 ☑
    nightwear X05 ☑
  bed linen (sheets) (spreads) (pillows) (mattress) — *see*
    Exposure, fire, uncontrolled, building, bed
  benzine X04 ☑
  clothes, clothing NEC (from controlled fire) X06.2 ☑
    from
      highly flammable material X04 ☑
  ether X04 ☑
    in operating room W40.1 ☑
  explosive material — *see* Explosion
  gasoline X04 ☑
  jewelry (plastic) (any) X06.0 ☑
  kerosene X04 ☑
  material
    explosive — *see* Explosion
    highly flammable with secondary explosion X04 ☑
  nightwear X05 ☑
  paraffin X04 ☑
  petrol X04 ☑
Immersion (accidental) (*see also* Drowning)
  hand or foot due to cold (excessive) X31 ☑
Implantation of quills of porcupine W55.89 ☑
Inanition (from) (hunger) X58 ☑
  thirst X58 ☑
Inappropriate operation performed
  correct operation on wrong side or body part (wrong
    side) (wrong site) Y65.53
  operation intended for another patient done on wrong
    patient Y65.52
  wrong operation performed on correct patient Y65.51
Inattention after, at birth (homicidal intent) (infantici-
  dal intent) X58 ☑

Incident, adverse
  device
    anesthesiology Y70.8
      accessory Y70.2
      diagnostic Y70.0
      miscellaneous Y70.8
      monitoring Y70.0
      prosthetic Y70.2
      rehabilitative Y70.1
      surgical Y70.3
      therapeutic Y70.1
    cardiovascular Y71.8
      accessory Y71.2
      diagnostic Y71.0
      miscellaneous Y71.8
      monitoring Y71.0
      prosthetic Y71.2
      rehabilitative Y71.1
      surgical Y71.3
      therapeutic Y71.1
    gastroenterology Y73.8
      accessory Y73.2
      diagnostic Y73.0
      miscellaneous Y73.8
      monitoring Y73.0
      prosthetic Y73.2
      rehabilitative Y73.1
      surgical Y73.3
      therapeutic Y73.1
    general
      hospital Y74.8
        accessory Y74.2
        diagnostic Y74.0
        miscellaneous Y74.8
        monitoring Y74.0
        prosthetic Y74.2
        rehabilitative Y74.1
        surgical Y74.3
        therapeutic Y74.1
      surgical Y81.8
        accessory Y81.2
        diagnostic Y81.0
        miscellaneous Y81.8
        monitoring Y81.0
        prosthetic Y81.2
        rehabilitative Y81.1
        surgical Y81.3
        therapeutic Y81.1
    gynecological Y76.8
      accessory Y76.2
      diagnostic Y76.0
      miscellaneous Y76.8
      monitoring Y76.0
      prosthetic Y76.2
      rehabilitative Y76.1
      surgical Y76.3
      therapeutic Y76.1
    medical Y82.9
      specified type NEC Y82.8
    neurological Y75.8
      accessory Y75.2
      diagnostic Y75.0
      miscellaneous Y75.8
      monitoring Y75.0
      prosthetic Y75.2
      rehabilitative Y75.1
      surgical Y75.3
      therapeutic Y75.1
    obstetrical Y76.8
      accessory Y76.2
      diagnostic Y76.0
      miscellaneous Y76.8
      monitoring Y76.0
      prosthetic Y76.2
      rehabilitative Y76.1
      surgical Y76.3
      therapeutic Y76.1
    ophthalmic Y77.8
      accessory Y77.2
      diagnostic Y77.0
      miscellaneous Y77.8
      monitoring Y77.0
      prosthetic Y77.2
      rehabilitative Y77.1
      surgical Y77.3
      therapeutic Y77.1
    orthopedic Y79.8
      accessory Y79.2

Incident, adverse — *continued*
  device — *continued*
    orthopedic — *continued*
      diagnostic Y79.0
      miscellaneous Y79.8
      monitoring Y79.0
      prosthetic Y79.2
      rehabilitative Y79.1
      surgical Y79.3
      therapeutic Y79.1
    otorhinolaryngological Y72.8
      accessory Y72.2
      diagnostic Y72.0
      miscellaneous Y72.8
      monitoring Y72.0
      prosthetic Y72.2
      rehabilitative Y72.1
      surgical Y72.3
      therapeutic Y72.1
    personal use Y74.8
      accessory Y74.2
      diagnostic Y74.0
      miscellaneous Y74.8
      monitoring Y74.0
      prosthetic Y74.2
      rehabilitative Y74.1
      surgical Y74.3
      therapeutic Y74.1
    physical medicine Y80.8
      accessory Y80.2
      diagnostic Y80.0
      miscellaneous Y80.8
      monitoring Y80.0
      prosthetic Y80.2
      rehabilitative Y80.1
      surgical Y80.3
      therapeutic Y80.1
    plastic surgical Y81.8
      accessory Y81.2
      diagnostic Y81.0
      miscellaneous Y81.8
      monitoring Y81.0
      prosthetic Y81.2
      rehabilitative Y81.1
      surgical Y81.3
      therapeutic Y81.1
    radiological Y78.8
      accessory Y78.2
      diagnostic Y78.0
      miscellaneous Y78.8
      monitoring Y78.0
      prosthetic Y78.2
      rehabilitative Y78.1
      surgical Y78.3
      therapeutic Y78.1
    urology Y73.8
      accessory Y73.2
      diagnostic Y73.0
      miscellaneous Y73.8
      monitoring Y73.0
      prosthetic Y73.2
      rehabilitative Y73.1
      surgical Y73.3
      therapeutic Y73.1
Incineration (accidental) — *see* Exposure, fire
Infanticide — *see* Assault
Infrasound waves (causing injury) W49.9 ☑
Ingestion
  foreign body (causing injury) (with obstruction) — *see*
    Foreign body, alimentary canal
  poisonous
    plant(s) X58 ☑
    substance NEC — *see* Table of Drugs and Chemicals
Inhalation
  excessively cold substance, man-made — *see* Expo-
    sure, cold, man-made
  food (any type) (into respiratory tract) (with asphyxia,
    obstruction respiratory tract, suffocation) — *see*
    categories T17 and T18 ☑
  foreign body — *see* Foreign body, aspiration
  gastric contents (with asphyxia, obstruction respiratory
    passage, suffocation) T17.81- ☑
  hot air or gases X14.0 ☑
  liquid air, hydrogen, nitrogen W93.12 ☑
    suicide (attempt) X83.2 ☑
  steam X13.0 ☑
    assault X98.0 ☑

Inhalation — *continued*
  steam — *continued*
    stated as undetermined whether accidental or intentional Y27.0 ☑
    suicide (attempt) X77.0 ☑
  toxic gas — *see* Table of Drugs and Chemicals
  vomitus (with asphyxia, obstruction respiratory passage, suffocation) T17.81- ☑
Injury, injured (accidental(ly)) NOS X58 ☑
  by, caused by, from
    assault — *see* Assault
    law-enforcing agent, police, in course of legal intervention — *see* Legal intervention
    suicide (attempt) X83.8 ☑
  due to, in
    civil insurrection — *see* War operations
    fight (*see also* Assault, fight) Y04.0 ☑
    war operations — *see* War operations
  homicide (*see also* Assault) Y09
  inflicted (by)
    in course of arrest (attempted), suppression of disturbance, maintenance of order, by law-enforcing agents — *see* Legal intervention
    other person
      stated as
        accidental X58 ☑
        intentional, homicide (attempt) — *see* Assault
        undetermined whether accidental or intentional Y33 ☑
  purposely (inflicted) by other person(s) — *see* Assault
  self-inflicted X83.8 ☑
    stated as accidental X58 ☑
  specified cause NEC X58 ☑
  undetermined whether accidental or intentional Y33 ☑
Insolation, effects X30 ☑
Insufficient nourishment X58 ☑
Interruption of respiration (by)
  food (lodged in esophagus) — *see* categories T17 and T18
  vomitus (lodged in esophagus) T17.81- ☑
Intervention, legal — *see* Legal intervention
Intoxication
  drug — *see* Table of Drugs and Chemicals
  poison — *see* Table of Drugs and Chemicals

J

Jammed (accidentally)
  between objects (moving) (stationary and moving) W23.0 ☑
  stationary W23.1 ☑
Jumped, jumping
  before moving object NEC X81.8 ☑
    motor vehicle X81.0 ☑
    subway train X81.1 ☑
    train X81.1 ☑
    undetermined whether accidental or intentional Y31 ☑
  from
    boat (into water) voluntarily, without accident (to or on boat) W16.712 ☑
      with
        accident to or on boat — *see* Accident, watercraft
        drowning or submersion W16.711 ☑
        suicide (attempt) X71.3 ☑
      striking bottom W16.722 ☑
        causing drowning W16.721 ☑
    building (*see also* Jumped, from, high place) W13.9 ☑
      burning (uncontrolled fire) X00.5 ☑
    high place NEC W17.89 ☑
      suicide (attempt) X80 ☑
      undetermined whether accidental or intentional Y30 ☑
    structure (*see also* Jumped, from, high place) W13.9 ☑
      burning (uncontrolled fire) X00.5 ☑
  into water W16.92 ☑
    causing drowning W16.91 ☑
    from, off watercraft — *see* Jumped, from, boat
    in
      natural body W16.612 ☑
        causing drowning W16.611 ☑

Jumped, jumping — *continued*
  into water — *continued*
    in — *continued*
      natural body — *continued*
        striking bottom W16.622 ☑
          causing drowning W16.621 ☑
      specified place NEC W16.812 ☑
        causing drowning W16.811 ☑
        striking
          bottom W16.822 ☑
            causing drowning W16.821 ☑
          wall W16.832 ☑
            causing drowning W16.831 ☑
      swimming pool W16.512 ☑
        causing drowning W16.511 ☑
        striking
          bottom W16.522 ☑
            causing drowning W16.521 ☑
          wall W16.532 ☑
            causing drowning W16.531 ☑
  suicide (attempt) X71.3 ☑

K

Kicked by
  animal NEC W55.82 ☑
  person(s) (accidentally) W50.1 ☑
    with intent to injure or kill Y04.0 ☑
    as, or caused by, a crowd or human stampede (with fall) W52 ☑
    assault Y04.0 ☑
    homicide (attempt) Y04.0 ☑
    in
      fight Y04.0 ☑
      legal intervention
        injuring
          bystander Y35.812 ☑
          law enforcement personnel Y35.811 ☑
          suspect Y35.813 ☑
Kicking against
  object W22.8 ☑
    sports equipment W21.9 ☑
    stationary wW22.09
      sports equipment W21.89 ☑
  person — *see* Striking against, person
  sports equipment W21.9 ☑
Killed, killing (accidentally) NOS (*see also* Injury) X58 ☑
  in
    action — *see* War operations
    brawl, fight (hand) (fists) (foot) Y04.0 ☑
      by weapon (*see also* Assault)
        cutting, piercing — *see* Assault, cutting or piercing instrument
        firearm — *see* Discharge, firearm, by type, homicide
  self
    stated as
      accident NOS X58 ☑
      suicide — *see* Suicide
      undetermined whether accidental or intentional Y33 ☑
Knocked down (accidentally) (by) NOS X58 ☑
  animal (not being ridden) NEC (*see also* Struck by, by type of animal)
  crowd or human stampede W52 ☑
  person W51 ☑
    in brawl, fight Y04.0 ☑
  transport vehicle NEC (*see also* Accident, transport) V09.9 ☑

L

Laceration NEC — *see* Injury
Lack of
  care (helpless person) (infant) (newborn) X58 ☑
  food except as result of abandonment or neglect X58 ☑
    due to abandonment or neglect X58 ☑
  water except as result of transport accident X58 ☑
    due to transport accident B — *see* Accident, transport, by type
    helpless person, infant, newborn X58 ☑
Landslide (falling on transport vehicle) X36.1 ☑
  caused by collapse of man-made structure X36.0 ☑
Late effect — *see* Sequelae

Legal
  execution (any method) — *see* Legal, intervention
  intervention (by)
    baton — *see* Legal, intervention, blunt object, baton
    bayonet — *see* Legal, intervention, sharp object, bayonet
    blow — *see* Legal, intervention, manhandling
    blunt object
      baton
        injuring
          bystander Y35.312 ☑
          law enforcement personnel Y35.311 ☑
          suspect Y35.313 ☑
      injuring
        bystander Y35.302 ☑
        law enforcement personnel Y35.301 ☑
        suspect Y35.303 ☑
      specified NEC
        injuring
          bystander Y35.392 ☑
          law enforcement personnel Y35.391 ☑
          suspect Y35.393 ☑
      stave
        injuring
          bystander Y35.392 ☑
          law enforcement personnel Y35.391 ☑
          suspect Y35.393 ☑
    bomb — *see* Legal, intervention, explosive
    cutting or piercing instrument — *see* Legal, intervention, sharp object
    dynamite — *see* Legal, intervention, explosive, dynamite
    explosive(s)
      dynamite
        injuring
          bystander Y35.112 ☑
          law enforcement personnel Y35.111 ☑
          suspect Y35.113 ☑
      grenade
        injuring
          bystander Y35.192 ☑
          law enforcement personnel Y35.191 ☑
          suspect Y35.193 ☑
      injuring
        bystander Y35.102 ☑
        law enforcement personnel Y35.101 ☑
        suspect Y35.103 ☑
      mortar bomb
        injuring
          bystander Y35.192 ☑
          law enforcement personnel Y35.191 ☑
          suspect Y35.193 ☑
      shell
        injuring
          bystander Y35.122 ☑
          law enforcement personnel Y35.121 ☑
          suspect Y35.123 ☑
      specified NEC
        injuring
          bystander Y35.192 ☑
          law enforcement personnel Y35.191 ☑
          suspect Y35.193 ☑
    firearm(s) (discharge)
      handgun
        injuring
          bystander Y35.022 ☑
          law enforcement personnel Y35.021 ☑
          suspect Y35.023 ☑
      injuring
        bystander Y35.002 ☑
        law enforcement personnel Y35.001 ☑
        suspect Y35.003 ☑
      machine gun
        injuring
          bystander Y35.012 ☑
          law enforcement personnel Y35.011 ☑
          suspect Y35.013 ☑
      rifle pellet
        injuring
          bystander Y35.032 ☑
          law enforcement personnel Y35.031 ☑
          suspect Y35.033 ☑
      rubber bullet
        injuring
          bystander Y35.042 ☑
          law enforcement personnel Y35.041 ☑

Legal — *continued*
  intervention — *continued*
    firearm(s) — *continued*
      rubber bullet — *continued*
        injuring — *continued*
          suspect Y35.043 ☑
      shotgun — *see* Legal, intervention, firearm, specified NEC
      specified NEC
        injuring
          bystander Y35.092 ☑
          law enforcement personnel Y35.091 ☑
          suspect Y35.093 ☑
    gas (asphyxiation) (poisoning)
      injuring
        bystander Y35.202 ☑
        law enforcement personnel Y35.201 ☑
        suspect Y35.203 ☑
      specified NEC
        injuring
          bystander Y35.292 ☑
          law enforcement personnel Y35.291 ☑
          suspect Y35.293 ☑
      tear gas
        injuring
          bystander Y35.212 ☑
          law enforcement personnel Y35.211 ☑
          suspect Y35.213 ☑
    grenade — *see* Legal, intervention, explosive, grenade
    injuring
      bystander Y35.92 ☑
      law enforcement personnel Y35.91 ☑
      suspect Y35.93 ☑
    late effect (of) — *see* with 7th character S Y35 ☑
    manhandling
      injuring
        bystander Y35.812 ☑
        law enforcement personnel Y35.811 ☑
        suspect Y35.813 ☑
    sequelae (of) — *see* with 7th character S Y35 ☑
    sharp objects
      bayonet
        injuring
          bystander Y35.412 ☑
          law enforcement personnel Y35.411 ☑
          suspect Y35.413 ☑
      injuring
        bystander Y35.402 ☑
        law enforcement personnel Y35.401 ☑
        suspect Y35.403 ☑
      specified NEC
        injuring
          bystander Y35.492 ☑
          law enforcement personnel Y35.491 ☑
          suspect Y35.493 ☑
    specified means NEC
      injuring
        bystander Y35.892 ☑
        law enforcement personnel Y35.891 ☑
        suspect Y35.893 ☑
    stabbing — *see* Legal, intervention, sharp object
    stave — *see* Legal, intervention, blunt object, stave
    tear gas — *see* Legal, intervention, gas, tear gas
    truncheon — *see* Legal, intervention, blunt object, stave
Lightning (shock) (stroke) (struck by) — *see* subcategory T75.0 ☑
  causing fire — *see* Exposure, fire
Loss of control (transport vehicle) NEC — *see* Accident, transport
Lost at sea NOS — *see* Drowning, due to, fall overboard
Low
  pressure (effects) — *see* Air, pressure, low
  temperature (effects) — *see* Exposure, cold
Lying before train, vehicle or other moving object X81.8
  subway train X81.1 ☑
  train X81.1 ☑
  undetermined whether accidental or intentional Y31 ☑
Lynching — *see* Assault

M

Malfunction (mechanism or component) (of)

Malfunction — *continued*
  firearm W34.10 ☑
    airgun W34.110 ☑
    BB gun W34.110 ☑
    gas, air or spring-operated gun NEC W34.118 ☑
    handgun W32.1 ☑
    hunting rifle W33.12 ☑
    larger firearm W33.10 ☑
      specified NEC W33.19 ☑
    machine gun W33.13 ☑
    paintball gun W34.111 ☑
    pellet gun W34.110 ☑
    shotgun W33.11 ☑
    specified NEC W34.19 ☑
    Very pistol [flare] W34.19 ☑
  handgun — *see* Malfunction, firearm, handgun
Maltreatment — *see* Perpetrator
Mangled (accidentally) NOS X58
Manhandling (in brawl, fight) Y04.0 ☑
  legal intervention — *see* Legal, intervention, manhandling
Manslaughter (nonaccidental) — *see* Assault
Mauled by animal NEC W55.89 ☑
Medical procedure, complication of (delayed or as an abnormal reaction without mention of misadventure) — *see* Complication of or following, by specified type of procedure
  due to or as a result of misadventure — *see* Misadventure
Melting (due to fire) (*see also* Exposure, fire)
  apparel NEC X06.3
  clothes, clothing NEC X06.3
    nightwear X05
  fittings or furniture (burning building) (uncontrolled fire) X00.8 ☑
  nightwear X05
  plastic jewelry X06.1
Mental cruelty X58
Military operations (injuries to military and civilians occuring during peacetime on military property and during routine military exercises and operations) (by) (from) (involving) Y37.90- ☑
  air blast Y37.20- ☑
  aircraft
    destruction — *see* Military operations, destruction of aircraft
    airway restriction — *see* Military operations, restriction of airways
    asphyxiation — *see* Military operations, restriction of airways
  biological weapons Y37.6X- ☑
  blast Y37.20- ☑
  blast fragments Y37.20- ☑
  blast wave Y37.20- ☑
  blast wind Y37.20- ☑
  bomb Y37.20- ☑
    dirty Y37.50- ☑
    gasoline Y37.31- ☑
    incendiary Y37.31- ☑
    petrol Y37.31- ☑
  bullet Y37.43- ☑
    incendiary Y37.32- ☑
    rubber Y37.41- ☑
  chemical weapons Y37.7X- ☑
  combat
    hand to hand (unarmed) combat Y37.44- ☑
    using blunt or piercing object Y37.45- ☑
  conflagration — *see* Military operations, fire
  conventional warfare NEC Y37.49- ☑
  depth-charge Y37.01- ☑
  destruction of aircraft Y37.10- ☑
    due to
      air to air missile Y37.11- ☑
      collision with other aircraft Y37.12- ☑
      detonation (accidental) of onboard munitions and explosives Y37.14- ☑
      enemy fire or explosives Y37.11- ☑
      explosive piaced on aircraft Y37.11- ☑
      onboard fire Y37.13- ☑
      rocket propelled grenade [RPG] Y37.11- ☑
      small arms fire Y37.11- ☑
      surface to air missile Y37.11- ☑
    specified NEC Y37.19- ☑
  detonation (accidental) of
    onboard marine weapons Y37.05- ☑

Military operations — *continued*
  detonation of — *continued*
    own munitions or munitions launch device Y37.24- ☑
  dirty bomb Y37.50- ☑
  explosion (of) Y37.20- ☑
    aerial bomb Y37.21- ☑
    bomb NOS (*see also* Military operations, bomb(s)) Y37.20- ☑
    fragments Y37.20- ☑
    grenade Y37.29- ☑
    guided missile Y37.22- ☑
    improvised explosive device [IED] (person-borne) (roadside) (vehicle-borne) Y37.23- ☑
    land mine Y37.29- ☑
    marine mine (at sea) (in harbor) Y37.02- ☑
    marine weapon Y37.00- ☑
      specified NEC Y37.09- ☑
    own munitions or munitions launch device (accidental) Y37.24- ☑
    sea-based artillery shell Y37.03- ☑
    specified NEC Y37.29- ☑
    torpedo Y37.04- ☑
  fire Y37.30- ☑
    specified NEC Y37.39- ☑
  firearms
    discharge Y37.43- ☑
    pellets Y37.42- ☑
  flamethrower Y37.33- ☑
  fragments (from) (of)
    improvised explosive device [IED] (person-borne) (roadside) (vehicle-borne) Y37.26- ☑
    munitions Y37.25- ☑
    specified NEC Y37.29- ☑
    weapons Y37.27- ☑
  friendly fire Y37.92- ☑
  hand to hand (unarmed) combat Y37.44- ☑
  hot substances — *see* Military operations, fire
  incendiary bullet Y37.32- ☑
  nuclear weapon (effects of) Y37.50- ☑
    acute radiation exposure Y37.54- ☑
    blast pressure Y37.51- ☑
    direct blast Y37.51- ☑
    direct heat Y37.53- ☑
    fallout exposure Y37.54- ☑
    fireball Y37.53- ☑
    indirect blast (struck or crushed by blast debris) (being thrown by blast) Y37.52- ☑
    ionizing radiation (immediate exposure) Y37.54- ☑
    nuclear radiation Y37.54- ☑
    radiation
      ionizing (immediate exposure) Y37.54- ☑
      nuclear Y37.54- ☑
      thermal Y37.53- ☑
    secondary effects Y37.54- ☑
    specified NEC Y37.59- ☑
    thermal radiation Y37.53- ☑
  restriction of air (airway)
    intentional Y37.46- ☑
    unintentional Y37.47- ☑
  rubber bullets Y37.41- ☑
  shrapnel NOS Y37.29- ☑
  suffocation –– *see* Military operations, restriction of airways
  unconventional warfare NEC Y37.7X- ☑
  underwater blast NOS Y37.00- ☑
  warfare
    conventional NEC Y37.49- ☑
    unconventional NEC Y37.7X- ☑
  weapon of mass destruction [WMD] Y37.91- ☑
  weapons
    biological weapons Y37.6X- ☑
    chemical Y37.7X- ☑
    nuclear (effects of) Y37.50- ☑
      acute radiation exposure Y37.54- ☑
      blast pressure Y37.51- ☑
      direct blast Y37.51- ☑
      direct heat Y37.53- ☑
      fallout exposure Y37.54- ☑
      fireball Y37.53- ☑
      indirect blast (struck or crushed by blast debris) (being thrown by blast) Y37.52- ☑
      radiation
        ionizing (immediate exposure) Y37.54- ☑
        nuclear Y37.54- ☑
        thermal Y37.53- ☑

Military operations — continued
weapons — continued
nuclear — continued
secondary effects Y37.54- ☑
specified NEC Y37.59- ☑
of mass destruction [WMD] Y37.91- ☑
Misadventure(s) to patient(s) during surgical or medical care Y69
contaminated medical or biological substance (blood, drug, fluid) Y64.9
administered (by) NEC Y64.9
immunization Y64.1
infusion Y64.0
injection Y64.1
specified means NEC Y64.8
transfusion Y64.0
vaccination Y64.1
excessive amount of blood or other fluid during transfusion or infusion Y63.0
failure
in dosage Y63.9
electroshock therapy Y63.4
inappropriate temperature (too hot or too cold) in local application and packing Y63.5
infusion
excessive amount of fluid Y63.0
incorrect dilution of fluid Y63.1
insulin-shock therapy Y63.4
nonadministration of necessary drug or biological substance Y63.6
overdose — see Table of Drugs and Chemicals
radiation, in therapy Y63.2
radiation
overdose Y63.2
specified procedure NEC Y63.8
transfusion
excessive amount of blood Y63.0
mechanical, of instrument or apparatus (any) (during any procedure) Y65.8
sterile precautions (during procedure) Y62.9
aspiration of fluid or tissue (by puncture or catheterization, except heart) Y62.6
biopsy (except needle aspiration) Y62.8
needle (aspirating) Y62.6
blood sampling Y62.6
catheterization Y62.6
heart Y62.5
dialysis (kidney) Y62.2
endoscopic examination Y62.4
enema Y62.8
immunization Y62.3
infusion Y62.1
injection Y62.3
needle biopsy Y62.6
paracentesis (abdominal) (thoracic) Y62.6
perfusion Y62.2
puncture (lumbar) Y62.6
removal of catheter or packing Y62.8
specified procedure NEC Y62.8
surgical operation Y62.0
transfusion Y62.1
vaccination Y62.3
suture or ligature during surgical procedure Y65.2
to introduce or to remove tube or instrument B — see Failure, to
hemorrhage — see Index to Diseases and Injuries, Complication(s)
inadvertent exposure of patient to radiation Y63.3
inappropriate
operation performed — see Inappropriate operation performed
temperature (too hot or too cold) in local application or packing Y63.5
infusion (see also Misadventure, by type, infusion) Y69
excessive amount of fluid Y63.0
incorrect dilution of fluid Y63.1
wrong fluid Y65.1
mismatched blood in transfusion Y65.0
nonadministration of necessary drug or biological substance
overdose — see Table of Drugs and Chemicals
radiation (in therapy) Y63.2
perforation — see Index to Diseases and Injuries, Complication(s)
performance of inappropriate operation — see Inappropriate operation performed
puncture — see Index to Diseases and Injuries, Complication(s)

Misadventure(s) to patient(s) during surgical or medical care — continued
specified type NEC Y65.8
failure
suture or ligature during surgical operation Y65.2
to introduce or to remove tube or instrument B — see Failure, to
infusion of wrong fluid Y65.1
performance of inappropriate operation — see Inappropriate operation performed
transfusion of mismatched blood Y65.0
wrong
fluid in infusion Y65.1
placement of endotracheal tube during anesthetic procedure Y65.3
transfusion — see Misadventure, by type, transfusion
excessive amount of blood Y63.0
mismatched blood Y65.0
wrong
drug given in error — see Table of Drugs and Chemicals
fluid in infusion Y65.1
placement of endotracheal tube during anesthetic procedure Y65.3
Mismatched blood in transfusion Y65.0
Motion sickness T75.3 ☑
Mountain sickness W94.11 ☑
Mudslide (of cataclysmic nature) — see Landslide
Murder (attempt) — see Assault

N

Nail, contact with W45.0 ☑
gun W29.4 ☑
Neglect (criminal) (homicidal intent) X58 ☑
Noise (causing injury) (pollution) W42.9 ☑
supersonic W42.0 ☑
Nonadministration (of)
drug or biological substance (necessary) Y63.6
surgical and medical care Y66
Nosocomial condition Y95

O

Object
falling
from, in, on, hitting
machinery — see Contact, with, by type of machine
set in motion by
accidental explosion or rupture of pressure vessel W38 ☑
firearm — see Discharge, firearm, by type
machine(ry) — see Contact, with, by type of machine
Overdose (drug) — see Table of Drugs and Chemicals
radiation Y63.2
Overexertion — see category Y93 ☑
Overexposure (accidental) (to)
cold (see also Exposure, cold) X31 ☑
due to man-made conditions — see Exposure, cold, man-made
heat (see also Heat) X30 ☑
radiation — see Radiation
radioactivity W88.0 ☑
sun (sunburn) X32 ☑
weather NEC — see Forces of nature
wind NEC — see Forces of nature
Overheated — see Heat
Overturning (accidental)
machinery — see Contact, with, by type of machine
transport vehicle NEC (see also Accident, transport) V89.9 ☑
watercraft (causing drowning, submersion) (see also Drowning, due to, accident to, watercraft, overturning)
causing injury except drowning or submersion B — see Accident, watercraft, causing, injury NEC

P

Parachute descent (voluntary) (without accident to aircraft) V97.29 ☑

Parachute descent — continued
due to accident to aircraft — see Accident, transport, aircraft
Pecked by bird W61.99 ☑
Perforation during medical or surgical treatment as misadventure — see Index to Diseases and Injuries, Complication(s)
Perpetrator, perpetration, of assault, maltreatment and neglect (by) Y07.9
boyfriend Y07.03
brother Y07.410
stepbrother Y07.435
coach Y07.53
cousin
female Y07.491
male Y07.490
daycare provider Y07.519
at-home
adult care Y07.512
childcare Y07.510
care center
adult care Y07.513
childcare Y07.511
family member NEC Y07.499
father Y07.11
adoptive Y07.13
foster Y07.420
stepfather Y07.430
foster father Y07.420
foster mother Y07.421
girl friend Y07.04
healthcare provider Y07.529
mental health Y07.521
specified NEC Y07.528
husband Y07.01
instructor Y07.53
mother Y07.12
adoptive Y07.14
foster Y07.421
stepmother Y07.433
nonfamily member Y07.50
specified NEC Y07.59
nurse Y07.528
occupational therapist Y07.528
partner of parent
female Y07.434
male Y07.432
physical therapist Y07.528
sister Y07.411
speech therapist Y07.528
stepbrother Y07.435
stepfather Y07.430
stepmother Y07.433
stepsister Y07.436
teacher Y07.53
wife Y07.02
Piercing — see Contact, with, by type of object or machine
Pinched
between objects (moving) (stationary and moving) W23.0 ☑
stationary W23.1 ☑
Pinned under machine(ry) — see Contact, with, by type of machine
Place of occurrence Y92.9
abandoned house Y92.89
airplane Y92.813
airport Y92.520
ambulatory health services establishment NEC Y92.538
ambulatory surgery center Y92.530
amusement park Y92.831
apartment (co-op) — see Place of occurrence, residence, apartment
assembly hall Y92.29
bank Y92.510
barn Y92.71
baseball field Y92.320
basketball court Y92.310
beach Y92.832
boarding house — see Place of occurrence, residence, boarding house
boat Y92.814
bowling alley Y92.39
bridge Y92.89
building under construction Y92.61
bus Y92.811
station Y92.521
cafe Y92.511

Place of occurrence — *continued*
    campsite Y92.833
    campus — *see* Place of occurrence, school
    canal Y92.89
    car Y92.810
    casino Y92.59
    children's home — *see* Place of occurrence, residence, institutional, orphanage
    church Y92.22
    cinema Y92.26
    clubhouse Y92.29
    coal pit Y92.64
    college (community) Y92.214
    condominium — *see* Place of occurrence, residence, apartment
    construction area — *see* Place of occurrence, industrial and construction area
    convalescent home — *see* Place of occurrence, residence, institutional, nursing home
    court-house Y92.240
    cricket ground Y92.328
    cultural building Y92.258
        art gallery Y92.250
        museum Y92.251
        music hall Y92.252
        opera house Y92.253
        specified NEC Y92.258
        theater Y92.254
    dancehall Y92.252
    day nursery Y92.210
    dentist office Y92.531
    derelict house Y92.89
    desert Y92.820
    dockyard Y92.62
    dock NOS Y92.89
    doctor's office Y92.531
    dormitory — *see* Place of occurrence, residence, institutional, school dormitory
    dry dock Y92.62
    factory (building) (premises) Y92.63
    farm (land under cultivation) (outbuildings) Y92.79
        barn Y92.71
        chicken coop Y92.72
        field Y92.73
        hen house Y92.72
        house — *see* Place of occurrence, residence, house
        orchard Y92.74
        specified NEC Y92.79
    football field Y92.321
    forest Y92.821
    freeway Y92.411
    gallery Y92.250
    garage (commercial) Y92.59
        boarding house Y92.044
        military base Y92.135
        mobile home Y92.025
        nursing home Y92.124
        orphanage Y92.114
        private house Y92.015
        reform school Y92.155
    gas station Y92.524
    gasworks Y92.69
    golf course Y92.39
    gravel pit Y92.64
    grocery Y92.512
    gymnasium Y92.39
    handball court Y92.318
    harbor Y92.89
    harness racing course Y92.39
    healthcare provider office Y92.531
    highway (interstate) Y92.411
    hill Y92.828
    hockey rink Y92.330
    home — *see* Place of occurrence, residence
    hospice — *see* Place of occurrence, residence, institutional, nursing home
    hospital Y92.239
        cafeteria Y92.233
        corridor Y92.232
        operating room Y92.234
        patient
            bathroom Y92.231
            room Y92.230
        specified NEC Y92.238
    hotel Y92.59
    house (*see also* Place of occurrence, residence)
        abandoned Y92.89
        under construction Y92.61

Place of occurrence — *continued*
    industrial and construction area (yard) Y92.69
        building under construction Y92.61
        dock Y92.62
        dry dock Y92.62
        factory Y92.63
        gasworks Y92.69
        mine Y92.64
        oil rig Y92.65
        pit Y92.64
        power station Y92.69
        shipyard Y92.62
        specified NEC Y92.69
        tunnel under construction Y92.69
        workshop Y92.69
    kindergarten Y92.211
    lacrosse field Y92.328
    lake Y92.828
    library Y92.241
    mall Y92.59
    market Y92.512
    marsh Y92.828
    military
        base — *see* Place of occurrence, residence, institutional, military base
        training ground Y92.84
    mine Y92.64
    mosque Y92.22
    motel Y92.59
    motorway (interstate) Y92.411
    mountain Y92.828
    movie-house Y92.26
    museum Y92.251
    music-hall Y92.252
    not applicable Y92.9
    nuclear power station Y92.69
    nursing home — *see* Place of occurrence, residence, institutional, nursing home
    office building Y92.59
    offshore installation Y92.65
    oil rig Y92.65
    old people's home — *see* Place of occurrence, residence, institutional, specified NEC
    opera-house Y92.253
    orphanage — *see* Place of occurrence, residence, institutional, orphanage
    outpatient surgery center Y92.530
    park (public) Y92.830
        amusement Y92.831
    parking garage Y92.89
        lot Y92.481
    pavement Y92.480
    physician office Y92.531
    polo field Y92.328
    pond Y92.828
    post office Y92.242
    power station Y92.69
    prairie Y92.828
    prison — *see* Place of occurrence, residence, institutional, prison
    public
        administration building Y92.248
            city hall Y92.243
            courthouse Y92.240
            library Y92.241
            post office Y92.242
            specified NEC Y92.248
        building NEC Y92.29
        hall Y92.29
        place NOS Y92.89
    race course Y92.39
    radio station Y92.59
    railway line (bridge) Y92.85
    ranch (outbuildings) — *see* Place of occurrence, farm
    recreation area Y92.838
        amusement park Y92.831
        beach Y92.832
        campsite Y92.833
        park (public) Y92.830
        seashore Y92.832
        specified NEC Y92.838
    reform school - — *see* Place of occurrence, residence, institutional, reform school
    religious institution Y92.22
    residence (non-institutional) (private) Y92.009
        apartment Y92.039
            bathroom Y92.031
            bedroom Y92.032

Place of occurrence — *continued*
    residence — *continued*
        apartment — *continued*
            kitchen Y92.030
            specified NEC Y92.038
        bathroom Y92.002
        bedroom Y92.003
        boarding house Y92.049
            bathroom Y92.041
            bedroom Y92.042
            driveway Y92.043
            garage Y92.044
            garden Y92.046
            kitchen Y92.040
            specified NEC Y92.048
            swimming pool Y92.045
            yard Y92.046
        dining room Y92.001
        garden Y92.007
        home Y92.009
        house, single family Y92.019
            bathroom Y92.012
            bedroom Y92.013
            dining room Y92.011
            driveway Y92.014
            garage Y92.015
            garden Y92.017
            kitchen Y92.010
            specified NEC Y92.018
            swimming pool Y92.016
            yard Y92.017
        institutional Y92.10
            children's home — *see* Place of occurrence, residence, institutional, orphanage
            hospice — *see* Place of occurrence, residence, institutional, nursing home
            military base Y92.139
                barracks Y92.133
                garage Y92.135
                garden Y92.137
                kitchen Y92.130
                mess hall Y92.131
                specified NEC Y92.138
                swimming pool Y92.136
                yard Y92.137
            nursing home Y92.129
                bathroom Y92.121
                bedroom Y92.122
                driveway Y92.123
                garage Y92.124
                garden Y92.126
                kitchen Y92.120
                specified NEC Y92.128
                swimming pool Y92.125
                yard Y92.126
            orphanage Y92.119
                bathroom Y92.111
                bedroom Y92.112
                driveway Y92.113
                garage Y92.114
                garden Y92.116
                kitchen Y92.110
                specified NEC Y92.118
                swimming pool Y92.115
                yard Y92.116
            prison Y92.149
                bathroom Y92.142
                cell Y92.143
                courtyard Y92.147
                dining room Y92.141
                kitchen Y92.140
                specified NEC Y92.148
                swimming pool Y92.146
            reform school Y92.159
                bathroom Y92.152
                bedroom Y92.153
                dining room Y92.151
                driveway Y92.154
                garage Y92.155
                garden Y92.157
                kitchen Y92.150
                specified NEC Y92.158
                swimming pool Y92.156
                yard Y92.157
            school dormitory Y92.169
                bathroom Y92.162
                bedroom Y92.163
                dining room Y92.161

External Causes Index

Place of occurrence — Prolonged

Place of occurrence — *continued*
  residence — *continued*
    institutional — *continued*
      school dormitory — *continued*
        kitchen Y92.160
        specified NEC Y92.168
      specified NEC Y92.199
        bathroom Y92.192
        bedroom Y92.193
        dining room Y92.191
        driveway Y92.194
        garage Y92.195
        garden Y92.197
        kitchen Y92.190
        specified NEC Y92.198
        swimming pool Y92.196
        yard Y92.197
    kitchen Y92.000
    mobile home Y92.029
      bathroom Y92.022
      bedroom Y92.023
      dining room Y92.021
      driveway Y92.024
      garage Y92.025
      garden Y92.027
      kitchen Y92.020
      specified NEC Y92.028
      swimming pool Y92.026
      yard Y92.027
    specified place in residence NEC Y92.009
    specified residence type NEC Y92.099
      bathroom Y92.091
      bedroom Y92.092
      driveway Y92.093
      garage Y92.094
      garden Y92.096
      kitchen Y92.090
      specified NEC Y92.098
      swimming pool Y92.095
      yard Y92.096
  restaurant Y92.511
  riding school Y92.39
  river Y92.828
  road Y92.488
  rodeo ring Y92.39
  rugby field Y92.328
  same day surgery center Y92.530
  sand pit Y92.64
  school (private) (public) (state) Y92.219
    college Y92.214
    daycare center Y92.210
    elementary school Y92.211
    high school Y92.213
    kindergarten Y92.211
    middle school Y92.212
    specified NEC Y92.218
    trace school Y92.218
    university Y92.214
    vocational school Y92.215
  sea (shore) Y92.832
  senior citizen center Y92.29
  service area
    airport Y92.520
    bus station Y92.521
    gas station Y92.524
    highway rest stop Y92.523
    railway station Y92.522
  shipyard Y92.62
  shop (commercial) Y92.513
  sidewalk Y92.480
  silo Y92.79
  skating rink (roller) Y92.331
    ice Y92.330
  slaughter house Y92.86
  soccer field Y92.322
  specified place NEC Y92.89
  sports area Y92.39
    athletic
      court Y92.318
        basketball Y92.310
        specified NEC Y92.318
        squash Y92.311
        tennis Y92.312
      field Y92.328
        baseball Y92.320
        cricket ground Y92.328
        football Y92.321
        hockey Y92.328

Place of occurrence — *continued*
  sports area — *continued*
    athletic — *continued*
      field — *continued*
        soccer Y92.322
        specified NEC Y92.328
    golf course Y92.39
    gymnasium Y92.39
    riding school Y92.39
    skating rink (roller) Y92.331
      ice Y92.330
    stadium Y92.39
    swimming pool Y92.34
  squash court Y92.311
  stadium Y92.39
  steeplechasing course Y92.39
  store Y92.512
  stream Y92.828
  street and highway Y92.410
    bike path Y92.482
    freeway Y92.411
    highway ramp Y92.415
    interstate highway Y92.411
    local residential or business street Y92.414
    motorway Y92.411
    parking lot Y92.481
    parkway Y92.412
    sidewalk Y92.480
    specified NEC Y92.488
    state road Y92.413
  subway car Y92.816
  supermarket Y92.512
  swamp Y92.828
  swimming pool (public) Y92.34
    private (at) Y92.095
      boarding house Y92.045
      military base Y92.136
      mobile home Y92.026
      nursing home Y92.125
      orphanage Y92.115
      prison Y92.146
      reform school Y92.156
      single family residence Y92.016
  synagogue Y92.22
  television station Y92.59
  tennis court Y92.312
  theater Y92.254
  trade area Y92.59
    bank Y92.510
    cafe Y92.511
    casino Y92.59
    garage Y92.59
    hotel Y92.59
    market Y92.512
    office building Y92.59
    radio station Y92.59
    restaurant Y92.511
    shop Y92.513
    shopping mall Y92.59
    store Y92.512
    supermarket Y92.512
    television station Y92.59
    warehouse Y92.59
  trailer park, residential — *see* Place of occurrence, residence, mobile home
  trailer site NOS Y92.89
  train Y92.815
    station Y92.522
  truck Y92.812
  tunnel under construction Y92.69
  university Y92.214
  urgent (health) care center Y92.532
  vehicle (transport) Y92.818
    airplane Y92.813
    boat Y92.814
    bus Y92.811
    car Y92.810
    specified NEC Y92.818
    subway car Y92.816
    train Y92.815
    truck Y92.812
  warehouse Y92.59
  water reservoir Y92.89
  wilderness area Y92.828
    desert Y92.820
    forest Y92.821
    marsh Y92.828
    mountain Y92.828

Place of occurrence — *continued*
  wilderness area — *continued*
    prairie Y92.828
    specified NEC Y92.828
    swamp Y92.828
  workshop Y92.69
  yard, private Y92.096
    boarding house Y92.046
    mobile home Y92.027
    single family house Y92.017
  youth center Y92.29
  zoo (zoological garden) Y92.834
Plumbism — *see* Table of Drugs and Chemicals, lead
Poisoning (accidental) (by) (*see also* Table of Drugs and Chemicals)
  by plant, thorns, spines, sharp leaves or other mechanisms NEC X58 ☑
  carbon monoxide
    generated by
      motor vehicle — *see* Accident, transport
      watercraft (in transit) (not in transit) V93.89 ☑
        ferry boat V93.81 ☑
        fishing boat V93.82 ☑
        jet skis V93.83 ☑
        liner V93.81 ☑
        merchant ship V93.80 ☑
        passenger ship V93.81 ☑
        powered craft NEC V93.83 ☑
  caused by injection of poisons into skin by plant thorns, spines, sharp leaves X58 ☑
    marine or sea plants (venomous) X58 ☑
  execution — *see* Legal, intervention, gas
  intervention
    by gas — *see* Legal, intervention, gas
    other specified means — *see* Legal, intervention, specified means NEC
  exhaust gas
    generated by
      motor vehicle — *see* Accident, transport
      watercraft (in transit) (not in transit) V93.89 ☑
        ferry boat V93.81 ☑
        fishing boat V93.82 ☑
        jet skis V93.83 ☑
        liner V93.81 ☑
        merchant ship V93.80 ☑
        passenger ship V93.81 ☑
        powered craft NEC V93.83 ☑
  fumes or smoke due to
    explosion (*see also* Explosion) W40.9 ☑
    fire — *see* Exposure, fire
    ignition — *see* Ignition
  gas
    in legal intervention — *see* Legal, intervention, gas
    legal execution — *see* Legal, intervention, gas
  in war operations — *see* War operations
  legal
Powder burn (by) (from)
  airgun W34.110 ☑
  BB gun W34.110 ☑
  firearm NEC W34.19 ☑
  gas, air or spring-operated gun NEC W34.118 ☑
  handgun W32.1 ☑
  hunting rifle W33.12 ☑
  larger firearm W33.10 ☑
    specified NEC W33.19 ☑
  machine gun W33.13 ☑
  paintball gun W34.111 ☑
  pellet gun W34.110 ☑
  shotgun W33.11 ☑
  Very pistol [flare] W34.19 ☑
Premature cessation (of) **surgical and medical care** Y66
Privation (food) (water) X58 ☑
Procedure (operation)
  correct, on wrong side or body part (wrong side) (wrong site) Y65.53
  intended for another patient done on wrong patient Y65.52
  performed on patient not scheduled for surgery Y65.52
  performed on wrong patient Y65.52
  wrong, performed on correct patient Y65.51
Prolonged
  sitting in transport vehicle — *see* Travel, by type of vehicle
  stay in
    high altitude as cause of anoxia, barodontalgia, barotitis or hypoxia W94.11 ☑

Prolonged — *continued*
  stay in — *continued*
    weightless environment X52 ☑
Pulling, excessive — *see category* Y93 ☑
Puncture, puncturing (*see also* Contact, with, by type of object or machine)
  by
    plant thorns, spines, sharp leaves or other mechanisms NEC W60 ☑
  during medical or surgical treatment as misadventure — *see* Index to Diseases and Injuries, Complication(s)
Pushed, pushing (accidental) (injury in) (overexertion)
    see category Y93 ☑
  by other person(s) (accidental) W51 ☑
    with fall W03 ☑
      due to ice or snow W00.0 ☑
    as, or caused by, a crowd or human stampede (with fall) W52 ☑
    before moving object NEC Y02.8 ☑
      motor vehicle Y02.0 ☑
      subway train Y02.1 ☑
      train Y02.1 ☑
    from
      high place NEC
        in accidental circumstances W17.89 ☑
        stated as
          intentional, homicide (attempt) Y01 ☑
          undetermined whether accidental or intentional Y30 ☑
      transport vehicle NEC (*see also* Accident, transport) V89.9 ☑
        stated as
          intentional, homicide (attempt) Y08.89 ☑

R

Radiation (exposure to)
  arc lamps W89.0 ☑
  atomic power plant (malfunction) NEC W88.1 ☑
  complication of or abnormal reaction to medical radiotherapy Y84.2
  electromagnetic, ionizing W88.0 ☑
  gamma rays W88.1 ☑
  in
    war operations (from or following nuclear explosion) — *see* War operations
  inadvertent exposure of patient (receiving test or therapy) Y63.3
  infrared (heaters and lamps) W90.1 ☑
    excessive heat from W92 ☑
  ionized, ionizing (particles, artificially accelerated)
    radioisotopes W88.1 ☑
    specified NEC W88.8 ☑
    x-rays W88.0 ☑
  isotopes, radioactive — *see* Radiation, radioactive isotopes
  laser(s) W90.2 ☑
    in war operations — *see* War operations
    misadventure in medical care Y63.2
  light sources (man-made visible and ultraviolet) W89.9 ☑
    natural X32 ☑
    specified NEC W89.8 ☑
    tanning bed W89.1 ☑
    welding light W89.0 ☑
  man-made visible light W89.9 ☑
    specified NEC W89.8 ☑
    tanning bed W89.1 ☑
    welding light W89.0 ☑
  microwave W90.8 ☑
  misadventure in medical or surgical procedure Y63.2
  natural NEC X39.08 ☑
    radon X39.01 ☑
  overdose (in medical or surgical procedure) Y63.2
  radar W90.0 ☑
  radioactive isotopes (any) W88.1 ☑
    atomic power plant malfunction W88.1 ☑
    misadventure in medical or surgical treatment Y63.2
  radiofrequency W90.0 ☑
  radium NEC W88.1 ☑
  sun X32 ☑
  ultraviolet (light) (man-made) W89.9 ☑
    natural X32 ☑

Radiation — *continued*
  ultraviolet — *continued*
    specified NEC W89.8 ☑
    tanning bed W89.1 ☑
    welding light W89.0 ☑
  welding arc, torch, or light W89.0 ☑
    excessive heat from W92 ☑
  x-rays (hard) (soft) W88.0 ☑
Range disease W94.11 ☑
Rape (attempted) T74.2- ☑
Rat bite W53.11 ☑
Reaction, abnormal to medical procedure (*see also* Complication of or following, by type of procedure) Y84.9
  with misadventure — *see* Misadventure
  biologicals — *see* Table of Drugs and Chemicals
  drugs — *see* Table of Drugs and Chemicals
  vaccine — *see* Table of Drugs and Chemicals
Recoil
  airgun W34.110 ☑
  BB gun W34.110 ☑
  firearm NEC W34.19 ☑
  gas, air or spring-operated gun NEC W34.118 ☑
  handgun W32.1 ☑
  hunting rifle W33.12 ☑
  larger firearm W33.10 ☑
    specified NEC W33.19 ☑
  machine gun W33.13 ☑
  paintball gun W34.111 ☑
  pellet W34.110 ☑
  shotgun W33.11 ☑
  Very pistol [flare] W34.19 ☑
Reduction in
  atmospheric pressure — *see* Air, pressure, change
Rock falling on or hitting (accidentally) (person) W20.8 ☑
  in cave-in W20.0 ☑
Run over (accidentally) (by)
  animal (not being ridden) NEC W55.89 ☑
  machinery — *see* Contact, with, by specified type of machine
  transport vehicle NEC (*see also* Accident, transport) V09.9 ☑
    intentional homicide (attempt) Y03.0 ☑
    motor NEC V09.20 ☑
      intentional homicide (attempt) Y03.0 ☑
Running
  before moving object X81.8 ☑
    motor vehicle X81.0 ☑
Running off, away
  animal (being ridden) (*see also* Accident, transport) V80.918 ☑
    not being ridden W55.89 ☑
  animal-drawn vehicle NEC (*see also* Accident, transport) V80.928 ☑
  highway, road(way), street
    transport vehicle NEC (*see also* Accident, transport) V89.9 ☑
Rupture pressurized devices — *see* Explosion, by type of device

S

Saturnism — *see* Table of Drugs and Chemicals, lead
Scald, scalding (accidental) (by) (from) (in) X19 ☑
  air (hot) X14.1 ☑
  gases (hot) X14.1 ☑
  homicide (attempt) — *see* Assault, burning, hot object
  inflicted by other person
    stated as intentional, homicide (attempt) — *see* Assault, burning, hot object
  liquid (boiling) (hot) NEC X12 ☑
    stated as undetermined whether accidental or intentional Y27.2 ☑
    suicide (attempt) X77.2 ☑
  local application of externally applied substance in medical or surgical care Y63.5
  metal (molten) (liquid) (hot) NEC X18 ☑
  self-inflicted X77.9 ☑
    stated as undetermined whether accidental or intentional Y27.8 ☑
  steam X13.1 ☑
    assault X98.0 ☑
    stated as undetermined whether accidental or intentional Y27.0 ☑
    suicide (attempt) X77.0 ☑

Scald, scalding — *continued*
  suicide (attempt) X77.9 ☑
  vapor (hot) X13.1 ☑
    assault X98.0 ☑
    stated as undetermined whether accidental or intentional Y27.0 ☑
    suicide (attempt) X77.0 ☑
Scratched by
  cat W55.03 ☑
  person(s) (accidentally) W50.4 ☑
    with intent to injure or kill Y04.0 ☑
    as, or caused by, a crowd or human stampede (with fall) W52 ☑
    assault Y04.0 ☑
    homicide (attempt) Y04.0 ☑
    in
      fight Y04.0 ☑
      legal intervention
        injuring
          bystander Y35.892 ☑
          law enforcement personnel Y35.891 ☑
          suspect Y35.893 ☑
Seasickness T75.3 ☑
Self-harm NEC (*see also* External cause by type, undetermined whether accidental or intentional)
  intentional — *see* Suicide
  poisoning NEC — *see* Table of Drugs and Chemicals, poisoning, accidental
Self-inflicted (injury) **NEC** (*see also* External cause by type, undetermined whether accidental or intentional)
  intentional — *see* Suicide
  poisoning NEC — *see* Table of Drugs and Chemicals, poisoning, accidental
Sequelae (of)
  accident NEC — *see* W00-X58 with 7th character S
  assault (homicidal) (any means) — *see* X92-Y08 with 7th character S
  homicide, attempt (any means) — *see* X92-Y08 with 7th character S
  injury undetermined whether accidentally or purposely inflicted — *see* Y21-Y33 with 7th character S
  intentional self-harm (classifiable to X71-X83) — *see* X71-X83 with 7th character S
  legal intervention — *see* with 7th character S Y35 ☑
  motor vehicle accident — *see* V00-V99 with 7th character S
  suicide, attempt (any means) — *see* X71-X83 with 7th character S
  transport accident — *see* V00-V99 with 7th character S
  war operations — *see* War operations
Shock
  electric — *see* Exposure, electric current
  from electric appliance (any) (faulty) W86.8 ☑
    domestic W86.0 ☑
    suicide (attempt) X83.1 ☑
Shooting, shot (accidental(ly)) (*see also* Discharge, firearm, by type)
  herself or himself — *see* Discharge, firearm by type, self-inflicted
  homicide (attempt) — *see* Discharge, firearm by type, homicide
  in war operations — *see* War operations
  inflicted by other person — *see* Discharge, firearm by type, homicide
    accidental — *see* Discharge, firearm, by type of firearm
  legal
    execution — *see* Legal, intervention, firearm
    intervention — *see* Legal, intervention, firearm
  self-inflicted — *see* Discharge, firearm by type, suicide
    accidental — *see* Discharge, firearm, by type of firearm
  suicide (attempt) — *see* Discharge, firearm by type, suicide
Shoving (accidentally) **by other person** — *see* Pushed, by other person
Sickness
  alpine W94.11 ☑
  motion — *see* Motion
  mountain W94.11 ☑
Sinking (accidental)
  watercraft (causing drowning, submersion) (*see also* Drowning, due to, accident to, watercraft, sinking)

External Causes Index

Sinking — Struck

Sinking — *continued*
  watercraft (*see also* Drowning, due to, accident to, watercraft, sinking) — *continued*
    causing injury except drowning or submersion B — *see* Accident, watercraft, causing, injury NEC
Siriasis X32 ☑
Slashed wrists — *see* Cut, self-inflicted
Slipping (accidental) (on same level) (with fall) W01.0 ☑
  without fall W18.40 ☑
    due to
      specified NEC W18.49 ☑
      stepping from one level to another W18.43 ☑
      stepping into hole or opening W18.42 ☑
      stepping on object W18.41 ☑
  on
    ice W00.0 ☑
      with skates — *see* Accident, transport, pedestrian, conveyance
    mud W01.0 ☑
    oil W01.0 ☑
    snow W00.0 ☑
      with skis — *see* Accident, transport, pedestrian, conveyance
    surface (slippery) (wet) NEC W01.0 ☑
Sliver, wood, contact with W45.8 ☑
Smoldering (due to fire) — *see* Exposure, fire
Sodomy (attempted) **by force** T74.2 ☑
Sound waves (causing injury) W42.9 ☑
  supersonic W42.0 ☑
Splinter, contact with W45.8 ☑
Stab, stabbing B — *see* Cut
Starvation X58 ☑
Status of external cause Y99.9
  child assisting in compensated work for family Y99.8
  civilian activity done for financial or other compensation Y99.0
  civilian activity done for income or pay Y99.0
  family member assisting in compensated work for other family member Y99.8
  hobby not done for income Y99.8
  leisure activity Y99.8
  military activity Y99.1
  off-duty activity of military personnel Y99.8
  recreation or sport not for income or while a student Y99.8
  specified NEC Y99.8
  student activity Y99.8
  volunteer activity Y99.2
Stepped on
  by
    animal (not being ridden) NEC W55.89 ☑
    crowd or human stampede W52 ☑
    person W50.0 ☑
Stepping on
  object W22.8 ☑
    with fall W18.31 ☑
    sports equipment W21.9 ☑
    stationary W22.09 ☑
      sports equipment W21.89 ☑
  person W51 ☑
    by crowd or human stampede W52 ☑
  sports equipment W21.9 ☑
Sting
  arthropod, nonvenomous W57 ☑
  insect, nonvenomous W57 ☑
Storm (cataclysmic) — *see* Forces of nature, cataclysmic storm
Straining, excessive — *see* category Y93 ☑
Strangling — *see* Strangulation
Strangulation (accidental) T71 ☑
Strenuous movements — *see* category Y93 ☑
Striking against
  airbag (automobile) W22.10 ☑
    driver side W22.11 ☑
    front passenger side W22.12 ☑
    specified NEC W22.19 ☑
  bottom when
    diving or jumping into water (in) W16.822 ☑
      causing drowning W16.821 ☑
      from boat W16.722 ☑
        causing drowning W16.721 ☑
      natural body W16.622 ☑
        causing drowning W16.821 ☑
      swimming pool W16.522 ☑
        causing drowning W16.521 ☑

Striking against — *continued*
  bottom when — *continued*
    falling into water (in) W16.322 ☑
      causing drowning W16.321 ☑
      fountain — *see* Striking against, bottom when, falling into water, specified NEC
      natural body W16.122 ☑
        causing drowning W16.121 ☑
      reservoir — *see* Striking against, bottom when, falling into water, specified NEC
      specified NEC W16.322 ☑
        causing drowning W16.321 ☑
      swimming pool W16.022 ☑
        causing drowning W16.021 ☑
  diving board (swimming-pool) W21.4 ☑
  object W22.8 ☑
    with
      drowning or submersion — *see* Drowning
      fall — *see* Fall, due to, bumping against, object
      caused by crowd or human stampede (with fall) W52
    furniture W22.03 ☑
    lamppost W22.02 ☑
    sports equipment W21.9 ☑
    stationary W22.09 ☑
      sports equipment W21.89 ☑
    wall W22.01 ☑
  person(s) W51 ☑
    with fall W03 ☑
      due to ice or snow W00.0 ☑
    as, or caused by, a crowd or human stampede (with fall) W52
    assault Y04.2 ☑
    homicide (attempt) Y04.2 ☑
  sports equipment W21.9 ☑
  wall (when) W22.01 ☑
    diving or jumping into water (in) W16.832 ☑
      causing drowning W16.831 ☑
      swimming pool W16.532 ☑
        causing drowning W16.531 ☑
    falling into water (in) W16.332 ☑
      causing drowning W16.331 ☑
      fountain — *see* Striking against, wall when, falling into water, specified NEC
      natural body W16.132 ☑
        causing drowning W16.131 ☑
      reservoir — *see* Striking against, wall when, falling into water, specified NEC
      specified NEC W16.332 ☑
        causing drowning W16.331 ☑
      swimming pool W16.032 ☑
        causing drowning W16.031 ☑
    swimming pool (when) W22.042 ☑
      causing drowning W22.041 ☑
      diving or jumping into water W16.532 ☑
        causing drowning W16.531 ☑
      falling into water W16.032 ☑
        causing drowning W16.031 ☑
Struck (accidentally) **by**
  airbag (automobile) W22.10 ☑
    driver side W22.11 ☑
    front passenger side W22.12 ☑
    specified NEC W22.19 ☑
  alligator W58.02 ☑
  animal (not being ridden) NEC W55.89 ☑
  avalanche — *see* Landslide
  ball (hit) (thrown) W21.00 ☑
    assault Y08.09 ☑
    baseball W21.03 ☑
    basketball W21.05 ☑
    football W21.01 ☑
    golf ball W21.04 ☑
    soccer W21.02 ☑
    softball W21.07 ☑
    specified NEC W21.09 ☑
    volleyball W21.06 ☑
  bat or racquet
    baseball bat W21.11 ☑
      assault Y08.02 ☑
    golf club W21.13 ☑
      assault Y08.09 ☑
    specified NEC W21.19 ☑
      assault Y08.09 ☑
    tennis racquet W21.12 ☑
      assault Y08.09 ☑
  bullet (*see also* Discharge, firearm by type)

Struck (accidentally) **by** — *continued*
  bullet (*see also* Discharge, firearm by type) — *continued*
    in war operations — *see* War operations
  crocodile W58.12 ☑
  dog W54.1 ☑
  flare, Very pistol — *see* Discharge, firearm NEC
  hailstones X39.8 ☑
  hockey (ice)
    field
      puck W21.221 ☑
      stick W21.211 ☑
    puck W21.220 ☑
    stick W21.210 ☑
      assault Y08.01 ☑
  landslide — *see* Landslide
  law-enforcement agent (on duty) — *see* Legal, intervention, manhandling
    with blunt object — *see* Legal, intervention, blunt object
  lightning T75.0 ☑
    causing fire — *see* Exposure, fire
  machine — *see* Contact, with, by type of machine
  mammal NEC W55.89 ☑
    marine W56.32 ☑
  marine animal W56.82 ☑
  missile
    firearm — *see* Discharge, firearm by type
    in war operations — *see* War operations, missile
  object W22.8 ☑
    blunt W22.8 ☑
      assault Y00 ☑
      suicide (attempt) X79 ☑
      undetermined whether accidental or intentional Y29 ☑
    falling W20.8 ☑
      from, in, on
        building W20.1 ☑
          burning (uncontrolled fire) X00.4 ☑
        cataclysmic
          earth surface movement NEC — *see* Landslide
          storm — *see* Forces of nature, cataclysmic storm
        cave-in W20.0 ☑
        earthquake X34 ☑
        machine (in operation) — *see* Contact, with, by type of machine
        structure W20.1 ☑
          burning X00.4 ☑
        transport vehicle (in motion) — *see* Accident, transport, by type of vehicle
        watercraft V93.49 ☑
          due to
            accident to craft V91.39 ☑
              powered craft V91.33 ☑
                ferry boat V91.31 ☑
                fishing boat V91.32 ☑
                jetskis V91.33 ☑
                liner V91.31 ☑
                merchant ship V91.30 ☑
                passenger ship V91.31 ☑
              unpowered craft V91.38 ☑
                canoe V91.35 ☑
                inflatable V91.36 ☑
                kayak V91.35 ☑
                sailboat V91.34 ☑
                surf-board V91.38 ☑
                windsurfer V91.38 ☑
            powered craft V93.43 ☑
              ferry boat V93.41 ☑
              fishing boat V93.42 ☑
              jetskis V93.43 ☑
              liner V93.41 ☑
              merchant ship V93.40 ☑
              passenger ship V93.41 ☑
            unpowered craft V93.48 ☑
              sailboat V93.44 ☑
              surf-board V93.48 ☑
              windsurfer V93.48 ☑
      moving NEC W20.8 ☑
    projected W20.8 ☑
      assault Y00 ☑
      in sports W21.9 ☑
        assault Y08.09 ☑
        ball W21.00 ☑

Struck (accidentally) **by** — *continued*
  object — *continued*
    projected — *continued*
      in sports — *continued*
        ball — *continued*
          baseball W21.03 ☑
          basketball W21.05 ☑
          football W21.01 ☑
          golf ball W21.04 ☑
          soccer W21.02 ☑
          softball W21.07 ☑
          specified NEC W21.09 ☑
          volleyball W21.06 ☑
        bat or racquet
          baseball bat W21.11 ☑
            assault Y08.02 ☑
          golf club W21.13 ☑
            assault Y08.09 ☑
          specified NEC W21.19 ☑
            assault Y08.09 ☑
          tennis racquet W21.12 ☑
            assault Y08.09 ☑
        hockey (ice)
          field
            puck W21.221 ☑
            stick W21.211 ☑
          puck W21.220 ☑
          stick W21.210 ☑
            assault Y08.01 ☑
        specified NEC W21.89 ☑
      set in motion by explosion — *see* Explosion
    thrown W20.8 ☑
      assault Y00 ☑
      in sports W21.9 ☑
        assault Y08.09 ☑
        ball W21.00 ☑
          baseball W21.03 ☑
          basketball W21.05 ☑
          football W21.01 ☑
          golf ball W21.04 ☑
          soccer W21.02 ☑
          soft ball W21.07 ☑
          specified NEC W21.09 ☑
          volleyball W21.06 ☑
        bat or racquet
          baseball bat W21.11 ☑
            assault Y08.02 ☑
          golf club W21.13 ☑
            assault Y08.09 ☑
          specified NEC W21.19 ☑
            assault Y08.09 ☑
          tennis racquet W21.12 ☑
            assault Y08.09 ☑
        hockey (ice)
          field
            puck W21.221 ☑
            stick W21.211 ☑
          puck W21.220 ☑
          stick W21.210 ☑
            assault Y08.01 ☑
        specified NEC W21.89 ☑
  other person(s) W50.0 ☑
    with
      blunt object W22.8 ☑
        intentional, homicide (attempt) Y00 ☑
        sports equipment W21.9 ☑
        undetermined whether accidental or intentional Y29 ☑
      fall W03 ☑
        due to ice or snow W00.0 ☑
    as, or caused by, a crowd or human stampede (with fall) W52 ☑
    assault Y04.2 ☑
    homicide (attempt) Y04.2 ☑
    in legal intervention
      injuring
        bystander Y35.812 ☑
        law enforcement personnel Y35.811 ☑
        suspect Y35.813 ☑
    sports equipment W21.9 ☑
  police (on duty) — *see* Legal, intervention, manhandling
    with blunt object — *see* Legal, intervention, blunt object
  sports equipment W21.9 ☑
    assault Y08.09 ☑

Struck (accidentally) **by** — *continued*
  sports equipment — *continued*
    ball W21.00 ☑
      baseball W21.03 ☑
      basketball W21.05 ☑
      football W21.01 ☑
      golf ball W21.04 ☑
      soccer W21.02 ☑
      soft ball W21.07 ☑
      specified NEC W21.09 ☑
      volleyball W21.06 ☑
    bat or racquet
      baseball bat W21.11 ☑
        assault Y08.02 ☑
      golf club W21.13 ☑
        assault Y08.09 ☑
      specified NEC W21.19 ☑
      tennis racquet W21.12 ☑
        assault Y08.09 ☑
    cleats (shoe) W21.31 ☑
    foot wear NEC W21.39 ☑
    football helmet W21.81 ☑
    hockey (ice)
      field
        puck W21.221 ☑
        stick W21.211 ☑
      puck W21.220 ☑
      stick W21.210 ☑
        assault Y08.01 ☑
    skate blades W21.32 ☑
    specified NEC W21.89 ☑
      assault Y08.09 ☑
  thunderbolt — *see* subcategory T75.0 ☑
    causing fire — *see* Exposure, fire
  transport vehicle NEC (*see also* Accident, transport) V09.9 ☑
    intentional, homicide (attempt) Y03.0 ☑
    motor NEC (*see also* Accident, transport) V09.20 ☑
      homicide Y03.0 ☑
  vehicle (transport) NEC — *see* Accident, transport, by type of vehicle
    stationary (falling from jack, hydraulic lift, ramp) W20.8 ☑

Stumbling
  without fall W18.40 ☑
    due to
      specified NEC W18.49 ☑
      stepping from one level to another W18.43 ☑
      stepping into hole or opening W18.42 ☑
      stepping on object W18.41 ☑
    over
      animal NEC W01.0 ☑
        with fall W18.09 ☑
      carpet, rug or (small) object W22.8 ☑
        with fall W18.09 ☑
      person W51 ☑
        with fall W03 ☑
          due to ice or snow W00.0 ☑
Submersion (accidental) — *see* Drowning
Suffocation (accidental) (by external means) (by pressure) (mechanical) (*see also* category) T71 ☑
  due to, by
    avalanche — *see* Landslide
    explosion — *see* Explosion
    fire — *see* Exposure, fire
    food, any type (aspiration) (ingestion) (inhalation) — *see* categories T17 and T18 ☑
    ignition — *see* Ignition
    landslide — *see* Landslide
    machine(ry) — *see* Contact, with, by type of machine
    vomitus (aspiration) (inhalation) T17.81- ☑
  in
    burning building X00.8 ☑
Suicide, suicidal (attempted) (by) X83.8 ☑
  blunt object X79 ☑
  burning, burns X76 ☑
    hot object X77.9 ☑
      fluid NEC X77.2 ☑
      household appliance X77.3 ☑
      specified NEC X77.8 ☑
      steam X77.0 ☑
      tap water X77.1 ☑
      vapors X77.0 ☑
  caustic substance — *see* Table of Drugs and Chemicals
  cold, extreme X83.2 ☑

Suicide, suicidal — *continued*
  collision of motor vehicle with
    motor vehicle X82.0 ☑
    specified NEC X82.8 ☑
    train X82.1 ☑
    tree X82.2 ☑
  crashing of aircraft X83.0 ☑
  cut (any part of body) X78.9 ☑
  cutting or piercing instrument X78.9 ☑
    dagger X78.2 ☑
    glass X78.0 ☑
    knife X78.1 ☑
    specified NEC X78.8 ☑
    sword X78.2 ☑
  drowning (in) X71.9 ☑
    bathtub X71.0 ☑
    natural water X71.3 ☑
    specified NEC X71.8 ☑
    swimming pool X71.1 ☑
      following fall X71.2 ☑
  electrocution X83.1 ☑
  explosive(s) (material) X75 ☑
  fire, flames X76 ☑
  firearm X74.9 ☑
    airgun X74.01 ☑
    handgun X72 ☑
    hunting rifle X73.1 ☑
    larger X73.9 ☑
      specified NEC X73.8 ☑
    machine gun X73.2 ☑
    shotgun X73.0 ☑
    specified NEC X74.8 ☑
  hanging X83.8 ☑
  hot object — *see* Suicide, burning, hot object
  jumping
    before moving object X81.8 ☑
      motor vehicle X81.0 ☑
      subway train X81.1 ☑
      train X81.1 ☑
    from high place X80 ☑
  late effect of attempt — *see* X71-X83 with 7th character S
  lying before moving object, train, vehicle X81.8 ☑
  poisoning — *see* Table of Drugs and Chemicals
  puncture (any part of body) — *see* Suicide, cutting or piercing instrument
  scald — *see* Suicide, burning, hot object
  sequelae of attempt — *see* X71-X83 with 7th character S
  sharp object (any) — *see* Suicide, cutting or piercing instrument
  shooting — *see* Suicide, firearm
  specified means NEC X83.8 ☑
  stab (any part of body) — *see* Suicide, cutting or piercing instrument
  steam, hot vapors X77.0 ☑
  strangulation X83.8 ☑
  submersion — *see* Suicide, drowning
  suffocation X83.8 ☑
  wound NEC X83.8 ☑
Sunstroke X32 ☑
Supersonic waves (causing injury) W42.0 ☑
Surgical procedure, complication of (delayed or as an abnormal reaction without mention of misadventure) (*see also* Complication of or following, by type of procedure)
  due to or as a result of misadventure — *see* Misadventure
Swallowed, swallowing
  foreign body — *see* Foreign body, alimentary canal
  poison — *see* Table of Drugs and Chemicals
  substance
    caustic or corrosive — *see* Table of Drugs and Chemicals
    poisonous — *see* Table of Drugs and Chemicals

T

Tackle in sport W03 ☑
Terrorism (involving) Y38.80 ☑
  biological weapons Y38.6X- ☑
  chemical weapons Y38.7X- ☑
  conflagration Y38.3X- ☑
  explosion Y38.2X- ☑
    destruction of aircraft Y38.1X- ☑
    marine weapons Y38.0X- ☑

Terrorism — *continued*
fire Y38.3X- ☑
firearms Y38.4X- ☑
hot substances Y38.5X- ☑
nuclear weapons Y38.5X- ☑
specified method NEC Y38.89- ☑
Thirst X58 ☑
Threat to breathing
aspiration — *see* Aspiration
due to cave-in, falling earth or substance NEC T71 ☑
Thrown (accidentally)
against part (any) of or object in transport vehicle (in motion) NEC (*see also* Accident, transport)
from
high place, homicide (attempt) Y01 ☑
machinery — *see* Contact, with, by type of machine
transport vehicle NEC (*see also* Accident, transport) V89.9 ☑
off — *see* Thrown, from
Thunderbolt — *see* subcategory T75.0 ☑
causing fire — *see* Exposure, fire
Tidal wave (any injury) NEC — *see* Forces of nature, tidal wave
Took
overdose (drug) — *see* Table of Drugs and Chemicals
poison — *see* Table of Drugs and Chemicals
Tornado (any injury) X37.1 ☑
Torrential rain (any injury) X37.8 ☑
Torture X58 ☑
Trampled by animal NEC W55.89 ☑
Trapped (accidentally)
between objects (moving) (stationary and moving) — *see* Caught
by part (any) of
motorcycle V29.88 ☑
pedal cycle V19.88 ☑
transport vehicle NEC (*see also* Accident, transport) V89.9 ☑
Travel (effects) (sickness) T75.3 ☑
Tree falling on or hitting (accidentally) (person) W20.8 ☑
Tripping
without fall W18.40 ☑
due to
specified NEC W18.49 ☑
stepping from one level to another W18.43 ☑
stepping into hole or opening W18.42 ☑
stepping on object W18.41 ☑
over
animal W01.0 ☑
with fall W01.0 ☑
carpet, rug or (small) object W22.8 ☑
with fall W18.09 ☑
person W51 ☑
with fall W03 ☑
due to ice or snow W00.0 ☑
Twisted by person(s) (accidentally) W50.2 ☑
with intent to injure or kill Y04.0 ☑
as, or caused by, a crowd or human stampede (with fall) W52 ☑
assault Y04.0 ☑
homicide (attempt) Y04.0 ☑
in
fight Y04.0 ☑
legal intervention — *see* Legal, intervention, manhandling
Twisting, excessive — *see* category Y93 ☑

U

Underdosing of necessary drugs, medicaments or biological substances Y63.6
Undetermined intent (contact) (exposure)
automobile collision Y32 ☑
blunt object Y29 ☑
drowning (submersion) (in) Y21.9 ☑
bathtub Y21.0 ☑
after fall Y21.1 ☑
natural water (lake) (ocean) (pond) (river) (stream) Y21.4 ☑
specified place NEC Y21.8 ☑
swimming pool Y21.2 ☑
after fall Y21.3 ☑
explosive material Y25 ☑
fall, jump or push from high place Y30 ☑
falling, lying or running before moving object Y31 ☑

Undetermined intent — *continued*
fire Y26 ☑
firearm discharge Y24.9 ☑
airgun (BB) (pellet) Y24.0 ☑
handgun (pistol) (revolver) Y22 ☑
hunting rifle Y23.1 ☑
larger Y23.9 ☑
hunting rifle Y23.1 ☑
machine gun Y23.3 ☑
military Y23.2 ☑
shotgun Y23.0 ☑
specified type NEC Y23.8 ☑
machine gun Y23.3 ☑
military Y23.2 ☑
shotgun Y23.0 ☑
specified type NEC Y24.8 ☑
Very pistol Y24.8 ☑
hot object Y27.9 ☑
fluid Y27.2 ☑
household appliance Y27.3 ☑
specified object NEC Y27.8 ☑
steam Y27.0 ☑
tap water Y27.1 ☑
vapor Y27.0 ☑
jump, fall or push from high place Y30 ☑
lying, falling or running before moving object Y31 ☑
motor vehicle crash Y32 ☑
push, fall or jump from high place Y30 ☑
running, falling or lying before moving object Y31 ☑
sharp object Y28.9 ☑
dagger Y28.2 ☑
glass Y28.0 ☑
knife Y28.1 ☑
specified object NEC Y28.8 ☑
sword Y28.2 ☑
smoke Y26 ☑
specified event NEC Y33 ☑

V

Vibration (causing injury) W49.9 ☑
Victim (of)
avalanche — *see* Landslide
earth movements NEC — *see* Forces of nature, earth movement
earthquake X34 ☑
flood — *see* Flood
landslide — *see* Landslide
lightning — *see* subcategory T75.0 ☑
causing fire — *see* Exposure, fire
storm (cataclysmic) NEC — *see* Forces of nature, cataclysmic storm
volcanic eruption X35 ☑
Volcanic eruption (any injury) X35 ☑
Vomitus, gastric contents in air passages (with asphyxia, obstruction or suffocation) T17.81- ☑

W

Walked into stationary object (any) W22.09 ☑
furniture W22.03 ☑
lamppost W22.02 ☑
wall W22.01 ☑
War operations (injuries to military personnel and civilians during war, civil insurrection and peacekeeping missions) (by) (from) (involving) Y36.90 ☑
after cessation of hostilities Y36.89- ☑
explosion (of)
bomb placed during war operations Y36.82- ☑
mine placed during war operations Y36.81- ☑
specified NEC Y36.88- ☑
air blast Y36.20- ☑
aircraft
destruction — *see* War operations, destruction of aircraft
airway restriction — *see* War operations, restriction of airways
asphyxiation — *see* War operations, restriction of airways
biological weapons Y36.6X- ☑
blast Y36.20- ☑
blast fragments Y36.20- ☑
blast wave Y36.20- ☑
blast wind Y36.20- ☑
bomb Y36.20- ☑

War operations — *continued*
bomb — *continued*
dirty Y36.50- ☑
gasoline Y36.31- ☑
incendiary Y36.31- ☑
petrol Y36.31- ☑
bullet Y36.43- ☑
incendiary Y36.32- ☑
rubber Y36.41- ☑
chemical weapons Y36.7X- ☑
combat
hand to hand (unarmed) combat Y36.44- ☑
using blunt or piercing object Y36.45- ☑
conflagration — *see* War operations, fire
conventional warfare NEC Y36.49- ☑
depth-charge Y36.01- ☑
destruction of aircraft Y36.10- ☑
due to
air to air missile Y36.11- ☑
collision with other aircraft Y36.12- ☑
detonation (accidental) of onboard munitions and explosives Y36.14- ☑
enemy fire or explosives Y36.11- ☑
explosive placed on aircraft Y36.11- ☑
onboard fire Y36.13- ☑
rocket propelled grenade [RPG] Y36.11- ☑
small arms fire Y36.11- ☑
surface to air missile Y36.11- ☑
specified NEC Y36.19- ☑
detonation (accidental) of
onboard marine weapons Y36.05- ☑
own munitions or munitions launch device Y36.24- ☑
dirty bomb Y36.50- ☑
explosion (of) Y36.20- ☑
aerial bomb Y36.21- ☑
after cessation of hostilities
bomb placed during war operations Y36.82- ☑
mine placed during war operations Y36.81- ☑
bomb NOS (*see also* War operations, bomb(s)) Y36.20- ☑
fragments Y36.20- ☑
grenade Y36.29- ☑
guided missile Y36.22- ☑
improvised explosive device [IED] (person-borne) (roadside) (vehicle-borne) Y36.23- ☑
land mine Y36.29- ☑
marine mine (at sea) (in harbor) Y36.02- ☑
marine weapon Y36.00- ☑
specified NEC Y36.09- ☑
own munitions or munitions launch device (accidental) Y36.24- ☑
sea-based artillery shell Y36.03- ☑
specified NEC Y36.29- ☑
torpedo Y36.04- ☑
fire Y36.30- ☑
specified NEC Y36.39- ☑
firearms
discharge Y36.43- ☑
pellets Y36.42- ☑
flamethrower Y36.33- ☑
fragments (from) (of)
improvised explosive device [IED] (person-borne) (roadside) (vehicle-borne) Y36.26- ☑
munitions Y36.25- ☑
specified NEC Y36.29- ☑
weapons Y36.27- ☑
friendly fire Y36.92 ☑
hand to hand (unarmed) combat Y36.44- ☑
hot substances — *see* War operations, fire
incendiary bullet Y36.32- ☑
nuclear weapon (effects of) Y36.50- ☑
acute radiation exposure Y36.54- ☑
blast pressure Y36.51- ☑
direct blast Y36.51- ☑
direct heat Y36.53- ☑
fallout exposure Y36.54- ☑
fireball Y36.53- ☑
indirect blast (struck or crushed by blast debris) (being thrown by blast) Y36.52- ☑
ionizing radiation (immediate exposure) Y36.54- ☑
nuclear radiation Y36.54- ☑
radiation
ionizing (immediate exposure) Y36.54- ☑
nuclear Y36.54- ☑
thermal Y36.53- ☑

☑ **Additional Character Required** — Refer to the Tabular List for Character Selection
▽ **Subterms under main terms may continue to next column or page**

War operations — *continued*
  nuclear weapon — *continued*
    secondary effects Y36.54- ☑
    specified NEC Y36.59- ☑
    thermal radiation Y36.53- ☑
  restriction of air (airway)
    intentional Y36.46- ☑
    unintentional Y36.47- ☑
  rubber bullets Y36.41- ☑
  shrapnel NOS Y36.29- ☑
  suffocation — *see* War operations, restriction of air-
    ways
  unconventional warfare NEC Y36.7X- ☑
  underwater blast NOS Y36.00- ☑
  warfare
    conventional NEC Y36.49- ☑
    unconventional NEC Y36.7X- ☑
  weapon of mass destruction [WMD] Y36.91 ☑
  weapons
    biological weapons Y36.6X- ☑

War operations — *continued*
  weapons — *continued*
    chemical Y36.7X- ☑
    nuclear (effects of) Y36.50- ☑
      acute radiation exposure Y36.54- ☑
      blast pressure Y36.51- ☑
      direct blast Y36.51- ☑
      direct heat Y36.53- ☑
      fallout exposure Y36.54- ☑
      fireball Y36.53- ☑
      indirect blast (struck or crushed by blast debris)
        (being thrown by blast) Y36.52- ☑
      radiation
        ionizing (immediate exposure) Y36.54- ☑
        nuclear Y36.54- ☑
        thermal Y36.53- ☑
      secondary effects Y36.54- ☑
      specified NEC Y36.59- ☑
    of mass destruction [WMD] Y36.91 ☑

Washed
  away by flood — *see* Flood
  off road by storm (transport vehicle) — *see* Forces of
    nature, cataclysmic storm
Weather exposure NEC — *see* Forces of nature
Weightlessness (causing injury) (effects of) (in spacecraft,
  real or simulated) X52 ☑
Work related condition Y99.0
Wound (accidental) NEC (*see also* Injury) X58 ☑
  battle (*see also* War operations) Y36.90 ☑
  gunshot — *see* Discharge, firearm by type
Wreck transport vehicle NEC (*see also* Accident, transport) V89.9 ☑
Wrong
  device implanted into correct surgical site Y65.51
  fluid in infusion Y65.1
  patient, procedure performed on Y65.52
  procedure (operation) on correct patient Y65.51

ICD-10-CM Tabular List of Diseases and Injuries

Chapter 1. Certain Infectious and Parasitic Diseases (A00-B99)

INCLUDES diseases generally recognized as communicable or transmissible

Use additional code to identify resistance to antimicrobial drugs (Z16.-)

EXCLUDES 1 certain localized infections—see body system-related chapters

EXCLUDES 2 carrier or suspected carrier of infectious disease (Z22.-)

infectious and parasitic diseases specific to the perinatal period (P35-P39)

infectious and parasitic diseases complicating pregnancy, childbirth and the puerperium (O98.-)

influenza and other acute respiratory infections (J00-J22)

This chapter contains the following blocks:

A00-A09	Intestinal infectious diseases
A15-A19	Tuberculosis
A20-A28	Certain zoonotic bacterial diseases
A30-A49	Other bacterial diseases
A50-A64	Infections with a predominantly sexual mode of transmission
A65-A69	Other spirochetal diseases
A70-A74	Other diseases caused by chlamydiae
A75-A79	Rickettsioses
A80-A89	Viral infections of the central nervous system
A90-A99	Arthropod-borne viral fevers and viral hemorrhagic fevers
B00-B09	Viral infections characterized by skin and mucous membrane lesions
B10	Other human herpesviruses
B15-B19	Viral hepatitis
B20	Human immunodeficiency virus [HIV] disease
B25-B34	Other viral diseases
B35-B49	Mycoses
B50-B64	Protozoal diseases
B65-B83	Helminthiases
B85-B89	Pediculosis, acariasis and other infestations
B90-B94	Sequelae of infectious and parasitic diseases
B95-B97	Bacterial and viral infectious agents
B99	Other infectious diseases

Intestinal Infectious Diseases (A00-A09)

✓4ᵗʰ A00 Cholera

A00.0 Cholera due to Vibrio cholerae 01, biovar cholerae
Classical cholera

A00.1 Cholera due to Vibrio cholerae 01, biovar eltor
Cholera eltor

A00.9 Cholera, unspecified

✓4ᵗʰ A01 Typhoid and paratyphoid fevers

✓5ᵗʰ A01.0 Typhoid fever
Infection due to Salmonella typhi

A01.00 Typhoid fever, unspecified

A01.01 Typhoid meningitis

A01.02 Typhoid fever with heart involvement
Typhoid endocarditis
Typhoid myocarditis

A01.03 Typhoid pneumonia

A01.04 Typhoid arthritis

A01.05 Typhoid osteomyelitis

A01.09 Typhoid fever with other complications

A01.1 Paratyphoid fever A

A01.2 Paratyphoid fever B

A01.3 Paratyphoid fever C

A01.4 Paratyphoid fever, unspecified
Infection due to Salmonella paratyphi NOS

✓4ᵗʰ A02 Other salmonella infections

INCLUDES infection or foodborne intoxication due to any Salmonella species other than S. typhi and S. paratyphi

A02.0 Salmonella enteritis
Salmonellosis

A02.1 Salmonella sepsis

✓5ᵗʰ A02.2 Localized salmonella infections

A02.20 Localized salmonella infection, unspecified

A02.21 Salmonella meningitis

A02.22 Salmonella pneumonia

A02.23 Salmonella arthritis

A02.24 Salmonella osteomyelitis

A02.25 Salmonella pyelonephritis
Salmonella tubulo-interstitial nephropathy

A02.29 Salmonella with other localized infection

A02.8 Other specified salmonella infections

A02.9 Salmonella infection, unspecified

✓4ᵗʰ A03 Shigellosis

A03.0 Shigellosis due to Shigella dysenteriae
Group A shigellosis [Shiga-Kruse dysentery]

A03.1 Shigellosis due to Shigella flexneri
Group B shigellosis

A03.2 Shigellosis due to Shigella boydii
Group C shigellosis

A03.3 Shigellosis due to Shigella sonnei
Group D shigellosis

A03.8 Other shigellosis

A03.9 Shigellosis, unspecified
Bacillary dysentery NOS

✓4ᵗʰ A04 Other bacterial intestinal infections

EXCLUDES 1 bacterial foodborne intoxications, NEC (A05.-)
tuberculous enteritis (A18.32)

A04.0 Enteropathogenic Escherichia coli infection

A04.1 Enterotoxigenic Escherichia coli infection

A04.2 Enteroinvasive Escherichia coli infection

A04.3 Enterohemorrhagic Escherichia coli infection

A04.4 Other intestinal Escherichia coli infections
Escherichia coli enteritis NOS

A04.5 Campylobacter enteritis

A04.6 Enteritis due to Yersinia enterocolitica
EXCLUDES 1 extraintestinal yersiniosis (A28.2)

A04.7 Enterocolitis due to Clostridium difficile
Foodborne intoxication by Clostridium difficile
Pseudomembraneous colitis

A04.8 Other specified bacterial intestinal infections

A04.9 Bacterial intestinal infection, unspecified
Bacterial enteritis NOS

✓4ᵗʰ A05 Other bacterial foodborne intoxications, not elsewhere classified

EXCLUDES 1 Clostridium difficile foodborne intoxication and infection (A04.7)
Escherichia coli infection (A04.0-A04.4)
listeriosis (A32.-)
salmonella foodborne intoxication and infection (A02.-)
toxic effect of noxious foodstuffs (T61-T62)

A05.0 Foodborne staphylococcal intoxication

A05.1 Botulism food poisoning
Botulism NOS
Classical foodborne intoxication due to Clostridium botulinum
EXCLUDES 1 infant botulism (A48.51)
wound botulism (A48.52)

A05.2 Foodborne Clostridium perfringens [Clostridium welchii] intoxication
Enteritis necroticans
Pig-bel

A05.3 Foodborne Vibrio parahaemolyticus intoxication

A05.4 Foodborne Bacillus cereus intoxication

A05.5 Foodborne Vibrio vulnificus intoxication

A05.8 Other specified bacterial foodborne intoxications

A05.9 Bacterial foodborne intoxication, unspecified

✓4ᵗʰ A06 Amebiasis

INCLUDES infection due to Entamoeba histolytica
EXCLUDES 1 other protozoal intestinal diseases (A07.-)
EXCLUDES 2 acanthamebiasis (B60.1-)
Naegleriasis (B60.2)

A06.0 Acute amebic dysentery
Acute amebiasis
Intestinal amebiasis NOS

A06.1 Chronic intestinal amebiasis

A06.2 Amebic nondysenteric colitis

A06.3 Ameboma of intestine
Ameboma NOS

A06.4 Amebic liver abscess
Hepatic amebiasis

A06.5 Amebic lung abscess
Amebic abscess of lung (and liver)

A06.6 Amebic brain abscess
Amebic abscess of brain (and liver) (and lung)

✓ Additional Character Required ✓7ᵗʰ Xtension Alert Unspecified Dx Other Specified Dx Manifestation ▶◀ Revised Text ● New Code ▲ Revised Code Title

ICD-10-CM Draft (2015)

423

Certain Infectious and Parasitic Diseases

A06.7–A18.12

A06.7   Cutaneous **ambeiasis**

✓5ᵗʰ   A06.8   **Amebic infection of other sites**

    A06.81   **Amebic** cystitis

    A06.82   Other amebic genitourinary infections
       Amebic balanitis
       Amebic vesiculitis
       Amebic vulvovaginitis

    A06.89   **Other amebic infections**
       Amebic appendicitis
       Amebic splenic abscess

A06.9   **Amebiasis, unspecified**

✓4ᵗʰ   A07   **Other protozoal intestinal diseases**

    A07.0   **Balantidiasis**
       Balantidial dysentery

    A07.1   **Giardiasis [lambliasis]**

    A07.2   **Cryptosporidiosis**

    A07.3   **Isosporiasis**
       Infection due to Isospora belli and Isospora hominis
       Intestinal coccidiosis
       Isosporosis

    A07.4   **Cyclosporiasis**

    A07.8   Other specified protozoal intestinal diseases
       Intestinal microsporidiosis
       Intestinal trichomoniasis
       Sarcocystosis
       Sarcosporidiosis

    A07.9   **Protozoal intestinal disease, unspecified**
       Flagellate diarrhea   Protozoal diarrhea
       Protozoal colitis   Protozoal dysentery

✓4ᵗʰ   A08   **Viral and other specified intestinal infections**
      EXCLUDES1   *influenza with involvement of gastrointestinal tract (J09.X3, J10.2, J11.2)*

    A08.0   **Rotaviral enteritis**

✓5ᵗʰ   A08.1   **Acute gastroenteropathy due to Norwalk agent and other small round viruses**

    A08.11   **Acute gastroenteropathy due to** Norwalk agent
       Acute gastroenteropathy due to Norovirus
       Acute gastroenteropathy due to Norwalk-like agent

    A08.19   **Acute gastroenteropathy due to** other small round viruses
       Acute gastroenteropathy due to small round virus [SRV] NOS

    A08.2   **Adenoviral enteritis**

✓5ᵗʰ   A08.3   Other viral enteritis

    A08.31   **Calicivirus enteritis**

    A08.32   **Astrovirus enteritis**

    A08.39   **Other viral enteritis**
       Coxsackie virus enteritis
       Echovirus enteritis
       Enterovirus enteritis NEC
       Torovirus enteritis

    A08.4   **Viral intestinal infection, unspecified**
       Viral enteritis NOS
       Viral gastroenteritis NOS
       Viral gastroenteropathy NOS

    A08.8   Other specified intestinal infections

A09   **Infectious gastroenteritis and colitis, unspecified**
       Infectious colitis NOS
       Infectious enteritis NOS
       Infectious gastroenteritis NOS
      EXCLUDES1   *colitis NOS (K52.9)*
           diarrhea NOS (R19.7)
           enteritis NOS (K52.9)
           gastroenteritis NOS (K52.9)
           noninfective gastroenteritis and colitis, unspecified (K52.9)

Tuberculosis (A15-A19)

INCLUDES   infections due to Mycobacterium tuberculosis and Mycobacterium bovis

EXCLUDES1   *congenital tuberculosis (P37.0)*
      nonspecific reaction to test for tuberculosis without active tuberculosis (R76.1-)
      pneumoconiosis associated with tuberculosis, any type in A15 (J65)
      positive PPD (R76.11)
      positive tuberculin skin test without active tuberculosis (R76.11)
      sequelae of tuberculosis (B90.-)
      silicotuberculosis (J65)

✓4ᵗʰ   A15   **Respiratory** tuberculosis

    A15.0   **Tuberculosis of lung**
       Tuberculous bronchiectasis
       Tuberculous fibrosis of lung
       Tuberculous pneumonia
       Tuberculous pneumothorax

    A15.4   **Tuberculosis of intrathoracic lymph nodes**
       Tuberculosis of hilar lymph nodes
       Tuberculosis of mediastinal lymph nodes
       Tuberculosis of tracheobronchial lymph nodes
      EXCLUDES1   *tuberculosis specified as primary (A15.7)*

    A15.5   **Tuberculosis of larynx, trachea and bronchus**
       Tuberculosis of bronchus
       Tuberculosis of glottis
       Tuberculosis of larynx
       Tuberculosis of trachea

    A15.6   **Tuberculous pleurisy**
       Tuberculosis of pleura Tuberculous empyema
      EXCLUDES1   *primary respiratory tuberculosis (A15.7)*

    A15.7   **Primary respiratory tuberculosis**

    A15.8   **Other respiratory tuberculosis**
       Mediastinal tuberculosis
       Nasopharyngeal tuberculosis
       Tuberculosis of nose
       Tuberculosis of sinus [any nasal]

    A15.9   **Respiratory tuberculosis unspecified**

✓4ᵗʰ   A17   **Tuberculosis of nervous system**

    A17.0   **Tuberculous meningitis**
       Tuberculosis of meninges (cerebral)(spinal)
       Tuberculous leptomeningitis
      EXCLUDES1   *tuberculous meningoencephalitis (A17.82)*

    A17.1   Meningeal tuberculoma
       Tuberculoma of meninges (cerebral) (spinal)
      EXCLUDES2   *tuberculoma of brain and spinal cord (A17.81)*

✓5ᵗʰ   A17.8   Other tuberculosis of nervous system

    A17.81   **Tuberculoma of brain and spinal cord**
       Tuberculous abscess of brain and spinal cord

    A17.82   **Tuberculous meningoencephalitis**
       Tuberculous myelitis

    A17.83   **Tuberculous neuritis**
       Tuberculous mononeuropathy

    A17.89   **Other tuberculosis of nervous system**
       Tuberculous polyneuropathy

    A17.9   **Tuberculosis of nervous system, unspecified**

✓4ᵗʰ   A18   **Tuberculosis of other organs**

✓5ᵗʰ   A18.0   **Tuberculosis of bones and joints**

    A18.01   **Tuberculosis of spine**
       Pott's disease or curvature of spine
       Tuberculous arthritis
       Tuberculous osteomyelitis of spine
       Tuberculous spondylitis

    A18.02   **Tuberculous arthritis of other joints**
       Tuberculosis of hip (joint)
       Tuberculosis of knee (joint)

    A18.03   **Tuberculosis of other bones**
       Tuberculous mastoiditis
       Tuberculous osteomyelitis

    A18.09   Other musculoskeletal tuberculosis
       Tuberculous myositis
       Tuberculous synovitis
       Tuberculous tenosynovitis

✓5ᵗʰ   A18.1   **Tuberculosis of genitourinary system**

    A18.10   **Tuberculosis of genitourinary system, unspecified**

    A18.11   **Tuberculosis of kidney and ureter**

    A18.12   **Tuberculosis of bladder**

EXCLUDES1 Not coded here   EXCLUDES2 Not included here   N Newborn Age: 0   P Pediatric Age: 0-17   M Maternity Age: 12-55   A Adult Age: 15-124

424   ICD-10-CM Draft (2015)

A18.13   **Tuberculosis of** other urinary organs
Tuberculous urethritis

A18.14   **Tuberculosis of** prostate   A♂

A18.15   **Tuberculosis of** other male genital organs   ♂

A18.16   **Tuberculosis of** cervix   ♀

A18.17   **Tuberculosis female** pelvic inflammatory disease   ♀
Tuberculous endometritis
Tuberculous oophoritis and salpingitis

A18.18   **Tuberculosis of** other female genital organs   ♀
Tuberculous ulceration of vulva

A18.2   **Tuberculous** peripheral lymphadenopathy
Tuberculous adenitis
   EXCLUDES 2   *tuberculosis of bronchial and mediastinal lymph nodes (A15.4)*
          tuberculosis of mesenteric and retroperitoneal lymph nodes (A18.39)
          tuberculous tracheobronchial adenopathy (A15.4)

✓5th **A18.3**   **Tuberculosis of** intestines, peritoneum and mesenteric glands

A18.31   **Tuberculous** peritonitis
Tuberculous ascites

A18.32   **Tuberculous** enteritis
Tuberculosis of anus and rectum
Tuberculosis of intestine (large) (small)

A18.39   Retroperitoneal **tuberculosis**
Tuberculosis of mesenteric glands
Tuberculosis of retroperitoneal (lymph glands)

A18.4   **Tuberculosis of** skin and subcutaneous tissue
Erythema induratum, tuberculous
Lupus excedens
Lupus vulgaris NOS
Lupus vulgaris of eyelid
Scrofuloderma
Tuberculosis of external ear
   EXCLUDES 2   *lupus erythematosus (L93.-)*
          lupus NOS (M32.9)
          systemic (M32.-)

✓5th **A18.5**   **Tuberculosis of** eye
   EXCLUDES 2   *lupus vulgaris of eyelid (A18.4)*

A18.50   Tuberculosis of eye, **unspecified**

A18.51   **Tuberculous** episcleritis

A18.52   **Tuberculous** keratitis
Tuberculous interstitial keratitis
Tuberculous keratoconjunctivitis (interstitial) (phlyctenular)

A18.53   **Tuberculous** chorioretinitis

A18.54   **Tuberculous** iridocyclitis

A18.59   Other tuberculosis of eye
Tuberculous conjunctivitis

A18.6   **Tuberculosis of (inner) (middle)** ear
Tuberculous otitis media
   EXCLUDES 2   *tuberculosis of external ear (A18.4)*
          tuberculous mastoiditis (A18.03)

A18.7   **Tuberculosis of** adrenal glands
Tuberculous Addison's disease

✓5th **A18.8**   **Tuberculosis of** other specified organs

A18.81   **Tuberculosis of** thyroid gland

A18.82   **Tuberculosis of** other endocrine glands
Tuberculosis of pituitary gland
Tuberculosis of thymus gland

A18.83   **Tuberculosis of** digestive tract organs**, not elsewhere classified**
   EXCLUDES 1   *tuberculosis of intestine (A18.32)*

A18.84   **Tuberculosis of** heart
Tuberculous cardiomyopathy
Tuberculous endocarditis
Tuberculous myocarditis
Tuberculous pericarditis

A18.85   **Tuberculosis of** spleen

A18.89   Tuberculosis of other sites
Tuberculosis of muscle
Tuberculous cerebral arteritis

✓4th **A19**   **Miliary tuberculosis**
   INCLUDES   disseminated tuberculosis
          generalized tuberculosis
          tuberculous polyserositis

A19.0   **Acute miliary tuberculosis of a** single specified site

A19.1   **Acute miliary tuberculosis of** multiple sites

A19.2   **Acute miliary tuberculosis, unspecified**

A19.8   Other miliary tuberculosis

A19.9   **Miliary tuberculosis, unspecified**

Certain zoonotic bacterial diseases (A20-A28)

✓4th **A20**   **Plague**
   INCLUDES   infection due to Yersinia pestis

A20.0   Bubonic **plague**

A20.1   Cellulocutaneous **plague**

A20.2   Pneumonic **plague**

A20.3   **Plague** meningitis

A20.7   Septicemic **plague**

A20.8   Other forms of plague
Abortive plague
Asymptomatic plague
Pestis minor

A20.9   **Plague, unspecified**

✓4th **A21**   **Tularemia**
   INCLUDES   deer-fly fever
          infection due to Francisella tularensis
          rabbit fever

A21.0   Ulceroglandular **tularemia**

A21.1   Oculoglandular **tularemia**
Ophthalmic tularemia

A21.2   Pulmonary **tularemia**

A21.3   Gastrointestinal **tularemia**
Abdominal tularemia

A21.7   Generalized **tularemia**

A21.8   Other forms of tularemia

A21.9   Tularemia, **unspecified**

✓4th **A22**   **Anthrax**
   INCLUDES   infection due to Bacillus anthracis

A22.0   Cutaneous **anthrax**
Malignant carbuncle
Malignant pustule

A22.1   Pulmonary **anthrax**
Inhalation anthrax
Ragpicker's disease
Woolsorter's disease

A22.2   Gastrointestinal **anthrax**

A22.7   **Anthrax** sepsis

A22.8   Other forms of anthrax
Anthrax meningitis

A22.9   **Anthrax, unspecified**

✓4th **A23**   **Brucellosis**
Malta fever
Mediterranean fever
Undulant fever

A23.0   **Brucellosis due to** Brucella melitensis

A23.1   **Brucellosis due to** Brucella abortus

A23.2   **Brucellosis due to** Brucella suis

A23.3   **Brucellosis due to** Brucella canis

A23.8   Other brucellosis

A23.9   **Brucellosis, unspecified**

✓4th **A24**   **Glanders and melioidosis**

A24.0   Glanders
Infection due to Pseudomonas mallei
Malleus

A24.1   Acute and fulminating **melioidosis**
Melioidosis pneumonia
Melioidosis sepsis

A24.2   Subacute and chronic **melioidosis**

A24.3   Other melioidosis

A24.9   Melioidosis, unspecified
Infection due to Pseudomonas pseudomallei NOS
Whitmore's disease

✓4th **A25**   **Rat-bite fevers**

A25.0   Spirillosis
Sodoku

A25.1   Streptobacillosis
Epidemic arthritic erythema
Haverhill fever
Streptobacillary rat-bite fever

A25.9   Rat-bite fever, unspecified

☑ Additional Character Required   ✓x.7th Xtension Alert   Unspecified Dx   Other Specified Dx   Manifestation   ▶◀ Revised Text   ● New Code   ▲ Revised Code Title

ICD-10-CM Draft (2015)   **425**

Certain Infectious and Parasitic Diseases

A26–A39.53

✓4ᵗʰ **A26 Erysipeloid**

A26.0 Cutaneous **erysipeloid**
    Erythema migrans

A26.7 Erysipelothrix sepsis

A26.8 Other forms of erysipeloid

A26.9 Erysipeloid, unspecified

✓4ᵗʰ **A27 Leptospirosis**

A27.0 Leptospirosis icterohemorrhagica
    Leptospiral or spirochetal jaundice (hemorrhagic)
    Weil's disease

✓5ᵗʰ **A27.8** Other forms of leptospirosis

A27.81 Aseptic meningitis in leptospirosis

A27.89 Other forms of leptospirosis

A27.9 Leptospirosis, unspecified

✓4ᵗʰ **A28 Other zoonotic bacterial diseases, not elsewhere classified**

A28.0 Pasteurellosis

A28.1 Cat-scratch disease
    Cat-scratch fever

A28.2 Extraintestinal yersiniosis
    EXCLUDES 1   enteritis due to Yersinia enterocolitica (A04.6)
               plague (A20.-)

A28.8 Other specified zoonotic bacterial diseases, not elsewhere classified

A28.9 Zoonotic bacterial disease, unspecified

Other bacterial diseases (A30-A49)

✓4ᵗʰ **A30 Leprosy [Hansen's disease]**
    INCLUDES   infection due to Mycobacterium leprae
    EXCLUDES 1   sequelae of leprosy (B92)

A30.0 Indeterminate **leprosy**
    I leprosy

A30.1 Tuberculoid **leprosy**
    TT leprosy

A30.2 Borderline tuberculoid **leprosy**
    BT leprosy

A30.3 Borderline **leprosy**
    BB leprosy

A30.4 Borderline lepromatous **leprosy**
    BL leprosy

A30.5 Lepromatous **leprosy**
    LL leprosy

A30.8 Other forms of leprosy

A30.9 Leprosy, unspecified

✓4ᵗʰ **A31 Infection due to other mycobacteria**
    EXCLUDES 2   leprosy (A30.-)
               tuberculosis (A15-A19)

A31.0 Pulmonary **mycobacterial infection**
    Infection due to Mycobacterium avium
    Infection due to Mycobacterium intracellulare [Battey bacillus]
    Infection due to Mycobacterium kansasii

A31.1 Cutaneous **mycobacterial infection**
    Buruli ulcer
    Infection due to Mycobacterium marinum
    Infection due to Mycobacterium ulcerans

A31.2 Disseminated mycobacterium avium-intracellulare complex (DMAC)
    MAC sepsis

A31.8 Other mycobacterial infections

A31.9 Mycobacterial infection, unspecified
    Atypical mycobacterial infection NOS
    Mycobacteriosis NOS

✓4ᵗʰ **A32 Listeriosis**
    INCLUDES   listerial foodborne infection
    EXCLUDES 1   neonatal (disseminated) listeriosis (P37.2)

A32.0 Cutaneous **listeriosis**

✓5ᵗʰ **A32.1** Listerial meningitis and meningoencephalitis

A32.11 Listerial meningitis

A32.12 Listerial meningoencephalitis

A32.7 Listerial sepsis

✓5ᵗʰ **A32.8** Other forms of listeriosis

A32.81 Oculoglandular **listeriosis**

A32.82 Listerial endocarditis

A32.89 Other forms of listeriosis
    Listerial cerebral arteritis

A32.9 Listeriosis, unspecified

A33 Tetanus neonatorum   N

A34 Obstetrical tetanus   M♀

A35 Other tetanus
    Tetanus NOS
    EXCLUDES 1   obstetrical tetanus (A34)
               tetanus neonatorum (A33)

✓4ᵗʰ **A36 Diphtheria**

A36.0 Pharyngeal **diphtheria**
    Diphtheritic membranous angina
    Tonsillar diphtheria

A36.1 Nasopharyngeal **diphtheria**

A36.2 Laryngeal **diphtheria**
    Diphtheritic laryngotracheitis

A36.3 Cutaneous **diphtheria**
    EXCLUDES 2   erythrasma (L08.1)

✓5ᵗʰ **A36.8** Other **diphtheria**

A36.81 Diphtheritic cardiomyopathy
    Diphtheritic myocarditis

A36.82 Diphtheritic radiculomyelitis

A36.83 Diphtheritic polyneuritis

A36.84 Diphtheritic tubulo-interstitial nephropathy

A36.85 Diphtheritic cystitis

A36.86 Diphtheritic conjunctivitis

A36.89 Other diphtheritic complications
    Diphtheritic peritonitis

A36.9 Diphtheria, unspecified

✓4ᵗʰ **A37 Whooping cough**

✓5ᵗʰ **A37.0** Whooping cough due to Bordetella pertussis

A37.00 Whooping cough due to Bordetella pertussis without pneumonia

A37.01 Whooping cough due to Bordetella pertussis with pneumonia

✓5ᵗʰ **A37.1** Whooping cough due to Bordetella parapertussis

A37.10 Whooping cough due to Bordetella parapertussis without pneumonia

A37.11 Whooping cough due to Bordetella parapertussis with pneumonia

✓5ᵗʰ **A37.8** Whooping cough due to other Bordetella species

A37.80 Whooping cough due to other Bordetella species without pneumonia

A37.81 Whooping cough due to other Bordetella species with pneumonia

✓5ᵗʰ **A37.9** Whooping cough, unspecified species

A37.90 Whooping cough, unspecified species without pneumonia

A37.91 Whooping cough, unspecified species with pneumonia

✓4ᵗʰ **A38 Scarlet fever**
    INCLUDES   scarlatina
    EXCLUDES 2   streptococcal sore throat (J02.0)

A38.0 Scarlet fever with otitis media

A38.1 Scarlet fever with myocarditis

A38.8 Scarlet fever with other complications

A38.9 Scarlet fever, uncomplicated
    Scarlet fever, NOS

✓4ᵗʰ **A39 Meningococcal infection**

A39.0 Meningococcal meningitis

A39.1 Waterhouse-Friderichsen syndrome
    Meningococcal hemorrhagic adrenalitis
    Meningococcic adrenal syndrome

A39.2 Acute meningococcemia

A39.3 Chronic meningococcemia

A39.4 Meningococcemia, unspecified

✓5ᵗʰ **A39.5** Meningococcal heart disease

A39.50 Meningococcal carditis, unspecified

A39.51 Meningococcal endocarditis

A39.52 Meningococcal myocarditis

A39.53 Meningococcal pericarditis

EXCLUDES 1 Not coded here   EXCLUDES 2 Not included here   N Newborn Age: 0   P Pediatric Age: 0-17   M Maternity Age: 12-55   A Adult Age: 15-124

426   ICD-10-CM Draft (2015)

Certain Infectious and Parasitic Diseases

A39.8–A49.9

✓5ᵗʰ **A39.8** Other **meningococcal infections**
    A39.81 Meningococcal **encephalitis**
    A39.82 Meningococcal **retrobulbar neuritis**
    A39.83 Meningococcal **arthritis**
    A39.84 Postmeningococcal **arthritis**
    A39.89 Other meningococcal infections
        Meningococcal conjunctivitis
  A39.9 **Meningococcal infection, unspecified**
    Meningococcal disease NOS

✓4ᵗʰ **A40** **Streptococcal sepsis**
  Code first: postprocedural streptococcal sepsis (T81.4)
    streptococcal sepsis during labor (O75.3)
    streptococcal sepsis following abortion or ectopic or molar
      pregnancy (O03-O07, O08.0)
    streptococcal sepsis following immunization (T88.0)
    streptococcal sepsis following infusion, transfusion or
      therapeutic injection (T80.2-)
    EXCLUDES 1 neonatal (P36.0-P36.1)
      puerperal sepsis (O85)
      sepsis due to Streptococcus, group D (A41.81)
  A40.0 Sepsis due to streptococcus, **group A**
  A40.1 Sepsis due to streptococcus, **group B**
  A40.3 Sepsis due to **Streptococcus pneumoniae**
    Pneumococcal sepsis
  A40.8 Other streptococcal sepsis
  A40.9 **Streptococcal sepsis, unspecified**

✓4ᵗʰ **A41** **Other sepsis**
  Code first: postprocedural sepsis (T81.4)
    sepsis during labor (O75.3)
    sepsis following abortion, ectopic or molar pregnancy
      (O03-O07, O08.0)
    sepsis following immunization (T88.0)
    sepsis following infusion, transfusion or therapeutic injection
      (T80.2-)
    EXCLUDES 1 bacteremia NOS (R78.81)
      neonatal (P36.-)
      puerperal sepsis (O85)
      sepsis NOS (A41.9)
      streptococcal sepsis (A40.-)
    EXCLUDES 2 sepsis (due to) (in) actinomycotic (A42.7)
      sepsis (due to) (in) anthrax (A22.7)
      sepsis (due to) (in) candidal (B37.7)
      sepsis (due to) (in) Erysipelothrix (A26.7)
      sepsis (due to) (in) extraintestinal yersiniosis (A28.2)
      sepsis (due to) (in) gonococcal (A54.86)
      sepsis (due to) (in) herpesviral (B00.7)
      sepsis (due to) (in) listerial (A32.7)
      sepsis (due to) (in) melioidosis (A24.1)
      sepsis (due to) (in) meningococcal (A39.2-A39.4)
      sepsis (due to) (in) plague (A20.7)
      sepsis (due to) (in) tularemia (A21.7)
      toxic shock syndrome (A48.3)
    AHA: 2014, 2Q, 13
  ✓5ᵗʰ **A41.0** Sepsis due to **Staphylococcus aureus**
    A41.01 Sepsis due to **methicillin susceptible Staphylococcus aureus**
      MSSA sepsis
      Staphylococcus aureus sepsis NOS
    A41.02 Sepsis due to **methicillin resistant Staphylococcus aureus**
  A41.1 **Sepsis due to other specified staphylococcus**
    Coagulase negative staphylococcus sepsis
  A41.2 **Sepsis due to unspecified staphylococcus**
  A41.3 Sepsis due to **Hemophilus influenzae**
  A41.4 Sepsis due to **anaerobes**
    EXCLUDES 1 gas gangrene (A48.0)
  ✓5ᵗʰ **A41.5** Sepsis due to other **Gram-negative organisms**
    A41.50 **Gram-negative sepsis, unspecified**
      Gram-negative sepsis NOS
    A41.51 Sepsis due to **Escherichia coli [E. coli]**
    A41.52 Sepsis due to **Pseudomonas**
      Pseudomonas aeroginosa
    A41.53 Sepsis due to **Serratia**
    A41.59 Other **Gram-negative sepsis**
  ✓5ᵗʰ **A41.8** Other **specified sepsis**
    A41.81 Sepsis due to **Enterococcus**
    A41.89 Other specified sepsis

  A41.9 **Sepsis, unspecified organism**
    Septicemia NOS

✓4ᵗʰ **A42** **Actinomycosis**
  EXCLUDES 1 actinomycetoma (B47.1)
  A42.0 **Pulmonary actinomycosis**
  A42.1 **Abdominal actinomycosis**
  A42.2 **Cervicofacial actinomycosis**
  A42.7 Actinomycotic **sepsis**
  ✓5ᵗʰ **A42.8** **Other forms of actinomycosis**
    A42.81 Actinomycotic **meningitis**
    A42.82 Actinomycotic **encephalitis**
    A42.89 Other forms of actinomycosis
  A42.9 **Actinomycosis, unspecified**

✓4ᵗʰ **A43** **Nocardiosis**
  A43.0 **Pulmonary nocardiosis**
  A43.1 **Cutaneous nocardiosis**
  A43.8 Other forms of nocardiosis
  A43.9 **Nocardiosis, unspecified**

✓4ᵗʰ **A44** **Bartonellosis**
  A44.0 Systemic **bartonellosis**
    Oroya fever
  A44.1 Cutaneous and mucocutaneous **bartonellosis**
    Verruga peruana
  A44.8 Other forms of bartonellosis
  A44.9 **Bartonellosis, unspecified**

  A46 **Erysipelas**
  EXCLUDES 1 postpartum or puerperal erysipelas (O86.89)

✓4ᵗʰ **A48** **Other bacterial diseases, not elsewhere classified**
  EXCLUDES 1 actinomycetoma (B47.1)
  A48.0 **Gas gangrene**
    Clostridial cellulitis
    Clostridial myonecrosis
  A48.1 **Legionnaires' disease**
  A48.2 **Nonpneumonic Legionnaires' disease [Pontiac fever]**
  A48.3 **Toxic shock syndrome**
    Use additional code to identify the organism (B95, B96)
    EXCLUDES 1 endotoxic shock NOS (R57.8)
      sepsis NOS (A41.9)
  A48.4 **Brazilian purpuric fever**
    Systemic Hemophilus aegyptius infection
  ✓5ᵗʰ **A48.5** **Other specified botulism**
    Non-foodborne intoxication due to toxins of Clostridium
      botulinum [C. botulinum]
    EXCLUDES 1 food poisoning due to toxins of Clostridium botulinum
      (A05.1)
    A48.51 **Infant botulism**   P
    A48.52 **Wound botulism**
      Non-foodborne botulism NOS
      Use additional code for associated wound
  A48.8 **Other specified bacterial diseases**

✓4ᵗʰ **A49** **Bacterial infection of unspecified site**
  EXCLUDES 1 bacterial agents as the cause of diseases classified elsewhere
    (B95-B96)
    chlamydial infection NOS (A74.9)
    meningococcal infection NOS (A39.9)
    rickettsial infection NOS (A79.9)
    spirochetal infection NOS (A69.9)
  ✓5ᵗʰ **A49.0** **Staphylococcal infection, unspecified site**
    A49.01 **Methicillin susceptible Staphylococcus aureus infection, unspecified site**
      Methicillin susceptible Staphylococcus aureus (MSSA) infection
      Staphylococcus aureus infection NOS
    A49.02 **Methicillin resistant Staphylococcus aureus infection, unspecified site**
      Methicillin resistant Staphylococcus aureus (MRSA) infection
  A49.1 **Streptococcal infection, unspecified site**
  A49.2 **Hemophilus influenzae infection, unspecified site**
  A49.3 **Mycoplasma infection, unspecified site**
  A49.8 Other bacterial infections of unspecified site
  A49.9 **Bacterial infection, unspecified**
    EXCLUDES 1 bacteremia NOS (R78.81)

✓ Additional Character Required   ✓7ᵗʰ Xtension Alert   Unspecified Dx   Other Specified Dx   Manifestation   ▶◀ Revised Text   ● New Code   ▲ Revised Code Title

Certain Infectious and Parasitic Diseases

A50–A52.75

Infections with a predominantly sexual mode of transmission (A50-A64)

EXCLUDES 1   human immunodeficiency virus [HIV] disease (B20)
nonspecific and nongonococcal urethritis (N34.1)
Reiter's disease (M02.3-)

✓4th A50   Congenital syphilis

  ✓5th A50.0   Early congenital syphilis, symptomatic
       Any congenital syphilitic condition specified as early or manifest less than two years after birth.

    A50.01   Early congenital syphilitic oculopathy

    A50.02   Early congenital syphilitic osteochondropathy

    A50.03   Early congenital syphilitic pharyngitis
       Early congenital syphilitic laryngitis

    A50.04   Early congenital syphilitic pneumonia

    A50.05   Early congenital syphilitic rhinitis

    A50.06   Early cutaneous congenital syphilis

    A50.07   Early mucocutaneous congenital syphilis

    A50.08   Early visceral congenital syphilis

    A50.09   Other early congenital syphilis, symptomatic

  A50.1   Early congenital syphilis, latent
       Congenital syphilis without clinical manifestations, with positive serological reaction and negative spinal fluid test, less than two years after birth.

  A50.2   Early congenital syphilis, unspecified
       Congenital syphilis NOS less than two years after birth.

  ✓5th A50.3   Late congenital syphilitic oculopathy
       EXCLUDES 1   Hutchinson's triad (A50.53)

    A50.30   Late congenital syphilitic oculopathy, unspecified

    A50.31   Late congenital syphilitic interstitial keratitis

    A50.32   Late congenital syphilitic chorioretinitis

    A50.39   Other late congenital syphilitic oculopathy

  ✓5th A50.4   Late congenital neurosyphilis [juvenile neurosyphilis]
       Use additional code to identify any associated mental disorder
       EXCLUDES 1   Hutchinson's triad (A50.53)

    A50.40   Late congenital neurosyphilis, unspecified
       Juvenile neurosyphilis NOS

    A50.41   Late congenital syphilitic meningitis

    A50.42   Late congenital syphilitic encephalitis

    A50.43   Late congenital syphilitic polyneuropathy

    A50.44   Late congenital syphilitic optic nerve atrophy

    A50.45   Juvenile general paresis
       Dementia paralytica juvenilis
       Juvenile tabetoparetic neurosyphilis

    A50.49   Other late congenital neurosyphilis
       Juvenile tabes dorsalis

  ✓5th A50.5   Other late congenital syphilis, symptomatic
       Any congenital syphilitic condition specified as late or manifest two years or more after birth.

    A50.51   Clutton's joints

    A50.52   Hutchinson's teeth

    A50.53   Hutchinson's triad

    A50.54   Late congenital cardiovascular syphilis

    A50.55   Late congenital syphilitic arthropathy

    A50.56   Late congenital syphilitic osteochondropathy

    A50.57   Syphilitic saddle nose

    A50.59   Other late congenital syphilis, symptomatic

  A50.6   Late congenital syphilis, latent
       Congenital syphilis without clinical manifestations, with positive serological reaction and negative spinal fluid test, two years or more after birth.

  A50.7   Late congenital syphilis, unspecified
       Congenital syphilis NOS two years or more after birth.

  A50.9   Congenital syphilis, unspecified

✓4th A51   Early syphilis

  A51.0   Primary genital syphilis
       Syphilitic chancre NOS

  A51.1   Primary anal syphilis

  A51.2   Primary syphilis of other sites

  ✓5th A51.3   Secondary syphilis of skin and mucous membranes

    A51.31   Condyloma latum

    A51.32   Syphilitic alopecia

    A51.39   Other secondary syphilis of skin
       Syphilitic leukoderma
       Syphilitic mucous patch
       EXCLUDES 1   late syphilitic leukoderma (A52.79)

  ✓5th A51.4   Other secondary syphilis

    A51.41   Secondary syphilitic meningitis

    A51.42   Secondary syphilitic female pelvic disease ♀

    A51.43   Secondary syphilitic oculopathy
       Secondary syphilitic chorioretinitis
       Secondary syphilitic iridocyclitis, iritis
       Secondary syphilitic uveitis

    A51.44   Secondary syphilitic nephritis

    A51.45   Secondary syphilitic hepatitis

    A51.46   Secondary syphilitic osteopathy

    A51.49   Other secondary syphilitic conditions
       Secondary syphilitic lymphadenopathy
       Secondary syphilitic myositis

  A51.5   Early syphilis, latent
       Syphilis (acquired) without clinical manifestations, with positive serological reaction and negative spinal fluid test, less than two years after infection.

  A51.9   Early syphilis, unspecified

✓4th A52   Late syphilis

  ✓5th A52.0   Cardiovascular and cerebrovascular syphilis

    A52.00   Cardiovascular syphilis, unspecified

    A52.01   Syphilitic aneurysm of aorta

    A52.02   Syphilitic aortitis

    A52.03   Syphilitic endocarditis
       Syphilitic aortic valve incompetence or stenosis
       Syphilitic mitral valve stenosis
       Syphilitic pulmonary valve regurgitation

    A52.04   Syphilitic cerebral arteritis

    A52.05   Other cerebrovascular syphilis
       Syphilitic cerebral aneurysm (ruptured) (non-ruptured)
       Syphilitic cerebral thrombosis

    A52.06   Other syphilitic heart involvement
       Syphilitic coronary artery disease
       Syphilitic myocarditis
       Syphilitic pericarditis

    A52.09   Other cardiovascular syphilis

  ✓5th A52.1   Symptomatic neurosyphilis

    A52.10   Symptomatic neurosyphilis, unspecified

    A52.11   Tabes dorsalis
       Locomotor ataxia (progressive)
       Tabetic neurosyphilis

    A52.12   Other cerebrospinal syphilis

    A52.13   Late syphilitic meningitis

    A52.14   Late syphilitic encephalitis

    A52.15   Late syphilitic neuropathy
       Late syphilitic acoustic neuritis
       Late syphilitic optic (nerve) atrophy
       Late syphilitic polyneuropathy
       Late syphilitic retrobulbar neuritis

    A52.16   Charcôt's arthropathy (tabetic)

    A52.17   General paresis
       Dementia paralytica

    A52.19   Other symptomatic neurosyphilis
       Syphilitic parkinsonism

  A52.2   Asymptomatic neurosyphilis

  A52.3   Neurosyphilis, unspecified
       Gumma (syphilitic)
       Syphilis (late)
       Syphiloma

  ✓5th A52.7   Other symptomatic late syphilis

    A52.71   Late syphilitic oculopathy
       Late syphilitic chorioretinitis
       Late syphilitic episcleritis

    A52.72   Syphilis of lung and bronchus

    A52.73   Symptomatic late syphilis of other respiratory organs

    A52.74   Syphilis of liver and other viscera
       Late syphilitic peritonitis

    A52.75   Syphilis of kidney and ureter
       Syphilitic glomerular disease

EXCLUDES 1 Not coded here   **EXCLUDES 2** Not included here   **N** Newborn Age: 0   **P** Pediatric Age: 0-17   **M** Maternity Age: 12-55   **A** Adult Age: 15-124

428   ICD-10-CM Draft (2015)

A52.76 **Other genitourinary symptomatic late syphilis**
Late syphilitic female pelvic inflammatory disease

A52.77 **Syphilis of bone and joint**

A52.78 **Syphilis of other musculoskeletal tissue**
Late syphilitic bursitis
Syphilis [stage unspecified] of bursa
Syphilis [stage unspecified] of muscle
Syphilis [stage unspecified] of synovium
Syphilis [stage unspecified] of tendon

A52.79 **Other symptomatic late syphilis**
Late syphilitic leukoderma
Syphilis of adrenal gland
Syphilis of pituitary gland
Syphilis of thyroid gland
Syphilitic splenomegaly
EXCLUDES 1 *syphilitic leukoderma (secondary) (A51.39)*

A52.8 **Late syphilis, latent**
Syphilis (acquired) without clinical manifestations, with positive serological reaction and negative spinal fluid test, two years or more after infection

A52.9 **Late syphilis, unspecified**

✓4ᵗʰ **A53 Other and unspecified syphilis**

A53.0 **Latent syphilis, unspecified as early or late**
Latent syphilis NOS
Positive serological reaction for syphilis

A53.9 **Syphilis, unspecified**
Infection due to Treponema pallidum NOS
Syphilis (acquired) NOS
EXCLUDES 1 *syphilis NOS under two years of age (A50.2)*

✓4ᵗʰ **A54 Gonococcal infection**

✓5ᵗʰ A54.0 **Gonococcal infection of lower genitourinary tract without periurethral or accessory gland abscess**
EXCLUDES 1 *gonococcal infection with genitourinary gland abscess (A54.1)*
gonococcal infection with periurethral abscess (A54.1)

A54.00 **Gonococcal infection of lower genitourinary tract, unspecified**

A54.01 **Gonococcal cystitis and urethritis, unspecified**

A54.02 **Gonococcal vulvovaginitis, unspecified** ♀

A54.03 **Gonococcal cervicitis, unspecified** ♀

A54.09 **Other gonococcal infection of lower genitourinary tract**

A54.1 **Gonococcal infection of lower genitourinary tract with periurethral and accessory gland abscess**
Gonococcal Bartholin's gland abscess

✓5ᵗʰ A54.2 **Gonococcal pelviperitonitis and other gonococcal genitourinary infection**

A54.21 **Gonococcal infection of kidney and ureter**

A54.22 **Gonococcal prostatitis** ♂

A54.23 **Gonococcal infection of other male genital organs** ♂
Gonococcal epididymitis
Gonococcal orchitis

A54.24 **Gonococcal female pelvic inflammatory disease** ♀
Gonococcal pelviperitonitis
EXCLUDES 1 *gonococcal peritonitis (A54.85)*

A54.29 **Other gonococcal genitourinary infections**

✓5ᵗʰ A54.3 **Gonococcal infection of eye**

A54.30 **Gonococcal infection of eye, unspecified**

A54.31 **Gonococcal conjunctivitis**
Ophthalmia neonatorum due to gonococcus

A54.32 **Gonococcal iridocyclitis**

A54.33 **Gonococcal keratitis**

A54.39 **Other gonococcal eye infection**
Gonococcal endophthalmia

✓5ᵗʰ A54.4 **Gonococcal infection of musculoskeletal system**

A54.40 **Gonococcal infection of musculoskeletal system, unspecified**

A54.41 **Gonococcal spondylopathy**

A54.42 **Gonococcal arthritis**
EXCLUDES 2 *gonococcal infection of spine (A54.41)*

A54.43 **Gonococcal osteomyelitis**
EXCLUDES 2 *gonococcal infection of spine (A54.41)*

A54.49 **Gonococcal infection of other musculoskeletal tissue**
Gonococcal bursitis
Gonococcal myositis
Gonococcal synovitis
Gonococcal tenosynovitis

A54.5 **Gonococcal pharyngitis**

A54.6 **Gonococcal infection of anus and rectum**

✓5ᵗʰ A54.8 **Other gonococcal infections**

A54.81 **Gonococcal meningitis**

A54.82 **Gonococcal brain abscess**

A54.83 **Gonococcal heart infection**
Gonococcal endocarditis
Gonococcal myocarditis
Gonococcal pericarditis

A54.84 **Gonococcal pneumonia**

A54.85 **Gonococcal peritonitis**
EXCLUDES 1 *gonococcal pelviperitonitis (A54.24)*

A54.86 **Gonococcal sepsis**

A54.89 **Other gonococcal infections**
Gonococcal keratoderma
Gonococcal lymphadenitis

A54.9 **Gonococcal infection, unspecified**

A55 Chlamydial lymphogranuloma (venereum)
Climatic or tropical bubo
Durand-Nicolas-Favre disease
Esthiomene
Lymphogranuloma inguinale

✓4ᵗʰ **A56 Other sexually transmitted chlamydial diseases**
INCLUDES sexually transmitted diseases due to Chlamydia trachomatis
EXCLUDES 1 *neonatal chlamydial conjunctivitis (P39.1)*
neonatal chlamydial pneumonia (P23.1)
EXCLUDES 2 *chlamydial lymphogranuloma (A55)*
conditions classified to A74-

✓5ᵗʰ A56.0 **Chlamydial infection of lower genitourinary tract**

A56.00 **Chlamydial infection of lower genitourinary tract, unspecified**

A56.01 **Chlamydial cystitis and urethritis**

A56.02 **Chlamydial vulvovaginitis** ♀

A56.09 **Other chlamydial infection of lower genitourinary tract**
Chlamydial cervicitis

✓5ᵗʰ A56.1 **Chlamydial infection of pelviperitoneum and other genitourinary organs**

A56.11 **Chlamydial female pelvic inflammatory disease** ♀

A56.19 **Other chlamydial genitourinary infection**
Chlamydial epididymitis
Chlamydial orchitis

A56.2 **Chlamydial infection of genitourinary tract, unspecified**

A56.3 **Chlamydial infection of anus and rectum**

A56.4 **Chlamydial infection of pharynx**

A56.8 **Sexually transmitted chlamydial infection of other sites**

A57 Chancroid
Ulcus molle

A58 Granuloma inguinale
Donovanosis

✓4ᵗʰ **A59 Trichomoniasis**
EXCLUDES 2 *intestinal trichomoniasis (A07.8)*

✓5ᵗʰ A59.0 **Urogenital trichomoniasis**

A59.00 **Urogenital trichomoniasis, unspecified**
Fluor (vaginalis) due to Trichomonas
Leukorrhea (vaginalis) due to Trichomonas

A59.01 **Trichomonal vulvovaginitis** ♀

A59.02 **Trichomonal prostatitis** ♂

A59.03 **Trichomonal cystitis and urethritis**

A59.09 **Other urogenital trichomoniasis**
Trichomonas cervicitis

A59.8 **Trichomoniasis of other sites**

A59.9 **Trichomoniasis, unspecified**

✓4ᵗʰ **A60 Anogenital herpesviral [herpes simplex] infections**

✓5ᵗʰ A60.0 **Herpesviral infection of genitalia and urogenital tract**

A60.00 **Herpesviral infection of urogenital system, unspecified**

A60.01 **Herpesviral infection of penis** ♂

A60.02 **Herpesviral infection of other male genital organs** ♂

A60.03 **Herpesviral cervicitis** ♀

☑ Additional Character Required   ✓x7ᵗʰ Xtension Alert   Unspecified Dx   Other Specified Dx   Manifestation   ▶◀ Revised Text   ● New Code   ▲ Revised Code Title

Certain Infectious and Parasitic Diseases

A60.04–A75.1

A60.04   Herpesviral vulvovaginitis   ♀
Herpesviral [herpes simplex] ulceration
Herpesviral [herpes simplex] vaginitis
Herpesviral [herpes simplex] vulvitis

A60.09   Herpesviral infection of other urogenital tract

A60.1   Herpesviral infection of perianal skin and rectum

A60.9   Anogenital herpesviral infection, unspecified

✓4ᵗʰ **A63   Other predominantly sexually transmitted diseases, not elsewhere classified**
EXCLUDES 2   *molluscum contagiosum (B08.1)*
papilloma of cervix (D26.0)

A63.0   Anogenital (venereal) warts
Anogenital warts due to (human) papillomavirus [HPV]
Condyloma acuminatum

A63.8   Other specified predominantly sexually transmitted diseases

A64   Unspecified sexually transmitted disease

Other spirochetal diseases (A65-A69)

EXCLUDES 2   *leptospirosis (A27.-)*
syphilis (A50-A53)

A65   Nonvenereal syphilis
Bejel   Njovera
Endemic syphilis

✓4ᵗʰ **A66   Yaws**
INCLUDES   bouba
frambesia (tropica)
pian

A66.0   Initial lesions of yaws
Chancre of yaws
Frambesia, initial or primary
Initial frambesial ulcer
Mother yaw

A66.1   Multiple papillomata and wet crab yaws
Frambesioma
Pianoma
Plantar or palmar papilloma of yaws

A66.2   Other early skin lesions of yaws
Cutaneous yaws, less than five years after infection
Early yaws (cutaneous) (macular) (maculopapular)
(micropapular) (papular)
Frambeside of early yaws

A66.3   Hyperkeratosis of yaws
Ghoul hand
Hyperkeratosis, palmar or plantar (early) (late) due to yaws
Worm-eaten soles

A66.4   Gummata and ulcers of yaws
Gummatous frambeside
Nodular late yaws (ulcerated)

A66.5   Gangosa
Rhinopharyngitis mutilans

A66.6   Bone and joint lesions of yaws
Yaws ganglion   Yaws hydrarthrosis
Yaws goundou   Yaws osteitis
Yaws gumma, bone   Yaws periostitis (hypertrophic)
Yaws gummatous osteitis
or periostitis

A66.7   Other manifestations of yaws
Juxta-articular nodules of yaws
Mucosal yaws

A66.8   Latent yaws
Yaws without clinical manifestations, with positive serology

A66.9   Yaws, unspecified

✓4ᵗʰ **A67   Pinta [carate]**

A67.0   Primary lesions of pinta
Chancre (primary) of pinta
Papule (primary) of pinta

A67.1   Intermediate lesions of pinta
Erythematous plaques of pinta
Hyperchromic lesions of pinta
Hyperkeratosis of pinta
Pintids

A67.2   Late lesions of pinta
Achromic skin lesions of pinta
Cicatricial skin lesions of pinta
Dyschromic skin lesions of pinta

A67.3   Mixed lesions of pinta
Achromic with hyperchromic skin lesions of pinta [carate]

A67.9   Pinta, unspecified

✓4ᵗʰ **A68   Relapsing fevers**
INCLUDES   recurrent fever
EXCLUDES 2   *Lyme disease (A69.2-)*

A68.0   Louse-borne relapsing fever
Relapsing fever due to Borrelia recurrentis

A68.1   Tick-borne relapsing fever
Relapsing fever due to any Borrelia species other than Borrelia recurrentis

A68.9   Relapsing fever, unspecified

✓4ᵗʰ **A69   Other spirochetal infections**

A69.0   Necrotizing ulcerative stomatitis
Cancrum oris
Fusospirochetal gangrene
Noma
Stomatitis gangrenosa

A69.1   Other Vincent's infections
Fusospirochetal pharyngitis
Necrotizing ulcerative (acute) gingivitis
Necrotizing ulcerative (acute) gingivostomatitis
Spirochetal stomatitis
Trench mouth
Vincent's angina
Vincent's gingivitis

✓5ᵗʰ **A69.2   Lyme disease**
Erythema chronicum migrans due to Borrelia burgdorferi

A69.20   Lyme disease, unspecified

A69.21   Meningitis due to Lyme disease

A69.22   Other neurologic disorders in Lyme disease
Cranial neuritis
Meningoencephalitis
Polyneuropathy

A69.23   Arthritis due to Lyme disease

A69.29   Other conditions associated with Lyme disease
Myopericarditis due to Lyme disease

A69.8   Other specified spirochetal infections

A69.9   Spirochetal infection, unspecified

Other diseases caused by chlamydiae (A70-A74)

EXCLUDES 1   *sexually transmitted chlamydial diseases (A55-A56)*

A70   Chlamydia psittaci infections
Ornithosis
Parrot fever
Psittacosis

✓4ᵗʰ **A71   Trachoma**
EXCLUDES 1   *sequelae of trachoma (B94.0)*

A71.0   Initial stage of trachoma
Trachoma dubium

A71.1   Active stage of trachoma
Granular conjunctivitis (trachomatous)
Trachomatous follicular conjunctivitis
Trachomatous pannus

A71.9   Trachoma, unspecified

✓4ᵗʰ **A74   Other diseases caused by chlamydiae**
EXCLUDES 1   *neonatal chlamydial conjunctivitis (P39.1)*
neonatal chlamydial pneumonia (P23.1)
Reiter's disease (M02.3-)
sexually transmitted chlamydial diseases (A55-A56)
EXCLUDES 2   *chlamydial pneumonia (J16.0)*

A74.0   Chlamydial conjunctivitis
Paratrachoma

✓5ᵗʰ **A74.8   Other chlamydial diseases**

A74.81   Chlamydial peritonitis

A74.89   Other chlamydial diseases

A74.9   Chlamydial infection, unspecified
Chlamydiosis NOS

Rickettsioses (A75-A79)

✓4ᵗʰ **A75   Typhus fever**
EXCLUDES 1   *rickettsiosis due to Ehrlichia sennetsu (A79.81)*

A75.0   Epidemic louse-borne typhus fever due to Rickettsia prowazekii
Classical typhus (fever)
Epidemic (louse-borne) typhus

A75.1   Recrudescent typhus [Brill's disease]
Brill-Zinsser disease

EXCLUDES 1 Not coded here   EXCLUDES 2 Not included here   N Newborn Age: 0   P Pediatric Age: 0-17   M Maternity Age: 12-55   A Adult Age: 15-124

430   ICD-10-CM Draft (2015)

A75.2 **Typhus fever due to** Rickettsia typhi
Murine (flea-borne) typhus

A75.3 **Typhus fever due to** Rickettsia tsutsugamushi
Scrub (mite-borne) typhus
Tsutsugamushi fever

A75.9 **Typhus fever, unspecified**
Typhus (fever) NOS

✓4ᵗʰ **A77** **Spotted fever [tick-borne rickettsioses]**

A77.0 **Spotted fever due to** Rickettsia rickettsii
Rocky Mountain spotted fever
Sao Paulo fever

A77.1 **Spotted fever due to** Rickettsia conorii
African tick typhus
Boutonneuse fever
India tick typhus
Kenya tick typhus
Marseilles fever
Mediterranean tick fever

A77.2 **Spotted fever due to** Rickettsia siberica
North Asian tick fever
Siberian tick typhus

A77.3 **Spotted fever due to** Rickettsia australis
Queensland tick typhus

✓5ᵗʰ **A77.4** **Ehrlichiosis**
EXCLUDES 1   Rickettsiosis due to Ehrlichia sennetsu (A79.81)
A77.40 **Ehrlichiosis, unspecified**
A77.41 **Ehrlichiosis** chafeensis [E. chafeensis]
A77.49 **Other ehrlichiosis**

A77.8 **Other spotted fevers**

A77.9 **Spotted fever, unspecified**
Tick-borne typhus NOS

A78 **Q fever**
Infection due to Coxiella burnetii
Nine Mile fever
Quadrilateral fever

✓4ᵗʰ **A79** **Other rickettsioses**

A79.0 **Trench fever**
Quintan fever
Wolhynian fever

A79.1 **Rickettsialpox due to** Rickettsia akari
Kew Garden fever
Vesicular rickettsiosis

✓5ᵗʰ **A79.8** **Other** specified rickettsioses
A79.81 **Rickettsiosis due to** Ehrlichia sennetsu
A79.89 **Other specified rickettsioses**

A79.9 **Rickettsiosis, unspecified**
Rickettsial infection NOS

Viral and prion infections of the central nervous system (A80-A89)

EXCLUDES 1   postpolio syndrome (G14)
sequelae of poliomyelitis (B91)
sequelae of viral encephalitis (B94.1)

✓4ᵗʰ **A80** **Acute poliomyelitis**

A80.0 **Acute paralytic poliomyelitis,** vaccine-associated

A80.1 **Acute paralytic poliomyelitis,** wild virus, imported

A80.2 **Acute paralytic poliomyelitis,** wild virus, indigenous

✓5ᵗʰ **A80.3** **Acute paralytic poliomyelitis,** other and unspecified
A80.30 **Acute paralytic poliomyelitis, unspecified**
A80.39 **Other acute paralytic poliomyelitis**

A80.4 **Acute** nonparalytic poliomyelitis

A80.9 **Acute poliomyelitis, unspecified**

✓4ᵗʰ **A81** **Atypical virus infections of central nervous system**
INCLUDES   diseases of the central nervous system caused by prions
Use additional code to identify:
dementia with behavioral disturbance (F02.81)
dementia without behavioral disturbance (F02.80)

✓5ᵗʰ **A81.0** **Creutzfeldt-Jakob disease**
A81.00 **Creutzfeldt-Jakob disease, unspecified**
Jakob-Creutzfeldt disease, unspecified
A81.01 **Variant** Creutzfeldt-Jakob disease
vCJD

A81.09 **Other Creutzfeldt-Jakob disease**
CJD
Familial Creutzfeldt-Jakob disease
Iatrogenic Creutzfeldt-Jakob disease
Sporadic Creutzfeldt-Jakob disease
Subacute spongiform encephalopathy (with dementia)

A81.1 **Subacute sclerosing panencephalitis**
Dawson's inclusion body encephalitis
Van Bogaert's sclerosing leukoencephalopathy

A81.2 **Progressive multifocal leukoencephalopathy**
Multifocal leukoencephalopathy NOS

✓5ᵗʰ **A81.8** **Other atypical virus infections of central nervous system**
A81.81 **Kuru**
A81.82 **Gerstmann-Sträussler-Scheinker syndrome**
GSS syndrome
A81.83 **Fatal familial insomnia**
FFI
A81.89 **Other atypical virus infections of central nervous system**

A81.9 **Atypical virus infection of central nervous system, unspecified**
Prion diseases of the central nervous system NOS

✓4ᵗʰ **A82** **Rabies**

A82.0 **Sylvatic rabies**

A82.1 **Urban rabies**

A82.9 **Rabies, unspecified**

✓4ᵗʰ **A83** **Mosquito-borne viral encephalitis**
INCLUDES   mosquito-borne viral meningoencephalitis
EXCLUDES 2   Venezuelan equine encephalitis (A92.2)
West Nile fever (A92.3-)
West Nile virus (A92.3-)

A83.0 **Japanese encephalitis**

A83.1 **Western equine encephalitis**

A83.2 **Eastern equine encephalitis**

A83.3 **St Louis encephalitis**

A83.4 **Australian encephalitis**
Kunjin virus disease

A83.5 **California encephalitis**
California meningoencephalitis
La Crosse encephalitis

A83.6 **Rocio virus disease**

A83.8 **Other mosquito-borne viral encephalitis**

A83.9 **Mosquito-borne viral encephalitis, unspecified**

✓4ᵗʰ **A84** **Tick-borne viral encephalitis**
INCLUDES   tick-borne viral meningoencephalitis

A84.0 **Far Eastern tick-borne encephalitis [Russian spring-summer encephalitis]**

A84.1 **Central European tick-borne encephalitis**

A84.8 **Other tick-borne viral encephalitis**
Louping ill
Powassan virus disease

A84.9 **Tick-borne viral encephalitis, unspecified**

✓4ᵗʰ **A85** **Other viral encephalitis, not elsewhere classified**
INCLUDES   specified viral encephalomyelitis NEC
specified viral meningoencephalitis NEC
EXCLUDES 1   benign myalgic encephalomyelitis (G93.3)
encephalitis due to cytomegalovirus (B25.8)
encephalitis due to herpesvirus NEC (B10.0-)
encephalitis due to herpesvirus [herpes simplex] (B00.4)
encephalitis due to measles virus (B05.0)
encephalitis due to mumps virus (B26.2)
encephalitis due to poliomyelitis virus (A80.-)
encephalitis due to zoster (B02.0)
lymphocytic choriomeningitis (A87.2)

A85.0 **Enteroviral encephalitis**
Enteroviral encephalomyelitis

A85.1 **Adenoviral encephalitis**
Adenoviral meningoencephalitis

A85.2 **Arthropod-borne viral encephalitis, unspecified**
EXCLUDES 1   West nile virus with encephalitis (A92.31)

A85.8 **Other specified viral encephalitis**
Encephalitis lethargica
Von Economo-Cruchet disease

Certain Infectious and Parasitic Diseases

A86–B00.9

A86 Unspecified viral encephalitis
Viral encephalomyelitis NOS
Viral meningoencephalitis NOS

✓4ᵗʰ **A87 Viral meningitis**
> EXCLUDES 1   meningitis due to herpesvirus [herpes simplex] (B00.3)
> meningitis due to measles virus (B05.1)
> meningitis due to mumps virus (B26.1)
> meningitis due to poliomyelitis virus (A80.-)
> meningitis due to zoster (B02.1)

A87.0 Enteroviral meningitis
Coxsackievirus meningitis
Echovirus meningitis

A87.1 Adenoviral meningitis

A87.2 Lymphocytic choriomeningitis
Lymphocytic meningoencephalitis

A87.8 Other viral meningitis

A87.9 Viral meningitis, unspecified

✓4ᵗʰ **A88 Other viral infections of central nervous system, not elsewhere classified**
> EXCLUDES 1   viral encephalitis NOS (A86)
> viral meningitis NOS (A87.9)

A88.0 Enteroviral exanthematous fever [Boston exanthem]

A88.1 Epidemic vertigo

A88.8 Other specified viral infections of central nervous system

A89 Unspecified viral infection of central nervous system

Arthropod-borne viral fevers and viral hemorrhagic fevers (A90-A99)

A90 Dengue fever [classical dengue]
> EXCLUDES 1   dengue hemorrhagic fever (A91)

A91 Dengue hemorrhagic fever

✓4ᵗʰ **A92 Other mosquito-borne viral fevers**
> EXCLUDES 1   Ross River disease (B33.1)

A92.0 Chikungunya virus disease
Chikungunya (hemorrhagic) fever

A92.1 O'nyong-nyong fever

A92.2 Venezuelan equine fever
Venezuelan equine encephalitis
Venezuelan equine encephalomyelitis virus disease

✓5ᵗʰ **A92.3 West Nile virus infection**
West Nile fever

A92.30 West Nile virus infection, unspecified
West Nile fever NOS
West Nile fever without complications
West Nile virus NOS

A92.31 West Nile virus infection with encephalitis
West Nile encephalitis
West Nile encephalomyelitis

A92.32 West Nile virus infection with other neurologic manifestation
Use additional code to specify the neurologic manifestation

A92.39 West Nile virus infection with other complications
Use additional code to specify the other conditions

A92.4 Rift Valley fever

A92.8 Other specified mosquito-borne viral fevers

A92.9 Mosquito-borne viral fever, unspecified

✓4ᵗʰ **A93 Other arthropod-borne viral fevers, not elsewhere classified**

A93.0 Oropouche virus disease
Oropouche fever

A93.1 Sandfly fever
Pappataci fever
Phlebotomus fever

A93.2 Colorado tick fever

A93.8 Other specified arthropod-borne viral fevers
Piry virus disease
Vesicular stomatitis virus disease [Indiana fever]

A94 Unspecified arthropod-borne viral fever
Arboviral fever NOS
Arbovirus infection NOS

✓4ᵗʰ **A95 Yellow fever**

A95.0 Sylvatic yellow fever
Jungle yellow fever

A95.1 Urban yellow fever

A95.9 Yellow fever, unspecified

✓4ᵗʰ **A96 Arenaviral hemorrhagic fever**

A96.0 Junin hemorrhagic fever
Argentinian hemorrhagic fever

A96.1 Machupo hemorrhagic fever
Bolivian hemorrhagic fever

A96.2 Lassa fever

A96.8 Other arenaviral hemorrhagic fevers

A96.9 Arenaviral hemorrhagic fever, unspecified

✓4ᵗʰ **A98 Other viral hemorrhagic fevers, not elsewhere classified**
> EXCLUDES 1   chikungunya hemorrhagic fever (A92.0)
> dengue hemorrhagic fever (A91)

A98.0 Crimean-Congo hemorrhagic fever
Central Asian hemorrhagic fever

A98.1 Omsk hemorrhagic fever

A98.2 Kyasanur Forest disease

A98.3 Marburg virus disease

A98.4 Ebola virus disease

A98.5 Hemorrhagic fever with renal syndrome
Epidemic hemorrhagic fever
Korean hemorrhagic fever
Russian hemorrhagic fever
Hantaan virus disease
Hantavirus disease with renal manifestations
Nephropathia epidemica
Songo fever
> EXCLUDES 1   hantavirus (cardio)-pulmonary syndrome (B33.4)

A98.8 Other specified viral hemorrhagic fevers

A99 Unspecified viral hemorrhagic fever

Viral infections characterized by skin and mucous membrane lesions (B00-B09)

✓4ᵗʰ **B00 Herpesviral [herpes simplex] infections**
> EXCLUDES 1   congenital herpesviral infections (P35.2)
> EXCLUDES 2   anogenital herpesviral infection (A60.-)
> gammaherpesviral mononucleosis (B27.0-)
> herpangina (B08.5)

B00.0 Eczema herpeticum
Kaposi's varicelliform eruption

B00.1 Herpesviral vesicular dermatitis
Herpes simplex facialis
Herpes simplex labialis
Herpes simplex otitis externa
Vesicular dermatitis of ear
Vesicular dermatitis of lip

B00.2 Herpesviral gingivostomatitis and pharyngotonsillitis
Herpesviral pharyngitis

B00.3 Herpesviral meningitis

B00.4 Herpesviral encephalitis
Herpesviral meningoencephalitis
Simian B disease
> EXCLUDES 1   herpesviral encephalitis due to herpesvirus 6 and 7 (B10.01, B10.09)
> non-simplex herpesviral encephalitis (B10.0-)

✓5ᵗʰ **B00.5 Herpesviral ocular disease**

B00.50 Herpesviral ocular disease, unspecified

B00.51 Herpesviral iridocyclitis
Herpesviral iritis
Herpesviral uveitis, anterior

B00.52 Herpesviral keratitis
Herpesviral keratoconjunctivitis

B00.53 Herpesviral conjunctivitis

B00.59 Other herpesviral disease of eye
Herpesviral dermatitis of eyelid

B00.7 Disseminated herpesviral disease
Herpesviral sepsis

✓5ᵗʰ **B00.8 Other forms of herpesviral infections**

B00.81 Herpesviral hepatitis

B00.82 Herpes simplex myelitis

B00.89 Other herpesviral infection
Herpesviral whitlow

B00.9 Herpesviral infection, unspecified
Herpes simplex infection NOS

| EXCLUDES 1 Not coded here | EXCLUDES 2 Not included here | N Newborn Age: 0 | P Pediatric Age: 0-17 | M Maternity Age: 12-55 | A Adult Age: 15-124 |

432   ICD-10-CM Draft (2015)

✓4th **B01 Varicella [chickenpox]**

    B01.0 Varicella meningitis

    ✓5th **B01.1 Varicella** encephalitis, myelitis and encephalomyelitis
        Postchickenpox encephalitis, myelitis and encephalomyelitis

        B01.11 Varicella encephalitis and encephalomyelitis
            Postchickenpox encephalitis and encephalomyelitis

        B01.12 Varicella myelitis
            Postchickenpox myelitis

    B01.2 Varicella pneumonia

    ✓5th **B01.8 Varicella with** other complications

        B01.81 Varicella keratitis

        B01.89 Other varicella complications

    B01.9 Varicella without complication
        Varicella NOS

✓4th **B02 Zoster [herpes zoster]**

    INCLUDES shingles
               zona

    B02.0 Zoster encephalitis
        Zoster meningoencephalitis

    B02.1 Zoster meningitis

    ✓5th **B02.2 Zoster with** other nervous system **involvement**

        B02.21 Postherpetic geniculate ganglionitis

        B02.22 Postherpetic trigeminal neuralgia

        B02.23 Postherpetic polyneuropathy

        B02.24 Postherpetic myelitis
            Herpes zoster myelitis

        B02.29 Other postherpetic nervous system involvement
            Postherpetic radiculopathy

    ✓5th **B02.3 Zoster** ocular **disease**

        B02.30 Zoster ocular disease, unspecified

        B02.31 Zoster conjunctivitis

        B02.32 Zoster iridocyclitis

        B02.33 Zoster keratitis
            Herpes zoster keratoconjunctivitis

        B02.34 Zoster scleritis

        B02.39 Other herpes zoster eye disease
            Zoster blepharitis

    B02.7 Disseminated zoster

    B02.8 Zoster with other complications
        Herpes zoster otitis externa

    B02.9 Zoster without complications
        Zoster NOS

  B03 Smallpox

    NOTE   In 1980 the 33rd World Health Assembly declared that smallpox had been eradicated.
           The classification is maintained for surveillance purposes.

  B04 Monkeypox

✓4th **B05 Measles**

    INCLUDES morbilli
    EXCLUDES1 subacute sclerosing panencephalitis (A81.1)

    B05.0 Measles complicated by encephalitis
        Postmeasles encephalitis

    B05.1 Measles complicated by meningitis
        Postmeasles meningitis

    B05.2 Measles complicated by pneumonia
        Postmeasles pneumonia

    B05.3 Measles complicated by otitis media
        Postmeasles otitis media

    B05.4 Measles with intestinal **complications**

    ✓5th **B05.8 Measles with** other **complications**

        B05.81 Measles keratitis and keratoconjunctivitis

        B05.89 Other measles complications

    B05.9 Measles without complication
        Measles NOS

✓4th **B06 Rubella [German measles]**

    EXCLUDES1 congenital rubella (P35.0)

    ✓5th **B06.0 Rubella with** neurological **complications**

        B06.00 Rubella with neurological complication, unspecified

        B06.01 Rubella encephalitis
            Rubella meningoencephalitis

        B06.02 Rubella meningitis

        B06.09 Other neurological complications of rubella

    ✓5th **B06.8 Rubella with** other complications

        B06.81 Rubella pneumonia

        B06.82 Rubella arthritis

        B06.89 Other rubella complications

    B06.9 Rubella without complication
        Rubella NOS

✓4th **B07 Viral warts**

    INCLUDES verruca simplex
              verruca vulgaris
              viral warts due to human papillomavirus
    EXCLUDES2 anogenital (venereal) warts (A63.0)
              papilloma of bladder (D41.4)
              papilloma of cervix (D26.0)
              papilloma larynx (D14.1)

    B07.0 Plantar wart
        Verruca plantaris

    B07.8 Other viral warts
        Common wart
        Flat wart
        Verruca plana

    B07.9 Viral wart, unspecified

✓4th **B08 Other viral infections characterized by skin and mucous membrane lesions, not elsewhere classified**

    EXCLUDES1 vesicular stomatitis virus disease (A93.8)

    ✓5th **B08.0 Other orthopoxvirus infections**

        EXCLUDES2 monkeypox (B04)

        ✓6th **B08.01 Cowpox and vaccinia not from vaccine**

            B08.010 Cowpox

            B08.011 Vaccinia not from vaccine
                EXCLUDES1 vaccinia (from vaccination) (generalized) (T88.1)

        B08.02 Orf virus disease
            Contagious pustular dermatitis
            Ecthyma contagiosum

        B08.03 Pseudocowpox [milker's node]

        B08.04 Paravaccinia, unspecified

        B08.09 Other orthopoxvirus infections
            Orthopoxvirus infection NOS

    B08.1 Molluscum contagiosum

    ✓5th **B08.2 Exanthema subitum [sixth disease]**
        Roseola infantum

        B08.20 Exanthema subitum [sixth disease], unspecified P
            Roseola infantum, unspecified

        B08.21 Exanthema subitum [sixth disease] due to human P **herpesvirus 6**
            Roseola infantum due to human herpesvirus 6

        B08.22 Exanthema subitum [sixth disease] due to human P **herpesvirus 7**
            Roseola infantum due to human herpesvirus 7

    B08.3 Erythema infectiosum [fifth disease]

    B08.4 Enteroviral vesicular stomatitis with exanthem
        Hand, foot and mouth disease

    B08.5 Enteroviral vesicular pharyngitis
        Herpangina

    ✓5th **B08.6 Parapoxvirus infections**

        B08.60 Parapoxvirus infection, unspecified

        B08.61 Bovine stomatitis

        B08.62 Sealpox

        B08.69 Other parapoxvirus infections

    ✓5th **B08.7 Yatapoxvirus infections**

        B08.70 Yatapoxvirus infection, unspecified

        B08.71 Tanapox virus disease

        B08.72 Yaba pox virus disease
            Yaba monkey tumor disease

        B08.79 Other yatapoxvirus infections

    B08.8 Other specified viral infections characterized by skin and mucous membrane lesions
        Enteroviral lymphonodular pharyngitis
        Foot-and-mouth disease
        Poxvirus NEC

  B09 Unspecified viral infection characterized by skin and mucous membrane lesions
    Viral enanthema NOS
    Viral exanthema NOS

✓ Additional Character Required   ✓x7th Xtension Alert   Unspecified Dx   Other Specified Dx   Manifestation   ▶◀ Revised Text   ● New Code   ▲ Revised Code Title

Other human herpesviruses (B10)

✓4th B10　Other human herpesviruses
    EXCLUDES 2 *cytomegalovirus (B25.9)*
          Epstein-Barr virus (B27.0-)
          herpes NOS (B00.9)
          herpes simplex (B00.-)
          herpes zoster (B02.-)
          human herpesvirus NOS (B00.-)
          human herpesvirus 1 and 2 (B00.-)
          human herpesvirus 3 (B01.-, B02.-)
          human herpesvirus 4 (B27.0-)
          human herpesvirus 5 (B25.-)
          varicella (B01.-)
          zoster (B02.-)

✓5th B10.0　Other human herpesvirus encephalitis
    EXCLUDES 2 *herpes encephalitis NOS (B00.4)*
          herpes simplex encephalitis (B00.4)
          human herpesvirus encephalitis (B00.4)
          simian B herpes virus encephalitis (B00.4)

    B10.01　Human herpesvirus 6 encephalitis
    B10.09　Other human herpesvirus encephalitis
        Human herpesvirus 7 encephalitis

✓5th B10.8　Other human herpesvirus infection
    B10.81　Human herpesvirus 6 infection
    B10.82　Human herpesvirus 7 infection
    B10.89　Other human herpesvirus infection
        Human herpesvirus 8 infection
        Kaposi's sarcoma-associated herpesvirus infection

Viral hepatitis (B15-B19)

    EXCLUDES 1 *sequelae of viral hepatitis (B94.2)*
    EXCLUDES 2 *cytomegaloviral hepatitis (B25.1)*
          herpesviral [herpes simplex] hepatitis (B00.81)

✓4th B15　Acute hepatitis A
    B15.0　Hepatitis A with hepatic coma
    B15.9　Hepatitis A without hepatic coma
        Hepatitis A (acute)(viral) NOS

✓4th B16　Acute hepatitis B
    B16.0　Acute hepatitis B with delta-agent with hepatic coma
    B16.1　Acute hepatitis B with delta-agent without hepatic coma
    B16.2　Acute hepatitis B without delta-agent with hepatic coma
    B16.9　Acute hepatitis B without delta-agent and without hepatic coma
        Hepatitis B (acute) (viral) NOS

✓4th B17　Other acute viral hepatitis
    B17.0　Acute delta-(super) infection of hepatitis B carrier
    ✓5th B17.1　Acute hepatitis C
        B17.10　Acute hepatitis C without hepatic coma
            Acute hepatitis C NOS
        B17.11　Acute hepatitis C with hepatic coma
    B17.2　Acute hepatitis E
    B17.8　Other specified acute viral hepatitis
        Hepatitis non-A non-B (acute) (viral) NEC
    B17.9　Acute viral hepatitis, unspecified
        Acute hepatitis NOS

✓4th B18　Chronic viral hepatitis
    B18.0　Chronic viral hepatitis B with delta-agent
    B18.1　Chronic viral hepatitis B without delta-agent
        Chronic (viral) hepatitis B
    B18.2　Chronic viral hepatitis C
    B18.8　Other chronic viral hepatitis
    B18.9　Chronic viral hepatitis, unspecified

✓4th B19　Unspecified viral hepatitis
    B19.0　Unspecified viral hepatitis with hepatic coma
    ✓5th B19.1　Unspecified viral hepatitis B
        B19.10　Unspecified viral hepatitis B without hepatic coma
            Unspecified viral hepatitis B NOS
        B19.11　Unspecified viral hepatitis B with hepatic coma
    ✓5th B19.2　Unspecified viral hepatitis C
        B19.20　Unspecified viral hepatitis C without hepatic coma
            Viral hepatitis C NOS
        B19.21　Unspecified viral hepatitis C with hepatic coma

    B19.9　Unspecified viral hepatitis without hepatic coma
        Viral hepatitis NOS

Human immunodeficiency virus [HIV] disease (B20)

B20　Human immunodeficiency virus [HIV] disease
    INCLUDES acquired immune deficiency syndrome [AIDS]
          AIDS-related complex [ARC]
          HIV infection, symptomatic
    Code first human immunodeficiency virus [HIV] disease complicating
        pregnancy, childbirth and the puerperium, if applicable (O98.7-)
    Use additional code(s) to identify all manifestations of HIV infection
    EXCLUDES 1 *asymptomatic human immunodeficiency virus [HIV] infection*
            status (Z21)
          exposure to HIV virus (Z20.6)
          inconclusive serologic evidence of HIV (R75)

Other viral diseases (B25-B34)

✓4th B25　Cytomegaloviral disease
    EXCLUDES 1 *congenital cytomegalovirus infection (P35.1)*
            cytomegaloviral mononucleosis (B27.1-)
    B25.0　Cytomegaloviral pneumonitis
    B25.1　Cytomegaloviral hepatitis
    B25.2　Cytomegaloviral pancreatitis
    B25.8　Other cytomegaloviral diseases
        Cytomegaloviral encephalitis
    B25.9　Cytomegaloviral disease, unspecified

✓4th B26　Mumps
    INCLUDES epidemic parotitis
          infectious parotitis
    B26.0　Mumps orchitis   ♂
    B26.1　Mumps meningitis
    B26.2　Mumps encephalitis
    B26.3　Mumps pancreatitis
    ✓5th B26.8　Mumps with other complications
        B26.81　Mumps hepatitis
        B26.82　Mumps myocarditis
        B26.83　Mumps nephritis
        B26.84　Mumps polyneuropathy
        B26.85　Mumps arthritis
        B26.89　Other mumps complications
    B26.9　Mumps without complication
        Mumps NOS
        Mumps parotitis NOS

✓4th B27　Infectious mononucleosis
    INCLUDES glandular fever
          monocytic angina
          Pfeiffer's disease
    ✓5th B27.0　Gammaherpesviral mononucleosis
        Mononucleosis due to Epstein-Barr virus
        B27.00　Gammaherpesviral mononucleosis without complication
        B27.01　Gammaherpesviral mononucleosis with polyneuropathy
        B27.02　Gammaherpesviral mononucleosis with meningitis
        B27.09　Gammaherpesviral mononucleosis with other complications
            Hepatomegaly in gammaherpesviral mononucleosis
    ✓5th B27.1　Cytomegaloviral mononucleosis
        B27.10　Cytomegaloviral mononucleosis without complications
        B27.11　Cytomegaloviral mononucleosis with polyneuropathy
        B27.12　Cytomegaloviral mononucleosis with meningitis
        B27.19　Cytomegaloviral mononucleosis with other complication
            Hepatomegaly in cytomegaloviral mononucleosis
    ✓5th B27.8　Other infectious mononucleosis
        B27.80　Other infectious mononucleosis without complication
        B27.81　Other infectious mononucleosis with polyneuropathy
        B27.82　Other infectious mononucleosis with meningitis

EXCLUDES 1 Not coded here   *EXCLUDES 2* Not included here   N Newborn Age: 0   P Pediatric Age: 0-17   M Maternity Age: 12-55   A Adult Age: 15-124

434   ICD-10-CM Draft (2015)

B27.89　Other infectious mononucleosis with other complication
　Hepatomegaly in other infectious mononucleosis

☑5ᵗʰ **B27.9**　Infectious mononucleosis, unspecified

B27.90　Infectious mononucleosis, unspecified without complication

B27.91　Infectious mononucleosis, unspecified with polyneuropathy

B27.92　Infectious mononucleosis, unspecified with meningitis

B27.99　Infectious mononucleosis, unspecified with other complication
　Hepatomegaly in unspecified infectious mononucleosis

☑4ᵗʰ **B30**　Viral conjunctivitis
　EXCLUDES1　herpesviral [herpes simplex] ocular disease (B00.5)
　　ocular zoster (B02.3)

B30.0　Keratoconjunctivitis due to adenovirus
　Epidemic keratoconjunctivitis
　Shipyard eye

B30.1　Conjunctivitis due to adenovirus
　Acute adenoviral follicular conjunctivitis
　Swimming-pool conjunctivitis

B30.2　Viral pharyngoconjunctivitis

B30.3　Acute epidemic hemorrhagic conjunctivitis (enteroviral)
　Conjunctivitis due to coxsackievirus 24
　Conjunctivitis due to enterovirus 70
　Hemorrhagic conjunctivitis (acute)(epidemic)

B30.8　Other viral conjunctivitis
　Newcastle conjunctivitis

B30.9　Viral conjunctivitis, unspecified

☑4ᵗʰ **B33**　Other viral diseases, not elsewhere classified

B33.0　Epidemic myalgia
　Bornholm disease

B33.1　Ross River disease
　Epidemic polyarthritis and exanthema
　Ross River fever

☑5ᵗʰ **B33.2**　Viral carditis
　Coxsackie (virus) carditis

B33.20　Viral carditis, unspecified

B33.21　Viral endocarditis

B33.22　Viral myocarditis

B33.23　Viral pericarditis

B33.24　Viral cardiomyopathy

B33.3　Retrovirus infections, not elsewhere classified
　Retrovirus infection NOS

B33.4　Hantavirus (cardio)-pulmonary syndrome [HPS] [HCPS]
　Hantavirus disease with pulmonary manifestations
　Sin nombre virus disease
　Use additional code to identify any associated acute kidney failure (N17.9)
　EXCLUDES1　hantavirus disease with renal manifestations (A98.5)
　　hemorrhagic fever with renal manifestations (A98.5)

B33.8　Other specified viral diseases
　EXCLUDES1　anogenital human papillomavirus infection (A63.0)
　　viral warts due to human papillomavirus infection (B07)

☑4ᵗʰ **B34**　Viral infection of unspecified site
　EXCLUDES1　anogenital human papillomavirus infection (A63.0)
　　cytomegaloviral disease NOS (B25.9)
　　herpesvirus [herpes simplex] infection NOS (B00.9)
　　retrovirus infection NOS (B33.3)
　　viral agents as the cause of diseases classified elsewhere (B97.-)
　　viral warts due to human papillomavirus infection (B07)

B34.0　Adenovirus infection, unspecified

B34.1　Enterovirus infection, unspecified
　Coxsackievirus infection NOS
　Echovirus infection NOS

B34.2　Coronavirus infection, unspecified
　EXCLUDES1　pneumonia due to SARS-associated coronavirus (J12.81)

B34.3　Parvovirus infection, unspecified

B34.4　Papovavirus infection, unspecified

B34.8　Other viral infections of unspecified site

B34.9　Viral infection, unspecified
　Viremia NOS

Mycoses (B35-B49)

EXCLUDES2　hypersensitivity pneumonitis due to organic dust (J67.-)
　mycosis fungoides (C84.0-)

☑4ᵗʰ **B35**　Dermatophytosis
　INCLUDES　favus
　　infections due to species of Epidermophyton, Micro-sporum and Trichophyton
　　tinea, any type except those in B36-

B35.0　Tinea barbae and tinea capitis
　Beard ringworm
　Kerion
　Scalp ringworm
　Sycosis, mycotic

B35.1　Tinea unguium
　Dermatophytic onychia
　Dermatophytosis of nail
　Onychomycosis
　Ringworm of nails

B35.2　Tinea manuum
　Dermatophytosis of hand
　Hand ringworm

B35.3　Tinea pedis
　Athlete's foot
　Dermatophytosis of foot
　Foot ringworm

B35.4　Tinea corporis
　Ringworm of the body

B35.5　Tinea imbricata
　Tokelau

B35.6　Tinea cruris
　Dhobi itch
　Groin ringworm
　Jock itch

B35.8　Other dermatophytoses
　Disseminated dermatophytosis
　Granulomatous dermatophytosis

B35.9　Dermatophytosis, unspecified
　Ringworm NOS

☑4ᵗʰ **B36**　Other superficial mycoses

B36.0　Pityriasis versicolor
　Tinea flava
　Tinea versicolor

B36.1　Tinea nigra
　Keratomycosis nigricans palmaris
　Microsporosis nigra
　Pityriasis nigra

B36.2　White piedra
　Tinea blanca

B36.3　Black piedra

B36.8　Other specified superficial mycoses

B36.9　Superficial mycosis, unspecified

☑4ᵗʰ **B37**　Candidiasis
　INCLUDES　candidosis
　　moniliasis
　EXCLUDES1　neonatal candidiasis (P37.5)

B37.0　Candidal stomatitis
　Oral thrush

B37.1　Pulmonary candidiasis
　Candidal bronchitis
　Candidal pneumonia

B37.2　Candidiasis of skin and nail
　Candidal onychia
　Candidal paronychia
　EXCLUDES2　diaper dermatitis (L22)

B37.3　Candidiasis of vulva and vagina　　　　♀
　Candidal vulvovaginitis
　Monilial vulvovaginitis
　Vaginal thrush

☑5ᵗʰ **B37.4**　Candidiasis of other urogenital sites

B37.41　Candidal cystitis and urethritis

B37.42　Candidal balanitis

B37.49　Other urogenital candidiasis
　Candidal pyelonephritis

B37.5　Candidal meningitis

B37.6　Candidal endocarditis

B37.7　Candidal sepsis
　Disseminated candidiasis
　Systemic candidiasis

☑ Additional Character Required　　✓x7ᵗʰ Xtension Alert　　Unspecified Dx　　Other Specified Dx　　Manifestation　　▶◀ Revised Text　　● New Code　　▲ Revised Code Title

Certain Infectious and Parasitic Diseases

B37.8–B49

✓5th **B37.8 Candidiasis of** other sites

    B37.81 Candidal esophagitis

    B37.82 Candidal enteritis

         Candidal proctitis

    B37.83 Candidal cheilitis

    B37.84 Candidal otitis externa

    B37.89 Other sites of candidiasis

         Candidal osteomyelitis

B37.9 Candidiasis, unspecified

     Thrush NOS

✓4th **B38 Coccidioidomycosis**

    B38.0 Acute pulmonary coccidioidomycosis

    B38.1 Chronic pulmonary coccidioidomycosis

    B38.2 Pulmonary coccidioidomycosis, unspecified

    B38.3 Cutaneous coccidioidomycosis

    B38.4 Coccidioidomycosis meningitis

    B38.7 Disseminated coccidioidomycosis

         Generalized coccidioidomycosis

  ✓5th **B38.8 Other forms of coccidioidomycosis**

    B38.81 Prostatic coccidioidomycosis   ♂

    B38.89 Other forms of coccidioidomycosis

    B38.9 Coccidioidomycosis, unspecified

✓4th **B39 Histoplasmosis**

     Code first associated AIDS (B20)

     Use additional code for any associated manifestations, such as:

       endocarditis (I39)

       meningitis (G02)

       pericarditis (I32)

       retinititis (H32)

    B39.0 Acute pulmonary histoplasmosis capsulati

    B39.1 Chronic pulmonary histoplasmosis capsulati

    B39.2 Pulmonary histoplasmosis capsulati, unspecified

    B39.3 Disseminated histoplasmosis capsulati

         Generalized histoplasmosis capsulati

    B39.4 Histoplasmosis capsulati, unspecified

         American histoplasmosis

    B39.5 Histoplasmosis duboisii

         African histoplasmosis

    B39.9 Histoplasmosis, unspecified

✓4th **B40 Blastomycosis**

    EXCLUDES1   Brazilian blastomycosis (B41.-)

               keloidal blastomycosis (B48.0)

    B40.0 Acute pulmonary blastomycosis

    B40.1 Chronic pulmonary blastomycosis

    B40.2 Pulmonary blastomycosis, unspecified

    B40.3 Cutaneous blastomycosis

    B40.7 Disseminated blastomycosis

         Generalized blastomycosis

  ✓5th **B40.8 Other forms of blastomycosis**

    B40.81 Blastomycotic meningoencephalitis

         Meningomyelitis due to blastomycosis

    B40.89 Other forms of blastomycosis

    B40.9 Blastomycosis, unspecified

✓4th **B41 Paracoccidioidomycosis**

    INCLUDES   Brazilian blastomycosis

               Lutz' disease

    B41.0 Pulmonary paracoccidioidomycosis

    B41.7 Disseminated paracoccidioidomycosis

         Generalized paracoccidioidomycosis

    B41.8 Other forms of paracoccidioidomycosis

    B41.9 Paracoccidioidomycosis, unspecified

✓4th **B42 Sporotrichosis**

    B42.0 Pulmonary sporotrichosis

    B42.1 Lymphocutaneous sporotrichosis

    B42.7 Disseminated sporotrichosis

         Generalized sporotrichosis

  ✓5th **B42.8 Other forms of sporotrichosis**

    B42.81 Cerebral sporotrichosis

         Meningitis due to sporotrichosis

    B42.82 Sporotrichosis arthritis

    B42.89 Other forms of sporotrichosis

    B42.9 Sporotrichosis, unspecified

✓4th **B43 Chromomycosis and pheomycotic abscess**

    B43.0 Cutaneous chromomycosis

         Dermatitis verrucosa

    B43.1 Pheomycotic brain abscess

         Cerebral chromomycosis

    B43.2 Subcutaneous pheomycotic abscess and cyst

    B43.8 Other forms of chromomycosis

    B43.9 Chromomycosis, unspecified

✓4th **B44 Aspergillosis**

    INCLUDES   aspergilloma

    B44.0 Invasive pulmonary aspergillosis

    B44.1 Other pulmonary aspergillosis

    B44.2 Tonsillar aspergillosis

    B44.7 Disseminated aspergillosis

         Generalized aspergillosis

  ✓5th **B44.8 Other forms of aspergillosis**

    B44.81 Allergic bronchopulmonary aspergillosis

    B44.89 Other forms of aspergillosis

    B44.9 Aspergillosis, unspecified

✓4th **B45 Cryptococcosis**

    B45.0 Pulmonary cryptococcosis

    B45.1 Cerebral cryptococcosis

         Cryptococcal meningitis

         Cryptococcosis meningocerebralis

    B45.2 Cutaneous cryptococcosis

    B45.3 Osseous cryptococcosis

    B45.7 Disseminated cryptococcosis

         Generalized cryptococcosis

    B45.8 Other forms of cryptococcosis

    B45.9 Cryptococcosis, unspecified

✓4th **B46 Zygomycosis**

    B46.0 Pulmonary mucormycosis

    B46.1 Rhinocerebral mucormycosis

    B46.2 Gastrointestinal mucormycosis

    B46.3 Cutaneous mucormycosis

         Subcutaneous mucormycosis

    B46.4 Disseminated mucormycosis

         Generalized mucormycosis

    B46.5 Mucormycosis, unspecified

    B46.8 Other zygomycoses

         Entomophthoromycosis

    B46.9 Zygomycosis, unspecified

         Phycomycosis NOS

✓4th **B47 Mycetoma**

    B47.0 Eumycetoma

         Madura foot, mycotic

         Maduromycosis

    B47.1 Actinomycetoma

    B47.9 Mycetoma, unspecified

         Madura foot NOS

✓4th **B48 Other mycoses, not elsewhere classified**

    B48.0 Lobomycosis

         Keloidal blastomycosis

         Lobo's disease

    B48.1 Rhinosporidiosis

    B48.2 Allescheriasis

         Infection due to Pseudallescheria boydii

         EXCLUDES1   eumycetoma (B47.0)

    B48.3 Geotrichosis

         Geotrichum stomatitis

    B48.4 Penicillosis

    B48.8 Other specified mycoses

         Adiaspiromycosis

         Infection of tissue and organs by Alternaria

         Infection of tissue and organs by Drechslera

         Infection of tissue and organs by Fusarium

         Infection of tissue and organs by saprophytic fungi NEC

         AHA: 2014, 2Q, 13

B49 Unspecified mycosis

     Fungemia NOS

EXCLUDES1 Not coded here   EXCLUDES2 Not included here   N Newborn Age: 0   P Pediatric Age: 0-17   M Maternity Age: 12-55   A Adult Age: 15-124

Protozoal diseases (B50-B64)

EXCLUDES 1 *amebiasis (A06.-)*
other protozoal intestinal diseases (A07.-)

✓4th **B50 Plasmodium falciparum malaria**
      INCLUDES mixed infections of Plasmodium falciparum with any other Plasmodium species

  B50.0 Plasmodium falciparum malaria with cerebral complications
      Cerebral malaria NOS

  B50.8 Other severe and complicated Plasmodium falciparum malaria
      Severe or complicated Plasmodium falciparum malaria NOS

  B50.9 Plasmodium falciparum malaria, unspecified

✓4th **B51 Plasmodium vivax malaria**
      INCLUDES mixed infections of Plasmodium vivax with other Plasmodium species, except Plasmodium falciparum
      EXCLUDES 1 *plasmodium vivax with Plasmodium falciparum (B50.-)*

  B51.0 Plasmodium vivax malaria with rupture of spleen

  B51.8 Plasmodium vivax malaria with other complications

  B51.9 Plasmodium vivax malaria without complication
      Plasmodium vivax malaria NOS

✓4th **B52 Plasmodium malariae malaria**
      INCLUDES mixed infections of Plasmodium malariae with other Plasmodium species, except Plasmodium falciparum and Plasmodium vivax
      EXCLUDES 1 *Plasmodium falciparum (B50.-)*
Plasmodium vivax (B51.-)

  B52.0 Plasmodium malariae malaria with nephropathy

  B52.8 Plasmodium malariae malaria with other complications

  B52.9 Plasmodium malariae malaria without complication
      Plasmodium malariae malaria NOS

✓4th **B53 Other specified malaria**

  B53.0 Plasmodium ovale malaria
      EXCLUDES 1 *Plasmodium ovale with Plasmodium falciparum (B50.-)*
Plasmodium ovale with Plasmodium malariae (B52.-)
Plasmodium ovale with Plasmodium vivax (B51.-)

  B53.1 Malaria due to simian plasmodia
      EXCLUDES 1 *Malaria due to simian plasmodia with Plasmodium falciparum (B50.-)*
Malaria due to simian plasmodia with Plasmodium malariae (B52.-)
Malaria due to simian plasmodia with Plasmodium ovale (B53.0)
Malaria due to simian plasmodia with Plasmodium vivax (B51.-)

  B53.8 Other malaria, not elsewhere classified

  B54 Unspecified malaria

✓4th **B55 Leishmaniasis**

  B55.0 Visceral leishmaniasis
      Kala-azar
      Post-kala-azar dermal leishmaniasis

  B55.1 Cutaneous leishmaniasis

  B55.2 Mucocutaneous leishmaniasis

  B55.9 Leishmaniasis, unspecified

✓4th **B56 African trypanosomiasis**

  B56.0 Gambiense trypanosomiasis
      Infection due to Trypanosoma brucei gambiense
      West African sleeping sickness

  B56.1 Rhodesiense trypanosomiasis
      East African sleeping sickness
      Infection due to Trypanosoma brucei rhodesiense

  B56.9 African trypanosomiasis, unspecified
      Sleeping sickness NOS

✓4th **B57 Chagas' disease**
      INCLUDES American trypanosomiasis
      infection due to Trypanosoma cruzi

  B57.0 Acute Chagas' disease with heart involvement
      Acute Chagas' disease with myocarditis

  B57.1 Acute Chagas' disease without heart involvement
      Acute Chagas' disease NOS

  B57.2 Chagas' disease (chronic) with heart involvement
      American trypanosomiasis NOS
      Chagas' disease (chronic) NOS
      Chagas' disease (chronic) with myocarditis
      Trypanosomiasis NOS

✓5th **B57.3 Chagas' disease (chronic) with digestive system involvement**

  B57.30 Chagas' disease with digestive system involvement, unspecified

  B57.31 Megaesophagus in Chagas' disease

  B57.32 Megacolon in Chagas' disease

  B57.39 Other digestive system involvement in Chagas' disease

✓5th **B57.4 Chagas' disease (chronic) with nervous system involvement**

  B57.40 Chagas' disease with nervous system involvement, unspecified

  B57.41 Meningitis in Chagas' disease

  B57.42 Meningoencephalitis in Chagas' disease

  B57.49 Other nervous system involvement in Chagas' disease

  B57.5 Chagas' disease (chronic) with other organ involvement

✓4th **B58 Toxoplasmosis**
      INCLUDES infection due to Toxoplasma gondii
      EXCLUDES 1 *congenital toxoplasmosis (P37.1)*

✓5th **B58.0 Toxoplasma oculopathy**

  B58.00 Toxoplasma oculopathy, unspecified

  B58.01 Toxoplasma chorioretinitis

  B58.09 Other toxoplasma oculopathy
      Toxoplasma uveitis

  B58.1 Toxoplasma hepatitis

  B58.2 Toxoplasma meningoencephalitis

  B58.3 Pulmonary toxoplasmosis

✓5th **B58.8 Toxoplasmosis with other organ involvement**

  B58.81 Toxoplasma myocarditis

  B58.82 Toxoplasma myositis

  B58.83 Toxoplasma tubulo-interstitial nephropathy
      Toxoplasma pyelonephritis

  B58.89 Toxoplasmosis with other organ involvement

  B58.9 Toxoplasmosis, unspecified

  B59 Pneumocystosis
      Pneumonia due to Pneumocystis carinii
      Pneumonia due to Pneumocystis jiroveci

✓4th **B60 Other protozoal diseases, not elsewhere classified**
      EXCLUDES 1 *cryptosporidiosis (A07.2)*
intestinal microsporidiosis (A07.8)
isosporiasis (A07.3)

  B60.0 Babesiosis
      Piroplasmosis

✓5th **B60.1 Acanthamebiasis**

  B60.10 Acanthamebiasis, unspecified

  B60.11 Meningoencephalitis due to Acanthamoeba (culbertsoni)

  B60.12 Conjunctivitis due to Acanthamoeba

  B60.13 Keratoconjunctivitis due to Acanthamoeba

  B60.19 Other acanthamebic disease

  B60.2 Naegleriasis
      Primary amebic meningoencephalitis

  B60.8 Other specified protozoal diseases
      Microsporidiosis

  B64 Unspecified protozoal disease

Helminthiases (B65-B83)

✓4th **B65 Schistosomiasis [bilharziasis]**
      INCLUDES snail fever

  B65.0 Schistosomiasis due to Schistosoma haematobium [urinary schistosomiasis]

  B65.1 Schistosomiasis due to Schistosoma mansoni [intestinal schistosomiasis]

  B65.2 Schistosomiasis due to Schistosoma japonicum
      Asiatic schistosomiasis

  B65.3 Cercarial dermatitis
      Swimmer's itch

  B65.8 Other schistosomiasis
      Infection due to Schistosoma intercalatum
      Infection due to Schistosoma mattheei
      Infection due to Schistosoma mekongi

  B65.9 Schistosomiasis, unspecified

✓ Additional Character Required   VX7th Xtension Alert   Unspecified Dx   Other Specified Dx   Manifestation   ►◄ Revised Text   ● New Code   ▲ Revised Code Title

Certain Infectious and Parasitic Diseases   B50–B65.9

✓4ᵗʰ **B66 Other fluke infections**

B66.0 Opisthorchiasis
Infection due to cat liver fluke
Infection due to Opisthorchis (felineus)(viverrini)

B66.1 Clonorchiasis
Chinese liver fluke disease
Infection due to Clonorchis sinensis
Oriental liver fluke disease

B66.2 Dicroceliasis
Infection due to Dicrocoelium dendriticum
Lancet fluke infection

B66.3 Fascioliasis
Infection due to Fasciola gigantica
Infection due to Fasciola hepatica
Infection due to Fasciola indica
Sheep liver fluke disease

B66.4 Paragonimiasis
Infection due to Paragonimus species
Lung fluke disease
Pulmonary distomiasis

B66.5 Fasciolopsiasis
Infection due to Fasciolopsis buski
Intestinal distomiasis

B66.8 Other specified fluke infections
Echinostomiasis
Heterophyiasis
Metagonimiasis
Nanophyetiasis
Watsoniasis

B66.9 Fluke infection, unspecified

✓4ᵗʰ **B67 Echinococcosis**
INCLUDES hydatidosis

B67.0 Echinococcus granulosus infection of liver

B67.1 Echinococcus granulosus infection of lung

B67.2 Echinococcus granulosus infection of bone

✓5ᵗʰ **B67.3 Echinococcus granulosus infection, other and multiple sites**

B67.31 Echinococcus granulosus infection, thyroid gland

B67.32 Echinococcus granulosus infection, multiple sites

B67.39 Echinococcus granulosus infection, other sites

B67.4 Echinococcus granulosus infection, unspecified
Dog tapeworm (infection)

B67.5 Echinococcus multilocularis infection of liver

✓5ᵗʰ **B67.6 Echinococcus multilocularis infection, other and multiple sites**

B67.61 Echinococcus multilocularis infection, multiple sites

B67.69 Echinococcus multilocularis infection, other sites

B67.7 Echinococcus multilocularis infection, unspecified

B67.8 Echinococcosis, unspecified, of liver

✓5ᵗʰ **B67.9 Echinococcosis, other and unspecified**

B67.90 Echinococcosis, unspecified
Echinococcosis NOS

B67.99 Other echinococcosis

✓4ᵗʰ **B68 Taeniasis**
EXCLUDES 1 cysticercosis (B69.-)

B68.0 Taenia solium taeniasis
Pork tapeworm (infection)

B68.1 Taenia saginata taeniasis
Beef tapeworm (infection)
Infection due to adult tapeworm Taenia saginata

B68.9 Taeniasis, unspecified

✓4ᵗʰ **B69 Cysticercosis**
INCLUDES cysticerciasis infection due to larval form of Taenia solium

B69.0 Cysticercosis of central nervous system

B69.1 Cysticercosis of eye

✓5ᵗʰ **B69.8 Cysticercosis of other sites**

B69.81 Myositis in cysticercosis

B69.89 Cysticercosis of other sites

B69.9 Cysticercosis, unspecified

✓4ᵗʰ **B70 Diphyllobothriasis and sparganosis**

B70.0 Diphyllobothriasis
Diphyllobothrium (adult) (latum) (pacificum) infection
Fish tapeworm (infection)
EXCLUDES 2 larval diphyllobothriasis (B70.1)

B70.1 Sparganosis
Infection due to Sparganum (mansoni) (proliferum)
Infection due to Spirometra larva
Larval diphyllobothriasis
Spirometrosis

✓4ᵗʰ **B71 Other cestode infections**

B71.0 Hymenolepiasis
Dwarf tapeworm infection
Rat tapeworm (infection)

B71.1 Dipylidiasis

B71.8 Other specified cestode infections
Coenurosis

B71.9 Cestode infection, unspecified
Tapeworm (infection) NOS

B72 Dracunculiasis
INCLUDES guinea worm infection
infection due to Dracunculus medinensis

✓4ᵗʰ **B73 Onchocerciasis**
INCLUDES onchocerca volvulus infection
onchocercosis
river blindness

✓5ᵗʰ **B73.0 Onchocerciasis with eye disease**

B73.00 Onchocerciasis with eye involvement, unspecified

B73.01 Onchocerciasis with endophthalmitis

B73.02 Onchocerciasis with glaucoma

B73.09 Onchocerciasis with other eye involvement
Infestation of eyelid due to onchocerciasis

B73.1 Onchocerciasis without eye disease

✓4ᵗʰ **B74 Filariasis**
EXCLUDES 2 onchocerciasis (B73)
tropical (pulmonary) eosinophilia NOS (J82)

B74.0 Filariasis due to Wuchereria bancrofti
Bancroftian elephantiasis
Bancroftian filariasis

B74.1 Filariasis due to Brugia malayi

B74.2 Filariasis due to Brugia timori

B74.3 Loiasis
Calabar swelling
Eyeworm disease of Africa
Loa loa infection

B74.4 Mansonelliasis
Infection due to Mansonella ozzardi
Infection due to Mansonella perstans
Infection due to Mansonella streptocerca

B74.8 Other filariases
Dirofilariasis

B74.9 Filariasis, unspecified

B75 Trichinellosis
INCLUDES infection due to Trichinella species
trichiniasis

✓4ᵗʰ **B76 Hookworm diseases**
INCLUDES uncinariasis

B76.0 Ancylostomiasis
Infection due to Ancylostoma species

B76.1 Necatoriasis
Infection due to Necator americanus

B76.8 Other hookworm diseases

B76.9 Hookworm disease, unspecified
Cutaneous larva migrans NOS

✓4ᵗʰ **B77 Ascariasis**
INCLUDES ascaridiasis
roundworm infection

B77.0 Ascariasis with intestinal complications

✓5ᵗʰ **B77.8 Ascariasis with other complications**

B77.81 Ascariasis pneumonia

B77.89 Ascariasis with other complications

B77.9 Ascariasis, unspecified

✓4ᵗʰ **B78 Strongyloidiasis**
EXCLUDES 1 trichostrongyliasis (B81.2)

B78.0 Intestinal strongyloidiasis

B78.1 Cutaneous strongyloidiasis

B78.7 Disseminated strongyloidiasis

B78.9 Strongyloidiasis, unspecified

EXCLUDES 1 Not coded here   EXCLUDES 2 Not included here   N Newborn Age: 0   P Pediatric Age: 0-17   M Maternity Age: 12-55   A Adult Age: 15-124

438   ICD-10-CM Draft (2015)

B79 Trichuriasis
> INCLUDES   trichocephaliasis
> whipworm (disease)(infection)

B80 Enterobiasis
> INCLUDES   oxyuriasis
> pinworm infection
> threadworm infection

✓4th B81 Other intestinal helminthiases, not elsewhere classified
> EXCLUDES 1   angiostrongyliasis due to Parastrongylus cantonensis (B83.2)

B81.0 Anisakiasis
> Infection due to Anisakis larva

B81.1 Intestinal capillariasis
> Capillariasis NOS
> Infection due to Capillaria philippinensis
> EXCLUDES 2   hepatic capillariasis (B83.8)

B81.2 Trichostrongyliasis

B81.3 Intestinal angiostrongyliasis
> Angiostrongyliasis due to Parastrongylus costaricensis

B81.4 Mixed intestinal helminthiases
> Infection due to intestinal helminths classified to more than one of the categories B65.0-B81.3 and B81.8
> Mixed helminthiasis NOS

B81.8 Other specified intestinal helminthiases
> Infection due to Oesophagostomum species [esophagostomiasis]
> Infection due to Ternidens diminutus [ternidensiasis]

✓4th B82 Unspecified intestinal parasitism

B82.0 Intestinal helminthiasis, unspecified

B82.9 Intestinal parasitism, unspecified

✓4th B83 Other helminthiases
> EXCLUDES 1   capillariasis NOS (B81.1)
> EXCLUDES 2   intestinal capillariasis (B81.1)

B83.0 Visceral larva migrans
> Toxocariasis

B83.1 Gnathostomiasis
> Wandering swelling

B83.2 Angiostrongyliasis due to Parastrongylus cantonensis
> Eosinophilic meningoencephalitis due to Parastrongylus cantonensis
> EXCLUDES 2   intestinal angiostrongyliasis (B81.3)

B83.3 Syngamiasis
> Syngamosis

B83.4 Internal hirudiniasis
> EXCLUDES 2   external hirudiniasis (B88.3)

B83.8 Other specified helminthiases
> Acanthocephaliasis
> Gongylonemiasis
> Hepatic capillariasis
> Metastrongyliasis
> Thelaziasis

B83.9 Helminthiasis, unspecified
> Worms NOS
> EXCLUDES 1   intestinal helminthiasis NOS (B82.0)

Pediculosis, acariasis and other infestations (B85-B89)

✓4th B85 Pediculosis and phthiriasis

B85.0 Pediculosis due to Pediculus humanus capitis
> Head-louse infestation

B85.1 Pediculosis due to Pediculus humanus corporis
> Body-louse infestation

B85.2 Pediculosis, unspecified

B85.3 Phthiriasis
> Infestation by crab-louse
> Infestation by Phthirus pubis

B85.4 Mixed pediculosis and phthiriasis
> Infestation classifiable to more than one of the categories B85.0-B85.3

B86 Scabies
> Sarcoptic itch

✓4th B87 Myiasis
> INCLUDES   infestation by larva of flies

B87.0 Cutaneous myiasis
> Creeping myiasis

B87.1 Wound myiasis
> Traumatic myiasis

B87.2 Ocular myiasis

B87.3 Nasopharyngeal myiasis
> Laryngeal myiasis

B87.4 Aural myiasis

✓5th B87.8 Myiasis of other sites

B87.81 Genitourinary myiasis

B87.82 Intestinal myiasis

B87.89 Myiasis of other sites

B87.9 Myiasis, unspecified

✓4th B88 Other infestations

B88.0 Other acariasis
> Acarine dermatitis
> Dermatitis due to Demodex species
> Dermatitis due to Dermanyssus gallinae
> Dermatitis due to Liponyssoides sanguineus
> Trombiculosis
> EXCLUDES 2   scabies (B86)

B88.1 Tungiasis [sandflea infestation]

B88.2 Other arthropod infestations
> Scarabiasis

B88.3 External hirudiniasis
> Leech infestation NOS
> EXCLUDES 2   internal hirudiniasis (B83.4)

B88.8 Other specified infestations
> Ichthyoparasitism due to Vandellia cirrhosa
> Linguatulosis
> Porocephaliasis

B88.9 Infestation, unspecified
> Infestation (skin) NOS
> Infestation by mites NOS
> Skin parasites NOS

B89 Unspecified parasitic disease

Sequelae of infectious and parasitic diseases (B90-B94)

> NOTE   Categories B90-B94 are to be used to indicate conditions in categories A00-B89 as the cause of sequelae, which are themselves classified elsewhere. The "sequelae" include conditions specified as such; they also include residuals of diseases classifiable to the above categories if there is evidence that the disease itself is no longer present. Codes from these categories are not to be used for chronic infections. Code chronic current infections to active infectious disease as appropriate.

Code first condition resulting from (sequela) the infectious or parasitic disease

✓4th B90 Sequelae of tuberculosis

B90.0 Sequelae of central nervous system tuberculosis

B90.1 Sequelae of genitourinary tuberculosis

B90.2 Sequelae of tuberculosis of bones and joints

B90.8 Sequelae of tuberculosis of other organs
> EXCLUDES 2   sequelae of respiratory tuberculosis (B90.9)

B90.9 Sequelae of respiratory and unspecified tuberculosis
> Sequelae of tuberculosis NOS

B91 Sequelae of poliomyelitis
> EXCLUDES 1   postpolio syndrome (G14)

B92 Sequelae of leprosy

✓4th B94 Sequelae of other and unspecified infectious and parasitic diseases

B94.0 Sequelae of trachoma

B94.1 Sequelae of viral encephalitis

B94.2 Sequelae of viral hepatitis

B94.8 Sequelae of other specified infectious and parasitic diseases

B94.9 Sequelae of unspecified infectious and parasitic disease

Bacterial and viral infectious agents (B95-B97)

> NOTE   These categories are provided for use as supplementary or additional codes to identify the infectious agent(s) in diseases classified elsewhere.

✓4th B95 Streptococcus, Staphylococcus, and Enterococcus as the cause of diseases classified elsewhere

B95.0 Streptococcus, group A, as the cause of diseases classified elsewhere

B95.1 Streptococcus, group B, as the cause of diseases classified elsewhere

B95.2 Enterococcus as the cause of diseases classified elsewhere

---

✓ Additional Character Required   ✓x7th Xtension Alert   Unspecified Dx   Other Specified Dx   Manifestation   ►◄ Revised Text   ● New Code   ▲ Revised Code Title

Certain Infectious and Parasitic Diseases

B95.3–B99.9

B95.3 Streptococcus pneumoniae as the cause of diseases classified elsewhere

B95.4 Other streptococcus as the cause of diseases classified elsewhere

B95.5 Unspecified streptococcus as the cause of diseases classified elsewhere

✓5th **B95.6** Staphylococcus aureus as the cause of diseases classified elsewhere

     B95.61 Methicillin susceptible Staphylococcus aureus infection as the cause of diseases classified elsewhere
         Methicillin susceptible Staphylococcus aureus (MSSA) infection as the cause of diseases classified elsewhere
         Staphylococcus aureus infection NOS as the cause of diseases classified elsewhere

     B95.62 Methicillin resistant Staphylococcus aureus infection as the cause of diseases classified elsewhere
         Methicillin resistant Staphylococcus aureus (MRSA) infection as the cause of diseases classified elsewhere

B95.7 Other staphylococcus as the cause of diseases classified elsewhere

B95.8 Unspecified staphylococcus as the cause of diseases classified elsewhere

✓4th **B96** Other bacterial agents as the cause of diseases classified elsewhere

     B96.0 Mycoplasma pneumoniae [M. pneumoniae] as the cause of diseases classified elsewhere
         Pleuro-pneumonia-like-organism [PPLO]

     B96.1 Klebsiella pneumoniae [K. pneumoniae] as the cause of diseases classified elsewhere

✓5th **B96.2** Escherichia coli [E. coli] as the cause of diseases classified elsewhere

     B96.20 Unspecified Escherichia coli [E. coli] as the cause of diseases classified elsewhere
         Escherichia coli [E. coli] NOS

     B96.21 Shiga toxin-producing Escherichia coli [E. coli] (STEC) O157 as the cause of diseases classified elsewhere
         E. coli O157:H- (nonmotile) with confirmation of Shiga toxin
         E. coli O157 with confirmation of Shiga toxin when H antigen is unknown, or is not H7
         O157:H7 Escherichia coli [E.coli] with or without confirmation of Shiga toxin-production
         Shiga toxin-producing Escherichia coli [E.coli] O157:H7 with or without confirmation of Shiga toxin-production
         STEC O157:H7 with or without confirmation of Shiga toxin-production

     B96.22 Other specified Shiga toxin-producing Escherichia coli [E. coli] (STEC) as the cause of diseases classified elsewhere
         Non-O157 Shiga toxin-producing Escherichia coli [E.coli]
         Non-O157 Shiga toxin-producing Escherichia coli [E.coli] with known O group

     B96.23 Unspecified Shiga toxin-producing Escherichia coli [E. coli] (STEC) as the cause of diseases classified elsewhere
         Shiga toxin-producing Escherichia coli [E. coli] with unspecified O group
         STEC NOS

     B96.29 Other Escherichia coli [E. coli] as the cause of diseases classified elsewhere
         Non-Shiga toxin-producing E. coli

     B96.3 Hemophilus influenzae [H. influenzae] as the cause of diseases classified elsewhere

     B96.4 Proteus (mirabilis) (morganii) as the cause of diseases classified elsewhere

     B96.5 Pseudomonas (aeruginosa) (mallei) (pseudomallei) as the cause of diseases classified elsewhere

     B96.6 Bacteroides fragilis [B. fragilis] as the cause of diseases classified elsewhere

     B96.7 Clostridium perfringens [C. perfringens] as the cause of diseases classified elsewhere

✓5th **B96.8** Other specified bacterial agents as the cause of diseases classified elsewhere

     B96.81 Helicobacter pylori [H. pylori] as the cause of diseases classified elsewhere

     B96.82 Vibrio vulnificus as the cause of diseases classified elsewhere

     B96.89 Other specified bacterial agents as the cause of diseases classified elsewhere

✓4th **B97** Viral agents as the cause of diseases classified elsewhere

     B97.0 Adenovirus as the cause of diseases classified elsewhere

✓5th **B97.1** Enterovirus as the cause of diseases classified elsewhere

     B97.10 Unspecified enterovirus as the cause of diseases classified elsewhere

     B97.11 Coxsackievirus as the cause of diseases classified elsewhere

     B97.12 Echovirus as the cause of diseases classified elsewhere

     B97.19 Other enterovirus as the cause of diseases classified elsewhere

✓5th **B97.2** Coronavirus as the cause of diseases classified elsewhere

     B97.21 SARS-associated coronavirus as the cause of diseases classified elsewhere
         EXCLUDES 1 pneumonia due to SARS-associated coronavirus (J12.81)

     B97.29 Other coronavirus as the cause of diseases classified elsewhere

✓5th **B97.3** Retrovirus as the cause of diseases classified elsewhere
     EXCLUDES 1 human immunodeficiency virus [HIV} disease (B20)

     B97.30 Unspecified retrovirus as the cause of diseases classified elsewhere

     B97.31 Lentivirus as the cause of diseases classified elsewhere

     B97.32 Oncovirus as the cause of diseases classified elsewhere

     B97.33 Human T-cell lymphotrophic virus, type I [HTLV-I] as the cause of diseases classified elsewhere

     B97.34 Human T-cell lymphotrophic virus, type II [HTLV-II] as the cause of diseases classified elsewhere

     B97.35 Human immunodeficiency virus, type 2 [HIV 2] as the cause of diseases classified elsewhere

     B97.39 Other retrovirus as the cause of diseases classified elsewhere

     B97.4 Respiratory syncytial virus as the cause of diseases classified elsewhere

     B97.5 Reovirus as the cause of diseases classified elsewhere

     B97.6 Parvovirus as the cause of diseases classified elsewhere

     B97.7 Papillomavirus as the cause of diseases classified elsewhere

✓5th **B97.8** Other viral agents as the cause of diseases classified elsewhere

     B97.81 Human metapneumovirus as the cause of diseases classified elsewhere

     B97.89 Other viral agents as the cause of diseases classified elsewhere

Other infectious diseases (B99)

✓4th **B99** Other and unspecified infectious diseases

     B99.8 Other infectious disease

     B99.9 Unspecified infectious disease

EXCLUDES 1 Not coded here   **EXCLUDES 2** Not included here   N Newborn Age: 0   P Pediatric Age: 0-17   M Maternity Age: 12-55   A Adult Age: 15-124

Chapter 2. Neoplasms (C00-D49)

NOTE

Functional activity

All neoplasms are classified in this chapter, whether they are functionally active or not. An additional code from Chapter 4 may be used, to identify functional activity associated with any neoplasm.

Morphology [Histology]

Chapter 2 classifies neoplasms primarily by site (topography), with broad groupings for behavior, malignant, in situ, benign, etc. The Table of Neoplasms should be used to identify the correct topography code. In a few cases, such as for malignant melanoma and certain neuroendocrine tumors, the morphology (histologic type) is included in the category and codes.

Primary malignant neoplasms overlapping site boundaries

A primary malignant neoplasm that overlaps two or more contiguous (next to each other) sites should be classified to the subcategory/code .8 ("overlapping lesion"), unless the combination is specifically indexed elsewhere. For multiple neoplasms of the same site that are not contiguous, such as tumors in different quadrants of the same breast, codes for each site should be assigned.

Malignant neoplasm of ectopic tissue

Malignant neoplasms of ectopic tissue are to be coded to the site mentioned, e.g., ectopic pancreatic malignant neoplasms are coded to pancreas, unspecified (C25.9).

This chapter contains the following blocks:

C00-C14   Malignant neoplasms of lip, oral cavity and pharynx
C15-C26   Malignant neoplasms of digestive organs
C30-C39   Malignant neoplasms of respiratory and intrathoracic organs
C40-C41   Malignant neoplasms of bone and articular cartilage
C43-C44   Melanoma and other malignant neoplasms of skin
C45-C49   Malignant neoplasms of mesothelial and soft tissue
C50   Malignant neoplasms of breast
C51-C58   Malignant neoplasms of female genital organs
C60-C63   Malignant neoplasms of male genital organs
C64-C68   Malignant neoplasms of urinary tract
C69-C72   Malignant neoplasms of eye, brain and other parts of central nervous system
C73-C75   Malignant neoplasms of thyroid and other endocrine glands
C7A   Malignant neuroendocrine tumors
C7B   Secondary neuroendocrine tumors
C76-C80   Malignant neoplasms of ill-defined, other secondary and unspecified sites
C81-C96   Malignant neoplasms of lymphoid, hematopoietic and related tissue
D00-D09   In situ neoplasms
D10-D36   Benign neoplasms, except benign neuroendocrine tumors
D3A   Benign neuroendocrine tumors
D37-D48   Neoplasms of uncertain behavior, polycythemia vera and myelodysplastic syndromes
D49   Neoplasms of unspecified behavior

MALIGNANT NEOPLASMS (C00-C96)

NOTE Malignant neoplasms, stated or presumed to be primary (of specified sites), and certain specified histologies, except neuroendocrine, and of lymphoid, hematopoietic and related tissue (C00-C75).

Malignant neoplasms of lip, oral cavity and pharynx (C00-C14)

☑4ᵗʰ **C00   Malignant neoplasm of lip**
   Use additional code to identify:
      alcohol abuse and dependence (F10.-)
      history of tobacco use (Z87.891)
      tobacco dependence (F17.-)
      tobacco use (Z72.0)
   EXCLUDES 1 malignant melanoma of lip (C43.0)
                   Merkel cell carcinoma of lip (C4A.0)
                   other and unspecified malignant neoplasm of skin of lip (C44.0-)

   C00.0   Malignant neoplasm of external upper lip
      Malignant neoplasm of lipstick area of upper lip
      Malignant neoplasm of upper lip NOS
      Malignant neoplasm of vermilion border of upper lip

   C00.1   Malignant neoplasm of external lower lip
      Malignant neoplasm of lower lip NOS
      Malignant neoplasm of lipstick area of lower lip
      Malignant neoplasm of vermilion border of lower lip

   C00.2   Malignant neoplasm of external lip, unspecified
      Malignant neoplasm of vermilion border of lip NOS

   C00.3   Malignant neoplasm of upper lip, inner aspect
      Malignant neoplasm of buccal aspect of upper lip
      Malignant neoplasm of frenulum of upper lip
      Malignant neoplasm of mucosa of upper lip
      Malignant neoplasm of oral aspect of upper lip

   C00.4   Malignant neoplasm of lower lip, inner aspect
      Malignant neoplasm of buccal aspect of lower lip
      Malignant neoplasm of frenulum of lower lip
      Malignant neoplasm of mucosa of lower lip
      Malignant neoplasm of oral aspect of lower lip

   C00.5   Malignant neoplasm of lip, unspecified, inner aspect
      Malignant neoplasm of buccal aspect of lip, unspecified
      Malignant neoplasm of frenulum of lip, unspecified
      Malignant neoplasm of mucosa of lip, unspecified
      Malignant neoplasm of oral aspect of lip, unspecified

   C00.6   Malignant neoplasm of commissure of lip, unspecified

   C00.8   Malignant neoplasm of overlapping sites of lip

   C00.9   Malignant neoplasm of lip, unspecified

C01   Malignant neoplasm of base of tongue
   Malignant neoplasm of dorsal surface of base of tongue
   Malignant neoplasm of fixed part of tongue NOS
   Malignant neoplasm of posterior third of tongue
   Use additional code to identify:
      alcohol abuse and dependence (F10.-)
      history of tobacco use (Z87.891)
      tobacco dependence (F17.-)
      tobacco use (Z72.0)

☑4ᵗʰ **C02   Malignant neoplasm of other and unspecified parts of tongue**
   Use additional code to identify:
      alcohol abuse and dependence (F10.-)
      history of tobacco use (Z87.891)
      tobacco dependence (F17.-)
      tobacco use (Z72.0)

   C02.0   Malignant neoplasm of dorsal surface of tongue
      Malignant neoplasm of anterior two-thirds of tongue, dorsal surface
      EXCLUDES 2 malignant neoplasm of dorsal surface of base of tongue (C01)

   C02.1   Malignant neoplasm of border of tongue
      Malignant neoplasm of tip of tongue

   C02.2   Malignant neoplasm of ventral surface of tongue
      Malignant neoplasm of anterior two-thirds of tongue, ventral surface
      Malignant neoplasm of frenulum linguae

   C02.3   Malignant neoplasm of anterior two-thirds of tongue, part unspecified
      Malignant neoplasm of middle third of tongue NOS
      Malignant neoplasm of mobile part of tongue NOS

   C02.4   Malignant neoplasm of lingual tonsil
      EXCLUDES 2 malignant neoplasm of tonsil NOS (C09.9)

   C02.8   Malignant neoplasm of overlapping sites of tongue
      Malignant neoplasm of two or more contiguous sites of tongue

   C02.9   Malignant neoplasm of tongue, unspecified

☑4ᵗʰ **C03   Malignant neoplasm of gum**
   INCLUDES malignant neoplasm of alveolar (ridge) mucosa
                 malignant neoplasm of gingiva
   Use additional code to identify:
      alcohol abuse and dependence (F10.-)
      history of tobacco use (Z87.891)
      tobacco dependence (F17.-)
      tobacco use (Z72.0)
   EXCLUDES 2 malignant odontogenic neoplasms (C41.0-C41.1)

   C03.0   Malignant neoplasm of upper gum

   C03.1   Malignant neoplasm of lower gum

   C03.9   Malignant neoplasm of gum, unspecified

☑4ᵗʰ **C04   Malignant neoplasm of floor of mouth**
   Use additional code to identify:
      alcohol abuse and dependence (F10.-)
      history of tobacco use (Z87.891)
      tobacco dependence (F17.-)
      tobacco use (Z72.0)

   C04.0   Malignant neoplasm of anterior floor of mouth
      Malignant neoplasm of anterior to the premolar-canine junction

   C04.1   Malignant neoplasm of lateral floor of mouth

   C04.8   Malignant neoplasm of overlapping sites of floor of mouth

   C04.9   Malignant neoplasm of floor of mouth, unspecified

C00–C04.9

☑ Additional Character Required   ✗7ᵗʰ Xtension Alert   Unspecified Dx   Other Specified Dx   Manifestation   ▶◀ Revised Text   ● New Code   ▲ Revised Code Title

Neoplasms

C05–C12

✓4ᵗʰ **C05** **Malignant neoplasm of palate**
Use additional code to identify:
alcohol abuse and dependence (F10.-)
history of tobacco use (Z87.891)
tobacco dependence (F17.-)
tobacco use (Z72.0)
EXCLUDES 1   Kaposi's sarcoma of palate (C46.2)

C05.0 **Malignant neoplasm of hard palate**

C05.1 **Malignant neoplasm of soft palate**
EXCLUDES 2   malignant neoplasm of nasopharyngeal surface of soft palate (C11.3)

C05.2 **Malignant neoplasm of uvula**

C05.8 **Malignant neoplasm of overlapping sites of palate**

C05.9 **Malignant neoplasm of palate, unspecified**
Malignant neoplasm of roof of mouth

✓4ᵗʰ **C06** **Malignant neoplasm of other and unspecified parts of mouth**
Use additional code to identify:
alcohol abuse and dependence (F10.-)
history of tobacco use (Z87.891)
tobacco dependence (F17.-)
tobacco use (Z72.0)

C06.0 **Malignant neoplasm of cheek mucosa**
Malignant neoplasm of buccal mucosa NOS
Malignant neoplasm of internal cheek

C06.1 **Malignant neoplasm of vestibule of mouth**
Malignant neoplasm of buccal sulcus (upper) (lower)
Malignant neoplasm of labial sulcus (upper) (lower)

C06.2 **Malignant neoplasm of retromolar area**

✓5ᵗʰ **C06.8** **Malignant neoplasm of overlapping sites of other and unspecified parts of mouth**

C06.80 **Malignant neoplasm of overlapping sites of unspecified parts of mouth**

C06.89 **Malignant neoplasm of overlapping sites of other parts of mouth**
"book leaf" neoplasm [ventral surface of tongue and floor of mouth]

C06.9 **Malignant neoplasm of mouth, unspecified**
Malignant neoplasm of minor salivary gland, unspecified site
Malignant neoplasm of oral cavity NOS

C07 **Malignant neoplasm of parotid gland**
Use additional code to identify:
alcohol abuse and dependence (F10.-)
exposure to environmental tobacco smoke (Z77.22)
exposure to tobacco smoke in the perinatal period (P96.81)
history of tobacco use (Z87.891)
occupational exposure to environmental tobacco smoke (Z57.31)
tobacco dependence (F17.-)
tobacco use (Z72.0)

✓4ᵗʰ **C08** **Malignant neoplasm of other and unspecified major salivary glands**
INCLUDES   malignant neoplasm of salivary ducts
Use additional code to identify:
alcohol abuse and dependence (F10.-)
exposure to environmental tobacco smoke (Z77.22)
exposure to tobacco smoke in the perinatal period (P96.81)
history of tobacco use (Z87.891)
occupational exposure to environmental tobacco smoke (Z57.31)
tobacco dependence (F17.-)
tobacco use (Z72.0)
EXCLUDES 1   malignant neoplasms of specified minor salivary glands which are classified according to their anatomical location
EXCLUDES 2   malignant neoplasms of minor salivary glands NOS (C06.9)
malignant neoplasm of parotid gland (C07)

C08.0 **Malignant neoplasm of submandibular gland**
Malignant neoplasm of submaxillary gland

C08.1 **Malignant neoplasm of sublingual gland**

C08.9 **Malignant neoplasm of major salivary gland, unspecified**
Malignant neoplasm of salivary gland (major) NOS

✓4ᵗʰ **C09** **Malignant neoplasm of tonsil**
Use additional code to identify:
alcohol abuse and dependence (F10.-)
exposure to environmental tobacco smoke (Z77.22)
exposure to tobacco smoke in the perinatal period (P96.81)
history of tobacco use (Z87.891)
occupational exposure to environmental tobacco smoke (Z57.31)
tobacco dependence (F17.-)
tobacco use (Z72.0)
EXCLUDES 2   malignant neoplasm of lingual tonsil (C02.4)
malignant neoplasm of pharyngeal tonsil (C11.1)

C09.0 **Malignant neoplasm of tonsillar fossa**

C09.1 **Malignant neoplasm of tonsillar pillar (anterior) (posterior)**

C09.8 **Malignant neoplasm of overlapping sites of tonsil**

C09.9 **Malignant neoplasm of tonsil, unspecified**
Malignant neoplasm of tonsil NOS
Malignant neoplasm of faucial tonsils
Malignant neoplasm of palatine tonsils

✓4ᵗʰ **C10** **Malignant neoplasm of oropharynx**
Use additional code to identify:
alcohol abuse and dependence (F10.-)
exposure to environmental tobacco smoke (Z77.22)
exposure to tobacco smoke in the perinatal period (P96.81)
history of tobacco use (Z87.891)
occupational exposure to environmental tobacco smoke (Z57.31)
tobacco dependence (F17.-)
tobacco use (Z72.0)
EXCLUDES 2   malignant neoplasm of tonsil (C09.-)

C10.0 **Malignant neoplasm of vallecula**

C10.1 **Malignant neoplasm of anterior surface of epiglottis**
Malignant neoplasm of epiglottis, free border [margin]
Malignant neoplasm of glossoepiglottic fold(s)
EXCLUDES 2   malignant neoplasm of epiglottis (suprahyoid portion) NOS (C32.1)

C10.2 **Malignant neoplasm of lateral wall of oropharynx**

C10.3 **Malignant neoplasm of posterior wall of oropharynx**

C10.4 **Malignant neoplasm of branchial cleft**
Malignant neoplasm of branchial cyst [site of neoplasm]

C10.8 **Malignant neoplasm of overlapping sites of oropharynx**
Malignant neoplasm of junctional region of oropharynx

C10.9 **Malignant neoplasm of oropharynx, unspecified**

✓4ᵗʰ **C11** **Malignant neoplasm of nasopharynx**
Use additional code to identify:
exposure to environmental tobacco smoke (Z77.22)
exposure to tobacco smoke in the perinatal period (P96.81)
history of tobacco use (Z87.891)
occupational exposure to environmental tobacco smoke (Z57.31)
tobacco dependence (F17.-)
tobacco use (Z72.0)

C11.0 **Malignant neoplasm of superior wall of nasopharynx**
Malignant neoplasm of roof of nasopharynx

C11.1 **Malignant neoplasm of posterior wall of nasopharynx**
Malignant neoplasm of adenoid
Malignant neoplasm of pharyngeal tonsil

C11.2 **Malignant neoplasm of lateral wall of nasopharynx**
Malignant neoplasm of fossa of Rosenmüller
Malignant neoplasm of opening of auditory tube
Malignant neoplasm of pharyngeal recess

C11.3 **Malignant neoplasm of anterior wall of nasopharynx**
Malignant neoplasm of floor of nasopharynx
Malignant neoplasm of nasopharyngeal (anterior) (posterior) surface of soft palate
Malignant neoplasm of posterior margin of nasal choana
Malignant neoplasm of posterior margin of nasal septum

C11.8 **Malignant neoplasm of overlapping sites of nasopharynx**

C11.9 **Malignant neoplasm of nasopharynx, unspecified**
Malignant neoplasm of nasopharyngeal wall NOS

C12 **Malignant neoplasm of pyriform sinus**
Malignant neoplasm of pyriform fossa
Use additional code to identify:
exposure to environmental tobacco smoke (Z77.22)
exposure to tobacco smoke in the perinatal period (P96.81)
history of tobacco use (Z87.891)
occupational exposure to environmental tobacco smoke (Z57.31)
tobacco dependence (F17.-)
tobacco use (Z72.0)

EXCLUDES 1 Not coded here   EXCLUDES 2 Not included here   N Newborn Age: 0   P Pediatric Age: 0-17   M Maternity Age: 12-55   A Adult Age: 15-124

442   ICD-10-CM Draft (2015)

☑4ᵗʰ **C13 Malignant neoplasm of hypopharynx**
Use additional code to identify:
exposure to environmental tobacco smoke (Z77.22)
exposure to tobacco smoke in the perinatal period (P96.81)
history of tobacco use (Z87.891)
occupational exposure to environmental tobacco smoke (Z57.31)
tobacco dependence (F17.-)
tobacco use (Z72.0)
EXCLUDES 2 *malignant neoplasm of pyriform sinus (C12)*

C13.0 Malignant neoplasm of postcricoid region

C13.1 Malignant neoplasm of aryepiglottic fold, hypopharyngeal aspect
Malignant neoplasm of aryepiglottic fold, marginal zone
Malignant neoplasm of aryepiglottic fold NOS
Malignant neoplasm of interarytenoid fold, marginal zone
Malignant neoplasm of interarytenoid fold NOS
EXCLUDES 2 *malignant neoplasm of aryepiglottic fold or interarytenoid fold, laryngeal aspect (C32.1)*

C13.2 Malignant neoplasm of posterior wall of hypopharynx

C13.8 Malignant neoplasm of overlapping sites of hypopharynx

C13.9 Malignant neoplasm of hypopharynx, unspecified
Malignant neoplasm of hypopharyngeal wall NOS

☑4ᵗʰ **C14 Malignant neoplasm of other and ill-defined sites in the lip, oral cavity and pharynx**
Use additional code to identify:
alcohol abuse and dependence (F10.-)
exposure to environmental tobacco smoke (Z77.22)
exposure to tobacco smoke in the perinatal period (P96.81)
history of tobacco use (Z87.891)
occupational exposure to environmental tobacco smoke (Z57.31)
tobacco dependence (F17.-)
tobacco use (Z72.0)
EXCLUDES 1 *malignant neoplasm of oral cavity NOS (C06.9)*

C14.0 Malignant neoplasm of pharynx, unspecified

C14.2 Malignant neoplasm of Waldeyer's ring

C14.8 Malignant neoplasm of overlapping sites of lip, oral cavity and pharynx
Primary malignant neoplasm of two or more contiguous sites of lip, oral cavity and pharynx
EXCLUDES 1 *"book leaf" neoplasm [ventral surface of tongue and floor of mouth] (C06.89)*

Malignant neoplasms of digestive organs (C15-C26)
EXCLUDES 1 *Kaposi's sarcoma of gastrointestinal sites (C46.4)*

☑4ᵗʰ **C15 Malignant neoplasm of esophagus**
Use additional code to identify:
alcohol abuse and dependence (F10.-)

C15.3 Malignant neoplasm of upper third of esophagus

C15.4 Malignant neoplasm of middle third of esophagus

C15.5 Malignant neoplasm of lower third of esophagus
EXCLUDES 1 *malignant neoplasm of cardio-esophageal junction (C16.0)*

C15.8 Malignant neoplasm of overlapping sites of esophagus

C15.9 Malignant neoplasm of esophagus, unspecified

☑4ᵗʰ **C16 Malignant neoplasm of stomach**
Use additional code to identify:
alcohol abuse and dependence (F10.-)
EXCLUDES 2 *malignant carcinoid tumor of the stomach (C7A.092)*

C16.0 Malignant neoplasm of cardia
Malignant neoplasm of cardiac orifice
Malignant neoplasm of cardio-esophageal junction
Malignant neoplasm of esophagus and stomach
Malignant neoplasm of gastro-esophageal junction

C16.1 Malignant neoplasm of fundus of stomach

C16.2 Malignant neoplasm of body of stomach

C16.3 Malignant neoplasm of pyloric antrum
Malignant neoplasm of gastric antrum

C16.4 Malignant neoplasm of pylorus
Malignant neoplasm of prepylorus
Malignant neoplasm of pyloric canal

C16.5 Malignant neoplasm of lesser curvature of stomach, unspecified
Malignant neoplasm of lesser curvature of stomach, not classifiable to C16.1-C16.4

C16.6 Malignant neoplasm of greater curvature of stomach, unspecified
Malignant neoplasm of greater curvature of stomach, not classifiable to C16.0-C16.4

C16.8 Malignant neoplasm of overlapping sites of stomach

C16.9 Malignant neoplasm of stomach, unspecified
Gastric cancer NOS

☑4ᵗʰ **C17 Malignant neoplasm of small intestine**
EXCLUDES 1 *malignant carcinoid tumors of the small intestine (C7A.01)*

C17.0 Malignant neoplasm of duodenum

C17.1 Malignant neoplasm of jejunum

C17.2 Malignant neoplasm of ileum
EXCLUDES 1 *malignant neoplasm of ileocecal valve (C18.0)*

C17.3 Meckel's diverticulum, malignant
EXCLUDES 1 *Meckel's diverticulum, congenital (Q43.0)*

C17.8 Malignant neoplasm of overlapping sites of small intestine

C17.9 Malignant neoplasm of small intestine, unspecified

☑4ᵗʰ **C18 Malignant neoplasm of colon**
EXCLUDES 1 *malignant carcinoid tumors of the colon (C7A.02-)*

C18.0 Malignant neoplasm of cecum
Malignant neoplasm of ileocecal valve

C18.1 Malignant neoplasm of appendix

C18.2 Malignant neoplasm of ascending colon

C18.3 Malignant neoplasm of hepatic flexure

C18.4 Malignant neoplasm of transverse colon

C18.5 Malignant neoplasm of splenic flexure

C18.6 Malignant neoplasm of descending colon

C18.7 Malignant neoplasm of sigmoid colon
Malignant neoplasm of sigmoid (flexure)
EXCLUDES 1 *malignant neoplasm of rectosigmoid junction (C19)*

C18.8 Malignant neoplasm of overlapping sites of colon

C18.9 Malignant neoplasm of colon, unspecified
Malignant neoplasm of large intestine NOS

C19 Malignant neoplasm of rectosigmoid junction
Malignant neoplasm of colon with rectum
Malignant neoplasm of rectosigmoid (colon)
EXCLUDES 1 *malignant carcinoid tumors of the colon (C7A.02-)*

C20 Malignant neoplasm of rectum
Malignant neoplasm of rectal ampulla
EXCLUDES 1 *malignant carcinoid tumor of the rectum (C7A.026)*

☑4ᵗʰ **C21 Malignant neoplasm of anus and anal canal**
EXCLUDES 2 *malignant carcinoid tumors of the colon (C7A.02-)*
malignant melanoma of anal margin (C43.51)
malignant melanoma of anal skin (C43.51)
malignant melanoma of perianal skin (C43.51)
other and unspecified malignant neoplasm of anal margin (C44.500, C44.510, C44.520, C44.590)
other and unspecified malignant neoplasm of anal skin (C44.500, C44.510, C44.520, C44.590)
other and unspecified malignant neoplasm of perianal skin (C44.500, C44.510, C44.520, C44.590)

C21.0 Malignant neoplasm of anus, unspecified

C21.1 Malignant neoplasm of anal canal
Malignant neoplasm of anal sphincter

C21.2 Malignant neoplasm of cloacogenic zone

C21.8 Malignant neoplasm of overlapping sites of rectum, anus and anal canal
Malignant neoplasm of anorectal junction
Malignant neoplasm of anorectum
Primary malignant neoplasm of two or more contiguous sites of rectum, anus and anal canal

☑4ᵗʰ **C22 Malignant neoplasm of liver and intrahepatic bile ducts**
Use additional code to identify:
alcohol abuse and dependence (F10.-)
hepatitis B (B16.-, B18.0-B18.1)
hepatitis C (B17.1-, B18.2)
EXCLUDES 1 *malignant neoplasm of biliary tract NOS (C24.9)*
secondary malignant neoplasm of liver and intrahepatic bile duct (C78.7)

C22.0 Liver cell carcinoma
Hepatocellular carcinoma
Hepatoma

C22.1 Intrahepatic bile duct carcinoma
Cholangiocarcinoma
EXCLUDES 1 *malignant neoplasm of hepatic duct (C24.0)*

C22.2 Hepatoblastoma

C22.3 Angiosarcoma of liver
Kupffer cell sarcoma

C22.4 Other sarcomas of liver

☑ Additional Character Required   ✗x7ᵗʰ Xtension Alert   Unspecified Dx   Other Specified Dx   Manifestation   ►◄ Revised Text   ● New Code   ▲ Revised Code Title

Neoplasms

C22.7–C34.01

C22.7 Other specified carcinomas of liver

C22.8 Malignant neoplasm of liver, primary, unspecified as to type

C22.9 Malignant neoplasm of liver, not specified as primary or secondary

C23 Malignant neoplasm of gallbladder

C24 Malignant neoplasm of other and unspecified parts of biliary tract
> EXCLUDES 1   *malignant neoplasm of intrahepatic bile duct (C22.1)*

C24.0 Malignant neoplasm of extrahepatic bile duct
Malignant neoplasm of biliary duct or passage NOS
Malignant neoplasm of common bile duct
Malignant neoplasm of cystic duct
Malignant neoplasm of hepatic duct

C24.1 Malignant neoplasm of ampulla of Vater

C24.8 Malignant neoplasm of overlapping sites of biliary tract
Malignant neoplasm involving both intrahepatic and extrahepatic bile ducts
Primary malignant neoplasm of two or more contiguous sites of biliary tract

C24.9 Malignant neoplasm of biliary tract, unspecified

C25 Malignant neoplasm of pancreas
Use additional code to identify:
alcohol abuse and dependence (F10.-)

C25.0 Malignant neoplasm of head of pancreas

C25.1 Malignant neoplasm of body of pancreas

C25.2 Malignant neoplasm of tail of pancreas

C25.3 Malignant neoplasm of pancreatic duct

C25.4 Malignant neoplasm of endocrine pancreas
Malignant neoplasm of islets of Langerhans
Use additional code to identify any functional activity

C25.7 Malignant neoplasm of other parts of pancreas
Malignant neoplasm of neck of pancreas

C25.8 Malignant neoplasm of overlapping sites of pancreas

C25.9 Malignant neoplasm of pancreas, unspecified

C26 Malignant neoplasm of other and ill-defined digestive organs
> EXCLUDES 1   *malignant neoplasm of peritoneum and retroperitoneum (C48.-)*

C26.0 Malignant neoplasm of intestinal tract, part unspecified
Malignant neoplasm of intestine NOS

C26.1 Malignant neoplasm of spleen
> EXCLUDES 1   *Hodgkin lymphoma (C81.-)*
> *non-Hodgkin lymphoma (C82-C85)*

C26.9 Malignant neoplasm of ill-defined sites within the digestive system
Malignant neoplasm of alimentary canal or tract NOS
Malignant neoplasm of gastrointestinal tract NOS
> EXCLUDES 1   *malignant neoplasm of abdominal NOS (C76.2)*
> *malignant neoplasm of intra-abdominal NOS (C76.2)*

Malignant neoplasms of respiratory and intrathoracic organs (C30-C39)

> INCLUDES   malignant neoplasm of middle ear
> EXCLUDES 1   *mesothelioma (C45.-)*

C30 Malignant neoplasm of nasal cavity and middle ear

C30.0 Malignant neoplasm of nasal cavity
Malignant neoplasm of cartilage of nose
Malignant neoplasm of nasal concha
Malignant neoplasm of internal nose
Malignant neoplasm of septum of nose
Malignant neoplasm of vestibule of nose
> EXCLUDES 1   *malignant melanoma of skin of nose (C43.31)*
> *malignant neoplasm of nasal bone (C41.0)*
> *malignant neoplasm of nose NOS (C76.0)*
> *malignant neoplasm of olfactory bulb (C72.2-)*
> *malignant neoplasm of posterior margin of nasal septum and choana (C11.3)*
> *malignant neoplasm of turbinates (C41.0)*
> *other and unspecified malignant neoplasm of skin of nose (C44.301, C44.311, C44.321, C44.391)*

C30.1 Malignant neoplasm of middle ear
Malignant neoplasm of antrum tympanicum
Malignant neoplasm of auditory tube
Malignant neoplasm of eustachian tube
Malignant neoplasm of inner ear
Malignant neoplasm of mastoid air cells
Malignant neoplasm of tympanic cavity
> EXCLUDES 1   *malignant melanoma of skin of (external) ear (C43.2-)*
> *malignant neoplasm of auricular canal (external) (C43.2-,C44.2-)*
> *malignant neoplasm of bone of ear (meatus) (C41.0)*
> *malignant neoplasm of cartilage of ear (C49.0)*
> *other and unspecified malignant neoplasm of skin of (external) ear (C44.2-)*

C31 Malignant neoplasm of accessory sinuses

C31.0 Malignant neoplasm of maxillary sinus
Malignant neoplasm of antrum (Highmore) (maxillary)

C31.1 Malignant neoplasm of ethmoidal sinus

C31.2 Malignant neoplasm of frontal sinus

C31.3 Malignant neoplasm of sphenoid sinus

C31.8 Malignant neoplasm of overlapping sites of accessory sinuses

C31.9 Malignant neoplasm of accessory sinus, unspecified

C32 Malignant neoplasm of larynx
Use additional code to identify:
alcohol abuse and dependence (F10.-)
exposure to environmental tobacco smoke (Z77.22)
exposure to tobacco smoke in the perinatal period (P96.81)
history of tobacco use (Z87.891)
occupational exposure to environmental tobacco smoke (Z57.31)
tobacco dependence (F17.-)
tobacco use (Z72.0)

C32.0 Malignant neoplasm of glottis
Malignant neoplasm of intrinsic larynx
Malignant neoplasm of laryngeal commissure (anterior)(posterior)
Malignant neoplasm of vocal cord (true) NOS

C32.1 Malignant neoplasm of supraglottis
Malignant neoplasm of aryepiglottic fold or interarytenoid fold, laryngeal aspect
Malignant neoplasm of epiglottis (suprahyoid portion) NOS
Malignant neoplasm of extrinsic larynx
Malignant neoplasm of false vocal cord
Malignant neoplasm of posterior (laryngeal) surface of epiglottis
Malignant neoplasm of ventricular bands
> EXCLUDES 2   *malignant neoplasm of anterior surface of epiglottis (C10.1)*
> *malignant neoplasm of aryepiglottic fold or interarytenoid fold, hypopharyngeal aspect (C13.1)*
> *malignant neoplasm of aryepiglottic fold or interarytenoid fold, marginal zone (C13.1)*
> *malignant neoplasm of aryepiglottic fold or interarytenoid fold NOS (C13.1)*

C32.2 Malignant neoplasm of subglottis

C32.3 Malignant neoplasm of laryngeal cartilage

C32.8 Malignant neoplasm of overlapping sites of larynx

C32.9 Malignant neoplasm of larynx, unspecified

C33 Malignant neoplasm of trachea
Use additional code to identify:
exposure to environmental tobacco smoke (Z77.22)
exposure to tobacco smoke in the perinatal period (P96.81)
history of tobacco use (Z87.891)
occupational exposure to environmental tobacco smoke (Z57.31)
tobacco dependence (F17.-)
tobacco use (Z72.0)

C34 Malignant neoplasm of bronchus and lung
Use additional code to identify:
exposure to environmental tobacco smoke (Z77.22)
exposure to tobacco smoke in the perinatal period (P96.81)
history of tobacco use (Z87.891)
occupational exposure to environmental tobacco smoke (Z57.31)
tobacco dependence (F17.-)
tobacco use (Z72.0)
> EXCLUDES 1   *Kaposi's sarcoma of lung (C46.5-)*
> *malignant carcinoid tumor of the bronchus and lung (C7A.090)*

C34.0 Malignant neoplasm of main bronchus
Malignant neoplasm of carina
Malignant neoplasm of hilus (of lung)

C34.00 Malignant neoplasm of unspecified main bronchus

C34.01 Malignant neoplasm of right main bronchus

EXCLUDES 1 Not coded here   EXCLUDES 2 Not included here   N Newborn Age: 0   P Pediatric Age: 0-17   M Maternity Age: 12-55   A Adult Age: 15-124

444   ICD-10-CM Draft (2015)

C34.02 **Malignant neoplasm of** left **main bronchus**

✓5ᵗʰ C34.1 **Malignant neoplasm of** upper lobe, **bronchus or lung**

C34.10 **Malignant neoplasm of upper lobe, unspecified bronchus or lung**

C34.11 **Malignant neoplasm of upper lobe,** right **bronchus or lung**

C34.12 **Malignant neoplasm of upper lobe,** left **bronchus or lung**

✓5ᵗʰ C34.2 **Malignant neoplasm of** middle lobe, **bronchus or lung**

✓5ᵗʰ C34.3 **Malignant neoplasm of lower lobe, bronchus or lung**

C34.30 **Malignant neoplasm of lower lobe, unspecified bronchus or lung**

C34.31 **Malignant neoplasm of lower lobe,** right **bronchus or lung**

C34.32 **Malignant neoplasm of lower lobe,** left **bronchus or lung**

✓5ᵗʰ C34.8 **Malignant neoplasm of** overlapping sites **of bronchus and lung**

C34.80 **Malignant neoplasm of overlapping sites of unspecified bronchus and lung**

C34.81 **Malignant neoplasm of overlapping sites of** right **bronchus and lung**

C34.82 **Malignant neoplasm of overlapping sites of** left **bronchus and lung**

✓5ᵗʰ C34.9 **Malignant neoplasm of** unspecified **part of bronchus or lung**

C34.90 **Malignant neoplasm of unspecified part of unspecified bronchus or lung**
Lung cancer NOS

C34.91 **Malignant neoplasm of unspecified part of** right **bronchus or lung**

C34.92 **Malignant neoplasm of unspecified part of** left **bronchus or lung**

C37 **Malignant neoplasm of** thymus
EXCLUDES 1   *malignant carcinoid tumor of the thymus (C7A.091)*

✓4ᵗʰ C38 **Malignant neoplasm of** heart, mediastinum and pleura
EXCLUDES 1   *mesothelioma (C45.-)*

C38.0 **Malignant neoplasm of** heart
Malignant neoplasm of pericardium
EXCLUDES 1   *malignant neoplasm of great vessels (C49.3)*

C38.1 **Malignant neoplasm of** anterior mediastinum

C38.2 **Malignant neoplasm of** posterior mediastinum

C38.3 **Malignant neoplasm of** mediastinum, **part unspecified**

C38.4 **Malignant neoplasm of** pleura

C38.8 **Malignant neoplasm of** overlapping sites **of heart, mediastinum and pleura**

✓4ᵗʰ C39 **Malignant neoplasm of** other and ill-defined sites in the respiratory system and intrathoracic organs
Use additional code to identify:
exposure to environmental tobacco smoke (Z77.22)
exposure to tobacco smoke in the perinatal period (P96.81)
history of tobacco use (Z87.891)
occupational exposure to environmental tobacco smoke (Z57.31)
tobacco dependence (F17.-)
tobacco use (Z72.0)
EXCLUDES 1   *intrathoracic malignant neoplasm NOS (C76.1)*
thoracic malignant neoplasm NOS (C76.1)

C39.0 **Malignant neoplasm of** upper **respiratory tract, part unspecified**

C39.9 **Malignant neoplasm of** lower **respiratory tract, part unspecified**
Malignant neoplasm of respiratory tract NOS

Malignant neoplasms of bone and articular cartilage (C40-C41)
INCLUDES   malignant neoplasm of cartilage (articular) (joint)
malignant neoplasm of periosteum
EXCLUDES 1   *malignant neoplasm of bone marrow NOS (C96.9)*
malignant neoplasm of synovia (C49.-)

✓4ᵗʰ C40 **Malignant neoplasm of** bone and articular cartilage of limbs
Use additional code to identify major osseous defect, if applicable (M89.7-)

✓5ᵗʰ C40.0 **Malignant neoplasm of** scapula and long bones of upper limb

C40.00 **Malignant neoplasm of scapula and long bones of unspecified upper limb**

C40.01 **Malignant neoplasm of scapula and long bones of** right **upper limb**

C40.02 **Malignant neoplasm of scapula and long bones of** left **upper limb**

✓5ᵗʰ C40.1 **Malignant neoplasm of** short bones of upper limb

C40.10 **Malignant neoplasm of short bones of unspecified upper limb**

C40.11 **Malignant neoplasm of short bones of** right **upper limb**

C40.12 **Malignant neoplasm of short bones of** left **upper limb**

✓5ᵗʰ C40.2 **Malignant neoplasm of** long bones of lower limb

C40.20 **Malignant neoplasm of long bones of unspecified lower limb**

C40.21 **Malignant neoplasm of long bones of** right **lower limb**

C40.22 **Malignant neoplasm of long bones of** left **lower limb**

✓5ᵗʰ C40.3 **Malignant neoplasm of** short bones of lower limb

C40.30 **Malignant neoplasm of short bones of unspecified lower limb**

C40.31 **Malignant neoplasm of short bones of** right **lower limb**

C40.32 **Malignant neoplasm of short bones of** left **lower limb**

✓5ᵗʰ C40.8 **Malignant neoplasm of** overlapping sites **of bone and articular cartilage of limb**

C40.80 **Malignant neoplasm of overlapping sites of bone and articular cartilage of unspecified limb**

C40.81 **Malignant neoplasm of overlapping sites of bone and articular cartilage of** right **limb**

C40.82 **Malignant neoplasm of overlapping sites of bone and articular cartilage of** left **limb**

✓5ᵗʰ C40.9 **Malignant neoplasm of** unspecified **bones and articular cartilage of limb**

C40.90 **Malignant neoplasm of unspecified bones and articular cartilage of unspecified limb**

C40.91 **Malignant neoplasm of unspecified bones and articular cartilage of** right **limb**

C40.92 **Malignant neoplasm of unspecified bones and articular cartilage of** left **limb**

✓4ᵗʰ C41 **Malignant neoplasm of bone and articular cartilage of other and unspecified sites**
EXCLUDES 1   *malignant neoplasm of bones of limbs (C40.-)*
malignant neoplasm of cartilage of ear (C49.0)
malignant neoplasm of cartilage of eyelid (C49.0)
malignant neoplasm of cartilage of larynx (C32.3)
malignant neoplasm of cartilage of limbs (C40.-)
malignant neoplasm of cartilage of nose (C30.0)

C41.0 **Malignant neoplasm of bones of** skull and face
Malignant neoplasm of maxilla (superior)
Malignant neoplasm of orbital bone
EXCLUDES 2   *carcinoma, any type except intraosseous or odontogenic of:*
maxillary sinus (C31.0)
upper jaw (C03.0)
malignant neoplasm of jaw bone (lower) (C41.1)

C41.1 **Malignant neoplasm of** mandible
Malignant neoplasm of inferior maxilla
Malignant neoplasm of lower jaw bone
EXCLUDES 2   *carcinoma, any type except intraosseous or odontogenic of:*
jaw NOS (C03.9)
lower (C03.1)
malignant neoplasm of upper jaw bone (C41.0)

C41.2 **Malignant neoplasm of** vertebral column
EXCLUDES 1   *malignant neoplasm of sacrum and coccyx (C41.4)*

C41.3 **Malignant neoplasm of** ribs, sternum and clavicle

C41.4 **Malignant neoplasm of** pelvic bones, sacrum and coccyx

C41.9 **Malignant neoplasm of** bone and articular cartilage, **unspecified**

✓ Additional Character Required   ✓x7ᵗʰ Xtension Alert   Unspecified Dx   Other Specified Dx   Manifestation   ▶◀ Revised Text   ● New Code   ▲ Revised Code Title

Neoplasms

C43–C44.192

Melanoma and other malignant neoplasms of skin (C43-C44)

✓4ᵗʰ **C43** Malignant melanoma of skin

    EXCLUDES 1   melanoma in situ (D03.-)

    EXCLUDES 2   malignant melanoma of skin of genital organs (C51-C52, C60.-, C63.-)

         Merkel cell carcinoma (C4A.-)

         sites other than skin—code to malignant neoplasm of the site

     C43.0   Malignant melanoma of lip

         EXCLUDES 1   malignant neoplasm of vermilion border of lip (C00.0-C00.2)

     ✓5ᵗʰ **C43.1**   Malignant melanoma of eyelid, including canthus

         C43.10   Malignant melanoma of unspecified eyelid, including canthus

         C43.11   Malignant melanoma of right eyelid, including canthus

         C43.12   Malignant melanoma of left eyelid, including canthus

     ✓5ᵗʰ **C43.2**   Malignant melanoma of ear and external auricular canal

         C43.20   Malignant melanoma of unspecified ear and external auricular canal

         C43.21   Malignant melanoma of right ear and external auricular canal

         C43.22   Malignant melanoma of left ear and external auricular canal

     ✓5ᵗʰ **C43.3**   Malignant melanoma of other and unspecified parts of face

         C43.30   Malignant melanoma of unspecified part of face

         C43.31   Malignant melanoma of nose

         C43.39   Malignant melanoma of other parts of face

     C43.4   Malignant melanoma of scalp and neck

     ✓5ᵗʰ **C43.5**   Malignant melanoma of trunk

         EXCLUDES 2   malignant neoplasm of anus NOS (C21.0)

                 malignant neoplasm of scrotum (C63.2)

         C43.51   Malignant melanoma of anal skin

                 Malignant melanoma of anal margin

                 Malignant melanoma of perianal skin

         C43.52   Malignant melanoma of skin of breast

         C43.59   Malignant melanoma of other part of trunk

     ✓5ᵗʰ **C43.6**   Malignant melanoma of upper limb, including shoulder

         C43.60   Malignant melanoma of unspecified upper limb, including shoulder

         C43.61   Malignant melanoma of right upper limb, including shoulder

         C43.62   Malignant melanoma of left upper limb, including shoulder

     ✓5ᵗʰ **C43.7**   Malignant melanoma of lower limb, including hip

         C43.70   Malignant melanoma of unspecified lower limb, including hip

         C43.71   Malignant melanoma of right lower limb, including hip

         C43.72   Malignant melanoma of left lower limb, including hip

     C43.8   Malignant melanoma of overlapping sites of skin

     C43.9   Malignant melanoma of skin, unspecified

         Malignant melanoma of unspecified site of skin

✓4ᵗʰ **C4A** Merkel cell carcinoma

     C4A.0   Merkel cell carcinoma of lip

         EXCLUDES 1   malignant neoplasm of vermilion border of lip (C00.0-C00.2)

     ✓5ᵗʰ **C4A.1**   Merkel cell carcinoma of eyelid, including canthus

         C4A.10   Merkel cell carcinoma of unspecified eyelid, including canthus

         C4A.11   Merkel cell carcinoma of right eyelid, including canthus

         C4A.12   Merkel cell carcinoma of left eyelid, including canthus

     ✓5ᵗʰ **C4A.2**   Merkel cell carcinoma of ear and external auricular canal

         C4A.20   Merkel cell carcinoma of unspecified ear and external auricular canal

         C4A.21   Merkel cell carcinoma of right ear and external auricular canal

         C4A.22   Merkel cell carcinoma of left ear and external auricular canal

     ✓5ᵗʰ **C4A.3**   Merkel cell carcinoma of other and unspecified parts of face

         C4A.30   Merkel cell carcinoma of unspecified part of face

         C4A.31   Merkel cell carcinoma of nose

         C4A.39   Merkel cell carcinoma of other parts of face

     C4A.4   Merkel cell carcinoma of scalp and neck

     ✓5ᵗʰ **C4A.5**   Merkel cell carcinoma of trunk

         EXCLUDES 2   malignant neoplasm of anus NOS (C21.0)

                 malignant neoplasm of scrotum (C63.2)

         C4A.51   Merkel cell carcinoma of anal skin

                 Merkel cell carcinoma of anal margin

                 Merkel cell carcinoma of perianal skin

         C4A.52   Merkel cell carcinoma of skin of breast

         C4A.59   Merkel cell carcinoma of other part of trunk

     ✓5ᵗʰ **C4A.6**   Merkel cell carcinoma of upper limb, including shoulder

         C4A.60   Merkel cell carcinoma of unspecified upper limb, including shoulder

         C4A.61   Merkel cell carcinoma of right upper limb, including shoulder

         C4A.62   Merkel cell carcinoma of left upper limb, including shoulder

     ✓5ᵗʰ **C4A.7**   Merkel cell carcinoma of lower limb, including hip

         C4A.70   Merkel cell carcinoma of unspecified lower limb, including hip

         C4A.71   Merkel cell carcinoma of right lower limb, including hip

         C4A.72   Merkel cell carcinoma of left lower limb, including hip

     C4A.8   Merkel cell carcinoma of overlapping sites

     C4A.9   Merkel cell carcinoma, unspecified

         Merkel cell carcinoma of unspecified site

✓4ᵗʰ **C44** Other and unspecified malignant neoplasm of skin

     INCLUDES   malignant neoplasm of sebaceous glands

               malignant neoplasm of sweat glands

     EXCLUDES 1   Kaposi's sarcoma of skin (C46.0)

               malignant melanoma of skin (C43.-)

               malignant neoplasm of skin of genital organs (C51-C52, C60-, C63.2)

               Merkel cell carcinoma (C4A.-)

     ✓5ᵗʰ **C44.0**   Other and unspecified malignant neoplasm of skin of lip

         EXCLUDES 1   malignant neoplasm of lip (C00.-)

         C44.00   Unspecified malignant neoplasm of skin of lip

         C44.01   Basal cell carcinoma of skin of lip

         C44.02   Squamous cell carcinoma of skin of lip

         C44.09   Other specified malignant neoplasm of skin of lip

     ✓5ᵗʰ **C44.1**   Other and unspecified malignant neoplasm of skin of eyelid, including canthus

         EXCLUDES 1   connective tissue of eyelid (C49.0)

         ✓6ᵗʰ **C44.10**   Unspecified malignant neoplasm of skin of eyelid, including canthus

                 C44.101   Unspecified malignant neoplasm of skin of unspecified eyelid, including canthus

                 C44.102   Unspecified malignant neoplasm of skin of right eyelid, including canthus

                 C44.109   Unspecified malignant neoplasm of skin of left eyelid, including canthus

         ✓6ᵗʰ **C44.11**   Basal cell carcinoma of skin of eyelid, including canthus

                 C44.111   Basal cell carcinoma of skin of unspecified eyelid, including canthus

                 C44.112   Basal cell carcinoma of skin of right eyelid, including canthus

                 C44.119   Basal cell carcinoma of skin of left eyelid, including canthus

         ✓6ᵗʰ **C44.12**   Squamous cell carcinoma of skin of eyelid, including canthus

                 C44.121   Squamous cell carcinoma of skin of unspecified eyelid, including canthus

                 C44.122   Squamous cell carcinoma of skin of right eyelid, including canthus

                 C44.129   Squamous cell carcinoma of skin of left eyelid, including canthus

         ✓6ᵗʰ **C44.19**   Other specified malignant neoplasm of skin of eyelid, including canthus

                 C44.191   Other specified malignant neoplasm of skin of unspecified eyelid, including canthus

                 C44.192   Other specified malignant neoplasm of skin of right eyelid, including canthus

EXCLUDES 1 Not coded here   EXCLUDES 2 Not included here   N Newborn Age: 0   P Pediatric Age: 0-17   M Maternity Age: 12-55   A Adult Age: 15-124

446   ICD-10-CM Draft (2015)

C44.199   Other specified malignant neoplasm of skin of left eyelid, including canthus

☑5ᵗʰ **C44.2**   Other and unspecified malignant neoplasm of skin of ear and external auricular canal

EXCLUDES 1   *connective tissue of ear (C49.0)*

☑6ᵗʰ **C44.20**   Unspecified malignant neoplasm of skin of ear and external auricular canal

C44.201   Unspecified malignant neoplasm of skin of unspecified ear and external auricular canal

C44.202   Unspecified malignant neoplasm of skin of right ear and external auricular canal

C44.209   Unspecified malignant neoplasm of skin of left ear and external auricular canal

☑6ᵗʰ **C44.21**   Basal cell carcinoma of skin of ear and external auricular canal

C44.211   Basal cell carcinoma of skin of unspecified ear and external auricular canal

C44.212   Basal cell carcinoma of skin of right ear and external auricular canal

C44.219   Basal cell carcinoma of skin of left ear and external auricular canal

☑6ᵗʰ **C44.22**   Squamous cell carcinoma of skin of ear and external auricular canal

C44.221   Squamous cell carcinoma of skin of unspecified ear and external auricular canal

C44.222   Squamous cell carcinoma of skin of right ear and external auricular canal

C44.229   Squamous cell carcinoma of skin of left ear and external auricular canal

☑6ᵗʰ **C44.29**   Other specified malignant neoplasm of skin of ear and external auricular canal

C44.291   Other specified malignant neoplasm of skin of unspecified ear and external auricular canal

C44.292   Other specified malignant neoplasm of skin of right ear and external auricular canal

C44.299   Other specified malignant neoplasm of skin of left ear and external auricular canal

☑5ᵗʰ **C44.3**   Other and unspecified malignant neoplasm of skin of other and unspecified parts of face

☑6ᵗʰ **C44.30**   Unspecified malignant neoplasm of skin of other and unspecified parts of face

C44.300   Unspecified malignant neoplasm of skin of unspecified part of face

C44.301   Unspecified malignant neoplasm of skin of nose

C44.309   Unspecified malignant neoplasm of skin of other parts of face

☑6ᵗʰ **C44.31**   Basal cell carcinoma of skin of other and unspecified parts of face

C44.310   Basal cell carcinoma of skin of unspecified parts of face

C44.311   Basal cell carcinoma of skin of nose

C44.319   Basal cell carcinoma of skin of other parts of face

☑6ᵗʰ **C44.32**   Squamous cell carcinoma of skin of other and unspecified parts of face

C44.320   Squamous cell carcinoma of skin of unspecified parts of face

C44.321   Squamous cell carcinoma of skin of nose

C44.329   Squamous cell carcinoma of skin of other parts of face

☑6ᵗʰ **C44.39**   Other specified malignant neoplasm of skin of other and unspecified parts of face

C44.390   Other specified malignant neoplasm of skin of unspecified parts of face

C44.391   Other specified malignant neoplasm of skin of nose

C44.399   Other specified malignant neoplasm of skin of other parts of face

☑5ᵗʰ **C44.4**   Other and unspecified malignant neoplasm of skin of scalp and neck

C44.40   Unspecified malignant neoplasm of skin of scalp and neck

C44.41   Basal cell carcinoma of skin of scalp and neck

C44.42   Squamous cell carcinoma of skin of scalp and neck

C44.49   Other specified malignant neoplasm of skin of scalp and neck

☑5ᵗʰ **C44.5**   Other and unspecified malignant neoplasm of skin of trunk

EXCLUDES 1   *anus NOS (C21.0)*
            scrotum (C63.2)

☑6ᵗʰ **C44.50**   Unspecified malignant neoplasm of skin of trunk

C44.500   Unspecified malignant neoplasm of anal skin
            Unspecified malignant neoplasm of anal margin
            Unspecified malignant neoplasm of perianal skin

C44.501   Unspecified malignant neoplasm of skin of breast

C44.509   Unspecified malignant neoplasm of skin of other part of trunk

☑6ᵗʰ **C44.51**   Basal cell carcinoma of skin of trunk

C44.510   Basal cell carcinoma of anal skin
            Basal cell carcinoma of anal margin
            Basal cell carcinoma of perianal skin

C44.511   Basal cell carcinoma of skin of breast

C44.519   Basal cell carcinoma of skin of other part of trunk

☑6ᵗʰ **C44.52**   Squamous cell carcinoma of skin of trunk

C44.520   Squamous cell carcinoma of anal skin
            Squamous cell carcinoma of anal margin
            Squamous cell carcinoma of perianal skin

C44.521   Squamous cell carcinoma of skin of breast

C44.529   Squamous cell carcinoma of skin of other part of trunk

☑6ᵗʰ **C44.59**   Other specified malignant neoplasm of skin of trunk

C44.590   Other specified malignant neoplasm of anal skin
            Other specified malignant neoplasm of anal margin
            Other specified malignant neoplasm of perianal skin

C44.591   Other specified malignant neoplasm of skin of breast

C44.599   Other specified malignant neoplasm of skin of other part of trunk

☑5ᵗʰ **C44.6**   Other and unspecified malignant neoplasm of skin of upper limb, including shoulder

☑6ᵗʰ **C44.60**   Unspecified malignant neoplasm of skin of upper limb, including shoulder

C44.601   Unspecified malignant neoplasm of skin of unspecified upper limb, including shoulder

C44.602   Unspecified malignant neoplasm of skin of right upper limb, including shoulder

C44.609   Unspecified malignant neoplasm of skin of left upper limb, including shoulder

☑6ᵗʰ **C44.61**   Basal cell carcinoma of skin of upper limb, including shoulder

C44.611   Basal cell carcinoma of skin of unspecified upper limb, including shoulder

C44.612   Basal cell carcinoma of skin of right upper limb, including shoulder

C44.619   Basal cell carcinoma of skin of left upper limb, including shoulder

☑6ᵗʰ **C44.62**   Squamous cell carcinoma of skin of upper limb, including shoulder

C44.621   Squamous cell carcinoma of skin of unspecified upper limb, including shoulder

C44.622   Squamous cell carcinoma of skin of right upper limb, including shoulder

C44.629   Squamous cell carcinoma of skin of left upper limb, including shoulder

☑6ᵗʰ **C44.69**   Other specified malignant neoplasm of skin of upper limb, including shoulder

C44.691   Other specified malignant neoplasm of skin of unspecified upper limb, including shoulder

C44.692   Other specified malignant neoplasm of skin of right upper limb, including shoulder

☑ Additional Character Required   ⁷ᵗʰ Xtension Alert   Unspecified Dx   Other Specified Dx   Manifestation   ►◄ Revised Text   ● New Code   ▲ Revised Code Title

ICD-10-CM Draft (2015)   447

Neoplasms

C44.699–C48.8

C44.699 Other specified malignant neoplasm of skin of left upper limb, including shoulder

✓5ᵗʰ **C44.7 Other and unspecified malignant neoplasm of skin of lower limb, including hip**

   ✓6ᵗʰ **C44.70 Unspecified malignant neoplasm of skin of lower limb, including hip**

     C44.701 Unspecified malignant neoplasm of skin of unspecified lower limb, including hip

     C44.702 Unspecified malignant neoplasm of skin of right lower limb, including hip

     C44.709 Unspecified malignant neoplasm of skin of left lower limb, including hip

   ✓6ᵗʰ **C44.71 Basal cell carcinoma of skin of lower limb, including hip**

     C44.711 Basal cell carcinoma of skin of unspecified lower limb, including hip

     C44.712 Basal cell carcinoma of skin of right lower limb, including hip

     C44.719 Basal cell carcinoma of skin of left lower limb, including hip

   ✓6ᵗʰ **C44.72 Squamous cell carcinoma of skin of lower limb, including hip**

     C44.721 Squamous cell carcinoma of skin of unspecified lower limb, including hip

     C44.722 Squamous cell carcinoma of skin of right lower limb, including hip

     C44.729 Squamous cell carcinoma of skin of left lower limb, including hip

   ✓6ᵗʰ **C44.79 Other specified malignant neoplasm of skin of lower limb, including hip**

     C44.791 Other specified malignant neoplasm of skin of unspecified lower limb, including hip

     C44.792 Other specified malignant neoplasm of skin of right lower limb, including hip

     C44.799 Other specified malignant neoplasm of skin of left lower limb, including hip

✓5ᵗʰ **C44.8 Other and unspecified malignant neoplasm of overlapping sites of skin**

   C44.80 Unspecified malignant neoplasm of overlapping sites of skin

   C44.81 Basal cell carcinoma of overlapping sites of skin

   C44.82 Squamous cell carcinoma of overlapping sites of skin

   C44.89 Other specified malignant neoplasm of overlapping sites of skin

✓5ᵗʰ **C44.9 Other and unspecified malignant neoplasm of skin, unspecified**

   C44.90 Unspecified malignant neoplasm of skin, unspecified
     Malignant neoplasm of unspecified site of skin

   C44.91 Basal cell carcinoma of skin, unspecified

   C44.92 Squamous cell carcinoma of skin, unspecified

   C44.99 Other specified malignant neoplasm of skin, unspecified

Malignant neoplasms of mesothelial and soft tissue (C45-C49)

✓4ᵗʰ **C45 Mesothelioma**

   C45.0 Mesothelioma of pleura
     EXCLUDES 1 other malignant neoplasm of pleura (C38.4)

   C45.1 Mesothelioma of peritoneum
     Mesothelioma of cul-de-sac
     Mesothelioma of mesentery
     Mesothelioma of mesocolon
     Mesothelioma of omentum
     Mesothelioma of peritoneum (parietal) (pelvic)
     EXCLUDES 1 other malignant neoplasm of soft tissue of peritoneum (C48.-)

   C45.2 Mesothelioma of pericardium
     EXCLUDES 1 other malignant neoplasm of pericardium (C38.0)

   C45.7 Mesothelioma of other sites

   C45.9 Mesothelioma, unspecified

✓4ᵗʰ **C46 Kaposi's sarcoma**
   Code first any human immunodeficiency virus [HIV] disease (B20)

   C46.0 Kaposi's sarcoma of skin

   C46.1 Kaposi's sarcoma of soft tissue
     Kaposi's sarcoma of blood vessel
     Kaposi's sarcoma of connective tissue
     Kaposi's sarcoma of fascia
     Kaposi's sarcoma of ligament
     Kaposi's sarcoma of lymphatic(s) NEC
     Kaposi's sarcoma of muscle
     EXCLUDES 2 Kaposi's sarcoma of lymph glands and nodes (C46.3)

   C46.2 Kaposi's sarcoma of palate

   C46.3 Kaposi's sarcoma of lymph nodes

   C46.4 Kaposi's sarcoma of gastrointestinal sites

   ✓5ᵗʰ **C46.5 Kaposi's sarcoma of lung**

     C46.50 Kaposi's sarcoma of unspecified lung

     C46.51 Kaposi's sarcoma of right lung

     C46.52 Kaposi's sarcoma of left lung

   C46.7 Kaposi's sarcoma of other sites

   C46.9 Kaposi's sarcoma, unspecified
     Kaposi's sarcoma of unspecified site

✓4ᵗʰ **C47 Malignant neoplasm of peripheral nerves and autonomic nervous system**
   INCLUDES malignant neoplasm of sympathetic and parasympathetic nerves and ganglia
   EXCLUDES 1 Kaposi's sarcoma of soft tissue (C46.1)

   C47.0 Malignant neoplasm of peripheral nerves of head, face and neck
     EXCLUDES 1 malignant neoplasm of peripheral nerves of orbit (C69.6-)

   ✓5ᵗʰ **C47.1 Malignant neoplasm of peripheral nerves of upper limb, including shoulder**

     C47.10 Malignant neoplasm of peripheral nerves of unspecified upper limb, including shoulder

     C47.11 Malignant neoplasm of peripheral nerves of right upper limb, including shoulder

     C47.12 Malignant neoplasm of peripheral nerves of left upper limb, including shoulder

   ✓5ᵗʰ **C47.2 Malignant neoplasm of peripheral nerves of lower limb, including hip**

     C47.20 Malignant neoplasm of peripheral nerves of unspecified lower limb, including hip

     C47.21 Malignant neoplasm of peripheral nerves of right lower limb, including hip

     C47.22 Malignant neoplasm of peripheral nerves of left lower limb, including hip

   C47.3 Malignant neoplasm of peripheral nerves of thorax

   C47.4 Malignant neoplasm of peripheral nerves of abdomen

   C47.5 Malignant neoplasm of peripheral nerves of pelvis

   C47.6 Malignant neoplasm of peripheral nerves of trunk, unspecified
     Malignant neoplasm of peripheral nerves of unspecified part of trunk

   C47.8 Malignant neoplasm of overlapping sites of peripheral nerves and autonomic nervous system

   C47.9 Malignant neoplasm of peripheral nerves and autonomic nervous system, unspecified
     Malignant neoplasm of unspecified site of peripheral nerves and autonomic nervous system

✓4ᵗʰ **C48 Malignant neoplasm of retroperitoneum and peritoneum**
   EXCLUDES 1 Kaposi's sarcoma of connective tissue (C46.1)
      mesothelioma (C45.-)

   C48.0 Malignant neoplasm of retroperitoneum

   C48.1 Malignant neoplasm of specified parts of peritoneum
     Malignant neoplasm of cul-de-sac
     Malignant neoplasm of mesentery
     Malignant neoplasm of mesocolon
     Malignant neoplasm of omentum
     Malignant neoplasm of parietal peritoneum
     Malignant neoplasm of pelvic peritoneum

   C48.2 Malignant neoplasm of peritoneum, unspecified

   C48.8 Malignant neoplasm of overlapping sites of retroperitoneum and peritoneum

EXCLUDES 1 Not coded here   *EXCLUDES 2* Not included here   N Newborn Age: 0   P Pediatric Age: 0-17   M Maternity Age: 12-55   A Adult Age: 15-124

448   ICD-10-CM Draft (2015)

✓4th **C49 Malignant neoplasm of** other connective and soft tissue

   INCLUDES   malignant neoplasm of blood vessel
           malignant neoplasm of bursa
           malignant neoplasm of cartilage
           malignant neoplasm of fascia
           malignant neoplasm of fat
           malignant neoplasm of ligament, except uterine
           malignant neoplasm of lymphatic vessel
           malignant neoplasm of muscle
           malignant neoplasm of synovia
           malignant neoplasm of tendon (sheath)

    EXCLUDES 1   *malignant neoplasm of cartilage (of):*
           articular (C40-C41)
           larynx (C32.3)
           nose (C30.0)
           malignant neoplasm of connective tissue of breast (C50.-)

    EXCLUDES 2   *Kaposi's sarcoma of soft tissue (C46.1)*
           malignant neoplasm of heart (C38.0)
           malignant neoplasm of peripheral nerves and autonomic
              nervous system (C47.-)
           malignant neoplasm of peritoneum (C48.2)
           malignant neoplasm of retroperitoneum (C48.0)
           malignant neoplasm of uterine ligament (C57.3)
           mesothelioma (C45.-)

C49.0 Malignant neoplasm of connective and soft tissue of head, face and neck
     Malignant neoplasm of connective tissue of ear
     Malignant neoplasm of connective tissue of eyelid
    EXCLUDES 1   *connective tissue of orbit (C69.6-)*

✓5th **C49.1 Malignant neoplasm of connective and soft tissue of** upper limb, including shoulder

   C49.10 Malignant neoplasm of connective and soft tissue of unspecified upper limb, including shoulder

   C49.11 Malignant neoplasm of connective and soft tissue of right **upper limb, including shoulder**

   C49.12 Malignant neoplasm of connective and soft tissue of left **upper limb, including shoulder**

✓5th **C49.2 Malignant neoplasm of connective and soft tissue of** lower limb, including hip

   C49.20 Malignant neoplasm of connective and soft tissue of unspecified lower limb, including hip

   C49.21 Malignant neoplasm of connective and soft tissue of right **lower limb, including hip**

   C49.22 Malignant neoplasm of connective and soft tissue of left **lower limb, including hip**

C49.3 Malignant neoplasm of connective and soft tissue of thorax
     Malignant neoplasm of axilla
     Malignant neoplasm of diaphragm
     Malignant neoplasm of great vessels
    EXCLUDES 1   *malignant neoplasm of breast (C50.-)*
           malignant neoplasm of heart (C38.0)
           malignant neoplasm of mediastinum (C38.1-C38.3)
           malignant neoplasm of thymus (C37)

C49.4 Malignant neoplasm of connective and soft tissue of abdomen
     Malignant neoplasm of abdominal wall
     Malignant neoplasm of hypochondrium

C49.5 Malignant neoplasm of connective and soft tissue of pelvis
     Malignant neoplasm of buttock
     Malignant neoplasm of groin
     Malignant neoplasm of perineum

C49.6 Malignant neoplasm of connective and soft tissue of trunk, unspecified
     Malignant neoplasm of back NOS

C49.8 Malignant neoplasm of overlapping sites **of connective and soft tissue**
     Primary malignant neoplasm of two or more contiguous sites of connective and soft tissue

C49.9 Malignant neoplasm of connective and soft tissue, unspecified

Malignant neoplasms of breast (C50)

✓4th **C50 Malignant neoplasm of** breast

   INCLUDES   connective tissue of breast
           Paget's disease of breast
           Paget's disease of nipple
   Use additional code to identify estrogen receptor status (Z17.0, Z17.1)
    EXCLUDES 1   *skin of breast (C44.501, C44.511, C44.521, C44.591)*

✓5th **C50.0 Malignant neoplasm of** nipple and areola

  ✓6th **C50.01 Malignant neoplasm of nipple and areola,** female
    C50.011 Malignant neoplasm of nipple and areola, right **female breast** ♀
    C50.012 Malignant neoplasm of nipple and areola, left **female breast** ♀
    C50.019 Malignant neoplasm of nipple and areola, unspecified female breast ♀

  ✓6th **C50.02 Malignant neoplasm of nipple and areola,** male
    C50.021 Malignant neoplasm of nipple and areola, right **male breast** ♂
    C50.022 Malignant neoplasm of nipple and areola, left **male breast** ♂
    C50.029 Malignant neoplasm of nipple and areola, unspecified male breast ♂

✓5th **C50.1 Malignant neoplasm of** central portion **of breast**

  ✓6th **C50.11 Malignant neoplasm of central portion of breast,** female
    C50.111 Malignant neoplasm of central portion of right **female breast** ♀
    C50.112 Malignant neoplasm of central portion of left **female breast** ♀
    C50.119 Malignant neoplasm of central portion of unspecified female breast ♀

  ✓6th **C50.12 Malignant neoplasm of central portion of breast,** male
    C50.121 Malignant neoplasm of central portion of right **male breast** ♂
    C50.122 Malignant neoplasm of central portion of left **male breast** ♂
    C50.129 Malignant neoplasm of central portion of unspecified male breast ♂

✓5th **C50.2 Malignant neoplasm of** upper-inner quadrant **of breast**

  ✓6th **C50.21 Malignant neoplasm of upper-inner quadrant of breast,** female
    C50.211 Malignant neoplasm of upper-inner quadrant of right **female breast** ♀
    C50.212 Malignant neoplasm of upper-inner quadrant of left **female breast** ♀
    C50.219 Malignant neoplasm of upper-inner quadrant of unspecified female breast ♀

  ✓6th **C50.22 Malignant neoplasm of upper-inner quadrant of breast,** male
    C50.221 Malignant neoplasm of upper-inner quadrant of right **male breast** ♂
    C50.222 Malignant neoplasm of upper-inner quadrant of left **male breast** ♂
    C50.229 Malignant neoplasm of upper-inner quadrant of unspecified male breast ♂

✓5th **C50.3 Malignant neoplasm of** lower-inner quadrant **of breast**

  ✓6th **C50.31 Malignant neoplasm of lower-inner quadrant of breast,** female
    C50.311 Malignant neoplasm of lower-inner quadrant of right **female breast** ♀
    C50.312 Malignant neoplasm of lower-inner quadrant of left **female breast** ♀
    C50.319 Malignant neoplasm of lower-inner quadrant of unspecified female breast ♀

  ✓6th **C50.32 Malignant neoplasm of lower-inner quadrant of breast,** male
    C50.321 Malignant neoplasm of lower-inner quadrant of right **male breast** ♂
    C50.322 Malignant neoplasm of lower-inner quadrant of left **male breast** ♂
    C50.329 Malignant neoplasm of lower-inner quadrant of unspecified male breast ♂

☑ Additional Character Required   ✓x7th Xtension Alert   Unspecified Dx   Other Specified Dx   Manifestation   ►◄ Revised Text   ● New Code   ▲ Revised Code Title

Neoplasms

C50.4–C57.7

✓5ᵗʰ **C50.4** Malignant neoplasm of upper-outer quadrant of breast
- ✓6ᵗʰ **C50.41** Malignant neoplasm of upper-outer quadrant of breast, female
  - **C50.411** Malignant neoplasm of upper-outer quadrant of right female breast ♀
  - **C50.412** Malignant neoplasm of upper-outer quadrant of left female breast ♀
  - **C50.419** Malignant neoplasm of upper-outer quadrant of unspecified female breast ♀
- ✓6ᵗʰ **C50.42** Malignant neoplasm of upper-outer quadrant of breast, male
  - **C50.421** Malignant neoplasm of upper-outer quadrant of right male breast ♂
  - **C50.422** Malignant neoplasm of upper-outer quadrant of left male breast ♂
  - **C50.429** Malignant neoplasm of upper-outer quadrant of unspecified male breast ♂

✓5ᵗʰ **C50.5** Malignant neoplasm of lower-outer quadrant of breast
- ✓6ᵗʰ **C50.51** Malignant neoplasm of lower-outer quadrant of breast, female
  - **C50.511** Malignant neoplasm of lower-outer quadrant of right female breast ♀
  - **C50.512** Malignant neoplasm of lower-outer quadrant of left female breast ♀
  - **C50.519** Malignant neoplasm of lower-outer quadrant of unspecified female breast ♀
- ✓6ᵗʰ **C50.52** Malignant neoplasm of lower-outer quadrant of breast, male
  - **C50.521** Malignant neoplasm of lower-outer quadrant of right male breast ♂
  - **C50.522** Malignant neoplasm of lower-outer quadrant of left male breast ♂
  - **C50.529** Malignant neoplasm of lower-outer quadrant of unspecified male breast ♂

✓5ᵗʰ **C50.6** Malignant neoplasm of axillary tail of breast
- ✓6ᵗʰ **C50.61** Malignant neoplasm of axillary tail of breast, female
  - **C50.611** Malignant neoplasm of axillary tail of right female breast ♀
  - **C50.612** Malignant neoplasm of axillary tail of left female breast ♀
  - **C50.619** Malignant neoplasm of axillary tail of unspecified female breast ♀
- ✓6ᵗʰ **C50.62** Malignant neoplasm of axillary tail of breast, male
  - **C50.621** Malignant neoplasm of axillary tail of right male breast ♂
  - **C50.622** Malignant neoplasm of axillary tail of left male breast ♂
  - **C50.629** Malignant neoplasm of axillary tail of unspecified male breast ♂

✓5ᵗʰ **C50.8** Malignant neoplasm of overlapping sites of breast
- ✓6ᵗʰ **C50.81** Malignant neoplasm of overlapping sites of breast, female
  - **C50.811** Malignant neoplasm of overlapping sites of right female breast ♀
  - **C50.812** Malignant neoplasm of overlapping sites of left female breast ♀
  - **C50.819** Malignant neoplasm of overlapping sites of unspecified female breast ♀
- ✓6ᵗʰ **C50.82** Malignant neoplasm of overlapping sites of breast, male
  - **C50.821** Malignant neoplasm of overlapping sites of right male breast ♂
  - **C50.822** Malignant neoplasm of overlapping sites of left male breast ♂
  - **C50.829** Malignant neoplasm of overlapping sites of unspecified male breast ♂

✓5ᵗʰ **C50.9** Malignant neoplasm of breast of unspecified site
- ✓6ᵗʰ **C50.91** Malignant neoplasm of breast of unspecified site, female
  - **C50.911** Malignant neoplasm of unspecified site of right female breast ♀
  - **C50.912** Malignant neoplasm of unspecified site of left female breast ♀
  - **C50.919** Malignant neoplasm of unspecified site of unspecified female breast ♀
- ✓6ᵗʰ **C50.92** Malignant neoplasm of breast of unspecified site, male
  - **C50.921** Malignant neoplasm of unspecified site of right male breast ♂
  - **C50.922** Malignant neoplasm of unspecified site of left male breast ♂
  - **C50.929** Malignant neoplasm of unspecified site of unspecified male breast ♂

Malignant neoplasms of female genital organs (C51-C58)

INCLUDES malignant neoplasm of skin of female genital organs

✓4ᵗʰ **C51** Malignant neoplasm of vulva
EXCLUDES 1 carcinoma in situ of vulva (D07.1)
- **C51.0** Malignant neoplasm of labium majus ♀
  Malignant neoplasm of Bartholin's [greater vestibular] gland
- **C51.1** Malignant neoplasm of labium minus ♀
- **C51.2** Malignant neoplasm of clitoris ♀
- **C51.8** Malignant neoplasm of overlapping sites of vulva ♀
- **C51.9** Malignant neoplasm of vulva, unspecified ♀
  Malignant neoplasm of external female genitalia NOS
  Malignant neoplasm of pudendum

C52 Malignant neoplasm of vagina ♀
EXCLUDES 1 carcinoma in situ of vagina (D07.2)

✓4ᵗʰ **C53** Malignant neoplasm of cervix uteri
EXCLUDES 1 carcinoma in situ of cervix uteri (D06.-)
- **C53.0** Malignant neoplasm of endocervix ♀
- **C53.1** Malignant neoplasm of exocervix ♀
- **C53.8** Malignant neoplasm of overlapping sites of cervix uteri ♀
- **C53.9** Malignant neoplasm of cervix uteri, unspecified ♀

✓4ᵗʰ **C54** Malignant neoplasm of corpus uteri
- **C54.0** Malignant neoplasm of isthmus uteri ♀
  Malignant neoplasm of lower uterine segment
- **C54.1** Malignant neoplasm of endometrium ♀
- **C54.2** Malignant neoplasm of myometrium ♀
- **C54.3** Malignant neoplasm of fundus uteri ♀
- **C54.8** Malignant neoplasm of overlapping sites of corpus uteri ♀
- **C54.9** Malignant neoplasm of corpus uteri, unspecified ♀

C55 Malignant neoplasm of uterus, part unspecified ♀

✓4ᵗʰ **C56** Malignant neoplasm of ovary
Use additional code to identify any functional activity
- **C56.1** Malignant neoplasm of right ovary ♀
- **C56.2** Malignant neoplasm of left ovary ♀
- **C56.9** Malignant neoplasm of unspecified ovary ♀

✓4ᵗʰ **C57** Malignant neoplasm of other and unspecified female genital organs
- ✓5ᵗʰ **C57.0** Malignant neoplasm of fallopian tube
  Malignant neoplasm of oviduct
  Malignant neoplasm of uterine tube
  - **C57.00** Malignant neoplasm of unspecified fallopian tube ♀
  - **C57.01** Malignant neoplasm of right fallopian tube ♀
  - **C57.02** Malignant neoplasm of left fallopian tube ♀
- ✓5ᵗʰ **C57.1** Malignant neoplasm of broad ligament
  - **C57.10** Malignant neoplasm of unspecified broad ligament ♀
  - **C57.11** Malignant neoplasm of right broad ligament ♀
  - **C57.12** Malignant neoplasm of left broad ligament ♀
- ✓5ᵗʰ **C57.2** Malignant neoplasm of round ligament
  - **C57.20** Malignant neoplasm of unspecified round ligament ♀
  - **C57.21** Malignant neoplasm of right round ligament ♀
  - **C57.22** Malignant neoplasm of left round ligament ♀
- **C57.3** Malignant neoplasm of parametrium ♀
  Malignant neoplasm of uterine ligament NOS
- **C57.4** Malignant neoplasm of uterine adnexa, unspecified ♀
- **C57.7** Malignant neoplasm of other specified female genital organs ♀
  Malignant neoplasm of wolffian body or duct

EXCLUDES 1 Not coded here   EXCLUDES 2 Not included here   N Newborn Age: 0   P Pediatric Age: 0-17   M Maternity Age: 12-55   A Adult Age: 15-124

450   ICD-10-CM Draft (2015)

C57.8　Malignant neoplasm of overlapping sites **of female** ♀
genital organs
　　Primary malignant neoplasm of two or more contiguous sites of
　　the female genital organs whose point of origin cannot be
　　determined
　　Primary tubo-ovarian malignant neoplasm whose point of origin
　　cannot be determined
　　Primary utero-ovarian malignant neoplasm whose point of
　　origin cannot be determined

C57.9　Malignant neoplasm of female genital organ, unspecified ♀
　　Malignant neoplasm of female genitourinary tract NOS

C58　Malignant neoplasm of placenta ♀
　　INCLUDES　choriocarcinoma NOS
　　　　　　　chorionepithelioma NOS
　　EXCLUDES 1　chorioadenoma (destruens) (D39.2)
　　　　　　　hydatidiform mole NOS (O01.9)
　　　　　　　invasive hydatidiform mole (D39.2)
　　　　　　　male choriocarcinoma NOS (C62.9-)
　　　　　　　malignant hydatidiform mole (D39.2)

Malignant neoplasms of male genital organs (C60-C63)

INCLUDES　malignant neoplasm of skin of male genital organs

✓4ᵗʰ **C60　Malignant neoplasm of** penis

C60.0　Malignant neoplasm of prepuce ♂
　　Malignant neoplasm of foreskin

C60.1　Malignant neoplasm of glans penis ♂

C60.2　Malignant neoplasm of body **of penis** ♂
　　Malignant neoplasm of corpus cavernosum

C60.8　Malignant neoplasm of overlapping sites **of penis** ♂

C60.9　Malignant neoplasm of penis, unspecified ♂
　　Malignant neoplasm of skin of penis NOS

C61　Malignant neoplasm of prostate ♂
　　EXCLUDES 1　malignant neoplasm of seminal vesicle (C63.7)

✓4ᵗʰ **C62　Malignant neoplasm of** testis
　　Use additional code to identify any functional activity

✓5ᵗʰ **C62.0　Malignant neoplasm of** undescended **testis**
　　Malignant neoplasm of ectopic testis
　　Malignant neoplasm of retained testis

C62.00　Malignant neoplasm of unspecified undescended ♂
testis

C62.01　Malignant neoplasm of undescended right **testis** ♂

C62.02　Malignant neoplasm of undescended left **testis** ♂

✓5ᵗʰ **C62.1　Malignant neoplasm of** descended **testis**
　　Malignant neoplasm of scrotal testis

C62.10　Malignant neoplasm of unspecified descended ♂
testis

C62.11　Malignant neoplasm of descended right **testis** ♂

C62.12　Malignant neoplasm of descended left **testis** ♂

✓5ᵗʰ **C62.9　Malignant neoplasm of testis,** unspecified whether
descended or undescended

C62.90　Malignant neoplasm of unspecified testis, ♂
unspecified whether descended or undescended
　　Malignant neoplasm of testis NOS

C62.91　Malignant neoplasm of right **testis, unspecified** ♂
whether descended or undescended

C62.92　Malignant neoplasm of left **testis, unspecified** ♂
whether descended or undescended

✓4ᵗʰ **C63　Malignant neoplasm of** other and unspecified male genital
organs

✓5ᵗʰ **C63.0　Malignant neoplasm of** epididymis

C63.00　Malignant neoplasm of unspecified epididymis ♂

C63.01　Malignant neoplasm of right **epididymis** ♂

C63.02　Malignant neoplasm of left **epididymis** ♂

✓5ᵗʰ **C63.1　Malignant neoplasm of** spermatic cord

C63.10　Malignant neoplasm of unspecified spermatic ♂
cord

C63.11　Malignant neoplasm of right **spermatic cord** ♂

C63.12　Malignant neoplasm of left **spermatic cord** ♂

C63.2　Malignant neoplasm of scrotum ♂
　　Malignant neoplasm of skin of scrotum

C63.7　Malignant neoplasm of other specified **male genital** ♂
organs
　　Malignant neoplasm of seminal vesicle
　　Malignant neoplasm of tunica vaginalis

C63.8　Malignant neoplasm of overlapping sites **of male genital** ♂
organs
　　Primary malignant neoplasm of two or more contiguous sites of
　　male genital organs whose point of origin cannot be
　　determined

C63.9　Malignant neoplasm of male genital organ, unspecified ♂
　　Malignant neoplasm of male genitourinary tract NOS

Malignant neoplasms of urinary tract (C64-C68)

✓4ᵗʰ **C64　Malignant neoplasm of** kidney, except renal pelvis
　　EXCLUDES 1　malignant carcinoid tumor of the kidney (C7A.093)
　　　　　　　malignant neoplasm of renal calyces (C65.-)
　　　　　　　malignant neoplasm of renal pelvis (C65.-)

C64.1　Malignant neoplasm of right **kidney, except renal pelvis**

C64.2　Malignant neoplasm of left **kidney, except renal pelvis**

C64.9　Malignant neoplasm of unspecified kidney, except renal
pelvis

✓4ᵗʰ **C65　Malignant neoplasm of** renal pelvis
　　INCLUDES　malignant neoplasm of pelviureteric junction
　　　　　　　malignant neoplasm of renal calyces

C65.1　Malignant neoplasm of right **renal pelvis**

C65.2　Malignant neoplasm of left **renal pelvis**

C65.9　Malignant neoplasm of unspecified renal pelvis

✓4ᵗʰ **C66　Malignant neoplasm of** ureter
　　EXCLUDES 1　malignant neoplasm of ureteric orifice of bladder (C67.6)

C66.1　Malignant neoplasm of right **ureter**

C66.2　Malignant neoplasm of left **ureter**

C66.9　Malignant neoplasm of unspecified ureter

✓4ᵗʰ **C67　Malignant neoplasm of** bladder

C67.0　Malignant neoplasm of trigone **of bladder**

C67.1　Malignant neoplasm of dome **of bladder**

C67.2　Malignant neoplasm of lateral wall **of bladder**

C67.3　Malignant neoplasm of anterior wall **of bladder**

C67.4　Malignant neoplasm of posterior wall **of bladder**

C67.5　Malignant neoplasm of bladder neck
　　Malignant neoplasm of internal urethral orifice

C67.6　Malignant neoplasm of ureteric orifice

C67.7　Malignant neoplasm of urachus

C67.8　Malignant neoplasm of overlapping sites **of bladder**

C67.9　Malignant neoplasm of bladder, unspecified

✓4ᵗʰ **C68　Malignant neoplasm of** other and unspecified urinary organs
　　EXCLUDES 1　malignant neoplasm of female genitourinary tract NOS (C57.9)
　　　　　　　malignant neoplasm of male genitourinary tract NOS (C63.9)

C68.0　Malignant neoplasm of urethra
　　EXCLUDES 1　malignant neoplasm of urethral orifice of bladder
　　　　　　　(C67.5)

C68.1　Malignant neoplasm of paraurethral glands

C68.8　Malignant neoplasm of overlapping sites **of urinary organs**
　　Primary malignant neoplasm of two or more contiguous sites of
　　urinary organs whose point of origin cannot be determined

C68.9　Malignant neoplasm of urinary organ, unspecified
　　Malignant neoplasm of urinary system NOS

Malignant neoplasms of eye, brain and other parts of central nervous system (C69-C72)

✓4ᵗʰ **C69　Malignant neoplasm of** eye and adnexa
　　EXCLUDES 1　malignant neoplasm of connective tissue of eyelid (C49.0)
　　　　　　　malignant neoplasm of eyelid (skin) (C43.1-, C44.1-)
　　　　　　　malignant neoplasm of optic nerve (C72.3-)

✓5ᵗʰ **C69.0　Malignant neoplasm of** conjunctiva

C69.00　Malignant neoplasm of unspecified conjunctiva

C69.01　Malignant neoplasm of right **conjunctiva**

C69.02　Malignant neoplasm of left **conjunctiva**

✓5ᵗʰ **C69.1　Malignant neoplasm of** cornea

C69.10　Malignant neoplasm of unspecified cornea

C69.11　Malignant neoplasm of right **cornea**

C69.12　Malignant neoplasm of left **cornea**

✓ Additional Character Required　　✓x7ᵗʰ Xtension Alert　　Unspecified Dx　　Other Specified Dx　　Manifestation　　▶◀ Revised Text　　● New Code　　▲ Revised Code Title

ICD-10-CM Draft (2015)　　　　　　　　　　　　　　　　　　　　　　　　　　　　　　　　　　　　451

C69.2 Malignant neoplasm of retina
EXCLUDES 1   dark area on retina (D49.81)
neoplasm of unspecified behavior of retina and choroid (D49.81)
retinal freckle (D49.81)

C69.20   Malignant neoplasm of unspecified retina
C69.21   Malignant neoplasm of right retina
C69.22   Malignant neoplasm of left retina

C69.3 Malignant neoplasm of choroid
C69.30   Malignant neoplasm of unspecified choroid
C69.31   Malignant neoplasm of right choroid
C69.32   Malignant neoplasm of left choroid

C69.4 Malignant neoplasm of ciliary body
C69.40   Malignant neoplasm of unspecified ciliary body
C69.41   Malignant neoplasm of right ciliary body
C69.42   Malignant neoplasm of left ciliary body

C69.5 Malignant neoplasm of lacrimal gland and duct
Malignant neoplasm of lacrimal sac
Malignant neoplasm of nasolacrimal duct
C69.50   Malignant neoplasm of unspecified lacrimal gland and duct
C69.51   Malignant neoplasm of right lacrimal gland and duct
C69.52   Malignant neoplasm of left lacrimal gland and duct

C69.6 Malignant neoplasm of orbit
Malignant neoplasm of connective tissue of orbit
Malignant neoplasm of extraocular muscle
Malignant neoplasm of peripheral nerves of orbit
Malignant neoplasm of retrobulbar tissue
Malignant neoplasm of retro-ocular tissue
EXCLUDES 1   malignant neoplasm of orbital bone (C41.0)
C69.60   Malignant neoplasm of unspecified orbit
C69.61   Malignant neoplasm of right orbit
C69.62   Malignant neoplasm of left orbit

C69.8 Malignant neoplasm of overlapping sites of eye and adnexa
C69.80   Malignant neoplasm of overlapping sites of unspecified eye and adnexa
C69.81   Malignant neoplasm of overlapping sites of right eye and adnexa
C69.82   Malignant neoplasm of overlapping sites of left eye and adnexa

C69.9 Malignant neoplasm of unspecified site of eye
Malignant neoplasm of eyeball
C69.90   Malignant neoplasm of unspecified site of unspecified eye
C69.91   Malignant neoplasm of unspecified site of right eye
C69.92   Malignant neoplasm of unspecified site of left eye

C70 Malignant neoplasm of meninges
C70.0   Malignant neoplasm of cerebral meninges
C70.1   Malignant neoplasm of spinal meninges
C70.9   Malignant neoplasm of meninges, unspecified

C71 Malignant neoplasm of brain
EXCLUDES 1   malignant neoplasm of cranial nerves (C72.2-C72.5)
retrobulbar malignant neoplasm (C69.6-)
C71.0   Malignant neoplasm of cerebrum, except lobes and ventricles
Malignant neoplasm of supratentorial NOS
C71.1   Malignant neoplasm of frontal lobe
C71.2   Malignant neoplasm of temporal lobe
C71.3   Malignant neoplasm of parietal lobe
C71.4   Malignant neoplasm of occipital lobe
C71.5   Malignant neoplasm of cerebral ventricle
EXCLUDES 1   malignant neoplasm of fourth cerebral ventricle (C71.7)
C71.6   Malignant neoplasm of cerebellum
C71.7   Malignant neoplasm of brain stem
Malignant neoplasm of fourth cerebral ventricle
Infratentorial malignant neoplasm NOS
C71.8   Malignant neoplasm of overlapping sites of brain
C71.9   Malignant neoplasm of brain, unspecified

C72 Malignant neoplasm of spinal cord, cranial nerves and other parts of central nervous system
EXCLUDES 1   malignant neoplasm of meninges (C70.-)
malignant neoplasm of peripheral nerves and autonomic nervous system (C47.-)
C72.0   Malignant neoplasm of spinal cord

C72.1   Malignant neoplasm of cauda equina

C72.2 Malignant neoplasm of olfactory nerve
Malignant neoplasm of olfactory bulb
C72.20   Malignant neoplasm of unspecified olfactory nerve
C72.21   Malignant neoplasm of right olfactory nerve
C72.22   Malignant neoplasm of left olfactory nerve

C72.3 Malignant neoplasm of optic nerve
C72.30   Malignant neoplasm of unspecified optic nerve
C72.31   Malignant neoplasm of right optic nerve
C72.32   Malignant neoplasm of left optic nerve

C72.4 Malignant neoplasm of acoustic nerve
C72.40   Malignant neoplasm of unspecified acoustic nerve
C72.41   Malignant neoplasm of right acoustic nerve
C72.42   Malignant neoplasm of left acoustic nerve

C72.5 Malignant neoplasm of other and unspecified cranial nerves
C72.50   Malignant neoplasm of unspecified cranial nerve
Malignant neoplasm of cranial nerve NOS
C72.59   Malignant neoplasm of other cranial nerves
C72.9   Malignant neoplasm of central nervous system, unspecified
Malignant neoplasm of unspecified site of central nervous system
Malignant neoplasm of nervous system NOS

Malignant neoplasms of thyroid and other endocrine glands (C73-C75)

C73 Malignant neoplasm of thyroid gland
Use additional code to identify any functional activity

C74 Malignant neoplasm of adrenal gland
C74.0 Malignant neoplasm of cortex of adrenal gland
C74.00   Malignant neoplasm of cortex of unspecified adrenal gland
C74.01   Malignant neoplasm of cortex of right adrenal gland
C74.02   Malignant neoplasm of cortex of left adrenal gland
C74.1 Malignant neoplasm of medulla of adrenal gland
C74.10   Malignant neoplasm of medulla of unspecified adrenal gland
C74.11   Malignant neoplasm of medulla of right adrenal gland
C74.12   Malignant neoplasm of medulla of left adrenal gland
C74.9 Malignant neoplasm of unspecified part of adrenal gland
C74.90   Malignant neoplasm of unspecified part of unspecified adrenal gland
C74.91   Malignant neoplasm of unspecified part of right adrenal gland
C74.92   Malignant neoplasm of unspecified part of left adrenal gland

C75 Malignant neoplasm of other endocrine glands and related structures
EXCLUDES 1   malignant carcinoid tumors (C7A.0-)
malignant neoplasm of adrenal gland (C74.-)
malignant neoplasm of endocrine pancreas (C25.4)
malignant neoplasm of islets of Langerhans (C25.4)
malignant neoplasm of ovary (C56.-)
malignant neoplasm of testis (C62.-)
malignant neoplasm of thymus (C37)
malignant neoplasm of thyroid gland (C73)
malignant neuroendocrine tumors (C7A.-)
C75.0   Malignant neoplasm of parathyroid gland
C75.1   Malignant neoplasm of pituitary gland
C75.2   Malignant neoplasm of craniopharyngeal duct
C75.3   Malignant neoplasm of pineal gland
C75.4   Malignant neoplasm of carotid body
C75.5   Malignant neoplasm of aortic body and other paraganglia
C75.8   Malignant neoplasm with pluriglandular involvement, unspecified
C75.9   Malignant neoplasm of endocrine gland, unspecified

Malignant neuroendocrine tumors (C7A)

☑4ᵗʰ **C7A   Malignant** neuroendocrine tumors
Code also any associated multiple endocrine neoplasia [MEN]
   syndromes (E31.2-)
Use additional code to identify any associated endocrine syndrome,
   such as:
   carcinoid syndrome (E34.0)
EXCLUDES 2   *malignant pancreatic islet cell tumors (C25.4)*
   Merkel cell carcinoma (C4A.-)

☑5ᵗʰ **C7A.0   Malignant** carcinoid tumors

   C7A.00   Malignant carcinoid tumor of unspecified site

   ☑6ᵗʰ **C7A.01   Malignant** carcinoid tumors of the small intestine

   **C7A.010   Malignant carcinoid tumor of the
      duodenum**

   C7A.011   Malignant carcinoid tumor of the jejunum

   C7A.012   Malignant carcinoid tumor of the ileum

   **C7A.019   Malignant carcinoid tumor of the small
      intestine, unspecified portion**

   ☑6ᵗʰ **C7A.02   Malignant** carcinoid tumors of the appendix, large
      intestine, and rectum

   **C7A.020   Malignant carcinoid tumor of the
      appendix**

   C7A.021   Malignant carcinoid tumor of the cecum

   **C7A.022   Malignant carcinoid tumor of the
      ascending colon**

   **C7A.023   Malignant carcinoid tumor of the
      transverse colon**

   **C7A.024   Malignant carcinoid tumor of the
      descending colon**

   C7A.025   Malignant carcinoid tumor of the sigmoid
      colon

   C7A.026   Malignant carcinoid tumor of the rectum

   **C7A.029   Malignant carcinoid tumor of the large
      intestine, unspecified portion**
      Malignant carcinoid tumor of the colon
         NOS

   ☑6ᵗʰ **C7A.09   Malignant** carcinoid tumors of other sites

   **C7A.090   Malignant carcinoid tumor of the
      bronchus and lung**

   C7A.091   Malignant carcinoid tumor of the thymus

   C7A.092   Malignant carcinoid tumor of the stomach

   C7A.093   Malignant carcinoid tumor of the kidney

   C7A.094   Malignant carcinoid tumor of the foregut
      NOS

   C7A.095   Malignant carcinoid tumor of the midgut
      NOS

   C7A.096   Malignant carcinoid tumor of the hindgut
      NOS

   C7A.098   Malignant carcinoid tumors of other sites

C7A.1   Malignant poorly differentiated neuroendocrine tumors
   High grade neuroendocrine carcinoma, any site
   Malignant poorly differentiated neuroendocrine tumor NOS
   Malignant poorly differentiated neuroendocrine carcinoma, any
      site

C7A.8   Other malignant neuroendocrine tumors

Secondary neuroendocrine tumors (C7B)

☑4ᵗʰ **C7B   Secondary** neuroendocrine tumors
Use additional code to identify any functional activity

☑5ᵗʰ **C7B.0   Secondary** carcinoid tumors

   C7B.00   Secondary carcinoid tumors, unspecified site

   C7B.01   Secondary carcinoid tumors of distant lymph nodes

   C7B.02   Secondary carcinoid tumors of liver

   C7B.03   Secondary carcinoid tumors of bone

   C7B.04   Secondary carcinoid tumors of peritoneum
      Mesentery metastasis of carcinoid tumor

   C7B.09   Secondary carcinoid tumors of other sites

C7B.1   Secondary Merkel cell carcinoma
   Merkel cell carcinoma nodal presentation
   Merkel cell carcinoma visceral metastatic presentation

C7B.8   Other secondary neuroendocrine tumors

Malignant neoplasms of ill-defined, other secondary and unspecified sites (C76-C80)

☑4ᵗʰ **C76   Malignant neoplasm of** other and ill-defined sites
EXCLUDES 1   *malignant neoplasm of female genitourinary tract NOS (C57.9)*
   malignant neoplasm of male genitourinary tract NOS (C63.9)
   *malignant neoplasm of lymphoid, hematopoietic and related
      tissue (C81-C96)*
   malignant neoplasm of skin (C44.-)
   malignant neoplasm of unspecified site NOS (C80.1)

C76.0   Malignant neoplasm of head, face and neck
   Malignant neoplasm of cheek NOS
   Malignant neoplasm of nose NOS

C76.1   Malignant neoplasm of thorax
   Intrathoracic malignant neoplasm NOS
   Malignant neoplasm of axilla NOS
   Thoracic malignant neoplasm NOS

C76.2   Malignant neoplasm of abdomen

C76.3   Malignant neoplasm of pelvis
   Malignant neoplasm of groin NOS
   Malignant neoplasm of sites overlapping systems within the
      pelvis
   Rectovaginal (septum) malignant neoplasm
   Rectovesical (septum) malignant neoplasm

☑5ᵗʰ **C76.4   Malignant neoplasm of** upper limb

   C76.40   Malignant neoplasm of unspecified upper limb

   C76.41   Malignant neoplasm of right upper limb

   C76.42   Malignant neoplasm of left upper limb

☑5ᵗʰ **C76.5   Malignant neoplasm of** lower limb

   C76.50   Malignant neoplasm of unspecified lower limb

   C76.51   Malignant neoplasm of right lower limb

   C76.52   Malignant neoplasm of left lower limb

C76.8   Malignant neoplasm of other specified ill-defined sites
   Malignant neoplasm of overlapping ill-defined sites

☑4ᵗʰ **C77   Secondary and unspecified** malignant neoplasm of lymph nodes
EXCLUDES 1   *malignant neoplasm of lymph nodes, specified as primary
      (C81-C86, C88, C96.-)*
   mesentery metastasis of carcinoid tumor (C7B.04)
   secondary carcinoid tumors of distant lymph nodes (C7B.01)

**C77.0   Secondary and unspecified malignant neoplasm of lymph
      nodes of** head, face and neck
   Secondary and unspecified malignant neoplasm of
      supraclavicular lymph nodes

C77.1   Secondary and unspecified malignant neoplasm of
      intrathoracic lymph nodes

C77.2   Secondary and unspecified malignant neoplasm of
      intra-abdominal lymph nodes

C77.3   Secondary and unspecified malignant neoplasm of axilla and
      upper limb lymph nodes
   Secondary and unspecified malignant neoplasm of pectoral
      lymph nodes

C77.4   Secondary and unspecified malignant neoplasm of inguinal
      and lower limb lymph nodes

C77.5   Secondary and unspecified malignant neoplasm of
      intrapelvic lymph nodes

C77.8   Secondary and unspecified malignant neoplasm of lymph
      nodes of multiple regions

C77.9   Secondary and unspecified malignant neoplasm of lymph
      node, unspecified

☑4ᵗʰ **C78   Secondary** malignant neoplasm of respiratory and digestive
      organs
EXCLUDES 1   *lymph node metastases (C77.0)*
   secondary carcinoid tumors of liver (C7B.02)
   secondary carcinoid tumors of peritoneum (C7B.04)

☑5ᵗʰ **C78.0   Secondary malignant neoplasm of** lung

   C78.00   Secondary malignant neoplasm of unspecified lung

   C78.01   Secondary malignant neoplasm of right lung

   C78.02   Secondary malignant neoplasm of left lung

C78.1   Secondary malignant neoplasm of mediastinum

C78.2   Secondary malignant neoplasm of pleura

☑5ᵗʰ **C78.3   Secondary malignant neoplasm of** other and unspecified
      respiratory organs

   **C78.30   Secondary malignant neoplasm of unspecified
      respiratory organ**

   **C78.39   Secondary malignant neoplasm of other respiratory
      organs**

C78.4   Secondary malignant neoplasm of small intestine

☑ Additional Character Required   √x7ᵗʰ Xtension Alert   Unspecified Dx   Other Specified Dx   Manifestation   ►◄ Revised Text   ● New Code   ▲ Revised Code Title

ICD-10-CM Draft (2015)   453

C78.5   Secondary malignant neoplasm of large intestine and rectum

C78.6   Secondary malignant neoplasm of retroperitoneum and peritoneum

C78.7   Secondary malignant neoplasm of liver and intrahepatic bile duct

✓5ᵗʰ **C78.8**   Secondary malignant neoplasm of other and unspecified digestive organs

   C78.80   Secondary malignant neoplasm of unspecified digestive organ

   C78.89   Secondary malignant neoplasm of other digestive organs

✓4ᵗʰ **C79**   Secondary malignant neoplasm of other and unspecified sites

   EXCLUDES 1   lymph node metastases (C77.0)
               secondary carcinoid tumors (C7B.-)
               secondary neuroendocrine tumors (C7B.-)

✓5ᵗʰ **C79.0**   Secondary malignant neoplasm of kidney and renal pelvis

   C79.00   Secondary malignant neoplasm of unspecified kidney and renal pelvis

   C79.01   Secondary malignant neoplasm of right kidney and renal pelvis

   C79.02   Secondary malignant neoplasm of left kidney and renal pelvis

✓5ᵗʰ **C79.1**   Secondary malignant neoplasm of bladder and other and unspecified urinary organs

   C79.10   Secondary malignant neoplasm of unspecified urinary organs

   C79.11   Secondary malignant neoplasm of bladder

   C79.19   Secondary malignant neoplasm of other urinary organs

C79.2   Secondary malignant neoplasm of skin

   EXCLUDES 1   secondary Merkel cell carcinoma (C7B.1)

✓5ᵗʰ **C79.3**   Secondary malignant neoplasm of brain and cerebral meninges

   C79.31   Secondary malignant neoplasm of brain

   C79.32   Secondary malignant neoplasm of cerebral meninges

✓5ᵗʰ **C79.4**   Secondary malignant neoplasm of other and unspecified parts of nervous system

   C79.40   Secondary malignant neoplasm of unspecified part of nervous system

   C79.49   Secondary malignant neoplasm of other parts of nervous system

✓5ᵗʰ **C79.5**   Secondary malignant neoplasm of bone and bone marrow

   EXCLUDES 1   secondary carcinoid tumors of bone (C7B.03)

   C79.51   Secondary malignant neoplasm of bone

   C79.52   Secondary malignant neoplasm of bone marrow

✓5ᵗʰ **C79.6**   Secondary malignant neoplasm of ovary

   C79.60   Secondary malignant neoplasm of unspecified ovary ♀

   C79.61   Secondary malignant neoplasm of right ovary ♀

   C79.62   Secondary malignant neoplasm of left ovary ♀

✓5ᵗʰ **C79.7**   Secondary malignant neoplasm of adrenal gland

   C79.70   Secondary malignant neoplasm of unspecified adrenal gland

   C79.71   Secondary malignant neoplasm of right adrenal gland

   C79.72   Secondary malignant neoplasm of left adrenal gland

✓5ᵗʰ **C79.8**   Secondary malignant neoplasm of other specified sites

   C79.81   Secondary malignant neoplasm of breast

   C79.82   Secondary malignant neoplasm of genital organs

   C79.89   Secondary malignant neoplasm of other specified sites

C79.9   Secondary malignant neoplasm of unspecified site

   Metastatic cancer NOS
   Metastatic disease NOS

   EXCLUDES 1   carcinomatosis NOS (C80.0)
               generalized cancer NOS (C80.0)
               malignant (primary) neoplasm of unspecified site (C80.1)

✓4ᵗʰ **C80**   Malignant neoplasm without specification of site

   EXCLUDES 1   malignant carcinoid tumor of unspecified site (C7A.00)
               malignant neoplasm of specified multiple sites—code to each site

C80.0   Disseminated malignant neoplasm, unspecified

   Carcinomatosis NOS
   Generalized cancer, unspecified site (primary) (secondary)
   Generalized malignancy, unspecified site (primary) (secondary)

C80.1   Malignant (primary) neoplasm, unspecified

   Cancer NOS
   Cancer unspecified site (primary)
   Carcinoma unspecified site (primary)
   Malignancy unspecified site (primary)

   EXCLUDES 1   secondary malignant neoplasm of unspecified site (C79.9)

C80.2   Malignant neoplasm associated with transplanted organ

   Code first complication of transplanted organ (T86.-)
   Use additional code to identify the specific malignancy

Malignant neoplasms of lymphoid, hematopoietic and related tissue (C81-C96)

   EXCLUDES 2   Kaposi's sarcoma of lymph nodes (C46.3)
               secondary and unspecified neoplasm of lymph nodes (C77.-)
               secondary neoplasm of bone marrow (C79.52)
               secondary neoplasm of spleen (C78.89)

✓4ᵗʰ **C81**   Hodgkin lymphoma

   EXCLUDES 1   personal history of Hodgkin lymphoma (Z85.71)

✓5ᵗʰ **C81.0**   Nodular lymphocyte predominant Hodgkin lymphoma

   C81.00   Nodular lymphocyte predominant Hodgkin lymphoma, unspecified site

   C81.01   Nodular lymphocyte predominant Hodgkin lymphoma, lymph nodes of head, face, and neck

   C81.02   Nodular lymphocyte predominant Hodgkin lymphoma, intrathoracic lymph nodes

   C81.03   Nodular lymphocyte predominant Hodgkin lymphoma, intra-abdominal lymph nodes

   C81.04   Nodular lymphocyte predominant Hodgkin lymphoma, lymph nodes of axilla and upper limb

   C81.05   Nodular lymphocyte predominant Hodgkin lymphoma, lymph nodes of inguinal region and lower limb

   C81.06   Nodular lymphocyte predominant Hodgkin lymphoma, intrapelvic lymph nodes

   C81.07   Nodular lymphocyte predominant Hodgkin lymphoma, spleen

   C81.08   Nodular lymphocyte predominant Hodgkin lymphoma, lymph nodes of multiple sites

   C81.09   Nodular lymphocyte predominant Hodgkin lymphoma, extranodal and solid organ sites

✓5ᵗʰ **C81.1**   Nodular sclerosis classical Hodgkin lymphoma

   C81.10   Nodular sclerosis classical Hodgkin lymphoma, unspecified site

   C81.11   Nodular sclerosis classical Hodgkin lymphoma, lymph nodes of head, face, and neck

   C81.12   Nodular sclerosis classical Hodgkin lymphoma, intrathoracic lymph nodes

   C81.13   Nodular sclerosis classical Hodgkin lymphoma, intra-abdominal lymph nodes

   C81.14   Nodular sclerosis classical Hodgkin lymphoma, lymph nodes of axilla and upper limb

   C81.15   Nodular sclerosis classical Hodgkin lymphoma, lymph nodes of inguinal region and lower limb

   C81.16   Nodular sclerosis classical Hodgkin lymphoma, intrapelvic lymph nodes

   C81.17   Nodular sclerosis classical Hodgkin lymphoma, spleen

   C81.18   Nodular sclerosis classical Hodgkin lymphoma, lymph nodes of multiple sites

   C81.19   Nodular sclerosis classical Hodgkin lymphoma, extranodal and solid organ sites

✓5ᵗʰ **C81.2**   Mixed cellularity classical Hodgkin lymphoma

   C81.20   Mixed cellularity classical Hodgkin lymphoma, unspecified site

   C81.21   Mixed cellularity classical Hodgkin lymphoma, lymph nodes of head, face, and neck

   C81.22   Mixed cellularity classical Hodgkin lymphoma, intrathoracic lymph nodes

EXCLUDES 1 Not coded here   EXCLUDES 2 Not included here   N Newborn Age: 0   P Pediatric Age: 0-17   M Maternity Age: 12-55   A Adult Age: 15-124

454   ICD-10-CM Draft (2015)

C81.23 Mixed cellularity classical Hodgkin lymphoma, intra-abdominal lymph nodes

C81.24 Mixed cellularity classical Hodgkin lymphoma, lymph nodes of axilla and upper limb

C81.25 Mixed cellularity classical Hodgkin lymphoma, lymph nodes of inguinal region and lower limb

C81.26 Mixed cellularity classical Hodgkin lymphoma, intrapelvic lymph nodes

C81.27 Mixed cellularity classical Hodgkin lymphoma, spleen

C81.28 Mixed cellularity classical Hodgkin lymphoma, lymph nodes of multiple sites

C81.29 Mixed cellularity classical Hodgkin lymphoma, extranodal and solid organ sites

√5ᵗʰ **C81.3 Lymphocyte-depleted classical Hodgkin lymphoma**

C81.30 Lymphocyte-depleted classical Hodgkin lymphoma, unspecified site

C81.31 Lymphocyte-depleted classical Hodgkin lymphoma, lymph nodes of head, face, and neck

C81.32 Lymphocyte-depleted classical Hodgkin lymphoma, intrathoracic lymph nodes

C81.33 Lymphocyte-depleted classical Hodgkin lymphoma, intra-abdominal lymph nodes

C81.34 Lymphocyte-depleted classical Hodgkin lymphoma, lymph nodes of axilla and upper limb

C81.35 Lymphocyte-depleted classical Hodgkin lymphoma, lymph nodes of inguinal region and lower limb

C81.36 Lymphocyte-depleted classical Hodgkin lymphoma, intrapelvic lymph nodes

C81.37 Lymphocyte-depleted classical Hodgkin lymphoma, spleen

C81.38 Lymphocyte-depleted classical Hodgkin lymphoma, lymph nodes of multiple sites

C81.39 Lymphocyte-depleted classical Hodgkin lymphoma, extranodal and solid organ sites

√5ᵗʰ **C81.4 Lymphocyte-rich classical Hodgkin lymphoma**
EXCLUDES 1 nodular lymphocyte predominant Hodgkin lymphoma (C81.0-)

C81.40 Lymphocyte-rich classical Hodgkin lymphoma, unspecified site

C81.41 Lymphocyte-rich classical Hodgkin lymphoma, lymph nodes of head, face, and neck

C81.42 Lymphocyte-rich classical Hodgkin lymphoma, intrathoracic lymph nodes

C81.43 Lymphocyte-rich classical Hodgkin lymphoma, intra-abdominal lymph nodes

C81.44 Lymphocyte-rich classical Hodgkin lymphoma, lymph nodes of axilla and upper limb

C81.45 Lymphocyte-rich classical Hodgkin lymphoma, lymph nodes of inguinal region and lower limb

C81.46 Lymphocyte-rich classical Hodgkin lymphoma, intrapelvic lymph nodes

C81.47 Lymphocyte-rich classical Hodgkin lymphoma, spleen

C81.48 Lymphocyte-rich classical Hodgkin lymphoma, lymph nodes of multiple sites

C81.49 Lymphocyte-rich classical Hodgkin lymphoma, extranodal and solid organ sites

√5ᵗʰ **C81.7 Other classical Hodgkin lymphoma**
Classical Hodgkin lymphoma NOS

C81.70 Other classical Hodgkin lymphoma, unspecified site

C81.71 Other classical Hodgkin lymphoma, lymph nodes of head, face, and neck

C81.72 Other classical Hodgkin lymphoma, intrathoracic lymph nodes

C81.73 Other classical Hodgkin lymphoma, intra-abdominal lymph nodes

C81.74 Other classical Hodgkin lymphoma, lymph nodes of axilla and upper limb

C81.75 Other classical Hodgkin lymphoma, lymph nodes of inguinal region and lower limb

C81.76 Other classical Hodgkin lymphoma, intrapelvic lymph nodes

C81.77 Other classical Hodgkin lymphoma, spleen

C81.78 Other classical Hodgkin lymphoma, lymph nodes of multiple sites

C81.79 Other classical Hodgkin lymphoma, extranodal and solid organ sites

√5ᵗʰ **C81.9 Hodgkin lymphoma, unspecified**

C81.90 Hodgkin lymphoma, unspecified, unspecified site

C81.91 Hodgkin lymphoma, unspecified, lymph nodes of head, face, and neck

C81.92 Hodgkin lymphoma, unspecified, intrathoracic lymph nodes

C81.93 Hodgkin lymphoma, unspecified, intra-abdominal lymph nodes

C81.94 Hodgkin lymphoma, unspecified, lymph nodes of axilla and upper limb

C81.95 Hodgkin lymphoma, unspecified, lymph nodes of inguinal region and lower limb

C81.96 Hodgkin lymphoma, unspecified, intrapelvic lymph nodes

C81.97 Hodgkin lymphoma, unspecified, spleen

C81.98 Hodgkin lymphoma, unspecified, lymph nodes of multiple sites

C81.99 Hodgkin lymphoma, unspecified, extranodal and solid organ sites

√4ᵗʰ **C82 Follicular lymphoma**
INCLUDES follicular lymphoma with or without diffuse areas
EXCLUDES 1 mature T/NK-cell lymphomas (C84.-)
personal history of non-Hodgkin lymphoma (Z85.72)

√5ᵗʰ **C82.0 Follicular lymphoma grade I**

C82.00 Follicular lymphoma grade I, unspecified site

C82.01 Follicular lymphoma grade I, lymph nodes of head, face, and neck

C82.02 Follicular lymphoma grade I, intrathoracic lymph nodes

C82.03 Follicular lymphoma grade I, intra-abdominal lymph nodes

C82.04 Follicular lymphoma grade I, lymph nodes of axilla and upper limb

C82.05 Follicular lymphoma grade I, lymph nodes of inguinal region and lower limb

C82.06 Follicular lymphoma grade I, intrapelvic lymph nodes

C82.07 Follicular lymphoma grade I, spleen

C82.08 Follicular lymphoma grade I, lymph nodes of multiple sites

C82.09 Follicular lymphoma grade I, extranodal and solid organ sites

√5ᵗʰ **C82.1 Follicular lymphoma grade II**

C82.10 Follicular lymphoma grade II, unspecified site

C82.11 Follicular lymphoma grade II, lymph nodes of head, face, and neck

C82.12 Follicular lymphoma grade II, intrathoracic lymph nodes

C82.13 Follicular lymphoma grade II, intra-abdominal lymph nodes

C82.14 Follicular lymphoma grade II, lymph nodes of axilla and upper limb

C82.15 Follicular lymphoma grade II, lymph nodes of inguinal region and lower limb

C82.16 Follicular lymphoma grade II, intrapelvic lymph nodes

C82.17 Follicular lymphoma grade II, spleen

C82.18 Follicular lymphoma grade II, lymph nodes of multiple sites

C82.19 Follicular lymphoma grade II, extranodal and solid organ sites

√5ᵗʰ **C82.2 Follicular lymphoma grade III, unspecified**

C82.20 Follicular lymphoma grade III, unspecified, unspecified site

C82.21 Follicular lymphoma grade III, unspecified, lymph nodes of head, face, and neck

C82.22 Follicular lymphoma grade III, unspecified, intrathoracic lymph nodes

C82.23 Follicular lymphoma grade III, unspecified, intra-abdominal lymph nodes

C82.24 Follicular lymphoma grade III, unspecified, lymph nodes of axilla and upper limb

C82.25 Follicular lymphoma grade III, unspecified, lymph nodes of inguinal region and lower limb

Neoplasms

C82.26–C83.09

C82.26   Follicular lymphoma grade III, unspecified, intrapelvic lymph nodes

C82.27   Follicular lymphoma grade III, unspecified, spleen

C82.28   Follicular lymphoma grade III, unspecified, lymph nodes of multiple sites

C82.29   Follicular lymphoma grade III, unspecified, extranodal and solid organ sites

✓5ᵗʰ **C82.3   Follicular lymphoma grade IIIa**

C82.30   **Follicular lymphoma grade IIIa, unspecified site**

C82.31   **Follicular lymphoma grade IIIa, lymph nodes of head, face, and neck**

C82.32   **Follicular lymphoma grade IIIa, intrathoracic lymph nodes**

C82.33   **Follicular lymphoma grade IIIa, intra-abdominal lymph nodes**

C82.34   **Follicular lymphoma grade IIIa, lymph nodes of axilla and upper limb**

C82.35   **Follicular lymphoma grade IIIa, lymph nodes of inguinal region and lower limb**

C82.36   **Follicular lymphoma grade IIIa, intrapelvic lymph nodes**

C82.37   **Follicular lymphoma grade IIIa, spleen**

C82.38   **Follicular lymphoma grade IIIa, lymph nodes of multiple sites**

C82.39   **Follicular lymphoma grade IIIa, extranodal and solid organ sites**

✓5ᵗʰ **C82.4   Follicular lymphoma grade IIIb**

C82.40   **Follicular lymphoma grade IIIb, unspecified site**

C82.41   **Follicular lymphoma grade IIIb, lymph nodes of head, face, and neck**

C82.42   **Follicular lymphoma grade IIIb, intrathoracic lymph nodes**

C82.43   **Follicular lymphoma grade IIIb, intra-abdominal lymph nodes**

C82.44   **Follicular lymphoma grade IIIb, lymph nodes of axilla and upper limb**

C82.45   **Follicular lymphoma grade IIIb, lymph nodes of inguinal region and lower limb**

C82.46   **Follicular lymphoma grade IIIb, intrapelvic lymph nodes**

C82.47   **Follicular lymphoma grade IIIb, spleen**

C82.48   **Follicular lymphoma grade IIIb, lymph nodes of multiple sites**

C82.49   **Follicular lymphoma grade IIIb, extranodal and solid organ sites**

✓5ᵗʰ **C82.5   Diffuse follicle center lymphoma**

C82.50   **Diffuse follicle center lymphoma, unspecified site**

C82.51   **Diffuse follicle center lymphoma, lymph nodes of head, face, and neck**

C82.52   **Diffuse follicle center lymphoma, intrathoracic lymph nodes**

C82.53   **Diffuse follicle center lymphoma, intra-abdominal lymph nodes**

C82.54   **Diffuse follicle center lymphoma, lymph nodes of axilla and upper limb**

C82.55   **Diffuse follicle center lymphoma, lymph nodes of inguinal region and lower limb**

C82.56   **Diffuse follicle center lymphoma, intrapelvic lymph nodes**

C82.57   **Diffuse follicle center lymphoma, spleen**

C82.58   **Diffuse follicle center lymphoma, lymph nodes of multiple sites**

C82.59   **Diffuse follicle center lymphoma, extranodal and solid organ sites**

✓5ᵗʰ **C82.6   Cutaneous follicle center lymphoma**

C82.60   **Cutaneous follicle center lymphoma, unspecified site**

C82.61   **Cutaneous follicle center lymphoma, lymph nodes of head, face, and neck**

C82.62   **Cutaneous follicle center lymphoma, intrathoracic lymph nodes**

C82.63   **Cutaneous follicle center lymphoma, intra-abdominal lymph nodes**

C82.64   **Cutaneous follicle center lymphoma, lymph nodes of axilla and upper limb**

C82.65   **Cutaneous follicle center lymphoma, lymph nodes of inguinal region and lower limb**

C82.66   **Cutaneous follicle center lymphoma, intrapelvic lymph nodes**

C82.67   **Cutaneous follicle center lymphoma, spleen**

C82.68   **Cutaneous follicle center lymphoma, lymph nodes of multiple sites**

C82.69   **Cutaneous follicle center lymphoma, extranodal and solid organ sites**

✓5ᵗʰ **C82.8   Other types of follicular lymphoma**

C82.80   **Other types of follicular lymphoma, unspecified site**

C82.81   **Other types of follicular lymphoma, lymph nodes of head, face, and neck**

C82.82   **Other types of follicular lymphoma, intrathoracic lymph nodes**

C82.83   **Other types of follicular lymphoma, intra-abdominal lymph nodes**

C82.84   **Other types of follicular lymphoma, lymph nodes of axilla and upper limb**

C82.85   **Other types of follicular lymphoma, lymph nodes of inguinal region and lower limb**

C82.86   **Other types of follicular lymphoma, intrapelvic lymph nodes**

C82.87   **Other types of follicular lymphoma, spleen**

C82.88   **Other types of follicular lymphoma, lymph nodes of multiple sites**

C82.89   **Other types of follicular lymphoma, extranodal and solid organ sites**

✓5ᵗʰ **C82.9   Follicular lymphoma, unspecified**

C82.90   **Follicular lymphoma, unspecified, unspecified site**

C82.91   **Follicular lymphoma, unspecified, lymph nodes of head, face, and neck**

C82.92   **Follicular lymphoma, unspecified, intrathoracic lymph nodes**

C82.93   **Follicular lymphoma, unspecified, intra-abdominal lymph nodes**

C82.94   **Follicular lymphoma, unspecified, lymph nodes of axilla and upper limb**

C82.95   **Follicular lymphoma, unspecified, lymph nodes of inguinal region and lower limb**

C82.96   **Follicular lymphoma, unspecified, intrapelvic lymph nodes**

C82.97   **Follicular lymphoma, unspecified, spleen**

C82.98   **Follicular lymphoma, unspecified, lymph nodes of multiple sites**

C82.99   **Follicular lymphoma, unspecified, extranodal and solid organ sites**

✓4ᵗʰ **C83   Non-follicular lymphoma**

EXCLUDES 1   personal history of non-Hodgkin lymphoma (Z85.72)

✓5ᵗʰ **C83.0   Small cell B-cell lymphoma**

Lymphoplasmacytic lymphoma
Nodal marginal zone lymphoma
Non-leukemic variant of B-CLL
Splenic marginal zone lymphoma

EXCLUDES 1   chronic lymphocytic leukemia (C91.1)
mature T/NK-cell lymphomas (C84.-)
Waldenström macroglobulinemia (C88.0)

C83.00   **Small cell B-cell lymphoma, unspecified site**

C83.01   **Small cell B-cell lymphoma, lymph nodes of head, face, and neck**

C83.02   **Small cell B-cell lymphoma, intrathoracic lymph nodes**

C83.03   **Small cell B-cell lymphoma, intra-abdominal lymph nodes**

C83.04   **Small cell B-cell lymphoma, lymph nodes of axilla and upper limb**

C83.05   **Small cell B-cell lymphoma, lymph nodes of inguinal region and lower limb**

C83.06   **Small cell B-cell lymphoma, intrapelvic lymph nodes**

C83.07   **Small cell B-cell lymphoma, spleen**

C83.08   **Small cell B-cell lymphoma, lymph nodes of multiple sites**

C83.09   **Small cell B-cell lymphoma, extranodal and solid organ sites**

EXCLUDES 1 Not coded here   EXCLUDES 2 Not included here   N Newborn Age: 0   P Pediatric Age: 0-17   M Maternity Age: 12-55   A Adult Age: 15-124

456   ICD-10-CM Draft (2015)

☑5th **C83.1** Mantle cell lymphoma
Centrocytic lymphoma
Malignant lymphomatous polyposis

C83.10 **Mantle cell lymphoma, unspecified site**

C83.11 **Mantle cell lymphoma, lymph nodes of** head, face, and neck

C83.12 **Mantle cell lymphoma, intrathoracic lymph nodes**

C83.13 **Mantle cell lymphoma, intra-abdominal lymph nodes**

C83.14 **Mantle cell lymphoma, lymph nodes of** axilla and upper limb

C83.15 **Mantle cell lymphoma, lymph nodes of** inguinal region and lower limb

C83.16 **Mantle cell lymphoma, intrapelvic lymph nodes**

C83.17 **Mantle cell lymphoma, spleen**

C83.18 **Mantle cell lymphoma, lymph nodes of** multiple sites

C83.19 **Mantle cell lymphoma, extranodal and solid organ sites**

☑5th **C83.3** Diffuse large B-cell lymphoma
Anaplastic diffuse large B-cell lymphoma
CD30-positive diffuse large B-cell lymphoma
Centroblastic diffuse large B-cell lymphoma
Diffuse large B-cell lymphoma, subtype not specified
Immunoblastic diffuse large B-cell lymphoma
Plasmablastic diffuse large B-cell lymphoma
T-cell rich diffuse large B-cell lymphoma
EXCLUDES 1 *mature T/NK-cell lymphomas (C84.-)*
mediastinal (thymic) large B-cell lymphoma (C85.2-)

C83.30 **Diffuse large B-cell lymphoma, unspecified site**

C83.31 **Diffuse large B-cell lymphoma, lymph nodes of** head, face, and neck

C83.32 **Diffuse large B-cell lymphoma, intrathoracic lymph nodes**

C83.33 **Diffuse large B-cell lymphoma, intra-abdominal lymph nodes**

C83.34 **Diffuse large B-cell lymphoma, lymph nodes of** axilla and upper limb

C83.35 **Diffuse large B-cell lymphoma, lymph nodes of** inguinal region and lower limb

C83.36 **Diffuse large B-cell lymphoma, intrapelvic lymph nodes**

C83.37 **Diffuse large B-cell lymphoma, spleen**

C83.38 **Diffuse large B-cell lymphoma, lymph nodes of** multiple sites

C83.39 **Diffuse large B-cell lymphoma, extranodal and solid organ sites**

☑5th **C83.5** Lymphoblastic (diffuse) lymphoma
B-precursor lymphoma
Lymphoblastic B-cell lymphoma
Lymphoblastic lymphoma NOS
Lymphoblastic T-cell lymphoma
T-precursor lymphoma

C83.50 **Lymphoblastic (diffuse) lymphoma, unspecified site**

C83.51 **Lymphoblastic (diffuse) lymphoma, lymph nodes of** head, face, and neck

C83.52 **Lymphoblastic (diffuse) lymphoma, intrathoracic lymph nodes**

C83.53 **Lymphoblastic (diffuse) lymphoma, intra-abdominal lymph nodes**

C83.54 **Lymphoblastic (diffuse) lymphoma, lymph nodes of** axilla and upper limb

C83.55 **Lymphoblastic (diffuse) lymphoma, lymph nodes of** inguinal region and lower limb

C83.56 **Lymphoblastic (diffuse) lymphoma, intrapelvic lymph nodes**

C83.57 **Lymphoblastic (diffuse) lymphoma, spleen**

C83.58 **Lymphoblastic (diffuse) lymphoma, lymph nodes of** multiple sites

C83.59 **Lymphoblastic (diffuse) lymphoma, extranodal and solid organ sites**

☑5th **C83.7** Burkitt lymphoma
Atypical Burkitt lymphoma
Burkitt-like lymphoma
EXCLUDES 1 *mature B-cell leukemia Burkitt type (C91.A-)*

C83.70 **Burkitt lymphoma, unspecified site**

C83.71 **Burkitt lymphoma, lymph nodes of** head, face, and neck

C83.72 **Burkitt lymphoma, intrathoracic lymph nodes**

C83.73 **Burkitt lymphoma, intra-abdominal lymph nodes**

C83.74 **Burkitt lymphoma, lymph nodes of** axilla and upper limb

C83.75 **Burkitt lymphoma, lymph nodes of** inguinal region and lower limb

C83.76 **Burkitt lymphoma, intrapelvic lymph nodes**

C83.77 **Burkitt lymphoma, spleen**

C83.78 **Burkitt lymphoma, lymph nodes of** multiple sites

C83.79 **Burkitt lymphoma, extranodal and solid organ sites**

☑5th **C83.8** Other non-follicular lymphoma
Intravascular large B-cell lymphoma
Lymphoid granulomatosis
Primary effusion B-cell lymphoma
EXCLUDES 1 *mediastinal (thymic) large B-cell lymphoma (C85.2-)*
T-cell rich B-cell lymphoma (C83.3-)

C83.80 **Other non-follicular lymphoma, unspecified site**

C83.81 **Other non-follicular lymphoma, lymph nodes of** head, face, and neck

C83.82 **Other non-follicular lymphoma, intrathoracic lymph nodes**

C83.83 **Other non-follicular lymphoma, intra-abdominal lymph nodes**

C83.84 **Other non-follicular lymphoma, lymph nodes of** axilla and upper limb

C83.85 **Other non-follicular lymphoma, lymph nodes of** inguinal region and lower limb

C83.86 **Other non-follicular lymphoma, intrapelvic lymph nodes**

C83.87 **Other non-follicular lymphoma, spleen**

C83.88 **Other non-follicular lymphoma, lymph nodes of** multiple sites

C83.89 **Other non-follicular lymphoma, extranodal and solid organ sites**

☑5th **C83.9** Non-follicular (diffuse) lymphoma, unspecified

C83.90 **Non-follicular (diffuse) lymphoma, unspecified, unspecified site**

C83.91 **Non-follicular (diffuse) lymphoma, unspecified, lymph nodes of** head, face, and neck

C83.92 **Non-follicular (diffuse) lymphoma, unspecified, intrathoracic lymph nodes**

C83.93 **Non-follicular (diffuse) lymphoma, unspecified, intra-abdominal lymph nodes**

C83.94 **Non-follicular (diffuse) lymphoma, unspecified, lymph nodes of** axilla and upper limb

C83.95 **Non-follicular (diffuse) lymphoma, unspecified, lymph nodes of** inguinal region and lower limb

C83.96 **Non-follicular (diffuse) lymphoma, unspecified, intrapelvic lymph nodes**

C83.97 **Non-follicular (diffuse) lymphoma, unspecified, spleen**

C83.98 **Non-follicular (diffuse) lymphoma, unspecified, lymph nodes of** multiple sites

C83.99 **Non-follicular (diffuse) lymphoma, unspecified, extranodal and solid organ sites**

☑4th **C84** **Mature T/NK-cell lymphomas**
EXCLUDES 1 *personal history of non-Hodgkin lymphoma (Z85.72)*

☑5th **C84.0** **Mycosis fungoides**
EXCLUDES 1 *peripheral T-cell lymphoma, not classified (C84.4-)*

C84.00 **Mycosis fungoides, unspecified site**

C84.01 **Mycosis fungoides, lymph nodes of** head, face, and neck

C84.02 **Mycosis fungoides, intrathoracic lymph nodes**

C84.03 **Mycosis fungoides, intra-abdominal lymph nodes**

C84.04 **Mycosis fungoides, lymph nodes of** axilla and upper limb

C84.05 **Mycosis fungoides, lymph nodes of** inguinal region and lower limb

C84.06 **Mycosis fungoides, intrapelvic lymph nodes**

C84.07 **Mycosis fungoides, spleen**

C84.08 **Mycosis fungoides, lymph nodes of** multiple sites

C84.09 **Mycosis fungoides, extranodal and solid organ sites**

☑5th **C84.1** Sézary disease

C84.10 **Sézary disease, unspecified site**

C84.11 **Sézary disease, lymph nodes of** head, face, and neck

☑ Additional Character Required   ☑x7th Xtension Alert   Unspecified Dx   Other Specified Dx   Manifestation   ▶◀ Revised Text   ● New Code   ▲ Revised Code Title

ICD-10-CM Draft (2015)   457

C83.1–C84.11

C84.12   Sézary disease, intrathoracic lymph nodes

C84.13   Sézary disease, intra-abdominal lymph nodes

C84.14   Sézary disease, lymph nodes of axilla and upper limb

C84.15   Sézary disease, lymph nodes of inguinal region and lower limb

C84.16   Sézary disease, intrapelvic lymph nodes

C84.17   Sézary disease, spleen

C84.18   Sézary disease, lymph nodes of multiple sites

C84.19   Sézary disease, extranodal and solid organ sites

✓5ᵗʰ **C84.4**   **Peripheral T-cell lymphoma, not classified**
Lennert's lymphoma
Lymphoepithelioid lymphoma
Mature T-cell lymphoma, not elsewhere classified

C84.40   **Peripheral T-cell lymphoma, not classified, unspecified site**

C84.41   **Peripheral T-cell lymphoma, not classified, lymph nodes of head, face, and neck**

C84.42   **Peripheral T-cell lymphoma, not classified, intrathoracic lymph nodes**

C84.43   **Peripheral T-cell lymphoma, not classified, intra-abdominal lymph nodes**

C84.44   **Peripheral T-cell lymphoma, not classified, lymph nodes of axilla and upper limb**

C84.45   **Peripheral T-cell lymphoma, not classified, lymph nodes of inguinal region and lower limb**

C84.46   **Peripheral T-cell lymphoma, not classified, intrapelvic lymph nodes**

C84.47   **Peripheral T-cell lymphoma, not classified, spleen**

C84.48   **Peripheral T-cell lymphoma, not classified, lymph nodes of multiple sites**

C84.49   **Peripheral T-cell lymphoma, not classified, extranodal and solid organ sites**

✓5ᵗʰ **C84.6**   **Anaplastic large cell lymphoma, ALK-positive**
Anaplastic large cell lymphoma, CD30-positive

C84.60   **Anaplastic large cell lymphoma, ALK-positive, unspecified site**

C84.61   **Anaplastic large cell lymphoma, ALK-positive, lymph nodes of head, face, and neck**

C84.62   **Anaplastic large cell lymphoma, ALK-positive, intrathoracic lymph nodes**

C84.63   **Anaplastic large cell lymphoma, ALK-positive, intra-abdominal lymph nodes**

C84.64   **Anaplastic large cell lymphoma, ALK-positive, lymph nodes of axilla and upper limb**

C84.65   **Anaplastic large cell lymphoma, ALK-positive, lymph nodes of inguinal region and lower limb**

C84.66   **Anaplastic large cell lymphoma, ALK-positive, intrapelvic lymph nodes**

C84.67   **Anaplastic large cell lymphoma, ALK-positive, spleen**

C84.68   **Anaplastic large cell lymphoma, ALK-positive, lymph nodes of multiple sites**

C84.69   **Anaplastic large cell lymphoma, ALK-positive, extranodal and solid organ sites**

✓5ᵗʰ **C84.7**   **Anaplastic large cell lymphoma, ALK-negative**
EXCLUDES 1   primary cutaneous CD30-positive T-cell proliferations (C86.6-)

C84.70   **Anaplastic large cell lymphoma, ALK-negative, unspecified site**

C84.71   **Anaplastic large cell lymphoma, ALK-negative, lymph nodes of head, face, and neck**

C84.72   **Anaplastic large cell lymphoma, ALK-negative, intrathoracic lymph nodes**

C84.73   **Anaplastic large cell lymphoma, ALK-negative, intra-abdominal lymph nodes**

C84.74   **Anaplastic large cell lymphoma, ALK-negative, lymph nodes of axilla and upper limb**

C84.75   **Anaplastic large cell lymphoma, ALK-negative, lymph nodes of inguinal region and lower limb**

C84.76   **Anaplastic large cell lymphoma, ALK-negative, intrapelvic lymph nodes**

C84.77   **Anaplastic large cell lymphoma, ALK-negative, spleen**

C84.78   **Anaplastic large cell lymphoma, ALK-negative, lymph nodes of multiple sites**

C84.79   **Anaplastic large cell lymphoma, ALK-negative, extranodal and solid organ sites**

✓5ᵗʰ **C84.A**   **Cutaneous T-cell lymphoma, unspecified**

C84.A0   **Cutaneous T-cell lymphoma, unspecified, unspecified site**

C84.A1   **Cutaneous T-cell lymphoma, unspecified lymph nodes of head, face, and neck**

C84.A2   **Cutaneous T-cell lymphoma, unspecified, intrathoracic lymph nodes**

C84.A3   **Cutaneous T-cell lymphoma, unspecified, intra-abdominal lymph nodes**

C84.A4   **Cutaneous T-cell lymphoma, unspecified, lymph nodes of axilla and upper limb**

C84.A5   **Cutaneous T-cell lymphoma, unspecified, lymph nodes of inguinal region and lower limb**

C84.A6   **Cutaneous T-cell lymphoma, unspecified, intrapelvic lymph nodes**

C84.A7   **Cutaneous T-cell lymphoma, unspecified, spleen**

C84.A8   **Cutaneous T-cell lymphoma, unspecified, lymph nodes of multiple sites**

C84.A9   **Cutaneous T-cell lymphoma, unspecified, extranodal and solid organ sites**

✓5ᵗʰ **C84.Z**   **Other mature T/NK-cell lymphomas**
NOTE   If T-cell lineage or involvement is mentioned in conjunction with a specific lymphoma, code to the more specific description.
EXCLUDES 1   angioimmunoblastic T-cell lymphoma (C86.5)
blastic NK-cell lymphoma (C86.4)
enteropathy-type T-cell lymphoma (C86.2)
extranodal NK-cell lymphoma, nasal type (C86.0)
hepatosplenic T-cell lymphoma (C86.1)
primary cutaneous CD30-positive T-cell proliferations (C86.6)
subcutaneous panniculitis-like T-cell lymphoma (C86.3)
T-cell leukemia (C91.1-)

C84.Z0   **Other mature T/NK-cell lymphomas, unspecified site**

C84.Z1   **Other mature T/NK-cell lymphomas, lymph nodes of head, face, and neck**

C84.Z2   **Other mature T/NK-cell lymphomas, intrathoracic lymph nodes**

C84.Z3   **Other mature T/NK-cell lymphomas, intra-abdominal lymph nodes**

C84.Z4   **Other mature T/NK-cell lymphomas, lymph nodes of axilla and upper limb**

C84.Z5   **Other mature T/NK-cell lymphomas, lymph nodes of inguinal region and lower limb**

C84.Z6   **Other mature T/NK-cell lymphomas, intrapelvic lymph nodes**

C84.Z7   **Other mature T/NK-cell lymphomas, spleen**

C84.Z8   **Other mature T/NK-cell lymphomas, lymph nodes of multiple sites**

C84.Z9   **Other mature T/NK-cell lymphomas, extranodal and solid organ sites**

✓5ᵗʰ **C84.9**   **Mature T/NK-cell lymphomas, unspecified**
NK/T cell lymphoma NOS
EXCLUDES 1   mature T-cell lymphoma, not elsewhere classified (C84.4-)

C84.90   **Mature T/NK-cell lymphomas, unspecified, unspecified site**

C84.91   **Mature T/NK-cell lymphomas, unspecified, lymph nodes of head, face, and neck**

C84.92   **Mature T/NK-cell lymphomas, unspecified, intrathoracic lymph nodes**

C84.93   **Mature T/NK-cell lymphomas, unspecified, intra-abdominal lymph nodes**

C84.94   **Mature T/NK-cell lymphomas, unspecified, lymph nodes of axilla and upper limb**

C84.95   **Mature T/NK-cell lymphomas, unspecified, lymph nodes of inguinal region and lower limb**

C84.96   **Mature T/NK-cell lymphomas, unspecified, intrapelvic lymph nodes**

C84.97   **Mature T/NK-cell lymphomas, unspecified, spleen**

C84.98   **Mature T/NK-cell lymphomas, unspecified, lymph nodes of multiple sites**

C84.99   **Mature T/NK-cell lymphomas, unspecified, extranodal and solid organ sites**

✓4ᵗʰ **C85 Other specified and unspecified types of non-Hodgkin lymphoma**

> **EXCLUDES 1** *other specified types of T/NK-cell lymphoma (C86.-)*
> *personal history of non-Hodgkin lymphoma (Z85.72)*

✓5ᵗʰ **C85.1 Unspecified B-cell lymphoma**

> **NOTE** If B-cell lineage or involvement is mentioned in conjunction with a specific lymphoma, code to the more specific description.

C85.10 Unspecified B-cell lymphoma, unspecified site

C85.11 Unspecified B-cell lymphoma, lymph nodes of head, face, and neck

C85.12 Unspecified B-cell lymphoma, intrathoracic lymph nodes

C85.13 Unspecified B-cell lymphoma, intra-abdominal lymph nodes

C85.14 Unspecified B-cell lymphoma, lymph nodes of axilla and upper limb

C85.15 Unspecified B-cell lymphoma, lymph nodes of inguinal region and lower limb

C85.16 Unspecified B-cell lymphoma, intrapelvic lymph nodes

C85.17 Unspecified B-cell lymphoma, spleen

C85.18 Unspecified B-cell lymphoma, lymph nodes of multiple sites

C85.19 Unspecified B-cell lymphoma, extranodal and solid organ sites

✓5ᵗʰ **C85.2 Mediastinal (thymic) large B-cell lymphoma**

C85.20 Mediastinal (thymic) large B-cell lymphoma, unspecified site

C85.21 Mediastinal (thymic) large B-cell lymphoma, lymph nodes of head, face, and neck

C85.22 Mediastinal (thymic) large B-cell lymphoma, intrathoracic lymph nodes

C85.23 Mediastinal (thymic) large B-cell lymphoma, intra-abdominal lymph nodes

C85.24 Mediastinal (thymic) large B-cell lymphoma, lymph nodes of axilla and upper limb

C85.25 Mediastinal (thymic) large B-cell lymphoma, lymph nodes of inguinal region and lower limb

C85.26 Mediastinal (thymic) large B-cell lymphoma, intrapelvic lymph nodes

C85.27 Mediastinal (thymic) large B-cell lymphoma, spleen

C85.28 Mediastinal (thymic) large B-cell lymphoma, lymph nodes of multiple sites

C85.29 Mediastinal (thymic) large B-cell lymphoma, extranodal and solid organ sites

✓5ᵗʰ **C85.8 Other specified types of non-Hodgkin lymphoma**

C85.80 Other specified types of non-Hodgkin lymphoma, unspecified site

C85.81 Other specified types of non-Hodgkin lymphoma, lymph nodes of head, face, and neck

C85.82 Other specified types of non-Hodgkin lymphoma, intrathoracic lymph nodes

C85.83 Other specified types of non-Hodgkin lymphoma, intra-abdominal lymph nodes

C85.84 Other specified types of non-Hodgkin lymphoma, lymph nodes of axilla and upper limb

C85.85 Other specified types of non-Hodgkin lymphoma, lymph nodes of inguinal region and lower limb

C85.86 Other specified types of non-Hodgkin lymphoma, intrapelvic lymph nodes

C85.87 Other specified types of non-Hodgkin lymphoma, spleen

C85.88 Other specified types of non-Hodgkin lymphoma, lymph nodes of multiple sites

C85.89 Other specified types of non-Hodgkin lymphoma, extranodal and solid organ sites

✓5ᵗʰ **C85.9 Non-Hodgkin lymphoma, unspecified**

Lymphoma NOS
Malignant lymphoma NOS
Non-Hodgkin lymphoma NOS

C85.90 Non-Hodgkin lymphoma, unspecified, unspecified site

C85.91 Non-Hodgkin lymphoma, unspecified, lymph nodes of head, face, and neck

C85.92 Non-Hodgkin lymphoma, unspecified, intrathoracic lymph nodes

C85.93 Non-Hodgkin lymphoma, unspecified, intra-abdominal lymph nodes

C85.94 Non-Hodgkin lymphoma, unspecified, lymph nodes of axilla and upper limb

C85.95 Non-Hodgkin lymphoma, unspecified, lymph nodes of inguinal region and lower limb

C85.96 Non-Hodgkin lymphoma, unspecified, intrapelvic lymph nodes

C85.97 Non-Hodgkin lymphoma, unspecified, spleen

C85.98 Non-Hodgkin lymphoma, unspecified, lymph nodes of multiple sites

C85.99 Non-Hodgkin lymphoma, unspecified, extranodal and solid organ sites

✓4ᵗʰ **C86 Other specified types of T/NK-cell lymphoma**

> **EXCLUDES 1** *anaplastic large cell lymphoma, ALK negative (C84.7-)*
> *anaplastic large cell lymphoma, ALK positive (C84.6-)*
> *mature T/NK-cell lymphomas (C84.-)*
> *other specified types of non-Hodgkin lymphoma (C85.8-)*

C86.0 Extranodal NK/T-cell lymphoma, nasal type

C86.1 Hepatosplenic T-cell lymphoma
Alpha-beta and gamma delta types

C86.2 Enteropathy-type (intestinal) T-cell lymphoma
Enteropathy associated T-cell lymphoma

C86.3 Subcutaneous panniculitis-like T-cell lymphoma

C86.4 Blastic NK-cell lymphoma

C86.5 Angioimmunoblastic T-cell lymphoma
Angioimmunoblastic lymphadenopathy with dysproteinemia [AILD]

C86.6 Primary cutaneous CD30-positive T-cell proliferations
Lymphomatoid papulosis
Primary cutaneous anaplastic large cell lymphoma
Primary cutaneous CD30-positive large T-cell lymphoma

✓4ᵗʰ **C88 Malignant immunoproliferative diseases and certain other B-cell lymphomas**

> **EXCLUDES 1** *B-cell lymphoma, unspecified (C85.1-)*
> *personal history of other malignant neoplasms of lymphoid, hematopoietic and related tissues (Z85.79)*

C88.0 Waldenström macroglobulinemia
Lymphoplasmacytic lymphoma with IgM-production
Macroglobulinemia (idiopathic) (primary)
> **EXCLUDES 1** *small cell B-cell lymphoma (C83.0)*

C88.2 Heavy chain disease
Franklin disease
Gamma heavy chain disease
Mu heavy chain disease

C88.3 Immunoproliferative small intestinal disease
Alpha heavy chain disease
Mediterranean lymphoma

C88.4 Extranodal marginal zone B-cell lymphoma of mucosa-associated lymphoid tissue [MALT-lymphoma]
Lymphoma of skin-associated lymphoid tissue [SALT-lymphoma]
Lymphoma of bronchial-associated lymphoid tissue [BALT-lymphoma]
> **EXCLUDES 1** *high malignant (diffuse large B-cell) lymphoma (C83.3-)*

C88.8 Other malignant immunoproliferative diseases

C88.9 Malignant immunoproliferative disease, unspecified
Immunoproliferative disease NOS

✓4ᵗʰ **C90 Multiple myeloma and malignant plasma cell neoplasms**

> **EXCLUDES 1** *personal history of other malignant neoplasms of lymphoid, hematopoietic and related tissues (Z85.79)*

✓5ᵗʰ **C90.0 Multiple myeloma**
Kahler's disease   Myelomatosis
Medullary plasmacytoma   Plasma cell myeloma
> **EXCLUDES 1** *solitary myeloma (C90.3-)*
> *solitary plasmacytoma (C90.3-)*

C90.00 Multiple myeloma not having achieved remission
Multiple myeloma with failed remission
Multiple myeloma NOS

C90.01 Multiple myeloma in remission

C90.02 Multiple myeloma in relapse

✓5ᵗʰ **C90.1 Plasma cell leukemia**
Plasmacytic leukemia

C90.10 Plasma cell leukemia not having achieved remission
Plasma cell leukemia with failed remission
Plasma cell leukemia NOS

✓ Additional Character Required   ✓7ᵗʰ Xtension Alert   Unspecified Dx   Other Specified Dx   Manifestation   ►◄ Revised Text   ● New Code   ▲ Revised Code Title

ICD-10-CM Draft (2015)   **459**

Neoplasms

C90.11-C92.12

C90.11   **Plasma cell leukemia** in remission

C90.12   **Plasma cell leukemia** in relapse

√5th **C90.2**   **Extramedullary plasmacytoma**

   C90.20   **Extramedullary plasmacytoma** not having achieved remission

     Extramedullary plasmacytoma with failed remission

     Extramedullary plasmacytoma NOS

   C90.21   **Extramedullary plasmacytoma** in remission

   C90.22   **Extramedullary plasmacytoma** in relapse

√5th **C90.3**   **Solitary plasmacytoma**

   Localized malignant plasma cell tumor NOS

   Plasmacytoma NOS

   Solitary myeloma

   C90.30   **Solitary plasmacytoma** not having achieved remission

     Solitary plasmacytoma with failed remission

     Solitary plasmacytoma NOS

   C90.31   **Solitary plasmacytoma** in remission

   C90.32   **Solitary plasmacytoma** in relapse

√4th **C91**   **Lymphoid leukemia**

   EXCLUDES1   *personal history of leukemia (Z85.6)*

√5th **C91.0**   **Acute lymphoblastic leukemia [ALL]**

   NOTE   Code C91.0 should only be used for T-cell and B-cell precursor leukemia.

   C91.00   **Acute lymphoblastic leukemia** not having achieved remission

     Acute lymphoblastic leukemia with failed remission

     Acute lymphoblastic leukemia NOS

   C91.01   **Acute lymphoblastic leukemia,** in remission

   C91.02   **Acute lymphoblastic leukemia,** in relapse

√5th **C91.1**   **Chronic lymphocytic leukemia of B-cell type**

   Lymphoplasmacytic leukemia

   Richter syndrome

   EXCLUDES1   *lymphoplasmacytic lymphoma (C83.0-)*

   C91.10   **Chronic lymphocytic leukemia of B-cell type** not having achieved remission

     Chronic lymphocytic leukemia of B-cell type with failed remission

     Chronic lymphocytic leukemia of B-cell type NOS

   C91.11   **Chronic lymphocytic leukemia of B-cell type** in remission

   C91.12   **Chronic lymphocytic leukemia of B-cell type** in relapse

√5th **C91.3**   **Prolymphocytic leukemia of B-cell type**

   C91.30   **Prolymphocytic leukemia of B-cell type** not having achieved remission

     Prolymphocytic leukemia of B-cell type with failed remission

     Prolymphocytic leukemia of B-cell type NOS

   C91.31   **Prolymphocytic leukemia of B-cell type,** in remission

   C91.32   **Prolymphocytic leukemia of B-cell type,** in relapse

√5th **C91.4**   **Hairy cell leukemia**

   Leukemic reticuloendotheliosis

   C91.40   **Hairy cell leukemia** not having achieved remission

     Hairy cell leukemia with failed remission

     Hairy cell leukemia NOS

   C91.41   **Hairy cell leukemia,** in remission

   C91.42   **Hairy cell leukemia,** in relapse

√5th **C91.5**   **Adult T-cell lymphoma/leukemia (HTLV-1-associated)**

   Acute variant of adult T-cell lymphoma/leukemia (HTLV-1-associated)

   Chronic variant of adult T-cell lymphoma/leukemia (HTLV-1-associated)

   Lymphomatoid variant of adult T-cell lymphoma/leukemia (HTLV-1-associated)

   Smouldering variant of adult T-cell lymphoma/leukemia (HTLV-1-associated)

   C91.50   **Adult T-cell lymphoma/leukemia (HTLV-1-associated)** not having achieved remission   A

     Adult T-cell lymphoma/leukemia (HTLV-1-associated) with failed remission

     Adult T-cell lymphoma/leukemia (HTLV-1-associated) NOS

   C91.51   **Adult T-cell lymphoma/leukemia (HTLV-1-associated), in remission**   A

   C91.52   **Adult T-cell lymphoma/leukemia (HTLV-1-associated), in relapse**   A

√5th **C91.6**   **Prolymphocytic leukemia of T-cell type**

   C91.60   **Prolymphocytic leukemia of T-cell type** not having achieved remission

     Prolymphocytic leukemia of T-cell type with failed remission

     Prolymphocytic leukemia of T-cell type NOS

   C91.61   **Prolymphocytic leukemia of T-cell type, in remission**

   C91.62   **Prolymphocytic leukemia of T-cell type, in relapse**

√5th **C91.A**   **Mature B-cell leukemia Burkitt-type**

   EXCLUDES1   *Burkitt lymphoma (C83.7-)*

   C91.A0   **Mature B-cell leukemia Burkitt-type** not having achieved remission

     Mature B-cell leukemia Burkitt-type with failed remission

     Mature B-cell leukemia Burkitt-type NOS

   C91.A1   **Mature B-cell leukemia Burkitt-type, in remission**

   C91.A2   **Mature B-cell leukemia Burkitt-type, in relapse**

√5th **C91.Z**   **Other lymphoid leukemia**

   T-cell large granular lymphocytic leukemia (associated with rheumatoid arthritis)

   C91.Z0   **Other lymphoid leukemia** not having achieved remission

     Other lymphoid leukemia with failed remission

     Other lymphoid leukemia NOS

   C91.Z1   **Other lymphoid leukemia, in remission**

   C91.Z2   **Other lymphoid leukemia, in relapse**

√5th **C91.9**   **Lymphoid leukemia, unspecified**

   C91.90   **Lymphoid leukemia, unspecified** not having achieved remission

     Lymphoid leukemia with failed remission

     Lymphoid leukemia NOS

   C91.91   **Lymphoid leukemia, unspecified, in remission**

   C91.92   **Lymphoid leukemia, unspecified, in relapse**

√4th **C92**   **Myeloid leukemia**

   INCLUDES   granulocytic leukemia

         myelogenous leukemia

   EXCLUDES1   *personal history of leukemia (Z85.6)*

√5th **C92.0**   **Acute myeloblastic leukemia**

   Acute myeloblastic leukemia, minimal differentiation

   Acute myeloblastic leukemia (with maturation)

   Acute myeloblastic leukemia 1/ETO

   Acute myeloblastic leukemia M0

   Acute myeloblastic leukemia M1

   Acute myeloblastic leukemia M2

   Acute myeloblastic leukemia with t(8;21)

   Acute myeloblastic leukemia (without a FAB classification) NOS

   Refractory anemia with excess blasts in transformation [RAEB T]

   EXCLUDES1   *acute exacerbation of chronic myeloid leukemia (C92.10)*

         refractory anemia with excess of blasts not in transformation (D46.2-)

   C92.00   **Acute myeloblastic leukemia,** not having achieved remission

     Acute myeloblastic leukemia with failed remission

     Acute myeloblastic leukemia NOS

   C92.01   **Acute myeloblastic leukemia,** in remission

   C92.02   **Acute myeloblastic leukemia,** in relapse

√5th **C92.1**   **Chronic myeloid leukemia, BCR/ABL-positive**

   Chronic myelogenous leukemia, Philadelphia chromosome (Ph1) positive

   Chronic myelogenous leukemia, t(9;22) (q34;q11)

   Chronic myelogenous leukemia with crisis of blast cells

   EXCLUDES1   *atypical chronic myeloid leukemia BCR/ABL-negative (C92.2-)*

         chronic myelomonocytic leukemia (C93.1-)

         chronic myeloproliferative disease (D47.1)

   C92.10   **Chronic myeloid leukemia, BCR/ABL-positive,** not having achieved remission

     Chronic myeloid leukemia, BCR/ABL-positive with failed remission

     Chronic myeloid leukemia, BCR/ABL-positive NOS

   C92.11   **Chronic myeloid leukemia, BCR/ABL-positive,** in remission

   C92.12   **Chronic myeloid leukemia, BCR/ABL-positive,** in relapse

EXCLUDES1 Not coded here   EXCLUDES2 Not included here   N Newborn Age: 0   P Pediatric Age: 0-17   M Maternity Age: 12-55   A Adult Age: 15-124

460   ICD-10-CM Draft (2015)

☑5ᵗʰ **C92.2** Atypical chronic **myeloid leukemia, BCR/ABL-negative**

    C92.20 **Atypical chronic myeloid leukemia, BCR/ABL-negative,** not having achieved remission
         Atypical chronic myeloid leukemia, BCR/ABL-negative with failed remission
         Atypical chronic myeloid leukemia, BCR/ABL-negative NOS

    C92.21 **Atypical chronic myeloid leukemia, BCR/ABL-negative,** in remission

    C92.22 **Atypical chronic myeloid leukemia, BCR/ABL-negative,** in relapse

☑5ᵗʰ **C92.3** Myeloid sarcoma
     A malignant tumor of immature myeloid cells
     Chloroma
     Granulocytic sarcoma

    C92.30 **Myeloid sarcoma,** not having achieved remission
         Myeloid sarcoma with failed remission
         Myeloid sarcoma NOS

    C92.31 **Myeloid sarcoma,** in remission

    C92.32 **Myeloid sarcoma,** in relapse

☑5ᵗʰ **C92.4** Acute promyelocytic **leukemia**
     AML M3
     AML Me with t(15;17) and variants

    C92.40 **Acute promyelocytic leukemia,** not having achieved remission
         Acute promyelocytic leukemia with failed remission
         Acute promyelocytic leukemia NOS

    C92.41 **Acute promyelocytic leukemia,** in remission

    C92.42 **Acute promyelocytic leukemia,** in relapse

☑5ᵗʰ **C92.5** Acute myelomonocytic **leukemia**
     AML M4
     AML M4 Eo with inv(16) or t(16;16)

    C92.50 **Acute myelomonocytic leukemia,** not having achieved remission
         Acute myelomonocytic leukemia with failed remission
         Acute myelomonocytic leukemia NOS

    C92.51 **Acute myelomonocytic leukemia,** in remission

    C92.52 **Acute myelomonocytic leukemia,** in relapse

☑5ᵗʰ **C92.6** Acute myeloid **leukemia with** multilineage **dysplasia**
     Acute myeloid leukemia with variation of MLL-gene

    C92.60 **Acute myeloid leukemia with 11q23-abnormality** not having achieved remission
         Acute myeloid leukemia with 11q23-abnormality with failed remission
         Acute myeloid leukemia with 11q23-abnormality NOS

    C92.61 **Acute myeloid leukemia with 11q23-abnormality** in remission

    C92.62 **Acute myeloid leukemia with 11q23-abnormality** in relapse

☑5ᵗʰ **C92.A** Acute myeloid **leukemia with** multilineage dysplasia
     Acute myeloid leukemia with dysplasia of remaining hematopoesis and/or myelodysplastic disease in its history

    C92.A0 **Acute myeloid leukemia with multilineage dysplasia,** not having achieved remission
         Acute myeloid leukemia with multilineage dysplasia with failed remission
         Acute myeloid leukemia with multilineage dysplasia NOS

    C92.A1 **Acute myeloid leukemia with multilineage dysplasia,** in remission

    C92.A2 **Acute myeloid leukemia with multilineage dysplasia,** in relapse

☑5ᵗʰ **C92.Z** Other **myeloid leukemia**

    C92.Z0 **Other myeloid leukemia** not having achieved remission
         Myeloid leukemia NEC with failed remission
         Myeloid leukemia NEC

    C92.Z1 **Other myeloid leukemia,** in remission

    C92.Z2 **Other myeloid leukemia,** in relapse

☑5ᵗʰ **C92.9** Myeloid **leukemia,** unspecified

    C92.90 **Myeloid leukemia, unspecified,** not having achieved remission
         Myeloid leukemia, unspecified with failed remission
         Myeloid leukemia, unspecified NOS

    C92.91 **Myeloid leukemia, unspecified** in remission

    C92.92 **Myeloid leukemia, unspecified** in relapse

☑4ᵗʰ **C93** **Monocytic leukemia**
     INCLUDES monocytoid leukemia
     EXCLUDES 1 *personal history of leukemia (Z85.6)*

☑5ᵗʰ **C93.0** Acute **monoblastic/monocytic leukemia**
     AML M5   AML M5b
     AML M5a

    C93.00 **Acute monoblastic/monocytic leukemia,** not having achieved remission
         Acute monoblastic/monocytic leukemia with failed remission
         Acute monoblastic/monocytic leukemia NOS

    C93.01 **Acute monoblastic/monocytic leukemia,** in remission

    C93.02 **Acute monoblastic/monocytic leukemia,** in relapse

☑5ᵗʰ **C93.1** Chronic **myelomonocytic leukemia**
     Chronic monocytic leukemia
     CMML-1
     CMML-2
     CMML with eosinophilia

    C93.10 **Chronic myelomonocytic leukemia** not having achieved remission
         Chronic myelomonocytic leukemia with failed remission
         Chronic myelomonocytic leukemia NOS

    C93.11 **Chronic myelomonocytic leukemia,** in remission

    C93.12 **Chronic myelomonocytic leukemia,** in relapse

☑5ᵗʰ **C93.3** Juvenile **myelomonocytic leukemia**

    C93.30 **Juvenile myelomonocytic leukemia,** not having achieved remission   P
         Juvenile myelomonocytic leukemia with failed remission
         Juvenile myelomonocytic leukemia NOS

    C93.31 **Juvenile myelomonocytic leukemia,** in remission   P

    C93.32 **Juvenile myelomonocytic leukemia,** in relapse   P

☑5ᵗʰ **C93.Z** Other **monocytic leukemia**

    C93.Z0 **Other monocytic leukemia,** not having achieved remission
         Other monocytic leukemia NOS

    C93.Z1 **Other monocytic leukemia,** in remission

    C93.Z2 **Other monocytic leukemia,** in relapse

☑5ᵗʰ **C93.9** Monocytic **leukemia,** unspecified

    C93.90 **Monocytic leukemia, unspecified,** not having achieved remission
         Monocytic leukemia, unspecified with failed remission
         Monocytic leukemia, unspecified NOS

    C93.91 **Monocytic leukemia, unspecified** in remission

    C93.92 **Monocytic leukemia, unspecified** in relapse

☑4ᵗʰ **C94** **Other leukemias of** specified cell type
     EXCLUDES 1 *leukemic reticuloendotheliosis (C91.4-)*
         myelodysplastic syndromes (D46.-)
         personal history of leukemia (Z85.6)
         plasma cell leukemia (C90.1-)

☑5ᵗʰ **C94.0** Acute **erythroid leukemia**
     Acute myeloid leukemia M6(a)(b)
     Erythroleukemia

    C94.00 **Acute erythroid leukemia,** not having achieved remission
         Acute erythroid leukemia with failed remission
         Acute erythroid leukemia NOS

    C94.01 **Acute erythroid leukemia,** in remission

    C94.02 **Acute erythroid leukemia,** in relapse

☑5ᵗʰ **C94.2** Acute **megakaryoblastic leukemia**
     Acute myeloid leukemia M7
     Acute megakaryocytic leukemia

    C94.20 **Acute megakaryoblastic leukemia** not having achieved remission
         Acute megakaryoblastic leukemia with failied remission
         Acute megakaryoblastic leukemia NOS

    C94.21 **Acute megakaryoblastic leukemia,** in remission

    C94.22 **Acute megakaryoblastic leukemia,** in relapse

☑5ᵗʰ **C94.3** Mast **cell leukemia**

    C94.30 **Mast cell leukemia** not having achieved remission
         Mast cell leukemia with failed remission
         Mast cell leukemia NOS

    C94.31 **Mast cell leukemia,** in remission

    C94.32 **Mast cell leukemia,** in relapse

☑ Additional Character Required   ☑x7ᵗʰ Xtension Alert   Unspecified Dx   Other Specified Dx   Manifestation   ►◄ Revised Text   ● New Code   ▲ Revised Code Title

Neoplasms

C94.4–D01.5

☑5ᵗʰ **C94.4 Acute panmyelosis with myelofibrosis**
Acute myelofibrosis
EXCLUDES 1 *myelofibrosis NOS (D75.81)*
secondary myelofibrosis NOS (D75.81)

     C94.40 Acute panmyelosis with myelofibrosis not having achieved remission
Acute myelofibrosis NOS
Acute panmyelosis with myelofibrosis with failed remission
Acute panmyelosis NOS

     C94.41 Acute panmyelosis with myelofibrosis, in remission

     C94.42 Acute panmyelosis with myelofibrosis, in relapse

C94.6 Myelodysplastic disease, not classified
Myeloproliferative disease, not classified

☑5ᵗʰ **C94.8 Other specified leukemias**
Aggressive NK-cell leukemia
Acute basophilic leukemia

     C94.80 Other specified leukemias not having achieved remission
Other specified leukemia with failed remission
Other specified leukemias NOS

     C94.81 Other specified leukemias, in remission

     C94.82 Other specified leukemias, in relapse

☑4ᵗʰ **C95 Leukemia of unspecified cell type**
EXCLUDES 1 *personal history of leukemia (Z85.6)*

☑5ᵗʰ **C95.0 Acute leukemia of unspecified cell type**
Acute bilineal leukemia
Acute mixed lineage leukemia
Biphenotypic acute leukemia
Stem cell leukemia of unclear lineage
EXCLUDES 1 *acute exacerbation of unspecified chronic leukemia (C95.10)*

     C95.00 Acute leukemia of unspecified cell type not having achieved remission
Acute leukemia of unspecified cell type with failed remission
Acute leukemia NOS

     C95.01 Acute leukemia of unspecified cell type, in remission

     C95.02 Acute leukemia of unspecified cell type, in relapse

☑5ᵗʰ **C95.1 Chronic leukemia of unspecified cell type**

     C95.10 Chronic leukemia of unspecified cell type not having achieved remission
Chronic leukemia of unspecified cell type with failed remission
Chronic leukemia NOS

     C95.11 Chronic leukemia of unspecified cell type, in remission

     C95.12 Chronic leukemia of unspecified cell type, in relapse

☑5ᵗʰ **C95.9 Leukemia, unspecified**

     C95.90 Leukemia, unspecified not having achieved remission
Leukemia, unspecified with failed remission
Leukemia NOS

     C95.91 Leukemia, unspecified, in remission

     C95.92 Leukemia, unspecified, in relapse

☑4ᵗʰ **C96 Other and unspecified malignant neoplasms of lymphoid, hematopoietic and related tissue**
EXCLUDES 1 *personal history of other malignant neoplasms of lymphoid, hematopoietic and related tissues (Z85.79)*

C96.0 Multifocal and multisystemic (disseminated) Langerhans-cell histiocytosis
Histiocytosis X, multisystemic
Letterer-Siwe disease
EXCLUDES 1 *adult pulmonary Langerhans cell histiocytosis (J84.82)*
multifocal and unisystemic Langerhans-cell histiocytosis (C96.5)
unifocal Langerhans-cell histiocytosis (C96.6)

C96.2 Malignant mast cell tumor
Aggressive systemic mastocytosis
Mast cell sarcoma
EXCLUDES 1 *indolent mastocytosis (D47.0)*
mast cell leukemia (C94.30)
mastocytosis (congenital) (cutaneous) (Q82.2)

C96.4 Sarcoma of dendritic cells (accessory cells)
Follicular dendritic cell sarcoma
Interdigitating dendritic cell sarcoma
Langerhans cell sarcoma

C96.5 Multifocal and unisystemic Langerhans-cell histiocytosis
Hand-Schüller-Christian disease
Histiocytosis X, multifocal
EXCLUDES 1 *multifocal and multisystemic (disseminated) Langerhans-cell histiocytosis (C96.0)*
unifocal Langerhans-cell histiocytosis (C96.6)

C96.6 Unifocal Langerhans-cell histiocytosis
Eosinophilic granuloma
Histiocytosis X, unifocal
Histiocytosis X NOS
Langerhans-cell histiocytosis NOS
EXCLUDES 1 *multifocal and multisysemic (disseminated) Langerhans-cell histiocytosis (C96.0)*
multifocal and unisystemic Langerhans-cell histiocytosis (C96.5)

C96.A Histiocytic sarcoma
Malignant histiocytosis

C96.Z Other specified malignant neoplasms of lymphoid, hematopoietic and related tissue

C96.9 Malignant neoplasm of lymphoid, hematopoietic and related tissue, unspecified

In situ neoplasms (D00-D09)

INCLUDES Bowen's disease
erythroplasia
grade III intraepithelial neoplasia
Queyrat's erythroplasia

☑4ᵗʰ **D00 Carcinoma in situ of oral cavity, esophagus and stomach**
EXCLUDES 1 *melanoma in situ (D03.-)*

☑5ᵗʰ **D00.0 Carcinoma in situ of lip, oral cavity and pharynx**
Use additional code to identify:
exposure to environmental tobacco smoke (Z77.22)
exposure to tobacco smoke in the perinatal period (P96.81)
history of tobacco use (Z87.891)
occupational exposure to environmental tobacco smoke (Z57.31)
tobacco dependence (F17.-)
tobacco use (Z72.0)
EXCLUDES 1 *carcinoma in situ of aryepiglottic fold or interarytenoid fold, laryngeal aspect (D02.0)*
carcinoma in situ of epiglottis NOS (D02.0)
carcinoma in situ of epiglottis suprahyoid portion (D02.0)
carcinoma in situ of skin of lip (D03.0, D04.0)

     D00.00 Carcinoma in situ of oral cavity, unspecified site

     D00.01 Carcinoma in situ of labial mucosa and vermilion border

     D00.02 Carcinoma in situ of buccal mucosa

     D00.03 Carcinoma in situ of gingiva and edentulous alveolar ridge

     D00.04 Carcinoma in situ of soft palate

     D00.05 Carcinoma in situ of hard palate

     D00.06 Carcinoma in situ of floor of mouth

     D00.07 Carcinoma in situ of tongue

     D00.08 Carcinoma in situ of pharynx
Carcinoma in situ of aryepiglottic fold NOS
Carcinoma in situ of hypopharyngeal aspect of aryepiglottic fold
Carcinoma in situ of marginal zone of aryepiglottic fold

D00.1 Carcinoma in situ of esophagus

D00.2 Carcinoma in situ of stomach

☑4ᵗʰ **D01 Carcinoma in situ of other and unspecified digestive organs**
EXCLUDES 1 *melanoma in situ (D03.-)*

D01.0 Carcinoma in situ of colon
EXCLUDES 1 *carcinoma in situ of rectosigmoid junction (D01.1)*

D01.1 Carcinoma in situ of rectosigmoid junction

D01.2 Carcinoma in situ of rectum

D01.3 Carcinoma in situ of anus and anal canal
EXCLUDES 1 *carcinoma in situ of anal margin (D04.5)*
carcinoma in situ of anal skin (D04.5)
carcinoma in situ of perianal skin (D04.5)

☑5ᵗʰ **D01.4 Carcinoma in situ of other and unspecified parts of intestine**
EXCLUDES 1 *carcinoma in situ of ampulla of Vater (D01.5)*

     D01.40 Carcinoma in situ of unspecified part of intestine

     D01.49 Carcinoma in situ of other parts of intestine

D01.5 Carcinoma in situ of liver, gallbladder and bile ducts
Carcinoma in situ of ampulla of Vater

EXCLUDES 1 Not coded here   **EXCLUDES 2** Not included here   N Newborn Age: 0   P Pediatric Age: 0-17   M Maternity Age: 12-55   A Adult Age: 15-124

D01.7   Carcinoma in situ of other specified digestive organs
Carcinoma in situ of pancreas

D01.9   Carcinoma in situ of digestive organ, unspecified

✓4ᵗʰ **D02**   **Carcinoma in situ of middle ear and respiratory system**
Use additional code to identify:
exposure to environmental tobacco smoke (Z77.22)
exposure to tobacco smoke in the perinatal period (P96.81)
history of tobacco use (Z87.891)
occupational exposure to environmental tobacco smoke (Z57.31)
tobacco dependence (F17.-)
tobacco use (Z72.0)
EXCLUDES 1   *melanoma in situ (D03.-)*

D02.0   Carcinoma in situ of larynx
Carcinoma in situ of aryepiglottic fold or interarytenoid fold, laryngeal aspect
Carcinoma in situ of epiglottis (suprahyoid portion)
EXCLUDES 1   *carcinoma in situ of aryepiglottic fold or interarytenoid fold NOS (D00.08)*
carcinoma in situ of hypopharyngeal aspect (D00.08)
carcinoma in situ of marginal zone (D00.08)

D02.1   Carcinoma in situ of trachea

✓5ᵗʰ **D02.2**   Carcinoma in situ of bronchus and lung

D02.20   Carcinoma in situ of unspecified bronchus and lung

D02.21   Carcinoma in situ of right bronchus and lung

D02.22   Carcinoma in situ of left bronchus and lung

D02.3   Carcinoma in situ of other parts of respiratory system
Carcinoma in situ of accessory sinuses
Carcinoma in situ of middle ear
Carcinoma in situ of nasal cavities
EXCLUDES 1   *carcinoma in situ of ear (external) (skin) (D04.2-)*
carcinoma in situ of nose NOS (D09.8)
carcinoma in situ of skin of nose (D04.3)

D02.4   Carcinoma in situ of respiratory system, unspecified

✓4ᵗʰ **D03**   **Melanoma in situ**

D03.0   Melanoma in situ of lip

✓5ᵗʰ **D03.1**   Melanoma in situ of eyelid, including canthus

D03.10   Melanoma in situ of unspecified eyelid, including canthus

D03.11   Melanoma in situ of right eyelid, including canthus

D03.12   Melanoma in situ of left eyelid, including canthus

✓5ᵗʰ **D03.2**   Melanoma in situ of ear and external auricular canal

D03.20   Melanoma in situ of unspecified ear and external auricular canal

D03.21   Melanoma in situ of right ear and external auricular canal

D03.22   Melanoma in situ of left ear and external auricular canal

✓5ᵗʰ **D03.3**   Melanoma in situ of other and unspecified parts of face

D03.30   Melanoma in situ of unspecified part of face

D03.39   Melanoma in situ of other parts of face

D03.4   Melanoma in situ of scalp and neck

✓5ᵗʰ **D03.5**   Melanoma in situ of trunk

D03.51   Melanoma in situ of anal skin
Melanoma in situ of anal margin
Melanoma in situ of perianal skin

D03.52   Melanoma in situ of breast (skin) (soft tissue)

D03.59   Melanoma in situ of other part of trunk

✓5ᵗʰ **D03.6**   Melanoma in situ of upper limb, including shoulder

D03.60   Melanoma in situ of unspecified upper limb, including shoulder

D03.61   Melanoma in situ of right upper limb, including shoulder

D03.62   Melanoma in situ of left upper limb, including shoulder

✓5ᵗʰ **D03.7**   Melanoma in situ of lower limb, including hip

D03.70   Melanoma in situ of unspecified lower limb, including hip

D03.71   Melanoma in situ of right lower limb, including hip

D03.72   Melanoma in situ of left lower limb, including hip

D03.8   Melanoma in situ of other sites
Melanoma in situ of scrotum
EXCLUDES 1   *carcinoma in situ of scrotum (D07.61)*

D03.9   Melanoma in situ, unspecified

✓4ᵗʰ **D04**   **Carcinoma in situ of skin**
EXCLUDES 1   *erythroplasia of Queyrat (penis) NOS (D07.4)*
melanoma in situ (D03.-)

D04.0   Carcinoma in situ of skin of lip
EXCLUDES 1   *carcinoma in situ of vermilion border of lip (D00.01)*

✓5ᵗʰ **D04.1**   Carcinoma in situ of skin of eyelid, including canthus

D04.10   Carcinoma in situ of skin of unspecified eyelid, including canthus

D04.11   Carcinoma in situ of skin of right eyelid, including canthus

D04.12   Carcinoma in situ of skin of left eyelid, including canthus

✓5ᵗʰ **D04.2**   Carcinoma in situ of skin of ear and external auricular canal

D04.20   Carcinoma in situ of skin of unspecified ear and external auricular canal

D04.21   Carcinoma in situ of skin of right ear and external auricular canal

D04.22   Carcinoma in situ of skin of left ear and external auricular canal

✓5ᵗʰ **D04.3**   Carcinoma in situ of skin of other and unspecified parts of face

D04.30   Carcinoma in situ of skin of unspecified part of face

D04.39   Carcinoma in situ of skin of other parts of face

D04.4   Carcinoma in situ of skin of scalp and neck

D04.5   Carcinoma in situ of skin of trunk
Carcinoma in situ of anal margin
Carcinoma in situ of anal skin
Carcinoma in situ of perianal skin
Carcinoma in situ of skin of breast
EXCLUDES 1   *carcinoma in situ of anus NOS (D01.3)*
carcinoma in situ of scrotum (D07.61)
carcinoma in situ of skin of genital organs (D07.-)

✓5ᵗʰ **D04.6**   Carcinoma in situ of skin of upper limb, including shoulder

D04.60   Carcinoma in situ of skin of unspecified upper limb, including shoulder

D04.61   Carcinoma in situ of skin of right upper limb, including shoulder

D04.62   Carcinoma in situ of skin of left upper limb, including shoulder

✓5ᵗʰ **D04.7**   Carcinoma in situ of skin of lower limb, including hip

D04.70   Carcinoma in situ of skin of unspecified lower limb, including hip

D04.71   Carcinoma in situ of skin of right lower limb, including hip

D04.72   Carcinoma in situ of skin of left lower limb, including hip

D04.8   Carcinoma in situ of skin of other sites

D04.9   Carcinoma in situ of skin, unspecified

✓4ᵗʰ **D05**   **Carcinoma in situ of breast**
EXCLUDES 1   *carcinoma in situ of skin of breast (D04.5)*
melanoma in situ of breast (skin) (D03.5)
Paget's disease of breast or nipple (C50.-)

✓5ᵗʰ **D05.0**   Lobular carcinoma in situ of breast

D05.00   Lobular carcinoma in situ of unspecified breast

D05.01   Lobular carcinoma in situ of right breast

D05.02   Lobular carcinoma in situ of left breast

✓5ᵗʰ **D05.1**   Intraductal carcinoma in situ of breast

D05.10   Intraductal carcinoma in situ of unspecified breast

D05.11   Intraductal carcinoma in situ of right breast

D05.12   Intraductal carcinoma in situ of left breast

✓5ᵗʰ **D05.8**   Other specified type of carcinoma in situ of breast

D05.80   Other specified type of carcinoma in situ of unspecified breast

D05.81   Other specified type of carcinoma in situ of right breast

D05.82   Other specified type of carcinoma in situ of left breast

✓5ᵗʰ **D05.9**   Unspecified type of carcinoma in situ of breast

D05.90   Unspecified type of carcinoma in situ of unspecified breast

D05.91   Unspecified type of carcinoma in situ of right breast

D05.92   Unspecified type of carcinoma in situ of left breast

---

✓ Additional Character Required   ✓x7ᵗʰ Xtension Alert   Unspecified Dx   Other Specified Dx   Manifestation   ▶◀ Revised Text   ● New Code   ▲ Revised Code Title

Neoplasms

D06–D13.2

✓4ᵗʰ **D06 Carcinoma in situ of** cervix uteri
> INCLUDES cervical adenocarcinoma in situ
> cervical intraepithelial glandular neoplasia
> cervical intraepithelial neoplasia III [CIN III]
> severe dysplasia of cervix uteri
> EXCLUDES 1 cervical intraepithelial neoplasia II [CIN II] (N87.1)
> cytologic evidence of malignancy of cervix without histologic
>   confirmation (R87.614)
> high grade squamous intraepithelial lesion (HGSIL) of cervix
>   (R87.613)
> melanoma in situ of cervix (D03.5)
> moderate cervical dysplasia (N87.1)

　　D06.0 **Carcinoma in situ of** endocervix　　　　　♀
　　D06.1 **Carcinoma in situ of** exocervix　　　　　♀
　　D06.7 **Carcinoma in situ of other** parts **of cervix**　♀
　　D06.9 **Carcinoma in situ of cervix, unspecified**　♀

✓4ᵗʰ **D07 Carcinoma in situ of** other and unspecified genital organs
> EXCLUDES 1 melanoma in situ of trunk (D03.5)

　　D07.0 **Carcinoma in situ of** endometrium　　　♀
　　D07.1 **Carcinoma in situ of** vulva　　　　　　♀
　　　　　Severe dysplasia of vulva
　　　　　Vulvar intraepithelial neoplasia III [VIN III]
> EXCLUDES 1 moderate dysplasia of vulva (N90.1)
> vulvar intraepithelial neoplasia II [VIN II] (N90.1)

　　D07.2 **Carcinoma in situ of** vagina　　　　　　♀
　　　　　Severe dysplasia of vagina
　　　　　Vaginal intraepithelial neoplasia III [VAIN III]
> EXCLUDES 1 moderate dysplasia of vagina (N89.1)
> vaginal intraepithelial neoplasia II [VIN II] (N89.1)

✓5ᵗʰ D07.3 **Carcinoma in situ of** other and unspecified female genital
　　　　　organs
　　　　D07.30 **Carcinoma in situ of unspecified female**　♀
　　　　　　　genital organs
　　　　D07.39 **Carcinoma in situ of other female genital**　♀
　　　　　　　organs

　　D07.4 **Carcinoma in situ of** penis　　　　　　♂
　　　　　Erythroplasia of Queyrat NOS
　　D07.5 **Carcinoma in situ of** prostate　　　　　♂
　　　　　Prostatic intraepithelial neoplasia III (PIN III)
　　　　　Severe dysplasia of prostate
> EXCLUDES 1 dysplasia (mild) (moderate) of prostate (N42.3)

✓5ᵗʰ D07.6 **Carcinoma in situ of** other and unspecified male genital
　　　　　organs
　　　　D07.60 **Carcinoma in situ of unspecified male genital**　♂
　　　　　　　organs
　　　　D07.61 **Carcinoma in situ of** scrotum　　　　♂
　　　　D07.69 **Carcinoma in situ of other male genital organs**　♂

✓4ᵗʰ **D09 Carcinoma in situ of** other and unspecified sites
> EXCLUDES 1 melanoma in situ (D03.-)

　　D09.0 **Carcinoma in situ of** bladder
✓5ᵗʰ D09.1 **Carcinoma in situ of other and unspecified** urinary organs
　　　　D09.10 **Carcinoma in situ of unspecified urinary organ**
　　　　D09.19 **Carcinoma in situ of other urinary organs**
✓5ᵗʰ D09.2 **Carcinoma in situ of** eye
> EXCLUDES 1 carcinoma in situ of skin of eyelid (D04.1-)
　　　　D09.20 **Carcinoma in situ of unspecified eye**
　　　　D09.21 **Carcinoma in situ of** right **eye**
　　　　D09.22 **Carcinoma in situ of** left **eye**
　　D09.3 **Carcinoma in situ of** thyroid and other endocrine glands
> EXCLUDES 1 carcinoma in situ of endocrine pancreas (D01.7)
> carcinoma in situ of ovary (D07.39)
> carcinoma in situ of testis (D07.69)
　　D09.8 **Carcinoma in situ of other specified sites**
　　D09.9 **Carcinoma in situ, unspecified**

Benign neoplasms, except benign
neuroendocrine tumors (D10-D36)

✓4ᵗʰ **D10 Benign neoplasm of** mouth and pharynx
　　D10.0 **Benign neoplasm of** lip
　　　　　Benign neoplasm of lip (frenulum) (inner aspect) (mucosa)
　　　　　　(vermilion border)
> EXCLUDES 1 benign neoplasm of skin of lip (D22.0, D23.0)
　　D10.1 **Benign neoplasm of** tongue
　　　　　Benign neoplasm of lingual tonsil
　　D10.2 **Benign neoplasm of** floor **of mouth**

✓5ᵗʰ D10.3 Other and unspecified parts of mouth
　　　　D10.30 **Benign neoplasm of unspecified part of** mouth
　　　　D10.39 **Benign neoplasm of other parts of** mouth
　　　　　　　Benign neoplasm of minor salivary gland NOS
> EXCLUDES 1 benign odontogenic neoplasms
>   (D16.4-D16.5)
> benign neoplasm of mucosa of lip (D10.0)
> benign neoplasm of nasopharyngeal surface
>   of soft palate (D10.6)

　　D10.4 **Benign neoplasm of** tonsil
　　　　　Benign neoplasm of tonsil (faucial) (palatine)
> EXCLUDES 1 benign neoplasm of lingual tonsil (D10.1)
> benign neoplasm of pharyngeal tonsil (D10.6)
> benign neoplasm of tonsillar fossa (D10.5)
> benign neoplasm of tonsillar pillars (D10.5)

　　D10.5 **Benign neoplasm of other parts of** oropharynx
　　　　　Benign neoplasm of epiglottis, anterior aspect
　　　　　Benign neoplasm of tonsillar fossa
　　　　　Benign neoplasm of tonsillar pillars
　　　　　Benign neoplasm of vallecula
> EXCLUDES 1 benign neoplasm of epiglottis NOS (D14.1)
> benign neoplasm of epiglottis, suprahyoid portion
>   (D14.1)

　　D10.6 **Benign neoplasm of** nasopharynx
　　　　　Benign neoplasm of pharyngeal tonsil
　　　　　Benign neoplasm of posterior margin of septum and choanae
　　D10.7 **Benign neoplasm of** hypopharynx
　　D10.9 **Benign neoplasm of pharynx, unspecified**

✓4ᵗʰ **D11 Benign neoplasm of** major salivary glands
> EXCLUDES 1 benign neoplasms of specified minor salivary glands which are
>   classified according to their anatomical location
> benign neoplasms of minor salivary glands NOS (D10.39)

　　D11.0 **Benign neoplasm of** parotid gland
　　D11.7 **Benign neoplasm of other major salivary glands**
　　　　　Benign neoplasm of sublingual salivary gland
　　　　　Benign neoplasm of submandibular salivary gland
　　D11.9 **Benign neoplasm of major salivary gland, unspecified**

✓4ᵗʰ **D12 Benign neoplasm of** colon, rectum, anus and anal canal
> EXCLUDES 1 benign carcinoid tumors of the large intestine, and rectum
>   (D3A.02-)

　　D12.0 **Benign neoplasm of** cecum
　　　　　Benign neoplasm of ileocecal valve
　　D12.1 **Benign neoplasm of** appendix
> EXCLUDES 1 benign carcinoid tumor of the appendix (D3A.020)
　　D12.2 **Benign neoplasm of** ascending colon
　　D12.3 **Benign neoplasm of** transverse colon
　　　　　Benign neoplasm of hepatic flexure
　　　　　Benign neoplasm of splenic flexure
　　D12.4 **Benign neoplasm of** descending colon
　　D12.5 **Benign neoplasm of** sigmoid colon
　　D12.6 **Benign neoplasm of colon, unspecified**
　　　　　Adenomatosis of colon
　　　　　Benign neoplasm of large intestine NOS
　　　　　Polyposis (hereditary) of colon
> EXCLUDES 1 inflammatory polyp of colon (K51.4-)
> polyp of colon NOS (K63.5)
　　D12.7 **Benign neoplasm of** rectosigmoid junction
　　D12.8 **Benign neoplasm of** rectum
> EXCLUDES 1 benign carcinoid tumor of the rectum (D3A.026)
　　D12.9 **Benign neoplasm of** anus and anal canal
　　　　　Benign neoplasm of anus NOS
> EXCLUDES 1 benign neoplasm of anal margin (D22.5, D23.5)
> benign neoplasm of anal skin (D22.5, D23.5)
> benign neoplasm of perianal skin (D22.5, D23.5)

✓4ᵗʰ **D13 Benign neoplasm of** other and ill-defined parts of digestive
　　　system
> EXCLUDES 1 benign stromal tumors of digestive system (D21.4)
　　D13.0 **Benign neoplasm of** esophagus
　　D13.1 **Benign neoplasm of** stomach
> EXCLUDES 1 benign carcinoid tumor of the stomach (D3A.092)
　　D13.2 **Benign neoplasm of** duodenum
> EXCLUDES 1 benign carcinoid tumor of the duodenum (D3A.010)

☑5ᵗʰ D13.3 Benign neoplasm of other and unspecified parts of small intestine

    EXCLUDES 1   *benign carcinoid tumors of the small intestine (D3A.01-)*
              benign neoplasm of ileocecal valve (D12.0)

    D13.30 Benign neoplasm of unspecified part of small intestine

    D13.39 Benign neoplasm of other parts of small intestine

D13.4 Benign neoplasm of liver
    Benign neoplasm of intrahepatic bile ducts

D13.5 Benign neoplasm of extrahepatic bile ducts

D13.6 Benign neoplasm of pancreas
    EXCLUDES 1   *benign neoplasm of endocrine pancreas (D13.7)*

D13.7 Benign neoplasm of endocrine pancreas
    Islet cell tumor
    Benign neoplasm of islets of Langerhans
    Use additional code to identify any functional activity

D13.9 Benign neoplasm of ill-defined sites **within the digestive system**
    Benign neoplasm of digestive system NOS
    Benign neoplasm of intestine NOS
    Benign neoplasm of spleen

☑4ᵗʰ D14 Benign neoplasm of middle ear and respiratory system

D14.0 Benign neoplasm of middle ear, nasal cavity and accessory sinuses
    Benign neoplasm of cartilage of nose
    EXCLUDES 1   *benign neoplasm of auricular canal (external) (D22.2-, D23.2-)*
              benign neoplasm of bone of ear (D16.4)
              benign neoplasm of bone of nose (D16.4)
              benign neoplasm of cartilage of ear (D21.0)
              benign neoplasm of ear (external)(skin) (D22.2-, D23.2-)
              benign neoplasm of nose NOS (D36.7)
              benign neoplasm of skin of nose (D22.39, D23.39)
              benign neoplasm of olfactory bulb (D33.3)
              benign neoplasm of posterior margin of septum and choanae (D10.6)
              polyp of accessory sinus (J33.8)
              polyp of ear (middle) (H74.4)
              polyp of nasal (cavity) (J33.-)

D14.1 Benign neoplasm of larynx
    Adenomatous polyp of larynx
    Benign neoplasm of epiglottis (suprahyoid portion)
    EXCLUDES 1   *benign neoplasm of epiglottis, anterior aspect (D10.5)*
              polyp (nonadenomatous) of vocal cord or larynx (J38.1)

D14.2 Benign neoplasm of trachea

☑5ᵗʰ D14.3 Benign neoplasm of bronchus and lung
    EXCLUDES 1   *benign carcinoid tumor of the bronchus and lung (D3A.090)*

    D14.30 Benign neoplasm of unspecified bronchus and lung

    D14.31 Benign neoplasm of right **bronchus and lung**

    D14.32 Benign neoplasm of left **bronchus and lung**

D14.4 Benign neoplasm of respiratory system, unspecified

☑4ᵗʰ D15 Benign neoplasm of other and unspecified intrathoracic organs
    EXCLUDES 1   *benign neoplasm of mesothelial tissue (D19.-)*

D15.0 Benign neoplasm of thymus
    EXCLUDES 1   *benign carcinoid tumor of the thymus (D3A.091)*

D15.1 Benign neoplasm of heart
    EXCLUDES 1   *benign neoplasm of great vessels (D21.3)*

D15.2 Benign neoplasm of mediastinum

D15.7 Benign neoplasm of other specified intrathoracic organs

D15.9 Benign neoplasm of intrathoracic organ, unspecified

☑4ᵗʰ D16 Benign neoplasm of bone and articular cartilage
    EXCLUDES 1   *benign neoplasm of connective tissue of ear (D21.0)*
              benign neoplasm of connective tissue of eyelid (D21.0)
              benign neoplasm of connective tissue of larynx (D14.1)
              benign neoplasm of connective tissue of nose (D14.0)
              benign neoplasm of synovia (D21.-)

☑5ᵗʰ D16.0 Benign neoplasm of scapula and long bones of upper limb

    D16.00 Benign neoplasm of scapula and long bones of unspecified upper limb

    D16.01 Benign neoplasm of scapula and long bones of right **upper limb**

    D16.02 Benign neoplasm of scapula and long bones of left **upper limb**

☑5ᵗʰ D16.1 Benign neoplasm of short bones of upper limb

    D16.10 Benign neoplasm of short bones of unspecified upper limb

    D16.11 Benign neoplasm of short bones of right **upper limb**

    D16.12 Benign neoplasm of short bones of left **upper limb**

☑5ᵗʰ D16.2 Benign neoplasm of long bones of lower limb

    D16.20 Benign neoplasm of long bones of unspecified lower limb

    D16.21 Benign neoplasm of long bones of right **lower limb**

    D16.22 Benign neoplasm of long bones of left **lower limb**

☑5ᵗʰ D16.3 Benign neoplasm of short bones of lower limb

    D16.30 Benign neoplasm of short bones of unspecified lower limb

    D16.31 Benign neoplasm of short bones of right **lower limb**

    D16.32 Benign neoplasm of short bones of left **lower limb**

D16.4 Benign neoplasm of bones of skull and face
    Benign neoplasm of maxilla (superior)
    Benign neoplasm of orbital bone
    Keratocyst of maxilla
    Keratocystic odontogenic tumor of maxilla
    EXCLUDES 1   *benign neoplasm of lower jaw bone (D16.5)*

D16.5 Benign neoplasm of lower jaw bone
    Keratocyst of mandible
    Keratocystic odontogenic tumor of mandible

D16.6 Benign neoplasm of vertebral column
    EXCLUDES 1   *benign neoplasm of sacrum and coccyx (D16.8)*

D16.7 Benign neoplasm of ribs, sternum and clavicle

D16.8 Benign neoplasm of pelvic bones, sacrum and coccyx

D16.9 Benign neoplasm of bone and articular cartilage, unspecified

☑4ᵗʰ D17 Benign lipomatous **neoplasm**

D17.0 Benign lipomatous neoplasm of skin and subcutaneous tissue of head, face and neck

D17.1 Benign lipomatous neoplasm of skin and subcutaneous tissue of trunk

☑5ᵗʰ D17.2 Benign lipomatous neoplasm of skin and subcutaneous tissue of limb

    D17.20 Benign lipomatous neoplasm of skin and subcutaneous tissue of unspecified limb

    D17.21 Benign lipomatous neoplasm of skin and subcutaneous tissue of right arm

    D17.22 Benign lipomatous neoplasm of skin and subcutaneous tissue of left arm

    D17.23 Benign lipomatous neoplasm of skin and subcutaneous tissue of right leg

    D17.24 Benign lipomatous neoplasm of skin and subcutaneous tissue of left leg

☑5ᵗʰ D17.3 Benign lipomatous neoplasm of skin and subcutaneous tissue of other and unspecified sites

    D17.30 Benign lipomatous neoplasm of skin and subcutaneous tissue of unspecified sites

    D17.39 Benign lipomatous neoplasm of skin and subcutaneous tissue of other sites

D17.4 Benign lipomatous neoplasm of intrathoracic organs

D17.5 Benign lipomatous neoplasm of intra-abdominal organs
    EXCLUDES 1   *benign lipomatous neoplasm of peritoneum and retroperitoneum (D17.79)*

D17.6 Benign lipomatous neoplasm of spermatic cord   ♂

☑5ᵗʰ D17.7 Benign lipomatous neoplasm of other sites

    D17.71 Benign lipomatous neoplasm of kidney

    D17.72 Benign lipomatous neoplasm of other genitourinary organ

    D17.79 Benign lipomatous neoplasm of other sites
        Benign lipomatous neoplasm of peritoneum
        Benign lipomatous neoplasm of retroperitoneum

D17.9 Benign lipomatous neoplasm, unspecified
    Lipoma NOS

☑4ᵗʰ D18 Hemangioma and lymphangioma, any site
    EXCLUDES 1   *benign neoplasm of glomus jugulare (D35.6)*
              blue or pigmented nevus (D22.-)
              nevus NOS (D22.-)
              vascular nevus (Q82.5)

☑5ᵗʰ D18.0 Hemangioma
    Angioma NOS
    Cavernous nevus

    D18.00 Hemangioma unspecified site

☑ Additional Character Required   ✗x7ᵗʰ Xtension Alert   Unspecified Dx   Other Specified Dx   Manifestation   ►◄ Revised Text   ● New Code   ▲ Revised Code Title

Neoplasms

D18.01–D23.39

> **D18.01 Hemangioma of** skin and subcutaneous tissue
>
> **D18.02 Hemangioma of** intracranial structures
>
> **D18.03 Hemangioma of** intra-abdominal structures
>
> **D18.09 Hemangioma of other sites**

D18.1 Lymphangioma, any site

✓4ᵗʰ **D19 Benign neoplasm of** mesothelial tissue

D19.0 Benign neoplasm of mesothelial tissue of pleura

D19.1 Benign neoplasm of mesothelial tissue of peritoneum

D19.7 Benign neoplasm of mesothelial tissue of other sites

D19.9 Benign neoplasm of mesothelial tissue, unspecified
  Benign mesothelioma NOS

✓4ᵗʰ **D20 Benign neoplasm of soft tissue of** retroperitoneum and peritoneum

  EXCLUDES 1 *benign lipomatous neoplasm of peritoneum and retroperitoneum (D17.79)*
  benign neoplasm of mesothelial tissue (D19.-)

D20.0 Benign neoplasm of soft tissue of retroperitoneum

D20.1 Benign neoplasm of soft tissue of peritoneum

✓4ᵗʰ **D21 Other benign neoplasms of** connective and other soft tissue

  INCLUDES   benign neoplasm of blood vessel
  benign neoplasm of bursa
  benign neoplasm of cartilage
  benign neoplasm of fascia
  benign neoplasm of fat
  benign neoplasm of ligament, except uterine
  benign neoplasm of lymphatic channel
  benign neoplasm of muscle
  benign neoplasm of synovia
  benign neoplasm of tendon (sheath)
  benign stromal tumors

  EXCLUDES 1 *benign neoplasm of articular cartilage (D16.-)*
  benign neoplasm of cartilage of larynx (D14.1)
  benign neoplasm of cartilage of nose (D14.0)
  benign neoplasm of connective tissue of breast (D24.-)
  benign neoplasm of peripheral nerves and autonomic nervous system (D36.1-)
  benign neoplasm of peritoneum (D20.1)
  benign neoplasm of retroperitoneum (D20.0)
  benign neoplasm of uterine ligament, any (D28.2)
  benign neoplasm of vascular tissue (D18.-)
  hemangioma (D18.0-)
  lipomatous neoplasm (D17.-)
  lymphangioma (D18.1)
  uterine leiomyoma (D25.-)

D21.0 Benign neoplasm of connective and other soft tissue of head, face and neck
  Benign neoplasm of connective tissue of ear
  Benign neoplasm of connective tissue of eyelid
  EXCLUDES 1 *benign neoplasm of connective tissue of orbit (D31.6-)*

✓5ᵗʰ **D21.1 Benign neoplasm of connective and other soft tissue of** upper limb, including shoulder

  D21.10 Benign neoplasm of connective and other soft tissue of unspecified upper limb, including shoulder

  D21.11 Benign neoplasm of connective and other soft tissue of right **upper limb, including shoulder**

  D21.12 Benign neoplasm of connective and other soft tissue of left **upper limb, including shoulder**

✓5ᵗʰ **D21.2 Benign neoplasm of connective and other soft tissue of** lower limb, including hip

  D21.20 Benign neoplasm of connective and other soft tissue of unspecified lower limb, including hip

  D21.21 Benign neoplasm of connective and other soft tissue of right **lower limb, including hip**

  D21.22 Benign neoplasm of connective and other soft tissue of left **lower limb, including hip**

D21.3 Benign neoplasm of connective and other soft tissue of thorax
  Benign neoplasm of axilla
  Benign neoplasm of diaphragm
  Benign neoplasm of great vessels
  EXCLUDES 1 *benign neoplasm of heart (D15.1)*
  benign neoplasm of mediastinum (D15.2)
  benign neoplasm of thymus (D15.0)

D21.4 Benign neoplasm of connective and other soft tissue of abdomen
  Benign stromal tumors of abdomen

D21.5 Benign neoplasm of connective and other soft tissue of pelvis
  EXCLUDES 1 *benign neoplasm of any uterine ligament (D28.2)*
  uterine leiomyoma (D25.-)

D21.6 Benign neoplasm of connective and other soft tissue of trunk, unspecified
  Benign neoplasm of back NOS

D21.9 Benign neoplasm of connective and other soft tissue, unspecified

✓4ᵗʰ **D22 Melanocytic nevi**
  INCLUDES   atypical nevus
  blue hairy pigmented nevus
  nevus NOS

D22.0 Melanocytic nevi of lip

✓5ᵗʰ **D22.1 Melanocytic nevi of** eyelid, including canthus

  D22.10 Melanocytic nevi of unspecified eyelid, including canthus

  D22.11 Melanocytic nevi of right **eyelid, including canthus**

  D22.12 Melanocytic nevi of left **eyelid, including canthus**

✓5ᵗʰ **D22.2 Melanocytic nevi of** ear and external auricular canal

  D22.20 Melanocytic nevi of unspecified ear and external auricular canal

  D22.21 Melanocytic nevi of right **ear and external auricular canal**

  D22.22 Melanocytic nevi of left **ear and external auricular canal**

✓5ᵗʰ **D22.3 Melanocytic nevi of** other and unspecified parts of face

  D22.30 Melanocytic nevi of unspecified part of face

  D22.39 Melanocytic nevi of other parts of face

D22.4 Melanocytic nevi of scalp and neck

D22.5 Melanocytic nevi of trunk
  Melanocytic nevi of anal margin
  Melanocytic nevi of anal skin
  Melanocytic nevi of perianal skin
  Melanocytic nevi of skin of breast

✓5ᵗʰ **D22.6 Melanocytic nevi of** upper limb, including shoulder

  D22.60 Melanocytic nevi of unspecified upper limb, including shoulder

  D22.61 Melanocytic nevi of right **upper limb, including shoulder**

  D22.62 Melanocytic nevi of left **upper limb, including shoulder**

✓5ᵗʰ **D22.7 Melanocytic nevi of** lower limb, including hip

  D22.70 Melanocytic nevi of unspecified lower limb, including hip

  D22.71 Melanocytic nevi of right **lower limb, including hip**

  D22.72 Melanocytic nevi of left **lower limb, including hip**

D22.9 Melanocytic nevi, unspecified

✓4ᵗʰ **D23 Other benign neoplasms of** skin
  INCLUDES   benign neoplasm of hair follicles
  benign neoplasm of sebaceous glands
  benign neoplasm of sweat glands
  EXCLUDES 1 *benign lipomatous neoplasms of skin (D17.0-D17.3)*
  melanocytic nevi (D22.-)

D23.0 Other benign neoplasm of skin of lip
  EXCLUDES 1 *benign neoplasm of vermilion border of lip (D10.0)*

✓5ᵗʰ **D23.1 Other benign neoplasm of skin of** eyelid, including canthus

  D23.10 Other benign neoplasm of skin of unspecified eyelid, including canthus

  D23.11 Other benign neoplasm of skin of right **eyelid, including canthus**

  D23.12 Other benign neoplasm of skin of left **eyelid, including canthus**

✓5ᵗʰ **D23.2 Other benign neoplasm of skin of** ear and external auricular canal

  D23.20 Other benign neoplasm of skin of unspecified ear and external auricular canal

  D23.21 Other benign neoplasm of skin of right **ear and external auricular canal**

  D23.22 Other benign neoplasm of skin of left **ear and external auricular canal**

✓5ᵗʰ **D23.3 Other benign neoplasm of skin of** other and unspecified parts of face

  D23.30 Other benign neoplasm of skin of unspecified part of face

  D23.39 Other benign neoplasm of skin of other parts of face

EXCLUDES 1 Not coded here   EXCLUDES 2 Not included here   N Newborn Age: 0   P Pediatric Age: 0-17   M Maternity Age: 12-55   A Adult Age: 15-124

466   ICD-10-CM Draft (2015)

D23.4 Other benign neoplasm of skin of scalp and neck

D23.5 Other benign neoplasm of skin of trunk
Other benign neoplasm of anal margin
Other benign neoplasm of anal skin
Other benign neoplasm of perianal skin
Other benign neoplasm of skin of breast
EXCLUDES 1 benign neoplasm of anus NOS (D12.9)

✓5ᵗʰ **D23.6** Other benign neoplasm of skin of upper limb, including shoulder
D23.60 Other benign neoplasm of skin of unspecified upper limb, including shoulder
D23.61 Other benign neoplasm of skin of right upper limb, including shoulder
D23.62 Other benign neoplasm of skin of left upper limb, including shoulder

✓5ᵗʰ **D23.7** Other benign neoplasm of skin of lower limb, including hip
D23.70 Other benign neoplasm of skin of unspecified lower limb, including hip
D23.71 Other benign neoplasm of skin of right lower limb, including hip
D23.72 Other benign neoplasm of skin of left lower limb, including hip

D23.9 Other benign neoplasm of skin, unspecified

✓4ᵗʰ **D24 Benign neoplasm of breast**
INCLUDES benign neoplasm of connective tissue of breast
benign neoplasm of soft parts of breast
fibroadenoma of breast
EXCLUDES 2 adenofibrosis of breast (N60.2)
benign cyst of breast (N60.-)
benign mammary dysplasia (N60.-)
benign neoplasm of skin of breast (D22.5, D23.5)
fibrocystic disease of breast (N60.-)

D24.1 Benign neoplasm of right breast
D24.2 Benign neoplasm of left breast
D24.9 Benign neoplasm of unspecified breast

✓4ᵗʰ **D25 Leiomyoma of uterus**
INCLUDES uterine fibroid
uterine fibromyoma
uterine myoma

D25.0 Submucous leiomyoma of uterus ♀
D25.1 Intramural leiomyoma of uterus ♀
Interstitial leiomyoma of uterus
D25.2 Subserosal leiomyoma of uterus ♀
Subperitoneal leiomyoma of uterus
D25.9 Leiomyoma of uterus, unspecified ♀

✓4ᵗʰ **D26 Other benign neoplasms of uterus**
D26.0 Other benign neoplasm of cervix uteri ♀
D26.1 Other benign neoplasm of corpus uteri ♀
D26.7 Other benign neoplasm of other parts of uterus ♀
D26.9 Other benign neoplasm of uterus, unspecified ♀

✓4ᵗʰ **D27 Benign neoplasm of ovary**
Use additional code to identify any functional activity
EXCLUDES 2 corpus albicans cyst (N83.2)
corpus luteum cyst (N83.1)
endometrial cyst (N80.1)
follicular (atretic) cyst (N83.0)
graafian follicle cyst (N83.0)
ovarian cyst NEC (N83.2)
ovarian retention cyst (N83.2)

D27.0 Benign neoplasm of right ovary ♀
D27.1 Benign neoplasm of left ovary ♀
D27.9 Benign neoplasm of unspecified ovary ♀

✓4ᵗʰ **D28 Benign neoplasm of other and unspecified female genital organs**
INCLUDES adenomatous polyp
benign neoplasm of skin of female genital organs
benign teratoma
EXCLUDES 1 epoophoron cyst (Q50.5)
fimbrial cyst (Q50.4)
Gartner's duct cyst (Q52.4)
parovarian cyst (Q50.5)

D28.0 Benign neoplasm of vulva ♀
D28.1 Benign neoplasm of vagina ♀
D28.2 Benign neoplasm of uterine tubes and ligaments ♀
Benign neoplasm of fallopian tube
Benign neoplasm of uterine ligament (broad) (round)

D28.7 Benign neoplasm of other specified female genital organs ♀
D28.9 Benign neoplasm of female genital organ, unspecified ♀

✓4ᵗʰ **D29 Benign neoplasm of male genital organs**
INCLUDES benign neoplasm of skin of male genital organs
D29.0 Benign neoplasm of penis ♂
D29.1 Benign neoplasm of prostate ♂
EXCLUDES 1 enlarged prostate (N40.-)

✓5ᵗʰ **D29.2** Benign neoplasm of testis
Use additional code to identify any functional activity
D29.20 Benign neoplasm of unspecified testis ♂
D29.21 Benign neoplasm of right testis ♂
D29.22 Benign neoplasm of left testis ♂

✓5ᵗʰ **D29.3** Benign neoplasm of epididymis
D29.30 Benign neoplasm of unspecified epididymis ♂
D29.31 Benign neoplasm of right epididymis ♂
D29.32 Benign neoplasm of left epididymis ♂

D29.4 Benign neoplasm of scrotum ♂
Benign neoplasm of skin of scrotum

D29.8 Benign neoplasm of other specified male genital organs ♂
Benign neoplasm of seminal vesicle
Benign neoplasm of spermatic cord
Benign neoplasm of tunica vaginalis

D29.9 Benign neoplasm of male genital organ, unspecified ♂

✓4ᵗʰ **D30 Benign neoplasm of urinary organs**
✓5ᵗʰ **D30.0** Benign neoplasm of kidney
EXCLUDES 1 benign carcinoid tumor of the kidney (D3A.093)
benign neoplasm of renal calyces (D30.1-)
benign neoplasm of renal pelvis (D30.1-)
D30.00 Benign neoplasm of unspecified kidney
D30.01 Benign neoplasm of right kidney
D30.02 Benign neoplasm of left kidney

✓5ᵗʰ **D30.1** Benign neoplasm of renal pelvis
D30.10 Benign neoplasm of unspecified renal pelvis
D30.11 Benign neoplasm of right renal pelvis
D30.12 Benign neoplasm of left renal pelvis

✓5ᵗʰ **D30.2** Benign neoplasm of ureter
EXCLUDES 1 benign neoplasm of ureteric orifice of bladder (D30.3)
D30.20 Benign neoplasm of unspecified ureter
D30.21 Benign neoplasm of right ureter
D30.22 Benign neoplasm of left ureter

D30.3 Benign neoplasm of bladder
Benign neoplasm of ureteric orifice of bladder
Benign neoplasm of urethral orifice of bladder

D30.4 Benign neoplasm of urethra
EXCLUDES 1 benign neoplasm of urethral orifice of bladder (D30.3)

D30.8 Benign neoplasm of other specified urinary organs
Benign neoplasm of paraurethral glands

D30.9 Benign neoplasm of urinary organ, unspecified
Benign neoplasm of urinary system NOS

✓4ᵗʰ **D31 Benign neoplasm of eye and adnexa**
EXCLUDES 1 benign neoplasm of connective tissue of eyelid (D21.0)
benign neoplasm of optic nerve (D33.3)
benign neoplasm of skin of eyelid (D22.1-, D23.1-)

✓5ᵗʰ **D31.0** Benign neoplasm of conjunctiva
D31.00 Benign neoplasm of unspecified conjunctiva
D31.01 Benign neoplasm of right conjunctiva
D31.02 Benign neoplasm of left conjunctiva

✓5ᵗʰ **D31.1** Benign neoplasm of cornea
D31.10 Benign neoplasm of unspecified cornea
D31.11 Benign neoplasm of right cornea
D31.12 Benign neoplasm of left cornea

✓5ᵗʰ **D31.2** Benign neoplasm of retina
EXCLUDES 1 dark area on retina (D49.81)
hemangioma of retina (D49.81)
neoplasm of unspecified behavior of retina and choroid (D49.81)
retinal freckle (D49.81)
D31.20 Benign neoplasm of unspecified retina
D31.21 Benign neoplasm of right retina
D31.22 Benign neoplasm of left retina

✓5ᵗʰ **D31.3** Benign neoplasm of choroid
D31.30 Benign neoplasm of unspecified choroid

D23.4–D31.30

✓ Additional Character Required   ✓x7ᵗʰ Xtension Alert   Unspecified Dx   Other Specified Dx   Manifestation   ▶◀ Revised Text   ● New Code   ▲ Revised Code Title

Neoplasms

D31.31–D3A.029

        D31.31 **Benign neoplasm of** right **choroid**

        D31.32 **Benign neoplasm of** left **choroid**

✓5ᵗʰ **D31.4** **Benign neoplasm of** ciliary body

        D31.40 **Benign neoplasm of unspecified ciliary body**

        D31.41 **Benign neoplasm of** right **ciliary body**

        D31.42 **Benign neoplasm of** left **ciliary body**

✓5ᵗʰ **D31.5** **Benign neoplasm of** lacrimal gland and duct

        Benign neoplasm of lacrimal sac

        Benign neoplasm of nasolacrimal duct

        D31.50 **Benign neoplasm of unspecified lacrimal gland and duct**

        D31.51 **Benign neoplasm of** right **lacrimal gland and duct**

        D31.52 **Benign neoplasm of** left **lacrimal gland and duct**

✓5ᵗʰ **D31.6** **Benign neoplasm of unspecified site of** orbit

        Benign neoplasm of connective tissue of orbit

        Benign neoplasm of extraocular muscle

        Benign neoplasm of peripheral nerves of orbit

        Benign neoplasm of retrobulbar tissue

        Benign neoplasm of retro-ocular tissue

        EXCLUDES 1 *benign neoplasm of orbital bone (D16.4)*

        D31.60 **Benign neoplasm of unspecified site of unspecified orbit**

        D31.61 **Benign neoplasm of unspecified site of** right **orbit**

        D31.62 **Benign neoplasm of unspecified site of** left **orbit**

✓5ᵗʰ **D31.9** **Benign neoplasm of** unspecified part of eye

        Benign neoplasm of eyeball

        D31.90 **Benign neoplasm of unspecified part of unspecified eye**

        D31.91 **Benign neoplasm of unspecified part of** right **eye**

        D31.92 **Benign neoplasm of unspecified part of** left **eye**

✓4ᵗʰ **D32** **Benign neoplasm of** meninges

        D32.0 **Benign neoplasm of** cerebral **meninges**

        D32.1 **Benign neoplasm of** spinal **meninges**

        D32.9 **Benign neoplasm of meninges, unspecified**

            Meningioma NOS

✓4ᵗʰ **D33** **Benign neoplasm of** brain and other parts of central nervous system

        EXCLUDES 1 *angioma (D18.0-)*

            benign neoplasm of meninges (D32.-)

            benign neoplasm of peripheral nerves and autonomic nervous system (D36.1-)

            hemangioma (D18.0-)

            neurofibromatosis (Q85.0-)

            retro-ocular benign neoplasm (D31.6-)

        D33.0 **Benign neoplasm of** brain, supratentorial

            Benign neoplasm of cerebral ventricle

            Benign neoplasm of cerebrum

            Benign neoplasm of frontal lobe

            Benign neoplasm of occipital lobe

            Benign neoplasm of parietal lobe

            Benign neoplasm of temporal lobe

            EXCLUDES 1 *benign neoplasm of fourth ventricle (D33.1)*

        D33.1 **Benign neoplasm of** brain, infratentorial

            Benign neoplasm of brain stem

            Benign neoplasm of cerebellum

            Benign neoplasm of fourth ventricle

        D33.2 **Benign neoplasm of brain, unspecified**

        D33.3 **Benign neoplasm of** cranial nerves

            Benign neoplasm of olfactory bulb

        D33.4 **Benign neoplasm of** spinal cord

        D33.7 **Benign neoplasm of other specified parts of central nervous system**

        D33.9 **Benign neoplasm of central nervous system, unspecified**

            Benign neoplasm of nervous system (central) NOS

      D34 **Benign neoplasm of** thyroid gland

        Use additional code to identify any functional activity

✓4ᵗʰ **D35** **Benign neoplasm of** other and unspecified endocrine glands

        Use additional code to identify any functional activity

        EXCLUDES 1 *benign neoplasm of endocrine pancreas (D13.7)*

            benign neoplasm of ovary (D27.-)

            benign neoplasm of testis (D29.2-)

            benign neoplasm of thymus (D15.0)

✓5ᵗʰ **D35.0** **Benign neoplasm of** adrenal gland

        D35.00 **Benign neoplasm of unspecified adrenal gland**

        D35.01 **Benign neoplasm of** right **adrenal gland**

        D35.02 **Benign neoplasm of** left **adrenal gland**

        D35.1 **Benign neoplasm of** parathyroid gland

        D35.2 **Benign neoplasm of** pituitary gland

        D35.3 **Benign neoplasm of** craniopharyngeal duct

        D35.4 **Benign neoplasm of** pineal gland

        D35.5 **Benign neoplasm of** carotid body

        D35.6 **Benign neoplasm of** aortic body and other paraganglia

            Benign tumor of glomus jugulare

        D35.7 **Benign neoplasm of other specified endocrine glands**

        D35.9 **Benign neoplasm of endocrine gland, unspecified**

            Benign neoplasm of unspecified endocrine gland

✓4ᵗʰ **D36** **Benign neoplasm of** other and unspecified sites

        D36.0 **Benign neoplasm of** lymph nodes

            EXCLUDES 1 *lymphangioma (D18.1)*

✓5ᵗʰ **D36.1** **Benign neoplasm of** peripheral nerves and autonomic nervous system

        EXCLUDES 1 *benign neoplasm of peripheral nerves of orbit (D31.6-)*

            neurofibromatosis (Q85.0-)

        D36.10 **Benign neoplasm of peripheral nerves and autonomic nervous system, unspecified**

        D36.11 **Benign neoplasm of peripheral nerves and autonomic nervous system of** face, head, and neck

        D36.12 **Benign neoplasm of peripheral nerves and autonomic nervous system,** upper limb, including shoulder

        D36.13 **Benign neoplasm of peripheral nerves and autonomic nervous system of** lower limb, including hip

        D36.14 **Benign neoplasm of peripheral nerves and autonomic nervous system of** thorax

        D36.15 **Benign neoplasm of peripheral nerves and autonomic nervous system of** abdomen

        D36.16 **Benign neoplasm of peripheral nerves and autonomic nervous system of** pelvis

        D36.17 **Benign neoplasm of peripheral nerves and autonomic nervous system of** trunk, unspecified

        D36.7 **Benign neoplasm of other specified sites**

            Benign neoplasm of nose NOS

        D36.9 **Benign neoplasm, unspecified site**

Benign neuroendocrine tumors (D3A)

✓4ᵗʰ **D3A** **Benign neuroendocrine tumors**

        Code also any associated multiple endocrine neoplasia [MEN] syndromes (E31.2-)

        Use additional code to identify any associated endocrine syndrome, such as:

            carcinoid syndrome (E34.0)

        EXCLUDES 2 *benign pancreatic islet cell tumors (D13.7)*

✓5ᵗʰ **D3A.0** **Benign** carcinoid tumors

        D3A.00 **Benign carcinoid tumor of unspecified site**

            Carcinoid tumor NOS

        ✓6ᵗʰ D3A.01 **Benign carcinoid tumors of the** small intestine

            D3A.010 **Benign carcinoid tumor of the** duodenum

            D3A.011 **Benign carcinoid tumor of the** jejunum

            D3A.012 **Benign carcinoid tumor of the** ileum

            D3A.019 **Benign carcinoid tumor of the small intestine, unspecified portion**

        ✓6ᵗʰ D3A.02 **Benign carcinoid tumors of the** appendix, large intestine, and rectum

            D3A.020 **Benign carcinoid tumor of the** appendix

            D3A.021 **Benign carcinoid tumor of the** cecum

            D3A.022 **Benign carcinoid tumor of the** ascending colon

            D3A.023 **Benign carcinoid tumor of the** transverse colon

            D3A.024 **Benign carcinoid tumor of the** descending colon

            D3A.025 **Benign carcinoid tumor of the** sigmoid colon

            D3A.026 **Benign carcinoid tumor of the** rectum

            D3A.029 **Benign carcinoid tumor of the large intestine, unspecified portion**

               Benign carcinoid tumor of the colon NOS

EXCLUDES 1 Not coded here   **EXCLUDES 2** Not included here   N Newborn Age: 0   P Pediatric Age: 0-17   M Maternity Age: 12-55   A Adult Age: 15-124

468   ICD-10-CM Draft (2015)

☑6ᵗʰ **D3A.09** Benign carcinoid tumors of other sites

    D3A.090 Benign carcinoid tumor of the bronchus and lung

    D3A.091 Benign carcinoid tumor of the thymus

    D3A.092 Benign carcinoid tumor of the stomach

    D3A.093 Benign carcinoid tumor of the kidney

    D3A.094 Benign carcinoid tumor of the foregut NOS

    D3A.095 Benign carcinoid tumor of the midgut NOS

    D3A.096 Benign carcinoid tumor of the hindgut NOS

    D3A.098 Benign carcinoid tumors of other sites

D3A.8 Other benign neuroendocrine tumors

    Neuroendocrine tumor NOS

Neoplasms of uncertain behavior, polycythemia vera and myelodysplastic syndromes (D37-D48)

NOTE Categories D37-D44, and D48 classify by site neoplasms of uncertain behavior, i.e., histologic confirmation whether the neoplasm is malignant or benign cannot be made.

EXCLUDES 1 neoplasms of unspecified behavior (D49.-)

☑4ᵗʰ **D37** Neoplasm of uncertain behavior of oral cavity and digestive organs

    EXCLUDES 1 stromal tumors of uncertain behavior of digestive system (D48.1)

☑6ᵗʰ **D37.0** Neoplasm of uncertain behavior of lip, oral cavity and pharynx

    EXCLUDES 1 neoplasm of uncertain behavior of aryepiglottic fold or interarytenoid fold, laryngeal aspect (D38.0)

    neoplasm of uncertain behavior of epiglottis NOS (D38.0)

    neoplasm of uncertain behavior of skin of lip (D48.5)

    neoplasm of uncertain behavior of suprahyoid portion of epiglottis (D38.0)

    D37.01 Neoplasm of uncertain behavior of lip

        Neoplasm of uncertain behavior of vermilion border of lip

    D37.02 Neoplasm of uncertain behavior of tongue

☑6ᵗʰ   **D37.03** Neoplasm of uncertain behavior of the major salivary glands

        D37.030 Neoplasm of uncertain behavior of the parotid salivary glands

        D37.031 Neoplasm of uncertain behavior of the sublingual salivary glands

        D37.032 Neoplasm of uncertain behavior of the submandibular salivary glands

        D37.039 Neoplasm of uncertain behavior of the major salivary glands, unspecified

    D37.04 Neoplasm of uncertain behavior of the minor salivary glands

        Neoplasm of uncertain behavior of submucosal salivary glands of lip

        Neoplasm of uncertain behavior of submucosal salivary glands of cheek

        Neoplasm of uncertain behavior of submucosal salivary glands of hard palate

        Neoplasm of uncertain behavior of submucosal salivary glands of soft palate

    D37.05 Neoplasm of uncertain behavior of pharynx

        Neoplasm of uncertain behavior of aryepiglottic fold of pharynx NOS

        Neoplasm of uncertain behavior of hypopharyngeal aspect of aryepiglottic fold of pharynx

        Neoplasm of uncertain behavior of marginal zone of aryepiglottic fold of pharynx

    D37.09 Neoplasm of uncertain behavior of other specified sites of the oral cavity

D37.1 Neoplasm of uncertain behavior of stomach

D37.2 Neoplasm of uncertain behavior of small intestine

D37.3 Neoplasm of uncertain behavior of appendix

D37.4 Neoplasm of uncertain behavior of colon

D37.5 Neoplasm of uncertain behavior of rectum

    Neoplasm of uncertain behavior of rectosigmoid junction

D37.6 Neoplasm of uncertain behavior of liver, gallbladder and bile ducts

    Neoplasm of uncertain behavior of ampulla of Vater

D37.8 Neoplasm of uncertain behavior of other specified digestive organs

    Neoplasm of uncertain behavior of anal canal

    Neoplasm of uncertain behavior of anal sphincter

    Neoplasm of uncertain behavior of anus NOS

    Neoplasm of uncertain behavior of esophagus

    Neoplasm of uncertain behavior of intestine NOS

    Neoplasm of uncertain behavior of pancreas

    EXCLUDES 1 neoplasm of uncertain behavior of anal margin (D48.5)

    neoplasm of uncertain behavior of anal skin (D48.5)

    neoplasm of uncertain behavior of perianal skin (D48.5)

D37.9 Neoplasm of uncertain behavior of digestive organ, unspecified

☑4ᵗʰ **D38** Neoplasm of uncertain behavior of middle ear and respiratory and intrathoracic organs

    EXCLUDES 1 neoplasm of uncertain behavior of heart (D48.7)

D38.0 Neoplasm of uncertain behavior of larynx

    Neoplasm of uncertain behavior of aryepiglottic fold or interarytenoid fold, laryngeal aspect

    Neoplasm of uncertain behavior of epiglottis (suprahyoid portion)

    EXCLUDES 1 neoplasm of uncertain behavior of aryepiglottic fold or interarytenoid fold NOS (D37.05)

    neoplasm of uncertain behavior of hypopharyngeal aspect of aryepiglottic fold (D37.05)

    neoplasm of uncertain behavior of marginal zone of aryepiglottic fold (D37.05)

D38.1 Neoplasm of uncertain behavior of trachea, bronchus and lung

D38.2 Neoplasm of uncertain behavior of pleura

D38.3 Neoplasm of uncertain behavior of mediastinum

D38.4 Neoplasm of uncertain behavior of thymus

D38.5 Neoplasm of uncertain behavior of other respiratory organs

    Neoplasm of uncertain behavior of accessory sinuses

    Neoplasm of uncertain behavior of cartilage of nose

    Neoplasm of uncertain behavior of middle ear

    Neoplasm of uncertain behavior of nasal cavities

    EXCLUDES 1 neoplasm of uncertain behavior of ear (external) (skin) (D48.5)

    neoplasm of uncertain behavior of nose NOS (D48.7)

    neoplasm of uncertain behavior of skin of nose (D48.5)

D38.6 Neoplasm of uncertain behavior of respiratory organ, unspecified

☑4ᵗʰ **D39** Neoplasm of uncertain behavior of female genital organs

D39.0 Neoplasm of uncertain behavior of uterus   ♀

☑5ᵗʰ **D39.1** Neoplasm of uncertain behavior of ovary

    Use additional code to identify any functional activity

    D39.10 Neoplasm of uncertain behavior of unspecified ovary   ♀

    D39.11 Neoplasm of uncertain behavior of right ovary   ♀

    D39.12 Neoplasm of uncertain behavior of left ovary   ♀

D39.2 Neoplasm of uncertain behavior of placenta   ♀

    Chorioadenoma destruens

    Invasive hydatidiform mole

    Malignant hydatidiform mole

    EXCLUDES 1 hydatidiform mole NOS (O01.9)

D39.8 Neoplasm of uncertain behavior of other specified female genital organs   ♀

    Neoplasm of uncertain behavior of skin of female genital organs

D39.9 Neoplasm of uncertain behavior of female genital organ, unspecified   ♀

☑4ᵗʰ **D40** Neoplasm of uncertain behavior of male genital organs

D40.0 Neoplasm of uncertain behavior of prostate   ♂

☑5ᵗʰ **D40.1** Neoplasm of uncertain behavior of testis

    D40.10 Neoplasm of uncertain behavior of unspecified testis   ♂

    D40.11 Neoplasm of uncertain behavior of right testis   ♂

    D40.12 Neoplasm of uncertain behavior of left testis   ♂

D40.8 Neoplasm of uncertain behavior of other specified male genital organs   ♂

    Neoplasm of uncertain behavior of skin of male genital organs

D40.9 Neoplasm of uncertain behavior of male genital organ, unspecified   ♂

☑ Additional Character Required   ✓x7ᵗʰ Xtension Alert   Unspecified Dx   Other Specified Dx   Manifestation   ►◄ Revised Text   ● New Code   ▲ Revised Code Title

ICD-10-CM Draft (2015)   469

Neoplasms

D41–D47.9

✓4ᵗʰ **D41 Neoplasm of uncertain behavior of** urinary organs

  ✓5ᵗʰ **D41.0 Neoplasm of uncertain behavior of** kidney
    EXCLUDES 1 *neoplasm of uncertain behavior of renal pelvis (D41.1-)*

    D41.00 Neoplasm of uncertain behavior of unspecified kidney
    D41.01 Neoplasm of uncertain behavior of right **kidney**
    D41.02 Neoplasm of uncertain behavior of left **kidney**

  ✓5ᵗʰ **D41.1 Neoplasm of uncertain behavior of** renal pelvis
    D41.10 Neoplasm of uncertain behavior of unspecified renal pelvis
    D41.11 Neoplasm of uncertain behavior of right **renal pelvis**
    D41.12 Neoplasm of uncertain behavior of left **renal pelvis**

  ✓5ᵗʰ **D41.2 Neoplasm of uncertain behavior of** ureter
    D41.20 Neoplasm of uncertain behavior of unspecified ureter
    D41.21 Neoplasm of uncertain behavior of right **ureter**
    D41.22 Neoplasm of uncertain behavior of left **ureter**

  D41.3 Neoplasm of uncertain behavior of urethra
  D41.4 Neoplasm of uncertain behavior of bladder
  D41.8 Neoplasm of uncertain behavior of other specified urinary organs
  D41.9 Neoplasm of uncertain behavior of unspecified urinary organ

✓4ᵗʰ **D42 Neoplasm of uncertain behavior of** meninges

  D42.0 Neoplasm of uncertain behavior of cerebral **meninges**
  D42.1 Neoplasm of uncertain behavior of spinal **meninges**
  D42.9 Neoplasm of uncertain behavior of meninges, unspecified

✓4ᵗʰ **D43 Neoplasm of uncertain behavior of** brain and central nervous system
  EXCLUDES 1 *neoplasm of uncertain behavior of peripheral nerves and autonomic nervous system (D48.2)*

  D43.0 Neoplasm of uncertain behavior of brain, supratentorial
    Neoplasm of uncertain behavior of cerebral ventricle
    Neoplasm of uncertain behavior of cerebrum
    Neoplasm of uncertain behavior of frontal lobe
    Neoplasm of uncertain behavior of occipital lobe
    Neoplasm of uncertain behavior of parietal lobe
    Neoplasm of uncertain behavior of temporal lobe
    EXCLUDES 1 *neoplasm of uncertain behavior of fourth ventricle (D43.1)*

  D43.1 Neoplasm of uncertain behavior of brain, infratentorial
    Neoplasm of uncertain behavior of brain stem
    Neoplasm of uncertain behavior of cerebellum
    Neoplasm of uncertain behavior of fourth ventricle

  D43.2 Neoplasm of uncertain behavior of brain, unspecified
  D43.3 Neoplasm of uncertain behavior of cranial nerves
  D43.4 Neoplasm of uncertain behavior of spinal cord
  D43.8 Neoplasm of uncertain behavior of other specified parts of central nervous system
  D43.9 Neoplasm of uncertain behavior of central nervous system, unspecified
    Neoplasm of uncertain behavior of nervous system (central) NOS

✓4ᵗʰ **D44 Neoplasm of uncertain behavior of** endocrine glands
  EXCLUDES 1 *multiple endocrine adenomatosis (E31.2-)*
    multiple endocrine neoplasia (E31.2-)
    neoplasm of uncertain behavior of endocrine pancreas (D37.8)
    neoplasm of uncertain behavior of ovary (D39.1-)
    neoplasm of uncertain behavior of testis (D40.1-)
    neoplasm of uncertain behavior of thymus (D38.4)

  D44.0 Neoplasm of uncertain behavior of thyroid gland

  ✓5ᵗʰ **D44.1 Neoplasm of uncertain behavior of** adrenal gland
    Use additional code to identify any functional activity
    D44.10 Neoplasm of uncertain behavior of unspecified adrenal gland
    D44.11 Neoplasm of uncertain behavior of right **adrenal gland**
    D44.12 Neoplasm of uncertain behavior of left **adrenal gland**

  D44.2 Neoplasm of uncertain behavior of parathyroid gland
  D44.3 Neoplasm of uncertain behavior of pituitary gland
    Use additional code to identify any functional activity
  D44.4 Neoplasm of uncertain behavior of craniopharyngeal duct
  D44.5 Neoplasm of uncertain behavior of pineal gland
  D44.6 Neoplasm of uncertain behavior of carotid body

  D44.7 Neoplasm of uncertain behavior of aortic body and other paraganglia
  D44.9 Neoplasm of uncertain behavior of unspecified endocrine gland

D45 Polycythemia vera
  EXCLUDES 1 *familial polycythemia (D75.0)*
    secondary polycythemia (D75.1)

✓4ᵗʰ **D46 Myelodysplastic syndromes**
  Use additional code for adverse effect, if applicable, to identify drug (T36-T50 with fifth or sixth character 5)
  EXCLUDES 2 *drug-induced aplastic anemia (D61.1)*

  D46.0 Refractory anemia without ring sideroblasts, **so stated**
    Refractory anemia without sideroblasts, without excess of blasts

  D46.1 Refractory anemia with ring sideroblasts
    RARS

  ✓5ᵗʰ **D46.2 Refractory anemia** with excess of blasts
    D46.20 Refractory anemia with excess of blasts, unspecified
      RAEB NOS
    D46.21 Refractory anemia with excess of blasts 1
      RAEB 1
    D46.22 Refractory anemia with excess of blasts 2
      RAEB 2

  D46.A Refractory cytopenia with multilineage dysplasia
  D46.B Refractory cytopenia with multilineage dysplasia and ring sideroblasts
    RCMD RS
  D46.C Myelodysplastic syndrome with isolated del(5q) chromosomal abnormality
    Myelodysplastic syndrome with 5q deletion
    5q minus syndrome NOS
  D46.4 Refractory anemia, unspecified
  D46.Z Other myelodysplastic syndromes
    EXCLUDES 1 *chronic myelomonocytic leukemia (C93.1-)*
  D46.9 Myelodysplastic syndrome, unspecified
    Myelodysplasia NOS

✓4ᵗʰ **D47 Other neoplasms of uncertain behavior of** lymphoid, hematopoietic and related tissue

  D47.0 Histiocytic and mast cell tumors of uncertain behavior
    Indolent systemic mastocytosis
    Mast cell tumor NOS
    Mastocytoma NOS
    EXCLUDES 1 *malignant mast cell tumor (C96.2)*
    mastocytosis (congenital) (cutaneous) (Q82.2)

  D47.1 Chronic myeloproliferative disease
    Chronic neutrophilic leukemia
    Myeloproliferative disease, unspecified
    EXCLUDES 1 *atypical chronic myeloid leukemia BCR/ABL-negative (C92.2-)*
    chronic myeloid leukemia BCR/ABL-positive (C92.1-)
    myelofibrosis NOS (D75.81)
    myelophthisic anemia (D61.82)
    myelophthisis (D61.82)
    secondary myelofibrosis NOS (D75.81)

  D47.2 Monoclonal gammopathy
    Monoclonal gammopathy of undetermined significance [MGUS]

  D47.3 Essential (hemorrhagic) thrombocythemia
    Essential thrombocytosis
    Idiopathic hemorrhagic thrombocythemia

  D47.4 Osteomyelofibrosis
    Chronic idiopathic myelofibrosis
    Myelofibrosis (idiopathic) (with myeloid metaplasia)
    Myelosclerosis (megakaryocytic) with myeloid metaplasia
    Secondary myelofibrosis in myeloproliferative disease
    EXCLUDES 1 *acute myelofibrosis (C94.4-)*

  ✓5ᵗʰ **D47.Z Other** specified neoplasms of uncertain behavior of lymphoid, hematopoietic and related tissue
    D47.Z1 Post-transplant lymphoproliferative disorder (PTLD)
      Code first complications of transplanted organs and tissue (T86.-)
    D47.Z9 Other specified neoplasms of uncertain behavior of lymphoid, hematopoietic and related tissue
      Histiocytic tumors of uncertain behavior

  D47.9 Neoplasm of uncertain behavior of lymphoid, hematopoietic and related tissue, unspecified
    Lymphoproliferative disease NOS

EXCLUDES 1 Not coded here   EXCLUDES 2 Not included here   N Newborn Age: 0   P Pediatric Age: 0-17   M Maternity Age: 12-55   A Adult Age: 15-124

470   ICD-10-CM Draft (2015)

☑4ᵗʰ D48　Neoplasm of uncertain behavior of other and unspecified sites

> EXCLUDES 1　*neurofibromatosis (nonmalignant) (Q85.Ø-)*

D48.Ø　Neoplasm of uncertain behavior of bone and articular cartilage

> EXCLUDES 1　*neoplasm of uncertain behavior of cartilage of ear (D48.1)*
> *neoplasm of uncertain behavior of cartilage of larynx (D38.Ø)*
> *neoplasm of uncertain behavior of cartilage of nose (D38.5)*
> *neoplasm of uncertain behavior of connective tissue of eyelid (D48.1)*
> *neoplasm of uncertain behavior of synovia (D48.1)*

D48.1　Neoplasm of uncertain behavior of connective and other soft tissue

Neoplasm of uncertain behavior of connective tissue of ear
Neoplasm of uncertain behavior of connective tissue of eyelid
Stromal tumors of uncertain behavior of digestive system

> EXCLUDES 1　*neoplasm of uncertain behavior of articular cartilage (D48.Ø)*
> *neoplasm of uncertain behavior of cartilage of larynx (D38.Ø)*
> *neoplasm of uncertain behavior of cartilage of nose (D38.5)*
> *neoplasm of uncertain behavior of connective tissue of breast (D48.6-)*

D48.2　Neoplasm of uncertain behavior of peripheral nerves and autonomic nervous system

> EXCLUDES 1　*neoplasm of uncertain behavior of peripheral nerves of orbit (D48.7)*

D48.3　Neoplasm of uncertain behavior of retroperitoneum

D48.4　Neoplasm of uncertain behavior of peritoneum

D48.5　Neoplasm of uncertain behavior of skin

Neoplasm of uncertain behavior of anal margin
Neoplasm of uncertain behavior of anal skin
Neoplasm of uncertain behavior of perianal skin
Neoplasm of uncertain behavior of skin of breast

> EXCLUDES 1　*neoplasm of uncertain behavior of anus NOS (D37.8)*
> *neoplasm of uncertain behavior of skin of genital organs (D39.8, D4Ø.8)*
> *neoplasm of uncertain behavior of vermilion border of lip (D37.Ø)*

☑5ᵗʰ D48.6　Neoplasm of uncertain behavior of breast

Neoplasm of uncertain behavior of connective tissue of breast
Cystosarcoma phyllodes

> EXCLUDES 1　*neoplasm of uncertain behavior of skin of breast (D48.5)*

D48.6Ø　Neoplasm of uncertain behavior of unspecified breast

D48.61　Neoplasm of uncertain behavior of right breast

D48.62　Neoplasm of uncertain behavior of left breast

D48.7　Neoplasm of uncertain behavior of other specified sites

Neoplasm of uncertain behavior of eye
Neoplasm of uncertain behavior of heart
Neoplasm of uncertain behavior of peripheral nerves of orbit

> EXCLUDES 1　*neoplasm of uncertain behavior of connective tissue (D48.1)*
> *neoplasm of uncertain behavior of skin of eyelid (D48.5)*

D48.9　Neoplasm of uncertain behavior, unspecified

Neoplasms of uncertain behavior (D49)

☑4ᵗʰ D49　Neoplasms of unspecified behavior

> NOTE　Category D49 classifies by site neoplasms of unspecified morphology and behavior. The term "mass", unless otherwise stated, is not to be regarded as a neoplastic growth.
> INCLUDES　"growth" NOS
> neoplasm NOS
> new growth NOS
> tumor NOS
> EXCLUDES 1　*neoplasms of uncertain behavior (D37-D44, D48)*

D49.Ø　Neoplasm of unspecified behavior of digestive system

> EXCLUDES 1　*neoplasm of unspecified behavior of margin of anus (D49.2)*
> *neoplasm of unspecified behavior of perianal skin (D49.2)*
> *neoplasm of unspecified behavior of skin of anus (D49.2)*

D49.1　Neoplasm of unspecified behavior of respiratory system

D49.2　Neoplasm of unspecified behavior of bone, soft tissue, and skin

> EXCLUDES 1　*neoplasm of unspecified behavior of anal canal (D49.Ø)*
> *neoplasm of unspecified behavior of anus NOS (D49.Ø)*
> *neoplasm of unspecified behavior of bone marrow (D49.89)*
> *neoplasm of unspecified behavior of cartilage of larynx (D49.1)*
> *neoplasm of unspecified behavior of cartilage of nose (D49.1)*
> *neoplasm of unspecified behavior of connective tissue of breast (D49.3)*
> *neoplasm of unspecified behavior of skin of genital organs (D49.5)*
> *neoplasm of unspecified behavior of vermilion border of lip (D49.Ø)*

D49.3　Neoplasm of unspecified behavior of breast

> EXCLUDES 1　*neoplasm of unspecified behavior of skin of breast (D49.2)*

D49.4　Neoplasm of unspecified behavior of bladder

D49.5　Neoplasm of unspecified behavior of other genitourinary organs

D49.6　Neoplasm of unspecified behavior of brain

> EXCLUDES 1　*neoplasm of unspecified behavior of cerebral meninges (D49.7)*
> *neoplasm of unspecified behavior of cranial nerves (D49.7)*

D49.7　Neoplasm of unspecified behavior of endocrine glands and other parts of nervous system

> EXCLUDES 1　*neoplasm of unspecified behavior of peripheral, sympathetic, and parasympathetic nerves and ganglia (D49.2)*

☑5ᵗʰ D49.8　Neoplasm of unspecified behavior of other specified sites

> EXCLUDES 1　*neoplasm of unspecified behavior of eyelid (skin) (D49.2)*
> *neoplasm of unspecified behavior of eyelid cartilage (D49.2)*
> *neoplasm of unspecified behavior of great vessels (D49.2)*
> *neoplasm of unspecified behavior of optic nerve (D49.7)*

D49.81　Neoplasm of unspecified behavior of retina and choroid

Dark area on retina
Retinal freckle

D49.89　Neoplasm of unspecified behavior of other specified sites

D49.9　Neoplasm of unspecified behavior of unspecified site

☑ Additional Character Required　　☑7ᵗʰ Xtension Alert　　Unspecified Dx　　Other Specified Dx　　Manifestation　　▶◀ Revised Text　　● New Code　　▲ Revised Code Title

Chapter 3. Diseases of the Blood and Blood-forming Organs and Certain Disorders Involving the Immune Mechanism (D50-D89)

EXCLUDES 2   autoimmune disease (systemic) NOS (M35.9)
certain conditions originating in the perinatal period (P00-P96)
complications of pregnancy, childbirth and the puerperium (O00-O9A)
congenital malformations, deformations and chromosomal abnormalities (Q00-Q99)
endocrine, nutritional and metabolic diseases (E00-E88)
human immunodeficiency virus [HIV] disease (B20)
injury, poisoning and certain other consequences of external causes (S00-T88)
neoplasms (C00-D49)
symptoms, signs and abnormal clinical and laboratory findings, not elsewhere classified (R00-R94)

This chapter contains the following blocks:

D50-D53   Nutritional anemias
D55-D59   Hemolytic anemias
D60-D64   Aplastic and other anemias and other bone marrow failure syndromes
D65-D69   Coagulation defects, purpura and other hemorrhagic conditions
D70-D77   Other disorders of blood and blood-forming organs
D78   Intraoperative and postprocedural complications of the spleen
D80-D89   Certain disorders involving the immune mechanism

Nutritional anemias (D50-D53)

✓4ᵗʰ D50   Iron deficiency anemia
INCLUDES   asiderotic anemia
hypochromic anemia

D50.0   Iron deficiency anemia secondary to blood loss (chronic)
Posthemorrhagic anemia (chronic)
EXCLUDES 1   acute posthemorrhagic anemia (D62)
congenital anemia from fetal blood loss (P61.3)

D50.1   Sideropenic dysphagia
Kelly-Paterson syndrome
Plummer-Vinson syndrome

D50.8   Other iron deficiency anemias
Iron deficiency anemia due to inadequate dietary iron intake

D50.9   Iron deficiency anemia, unspecified

✓4ᵗʰ D51   Vitamin B12 deficiency anemia
EXCLUDES 1   vitamin B12 deficiency (E53.8)

D51.0   Vitamin B12 deficiency anemia due to intrinsic factor deficiency
Addison anemia
Biermer anemia
Pernicious (congenital) anemia
Congenital intrinsic factor deficiency

D51.1   Vitamin B12 deficiency anemia due to selective vitamin B12 malabsorption with proteinuria
Imerslund (Gräsbeck) syndrome
Megaloblastic hereditary anemia

D51.2   Transcobalamin II deficiency

D51.3   Other dietary vitamin B12 deficiency anemia
Vegan anemia

D51.8   Other vitamin B12 deficiency anemias

D51.9   Vitamin B12 deficiency anemia, unspecified

✓4ᵗʰ D52   Folate deficiency anemia
EXCLUDES 1   folate deficiency without anemia (E53.8)

D52.0   Dietary folate deficiency anemia
Nutritional megaloblastic anemia

D52.1   Drug-induced folate deficiency anemia
Use additional code for adverse effect, if applicable, to identify drug (T36-T50 with fifth or sixth character 5)

D52.8   Other folate deficiency anemias

D52.9   Folate deficiency anemia, unspecified
Folic acid deficiency anemia NOS

✓4ᵗʰ D53   Other nutritional anemias
INCLUDES   megaloblastic anemia unresponsive to vitamin B12 or folate therapy

D53.0   Protein deficiency anemia
Amino-acid deficiency anemia
Orotaciduric anemia
EXCLUDES 1   Lesch-Nyhan syndrome (E79.1)

D53.1   Other megaloblastic anemias, not elsewhere classified
Megaloblastic anemia NOS
EXCLUDES 1   Di Guglielmo's disease (C94.0)

D53.2   Scorbutic anemia
EXCLUDES 1   scurvy (E54)

D53.8   Other specified nutritional anemias
Anemia associated with deficiency of copper
Anemia associated with deficiency of molybdenum
Anemia associated with deficiency of zinc
EXCLUDES 1   nutritional deficiencies without anemia, such as:
copper deficiency NOS (E61.0)
molybdenum deficiency NOS (E61.5)
zinc deficiency NOS (E60)

D53.9   Nutritional anemia, unspecified
Simple chronic anemia
EXCLUDES 1   anemia NOS (D64.9)

Hemolytic anemias (D55-D59)

✓4ᵗʰ D55   Anemia due to enzyme disorders
EXCLUDES 1   drug-induced enzyme deficiency anemia (D59.2)

D55.0   Anemia due to glucose-6-phosphate dehydrogenase [G6PD] deficiency
Favism
G6PD deficiency anemia

D55.1   Anemia due to other disorders of glutathione metabolism
Anemia (due to) enzyme deficiencies, except G6PD, related to the hexose monophosphate [HMP] shunt pathway
Anemia (due to) hemolytic nonspherocytic (hereditary), type I

D55.2   Anemia due to disorders of glycolytic enzymes
Hemolytic nonspherocytic (hereditary) anemia, type II
Hexokinase deficiency anemia
Pyruvate kinase [PK] deficiency anemia
Triose-phosphate isomerase deficiency anemia
EXCLUDES 1   disorders of glycolysis not associated with anemia (E74.8)

D55.3   Anemia due to disorders of nucleotide metabolism

D55.8   Other anemias due to enzyme disorders

D55.9   Anemia due to enzyme disorder, unspecified

✓4ᵗʰ D56   Thalassemia
EXCLUDES 1   sickle-cell thalassemia (D57.4-)

D56.0   Alpha thalassemia
Alpha thalassemia major
Hemoglobin H Constant Spring
Hemoglobin H disease
Hydrops fetalis due to alpha thalassemia
Severe alpha thalassemia
Triple gene defect alpha thalassemia
Use additional code, if applicable, for hydrops fetalis due to alpha thalassemia (P56.99)
EXCLUDES 1   alpha thalassemia trait or minor (D56.3)
asymptomatic alpha thalassemia (D56.3)
hydrops fetalis due to isoimmunization (P56.0)
hydrops fetalis not due to immune hemolysis (P83.2)

D56.1   Beta thalassemia
Beta thalassemia major
Cooley's anemia
Homozygous beta thalassemia
Severe beta thalassemia
Thalassemia intermedia
Thalassemia major
EXCLUDES 1   beta thalassemia minor (D56.3)
beta thalassemia trait (D56.3)
delta-beta thalassemia (D56.2)
hemoglobin E-beta thalassemia (D56.5)
sickle-cell beta thalassemia (D57.4-)

D56.2   Delta-beta thalassemia
Homozygous delta-beta thalassemia
EXCLUDES 1   delta-beta thalassemia minor (D56.3)
delta-beta thalassemia trait (D56.3)

D56.3   Thalassemia minor
Alpha thalassemia minor
Alpha thalassemia silent carrier
Alpha thalassemia trait
Beta thalassemia minor
Beta thalassemia trait
Delta-beta thalassemia minor
Delta-beta thalassemia trait
Thalassemia trait NOS
EXCLUDES 1   alpha thalassemia (D56.0)
beta thalassemia (D56.1)
delta-beta thalassemia (D56.2)
hemoglobin E-beta thalassemia (D56.5)
sickle-cell trait (D57.3)

EXCLUDES 1 Not coded here   EXCLUDES 2 Not included here   N Newborn Age: 0   P Pediatric Age: 0-17   M Maternity Age: 12-55   A Adult Age: 15-124

472   ICD-10-CM Draft (2015)

D56.4 Hereditary persistence of fetal hemoglobin [HPFH]

D56.5 Hemoglobin E-beta thalassemia
> EXCLUDES 1   *beta thalassemia (D56.1)*
> *beta thalassemia minor (D56.3)*
> *beta thalassemia trait (D56.3)*
> *delta-beta thalassemia (D56.2)*
> *delta-beta thalassemia trait (D56.3)*
> *hemoglobin E disease (D58.2)*
> *other hemoglobinopathies (D58.2)*
> *sickle-cell beta thalassemia (D57.4-)*

D56.8 Other thalassemias
Dominant thalassemia
Hemoglobin C thalassemia
Mixed thalassemia
Thalassemia with other hemoglobinopathy
> EXCLUDES 1   *hemoglobin C disease (D58.2)*
> *hemoglobin E disease (D58.2)*
> *other hemoglobinopathies (D58.2)*
> *sickle-cell anemia (D57.-)*
> *sickle-cell thalassemia (D57.4)*

D56.9 Thalassemia, unspecified
Mediterranean anemia (with other hemoglobinopathy)

✓4ᵗʰ **D57** Sickle-cell disorders
Use additional code for any associated fever (R50.81)
> EXCLUDES 1   *other hemoglobinopathies (D58.-)*

✓5ᵗʰ **D57.0** Hb-SS disease with crisis
Sickle-cell disease NOS with crisis
Hb-SS disease with vasoocclusive pain

D57.00 Hb-SS disease with crisis, unspecified

D57.01 Hb-SS disease with acute chest syndrome

D57.02 Hb-SS disease with splenic sequestration

D57.1 Sickle-cell disease without crisis
Hb-SS disease without crisis
Sickle-cell anemia NOS
Sickle-cell disease NOS
Sickle-cell disorder NOS

✓5ᵗʰ **D57.2** Sickle-cell/Hb-C disease
Hb-SC disease
Hb-S/Hb-C disease

D57.20 Sickle-cell/Hb-C disease without crisis

✓6ᵗʰ **D57.21** Sickle-cell/Hb-C disease with crisis

D57.211 Sickle-cell/Hb-C disease with acute chest syndrome

D57.212 Sickle-cell/Hb-C disease with splenic sequestration

D57.219 Sickle-cell/Hb-C disease with crisis, unspecified
Sickle-cell/Hb-C disease with crisis NOS

D57.3 Sickle-cell trait
Hb-S trait
Heterozygous hemoglobin S

✓5ᵗʰ **D57.4** Sickle-cell thalassemia
Sickle-cell beta thalassemia
Thalassemia Hb-S disease

D57.40 Sickle-cell thalassemia without crisis
Microdrepanocytosis
Sickle-cell thalassemia NOS

✓6ᵗʰ **D57.41** Sickle-cell thalassemia with crisis
Sickle-cell thalassemia with vasoocclusive pain

D57.411 Sickle-cell thalassemia with acute chest syndrome

D57.412 Sickle-cell thalassemia with splenic sequestration

D57.419 Sickle-cell thalassemia with crisis, unspecified
Sickle-cell thalassemia with crisis NOS

✓5ᵗʰ **D57.8** Other sickle-cell disorders
Hb-SD disease
Hb-SE disease

D57.80 Other sickle-cell disorders without crisis

✓6ᵗʰ **D57.81** Other sickle-cell disorders with crisis

D57.811 Other sickle-cell disorders with acute chest syndrome

D57.812 Other sickle-cell disorders with splenic sequestration

D57.819 Other sickle-cell disorders with crisis, unspecified
Other sickle-cell disorders with crisis NOS

✓4ᵗʰ **D58** Other hereditary hemolytic anemias
> EXCLUDES 1   *hemolytic anemia of the newborn (P55.-)*

D58.0 Hereditary spherocytosis
Acholuric (familial) jaundice
Congenital (spherocytic) hemolytic icterus
Minkowski-Chauffard syndrome

D58.1 Hereditary elliptocytosis
Elliptocytosis (congenital)
Ovalocytosis (congenital) (hereditary)

D58.2 Other hemoglobinopathies
Abnormal hemoglobin NOS
Congenital Heinz body anemia
Hb-C disease
Hb-D disease
Hb-E disease
Hemoglobinopathy NOS
Unstable hemoglobin hemolytic disease
> EXCLUDES 1   *familial polycythemia (D75.0)*
> *Hb-M disease (D74.0)*
> *hemoglobin E-beta thalassemia (D56.5)*
> *hereditary persistence of fetal hemoglobin [HPFH] (D56.4)*
> *high-altitude polycythemia (D75.1)*
> *methemoglobinemia (D74.-)*
> *other hemoglobinopathies with thalassemia (D56.8)*

D58.8 Other specified hereditary hemolytic anemias
Stomatocytosis

D58.9 Hereditary hemolytic anemia, unspecified

✓4ᵗʰ **D59** Acquired hemolytic anemia

D59.0 Drug-induced autoimmune hemolytic anemia
Use additional code for adverse effect, if applicable, to identify drug (T36-T50 with fifth or sixth character 5)

D59.1 Other autoimmune hemolytic anemias
Autoimmune hemolytic disease (cold type) (warm type)
Chronic cold hemagglutinin disease
Cold agglutinin disease
Cold agglutinin hemoglobinuria
Cold type (secondary) (symptomatic) hemolytic anemia
Warm type (secondary) (symptomatic) hemolytic anemia
> EXCLUDES 1   *Evans syndrome (D69.41)*
> *hemolytic disease of newborn (P55.-)*
> *paroxysmal cold hemoglobinuria (D59.6)*

D59.2 Drug-induced nonautoimmune hemolytic anemia
Drug-induced enzyme deficiency anemia
Use additional code for adverse effect, if applicable, to identify drug (T36-T50 with fifth or sixth character 5)

D59.3 Hemolytic-uremic syndrome
Use additional code to identify associated:
E. coli infection (B96.2-)
Pneumococcal pneumonia (J13)
Shigella dysenteriae (A03.9)

D59.4 Other nonautoimmune hemolytic anemias
Mechanical hemolytic anemia
Microangiopathic hemolytic anemia
Toxic hemolytic anemia

D59.5 Paroxysmal nocturnal hemoglobinuria [Marchiafava-Micheli]
> EXCLUDES 1   *hemoglobinuria NOS (R82.3)*

D59.6 Hemoglobinuria due to hemolysis from other external causes
Hemoglobinuria from exertion
March hemoglobinuria
Paroxysmal cold hemoglobinuria
Use additional code (Chapter 20) to identify external cause
> EXCLUDES 1   *hemoglobinuria NOS (R82.3)*

D59.8 Other acquired hemolytic anemias

D59.9 Acquired hemolytic anemia, unspecified
Idiopathic hemolytic anemia, chronic

Aplastic and other anemias and other bone marrow failure syndromes (D60-D64)

✓4ᵗʰ **D60** Acquired pure red cell aplasia [erythroblastopenia]
> INCLUDES   red cell aplasia (acquired) (adult) (with thymoma)
> EXCLUDES 1   *congenital red cell aplasia (D61.01)*

D60.0 Chronic acquired pure red cell aplasia

D60.1 Transient acquired pure red cell aplasia

D60.8 Other acquired pure red cell aplasias

D60.9 Acquired pure red cell aplasia, unspecified

✓ Additional Character Required   ✓x7ᵗʰ Xtension Alert   Unspecified Dx   Other Specified Dx   Manifestation   ►◄ Revised Text   ● New Code   ▲ Revised Code Title

Diseases of the Blood and Blood-forming Organs

D61–D68.0

☑4ᵗʰ **D61 Other aplastic anemias and other bone marrow failure syndromes**
> EXCLUDES 1   *neutropenia (D70.-)*

☑5ᵗʰ **D61.0 Constitutional aplastic anemia**

D61.01 Constitutional (pure) red blood cell aplasia
Blackfan-Diamond syndrome
Congenital (pure) red cell aplasia
Familial hypoplastic anemia
Primary (pure) red cell aplasia
Red cell (pure) aplasia of infants
> EXCLUDES 1   *acquired red cell aplasia (D60.9)*

D61.09 Other constitutional aplastic anemia
Fanconi's anemia
Pancytopenia with malformations

D61.1 Drug-induced aplastic anemia
Use additional code for adverse effect, if applicable, to identify drug (T36-T50 with fifth or sixth character 5)

D61.2 Aplastic anemia due to other external agents
Code first, if applicable, toxic effects of substances chiefly nonmedicinal as to source (T51-T65)

D61.3 Idiopathic aplastic anemia

☑5ᵗʰ **D61.8 Other specified aplastic anemias and other bone marrow failure syndromes**

☑6ᵗʰ **D61.81 Pancytopenia**
> EXCLUDES 1   *pancytopenia (due to) (with) aplastic anemia (D61.9)*
> *pancytopenia (due to) (with) bone marrow infiltration (D61.82)*
> *pancytopenia (due to) (with) congenital (pure) red cell aplasia (D61.01)*
> *pancytopenia (due to) (with) hairy cell leukemia (C91.4-)*
> *pancytopenia (due to) (with) human immunodeficiency virus disease (B20)*
> *pancytopenia (due to) (with) leukoerythroblastic anemia (D61.82)*
> *pancytopenia (due to) (with) myelodysplastic syndromes (D46.-)*
> *pancytopenia (due to) (with) myeloproliferative disease (D47.1)*

D61.810 Antineoplastic chemotherapy induced pancytopenia
> EXCLUDES 2   *aplastic anemia due to antineoplastic chemotherapy (D61.1)*

D61.811 Other drug-induced pancytopenia
> EXCLUDES 2   *aplastic anemia due to drugs (D61.1)*

D61.818 Other pancytopenia

D61.82 Myelophthisis
Leukoerythroblastic anemia
Myelophthisic anemia
Panmyelophthisis
Code also the underlying disorder, such as:
malignant neoplasm of breast (C50.-)
tuberculosis (A15.-)
> EXCLUDES 1   *idiopathic myelofibrosis (D47.1)*
> *myelofibrosis NOS (D75.81)*
> *myelofibrosis with myeloid metaplasia (D47.4)*
> *primary myelofibrosis (D47.1)*
> *secondary myelofibrosis (D75.81)*

D61.89 Other specified aplastic anemias and other bone marrow failure syndromes

D61.9 Aplastic anemia, unspecified
Hypoplastic anemia NOS
Medullary hypoplasia

D62 Acute posthemorrhagic anemia
> EXCLUDES 1   *anemia due to chronic blood loss (D50.0)*
> *blood loss anemia NOS (D50.0)*
> *congenital anemia from fetal blood loss (P61.3)*

☑4ᵗʰ **D63 Anemia in chronic diseases classified elsewhere**

D63.0 Anemia in neoplastic disease
Code first neoplasm (C00-D49)
> EXCLUDES 1   *anemia due to antineoplastic chemotherapy (D64.81)*
> *aplastic anemia due to antineoplastic chemotherapy (D61.1)*

D63.1 Anemia in chronic kidney disease
Erythropoietin resistant anemia (EPO resistant anemia)
Code first underlying chronic kidney disease (CKD) (N18.-)

D63.8 Anemia in other chronic diseases classified elsewhere
Code first underlying disease, such as:
diphyllobothriasis (B70.0)
hookworm disease (B76.0-B76.9)
hypothyroidism (E00.0-E03.9)
malaria (B50.0-B54)
symptomatic late syphilis (A52.79)
tuberculosis (A18.89)

☑4ᵗʰ **D64 Other anemias**
> EXCLUDES 1   *refractory anemia (D46.-)*
> *refractory anemia with excess blasts in transformation [RAEB T] (C92.0-)*

D64.0 Hereditary sideroblastic anemia
Sex-linked hypochromic sideroblastic anemia

D64.1 Secondary sideroblastic anemia due to disease
Code first underlying disease

D64.2 Secondary sideroblastic anemia due to drugs and toxins
Code first poisoning due to drug or toxin, if applicable (T36-T65 with fifth or sixth character 1-4 or 6)
Use additional code for adverse effect, if applicable, to identify drug (T36-T50 with fifth or sixth character 5)

D64.3 Other sideroblastic anemias
Sideroblastic anemia NOS
Pyridoxine-responsive sideroblastic anemia NEC

D64.4 Congenital dyserythropoietic anemia
Dyshematopoietic anemia (congenital)
> EXCLUDES 1   *Blackfan-Diamond syndrome (D61.01)*
> *Di Guglielmo's disease (C94.0)*

☑5ᵗʰ **D64.8 Other specified anemias**

D64.81 Anemia due to antineoplastic chemotherapy
Antineoplastic chemotherapy induced anemia
> EXCLUDES 1   *anemia in neoplastic disease (D63.0)*
> *aplastic anemia due to antineoplastic chemotherapy (D61.1)*

D64.89 Other specified anemias
Infantile pseudoleukemia

D64.9 Anemia, unspecified

Coagulation defects, purpura and other hemorrhagic conditions (D65-D69)

D65 Disseminated intravascular coagulation [defibrination syndrome]
Afibrinogenemia, acquired
Consumption coagulopathy
Diffuse or disseminated intravascular coagulation [DIC]
Fibrinolytic hemorrhage, acquired
Fibrinolytic purpura
Purpura fulminans
> EXCLUDES 1   *disseminated intravascular coagulation (complicating):*
> *abortion or ectopic or molar pregnancy (O00-O07, O08.1)*
> *in newborn (P60)*
> *pregnancy, childbirth and the puerperium (O45.0, O46.0, O67.0, O72.3)*

D66 Hereditary factor VIII deficiency
Classical hemophilia
Deficiency factor VIII (with functional defect)
Hemophilia A
Hemophilia NOS
> EXCLUDES 1   *factor VIII deficiency with vascular defect (D68.0)*

D67 Hereditary factor IX deficiency
Christmas disease
Factor IX deficiency (with functional defect)
Hemophilia B
Plasma thromboplastin component [PTC] deficiency

☑4ᵗʰ **D68 Other coagulation defects**
> EXCLUDES 1   *abnormal coagulation profile (R79.1)*
> *coagulation defects complicating abortion or ectopic or molar pregnancy (O00-O07, O08.1)*
> *coagulation defects complicating pregnancy, childbirth and the puerperium (O45.0, O46.0, O67.0, O72.3)*

D68.0 Von Willebrand's disease
Angiohemophilia
Factor VIII deficiency with vascular defect
Vascular hemophilia
> EXCLUDES 1   *capillary fragility (hereditary) (D69.8)*
> *factor VIII deficiency NOS (D66)*
> *factor VIII deficiency with functional defect (D66)*

EXCLUDES 1 Not coded here   EXCLUDES 2 Not included here   N Newborn Age: 0   P Pediatric Age: 0-17   M Maternity Age: 12-55   A Adult Age: 15-124

D68.1 Hereditary factor XI deficiency
Hemophilia C
Plasma thromboplastin antecedent [PTA] deficiency
Rosenthal's disease

D68.2 Hereditary deficiency of other clotting factors
AC globulin deficiency
Congenital afibrinogenemia
Deficiency of factor I [fibrinogen]
Deficiency of factor II [prothrombin]
Deficiency of factor V [labile]
Deficiency of factor VII [stable]
Deficiency of factor X [Stuart-Prower]
Deficiency of factor XII [Hageman]
Deficiency of factor XIII [fibrin stabilizing]
Dysfibrinogenemia (congenital)
Hypoproconvertinemia
Owren's disease
Proaccelerin deficiency

√5ᵗʰ **D68.3 Hemorrhagic disorder due to circulating anticoagulants**

√6ᵗʰ **D68.31 Hemorrhagic disorder due to intrinsic circulating anticoagulants, antibodies, or inhibitors**

D68.311 Acquired hemophilia
Autoimmune hemophilia
Autoimmune inhibitors to clotting factors
Secondary hemophilia

D68.312 Antiphospholipid antibody with hemorrhagic disorder
Lupus anticoagulant (LAC) with hemorrhagic disorder
Systemic lupus erythematosus [SLE] inhibitor with hemorrhagic disorder
EXCLUDES 1 *antiphospholipid antibody, finding without diagnosis (R76.0)*
antiphospholipid antibody syndrome (D68.61)
antiphospholipid antibody with hypercoagulable state (D68.61)
lupus anticoagulant (LAC) finding without diagnosis (R76.0)
lupus anticoagulant (LAC) with hypercoagulable state (D68.62)
systemic lupus erythematosus [SLE] inhibitor finding without diagnosis (R76.0)
systemic lupus erythematosus [SLE] inhibitor with hypercoagulable state (D68.62)

D68.318 Other hemorrhagic disorder due to intrinsic circulating anticoagulants, antibodies, or inhibitors
Antithromboplastinemia
Antithromboplastinogenemia
Hemorrhagic disorder due to intrinsic increase in antithrombin
Hemorrhagic disorder due to intrinsic increase in anti-VIIIa
Hemorrhagic disorder due to intrinsic increase in anti-IXa
Hemorrhagic disorder due to intrinsic increase in anti-XIa

D68.32 Hemorrhagic disorder due to extrinsic circulating anticoagulants
Drug-induced hemorrhagic disorder
Hemorrhagic disorder due to increase in anti-IIa
Hemorrhagic disorder due to increase in anti-Xa
Hyperheparinemia
Use additional code for adverse effect, if applicable, to identify drug (T45.515, T45.525)

D68.4 Acquired coagulation factor deficiency
Deficiency of coagulation factor due to liver disease
Deficiency of coagulation factor due to vitamin K deficiency
EXCLUDES 1 *vitamin K deficiency of newborn (P53)*

√5ᵗʰ **D68.5 Primary thrombophilia**
Primary hypercoagulable states
EXCLUDES 1 *antiphospholipid syndrome (D68.61)*
lupus anticoagulant (D68.62)
secondary activated protein C resistance (D68.69)
secondary antiphospholipid antibody syndrome (D68.69)
secondary lupus anticoagulant with hypercoagulable state (D68.69)
secondary systemic lupus erythematosus [SLE] inhibitor with hypercoagulable state (D68.69)
systemic lupus erythematosus [SLE] inhibitor finding without diagnosis (R76.0)
systemic lupus erythematosus [SLE] inhibitor with hemorrhagic disorder (D68.312)
thrombotic thrombocytopenic purpura (M31.1)

D68.51 Activated protein C resistance
Factor V Leiden mutation

D68.52 Prothrombin gene mutation

D68.59 Other primary thrombophilia
Antithrombin III deficiencyProtein C deficiency
Hypercoagulable state NOSProtein S deficiency
Primary hypercoagulable Thrombophilia NOS state NEC
Primary thrombophilia NEC

√5ᵗʰ **D68.6 Other thrombophilia**
Other hypercoagulable states
EXCLUDES 1 *diffuse or disseminated intravascular coagulation [DIC] (D65)*
heparin induced thrombocytopenia (HIT) (D75.82)
hyperhomocysteinemia (E72.11)

D68.61 Antiphospholipid syndrome
Anticardiolipin syndrome
Antiphospholipid antibody syndrome
EXCLUDES 1 *antiphospholipid antibody, finding without diagnosis (R76.0)*
antiphospholipid antibody with hemorrhagic disorder (D68.312)
lupus anticoagulant syndrome (D68.62)

D68.62 Lupus anticoagulant syndrome
Lupus anticoagulant
Presence of systemic lupus erythematosus [SLE] inhibitor
EXCLUDES 1 *anticardiolipin syndrome (D68.61)*
antiphospholipid syndrome (D68.61)
lupus anticoagulant (LAC) finding without diagnosis (R79.0)
lupus anticoagulant (LAC) with hemorrhagic disorder (D68.312)

D68.69 Other thrombophilia
Hypercoagulable states NEC
Secondary hypercoagulable state NOS

D68.8 Other specified coagulation defects
EXCLUDES 1 *hemorrhagic disease of newborn (P53)*

D68.9 Coagulation defect, unspecified

√4ᵗʰ **D69 Purpura and other hemorrhagic conditions**
EXCLUDES 1 *benign hypergammaglobulinemic purpura (D89.0)*
cryoglobulinemic purpura (D89.1)
essential (hemorrhagic) thrombocythemia (D47.3)
hemorrhagic thrombocythemia (D47.3)
purpura fulminans (D65)
thrombotic thrombocytopenic purpura (M31.1)
Waldenström hypergammaglobulinemic purpura (D89.0)

D69.0 Allergic purpura
Allergic vasculitis
Nonthrombocytopenic hemorrhagic purpura
Nonthrombocytopenic idiopathic purpura
Purpura anaphylactoid
Purpura Henoch(-Schönlein)
Purpura rheumatica
Vascular purpura
EXCLUDES 1 *thrombocytopenic hemorrhagic purpura (D69.3)*

D69.1 Qualitative platelet defects
Bernard-Soulier [giant platelet] syndrome
Glanzmann's disease
Grey platelet syndrome
Thromboasthenia (hemorrhagic) (hereditary)
Thrombocytopathy
EXCLUDES 1 *von Willebrand's disease (D68.0)*

D69.2 Other nonthrombocytopenic purpura
Purpura NOS   Senile purpura
Purpura simplex

☑ Additional Character Required   √x7ᵗʰ Xtension Alert   Unspecified Dx   Other Specified Dx   Manifestation   ▶◀ Revised Text   ● New Code   ▲ Revised Code Title

Diseases of the Blood and Blood-forming Organs

D69.3–D73.81

D69.3 Immune thrombocytopenic purpura
Hemorrhagic (thrombocytopenic) purpura
Idiopathic thrombocytopenic purpura
Tidal platelet dysgenesis

☑5ᵗʰ **D69.4 Other primary thrombocytopenia**
EXCLUDES 1 *transient neonatal thrombocytopenia (P61.0)*
Wiskott-Aldrich syndrome (D82.0)

D69.41 Evans syndrome

D69.42 Congenital and hereditary thrombocytopenia purpura
Congenital thrombocytopenia
Hereditary thrombocytopenia
Code first congenital or hereditary disorder, such as: thrombocytopenia with absent radius (TAR syndrome) (Q87.2)

D69.49 Other primary thrombocytopenia
Megakaryocytic hypoplasia
Primary thrombocytopenia NOS

☑5ᵗʰ **D69.5 Secondary thrombocytopenia**
EXCLUDES 1 *heparin induced thrombocytopenia (HIT) (D75.82)*
transient thrombocytopenia of newborn (P61.0)

D69.51 Posttransfusion purpura
Posttransfusion purpura from whole blood (fresh) or blood products
PTP

D69.59 Other secondary thrombocytopenia

D69.6 Thrombocytopenia, unspecified

D69.8 Other specified hemorrhagic conditions
Capillary fragility (hereditary)   Vascular pseudohemophilia

D69.9 Hemorrhagic condition, unspecified

Other disorders of blood and blood-forming organs (D70-D77)

☑4ᵗʰ **D70 Neutropenia**
INCLUDES   agranulocytosis
decreased absolute neurophile count (ANC)
Use additional code for any associated:
fever (R50.81)
mucositis (J34.81, K12.3-, K92.81, N76.81)
EXCLUDES 1 *neutropenic splenomegaly (D73.81)*
transient neonatal neutropenia (P61.5)

D70.0 Congenital agranulocytosis
Congenital neutropenia
Infantile genetic agranulocytosis
Kostmann's disease

D70.1 Agranulocytosis secondary to cancer chemotherapy
Code also underlying neoplasm
Use additional code for adverse effect, if applicable, to identify drug (T45.1X5)

D70.2 Other drug-induced agranulocytosis
Use additional code for adverse effect, if applicable, to identify drug (T36-T50 with fifth or sixth character 5)

D70.3 Neutropenia due to infection

D70.4 Cyclic neutropenia
Cyclic hematopoiesis
Periodic neutropenia

D70.8 Other neutropenia

D70.9 Neutropenia, unspecified

D71 Functional disorders of polymorphonuclear neutrophils
Cell membrane receptor complex [CR3] defect
Chronic (childhood) granulomatous disease
Congenital dysphagocytosis
Progressive septic granulomatosis

☑4ᵗʰ **D72 Other disorders of white blood cells**
EXCLUDES 1 *basophilia (D72.824)*
immunity disorders (D80-D89)
neutropenia (D70)
preleukemia (syndrome) (D46.9)

D72.0 Genetic anomalies of leukocytes
Alder (granulation) (granulocyte) anomaly
Alder syndrome
Hereditary leukocytic hypersegmentation
Hereditary leukocytic hyposegmentation
Hereditary leukomelanopathy
May-Hegglin (granulation) (granulocyte) anomaly
May-Hegglin syndrome
Pelger-Huët (granulation) (granulocyte) anomaly
Pelger-Huët syndrome
EXCLUDES 1 *Chédiak (-Steinbrinck)-Higashi syndrome (E70.330)*

D72.1 Eosinophilia
Allergic eosinophilia
Hereditary eosinophilia
EXCLUDES 1 *Löffler's syndrome (J82)*
pulmonary eosinophilia (J82)

☑5ᵗʰ **D72.8 Other specified disorders of white blood cells**
EXCLUDES 1 *leukemia (C91-C95)*

☑6ᵗʰ **D72.81 Decreased white blood cell count**
EXCLUDES 1 *neutropenia (D70.-)*

D72.810 Lymphocytopenia
Decreased lymphocytes

D72.818 Other decreased white blood cell count
Basophilic leukopenia
Eosinophilic leukopenia
Monocytopenia
Other decreased leukocytes
Plasmacytopenia

D72.819 Decreased white blood cell count, unspecified
Decreased leukocytes, unspecified
Leukocytopenia, unspecified
Leukopenia
EXCLUDES 1 *malignant leukopenia (D70.9)*

☑6ᵗʰ **D72.82 Elevated white blood cell count**
EXCLUDES 1 *eosinophilia (D72.1)*

D72.820 Lymphocytosis (symptomatic)
Elevated lymphocytes

D72.821 Monocytosis (symptomatic)
EXCLUDES 1 *infectious mononucleosis (B27.-)*

D72.822 Plasmacytosis

D72.823 Leukemoid reaction
Basophilic leukemoid reaction
Leukemoid reaction NOS
Lymphocytic leukemoid reaction
Monocytic leukemoid reaction
Myelocytic leukemoid reaction
Neutrophilic leukemoid reaction

D72.824 Basophilia

D72.825 Bandemia
Bandemia without diagnosis of specific infection
EXCLUDES 1 *confirmed infection—code to infection*
leukemia (C91.-, C92.-, C93.-, C94.-, C95.-)

D72.828 Other elevated white blood cell count

D72.829 Elevated white blood cell count, unspecified
Elevated leukocytes, unspecified
Leukocytosis, unspecified

D72.89 Other specified disorders of white blood cells
Abnormality of white blood cells NEC

D72.9 Disorder of white blood cells, unspecified
Abnormal leukocyte differential NOS

☑4ᵗʰ **D73 Diseases of spleen**

D73.0 Hyposplenism
Atrophy of spleen
EXCLUDES 1 *asplenia (congenital) (Q89.01)*
postsurgical absence of spleen (Z90.81)

D73.1 Hypersplenism
EXCLUDES 1 *neutropenic splenomegaly (D73.81)*
primary splenic neutropenia (D73.81)
splenitis, splenomegaly in late syphilis (A52.79)
splenitis, splenomegaly in tuberculosis (A18.85)
splenomegaly NOS (R16.1)
splenomegaly congenital (Q89.0)

D73.2 Chronic congestive splenomegaly

D73.3 Abscess of spleen

D73.4 Cyst of spleen

D73.5 Infarction of spleen
Splenic rupture, nontraumatic
Torsion of spleen
EXCLUDES 1 *rupture of spleen due to Plasmodium vivax malaria (B51.0)*
traumatic rupture of spleen (S36.03-)

☑5ᵗʰ **D73.8 Other diseases of spleen**

D73.81 Neutropenic splenomegaly
Werner-Schultz disease

EXCLUDES 1 Not coded here   EXCLUDES 2 Not included here   N Newborn Age: 0   P Pediatric Age: 0-17   M Maternity Age: 12-55   A Adult Age: 15-124

D73.89 **Other diseases of spleen**
Fibrosis of spleen NOS
Perisplenitis
Splenitis NOS

D73.9 **Disease of spleen, unspecified**

☑4th **D74 Methemoglobinemia**

D74.0 **Congenital** methemoglobinemia
Congenital NADH-methemoglobin reductase deficiency
Hemoglobin-M [Hb-M] disease
Methemoglobinemia, hereditary

D74.8 **Other methemoglobinemias**
Acquired methemoglobinemia (with sulfhemoglobinemia)
Toxic methemoglobinemia

D74.9 **Methemoglobinemia, unspecified**

☑4th **D75 Other and unspecified diseases of blood and blood-forming organs**
EXCLUDES 2   acute lymphadenitis (L04.-)
chronic lymphadenitis (I88.1)
enlarged lymph nodes (R59.-)
hypergammaglobulinemia NOS (D89.2)
lymphadenitis NOS (I88.9)
mesenteric lymphadenitis (acute) (chronic) (I88.0)

D75.0 **Familial erythrocytosis**
Benign polycythemia
Familial polycythemia
EXCLUDES 1   hereditary ovalocytosis (D58.1)

D75.1 **Secondary polycythemia**
Acquired polycythemia
Emotional polycythemia
Erythrocytosis NOS
Hypoxemic polycythemia
Nephrogenous polycythemia
Polycythemia due to erythropoietin
Polycythemia due to fall in plasma volume
Polycythemia due to high altitude
Polycythemia due to stress
Polycythemia NOS
Relative polycythemia
EXCLUDES 1   polycythemia neonatorum (P61.1)
polycythemia vera (D45)

☑5th D75.8 **Other specified diseases of blood and blood-forming organs**

D75.81 **Myelofibrosis**
Myelofibrosis NOS
Secondary myelofibrosis NOS
Code first the underlying disorder, such as:
malignant neoplasm of breast (C50.-)
Use additional code, if applicable, for associated therapy-related myelodysplastic syndrome (D46.-)
Use additional code for adverse effect, if applicable, to identify drug (T45.1X5)
EXCLUDES 1   acute myelofibrosis (C94.4-)
idiopathic myelofibrosis (D47.1)
leukoerythroblastic anemia (D61.82)
myelofibrosis with myeloid metaplasia (D47.4)
myelophthisic anemia (D61.82)
myelophthisis (D61.82)
primary myelofibrosis (D47.1)

D75.82 **Heparin induced thrombocytopenia (HIT)**

D75.89 **Other specified diseases of blood and blood-forming organs**

D75.9 **Disease of blood and blood-forming organs, unspecified**

☑4th **D76 Other specified diseases with participation of lymphoreticular and reticulohistiocytic tissue**
EXCLUDES 1   (Abt-) Letterer-Siwe disease (C96.0)
eosinophilic granuloma (C96.6)
Hand-Schüller-Christian disease (C96.5)
histiocytic sarcoma (C96.A)
histiocytosis X, multifocal (C96.5)
histiocytosis X, unifocal (C96.6)
Langerhans-cell histiocytosis, multifocal (C96.5)
Langerhans-cell histiocytosis NOS (C96.6)
Langerhans-cell histiocytosis, unifocal (C96.6)
leukemic reticuloendotheliosis or reticulosis (C91.4-)
lipomelanotic reticuloendotheliosis or reticulosis (I89.8)
malignant histiocytosis (C96.A)

D76.1 **Hemophagocytic lymphohistiocytosis**
Familial hemophagocytic reticulosis
Histiocytoses of mononuclear phagocytes

D76.2 **Hemophagocytic syndrome, infection-associated**
Use additional code to identify infectious agent or disease

D76.3 **Other histiocytosis syndromes**
Reticulohistiocytoma (giant-cell)
Sinus histiocytosis with massive lymphadenopathy
Xanthogranuloma

D77 *Other disorders of blood and blood-forming organs in diseases classified elsewhere*
Code first underlying disease, such as:
amyloidosis (E85.-)
congenital early syphilis (A50.0)
echinococcosis (B67.0-B67.9)
malaria (B50.0-B54)
schistosomiasis [bilharziasis] (B65.0-B65.9)
vitamin C deficiency (E54)
EXCLUDES 1   *rupture of spleen due to Plasmodium vivax malaria (B51.0)*
splenitis, splenomegaly in late syphilis (A52.79)
splenitis, splenomegaly in tuberculosis (A18.85)

Intraoperative and postprocedural complications of the spleen (D78)

☑4th **D78 Intraoperative and postprocedural complications of the spleen**

☑5th D78.0 **Intraoperative hemorrhage and hematoma of the spleen complicating a procedure**
EXCLUDES 1   *intraoperative hemorrhage and hematoma of the spleen due to accidental puncture or laceration during a procedure (D78.1-)*

D78.01 **Intraoperative hemorrhage and hematoma of the spleen complicating a procedure on the spleen**

D78.02 **Intraoperative hemorrhage and hematoma of the spleen complicating other procedure**

☑5th D78.1 **Accidental puncture and laceration of the spleen during a procedure**

D78.11 **Accidental puncture and laceration of the spleen during a procedure on the spleen**

D78.12 **Accidental puncture and laceration of the spleen during other procedure**

☑5th D78.2 **Postprocedural hemorrhage and hematoma of the spleen following a procedure**

D78.21 **Postprocedural hemorrhage and hematoma of the spleen following a procedure on the spleen**

D78.22 **Postprocedural hemorrhage and hematoma of the spleen following other procedure**

☑5th D78.8 **Other intraoperative and postprocedural complications of the spleen**
Use additional code, if applicable, to further specify disorder

D78.81 **Other intraoperative complications of the spleen**

D78.89 **Other postprocedural complications of the spleen**

Certain disorders involving the immune mechanism (D80-D89)

INCLUDES   defects in the complement system
immunodeficiency disorders, except human immunodeficiency virus [HIV] disease
sarcoidosis
EXCLUDES 1   *autoimmune disease (systemic) NOS (M35.9)*
functional disorders of polymorphonuclear neutrophils (D71)
human immunodeficiency virus [HIV] disease (B20)

☑4th **D80 Immunodeficiency with predominantly antibody defects**

D80.0 **Hereditary hypogammaglobulinemia**
Autosomal recessive agammaglobulinemia (Swiss type)
X-linked agammaglobulinemia [Bruton] (with growth hormone deficiency)

D80.1 **Nonfamilial hypogammaglobulinemia**
Agammaglobulinemia with immunoglobulin-bearing B-lymphocytes
Common variable agammaglobulinemia [CVAgamma]
Hypogammaglobulinemia NOS

D80.2 **Selective deficiency of immunoglobulin A [IgA]**

D80.3 **Selective deficiency of immunoglobulin G [IgG] subclasses**

D80.4 **Selective deficiency of immunoglobulin M [IgM]**

D80.5 **Immunodeficiency with increased immunoglobulin M [IgM]**

D80.6 **Antibody deficiency with near-normal immunoglobulins or with hyperimmunoglobulinemia**

D80.7 **Transient hypogammaglobulinemia of infancy**   N

D80.8 **Other immunodeficiencies with predominantly antibody defects**
Kappa light chain deficiency

☑ Additional Character Required   ✓x7th Xtension Alert   Unspecified Dx   Other Specified Dx   Manifestation   ►◄ Revised Text   ● New Code   ▲ Revised Code Title

Diseases of the Blood and Blood-forming Organs

D80.9–D89.9

D80.9 Immunodeficiency with predominantly antibody defects, unspecified

✓4ᵗʰ D81 Combined immunodeficiencies

> **EXCLUDES 1** *autosomal recessive agammaglobulinemia (Swiss type) (D80.0)*

D81.0 Severe combined immunodeficiency [SCID] with reticular dysgenesis

D81.1 Severe combined immunodeficiency [SCID] with low T- and B-cell numbers

D81.2 Severe combined immunodeficiency [SCID] with low or normal B-cell numbers

D81.3 Adenosine deaminase [ADA] deficiency

D81.4 Nezelof's syndrome

D81.5 Purine nucleoside phosphorylase [PNP] deficiency

D81.6 Major histocompatibility complex class I deficiency
> Bare lymphocyte syndrome

D81.7 Major histocompatibility complex class II deficiency

✓5ᵗʰ D81.8 Other combined immunodeficiencies

> **✓6ᵗʰ D81.81 Biotin-dependent carboxylase deficiency**
> > Multiple carboxylase deficiency
> > **EXCLUDES 1** *biotin-dependent carboxylase deficiency due to dietary deficiency of biotin (E53.8)*
>
> > **D81.810 Biotinidase deficiency**
> > **D81.818 Other biotin-dependent carboxylase deficiency**
> > > Holocarboxylase synthetase deficiency
> > > Other multiple carboxylase deficiency
> > **D81.819 Biotin-dependent carboxylase deficiency, unspecified**
> > > Multiple carboxylase deficiency, unspecified
>
> **D81.89 Other combined immunodeficiencies**

D81.9 Combined immunodeficiency, unspecified
> Severe combined immunodeficiency disorder [SCID] NOS

✓4ᵗʰ D82 Immunodeficiency associated with other major defects

> **EXCLUDES 1** *ataxia telangiectasia [Louis-Bar] (G11.3)*

D82.0 Wiskott-Aldrich syndrome
> Immunodeficiency with thrombocytopenia and eczema

D82.1 Di George's syndrome
> Pharyngeal pouch syndrome   Thymic aplasia or hypoplasia
> Thymic alymphoplasia   with immunodeficiency

D82.2 Immunodeficiency with short-limbed stature

D82.3 Immunodeficiency following hereditary defective response to Epstein-Barr virus
> X-linked lymphoproliferative disease

D82.4 Hyperimmunoglobulin E [IgE] syndrome

D82.8 Immunodeficiency associated with other specified major defects

D82.9 Immunodeficiency associated with major defect, unspecified

✓4ᵗʰ D83 Common variable immunodeficiency

D83.0 Common variable immunodeficiency with predominant abnormalities of B-cell numbers and function

D83.1 Common variable immunodeficiency with predominant immunoregulatory T-cell disorders

D83.2 Common variable immunodeficiency with autoantibodies to B- or T-cells

D83.8 Other common variable immunodeficiencies

D83.9 Common variable immunodeficiency, unspecified

✓4ᵗʰ D84 Other immunodeficiencies

D84.0 Lymphocyte function antigen-1 [LFA-1] defect

D84.1 Defects in the complement system
> C1 esterase inhibitor [C1-INH] deficiency

D84.8 Other specified immunodeficiencies

D84.9 Immunodeficiency, unspecified

✓4ᵗʰ D86 Sarcoidosis

D86.0 Sarcoidosis of lung

D86.1 Sarcoidosis of lymph nodes

D86.2 Sarcoidosis of lung with sarcoidosis of lymph nodes

D86.3 Sarcoidosis of skin

✓5ᵗʰ D86.8 Sarcoidosis of other sites

> **D86.81 Sarcoid meningitis**
> **D86.82 Multiple cranial nerve palsies in sarcoidosis**
> **D86.83 Sarcoid iridocyclitis**
> **D86.84 Sarcoid pyelonephritis**
> > Tubulo-interstitial nephropathy in sarcoidosis
> **D86.85 Sarcoid myocarditis**
> **D86.86 Sarcoid arthropathy**
> > Polyarthritis in sarcoidosis
> **D86.87 Sarcoid myositis**
> **D86.89 Sarcoidosis of other sites**
> > Hepatic granulomaUveoparotid fever [Heerfordt]

D86.9 Sarcoidosis, unspecified

✓4ᵗʰ D89 Other disorders involving the immune mechanism, not elsewhere classified

> **EXCLUDES 1** *hyperglobulinemia NOS (R77.1)*
> *monoclonal gammopathy (of undetermined significance) (D47.2)*
> **EXCLUDES 2** *transplant failure and rejection (T86.-)*

D89.0 Polyclonal hypergammaglobulinemia
> Benign hypergammaglobulinemic purpura
> Polyclonal gammopathy NOS

D89.1 Cryoglobulinemia
> Cryoglobulinemic purpura   Mixed cryoglobulinemia
> Cryoglobulinemic vasculitis   Primary cryoglobulinemia
> Essential cryoglobulinemia   Secondary cryoglobulinemia
> Idiopathic cryoglobulinemia

D89.2 Hypergammaglobulinemia, unspecified

D89.3 Immune reconstitution syndrome
> Immune reconstitution inflammatory syndrome [IRIS]
> Use additional code for adverse effect, if applicable, to identify drug (T36-T50 with fifth or sixth character 5)

✓5ᵗʰ D89.8 Other specified disorders involving the immune mechanism, not elsewhere classified

> **✓6ᵗʰ D89.81 Graft-versus-host disease**
> > Code first underlying cause, such as:
> > complications of transplanted organs and tissue (T86.-)
> > complications of blood transfusion (T80.89)
> > Use additional code to identify associated manifestations, such as:
> > desquamative dermatitis (L30.8)
> > diarrhea (R19.7)
> > elevated bilirubin (R17)
> > hair loss (L65.9)
> >
> > **D89.810 Acute graft-versus-host disease**
> > **D89.811 Chronic graft-versus-host disease**
> > **D89.812 Acute on chronic graft-versus-host disease**
> > **D89.813 Graft-versus-host disease, unspecified**
>
> **D89.82 Autoimmune lymphoproliferative syndrome [ALPS]**
> **D89.89 Other specified disorders involving the immune mechanism, not elsewhere classified**
> > **EXCLUDES 1** *human immunodeficiency virus disease (B20)*

D89.9 Disorder involving the immune mechanism, unspecified
> Immune disease NOS

EXCLUDES 1 Not coded here   **EXCLUDES 2** Not included here   **N** Newborn Age: 0   **P** Pediatric Age: 0-17   **M** Maternity Age: 12-55   **A** Adult Age: 15-124

478   ICD-10-CM Draft (2015)

Chapter 4. Endocrine, Nutritional and Metabolic Diseases (E00-E89)

NOTE All neoplasms, whether functionally active or not, are classified in Chapter 2. Appropriate codes in this chapter (i.e. E05.8, E07.0, E16-E31, E34-) may be used as additional codes to indicate either functional activity by neoplasms and ectopic endocrine tissue or hyperfunction and hypofunction of endocrine glands associated with neoplasms and other conditions classified elsewhere.

EXCLUDES 1 *transitory endocrine and metabolic disorders specific to newborn (P70-P74)*

This chapter contains the following blocks:

E00-E07	Disorders of thyroid gland
E08-E13	Diabetes mellitus
E15-E16	Other disorders of glucose regulation and pancreatic internal secretion
E20-E35	Disorders of other endocrine glands
E36	Intraoperative complications of endocrine system
E40-E46	Malnutrition
E50-E64	Other nutritional deficiencies
E65-E68	Overweight, obesity and other hyperalimentation
E70-E88	Metabolic disorders
E89	Postprocedural endocrine and metabolic complications and disorders, not elsewhere classified

Disorders of thyroid gland (E00-E07)

✓4ᵗʰ **E00 Congenital iodine-deficiency syndrome**
Use additional code (F70-F79) to identify associated intellectual disabilities
EXCLUDES 1 *subclinical iodine-deficiency hypothyroidism (E02)*

E00.0 Congenital iodine-deficiency syndrome, neurological type
Endemic cretinism, neurological type

E00.1 Congenital iodine-deficiency syndrome, myxedematous type
Endemic hypothyroid cretinism
Endemic cretinism, myxedematous type

E00.2 Congenital iodine-deficiency syndrome, mixed type
Endemic cretinism, mixed type

E00.9 Congenital iodine-deficiency syndrome, unspecified
Congenital iodine-deficiency hypothyroidism NOS
Endemic cretinism NOS

✓4ᵗʰ **E01 Iodine-deficiency related thyroid disorders and allied conditions**
EXCLUDES 1 *congenital iodine-deficiency syndrome (E00.-)*
subclinical iodine-deficiency hypothyroidism (E02)

E01.0 Iodine-deficiency related diffuse (endemic) goiter

E01.1 Iodine-deficiency related multinodular (endemic) goiter
Iodine-deficiency related nodular goiter

E01.2 Iodine-deficiency related (endemic) goiter, unspecified
Endemic goiter NOS

E01.8 Other iodine-deficiency related thyroid disorders and allied conditions
Acquired iodine-deficiency hypothyroidism NOS

E02 Subclinical iodine-deficiency hypothyroidism

✓4ᵗʰ **E03 Other hypothyroidism**
EXCLUDES 1 *iodine-deficiency related hypothyroidism (E00-E02)*
postprocedural hypothyroidism (E89.0)

E03.0 Congenital hypothyroidism with diffuse goiter
Congenital parenchymatous goiter (nontoxic)
Congenital goiter (nontoxic) NOS
EXCLUDES 1 *transitory congenital goiter with normal function (P72.0)*

E03.1 Congenital hypothyroidism without goiter
Aplasia of thyroid (with myxedema)
Congenital atrophy of thyroid
Congenital hypothyroidism NOS

E03.2 Hypothyroidism due to medicaments and other exogenous substances
Code first poisoning due to drug or toxin, if applicable (T36-T65 with fifth or sixth character 1-4 or 6)
Use additional code for adverse effect, if applicable, to identify drug (T36-T50 with fifth or sixth character 5)

E03.3 Postinfectious hypothyroidism

E03.4 Atrophy of thyroid (acquired)
EXCLUDES 1 *congenital atrophy of thyroid (E03.1)*

E03.5 Myxedema coma

E03.8 Other specified hypothyroidism

E03.9 Hypothyroidism, unspecified
Myxedema NOS

✓4ᵗʰ **E04 Other nontoxic goiter**
EXCLUDES 1 *congenital goiter (NOS) (diffuse) (parenchymatous) (E03.0)*
iodine-deficiency related goiter (E00-E02)

E04.0 Nontoxic diffuse goiter
Diffuse (colloid) nontoxic goiter
Simple nontoxic goiter

E04.1 Nontoxic single thyroid nodule
Colloid nodule (cystic) (thyroid)
Nontoxic uninodular goiter
Thyroid (cystic) nodule NOS

E04.2 Non toxic multinodular goiter
Cystic goiter NOS
Multinodular (cystic) goiter NOS

E04.8 Other specified nontoxic goiter

E04.9 Nontoxic goiter, unspecified
Goiter NOS
Nodular goiter (nontoxic) NOS

✓4ᵗʰ **E05 Thyrotoxicosis [hyperthyroidism]**
EXCLUDES 1 *chronic thyroiditis with transient thyrotoxicosis (E06.2)*
neonatal thyrotoxicosis (P72.1)

✓5ᵗʰ **E05.0 Thyrotoxicosis with diffuse goiter**
Exophthalmic or toxic goiter NOS
Graves' disease
Toxic diffuse goiter

E05.00 Thyrotoxicosis with diffuse goiter without thyrotoxic crisis or storm

E05.01 Thyrotoxicosis with diffuse goiter with thyrotoxic crisis or storm

✓5ᵗʰ **E05.1 Thyrotoxicosis with toxic single thyroid nodule**
Thyrotoxicosis with toxic uninodular goiter

E05.10 Thyrotoxicosis with toxic single thyroid nodule without thyrotoxic crisis or storm

E05.11 Thyrotoxicosis with toxic single thyroid nodule with thyrotoxic crisis or storm

✓5ᵗʰ **E05.2 Thyrotoxicosis with toxic multinodular goiter**
Toxic nodular goiter NOS

E05.20 Thyrotoxicosis with toxic multinodular goiter without thyrotoxic crisis or storm

E05.21 Thyrotoxicosis with toxic multinodular goiter with thyrotoxic crisis or storm

✓5ᵗʰ **E05.3 Thyrotoxicosis from ectopic thyroid tissue**

E05.30 Thyrotoxicosis from ectopic thyroid tissue without thyrotoxic crisis or storm

E05.31 Thyrotoxicosis from ectopic thyroid tissue with thyrotoxic crisis or storm

✓5ᵗʰ **E05.4 Thyrotoxicosis factitia**

E05.40 Thyrotoxicosis factitia without thyrotoxic crisis or storm

E05.41 Thyrotoxicosis factitia with thyrotoxic crisis or storm

✓5ᵗʰ **E05.8 Other thyrotoxicosis**
Overproduction of thyroid-stimulating hormone

E05.80 Other thyrotoxicosis without thyrotoxic crisis or storm

E05.81 Other thyrotoxicosis with thyrotoxic crisis or storm

✓5ᵗʰ **E05.9 Thyrotoxicosis, unspecified**
Hyperthyroidism NOS

E05.90 Thyrotoxicosis, unspecified without thyrotoxic crisis or storm

E05.91 Thyrotoxicosis, unspecified with thyrotoxic crisis or storm

✓4ᵗʰ **E06 Thyroiditis**
EXCLUDES 1 *postpartum thyroiditis (O90.5)*

E06.0 Acute thyroiditis
Abscess of thyroid
Pyogenic thyroiditis
Suppurative thyroiditis
Use additional code (B95-B97) to identify infectious agent

E06.1 Subacute thyroiditis
de Quervain thyroiditis
Giant-cell thyroiditis
Granulomatous thyroiditis
Nonsuppurative thyroiditis
Viral thyroiditis
EXCLUDES 1 *autoimmune thyroiditis (E06.3)*

E06.2 Chronic thyroiditis with transient thyrotoxicosis
EXCLUDES 1 *autoimmune thyroiditis (E06.3)*

E06.3 Autoimmune thyroiditis
Hashimoto's thyroiditis
Hashitoxicosis (transient)
Lymphadenoid goiter
Lymphocytic thyroiditis
Struma lymphomatosa

✓ Additional Character Required   ✓x7ᵗʰ Xtension Alert   Unspecified Dx   Other Specified Dx   Manifestation   ▶◀ Revised Text   ● New Code   ▲ Revised Code Title

E06.4 **Drug-induced** thyroiditis
Use additional code for adverse effect, if applicable, to identify drug (T36-T50 with fifth or sixth character 5)

E06.5 Other chronic thyroiditis
Chronic fibrous thyroiditis   Ligneous thyroiditis
Chronic thyroiditis NOS   Riedel thyroiditis

E06.9 **Thyroiditis, unspecified**

✓4th **E07 Other disorders of thyroid**

E07.0 **Hypersecretion of calcitonin**
C-cell hyperplasia of thyroid
Hypersecretion of thyrocalcitonin

E07.1 **Dyshormogenetic goiter**
Familial dyshormogenetic goiter
Pendred's syndrome
EXCLUDES1   transitory congenital goiter with normal function (P72.0)

✓5th E07.8 Other specified disorders of thyroid
E07.81 **Sick-euthyroid syndrome**
Euthyroid sick-syndrome

E07.89 **Other specified disorders of thyroid**
Abnormality of thyroid-binding globulin
Hemorrhage of thyroid
Infarction of thyroid

E07.9 **Disorder of thyroid, unspecified**

Diabetes mellitus (E08-E13)

✓4th **E08 Diabetes mellitus due to underlying condition**
Code first the underlying condition, such as:
congenital rubella (P35.0)
cushing's syndrome (E24.-)
cystic fibrosis (E84.-)
malignant neoplasm (C00-C96)
malnutrition (E40-E46)
pancreatitis and other diseases of the pancreas (K85.-, K86.-)
Use additional code to identify any insulin use (Z79.4)
EXCLUDES1   drug or chemical induced diabetes mellitus (E09.-)
gestational diabetes (O24.4-)
neonatal diabetes mellitus (P70.2)
postpancreatectomy diabetes mellitus (E13.-)
postprocedural diabetes mellitus (E13.-)
secondary diabetes mellitus NEC (E13.-)
type 1 diabetes mellitus (E10.-)
type 2 diabetes mellitus (E11.-)
AHA: 2013, 4Q, 114; 2013, 3Q, 20

✓5th E08.0 Diabetes mellitus due to underlying condition with hyperosmolarity
E08.00 **Diabetes mellitus due to underlying condition with hyperosmolarity without nonketotic hyperglycemic-hyperosmolar coma (NKHHC)**

E08.01 **Diabetes mellitus due to underlying condition with hyperosmolarity with coma**

✓5th E08.1 Diabetes mellitus due to underlying condition with ketoacidosis
E08.10 **Diabetes mellitus due to underlying condition with ketoacidosis without coma**

E08.11 **Diabetes mellitus due to underlying condition with ketoacidosis with coma**

✓5th E08.2 Diabetes mellitus due to underlying condition with kidney complications
E08.21 **Diabetes mellitus due to underlying condition with diabetic nephropathy**
Diabetes mellitus due to underlying condition with intercapillary glomerulosclerosis
Diabetes mellitus due to underlying condition with intracapillary glomerulonephrosis
Diabetes mellitus due to underlying condition with Kimmelstiel-Wilson disease

E08.22 **Diabetes mellitus due to underlying condition with diabetic chronic kidney disease**
Use additional code to identify stage of chronic kidney disease (N18.1-N18.6)

E08.29 **Diabetes mellitus due to underlying condition with other diabetic kidney complication**
Renal tubular degeneration in diabetes mellitus due to underlying condition

✓5th E08.3 Diabetes mellitus due to underlying condition with ophthalmic complications
✓6th E08.31 **Diabetes mellitus due to underlying condition with unspecified diabetic retinopathy**

E08.311 **Diabetes mellitus due to underlying condition with unspecified diabetic retinopathy with macular edema**

E08.319 **Diabetes mellitus due to underlying condition with unspecified diabetic retinopathy without macular edema**

✓6th E08.32 **Diabetes mellitus due to underlying condition with mild nonproliferative diabetic retinopathy**
Diabetes mellitus due to underlying condition with nonproliferative diabetic retinopathy NOS
E08.321 **Diabetes mellitus due to underlying condition with mild nonproliferative diabetic retinopathy with macular edema**

E08.329 **Diabetes mellitus due to underlying condition with mild nonproliferative diabetic retinopathy without macular edema**

✓6th E08.33 **Diabetes mellitus due to underlying condition with moderate nonproliferative diabetic retinopathy**
E08.331 **Diabetes mellitus due to underlying condition with moderate nonproliferative diabetic retinopathy with macular edema**

E08.339 **Diabetes mellitus due to underlying condition with moderate nonproliferative diabetic retinopathy without macular edema**

✓6th E08.34 **Diabetes mellitus due to underlying condition with severe nonproliferative diabetic retinopathy**
E08.341 **Diabetes mellitus due to underlying condition with severe nonproliferative diabetic retinopathy with macular edema**

E08.349 **Diabetes mellitus due to underlying condition with severe nonproliferative diabetic retinopathy without macular edema**

✓6th E08.35 **Diabetes mellitus due to underlying condition with proliferative diabetic retinopathy**
E08.351 **Diabetes mellitus due to underlying condition with proliferative diabetic retinopathy with macular edema**

E08.359 **Diabetes mellitus due to underlying condition with proliferative diabetic retinopathy without macular edema**

E08.36 **Diabetes mellitus due to underlying condition with diabetic cataract**

E08.39 **Diabetes mellitus due to underlying condition with other diabetic ophthalmic complication**
Use additional code to identify manifestation, such as: diabetic glaucoma (H40-H42)

✓5th E08.4 Diabetes mellitus due to underlying condition with neurological complications
E08.40 **Diabetes mellitus due to underlying condition with diabetic neuropathy, unspecified**

E08.41 **Diabetes mellitus due to underlying condition with diabetic mononeuropathy**

E08.42 **Diabetes mellitus due to underlying condition with diabetic polyneuropathy**
Diabetes mellitus due to underlying condition with diabetic neuralgia

E08.43 **Diabetes mellitus due to underlying condition with diabetic autonomic (poly)neuropathy**
Diabetes mellitus due to underlying condition with diabetic gastroparesis
AHA: 2013, 4Q, 114

E08.44 **Diabetes mellitus due to underlying condition with diabetic amyotrophy**

E08.49 **Diabetes mellitus due to underlying condition with other diabetic neurological complication**

✓5th E08.5 Diabetes mellitus due to underlying condition with circulatory complications
E08.51 **Diabetes mellitus due to underlying condition with diabetic peripheral angiopathy without gangrene**

E08.52 **Diabetes mellitus due to underlying condition with diabetic peripheral angiopathy with gangrene**
Diabetes mellitus due to underlying condition with diabetic gangrene

E08.59 **Diabetes mellitus due to underlying condition with other circulatory complications**

EXCLUDES1 Not coded here   EXCLUDES2 Not included here   N Newborn Age: 0   P Pediatric Age: 0-17   M Maternity Age: 12-55   A Adult Age: 15-124

480   ICD-10-CM Draft (2015)

☑5ᵗʰ **E08.6 Diabetes mellitus due to underlying condition with** other specified complications

　☑6ᵗʰ **E08.61 Diabetes mellitus due to underlying condition with** diabetic arthropathy

　　E08.610 Diabetes mellitus due to underlying condition with diabetic neuropathic arthropathy

　　　Diabetes mellitus due to underlying condition with Charcôt's joints

　　E08.618 Diabetes mellitus due to underlying condition with other diabetic arthropathy

　☑6ᵗʰ **E08.62 Diabetes mellitus due to underlying condition with** skin complications

　　E08.620 Diabetes mellitus due to underlying condition with diabetic dermatitis

　　　Diabetes mellitus due to underlying condition with diabetic necrobiosis lipoidica

　　E08.621 Diabetes mellitus due to underlying condition with foot ulcer

　　　Use additional code to identify site of ulcer (L97.4-, L97.5-)

　　E08.622 Diabetes mellitus due to underlying condition with other skin ulcer

　　　Use additional code to identify site of ulcer (L97.1-L97.9, L98.41-L98.49)

　　E08.628 Diabetes mellitus due to underlying condition with other skin complications

　☑6ᵗʰ **E08.63 Diabetes mellitus due to underlying condition with** oral complications

　　E08.630 Diabetes mellitus due to underlying condition with periodontal disease

　　E08.638 Diabetes mellitus due to underlying condition with other oral complications

　☑6ᵗʰ **E08.64 Diabetes mellitus due to underlying condition with** hypoglycemia

　　E08.641 Diabetes mellitus due to underlying condition with hypoglycemia with coma

　　E08.649 Diabetes mellitus due to underlying condition with hypoglycemia without coma

　　E08.65 Diabetes mellitus due to underlying condition with hyperglycemia

　　E08.69 Diabetes mellitus due to underlying condition with other specified complication

　　　Use additional code to identify complication

　E08.8 Diabetes mellitus due to underlying condition with unspecified complications

　E08.9 Diabetes mellitus due to underlying condition without complications

☑4ᵗʰ **E09 Drug or chemical induced diabetes mellitus**

　Code first poisoning due to drug or toxin, if applicable (T36-T65 with fifth or sixth character 1-4 or 6)

　Use additional code for adverse effect, if applicable, to identify drug (T36-T50 with fifth or sixth character 5)

　Use additional code to identify any insulin use (Z79.4)

　EXCLUDES 1 *diabetes mellitus due to underlying condition (E08.-)*
　　gestational diabetes (O24.4-)
　　neonatal diabetes mellitus (P70.2)
　　postpancreatectomy diabetes mellitus (E13.-)
　　postprocedural diabetes mellitus (E13.-)
　　secondary diabetes mellitus NEC (E13.-)
　　type 1 diabetes mellitus (E10.-)
　　type 2 diabetes mellitus (E11.-)

　AHA: 2013, 4Q, 114; 2013, 3Q, 20

☑5ᵗʰ **E09.0 Drug or chemical induced diabetes mellitus with** hyperosmolarity

　　E09.00 Drug or chemical induced diabetes mellitus with hyperosmolarity without nonketotic hyperglycemic-hyperosmolar coma **(NKHHC)**

　　E09.01 Drug or chemical induced diabetes mellitus with hyperosmolarity with coma

☑5ᵗʰ **E09.1 Drug or chemical induced diabetes mellitus with** ketoacidosis

　　E09.10 Drug or chemical induced diabetes mellitus with ketoacidosis without coma

　　E09.11 Drug or chemical induced diabetes mellitus with ketoacidosis with coma

☑5ᵗʰ **E09.2 Drug or chemical induced diabetes mellitus with** kidney complications

　E09.21 Drug or chemical induced diabetes mellitus with diabetic nephropathy

　　Drug or chemical induced diabetes mellitus with intercapillary glomerulosclerosis
　　Drug or chemical induced diabetes mellitus with intracapillary glomerulonephrosis
　　Drug or chemical induced diabetes mellitus with Kimmelstiel-Wilson disease

　E09.22 Drug or chemical induced diabetes mellitus with diabetic chronic kidney disease

　　Use additional code to identify stage of chronic kidney disease (N18.1-N18.6)

　E09.29 Drug or chemical induced diabetes mellitus with other diabetic kidney complication

　　Drug or chemical induced diabetes mellitus with renal tubular degeneration

☑5ᵗʰ **E09.3 Drug or chemical induced diabetes mellitus with** ophthalmic complications

　☑6ᵗʰ **E09.31 Drug or chemical induced diabetes mellitus with** unspecified diabetic retinopathy

　　E09.311 Drug or chemical induced diabetes mellitus with unspecified diabetic retinopathy with macular edema

　　E09.319 Drug or chemical induced diabetes mellitus with unspecified diabetic retinopathy without macular edema

　☑6ᵗʰ **E09.32 Drug or chemical induced diabetes mellitus with** mild nonproliferative **diabetic retinopathy**

　　Drug or chemical induced diabetes mellitus with nonproliferative diabetic retinopathy NOS

　　E09.321 Drug or chemical induced diabetes mellitus with mild nonproliferative diabetic retinopathy with macular edema

　　E09.329 Drug or chemical induced diabetes mellitus with mild nonproliferative diabetic retinopathy without macular edema

　☑6ᵗʰ **E09.33 Drug or chemical induced diabetes mellitus with** moderate nonproliferative **diabetic retinopathy**

　　E09.331 Drug or chemical induced diabetes mellitus with moderate nonproliferative diabetic retinopathy with macular edema

　　E09.339 Drug or chemical induced diabetes mellitus with moderate nonproliferative diabetic retinopathy without macular edema

　☑6ᵗʰ **E09.34 Drug or chemical induced diabetes mellitus with** severe nonproliferative **diabetic retinopathy**

　　E09.341 Drug or chemical induced diabetes mellitus with severe nonproliferative diabetic retinopathy with macular edema

　　E09.349 Drug or chemical induced diabetes mellitus with severe nonproliferative diabetic retinopathy without macular edema

　☑6ᵗʰ **E09.35 Drug or chemical induced diabetes mellitus with** proliferative **diabetic retinopathy**

　　E09.351 Drug or chemical induced diabetes mellitus with proliferative diabetic retinopathy with macular edema

　　E09.359 Drug or chemical induced diabetes mellitus with proliferative diabetic retinopathy without macular edema

　E09.36 Drug or chemical induced diabetes mellitus with diabetic cataract

　E09.39 Drug or chemical induced diabetes mellitus with other diabetic ophthalmic complication

　　Use additional code to identify manifestation, such as: diabetic glaucoma (H40-H42)

☑5ᵗʰ **E09.4 Drug or chemical induced diabetes mellitus with** neurological complications

　E09.40 Drug or chemical induced diabetes mellitus with neurological complications with diabetic neuropathy, unspecified

　E09.41 Drug or chemical induced diabetes mellitus with neurological complications with diabetic mononeuropathy

☑ Additional Character Required　　✓x7ᵗʰ Xtension Alert　　Unspecified Dx　　Other Specified Dx　　Manifestation　　▶◀ Revised Text　　● New Code　　▲ Revised Code Title

E09.42 **Drug or chemical induced diabetes mellitus with neurological complications with diabetic polyneuropathy**
Drug or chemical induced diabetes mellitus with diabetic neuralgia

E09.43 **Drug or chemical induced diabetes mellitus with neurological complications with diabetic autonomic (poly)neuropathy**
Drug or chemical induced diabetes mellitus with diabetic gastroparesis
AHA: 2013, 4Q, 114

E09.44 **Drug or chemical induced diabetes mellitus with neurological complications with diabetic amyotrophy**

E09.49 **Drug or chemical induced diabetes mellitus with neurological complications with other diabetic neurological complication**

✓5ᵗʰ **E09.5** **Drug or chemical induced diabetes mellitus with circulatory complications**

E09.51 **Drug or chemical induced diabetes mellitus with diabetic peripheral angiopathy without gangrene**

E09.52 **Drug or chemical induced diabetes mellitus with diabetic peripheral angiopathy with gangrene**
Drug or chemical induced diabetes mellitus with diabetic gangrene

E09.59 **Drug or chemical induced diabetes mellitus with other circulatory complications**

✓5ᵗʰ **E09.6** **Drug or chemical induced diabetes mellitus with other specified complications**

✓6ᵗʰ **E09.61** **Drug or chemical induced diabetes mellitus with diabetic arthropathy**

E09.610 **Drug or chemical induced diabetes mellitus with diabetic neuropathic arthropathy**
Drug or chemical induced diabetes mellitus with Charcôt's joints

E09.618 **Drug or chemical induced diabetes mellitus with other diabetic arthropathy**

✓6ᵗʰ **E09.62** **Drug or chemical induced diabetes mellitus with skin complications**

E09.620 **Drug or chemical induced diabetes mellitus with diabetic dermatitis**
Drug or chemical induced diabetes mellitus with diabetic necrobiosis lipoidica

E09.621 **Drug or chemical induced diabetes mellitus with foot ulcer**
Use additional code to identify site of ulcer (L97.4-, L97.5-)

E09.622 **Drug or chemical induced diabetes mellitus with other skin ulcer**
Use additional code to identify site of ulcer (L97.1-L97.9, L98.41-L98.49)

E09.628 **Drug or chemical induced diabetes mellitus with other skin complications**

✓6ᵗʰ **E09.63** **Drug or chemical induced diabetes mellitus with oral complications**

E09.630 **Drug or chemical induced diabetes mellitus with periodontal disease**

E09.638 **Drug or chemical induced diabetes mellitus with other oral complications**

✓6ᵗʰ **E09.64** **Drug or chemical induced diabetes mellitus with hypoglycemia**

E09.641 **Drug or chemical induced diabetes mellitus with hypoglycemia with coma**

E09.649 **Drug or chemical induced diabetes mellitus with hypoglycemia without coma**

E09.65 **Drug or chemical induced diabetes mellitus with hyperglycemia**

E09.69 **Drug or chemical induced diabetes mellitus with other specified complication**
Use additional code to identify complication

E09.8 **Drug or chemical induced diabetes mellitus with unspecified complications**

E09.9 **Drug or chemical induced diabetes mellitus without complications**

✓4ᵗʰ **E10** **Type 1 diabetes mellitus**
INCLUDES brittle diabetes (mellitus)
diabetes (mellitus) due to autoimmune process
diabetes (mellitus) due to immune mediated pancreatic islet beta-cell destruction
idiopathic diabetes (mellitus)
juvenile onset diabetes (mellitus)
ketosis-prone diabetes (mellitus)

EXCLUDES 1 *diabetes mellitus due to underlying condition (E08.-)*
drug or chemical induced diabetes mellitus (E09.-)
gestational diabetes (O24.4-)
hyperglycemia NOS (R73.9)
neonatal diabetes mellitus (P70.2)
postpancreatectomy diabetes mellitus (E13.-)
postprocedural diabetes mellitus (E13.-)
secondary diabetes mellitus NEC (E13.-)
type 2 diabetes mellitus (E11.-)
AHA: 2013, 4Q, 114; 2013, 3Q, 20

✓5ᵗʰ **E10.1** **Type 1 diabetes mellitus with ketoacidosis**
AHA: 2013, 3Q, 20

E10.10 **Type 1 diabetes mellitus with ketoacidosis without coma**

E10.11 **Type 1 diabetes mellitus with ketoacidosis with coma**

✓5ᵗʰ **E10.2** **Type 1 diabetes mellitus with kidney complications**

E10.21 **Type 1 diabetes mellitus with diabetic nephropathy**
Type 1 diabetes mellitus with intercapillary glomerulosclerosis
Type 1 diabetes mellitus with intracapillary glomerulonephrosis
Type 1 diabetes mellitus with Kimmelstiel-Wilson disease

E10.22 **Type 1 diabetes mellitus with diabetic chronic kidney disease**
Use additional code to identify stage of chronic kidney disease (N18.1-N18.6)

E10.29 **Type 1 diabetes mellitus with other diabetic kidney complication**
Type 1 diabetes mellitus with renal tubular degeneration

✓5ᵗʰ **E10.3** **Type 1 diabetes mellitus with ophthalmic complications**

✓6ᵗʰ **E10.31** **Type 1 diabetes mellitus with unspecified diabetic retinopathy**

E10.311 **Type 1 diabetes mellitus with unspecified diabetic retinopathy with macular edema**

E10.319 **Type 1 diabetes mellitus with unspecified diabetic retinopathy without macular edema**

✓6ᵗʰ **E10.32** **Type 1 diabetes mellitus with mild nonproliferative diabetic retinopathy**
Type 1 diabetes mellitus with nonproliferative diabetic retinopathy NOS

E10.321 **Type 1 diabetes mellitus with mild nonproliferative diabetic retinopathy with macular edema**

E10.329 **Type 1 diabetes mellitus with mild nonproliferative diabetic retinopathy without macular edema**

✓6ᵗʰ **E10.33** **Type 1 diabetes mellitus with moderate nonproliferative diabetic retinopathy**

E10.331 **Type 1 diabetes mellitus with moderate nonproliferative diabetic retinopathy with macular edema**

E10.339 **Type 1 diabetes mellitus with moderate nonproliferative diabetic retinopathy without macular edema**

✓6ᵗʰ **E10.34** **Type 1 diabetes mellitus with severe nonproliferative diabetic retinopathy**

E10.341 **Type 1 diabetes mellitus with severe nonproliferative diabetic retinopathy with macular edema**

E10.349 **Type 1 diabetes mellitus with severe nonproliferative diabetic retinopathy without macular edema**

✓6ᵗʰ **E10.35** **Type 1 diabetes mellitus with proliferative diabetic retinopathy**

E10.351 **Type 1 diabetes mellitus with proliferative diabetic retinopathy with macular edema**

Endocrine, Nutritional and Metabolic Diseases

E10.359–E11.36

E10.359 **Type 1 diabetes mellitus with proliferative diabetic retinopathy** without macular edema

E10.36 **Type 1 diabetes mellitus with diabetic** cataract

E10.39 **Type 1 diabetes mellitus with other diabetic ophthalmic complication**
Use additional code to identify manifestation, such as: diabetic glaucoma (H40-H42)

✓5ᵗʰ E10.4 **Type 1 diabetes mellitus with** neurological complications

E10.40 **Type 1 diabetes mellitus with diabetic neuropathy, unspecified**

E10.41 **Type 1 diabetes mellitus with diabetic mononeuropathy**

E10.42 **Type 1 diabetes mellitus with diabetic polyneuropathy**
Type 1 diabetes mellitus with diabetic neuralgia

E10.43 **Type 1 diabetes mellitus with diabetic autonomic (poly)neuropathy**
Type 1 diabetes mellitus with diabetic gastroparesis
AHA: 2013, 4Q, 114

E10.44 **Type 1 diabetes mellitus with diabetic amyotrophy**

E10.49 **Type 1 diabetes mellitus with other diabetic neurological complication**

✓5ᵗʰ E10.5 **Type 1 diabetes mellitus with** circulatory complications

E10.51 **Type 1 diabetes mellitus with diabetic peripheral angiopathy without gangrene**

E10.52 **Type 1 diabetes mellitus with diabetic peripheral angiopathy with gangrene**
Type 1 diabetes mellitus with diabetic gangrene

E10.59 **Type 1 diabetes mellitus with other circulatory complications**

✓5ᵗʰ E10.6 **Type 1 diabetes mellitus with** other specified complications

✓6ᵗʰ E10.61 **Type 1 diabetes mellitus with diabetic** arthropathy

E10.610 **Type 1 diabetes mellitus with diabetic neuropathic arthropathy**
Type 1 diabetes mellitus with Charcôt's joints

E10.618 **Type 1 diabetes mellitus with other diabetic arthropathy**

✓6ᵗʰ E10.62 **Type 1 diabetes mellitus with** skin complications

E10.620 **Type 1 diabetes mellitus with diabetic dermatitis**
Type 1 diabetes mellitus with diabetic necrobiosis lipoidica

E10.621 **Type 1 diabetes mellitus with** foot ulcer
Use additional code to identify site of ulcer (L97.4-, L97.5-)

E10.622 **Type 1 diabetes mellitus with** other skin ulcer
Use additional code to identify site of ulcer (L97.1-L97.9, L98.41-L98.49)

E10.628 **Type 1 diabetes mellitus with other skin complications**

✓6ᵗʰ E10.63 **Type 1 diabetes mellitus with** oral complications

E10.630 **Type 1 diabetes mellitus with** periodontal disease

E10.638 **Type 1 diabetes mellitus with other oral complications**

✓6ᵗʰ E10.64 **Type 1 diabetes mellitus with** hypoglycemia

E10.641 **Type 1 diabetes mellitus with hypoglycemia** with coma

E10.649 **Type 1 diabetes mellitus with hypoglycemia** without coma

E10.65 **Type 1 diabetes mellitus with** hyperglycemia
AHA: 2013, 3Q, 20

E10.69 **Type 1 diabetes mellitus with other specified complication**
Use additional code to identify complication

E10.8 **Type 1 diabetes mellitus with unspecified** complications

E10.9 **Type 1 diabetes mellitus** without complications

✓4ᵗʰ **E11 Type 2 diabetes mellitus**
INCLUDES diabetes (mellitus) due to insulin secretory defect
diabetes NOS
insulin resistant diabetes (mellitus)
Use additional code to identify any insulin use (Z79.4)
EXCLUDES 1 *diabetes mellitus due to underlying condition (E08.-)*
drug or chemical induced diabetes mellitus (E09.-)
gestational diabetes (O24.4-)
neonatal diabetes mellitus (P70.2)
postpancreatectomy diabetes mellitus (E13.-)
postprocedural diabetes mellitus (E13.-)
secondary diabetes mellitus NEC (E13.-)
type 1 diabetes mellitus (E10.-)
AHA: 2013, 4Q, 114; 2013, 3Q, 20; 2013, 1Q, 26

✓5ᵗʰ E11.0 **Type 2 diabetes mellitus with** hyperosmolarity

E11.00 **Type 2 diabetes mellitus with hyperosmolarity** without nonketotic hyperglycemic-hyperosmolar coma (NKHHC)

E11.01 **Type 2 diabetes mellitus with hyperosmolarity** with coma

✓5ᵗʰ E11.2 **Type 2 diabetes mellitus with** kidney complications

E11.21 **Type 2 diabetes mellitus with diabetic** nephropathy
Type 2 diabetes mellitus with intercapillary glomerulosclerosis
Type 2 diabetes mellitus with intracapillary glomerulonephrosis
Type 2 diabetes mellitus with Kimmelstiel-Wilson disease

E11.22 **Type 2 diabetes mellitus with diabetic** chronic kidney disease
Use additional code to identify stage of chronic kidney disease (N18.1-N18.6)

E11.29 **Type 2 diabetes mellitus with other diabetic kidney complication**
Type 2 diabetes mellitus with renal tubular degeneration

✓5ᵗʰ E11.3 **Type 2 diabetes mellitus with** ophthalmic complications

✓6ᵗʰ E11.31 **Type 2 diabetes mellitus with unspecified** diabetic retinopathy

E11.311 **Type 2 diabetes mellitus with unspecified diabetic retinopathy** with macular edema

E11.319 **Type 2 diabetes mellitus with unspecified diabetic retinopathy** without macular edema

✓6ᵗʰ E11.32 **Type 2 diabetes mellitus with** mild nonproliferative diabetic retinopathy
Type 2 diabetes mellitus with nonproliferative diabetic retinopathy NOS

E11.321 **Type 2 diabetes mellitus with mild nonproliferative diabetic retinopathy with macular edema**

E11.329 **Type 2 diabetes mellitus with mild nonproliferative diabetic retinopathy without macular edema**

✓6ᵗʰ E11.33 **Type 2 diabetes mellitus with** moderate nonproliferative diabetic retinopathy

E11.331 **Type 2 diabetes mellitus with moderate nonproliferative diabetic retinopathy with macular edema**

E11.339 **Type 2 diabetes mellitus with moderate nonproliferative diabetic retinopathy without macular edema**

✓6ᵗʰ E11.34 **Type 2 diabetes mellitus with** severe nonproliferative diabetic retinopathy

E11.341 **Type 2 diabetes mellitus with severe nonproliferative diabetic retinopathy with macular edema**

E11.349 **Type 2 diabetes mellitus with severe nonproliferative diabetic retinopathy without macular edema**

✓6ᵗʰ E11.35 **Type 2 diabetes mellitus with** proliferative diabetic retinopathy

E11.351 **Type 2 diabetes mellitus with proliferative diabetic retinopathy** with macular edema

E11.359 **Type 2 diabetes mellitus with proliferative diabetic retinopathy** without macular edema

E11.36 **Type 2 diabetes mellitus with diabetic** cataract

Endocrine, Nutritional and Metabolic Diseases

E11.39–E13.349

E11.39   **Type 2 diabetes mellitus with other diabetic ophthalmic complication**
Use additional code to identify manifestation, such as: diabetic glaucoma (H40-H42)

✓5ᵗʰ **E11.4**   **Type 2 diabetes mellitus with neurological complications**

E11.40   **Type 2 diabetes mellitus with diabetic neuropathy, unspecified**
AHA: 2013, 4Q, 129

E11.41   **Type 2 diabetes mellitus with diabetic mononeuropathy**

E11.42   **Type 2 diabetes mellitus with diabetic polyneuropathy**
Type 2 diabetes mellitus with diabetic neuralgia

E11.43   **Type 2 diabetes mellitus with diabetic autonomic (poly)neuropathy**
Type 2 diabetes mellitus with diabetic gastroparesis
AHA: 2013, 4Q, 114

E11.44   **Type 2 diabetes mellitus with diabetic amyotrophy**

E11.49   **Type 2 diabetes mellitus with other diabetic neurological complication**

✓5ᵗʰ **E11.5**   **Type 2 diabetes mellitus with circulatory complications**

E11.51   **Type 2 diabetes mellitus with diabetic peripheral angiopathy without gangrene**

E11.52   **Type 2 diabetes mellitus with diabetic peripheral angiopathy with gangrene**
Type 2 diabetes mellitus with diabetic gangrene

E11.59   **Type 2 diabetes mellitus with other circulatory complications**

✓5ᵗʰ **E11.6**   **Type 2 diabetes mellitus with other specified complications**

✓6ᵗʰ **E11.61**   **Type 2 diabetes mellitus with diabetic arthropathy**

E11.610   **Type 2 diabetes mellitus with diabetic neuropathic arthropathy**
Type 2 diabetes mellitus with Charcôt's joints

E11.618   **Type 2 diabetes mellitus with other diabetic arthropathy**

✓6ᵗʰ **E11.62**   **Type 2 diabetes mellitus with skin complications**

E11.620   **Type 2 diabetes mellitus with diabetic dermatitis**
Type 2 diabetes mellitus with diabetic necrobiosis lipoidica

E11.621   **Type 2 diabetes mellitus with foot ulcer**
Use additional code to identify site of ulcer (L97.4-, L97.5-)

E11.622   **Type 2 diabetes mellitus with other skin ulcer**
Use additional code to identify site of ulcer (L97.1-L97.9, L98.41-L98.49)

E11.628   **Type 2 diabetes mellitus with other skin complications**

✓6ᵗʰ **E11.63**   **Type 2 diabetes mellitus with oral complications**

E11.630   **Type 2 diabetes mellitus with periodontal disease**

E11.638   **Type 2 diabetes mellitus with other oral complications**

✓6ᵗʰ **E11.64**   **Type 2 diabetes mellitus with hypoglycemia**

E11.641   **Type 2 diabetes mellitus with hypoglycemia with coma**

E11.649   **Type 2 diabetes mellitus with hypoglycemia without coma**

E11.65   **Type 2 diabetes mellitus with hyperglycemia**
AHA: 2013, 3Q, 20

E11.69   **Type 2 diabetes mellitus with other specified complication**
Use additional code to identify complication

E11.8   **Type 2 diabetes mellitus with unspecified complications**

E11.9   **Type 2 diabetes mellitus without complications**

✓4ᵗʰ **E13**   **Other specified diabetes mellitus**
Diabetes mellitus due to genetic defects of beta-cell function
Diabetes mellitus due to genetic defects in insulin action
Postpancreatectomy diabetes mellitus
Postprocedural diabetes mellitus
Secondary diabetes mellitus NEC
Use additional code to identify any insulin use (Z79.4)
EXCLUDES 1   diabetes (mellitus) due to autoimmune process (E10.-)
diabetes (mellitus) due to immune mediated pancreatic islet beta-cell destruction (E10.-)
diabetes mellitus due to underlying condition (E08.-)
drug or chemical induced diabetes mellitus (E09.-)
gestational diabetes (O24.4-)
neonatal diabetes mellitus (P70.2)
type 2 diabetes mellitus (E11.-)
AHA: 2013, 4Q, 114; 2013, 3Q, 20

✓5ᵗʰ **E13.0**   **Other specified diabetes mellitus with hyperosmolarity**

E13.00   **Other specified diabetes mellitus with hyperosmolarity without nonketotic hyperglycemic-hyperosmolar coma (NKHHC)**

E13.01   **Other specified diabetes mellitus with hyperosmolarity with coma**

✓5ᵗʰ **E13.1**   **Other specified diabetes mellitus with ketoacidosis**
AHA: 2013, 1Q, 26

E13.10   **Other specified diabetes mellitus with ketoacidosis without coma**

E13.11   **Other specified diabetes mellitus with ketoacidosis with coma**

✓5ᵗʰ **E13.2**   **Other specified diabetes mellitus with kidney complications**

E13.21   **Other specified diabetes mellitus with diabetic nephropathy**
Other specified diabetes mellitus with intercapillary glomerulosclerosis
Other specified diabetes mellitus with intracapillary glomerulonephrosis
Other specified diabetes mellitus with Kimmelstiel-Wilson disease

E13.22   **Other specified diabetes mellitus with diabetic chronic kidney disease**
Use additional code to identify stage of chronic kidney disease (N18.1-N18.6)

E13.29   **Other specified diabetes mellitus with other diabetic kidney complication**
Other specified diabetes mellitus with renal tubular degeneration

✓5ᵗʰ **E13.3**   **Other specified diabetes mellitus with ophthalmic complications**

✓6ᵗʰ **E13.31**   **Other specified diabetes mellitus with unspecified diabetic retinopathy**

E13.311   **Other specified diabetes mellitus with unspecified diabetic retinopathy with macular edema**

E13.319   **Other specified diabetes mellitus with unspecified diabetic retinopathy without macular edema**

✓6ᵗʰ **E13.32**   **Other specified diabetes mellitus with mild nonproliferative diabetic retinopathy**
Other specified diabetes mellitus with nonproliferative diabetic retinopathy NOS

E13.321   **Other specified diabetes mellitus with mild nonproliferative diabetic retinopathy with macular edema**

E13.329   **Other specified diabetes mellitus with mild nonproliferative diabetic retinopathy without macular edema**

✓6ᵗʰ **E13.33**   **Other specified diabetes mellitus with moderate nonproliferative diabetic retinopathy**

E13.331   **Other specified diabetes mellitus with moderate nonproliferative diabetic retinopathy with macular edema**

E13.339   **Other specified diabetes mellitus with moderate nonproliferative diabetic retinopathy without macular edema**

✓6ᵗʰ **E13.34**   **Other specified diabetes mellitus with severe nonproliferative diabetic retinopathy**

E13.341   **Other specified diabetes mellitus with severe nonproliferative diabetic retinopathy with macular edema**

E13.349   **Other specified diabetes mellitus with severe nonproliferative diabetic retinopathy without macular edema**

EXCLUDES 1 Not coded here   **EXCLUDES 2** Not included here   **N** Newborn Age: 0   **P** Pediatric Age: 0-17   **M** Maternity Age: 12-55   **A** Adult Age: 15-124

484   ICD-10-CM Draft (2015)

✓6ᵗʰ **E13.35 Other specified diabetes mellitus with proliferative diabetic retinopathy**
- **E13.351 Other specified diabetes mellitus with proliferative diabetic retinopathy with macular edema**
- **E13.359 Other specified diabetes mellitus with proliferative diabetic retinopathy without macular edema**

E13.36 Other specified diabetes mellitus with diabetic cataract

E13.39 Other specified diabetes mellitus with other diabetic ophthalmic complication
Use additional code to identify manifestation, such as: diabetic glaucoma (H40-H42)

✓5ᵗʰ **E13.4 Other specified diabetes mellitus with neurological complications**
- **E13.40 Other specified diabetes mellitus with diabetic neuropathy, unspecified**
- **E13.41 Other specified diabetes mellitus with diabetic mononeuropathy**
- **E13.42 Other specified diabetes mellitus with diabetic polyneuropathy**
  Other specified diabetes mellitus with diabetic neuralgia
- **E13.43 Other specified diabetes mellitus with diabetic autonomic (poly)neuropathy**
  Other specified diabetes mellitus with diabetic gastroparesis
  AHA: 2013, 4Q, 114
- **E13.44 Other specified diabetes mellitus with diabetic amyotrophy**
- **E13.49 Other specified diabetes mellitus with other diabetic neurological complication**

✓5ᵗʰ **E13.5 Other specified diabetes mellitus with circulatory complications**
- **E13.51 Other specified diabetes mellitus with diabetic peripheral angiopathy without gangrene**
- **E13.52 Other specified diabetes mellitus with diabetic peripheral angiopathy with gangrene**
  Other specified diabetes mellitus with diabetic gangrene
- **E13.59 Other specified diabetes mellitus with other circulatory complications**

✓5ᵗʰ **E13.6 Other specified diabetes mellitus with other specified complications**
- ✓6ᵗʰ **E13.61 Other specified diabetes mellitus with diabetic arthropathy**
  - **E13.610 Other specified diabetes mellitus with diabetic neuropathic arthropathy**
    Other specified diabetes mellitus with Charcôt's joints
  - **E13.618 Other specified diabetes mellitus with other diabetic arthropathy**
- ✓6ᵗʰ **E13.62 Other specified diabetes mellitus with skin complications**
  - **E13.620 Other specified diabetes mellitus with diabetic dermatitis**
    Other specified diabetes mellitus with diabetic necrobiosis lipoidica
  - **E13.621 Other specified diabetes mellitus with foot ulcer**
    Use additional code to identify site of ulcer (L97.4-, L97.5-)
  - **E13.622 Other specified diabetes mellitus with other skin ulcer**
    Use additional code to identify site of ulcer (L97.1-L97.9, L98.41-L98.49)
  - **E13.628 Other specified diabetes mellitus with other skin complications**
- ✓6ᵗʰ **E13.63 Other specified diabetes mellitus with oral complications**
  - **E13.630 Other specified diabetes mellitus with periodontal disease**
  - **E13.638 Other specified diabetes mellitus with other oral complications**
- ✓6ᵗʰ **E13.64 Other specified diabetes mellitus with hypoglycemia**
  - **E13.641 Other specified diabetes mellitus with hypoglycemia with coma**

- **E13.649 Other specified diabetes mellitus with hypoglycemia without coma**
- **E13.65 Other specified diabetes mellitus with hyperglycemia**
- **E13.69 Other specified diabetes mellitus with other specified complication**
  Use additional code to identify complication

E13.8 Other specified diabetes mellitus with unspecified complications

E13.9 Other specified diabetes mellitus without complications

Other disorders of glucose regulation and pancreatic internal secretion (E15-E16)

E15 Nondiabetic hypoglycemic coma
INCLUDES drug-induced insulin coma in nondiabetic
hyperinsulinism with hypoglycemic coma
hypoglycemic coma NOS

✓4ᵗʰ **E16 Other disorders of pancreatic internal secretion**
- **E16.0 Drug-induced hypoglycemia without coma**
  Use additional code for adverse effect, if applicable, to identify drug (T36-T50 with fifth or sixth character 5)
- **E16.1 Other hypoglycemia**
  Functional hyperinsulinism
  Functional nonhyperinsulinemic hypoglycemia
  Hyperinsulinism NOS
  Hyperplasia of pancreatic islet beta cells NOS
  EXCLUDES 1 hypoglycemia in infant of diabetic mother (P70.1)
  neonatal hypoglycemia (P70.4)
- **E16.2 Hypoglycemia, unspecified**
- **E16.3 Increased secretion of glucagon**
  Hyperplasia of pancreatic endocrine cells with glucagon excess
- **E16.4 Increased secretion of gastrin**
  Hypergastrinemia
  Hyperplasia of pancreatic endocrine cells with gastrin excess
  Zollinger-Ellison syndrome
- **E16.8 Other specified disorders of pancreatic internal secretion**
  Increased secretion from endocrine pancreas of growth hormone-releasing hormone
  Increased secretion from endocrine pancreas of pancreatic polypeptide
  Increased secretion from endocrine pancreas of somatostatin
  Increased secretion from endocrine pancreas of vasoactive-intestinal polypeptide
- **E16.9 Disorder of pancreatic internal secretion, unspecified**
  Islet-cell hyperplasia NOS
  Pancreatic endocrine cell hyperplasia NOS

Disorders of other endocrine glands (E20-E35)

EXCLUDES 1 galactorrhea (N64.3)
gynecomastia (N62)

✓4ᵗʰ **E20 Hypoparathyroidism**
EXCLUDES 1 Di George's syndrome (D82.1)
postprocedural hypoparathyroidism (E89.2)
tetany NOS (R29.0)
transitory neonatal hypoparathyroidism (P71.4)
- **E20.0 Idiopathic hypoparathyroidism**
- **E20.1 Pseudohypoparathyroidism**
- **E20.8 Other hypoparathyroidism**
- **E20.9 Hypoparathyroidism, unspecified**
  Parathyroid tetany

✓4ᵗʰ **E21 Hyperparathyroidism and other disorders of parathyroid gland**
EXCLUDES 1 adult osteomalacia (M83.-)
ectopic hyperparathyroidism (E34.2)
familial hypocalciuric hypercalcemia (E83.52)
hungry bone syndrome (E83.81)
infantile and juvenile osteomalacia (E55.0)
- **E21.0 Primary hyperparathyroidism**
  Hyperplasia of parathyroid
  Osteitis fibrosa cystica generalisata [von Recklinghausen's disease of bone]
- **E21.1 Secondary hyperparathyroidism, not elsewhere classified**
  EXCLUDES 1 secondary hyperparathyroidism of renal origin (N25.81)
- **E21.2 Other hyperparathyroidism**
  Tertiary hyperparathyroidism
  EXCLUDES 1 familial hypocalciuric hypercalcemia (E83.52)
- **E21.3 Hyperparathyroidism, unspecified**
- **E21.4 Other specified disorders of parathyroid gland**

✓ Additional Character Required ✓x7ᵗʰ Xtension Alert Unspecified Dx Other Specified Dx Manifestation ►◄ Revised Text ● New Code ▲ Revised Code Title

Endocrine, Nutritional and Metabolic Diseases

E21.5–E28.2

E21.5 Disorder of parathyroid gland, unspecified

✓4ᵗʰ E22 Hyperfunction of pituitary gland
EXCLUDES 1   *Cushing's syndrome (E24.-)*
Nelson's syndrome (E24.1)
overproduction of ACTH not associated with Cushing's disease (E27.0)
overproduction of pituitary ACTH (E24.0)
overproduction of thyroid-stimulating hormone (E05.8-)

E22.0 Acromegaly and pituitary gigantism
Overproduction of growth hormone
EXCLUDES 1   *constitutional gigantism (E34.4)*
constitutional tall stature (E34.4)
increased secretion from endocrine pancreas of growth hormone-releasing hormone (E16.8)

E22.1 Hyperprolactinemia
Use additional code for adverse effect, if applicable, to identify drug (T36-T50 with fifth or sixth character 5)

E22.2 Syndrome of inappropriate secretion of antidiuretic hormone

E22.8 Other hyperfunction of pituitary gland
Central precocious puberty

E22.9 Hyperfunction of pituitary gland, unspecified

✓4ᵗʰ E23 Hypofunction and other disorders of the pituitary gland
INCLUDES   the listed conditions whether the disorder is in the pituitary or the hypothalamus
EXCLUDES 1   *postprocedural hypopituitarism (E89.3)*

E23.0 Hypopituitarism
Fertile eunuch syndrome
Hypogonadotropic hypogonadism
Idiopathic growth hormone deficiency
Isolated deficiency of gonadotropin
Isolated deficiency of growth hormone
Isolated deficiency of pituitary hormone
Kallmann's syndrome
Lorain-Levi short stature
Necrosis of pituitary gland (postpartum)
Panhypopituitarism
Pituitary cachexia
Pituitary insufficiency NOS
Pituitary short stature
Sheehan's syndrome
Simmonds' disease

E23.1 Drug-induced hypopituitarism
Use additional code for adverse effect, if applicable, to identify drug (T36-T50 with fifth or sixth character 5)

E23.2 Diabetes insipidus
EXCLUDES 1   *nephrogenic diabetes insipidus (N25.1)*

E23.3 Hypothalamic dysfunction, not elsewhere classified
EXCLUDES 1   *Prader-Willi syndrome (Q87.1)*
Russell-Silver syndrome (Q87.1)

E23.6 Other disorders of pituitary gland
Abscess of pituitary   Adiposogenital dystrophy

E23.7 Disorder of pituitary gland, unspecified

✓4ᵗʰ E24 Cushing's syndrome
EXCLUDES 1   *congenital adrenal hyperplasia (E25.0)*

E24.0 Pituitary-dependent Cushing's disease
Overproduction of pituitary ACTH
Pituitary-dependent hypercorticalism

E24.1 Nelson's syndrome

E24.2 Drug-induced Cushing's syndrome
Use additional code for adverse effect, if applicable, to identify drug (T36-T50 with fifth or sixth character 5)

E24.3 Ectopic ACTH syndrome

E24.4 Alcohol-induced pseudo-Cushing's syndrome

E24.8 Other Cushing's syndrome

E24.9 Cushing's syndrome, unspecified

✓4ᵗʰ E25 Adrenogenital disorders
INCLUDES   adrenogenital syndromes, virilizing or feminizing, whether acquired or due to adrenal hyperplasia
consequent on inborn enzyme defects in hormone synthesis
female adrenal pseudohermaphroditism
female heterosexual precocious pseudopuberty
male isosexual precocious pseudopuberty
male macrogenitosomia praecox
male sexual precocity with adrenal hyperplasia
male virilization (female)
EXCLUDES 1   *indeterminate sex and pseudohermaphroditism (Q56)*
chromosomal abnormalities (Q90-Q99)

E25.0 Congenital adrenogenital disorders associated with enzyme deficiency
Congenital adrenal hyperplasia
21-Hydroxylase deficiency
Salt-losing congenital adrenal hyperplasia

E25.8 Other adrenogenital disorders
Idiopathic adrenogenital disorder
Use additional code for adverse effect, if applicable, to identify drug (T36-T50 with fifth or sixth character 5)

E25.9 Adrenogenital disorder, unspecified
Adrenogenital syndrome NOS

✓4ᵗʰ E26 Hyperaldosteronism

✓5ᵗʰ E26.0 Primary hyperaldosteronism

    E26.01 Conn's syndrome
Code also adrenal adenoma (D35.0-)

    E26.02 Glucocorticoid-remediable aldosteronism
Familial aldosteronism type I

    E26.09 Other primary hyperaldosteronism
Primary aldosteronism due to adrenal hyperplasia (bilateral)

E26.1 Secondary hyperaldosteronism

✓5ᵗʰ E26.8 Other hyperaldosteronism

    E26.81 Bartter's syndrome

    E26.89 Other hyperaldosteronism

E26.9 Hyperaldosteronism, unspecified
Aldosteronism NOS   Hyperaldosteronism NOS

✓4ᵗʰ E27 Other disorders of adrenal gland

E27.0 Other adrenocortical overactivity
Overproduction of ACTH, not associated with Cushing's disease
Premature adrenarche
EXCLUDES 1   *Cushing's syndrome (E24.-)*

E27.1 Primary adrenocortical insufficiency
Addison's disease
Autoimmune adrenalitis
EXCLUDES 1   *Addison only phenotype adrenoleukodystrophy (E71.528)*
amyloidosis (E85.-)
tuberculous Addison's disease (A18.7)
Waterhouse-Friderichsen syndrome (A39.1)

E27.2 Addisonian crisis
Adrenal crisis
Adrenocortical crisis

E27.3 Drug-induced adrenocortical insufficiency
Use additional code for adverse effect, if applicable, to identify drug (T36-T50 with fifth or sixth character 5)

✓5ᵗʰ E27.4 Other and unspecified adrenocortical insufficiency
EXCLUDES 1   *adrenoleukodystrophy [Addison-Schilder] (E71.528)*
Waterhouse-Friderichsen syndrome (A39.1)

    E27.40 Unspecified adrenocortical insufficiency
Adrenocortical insufficiency NOS
Hypoaldosteronism

    E27.49 Other adrenocortical insufficiency
Adrenal hemorrhage
Adrenal infarction

E27.5 Adrenomedullary hyperfunction
Adrenomedullary hyperplasia
Catecholamine hypersecretion

E27.8 Other specified disorders of adrenal gland
Abnormality of cortisol-binding globulin

E27.9 Disorder of adrenal gland, unspecified

✓4ᵗʰ E28 Ovarian dysfunction
EXCLUDES 1   *isolated gonadotropin deficiency (E23.0)*
postprocedural ovarian failure (E89.4-)

E28.0 Estrogen excess   ♀
Use additional code for adverse effect, if applicable, to identify drug (T36-T50 with fifth or sixth character 5)

E28.1 Androgen excess   ♀
Hypersecretion of ovarian androgens
Use additional code for adverse effect, if applicable, to identify drug (T36-T50 with fifth or sixth character 5)

E28.2 Polycystic ovarian syndrome   ♀
Sclerocystic ovary syndrome
Stein-Leventhal syndrome

EXCLUDES 1 Not coded here   EXCLUDES 2 Not included here   N Newborn Age: 0   P Pediatric Age: 0-17   M Maternity Age: 12-55   A Adult Age: 15-124

√5ᵗʰ **E28.3** **Primary ovarian failure**
EXCLUDES 1 *pure gonadal dysgenesis (Q99.1)*
Turner's syndrome (Q96.-)

√6ᵗʰ **E28.31** **Premature** menopause

E28.310 **Symptomatic** **premature menopause** 🅐♀
Symptoms such as flushing, sleeplessness, headache, lack of concentration, associated with premature menopause

E28.319 **Asymptomatic** **premature menopause** 🅐♀
Premature menopause NOS

E28.39 **Other primary ovarian failure** ♀
Decreased estrogen
Resistant ovary syndrome

E28.8 **Other ovarian dysfunction** ♀
Ovarian hyperfunction NOS
EXCLUDES 1 *postprocedural ovarian failure (E89.4-)*

E28.9 **Ovarian dysfunction, unspecified** ♀

√4ᵗʰ **E29** **Testicular dysfunction**
EXCLUDES 1 *androgen insensitivity syndrome (E34.5-)*
azoospermia or oligospermia NOS (N46.0-N46.1)
isolated gonadotropin deficiency (E23.0)
Klinefelter's syndrome (Q98.0-Q98.2, Q98.4)

E29.0 **Testicular** **hyperfunction** ♂
Hypersecretion of testicular hormones

E29.1 **Testicular** hypofunction ♂
Defective biosynthesis of testicular androgen NOS
5-delta-Reductase deficiency (with male pseudohermaphroditism)
Testicular hypogonadism NOS
Use additional code for adverse effect, if applicable, to identify drug (T36-T50 with fifth or sixth character 5)
EXCLUDES 1 *postprocedural testicular hypofunction (E89.5)*

E29.8 **Other testicular dysfunction** ♂

E29.9 **Testicular dysfunction, unspecified** ♂

√4ᵗʰ **E30** **Disorders of puberty, not elsewhere classified**

E30.0 **Delayed** puberty
Constitutional delay of puberty
Delayed sexual development

E30.1 **Precocious** puberty 🅟
Precocious menstruation
EXCLUDES 1 *Albright (-McCune) (-Sternberg) syndrome (Q78.1)*
central precocious puberty (E22.8)
congenital adrenal hyperplasia (E25.0)
female heterosexual precocious pseudopuberty (E25.-)
male isosexual precocious pseudopuberty (E25.-)

E30.8 **Other disorders of puberty** 🅟
Premature thelarche

E30.9 **Disorder of puberty, unspecified**

√4ᵗʰ **E31** **Polyglandular dysfunction**
EXCLUDES 1 *ataxia telangiectasia [Louis-Bar] (G11.3)*
dystrophia myotonica [Steinert] (G71.11)
pseudohypoparathyroidism (E20.1)

E31.0 **Autoimmune** polyglandular **failure**
Schmidt's syndrome

E31.1 **Polyglandular** hyperfunction
EXCLUDES 1 *multiple endocrine adenomatosis (E31.2-)*
multiple endocrine neoplasia (E31.2-)

√5ᵗʰ **E31.2** **Multiple endocrine neoplasia [MEN] syndromes**
Multiple endocrine adenomatosis
Code also any associated malignancies and other conditions associated with the syndromes

E31.20 **Multiple endocrine neoplasia [MEN] syndrome, unspecified**
Multiple endocrine adenomatosis NOS
Multiple endocrine neoplasia [MEN] syndrome NOS

E31.21 **Multiple endocrine neoplasia [MEN]** type I
Wermer's syndrome

E31.22 **Multiple endocrine neoplasia [MEN]** type IIA
Sipple's syndrome

E31.23 **Multiple endocrine neoplasia [MEN]** type IIB

E31.8 **Other polyglandular dysfunction**

E31.9 **Polyglandular dysfunction, unspecified**

√4ᵗʰ **E32** **Diseases of thymus**
EXCLUDES 1 *aplasia or hypoplasia of thymus with immunodeficiency (D82.1)*
myasthenia gravis (G70.0)

E32.0 **Persistent hyperplasia** of thymus
Hypertrophy of thymus

E32.1 **Abscess** of thymus

E32.8 **Other diseases of thymus**
EXCLUDES 1 *aplasia or hypoplasia with immunodeficiency (D82.1)*
thymoma (D15.0)

E32.9 **Disease of thymus, unspecified**

√4ᵗʰ **E34** **Other endocrine disorders**
EXCLUDES 1 *pseudohypoparathyroidism (E20.1)*

E34.0 **Carcinoid syndrome**
NOTE   May be used as an additional code to identify functional activity associated with a carcinoid tumor.

E34.1 **Other hypersecretion of intestinal hormones**

E34.2 **Ectopic hormone secretion, not elsewhere classified**
EXCLUDES 1 *ectopic ACTH syndrome (E24.3)*

E34.3 **Short stature due to endocrine disorder**
Constitutional short stature
Laron-type short stature
EXCLUDES 1 *achondroplastic short stature (Q77.4)*
hypochondroplastic short stature (Q77.4)
nutritional short stature (E45)
pituitary short stature (E23.0)
progeria (E34.8)
renal short stature (N25.0)
Russell-Silver syndrome (Q87.1)
short-limbed stature with immunodeficiency (D82.2)
short stature in specific dysmorphic syndromes— code to syndrome—see Alphabetical Index
short stature NOS (R62.52)

E34.4 **Constitutional tall stature**
Constitutional gigantism

√5ᵗʰ **E34.5** **Androgen insensitivity syndrome**

E34.50 **Androgen insensitivity syndrome, unspecified**
Androgen insensitivity NOS

E34.51 **Complete** **androgen insensitivity syndrome**
Complete androgen insensitivity
de Quervain syndrome
Goldberg-Maxwell syndrome

E34.52 **Partial** **androgen insensitivity syndrome**
Partial androgen insensitivity
Reifenstein syndrome

E34.8 **Other specified endocrine disorders**
Pineal gland dysfunction
Progeria
EXCLUDES 2 *pseudohypoparathyroidism (E20.1)*

E34.9 **Endocrine disorder, unspecified**
Endocrine disturbance NOS
Hormone disturbance NOS

E35 **Disorders of endocrine glands in diseases classified elsewhere**
Code first underlying disease, such as:
late congenital syphilis of thymus gland [Dubois disease] (A50.5)
Use additional code, if applicable, to identify:
sequelae of tuberculosis of other organs (B90.8)
EXCLUDES 1 *Echinococcus granulosus infection of thyroid gland (B67.3)*
meningococcal hemorrhagic adrenalitis (A39.1)
syphilis of endocrine gland (A52.79)
tuberculosis of adrenal gland, except calcification (A18.7)
tuberculosis of endocrine gland NEC (A18.82)
tuberculosis of thyroid gland (A18.81)
Waterhouse-Friderichsen syndrome (A39.1)

√4ᵗʰ **E36** **Intraoperative complications of endocrine system**
EXCLUDES 2 *postprocedural endocrine and metabolic complications and disorders, not elsewhere classified (E89.-)*

√5ᵗʰ **E36.0** **Intraoperative hemorrhage and hematoma of an endocrine system organ or structure complicating a procedure**
EXCLUDES 1 *intraoperative hemorrhage and hematoma of an endocrine system organ or structure due to accidental puncture or laceration during a procedure (E36.1-)*

E36.01 **Intraoperative hemorrhage and hematoma of an endocrine system organ or structure complicating an endocrine system procedure**

E36.02 **Intraoperative hemorrhage and hematoma of an endocrine system organ or structure complicating other procedure**

✓ Additional Character Required   √x7ᵗʰ Xtension Alert   Unspecified Dx   Other Specified Dx   Manifestation   ►◄ Revised Text   ● New Code   ▲ Revised Code Title

ICD-10-CM Draft (2015)   487

Endocrine, Nutritional and Metabolic Diseases

E28.3–E36.02

Endocrine, Nutritional and Metabolic Diseases

E36.1–E61.9

√5ᵗʰ **E36.1** Accidental puncture and laceration of an endocrine system organ or structure during a procedure

    E36.11 Accidental puncture and laceration of an endocrine system organ or structure during an endocrine system procedure

    E36.12 Accidental puncture and laceration of an endocrine system organ or structure during other procedure

E36.8 Other intraoperative complications of endocrine system
    Use additional code, if applicable, to further specify disorder

Malnutrition (E40-E46)

EXCLUDES 1   intestinal malabsorption (K90.-)
       sequelae of protein-calorie malnutrition (E64.0)
EXCLUDES 2   nutritional anemias (D50-D53)
       starvation (T73.0)

E40 **Kwashiorkor**
    Severe malnutrition with nutritional edema with dyspigmentation of skin and hair
    EXCLUDES 1   marasmic kwashiorkor (E42)

E41 **Nutritional marasmus**
    Severe malnutrition with marasmus
    EXCLUDES 1   marasmic kwashiorkor (E42)

E42 **Marasmic kwashiorkor**
    Intermediate form severe protein-calorie malnutrition
    Severe protein-calorie malnutrition with signs of both kwashiorkor and marasmus

E43 **Unspecified severe protein-calorie malnutrition**
    Starvation edema

√4ᵗʰ **E44** **Protein-calorie malnutrition of moderate and mild degree**
    E44.0 Moderate protein-calorie malnutrition
    E44.1 Mild protein-calorie malnutrition

E45 **Retarded development following protein-calorie malnutrition**
    Nutritional short stature
    Nutritional stunting
    Physical retardation due to malnutrition

E46 **Unspecified protein-calorie malnutrition**
    Malnutrition NOS
    Protein-calorie imbalance NOS
    EXCLUDES 1   nutritional deficiency NOS (E63.9)

Other nutritional deficiencies (E50-E64)

EXCLUDES 2   nutritional anemias (D50-D53)

√4ᵗʰ **E50** **Vitamin A deficiency**
    EXCLUDES 1   sequelae of vitamin A deficiency (E64.1)

    E50.0 Vitamin A deficiency with conjunctival xerosis

    E50.1 Vitamin A deficiency with Bitot's spot and conjunctival xerosis
        Bitot's spot in the young child

    E50.2 Vitamin A deficiency with corneal xerosis

    E50.3 Vitamin A deficiency with corneal ulceration and xerosis

    E50.4 Vitamin A deficiency with keratomalacia

    E50.5 Vitamin A deficiency with night blindness

    E50.6 Vitamin A deficiency with xerophthalmic scars of cornea

    E50.7 Other ocular manifestations of vitamin A deficiency
        Xerophthalmia NOS

    E50.8 Other manifestations of vitamin A deficiency
        Follicular keratosis
        Xeroderma

    E50.9 Vitamin A deficiency, unspecified
        Hypovitaminosis A NOS

√4ᵗʰ **E51** **Thiamine deficiency**
    EXCLUDES 1   sequelae of thiamine deficiency (E64.8)

    √5ᵗʰ **E51.1** Beriberi

        E51.11 Dry beriberi
           Beriberi NOS
           Beriberi with polyneuropathy

        E51.12 Wet beriberi
           Beriberi with cardiovascular manifestations
           Cardiovascular beriberi
           Shoshin disease

    E51.2 Wernicke's encephalopathy

    E51.8 Other manifestations of thiamine deficiency

    E51.9 Thiamine deficiency, unspecified

E52 **Niacin deficiency [pellagra]**
    Niacin (-tryptophan) deficiency
    Nicotinamide deficiency
    Pellagra (alcoholic)
    EXCLUDES 1   sequelae of niacin deficiency (E64.8)

√4ᵗʰ **E53** **Deficiency of other B group vitamins**
    EXCLUDES 1   sequelae of vitamin B deficiency (E64.8)

    E53.0 Riboflavin deficiency
        Ariboflavinosis
        Vitamin B2 deficiency

    E53.1 Pyridoxine deficiency
        Vitamin B6 deficiency
        EXCLUDES 1   pyridoxine-responsive sideroblastic anemia (D64.3)

    E53.8 Deficiency of other specified B group vitamins
        Biotin deficiency   Folic acid deficiency
        Cyanocobalamin deficiency   Pantothenic acid deficiency
        Folate deficiency   Vitamin B12 deficiency
        EXCLUDES 1   folate deficiency anemia (D52.-)
                vitamin B12 deficiency anemia (D51.-)

    E53.9 Vitamin B deficiency, unspecified

E54 **Ascorbic acid deficiency**
    Deficiency of vitamin C
    Scurvy
    EXCLUDES 1   scorbutic anemia (D53.2)
           sequelae of vitamin C deficiency (E64.2)

√4ᵗʰ **E55** **Vitamin D deficiency**
    EXCLUDES 1   adult osteomalacia (M83.-)
           osteoporosis (M80.-)
           sequelae of rickets (E64.3)

    E55.0 Rickets, active
        Infantile osteomalacia
        Juvenile osteomalacia
        EXCLUDES 1   celiac rickets (K90.0)
                Crohn's rickets (K50.-)
                hereditary vitamin D-dependent rickets (E83.32)
                inactive rickets (E64.3)
                renal rickets (N25.0)
                sequelae of rickets (E64.3)
                vitamin D-resistant rickets (E83.31)

    E55.9 Vitamin D deficiency, unspecified
        Avitaminosis D

√4ᵗʰ **E56** **Other vitamin deficiencies**
    EXCLUDES 1   sequelae of other vitamin deficiencies (E64.8)

    E56.0 Deficiency of vitamin E

    E56.1 Deficiency of vitamin K
        EXCLUDES 1   deficiency of coagulation factor due to vitamin K deficiency (D68.4)
                vitamin K deficiency of newborn (P53)

    E56.8 Deficiency of other vitamins

    E56.9 Vitamin deficiency, unspecified

E58 **Dietary calcium deficiency**
    EXCLUDES 1   disorders of calcium metabolism (E83.5-)
           sequelae of calcium deficiency (E64.8)

E59 **Dietary selenium deficiency**
    Keshan disease
    EXCLUDES 1   sequelae of selenium deficiency (E64.8)

E60 **Dietary zinc deficiency**

√4ᵗʰ **E61** **Deficiency of other nutrient elements**
    Use additional code for adverse effect, if applicable, to identify drug (T36-T50 with fifth or sixth character 5)
    EXCLUDES 1   disorders of mineral metabolism (E83.-)
           iodine deficiency related thyroid disorders (E00-E02)
           sequelae of malnutrition and other nutritional deficiencies (E64.-)

    E61.0 Copper deficiency

    E61.1 Iron deficiency
        EXCLUDES 1   iron deficiency anemia (D50.-)

    E61.2 Magnesium deficiency

    E61.3 Manganese deficiency

    E61.4 Chromium deficiency

    E61.5 Molybdenum deficiency

    E61.6 Vanadium deficiency

    E61.7 Deficiency of multiple nutrient elements

    E61.8 Deficiency of other specified nutrient elements

    E61.9 Deficiency of nutrient element, unspecified

EXCLUDES 1 Not coded here   EXCLUDES 2 Not included here   N Newborn Age: 0   P Pediatric Age: 0-17   M Maternity Age: 12-55   A Adult Age: 15-124

488   ICD-10-CM Draft (2015)

☑4ᵗʰ **E63 Other nutritional deficiencies**

> **EXCLUDES 1** *dehydration (E86.0)*
> *failure to thrive, adult (R62.7)*
> *failure to thrive, child (R62.51)*
> *feeding problems in newborn (P92.-)*
> *sequelae of malnutrition and other nutritional deficiencies (E64.-)*

     E63.0 Essential fatty acid [EFA] deficiency

     E63.1 Imbalance of constituents of food intake

     E63.8 Other specified nutritional deficiencies

     E63.9 Nutritional deficiency, unspecified

☑4ᵗʰ **E64 Sequelae of malnutrition and other nutritional deficiencies**

> **NOTE** This category is to be used to indicate conditions in categories E43, E44, E46, E50-E63 as the cause of sequelae, which are themselves classified elsewhere. The 'sequelae' include conditions specified as such; they also include the late effects of diseases classifiable to the above categories if the disease itself is no longer present.

> Code first condition resulting from (sequela) of malnutrition and other nutritional deficiencies

     E64.0 Sequelae of protein-calorie malnutrition

> **EXCLUDES 2** *retarded development following protein-calorie malnutrition (E45)*

     E64.1 Sequelae of vitamin A deficiency

     E64.2 Sequelae of vitamin C deficiency

     E64.3 Sequelae of rickets

     E64.8 Sequelae of other nutritional deficiencies

     E64.9 Sequelae of unspecified nutritional deficiency

Overweight, obesity and other hyperalimentation (E65-E68)

E65 Localized adiposity

> Fat pad

☑4ᵗʰ **E66 Overweight and obesity**

> Code first obesity complicating pregnancy, childbirth and the puerperium, if applicable (O99.21-)
> Use additional code to identify body mass index (BMI), if known (Z68.-)

> **EXCLUDES 1** *adiposogenital dystrophy (E23.6)*
> *lipomatosis NOS (E88.2)*
> *lipomatosis dolorosa [Dercum] (E88.2)*
> *Prader-Willi syndrome (Q87.1)*

☑5ᵗʰ   **E66.0** Obesity due to excess calories

       E66.01 Morbid (severe) obesity due to excess calories

> **EXCLUDES 1** *morbid (severe) obesity with alveolar hypoventilation (E66.2)*

       E66.09 Other obesity due to excess calories

     E66.1 Drug-induced obesity

> Use additional code for adverse effect, if applicable, to identify drug (T36-T50 with fifth or sixth character 5)

     E66.2 Morbid (severe) obesity with alveolar hypoventilation

> Pickwickian syndrome

     E66.3 Overweight

     E66.8 Other obesity

     E66.9 Obesity, unspecified

> Obesity NOS

☑4ᵗʰ **E67 Other hyperalimentation**

> **EXCLUDES 1** *hyperalimentation NOS (R63.2)*
> *sequelae of hyperalimentation (E68)*

     E67.0 Hypervitaminosis A

     E67.1 Hypercarotinemia

     E67.2 Megavitamin-B6 syndrome

     E67.3 Hypervitaminosis D

     E67.8 Other specified hyperalimentation

E68 Sequelae of hyperalimentation

> Code first condition resulting from (sequela) of hyperalimentation

Metabolic disorders (E70-E88)

> **EXCLUDES 1** *androgen insensitivity syndrome (E34.5-)*
> *congenital adrenal hyperplasia (E25.0)*
> *Ehlers-Danlos syndrome (Q79.6)*
> *hemolytic anemias attributable to enzyme disorders (D55.-)*
> *Marfan's syndrome (Q87.4)*
> *5-alpha-reductase deficiency (E29.1)*

☑4ᵗʰ **E70 Disorders of aromatic amino-acid metabolism**

     E70.0 Classical phenylketonuria

     E70.1 Other hyperphenylalaninemias

☑5ᵗʰ   **E70.2** Disorders of tyrosine metabolism

> **EXCLUDES 1** *transitory tyrosinemia of newborn (P74.5)*

       E70.20 Disorder of tyrosine metabolism, unspecified

       E70.21 Tyrosinemia

> Hypertyrosinemia

       E70.29 Other disorders of tyrosine metabolism

> Alkaptonuria   Ochronosis

☑5ᵗʰ   **E70.3** Albinism

       E70.30 Albinism, unspecified

☑6ᵗʰ   **E70.31** Ocular albinism

         E70.310 X-linked ocular albinism

         E70.311 Autosomal recessive ocular albinism

         E70.318 Other ocular albinism

         E70.319 Ocular albinism, unspecified

☑6ᵗʰ   **E70.32** Oculocutaneous albinism

> **EXCLUDES 1** *Chediak-Higashi syndrome (E70.330)*
> *Hermansky-Pudlak syndrome (E70.331)*

         E70.320 Tyrosinase negative oculocutaneous albinism

> Albinism I
> Oculocutaneous albinism ty-neg

         E70.321 Tyrosinase positive oculocutaneous albinism

> Albinism II
> Oculocutaneous albinism ty-pos

         E70.328 Other oculocutaneous albinism

> Cross syndrome

         E70.329 Oculocutaneous albinism, unspecified

☑6ᵗʰ   **E70.33** Albinism with hematologic abnormality

         E70.330 Chediak-Higashi syndrome

         E70.331 Hermansky-Pudlak syndrome

         E70.338 Other albinism with hematologic abnormality

         E70.339 Albinism with hematologic abnormality, unspecified

       E70.39 Other specified albinism

> Piebaldism

☑5ᵗʰ   **E70.4** Disorders of histidine metabolism

       E70.40 Disorders of histidine metabolism, unspecified

       E70.41 Histidinemia

       E70.49 Other disorders of histidine metabolism

     E70.5 Disorders of tryptophan metabolism

     E70.8 Other disorders of aromatic amino-acid metabolism

     E70.9 Disorder of aromatic amino-acid metabolism, unspecified

☑4ᵗʰ **E71 Disorders of branched-chain amino-acid metabolism and fatty-acid metabolism**

     E71.0 Maple-syrup-urine disease

☑5ᵗʰ   **E71.1** Other disorders of branched-chain amino-acid metabolism

☑6ᵗʰ   **E71.11** Branched-chain organic acidurias

         E71.110 Isovaleric acidemia

         E71.111 3-methylglutaconic aciduria

         E71.118 Other branched-chain organic acidurias

☑6ᵗʰ   **E71.12** Disorders of propionate metabolism

         E71.120 Methylmalonic acidemia

         E71.121 Propionic acidemia

         E71.128 Other disorders of propionate metabolism

       E71.19 Other disorders of branched-chain amino-acid metabolism

> Hyperleucine-isoleucinemia
> Hypervalinemia

     E71.2 Disorder of branched-chain amino-acid metabolism, unspecified

---

✔ Additional Character Required   ✓x7ᵗʰ Xtension Alert   Unspecified Dx   Other Specified Dx   Manifestation   ►◄ Revised Text   ● New Code   ▲ Revised Code Title

ICD-10-CM Draft (2015)   **489**

Endocrine, Nutritional and Metabolic Diseases   **E71.3–E73.1**

✓5th **E71.3** **Disorders of fatty-acid metabolism**
- EXCLUDES 1   *peroxisomal disorders (E71.5)*
  Refsum's disease (G60.1)
  Schilder's disease (G37.0)
- EXCLUDES 2   *carnitine deficiency due to inborn error of metabolism (E71.42)*

    E71.30 **Disorder of fatty-acid metabolism, unspecified**

✓6th   **E71.31** **Disorders of fatty-acid oxidation**
- **E71.310** **Long chain/very long chain acyl CoA dehydrogenase deficiency**
  - LCAD   VLCAD
- **E71.311** **Medium chain acyl CoA dehydrogenase deficiency**
  - MCAD
- **E71.312** **Short chain acyl CoA dehydrogenase deficiency**
  - SCAD
- **E71.313** **Glutaric aciduria type II**
  - Glutaric aciduria type II A
  - Glutaric aciduria type II B
  - Glutaric aciduria type II C
  - EXCLUDES 1   *glutaric aciduria (type 1) NOS (E72.3)*
- **E71.314** **Muscle carnitine palmitoyltransferase deficiency**
- **E71.318** **Other disorders of fatty-acid oxidation**

    E71.32 **Disorders of ketone metabolism**

    E71.39 **Other disorders of fatty-acid metabolism**

✓5th **E71.4** **Disorders of carnitine metabolism**
- EXCLUDES 1   *muscle carnitine palmitoyltransferase deficiency (E71.314)*

    E71.40 **Disorder of carnitine metabolism, unspecified**

    E71.41 **Primary carnitine deficiency**

    E71.42 **Carnitine deficiency due to inborn errors of metabolism**
- Code also associated inborn error or metabolism

    E71.43 **Iatrogenic carnitine deficiency**
- Carnitine deficiency due to hemodialysis
- Carnitine deficiency due to Valproic acid therapy

✓6th   **E71.44** **Other secondary carnitine deficiency**
- **E71.440** **Ruvalcaba-Myhre-Smith syndrome**
- **E71.448** **Other secondary carnitine deficiency**

✓5th **E71.5** **Peroxisomal disorders**
- EXCLUDES 1   *Schilder's disease (G37.0)*

    E71.50 **Peroxisomal disorder, unspecified**

✓6th   **E71.51** **Disorders of peroxisome biogenesis**
- Group 1 peroxisomal disorders
- EXCLUDES 1   *Refsum's disease (G60.1)*
- **E71.510** **Zellweger syndrome**
- **E71.511** **Neonatal adrenoleukodystrophy** N
  - EXCLUDES 1   *X-linked adrenoleuko- dystrophy (E71.52-)*
- **E71.518** **Other disorders of peroxisome biogenesis**

✓6th   **E71.52** **X-linked adrenoleukodystrophy**
- **E71.520** **Childhood cerebral X-linked adrenoleukodystrophy**
- **E71.521** **Adolescent X-linked adrenoleukodystrophy**
- **E71.522** **Adrenomyeloneuropathy**
- **E71.528** **Other X-linked adrenoleukodystrophy**
  - Addison only phenotype adrenoleukodystrophy
  - Addison-Schilder adrenoleukodystrophy
- **E71.529** **X-linked adrenoleukodystrophy, unspecified type**

    E71.53 **Other group 2 peroxisomal disorders**

✓6th   **E71.54** **Other peroxisomal disorders**
- **E71.540** **Rhizomelic chondrodysplasia punctata**
  - EXCLUDES 1   *chondrodysplasia punctata NOS (Q77.3)*
- **E71.541** **Zellweger-like syndrome**
- **E71.542** **Other group 3 peroxisomal disorders**
- **E71.548** **Other peroxisomal disorders**

✓4th **E72** **Other disorders of amino-acid metabolism**
- EXCLUDES 1   *disorders of:*
  aromatic amino-acid metabolism (E70.-)
  branched-chain amino-acid metabolism (E71.0-E71.2)
  fatty-acid metabolism (E71.3)
  purine and pyrimidine metabolism (E79.-)
  gout (M1A.-, M10.-)

✓5th **E72.0** **Disorders of amino-acid transport**
- EXCLUDES 1   *disorders of tryptophan metabolism (E70.5)*

    E72.00 **Disorders of amino-acid transport, unspecified**

    E72.01 **Cystinuria**

    E72.02 **Hartnup's disease**

    E72.03 **Lowe's syndrome**
- Use additional code for associated glaucoma (H42)

    E72.04 **Cystinosis**
- Fanconi (-de Toni) (-Debré) syndrome with cystinosis
- EXCLUDES 1   *Fanconi (-de Toni) (-Debré) syndrome without cystinosis (E72.09)*

    E72.09 **Other disorders of amino-acid transport**
- Fanconi (-de Toni) (-Debré) syndrome, unspecified

✓5th **E72.1** **Disorders of sulfur-bearing amino-acid metabolism**
- EXCLUDES 1   *cystinosis (E72.04)*
  cystinuria (E72.01)
  transcobalamin II deficiency (D51.2)

    E72.10 **Disorders of sulfur-bearing amino-acid metabolism, unspecified**

    E72.11 **Homocystinuria**
- Cystathionine synthase deficiency

    E72.12 **Methylenetetrahydrofolate reductase deficiency**

    E72.19 **Other disorders of sulfur-bearing amino-acid metabolism**
- Cystathioninuria
- Methioninemia
- Sulfite oxidase deficiency

✓5th **E72.2** **Disorders of urea cycle metabolism**
- EXCLUDES 1   *disorders of ornithine metabolism (E72.4)*

    E72.20 **Disorder of urea cycle metabolism, unspecified**
- Hyperammonemia
- EXCLUDES 1   *hyperammonemia- hyperornithinemia-homocitrullinemia syndrome (E72.4)*
  transient hyperammonemia of newborn (P74.6)

    E72.21 **Argininemia**

    E72.22 **Arginosuccinic aciduria**

    E72.23 **Citrullinemia**

    E72.29 **Other disorders of urea cycle metabolism**

    E72.3 **Disorders of lysine and hydroxylysine metabolism**
- Glutaric aciduria NOS   Hydroxylysinemia
- Glutaric aciduria (type I)   Hyperlysinemia
- EXCLUDES 1   *glutaric aciduria type II (E71.313)*
  Refsum's disease (G60.1)
  Zellweger syndrome (E71.510)

    E72.4 **Disorders of ornithine metabolism**
- Hyperammonemia-hyperornithinemia-homocitrullinemia syndrome
- Ornithinemia (types I, II)
- Ornithine transcarbamylase deficiency
- EXCLUDES 1   *hereditary choroidal dystrophy (H31.2-)*

✓5th **E72.5** **Disorders of glycine metabolism**
- **E72.50** **Disorder of glycine metabolism, unspecified**
- **E72.51** **Non-ketotic hyperglycinemia**
- **E72.52** **Trimethylaminuria**
- **E72.53** **Hyperoxaluria**
  - Oxalosis
  - Oxaluria
- **E72.59** **Other disorders of glycine metabolism**
  - D-glycericacidemia
  - Hyperhydroxyprolinemia
  - Hyperprolinemia (types I, II)
  - Sarcosinemia

    E72.8 **Other specified disorders of amino-acid metabolism**
- Disorders of beta-amino-acid metabolism
- Disorders of gamma-glutamyl cycle

    E72.9 **Disorder of amino-acid metabolism, unspecified**

✓4th **E73** **Lactose intolerance**

    E73.0 **Congenital lactase deficiency**

    E73.1 **Secondary lactase deficiency**

EXCLUDES 1 Not coded here   EXCLUDES 2 Not included here   N Newborn Age: 0   P Pediatric Age: 0-17   M Maternity Age: 12-55   A Adult Age: 15-124

490   ICD-10-CM Draft (2015)

E73.8　**Other lactose intolerance**

E73.9　**Lactose intolerance, unspecified**

✓4th **E74**　**Other disorders of carbohydrate metabolism**
　　EXCLUDES 1　*diabetes mellitus (E08-E13)*
　　　　　　hypoglycemia NOS (E16.2)
　　　　　　increased secretion of glucagon (E16.3)
　　　　　　mucopolysaccharidosis (E76.0-E76.3)

✓5th **E74.0**　Glycogen storage **disease**

　　E74.00　**Glycogen storage disease, unspecified**

　　E74.01　**von Gierke disease**
　　　　　　Type I glycogen storage disease

　　E74.02　**Pompe disease**
　　　　　　Cardiac glycogenosis
　　　　　　Type II glycogen storage disease

　　E74.03　**Cori disease**
　　　　　　Forbes disease
　　　　　　Type III glycogen storage disease

　　E74.04　**McArdle disease**
　　　　　　Type V glycogen storage disease

　　E74.09　**Other glycogen storage disease**
　　　　　　Andersen disease
　　　　　　Hers disease
　　　　　　Tauri disease
　　　　　　Glycogen storage disease, types 0, IV, VI-XI
　　　　　　Liver phosphorylase deficiency
　　　　　　Muscle phosphofructokinase deficiency

✓5th **E74.1**　Disorders of **fructose** metabolism
　　　　EXCLUDES 1　*muscle phosphofructokinase deficiency (E74.09)*

　　E74.10　**Disorder of fructose metabolism, unspecified**

　　E74.11　**Essential fructosuria**
　　　　　　Fructokinase deficiency

　　E74.12　**Hereditary fructose intolerance**
　　　　　　Fructosemia

　　E74.19　**Other disorders of fructose metabolism**
　　　　　　Fructose-1, 6-diphosphatase deficiency

✓5th **E74.2**　Disorders of **galactose** metabolism

　　E74.20　**Disorders of galactose metabolism, unspecified**

　　E74.21　**Galactosemia**

　　E74.29　**Other disorders of galactose metabolism**
　　　　　　Galactokinase deficiency

✓5th **E74.3**　Other disorders of **intestinal carbohydrate absorption**
　　　　EXCLUDES 2　*lactose intolerance (E73.-)*

　　E74.31　**Sucrase-isomaltase deficiency**

　　E74.39　**Other disorders of intestinal carbohydrate absorption**
　　　　　　Disorder of intestinal carbohydrate absorption NOS
　　　　　　Glucose-galactose malabsorption
　　　　　　Sucrase deficiency

　E74.4　**Disorders of pyruvate metabolism and gluconeogenesis**
　　　　Deficiency of phosphoenolpyruvate carboxykinase
　　　　Deficiency of pyruvate carboxylase
　　　　Deficiency of pyruvate dehydrogenase
　　　　EXCLUDES 1　*disorders of pyruvate metabolism and gluconeogenesis with anemia (D55.-)*
　　　　　　Leigh's syndrome (G31.82)

　E74.8　**Other specified disorders of carbohydrate metabolism**
　　　　Essential pentosuria
　　　　Renal glycosuria

　E74.9　**Disorder of carbohydrate metabolism, unspecified**

✓4th **E75**　**Disorders of sphingolipid metabolism and other lipid storage disorders**
　　EXCLUDES 1　*mucolipidosis, types I-III (E77.0-E77.1)*
　　　　　　Refsum's disease (G60.1)

✓5th **E75.0**　GM2 gangliosidosis

　　E75.00　**GM2 gangliosidosis, unspecified**

　　E75.01　**Sandhoff disease**

　　E75.02　**Tay-Sachs disease**

　　E75.09　**Other GM2 gangliosidosis**
　　　　　　Adult GM2 gangliosidosis
　　　　　　Juvenile GM2 gangliosidosis

✓5th **E75.1**　**Other and unspecified gangliosidosis**

　　E75.10　**Unspecified gangliosidosis**
　　　　　　Gangliosidosis NOS

　　E75.11　**Mucolipidosis IV**

　　E75.19　**Other gangliosidosis**
　　　　　　GM1 gangliosidosis
　　　　　　GM3 gangliosidosis

✓5th **E75.2**　**Other sphingolipidosis**
　　　　EXCLUDES 1　*adrenoleukodystrophy [Addison-Schilder] (E71.528)*

　　E75.21　**Fabry (-Anderson) disease**

　　E75.22　**Gaucher disease**

　　E75.23　**Krabbe disease**

✓6th **E75.24**　**Niemann-Pick disease**

　　　　E75.240　**Niemann-Pick disease type A**

　　　　E75.241　**Niemann-Pick disease type B**

　　　　E75.242　**Niemann-Pick disease type C**

　　　　E75.243　**Niemann-Pick disease type D**

　　　　E75.248　**Other Niemann-Pick disease**

　　　　E75.249　**Niemann-Pick disease, unspecified**

　　E75.25　**Metachromatic leukodystrophy**

　　E75.29　**Other sphingolipidosis**
　　　　　　Farber's syndrome
　　　　　　Sulfatase deficiency
　　　　　　Sulfatide lipidosis

　E75.3　**Sphingolipidosis, unspecified**

　E75.4　**Neuronal ceroid lipofuscinosis**
　　　　Batten disease　　　　　　　　Kufs disease
　　　　Bielschowsky-Jansky disease　　Spielmeyer-Vogt disease

　E75.5　**Other lipid storage disorders**
　　　　Cerebrotendinous cholesterosis [van Bogaert-Scherer-Epstein]
　　　　Wolman's disease

　E75.6　**Lipid storage disorder, unspecified**

✓4th **E76**　**Disorders of glycosaminoglycan metabolism**

✓5th **E76.0**　**Mucopolysaccharidosis, type I**

　　E76.01　**Hurler's syndrome**

　　E76.02　**Hurler-Scheie syndrome**

　　E76.03　**Scheie's syndrome**

　E76.1　**Mucopolysaccharidosis, type II**
　　　　Hunter's syndrome

✓5th **E76.2**　**Other mucopolysaccharides**

✓6th **E76.21**　**Morquio mucopolysaccharides**

　　　　E76.210　**Morquio A mucopolysaccharides**
　　　　　　　Classic Morquio syndrome
　　　　　　　Morquio syndrome A
　　　　　　　Mucopolysaccharidosis, type IVA

　　　　E76.211　**Morquio B mucopolysaccharides**
　　　　　　　Morquio-like mucopolysaccharides
　　　　　　　Morquio-like syndrome
　　　　　　　Morquio syndrome B
　　　　　　　Mucopolysaccharidosis, type IVB

　　　　E76.219　**Morquio mucopolysaccharides, unspecified**
　　　　　　　Morquio syndrome
　　　　　　　Mucopolysaccharidosis, type IV

　　E76.22　**Sanfilippo mucopolysaccharides**
　　　　　　Mucopolysaccharidosis, type III (A) (B) (C) (D)
　　　　　　Sanfilippo A syndrome
　　　　　　Sanfilippo B syndrome
　　　　　　Sanfilippo C syndrome
　　　　　　Sanfilippo D syndrome

　　E76.29　**Other mucopolysaccharides**
　　　　　　beta-Glucuronidase deficiency
　　　　　　Maroteaux-Lamy (mild) (severe) syndrome
　　　　　　Mucopolysaccharidosis, types VI, VII

　E76.3　**Mucopolysaccharidosis, unspecified**

　E76.8　**Other disorders of glucosaminoglycan metabolism**

　E76.9　**Glucosaminoglycan metabolism disorder, unspecified**

✓4th **E77**　**Disorders of glycoprotein metabolism**

　E77.0　**Defects in post-translational modification of lysosomal enzymes**
　　　　Mucolipidosis II [I-cell disease]
　　　　Mucolipidosis III [pseudo-Hurler polydystrophy]

　E77.1　**Defects in glycoprotein degradation**
　　　　Aspartylglucosaminuria
　　　　Fucosidosis
　　　　Mannosidosis
　　　　Sialidosis [mucolipidosis I]

　E77.8　**Other disorders of glycoprotein metabolism**

　E77.9　**Disorder of glycoprotein metabolism, unspecified**

✓ Additional Character Required　　✓x7th Xtension Alert　　Unspecified Dx　　Other Specified Dx　　Manifestation　　►◄ Revised Text　　● New Code　　▲ Revised Code Title

ICD-10-CM Draft (2015)　　　　　　　　　　　　　　　　　　　　　　　　　　　　491

✓4ᵗʰ **E78** **Disorders of lipoprotein metabolism and other lipidemias**
     EXCLUDES 1   *sphingolipidosis (E75.0-E75.3)*

     E78.0 **Pure hypercholesterolemia**
         Familial hypercholesterolemia
         Fredrickson's hyperlipoproteinemia, type IIa
         Hyperbetalipoproteinemia
         Hyperlipidemia, Group A
         Low-density-lipoprotein-type [LDL] hyperlipoproteinemia

     E78.1 **Pure hyperglyceridemia**
         Elevated fasting triglycerides
         Endogenous hyperglyceridemia
         Fredrickson's hyperlipoproteinemia, type IV
         Hyperlipidemia, group B
         Hyperprebetalipoproteinemia
         Very-low-density-lipoprotein-type [VLDL] hyperlipoproteinemia

     E78.2 **Mixed hyperlipidemia**
         Broad- or floating-betalipoproteinemia
         Combined hyperlipidemia NOS
         Elevated cholesterol with elevated triglycerides NEC
         Fredrickson's hyperlipoproteinemia, type IIb or III
         Hyperbetalipoproteinemia with prebetalipoproteinemia
         Hypercholesteremia with endogenous hyperglyceridemia
         Hyperlipidemia, group C
         Tubo-eruptive xanthoma
         Xanthoma tuberosum
         EXCLUDES 1   *cerebrotendinous cholesterosis [van Bogaert-Scherer-Epstein] (E75.5)*
                   familial combined hyperlipidemia (E78.4)

     E78.3 **Hyperchylomicronemia**
         Chylomicron retention disease
         Fredrickson's hyperlipoproteinemia, type I or V
         Hyperlipidemia, group D
         Mixed hyperglyceridemia

     E78.4 **Other hyperlipidemia**
         Familial combined hyperlipidemia

     E78.5 **Hyperlipidemia, unspecified**

     E78.6 **Lipoprotein deficiency**
         Abetalipoproteinemia
         Depressed HDL cholesterol
         High-density lipoprotein deficiency
         Hypoalphalipoproteinemia
         Hypobetalipoproteinemia (familial)
         Lecithin cholesterol acyltransferase deficiency
         Tangier disease

✓5ᵗʰ   **E78.7** **Disorders of bile acid and cholesterol metabolism**
         EXCLUDES 1   *Niemann-Pick disease type C (E75.242)*

         E78.70 **Disorder of bile acid and cholesterol metabolism, unspecified**

         E78.71 **Barth syndrome**

         E78.72 **Smith-Lemli-Opitz syndrome**

         E78.79 **Other disorders of bile acid and cholesterol metabolism**

✓5ᵗʰ   **E78.8** **Other disorders of lipoprotein metabolism**
         E78.81 **Lipoid dermatoarthritis**
         E78.89 **Other lipoprotein metabolism disorders**

     E78.9 **Disorder of lipoprotein metabolism, unspecified**

✓4ᵗʰ **E79** **Disorders of purine and pyrimidine metabolism**
     EXCLUDES 1   *Ataxia-telangiectasia (Q87.1)*
                   Bloom's syndrome (Q82.8)
                   Cockayne's syndrome (Q87.1)
                   calculus of kidney (N20.0)
                   combined immunodeficiency disorders (D81.-)
                   Fanconi's anemia (D61.09)
                   gout (M1A.-, M10.-)
                   orotaciduric anemia (D53.0)
                   progeria (E34.8)
                   Werner's syndrome (E34.8)
                   xeroderma pigmentosum (Q82.1)

     E79.0 **Hyperuricemia without signs of inflammatory arthritis and tophaceous disease**
         Asymptomatic hyperuricemia

     E79.1 **Lesch-Nyhan syndrome**
         HGPRT deficiency

     E79.2 **Myoadenylate deaminase deficiency**

     E79.8 **Other disorders of purine and pyrimidine metabolism**
         Hereditary xanthinuria

     E79.9 **Disorder of purine and pyrimidine metabolism, unspecified**

✓4ᵗʰ **E80** **Disorders of porphyrin and bilirubin metabolism**
     INCLUDES   defects of catalase and peroxidase

     E80.0 **Hereditary erythropoietic porphyria**
         Congenital erythropoietic porphyria
         Erythropoietic protoporphyria

     E80.1 **Porphyria cutanea tarda**

✓5ᵗʰ   **E80.2** **Other and unspecified porphyria**
         E80.20 **Unspecified porphyria**
             Porphyria NOS

         E80.21 **Acute intermittent (hepatic) porphyria**

         E80.29 **Other porphyria**
             Hereditary coproporphyria

     E80.3 **Defects of catalase and peroxidase**
         Acatalasia [Takahara]

     E80.4 **Gilbert syndrome**

     E80.5 **Crigler-Najjar syndrome**

     E80.6 **Other disorders of bilirubin metabolism**
         Dubin-Johnson syndrome
         Rotor's syndrome

     E80.7 **Disorder of bilirubin metabolism, unspecified**

✓4ᵗʰ **E83** **Disorders of mineral metabolism**
     EXCLUDES 1   *dietary mineral deficiency (E58-E61)*
                   parathyroid disorders (E20-E21)
                   vitamin D deficiency (E55.-)

✓5ᵗʰ   **E83.0** **Disorders of copper metabolism**
         E83.00 **Disorder of copper metabolism, unspecified**

         E83.01 **Wilson's disease**
             Code also associated Kayser Fleischer ring (H18.04-)

         E83.09 **Other disorders of copper metabolism**
             Menkes' (kinky hair) (steely hair) disease

✓5ᵗʰ   **E83.1** **Disorders of iron metabolism**
         EXCLUDES 1   *iron deficiency anemia (D50.-)*
                       sideroblastic anemia (D64.0-D64.3)

         E83.10 **Disorder of iron metabolism, unspecified**

     ✓6ᵗʰ   **E83.11** **Hemochromatosis**
         E83.110 **Hereditary hemochromatosis**
             Bronzed diabetes
             Pigmentary cirrhosis (of liver)
             Primary (hereditary) hemochromatosis

         E83.111 **Hemochromatosis due to repeated red blood cell transfusions**
             Iron overload due to repeated red blood cell transfusions
             Transfusion (red blood cell) associated hemochromatosis

         E83.118 **Other hemochromatosis**

         E83.119 **Hemochromatosis, unspecified**

         E83.19 **Other disorders of iron metabolism**
             Use additional code, if applicable, for idiopathic pulmonary hemosiderosis (J84.03)

     E83.2 **Disorders of zinc metabolism**
         Acrodermatitis enteropathica

✓5ᵗʰ   **E83.3** **Disorders of phosphorus metabolism and phosphatases**
         EXCLUDES 1   *adult osteomalacia (M83.-)*
                       osteoporosis (M80.-)

         E83.30 **Disorder of phosphorus metabolism, unspecified**

         E83.31 **Familial hypophosphatemia**
             Vitamin D-resistant osteomalacia
             Vitamin D-resistant rickets
             EXCLUDES 1   *vitamin D-deficiency rickets (E55.0)*

         E83.32 **Hereditary vitamin D-dependent rickets (type 1) (type 2)**
             25-hydroxyvitamin D 1-alpha-hydroxylase deficiency
             Pseudovitamin D deficiency
             Vitamin D receptor defect

         E83.39 **Other disorders of phosphorus metabolism**
             Acid phosphatase deficiency
             Hypophosphatasia

✓5ᵗʰ   **E83.4** **Disorders of magnesium metabolism**
         E83.40 **Disorders of magnesium metabolism, unspecified**
         E83.41 **Hypermagnesemia**
         E83.42 **Hypomagnesemia**
         E83.49 **Other disorders of magnesium metabolism**

EXCLUDES 1 Not coded here   EXCLUDES 2 Not included here   N Newborn Age: 0   P Pediatric Age: 0-17   M Maternity Age: 12-55   A Adult Age: 15-124

492   ICD-10-CM Draft (2015)

E83.5 ✓5th **Disorders of calcium metabolism**
  EXCLUDES 1 *chondrocalcinosis (M11.1-M11.2)*
  hungry bone syndrome (E83.81)
  hyperparathyroidism (E21.0-E21.3)
  E83.50 Unspecified disorder of calcium metabolism
  E83.51 Hypocalcemia
  E83.52 Hypercalcemia
    Familial hypocalciuric hypercalcemia
  E83.59 Other disorders of calcium metabolism
    Idiopathic hypercalciuria

E83.8 ✓5th **Other disorders of mineral metabolism**
  E83.81 Hungry bone syndrome
  E83.89 Other disorders of mineral metabolism

E83.9 Disorder of mineral metabolism, unspecified

✓4th **E84 Cystic fibrosis**
  INCLUDES mucoviscidosis
  E84.0 Cystic fibrosis with pulmonary manifestations
    Use additional code to identify any infectious organism present, such as:
    Pseudomonas (B96.5)
  E84.1 ✓5th **Cystic fibrosis with intestinal manifestations**
    E84.11 Meconium ileus in cystic fibrosis N
      EXCLUDES 1 *meconium ileus not due to cystic fibrosis (P76.0)*
    E84.19 Cystic fibrosis with other intestinal manifestations
      Distal intestinal obstruction syndrome
  E84.8 Cystic fibrosis with other manifestations
  E84.9 Cystic fibrosis, unspecified

✓4th **E85 Amyloidosis**
  EXCLUDES 1 *Alzheimer's disease (G30.0-)*
  E85.0 Non-neuropathic heredofamilial amyloidosis
    Familial Mediterranean fever
    Hereditary amyloid nephropathy
  E85.1 Neuropathic heredofamilial amyloidosis
    Amyloid polyneuropathy (Portuguese)
    AHA: 2012, 4Q, 99
  E85.2 Heredofamilial amyloidosis, unspecified
  E85.3 Secondary systemic amyloidosis
    Hemodialysis-associated amyloidosis
  E85.4 Organ-limited amyloidosis
    Localized amyloidosis
  E85.8 Other amyloidosis
  E85.9 Amyloidosis, unspecified

✓4th **E86 Volume depletion**
  EXCLUDES 1 *dehydration of newborn (P74.1)*
  hypovolemic shock NOS (R57.1)
  postprocedural hypovolemic shock (T81.19)
  traumatic hypovolemic shock (T79.4)
  E86.0 Dehydration
    AHA: 2014, 1Q, 7
  E86.1 Hypovolemia
    Depletion of volume of plasma
  E86.9 Volume depletion, unspecified

✓4th **E87 Other disorders of fluid, electrolyte and acid-base balance**
  EXCLUDES 1 *diabetes insipidus (E23.2)*
  electrolyte imbalance associated with hyperemesis gravidarum (O21.1)
  electrolyte imbalance following ectopic or molar pregnancy (O08.5)
  familial periodic paralysis (G72.3)
  E87.0 Hyperosmolality and hypernatremia
    Sodium [Na] excess
    Sodium [Na] overload
    AHA: 2014, 1Q, 7
  E87.1 Hypo-osmolality and hyponatremia
    Sodium [Na] deficiency
    EXCLUDES 1 *syndrome of inappropriate secretion of antidiuretic hormone (E22.2)*
    AHA: 2014, 1Q, 7
  E87.2 Acidosis
    Acidosis NOS   Metabolic acidosis
    Lactic acidosis   Respiratory acidosis
    EXCLUDES 1 *diabetic acidosis—see categories E08-E10, E13 with ketoacidosis*

E87.3 Alkalosis
  Alkalosis NOS   Respiratory alkalosis
  Metabolic alkalosis
E87.4 Mixed disorder of acid-base balance
E87.5 Hyperkalemia
  Potassium [K] excess   Potassium [K] overload
E87.6 Hypokalemia
  Potassium [K] deficiency
✓5th **E87.7 Fluid overload**
  EXCLUDES 1 *edema NOS (R60.9)*
  fluid retention (R60.9)
  E87.70 Fluid overload, unspecified
  E87.71 Transfusion associated circulatory overload
    Fluid overload due to transfusion (blood) (blood components)
    TACO
  E87.79 Other fluid overload
E87.8 Other disorders of electrolyte and fluid balance, not elsewhere classified
  Electrolyte imbalance NOS
  Hyperchloremia
  Hypochloremia

✓4th **E88 Other and unspecified metabolic disorders**
  Use additional codes for associated conditions
  EXCLUDES 1 *histiocytosis X (chronic) (C96.6)*
  ✓5th **E88.0 Disorders of plasma-protein metabolism, not elsewhere classified**
    EXCLUDES 1 *disorder of lipoprotein metabolism (E78.-)*
    monoclonal gammopathy (of undetermined significance) (D47.2)
    polyclonal hypergammaglobulinemia (D89.0)
    Waldenström's macroglobulinemia (C88.0)
    E88.01 Alpha-1-antitrypsin deficiency
      AAT deficiency
    E88.09 Other disorders of plasma-protein metabolism, not elsewhere classified
      Bisalbuminemia
  E88.1 Lipodystrophy, not elsewhere classified
    Lipodystrophy NOS
    EXCLUDES 1 *Whipple's disease (K90.81)*
  E88.2 Lipomatosis, not elsewhere classified
    Lipomatosis NOS
    Lipomatosis (Check) dolorosa [Dercum]
  E88.3 Tumor lysis syndrome
    Tumor lysis syndrome (spontaneous)
    Tumor lysis syndrome following antineoplastic drug chemotherapy
    Use additional code for adverse effect, if applicable, to identify drug (T45.1X5)
  ✓5th **E88.4 Mitochondrial metabolism disorders**
    EXCLUDES 1 *disorders of pyruvate metabolism (E74.4)*
    Kearns-Sayre syndrome (H49.81)
    Leber's disease (H47.22)
    Leigh's encephalopathy (G31.82)
    Mitochondrial myopathy, NEC (G71.3)
    Reye's syndrome (G93.7)
    E88.40 Mitochondrial metabolism disorder, unspecified
    E88.41 MELAS syndrome
      Mitochondrial myopathy, encephalopathy, lactic acidosis and stroke-like episodes
    E88.42 MERRF syndrome
      Myoclonic epilepsy associated with ragged-red fibers
      Code also myoclonic epilepsy (G40.3-)
    E88.49 Other mitochondrial metabolism disorders
  ✓5th **E88.8 Other specified metabolic disorders**
    E88.81 Metabolic syndrome
      Dysmetabolic syndrome X
      Use additional codes for associated manifestations, such as:
      obesity (E66.-)
    E88.89 Other specified metabolic disorders
      Launois-Bensaude adenolipomatosis
      EXCLUDES 1 *adult pulmonary Langerhans cell histiocytosis (J84.82)*
  E88.9 Metabolic disorder, unspecified

Endocrine, Nutritional and Metabolic Diseases

E89–E89.89

✓4ᵗʰ **E89 Postprocedural endocrine and metabolic complications and disorders, not elsewhere classified**

> **EXCLUDES 2** *intraoperative complications of endocrine system organ or structure (E36.0-, E36.1-, E36.8)*

E89.0 Postprocedural hypothyroidism
Postirradiation hypothyroidism
Postsurgical hypothyroidism

E89.1 Postprocedural hypoinsulinemia
Postpancreatectomy hyperglycemia
Postsurgical hypoinsulinemia
Use additional code, if applicable, to identify:
  acquired absence of pancreas (Z90.41-)
  diabetes mellitus (postpancreatectomy) (postprocedural) (E13.-)
  insulin use (Z79.4)

> **EXCLUDES 1** *transient postprocedural hyperglycemia (R73.9)*
> *transient postprocedural hypoglycemia (E16.2)*

E89.2 Postprocedural hypoparathyroidism
Parathyroprival tetany

E89.3 Postprocedural hypopituitarism
Postirradiation hypopituitarism

✓5ᵗʰ **E89.4 Postprocedural ovarian failure**

E89.40 Asymptomatic postprocedural ovarian failure ♀
Postprocedural ovarian failure NOS

E89.41 Symptomatic postprocedural ovarian failure ♀
Symptoms such as flushing, sleeplessness, headache, lack of concentration, associated with postprocedural menopause

E89.5 Postprocedural testicular hypofunction ♂

E89.6 Postprocedural adrenocortical (-medullary) hypofunction

✓5ᵗʰ **E89.8 Other postprocedural endocrine and metabolic complications and disorders**

✓6ᵗʰ **E89.81 Postprocedural hemorrhage and hematoma of an endocrine system organ or structure following a procedure**

E89.810 Postprocedural hemorrhage and hematoma of an endocrine system organ or structure following an endocrine system procedure

E89.811 Postprocedural hemorrhage and hematoma of an endocrine system organ or structure following other procedure

E89.89 Other postprocedural endocrine and metabolic complications and disorders
Use additional code, if applicable, to further specify disorder

EXCLUDES 1 Not coded here   **EXCLUDES 2** Not included here   N Newborn Age: 0   P Pediatric Age: 0-17   M Maternity Age: 12-55   A Adult Age: 15-124

494
ICD-10-CM Draft (2015)

Chapter 5. Mental, Behavioral, and Neurodevelopmental Disorders (F01-F99)

INCLUDES disorders of psychological development
EXCLUDES 2 *symptoms, signs and abnormal clinical laboratory findings, not elsewhere classified (R00-R99)*

This chapter contains the following blocks:

F01-F09   Mental disorders due to known physiological conditions
F10-F19   Mental and behavioral disorders due to psychoactive substance use
F20-F29   Schizophrenia, schizotypal, delusional, and other non-mood psychotic disorders
F30-F39   Mood [affective] disorders
F40-F48   Anxiety, dissociative, stress-related, somatoform and other nonpsychotic mental disorders
F50-F59   Behavioral syndromes associated with physiological disturbances and physical factors
F60-F69   Disorders of adult personality and behavior
F70-F79   Intellectual disabilities
F80-F89   Pervasive and specific developmental disorders
F90-F98   Behavioral and emotional disorders with onset usually occurring in childhood and adolescence
F99   Unspecified mental disorder

Mental disorders due to known physiological conditions (F01-F09)

NOTE   This block comprises a range of mental disorders grouped together on the basis of their having in common a demonstrable etiology in cerebral disease, brain injury, or other insult leading to cerebral dysfunction. The dysfunction may be primary, as in diseases, injuries, and insults that affect the brain directly and selectively; or secondary, as in systemic diseases and disorders that attack the brain only as one of the multiple organs or systems of the body that are involved.

✓4th **F01 Vascular dementia**

Vascular dementia as a result of infarction of the brain due to vascular disease, including hypertensive cerebrovascular disease.
INCLUDES arteriosclerotic dementia
Code first the underlying physiological condition or sequelae of cerebrovascular disease.

✓5th **F01.5 Vascular dementia**

F01.50   **Vascular dementia** without behavioral disturbance   A

F01.51   **Vascular dementia** with behavioral disturbance   A
Vascular dementia with aggressive behavior
Vascular dementia with combative behavior
Vascular dementia with violent behavior
Use additional code, if applicable, to identify wandering in vascular dementia (Z91.83)

✓4th **F02 Dementia in other diseases classified elsewhere**

Code first the underlying physiological condition, such as:
Alzheimer's (G30.-)
cerebral lipidosis (E75.4)
Creutzfeldt-Jakob disease (A81.0-)
dementia with Lewy bodies (G31.83)
epilepsy and recurrent seizures (G40.-)
frontotemporal dementia (G31.09)
hepatolenticular degeneration (E83.0)
human immunodeficiency virus [HIV] disease (B20)
hypercalcemia (E83.52)
hypothyroidism, acquired (E00-E03.-)
intoxications (T36-T65)
Jakob-Creutzfeldt disease (A81.0-)
multiple sclerosis (G35)
neurosyphilis (A52.17)
niacin deficiency [pellagra] (E52)
Parkinson's disease (G20)
Pick's disease (G31.01)
polyarteritis nodosa (M30.0)
systemic lupus erythematosus (M32.-)
trypanosomiasis (B56.-, B57.-)
vitamin B deficiency (E53.8)
EXCLUDES 1 *dementia with Parkinsonism (G31.83)*
EXCLUDES 2 *dementia in alcohol and psychoactive substance disorders (F10-F19, with .17, .27, .97)*
vascular dementia (F01.5-)

✓5th **F02.8 Dementia in other diseases classified elsewhere**

F02.80   ***Dementia in other diseases classified elsewhere without behavioral disturbance***
Dementia in other diseases classified elsewhere NOS

F02.81   ***Dementia in other diseases classified elsewhere with behavioral disturbance***
Dementia in other diseases classified elsewhere with aggressive behavior
Dementia in other diseases classified elsewhere with combative behavior
Dementia in other diseases classified elsewhere with violent behavior
Use additional code, if applicable, to identify wandering in dementia in conditions classified elsewhere (Z91.83)

✓4th **F03 Unspecified dementia**

Presenile dementia NOS
Presenile psychosis NOS
Primary degenerative dementia NOS
Senile dementia NOS
Senile dementia depressed or paranoid type
Senile psychosis NOS
EXCLUDES 1 *senility NOS (R41.81)*
EXCLUDES 2 *mild memory disturbance due to known physiological condition (F06.8)*
senile dementia with delirium or acute confusional state (F05)

✓5th **F03.9 Unspecified dementia**

F03.90   **Unspecified dementia** without behavioral disturbance   A
Dementia NOS
AHA: 2012, 4Q, 92

F03.91   **Unspecified dementia** with behavioral disturbance   A
Unspecified dementia with aggressive behavior
Unspecified dementia with combative behavior
Unspecified dementia with violent behavior
Use additional code, if applicable, to identify wandering in unspecified dementia (Z91.83)

F04 Amnestic disorder due to known physiological condition

Korsakov's psychosis or syndrome, nonalcoholic
Code first the underlying physiological condition
EXCLUDES 1 *amnesia NOS (R41.3)*
anterograde amnesia (R41.1)
dissociative amnesia (F44.0)
retrograde amnesia (R41.2)
EXCLUDES 2 *alcohol-induced or unspecified Korsakov's syndrome (F10.26, F10.96)*
Korsakov's syndrome induced by other psychoactive substances (F13.26, F13.96, F19.16, F19.26, F19.96)

F05 Delirium due to known physiological condition

Acute or subacute brain syndrome
Acute or subacute confusional state (nonalcoholic)
Acute or subacute infective psychosis
Acute or subacute organic reaction
Acute or subacute psycho-organic syndrome
Delirium of mixed etiology
Delirium superimposed on dementia
Sundowning
Code first the underlying physiological condition
EXCLUDES 1 *delirium NOS (R41.0)*
EXCLUDES 2 *delirium tremens alcohol-induced or unspecified (F10.231, F10.921)*

✓4th **F06 Other mental disorders due to known physiological condition**

INCLUDES mental disorders due to endocrine disorder
mental disorders due to exogenous hormone
mental disorders due to exogenous toxic substance
mental disorders due to primary cerebral disease
mental disorders due to somatic illness
mental disorders due to systemic disease affecting the brain
Code first the underlying physiological condition
EXCLUDES 1 *unspecified dementia (F03)*
EXCLUDES 2 *delirium due to known physiological condition (F05)*
dementia as classified in F01-F02
other mental disorders associated with alcohol and other psychoactive substances (F10-F19)

F06.0   **Psychotic disorder** with hallucinations **due to known physiological condition**
Organic hallucinatory state (nonalcoholic)
EXCLUDES 2 *hallucinations and perceptual disturbance induced by alcohol and other psychoactive substances (F10-F19 with .151, .251, .951)*
schizophrenia (F20.-)

✓ Additional Character Required   ✓x7th Xtension Alert   Unspecified Dx   Other Specified Dx   Manifestation   ▶◀ Revised Text   ● New Code   ▲ Revised Code Title

ICD-10-CM Draft (2015)   **495**

Mental, Behavioral, and Neurodevelopmental Disorders

F06.1–F10.27

F06.1 Catatonic disorder due to known physiological condition
- EXCLUDES 1   *catatonic stupor (R40.1)*
  stupor NOS (R40.1)
- EXCLUDES 2   *catatonic schizophrenia (F20.2)*
  dissociative stupor (F44.2)

F06.2 Psychotic disorder with delusions due to known physiological condition
- Paranoid and paranoid-hallucinatory organic states
- Schizophrenia-like psychosis in epilepsy
- EXCLUDES 2   *alcohol and drug-induced psychotic disorder (F10-F19 with .150, .250, .950)*
  brief psychotic disorder (F23)
  delusional disorder (F22)
  schizophrenia (F20.-)

✓5ᵗʰ **F06.3** Mood disorder due to known physiological condition
- EXCLUDES 2   *mood disorders due to alcohol and other psychoactive substances (F10-F19 with .14, .24, .94)*
  mood disorders, not due to known physiological condition or unspecified (F30-F39)

   F06.30 Mood disorder due to known physiological condition, unspecified

   F06.31 Mood disorder due to known physiological condition with depressive features

   F06.32 Mood disorder due to known physiological condition with major depressive-like episode

   F06.33 Mood disorder due to known physiological condition with manic features

   F06.34 Mood disorder due to known physiological condition with mixed features

F06.4 Anxiety disorder due to known physiological condition
- EXCLUDES 2   *anxiety disorders due to alcohol and other psychoactive substances (F10-F19 with .180, .280, .980)*
  anxiety disorders, not due to known physiological condition or unspecified (F40.-, F41.-)

F06.8 Other specified mental disorders due to known physiological condition
- Epileptic psychosis NOS
- Organic dissociative disorder
- Organic emotionally labile [asthenic] disorder

✓4ᵗʰ **F07** Personality and behavioral disorders due to known physiological condition
- Code first the underlying physiological condition

   F07.0 Personality change due to known physiological condition
- Frontal lobe syndrome
- Limbic epilepsy personality syndrome
- Lobotomy syndrome
- Organic personality disorder
- Organic pseudopsychopathic personality
- Organic pseudoretarded personality
- Postleucotomy syndrome
- Code first underlying physiological condition
  - EXCLUDES 1   *mild cognitive impairment (G31.84)*
    postconcussional syndrome (F07.81)
    postencephalitic syndrome (F07.89)
    signs and symptoms involving emotional state (R45.-)
  - EXCLUDES 2   *specific personality disorder (F60.-)*

✓5ᵗʰ **F07.8** Other personality and behavioral disorders due to known physiological condition

   F07.81 Postconcussional syndrome
- Postcontusional syndrome (encephalopathy)
- Post-traumatic brain syndrome, nonpsychotic
- Use additional code to identify associated post-traumatic headache, if applicable (G44.3-)
  - EXCLUDES 1   *current concussion (brain) (S06.0-)*
    postencephalitic syndrome (F07.89)

   F07.89 Other personality and behavioral disorders due to known physiological condition
- Postencephalitic syndrome
- Right hemispheric organic affective disorder

F07.9 Unspecified personality and behavioral disorder due to known physiological condition
- Organic psychosyndrome

F09 Unspecified mental disorder due to known physiological condition
- Mental disorder NOS due to known physiological condition
- Organic brain syndrome NOS
- Organic mental disorder NOS
- Organic psychosis NOS
- Symptomatic psychosis NOS
- Code first the underlying physiological condition
  - EXCLUDES 1   *psychosis NOS (F29)*

Mental and behavioral disorders due to psychoactive substance use (F10-F19)

✓4ᵗʰ **F10** Alcohol related disorders
- Use additional code for blood alcohol level, if applicable (Y90.-)

✓5ᵗʰ **F10.1** Alcohol abuse
- EXCLUDES 1   *alcohol dependence (F10.2-)*
  alcohol use, unspecified (F10.9-)

   F10.10 Alcohol abuse, uncomplicated

✓6ᵗʰ **F10.12** Alcohol abuse with intoxication

   F10.120 Alcohol abuse with intoxication, uncomplicated

   F10.121 Alcohol abuse with intoxication delirium

   F10.129 Alcohol abuse with intoxication, unspecified

   F10.14 Alcohol abuse with alcohol-induced mood disorder

✓6ᵗʰ **F10.15** Alcohol abuse with alcohol-induced psychotic disorder

   F10.150 Alcohol abuse with alcohol-induced psychotic disorder with delusions

   F10.151 Alcohol abuse with alcohol-induced psychotic disorder with hallucinations

   F10.159 Alcohol abuse with alcohol-induced psychotic disorder, unspecified

✓6ᵗʰ **F10.18** Alcohol abuse with other alcohol-induced disorders

   F10.180 Alcohol abuse with alcohol-induced anxiety disorder

   F10.181 Alcohol abuse with alcohol-induced sexual dysfunction

   F10.182 Alcohol abuse with alcohol-induced sleep disorder

   F10.188 Alcohol abuse with other alcohol-induced disorder

   F10.19 Alcohol abuse with unspecified alcohol-induced disorder

✓5ᵗʰ **F10.2** Alcohol dependence
- EXCLUDES 1   *alcohol abuse (F10.1-)*
  alcohol use, unspecified (F10.9-)
- EXCLUDES 2   *toxic effect of alcohol (T51.0-)*

   F10.20 Alcohol dependence, uncomplicated

   F10.21 Alcohol dependence, in remission

✓6ᵗʰ **F10.22** Alcohol dependence with intoxication
- Acute drunkenness (in alcoholism)
  - EXCLUDES 1   *alcohol dependence with withdrawal (F10.23-)*

   F10.220 Alcohol dependence with intoxication, uncomplicated

   F10.221 Alcohol dependence with intoxication delirium

   F10.229 Alcohol dependence with intoxication, unspecified

✓6ᵗʰ **F10.23** Alcohol dependence with withdrawal
- EXCLUDES 1   *Alcohol dependence with intoxication (F10.22-)*

   F10.230 Alcohol dependence with withdrawal, uncomplicated

   F10.231 Alcohol dependence with withdrawal delirium

   F10.232 Alcohol dependence with withdrawal with perceptual disturbance

   F10.239 Alcohol dependence with withdrawal, unspecified

   F10.24 Alcohol dependence with alcohol-induced mood disorder

✓6ᵗʰ **F10.25** Alcohol dependence with alcohol-induced psychotic disorder

   F10.250 Alcohol dependence with alcohol-induced psychotic disorder with delusions

   F10.251 Alcohol dependence with alcohol-induced psychotic disorder with hallucinations

   F10.259 Alcohol dependence with alcohol-induced psychotic disorder, unspecified

   F10.26 Alcohol dependence with alcohol-induced persisting amnestic disorder

   F10.27 Alcohol dependence with alcohol-induced persisting dementia

---

EXCLUDES 1 Not coded here   EXCLUDES 2 Not included here   N Newborn Age: 0   P Pediatric Age: 0-17   M Maternity Age: 12-55   A Adult Age: 15-124

✓6th F10.28　Alcohol dependence with other alcohol-induced disorders

F10.280　Alcohol dependence with alcohol-induced anxiety disorder

F10.281　Alcohol dependence with alcohol-induced sexual dysfunction

F10.282　Alcohol dependence with alcohol-induced sleep disorder

F10.288　Alcohol dependence with other alcohol-induced disorder

F10.29　Alcohol dependence with unspecified alcohol-induced disorder

✓5th F10.9　Alcohol use, unspecified

EXCLUDES 1　alcohol abuse (F10.1-)
alcohol dependence (F10.2-)

✓6th F10.92　Alcohol use, unspecified with intoxication

F10.920　Alcohol use, unspecified with intoxication, uncomplicated

F10.921　Alcohol use, unspecified with intoxication delirium

F10.929　Alcohol use, unspecified with intoxication, unspecified

F10.94　Alcohol use, unspecified with alcohol-induced mood disorder

✓6th F10.95　Alcohol use, unspecified with alcohol-induced psychotic disorder

F10.950　Alcohol use, unspecified with alcohol-induced psychotic disorder with delusions

F10.951　Alcohol use, unspecified with alcohol-induced psychotic disorder with hallucinations

F10.959　Alcohol use, unspecified with alcohol-induced psychotic disorder, unspecified

F10.96　Alcohol use, unspecified with alcohol-induced persisting amnestic disorder

F10.97　Alcohol use, unspecified with alcohol-induced persisting dementia

✓6th F10.98　Alcohol use, unspecified with other alcohol-induced disorders

F10.980　Alcohol use, unspecified with alcohol-induced anxiety disorder

F10.981　Alcohol use, unspecified with alcohol-induced sexual dysfunction

F10.982　Alcohol use, unspecified with alcohol-induced sleep disorder

F10.988　Alcohol use, unspecified with other alcohol-induced disorder

F10.99　Alcohol use, unspecified with unspecified alcohol-induced disorder

✓4th F11　Opioid related disorders

✓5th F11.1　Opioid abuse

EXCLUDES 1　opioid dependence (F11.2-)
opioid use, unspecified (F11.9-)

F11.10　Opioid abuse, uncomplicated

✓6th F11.12　Opioid abuse with intoxication

F11.120　Opioid abuse with intoxication, uncomplicated

F11.121　Opioid abuse with intoxication delirium

F11.122　Opioid abuse with intoxication with perceptual disturbance

F11.129　Opioid abuse with intoxication, unspecified

F11.14　Opioid abuse with opioid-induced mood disorder

✓6th F11.15　Opioid abuse with opioid-induced psychotic disorder

F11.150　Opioid abuse with opioid-induced psychotic disorder with delusions

F11.151　Opioid abuse with opioid-induced psychotic disorder with hallucinations

F11.159　Opioid abuse with opioid-induced psychotic disorder, unspecified

✓6th F11.18　Opioid abuse with other opioid-induced disorder

F11.181　Opioid abuse with opioid-induced sexual dysfunction

F11.182　Opioid abuse with opioid-induced sleep disorder

F11.188　Opioid abuse with other opioid-induced disorder

F11.19　Opioid abuse with unspecified opioid-induced disorder

✓5th F11.2　Opioid dependence

EXCLUDES 1　opioid abuse (F11.1-)
opioid use, unspecified (F11.9-)

EXCLUDES 2　opioid poisoning (T40.0-T40.2-)

F11.20　Opioid dependence, uncomplicated

F11.21　Opioid dependence, in remission

✓6th F11.22　Opioid dependence with intoxication

EXCLUDES 1　opioid dependence with withdrawal (F11.23)

F11.220　Opioid dependence with intoxication, uncomplicated

F11.221　Opioid dependence with intoxication delirium

F11.222　Opioid dependence with intoxication with perceptual disturbance

F11.229　Opioid dependence with intoxication, unspecified

F11.23　Opioid dependence with withdrawal

EXCLUDES 1　opioid dependence with intoxication (F11.22-)

F11.24　Opioid dependence with opioid-induced mood disorder

✓6th F11.25　Opioid dependence with opioid-induced psychotic disorder

F11.250　Opioid dependence with opioid-induced psychotic disorder with delusions

F11.251　Opioid dependence with opioid-induced psychotic disorder with hallucinations

F11.259　Opioid dependence with opioid-induced psychotic disorder, unspecified

✓6th F11.28　Opioid dependence with other opioid-induced disorder

F11.281　Opioid dependence with opioid-induced sexual dysfunction

F11.282　Opioid dependence with opioid-induced sleep disorder

F11.288　Opioid dependence with other opioid-induced disorder

F11.29　Opioid dependence with unspecified opioid-induced disorder

✓5th F11.9　Opioid use, unspecified

EXCLUDES 1　opioid abuse (F11.1-)
opioid dependence (F11.2-)

F11.90　Opioid use, unspecified, uncomplicated

✓6th F11.92　Opioid use, unspecified with intoxication

EXCLUDES 1　opioid use, unspecified with withdrawal (F11.93)

F11.920　Opioid use, unspecified with intoxication, uncomplicated

F11.921　Opioid use, unspecified with intoxication delirium

F11.922　Opioid use, unspecified with intoxication with perceptual disturbance

F11.929　Opioid use, unspecified with intoxication, unspecified

F11.93　Opioid use, unspecified with withdrawal

EXCLUDES 1　opioid use, unspecified with intoxication (F11.92-)

F11.94　Opioid use, unspecified with opioid-induced mood disorder

✓6th F11.95　Opioid use, unspecified with opioid-induced psychotic disorder

F11.950　Opioid use, unspecified with opioid-induced psychotic disorder with delusions

F11.951　Opioid use, unspecified with opioid-induced psychotic disorder with hallucinations

F11.959　Opioid use, unspecified with opioid-induced psychotic disorder, unspecified

✔ Additional Character Required　　✓x7th Xtension Alert　　Unspecified Dx　　Other Specified Dx　　Manifestation　　►◄ Revised Text　　● New Code　　▲ Revised Code Title

ICD-10-CM Draft (2015)　　　　　　497

✓6ᵗʰ F11.98 Opioid use, unspecified with other specified opioid-induced disorder
- F11.981 Opioid use, unspecified with opioid-induced sexual dysfunction
- F11.982 Opioid use, unspecified with opioid-induced sleep disorder
- F11.988 Opioid use, unspecified with other opioid-induced disorder

F11.99 Opioid use, unspecified with unspecified opioid-induced disorder

✓4ᵗʰ F12 Cannabis related disorders
INCLUDES marijuana

✓5ᵗʰ F12.1 Cannabis abuse
EXCLUDES 1 cannabis dependence (F12.2-)
cannabis use, unspecified (F12.9-)

F12.10 Cannabis abuse, uncomplicated

✓6ᵗʰ F12.12 Cannabis abuse with intoxication
- F12.120 Cannabis abuse with intoxication, uncomplicated
- F12.121 Cannabis abuse with intoxication delirium
- F12.122 Cannabis abuse with intoxication with perceptual disturbance
- F12.129 Cannabis abuse with intoxication, unspecified

✓6ᵗʰ F12.15 Cannabis abuse with psychotic disorder
- F12.150 Cannabis abuse with psychotic disorder with delusions
- F12.151 Cannabis abuse with psychotic disorder with hallucinations
- F12.159 Cannabis abuse with psychotic disorder, unspecified

✓6ᵗʰ F12.18 Cannabis abuse with other cannabis-induced disorder
- F12.180 Cannabis abuse with cannabis-induced anxiety disorder
- F12.188 Cannabis abuse with other cannabis-induced disorder

F12.19 Cannabis abuse with unspecified cannabis-induced disorder

✓5ᵗʰ F12.2 Cannabis dependence
EXCLUDES 1 cannabis abuse (F12.1-)
cannabis use, unspecified (F12.9-)
EXCLUDES 2 cannabis poisoning (T40.7-)

F12.20 Cannabis dependence, uncomplicated

F12.21 Cannabis dependence, in remission

✓6ᵗʰ F12.22 Cannabis dependence with intoxication
- F12.220 Cannabis dependence with intoxication, uncomplicated
- F12.221 Cannabis dependence with intoxication delirium
- F12.222 Cannabis dependence with intoxication with perceptual disturbance
- F12.229 Cannabis dependence with intoxication, unspecified

✓6ᵗʰ F12.25 Cannabis dependence with psychotic disorder
- F12.250 Cannabis dependence with psychotic disorder with delusions
- F12.251 Cannabis dependence with psychotic disorder with hallucinations
- F12.259 Cannabis dependence with psychotic disorder, unspecified

✓6ᵗʰ F12.28 Cannabis dependence with other cannabis-induced disorder
- F12.280 Cannabis dependence with cannabis-induced anxiety disorder
- F12.288 Cannabis dependence with other cannabis-induced disorder

F12.29 Cannabis dependence with unspecified cannabis-induced disorder

✓5ᵗʰ F12.9 Cannabis use, unspecified
EXCLUDES 1 cannabis abuse (F12.1-)
cannabis dependence (F12.2-)

F12.90 Cannabis use, unspecified, uncomplicated

✓6ᵗʰ F12.92 Cannabis use, unspecified with intoxication
- F12.920 Cannabis use, unspecified with intoxication, uncomplicated

- F12.921 Cannabis use, unspecified with intoxication delirium
- F12.922 Cannabis use, unspecified with intoxication with perceptual disturbance
- F12.929 Cannabis use, unspecified with intoxication, unspecified

✓6ᵗʰ F12.95 Cannabis use, unspecified with psychotic disorder
- F12.950 Cannabis use, unspecified with psychotic disorder with delusions
- F12.951 Cannabis use, unspecified with psychotic disorder with hallucinations
- F12.959 Cannabis use, unspecified with psychotic disorder, unspecified

✓6ᵗʰ F12.98 Cannabis use, unspecified with other cannabis-induced disorder
- F12.980 Cannabis use, unspecified with anxiety disorder
- F12.988 Cannabis use, unspecified with other cannabis-induced disorder

F12.99 Cannabis use, unspecified with unspecified cannabis-induced disorder

✓4ᵗʰ F13 Sedative, hypnotic, or anxiolytic related disorders

✓5ᵗʰ F13.1 Sedative, hypnotic or anxiolytic-related abuse
EXCLUDES 1 sedative, hypnotic or anxiolytic-related dependence (F13.2-)
sedative, hypnotic, or anxiolytic use, unspecified (F13.9-)

F13.10 Sedative, hypnotic or anxiolytic abuse, uncomplicated

✓6ᵗʰ F13.12 Sedative, hypnotic or anxiolytic abuse with intoxication
- F13.120 Sedative, hypnotic or anxiolytic abuse with intoxication, uncomplicated
- F13.121 Sedative, hypnotic or anxiolytic abuse with intoxication delirium
- F13.129 Sedative, hypnotic or anxiolytic abuse with intoxication, unspecified

F13.14 Sedative, hypnotic or anxiolytic abuse with sedative, hypnotic or anxiolytic-induced mood disorder

✓6ᵗʰ F13.15 Sedative, hypnotic or anxiolytic abuse with sedative, hypnotic or anxiolytic-induced psychotic disorder
- F13.150 Sedative, hypnotic or anxiolytic abuse with sedative, hypnotic or anxiolytic-induced psychotic disorder with delusions
- F13.151 Sedative, hypnotic or anxiolytic abuse with sedative, hypnotic or anxiolytic-induced psychotic disorder with hallucinations
- F13.159 Sedative, hypnotic or anxiolytic abuse with sedative, hypnotic or anxiolytic-induced psychotic disorder, unspecified

✓6ᵗʰ F13.18 Sedative, hypnotic or anxiolytic abuse with other sedative, hypnotic or anxiolytic-induced disorders
- F13.180 Sedative, hypnotic or anxiolytic abuse with sedative, hypnotic or anxiolytic-induced anxiety disorder
- F13.181 Sedative, hypnotic or anxiolytic abuse with sedative, hypnotic or anxiolytic-induced sexual dysfunction
- F13.182 Sedative, hypnotic or anxiolytic abuse with sedative, hypnotic or anxiolytic-induced sleep disorder
- F13.188 Sedative, hypnotic or anxiolytic abuse with other sedative, hypnotic or anxiolytic-induced disorder

F13.19 Sedative, hypnotic or anxiolytic abuse with unspecified sedative, hypnotic or anxiolytic-induced disorder

✓5ᵗʰ F13.2 Sedative, hypnotic or anxiolytic-related dependence
EXCLUDES 1 sedative, hypnotic or anxiolytic-related abuse (F13.1-)
sedative, hypnotic, or anxiolytic use, unspecified (F13.9-)
EXCLUDES 2 sedative, hypnotic, or anxiolytic poisoning (T42.-)

F13.20 Sedative, hypnotic or anxiolytic dependence, uncomplicated

F13.21 Sedative, hypnotic or anxiolytic dependence, in remission

EXCLUDES 1 Not coded here   EXCLUDES 2 Not included here   N Newborn Age: 0   P Pediatric Age: 0-17   M Maternity Age: 12-55   A Adult Age: 15-124

498   ICD-10-CM Draft (2015)

☑6ᵗʰ **F13.22** Sedative, hypnotic or anxiolytic dependence with intoxication
> EXCLUDES 1   *sedative, hypnotic or anxiolytic dependence with withdrawal (F13.23-)*

     F13.220 Sedative, hypnotic or anxiolytic dependence with intoxication, uncomplicated

     F13.221 Sedative, hypnotic or anxiolytic dependence with intoxication delirium

     F13.229 Sedative, hypnotic or anxiolytic dependence with intoxication, unspecified

☑6ᵗʰ **F13.23** Sedative, hypnotic or anxiolytic dependence with withdrawal
> EXCLUDES 1   *sedative, hypnotic or anxiolytic dependence with intoxication (F13.22-)*

     F13.230 Sedative, hypnotic or anxiolytic dependence with withdrawal, uncomplicated

     F13.231 Sedative, hypnotic or anxiolytic dependence with withdrawal delirium

     F13.232 Sedative, hypnotic or anxiolytic dependence with withdrawal with perceptual disturbance

     F13.239 Sedative, hypnotic or anxiolytic dependence with withdrawal, unspecified

F13.24 Sedative, hypnotic or anxiolytic dependence with sedative, hypnotic or anxiolytic-induced mood disorder

☑6ᵗʰ **F13.25** Sedative, hypnotic or anxiolytic dependence with sedative, hypnotic or anxiolytic-induced psychotic disorder

     F13.250 Sedative, hypnotic or anxiolytic dependence with sedative, hypnotic or anxiolytic-induced psychotic disorder with delusions

     F13.251 Sedative, hypnotic or anxiolytic dependence with sedative, hypnotic or anxiolytic-induced psychotic disorder with hallucinations

     F13.259 Sedative, hypnotic or anxiolytic dependence with sedative, hypnotic or anxiolytic-induced psychotic disorder, unspecified

F13.26 Sedative, hypnotic or anxiolytic dependence with sedative, hypnotic or anxiolytic-induced persisting amnestic disorder

F13.27 Sedative, hypnotic or anxiolytic dependence with sedative, hypnotic or anxiolytic-induced persisting dementia

☑6ᵗʰ **F13.28** Sedative, hypnotic or anxiolytic dependence with other sedative, hypnotic or anxiolytic-induced disorders

     F13.280 Sedative, hypnotic or anxiolytic dependence with sedative, hypnotic or anxiolytic-induced anxiety disorder

     F13.281 Sedative, hypnotic or anxiolytic dependence with sedative, hypnotic or anxiolytic-induced sexual dysfunction

     F13.282 Sedative, hypnotic or anxiolytic dependence with sedative, hypnotic or anxiolytic-induced sleep disorder

     F13.288 Sedative, hypnotic or anxiolytic dependence with other sedative, hypnotic or anxiolytic-induced disorder

F13.29 Sedative, hypnotic or anxiolytic dependence with unspecified sedative, hypnotic or anxiolytic-induced disorder

☑5ᵗʰ **F13.9** Sedative, hypnotic or anxiolytic-related use, unspecified
> EXCLUDES 1   *sedative, hypnotic or anxiolytic-related abuse (F13.1-)*
> *sedative, hypnotic or anxiolytic-related dependence (F13.2-)*

     F13.90 Sedative, hypnotic, or anxiolytic use, unspecified, uncomplicated

☑6ᵗʰ **F13.92** Sedative, hypnotic or anxiolytic use, unspecified with intoxication
> EXCLUDES 1   *sedative, hypnotic or anxiolytic use, unspecified with withdrawal (F13.93-)*

     F13.920 Sedative, hypnotic or anxiolytic use, unspecified with intoxication, uncomplicated

     F13.921 Sedative, hypnotic or anxiolytic use, unspecified with intoxication delirium

     F13.929 Sedative, hypnotic or anxiolytic use, unspecified with intoxication, unspecified

☑6ᵗʰ **F13.93** Sedative, hypnotic or anxiolytic use, unspecified with withdrawal
> EXCLUDES 1   *sedative, hypnotic or anxiolytic use, unspecified with intoxication (F13.92-)*

     F13.930 Sedative, hypnotic or anxiolytic use, unspecified with withdrawal, uncomplicated

     F13.931 Sedative, hypnotic or anxiolytic use, unspecified with withdrawal delirium

     F13.932 Sedative, hypnotic or anxiolytic use, unspecified with withdrawal with perceptual disturbances

     F13.939 Sedative, hypnotic or anxiolytic use, unspecified with withdrawal, unspecified

F13.94 Sedative, hypnotic or anxiolytic use, unspecified with sedative, hypnotic or anxiolytic-induced mood disorder

☑6ᵗʰ **F13.95** Sedative, hypnotic or anxiolytic use, unspecified with sedative, hypnotic or anxiolytic-induced psychotic disorder

     F13.950 Sedative, hypnotic or anxiolytic use, unspecified with sedative, hypnotic or anxiolytic-induced psychotic disorder with delusions

     F13.951 Sedative, hypnotic or anxiolytic use, unspecified with sedative, hypnotic or anxiolytic-induced psychotic disorder with hallucinations

     F13.959 Sedative, hypnotic or anxiolytic use, unspecified with sedative, hypnotic or anxiolytic-induced psychotic disorder, unspecified

F13.96 Sedative, hypnotic or anxiolytic use, unspecified with sedative, hypnotic or anxiolytic-induced persisting amnestic disorder

F13.97 Sedative, hypnotic or anxiolytic use, unspecified with sedative, hypnotic or anxiolytic-induced persisting dementia

☑6ᵗʰ **F13.98** Sedative, hypnotic or anxiolytic use, unspecified with other sedative, hypnotic or anxiolytic-induced disorders

     F13.980 Sedative, hypnotic or anxiolytic use, unspecified with sedative, hypnotic or anxiolytic-induced anxiety disorder

     F13.981 Sedative, hypnotic or anxiolytic use, unspecified with sedative, hypnotic or anxiolytic-induced sexual dysfunction

     F13.982 Sedative, hypnotic or anxiolytic use, unspecified with sedative, hypnotic or anxiolytic-induced sleep disorder

     F13.988 Sedative, hypnotic or anxiolytic use, unspecified with other sedative, hypnotic or anxiolytic-induced disorder

F13.99 Sedative, hypnotic or anxiolytic use, unspecified with unspecified sedative, hypnotic or anxiolytic-induced disorder

☑4ᵗʰ **F14** **Cocaine related disorders**
> EXCLUDES 2   *other stimulant-related disorders (F15.-)*

☑5ᵗʰ **F14.1** Cocaine abuse
> EXCLUDES 1   *cocaine dependence (F14.2-)*
> *cocaine use, unspecified (F14.9-)*

     F14.10 Cocaine abuse, uncomplicated

☑6ᵗʰ   **F14.12** Cocaine abuse with intoxication

         F14.120 Cocaine abuse with intoxication, uncomplicated

         F14.121 Cocaine abuse with intoxication with delirium

☑ Additional Character Required   √x7ᵗʰ *X*tension Alert   Unspecified Dx   Other Specified Dx   Manifestation   ►◄ Revised Text   ● New Code   ▲ Revised Code Title

ICD-10-CM Draft (2015)   499

Mental, Behavioral, and Neurodevelopmental Disorders

F14.122–F15.21

         F14.122   Cocaine abuse with intoxication with perceptual disturbance

         F14.129   Cocaine abuse with intoxication, unspecified

     F14.14   Cocaine abuse with cocaine-induced mood disorder

√6th   **F14.15**   Cocaine abuse with cocaine-induced psychotic disorder

         F14.150   Cocaine abuse with cocaine-induced psychotic disorder with delusions

         F14.151   Cocaine abuse with cocaine-induced psychotic disorder with hallucinations

         F14.159   Cocaine abuse with cocaine-induced psychotic disorder, unspecified

√6th   **F14.18**   Cocaine abuse with other cocaine-induced disorder

         F14.180   Cocaine abuse with cocaine-induced anxiety disorder

         F14.181   Cocaine abuse with cocaine-induced sexual dysfunction

         F14.182   Cocaine abuse with cocaine-induced sleep disorder

         F14.188   Cocaine abuse with other cocaine-induced disorder

     F14.19   Cocaine abuse with unspecified cocaine-induced disorder

√5th   **F14.2**   **Cocaine dependence**

     EXCLUDES 1   *cocaine abuse (F14.1-)*
         cocaine use, unspecified (F14.9-)
     EXCLUDES 2   *cocaine poisoning (T40.5-)*

     F14.20   Cocaine dependence, uncomplicated

     F14.21   Cocaine dependence, in remission

√6th   **F14.22**   Cocaine dependence with intoxication

         EXCLUDES 1   *cocaine dependence with withdrawal (F14.23)*

         F14.220   Cocaine dependence with intoxication, uncomplicated

         F14.221   Cocaine dependence with intoxication delirium

         F14.222   Cocaine dependence with intoxication with perceptual disturbance

         F14.229   Cocaine dependence with intoxication, unspecified

     F14.23   Cocaine dependence with withdrawal

         EXCLUDES 1   *cocaine dependence with intoxication (F14.22-)*

     F14.24   Cocaine dependence with cocaine-induced mood disorder

√6th   **F14.25**   Cocaine dependence with cocaine-induced psychotic disorder

         F14.250   Cocaine dependence with cocaine-induced psychotic disorder with delusions

         F14.251   Cocaine dependence with cocaine-induced psychotic disorder with hallucinations

         F14.259   Cocaine dependence with cocaine-induced psychotic disorder, unspecified

√6th   **F14.28**   Cocaine dependence with other cocaine-induced disorder

         F14.280   Cocaine dependence with cocaine-induced anxiety disorder

         F14.281   Cocaine dependence with cocaine-induced sexual dysfunction

         F14.282   Cocaine dependence with cocaine-induced sleep disorder

         F14.288   Cocaine dependence with other cocaine-induced disorder

     F14.29   Cocaine dependence with unspecified cocaine-induced disorder

√5th   **F14.9**   **Cocaine use, unspecified**

     EXCLUDES 1   *cocaine abuse (F14.1-)*
         cocaine dependence (F14.2-)

     F14.90   Cocaine use, unspecified, uncomplicated

√6th   **F14.92**   Cocaine use, unspecified with intoxication

         F14.920   Cocaine use, unspecified with intoxication, uncomplicated

         F14.921   Cocaine use, unspecified with intoxication delirium

         F14.922   Cocaine use, unspecified with intoxication with perceptual disturbance

         F14.929   Cocaine use, unspecified with intoxication, unspecified

     F14.94   Cocaine use, unspecified with cocaine-induced mood disorder

√6th   **F14.95**   Cocaine use, unspecified with cocaine-induced psychotic disorder

         F14.950   Cocaine use, unspecified with cocaine-induced psychotic disorder with delusions

         F14.951   Cocaine use, unspecified with cocaine-induced psychotic disorder with hallucinations

         F14.959   Cocaine use, unspecified with cocaine-induced psychotic disorder, unspecified

√6th   **F14.98**   Cocaine use, unspecified with other specified cocaine-induced disorder

         F14.980   Cocaine use, unspecified with cocaine-induced anxiety disorder

         F14.981   Cocaine use, unspecified with cocaine-induced sexual dysfunction

         F14.982   Cocaine use, unspecified with cocaine-induced sleep disorder

         F14.988   Cocaine use, unspecified with other cocaine-induced disorder

     F14.99   Cocaine use, unspecified with unspecified cocaine-induced disorder

√4th   **F15**   **Other stimulant related disorders**

     INCLUDES   amphetamine-related disorders
         caffeine
     EXCLUDES 2   *cocaine-related disorders (F14.-)*

√5th   **F15.1**   **Other stimulant abuse**

     EXCLUDES 1   *other stimulant dependence (F15.2-)*
         other stimulant use, unspecified (F15.9-)

     F15.10   Other stimulant abuse, uncomplicated

√6th   **F15.12**   Other stimulant abuse with intoxication

         F15.120   Other stimulant abuse with intoxication, uncomplicated

         F15.121   Other stimulant abuse with intoxication delirium

         F15.122   Other stimulant abuse with intoxication with perceptual disturbance

         F15.129   Other stimulant abuse with intoxication, unspecified

     F15.14   Other stimulant abuse with stimulant-induced mood disorder

√6th   **F15.15**   Other stimulant abuse with stimulant-induced psychotic disorder

         F15.150   Other stimulant abuse with stimulant-induced psychotic disorder with delusions

         F15.151   Other stimulant abuse with stimulant-induced psychotic disorder with hallucinations

         F15.159   Other stimulant abuse with stimulant-induced psychotic disorder, unspecified

√6th   **F15.18**   Other stimulant abuse with other stimulant-induced disorder

         F15.180   Other stimulant abuse with stimulant-induced anxiety disorder

         F15.181   Other stimulant abuse with stimulant-induced sexual dysfunction

         F15.182   Other stimulant abuse with stimulant-induced sleep disorder

         F15.188   Other stimulant abuse with other stimulant-induced disorder

     F15.19   Other stimulant abuse with unspecified stimulant-induced disorder

√5th   **F15.2**   **Other stimulant dependence**

     EXCLUDES 1   *other stimulant abuse (F15.1-)*
         other stimulant use, unspecified (F15.9-)

     F15.20   Other stimulant dependence, uncomplicated

     F15.21   Other stimulant dependence, in remission

EXCLUDES 1 Not coded here   **EXCLUDES 2** Not included here   **N** Newborn Age: 0   **P** Pediatric Age: 0-17   **M** Maternity Age: 12-55   **A** Adult Age: 15-124

500   ICD-10-CM Draft (2015)

✓6th **F15.22** **Other stimulant dependence with intoxication**
> EXCLUDES 1 *other stimulant dependence with withdrawal (F15.23)*

F15.220 **Other stimulant dependence with intoxication, uncomplicated**

F15.221 **Other stimulant dependence with intoxication delirium**

F15.222 **Other stimulant dependence with intoxication with perceptual disturbance**

F15.229 **Other stimulant dependence with intoxication, unspecified**

F15.23 **Other stimulant dependence with withdrawal**
> EXCLUDES 1 *other stimulant dependence with intoxication (F15.22-)*

F15.24 **Other stimulant dependence with stimulant-induced mood disorder**

✓6th **F15.25** **Other stimulant dependence with stimulant-induced psychotic disorder**

F15.250 **Other stimulant dependence with stimulant-induced psychotic disorder with delusions**

F15.251 **Other stimulant dependence with stimulant-induced psychotic disorder with hallucinations**

F15.259 **Other stimulant dependence with stimulant-induced psychotic disorder, unspecified**

✓6th **F15.28** **Other stimulant dependence with other stimulant-induced disorder**

F15.280 **Other stimulant dependence with stimulant-induced anxiety disorder**

F15.281 **Other stimulant dependence with stimulant-induced sexual dysfunction**

F15.282 **Other stimulant dependence with stimulant-induced sleep disorder**

F15.288 **Other stimulant dependence with other stimulant-induced disorder**

F15.29 **Other stimulant dependence with unspecified stimulant-induced disorder**

✓5th **F15.9** **Other stimulant use, unspecified**
> EXCLUDES 1 *other stimulant abuse (F15.1-)*
> *other stimulant dependence (F15.2-)*

F15.90 **Other stimulant use, unspecified, uncomplicated**

✓6th **F15.92** **Other stimulant use, unspecified with intoxication**
> EXCLUDES 1 *other stimulant use, unspecified with withdrawal (F15.93)*

F15.920 **Other stimulant use, unspecified with intoxication, uncomplicated**

F15.921 **Other stimulant use, unspecified with intoxication delirium**

F15.922 **Other stimulant use, unspecified with intoxication with perceptual disturbance**

F15.929 **Other stimulant use, unspecified with intoxication, unspecified**

F15.93 **Other stimulant use, unspecified with withdrawal**
> EXCLUDES 1 *other stimulant use, unspecified with intoxication (F15.92-)*

F15.94 **Other stimulant use, unspecified with stimulant-induced mood disorder**

✓6th **F15.95** **Other stimulant use, unspecified with stimulant-induced psychotic disorder**

F15.950 **Other stimulant use, unspecified with stimulant-induced psychotic disorder with delusions**

F15.951 **Other stimulant use, unspecified with stimulant-induced psychotic disorder with hallucinations**

F15.959 **Other stimulant use, unspecified with stimulant-induced psychotic disorder, unspecified**

✓6th **F15.98** **Other stimulant use, unspecified with other stimulant-induced disorder**

F15.980 **Other stimulant use, unspecified with stimulant-induced anxiety disorder**

F15.981 **Other stimulant use, unspecified with stimulant-induced sexual dysfunction**

F15.982 **Other stimulant use, unspecified with stimulant-induced sleep disorder**

F15.988 **Other stimulant use, unspecified with other stimulant-induced disorder**

F15.99 **Other stimulant use, unspecified with unspecified stimulant-induced disorder**

✓4th **F16** **Hallucinogen related disorders**
> INCLUDES ecstasy
> PCP
> phencyclidine

✓5th **F16.1** **Hallucinogen abuse**
> EXCLUDES 1 *hallucinogen dependence (F16.2-)*
> *hallucinogen use, unspecified (F16.9-)*

F16.10 **Hallucinogen abuse, uncomplicated**

✓6th **F16.12** **Hallucinogen abuse with intoxication**

F16.120 **Hallucinogen abuse with intoxication, uncomplicated**

F16.121 **Hallucinogen abuse with intoxication with delirium**

F16.122 **Hallucinogen abuse with intoxication with perceptual disturbance**

F16.129 **Hallucinogen abuse with intoxication, unspecified**

F16.14 **Hallucinogen abuse with hallucinogen-induced mood disorder**

✓6th **F16.15** **Hallucinogen abuse with hallucinogen-induced psychotic disorder**

F16.150 **Hallucinogen abuse with hallucinogen-induced psychotic disorder with delusions**

F16.151 **Hallucinogen abuse with hallucinogen-induced psychotic disorder with hallucinations**

F16.159 **Hallucinogen abuse with hallucinogen-induced psychotic disorder, unspecified**

✓6th **F16.18** **Hallucinogen abuse with other hallucinogen-induced disorder**

F16.180 **Hallucinogen abuse with hallucinogen-induced anxiety disorder**

F16.183 **Hallucinogen abuse with hallucinogen persisting perception disorder (flashbacks)**

F16.188 **Hallucinogen abuse with other hallucinogen-induced disorder**

F16.19 **Hallucinogen abuse with unspecified hallucinogen-induced disorder**

✓5th **F16.2** **Hallucinogen dependence**
> EXCLUDES 1 *hallucinogen abuse (F16.1-)*
> *hallucinogen use, unspecified (F16.9-)*

F16.20 **Hallucinogen dependence, uncomplicated**

F16.21 **Hallucinogen dependence, in remission**

✓6th **F16.22** **Hallucinogen dependence with intoxication**

F16.220 **Hallucinogen dependence with intoxication, uncomplicated**

F16.221 **Hallucinogen dependence with intoxication with delirium**

F16.229 **Hallucinogen dependence with intoxication, unspecified**

F16.24 **Hallucinogen dependence with hallucinogen-induced mood disorder**

✓6th **F16.25** **Hallucinogen dependence with hallucinogen-induced psychotic disorder**

F16.250 **Hallucinogen dependence with hallucinogen-induced psychotic disorder with delusions**

F16.251 **Hallucinogen dependence with hallucinogen-induced psychotic disorder with hallucinations**

F16.259 **Hallucinogen dependence with hallucinogen-induced psychotic disorder, unspecified**

✓6th **F16.28** **Hallucinogen dependence with other hallucinogen-induced disorder**

F16.280 **Hallucinogen dependence with hallucinogen-induced anxiety disorder**

F16.283 **Hallucinogen dependence with hallucinogen persisting perception disorder (flashbacks)**

✓ Additional Character Required   ✓x7th Xtension Alert   Unspecified Dx   Other Specified Dx   Manifestation   ►◄ Revised Text   ● New Code   ▲ Revised Code Title

Mental, Behavioral, and Neurodevelopmental Disorders

F16.288–F18.27

F16.288   Hallucinogen dependence with other hallucinogen-induced disorder

F16.29   Hallucinogen dependence with unspecified hallucinogen-induced disorder

√5ᵗʰ   F16.9   Hallucinogen use, unspecified
> EXCLUDES 1   hallucinogen abuse (F16.1-)
> hallucinogen dependence (F16.2-)

F16.90   Hallucinogen use, unspecified, uncomplicated

√6ᵗʰ   F16.92   Hallucinogen use, unspecified with intoxication

F16.920   Hallucinogen use, unspecified with intoxication, uncomplicated

F16.921   Hallucinogen use, unspecified with intoxication with delirium

F16.929   Hallucinogen use, unspecified with intoxication, unspecified

F16.94   Hallucinogen use, unspecified with hallucinogen-induced mood disorder

√6ᵗʰ   F16.95   Hallucinogen use, unspecified with hallucinogen-induced psychotic disorder

F16.950   Hallucinogen use, unspecified with hallucinogen-induced psychotic disorder with delusions

F16.951   Hallucinogen use, unspecified with hallucinogen-induced psychotic disorder with hallucinations

F16.959   Hallucinogen use, unspecified with hallucinogen-induced psychotic disorder, unspecified

√6ᵗʰ   F16.98   Hallucinogen use, unspecified with other specified hallucinogen-induced disorder

F16.980   Hallucinogen use, unspecified with hallucinogen-induced anxiety disorder

F16.983   Hallucinogen use, unspecified with hallucinogen persisting perception disorder (flashbacks)

F16.988   Hallucinogen use, unspecified with other hallucinogen-induced disorder

F16.99   Hallucinogen use, unspecified with unspecified hallucinogen-induced disorder

√4ᵗʰ   **F17   Nicotine dependence**
> EXCLUDES 1   history of tobacco dependence (Z87.891)
> tobacco use NOS (Z72.0)
> EXCLUDES 2   tobacco use (smoking) during pregnancy, childbirth and the puerperium (O99.33-)
> toxic effect of nicotine (T65.2-)

AHA: 2013, 4Q, 108-109

√5ᵗʰ   F17.2   Nicotine dependence

√6ᵗʰ   F17.20   Nicotine dependence, unspecified

F17.200   Nicotine dependence, unspecified, uncomplicated

F17.201   Nicotine dependence, unspecified, in remission

F17.203   Nicotine dependence unspecified, with withdrawal

F17.208   Nicotine dependence, unspecified, with other nicotine-induced disorders

F17.209   Nicotine dependence, unspecified, with unspecified nicotine-induced disorders

√6ᵗʰ   F17.21   Nicotine dependence, cigarettes

F17.210   Nicotine dependence, cigarettes, uncomplicated

F17.211   Nicotine dependence, cigarettes, in remission

F17.213   Nicotine dependence, cigarettes, with withdrawal

F17.218   Nicotine dependence, cigarettes, with other nicotine-induced disorders

F17.219   Nicotine dependence, cigarettes, with unspecified nicotine-induced disorders

√6ᵗʰ   F17.22   Nicotine dependence, chewing tobacco

F17.220   Nicotine dependence, chewing tobacco, uncomplicated

F17.221   Nicotine dependence, chewing tobacco, in remission

F17.223   Nicotine dependence, chewing tobacco, with withdrawal

F17.228   Nicotine dependence, chewing tobacco, with other nicotine-induced disorders

F17.229   Nicotine dependence, chewing tobacco, with unspecified nicotine-induced disorders

√6ᵗʰ   F17.29   Nicotine dependence, other tobacco product

F17.290   Nicotine dependence, other tobacco product, uncomplicated

F17.291   Nicotine dependence, other tobacco product, in remission

F17.293   Nicotine dependence, other tobacco product, with withdrawal

F17.298   Nicotine dependence, other tobacco product, with other nicotine-induced disorders

F17.299   Nicotine dependence, other tobacco product, with unspecified nicotine-induced disorders

√4ᵗʰ   **F18   Inhalant related disorders**
> INCLUDES   volatile solvents

√5ᵗʰ   F18.1   Inhalant abuse
> EXCLUDES 1   inhalant dependence (F18.2-)
> inhalant use, unspecified (F18.9-)

F18.10   Inhalant abuse, uncomplicated

√6ᵗʰ   F18.12   Inhalant abuse with intoxication

F18.120   Inhalant abuse with intoxication, uncomplicated

F18.121   Inhalant abuse with intoxication delirium

F18.129   Inhalant abuse with intoxication, unspecified

F18.14   Inhalant abuse with inhalant-induced mood disorder

√6ᵗʰ   F18.15   Inhalant abuse with inhalant-induced psychotic disorder

F18.150   Inhalant abuse with inhalant-induced psychotic disorder with delusions

F18.151   Inhalant abuse with inhalant-induced psychotic disorder with hallucinations

F18.159   Inhalant abuse with inhalant-induced psychotic disorder, unspecified

F18.17   Inhalant abuse with inhalant-induced dementia

√6ᵗʰ   F18.18   Inhalant abuse with other inhalant-induced disorders

F18.180   Inhalant abuse with inhalant-induced anxiety disorder

F18.188   Inhalant abuse with other inhalant-induced disorder

F18.19   Inhalant abuse with unspecified inhalant-induced disorder

√5ᵗʰ   F18.2   Inhalant dependence
> EXCLUDES 1   inhalant abuse (F18.1-)
> inhalant use, unspecified (F18.9-)

F18.20   Inhalant dependence, uncomplicated

F18.21   Inhalant dependence, in remission

√6ᵗʰ   F18.22   Inhalant dependence with intoxication

F18.220   Inhalant dependence with intoxication, uncomplicated

F18.221   Inhalant dependence with intoxication delirium

F18.229   Inhalant dependence with intoxication, unspecified

F18.24   Inhalant dependence with inhalant-induced mood disorder

√6ᵗʰ   F18.25   Inhalant dependence with inhalant-induced psychotic disorder

F18.250   Inhalant dependence with inhalant-induced psychotic disorder with delusions

F18.251   Inhalant dependence with inhalant-induced psychotic disorder with hallucinations

F18.259   Inhalant dependence with inhalant-induced psychotic disorder, unspecified

F18.27   Inhalant dependence with inhalant-induced dementia

EXCLUDES 1 Not coded here   EXCLUDES 2 Not included here   N Newborn Age: 0   P Pediatric Age: 0-17   M Maternity Age: 12-55   A Adult Age: 15-124

502   ICD-10-CM Draft (2015)

✓6ᵗʰ **F18.28 Inhalant dependence with** other **inhalant-induced disorders**

F18.280 **Inhalant dependence with inhalant-induced** anxiety disorder

F18.288 **Inhalant dependence with other inhalant-induced disorder**

F18.29 **Inhalant dependence with unspecified inhalant-induced disorder**

✓5ᵗʰ **F18.9 Inhalant use,** unspecified

EXCLUDES 1   *inhalant abuse (F18.1-)*
inhalant dependence (F18.2-)

F18.90 **Inhalant use, unspecified, uncomplicated**

✓6ᵗʰ F18.92 **Inhalant use, unspecified with** intoxication

F18.920 **Inhalant use, unspecified with intoxication,** uncomplicated

F18.921 **Inhalant use, unspecified with intoxication with** delirium

F18.929 **Inhalant use, unspecified with intoxication, unspecified**

F18.94 **Inhalant use, unspecified with inhalant-induced** mood disorder

✓6ᵗʰ F18.95 **Inhalant use, unspecified with inhalant-induced** psychotic disorder

F18.950 **Inhalant use, unspecified with inhalant-induced psychotic disorder with** delusions

F18.951 **Inhalant use, unspecified with inhalant-induced psychotic disorder with** hallucinations

F18.959 **Inhalant use, unspecified with inhalant-induced psychotic disorder, unspecified**

F18.97 **Inhalant use, unspecified with inhalant-induced** persisting dementia

✓6ᵗʰ F18.98 **Inhalant use, unspecified with** other **inhalant-induced disorders**

F18.980 **Inhalant use, unspecified with inhalant-induced** anxiety disorder

F18.988 **Inhalant use, unspecified with other inhalant-induced disorder**

F18.99 **Inhalant use, unspecified with unspecified inhalant-induced disorder**

✓4ᵗʰ **F19** Other psychoactive **substance related disorders**

INCLUDES   polysubstance drug use (indiscriminate drug use)

✓5ᵗʰ **F19.1 Other psychoactive substance** abuse

EXCLUDES 1   *other psychoactive substance dependence (F19.2-)*
other psychoactive substance use, unspecified (F19.9-)

F19.10 **Other psychoactive substance abuse,** uncomplicated

✓6ᵗʰ F19.12 **Other psychoactive substance abuse with** intoxication

F19.120 **Other psychoactive substance abuse with intoxication,** uncomplicated

F19.121 **Other psychoactive substance abuse with intoxication** delirium

F19.122 **Other psychoactive substance abuse with intoxication with** perceptual disturbances

F19.129 **Other psychoactive substance abuse with intoxication, unspecified**

F19.14 **Other psychoactive substance abuse with psychoactive substance-induced** mood disorder

✓6ᵗʰ F19.15 **Other psychoactive substance abuse with psychoactive substance-induced** psychotic disorder

F19.150 **Other psychoactive substance abuse with psychoactive substance-induced psychotic disorder with** delusions

F19.151 **Other psychoactive substance abuse with psychoactive substance-induced psychotic disorder with** hallucinations

F19.159 **Other psychoactive substance abuse with psychoactive substance-induced psychotic disorder, unspecified**

F19.16 **Other psychoactive substance abuse with psychoactive substance-induced** persisting amnestic disorder

F19.17 **Other psychoactive substance abuse with psychoactive substance-induced** persisting dementia

✓6ᵗʰ **F19.18 Other psychoactive substance abuse with** other **psychoactive substance-induced disorders**

F19.180 **Other psychoactive substance abuse with psychoactive substance-induced** anxiety disorder

F19.181 **Other psychoactive substance abuse with psychoactive substance-induced** sexual dysfunction

F19.182 **Other psychoactive substance abuse with psychoactive substance-induced** sleep disorder

F19.188 **Other psychoactive substance abuse with other psychoactive substance-induced disorder**

F19.19 **Other psychoactive substance abuse with unspecified psychoactive substance-induced disorder**

✓5ᵗʰ **F19.2 Other psychoactive substance** dependence

EXCLUDES 1   *other psychoactive substance abuse (F19.1-)*
other psychoactive substance use, unspecified (F19.9-)

F19.20 **Other psychoactive substance dependence, uncomplicated**

F19.21 **Other psychoactive substance dependence,** in remission

✓6ᵗʰ F19.22 **Other psychoactive substance dependence with** intoxication

EXCLUDES 1   *other psychoactive substance dependence with withdrawal (F19.23-)*

F19.220 **Other psychoactive substance dependence with intoxication,** uncomplicated

F19.221 **Other psychoactive substance dependence with intoxication** delirium

F19.222 **Other psychoactive substance dependence with intoxication with** perceptual disturbance

F19.229 **Other psychoactive substance dependence with intoxication, unspecified**

✓6ᵗʰ F19.23 **Other psychoactive substance dependence with** withdrawal

EXCLUDES 1   *other psychoactive substance dependence with intoxication (F19.22-)*

F19.230 **Other psychoactive substance dependence with withdrawal,** uncomplicated

F19.231 **Other psychoactive substance dependence with withdrawal** delirium

F19.232 **Other psychoactive substance dependence with withdrawal with** perceptual disturbance

F19.239 **Other psychoactive substance dependence with withdrawal, unspecified**

F19.24 **Other psychoactive substance dependence with psychoactive substance-induced** mood disorder

✓6ᵗʰ F19.25 **Other psychoactive substance dependence with psychoactive substance-induced** psychotic disorder

F19.250 **Other psychoactive substance dependence with psychoactive substance-induced psychotic disorder with** delusions

F19.251 **Other psychoactive substance dependence with psychoactive substance-induced psychotic disorder with** hallucinations

F19.259 **Other psychoactive substance dependence with psychoactive substance-induced psychotic disorder, unspecified**

F19.26 **Other psychoactive substance dependence with psychoactive substance-induced** persisting amnestic disorder

F19.27 **Other psychoactive substance dependence with psychoactive substance-induced** persisting dementia

✓6ᵗʰ F19.28 **Other psychoactive substance dependence with** other **psychoactive substance-induced disorders**

F19.280 **Other psychoactive substance dependence with psychoactive substance-induced** anxiety disorder

---

✓ Additional Character Required   ✓x7ᵗʰ Xtension Alert   Unspecified Dx   Other Specified Dx   Manifestation   ▶◀ Revised Text   ● New Code   ▲ Revised Code Title

ICD-10-CM Draft (2015)   503

F19.281 Other psychoactive substance dependence with psychoactive substance-induced sexual dysfunction

F19.282 Other psychoactive substance dependence with psychoactive substance-induced sleep disorder

F19.288 Other psychoactive substance dependence with other psychoactive substance-induced disorder

F19.29 Other psychoactive substance dependence with unspecified psychoactive substance-induced disorder

✓5ᵗʰ **F19.9** Other psychoactive substance use, unspecified
> EXCLUDES 1   other psychoactive substance abuse (F19.1-)
>   other psychoactive substance dependence (F19.2-)

F19.90 Other psychoactive substance use, unspecified, uncomplicated

✓6ᵗʰ **F19.92** Other psychoactive substance use, unspecified with intoxication
> EXCLUDES 1   other psychoactive substance use, unspecified with withdrawal (F19.93)

F19.920 Other psychoactive substance use, unspecified with intoxication, uncomplicated

F19.921 Other psychoactive substance use, unspecified with intoxication with delirium

F19.922 Other psychoactive substance use, unspecified with intoxication with perceptual disturbance

F19.929 Other psychoactive substance use, unspecified with intoxication, unspecified

✓6ᵗʰ **F19.93** Other psychoactive substance use, unspecified with withdrawal
> EXCLUDES 1   other psychoactive substance use, unspecified with intoxication (F19.92-)

F19.930 Other psychoactive substance use, unspecified with withdrawal, uncomplicated

F19.931 Other psychoactive substance use, unspecified with withdrawal delirium

F19.932 Other psychoactive substance use, unspecified with withdrawal with perceptual disturbance

F19.939 Other psychoactive substance use, unspecified with withdrawal, unspecified

F19.94 Other psychoactive substance use, unspecified with psychoactive substance-induced mood disorder

✓6ᵗʰ **F19.95** Other psychoactive substance use, unspecified with psychoactive substance-induced psychotic disorder

F19.950 Other psychoactive substance use, unspecified with psychoactive substance-induced psychotic disorder with delusions

F19.951 Other psychoactive substance use, unspecified with psychoactive substance-induced psychotic disorder with hallucinations

F19.959 Other psychoactive substance use, unspecified with psychoactive substance-induced psychotic disorder, unspecified

F19.96 Other psychoactive substance use, unspecified with psychoactive substance-induced persisting amnestic disorder

F19.97 Other psychoactive substance use, unspecified with psychoactive substance-induced persisting dementia

✓6ᵗʰ **F19.98** Other psychoactive substance use, unspecified with other psychoactive substance-induced disorders

F19.980 Other psychoactive substance use, unspecified with psychoactive substance-induced anxiety disorder

F19.981 Other psychoactive substance use, unspecified with psychoactive substance-induced sexual dysfunction

F19.982 Other psychoactive substance use, unspecified with psychoactive substance-induced sleep disorder

F19.988 Other psychoactive substance use, unspecified with other psychoactive substance-induced disorder

F19.99 Other psychoactive substance use, unspecified with unspecified psychoactive substance-induced disorder

Schizophrenia, schizotypal, delusional, and other non-mood psychotic disorders (F20-F29)

✓4ᵗʰ **F20** Schizophrenia
> EXCLUDES 1   brief psychotic disorder (F23)
>   cyclic schizophrenia (F25.0)
>   mood [affective] disorders with psychotic symptoms (F30.2, F31.2, F31.5, F31.64, F32.3, F33.3)
>   schizoaffective disorder (F25.-)
>   schizophrenic reaction NOS (F23)
> EXCLUDES 2   schizophrenic reaction in:
>   alcoholism (F10.15-, F10.25-, F10.95-)
>   brain disease (F06.2)
>   epilepsy (F06.2)
>   psychoactive drug use (F11-F19 with .15..25, .95)
>   schizotypal disorder (F21)

F20.0 Paranoid schizophrenia
Paraphrenic schizophrenia
> EXCLUDES 1   involutional paranoid state (F22)
>   paranoia (F22)

F20.1 Disorganized schizophrenia
Hebephrenic schizophrenia
Hebephrenia

F20.2 Catatonic schizophrenia
Schizophrenic catalepsy
Schizophrenic catatonia
Schizophrenic flexibilitas cerea
> EXCLUDES 1   catatonic stupor (R40.1)

F20.3 Undifferentiated schizophrenia
Atypical schizophrenia
> EXCLUDES 1   acute schizophrenia-like psychotic disorder (F23)
> EXCLUDES 2   post-schizophrenic depression (F32.8)

F20.5 Residual schizophrenia
Restzustand (schizophrenic)
Schizophrenic residual state

✓5ᵗʰ **F20.8** Other schizophrenia

F20.81 Schizophreniform disorder
Schizophreniform psychosis NOS

F20.89 Other schizophrenia
Cenesthopathic schizophrenia
Simple schizophrenia

F20.9 Schizophrenia, unspecified

F21 Schizotypal disorder
Borderline schizophrenia   Prodromal schizophrenia
Latent schizophrenia   Pseudoneurotic schizophrenia
Latent schizophrenic reaction   Pseudopsychopathic schizophrenia
Prepsychotic schizophrenia   Schizotypal personality disorder
> EXCLUDES 2   Asperger's syndrome (F84.5)
>   schizoid personality disorder (F60.1)

F22 Delusional disorders
Delusional dysmorphophobia   Paranoid psychosis
Involutional paranoid state   Paranoid state
Paranoia   Paraphrenia (late)
Paranoia querulans   Sensitiver Beziehungswahn
> EXCLUDES 1   mood [affective] disorders with psychotic symptoms (F30.2, F31.2, F31.5, F31.64, F32.3, F33.3)
>   paranoid schizophrenia (F20.0)
> EXCLUDES 2   paranoid personality disorder (F60.0)
>   paranoid psychosis, psychogenic (F23)
>   paranoid reaction (F23)

F23 Brief psychotic disorder
Paranoid reaction
Psychogenic paranoid psychosis
> EXCLUDES 2   mood [affective] disorders with psychotic symptoms (F30.2, F31.2, F31.5, F31.64, F32.3, F33.3)

F24 Shared psychotic disorder
Folie à deux
Induced paranoid disorder
Induced psychotic disorder

EXCLUDES 1 Not coded here   EXCLUDES 2 Not included here   N Newborn Age: 0   P Pediatric Age: 0-17   M Maternity Age: 12-55   A Adult Age: 15-124

504   ICD-10-CM Draft (2015)

✓4th **F25 Schizoaffective disorders**

> EXCLUDES 1 *mood [affective] disorders with psychotic symptoms (F30.2, F31.2, F31.5, F31.64, F32.3, F33.3)*
> *schizophrenia (F20.-)*

F25.0 Schizoaffective disorder, bipolar type
Cyclic schizophrenia
Schizoaffective disorder, manic type
Schizoaffective disorder, mixed type
Schizoaffective psychosis, bipolar type
Schizophreniform psychosis, manic type

F25.1 Schizoaffective disorder, depressive type
Schizoaffective psychosis, depressive type
Schizophreniform psychosis, depressive type

F25.8 Other schizoaffective disorders

F25.9 Schizoaffective disorder, unspecified
Schizoaffective psychosis NOS

F28 Other psychotic disorder not due to a substance or known physiological condition
Chronic hallucinatory psychosis

F29 Unspecified psychosis not due to a substance or known physiological condition
Psychosis NOS

> EXCLUDES 1 *mental disorder NOS (F99)*
> *unspecified mental disorder due to known physiological condition (F09)*

Mood [affective] disorders (F30-F39)

✓4th **F30 Manic episode**

> INCLUDES bipolar disorder, single manic episode
> mixed affective episode
> EXCLUDES 1 *bipolar disorder (F31.-)*
> *major depressive disorder, recurrent (F33.-)*
> *major depressive disorder, single episode (F32.-)*

✓5th **F30.1 Manic episode without psychotic symptoms**

F30.10 Manic episode without psychotic symptoms, unspecified

F30.11 Manic episode without psychotic symptoms, mild

F30.12 Manic episode without psychotic symptoms, moderate

F30.13 Manic episode, severe, without psychotic symptoms

F30.2 Manic episode, severe with psychotic symptoms
Manic stupor
Mania with mood-congruent psychotic symptoms
Mania with mood-incongruent psychotic symptoms

F30.3 Manic episode in partial remission

F30.4 Manic episode in full remission

F30.8 Other manic episodes
Hypomania

F30.9 Manic episode, unspecified
Mania NOS

✓4th **F31 Bipolar disorder**

> INCLUDES manic-depressive illness
> manic-depressive psychosis
> manic-depressive reaction
> EXCLUDES 1 *bipolar disorder, single manic episode (F30.-)*
> *major depressive disorder, single episode (F32.-)*
> *major depressive disorder, recurrent (F33.-)*
> EXCLUDES 2 *cyclothymia (F34.0)*

F31.0 Bipolar disorder, current episode hypomanic

✓5th **F31.1 Bipolar disorder, current episode manic without psychotic features**

F31.10 Bipolar disorder, current episode manic without psychotic features, unspecified

F31.11 Bipolar disorder, current episode manic without psychotic features, mild

F31.12 Bipolar disorder, current episode manic without psychotic features, moderate

F31.13 Bipolar disorder, current episode manic without psychotic features, severe

F31.2 Bipolar disorder, current episode manic severe with psychotic features
Bipolar disorder, current episode manic with mood-congruent psychotic symptoms
Bipolar disorder, current episode manic with mood-incongruent psychotic symptoms

✓5th **F31.3 Bipolar disorder, current episode depressed, mild or moderate severity**

F31.30 Bipolar disorder, current episode depressed, mild or moderate severity, unspecified

F31.31 Bipolar disorder, current episode depressed, mild

F31.32 Bipolar disorder, current episode depressed, moderate

F31.4 Bipolar disorder, current episode depressed, severe, without psychotic features

F31.5 Bipolar disorder, current episode depressed, severe, with psychotic features
Bipolar disorder, current episode depressed with mood-incongruent psychotic symptoms
Bipolar disorder, current episode depressed with mood-congruent psychotic symptoms

✓5th **F31.6 Bipolar disorder, current episode mixed**

F31.60 Bipolar disorder, current episode mixed, unspecified

F31.61 Bipolar disorder, current episode mixed, mild

F31.62 Bipolar disorder, current episode mixed, moderate

F31.63 Bipolar disorder, current episode mixed, severe, without psychotic features

F31.64 Bipolar disorder, current episode mixed, severe, with psychotic features
Bipolar disorder, current episode mixed with mood-congruent psychotic symptoms
Bipolar disorder, current episode mixed with mood-incongruent psychotic symptoms

✓5th **F31.7 Bipolar disorder, currently in remission**

F31.70 Bipolar disorder, currently in remission, most recent episode unspecified

F31.71 Bipolar disorder, in partial remission, most recent episode hypomanic

F31.72 Bipolar disorder, in full remission, most recent episode hypomanic

F31.73 Bipolar disorder, in partial remission, most recent episode manic

F31.74 Bipolar disorder, in full remission, most recent episode manic

F31.75 Bipolar disorder, in partial remission, most recent episode depressed

F31.76 Bipolar disorder, in full remission, most recent episode depressed

F31.77 Bipolar disorder, in partial remission, most recent episode mixed

F31.78 Bipolar disorder, in full remission, most recent episode mixed

✓5th **F31.8 Other bipolar disorders**

F31.81 Bipolar II disorder

F31.89 Other bipolar disorder
Recurrent manic episodes NOS

F31.9 Bipolar disorder, unspecified

✓4th **F32 Major depressive disorder, single episode**

> INCLUDES single episode of agitated depression
> single episode of depressive reaction
> single episode of major depression
> single episode of psychogenic depression
> single episode of reactive depression
> single episode of vital depression
> EXCLUDES 1 *bipolar disorder (F31.-)*
> *manic episode (F30.-)*
> *recurrent depressive disorder (F33.-)*
> EXCLUDES 2 *adjustment disorder (F43.2)*

F32.0 Major depressive disorder, single episode, mild

F32.1 Major depressive disorder, single episode, moderate

F32.2 Major depressive disorder, single episode, severe without psychotic features

F32.3 Major depressive disorder, single episode, severe with psychotic features
Single episode of major depression with mood-congruent psychotic symptoms
Single episode of major depression with mood-incongruent psychotic symptoms
Single episode of major depression with psychotic symptoms
Single episode of psychogenic depressive psychosis
Single episode of psychotic depression
Single episode of reactive depressive psychosis

F32.4 Major depressive disorder, single episode, in partial remission

---

✓ Additional Character Required   ✓x7th Xtension Alert   Unspecified Dx   Other Specified Dx   Manifestation   ►◄ Revised Text   ● New Code   ▲ Revised Code Title

F32.5 **Major depressive disorder, single episode, in full remission**

F32.8 **Other depressive episodes**
Atypical depression
Post-schizophrenic depression
Single episode of 'masked' depression NOS

F32.9 **Major depressive disorder, single episode, unspecified**
Depression NOS
Depressive disorder NOS
Major depression NOS
AHA: 2013, 4Q, 107

✓4ᵗʰ **F33** **Major depressive disorder, recurrent**
Recurrent episodes of depressive reaction
Recurrent episodes of endogenous depression
Recurrent episodes of major depression
Recurrent episodes of psychogenic depression
Recurrent episodes of reactive depression
Recurrent episodes of seasonal depressive disorder
Recurrent episodes of vital depression
EXCLUDES 1 *bipolar disorder (F31.-)*
manic episode (F30.-)

F33.0 **Major depressive disorder, recurrent, mild**

F33.1 **Major depressive disorder, recurrent, moderate**

F33.2 **Major depressive disorder, recurrent, severe without psychotic features**

F33.3 **Major depressive disorder, recurrent, severe with psychotic symptoms**
Endogenous depression with psychotic symptoms
Recurrent severe episodes of major depression with mood-congruent psychotic symptoms
Recurrent severe episodes of major depression with mood-incongruent psychotic symptoms
Recurrent severe episodes of major depression with psychotic symptoms
Recurrent severe episodes of psychogenic depressive psychosis
Recurrent severe episodes of psychotic depression
Recurrent severe episodes of reactive depressive psychosis

✓5ᵗʰ **F33.4** **Major depressive disorder, recurrent, in remission**

F33.40 **Major depressive disorder, recurrent, in remission, unspecified**

F33.41 **Major depressive disorder, recurrent, in partial remission**

F33.42 **Major depressive disorder, recurrent, in full remission**

F33.8 **Other recurrent depressive disorders**
Recurrent brief depressive episodes

F33.9 **Major depressive disorder, recurrent, unspecified**
Monopolar depression NOS

✓4ᵗʰ **F34** **Persistent mood [affective] disorders**

F34.0 **Cyclothymic disorder**
Affective personality disorder
Cycloid personality
Cyclothymia
Cyclothymic personality

F34.1 **Dysthymic disorder**
Depressive neurosis
Depressive personality disorder
Dysthymia
Neurotic depression
Persistent anxiety depression
EXCLUDES 2 *anxiety depression (mild or not persistent) (F41.8)*

F34.8 **Other persistent mood [affective] disorders**

F34.9 **Persistent mood [affective] disorder, unspecified**

F39 **Unspecified mood [affective] disorder**
Affective psychosis NOS

Anxiety, dissociative, stress-related, somatoform and other nonpsychotic mental disorders (F40-F48)

✓4ᵗʰ **F40** **Phobic anxiety disorders**

✓5ᵗʰ **F40.0** **Agoraphobia**

F40.00 **Agoraphobia, unspecified**

F40.01 **Agoraphobia with panic disorder**
Panic disorder with agoraphobia
EXCLUDES 1 *panic disorder without agoraphobia (F41.0)*

F40.02 **Agoraphobia without panic disorder**

✓5ᵗʰ **F40.1** **Social phobias**
Anthropophobia
Social anxiety disorder of childhood
Social neurosis

F40.10 **Social phobia, unspecified**

F40.11 **Social phobia, generalized**

✓5ᵗʰ **F40.2** **Specific (isolated) phobias**
EXCLUDES 2 *dysmorphophobia (nondelusional) (F45.22)*
nosophobia (F45.22)

✓6ᵗʰ **F40.21** **Animal type phobia**

F40.210 **Arachnophobia**
Fear of spiders

F40.218 **Other animal type phobia**

✓6ᵗʰ **F40.22** **Natural environment type phobia**

F40.220 **Fear of thunderstorms**

F40.228 **Other natural environment type phobia**

✓6ᵗʰ **F40.23** **Blood, injection, injury type phobia**

F40.230 **Fear of blood**

F40.231 **Fear of injections and transfusions**

F40.232 **Fear of other medical care**

F40.233 **Fear of injury**

✓6ᵗʰ **F40.24** **Situational type phobia**

F40.240 **Claustrophobia**

F40.241 **Acrophobia**

F40.242 **Fear of bridges**

F40.243 **Fear of flying**

F40.248 **Other situational type phobia**

✓6ᵗʰ **F40.29** **Other specified phobia**

F40.290 **Androphobia**
Fear of men

F40.291 **Gynephobia**
Fear of women

F40.298 **Other specified phobia**

F40.8 **Other phobic anxiety disorders**
Phobic anxiety disorder of childhood

F40.9 **Phobic anxiety disorder, unspecified**
Phobia NOS
Phobic state NOS

✓4ᵗʰ **F41** **Other anxiety disorders**
EXCLUDES 2 *anxiety in:*
acute stress reaction (F43.0)
transient adjustment reaction (F43.2)
neurasthenia (F48.8)
psychophysiologic disorders (F45.-)
separation anxiety (F93.0)

F41.0 **Panic disorder [episodic paroxysmal anxiety] without agoraphobia**
Panic attack   Panic state
EXCLUDES 1 *panic disorder with agoraphobia (F40.01)*

F41.1 **Generalized anxiety disorder**
Anxiety neurosis   Anxiety state
Anxiety reaction   Overanxious disorder
EXCLUDES 2 *neurasthenia (F48.8)*

F41.3 **Other mixed anxiety disorders**

F41.8 **Other specified anxiety disorders**
Anxiety depression (mild or not persistent)
Anxiety hysteria
Mixed anxiety and depressive disorder

F41.9 **Anxiety disorder, unspecified**
Anxiety NOS

F42 **Obsessive-compulsive disorder**
Anancastic neurosis
Obsessive-compulsive neurosis
EXCLUDES 2 *obsessive-compulsive personality (disorder) (F60.5)*
obsessive-compulsive symptoms occurring in depression (F32-F33)
obsessive-compulsive symptoms occurring in schizophrenia (F20.-)

✓4ᵗʰ **F43** **Reaction to severe stress, and adjustment disorders**

F43.0 **Acute stress reaction**
Acute crisis reaction
Acute reaction to stress
Combat and operational stress reaction
Combat fatigue
Crisis state
Psychic shock

EXCLUDES 1 Not coded here   *EXCLUDES 2* Not included here   N Newborn Age: 0   P Pediatric Age: 0-17   M Maternity Age: 12-55   A Adult Age: 15-124

506   ICD-10-CM Draft (2015)

✓5ᵗʰ **F43.1** **Post-traumatic stress disorder (PTSD)**
Traumatic neurosis

    F43.10 **Post-traumatic stress disorder, unspecified**

    F43.11 **Post-traumatic stress disorder, acute**

    F43.12 **Post-traumatic stress disorder, chronic**

✓5ᵗʰ **F43.2** **Adjustment disorders**
Culture shock
Grief reaction
Hospitalism in children
EXCLUDES 2 *separation anxiety disorder of childhood (F93.0)*

    F43.20 **Adjustment disorder, unspecified**

    F43.21 **Adjustment disorder with depressed mood**
        AHA: 2014, 1Q, 25

    F43.22 **Adjustment disorder with anxiety**

    F43.23 **Adjustment disorder with mixed anxiety and depressed mood**

    F43.24 **Adjustment disorder with disturbance of conduct**

    F43.25 **Adjustment disorder with mixed disturbance of emotions and conduct**

    F43.29 **Adjustment disorder with other symptoms**

    F43.8 **Other reactions to severe stress**

    F43.9 **Reaction to severe stress, unspecified**

✓4ᵗʰ **F44** **Dissociative and conversion disorders**
    INCLUDES conversion hysteria
              conversion reaction
              hysteria
              hysterical psychosis
    EXCLUDES 2 *malingering [conscious simulation] (Z76.5)*

    F44.0 **Dissociative amnesia**
        EXCLUDES 1 *amnesia NOS (R41.3)*
                 anterograde amnesia (R41.1)
                 retrograde amnesia (R41.2)
        EXCLUDES 2 *alcohol-or other psychoactive substance-induced amnestic disorder (F10, F13, F19 with .26, .96)*
                 amnestic disorder due to known physiological condition (F04)
                 postictal amnesia in epilepsy (G40.-)

    F44.1 **Dissociative fugue**
        EXCLUDES 2 *postictal fugue in epilepsy (G40.-)*

    F44.2 **Dissociative stupor**
        EXCLUDES 1 *catatonic stupor (R40.1)*
                 stupor NOS (R40.1)
        EXCLUDES 2 *catatonic disorder due to known physiological condition (F06.1)*
                 depressive stupor (F32, F33)
                 manic stupor (F30, F31)

    F44.4 **Conversion disorder with motor symptom or deficit**
Dissociative motor disorders
Psychogenic aphonia
Psychogenic dysphonia

    F44.5 **Conversion disorder with seizures or convulsions**
Dissociative convulsions

    F44.6 **Conversion disorder with sensory symptom or deficit**
Dissociative anesthesia and sensory loss
Psychogenic deafness

    F44.7 **Conversion disorder with mixed symptom presentation**

✓5ᵗʰ **F44.8** **Other dissociative and conversion disorders**

    F44.81 **Dissociative identity disorder**
Multiple personality disorder

    F44.89 **Other dissociative and conversion disorders**
Ganser's syndrome
Psychogenic confusion
Psychogenic twilight state
Trance and possession disorders

    F44.9 **Dissociative and conversion disorder, unspecified**
Dissociative disorder NOS

✓4ᵗʰ **F45** **Somatoform disorders**
    EXCLUDES 2 *dissociative and conversion disorders (F44.-)*
                 factitious disorders (F68.1-)
                 hair-plucking (F63.3)
                 lalling (F80.0)
                 lisping (F80.0)
                 malingering [conscious simulation] (Z76.5)
                 nail-biting (F98.8)
                 psychological or behavioral factors associated with disorders or diseases classified elsewhere (F54)
                 sexual dysfunction, not due to a substance or known physiological condition (F52.-)
                 thumb-sucking (F98.8)
                 tic disorders (in childhood and adolescence) (F95.-)
                 Tourette's syndrome (F95.2)
                 trichotillomania (F63.3)

    F45.0 **Somatization disorder**
Briquet's disorder
Multiple psychosomatic disorder

    F45.1 **Undifferentiated somatoform disorder**
Undifferentiated psychosomatic disorder

✓5ᵗʰ **F45.2** **Hypochondriacal disorders**
        EXCLUDES 2 *delusional dysmorphophobia (F22)*
                 fixed delusions about bodily functions or shape (F22)

    F45.20 **Hypochondriacal disorder, unspecified**

    F45.21 **Hypochondriasis**
Hypochondriacal neurosis

    F45.22 **Body dysmorphic disorder**
Dysmorphophobia (nondelusional)
Nosophobia

    F45.29 **Other hypochondriacal disorders**

✓5ᵗʰ **F45.4** **Pain disorders related to psychological factors**
        EXCLUDES 1 *pain NOS (R52)*

    F45.41 **Pain disorder exclusively related to psychological factors**
Somatoform pain disorder (persistent)

    F45.42 **Pain disorder with related psychological factors**
Code also associated acute or chronic pain (G89.-)

    F45.8 **Other somatoform disorders**
Psychogenic dysmenorrhea
Psychogenic dysphagia, including "globus hystericus"
Psychogenic pruritus
Psychogenic torticollis
Somatoform autonomic dysfunction
Teeth grinding
        EXCLUDES 1 *sleep related teeth grinding (G47.63)*

    F45.9 **Somatoform disorder, unspecified**
Psychosomatic disorder NOS

✓4ᵗʰ **F48** **Other nonpsychotic mental disorders**

    F48.1 **Depersonalization-derealization syndrome**

    F48.2 **Pseudobulbar affect**
Involuntary emotional expression disorder
Code first underlying cause, if known, such as:
    amyotrophic lateral sclerosis (G12.21)
    multiple sclerosis (G35)
    sequelae of cerebrovascular disease (I69.-)
    sequelae of traumatic intracranial injury (S06.-)

    F48.8 **Other specified nonpsychotic mental disorders**
Dhat syndrome
Neurasthenia
Occupational neurosis, including writer's cramp
Psychasthenia
Psychasthenic neurosis
Psychogenic syncope

    F48.9 **Nonpsychotic mental disorder, unspecified**
Neurosis NOS

Behavioral syndromes associated with physiological disturbances and physical factors (F50-F59)

✓4ᵗʰ **F50** **Eating disorders**
    EXCLUDES 1 *anorexia NOS (R63.0)*
                 feeding difficulties (R63.3)
                 polyphagia (R63.2)
    EXCLUDES 2 *feeding disorder in infancy or childhood (F98.2-)*

✓5ᵗʰ **F50.0** **Anorexia nervosa**
        EXCLUDES 1 *loss of appetite (R63.0)*
                 psychogenic loss of appetite (F50.8)

    F50.00 **Anorexia nervosa, unspecified**

    F50.01 **Anorexia nervosa, restricting type**

☑ Additional Character Required   ✓ˣ⁷ᵗʰ Xtension Alert   Unspecified Dx   Other Specified Dx   Manifestation   ▶◀ Revised Text   ● New Code   ▲ Revised Code Title

Mental, Behavioral, and Neurodevelopmental Disorders

F50.02–F60.0

    F50.02   **Anorexia nervosa, binge eating/purging type**
           EXCLUDES 1   *bulimia nervosa (F50.2)*

   F50.2   **Bulimia nervosa**
        Bulimia NOS
        Hyperorexia nervosa
        EXCLUDES 1   *anorexia nervosa, binge eating/purging type (F50.02)*

   F50.8   **Other eating disorders**
        Pica in adults
        Psychogenic loss of appetite
        EXCLUDES 2   *pica of infancy and childhood (F98.3)*

   F50.9   **Eating disorder, unspecified**
        Atypical anorexia nervosa
        Atypical bulimia nervosa

✓4ᵗʰ **F51**   **Sleep disorders not due to a substance or known physiological condition**
       EXCLUDES 2   *organic sleep disorders (G47.-)*

  ✓5ᵗʰ **F51.0**   **Insomnia not due to a substance or known physiological condition**
         EXCLUDES 2   *alcohol related insomnia (F10.182, F10.282, F10.982)*
                     drug-related insomnia (F11.182, F11.282, F11.982,
                           F13.182, F13.282, F13.982, F14.182, F14.282,
                           F14.982, F15.182, F15.282, F15.982, F19.182,
                           F19.282, F19.982)
                     insomnia NOS (G47.0-)
                     insomnia due to known physiological condition
                         (G47.0-)
                     organic insomnia (G47.0-)
                     sleep deprivation (Z72.820)

     F51.01   **Primary insomnia**
          Idiopathic insomnia

     F51.02   **Adjustment insomnia**

     F51.03   **Paradoxical insomnia**

     F51.04   **Psychophysiologic insomnia**

     F51.05   **Insomnia due to other mental disorder**
          Code also associated mental disorder

     F51.09   **Other insomnia not due to a substance or known physiological condition**

  ✓5ᵗʰ **F51.1**   **Hypersomnia not due to a substance or known physiological condition**
         EXCLUDES 2   *alcohol related hypersomnia (F10.182, F10.282,*
                     F10.982)
                     drug-related hypersomnia (F11.182, F11.282, F11.982,
                           F13.182, F13.282, F13.982, F14.182, F14.282,
                           F14.982, F15.182, F15.282, F15.982, F19.182,
                           F19.282, F19.982)
                     hypersomnia NOS (G47.10)
                     hypersomnia due to known physiological condition
                         (G47.10)
                     idiopathic hypersomnia (G47.11, G47.12)
                     narcolepsy (G47.4-)

     F51.11   **Primary hypersomnia**

     F51.12   **Insufficient sleep syndrome**
          EXCLUDES 1   *sleep deprivation (Z72.820)*

     F51.13   **Hypersomnia due to other mental disorder**
          Code also associated mental disorder

     F51.19   **Other hypersomnia not due to a substance or known physiological condition**

   F51.3   **Sleepwalking [somnambulism]**

   F51.4   **Sleep terrors [night terrors]**

   F51.5   **Nightmare disorder**
        Dream anxiety disorder

   F51.8   **Other sleep disorders not due to a substance or known physiological condition**

   F51.9   **Sleep disorder not due to a substance or known physiological condition, unspecified**
        Emotional sleep disorder NOS

✓4ᵗʰ **F52**   **Sexual dysfunction not due to a substance or known physiological condition**
       EXCLUDES 2   *Dhat syndrome (F48.8)*

   F52.0   **Hypoactive sexual desire disorder**
        Anhedonia (sexual)
        Lack or loss of sexual desire
        EXCLUDES 1   *decreased libido (R68.82)*

   F52.1   **Sexual aversion disorder**
        Sexual aversion and lack of sexual enjoyment

  ✓5ᵗʰ **F52.2**   **Sexual arousal disorders**
        Failure of genital response

     F52.21   **Male erectile disorder**   ♂
          Psychogenic impotence
          EXCLUDES 1   *impotence of organic origin (N52.-)*
                     impotence NOS (N52.-)

     F52.22   **Female sexual arousal disorder**   ♀
          Frigidity

  ✓5ᵗʰ **F52.3**   **Orgasmic disorder**
        Inhibited orgasm
        Psychogenic anorgasmy

     F52.31   **Female orgasmic disorder**   ♀

     F52.32   **Male orgasmic disorder**   ♂

   F52.4   **Premature ejaculation**   ♂

   F52.5   **Vaginismus not due to a substance or known physiological condition**   ♀
        Psychogenic vaginismus
        EXCLUDES 2   *vaginismus (due to a known physiological condition)*
                     (N94.2)

   F52.6   **Dyspareunia not due to a substance or known physiological condition**   ♀
        Psychogenic dyspareunia
        EXCLUDES 2   *dyspareunia (due to a known physiological condition)*
                     (N94.1)

   F52.8   **Other sexual dysfunction not due to a substance or known physiological condition**
        Excessive sexual drive
        Nymphomania
        Satyriasis

   F52.9   **Unspecified sexual dysfunction not due to a substance or known physiological condition**
        Sexual dysfunction NOS

F53   **Puerperal psychosis**   ♀
       Postpartum depression
       EXCLUDES 1   *mood disorders with psychotic features (F30.2, F31.2, F31.5,*
                   F31.64, F32.3, F33.3)
                postpartum dysphoria (O90.6)
                psychosis in schizophrenia, schizotypal, delusional, and other
                    psychotic disorders (F20-F29)

F54   *Psychological and behavioral factors associated with disorders or diseases classified elsewhere*
       Psychological factors affecting physical conditions
       Code first the associated physical disorder, such as:
         asthma (J45.-)
         dermatitis (L23-L25)
         gastric ulcer (K25.-)
         mucous colitis (K58.-)
         ulcerative colitis (K51.-)
         urticaria (L50.-)
       EXCLUDES 2   *tension-type headache (G44.2)*

✓4ᵗʰ **F55**   **Abuse of non-psychoactive substances**
       EXCLUDES 2   *abuse of psychoactive substances (F10-F19)*

   F55.0   **Abuse of antacids**

   F55.1   **Abuse of herbal or folk remedies**

   F55.2   **Abuse of laxatives**

   F55.3   **Abuse of steroids or hormones**

   F55.4   **Abuse of vitamins**

   F55.8   **Abuse of other non-psychoactive substances**

F59   **Unspecified behavioral syndromes associated with physiological disturbances and physical factors**
       Psychogenic physiological dysfunction NOS

Disorders of adult personality and behavior (F60-F69)

✓4ᵗʰ **F60**   **Specific personality disorders**

   F60.0   **Paranoid personality disorder**
        Expansive paranoid personality (disorder)
        Fanatic personality (disorder)
        Paranoid personality (disorder)
        Querulant personality (disorder)
        Sensitive paranoid personality (disorder)
       EXCLUDES 2   *paranoia (F22)*
                   paranoia querulans (F22)
                   paranoid psychosis (F22)
                   paranoid schizophrenia (F20.0)
                   paranoid state (F22)

EXCLUDES 1   Not coded here   EXCLUDES 2   Not included here   N Newborn Age: 0   P Pediatric Age: 0-17   M Maternity Age: 12-55   A Adult Age: 15-124

508   ICD-10-CM Draft (2015)

F60.1 Schizoid personality disorder
> *EXCLUDES 2* *Asperger's syndrome (F84.5)*
> *delusional disorder (F22)*
> *schizoid disorder of childhood (F84.5)*
> *schizophrenia (F20.-)*
> *schizotypal disorder (F21)*

F60.2 Antisocial personality disorder
Amoral personality (disorder)
Asocial personality (disorder)
Dissocial personality disorder
Psychopathic personality (disorder)
Sociopathic personality (disorder)
> *EXCLUDES 1* *conduct disorders (F91.-)*
> *EXCLUDES 2* *borderline personality disorder (F60.3)*

F60.3 Borderline personality disorder
Aggressive personality (disorder)
Emotionally unstable personality disorder
Explosive personality (disorder)
> *EXCLUDES 2* *antisocial personality disorder (F60.2)*

F60.4 Histrionic personality disorder
Hysterical personality (disorder)
Psychoinfantile personality (disorder)

F60.5 Obsessive-compulsive personality disorder
Anankastic personality (disorder)
Compulsive personality (disorder)
Obsessional personality (disorder)
> *EXCLUDES 2* *obsessive-compulsive disorder (F42)*

F60.6 Avoidant personality disorder
Anxious personality disorder

F60.7 Dependent personality disorder
Asthenic personality (disorder)
Inadequate personality (disorder)
Passive personality (disorder)

✓5ᵗʰ F60.8 Other specific personality disorders
> **F60.81 Narcissistic personality disorder**
> **F60.89 Other specific personality disorders**
> Eccentric personality disorder
> "Haltlose" type personality disorder
> Immature personality disorder
> Passive-aggressive personality disorder
> Psychoneurotic personality disorder
> Self-defeating personality disorder

F60.9 Personality disorder, unspecified
Character disorder NOS
Character neurosis NOS
Pathological personality NOS

✓4ᵗʰ F63 Impulse disorders
> *EXCLUDES 2* *habitual excessive use of alcohol or psychoactive substances (F10-F19)*
> *impulse disorders involving sexual behavior (F65.-)*

F63.0 Pathological gambling
Compulsive gambling
> *EXCLUDES 1* *gambling and betting NOS (Z72.6)*
> *EXCLUDES 2* *excessive gambling by manic patients (F30, F31)*
> *gambling in antisocial personality disorder (F60.2)*

F63.1 Pyromania
Pathological fire-setting
> *EXCLUDES 2* *fire-setting (by) (in):*
> *adult with antisocial personality disorder (F60.2)*
> *alcohol or psychoactive substance intoxication (F10-F19)*
> *conduct disorders (F91.-)*
> *mental disorders due to known physiological condition (F01-F09)*
> *schizophrenia (F20.-)*

F63.2 Kleptomania
Pathological stealing
> *EXCLUDES 1* *shoplifting as the reason for observation for suspected mental disorder (Z03.8)*
> *EXCLUDES 2* *depressive disorder with stealing (F31-F33)*
> *stealing due to underlying mental condition—code to mental condition*
> *stealing in mental disorders due to known physiological condition (F01-F09)*

F63.3 Trichotillomania
Hair plucking
> *EXCLUDES 2* *other stereotyped movement disorder (F98.4)*

✓5ᵗʰ F63.8 Other impulse disorders
> **F63.81 Intermittent explosive disorder**
> **F63.89 Other impulse disorders**

F63.9 Impulse disorder, unspecified
Impulse control disorder NOS

✓4ᵗʰ F64 Gender identity disorders
F64.1 Gender identity disorder in adolescence and adulthood
Dual role transvestism
Transsexualism
Use additional code to identify sex reassignment status (Z87.890)
> *EXCLUDES 1* *gender identity disorder in childhood (F64.2)*
> *EXCLUDES 2* *fetishistic transvestism (F65.1)*

F64.2 Gender identity disorder of childhood
> *EXCLUDES 1* *gender identity disorder in adolescence and adulthood (F64.1)*
> *EXCLUDES 2* *sexual maturation disorder (F66)*

F64.8 Other gender identity disorders
F64.9 Gender identity disorder, unspecified
Gender-role disorder NOS

✓4ᵗʰ F65 Paraphilias
F65.0 Fetishism
F65.1 Transvestic fetishism
Fetishistic transvestism
F65.2 Exhibitionism
F65.3 Voyeurism
F65.4 Pedophilia
✓5ᵗʰ F65.5 Sadomasochism
> **F65.50 Sadomasochism, unspecified**
> **F65.51 Sexual masochism**
> **F65.52 Sexual sadism**
✓5ᵗʰ F65.8 Other paraphilias
> **F65.81 Frotteurism**
> **F65.89 Other paraphilias**
> Necrophilia
F65.9 Paraphilia, unspecified
Sexual deviation NOS

F66 Other sexual disorders
Sexual maturation disorder
Sexual relationship disorder

✓4ᵗʰ F68 Other disorders of adult personality and behavior
✓5ᵗʰ F68.1 Factitious disorder
Compensation neurosis
Elaboration of physical symptoms for psychological reasons
Hospital hopper syndrome
Münchhausen's syndrome
Peregrinating patient
> *EXCLUDES 2* *factitial dermatitis (L98.1)*
> *person feigning illness (with obvious motivation) (Z76.5)*

> **F68.10 Factitious disorder, unspecified**
> **F68.11 Factitious disorder with predominantly psychological signs and symptoms**
> **F68.12 Factitious disorder with predominantly physical signs and symptoms**
> **F68.13 Factitious disorder with combined psychological and physical signs and symptoms**
F68.8 Other specified disorders of adult personality and behavior

F69 Unspecified disorder of adult personality and behavior

Intellectual Disabilities (F70-F79)
Code first any associated physical or developmental disorders
> *EXCLUDES 1* *borderline intellectual functioning, IQ above 70 to 84 (R41.83)*

F70 Mild intellectual disabilities
IQ level 50-55 to approximately 70
Mild mental subnormality

F71 Moderate intellectual disabilities
IQ level 35-40 to 50-55
Moderate mental subnormality

F72 Severe intellectual disabilities
IQ 20-25 to 35-40
Severe mental subnormality

F73 Profound intellectual disabilities
IQ level below 20-25
Profound mental subnormality

F78   **Other intellectual disabilities**

F79   **Unspecified intellectual disabilities**
Mental deficiency NOS
Mental subnormality NOS

Pervasive and specific developmental disorders (F80-F89)

✓4ᵗʰ **F80**   **Specific developmental disorders of speech and language**

     F80.0   **Phonological disorder**
Dyslalia
Functional speech articulation disorder
Lalling
Lisping
Phonological developmental disorder
Speech articulation developmental disorder
EXCLUDES 1   *speech articulation impairment due to aphasia NOS (R47.01)*
          speech articulation impairment due to apraxia (R48.2)
EXCLUDES 2   *speech articulation impairment due to hearing loss (F80.4)*
          speech articulation impairment due to intellectual disabilities (F70-F79)
          speech articulation impairment with expressive language developmental disorder (F80.1)
          speech articulation impairment with mixed receptive expressive language developmental disorder (F80.2)

     F80.1   **Expressive language disorder**
Developmental dysphasia or aphasia, expressive type
EXCLUDES 1   *dysphasia and aphasia NOS (R47.-)*
          mixed receptive-expressive language disorder (F80.2)
EXCLUDES 2   *acquired aphasia with epilepsy [Landau-Kleffner] (G40.80-)*
          intellectual disabilities (F70-F79)
          pervasive developmental disorders (F84.-)
          selective mutism (F94.0)

     F80.2   **Mixed receptive-expressive language disorder**
Developmental dysphasia or aphasia, receptive type
Developmental Wernicke's aphasia
EXCLUDES 1   *central auditory processing disorder (H93.25)*
          dysphasia or aphasia NOS (R47.-)
          expressive language disorder (F80.1)
          expressive type dysphasia or aphasia (F80.1)
          word deafness (H93.25)
EXCLUDES 2   *acquired aphasia with epilepsy [Landau-Kleffner] (G40.80-)*
          intellectual disabilities (F70-F79)
          pervasive developmental disorders (F84.-)
          selective mutism (F94.0)

     F80.4   **Speech and language development delay due to hearing loss**
Code also type of hearing loss (H90.-, H91.-)

     ✓5ᵗʰ **F80.8**   **Other developmental disorders of speech and language**

         F80.81   **Childhood onset fluency disorder**
Cluttering NOS
Stuttering NOS
EXCLUDES 1   *adult onset fluency disorder (F98.5)*
          fluency disorder in conditions classified elsewhere (R47.82)
          fluency disorder (stuttering) following cerebrovascular disease (I69. with final characters-23)

         F80.89   **Other developmental disorders of speech and language**

     F80.9   **Developmental disorder of speech and language, unspecified**
Communication disorder NOS
Language disorder NOS

✓4ᵗʰ **F81**   **Specific developmental disorders of scholastic skills**

     F81.0   **Specific reading disorder**
"Backward reading"
Developmental dyslexia
Specific reading retardation
EXCLUDES 1   *alexia NOS (R48.0)*
          dyslexia NOS (R48.0)

     F81.2   **Mathematics disorder**
Developmental acalculia
Developmental arithmetical disorder
Developmental Gerstmann's syndrome
EXCLUDES 1   *acalculia NOS (R48.8)*
EXCLUDES 2   *arithmetical difficulties associated with a reading disorder (F81.0)*
          arithmetical difficulties associated with a spelling disorder (F81.81)
          arithmetical difficulties due to inadequate teaching (Z55.8)

     ✓5ᵗʰ **F81.8**   **Other developmental disorders of scholastic skills**

         F81.81   **Disorder of written expression**
Specific spelling disorder

         F81.89   **Other developmental disorders of scholastic skills**

     F81.9   **Developmental disorder of scholastic skills, unspecified**
Knowledge acquisition disability NOS
Learning disability NOS
Learning disorder NOS

F82   **Specific developmental disorder of motor function**
Clumsy child syndrome
Developmental coordination disorder
Developmental dyspraxia
EXCLUDES 1   *abnormalities of gait and mobility (R26.-)*
          lack of coordination (R27.-)
EXCLUDES 2   *lack of coordination secondary to intellectual disabilities (F70-F79)*

✓4ᵗʰ **F84**   **Pervasive developmental disorders**
Use additional code to identify any associated medical condition and intellectual disabilities

     F84.0   **Autistic disorder**
Infantile autism
Infantile psychosis
Kanner's syndrome
EXCLUDES 1   *Asperger's syndrome (F84.5)*

     F84.2   **Rett's syndrome**
EXCLUDES 1   *Asperger's syndrome (F84.5)*
          Autistic disorder (F84.0)
          Other childhood disintegrative disorder (F84.3)

     F84.3   **Other childhood disintegrative disorder**   P
Dementia infantilis
Disintegrative psychosis
Heller's syndrome
Symbiotic psychosis
Use additional code to identify any associated neurological condition
EXCLUDES 1   *Asperger's syndrome (F84.5)*
          Autistic disorder (F84.0)
          Rett's syndrome (F84.2)

     F84.5   **Asperger's syndrome**
Asperger's disorder
Autistic psychopathy
Schizoid disorder of childhood

     F84.8   **Other pervasive developmental disorders**
Overactive disorder associated with intellectual disabilities and stereotyped movements

     F84.9   **Pervasive developmental disorder, unspecified**
Atypical autism

F88   **Other disorders of psychological development**
Developmental agnosia

F89   **Unspecified disorder of psychological development**
Developmental disorder NOS

Behavioral and emotional disorders with onset usually occurring in childhood and adolescence (F90-F98)

NOTE   Codes within categories F90-F98 may be used regardless of the age of a patient. These disorders generally have onset within the childhood or adolescent years, but may continue throughout life or not be diagnosed until adulthood.

✓4ᵗʰ **F90**   **Attention-deficit hyperactivity disorders**
INCLUDES   attention deficit disorder with hyperactivity
          attention deficit syndrome with hyperactivity
EXCLUDES 2   *anxiety disorders (F40.-, F41.-)*
          mood [affective] disorders (F30-F39)
          pervasive developmental disorders (F84.-)
          schizophrenia (F20.-)

     F90.0   **Attention-deficit hyperactivity disorder, predominantly inattentive type**

EXCLUDES 1 Not coded here   *EXCLUDES 2* Not included here   N Newborn Age: 0   P Pediatric Age: 0-17   M Maternity Age: 12-55   A Adult Age: 15-124

510   ICD-10-CM Draft (2015)

F90.1 **Attention-deficit hyperactivity disorder, predominantly hyperactive type**

F90.2 **Attention-deficit hyperactivity disorder, combined type**

F90.8 **Attention-deficit hyperactivity disorder, other type**

F90.9 **Attention-deficit hyperactivity disorder, unspecified type**
Attention-deficit hyperactivity disorder of childhood or adolescence NOS
Attention-deficit hyperactivity disorder NOS

✓4ᵗʰ **F91** **Conduct disorders**
> EXCLUDES 1   *antisocial behavior (Z72.81-)*
> *antisocial personality disorder (F60.2)*
> EXCLUDES 2   *conduct problems associated with attention-deficit hyperactivity disorder (F90.-)*
> *mood [affective] disorders (F30-F39)*
> *pervasive developmental disorders (F84.-)*
> *schizophrenia (F20.-)*

F91.0 **Conduct disorder confined to family context**

F91.1 **Conduct disorder, childhood-onset type**
Unsocialized conduct disorder
Conduct disorder, solitary aggressive type
Unsocialized aggressive disorder

F91.2 **Conduct disorder, adolescent-onset type**
Socialized conduct disorder
Conduct disorder, group type

F91.3 **Oppositional defiant disorder**

F91.8 **Other conduct disorders**

F91.9 **Conduct disorder, unspecified**
Behavioral disorder NOS
Conduct disorder NOS
Disruptive behavior disorder NOS

✓4ᵗʰ **F93** **Emotional disorders with onset specific to childhood**

F93.0 **Separation anxiety disorder of childhood**   ▣
> EXCLUDES 2   *mood [affective] disorders (F30-F39)*
> *nonpsychotic mental disorders (F40-F48)*
> *phobic anxiety disorder of childhood (F40.8)*
> *social phobia (F40.1)*

F93.8 **Other childhood emotional disorders**   ▣
Identity disorder
> EXCLUDES 2   *gender identity disorder of childhood (F64.2)*

F93.9 **Childhood emotional disorder, unspecified**   ▣

✓4ᵗʰ **F94** **Disorders of social functioning with onset specific to childhood and adolescence**

F94.0 **Selective mutism**
Elective mutism
> EXCLUDES 2   *pervasive developmental disorders (F84.-)*
> *schizophrenia (F20.-)*
> *specific developmental disorders of speech and language (F80.-)*
> *transient mutism as part of separation anxiety in young children (F93.0)*

F94.1 **Reactive attachment disorder of childhood**   ▣
Use additional code to identify any associated failure to thrive or growth retardation
> EXCLUDES 1   *disinhibited attachment disorder of childhood (F94.1)*
> *normal variation in pattern of selective attachment*
> EXCLUDES 2   *Asperger's syndrome (F84.5)*
> *maltreatment syndromes (T74.-)*
> *sexual or physical abuse in childhood, resulting in psychosocial problems (Z62.81-)*

F94.2 **Disinhibited attachment disorder of childhood**   ▣
Affectionless psychopathy
Institutional syndrome
> EXCLUDES 1   *reactive attachment disorder of childhood (F94.1)*
> EXCLUDES 2   *Asperger's syndrome (F84.5)*
> *attention-deficit hyperactivity disorders (F90.-)*
> *hospitalism in children (F43.2-)*

F94.8 **Other childhood disorders of social functioning**   ▣

F94.9 **Childhood disorder of social functioning, unspecified**   ▣

✓4ᵗʰ **F95** **Tic disorder**

F95.0 **Transient tic disorder**

F95.1 **Chronic motor or vocal tic disorder**

F95.2 **Tourette's disorder**
Combined vocal and multiple motor tic disorder [de la Tourette]
Tourette's syndrome

F95.8 **Other tic disorders**

F95.9 **Tic disorder, unspecified**
Tic NOS

✓4ᵗʰ **F98** **Other behavioral and emotional disorders with onset usually occurring in childhood and adolescence**
> EXCLUDES 2   *breath-holding spells (R06.89)*
> *gender identity disorder of childhood (F64.2)*
> *Kleine-Levin syndrome (G47.13)*
> *obsessive-compulsive disorder (F42)*
> *sleep disorders not due to a substance or known physiological condition (F51.-)*

F98.0 **Enuresis not due to a substance or known physiological condition**
Enuresis (primary) (secondary) of nonorganic origin
Functional enuresis
Psychogenic enuresis
Urinary incontinence of nonorganic origin
> EXCLUDES 1   *enuresis NOS (R32)*

F98.1 **Encopresis not due to a substance or known physiological condition**
Functional encopresis
Incontinence of feces of nonorganic origin
Psychogenic encopresis
Use additional code to identify the cause of any coexisting constipation
> EXCLUDES 1   *encopresis NOS (R15.-)*

✓5ᵗʰ **F98.2** **Other feeding disorders of infancy and childhood**
> EXCLUDES 1   *feeding difficulties (R63.3)*
> EXCLUDES 2   *anorexia nervosa and other eating disorders (F50.-)*
> *feeding problems of newborn (P92.-)*
> *pica of infancy or childhood (F98.3)*

F98.21 **Rumination disorder of infancy**   ▣

F98.29 **Other feeding disorders of infancy and early childhood**   ▣

F98.3 **Pica of infancy and childhood**   ▣

F98.4 **Stereotyped movement disorders**
Stereotype/habit disorder
> EXCLUDES 1   *abnormal involuntary movements (R25.-)*
> EXCLUDES 2   *compulsions in obsessive-compulsive disorder (F42)*
> *hair plucking (F63.3)*
> *movement disorders of organic origin (G20-G25)*
> *nail-biting (F98.8)*
> *nose-picking (F98.8)*
> *stereotypies that are part of a broader psychiatric condition (F01-F95)*
> *thumb-sucking (F98.8)*
> *tic disorders (F95.-)*
> *trichotillomania (F63.3)*

F98.5 **Adult onset fluency disorder**
> EXCLUDES 1   *childhood onset fluency disorder (F80.81)*
> *dysphasia (R47.02)*
> *fluency disorder in conditions classified elsewhere (R47.82)*
> *fluency disorder (stuttering) following cerebrovascular disease (I69. with final characters -23)*
> *tic disorders (F95.-)*

F98.8 **Other specified behavioral and emotional disorders with onset usually occurring in childhood and adolescence**   ▣
Excessive masturbation
Nail-biting
Nose-picking
Thumb-sucking

F98.9 **Unspecified behavioral and emotional disorders with onset usually occurring in childhood and adolescence**   ▣

Unspecified mental disorder (F99)

F99 **Mental disorder, not otherwise specified**
Mental illness NOS
> EXCLUDES 1   *unspecified mental disorder due to known physiological condition (F09)*

✓ Additional Character Required   ✓x7ᵗʰ Xtension Alert   Unspecified Dx   Other Specified Dx   Manifestation   ►◄ Revised Text   ● New Code   ▲ Revised Code Title

Diseases of the Nervous System

G00–G04.32

Chapter 6. Diseases of the Nervous System (G00-G99)

EXCLUDES 2   *certain conditions originating in the perinatal period (P04-P96)*
certain infectious and parasitic diseases (A00-B99)
complications of pregnancy, childbirth and the puerperium (O00-O9A)
congenital malformations, deformations, and chromosomal abnormalities (Q00-Q99)
endocrine, nutritional and metabolic diseases (E00-E88)
injury, poisoning and certain other consequences of external causes (S00-T88)
neoplasms (C00-D49)
symptoms, signs and abnormal clinical and laboratory findings, not elsewhere classified (R00-R94)

This chapter contains the following blocks:

G00-G09	Inflammatory diseases of the central nervous system
G10-G14	Systemic atrophies primarily affecting the central nervous system
G20-G26	Extrapyramidal and movement disorders
G30-G32	Other degenerative diseases of the nervous system
G35-G37	Demyelinating diseases of the central nervous system
G40-G47	Episodic and paroxysmal disorders
G50-G59	Nerve, nerve root and plexus disorders
G60-G65	Polyneuropathies and other disorders of the peripheral nervous system
G70-G73	Diseases of myoneural junction and muscle
G80-G83	Cerebral palsy and other paralytic syndromes
G89-G99	Other disorders of the nervous system

Inflammatory diseases of the central nervous system (G00-G09)

✓4ᵗʰ **G00 Bacterial meningitis, not elsewhere classified**
INCLUDES   bacterial arachnoiditis
bacterial leptomeningitis
bacterial meningitis
bacterial pachymeningitis
EXCLUDES 1   *bacterial:*
meningoencephalitis (G04.2)
meningomyelitis (G04.2)

G00.0 Hemophilus meningitis
Meningitis due to Hemophilus influenzae

G00.1 Pneumococcal meningitis

G00.2 Streptococcal meningitis
Use additional code to further identify organism (B95.0-B95.5)

G00.3 Staphylococcal meningitis
Use additional code to further identify organism (B95.61-B95.8)

G00.8 Other bacterial meningitis
Meningitis due to Escherichia coli
Meningitis due to Friedländer's bacillus
Meningitis due to Klebsiella
Use additional code to further identify organism (B96.-)

G00.9 Bacterial meningitis, unspecified
Meningitis due to gram-negative bacteria, unspecified
Purulent meningitis NOS
Pyogenic meningitis NOS
Suppurative meningitis NOS

G01 *Meningitis in bacterial diseases classified elsewhere*
Code first underlying disease
EXCLUDES 1   *meningitis (in):*
gonococcal (A54.81)
leptospirosis (A27.81)
listeriosis (A32.11)
Lyme disease (A69.21)
meningococcal (A39.0)
neurosyphilis (A52.13)
tuberculosis (A17.0)
meningoencephalitis and meningomyelitis in bacterial diseases classified elsewhere (G05)

G02 *Meningitis in other infectious and parasitic diseases classified elsewhere*
Code first underlying disease, such as:
African trypanosomiasis (B56.-)
poliovirus infection (A80.-)
EXCLUDES 1   *candidal meningitis (B37.5)*
coccidioidomycosis meningitis (B38.4)
cryptococcal meningitis (B45.1)
herpesviral [herpes simplex] meningitis (B00.3)
infectious mononucleosis complicated by meningitis (B27.- with fourth character 2)
measles complicated by meningitis (B05.1)
meningoencephalitis and meningomyelitis in other infectious and parasitic diseases classified elsewhere (G05)
mumps meningitis (B26.1)
rubella meningitis (B06.02)
varicella [chickenpox] meningitis (B01.0)
zoster meningitis (B02.1)

✓4ᵗʰ **G03 Meningitis due to other and unspecified causes**
INCLUDES   arachnoiditis NOS
leptomeningitis NOS
meningitis NOS
pachymeningitis NOS
EXCLUDES 1   *meningoencephalitis (G04.-)*
meningomyelitis (G04.-)

G03.0 Nonpyogenic meningitis
Aseptic meningitis
Nonbacterial meningitis

G03.1 Chronic meningitis

G03.2 Benign recurrent meningitis [Mollaret]

G03.8 Meningitis due to other specified causes

G03.9 Meningitis, unspecified
Arachnoiditis (spinal) NOS

✓4ᵗʰ **G04 Encephalitis, myelitis and encephalomyelitis**
INCLUDES   acute ascending myelitis
meningoencephalitis
meningomyelitis
EXCLUDES 1   *encephalopathy NOS (G93.40)*
EXCLUDES 2   *acute transverse myelitis (G37.3-)*
alcoholic encephalopathy (G31.2)
benign myalgic encephalomyelitis (G93.3)
multiple sclerosis (G35)
subacute necrotizing myelitis (G37.4)
toxic encephalitis (G92)
toxic encephalopathy (G92)

✓5ᵗʰ **G04.0 Acute disseminated encephalitis and encephalomyelitis (ADEM)**
EXCLUDES 1   *acute necrotizing hemorrhagic encephalopathy (G04.3-)*
other noninfectious acute disseminated encephalomyelitis (noninfectious ADEM) (G04.81)

G04.00 Acute disseminated encephalitis and encephalomyelitis, unspecified

G04.01 Postinfectious acute disseminated encephalitis and encephalomyelitis (postinfectious ADEM)
EXCLUDES 1   *post chickenpox encephalitis (B01.1)*
post measles encephalitis (B05.0)
post measles myelitis (B05.1)

G04.02 Postimmunization acute disseminated encephalitis, myelitis and encephalomyelitis
Encephalitis, postimmunization
Encephalomyelitis, postimmunization
Use additional code to identify the vaccine (T50.A-, T50.B-, T50.Z-)

G04.1 Tropical spastic paraplegia

G04.2 Bacterial meningoencephalitis and meningomyelitis, not elsewhere classified

✓5ᵗʰ **G04.3 Acute necrotizing hemorrhagic encephalopathy**
EXCLUDES 1   *acute disseminated encephalitis and encephalomyelitis (G04.0-)*

G04.30 Acute necrotizing hemorrhagic encephalopathy, unspecified

G04.31 Postinfectious acute necrotizing hemorrhagic encephalopathy

G04.32 Postimmunization acute necrotizing hemorrhagic encephalopathy
Use additional code to identify the vaccine (T50.A-, T50.B-, T50.Z-)

EXCLUDES 1 Not coded here   EXCLUDES 2 Not included here   N Newborn Age: 0   P Pediatric Age: 0-17   M Maternity Age: 12-55   A Adult Age: 15-124

512   ICD-10-CM Draft (2015)

G04.39 **Other acute necrotizing hemorrhagic encephalopathy**
Code also underlying etiology, if applicable

✓5ᵗʰ G04.8 **Other encephalitis, myelitis and encephalomyelitis**
Code also any associated seizure (G40.-, R56.9)

    G04.81 **Other encephalitis and encephalomyelitis**
Noninfectious acute disseminated encephalomyelitis (noninfectious ADEM)

    G04.89 **Other myelitis**

✓5ᵗʰ G04.9 **Encephalitis, myelitis and encephalomyelitis, unspecified**

    G04.90 **Encephalitis and encephalomyelitis, unspecified**
Ventriculitis (cerebral) NOS

    G04.91 **Myelitis, unspecified**

✓4ᵗʰ **G05 Encephalitis, myelitis and encephalomyelitis in diseases classified elsewhere**
Code first underlying disease, such as:
human immunodeficiency virus [HIV] disease (B20)
poliovirus (A80.-)
suppurative otitis media (H66.01-H66.4)
trichinellosis (B75)

    EXCLUDES 1 *adenoviral encephalitis, myelitis and encephalomyelitis (A85.1)*
congenital toxoplasmosis encephalitis, myelitis and encephalomyelitis (P37.1)
cytomegaloviral encephalitis, myelitis and encephalomyelitis (B25.8)
encephalitis, myelitis and encephalomyelitis (in) measles (B05.0)
encephalitis, myelitis and encephalomyelitis (in) systemic lupus erythematosus (M32.19)
enteroviral encephalitis, myelitis and encephalomyelitis (A85.0)
eosinophilic meningoencephalitis (B83.2)
herpesviral [herpes simplex] encephalitis, myelitis and encephalomyelitis (B00.4)
listerial encephalitis, myelitis and encephalomyelitis (A32.12)
meningococcal encephalitis, myelitis and encephalomyelitis (A39.81)
mumps encephalitis, myelitis and encephalomyelitis (B26.2)
postchickenpox encephalitis, myelitis and encephalomyelitis (B01.1-)
rubella encephalitis, myelitis and encephalomyelitis (B06.01)
toxoplasmosis encephalitis, myelitis and encephalomyelitis (B58.2)
zoster encephalitis, myelitis and encephalomyelitis (B02.0)

  G05.3 Encephalitis and encephalomyelitis in diseases classified elsewhere
Meningoencephalitis in diseases classified elsewhere

  G05.4 Myelitis in diseases classified elsewhere
Meningomyelitis in diseases classified elsewhere

✓4ᵗʰ **G06 Intracranial and intraspinal abscess and granuloma**
Use additional code (B95-B97) to identify infectious agent

  G06.0 **Intracranial abscess and granuloma**
Brain [any part] abscess (embolic)
Cerebellar abscess (embolic)
Cerebral abscess (embolic)
Intracranial epidural abscess or granuloma
Intracranial extradural abscess or granuloma
Intracranial subdural abscess or granuloma
Otogenic abscess (embolic)

    EXCLUDES 1 *tuberculous intracranial abscess and granuloma (A17.81)*

  G06.1 **Intraspinal abscess and granuloma**
Abscess (embolic) of spinal cord [any part]
Intraspinal epidural abscess or granuloma
Intraspinal extradural abscess or granuloma
Intraspinal subdural abscess or granuloma

    EXCLUDES 1 *tuberculous intraspinal abscess and granuloma (A17.81)*

  G06.2 **Extradural and subdural abscess, unspecified**

G07 Intracranial and intraspinal abscess and granuloma in diseases classified elsewhere
Code first underlying disease, such as:
schistosomiasis granuloma of brain (B65.-)

    EXCLUDES 1 *abscess of brain:*
amebic (A06.6)
chromomycotic (B43.1)
gonococcal (A54.82)
tuberculous (A17.81)
tuberculoma of meninges (A17.1)

G08 Intracranial and intraspinal phlebitis and thrombophlebitis
Septic embolism of intracranial or intraspinal venous sinuses and veins
Septic endophlebitis of intracranial or intraspinal venous sinuses and veins
Septic phlebitis of intracranial or intraspinal venous sinuses and veins
Septic thrombophlebitis of intracranial or intraspinal venous sinuses and veins
Septic thrombosis of intracranial or intraspinal venous sinuses and veins

  EXCLUDES 1 *intracranial phlebitis and thrombophlebitis complicating:*
abortion, ectopic or molar pregnancy (O00-O07, O08.7)
pregnancy, childbirth and the puerperium (O22.5, O87.3)
nonpyogenic intracranial phlebitis and thrombophlebitis (I67.6)

  EXCLUDES 2 *intracranial phlebitis and thrombophlebitis complicating nonpyogenic intraspinal phlebitis and thrombophlebitis (G95.1)*

G09 Sequelae of inflammatory diseases of central nervous system
NOTE Category G09 is to be used to indicate conditions whose primary classification is to G00-G08 as the cause of sequelae, themselves classifiable elsewhere. The "sequelae" include conditions specified as residuals.
Code first condition resulting from (sequela) of inflammatory diseases of central nervous system

Systemic atrophies primarily affecting the central nervous system (G10-G14)

G10 Huntington's disease
Huntington's chorea
Huntington's dementia

✓4ᵗʰ **G11 Hereditary ataxia**
  EXCLUDES 2 *cerebral palsy (G80.-)*
hereditary and idiopathic neuropathy (G60.-)
metabolic disorders (E70-E88)

  G11.0 **Congenital nonprogressive ataxia**

  G11.1 **Early-onset cerebellar ataxia**
Early-onset cerebellar ataxia with essential tremor
Early-onset cerebellar ataxia with myoclonus [Hunt's ataxia]
Early-onset cerebellar ataxia with retained tendon reflexes
Friedreich's ataxia (autosomal recessive)
X-linked recessive spinocerebellar ataxia

  G11.2 **Late-onset cerebellar ataxia** ▲

  G11.3 **Cerebellar ataxia with defective DNA repair**
Ataxia telangiectasia [Louis-Bar]
    EXCLUDES 2 *Cockayne's syndrome (Q87.1)*
other disorders of purine and pyrimidine metabolism (E79.-)
xeroderma pigmentosum (Q82.1)

  G11.4 **Hereditary spastic paraplegia**

  G11.8 **Other hereditary ataxias**

  G11.9 **Hereditary ataxia, unspecified**
Hereditary cerebellar ataxia NOS
Hereditary cerebellar degeneration
Hereditary cerebellar disease
Hereditary cerebellar syndrome

✓4ᵗʰ **G12 Spinal muscular atrophy and related syndromes**

  G12.0 **Infantile spinal muscular atrophy, type I [Werdnig-Hoffman]**

  G12.1 **Other inherited spinal muscular atrophy**
Adult form spinal muscular atrophy
Childhood form, type II spinal muscular atrophy
Distal spinal muscular atrophy
Juvenile form, type III spinal muscular atrophy [Kugelberg-Welander]
Progressive bulbar palsy of childhood [Fazio-Londe]
Scapuloperoneal form spinal muscular atrophy

  ✓5ᵗʰ G12.2 **Motor neuron disease**

    G12.20 **Motor neuron disease, unspecified**

    G12.21 **Amyotrophic lateral sclerosis** ▲
Progressive spinal muscle atrophy

    G12.22 **Progressive bulbar palsy**

    G12.29 **Other motor neuron disease**
Familial motor neuron disease
Primary lateral sclerosis

  G12.8 **Other spinal muscular atrophies and related syndromes**

  G12.9 **Spinal muscular atrophy, unspecified**

☑ Additional Character Required   ✓x7ᵗʰ Xtension Alert   Unspecified Dx   Other Specified Dx   Manifestation   ▶◀ Revised Text   ● New Code   ▲ Revised Code Title

ICD-10-CM Draft (2015)   513

Diseases of the Nervous System

✓4ᵗʰ **G13 Systemic atrophies primarily affecting central nervous system in diseases classified elsewhere**

G13.0 Paraneoplastic neuromyopathy and neuropathy
Carcinomatous neuromyopathy
Sensorial paraneoplastic neuropathy [Denny Brown]
Code first underlying neoplasm (C00-D49)

G13.1 Other systemic atrophy primarily affecting central nervous system in neoplastic disease
Paraneoplastic limbic encephalopathy
Code first underlying neoplasm (C00-D49)

G13.2 Systemic atrophy primarily affecting the central nervous system in myxedema
Code first underlying disease, such as:
hypothyroidism (E03.-)
myxedematous congenital iodine deficiency (E00.1)

G13.8 Systemic atrophy primarily affecting central nervous system in other diseases classified elsewhere
Code first underlying disease

G14 Postpolio syndrome
Postpolio myelitic syndrome
EXCLUDES 1 *sequelae of poliomyelitis (B91)*

Extrapyramidal and movement disorders (G20-G26)

G20 Parkinson's disease
Hemiparkinsonism
Idiopathic Parkinsonism or Parkinson's disease
Paralysis agitans
Parkinsonism or Parkinson's disease NOS
Primary Parkinsonism or Parkinson's disease
EXCLUDES 1 *dementia with Parkinsonism (G31.83)*

✓4ᵗʰ **G21 Secondary parkinsonism**
EXCLUDES 1 *dementia with Parkinsonism (G31.83)*
Huntington's disease (G10)
Shy-Drager syndrome (G90.3)
syphilitic Parkinsonism (A52.19)

G21.0 Malignant neuroleptic syndrome
Use additional code for adverse effect, if applicable, to identify drug (T43.3X5, T43.4X5, T43.505, T43.595)
EXCLUDES 1 *neuroleptic induced parkinsonism (G21.11)*

✓5ᵗʰ **G21.1 Other drug-induced secondary parkinsonism**
G21.11 Neuroleptic induced parkinsonism
Use additional code for adverse effect, if applicable, to identify drug (T43.3X5, T43.4X5, T43.505, T43.595)
EXCLUDES 1 *malignant neuroleptic syndrome (G21.0)*
G21.19 Other drug induced secondary parkinsonism
Use additional code for adverse effect, if applicable, to identify drug (T36-T50 with fifth or sixth character 5)

G21.2 Secondary parkinsonism due to other external agents
Code first (T51-T65) to identify external agent
G21.3 Postencephalitic parkinsonism
G21.4 Vascular parkinsonism
G21.8 Other secondary parkinsonism
G21.9 Secondary parkinsonism, unspecified

✓4ᵗʰ **G23 Other degenerative diseases of basal ganglia**
EXCLUDES 2 *multi-system degeneration of the autonomic nervous system (G90.3)*
G23.0 Hallervorden-Spatz disease
Pigmentary pallidal degeneration
G23.1 Progressive supranuclear ophthalmoplegia [Steele-Richardson-Olszewski]
Progressive supranuclear palsy
G23.2 Striatonigral degeneration
G23.8 Other specified degenerative diseases of basal ganglia
Calcification of basal ganglia
G23.9 Degenerative disease of basal ganglia, unspecified

✓4ᵗʰ **G24 Dystonia**
INCLUDES dyskinesia
EXCLUDES 2 *athetoid cerebral palsy (G80.3)*
✓5ᵗʰ **G24.0 Drug induced dystonia**
Use additional code code for adverse effect, if applicable, to identify drug (T36-T50 with fifth or sixth character5)

G24.01 Drug induced subacute dyskinesia
Drug induced blepharospasm
Drug induced orofacial dyskinesia
Neuroleptic induced tardive dyskinesia
Tardive dyskinesia
G24.02 Drug induced acute dystonia
Acute dystonic reaction to drugs
Neuroleptic induced acute dystonia
G24.09 Other drug induced dystonia
G24.1 Genetic torsion dystonia
Dystonia deformans progressiva
Dystonia musculorum deformans
Familial torsion dystonia
Idiopathic familial dystonia
Idiopathic (torsion) dystonia NOS
(Schwalbe-) Ziehen-Oppenheim disease
G24.2 Idiopathic nonfamilial dystonia
G24.3 Spasmodic torticollis
EXCLUDES 1 *congenital torticollis (Q68.0)*
hysterical torticollis (F44.4)
ocular torticollis (R29.891)
psychogenic torticollis (F45.8)
torticollis NOS (M43.6)
traumatic recurrent torticollis (S13.4)
G24.4 Idiopathic orofacial dystonia
Orofacial dyskinesia
EXCLUDES 1 *drug induced orofacial dyskinesia (G24.01)*
G24.5 Blepharospasm
EXCLUDES 1 *drug induced blepharospasm (G24.01)*
G24.8 Other dystonia
Acquired torsion dystonia NOS
G24.9 Dystonia, unspecified
Dyskinesia NOS

✓4ᵗʰ **G25 Other extrapyramidal and movement disorders**
EXCLUDES 2 *sleep related movement disorders (G47.6-)*
G25.0 Essential tremor
Familial tremor
EXCLUDES 1 *tremor NOS (R25.1)*
G25.1 Drug-induced tremor
Use additional code for adverse effect, if applicable, to identify drug (T36-T50 with fifth or sixth character 5)
G25.2 Other specified forms of tremor
Intention tremor
G25.3 Myoclonus
Drug-induced myoclonus
Palatal myoclonus
Use additional code for adverse effect, if applicable, to identify drug (T36-T50 with fifth or sixth character 5)
EXCLUDES 1 *facial myokymia (G51.4)*
myoclonic epilepsy (G40.-)
G25.4 Drug-induced chorea
Use additional code for adverse effect, if applicable, to identify drug (T36-T50 with fifth or sixth character 5)
G25.5 Other chorea
Chorea NOS
EXCLUDES 1 *chorea NOS with heart involvement (I02.0)*
Huntington's chorea (G10)
rheumatic chorea (I02.-)
Sydenham's chorea (I02.-)
✓5ᵗʰ **G25.6 Drug induced tics and other tics of organic origin**
G25.61 Drug induced tics
Use additional code for adverse effect, if applicable, to identify drug (T36-T50 with fifth or sixth character 5)
G25.69 Other tics of organic origin
EXCLUDES 1 *habit spasm (F95.9)*
tic NOS (F95.9)
Tourette's syndrome (F95.2)
✓5ᵗʰ **G25.7 Other and unspecified drug induced movement disorders**
Use additional code for adverse effect, if applicable, to identify drug (T36-T50 with fifth or sixth character 5)
G25.70 Drug induced movement disorder, unspecified
G25.71 Drug induced akathisia
Drug induced acathisia
Neuroleptic induced acute akathisia
G25.79 Other drug induced movement disorders
✓5ᵗʰ **G25.8 Other specified extrapyramidal and movement disorders**
G25.81 Restless legs syndrome

G25.82   **Stiff-man syndrome**

G25.83   **Benign shuddering attacks**

G25.89   **Other specified extrapyramidal and movement disorders**

G25.9   **Extrapyramidal and movement disorder, unspecified**

G26   *Extrapyramidal and movement disorders in diseases classified elsewhere*
      Code first underlying disease

Other degenerative diseases of the nervous system (G30-G32)

✓4ᵗʰ **G30   Alzheimer's disease**

INCLUDES   Alzheimer's dementia senile and presenile forms
Use additional code to identify:
delirium, if applicable (FØ5)
dementia with behavioral disturbance (FØ2.81)
dementia without behavioral disturbance (FØ2.8Ø)

EXCLUDES 1   *senile degeneration of brain NEC (G31.1)*
senile dementia NOS (FØ3)
senility NOS (R41.81)

G30.0   **Alzheimer's disease with early onset**

G30.1   **Alzheimer's disease with late onset**   Ⓐ

G30.8   **Other Alzheimer's disease**

G30.9   **Alzheimer's disease, unspecified**
        AHA: 2012, 4Q, 95

✓4ᵗʰ **G31   Other degenerative diseases of nervous system, not elsewhere classified**

Use additional code to identify:
dementia with behavioral disturbance (FØ2.81)
dementia without behavioral disturbance (FØ2.8Ø)

EXCLUDES 2   *Reye's syndrome (G93.7)*

✓5ᵗʰ   G31.Ø   **Frontotemporal dementia**

G31.01   **Pick's disease**
         Primary progressive aphasia
         Progressive isolated aphasia

G31.09   **Other frontotemporal dementia**
         Frontal dementia

G31.1   **Senile degeneration of brain, not elsewhere classified**
        EXCLUDES 1   *Alzheimer's disease (G3Ø.-)*
        senility NOS (R41.81)

G31.2   **Degeneration of nervous system due to alcohol**
        Alcoholic cerebellar ataxia
        Alcoholic cerebellar degeneration
        Alcoholic cerebral degeneration
        Alcoholic encephalopathy
        Dysfunction of the autonomic nervous system due to alcohol
        Code also associated alcoholism (F1Ø.-)

✓5ᵗʰ   G31.8   **Other specified degenerative diseases of nervous system**

G31.81   **Alpers disease**
         Grey-matter degeneration

G31.82   **Leigh's disease**
         Subacute necrotizing encephalopathy

G31.83   **Dementia with Lewy bodies**
         Dementia with Parkinsonism
         Lewy body dementia
         Lewy body disease

G31.84   **Mild cognitive impairment, so stated**
         EXCLUDES 1   *age related cognitive decline (R41.81)*
         altered mental status (R41.82)
         cerebral degeneration (G31.9)
         change in mental status (R41.82)
         cognitive deficits following (sequelae of)
         cerebral hemorrhage or infarction
         (I69.Ø1, I69.11, I69.21, I69.31, I69.81,
         I69.91)
         cognitive impairment due to intracranial or
         head injury (SØ6.-)
         dementia (FØ1.-, FØ2.-, FØ3)
         mild memory disturbance (FØ6.8)
         neurologic neglect syndrome (R41.4)
         personality change, nonpsychotic (F68.8)

G31.85   **Corticobasal degeneration**

G31.89   **Other specified degenerative diseases of nervous system**

G31.9   **Degenerative disease of nervous system, unspecified**

✓4ᵗʰ **G32   Other degenerative disorders of nervous system in diseases classified elsewhere**

G32.Ø   *Subacute combined degeneration of spinal cord in diseases classified elsewhere*
        Dana-Putnam syndrome
        Sclerosis of spinal cord (combined) (dorsolateral) (posterolateral)
        Code first underlying disease, such as:
        vitamin B12 deficiency (E53.8)
        vitamin B12 deficiency:
        anemia (D51.9)
        dietary (D51.3)
        pernicious (D51.Ø)
        EXCLUDES 1   *syphilitic combined degeneration of spinal cord (A52.11)*

✓5ᵗʰ   G32.8   **Other specified degenerative disorders of nervous system in diseases classified elsewhere**
        Code first underlying disease, such as:
        amyloidosis cerebral degeneration (E85.-)
        cerebral degeneration (due to) hypothyroidism (EØØ.Ø-EØ3.9)
        cerebral degeneration (due to) neoplasm (CØØ-D49)
        cerebral degeneration (due to) vitamin B deficiency, except thiamine (E52-E53.-)
        EXCLUDES 1   *superior hemorrhagic polioencephalitis [Wernicke's encephalopathy] (E51.2)*

G32.81   *Cerebellar ataxia in diseases classified elsewhere*
         Code first underlying disease, such as:
         celiac disease (with gluten ataxia) (K9Ø.Ø)
         cerebellar ataxia (in) neoplastic disease (paraneoplastic cerebellar degeneration) (CØØ-D49)
         non-celiac gluten ataxia (M35.9)
         EXCLUDES 1   *systemic atrophy primarily affecting the central nervous system in alcoholic cerebellar ataxia (G31.2)*
         systemic atrophy primarily affecting the central nervous system in myxedema (G13.2)

G32.89   *Other specified degenerative disorders of nervous system in diseases classified elsewhere*
         Degenerative encephalopathy in diseases classified elsewhere

Demyelinating diseases of the central nervous system (G35-G37)

G35   Multiple sclerosis
Disseminated multiple sclerosis
Generalized multiple sclerosis
Multiple sclerosis NOS
Multiple sclerosis of brain stem
Multiple sclerosis of cord

✓4ᵗʰ **G36   Other acute disseminated demyelination**
EXCLUDES 1   *postinfectious encephalitis and encephalomyelitis NOS (GØ4.Ø1)*

G36.Ø   **Neuromyelitis optica [Devic]**
        Demyelination in optic neuritis
        EXCLUDES 1   *optic neuritis NOS (H46)*

G36.1   **Acute and subacute hemorrhagic leukoencephalitis [Hurst]**

G36.8   **Other specified acute disseminated demyelination**

G36.9   **Acute disseminated demyelination, unspecified**

✓4ᵗʰ **G37   Other demyelinating diseases of central nervous system**

G37.Ø   **Diffuse sclerosis of central nervous system**
        Periaxial encephalitis
        Schilder's disease
        EXCLUDES 1   *X linked adrenoleukodystrophy (E71.52-)*

G37.1   **Central demyelination of corpus callosum**

G37.2   **Central pontine myelinolysis**

G37.3   **Acute transverse myelitis in demyelinating disease of central nervous system**
        Acute transverse myelitis NOS
        Acute transverse myelopathy
        EXCLUDES 1   *multiple sclerosis (G35)*
        neuromyelitis optica [Devic] (G36.Ø)

G37.4   **Subacute necrotizing myelitis of central nervous system**

G37.5   **Concentric sclerosis [Balo] of central nervous system**

G37.8   **Other specified demyelinating diseases of central nervous system**

G37.9   **Demyelinating disease of central nervous system, unspecified**

Diseases of the Nervous System

G40–G40.A11

Episodic and paroxysmal disorders (G40-G47)

✓4ᵗʰ G40 Epilepsy and recurrent seizures

> **NOTE** The following terms are to be considered equivalent to intractable: pharmacoresistant (pharmacologically resistant), treatment resistant, refractory (medically) and poorly controlled

> **EXCLUDES 1** conversion disorder with seizures (F44.5)
> convulsions NOS (R56.9)
> hippocampal sclerosis (G93.81)
> mesial temporal sclerosis (G93.81)
> post traumatic seizures (R56.1)
> seizure (convulsive) NOS (R56.9)
> seizure of newborn (P90)
> temporal sclerosis (G93.81)
> Todd's paralysis (G83.8)

✓5ᵗʰ G40.0 Localization-related (focal) (partial) idiopathic epilepsy and epileptic syndromes with seizures of localized onset
> Benign childhood epilepsy with centrotemporal EEG spikes
> Childhood epilepsy with occipital EEG paroxysms
> **EXCLUDES 1** adult onset localization-related epilepsy (G40.1-, G40.2-)

> **✓6ᵗʰ G40.00 Localization-related (focal) (partial) idiopathic epilepsy and epileptic syndromes with seizures of localized onset, not intractable**
> > Localization-related (focal) (partial) idiopathic epilepsy and epileptic syndromes with seizures of localized onset without intractability
> >
> > **G40.001 Localization-related (focal) (partial) idiopathic epilepsy and epileptic syndromes with seizures of localized onset, not intractable, with status epilepticus**
> >
> > **G40.009 Localization-related (focal) (partial) idiopathic epilepsy and epileptic syndromes with seizures of localized onset, not intractable, without status epilepticus**
> > > Localization-related (focal) (partial) idiopathic epilepsy and epileptic syndromes with seizures of localized onset NOS

> **✓6ᵗʰ G40.01 Localization-related (focal) (partial) idiopathic epilepsy and epileptic syndromes with seizures of localized onset, intractable**
> > **G40.011 Localization-related (focal) (partial) idiopathic epilepsy and epileptic syndromes with seizures of localized onset, intractable, with status epilepticus**
> >
> > **G40.019 Localization-related (focal) (partial) idiopathic epilepsy and epileptic syndromes with seizures of localized onset, intractable, without status epilepticus**

✓5ᵗʰ G40.1 Localization-related (focal) (partial) symptomatic epilepsy and epileptic syndromes with simple partial seizures
> Attacks without alteration of consciousness
> Epilepsia partialis continua [Kozhevnikof]
> Simple partial seizures developing into secondarily generalized seizures

> **✓6ᵗʰ G40.10 Localization-related (focal) (partial) symptomatic epilepsy and epileptic syndromes with simple partial seizures, not intractable**
> > Localization-related (focal) (partial) symptomatic epilepsy and epileptic syndromes with simple partial seizures without intractability
> >
> > **G40.101 Localization-related (focal) (partial) symptomatic epilepsy and epileptic syndromes with simple partial seizures, not intractable, with status epilepticus**
> >
> > **G40.109 Localization-related (focal) (partial) symptomatic epilepsy and epileptic syndromes with simple partial seizures, not intractable, without status epilepticus**
> > > Localization-related (focal) (partial) symptomatic epilepsy and epileptic syndromes with simple partial seizures NOS

> **✓6ᵗʰ G40.11 Localization-related (focal) (partial) symptomatic epilepsy and epileptic syndromes with simple partial seizures, intractable**
> > **G40.111 Localization-related (focal) (partial) symptomatic epilepsy and epileptic syndromes with simple partial seizures, intractable, with status epilepticus**
> >
> > **G40.119 Localization-related (focal) (partial) symptomatic epilepsy and epileptic syndromes with simple partial seizures, intractable, without status epilepticus**

✓5ᵗʰ G40.2 Localization-related (focal) (partial) symptomatic epilepsy and epileptic syndromes with complex partial seizures
> Attacks with alteration of consciousness, often with automatisms
> Complex partial seizures developing into secondarily generalized seizures

> **✓6ᵗʰ G40.20 Localization-related (focal) (partial) symptomatic epilepsy and epileptic syndromes with complex partial seizures, not intractable**
> > Localization-related (focal) (partial) symptomatic epilepsy and epileptic syndromes with complex partial seizures without intractability
> >
> > **G40.201 Localization-related (focal) (partial) symptomatic epilepsy and epileptic syndromes with complex partial seizures, not intractable, with status epilepticus**
> >
> > **G40.209 Localization-related (focal) (partial) symptomatic epilepsy and epileptic syndromes with complex partial seizures, not intractable, without status epilepticus**
> > > Localization-related (focal) (partial) symptomatic epilepsy and epileptic syndromes with complex partial seizures NOS

> **✓6ᵗʰ G40.21 Localization-related (focal) (partial) symptomatic epilepsy and epileptic syndromes with complex partial seizures, intractable**
> > **G40.211 Localization-related (focal) (partial) symptomatic epilepsy and epileptic syndromes with complex partial seizures, intractable, with status epilepticus**
> >
> > **G40.219 Localization-related (focal) (partial) symptomatic epilepsy and epileptic syndromes with complex partial seizures, intractable, without status epilepticus**

✓5ᵗʰ G40.3 Generalized idiopathic epilepsy and epileptic syndromes
> Code also MERRF syndrome, if applicable (E88.42)

> **✓6ᵗʰ G40.30 Generalized idiopathic epilepsy and epileptic syndromes, not intractable**
> > Generalized idiopathic epilepsy and epileptic syndromes without intractability
> >
> > **G40.301 Generalized idiopathic epilepsy and epileptic syndromes, not intractable, with status epilepticus**
> >
> > **G40.309 Generalized idiopathic epilepsy and epileptic syndromes, not intractable, without status epilepticus**
> > > Generalized idiopathic epilepsy and epileptic syndromes NOS

> **✓6ᵗʰ G40.31 Generalized idiopathic epilepsy and epileptic syndromes, intractable**
> > **G40.311 Generalized idiopathic epilepsy and epileptic syndromes, intractable, with status epilepticus**
> >
> > **G40.319 Generalized idiopathic epilepsy and epileptic syndromes, intractable, without status epilepticus**

✓5ᵗʰ G40.A Absence epileptic syndrome
> Childhood absence epilepsy [pyknolepsy]
> Juvenile absence epilepsy
> Absence epileptic syndrome, NOS

> **✓6ᵗʰ G40.A0 Absence epileptic syndrome, not intractable**
> > **G40.A01 Absence epileptic syndrome, not intractable, with status epilepticus**
> >
> > **G40.A09 Absence epileptic syndrome, not intractable, without status epilepticus**

> **✓6ᵗʰ G40.A1 Absence epileptic syndrome, intractable**
> > **G40.A11 Absence epileptic syndrome, intractable, with status epilepticus**

EXCLUDES 1 Not coded here   **EXCLUDES 2** Not included here   **N** Newborn Age: 0   **P** Pediatric Age: 0-17   **M** Maternity Age: 12-55   **A** Adult Age: 15-124

516   ICD-10-CM Draft (2015)

G40.A19   **Absence epileptic syndrome, intractable, without status epilepticus**

✓5th **G40.B**   Juvenile myoclonic epilepsy [impulsive petit mal]

✓6th **G40.B0**   **Juvenile myoclonic epilepsy,** not intractable

G40.B01   **Juvenile myoclonic epilepsy, not intractable, with status epilepticus**

G40.B09   **Juvenile myoclonic epilepsy, not intractable, without status epilepticus**

✓6th **G40.B1**   **Juvenile myoclonic epilepsy,** intractable

G40.B11   **Juvenile myoclonic epilepsy, intractable, with status epilepticus**

G40.B19   **Juvenile myoclonic epilepsy, intractable, without status epilepticus**

✓5th **G40.4**   Other generalized epilepsy and epileptic syndromes

    Epilepsy with grand mal seizures on awakening
    Epilepsy with myoclonic absences
    Epilepsy with myoclonic-astatic seizures
    Grand mal seizure NOS
    Nonspecific atonic epileptic seizures
    Nonspecific clonic epileptic seizures
    Nonspecific myoclonic epileptic seizures
    Nonspecific tonic epileptic seizures
    Nonspecific tonic-clonic epileptic seizures
    Symptomatic early myoclonic encephalopathy

✓6th **G40.40**   **Other generalized epilepsy and epileptic syndromes,** not intractable

    Other generalized epilepsy and epileptic syndromes without intractability
    Other generalized epilepsy and epileptic syndromes NOS

G40.401   **Other generalized epilepsy and epileptic syndromes, not intractable, with status epilepticus**

G40.409   **Other generalized epilepsy and epileptic syndromes, not intractable, without status epilepticus**

✓6th **G40.41**   **Other generalized epilepsy and epileptic syndromes,** intractable

G40.411   **Other generalized epilepsy and epileptic syndromes, intractable, with status epilepticus**

G40.419   **Other generalized epilepsy and epileptic syndromes, intractable, without status epilepticus**

✓5th **G40.5**   Epileptic seizures related to external causes

    Epileptic seizures related to alcohol
    Epileptic seizures related to drugs
    Epileptic seizures related to hormonal changes
    Epileptic seizures related to sleep deprivation
    Epileptic seizures related to stress
    Code also, if applicable, associated epilepsy and recurrent seizures (G40.-)
    Use additional code for adverse effect, if applicable, to identify drug (T36-T50 with fifth or sixth character 5)

✓6th **G40.50**   **Epileptic seizures related to external causes,** not intractable

G40.501   **Epileptic seizures related to external causes, not intractable, with status epilepticus**

G40.509   **Epileptic seizures related to external causes, not intractable, without status epilepticus**
    Epileptic seizures related to external causes, NOS

✓5th **G40.8**   Other epilepsy and recurrent seizures

    Epilepsies and epileptic syndromes undetermined as to whether they are focal or generalized
    Landau-Kleffner syndrome

✓6th **G40.80**   **Other epilepsy**

G40.801   **Other epilepsy, not intractable, with status epilepticus**
    Other epilepsy without intractability with status epilepticus

G40.802   **Other epilepsy, not intractable, without status epilepticus**
    Other epilepsy without intractability without status epilepticus

G40.803   **Other epilepsy, intractable, with status epilepticus**

G40.804   **Other epilepsy, intractable,** without status epilepticus

✓6th **G40.81**   **Lennox-Gastaut syndrome**

G40.811   **Lennox-Gastaut syndrome,** not intractable, with status epilepticus

G40.812   **Lennox-Gastaut syndrome,** not intractable, without status epilepticus

G40.813   **Lennox-Gastaut syndrome,** intractable, with status epilepticus

G40.814   **Lennox-Gastaut syndrome,** intractable, without status epilepticus

✓6th **G40.82**   **Epileptic spasms**

    Infantile spasms
    Salaam attacks
    West's syndrome

G40.821   **Epileptic spasms,** not intractable, **with status epilepticus**

G40.822   **Epileptic spasms,** not intractable, **without status epilepticus**

G40.823   **Epileptic spasms,** intractable, **with status epilepticus**

G40.824   **Epileptic spasms,** intractable, **without status epilepticus**

G40.89   **Other seizures**
    EXCLUDES 1   *post traumatic seizures (R56.1)*
    recurrent seizures NOS (G40.909)
    seizure NOS (R56.9)

✓5th **G40.9**   Epilepsy, unspecified

✓6th **G40.90**   **Epilepsy, unspecified,** not intractable
    Epilepsy, unspecified, without intractability

G40.901   **Epilepsy, unspecified, not intractable, with status epilepticus**

G40.909   **Epilepsy, unspecified, not intractable, without status epilepticus**
    Epilepsy NOS
    Epileptic convulsions NOS
    Epileptic fits NOS
    Epileptic seizures NOS
    Recurrent seizures NOS
    Seizure disorder NOS

✓6th **G40.91**   **Epilepsy, unspecified,** intractable
    Intractable seizure disorder NOS

G40.911   **Epilepsy, unspecified, intractable,** with status epilepticus

G40.919   **Epilepsy, unspecified, intractable,** without status epilepticus

✓4th **G43**   **Migraine**
    NOTE   The following terms are to be considered equivalent to intractable: pharmacoresistant (pharmacologically resistant), treatment resistant, refractory (medically) and poorly controlled.
    Use additional code for adverse effect, if applicable, to identify drug (T36-T50 with fifth or sixth character 5)
    EXCLUDES 1   *headache NOS (R51)*
    lower half migraine (G44.00)
    EXCLUDES 2   *headache syndromes (G44.-)*

✓5th **G43.0**   Migraine without aura
    Common migraine
    EXCLUDES 1   *chronic migraine without aura (G43.7-)*

✓6th **G43.00**   **Migraine without aura,** not intractable
    Migraine without aura without mention of refractory migraine

G43.001   **Migraine without aura, not intractable, with status migrainosus**

G43.009   **Migraine without aura, not intractable, without status migrainosus**
    Migraine without aura NOS

✓6th **G43.01**   **Migraine without aura,** intractable
    Migraine without aura with refractory migraine

G43.011   **Migraine without aura, intractable, with status migrainosus**

G43.019   **Migraine without aura, intractable, without status migrainosus**

✓ Additional Character Required   ✓x7th Xtension Alert   Unspecified Dx   Other Specified Dx   Manifestation   ►◄ Revised Text   ● New Code   ▲ Revised Code Title

ICD-10-CM Draft (2015)   **517**

Diseases of the Nervous System

G43.1–G43.821

✓5ᵗʰ **G43.1** **Migraine** with aura
Basilar migraine
Classical migraine
Migraine equivalents
Migraine preceded or accompanied by transient focal
  neurological phenomena
Migraine triggered seizures
Migraine with acute-onset aura
Migraine with aura without headache (migraine equivalents)
Migraine with prolonged aura
Migraine with typical aura
Retinal migraine
Code also any associated seizure (G40.-, R56.9)
EXCLUDES 1 persistent migraine aura (G43.5-, G43.6-)

✓6ᵗʰ **G43.10** **Migraine with aura,** not intractable
Migraine with aura without mention of refractory
  migraine

G43.101 **Migraine with aura, not intractable,** with
  status migrainosus

G43.109 **Migraine with aura, not intractable,**
  without status migrainosus
  Migraine with aura NOS

✓6ᵗʰ **G43.11** **Migraine with aura,** intractable
Migraine with aura with refractory migraine

G43.111 **Migraine with aura, intractable,** with
  status migrainosus

G43.119 **Migraine with aura, intractable,** without
  status migrainosus

✓5ᵗʰ **G43.4** **Hemiplegic** migraine
Familial migraine
Sporadic migraine

✓6ᵗʰ **G43.40** **Hemiplegic migraine,** not intractable
Hemiplegic migraine without refractory migraine

G43.401 **Hemiplegic migraine, not intractable,** with
  status migrainosus

G43.409 **Hemiplegic migraine, not intractable,**
  without status migrainosus
  Hemiplegic migraine NOS

✓6ᵗʰ **G43.41** **Hemiplegic migraine,** intractable
Hemiplegic migraine with refractory migraine

G43.411 **Hemiplegic migraine, intractable,** with
  status migrainosus

G43.419 **Hemiplegic migraine, intractable,** without
  status migrainosus

✓5ᵗʰ **G43.5** **Persistent** migraine aura without cerebral infarction

✓6ᵗʰ **G43.50** **Persistent migraine aura without cerebral infarction,**
  not intractable
  Persistent migraine aura without cerebral infarction,
    without refractory migraine

G43.501 **Persistent migraine aura without cerebral
  infarction, not intractable,** with status
  migrainosus

G43.509 **Persistent migraine aura without cerebral
  infarction, not intractable,** without status
  migrainosus
  Persistent migraine aura NOS

✓6ᵗʰ **G43.51** **Persistent migraine aura without cerebral infarction,**
  intractable
  Persistent migraine aura without cerebral infarction,
    with refractory migraine

G43.511 **Persistent migraine aura without cerebral
  infarction, intractable,** with status
  migrainosus

G43.519 **Persistent migraine aura without cerebral
  infarction, intractable,** without status
  migrainosus

✓5ᵗʰ **G43.6** **Persistent** migraine aura with cerebral infarction
Code also the type of cerebral infarction (I63.-)

✓6ᵗʰ **G43.60** **Persistent migraine aura with cerebral infarction,**
  not intractable
  Persistent migraine aura with cerebral infarction,
    without refractory migraine

G43.601 **Persistent migraine aura with cerebral
  infarction, not intractable,** with status
  migrainosus

G43.609 **Persistent migraine aura with cerebral
  infarction, not intractable,** without status
  migrainosus

✓6ᵗʰ **G43.61** **Persistent migraine aura with cerebral infarction,**
  intractable
  Persistent migraine aura with cerebral infarction, with
    refractory migraine

G43.611 **Persistent migraine aura with cerebral
  infarction, intractable,** with status
  migrainosus

G43.619 **Persistent migraine aura with cerebral
  infarction, intractable,** without status
  migrainosus

✓5ᵗʰ **G43.7** **Chronic** migraine without aura
Transformed migraine
EXCLUDES 1 migraine without aura (G43.0-)

✓6ᵗʰ **G43.70** **Chronic migraine without aura,** not intractable
Chronic migraine without aura, without refractory
  migraine

G43.701 **Chronic migraine without aura, not
  intractable,** with status migrainosus

G43.709 **Chronic migraine without aura, not
  intractable,** without status migrainosus
  Chronic migraine without aura NOS

✓6ᵗʰ **G43.71** **Chronic migraine without aura,** intractable
Chronic migraine without aura, with refractory
  migraine

G43.711 **Chronic migraine without aura,
  intractable,** with status migrainosus

G43.719 **Chronic migraine without aura,
  intractable,** without status migrainosus

✓5ᵗʰ **G43.A** **Cyclical vomiting**

G43.A0 **Cyclical vomiting,** not intractable
Cyclical vomiting, without refractory migraine

G43.A1 **Cyclical vomiting,** intractable
Cyclical vomiting, with refractory migraine

✓5ᵗʰ **G43.B** **Ophthalmoplegic** migraine

G43.B0 **Ophthalmoplegic migraine,** not intractable
Ophthalmoplegic migraine, without refractory
  migraine

G43.B1 **Ophthalmoplegic migraine,** intractable
Ophthalmoplegic migraine, with refractory migraine

✓5ᵗʰ **G43.C** **Periodic headache** syndromes in child or adult

G43.C0 **Periodic headache syndromes in child or adult,** not
  intractable
  Periodic headache syndromes in child or adult,
    without refractory migraine

G43.C1 **Periodic headache syndromes in child or adult,**
  intractable
  Periodic headache syndromes in child or adult, with
    refractory migraine

✓5ᵗʰ **G43.D** **Abdominal** migraine

G43.D0 **Abdominal migraine,** not intractable
Abdominal migraine, without refractory migraine

G43.D1 **Abdominal migraine,** intractable
Abdominal migraine, with refractory migraine

✓5ᵗʰ **G43.8** **Other** migraine

✓6ᵗʰ **G43.80** **Other migraine,** not intractable
Other migraine, without refractory migraine

G43.801 **Other migraine, not intractable,** with
  status migrainosus

G43.809 **Other migraine, not intractable,** without
  status migrainosus

✓6ᵗʰ **G43.81** **Other migraine,** intractable
Other migraine, with refractory migraine

G43.811 **Other migraine, intractable,** with status
  migrainosus

G43.819 **Other migraine, intractable,** without
  status migrainosus

✓6ᵗʰ **G43.82** **Menstrual** migraine, not intractable
Menstrual headache, not intractable
Menstrual migraine, without refractory migraine
Menstrually related migraine, not intractable
Pre-menstrual headache, not intractable
Pre-menstrual migraine, not intractable
Pure menstrual migraine, not intractable
Code also associated premenstrual tension syndrome
  (N94.3)

G43.821 **Menstrual migraine, not intractable,**   ♀
  with status migrainosus

EXCLUDES 1 Not coded here   **EXCLUDES 2** Not included here   **N** Newborn Age: 0   **P** Pediatric Age: 0-17   **M** Maternity Age: 12-55   **A** Adult Age: 15-124

518   ICD-10-CM Draft (2015)

G43.829   **Menstrual migraine, not intractable,**   ♀
           without status migrainosus
           Menstrual migraine NOS

√6ᵗʰ   G43.83   Menstrual migraine, intractable
           Menstrual headache, intractable
           Menstrual migraine, with refractory migraine
           Menstrually related migraine, intractable
           Pre-menstrual headache, intractable
           Pre-menstrual migraine, intractable
           Pure menstrual migraine, intractable
           Code also associated premenstrual tension syndrome
               (N94.3)

G43.831   **Menstrual migraine, intractable, with**   ♀
           status migrainosus

G43.839   **Menstrual migraine, intractable,**   ♀
           without status migrainosus

√5ᵗʰ   G43.9   Migraine, unspecified

√6ᵗʰ   G43.90   **Migraine, unspecified,** not intractable
           Migraine, unspecified, without refractory migraine

G43.901   **Migraine, unspecified, not intractable,**
           with status migrainosus
           Status migrainosus NOS

G43.909   **Migraine, unspecified, not intractable,**
           without status migrainosus
           Migraine NOS

√6ᵗʰ   G43.91   **Migraine, unspecified,** intractable
           Migraine, unspecified, with refractory migraine

G43.911   **Migraine, unspecified, intractable,**
           with status migrainosus

G43.919   **Migraine, unspecified, intractable,**
           without status migrainosus

√4ᵗʰ   **G44**   Other headache **syndromes**
           EXCLUDES 1   headache NOS (R51)
           EXCLUDES 2   atypical facial pain (G50.1)
                       headache due to lumbar puncture (G97.1)
                       migraines (G43.-)
                       trigeminal neuralgia (G50.0)

√5ᵗʰ   **G44.0**   Cluster headaches **and other trigeminal autonomic**
           cephalgias (TAC)

√6ᵗʰ   G44.00   **Cluster headache syndrome,** unspecified
           Ciliary neuralgia
           Cluster headache NOS
           Histamine cephalgia
           Lower half migraine
           Migrainous neuralgia

G44.001   **Cluster headache syndrome, unspecified,**
           intractable

G44.009   **Cluster headache syndrome, unspecified,**
           not intractable
           Cluster headache syndrome NOS

√6ᵗʰ   G44.01   Episodic **cluster headache**
           G44.011   **Episodic cluster headache,** intractable
           G44.019   **Episodic cluster headache,** not intractable
                     Episodic cluster headache NOS

√6ᵗʰ   G44.02   Chronic **cluster headache**
           G44.021   **Chronic cluster headache,** intractable
           G44.029   **Chronic cluster headache,** not intractable
                     Chronic cluster headache NOS

√6ᵗʰ   G44.03   Episodic **paroxysmal hemicrania**
           Paroxysmal hemicrania NOS
           G44.031   **Episodic paroxysmal hemicrania,**
                     intractable
           G44.039   **Episodic paroxysmal hemicrania,** not
                     intractable
                     Episodic paroxysmal hemicrania NOS

√6ᵗʰ   G44.04   Chronic **paroxysmal hemicrania**
           G44.041   **Chronic paroxysmal hemicrania,**
                     intractable
           G44.049   **Chronic paroxysmal hemicrania,** not
                     intractable
                     Chronic paroxysmal hemicrania NOS

√6ᵗʰ   G44.05   Short lasting unilateral **neuralgiform headache with**
           conjunctival injection and tearing (SUNCT)
           G44.051   **Short lasting unilateral neuralgiform**
                     headache with conjunctival injection and
                     tearing (SUNCT), intractable

G44.059   **Short lasting unilateral neuralgiform**
           headache with conjunctival injection and
           tearing (SUNCT), not intractable
           Short lasting unilateral neuralgiform
               headache with conjunctival injection
               and tearing (SUNCT) NOS

√6ᵗʰ   G44.09   Other trigeminal autonomic cephalgias **(TAC)**

G44.091   **Other trigeminal autonomic cephalgias**
           (TAC), intractable

G44.099   **Other trigeminal autonomic cephalgias**
           syndrome (TAC), not intractable

G44.1   Vascular **headache, not elsewhere classified**
           EXCLUDES 2   cluster headache (G44.0)
                       complicated headache syndromes (G44.5-)
                       drug-induced headache (G44.4-)
                       migraine (G43.-)
                       other specified headache syndromes (G44.8-)
                       post-traumatic headache (G44.3-)
                       tension-type headache (G44.2-)

√5ᵗʰ   G44.2   Tension-type **headache**

√6ᵗʰ   G44.20   **Tension-type headache,** unspecified

G44.201   **Tension-type headache, unspecified,**
           intractable

G44.209   **Tension-type headache, unspecified,**
           not intractable
           Tension headache NOS

√6ᵗʰ   G44.21   Episodic **tension-type headache**

G44.211   **Episodic tension-type headache,**
           intractable

G44.219   **Episodic tension-type headache,** not
           intractable
           Episodic tension-type headache NOS

√6ᵗʰ   G44.22   Chronic **tension-type headache**

G44.221   **Chronic tension-type headache,**
           intractable

G44.229   **Chronic tension-type headache,** not
           intractable
           Chronic tension-type headache NOS

√5ᵗʰ   G44.3   Post-traumatic **headache**

√6ᵗʰ   G44.30   **Post-traumatic headache,** unspecified

G44.301   **Post-traumatic headache, unspecified,**
           intractable

G44.309   **Post-traumatic headache, unspecified,**
           not intractable
           Post-traumatic headache NOS

√6ᵗʰ   G44.31   Acute **post-traumatic headache**

G44.311   **Acute post-traumatic headache,**
           intractable

G44.319   **Acute post-traumatic headache,** not
           intractable
           Acute post-traumatic headache NOS

√6ᵗʰ   G44.32   Chronic **post-traumatic headache**

G44.321   **Chronic post-traumatic headache,**
           intractable

G44.329   **Chronic post-traumatic headache,** not
           intractable
           Chronic post-traumatic headache NOS

√5ᵗʰ   G44.4   Drug-induced **headache, not elsewhere classified**
           Medication overuse headache
           Use additional code for adverse effect, if applicable, to identify
               drug (T36-T50 with fifth or sixth character 5)

G44.40   **Drug-induced headache, not elsewhere classified,**
           not intractable

G44.41   **Drug-induced headache, not elsewhere classified,**
           intractable

√5ᵗʰ   G44.5   Complicated **headache syndromes**

G44.51   Hemicrania continua

G44.52   New daily persistent headache (NDPH)

G44.53   Primary thunderclap **headache**

G44.59   Other complicated headache syndrome

√5ᵗʰ   G44.8   Other specified **headache syndromes**

G44.81   Hypnic **headache**

G44.82   Headache associated with sexual activity
           Orgasmic headache
           Preorgasmic headache

G44.83   Primary cough **headache**

G44.84   Primary exertional **headache**

Diseases of the Nervous System

G44.85–G47.53

G44.85   Primary stabbing headache

G44.89   Other headache syndrome

✓4ᵗʰ **G45**   **Transient cerebral ischemic attacks and related syndromes**

> EXCLUDES 1   neonatal cerebral ischemia (P91.0)
> transient retinal artery occlusion (H34.0-)

G45.0   **Vertebro-basilar artery syndrome**

G45.1   **Carotid artery syndrome (hemispheric)**

G45.2   **Multiple and bilateral precerebral artery syndromes**

G45.3   **Amaurosis fugax**

G45.4   **Transient global amnesia**

> EXCLUDES 1   amnesia NOS (R41.3)

G45.8   **Other transient cerebral ischemic attacks and related syndromes**

G45.9   **Transient cerebral ischemic attack, unspecified**

> Spasm of cerebral artery
> TIA
> Transient cerebral ischemia NOS

✓4ᵗʰ **G46**   **Vascular syndromes of brain in cerebrovascular diseases**

> Code first underlying cerebrovascular disease (I60-I69)

G46.0   **Middle cerebral artery syndrome**

G46.1   **Anterior cerebral artery syndrome**

G46.2   **Posterior cerebral artery syndrome**

G46.3   **Brain stem stroke syndrome**

> Benedikt syndrome
> Claude syndrome
> Foville syndrome
> Millard-Gubler syndrome
> Wallenberg syndrome
> Weber syndrome

G46.4   **Cerebellar stroke syndrome**

G46.5   **Pure motor lacunar syndrome**

G46.6   **Pure sensory lacunar syndrome**

G46.7   **Other lacunar syndromes**

G46.8   **Other vascular syndromes of brain in cerebrovascular diseases**

✓4ᵗʰ **G47**   **Sleep disorders**

> EXCLUDES 2   nightmares (F51.5)
> nonorganic sleep disorders (F51.-)
> sleep terrors (F51.4)
> sleepwalking (F51.3)

✓5ᵗʰ **G47.0**   **Insomnia**

> EXCLUDES 2   alcohol related insomnia (F10.182, F10.282, F10.982)
> drug-related insomnia (F11.182, F11.282, F11.982, F13.182, F13.282, F13.982, F14.182, F14.282, F14.982, F15.182, F15.282, F15.982, F19.182, F19.282, F19.982)
> idiopathic insomnia (F51.01)
> insomnia due to a mental disorder (F51.05)
> insomnia not due to a substance or known physiological condition (F51.0-)
> nonorganic insomnia (F51.0-)
> primary insomnia (F51.01)
> sleep apnea (G47.3-)

G47.00   **Insomnia, unspecified**

> Insomnia NOS

G47.01   **Insomnia due to medical condition**

> Code also associated medical condition

G47.09   **Other insomnia**

✓5ᵗʰ **G47.1**   **Hypersomnia**

> EXCLUDES 2   alcohol-related hypersomnia (F10.182, F10.282, F10.982)
> drug-related hypersomnia (F11.182, F11.282, F11.982, F13.182, F13.282, F13.982, F14.182, F14.282, F14.982, F15.182, F15.282, F15.982, F19.182, F19.282, F19.982)
> hypersomnia due to a mental disorder (F51.13)
> hypersomnia not due to a substance or known physiological condition (F51.1-)
> primary hypersomnia (F51.11)
> sleep apnea (G47.3-)

G47.10   **Hypersomnia, unspecified**

> Hypersomnia NOS

G47.11   **Idiopathic hypersomnia with long sleep time**

> Idiopathic hypersomnia NOS

G47.12   **Idiopathic hypersomnia without long sleep time**

G47.13   **Recurrent hypersomnia**

> Kleine-Levin syndrome
> Menstrual related hypersomnia

G47.14   **Hypersomnia due to medical condition**

> Code also associated medical condition

G47.19   **Other hypersomnia**

✓5ᵗʰ **G47.2**   **Circadian rhythm sleep disorders**

> Disorders of the sleep wake schedule
> Inversion of nyctohemeral rhythm
> Inversion of sleep rhythm

G47.20   **Circadian rhythm sleep disorder, unspecified type**

> Sleep wake schedule disorder NOS

G47.21   **Circadian rhythm sleep disorder, delayed sleep phase type**

> Delayed sleep phase syndrome

G47.22   **Circadian rhythm sleep disorder, advanced sleep phase type**

G47.23   **Circadian rhythm sleep disorder, irregular sleep wake type**

> Irregular sleep-wake pattern

G47.24   **Circadian rhythm sleep disorder, free running type**

G47.25   **Circadian rhythm sleep disorder, jet lag type**

G47.26   **Circadian rhythm sleep disorder, shift work type**

G47.27   *Circadian rhythm sleep disorder in conditions classified elsewhere*

> *Code first underlying condition*

G47.29   **Other circadian rhythm sleep disorder**

✓5ᵗʰ **G47.3**   **Sleep apnea**

> Code also any associated underlying condition
>
> EXCLUDES 1   apnea NOS (R06.81)
> Cheyne-Stokes breathing (R06.3)
> pickwickian syndrome (E66.2)
> sleep apnea of newborn (P28.3)

G47.30   **Sleep apnea, unspecified**

> Sleep apnea NOS

G47.31   **Primary central sleep apnea**

G47.32   **High altitude periodic breathing**

G47.33   **Obstructive sleep apnea (adult) (pediatric)**

> EXCLUDES 1   obstructive sleep apnea of newborn (P28.3)

G47.34   **Idiopathic sleep related nonobstructive alveolar hypoventilation**

> Sleep related hypoxia

G47.35   **Congenital central alveolar hypoventilation syndrome**

G47.36   *Sleep related hypoventilation in conditions classified elsewhere*

> Sleep related hypoxemia in conditions classified elsewhere
> *Code first underlying condition*

G47.37   *Central sleep apnea in conditions classified elsewhere*

> *Code first underlying condition*

G47.39   **Other sleep apnea**

✓5ᵗʰ **G47.4**   **Narcolepsy and cataplexy**

    ✓6ᵗʰ **G47.41**   **Narcolepsy**

> **G47.411**   **Narcolepsy with cataplexy**
>
> **G47.419**   **Narcolepsy without cataplexy**
> Narcolepsy NOS

    ✓6ᵗʰ **G47.42**   **Narcolepsy in conditions classified elsewhere**

> *Code first underlying condition*
>
> **G47.421**   *Narcolepsy in conditions classified elsewhere with cataplexy*
>
> **G47.429**   *Narcolepsy in conditions classified elsewhere without cataplexy*

✓5ᵗʰ **G47.5**   **Parasomnia**

> EXCLUDES 1   alcohol induced parasomnia (F10.182, F10.282, F10.982)
> drug induced parasomnia (F11.182, F11.282, F11.982, F13.182, F13.282, F13.982, F14.182, F14.282, F14.982, F15.182, F15.282, F15.982, F19.182, F19.282, F19.982)
> parasomnia not due to a substance or known physiological condition (F51.8)

G47.50   **Parasomnia, unspecified**

> Parasomnia NOS

G47.51   **Confusional arousals**

G47.52   **REM sleep behavior disorder**

G47.53   **Recurrent isolated sleep paralysis**

EXCLUDES 1 Not coded here   EXCLUDES 2 Not included here   N Newborn Age: 0   P Pediatric Age: 0-17   M Maternity Age: 12-55   A Adult Age: 15-124

520   ICD-10-CM Draft (2015)

G47.54 *Parasomnia in conditions classified elsewhere*
  Code first underlying condition

G47.59 **Other parasomnia**

✓5ᵗʰ G47.6 **Sleep related movement disorders**
  EXCLUDES 2 *restless legs syndrome (G25.81)*

G47.61 **Periodic limb movement disorder**

G47.62 **Sleep related leg cramps**

G47.63 **Sleep related bruxism**
  EXCLUDES 1 *psychogenic bruxism (F45.8)*

G47.69 **Other sleep related movement disorders**

G47.8 **Other sleep disorders**

G47.9 **Sleep disorder, unspecified**
  Sleep disorder NOS

Nerve, nerve root and plexus disorders (G50-G59)

EXCLUDES 1 *current traumatic nerve, nerve root and plexus disorders—see Injury,*
  nerve by body region
  neuralgia NOS (M79.2)
  neuritis NOS (M79.2)
  peripheral neuritis in pregnancy (O26.82-)
  radiculitis NOS (M54.1-)

✓4ᵗʰ G50 **Disorders of trigeminal nerve**
  INCLUDES disorders of 5th cranial nerve

G50.0 **Trigeminal neuralgia**
  Syndrome of paroxysmal facial pain
  Tic douloureux

G50.1 **Atypical facial pain**

G50.8 **Other disorders of trigeminal nerve**

G50.9 **Disorder of trigeminal nerve, unspecified**

✓4ᵗʰ G51 **Facial nerve disorders**
  INCLUDES disorders of 7th cranial nerve

G51.0 **Bell's palsy**
  Facial palsy

G51.1 **Geniculate ganglionitis**
  EXCLUDES 1 *postherpetic geniculate ganglionitis (B02.21)*

G51.2 **Melkersson's syndrome**
  Melkersson-Rosenthal syndrome

G51.3 **Clonic hemifacial spasm**

G51.4 **Facial myokymia**

G51.8 **Other disorders of facial nerve**

G51.9 **Disorder of facial nerve, unspecified**

✓4ᵗʰ G52 **Disorders of other cranial nerves**
  EXCLUDES 2 *disorders of acoustic [8th] nerve (H93.3)*
  disorders of optic [2nd] nerve (H46, H47.0)
  paralytic strabismus due to nerve palsy (H49.0-H49.2)

G52.0 **Disorders of olfactory nerve**
  Disorders of 1st cranial nerve

G52.1 **Disorders of glossopharyngeal nerve**
  Disorder of 9th cranial nerve
  Glossopharyngeal neuralgia

G52.2 **Disorders of vagus nerve**
  Disorders of pneumogastric [10th] nerve

G52.3 **Disorders of hypoglossal nerve**
  Disorders of 12th cranial nerve

G52.7 **Disorders of multiple cranial nerves**
  Polyneuritis cranialis

G52.8 **Disorders of other specified cranial nerves**

G52.9 **Cranial nerve disorder, unspecified**

G53 *Cranial nerve disorders in diseases classified elsewhere*
  Code first underlying disease, such as:
  neoplasm (C00-D49)
  EXCLUDES 1 *multiple cranial nerve palsy in sarcoidosis (D86.82)*
  multiple cranial nerve palsy in syphilis (A52.15)
  postherpetic geniculate ganglionitis (B02.21)
  postherpetic trigeminal neuralgia (B02.22)

✓4ᵗʰ G54 **Nerve root and plexus disorders**
  EXCLUDES 1 *current traumatic nerve root and plexus disorders—see nerve*
  injury by body region
  intervertebral disc disorders (M50-M51)
  neuralgia or neuritis NOS (M79.2)
  neuritis or radiculitis brachial NOS (M54.13)
  neuritis or radiculitis lumbar NOS (M54.16)
  neuritis or radiculitis lumbosacral NOS (M54.17)
  neuritis or radiculitis thoracic NOS (M54.14)
  radiculitis NOS (M54.10)
  radiculopathy NOS (M54.10)
  spondylosis (M47.-)

G54.0 **Brachial plexus disorders**
  Thoracic outlet syndrome

G54.1 **Lumbosacral plexus disorders**

G54.2 **Cervical root disorders, not elsewhere classified**

G54.3 **Thoracic root disorders, not elsewhere classified**

G54.4 **Lumbosacral root disorders, not elsewhere classified**

G54.5 **Neuralgic amyotrophy**
  Parsonage-Aldren-Turner syndrome
  Shoulder-girdle neuritis
  EXCLUDES 1 *neuralgic amyotrophy in diabetes mellitus (E08-E13*
  with .44)

G54.6 **Phantom limb syndrome with pain**

G54.7 **Phantom limb syndrome without pain**
  Phantom limb syndrome NOS

G54.8 **Other nerve root and plexus disorders**

G54.9 **Nerve root and plexus disorder, unspecified**

G55 *Nerve root and plexus compressions in diseases classified elsewhere*
  Code first underlying disease, such as:
  neoplasm (C00-D49)
  EXCLUDES 1 *nerve root compression (due to) (in) ankylosing spondylitis*
  (M45.-)
  nerve root compression (due to) (in) dorsopathies (M53.-, M54.-)
  nerve root compression (due to) (in) intervertebral disc
  disorders (M50.1-, M51.1-)
  nerve root compression (due to) (in) spondylopathies
  (M46.-, M48.-)

✓4ᵗʰ G56 **Mononeuropathies of upper limb**
  EXCLUDES 1 *current traumatic nerve disorder—see nerve injury by body*
  region

✓5ᵗʰ G56.0 **Carpal tunnel syndrome**

G56.00 **Carpal tunnel syndrome, unspecified upper limb**

G56.01 **Carpal tunnel syndrome, right upper limb**

G56.02 **Carpal tunnel syndrome, left upper limb**

✓5ᵗʰ G56.1 **Other lesions of median nerve**

G56.10 **Other lesions of median nerve, unspecified upper limb**

G56.11 **Other lesions of median nerve, right upper limb**

G56.12 **Other lesions of median nerve, left upper limb**

✓5ᵗʰ G56.2 **Lesion of ulnar nerve**
  Tardy ulnar nerve palsy

G56.20 **Lesion of ulnar nerve, unspecified upper limb**

G56.21 **Lesion of ulnar nerve, right upper limb**

G56.22 **Lesion of ulnar nerve, left upper limb**

✓5ᵗʰ G56.3 **Lesion of radial nerve**

G56.30 **Lesion of radial nerve, unspecified upper limb**

G56.31 **Lesion of radial nerve, right upper limb**

G56.32 **Lesion of radial nerve, left upper limb**

✓5ᵗʰ G56.4 **Causalgia of upper limb**
  Complex regional pain syndrome II of upper limb
  EXCLUDES 1 *complex regional pain syndrome I of lower limb*
  (G90.52-)
  complex regional pain syndrome I of upper limb
  (G90.51-)
  complex regional pain syndrome II of lower limb
  (G57.7-)
  reflex sympathetic dystrophy of lower limb (G90.52-)
  reflex sympathetic dystrophy of upper limb (G90.51-)

G56.40 **Causalgia of unspecified upper limb**

G56.41 **Causalgia of right upper limb**

G56.42 **Causalgia of left upper limb**

✓ Additional Character Required ✓x7ᵗʰ Xtension Alert Unspecified Dx Other Specified Dx Manifestation ►◄ Revised Text ● New Code ▲ Revised Code Title

ICD-10-CM Draft (2015) **521**

Diseases of the Nervous System

G56.8–G62.9

✓5ᵗʰ **G56.8** Other specified mononeuropathies of upper limb
Interdigital neuroma of upper limb

     G56.80 Other specified mononeuropathies of unspecified upper limb

     G56.81 Other specified mononeuropathies of right upper limb

     G56.82 Other specified mononeuropathies of left upper limb

✓5ᵗʰ **G56.9** Unspecified mononeuropathy of upper limb

     G56.90 Unspecified mononeuropathy of unspecified upper limb

     G56.91 Unspecified mononeuropathy of right upper limb

     G56.92 Unspecified mononeuropathy of left upper limb

✓4ᵗʰ **G57 Mononeuropathies of lower limb**

     EXCLUDES 1   current traumatic nerve disorder—see nerve injury by body region

✓5ᵗʰ **G57.0** Lesion of sciatic nerve

     EXCLUDES 1   sciatica NOS (M54.3-)

     EXCLUDES 2   sciatica attributed to intervertebral disc disorder (M51.1-)

     G57.00 Lesion of sciatic nerve, unspecified lower limb

     G57.01 Lesion of sciatic nerve, right lower limb

     G57.02 Lesion of sciatic nerve, left lower limb

✓5ᵗʰ **G57.1** Meralgia paresthetica
Lateral cutaneous nerve of thigh syndrome

     G57.10 Meralgia paresthetica, unspecified lower limb

     G57.11 Meralgia paresthetica, right lower limb

     G57.12 Meralgia paresthetica, left lower limb

✓5ᵗʰ **G57.2** Lesion of femoral nerve

     G57.20 Lesion of femoral nerve, unspecified lower limb

     G57.21 Lesion of femoral nerve, right lower limb

     G57.22 Lesion of femoral nerve, left lower limb

✓5ᵗʰ **G57.3** Lesion of lateral popliteal nerve
Peroneal nerve palsy

     G57.30 Lesion of lateral popliteal nerve, unspecified lower limb

     G57.31 Lesion of lateral popliteal nerve, right lower limb

     G57.32 Lesion of lateral popliteal nerve, left lower limb

✓5ᵗʰ **G57.4** Lesion of medial popliteal nerve

     G57.40 Lesion of medial popliteal nerve, unspecified lower limb

     G57.41 Lesion of medial popliteal nerve, right lower limb

     G57.42 Lesion of medial popliteal nerve, left lower limb

✓5ᵗʰ **G57.5** Tarsal tunnel syndrome

     G57.50 Tarsal tunnel syndrome, unspecified lower limb

     G57.51 Tarsal tunnel syndrome, right lower limb

     G57.52 Tarsal tunnel syndrome, left lower limb

✓5ᵗʰ **G57.6** Lesion of plantar nerve
Morton's metatarsalgia

     G57.60 Lesion of plantar nerve, unspecified lower limb

     G57.61 Lesion of plantar nerve, right lower limb

     G57.62 Lesion of plantar nerve, left lower limb

✓5ᵗʰ **G57.7** Causalgia of lower limb
Complex regional pain syndrome II of lower limb

     EXCLUDES 1   complex regional pain syndrome I of lower limb (G90.52-)
            complex regional pain syndrome I of upper limb (G90.51-)
            complex regional pain syndrome II of upper limb (G56.4-)
            reflex sympathetic dystrophy of lower limb (G90.52-)
            reflex sympathetic dystrophy of upper limb (G90.51-)

     G57.70 Causalgia of unspecified lower limb

     G57.71 Causalgia of right lower limb

     G57.72 Causalgia of left lower limb

✓5ᵗʰ **G57.8** Other specified mononeuropathies of lower limb
Interdigital neuroma of lower limb

     G57.80 Other specified mononeuropathies of unspecified lower limb

     G57.81 Other specified mononeuropathies of right lower limb

     G57.82 Other specified mononeuropathies of left lower limb

✓5ᵗʰ **G57.9** Unspecified mononeuropathy of lower limb

     G57.90 Unspecified mononeuropathy of unspecified lower limb

     G57.91 Unspecified mononeuropathy of right lower limb

     G57.92 Unspecified mononeuropathy of left lower limb

✓4ᵗʰ **G58 Other mononeuropathies**

     G58.0 Intercostal neuropathy

     G58.7 Mononeuritis multiplex

     G58.8 Other specified mononeuropathies

     G58.9 Mononeuropathy, unspecified

G59 *Mononeuropathy in diseases classified elsewhere*
     Code first underlying disease

     EXCLUDES 1   *diabetic mononeuropathy (E08-E13 with .41)*
            syphilitic nerve paralysis (A52.19)
            syphilitic neuritis (A52.15)
            tuberculous mononeuropathy (A17.83)

Polyneuropathies and other disorders of the peripheral nervous system (G60-G65)

     EXCLUDES 1   *neuralgia NOS (M79.2)*
            neuritis NOS (M79.2)
            peripheral neuritis in pregnancy (O26.82-)
            radiculitis NOS (M54.10)

✓4ᵗʰ **G60 Hereditary and idiopathic neuropathy**

     G60.0 Hereditary motor and sensory neuropathy
         Charcôt-Marie-Tooth disease
         Déjérine-Sottas disease
         Hereditary motor and sensory neuropathy, types I-IV
         Hypertrophic neuropathy of infancy
         Peroneal muscular atrophy (axonal type) (hypertrophic type)
         Roussy-Levy syndrome

     G60.1 Refsum's disease
         Infantile Refsum disease

     G60.2 Neuropathy in association with hereditary ataxia

     G60.3 Idiopathic progressive neuropathy

     G60.8 Other hereditary and idiopathic neuropathies
         Dominantly inherited sensory neuropathy
         Morvan's disease
         Nelaton's syndrome
         Recessively inherited sensory neuropathy

     G60.9 Hereditary and idiopathic neuropathy, unspecified

✓4ᵗʰ **G61 Inflammatory polyneuropathy**

     G61.0 Guillain-Barre syndrome
         Acute (post-)infective polyneuritis
         Miller Fisher syndrome
         AHA: 2014, 2Q, 4

     G61.1 Serum neuropathy
         Use additional code for adverse effect, if applicable, to identify serum (T50.-)

✓5ᵗʰ   **G61.8** Other inflammatory polyneuropathies

     G61.81 Chronic inflammatory demyelinating polyneuritis

     G61.89 Other inflammatory polyneuropathies

     G61.9 Inflammatory polyneuropathy, unspecified

✓4ᵗʰ **G62 Other and unspecified polyneuropathies**

     G62.0 Drug-induced polyneuropathy
         Use additional code for adverse effect, if applicable, to identify drug (T36-T50 with fifth or sixth character 5)

     G62.1 Alcoholic polyneuropathy

     G62.2 Polyneuropathy due to other toxic agents
         Code first (T51-T65) to identify toxic agent

✓5ᵗʰ   **G62.8** Other specified polyneuropathies

     G62.81 Critical illness polyneuropathy
         Acute motor neuropathy

     G62.82 Radiation-induced polyneuropathy
         Use additional external cause code (W88-W90, X39.0-) to identify cause

     G62.89 Other specified polyneuropathies

     G62.9 Polyneuropathy, unspecified
         Neuropathy NOS

EXCLUDES 1 Not coded here   EXCLUDES 2 Not included here   N Newborn Age: 0   P Pediatric Age: 0-17   M Maternity Age: 12-55   A Adult Age: 15-124

522   ICD-10-CM Draft (2015)

G63   Polyneuropathy in diseases classified elsewhere
Code first underlying disease, such as:
*   amyloidosis (E85.-)*
*   endocrine disease, except diabetes (E00-E07, E15-E16, E20-E34)*
*   metabolic diseases (E70-E88)*
*   neoplasm (C00-D49)*
*   nutritional deficiency (E40-E64)*
EXCLUDES 1   *polyneuropathy (in):*
*   diabetes mellitus (E08-E13 with .42)*
*   diphtheria (A36.83)*
*   infectious mononucleosis (B27.0-B27.9 with 1)*
*   Lyme disease (A69.22)*
*   mumps (B26.84)*
*   postherpetic (B02.23)*
*   rheumatoid arthritis (M05.33)*
*   scleroderma (M34.83)*
*   systemic lupus erythematosus (M32.19)*
AHA: 2012, 4Q, 99

G64   Other disorders of peripheral nervous system
Disorder of peripheral nervous system NOS

☑4th **G65   Sequelae of inflammatory and toxic polyneuropathies**
Code first condition resulting from (sequela) of inflammatory and toxic polyneuropathies

G65.0   Sequelae of Guillain-Barré syndrome

G65.1   Sequelae of other inflammatory polyneuropathy

G65.2   Sequelae of toxic polyneuropathy

Diseases of myoneural junction and muscle (G70-G73)

☑4th **G70   Myasthenia gravis and other myoneural disorders**
EXCLUDES 1   *botulism (A05.1, A48.51-A48.52)*
transient neonatal myasthenia gravis (P94.0)

☑5th **G70.0   Myasthenia gravis**

G70.00   Myasthenia gravis without (acute) exacerbation
Myasthenia gravis NOS

G70.01   Myasthenia gravis with (acute) exacerbation
Myasthenia gravis in crisis

G70.1   Toxic myoneural disorders
Code first (T51-T65) to identify toxic agent

G70.2   Congenital and developmental myasthenia

☑5th **G70.8   Other specified myoneural disorders**

G70.80   Lambert-Eaton syndrome, unspecified
Lambert-Eaton syndrome NOS

G70.81   Lambert-Eaton syndrome in disease classified elsewhere
Code first underlying disease
EXCLUDES 1   *Lambert-Eaton syndrome in neoplastic disease (G73.1)*

G70.89   Other specified myoneural disorders

G70.9   Myoneural disorder, unspecified

☑4th **G71   Primary disorders of muscles**
EXCLUDES 2   *arthrogryposis multiplex congenita (Q74.3)*
metabolic disorders (E70-E88)
myositis (M60.-)

G71.0   Muscular dystrophy
Autosomal recessive, childhood type, muscular dystrophy resembling Duchenne or Becker muscular dystrophy
Benign [Becker] muscular dystrophy
Benign scapuloperoneal muscular dystrophy with early contractures [Emery-Dreifuss]
Congenital muscular dystrophy NOS
Congenital muscular dystrophy with specific morphological abnormalities of the muscle fiber
Distal muscular dystrophy
Facioscapulohumeral muscular dystrophy
Limb-girdle muscular dystrophy
Ocular muscular dystrophy
Oculopharyngeal muscular dystrophy
Scapuloperoneal muscular dystrophy
Severe [Duchenne] muscular dystrophy

☑5th **G71.1   Myotonic disorders**

G71.11   Myotonic muscular dystrophy
Dystrophia myotonica [Steinert]
Myotonia atrophica
Myotonic dystrophy
Proximal myotonic myopathy (PROMM)
Steinert disease

G71.12   Myotonia congenita
Acetazolamide responsive myotonia congenita
Dominant myotonia congenita [Thomsen disease]
Myotonia levior
Recessive myotonia congenita [Becker disease]

G71.13   Myotonic chondrodystrophy
Chondrodystrophic myotonia
Congenital myotonic chondrodystrophy
Schwartz-Jampel disease

G71.14   Drug induced myotonia
Use additional code for adverse effect, if applicable, to identify drug (T36-T50 with fifth or sixth character 5)

G71.19   Other specified myotonic disorders
Myotonia fluctuans
Myotonia permanens
Neuromyotonia [Isaacs]
Paramyotonia congenita (of von Eulenburg)
Pseudomyotonia
Symptomatic myotonia

G71.2   Congenital myopathies
Central core disease
Fiber-type disproportion
Minicore disease
Multicore disease
Myotubular (centronuclear) myopathy
Nemaline myopathy
EXCLUDES 1   *arthrogryposis multiplex congenita (Q74.3)*

G71.3   Mitochondrial myopathy, not elsewhere classified
EXCLUDES 1   *Kearns-Sayre syndrome (H49.81)*
Leber's disease (H47.21)
Leigh's encephalopathy (G31.82)
mitochondrial metabolism disorders (E88.4-)
Reye's syndrome (G93.7)

G71.8   Other primary disorders of muscles

G71.9   Primary disorder of muscle, unspecified
Hereditary myopathy NOS

☑4th **G72   Other and unspecified myopathies**
EXCLUDES 1   *arthrogryposis multiplex congenita (Q74.3)*
dermatopolymyositis (M33.-)
ischemic infarction of muscle (M62.2-)
myositis (M60.-)
polymyositis (M33.2-)

G72.0   Drug-induced myopathy
Use additional code for adverse effect, if applicable, to identify drug (T36-T50 with fifth or sixth character 5)

G72.1   Alcoholic myopathy
Use additional code to identify alcoholism (F10.-)

G72.2   Myopathy due to other toxic agents
Code first (T51-T65) to identify toxic agent

G72.3   Periodic paralysis
Familial periodic paralysis
Hyperkalemic periodic paralysis (familial)
Hypokalemic periodic paralysis (familial)
Myotonic periodic paralysis (familial)
Normokalemic paralysis (familial)
Potassium sensitive periodic paralysis
EXCLUDES 1   *paramyotonia congenita (of von Eulenburg) (G71.19)*

☑5th **G72.4   Inflammatory and immune myopathies, not elsewhere classified**

G72.41   Inclusion body myositis [IBM]

G72.49   Other inflammatory and immune myopathies, not elsewhere classified
Inflammatory myopathy NOS

☑5th **G72.8   Other specified myopathies**

G72.81   Critical illness myopathy
Acute necrotizing myopathy
Acute quadriplegic myopathy
Intensive care (ICU) myopathy
Myopathy of critical illness

G72.89   Other specified myopathies

G72.9   Myopathy, unspecified

☑4th **G73   Disorders of myoneural junction and muscle in diseases classified elsewhere**

G73.1   Lambert-Eaton syndrome in neoplastic disease
Code first underlying neoplasm (C00-D49)
EXCLUDES 1   *Lambert-Eaton syndrome not associated with neoplasm (G70.80-G70.81)*

G73.3 Myasthenic syndromes in other diseases classified elsewhere
Code first underlying disease, such as:
neoplasm (C00-D49)
thyrotoxicosis (E05.-)

G73.7 Myopathy in diseases classified elsewhere
Code first underlying disease, such as:
hyperparathyroidism (E21.0, E21.3)
hypoparathyroidism (E20.-)
glycogen storage disease (E74.0)
lipid storage disorders (E75.-)
EXCLUDES 1 myopathy in:
rheumatoid arthritis (M05.4-)
sarcoidosis (D86.87)
scleroderma (M34.82)
sicca syndrome [Sjögren] (M35.03)
systemic lupus erythematosus (M32.19)

Cerebral palsy and other paralytic syndromes (G80-G83)

☑4th **G80 Cerebral palsy**
EXCLUDES 1 hereditary spastic paraplegia (G11.4)

G80.0 Spastic quadriplegic cerebral palsy
Congenital spastic paralysis (cerebral)

G80.1 Spastic diplegic cerebral palsy
Spastic cerebral palsy NOS

G80.2 Spastic hemiplegic cerebral palsy

G80.3 Athetoid cerebral palsy
Double athetosis (syndrome)
Dyskinetic cerebral palsy
Dystonic cerebral palsy
Vogt disease

G80.4 Ataxic cerebral palsy

G80.8 Other cerebral palsy
Mixed cerebral palsy syndromes

G80.9 Cerebral palsy, unspecified
Cerebral palsy NOS

☑4th **G81 Hemiplegia and hemiparesis**
NOTE This category is to be used only when hemiplegia (complete)(incomplete) is reported without further specification, or is stated to be old or longstanding but of unspecified cause. The category is also for use in multiple coding to identify these types of hemiplegia resulting from any cause.
EXCLUDES 1 congenital cerebral palsy (G80.-)
hemiplegia and hemiparesis due to sequela of cerebrovascular disease (I69.05-, I69.15-, I69.25-, I69.35-, I69.85-, I69.95-)

☑5th **G81.0 Flaccid hemiplegia**
G81.00 Flaccid hemiplegia affecting unspecified side
G81.01 Flaccid hemiplegia affecting right dominant side
G81.02 Flaccid hemiplegia affecting left dominant side
G81.03 Flaccid hemiplegia affecting right nondominant side
G81.04 Flaccid hemiplegia affecting left nondominant side

☑5th **G81.1 Spastic hemiplegia**
G81.10 Spastic hemiplegia affecting unspecified side
G81.11 Spastic hemiplegia affecting right dominant side
G81.12 Spastic hemiplegia affecting left dominant side
G81.13 Spastic hemiplegia affecting right nondominant side
G81.14 Spastic hemiplegia affecting left nondominant side

☑5th **G81.9 Hemiplegia, unspecified**
AHA: 2014, 1Q, 23
G81.90 Hemiplegia, unspecified affecting unspecified side
G81.91 Hemiplegia, unspecified affecting right dominant side
G81.92 Hemiplegia, unspecified affecting left dominant side
G81.93 Hemiplegia, unspecified affecting right nondominant side
G81.94 Hemiplegia, unspecified affecting left nondominant side

☑4th **G82 Paraplegia (paraparesis) and quadriplegia (quadriparesis)**
NOTE This category is to be used only when the listed conditions are reported without further specification, or are stated to be old or longstanding but of unspecified cause. The category is also for use in multiple coding to identify these conditions resulting from any cause
EXCLUDES 1 congenital cerebral palsy (G80.-)
functional quadriplegia (R53.2)
hysterical paralysis (F44.4)

☑5th **G82.2 Paraplegia**
Paralysis of both lower limbs NOS
Paraparesis (lower) NOS
Paraplegia (lower) NOS
G82.20 Paraplegia, unspecified
G82.21 Paraplegia, complete
G82.22 Paraplegia, incomplete

☑5th **G82.5 Quadriplegia**
G82.50 Quadriplegia, unspecified
G82.51 Quadriplegia, C1-C4 complete
G82.52 Quadriplegia, C1-C4 incomplete
G82.53 Quadriplegia, C5-C7 complete
G82.54 Quadriplegia, C5-C7 incomplete

☑4th **G83 Other paralytic syndromes**
NOTE This category is to be used only when the listed conditions are reported without further specification, or are stated to be old or longstanding but of unspecified cause. The category is also for use in multiple coding to identify these conditions resulting from any cause.
INCLUDES paralysis (complete) (incomplete), except as in G80-G82

G83.0 Diplegia of upper limbs
Diplegia (upper)
Paralysis of both upper limbs

☑5th **G83.1 Monoplegia of lower limb**
Paralysis of lower limb
EXCLUDES 1 monoplegia of lower limbs due to sequela of cerebrovascular disease (I69.04-, I69.14-, I69.24-, I69.34-, I69.84-, I69.94-)
G83.10 Monoplegia of lower limb affecting unspecified side
G83.11 Monoplegia of lower limb affecting right dominant side
G83.12 Monoplegia of lower limb affecting left dominant side
G83.13 Monoplegia of lower limb affecting right nondominant side
G83.14 Monoplegia of lower limb affecting left nondominant side

☑5th **G83.2 Monoplegia of upper limb**
Paralysis of upper limb
EXCLUDES 1 monoplegia of upper limbs due to sequela of cerebrovascular disease (I69.03-, I69.13-, I69.23-, I69.33-, I69.83-, I69.93-)
G83.20 Monoplegia of upper limb affecting unspecified side
G83.21 Monoplegia of upper limb affecting right dominant side
G83.22 Monoplegia of upper limb affecting left dominant side
G83.23 Monoplegia of upper limb affecting right nondominant side
G83.24 Monoplegia of upper limb affecting left nondominant side

☑5th **G83.3 Monoplegia, unspecified**
G83.30 Monoplegia, unspecified affecting unspecified side
G83.31 Monoplegia, unspecified affecting right dominant side
G83.32 Monoplegia, unspecified affecting left dominant side
G83.33 Monoplegia, unspecified affecting right nondominant side
G83.34 Monoplegia, unspecified affecting left nondominant side

G83.4 Cauda equina syndrome
Neurogenic bladder due to cauda equina syndrome
EXCLUDES 1 cord bladder NOS (G95.89)
neurogenic bladder NOS (N31.9)

G83.5 Locked-in state

EXCLUDES 1 Not coded here   EXCLUDES 2 Not included here   N Newborn Age: 0   P Pediatric Age: 0-17   M Maternity Age: 12-55   A Adult Age: 15-124

524   ICD-10-CM Draft (2015)

☑5ᵗʰ **G83.8 Other specified paralytic syndromes**
    EXCLUDES 1 *paralytic syndromes due to current spinal cord injury—code to spinal cord injury (S14, S24, S34)*

    G83.81 Brown-Séquard syndrome
    G83.82 Anterior cord syndrome
    G83.83 Posterior cord syndrome
    G83.84 Todd's paralysis (postepileptic)
    G83.89 Other specified paralytic syndromes
G83.9 Paralytic syndrome, unspecified

Other disorders of the nervous system (G89-G99)

☑4ᵗʰ **G89 Pain, not elsewhere classified**
    Code also related psychological factors associated with pain (F45.42)
    EXCLUDES 1 *generalized pain NOS (R52)*
        pain disorders exclusively related to psychological factors (F45.41)
        pain NOS (R52)
    EXCLUDES 2 *atypical face pain (G50.1)*
        headache syndromes (G44.-)
        localized pain, unspecified type—code to pain by site, such as:
          abdomen pain (R10.-)
          back pain (M54.9)
          breast pain (N64.4)
          chest pain (R07.1-R07.9)
          ear pain (H92.0-)
          eye pain (H57.1)
          headache (R51)
          joint pain (M25.5-)
          limb pain (M79.6-)
          lumbar region pain (M54.5)
          painful urination (R30.9)
          pelvic and perineal pain (R10.2)
          renal colic (N23)
          shoulder pain (M25.51-)
          spine pain (M54.-)
          throat pain (R07.0)
          tongue pain (K14.6)
          tooth pain (K08.8)
         migraines (G43.-)
        myalgia (M79.1)
        pain from prosthetic devices, implants, and grafts (T82.84, T83.84, T84.84, T85.84)
        phantom limb syndrome with pain (G54.6)
        vulvar vestibulitis (N94.810)
        vulvodynia (N94.81-)

G89.0 Central pain syndrome
    Déjérine-Roussy syndrome
    Myelopathic pain syndrome
    Thalamic pain syndrome (hyperesthetic)

☑5ᵗʰ **G89.1 Acute pain, not elsewhere classified**
    G89.11 Acute pain due to trauma
    G89.12 Acute post-thoracotomy pain
      Post-thoracotomy pain NOS
    G89.18 Other acute postprocedural pain
      Postoperative pain NOS
      Postprocedural pain NOS

☑5ᵗʰ **G89.2 Chronic pain, not elsewhere classified**
    EXCLUDES 1 *causalgia, lower limb (G57.7-)*
        causalgia, upper limb (G56.4-)
        central pain syndrome (G89.0)
        chronic pain syndrome (G89.4)
        complex regional pain syndrome II, lower limb (G57.7-)
        complex regional pain syndrome II, upper limb (G56.4-)
        neoplasm related chronic pain (G89.3)
        reflex sympathetic dystrophy (G90.5-)

    G89.21 Chronic pain due to trauma
    G89.22 Chronic post-thoracotomy pain
    G89.28 Other chronic postprocedural pain
      Other chronic postoperative pain
    G89.29 Other chronic pain

G89.3 Neoplasm related pain (acute) (chronic)
    Cancer associated pain
    Pain due to malignancy (primary) (secondary)
    Tumor associated pain

G89.4 Chronic pain syndrome
    Chronic pain associated with significant psychosocial dysfunction

---

☑4ᵗʰ **G90 Disorders of autonomic nervous system**
    EXCLUDES 1 *dysfunction of the autonomic nervous system due to alcohol (G31.2)*

☑5ᵗʰ **G90.0 Idiopathic peripheral autonomic neuropathy**
    G90.01 Carotid sinus syncope
      Carotid sinus syndrome
    G90.09 Other idiopathic peripheral autonomic neuropathy
      Idiopathic peripheral autonomic neuropathy NOS

G90.1 Familial dysautonomia [Riley-Day]
G90.2 Horner's syndrome
    Bernard(-Horner) syndrome
    Cervical sympathetic dystrophy or paralysis
G90.3 Multi-system degeneration of the autonomic nervous system
    Neurogenic orthostatic hypotension [Shy-Drager]
    EXCLUDES 1 *orthostatic hypotension NOS (I95.1)*
G90.4 Autonomic dysreflexia
    Use additional code to identify the cause, such as:
      fecal impaction (K56.41)
      pressure ulcer (pressure area) (L89.-)
      urinary tract infection (N39.0)

☑5ᵗʰ **G90.5 Complex regional pain syndrome I (CRPS I)**
    Reflex sympathetic dystrophy
    EXCLUDES 1 *causalgia of lower limb (G57.7-)*
        causalgia of upper limb (G56.4-)
        complex regional pain syndrome II of lower limb (G57.7-)
        complex regional pain syndrome II of upper limb (G56.4-)

    G90.50 Complex regional pain syndrome I, unspecified
    ☑6ᵗʰ **G90.51 Complex regional pain syndrome I of upper limb**
      G90.511 Complex regional pain syndrome I of right upper limb
      G90.512 Complex regional pain syndrome I of left upper limb
      G90.513 Complex regional pain syndrome I of upper limb, bilateral
      G90.519 Complex regional pain syndrome I of unspecified upper limb
    ☑6ᵗʰ **G90.52 Complex regional pain syndrome I of lower limb**
      G90.521 Complex regional pain syndrome I of right lower limb
      G90.522 Complex regional pain syndrome I of left lower limb
      G90.523 Complex regional pain syndrome I of lower limb, bilateral
      G90.529 Complex regional pain syndrome I of unspecified lower limb
    G90.59 Complex regional pain syndrome I of other specified site

G90.8 Other disorders of autonomic nervous system
G90.9 Disorder of the autonomic nervous system, unspecified

☑4ᵗʰ **G91 Hydrocephalus**
    INCLUDES acquired hydrocephalus
    EXCLUDES 1 *Arnold-Chiari syndrome with hydrocephalus (Q07.-)*
        congenital hydrocephalus (Q03.-)
        spina bifida with hydrocephalus (Q05.-)

G91.0 Communicating hydrocephalus
    Secondary normal pressure hydrocephalus
G91.1 Obstructive hydrocephalus
G91.2 (Idiopathic) normal pressure hydrocephalus
    Normal pressure hydrocephalus NOS
G91.3 Post-traumatic hydrocephalus, unspecified
G91.4 Hydrocephalus in diseases classified elsewhere
    Code first underlying condition, such as:
      congenital syphilis (A50.4-)
      neoplasm (C00-D49)
    EXCLUDES 1 *hydrocephalus due to congenital toxoplasmosis (P37.1)*
G91.8 Other hydrocephalus
G91.9 Hydrocephalus, unspecified

G92 Toxic encephalopathy
    Toxic encephalitis
    Toxic metabolic encephalopathy
    Code first (T51-T65) to identify toxic agent

☑ Additional Character Required   ✗7ᵗʰ X'tension Alert   Unspecified Dx   Other Specified Dx   Manifestation   ▶◀ Revised Text   ● New Code   ▲ Revised Code Title

Diseases of the Nervous System

G93–G98.8

✓4th **G93** **Other disorders of brain**

G93.0 **Cerebral cysts**
Arachnoid cyst
Porencephalic cyst, acquired
EXCLUDES 1   *acquired periventricular cysts of newborn (P91.1)*
congenital cerebral cysts (Q04.6)

G93.1 **Anoxic brain damage, not elsewhere classified**
EXCLUDES 1   *cerebral anoxia due to anesthesia during labor and delivery (O74.3)*
cerebral anoxia due to anesthesia during the puerperium (O89.2)
neonatal anoxia (P84)

G93.2 **Benign intracranial hypertension**
EXCLUDES 1   *hypertensive encephalopathy (I67.4)*

G93.3 **Postviral fatigue syndrome**
Benign myalgic encephalomyelitis
EXCLUDES 1   *chronic fatigue syndrome NOS (R53.82)*

✓5th **G93.4** **Other and unspecified encephalopathy**
EXCLUDES 1   *alcoholic encephalopathy (G31.2)*
encephalopathy in diseases classified elsewhere (G94)
hypertensive encephalopathy (I67.4)
toxic (metabolic) encephalopathy (G92)

G93.40 **Encephalopathy, unspecified**

G93.41 **Metabolic encephalopathy**
Septic encephalopathy

G93.49 **Other encephalopathy**
Encephalopathy NEC

G93.5 **Compression of brain**
Arnold-Chiari type 1 compression of brain
Compression of brain (stem)
Herniation of brain (stem)
EXCLUDES 1   *diffuse traumatic compression of brain (S06.2-)*
focal traumatic compression of brain (S06.3-)

G93.6 **Cerebral edema**
EXCLUDES 1   *cerebral edema due to birth injury (P11.0)*
traumatic cerebral edema (S06.1-)

G93.7 **Reye's syndrome**   P
Code first (T39.0-), if salicylates-induced

✓5th **G93.8** **Other specified disorders of brain**

G93.81 **Temporal sclerosis**
Hippocampal sclerosis
Mesial temporal sclerosis

G93.82 **Brain death**

G93.89 **Other specified disorders of brain**
Postradiation encephalopathy

G93.9 **Disorder of brain, unspecified**

G94 **Other disorders of brain in diseases classified elsewhere**
Code first underlying disease
EXCLUDES 1   *encephalopathy in congenital syphilis (A50.49)*
encephalopathy in influenza (J09.X9, J10.81, J11.81)
encephalopathy in syphilis (A52.19)
hydrocephalus in diseases classified elsewhere (G91.4)

✓4th **G95** **Other and unspecified diseases of spinal cord**
EXCLUDES 2   *myelitis (G04.-)*

G95.0 **Syringomyelia and syringobulbia**

✓5th **G95.1** **Vascular myelopathies**
EXCLUDES 2   *intraspinal phlebitis and thrombophlebitis, except non-pyogenic (G08)*

G95.11 **Acute infarction of spinal cord (embolic) (nonembolic)**
Anoxia of spinal cord
Arterial thrombosis of spinal cord

G95.19 **Other vascular myelopathies**
Edema of spinal cord
Hematomyelia
Nonpyogenic intraspinal phlebitis and thrombophlebitis
Subacute necrotic myelopathy

✓5th **G95.2** **Other and unspecified cord compression**

G95.20 **Unspecified cord compression**

G95.29 **Other cord compression**

✓5th **G95.8** **Other specified diseases of spinal cord**
EXCLUDES 1   *neurogenic bladder NOS (N31.9)*
neurogenic bladder due to cauda equina syndrome (G83.4)
neuromuscular dysfunction of bladder without spinal cord lesion (N31.-)

G95.81 **Conus medullaris syndrome**

G95.89 **Other specified diseases of spinal cord**
Cord bladder NOS
Drug-induced myelopathy
Radiation-induced myelopathy
EXCLUDES 1   *myelopathy NOS (G95.9)*

G95.9 **Disease of spinal cord, unspecified**
Myelopathy NOS

✓4th **G96** **Other disorders of central nervous system**

G96.0 **Cerebrospinal fluid leak**
EXCLUDES 1   *cerebrospinal fluid leak from spinal puncture (G97.0)*

✓5th **G96.1** **Disorders of meninges, not elsewhere classified**

G96.11 **Dural tear**
EXCLUDES 1   *accidental puncture or laceration of dura during a procedure (G97.41)*

G96.12 **Meningeal adhesions (cerebral) (spinal)**

G96.19 **Other disorders of meninges, not elsewhere classified**

G96.8 **Other specified disorders of central nervous system**

G96.9 **Disorder of central nervous system, unspecified**

✓4th **G97** **Intraoperative and postprocedural complications and disorders of nervous system, not elsewhere classified**
EXCLUDES 2   *intraoperative and postprocedural cerebrovascular infarction (I97.81-, I97.82-)*

G97.0 **Cerebrospinal fluid leak from spinal puncture**

G97.1 **Other reaction to spinal and lumbar puncture**
Headache due to lumbar puncture

G97.2 **Intracranial hypotension following ventricular shunting**

✓5th **G97.3** **Intraoperative hemorrhage and hematoma of a nervous system organ or structure complicating a procedure**
EXCLUDES 1   *intraoperative hemorrhage and hematoma of a nervous system organ or structure due to accidental puncture and laceration during a procedure (G97.4-)*

G97.31 **Intraoperative hemorrhage and hematoma of a nervous system organ or structure complicating a nervous system procedure**

G97.32 **Intraoperative hemorrhage and hematoma of a nervous system organ or structure complicating other procedure**

✓5th **G97.4** **Accidental puncture and laceration of a nervous system organ or structure during a procedure**

G97.41 **Accidental puncture or laceration of dura during a procedure**
Incidental (inadvertent) durotomy

G97.48 **Accidental puncture and laceration of other nervous system organ or structure during a nervous system procedure**

G97.49 **Accidental puncture and laceration of other nervous system organ or structure during other procedure**

✓5th **G97.5** **Postprocedural hemorrhage and hematoma of a nervous system organ or structure following a procedure**

G97.51 **Postprocedural hemorrhage and hematoma of a nervous system organ or structure following a nervous system procedure**

G97.52 **Postprocedural hemorrhage and hematoma of a nervous system organ or structure following other procedure**

✓5th **G97.8** **Other intraoperative and postprocedural complications and disorders of nervous system**
Use additional code to further specify disorder

G97.81 **Other intraoperative complications of nervous system**

G97.82 **Other postprocedural complications and disorders of nervous system**

✓4th **G98** **Other disorders of nervous system not elsewhere classified**
INCLUDES   nervous system disorder NOS

G98.0 **Neurogenic arthritis, not elsewhere classified**
Nonsyphilitic neurogenic arthropathy NEC
Nonsyphilitic neurogenic spondylopathy NEC
EXCLUDES 1   *spondylopathy (in):*
syringomyelia and syringobulbia (G95.0)
tabes dorsalis (A52.11)

G98.8 **Other disorders of nervous system**
Nervous system disorder NOS

EXCLUDES 1 Not coded here   *EXCLUDES 2* Not included here   N Newborn Age: 0   P Pediatric Age: 0-17   M Maternity Age: 12-55   A Adult Age: 15-124

526   ICD-10-CM Draft (2015)

✓4ᵗʰ **G99 Other disorders of nervous system in diseases classified elsewhere**

G99.0 *Autonomic neuropathy in diseases classified elsewhere*

> Code first underlying disease, such as:
> > amyloidosis (E85.-)
> > gout (M1A.-, M10.-)
> > hyperthyroidism (E05.-)
> EXCLUDES 1 diabetic autonomic neuropathy (E08-E13 with .43)

G99.2 *Myelopathy in diseases classified elsewhere*

> Code first underlying disease, such as:
> > neoplasm (C00-D49)
> EXCLUDES 1 myelopathy in:
> > > intervertebral disease (M50.0-, M51.0-)
> > > spondylosis (M47.0-, M47.1-)

G99.8 *Other specified disorders of nervous system in diseases classified elsewhere*

> Code first underlying disorder, such as:
> > amyloidosis (E85.-)
> > avitaminosis (E56.9)
> EXCLUDES 1 nervous system involvement in:
> > > cysticercosis (B69.0)
> > > rubella (B06.0-)
> > > syphilis (A52.1-)

DRAFT

☑ Additional Character Required   ✓×7ᵗʰ Xtension Alert   Unspecified Dx   Other Specified Dx   Manifestation   ▶◀ Revised Text   ● New Code   ▲ Revised Code Title

Diseases of the Eye and Adnexa

H00-H01.129

Chapter 7. Diseases of the Eye and Adnexa (H00-H59)

NOTE   Use an external cause code following the code for the eye condition, if applicable, to identify the cause of the eye condition.

EXCLUDES 2   *certain conditions originating in the perinatal period (P04-P96)*
certain infectious and parasitic diseases (A00-B99)
complications of pregnancy, childbirth and the puerperium (O00-O9A)
congenital malformations, deformations, and chromosomal abnormalities (Q00-Q99)
diabetes mellitus related eye conditions (E09.3-, E10.3-, E11.3-, E13.3-)
endocrine, nutritional and metabolic diseases (E00-E88)
injury (trauma) of eye and orbit (S05.-)
injury, poisoning and certain other consequences of external causes (S00-T88)
neoplasms (C00-D49)
symptoms, signs and abnormal clinical and laboratory findings, not elsewhere classified (R00-R94)
syphilis related eye disorders (A50.01, A50.3-, A51.43, A52.71)

This chapter contains the following blocks:

H00-H05	Disorders of eyelid, lacrimal system and orbit
H10-H11	Disorders of conjunctiva
H15-H22	Disorders of sclera, cornea, iris and ciliary body
H25-H28	Disorders of lens
H30-H36	Disorders of choroid and retina
H40-H42	Glaucoma
H43-H44	Disorders of vitreous body and globe
H46-H47	Disorders of optic nerve and visual pathways
H49-H52	Disorders of ocular muscles, binocular movement, accommodation and refraction
H53-H54	Visual disturbances and blindness
H55-H57	Other disorders of eye and adnexa
H59	Intraoperative and postprocedural complications and disorders of eye and adnexa, not elsewhere classified

Disorders of eyelid, lacrimal system and orbit (H00-H05)

EXCLUDES 2   *open wound of eyelid (S01.1-)*
superficial injury of eyelid (S00.1-, S00.2-)

✓4ᵗʰ H00 Hordeolum and chalazion

  ✓5ᵗʰ H00.0 Hordeolum (externum) (internum) of eyelid

    ✓6ᵗʰ H00.01 Hordeolum externum
Hordeolum NOS
Stye
- H00.011 Hordeolum externum right upper eyelid
- H00.012 Hordeolum externum right lower eyelid
- H00.013 Hordeolum externum right eye, unspecified eyelid
- H00.014 Hordeolum externum left upper eyelid
- H00.015 Hordeolum externum left lower eyelid
- H00.016 Hordeolum externum left eye, unspecified eyelid
- H00.019 Hordeolum externum unspecified eye, unspecified eyelid

    ✓6ᵗʰ H00.02 Hordeolum internum
Infection of meibomian gland
- H00.021 Hordeolum internum right upper eyelid
- H00.022 Hordeolum internum right lower eyelid
- H00.023 Hordeolum internum right eye, unspecified eyelid
- H00.024 Hordeolum internum left upper eyelid
- H00.025 Hordeolum internum left lower eyelid
- H00.026 Hordeolum internum left eye, unspecified eyelid
- H00.029 Hordeolum internum unspecified eye, unspecified eyelid

    ✓6ᵗʰ H00.03 Abscess of eyelid
Furuncle of eyelid
- H00.031 Abscess of right upper eyelid
- H00.032 Abscess of right lower eyelid
- H00.033 Abscess of eyelid right eye, unspecified eyelid
- H00.034 Abscess of left upper eyelid
- H00.035 Abscess of left lower eyelid
- H00.036 Abscess of eyelid left eye, unspecified eyelid
- H00.039 Abscess of eyelid unspecified eye, unspecified eyelid

  ✓5ᵗʰ H00.1 Chalazion
Meibomian (gland) cyst
EXCLUDES 2 *infected meibomian gland (H00.02-)*
- H00.11 Chalazion right upper eyelid
- H00.12 Chalazion right lower eyelid
- H00.13 Chalazion right eye, unspecified eyelid
- H00.14 Chalazion left upper eyelid
- H00.15 Chalazion left lower eyelid
- H00.16 Chalazion left eye, unspecified eyelid
- H00.19 Chalazion unspecified eye, unspecified eyelid

✓4ᵗʰ H01 Other inflammation of eyelid

  ✓5ᵗʰ H01.0 Blepharitis
EXCLUDES 1 *blepharoconjunctivitis (H10.5-)*

    ✓6ᵗʰ H01.00 Unspecified blepharitis
- H01.001 Unspecified blepharitis right upper eyelid
- H01.002 Unspecified blepharitis right lower eyelid
- H01.003 Unspecified blepharitis right eye, unspecified eyelid
- H01.004 Unspecified blepharitis left upper eyelid
- H01.005 Unspecified blepharitis left lower eyelid
- H01.006 Unspecified blepharitis left eye, unspecified eyelid
- H01.009 Unspecified blepharitis unspecified eye, unspecified eyelid

    ✓6ᵗʰ H01.01 Ulcerative blepharitis
- H01.011 Ulcerative blepharitis right upper eyelid
- H01.012 Ulcerative blepharitis right lower eyelid
- H01.013 Ulcerative blepharitis right eye, unspecified eyelid
- H01.014 Ulcerative blepharitis left upper eyelid
- H01.015 Ulcerative blepharitis left lower eyelid
- H01.016 Ulcerative blepharitis left eye, unspecified eyelid
- H01.019 Ulcerative blepharitis unspecified eye, unspecified eyelid

    ✓6ᵗʰ H01.02 Squamous blepharitis
- H01.021 Squamous blepharitis right upper eyelid
- H01.022 Squamous blepharitis right lower eyelid
- H01.023 Squamous blepharitis right eye, unspecified eyelid
- H01.024 Squamous blepharitis left upper eyelid
- H01.025 Squamous blepharitis left lower eyelid
- H01.026 Squamous blepharitis left eye, unspecified eyelid
- H01.029 Squamous blepharitis unspecified eye, unspecified eyelid

  ✓5ᵗʰ H01.1 Noninfectious dermatoses of eyelid

    ✓6ᵗʰ H01.11 Allergic dermatitis of eyelid
Contact dermatitis of eyelid
- H01.111 Allergic dermatitis of right upper eyelid
- H01.112 Allergic dermatitis of right lower eyelid
- H01.113 Allergic dermatitis of right eye, unspecified eyelid
- H01.114 Allergic dermatitis of left upper eyelid
- H01.115 Allergic dermatitis of left lower eyelid
- H01.116 Allergic dermatitis of left eye, unspecified eyelid
- H01.119 Allergic dermatitis of unspecified eye, unspecified eyelid

    ✓6ᵗʰ H01.12 Discoid lupus erythematosus of eyelid
- H01.121 Discoid lupus erythematosus of right upper eyelid
- H01.122 Discoid lupus erythematosus of right lower eyelid
- H01.123 Discoid lupus erythematosus of right eye, unspecified eyelid
- H01.124 Discoid lupus erythematosus of left upper eyelid
- H01.125 Discoid lupus erythematosus of left lower eyelid
- H01.126 Discoid lupus erythematosus of left eye, unspecified eyelid
- H01.129 Discoid lupus erythematosus of unspecified eye, unspecified eyelid

EXCLUDES 1 Not coded here   **EXCLUDES 2** Not included here   **N** Newborn Age: 0   **P** Pediatric Age: 0-17   **M** Maternity Age: 12-55   **A** Adult Age: 15-124

528   ICD-10-CM Draft (2015)

✓6ᵗʰ **H01.13** Eczematous dermatitis of eyelid

H01.131 **Eczematous dermatitis of** right upper **eyelid**

H01.132 **Eczematous dermatitis of** right lower **eyelid**

H01.133 **Eczematous dermatitis of** right eye, **unspecified eyelid**

H01.134 **Eczematous dermatitis of** left upper **eyelid**

H01.135 **Eczematous dermatitis of** left lower **eyelid**

H01.136 **Eczematous dermatitis of** left eye, **unspecified eyelid**

H01.139 **Eczematous dermatitis of unspecified eye, unspecified eyelid**

✓6ᵗʰ **H01.14** Xeroderma of eyelid

H01.141 **Xeroderma of** right upper **eyelid**

H01.142 **Xeroderma of** right lower **eyelid**

H01.143 **Xeroderma of** right eye, **unspecified eyelid**

H01.144 **Xeroderma of** left upper **eyelid**

H01.145 **Xeroderma of** left lower **eyelid**

H01.146 **Xeroderma of** left eye, **unspecified eyelid**

H01.149 **Xeroderma of unspecified eye, unspecified eyelid**

H01.8 Other specified inflammations of eyelid

H01.9 Unspecified inflammation of eyelid
Inflammation of eyelid NOS

✓4ᵗʰ **H02 Other disorders of eyelid**

EXCLUDES 1 *congenital malformations of eyelid (Q10.0-Q10.3)*

✓5ᵗʰ **H02.0 Entropion and trichiasis of eyelid**

✓6ᵗʰ **H02.00** Unspecified entropion of eyelid

H02.001 **Unspecified entropion of** right upper **eyelid**

H02.002 **Unspecified entropion of** right lower **eyelid**

H02.003 **Unspecified entropion of** right eye, **unspecified eyelid**

H02.004 **Unspecified entropion of** left upper **eyelid**

H02.005 **Unspecified entropion of** left lower **eyelid**

H02.006 **Unspecified entropion of** left eye, **unspecified eyelid**

H02.009 **Unspecified entropion of unspecified eye, unspecified eyelid**

✓6ᵗʰ **H02.01** Cicatricial entropion of eyelid

H02.011 **Cicatricial entropion of** right upper **eyelid**

H02.012 **Cicatricial entropion of** right lower **eyelid**

H02.013 **Cicatricial entropion of** right eye, **unspecified eyelid**

H02.014 **Cicatricial entropion of** left upper **eyelid**

H02.015 **Cicatricial entropion of** left lower **eyelid**

H02.016 **Cicatricial entropion of** left eye, **unspecified eyelid**

H02.019 **Cicatricial entropion of unspecified eye, unspecified eyelid**

✓6ᵗʰ **H02.02** Mechanical entropion of eyelid

H02.021 **Mechanical entropion of** right upper **eyelid**

H02.022 **Mechanical entropion of** right lower **eyelid**

H02.023 **Mechanical entropion of** right eye, **unspecified eyelid**

H02.024 **Mechanical entropion of** left upper **eyelid**

H02.025 **Mechanical entropion of** left lower **eyelid**

H02.026 **Mechanical entropion of** left eye, **unspecified eyelid**

H02.029 **Mechanical entropion of unspecified eye, unspecified eyelid**

✓6ᵗʰ **H02.03** Senile entropion of eyelid

H02.031 **Senile entropion of** right upper **eyelid** Ⓐ

H02.032 **Senile entropion of** right lower **eyelid** Ⓐ

H02.033 **Senile entropion of** right eye, **unspecified eyelid** Ⓐ

H02.034 **Senile entropion of** left upper **eyelid** Ⓐ

H02.035 **Senile entropion of** left lower **eyelid** Ⓐ

H02.036 **Senile entropion of** left eye, **unspecified eyelid** Ⓐ

H02.039 **Senile entropion of unspecified eye, unspecified eyelid** Ⓐ

✓6ᵗʰ **H02.04** Spastic entropion of eyelid

H02.041 **Spastic entropion of** right upper **eyelid**

H02.042 **Spastic entropion of** right lower **eyelid**

H02.043 **Spastic entropion of** right eye, **unspecified eyelid**

H02.044 **Spastic entropion of** left upper **eyelid**

H02.045 **Spastic entropion of** left lower **eyelid**

H02.046 **Spastic entropion of** left eye, **unspecified eyelid**

H02.049 **Spastic entropion of unspecified eye, unspecified eyelid**

✓6ᵗʰ **H02.05** Trichiasis without entropian

H02.051 **Trichiasis without entropian** right upper **eyelid**

H02.052 **Trichiasis without entropian** right lower **eyelid**

H02.053 **Trichiasis without entropian** right eye, **unspecified eyelid**

H02.054 **Trichiasis without entropian** left upper **eyelid**

H02.055 **Trichiasis without entropian** left lower **eyelid**

H02.056 **Trichiasis without entropian** left eye, **unspecified eyelid**

H02.059 **Trichiasis without entropian unspecified eye, unspecified eyelid**

✓5ᵗʰ **H02.1 Ectropion of eyelid**

✓6ᵗʰ **H02.10** Unspecified ectropion of eyelid

H02.101 **Unspecified ectropion of** right upper **eyelid**

H02.102 **Unspecified ectropion of** right lower **eyelid**

H02.103 **Unspecified ectropion of** right eye, **unspecified eyelid**

H02.104 **Unspecified ectropion of** left upper **eyelid**

H02.105 **Unspecified ectropion of** left lower **eyelid**

H02.106 **Unspecified ectropion of** left eye, **unspecified eyelid**

H02.109 **Unspecified ectropion of unspecified eye, unspecified eyelid**

✓6ᵗʰ **H02.11** Cicatricial ectropion of eyelid

H02.111 **Cicatricial ectropion of** right upper **eyelid**

H02.112 **Cicatricial ectropion of** right lower **eyelid**

H02.113 **Cicatricial ectropion of** right eye, **unspecified eyelid**

H02.114 **Cicatricial ectropion of** left upper **eyelid**

H02.115 **Cicatricial ectropion of** left lower **eyelid**

H02.116 **Cicatricial ectropion of** left eye, **unspecified eyelid**

H02.119 **Cicatricial ectropion of unspecified eye, unspecified eyelid**

✓6ᵗʰ **H02.12** Mechanical ectropion of eyelid

H02.121 **Mechanical ectropion of** right upper **eyelid**

H02.122 **Mechanical ectropion of** right lower **eyelid**

H02.123 **Mechanical ectropion of** right eye, **unspecified eyelid**

H02.124 **Mechanical ectropion of** left upper **eyelid**

H02.125 **Mechanical ectropion of** left lower **eyelid**

H02.126 **Mechanical ectropion of** left eye, **unspecified eyelid**

H02.129 **Mechanical ectropion of unspecified eye, unspecified eyelid**

✓6ᵗʰ **H02.13** Senile ectropion of eyelid

H02.131 **Senile ectropion of** right upper **eyelid** Ⓐ

H02.132 **Senile ectropion of** right lower **eyelid** Ⓐ

H02.133 **Senile ectropion of** right eye, **unspecified eyelid** Ⓐ

H02.134 **Senile ectropion of** left upper **eyelid** Ⓐ

H02.135 **Senile ectropion of** left lower **eyelid** Ⓐ

H02.136 **Senile ectropion of** left eye, **unspecified eyelid** Ⓐ

H02.139 **Senile ectropion of unspecified eye, unspecified eyelid** Ⓐ

✓6ᵗʰ **H02.14** Spastic ectropion of eyelid

H02.141 **Spastic ectropion of** right upper **eyelid**

H02.142 **Spastic ectropion of** right lower **eyelid**

☑ Additional Character Required   ✓x7ᵗʰ Xtension Alert   Unspecified Dx   Other Specified Dx   Manifestation   ►◄ Revised Text   ● New Code   ▲ Revised Code Title

ICD-10-CM Draft (2015)   529

Diseases of the Eye and Adnexa

H02.143–H02.65

H02.143   Spastic ectropion of right eye, unspecified eyelid

H02.144   Spastic ectropion of left upper eyelid

H02.145   Spastic ectropion of left lower eyelid

H02.146   Spastic ectropion of left eye, unspecified eyelid

H02.149   Spastic ectropion of unspecified eye, unspecified eyelid

✓5th **H02.2 Lagophthalmos**

  ✓6th **H02.20**   Unspecified lagophthalmos

H02.201   Unspecified lagophthalmos right upper eyelid

H02.202   Unspecified lagophthalmos right lower eyelid

H02.203   Unspecified lagophthalmos right eye, unspecified eyelid

H02.204   Unspecified lagophthalmos left upper eyelid

H02.205   Unspecified lagophthalmos left lower eyelid

H02.206   Unspecified lagophthalmos left eye, unspecified eyelid

H02.209   Unspecified lagophthalmos unspecified eye, unspecified eyelid

  ✓6th **H02.21**   Cicatricial lagophthalmos

H02.211   Cicatricial lagophthalmos right upper eyelid

H02.212   Cicatricial lagophthalmos right lower eyelid

H02.213   Cicatricial lagophthalmos right eye, unspecified eyelid

H02.214   Cicatricial lagophthalmos left upper eyelid

H02.215   Cicatricial lagophthalmos left lower eyelid

H02.216   Cicatricial lagophthalmos left eye, unspecified eyelid

H02.219   Cicatricial lagophthalmos unspecified eye, unspecified eyelid

  ✓6th **H02.22**   Mechanical lagophthalmos

H02.221   Mechanical lagophthalmos right upper eyelid

H02.222   Mechanical lagophthalmos right lower eyelid

H02.223   Mechanical lagophthalmos right eye, unspecified eyelid

H02.224   Mechanical lagophthalmos left upper eyelid

H02.225   Mechanical lagophthalmos left lower eyelid

H02.226   Mechanical lagophthalmos left eye, unspecified eyelid

H02.229   Mechanical lagophthalmos unspecified eye, unspecified eyelid

  ✓6th **H02.23**   Paralytic lagophthalmos

H02.231   Paralytic lagophthalmos right upper eyelid

H02.232   Paralytic lagophthalmos right lower eyelid

H02.233   Paralytic lagophthalmos right eye, unspecified eyelid

H02.234   Paralytic lagophthalmos left upper eyelid

H02.235   Paralytic lagophthalmos left lower eyelid

H02.236   Paralytic lagophthalmos left eye, unspecified eyelid

H02.239   Paralytic lagophthalmos unspecified eye, unspecified eyelid

✓5th **H02.3 Blepharochalasis**
     Pseudoptosis

H02.30   Blepharochalasis unspecified eye, unspecified eyelid

H02.31   Blepharochalasis right upper eyelid

H02.32   Blepharochalasis right lower eyelid

H02.33   Blepharochalasis right eye, unspecified eyelid

H02.34   Blepharochalasis left upper eyelid

H02.35   Blepharochalasis left lower eyelid

H02.36   Blepharochalasis left eye, unspecified eyelid

✓5th **H02.4 Ptosis of eyelid**

  ✓6th **H02.40**   Unspecified ptosis of eyelid

H02.401   Unspecified ptosis of right eyelid

H02.402   Unspecified ptosis of left eyelid

H02.403   Unspecified ptosis of bilateral eyelids

H02.409   Unspecified ptosis of unspecified eyelid

  ✓6th **H02.41**   Mechanical ptosis of eyelid

H02.411   Mechanical ptosis of right eyelid

H02.412   Mechanical ptosis of left eyelid

H02.413   Mechanical ptosis of bilateral eyelids

H02.419   Mechanical ptosis of unspecified eyelid

  ✓6th **H02.42**   Myogenic ptosis of eyelid

H02.421   Myogenic ptosis of right eyelid

H02.422   Myogenic ptosis of left eyelid

H02.423   Myogenic ptosis of bilateral eyelids

H02.429   Myogenic ptosis of unspecified eyelid

  ✓6th **H02.43**   Paralytic ptosis of eyelid
       Neurogenic ptosis of eyelid

H02.431   Paralytic ptosis of right eyelid

H02.432   Paralytic ptosis of left eyelid

H02.433   Paralytic ptosis of bilateral eyelids

H02.439   Paralytic ptosis unspecified eyelid

✓5th **H02.5 Other disorders affecting eyelid function**
     EXCLUDES 2   blepharospasm (G24.5)
                 organic tic (G25.69)
                 psychogenic tic (F95.-)

  ✓6th **H02.51**   Abnormal innervation syndrome

H02.511   Abnormal innervation syndrome right upper eyelid

H02.512   Abnormal innervation syndrome right lower eyelid

H02.513   Abnormal innervation syndrome right eye, unspecified eyelid

H02.514   Abnormal innervation syndrome left upper eyelid

H02.515   Abnormal innervation syndrome left lower eyelid

H02.516   Abnormal innervation syndrome left eye, unspecified eyelid

H02.519   Abnormal innervation syndrome unspecified eye, unspecified eyelid

  ✓6th **H02.52**   Blepharophimosis
       Ankyloblepharon

H02.521   Blepharophimosis right upper eyelid

H02.522   Blepharophimosis right lower eyelid

H02.523   Blepharophimosis right eye, unspecified eyelid

H02.524   Blepharophimosis left upper eyelid

H02.525   Blepharophimosis left lower eyelid

H02.526   Blepharophimosis left eye, unspecified eyelid

H02.529   Blepharophimosis unspecified eye, unspecified lid

  ✓6th **H02.53**   Eyelid retraction
       Eyelid lag

H02.531   Eyelid retraction right upper eyelid

H02.532   Eyelid retraction right lower eyelid

H02.533   Eyelid retraction right eye, unspecified eyelid

H02.534   Eyelid retraction left upper eyelid

H02.535   Eyelid retraction left lower eyelid

H02.536   Eyelid retraction left eye, unspecified eyelid

H02.539   Eyelid retraction unspecified eye, unspecified lid

H02.59   Other disorders affecting eyelid function
       Deficient blink reflex
       Sensory disorders

✓5th **H02.6 Xanthelasma of eyelid**

H02.60   Xanthelasma of unspecified eye, unspecified eyelid

H02.61   Xanthelasma of right upper eyelid

H02.62   Xanthelasma of right lower eyelid

H02.63   Xanthelasma of right eye, unspecified eyelid

H02.64   Xanthelasma of left upper eyelid

H02.65   Xanthelasma of left lower eyelid

EXCLUDES 1 Not coded here   EXCLUDES 2 Not included here   N Newborn Age: 0   P Pediatric Age: 0-17   M Maternity Age: 12-55   A Adult Age: 15-124

H02.66 **Xanthelasma of** left eye, **unspecified eyelid**

✓5ᵗʰ H02.7 **Other and unspecified degenerative disorders of eyelid and periocular area**

H02.70 **Unspecified degenerative disorders of eyelid and periocular area**

✓6ᵗʰ H02.71 Chloasma **of eyelid and periocular area**
Dyspigmentation of eyelid
Hyperpigmentation of eyelid

H02.711 **Chloasma of** right upper **eyelid and periocular area**

H02.712 **Chloasma of** right lower **eyelid and periocular area**

H02.713 **Chloasma of** right eye, unspecified eyelid and periocular area

H02.714 **Chloasma of** left upper **eyelid and periocular area**

H02.715 **Chloasma of** left lower **eyelid and periocular area**

H02.716 **Chloasma of** left eye, unspecified eyelid and periocular area

H02.719 **Chloasma of unspecified eye, unspecified eyelid and periocular area**

✓6ᵗʰ H02.72 Madarosis **of eyelid and periocular area**
Hypotrichosis of eyelid

H02.721 **Madarosis of** right upper **eyelid and periocular area**

H02.722 **Madarosis of** right lower **eyelid and periocular area**

H02.723 **Madarosis of** right eye, unspecified eyelid and periocular area

H02.724 **Madarosis of** left upper **eyelid and periocular area**

H02.725 **Madarosis of** left lower **eyelid and periocular area**

H02.726 **Madarosis of** left eye, unspecified eyelid and periocular area

H02.729 **Madarosis of unspecified eye, unspecified eyelid and periocular area**

✓6ᵗʰ H02.73 Vitiligo **of eyelid and periocular area**
Hypopigmentation of eyelid

H02.731 **Vitiligo of** right upper **eyelid and periocular area**

H02.732 **Vitiligo of** right lower **eyelid and periocular area**

H02.733 **Vitiligo of** right eye, unspecified eyelid and periocular area

H02.734 **Vitiligo of** left upper **eyelid and periocular area**

H02.735 **Vitiligo of** left lower **eyelid and periocular area**

H02.736 **Vitiligo of** left eye, unspecified eyelid and periocular area

H02.739 **Vitiligo of unspecified eye, unspecified eyelid and periocular area**

H02.79 **Other degenerative disorders of eyelid and periocular area**

✓5ᵗʰ H02.8 **Other specified disorders of eyelid**

✓6ᵗʰ H02.81 **Retained foreign body in eyelid**
Use additional code to identify the type of retained foreign body (Z18.-)
EXCLUDES 1 laceration of eyelid with foreign body (S01.12-)
retained intraocular foreign body (H44.6-, H44.7-)
superficial foreign body of eyelid and periocular area (S00.25-)

H02.811 **Retained foreign body in** right upper **eyelid**

H02.812 **Retained foreign body in** right lower **eyelid**

H02.813 **Retained foreign body in** right eye, unspecified eyelid

H02.814 **Retained foreign body in** left upper **eyelid**

H02.815 **Retained foreign body in** left lower **eyelid**

H02.816 **Retained foreign body in** left eye, unspecified eyelid

H02.819 **Retained foreign body in unspecified eye, unspecified eyelid**

✓6ᵗʰ H02.82 Cysts **of eyelid**
Sebaceous cyst of eyelid

H02.821 **Cysts of** right upper **eyelid**

H02.822 **Cysts of** right lower **eyelid**

H02.823 **Cysts of** right eye, unspecified eyelid

H02.824 **Cysts of** left upper **eyelid**

H02.825 **Cysts of** left lower **eyelid**

H02.826 **Cysts of** left eye, unspecified eyelid

H02.829 **Cysts of unspecified eye, unspecified eyelid**

✓6ᵗʰ H02.83 Dermatochalasis **of eyelid**

H02.831 **Dermatochalasis of** right upper **eyelid**

H02.832 **Dermatochalasis of** right lower **eyelid**

H02.833 **Dermatochalasis of** right eye, unspecified eyelid

H02.834 **Dermatochalasis of** left upper **eyelid**

H02.835 **Dermatochalasis of** left lower **eyelid**

H02.836 **Dermatochalasis of** left eye, unspecified eyelid

H02.839 **Dermatochalasis of unspecified eye, unspecified eyelid**

✓6ᵗʰ H02.84 Edema **of eyelid**
Hyperemia of eyelid

H02.841 **Edema of** right upper **eyelid**

H02.842 **Edema of** right lower **eyelid**

H02.843 **Edema of** right eye, unspecified eyelid

H02.844 **Edema of** left upper **eyelid**

H02.845 **Edema of** left lower **eyelid**

H02.846 **Edema of** left eye, unspecified eyelid

H02.849 **Edema of unspecified eye, unspecified eyelid**

✓6ᵗʰ H02.85 Elephantiasis **of eyelid**

H02.851 **Elephantiasis of** right upper **eyelid**

H02.852 **Elephantiasis of** right lower **eyelid**

H02.853 **Elephantiasis of** right eye, unspecified eyelid

H02.854 **Elephantiasis of** left upper **eyelid**

H02.855 **Elephantiasis of** left lower **eyelid**

H02.856 **Elephantiasis of** left eye, unspecified eyelid

H02.859 **Elephantiasis of unspecified eye, unspecified eyelid**

✓6ᵗʰ H02.86 Hypertrichosis **of eyelid**

H02.861 **Hypertrichosis of** right upper **eyelid**

H02.862 **Hypertrichosis of** right lower **eyelid**

H02.863 **Hypertrichosis of** right eye, unspecified eyelid

H02.864 **Hypertrichosis of** left upper **eyelid**

H02.865 **Hypertrichosis of** left lower **eyelid**

H02.866 **Hypertrichosis of** left eye, unspecified eyelid

H02.869 **Hypertrichosis of unspecified eye, unspecified eyelid**

✓6ᵗʰ H02.87 Vascular anomalies **of eyelid**

H02.871 **Vascular anomalies of** right upper **eyelid**

H02.872 **Vascular anomalies of** right lower **eyelid**

H02.873 **Vascular anomalies of** right eye, unspecified eyelid

H02.874 **Vascular anomalies of** left upper **eyelid**

H02.875 **Vascular anomalies of** left lower **eyelid**

H02.876 **Vascular anomalies of** left eye, unspecified eyelid

H02.879 **Vascular anomalies of unspecified eye, unspecified eyelid**

H02.89 **Other specified disorders of eyelid**
Hemorrhage of eyelid

H02.9 **Unspecified disorder of eyelid**
Disorder of eyelid NOS

✓4ᵗʰ H04 **Disorders of lacrimal system**
EXCLUDES 1 congenital malformations of lacrimal system (Q10.4-Q10.6)

✓5ᵗʰ H04.0 **Dacryoadenitis**

✓6ᵗʰ H04.00 Unspecified **dacryoadenitis**

H04.001 **Unspecified dacryoadenitis,** right **lacrimal gland**

Diseases of the Eye and Adnexa

H04.002–H04.419

H04.002　Unspecified dacryoadenitis, left lacrimal gland

H04.003　Unspecified dacryoadenitis, bilateral lacrimal glands

H04.009　Unspecified dacryoadenitis, unspecified lacrimal gland

✓6ᵗʰ H04.01　Acute dacryoadenitis

H04.011　Acute dacryoadenitis, right lacrimal gland

H04.012　Acute dacryoadenitis, left lacrimal gland

H04.013　Acute dacryoadenitis, bilateral lacrimal glands

H04.019　Acute dacryoadenitis, unspecified lacrimal gland

✓6ᵗʰ H04.02　Chronic dacryoadenitis

H04.021　Chronic dacryoadenitis, right lacrimal gland

H04.022　Chronic dacryoadenitis, left lacrimal gland

H04.023　Chronic dacryoadenitis, bilateral lacrimal glands

H04.029　Chronic dacryoadenitis, unspecified lacrimal gland

✓6ᵗʰ H04.03　Chronic enlargement of lacrimal gland

H04.031　Chronic enlargement of right lacrimal gland

H04.032　Chronic enlargement of left lacrimal gland

H04.033　Chronic enlargement of bilateral lacrimal glands

H04.039　Chronic enlargement of unspecified lacrimal gland

✓5ᵗʰ H04.1　Other disorders of lacrimal gland

✓6ᵗʰ H04.11　Dacryops

H04.111　Dacryops of right lacrimal gland

H04.112　Dacryops of left lacrimal gland

H04.113　Dacryops of bilateral lacrimal glands

H04.119　Dacryops of unspecified lacrimal gland

✓6ᵗʰ H04.12　Dry eye syndrome
　　　　　Tear film insufficiency, NOS

H04.121　Dry eye syndrome of right lacrimal gland

H04.122　Dry eye syndrome of left lacrimal gland

H04.123　Dry eye syndrome of bilateral lacrimal glands

H04.129　Dry eye syndrome of unspecified lacrimal gland

✓6ᵗʰ H04.13　Lacrimal cyst
　　　　　Lacrimal cystic degeneration

H04.131　Lacrimal cyst, right lacrimal gland

H04.132　Lacrimal cyst, left lacrimal gland

H04.133　Lacrimal cyst, bilateral lacrimal glands

H04.139　Lacrimal cyst, unspecified lacrimal gland

✓6ᵗʰ H04.14　Primary lacrimal gland atrophy

H04.141　Primary lacrimal gland atrophy, right lacrimal gland

H04.142　Primary lacrimal gland atrophy, left lacrimal gland

H04.143　Primary lacrimal gland atrophy, bilateral lacrimal glands

H04.149　Primary lacrimal gland atrophy, unspecified lacrimal gland

✓6ᵗʰ H04.15　Secondary lacrimal gland atrophy

H04.151　Secondary lacrimal gland atrophy, right lacrimal gland

H04.152　Secondary lacrimal gland atrophy, left lacrimal gland

H04.153　Secondary lacrimal gland atrophy, bilateral lacrimal glands

H04.159　Secondary lacrimal gland atrophy, unspecified lacrimal gland

✓6ᵗʰ H04.16　Lacrimal gland dislocation

H04.161　Lacrimal gland dislocation, right lacrimal gland

H04.162　Lacrimal gland dislocation, left lacrimal gland

H04.163　Lacrimal gland dislocation, bilateral lacrimal glands

H04.169　Lacrimal gland dislocation, unspecified lacrimal gland

H04.19　Other specified disorders of lacrimal gland

✓5ᵗʰ H04.2　Epiphora

✓6ᵗʰ H04.20　Unspecified epiphora

H04.201　Unspecified epiphora, right lacrimal gland

H04.202　Unspecified epiphora, left lacrimal gland

H04.203　Unspecified epiphora, bilateral lacrimal glands

H04.209　Unspecified epiphora, unspecified lacrimal gland

✓6ᵗʰ H04.21　Epiphora due to excess lacrimation

H04.211　Epiphora due to excess lacrimation, right lacrimal gland

H04.212　Epiphora due to excess lacrimation, left lacrimal gland

H04.213　Epiphora due to excess lacrimation, bilateral lacrimal glands

H04.219　Epiphora due to excess lacrimation, unspecified lacrimal gland

✓6ᵗʰ H04.22　Epiphora due to insufficient drainage

H04.221　Epiphora due to insufficient drainage, right lacrimal gland

H04.222　Epiphora due to insufficient drainage, left lacrimal gland

H04.223　Epiphora due to insufficient drainage, bilateral lacrimal glands

H04.229　Epiphora due to insufficient drainage, unspecified lacrimal gland

✓5ᵗʰ H04.3　Acute and unspecified inflammation of lacrimal passages
　　　EXCLUDES 1　neonatal dacryocystitis (P39.1)

✓6ᵗʰ H04.30　Unspecified dacryocystitis

H04.301　Unspecified dacryocystitis of right lacrimal passage

H04.302　Unspecified dacryocystitis of left lacrimal passage

H04.303　Unspecified dacryocystitis of bilateral lacrimal passages

H04.309　Unspecified dacryocystitis of unspecified lacrimal passage

✓6ᵗʰ H04.31　Phlegmonous dacryocystitis

H04.311　Phlegmonous dacryocystitis of right lacrimal passage

H04.312　Phlegmonous dacryocystitis of left lacrimal passage

H04.313　Phlegmonous dacryocystitis of bilateral lacrimal passages

H04.319　Phlegmonous dacryocystitis of unspecified lacrimal passage

✓6ᵗʰ H04.32　Acute dacryocystitis
　　　　　Acute dacryopericystitis

H04.321　Acute dacryocystitis of right lacrimal passage

H04.322　Acute dacryocystitis of left lacrimal passage

H04.323　Acute dacryocystitis of bilateral lacrimal passages

H04.329　Acute dacryocystitis of unspecified lacrimal passage

✓6ᵗʰ H04.33　Acute lacrimal canaliculitis

H04.331　Acute lacrimal canaliculitis of right lacrimal passage

H04.332　Acute lacrimal canaliculitis of left lacrimal passage

H04.333　Acute lacrimal canaliculitis of bilateral lacrimal passages

H04.339　Acute lacrimal canaliculitis of unspecified lacrimal passage

✓5ᵗʰ H04.4　Chronic inflammation of lacrimal passages

✓6ᵗʰ H04.41　Chronic dacryocystitis

H04.411　Chronic dacryocystitis of right lacrimal passage

H04.412　Chronic dacryocystitis of left lacrimal passage

H04.413　Chronic dacryocystitis of bilateral lacrimal passages

H04.419　Chronic dacryocystitis of unspecified lacrimal passage

EXCLUDES 1 Not coded here　　EXCLUDES 2 Not included here　　N Newborn Age: 0　　P Pediatric Age: 0-17　　M Maternity Age: 12-55　　A Adult Age: 15-124

532　　　　　　　　　　　　　　　　　　　　　　　　　　　　　　　　ICD-10-CM Draft (2015)

√6ᵗʰ **H04.42** Chronic lacrimal canaliculitis
- **H04.421 Chronic lacrimal canaliculitis of** right **lacrimal passage**
- **H04.422 Chronic lacrimal canaliculitis of** left **lacrimal passage**
- **H04.423 Chronic lacrimal canaliculitis of** bilateral **lacrimal passages**
- **H04.429 Chronic lacrimal canaliculitis of unspecified lacrimal passage**

√6ᵗʰ **H04.43** Chronic lacrimal mucocele
- **H04.431 Chronic lacrimal mucocele of** right **lacrimal passage**
- **H04.432 Chronic lacrimal mucocele of** left **lacrimal passage**
- **H04.433 Chronic lacrimal mucocele of** bilateral **lacrimal passages**
- **H04.439 Chronic lacrimal mucocele of unspecified lacrimal passage**

√5ᵗʰ **H04.5 Stenosis and insufficiency of lacrimal passages**

√6ᵗʰ **H04.51** Dacryolith
- **H04.511 Dacryolith of** right **lacrimal passage**
- **H04.512 Dacryolith of** left **lacrimal passage**
- **H04.513 Dacryolith of** bilateral **lacrimal passages**
- **H04.519 Dacryolith of unspecified lacrimal passage**

√6ᵗʰ **H04.52** Eversion of lacrimal punctum
- **H04.521 Eversion of** right **lacrimal punctum**
- **H04.522 Eversion of** left **lacrimal punctum**
- **H04.523 Eversion of** bilateral **lacrimal punctum**
- **H04.529 Eversion of unspecified lacrimal punctum**

√6ᵗʰ **H04.53** Neonatal obstruction of nasolacrimal duct

　　EXCLUDES 1　*congenital stenosis and stricture of lacrimal duct (Q10.5)*
- **H04.531 Neonatal obstruction of** right **nasolacrimal duct** Ⓝ
- **H04.532 Neonatal obstruction of** left **nasolacrimal duct** Ⓝ
- **H04.533 Neonatal obstruction of** bilateral **nasolacrimal duct** Ⓝ
- **H04.539 Neonatal obstruction of unspecified nasolacrimal duct** Ⓝ

√6ᵗʰ **H04.54** Stenosis of lacrimal canaliculi
- **H04.541 Stenosis of** right **lacrimal canaliculi**
- **H04.542 Stenosis of** left **lacrimal canaliculi**
- **H04.543 Stenosis of** bilateral **lacrimal canaliculi**
- **H04.549 Stenosis of unspecified lacrimal canaliculi**

√6ᵗʰ **H04.55** Acquired stenosis of nasolacrimal duct
- **H04.551 Acquired stenosis of** right **nasolacrimal duct**
- **H04.552 Acquired stenosis of** left **nasolacrimal duct**
- **H04.553 Acquired stenosis of** bilateral **nasolacrimal duct**
- **H04.559 Acquired stenosis of unspecified nasolacrimal duct**

√6ᵗʰ **H04.56** Stenosis of lacrimal punctum
- **H04.561 Stenosis of** right **lacrimal punctum**
- **H04.562 Stenosis of** left **lacrimal punctum**
- **H04.563 Stenosis of** bilateral **lacrimal punctum**
- **H04.569 Stenosis of unspecified lacrimal punctum**

√6ᵗʰ **H04.57** Stenosis of lacrimal sac
- **H04.571 Stenosis of** right **lacrimal sac**
- **H04.572 Stenosis of** left **lacrimal sac**
- **H04.573 Stenosis of** bilateral **lacrimal sac**
- **H04.579 Stenosis of unspecified lacrimal sac**

√5ᵗʰ **H04.6 Other changes of lacrimal passages**

√6ᵗʰ **H04.61** Lacrimal fistula
- **H04.611 Lacrimal fistula** right **lacrimal passage**
- **H04.612 Lacrimal fistula** left **lacrimal passage**
- **H04.613 Lacrimal fistula** bilateral **lacrimal passages**
- **H04.619 Lacrimal fistula unspecified lacrimal passage**

H04.69 Other changes of lacrimal passages

√6ᵗʰ **H04.8 Other disorders of lacrimal system**

√6ᵗʰ **H04.81 Granuloma of lacrimal passages**
- **H04.811 Granuloma of** right **lacrimal passage**
- **H04.812 Granuloma of** left **lacrimal passage**
- **H04.813 Granuloma of** bilateral **lacrimal passages**
- **H04.819 Granuloma of unspecified lacrimal passage**

H04.89 Other disorders of lacrimal system

H04.9 Disorder of lacrimal system, unspecified

√4ᵗʰ **H05 Disorders of orbit**

　　EXCLUDES 1　*congenital malformation of orbit (Q10.7)*

√5ᵗʰ **H05.0 Acute inflammation of orbit**

H05.00 Unspecified acute inflammation of orbit

√6ᵗʰ **H05.01** Cellulitis of orbit
　　Abscess of orbit
- **H05.011 Cellulitis of** right **orbit**
- **H05.012 Cellulitis of** left **orbit**
- **H05.013 Cellulitis of** bilateral **orbits**
- **H05.019 Cellulitis of unspecified orbit**

√6ᵗʰ **H05.02** Osteomyelitis of orbit
- **H05.021 Osteomyelitis of** right **orbit**
- **H05.022 Osteomyelitis of** left **orbit**
- **H05.023 Osteomyelitis of** bilateral **orbits**
- **H05.029 Osteomyelitis of unspecified orbit**

√6ᵗʰ **H05.03** Periostitis of orbit
- **H05.031 Periostitis of** right **orbit**
- **H05.032 Periostitis of** left **orbit**
- **H05.033 Periostitis of** bilateral **orbits**
- **H05.039 Periostitis of unspecified orbit**

√6ᵗʰ **H05.04** Tenonitis of orbit
- **H05.041 Tenonitis of** right **orbit**
- **H05.042 Tenonitis of** left **orbit**
- **H05.043 Tenonitis of** bilateral **orbits**
- **H05.049 Tenonitis of unspecified orbit**

√5ᵗʰ **H05.1** Chronic inflammatory disorders of orbit

H05.10 Unspecified chronic inflammatory disorders of orbit

√6ᵗʰ **H05.11** Granuloma of orbit
　　Pseudotumor (inflammatory) of orbit
- **H05.111 Granuloma of** right **orbit**
- **H05.112 Granuloma of** left **orbit**
- **H05.113 Granuloma of** bilateral **orbits**
- **H05.119 Granuloma of unspecified orbit**

√6ᵗʰ **H05.12** Orbital myositis
- **H05.121 Orbital myositis,** right **orbit**
- **H05.122 Orbital myositis,** left **orbit**
- **H05.123 Orbital myositis,** bilateral
- **H05.129 Orbital myositis, unspecified orbit**

√5ᵗʰ **H05.2** Exophthalmic conditions

H05.20 Unspecified exophthalmos

√6ᵗʰ **H05.21** Displacement (lateral) of globe
- **H05.211 Displacement (lateral) of globe,** right eye
- **H05.212 Displacement (lateral) of globe,** left eye
- **H05.213 Displacement (lateral) of globe,** bilateral
- **H05.219 Displacement (lateral) of globe, unspecified eye**

√6ᵗʰ **H05.22** Edema of orbit
　　Orbital congestion
- **H05.221 Edema of** right **orbit**
- **H05.222 Edema of** left **orbit**
- **H05.223 Edema of** bilateral **orbit**
- **H05.229 Edema of unspecified orbit**

√6ᵗʰ **H05.23** Hemorrhage of orbit
- **H05.231 Hemorrhage of** right **orbit**
- **H05.232 Hemorrhage of** left **orbit**
- **H05.233 Hemorrhage of** bilateral **orbit**
- **H05.239 Hemorrhage of unspecified orbit**

√6ᵗʰ **H05.24** Constant exophthalmos
- **H05.241 Constant exophthalmos,** right eye
- **H05.242 Constant exophthalmos,** left eye
- **H05.243 Constant exophthalmos,** bilateral
- **H05.249 Constant exophthalmos, unspecified eye**

√6ᵗʰ **H05.25** Intermittent exophthalmos
- **H05.251 Intermittent exophthalmos,** right eye
- **H05.252 Intermittent exophthalmos,** left eye

✔ Additional Character Required　　　√x7ᵗʰ Xtension Alert　　Unspecified Dx　　Other Specified Dx　　Manifestation　　►◄ Revised Text　　● New Code　　▲ Revised Code Title

Diseases of the Eye and Adnexa

H05.253–H10.222

H05.253   Intermittent exophthalmos, bilateral

H05.259   Intermittent exophthalmos, unspecified eye

✓6ᵗʰ   **H05.26**   Pulsating exophthalmos

H05.261   Pulsating exophthalmos, right eye

H05.262   Pulsating exophthalmos, left eye

H05.263   Pulsating exophthalmos, bilateral

H05.269   Pulsating exophthalmos, unspecified eye

✓5ᵗʰ   **H05.3**   **Deformity of orbit**

> EXCLUDES 1   congenital deformity of orbit (Q10.7)
> hypertelorism (Q75.2)

H05.30   Unspecified deformity of orbit

✓6ᵗʰ   **H05.31**   Atrophy of orbit

H05.311   Atrophy of right orbit

H05.312   Atrophy of left orbit

H05.313   Atrophy of bilateral orbit

H05.319   Atrophy of unspecified orbit

✓6ᵗʰ   **H05.32**   Deformity of orbit due to bone disease

> Code also associated bone disease

H05.321   Deformity of right orbit due to bone disease

H05.322   Deformity of left orbit due to bone disease

H05.323   Deformity of bilateral orbits due to bone disease

H05.329   Deformity of unspecified orbit due to bone disease

✓6ᵗʰ   **H05.33**   Deformity of orbit due to trauma or surgery

H05.331   Deformity of right orbit due to trauma or surgery

H05.332   Deformity of left orbit due to trauma or surgery

H05.333   Deformity of bilateral orbits due to trauma or surgery

H05.339   Deformity of unspecified orbit due to trauma or surgery

✓6ᵗʰ   **H05.34**   Enlargement of orbit

H05.341   Enlargement of right orbit

H05.342   Enlargement of left orbit

H05.343   Enlargement of bilateral orbits

H05.349   Enlargement of unspecified orbit

✓6ᵗʰ   **H05.35**   Exostosis of orbit

H05.351   Exostosis of right orbit

H05.352   Exostosis of left orbit

H05.353   Exostosis of bilateral orbits

H05.359   Exostosis of unspecified orbit

✓5ᵗʰ   **H05.4**   **Enophthalmos**

✓6ᵗʰ   **H05.40**   Unspecified enophthalmos

H05.401   Unspecified enophthalmos, right eye

H05.402   Unspecified enophthalmos, left eye

H05.403   Unspecified enophthalmos, bilateral

H05.409   Unspecified enophthalmos, unspecified eye

✓6ᵗʰ   **H05.41**   Enophthalmos due to atrophy of orbital tissue

H05.411   Enophthalmos due to atrophy of orbital tissue, right eye

H05.412   Enophthalmos due to atrophy of orbital tissue, left eye

H05.413   Enophthalmos due to atrophy of orbital tissue, bilateral

H05.419   Enophthalmos due to atrophy of orbital tissue, unspecified eye

✓6ᵗʰ   **H05.42**   Enophthalmos due to trauma or surgery

H05.421   Enophthalmos due to trauma or surgery, right eye

H05.422   Enophthalmos due to trauma or surgery, left eye

H05.423   Enophthalmos due to trauma or surgery, bilateral

H05.429   Enophthalmos due to trauma or surgery, unspecified eye

✓5ᵗʰ   **H05.5**   **Retained (old) foreign body following penetrating wound of orbit**

> Retrobulbar foreign body
> Use additional code to identify the type of retained foreign body (Z18.-)
>
> EXCLUDES 1   current penetrating wound of orbit (S05.4-)
>
> EXCLUDES 2   retained foreign body of eyelid (H02.81-)
> retained intraocular foreign body (H44.6-, H44.7-)

H05.50   Retained (old) foreign body following penetrating wound of unspecified orbit

H05.51   Retained (old) foreign body following penetrating wound of right orbit

H05.52   Retained (old) foreign body following penetrating wound of left orbit

H05.53   Retained (old) foreign body following penetrating wound of bilateral orbits

✓5ᵗʰ   **H05.8**   **Other disorders of orbit**

✓6ᵗʰ   **H05.81**   Cyst of orbit

> Encephalocele of orbit

H05.811   Cyst of right orbit

H05.812   Cyst of left orbit

H05.813   Cyst of bilateral orbits

H05.819   Cyst of unspecified orbit

✓6ᵗʰ   **H05.82**   Myopathy of extraocular muscles

H05.821   Myopathy of extraocular muscles, right orbit

H05.822   Myopathy of extraocular muscles, left orbit

H05.823   Myopathy of extraocular muscles, bilateral

H05.829   Myopathy of extraocular muscles, unspecified orbit

H05.89   Other disorders of orbit

H05.9   **Unspecified disorder of orbit**

Disorders of conjunctiva (H10-H11)

✓4ᵗʰ   **H10**   **Conjunctivitis**

> EXCLUDES 1   keratoconjunctivitis (H16.2-)

✓5ᵗʰ   **H10.0**   Mucopurulent conjunctivitis

✓6ᵗʰ   **H10.01**   Acute follicular conjunctivitis

H10.011   Acute follicular conjunctivitis, right eye

H10.012   Acute follicular conjunctivitis, left eye

H10.013   Acute follicular conjunctivitis, bilateral

H10.019   Acute follicular conjunctivitis, unspecified eye

✓6ᵗʰ   **H10.02**   Other mucopurulent conjunctivitis

H10.021   Other mucopurulent conjunctivitis, right eye

H10.022   Other mucopurulent conjunctivitis, left eye

H10.023   Other mucopurulent conjunctivitis, bilateral

H10.029   Other mucopurulent conjunctivitis, unspecified eye

✓5ᵗʰ   **H10.1**   Acute atopic conjunctivitis

> Acute papillary conjunctivitis

H10.10   Acute atopic conjunctivitis, unspecified eye

H10.11   Acute atopic conjunctivitis, right eye

H10.12   Acute atopic conjunctivitis, left eye

H10.13   Acute atopic conjunctivitis, bilateral

✓5ᵗʰ   **H10.2**   Other acute conjunctivitis

✓6ᵗʰ   **H10.21**   Acute toxic conjunctivitis

> Acute chemical conjunctivitis
> Code first (T51-T65) to identify chemical and intent
>
> EXCLUDES 1   burn and corrosion of eye and adnexa (T26.-)

H10.211   Acute toxic conjunctivitis, right eye

H10.212   Acute toxic conjunctivitis, left eye

H10.213   Acute toxic conjunctivitis, bilateral

H10.219   Acute toxic conjunctivitis, unspecified eye

✓6ᵗʰ   **H10.22**   Pseudomembranous conjunctivitis

H10.221   Pseudomembranous conjunctivitis, right eye

H10.222   Pseudomembranous conjunctivitis, left eye

EXCLUDES 1 Not coded here   EXCLUDES 2 Not included here   N Newborn Age: 0   P Pediatric Age: 0-17   M Maternity Age: 12-55   A Adult Age: 15-124

534   ICD-10-CM Draft (2015)

H10.223　Pseudomembranous conjunctivitis, bilateral

H10.229　Pseudomembranous conjunctivitis, unspecified eye

✓6ᵗʰ H10.23　Serous conjunctivitis, except viral
EXCLUDES 1　viral conjunctivitis (B30.-)

H10.231　Serous conjunctivitis, except viral, right eye

H10.232　Serous conjunctivitis, except viral, left eye

H10.233　Serous conjunctivitis, except viral, bilateral

H10.239　Serous conjunctivitis, except viral, unspecified eye

✓5ᵗʰ H10.3　Unspecified acute conjunctivitis
EXCLUDES 1　ophthalmia neonatorum NOS (P39.1)

H10.30　Unspecified acute conjunctivitis, unspecified eye

H10.31　Unspecified acute conjunctivitis, right eye

H10.32　Unspecified acute conjunctivitis, left eye

H10.33　Unspecified acute conjunctivitis, bilateral

✓5ᵗʰ H10.4　Chronic conjunctivitis

✓6ᵗʰ H10.40　Unspecified chronic conjunctivitis

H10.401　Unspecified chronic conjunctivitis, right eye

H10.402　Unspecified chronic conjunctivitis, left eye

H10.403　Unspecified chronic conjunctivitis, bilateral

H10.409　Unspecified chronic conjunctivitis, unspecified eye

✓6ᵗʰ H10.41　Chronic giant papillary conjunctivitis

H10.411　Chronic giant papillary conjunctivitis, right eye

H10.412　Chronic giant papillary conjunctivitis, left eye

H10.413　Chronic giant papillary conjunctivitis, bilateral

H10.419　Chronic giant papillary conjunctivitis, unspecified eye

✓6ᵗʰ H10.42　Simple chronic conjunctivitis

H10.421　Simple chronic conjunctivitis, right eye

H10.422　Simple chronic conjunctivitis, left eye

H10.423　Simple chronic conjunctivitis, bilateral

H10.429　Simple chronic conjunctivitis, unspecified eye

✓6ᵗʰ H10.43　Chronic follicular conjunctivitis

H10.431　Chronic follicular conjunctivitis, right eye

H10.432　Chronic follicular conjunctivitis, left eye

H10.433　Chronic follicular conjunctivitis, bilateral

H10.439　Chronic follicular conjunctivitis, unspecified eye

H10.44　Vernal conjunctivitis
EXCLUDES 1　vernal keratoconjunctivitis with limbar and corneal involvement (H16.26-)

H10.45　Other chronic allergic conjunctivitis

✓5ᵗʰ H10.5　Blepharoconjunctivitis

✓6ᵗʰ H10.50　Unspecified blepharoconjunctivitis

H10.501　Unspecified blepharoconjunctivitis, right eye

H10.502　Unspecified blepharoconjunctivitis, left eye

H10.503　Unspecified blepharoconjunctivitis, bilateral

H10.509　Unspecified blepharoconjunctivitis, unspecified eye

✓6ᵗʰ H10.51　Ligneous conjunctivitis

H10.511　Ligneous conjunctivitis, right eye

H10.512　Ligneous conjunctivitis, left eye

H10.513　Ligneous conjunctivitis, bilateral

H10.519　Ligneous conjunctivitis, unspecified eye

✓6ᵗʰ H10.52　Angular blepharoconjunctivitis

H10.521　Angular blepharoconjunctivitis, right eye

H10.522　Angular blepharoconjunctivitis, left eye

H10.523　Angular blepharoconjunctivitis, bilateral

H10.529　Angular blepharoconjunctivitis, unspecified eye

✓6ᵗʰ H10.53　Contact blepharoconjunctivitis

H10.531　Contact blepharoconjunctivitis, right eye

H10.532　Contact blepharoconjunctivitis, left eye

H10.533　Contact blepharoconjunctivitis, bilateral

H10.539　Contact blepharoconjunctivitis, unspecified eye

✓5ᵗʰ H10.8　Other conjunctivitis

✓6ᵗʰ H10.81　Pingueculitis
EXCLUDES 1　pinguecula (H11.15-)

H10.811　Pingueculitis, right eye

H10.812　Pingueculitis, left eye

H10.813　Pingueculitis, bilateral

H10.819　Pingueculitis, unspecified eye

H10.89　Other conjunctivitis

H10.9　Unspecified conjunctivitis

✓4ᵗʰ H11　Other disorders of conjunctiva
EXCLUDES 1　keratoconjunctivitis (H16.2-)

✓5ᵗʰ H11.0　Pterygium of eye
EXCLUDES 1　pseudopterygium (H11.81-)

✓6ᵗʰ H11.00　Unspecified pterygium of eye

H11.001　Unspecified pterygium of right eye

H11.002　Unspecified pterygium of left eye

H11.003　Unspecified pterygium of eye, bilateral

H11.009　Unspecified pterygium of unspecified eye

✓6ᵗʰ H11.01　Amyloid pterygium

H11.011　Amyloid pterygium of right eye

H11.012　Amyloid pterygium of left eye

H11.013　Amyloid pterygium of eye, bilateral

H11.019　Amyloid pterygium of unspecified eye

✓6ᵗʰ H11.02　Central pterygium of eye

H11.021　Central pterygium of right eye

H11.022　Central pterygium of left eye

H11.023　Central pterygium of eye, bilateral

H11.029　Central pterygium of unspecified eye

✓6ᵗʰ H11.03　Double pterygium of eye

H11.031　Double pterygium of right eye

H11.032　Double pterygium of left eye

H11.033　Double pterygium of eye, bilateral

H11.039　Double pterygium of unspecified eye

✓6ᵗʰ H11.04　Peripheral pterygium of eye, stationary

H11.041　Peripheral pterygium, stationary, right eye

H11.042　Peripheral pterygium, stationary, left eye

H11.043　Peripheral pterygium, stationary, bilateral

H11.049　Peripheral pterygium, stationary, unspecified eye

✓6ᵗʰ H11.05　Peripheral pterygium of eye, progressive

H11.051　Peripheral pterygium, progressive, right eye

H11.052　Peripheral pterygium, progressive, left eye

H11.053　Peripheral pterygium, progressive, bilateral

H11.059　Peripheral pterygium, progressive, unspecified eye

✓6ᵗʰ H11.06　Recurrent pterygium of eye

H11.061　Recurrent pterygium of right eye

H11.062　Recurrent pterygium of left eye

H11.063　Recurrent pterygium of eye, bilateral

H11.069　Recurrent pterygium of unspecified eye

✓5ᵗʰ H11.1　Conjunctival degenerations and deposits
EXCLUDES 2　pseudopterygium (H11.81)

H11.10　Unspecified conjunctival degenerations

✓6ᵗʰ H11.11　Conjunctival deposits

H11.111　Conjunctival deposits, right eye

H11.112　Conjunctival deposits, left eye

H11.113　Conjunctival deposits, bilateral

H11.119　Conjunctival deposits, unspecified eye

✓6ᵗʰ H11.12　Conjunctival concretions

H11.121　Conjunctival concretions, right eye

H11.122　Conjunctival concretions, left eye

H11.123　Conjunctival concretions, bilateral

✓ Additional Character Required　　v x 7ᵗʰ Xtension Alert　　Unspecified Dx　　Other Specified Dx　　Manifestation　　▶◀ Revised Text　　● New Code　　▲ Revised Code Title

ICD-10-CM Draft (2015)　　　　　535

Diseases of the Eye and Adnexa

H11.129–H15.109

H11.129   **Conjunctival concretions, unspecified eye**

✓6ᵗʰ **H11.13**   **Conjunctival** pigmentations
Conjunctival argyrosis [argyria]
- H11.131   **Conjunctival pigmentations,** right **eye**
- H11.132   **Conjunctival pigmentations,** left **eye**
- H11.133   **Conjunctival pigmentations,** bilateral
- H11.139   **Conjunctival pigmentations, unspecified eye**

✓6ᵗʰ **H11.14**   **Conjunctival xerosis,** unspecified
EXCLUDES 1   *xerosis of conjunctiva due to vitamin A deficiency (E50.0, E50.1)*
- H11.141   **Conjunctival xerosis, unspecified,** right **eye**
- H11.142   **Conjunctival xerosis , unspecified,** left **eye**
- H11.143   **Conjunctival xerosis, unspecified,** bilateral
- H11.149   **Conjunctival xerosis, unspecified, unspecified eye**

✓6ᵗʰ **H11.15**   Pinguecula
EXCLUDES 1   *pingueculitis (H10.81-)*
- H11.151   **Pinguecula,** right **eye**
- H11.152   **Pinguecula,** left **eye**
- H11.153   **Pinguecula,** bilateral
- H11.159   **Pinguecula, unspecified eye**

✓5ᵗʰ **H11.2**   **Conjunctival scars**

✓6ᵗʰ **H11.21**   **Conjunctival** adhesions and strands **(localized)**
- H11.211   **Conjunctival adhesions and strands (localized),** right **eye**
- H11.212   **Conjunctival adhesions and strands (localized),** left **eye**
- H11.213   **Conjunctival adhesions and strands (localized),** bilateral
- H11.219   **Conjunctival adhesions and strands (localized), unspecified eye**

✓6ᵗʰ **H11.22**   **Conjunctival** granuloma
- H11.221   **Conjunctival granuloma,** right **eye**
- H11.222   **Conjunctival granuloma,** left **eye**
- H11.223   **Conjunctival granuloma,** bilateral
- H11.229   **Conjunctival granuloma, unspecified**

✓6ᵗʰ **H11.23**   Symblepharon
- H11.231   **Symblepharon,** right **eye**
- H11.232   **Symblepharon,** left **eye**
- H11.233   **Symblepharon,** bilateral
- H11.239   **Symblepharon, unspecified eye**

✓6ᵗʰ **H11.24**   Scarring of conjunctiva
- H11.241   **Scarring of conjunctiva,** right **eye**
- H11.242   **Scarring of conjunctiva,** left **eye**
- H11.243   **Scarring of conjunctiva,** bilateral
- H11.249   **Scarring of conjunctiva, unspecified eye**

✓5ᵗʰ **H11.3**   **Conjunctival hemorrhage**
Subconjunctival hemorrhage
- H11.30   **Conjunctival hemorrhage, unspecified eye**
- H11.31   **Conjunctival hemorrhage,** right **eye**
- H11.32   **Conjunctival hemorrhage,** left **eye**
- H11.33   **Conjunctival hemorrhage,** bilateral

✓5ᵗʰ **H11.4**   **Other conjunctival vascular disorders and cysts**

✓6ᵗʰ **H11.41**   Vascular abnormalities **of conjunctiva**
Conjunctival aneurysm
- H11.411   **Vascular abnormalities of conjunctiva,** right **eye**
- H11.412   **Vascular abnormalities of conjunctiva,** left **eye**
- H11.413   **Vascular abnormalities of conjunctiva,** bilateral
- H11.419   **Vascular abnormalities of conjunctiva, unspecified eye**

✓6ᵗʰ **H11.42**   **Conjunctival** edema
- H11.421   **Conjunctival edema,** right **eye**
- H11.422   **Conjunctival edema,** left **eye**
- H11.423   **Conjunctival edema,** bilateral
- H11.429   **Conjunctival edema, unspecified eye**

✓6ᵗʰ **H11.43**   **Conjunctival** hyperemia
- H11.431   **Conjunctival hyperemia,** right **eye**
- H11.432   **Conjunctival hyperemia,** left **eye**
- H11.433   **Conjunctival hyperemia,** bilateral

H11.439   **Conjunctival hyperemia, unspecified eye**

✓6ᵗʰ **H11.44**   **Conjunctival** cysts
- H11.441   **Conjunctival cysts,** right **eye**
- H11.442   **Conjunctival cysts,** left **eye**
- H11.443   **Conjunctival cysts,** bilateral
- H11.449   **Conjunctival cysts, unspecified eye**

✓5ᵗʰ **H11.8**   **Other specified disorders of conjunctiva**

✓6ᵗʰ **H11.81**   **Pseudopterygium of conjunctiva**
- H11.811   **Pseudopterygium of conjunctiva,** right **eye**
- H11.812   **Pseudopterygium of conjunctiva,** left **eye**
- H11.813   **Pseudopterygium of conjunctiva,** bilateral
- H11.819   **Pseudopterygium of conjunctiva, unspecified eye**

✓6ᵗʰ **H11.82**   **Conjunctivochalasis**
- H11.821   **Conjunctivochalasis,** right **eye**
- H11.822   **Conjunctivochalasis,** left **eye**
- H11.823   **Conjunctivochalasis,** bilateral
- H11.829   **Conjunctivochalasis, unspecified eye**

H11.89   **Other specified disorders of conjunctiva**

H11.9   **Unspecified disorder of conjunctiva**

Disorders of sclera, cornea, iris and ciliary body (H15-H22)

✓4ᵗʰ **H15**   **Disorders of sclera**

✓5ᵗʰ **H15.0**   **Scleritis**

✓6ᵗʰ **H15.00**   Unspecified scleritis
- H15.001   **Unspecified scleritis,** right **eye**
- H15.002   **Unspecified scleritis,** left **eye**
- H15.003   **Unspecified scleritis,** bilateral
- H15.009   **Unspecified scleritis, unspecified eye**

✓6ᵗʰ **H15.01**   Anterior scleritis
- H15.011   **Anterior scleritis,** right **eye**
- H15.012   **Anterior scleritis,** left **eye**
- H15.013   **Anterior scleritis,** bilateral
- H15.019   **Anterior scleritis, unspecified eye**

✓6ᵗʰ **H15.02**   Brawny scleritis
- H15.021   **Brawny scleritis,** right **eye**
- H15.022   **Brawny scleritis,** left **eye**
- H15.023   **Brawny scleritis,** bilateral
- H15.029   **Brawny scleritis, unspecified eye**

✓6ᵗʰ **H15.03**   Posterior scleritis
Sclerotenonitis
- H15.031   **Posterior scleritis,** right **eye**
- H15.032   **Posterior scleritis,** left **eye**
- H15.033   **Posterior scleritis,** bilateral
- H15.039   **Posterior scleritis, unspecified eye**

✓6ᵗʰ **H15.04**   **Scleritis with** corneal involvement
- H15.041   **Scleritis with corneal involvement,** right **eye**
- H15.042   **Scleritis with corneal involvement,** left **eye**
- H15.043   **Scleritis with corneal involvement,** bilateral
- H15.049   **Scleritis with corneal involvement, unspecified eye**

✓6ᵗʰ **H15.05**   Scleromalacia perforans
- H15.051   **Scleromalacia perforans,** right **eye**
- H15.052   **Scleromalacia perforans,** left **eye**
- H15.053   **Scleromalacia perforans,** bilateral
- H15.059   **Scleromalacia perforans, unspecified eye**

✓6ᵗʰ **H15.09**   Other scleritis
Scleral abscess
- H15.091   **Other scleritis,** right **eye**
- H15.092   **Other scleritis,** left **eye**
- H15.093   **Other scleritis,** bilateral
- H15.099   **Other scleritis, unspecified eye**

✓5ᵗʰ **H15.1**   **Episcleritis**

✓6ᵗʰ **H15.10**   Unspecified episcleritis
- H15.101   **Unspecified episcleritis,** right **eye**
- H15.102   **Unspecified episcleritis,** left **eye**
- H15.103   **Unspecified episcleritis,** bilateral
- H15.109   **Unspecified episcleritis, unspecified eye**

EXCLUDES 1 Not coded here   EXCLUDES 2 Not included here   N Newborn Age: 0   P Pediatric Age: 0-17   M Maternity Age: 12-55   A Adult Age: 15-124

✓6ᵗʰ **H15.11** Episcleritis periodica fugax
    H15.111 Episcleritis periodica fugax, right eye
    H15.112 Episcleritis periodica fugax, left eye
    H15.113 Episcleritis periodica fugax, bilateral
    H15.119 Episcleritis periodica fugax, unspecified eye

✓6ᵗʰ **H15.12** Nodular episcleritis
    H15.121 Nodular episcleritis, right eye
    H15.122 Nodular episcleritis, left eye
    H15.123 Nodular episcleritis, bilateral
    H15.129 Nodular episcleritis, unspecified eye

✓5ᵗʰ **H15.8 Other disorders of sclera**
    EXCLUDES 2 blue sclera (Q13.5)
                 degenerative myopia (H44.2-)

✓6ᵗʰ **H15.81** Equatorial staphyloma
    H15.811 Equatorial staphyloma, right eye
    H15.812 Equatorial staphyloma, left eye
    H15.813 Equatorial staphyloma, bilateral
    H15.819 Equatorial staphyloma, unspecified eye

✓6ᵗʰ **H15.82** Localized anterior staphyloma
    H15.821 Localized anterior staphyloma, right eye
    H15.822 Localized anterior staphyloma, left eye
    H15.823 Localized anterior staphyloma, bilateral
    H15.829 Localized anterior staphyloma, unspecified eye

✓6ᵗʰ **H15.83** Staphyloma posticum
    H15.831 Staphyloma posticum, right eye
    H15.832 Staphyloma posticum, left eye
    H15.833 Staphyloma posticum, bilateral
    H15.839 Staphyloma posticum, unspecified eye

✓6ᵗʰ **H15.84** Scleral ectasia
    H15.841 Scleral ectasia, right eye
    H15.842 Scleral ectasia, left eye
    H15.843 Scleral ectasia, bilateral
    H15.849 Scleral ectasia, unspecified eye

✓6ᵗʰ **H15.85** Ring staphyloma
    H15.851 Ring staphyloma, right eye
    H15.852 Ring staphyloma, left eye
    H15.853 Ring staphyloma, bilateral
    H15.859 Ring staphyloma, unspecified eye

    H15.89 Other disorders of sclera

H15.9 Unspecified disorder of sclera

✓4ᵗʰ **H16 Keratitis**

✓5ᵗʰ **H16.0 Corneal ulcer**

✓6ᵗʰ **H16.00** Unspecified corneal ulcer
    H16.001 Unspecified corneal ulcer, right eye
    H16.002 Unspecified corneal ulcer, left eye
    H16.003 Unspecified corneal ulcer, bilateral
    H16.009 Unspecified corneal ulcer, unspecified eye

✓6ᵗʰ **H16.01** Central corneal ulcer
    H16.011 Central corneal ulcer, right eye
    H16.012 Central corneal ulcer, left eye
    H16.013 Central corneal ulcer, bilateral
    H16.019 Central corneal ulcer, unspecified eye

✓6ᵗʰ **H16.02** Ring corneal ulcer
    H16.021 Ring corneal ulcer, right eye
    H16.022 Ring corneal ulcer, left eye
    H16.023 Ring corneal ulcer, bilateral
    H16.029 Ring corneal ulcer, unspecified eye

✓6ᵗʰ **H16.03** Corneal ulcer with hypopyon
    H16.031 Corneal ulcer with hypopyon, right eye
    H16.032 Corneal ulcer with hypopyon, left eye
    H16.033 Corneal ulcer with hypopyon, bilateral
    H16.039 Corneal ulcer with hypopyon, unspecified eye

✓6ᵗʰ **H16.04** Marginal corneal ulcer
    H16.041 Marginal corneal ulcer, right eye
    H16.042 Marginal corneal ulcer, left eye
    H16.043 Marginal corneal ulcer, bilateral
    H16.049 Marginal corneal ulcer, unspecified eye

✓6ᵗʰ **H16.05** Mooren's corneal ulcer
    H16.051 Mooren's corneal ulcer, right eye
    H16.052 Mooren's corneal ulcer, left eye
    H16.053 Mooren's corneal ulcer, bilateral
    H16.059 Mooren's corneal ulcer, unspecified eye

✓6ᵗʰ **H16.06** Mycotic corneal ulcer
    H16.061 Mycotic corneal ulcer, right eye
    H16.062 Mycotic corneal ulcer, left eye
    H16.063 Mycotic corneal ulcer, bilateral
    H16.069 Mycotic corneal ulcer, unspecified eye

✓6ᵗʰ **H16.07** Perforated corneal ulcer
    H16.071 Perforated corneal ulcer, right eye
    H16.072 Perforated corneal ulcer, left eye
    H16.073 Perforated corneal ulcer, bilateral
    H16.079 Perforated corneal ulcer, unspecified eye

✓5ᵗʰ **H16.1 Other and unspecified superficial keratitis without conjunctivitis**

✓6ᵗʰ **H16.10** Unspecified superficial keratitis
    H16.101 Unspecified superficial keratitis, right eye
    H16.102 Unspecified superficial keratitis, left eye
    H16.103 Unspecified superficial keratitis, bilateral
    H16.109 Unspecified superficial keratitis, unspecified eye

✓6ᵗʰ **H16.11** Macular keratitis
    Areolar keratitis
    Nummular keratitis
    Stellate keratitis
    Striate keratitis
    H16.111 Macular keratitis, right eye
    H16.112 Macular keratitis, left eye
    H16.113 Macular keratitis, bilateral
    H16.119 Macular keratitis, unspecified eye

✓6ᵗʰ **H16.12** Filamentary keratitis
    H16.121 Filamentary keratitis, right eye
    H16.122 Filamentary keratitis, left eye
    H16.123 Filamentary keratitis, bilateral
    H16.129 Filamentary keratitis, unspecified eye

✓6ᵗʰ **H16.13** Photokeratitis
    Snow blindness
    Welders keratitis
    H16.131 Photokeratitis, right eye
    H16.132 Photokeratitis, left eye
    H16.133 Photokeratitis, bilateral
    H16.139 Photokeratitis, unspecified eye

✓6ᵗʰ **H16.14** Punctate keratitis
    H16.141 Punctate keratitis, right eye
    H16.142 Punctate keratitis, left eye
    H16.143 Punctate keratitis, bilateral
    H16.149 Punctate keratitis, unspecified eye

✓5ᵗʰ **H16.2 Keratoconjunctivitis**

✓6ᵗʰ **H16.20** Unspecified keratoconjunctivitis
    Superficial keratitis with conjunctivitis NOS
    H16.201 Unspecified keratoconjunctivitis, right eye
    H16.202 Unspecified keratoconjunctivitis, left eye
    H16.203 Unspecified keratoconjunctivitis, bilateral
    H16.209 Unspecified keratoconjunctivitis, unspecified eye

✓6ᵗʰ **H16.21** Exposure keratoconjunctivitis
    H16.211 Exposure keratoconjunctivitis, right eye
    H16.212 Exposure keratoconjunctivitis, left eye
    H16.213 Exposure keratoconjunctivitis, bilateral
    H16.219 Exposure keratoconjunctivitis, unspecified eye

✓6ᵗʰ **H16.22** Keratoconjunctivitis sicca, not specified as Sjögren's
    EXCLUDES 1 Sjögren's syndrome (M35.01)
    H16.221 Keratoconjunctivitis sicca, not specified as Sjögren's, right eye
    H16.222 Keratoconjunctivitis sicca, not specified as Sjögren's, left eye
    H16.223 Keratoconjunctivitis sicca, not specified as Sjögren's, bilateral
    H16.229 Keratoconjunctivitis sicca, not specified as Sjögren's, unspecified eye

✓6ᵗʰ **H16.23** Neurotrophic **keratoconjunctivitis**
- **H16.231** Neurotrophic keratoconjunctivitis, right eye
- **H16.232** Neurotrophic keratoconjunctivitis, left eye
- **H16.233** Neurotrophic keratoconjunctivitis, bilateral
- **H16.239** Neurotrophic keratoconjunctivitis, unspecified eye

✓6ᵗʰ **H16.24** Ophthalmia nodosa
- **H16.241** Ophthalmia nodosa, right eye
- **H16.242** Ophthalmia nodosa, left eye
- **H16.243** Ophthalmia nodosa, bilateral
- **H16.249** Ophthalmia nodosa, unspecified eye

✓6ᵗʰ **H16.25** Phlyctenular **keratoconjunctivitis**
- **H16.251** Phlyctenular keratoconjunctivitis, right eye
- **H16.252** Phlyctenular keratoconjunctivitis, left eye
- **H16.253** Phlyctenular keratoconjunctivitis, bilateral
- **H16.259** Phlyctenular keratoconjunctivitis, unspecified eye

✓6ᵗʰ **H16.26** Vernal **keratoconjunctivitis, with** limbar and corneal involvement
> **EXCLUDES 1** *vernal conjunctivitis without limbar and corneal involvement (H10.44)*
- **H16.261** Vernal keratoconjunctivitis, with limbar and corneal involvement, right eye
- **H16.262** Vernal keratoconjunctivitis, with limbar and corneal involvement, left eye
- **H16.263** Vernal keratoconjunctivitis, with limbar and corneal involvement, bilateral
- **H16.269** Vernal keratoconjunctivitis, with limbar and corneal involvement, unspecified eye

✓6ᵗʰ **H16.29** Other **keratoconjunctivitis**
- **H16.291** Other keratoconjunctivitis, right eye
- **H16.292** Other keratoconjunctivitis, left eye
- **H16.293** Other keratoconjunctivitis, bilateral
- **H16.299** Other keratoconjunctivitis, unspecified eye

✓5ᵗʰ **H16.3** Interstitial and deep keratitis

✓6ᵗʰ **H16.30** Unspecified interstitial keratitis
- **H16.301** Unspecified interstitial keratitis, right eye
- **H16.302** Unspecified interstitial keratitis, left eye
- **H16.303** Unspecified interstitial keratitis, bilateral
- **H16.309** Unspecified interstitial keratitis, unspecified eye

✓6ᵗʰ **H16.31** Corneal **abscess**
- **H16.311** Corneal abscess, right eye
- **H16.312** Corneal abscess, left eye
- **H16.313** Corneal abscess, bilateral
- **H16.319** Corneal abscess, unspecified eye

✓6ᵗʰ **H16.32** Diffuse **interstitial keratitis**
Cogan's syndrome
- **H16.321** Diffuse interstitial keratitis, right eye
- **H16.322** Diffuse interstitial keratitis, left eye
- **H16.323** Diffuse interstitial keratitis, bilateral
- **H16.329** Diffuse interstitial keratitis, unspecified eye

✓6ᵗʰ **H16.33** Sclerosing **keratitis**
- **H16.331** Sclerosing keratitis, right eye
- **H16.332** Sclerosing keratitis, left eye
- **H16.333** Sclerosing keratitis, bilateral
- **H16.339** Sclerosing keratitis, unspecified eye

✓6ᵗʰ **H16.39** Other **interstitial and deep keratitis**
- **H16.391** Other interstitial and deep keratitis, right eye
- **H16.392** Other interstitial and deep keratitis, left eye
- **H16.393** Other interstitial and deep keratitis, bilateral
- **H16.399** Other interstitial and deep keratitis, unspecified eye

✓5ᵗʰ **H16.4** Corneal neovascularization

✓6ᵗʰ **H16.40** Unspecified corneal neovascularization
- **H16.401** Unspecified corneal neovascularization, right eye
- **H16.402** Unspecified corneal neovascularization, left eye
- **H16.403** Unspecified corneal neovascularization, bilateral
- **H16.409** Unspecified corneal neovascularization, unspecified eye

✓6ᵗʰ **H16.41** Ghost vessels (corneal)
- **H16.411** Ghost vessels (corneal), right eye
- **H16.412** Ghost vessels (corneal), left eye
- **H16.413** Ghost vessels (corneal), bilateral
- **H16.419** Ghost vessels (corneal), unspecified eye

✓6ᵗʰ **H16.42** Pannus (corneal)
- **H16.421** Pannus (corneal), right eye
- **H16.422** Pannus (corneal), left eye
- **H16.423** Pannus (corneal), bilateral
- **H16.429** Pannus (corneal), unspecified eye

✓6ᵗʰ **H16.43** Localized vascularization of cornea
- **H16.431** Localized vascularization of cornea, right eye
- **H16.432** Localized vascularization of cornea, left eye
- **H16.433** Localized vascularization of cornea, bilateral
- **H16.439** Localized vascularization of cornea, unspecified eye

✓6ᵗʰ **H16.44** Deep vascularization of cornea
- **H16.441** Deep vascularization of cornea, right eye
- **H16.442** Deep vascularization of cornea, left eye
- **H16.443** Deep vascularization of cornea, bilateral
- **H16.449** Deep vascularization of cornea, unspecified eye

H16.8 Other keratitis

H16.9 Unspecified keratitis

✓4ᵗʰ **H17 Corneal scars and opacities**

✓5ᵗʰ **H17.0** Adherent leukoma
- **H17.00** Adherent leukoma, unspecified eye
- **H17.01** Adherent leukoma, right eye
- **H17.02** Adherent leukoma, left eye
- **H17.03** Adherent leukoma, bilateral

✓5ᵗʰ **H17.1** Central corneal opacity
- **H17.10** Central corneal opacity, unspecified eye
- **H17.11** Central corneal opacity, right eye
- **H17.12** Central corneal opacity, left eye
- **H17.13** Central corneal opacity, bilateral

✓5ᵗʰ **H17.8** Other corneal scars and opacities

✓6ᵗʰ **H17.81** Minor opacity of cornea
Corneal nebula
- **H17.811** Minor opacity of cornea, right eye
- **H17.812** Minor opacity of cornea, left eye
- **H17.813** Minor opacity of cornea, bilateral
- **H17.819** Minor opacity of cornea, unspecified eye

✓6ᵗʰ **H17.82** Peripheral opacity of cornea
- **H17.821** Peripheral opacity of cornea, right eye
- **H17.822** Peripheral opacity of cornea, left eye
- **H17.823** Peripheral opacity of cornea, bilateral
- **H17.829** Peripheral opacity of cornea, unspecified eye

- **H17.89** Other corneal scars and opacities

H17.9 Unspecified corneal scar and opacity

✓4ᵗʰ **H18 Other disorders of cornea**

✓5ᵗʰ **H18.0** Corneal pigmentations and deposits

✓6ᵗʰ **H18.00** Unspecified corneal deposit
- **H18.001** Unspecified corneal deposit, right eye
- **H18.002** Unspecified corneal deposit, left eye
- **H18.003** Unspecified corneal deposit, bilateral
- **H18.009** Unspecified corneal deposit, unspecified eye

EXCLUDES 1 Not coded here **EXCLUDES 2** Not included here N Newborn Age: 0 P Pediatric Age: 0-17 M Maternity Age: 12-55 A Adult Age: 15-124

538

ICD-10-CM Draft (2015)

✓6ᵗʰ **H18.01** Anterior **corneal pigmentations**
Staehli's line
 H18.011 **Anterior corneal pigmentations,** right **eye**
 H18.012 **Anterior corneal pigmentations,** left **eye**
 H18.013 **Anterior corneal pigmentations,** bilateral
 H18.019 **Anterior corneal pigmentations, unspecified eye**

✓6ᵗʰ **H18.02** Argentous **corneal deposits**
 H18.021 **Argentous corneal deposits,** right **eye**
 H18.022 **Argentous corneal deposits,** left **eye**
 H18.023 **Argentous corneal deposits,** bilateral
 H18.029 **Argentous corneal deposits, unspecified eye**

✓6ᵗʰ **H18.03** **Corneal deposits in** metabolic disorders
Code also associated metabolic disorder
 H18.031 **Corneal deposits in metabolic disorders,** right **eye**
 H18.032 **Corneal deposits in metabolic disorders,** left **eye**
 H18.033 **Corneal deposits in metabolic disorders,** bilateral
 H18.039 **Corneal deposits in metabolic disorders, unspecified eye**

✓6ᵗʰ **H18.04** Kayser-Fleischer **ring**
Code also associated Wilson's disease (E83.01)
 H18.041 **Kayser-Fleischer ring,** right **eye**
 H18.042 **Kayser-Fleischer ring,** left **eye**
 H18.043 **Kayser-Fleischer ring,** bilateral
 H18.049 **Kayser-Fleischer ring, unspecified eye**

✓6ᵗʰ **H18.05** Posterior **corneal pigmentations**
Krukenberg's spindle
 H18.051 **Posterior corneal pigmentations,** right **eye**
 H18.052 **Posterior corneal pigmentations,** left **eye**
 H18.053 **Posterior corneal pigmentations,** bilateral
 H18.059 **Posterior corneal pigmentations, unspecified eye**

✓6ᵗʰ **H18.06** Stromal **corneal pigmentations**
Hematocornea
 H18.061 **Stromal corneal pigmentations,** right **eye**
 H18.062 **Stromal corneal pigmentations,** left **eye**
 H18.063 **Stromal corneal pigmentations,** bilateral
 H18.069 **Stromal corneal pigmentations, unspecified eye**

✓5ᵗʰ **H18.1** **Bullous keratopathy**
 H18.10 **Bullous keratopathy, unspecified eye**
 H18.11 **Bullous keratopathy,** right **eye**
 H18.12 **Bullous keratopathy,** left **eye**
 H18.13 **Bullous keratopathy,** bilateral

✓5ᵗʰ **H18.2** **Other and unspecified corneal edema**
 H18.20 **Unspecified corneal edema**
 ✓6ᵗʰ **H18.21** **Corneal edema** secondary to contact lens
  EXCLUDES 2 other corneal disorders due to contact lens (H18.82-)
  H18.211 **Corneal edema secondary to contact lens,** right **eye**
  H18.212 **Corneal edema secondary to contact lens,** left **eye**
  H18.213 **Corneal edema secondary to contact lens,** bilateral
  H18.219 **Corneal edema secondary to contact lens, unspecified eye**
 ✓6ᵗʰ **H18.22** Idiopathic **corneal edema**
  H18.221 **Idiopathic corneal edema,** right **eye**
  H18.222 **Idiopathic corneal edema,** left **eye**
  H18.223 **Idiopathic corneal edema,** bilateral
  H18.229 **Idiopathic corneal edema, unspecified eye**
 ✓6ᵗʰ **H18.23** Secondary **corneal edema**
  H18.231 **Secondary corneal edema,** right **eye**
  H18.232 **Secondary corneal edema,** left **eye**
  H18.233 **Secondary corneal edema,** bilateral
  H18.239 **Secondary corneal edema, unspecified eye**

✓5ᵗʰ **H18.3** **Changes of corneal membranes**
 H18.30 **Unspecified corneal membrane change**

✓6ᵗʰ **H18.31** **Folds and rupture in** Bowman's membrane
 H18.311 **Folds and rupture in Bowman's membrane,** right **eye**
 H18.312 **Folds and rupture in Bowman's membrane,** left **eye**
 H18.313 **Folds and rupture in Bowman's membrane,** bilateral
 H18.319 **Folds and rupture in Bowman's membrane, unspecified eye**

✓6ᵗʰ **H18.32** Folds **in** Descemet's **membrane**
 H18.321 **Folds in Descemet's membrane,** right **eye**
 H18.322 **Folds in Descemet's membrane,** left **eye**
 H18.323 **Folds in Descemet's membrane,** bilateral
 H18.329 **Folds in Descemet's membrane, unspecified eye**

✓6ᵗʰ **H18.33** Rupture **in** Descemet's **membrane**
 H18.331 **Rupture in Descemet's membrane,** right **eye**
 H18.332 **Rupture in Descemet's membrane,** left **eye**
 H18.333 **Rupture in Descemet's membrane,** bilateral
 H18.339 **Rupture in Descemet's membrane, unspecified eye**

✓5ᵗʰ **H18.4** **Corneal degeneration**
 EXCLUDES 1 Mooren's ulcer (H16.0-)
  recurrent erosion of cornea (H18.83-)
 H18.40 **Unspecified corneal degeneration**
 ✓6ᵗʰ **H18.41** Arcus **senilis**
  Senile corneal changes
  H18.411 **Arcus senilis,** right **eye**
  H18.412 **Arcus senilis,** left **eye**
  H18.413 **Arcus senilis,** bilateral
  H18.419 **Arcus senilis, unspecified eye**
 ✓6ᵗʰ **H18.42** Band **keratopathy**
  H18.421 **Band keratopathy,** right **eye**
  H18.422 **Band keratopathy,** left **eye**
  H18.423 **Band keratopathy,** bilateral
  H18.429 **Band keratopathy, unspecified eye**
 H18.43 **Other calcerous corneal degeneration**
 ✓6ᵗʰ **H18.44** **Keratomalacia**
  EXCLUDES 1 keratomalacia due to vitamin A deficiency (E50.4)
  H18.441 **Keratomalacia,** right **eye**
  H18.442 **Keratomalacia,** left **eye**
  H18.443 **Keratomalacia,** bilateral
  H18.449 **Keratomalacia, unspecified eye**
 ✓6ᵗʰ **H18.45** Nodular **corneal degeneration**
  H18.451 **Nodular corneal degeneration,** right **eye**
  H18.452 **Nodular corneal degeneration,** left **eye**
  H18.453 **Nodular corneal degeneration,** bilateral
  H18.459 **Nodular corneal degeneration, unspecified eye**
 ✓6ᵗʰ **H18.46** Peripheral **corneal degeneration**
  H18.461 **Peripheral corneal degeneration,** right **eye**
  H18.462 **Peripheral corneal degeneration,** left **eye**
  H18.463 **Peripheral corneal degeneration,** bilateral
  H18.469 **Peripheral corneal degeneration, unspecified eye**
 H18.49 **Other corneal degeneration**

✓5ᵗʰ **H18.5** **Hereditary corneal dystrophies**
 H18.50 **Unspecified hereditary corneal dystrophies**
 H18.51 Endothelial **corneal dystrophy**
  Fuchs' dystrophy
 H18.52 Epithelial (juvenile) **corneal dystrophy**
 H18.53 Granular **corneal dystrophy**
 H18.54 Lattice **corneal dystrophy**
 H18.55 Macular **corneal dystrophy**
 H18.59 **Other hereditary corneal dystrophies**

✓5ᵗʰ **H18.6** **Keratoconus**
 ✓6ᵗʰ **H18.60** **Keratoconus,** unspecified
  H18.601 **Keratoconus, unspecified,** right **eye**
  H18.602 **Keratoconus, unspecified,** left **eye**

☑ Additional Character Required   ✓x7ᵗʰ Xtension Alert   Unspecified Dx   Other Specified Dx   Manifestation   ▶◀ Revised Text   ● New Code   ▲ Revised Code Title

H18.603 **Keratoconus, unspecified, bilateral**
H18.609 **Keratoconus, unspecified, unspecified eye**
√6th H18.61 **Keratoconus, stable**
H18.611 **Keratoconus, stable, right eye**
H18.612 **Keratoconus, stable, left eye**
H18.613 **Keratoconus, stable, bilateral**
H18.619 **Keratoconus, stable, unspecified eye**
√6th H18.62 **Keratoconus, unstable**
Acute hydrops
H18.621 **Keratoconus, unstable, right eye**
H18.622 **Keratoconus, unstable, left eye**
H18.623 **Keratoconus, unstable, bilateral**
H18.629 **Keratoconus, unstable, unspecified eye**
√5th H18.7 **Other and unspecified corneal deformities**
EXCLUDES1 congenital malformations of cornea (Q13.3-Q13.4)
H18.70 **Unspecified corneal deformity**
√6th H18.71 **Corneal ectasia**
H18.711 **Corneal ectasia, right eye**
H18.712 **Corneal ectasia, left eye**
H18.713 **Corneal ectasia, bilateral**
H18.719 **Corneal ectasia, unspecified eye**
√6th H18.72 **Corneal staphyloma**
H18.721 **Corneal staphyloma, right eye**
H18.722 **Corneal staphyloma, left eye**
H18.723 **Corneal staphyloma, bilateral**
H18.729 **Corneal staphyloma, unspecified eye**
√6th H18.73 **Descemetocele**
H18.731 **Descemetocele, right eye**
H18.732 **Descemetocele, left eye**
H18.733 **Descemetocele, bilateral**
H18.739 **Descemetocele, unspecified eye**
√6th H18.79 **Other corneal deformities**
H18.791 **Other corneal deformities, right eye**
H18.792 **Other corneal deformities, left eye**
H18.793 **Other corneal deformities, bilateral**
H18.799 **Other corneal deformities, unspecified eye**
√5th H18.8 **Other specified disorders of cornea**
√6th H18.81 **Anesthesia and hypoesthesia of cornea**
H18.811 **Anesthesia and hypoesthesia of cornea, right eye**
H18.812 **Anesthesia and hypoesthesia of cornea, left eye**
H18.813 **Anesthesia and hypoesthesia of cornea, bilateral**
H18.819 **Anesthesia and hypoesthesia of cornea, unspecified eye**
√6th H18.82 **Corneal disorder due to contact lens**
EXCLUDES2 corneal edema due to contact lens (H18.21-)
H18.821 **Corneal disorder due to contact lens, right eye**
H18.822 **Corneal disorder due to contact lens, left eye**
H18.823 **Corneal disorder due to contact lens, bilateral**
H18.829 **Corneal disorder due to contact lens, unspecified eye**
√6th H18.83 **Recurrent erosion of cornea**
H18.831 **Recurrent erosion of cornea, right eye**
H18.832 **Recurrent erosion of cornea, left eye**
H18.833 **Recurrent erosion of cornea, bilateral**
H18.839 **Recurrent erosion of cornea, unspecified eye**
√6th H18.89 **Other specified disorders of cornea**
H18.891 **Other specified disorders of cornea, right eye**
H18.892 **Other specified disorders of cornea, left eye**
H18.893 **Other specified disorders of cornea, bilateral**
H18.899 **Other specified disorders of cornea, unspecified eye**
H18.9 **Unspecified disorder of cornea**

√4th H20 **Iridocyclitis**
√5th H20.0 **Acute and subacute iridocyclitis**
Acute anterior uveitis
Acute cyclitis
Acute iritis
Subacute anterior uveitis
Subacute cyclitis
Subacute iritis
EXCLUDES1 iridocyclitis, iritis, uveitis (due to) (in) diabetes mellitus (E08-E13 with .39)
iridocyclitis, iritis, uveitis (due to) (in) diphtheria (A36.89)
iridocyclitis, iritis, uveitis (due to) (in) gonococcal (A54.32)
iridocyclitis, iritis, uveitis (due to) (in) herpes (simplex) (B00.51)
iridocyclitis, iritis, uveitis (due to) (in) herpes zoster (B02.32)
iridocyclitis, iritis, uveitis (due to) (in) late congenital syphilis (A50.39)
iridocyclitis, iritis, uveitis (due to) (in) late syphilis (A52.71)
iridocyclitis, iritis, uveitis (due to) (in) sarcoidosis (D86.83)
iridocyclitis, iritis, uveitis (due to) (in) syphilis (A51.43)
iridocyclitis, iritis, uveitis (due to) (in) toxoplasmosis (B58.09)
iridocyclitis, iritis, uveitis (due to) (in) tuberculosis (A18.54)
H20.00 **Unspecified acute and subacute iridocyclitis**
√6th H20.01 **Primary iridocyclitis**
H20.011 **Primary iridocyclitis, right eye**
H20.012 **Primary iridocyclitis, left eye**
H20.013 **Primary iridocyclitis, bilateral**
H20.019 **Primary iridocyclitis, unspecified eye**
√6th H20.02 **Recurrent acute iridocyclitis**
H20.021 **Recurrent acute iridocyclitis, right eye**
H20.022 **Recurrent acute iridocyclitis, left eye**
H20.023 **Recurrent acute iridocyclitis, bilateral**
H20.029 **Recurrent acute iridocyclitis, unspecified eye**
√6th H20.03 **Secondary infectious iridocyclitis**
H20.031 **Secondary infectious iridocyclitis, right eye**
H20.032 **Secondary infectious iridocyclitis, left eye**
H20.033 **Secondary infectious iridocyclitis, bilateral**
H20.039 **Secondary infectious iridocyclitis, unspecified eye**
√6th H20.04 **Secondary noninfectious iridocyclitis**
H20.041 **Secondary noninfectious iridocyclitis, right eye**
H20.042 **Secondary noninfectious iridocyclitis, left eye**
H20.043 **Secondary noninfectious iridocyclitis, bilateral**
H20.049 **Secondary noninfectious iridocyclitis, unspecified eye**
√6th H20.05 **Hypopyon**
H20.051 **Hypopyon, right eye**
H20.052 **Hypopyon, left eye**
H20.053 **Hypopyon, bilateral**
H20.059 **Hypopyon, unspecified eye**
√5th H20.1 **Chronic iridocyclitis**
Use additional code for any associated cataract (H26.21-)
EXCLUDES2 posterior cyclitis (H30.2-)
H20.10 **Chronic iridocyclitis, unspecified eye**
H20.11 **Chronic iridocyclitis, right eye**
H20.12 **Chronic iridocyclitis, left eye**
H20.13 **Chronic iridocyclitis, bilateral**
√5th H20.2 **Lens-induced iridocyclitis**
H20.20 **Lens-induced iridocyclitis, unspecified eye**
H20.21 **Lens-induced iridocyclitis, right eye**
H20.22 **Lens-induced iridocyclitis, left eye**
H20.23 **Lens-induced iridocyclitis, bilateral**

✓5ᵗʰ H20.8 Other iridocyclitis
> **EXCLUDES 2** glaucomatocyclitis crises (H40.4-)
> posterior cyclitis (H30.2-)
> sympathetic uveitis (H44.13-)

✓6ᵗʰ H20.81 Fuchs' heterochromic cyclitis
- H20.811 Fuchs' heterochromic cyclitis, right eye
- H20.812 Fuchs' heterochromic cyclitis, left eye
- H20.813 Fuchs' heterochromic cyclitis, bilateral
- H20.819 Fuchs' heterochromic cyclitis, unspecified eye

✓6ᵗʰ H20.82 Vogt-Koyanagi syndrome
- H20.821 Vogt-Koyanagi syndrome, right eye
- H20.822 Vogt-Koyanagi syndrome, left eye
- H20.823 Vogt-Koyanagi syndrome, bilateral
- H20.829 Vogt-Koyanagi syndrome, unspecified eye

H20.9 Unspecified iridocyclitis
> Uveitis NOS

✓4ᵗʰ H21 Other disorders of iris and ciliary body
> **EXCLUDES 2** sympathetic uveitis (H44.1-)

✓5ᵗʰ H21.0 Hyphema
> **EXCLUDES 1** traumatic hyphema (S05.1-)
- H21.00 Hyphema, unspecified eye
- H21.01 Hyphema, right eye
- H21.02 Hyphema, left eye
- H21.03 Hyphema, bilateral

✓5ᵗʰ H21.1 Other vascular disorders of iris and ciliary body
> Neovascularization of iris or ciliary body
> Rubeosis iridis
> Rubeosis of iris

✓6ᵗʰ H21.1X Other vascular disorders of iris and ciliary body
- H21.1X1 Other vascular disorders of iris and ciliary body, right eye
- H21.1X2 Other vascular disorders of iris and ciliary body, left eye
- H21.1X3 Other vascular disorders of iris and ciliary body, bilateral
- H21.1X9 Other vascular disorders of iris and ciliary body, unspecified eye

✓5ᵗʰ H21.2 Degeneration of iris and ciliary body

✓6ᵗʰ H21.21 Degeneration of chamber angle
- H21.211 Degeneration of chamber angle, right eye
- H21.212 Degeneration of chamber angle, left eye
- H21.213 Degeneration of chamber angle, bilateral
- H21.219 Degeneration of chamber angle, unspecified eye

✓6ᵗʰ H21.22 Degeneration of ciliary body
- H21.221 Degeneration of ciliary body, right eye
- H21.222 Degeneration of ciliary body, left eye
- H21.223 Degeneration of ciliary body, bilateral
- H21.229 Degeneration of ciliary body, unspecified eye

✓6ᵗʰ H21.23 Degeneration of iris (pigmentary)
> Translucency of iris
- H21.231 Degeneration of iris (pigmentary), right eye
- H21.232 Degeneration of iris (pigmentary), left eye
- H21.233 Degeneration of iris (pigmentary), bilateral
- H21.239 Degeneration of iris (pigmentary), unspecified eye

✓6ᵗʰ H21.24 Degeneration of pupillary margin
- H21.241 Degeneration of pupillary margin, right eye
- H21.242 Degeneration of pupillary margin, left eye
- H21.243 Degeneration of pupillary margin, bilateral
- H21.249 Degeneration of pupillary margin, unspecified eye

✓6ᵗʰ H21.25 Iridoschisis
- H21.251 Iridoschisis, right eye
- H21.252 Iridoschisis, left eye
- H21.253 Iridoschisis, bilateral
- H21.259 Iridoschisis, unspecified eye

✓6ᵗʰ H21.26 Iris atrophy (essential) (progressive)
- H21.261 Iris atrophy (essential) (progressive), right eye
- H21.262 Iris atrophy (essential) (progressive), left eye
- H21.263 Iris atrophy (essential) (progressive), bilateral
- H21.269 Iris atrophy (essential) (progressive), unspecified eye

✓6ᵗʰ H21.27 Miotic pupillary cyst
- H21.271 Miotic pupillary cyst, right eye
- H21.272 Miotic pupillary cyst, left eye
- H21.273 Miotic pupillary cyst, bilateral
- H21.279 Miotic pupillary cyst, unspecified eye

H21.29 Other iris atrophy

✓5ᵗʰ H21.3 Cyst of iris, ciliary body and anterior chamber
> **EXCLUDES 2** miotic pupillary cyst (H21.27-)

✓6ᵗʰ H21.30 Idiopathic cysts of iris, ciliary body or anterior chamber
> Cyst of iris, ciliary body or anterior chamber NOS
- H21.301 Idiopathic cysts of iris, ciliary body or anterior chamber, right eye
- H21.302 Idiopathic cysts of iris, ciliary body or anterior chamber, left eye
- H21.303 Idiopathic cysts of iris, ciliary body or anterior chamber, bilateral
- H21.309 Idiopathic cysts of iris, ciliary body or anterior chamber, unspecified eye

✓6ᵗʰ H21.31 Exudative cysts of iris or anterior chamber
- H21.311 Exudative cysts of iris or anterior chamber, right eye
- H21.312 Exudative cysts of iris or anterior chamber, left eye
- H21.313 Exudative cysts of iris or anterior chamber, bilateral
- H21.319 Exudative cysts of iris or anterior chamber, unspecified eye

✓6ᵗʰ H21.32 Implantation cysts of iris, ciliary body or anterior chamber
- H21.321 Implantation cysts of iris, ciliary body or anterior chamber, right eye
- H21.322 Implantation cysts of iris, ciliary body or anterior chamber, left eye
- H21.323 Implantation cysts of iris, ciliary body or anterior chamber, bilateral
- H21.329 Implantation cysts of iris, ciliary body or anterior chamber, unspecified eye

✓6ᵗʰ H21.33 Parasitic cyst of iris, ciliary body or anterior chamber
- H21.331 Parasitic cyst of iris, ciliary body or anterior chamber, right eye
- H21.332 Parasitic cyst of iris, ciliary body or anterior chamber, left eye
- H21.333 Parasitic cyst of iris, ciliary body or anterior chamber, bilateral
- H21.339 Parasitic cyst of iris, ciliary body or anterior chamber, unspecified eye

✓6ᵗʰ H21.34 Primary cyst of pars plana
- H21.341 Primary cyst of pars plana, right eye
- H21.342 Primary cyst of pars plana, left eye
- H21.343 Primary cyst of pars plana, bilateral
- H21.349 Primary cyst of pars plana, unspecified eye

✓6ᵗʰ H21.35 Exudative cyst of pars plana
- H21.351 Exudative cyst of pars plana, right eye
- H21.352 Exudative cyst of pars plana, left eye
- H21.353 Exudative cyst of pars plana, bilateral
- H21.359 Exudative cyst of pars plana, unspecified eye

✓5ᵗʰ H21.4 Pupillary membranes
> Iris bombé   Pupillary seclusion
> Pupillary occlusion
> **EXCLUDES 1** congenital pupillary membranes (Q13.8)
- H21.40 Pupillary membranes, unspecified eye
- H21.41 Pupillary membranes, right eye
- H21.42 Pupillary membranes, left eye
- H21.43 Pupillary membranes, bilateral

✓ Additional Character Required   ✓x7ᵗʰ Xtension Alert   Unspecified Dx   Other Specified Dx   Manifestation   ►◄ Revised Text   ● New Code   ▲ Revised Code Title

Diseases of the Eye and Adnexa

H21.5–H26.013

✓5ᵗʰ **H21.5 Other and unspecified adhesions and disruptions of iris and ciliary body**
- EXCLUDES 1   corectopia (Q13.2)

  ✓6ᵗʰ **H21.50 Unspecified adhesions of iris**
    Synechia (iris) NOS
    H21.501 Unspecified adhesions of iris, right eye
    H21.502 Unspecified adhesions of iris, left eye
    H21.503 Unspecified adhesions of iris, bilateral
    H21.509 Unspecified adhesions of iris and ciliary body, unspecified eye

  ✓6ᵗʰ **H21.51 Anterior synechiae (iris)**
    H21.511 Anterior synechiae (iris), right eye
    H21.512 Anterior synechiae (iris), left eye
    H21.513 Anterior synechiae (iris), bilateral
    H21.519 Anterior synechiae (iris), unspecified eye

  ✓6ᵗʰ **H21.52 Goniosynechiae**
    H21.521 Goniosynechiae, right eye
    H21.522 Goniosynechiae, left eye
    H21.523 Goniosynechiae, bilateral
    H21.529 Goniosynechiae, unspecified eye

  ✓6ᵗʰ **H21.53 Iridodialysis**
    H21.531 Iridodialysis, right eye
    H21.532 Iridodialysis, left eye
    H21.533 Iridodialysis, bilateral
    H21.539 Iridodialysis, unspecified eye

  ✓6ᵗʰ **H21.54 Posterior synechiae (iris)**
    H21.541 Posterior synechiae (iris), right eye
    H21.542 Posterior synechiae (iris), left eye
    H21.543 Posterior synechiae (iris), bilateral
    H21.549 Posterior synechiae (iris), unspecified eye

  ✓6ᵗʰ **H21.55 Recession of chamber angle**
    H21.551 Recession of chamber angle, right eye
    H21.552 Recession of chamber angle, left eye
    H21.553 Recession of chamber angle, bilateral
    H21.559 Recession of chamber angle, unspecified eye

  ✓6ᵗʰ **H21.56 Pupillary abnormalities**
    Deformed pupil
    Ectopic pupil
    Rupture of sphincter, pupil
    EXCLUDES 1   congenital deformity of pupil (Q13.2-)
    H21.561 Pupillary abnormality, right eye
    H21.562 Pupillary abnormality, left eye
    H21.563 Pupillary abnormality, bilateral
    H21.569 Pupillary abnormality, unspecified eye

✓5ᵗʰ **H21.8 Other specified disorders of iris and ciliary body**
  H21.81 Floppy iris syndrome
    Intraoperative floppy iris syndrome (IFIS)
    Use additional code for adverse effect, if applicable, to identify drug (T36-T50 with fifth or sixth character 5)
  H21.82 Plateau iris syndrome (post-iridectomy) (postprocedural)
  H21.89 Other specified disorders of iris and ciliary body
H21.9 Unspecified disorder of iris and ciliary body

H22 Disorders of iris and ciliary body in diseases classified elsewhere
  Code first underlying disease, such as:
    gout (M1A.-, M10.-)
    leprosy (A30.-)
    parasitic disease (B89)

Disorders of lens (H25-H28)

✓4ᵗʰ **H25 Age-related cataract**
  Senile cataract
  EXCLUDES 2   capsular glaucoma with pseudoexfoliation of lens (H40.1-)

  ✓5ᵗʰ **H25.0 Age-related incipient cataract**
    ✓6ᵗʰ **H25.01 Cortical age-related cataract**
      H25.011 Cortical age-related cataract, right eye Ⓐ
      H25.012 Cortical age-related cataract, left eye Ⓐ
      H25.013 Cortical age-related cataract, bilateral Ⓐ
      H25.019 Cortical age-related cataract, unspecified eye Ⓐ
    ✓6ᵗʰ **H25.03 Anterior subcapsular polar age-related cataract**

      H25.031 Anterior subcapsular polar age-related cataract, right eye Ⓐ
      H25.032 Anterior subcapsular polar age-related cataract, left eye Ⓐ
      H25.033 Anterior subcapsular polar age-related cataract, bilateral Ⓐ
      H25.039 Anterior subcapsular polar age-related cataract, unspecified eye Ⓐ

    ✓6ᵗʰ **H25.04 Posterior subcapsular polar age-related cataract**
      H25.041 Posterior subcapsular polar age-related cataract, right eye Ⓐ
      H25.042 Posterior subcapsular polar age-related cataract, left eye Ⓐ
      H25.043 Posterior subcapsular polar age-related cataract, bilateral Ⓐ
      H25.049 Posterior subcapsular polar age-related cataract, unspecified eye Ⓐ

    ✓6ᵗʰ **H25.09 Other age-related incipient cataract**
      Coronary age-related cataract
      Punctate age-related cataract
      Water clefts
      H25.091 Other age-related incipient cataract, right eye Ⓐ
      H25.092 Other age-related incipient cataract, left eye Ⓐ
      H25.093 Other age-related incipient cataract, bilateral Ⓐ
      H25.099 Other age-related incipient cataract, unspecified eye Ⓐ

  ✓5ᵗʰ **H25.1 Age-related nuclear cataract**
    Cataracta brunescens
    Nuclear sclerosis cataract
    H25.10 Age-related nuclear cataract, unspecified eye Ⓐ
    H25.11 Age-related nuclear cataract, right eye Ⓐ
    H25.12 Age-related nuclear cataract, left eye Ⓐ
    H25.13 Age-related nuclear cataract, bilateral Ⓐ

  ✓5ᵗʰ **H25.2 Age-related cataract, morgagnian type**
    Age-related hypermature cataract
    H25.20 Age-related cataract, morgagnian type, unspecified eye Ⓐ
    H25.21 Age-related cataract, morgagnian type, right eye Ⓐ
    H25.22 Age-related cataract, morgagnian type, left eye Ⓐ
    H25.23 Age-related cataract, morgagnian type, bilateral Ⓐ

  ✓5ᵗʰ **H25.8 Other age-related cataract**
    ✓6ᵗʰ **H25.81 Combined forms of age-related cataract**
      H25.811 Combined forms of age-related cataract, right eye Ⓐ
      H25.812 Combined forms of age-related cataract, left eye Ⓐ
      H25.813 Combined forms of age-related cataract, bilateral Ⓐ
      H25.819 Combined forms of age-related cataract, unspecified eye Ⓐ
    H25.89 Other age-related cataract Ⓐ
  H25.9 Unspecified age-related cataract Ⓐ

✓4ᵗʰ **H26 Other cataract**
  EXCLUDES 1   congenital cataract (Q12.0)
  ✓5ᵗʰ **H26.0 Infantile and juvenile cataract**
    ✓6ᵗʰ **H26.00 Unspecified infantile and juvenile cataract**
      H26.001 Unspecified infantile and juvenile cataract, right eye Ⓟ
      H26.002 Unspecified infantile and juvenile cataract, left eye Ⓟ
      H26.003 Unspecified infantile and juvenile cataract, bilateral Ⓟ
      H26.009 Unspecified infantile and juvenile cataract, unspecified eye Ⓟ

    ✓6ᵗʰ **H26.01 Infantile and juvenile cortical, lamellar, or zonular cataract**
      H26.011 Infantile and juvenile cortical, lamellar, or zonular cataract, right eye Ⓟ
      H26.012 Infantile and juvenile cortical, lamellar, or zonular cataract, left eye Ⓟ
      H26.013 Infantile and juvenile cortical, lamellar, or zonular cataract, bilateral Ⓟ

EXCLUDES 1 Not coded here   EXCLUDES 2 Not included here   Ⓝ Newborn Age: 0   Ⓟ Pediatric Age: 0-17   Ⓜ Maternity Age: 12-55   Ⓐ Adult Age: 15-124

542   ICD-10-CM Draft (2015)

H26.019 **Infantile and juvenile cortical, lamellar, or zonular cataract, unspecified eye** P

✓6ᵗʰ **H26.03** Infantile and juvenile nuclear cataract

  H26.031 **Infantile and juvenile nuclear cataract, right eye** P

  H26.032 **Infantile and juvenile nuclear cataract, left eye** P

  H26.033 **Infantile and juvenile nuclear cataract, bilateral** P

  H26.039 **Infantile and juvenile nuclear cataract, unspecified eye** P

✓6ᵗʰ **H26.04** Anterior subcapsular polar infantile and juvenile cataract

  H26.041 **Anterior subcapsular polar infantile and juvenile cataract, right eye** P

  H26.042 **Anterior subcapsular polar infantile and juvenile cataract, left eye** P

  H26.043 **Anterior subcapsular polar infantile and juvenile cataract, bilateral** P

  H26.049 **Anterior subcapsular polar infantile and juvenile cataract, unspecified eye** P

✓6ᵗʰ **H26.05** Posterior subcapsular polar infantile and juvenile cataract

  H26.051 **Posterior subcapsular polar infantile and juvenile cataract, right eye** P

  H26.052 **Posterior subcapsular polar infantile and juvenile cataract, left eye** P

  H26.053 **Posterior subcapsular polar infantile and juvenile cataract, bilateral** P

  H26.059 **Posterior subcapsular polar infantile and juvenile cataract, unspecified eye** P

✓6ᵗʰ **H26.06** Combined forms of infantile and juvenile cataract

  H26.061 **Combined forms of infantile and juvenile cataract, right eye** P

  H26.062 **Combined forms of infantile and juvenile cataract, left eye** P

  H26.063 **Combined forms of infantile and juvenile cataract, bilateral** P

  H26.069 **Combined forms of infantile and juvenile cataract, unspecified eye** P

  H26.09 **Other infantile and juvenile cataract** P

✓5ᵗʰ **H26.1** Traumatic cataract

  Use additional code (Chapter 20) to identify external cause

✓6ᵗʰ **H26.10** Unspecified traumatic cataract

  H26.101 **Unspecified traumatic cataract, right eye**

  H26.102 **Unspecified traumatic cataract, left eye**

  H26.103 **Unspecified traumatic cataract, bilateral**

  H26.109 **Unspecified traumatic cataract, unspecified eye**

✓6ᵗʰ **H26.11** Localized traumatic opacities

  H26.111 **Localized traumatic opacities, right eye**

  H26.112 **Localized traumatic opacities, left eye**

  H26.113 **Localized traumatic opacities, bilateral**

  H26.119 **Localized traumatic opacities, unspecified eye**

✓6ᵗʰ **H26.12** Partially resolved traumatic cataract

  H26.121 **Partially resolved traumatic cataract, right eye**

  H26.122 **Partially resolved traumatic cataract, left eye**

  H26.123 **Partially resolved traumatic cataract, bilateral**

  H26.129 **Partially resolved traumatic cataract, unspecified eye**

✓6ᵗʰ **H26.13** Total traumatic cataract

  H26.131 **Total traumatic cataract, right eye**

  H26.132 **Total traumatic cataract, left eye**

  H26.133 **Total traumatic cataract, bilateral**

  H26.139 **Total traumatic cataract, unspecified eye**

✓5ᵗʰ **H26.2** Complicated cataract

  H26.20 **Unspecified complicated cataract**

    Cataracta complicata NOS

✓6ᵗʰ **H26.21** Cataract with neovascularization

    Code also associated condition, such as:
    chronic iridocyclitis (H20.1-)

  H26.211 **Cataract with neovascularization, right eye**

  H26.212 **Cataract with neovascularization, left eye**

  H26.213 **Cataract with neovascularization, bilateral**

  H26.219 **Cataract with neovascularization, unspecified eye**

✓6ᵗʰ **H26.22** Cataract secondary to ocular disorders (degenerative) (inflammatory)

    Code also associated ocular disorder

  H26.221 **Cataract secondary to ocular disorders (degenerative) (inflammatory), right eye**

  H26.222 **Cataract secondary to ocular disorders (degenerative) (inflammatory), left eye**

  H26.223 **Cataract secondary to ocular disorders (degenerative) (inflammatory), bilateral**

  H26.229 **Cataract secondary to ocular disorders (degenerative) (inflammatory), unspecified eye**

✓6ᵗʰ **H26.23** Glaucomatous flecks (subcapsular)

    Code first underlying glaucoma (H40-H42)

  H26.231 **Glaucomatous flecks (subcapsular), right eye**

  H26.232 **Glaucomatous flecks (subcapsular), left eye**

  H26.233 **Glaucomatous flecks (subcapsular), bilateral**

  H26.239 **Glaucomatous flecks (subcapsular), unspecified eye**

✓5ᵗʰ **H26.3** Drug-induced cataract

  Toxic cataract

  Use additional code for adverse effect, if applicable, to identify drug (T36-T50 with fifth or sixth character 5)

  H26.30 **Drug-induced cataract, unspecified eye**

  H26.31 **Drug-induced cataract, right eye**

  H26.32 **Drug-induced cataract, left eye**

  H26.33 **Drug-induced cataract, bilateral**

✓5ᵗʰ **H26.4** Secondary cataract

  H26.40 **Unspecified secondary cataract**

✓6ᵗʰ **H26.41** Soemmering's ring

  H26.411 **Soemmering's ring, right eye**

  H26.412 **Soemmering's ring, left eye**

  H26.413 **Soemmering's ring, bilateral**

  H26.419 **Soemmering's ring, unspecified eye**

✓6ᵗʰ **H26.49** Other secondary cataract

  H26.491 **Other secondary cataract, right eye**

  H26.492 **Other secondary cataract, left eye**

  H26.493 **Other secondary cataract, bilateral**

  H26.499 **Other secondary cataract, unspecified eye**

H26.8 **Other specified cataract**

H26.9 **Unspecified cataract**

✓4ᵗʰ **H27** Other disorders of lens

  EXCLUDES 1 *congenital lens malformations (Q12.-)*
    mechanical complications of intraocular lens implant (T85.2)
    pseudophakia (Z96.1)

✓5ᵗʰ **H27.0** Aphakia

  Acquired absence of lens

  Acquired aphakia

  Aphakia due to trauma

  EXCLUDES 1 *cataract extraction status (Z98.4-)*
    congenital absence of lens (Q12.3)
    congenital aphakia (Q12.3)

  H27.00 **Aphakia, unspecified eye**

  H27.01 **Aphakia, right eye**

  H27.02 **Aphakia, left eye**

  H27.03 **Aphakia, bilateral**

✓5ᵗʰ **H27.1** Dislocation of lens

  H27.10 **Unspecified dislocation of lens**

✓6ᵗʰ **H27.11** Subluxation of lens

  H27.111 **Subluxation of lens, right eye**

  H27.112 **Subluxation of lens, left eye**

  H27.113 **Subluxation of lens, bilateral**

  H27.119 **Subluxation of lens, unspecified eye**

✓6ᵗʰ **H27.12** Anterior dislocation of lens

  H27.121 **Anterior dislocation of lens, right eye**

  H27.122 **Anterior dislocation of lens, left eye**

☑ Additional Character Required   ✓x7ᵗʰ *X*tension Alert   Unspecified Dx   Other Specified Dx   Manifestation   ▶◀ Revised Text   ● New Code   ▲ Revised Code Title

H27.123　**Anterior dislocation of lens,** bilateral
H27.129　**Anterior dislocation of lens, unspecified eye**

✓6ᵗʰ **H27.13**　**Posterior dislocation of lens**
　　　H27.131　**Posterior dislocation of lens,** right eye
　　　H27.132　**Posterior dislocation of lens,** left eye
　　　H27.133　**Posterior dislocation of lens,** bilateral
　　　H27.139　**Posterior dislocation of lens, unspecified eye**

H27.8　**Other specified disorders of lens**

H27.9　**Unspecified disorder of lens**

H28　*Cataract in diseases classified elsewhere*
　　Code first underlying disease, such as:
　　　hypoparathyroidism (E20.-)
　　　myotonia (G71.1-)
　　　myxedema (E03.-)
　　　protein-calorie malnutrition (E40-E46)
　　EXCLUDES 1　*cataract in diabetes mellitus (E08.36, E09.36, E10.36, E11.36, E13.36)*

Disorders of choroid and retina (H30-H36)

✓4ᵗʰ **H30**　**Chorioretinal inflammation**

✓5ᵗʰ **H30.0**　**Focal** chorioretinal inflammation
　　Focal chorioretinitis
　　Focal choroiditis
　　Focal retinitis
　　Focal retinochoroiditis

　✓6ᵗʰ **H30.00**　**Unspecified** focal chorioretinal inflammation
　　　Focal chorioretinitis NOS
　　　Focal choroiditis NOS
　　　Focal retinitis NOS
　　　Focal retinochoroiditis NOS
　　　H30.001　**Unspecified focal chorioretinal inflammation,** right eye
　　　H30.002　**Unspecified focal chorioretinal inflammation,** left eye
　　　H30.003　**Unspecified focal chorioretinal inflammation,** bilateral
　　　H30.009　**Unspecified focal chorioretinal inflammation, unspecified eye**

　✓6ᵗʰ **H30.01**　**Focal chorioretinal inflammation,** juxtapapillary
　　　H30.011　**Focal chorioretinal inflammation, juxtapapillary,** right eye
　　　H30.012　**Focal chorioretinal inflammation, juxtapapillary,** left eye
　　　H30.013　**Focal chorioretinal inflammation, juxtapapillary,** bilateral
　　　H30.019　**Focal chorioretinal inflammation, juxtapapillary, unspecified eye**

　✓6ᵗʰ **H30.02**　**Focal chorioretinal inflammation of** posterior pole
　　　H30.021　**Focal chorioretinal inflammation of posterior pole,** right eye
　　　H30.022　**Focal chorioretinal inflammation of posterior pole,** left eye
　　　H30.023　**Focal chorioretinal inflammation of posterior pole,** bilateral
　　　H30.029　**Focal chorioretinal inflammation of posterior pole, unspecified eye**

　✓6ᵗʰ **H30.03**　**Focal chorioretinal inflammation,** peripheral
　　　H30.031　**Focal chorioretinal inflammation, peripheral,** right eye
　　　H30.032　**Focal chorioretinal inflammation, peripheral,** left eye
　　　H30.033　**Focal chorioretinal inflammation, peripheral,** bilateral
　　　H30.039　**Focal chorioretinal inflammation, peripheral, unspecified eye**

　✓6ᵗʰ **H30.04**　**Focal chorioretinal inflammation,** macular or paramacular
　　　H30.041　**Focal chorioretinal inflammation, macular or paramacular,** right eye
　　　H30.042　**Focal chorioretinal inflammation, macular or paramacular,** left eye
　　　H30.043　**Focal chorioretinal inflammation, macular or paramacular,** bilateral
　　　H30.049　**Focal chorioretinal inflammation, macular or paramacular, unspecified eye**

✓5ᵗʰ **H30.1**　**Disseminated** chorioretinal inflammation
　　Disseminated chorioretinitis
　　Disseminated choroiditis
　　Disseminated retinitis
　　Disseminated retinochoroiditis
　　EXCLUDES 2　*exudative retinopathy (H35.02-)*

　✓6ᵗʰ **H30.10**　**Unspecified** disseminated chorioretinal inflammation
　　　Disseminated chorioretinitis NOS
　　　Disseminated choroiditis NOS
　　　Disseminated retinitis NOS
　　　Disseminated retinochoroiditis NOS
　　　H30.101　**Unspecified disseminated chorioretinal inflammation,** right eye
　　　H30.102　**Unspecified disseminated chorioretinal inflammation,** left eye
　　　H30.103　**Unspecified disseminated chorioretinal inflammation,** bilateral
　　　H30.109　**Unspecified disseminated chorioretinal inflammation, unspecified eye**

　✓6ᵗʰ **H30.11**　**Disseminated chorioretinal inflammation of** posterior pole
　　　H30.111　**Disseminated chorioretinal inflammation of posterior pole,** right eye
　　　H30.112　**Disseminated chorioretinal inflammation of posterior pole,** left eye
　　　H30.113　**Disseminated chorioretinal inflammation of posterior pole,** bilateral
　　　H30.119　**Disseminated chorioretinal inflammation of posterior pole, unspecified eye**

　✓6ᵗʰ **H30.12**　**Disseminated chorioretinal inflammation,** peripheral
　　　H30.121　**Disseminated chorioretinal inflammation, peripheral** right eye
　　　H30.122　**Disseminated chorioretinal inflammation, peripheral, left eye**
　　　H30.123　**Disseminated chorioretinal inflammation, peripheral,** bilateral
　　　H30.129　**Disseminated chorioretinal inflammation, peripheral, unspecified eye**

　✓6ᵗʰ **H30.13**　**Disseminated chorioretinal inflammation,** generalized
　　　H30.131　**Disseminated chorioretinal inflammation, generalized,** right eye
　　　H30.132　**Disseminated chorioretinal inflammation, generalized,** left eye
　　　H30.133　**Disseminated chorioretinal inflammation, generalized,** bilateral
　　　H30.139　**Disseminated chorioretinal inflammation, generalized, unspecified eye**

　✓6ᵗʰ **H30.14**　**Acute posterior multifocal placoid pigment epitheliopathy**
　　　H30.141　**Acute posterior multifocal placoid pigment epitheliopathy,** right eye
　　　H30.142　**Acute posterior multifocal placoid pigment epitheliopathy,** left eye
　　　H30.143　**Acute posterior multifocal placoid pigment epitheliopathy,** bilateral
　　　H30.149　**Acute posterior multifocal placoid pigment epitheliopathy, unspecified eye**

✓5ᵗʰ **H30.2**　**Posterior cyclitis**
　　Pars planitis
　　H30.20　**Posterior cyclitis, unspecified eye**
　　H30.21　**Posterior cyclitis,** right eye
　　H30.22　**Posterior cyclitis,** left eye
　　H30.23　**Posterior cyclitis,** bilateral

✓5ᵗʰ **H30.8**　**Other** chorioretinal inflammations

　✓6ᵗʰ **H30.81**　**Harada's disease**
　　　H30.811　**Harada's disease,** right eye
　　　H30.812　**Harada's disease,** left eye
　　　H30.813　**Harada's disease,** bilateral
　　　H30.819　**Harada's disease, unspecified eye**

　✓6ᵗʰ **H30.89**　**Other** chorioretinal inflammations
　　　H30.891　**Other chorioretinal inflammations,** right eye
　　　H30.892　**Other chorioretinal inflammations,** left eye

H30.893 **Other chorioretinal inflammations, bilateral**

H30.899 **Other chorioretinal inflammations, unspecified eye**

✓5ᵗʰ H30.9 Unspecified chorioretinal inflammation
Chorioretinitis NOS Retinitis NOS
Choroiditis NOS Retinochoroiditis NOS
Neuroretinitis NOS

H30.90 **Unspecified chorioretinal inflammation, unspecified eye**

H30.91 **Unspecified chorioretinal inflammation, right eye**

H30.92 **Unspecified chorioretinal inflammation, left eye**

H30.93 **Unspecified chorioretinal inflammation, bilateral**

✓4ᵗʰ **H31 Other disorders of choroid**

✓5ᵗʰ **H31.0 Chorioretinal scars**
EXCLUDES 2 *postsurgical chorioretinal scars (H59.81-)*

✓6ᵗʰ H31.00 Unspecified chorioretinal scars

H31.001 **Unspecified chorioretinal scars, right eye**

H31.002 **Unspecified chorioretinal scars, left eye**

H31.003 **Unspecified chorioretinal scars, bilateral**

H31.009 **Unspecified chorioretinal scars, unspecified eye**

✓6ᵗʰ H31.01 **Macula scars of posterior pole (postinflammatory) (post-traumatic)**
EXCLUDES 1 *postprocedural chorioretinal scar (H59.81-)*

H31.011 **Macula scars of posterior pole (postinflammatory) (post-traumatic), right eye**

H31.012 **Macula scars of posterior pole (postinflammatory) (post-traumatic), left eye**

H31.013 **Macula scars of posterior pole (postinflammatory) (post-traumatic), bilateral**

H31.019 **Macula scars of posterior pole (postinflammatory) (post-traumatic), unspecified eye**

✓6ᵗʰ H31.02 **Solar retinopathy**

H31.021 **Solar retinopathy, right eye**

H31.022 **Solar retinopathy, left eye**

H31.023 **Solar retinopathy, bilateral**

H31.029 **Solar retinopathy, unspecified eye**

✓6ᵗʰ H31.09 **Other chorioretinal scars**

H31.091 **Other chorioretinal scars, right eye**

H31.092 **Other chorioretinal scars, left eye**

H31.093 **Other chorioretinal scars, bilateral**

H31.099 **Other chorioretinal scars, unspecified eye**

✓5ᵗʰ **H31.1 Choroidal degeneration**
EXCLUDES 2 *angioid streaks of macula (H35.33)*

✓6ᵗʰ H31.10 Unspecified choroidal degeneration
Choroidal sclerosis NOS

H31.101 **Choroidal degeneration, unspecified, right eye**

H31.102 **Choroidal degeneration, unspecified, left eye**

H31.103 **Choroidal degeneration, unspecified, bilateral**

H31.109 **Choroidal degeneration, unspecified, unspecified eye**

✓6ᵗʰ H31.11 Age-related choroidal atrophy

H31.111 **Age-related choroidal atrophy, right eye** Ⓐ

H31.112 **Age-related choroidal atrophy, left eye** Ⓐ

H31.113 **Age-related choroidal atrophy, bilateral** Ⓐ

H31.119 **Age-related choroidal atrophy, unspecified eye** Ⓐ

✓6ᵗʰ H31.12 Diffuse secondary atrophy of choroid

H31.121 **Diffuse secondary atrophy of choroid, right eye**

H31.122 **Diffuse secondary atrophy of choroid, left eye**

H31.123 **Diffuse secondary atrophy of choroid, bilateral**

H31.129 **Diffuse secondary atrophy of choroid, unspecified eye**

✓5ᵗʰ H31.2 **Hereditary choroidal dystrophy**
EXCLUDES 2 *hyperornithinemia (E72.4)*
ornithinemia (E72.4)

H31.20 **Hereditary choroidal dystrophy, unspecified**

H31.21 **Choroideremia**

H31.22 **Choroidal dystrophy (central areolar) (generalized) (peripapillary)**

H31.23 **Gyrate atrophy, choroid**

H31.29 **Other hereditary choroidal dystrophy**

✓5ᵗʰ **H31.3 Choroidal hemorrhage and rupture**

✓6ᵗʰ H31.30 Unspecified choroidal hemorrhage

H31.301 **Unspecified choroidal hemorrhage, right eye**

H31.302 **Unspecified choroidal hemorrhage, left eye**

H31.303 **Unspecified choroidal hemorrhage, bilateral**

H31.309 **Unspecified choroidal hemorrhage, unspecified eye**

✓6ᵗʰ H31.31 Expulsive choroidal hemorrhage

H31.311 **Expulsive choroidal hemorrhage, right eye**

H31.312 **Expulsive choroidal hemorrhage, left eye**

H31.313 **Expulsive choroidal hemorrhage, bilateral**

H31.319 **Expulsive choroidal hemorrhage, unspecified eye**

✓6ᵗʰ H31.32 Choroidal rupture

H31.321 **Choroidal rupture, right eye**

H31.322 **Choroidal rupture, left eye**

H31.323 **Choroidal rupture, bilateral**

H31.329 **Choroidal rupture, unspecified eye**

✓5ᵗʰ **H31.4 Choroidal detachment**

✓6ᵗʰ H31.40 Unspecified choroidal detachment

H31.401 **Unspecified choroidal detachment, right eye**

H31.402 **Unspecified choroidal detachment, left eye**

H31.403 **Unspecified choroidal detachment, bilateral**

H31.409 **Unspecified choroidal detachment, unspecified eye**

✓6ᵗʰ H31.41 Hemorrhagic choroidal detachment

H31.411 **Hemorrhagic choroidal detachment, right eye**

H31.412 **Hemorrhagic choroidal detachment, left eye**

H31.413 **Hemorrhagic choroidal detachment, bilateral**

H31.419 **Hemorrhagic choroidal detachment, unspecified eye**

✓6ᵗʰ H31.42 Serous choroidal detachment

H31.421 **Serous choroidal detachment, right eye**

H31.422 **Serous choroidal detachment, left eye**

H31.423 **Serous choroidal detachment, bilateral**

H31.429 **Serous choroidal detachment, unspecified eye**

H31.8 **Other specified disorders of choroid**

H31.9 **Unspecified disorder of choroid**

H32 **Chorioretinal disorders in diseases classified elsewhere**
Code first underlying disease, such as:
congenital toxoplasmosis (P37.1)
histoplasmosis (B39.-)
leprosy (A30.-)
EXCLUDES 1 *chorioretinitis (in):*
toxoplasmosis (acquired) (B58.01)
tuberculosis (A18.53)

✓4ᵗʰ **H33 Retinal detachments and breaks**
EXCLUDES 1 *detachment of retinal pigment epithelium (H35.72-, H35.73-)*

✓5ᵗʰ **H33.0 Retinal detachment with retinal break**
Rhegmatogenous retinal detachment
EXCLUDES 1 *serous retinal detachment (without retinal break) (H33.2-)*

✓6ᵗʰ H33.00 Unspecified retinal detachment with retinal break

H33.001 **Unspecified retinal detachment with retinal break, right eye**

✓ Additional Character Required ✓x7ᵗʰ *X*tension Alert Unspecified Dx Other Specified Dx Manifestation ▶◀ Revised Text ● New Code ▲ Revised Code Title

H33.002 **Unspecified retinal detachment with retinal break, left eye**
H33.003 **Unspecified retinal detachment with retinal break, bilateral**
H33.009 **Unspecified retinal detachment with retinal break, unspecified eye**

✓6th H33.01 **Retinal detachment with single break**
H33.011 **Retinal detachment with single break, right eye**
H33.012 **Retinal detachment with single break, left eye**
H33.013 **Retinal detachment with single break, bilateral**
H33.019 **Retinal detachment with single break, unspecified eye**

✓6th H33.02 **Retinal detachment with multiple breaks**
H33.021 **Retinal detachment with multiple breaks, right eye**
H33.022 **Retinal detachment with multiple breaks, left eye**
H33.023 **Retinal detachment with multiple breaks, bilateral**
H33.029 **Retinal detachment with multiple breaks, unspecified eye**

✓6th H33.03 **Retinal detachment with giant retinal tear**
H33.031 **Retinal detachment with giant retinal tear, right eye**
H33.032 **Retinal detachment with giant retinal tear, left eye**
H33.033 **Retinal detachment with giant retinal tear, bilateral**
H33.039 **Retinal detachment with giant retinal tear, unspecified eye**

✓6th H33.04 **Retinal detachment with retinal dialysis**
H33.041 **Retinal detachment with retinal dialysis, right eye**
H33.042 **Retinal detachment with retinal dialysis, left eye**
H33.043 **Retinal detachment with retinal dialysis, bilateral**
H33.049 **Retinal detachment with retinal dialysis, unspecified eye**

✓6th H33.05 **Total retinal detachment**
H33.051 **Total retinal detachment, right eye**
H33.052 **Total retinal detachment, left eye**
H33.053 **Total retinal detachment, bilateral**
H33.059 **Total retinal detachment, unspecified eye**

✓5th H33.1 **Retinoschisis and retinal cysts**
EXCLUDES 1 *congenital retinoschisis (Q14.1)*
microcystoid degeneration of retina (H35.42-)

✓6th H33.10 **Unspecified retinoschisis**
H33.101 **Unspecified retinoschisis, right eye**
H33.102 **Unspecified retinoschisis, left eye**
H33.103 **Unspecified retinoschisis, bilateral**
H33.109 **Unspecified retinoschisis, unspecified eye**

✓6th H33.11 **Cyst of ora serrata**
H33.111 **Cyst of ora serrata, right eye**
H33.112 **Cyst of ora serrata, left eye**
H33.113 **Cyst of ora serrata, bilateral**
H33.119 **Cyst of ora serrata, unspecified eye**

✓6th H33.12 **Parasitic cyst of retina**
H33.121 **Parasitic cyst of retina, right eye**
H33.122 **Parasitic cyst of retina, left eye**
H33.123 **Parasitic cyst of retina, bilateral**
H33.129 **Parasitic cyst of retina, unspecified eye**

✓6th H33.19 **Other retinoschisis and retinal cysts**
Pseudocyst of retina
H33.191 **Other retinoschisis and retinal cysts, right eye**
H33.192 **Other retinoschisis and retinal cysts, left eye**
H33.193 **Other retinoschisis and retinal cysts, bilateral**
H33.199 **Other retinoschisis and retinal cysts, unspecified eye**

✓5th H33.2 **Serous retinal detachment**
Retinal detachment NOS
Retinal detachment without retinal break
EXCLUDES 1 *central serous chorioretinopathy (H35.71-)*
H33.20 **Serous retinal detachment, unspecified eye**
H33.21 **Serous retinal detachment, right eye**
H33.22 **Serous retinal detachment, left eye**
H33.23 **Serous retinal detachment, bilateral**

✓5th H33.3 **Retinal breaks without detachment**
EXCLUDES 1 *chorioretinal scars after surgery for detachment (H59.81-)*
peripheral retinal degeneration without break (H35.4-)

✓6th H33.30 **Unspecified retinal break**
H33.301 **Unspecified retinal break, right eye**
H33.302 **Unspecified retinal break, left eye**
H33.303 **Unspecified retinal break, bilateral**
H33.309 **Unspecified retinal break, unspecified eye**

✓6th H33.31 **Horseshoe tear of retina without detachment**
Operculum of retina without detachment
H33.311 **Horseshoe tear of retina without detachment, right eye**
H33.312 **Horseshoe tear of retina without detachment, left eye**
H33.313 **Horseshoe tear of retina without detachment, bilateral**
H33.319 **Horseshoe tear of retina without detachment, unspecified eye**

✓6th H33.32 **Round hole of retina without detachment**
H33.321 **Round hole, right eye**
H33.322 **Round hole, left eye**
H33.323 **Round hole, bilateral**
H33.329 **Round hole, unspecified eye**

✓6th H33.33 **Multiple defects of retina without detachment**
H33.331 **Multiple defects of retina without detachment, right eye**
H33.332 **Multiple defects of retina without detachment, left eye**
H33.333 **Multiple defects of retina without detachment, bilateral**
H33.339 **Multiple defects of retina without detachment, unspecified eye**

✓5th H33.4 **Traction detachment of retina**
Proliferative vitreo-retinopathy with retinal detachment
H33.40 **Traction detachment of retina, unspecified eye**
H33.41 **Traction detachment of retina, right eye**
H33.42 **Traction detachment of retina, left eye**
H33.43 **Traction detachment of retina, bilateral**
H33.8 **Other retinal detachments**

✓4th H34 **Retinal vascular occlusions**
EXCLUDES 1 *amaurosis fugax (G45.3)*

✓5th H34.0 **Transient retinal artery occlusion**
H34.00 **Transient retinal artery occlusion, unspecified eye**
H34.01 **Transient retinal artery occlusion, right eye**
H34.02 **Transient retinal artery occlusion, left eye**
H34.03 **Transient retinal artery occlusion, bilateral**

✓5th H34.1 **Central retinal artery occlusion**
H34.10 **Central retinal artery occlusion, unspecified eye**
H34.11 **Central retinal artery occlusion, right eye**
H34.12 **Central retinal artery occlusion, left eye**
H34.13 **Central retinal artery occlusion, bilateral**

✓5th H34.2 **Other retinal artery occlusions**
✓6th H34.21 **Partial retinal artery occlusion**
Hollenhorst's plaque
Retinal microembolism
H34.211 **Partial retinal artery occlusion, right eye**
H34.212 **Partial retinal artery occlusion, left eye**
H34.213 **Partial retinal artery occlusion, bilateral**
H34.219 **Partial retinal artery occlusion, unspecified eye**

✓6th H34.23 **Retinal artery branch occlusion**
H34.231 **Retinal artery branch occlusion, right eye**
H34.232 **Retinal artery branch occlusion, left eye**
H34.233 **Retinal artery branch occlusion, bilateral**

H34.239　**Retinal artery branch occlusion, unspecified eye**

✓5ᵗʰ H34.8　Other retinal vascular occlusions

✓6ᵗʰ H34.81　Central retinal vein occlusion
H34.811　Central retinal vein occlusion, right eye
H34.812　Central retinal vein occlusion, left eye
H34.813　Central retinal vein occlusion, bilateral
H34.819　**Central retinal vein occlusion, unspecified eye**

✓6ᵗʰ H34.82　Venous engorgement
Incipient retinal vein occlusion
Partial retinal vein occlusion
H34.821　Venous engorgement, right eye
H34.822　Venous engorgement, left eye
H34.823　Venous engorgement, bilateral
H34.829　**Venous engorgement, unspecified eye**

✓6ᵗʰ H34.83　Tributary (branch) retinal vein occlusion
H34.831　Tributary (branch) retinal vein occlusion, right eye
H34.832　Tributary (branch) retinal vein occlusion, left eye
H34.833　Tributary (branch) retinal vein occlusion, bilateral
H34.839　**Tributary (branch) retinal vein occlusion, unspecified eye**

H34.9　Unspecified retinal vascular occlusion

✓4ᵗʰ **H35　Other retinal disorders**
EXCLUDES 2　diabetic retinal disorders (E08.311- E08.359, E09.311- E09.359, E10.311- E10.359, E11.311- E11.359, E13.311- E13.359)

✓5ᵗʰ H35.0　Background retinopathy and retinal vascular changes
Code also any associated hypertension (I10.-)

H35.00　**Unspecified background retinopathy**

✓6ᵗʰ H35.01　Changes in retinal vascular appearance
Retinal vascular sheathing
H35.011　Changes in retinal vascular appearance, right eye
H35.012　Changes in retinal vascular appearance, left eye
H35.013　Changes in retinal vascular appearance, bilateral
H35.019　**Changes in retinal vascular appearance, unspecified eye**

✓6ᵗʰ H35.02　Exudative retinopathy
Coats retinopathy
H35.021　Exudative retinopathy, right eye
H35.022　Exudative retinopathy, left eye
H35.023　Exudative retinopathy, bilateral
H35.029　**Exudative retinopathy, unspecified eye**

✓6ᵗʰ H35.03　Hypertensive retinopathy
H35.031　Hypertensive retinopathy, right eye
H35.032　Hypertensive retinopathy, left eye
H35.033　Hypertensive retinopathy, bilateral
H35.039　**Hypertensive retinopathy, unspecified eye**

✓6ᵗʰ H35.04　Retinal micro-aneurysms, unspecified
H35.041　Retinal micro-aneurysms, unspecified, right eye
H35.042　Retinal micro-aneurysms, unspecified, left eye
H35.043　Retinal micro-aneurysms, unspecified, bilateral
H35.049　**Retinal micro-aneurysms, unspecified, unspecified eye**

✓6ᵗʰ H35.05　Retinal neovascularization, unspecified
H35.051　Retinal neovascularization, unspecified, right eye
H35.052　Retinal neovascularization, unspecified, left eye
H35.053　Retinal neovascularization, unspecified, bilateral
H35.059　**Retinal neovascularization, unspecified, unspecified eye**

✓6ᵗʰ H35.06　Retinal vasculitis
Eales diseaseRetinal perivasculitis
H35.061　Retinal vasculitis, right eye

H35.062　Retinal vasculitis, left eye
H35.063　Retinal vasculitis, bilateral
H35.069　**Retinal vasculitis, unspecified eye**

✓6ᵗʰ H35.07　Retinal telangiectasis
H35.071　Retinal telangiectasis, right eye
H35.072　Retinal telangiectasis, left eye
H35.073　Retinal telangiectasis, bilateral
H35.079　**Retinal telangiectasis, unspecified eye**

H35.09　**Other intraretinal microvascular abnormalities**
Retinal varices

✓5ᵗʰ H35.1　Retinopathy of prematurity

✓6ᵗʰ H35.10　Retinopathy of prematurity, unspecified
Retinopathy of prematurity NOS
H35.101　Retinopathy of prematurity, unspecified, right eye
H35.102　Retinopathy of prematurity, unspecified, left eye
H35.103　Retinopathy of prematurity, unspecified, bilateral
H35.109　**Retinopathy of prematurity, unspecified, unspecified eye**

✓6ᵗʰ H35.11　Retinopathy of prematurity, stage 0
H35.111　Retinopathy of prematurity, stage 0, right eye
H35.112　Retinopathy of prematurity, stage 0, left eye
H35.113　Retinopathy of prematurity, stage 0, bilateral
H35.119　**Retinopathy of prematurity, stage 0, unspecified eye**

✓6ᵗʰ H35.12　Retinopathy of prematurity, stage 1
H35.121　Retinopathy of prematurity, stage 1, right eye
H35.122　Retinopathy of prematurity, stage 1, left eye
H35.123　Retinopathy of prematurity, stage 1, bilateral
H35.129　**Retinopathy of prematurity, stage 1, unspecified eye**

✓6ᵗʰ H35.13　Retinopathy of prematurity, stage 2
H35.131　Retinopathy of prematurity, stage 2, right eye
H35.132　Retinopathy of prematurity, stage 2, left eye
H35.133　Retinopathy of prematurity, stage 2, bilateral
H35.139　**Retinopathy of prematurity, stage 2, unspecified eye**

✓6ᵗʰ H35.14　Retinopathy of prematurity, stage 3
H35.141　Retinopathy of prematurity, stage 3, right eye
H35.142　Retinopathy of prematurity, stage 3, left eye
H35.143　Retinopathy of prematurity, stage 3, bilateral
H35.149　**Retinopathy of prematurity, stage 3, unspecified eye**

✓6ᵗʰ H35.15　Retinopathy of prematurity, stage 4
H35.151　Retinopathy of prematurity, stage 4, right eye
H35.152　Retinopathy of prematurity, stage 4, left eye
H35.153　Retinopathy of prematurity, stage 4, bilateral
H35.159　**Retinopathy of prematurity, stage 4, unspecified eye**

✓6ᵗʰ H35.16　Retinopathy of prematurity, stage 5
H35.161　Retinopathy of prematurity, stage 5, right eye
H35.162　Retinopathy of prematurity, stage 5, left eye
H35.163　Retinopathy of prematurity, stage 5, bilateral
H35.169　**Retinopathy of prematurity, stage 5, unspecified eye**

✓6ᵗʰ **H35.17** Retrolental fibroplasia
- **H35.171** Retrolental fibroplasia, right eye
- **H35.172** Retrolental fibroplasia, left eye
- **H35.173** Retrolental fibroplasia, bilateral
- **H35.179** Retrolental fibroplasia, unspecified eye

✓5ᵗʰ **H35.2** Other non-diabetic proliferative retinopathy
Proliferative vitreo-retinopathy
> EXCLUDES 1   proliferative vitreo-retinopathy with retinal detachment (H33.4-)

- **H35.20** Other non-diabetic proliferative retinopathy, unspecified eye
- **H35.21** Other non-diabetic proliferative retinopathy, right eye
- **H35.22** Other non-diabetic proliferative retinopathy, left eye
- **H35.23** Other non-diabetic proliferative retinopathy, bilateral

✓5ᵗʰ **H35.3** Degeneration of macula and posterior pole
- **H35.30** Unspecified macular degeneration   A
  Age-related macular degeneration
- **H35.31** Nonexudative age-related macular degeneration   A
  Atrophic age-related macular degeneration
- **H35.32** Exudative age-related macular degeneration   A
- **H35.33** Angioid streaks of macula

✓6ᵗʰ **H35.34** Macular cyst, hole, or pseudohole
- **H35.341** Macular cyst, hole, or pseudohole, right eye
- **H35.342** Macular cyst, hole, or pseudohole, left eye
- **H35.343** Macular cyst, hole, or pseudohole, bilateral
- **H35.349** Macular cyst, hole, or pseudohole, unspecified eye

✓6ᵗʰ **H35.35** Cystoid macular degeneration
> EXCLUDES 1   cystoid macular edema following cataract surgery (H59.03-)

- **H35.351** Cystoid macular degeneration, right eye
- **H35.352** Cystoid macular degeneration, left eye
- **H35.353** Cystoid macular degeneration, bilateral
- **H35.359** Cystoid macular degeneration, unspecified eye

✓6ᵗʰ **H35.36** Drusen (degenerative) of macula
- **H35.361** Drusen (degenerative) of macula, right eye
- **H35.362** Drusen (degenerative) of macula, left eye
- **H35.363** Drusen (degenerative) of macula, bilateral
- **H35.369** Drusen (degenerative) of macula, unspecified eye

✓6ᵗʰ **H35.37** Puckering of macula
- **H35.371** Puckering of macula, right eye
- **H35.372** Puckering of macula, left eye
- **H35.373** Puckering of macula, bilateral
- **H35.379** Puckering of macula, unspecified eye

✓6ᵗʰ **H35.38** Toxic maculopathy
Code first poisoning due to drug or toxin, if applicable (T36-T65 with fifth or sixth character 1-4 or 6)
Use additional code for adverse effect, if applicable, to identify drug (T36-T50 with fifth or sixth character 5)
- **H35.381** Toxic maculopathy, right eye
- **H35.382** Toxic maculopathy, left eye
- **H35.383** Toxic maculopathy, bilateral
- **H35.389** Toxic maculopathy, unspecified eye

✓5ᵗʰ **H35.4** Peripheral retinal degeneration
> EXCLUDES 1   hereditary retinal degeneration (dystrophy) (H35.5-)
> peripheral retinal degeneration with retinal break (H33.3-)

- **H35.40** Unspecified peripheral retinal degeneration

✓6ᵗʰ **H35.41** Lattice degeneration of retina
Palisade degeneration of retina
- **H35.411** Lattice degeneration of retina, right eye
- **H35.412** Lattice degeneration of retina, left eye
- **H35.413** Lattice degeneration of retina, bilateral
- **H35.419** Lattice degeneration of retina, unspecified eye

✓6ᵗʰ **H35.42** Microcystoid degeneration of retina
- **H35.421** Microcystoid degeneration of retina, right eye
- **H35.422** Microcystoid degeneration of retina, left eye
- **H35.423** Microcystoid degeneration of retina, bilateral
- **H35.429** Microcystoid degeneration of retina, unspecified eye

✓6ᵗʰ **H35.43** Paving stone degeneration of retina
- **H35.431** Paving stone degeneration of retina, right eye
- **H35.432** Paving stone degeneration of retina, left eye
- **H35.433** Paving stone degeneration of retina, bilateral
- **H35.439** Paving stone degeneration of retina, unspecified eye

✓6ᵗʰ **H35.44** Age-related reticular degeneration of retina
- **H35.441** Age-related reticular degeneration of retina, right eye   A
- **H35.442** Age-related reticular degeneration of retina, left eye   A
- **H35.443** Age-related reticular degeneration of retina, bilateral   A
- **H35.449** Age-related reticular degeneration of retina, unspecified eye   A

✓6ᵗʰ **H35.45** Secondary pigmentary degeneration
- **H35.451** Secondary pigmentary degeneration, right eye
- **H35.452** Secondary pigmentary degeneration, left eye
- **H35.453** Secondary pigmentary degeneration, bilateral
- **H35.459** Secondary pigmentary degeneration, unspecified eye

✓6ᵗʰ **H35.46** Secondary vitreoretinal degeneration
- **H35.461** Secondary vitreoretinal degeneration, right eye
- **H35.462** Secondary vitreoretinal degeneration, left eye
- **H35.463** Secondary vitreoretinal degeneration, bilateral
- **H35.469** Secondary vitreoretinal degeneration, unspecified eye

✓5ᵗʰ **H35.5** Hereditary retinal dystrophy
> EXCLUDES 1   dystrophies primarily involving Bruch's membrane (H31.1-)

- **H35.50** Unspecified hereditary retinal dystrophy
- **H35.51** Vitreoretinal dystrophy
- **H35.52** Pigmentary retinal dystrophy
  Albipunctate retinal dystrophy
  Retinitis pigmentosa
  Tapetoretinal dystrophy
- **H35.53** Other dystrophies primarily involving the sensory retina
  Stargardt's disease
- **H35.54** Dystrophies primarily involving the retinal pigment epithelium
  Vitelliform retinal dystrophy

✓5ᵗʰ **H35.6** Retinal hemorrhage
- **H35.60** Retinal hemorrhage, unspecified eye
- **H35.61** Retinal hemorrhage, right eye
- **H35.62** Retinal hemorrhage, left eye
- **H35.63** Retinal hemorrhage, bilateral

✓5ᵗʰ **H35.7** Separation of retinal layers
> EXCLUDES 1   retinal detachment (serous) (H33.2-)
> rhegmatogenous retinal detachment (H33.0-)

- **H35.70** Unspecified separation of retinal layers

✓6ᵗʰ **H35.71** Central serous chorioretinopathy
- **H35.711** Central serous chorioretinopathy, right eye
- **H35.712** Central serous chorioretinopathy, left eye
- **H35.713** Central serous chorioretinopathy, bilateral
- **H35.719** Central serous chorioretinopathy, unspecified eye

---

EXCLUDES 1 Not coded here   EXCLUDES 2 Not included here   N Newborn Age: 0   P Pediatric Age: 0-17   M Maternity Age: 12-55   A Adult Age: 15-124

✓6ᵗʰ **H35.72** Serous **detachment of retinal pigment epithelium**

    H35.721 Serous detachment of retinal pigment epithelium, right eye

    H35.722 Serous detachment of retinal pigment epithelium, left eye

    H35.723 Serous detachment of retinal pigment epithelium, bilateral

    H35.729 Serous detachment of retinal pigment epithelium, unspecified eye

✓6ᵗʰ **H35.73** Hemorrhagic **detachment of retinal pigment epithelium**

    H35.731 Hemorrhagic detachment of retinal pigment epithelium, right eye

    H35.732 Hemorrhagic detachment of retinal pigment epithelium, left eye

    H35.733 Hemorrhagic detachment of retinal pigment epithelium, bilateral

    H35.739 Hemorrhagic detachment of retinal pigment epithelium, unspecified eye

✓5ᵗʰ **H35.8** **Other specified retinal disorders**

    EXCLUDES 2 retinal hemorrhage (H35.6-)

    H35.81 **Retinal edema**

        Retinal cotton wool spots

    H35.82 **Retinal ischemia**

    H35.89 Other specified retinal disorders

H35.9 **Unspecified retinal disorder**

H36 *Retinal disorders in diseases classified elsewhere*

    Code first underlying disease, such as:
      lipid storage disorders (E75.-)
      sickle-cell disorders (D57.-)

    EXCLUDES 1 *arteriosclerotic retinopathy (H35.Ø-)*
              diabetic retinopathy (EØ8.3-, EØ9.3-, E1Ø.3-, E11.3-, E13.3-)

Glaucoma (H4Ø-H42)

✓4ᵗʰ **H4Ø** **Glaucoma**

    EXCLUDES 1 *absolute glaucoma (H44.51-)*
              congenital glaucoma (Q15.Ø)
              traumatic glaucoma due to birth injury (P15.3)

✓5ᵗʰ **H4Ø.Ø** **Glaucoma** suspect

  ✓6ᵗʰ **H4Ø.ØØ** **Preglaucoma, unspecified**

    H4Ø.ØØ1 **Preglaucoma, unspecified, right eye**

    H4Ø.ØØ2 **Preglaucoma, unspecified, left eye**

    H4Ø.ØØ3 **Preglaucoma, unspecified, bilateral**

    H4Ø.ØØ9 **Preglaucoma, unspecified, unspecified eye**

  ✓6ᵗʰ **H4Ø.Ø1** Open angle **with borderline findings, low risk**

    Open angle, low risk

    H4Ø.Ø11 **Open angle with borderline findings, low risk, right eye**

    H4Ø.Ø12 **Open angle with borderline findings, low risk, left eye**

    H4Ø.Ø13 **Open angle with borderline findings, low risk, bilateral**

    H4Ø.Ø19 **Open angle with borderline findings, low risk, unspecified eye**

  ✓6ᵗʰ **H4Ø.Ø2** Open angle **with borderline findings, high risk**

    Open angle, high risk

    H4Ø.Ø21 **Open angle with borderline findings, high risk, right eye**

    H4Ø.Ø22 **Open angle with borderline findings, high risk, left eye**

    H4Ø.Ø23 **Open angle with borderline findings, high risk, bilateral**

    H4Ø.Ø29 **Open angle with borderline findings, high risk, unspecified eye**

  ✓6ᵗʰ **H4Ø.Ø3** Anatomical narrow **angle**

    Primary angle closure suspect

    H4Ø.Ø31 **Anatomical narrow angle, right eye**

    H4Ø.Ø32 **Anatomical narrow angle, left eye**

    H4Ø.Ø33 **Anatomical narrow angle, bilateral**

    H4Ø.Ø39 **Anatomical narrow angle, unspecified eye**

  ✓6ᵗʰ **H4Ø.Ø4** **Steroid responder**

    H4Ø.Ø41 **Steroid responder, right eye**

    H4Ø.Ø42 **Steroid responder, left eye**

    H4Ø.Ø43 **Steroid responder, bilateral**

    H4Ø.Ø49 **Steroid responder, unspecified eye**

  ✓6ᵗʰ **H4Ø.Ø5** Ocular hypertension

    H4Ø.Ø51 **Ocular hypertension, right eye**

    H4Ø.Ø52 **Ocular hypertension, left eye**

    H4Ø.Ø53 **Ocular hypertension, bilateral**

    H4Ø.Ø59 **Ocular hypertension, unspecified eye**

  ✓6ᵗʰ **H4Ø.Ø6** Primary angle closure without glaucoma damage

    H4Ø.Ø61 **Primary angle closure without glaucoma damage, right eye**

    H4Ø.Ø62 **Primary angle closure without glaucoma damage, left eye**

    H4Ø.Ø63 **Primary angle closure without glaucoma damage, bilateral**

    H4Ø.Ø69 **Primary angle closure without glaucoma damage, unspecified eye**

✓5ᵗʰ **H4Ø.1** **Open-angle glaucoma**

    One of the following 7th characters is to be assigned to each code in subcategories H4Ø.1Ø, H4Ø.11, H4Ø.12-, H4Ø.13-, and H4Ø.14- to designate the stage of glaucoma.
    Ø   stage unspecified
    1   mild stage
    2   moderate stage
    3   severe stage
    4   indeterminate stage

  ✓x7ᵗʰ **H4Ø.1Ø** **Unspecified open-angle glaucoma**

  ✓x7ᵗʰ **H4Ø.11** Primary **open-angle glaucoma**

    Chronic simple glaucoma

  ✓6ᵗʰ **H4Ø.12** Low-tension **glaucoma**

    ✓7ᵗʰ **H4Ø.121** **Low-tension glaucoma, right eye**

    ✓7ᵗʰ **H4Ø.122** **Low-tension glaucoma, left eye**

    ✓7ᵗʰ **H4Ø.123** **Low-tension glaucoma, bilateral**

    ✓7ᵗʰ **H4Ø.129** **Low-tension glaucoma, unspecified eye**

  ✓6ᵗʰ **H4Ø.13** Pigmentary **glaucoma**

    ✓7ᵗʰ **H4Ø.131** **Pigmentary glaucoma, right eye**

    ✓7ᵗʰ **H4Ø.132** **Pigmentary glaucoma, left eye**

    ✓7ᵗʰ **H4Ø.133** **Pigmentary glaucoma, bilateral**

    ✓7ᵗʰ **H4Ø.139** **Pigmentary glaucoma, unspecified eye**

  ✓6ᵗʰ **H4Ø.14** Capsular glaucoma with pseudoexfoliation **of lens**

    ✓7ᵗʰ **H4Ø.141** **Capsular glaucoma with pseudoexfoliation of lens, right eye**

    ✓7ᵗʰ **H4Ø.142** **Capsular glaucoma with pseudoexfoliation of lens, left eye**

    ✓7ᵗʰ **H4Ø.143** **Capsular glaucoma with pseudoexfoliation of lens, bilateral**

    ✓7ᵗʰ **H4Ø.149** **Capsular glaucoma with pseudoexfoliation of lens, unspecified eye**

  ✓6ᵗʰ **H4Ø.15** Residual stage **of open-angle glaucoma**

    H4Ø.151 **Residual stage of open-angle glaucoma, right eye**

    H4Ø.152 **Residual stage of open-angle glaucoma, left eye**

    H4Ø.153 **Residual stage of open-angle glaucoma, bilateral**

    H4Ø.159 **Residual stage of open-angle glaucoma, unspecified eye**

✓5ᵗʰ **H4Ø.2** **Primary angle-closure glaucoma**

    EXCLUDES 1 *aqueous misdirection (H4Ø.83-)*
              malignant glaucoma (H4Ø.83-)

    One of the following 7th characters is to be assigned to each code in subcategories H4Ø.2Ø and H4Ø.22- to designate the stage of glaucoma.
    Ø   stage unspecified
    1   mild stage
    2   moderate stage
    3   severe stage
    4   indeterminate stage

  ✓x7ᵗʰ **H4Ø.2Ø** **Unspecified primary angle-closure glaucoma**

  ✓6ᵗʰ **H4Ø.21** Acute **angle-closure glaucoma**

    Acute angle-closure glaucoma attack
    Acute angle-closure glaucoma crisis

    H4Ø.211 **Acute angle-closure glaucoma, right eye**

    H4Ø.212 **Acute angle-closure glaucoma, left eye**

    H4Ø.213 **Acute angle-closure glaucoma, bilateral**

✓ Additional Character Required   ✓x7ᵗʰ Xtension Alert   Unspecified Dx   Other Specified Dx   Manifestation   ►◄ Revised Text   ● New Code   ▲ Revised Code Title

H40.219 **Acute angle-closure glaucoma, unspecified eye**

√6ᵗʰ H40.22 Chronic **angle-closure glaucoma**
Chronic primary angle-closure glaucoma

√7ᵗʰ H40.221 **Chronic angle-closure glaucoma,** right **eye**

√7ᵗʰ H40.222 **Chronic angle-closure glaucoma,** left **eye**

√7ᵗʰ H40.223 **Chronic angle-closure glaucoma,** bilateral

√7ᵗʰ H40.229 **Chronic angle-closure glaucoma, unspecified eye**

√6ᵗʰ H40.23 Intermittent **angle-closure glaucoma**

H40.231 **Intermittent angle-closure glaucoma,** right **eye**

H40.232 **Intermittent angle-closure glaucoma,** left **eye**

H40.233 **Intermittent angle-closure glaucoma, bilateral**

H40.239 **Intermittent angle-closure glaucoma, unspecified eye**

√6ᵗʰ H40.24 Residual stage **of angle-closure glaucoma**

H40.241 **Residual stage of angle-closure glaucoma,** right **eye**

H40.242 **Residual stage of angle-closure glaucoma,** left **eye**

H40.243 **Residual stage of angle-closure glaucoma, bilateral**

H40.249 **Residual stage of angle-closure glaucoma, unspecified eye**

√5ᵗʰ H40.3 Glaucoma secondary to eye trauma
Code also underlying condition

> One of the following 7th characters is to be assigned to each code in subcategory H40.3- to designate the stage of glaucoma.
> Ø   stage unspecified
> 1   mild stage
> 2   moderate stage
> 3   severe stage
> 4   indeterminate stage

√x7ᵗʰ H40.30 **Glaucoma secondary to eye trauma, unspecified eye**

√x7ᵗʰ H40.31 **Glaucoma secondary to eye trauma,** right **eye**

√x7ᵗʰ H40.32 **Glaucoma secondary to eye trauma,** left **eye**

√x7ᵗʰ H40.33 **Glaucoma secondary to eye trauma,** bilateral

√5ᵗʰ H40.4 Glaucoma secondary to eye inflammation
Code also underlying condition

> One of the following 7th characters is to be assigned to each code in subcategory H40.4- to designate the stage of glaucoma.
> Ø   stage unspecified
> 1   mild stage
> 2   moderate stage
> 3   severe stage
> 4   indeterminate stage

√x7ᵗʰ H40.40 **Glaucoma secondary to eye inflammation, unspecified eye**

√x7ᵗʰ H40.41 **Glaucoma secondary to eye inflammation,** right **eye**

√x7ᵗʰ H40.42 **Glaucoma secondary to eye inflammation,** left **eye**

√x7ᵗʰ H40.43 **Glaucoma secondary to eye inflammation,** bilateral

√5ᵗʰ H40.5 Glaucoma secondary to other eye disorders
Code also underlying eye disorder

> One of the following 7th characters is to be assigned to each code in subcategory H40.5- to designate the stage of glaucoma.
> Ø   stage unspecified
> 1   mild stage
> 2   moderate stage
> 3   severe stage
> 4   indeterminate stage

√x7ᵗʰ H40.50 **Glaucoma secondary to other eye disorders, unspecified eye**

√x7ᵗʰ H40.51 **Glaucoma secondary to other eye disorders,** right **eye**

√x7ᵗʰ H40.52 **Glaucoma secondary to other eye disorders,** left **eye**

√x7ᵗʰ H40.53 **Glaucoma secondary to other eye disorders,** bilateral

√5ᵗʰ H40.6 Glaucoma secondary to **drugs**
Use additional code for adverse effect, if applicable, to identify drug (T36-T50 with fifth or sixth character 5)

> One of the following 7th characters is to be assigned to each code in subcategory H40.6- to designate the stage of glaucoma.
> Ø   stage unspecified
> 1   mild stage
> 2   moderate stage
> 3   severe stage
> 4   indeterminate stage

√x7ᵗʰ H40.60 **Glaucoma secondary to drugs, unspecified eye**

√x7ᵗʰ H40.61 **Glaucoma secondary to drugs,** right **eye**

√x7ᵗʰ H40.62 **Glaucoma secondary to drugs,** left **eye**

√x7ᵗʰ H40.63 **Glaucoma secondary to drugs,** bilateral

√5ᵗʰ H40.8 Other **glaucoma**

√6ᵗʰ H40.81 **Glaucoma with** increased episcleral venous pressure

H40.811 **Glaucoma with increased episcleral venous pressure,** right **eye**

H40.812 **Glaucoma with increased episcleral venous pressure,** left **eye**

H40.813 **Glaucoma with increased episcleral venous pressure,** bilateral

H40.819 **Glaucoma with increased episcleral venous pressure, unspecified eye**

√6ᵗʰ H40.82 Hypersecretion **glaucoma**

H40.821 **Hypersecretion glaucoma,** right **eye**

H40.822 **Hypersecretion glaucoma,** left **eye**

H40.823 **Hypersecretion glaucoma,** bilateral

H40.829 **Hypersecretion glaucoma, unspecified eye**

√6ᵗʰ H40.83 Aqueous misdirection
Malignant glaucoma

H40.831 **Aqueous misdirection,** right **eye**

H40.832 **Aqueous misdirection,** left **eye**

H40.833 **Aqueous misdirection,** bilateral

H40.839 **Aqueous misdirection, unspecified eye**

H40.89 **Other specified glaucoma**

H40.9 **Unspecified glaucoma**

H42   Glaucoma in diseases classified elsewhere
Code first underlying condition, such as:
amyloidosis (E85.-)
aniridia (Q13.1)
Lowe's syndrome (E72.Ø3)
Reiger's anomaly (Q13.81)
specified metabolic disorder (E70-E88)
EXCLUDES 1 glaucoma (in):
diabetes mellitus (EØ8.39, EØ9.39, E1Ø.39, E11.39, E13.39)
onchocerciasis (B73.Ø2)
syphilis (A52.71)
tuberculous (A18.59)

Disorders of vitreous body and globe (H43-H44)

√4ᵗʰ **H43 Disorders of vitreous body**

√5ᵗʰ H43.Ø Vitreous prolapse
EXCLUDES 1 traumatic vitreous prolapse (SØ5.2-)
vitreous syndrome following cataract surgery (H59.Ø-)

H43.ØØ **Vitreous prolapse, unspecified eye**

H43.Ø1 **Vitreous prolapse,** right **eye**

H43.Ø2 **Vitreous prolapse,** left **eye**

H43.Ø3 **Vitreous prolapse,** bilateral

√5ᵗʰ H43.1 Vitreous hemorrhage

H43.1Ø **Vitreous hemorrhage, unspecified eye**

H43.11 **Vitreous hemorrhage,** right **eye**

H43.12 **Vitreous hemorrhage,** left **eye**

H43.13 **Vitreous hemorrhage,** bilateral

√5ᵗʰ H43.2 Crystalline deposits in vitreous body

H43.2Ø **Crystalline deposits in vitreous body, unspecified eye**

H43.21 **Crystalline deposits in vitreous body,** right **eye**

H43.22 **Crystalline deposits in vitreous body,** left **eye**

H43.23 **Crystalline deposits in vitreous body,** bilateral

EXCLUDES 1 Not coded here   EXCLUDES 2 Not included here   N Newborn Age: Ø   P Pediatric Age: Ø-17   M Maternity Age: 12-55   A Adult Age: 15-124

550   ICD-10-CM Draft (2015)

√5ᵗʰ **H43.3** Other vitreous opacities

  √6ᵗʰ **H43.31** Vitreous membranes and strands
    H43.311 Vitreous membranes and strands, right eye
    H43.312 Vitreous membranes and strands, left eye
    H43.313 Vitreous membranes and strands, bilateral
    H43.319 Vitreous membranes and strands, unspecified eye

  √6ᵗʰ **H43.39** Other vitreous opacities
    Vitreous floaters
    H43.391 Other vitreous opacities, right eye
    H43.392 Other vitreous opacities, left eye
    H43.393 Other vitreous opacities, bilateral
    H43.399 Other vitreous opacities, unspecified eye

√5ᵗʰ **H43.8** Other disorders of vitreous body
    EXCLUDES 1   proliferative vitreo-retinopathy with retinal detachment (H33.4-)
    EXCLUDES 2   vitreous abscess (H44.02-)

  √6ᵗʰ **H43.81** Vitreous degeneration
    Vitreous detachment
    H43.811 Vitreous degeneration, right eye
    H43.812 Vitreous degeneration, left eye
    H43.813 Vitreous degeneration, bilateral
    H43.819 Vitreous degeneration, unspecified eye

  √6ᵗʰ **H43.82** Vitreomacular adhesion
    Vitreomacular traction
    H43.821 Vitreomacular adhesion, right eye   🅐
    H43.822 Vitreomacular adhesion, left eye   🅐
    H43.823 Vitreomacular adhesion, bilateral   🅐
    H43.829 Vitreomacular adhesion, unspecified eye   🅐

  H43.89 Other disorders of vitreous body

  H43.9 Unspecified disorder of vitreous body

√4ᵗʰ **H44** Disorders of globe
    INCLUDES   disorders affecting multiple structures of eye

  √5ᵗʰ **H44.0** Purulent endophthalmitis
    Use additional code to identify organism
    EXCLUDES 1   bleb associated endophthalmitis (H59.4-)

    √6ᵗʰ **H44.00** Unspecified purulent endophthalmitis
      H44.001 Unspecified purulent endophthalmitis, right eye
      H44.002 Unspecified purulent endophthalmitis, left eye
      H44.003 Unspecified purulent endophthalmitis, bilateral
      H44.009 Unspecified purulent endophthalmitis, unspecified eye

    √6ᵗʰ **H44.01** Panophthalmitis (acute)
      H44.011 Panophthalmitis (acute), right eye
      H44.012 Panophthalmitis (acute), left eye
      H44.013 Panophthalmitis (acute), bilateral
      H44.019 Panophthalmitis (acute), unspecified eye

    √6ᵗʰ **H44.02** Vitreous abscess (chronic)
      H44.021 Vitreous abscess (chronic), right eye
      H44.022 Vitreous abscess (chronic), left eye
      H44.023 Vitreous abscess (chronic), bilateral
      H44.029 Vitreous abscess (chronic), unspecified eye

  √5ᵗʰ **H44.1** Other endophthalmitis
    EXCLUDES 1   bleb associated endophthalmitis (H59.4-)
    EXCLUDES 2   ophthalmia nodosa (H16.2-)

    √6ᵗʰ **H44.11** Panuveitis
      H44.111 Panuveitis, right eye
      H44.112 Panuveitis, left eye
      H44.113 Panuveitis, bilateral
      H44.119 Panuveitis, unspecified eye

    √6ᵗʰ **H44.12** Parasitic endophthalmitis, unspecified
      H44.121 Parasitic endophthalmitis, unspecified, right eye
      H44.122 Parasitic endophthalmitis, unspecified, left eye
      H44.123 Parasitic endophthalmitis, unspecified, bilateral

      H44.129 Parasitic endophthalmitis, unspecified, unspecified eye

    √6ᵗʰ **H44.13** Sympathetic uveitis
      H44.131 Sympathetic uveitis, right eye
      H44.132 Sympathetic uveitis, left eye
      H44.133 Sympathetic uveitis, bilateral
      H44.139 Sympathetic uveitis, unspecified eye

    H44.19 Other endophthalmitis

  √5ᵗʰ **H44.2** Degenerative myopia
    Malignant myopia
    H44.20 Degenerative myopia, unspecified eye
    H44.21 Degenerative myopia, right eye
    H44.22 Degenerative myopia, left eye
    H44.23 Degenerative myopia, bilateral

  √5ᵗʰ **H44.3** Other and unspecified degenerative disorders of globe
    H44.30 Unspecified degenerative disorder of globe

    √6ᵗʰ **H44.31** Chalcosis
      H44.311 Chalcosis, right eye
      H44.312 Chalcosis, left eye
      H44.313 Chalcosis, bilateral
      H44.319 Chalcosis, unspecified eye

    √6ᵗʰ **H44.32** Siderosis of eye
      H44.321 Siderosis of eye, right eye
      H44.322 Siderosis of eye, left eye
      H44.323 Siderosis of eye, bilateral
      H44.329 Siderosis of eye, unspecified eye

    √6ᵗʰ **H44.39** Other degenerative disorders of globe
      H44.391 Other degenerative disorders of globe, right eye
      H44.392 Other degenerative disorders of globe, left eye
      H44.393 Other degenerative disorders of globe, bilateral
      H44.399 Other degenerative disorders of globe, unspecified eye

  √5ᵗʰ **H44.4** Hypotony of eye
    H44.40 Unspecified hypotony of eye

    √6ᵗʰ **H44.41** Flat anterior chamber hypotony of eye
      H44.411 Flat anterior chamber hypotony of right eye
      H44.412 Flat anterior chamber hypotony of left eye
      H44.413 Flat anterior chamber hypotony of eye, bilateral
      H44.419 Flat anterior chamber hypotony of unspecified eye

    √6ᵗʰ **H44.42** Hypotony of eye due to ocular fistula
      H44.421 Hypotony of right eye due to ocular fistula
      H44.422 Hypotony of left eye due to ocular fistula
      H44.423 Hypotony of eye due to ocular fistula, bilateral
      H44.429 Hypotony of unspecified eye due to ocular fistula

    √6ᵗʰ **H44.43** Hypotony of eye due to other ocular disorders
      H44.431 Hypotony of eye due to other ocular disorders, right eye
      H44.432 Hypotony of eye due to other ocular disorders, left eye
      H44.433 Hypotony of eye due to other ocular disorders, bilateral
      H44.439 Hypotony of eye due to other ocular disorders, unspecified eye

    √6ᵗʰ **H44.44** Primary hypotony of eye
      H44.441 Primary hypotony of right eye
      H44.442 Primary hypotony of left eye
      H44.443 Primary hypotony of eye, bilateral
      H44.449 Primary hypotony of unspecified eye

  √5ᵗʰ **H44.5** Degenerated conditions of globe
    H44.50 Unspecified degenerated conditions of globe

    √6ᵗʰ **H44.51** Absolute glaucoma
      H44.511 Absolute glaucoma, right eye
      H44.512 Absolute glaucoma, left eye
      H44.513 Absolute glaucoma, bilateral
      H44.519 Absolute glaucoma, unspecified eye

Diseases of the Eye and Adnexa

H44.52–H44.749

√6th **H44.52 Atrophy of globe**
Phthisis bulbi
H44.521 Atrophy of globe, right **eye**
H44.522 Atrophy of globe, left **eye**
H44.523 Atrophy of globe, bilateral
H44.529 Atrophy of globe, unspecified eye

√6th **H44.53 Leucocoria**
H44.531 Leucocoria, right **eye**
H44.532 Leucocoria, left **eye**
H44.533 Leucocoria, bilateral
H44.539 Leucocoria, unspecified eye

√5th **H44.6 Retained (old) intraocular foreign body,** magnetic
Use additional code to identify magnetic foreign body (Z18.11)
EXCLUDES 1 *current intraocular foreign body (S05.-)*
EXCLUDES 2 *retained foreign body in eyelid (H02.81-)*
retained (old) foreign body following penetrating wound of orbit (H05.5-)
retained (old) intraocular foreign body, nonmagnetic (H44.7-)

√6th **H44.60** Unspecified **retained (old) intraocular foreign body, magnetic**
H44.601 Unspecified retained (old) intraocular foreign body, magnetic, right **eye**
H44.602 Unspecified retained (old) intraocular foreign body, magnetic, left **eye**
H44.603 Unspecified retained (old) intraocular foreign body, magnetic, bilateral
H44.609 Unspecified retained (old) intraocular foreign body, magnetic, unspecified eye

√6th **H44.61 Retained (old) magnetic foreign body in** anterior chamber
H44.611 Retained (old) magnetic foreign body in anterior chamber, right **eye**
H44.612 Retained (old) magnetic foreign body in anterior chamber, left **eye**
H44.613 Retained (old) magnetic foreign body in anterior chamber, bilateral
H44.619 Retained (old) magnetic foreign body in anterior chamber, unspecified eye

√6th **H44.62 Retained (old) magnetic foreign body in** iris or ciliary body
H44.621 Retained (old) magnetic foreign body in iris or ciliary body, right **eye**
H44.622 Retained (old) magnetic foreign body in iris or ciliary body, left **eye**
H44.623 Retained (old) magnetic foreign body in iris or ciliary body, bilateral
H44.629 Retained (old) magnetic foreign body in iris or ciliary body, unspecified eye

√6th **H44.63 Retained (old) magnetic foreign body in** lens
H44.631 Retained (old) magnetic foreign body in lens, right **eye**
H44.632 Retained (old) magnetic foreign body in lens, left **eye**
H44.633 Retained (old) magnetic foreign body in lens, bilateral
H44.639 Retained (old) magnetic foreign body in lens, unspecified eye

√6th **H44.64 Retained (old) magnetic foreign body in** posterior wall of globe
H44.641 Retained (old) magnetic foreign body in posterior wall of globe, right **eye**
H44.642 Retained (old) magnetic foreign body in posterior wall of globe, left **eye**
H44.643 Retained (old) magnetic foreign body in posterior wall of globe, bilateral
H44.649 Retained (old) magnetic foreign body in posterior wall of globe, unspecified eye

√6th **H44.65 Retained (old) magnetic foreign body in** vitreous body
H44.651 Retained (old) magnetic foreign body in vitreous body, right **eye**
H44.652 Retained (old) magnetic foreign body in vitreous body, left **eye**
H44.653 Retained (old) magnetic foreign body in vitreous body, bilateral

H44.659 Retained (old) magnetic foreign body in vitreous body, unspecified eye

√6th **H44.69 Retained (old) intraocular foreign body, magnetic, in** other or multiple sites
H44.691 Retained (old) intraocular foreign body, magnetic, in other or multiple sites, right **eye**
H44.692 Retained (old) intraocular foreign body, magnetic, in other or multiple sites, left **eye**
H44.693 Retained (old) intraocular foreign body, magnetic, in other or multiple sites, bilateral
H44.699 Retained (old) intraocular foreign body, magnetic, in other or multiple sites, unspecified eye

√5th **H44.7 Retained (old) intraocular foreign body,** nonmagnetic
Use additional code to identify nonmagnetic foreign body (Z18.01-Z18.10, Z18.12, Z18.2-Z18.9)
EXCLUDES 1 *current intraocular foreign body (S05.-)*
EXCLUDES 2 *retained foreign body in eyelid (H02.81-)*
retained (old) foreign body following penetrating wound of orbit (H05.5-)
retained (old) intraocular foreign body, magnetic (H44.6-)

√6th **H44.70** Unspecified **retained (old) intraocular foreign body, nonmagnetic**
H44.701 Unspecified retained (old) intraocular foreign body, nonmagnetic, right **eye**
H44.702 Unspecified retained (old) intraocular foreign body, nonmagnetic, left **eye**
H44.703 Unspecified retained (old) intraocular foreign body, nonmagnetic, bilateral
H44.709 Unspecified retained (old) intraocular foreign body, nonmagnetic, unspecified eye
Retained (old) intraocular foreign body NOS

√6th **H44.71 Retained (nonmagnetic) (old) foreign body in** anterior chamber
H44.711 Retained (nonmagnetic) (old) foreign body in anterior chamber, right **eye**
H44.712 Retained (nonmagnetic) (old) foreign body in anterior chamber, left **eye**
H44.713 Retained (nonmagnetic) (old) foreign body in anterior chamber, bilateral
H44.719 Retained (nonmagnetic) (old) foreign body in anterior chamber, unspecified eye

√6th **H44.72 Retained (nonmagnetic) (old) foreign body in** iris or ciliary body
H44.721 Retained (nonmagnetic) (old) foreign body in iris or ciliary body, right **eye**
H44.722 Retained (nonmagnetic) (old) foreign body in iris or ciliary body, left **eye**
H44.723 Retained (nonmagnetic) (old) foreign body in iris or ciliary body, bilateral
H44.729 Retained (nonmagnetic) (old) foreign body in iris or ciliary body, unspecified eye

√6th **H44.73 Retained (nonmagnetic) (old) foreign body in** lens
H44.731 Retained (nonmagnetic) (old) foreign body in lens, right **eye**
H44.732 Retained (nonmagnetic) (old) foreign body in lens, left **eye**
H44.733 Retained (nonmagnetic) (old) foreign body in lens, bilateral
H44.739 Retained (nonmagnetic) (old) foreign body in lens, unspecified eye

√6th **H44.74 Retained (nonmagnetic) (old) foreign body in** posterior wall of globe
H44.741 Retained (nonmagnetic) (old) foreign body in posterior wall of globe, right **eye**
H44.742 Retained (nonmagnetic) (old) foreign body in posterior wall of globe, left **eye**
H44.743 Retained (nonmagnetic) (old) foreign body in posterior wall of globe, bilateral
H44.749 Retained (nonmagnetic) (old) foreign body in posterior wall of globe, unspecified eye

EXCLUDES 1 Not coded here   EXCLUDES 2 Not included here   N Newborn Age: 0   P Pediatric Age: 0-17   M Maternity Age: 12-55   A Adult Age: 15-124

552   ICD-10-CM Draft (2015)

√6ᵗʰ **H44.75** Retained (nonmagnetic) (old) foreign body in vitreous body

    H44.751 Retained (nonmagnetic) (old) foreign body in vitreous body, right eye

    H44.752 Retained (nonmagnetic) (old) foreign body in vitreous body, left eye

    H44.753 Retained (nonmagnetic) (old) foreign body in vitreous body, bilateral

    H44.759 Retained (nonmagnetic) (old) foreign body in vitreous body, unspecified eye

√6ᵗʰ **H44.79** Retained (old) intraocular foreign body, nonmagnetic, in other or multiple sites

    H44.791 Retained (old) intraocular foreign body, nonmagnetic, in other or multiple sites, right eye

    H44.792 Retained (old) intraocular foreign body, nonmagnetic, in other or multiple sites, left eye

    H44.793 Retained (old) intraocular foreign body, nonmagnetic, in other or multiple sites, bilateral

    H44.799 Retained (old) intraocular foreign body, nonmagnetic, in other or multiple sites, unspecified eye

√5ᵗʰ **H44.8** Other disorders of globe

  √6ᵗʰ **H44.81** Hemophthalmos

    H44.811 Hemophthalmos, right eye

    H44.812 Hemophthalmos, left eye

    H44.813 Hemophthalmos, bilateral

    H44.819 Hemophthalmos, unspecified eye

  √6ᵗʰ **H44.82** Luxation of globe

    H44.821 Luxation of globe, right eye

    H44.822 Luxation of globe, left eye

    H44.823 Luxation of globe, bilateral

    H44.829 Luxation of globe, unspecified eye

  H44.89 Other disorders of globe

 H44.9 Unspecified disorder of globe

Disorders of optic nerve and visual pathways (H46-H47)

√4ᵗʰ **H46** Optic neuritis

  EXCLUDES 2   ischemic optic neuropathy (H47.01-)
            neuromyelitis optica [Devic] (G36.0)

 √5ᵗʰ **H46.0** Optic papillitis

    H46.00 Optic papillitis, unspecified eye

    H46.01 Optic papillitis, right eye

    H46.02 Optic papillitis, left eye

    H46.03 Optic papillitis, bilateral

 √5ᵗʰ **H46.1** Retrobulbar neuritis

    Retrobulbar neuritis NOS

    EXCLUDES 1   syphilitic retrobulbar neuritis (A52.15)

    H46.10 Retrobulbar neuritis, unspecified eye

    H46.11 Retrobulbar neuritis, right eye

    H46.12 Retrobulbar neuritis, left eye

    H46.13 Retrobulbar neuritis, bilateral

 H46.2 Nutritional optic neuropathy

 H46.3 Toxic optic neuropathy

    Code first (T51-T65) to identify cause

 H46.8 Other optic neuritis

 H46.9 Unspecified optic neuritis

√4ᵗʰ **H47** Other disorders of optic [2nd] nerve and visual pathways

 √5ᵗʰ **H47.0** Disorders of optic nerve, not elsewhere classified

  √6ᵗʰ **H47.01** Ischemic optic neuropathy

    H47.011 Ischemic optic neuropathy, right eye

    H47.012 Ischemic optic neuropathy, left eye

    H47.013 Ischemic optic neuropathy, bilateral

    H47.019 Ischemic optic neuropathy, unspecified eye

  √6ᵗʰ **H47.02** Hemorrhage in optic nerve sheath

    H47.021 Hemorrhage in optic nerve sheath, right eye

    H47.022 Hemorrhage in optic nerve sheath, left eye

    H47.023 Hemorrhage in optic nerve sheath, bilateral

    H47.029 Hemorrhage in optic nerve sheath, unspecified eye

  √6ᵗʰ **H47.03** Optic nerve hypoplasia

    H47.031 Optic nerve hypoplasia, right eye

    H47.032 Optic nerve hypoplasia, left eye

    H47.033 Optic nerve hypoplasia, bilateral

    H47.039 Optic nerve hypoplasia, unspecified eye

  √6ᵗʰ **H47.09** Other disorders of optic nerve, not elsewhere classified

    Compression of optic nerve

    H47.091 Other disorders of optic nerve, not elsewhere classified, right eye

    H47.092 Other disorders of optic nerve, not elsewhere classified, left eye

    H47.093 Other disorders of optic nerve, not elsewhere classified, bilateral

    H47.099 Other disorders of optic nerve, not elsewhere classified, unspecified eye

√5ᵗʰ **H47.1** Papilledema

  H47.10 Unspecified papilledema

  H47.11 Papilledema associated with increased intracranial pressure

  H47.12 Papilledema associated with decreased ocular pressure

  H47.13 Papilledema associated with retinal disorder

 √6ᵗʰ **H47.14** Foster-Kennedy syndrome

    H47.141 Foster-Kennedy syndrome, right eye

    H47.142 Foster-Kennedy syndrome, left eye

    H47.143 Foster-Kennedy syndrome, bilateral

    H47.149 Foster-Kennedy syndrome, unspecified eye

√5ᵗʰ **H47.2** Optic atrophy

  H47.20 Unspecified optic atrophy

 √6ᵗʰ **H47.21** Primary optic atrophy

    H47.211 Primary optic atrophy, right eye

    H47.212 Primary optic atrophy, left eye

    H47.213 Primary optic atrophy, bilateral

    H47.219 Primary optic atrophy, unspecified eye

  H47.22 Hereditary optic atrophy

    Leber's optic atrophy

 √6ᵗʰ **H47.23** Glaucomatous optic atrophy

    H47.231 Glaucomatous optic atrophy, right eye

    H47.232 Glaucomatous optic atrophy, left eye

    H47.233 Glaucomatous optic atrophy, bilateral

    H47.239 Glaucomatous optic atrophy, unspecified eye

 √6ᵗʰ **H47.29** Other optic atrophy

    Temporal pallor of optic disc

    H47.291 Other optic atrophy, right eye

    H47.292 Other optic atrophy, left eye

    H47.293 Other optic atrophy, bilateral

    H47.299 Other optic atrophy, unspecified eye

√5ᵗʰ **H47.3** Other disorders of optic disc

 √6ᵗʰ **H47.31** Coloboma of optic disc

    H47.311 Coloboma of optic disc, right eye

    H47.312 Coloboma of optic disc, left eye

    H47.313 Coloboma of optic disc, bilateral

    H47.319 Coloboma of optic disc, unspecified eye

 √6ᵗʰ **H47.32** Drusen of optic disc

    H47.321 Drusen of optic disc, right eye

    H47.322 Drusen of optic disc, left eye

    H47.323 Drusen of optic disc, bilateral

    H47.329 Drusen of optic disc, unspecified eye

 √6ᵗʰ **H47.33** Pseudopapilledema of optic disc

    H47.331 Pseudopapilledema of optic disc, right eye

    H47.332 Pseudopapilledema of optic disc, left eye

    H47.333 Pseudopapilledema of optic disc, bilateral

    H47.339 Pseudopapilledema of optic disc, unspecified eye

 √6ᵗʰ **H47.39** Other disorders of optic disc

    H47.391 Other disorders of optic disc, right eye

    H47.392 Other disorders of optic disc, left eye

    H47.393 Other disorders of optic disc, bilateral

☑ Additional Character Required   √x7ᵗʰ Xtension Alert   Unspecified Dx   Other Specified Dx   Manifestation   ►◄ Revised Text   ● New Code   ▲ Revised Code Title

Diseases of the Eye and Adnexa

H47.399–H50.032

     H47.399   **Other disorders of optic disc, unspecified eye**

✓5th **H47.4 Disorders of optic chiasm**
       Code also underlying condition

     H47.41   **Disorders of optic chiasm in (due to)** inflammatory disorders

     H47.42   **Disorders of optic chiasm in (due to)** neoplasm

     H47.43   **Disorders of optic chiasm in (due to)** vascular disorders

     H47.49   **Disorders of optic chiasm in (due to) other** disorders

✓5th **H47.5 Disorders of other visual pathways**
       Disorders of optic tracts, geniculate nuclei and optic radiations
       Code also underlying condition

     ✓6th H47.51   **Disorders of visual pathways in (due to)** inflammatory disorders

       H47.511   **Disorders of visual pathways in (due to) inflammatory disorders, right side**

       H47.512   **Disorders of visual pathways in (due to) inflammatory disorders, left side**

       H47.519   **Disorders of visual pathways in (due to) inflammatory disorders, unspecified side**

     ✓6th H47.52   **Disorders of visual pathways in (due to)** neoplasm

       H47.521   **Disorders of visual pathways in (due to) neoplasm, right side**

       H47.522   **Disorders of visual pathways in (due to) neoplasm, left side**

       H47.529   **Disorders of visual pathways in (due to) neoplasm, unspecified side**

     ✓6th H47.53   **Disorders of visual pathways in (due to)** vascular disorders

       H47.531   **Disorders of visual pathways in (due to) vascular disorders, right side**

       H47.532   **Disorders of visual pathways in (due to) vascular disorders, left side**

       H47.539   **Disorders of visual pathways in (due to) vascular disorders, unspecified side**

✓5th **H47.6 Disorders of visual cortex**
       Code also underlying condition
       EXCLUDES 1   injury to visual cortex S04.04

     ✓6th H47.61   Cortical blindness

       H47.611   **Cortical blindness, right side of brain**

       H47.612   **Cortical blindness, left side of brain**

       H47.619   **Cortical blindness, unspecified side of brain**

     ✓6th H47.62   **Disorders of visual cortex in (due to)** inflammatory disorders

       H47.621   **Disorders of visual cortex in (due to) inflammatory disorders, right side of brain**

       H47.622   **Disorders of visual cortex in (due to) inflammatory disorders, left side of brain**

       H47.629   **Disorders of visual cortex in (due to) inflammatory disorders, unspecified side of brain**

     ✓6th H47.63   **Disorders of visual cortex in (due to)** neoplasm

       H47.631   **Disorders of visual cortex in (due to) neoplasm, right side of brain**

       H47.632   **Disorders of visual cortex in (due to) neoplasm, left side of brain**

       H47.639   **Disorders of visual cortex in (due to) neoplasm, unspecified side of brain**

     ✓6th H47.64   **Disorders of visual cortex in (due to)** vascular disorders

       H47.641   **Disorders of visual cortex in (due to) vascular disorders, right side of brain**

       H47.642   **Disorders of visual cortex in (due to) vascular disorders, left side of brain**

       H47.649   **Disorders of visual cortex in (due to) vascular disorders, unspecified side of brain**

   H47.9   **Unspecified disorder of visual pathways**

Disorders of ocular muscles, binocular movement, accommodation and refraction (H49-H52)

     EXCLUDES 2   nystagmus and other irregular eye movements (H55)

✓4th **H49 Paralytic strabismus**
     EXCLUDES 2   internal ophthalmoplegia (H52.51-)
             internuclear ophthalmoplegia (H51.2-)
             progressive supranuclear ophthalmoplegia (G23.1)

   ✓5th H49.0   Third [oculomotor] nerve palsy

     H49.00   **Third [oculomotor] nerve palsy, unspecified eye**

     H49.01   **Third [oculomotor] nerve palsy, right eye**

     H49.02   **Third [oculomotor] nerve palsy, left eye**

     H49.03   **Third [oculomotor] nerve palsy, bilateral**

   ✓5th H49.1   Fourth [trochlear] nerve palsy

     H49.10   **Fourth [trochlear] nerve palsy, unspecified eye**

     H49.11   **Fourth [trochlear] nerve palsy, right eye**

     H49.12   **Fourth [trochlear] nerve palsy, left eye**

     H49.13   **Fourth [trochlear] nerve palsy, bilateral**

   ✓5th H49.2   Sixth [abducent] nerve palsy

     H49.20   **Sixth [abducent] nerve palsy, unspecified eye**

     H49.21   **Sixth [abducent] nerve palsy, right eye**

     H49.22   **Sixth [abducent] nerve palsy, left eye**

     H49.23   **Sixth [abducent] nerve palsy, bilateral**

   ✓5th H49.3   Total (external) ophthalmoplegia

     H49.30   **Total (external) ophthalmoplegia, unspecified eye**

     H49.31   **Total (external) ophthalmoplegia, right eye**

     H49.32   **Total (external) ophthalmoplegia, left eye**

     H49.33   **Total (external) ophthalmoplegia, bilateral**

   ✓5th H49.4   Progressive external ophthalmoplegia
     EXCLUDES 1   Kearns-Sayre syndrome (H49.81-)

     H49.40   **Progressive external ophthalmoplegia, unspecified eye**

     H49.41   **Progressive external ophthalmoplegia, right eye**

     H49.42   **Progressive external ophthalmoplegia, left eye**

     H49.43   **Progressive external ophthalmoplegia, bilateral**

   ✓5th H49.8   Other paralytic strabismus

     ✓6th H49.81   Kearns-Sayre syndrome
         Progressive external ophthalmoplegia with pigmentary retinopathy
         Use additional code for other manifestation, such as: heart block (I45.9)

       H49.811   **Kearns-Sayre syndrome, right eye**

       H49.812   **Kearns-Sayre syndrome, left eye**

       H49.813   **Kearns-Sayre syndrome, bilateral**

       H49.819   **Kearns-Sayre syndrome, unspecified eye**

     ✓6th H49.88   **Other paralytic strabismus**
         External ophthalmoplegia NOS

       H49.881   **Other paralytic strabismus, right eye**

       H49.882   **Other paralytic strabismus, left eye**

       H49.883   **Other paralytic strabismus, bilateral**

       H49.889   **Other paralytic strabismus, unspecified eye**

   H49.9   **Unspecified paralytic strabismus**

✓4th **H50 Other strabismus**

   ✓5th H50.0   Esotropia
       Convergent concomitant strabismus
       EXCLUDES 1   intermittent esotropia (H50.31-, H50.32)

     H50.00   **Unspecified esotropia**

     ✓6th H50.01   Monocular esotropia

       H50.011   **Monocular esotropia, right eye**

       H50.012   **Monocular esotropia, left eye**

     ✓6th H50.02   **Monocular esotropia with** A pattern

       H50.021   **Monocular esotropia with A pattern, right eye**

       H50.022   **Monocular esotropia with A pattern, left eye**

     ✓6th H50.03   **Monocular esotropia with** V pattern

       H50.031   **Monocular esotropia with V pattern, right eye**

       H50.032   **Monocular esotropia with V pattern, left eye**

EXCLUDES 1 Not coded here   EXCLUDES 2 Not included here   N Newborn Age: 0   P Pediatric Age: 0-17   M Maternity Age: 12-55   A Adult Age: 15-124

554   ICD-10-CM Draft (2015)

✓6th **H50.04 Monocular esotropia with** other noncomitancies
 H50.041 Monocular esotropia with other noncomitancies, right **eye**
 H50.042 Monocular esotropia with other noncomitancies, left **eye**
 H50.05 Alternating **esotropia**
 H50.06 Alternating esotropia with A **pattern**
 H50.07 Alternating esotropia with V **pattern**
 H50.08 Alternating esotropia with other noncomitancies

✓5th **H50.1 Exotropia**
 Divergent concomitant strabismus
 EXCLUDES 1 intermittent exotropia (H50.33-, H50.34)
 H50.10 Unspecified exotropia
✓6th **H50.11** Monocular **exotropia**
 H50.111 Monocular exotropia, right **eye**
 H50.112 Monocular exotropia, left **eye**
✓6th **H50.12 Monocular exotropia with** A **pattern**
 H50.121 Monocular exotropia with A pattern, right **eye**
 H50.122 Monocular exotropia with A pattern, left **eye**
✓6th **H50.13 Monocular exotropia with** V **pattern**
 H50.131 Monocular exotropia with V pattern, right **eye**
 H50.132 Monocular exotropia with V pattern, left **eye**
✓6th **H50.14 Monocular exotropia with** other noncomitancies
 H50.141 Monocular exotropia with other noncomitancies, right **eye**
 H50.142 Monocular exotropia with other noncomitancies, left **eye**
 H50.15 Alternating **exotropia**
 H50.16 Alternating exotropia with A **pattern**
 H50.17 Alternating exotropia with V **pattern**
 H50.18 Alternating exotropia with other noncomitancies

✓5th **H50.2 Vertical strabismus**
 Hypertropia
 H50.21 Vertical strabismus, right **eye**
 H50.22 Vertical strabismus, left **eye**

✓5th **H50.3 Intermittent heterotropia**
 H50.30 Unspecified intermittent heterotropia
✓6th **H50.31 Intermittent** monocular esotropia
 H50.311 Intermittent monocular esotropia, right **eye**
 H50.312 Intermittent monocular esotropia, left **eye**
 H50.32 Intermittent alternating **esotropia**
✓6th **H50.33 Intermittent** monocular exotropia
 H50.331 Intermittent monocular exotropia, right **eye**
 H50.332 Intermittent monocular exotropia, left **eye**
 H50.34 Intermittent alternating **exotropia**

✓5th **H50.4 Other and unspecified heterotropia**
 H50.40 Unspecified heterotropia
✓6th **H50.41** Cyclotropia
 H50.411 Cyclotropia, right **eye**
 H50.412 Cyclotropia, left **eye**
 H50.42 Monofixation **syndrome**
 H50.43 Accommodative component in esotropia

✓5th **H50.5 Heterophoria**
 H50.50 Unspecified heterophoria
 H50.51 Esophoria
 H50.52 Exophoria
 H50.53 Vertical **heterophoria**
 H50.54 Cyclophoria
 H50.55 Alternating **heterophoria**

✓5th **H50.6 Mechanical strabismus**
 H50.60 Mechanical strabismus, unspecified
✓6th **H50.61** Brown's sheath **syndrome**
 H50.611 Brown's sheath syndrome, right **eye**
 H50.612 Brown's sheath syndrome, left **eye**

 H50.69 Other mechanical strabismus
 Strabismus due to adhesions
 Traumatic limitation of duction of eye muscle
✓5th **H50.8 Other specified strabismus**
✓6th **H50.81 Duane's syndrome**
 H50.811 Duane's syndrome, right **eye**
 H50.812 Duane's syndrome, left **eye**
 H50.89 Other specified strabismus
 H50.9 Unspecified strabismus

✓4th **H51 Other disorders of binocular movement**
 H51.0 Palsy (spasm) of conjugate gaze
✓5th **H51.1 Convergence insufficiency and excess**
 H51.11 Convergence insufficiency
 H51.12 Convergence excess
✓5th **H51.2 Internuclear ophthalmoplegia**
 H51.20 Internuclear ophthalmoplegia, unspecified eye
 H51.21 Internuclear ophthalmoplegia, right **eye**
 H51.22 Internuclear ophthalmoplegia, left **eye**
 H51.23 Internuclear ophthalmoplegia, bilateral
 H51.8 Other specified disorders of binocular movement
 H51.9 Unspecified disorder of binocular movement

✓4th **H52 Disorders of refraction and accommodation**
✓5th **H52.0 Hypermetropia**
 H52.00 Hypermetropia, unspecified eye
 H52.01 Hypermetropia, right **eye**
 H52.02 Hypermetropia, left **eye**
 H52.03 Hypermetropia, bilateral
✓5th **H52.1 Myopia**
 EXCLUDES 1 degenerative myopia (H44.2-)
 H52.10 Myopia, unspecified eye
 H52.11 Myopia, right **eye**
 H52.12 Myopia, left **eye**
 H52.13 Myopia, bilateral
✓5th **H52.2 Astigmatism**
✓6th **H52.20** Unspecified **astigmatism**
 H52.201 Unspecified astigmatism, right **eye**
 H52.202 Unspecified astigmatism, left **eye**
 H52.203 Unspecified astigmatism, bilateral
 H52.209 Unspecified astigmatism, unspecified eye
✓6th **H52.21** Irregular **astigmatism**
 H52.211 Irregular astigmatism, right **eye**
 H52.212 Irregular astigmatism, left **eye**
 H52.213 Irregular astigmatism, bilateral
 H52.219 Irregular astigmatism, unspecified eye
✓6th **H52.22** Regular **astigmatism**
 H52.221 Regular astigmatism, right **eye**
 H52.222 Regular astigmatism, left **eye**
 H52.223 Regular astigmatism, bilateral
 H52.229 Regular astigmatism, unspecified eye
✓5th **H52.3 Anisometropia and aniseikonia**
 H52.31 Anisometropia
 H52.32 Aniseikonia
 H52.4 Presbyopia
✓5th **H52.5 Disorders of accommodation**
✓6th **H52.51** Internal ophthalmoplegia (complete) (total)
 H52.511 Internal ophthalmoplegia (complete) (total), right **eye**
 H52.512 Internal ophthalmoplegia (complete) (total), left **eye**
 H52.513 Internal ophthalmoplegia (complete) (total), bilateral
 H52.519 Internal ophthalmoplegia (complete) (total), unspecified eye
✓6th **H52.52** Paresis **of accommodation**
 H52.521 Paresis of accommodation, right **eye**
 H52.522 Paresis of accommodation, left **eye**
 H52.523 Paresis of accommodation, bilateral
 H52.529 Paresis of accommodation, unspecified eye

✔ Additional Character Required ✓x7th Xtension Alert Unspecified Dx Other Specified Dx Manifestation ►◄ Revised Text ● New Code ▲ Revised Code Title

✓6ᵗʰ **H52.53** Spasm of accommodation
    H52.531 Spasm of accommodation, right eye
    H52.532 Spasm of accommodation, left eye
    H52.533 Spasm of accommodation, bilateral
    H52.539 Spasm of accommodation, unspecified eye

H52.6 Other disorders of refraction
H52.7 Unspecified disorder of refraction

Visual disturbances and blindness (H53-H54)

✓4ᵗʰ **H53** Visual disturbances

✓5ᵗʰ **H53.0** Amblyopia ex anopsia
    EXCLUDES 1   amblyopia due to vitamin A deficiency (E50.5)

✓6ᵗʰ **H53.00** Unspecified amblyopia
    H53.001 Unspecified amblyopia, right eye
    H53.002 Unspecified amblyopia, left eye
    H53.003 Unspecified amblyopia, bilateral
    H53.009 Unspecified amblyopia, unspecified eye

✓6ᵗʰ **H53.01** Deprivation amblyopia
    H53.011 Deprivation amblyopia, right eye
    H53.012 Deprivation amblyopia, left eye
    H53.013 Deprivation amblyopia, bilateral
    H53.019 Deprivation amblyopia, unspecified eye

✓6ᵗʰ **H53.02** Refractive amblyopia
    H53.021 Refractive amblyopia, right eye
    H53.022 Refractive amblyopia, left eye
    H53.023 Refractive amblyopia, bilateral
    H53.029 Refractive amblyopia, unspecified eye

✓6ᵗʰ **H53.03** Strabismic amblyopia
    EXCLUDES 1   strabismus (H50.-)
    H53.031 Strabismic amblyopia, right eye
    H53.032 Strabismic amblyopia, left eye
    H53.033 Strabismic amblyopia, bilateral
    H53.039 Strabismic amblyopia, unspecified eye

✓5ᵗʰ **H53.1** Subjective visual disturbances
    EXCLUDES 1   subjective visual disturbances due to vitamin A deficiency (E50.5)
          visual hallucinations (R44.1)

    H53.10 Unspecified subjective visual disturbances
    H53.11 Day blindness
         Hemeralopia

✓6ᵗʰ **H53.12** Transient visual loss
         Scintillating scotoma
    EXCLUDES 1   amaurosis fugax (G45.3-)
          transient retinal artery occlusion (H34.0-)
    H53.121 Transient visual loss, right eye
    H53.122 Transient visual loss, left eye
    H53.123 Transient visual loss, bilateral
    H53.129 Transient visual loss, unspecified eye

✓6ᵗʰ **H53.13** Sudden visual loss
    H53.131 Sudden visual loss, right eye
    H53.132 Sudden visual loss, left eye
    H53.133 Sudden visual loss, bilateral
    H53.139 Sudden visual loss, unspecified eye

✓6ᵗʰ **H53.14** Visual discomfort
         Asthenopia
         Photophobia
    H53.141 Visual discomfort, right eye
    H53.142 Visual discomfort, left eye
    H53.143 Visual discomfort, bilateral
    H53.149 Visual discomfort, unspecified
    H53.15 Visual distortions of shape and size
         Metamorphopsia
    H53.16 Psychophysical visual disturbances
    H53.19 Other subjective visual disturbances
         Visual halos

H53.2 Diplopia
     Double vision

✓5ᵗʰ **H53.3** Other and unspecified disorders of binocular vision
    H53.30 Unspecified disorder of binocular vision
    H53.31 Abnormal retinal correspondence
    H53.32 Fusion with defective stereopsis
    H53.33 Simultaneous visual perception without fusion

    H53.34 Suppression of binocular vision

✓5ᵗʰ **H53.4** Visual field defects
    H53.40 Unspecified visual field defects

✓6ᵗʰ **H53.41** Scotoma involving central area
         Central scotoma
    H53.411 Scotoma involving central area, right eye
    H53.412 Scotoma involving central area, left eye
    H53.413 Scotoma involving central area, bilateral
    H53.419 Scotoma involving central area, unspecified eye

✓6ᵗʰ **H53.42** Scotoma of blind spot area
         Enlarged blind spot
    H53.421 Scotoma of blind spot area, right eye
    H53.422 Scotoma of blind spot area, left eye
    H53.423 Scotoma of blind spot area, bilateral
    H53.429 Scotoma of blind spot area, unspecified eye

✓6ᵗʰ **H53.43** Sector or arcuate defects
         Arcuate scotoma
         Bjerrum scotoma
    H53.431 Sector or arcuate defects, right eye
    H53.432 Sector or arcuate defects, left eye
    H53.433 Sector or arcuate defects, bilateral
    H53.439 Sector or arcuate defects, unspecified eye

✓6ᵗʰ **H53.45** Other localized visual field defect
         Peripheral visual field defect
         Ring scotoma NOS
         Scotoma NOS
    H53.451 Other localized visual field defect, right eye
    H53.452 Other localized visual field defect, left eye
    H53.453 Other localized visual field defect, bilateral
    H53.459 Other localized visual field defect, unspecified eye

✓6ᵗʰ **H53.46** Homonymous bilateral field defects
         Homonymous hemianopia
         Homonymous hemianopsia
         Quadrant anopia
         Quadrant anopsia
    H53.461 Homonymous bilateral field defects, right side
    H53.462 Homonymous bilateral field defects, left side
    H53.469 Homonymous bilateral field defects, unspecified side
         Homonymous bilateral field defects NOS
    H53.47 Heteronymous bilateral field defects
         Heteronymous hemianop(s)ia

✓6ᵗʰ **H53.48** Generalized contraction of visual field
    H53.481 Generalized contraction of visual field, right eye
    H53.482 Generalized contraction of visual field, left eye
    H53.483 Generalized contraction of visual field, bilateral
    H53.489 Generalized contraction of visual field, unspecified eye

✓5ᵗʰ **H53.5** Color vision deficiencies
         Color blindness
    EXCLUDES 2   day blindness (H53.11)
    H53.50 Unspecified color vision deficiencies
         Color blindness NOS
    H53.51 Achromatopsia
    H53.52 Acquired color vision deficiency
    H53.53 Deuteranomaly
         Deuteranopia
    H53.54 Protanomaly
         Protanopia
    H53.55 Tritanomaly
         Tritanopia
    H53.59 Other color vision deficiencies

✓5ᵗʰ **H53.6** Night blindness
    EXCLUDES 1   night blindness due to vitamin A deficiency (E50.5)
    H53.60 Unspecified night blindness
    H53.61 Abnormal dark adaptation curve

EXCLUDES 1 Not coded here   EXCLUDES 2 Not included here   N Newborn Age: 0   P Pediatric Age: 0-17   M Maternity Age: 12-55   A Adult Age: 15-124

556   ICD-10-CM Draft (2015)

H53.62   Acquired **night blindness**

H53.63   Congenital **night blindness**

H53.69   **Other night blindness**

✓5th   **H53.7 Vision** sensitivity **deficiencies**

H53.71   Glare **sensitivity**

H53.72   Impaired contrast **sensitivity**

H53.8 Other visual disturbances

H53.9 Unspecified visual disturbance

✓4th   **H54 Blindness and low vision**

> **NOTE**   For definition of visual impairment categories see table below
>
> Code first any associated underlying cause of the blindness
>
> **EXCLUDES 1**   amaurosis fugax (G45.3)

H54.0 Blindness, both eyes

Visual impairment categories 3, 4, 5 in both eyes.

✓5th   **H54.1 Blindness,** one eye, low vision other eye

Visual impairment categories 3, 4, 5 in one eye, with categories 1 or 2 in the other eye.

H54.10   **Blindness, one eye, low vision other eye, unspecified eyes**

H54.11   **Blindness,** right **eye, low vision** left **eye**

H54.12   **Blindness,** left **eye, low vision** right **eye**

H54.2 Low vision, both eyes

Visual impairment categories 1 or 2 in both eyes.

H54.3 Unqualified visual loss, both eyes

Visual impairment category 9 in both eyes.

✓5th   **H54.4 Blindness,** one eye

Visual impairment categories 3, 4, 5 in one eye [normal vision in other eye]

H54.40   **Blindness, one eye, unspecified eye**

H54.41   **Blindness,** right **eye, normal vision** left **eye**

H54.42   **Blindness,** left **eye, normal vision** right **eye**

✓5th   **H54.5 Low vision,** one eye

Visual impairment categories 1 or 2 in one eye [normal vision in other eye].

H54.50   **Low vision, one eye, unspecified eye**

H54.51   **Low vision,** right **eye, normal vision** left **eye**

H54.52   **Low vision,** left **eye, normal vision** right **eye**

✓5th   **H54.6 Unqualified visual loss,** one eye

Visual impairment category 9 in one eye [normal vision in other eye].

H54.60   **Unqualified visual loss, one eye, unspecified**

H54.61   **Unqualified visual loss,** right **eye, normal vision** left **eye**

H54.62   **Unqualified visual loss,** left **eye, normal vision** right **eye**

H54.7 Unspecified visual loss

Visual impairment category 9 NOS

H54.8 Legal blindness, as defined in USA

Blindness NOS according to USA definition

> **EXCLUDES 1**   legal blindness with specification of impairment level (H54.0-H54.7)

> **NOTE**   The following table gives a classification of severity of visual impairment recommended by a WHO Study Group on the Prevention of Blindness, Geneva, 6-10 November l972.
>
> The term "low vision" in category H54 comprises categories 1 and 2 of the table, the term "blindness" categories 3, 4 and 5, and the term "unqualified visual loss" category 9.
>
> If the extent of the visual field is taken into account, patients with a field no greater than 10 but greater than 5 around central fixation should be placed in category 3 and patients with a field no category greater than 5 around central fixation should be placed in 4, even if the central acuity is not impaired.

Category of visual impairment	Visual acuity with best possible correction	
	Maximum less than:	**Minimum equal to or better than:**
1	6/18 3/10 (0.3) 20/70	6/60 1/10 (0.1) 20/200
2	6/60 1/10 (0.1) 20/200	3/60 1/20 (0.5) 20/400
3	3/60 1/20 (0.05) 20/400	1/60 (finger counting at one meter) 1/50 (0.02) 5/300 (20/1200)
4	1/60 (finger counting at one meter) 1/50 (0.02) 5/300	Light perception
5	No light perception	
9	Undetermined or unspecified	

Other disorders of eye and adnexa (H55-H59)

✓4th   **H55 Nystagmus and other** irregular eye movements

✓5th   **H55.0 Nystagmus**

H55.00   **Unspecified nystagmus**

H55.01   Congenital **nystagmus**

H55.02   Latent **nystagmus**

H55.03   Visual deprivation **nystagmus**

H55.04   Dissociated **nystagmus**

H55.09   **Other forms of nystagmus**

✓5th   **H55.8 Other irregular eye movements**

H55.81   Saccadic **eye movements**

H55.89   **Other irregular eye movements**

✓4th   **H57 Other disorders of eye and adnexa**

✓5th   **H57.0 Anomalies of pupillary function**

H57.00   **Unspecified anomaly of pupillary function**

H57.01   **Argyll Robertson pupil, atypical**

> **EXCLUDES 1**   syphilitic Argyll Robertson pupil (A52.19)

H57.02   **Anisocoria**

H57.03   **Miosis**

H57.04   **Mydriasis**

✓6th   H57.05   **Tonic pupil**

H57.051   **Tonic pupil,** right **eye**

H57.052   **Tonic pupil,** left **eye**

H57.053   **Tonic pupil,** bilateral

H57.059   **Tonic pupil, unspecified eye**

H57.09   **Other anomalies of pupillary function**

✓5th   **H57.1 Ocular pain**

H57.10   **Ocular pain, unspecified eye**

H57.11   **Ocular pain,** right **eye**

H57.12   **Ocular pain,** left **eye**

H57.13   **Ocular pain,** bilateral

H57.8 Other specified disorders of eye and adnexa

H57.9 Unspecified disorder of eye and adnexa

✓4th   **H59 Intraoperative and postprocedural complications and disorders of eye and adnexa, not elsewhere classified**

> **EXCLUDES 1**   mechanical complication of intraocular lens (T85.2)
> mechanical complication of other ocular prosthetic devices, implants and grafts (T85.3)
> pseudophakia (Z96.1)
> secondary cataracts (H26.4-)

✓5th   **H59.0 Disorders of the eye** following cataract surgery

✓6th   H59.01   **Keratopathy (bullous aphakic) following cataract surgery**

Vitreal corneal syndrome

Vitreous (touch) syndrome

H59.011   **Keratopathy (bullous aphakic) following cataract surgery,** right **eye**

H59.012   **Keratopathy (bullous aphakic) following cataract surgery,** left **eye**

☑ Additional Character Required   ✓x7th Xtension Alert   Unspecified Dx   Other Specified Dx   Manifestation   ►◄ Revised Text   ● New Code   ▲ Revised Code Title

ICD-10-CM Draft (2015)   **557**

Diseases of the Eye and Adnexa

H59.013–H59.89

H59.013   **Keratopathy (bullous aphakic) following cataract surgery, bilateral**

H59.019   **Keratopathy (bullous aphakic) following cataract surgery, unspecified eye**

√6ᵗʰ **H59.02**   Cataract (lens) fragments in eye following cataract surgery

H59.021   **Cataract (lens) fragments in eye following cataract surgery, right eye**

H59.022   **Cataract (lens) fragments in eye following cataract surgery, left eye**

H59.023   **Cataract (lens) fragments in eye following cataract surgery, bilateral**

H59.029   **Cataract (lens) fragments in eye following cataract surgery, unspecified eye**

√6ᵗʰ **H59.03**   Cystoid macular edema following cataract surgery

H59.031   **Cystoid macular edema following cataract surgery, right eye**

H59.032   **Cystoid macular edema following cataract surgery, left eye**

H59.033   **Cystoid macular edema following cataract surgery, bilateral**

H59.039   **Cystoid macular edema following cataract surgery, unspecified eye**

√6ᵗʰ **H59.09**   Other disorders of the eye following cataract surgery

H59.091   **Other disorders of the right eye following cataract surgery**

H59.092   **Other disorders of the left eye following cataract surgery**

H59.093   **Other disorders of the eye following cataract surgery, bilateral**

H59.099   **Other disorders of unspecified eye following cataract surgery**

√5ᵗʰ **H59.1**   Intraoperative hemorrhage and hematoma of eye and adnexa complicating a procedure

> **EXCLUDES 1**   *intraoperative hemorrhage and hematoma of eye and adnexa due to accidental puncture or laceration during a procedure (H59.2-)*

√6ᵗʰ **H59.11**   Intraoperative hemorrhage and hematoma of eye and adnexa complicating an ophthalmic procedure

H59.111   **Intraoperative hemorrhage and hematoma of right eye and adnexa complicating an ophthalmic procedure**

H59.112   **Intraoperative hemorrhage and hematoma of left eye and adnexa complicating an ophthalmic procedure**

H59.113   **Intraoperative hemorrhage and hematoma of eye and adnexa complicating an ophthalmic procedure, bilateral**

H59.119   **Intraoperative hemorrhage and hematoma of unspecified eye and adnexa complicating an ophthalmic procedure**

√6ᵗʰ **H59.12**   Intraoperative hemorrhage and hematoma of eye and adnexa complicating other procedure

H59.121   **Intraoperative hemorrhage and hematoma of right eye and adnexa complicating other procedure**

H59.122   **Intraoperative hemorrhage and hematoma of left eye and adnexa complicating other procedure**

H59.123   **Intraoperative hemorrhage and hematoma of eye and adnexa complicating other procedure, bilateral**

H59.129   **Intraoperative hemorrhage and hematoma of unspecified eye and adnexa complicating other procedure**

√5ᵗʰ **H59.2**   Accidental puncture and laceration of eye and adnexa during a procedure

√6ᵗʰ **H59.21**   Accidental puncture and laceration of eye and adnexa during an ophthalmic procedure

H59.211   **Accidental puncture and laceration of right eye and adnexa during an ophthalmic procedure**

H59.212   **Accidental puncture and laceration of left eye and adnexa during an ophthalmic procedure**

H59.213   **Accidental puncture and laceration of eye and adnexa during an ophthalmic procedure, bilateral**

H59.219   **Accidental puncture and laceration of unspecified eye and adnexa during an ophthalmic procedure**

√6ᵗʰ **H59.22**   Accidental puncture and laceration of eye and adnexa during other procedure

H59.221   **Accidental puncture and laceration of right eye and adnexa during other procedure**

H59.222   **Accidental puncture and laceration of left eye and adnexa during other procedure**

H59.223   **Accidental puncture and laceration of eye and adnexa during other procedure, bilateral**

H59.229   **Accidental puncture and laceration of unspecified eye and adnexa during other procedure**

√5ᵗʰ **H59.3**   Postprocedural hemorrhage and hematoma of eye and adnexa following a procedure

√6ᵗʰ **H59.31**   Postprocedural hemorrhage and hematoma of eye and adnexa following an ophthalmic procedure

H59.311   **Postprocedural hemorrhage and hematoma of right eye and adnexa following an ophthalmic procedure**

H59.312   **Postprocedural hemorrhage and hematoma of left eye and adnexa following an ophthalmic procedure**

H59.313   **Postprocedural hemorrhage and hematoma of eye and adnexa following an ophthalmic procedure, bilateral**

H59.319   **Postprocedural hemorrhage and hematoma of unspecified eye and adnexa following an ophthalmic procedure**

√6ᵗʰ **H59.32**   Postprocedural hemorrhage and hematoma of eye and adnexa following other procedure

H59.321   **Postprocedural hemorrhage and hematoma of right eye and adnexa following other procedure**

H59.322   **Postprocedural hemorrhage and hematoma of left eye and adnexa following other procedure**

H59.323   **Postprocedural hemorrhage and hematoma of eye and adnexa following other procedure, bilateral**

H59.329   **Postprocedural hemorrhage and hematoma of unspecified eye and adnexa following other procedure**

√5ᵗʰ **H59.4**   Inflammation (infection) of postprocedural bleb

Postprocedural blebitis

> **EXCLUDES 1**   *filtering (vitreous) bleb after glaucoma surgery status (Z98.83)*

H59.40   **Inflammation (infection) of postprocedural bleb, unspecified**

H59.41   **Inflammation (infection) of postprocedural bleb, stage 1**

H59.42   **Inflammation (infection) of postprocedural bleb, stage 2**

H59.43   **Inflammation (infection) of postprocedural bleb, stage 3**

Bleb endophthalmitis

√5ᵗʰ **H59.8**   Other intraoperative and postprocedural complications and disorders of eye and adnexa, not elsewhere classified

√6ᵗʰ **H59.81**   Chorioretinal scars after surgery for detachment

H59.811   **Chorioretinal scars after surgery for detachment, right eye**

H59.812   **Chorioretinal scars after surgery for detachment, left eye**

H59.813   **Chorioretinal scars after surgery for detachment, bilateral**

H59.819   **Chorioretinal scars after surgery for detachment, unspecified eye**

H59.88   **Other intraoperative complications of eye and adnexa, not elsewhere classified**

H59.89   **Other postprocedural complications and disorders of eye and adnexa, not elsewhere classified**

EXCLUDES 1 Not coded here   **EXCLUDES 2** Not included here   N Newborn Age: 0   P Pediatric Age: 0-17   M Maternity Age: 12-55   A Adult Age: 15-124

558   ICD-10-CM Draft (2015)

Chapter 8. Diseases of the Ear and Mastoid Process (H60-H95)

NOTE Use an external cause code following the code for the ear condition, if applicable, to identify the cause of the ear condition.

EXCLUDES 2 *certain conditions originating in the perinatal period (P04-P96)*
certain infectious and parasitic diseases (A00-B99)
complications of pregnancy, childbirth and the puerperium (O00-O9A)
congenital malformations, deformations and chromosomal abnormalities (Q00-Q99)
endocrine, nutritional and metabolic diseases (E00-E88)
injury, poisoning and certain other consequences of external causes (S00-T88)
neoplasms (C00-D49)
symptoms, signs and abnormal clinical and laboratory findings, not elsewhere classified (R00-R94)

This chapter contains the following blocks:
H60-H62　Diseases of external ear
H65-H75　Diseases of middle ear and mastoid
H80-H83　Diseases of inner ear
H90-H94　Other disorders of ear
H95　　　Intraoperative and postprocedural complications and disorders of ear and mastoid process, not elsewhere classified

Diseases of external ear (H60-H62)

✓4ᵗʰ **H60　Otitis externa**

✓5ᵗʰ **H60.0　Abscess of external ear**
　　Boil of external ear
　　Carbuncle of auricle or external auditory canal
　　Furuncle of external ear

　　H60.00　Abscess of external ear, unspecified ear
　　H60.01　Abscess of right external ear
　　H60.02　Abscess of left external ear
　　H60.03　Abscess of external ear, bilateral

✓5ᵗʰ **H60.1　Cellulitis of external ear**
　　Cellulitis of auricle
　　Cellulitis of external auditory canal

　　H60.10　Cellulitis of external ear, unspecified ear
　　H60.11　Cellulitis of right external ear
　　H60.12　Cellulitis of left external ear
　　H60.13　Cellulitis of external ear, bilateral

✓5ᵗʰ **H60.2　Malignant otitis externa**
　　H60.20　Malignant otitis externa, unspecified ear
　　H60.21　Malignant otitis externa, right ear
　　H60.22　Malignant otitis externa, left ear
　　H60.23　Malignant otitis externa, bilateral

✓5ᵗʰ **H60.3　Other infective otitis externa**

　　✓6ᵗʰ **H60.31　Diffuse otitis externa**
　　　　H60.311　Diffuse otitis externa, right ear
　　　　H60.312　Diffuse otitis externa, left ear
　　　　H60.313　Diffuse otitis externa, bilateral
　　　　H60.319　Diffuse otitis externa, unspecified ear

　　✓6ᵗʰ **H60.32　Hemorrhagic otitis externa**
　　　　H60.321　Hemorrhagic otitis externa, right ear
　　　　H60.322　Hemorrhagic otitis externa, left ear
　　　　H60.323　Hemorrhagic otitis externa, bilateral
　　　　H60.329　Hemorrhagic otitis externa, unspecified ear

　　✓6ᵗʰ **H60.33　Swimmer's ear**
　　　　H60.331　Swimmer's ear, right ear
　　　　H60.332　Swimmer's ear, left ear
　　　　H60.333　Swimmer's ear, bilateral
　　　　H60.339　Swimmer's ear, unspecified ear

　　✓6ᵗʰ **H60.39　Other infective otitis externa**
　　　　H60.391　Other infective otitis externa, right ear
　　　　H60.392　Other infective otitis externa, left ear
　　　　H60.393　Other infective otitis externa, bilateral
　　　　H60.399　Other infective otitis externa, unspecified ear

✓5ᵗʰ **H60.4　Cholesteatoma of external ear**
　　Keratosis obturans of external ear (canal)
　　EXCLUDES 2 *cholesteatoma of middle ear (H71.-)*
　　　　recurrent cholesteatoma of postmastoidectomy cavity (H95.0-)

　　H60.40　Cholesteatoma of external ear, unspecified ear

H60.41　Cholesteatoma of right external ear
H60.42　Cholesteatoma of left external ear
H60.43　Cholesteatoma of external ear, bilateral

✓5ᵗʰ **H60.5　Acute noninfective otitis externa**

　　✓6ᵗʰ **H60.50　Unspecified acute noninfective otitis externa**
　　　　Acute otitis externa NOS
　　　　H60.501　Unspecified acute noninfective otitis externa, right ear
　　　　H60.502　Unspecified acute noninfective otitis externa, left ear
　　　　H60.503　Unspecified acute noninfective otitis externa, bilateral
　　　　H60.509　Unspecified acute noninfective otitis externa, unspecified ear

　　✓6ᵗʰ **H60.51　Acute actinic otitis externa**
　　　　H60.511　Acute actinic otitis externa, right ear
　　　　H60.512　Acute actinic otitis externa, left ear
　　　　H60.513　Acute actinic otitis externa, bilateral
　　　　H60.519　Acute actinic otitis externa, unspecified ear

　　✓6ᵗʰ **H60.52　Acute chemical otitis externa**
　　　　H60.521　Acute chemical otitis externa, right ear
　　　　H60.522　Acute chemical otitis externa, left ear
　　　　H60.523　Acute chemical otitis externa, bilateral
　　　　H60.529　Acute chemical otitis externa, unspecified ear

　　✓6ᵗʰ **H60.53　Acute contact otitis externa**
　　　　H60.531　Acute contact otitis externa, right ear
　　　　H60.532　Acute contact otitis externa, left ear
　　　　H60.533　Acute contact otitis externa, bilateral
　　　　H60.539　Acute contact otitis externa, unspecified ear

　　✓6ᵗʰ **H60.54　Acute eczematoid otitis externa**
　　　　H60.541　Acute eczematoid otitis externa, right ear
　　　　H60.542　Acute eczematoid otitis externa, left ear
　　　　H60.543　Acute eczematoid otitis externa, bilateral
　　　　H60.549　Acute eczematoid otitis externa, unspecified ear

　　✓6ᵗʰ **H60.55　Acute reactive otitis externa**
　　　　H60.551　Acute reactive otitis externa, right ear
　　　　H60.552　Acute reactive otitis externa, left ear
　　　　H60.553　Acute reactive otitis externa, bilateral
　　　　H60.559　Acute reactive otitis externa, unspecified ear

　　✓6ᵗʰ **H60.59　Other noninfective acute otitis externa**
　　　　H60.591　Other noninfective acute otitis externa, right ear
　　　　H60.592　Other noninfective acute otitis externa, left ear
　　　　H60.593　Other noninfective acute otitis externa, bilateral
　　　　H60.599　Other noninfective acute otitis externa, unspecified ear

✓5ᵗʰ **H60.6　Unspecified chronic otitis externa**
　　H60.60　Unspecified chronic otitis externa, unspecified ear
　　H60.61　Unspecified chronic otitis externa, right ear
　　H60.62　Unspecified chronic otitis externa, left ear
　　H60.63　Unspecified chronic otitis externa, bilateral

✓5ᵗʰ **H60.8　Other otitis externa**

　　✓6ᵗʰ **H60.8X　Other otitis externa**
　　　　H60.8X1　Other otitis externa, right ear
　　　　H60.8X2　Other otitis externa, left ear
　　　　H60.8X3　Other otitis externa, bilateral
　　　　H60.8X9　Other otitis externa, unspecified ear

✓5ᵗʰ **H60.9　Unspecified otitis externa**
　　H60.90　Unspecified otitis externa, unspecified ear
　　H60.91　Unspecified otitis externa, right ear
　　H60.92　Unspecified otitis externa, left ear
　　H60.93　Unspecified otitis externa, bilateral

✓4th **H61 Other disorders of external ear**

✓5th **H61.0 Chondritis and perichondritis of external ear**
Chondrodermatitis nodularis chronica helicis
Perichondritis of auricle
Perichondritis of pinna

     ✓6th **H61.00 Unspecified perichondritis of external ear**
         H61.001 **Unspecified perichondritis of right external ear**
         H61.002 **Unspecified perichondritis of left external ear**
         H61.003 **Unspecified perichondritis of external ear, bilateral**
         H61.009 **Unspecified perichondritis of external ear, unspecified ear**

     ✓6th **H61.01 Acute perichondritis of external ear**
         H61.011 **Acute perichondritis of right external ear**
         H61.012 **Acute perichondritis of left external ear**
         H61.013 **Acute perichondritis of external ear, bilateral**
         H61.019 **Acute perichondritis of external ear, unspecified ear**

     ✓6th **H61.02 Chronic perichondritis of external ear**
         H61.021 **Chronic perichondritis of right external ear**
         H61.022 **Chronic perichondritis of left external ear**
         H61.023 **Chronic perichondritis of external ear, bilateral**
         H61.029 **Chronic perichondritis of external ear, unspecified ear**

     ✓6th **H61.03 Chondritis of external ear**
         Chondritis of auricle
         Chondritis of pinna
         H61.031 **Chondritis of right external ear**
         H61.032 **Chondritis of left external ear**
         H61.033 **Chondritis of external ear, bilateral**
         H61.039 **Chondritis of external ear, unspecified ear**

✓5th **H61.1 Noninfective disorders of pinna**
     EXCLUDES 2   *cauliflower ear (M95.1-)*
           gouty tophi of ear (M1A.-)

     ✓6th **H61.10 Unspecified noninfective disorders of pinna**
         Disorder of pinna NOS
         H61.101 **Unspecified noninfective disorders of pinna, right ear**
         H61.102 **Unspecified noninfective disorders of pinna, left ear**
         H61.103 **Unspecified noninfective disorders of pinna, bilateral**
         H61.109 **Unspecified noninfective disorders of pinna, unspecified ear**

     ✓6th **H61.11 Acquired deformity of pinna**
         Acquired deformity of auricle
         EXCLUDES 2   *cauliflower ear (M95.1-)*
         H61.111 **Acquired deformity of pinna, right ear**
         H61.112 **Acquired deformity of pinna, left ear**
         H61.113 **Acquired deformity of pinna, bilateral**
         H61.119 **Acquired deformity of pinna, unspecified ear**

     ✓6th **H61.12 Hematoma of pinna**
         Hematoma of auricle
         H61.121 **Hematoma of pinna, right ear**
         H61.122 **Hematoma of pinna, left ear**
         H61.123 **Hematoma of pinna, bilateral**
         H61.129 **Hematoma of pinna, unspecified ear**

     ✓6th **H61.19 Other noninfective disorders of pinna**
         H61.191 **Noninfective disorders of pinna, right ear**
         H61.192 **Noninfective disorders of pinna, left ear**
         H61.193 **Noninfective disorders of pinna, bilateral**
         H61.199 **Noninfective disorders of pinna, unspecified ear**

✓5th **H61.2 Impacted cerumen**
     Wax in ear
     H61.20 **Impacted cerumen, unspecified ear**
     H61.21 **Impacted cerumen, right ear**
     H61.22 **Impacted cerumen, left ear**
     H61.23 **Impacted cerumen, bilateral**

✓5th **H61.3 Acquired stenosis of external ear canal**
     Collapse of external ear canal
     EXCLUDES 1   *postprocedural stenosis of external ear canal (H95.81-)*

     ✓6th **H61.30 Acquired stenosis of external ear canal, unspecified**
         H61.301 **Acquired stenosis of right external ear canal, unspecified**
         H61.302 **Acquired stenosis of left external ear canal, unspecified**
         H61.303 **Acquired stenosis of external ear canal, unspecified, bilateral**
         H61.309 **Acquired stenosis of external ear canal, unspecified, unspecified ear**

     ✓6th **H61.31 Acquired stenosis of external ear canal secondary to trauma**
         H61.311 **Acquired stenosis of right external ear canal secondary to trauma**
         H61.312 **Acquired stenosis of left external ear canal secondary to trauma**
         H61.313 **Acquired stenosis of external ear canal secondary to trauma, bilateral**
         H61.319 **Acquired stenosis of external ear canal secondary to trauma, unspecified ear**

     ✓6th **H61.32 Acquired stenosis of external ear canal secondary to inflammation and infection**
         H61.321 **Acquired stenosis of right external ear canal secondary to inflammation and infection**
         H61.322 **Acquired stenosis of left external ear canal secondary to inflammation and infection**
         H61.323 **Acquired stenosis of external ear canal secondary to inflammation and infection, bilateral**
         H61.329 **Acquired stenosis of external ear canal secondary to inflammation and infection, unspecified ear**

     ✓6th **H61.39 Other acquired stenosis of external ear canal**
         H61.391 **Other acquired stenosis of right external ear canal**
         H61.392 **Other acquired stenosis of left external ear canal**
         H61.393 **Other acquired stenosis of external ear canal, bilateral**
         H61.399 **Other acquired stenosis of external ear canal, unspecified ear**

✓5th **H61.8 Other specified disorders of external ear**
     ✓6th **H61.81 Exostosis of external canal**
         H61.811 **Exostosis of right external canal**
         H61.812 **Exostosis of left external canal**
         H61.813 **Exostosis of external canal, bilateral**
         H61.819 **Exostosis of external canal, unspecified ear**

     ✓6th **H61.89 Other specified disorders of external ear**
         H61.891 **Other specified disorders of right external ear**
         H61.892 **Other specified disorders of left external ear**
         H61.893 **Other specified disorders of external ear, bilateral**
         H61.899 **Other specified disorders of external ear, unspecified ear**

✓5th **H61.9 Disorder of external ear, unspecified**
     H61.90 **Disorder of external ear, unspecified, unspecified ear**
     H61.91 **Disorder of right external ear, unspecified**
     H61.92 **Disorder of left external ear, unspecified**
     H61.93 **Disorder of external ear, unspecified, bilateral**

✓4th **H62 Disorders of external ear in diseases classified elsewhere**

✓5th **H62.4 Otitis externa in other diseases classified elsewhere**
     Code first underlying disease, such as:
         erysipelas (A46)
         impetigo (L01.0)
     EXCLUDES 1   *otitis externa (in):*
         candidiasis (B37.84)
         herpes viral [herpes simplex] (B00.1)
         herpes zoster (B02.8)
     H62.40 ***Otitis externa in other diseases classified elsewhere, unspecified ear***

EXCLUDES 1 Not coded here   EXCLUDES 2 Not included here   N Newborn Age: 0   P Pediatric Age: 0-17   M Maternity Age: 12-55   A Adult Age: 15-124

560   ICD-10-CM Draft (2015)

H62.41 *Otitis externa in other diseases classified elsewhere, right ear*

H62.42 *Otitis externa in other diseases classified elsewhere, left ear*

H62.43 *Otitis externa in other diseases classified elsewhere, bilateral*

✓5ᵗʰ H62.8 **Other disorders of external ear in diseases classified elsewhere**

Code first underlying disease, such as:
gout (M1A.-, M1Ø.-)

✓6ᵗʰ H62.8X **Other disorders of external ear in diseases classified elsewhere**

H62.8X1 *Other disorders of right external ear in diseases classified elsewhere*

H62.8X2 *Other disorders of left external ear in diseases classified elsewhere*

H62.8X3 *Other disorders of external ear in diseases classified elsewhere, bilateral*

H62.8X9 *Other disorders of external ear in diseases classified elsewhere, unspecified ear*

Diseases of middle ear and mastoid (H65-H75)

✓4ᵗʰ H65 **Nonsuppurative otitis media**

INCLUDES nonsuppurative otitis media with myringitis

Use additional code for any associated perforated tympanic membrane (H72.-)
Use additional code to identify:
exposure to environmental tobacco smoke (Z77.22)
exposure to tobacco smoke in the perinatal period (P96.81)
history of tobacco use (Z87.891)
occupational exposure to environmental tobacco smoke (Z57.31)
tobacco dependence (F17.-)
tobacco use (Z72.Ø)

✓5ᵗʰ H65.Ø Acute serous **otitis media**

Acute and subacute secretory otitis

H65.ØØ **Acute serous otitis media, unspecified ear**

H65.Ø1 **Acute serous otitis media, right ear**

H65.Ø2 **Acute serous otitis media, left ear**

H65.Ø3 **Acute serous otitis media, bilateral**

H65.Ø4 **Acute serous otitis media, recurrent, right ear**

H65.Ø5 **Acute serous otitis media, recurrent, left ear**

H65.Ø6 **Acute serous otitis media, recurrent, bilateral**

H65.Ø7 **Acute serous otitis media, recurrent, unspecified ear**

✓5ᵗʰ H65.1 Other acute **nonsuppurative otitis media**

EXCLUDES 1 otitic barotrauma (T7Ø.Ø)
otitis media (acute) NOS (H66.9)

✓6ᵗʰ H65.11 Acute and subacute allergic **otitis media (mucoid) (sanguinous) (serous)**

H65.111 **Acute and subacute allergic otitis media (mucoid) (sanguinous) (serous), right ear**

H65.112 **Acute and subacute allergic otitis media (mucoid) (sanguinous) (serous), left ear**

H65.113 **Acute and subacute allergic otitis media (mucoid) (sanguinous) (serous), bilateral**

H65.114 **Acute and subacute allergic otitis media (mucoid) (sanguinous) (serous), recurrent, right ear**

H65.115 **Acute and subacute allergic otitis media (mucoid) (sanguinous) (serous), recurrent, left ear**

H65.116 **Acute and subacute allergic otitis media (mucoid) (sanguinous) (serous), recurrent, bilateral**

H65.117 **Acute and subacute allergic otitis media (mucoid) (sanguinous) (serous), recurrent, unspecified ear**

H65.119 **Acute and subacute allergic otitis media (mucoid) (sanguinous) (serous), unspecified ear**

✓6ᵗʰ H65.19 Other acute **nonsuppurative otitis media**

Acute and subacute mucoid otitis media
Acute and subacute nonsuppurative otitis media NOS
Acute and subacute sanguinous otitis media
Acute and subacute seromucinous otitis media

H65.191 **Other acute nonsuppurative otitis media, right ear**

H65.192 **Other acute nonsuppurative otitis media, left ear**

H65.193 **Other acute nonsuppurative otitis media, bilateral**

H65.194 **Other acute nonsuppurative otitis media, recurrent, right ear**

H65.195 **Other acute nonsuppurative otitis media, recurrent, left ear**

H65.196 **Other acute nonsuppurative otitis media, recurrent, bilateral**

H65.197 **Other acute nonsuppurative otitis media recurrent, unspecified ear**

H65.199 **Other acute nonsuppurative otitis media, unspecified ear**

✓5ᵗʰ H65.2 Chronic serous **otitis media**

Chronic tubotympanal catarrh

H65.2Ø **Chronic serous otitis media, unspecified ear**

H65.21 **Chronic serous otitis media, right ear**

H65.22 **Chronic serous otitis media, left ear**

H65.23 **Chronic serous otitis media, bilateral**

✓5ᵗʰ H65.3 Chronic mucoid **otitis media**

Chronic mucinous otitis media
Chronic secretory otitis media
Glue ear
Chronic transudative otitis media

EXCLUDES 1 adhesive middle ear disease (H74.1)

H65.3Ø **Chronic mucoid otitis media, unspecified ear**

H65.31 **Chronic mucoid otitis media, right ear**

H65.32 **Chronic mucoid otitis media, left ear**

H65.33 **Chronic mucoid otitis media, bilateral**

✓5ᵗʰ H65.4 Other chronic **nonsuppurative otitis media**

✓6ᵗʰ H65.41 Chronic allergic **otitis media**

H65.411 **Chronic allergic otitis media, right ear**

H65.412 **Chronic allergic otitis media, left ear**

H65.413 **Chronic allergic otitis media, bilateral**

H65.419 **Chronic allergic otitis media, unspecified ear**

✓6ᵗʰ H65.49 Other chronic **nonsuppurative otitis media**

Chronic exudative otitis media
Chronic nonsuppurative otitis media NOS
Chronic otitis media with effusion (nonpurulent)
Chronic seromucinous otitis media

H65.491 **Other chronic nonsuppurative otitis media, right ear**

H65.492 **Other chronic nonsuppurative otitis media, left ear**

H65.493 **Other chronic nonsuppurative otitis media, bilateral**

H65.499 **Other chronic nonsuppurative otitis media, unspecified ear**

✓5ᵗʰ H65.9 Unspecified **nonsuppurative otitis media**

Allergic otitis media NOS
Catarrhal otitis media NOS
Exudative otitis media NOS
Mucoid otitis media NOS
Otitis media with effusion (nonpurulent) NOS
Secretory otitis media NOS
Seromucinous otitis media NOS
Serous otitis media NOS
Transudative otitis media NOS

H65.9Ø **Unspecified nonsuppurative otitis media, unspecified ear**

H65.91 **Unspecified nonsuppurative otitis media, right ear**

H65.92 **Unspecified nonsuppurative otitis media, left ear**

H65.93 **Unspecified nonsuppurative otitis media, bilateral**

✓4ᵗʰ H66 **Suppurative and unspecified otitis media**

INCLUDES suppurative and unspecified otitis media with myringitis

Use additional code to identify:
exposure to environmental tobacco smoke (Z77.22)
exposure to tobacco smoke in the perinatal period (P96.81)
history of tobacco use (Z87.891)
occupational exposure to environmental tobacco smoke (Z57.31)
tobacco dependence (F17.-)
tobacco use (Z72.Ø)

✓5ᵗʰ H66.Ø Acute suppurative **otitis media**

✓6ᵗʰ H66.ØØ **Acute suppurative otitis media without spontaneous rupture of ear drum**

H66.ØØ1 **Acute suppurative otitis media without spontaneous rupture of ear drum, right ear**

✓ Additional Character Required   ✓7ᵗʰ Xtension Alert   Unspecified Dx   Other Specified Dx   Manifestation   ►◄ Revised Text   ● New Code   ▲ Revised Code Title

Diseases of the Ear and Mastoid Process

H66.002–H68.112

H66.002   **Acute suppurative otitis media without spontaneous rupture of ear drum, left ear**

H66.003   **Acute suppurative otitis media without spontaneous rupture of ear drum, bilateral**

H66.004   **Acute suppurative otitis media without spontaneous rupture of ear drum, recurrent, right ear**

H66.005   **Acute suppurative otitis media without spontaneous rupture of ear drum, recurrent, left ear**

H66.006   **Acute suppurative otitis media without spontaneous rupture of ear drum, recurrent, bilateral**

H66.007   **Acute suppurative otitis media without spontaneous rupture of ear drum, recurrent, unspecified ear**

H66.009   **Acute suppurative otitis media without spontaneous rupture of ear drum, unspecified ear**

✓6th **H66.01 Acute suppurative otitis media with spontaneous rupture of ear drum**

H66.011   **Acute suppurative otitis media with spontaneous rupture of ear drum, right ear**

H66.012   **Acute suppurative otitis media with spontaneous rupture of ear drum, left ear**

H66.013   **Acute suppurative otitis media with spontaneous rupture of ear drum, bilateral**

H66.014   **Acute suppurative otitis media with spontaneous rupture of ear drum, recurrent, right ear**

H66.015   **Acute suppurative otitis media with spontaneous rupture of ear drum, recurrent, left ear**

H66.016   **Acute suppurative otitis media with spontaneous rupture of ear drum, recurrent, bilateral**

H66.017   **Acute suppurative otitis media with spontaneous rupture of ear drum, recurrent, unspecified ear**

H66.019   **Acute suppurative otitis media with spontaneous rupture of ear drum, unspecified ear**

✓5th **H66.1 Chronic tubotympanic suppurative otitis media**
Benign chronic suppurative otitis media
Chronic tubotympanic disease
Use additional code for any associated perforated tympanic membrane (H72.-)

H66.10   **Chronic tubotympanic suppurative otitis media, unspecified**

H66.11   **Chronic tubotympanic suppurative otitis media, right ear**

H66.12   **Chronic tubotympanic suppurative otitis media, left ear**

H66.13   **Chronic tubotympanic suppurative otitis media, bilateral**

✓5th **H66.2 Chronic atticoantral suppurative otitis media**
Chronic atticoantral disease
Use additional code for any associated perforated tympanic membrane (H72.-)

H66.20   **Chronic atticoantral suppurative otitis media, unspecified ear**

H66.21   **Chronic atticoantral suppurative otitis media, right ear**

H66.22   **Chronic atticoantral suppurative otitis media, left ear**

H66.23   **Chronic atticoantral suppurative otitis media, bilateral**

✓5th **H66.3 Other chronic suppurative otitis media**
Chronic suppurative otitis media NOS
Use additional code for any associated perforated tympanic membrane (H72.-)
EXCLUDES 1   tuberculous otitis media (A18.6)

✓6th **H66.3X Other chronic suppurative otitis media**

H66.3X1   **Other chronic suppurative otitis media, right ear**

H66.3X2   **Other chronic suppurative otitis media, left ear**

H66.3X3   **Other chronic suppurative otitis media, bilateral**

H66.3X9   **Other chronic suppurative otitis media, unspecified ear**

✓5th **H66.4 Suppurative otitis media, unspecified**
Purulent otitis media NOS
Use additional code for any associated perforated tympanic membrane (H72.-)

H66.40   **Suppurative otitis media, unspecified, unspecified ear**

H66.41   **Suppurative otitis media, unspecified, right ear**

H66.42   **Suppurative otitis media, unspecified, left ear**

H66.43   **Suppurative otitis media, unspecified, bilateral**

✓5th **H66.9 Otitis media, unspecified**
Otitis media NOS
Acute otitis media NOS
Chronic otitis media NOS
Use additional code for any associated perforated tympanic membrane (H72.-)

H66.90   **Otitis media, unspecified, unspecified ear**

H66.91   **Otitis media, unspecified, right ear**

H66.92   **Otitis media, unspecified, left ear**

H66.93   **Otitis media, unspecified, bilateral**

✓4th **H67 Otitis media in diseases classified elsewhere**
Code first underlying disease, such as:
viral disease NEC (B00-B34)
Use additional code for any associated perforated tympanic membrane (H72.-)
EXCLUDES 1   otitis media in:
influenza (J09.X9, J10.83, J11.83)
measles (B05.3)
scarlet fever (A38.0)
tuberculosis (A18.6)

H67.1   *Otitis media in diseases classified elsewhere, right ear*

H67.2   *Otitis media in diseases classified elsewhere, left ear*

H67.3   *Otitis media in diseases classified elsewhere, bilateral*

H67.9   *Otitis media in diseases classified elsewhere, unspecified ear*

✓4th **H68 Eustachian salpingitis and obstruction**

✓5th **H68.0 Eustachian salpingitis**

✓6th **H68.00 Unspecified Eustachian salpingitis**

H68.001   **Unspecified Eustachian salpingitis, right ear**

H68.002   **Unspecified Eustachian salpingitis, left ear**

H68.003   **Unspecified Eustachian salpingitis, bilateral**

H68.009   **Unspecified Eustachian salpingitis, unspecified ear**

✓6th **H68.01 Acute Eustachian salpingitis**

H68.011   **Acute Eustachian salpingitis, right ear**

H68.012   **Acute Eustachian salpingitis, left ear**

H68.013   **Acute Eustachian salpingitis, bilateral**

H68.019   **Acute Eustachian salpingitis, unspecified ear**

✓6th **H68.02 Chronic Eustachian salpingitis**

H68.021   **Chronic Eustachian salpingitis, right ear**

H68.022   **Chronic Eustachian salpingitis, left ear**

H68.023   **Chronic Eustachian salpingitis, bilateral**

H68.029   **Chronic Eustachian salpingitis, unspecified ear**

✓5th **H68.1 Obstruction of Eustachian tube**
Stenosis of Eustachian tube   Stricture of Eustachian tube

✓6th **H68.10 Unspecified obstruction of Eustachian tube**

H68.101   **Unspecified obstruction of Eustachian tube, right ear**

H68.102   **Unspecified obstruction of Eustachian tube, left ear**

H68.103   **Unspecified obstruction of Eustachian tube, bilateral**

H68.109   **Unspecified obstruction of Eustachian tube, unspecified ear**

✓6th **H68.11 Osseous obstruction of Eustachian tube**

H68.111   **Osseous obstruction of Eustachian tube, right ear**

H68.112   **Osseous obstruction of Eustachian tube, left ear**

EXCLUDES 1 Not coded here   EXCLUDES 2 Not included here   N Newborn Age: 0   P Pediatric Age: 0-17   M Maternity Age: 12-55   A Adult Age: 15-124

562   ICD-10-CM Draft (2015)

H68.113   **Osseous obstruction of Eustachian tube,** bilateral

H68.119   **Osseous obstruction of Eustachian tube, unspecified ear**

✓6th   **H68.12**   Intrinsic cartilagenous obstruction of Eustachian tube

H68.121   **Intrinsic cartilagenous obstruction of Eustachian tube,** right **ear**

H68.122   **Intrinsic cartilagenous obstruction of Eustachian tube,** left **ear**

H68.123   **Intrinsic cartilagenous obstruction of Eustachian tube,** bilateral

H68.129   **Intrinsic cartilagenous obstruction of Eustachian tube, unspecified ear**

✓6th   **H68.13**   Extrinsic cartilagenous obstruction of Eustachian tube

Compression of Eustachian tube

H68.131   **Extrinsic cartilagenous obstruction of Eustachian tube,** right **ear**

H68.132   **Extrinsic cartilagenous obstruction of Eustachian tube,** left **ear**

H68.133   **Extrinsic cartilagenous obstruction of Eustachian tube,** bilateral

H68.139   **Extrinsic cartilagenous obstruction of Eustachian tube, unspecified ear**

✓4th   **H69**   **Other and unspecified disorders of Eustachian tube**

✓5th   **H69.0**   Patulous **Eustachian tube**

H69.00   **Patulous Eustachian tube, unspecified ear**

H69.01   **Patulous Eustachian tube,** right **ear**

H69.02   **Patulous Eustachian tube,** left **ear**

H69.03   **Patulous Eustachian tube,** bilateral

✓5th   **H69.8**   Other specified **disorders of Eustachian tube**

H69.80   **Other specified disorders of Eustachian tube, unspecified ear**

H69.81   **Other specified disorders of Eustachian tube,** right **ear**

H69.82   **Other specified disorders of Eustachian tube,** left **ear**

H69.83   **Other specified disorders of Eustachian tube,** bilateral

✓5th   **H69.9**   Unspecified **Eustachian tube disorder**

H69.90   **Unspecified Eustachian tube disorder, unspecified ear**

H69.91   **Unspecified Eustachian tube disorder,** right **ear**

H69.92   **Unspecified Eustachian tube disorder,** left **ear**

H69.93   **Unspecified Eustachian tube disorder,** bilateral

✓4th   **H70**   **Mastoiditis and related conditions**

✓5th   **H70.0**   Acute **mastoiditis**

Abscess of mastoid
Empyema of mastoid

✓6th   **H70.00**   **Acute mastoiditis** without complications

H70.001   **Acute mastoiditis without complications,** right **ear**

H70.002   **Acute mastoiditis without complications,** left **ear**

H70.003   **Acute mastoiditis without complications,** bilateral

H70.009   **Acute mastoiditis without complications, unspecified ear**

✓6th   **H70.01**   Subperiosteal abscess **of mastoid**

H70.011   **Subperiosteal abscess of mastoid,** right **ear**

H70.012   **Subperiosteal abscess of mastoid,** left **ear**

H70.013   **Subperiosteal abscess of mastoid,** bilateral

H70.019   **Subperiosteal abscess of mastoid, unspecified ear**

✓6th   **H70.09**   Acute mastoiditis with other complications

H70.091   **Acute mastoiditis with other complications,** right **ear**

H70.092   **Acute mastoiditis with other complications,** left **ear**

H70.093   **Acute mastoiditis with other complications,** bilateral

H70.099   **Acute mastoiditis with other complications, unspecified ear**

✓5th   **H70.1**   Chronic **mastoiditis**

Caries of mastoid
Fistula of mastoid

> **EXCLUDES 1**   *tuberculous mastoiditis (A18.03)*

H70.10   **Chronic mastoiditis, unspecified ear**

H70.11   **Chronic mastoiditis,** right **ear**

H70.12   **Chronic mastoiditis,** left **ear**

H70.13   **Chronic mastoiditis,** bilateral

✓5th   **H70.2**   Petrositis

Inflammation of petrous bone

✓6th   **H70.20**   Unspecified **petrositis**

H70.201   **Unspecified petrositis,** right **ear**

H70.202   **Unspecified petrositis,** left **ear**

H70.203   **Unspecified petrositis,** bilateral

H70.209   **Unspecified petrositis, unspecified ear**

✓6th   **H70.21**   Acute **petrositis**

H70.211   **Acute petrositis,** right **ear**

H70.212   **Acute petrositis,** left **ear**

H70.213   **Acute petrositis,** bilateral

H70.219   **Acute petrositis, unspecified ear**

✓6th   **H70.22**   Chronic **petrositis**

H70.221   **Chronic petrositis,** right **ear**

H70.222   **Chronic petrositis,** left **ear**

H70.223   **Chronic petrositis,** bilateral

H70.229   **Chronic petrositis, unspecified ear**

✓5th   **H70.8**   **Other mastoiditis and related conditions**

> **EXCLUDES 1**   *preauricular sinus and cyst (Q18.1)*
> *sinus, fistula, and cyst of branchial cleft (Q18.0)*

✓6th   **H70.81**   Postauricular fistula

H70.811   **Postauricular fistula,** right **ear**

H70.812   **Postauricular fistula,** left **ear**

H70.813   **Postauricular fistula,** bilateral

H70.819   **Postauricular fistula, unspecified ear**

✓6th   **H70.89**   Other **mastoiditis and related conditions**

H70.891   **Other mastoiditis and related conditions,** right **ear**

H70.892   **Other mastoiditis and related conditions,** left **ear**

H70.893   **Other mastoiditis and related conditions,** bilateral

H70.899   **Other mastoiditis and related conditions, unspecified ear**

✓5th   **H70.9**   Unspecified **mastoiditis**

H70.90   **Unspecified mastoiditis, unspecified ear**

H70.91   **Unspecified mastoiditis,** right **ear**

H70.92   **Unspecified mastoiditis,** left **ear**

H70.93   **Unspecified mastoiditis,** bilateral

✓4th   **H71**   **Cholesteatoma of middle ear**

> **EXCLUDES 2**   *cholesteatoma of external ear (H60.4-)*
> *recurrent cholesteatoma of postmastoidectomy cavity (H95.0-)*

✓5th   **H71.0**   Cholesteatoma of **attic**

H71.00   **Cholesteatoma of attic, unspecified ear**

H71.01   **Cholesteatoma of attic,** right **ear**

H71.02   **Cholesteatoma of attic,** left **ear**

H71.03   **Cholesteatoma of attic,** bilateral

✓5th   **H71.1**   **Cholesteatoma of** tympanum

H71.10   **Cholesteatoma of tympanum, unspecified ear**

H71.11   **Cholesteatoma of tympanum,** right **ear**

H71.12   **Cholesteatoma of tympanum,** left **ear**

H71.13   **Cholesteatoma of tympanum,** bilateral

✓5th   **H71.2**   **Cholesteatoma of** mastoid

H71.20   **Cholesteatoma of mastoid, unspecified ear**

H71.21   **Cholesteatoma of mastoid,** right **ear**

H71.22   **Cholesteatoma of mastoid,** left **ear**

H71.23   **Cholesteatoma of mastoid,** bilateral

✓5th   **H71.3**   Diffuse cholesteatosis

H71.30   **Diffuse cholesteatosis, unspecified ear**

H71.31   **Diffuse cholesteatosis,** right **ear**

H71.32   **Diffuse cholesteatosis,** left **ear**

H71.33   **Diffuse cholesteatosis,** bilateral

✓ Additional Character Required   ✓x7th Xtension Alert   Unspecified Dx   Other Specified Dx   Manifestation   ►◄ Revised Text   ● New Code   ▲ Revised Code Title

✓5th **H71.9** Unspecified **cholesteatoma**

    H71.90 **Unspecified cholesteatoma, unspecified ear**

    H71.91 **Unspecified cholesteatoma,** right **ear**

    H71.92 **Unspecified cholesteatoma,** left **ear**

    H71.93 **Unspecified cholesteatoma,** bilateral

✓4th **H72** **Perforation of tympanic membrane**

    INCLUDES persistent post-traumatic perforation of ear drum

              postinflammatory perforation of ear drum

    Code first any associated otitis media (H65.-, H66.1-, H66.2-, H66.3-, H66.4-, H66.9-, H67.-)

    EXCLUDES 1 *acute suppurative otitis media with rupture of the tympanic membrane (H66.01-)*

              traumatic rupture of ear drum (S09.2-)

✓5th **H72.0** Central **perforation of tympanic membrane**

    H72.00 **Central perforation of tympanic membrane, unspecified ear**

    H72.01 **Central perforation of tympanic membrane,** right **ear**

    H72.02 **Central perforation of tympanic membrane,** left **ear**

    H72.03 **Central perforation of tympanic membrane,** bilateral

✓5th **H72.1** Attic **perforation of tympanic membrane**

    Perforation of pars flaccida

    H72.10 **Attic perforation of tympanic membrane, unspecified ear**

    H72.11 **Attic perforation of tympanic membrane,** right **ear**

    H72.12 **Attic perforation of tympanic membrane,** left **ear**

    H72.13 **Attic perforation of tympanic membrane,** bilateral

✓5th **H72.2** **Other marginal perforations of tympanic membrane**

    ✓6th **H72.2X** Other marginal **perforations of tympanic membrane**

        H72.2X1 **Other marginal perforations of tympanic membrane,** right **ear**

        H72.2X2 **Other marginal perforations of tympanic membrane,** left **ear**

        H72.2X3 **Other marginal perforations of tympanic membrane,** bilateral

        H72.2X9 **Other marginal perforations of tympanic membrane, unspecified ear**

✓5th **H72.8** Other **perforations of tympanic membrane**

    ✓6th **H72.81** Multiple **perforations of tympanic membrane**

        H72.811 **Multiple perforations of tympanic membrane,** right **ear**

        H72.812 **Multiple perforations of tympanic membrane,** left **ear**

        H72.813 **Multiple perforations of tympanic membrane,** bilateral

        H72.819 **Multiple perforations of tympanic membrane, unspecified ear**

    ✓6th **H72.82** Total **perforations of tympanic membrane**

        H72.821 **Total perforations of tympanic membrane,** right **ear**

        H72.822 **Total perforations of tympanic membrane,** left **ear**

        H72.823 **Total perforations of tympanic membrane,** bilateral

        H72.829 **Total perforations of tympanic membrane, unspecified ear**

✓5th **H72.9** Unspecified **perforation of tympanic membrane**

    H72.90 **Unspecified perforation of tympanic membrane, unspecified ear**

    H72.91 **Unspecified perforation of tympanic membrane,** right **ear**

    H72.92 **Unspecified perforation of tympanic membrane,** left **ear**

    H72.93 **Unspecified perforation of tympanic membrane,** bilateral

✓4th **H73** **Other disorders of tympanic membrane**

    ✓5th **H73.0** Acute **myringitis**

        EXCLUDES 1 *acute myringitis with otitis media (H65, H66)*

        ✓6th **H73.00** Unspecified **acute myringitis**

            Acute tympanitis NOS

            H73.001 **Acute myringitis,** right **ear**

            H73.002 **Acute myringitis,** left **ear**

            H73.003 **Acute myringitis,** bilateral

            H73.009 **Acute myringitis, unspecified ear**

✓6th **H73.01** Bullous **myringitis**

    H73.011 **Bullous myringitis,** right **ear**

    H73.012 **Bullous myringitis,** left **ear**

    H73.013 **Bullous myringitis,** bilateral

    H73.019 **Bullous myringitis, unspecified ear**

✓6th **H73.09** Other **acute myringitis**

    H73.091 **Other acute myringitis,** right **ear**

    H73.092 **Other acute myringitis,** left **ear**

    H73.093 **Other acute myringitis,** bilateral

    H73.099 **Other acute myringitis, unspecified ear**

✓5th **H73.1** Chronic **myringitis**

    Chronic tympanitis

    EXCLUDES 1 *chronic myringitis with otitis media (H65, H66)*

    H73.10 **Chronic myringitis, unspecified ear**

    H73.11 **Chronic myringitis,** right **ear**

    H73.12 **Chronic myringitis,** left **ear**

    H73.13 **Chronic myringitis,** bilateral

✓5th **H73.2** Unspecified **myringitis**

    H73.20 **Unspecified myringitis, unspecified ear**

    H73.21 **Unspecified myringitis,** right **ear**

    H73.22 **Unspecified myringitis,** left **ear**

    H73.23 **Unspecified myringitis,** bilateral

✓5th **H73.8** **Other specified disorders of tympanic membrane**

    ✓6th **H73.81** Atrophic flaccid **tympanic membrane**

        H73.811 **Atrophic flaccid tympanic membrane,** right **ear**

        H73.812 **Atrophic flaccid tympanic membrane,** left **ear**

        H73.813 **Atrophic flaccid tympanic membrane,** bilateral

        H73.819 **Atrophic flaccid tympanic membrane, unspecified ear**

    ✓6th **H73.82** Atrophic nonflaccid **tympanic membrane**

        H73.821 **Atrophic nonflaccid tympanic membrane,** right **ear**

        H73.822 **Atrophic nonflaccid tympanic membrane,** left **ear**

        H73.823 **Atrophic nonflaccid tympanic membrane,** bilateral

        H73.829 **Atrophic nonflaccid tympanic membrane, unspecified ear**

    ✓6th **H73.89** Other **specified disorders of tympanic membrane**

        H73.891 **Other specified disorders of tympanic membrane,** right **ear**

        H73.892 **Other specified disorders of tympanic membrane,** left **ear**

        H73.893 **Other specified disorders of tympanic membrane,** bilateral

        H73.899 **Other specified disorders of tympanic membrane, unspecified ear**

✓5th **H73.9** Unspecified **disorder of tympanic membrane**

    H73.90 **Unspecified disorder of tympanic membrane, unspecified ear**

    H73.91 **Unspecified disorder of tympanic membrane,** right **ear**

    H73.92 **Unspecified disorder of tympanic membrane,** left **ear**

    H73.93 **Unspecified disorder of tympanic membrane,** bilateral

✓4th **H74** **Other disorders of middle ear mastoid**

    EXCLUDES 2 *mastoiditis (H70.-)*

    ✓5th **H74.0** **Tympanosclerosis**

        H74.01 **Tympanosclerosis,** right **ear**

        H74.02 **Tympanosclerosis,** left **ear**

        H74.03 **Tympanosclerosis,** bilateral

        H74.09 **Tympanosclerosis, unspecified ear**

    ✓5th **H74.1** **Adhesive middle ear disease**

        Adhesive otitis

        EXCLUDES 1 *glue ear (H65.3-)*

        H74.11 **Adhesive** right **middle ear disease**

        H74.12 **Adhesive** left **middle ear disease**

        H74.13 **Adhesive middle ear disease,** bilateral

        H74.19 **Adhesive middle ear disease, unspecified ear**

EXCLUDES 1 Not coded here   EXCLUDES 2 Not included here   N Newborn Age: 0   P Pediatric Age: 0-17   M Maternity Age: 12-55   A Adult Age: 15-124

564   ICD-10-CM Draft (2015)

✓5th **H74.2** Discontinuity and dislocation of ear ossicles

    H74.20 **Discontinuity and dislocation of ear ossicles, unspecified ear**

    H74.21 Discontinuity and dislocation of right ear ossicles

    H74.22 Discontinuity and dislocation of left ear ossicles

    H74.23 Discontinuity and dislocation of ear ossicles, bilateral

✓5th **H74.3** Other acquired abnormalities of ear ossicles

    ✓6th **H74.31** Ankylosis of ear ossicles

        H74.311 Ankylosis of ear ossicles, right ear

        H74.312 Ankylosis of ear ossicles, left ear

        H74.313 Ankylosis of ear ossicles, bilateral

        H74.319 Ankylosis of ear ossicles, unspecified ear

    ✓6th **H74.32** Partial loss of ear ossicles

        H74.321 Partial loss of ear ossicles, right ear

        H74.322 Partial loss of ear ossicles, left ear

        H74.323 Partial loss of ear ossicles, bilateral

        H74.329 Partial loss of ear ossicles, unspecified ear

    ✓6th **H74.39** Other acquired abnormalities of ear ossicles

        H74.391 **Other acquired abnormalities of right ear ossicles**

        H74.392 **Other acquired abnormalities of left ear ossicles**

        H74.393 **Other acquired abnormalities of ear ossicles, bilateral**

        H74.399 **Other acquired abnormalities of ear ossicles, unspecified ear**

✓5th **H74.4** Polyp of middle ear

    H74.40 **Polyp of middle ear, unspecified ear**

    H74.41 Polyp of right middle ear

    H74.42 Polyp of left middle ear

    H74.43 Polyp of middle ear, bilateral

✓5th **H74.8** Other specified disorders of middle ear and mastoid

    ✓6th **H74.8X** Other specified disorders of middle ear and mastoid

        H74.8X1 **Other specified disorders of right middle ear and mastoid**

        H74.8X2 **Other specified disorders of left middle ear and mastoid**

        H74.8X3 **Other specified disorders of middle ear and mastoid, bilateral**

        H74.8X9 **Other specified disorders of middle ear and mastoid, unspecified ear**

✓5th **H74.9** Unspecified disorder of middle ear and mastoid

    H74.90 **Unspecified disorder of middle ear and mastoid, unspecified ear**

    H74.91 **Unspecified disorder of right middle ear and mastoid**

    H74.92 Unspecified disorder of left middle ear and mastoid

    H74.93 **Unspecified disorder of middle ear and mastoid, bilateral**

✓4th **H75** **Other disorders of middle ear and mastoid in diseases classified elsewhere**

    Code first underlying disease

    ✓5th **H75.0** **Mastoiditis in infectious and parasitic diseases classified elsewhere**

        EXCLUDES 1 *mastoiditis (in):*

            syphilis (A52.77)

            tuberculosis (A18.03)

        H75.00 *Mastoiditis in infectious and parasitic diseases classified elsewhere, unspecified ear*

        H75.01 *Mastoiditis in infectious and parasitic diseases classified elsewhere, right ear*

        H75.02 *Mastoiditis in infectious and parasitic diseases classified elsewhere, left ear*

        H75.03 *Mastoiditis in infectious and parasitic diseases classified elsewhere, bilateral*

    ✓5th **H75.8** **Other specified disorders of middle ear and mastoid in diseases classified elsewhere**

        H75.80 *Other specified disorders of middle ear and mastoid in diseases classified elsewhere, unspecified ear*

        H75.81 *Other specified disorders of right middle ear and mastoid in diseases classified elsewhere*

        H75.82 *Other specified disorders of left middle ear and mastoid in diseases classified elsewhere*

        H75.83 *Other specified disorders of middle ear and mastoid in diseases classified elsewhere, bilateral*

Diseases of inner ear (H80-H83)

✓4th **H80** **Otosclerosis**

    INCLUDES Otospongiosis

    ✓5th **H80.0** Otosclerosis involving oval window, nonobliterative

        H80.00 **Otosclerosis involving oval window, nonobliterative, unspecified ear**

        H80.01 **Otosclerosis involving oval window, nonobliterative, right ear**

        H80.02 **Otosclerosis involving oval window, nonobliterative, left ear**

        H80.03 **Otosclerosis involving oval window, nonobliterative, bilateral**

    ✓5th **H80.1** Otosclerosis involving oval window, obliterative

        H80.10 **Otosclerosis involving oval window, obliterative, unspecified ear**

        H80.11 **Otosclerosis involving oval window, obliterative, right ear**

        H80.12 **Otosclerosis involving oval window, obliterative, left ear**

        H80.13 **Otosclerosis involving oval window, obliterative, bilateral**

    ✓5th **H80.2** Cochlear otosclerosis

        Otosclerosis involving otic capsule

        Otosclerosis involving round window

        H80.20 **Cochlear otosclerosis, unspecified ear**

        H80.21 **Cochlear otosclerosis, right ear**

        H80.22 **Cochlear otosclerosis, left ear**

        H80.23 **Cochlear otosclerosis, bilateral**

    ✓5th **H80.8** Other otosclerosis

        H80.80 **Other otosclerosis, unspecified ear**

        H80.81 **Other otosclerosis, right ear**

        H80.82 **Other otosclerosis, left ear**

        H80.83 **Other otosclerosis, bilateral**

    ✓5th **H80.9** Unspecified otosclerosis

        H80.90 **Unspecified otosclerosis, unspecified ear**

        H80.91 **Unspecified otosclerosis, right ear**

        H80.92 **Unspecified otosclerosis, left ear**

        H80.93 **Unspecified otosclerosis, bilateral**

✓4th **H81** **Disorders of vestibular function**

    EXCLUDES 1 *epidemic vertigo (A88.1)*

            vertigo NOS (R42)

    ✓5th **H81.0** Ménière's disease

        Labyrinthine hydrops

        Ménière's syndrome or vertigo

        H81.01 Ménière's disease, right ear

        H81.02 Ménière's disease, left ear

        H81.03 Ménière's disease, bilateral

        H81.09 Ménière's disease, unspecified ear

    ✓5th **H81.1** Benign paroxysmal vertigo

        H81.10 **Benign paroxysmal vertigo, unspecified ear**

        H81.11 Benign paroxysmal vertigo, right ear

        H81.12 Benign paroxysmal vertigo, left ear

        H81.13 Benign paroxysmal vertigo, bilateral

    ✓5th **H81.2** Vestibular neuronitis

        H81.20 **Vestibular neuronitis, unspecified ear**

        H81.21 Vestibular neuronitis, right ear

        H81.22 Vestibular neuronitis, left ear

        H81.23 Vestibular neuronitis, bilateral

    ✓5th **H81.3** Other peripheral vertigo

        ✓6th **H81.31** Aural vertigo

            H81.311 Aural vertigo, right ear

            H81.312 Aural vertigo, left ear

            H81.313 Aural vertigo, bilateral

            H81.319 Aural vertigo, unspecified ear

        ✓6th **H81.39** Other peripheral vertigo

            Lermoyez' syndrome

            Otogenic vertigo

            Peripheral vertigo NOS

            H81.391 **Other peripheral vertigo, right ear**

☑ Additional Character Required   ✓x7th Xtension Alert   Unspecified Dx   Other Specified Dx   Manifestation   ▶◀ Revised Text   ● New Code   ▲ Revised Code Title

ICD-10-CM Draft (2015)   **565**

Diseases of the Ear and Mastoid Process

H81.392–H91.21

H81.392   **Other peripheral vertigo, left ear**

H81.393   **Other peripheral vertigo, bilateral**

H81.399   **Other peripheral vertigo, unspecified ear**

✓5ᵗʰ **H81.4 Vertigo of central origin**
Central positional nystagmus

    H81.41   **Vertigo of central origin, right ear**

    H81.42   **Vertigo of central origin, left ear**

    H81.43   **Vertigo of central origin, bilateral**

    H81.49   **Vertigo of central origin, unspecified ear**

✓5ᵗʰ **H81.8 Other disorders of vestibular function**

   ✓6ᵗʰ **H81.8X**   **Other disorders of vestibular function**

     H81.8X1   **Other disorders of vestibular function, right ear**

     H81.8X2   **Other disorders of vestibular function, left ear**

     H81.8X3   **Other disorders of vestibular function, bilateral**

     H81.8X9   **Other disorders of vestibular function, unspecified ear**

✓5ᵗʰ **H81.9 Unspecified disorder of vestibular function**
Vertiginous syndrome NOS

    H81.90   **Unspecified disorder of vestibular function, unspecified ear**

    H81.91   **Unspecified disorder of vestibular function, right ear**

    H81.92   **Unspecified disorder of vestibular function, left ear**

    H81.93   **Unspecified disorder of vestibular function, bilateral**

✓4ᵗʰ **H82 Vertiginous syndromes in diseases classified elsewhere**
Code first underlying disease
EXCLUDES 1 *epidemic vertigo (A88.1)*

    H82.1   ***Vertiginous syndromes in diseases classified elsewhere, right ear***

    H82.2   ***Vertiginous syndromes in diseases classified elsewhere, left ear***

    H82.3   ***Vertiginous syndromes in diseases classified elsewhere, bilateral***

    H82.9   ***Vertiginous syndromes in diseases classified elsewhere, unspecified ear***

✓4ᵗʰ **H83 Other diseases of inner ear**

   ✓5ᵗʰ **H83.0 Labyrinthitis**

    H83.01   **Labyrinthitis, right ear**

    H83.02   **Labyrinthitis, left ear**

    H83.03   **Labyrinthitis, bilateral**

    H83.09   **Labyrinthitis, unspecified ear**

   ✓5ᵗʰ **H83.1 Labyrinthine fistula**

    H83.11   **Labyrinthine fistula, right ear**

    H83.12   **Labyrinthine fistula, left ear**

    H83.13   **Labyrinthine fistula, bilateral**

    H83.19   **Labyrinthine fistula, unspecified ear**

   ✓5ᵗʰ **H83.2 Labyrinthine dysfunction**
Labyrinthine hypersensitivity
Labyrinthine hypofunction
Labyrinthine loss of function

    ✓6ᵗʰ **H83.2X**   **Labyrinthine dysfunction**

     H83.2X1   **Labyrinthine dysfunction, right ear**

     H83.2X2   **Labyrinthine dysfunction, left ear**

     H83.2X3   **Labyrinthine dysfunction, bilateral**

     H83.2X9   **Labyrinthine dysfunction, unspecified ear**

   ✓5ᵗʰ **H83.3 Noise effects on inner ear**
Acoustic trauma of inner ear
Noise-induced hearing loss of inner ear

    ✓6ᵗʰ **H83.3X**   **Noise effects on inner ear**

     H83.3X1   **Noise effects on right inner ear**

     H83.3X2   **Noise effects on left inner ear**

     H83.3X3   **Noise effects on inner ear, bilateral**

     H83.3X9   **Noise effects on inner ear, unspecified ear**

   ✓5ᵗʰ **H83.8 Other specified diseases of inner ear**

    ✓6ᵗʰ **H83.8X**   **Other specified diseases of inner ear**

     H83.8X1   **Other specified diseases of right inner ear**

     H83.8X2   **Other specified diseases of left inner ear**

     H83.8X3   **Other specified diseases of inner ear, bilateral**

     H83.8X9   **Other specified diseases of inner ear, unspecified ear**

✓5ᵗʰ **H83.9 Unspecified disease of inner ear**

    H83.90   **Unspecified disease of inner ear, unspecified ear**

    H83.91   **Unspecified disease of right inner ear**

    H83.92   **Unspecified disease of left inner ear**

    H83.93   **Unspecified disease of inner ear, bilateral**

Other disorders of ear (H90-H94)

✓4ᵗʰ **H90 Conductive and sensorineural hearing loss**
EXCLUDES 1 *deaf nonspeaking NEC (H91.3)*
deafness NOS (H91.9-)
hearing loss NOS (H91.9-)
noise-induced hearing loss (H83.3-)
ototoxic hearing loss (H91.0-)
sudden (idiopathic) hearing loss (H91.2-)

   H90.0 Conductive hearing loss, bilateral

   ✓5ᵗʰ **H90.1 Conductive hearing loss, unilateral with unrestricted hearing on the contralateral side**

    H90.11   **Conductive hearing loss, unilateral, right ear, with unrestricted hearing on the contralateral side**

    H90.12   **Conductive hearing loss, unilateral, left ear, with unrestricted hearing on the contralateral side**

   H90.2 Conductive hearing loss, unspecified
Conductive deafness NOS

   H90.3 Sensorineural hearing loss, bilateral

   ✓5ᵗʰ **H90.4 Sensorineural hearing loss, unilateral with unrestricted hearing on the contralateral side**

    H90.41   **Sensorineural hearing loss, unilateral, right ear, with unrestricted hearing on the contralateral side**

    H90.42   **Sensorineural hearing loss, unilateral, left ear, with unrestricted hearing on the contralateral side**

   H90.5 Unspecified sensorineural hearing loss
Central hearing loss NOS
Congenital deafness NOS
Neural hearing loss NOS
Perceptive hearing loss NOS
Sensorineural deafness NOS
Sensory hearing loss NOS
EXCLUDES 1 *abnormal auditory perception (H93.2-)*
psychogenic deafness (F44.6)

   H90.6 Mixed conductive and sensorineural hearing loss, bilateral

   ✓5ᵗʰ **H90.7 Mixed conductive and sensorineural hearing loss, unilateral with unrestricted hearing on the contralateral side**

    H90.71   **Mixed conductive and sensorineural hearing loss, unilateral, right ear, with unrestricted hearing on the contralateral side**

    H90.72   **Mixed conductive and sensorineural hearing loss, unilateral, left ear, with unrestricted hearing on the contralateral side**

   H90.8 Mixed conductive and sensorineural hearing loss, unspecified

✓4ᵗʰ **H91 Other and unspecified hearing loss**
EXCLUDES 1 *abnormal auditory perception (H93.2-)*
hearing loss as classified in H90-
impacted cerumen (H61.2-)
noise-induced hearing loss (H83.3-)
psychogenic deafness (F44.6)
transient ischemic deafness (H93.01-)

   ✓5ᵗʰ **H91.0 Ototoxic hearing loss**
Code first poisoning due to drug or toxin, if applicable (T36-T65 with fifth or sixth character 1-4 or 6)
Use additional code for adverse effect, if applicable, to identify drug (T36-T50 with fifth or sixth character 5)

    H91.01   **Ototoxic hearing loss, right ear**

    H91.02   **Ototoxic hearing loss, left ear**

    H91.03   **Ototoxic hearing loss, bilateral**

    H91.09   **Ototoxic hearing loss, unspecified ear**

   ✓5ᵗʰ **H91.1 Presbycusis**
Presbyacusia

    H91.10   **Presbycusis, unspecified ear**

    H91.11   **Presbycusis, right ear**

    H91.12   **Presbycusis, left ear**

    H91.13   **Presbycusis, bilateral**

   ✓5ᵗʰ **H91.2 Sudden idiopathic hearing loss**
Sudden hearing loss NOS

    H91.20   **Sudden idiopathic hearing loss, unspecified ear**

    H91.21   **Sudden idiopathic hearing loss, right ear**

EXCLUDES 1 Not coded here   **EXCLUDES 2** Not included here   N Newborn Age: 0   P Pediatric Age: 0-17   M Maternity Age: 12-55   A Adult Age: 15-124

566   ICD-10-CM Draft (2015)

H91.22 Sudden idiopathic hearing loss, left ear
H91.23 Sudden idiopathic hearing loss, bilateral
H91.3 Deaf nonspeaking, not elsewhere classified

✓5ᵗʰ H91.8 Other specified hearing loss

  ✓6ᵗʰ H91.8X Other specified hearing loss
    H91.8X1 Other specified hearing loss, right ear
    H91.8X2 Other specified hearing loss, left ear
    H91.8X3 Other specified hearing loss, bilateral
    H91.8X9 Other specified hearing loss, unspecified ear

✓5ᵗʰ H91.9 Unspecified hearing loss
  Deafness NOS
  High frequency deafness
  Low frequency deafness
  H91.90 Unspecified hearing loss, unspecified ear
  H91.91 Unspecified hearing loss, right ear
  H91.92 Unspecified hearing loss, left ear
  H91.93 Unspecified hearing loss, bilateral

✓4ᵗʰ **H92 Otalgia and effusion of ear**

  ✓5ᵗʰ H92.0 Otalgia
    H92.01 Otalgia, right ear
    H92.02 Otalgia, left ear
    H92.03 Otalgia, bilateral
    H92.09 Otalgia, unspecified ear

  ✓5ᵗʰ H92.1 Otorrhea
    EXCLUDES 1 leakage of cerebrospinal fluid through ear (G96.0)
    H92.10 Otorrhea, unspecified ear
    H92.11 Otorrhea, right ear
    H92.12 Otorrhea, left ear
    H92.13 Otorrhea, bilateral

  ✓5ᵗʰ H92.2 Otorrhagia
    EXCLUDES 1 traumatic otorrhagia—code to injury
    H92.20 Otorrhagia, unspecified ear
    H92.21 Otorrhagia, right ear
    H92.22 Otorrhagia, left ear
    H92.23 Otorrhagia, bilateral

✓4ᵗʰ **H93 Other disorders of ear, not elsewhere classified**

  ✓5ᵗʰ H93.0 Degenerative and vascular disorders of ear
    EXCLUDES 1 presbycusis (H91.1)

    ✓6ᵗʰ H93.01 Transient ischemic deafness
      H93.011 Transient ischemic deafness, right ear
      H93.012 Transient ischemic deafness, left ear
      H93.013 Transient ischemic deafness, bilateral
      H93.019 Transient ischemic deafness, unspecified ear

    ✓6ᵗʰ H93.09 Unspecified degenerative and vascular disorders of ear
      H93.091 Unspecified degenerative and vascular disorders of right ear
      H93.092 Unspecified degenerative and vascular disorders of left ear
      H93.093 Unspecified degenerative and vascular disorders of ear, bilateral
      H93.099 Unspecified degenerative and vascular disorders of unspecified ear

  ✓5ᵗʰ H93.1 Tinnitus
    H93.11 Tinnitus, right ear
    H93.12 Tinnitus, left ear
    H93.13 Tinnitus, bilateral
    H93.19 Tinnitus, unspecified ear

  ✓5ᵗʰ H93.2 Other abnormal auditory perceptions
    EXCLUDES 2 auditory hallucinations (R44.0)

    ✓6ᵗʰ H93.21 Auditory recruitment
      H93.211 Auditory recruitment, right ear
      H93.212 Auditory recruitment, left ear
      H93.213 Auditory recruitment, bilateral
      H93.219 Auditory recruitment, unspecified ear

    ✓6ᵗʰ H93.22 Diplacusis
      H93.221 Diplacusis, right ear
      H93.222 Diplacusis, left ear
      H93.223 Diplacusis, bilateral

      H93.229 Diplacusis, unspecified ear

    ✓6ᵗʰ H93.23 Hyperacusis
      H93.231 Hyperacusis, right ear
      H93.232 Hyperacusis, left ear
      H93.233 Hyperacusis, bilateral
      H93.239 Hyperacusis, unspecified ear

    ✓6ᵗʰ H93.24 Temporary auditory threshold shift
      H93.241 Temporary auditory threshold shift, right ear
      H93.242 Temporary auditory threshold shift, left ear
      H93.243 Temporary auditory threshold shift, bilateral
      H93.249 Temporary auditory threshold shift, unspecified ear

    H93.25 Central auditory processing disorder
      Congenital auditory imperception
      Word deafness
      EXCLUDES 1 mixed receptive-expressive language disorder (F80.2)

    ✓6ᵗʰ H93.29 Other abnormal auditory perceptions
      H93.291 Other abnormal auditory perceptions, right ear
      H93.292 Other abnormal auditory perceptions, left ear
      H93.293 Other abnormal auditory perceptions, bilateral
      H93.299 Other abnormal auditory perceptions, unspecified ear

  ✓5ᵗʰ H93.3 Disorders of acoustic nerve
    Disorder of 8th cranial nerve
    EXCLUDES 1 acoustic neuroma (D33.3)
      syphilitic acoustic neuritis (A52.15)

    ✓6ᵗʰ H93.3X Disorders of acoustic nerve
      H93.3X1 Disorders of right acoustic nerve
      H93.3X2 Disorders of left acoustic nerve
      H93.3X3 Disorders of bilateral acoustic nerves
      H93.3X9 Disorders of unspecified acoustic nerve

  ✓5ᵗʰ H93.8 Other specified disorders of ear

    ✓6ᵗʰ H93.8X Other specified disorders of ear
      H93.8X1 Other specified disorders of right ear
      H93.8X2 Other specified disorders of left ear
      H93.8X3 Other specified disorders of ear, bilateral
      H93.8X9 Other specified disorders of ear, unspecified ear

  ✓5ᵗʰ H93.9 Unspecified disorder of ear
    H93.90 Unspecified disorder of ear, unspecified ear
    H93.91 Unspecified disorder of right ear
    H93.92 Unspecified disorder of left ear
    H93.93 Unspecified disorder of ear, bilateral

✓4ᵗʰ **H94 Other disorders of ear in diseases classified elsewhere**

  ✓5ᵗʰ H94.0 Acoustic neuritis in infectious and parasitic diseases classified elsewhere
    Code first underlying disease, such as:
      parasitic disease (B65-B89)
    EXCLUDES 1 acoustic neuritis (in):
      herpes zoster (B02.29)
      syphilis (A52.15)

    H94.00 *Acoustic neuritis in infectious and parasitic diseases classified elsewhere, unspecified ear*
    H94.01 *Acoustic neuritis in infectious and parasitic diseases classified elsewhere, right ear*
    H94.02 *Acoustic neuritis in infectious and parasitic diseases classified elsewhere, left ear*
    H94.03 *Acoustic neuritis in infectious and parasitic diseases classified elsewhere, bilateral*

  ✓5ᵗʰ H94.8 Other specified disorders of ear in diseases classified elsewhere
    Code first underlying disease, such as:
      congenital syphilis (A50.0)
    EXCLUDES 1 aural myiasis (B87.4)
      syphilitic labyrinthitis (A52.79)

    H94.80 *Other specified disorders of ear in diseases classified elsewhere, unspecified ear*

☑ Additional Character Required   ✓ₓ7ᵗʰ Xtension Alert   Unspecified Dx   Other Specified Dx   Manifestation   ►◄ Revised Text   ● New Code   ▲ Revised Code Title

H94.81   **Other specified disorders of right ear in diseases classified elsewhere**

H94.82   **Other specified disorders of left ear in diseases classified elsewhere**

H94.83   **Other specified disorders of ear in diseases classified elsewhere, bilateral**

Intraoperative and postprocedural complications and disorders of ear and mastoid process, not elsewhere classified (H95)

✓4ᵗʰ **H95**   **Intraoperative and postprocedural complications and disorders of ear and mastoid process, not elsewhere classified**

    ✓5ᵗʰ **H95.0**   **Recurrent cholesteatoma of postmastoidectomy cavity**

       H95.00   **Recurrent cholesteatoma of postmastoidectomy cavity, unspecified ear**

       H95.01   **Recurrent cholesteatoma of postmastoidectomy cavity, right ear**

       H95.02   **Recurrent cholesteatoma of postmastoidectomy cavity, left ear**

       H95.03   **Recurrent cholesteatoma of postmastoidectomy cavity, bilateral ears**

    ✓5ᵗʰ **H95.1**   **Other disorders of ear and mastoid process following mastoidectomy**

       ✓6ᵗʰ H95.11   **Chronic inflammation of postmastoidectomy cavity**

          H95.111   **Chronic inflammation of postmastoidectomy cavity, right ear**

          H95.112   **Chronic inflammation of postmastoidectomy cavity, left ear**

          H95.113   **Chronic inflammation of postmastoidectomy cavity, bilateral ears**

          H95.119   **Chronic inflammation of postmastoidectomy cavity, unspecified ear**

       ✓6ᵗʰ H95.12   **Granulation of postmastoidectomy cavity**

          H95.121   **Granulation of postmastoidectomy cavity, right ear**

          H95.122   **Granulation of postmastoidectomy cavity, left ear**

          H95.123   **Granulation of postmastoidectomy cavity, bilateral ears**

          H95.129   **Granulation of postmastoidectomy cavity, unspecified ear**

       ✓6ᵗʰ H95.13   **Mucosal cyst of postmastoidectomy cavity**

          H95.131   **Mucosal cyst of postmastoidectomy cavity, right ear**

          H95.132   **Mucosal cyst of postmastoidectomy cavity, left ear**

          H95.133   **Mucosal cyst of postmastoidectomy cavity, bilateral ears**

          H95.139   **Mucosal cyst of postmastoidectomy cavity, unspecified ear**

       ✓6ᵗʰ H95.19   **Other disorders following mastoidectomy**

          H95.191   **Other disorders following mastoidectomy, right ear**

          H95.192   **Other disorders following mastoidectomy, left ear**

          H95.193   **Other disorders following mastoidectomy, bilateral ears**

          H95.199   **Other disorders following mastoidectomy, unspecified ear**

    ✓5ᵗʰ **H95.2**   **Intraoperative hemorrhage and hematoma of ear and mastoid process complicating a procedure**

       EXCLUDES 1   *intraoperative hemorrhage and hematoma of ear and mastoid process due to accidental puncture or laceration during a procedure (H95.3-)*

       H95.21   **Intraoperative hemorrhage and hematoma of ear and mastoid process complicating a procedure on the ear and mastoid process**

       H95.22   **Intraoperative hemorrhage and hematoma of ear and mastoid process complicating other procedure**

    ✓5ᵗʰ **H95.3**   **Accidental puncture and laceration of ear and mastoid process during a procedure**

       H95.31   **Accidental puncture and laceration of the ear and mastoid process during a procedure on the ear and mastoid process**

       H95.32   **Accidental puncture and laceration of the ear and mastoid process during other procedure**

    ✓5ᵗʰ **H95.4**   **Postprocedural hemorrhage and hematoma of ear and mastoid process following a procedure**

       H95.41   **Postprocedural hemorrhage and hematoma of ear and mastoid process following a procedure on the ear and mastoid process**

       H95.42   **Postprocedural hemorrhage and hematoma of ear and mastoid process following other procedure**

    ✓5ᵗʰ **H95.8**   **Other intraoperative and postprocedural complications and disorders of the ear and mastoid process, not elsewhere classified**

       EXCLUDES 2   *postprocedural complications and disorders following mastoidectomy (H95.0-, H95.1-)*

       ✓6ᵗʰ H95.81   **Postprocedural stenosis of external ear canal**

          H95.811   **Postprocedural stenosis of right external ear canal**

          H95.812   **Postprocedural stenosis of left external ear canal**

          H95.813   **Postprocedural stenosis of external ear canal, bilateral**

          H95.819   **Postprocedural stenosis of unspecified external ear canal**

       H95.88   **Other intraoperative complications and disorders of the ear and mastoid process, not elsewhere classified**

          Use additional code, if applicable, to further specify disorder

       H95.89   **Other postprocedural complications and disorders of the ear and mastoid process, not elsewhere classified**

          Use additional code, if applicable, to further specify disorder

EXCLUDES 1 Not coded here   **EXCLUDES 2** Not included here   N Newborn Age: 0   P Pediatric Age: 0-17   M Maternity Age: 12-55   A Adult Age: 15-124

568   ICD-10-CM Draft (2015)

Chapter 9. Diseases of the Circulatory System(I00-I99)

EXCLUDES 2　certain conditions originating in the perinatal period (P04-P96)
certain infectious and parasitic diseases (A00-B99)
complications of pregnancy, childbirth and the puerperium (O00-O9A)
congenital malformations, deformations, and chromosomal abnormalities (Q00-Q99)
endocrine, nutritional and metabolic diseases (E00-E88)
injury, poisoning and certain other consequences of external causes (S00-T88)
neoplasms (C00-D49)
symptoms, signs and abnormal clinical and laboratory findings, not elsewhere classified (R00-R94)
systemic connective tissue disorders (M30-M36)
transient cerebral ischemic attacks and related syndromes (G45.-)

This chapter contains the following blocks:

I00-I02	Acute rheumatic fever
I05-I09	Chronic rheumatic heart diseases
I10-I15	Hypertensive diseases
I20-I25	Ischemic heart diseases
I26-I28	Pulmonary heart disease and diseases of pulmonary circulation
I30-I52	Other forms of heart disease
I60-I69	Cerebrovascular diseases
I70-I79	Diseases of arteries, arterioles and capillaries
I80-I89	Diseases of veins, lymphatic vessels and lymph nodes, not elsewhere classified
I95-I99	Other and unspecified disorders of the circulatory system

Acute rheumatic fever (I00-I02)

I00　**Rheumatic fever without heart involvement**
　INCLUDES　arthritis, rheumatic, acute or subacute
　EXCLUDES 1　rheumatic fever with heart involvement (I01.0-I01.9)

✓4th I01　**Rheumatic fever with heart involvement**
　EXCLUDES 1　chronic diseases of rheumatic origin (I05-I09) unless rheumatic fever is also present or there is evidence of reactivation or activity of the rheumatic process.

　I01.0　**Acute rheumatic pericarditis**
　　Any condition in I00 with pericarditis
　　Rheumatic pericarditis (acute)
　　EXCLUDES 1　acute pericarditis not specified as rheumatic (I30.-)

　I01.1　**Acute rheumatic endocarditis**
　　Any condition in I00 with endocarditis or valvulitis
　　Acute rheumatic valvulitis

　I01.2　**Acute rheumatic myocarditis**
　　Any condition in I00 with myocarditis

　I01.8　**Other acute rheumatic heart disease**
　　Any condition in I00 with other or multiple types of heart involvement
　　Acute rheumatic pancarditis

　I01.9　**Acute rheumatic heart disease, unspecified**
　　Any condition in I00 with unspecified type of heart involvement
　　Rheumatic carditis, acute
　　Rheumatic heart disease, active or acute

✓4th I02　**Rheumatic chorea**
　INCLUDES　Sydenham's chorea
　EXCLUDES 1　chorea NOS (G25.5)
　　　　　　　Huntington's chorea (G10)

　I02.0　**Rheumatic chorea with heart involvement**
　　Chorea NOS with heart involvement
　　Rheumatic chorea with heart involvement of any type classifiable under I01-

　I02.9　**Rheumatic chorea without heart involvement**
　　Rheumatic chorea NOS

Chronic rheumatic heart diseases (I05-I09)

✓4th I05　**Rheumatic mitral valve diseases**
　INCLUDES　conditions classifiable to both I05.0 and I05.2-I05.9, whether specified as rheumatic or not
　EXCLUDES 1　mitral valve disease specified as nonrheumatic (I34.-)
　　　　　　　mitral valve disease with aortic and/or tricuspid valve involvement (I08.-)

　I05.0　**Rheumatic mitral stenosis**
　　Mitral (valve) obstruction (rheumatic)

　I05.1　**Rheumatic mitral insufficiency**
　　Rheumatic mitral incompetence
　　Rheumatic mitral regurgitation
　　EXCLUDES 1　mitral insufficiency not specified as rheumatic (I34.0)

　I05.2　**Rheumatic mitral stenosis with insufficiency**
　　Rheumatic mitral stenosis with incompetence or regurgitation

　I05.8　**Other rheumatic mitral valve diseases**
　　Rheumatic mitral (valve) failure

　I05.9　**Rheumatic mitral valve disease, unspecified**
　　Rheumatic mitral (valve) disorder (chronic) NOS

✓4th I06　**Rheumatic aortic valve diseases**
　EXCLUDES 1　aortic valve disease not specified as rheumatic (I35.-)
　　　　　　　aortic valve disease with mitral and/or tricuspid valve involvement (I08.-)

　I06.0　**Rheumatic aortic stenosis**
　　Rheumatic aortic (valve) obstruction

　I06.1　**Rheumatic aortic insufficiency**
　　Rheumatic aortic incompetence
　　Rheumatic aortic regurgitation

　I06.2　**Rheumatic aortic stenosis with insufficiency**
　　Rheumatic aortic stenosis with incompetence or regurgitation

　I06.8　**Other rheumatic aortic valve diseases**

　I06.9　**Rheumatic aortic valve disease, unspecified**
　　Rheumatic aortic (valve) disease NOS

✓4th I07　**Rheumatic tricuspid valve diseases**
　INCLUDES　rheumatic tricuspid valve diseases specified as rheumatic or unspecified
　EXCLUDES 1　tricuspid valve disease specified as nonrheumatic (I36.-)
　　　　　　　tricuspid valve disease with aortic and/or mitral valve involvement (I08.-)

　I07.0　**Rheumatic tricuspid stenosis**
　　Tricuspid (valve) stenosis (rheumatic)

　I07.1　**Rheumatic tricuspid insufficiency**
　　Tricuspid (valve) insufficiency (rheumatic)

　I07.2　**Rheumatic tricuspid stenosis and insufficiency**

　I07.8　**Other rheumatic tricuspid valve diseases**

　I07.9　**Rheumatic tricuspid valve disease, unspecified**
　　Rheumatic tricuspid valve disorder NOS

✓4th I08　**Multiple valve diseases**
　INCLUDES　multiple valve diseases specified as rheumatic or unspecified
　EXCLUDES 1　endocarditis, valve unspecified (I38)
　　　　　　　multiple valve disease specified a nonrheumatic (I34.-, I35.-, I36.-, I37.-, I38.-, Q22.-, Q23.-, Q24.8-)
　　　　　　　rheumatic valve disease NOS (I09.1)

　I08.0　**Rheumatic disorders of both mitral and aortic valves**
　　Involvement of both mitral and aortic valves specified as rheumatic or unspecified

　I08.1　**Rheumatic disorders of both mitral and tricuspid valves**

　I08.2　**Rheumatic disorders of both aortic and tricuspid valves**

　I08.3　**Combined rheumatic disorders of mitral, aortic and tricuspid valves**

　I08.8　**Other rheumatic multiple valve diseases**

　I08.9　**Rheumatic multiple valve disease, unspecified**

✓4th I09　**Other rheumatic heart diseases**

　I09.0　**Rheumatic myocarditis**
　　EXCLUDES 1　myocarditis not specified as rheumatic (I51.4)

　I09.1　**Rheumatic diseases of endocardium, valve unspecified**
　　Rheumatic endocarditis (chronic)
　　Rheumatic valvulitis (chronic)
　　EXCLUDES 1　endocarditis, valve unspecified (I38)

　I09.2　**Chronic rheumatic pericarditis**
　　Adherent pericardium, rheumatic
　　Chronic rheumatic mediastinopericarditis
　　Chronic rheumatic myopericarditis
　　EXCLUDES 1　chronic pericarditis not specified as rheumatic (I31.-)

　✓5th I09.8　**Other specified rheumatic heart diseases**

　　I09.81　**Rheumatic heart failure**
　　　Use additional code to identify type of heart failure (I50.-)

　　I09.89　**Other specified rheumatic heart diseases**
　　　Rheumatic disease of pulmonary valve

　I09.9　**Rheumatic heart disease, unspecified**
　　Rheumatic carditis
　　EXCLUDES 1　rheumatoid carditis (M05.31)

✓ Additional Character Required　　✓x7th Xtension Alert　　Unspecified Dx　　Other Specified Dx　　Manifestation　　►◄ Revised Text　　● New Code　　▲ Revised Code Title

Diseases of the Circulatory System *(left margin)*

I10–I21.02 *(left margin)*

Hypertensive diseases (I10-I15)

Use additional code to identify:
exposure to environmental tobacco smoke (Z77.22)
history of tobacco use (Z87.891)
occupational exposure to environmental tobacco smoke (Z57.31)
tobacco dependence (F17.-)
tobacco use (Z72.0)
EXCLUDES 1   *hypertensive disease complicating pregnancy, childbirth and the*
puerperium (O10-O11, O13-O16)
neonatal hypertension (P29.2)
primary pulmonary hypertension (I27.0)

I10   Essential (primary) hypertension
INCLUDES   high blood pressure
hypertension (arterial) (benign) (essential) (malignant)
(primary) (systemic)
EXCLUDES 1   *hypertensive disease complicating pregnancy, childbirth and*
the puerperium (O10-O11, O13-O16)
EXCLUDES 2   *essential (primary) hypertension involving vessels of brain*
(I60-I69)
essential (primary) hypertension involving vessels of eye
(H35.0-)

✓4ᵗʰ I11   Hypertensive heart disease
INCLUDES   any condition in I51.4-I51.9 due to hypertension

I11.0   Hypertensive heart disease with heart failure
Hypertensive heart failure
Use additional code to identify type of heart failure (I50.-)

I11.9   Hypertensive heart disease without heart failure
Hypertensive heart disease NOS

✓4ᵗʰ I12   Hypertensive chronic kidney disease
INCLUDES   any condition in N18- and N26- due to hypertension
arteriosclerosis of kidney
arteriosclerotic nephritis (chronic) (interstitial)
hypertensive nephropathy
nephrosclerosis
EXCLUDES 1   *hypertension due to kidney disease (I15.0, I15.1)*
renovascular hypertension (I15.0)
secondary hypertension (I15.-)
EXCLUDES 2   *acute kidney failure (N17.-)*

**I12.0   Hypertensive chronic kidney disease with stage 5
chronic kidney disease or end stage renal disease**
Use additional code to identify the stage of chronic kidney
disease (N18.5, N18.6)

**I12.9   Hypertensive chronic kidney disease with stage 1 through
stage 4 chronic kidney disease, or unspecified chronic kidney
disease**
Hypertensive chronic kidney disease NOS
Hypertensive renal disease NOS
Use additional code to identify the stage of chronic kidney
disease (N18.1-N18.4, N18.9)

✓4ᵗʰ I13   Hypertensive heart and chronic kidney disease
INCLUDES   any condition in I11- with any condition in I12-
cardiorenal disease
cardiovascular renal disease

**I13.0   Hypertensive heart and chronic kidney disease with heart
failure and stage 1 through stage 4 chronic kidney disease, or
unspecified chronic kidney disease**
Use additional code to identify type of heart failure (I50.-)
Use additional code to identify stage of chronic kidney disease
(N18.1-N18.4, N18.9)

**✓5ᵗʰ I13.1   Hypertensive heart and chronic kidney disease without heart
failure**

**I13.10   Hypertensive heart and chronic kidney disease
without heart failure, with stage 1 through stage 4
chronic kidney disease, or unspecified chronic
kidney disease**
Hypertensive heart disease and hypertensive chronic
kidney disease NOS
Use additional code to identify the stage of chronic
kidney disease (N18.1-N18.4, N18.9)

**I13.11   Hypertensive heart and chronic kidney disease
without heart failure, with stage 5 chronic kidney
disease, or end stage renal disease**
Use additional code to identify the stage of chronic
kidney disease (N18.5, N18.6)

**I13.2   Hypertensive heart and chronic kidney disease with heart
failure and with stage 5 chronic kidney disease, or end stage
renal disease**
Use additional code to identify type of heart failure (I50.-)
Use additional code to identify the stage of chronic kidney
disease (N18.5, N18.6)

✓4ᵗʰ I15   Secondary hypertension
Code also underlying condition
EXCLUDES 1   *postprocedural hypertension (I97.3)*
EXCLUDES 2   *secondary hypertension involving vessels of brain (I60-I69)*
secondary hypertension involving vessels of eye (H35.0-)

I15.0   Renovascular hypertension
I15.1   Hypertension secondary to other renal disorders
I15.2   Hypertension secondary to endocrine disorders
I15.8   Other secondary hypertension
I15.9   Secondary hypertension, unspecified

Ischemic heart diseases (I20-I25)

Use additional code to identify presence of hypertension (I10-I15)

✓4ᵗʰ I20   Angina pectoris
Use additional code to identify:
exposure to environmental tobacco smoke (Z77.22)
history of tobacco use (Z87.891)
occupational exposure to environmental tobacco smoke (Z57.31)
tobacco dependence (F17.-)
tobacco use (Z72.0)
EXCLUDES 1   *angina pectoris with atherosclerotic heart disease of native*
coronary arteries (I25.1-)
atherosclerosis of coronary artery bypass graft(s) and coronary
artery of transplanted heart with angina pectoris (I25.7-)
postinfarction angina (I23.7)

I20.0   Unstable angina
Accelerated angina
Crescendo angina
De novo effort angina
Intermediate coronary syndrome
Preinfarction syndrome
Worsening effort angina

I20.1   Angina pectoris with documented spasm
Angiospastic angina
Prinzmetal angina
Spasm-induced angina
Variant angina

I20.8   Other forms of angina pectoris
Angina equivalent
Angina of effort
Coronary slow flow syndrome
Stenocardia
Use additional code(s) for symptoms associated with angina
equivalent

I20.9   Angina pectoris, unspecified
Angina NOS
Anginal syndrome
Cardiac angina
Ischemic chest pain

✓4ᵗʰ I21   ST elevation (STEMI) and non-ST elevation (NSTEMI) myocardial infarction
INCLUDES   cardiac infarction
coronary (artery) embolism
coronary (artery) occlusion
coronary (artery) rupture
coronary (artery) thrombosis
infarction of heart, myocardium, or ventricle
myocardial infarction specified as acute or with a stated
duration of 4 weeks (28 days) or less from onset
Use additional code, if applicable, to identify:
exposure to environmental tobacco smoke (Z77.22)
history of tobacco use (Z87.891)
occupational exposure to environmental tobacco smoke (Z57.31)
status post administration of tPA (rtPA) in a different facility within
the last 24 hours prior to admission to current facility (Z92.82)
tobacco dependence (F17.-)
tobacco use (Z72.0)
EXCLUDES 2   *old myocardial infarction (I25.2)*
postmyocardial infarction syndrome (I24.1)
subsequent myocardial infarction (I22.-)
AHA: 2013, 1Q, 25; 2012, 4Q, 96, 102-103

✓5ᵗʰ I21.0   ST elevation (STEMI) myocardial infarction of anterior wall

**I21.01   ST elevation (STEMI) myocardial infarction involving
left main coronary artery**

**I21.02   ST elevation (STEMI) myocardial infarction involving
left anterior descending coronary artery**
ST elevation (STEMI) myocardial infarction involving
diagonal coronary artery
AHA: 2013, 1Q, 25

EXCLUDES 1 Not coded here   EXCLUDES 2 Not included here   N Newborn Age: 0   P Pediatric Age: 0-17   M Maternity Age: 12-55   A Adult Age: 15-124

I21.09 ST elevation (STEMI) myocardial infarction involving other coronary artery of anterior wall
Acute transmural myocardial infarction of anterior wall
Anteroapical transmural (Q wave) infarction (acute)
Anterolateral transmural (Q wave) infarction (acute)
Anteroseptal transmural (Q wave) infarction (acute)
Transmural (Q wave) infarction (acute) (of) anterior (wall) NOS
AHA: 2012, 4Q, 102-103

√5ᵗʰ **I21.1 ST elevation (STEMI) myocardial infarction of inferior wall**

I21.11 ST elevation (STEMI) myocardial infarction involving right coronary artery
Inferoposterior transmural (Q wave) infarction (acute)

I21.19 ST elevation (STEMI) myocardial infarction involving other coronary artery of inferior wall
Acute transmural myocardial infarction of inferior wall
Inferolateral transmural (Q wave) infarction (acute)
Transmural (Q wave) infarction (acute) (of) diaphragmatic wall
Transmural (Q wave) infarction (acute) (of) inferior (wall) NOS
EXCLUDES 2 ST elevation (STEMI) myocardial infarction involving left circumflex coronary artery (I21.21)
AHA: 2012, 4Q, 96

√5ᵗʰ **I21.2 ST elevation (STEMI) myocardial infarction of other sites**

I21.21 ST elevation (STEMI) myocardial infarction involving left circumflex coronary artery
ST elevation (STEMI) myocardial infarction involving oblique marginal coronary artery

I21.29 ST elevation (STEMI) myocardial infarction involving other sites
Acute transmural myocardial infarction of other sites
Apical-lateral transmural (Q wave) infarction (acute)
Basal-lateral transmural (Q wave) infarction (acute)
High lateral transmural (Q wave) infarction (acute)
Lateral (wall) NOS transmural (Q wave) infarction (acute)
Posterior (true) transmural (Q wave) infarction (acute)
Posterobasal transmural (Q wave) infarction (acute)
Posterolateral transmural (Q wave) infarction (acute)
Posteroseptal transmural (Q wave) infarction (acute)
Septal transmural (Q wave) infarction (acute) NOS

I21.3 ST elevation (STEMI) myocardial infarction of unspecified site
Acute transmural myocardial infarction of unspecified site
Myocardial infarction (acute) NOS
Transmural (Q wave) myocardial infarction NOS

I21.4 Non-ST elevation (NSTEMI) myocardial infarction
Acute subendocardial myocardial infarction
Non-Q wave myocardial infarction NOS
Nontransmural myocardial infarction NOS

√4ᵗʰ **I22 Subsequent ST elevation (STEMI) and non-ST elevation (NSTEMI) myocardial infarction**
INCLUDES acute myocardial infarction occurring within four weeks (28 days) of a previous acute myocardial infarction, regardless of site
cardiac infarction
coronary (artery) embolism
coronary (artery) occlusion
coronary (artery) rupture
coronary (artery) thrombosis
infarction of heart, myocardium, or ventricle
recurrent myocardial infarction
reinfarction of myocardium
rupture of heart, myocardium, or ventricle
Use additional code, if applicable, to identify:
exposure to environmental tobacco smoke (Z77.22)
history of tobacco use (Z87.891)
occupational exposure to environmental tobacco smoke (Z57.31)
status post administration of tPA (rtPA) in a different facility within the last 24 hours prior to admission to current facility (Z92.82)
tobacco dependence (F17.-)
tobacco use (Z72.0)
AHA: 2013, 1Q, 25; 2012, 4Q, 97, 102-103

I22.0 Subsequent ST elevation (STEMI) myocardial infarction of anterior wall
Subsequent acute transmural myocardial infarction of anterior wall
Subsequent transmural (Q wave) infarction (acute)(of) anterior (wall) NOS
Subsequent anteroapical transmural (Q wave) infarction (acute)
Subsequent anterolateral transmural (Q wave) infarction (acute)
Subsequent anteroseptal transmural (Q wave) infarction (acute)

I22.1 Subsequent ST elevation (STEMI) myocardial infarction of inferior wall
Subsequent acute transmural myocardial infarction of inferior wall
Subsequent transmural (Q wave) infarction (acute)(of) diaphragmatic wall
Subsequent transmural (Q wave) infarction (acute)(of) inferior (wall) NOS
Subsequent inferolateral transmural (Q wave) infarction (acute)
Subsequent inferoposterior transmural (Q wave) infarction (acute)
AHA: 2012, 4Q, 102

I22.2 Subsequent non-ST elevation (NSTEMI) myocardial infarction
Subsequent acute subendocardial myocardial infarction
Subsequent non-Q wave myocardial infarction NOS
Subsequent nontransmural myocardial infarction NOS

I22.8 Subsequent ST elevation (STEMI) myocardial infarction of other sites
Subsequent acute transmural myocardial infarction of other sites
Subsequent apical-lateral transmural (Q wave) myocardial infarction (acute)
Subsequent basal-lateral transmural (Q wave) myocardial infarction (acute)
Subsequent high lateral transmural (Q wave) myocardial infarction (acute)
Subsequent transmural (Q wave) myocardial infarction (acute)(of) lateral (wall) NOS
Subsequent posterior (true)transmural (Q wave) myocardial infarction (acute)
Subsequent posterobasal transmural (Q wave) myocardial infarction (acute)
Subsequent posterolateral transmural (Q wave) myocardial infarction (acute)
Subsequent posteroseptal transmural (Q wave) myocardial infarction (acute)
Subsequent septal NOS transmural (Q wave) myocardial infarction (acute)

I22.9 Subsequent ST elevation (STEMI) myocardial infarction of unspecified site
Subsequent acute myocardial infarction of unspecified site
Subsequent myocardial infarction (acute) NOS

√4ᵗʰ **I23 Certain current complications following ST elevation (STEMI) and non-ST elevation (NSTEMI) myocardial infarction (within the 28 day period)**

I23.0 Hemopericardium as current complication following acute myocardial infarction 🅐
EXCLUDES 1 hemopericardium not specified as current complication following acute myocardial infarction (I31.2)

I23.1 Atrial septal defect as current complication following acute myocardial infarction 🅐
EXCLUDES 1 acquired atrial septal defect not specified as current complication following acute myocardial infarction (I51.0)

I23.2 Ventricular septal defect as current complication following acute myocardial infarction 🅐
EXCLUDES 1 acquired ventricular septal defect not specified as current complication following acute myocardial infarction (I51.0)

I23.3 Rupture of cardiac wall without hemopericardium as current complication following acute myocardial infarction 🅐

I23.4 Rupture of chordae tendineae as current complication following acute myocardial infarction 🅐
EXCLUDES 1 rupture of chordae tendineae not specified as current complication following acute myocardial infarction (I51.1)

I23.5 Rupture of papillary muscle as current complication following acute myocardial infarction 🅐
EXCLUDES 1 rupture of papillary muscle not specified as current complication following acute myocardial infarction (I51.2)

I23.6 Thrombosis of atrium, auricular appendage, and ventricle as current complications following acute myocardial infarction 🅐
EXCLUDES 1 thrombosis of atrium, auricular appendage, and ventricle not specified as current complication following acute myocardial infarction (I51.3)

I23.7 Postinfarction angina 🅐

I23.8 Other current complications following acute myocardial infarction 🅐

✓4ᵗʰ I24 Other acute ischemic heart diseases
> EXCLUDES1   *angina pectoris (I20.-)*
> *transient myocardial ischemia in newborn (P29.4)*

I24.0 Acute coronary thrombosis not resulting in myocardial infarction
> Acute coronary (artery) (vein) embolism not resulting in myocardial infarction
> Acute coronary (artery) (vein) occlusion not resulting in myocardial infarction
> Acute coronary (artery) (vein) thromboembolism not resulting in myocardial infarction
> EXCLUDES1   *atherosclerotic heart disease (I25.1-)*
> **AHA:** 2013, 1Q, 24

I24.1 Dressler's syndrome
> Postmyocardial infarction syndrome
> EXCLUDES1   *postinfarction angina (I23.7)*

I24.8 Other forms of acute ischemic heart disease

I24.9 Acute ischemic heart disease, unspecified
> EXCLUDES1   *ischemic heart disease (chronic) NOS (I25.9)*

✓4ᵗʰ I25 Chronic ischemic heart disease
> Use additional code to identify:
> chronic total occlusion of coronary artery (I25.82)
> exposure to environmental tobacco smoke (Z77.22)
> history of tobacco use (Z87.891)
> occupational exposure to environmental tobacco smoke (Z57.31)
> tobacco dependence (F17.-)
> tobacco use (Z72.0)

I25.1 Atherosclerotic heart disease of native coronary artery
> Atherosclerotic cardiovascular disease
> Coronary (artery) atheroma
> Coronary (artery) atherosclerosis
> Coronary (artery) disease
> Coronary (artery) sclerosis
> Use additional code, if applicable, to identify:
> coronary atherosclerosis due to calcified coronary lesion (I25.84)
> coronary atherosclerosis due to lipid rich plaque (I25.83)
> EXCLUDES2   *atheroembolism (I75.-)*
> *atherosclerosis of coronary artery bypass graft(s) and transplanted heart (I25.7-)*

I25.10 Atherosclerotic heart disease of native coronary artery without angina pectoris 🄰
> Atherosclerotic heart disease NOS
> **AHA:** 2012, 4Q, 92

✓6ᵗʰ I25.11 Atherosclerotic heart disease of native coronary artery with angina pectoris

I25.110 Atherosclerotic heart disease of native coronary artery with unstable angina pectoris 🄰
> EXCLUDES1   *unstable angina without atherosclerotic heart disease (I20.0)*

I25.111 Atherosclerotic heart disease of native coronary artery with angina pectoris with documented spasm 🄰
> EXCLUDES1   *angina pectoris with documented spasm without atherosclerotic heart disease (I20.1)*

I25.118 Atherosclerotic heart disease of native coronary artery with other forms of angina pectoris 🄰
> EXCLUDES1   *other forms of angina pectoris without atherosclerotic heart disease (I20.8)*

I25.119 Atherosclerotic heart disease of native coronary artery with unspecified angina pectoris 🄰
> Atherosclerotic heart disease with angina NOS
> Atherosclerotic heart disease with ischemic chest pain
> EXCLUDES1   *unspecified angina pectoris without atherosclerotic heart disease (I20.9)*

I25.2 Old myocardial infarction
> Healed myocardial infarction
> Past myocardial infarction diagnosed by ECG or other investigation, but currently presenting no symptoms

I25.3 Aneurysm of heart
> Mural aneurysm
> Ventricular aneurysm

✓5ᵗʰ I25.4 Coronary artery aneurysm and dissection

I25.41 Coronary artery aneurysm
> Coronary arteriovenous fistula, acquired
> EXCLUDES1   *congenital coronary (artery) aneurysm (Q24.5)*

I25.42 Coronary artery dissection

I25.5 Ischemic cardiomyopathy
> EXCLUDES2   *coronary atherosclerosis (I25.1-, I25.7-)*

I25.6 Silent myocardial ischemia

✓5ᵗʰ I25.7 Atherosclerosis of coronary artery bypass graft(s) and coronary artery of transplanted heart with angina pectoris
> Use additional code, if applicable, to identify:
> coronary atherosclerosis due to calcified coronary lesion (I25.84)
> coronary atherosclerosis due to lipid rich plaque (I25.83)
> EXCLUDES1   *atherosclerosis of bypass graft(s) of transplanted heart without angina pectoris (I25.812)*
> *atherosclerosis of coronary artery bypass graft(s) without angina pectoris (I25.810)*
> *atherosclerosis of native coronary artery of transplanted heart without angina pectoris (I25.811)*
> *embolism or thrombus of coronary artery bypass graft(s) (T82.8-)*

✓6ᵗʰ I25.70 Atherosclerosis of coronary artery bypass graft(s), unspecified, with angina pectoris

I25.700 Atherosclerosis of coronary artery bypass graft(s), unspecified, with unstable angina pectoris 🄰
> EXCLUDES1   *unstable angina pectoris without atherosclerosis of coronary artery bypass graft (I20.0)*

I25.701 Atherosclerosis of coronary artery bypass graft(s), unspecified, with angina pectoris with documented spasm 🄰
> EXCLUDES1   *angina pectoris with documented spasm without atherosclerosis of coronary artery bypass graft (I20.1)*

I25.708 Atherosclerosis of coronary artery bypass graft(s), unspecified, with other forms of angina pectoris 🄰
> EXCLUDES1   *other forms of angina pectoris without atherosclerosis of coronary artery bypass graft (I20.8)*

I25.709 Atherosclerosis of coronary artery bypass graft(s), unspecified, with unspecified angina pectoris 🄰
> EXCLUDES1   *unspecified angina pectoris without atherosclerosis of coronary artery bypass graft (I20.9)*

✓6ᵗʰ I25.71 Atherosclerosis of autologous vein coronary artery bypass graft(s) with angina pectoris

I25.710 Atherosclerosis of autologous vein coronary artery bypass graft(s) with unstable angina pectoris 🄰
> EXCLUDES1   *unstable angina without atherosclerosis of autologous vein coronary artery bypass graft(s) (I20.0)*

I25.711 Atherosclerosis of autologous vein coronary artery bypass graft(s) with angina pectoris with documented spasm 🄰
> EXCLUDES1   *angina pectoris with documented spasm without atherosclerosis of autologous vein coronary artery bypass graft(s) (I20.1)*

I25.718 Atherosclerosis of autologous vein coronary artery bypass graft(s) with other forms of angina pectoris 🄰
> EXCLUDES1   *other forms of angina pectoris without atherosclerosis of autologous vein coronary artery bypass graft(s) (I20.8)*

EXCLUDES1 Not coded here   EXCLUDES2 Not included here   🄽 Newborn Age: 0   🄿 Pediatric Age: 0-17   🄼 Maternity Age: 12-55   🄰 Adult Age: 15-124

572   ICD-10-CM Draft (2015)

I25.719　**Atherosclerosis of autologous vein coronary artery bypass graft(s) with unspecified angina pectoris** 🅐
  EXCLUDES 1　unspecified angina pectoris without atherosclerosis of autologous vein coronary artery bypass graft(s) (I20.9)

✓6ᵗʰ **I25.72**　**Atherosclerosis of autologous artery coronary artery bypass graft(s) with angina pectoris**
　Atherosclerosis of internal mammary artery graft with angina pectoris

I25.720　**Atherosclerosis of autologous artery coronary artery bypass graft(s) with unstable angina pectoris** 🅐
  EXCLUDES 1　unstable angina without atherosclerosis of autologous artery coronary artery bypass graft(s) (I20.0)

I25.721　**Atherosclerosis of autologous artery coronary artery bypass graft(s) with angina pectoris with documented spasm** 🅐
  EXCLUDES 1　angina pectoris with documented spasm without atherosclerosis of autologous artery coronary artery bypass graft(s) (I20.1)

I25.728　**Atherosclerosis of autologous artery coronary artery bypass graft(s) with other forms of angina pectoris** 🅐
  EXCLUDES 1　other forms of angina pectoris without atherosclerosis of autologous artery coronary artery bypass graft(s) (I20.8)

I25.729　**Atherosclerosis of autologous artery coronary artery bypass graft(s) with unspecified angina pectoris** 🅐
  EXCLUDES 1　unspecified angina pectoris without atherosclerosis of autologous artery coronary artery bypass graft(s) (I20.9)

✓6ᵗʰ **I25.73**　**Atherosclerosis of nonautologous biological coronary artery bypass graft(s) with angina pectoris**

I25.730　**Atherosclerosis of nonautologous biological coronary artery bypass graft(s) with unstable angina pectoris** 🅐
  EXCLUDES 1　unstable angina without atherosclerosis of nonautologous biological coronary artery bypass graft(s) (I20.0)

I25.731　**Atherosclerosis of nonautologous biological coronary artery bypass graft(s) with angina pectoris with documented spasm** 🅐
  EXCLUDES 1　angina pectoris with documented spasm without atherosclerosis of nonautologous biological coronary artery bypass graft(s) (I20.1)

I25.738　**Atherosclerosis of nonautologous biological coronary artery bypass graft(s) with other forms of angina pectoris** 🅐
  EXCLUDES 1　other forms of angina pectoris without atherosclerosis of nonautologous biological coronary artery bypass graft(s) (I20.8)

I25.739　**Atherosclerosis of nonautologous biological coronary artery bypass graft(s) with unspecified angina pectoris** 🅐
  EXCLUDES 1　unspecified angina pectoris without atherosclerosis of nonautologous biological coronary artery bypass graft(s) (I20.9)

✓6ᵗʰ **I25.75**　**Atherosclerosis of native coronary artery of transplanted heart with angina pectoris**
  EXCLUDES 1　atherosclerosis of native coronary artery of transplanted heart without angina pectoris (I25.811)

I25.750　**Atherosclerosis of native coronary artery of transplanted heart with unstable angina**

I25.751　**Atherosclerosis of native coronary artery of transplanted heart with angina pectoris with documented spasm**

I25.758　**Atherosclerosis of native coronary artery of transplanted heart with other forms of angina pectoris**

I25.759　**Atherosclerosis of native coronary artery of transplanted heart with unspecified angina pectoris**

✓6ᵗʰ **I25.76**　**Atherosclerosis of bypass graft of coronary artery of transplanted heart with angina pectoris**
  EXCLUDES 1　atherosclerosis of bypass graft of coronary artery of transplanted heart without angina pectoris (I25.812)

I25.760　**Atherosclerosis of bypass graft of coronary artery of transplanted heart with unstable angina** 🅐

I25.761　**Atherosclerosis of bypass graft of coronary artery of transplanted heart with angina pectoris with documented spasm** 🅐

I25.768　**Atherosclerosis of bypass graft of coronary artery of transplanted heart with other forms of angina pectoris** 🅐

I25.769　**Atherosclerosis of bypass graft of coronary artery of transplanted heart with unspecified angina pectoris** 🅐

✓6ᵗʰ **I25.79**　**Atherosclerosis of other coronary artery bypass graft(s) with angina pectoris**

I25.790　**Atherosclerosis of other coronary artery bypass graft(s) with unstable angina pectoris** 🅐
  EXCLUDES 1　unstable angina without atherosclerosis of other coronary artery bypass graft(s) (I20.0)

I25.791　**Atherosclerosis of other coronary artery bypass graft(s) with angina pectoris with documented spasm** 🅐
  EXCLUDES 1　angina pectoris with documented spasm without atherosclerosis of other coronary artery bypass graft(s) (I20.1)

I25.798　**Atherosclerosis of other coronary artery bypass graft(s) with other forms of angina pectoris** 🅐
  EXCLUDES 1　other forms of angina pectoris without atherosclerosis of other coronary artery bypass graft(s) (I20.8)

I25.799　**Atherosclerosis of other coronary artery bypass graft(s) with unspecified angina pectoris** 🅐
  EXCLUDES 1　unspecified angina pectoris without atherosclerosis of other coronary artery bypass graft(s) (I20.9)

✓5ᵗʰ **I25.8**　**Other forms of chronic ischemic heart disease**

✓6ᵗʰ **I25.81**　**Atherosclerosis of other coronary vessels without angina pectoris**
　Use additional code, if applicable, to identify:
　　coronary atherosclerosis due to calcified coronary lesion (I25.84)
　　coronary atherosclerosis due to lipid rich plaque (I25.83)
  EXCLUDES 1　atherosclerotic heart disease of native coronary artery without angina pectoris (I25.10)

I25.810　**Atherosclerosis of coronary artery bypass graft(s) without angina pectoris** 🅐
　Atherosclerosis of coronary artery bypass graft NOS
  EXCLUDES 1　atherosclerosis of coronary bypass graft(s) with angina pectoris (I25.70--I25.73-, I25.79-)

☑ Additional Character Required　　✓x7ᵗʰ Xtension Alert　　Unspecified Dx　　Other Specified Dx　　Manifestation　　▶◀ Revised Text　　● New Code　　▲ Revised Code Title

Diseases of the Circulatory System

I25.811–I31.4

I25.811   **Atherosclerosis of** native **coronary artery of** transplanted heart **without angina pectoris**

Atherosclerosis of native coronary artery of transplanted heart NOS

EXCLUDES 1   *atherosclerosis of native coronary artery of transplanted heart with angina pectoris (I25.75-)*

I25.812   **Atherosclerosis of** bypass graft **of coronary artery of** transplanted heart **without angina pectoris** 🅰

Atherosclerosis of bypass graft of transplanted heart NOS

EXCLUDES 1   *atherosclerosis of bypass graft of transplanted heart with angina pectoris (I25.76)*

I25.82   **Chronic total occlusion** of coronary artery

Complete occlusion of coronary artery

Total occlusion of coronary artery

Code first coronary atherosclerosis (I25.1-, I25.7-, I25.81-)

EXCLUDES 1   *acute coronary occlusion with myocardial infarction (I21.-, I22.-)*

acute coronary occlusion without myocardial infarction (I24.0)

I25.83   **Coronary atherosclerosis due to** lipid rich plaque 🅰

Code first coronary atherosclerosis (I25.1-, I25.7-, I25.81-)

I25.84   **Coronary atherosclerosis due to** calcified coronary lesion

Coronary atherosclerosis due to severely calcified coronary lesion

Code first coronary atherosclerosis (I25.1-, I25.7-, I25.81-)

I25.89   **Other forms of chronic ischemic heart disease**

I25.9   **Chronic ischemic heart disease, unspecified**

Ischemic heart disease (chronic) NOS

Pulmonary heart disease and diseases of pulmonary circulation (I26-I28)

✓4ᵗʰ **I26**   **Pulmonary embolism**

Pulmonary (acute) (artery)(vein) infarction

Pulmonary (acute) (artery)(vein) thromboembolism

Pulmonary (acute) (artery)(vein) thrombosis

EXCLUDES 2   *chronic pulmonary embolism (I27.82)*

personal history of pulmonary embolism (Z86.711)

pulmonary embolism due to trauma (T79.0, T79.1)

pulmonary embolism due to complications of surgical and medical care (T80.0, T81.7-, T82.8-)

pulmonary embolism complicating abortion, ectopic or molar pregnancy (O00-O07, O08.2)

pulmonary embolism complicating pregnancy, childbirth and the puerperium (O88.-)

septic (non-pulmonary) arterial embolism (I76)

✓5ᵗʰ **I26.0**   **Pulmonary embolism** with acute cor pulmonale

I26.01   Septic **pulmonary embolism with acute cor pulmonale**

Code first underlying infection

I26.02   Saddle **embolus of pulmonary artery with acute cor pulmonale**

I26.09   **Other pulmonary embolism with acute cor pulmonale**

Acute cor pulmonale NOS

✓5ᵗʰ **I26.9**   **Pulmonary embolism** without acute cor pulmonale

I26.90   Septic **pulmonary embolism without acute cor pulmonale**

Code first underlying infection

I26.92   Saddle **embolus of pulmonary artery without acute cor pulmonale**

I26.99   **Other pulmonary embolism without acute cor pulmonale**

Acute pulmonary embolism NOS

Pulmonary embolism NOS

✓4ᵗʰ **I27**   **Other pulmonary heart diseases**

I27.0   **Primary pulmonary hypertension**

EXCLUDES 1   *pulmonary hypertension NOS (I27.2)*

secondary pulmonary hypertension (I27.2)

I27.1   **Kyphoscoliotic heart disease**

I27.2   **Other secondary pulmonary hypertension**

Pulmonary hypertension NOS

Code also associated underlying condition

✓5ᵗʰ **I27.8**   **Other specified pulmonary heart diseases**

I27.81   **Cor pulmonale (chronic)**

Cor pulmonale NOS

EXCLUDES 1   *acute cor pulmonale (I26.0-)*

I27.82   **Chronic pulmonary embolism**

Use additional code, if applicable, for associated long-term (current) use of anticoagulants (Z79.01)

EXCLUDES 1   *personal history of pulmonary embolism (Z86.711)*

I27.89   **Other specified pulmonary heart diseases**

Eisenmenger's complex

Eisenmenger's syndrome

EXCLUDES 1   *Eisenmenger's defect (Q21.8)*

I27.9   **Pulmonary heart disease, unspecified**

Chronic cardiopulmonary disease

✓4ᵗʰ **I28**   **Other diseases of pulmonary vessels**

I28.0   **Arteriovenous fistula of pulmonary vessels**

EXCLUDES 1   *congenital arteriovenous fistula (Q25.72)*

I28.1   **Aneurysm of pulmonary artery**

EXCLUDES 1   *congenital aneurysm (Q25.79)*

congenital arteriovenous aneurysm (Q25.72)

I28.8   **Other diseases of pulmonary vessels**

Pulmonary arteritis

Pulmonary endarteritis

Rupture of pulmonary vessels

Stenosis of pulmonary vessels

Stricture of pulmonary vessels

I28.9   **Disease of pulmonary vessels, unspecified**

Other forms of heart disease (I30-I52)

✓4ᵗʰ **I30**   **Acute pericarditis**

INCLUDES   acute mediastinopericarditis

acute myopericarditis

acute pericardial effusion

acute pleuropericarditis

acute pneumopericarditis

EXCLUDES 1   *Dressler's syndrome (I24.1)*

rheumatic pericarditis (acute) (I01.0)

I30.0   **Acute** nonspecific idiopathic **pericarditis**

I30.1   Infective **pericarditis**

Pneumococcal pericarditis

Pneumopyopericardium

Purulent pericarditis

Pyopericarditis

Pyopericardium

Pyopneumopericardium

Staphylococcal pericarditis

Streptococcal pericarditis

Suppurative pericarditis

Viral pericarditis

Use additional code (B95-B97) to identify infectious agent

I30.8   **Other forms of acute pericarditis**

I30.9   **Acute pericarditis, unspecified**

✓4ᵗʰ **I31**   **Other diseases of pericardium**

EXCLUDES 1   *diseases of pericardium specified as rheumatic (I09.2)*

postcardiotomy syndrome (I97.0)

traumatic injury to pericardium (S26.-)

I31.0   **Chronic** adhesive **pericarditis**

Accretio cordis

Adherent pericardium

Adhesive mediastinopericarditis

I31.1   **Chronic** constrictive **pericarditis**

Concretio cordis

Pericardial calcification

I31.2   **Hemopericardium, not elsewhere classified**

EXCLUDES 1   *hemopericardium as current complication following acute myocardial infarction (I23.0)*

I31.3   **Pericardial effusion (noninflammatory)**

Chylopericardium

EXCLUDES 1   *acute pericardial effusion (I30.9)*

I31.4   **Cardiac tamponade**

Code first underlying cause

EXCLUDES 1 Not coded here   *EXCLUDES 2* Not included here   🄽 Newborn Age: 0   🄿 Pediatric Age: 0-17   🄼 Maternity Age: 12-55   🄰 Adult Age: 15-124

574   ICD-10-CM Draft (2015)

I31.8 **Other specified diseases of pericardium**
Epicardial plaques
Focal pericardial adhesions

I31.9 **Disease of pericardium, unspecified**
Pericarditis (chronic) NOS

I32 *Pericarditis in diseases classified elsewhere*
Code first underlying disease
EXCLUDES 1 *pericarditis (in):*
coxsackie (virus) (B33.23)
gonococcal (A54.83)
meningococcal (A39.53)
rheumatoid (arthritis) (M05.31)
syphilitic (A52.06)
systemic lupus erythematosus (M32.12)
tuberculosis (A18.84)

✓4ᵗʰ **I33** **Acute and subacute endocarditis**
EXCLUDES 1 *acute rheumatic endocarditis (I01.1)*
endocarditis NOS (I38)

I33.0 **Acute and subacute infective endocarditis**
Bacterial endocarditis (acute) (subacute)
Infective endocarditis (acute) (subacute) NOS
Endocarditis lenta (acute) (subacute)
Malignant endocarditis (acute) (subacute)
Purulent endocarditis (acute) (subacute)
Septic endocarditis (acute) (subacute)
Ulcerative endocarditis (acute) (subacute)
Vegetative endocarditis (acute) (subacute)
Use additional code (B95-B97) to identify infectious agent

I33.9 **Acute and subacute endocarditis, unspecified**
Acute endocarditis NOS
Acute myoendocarditis NOS
Acute periendocarditis NOS
Subacute endocarditis NOS
Subacute myoendocarditis NOS
Subacute periendocarditis NOS

✓4ᵗʰ **I34** **Nonrheumatic mitral valve disorders**
EXCLUDES 1 *mitral valve disease (I05.9)*
mitral valve failure (I05.8)
mitral valve stenosis (I05.0)
mitral valve disorder of unspecified cause with diseases of aortic and/or tricuspid valve(s) (I08.-)
mitral valve disorder of unspecified cause with mitral stenosis or obstruction (I05.0)
mitral valve disorder specified as congenital (Q23.2, Q23.3)
mitral valve disorder specified as rheumatic (I05.-)

I34.0 **Nonrheumatic mitral (valve) insufficiency**
Nonrheumatic mitral (valve) incompetence NOS
Nonrheumatic mitral (valve) regurgitation NOS

I34.1 **Nonrheumatic mitral (valve) prolapse**
Floppy nonrheumatic mitral valve syndrome
EXCLUDES 1 *Marfan's syndrome (Q87.4-)*

I34.2 **Nonrheumatic mitral (valve) stenosis**

I34.8 **Other nonrheumatic mitral valve disorders**

I34.9 **Nonrheumatic mitral valve disorder, unspecified**

✓4ᵗʰ **I35** **Nonrheumatic aortic valve disorders**
EXCLUDES 1 *aortic valve disorder of unspecified cause but with diseases of mitral and/or tricuspid valve(s) (I08.-)*
aortic valve disorder specified as congenital (Q23.0, Q23.1)
aortic valve disorder specified as rheumatic (I06.-)
hypertrophic subaortic stenosis (I42.1)

I35.0 **Nonrheumatic aortic (valve) stenosis**

I35.1 **Nonrheumatic aortic (valve) insufficiency**
Nonrheumatic aortic (valve) incompetence NOS
Nonrheumatic aortic (valve) regurgitation NOS

I35.2 **Nonrheumatic aortic (valve) stenosis with insufficiency**

I35.8 **Other nonrheumatic aortic valve disorders**

I35.9 **Nonrheumatic aortic valve disorder, unspecified**

✓4ᵗʰ **I36** **Nonrheumatic tricuspid valve disorders**
EXCLUDES 1 *tricuspid valve disorders of unspecified cause (I07.-)*
tricuspid valve disorders specified as congenital (Q22.4, Q22.8, Q22.9)
tricuspid valve disorders specified as rheumatic (I07.-)
tricuspid valve disorders with aortic and/or mitral valve involvement (I08.-)

I36.0 **Nonrheumatic tricuspid (valve) stenosis**

I36.1 **Nonrheumatic tricuspid (valve) insufficiency**
Nonrheumatic tricuspid (valve) incompetence
Nonrheumatic tricuspid (valve) regurgitation

I36.2 **Nonrheumatic tricuspid (valve) stenosis with insufficiency**

I36.8 **Other nonrheumatic tricuspid valve disorders**

I36.9 **Nonrheumatic tricuspid valve disorder, unspecified**

✓4ᵗʰ **I37** **Nonrheumatic pulmonary valve disorders**
EXCLUDES 1 *pulmonary valve disorder specified as congenital (Q22.1, Q22.2, Q22.3)*
pulmonary valve disorder specified as rheumatic (I09.89)

I37.0 **Nonrheumatic pulmonary valve stenosis**

I37.1 **Nonrheumatic pulmonary valve insufficiency**
Nonrheumatic pulmonary valve incompetence
Nonrheumatic pulmonary valve regurgitation

I37.2 **Nonrheumatic pulmonary valve stenosis with insufficiency**

I37.8 **Other nonrheumatic pulmonary valve disorders**

I37.9 **Nonrheumatic pulmonary valve disorder, unspecified**

I38 **Endocarditis, valve unspecified**
INCLUDES endocarditis (chronic) NOS
valvular incompetence NOS
valvular insufficiency NOS
valvular regurgitation NOS
valvular stenosis NOS
valvulitis (chronic) NOS
EXCLUDES 1 *congenital insufficiency of cardiac valve NOS (Q24.8)*
congenital stenosis of cardiac valve NOS (Q24.8)
endocardial fibroelastosis (I42.4)
endocarditis specified as rheumatic (I09.1)

I39 *Endocarditis and heart valve disorders in diseases classified elsewhere*
Code first underlying disease, such as:
Q fever (A78)
EXCLUDES 1 *endocardial involvement in:*
candidiasis (B37.6)
gonococcal infection (A54.83)
Libman-Sacks disease (M32.11)
listerosis (A32.82)
meningococcal infection (A39.51)
rheumatoid arthritis (M05.31)
syphilis (A52.03)
tuberculosis (A18.84)
typhoid fever (A01.02)

✓4ᵗʰ **I40** **Acute myocarditis**
INCLUDES subacute myocarditis
EXCLUDES 1 *acute rheumatic myocarditis (I01.2)*

I40.0 **Infective myocarditis**
Septic myocarditis
Use additional code (B95-B97) to identify infectious agent

I40.1 **Isolated myocarditis**
Fiedler's myocarditis
Giant cell myocarditis
Idiopathic myocarditis

I40.8 **Other acute myocarditis**

I40.9 **Acute myocarditis, unspecified**

I41 *Myocarditis in diseases classified elsewhere*
Code first underlying disease, such as:
typhus (A75.0-A75.9)
EXCLUDES 1 *myocarditis (in):*
Chagas' disease (chronic) (B57.2)
acute (B57.0)
coxsackie (virus) infection (B33.22)
diphtheritic (A36.81)
gonococcal (A54.83)
influenzal (J09.X9, J10.82, J11.82)
meningococcal (A39.52)
mumps (B26.82)
rheumatoid arthritis (M05.31)
sarcoid (D86.85)
syphilis (A52.06)
toxoplasmosis (B58.81)
tuberculous (A18.84)

✓4ᵗʰ **I42** **Cardiomyopathy**
INCLUDES myocardiopathy
Code first pre-existing cardiomyopathy complicating pregnancy and puerperium (O99.4)
EXCLUDES 1 *ischemic cardiomyopathy (I25.5)*
peripartum cardiomyopathy (O90.3)
EXCLUDES 2 *ventricular hypertrophy (I51.7)*

I42.0 **Dilated cardiomyopathy**
Congestive cardiomyopathy

I42.1 **Obstructive hypertrophic cardiomyopathy**
Hypertrophic subaortic stenosis (idiopathic)

☑ Additional Character Required   ✓⁷ᵗʰ Xtension Alert   Unspecified Dx   Other Specified Dx   Manifestation   ▶◀ Revised Text   ● New Code   ▲ Revised Code Title

Diseases of the Circulatory System

I42.2–I49.9

I42.2 Other hypertrophic cardiomyopathy
Nonobstructive hypertrophic cardiomyopathy

I42.3 Endomyocardial (eosinophilic) disease
Endomyocardial (tropical) fibrosis
Löffler's endocarditis

I42.4 Endocardial fibroelastosis
Congenital cardiomyopathy
Elastomyofibrosis

I42.5 Other restrictive cardiomyopathy
Constrictive cardiomyopathy NOS

I42.6 Alcoholic cardiomyopathy
Code also presence of alcoholism (F10.-)

I42.7 Cardiomyopathy due to drug and external agent
Code first poisoning due to drug or toxin, if applicable (T36-T65 with fifth or sixth character 1-4 or 6)
Use additional code for adverse effect, if applicable, to identify drug (T36-T50 with fifth or sixth character 5)

I42.8 Other cardiomyopathies

I42.9 Cardiomyopathy, unspecified
Cardiomyopathy (primary) (secondary) NOS

I43 Cardiomyopathy in diseases classified elsewhere
Code first underlying disease, such as:
amyloidosis (E85.-)
glycogen storage disease (E74.0)
gout (M10.0-)
thyrotoxicosis (E05.0-E05.9-)
EXCLUDES 1   cardiomyopathy (in):
coxsackie (virus) (B33.24)
diphtheria (A36.81)
sarcoidosis (D86.85)
tuberculosis (A18.84)

✓4ᵗʰ I44 Atrioventricular and left bundle-branch block

I44.0 Atrioventricular block, first degree

I44.1 Atrioventricular block, second degree
Atrioventricular block, type I and II
Möbitz block, type I and II
Second degree block, type I and II
Wenckebach's block

I44.2 Atrioventricular block, complete
Complete heart block NOS
Third degree block

✓5ᵗʰ I44.3 Other and unspecified atrioventricular block
Atrioventricular block NOS

     I44.30 Unspecified atrioventricular block

     I44.39 Other atrioventricular block

I44.4 Left anterior fascicular block

I44.5 Left posterior fascicular block

✓5ᵗʰ I44.6 Other and unspecified fascicular block

     I44.60 Unspecified fascicular block
Left bundle-branch hemiblock NOS

     I44.69 Other fascicular block

I44.7 Left bundle-branch block, unspecified

✓4ᵗʰ I45 Other conduction disorders

I45.0 Right fascicular block

✓5ᵗʰ I45.1 Other and unspecified right bundle-branch block

     I45.10 Unspecified right bundle-branch block
Right bundle-branch block NOS

     I45.19 Other right bundle-branch block

I45.2 Bifascicular block

I45.3 Trifascicular block

I45.4 Nonspecific intraventricular block
Bundle-branch block NOS

I45.5 Other specified heart block
Sinoatrial block
Sinoauricular block
EXCLUDES 1   heart block NOS (I45.9)

I45.6 Pre-excitation syndrome
Accelerated atrioventricular conduction
Accessory atrioventricular conduction
Anomalous atrioventricular excitation
Lown-Ganong-Levine syndrome
Pre-excitation atrioventricular conduction
Wolff-Parkinson-White syndrome

✓5ᵗʰ I45.8 Other specified conduction disorders

     I45.81 Long QT syndrome

     I45.89 Other specified conduction disorders
Atrioventricular [AV] dissociation
Interference dissociation
Isorhythmic dissociation
Nonparoxysmal AV nodal tachycardia
AHA: 2013, 2Q, 31

I45.9 Conduction disorder, unspecified
Heart block NOS
Stokes-Adams syndrome

✓4ᵗʰ I46 Cardiac arrest
EXCLUDES 1   cardiogenic shock (R57.0)

I46.2 Cardiac arrest due to underlying cardiac condition
Code first underlying cardiac condition

I46.8 Cardiac arrest due to other underlying condition
Code first underlying condition

I46.9 Cardiac arrest, cause unspecified

✓4ᵗʰ I47 Paroxysmal tachycardia
Code first tachycardia complicating:
abortion or ectopic or molar pregnancy (O00-O07, O08.8)
obstetric surgery and procedures (O75.4)
EXCLUDES 1   tachycardia NOS (R00.0)
sinoauricular tachycardia NOS (R00.0)
sinus [sinusal] tachycardia NOS (R00.0)

I47.0 Re-entry ventricular arrhythmia

I47.1 Supraventricular tachycardia
Atrial (paroxysmal) tachycardia
Atrioventricular [AV] (paroxysmal) tachycardia
Atrioventricular re-entrant (nodal) tachycardia [AVNRT] [AVRT]
Junctional (paroxysmal) tachycardia
Nodal (paroxysmal) tachycardia

I47.2 Ventricular tachycardia
AHA: 2013, 3Q, 23

I47.9 Paroxysmal tachycardia, unspecified
Bouveret (-Hoffman) syndrome

✓4ᵗʰ I48 Atrial fibrillation and flutter

I48.0 Paroxysmal atrial fibrillation

I48.1 Persistent atrial fibrillation

I48.2 Chronic atrial fibrillation
Permanent atrial fibrillation

I48.3 Typical atrial flutter
Type I atrial flutter

I48.4 Atypical atrial flutter
Type II atrial flutter

✓5ᵗʰ I48.9 Unspecified atrial fibrillation and atrial flutter

     I48.91 Unspecified atrial fibrillation

     I48.92 Unspecified atrial flutter

✓4ᵗʰ I49 Other cardiac arrhythmias
Code first cardiac arrhythmia complicating:
abortion or ectopic or molar pregnancy (O00-O07, O08.8)
obstetric surgery and procedures (O75.4)
EXCLUDES 1   bradycardia NOS (R00.1)
neonatal dysrhythmia (P29.1-)
sinoatrial bradycardia (R00.1)
sinus bradycardia (R00.1)
vagal bradycardia (R00.1)

✓5ᵗʰ I49.0 Ventricular fibrillation and flutter

     I49.01 Ventricular fibrillation

     I49.02 Ventricular flutter

I49.1 Atrial premature depolarization
Atrial premature beats

I49.2 Junctional premature depolarization

I49.3 Ventricular premature depolarization

✓5ᵗʰ I49.4 Other and unspecified premature depolarization

     I49.40 Unspecified premature depolarization
Premature beats NOS

     I49.49 Other premature depolarization
Ectopic beats Extrasystolic arrhythmias
Extrasystoles Premature contractions

I49.5 Sick sinus syndrome
Tachycardia-bradycardia syndrome

I49.8 Other specified cardiac arrhythmias
Coronary sinus rhythm disorder
Ectopic rhythm disorder
Nodal rhythm disorder

I49.9 Cardiac arrhythmia, unspecified
Arrhythmia (cardiac) NOS

EXCLUDES 1 Not coded here   EXCLUDES 2 Not included here   N Newborn Age: 0   P Pediatric Age: 0-17   M Maternity Age: 12-55   A Adult Age: 15-124

✓4th **I50**   **Heart failure**

Code first:
- heart failure complicating abortion or ectopic or molar pregnancy (O00-O07, O08.8)
- heart failure following surgery (I97.13-)
- heart failure due to hypertension (I11.0)
- heart failure due to hypertension with chronic kidney disease (I13.-)
- obstetric surgery and procedures (O75.4)
- rheumatic heart failure (I09.81)

EXCLUDES 1   cardiac arrest (I46.-)
         neonatal cardiac failure (P29.0)

AHA: 2014, 1Q, 25; 2013, 2Q, 33

I50.1   **Left ventricular failure**
- Cardiac asthma
- Edema of lung with heart disease NOS
- Edema of lung with heart failure
- Left heart failure
- Pulmonary edema with heart disease NOS
- Pulmonary edema with heart failure

EXCLUDES 1   edema of lung without heart disease or heart failure (J81.-)
         pulmonary edema without heart disease or failure (J81.-)

✓5th **I50.2**   **Systolic (congestive) heart failure**

EXCLUDES 1   combined systolic (congestive) and diastolic (congestive) heart failure (I50.4-)

   I50.20   **Unspecified systolic (congestive) heart failure**

   I50.21   **Acute systolic (congestive) heart failure**

   I50.22   **Chronic systolic (congestive) heart failure**

   I50.23   **Acute on chronic systolic (congestive) heart failure**

✓5th **I50.3**   **Diastolic (congestive) heart failure**

EXCLUDES 1   combined systolic (congestive) and diastolic (congestive) heart failure (I50.4-)

   I50.30   **Unspecified diastolic (congestive) heart failure**

   I50.31   **Acute diastolic (congestive) heart failure**

   I50.32   **Chronic diastolic (congestive) heart failure**

   I50.33   **Acute on chronic diastolic (congestive) heart failure**

✓5th **I50.4**   **Combined systolic (congestive) and diastolic (congestive) heart failure**

   I50.40   **Unspecified combined systolic (congestive) and diastolic (congestive) heart failure**

   I50.41   **Acute combined systolic (congestive) and diastolic (congestive) heart failure**

   I50.42   **Chronic combined systolic (congestive) and diastolic (congestive) heart failure**

   I50.43   **Acute on chronic combined systolic (congestive) and diastolic (congestive) heart failure**

I50.9   **Heart failure, unspecified**
- Biventricular (heart) failure NOS
- Cardiac, heart or myocardial failure NOS
- Congestive heart disease
- Congestive heart failure NOS
- Right ventricular failure (secondary to left heart failure)

EXCLUDES 1   fluid overload (E87.70)

AHA: 2012, 4Q, 92

✓4th **I51**   **Complications and ill-defined descriptions of heart disease**

EXCLUDES 1   any condition in I51.4-I51.9 due to hypertension (I11.-)
         any condition in I51.4-I51.9 due to hypertension and chronic kidney disease (I13.-)
         heart disease specified as rheumatic (I00-I09)

I51.0   **Cardiac septal defect, acquired**   A
- Acquired septal atrial defect (old)
- Acquired septal auricular defect (old)
- Acquired septal ventricular defect (old)

EXCLUDES 1   cardiac septal defect as current complication following acute myocardial infarction (I23.1, I23.2)

I51.1   **Rupture of chordae tendineae, not elsewhere classified**

EXCLUDES 1   rupture of chordae tendineae as current complication following acute myocardial infarction (I23.4)

I51.2   **Rupture of papillary muscle, not elsewhere classified**

EXCLUDES 1   rupture of papillary muscle as current complication following acute myocardial infarction (I23.5)

I51.3   **Intracardiac thrombosis, not elsewhere classified**   A
- Apical thrombosis (old)   Mural thrombosis (old)
- Atrial thrombosis (old)   Ventricular thrombosis (old)
- Auricular thrombosis (old)

EXCLUDES 1   intracardiac thrombosis as current complication following acute myocardial infarction (I23.6)

AHA: 2013, 1Q, 24

I51.4   **Myocarditis, unspecified**
- Chronic (interstitial) myocarditis
- Myocardial fibrosis
- Myocarditis NOS

EXCLUDES 1   acute or subacute myocarditis (I40.-)

I51.5   **Myocardial degeneration**
- Fatty degeneration of heart or myocardium
- Myocardial disease
- Senile degeneration of heart or myocardium

I51.7   **Cardiomegaly**
- Cardiac dilatation
- Cardiac hypertrophy
- Ventricular dilatation

✓5th **I51.8**   **Other ill-defined heart diseases**

   I51.81   **Takotsubo syndrome**
- Reversible left ventricular dysfunction following sudden emotional stress
- Stress induced cardiomyopathy
- Takotsubo cardiomyopathy
- Transient left ventricular apical ballooning syndrome

   I51.89   **Other ill-defined heart diseases**
- Carditis (acute)(chronic)
- Pancarditis (acute)(chronic)

I51.9   **Heart disease, unspecified**

I52   *Other heart disorders in diseases classified elsewhere*

Code first underlying disease, such as:
- congenital syphilis (A50.5)
- mucopolysaccharidosis (E76.3)
- schistosomiasis (B65.0-B65.9)

EXCLUDES 1   heart disease (in):
- gonococcal infection (A54.83)
- meningococcal infection (A39.50)
- rheumatoid arthritis (M05.31)
- syphilis (A52.06)

Cerebrovascular diseases (I60-I69)

Use additional code to identify presence of:
- alcohol abuse and dependence (F10.-)
- exposure to environmental tobacco smoke (Z77.22)
- history of tobacco use (Z87.891)
- hypertension (I10-I15)
- occupational exposure to environmental tobacco smoke (Z57.31)
- tobacco dependence (F17.-)
- tobacco use (Z72.0)

EXCLUDES 1   transient cerebral ischemic attacks and related syndromes (G45.-)
         traumatic intracranial hemorrhage (S06.-)

AHA: 2012, 4Q, 91-92

✓4th **I60**   **Nontraumatic subarachnoid hemorrhage**

INCLUDES   ruptured cerebral aneurysm

EXCLUDES 1   sequelae of subarachnoid hemorrhage (I69.0-)
         syphilitic ruptured cerebral aneurysm (A52.05)

✓5th **I60.0**   **Nontraumatic subarachnoid hemorrhage from carotid siphon and bifurcation**

   I60.00   **Nontraumatic subarachnoid hemorrhage from unspecified carotid siphon and bifurcation**

   I60.01   **Nontraumatic subarachnoid hemorrhage from right carotid siphon and bifurcation**

   I60.02   **Nontraumatic subarachnoid hemorrhage from left carotid siphon and bifurcation**

✓5th **I60.1**   **Nontraumatic subarachnoid hemorrhage from middle cerebral artery**

   I60.10   **Nontraumatic subarachnoid hemorrhage from unspecified middle cerebral artery**

   I60.11   **Nontraumatic subarachnoid hemorrhage from right middle cerebral artery**

   I60.12   **Nontraumatic subarachnoid hemorrhage from left middle cerebral artery**

✓5th **I60.2**   **Nontraumatic subarachnoid hemorrhage from anterior communicating artery**

   I60.20   **Nontraumatic subarachnoid hemorrhage from unspecified anterior communicating artery**

   I60.21   **Nontraumatic subarachnoid hemorrhage from right anterior communicating artery**

   I60.22   **Nontraumatic subarachnoid hemorrhage from left anterior communicating artery**

✓5th **I60.3**   **Nontraumatic subarachnoid hemorrhage from posterior communicating artery**

   I60.30   **Nontraumatic subarachnoid hemorrhage from unspecified posterior communicating artery**

✔ Additional Character Required   ✓x7th Xtension Alert   Unspecified Dx   Other Specified Dx   Manifestation   ►◄ Revised Text   ● New Code   ▲ Revised Code Title

Diseases of the Circulatory System

I60.31–I63.322

I60.31 Nontraumatic subarachnoid hemorrhage from right posterior communicating artery

I60.32 Nontraumatic subarachnoid hemorrhage from left posterior communicating artery

I60.4 Nontraumatic subarachnoid hemorrhage from basilar artery

✓5ᵗʰ I60.5 Nontraumatic subarachnoid hemorrhage from vertebral artery

I60.50 Nontraumatic subarachnoid hemorrhage from unspecified vertebral artery

I60.51 Nontraumatic subarachnoid hemorrhage from right vertebral artery

I60.52 Nontraumatic subarachnoid hemorrhage from left vertebral artery

I60.6 Nontraumatic subarachnoid hemorrhage from other intracranial arteries

I60.7 Nontraumatic subarachnoid hemorrhage from unspecified intracranial artery

Ruptured (congenital) berry aneurysm
Ruptured (congenital) cerebral aneurysm
Subarachnoid hemorrhage (nontraumatic) from cerebral artery NOS
Subarachnoid hemorrhage (nontraumatic) from communicating artery NOS

EXCLUDES 1 berry aneurysm, nonruptured (I67.1)

I60.8 Other nontraumatic subarachnoid hemorrhage

Meningeal hemorrhage
Rupture of cerebral arteriovenous malformation

I60.9 Nontraumatic subarachnoid hemorrhage, unspecified

✓4ᵗʰ I61 Nontraumatic intracerebral hemorrhage

EXCLUDES 1 sequelae of intracerebral hemorrhage (I69.1-)

I61.0 Nontraumatic intracerebral hemorrhage in hemisphere, subcortical

Deep intracerebral hemorrhage (nontraumatic)

I61.1 Nontraumatic intracerebral hemorrhage in hemisphere, cortical

Cerebral lobe hemorrhage (nontraumatic)
Superficial intracerebral hemorrhage (nontraumatic)

I61.2 Nontraumatic intracerebral hemorrhage in hemisphere, unspecified

I61.3 Nontraumatic intracerebral hemorrhage in brain stem

I61.4 Nontraumatic intracerebral hemorrhage in cerebellum

I61.5 Nontraumatic intracerebral hemorrhage, intraventricular

I61.6 Nontraumatic intracerebral hemorrhage, multiple localized

I61.8 Other nontraumatic intracerebral hemorrhage

I61.9 Nontraumatic intracerebral hemorrhage, unspecified

✓4ᵗʰ I62 Other and unspecified nontraumatic intracranial hemorrhage

EXCLUDES 1 sequelae of intracranial hemorrhage (I69.2)

✓5ᵗʰ I62.0 Nontraumatic subdural hemorrhage

I62.00 Nontraumatic subdural hemorrhage, unspecified

I62.01 Nontraumatic acute subdural hemorrhage

I62.02 Nontraumatic subacute subdural hemorrhage

I62.03 Nontraumatic chronic subdural hemorrhage

I62.1 Nontraumatic extradural hemorrhage

Nontraumatic epidural hemorrhage

I62.9 Nontraumatic intracranial hemorrhage, unspecified

✓4ᵗʰ I63 Cerebral infarction

INCLUDES occlusion and stenosis of cerebral and precerebral arteries, resulting in cerebral infarction

Use additional code, if applicable, to identify status post administration of tPA (rtPA) in a different facility within the last 24 hours prior to admission to current facility (Z92.82)

EXCLUDES 1 sequelae of cerebral infarction (I69.3-)

AHA: 2014, 1Q, 23

✓5ᵗʰ I63.0 Cerebral infarction due to thrombosis of precerebral arteries

I63.00 Cerebral infarction due to thrombosis of unspecified precerebral artery

✓6ᵗʰ I63.01 Cerebral infarction due to thrombosis of vertebral artery

I63.011 Cerebral infarction due to thrombosis of right vertebral artery

I63.012 Cerebral infarction due to thrombosis of left vertebral artery

I63.019 Cerebral infarction due to thrombosis of unspecified vertebral artery

I63.02 Cerebral infarction due to thrombosis of basilar artery

✓6ᵗʰ I63.03 Cerebral infarction due to thrombosis of carotid artery

I63.031 Cerebral infarction due to thrombosis of right carotid artery

I63.032 Cerebral infarction due to thrombosis of left carotid artery

I63.039 Cerebral infarction due to thrombosis of unspecified carotid artery

I63.09 Cerebral infarction due to thrombosis of other precerebral artery

✓5ᵗʰ I63.1 Cerebral infarction due to embolism of precerebral arteries

I63.10 Cerebral infarction due to embolism of unspecified precerebral artery

✓6ᵗʰ I63.11 Cerebral infarction due to embolism of vertebral artery

I63.111 Cerebral infarction due to embolism of right vertebral artery

I63.112 Cerebral infarction due to embolism of left vertebral artery

I63.119 Cerebral infarction due to embolism of unspecified vertebral artery

I63.12 Cerebral infarction due to embolism of basilar artery

✓6ᵗʰ I63.13 Cerebral infarction due to embolism of carotid artery

I63.131 Cerebral infarction due to embolism of right carotid artery

I63.132 Cerebral infarction due to embolism of left carotid artery

I63.139 Cerebral infarction due to embolism of unspecified carotid artery

I63.19 Cerebral infarction due to embolism of other precerebral artery

✓5ᵗʰ I63.2 Cerebral infarction due to unspecified occlusion or stenosis of precerebral arteries

I63.20 Cerebral infarction due to unspecified occlusion or stenosis of unspecified precerebral arteries

✓6ᵗʰ I63.21 Cerebral infarction due to unspecified occlusion or stenosis of vertebral arteries

I63.211 Cerebral infarction due to unspecified occlusion or stenosis of right vertebral arteries

I63.212 Cerebral infarction due to unspecified occlusion or stenosis of left vertebral arteries

I63.219 Cerebral infarction due to unspecified occlusion or stenosis of unspecified vertebral arteries

I63.22 Cerebral infarction due to unspecified occlusion or stenosis of basilar arteries

✓6ᵗʰ I63.23 Cerebral infarction due to unspecified occlusion or stenosis of carotid arteries

I63.231 Cerebral infarction due to unspecified occlusion or stenosis of right carotid arteries

I63.232 Cerebral infarction due to unspecified occlusion or stenosis of left carotid arteries

I63.239 Cerebral infarction due to unspecified occlusion or stenosis of unspecified carotid arteries

I63.29 Cerebral infarction due to unspecified occlusion or stenosis of other precerebral arteries

✓5ᵗʰ I63.3 Cerebral infarction due to thrombosis of cerebral arteries

I63.30 Cerebral infarction due to thrombosis of unspecified cerebral artery

✓6ᵗʰ I63.31 Cerebral infarction due to thrombosis of middle cerebral artery

I63.311 Cerebral infarction due to thrombosis of right middle cerebral artery

I63.312 Cerebral infarction due to thrombosis of left middle cerebral artery

I63.319 Cerebral infarction due to thrombosis of unspecified middle cerebral artery

✓6ᵗʰ I63.32 Cerebral infarction due to thrombosis of anterior cerebral artery

I63.321 Cerebral infarction due to thrombosis of right anterior cerebral artery

I63.322 Cerebral infarction due to thrombosis of left anterior cerebral artery

---

EXCLUDES 1 Not coded here   EXCLUDES 2 Not included here   N Newborn Age: 0   P Pediatric Age: 0-17   M Maternity Age: 12-55   A Adult Age: 15-124

I63.329　Cerebral infarction due to thrombosis of unspecified anterior cerebral artery

√6ᵗʰ I63.33　Cerebral infarction due to thrombosis of posterior cerebral artery

I63.331　Cerebral infarction due to thrombosis of right posterior cerebral artery

I63.332　Cerebral infarction due to thrombosis of left posterior cerebral artery

I63.339　Cerebral infarction due to thrombosis of unspecified posterior cerebral artery

√6ᵗʰ I63.34　Cerebral infarction due to thrombosis of cerebellar artery

I63.341　Cerebral infarction due to thrombosis of right cerebellar artery

I63.342　Cerebral infarction due to thrombosis of left cerebellar artery

I63.349　Cerebral infarction due to thrombosis of unspecified cerebellar artery

I63.39　Cerebral infarction due to thrombosis of other cerebral artery

√5ᵗʰ I63.4　Cerebral infarction due to embolism of cerebral arteries

I63.40　Cerebral infarction due to embolism of unspecified cerebral artery

√6ᵗʰ I63.41　Cerebral infarction due to embolism of middle cerebral artery

I63.411　Cerebral infarction due to embolism of right middle cerebral artery

I63.412　Cerebral infarction due to embolism of left middle cerebral artery

I63.419　Cerebral infarction due to embolism of unspecified middle cerebral artery

√6ᵗʰ I63.42　Cerebral infarction due to embolism of anterior cerebral artery

I63.421　Cerebral infarction due to embolism of right anterior cerebral artery

I63.422　Cerebral infarction due to embolism of left anterior cerebral artery

I63.429　Cerebral infarction due to embolism of unspecified anterior cerebral artery

√6ᵗʰ I63.43　Cerebral infarction due to embolism of posterior cerebral artery

I63.431　Cerebral infarction due to embolism of right posterior cerebral artery

I63.432　Cerebral infarction due to embolism of left posterior cerebral artery

I63.439　Cerebral infarction due to embolism of unspecified posterior cerebral artery

√6ᵗʰ I63.44　Cerebral infarction due to embolism of cerebellar artery

I63.441　Cerebral infarction due to embolism of right cerebellar artery

I63.442　Cerebral infarction due to embolism of left cerebellar artery

I63.449　Cerebral infarction due to embolism of unspecified cerebellar artery

I63.49　Cerebral infarction due to embolism of other cerebral artery

√5ᵗʰ I63.5　Cerebral infarction due to unspecified occlusion or stenosis of cerebral arteries

I63.50　Cerebral infarction due to unspecified occlusion or stenosis of unspecified cerebral artery

√6ᵗʰ I63.51　Cerebral infarction due to unspecified occlusion or stenosis of middle cerebral artery

I63.511　Cerebral infarction due to unspecified occlusion or stenosis of right middle cerebral artery

I63.512　Cerebral infarction due to unspecified occlusion or stenosis of left middle cerebral artery

I63.519　Cerebral infarction due to unspecified occlusion or stenosis of unspecified middle cerebral artery

√6ᵗʰ I63.52　Cerebral infarction due to unspecified occlusion or stenosis of anterior cerebral artery

I63.521　Cerebral infarction due to unspecified occlusion or stenosis of right anterior cerebral artery

I63.522　Cerebral infarction due to unspecified occlusion or stenosis of left anterior cerebral artery

I63.529　Cerebral infarction due to unspecified occlusion or stenosis of unspecified anterior cerebral artery

√6ᵗʰ I63.53　Cerebral infarction due to unspecified occlusion or stenosis of posterior cerebral artery

I63.531　Cerebral infarction due to unspecified occlusion or stenosis of right posterior cerebral artery

I63.532　Cerebral infarction due to unspecified occlusion or stenosis of left posterior cerebral artery

I63.539　Cerebral infarction due to unspecified occlusion or stenosis of unspecified posterior cerebral artery

√6ᵗʰ I63.54　Cerebral infarction due to unspecified occlusion or stenosis of cerebellar artery

I63.541　Cerebral infarction due to unspecified occlusion or stenosis of right cerebellar artery

I63.542　Cerebral infarction due to unspecified occlusion or stenosis of left cerebellar artery

I63.549　Cerebral infarction due to unspecified occlusion or stenosis of unspecified cerebellar artery

I63.59　Cerebral infarction due to unspecified occlusion or stenosis of other cerebral artery

I63.6　Cerebral infarction due to cerebral venous thrombosis, nonpyogenic

I63.8　Other cerebral infarction

I63.9　Cerebral infarction, unspecified
Stroke NOS

√4ᵗʰ I65　Occlusion and stenosis of precerebral arteries, not resulting in cerebral infarction

INCLUDES　embolism of precerebral artery
narrowing of precerebral artery
obstruction (complete) (partial) of precerebral artery
thrombosis of precerebral artery

EXCLUDES 1　insufficiency, NOS, of precerebral artery (G45.-)
insufficiency of precerebral arteries causing cerebral infarction (I63.0-I63.2)

√5ᵗʰ I65.0　Occlusion and stenosis of vertebral artery

I65.01　Occlusion and stenosis of right vertebral artery

I65.02　Occlusion and stenosis of left vertebral artery

I65.03　Occlusion and stenosis of bilateral vertebral arteries

I65.09　Occlusion and stenosis of unspecified vertebral artery

I65.1　Occlusion and stenosis of basilar artery

√5ᵗʰ I65.2　Occlusion and stenosis of carotid artery

I65.21　Occlusion and stenosis of right carotid artery

I65.22　Occlusion and stenosis of left carotid artery

I65.23　Occlusion and stenosis of bilateral carotid arteries

I65.29　Occlusion and stenosis of unspecified carotid artery

I65.8　Occlusion and stenosis of other precerebral arteries

I65.9　Occlusion and stenosis of unspecified precerebral artery
Occlusion and stenosis of precerebral artery NOS

√4ᵗʰ I66　Occlusion and stenosis of cerebral arteries, not resulting in cerebral infarction

INCLUDES　embolism of cerebral artery
narrowing of cerebral artery
obstruction (complete) (partial) of cerebral artery
thrombosis of cerebral artery

EXCLUDES 1　occlusion and stenosis of cerebral artery causing cerebral infarction (I63.3-I63.5)

√6ᵗʰ I66.0　Occlusion and stenosis of middle cerebral artery

I66.01　Occlusion and stenosis of right middle cerebral artery

I66.02　Occlusion and stenosis of left middle cerebral artery

I66.03　Occlusion and stenosis of bilateral middle cerebral arteries

I66.09　Occlusion and stenosis of unspecified middle cerebral artery

---

☑ Additional Character Required　　√x7ᵗʰ Xtension Alert　　Unspecified Dx　　Other Specified Dx　　Manifestation　　▶◀ Revised Text　　● New Code　　▲ Revised Code Title

Diseases of the Circulatory System

I66.1–I69.052

✓5ᵗʰ **I66.1   Occlusion and stenosis of anterior cerebral artery**
> **I66.11   Occlusion and stenosis of right anterior cerebral artery**
> **I66.12   Occlusion and stenosis of left anterior cerebral artery**
> **I66.13   Occlusion and stenosis of bilateral anterior cerebral arteries**
> **I66.19   Occlusion and stenosis of unspecified anterior cerebral artery**

✓5ᵗʰ **I66.2   Occlusion and stenosis of posterior cerebral artery**
> **I66.21   Occlusion and stenosis of right posterior cerebral artery**
> **I66.22   Occlusion and stenosis of left posterior cerebral artery**
> **I66.23   Occlusion and stenosis of bilateral posterior cerebral arteries**
> **I66.29   Occlusion and stenosis of unspecified posterior cerebral artery**

I66.3   Occlusion and stenosis of cerebellar arteries

I66.8   Occlusion and stenosis of other cerebral arteries
> Occlusion and stenosis of perforating arteries

I66.9   Occlusion and stenosis of unspecified cerebral artery

✓4ᵗʰ **I67   Other cerebrovascular diseases**
> EXCLUDES 1   *sequelae of the listed conditions (I69.8)*

I67.0   Dissection of cerebral arteries, nonruptured
> EXCLUDES 1   *ruptured cerebral arteries (I60.7)*

I67.1   Cerebral aneurysm, nonruptured
> Cerebral aneurysm NOS
> Cerebral arteriovenous fistula, acquired
> Internal carotid artery aneurysm, intracranial portion
> Internal carotid artery aneurysm, NOS
> EXCLUDES 1   *congenital cerebral aneurysm, nonruptured (Q28.-)*
> *ruptured cerebral aneurysm (I60.7)*

I67.2   Cerebral atherosclerosis   Ⓐ
> Atheroma of cerebral and precerebral arteries

I67.3   Progressive vascular leukoencephalopathy
> Binswanger's disease

I67.4   Hypertensive encephalopathy

I67.5   Moyamoya disease

I67.6   Nonpyogenic thrombosis of intracranial venous system
> Nonpyogenic thrombosis of cerebral vein
> Nonpyogenic thrombosis of intracranial venous sinus
> EXCLUDES 1   *nonpyogenic thrombosis of intracranial venous system causing infarction (I63.6)*

I67.7   Cerebral arteritis, not elsewhere classified
> Granulomatous angiitis of the nervous system
> EXCLUDES 1   *allergic granulomatous angiitis (M30.1)*

✓5ᵗʰ **I67.8   Other specified cerebrovascular diseases**
> **I67.81   Acute cerebrovascular insufficiency**
> > Acute cerebrovascular insufficiency unspecified as to location or reversibility
> **I67.82   Cerebral ischemia**
> > Chronic cerebral ischemia
> **I67.83   Posterior reversible encephalopathy syndrome**
> > PRES
> ✓6ᵗʰ **I67.84   Cerebral vasospasm and vasoconstriction**
> > **I67.841   Reversible cerebrovascular vasoconstriction syndrome**
> > > Call-Fleming syndrome
> > > Code first underlying condition, if applicable, such as eclampsia (O15.00-O15.9)
> > **I67.848   Other cerebrovascular vasospasm and vasoconstriction**
> **I67.89   Other cerebrovascular disease**

I67.9   Cerebrovascular disease, unspecified

✓4ᵗʰ **I68   Cerebrovascular disorders in diseases classified elsewhere**
> **I68.0   Cerebral amyloid angiopathy**
> > Code first underlying amyloidosis (E85.-)
> **I68.2   Cerebral arteritis in other diseases classified elsewhere**
> > Code first underlying disease
> > EXCLUDES 1   *cerebral arteritis (in):*
> > *listerosis (A32.89)*
> > *systemic lupus erythematosus (M32.19)*
> > *syphilis (A52.04)*
> > *tuberculosis (A18.89)*

I68.8   Other cerebrovascular disorders in diseases classified elsewhere
> Code first underlying disease
> EXCLUDES 1   *syphilitic cerebral aneurysm (A52.05)*

✓4ᵗʰ **I69   Sequelae of cerebrovascular disease**
> **NOTE**   Category I69 is to be used to indicate conditions in I60-I67 as the cause of sequelae. The "sequelae" include conditions specified as such or as residuals which may occur at any time after the onset of the causal condition
> EXCLUDES 1   *personal history of cerebral infarction without residual deficit (Z86.73)*
> *personal history of prolonged reversible ischemic neurologic deficit (PRIND) (Z86.73)*
> *personal history of reversible ischemic neurologcial deficit (RIND) (Z86.73)*
> *sequelae of traumatic intracranial injury (S06.-)*
> *transient ischemic attack (TIA) (G45.9)*
> AHA: 2012, 4Q, 106

✓5ᵗʰ **I69.0   Sequelae of nontraumatic subarachnoid hemorrhage**
> **I69.00   Unspecified sequelae of nontraumatic subarachnoid hemorrhage**
> **I69.01   Cognitive deficits following nontraumatic subarachnoid hemorrhage**
> ✓6ᵗʰ **I69.02   Speech and language deficits following nontraumatic subarachnoid hemorrhage**
> > **I69.020   Aphasia following nontraumatic subarachnoid hemorrhage**
> > **I69.021   Dysphasia following nontraumatic subarachnoid hemorrhage**
> > **I69.022   Dysarthria following nontraumatic subarachnoid hemorrhage**
> > **I69.023   Fluency disorder following nontraumatic subarachnoid hemorrhage**
> > > Stuttering following nontraumatic subarachnoid hemorrhage
> > **I69.028   Other speech and language deficits following nontraumatic subarachnoid hemorrhage**
> ✓6ᵗʰ **I69.03   Monoplegia of upper limb following nontraumatic subarachnoid hemorrhage**
> > **I69.031   Monoplegia of upper limb following nontraumatic subarachnoid hemorrhage affecting right dominant side**
> > **I69.032   Monoplegia of upper limb following nontraumatic subarachnoid hemorrhage affecting left dominant side**
> > **I69.033   Monoplegia of upper limb following nontraumatic subarachnoid hemorrhage affecting right non-dominant side**
> > **I69.034   Monoplegia of upper limb following nontraumatic subarachnoid hemorrhage affecting left non-dominant side**
> > **I69.039   Monoplegia of upper limb following nontraumatic subarachnoid hemorrhage affecting unspecified side**
> ✓6ᵗʰ **I69.04   Monoplegia of lower limb following nontraumatic subarachnoid hemorrhage**
> > **I69.041   Monoplegia of lower limb following nontraumatic subarachnoid hemorrhage affecting right dominant side**
> > **I69.042   Monoplegia of lower limb following nontraumatic subarachnoid hemorrhage affecting left dominant side**
> > **I69.043   Monoplegia of lower limb following nontraumatic subarachnoid hemorrhage affecting right non-dominant side**
> > **I69.044   Monoplegia of lower limb following nontraumatic subarachnoid hemorrhage affecting left non-dominant side**
> > **I69.049   Monoplegia of lower limb following nontraumatic subarachnoid hemorrhage affecting unspecified side**
> ✓6ᵗʰ **I69.05   Hemiplegia and hemiparesis following nontraumatic subarachnoid hemorrhage**
> > **I69.051   Hemiplegia and hemiparesis following nontraumatic subarachnoid hemorrhage affecting right dominant side**
> > **I69.052   Hemiplegia and hemiparesis following nontraumatic subarachnoid hemorrhage affecting left dominant side**

I69.053   **Hemiplegia and hemiparesis following nontraumatic subarachnoid hemorrhage affecting** right non-dominant **side**

I69.054   **Hemiplegia and hemiparesis following nontraumatic subarachnoid hemorrhage affecting** left non-dominant **side**

I69.059   **Hemiplegia and hemiparesis following nontraumatic subarachnoid hemorrhage affecting unspecified side**

√6ᵗʰ **I69.06**   Other paralytic syndrome **following nontraumatic subarachnoid hemorrhage**

    Use additional code to identify type of paralytic syndrome, such as:
      locked-in state (G83.5)
      quadriplegia (G82.5-)

    EXCLUDES 1   *hemiplegia/hemiparesis following nontraumatic subarachnoid hemorrhage (I69.05-)*
      monoplegia of lower limb following nontraumatic subarachnoid hemorrhage (I69.04-)
      monoplegia of upper limb following nontraumatic subarachnoid hemorrhage (I69.03-)

I69.061   **Other paralytic syndrome following nontraumatic subarachnoid hemorrhage affecting** right dominant **side**

I69.062   **Other paralytic syndrome following nontraumatic subarachnoid hemorrhage affecting** left dominant **side**

I69.063   **Other paralytic syndrome following nontraumatic subarachnoid hemorrhage affecting** right non-dominant **side**

I69.064   **Other paralytic syndrome following nontraumatic subarachnoid hemorrhage affecting** left non-dominant **side**

I69.065   **Other paralytic syndrome following nontraumatic subarachnoid hemorrhage, bilateral**

I69.069   **Other paralytic syndrome following nontraumatic subarachnoid hemorrhage affecting unspecified side**

√6ᵗʰ **I69.09**   Other **sequelae of nontraumatic subarachnoid hemorrhage**

I69.090   Apraxia **following nontraumatic subarachnoid hemorrhage**

I69.091   Dysphagia **following nontraumatic subarachnoid hemorrhage**
    Use additional code to identify the type of dysphagia, if known (R13.1-)

I69.092   Facial weakness **following nontraumatic subarachnoid hemorrhage**
    Facial droop following nontraumatic subarachnoid hemorrhage

I69.093   Ataxia **following nontraumatic subarachnoid hemorrhage**

I69.098   **Other sequelae following nontraumatic subarachnoid hemorrhage**
    Alterations of sensation following nontraumatic subarachnoid hemorrhage
    Disturbance of vision following nontraumatic subarachnoid hemorrhage
    Use additional code to identify the sequelae

√5ᵗʰ **I69.1**   **Sequelae of nontraumatic** intracerebral **hemorrhage**

I69.10   **Unspecified sequelae of nontraumatic intracerebral hemorrhage**

I69.11   Cognitive deficits **following nontraumatic intracerebral hemorrhage**

√6ᵗʰ **I69.12**   Speech **and** language deficits **following nontraumatic intracerebral hemorrhage**

I69.120   Aphasia **following nontraumatic intracerebral hemorrhage**

I69.121   Dysphasia **following nontraumatic intracerebral hemorrhage**

I69.122   Dysarthria **following nontraumatic intracerebral hemorrhage**

I69.123   Fluency disorder **following nontraumatic intracerebral hemorrhage**
    Stuttering following nontraumatic subarachnoid hemorrhage

I69.128   **Other speech and language deficits following nontraumatic intracerebral hemorrhage**

√6ᵗʰ **I69.13**   Monoplegia **of** upper limb **following nontraumatic intracerebral hemorrhage**

I69.131   **Monoplegia of upper limb following nontraumatic intracerebral hemorrhage affecting** right dominant **side**

I69.132   **Monoplegia of upper limb following nontraumatic intracerebral hemorrhage affecting** left dominant **side**

I69.133   **Monoplegia of upper limb following nontraumatic intracerebral hemorrhage affecting** right non-dominant **side**

I69.134   **Monoplegia of upper limb following nontraumatic intracerebral hemorrhage affecting** left non-dominant **side**

I69.139   **Monoplegia of upper limb following nontraumatic intracerebral hemorrhage affecting unspecified side**

√6ᵗʰ **I69.14**   Monoplegia **of** lower limb **following nontraumatic intracerebral hemorrhage**

I69.141   **Monoplegia of lower limb following nontraumatic intracerebral hemorrhage affecting** right dominant **side**

I69.142   **Monoplegia of lower limb following nontraumatic intracerebral hemorrhage affecting** left dominant **side**

I69.143   **Monoplegia of lower limb following nontraumatic intracerebral hemorrhage affecting** right non-dominant **side**

I69.144   **Monoplegia of lower limb following nontraumatic intracerebral hemorrhage affecting** left non-dominant **side**

I69.149   **Monoplegia of lower limb following nontraumatic intracerebral hemorrhage affecting unspecified side**

√6ᵗʰ **I69.15**   Hemiplegia **and** hemiparesis **following nontraumatic intracerebral hemorrhage**

I69.151   **Hemiplegia and hemiparesis following nontraumatic intracerebral hemorrhage affecting** right dominant **side**

I69.152   **Hemiplegia and hemiparesis following nontraumatic intracerebral hemorrhage affecting** left dominant **side**

I69.153   **Hemiplegia and hemiparesis following nontraumatic intracerebral hemorrhage affecting** right non-dominant **side**

I69.154   **Hemiplegia and hemiparesis following nontraumatic intracerebral hemorrhage affecting** left non-dominant **side**

I69.159   **Hemiplegia and hemiparesis following nontraumatic intracerebral hemorrhage affecting unspecified side**

√6ᵗʰ **I69.16**   Other paralytic syndrome **following nontraumatic intracerebral hemorrhage**

    Use additional code to identify type of paralytic syndrome, such as:
      locked-in state (G83.5)
      quadriplegia (G82.5-)

    EXCLUDES 1   *hemiplegia/hemiparesis following nontraumatic intracerebral hemorrhage (I69.15-)*
      monoplegia of lower limb following nontraumatic intracerebral hemorrhage (I69.14-)
      monoplegia of upper limb following nontraumatic intracerebral hemorrhage (I69.13-)

I69.161   **Other paralytic syndrome following nontraumatic intracerebral hemorrhage affecting** right dominant **side**

I69.162   **Other paralytic syndrome following nontraumatic intracerebral hemorrhage affecting** left dominant **side**

I69.163   **Other paralytic syndrome following nontraumatic intracerebral hemorrhage affecting** right non-dominant **side**

I69.164   **Other paralytic syndrome following nontraumatic intracerebral hemorrhage affecting** left non-dominant **side**

☑ Additional Character Required   √x7ᵗʰ Xtension Alert   Unspecified Dx   Other Specified Dx   Manifestation   ▶◀ Revised Text   ● New Code   ▲ Revised Code Title

I69.165 **Other paralytic syndrome following nontraumatic intracerebral hemorrhage, bilateral**

I69.169 **Other paralytic syndrome following nontraumatic intracerebral hemorrhage affecting unspecified side**

✓6ᵗʰ I69.19 Other **sequelae of nontraumatic intracerebral hemorrhage**

I69.190 Apraxia **following nontraumatic intracerebral hemorrhage**

I69.191 Dysphagia **following nontraumatic intracerebral hemorrhage**
  Use additional code to identify the type of dysphagia, if known (R13.1-)

I69.192 Facial weakness **following nontraumatic intracerebral hemorrhage**
  Facial droop following nontraumatic intracerebral hemorrhage

I69.193 Ataxia **following nontraumatic intracerebral hemorrhage**

I69.198 **Other sequelae of nontraumatic intracerebral hemorrhage**
  Alteration of sensations following nontraumatic intracerebral hemorrhage
  Disturbance of vision following nontraumatic intracerebral hemorrhage
  Use additional code to identify the sequelae

✓5ᵗʰ **I69.2 Sequelae of other nontraumatic** intracranial **hemorrhage**

I69.20 **Unspecified sequelae of other nontraumatic intracranial hemorrhage**

I69.21 Cognitive deficits **following other nontraumatic intracranial hemorrhage**

✓6ᵗʰ I69.22 Speech **and** language deficits **following other nontraumatic intracranial hemorrhage**

I69.220 Aphasia **following other nontraumatic intracranial hemorrhage**

I69.221 Dysphasia **following other nontraumatic intracranial hemorrhage**

I69.222 Dysarthria **following other nontraumatic intracranial hemorrhage**

I69.223 Fluency **disorder following other nontraumatic intracranial hemorrhage**
  Stuttering following nontraumatic subarachnoid hemorrhage

I69.228 **Other speech and language deficits following other nontraumatic intracranial hemorrhage**

✓6ᵗʰ I69.23 Monoplegia **of** upper limb **following other nontraumatic intracranial hemorrhage**

I69.231 **Monoplegia of upper limb following other nontraumatic intracranial hemorrhage affecting** right dominant **side**

I69.232 **Monoplegia of upper limb following other nontraumatic intracranial hemorrhage affecting** left dominant **side**

I69.233 **Monoplegia of upper limb following other nontraumatic intracranial hemorrhage affecting** right non-dominant **side**

I69.234 **Monoplegia of upper limb following other nontraumatic intracranial hemorrhage affecting** left non-dominant **side**

I69.239 **Monoplegia of upper limb following other nontraumatic intracranial hemorrhage affecting unspecified side**

✓6ᵗʰ I69.24 Monoplegia **of** lower limb **following other nontraumatic intracranial hemorrhage**

I69.241 **Monoplegia of lower limb following other nontraumatic intracranial hemorrhage affecting** right dominant **side**

I69.242 **Monoplegia of lower limb following other nontraumatic intracranial hemorrhage affecting** left dominant **side**

I69.243 **Monoplegia of lower limb following other nontraumatic intracranial hemorrhage affecting** right non-dominant **side**

I69.244 **Monoplegia of lower limb following other nontraumatic intracranial hemorrhage affecting** left non-dominant **side**

I69.249 **Monoplegia of lower limb following other nontraumatic intracranial hemorrhage affecting unspecified side**

✓6ᵗʰ I69.25 Hemiplegia **and** hemiparesis **following other nontraumatic intracranial hemorrhage**

I69.251 **Hemiplegia and hemiparesis following other nontraumatic intracranial hemorrhage affecting** right dominant **side**

I69.252 **Hemiplegia and hemiparesis following other nontraumatic intracranial hemorrhage affecting** left dominant **side**

I69.253 **Hemiplegia and hemiparesis following other nontraumatic intracranial hemorrhage affecting** right non-dominant **side**

I69.254 **Hemiplegia and hemiparesis following other nontraumatic intracranial hemorrhage affecting** left non-dominant **side**

I69.259 **Hemiplegia and hemiparesis following other nontraumatic intracranial hemorrhage affecting unspecified side**

✓6ᵗʰ I69.26 Other paralytic syndrome **following other nontraumatic intracranial hemorrhage**
  Use additional code to identify type of paralytic syndrome, such as:
  locked-in state (G83.5)
  quadriplegia (G82.5-)
  EXCLUDES 1 *hemiplegia/hemiparesis following other nontraumatic intracranial hemorrhage (I69.25-)*
  monoplegia of lower limb following other nontraumatic intracranial hemorrhage (I69.24-)
  monoplegia of upper limb following other nontraumatic intracranial hemorrhage (I69.23-)

I69.261 **Other paralytic syndrome following other nontraumatic intracranial hemorrhage affecting** right dominant **side**

I69.262 **Other paralytic syndrome following other nontraumatic intracranial hemorrhage affecting** left dominant **side**

I69.263 **Other paralytic syndrome following other nontraumatic intracranial hemorrhage affecting** right non-dominant **side**

I69.264 **Other paralytic syndrome following other nontraumatic intracranial hemorrhage affecting** left non-dominant **side**

I69.265 **Other paralytic syndrome following other nontraumatic intracranial hemorrhage, bilateral**

I69.269 **Other paralytic syndrome following other nontraumatic intracranial hemorrhage affecting unspecified side**

✓6ᵗʰ I69.29 Other sequelae **of other nontraumatic intracranial hemorrhage**

I69.290 Apraxia **following other nontraumatic intracranial hemorrhage**

I69.291 Dysphagia **following other nontraumatic intracranial hemorrhage**
  Use additional code to identify the type of dysphagia, if known (R13.1-)

I69.292 Facial weakness **following other nontraumatic intracranial hemorrhage**
  Facial droop following other nontraumatic intracranial hemorrhage

I69.293 Ataxia **following other nontraumatic intracranial hemorrhage**

I69.298 **Other sequelae of other nontraumatic intracranial hemorrhage**
  Alteration of sensation following other nontraumatic intracranial hemorrhage
  Disturbance of vision following other nontraumatic intracranial hemorrhage
  Use additional code to identify the sequelae

✓5ᵗʰ **I69.3 Sequelae of** cerebral infarction
  Sequelae of stroke NOS
  AHA: 2013, 4Q, 127-128; 2012, 4Q, 92, 94

I69.30 **Unspecified sequelae of cerebral infarction**

I69.31 Cognitive **deficits following cerebral infarction**

EXCLUDES 1 Not coded here   **EXCLUDES 2** Not included here   Ⓝ Newborn Age: 0   Ⓟ Pediatric Age: 0-17   Ⓜ Maternity Age: 12-55   Ⓐ Adult Age: 15-124

582   ICD-10-CM Draft (2015)

☑6ᵗʰ **I69.32** Speech and language deficits following cerebral infarction
- **I69.320** Aphasia following cerebral infarction
- **I69.321** Dysphasia following cerebral infarction
  AHA: 2012, 4Q, 91
- **I69.322** Dysarthria following cerebral infarction
- **I69.323** Fluency disorder following cerebral infarction
  Stuttering following nontraumatic subarachnoid hemorrhage
- **I69.328** Other speech and language deficits following cerebral infarction

☑6ᵗʰ **I69.33** Monoplegia of upper limb following cerebral infarction
- **I69.331** Monoplegia of upper limb following cerebral infarction affecting right dominant side
- **I69.332** Monoplegia of upper limb following cerebral infarction affecting left dominant side
- **I69.333** Monoplegia of upper limb following cerebral infarction affecting right non-dominant side
- **I69.334** Monoplegia of upper limb following cerebral infarction affecting left non-dominant side
- **I69.339** Monoplegia of upper limb following cerebral infarction affecting unspecified side

☑6ᵗʰ **I69.34** Monoplegia of lower limb following cerebral infarction
- **I69.341** Monoplegia of lower limb following cerebral infarction affecting right dominant side
- **I69.342** Monoplegia of lower limb following cerebral infarction affecting left dominant side
- **I69.343** Monoplegia of lower limb following cerebral infarction affecting right non-dominant side
- **I69.344** Monoplegia of lower limb following cerebral infarction affecting left non-dominant side
- **I69.349** Monoplegia of lower limb following cerebral infarction affecting unspecified side

☑6ᵗʰ **I69.35** Hemiplegia and hemiparesis following cerebral infarction
- **I69.351** Hemiplegia and hemiparesis following cerebral infarction affecting right dominant side
- **I69.352** Hemiplegia and hemiparesis following cerebral infarction affecting left dominant side
- **I69.353** Hemiplegia and hemiparesis following cerebral infarction affecting right non-dominant side
- **I69.354** Hemiplegia and hemiparesis following cerebral infarction affecting left non-dominant side
  AHA: 2012, 4Q, 91
- **I69.359** Hemiplegia and hemiparesis following cerebral infarction affecting unspecified side

☑6ᵗʰ **I69.36** Other paralytic syndrome following cerebral infarction
  Use additional code to identify type of paralytic syndrome, such as:
  locked-in state (G83.5)
  quadriplegia (G82.5-)
  EXCLUDES 1 hemiplegia/hemiparesis following cerebral infarction (I69.35-)
  monoplegia of lower limb following cerebral infarction (I69.34-)
  monoplegia of upper limb following cerebral infarction (I69.33-)
- **I69.361** Other paralytic syndrome following cerebral infarction affecting right dominant side

- **I69.362** Other paralytic syndrome following cerebral infarction affecting left dominant side
- **I69.363** Other paralytic syndrome following cerebral infarction affecting right non-dominant side
- **I69.364** Other paralytic syndrome following cerebral infarction affecting left non-dominant side
- **I69.365** Other paralytic syndrome following cerebral infarction, bilateral
- **I69.369** Other paralytic syndrome following cerebral infarction affecting unspecified side

☑6ᵗʰ **I69.39** Other sequelae of cerebral infarction
- **I69.390** Apraxia following cerebral infarction
- **I69.391** Dysphagia following cerebral infarction
  Use additional code to identify the type of dysphagia, if known (R13.1-)
- **I69.392** Facial weakness following cerebral infarction
  Facial droop following cerebral infarction
- **I69.393** Ataxia following cerebral infarction
- **I69.398** Other sequelae of cerebral infarction
  Alteration of sensation following cerebral infarction
  Disturbance of vision following cerebral infarction
  Use additional code to identify the sequelae

☑5ᵗʰ **I69.8** Sequelae of other cerebrovascular diseases
  EXCLUDES 1 sequelae of traumatic intracranial injury (S06.-)
- **I69.80** Unspecified sequelae of other cerebrovascular disease
- **I69.81** Cognitive deficits following other cerebrovascular disease

☑6ᵗʰ **I69.82** Speech and language deficits following other cerebrovascular disease
- **I69.820** Aphasia following other cerebrovascular disease
- **I69.821** Dysphasia following other cerebrovascular disease
- **I69.822** Dysarthria following other cerebrovascular disease
- **I69.823** Fluency disorder following other cerebrovascular disease
  Stuttering following nontraumatic subarachnoid hemorrhage
- **I69.828** Other speech and language deficits following other cerebrovascular disease

☑6ᵗʰ **I69.83** Monoplegia of upper limb following other cerebrovascular disease
- **I69.831** Monoplegia of upper limb following other cerebrovascular disease affecting right dominant side
- **I69.832** Monoplegia of upper limb following other cerebrovascular disease affecting left dominant side
- **I69.833** Monoplegia of upper limb following other cerebrovascular disease affecting right non-dominant side
- **I69.834** Monoplegia of upper limb following other cerebrovascular disease affecting left non-dominant side
- **I69.839** Monoplegia of upper limb following other cerebrovascular disease affecting unspecified side

☑6ᵗʰ **I69.84** Monoplegia of lower limb following other cerebrovascular disease
- **I69.841** Monoplegia of lower limb following other cerebrovascular disease affecting right dominant side
- **I69.842** Monoplegia of lower limb following other cerebrovascular disease affecting left dominant side
- **I69.843** Monoplegia of lower limb following other cerebrovascular disease affecting right non-dominant side

Diseases of the Circulatory System

I69.844–I69.96

I69.844   **Monoplegia of lower limb following other cerebrovascular disease affecting** left non-dominant **side**

I69.849   **Monoplegia of lower limb following other cerebrovascular disease affecting unspecified side**

✓6ᵗʰ   **I69.85**   Hemiplegia and hemiparesis following other cerebrovascular disease

I69.851   **Hemiplegia and hemiparesis following other cerebrovascular disease affecting** right dominant **side**

I69.852   **Hemiplegia and hemiparesis following other cerebrovascular disease affecting** left dominant **side**

I69.853   **Hemiplegia and hemiparesis following other cerebrovascular disease affecting** right non-dominant **side**

I69.854   **Hemiplegia and hemiparesis following other cerebrovascular disease affecting** left non-dominant **side**

I69.859   **Hemiplegia and hemiparesis following other cerebrovascular disease affecting unspecified side**

✓6ᵗʰ   **I69.86**   Other paralytic syndrome following other cerebrovascular disease

Use additional code to identify type of paralytic syndrome, such as:
locked-in state (G83.5)
quadriplegia (G82.5-)

EXCLUDES 1   *hemiplegia/hemiparesis following other cerebrovascular disease (I69.85-)*
monoplegia of lower limb following other cerebrovascular disease (I69.84-)
monoplegia of upper limb following other cerebrovascular disease (I69.83-)

I69.861   **Other paralytic syndrome following other cerebrovascular disease affecting** right dominant **side**

I69.862   **Other paralytic syndrome following other cerebrovascular disease affecting** left dominant **side**

I69.863   **Other paralytic syndrome following other cerebrovascular disease affecting** right non-dominant **side**

I69.864   **Other paralytic syndrome following other cerebrovascular disease affecting** left non-dominant **side**

I69.865   **Other paralytic syndrome following other cerebrovascular disease,** bilateral

I69.869   **Other paralytic syndrome other cerebrovascular disease affecting unspecified side**

✓6ᵗʰ   **I69.89**   Other sequelae of other cerebrovascular disease

I69.890   Apraxia **following other cerebrovascular disease**

I69.891   Dysphagia **following other cerebrovascular disease**

Use additional code to identify the type of dysphagia, if known (R13.1-)

I69.892   Facial weakness **following other cerebrovascular disease**

Facial droop following other cerebrovascular disease

I69.893   Ataxia **following other cerebrovascular disease**

I69.898   **Other sequelae of other cerebrovascular disease**

Alteration of sensation following other cerebrovascular disease
Disturbance of vision following other cerebrovascular disease
Use additional code to identify the sequelae

✓5ᵗʰ   **I69.9**   **Sequelae of** unspecified cerebrovascular diseases

EXCLUDES 1   *sequelae of stroke (I69.3)*
sequelae of traumatic intracranial injury (S06.-)

I69.90   **Unspecified sequelae of unspecified cerebrovascular disease**

I69.91   Cognitive deficits **following unspecified cerebrovascular disease**

✓6ᵗʰ   **I69.92**   Speech and language deficits **following unspecified cerebrovascular disease**

I69.920   Aphasia **following unspecified cerebrovascular disease**

I69.921   Dysphasia **following unspecified cerebrovascular disease**

I69.922   Dysarthria **following unspecified cerebrovascular disease**

I69.923   Fluency disorder **following unspecified cerebrovascular disease**

Stuttering following nontraumatic subarachnoid hemorrhage

I69.928   **Other speech and language deficits following unspecified cerebrovascular disease**

✓6ᵗʰ   **I69.93**   Monoplegia of upper limb **following unspecified cerebrovascular disease**

I69.931   **Monoplegia of upper limb following unspecified cerebrovascular disease affecting** right dominant **side**

I69.932   **Monoplegia of upper limb following unspecified cerebrovascular disease affecting** left dominant **side**

I69.933   **Monoplegia of upper limb following unspecified cerebrovascular disease affecting** right non-dominant **side**

I69.934   **Monoplegia of upper limb following unspecified cerebrovascular disease affecting** left non-dominant **side**

I69.939   **Monoplegia of upper limb following unspecified cerebrovascular disease affecting unspecified side**

✓6ᵗʰ   **I69.94**   Monoplegia of lower limb **following unspecified cerebrovascular disease**

I69.941   **Monoplegia of lower limb following unspecified cerebrovascular disease affecting** right dominant **side**

I69.942   **Monoplegia of lower limb following unspecified cerebrovascular disease affecting** left dominant **side**

I69.943   **Monoplegia of lower limb following unspecified cerebrovascular disease affecting** right non-dominant **side**

I69.944   **Monoplegia of lower limb following unspecified cerebrovascular disease affecting** left non-dominant **side**

I69.949   **Monoplegia of lower limb following unspecified cerebrovascular disease affecting unspecified side**

✓6ᵗʰ   **I69.95**   Hemiplegia and hemiparesis **following unspecified cerebrovascular disease**

I69.951   **Hemiplegia and hemiparesis following unspecified cerebrovascular disease affecting** right dominant **side**

I69.952   **Hemiplegia and hemiparesis following unspecified cerebrovascular disease affecting** left dominant **side**

I69.953   **Hemiplegia and hemiparesis following unspecified cerebrovascular disease affecting** right non-dominant **side**

I69.954   **Hemiplegia and hemiparesis following unspecified cerebrovascular disease affecting** left non-dominant **side**

I69.959   **Hemiplegia and hemiparesis following unspecified cerebrovascular disease affecting unspecified side**

✓6ᵗʰ   **I69.96**   Other paralytic syndrome **following unspecified cerebrovascular disease**

Use additional code to identify type of paralytic syndrome, such as:
locked-in state (G83.5)
quadriplegia (G82.5-)

EXCLUDES 1   *hemiplegia/hemiparesis following unspecified cerebrovascular disease (I69.95-)*
monoplegia of lower limb following unspecified cerebrovascular disease (I69.94-)
monoplegia of upper limb following unspecified cerebrovascular disease (I69.93-)

EXCLUDES 1 Not coded here   EXCLUDES 2 Not included here   N Newborn Age: 0   P Pediatric Age: 0-17   M Maternity Age: 12-55   A Adult Age: 15-124

584   ICD-10-CM Draft (2015)

I69.961   **Other paralytic syndrome following unspecified cerebrovascular disease affecting** right dominant **side**

I69.962   **Other paralytic syndrome following unspecified cerebrovascular disease affecting** left dominant **side**

I69.963   **Other paralytic syndrome following unspecified cerebrovascular disease affecting** right non-dominant **side**

I69.964   **Other paralytic syndrome following unspecified cerebrovascular disease affecting** left non-dominant **side**

I69.965   **Other paralytic syndrome following unspecified cerebrovascular disease, bilateral**

I69.969   **Other paralytic syndrome following unspecified cerebrovascular disease affecting unspecified side**

✓6ᵗʰ **I69.99**   Other **sequelae of unspecified cerebrovascular disease**

I69.99Ø   Apraxia **following unspecified cerebrovascular disease**

I69.991   Dysphagia **following unspecified cerebrovascular disease**
     Use additional code to identify the type of dysphagia, if known (R13.1-)

I69.992   Facial weakness **following unspecified cerebrovascular disease**
     Facial droop following unspecified cerebrovascular disease

I69.993   Ataxia **following unspecified cerebrovascular disease**

I69.998   **Other sequelae following unspecified cerebrovascular disease**
     Alteration in sensation following unspecified cerebrovascular disease
     Disturbance of vision following unspecified cerebrovascular disease
     Use additional code to identify the sequelae

Diseases of arteries, arterioles and capillaries (I7Ø-I79)

✓4ᵗʰ **I7Ø**   **Atherosclerosis**
   INCLUDES   arteriolosclerosis
            arterial degeneration
            arteriosclerosis
            arteriosclerotic vascular disease
            arteriovascular degeneration
            atheroma
            endarteritis deformans or obliterans
            senile arteritis
            senile endarteritis
            vascular degeneration
   Use additional code to identify:
     exposure to environmental tobacco smoke (Z77.22)
     history of tobacco use (Z87.891)
     occupational exposure to environmental tobacco smoke (Z57.31)
     tobacco dependence (F17.-)
     tobacco use (Z72.Ø)
   EXCLUDES 2   arteriosclerotic cardiovascular disease (I25.1-)
            arteriosclerotic heart disease (I25.1-)
            atheroembolism (I75.-)
            cerebral atherosclerosis (I67.2)
            coronary atherosclerosis (I25.1-)
            mesenteric atherosclerosis (K55.1)
            precerebral atherosclerosis (I67.2)
            primary pulmonary atherosclerosis (I27.Ø)

I7Ø.Ø   **Atherosclerosis of** aorta   🅰

I7Ø.1   **Atherosclerosis of** renal **artery**   🅰
   Goldblatt's kidney
   EXCLUDES 2   atherosclerosis of renal arterioles (I12.-)

✓5ᵗʰ **I7Ø.2**   **Atherosclerosis of** native **arteries of the** extremities
   Mönckeberg's (medial) sclerosis
   Use additional code, if applicable, to identify chronic total occlusion of artery of extremity (I7Ø.92)
   EXCLUDES 2   atherosclerosis of bypass graft of extremities (I7Ø.3Ø-I7Ø.79)

✓6ᵗʰ **I7Ø.2Ø**   Unspecified **atherosclerosis of native arteries of extremities**

I7Ø.2Ø1   **Unspecified atherosclerosis of native arteries of extremities,** right leg   🅰

I7Ø.2Ø2   **Unspecified atherosclerosis of native arteries of extremities,** left leg   🅰

I7Ø.2Ø3   **Unspecified atherosclerosis of native arteries of extremities,** bilateral legs   🅰

I7Ø.2Ø8   **Unspecified atherosclerosis of native arteries of extremities, other extremity**   🅰

I7Ø.2Ø9   **Unspecified atherosclerosis of native arteries of extremities, unspecified extremity**   🅰

✓6ᵗʰ **I7Ø.21**   **Atherosclerosis of native arteries of extremities with** intermittent claudication

I7Ø.211   **Atherosclerosis of native arteries of extremities with intermittent claudication,** right leg   🅰

I7Ø.212   **Atherosclerosis of native arteries of extremities with intermittent claudication,** left leg   🅰

I7Ø.213   **Atherosclerosis of native arteries of extremities with intermittent claudication,** bilateral legs   🅰

I7Ø.218   **Atherosclerosis of native arteries of extremities with intermittent claudication, other extremity**   🅰

I7Ø.219   **Atherosclerosis of native arteries of extremities with intermittent claudication, unspecified extremity**   🅰

✓6ᵗʰ **I7Ø.22**   **Atherosclerosis of native arteries of extremities with** rest pain
   INCLUDES   any condition classifiable to I7Ø.21-

I7Ø.221   **Atherosclerosis of native arteries of extremities with rest pain,** right leg   🅰

I7Ø.222   **Atherosclerosis of native arteries of extremities with rest pain,** left leg   🅰

I7Ø.223   **Atherosclerosis of native arteries of extremities with rest pain,** bilateral legs   🅰

I7Ø.228   **Atherosclerosis of native arteries of extremities with rest pain, other extremity**   🅰

I7Ø.229   **Atherosclerosis of native arteries of extremities with rest pain, unspecified extremity**   🅰

✓6ᵗʰ **I7Ø.23**   **Atherosclerosis of native arteries of** right leg **with** ulceration
   INCLUDES   any condition classifiable to I7Ø.211 and I7Ø.221
   Use additional code to identify severity of ulcer (L97.-)

I7Ø.231   **Atherosclerosis of native arteries of right leg with ulceration of** thigh   🅰

I7Ø.232   **Atherosclerosis of native arteries of right leg with ulceration of** calf   🅰

I7Ø.233   **Atherosclerosis of native arteries of right leg with ulceration of** ankle   🅰

I7Ø.234   **Atherosclerosis of native arteries of right leg with ulceration of** heel and midfoot   🅰
     Atherosclerosis of native arteries of right leg with ulceration of plantar surface of midfoot

I7Ø.235   **Atherosclerosis of native arteries of right leg with ulceration of other** part of foot   🅰
     Atherosclerosis of native arteries of right leg extremities with ulceration of toe

I7Ø.238   **Atherosclerosis of native arteries of right leg with ulceration of other part of lower right leg**   🅰

I7Ø.239   **Atherosclerosis of native arteries of right leg with ulceration of unspecified site**   🅰

✓6ᵗʰ **I7Ø.24**   **Atherosclerosis of native arteries of** left leg **with** ulceration
   INCLUDES   any condition classifiable to I7Ø.212 and I7Ø.222
   Use additional code to identify severity of ulcer (L97.-)

I7Ø.241   **Atherosclerosis of native arteries of left leg with ulceration of** thigh   🅰

I7Ø.242   **Atherosclerosis of native arteries of left leg with ulceration of** calf   🅰

I7Ø.243   **Atherosclerosis of native arteries of left leg with ulceration of** ankle   🅰

✓ Additional Character Required   ✓ₓ7ᵗʰ Xtension Alert   Unspecified Dx   Other Specified Dx   Manifestation   ►◄ Revised Text   ● New Code   ▲ Revised Code Title

ICD-1Ø-CM Draft (2Ø15)   **585**

Diseases of the Circulatory System

I70.244–I70.343

I70.244   **Atherosclerosis of native arteries of left leg with ulceration of** heel and midfoot 🅰
Atherosclerosis of native arteries of left leg with ulceration of plantar surface of midfoot

I70.245   **Atherosclerosis of native arteries of left leg with ulceration of other** part of foot 🅰
Atherosclerosis of native arteries of left leg extremities with ulceration of toe

I70.248   **Atherosclerosis of native arteries of left leg with ulceration of other** part of lower left leg 🅰

I70.249   **Atherosclerosis of native arteries of left leg with ulceration of unspecified site** 🅰

I70.25   **Atherosclerosis of native arteries of other** extremities **with** ulceration 🅰
   INCLUDES   any condition classifiable to I70.218 and I70.228
   Use additional code to identify the severity of the ulcer (L98.49-)

✓6th **I70.26**   **Atherosclerosis of native arteries of extremities with** gangrene
   INCLUDES   any condition classifiable to I70.21-, I70.22-, I70.23-, I70.24-, and I70.25-
   Use additional code to identify the severity of any ulcer (L97.-, L98.49-), if applicable

I70.261   **Atherosclerosis of native arteries of extremities with gangrene,** right leg 🅰

I70.262   **Atherosclerosis of native arteries of extremities with gangrene,** left leg 🅰

I70.263   **Atherosclerosis of native arteries of extremities with gangrene,** bilateral legs 🅰

I70.268   **Atherosclerosis of native arteries of extremities with gangrene, other extremity** 🅰

I70.269   **Atherosclerosis of native arteries of extremities with gangrene, unspecified extremity** 🅰

✓6th **I70.29**   Other **atherosclerosis of native arteries of extremities**

I70.291   **Other atherosclerosis of native arteries of extremities,** right leg 🅰

I70.292   **Other atherosclerosis of native arteries of extremities,** left leg 🅰

I70.293   **Other atherosclerosis of native arteries of extremities,** bilateral legs 🅰

I70.298   **Other atherosclerosis of native arteries of extremities, other extremity** 🅰

I70.299   **Other atherosclerosis of native arteries of extremities, unspecified extremity** 🅰

✓5th **I70.3**   **Atherosclerosis of** unspecified type of bypass graft(s) **of the** extremities
   Use additional code, if applicable, to identify chronic total occlusion of artery of extremity (I70.92)
   EXCLUDES 1   *embolism or thrombus of bypass graft(s) of extremities (T82.8-)*

✓6th **I70.30**   Unspecified **atherosclerosis of unspecified type of bypass graft(s) of the extremities**

I70.301   **Unspecified atherosclerosis of unspecified type of bypass graft(s) of the extremities,** right leg 🅰

I70.302   **Unspecified atherosclerosis of unspecified type of bypass graft(s) of the extremities,** left leg 🅰

I70.303   **Unspecified atherosclerosis of unspecified type of bypass graft(s) of the extremities,** bilateral legs 🅰

I70.308   **Unspecified atherosclerosis of unspecified type of bypass graft(s) of the extremities, other extremity** 🅰

I70.309   **Unspecified atherosclerosis of unspecified type of bypass graft(s) of the extremities, unspecified extremity** 🅰

✓6th **I70.31**   **Atherosclerosis of unspecified type of bypass graft(s) of the extremities with** intermittent claudication

I70.311   **Atherosclerosis of unspecified type of bypass graft(s) of the extremities with intermittent claudication,** right leg 🅰

I70.312   **Atherosclerosis of unspecified type of bypass graft(s) of the extremities with intermittent claudication,** left leg 🅰

I70.313   **Atherosclerosis of unspecified type of bypass graft(s) of the extremities with intermittent claudication,** bilateral legs 🅰

I70.318   **Atherosclerosis of unspecified type of bypass graft(s) of the extremities with intermittent claudication, other extremity** 🅰

I70.319   **Atherosclerosis of unspecified type of bypass graft(s) of the extremities with intermittent claudication, unspecified extremity** 🅰

✓6th **I70.32**   **Atherosclerosis of unspecified type of bypass graft(s) of the extremities with** rest pain
   INCLUDES   any condition classifiable to I70.31-

I70.321   **Atherosclerosis of unspecified type of bypass graft(s) of the extremities with rest pain,** right leg 🅰

I70.322   **Atherosclerosis of unspecified type of bypass graft(s) of the extremities with rest pain,** left leg 🅰

I70.323   **Atherosclerosis of unspecified type of bypass graft(s) of the extremities with rest pain,** bilateral legs 🅰

I70.328   **Atherosclerosis of unspecified type of bypass graft(s) of the extremities with rest pain, other extremity** 🅰

I70.329   **Atherosclerosis of unspecified type of bypass graft(s) of the extremities with rest pain, unspecified extremity** 🅰

✓6th **I70.33**   **Atherosclerosis of unspecified type of bypass graft(s) of the** right leg **with** ulceration
   INCLUDES   any condition classifiable to I70.311 and I70.321
   Use additional code to identify severity of ulcer (L97.-)

I70.331   **Atherosclerosis of unspecified type of bypass graft(s) of the right leg with ulceration of** thigh 🅰

I70.332   **Atherosclerosis of unspecified type of bypass graft(s) of the right leg with ulceration of** calf 🅰

I70.333   **Atherosclerosis of unspecified type of bypass graft(s) of the right leg with ulceration of** ankle 🅰

I70.334   **Atherosclerosis of unspecified type of bypass graft(s) of the right leg with ulceration of** heel and midfoot 🅰
Atherosclerosis of unspecified type of bypass graft(s) of right leg with ulceration of plantar surface of midfoot

I70.335   **Atherosclerosis of unspecified type of bypass graft(s) of the right leg with ulceration of other** part of foot 🅰
Atherosclerosis of unspecified type of bypass graft(s) of the right leg with ulceration of toe

I70.338   **Atherosclerosis of unspecified type of bypass graft(s) of the right leg with ulceration of other** part of lower leg 🅰

I70.339   **Atherosclerosis of unspecified type of bypass graft(s) of the right leg with ulceration of unspecified site** 🅰

✓6th **I70.34**   **Atherosclerosis of unspecified type of bypass graft(s) of the** left leg **with** ulceration
   INCLUDES   any condition classifiable to I70.312 and I70.322
   Use additional code to identify severity of ulcer (L97.-)

I70.341   **Atherosclerosis of unspecified type of bypass graft(s) of the left leg with ulceration of** thigh 🅰

I70.342   **Atherosclerosis of unspecified type of bypass graft(s) of the left leg with ulceration of** calf 🅰

I70.343   **Atherosclerosis of unspecified type of bypass graft(s) of the left leg with ulceration of** ankle 🅰

EXCLUDES 1 Not coded here   EXCLUDES 2 Not included here   N Newborn Age: 0   P Pediatric Age: 0-17   M Maternity Age: 12-55   A Adult Age: 15-124

586   ICD-10-CM Draft (2015)

I70.344　**Atherosclerosis of unspecified type of bypass graft(s) of the left leg with ulceration of** heel and midfoot 🅐
　　Atherosclerosis of unspecified type of bypass graft(s) of left leg with ulceration of plantar surface of midfoot

I70.345　**Atherosclerosis of unspecified type of bypass graft(s) of the left leg with ulceration of other** part of foot 🅐
　　Atherosclerosis of unspecified type of bypass graft(s) of the left leg with ulceration of toe

I70.348　**Atherosclerosis of unspecified type of bypass graft(s) of the left leg with ulceration of other** part of lower leg 🅐

I70.349　**Atherosclerosis of unspecified type of bypass graft(s) of the left leg with ulceration of unspecified site** 🅐

I70.35　**Atherosclerosis of unspecified type of bypass graft(s) of other extremity with** ulceration 🅐
　INCLUDES　any condition classifiable to I70.318 and I70.328
　Use additional code to identify severity of ulcer (L98.49-)

✓6ᵗʰ　I70.36　**Atherosclerosis of unspecified type of bypass graft(s) of the extremities with** gangrene
　INCLUDES　any condition classifiable to I70.31-, I70.32-, I70.33-, I70.34-, I70.35
　Use additional code to identify the severity of any ulcer (L97.-, L98.49-), if applicable

I70.361　**Atherosclerosis of unspecified type of bypass graft(s) of the extremities with gangrene,** right leg 🅐

I70.362　**Atherosclerosis of unspecified type of bypass graft(s) of the extremities with gangrene,** left leg 🅐

I70.363　**Atherosclerosis of unspecified type of bypass graft(s) of the extremities with gangrene,** bilateral legs 🅐

I70.368　**Atherosclerosis of unspecified type of bypass graft(s) of the extremities with gangrene, other extremity** 🅐

I70.369　**Atherosclerosis of unspecified type of bypass graft(s) of the extremities with gangrene, unspecified extremity** 🅐

✓6ᵗʰ　I70.39　Other **atherosclerosis of unspecified type of bypass graft(s) of the extremities**

I70.391　**Other atherosclerosis of unspecified type of bypass graft(s) of the extremities,** right leg 🅐

I70.392　**Other atherosclerosis of unspecified type of bypass graft(s) of the extremities,** left leg 🅐

I70.393　**Other atherosclerosis of unspecified type of bypass graft(s) of the extremities,** bilateral legs 🅐

I70.398　**Other atherosclerosis of unspecified type of bypass graft(s) of the extremities, other extremity** 🅐

I70.399　**Other atherosclerosis of unspecified type of bypass graft(s) of the extremities, unspecified extremity** 🅐

✓5ᵗʰ　I70.4　**Atherosclerosis of** autologous vein bypass graft(s) **of the extremities**
　Use additional code, if applicable, to identify chronic total occlusion of artery of extremity (I70.92)

✓6ᵗʰ　I70.40　Unspecified **atherosclerosis of autologous vein bypass graft(s) of the extremities**

I70.401　**Unspecified atherosclerosis of autologous vein bypass graft(s) of the extremities,** right leg 🅐

I70.402　**Unspecified atherosclerosis of autologous vein bypass graft(s) of the extremities,** left leg 🅐

I70.403　**Unspecified atherosclerosis of autologous vein bypass graft(s) of the extremities,** bilateral legs 🅐

I70.408　**Unspecified atherosclerosis of autologous vein bypass graft(s) of the extremities, other extremity** 🅐

I70.409　**Unspecified atherosclerosis of autologous vein bypass graft(s) of the extremities, unspecified extremity** 🅐

✓6ᵗʰ　I70.41　**Atherosclerosis of autologous vein bypass graft(s) of the extremities with** intermittent claudication

I70.411　**Atherosclerosis of autologous vein bypass graft(s) of the extremities with intermittent claudication,** right leg 🅐

I70.412　**Atherosclerosis of autologous vein bypass graft(s) of the extremities with intermittent claudication,** left leg 🅐

I70.413　**Atherosclerosis of autologous vein bypass graft(s) of the extremities with intermittent claudication,** bilateral legs 🅐

I70.418　**Atherosclerosis of autologous vein bypass graft(s) of the extremities with intermittent claudication, other extremity** 🅐

I70.419　**Atherosclerosis of autologous vein bypass graft(s) of the extremities with intermittent claudication, unspecified extremity** 🅐

✓6ᵗʰ　I70.42　**Atherosclerosis of autologous vein bypass graft(s) of the extremities with** rest pain
　INCLUDES　any condition classifiable to I70.41-

I70.421　**Atherosclerosis of autologous vein bypass graft(s) of the extremities with rest pain,** right leg 🅐

I70.422　**Atherosclerosis of autologous vein bypass graft(s) of the extremities with rest pain,** left leg 🅐

I70.423　**Atherosclerosis of autologous vein bypass graft(s) of the extremities with rest pain,** bilateral legs 🅐

I70.428　**Atherosclerosis of autologous vein bypass graft(s) of the extremities with rest pain, other extremity** 🅐

I70.429　**Atherosclerosis of autologous vein bypass graft(s) of the extremities with rest pain, unspecified extremity** 🅐

✓6ᵗʰ　I70.43　**Atherosclerosis of autologous vein bypass graft(s) of the** right leg **with** ulceration
　INCLUDES　any condition classifiable to I70.411 and I70.421
　Use additional code to identify severity of ulcer (L97.-)

I70.431　**Atherosclerosis of autologous vein bypass graft(s) of the right leg with ulceration of** thigh 🅐

I70.432　**Atherosclerosis of autologous vein bypass graft(s) of the right leg with ulceration of** calf 🅐

I70.433　**Atherosclerosis of autologous vein bypass graft(s) of the right leg with ulceration of** ankle 🅐

I70.434　**Atherosclerosis of autologous vein bypass graft(s) of the right leg with ulceration of** heel and midfoot 🅐
　　Atherosclerosis of autologous vein bypass graft(s) of right leg with ulceration of plantar surface of midfoot

I70.435　**Atherosclerosis of autologous vein bypass graft(s) of the right leg with ulceration of other** part of foot 🅐
　　Atherosclerosis of autologous vein bypass graft(s) of right leg with ulceration of toe

I70.438　**Atherosclerosis of autologous vein bypass graft(s) of the right leg with ulceration of other** part of lower leg 🅐

I70.439　**Atherosclerosis of autologous vein bypass graft(s) of the right leg with ulceration of unspecified site** 🅐

✓6ᵗʰ　I70.44　**Atherosclerosis of autologous vein bypass graft(s) of the** left leg **with** ulceration
　INCLUDES　any condition classifiable to I70.412 and I70.422
　Use additional code to identify severity of ulcer (L97.-)

I70.441　**Atherosclerosis of autologous vein bypass graft(s) of the left leg with ulceration of** thigh 🅐

I70.442　**Atherosclerosis of autologous vein bypass graft(s) of the left leg with ulceration of** calf 🅐

✓ Additional Character Required　　✓x7ᵗʰ Xtension Alert　　Unspecified Dx　　Other Specified Dx　　Manifestation　　▶◀ Revised Text　　● New Code　　▲ Revised Code Title

ICD-10-CM Draft (2015)　　　　587

Diseases of the Circulatory System

I70.443–I70.538

I70.443   Atherosclerosis of autologous vein bypass graft(s) of the left leg with ulceration of ankle   A

I70.444   Atherosclerosis of autologous vein bypass graft(s) of the left leg with ulceration of heel and midfoot   A
> Atherosclerosis of autologous vein bypass graft(s) of left leg with ulceration of plantar surface of midfoot

I70.445   Atherosclerosis of autologous vein bypass graft(s) of the left leg with ulceration of other part of foot   A
> Atherosclerosis of autologous vein bypass graft(s) of left leg with ulceration of toe

I70.448   Atherosclerosis of autologous vein bypass graft(s) of the left leg with ulceration of other part of lower leg   A

I70.449   Atherosclerosis of autologous vein bypass graft(s) of the left leg with ulceration of unspecified site   A

I70.45   Atherosclerosis of autologous vein bypass graft(s) of other extremity with ulceration   A
> INCLUDES   any condition classifiable to I70.418, I70.428, and I70.438
> Use additional code to identify severity of ulcer (L98.49)

√6ᵗʰ I70.46   Atherosclerosis of autologous vein bypass graft(s) of the extremities with gangrene
> INCLUDES   any condition classifiable to I70.41-, I70.42-, and I70.43-, I70.44-, I70.45
> Use additional code to identify the severity of any ulcer (L97.-, L98.49-), if applicable

I70.461   Atherosclerosis of autologous vein bypass graft(s) of the extremities with gangrene, right leg   A

I70.462   Atherosclerosis of autologous vein bypass graft(s) of the extremities with gangrene, left leg   A

I70.463   Atherosclerosis of autologous vein bypass graft(s) of the extremities with gangrene, bilateral legs   A

I70.468   Atherosclerosis of autologous vein bypass graft(s) of the extremities with gangrene, other extremity   A

I70.469   Atherosclerosis of autologous vein bypass graft(s) of the extremities with gangrene, unspecified extremity   A

√6ᵗʰ I70.49   Other atherosclerosis of autologous vein bypass graft(s) of the extremities

I70.491   Other atherosclerosis of autologous vein bypass graft(s) of the extremities, right leg   A

I70.492   Other atherosclerosis of autologous vein bypass graft(s) of the extremities, left leg   A

I70.493   Other atherosclerosis of autologous vein bypass graft(s) of the extremities, bilateral legs   A

I70.498   Other atherosclerosis of autologous vein bypass graft(s) of the extremities, other extremity   A

I70.499   Other atherosclerosis of autologous vein bypass graft(s) of the extremities, unspecified extremity   A

√5ᵗʰ I70.5   Atherosclerosis of nonautologous biological bypass graft(s) of the extremities
> Use additional code, if applicable, to identify chronic total occlusion of artery of extremity (I70.92)

√6ᵗʰ I70.50   Unspecified atherosclerosis of nonautologous biological bypass graft(s) of the extremities

I70.501   Unspecified atherosclerosis of nonautologous biological bypass graft(s) of the extremities, right leg   A

I70.502   Unspecified atherosclerosis of nonautologous biological bypass graft(s) of the extremities, left leg   A

I70.503   Unspecified atherosclerosis of nonautologous biological bypass graft(s) of the extremities, bilateral legs   A

I70.508   Unspecified atherosclerosis of nonautologous biological bypass graft(s) of the extremities, other extremity   A

I70.509   Unspecified atherosclerosis of nonautologous biological bypass graft(s) of the extremities, unspecified extremity   A

√6ᵗʰ I70.51   Atherosclerosis of nonautologous biological bypass graft(s) of the extremities with intermittent claudication

I70.511   Atherosclerosis of nonautologous biological bypass graft(s) of the extremities with intermittent claudication, right leg   A

I70.512   Atherosclerosis of nonautologous biological bypass graft(s) of the extremities with intermittent claudication, left leg   A

I70.513   Atherosclerosis of nonautologous biological bypass graft(s) of the extremities with intermittent claudication, bilateral legs   A

I70.518   Atherosclerosis of nonautologous biological bypass graft(s) of the extremities with intermittent claudication, other extremity   A

I70.519   Atherosclerosis of nonautologous biological bypass graft(s) of the extremities with intermittent claudication, unspecified extremity   A

√6ᵗʰ I70.52   Atherosclerosis of nonautologous biological bypass graft(s) of the extremities with rest pain
> INCLUDES   any condition classifiable to I70.51-

I70.521   Atherosclerosis of nonautologous biological bypass graft(s) of the extremities with rest pain, right leg   A

I70.522   Atherosclerosis of nonautologous biological bypass graft(s) of the extremities with rest pain, left leg   A

I70.523   Atherosclerosis of nonautologous biological bypass graft(s) of the extremities with rest pain, bilateral legs   A

I70.528   Atherosclerosis of nonautologous biological bypass graft(s) of the extremities with rest pain, other extremity   A

I70.529   Atherosclerosis of nonautologous biological bypass graft(s) of the extremities with rest pain, unspecified extremity   A

√6ᵗʰ I70.53   Atherosclerosis of nonautologous biological bypass graft(s) of the right leg with ulceration
> INCLUDES   any condition classifiable to I70.511 and I70.521
> Use additional code to identify severity of ulcer (L97.-)

I70.531   Atherosclerosis of nonautologous biological bypass graft(s) of the right leg with ulceration of thigh   A

I70.532   Atherosclerosis of nonautologous biological bypass graft(s) of the right leg with ulceration of calf   A

I70.533   Atherosclerosis of nonautologous biological bypass graft(s) of the right leg with ulceration of ankle   A

I70.534   Atherosclerosis of nonautologous biological bypass graft(s) of the right leg with ulceration of heel and midfoot   A
> Atherosclerosis of nonautologous biological bypass graft(s) of right leg with ulceration of plantar surface of midfoot

I70.535   Atherosclerosis of nonautologous biological bypass graft(s) of the right leg with ulceration of other part of foot   A
> Atherosclerosis of nonautologous biological bypass graft(s) of the right leg with ulceration of toe

I70.538   Atherosclerosis of nonautologous biological bypass graft(s) of the right leg with ulceration of other part of lower leg   A

EXCLUDES 1 Not coded here   EXCLUDES 2 Not included here   N Newborn Age: 0   P Pediatric Age: 0-17   M Maternity Age: 12-55   A Adult Age: 15-124

588   ICD-10-CM Draft (2015)

I70.539 Atherosclerosis of nonautologous biological bypass graft(s) of the right leg with ulceration of unspecified site ▲

✓6th **I70.54** Atherosclerosis of nonautologous biological bypass graft(s) of the left leg with ulceration

    INCLUDES any condition classifiable to I70.512 and I70.522

    Use additional code to identify severity of ulcer (L97.-)

I70.541 Atherosclerosis of nonautologous biological bypass graft(s) of the left leg with ulceration of thigh ▲

I70.542 Atherosclerosis of nonautologous biological bypass graft(s) of the left leg with ulceration of calf ▲

I70.543 Atherosclerosis of nonautologous biological bypass graft(s) of the left leg with ulceration of ankle ▲

I70.544 Atherosclerosis of nonautologous biological bypass graft(s) of the left leg with ulceration of heel and midfoot ▲

    Atherosclerosis of nonautologous biological bypass graft(s) of left leg with ulceration of plantar surface of midfoot

I70.545 Atherosclerosis of nonautologous biological bypass graft(s) of the left leg with ulceration of other part of foot ▲

    Atherosclerosis of nonautologous biological bypass graft(s) of the left leg with ulceration of toe

I70.548 Atherosclerosis of nonautologous biological bypass graft(s) of the left leg with ulceration of other part of lower leg ▲

I70.549 Atherosclerosis of nonautologous biological bypass graft(s) of the left leg with ulceration of unspecified site ▲

I70.55 Atherosclerosis of nonautologous biological bypass graft(s) of other extremity with ulceration ▲

    INCLUDES any condition classifiable to I70.518, I70.528, and I70.538

    Use additional code to identify severity of ulcer (L98.49)

✓6th **I70.56** Atherosclerosis of nonautologous biological bypass graft(s) of the extremities with gangrene

    INCLUDES any condition classifiable to I70.51-, I70.52-, and I70.53-, I70.54-, I70.55

    Use additional code to identify the severity of any ulcer (L97.-, L98.49-), if applicable

I70.561 Atherosclerosis of nonautologous biological bypass graft(s) of the extremities with gangrene, right leg ▲

I70.562 Atherosclerosis of nonautologous biological bypass graft(s) of the extremities with gangrene, left leg ▲

I70.563 Atherosclerosis of nonautologous biological bypass graft(s) of the extremities with gangrene, bilateral legs ▲

I70.568 Atherosclerosis of nonautologous biological bypass graft(s) of the extremities with gangrene, other extremity ▲

I70.569 Atherosclerosis of nonautologous biological bypass graft(s) of the extremities with gangrene, unspecified extremity ▲

✓6th **I70.59** Other atherosclerosis of nonautologous biological bypass graft(s) of the extremities

I70.591 Other atherosclerosis of nonautologous biological bypass graft(s) of the extremities, right leg ▲

I70.592 Other atherosclerosis of nonautologous biological bypass graft(s) of the extremities, left leg ▲

I70.593 Other atherosclerosis of nonautologous biological bypass graft(s) of the extremities, bilateral legs ▲

I70.598 Other atherosclerosis of nonautologous biological bypass graft(s) of the extremities, other extremity ▲

I70.599 Other atherosclerosis of nonautologous biological bypass graft(s) of the extremities, unspecified extremity ▲

✓5th **I70.6** Atherosclerosis of nonbiological bypass graft(s) of the extremities

    Use additional code, if applicable, to identify chronic total occlusion of artery of extremity (I70.92)

✓6th **I70.60** Unspecified atherosclerosis of nonbiological bypass graft(s) of the extremities

I70.601 Unspecified atherosclerosis of nonbiological bypass graft(s) of the extremities, right leg ▲

I70.602 Unspecified atherosclerosis of nonbiological bypass graft(s) of the extremities, left leg ▲

I70.603 Unspecified atherosclerosis of nonbiological bypass graft(s) of the extremities, bilateral legs ▲

I70.608 Unspecified atherosclerosis of nonbiological bypass graft(s) of the extremities, other extremity ▲

I70.609 Unspecified atherosclerosis of nonbiological bypass graft(s) of the extremities, unspecified extremity ▲

✓6th **I70.61** Atherosclerosis of nonbiological bypass graft(s) of the extremities with intermittent claudication

I70.611 Atherosclerosis of nonbiological bypass graft(s) of the extremities with intermittent claudication, right leg ▲

I70.612 Atherosclerosis of nonbiological bypass graft(s) of the extremities with intermittent claudication, left leg ▲

I70.613 Atherosclerosis of nonbiological bypass graft(s) of the extremities with intermittent claudication, bilateral legs ▲

I70.618 Atherosclerosis of nonbiological bypass graft(s) of the extremities with intermittent claudication, other extremity ▲

I70.619 Atherosclerosis of nonbiological bypass graft(s) of the extremities with intermittent claudication, unspecified extremity ▲

✓6th **I70.62** Atherosclerosis of nonbiological bypass graft(s) of the extremities with rest pain

    INCLUDES any condition classifiable to I70.61-

I70.621 Atherosclerosis of nonbiological bypass graft(s) of the extremities with rest pain, right leg ▲

I70.622 Atherosclerosis of nonbiological bypass graft(s) of the extremities with rest pain, left leg ▲

I70.623 Atherosclerosis of nonbiological bypass graft(s) of the extremities with rest pain, bilateral legs ▲

I70.628 Atherosclerosis of nonbiological bypass graft(s) of the extremities with rest pain, other extremity ▲

I70.629 Atherosclerosis of nonbiological bypass graft(s) of the extremities with rest pain, unspecified extremity ▲

✓6th **I70.63** Atherosclerosis of nonbiological bypass graft(s) of the right leg with ulceration

    INCLUDES any condition classifiable to I70.611 and I70.621

    Use additional code to identify severity of ulcer (L97.-)

I70.631 Atherosclerosis of nonbiological bypass graft(s) of the right leg with ulceration of thigh ▲

I70.632 Atherosclerosis of nonbiological bypass graft(s) of the right leg with ulceration of calf ▲

I70.633 Atherosclerosis of nonbiological bypass graft(s) of the right leg with ulceration of ankle ▲

I70.634 Atherosclerosis of nonbiological bypass graft(s) of the right leg with ulceration of heel and midfoot ▲

    Atherosclerosis of nonbiological bypass graft(s) of right leg with ulceration of plantar surface of midfoot

☑ Additional Character Required   ✓x7th Xtension Alert   Unspecified Dx   Other Specified Dx   Manifestation   ►◄ Revised Text   ● New Code   ▲ Revised Code Title

ICD-10-CM Draft (2015)   589

Diseases of the Circulatory System

I70.635–I70.733

I70.635   **Atherosclerosis of nonbiological bypass** A **graft(s) of the right leg with ulceration of other** part of foot

    Atherosclerosis of nonbiological bypass graft(s) of the right leg with ulceration of toe

I70.638   **Atherosclerosis of nonbiological bypass** A **graft(s) of the right leg with ulceration of other** part of lower leg

I70.639   **Atherosclerosis of nonbiological bypass** A **graft(s) of the right leg with ulceration of unspecified site**

✓6th **I70.64**   **Atherosclerosis of nonbiological bypass graft(s) of the** left leg **with** ulceration

    INCLUDES   any condition classifiable to I70.612 and I70.622

    Use additional code to identify severity of ulcer (L97.-)

I70.641   **Atherosclerosis of nonbiological bypass** A **graft(s) of the left leg with ulceration of** thigh

I70.642   **Atherosclerosis of nonbiological bypass** A **graft(s) of the left leg with ulceration of** calf

I70.643   **Atherosclerosis of nonbiological bypass** A **graft(s) of the left leg with ulceration of** ankle

I70.644   **Atherosclerosis of nonbiological bypass** A **graft(s) of the left leg with ulceration of** heel and midfoot

    Atherosclerosis of nonbiological bypass graft(s) of left leg with ulceration of plantar surface of midfoot

I70.645   **Atherosclerosis of nonbiological** A **bypassgraft(s) of the left leg with ulceration of other** part of foot

    Atherosclerosis of nonbiological bypass graft(s) of the left leg with ulceration of toe

I70.648   **Atherosclerosis of nonbiological** A **bypass graft(s) of the left leg with ulceration of other** part of lower leg

I70.649   **Atherosclerosis of nonbiological** A **bypass graft(s) of the left leg with ulceration of unspecified site**

I70.65   **Atherosclerosis of nonbiological bypass graft(s)** A **of other extremity with** ulceration

    INCLUDES   any condition classifiable to I70.618 and I70.628

    Use additional code to identify severity of ulcer (L98.49)

✓6th **I70.66**   **Atherosclerosis of nonbiological bypass graft(s) of the extremities with** gangrene

    INCLUDES   any condition classifiable to I70.61-, I70.62-, I70.63-, I70.64-, I70.65

    Use additional code to identify the severity of any ulcer (L97.-, L98.49-), if applicable

I70.661   **Atherosclerosis of nonbiological bypass** A **graft(s) of the extremities with gangrene,** right leg

I70.662   **Atherosclerosis of nonbiological bypass** A **graft(s) of the extremities with gangrene,** left leg

I70.663   **Atherosclerosis of nonbiological bypass** A **graft(s) of the extremities with gangrene,** bilateral legs

I70.668   **Atherosclerosis of nonbiological bypass** A **graft(s) of the extremities with gangrene, other extremity**

I70.669   **Atherosclerosis of nonbiological bypass** A **graft(s) of the extremities with gangrene, unspecified extremity**

✓6th **I70.69**   Other **atherosclerosis of nonbiological bypass graft(s) of the extremities**

I70.691   **Other atherosclerosis of nonbiological** A **bypass graft(s) of the extremities,** right leg

I70.692   **Other atherosclerosis of nonbiological** A **bypass graft(s) of the extremities,** left leg

I70.693   **Other atherosclerosis of nonbiological** A **bypass graft(s) of the extremities,** bilateral legs

I70.698   **Other atherosclerosis of nonbiological** A **bypass graft(s) of the extremities, other extremity**

I70.699   **Other atherosclerosis of nonbiological** A **bypass graft(s) of the extremities, unspecified extremity**

✓5th **I70.7**   **Atherosclerosis of** other **type of** bypass graft(s) **of the extremities**

    Use additional code, if applicable, to identify chronic total occlusion of artery of extremity (I70.92)

✓6th **I70.70**   Unspecified **atherosclerosis of other type of bypass graft(s) of the extremities**

I70.701   **Unspecified atherosclerosis of other** A **type of bypass graft(s) of the extremities,** right leg

I70.702   **Unspecified atherosclerosis of other** A **type of bypass graft(s) of the extremities,** left leg

I70.703   **Unspecified atherosclerosis of other** A **type of bypass graft(s) of the extremities,** bilateral legs

I70.708   **Unspecified atherosclerosis of other** A **type of bypass graft(s) of the extremities, other extremity**

I70.709   **Unspecified atherosclerosis of other** A **type of bypass graft(s) of the extremities, unspecified extremity**

✓6th **I70.71**   **Atherosclerosis of other type of bypass graft(s) of the extremities with** intermittent claudication

I70.711   **Atherosclerosis of other type of bypass** A **graft(s) of the extremities with intermittent claudication,** right leg

I70.712   **Atherosclerosis of other type of bypass** A **graft(s) of the extremities with intermittent claudication,** left leg

I70.713   **Atherosclerosis of other type of bypass** A **graft(s) of the extremities with intermittent claudication,** bilateral legs

I70.718   **Atherosclerosis of other type of bypass** A **graft(s) of the extremities with intermittent claudication, other extremity**

I70.719   **Atherosclerosis of other type of bypass** A **graft(s) of the extremities with intermittent claudication, unspecified extremity**

✓6th **I70.72**   **Atherosclerosis of other type of bypass graft(s) of the extremities with** rest pain

    INCLUDES   any condition classifiable to I70.71-

I70.721   **Atherosclerosis of other type of bypass** A **graft(s) of the extremities with rest pain,** right leg

I70.722   **Atherosclerosis of other type of bypass** A **graft(s) of the extremities with rest pain,** left leg

I70.723   **Atherosclerosis of other type of bypass** A **graft(s) of the extremities with rest pain,** bilateral legs

I70.728   **Atherosclerosis of other type of bypass** A **graft(s) of the extremities with rest pain, other extremity**

I70.729   **Atherosclerosis of other type of bypass** A **graft(s) of the extremities with rest pain, unspecified extremity**

✓6th **I70.73**   **Atherosclerosis of other type of bypass graft(s) of the** right leg **with** ulceration

    INCLUDES   any condition classifiable to I70.711 and I70.721

    Use additional code to identify severity of ulcer (L97.-)

I70.731   **Atherosclerosis of other type of bypass** A **graft(s) of the right leg with ulceration of** thigh

I70.732   **Atherosclerosis of other type of bypass** A **graft(s) of the right leg with ulceration of** calf

I70.733   **Atherosclerosis of other type of bypass** A **graft(s) of the right leg with ulceration of** ankle

EXCLUDES 1 Not coded here   EXCLUDES 2 Not included here   N Newborn Age: 0   P Pediatric Age: 0-17   M Maternity Age: 12-55   A Adult Age: 15-124

590   ICD-10-CM Draft (2015)

I70.734 Atherosclerosis of other type of bypass △
graft(s) of the right leg with ulceration
of heel and midfoot
　　Atherosclerosis of other type of bypass
　　graft(s) of right leg with ulceration of
　　plantar surface of midfoot

I70.735 Atherosclerosis of other type of bypass △
graft(s) of the right leg with ulceration
of other part of foot
　　Atherosclerosis of other type of bypass
　　graft(s) of right leg with ulceration of
　　toe

I70.738 Atherosclerosis of other type of bypass △
graft(s) of the right leg with ulceration
of other part of lower leg

I70.739 Atherosclerosis of other type of bypass △
graft(s) of the right leg with ulceration
of unspecified site

✓6th **I70.74** Atherosclerosis of other type of bypass graft(s) of
the left leg with ulceration
　　INCLUDES   any condition classifiable to I70.712 and
　　　　　　　I70.722
　　Use additional code to identify severity of ulcer (L97.-)

I70.741 Atherosclerosis of other type of bypass △
graft(s) of the left leg with ulceration
of thigh

I70.742 Atherosclerosis of other type of bypass △
graft(s) of the left leg with ulceration
of calf

I70.743 Atherosclerosis of other type of bypass △
graft(s) of the left leg with ulceration
of ankle

I70.744 Atherosclerosis of other type of bypass △
graft(s) of the left leg with ulceration
of heel and midfoot
　　Atherosclerosis of other type of bypass
　　graft(s) of left leg with ulceration of
　　plantar surface of midfoot

I70.745 Atherosclerosis of other type of bypass △
graft(s) of the left leg with ulceration
of other part of foot
　　Atherosclerosis of other type of bypass
　　graft(s) of left leg with ulceration of
　　toe

I70.748 Atherosclerosis of other type of bypass △
graft(s) of the left leg with ulceration
of other part of lower leg

I70.749 Atherosclerosis of other type of bypass △
graft(s) of the left leg with ulceration
of unspecified site

I70.75 Atherosclerosis of other type of bypass graft(s) △
of other extremity with ulceration
　　INCLUDES   any condition classifiable to I70.718 and
　　　　　　　I70.728
　　Use additional code to identify severity of ulcer
　　(L98.49)

✓6th **I70.76** Atherosclerosis of other type of bypass graft(s) of
the extremities with gangrene
　　INCLUDES   any condition classifiable to I70.71-, I70.72-,
　　　　　　　I70.73-, I70.74-, I70.75
　　Use additional code to identify the severity of any
　　ulcer (L97.-, L98.49-), if applicable

I70.761 Atherosclerosis of other type of bypass △
graft(s) of the extremities with gangrene,
right leg

I70.762 Atherosclerosis of other type of bypass △
graft(s) of the extremities with gangrene,
left leg

I70.763 Atherosclerosis of other type of bypass △
graft(s) of the extremities with gangrene,
bilateral legs

I70.768 Atherosclerosis of other type of bypass △
graft(s) of the extremities with gangrene,
other extremity

I70.769 Atherosclerosis of other type of bypass △
graft(s) of the extremities with gangrene,
unspecified extremity

✓6th **I70.79** Other atherosclerosis of other type of bypass graft(s)
of the extremities

I70.791 Other atherosclerosis of other type of △
bypass graft(s) of the extremities,
right leg

I70.792 Other atherosclerosis of other type of △
bypass graft(s) of the extremities, left leg

I70.793 Other atherosclerosis of other type of △
bypass graft(s) of the extremities,
bilateral legs

I70.798 Other atherosclerosis of other type of △
bypass graft(s) of the extremities, other
extremity

I70.799 Other atherosclerosis of other type of △
bypass graft(s) of the extremities,
unspecified extremity

I70.8 Atherosclerosis of other arteries △

✓5th **I70.9** Other and unspecified atherosclerosis

I70.90 Unspecified atherosclerosis △

I70.91 Generalized atherosclerosis △

I70.92 Chronic total occlusion of artery of the △
extremities
　　Complete occlusion of artery of the extremities
　　Total occlusion of artery of the extremities
　　Code first atherosclerosis of arteries of the extremities
　　(I70.2-, I70.3-, I70.4-, I70.5-, I70.6-, I70.7-)

✓4th **I71** Aortic aneurysm and dissection
　　EXCLUDES 1   aortic ectasia (I77.81-)
　　　　　　　　syphilitic aortic aneurysm (A52.01)
　　　　　　　　traumatic aortic aneurysm (S25.09, S35.09)

✓5th **I71.0** Dissection of aorta

I71.00 Dissection of unspecified site of aorta

I71.01 Dissection of thoracic aorta

I71.02 Dissection of abdominal aorta

I71.03 Dissection of thoracoabdominal aorta

I71.1 Thoracic aortic aneurysm, ruptured

I71.2 Thoracic aortic aneurysm, without rupture

I71.3 Abdominal aortic aneurysm, ruptured

I71.4 Abdominal aortic aneurysm, without rupture

I71.5 Thoracoabdominal aortic aneurysm, ruptured

I71.6 Thoracoabdominal aortic aneurysm, without rupture

I71.8 Aortic aneurysm of unspecified site, ruptured
　　Rupture of aorta NOS

I71.9 Aortic aneurysm of unspecified site, without rupture
　　Aneurysm of aorta
　　Dilatation of aorta
　　Hyaline necrosis of aorta

✓4th **I72** Other aneurysm
　　INCLUDES   aneurysm (cirsoid) (false) (ruptured)
　　EXCLUDES 2   acquired aneurysm (I77.0)
　　　　　　　　aneurysm (of) aorta (I71.-)
　　　　　　　　aneurysm (of) arteriovenous NOS (Q27.3-)
　　　　　　　　carotid artery dissection (I77.71)
　　　　　　　　cerebral (nonruptured) aneurysm (I67.1)
　　　　　　　　coronary aneurysm (I25.4)
　　　　　　　　coronary artery dissection (I25.42)
　　　　　　　　dissection of artery NEC (I77.79)
　　　　　　　　heart aneurysm (I25.3)
　　　　　　　　iliac artery dissection (I77.72)
　　　　　　　　pulmonary artery aneurysm (I28.1)
　　　　　　　　renal artery dissection (I77.73)
　　　　　　　　retinal aneurysm (H35.0)
　　　　　　　　ruptured cerebral aneurysm (I60.7)
　　　　　　　　varicose aneurysm (I77.0)
　　　　　　　　vertebral artery dissection (I77.74)

I72.0 Aneurysm of carotid artery
　　Aneurysm of common carotid artery
　　Aneurysm of external carotid artery
　　Aneurysm of internal carotid artery, extracranial portion
　　EXCLUDES 1   aneurysm of internal carotid artery, intracranial portion
　　　　　　　　(I67.1)
　　　　　　　　aneurysm of internal carotid artery NOS (I67.1)

I72.1 Aneurysm of artery of upper extremity

I72.2 Aneurysm of renal artery

I72.3 Aneurysm of iliac artery

I72.4 Aneurysm of artery of lower extremity

I72.8 Aneurysm of other specified arteries

I72.9 Aneurysm of unspecified site

☑ Additional Character Required　✓7th Xtension Alert　Unspecified Dx　Other Specified Dx　Manifestation　►◄ Revised Text　● New Code　▲ Revised Code Title

ICD-10-CM Draft (2015)　　591

✓4ᵗʰ **I73   Other peripheral vascular diseases**

EXCLUDES 2   *chilblains (T69.1)*
frostbite (T33- T34)
immersion hand or foot (T69.0-)
spasm of cerebral artery (G45.9)

✓5ᵗʰ **I73.0   Raynaud's syndrome**
Raynaud's disease
Raynaud's phenomenon (secondary)

I73.00   Raynaud's syndrome without gangrene

I73.01   Raynaud's syndrome with gangrene

I73.1   Thromboangiitis obliterans [Buerger's disease]

✓5ᵗʰ **I73.8   Other specified peripheral vascular diseases**

EXCLUDES 1   *diabetic (peripheral) angiopathy (E08-E13 with .51-.52)*

I73.81   Erythromelalgia

I73.89   Other specified peripheral vascular diseases
Acrocyanosis
Erythrocyanosis
Simple acroparesthesia [Schultze's type]
Vasomotor acroparesthesia [Nothnagel's type]

I73.9   Peripheral vascular disease, unspecified
Intermittent claudication
Peripheral angiopathy NOS
Spasm of artery

EXCLUDES 1   *atherosclerosis of the extremities (I70.2--I70.7-)*

✓4ᵗʰ **I74   Arterial embolism and thrombosis**
Embolic infarction
Embolic occlusion
Thrombotic infarction
Thrombotic occlusion
Code first:
embolism and thrombosis complicating abortion or ectopic or molar
    pregnancy (O00-O07, O08.2)
embolism and thrombosis complicating pregnancy, childbirth and
    the puerperium (O88.-)

EXCLUDES 2   *atheroembolism (I75.-)*
basilar embolism and thrombosis (I63.0-I63.2, I65.1)
carotid embolism and thrombosis (I63.0-I63.2, I65.2)
cerebral embolism and thrombosis (I63.3-I63.5, I66-)
coronary embolism and thrombosis (I21-I25)
mesenteric embolism and thrombosis (K55.0)
ophthalmic embolism and thrombosis (H34.-)
precerebral embolism and thrombosis NOS (I63.0-I63.2, I65.9)
pulmonary embolism and thrombosis (I26.-)
renal embolism and thrombosis (N28.0)
retinal embolism and thrombosis (H34.-)
septic embolism and thrombosis (I76)
vertebral embolism and thrombosis (I63.0-I63.2, I65.0)

✓5ᵗʰ **I74.0   Embolism and thrombosis of** abdominal aorta

I74.01   Saddle embolus of abdominal aorta

I74.09   Other arterial **embolism and thrombosis of abdominal aorta**
Aortic bifurcation syndrome
Aortoiliac obstruction
Leriche's syndrome

✓5ᵗʰ **I74.1   Embolism and thrombosis of** other and unspecified parts **of** aorta

I74.10   Embolism and thrombosis of unspecified parts of aorta

I74.11   Embolism and thrombosis of thoracic **aorta**

I74.19   Embolism and thrombosis of other parts of aorta

I74.2   Embolism and thrombosis of arteries of the upper extremities

I74.3   Embolism and thrombosis of arteries of the lower extremities

I74.4   Embolism and thrombosis of arteries of extremities, unspecified
Peripheral arterial embolism NOS

I74.5   Embolism and thrombosis of iliac **artery**

I74.8   Embolism and thrombosis of other arteries

I74.9   Embolism and thrombosis of unspecified artery

✓4ᵗʰ **I75   Atheroembolism**
Atherothrombotic microembolism
Cholesterol embolism

✓5ᵗʰ **I75.0   Atheroembolism of** extremities

✓6ᵗʰ **I75.01   Atheroembolism of** upper **extremity**

I75.011   Atheroembolism of right **upper extremity**

I75.012   Atheroembolism of left **upper extremity**

I75.013   Atheroembolism of bilateral **upper extremities**

I75.019   Atheroembolism of unspecified upper extremity

✓6ᵗʰ **I75.02   Atheroembolism of** lower **extremity**

I75.021   Atheroembolism of right **lower extremity**

I75.022   Atheroembolism of left **lower extremity**

I75.023   Atheroembolism of bilateral **lower extremities**

I75.029   Atheroembolism of unspecified lower extremity

✓5ᵗʰ **I75.8   Atheroembolism of** other sites

I75.81   Atheroembolism of kidney
Use additional code for any associated acute kidney
    failure and chronic kidney disease (N17.-, N18.-)

I75.89   Atheroembolism of other site

I76   Septic arterial embolism
Code first underlying infection, such as:
    infective endocarditis (I33.0)
    lung abscess (J85.-)
Use additional code to identify the site of the embolism (I74.-)

EXCLUDES 2   *septic pulmonary embolism (I26.01, I26.90)*

✓4ᵗʰ **I77   Other disorders of arteries and arterioles**

EXCLUDES 2   *collagen (vascular) diseases (M30-M36)*
hypersensitivity angiitis (M31.0)
pulmonary artery (I28.-)

I77.0   Arteriovenous fistula, acquired
Aneurysmal varix
Arteriovenous aneurysm, acquired

EXCLUDES 1   *arteriovenous aneurysm NOS (Q27.3-)*
presence of arteriovenous shunt (fistula) for dialysis
    (Z99.2)
traumatic—see injury of blood vessel by body region

EXCLUDES 2   *cerebral (I67.1)*
coronary (I25.4)

I77.1   Stricture of artery
Narrowing of artery

I77.2   Rupture of artery
Erosion of artery
Fistula of artery
Ulcer of artery

EXCLUDES 1   *traumatic rupture of artery—see injury of blood vessel*
    by body region

I77.3   Arterial fibromuscular dysplasia
Fibromuscular hyperplasia (of) carotid artery
Fibromuscular hyperplasia (of) renal artery

I77.4   Celiac artery compression syndrome

I77.5   Necrosis of artery

I77.6   Arteritis, unspecified
Aortitis NOS
Endarteritis NOS

EXCLUDES 1   *arteritis or endarteritis:*
    aortic arch (M31.4)
    cerebral NEC (I67.7)
    coronary (I25.89)
    deformans (I70.-)
    giant cell (M31.5., M31.6)
    obliterans (I70.-)
    senile (I70.-)

✓5ᵗʰ **I77.7   Other arterial dissection**

EXCLUDES 2   *dissection of aorta (I71.0-)*
dissection of coronary artery (I25.42)

I77.71   Dissection of carotid **artery**

I77.72   Dissection of iliac **artery**

I77.73   Dissection of renal **artery**

I77.74   Dissection of vertebral **artery**

I77.79   Dissection of other artery

✓5ᵗʰ **I77.8   Other specified disorders of arteries and arterioles**

✓6ᵗʰ **I77.81   Aortic ectasia**
Ectasis aorta

EXCLUDES 1   *aortic aneurysm and dissection (I71.0-)*

I77.810   Thoracic aortic ectasia

I77.811   Abdominal aortic ectasia

I77.812   Thoracoabdominal aortic ectasia

I77.819   Aortic ectasia, unspecified site

I77.89   Other specified disorders of arteries and arterioles

I77.9   Disorder of arteries and arterioles, unspecified

EXCLUDES 1 Not coded here   EXCLUDES 2 Not included here   N Newborn Age: 0   P Pediatric Age: 0-17   M Maternity Age: 12-55   A Adult Age: 15-124

592   ICD-10-CM Draft (2015)

✓4ᵗʰ **I78** **Diseases of capillaries**

I78.0 **Hereditary hemorrhagic telangiectasia**
Rendu-Osler-Weber disease

I78.1 **Nevus, non-neoplastic**
Araneus nevus
Senile nevus
Spider nevus
Stellar nevus
EXCLUDES 1　*nevus NOS (D22.-)*
　　　　　　vascular NOS (Q82.5)
EXCLUDES 2　*blue nevus (D22.-)*
　　　　　　flammeus nevus (Q82.5)
　　　　　　hairy nevus (D22.-)
　　　　　　melanocytic nevus (D22.-)
　　　　　　pigmented nevus (D22.-)
　　　　　　portwine nevus (Q82.5)
　　　　　　sanguineous nevus (Q82.5)
　　　　　　strawberry nevus (Q82.5)
　　　　　　verrucous nevus (Q82.5)

I78.8 **Other diseases of capillaries**

I78.9 **Disease of capillaries, unspecified**

✓4ᵗʰ **I79** **Disorders of arteries, arterioles and capillaries in diseases classified elsewhere**

I79.0 *Aneurysm of aorta in diseases classified elsewhere*
Code first underlying disease
EXCLUDES 1　*syphilitic aneurysm (A52.01)*

I79.1 *Aortitis in diseases classified elsewhere*
Code first underlying disease
EXCLUDES 1　*syphilitic aortitis (A52.02)*

I79.8 *Other disorders of arteries, arterioles and capillaries in diseases classified elsewhere*
Code first underlying disease, such as:
　　amyloidosis (E85.-)
EXCLUDES 1　*diabetic (peripheral) angiopathy (E08-E13 with .51-.52)*
　　　　　　syphilitic endarteritis (A52.09)
　　　　　　tuberculous endarteritis (A18.89)

Diseases of veins, lymphatic vessels and lymph nodes, not elsewhere classified. (I80-I89)

✓4ᵗʰ **I80** **Phlebitis and thrombophlebitis**
INCLUDES　endophlebitis
　　　　　inflammation, vein
　　　　　periphlebitis
　　　　　suppurative phlebitis
Code first:
　phlebitis and thrombophlebitis complicating abortion, ectopic or
　　molar pregnancy (O00-O07, O08.7)
　phlebitis and thrombophlebitis complicating pregnancy, childbirth
　　and the puerperium (O22.-, O87.-)
EXCLUDES 1　*venous embolism and thrombosis of lower extremities ((I82.4-,*
　　　　　　I82.5-, I82.81-)

✓5ᵗʰ **I80.0** **Phlebitis and thrombophlebitis of superficial vessels of lower extremities**
Phlebitis and thrombophlebitis of femoropopliteal vein

I80.00 **Phlebitis and thrombophlebitis of superficial vessels of unspecified lower extremity**

I80.01 **Phlebitis and thrombophlebitis of superficial vessels of right lower extremity**

I80.02 **Phlebitis and thrombophlebitis of superficial vessels of left lower extremity**

I80.03 **Phlebitis and thrombophlebitis of superficial vessels of lower extremities, bilateral**

✓5ᵗʰ **I80.1** **Phlebitis and thrombophlebitis of femoral vein**

I80.10 **Phlebitis and thrombophlebitis of unspecified femoral vein**

I80.11 **Phlebitis and thrombophlebitis of right femoral vein**

I80.12 **Phlebitis and thrombophlebitis of left femoral vein**

I80.13 **Phlebitis and thrombophlebitis of femoral vein, bilateral**

✓5ᵗʰ **I80.2** **Phlebitis and thrombophlebitis of other and unspecified deep vessels of lower extremities**

✓6ᵗʰ **I80.20** **Phlebitis and thrombophlebitis of unspecified deep vessels of lower extremities**

I80.201 **Phlebitis and thrombophlebitis of unspecified deep vessels of right lower extremity**

I80.202 **Phlebitis and thrombophlebitis of unspecified deep vessels of left lower extremity**

I80.203 **Phlebitis and thrombophlebitis of unspecified deep vessels of lower extremities, bilateral**

I80.209 **Phlebitis and thrombophlebitis of unspecified deep vessels of unspecified lower extremity**

✓6ᵗʰ **I80.21** **Phlebitis and thrombophlebitis of iliac vein**

I80.211 **Phlebitis and thrombophlebitis of right iliac vein**

I80.212 **Phlebitis and thrombophlebitis of left iliac vein**

I80.213 **Phlebitis and thrombophlebitis of iliac vein, bilateral**

I80.219 **Phlebitis and thrombophlebitis of unspecified iliac vein**

✓6ᵗʰ **I80.22** **Phlebitis and thrombophlebitis of popliteal vein**

I80.221 **Phlebitis and thrombophlebitis of right popliteal vein**

I80.222 **Phlebitis and thrombophlebitis of left popliteal vein**

I80.223 **Phlebitis and thrombophlebitis of popliteal vein, bilateral**

I80.229 **Phlebitis and thrombophlebitis of unspecified popliteal vein**

✓6ᵗʰ **I80.23** **Phlebitis and thrombophlebitis of tibial vein**

I80.231 **Phlebitis and thrombophlebitis of right tibial vein**

I80.232 **Phlebitis and thrombophlebitis of left tibial vein**

I80.233 **Phlebitis and thrombophlebitis of tibial vein, bilateral**

I80.239 **Phlebitis and thrombophlebitis of unspecified tibial vein**

✓6ᵗʰ **I80.29** **Phlebitis and thrombophlebitis of other deep vessels of lower extremities**

I80.291 **Phlebitis and thrombophlebitis of other deep vessels of right lower extremity**

I80.292 **Phlebitis and thrombophlebitis of other deep vessels of left lower extremity**

I80.293 **Phlebitis and thrombophlebitis of other deep vessels of lower extremity, bilateral**

I80.299 **Phlebitis and thrombophlebitis of other deep vessels of unspecified lower extremity**

I80.3 **Phlebitis and thrombophlebitis of lower extremities, unspecified**

I80.8 **Phlebitis and thrombophlebitis of other sites**

I80.9 **Phlebitis and thrombophlebitis of unspecified site**

I81 **Portal vein thrombosis**
Portal (vein) obstruction
EXCLUDES 2　*hepatic vein thrombosis (I82.0)*
　　　　　　phlebitis of portal vein (K75.1)

✓4ᵗʰ **I82** **Other venous embolism and thrombosis**
Code first venous embolism and thrombosis complicating:
　abortion, ectopic or molar pregnancy (O00-O07, O08.7)
　pregnancy, childbirth and the puerperium (O22.-, O87.-)
EXCLUDES 2　*venous embolism and thrombosis (of):*
　　　　　　cerebral (I63.6, I67.6)
　　　　　　coronary (I21-I25)
　　　　　　intracranial and intraspinal, septic or NOS (G08)
　　　　　　intracranial, nonpyogenic (I67.6)
　　　　　　intraspinal, nonpyogenic (G95.1)
　　　　　　mesenteric (K55.0)
　　　　　　portal (I81)
　　　　　　pulmonary (I26.-)

I82.0 **Budd-Chiari syndrome**
Hepatic vein thrombosis

I82.1 **Thrombophlebitis migrans**

✓5ᵗʰ **I82.2** **Embolism and thrombosis of vena cava and other thoracic veins**

✓6ᵗʰ **I82.21** **Embolism and thrombosis of superior vena cava**

I82.210 **Acute embolism and thrombosis of superior vena cava**
Embolism and thrombosis of superior vena cava NOS

✓ Additional Character Required　　✓x7ᵗʰ Xtension Alert　　Unspecified Dx　　Other Specified Dx　　Manifestation　　►◄ Revised Text　　● New Code　　▲ Revised Code Title

Diseases of the Circulatory System

I82.211–I82.512

I82.211   **Chronic** embolism and thrombosis of superior vena cava

✓6ᵗʰ **I82.22**   **Embolism and thrombosis of** inferior vena cava

    I82.220   **Acute** embolism and thrombosis of inferior vena cava
       Embolism and thrombosis of inferior vena cava NOS

    I82.221   **Chronic** embolism and thrombosis of inferior vena cava

✓6ᵗʰ **I82.29**   **Embolism and thrombosis of** other thoracic veins
      Embolism and thrombosis of brachiocephalic (innominate) vein

    I82.290   **Acute** embolism and thrombosis of other thoracic veins

    I82.291   **Chronic** embolism and thrombosis of other thoracic veins

I82.3   **Embolism and thrombosis of** renal vein

✓5ᵗʰ **I82.4**   **Acute** embolism and thrombosis of deep veins of lower extremity

✓6ᵗʰ **I82.40**   **Acute embolism and thrombosis of** unspecified deep veins of lower extremity
      Deep vein thrombosis NOS
      DVT NOS

      EXCLUDES 1   *acute embolism and thrombosis of unspecified deep veins of distal lower extremity (I82.4Z-)*
        acute embolism and thrombosis of unspecified deep veins of proximal lower extremity (I82.4Y-)

    I82.401   **Acute embolism and thrombosis of unspecified deep veins of** right **lower extremity**

    I82.402   **Acute embolism and thrombosis of unspecified deep veins of** left **lower extremity**

    I82.403   **Acute embolism and thrombosis of unspecified deep veins of lower extremity,** bilateral

    I82.409   **Acute embolism and thrombosis of unspecified deep veins of unspecified lower extremity**

✓6ᵗʰ **I82.41**   **Acute embolism and thrombosis of** femoral vein

    I82.411   **Acute embolism and thrombosis of** right **femoral vein**

    I82.412   **Acute embolism and thrombosis of** left **femoral vein**

    I82.413   **Acute embolism and thrombosis of femoral vein,** bilateral

    I82.419   **Acute embolism and thrombosis of unspecified femoral vein**

✓6ᵗʰ **I82.42**   **Acute embolism and thrombosis of** iliac vein

    I82.421   **Acute embolism and thrombosis of** right **iliac vein**

    I82.422   **Acute embolism and thrombosis of** left **iliac vein**

    I82.423   **Acute embolism and thrombosis of iliac vein,** bilateral

    I82.429   **Acute embolism and thrombosis of unspecified iliac vein**

✓6ᵗʰ **I82.43**   **Acute embolism and thrombosis of** popliteal vein

    I82.431   **Acute embolism and thrombosis of** right **popliteal vein**

    I82.432   **Acute embolism and thrombosis of** left **popliteal vein**

    I82.433   **Acute embolism and thrombosis of popliteal vein,** bilateral

    I82.439   **Acute embolism and thrombosis of unspecified popliteal vein**

✓6ᵗʰ **I82.44**   **Acute embolism and thrombosis of** tibial vein

    I82.441   **Acute embolism and thrombosis of** right **tibial vein**

    I82.442   **Acute embolism and thrombosis of** left **tibial vein**

    I82.443   **Acute embolism and thrombosis of tibial vein,** bilateral

    I82.449   **Acute embolism and thrombosis of unspecified tibial vein**

✓6ᵗʰ **I82.49**   **Acute embolism and thrombosis of** other specified deep vein of lower extremity

    I82.491   **Acute embolism and thrombosis of other specified deep vein of** right **lower extremity**

    I82.492   **Acute embolism and thrombosis of other specified deep vein of** left **lower extremity**

    I82.493   **Acute embolism and thrombosis of other specified deep vein of lower extremity,** bilateral

    I82.499   **Acute embolism and thrombosis of other specified deep vein of unspecified lower extremity**

✓6ᵗʰ **I82.4Y**   **Acute embolism and thrombosis of** unspecified **deep veins of** proximal lower extremity
      Acute embolism and thrombosis of deep vein of thigh NOS
      Acute embolism and thrombosis of deep vein of upper leg NOS

    I82.4Y1   **Acute embolism and thrombosis of unspecified deep veins of** right **proximal lower extremity**

    I82.4Y2   **Acute embolism and thrombosis of unspecified deep veins of** left **proximal lower extremity**

    I82.4Y3   **Acute embolism and thrombosis of unspecified deep veins of proximal lower extremity,** bilateral

    I82.4Y9   **Acute embolism and thrombosis of unspecified deep veins of unspecified proximal lower extremity**

✓6ᵗʰ **I82.4Z**   **Acute embolism and thrombosis of** unspecified **deep veins of** distal lower extremity
      Acute embolism and thrombosis of deep vein of calf NOS
      Acute embolism and thrombosis of deep vein of lower leg NOS

    I82.4Z1   **Acute embolism and thrombosis of unspecified deep veins of** right **distal lower extremity**

    I82.4Z2   **Acute embolism and thrombosis of unspecified deep veins of** left **distal lower extremity**

    I82.4Z3   **Acute embolism and thrombosis of unspecified deep veins of distal lower extremity,** bilateral

    I82.4Z9   **Acute embolism and thrombosis of unspecified deep veins of unspecified distal lower extremity**

✓5ᵗʰ **I82.5**   **Chronic** embolism and thrombosis of deep veins of lower extremity
      Use additional code, if applicable, for associated long-term (current) use of anticoagulants (Z79.01)

      EXCLUDES 1   *personal history of venous embolism and thrombosis (Z86.718)*

✓6ᵗʰ **I82.50**   **Chronic embolism and thrombosis of** unspecified **deep veins of** lower extremity

      EXCLUDES 1   *chronic embolism and thrombosis of unspecified deep veins of distal lower extremity (I82.5Z-)*
        chronic embolism and thrombosis of unspecified deep veins of proximal lower extremity (I82.5Y-)

    I82.501   **Chronic embolism and thrombosis of unspecified deep veins of** right **lower extremity**

    I82.502   **Chronic embolism and thrombosis of unspecified deep veins of** left **lower extremity**

    I82.503   **Chronic embolism and thrombosis of unspecified deep veins of lower extremity,** bilateral

    I82.509   **Chronic embolism and thrombosis of unspecified deep veins of unspecified lower extremity**

✓6ᵗʰ **I82.51**   **Chronic embolism and thrombosis of** femoral vein

    I82.511   **Chronic embolism and thrombosis of** right **femoral vein**

    I82.512   **Chronic embolism and thrombosis of** left **femoral vein**

EXCLUDES 1 Not coded here   **EXCLUDES 2** Not included here   **N** Newborn Age: 0   **P** Pediatric Age: 0-17   **M** Maternity Age: 12-55   **A** Adult Age: 15-124

594   ICD-10-CM Draft (2015)

I82.513 Chronic embolism and thrombosis of femoral vein, bilateral

I82.519 Chronic embolism and thrombosis of unspecified femoral vein

✓6ᵗʰ **I82.52** Chronic embolism and thrombosis of iliac vein

I82.521 Chronic embolism and thrombosis of right iliac vein

I82.522 Chronic embolism and thrombosis of left iliac vein

I82.523 Chronic embolism and thrombosis of iliac vein, bilateral

I82.529 Chronic embolism and thrombosis of unspecified iliac vein

✓6ᵗʰ **I82.53** Chronic embolism and thrombosis of popliteal vein

I82.531 Chronic embolism and thrombosis of right popliteal vein

I82.532 Chronic embolism and thrombosis of left popliteal vein

I82.533 Chronic embolism and thrombosis of popliteal vein, bilateral

I82.539 Chronic embolism and thrombosis of unspecified popliteal vein

✓6ᵗʰ **I82.54** Chronic embolism and thrombosis of tibial vein

I82.541 Chronic embolism and thrombosis of right tibial vein

I82.542 Chronic embolism and thrombosis of left tibial vein

I82.543 Chronic embolism and thrombosis of tibial vein, bilateral

I82.549 Chronic embolism and thrombosis of unspecified tibial vein

✓6ᵗʰ **I82.59** Chronic embolism and thrombosis of other specified deep vein of lower extremity

I82.591 Chronic embolism and thrombosis of other specified deep vein of right lower extremity

I82.592 Chronic embolism and thrombosis of other specified deep vein of left lower extremity

I82.593 Chronic embolism and thrombosis of other specified deep vein of lower extremity, bilateral

I82.599 Chronic embolism and thrombosis of other specified deep vein of unspecified lower extremity

✓6ᵗʰ **I82.5Y** Chronic embolism and thrombosis of unspecified deep veins of proximal lower extremity

Chronic embolism and thrombosis of deep veins of thigh NOS
Chronic embolism and thrombosis of deep veins of upper leg NOS

I82.5Y1 Chronic embolism and thrombosis of unspecified deep veins of right proximal lower extremity

I82.5Y2 Chronic embolism and thrombosis of unspecified deep veins of left proximal lower extremity

I82.5Y3 Chronic embolism and thrombosis of unspecified deep veins of proximal lower extremity, bilateral

I82.5Y9 Chronic embolism and thrombosis of unspecified deep veins of unspecified proximal lower extremity

✓6ᵗʰ **I82.5Z** Chronic embolism and thrombosis of unspecified deep veins of distal lower extremity

Chronic embolism and thrombosis of deep veins of calf NOS
Chronic embolism and thrombosis of deep veins of lower leg NOS

I82.5Z1 Chronic embolism and thrombosis of unspecified deep veins of right distal lower extremity

I82.5Z2 Chronic embolism and thrombosis of unspecified deep veins of left distal lower extremity

I82.5Z3 Chronic embolism and thrombosis of unspecified deep veins of distal lower extremity, bilateral

I82.5Z9 Chronic embolism and thrombosis of unspecified deep veins of unspecified distal lower extremity

✓5ᵗʰ **I82.6** Acute embolism and thrombosis of veins of upper extremity

✓6ᵗʰ **I82.60** Acute embolism and thrombosis of unspecified veins of upper extremity

I82.601 Acute embolism and thrombosis of unspecified veins of right upper extremity

I82.602 Acute embolism and thrombosis of unspecified veins of left upper extremity

I82.603 Acute embolism and thrombosis of unspecified veins of upper extremity, bilateral

I82.609 Acute embolism and thrombosis of unspecified veins of unspecified upper extremity

✓6ᵗʰ **I82.61** Acute embolism and thrombosis of superficial veins of upper extremity

Acute embolism and thrombosis of antecubital vein
Acute embolism and thrombosis of basilic vein
Acute embolism and thrombosis of cephalic vein

I82.611 Acute embolism and thrombosis of superficial veins of right upper extremity

I82.612 Acute embolism and thrombosis of superficial veins of left upper extremity

I82.613 Acute embolism and thrombosis of superficial veins of upper extremity, bilateral

I82.619 Acute embolism and thrombosis of superficial veins of unspecified upper extremity

✓6ᵗʰ **I82.62** Acute embolism and thrombosis of deep veins of upper extremity

Acute embolism and thrombosis of brachial vein
Acute embolism and thrombosis of radial vein
Acute embolism and thrombosis of ulnar vein

I82.621 Acute embolism and thrombosis of deep veins of right upper extremity

I82.622 Acute embolism and thrombosis of deep veins of left upper extremity

I82.623 Acute embolism and thrombosis of deep veins of upper extremity, bilateral

I82.629 Acute embolism and thrombosis of deep veins of unspecified upper extremity

✓5ᵗʰ **I82.7** Chronic embolism and thrombosis of veins of upper extremity

Use additional code, if applicable, for associated long-term (current) use of anticoagulants (Z79.01)

EXCLUDES 1 *personal history of venous embolism and thrombosis (Z86.718)*

✓6ᵗʰ **I82.70** Chronic embolism and thrombosis of unspecified veins of upper extremity

I82.701 Chronic embolism and thrombosis of unspecified veins of right upper extremity

I82.702 Chronic embolism and thrombosis of unspecified veins of left upper extremity

I82.703 Chronic embolism and thrombosis of unspecified veins of upper extremity, bilateral

I82.709 Chronic embolism and thrombosis of unspecified veins of unspecified upper extremity

✓6ᵗʰ **I82.71** Chronic embolism and thrombosis of superficial veins of upper extremity

Chronic embolism and thrombosis of antecubital vein
Chronic embolism and thrombosis of basilic vein
Chronic embolism and thrombosis of cephalic vein

I82.711 Chronic embolism and thrombosis of superficial veins of right upper extremity

I82.712 Chronic embolism and thrombosis of superficial veins of left upper extremity

I82.713 Chronic embolism and thrombosis of superficial veins of upper extremity, bilateral

I82.719 Chronic embolism and thrombosis of superficial veins of unspecified upper extremity

Diseases of the Circulatory System

I82.72–I83.022

☑6ᵗʰ **I82.72** **Chronic embolism and thrombosis of deep veins of upper extremity**
Chronic embolism and thrombosis of brachial vein
Chronic embolism and thrombosis of radial vein
Chronic embolism and thrombosis of ulnar vein

    I82.721 **Chronic embolism and thrombosis of deep veins of right upper extremity**

    I82.722 **Chronic embolism and thrombosis of deep veins of left upper extremity**

    I82.723 **Chronic embolism and thrombosis of deep veins of upper extremity, bilateral**

    I82.729 **Chronic embolism and thrombosis of deep veins of unspecified upper extremity**

☑5ᵗʰ **I82.A** **Embolism and thrombosis of axillary vein**

  ☑6ᵗʰ **I82.A1** **Acute embolism and thrombosis of axillary vein**

    I82.A11 **Acute embolism and thrombosis of right axillary vein**

    I82.A12 **Acute embolism and thrombosis of left axillary vein**

    I82.A13 **Acute embolism and thrombosis of axillary vein, bilateral**

    I82.A19 **Acute embolism and thrombosis of unspecified axillary vein**

  ☑6ᵗʰ **I82.A2** **Chronic embolism and thrombosis of axillary vein**

    I82.A21 **Chronic embolism and thrombosis of right axillary vein**

    I82.A22 **Chronic embolism and thrombosis of left axillary vein**

    I82.A23 **Chronic embolism and thrombosis of axillary vein, bilateral**

    I82.A29 **Chronic embolism and thrombosis of unspecified axillary vein**

☑5ᵗʰ **I82.B** **Embolism and thrombosis of subclavian vein**

  ☑6ᵗʰ **I82.B1** **Acute embolism and thrombosis of subclavian vein**

    I82.B11 **Acute embolism and thrombosis of right subclavian vein**

    I82.B12 **Acute embolism and thrombosis of left subclavian vein**

    I82.B13 **Acute embolism and thrombosis of subclavian vein, bilateral**

    I82.B19 **Acute embolism and thrombosis of unspecified subclavian vein**

  ☑6ᵗʰ **I82.B2** **Chronic embolism and thrombosis of subclavian vein**

    I82.B21 **Chronic embolism and thrombosis of right subclavian vein**

    I82.B22 **Chronic embolism and thrombosis of left subclavian vein**

    I82.B23 **Chronic embolism and thrombosis of subclavian vein, bilateral**

    I82.B29 **Chronic embolism and thrombosis of unspecified subclavian vein**

☑5ᵗʰ **I82.C** **Embolism and thrombosis of internal jugular vein**

  ☑6ᵗʰ **I82.C1** **Acute embolism and thrombosis of internal jugular vein**

    I82.C11 **Acute embolism and thrombosis of right internal jugular vein**

    I82.C12 **Acute embolism and thrombosis of left internal jugular vein**

    I82.C13 **Acute embolism and thrombosis of internal jugular vein, bilateral**

    I82.C19 **Acute embolism and thrombosis of unspecified internal jugular vein**

  ☑6ᵗʰ **I82.C2** **Chronic embolism and thrombosis of internal jugular vein**

    I82.C21 **Chronic embolism and thrombosis of right internal jugular vein**

    I82.C22 **Chronic embolism and thrombosis of left internal jugular vein**

    I82.C23 **Chronic embolism and thrombosis of internal jugular vein, bilateral**

    I82.C29 **Chronic embolism and thrombosis of unspecified internal jugular vein**

☑5ᵗʰ **I82.8** **Embolism and thrombosis of other specified veins**
Use additional code, if applicable, for associated long-term (current) use of anticoagulants (Z79.01)

  ☑6ᵗʰ **I82.81** **Embolism and thrombosis of superficial veins of lower extremities**
Embolism and thrombosis of saphenous vein (greater) (lesser)

    I82.811 **Embolism and thrombosis of superficial veins of right lower extremities**

    I82.812 **Embolism and thrombosis of superficial veins of left lower extremities**

    I82.813 **Embolism and thrombosis of superficial veins of lower extremities, bilateral**

    I82.819 **Embolism and thrombosis of superficial veins of unspecified lower extremities**

  ☑6ᵗʰ **I82.89** **Embolism and thrombosis of other specified veins**

    I82.890 **Acute embolism and thrombosis of other specified veins**

    I82.891 **Chronic embolism and thrombosis of other specified veins**

☑5ᵗʰ **I82.9** **Embolism and thrombosis of unspecified vein**

    I82.90 **Acute embolism and thrombosis of unspecified vein**
Embolism of vein NOS
Thrombosis (vein) NOS

    I82.91 **Chronic embolism and thrombosis of unspecified vein**

☑4ᵗʰ **I83** **Varicose veins of lower extremities**
  EXCLUDES 1 *varicose veins complicating pregnancy (O22.0-)*
           varicose veins complicating the puerperium (O87.4)

☑5ᵗʰ **I83.0** **Varicose veins of lower extremities with ulcer**
Use additional code to identify severity of ulcer (L97.-)

  ☑6ᵗʰ **I83.00** **Varicose veins of unspecified lower extremity with ulcer**

    I83.001 **Varicose veins of unspecified lower extremity with ulcer of thigh** 🅰

    I83.002 **Varicose veins of unspecified lower extremity with ulcer of calf** 🅰

    I83.003 **Varicose veins of unspecified lower extremity with ulcer of ankle** 🅰

    I83.004 **Varicose veins of unspecified lower extremity with ulcer of heel and midfoot** 🅰
Varicose veins of unspecified lower extremity with ulcer of plantar surface of midfoot

    I83.005 **Varicose veins of unspecified lower extremity with ulcer other part of foot** 🅰
Varicose veins of unspecified lower extremity with ulcer of toe

    I83.008 **Varicose veins of unspecified lower extremity with ulcer other part of lower leg** 🅰

    I83.009 **Varicose veins of unspecified lower extremity with ulcer of unspecified site** 🅰

  ☑6ᵗʰ **I83.01** **Varicose veins of right lower extremity with ulcer**

    I83.011 **Varicose veins of right lower extremity with ulcer of thigh** 🅰

    I83.012 **Varicose veins of right lower extremity with ulcer of calf** 🅰

    I83.013 **Varicose veins of right lower extremity with ulcer of ankle** 🅰

    I83.014 **Varicose veins of right lower extremity with ulcer of heel and midfoot** 🅰
Varicose veins of right lower extremity with ulcer of plantar surface of midfoot

    I83.015 **Varicose veins of right lower extremity with ulcer other part of foot** 🅰
Varicose veins of right lower extremity with ulcer of toe

    I83.018 **Varicose veins of right lower extremity with ulcer other part of lower leg** 🅰

    I83.019 **Varicose veins of right lower extremity with ulcer of unspecified site** 🅰

  ☑6ᵗʰ **I83.02** **Varicose veins of left lower extremity with ulcer**

    I83.021 **Varicose veins of left lower extremity with ulcer of thigh** 🅰

    I83.022 **Varicose veins of left lower extremity with ulcer of calf** 🅰

EXCLUDES 1 Not coded here   **EXCLUDES 2** Not included here   N Newborn Age: 0   P Pediatric Age: 0-17   M Maternity Age: 12-55   A Adult Age: 15-124

596   ICD-10-CM Draft (2015)

    I83.023   **Varicose veins of left lower extremity** ▲
                 with ulcer of ankle

    I83.024   **Varicose veins of left lower extremity** ▲
                 with ulcer of heel and midfoot
                 Varicose veins of left lower extremity with
                    ulcer of plantar surface of midfoot

    I83.025   **Varicose veins of left lower extremity** ▲
                 with ulcer other part of foot
                 Varicose veins of left lower extremity with
                    ulcer of toe

    I83.028   **Varicose veins of left lower extremity** ▲
                 with ulcer other part of lower leg

    I83.029   **Varicose veins of left lower extremity** ▲
                 with ulcer of unspecified site

✓5ᵗʰ **I83.1**   **Varicose veins of lower extremities with** inflammation
       Stasis dermatitis

   I83.10   **Varicose veins of unspecified lower extremity** ▲
           with inflammation

   I83.11   **Varicose veins of** right **lower extremity with** ▲
           inflammation

   I83.12   **Varicose veins of** left **lower extremity with** ▲
           inflammation

✓5ᵗʰ **I83.2**   **Varicose veins of lower extremities with both** ulcer and inflammation
       Use additional code to identify severity of ulcer (L97.-)

   ✓6ᵗʰ **I83.20**   **Varicose veins of** unspecified **lower extremity with both ulcer and inflammation**

       I83.201   **Varicose veins of unspecified lower** ▲
              extremity with both ulcer of thigh **and**
              inflammation

       I83.202   **Varicose veins of unspecified lower** ▲
              extremity with both ulcer of calf **and**
              inflammation

       I83.203   **Varicose veins of unspecified lower** ▲
              extremity with both ulcer of ankle **and**
              inflammation

       I83.204   **Varicose veins of unspecified lower** ▲
              extremity with both ulcer of heel and
              midfoot **and inflammation**
              Varicose veins of unspecified lower
                 extremity with both ulcer of plantar
                 surface of midfoot and inflammation

       I83.205   **Varicose veins of unspecified lower** ▲
              extremity with both ulcer of other
              part of foot **and inflammation**
              Varicose veins of unspecified lower
                 extremity with both ulcer of toe and
                 inflammation

       I83.208   **Varicose veins of unspecified lower** ▲
              extremity with both ulcer of other part
              of lower extremity **and inflammation**

       I83.209   **Varicose veins of unspecified lower** ▲
              extremity with both ulcer of unspecified
              site and inflammation

   ✓6ᵗʰ **I83.21**   **Varicose veins of** right **lower extremity with both ulcer and inflammation**

       I83.211   **Varicose veins of right lower extremity** ▲
              with both ulcer of thigh **and inflammation**

       I83.212   **Varicose veins of right lower extremity** ▲
              with both ulcer of calf **and inflammation**

       I83.213   **Varicose veins of right lower extremity** ▲
              with both ulcer of ankle **and inflammation**

       I83.214   **Varicose veins of right lower extremity** ▲
              with both ulcer of heel and midfoot **and**
              inflammation
              Varicose veins of right lower extremity with
                 both ulcer of plantar surface of
                 midfoot and inflammation

       I83.215   **Varicose veins of right lower extremity** ▲
              with both ulcer other part of foot **and**
              inflammation
              Varicose veins of right lower extremity with
                 both ulcer of toe and inflammation

       I83.218   **Varicose veins of right lower extremity** ▲
              with both ulcer of other part of lower
              extremity **and inflammation**

       I83.219   **Varicose veins of right lower extremity** ▲
              with both ulcer of unspecified site and
              inflammation

   ✓6ᵗʰ **I83.22**   **Varicose veins of** left **lower extremity with both ulcer and inflammation**

       I83.221   **Varicose veins of left lower extremity** ▲
              with both ulcer of thigh **and inflammation**

       I83.222   **Varicose veins of left lower extremity** ▲
              with both ulcer of calf **and inflammation**

       I83.223   **Varicose veins of left lower extremity** ▲
              with both ulcer of ankle **and inflammation**

       I83.224   **Varicose veins of left lower extremity** ▲
              with both ulcer of heel and midfoot **and**
              inflammation
              Varicose veins of left lower extremity with
                 both ulcer of plantar surface of
                 midfoot and inflammation

       I83.225   **Varicose veins of left lower extremity** ▲
              with both ulcer other part of foot **and**
              inflammation
              Varicose veins of left lower extremity with
                 both ulcer of toe and inflammation

       I83.228   **Varicose veins of left lower extremity** ▲
              with both ulcer of other part of lower
              extremity **and inflammation**

       I83.229   **Varicose veins of left lower extremity** ▲
              with both ulcer of unspecified site and
              inflammation

✓5ᵗʰ **I83.8**   **Varicose veins of lower extremities with** other complications

   ✓6ᵗʰ **I83.81**   **Varicose veins of lower extremities with** pain

       I83.811   **Varicose veins of** right **lower** ▲
              extremities with pain

       I83.812   **Varicose veins of** left **lower extremities** ▲
              with pain

       I83.813   **Varicose veins of** bilateral **lower** ▲
              extremities with pain

       I83.819   **Varicose veins of unspecified lower** ▲
              extremities with pain

   ✓6ᵗʰ **I83.89**   **Varicose veins of lower extremities with** other complications
          Varicose veins of lower extremities with edema
          Varicose veins of lower extremities with swelling

       I83.891   **Varicose veins of** right **lower** ▲
              extremities with other complications

       I83.892   **Varicose veins of** left **lower extremities** ▲
              with other complications

       I83.893   **Varicose veins of** bilateral **lower** ▲
              extremities with other complications

       I83.899   **Varicose veins of unspecified lower** ▲
              extremities with other complications

✓5ᵗʰ **I83.9**   Asymptomatic **varicose veins of lower extremities**
       Phlebectasia of lower extremities
       Varicose veins of lower extremities
       Varix of lower extremities

   I83.90   **Asymptomatic varicose veins of unspecified** ▲
           lower extremity
             Varicose veins NOS

   I83.91   **Asymptomatic varicose veins of** right **lower** ▲
           extremity

   I83.92   **Asymptomatic varicose veins of** left **lower** ▲
           extremity

   I83.93   **Asymptomatic varicose veins of** bilateral **lower** ▲
           extremities

✓4ᵗʰ **I85**   **Esophageal varices**
       Use additional code to identify:
       alcohol abuse and dependence (F10.-)

   ✓5ᵗʰ **I85.0**   **Esophageal varices**
          Idiopathic esophageal varices
          Primary esophageal varices

       I85.00   **Esophageal varices** without bleeding
             Esophageal varices NOS

       I85.01   **Esophageal varices** with bleeding

   ✓5ᵗʰ **I85.1**   **Secondary esophageal varices**
          Esophageal varices secondary to alcoholic liver disease
          Esophageal varices secondary to cirrhosis of liver
          Esophageal varices secondary to schistosomiasis
          Esophageal varices secondary to toxic liver disease
          Code first underlying disease

       I85.10   **Secondary esophageal varices** without bleeding

       I85.11   **Secondary esophageal varices** with bleeding

---

☑ Additional Character Required   ✓x7ᵗʰ Xtension Alert   Unspecified Dx   Other Specified Dx   Manifestation   ►◄ Revised Text   ● New Code   ▲ Revised Code Title

✓4th **I86 Varicose veins of other sites**
EXCLUDES 1 *varicose veins of unspecified site (I83.9-)*
EXCLUDES 2 *retinal varices (H35.0-)*

I86.0 Sublingual varices

I86.1 Scrotal varices ♂
Varicocele

I86.2 Pelvic varices

I86.3 Vulval varices ♀
EXCLUDES 1 *vulval varices complicating childbirth and the puerperium (O87.8)*
vulval varices complicating pregnancy (O22.1-)

I86.4 Gastric varices

I86.8 Varicose veins of other specified sites Ⓐ
Varicose ulcer of nasal septum

✓4th **I87 Other disorders of veins**

✓5th **I87.0 Postthrombotic syndrome**
Chronic venous hypertension due to deep vein thrombosis
Postphlebitic syndrome
EXCLUDES 1 *chronic venous hypertension without deep vein thrombosis (I87.3-)*

✓6th **I87.00 Postthrombotic syndrome without complications**
Asymptomatic postthrombotic syndrome
I87.001 Postthrombotic syndrome without complications of right lower extremity
I87.002 Postthrombotic syndrome without complications of left lower extremity
I87.003 Postthrombotic syndrome without complications of bilateral lower extremity
I87.009 Postthrombotic syndrome without complications of unspecified extremity
Postthrombotic syndrome NOS

✓6th **I87.01 Postthrombotic syndrome with ulcer**
Use additional code to specify site and severity of ulcer (L97.-)
I87.011 Postthrombotic syndrome with ulcer of right lower extremity
I87.012 Postthrombotic syndrome with ulcer of left lower extremity
I87.013 Postthrombotic syndrome with ulcer of bilateral lower extremity
I87.019 Postthrombotic syndrome with ulcer of unspecified lower extremity

✓6th **I87.02 Postthrombotic syndrome with inflammation**
I87.021 Postthrombotic syndrome with inflammation of right lower extremity
I87.022 Postthrombotic syndrome with inflammation of left lower extremity
I87.023 Postthrombotic syndrome with inflammation of bilateral lower extremity
I87.029 Postthrombotic syndrome with inflammation of unspecified lower extremity

✓6th **I87.03 Postthrombotic syndrome with ulcer and inflammation**
Use additional code to specify site and severity of ulcer (L97.-)
I87.031 Postthrombotic syndrome with ulcer and inflammation of right lower extremity
I87.032 Postthrombotic syndrome with ulcer and inflammation of left lower extremity
I87.033 Postthrombotic syndrome with ulcer and inflammation of bilateral lower extremity
I87.039 Postthrombotic syndrome with ulcer and inflammation of unspecified lower extremity

✓6th **I87.09 Postthrombotic syndrome with other complications**
I87.091 Postthrombotic syndrome with other complications of right lower extremity
I87.092 Postthrombotic syndrome with other complications of left lower extremity
I87.093 Postthrombotic syndrome with other complications of bilateral lower extremity
I87.099 Postthrombotic syndrome with other complications of unspecified lower extremity

I87.1 Compression of vein
Stricture of vein
Vena cava syndrome (inferior) (superior)
EXCLUDES 2 *compression of pulmonary vein (I28.8)*

I87.2 Venous insufficiency (chronic) (peripheral)

✓5th **I87.3 Chronic venous hypertension (idiopathic)**
Stasis edema
EXCLUDES 1 *chronic venous hypertension due to deep vein thrombosis (I87.0-)*
varicose veins of lower extremities (I83.-)

✓6th **I87.30 Chronic venous hypertension (idiopathic) without complications**
Asymptomatic chronic venous hypertension (idiopathic)
I87.301 Chronic venous hypertension (idiopathic) without complications of right lower extremity
I87.302 Chronic venous hypertension (idiopathic) without complications of left lower extremity
I87.303 Chronic venous hypertension (idiopathic) without complications of bilateral lower extremity
I87.309 Chronic venous hypertension (idiopathic) without complications of unspecified lower extremity
Chronic venous hypertension NOS

✓6th **I87.31 Chronic venous hypertension (idiopathic) with ulcer**
Use additional code to specify site and severity of ulcer (L97.-)
I87.311 Chronic venous hypertension (idiopathic) with ulcer of right lower extremity
I87.312 Chronic venous hypertension (idiopathic) with ulcer of left lower extremity
I87.313 Chronic venous hypertension (idiopathic) with ulcer of bilateral lower extremity
I87.319 Chronic venous hypertension (idiopathic) with ulcer of unspecified lower extremity

✓6th **I87.32 Chronic venous hypertension (idiopathic) with inflammation**
I87.321 Chronic venous hypertension (idiopathic) with inflammation of right lower extremity
I87.322 Chronic venous hypertension (idiopathic) with inflammation of left lower extremity
I87.323 Chronic venous hypertension (idiopathic) with inflammation of bilateral lower extremity
I87.329 Chronic venous hypertension (idiopathic) with inflammation of unspecified lower extremity

✓6th **I87.33 Chronic venous hypertension (idiopathic) with ulcer and inflammation**
Use additional code to specify site and severity of ulcer (L97.-)
I87.331 Chronic venous hypertension (idiopathic) with ulcer and inflammation of right lower extremity
I87.332 Chronic venous hypertension (idiopathic) with ulcer and inflammation of left lower extremity
I87.333 Chronic venous hypertension (idiopathic) with ulcer and inflammation of bilateral lower extremity
I87.339 Chronic venous hypertension (idiopathic) with ulcer and inflammation of unspecified lower extremity

✓6th **I87.39 Chronic venous hypertension (idiopathic) with other complications**
I87.391 Chronic venous hypertension (idiopathic) with other complications of right lower extremity
I87.392 Chronic venous hypertension (idiopathic) with other complications of left lower extremity
I87.393 Chronic venous hypertension (idiopathic) with other complications of bilateral lower extremity

---

EXCLUDES 1 Not coded here   EXCLUDES 2 Not included here   Ⓝ Newborn Age: 0   Ⓟ Pediatric Age: 0-17   Ⓜ Maternity Age: 12-55   Ⓐ Adult Age: 15-124

I87.399 **Chronic venous hypertension (idiopathic) with other complications of unspecified lower extremity**

I87.8 **Other specified disorders of veins**
Phlebosclerosis
Venofibrosis

I87.9 **Disorder of vein, unspecified**

☑4ᵗʰ **I88 Nonspecific lymphadenitis**
EXCLUDES 1 *acute lymphadenitis, except mesenteric (L04.-)*
enlarged lymph nodes NOS (R59.-)
human immunodeficiency virus [HIV] disease resulting in generalized lymphadenopathy (B20)

I88.0 **Nonspecific mesenteric lymphadenitis**
Mesenteric lymphadenitis (acute)(chronic)

I88.1 **Chronic lymphadenitis, except mesenteric**
Adenitis
Lymphadenitis

I88.8 **Other nonspecific lymphadenitis**

I88.9 **Nonspecific lymphadenitis, unspecified**
Lymphadenitis NOS

☑4ᵗʰ **I89 Other noninfective disorders of lymphatic vessels and lymph nodes**
EXCLUDES 1 *chylocele, tunica vaginalis (nonfilarial) NOS (N50.8)*
enlarged lymph nodes NOS (R59.-)
filarial chylocele (B74.-)
hereditary lymphedema (Q82.0)

I89.0 **Lymphedema, not elsewhere classified**
Elephantiasis (nonfilarial) NOS
Lymphangiectasis
Obliteration, lymphatic vessel
Praecox lymphedema
Secondary lymphedema
EXCLUDES 1 *postmastectomy lymphedema (I97.2)*

I89.1 **Lymphangitis**
Chronic lymphangitis
Lymphangitis NOS
Subacute lymphangitis
EXCLUDES 1 *acute lymphangitis (L03.-)*

I89.8 **Other specified noninfective disorders of lymphatic vessels and lymph nodes**
Chylocele (nonfilarial)
Chylous ascites
Chylous cyst
Lipomelanotic reticulosis
Lymph node or vessel fistula
Lymph node or vessel infarction
Lymph node or vessel rupture

I89.9 **Noninfective disorder of lymphatic vessels and lymph nodes, unspecified**
Disease of lymphatic vessels NOS

Other and unspecified disorders of the circulatory system (I95-I99)

☑4ᵗʰ **I95 Hypotension**
EXCLUDES 1 *cardiovascular collapse (R57.9)*
maternal hypotension syndrome (O26.5-)
nonspecific low blood pressure reading NOS (R03.1)

I95.0 **Idiopathic hypotension**

I95.1 **Orthostatic hypotension**
Hypotension, postural
EXCLUDES 1 *neurogenic orthostatic hypotension [Shy-Drager] (G90.3)*
orthostatic hypotension due to drugs (I95.2)

I95.2 **Hypotension due to drugs**
Orthostatic hypotension due to drugs
Use additional code for adverse effect, if applicable, to identify drug (T36-T50 with fifth or sixth character 5)

I95.3 **Hypotension of hemodialysis**
Intra-dialytic hypotension

☑5ᵗʰ I95.8 **Other hypotension**
I95.81 **Postprocedural hypotension**
I95.89 **Other hypotension**
Chronic hypotension

I95.9 **Hypotension, unspecified**

I96 Gangrene, not elsewhere classified
Gangrenous cellulitis
EXCLUDES 1 *gangrene in atherosclerosis of native arteries of the extremities (I70.26)*
gangrene in diabetes mellitus (E08-E13)
gangrene in hernia (K40.1, K40.4, K41.1, K41.4, K42.1, K43.1-, K44.1, K45.1, K46.1)
gangrene in other peripheral vascular diseases (I73.-)
gangrene of certain specified sites—see Alphabetical Index
gas gangrene (A48.0)
pyoderma gangrenosum (L88)
AHA: 2013, 2Q, 34

☑4ᵗʰ **I97 Intraoperative and postprocedural complications and disorders of circulatory system, not elsewhere classified**
EXCLUDES 2 *postprocedural shock (T81.1-)*

I97.0 **Postcardiotomy syndrome**

☑5ᵗʰ I97.1 **Other postprocedural cardiac functional disturbances**
EXCLUDES 2 *acute pulmonary insufficiency following thoracic surgery (J95.1)*
intraoperative cardiac functional disturbances (I97.7-)

☑6ᵗʰ I97.11 **Postprocedural cardiac insufficiency**
I97.110 **Postprocedural cardiac insufficiency following cardiac surgery**
I97.111 **Postprocedural cardiac insufficiency following other surgery**

☑6ᵗʰ I97.12 **Postprocedural cardiac arrest**
I97.120 **Postprocedural cardiac arrest following cardiac surgery**
I97.121 **Postprocedural cardiac arrest following other surgery**

☑6ᵗʰ I97.13 **Postprocedural heart failure**
Use additional code to identify the heart failure (I50.-)
I97.130 **Postprocedural heart failure following cardiac surgery**
I97.131 **Postprocedural heart failure following other surgery**

☑6ᵗʰ I97.19 **Other postprocedural cardiac functional disturbances**
Use additional code, if applicable, to further specify disorder
I97.190 **Other postprocedural cardiac functional disturbances following cardiac surgery**
I97.191 **Other postprocedural cardiac functional disturbances following other surgery**

I97.2 **Postmastectomy lymphedema syndrome** 🅰
Elephantiasis due to mastectomy
Obliteration of lymphatic vessels

I97.3 **Postprocedural hypertension**

☑5ᵗʰ I97.4 **Intraoperative hemorrhage and hematoma of a circulatory system organ or structure complicating a procedure**
EXCLUDES 1 *intraoperative hemorrhage and hematoma of a circulatory system organ or structure due to accidental puncture and laceration during a procedure (I97.5-)*
EXCLUDES 2 *intraoperative cerebrovascular hemorrhage complicating a procedure (G97.3-)*

☑6ᵗʰ I97.41 **Intraoperative hemorrhage and hematoma of a circulatory system organ or structure complicating a circulatory system procedure**
I97.410 **Intraoperative hemorrhage and hematoma of a circulatory system organ or structure complicating a cardiac catheterization**
I97.411 **Intraoperative hemorrhage and hematoma of a circulatory system organ or structure complicating a cardiac bypass**
I97.418 **Intraoperative hemorrhage and hematoma of a circulatory system organ or structure complicating other circulatory system procedure**

I97.42 **Intraoperative hemorrhage and hematoma of a circulatory system organ or structure complicating other procedure**

☑5ᵗʰ I97.5 **Accidental puncture and laceration of a circulatory system organ or structure during a procedure**
EXCLUDES 2 *accidental puncture and laceration of brain during a procedure (G97.4-)*

☑ Additional Character Required   ☑7ᵗʰ Xtension Alert   Unspecified Dx   Other Specified Dx   Manifestation   ►◄ Revised Text   ● New Code   ▲ Revised Code Title

Diseases of the Circulatory System

197.51–199.9

197.51 **Accidental puncture and laceration of a circulatory system organ or structure during a** circulatory system procedure

197.52 **Accidental puncture and laceration of a circulatory system organ or structure during** other procedure

☑5ᵗʰ **197.6** Postprocedural hemorrhage and hematoma **of a circulatory system organ or structure following a procedure**
    EXCLUDES 2 *postprocedural cerebrovascular hemorrhage complicating a procedure (G97.5-)*

  ☑6ᵗʰ **197.61** **Postprocedural hemorrhage and hematoma of a circulatory system organ or structure following a** circulatory system procedure

    197.610 **Postprocedural hemorrhage and hematoma of a circulatory system organ or structure following a** cardiac catheterization

    197.611 **Postprocedural hemorrhage and hematoma of a circulatory system organ or structure following** cardiac bypass

    197.618 **Postprocedural hemorrhage and hematoma of a circulatory system organ or structure following** other circulatory system procedure

  197.62 **Postprocedural hemorrhage and hematoma of a circulatory system organ or structure following other procedure**

☑5ᵗʰ **197.7** Intraoperative **cardiac** functional disturbances
    EXCLUDES 2 *acute pulmonary insufficiency following thoracic surgery (J95.1)*
             postprocedural cardiac functional disturbances (I97.1-)

  ☑6ᵗʰ **197.71** **Intraoperative** cardiac arrest

    197.710 **Intraoperative cardiac arrest during** cardiac surgery

    197.711 **Intraoperative cardiac arrest during** other surgery

  ☑6ᵗʰ **197.79** Other **intraoperative cardiac functional disturbances**
    Use additional code, if applicable, to further specify disorder

    197.790 **Other intraoperative cardiac functional disturbances during** cardiac surgery

    197.791 **Other intraoperative cardiac functional disturbances during** other surgery

☑5ᵗʰ **197.8** Other **intraoperative and postprocedural complications and disorders of the circulatory system, not elsewhere classified**
    Use additional code, if applicable, to further specify disorder

  ☑6ᵗʰ **197.81** Intraoperative **cerebrovascular infarction**

    197.810 **Intraoperative cerebrovascular infarction during** cardiac surgery

    197.811 **Intraoperative cerebrovascular infarction during** other surgery

  ☑6ᵗʰ **197.82** Postprocedural **cerebrovascular infarction**

    197.820 **Postprocedural cerebrovascular infarction during** cardiac surgery

    197.821 **Postprocedural cerebrovascular infarction during** other surgery

  197.88 **Other** intraoperative **complications of the circulatory system, not elsewhere classified**

  197.89 **Other** postprocedural **complications and disorders of the circulatory system, not elsewhere classified**

☑4ᵗʰ **199** **Other and unspecified disorders of circulatory system**

  199.8 **Other disorder of circulatory system**

  199.9 **Unspecified disorder of circulatory system**

EXCLUDES 1 Not coded here   *EXCLUDES 2* Not included here   Ⓝ Newborn Age: 0   Ⓟ Pediatric Age: 0-17   Ⓜ Maternity Age: 12-55   Ⓐ Adult Age: 15-124

600   ICD-10-CM Draft (2015)

Chapter 10. Diseases of the Respiratory System (J00-J99)

NOTE When a respiratory condition is described as occurring in more than one site and is not specifically indexed, it should be classified to the lower anatomic site (e.g. tracheobronchitis to bronchitis in J40).

Use additional code, where applicable, to identify:
exposure to environmental tobacco smoke (Z77.22)
exposure to tobacco smoke in the perinatal period (P96.81)
history of tobacco use (Z87.891)
occupational exposure to environmental tobacco smoke (Z57.31)
tobacco dependence (F17.-)
tobacco use (Z72.0)

EXCLUDES 2   *certain conditions originating in the perinatal period (P04-P96)*
certain infectious and parasitic diseases (A00-B99)
complications of pregnancy, childbirth and the puerperium (O00-O9A)
congenital malformations, deformations and chromosomal abnormalities (Q00-Q99)
endocrine, nutritional and metabolic diseases (E00-E88)
injury, poisoning and certain other consequences of external causes (S00-T88)
neoplasms (C00-D49)
smoke inhalation (T59.81-)
symptoms, signs and abnormal clinical and laboratory findings, not elsewhere classified (R00-R94)

This chapter contains the following blocks:
J00-J06   Acute upper respiratory infections
J09-J18   Influenza and pneumonia
J20-J22   Other acute lower respiratory infections
J30-J39   Other diseases of upper respiratory tract
J40-J47   Chronic lower respiratory diseases
J60-J70   Lung diseases due to external agents
J80-J84   Other respiratory diseases principally affecting the interstitium
J85-J86   Suppurative and necrotic conditions of the lower respiratory tract
J90-J94   Other diseases of the pleura
J95   Intraoperative and postprocedural complications and disorders of respiratory system, not elsewhere classified
J96-J99   Other diseases of the respiratory system

Acute upper respiratory infections (J00-J06)

EXCLUDES 1   *influenza virus with other respiratory manifestations (J09.X2, J10.1, J11.1)*

EXCLUDES 2   *chronic obstructive pulmonary disease with acute lower respiratory infection (J44.0)*

J00   Acute nasopharyngitis (common cold)
Acute rhinitis
Coryza (acute)
Infective nasopharyngitis NOS
Infective rhinitis
Nasal catarrh, acute
Nasopharyngitis NOS
EXCLUDES 1   *acute pharyngitis (J02.-)*
acute sore throat NOS (J02.9)
pharyngitis NOS (J02.9)
rhinitis NOS (J31.0)
sore throat NOS (J02.9)
EXCLUDES 2   *allergic rhinitis (J30.1-J30.9)*
chronic pharyngitis (J31.2)
chronic rhinitis (J31.0)
chronic sore throat (J31.2)
nasopharyngitis, chronic (J31.1)
vasomotor rhinitis (J30.0)

✓4th J01   Acute sinusitis
INCLUDES acute abscess of sinus
acute empyema of sinus
acute infection of sinus
acute inflammation of sinus
acute suppuration of sinus
Use additional code (B95-B97) to identify infectious agent
EXCLUDES 1   *sinusitis NOS (J32.9)*
EXCLUDES 2   *chronic sinusitis (J32.0-J32.8)*

✓5th J01.0   Acute maxillary sinusitis
Acute antritis
J01.00   Acute maxillary sinusitis, unspecified
J01.01   Acute recurrent maxillary sinusitis

✓5th J01.1   Acute frontal sinusitis
J01.10   Acute frontal sinusitis, unspecified
J01.11   Acute recurrent frontal sinusitis

✓5th J01.2   Acute ethmoidal sinusitis
J01.20   Acute ethmoidal sinusitis, unspecified

J01.21   Acute recurrent ethmoidal sinusitis

✓5th J01.3   Acute sphenoidal sinusitis
J01.30   Acute sphenoidal sinusitis, unspecified
J01.31   Acute recurrent sphenoidal sinusitis

✓5th J01.4   Acute pansinusitis
J01.40   Acute pansinusitis, unspecified
J01.41   Acute recurrent pansinusitis

✓5th J01.8   Other acute sinusitis
J01.80   Other acute sinusitis
Acute sinusitis involving more than one sinus but not pansinusitis
J01.81   Other acute recurrent sinusitis
Acute recurrent sinusitis involving more than one sinus but not pansinusitis

✓5th J01.9   Acute sinusitis, unspecified
J01.90   Acute sinusitis, unspecified
J01.91   Acute recurrent sinusitis, unspecified

✓4th J02   Acute pharyngitis
INCLUDES acute sore throat
EXCLUDES 1   *acute laryngopharyngitis (J06.0)*
peritonsillar abscess (J36)
pharyngeal abscess (J39.1)
retropharyngeal abscess (J39.0)
EXCLUDES 2   *chronic pharyngitis (J31.2)*

J02.0   Streptococcal pharyngitis
Septic pharyngitis
Streptococcal sore throat
EXCLUDES 2   *scarlet fever (A38.-)*

J02.8   Acute pharyngitis due to other specified organisms
Use additional code (B95-B97) to identify infectious agent
EXCLUDES 1   *acute pharyngitis due to coxsackie virus (B08.5)*
acute pharyngitis due to gonococcus (A54.5)
acute pharyngitis due to herpes [simplex] virus (B00.2)
acute pharyngitis due to infectious mononucleosis (B27.-)
enteroviral vesicular pharyngitis (B08.5)

J02.9   Acute pharyngitis, unspecified
Gangrenous pharyngitis (acute)
Infective pharyngitis (acute) NOS
Pharyngitis (acute) NOS
Sore throat (acute) NOS
Suppurative pharyngitis (acute)
Ulcerative pharyngitis (acute)

✓4th J03   Acute tonsillitis
EXCLUDES 1   *acute sore throat (J02.-)*
hypertrophy of tonsils (J35.1)
peritonsillar abscess (J36)
sore throat NOS (J02.9)
streptococcal sore throat (J02.0)
EXCLUDES 2   *chronic tonsillitis (J35.0)*

✓5th J03.0   Streptococcal tonsillitis
J03.00   Acute streptococcal tonsillitis, unspecified
J03.01   Acute recurrent streptococcal tonsillitis

✓5th J03.8   Acute tonsillitis due to other specified organisms
Use additional code (B95-B97) to identify infectious agent
EXCLUDES 1   *diphtheritic tonsillitis (A36.0)*
herpesviral pharyngotonsillitis (B00.2)
streptococcal tonsillitis (J03.0)
tuberculous tonsillitis (A15.8)
Vincent's tonsillitis (A69.1)
J03.80   Acute tonsillitis due to other specified organisms
J03.81   Acute recurrent tonsillitis due to other specified organisms

✓5th J03.9   Acute tonsillitis, unspecified
Follicular tonsillitis (acute)
Gangrenous tonsillitis (acute)
Infective tonsillitis (acute)
Tonsillitis (acute) NOS
Ulcerative tonsillitis (acute)
J03.90   Acute tonsillitis, unspecified
J03.91   Acute recurrent tonsillitis, unspecified

Diseases of the Respiratory System

J04–J11.Ø8

✓4th J04   Acute laryngitis and tracheitis
Use additional code (B95-B97) to identify infectious agent
EXCLUDES 1   *acute obstructive laryngitis [croup] and epiglottitis (J05.-)*
EXCLUDES 2   *laryngismus (stridulus) (J38.5)*

J04.Ø   Acute laryngitis
   Edematous laryngitis (acute)
   Laryngitis (acute) NOS
   Subglottic laryngitis (acute)
   Suppurative laryngitis (acute)
   Ulcerative laryngitis (acute)
   EXCLUDES 1   *acute obstructive laryngitis (J05.Ø)*
   EXCLUDES 2   *chronic laryngitis (J37.Ø)*

✓5th J04.1   Acute tracheitis
   Acute viral tracheitis
   Catarrhal tracheitis (acute)
   Tracheitis (acute) NOS
   EXCLUDES 2   *chronic tracheitis (J42)*

   J04.1Ø   Acute tracheitis without obstruction
   J04.11   Acute tracheitis with obstruction

J04.2   Acute laryngotracheitis
   Laryngotracheitis NOS
   Tracheitis (acute) with laryngitis (acute)
   EXCLUDES 1   *acute obstructive laryngotracheitis (J05.Ø)*
   EXCLUDES 2   *chronic laryngotracheitis (J37.1)*

✓5th J04.3   Supraglottitis, unspecified
   J04.3Ø   Supraglottitis, unspecified, without obstruction
   J04.31   Supraglottitis, unspecified, with obstruction

✓4th J05   Acute obstructive laryngitis [croup] and epiglottitis
Use additional code (B95-B97) to identify infectious agent

J05.Ø   Acute obstructive laryngitis [croup]
   Obstructive laryngitis (acute) NOS
   Obstructive laryngotracheitis NOS

✓5th J05.1   Acute epiglottitis
   EXCLUDES 2   *epiglottitis, chronic (J37.Ø)*

   J05.1Ø   Acute epiglottitis without obstruction
     Epiglottitis NOS
   J05.11   Acute epiglottitis with obstruction

✓4th J06   Acute upper respiratory infections of multiple and unspecified sites
   EXCLUDES 1   *acute respiratory infection NOS (J22)*
     streptococcal pharyngitis (J02.Ø)3

J06.Ø   Acute laryngopharyngitis

J06.9   Acute upper respiratory infection, unspecified
   Upper respiratory disease, acute
   Upper respiratory infection NOS

Influenza and pneumonia (J09-J18)

EXCLUDES 2   *allergic or eosinophilic pneumonia (J82)*
   aspiration pneumonia NOS (J69.Ø)
   congenital pneumonia (P23.9)
   lipid pneumonia (J69.1)
   meconium pneumonia (P24.Ø1)
   neonatal aspiration pneumonia (P24.-)
   pneumonia due to solids and liquids (J69.-)
   rheumatic pneumonia (IØØ)
   ventilator associated pneumonia (J95.851)

✓4th J09   Influenza due to certain identified influenza viruses
   EXCLUDES 1   *seasonal influenza due to other identified influenza virus (J10.-)*
     seasonal influenza due to unidentified influenza virus (J11.-)

✓5th J09.X   Influenza due to identified novel influenza A virus
   Avian influenza
   Bird influenza
   Influenza A/H5N1
   Influenza of other animal origin, not bird or swine
   Swine influenza virus (viruses that normally cause infections in pigs)

   J09.X1   Influenza due to identified novel influenza A virus with pneumonia
     Code also, if applicable, associated:
     lung abscess (J85.1)
     other specified type of pneumonia

   J09.X2   Influenza due to identified novel influenza A virus with other respiratory manifestations
     Influenza due to identified novel influenza A virus NOS
     Influenza due to identified novel influenza A virus with laryngitis
     Influenza due to identified novel influenza A virus with pharyngitis
     Influenza due to identified novel influenza A virus with upper respiratory symptoms
     Use additional code, if applicable, for associated:
     pleural effusion (J91.8)
     sinusitis (J01.-)

   J09.X3   Influenza due to identified novel influenza A virus with gastrointestinal manifestations
     Influenza due to identified novel influenza A virus gastroenteritis
     EXCLUDES 1   *'intestinal flu' [viral gastroenteritis] (A08.-)*

   J09.X9   Influenza due to identified novel influenza A virus with other manifestations
     Influenza due to identified novel influenza A virus with encephalopathy
     Influenza due to identified novel influenza A virus with myocarditis
     Influenza due to identified novel influenza A virus with otitis media
     Use additional code to identify manifestation

✓4th J10   Influenza due to other identified influenza virus
   EXCLUDES 1   *influenza due to avian influenza virus (J09.X-)*
     influenza due to swine flu (J09.X-)
     influenza due to unidentifed influenza virus (J11.-)

✓5th J10.Ø   Influenza due to other identified influenza virus with pneumonia
   Code also associated lung abscess, if applicable (J85.1)

   J10.ØØ   Influenza due to other identified influenza virus with unspecified type of pneumonia

   J10.Ø1   Influenza due to other identified influenza virus with the same other identified influenza virus pneumonia

   J10.Ø8   Influenza due to other identified influenza virus with other specified pneumonia
     Code also other specified type of pneumonia

J10.1   Influenza due to other identified influenza virus with other respiratory manifestations
   Influenza due to other identified influenza virus NOS
   Influenza due to other identified influenza virus with laryngitis
   Influenza due to other identified influenza virus with pharyngitis
   Influenza due to other identified influenza virus with upper respiratory symptoms
   Use additional code for associated pleural effusion, if applicable (J91.8)
   Use additional code for associated sinusitis, if applicable (J01.-)

J10.2   Influenza due to other identified influenza virus with gastrointestinal manifestations
   Influenza due to other identified influenza virus gastroenteritis
   EXCLUDES 1   *'intestinal flu' [viral gastroenteritis] (A08.-)*

✓5th J10.8   Influenza due to other identified influenza virus with other manifestations

   J10.81   Influenza due to other identified influenza virus with encephalopathy

   J10.82   Influenza due to other identified influenza virus with myocarditis

   J10.83   Influenza due to other identified influenza virus with otitis media
     Use additional code for any associated perforated tympanic membrane (H72.-)

   J10.89   Influenza due to other identified influenza virus with other manifestations
     Use additional codes to identify the manifestations

✓4th J11   Influenza due to unidentified influenza virus

✓5th J11.Ø   Influenza due to unidentified influenza virus with pneumonia
   Code also associated lung abscess, if applicable (J85.1)

   J11.ØØ   Influenza due to unidentified influenza virus with unspecified type of pneumonia
     Influenza with pneumonia NOS

   J11.Ø8   Influenza due to unidentified influenza virus with specified pneumonia
     Code also other specified type of pneumonia

EXCLUDES 1 Not coded here   *EXCLUDES 2* Not included here   N Newborn Age: Ø   P Pediatric Age: Ø-17   M Maternity Age: 12-55   A Adult Age: 15-124

602   ICD-1Ø-CM Draft (2Ø15)

J11.1 Influenza due to unidentified influenza virus with other respiratory manifestations
Influenza NOS
Influenzal laryngitis NOS
Influenzal pharyngitis NOS
Influenza with upper respiratory symptoms NOS
Use additional code for associated pleural effusion, if applicable (J91.8)
Use additional code for associated sinusitis, if applicable (J01.-)

J11.2 Influenza due to unidentified influenza virus with gastrointestinal manifestations
Influenza gastroenteritis NOS
EXCLUDES 1 *'intestinal flu' [viral gastroenteritis] (A08.-)*

✓5th **J11.8 Influenza due to unidentified influenza virus with other manifestations**

J11.81 Influenza due to unidentified influenza virus with encephalopathy
Influenzal encephalopathy NOS

J11.82 Influenza due to unidentified influenza virus with myocarditis
Influenzal myocarditis NOS

J11.83 Influenza due to unidentified influenza virus with otitis media
Influenzal otitis media NOS
Use additional code for any associated perforated tympanic membrane (H72.-)

J11.89 Influenza due to unidentified influenza virus with other manifestations
Use additional codes to identify the manifestations

✓4th **J12 Viral pneumonia, not elsewhere classified**
INCLUDES bronchopneumonia due to viruses other than influenza viruses
Code first associated influenza, if applicable (J09.X1, J10.0-, J11.0-)
Code also associated abscess, if applicable (J85.1)
EXCLUDES 1 *aspiration pneumonia due to anesthesia during labor and delivery (O74.0)*
aspiration pneumonia due to anesthesia during pregnancy (O29)
aspiration pneumonia due to anesthesia during puerperium (O89.0)
aspiration pneumonia due to solids and liquids (J69.-)
aspiration pneumonia NOS (J69.0)
congenital pneumonia (P23.0)
congenital rubella pneumonitis (P35.0)
interstitial pneumonia NOS (J84.9)
lipid pneumonia (J69.1)
neonatal aspiration pneumonia (P24.-)
AHA: 2013, 4Q, 118

J12.0 Adenoviral pneumonia

J12.1 Respiratory syncytial virus pneumonia

J12.2 Parainfluenza virus pneumonia

J12.3 Human metapneumovirus pneumonia

✓5th **J12.8 Other viral pneumonia**

J12.81 Pneumonia due to SARS-associated coronavirus
Severe acute respiratory syndrome NOS

J12.89 Other viral pneumonia

J12.9 Viral pneumonia, unspecified

J13 Pneumonia due to Streptococcus pneumoniae
Bronchopneumonia due to S. pneumoniae
Code first associated influenza, if applicable (J09.X1, J10.0-, J11.0-)
Code also associated lung abscess, if applicable (J85.1)
EXCLUDES 1 *congenital pneumonia due to S. pneumoniae (P23.6)*
lobar pneumonia, unspecified organism (J18.1)
pneumonia due to other streptococci (J15.3-J15.4)
AHA: 2013, 4Q, 118

J14 Pneumonia due to Hemophilus influenzae
Bronchopneumonia due to H. influenzae
Code first associated influenza, if applicable (J09.X1, J10.0-, J11.0-)
Code also associated lung abscess, if applicable (J85.1)
EXCLUDES 1 *congenital pneumonia due to H. influenzae (P23.6)*
AHA: 2013, 4Q, 118

✓4th **J15 Bacterial pneumonia, not elsewhere classified**
Bronchopneumonia due to bacteria other than S. pneumoniae and H. influenzae
Code first associated influenza, if applicable (J09.X1, J10.0-, J11.0-)
Code also associated lung abscess, if applicable (J85.1)
EXCLUDES 1 *chlamydial pneumonia (J16.0)*
congenital pneumonia (P23.-)
Legionnaires' disease (A48.1)
spirochetal pneumonia (A69.8)
AHA: 2013, 4Q, 118

J15.0 Pneumonia due to Klebsiella pneumoniae

J15.1 Pneumonia due to Pseudomonas

✓5th **J15.2 Pneumonia due to staphylococcus**

J15.20 Pneumonia due to staphylococcus, unspecified

✓6th **J15.21 Pneumonia due to Staphylococcus aureus**

J15.211 Pneumonia due to methicillin susceptible Staphylococcus aureus
MSSA pneumonia
Pneumonia due to Staphylococcus aureus NOS

J15.212 Pneumonia due to methicillin resistant Staphylococcus aureus

J15.29 Pneumonia due to other staphylococcus

J15.3 Pneumonia due to streptococcus, group B

J15.4 Pneumonia due to other streptococci
EXCLUDES 1 *pneumonia due to streptococcus, group B (J15.3)*
pneumonia due to Streptococcus pneumoniae (J13)

J15.5 Pneumonia due to Escherichia coli

J15.6 Pneumonia due to other aerobic Gram-negative bacteria
Pneumonia due to Serratia marcescens

J15.7 Pneumonia due to Mycoplasma pneumoniae

J15.8 Pneumonia due to other specified bacteria

J15.9 Unspecified bacterial pneumonia
Pneumonia due to gram-positive bacteria

✓4th **J16 Pneumonia due to other infectious organisms, not elsewhere classified**
Code first associated influenza, if applicable (J09.X1, J10.0-, J11.0-)
Code also associated lung abscess, if applicable (J85.1)
EXCLUDES 1 *congenital pneumonia (P23.-)*
ornithosis (A70)
pneumocystosis (B59)
pneumonia NOS (J18.9)
AHA: 2013, 4Q, 118

J16.0 Chlamydial pneumonia

J16.8 Pneumonia due to other specified infectious organisms

J17 Pneumonia in diseases classified elsewhere
Code first underlying disease, such as:
Q fever (A78)
rheumatic fever (I00)
schistosomiasis (B65.0-B65.9)
EXCLUDES 1 *candidial pneumonia (B37.1)*
chlamydial pneumonia (J16.0)
gonorrheal pneumonia (A54.84)
histoplasmosis pneumonia (B39.0-B39.2)
measles pneumonia (B05.2)
nocardiosis pneumonia (A43.0)
pneumocystosis (B59)
pneumonia due to Pneumocystis carinii (B59)
pneumonia due to Pneumocystis jiroveci (B59)
pneumonia in actinomycosis (A42.0)
pneumonia in anthrax (A22.1)
pneumonia in ascariasis (B77.81)
pneumonia in aspergillosis (B44.0-B44.1)
pneumonia in coccidioidomycosis (B38.0-B38.2)
pneumonia in cytomegalovirus disease (B25.0)
pneumonia in toxoplasmosis (B58.3)
rubella pneumonia (B06.81)
salmonella pneumonia (A02.22)
spirochetal infection NEC with pneumonia (A69.8)
tularemia pneumonia (A21.2)
typhoid fever with pneumonia (A01.03)
varicella pneumonia (B01.2)
whooping cough with pneumonia (A37 with fifth-character 1)
AHA: 2013, 4Q, 118

☑ Additional Character Required   ✓x7th Xtension Alert   Unspecified Dx   Other Specified Dx   Manifestation   ►◄ Revised Text   ● New Code   ▲ Revised Code Title

Diseases of the Respiratory System

J18–J32.8

J18 Pneumonia, unspecified organism

Code first associated influenza, if applicable (J09.X1, J10.0-, J11.0-)

EXCLUDES 1 abscess of lung with pneumonia (J85.1)
aspiration pneumonia due to anesthesia during labor and delivery (O74.0)
aspiration pneumonia due to anesthesia during pregnancy (O29)
aspiration pneumonia due to anesthesia during puerperium (O89.0)
aspiration pneumonia due to solids and liquids (J69.-)
aspiration pneumonia NOS (J69.0)
congenital pneumonia (P23.0)
drug-induced interstitial lung disorder (J70.2-J70.4)
interstitial pneumonia NOS (J84.9)
lipid pneumonia (J69.1)
neonatal aspiration pneumonia (P24.-)
pneumonitis due to external agents (J67-J70)
pneumonitis due to fumes and vapors (J68.0)
usual interstitial pneumonia (J84.17)

AHA: 2013, 4Q, 118

J18.0 Bronchopneumonia, unspecified organism

EXCLUDES 1 hypostatic bronchopneumonia (J18.2)
lipid pneumonia (J69.1)

EXCLUDES 2 acute bronchiolitis (J21.-)
chronic bronchiolitis (J44.9)

J18.1 Lobar pneumonia, unspecified organism

J18.2 Hypostatic pneumonia, unspecified organism
Hypostatic bronchopneumonia
Passive pneumonia

J18.8 Other pneumonia, unspecified organism

J18.9 Pneumonia, unspecified organism
AHA: 2013, 4Q, 119; 2012, 4Q, 94

Other acute lower respiratory infections (J20-J22)

EXCLUDES 2 chronic obstructive pulmonary disease with acute lower respiratory infection (J44.0)

J20 Acute bronchitis

INCLUDES acute and subacute bronchitis (with) bronchospasm
acute and subacute bronchitis (with) tracheitis
acute and subacute bronchitis (with) tracheobronchitis, acute
acute and subacute fibrinous bronchitis
acute and subacute membranous bronchitis
acute and subacute purulent bronchitis
acute and subacute septic bronchitis

EXCLUDES 1 bronchitis NOS (J40)
tracheobronchitis NOS (J40)

EXCLUDES 2 acute bronchitis with bronchiectasis (J47.0)
acute bronchitis with chronic obstructive asthma (J44.0)
acute bronchitis with chronic obstructive pulmonary disease (J44.0)
allergic bronchitis NOS (J45.909)
bronchitis due to chemicals, fumes and vapors (J68.0)
chronic bronchitis NOS (J42)
chronic mucopurulent bronchitis (J41.1)
chronic obstructive bronchitis (J44.-)
chronic obstructive tracheobronchitis (J44.-)
chronic simple bronchitis (J41.0)
chronic tracheobronchitis (J42)

J20.0 Acute bronchitis due to Mycoplasma pneumoniae

J20.1 Acute bronchitis due to Hemophilus influenzae

J20.2 Acute bronchitis due to streptococcus

J20.3 Acute bronchitis due to coxsackievirus

J20.4 Acute bronchitis due to parainfluenza virus

J20.5 Acute bronchitis due to respiratory syncytial virus

J20.6 Acute bronchitis due to rhinovirus

J20.7 Acute bronchitis due to echovirus

J20.8 Acute bronchitis due to other specified organisms

J20.9 Acute bronchitis, unspecified

J21 Acute bronchiolitis

Acute bronchiolitis with bronchospasm

EXCLUDES 2 respiratory bronchiolitis interstitial lung disease (J84.115)

J21.0 Acute bronchiolitis due to respiratory syncytial virus

J21.1 Acute bronchiolitis due to human metapneumovirus

J21.8 Acute bronchiolitis due to other specified organisms

J21.9 Acute bronchiolitis, unspecified
Bronchiolitis (acute)

EXCLUDES 1 chronic bronchiolitis (J44.-)

J22 Unspecified acute lower respiratory infection

Acute (lower) respiratory (tract) infection NOS

EXCLUDES 1 upper respiratory infection (acute) (J06.9)

Other diseases of upper respiratory tract (J30-J39)

J30 Vasomotor and allergic rhinitis

INCLUDES spasmodic rhinorrhea

EXCLUDES 1 allergic rhinitis with asthma (bronchial) (J45.909)
rhinitis NOS (J31.0)

J30.0 Vasomotor rhinitis

J30.1 Allergic rhinitis due to pollen
Allergy NOS due to pollen
Hay fever
Pollinosis

J30.2 Other seasonal allergic rhinitis

J30.5 Allergic rhinitis due to food

J30.8 Other allergic rhinitis

J30.81 Allergic rhinitis due to animal (cat) (dog) hair and dander

J30.89 Other allergic rhinitis
Perennial allergic rhinitis

J30.9 Allergic rhinitis, unspecified

J31 Chronic rhinitis, nasopharyngitis and pharyngitis

Use additional code to identify:
exposure to environmental tobacco smoke (Z77.22)
exposure to tobacco smoke in the perinatal period (P96.81)
history of tobacco use (Z87.891)
occupational exposure to environmental tobacco smoke (Z57.31)
tobacco dependence (F17.-)
tobacco use (Z72.0)

J31.0 Chronic rhinitis
Atrophic rhinitis (chronic)
Granulomatous rhinitis (chronic)
Hypertrophic rhinitis (chronic)
Obstructive rhinitis (chronic)
Ozena
Purulent rhinitis (chronic)
Rhinitis (chronic) NOS
Ulcerative rhinitis (chronic)

EXCLUDES 1 allergic rhinitis (J30.1-J30.9)
vasomotor rhinitis (J30.0)

J31.1 Chronic nasopharyngitis

EXCLUDES 2 acute nasopharyngitis (J00)

J31.2 Chronic pharyngitis
Atrophic pharyngitis (chronic)
Chronic sore throat
Granular pharyngitis (chronic)
Hypertrophic pharyngitis (chronic)

EXCLUDES 2 acute pharyngitis (J02.9)

J32 Chronic sinusitis

INCLUDES sinus abscess
sinus empyema
sinus infection
sinus suppuration

Use additional code to identify:
exposure to environmental tobacco smoke (Z77.22)
exposure to tobacco smoke in the perinatal period (P96.81)
history of tobacco use (Z87.891)
infectious agent (B95-B97)
occupational exposure to environmental tobacco smoke (Z57.31)
tobacco dependence (F17.-)
tobacco use (Z72.0)

EXCLUDES 2 acute sinusitis (J01.-)

J32.0 Chronic maxillary sinusitis
Antritis (chronic)
Maxillary sinusitis NOS

J32.1 Chronic frontal sinusitis
Frontal sinusitis NOS

J32.2 Chronic ethmoidal sinusitis
Ethmoidal sinusitis NOS

EXCLUDES 1 Woakes' ethmoiditis (J33.1)

J32.3 Chronic sphenoidal sinusitis
Sphenoidal sinusitis NOS

J32.4 Chronic pansinusitis
Pansinusitis NOS

J32.8 Other chronic sinusitis
Sinusitis (chronic) involving more than one sinus but not pansinusitis

EXCLUDES 1 Not coded here   EXCLUDES 2 Not included here   N Newborn Age: 0   P Pediatric Age: 0-17   M Maternity Age: 12-55   A Adult Age: 15-124

604   ICD-10-CM Draft (2015)

J32.9   **Chronic sinusitis, unspecified**
Sinusitis (chronic) NOS

✓4ᵗʰ J33   **Nasal polyp**
Use additional code to identify:
exposure to environmental tobacco smoke (Z77.22)
exposure to tobacco smoke in the perinatal period (P96.81)
history of tobacco use (Z87.891)
occupational exposure to environmental tobacco smoke (Z57.31)
tobacco dependence (F17.-)
tobacco use (Z72.0)
   EXCLUDES 1   adenomatous polyps (D14.0)

J33.0   **Polyp of nasal cavity**
Choanal polyp
Nasopharyngeal polyp

J33.1   **Polypoid sinus degeneration**
Woakes' syndrome or ethmoiditis

J33.8   **Other polyp of sinus**
Accessory polyp of sinus
Ethmoidal polyp of sinus
Maxillary polyp of sinus
Sphenoidal polyp of sinus

J33.9   **Nasal polyp, unspecified**

✓4ᵗʰ J34   **Other and unspecified disorders of nose and nasal sinuses**
   EXCLUDES 2   varicose ulcer of nasal septum (I86.8)

J34.0   **Abscess, furuncle and carbuncle of nose**
Cellulitis of nose
Necrosis of nose
Ulceration of nose

J34.1   **Cyst and mucocele of nose and nasal sinus**

J34.2   **Deviated nasal septum**
Deflection or deviation of septum (nasal) (acquired)
   EXCLUDES 1   congenital deviated nasal septum (Q67.4)

J34.3   **Hypertrophy of nasal turbinates**

✓5ᵗʰ J34.8   **Other specified disorders of nose and nasal sinuses**

J34.81   **Nasal mucositis (ulcerative)**
Code also type of associated therapy, such as:
antineoplastic and immunosuppressive drugs
(T45.1X-)
radiological procedure and radiotherapy (Y84.2)
   EXCLUDES 2   gastrointestinal mucositis (ulcerative)
(K92.81)
mucositis (ulcerative) of vagina and vulva
(N76.81)
oral mucositis (ulcerative) (K12.3-)

J34.89   **Other specified disorders of nose and nasal sinuses**
Perforation of nasal septum NOS
Rhinolith

J34.9   **Unspecified disorder of nose and nasal sinuses**

✓4ᵗʰ J35   **Chronic diseases of tonsils and adenoids**
Use additional code to identify:
exposure to environmental tobacco smoke (Z77.22)
exposure to tobacco smoke in the perinatal period (P96.81)
history of tobacco use (Z87.891)
occupational exposure to environmental tobacco smoke (Z57.31)
tobacco dependence (F17.-)
tobacco use (Z72.0)

✓5ᵗʰ J35.0   **Chronic tonsillitis and adenoiditis**
   EXCLUDES 2   acute tonsillitis (J03.-)

J35.01   **Chronic tonsillitis**

J35.02   **Chronic adenoiditis**

J35.03   **Chronic tonsillitis and adenoiditis**

J35.1   **Hypertrophy of tonsils**
Enlargement of tonsils
   EXCLUDES 1   hypertrophy of tonsils with tonsillitis (J35.0-)

J35.2   **Hypertrophy of adenoids**
Enlargement of adenoids
   EXCLUDES 1   hypertrophy of adenoids with adenoiditis (J35.0-)

J35.3   **Hypertrophy of tonsils with hypertrophy of adenoids**
   EXCLUDES 1   hypertrophy of tonsils and adenoids with tonsillitis and
adenoiditis (J35.03)

J35.8   **Other chronic diseases of tonsils and adenoids**
Adenoid vegetations
Amygdalolith
Calculus, tonsil
Cicatrix of tonsil (and adenoid)
Tonsillar tag
Ulcer of tonsil

J35.9   **Chronic disease of tonsils and adenoids, unspecified**
Disease (chronic) of tonsils and adenoids NOS

J36   **Peritonsillar abscess**
   INCLUDES   abscess of tonsil
peritonsillar cellulitis
quinsy
Use additional code (B95-B97) to identify infectious agent
   EXCLUDES 1   acute tonsillitis (J03.-)
chronic tonsillitis (J35.0)
retropharyngeal abscess (J39.0)
tonsillitis NOS (J03.9-)

✓4ᵗʰ J37   **Chronic laryngitis and laryngotracheitis**
Use additional code to identify:
exposure to environmental tobacco smoke (Z77.22)
exposure to tobacco smoke in the perinatal period (P96.81)
history of tobacco use (Z87.891)
infectious agent (B95-B97)
occupational exposure to environmental tobacco smoke (Z57.31)
tobacco dependence (F17.-)
tobacco use (Z72.0)

J37.0   **Chronic laryngitis**
Catarrhal laryngitis
Hypertrophic laryngitis
Sicca laryngitis
   EXCLUDES 2   acute laryngitis (J04.0)
obstructive (acute) laryngitis (J05.0)

J37.1   **Chronic laryngotracheitis**
Laryngitis, chronic, with tracheitis (chronic)
Tracheitis, chronic, with laryngitis
   EXCLUDES 1   chronic tracheitis (J42)
   EXCLUDES 2   acute laryngotracheitis (J04.2)
acute tracheitis (J04.1)

✓4ᵗʰ J38   **Diseases of vocal cords and larynx, not elsewhere classified**
Use additional code to identify:
exposure to environmental tobacco smoke (Z77.22)
exposure to tobacco smoke in the perinatal period (P96.81)
history of tobacco use (Z87.891)
occupational exposure to environmental tobacco smoke (Z57.31)
tobacco dependence (F17.-)
tobacco use (Z72.0)
   EXCLUDES 1   congenital laryngeal stridor (P28.89)
obstructive laryngitis (acute) (J05.0)
postprocedural subglottic stenosis (J95.5)
stridor (R06.1)
ulcerative laryngitis (J04.0)

✓5ᵗʰ J38.0   **Paralysis of vocal cords and larynx**
Laryngoplegia
Paralysis of glottis

J38.00   **Paralysis of vocal cords and larynx, unspecified**

J38.01   **Paralysis of vocal cords and larynx, unilateral**

J38.02   **Paralysis of vocal cords and larynx, bilateral**

J38.1   **Polyp of vocal cord and larynx**
   EXCLUDES 1   adenomatous polyps (D14.1)

J38.2   **Nodules of vocal cords**
Chorditis (fibrinous)(nodosa)(tuberosa)
Singer's nodes
Teacher's nodes

J38.3   **Other diseases of vocal cords**
Abscess of vocal cords
Cellulitis of vocal cords
Granuloma of vocal cords
Leukokeratosis of vocal cords
Leukoplakia of vocal cords

J38.4   **Edema of larynx**
Edema (of) glottis
Subglottic edema
Supraglottic edema
   EXCLUDES 1   acute obstructive laryngitis [croup] (J05.0)
edematous laryngitis (J04.0)

J38.5   **Laryngeal spasm**
Laryngismus (stridulus)

J38.6   **Stenosis of larynx**

J38.7   **Other diseases of larynx**
Abscess of larynx   Pachyderma of larynx
Cellulitis of larynx   Perichondritis of larynx
Disease of larynx NOS   Ulcer of larynx
Necrosis of larynx

✓ Additional Character Required   ✓x7ᵗʰ Xtension Alert   Unspecified Dx   Other Specified Dx   Manifestation   ►◄ Revised Text   ● New Code   ▲ Revised Code Title

Diseases of the Respiratory System *(side tab)*

J39–J44.9 *(side tab)*

☑4ᵗʰ **J39   Other diseases of upper respiratory tract**
> EXCLUDES 1   *acute respiratory infection NOS (J22)*
> *acute upper respiratory infection (J06.9)*
> *upper respiratory inflammation due to chemicals, gases, fumes or vapors (J68.2)*

J39.0   Retropharyngeal and parapharyngeal abscess
> Peripharyngeal abscess
> EXCLUDES 1   *peritonsillar abscess (J36)*

J39.1   Other abscess of pharynx
> Cellulitis of pharynx
> Nasopharyngeal abscess

J39.2   Other diseases of pharynx
> Cyst of pharynx
> Edema of pharynx
> EXCLUDES 2   *chronic pharyngitis (J31.2)*
> *ulcerative pharyngitis (J02.9)*

J39.3   Upper respiratory tract hypersensitivity reaction, site unspecified
> EXCLUDES 1   *hypersensitivity reaction of upper respiratory tract, such as:*
> *extrinsic allergic alveolitis (J67.9)*
> *pneumoconiosis (J60-J67.9)*

J39.8   Other specified diseases of upper respiratory tract

J39.9   Disease of upper respiratory tract, unspecified

Chronic lower respiratory diseases (J40-J47)

> EXCLUDES 1   *bronchitis due to chemicals, gases, fumes and vapors (J68.0)*
> EXCLUDES 2   *cystic fibrosis (E84.-)*

J40   Bronchitis, not specified as acute or chronic
> Bronchitis NOS
> Bronchitis with tracheitis NOS
> Catarrhal bronchitis
> Tracheobronchitis NOS
> Use additional code to identify:
>   exposure to environmental tobacco smoke (Z77.22)
>   exposure to tobacco smoke in the perinatal period (P96.81)
>   history of tobacco use (Z87.891)
>   occupational exposure to environmental tobacco smoke (Z57.31)
>   tobacco dependence (F17.-)
>   tobacco use (Z72.0)
> EXCLUDES 1   *acute bronchitis (J20.-)*
> *allergic bronchitis NOS (J45.909)*
> *asthmatic bronchitis NOS (J45.9-)*
> *bronchitis due to chemicals, gases, fumes and vapors (J68.0)*

☑4ᵗʰ **J41   Simple and mucopurulent chronic bronchitis**
> Use additional code to identify:
>   exposure to environmental tobacco smoke (Z77.22)
>   exposure to tobacco smoke in the perinatal period (P96.81)
>   history of tobacco use (Z87.891)
>   occupational exposure to environmental tobacco smoke (Z57.31)
>   tobacco dependence (F17.-)
>   tobacco use (Z72.0)
> EXCLUDES 1   *chronic bronchitis NOS (J42)*
> *chronic obstructive bronchitis (J44.-)*

J41.0   Simple chronic bronchitis

J41.1   Mucopurulent chronic bronchitis

J41.8   Mixed simple and mucopurulent chronic bronchitis

J42   Unspecified chronic bronchitis
> Chronic bronchitis NOS
> Chronic tracheitis
> Chronic tracheobronchitis
> Use additional code to identify:
>   exposure to environmental tobacco smoke (Z77.22)
>   exposure to tobacco smoke in the perinatal period (P96.81)
>   history of tobacco use (Z87.891)
>   occupational exposure to environmental tobacco smoke (Z57.31)
>   tobacco dependence (F17.-)
>   tobacco use (Z72.0)
> EXCLUDES 1   *chronic asthmatic bronchitis (J44.-)*
> *chronic bronchitis with airways obstruction (J44.-)*
> *chronic emphysematous bronchitis (J44.-)*
> *chronic obstructive pulmonary disease NOS (J44.9)*
> *simple and mucopurulent chronic bronchitis (J41.-)*

☑4ᵗʰ **J43   Emphysema**
> Use additional code to identify:
>   exposure to environmental tobacco smoke (Z77.22)
>   history of tobacco use (Z87.891)
>   occupational exposure to environmental tobacco smoke (Z57.31)
>   tobacco dependence (F17.-)
>   tobacco use (Z72.0)
> EXCLUDES 1   *compensatory emphysema (J98.3)*
> *emphysema due to inhalation of chemicals, gases, fumes or vapors (J68.4)*
> *emphysema with chronic (obstructive) bronchitis (J44.-)*
> *emphysematous (obstructive) bronchitis (J44.-)*
> *interstitial emphysema (J98.2)*
> *mediastinal emphysema (J98.2)*
> *neonatal interstitial emphysema (P25.0)*
> *surgical (subcutaneous) emphysema (T81.82)*
> *traumatic subcutaneous emphysema (T79.7)*

J43.0   Unilateral pulmonary emphysema [MacLeod's syndrome]
> Swyer-James syndrome
> Unilateral emphysema
> Unilateral hyperlucent lung
> Unilateral pulmonary artery functional hypoplasia
> Unilateral transparency of lung

J43.1   Panlobular emphysema
> Panacinar emphysema

J43.2   Centrilobular emphysema

J43.8   Other emphysema

J43.9   Emphysema, unspecified
> Bullous emphysema (lung)(pulmonary)
> Emphysema (lung)(pulmonary) NOS
> Emphysematous bleb
> Vesicular emphysema (lung)(pulmonary)

☑4ᵗʰ **J44   Other chronic obstructive pulmonary disease**
> INCLUDES   asthma with chronic obstructive pulmonary disease
> chronic asthmatic (obstructive) bronchitis
> chronic bronchitis with airways obstruction
> chronic bronchitis with emphysema
> chronic emphysematous bronchitis
> chronic obstructive asthma
> chronic obstructive bronchitis
> chronic obstructive tracheobronchitis
> Code also type of asthma, if applicable (J45.-)
> Use additional code to identify:
>   exposure to environmental tobacco smoke (Z77.22)
>   history of tobacco use (Z87.891)
>   occupational exposure to environmental tobacco smoke (Z57.31)
>   tobacco dependence (F17.-)
>   tobacco use (Z72.0)
> EXCLUDES 1   *bronchiectasis (J47.-)*
> *chronic bronchitis NOS (J42)*
> *chronic simple and mucopurulent bronchitis (J41.-)*
> *chronic tracheitis (J42)*
> *chronic tracheobronchitis (J42)*
> *emphysema without chronic bronchitis (J43.-)*
> *lung diseases due to external agents (J60-J70)*
> **AHA:** 2013, 4Q, 109

J44.0   Chronic obstructive pulmonary disease with acute lower respiratory infection
> Use additional code to identify the infection

J44.1   Chronic obstructive pulmonary disease with (acute) exacerbation
> Decompensated COPD
> Decompensated COPD with (acute) exacerbation
> EXCLUDES 2   *chronic obstructive pulmonary disease [COPD] with acute bronchitis (J44.0)*

J44.9   Chronic obstructive pulmonary disease, unspecified
> Chronic obstructive airway disease NOS
> Chronic obstructive lung disease NOS
> **AHA:** 2013, 4Q, 129

EXCLUDES 1 Not coded here   EXCLUDES 2 Not included here   N Newborn Age: 0   P Pediatric Age: 0-17   M Maternity Age: 12-55   A Adult Age: 15-124

✓4ᵗʰ J45 Asthma

> **INCLUDES** allergic (predominantly) asthma
> allergic bronchitis nos
> allergic rhinitis with asthma
> atopic asthma
> extrinsic allergic asthma
> hay fever with asthma
> idiosyncratic asthma
> intrinsic nonallergic asthma
> nonallergic asthma
>
> Use additional code to identify:
> exposure to environmental tobacco smoke (Z77.22)
> exposure to tobacco smoke in the perinatal period (P96.81)
> history of tobacco use (Z87.891)
> occupational exposure to environmental tobacco smoke (Z57.31)
> tobacco dependence (F17.-)
> tobacco use (Z72.0)
>
> **EXCLUDES 1** detergent asthma (J69.8)
> eosinophilic asthma (J82)
> lung diseases due to external agents (J60-J70)
> miner's asthma (J60)
> wheezing NOS (R06.2)
> wood asthma (J67.8)
>
> **EXCLUDES 2** asthma with chronic obstructive pulmonary disease (J44.9)
> chronic asthmatic (obstructive) bronchitis (J44.9)
> chronic obstructive asthma (J44.9)

  ✓5ᵗʰ J45.2 Mild intermittent asthma

    J45.20 Mild intermittent asthma, uncomplicated
Mild intermittent asthma NOS

    J45.21 Mild intermittent asthma with (acute) exacerbation

    J45.22 Mild intermittent asthma with status asthmaticus

  ✓5ᵗʰ J45.3 Mild persistent asthma

    J45.30 Mild persistent asthma, uncomplicated
Mild persistent asthma NOS

    J45.31 Mild persistent asthma with (acute) exacerbation

    J45.32 Mild persistent asthma with status asthmaticus

  ✓5ᵗʰ J45.4 Moderate persistent asthma

    J45.40 Moderate persistent asthma, uncomplicated
Moderate persistent asthma NOS

    J45.41 Moderate persistent asthma with (acute) exacerbation

    J45.42 Moderate persistent asthma with status asthmaticus

  ✓5ᵗʰ J45.5 Severe persistent asthma

    J45.50 Severe persistent asthma, uncomplicated
Severe persistent asthma NOS

    J45.51 Severe persistent asthma with (acute) exacerbation

    J45.52 Severe persistent asthma with status asthmaticus

  ✓5ᵗʰ J45.9 Other and unspecified asthma

    ✓6ᵗʰ J45.90 Unspecified asthma
Asthmatic bronchitis NOS
Childhood asthma NOS
Late onset asthma

      J45.901 Unspecified asthma with (acute) exacerbation

      J45.902 Unspecified asthma with status asthmaticus

      J45.909 Unspecified asthma, uncomplicated
Asthma NOS

    ✓6ᵗʰ J45.99 Other asthma

      J45.990 Exercise induced bronchospasm

      J45.991 Cough variant asthma

      J45.998 Other asthma

✓4ᵗʰ J47 Bronchiectasis

> **INCLUDES** bronchiolectasis
>
> Use additional code to identify:
> exposure to environmental tobacco smoke (Z77.22)
> exposure to tobacco smoke in the perinatal period (P96.81)
> history of tobacco use (Z87.891)
> occupational exposure to environmental tobacco smoke (Z57.31)
> tobacco dependence (F17.-)
> tobacco use (Z72.0)
>
> **EXCLUDES 1** congenital bronchiectasis (Q33.4)
> tuberculous bronchiectasis (current disease) (A15.0)

  J47.0 Bronchiectasis with acute lower respiratory infection
Bronchiectasis with acute bronchitis

  J47.1 Bronchiectasis with (acute) exacerbation

  J47.9 Bronchiectasis, uncomplicated
Bronchiectasis NOS

Lung diseases due to external agents (J60-J70)

> **EXCLUDES 2** asthma (J45.-)
> malignant neoplasm of bronchus and lung (C34.-)

J60 Coalworker's pneumoconiosis   ▲
Anthracosilicosis   Black lung disease
Anthracosis   Coalworker's lung

> **EXCLUDES 1** coalworker pneumoconiosis with tuberculosis, any type in A15 (J65)

J61 Pneumoconiosis due to asbestos and other mineral fibers   ▲
Asbestosis

> **EXCLUDES 1** pleural plaque with asbestosis (J92.0)
> pneumoconiosis with tuberculosis, any type in A15 (J65)

✓4ᵗʰ J62 Pneumoconiosis due to dust containing silica

> **INCLUDES** silicotic fibrosis (massive) of lung
>
> **EXCLUDES 1** pneumoconiosis with tuberculosis, any type in A15 (J65)

  J62.0 Pneumoconiosis due to talc dust

  J62.8 Pneumoconiosis due to other dust containing silica
Silicosis NOS

✓4ᵗʰ J63 Pneumoconiosis due to other inorganic dusts

> **EXCLUDES 1** pneumoconiosis with tuberculosis, any type in A15 (J65)

  J63.0 Aluminosis (of lung)

  J63.1 Bauxite fibrosis (of lung)

  J63.2 Berylliosis

  J63.3 Graphite fibrosis (of lung)

  J63.4 Siderosis

  J63.5 Stannosis

  J63.6 Pneumoconiosis due to other specified inorganic dusts

J64 Unspecified pneumoconiosis

> **EXCLUDES 1** pneumonoconiosis with tuberculosis, any type in A15 (J65)

J65 Pneumoconiosis associated with tuberculosis
Any condition in J60-J64 with tuberculosis, any type in A15
Silicotuberculosis

✓4ᵗʰ J66 Airway disease due to specific organic dust

> **EXCLUDES 2** allergic alveolitis (J67.-)
> asbestosis (J61)
> bagassosis (J67.1)
> farmer's lung (J67.0)
> hypersensitivity pneumonitis due to organic dust (J67.-)
> reactive airways dysfunction syndrome (J68.3)

  J66.0 Byssinosis
Airway disease due to cotton dust

  J66.1 Flax-dressers' disease

  J66.2 Cannabinosis

  J66.8 Airway disease due to other specific organic dusts

✓4ᵗʰ J67 Hypersensitivity pneumonitis due to organic dust

> **INCLUDES** allergic alveolitis and pneumonitis due to inhaled organic dust and particles of fungal, actinomycetic or other origin
>
> **EXCLUDES 1** pneumonitis due to inhalation of chemicals, gases, fumes or vapors (J68.0)

  J67.0 Farmer's lung
Harvester's lung   Moldy hay disease
Haymaker's lung

  J67.1 Bagassosis
Bagasse disease   Bagasse pneumonitis

  J67.2 Bird fancier's lung
Budgerigar fancier's disease or lung
Pigeon fancier's disease or lung

  J67.3 Suberosis
Corkhandler's disease or lung
Corkworker's disease or lung

  J67.4 Maltworker's lung
Alveolitis due to Aspergillus clavatus

  J67.5 Mushroom-worker's lung

  J67.6 Maple-bark-stripper's lung
Alveolitis due to Cryptostroma corticale
Cryptostromosis

  J67.7 Air conditioner and humidifier lung
Allergic alveolitis due to fungal, thermophilic actinomycetes and other organisms growing in ventilation [air conditioning] systems

  J67.8 Hypersensitivity pneumonitis due to other organic dusts
Cheese-washer's lung   Furrier's lung
Coffee-worker's lung   Sequoiosis
Fish-meal worker's lung

✔ Additional Character Required   ✓ˣ⁷ᵗʰ Xtension Alert   Unspecified Dx   Other Specified Dx   Manifestation   ▶◀ Revised Text   ● New Code   ▲ Revised Code Title

J67.9 **Hypersensitivity pneumonitis due to unspecified organic dust**
Allergic alveolitis (extrinsic) NOS
Hypersensitivity pneumonitis NOS

✓4th **J68** **Respiratory conditions due to inhalation of chemicals, gases, fumes and vapors**
Code first (T51-T65) to identify cause
Use additional code to identify associated respiratory conditions, such as:
   acute respiratory failure (J96.0-)

J68.0 **Bronchitis and pneumonitis** due to chemicals, gases, fumes and vapors
Chemical bronchitis (acute)

J68.1 **Pulmonary edema** due to chemicals, gases, fumes and vapors
Chemical pulmonary edema (acute) (chronic)
EXCLUDES 1   pulmonary edema (acute) (chronic) NOS (J81.-)

J68.2 **Upper respiratory inflammation** due to chemicals, gases, fumes and vapors, not elsewhere classified

J68.3 **Other** acute and subacute **respiratory conditions due to chemicals, gases, fumes and vapors**
Reactive airways dysfunction syndrome

J68.4 **Chronic respiratory** conditions due to chemicals, gases, fumes and vapors
Emphysema (diffuse) (chronic) due to inhalation of chemicals, gases, fumes and vapors
Obliterative bronchiolitis (chronic) (subacute) due to inhalation of chemicals, gases, fumes and vapors
Pulmonary fibrosis (chronic) due to inhalation of chemicals, gases, fumes and vapors
EXCLUDES 1   chronic pulmonary edema due to chemicals, gases, fumes and vapors (J68.1)

J68.8 **Other respiratory conditions due to chemicals, gases, fumes and vapors**

J68.9 **Unspecified respiratory condition due to chemicals, gases, fumes and vapors**

✓4th **J69** **Pneumonitis due to solids and liquids**
EXCLUDES 1   neonatal aspiration syndromes (P24.-)
postprocedural pneumonitis (J95.4)

J69.0 **Pneumonitis due to** inhalation of food and vomit
Aspiration pneumonia NOS
Aspiration pneumonia (due to) food (regurgitated)
Aspiration pneumonia (due to) gastric secretions
Aspiration pneumonia (due to) milk
Aspiration pneumonia (due to) vomit
Code also any associated foreign body in respiratory tract (T17.-)
EXCLUDES 1   chemical pneumonitis due to anesthesia (J95.4)
obstetric aspiration pneumonitis (O74.0)

J69.1 **Pneumonitis due to** inhalation of oils and essences
Exogenous lipoid pneumonia
Lipid pneumonia NOS
Code first (T51-T65) to identify substance
EXCLUDES 1   endogenous lipoid pneumonia (J84.89)

J69.8 **Pneumonitis due to inhalation of other** solids and liquids
Pneumonitis due to aspiration of blood
Pneumonitis due to aspiration of detergent
Code first (T51-T65) to identify substance

✓4th **J70** **Respiratory conditions due to other external agents**
J70.0 **Acute pulmonary manifestations due to** radiation
Radiation pneumonitis
Use additional code (W88-W90, X39.0-) to identify the external cause

J70.1 **Chronic and other pulmonary manifestations due to** radiation
Fibrosis of lung following radiation
Use additional code (W88-W90, X39.0-) to identify the external cause

J70.2 **Acute drug-induced interstitial lung** disorders
Use additional code for adverse effect, if applicable, to identify drug (T36-T50 with fifth or sixth character 5)
EXCLUDES 1   interstitial pneumonia NOS (J84.9)
lymphoid interstitial pneumonia (J84.2)

J70.3 **Chronic drug-induced interstitial lung** disorders
Use additional code for adverse effect, if applicable, to identify drug (T36-T50 with fifth or sixth character 5)
EXCLUDES 1   interstitial pneumonia NOS (J84.9)
lymphoid interstitial pneumonia (J84.2)

J70.4 **Drug-induced interstitial lung disorders, unspecified**
Use additional code for adverse effect, if applicable, to identify drug (T36-T50 with fifth or sixth character 5)
EXCLUDES 1   interstitial pneumonia NOS (J84.9)
lymphoid interstitial pneumonia (J84.2)

J70.5 **Respiratory conditions due to** smoke inhalation
Smoke inhalation NOS
EXCLUDES 1   smoke inhalation due to chemicals, gases, fumes and vapors (J68.9)
AHA: 2013, 4Q, 121

J70.8 **Respiratory conditions due to other specified external agents**
Code first (T51-T65) to identify the external agent

J70.9 **Respiratory conditions due to unspecified external agent**
Code first (T51-T65) to identify the external agent

Other respiratory diseases principally affecting the interstitium (J80-J84)

J80 **Acute respiratory distress syndrome**
Acute respiratory distress syndrome in adult or child
Adult hyaline membrane disease
EXCLUDES 1   respiratory distress syndrome in newborn (perinatal) (P22.0)

✓4th **J81** **Pulmonary edema**
Use additional code to identify:
   exposure to environmental tobacco smoke (Z77.22)
   history of tobacco use (Z87.891)
   occupational exposure to environmental tobacco smoke (Z57.31)
   tobacco dependence (F17.-)
   tobacco use (Z72.0)
EXCLUDES 1   chemical (acute) pulmonary edema (J68.1)
hypostatic pneumonia (J18.2)
passive pneumonia (J18.2)
pulmonary edema due to external agents (J60-J70)
pulmonary edema with heart disease NOS (I50.1)
pulmonary edema with heart failure (I50.1)

J81.0 **Acute pulmonary edema**
Acute edema of lung

J81.1 **Chronic pulmonary edema**
Pulmonary congestion (chronic) (passive)
Pulmonary edema NOS

J82 **Pulmonary eosinophilia, not elsewhere classified**
Allergic pneumonia
Eosinophilic asthma
Eosinophilic pneumonia
Löffler's pneumonia
Tropical (pulmonary) eosinophilia NOS
EXCLUDES 1   pulmonary eosinophilia due to aspergillosis (B44.-)
pulmonary eosinophilia due to drugs (J70.2-J70.4)
pulmonary eosinophilia due to specified parasitic infection (B50-B83)
pulmonary eosinophilia due to systemic connective tissue disorders (M30-M36)
pulmonary infiltrate NOS (R91.8)

✓4th **J84** **Other interstitial pulmonary diseases**
EXCLUDES 1   drug-induced interstitial lung disorders (J70.2-J70.4)
interstitial emphysema (J98.2)
lung diseases due to external agents (J60-J70)

✓5th **J84.0** **Alveolar and parieto-alveolar conditions**
J84.01 **Alveolar proteinosis**
J84.02 **Pulmonary alveolar microlithiasis**
J84.03 **Idiopathic pulmonary** hemosiderosis
Essential brown induration of lung
Code first underlying disease, such as:
disorders of iron metabolism (E83.1-)
EXCLUDES 1   acute idiopathic pulmonary hemorrhage in infants [AIPHI] (R04.81)

J84.09 **Other alveolar and parieto-alveolar conditions**

✓5th **J84.1** **Other interstitial pulmonary diseases with fibrosis**
EXCLUDES 1   pulmonary fibrosis (chronic) due to inhalation of chemicals, gases, fumes or vapors (J68.4)
pulmonary fibrosis (chronic) following radiation (J70.1)

J84.10 **Pulmonary fibrosis, unspecified**
Capillary fibrosis of lung
Cirrhosis of lung (chronic) NOS
Fibrosis of lung (atrophic) (chronic) (confluent) (massive) (perialveolar) (peribronchial) NOS
Induration of lung (chronic) NOS
Postinflammatory pulmonary fibrosis

✓6th **J84.11** **Idiopathic interstitial pneumonia**
EXCLUDES 1   lymphoid interstitial pneumonia (J84.2)
pneumocystis pneumonia (B59)

J84.111 **Idiopathic interstitial pneumonia, not otherwise specified**

EXCLUDES 1 Not coded here   *EXCLUDES 2* Not included here   ℕ Newborn Age: 0   ℙ Pediatric Age: 0-17   𝕄 Maternity Age: 12-55   𝔸 Adult Age: 15-124

608   ICD-10-CM Draft (2015)

J84.112   **Idiopathic** pulmonary fibrosis
     Cryptogenic fibrosing alveolitis
     Idiopathic fibrosing alveolitis

J84.113   **Idiopathic** non-specific interstitial **pneumonitis**
     EXCLUDES1   *non-specific interstitial pneumonia NOS, or due to known underlying cause (J84.89)*

J84.114   **Acute interstitial** pneumonitis
     Hamman-Rich syndrome
     EXCLUDES1   *pneumocystis pneumonia (B59)*

J84.115   **Respiratory bronchiolitis interstitial** lung disease

J84.116   **Cryptogenic organizing** pneumonia
     EXCLUDES1   *organizing pneumonia NOS, or due to known underlying cause (J84.89)*

J84.117   **Desquamative interstitial pneumonia**

J84.17   *Other interstitial pulmonary diseases with fibrosis in diseases classified elsewhere*
     Interstitial pneumonia (nonspecific) (usual) due to collagen vascular disease
     Interstitial pneumonia (nonspecific) (usual) in diseases classified elsewhere
     Organizing pneumonia due to collagen vascular disease
     Organizing pneumonia in diseases classified elsewhere
     Code first underlying disease, such as:
       progressive systemic sclerosis (M34.0)
       rheumatoid arthritis (M05.00-M06.9)
       systemic lupus erythematosis (M32.0-M32.9)

J84.2   **Lymphoid interstitial pneumonia**
     Lymphoid interstitial pneumonitis

✓5th   **J84.8**   Other specified **interstitial pulmonary diseases**
     EXCLUDES1   *exogenous lipoid pneumonia (J69.1)*
       unspecified lipoid pneumonia (J69.1)

     J84.81   **Lymphangioleiomyomatosis**   ♀
       Lymphangiomyomatosis

     J84.82   **Adult pulmonary Langerhans cell histiocytosis**   A
       Adult PLCH

     J84.83   **Surfactant mutations of the lung**

     ✓6th   **J84.84**   **Other interstitial lung diseases of childhood**
       J84.841   **Neuroendocrine cell hyperplasia of infancy**
       J84.842   **Pulmonary interstitial glycogenosis**
       J84.843   **Alveolar capillary dysplasia with vein misalignment**
       J84.848   **Other interstitial lung diseases of childhood**

     J84.89   **Other specified interstitial pulmonary diseases**
       Endogenous lipoid pneumonia
       Interstitial pneumonitis
       Non-specific interstitial pneumonitis NOS
       Organizing pneumonia due to known underlying cause
       Organizing pneumonia NOS
       Code first, if applicable:
         poisoning due to drug or toxin (T51-T65 with fifth or sixth character to indicate intent), for toxic pneumonopathy
         underlying cause of pneumonopathy, if known
       Use additional code, for adverse effect, to identify drug (T36-T50 with fifth or sixth character 5), if drug-induced
       EXCLUDES1   *cryptogenic organizing pneumonia (J84.116)*
         idiopathic non-specific interstitial pneumonitis (J84.113)
         lipoid pneumonia, exogenous or unspecified (J69.1)
         lymphoid interstitial pneumonia (J84.2)

J84.9   **Interstitial pulmonary disease, unspecified**
     Interstitial pneumonia NOS

Suppurative and necrotic conditions of the lower respiratory tract (J85-J86)

✓4th   **J85**   **Abscess of lung and mediastinum**
     Use additional code (B95-B97) to identify infectious agent.

     J85.0   **Gangrene** and necrosis **of lung**

     J85.1   **Abscess of lung** with pneumonia
       Code also the type of pneumonia

     J85.2   **Abscess of lung** without pneumonia
       Abscess of lung NOS

     J85.3   **Abscess of mediastinum**

✓4th   **J86**   **Pyothorax**
     Use additional code (B95-B97) to identify infectious agent
     EXCLUDES1   *abscess of lung (J85.-)*
       pyothorax due to tuberculosis (A15.6)

     J86.0   **Pyothorax** with fistula
       Bronchocutaneous fistula
       Bronchopleural fistula
       Hepatopleural fistula
       Mediastinal fistula
       Pleural fistula
       Thoracic fistula
       Any condition classifiable to J86.9 with fistula

     J86.9   **Pyothorax** without fistula
       Abscess of pleura   Pyopneumothorax
       Abscess of thorax   Septic pleurisy
       Empyema (chest) (lung) (pleura)   Seropurulent pleurisy
       Fibrinopurulent pleurisy   Suppurative pleurisy
       Purulent pleurisy

Other diseases of the pleura (J90-J94)

J90   **Pleural effusion, not elsewhere classified**
     Encysted pleurisy
     Pleural effusion NOS
     Pleurisy with effusion (exudative) (serous)
     EXCLUDES1   *chylous (pleural) effusion (J94.0)*
       malignant pleural effusion (J91.0))
       pleurisy NOS (R09.1)
       tuberculous pleural effusion (A15.6)

✓4th   **J91**   **Pleural effusion in conditions classified elsewhere**
     EXCLUDES2   *pleural effusion in heart failure (I50.-)*
       pleural effusion in systemic lupus erythematosus (M32.13)

     J91.0   *Malignant pleural effusion*
       Code first underlying neoplasm

     J91.8   *Pleural effusion in other conditions classified elsewhere*
       Code first underlying disease, such as:
         filariasis (B74.0-B74.9)
         influenza (J09.X2, J10.1, J11.1)

✓4th   **J92**   **Pleural plaque**
     INCLUDES   pleural thickening

     J92.0   **Pleural plaque** with presence of asbestos

     J92.9   **Pleural plaque** without asbestos
       Pleural plaque NOS

✓4th   **J93**   **Pneumothorax and air leak**
     EXCLUDES1   *congenital or perinatal pneumothorax (P25.1)*
       postprocedural air leak (J95.812)
       postprocedural pneumothorax (J95.811)
       traumatic pneumothorax (S27.0)
       tuberculous (current disease) pneumothorax (A15.-)
       pyopneumothorax (J86.-)

     J93.0   **Spontaneous tension pneumothorax**

     ✓5th   **J93.1**   Other spontaneous **pneumothorax**
       J93.11   Primary **spontaneous pneumothorax**
       J93.12   Secondary **spontaneous pneumothorax**
         Code first underlying condition, such as:
           catamenial pneumothorax due to endometriosis (N80.8)
           cystic fibrosis (E84.-)
           eosinophilic pneumonia (J82)
           lymphangioleiomyomatosis (J84.81)
           malignant neoplasm of bronchus and lung (C34.-)
           Marfan's syndrome (Q87.4)
           pneumonia due to Pneumocystis carinii (B59)
           secondary malignant neoplasm of lung (C78.0-)
           spontaneous rupture of the esophagus (K22.3)

     ✓5th   **J93.8**   Other pneumothorax **and air leak**
       J93.81   Chronic **pneumothorax**
       J93.82   Other air leak
         Persistent air leak
       J93.83   Other pneumothorax
         Acute pneumothorax
         Spontaneous pneumothorax NOS

     J93.9   **Pneumothorax, unspecified**
       Pneumothorax NOS

✓ Additional Character Required   ✓x7th Xtension Alert   Unspecified Dx   Other Specified Dx   Manifestation   ▶◀ Revised Text   ● New Code   ▲ Revised Code Title

☑4ᵗʰ **J94   Other pleural conditions**
    EXCLUDES 1 *pleurisy NOS (R09.1)*
          traumatic hemopneumothorax (S27.2)
          traumatic hemothorax (S27.1)
          tuberculous pleural conditions (current disease) (A15.-)

    J94.0   Chylous effusion
          Chyliform effusion

    J94.1   Fibrothorax

    J94.2   Hemothorax
          Hemopneumothorax

    J94.8   Other specified pleural conditions
          Hydropneumothorax
          Hydrothorax

    J94.9   Pleural condition, unspecified

Intraoperative and postprocedural complications and disorders of respiratory system, not elsewhere classified (J95)

☑4ᵗʰ **J95   Intraoperative and postprocedural complications and disorders of respiratory system, not elsewhere classified**
    EXCLUDES 2 *aspiration pneumonia (J69.-)*
          emphysema (subcutaneous) resulting from a procedure (T81.82)
          hypostatic pneumonia (J18.2)
          pulmonary manifestations due to radiation (J70.0- J70.1)

    ☑5ᵗʰ **J95.0   Tracheostomy complications**

        J95.00   Unspecified tracheostomy complication

        J95.01   Hemorrhage from tracheostomy stoma

        J95.02   Infection of tracheostomy stoma
            Use additional code to identify type of infection, such as:
               cellulitis of neck (L03.8)
               sepsis (A40, A41)

        J95.03   Malfunction of tracheostomy stoma
            Mechanical complication of tracheostomy stoma
            Obstruction of tracheostomy airway
            Tracheal stenosis due to tracheostomy

        J95.04   Tracheo-esophageal fistula following tracheostomy

        J95.09   Other tracheostomy complication

    J95.1   Acute pulmonary insufficiency following thoracic surgery
        EXCLUDES 2 *functional disturbances following cardiac surgery (I97.0, I97.1-)*

    J95.2   Acute pulmonary insufficiency following nonthoracic surgery
        EXCLUDES 2 *functional disturbances following cardiac surgery (I97.0, I97.1-)*

    J95.3   Chronic pulmonary insufficiency following surgery
        EXCLUDES 2 *functional disturbances following cardiac surgery (I97.0, I97.1-)*

    J95.4   Chemical pneumonitis due to anesthesia
        Mendelson's syndrome
        Postprocedural aspiration pneumonia
        Use additional code for adverse effect, if applicable, to identify drug (T41.- with fifth or sixth character 5)
        EXCLUDES 1 *aspiration pneumonitis due to anesthesia complicating labor and delivery (O74.0)*
             aspiration pneumonitis due to anesthesia complicating pregnancy (O29)
             aspiration pneumonitis due to anesthesia complicating the puerperium (O89.01)

    J95.5   Postprocedural subglottic stenosis

    ☑5ᵗʰ **J95.6   Intraoperative hemorrhage and hematoma of a respiratory system organ or structure complicating a procedure**
        EXCLUDES 1 *intraoperative hemorrhage and hematoma of a respiratory system organ or structure due to accidental puncture and laceration during procedure (J95.7-)*

        J95.61   Intraoperative hemorrhage and hematoma of a respiratory system organ or structure complicating a respiratory system procedure

        J95.62   Intraoperative hemorrhage and hematoma of a respiratory system organ or structure complicating other procedure

    ☑5ᵗʰ **J95.7   Accidental puncture and laceration of a respiratory system organ or structure during a procedure**
        EXCLUDES 2 *postprocedural pneumothorax (J95.811)*

        J95.71   Accidental puncture and laceration of a respiratory system organ or structure during a respiratory system procedure

        J95.72   Accidental puncture and laceration of a respiratory system organ or structure during other procedure

    ☑5ᵗʰ **J95.8   Other intraoperative and postprocedural complications and disorders of respiratory system, not elsewhere classified**

        ☑6ᵗʰ **J95.81   Postprocedural pneumothorax and air leak**

            J95.811   Postprocedural pneumothorax

            J95.812   Postprocedural air leak

        ☑6ᵗʰ **J95.82   Postprocedural respiratory failure**
            EXCLUDES 1 *respiratory failure in other conditions (J96.-)*

            J95.821   Acute postprocedural respiratory failure
               Postprocedural respiratory failure NOS

            J95.822   Acute and chronic postprocedural respiratory failure

        ☑6ᵗʰ **J95.83   Postprocedural hemorrhage and hematoma of a respiratory system organ or structure following a procedure**

            J95.830   Postprocedural hemorrhage and hematoma of a respiratory system organ or structure following a respiratory system procedure

            J95.831   Postprocedural hemorrhage and hematoma of a respiratory system organ or structure following other procedure

        J95.84   Transfusion-related acute lung injury (TRALI)

        ☑6ᵗʰ **J95.85   Complication of respirator [ventilator]**

            J95.850   Mechanical complication of respirator
               EXCLUDES 1 *encounter for respirator [ventilator] dependence during power failure (Z99.12)*

            J95.851   Ventilator associated pneumonia
               Ventilator associated pneumonitis
               Use additional code to identify the organism, if known (B95.-, B96.-, B97.-)
               EXCLUDES 1 *ventilator lung in newborn (P27.8)*

            J95.859   Other complication of respirator [ventilator]

        J95.88   Other intraoperative complications of respiratory system, not elsewhere classified

        J95.89   Other postprocedural complications and disorders of respiratory system, not elsewhere classified
            Use additional code to identify disorder, such as:
               aspiration pneumonia (J69.-)
               bacterial or viral pneumonia (J12-J18)
            EXCLUDES 2 *acute pulmonary insufficiency following thoracic surgery (J95.1)*
               postprocedural subglottic stenosis (J95.5)

Other diseases of the respiratory system (J96-J99)

☑4ᵗʰ **J96   Respiratory failure, not elsewhere classified**
    EXCLUDES 1 *acute respiratory distress syndrome (J80)*
          cardiorespiratory failure (R09.2)
          newborn respiratory distress syndrome (P22.0)
          postprocedural respiratory failure (J95.82-)
          respiratory arrest (R09.2)
          respiratory arrest of newborn (P28.81)
          respiratory failure of newborn (P28.5)

    ☑5ᵗʰ **J96.0   Acute respiratory failure**

        J96.00   Acute respiratory failure, unspecified whether with hypoxia or hypercapnia
            AHA: 2013, 4Q, 121

        J96.01   Acute respiratory failure with hypoxia

        J96.02   Acute respiratory failure with hypercapnia

    ☑5ᵗʰ **J96.1   Chronic respiratory failure**

        J96.10   Chronic respiratory failure, unspecified whether with hypoxia or hypercapnia

        J96.11   Chronic respiratory failure with hypoxia
            AHA: 2013, 4Q, 129

        J96.12   Chronic respiratory failure with hypercapnia

    ☑5ᵗʰ **J96.2   Acute and chronic respiratory failure**
        Acute on chronic respiratory failure

        J96.20   Acute and chronic respiratory failure, unspecified whether with hypoxia or hypercapnia

        J96.21   Acute and chronic respiratory failure with hypoxia

        J96.22   Acute and chronic respiratory failure with hypercapnia

EXCLUDES 1 Not coded here   **EXCLUDES 2** Not included here   **N** Newborn Age: 0   **P** Pediatric Age: 0-17   **M** Maternity Age: 12-55   **A** Adult Age: 15-124

610   ICD-10-CM Draft (2015)

✓5ᵗʰ **J96.9   Respiratory failure, unspecified**

J96.90   Respiratory failure, unspecified, unspecified whether with hypoxia or hypercapnia

J96.91   Respiratory failure, unspecified with hypoxia

J96.92   Respiratory failure, unspecified with hypercapnia

✓4ᵗʰ **J98   Other respiratory disorders**

Use additional code to identify:
exposure to environmental tobacco smoke (Z77.22)
exposure to tobacco smoke in the perinatal period (P96.81)
history of tobacco use (Z87.891)
occupational exposure to environmental tobacco smoke (Z57.31)
tobacco dependence (F17.-)
tobacco use (Z72.0)

EXCLUDES 1   *newborn apnea (P28.4)*
newborn sleep apnea (P28.3)

EXCLUDES 2   *apnea NOS (R06.81)*
sleep apnea (G47.3-)

✓5ᵗʰ **J98.0   Diseases of bronchus, not elsewhere classified**

J98.01   Acute bronchospasm

EXCLUDES 1   *acute bronchiolitis with bronchospasm (J21.-)*
acute bronchitis with bronchospasm (J20.-)
asthma (J45.-)
exercise induced bronchospasm (J45.990)

J98.09   Other diseases of bronchus, not elsewhere classified
Broncholithiasis
Calcification of bronchus
Stenosis of bronchus
Tracheobronchial collapse
Tracheobronchial dyskinesia
Ulcer of bronchus

✓5ᵗʰ **J98.1   Pulmonary collapse**

EXCLUDES 1   *therapeutic collapse of lung status (Z98.3)*

J98.11   Atelectasis

EXCLUDES 1   *newborn atelectasis*
tuberculous atelectasis (current disease) (A15)

J98.19   Other pulmonary collapse

J98.2   Interstitial emphysema
Mediastinal emphysema

EXCLUDES 1   *emphysema NOS (J43.9)*
emphysema in newborn (P25.0)
surgical emphysema (subcutaneous) (T81.82)
traumatic subcutaneous emphysema (T79.7)

J98.3   Compensatory emphysema

J98.4   Other disorders of lung
Calcification of lung
Cystic lung disease (acquired)
Lung disease NOS
Pulmolithiasis

EXCLUDES 1   *acute interstitial pneumonitis (J84.114)*
pulmonary insufficiency following surgery (J95.1-J95.2)

J98.5   Diseases of mediastinum, not elsewhere classified
Fibrosis of mediastinum
Hernia of mediastinum
Retraction of mediastinum
Mediastinitis

EXCLUDES 2   *abscess of mediastinum (J85.3)*

J98.6   Disorders of diaphragm
Diaphragmatitis
Paralysis of diaphragm
Relaxation of diaphragm

EXCLUDES 1   *congenital malformation of diaphragm NEC (Q79.1)*
congenital diaphragmatic hernia (Q79.0)

EXCLUDES 2   *diaphragmatic hernia (K44.-)*

J98.8   Other specified respiratory disorders

J98.9   Respiratory disorder, unspecified
Respiratory disease (chronic) NOS

J99   Respiratory disorders in diseases classified elsewhere

Code first underlying disease, such as:
amyloidosis (E85.-)
ankylosing spondylitis (M45)
congenital syphilis (A50.5)
cryoglobulinemia (D89.1)
early congenital syphilis (A50.0)
schistosomiasis (B65.0-B65.9)

EXCLUDES 1   *respiratory disorders in:*
amebiasis (A06.5)
blastomycosis (B40.0-B40.2)
candidiasis (B37.1)
coccidioidomycosis (B38.0-B38.2)
cystic fibrosis with pulmonary manifestations (E84.0)
dermatomyositis (M33.01, M33.11)
histoplasmosis (B39.0-B39.2)
late syphilis (A52.72, A52.73)
polymyositis (M33.21)
sicca syndrome (M35.02)
systemic lupus erythematosus (M32.13)
systemic sclerosis (M34.81)
Wegener's granulomatosis (M31.30-M31.31)

✓ Additional Character Required   ✓7ᵗʰ *X*tension Alert   Unspecified Dx   Other Specified Dx   Manifestation   ►◄ Revised Text   ● New Code   ▲ Revised Code Title

Diseases of the Digestive System *(left margin)*
K00–K03.5 *(left margin)*

Chapter 11. Diseases of the Digestive System (K00-K95)

EXCLUDES 2
- certain conditions originating in the perinatal period (P04-P96)
- certain infectious and parasitic diseases (A00-B99)
- complications of pregnancy, childbirth and the puerperium (O00-O9A)
- congenital malformations, deformations and chromosomal abnormalities (Q00-Q99)
- endocrine, nutritional and metabolic diseases (E00-E88)
- injury, poisoning and certain other consequences of external causes (S00-T88)
- neoplasms (C00-D49)
- symptoms, signs and abnormal clinical and laboratory findings, not elsewhere classified (R00-R94)

This chapter contains the following blocks:

K00-K14   Diseases of oral cavity and salivary glands
K20-K31   Diseases of esophagus, stomach and duodenum
K35-K38   Diseases of appendix
K40-K46   Hernia
K50-K52   Noninfective enteritis and colitis
K55-K64   Other diseases of intestines
K65-K68   Diseases of peritoneum and retroperitoneum
K70-K77   Diseases of liver
K80-K87   Disorders of gallbladder, biliary tract and pancreas
K90-K95   Other diseases of the digestive system

Diseases of oral cavity and salivary glands (K00-K14)

K00   Disorders of tooth development and eruption
EXCLUDES 2 embedded and impacted teeth (K01.-)

K00.0   Anodontia
- Hypodontia
- Oligodontia
- EXCLUDES 1 acquired absence of teeth (K08.1-)

K00.1   Supernumerary teeth
- Distomolar
- Fourth molar
- Mesiodens
- Paramolar
- Supplementary teeth
- EXCLUDES 2 supernumerary roots (K00.2)

K00.2   Abnormalities of size and form of teeth
- Concrescence of teeth
- Dens evaginatus
- Dens in dente
- Dens invaginatus
- Enamel pearls
- Fusion of teeth
- Gemination of teeth
- Macrodontia
- Microdontia
- Peg-shaped [conical] teeth
- Supernumerary roots
- Taurodontism
- Tuberculum paramolare
- EXCLUDES 1 abnormalities of teeth due to congenital syphilis (A50.5) tuberculum Carabelli, which is regarded as a normal variation and should not be coded

K00.3   Mottled teeth
- Dental fluorosis
- Mottling of enamel
- Nonfluoride enamel opacities
- EXCLUDES 2 deposits [accretions] on teeth (K03.6)

K00.4   Disturbances in tooth formation
- Aplasia and hypoplasia of cementum
- Dilaceration of tooth
- Enamel hypoplasia (neonatal) (postnatal) (prenatal)
- Regional odontodysplasia
- Turner's tooth
- EXCLUDES 1 Hutchinson's teeth and mulberry molars in congenital syphilis (A50.5)
- EXCLUDES 2 mottled teeth (K00.3)

K00.5   Hereditary disturbances in tooth structure, not elsewhere classified
- Amelogenesis imperfecta
- Dentinogenesis imperfecta
- Odontogenesis imperfecta
- Dentinal dysplasia
- Shell teeth

K00.6   Disturbances in tooth eruption
- Dentia praecox
- Natal tooth
- Neonatal tooth
- Premature eruption of tooth
- Premature shedding of primary [deciduous] tooth
- Prenatal teeth
- Retained [persistent] primary tooth
- EXCLUDES 2 embedded and impacted teeth (K01.-)

K00.7   Teething syndrome

K00.8   Other disorders of tooth development
- Color changes during tooth formation
- Intrinsic staining of teeth NOS
- EXCLUDES 2 posteruptive color changes (K03.7)

K00.9   Disorder of tooth development, unspecified
- Disorder of odontogenesis NOS

K01   Embedded and impacted teeth
EXCLUDES 1 abnormal position of fully erupted teeth (M26.3-)

K01.0   Embedded teeth

K01.1   Impacted teeth

K02   Dental caries
- Dental cavities
- Tooth decay

K02.3   Arrested dental caries
- Arrested coronal and root caries

K02.5   Dental caries on pit and fissure surface
- Dental caries on chewing surface of tooth

   K02.51   Dental caries on pit and fissure surface limited to enamel
- White spot lesions [initial caries] on pit and fissure surface of tooth

   K02.52   Dental caries on pit and fissure surface penetrating into dentin

   K02.53   Dental caries on pit and fissure surface penetrating into pulp

K02.6   Dental caries on smooth surface

   K02.61   Dental caries on smooth surface limited to enamel
- White spot lesions [initial caries] on smooth surface of tooth

   K02.62   Dental caries on smooth surface penetrating into dentin

   K02.63   Dental caries on smooth surface penetrating into pulp

K02.7   Dental root caries

K02.9   Dental caries, unspecified

K03   Other diseases of hard tissues of teeth
EXCLUDES 2 bruxism (F45.8)
- dental caries (K02.-)
- teeth-grinding NOS (F45.8)

K03.0   Excessive attrition of teeth
- Approximal wear of teeth
- Occlusal wear of teeth

K03.1   Abrasion of teeth
- Dentifrice abrasion of teeth
- Habitual abrasion of teeth
- Occupational abrasion of teeth
- Ritual abrasion of teeth
- Traditional abrasion of teeth
- Wedge defect NOS

K03.2   Erosion of teeth
- Erosion of teeth due to diet
- Erosion of teeth due to drugs and medicaments
- Erosion of teeth due to persistent vomiting
- Erosion of teeth NOS
- Idiopathic erosion of teeth
- Occupational erosion of teeth

K03.3   Pathological resorption of teeth
- Internal granuloma of pulp
- Resorption of teeth (external)

K03.4   Hypercementosis
- Cementation hyperplasia

K03.5   Ankylosis of teeth

EXCLUDES 1 Not coded here   EXCLUDES 2 Not included here   N Newborn Age: 0   P Pediatric Age: 0-17   M Maternity Age: 12-55   A Adult Age: 15-124

612   ICD-10-CM Draft (2015)

K03.6　Deposits [accretions] on teeth
Betel deposits [accretions] on teeth
Black deposits [accretions] on teeth
Extrinsic staining of teeth NOS
Green deposits [accretions] on teeth
Materia alba deposits [accretions] on teeth
Orange deposits [accretions] on teeth
Staining of teeth NOS
Subgingival dental calculus
Supragingival dental calculus
Tobacco deposits [accretions] on teeth

K03.7　Posteruptive color changes of dental hard tissues
EXCLUDES 2　deposits [accretions] on teeth (K03.6)

✓5th **K03.8　Other specified diseases of hard tissues of teeth**
　K03.81　Cracked tooth
　　EXCLUDES 1　asymptomatic craze lines in enamel—omit code
　　　broken or fractured tooth due to trauma (S02.5)
　K03.89　Other specified diseases of hard tissues of teeth
K03.9　Disease of hard tissues of teeth, unspecified

✓4th **K04　Diseases of pulp and periapical tissues**
K04.0　Pulpitis
Acute pulpitis
Chronic (hyperplastic) (ulcerative) pulpitis
Irreversible pulpitis
Reversible pulpitis

K04.1　Necrosis of pulp
Pulpal gangrene

K04.2　Pulp degeneration
Denticles
Pulpal calcifications
Pulpal stones

K04.3　Abnormal hard tissue formation in pulp
Secondary or irregular dentine

K04.4　Acute apical periodontitis of pulpal origin
Acute apical periodontitis NOS
EXCLUDES 1　acute periodontitis (K05.2-)

K04.5　Chronic apical periodontitis
Apical or periapical granuloma
Apical periodontitis NOS
EXCLUDES 1　chronic periodontitis (K05.3-)

K04.6　Periapical abscess with sinus
Dental abscess with sinus
Dentoalveolar abscess with sinus

K04.7　Periapical abscess without sinus
Dental abscess without sinus
Dentoalveolar abscess without sinus
Periapical abscess without sinus

K04.8　Radicular cyst
Apical (periodontal) cyst
Periapical cyst
Residual radicular cyst
EXCLUDES 2　lateral periodontal cyst (K09.0)

✓5th **K04.9　Other and unspecified diseases of pulp and periapical tissues**
　K04.90　Unspecified diseases of pulp and periapical tissues
　K04.99　Other diseases of pulp and periapical tissues

✓4th **K05　Gingivitis and periodontal diseases**
Use additional code to identify:
alcohol abuse and dependence (F10.-)
exposure to environmental tobacco smoke (Z77.22)
exposure to tobacco smoke in the perinatal period (P96.81)
history of tobacco use (Z87.891)
occupational exposure to environmental tobacco smoke (Z57.31)
tobacco dependence (F17.-)
tobacco use (Z72.0)

✓5th **K05.0　Acute gingivitis**
　EXCLUDES 1　acute necrotizing ulcerative gingivitis (A69.1)
　　herpesviral [herpes simplex] gingivostomatitis (B00.2)
　K05.00　Acute gingivitis, plaque induced
　　Acute gingivitis NOS
　K05.01　Acute gingivitis, non-plaque induced

✓5th **K05.1　Chronic gingivitis**
Desquamative gingivitis (chronic)
Gingivitis (chronic) NOS
Hyperplastic gingivitis (chronic)
Simple marginal gingivitis (chronic)
Ulcerative gingivitis (chronic)

　K05.10　Chronic gingivitis, plaque induced
　　Chronic gingivitis NOS
　　Gingivitis NOS
　K05.11　Chronic gingivitis, non-plaque induced

✓5th **K05.2　Aggressive periodontitis**
Acute pericoronitis
EXCLUDES 1　acute apical periodontitis (K04.4)
　periapical abscess (K04.7)
　periapical abscess with sinus (K04.6)

　K05.20　Aggressive periodontitis, unspecified
　K05.21　Aggressive periodontitis, localized
　　Periodontal abscess
　K05.22　Aggressive periodontitis, generalized

✓5th **K05.3　Chronic periodontitis**
Chronic pericoronitis
Complex periodontitis
Periodontitis NOS
Simplex periodontitis
EXCLUDES 1　chronic apical periodontitis (K04.5)

　K05.30　Chronic periodontitis, unspecified
　K05.31　Chronic periodontitis, localized
　K05.32　Chronic periodontitis, generalized

K05.4　Periodontosis
Juvenile periodontosis

K05.5　Other periodontal diseases
EXCLUDES 2　leukoplakia of gingiva (K13.21)

K05.6　Periodontal disease, unspecified

✓4th **K06　Other disorders of gingiva and edentulous alveolar ridge**
EXCLUDES 2　acute gingivitis (K05.0)
　atrophy of edentulous alveolar ridge (K08.2)
　chronic gingivitis (K05.1)
　gingivitis NOS (K05.1)

K06.0　Gingival recession
Gingival recession (generalized) (localized) (postinfective) (postprocedural)

K06.1　Gingival enlargement
Gingival fibromatosis

K06.2　Gingival and edentulous alveolar ridge lesions associated with trauma
Irritative hyperplasia of edentulous ridge [denture hyperplasia]
Use additional code (Chapter 20) to identify external cause or denture status (Z97.2)

K06.8　Other specified disorders of gingiva and edentulous alveolar ridge
Fibrous epulis
Flabby alveolar ridge
Giant cell epulis
Peripheral giant cell granuloma of gingiva
Pyogenic granuloma of gingiva
EXCLUDES 2　gingival cyst (K09.0)

K06.9　Disorder of gingiva and edentulous alveolar ridge, unspecified

✓4th **K08　Other disorders of teeth and supporting structures**
EXCLUDES 2　dentofacial anomalies [including malocclusion] (M26.-)
　disorders of jaw (M27.-)

K08.0　Exfoliation of teeth due to systemic causes
Code also underlying systemic condition

✓5th **K08.1　Complete loss of teeth**
Acquired loss of teeth, complete
EXCLUDES 1　congenital absence of teeth (K00.0)
　exfoliation of teeth due to systemic causes (K08.0)
　partial loss of teeth (K08.4-)

　✓6th **K08.10　Complete loss of teeth, unspecified cause**
　　K08.101　Complete loss of teeth, unspecified cause, class I
　　K08.102　Complete loss of teeth, unspecified cause, class II
　　K08.103　Complete loss of teeth, unspecified cause, class III
　　K08.104　Complete loss of teeth, unspecified cause, class IV
　　K08.109　Complete loss of teeth, unspecified cause, unspecified class
　　　Edentulism NOS

　✓6th **K08.11　Complete loss of teeth due to trauma**
　　K08.111　Complete loss of teeth due to trauma, class I

☑ Additional Character Required　　✓x7th Xtension Alert　　Unspecified Dx　　Other Specified Dx　　Manifestation　　▶◀ Revised Text　　● New Code　　▲ Revised Code Title

Diseases of the Digestive System

K08.112–K08.59

    K08.112   Complete loss of teeth due to trauma, class II

    K08.113   Complete loss of teeth due to trauma, class III

    K08.114   Complete loss of teeth due to trauma, class IV

    K08.119   Complete loss of teeth due to trauma, unspecified class

✓6ᵗʰ **K08.12**   Complete loss of teeth due to periodontal diseases

    K08.121   Complete loss of teeth due to periodontal diseases, class I

    K08.122   Complete loss of teeth due to periodontal diseases, class II

    K08.123   Complete loss of teeth due to periodontal diseases, class III

    K08.124   Complete loss of teeth due to periodontal diseases, class IV

    K08.129   Complete loss of teeth due to periodontal diseases, unspecified class

✓6ᵗʰ **K08.13**   Complete loss of teeth due to caries

    K08.131   Complete loss of teeth due to caries, class I

    K08.132   Complete loss of teeth due to caries, class II

    K08.133   Complete loss of teeth due to caries, class III

    K08.134   Complete loss of teeth due to caries, class IV

    K08.139   Complete loss of teeth due to caries, unspecified class

✓6ᵗʰ **K08.19**   Complete loss of teeth due to other specified cause

    K08.191   Complete loss of teeth due to other specified cause, class I

    K08.192   Complete loss of teeth due to other specified cause, class II

    K08.193   Complete loss of teeth due to other specified cause, class III

    K08.194   Complete loss of teeth due to other specified cause, class IV

    K08.199   Complete loss of teeth due to other specified cause, unspecified class

✓5ᵗʰ **K08.2**   Atrophy of edentulous alveolar ridge

    K08.20   Unspecified atrophy of edentulous alveolar ridge
Atrophy of the mandible NOS
Atrophy of the maxilla NOS

    K08.21   Minimal atrophy of the mandible
Minimal atrophy of the edentulous mandible

    K08.22   Moderate atrophy of the mandible
Moderate atrophy of the edentulous mandible

    K08.23   Severe atrophy of the mandible
Severe atrophy of the edentulous mandible

    K08.24   Minimal atrophy of maxilla
Minimal atrophy of the edentulous maxilla

    K08.25   Moderate atrophy of the maxilla
Moderate atrophy of the edentulous maxilla

    K08.26   Severe atrophy of the maxilla
Severe atrophy of the edentulous maxilla

K08.3   Retained dental root

✓5ᵗʰ **K08.4**   Partial loss of teeth
Acquired loss of teeth, partial
EXCLUDES 1   complete loss of teeth (K08.1-)
     congenital absence of teeth (K00.0)
EXCLUDES 2   exfoliation of teeth due to systemic causes (K08.0)

✓6ᵗʰ **K08.40**   Partial loss of teeth, unspecified cause

    K08.401   Partial loss of teeth, unspecified cause, class I

    K08.402   Partial loss of teeth, unspecified cause, class II

    K08.403   Partial loss of teeth, unspecified cause, class III

    K08.404   Partial loss of teeth, unspecified cause, class IV

    K08.409   Partial loss of teeth, unspecified cause, unspecified class
Tooth extraction status NOS

✓6ᵗʰ **K08.41**   Partial loss of teeth due to trauma

    K08.411   Partial loss of teeth due to trauma, class I

    K08.412   Partial loss of teeth due to trauma, class II

    K08.413   Partial loss of teeth due to trauma, class III

    K08.414   Partial loss of teeth due to trauma, class IV

    K08.419   Partial loss of teeth due to trauma, unspecified class

✓6ᵗʰ **K08.42**   Partial loss of teeth due to periodontal diseases

    K08.421   Partial loss of teeth due to periodontal diseases, class I

    K08.422   Partial loss of teeth due to periodontal diseases, class II

    K08.423   Partial loss of teeth due to periodontal diseases, class III

    K08.424   Partial loss of teeth due to periodontal diseases, class IV

    K08.429   Partial loss of teeth due to periodontal diseases, unspecified class

✓6ᵗʰ **K08.43**   Partial loss of teeth due to caries

    K08.431   Partial loss of teeth due to caries, class I

    K08.432   Partial loss of teeth due to caries, class II

    K08.433   Partial loss of teeth due to caries, class III

    K08.434   Partial loss of teeth due to caries, class IV

    K08.439   Partial loss of teeth due to caries, unspecified class

✓6ᵗʰ **K08.49**   Partial loss of teeth due to other specified cause

    K08.491   Partial loss of teeth due to other specified cause, class I

    K08.492   Partial loss of teeth due to other specified cause, class II

    K08.493   Partial loss of teeth due to other specified cause, class III

    K08.494   Partial loss of teeth due to other specified cause, class IV

    K08.499   Partial loss of teeth due to other specified cause, unspecified class

✓5ᵗʰ **K08.5**   Unsatisfactory restoration of tooth
Defective bridge, crown, filling
Defective dental restoration
EXCLUDES 1   dental restoration status (Z98.811)
EXCLUDES 2   endosseous dental implant failure (M27.6-)
     unsatisfactory endodontic treatment (M27.5-)

    K08.50   Unsatisfactory restoration of tooth, unspecified
Defective dental restoration NOS

    K08.51   Open restoration margins of tooth
Dental restoration failure of marginal integrity
Open margin on tooth restoration
Poor gingival margin to tooth restoration

    K08.52   Unrepairable overhanging of dental restorative materials
Overhanging of tooth restoration

✓6ᵗʰ **K08.53**   Fractured dental restorative material
EXCLUDES 1   cracked tooth (K03.81)
     traumatic fracture of tooth (S02.5)

    K08.530   Fractured dental restorative material without loss of material

    K08.531   Fractured dental restorative material with loss of material

    K08.539   Fractured dental restorative material, unspecified

    K08.54   Contour of existing restoration of tooth biologically incompatible with oral health
Dental restoration failure of periodontal anatomical integrity
Unacceptable contours of existing restoration of tooth
Unacceptable morphology of existing restoration of tooth

    K08.55   Allergy to existing dental restorative material
Use additional code to identify the specific type of allergy

    K08.56   Poor aesthetic of existing restoration of tooth
Dental restoration aesthetically inadequate or displeasing

    K08.59   Other unsatisfactory restoration of tooth
Other defective dental restoration

EXCLUDES 1 Not coded here   EXCLUDES 2 Not included here   N Newborn Age: 0   P Pediatric Age: 0-17   M Maternity Age: 12-55   A Adult Age: 15-124

614   ICD-10-CM Draft (2015)

K08.8   Other specified disorders of teeth and supporting structures
Enlargement of alveolar ridge NOS
Irregular alveolar process
Toothache NOS

K08.9   Disorder of teeth and supporting structures, unspecified

✓4ᵗʰ **K09   Cysts of oral region, not elsewhere classified**
INCLUDES   lesions showing histological features both of aneurysmal cyst and of another fibro-osseous lesion
EXCLUDES 2   cysts of jaw (M27.0-, M27.4-)
radicular cyst (K04.8)

K09.0   Developmental odontogenic cysts
Dentigerous cyst
Eruption cyst
Follicular cyst
Gingival cyst
Lateral periodontal cyst
Primordial cyst
EXCLUDES 2   keratocysts (D16.4, D16.5)
odontogenic keratocystic tumors (D16.4, D16.5)

K09.1   Developmental (nonodontogenic) cysts of oral region
Cyst (of) incisive canal
Cyst (of) palatine of papilla
Globulomaxillary cyst
Median palatal cyst
Nasoalveolar cyst
Nasolabial cyst
Nasopalatine duct cyst

K09.8   Other cysts of oral region, not elsewhere classified
Dermoid cyst
Epidermoid cyst
Lymphoepithelial cyst
Epstein's pearl

K09.9   Cyst of oral region, unspecified

✓4ᵗʰ **K11   Diseases of salivary glands**
Use additional code to identify:
alcohol abuse and dependence (F10.-)
exposure to environmental tobacco smoke (Z77.22)
exposure to tobacco smoke in the perinatal period (P96.81)
history of tobacco use (Z87.891)
occupational exposure to environmental tobacco smoke (Z57.31)
tobacco dependence (F17.-)
tobacco use (Z72.0)

K11.0   Atrophy of salivary gland

K11.1   Hypertrophy of salivary gland

✓5ᵗʰ **K11.2   Sialoadenitis**
Parotitis
EXCLUDES 1   epidemic parotitis (B26.-)
mumps (B26.-)
uveoparotid fever [Heerfordt] (D86.89)

K11.20   Sialoadenitis, unspecified

K11.21   Acute sialoadenitis
EXCLUDES 1   acute recurrent sialoadenitis (K11.22)

K11.22   Acute recurrent sialoadenitis

K11.23   Chronic sialoadenitis

K11.3   Abscess of salivary gland

K11.4   Fistula of salivary gland
EXCLUDES 1   congenital fistula of salivary gland (Q38.4)

K11.5   Sialolithiasis
Calculus of salivary gland or duct
Stone of salivary gland or duct

K11.6   Mucocele of salivary gland
Mucous extravasation cyst of salivary gland
Mucous retention cyst of salivary gland
Ranula

K11.7   Disturbances of salivary secretion
Hypoptyalism
Ptyalism
Xerostomia
EXCLUDES 2   dry mouth NOS (R68.2)

K11.8   Other diseases of salivary glands
Benign lymphoepithelial lesion of salivary gland
Mikulicz' disease
Necrotizing sialometaplasia
Sialectasia
Stenosis of salivary duct
Stricture of salivary duct
EXCLUDES 1   sicca syndrome [Sjögren] (M35.0-)

K11.9   Disease of salivary gland, unspecified
Sialoadenopathy NOS

✓4ᵗʰ **K12   Stomatitis and related lesions**
Use additional code to identify:
alcohol abuse and dependence (F10.-)
exposure to environmental tobacco smoke (Z77.22)
exposure to tobacco smoke in the perinatal period (P96.81)
history of tobacco use (Z87.891)
occupational exposure to environmental tobacco smoke (Z57.31)
tobacco dependence (F17.-)
tobacco use (Z72.0)
EXCLUDES 1   cancrum oris (A69.0)
cheilitis (K13.0)
gangrenous stomatitis (A69.0)
herpesviral [herpes simplex] gingivostomatitis (B00.2)
noma (A69.0)

K12.0   Recurrent oral aphthae
Aphthous stomatitis (major) (minor)
Bednar's aphthae
Periadenitis mucosa necrotica recurrens
Recurrent aphthous ulcer
Stomatitis herpetiformis

K12.1   Other forms of stomatitis
Stomatitis NOS   Ulcerative stomatitis
Denture stomatitis   Vesicular stomatitis
EXCLUDES 1   acute necrotizing ulcerative stomatitis (A69.1)
Vincent's stomatitis (A69.1)

K12.2   Cellulitis and abscess of mouth
Cellulitis of mouth (floor)
Submandibular abscess
EXCLUDES 2   abscess of salivary gland (K11.3)
abscess of tongue (K14.0)
periapical abscess (K04.6-K04.7)
periodontal abscess (K05.21)
peritonsillar abscess (J36)

✓5ᵗʰ **K12.3   Oral mucositis (ulcerative)**
Mucositis (oral) (oropharyneal)
EXCLUDES 2   gastrointestinal mucositis (ulcerative) (K92.81)
mucositis (ulcerative) of vagina and vulva (N76.81)
nasal mucositis (ulcerative) (J34.81)

K12.30   Oral mucositis (ulcerative), unspecified

K12.31   Oral mucositis (ulcerative) due to antineoplastic therapy
Use additional code for adverse effect, if applicable, to identify antineoplastic and immunosuppressive drugs (T45.1X5)
Use additional code for other antineoplastic therapy, such as:
radiological procedure and radiotherapy (Y84.2)

K12.32   Oral mucositis (ulcerative) due to other drugs
Use additional code for adverse effect, if applicable, to identify drug (T36-T50 with fifth or sixth character 5)

K12.33   Oral mucositis (ulcerative) due to radiation
Use additional external cause code (W88-W90, X39.0-) to identify cause

K12.39   Other oral mucositis (ulcerative)
Viral oral mucositis (ulcerative)

☑ Additional Character Required   ✓x7ᵗʰ Xtension Alert   Unspecified Dx   Other Specified Dx   Manifestation   ►◄ Revised Text   ● New Code   ▲ Revised Code Title

✓4th K13 Other diseases of lip and oral mucosa
> INCLUDES epithelial disturbances of tongue

Use additional code to identify:
alcohol abuse and dependence (F10.-)
exposure to environmental tobacco smoke (Z77.22)
exposure to tobacco smoke in the perinatal period (P96.81)
history of tobacco use (Z87.891)
occupational exposure to environmental tobacco smoke (Z57.31)
tobacco dependence (F17.-)
tobacco use (Z72.0)
> EXCLUDES 2 certain disorders of gingiva and edentulous alveolar ridge (K05-K06)
> cysts of oral region (K09.-)
> diseases of tongue (K14.-)
> stomatitis and related lesions (K12.-)

K13.0 Diseases of lips
Abscess of lips	Exfoliative cheilitis
Angular cheilitis	Fistula of lips
Cellulitis of lips	Glandular cheilitis
Cheilitis NOS	Hypertrophy of lips
Cheilodynia	Perlèche NEC
Cheilosis	

> EXCLUDES 1 ariboflavinosis (E53.0)
> cheilitis due to radiation-related disorders (L55-L59)
> congenital fistula of lips (Q38.0)
> congenital hypertrophy of lips (Q18.6)
> Perlèche due to candidiasis (B37.83)
> Perlèche due to riboflavin deficiency (E53.0)

K13.1 Cheek and lip biting

✓5th K13.2 Leukoplakia and other disturbances of oral epithelium, including tongue
> EXCLUDES 1 carcinoma in situ of oral epithelium (D00.0-)
> hairy leukoplakia (K13.3)

K13.21 Leukoplakia of oral mucosa, including tongue
Leukokeratosis of oral mucosa
Leukoplakia of gingiva, lips, tongue
> EXCLUDES 1 hairy leukoplakia (K13.3)
> leukokeratosis nicotina palati (K13.24)

K13.22 Minimal keratinized residual ridge mucosa
Minimal keratinization of alveolar ridge mucosa

K13.23 Excessive keratinized residual ridge mucosa
Excessive keratinization of alveolar ridge mucosa

K13.24 Leukokeratosis nicotina palati
Smoker's palate

K13.29 Other disturbances of oral epithelium, including tongue
Erythroplakia of mouth or tongue
Focal epithelial hyperplasia of mouth or tongue
Leukoedema of mouth or tongue
Other oral epithelium disturbances

K13.3 Hairy leukoplakia

K13.4 Granuloma and granuloma-like lesions of oral mucosa
Eosinophilic granuloma   Verrucous xanthoma
Granuloma pyogenicum

K13.5 Oral submucous fibrosis
Submucous fibrosis of tongue

K13.6 Irritative hyperplasia of oral mucosa
> EXCLUDES 2 irritative hyperplasia of edentulous ridge [denture hyperplasia] (K06.2)

✓5th K13.7 Other and unspecified lesions of oral mucosa

K13.70 Unspecified lesions of oral mucosa

K13.79 Other lesions of oral mucosa
Focal oral mucinosis

✓4th K14 Diseases of tongue
Use additional code to identify:
alcohol abuse and dependence (F10.-)
exposure to environmental tobacco smoke (Z77.22)
history of tobacco use (Z87.891)
occupational exposure to environmental tobacco smoke (Z57.31)
tobacco dependence (F17.-)
tobacco use (Z72.0)
> EXCLUDES 2 erythroplakia (K13.29)
> focal epithelial hyperplasia (K13.29)
> leukedema of tongue (K13.29)
> leukoplakia of tongue (K13.21)
> hairy leukoplakia (K13.3)
> macroglossia (congenital) (Q38.2)
> submucous fibrosis of tongue (K13.5)

K14.0 Glossitis
Abscess of tongue   Ulceration (traumatic) of tongue
> EXCLUDES 1 atrophic glossitis (K14.4)

K14.1 Geographic tongue
Benign migratory glossitis
Glossitis areata exfoliativa

K14.2 Median rhomboid glossitis

K14.3 Hypertrophy of tongue papillae
Black hairy tongue
Coated tongue
Hypertrophy of foliate papillae
Lingua villosa nigra

K14.4 Atrophy of tongue papillae
Atrophic glossitis

K14.5 Plicated tongue
Fissured tongue
Furrowed tongue
Scrotal tongue
> EXCLUDES 1 fissured tongue, congenital (Q38.3)

K14.6 Glossodynia
Glossopyrosis
Painful tongue

K14.8 Other diseases of tongue
Atrophy of tongue
Crenated tongue
Enlargement of tongue
Glossocele
Glossoptosis
Hypertrophy of tongue

K14.9 Disease of tongue, unspecified
Glossopathy NOS

Diseases of esophagus, stomach and duodenum (K20-K31)
> EXCLUDES 2 hiatus hernia (K44.-)

✓4th K20 Esophagitis
Use additional code to identify:
alcohol abuse and dependence (F10.-)
> EXCLUDES 1 erosion of esophagus (K22.1-)
> esophagitis with gastro-esophageal reflux disease (K21.0)
> reflux esophagitis (K21.0)
> ulcerative esophagitis (K22.1-)
> EXCLUDES 2 eosinophilic gastritis or gastroenteritis (K52.81)

K20.0 Eosinophilic esophagitis

K20.8 Other esophagitis
Abscess of esophagus

K20.9 Esophagitis, unspecified
Esophagitis NOS

✓4th K21 Gastro-esophageal reflux disease
> EXCLUDES 1 newborn esophageal reflux (P78.83)

K21.0 Gastro-esophageal reflux disease with esophagitis
Reflux esophagitis

K21.9 Gastro-esophageal reflux disease without esophagitis
Esophageal reflux NOS

✓4th K22 Other diseases of esophagus
> EXCLUDES 2 esophageal varices (I85.-)

K22.0 Achalasia of cardia
Achalasia NOS
Cardiospasm
> EXCLUDES 1 congenital cardiospasm (Q39.5)

✓5th K22.1 Ulcer of esophagus
Barrett's ulcer
Erosion of esophagus
Fungal ulcer of esophagus
Peptic ulcer of esophagus
Ulcer of esophagus due to ingestion of chemicals
Ulcer of esophagus due to ingestion of drugs and medicaments
Ulcerative esophagitis
Code first poisoning due to drug or toxin, if applicable (T36-T65 with fifth or sixth character 1-4 or 6)
Use additional code for adverse effect, if applicable, to identify drug (T36-T50 with fifth or sixth character 5)
> EXCLUDES 1 Barrett's esophagus (K22.7-)

K22.10 Ulcer of esophagus without bleeding
Ulcer of esophagus NOS

K22.11 Ulcer of esophagus with bleeding
> EXCLUDES 2 bleeding esophageal varices (I85.01, I85.11)

K22.2 Esophageal obstruction
Compression of esophagus
Constriction of esophagus
Stenosis of esophagus
Stricture of esophagus
> EXCLUDES 1 congenital stenosis or stricture of esophagus (Q39.3)

EXCLUDES 1 Not coded here   EXCLUDES 2 Not included here   N Newborn Age: 0   P Pediatric Age: 0-17   M Maternity Age: 12-55   A Adult Age: 15-124

616   ICD-10-CM Draft (2015)

K22.3   Perforation of esophagus
Rupture of esophagus
EXCLUDES 1   *traumatic perforation of (thoracic) esophagus (S27.8-)*

K22.4   Dyskinesia of esophagus
Corkscrew esophagus
Diffuse esophageal spasm
Spasm of esophagus
EXCLUDES 1   *cardiospasm (K22.0)*

K22.5   Diverticulum of esophagus, acquired
Esophageal pouch, acquired
EXCLUDES 1   *diverticulum of esophagus (congenital) (Q39.6)*

K22.6   Gastro-esophageal laceration-hemorrhage syndrome
Mallory-Weiss syndrome

✓5th **K22.7   Barrett's esophagus**
Barrett's disease
Barrett's syndrome
EXCLUDES 1   *Barrett's ulcer (K22.1)*
              malignant neoplasm of esophagus (C15.-)

    K22.70   Barrett's esophagus without dysplasia
Barrett's esophagus NOS

    ✓6th **K22.71   Barrett's esophagus with dysplasia**

        K22.710   Barrett's esophagus with low grade dysplasia

        K22.711   Barrett's esophagus with high grade dysplasia

        K22.719   Barrett's esophagus with dysplasia, unspecified

K22.8   Other specified diseases of esophagus
Hemorrhage of esophagus NOS
EXCLUDES 2   *esophageal varices (I85.-)*
              Paterson-Kelly syndrome (D50.1)

K22.9   Disease of esophagus, unspecified

K23   Disorders of esophagus in diseases classified elsewhere
Code first underlying disease, such as:
  congenital syphilis (A50.5)
EXCLUDES 1   *late syphilis (A52.79)*
              megaesophagus due to Chagas' disease (B57.31)
              tuberculosis (A18.83)

✓4th **K25   Gastric ulcer**
INCLUDES   erosion (acute) of stomach
            pylorus ulcer (peptic)
            stomach ulcer (peptic)
Use additional code to identify:
  alcohol abuse and dependence (F10.-)
EXCLUDES 1   *acute gastritis (K29.0-)*
              peptic ulcer NOS (K27.-)

K25.0   Acute gastric ulcer with hemorrhage

K25.1   Acute gastric ulcer with perforation

K25.2   Acute gastric ulcer with both hemorrhage and perforation

K25.3   Acute gastric ulcer without hemorrhage or perforation

K25.4   Chronic or unspecified gastric ulcer with hemorrhage

K25.5   Chronic or unspecified gastric ulcer with perforation

K25.6   Chronic or unspecified gastric ulcer with both hemorrhage and perforation

K25.7   Chronic gastric ulcer without hemorrhage or perforation

K25.9   Gastric ulcer, unspecified as acute or chronic, without hemorrhage or perforation

✓4th **K26   Duodenal ulcer**
INCLUDES   erosion (acute) of duodenum
            duodenum ulcer (peptic)
            postpyloric ulcer (peptic)
Use additional code to identify:
  alcohol abuse and dependence (F10.-)
EXCLUDES 1   *peptic ulcer NOS (K27.-)*

K26.0   Acute duodenal ulcer with hemorrhage

K26.1   Acute duodenal ulcer with perforation

K26.2   Acute duodenal ulcer with both hemorrhage and perforation

K26.3   Acute duodenal ulcer without hemorrhage or perforation

K26.4   Chronic or unspecified duodenal ulcer with hemorrhage

K26.5   Chronic or unspecified duodenal ulcer with perforation

K26.6   Chronic or unspecified duodenal ulcer with both hemorrhage and perforation

K26.7   Chronic duodenal ulcer without hemorrhage or perforation

K26.9   Duodenal ulcer, unspecified as acute or chronic, without hemorrhage or perforation

✓4th **K27   Peptic ulcer, site unspecified**
INCLUDES   gastroduodenal ulcer NOS
            peptic ulcer NOS
Use additional code to identify:
  alcohol abuse and dependence (F10.-)
EXCLUDES 1   *peptic ulcer of newborn (P78.82)*

K27.0   Acute peptic ulcer, site unspecified, with hemorrhage

K27.1   Acute peptic ulcer, site unspecified, with perforation

K27.2   Acute peptic ulcer, site unspecified, with both hemorrhage and perforation

K27.3   Acute peptic ulcer, site unspecified, without hemorrhage or perforation

K27.4   Chronic or unspecified peptic ulcer, site unspecified, with hemorrhage

K27.5   Chronic or unspecified peptic ulcer, site unspecified, with perforation

K27.6   Chronic or unspecified peptic ulcer, site unspecified, with both hemorrhage and perforation

K27.7   Chronic peptic ulcer, site unspecified, without hemorrhage or perforation

K27.9   Peptic ulcer, site unspecified, unspecified as acute or chronic, without hemorrhage or perforation

✓4th **K28   Gastrojejunal ulcer**
INCLUDES   anastomotic ulcer (peptic) or erosion
            gastrocolic ulcer (peptic) or erosion
            gastrointestinal ulcer (peptic) or erosion
            gastrojejunal ulcer (peptic) or erosion
            jejunal ulcer (peptic) or erosion
            marginal ulcer (peptic) or erosion
            stomal ulcer (peptic) or erosion
Use additional code to identify:
  alcohol abuse and dependence (F10.-)
EXCLUDES 1   *primary ulcer of small intestine (K63.3)*

K28.0   Acute gastrojejunal ulcer with hemorrhage

K28.1   Acute gastrojejunal ulcer with perforation

K28.2   Acute gastrojejunal ulcer with both hemorrhage and perforation

K28.3   Acute gastrojejunal ulcer without hemorrhage or perforation

K28.4   Chronic or unspecified gastrojejunal ulcer with hemorrhage

K28.5   Chronic or unspecified gastrojejunal ulcer with perforation

K28.6   Chronic or unspecified gastrojejunal ulcer with both hemorrhage and perforation

K28.7   Chronic gastrojejunal ulcer without hemorrhage or perforation

K28.9   Gastrojejunal ulcer, unspecified as acute or chronic, without hemorrhage or perforation

✓4th **K29   Gastritis and duodenitis**
EXCLUDES 1   *eosinophilic gastritis or gastroenteritis (K52.81)*
              Zollinger-Ellison syndrome (E16.4)

✓5th **K29.0   Acute gastritis**
Use additional code to identify:
  alcohol abuse and dependence (F10.-)
EXCLUDES 1   *erosion (acute) of stomach (K25.-)*

    K29.00   Acute gastritis without bleeding

    K29.01   Acute gastritis with bleeding

✓5th **K29.2   Alcoholic gastritis**
Use additional code to identify:
  alcohol abuse and dependence (F10.-)

    K29.20   Alcoholic gastritis without bleeding

    K29.21   Alcoholic gastritis with bleeding

✓5th **K29.3   Chronic superficial gastritis**

    K29.30   Chronic superficial gastritis without bleeding

    K29.31   Chronic superficial gastritis with bleeding

✓5th **K29.4   Chronic atrophic gastritis**
Gastric atrophy

    K29.40   Chronic atrophic gastritis without bleeding

    K29.41   Chronic atrophic gastritis with bleeding

✓5th **K29.5   Unspecified chronic gastritis**
Chronic antral gastritis
Chronic fundal gastritis

    K29.50   Unspecified chronic gastritis without bleeding

    K29.51   Unspecified chronic gastritis with bleeding

☑ Additional Character Required   ✓x7th Xtension Alert   Unspecified Dx   Other Specified Dx   Manifestation   ►◄ Revised Text   ● New Code   ▲ Revised Code Title

ICD-10-CM Draft (2015)   617

Diseases of the Digestive System

K29.6–K40.21

✓5th **K29.6** Other gastritis
Giant hypertrophic gastritis
Granulomatous gastritis
Ménétrier's disease

     K29.60 Other gastritis without bleeding
     K29.61 Other gastritis with bleeding

✓5th **K29.7** Gastritis, unspecified

     K29.70 Gastritis, unspecified, without bleeding
     K29.71 Gastritis, unspecified, with bleeding

✓5th **K29.8** Duodenitis

     K29.80 Duodenitis without bleeding
     K29.81 Duodenitis with bleeding

✓5th **K29.9** Gastroduodenitis, unspecified

     K29.90 Gastroduodenitis, unspecified, without bleeding
     K29.91 Gastroduodenitis, unspecified, with bleeding

K30 **Functional dyspepsia**
Indigestion
EXCLUDES 1   dyspepsia NOS (R10.13)
     heartburn (R12)
     nervous dyspepsia (F45.8)
     neurotic dyspepsia (F45.8)
     psychogenic dyspepsia (F45.8)

✓4th **K31** **Other diseases of stomach and duodenum**
INCLUDES   functional disorders of stomach
EXCLUDES 2   diabetic gastroparesis (E08.43, E09.43, E10.43, E11.43, E13.43)
     diverticulum of duodenum (K57.00-K57.13)

     K31.0 **Acute dilatation of stomach**
       Acute distention of stomach

     K31.1 **Adult hypertrophic pyloric stenosis**   A
       Pyloric stenosis NOS
       EXCLUDES 1   congenital or infantile pyloric stenosis (Q40.0)

     K31.2 **Hourglass stricture and stenosis of stomach**
       EXCLUDES 1   congenital hourglass stomach (Q40.2)
           hourglass contraction of stomach (K31.89)

     K31.3 **Pylorospasm, not elsewhere classified**
       EXCLUDES 1   congenital or infantile pylorospasm (Q40.0)
           neurotic pylorospasm (F45.8)
           psychogenic pylorospasm (F45.8)

     K31.4 **Gastric diverticulum**
       EXCLUDES 1   congenital diverticulum of stomach (Q40.2)

     K31.5 **Obstruction of duodenum**
       Constriction of duodenum
       Duodenal ileus (chronic)
       Stenosis of duodenum
       Stricture of duodenum
       Volvulus of duodenum
       EXCLUDES 1   congenital stenosis of duodenum (Q41.0)

     K31.6 **Fistula of stomach and duodenum**
       Gastrocolic fistula
       Gastrojejunocolic fistula

     K31.7 **Polyp of stomach and duodenum**
       EXCLUDES 1   adenomatous polyp of stomach (D13.1)

✓5th **K31.8** **Other specified diseases of stomach and duodenum**

     ✓6th **K31.81** **Angiodysplasia of stomach and duodenum**
         K31.811 **Angiodysplasia of stomach and duodenum with bleeding**
         K31.819 **Angiodysplasia of stomach and duodenum without bleeding**
            Angiodysplasia of stomach and duodenum NOS

     K31.82 **Dieulafoy lesion (hemorrhagic) of stomach and duodenum**
         EXCLUDES 2   Dieulafoy lesion of intestine (K63.81)

     K31.83 **Achlorhydria**

     K31.84 **Gastroparesis**
         Gastroparalysis
         Code first underlying disease, if known, such as:
           anorexia nervosa (F50.0-)
           diabetes mellitus (E08.43, E09.43, E10.43, E11.43, E13.43)
           scleroderma (M34.-)
         AHA: 2013, 4Q, 114

     K31.89 Other diseases of stomach and duodenum
     K31.9 **Disease of stomach and duodenum, unspecified**

Diseases of appendix (K35-K38)

✓4th **K35** **Acute appendicitis**

     K35.2 **Acute appendicitis with generalized peritonitis**
       Appendicitis (acute) with generalized (diffuse) peritonitis following rupture or perforation of appendix
       Perforated appendix NOS
       Ruptured appendix NOS

     K35.3 **Acute appendicitis with localized peritonitis**
       Acute appendicitis with or without perforation or rupture NOS
       Acute appendicitis with or without perforation or rupture with localized peritonitis
       Acute appendicitis with peritoneal abscess

     ✓5th **K35.8** Other and unspecified acute appendicitis
       K35.80 **Unspecified acute appendicitis**
         Acute appendicitis NOS
         Acute appendicitis without (localized) (generalized) peritonitis

       K35.89 Other acute appendicitis

K36 Other appendicitis
     Chronic appendicitis
     Recurrent appendicitis

K37 **Unspecified appendicitis**
     EXCLUDES 1   unspecified appendicitis with peritonitis (K35.2-K35.3)

✓4th **K38** **Other diseases of appendix**

     K38.0 **Hyperplasia of appendix**

     K38.1 **Appendicular concretions**
       Fecalith of appendix
       Stercolith of appendix

     K38.2 **Diverticulum of appendix**

     K38.3 **Fistula of appendix**

     K38.8 Other specified diseases of appendix
       Intussusception of appendix

     K38.9 **Disease of appendix, unspecified**

Hernia (K40-K46)

NOTE   Hernia with both gangrene and obstruction is classified to hernia with gangrene.
INCLUDES   acquired hernia
congenital [except diaphragmatic or hiatus] hernia
recurrent hernia

✓4th **K40** Inguinal hernia
INCLUDES   bubonocele
direct inguinal hernia
double inguinal hernia
indirect inguinal hernia
inguinal hernia NOS
oblique inguinal hernia
scrotal hernia

✓5th **K40.0** Bilateral inguinal hernia, with obstruction, without gangrene
     Inguinal hernia (bilateral) causing obstruction without gangrene
     Incarcerated inguinal hernia (bilateral) without gangrene
     Irreducible inguinal hernia (bilateral) without gangrene
     Strangulated inguinal hernia (bilateral) without gangrene

     K40.00 **Bilateral inguinal hernia, with obstruction, without gangrene, not specified as recurrent**
       Bilateral inguinal hernia, with obstruction, without gangrene NOS

     K40.01 **Bilateral inguinal hernia, with obstruction, without gangrene, recurrent**

✓5th **K40.1** Bilateral inguinal hernia, with gangrene

     K40.10 **Bilateral inguinal hernia, with gangrene, not specified as recurrent**
       Bilateral inguinal hernia, with gangrene NOS

     K40.11 **Bilateral inguinal hernia, with gangrene, recurrent**

✓5th **K40.2** Bilateral inguinal hernia, without obstruction or gangrene

     K40.20 **Bilateral inguinal hernia, without obstruction or gangrene, not specified as recurrent**
       Bilateral inguinal hernia NOS

     K40.21 **Bilateral inguinal hernia, without obstruction or gangrene, recurrent**

EXCLUDES 1 Not coded here   EXCLUDES 2 Not included here   N Newborn Age: 0   P Pediatric Age: 0-17   M Maternity Age: 12-55   A Adult Age: 15-124

618   ICD-10-CM Draft (2015)

√5ᵗʰ **K40.3** Unilateral **inguinal hernia,** with obstruction, without gangrene
Inguinal hernia (unilateral) causing obstruction without gangrene
Incarcerated inguinal hernia (unilateral) without gangrene
Irreducible inguinal hernia (unilateral) without gangrene
Strangulated inguinal hernia (unilateral) without gangrene

　　K40.30 **Unilateral inguinal hernia, with obstruction, without gangrene,** not specified as recurrent
Inguinal hernia, with obstruction NOS
Unilateral inguinal hernia, with obstruction, without gangrene NOS

　　K40.31 **Unilateral inguinal hernia, with obstruction, without gangrene,** recurrent

√5ᵗʰ **K40.4** Unilateral **inguinal hernia,** with gangrene

　　K40.40 **Unilateral inguinal hernia, with gangrene,** not specified as recurrent
Inguinal hernia with gangrene NOS
Unilateral inguinal hernia with gangrene NOS

　　K40.41 **Unilateral inguinal hernia, with gangrene,** recurrent

√5ᵗʰ **K40.9** Unilateral **inguinal hernia,** without obstruction or gangrene

　　K40.90 **Unilateral inguinal hernia, without obstruction or gangrene,** not specified as recurrent
Inguinal hernia NOS
Unilateral inguinal hernia NOS

　　K40.91 **Unilateral inguinal hernia, without obstruction or gangrene,** recurrent

√4ᵗʰ **K41** Femoral **hernia**

√5ᵗʰ **K41.0** Bilateral **femoral hernia,** with obstruction, without gangrene
Femoral hernia (bilateral) causing obstruction, without gangrene
Incarcerated femoral hernia (bilateral), without gangrene
Irreducible femoral hernia (bilateral), without gangrene
Strangulated femoral hernia (bilateral), without gangrene

　　K41.00 **Bilateral femoral hernia, with obstruction, without gangrene,** not specified as recurrent
Bilateral femoral hernia, with obstruction, without gangrene NOS

　　K41.01 **Bilateral femoral hernia, with obstruction, without gangrene,** recurrent

√5ᵗʰ **K41.1** Bilateral **femoral hernia,** with gangrene

　　K41.10 **Bilateral femoral hernia, with gangrene,** not specified as recurrent
Bilateral femoral hernia, with gangrene NOS

　　K41.11 **Bilateral femoral hernia, with gangrene,** recurrent

√5ᵗʰ **K41.2** Bilateral **femoral hernia,** without obstruction or gangrene

　　K41.20 **Bilateral femoral hernia, without obstruction or gangrene,** not specified as recurrent
Bilateral femoral hernia NOS

　　K41.21 **Bilateral femoral hernia, without obstruction or gangrene,** recurrent

√5ᵗʰ **K41.3** Unilateral **femoral hernia,** with obstruction, without gangrene
Femoral hernia (unilateral) causing obstruction, without gangrene
Incarcerated femoral hernia (unilateral), without gangrene
Irreducible femoral hernia (unilateral), without gangrene
Strangulated femoral hernia (unilateral), without gangrene

　　K41.30 **Unilateral femoral hernia, with obstruction, without gangrene,** not specified as recurrent
Femoral hernia, with obstruction NOS
Unilateral femoral hernia, with obstruction NOS

　　K41.31 **Unilateral femoral hernia, with obstruction, without gangrene,** recurrent

√5ᵗʰ **K41.4** Unilateral **femoral hernia,** with gangrene

　　K41.40 **Unilateral femoral hernia, with gangrene,** not specified as recurrent
Femoral hernia, with gangrene NOS
Unilateral femoral hernia, with gangrene NOS

　　K41.41 **Unilateral femoral hernia, with gangrene,** recurrent

√5ᵗʰ **K41.9** Unilateral **femoral hernia,** without obstruction or gangrene

　　K41.90 **Unilateral femoral hernia, without obstruction or gangrene,** not specified as recurrent
Femoral hernia NOS
Unilateral femoral hernia NOS

　　K41.91 **Unilateral femoral hernia, without obstruction or gangrene,** recurrent

√4ᵗʰ **K42** Umbilical **hernia**
　　INCLUDES　paraumbilical hernia
　　EXCLUDES 1　omphalocele (Q79.2)

　　K42.0 **Umbilical hernia** with obstruction, without gangrene
Umbilical hernia causing obstruction, without gangrene
Incarcerated umbilical hernia, without gangrene
Irreducible umbilical hernia, without gangrene
Strangulated umbilical hernia, without gangrene

　　K42.1 **Umbilical hernia** with gangrene
Gangrenous umbilical hernia

　　K42.9 **Umbilical hernia** without obstruction or gangrene
Umbilical hernia NOS

√4ᵗʰ **K43** Ventral **hernia**

　　K43.0 Incisional **hernia with obstruction,** without gangrene
Incisional hernia causing obstruction, without gangrene
Incarcerated incisional hernia, without gangrene
Irreducible incisional hernia, without gangrene
Strangulated incisional hernia, without gangrene

　　K43.1 Incisional **hernia** with gangrene
Gangrenous incisional hernia

　　K43.2 Incisional **hernia** without obstruction or gangrene
Incisional hernia NOS

　　K43.3 Parastomal **hernia with obstruction,** without gangrene
Incarcerated parastomal hernia, without gangrene
Irreducible parastomal hernia, without gangrene
Parastomal hernia causing obstruction, without gangrene
Strangulated parastomal hernia, without gangrene

　　K43.4 Parastomal **hernia** with gangrene
Gangrenous parastomal hernia

　　K43.5 Parastomal **hernia** without obstruction or gangrene
Parastomal hernia NOS

　　K43.6 **Other and unspecified ventral hernia with obstruction,** without gangrene
Epigastric hernia causing obstruction, without gangrene
Hypogastric hernia causing obstruction, without gangrene
Incarcerated epigastric hernia without gangrene
Incarcerated hypogastric hernia without gangrene
Incarcerated midline hernia without gangrene
Incarcerated spigelian hernia without gangrene
Incarcerated subxiphoid hernia without gangrene
Irreducible epigastric hernia without gangrene
Irreducible hypogastric hernia without gangrene
Irreducible midline hernia without gangrene
Irreducible spigelian hernia without gangrene
Irreducible subxiphoid hernia without gangrene
Midline hernia causing obstruction, without gangrene
Spigelian hernia causing obstruction, without gangrene
Strangulated epigastric hernia without gangrene
Strangulated hypogastric hernia without gangrene
Strangulated midline hernia without gangrene
Strangulated spigelian hernia without gangrene
Strangulated subxiphoid hernia without gangrene
Subxiphoid hernia causing obstruction, without gangrene

　　K43.7 **Other and unspecified ventral hernia** with gangrene
Any condition listed under K43.6 specified as gangrenous

　　K43.9 **Ventral hernia** without obstruction or gangrene
Epigastric hernia
Ventral hernia NOS

√4ᵗʰ **K44** Diaphragmatic **hernia**
　　INCLUDES　hiatus hernia (esophageal) (sliding)
　　　　　　　paraesophageal hernia
　　EXCLUDES 1　congenital diaphragmatic hernia (Q79.0)
　　　　　　　congenital hiatus hernia (Q40.1)

　　K44.0 **Diaphragmatic hernia** with obstruction, without gangrene
Diaphragmatic hernia causing obstruction
Incarcerated diaphragmatic hernia
Irreducible diaphragmatic hernia
Strangulated diaphragmatic hernia

　　K44.1 **Diaphragmatic hernia** with gangrene
Gangrenous diaphragmatic hernia

　　K44.9 **Diaphragmatic hernia** without obstruction or gangrene
Diaphragmatic hernia NOS

✔ Additional Character Required　　√7ᵗʰ Xtension Alert　　Unspecified Dx　　Other Specified Dx　　Manifestation　　►◄ Revised Text　　● New Code　　▲ Revised Code Title

ICD-10-CM Draft (2015)　　　　　　　　　　　　　　　　　　　　　　　　　　　　　　619

Diseases of the Digestive System

K45–K51.214

☑4ᵗʰ **K45 Other abdominal hernia**
  INCLUDES abdominal hernia, specified site NEC
      lumbar hernia
      obturator hernia
      pudendal hernia
      retroperitoneal hernia
      sciatic hernia

  K45.0 Other specified abdominal hernia with obstruction, without gangrene
      Other specified abdominal hernia causing obstruction
      Other specified incarcerated abdominal hernia
      Other specified irreducible abdominal hernia
      Other specified strangulated abdominal hernia

  K45.1 Other specified abdominal hernia with gangrene
      Any condition listed under K45 specified as gangrenous

  K45.8 Other specified abdominal hernia without obstruction or gangrene

☑4ᵗʰ **K46 Unspecified abdominal hernia**
  INCLUDES enterocele
      epiplocele
      hernia NOS
      interstitial hernia
      intestinal hernia
      intra-abdominal hernia
  EXCLUDES 1 vaginal enterocele (N81.5)

  K46.0 Unspecified abdominal hernia with obstruction, without gangrene
      Unspecified abdominal hernia causing obstruction
      Unspecified incarcerated abdominal hernia
      Unspecified irreducible abdominal hernia
      Unspecified strangulated abdominal hernia

  K46.1 Unspecified abdominal hernia with gangrene
      Any condition listed under K46 specified as gangrenous

  K46.9 Unspecified abdominal hernia without obstruction or gangrene
      Abdominal hernia NOS

Noninfective enteritis and colitis (K50-K52)

  INCLUDES noninfective inflammatory bowel disease
  EXCLUDES 1 irritable bowel syndrome (K58.-)
      megacolon (K59.3)

☑4ᵗʰ **K50 Crohn's disease [regional enteritis]**
  INCLUDES granulomatous enteritis
  Use additional code to identify manifestations, such as:
      pyoderma gangrenosum (L88)
  EXCLUDES 1 ulcerative colitis (K51.-)
  AHA: 2012, 4Q, 104

  ☑5ᵗʰ **K50.0 Crohn's disease of small intestine**
      Crohn's disease [regional enteritis] of duodenum
      Crohn's disease [regional enteritis] of ileum
      Crohn's disease [regional enteritis] of jejunum
      Regional ileitis
      Terminal ileitis
      EXCLUDES 1 Crohn's disease of both small and large intestine (K50.8-)

    K50.00 Crohn's disease of small intestine without complications

    ☑6ᵗʰ **K50.01 Crohn's disease of small intestine with complications**
      K50.011 Crohn's disease of small intestine with rectal bleeding
      K50.012 Crohn's disease of small intestine with intestinal obstruction
      K50.013 Crohn's disease of small intestine with fistula
      K50.014 Crohn's disease of small intestine with abscess
          AHA: 2012, 4Q, 104
      K50.018 Crohn's disease of small intestine with other complication
      K50.019 Crohn's disease of small intestine with unspecified complications

  ☑5ᵗʰ **K50.1 Crohn's disease of large intestine**
      Crohn's disease [regional enteritis] of colon
      Crohn's disease [regional enteritis] of large bowel
      Crohn's disease [regional enteritis] of rectum
      Granulomatous colitis
      Regional colitis
      EXCLUDES 1 Crohn's disease of both small and large intestine (K50.8)

    K50.10 Crohn's disease of large intestine without complications

  ☑6ᵗʰ **K50.11 Crohn's disease of large intestine with complications**
      K50.111 Crohn's disease of large intestine with rectal bleeding
      K50.112 Crohn's disease of large intestine with intestinal obstruction
      K50.113 Crohn's disease of large intestine with fistula
      K50.114 Crohn's disease of large intestine with abscess
      K50.118 Crohn's disease of large intestine with other complication
      K50.119 Crohn's disease of large intestine with unspecified complications

  ☑5ᵗʰ **K50.8 Crohn's disease of both small and large intestine**
    K50.80 Crohn's disease of both small and large intestine without complications

    ☑6ᵗʰ **K50.81 Crohn's disease of both small and large intestine with complications**
      K50.811 Crohn's disease of both small and large intestine with rectal bleeding
      K50.812 Crohn's disease of both small and large intestine with intestinal obstruction
      K50.813 Crohn's disease of both small and large intestine with fistula
      K50.814 Crohn's disease of both small and large intestine with abscess
      K50.818 Crohn's disease of both small and large intestine with other complication
      K50.819 Crohn's disease of both small and large intestine with unspecified complications

  ☑5ᵗʰ **K50.9 Crohn's disease, unspecified**
    K50.90 Crohn's disease, unspecified, without complications
        Crohn's disease NOS
        Regional enteritis NOS

    ☑6ᵗʰ **K50.91 Crohn's disease, unspecified, with complications**
      K50.911 Crohn's disease, unspecified, with rectal bleeding
      K50.912 Crohn's disease, unspecified, with intestinal obstruction
      K50.913 Crohn's disease, unspecified, with fistula
      K50.914 Crohn's disease, unspecified, with abscess
      K50.918 Crohn's disease, unspecified, with other complication
      K50.919 Crohn's disease, unspecified, with unspecified complications

☑4ᵗʰ **K51 Ulcerative colitis**
  Use additional code to identify manifestations, such as:
      pyoderma gangrenosum (L88)
  EXCLUDES 1 Crohn's disease [regional enteritis] (K50.-)

  ☑5ᵗʰ **K51.0 Ulcerative (chronic) pancolitis**
      Backwash ileitis
    K51.00 Ulcerative (chronic) pancolitis without complications
        Ulcerative (chronic) pancolitis NOS

    ☑6ᵗʰ **K51.01 Ulcerative (chronic) pancolitis with complications**
      K51.011 Ulcerative (chronic) pancolitis with rectal bleeding
      K51.012 Ulcerative (chronic) pancolitis with intestinal obstruction
      K51.013 Ulcerative (chronic) pancolitis with fistula
      K51.014 Ulcerative (chronic) pancolitis with abscess
      K51.018 Ulcerative (chronic) pancolitis with other complication
      K51.019 Ulcerative (chronic) pancolitis with unspecified complications

  ☑5ᵗʰ **K51.2 Ulcerative (chronic) proctitis**
    K51.20 Ulcerative (chronic) proctitis without complications
        Ulcerative (chronic) proctitis NOS

    ☑6ᵗʰ **K51.21 Ulcerative (chronic) proctitis with complications**
      K51.211 Ulcerative (chronic) proctitis with rectal bleeding
      K51.212 Ulcerative (chronic) proctitis with intestinal obstruction
      K51.213 Ulcerative (chronic) proctitis with fistula
      K51.214 Ulcerative (chronic) proctitis with abscess

EXCLUDES 1 Not coded here   EXCLUDES 2 Not included here   N Newborn Age: 0   P Pediatric Age: 0-17   M Maternity Age: 12-55   A Adult Age: 15-124

620   ICD-10-CM Draft (2015)

K51.218   Ulcerative (chronic) proctitis with other complication

K51.219   Ulcerative (chronic) proctitis with unspecified complications

✓5ᵗʰ **K51.3**   Ulcerative (chronic) rectosigmoiditis

     K51.30   Ulcerative (chronic) rectosigmoiditis without complications

        Ulcerative (chronic) rectosigmoiditis NOS

     ✓6ᵗʰ **K51.31**   Ulcerative (chronic) rectosigmoiditis with complications

        K51.311   Ulcerative (chronic) rectosigmoiditis with rectal bleeding

        K51.312   Ulcerative (chronic) rectosigmoiditis with intestinal obstruction

        K51.313   Ulcerative (chronic) rectosigmoiditis with fistula

        K51.314   Ulcerative (chronic) rectosigmoiditis with abscess

        K51.318   Ulcerative (chronic) rectosigmoiditis with other complication

        K51.319   Ulcerative (chronic) rectosigmoiditis with unspecified complications

✓5ᵗʰ **K51.4**   Inflammatory polyps of colon

     EXCLUDES 1   adenomatous polyp of colon (D12.6)
                   polyposis of colon (D12.6)
                   polyps of colon NOS (K63.5)

     K51.40   Inflammatory polyps of colon without complications

        Inflammatory polyps of colon NOS

     ✓6ᵗʰ **K51.41**   Inflammatory polyps of colon with complications

        K51.411   Inflammatory polyps of colon with rectal bleeding

        K51.412   Inflammatory polyps of colon with intestinal obstruction

        K51.413   Inflammatory polyps of colon with fistula

        K51.414   Inflammatory polyps of colon with abscess

        K51.418   Inflammatory polyps of colon with other complication

        K51.419   Inflammatory polyps of colon with unspecified complications

✓5ᵗʰ **K51.5**   Left sided colitis

     Left hemicolitis

     K51.50   Left sided colitis without complications

        Left sided colitis NOS

     ✓6ᵗʰ **K51.51**   Left sided colitis with complications

        K51.511   Left sided colitis with rectal bleeding

        K51.512   Left sided colitis with intestinal obstruction

        K51.513   Left sided colitis with fistula

        K51.514   Left sided colitis with abscess

        K51.518   Left sided colitis with other complication

        K51.519   Left sided colitis with unspecified complications

✓5ᵗʰ **K51.8**   Other ulcerative colitis

     K51.80   Other ulcerative colitis without complications

     ✓6ᵗʰ **K51.81**   Other ulcerative colitis with complications

        K51.811   Other ulcerative colitis with rectal bleeding

        K51.812   Other ulcerative colitis with intestinal obstruction

        K51.813   Other ulcerative colitis with fistula

        K51.814   Other ulcerative colitis with abscess

        K51.818   Other ulcerative colitis with other complication

        K51.819   Other ulcerative colitis with unspecified complications

✓5ᵗʰ **K51.9**   Ulcerative colitis, unspecified

     K51.90   Ulcerative colitis, unspecified, without complications

     ✓6ᵗʰ **K51.91**   Ulcerative colitis, unspecified, with complications

        K51.911   Ulcerative colitis, unspecified with rectal bleeding

        K51.912   Ulcerative colitis, unspecified with intestinal obstruction

        K51.913   Ulcerative colitis, unspecified with fistula

        K51.914   Ulcerative colitis, unspecified with abscess

        K51.918   Ulcerative colitis, unspecified with other complication

        K51.919   Ulcerative colitis, unspecified with unspecified complications

✓4ᵗʰ **K52**   Other and unspecified noninfective gastroenteritis and colitis

     K52.0   Gastroenteritis and colitis due to radiation

     K52.1   Toxic gastroenteritis and colitis

        Drug-induced gastroenteritis and colitis

        Code first (T51-T65) to identify toxic agent

        Use additional code for adverse effect, if applicable, to identify drug (T36-T50 with fifth or sixth character 5)

     K52.2   Allergic and dietetic gastroenteritis and colitis

        Food hypersensitivity gastroenteritis or colitis

        Use additional code to identify type of food allergy (Z91.01-, Z91.02-)

     ✓5ᵗʰ **K52.8**   Other specified noninfective gastroenteritis and colitis

        K52.81   Eosinophilic gastritis or gastroenteritis

           Eosinophilic enteritis

           EXCLUDES 1   eosinophilic esophagitis (K20.0)

        K52.82   Eosinophilic colitis

        K52.89   Other specified noninfective gastroenteritis and colitis

           Collagenous colitis

           Lymphocytic colitis

           Microscopic colitis (collagenous or lymphocytic)

     K52.9   Noninfective gastroenteritis and colitis, unspecified

        Colitis NOS   Ileitis NOS
        Enteritis NOS   Jejunitis NOS
        Gastroenteritis NOS   Sigmoiditis NOS

        EXCLUDES 1   diarrhea NOS (R19.7)
                   functional diarrhea (K59.1)
                   infectious gastroenteritis and colitis NOS (A09)
                   neonatal diarrhea (noninfective) (P78.3)
                   psychogenic diarrhea (F45.8)

Other diseases of intestines (K55-K64)

✓4ᵗʰ **K55**   Vascular disorders of intestine

     EXCLUDES 1   necrotizing enterocolitis of newborn (P77.-)

     K55.0   Acute vascular disorders of intestine

        Acute fulminant ischemic colitis

        Acute intestinal infarction

        Acute small intestine ischemia

        Infarction of appendices epiploicae

        Mesenteric (artery) (vein) embolism

        Mesenteric (artery) (vein) infarction

        Mesenteric (artery) (vein) thrombosis

        Necrosis of intestine

        Subacute ischemic colitis

     K55.1   Chronic vascular disorders of intestine

        Chronic ischemic colitis   Mesenteric atherosclerosis

        Chronic ischemic enteritis   Mesenteric vascular

        Chronic ischemic enterocolitis   insufficiency

        Ischemic stricture of intestine

     ✓5ᵗʰ **K55.2**   Angiodysplasia of colon

        K55.20   Angiodysplasia of colon without hemorrhage

        K55.21   Angiodysplasia of colon with hemorrhage

     K55.8   Other vascular disorders of intestine

     K55.9   Vascular disorder of intestine, unspecified

        Ischemic colitis

        Ischemic enteritis

        Ischemic enterocolitis

✓4ᵗʰ **K56**   Paralytic ileus and intestinal obstruction without hernia

     EXCLUDES 1   congenital stricture or stenosis of intestine (Q41-Q42)
                   cystic fibrosis with meconium ileus (E84.11)
                   intestinal obstruction with hernia (K40-K46)
                   ischemic stricture of intestine (K55.1)
                   meconium ileus NOS (P76.0)
                   neonatal intestinal obstructions classifiable to P76-
                   obstruction of duodenum (K31.5)
                   postprocedural intestinal obstruction (K91.3)
                   stenosis of anus or rectum (K62.4)

     K56.0   Paralytic ileus

        Paralysis of bowel

        Paralysis of colon

        Paralysis of intestine

        EXCLUDES 1   gallstone ileus (K56.3)
                   ileus NOS (K56.7)
                   obstructive ileus NOS (K56.69)

✓ Additional Character Required   ✓x7ᵗʰ Xtension Alert   Unspecified Dx   Other Specified Dx   Manifestation   ▶◀ Revised Text   ● New Code   ▲ Revised Code Title

Diseases of the Digestive System

K56.1–K59.4

K56.1 Intussusception
Intussusception or invagination of bowel
Intussusception or invagination of colon
Intussusception or invagination of intestine
Intussusception or invagination of rectum
EXCLUDES 2 intussusception of appendix (K38.8)

K56.2 Volvulus
Strangulation of colon or intestine
Torsion of colon or intestine
Twist of colon or intestine
EXCLUDES 2 volvulus of duodenum (K31.5)

K56.3 Gallstone ileus
Obstruction of intestine by gallstone

√5th **K56.4 Other impaction of intestine**

K56.41 Fecal impaction
EXCLUDES 1 constipation (K59.0-)
incomplete defecation (R15.0)

K56.49 Other impaction of intestine

K56.5 Intestinal adhesions [bands] with obstruction (postprocedural) (postinfection)
Abdominal hernia due to adhesions with obstruction
Peritoneal adhesions [bands] with intestinal obstruction (postprocedural) (postinfection)

√5th **K56.6 Other and unspecified intestinal obstruction**

K56.60 Unspecified intestinal obstruction
Intestinal obstruction NOS
EXCLUDES 1 intestinal obstruction due to specified condition—code to condition

K56.69 Other intestinal obstruction
Enterostenosis NOS
Obstructive ileus NOS
Occlusion of colon or intestine NOS
Stenosis of colon or intestine NOS
Stricture of colon or intestine NOS
EXCLUDES 1 intestinal obstruction due to specified condition—code to condition

K56.7 Ileus, unspecified
EXCLUDES 1 obstructive ileus (K56.69)

√4th **K57 Diverticular disease of intestine**
EXCLUDES 1 congenital diverticulum of intestine (Q43.8)
Meckel's diverticulum (Q43.0)
EXCLUDES 2 diverticulum of appendix (K38.2)

√5th **K57.0 Diverticulitis of** small intestine with perforation and abscess
Diverticulitis of small intestine with peritonitis
EXCLUDES 1 diverticulitis of both small and large intestine with perforation and abscess (K57.4-)

K57.00 Diverticulitis of small intestine with perforation and abscess without bleeding

K57.01 Diverticulitis of small intestine with perforation and abscess with bleeding

√5th **K57.1 Diverticular disease of** small intestine without perforation or abscess
EXCLUDES 1 diverticular disease of both small and large intestine without perforation or abscess (K57.5-)

K57.10 Diverticulosis of small intestine without perforation or abscess without bleeding
Diverticular disease of small intestine NOS

K57.11 Diverticulosis of small intestine without perforation or abscess with bleeding

K57.12 Diverticulitis of small intestine without perforation or abscess without bleeding

K57.13 Diverticulitis of small intestine without perforation or abscess with bleeding

√5th **K57.2 Diverticulitis of** large intestine with perforation and abscess
Diverticulitis of colon with peritonitis
EXCLUDES 1 diverticulitis of both small and large intestine with perforation and abscess (K57.4-)

K57.20 Diverticulitis of large intestine with perforation and abscess without bleeding

K57.21 Diverticulitis of large intestine with perforation and abscess with bleeding

√5th **K57.3 Diverticular disease of** large intestine without perforation or abscess
EXCLUDES 1 diverticular disease of both small and large intestine without perforation or abscess (K57.5-)

K57.30 Diverticulosis of large intestine without perforation or abscess without bleeding
Diverticular disease of colon NOS

K57.31 Diverticulosis of large intestine without perforation or abscess with bleeding

K57.32 Diverticulitis of large intestine without perforation or abscess without bleeding

K57.33 Diverticulitis of large intestine without perforation or abscess with bleeding

√5th **K57.4 Diverticulitis of both** small and large intestine with perforation and abscess
Diverticulitis of both small and large intestine with peritonitis

K57.40 Diverticulitis of both small and large intestine with perforation and abscess without bleeding

K57.41 Diverticulitis of both small and large intestine with perforation and abscess with bleeding

√5th **K57.5 Diverticular disease of** both small and large intestine without perforation or abscess

K57.50 Diverticulosis of both small and large intestine without perforation or abscess without bleeding
Diverticular disease of both small and large intestine NOS

K57.51 Diverticulosis of both small and large intestine without perforation or abscess with bleeding

K57.52 Diverticulitis of both small and large intestine without perforation or abscess without bleeding

K57.53 Diverticulitis of both small and large intestine without perforation or abscess with bleeding

√5th **K57.8 Diverticulitis of intestine,** part unspecified, with perforation and abscess
Diverticulitis of intestine NOS with peritonitis

K57.80 Diverticulitis of intestine, part unspecified, with perforation and abscess without bleeding

K57.81 Diverticulitis of intestine, part unspecified, with perforation and abscess with bleeding

√5th **K57.9 Diverticular disease of intestine,** part unspecified, without perforation or abscess

K57.90 Diverticulosis of intestine, part unspecified, without perforation or abscess without bleeding
Diverticular disease of intestine NOS

K57.91 Diverticulosis of intestine, part unspecified, without perforation or abscess with bleeding

K57.92 Diverticulitis of intestine, part unspecified, without perforation or abscess without bleeding

K57.93 Diverticulitis of intestine, part unspecified, without perforation or abscess with bleeding

√4th **K58 Irritable bowel syndrome**
INCLUDES irritable colon
spastic colon

K58.0 Irritable bowel syndrome with diarrhea

K58.9 Irritable bowel syndrome without diarrhea
Irritable bowel syndrome NOS

√4th **K59 Other functional intestinal disorders**
EXCLUDES 1 change in bowel habit NOS (R19.4)
intestinal malabsorption (K90.-)
psychogenic intestinal disorders (F45.8)
EXCLUDES 2 functional disorders of stomach (K31.-)

√5th **K59.0 Constipation**
EXCLUDES 1 fecal impaction (K56.41)
incomplete defecation (R15.0)

K59.00 Constipation, unspecified

K59.01 Slow transit constipation

K59.02 Outlet dysfunction constipation

K59.09 Other constipation

K59.1 Functional diarrhea
EXCLUDES 1 diarrhea NOS (R19.7)
irritable bowel syndrome with diarrhea (K58.0)

K59.2 Neurogenic bowel, not elsewhere classified

K59.3 Megacolon, not elsewhere classified
Dilatation of colon
Toxic megacolon
Code first (T51-T65) to identify toxic agent
EXCLUDES 1 congenital megacolon (aganglionic) (Q43.1)
megacolon (due to) (in) Chagas' disease (B57.32)
megacolon (due to) (in) Clostridium difficile (A04.7)
megacolon (due to) (in) Hirschsprung's disease (Q43.1)

K59.4 Anal spasm
Proctalgia fugax

K59.8 **Other specified functional intestinal disorders**
Atony of colon
Pseudo-obstruction (acute) (chronic) of intestine

K59.9 **Functional intestinal disorder, unspecified**

✓4ᵗʰ **K60** **Fissure and fistula of anal and rectal regions**
EXCLUDES 1 *fissure and fistula of anal and rectal regions with abscess or cellulitis (K61.-)*
EXCLUDES 2 *anal sphincter tear (healed) (nontraumatic) (old) (K62.81)*

K60.0 Acute **anal fissure**

K60.1 Chronic **anal fissure**

K60.2 **Anal fissure, unspecified**

K60.3 Anal **fistula**

K60.4 Rectal **fistula**
Fistula of rectum to skin
EXCLUDES 1 *rectovaginal fistula (N82.3)*
vesicorectal fistual (N32.1)

K60.5 Anorectal **fistula**

✓4ᵗʰ **K61** **Abscess of anal and rectal regions**
INCLUDES abscess of anal and rectal regions
cellulitis of anal and rectal regions

K61.0 Anal **abscess**
Perianal abscess
EXCLUDES 1 *intrasphincteric abscess (K61.4)*

K61.1 Rectal **abscess**
Perirectal abscess
EXCLUDES 1 *ischiorectal abscess (K61.3)*
AHA: 2012, 4Q, 104

K61.2 Anorectal **abscess**

K61.3 Ischiorectal **abscess**
Abscess of ischiorectal fossa

K61.4 Intrasphincteric **abscess**

✓4ᵗʰ **K62** **Other diseases of anus and rectum**
INCLUDES anal canal
EXCLUDES 2 *colostomy and enterostomy malfunction (K94.0-, K94.1-)*
fecal incontinence (R15.-)
hemorrhoids (K64.-)

K62.0 **Anal polyp**

K62.1 **Rectal polyp**
EXCLUDES 1 *adenomatous polyp (D12.8)*

K62.2 **Anal prolapse**
Prolapse of anal canal

K62.3 **Rectal prolapse**
Prolapse of rectal mucosa

K62.4 **Stenosis of anus and rectum**
Stricture of anus (sphincter)

K62.5 **Hemorrhage of anus and rectum**
EXCLUDES 1 *gastrointestinal bleeding NOS (K92.2)*
melena (K92.1)
neonatal rectal hemorrhage (P54.2)

K62.6 **Ulcer of anus and rectum**
Solitary ulcer of anus and rectum
Stercoral ulcer of anus and rectum
EXCLUDES 1 *fissure and fistula of anus and rectum (K60.-)*
ulcerative colitis (K51.-)

K62.7 **Radiation proctitis**
Use additional code to identify the type of radiation (W90.-)

✓5ᵗʰ **K62.8** **Other specified diseases of anus and rectum**
EXCLUDES 2 *ulcerative proctitis (K51.2)*

K62.81 **Anal sphincter tear (healed) (nontraumatic) (old)**
Tear of anus, nontraumatic
Use additional code for any associated fecal incontinence (R15.-)
EXCLUDES 2 *anal fissure (K60.-)*
anal sphincter tear (healed) (old) complicating delivery (O34.7-)
traumatic tear of anal sphincter (S31.831)

K62.82 **Dysplasia of anus**
Anal intraepithelial neoplasia I and II (AIN I and II) (histologically confirmed)
Dysplasia of anus NOS
Mild and moderate dysplasia of anus (histologically confirmed)
EXCLUDES 1 *abnormal results from anal cytologic examination without histologic confirmation (R85.61-)*
anal intraepithelial neoplasia III (D01.3)
carcinoma in situ of anus (D01.3)
HGSIL of anus (R85.613)
severe dysplasia of anus (D01.3)

K62.89 **Other specified diseases of anus and rectum**
Proctitis NOS
Use additional code for any associated fecal incontinence (R15.-)

K62.9 **Disease of anus and rectum, unspecified**

✓4ᵗʰ **K63** **Other diseases of intestine**

K63.0 Abscess **of intestine**
EXCLUDES 1 *abscess of intestine with Crohn's disease (K50.014, K50.114, K50.814, K50.914)*
abscess of intestine with diverticular disease (K57.0, K57.2, K57.4, K57.8)
abscess of intestine with ulcerative colitis (K51.014, K51.214, K51.314, K51.414, K51.514, K51.814, K51.914)
EXCLUDES 2 *abscess of anal and rectal regions (K61.-)*
abscess of appendix (K35.3)

K63.1 Perforation **of intestine (nontraumatic)**
Perforation (nontraumatic) of rectum
EXCLUDES 1 *perforation (nontraumatic) of duodenum (K26.-)*
perforation (nontraumatic) of intestine with diverticular disease (K57.0, K57.2, K57.4, K57.8)
EXCLUDES 2 *perforation (nontraumatic) of appendix (K35.2, K35.3)*

K63.2 Fistula **of intestine**
EXCLUDES 1 *fistula of duodenum (K31.6)*
fistula of intestine with Crohn's disease (K50.013, K50.113, K50.813, K50.913)
fistula of intestine with ulcerative colitis (K51.013, K51.213, K51.313, K51.413, K51.513, K51.813, K51.913)
EXCLUDES 2 *fistula of anal and rectal regions (K60.-)*
fistula of appendix (K38.3)
intestinal-genital fistula, female (N82.2-N82.4)
vesicointestinal fistula (N32.1)

K63.3 Ulcer **of intestine**
Primary ulcer of small intestine
EXCLUDES 1 *duodenal ulcer (K26.-)*
gastrointestinal ulcer (K28.-)
gastrojejunal ulcer (K28.-)
jejunal ulcer (K28.-)
peptic ulcer, site unspecified (K27.-)
ulcer of intestine with perforation (K63.1)
ulcer of anus or rectum (K62.6)
ulcerative colitis (K51.-)

K63.4 Enteroptosis

K63.5 Polyp **of colon**
EXCLUDES 1 *adenomatous polyp of colon (D12.6)*
inflammatory polyp of colon (K51.4-)
polyposis of colon (D12.6)

✓5ᵗʰ **K63.8** Other **specified diseases of intestine**

K63.81 **Dieulafoy lesion of intestine**
EXCLUDES 2 *Dieulafoy lesion of stomach and duodenum (K31.82)*

K63.89 **Other specified diseases of intestine**
AHA: 2013, 2Q, 31

K63.9 **Disease of intestine, unspecified**

✓4ᵗʰ **K64** **Hemorrhoids and perianal venous thrombosis**
INCLUDES piles
EXCLUDES 1 *hemorrhoids complicating childbirth and the puerperium (O87.2)*
hemorrhoids complicating pregnancy (O22.4)

K64.0 First degree **hemorrhoids**
Grade/stage I hemorrhoids
Hemorrhoids (bleeding) without prolapse outside of anal canal

K64.1 Second degree **hemorrhoids**
Grade/stage II hemorrhoids
Hemorrhoids (bleeding) that prolapse with straining, but retract spontaneously

---

✔ Additional Character Required   ✓x7ᵗʰ Xtension Alert   Unspecified Dx   Other Specified Dx   Manifestation   ▶◀ Revised Text   ● New Code   ▲ Revised Code Title

Diseases of the Digestive System

K64.2 Third degree hemorrhoids
Grade/stage III hemorrhoids
Hemorrhoids (bleeding) that prolapse with straining and require
manual replacement back inside anal canal

K64.3 Fourth degree hemorrhoids
Grade/stage IV hemorrhoids
Hemorrhoids (bleeding) with prolapsed tissue that cannot be
manually replaced

K64.4 Residual hemorrhoidal skin tags
External hemorrhoids, NOS
Skin tags of anus

K64.5 Perianal venous thrombosis
External hemorrhoids with thrombosis
Perianal hematoma
Thrombosed hemorrhoids NOS

K64.8 Other hemorrhoids
Internal hemorrhoids, without mention of degree
Prolapsed hemorrhoids, degree not specified

K64.9 Unspecified hemorrhoids
Hemorrhoids (bleeding) NOS
Hemorrhoids (bleeding) without mention of degree

Diseases of peritoneum and retroperitoneum (K65-K68)

✓4ᵗʰ K65 Peritonitis
Use additional code (B95-B97), to identify infectious agent
EXCLUDES 1   *acute appendicitis with generalized peritonitis (K35.2)*
aseptic peritonitis (T81.6)
benign paroxysmal peritonitis (E85.0)
chemical peritonitis (T81.6)
diverticulitis of both small and large intestine with peritonitis
(K57.4-)
diverticulitis of colon with peritonitis (K57.2-)
diverticulitis of intestine, NOS, with peritonitis (K57.8-)
diverticulitis of small intestine with peritonitis (K57.0-)
gonococcal peritonitis (A54.85)
neonatal peritonitis (P78.0-P78.1)
pelvic peritonitis, female (N73.3-N73.5)
periodic familial peritonitis (E85.0)
peritonitis due to talc or other foreign substance (T81.6)
peritonitis in chlamydia (A74.81)
peritonitis in diphtheria (A36.89)
peritonitis in syphilis (late) (A52.74)
peritonitis in tuberculosis (A18.31)
peritonitis with or following abortion or ectopic or molar
pregnancy (O00-O07, O08.0)
peritonitis with or following appendicitis (K35.-)
peritonitis with or following diverticular disease of intestine
(K57.-)
puerperal peritonitis (O85)
retroperitoneal infections (K68.-)

K65.0 Generalized (acute) peritonitis
Pelvic peritonitis (acute), male
Subphrenic peritonitis (acute)
Suppurative peritonitis (acute)

K65.1 Peritoneal abscess
Abdominopelvic abscess   Subdiaphragmatic abscess
Abscess (of) omentum   Subhepatic abscess
Abscess (of) peritoneum   Subphrenic abscess
Mesenteric abscess
Retrocecal abscess

K65.2 Spontaneous bacterial peritonitis
EXCLUDES 1   *bacterial peritonitis NOS (K65.9)*

K65.3 Choleperitonitis
Peritonitis due to bile

K65.4 Sclerosing mesenteritis
Fat necrosis of peritoneum
(Idiopathic) sclerosing mesenteric fibrosis
Mesenteric lipodystrophy
Mesenteric panniculitis
Retractile mesenteritis

K65.8 Other peritonitis
Chronic proliferative peritonitis
Peritonitis due to urine

K65.9 Peritonitis, unspecified
Bacterial peritonitis NOS
AHA: 2013, 2Q, 31

✓4ᵗʰ K66 Other disorders of peritoneum
EXCLUDES 2   *ascites (R18.-)*
peritoneal effusion (chronic) (R18.8)

K66.0 Peritoneal adhesions (postprocedural) (postinfection)
Adhesions (of) abdominal (wall)   Adhesions (of) omentum
Adhesions (of) diaphragm   Adhesions (of) stomach
Adhesions (of) intestine   Adhesive bands
Adhesions (of) male pelvis   Mesenteric adhesions
EXCLUDES 1   *female pelvic adhesions [bands] (N73.6)*
peritoneal adhesions with intestinal obstruction (K56.5)

K66.1 Hemoperitoneum
EXCLUDES 1   *traumatic hemoperitoneum (S36.8-)*

K66.8 Other specified disorders of peritoneum

K66.9 Disorder of peritoneum, unspecified

K67 Disorders of peritoneum in infectious diseases classified elsewhere
Code first underlying disease, such as :
congenital syphilis (A50.0)
helminthiasis (B65.0-B83.9)
EXCLUDES 1   *peritonitis in chlamydia (A74.81)*
peritonitis in diphtheria (A36.89)
peritonitis in gonococcal (A54.85)
peritonitis in syphilis (late) (A52.74)
peritonitis in tuberculosis (A18.31)

✓4ᵗʰ K68 Disorders of retroperitoneum

✓5ᵗʰ K68.1 Retroperitoneal abscess

K68.11 Postprocedural retroperitoneal abscess

K68.12 Psoas muscle abscess

K68.19 Other retroperitoneal abscess

K68.9 Other disorders of retroperitoneum

Diseases of liver (K70-K77)

EXCLUDES 1   *jaundice NOS (R17)*
EXCLUDES 2   *hemochromatosis (E83.11-)*
Reye's syndrome (G93.7)
viral hepatitis (B15-B19)
Wilson's disease (E83.0)

✓4ᵗʰ K70 Alcoholic liver disease
Use additional code to identify:
alcohol abuse and dependence (F10.-)

K70.0 Alcoholic fatty liver   🅰

✓5ᵗʰ K70.1 Alcoholic hepatitis

K70.10 Alcoholic hepatitis without ascites   🅰

K70.11 Alcoholic hepatitis with ascites   🅰

K70.2 Alcoholic fibrosis and sclerosis of liver   🅰

✓5ᵗʰ K70.3 Alcoholic cirrhosis of liver
Alcoholic cirrhosis NOS

K70.30 Alcoholic cirrhosis of liver without ascites   🅰

K70.31 Alcoholic cirrhosis of liver with ascites   🅰

✓5ᵗʰ K70.4 Alcoholic hepatic failure
Acute alcoholic hepatic failure
Alcoholic hepatic failure NOS
Chronic alcoholic hepatic failure
Subacute alcoholic hepatic failure

K70.40 Alcoholic hepatic failure without coma   🅰

K70.41 Alcoholic hepatic failure with coma   🅰

K70.9 Alcoholic liver disease, unspecified   🅰

✓4ᵗʰ K71 Toxic liver disease
INCLUDES   drug-induced idiosyncratic (unpredictable) liver disease
drug-induced toxic (predictable) liver disease
Code first poisoning due to drug or toxin, if applicable (T36-T65 with
fifth or sixth character 1-4 or 6)
Use additional code for adverse effect, if applicable, to identify drug
(T36-T50 with fifth or sixth character 5)
EXCLUDES 2   *alcoholic liver disease (K70.-)*
Budd-Chiari syndrome (I82.0)

K71.0 Toxic liver disease with cholestasis
Cholestasis with hepatocyte injury
"Pure" cholestasis

✓5ᵗʰ K71.1 Toxic liver disease with hepatic necrosis
Hepatic failure (acute) (chronic) due to drugs

K71.10 Toxic liver disease with hepatic necrosis, without coma

K71.11 Toxic liver disease with hepatic necrosis, with coma

K71.2 Toxic liver disease with acute hepatitis

K71.3 Toxic liver disease with chronic persistent hepatitis

EXCLUDES 1 Not coded here   *EXCLUDES 2* Not included here   Ⓝ Newborn Age: 0   Ⓟ Pediatric Age: 0-17   Ⓜ Maternity Age: 12-55   🅰 Adult Age: 15-124

624   ICD-10-CM Draft (2015)

K71.4 **Toxic liver disease with** chronic lobular hepatitis

√5ᵗʰ **K71.5** **Toxic liver disease with** chronic active hepatitis
Toxic liver disease with lupoid hepatitis

    K71.50 **Toxic liver disease with chronic active hepatitis** without ascites

    K71.51 **Toxic liver disease with chronic active hepatitis** with ascites

K71.6 **Toxic liver disease with** hepatitis, not elsewhere classified

K71.7 **Toxic liver disease with** fibrosis and cirrhosis **of liver**

K71.8 **Toxic liver disease with other disorders of liver**
Toxic liver disease with focal nodular hyperplasia
Toxic liver disease with hepatic granulomas
Toxic liver disease with peliosis hepatis
Toxic liver disease with veno-occlusive disease of liver

K71.9 **Toxic liver disease, unspecified**

√4ᵗʰ **K72** **Hepatic failure, not elsewhere classified**
INCLUDES   acute hepatitis NEC, with hepatic failure
fulminant hepatitis NEC, with hepatic failure
hepatic encephalopathy NOS
liver (cell) necrosis with hepatic failure
malignant hepatitis NEC, with hepatic failure
yellow liver atrophy or dystrophy
EXCLUDES 1   alcoholic hepatic failure (K70.4)
hepatic failure with toxic liver disease (K71.1-)
icterus of newborn (P55-P59)
postprocedural hepatic failure (K91.82)
viral hepatitis with hepatic coma (B15-B19)
EXCLUDES 2   hepatic failure complicating abortion or ectopic or molar
pregnancy (O00-O07, O08.8)
hepatic failure complicating pregnancy, childbirth and the
puerperium (O26.6-)

√5ᵗʰ **K72.0** Acute and subacute **hepatic failure**
AHA: 2014, 2Q, 13

    K72.00 **Acute and subacute hepatic failure** without coma

    K72.01 **Acute and subacute hepatic failure** with coma

√5ᵗʰ **K72.1** Chronic **hepatic failure**

    K72.10 **Chronic hepatic failure** without coma

    K72.11 **Chronic hepatic failure** with coma

√5ᵗʰ **K72.9** **Hepatic failure,** unspecified

    K72.90 **Hepatic failure, unspecified** without coma

    K72.91 **Hepatic failure, unspecified** with coma
Hepatic coma NOS

√4ᵗʰ **K73** **Chronic hepatitis, not elsewhere classified**
EXCLUDES 1   alcoholic hepatitis (chronic) (K70.1-)
drug-induced hepatitis (chronic) (K71.-)
granulomatous hepatitis (chronic) NEC (K75.3)
reactive, nonspecific hepatitis (chronic) (K75.2)
viral hepatitis (chronic) (B15-B19)

K73.0 **Chronic** persistent **hepatitis, not elsewhere classified**

K73.1 **Chronic** lobular **hepatitis, not elsewhere classified**

K73.2 **Chronic** active **hepatitis, not elsewhere classified**

K73.8 **Other chronic hepatitis, not elsewhere classified**

K73.9 **Chronic hepatitis, unspecified**

√4ᵗʰ **K74** **Fibrosis and cirrhosis of liver**
Code also, if applicable, viral hepatitis (acute) (chronic) (B15-B19)
EXCLUDES 1   alcoholic cirrhosis (of liver) (K70.3)
alcoholic fibrosis of liver (K70.2)
cardiac sclerosis of liver (K76.1)
cirrhosis (of liver) with toxic liver disease (K71.7)
congenital cirrhosis (of liver) (P78.81)
pigmentary cirrhosis (of liver) (E83.110)

K74.0 **Hepatic** fibrosis

K74.1 **Hepatic** sclerosis

K74.2 **Hepatic** fibrosis with hepatic sclerosis

K74.3 Primary biliary cirrhosis
Chronic nonsuppurative destructive cholangitis

K74.4 Secondary **biliary cirrhosis**

K74.5 **Biliary cirrhosis, unspecified**

√5ᵗʰ **K74.6** **Other and unspecified cirrhosis of liver**

    K74.60 **Unspecified cirrhosis of liver**
Cirrhosis (of liver) NOS

    K74.69 **Other cirrhosis of liver**
Cryptogenic cirrhosis (of liver)
Macronodular cirrhosis (of liver)
Micronodular cirrhosis (of liver)
Mixed type cirrhosis (of liver)
Portal cirrhosis (of liver)
Postnecrotic cirrhosis (of liver)

√4ᵗʰ **K75** **Other inflammatory liver diseases**
EXCLUDES 2   toxic liver disease (K71.-)

K75.0 **Abscess of liver**
Cholangitic hepatic abscess
Hematogenic hepatic abscess
Hepatic abscess NOS
Lymphogenic hepatic abscess
Pylephlebitic hepatic abscess
EXCLUDES 1   amebic liver abscess (A06.4)
cholangitis without liver abscess (K83.0)
pylephlebitis without liver abscess (K75.1)

K75.1 **Phlebitis of portal vein**
Pylephlebitis
EXCLUDES 1   pylephlebitic liver abscess (K75.0)

K75.2 **Nonspecific reactive hepatitis**
EXCLUDES 1   acute or subacute hepatitis (K72.0-)
chronic hepatitis NEC (K73.-)
viral hepatitis (B15-B19)

K75.3 **Granulomatous hepatitis, not elsewhere classified**
EXCLUDES 1   acute or subacute hepatitis (K72.0-)
chronic hepatitis NEC (K73.-)
viral hepatitis (B15-B19)

K75.4 **Autoimmune hepatitis**
Lupoid hepatitis NEC

√5ᵗʰ **K75.8** **Other specified inflammatory liver diseases**

    K75.81 **Nonalcoholic steatohepatitis (NASH)**

    K75.89 **Other specified inflammatory liver diseases**

K75.9 **Inflammatory liver disease, unspecified**
Hepatitis NOS
EXCLUDES 1   acute or subacute hepatitis (K72.0-)
chronic hepatitis NEC (K73.-)
viral hepatitis (B15-B19)

√4ᵗʰ **K76** **Other diseases of liver**
EXCLUDES 2   alcoholic liver disease (K70.-)
amyloid degeneration of liver (E85.-)
cystic disease of liver (congenital) (Q44.6)
hepatic vein thrombosis (I82.0)
hepatomegaly NOS (R16.0)
pigmentary cirrhosis (of liver) (E83.110)
portal vein thrombosis (I81)
toxic liver disease (K71.-)

K76.0 **Fatty (change of) liver, not elsewhere classified**
Nonalcoholic fatty liver disease (NAFLD)
EXCLUDES 1   nonalcoholic steatohepatitis (NASH) (K75.81)

K76.1 **Chronic passive congestion of liver**
Cardiac cirrhosis
Cardiac sclerosis

K76.2 **Central hemorrhagic necrosis of liver**
EXCLUDES 1   liver necrosis with hepatic failure (K72.-)

K76.3 **Infarction of liver**

K76.4 **Peliosis hepatis**
Hepatic angiomatosis

K76.5 **Hepatic veno-occlusive disease**
EXCLUDES 1   Budd-Chiari syndrome (I82.0)

K76.6 **Portal hypertension**
Use additional code for any associated complications, such as:
portal hypertensive gastropathy (K31.89)

K76.7 **Hepatorenal syndrome**
EXCLUDES 1   hepatorenal syndrome following labor and delivery
(O90.4)
postprocedural hepatorenal syndrome (K91.82)

√5ᵗʰ **K76.8** **Other specified diseases of liver**

    K76.81 **Hepatopulmonary syndrome**
Code first underlying liver disease, such as:
alcoholic cirrhosis of liver (K70.3-)
cirrhosis of liver without mention of alcohol (K74.6-)

    K76.89 **Other specified diseases of liver**
Cyst (simple) of liver
Focal nodular hyperplasia of liver
Hepatoptosis

K76.9 **Liver disease, unspecified**

☑ Additional Character Required   √x7ᵗʰ Xtension Alert   Unspecified Dx   Other Specified Dx   Manifestation   ▶◀ Revised Text   ● New Code   ▲ Revised Code Title

ICD-10-CM Draft (2015)   **625**

Diseases of the Digestive System

K77–K82.3

K77 Liver disorders in diseases classified elsewhere

Code first underlying disease, such as:
amyloidosis (E85.-)
congenital syphilis (A50.0, A50.5)
congenital toxoplasmosis (P37.1)
schistosomiasis (B65.0-B65.9)

EXCLUDES 1   alcoholic hepatitis (K70.1-)
alcoholic liver disease (K70-.)
cytomegaloviral hepatitis (B25.1)
herpesviral [herpes simplex] hepatitis (B00.81)
infectious mononucleosis with liver disease
(B27.0-B27.9 with .9)
mumps hepatitis (B26.81)
sarcoidosis with liver disease (D86.89)
secondary syphilis with liver disease (A51.45)
syphilis (late) with liver disease (A52.74)
toxoplasmosis (acquired) hepatitis (B58.1)
tuberculosis with liver disease (A18.83)

Disorders of gallbladder, biliary tract and pancreas (K80-K87)

✓4th K80 Cholelithiasis

EXCLUDES 1   retained cholelithiasis following cholecystectomy (K91.86)

✓5th K80.0 Calculus of gallbladder with acute cholecystitis
Any condition listed in K80.2 with acute cholecystitis

    K80.00 Calculus of gallbladder with acute cholecystitis without obstruction

    K80.01 Calculus of gallbladder with acute cholecystitis with obstruction

✓5th K80.1 Calculus of gallbladder with other cholecystitis

    K80.10 Calculus of gallbladder with chronic cholecystitis without obstruction
Cholelithiasis with cholecystitis NOS

    K80.11 Calculus of gallbladder with chronic cholecystitis with obstruction

    K80.12 Calculus of gallbladder with acute and chronic cholecystitis without obstruction

    K80.13 Calculus of gallbladder with acute and chronic cholecystitis with obstruction

    K80.18 Calculus of gallbladder with other cholecystitis without obstruction

    K80.19 Calculus of gallbladder with other cholecystitis with obstruction

✓5th K80.2 Calculus of gallbladder without cholecystitis
Cholecystolithiasis without cholecystitis
Cholelithiasis (without cholecystitis)
Colic (recurrent) of gallbladder (without cholecystitis)
Gallstone (impacted) of cystic duct (without cholecystitis)
Gallstone (impacted) of gallbladder (without cholecystitis)

    K80.20 Calculus of gallbladder without cholecystitis without obstruction

    K80.21 Calculus of gallbladder without cholecystitis with obstruction

✓5th K80.3 Calculus of bile duct with cholangitis
Any condition listed in K80.5 with cholangitis

    K80.30 Calculus of bile duct with cholangitis, unspecified, without obstruction

    K80.31 Calculus of bile duct with cholangitis, unspecified, with obstruction

    K80.32 Calculus of bile duct with acute cholangitis without obstruction

    K80.33 Calculus of bile duct with acute cholangitis with obstruction

    K80.34 Calculus of bile duct with chronic cholangitis without obstruction

    K80.35 Calculus of bile duct with chronic cholangitis with obstruction

    K80.36 Calculus of bile duct with acute and chronic cholangitis without obstruction

    K80.37 Calculus of bile duct with acute and chronic cholangitis with obstruction

✓5th K80.4 Calculus of bile duct with cholecystitis
Any condition listed in K80.5 with cholecystitis (with cholangitis)

    K80.40 Calculus of bile duct with cholecystitis, unspecified, without obstruction

    K80.41 Calculus of bile duct with cholecystitis, unspecified, with obstruction

    K80.42 Calculus of bile duct with acute cholecystitis without obstruction

    K80.43 Calculus of bile duct with acute cholecystitis with obstruction

    K80.44 Calculus of bile duct with chronic cholecystitis without obstruction

    K80.45 Calculus of bile duct with chronic cholecystitis with obstruction

    K80.46 Calculus of bile duct with acute and chronic cholecystitis without obstruction

    K80.47 Calculus of bile duct with acute and chronic cholecystitis with obstruction

✓5th K80.5 Calculus of bile duct without cholangitis or cholecystitis
Choledocholithiasis (without cholangitis or cholecystitis)
Gallstone (impacted) of bile duct NOS (without cholangitis or cholecystitis)
Gallstone (impacted) of common duct (without cholangitis or cholecystitis)
Gallstone (impacted) of hepatic duct (without cholangitis or cholecystitis)
Hepatic cholelithiasis (without cholangitis or cholecystitis)
Hepatic colic (recurrent) (without cholangitis or cholecystitis)

    K80.50 Calculus of bile duct without cholangitis or cholecystitis without obstruction

    K80.51 Calculus of bile duct without cholangitis or cholecystitis with obstruction

✓5th K80.6 Calculus of gallbladder and bile duct with cholecystitis

    K80.60 Calculus of gallbladder and bile duct with cholecystitis, unspecified, without obstruction

    K80.61 Calculus of gallbladder and bile duct with cholecystitis, unspecified, with obstruction

    K80.62 Calculus of gallbladder and bile duct with acute cholecystitis without obstruction

    K80.63 Calculus of gallbladder and bile duct with acute cholecystitis with obstruction

    K80.64 Calculus of gallbladder and bile duct with chronic cholecystitis without obstruction

    K80.65 Calculus of gallbladder and bile duct with chronic cholecystitis with obstruction

    K80.66 Calculus of gallbladder and bile duct with acute and chronic cholecystitis without obstruction

    K80.67 Calculus of gallbladder and bile duct with acute and chronic cholecystitis with obstruction

✓5th K80.7 Calculus of gallbladder and bile duct without cholecystitis

    K80.70 Calculus of gallbladder and bile duct without cholecystitis without obstruction

    K80.71 Calculus of gallbladder and bile duct without cholecystitis with obstruction

✓5th K80.8 Other cholelithiasis

    K80.80 Other cholelithiasis without obstruction

    K80.81 Other cholelithiasis with obstruction

✓4th K81 Cholecystitis

EXCLUDES 1   cholecystitis with cholelithiasis (K80.-)

K81.0 Acute cholecystitis
Abscess of gallbladder
Angiocholecystitis
Emphysematous (acute) cholecystitis
Empyema of gallbladder
Gangrene of gallbladder
Gangrenous cholecystitis
Suppurative cholecystitis

K81.1 Chronic cholecystitis

K81.2 Acute cholecystitis with chronic cholecystitis

K81.9 Cholecystitis, unspecified

✓4th K82 Other diseases of gallbladder

EXCLUDES 1   nonvisualization of gallbladder (R93.2)
postcholecystectomy syndrome (K91.5)

K82.0 Obstruction of gallbladder
Occlusion of cystic duct or gallbladder without cholelithiasis
Stenosis of cystic duct or gallbladder without cholelithiasis
Stricture of cystic duct or gallbladder without cholelithiasis
EXCLUDES 1   obstruction of gallbladder with cholelithiasis (K80.-)

K82.1 Hydrops of gallbladder
Mucocele of gallbladder

K82.2 Perforation of gallbladder
Rupture of cystic duct or gallbladder

K82.3 Fistula of gallbladder
Cholecystocolic fistula
Cholecystoduodenal fistula

EXCLUDES 1 Not coded here   EXCLUDES 2 Not included here   N Newborn Age: 0   P Pediatric Age: 0-17   M Maternity Age: 12-55   A Adult Age: 15-124

K82.4 Cholesterolosis of gallbladder
Strawberry gallbladder
EXCLUDES 1 *cholesterolosis of gallbladder with cholecystitis (K81.-)*
cholesterolosis of gallbladder with cholelithiasis (K80.-)

K82.8 Other specified diseases of gallbladder
Adhesions of cystic duct or gallbladder
Atrophy of cystic duct or gallbladder
Cyst of cystic duct or gallbladder
Dyskinesia of cystic duct or gallbladder
Hypertrophy of cystic duct or gallbladder
Nonfunctioning of cystic duct or gallbladder
Ulcer of cystic duct or gallbladder

K82.9 Disease of gallbladder, unspecified

✓4ᵗʰ **K83 Other diseases of biliary tract**
EXCLUDES 1 *postcholecystectomy syndrome (K91.5)*
EXCLUDES 2 *conditions involving the gallbladder (K81-K82)*
conditions involving the cystic duct (K81-K82)

K83.0 Cholangitis
Ascending cholangitis
Cholangitis NOS
Primary cholangitis
Recurrent cholangitis
Sclerosing cholangitis
Secondary cholangitis
Stenosing cholangitis
Suppurative cholangitis
EXCLUDES 1 *cholangitic liver abscess (K75.0)*
cholangitis with choledocholithiasis (K80.3-, K80.4-)
chronic nonsuppurative destructive cholangitis (K74.3)

K83.1 Obstruction of bile duct
Occlusion of bile duct without cholelithiasis
Stenosis of bile duct without cholelithiasis
Stricture of bile duct without cholelithiasis
EXCLUDES 1 *congenital obstruction of bile duct (Q44.3)*
obstruction of bile duct with cholelithiasis (K80.-)

K83.2 Perforation of bile duct
Rupture of bile duct

K83.3 Fistula of bile duct
Choledochoduodenal fistula

K83.4 Spasm of sphincter of Oddi

K83.5 Biliary cyst

K83.8 Other specified diseases of biliary tract
Adhesions of biliary tract
Atrophy of biliary tract
Hypertrophy of biliary tract
Ulcer of biliary tract

K83.9 Disease of biliary tract, unspecified

✓4ᵗʰ **K85 Acute pancreatitis**
Abscess of pancreas
Acute necrosis of pancreas
Acute (recurrent) pancreatitis
Gangrene of (gangrenous) pancreas
Hemorrhagic pancreatitis
Infective necrosis of pancreas
Subacute pancreatitis
Suppurative pancreatitis

K85.0 Idiopathic acute pancreatitis

K85.1 Biliary acute pancreatitis
Gallstone pancreatitis

K85.2 Alcohol induced acute pancreatitis
EXCLUDES 2 *alcohol induced chronic pancreatitis (K86.0)*

K85.3 Drug induced acute pancreatitis
Use additional code for adverse effect, if applicable, to identify drug (T36-T50 with fifth or sixth character 5)
Use additional code to identify drug abuse and dependence (F11.- F17.-)

K85.8 Other acute pancreatitis

K85.9 Acute pancreatitis, unspecified
Pancreatitis NOS

✓4ᵗʰ **K86 Other diseases of pancreas**
EXCLUDES 2 *fibrocystic disease of pancreas (E84.-)*
islet cell tumor (of pancreas) (D13.7)
pancreatic steatorrhea (K90.3)

K86.0 Alcohol-induced chronic pancreatitis
Use additional code to identify:
alcohol abuse and dependence (F10.-)
EXCLUDES 2 *alcohol induced acute pancreatitis (K85.2)*

K86.1 Other chronic pancreatitis
Chronic pancreatitis NOS
Infectious chronic pancreatitis
Recurrent chronic pancreatitis
Relapsing chronic pancreatitis

K86.2 Cyst of pancreas

K86.3 Pseudocyst of pancreas

K86.8 Other specified diseases of pancreas
Aseptic pancreatic necrosis
Atrophy of pancreas
Calculus of pancreas
Cirrhosis of pancreas
Fibrosis of pancreas
Pancreatic fat necrosis
Pancreatic infantilism
Pancreatic necrosis NOS

K86.9 Disease of pancreas, unspecified

K87 Disorders of gallbladder, biliary tract and pancreas in diseases classified elsewhere
Code first underlying disease
EXCLUDES 1 *cytomegaloviral pancreatitis (B25.2)*
mumps pancreatitis (B26.3)
syphilitic gallbladder (A52.74)
syphilitic pancreas (A52.74)
tuberculosis of gallbladder (A18.83)
tuberculosis of pancreas (A18.83)

Other diseases of the digestive system (K90-K95)

✓4ᵗʰ **K90 Intestinal malabsorption**
EXCLUDES 1 *intestinal malabsorption following gastrointestinal surgery (K91.2)*

K90.0 Celiac disease
Gluten-sensitive enteropathy
Idiopathic steatorrhea
Nontropical sprue
Use additional code for associated disorders including:
dermatitis herpetiformis (L13.0)
gluten ataxia (G32.81)

K90.1 Tropical sprue
Sprue NOS
Tropical steatorrhea

K90.2 Blind loop syndrome, not elsewhere classified
Blind loop syndrome NOS
EXCLUDES 1 *congenital blind loop syndrome (Q43.8)*
postsurgical blind loop syndrome (K91.2)

K90.3 Pancreatic steatorrhea

K90.4 Malabsorption due to intolerance, not elsewhere classified
Malabsorption due to intolerance to carbohydrate
Malabsorption due to intolerance to fat
Malabsorption due to intolerance to protein
Malabsorption due to intolerance to starch
EXCLUDES 2 *gluten-sensitive enteropathy (K90.0)*
lactose intolerance (E73.-)

✓5ᵗʰ **K90.8 Other intestinal malabsorption**
K90.81 Whipple's disease
K90.89 Other intestinal malabsorption

K90.9 Intestinal malabsorption, unspecified

✓4ᵗʰ **K91 Intraoperative and postprocedural complications and disorders of digestive system, not elsewhere classified**
EXCLUDES 2 *complications of artificial opening of digestive system (K94.-)*
complications of bariatric procedures (K95.-)
gastrojejunal ulcer (K28.-)
postprocedural (radiation) retroperitoneal abscess (K68.11)
radiation colitis (K52.0)
radiation gastroenteritis (K52.0)
radiation proctitis (K62.7)

K91.0 Vomiting following gastrointestinal surgery

K91.1 Postgastric surgery syndromes
Dumping syndrome
Postgastrectomy syndrome
Postvagotomy syndrome

K91.2 Postsurgical malabsorption, not elsewhere classified
Postsurgical blind loop syndrome
EXCLUDES 1 *malabsorption osteomalacia in adults (M83.2)*
malabsorption osteoporosis, postsurgical (M80.8-, M81.8)

K91.3 Postprocedural intestinal obstruction

K91.5 Postcholecystectomy syndrome

✓ Additional Character Required   ✓7ᵗʰ *X*tension Alert   Unspecified Dx   Other Specified Dx   Manifestation   ►◄ Revised Text   ● New Code   ▲ Revised Code Title

Diseases of the Digestive System

K91.6–K95.89

✓5ᵗʰ K91.6 Intraoperative hemorrhage and hematoma of a digestive system organ or structure complicating a procedure

> EXCLUDES 1   *intraoperative hemorrhage and hematoma of a digestive system organ or structure due to accidental puncture and laceration during a procedure (K91.7-)*

    K91.61 Intraoperative hemorrhage and hematoma of a digestive system organ or structure complicating a digestive sytem procedure

    K91.62 Intraoperative hemorrhage and hematoma of a digestive system organ or structure complicating other procedure

✓5ᵗʰ K91.7 Accidental puncture and laceration of a digestive system organ or structure during a procedure

    K91.71 Accidental puncture and laceration of a digestive system organ or structure during a digestive system procedure

    K91.72 Accidental puncture and laceration of a digestive system organ or structure during other procedure

✓5ᵗʰ K91.8 Other intraoperative and postprocedural complications and disorders of digestive system

    K91.81 Other intraoperative **complications of digestive system**

    K91.82 Postprocedural hepatic failure

    K91.83 Postprocedural hepatorenal syndrome

    ✓6ᵗʰ K91.84 Postprocedural hemorrhage and hematoma **of a digestive system organ or structure** following a procedure

        K91.840 Postprocedural hemorrhage and hematoma of a digestive system organ or structure following a digestive system procedure

        K91.841 Postprocedural hemorrhage and hematoma of a digestive system organ or structure following other procedure

    ✓6ᵗʰ K91.85 Complications of intestinal pouch

        K91.850 Pouchitis

             Inflammation of internal ileoanal pouch

        K91.858 Other complications of intestinal pouch

    K91.86 Retained cholelithiasis following cholecystectomy

    K91.89 Other postprocedural **complications and disorders of digestive system**

         Use additional code, if applicable, to further specify disorder

> EXCLUDES 2   *postprocedural retroperitoneal abscess (K68.11)*

✓4ᵗʰ K92 Other diseases of digestive system

> EXCLUDES 1   *neonatal gastrointestinal hemorrhage (P54.0-P54.3)*

    K92.0 Hematemesis

    K92.1 Melena

> EXCLUDES 1   *occult blood in feces (R19.5)*

    K92.2 Gastrointestinal hemorrhage, unspecified

         Gastric hemorrhage NOS

         Intestinal hemorrhage NOS

> EXCLUDES 1   *acute hemorrhagic gastritis (K29.01)*
> *hemorrhage of anus and rectum (K62.5)*
> *angiodysplasia of stomach with hemorrhage (K31.811)*
> *diverticular disease with hemorrhage (K57.-)*
> *gastritis and duodenitis with hemorrhage (K29.-)*
> *peptic ulcer with hemorrhage (K25-K28)*

    ✓5ᵗʰ K92.8 Other specified diseases of the digestive system

    K92.81 Gastrointestinal mucositis (ulcerative)

         Code also type of associated therapy, such as:

         antineoplastic and immunosuppressive drugs (T45.1X-)

         radiological procedure and radiotherapy (Y84.2)

> EXCLUDES 2   *mucositis (ulcerative) of vagina and vulva (N76.81)*
> *nasal mucositis (ulcerative) (J34.81)*
> *oral mucositis (ulcerative) (K12.3-)*

    K92.89 Other specified diseases of the digestive system

    K92.9 Disease of digestive system, unspecified

✓4ᵗʰ K94 Complications of artificial openings of the digestive system

    ✓5ᵗʰ K94.0 Colostomy complications

    K94.00 Colostomy complication, unspecified

    K94.01 Colostomy hemorrhage

    K94.02 Colostomy infection

         Use additional code to specify type of infection, such as:

         cellulitis of abdominal wall (L03.311)

         sepsis (A40-, A41-)

    K94.03 Colostomy malfunction

         Mechanical complication of colostomy

    K94.09 Other complications of colostomy

    ✓5ᵗʰ K94.1 Enterostomy complications

    K94.10 Enterostomy complication, unspecified

    K94.11 Enterostomy hemorrhage

    K94.12 Enterostomy infection

         Use additional code to specify type of infection, such as:

         cellulitis of abdominal wall (L03.311)

         sepsis (A40-, A41-)

    K94.13 Enterostomy malfunction

         Mechanical complication of enterostomy

    K94.19 Other complications of enterostomy

    ✓5ᵗʰ K94.2 Gastrostomy complications

    K94.20 Gastrostomy complication, unspecified

    K94.21 Gastrostomy hemorrhage

    K94.22 Gastrostomy infection

         Use additional code to specify type of infection, such as:

         cellulitis of abdominal wall (L03.311)

         sepsis (A40-, A41-)

    K94.23 Gastrostomy malfunction

         Mechanical complication of gastrostomy

    K94.29 Other complications of gastrostomy

    ✓5ᵗʰ K94.3 Esophagostomy complications

    K94.30 Esophagostomy complications, unspecified

    K94.31 Esophagostomy hemorrhage

    K94.32 Esophagostomy infection

         Use additional code to identify the infection

    K94.33 Esophagostomy malfunction

         Mechanical complication of esophagostomy

    K94.39 Other complications of esophagostom

✓4ᵗʰ K95 Complications of bariatric procedures

    ✓5ᵗʰ K95.0 Complications of gastric band procedure

    K95.01 Infection due to gastric band procedure

         Use additional code to specify type of infection or organism, such as:

         bacterial and viral infectious agents (B95.-, B96.-)

         cellulitis of abdominal wall (L03.311)

         sepsis (A40.-, A41.-)

    K95.09 Other complications of gastric band procedure

         Use additional code, if applicable, to further specify complication

    ✓5ᵗʰ K95.8 Complications of other bariatric procedure

> EXCLUDES 1   *complications of gastric band surgery (K95.0-)*

    K95.81 Infection due to other bariatric procedure

         Use additional code to specify type of infection or organism, such as:

         bacterial and viral infectious agents (B95.-, B96.-)

         cellulitis of abdominal wall (L03.311)

         sepsis (A40.-, A41.-)

    K95.89 Other complications of other bariatric procedure

         Use additional code, if applicable, to further specify complication

---

EXCLUDES 1 Not coded here   EXCLUDES 2 Not included here   N Newborn Age: 0   P Pediatric Age: 0-17   M Maternity Age: 12-55   A Adult Age: 15-124

628   ICD-10-CM Draft (2015)

Chapter 12. Diseases of the Skin and Subcutaneous Tissue (L00-L99)

EXCLUDES 2 *certain conditions originating in the perinatal period (P04-P96)*
certain infectious and parasitic diseases (A00-B99)
complications of pregnancy, childbirth and the puerperium (O00-O9A)
congenital malformations, deformations, and chromosomal abnormalities (Q00-Q99)
endocrine, nutritional and metabolic diseases (E00-E88)
lipomelanotic reticulosis (I89.8)
neoplasms (C00-D49)
symptoms, signs and abnormal clinical and laboratory findings, not elsewhere classified (R00-R94)
systemic connective tissue disorders (M30-M36)
viral warts (B07.-)

This chapter contains the following blocks:

L00-L08	Infections of the skin and subcutaneous tissue
L10-L14	Bullous disorders
L20-L30	Dermatitis and eczema
L40-L45	Papulosquamous disorders
L49-L54	Urticaria and erythema
L55-L59	Radiation-related disorders of the skin and subcutaneous tissue
L60-L75	Disorders of skin appendages
L76	Intraoperative and postprocedural complications of skin and subcutaneous tissue
L80-L99	Other disorders of the skin and subcutaneous tissue

Infections of the skin and subcutaneous tissue (L00-L08)

Use additional code (B95-B97) to identify infectious agent

EXCLUDES 2 *hordeolum (H00.0)*
infective dermatitis (L30.3)
local infections of skin classified in Chapter 1
lupus panniculitis (L93.2)
panniculitis NOS (M79.3)
panniculitis of neck and back (M54.0-)
Perlèche NOS (K13.0)
Perlèche due to candidiasis (B37.0)
Perlèche due to riboflavin deficiency (E53.0)
pyogenic granuloma (L98.0)
relapsing panniculitis [Weber-Christian] (M35.6)
viral warts (B07.-)
zoster (B02.-)

L00　Staphylococcal scalded skin syndrome
Ritter's disease
Use additional code to identify percentage of skin exfoliation (L49.-)
EXCLUDES 1 *bullous impetigo (L01.03)*
pemphigus neonatorum (L01.03)
toxic epidermal necrolysis [Lyell] (L51.2)

✓4ᵗʰ **L01　Impetigo**
EXCLUDES 1 *impetigo herpetiformis (L40.1)*

✓5ᵗʰ **L01.0　Impetigo**
Impetigo contagiosa　　　Impetigo vulgaris

L01.00　Impetigo, unspecified
Impetigo NOS

L01.01　Non-bullous impetigo

L01.02　Bockhart's impetigo
Impetigo follicularisSuperficial pustular
Perifolliculitis NOS　　perifolliculitis

L01.03　Bullous impetigo
Impetigo neonatorumPemphigus neonatorum

L01.09　Other impetigo
Ulcerative impetigo

L01.1　Impetiginization of other dermatoses

✓4ᵗʰ **L02　Cutaneous abscess, furuncle and carbuncle**
Use additional code to identify organism (B95-B96)
EXCLUDES 2 *abscess of anus and rectal regions (K61.-)*
abscess of female genital organs (external) (N76.4)
abscess of male genital organs (external) (N48.2, N49-)

✓5ᵗʰ **L02.0　Cutaneous abscess, furuncle and carbuncle of face**
EXCLUDES 2 *abscess of ear, external (H60.0)*
abscess of eyelid (H00.0)
abscess of head [any part, except face] (L02.8)
abscess of lacrimal gland (H04.0)
abscess of lacrimal passages (H04.3)
abscess of mouth (K12.2)
abscess of nose (J34.0)
abscess of orbit (H05.0)
submandibular abscess (K12.2)

L02.01　Cutaneous abscess of face

L02.02　Furuncle of face
Boil of face
Folliculitis of face

L02.03　Carbuncle of face

✓5ᵗʰ **L02.1　Cutaneous abscess, furuncle and carbuncle of neck**

L02.11　Cutaneous abscess of neck

L02.12　Furuncle of neck
Boil of neck
Folliculitis of neck

L02.13　Carbuncle of neck

✓5ᵗʰ **L02.2　Cutaneous abscess, furuncle and carbuncle of trunk**
EXCLUDES 1 *non-newborn omphalitis (L08.82)*
omphalitis of newborn (P38.-)
EXCLUDES 2 *abscess of breast (N61)*
abscess of buttocks (L02.3)
abscess of female external genital organs (N76.4)
abscess of hip (L02.4)
abscess of male external genital organs (N48.2, N49-)

✓6ᵗʰ **L02.21　Cutaneous abscess of trunk**

L02.211　Cutaneous abscess of abdominal wall

L02.212　Cutaneous abscess of back [any part, except buttock]

L02.213　Cutaneous abscess of chest wall

L02.214　Cutaneous abscess of groin

L02.215　Cutaneous abscess of perineum

L02.216　Cutaneous abscess of umbilicus

L02.219　Cutaneous abscess of trunk, unspecified

✓6ᵗʰ **L02.22　Furuncle of trunk**
Boil of trunk
Folliculitis of trunk

L02.221　Furuncle of abdominal wall

L02.222　Furuncle of back [any part, except buttock]

L02.223　Furuncle of chest wall

L02.224　Furuncle of groin

L02.225　Furuncle of perineum

L02.226　Furuncle of umbilicus

L02.229　Furuncle of trunk, unspecified

✓6ᵗʰ **L02.23　Carbuncle of trunk**

L02.231　Carbuncle of abdominal wall

L02.232　Carbuncle of back [any part, except buttock]

L02.233　Carbuncle of chest wall

L02.234　Carbuncle of groin

L02.235　Carbuncle of perineum

L02.236　Carbuncle of umbilicus

L02.239　Carbuncle of trunk, unspecified

✓5ᵗʰ **L02.3　Cutaneous abscess, furuncle and carbuncle of buttock**
EXCLUDES 1 *pilonidal cyst with abscess (L05.01)*

L02.31　Cutaneous abscess of buttock
Cutaneous abscess of gluteal region

L02.32　Furuncle of buttock
Boil of buttock
Folliculitis of buttock
Furuncle of gluteal region

L02.33　Carbuncle of buttock
Carbuncle of gluteal region

✓5ᵗʰ **L02.4　Cutaneous abscess, furuncle and carbuncle of limb**
EXCLUDES 2 *cutaneous abscess, furuncle and carbuncle of groin (L02.214, L02.224, L02.234)*
cutaneous abscess, furuncle and carbuncle of hand (L02.5-)
cutaneous abscess, furuncle and carbuncle of foot (L02.6-)

✓6ᵗʰ **L02.41　Cutaneous abscess of limb**

L02.411　Cutaneous abscess of right axilla

L02.412　Cutaneous abscess of left axilla

L02.413　Cutaneous abscess of right upper limb

L02.414　Cutaneous abscess of left upper limb

L02.415　Cutaneous abscess of right lower limb

L02.416　Cutaneous abscess of left lower limb

L02.419　Cutaneous abscess of limb, unspecified

✓6ᵗʰ **L02.42　Furuncle of limb**
Boil of limb
Folliculitis of limb

L02.421　Furuncle of right axilla

　　　　L02.422　**Furuncle of** left axilla
　　　　L02.423　**Furuncle of** right upper **limb**
　　　　L02.424　**Furuncle of** left upper **limb**
　　　　L02.425　**Furuncle of** right lower **limb**
　　　　L02.426　**Furuncle of** left lower **limb**
　　　　L02.429　**Furuncle of limb, unspecified**
　√6ᵗʰ　L02.43　Carbuncle **of limb**
　　　　L02.431　**Carbuncle of** right axilla
　　　　L02.432　**Carbuncle of** left axilla
　　　　L02.433　**Carbuncle of** right upper **limb**
　　　　L02.434　**Carbuncle of** left upper **limb**
　　　　L02.435　**Carbuncle of** right lower **limb**
　　　　L02.436　**Carbuncle of** left lower **limb**
　　　　L02.439　**Carbuncle of limb, unspecified**
√5ᵗʰ　L02.5　**Cutaneous abscess, furuncle and carbuncle of** hand
　√6ᵗʰ　L02.51　Cutaneous abscess **of hand**
　　　　L02.511　**Cutaneous abscess of** right **hand**
　　　　L02.512　**Cutaneous abscess of** left **hand**
　　　　L02.519　**Cutaneous abscess of unspecified hand**
　√6ᵗʰ　L02.52　Furuncle **hand**
　　　　　Boil of hand
　　　　　Folliculitis of hand
　　　　L02.521　**Furuncle** right **hand**
　　　　L02.522　**Furuncle** left **hand**
　　　　L02.529　**Furuncle unspecified hand**
　√6ᵗʰ　L02.53　Carbuncle **of hand**
　　　　L02.531　**Carbuncle of** right **hand**
　　　　L02.532　**Carbuncle of** left **hand**
　　　　L02.539　**Carbuncle of unspecified hand**
√5ᵗʰ　L02.6　**Cutaneous abscess, furuncle and carbuncle of** foot
　√6ᵗʰ　L02.61　Cutaneous abscess **of foot**
　　　　L02.611　**Cutaneous abscess of** right **foot**
　　　　L02.612　**Cutaneous abscess of** left **foot**
　　　　L02.619　**Cutaneous abscess of unspecified foot**
　√6ᵗʰ　L02.62　Furuncle **of foot**
　　　　　Boil of foot
　　　　　Folliculitis of foot
　　　　L02.621　**Furuncle of** right **foot**
　　　　L02.622　**Furuncle of** left **foot**
　　　　L02.629　**Furuncle of unspecified foot**
　√6ᵗʰ　L02.63　Carbuncle **of foot**
　　　　L02.631　**Carbuncle of** right **foot**
　　　　L02.632　**Carbuncle of** left **foot**
　　　　L02.639　**Carbuncle of unspecified foot**
√5ᵗʰ　L02.8　**Cutaneous abscess, furuncle and carbuncle of** other sites
　√6ᵗʰ　L02.81　Cutaneous abscess **of other sites**
　　　　L02.811　**Cutaneous abscess of** head **[any part, except face]**
　　　　L02.818　**Cutaneous abscess of other sites**
　√6ᵗʰ　L02.82　Furuncle **of other sites**
　　　　　Boil of other sites
　　　　　Folliculitis of other sites
　　　　L02.821　**Furuncle of head [any part, except face]**
　　　　L02.828　**Furuncle of other sites**
　√6ᵗʰ　L02.83　Carbuncle **of other sites**
　　　　L02.831　**Carbuncle of** head **[any part, except face]**
　　　　L02.838　**Carbuncle of other sites**
√5ᵗʰ　L02.9　**Cutaneous abscess, furuncle and carbuncle,** unspecified
　　　L02.91　Cutaneous abscess, **unspecified**
　　　L02.92　Furuncle, **unspecified**
　　　　　Boil NOS
　　　　　Furunculosis NOS
　　　L02.93　Carbuncle, **unspecified**

√4ᵗʰ　L03　**Cellulitis and acute lymphangitis**
　　　EXCLUDES 2　*cellulitis of anal and rectal region (K61.-)*
　　　　　cellulitis of external auditory canal (H60.1)
　　　　　cellulitis of eyelid (H00.03-)
　　　　　cellulitis of female external genital organs (N76.4)
　　　　　cellulitis of lacrimal apparatus (H04.3)
　　　　　cellulitis of male external genital organs (N48.2, N49-)
　　　　　cellulitis of mouth (K12.2)
　　　　　cellulitis of nose (J34.0)
　　　　　eosinophilic cellulitis [Wells] (L98.3)
　　　　　febrile neutrophilic dermatosis [Sweet] (L98.2)
　　　　　lymphangitis (chronic) (subacute) (I89.1)
　√5ᵗʰ　L03.0　**Cellulitis and acute lymphangitis of** finger and toe
　　　　　Infection of nail
　　　　　Onychia
　　　　　Paronychia
　　　　　Perionychia
　　√6ᵗʰ　L03.01　Cellulitis **of finger**
　　　　　　Felon
　　　　　　Whitlow
　　　　　　EXCLUDES 1　*herpetic whitlow (B00.89)*
　　　　　L03.011　**Cellulitis of** right **finger**
　　　　　L03.012　**Cellulitis of** left **finger**
　　　　　L03.019　**Cellulitis of unspecified finger**
　　√6ᵗʰ　L03.02　Acute lymphangitis **of finger**
　　　　　　Hangnail with lymphangitis of finger
　　　　　L03.021　**Acute lymphangitis of** right **finger**
　　　　　L03.022　**Acute lymphangitis of** left **finger**
　　　　　L03.029　**Acute lymphangitis of unspecified finger**
　　√6ᵗʰ　L03.03　Cellulitis **of** toe
　　　　　L03.031　**Cellulitis of** right **toe**
　　　　　L03.032　**Cellulitis of** left **toe**
　　　　　L03.039　**Cellulitis of unspecified toe**
　　√6ᵗʰ　L03.04　Acute lymphangitis **of** toe
　　　　　　Hangnail with lymphangitis of toe
　　　　　L03.041　**Acute lymphangitis of** right **toe**
　　　　　L03.042　**Acute lymphangitis of** left **toe**
　　　　　L03.049　**Acute lymphangitis of unspecified toe**
　√5ᵗʰ　L03.1　**Cellulitis and acute lymphangitis of** other parts **of limb**
　　√6ᵗʰ　L03.11　Cellulitis **of other parts of limb**
　　　　　EXCLUDES 2　*cellulitis of fingers (L03.01-)*
　　　　　　cellulitis of toes (L03.03-)
　　　　　　groin (L03.314)
　　　　　L03.111　**Cellulitis of** right axilla
　　　　　L03.112　**Cellulitis of** left axilla
　　　　　L03.113　**Cellulitis of** right upper limb
　　　　　L03.114　**Cellulitis of** left upper limb
　　　　　L03.115　**Cellulitis of** right lower limb
　　　　　L03.116　**Cellulitis of** left lower limb
　　　　　L03.119　**Cellulitis of unspecified part of limb**
　　√6ᵗʰ　L03.12　Acute lymphangitis **of other parts of limb**
　　　　　EXCLUDES 2　*acute lymphangitis of fingers (L03.02-)*
　　　　　　acute lymphangitis of groin (L03.324)
　　　　　　acute lymphangitis of toes (L03.04-)
　　　　　L03.121　**Acute lymphangitis of** right axilla
　　　　　L03.122　**Acute lymphangitis of** left axilla
　　　　　L03.123　**Acute lymphangitis of** right upper **limb**
　　　　　L03.124　**Acute lymphangitis of** left upper **limb**
　　　　　L03.125　**Acute lymphangitis of** right lower **limb**
　　　　　L03.126　**Acute lymphangitis of** left lower **limb**
　　　　　L03.129　**Acute lymphangitis of unspecified part of limb**
　√5ᵗʰ　L03.2　**Cellulitis and acute lymphangitis of** face and neck
　　√6ᵗʰ　L03.21　**Cellulitis and acute lymphangitis of** face
　　　　　L03.211　Cellulitis **of face**
　　　　　　EXCLUDES 2　*cellulitis of ear (H60.1-)*
　　　　　　　cellulitis of eyelid (H00.03-)
　　　　　　　cellulitis of head (L03.811)
　　　　　　　cellulitis of lacrimal apparatus (H04.3)
　　　　　　　cellulitis of lip (K13.0)
　　　　　　　cellulitis of mouth (K12.2)
　　　　　　　cellulitis of nose (internal) (J34.0)
　　　　　　　cellulitis of orbit (H05.0)
　　　　　　　cellulitis of scalp (L03.811)
　　　　　　AHA: 2013, 4Q, 123
　　　　　L03.212　Acute lymphangitis **of face**

EXCLUDES 1 Not coded here　　　EXCLUDES 2 Not included here　　　N Newborn Age: 0　　　P Pediatric Age: 0-17　　　M Maternity Age: 12-55　　　A Adult Age: 15-124

630　　　　　　　　　　　　　　　　　　　　　　　　　　　　　　ICD-10-CM Draft (2015)

✓6th **L03.22 Cellulitis and acute lymphangitis of** neck
    L03.221 Cellulitis of neck
    L03.222 Acute lymphangitis of neck

✓5th **L03.3 Cellulitis and acute lymphangitis of** trunk
  ✓6th **L03.31 Cellulitis of trunk**
    EXCLUDES 2 *cellulitis of anal and rectal regions (K61.-)*
        cellulitis of breast NOS (N61)
        cellulitis of female external genital organs (N76.4)
        cellulitis of male external genital organs (N48.2, N49-)
        omphalitis of newborn (P38.-)
        puerperal cellulitis of breast (O91.2)
    L03.311 Cellulitis of abdominal wall
      EXCLUDES 2 *cellulitis of umbilicus (L03.316)*
        cellulitis of groin (L03.314)
    L03.312 Cellulitis of back **[any part except buttock]**
    L03.313 Cellulitis of chest wall
    L03.314 Cellulitis of groin
    L03.315 Cellulitis of perineum
    L03.316 Cellulitis of umbilicus
    L03.317 Cellulitis of buttock
    L03.319 Cellulitis of trunk, unspecified
  ✓6th **L03.32 Acute lymphangitis of** trunk
    L03.321 Acute lymphangitis of abdominal wall
    L03.322 Acute lymphangitis of back **[any part except buttock]**
    L03.323 Acute lymphangitis of chest wall
    L03.324 Acute lymphangitis of groin
    L03.325 Acute lymphangitis of perineum
    L03.326 Acute lymphangitis of umbilicus
    L03.327 Acute lymphangitis of buttock
    L03.329 Acute lymphangitis of trunk, unspecified

✓5th **L03.8 Cellulitis and acute lymphangitis of** other sites
  ✓6th **L03.81 Cellulitis of** other sites
    L03.811 Cellulitis of head **[any part, except face]**
      Cellulitis of scalp
      EXCLUDES 2 *cellulitis of face (L03.211)*
    L03.818 Cellulitis of other sites
  ✓6th **L03.89 Acute lymphangitis of** other sites
    L03.891 Acute lymphangitis of head **[any part, except face]**
    L03.898 Acute lymphangitis of other sites

✓5th **L03.9 Cellulitis and acute lymphangitis, unspecified**
  L03.90 Cellulitis, unspecified
  L03.91 Acute lymphangitis, unspecified
    EXCLUDES 1 *lymphangitis NOS (I89.1)*

✓4th **L04 Acute lymphadenitis**
  INCLUDES abscess (acute) of lymph nodes, except mesenteric
    acute lymphadenitis, except mesenteric
  EXCLUDES 1 *chronic or subacute lymphadenitis, except mesenteric (I88.1)*
    enlarged lymph nodes (R59.-)
    human immunodeficiency virus [HIV] disease resulting in generalized lymphadenopathy (B20)
    lymphadenitis NOS (I88.9)
    nonspecific mesenteric lymphadenitis (I88.0)
  L04.0 Acute lymphadenitis of face, head and neck
  L04.1 Acute lymphadenitis of trunk
  L04.2 Acute lymphadenitis of upper limb
    Acute lymphadenitis of axilla
    Acute lymphadenitis of shoulder
  L04.3 Acute lymphadenitis of lower limb
    Acute lymphadenitis of hip
    EXCLUDES 2 *acute lymphadenitis of groin (L04.1)*
  L04.8 Acute lymphadenitis of other sites
  L04.9 Acute lymphadenitis, unspecified

✓4th **L05 Pilonidal cyst and sinus**
  ✓5th **L05.0 Pilonidal cyst and sinus** with abscess
    L05.01 Pilonidal cyst with abscess
      Parasacral dimple with abscess
      Pilonidal abscess
      Pilonidal dimple with abscess
      Postanal dimple with abscess

    L05.02 Pilonidal sinus **with abscess**
      Coccygeal fistula with abscess
      Coccygeal sinus with abscess
      Pilonidal fistula with abscess
  ✓5th **L05.9 Pilonidal cyst and sinus** without abscess
    L05.91 Pilonidal cyst **without abscess**
      Parasacral dimple
      Pilonidal dimple
      Postanal dimple
      Pilonidal cyst NOS
    L05.92 Pilonidal sinus **without abscess**
      Coccygeal fistula
      Coccygeal sinus without abscess
      Pilonidal fistula

✓4th **L08 Other local infections of skin and subcutaneous tissue**
  L08.0 Pyoderma
    Dermatitis gangrenosa
    Purulent dermatitis
    Septic dermatitis
    Suppurative dermatitis
    EXCLUDES 1 *pyoderma gangrenosum (L88)*
      pyoderma vegetans (L08.81)
  L08.1 Erythrasma
  ✓5th **L08.8 Other specified local infections of the skin and subcutaneous tissue**
    L08.81 Pyoderma vegetans
      EXCLUDES 1 *pyoderma gangrenosum (L88)*
      pyoderma NOS (L08.0)
    L08.82 Omphalitis not of newborn
      EXCLUDES 1 *omphalitis of newborn (P38.-)*
    L08.89 Other specified local infections of the skin and subcutaneous tissue
  L08.9 Local infection of the skin and subcutaneous tissue, unspecified

Bullous disorders (L10-L14)

EXCLUDES 1 *benign familial pemphigus [Hailey-Hailey] (Q82.8)*
  staphylococcal scalded skin syndrome (L00)
  toxic epidermal necrolysis [Lyell] (L51.2)

✓4th **L10 Pemphigus**
  EXCLUDES 1 *pemphigus neonatorum (L01.03)*
  L10.0 Pemphigus vulgaris
  L10.1 Pemphigus vegetans
  L10.2 Pemphigus foliaceous
  L10.3 Brazilian pemphigus [fogo selvagem]
  L10.4 Pemphigus erythematosus
    Senear-Usher syndrome
  L10.5 Drug-induced pemphigus
    Use additional code for adverse effect, if applicable, to identify drug (T36-T50 with fifth or sixth character 5)
  ✓5th **L10.8 Other pemphigus**
    L10.81 Paraneoplastic pemphigus
    L10.89 Other pemphigus
  L10.9 Pemphigus, unspecified

✓4th **L11 Other acantholytic disorders**
  L11.0 Acquired keratosis follicularis
    EXCLUDES 1 *keratosis follicularis (congenital) [Darier-White] (Q82.8)*
  L11.1 Transient acantholytic dermatosis [Grover]
  L11.8 Other specified acantholytic disorders
  L11.9 Acantholytic disorder, unspecified

✓4th **L12 Pemphigoid**
  EXCLUDES 1 *herpes gestationis (O26.4-)*
    impetigo herpetiformis (L40.1)
  L12.0 Bullous pemphigoid
  L12.1 Cicatricial pemphigoid
    Benign mucous membrane pemphigoid
  L12.2 Chronic bullous disease of childhood P
    Juvenile dermatitis herpetiformis
  ✓5th **L12.3 Acquired epidermolysis bullosa**
    EXCLUDES 1 *epidermolysis bullosa (congenital) (Q81.-)*
    L12.30 Acquired epidermolysis bullosa, unspecified
    L12.31 Epidermolysis bullosa due to drug
      Use additional code for adverse effect, if applicable, to identify drug (T36-T50 with fifth or sixth character 5)

✓ Additional Character Required   ✓x7th Xtension Alert   Unspecified Dx   Other Specified Dx   Manifestation   ►◄ Revised Text   ● New Code   ▲ Revised Code Title

ICD-10-CM Draft (2015)   681

Diseases of the Skin and Subcutaneous Tissue

L12.35–L25.2

L12.35   **Other acquired epidermolysis bullosa**

L12.8   **Other pemphigoid**

L12.9   **Pemphigoid, unspecified**

✓4ᵗʰ **L13**   **Other bullous disorders**

     L13.0   **Dermatitis herpetiformis**
         Duhring's disease
         Hydroa herpetiformis
         EXCLUDES 1   *juvenile dermatitis herpetiformis (L12.2)*
                    senile dermatitis herpetiformis (L12.0)

     L13.1   **Subcorneal pustular dermatitis**
         Sneddon-Wilkinson disease

     L13.8   **Other specified bullous disorders**

     L13.9   **Bullous disorder, unspecified**

L14   *Bullous disorders in diseases classified elsewhere*
         Code first underlying disease

Dermatitis and eczema (L20-L30)

NOTE   In this block the terms dermatitis and eczema are used synonymously and interchangeably.

EXCLUDES 2   *chronic (childhood) granulomatous disease (D71)*
         dermatitis gangrenosa (L08.0)
         dermatitis herpetiformis (L13.0)
         dry skin dermatitis (L85.3)
         factitial dermatitis (L98.1)
         perioral dermatitis (L71.0)
         radiation-related disorders of the skin and subcutaneous tissue (L55-L59)
         stasis dermatitis (I83.1-I83.2)

✓4ᵗʰ **L20**   **Atopic dermatitis**

     L20.0   Besnier's prurigo

✓5ᵗʰ   L20.8   **Other atopic dermatitis**
         EXCLUDES 2   *circumscribed neurodermatitis (L28.0)*

         L20.81   **Atopic neurodermatitis**
               Diffuse neurodermatitis

         L20.82   **Flexural eczema**

         L20.83   **Infantile (acute) (chronic) eczema**   P

         L20.84   **Intrinsic (allergic) eczema**

         L20.89   **Other atopic dermatitis**

     L20.9   **Atopic dermatitis, unspecified**

✓4ᵗʰ **L21**   **Seborrheic dermatitis**
         EXCLUDES 2   *infective dermatitis (L30.3)*
                seborrheic keratosis (L82.-)

     L21.0   **Seborrhea capitis**   P
         Cradle cap

     L21.1   **Seborrheic infantile dermatitis**   P

     L21.8   **Other seborrheic dermatitis**

     L21.9   **Seborrheic dermatitis, unspecified**
         Seborrhea NOS

L22   **Diaper dermatitis**
     Diaper erythema
     Diaper rash
     Psoriasiform diaper rash

✓4ᵗʰ **L23**   **Allergic contact dermatitis**
         EXCLUDES 1   *allergy NOS (T78.40)*
                contact dermatitis NOS (L25.9)
                dermatitis NOS (L30.9)
         EXCLUDES 2   *dermatitis due to substances taken internally (L27.-)*
                dermatitis of eyelid (H01.1-)
                diaper dermatitis (L22)
                eczema of external ear (H60.5-)
                irritant contact dermatitis (L24.-)
                perioral dermatitis (L71.0)
                radiation-related disorders of the skin and subcutaneous tissue (L55-L59)

     L23.0   **Allergic contact dermatitis due to metals**
         Allergic contact dermatitis due to chromium
         Allergic contact dermatitis due to nickel

     L23.1   **Allergic contact dermatitis due to adhesives**

     L23.2   **Allergic contact dermatitis due to cosmetics**

     L23.3   **Allergic contact dermatitis due to drugs in contact with skin**
         Use additional code for adverse effect, if applicable, to identify drug (T36-T50 with fifth or sixth character 5)
         EXCLUDES 2   *dermatitis due to ingested drugs and medicaments (L27.0-L27.1)*

     L23.4   **Allergic contact dermatitis due to dyes**

     L23.5   **Allergic contact dermatitis due to other chemical products**
         Allergic contact dermatitis due to cement
         Allergic contact dermatitis due to insecticide
         Allergic contact dermatitis due to plastic
         Allergic contact dermatitis due to rubber

     L23.6   **Allergic contact dermatitis due to food in contact with the skin**
         EXCLUDES 2   *dermatitis due to ingested food (L27.2)*

     L23.7   **Allergic contact dermatitis due to plants, except food**
         EXCLUDES 2   *allergy NOS due to pollen (J30.1)*

✓5ᵗʰ   L23.8   **Allergic contact dermatitis due to other agents**

         L23.81   **Allergic contact dermatitis due to animal (cat) (dog) dander**
               Allergic contact dermatitis due to animal (cat) (dog) hair

         L23.89   **Allergic contact dermatitis due to other agents**

     L23.9   **Allergic contact dermatitis, unspecified cause**
         Allergic contact eczema NOS

✓4ᵗʰ **L24**   **Irritant contact dermatitis**
         EXCLUDES 1   *allergy NOS (T78.40)*
                contact dermatitis NOS (L25.9)
                dermatitis NOS (L30.9)
         EXCLUDES 2   *allergic contact dermatitis (L23.-)*
                dermatitis due to substances taken internally (L27.-)
                dermatitis of eyelid (H01.1-)
                diaper dermatitis (L22)
                eczema of external ear (H60.5-)
                perioral dermatitis (L71.0)
                radiation-related disorders of the skin and subcutaneous tissue (L55-L59)

     L24.0   **Irritant contact dermatitis due to detergents**

     L24.1   **Irritant contact dermatitis due to oils and greases**

     L24.2   **Irritant contact dermatitis due to solvents**
         Irritant contact dermatitis due to chlorocompound
         Irritant contact dermatitis due to cyclohexane
         Irritant contact dermatitis due to ester
         Irritant contact dermatitis due to glycol
         Irritant contact dermatitis due to hydrocarbon
         Irritant contact dermatitis due to ketone

     L24.3   **Irritant contact dermatitis due to cosmetics**

     L24.4   **Irritant contact dermatitis due to drugs in contact with skin**
         Use additional code for adverse effect, if applicable, to identify drug (T36-T50 with fifth or sixth character 5)

     L24.5   **Irritant contact dermatitis due to other chemical products**
         Irritant contact dermatitis due to cement
         Irritant contact dermatitis due to insecticide
         Irritant contact dermatitis due to plastic
         Irritant contact dermatitis due to rubber

     L24.6   **Irritant contact dermatitis due to food in contact with skin**
         EXCLUDES 2   *dermatitis due to ingested food (L27.2)*

     L24.7   **Irritant contact dermatitis due to plants, except food**
         EXCLUDES 2   *allergy NOS to pollen (J30.1)*

✓5ᵗʰ   L24.8   **Irritant contact dermatitis due to other agents**

         L24.81   **Irritant contact dermatitis due to metals**
               Irritant contact dermatitis due to chromium
               Irritant contact dermatitis due to nickel

         L24.89   **Irritant contact dermatitis due to other agents**
               Irritant contact dermatitis due to dyes

     L24.9   **Irritant contact dermatitis, unspecified cause**
         Irritant contact eczema NOS

✓4ᵗʰ **L25**   **Unspecified contact dermatitis**
         EXCLUDES 1   *allergic contact dermatitis (L23.-)*
                allergy NOS (T78.40)
                dermatitis NOS (L30.9)
                irritant contact dermatitis (L24.-)
         EXCLUDES 2   *dermatitis due to ingested substances (L27.-)*
                dermatitis of eyelid (H01.1-)
                eczema of external ear (H60.5-)
                perioral dermatitis (L71.0)
                radiation-related disorders of the skin and subcutaneous tissue (L55-L59)

     L25.0   **Unspecified contact dermatitis due to cosmetics**

     L25.1   **Unspecified contact dermatitis due to drugs in contact with skin**
         Use additional code for adverse effect, if applicable, to identify drug (T36-T50 with fifth or sixth character 5)
         EXCLUDES 2   *dermatitis due to ingested drugs and medicaments (L27.0-L27.1)*

     L25.2   **Unspecified contact dermatitis due to dyes**

EXCLUDES 1 Not coded here   *EXCLUDES 2* Not included here   N Newborn Age: 0   P Pediatric Age: 0-17   M Maternity Age: 12-55   A Adult Age: 15-124

632   ICD-10-CM Draft (2015)

L25.3 **Unspecified contact dermatitis due to** other chemical products
    Unspecified contact dermatitis due to cement
    Unspecified contact dermatitis due to insecticide

L25.4 **Unspecified contact dermatitis due to** food in contact with skin
    EXCLUDES 2   *dermatitis due to ingested food (L27.2)*

L25.5 **Unspecified contact dermatitis due to** plants, except food
    EXCLUDES 1   *nettle rash (L50.9)*
    EXCLUDES 2   *allergy NOS due to pollen (J30.1)*

L25.8 **Unspecified contact dermatitis due to other** agents

L25.9 **Unspecified contact dermatitis, unspecified cause**
    Contact dermatitis (occupational) NOS
    Contact eczema (occupational) NOS

L26 Exfoliative **dermatitis**
    Hebra's pityriasis
    EXCLUDES 1   *Ritter's disease (L00)*

✓4ᵗʰ **L27** **Dermatitis** due to substances taken internally
    EXCLUDES 1   *allergy NOS (T78.40)*
    EXCLUDES 2   *adverse food reaction, except dermatitis (T78.0-T78.1)*
          contact dermatitis (L23-L25)
          drug photoallergic response (L56.1)
          drug phototoxic response (L56.0)
          urticaria (L50.-)

L27.0 Generalized **skin eruption due to** drugs and medicaments **taken internally**
    Use additional code for adverse effect, if applicable, to identify drug (T36-T50 with fifth or sixth character 5)

L27.1 Localized **skin eruption due to** drugs and medicaments **taken internally**
    Use additional code for adverse effect, if applicable, to identify drug (T36-T50 with fifth or sixth character 5)

L27.2 Dermatitis **due to ingested** food
    EXCLUDES 2   *dermatitis due to food in contact with skin (L23.6, L24.6, L25.4)*

L27.8 **Dermatitis due to other substances taken internally**

L27.9 **Dermatitis due to unspecified substance taken internally**

✓4ᵗʰ **L28** **Lichen simplex chronicus and prurigo**

L28.0 **Lichen simplex chronicus**
    Circumscribed neurodermatitis
    Lichen NOS

L28.1 **Prurigo nodularis**

L28.2 **Other prurigo**
    Prurigo NOS
    Prurigo Hebra
    Prurigo mitis
    Urticaria papulosa

✓4ᵗʰ **L29** **Pruritus**
    EXCLUDES 1   *neurotic excoriation (L98.1)*
          psychogenic pruritus (F45.8)

L29.0 **Pruritus** ani

L29.1 **Pruritus** scroti   ♂

L29.2 **Pruritus** vulvae   ♀

L29.3 Anogenital **pruritus, unspecified**

L29.8 **Other pruritus**

L29.9 **Pruritus, unspecified**
    Itch NOS

✓4ᵗʰ **L30** **Other and unspecified dermatitis**
    EXCLUDES 2   *contact dermatitis (L23-L25)*
          dry skin dermatitis (L85.3)
          small plaque parapsoriasis (L41.3)
          stasis dermatitis (I83.1-.2)

L30.0 **Nummular dermatitis**

L30.1 **Dyshidrosis [pompholyx]**

L30.2 **Cutaneous autosensitization**
    Candidid [levurid]
    Dermatophytid
    Eczematid

L30.3 **Infective dermatitis**
    Infectious eczematoid dermatitis

L30.4 **Erythema intertrigo**

L30.5 **Pityriasis alba**

L30.8 **Other specified dermatitis**

L30.9 **Dermatitis, unspecified**
    Eczema NOS

Papulosquamous disorders (L40-L45)

✓4ᵗʰ **L40** **Psoriasis**

L40.0 **Psoriasis** vulgaris
    Nummular psoriasis
    Plaque psoriasis

L40.1 Generalized pustular **psoriasis**
    Impetigo herpetiformis
    Von Zumbusch's disease

L40.2 **Acrodermatitis continua**

L40.3 **Pustulosis palmaris et plantaris**

L40.4 Guttate **psoriasis**

✓5ᵗʰ **L40.5** **Arthropathic** psoriasis

    L40.50 **Arthropathic psoriasis, unspecified**

    L40.51 Distal interphalangeal **psoriatic arthropathy**

    L40.52 **Psoriatic arthritis** mutilans

    L40.53 **Psoriatic** spondylitis

    L40.54 **Psoriatic** juvenile **arthropathy**

    L40.59 **Other psoriatic arthropathy**

L40.8 **Other psoriasis**
    Flexural psoriasis

L40.9 **Psoriasis, unspecified**

✓4ᵗʰ **L41** **Parapsoriasis**
    EXCLUDES 1   *poikiloderma vasculare atrophicans (L94.5)*

L41.0 **Pityriasis lichenoides et varioliformis acuta**
    Mucha-Habermann disease

L41.1 Pityriasis lichenoides chronica

L41.3 Small plaque **parapsoriasis**

L41.4 Large plaque **parapsoriasis**

L41.5 Retiform **parapsoriasis**

L41.8 **Other parapsoriasis**

L41.9 **Parapsoriasis, unspecified**

L42 **Pityriasis rosea**

✓4ᵗʰ **L43** **Lichen planus**
    EXCLUDES 1   *lichen planopilaris (L66.1)*

L43.0 Hypertrophic **lichen planus**

L43.1 Bullous **lichen planus**

L43.2 Lichenoid drug reaction
    Use additional code for adverse effect, if applicable, to identify drug (T36-T50 with fifth or sixth character 5)

L43.3 Subacute (active) lichen planus
    Lichen planus tropicus

L43.8 **Other lichen planus**

L43.9 **Lichen planus, unspecified**

✓4ᵗʰ **L44** **Other papulosquamous disorders**

L44.0 **Pityriasis rubra pilaris**

L44.1 **Lichen nitidus**

L44.2 **Lichen striatus**

L44.3 **Lichen ruber moniliformis**

L44.4 **Infantile papular acrodermatitis [Gianotti-Crosti]**   P

L44.8 **Other specified papulosquamous disorders**

L44.9 **Papulosquamous disorder, unspecified**

L45 *Papulosquamous disorders in diseases classified elsewhere*
    Code first underlying disease

Urticaria and erythema (L49-L54)

    EXCLUDES 1   *Lyme disease (A69.2-)*
          rosacea (L71.-)

✓4ᵗʰ **L49** **Exfoliation due to erythematous conditions according to extent of body surface involved**
    Code first erythematous condition causing exfoliation, such as:
        Ritter's disease (L00)
        (Staphylococcal) scalded skin syndrom (L00)
        Stevens-Johnson syndrome (L51.1)
        Stevens-Johnson syndrome-toxic epidermal necrolysis overlap syndrome (L51.3)
        toxic epidermal necrolysis (L51.2)

L49.0 **Exfoliation due to erythematous condition involving** less than 10 percent **of body surface**
    Exfoliation due to erythematous condition NOS

L49.1 **Exfoliation due to erythematous condition involving** 10-19 percent **of body surface**

✓ Additional Character Required   ✓x7ᵗʰ Xtension Alert   Unspecified Dx   Other Specified Dx   Manifestation   ▶◀ Revised Text   ● New Code   ▲ Revised Code Title

ICD-10-CM Draft (2015)   633

Diseases of the Skin and Subcutaneous Tissue

L49.2–L59.8

L49.2 **Exfoliation due to erythematous condition involving** 20-29 percent **of body surface**

L49.3 **Exfoliation due to erythematous condition involving** 30-39 percent **of body surface**

L49.4 **Exfoliation due to erythematous condition involving** 40-49 percent **of body surface**

L49.5 **Exfoliation due to erythematous condition involving** 50-59 percent **of body surface**

L49.6 **Exfoliation due to erythematous condition involving** 60-69 percent **of body surface**

L49.7 **Exfoliation due to erythematous condition involving** 70-79 percent **of body surface**

L49.8 **Exfoliation due to erythematous condition involving** 80-89 percent **of body surface**

L49.9 **Exfoliation due to erythematous condition involving** 90 or more percent **of body surface**

☑4ᵗʰ **L50** **Urticaria**

> **EXCLUDES 1**   *allergic contact dermatitis (L23.-)*
> *angioneurotic edema (T78.3)*
> *giant urticaria (T78.3)*
> *hereditary angio-edema (D84.1)*
> *Quincke's edema (T78.3)*
> *serum urticaria (T80.6-)*
> *solar urticaria (L56.3)*
> *urticaria neonatorum (P83.8)*
> *urticaria papulosa (L28.2)*
> *urticaria pigmentosa (Q82.2)*

L50.0 Allergic **urticaria**

L50.1 Idiopathic **urticaria**

L50.2 **Urticaria due to** cold and heat

L50.3 Dermatographic **urticaria**

L50.4 Vibratory **urticaria**

L50.5 Cholinergic **urticaria**

L50.6 Contact **urticaria**

L50.8 **Other urticaria**
> Chronic urticaria
> Recurrent periodic urticaria

L50.9 **Urticaria, unspecified**

☑4ᵗʰ **L51** **Erythema** multiforme

> Use additional code for adverse effect, if applicable, to identify drug (T36-T50 with fifth or sixth character 5)
> Use additional code to identify associated manifestations, such as:
> arthropathy associated with dermatological disorders (M14.8-)
> conjunctival edema (H11.42)
> conjunctivitis (H10.22-)
> corneal scars and opacities (H17.-)
> corneal ulcer (H16.0-)
> edema of eyelid (H02.84)
> inflammation of eyelid (H01.8)
> keratoconjunctivitis sicca (H16.22-)
> mechanical lagophthalmos (H02.22-)
> stomatitis (K12.-)
> symblepharon (H11.23-)
> Use additional code to identify percentage of skin exfoliation (L49.-)

> **EXCLUDES 1**   *staphylococcal scalded skin syndrome (L00)*
> *Ritter's disease (L00)*

L51.0 Nonbullous **erythema multiforme**

L51.1 Stevens-Johnson syndrome

L51.2 Toxic epidermal necrolysis [Lyell]

L51.3 Stevens-Johnson syndrome-toxic epidermal necrolysis overlap syndrome
> SJS-TEN overlap syndrome

L51.8 **Other erythema multiforme**

L51.9 **Erythema multiforme, unspecified**
> Erythema iris
> Erythema multiforme major NOS
> Erythema multiforme minor NOS
> Herpes iris

L52 **Erythema** nodosum

> **EXCLUDES 1**   *tuberculous erythema nodosum (A18.4)*

☑4ᵗʰ **L53** **Other erythematous conditions**

> **EXCLUDES 1**   *erythema ab igne (L59.0)*
> *erythema due to external agents in contact with skin (L23-L25)*
> *erythema intertrigo (L30.4)*

L53.0 **Toxic erythema**
> Code first poisoning due to drug or toxin, if applicable (T36-T65 with fifth or sixth character 1-4 or 6)
> Use additional code for adverse effect, if applicable, to identify drug (T36-T50 with fifth or sixth character 5)
> **EXCLUDES 1**   *neonatal erythema toxicum (P83.1)*

L53.1 **Erythema** annulare centrifugum

L53.2 **Erythema** marginatum

L53.3 Other chronic figurate **erythema**

L53.8 **Other specified erythematous conditions**

L53.9 **Erythematous condition, unspecified**
> Erythema NOS
> Erythroderma NOS

L54 *Erythema in diseases classified elsewhere*
> *Code first underlying disease*

Radiation-related disorders of the skin and subcutaneous tissue (L55-L59)

☑4ᵗʰ **L55** **Sunburn**

L55.0 **Sunburn of** first degree

L55.1 **Sunburn of** second degree

L55.2 **Sunburn of** third degree

L55.9 **Sunburn, unspecified**

☑4ᵗʰ **L56** **Other acute skin changes due to ultraviolet radiation**

> Use additional code to identify the source of the ultraviolet radiation (W89, X32)

L56.0 **Drug phototoxic response**
> Use additional code for adverse effect, if applicable, to identify drug (T36-T50 with fifth or sixth character 5)

L56.1 **Drug photoallergic response**
> Use additional code for adverse effect, if applicable, to identify drug (T36-T50 with fifth or sixth character 5)

L56.2 **Photocontact dermatitis [berloque dermatitis]**

L56.3 **Solar urticaria**

L56.4 **Polymorphous light eruption**

L56.5 **Disseminated superficial actinic porokeratosis (DSAP)**

L56.8 **Other specified acute skin changes due to ultraviolet radiation**

L56.9 **Acute skin change due to ultraviolet radiation, unspecified**

☑4ᵗʰ **L57** **Skin changes due to chronic exposure to nonionizing radiation**

> Use additional code to identify the source of the ultraviolet radiation (W89, X32)

L57.0 **Actinic keratosis**
> Keratosis NOS
> Senile keratosis
> Solar keratosis

L57.1 **Actinic reticuloid**

L57.2 **Cutis rhomboidalis nuchae**

L57.3 **Poikiloderma of Civatte**

L57.4 **Cutis laxa senilis**
> Elastosis senilis

L57.5 **Actinic granuloma**

L57.8 **Other skin changes due to chronic exposure to nonionizing radiation**
> Farmer's skin
> Sailor's skin
> Solar dermatitis

L57.9 **Skin changes due to chronic exposure to nonionizing radiation, unspecified**

☑4ᵗʰ **L58** **Radiodermatitis**

> Use additional code to identify the source of the radiation (W88, W90)

L58.0 Acute **radiodermatitis**

L58.1 Chronic **radiodermatitis**

L58.9 **Radiodermatitis, unspecified**

☑4ᵗʰ **L59** **Other disorders of skin and subcutaneous tissue related to radiation**

L59.0 **Erythema ab igne [dermatitis ab igne]**

L59.8 **Other specified disorders of the skin and subcutaneous tissue related to radiation**

EXCLUDES 1 Not coded here   **EXCLUDES 2** Not included here   N Newborn Age: 0   P Pediatric Age: 0-17   M Maternity Age: 12-55   A Adult Age: 15-124

634   ICD-10-CM Draft (2015)

L59.9   **Disorder of the skin and subcutaneous tissue related to radiation, unspecified**

Disorders of skin appendages (L60-L75)

EXCLUDES 1   *congenital malformations of integument (Q84.-)*

✓4th **L60   Nail disorders**

EXCLUDES 2   *clubbing of nails (R68.3)*
onychia and paronychia (L03.0-)

L60.0   **Ingrowing nail**

L60.1   **Onycholysis**

L60.2   **Onychogryphosis**

L60.3   **Nail dystrophy**

L60.4   **Beau's lines**

L60.5   **Yellow nail syndrome**

L60.8   **Other nail disorders**

L60.9   **Nail disorder, unspecified**

L62   Nail disorders in diseases classified elsewhere

Code first underlying disease, such as:
pachydermoperiostosis (M89.4-)

✓4th **L63   Alopecia areata**

L63.0   **Alopecia (capitis)** totalis

L63.1   **Alopecia** universalis

L63.2   **Ophiasis**

L63.8   **Other alopecia areata**

L63.9   **Alopecia areata, unspecified**

✓4th **L64   Androgenic alopecia**

INCLUDES   male-pattern baldness

L64.0   Drug-induced **androgenic alopecia**

Use additional code for adverse effect, if applicable, to identify drug (T36-T50 with fifth or sixth character 5)

L64.8   **Other androgenic alopecia**

L64.9   **Androgenic alopecia, unspecified**

✓4th **L65   Other nonscarring hair loss**

Use additional code for adverse effect, if applicable, to identify drug (T36-T50 with fifth or sixth character 5)

EXCLUDES 1   *trichotillomania (F63.3)*

L65.0   **Telogen effluvium**

L65.1   **Anagen effluvium**

L65.2   **Alopecia mucinosa**

L65.8   **Other specified nonscarring hair loss**

L65.9   **Nonscarring hair loss, unspecified**

Alopecia NOS

✓4th **L66   Cicatricial alopecia [scarring hair loss]**

L66.0   **Pseudopelade**

L66.1   **Lichen planopilaris**

Follicular lichen planus

L66.2   **Folliculitis decalvans**

L66.3   **Perifolliculitis capitis abscedens**

L66.4   **Folliculitis ulerythematosa reticulata**

L66.8   **Other cicatricial alopecia**

L66.9   **Cicatricial alopecia, unspecified**

✓4th **L67   Hair color and hair shaft abnormalities**

EXCLUDES 1   *monilethrix (Q84.1)*
pili annulati (Q84.1)
telogen effluvium (L65.0)

L67.0   **Trichorrhexis nodosa**

L67.1   **Variations in hair color**

Canities
Greyness, hair (premature)
Heterochromia of hair
Poliosis circumscripta, acquired
Poliosis NOS

L67.8   **Other hair color and hair shaft abnormalities**

Fragilitas crinium

L67.9   **Hair color and hair shaft abnormality, unspecified**

✓4th **L68   Hypertrichosis**

INCLUDES   excess hair

EXCLUDES 1   *congenital hypertrichosis (Q84.2)*
persistent lanugo (Q84.2)

L68.0   **Hirsutism**

L68.1   **Acquired hypertrichosis lanuginosa**

L68.2   **Localized hypertrichosis**

L68.3   **Polytrichia**

L68.8   **Other hypertrichosis**

L68.9   **Hypertrichosis, unspecified**

✓4th **L70   Acne**

EXCLUDES 2   *acne keloid (L73.0)*

L70.0   **Acne** vulgaris

L70.1   **Acne** conglobata

L70.2   **Acne** varioliformis

Acne necrotica miliaris

L70.3   **Acne** tropica

L70.4   Infantile **acne**   ℗

L70.5   Acné excoriée des jeunes filles

Picker's acne

L70.8   **Other acne**

L70.9   **Acne, unspecified**

✓4th **L71   Rosacea**

Use additional code for adverse effect, if applicable, to identify drug (T36-T50 with fifth or sixth character 5)

L71.0   **Perioral dermatitis**

L71.1   **Rhinophyma**

L71.8   **Other rosacea**

L71.9   **Rosacea, unspecified**

✓4th **L72   Follicular cysts of skin and subcutaneous tissue**

L72.0   **Epidermal cyst**

✓5th L72.1   **Pilar and trichodermal cyst**

L72.11   **Pilar cyst**

L72.12   **Trichodermal cyst**

Trichilemmal (proliferating) cyst

L72.2   **Steatocystoma multiplex**

L72.3   **Sebaceous cyst**

EXCLUDES 2   *pilar cyst (L72.11)*
trichilemmal (proliferating) cyst (L72.12)

L72.8   **Other follicular cysts of the skin and subcutaneous tissue**

L72.9   **Follicular cyst of the skin and subcutaneous tissue, unspecified**

✓4th **L73   Other follicular disorders**

L73.0   **Acne keloid**

L73.1   **Pseudofolliculitis barbae**

L73.2   **Hidradenitis suppurativa**

L73.8   **Other specified follicular disorders**

Sycosis barbae

L73.9   **Follicular disorder, unspecified**

✓4th **L74   Eccrine sweat disorders**

EXCLUDES 2   *generalized hyperhidrosis (R61)*

L74.0   **Miliaria** rubra

L74.1   **Miliaria** crystallina

L74.2   **Miliaria** profunda

Miliaria tropicalis

L74.3   **Miliaria, unspecified**

L74.4   **Anhidrosis**

Hypohidrosis

✓5th L74.5   **Focal hyperhidrosis**

✓6th L74.51   Primary **focal hyperhidrosis**

L74.510   **Primary focal hyperhidrosis,** axilla

L74.511   **Primary focal hyperhidrosis,** face

L74.512   **Primary focal hyperhidrosis,** palms

L74.513   **Primary focal hyperhidrosis,** soles

L74.519   **Primary focal hyperhidrosis, unspecified**

L74.52   Secondary **focal hyperhidrosis**

Frey's syndrome

L74.8   **Other eccrine sweat disorders**

L74.9   **Eccrine sweat disorder, unspecified**

Sweat gland disorder NOS

✓4th **L75   Apocrine sweat disorders**

EXCLUDES 1   *dyshidrosis (L30.1)*
hidradenitis suppurativa (L73.2)

L75.0   **Bromhidrosis**

L75.1   **Chromhidrosis**

L75.2   **Apocrine miliaria**

Fox-Fordyce disease

L75.8   **Other apocrine sweat disorders**

✓ Additional Character Required   ✓x7th Xtension Alert   Unspecified Dx   Other Specified Dx   Manifestation   ►◄ Revised Text   ● New Code   ▲ Revised Code Title

Diseases of the Skin and Subcutaneous Tissue

L59.9–L75.8

Diseases of the Skin and Subcutaneous Tissue

L75.9   Apocrine sweat disorder, unspecified

Intraoperative and postprocedural complications of skin and subcutaneous tissue (L76)

✓4th **L76   Intraoperative and postprocedural complications of skin and subcutaneous tissue**

    ✓5th **L76.0   Intraoperative hemorrhage and hematoma of skin and subcutaneous tissue complicating a procedure**

       EXCLUDES 1   intraoperative hemorrhage and hematoma of skin and subcutaneous tissue due to accidental puncture and laceration during a procedure (L76.1-)

       L76.01   Intraoperative hemorrhage and hematoma of skin and subcutaneous tissue complicating a dermatologic procedure

       L76.02   Intraoperative hemorrhage and hematoma of skin and subcutaneous tissue complicating other procedure

    ✓5th **L76.1   Accidental puncture and laceration of skin and subcutaneous tissue during a procedure**

       L76.11   Accidental puncture and laceration of skin and subcutaneous tissue during a dermatologic procedure

       L76.12   Accidental puncture and laceration of skin and subcutaneous tissue during other procedure

    ✓5th **L76.2   Postprocedural hemorrhage and hematoma of skin and subcutaneous tissue following a procedure**

       L76.21   Postprocedural hemorrhage and hematoma of skin and subcutaneous tissue following a dermatologic procedure

       L76.22   Postprocedural hemorrhage and hematoma of skin and subcutaneous tissue following other procedure

    ✓5th **L76.8   Other intraoperative and postprocedural complications of skin and subcutaneous tissue**

       Use additional code, if applicable, to further specify disorder

       L76.81   Other intraoperative complications of skin and subcutaneous tissue

       L76.82   Other postprocedural complications of skin and subcutaneous tissue

Other disorders of the skin and subcutaneous tissue (L80-L99)

L80   Vitiligo

    EXCLUDES 2   vitiligo of eyelids (H02.73-)
               vitiligo of vulva (N90.89)

✓4th **L81   Other disorders of pigmentation**

    EXCLUDES 1   birthmark NOS (Q82.5)
               Peutz-Jeghers syndrome (Q85.8)
    EXCLUDES 2   nevus—see Alphabetical Index

    L81.0   Postinflammatory hyperpigmentation

    L81.1   Chloasma

    L81.2   Freckles

    L81.3   Café au lait spots

    L81.4   Other melanin hyperpigmentation
       Lentigo

    L81.5   Leukoderma, not elsewhere classified

    L81.6   Other disorders of diminished melanin formation

    L81.7   Pigmented purpuric dermatosis
       Angioma serpiginosum

    L81.8   Other specified disorders of pigmentation
       Iron pigmentation
       Tattoo pigmentation

    L81.9   Disorder of pigmentation, unspecified

✓4th **L82   Seborrheic keratosis**

    INCLUDES   dermatosis papulosa nigra
             Leser-Trélat disease
    EXCLUDES 2   seborrheic dermatitis (L21.-)

    L82.0   Inflamed seborrheic keratosis

    L82.1   Other seborrheic keratosis
       Seborrheic keratosis NOS

L83   Acanthosis nigricans
    Confluent and reticulated papillomatosis

L84   Corns and callosities
    Callus
    Clavus

✓4th **L85   Other epidermal thickening**

    EXCLUDES 2   hypertrophic disorders of the skin (L91.-)

    L85.0   Acquired ichthyosis
       EXCLUDES 1   congenital ichthyosis (Q80.-)

    L85.1   Acquired keratosis [keratoderma] palmaris et plantaris
       EXCLUDES 1   inherited keratosis palmaris et plantaris (Q82.8)

    L85.2   Keratosis punctata (palmaris et plantaris)

    L85.3   Xerosis cutis
       Dry skin dermatitis

    L85.8   Other specified epidermal thickening
       Cutaneous horn

    L85.9   Epidermal thickening, unspecified

L86   ***Keratoderma in diseases classified elsewhere***

    Code first underlying disease, such as:
    Reiter's disease (M02.3-)
    EXCLUDES 1   gonococcal keratoderma (A54.89)
               gonococcal keratosis (A54.89)
               keratoderma due to vitamin A deficiency (E50.8)
               keratosis due to vitamin A deficiency (E50.8)
               xeroderma due to vitamin A deficiency (E50.8)

✓4th **L87   Transepidermal elimination disorders**

    EXCLUDES 1   granuloma annulare (perforating) (L92.0)

    L87.0   Keratosis follicularis et parafollicularis in cutem penetrans
       Hyperkeratosis follicularis penetrans
       Kyrle disease

    L87.1   Reactive perforating collagenosis

    L87.2   Elastosis perforans serpiginosa

    L87.8   Other transepidermal elimination disorders

    L87.9   Transepidermal elimination disorder, unspecified

L88   Pyoderma gangrenosum
    Phagedenic pyoderma
    EXCLUDES 1   dermatitis gangrenosa (L08.0)

✓4th **L89   Pressure ulcer**
    Bed sore
    Decubitus ulcer
    Plaster ulcer
    Pressure area
    Pressure sore
    Code first any associated gangrene (I96)
    EXCLUDES 2   decubitus (trophic) ulcer of cervix (uteri) (N86)
               diabetic ulcers (E08.621, E08.622, E09.621, E09.622, E10.621, E10.622, E11.621, E11.622, E13.621, E13.622)
               non-pressure chronic ulcer of skin (L97.-)
               skin infections (L00-L08)
               varicose ulcer (I83.0, I83.2)

    ✓5th **L89.0   Pressure ulcer of elbow**

       ✓6th **L89.00   Pressure ulcer of unspecified elbow**

          L89.000   Pressure ulcer of unspecified elbow, unstageable

          L89.001   Pressure ulcer of unspecified elbow, stage 1
             Healing pressure ulcer of unspecified elbow, stage 1
             Pressure pre-ulcer skin changes limited to persistent focal edema, unspecified elbow

          L89.002   Pressure ulcer of unspecified elbow, stage 2
             Healing pressure ulcer of unspecified elbow, stage 2
             Pressure ulcer with abrasion, blister, partial thickness skin loss involving epidermis and/or dermis, unspecified elbow

          L89.003   Pressure ulcer of unspecified elbow, stage 3
             Healing pressure ulcer of unspecified elbow, stage 3
             Pressure ulcer with full thickness skin loss involving damage or necrosis of subcutaneous tissue, unspecified elbow

          L89.004   Pressure ulcer of unspecified elbow, stage 4
             Healing pressure ulcer of unspecified elbow, stage 4
             Pressure ulcer with necrosis of soft tissues through to underlying muscle, tendon, or bone, unspecified elbow

EXCLUDES 1 Not coded here   *EXCLUDES 2* Not included here   N Newborn Age: 0   P Pediatric Age: 0-17   M Maternity Age: 12-55   A Adult Age: 15-124

636   ICD-10-CM Draft (2015)

L89.009 **Pressure ulcer of unspecified elbow, unspecified stage**
Healing pressure ulcer of elbow NOS
Healing pressure ulcer of unspecified elbow, unspecified stage

✓6th L89.01 **Pressure ulcer of** right elbow
L89.010 **Pressure ulcer of right elbow,** unstageable
L89.011 **Pressure ulcer of right elbow,** stage 1
Healing pressure ulcer of right elbow, stage 1
Pressure pre-ulcer skin changes limited to persistent focal edema, right elbow
L89.012 **Pressure ulcer of right elbow,** stage 2
Healing pressure ulcer of right elbow, stage 2
Pressure ulcer with abrasion, blister, partial thickness skin loss involving epidermis and/or dermis, right elbow
L89.013 **Pressure ulcer of right elbow,** stage 3
Healing pressure ulcer of right elbow, stage 3
Pressure ulcer with full thickness skin loss involving damage or necrosis of subcutaneous tissue, right elbow
L89.014 **Pressure ulcer of right elbow,** stage 4
Healing pressure ulcer of right elbow, stage 4
Pressure ulcer with necrosis of soft tissues through to underlying muscle, tendon, or bone, right elbow
L89.019 **Pressure ulcer of right elbow, unspecified stage**
Healing pressure right of elbow NOS
Healing pressure ulcer of unspecified elbow, unspecified stage

✓6th L89.02 **Pressure ulcer of** left elbow
L89.020 **Pressure ulcer of left elbow,** unstageable
L89.021 **Pressure ulcer of left elbow,** stage 1
Healing pressure ulcer of left elbow, stage 1
Pressure pre-ulcer skin changes limited to persistent focal edema, left elbow
L89.022 **Pressure ulcer of left elbow,** stage 2
Healing pressure ulcer of left elbow, stage 2
Pressure ulcer with abrasion, blister, partial thickness skin loss involving epidermis and/or dermis, left elbow
L89.023 **Pressure ulcer of left elbow,** stage 3
Healing pressure ulcer of left elbow, stage 3
Pressure ulcer with full thickness skin loss involving damage or necrosis of subcutaneous tissue, left elbow
L89.024 **Pressure ulcer of left elbow,** stage 4
Healing pressure ulcer of left elbow, stage 4
Pressure ulcer with necrosis of soft tissues through to underlying muscle, tendon, or bone, left elbow
L89.029 **Pressure ulcer of left elbow, unspecified stage**
Healing pressure ulcer of left of elbow NOS
Healing pressure ulcer of unspecified elbow, unspecified stage

✓5th L89.1 **Pressure ulcer of** back
✓6th L89.10 **Pressure ulcer of** unspecified part of back
L89.100 **Pressure ulcer of unspecified part of back,** unstageable
L89.101 **Pressure ulcer of unspecified part of back,** stage 1
Healing pressure ulcer of unspecified part of back, stage 1
Pressure pre-ulcer skin changes limited to persistent focal edema, unspecified part of back
L89.102 **Pressure ulcer of unspecified part of back,** stage 2
Healing pressure ulcer of unspecified part of back, stage 2
Pressure ulcer with abrasion, blister, partial thickness skin loss involving epidermis and/or dermis, unspecified part of back

L89.103 **Pressure ulcer of unspecified part of back,** stage 3
Healing pressure ulcer of unspecified part of back, stage 3
Pressure ulcer with full thickness skin loss involving damage or necrosis of subcutaneous tissue, unspecified part of back
L89.104 **Pressure ulcer of unspecified part of back,** stage 4
Healing pressure ulcer of unspecified part of back, stage 4
Pressure ulcer with necrosis of soft tissues through to underlying muscle, tendon, or bone, unspecified part of back
L89.109 **Pressure ulcer of unspecified part of back, unspecified stage**
Healing pressure ulcer of unspecified part of back NOS
Healing pressure ulcer of unspecified part of back, unspecified stage

✓6th L89.11 **Pressure ulcer of** right upper back
Pressure ulcer of right shoulder blade
L89.110 **Pressure ulcer of right upper back,** unstageable
L89.111 **Pressure ulcer of right upper back,** stage 1
Healing pressure ulcer of right upper back, stage 1
Pressure pre-ulcer skin changes limited to persistent focal edema, right upper back
L89.112 **Pressure ulcer of right upper back,** stage 2
Healing pressure ulcer of right upper back, stage 2
Pressure ulcer with abrasion, blister, partial thickness skin loss involving epidermis and/or dermis, right upper back
L89.113 **Pressure ulcer of right upper back,** stage 3
Healing pressure ulcer of right upper back, stage 3
Pressure ulcer with full thickness skin loss involving damage or necrosis of subcutaneous tissue, right upper back
L89.114 **Pressure ulcer of right upper back,** stage 4
Healing pressure ulcer of right upper back, stage 4
Pressure ulcer with necrosis of soft tissues through to underlying muscle, tendon, or bone, right upper back
L89.119 **Pressure ulcer of right upper back, unspecified stage**
Healing pressure ulcer of right upper back NOS
Healing pressure ulcer of right upper back, unspecified stage

✓6th L89.12 **Pressure ulcer of** left upper back
Pressure ulcer of left shoulder blade
L89.120 **Pressure ulcer of left upper back,** unstageable
L89.121 **Pressure ulcer of left upper back,** stage 1
Healing pressure ulcer of left upper back, stage 1
Pressure pre-ulcer skin changes limited to persistent focal edema, left upper back
L89.122 **Pressure ulcer of left upper back,** stage 2
Healing pressure ulcer of left upper back, stage 2
Pressure ulcer with abrasion, blister, partial thickness skin loss involving epidermis and/or dermis, left upper back
L89.123 **Pressure ulcer of left upper back,** stage 3
Healing pressure ulcer of left upper back, stage 3
Pressure ulcer with full thickness skin loss involving damage or necrosis of subcutaneous tissue, left upper back
L89.124 **Pressure ulcer of left upper back,** stage 4
Healing pressure ulcer of left upper back, stage 4
Pressure ulcer with necrosis of soft tissues through to underlying muscle, tendon, or bone, left upper back

Diseases of the Skin and Subcutaneous Tissue

L89.129–L89.214

L89.129 Pressure ulcer of left upper back, unspecified stage
Healing pressure ulcer of left upper back NOS
Healing pressure ulcer of left upper back, unspecified stage

✓6ᵗʰ **L89.13 Pressure ulcer of** right lower back

L89.130 Pressure ulcer of right lower back, unstageable

L89.131 Pressure ulcer of right lower back, stage 1
Healing pressure ulcer of right lower back, stage 1
Pressure pre-ulcer skin changes limited to persistent focal edema, right lower back

L89.132 Pressure ulcer of right lower back, stage 2
Healing pressure ulcer of right lower back, stage 2
Pressure ulcer with abrasion, blister, partial thickness skin loss involving epidermis and/or dermis, right lower back

L89.133 Pressure ulcer of right lower back, stage 3
Healing pressure ulcer of right lower back, stage 3
Pressure ulcer with full thickness skin loss involving damage or necrosis of subcutaneous tissue, right lower back

L89.134 Pressure ulcer of right lower back, stage 4
Healing pressure ulcer of right lower back, stage 4
Pressure ulcer with necrosis of soft tissues through to underlying muscle, tendon, or bone, right lower back

L89.139 Pressure ulcer of right lower back, unspecified stage
Healing pressure ulcer of right lower back NOS
Healing pressure ulcer of right lower back, unspecified stage

✓6ᵗʰ **L89.14 Pressure ulcer of** left lower back

L89.140 Pressure ulcer of left lower back, unstageable

L89.141 Pressure ulcer of left lower back, stage 1
Healing pressure ulcer of left lower back, stage 1
Pressure pre-ulcer skin changes limited to persistent focal edema, left lower back

L89.142 Pressure ulcer of left lower back, stage 2
Healing pressure ulcer of left lower back, stage 2
Pressure ulcer with abrasion, blister, partial thickness skin loss involving epidermis and/or dermis, left lower back

L89.143 Pressure ulcer of left lower back, stage 3
Healing pressure ulcer of left lower back, stage 3
Pressure ulcer with full thickness skin loss involving damage or necrosis of subcutaneous tissue, left lower back

L89.144 Pressure ulcer of left lower back, stage 4
Healing pressure ulcer of left lower back, stage 4
Pressure ulcer with necrosis of soft tissues through to underlying muscle, tendon, or bone, left lower back

L89.149 Pressure ulcer of left lower back, unspecified stage
Healing pressure ulcer of left lower back NOS
Healing pressure ulcer of left lower back, unspecified stage

✓6ᵗʰ **L89.15 Pressure ulcer of** sacral region
Pressure ulcer of coccyx
Pressure ulcer of tailbone

L89.150 Pressure ulcer of sacral region, unstageable

L89.151 Pressure ulcer of sacral region, stage 1
Healing pressure ulcer of sacral region, stage 1
Pressure pre-ulcer skin changes limited to persistent focal edema, sacral region

L89.152 Pressure ulcer of sacral region, stage 2
Healing pressure ulcer of sacral region, stage 2
Pressure ulcer with abrasion, blister, partial thickness skin loss involving epidermis and/or dermis, sacral region

L89.153 Pressure ulcer of sacral region, stage 3
Healing pressure ulcer of sacral region, stage 3
Pressure ulcer with full thickness skin loss involving damage or necrosis of subcutaneous tissue, sacral region

L89.154 Pressure ulcer of sacral region, stage 4
Healing pressure ulcer of sacral region, stage 4
Pressure ulcer with necrosis of soft tissues through to underlying muscle, tendon, or bone, sacral region

L89.159 Pressure ulcer of sacral region, unspecified stage
Healing pressure ulcer of sacral region NOS
Healing pressure ulcer of sacral region, unspecified stage

✓5ᵗʰ **L89.2 Pressure ulcer of** hip

✓6ᵗʰ **L89.20 Pressure ulcer of** unspecified hip

L89.200 Pressure ulcer of unspecified hip, unstageable

L89.201 Pressure ulcer of unspecified hip, stage 1
Healing pressure ulcer of unspecified hip, stage 1
Pressure pre-ulcer skin changes limited to persistent focal edema, unspecified hip

L89.202 Pressure ulcer of unspecified hip, stage 2
Healing pressure ulcer of unspecified hip, stage 2
Pressure ulcer with abrasion, blister, partial thickness skin loss involving epidermis and/or dermis, unspecified hip

L89.203 Pressure ulcer of unspecified hip, stage 3
Healing pressure ulcer of unspecified hip, stage 3
Pressure ulcer with full thickness skin loss involving damage or necrosis of subcutaneous tissue, unspecified hip

L89.204 Pressure ulcer of unspecified hip, stage 4
Healing pressure ulcer of unspecified hip, stage 4
Pressure ulcer with necrosis of soft tissues through to underlying muscle, tendon, or bone, unspecified hip

L89.209 Pressure ulcer of unspecified hip, unspecified stage
Healing pressure ulcer of unspecified hip NOS
Healing pressure ulcer of unspecified hip, unspecified stage

✓6ᵗʰ **L89.21 Pressure ulcer of** right hip

L89.210 Pressure ulcer of right hip, unstageable

L89.211 Pressure ulcer of right hip, stage 1
Healing pressure ulcer of right hip, stage 1
Pressure pre-ulcer skin changes limited to persistent focal edema, right hip

L89.212 Pressure ulcer of right hip, stage 2
Healing pressure ulcer of right hip, stage 2
Pressure ulcer with abrasion, blister, partial thickness skin loss involving epidermis and/or dermis, right hip

L89.213 Pressure ulcer of right hip, stage 3
Healing pressure ulcer of right hip, stage 3
Pressure ulcer with full thickness skin loss involving damage or necrosis of subcutaneous tissue, right hip

L89.214 Pressure ulcer of right hip, stage 4
Healing pressure ulcer of right hip, stage 4
Pressure ulcer with necrosis of soft tissues through to underlying muscle, tendon, or bone, right hip

EXCLUDES 1 Not coded here   **EXCLUDES 2** Not included here   N Newborn Age: 0   P Pediatric Age: 0-17   M Maternity Age: 12-55   A Adult Age: 15-124

638   ICD-10-CM Draft (2015)

L89.219 **Pressure ulcer of right hip, unspecified stage**
Healing pressure ulcer of right hip NOS
Healing pressure ulcer of right hip, unspecified stage

✓6th L89.22 **Pressure ulcer of** left hip
L89.220 **Pressure ulcer of left hip,** unstageable
L89.221 **Pressure ulcer of left hip,** stage 1
Healing pressure ulcer of left hip, stage 1
Pressure pre-ulcer skin changes limited to persistent focal edema, left hip
L89.222 **Pressure ulcer of left hip,** stage 2
Healing pressure ulcer of left hip, stage 2
Pressure ulcer with abrasion, blister, partial thickness skin loss involving epidermis and/or dermis, left hip
L89.223 **Pressure ulcer of left hip,** stage 3
Healing pressure ulcer of left hip, stage 3
Pressure ulcer with full thickness skin loss involving damage or necrosis of subcutaneous tissue, left hip
L89.224 **Pressure ulcer of left hip,** stage 4
Healing pressure ulcer of left hip, stage 4
Pressure ulcer with necrosis of soft tissues through to underlying muscle, tendon, or bone, left hip
L89.229 **Pressure ulcer of left hip, unspecified stage**
Healing pressure ulcer of left hip NOS
Healing pressure ulcer of left hip, unspecified stage

✓5th L89.3 **Pressure ulcer of** buttock
✓6th L89.30 **Pressure ulcer of** unspecified buttock
L89.300 **Pressure ulcer of unspecified buttock, unstageable**
L89.301 **Pressure ulcer of unspecified buttock,** stage 1
Healing pressure ulcer of unspecified buttock, stage 1
Pressure pre-ulcer skin changes limited to persistent focal edema, unspecified buttock
L89.302 **Pressure ulcer of unspecified buttock,** stage 2
Healing pressure ulcer of unspecified buttock, stage 2
Pressure ulcer with abrasion, blister, partial thickness skin loss involving epidermis and/or dermis, unspecified buttock
L89.303 **Pressure ulcer of unspecified buttock,** stage 3
Healing pressure ulcer of unspecified buttock, stage 3
Pressure ulcer with full thickness skin loss involving damage or necrosis of subcutaneous tissue, unspecified buttock
L89.304 **Pressure ulcer of unspecified buttock,** stage 4
Healing pressure ulcer of unspecified buttock, stage 4
Pressure ulcer with necrosis of soft tissues through to underlying muscle, tendon, or bone, unspecified buttock
L89.309 **Pressure ulcer of unspecified buttock, unspecified stage**
Healing pressure ulcer of unspecified buttock NOS
Healing pressure ulcer of unspecified buttock, unspecified stage

✓6th L89.31 **Pressure ulcer of** right buttock
L89.310 **Pressure ulcer of right buttock,** unstageable
L89.311 **Pressure ulcer of right buttock,** stage 1
Healing pressure ulcer of right buttock, stage 1
Pressure pre-ulcer skin changes limited to persistent focal edema, right buttock

L89.312 **Pressure ulcer of right buttock,** stage 2
Healing pressure ulcer of right buttock, stage 2
Pressure ulcer with abrasion, blister, partial thickness skin loss involving epidermis and/or dermis, right buttock
L89.313 **Pressure ulcer of right buttock,** stage 3
Healing pressure ulcer of right buttock, stage 3
Pressure ulcer with full thickness skin loss involving damage or necrosis of subcutaneous tissue, right buttock
L89.314 **Pressure ulcer of right buttock,** stage 4
Healing pressure ulcer of right buttock, stage 4
Pressure ulcer with necrosis of soft tissues through to underlying muscle, tendon, or bone, right buttock
L89.319 **Pressure ulcer of right buttock, unspecified stage**
Healing pressure ulcer of right buttock NOS
Healing pressure ulcer of right buttock, unspecified stage

✓6th L89.32 **Pressure ulcer of** left buttock
L89.320 **Pressure ulcer of left buttock,** unstageable
L89.321 **Pressure ulcer of left buttock,** stage 1
Healing pressure ulcer of left buttock, stage 1
Pressure pre-ulcer skin changes limited to persistent focal edema, left buttock
L89.322 **Pressure ulcer of left buttock,** stage 2
Healing pressure ulcer of left buttock, stage 2
Pressure ulcer with abrasion, blister, partial thickness skin loss involving epidermis and/or dermis, left buttock
L89.323 **Pressure ulcer of left buttock,** stage 3
Healing pressure ulcer of left buttock, stage 3
Pressure ulcer with full thickness skin loss involving damage or necrosis of subcutaneous tissue, left buttock
L89.324 **Pressure ulcer of left buttock,** stage 4
Healing pressure ulcer of left buttock, stage 4
Pressure ulcer with necrosis of soft tissues through to underlying muscle, tendon, or bone, left buttock
L89.329 **Pressure ulcer of left buttock, unspecified stage**
Healing pressure ulcer of left buttock NOS
Healing pressure ulcer of left buttock, unspecified stage

✓5th L89.4 **Pressure ulcer of contiguous site of** back, buttock and hip
L89.40 **Pressure ulcer of contiguous site of back, buttock and hip, unspecified stage**
Healing pressure ulcer of contiguous site of back, buttock and hip NOS
Healing pressure ulcer of contiguous site of back, buttock and hip, unspecified stage
L89.41 **Pressure ulcer of contiguous site of back, buttock and hip,** stage 1
Healing pressure ulcer of contiguous site of back, buttock and hip, stage 1
Pressure pre-ulcer skin changes limited to persistent focal edema, contiguous site of back, buttock and hip
L89.42 **Pressure ulcer of contiguous site of back, buttock and hip,** stage 2
Healing pressure ulcer of contiguous site of back, buttock and hip, stage 2
Pressure ulcer with abrasion, blister, partial thickness skin loss involving epidermis and/or dermis, contiguous site of back, buttock and hip
L89.43 **Pressure ulcer of contiguous site of back, buttock and hip,** stage 3
Healing pressure ulcer of contiguous site of back, buttock and hip, stage 3
Pressure ulcer with full thickness skin loss involving damage or necrosis of subcutaneous tissue, contiguous site of back, buttock and hip

L89.44   **Pressure ulcer of contiguous site of back, buttock and hip, stage 4**
Healing pressure ulcer of contiguous site of back, buttock and hip, stage 4
Pressure ulcer with necrosis of soft tissues through to underlying muscle, tendon, or bone, contiguous site of back, buttock and hip

L89.45   **Pressure ulcer of contiguous site of back, buttock and hip, unstageable**

✓5th **L89.5**   **Pressure ulcer of ankle**

   ✓6th **L89.50**   **Pressure ulcer of unspecified ankle**

     L89.500   **Pressure ulcer of unspecified ankle, unstageable**

     L89.501   **Pressure ulcer of unspecified ankle, stage 1**
Healing pressure ulcer of unspecified ankle, stage 1
Pressure pre-ulcer skin changes limited to persistent focal edema, unspecified ankle

     L89.502   **Pressure ulcer of unspecified ankle, stage 2**
Healing pressure ulcer of unspecified ankle, stage 2
Pressure ulcer with abrasion, blister, partial thickness skin loss involving epidermis and/or dermis, unspecified ankle

     L89.503   **Pressure ulcer of unspecified ankle, stage 3**
Healing pressure ulcer of unspecified ankle, stage 3
Pressure ulcer with full thickness skin loss involving damage or necrosis of subcutaneous tissue, unspecified ankle

     L89.504   **Pressure ulcer of unspecified ankle, stage 4**
Healing pressure ulcer of unspecified ankle, stage 4
Pressure ulcer with necrosis of soft tissues through to underlying muscle, tendon, or bone, unspecified ankle

     L89.509   **Pressure ulcer of unspecified ankle, unspecified stage**
Healing pressure ulcer of unspecified ankle NOS
Healing pressure ulcer of unspecified ankle, unspecified stage

   ✓6th **L89.51**   **Pressure ulcer of right ankle**

     L89.510   **Pressure ulcer of right ankle, unstageable**

     L89.511   **Pressure ulcer of right ankle, stage 1**
Healing pressure ulcer of right ankle, stage 1
Pressure pre-ulcer skin changes limited to persistent focal edema, right ankle

     L89.512   **Pressure ulcer of right ankle, stage 2**
Healing pressure ulcer of right ankle, stage 2
Pressure ulcer with abrasion, blister, partial thickness skin loss involving epidermis and/or dermis, right ankle

     L89.513   **Pressure ulcer of right ankle, stage 3**
Healing pressure ulcer of right ankle, stage 3
Pressure ulcer with full thickness skin loss involving damage or necrosis of subcutaneous tissue, right ankle

     L89.514   **Pressure ulcer of right ankle, stage 4**
Healing pressure ulcer of right ankle, stage 4
Pressure ulcer with necrosis of soft tissues through to underlying muscle, tendon, or bone, right ankle

     L89.519   **Pressure ulcer of right ankle, unspecified stage**
Healing pressure ulcer of right ankle NOS
Healing pressure ulcer of right ankle, unspecified stage

   ✓6th **L89.52**   **Pressure ulcer of left ankle**

     L89.520   **Pressure ulcer of left ankle, unstageable**

     L89.521   **Pressure ulcer of left ankle, stage 1**
Healing pressure ulcer of left ankle, stage 1
Pressure pre-ulcer skin changes limited to persistnt focal edema, left ankle

     L89.522   **Pressure ulcer of left ankle, stage 2**
Healing pressure ulcer of left ankle, stage 2
Pressure ulcer with abrasion, blister, partial thickness skin loss involving epidermis and/or dermis, left ankle

     L89.523   **Pressure ulcer of left ankle, stage 3**
Healing pressure ulcer of left ankle, stage 3
Pressure ulcer with full thickness skin loss involving damage or necrosis of subcutaneous tissue, left ankle

     L89.524   **Pressure ulcer of left ankle, stage 4**
Healing pressure ulcer of left ankle, stage 4
Pressure ulcer with necrosis of soft tissues through to underlying muscle, tendon, or bone, left ankle

     L89.529   **Pressure ulcer of left ankle, unspecified stage**
Healing pressure ulcer of left ankle NOS
Healing pressure ulcer of left ankle, unspecified stage

✓5th **L89.6**   **Pressure ulcer of heel**

   ✓6th **L89.60**   **Pressure ulcer of unspecified heel**

     L89.600   **Pressure ulcer of unspecified heel, unstageable**

     L89.601   **Pressure ulcer of unspecified heel, stage 1**
Healing pressure ulcer of unspecified heel, stage 1
Pressure pre-ulcer skin changes limited to persistent focal edema, unspecified heel

     L89.602   **Pressure ulcer of unspecified heel, stage 2**
Healing pressure ulcer of unspecified heel, stage 2
Pressure ulcer with abrasion, blister, partial thickness skin loss involving epidermis and/or dermis, unspecified heel

     L89.603   **Pressure ulcer of unspecified heel, stage 3**
Healing pressure ulcer of unspecified heel, stage 3
Pressure ulcer with full thickness skin loss involving damage or necrosis of subcutaneous tissue, unspecified heel

     L89.604   **Pressure ulcer of unspecified heel, stage 4**
Healing pressure ulcer of unspecified heel, stage 4
Pressure ulcer with necrosis of soft tissues through to underlying muscle, tendon, or bone, unspecified heel

     L89.609   **Pressure ulcer of unspecified heel, unspecified stage**
Healing pressure ulcer of unspecified heel NOS
Healing pressure ulcer of unspecified heel, unspecified stage

   ✓6th **L89.61**   **Pressure ulcer of right heel**

     L89.610   **Pressure ulcer of right heel, unstageable**

     L89.611   **Pressure ulcer of right heel, stage 1**
Healing pressure ulcer of right heel, stage 1
Pressure pre-ulcer skin changes limited to persistent focal edema, right heel

     L89.612   **Pressure ulcer of right heel, stage 2**
Healing pressure ulcer of right heel, stage 2
Pressure ulcer with abrasion, blister, partial thickness skin loss involving epidermis and/or dermis, right heel

     L89.613   **Pressure ulcer of right heel, stage 3**
Healing pressure ulcer of right heel, stage 3
Pressure ulcer with full thickness skin loss involving damage or necrosis of subcutaneous tissue, right heel

EXCLUDES 1 Not coded here   **EXCLUDES 2** Not included here   **N** Newborn Age: 0   **P** Pediatric Age: 0-17   **M** Maternity Age: 12-55   **A** Adult Age: 15-124

640   ICD-10-CM Draft (2015)

L89.614 **Pressure ulcer of right heel, stage 4**
Healing pressure ulcer of right heel, stage 4
Pressure ulcer with necrosis of soft tissues through to underlying muscle, tendon, or bone, right heel

L89.619 **Pressure ulcer of right heel, unspecified stage**
Healing pressure ulcer of right heel NOS
Healing pressure ulcer of unspecified heel, right stage

✓6th **L89.62 Pressure ulcer of left heel**

L89.620 **Pressure ulcer of left heel, unstageable**

L89.621 **Pressure ulcer of left heel, stage 1**
Healing pressure ulcer of left heel, stage 1
Pressure pre-ulcer skin changes limited to persistent focal edema, left heel

L89.622 **Pressure ulcer of left heel, stage 2**
Healing pressure ulcer of left heel, stage 2
Pressure ulcer with abrasion, blister, partial thickness skin loss involving epidermis and/or dermis, left heel

L89.623 **Pressure ulcer of left heel, stage 3**
Healing pressure ulcer of left heel, stage 3
Pressure ulcer with full thickness skin loss involving damage or necrosis of subcutaneous tissue, left heel

L89.624 **Pressure ulcer of left heel, stage 4**
Healing pressure ulcer of left heel, stage 4
Pressure ulcer with necrosis of soft tissues through to underlying muscle, tendon, or bone, left heel

L89.629 **Pressure ulcer of left heel, unspecified stage**
Healing pressure ulcer of left heel NOS
Healing pressure ulcer of left heel, unspecified stage

✓5th **L89.8 Pressure ulcer of other site**

✓6th **L89.81 Pressure ulcer of head**
Pressure ulcer of face

L89.810 **Pressure ulcer of head, unstageable**

L89.811 **Pressure ulcer of head, stage 1**
Healing pressure ulcer of head, stage 1
Pressure pre-ulcer skin changes limited to persistent focal edema, head

L89.812 **Pressure ulcer of head, stage 2**
Healing pressure ulcer of head, stage 2
Pressure ulcer with abrasion, blister, partial thickness skin loss involving epidermis and/or dermis, head

L89.813 **Pressure ulcer of head, stage 3**
Healing pressure ulcer of head, stage 3
Pressure ulcer with full thickness skin loss involving damage or necrosis of subcutaneous tissue, head

L89.814 **Pressure ulcer of head, stage 4**
Healing pressure ulcer of head, stage 4
Pressure ulcer with necrosis of soft tissues through to underlying muscle, tendon, or bone, head

L89.819 **Pressure ulcer of head, unspecified stage**
Healing pressure ulcer of head NOS
Healing pressure ulcer of head, unspecified stage

✓6th **L89.89 Pressure ulcer of other site**

L89.890 **Pressure ulcer of other site, unstageable**

L89.891 **Pressure ulcer of other site, stage 1**
Healing pressure ulcer of other site, stage 1
Pressure pre-ulcer skin changes limited to persistent focal edema, other site

L89.892 **Pressure ulcer of other site, stage 2**
Healing pressure ulcer of other site, stage 2
Pressure ulcer with abrasion, blister, partial thickness skin loss involving epidermis and/or dermis, other site

L89.893 **Pressure ulcer of other site, stage 3**
Healing pressure ulcer of other site, stage 3
Pressure ulcer with full thickness skin loss involving damage or necrosis of subcutaneous tissue, other site

L89.894 **Pressure ulcer of other site, stage 4**
Healing pressure ulcer of other site, stage 4
Pressure ulcer with necrosis of soft tissues through to underlying muscle, tendon, or bone, other site

L89.899 **Pressure ulcer of other site, unspecified stage**
Healing pressure ulcer of other site NOS
Healing pressure ulcer of other site, unspecified stage

✓5th **L89.9 Pressure ulcer of unspecified site**

L89.90 **Pressure ulcer of unspecified site, unspecified stage**
Healing pressure ulcer of unspecified site NOS
Healing pressure ulcer of unspecified site, unspecified stage

L89.91 **Pressure ulcer of unspecified site, stage 1**
Healing pressure ulcer of unspecified site, stage 1
Pressure pre-ulcer skin changes limited to persistent focal edema, unspecified site

L89.92 **Pressure ulcer of unspecified site, stage 2**
Healing pressure ulcer of unspecified site, stage 2
Pressure ulcer with abrasion, blister, partial thickness skin loss involving epidermis and/or dermis, unspecified site

L89.93 **Pressure ulcer of unspecified site, stage 3**
Healing pressure ulcer of unspecified site, stage 3
Pressure ulcer with full thickness skin loss involving damage or necrosis of subcutaneous tissue, unspecified site

L89.94 **Pressure ulcer of unspecified site, stage 4**
Healing pressure ulcer of unspecified site, stage 4
Pressure ulcer with necrosis of soft tissues through to underlying muscle, tendon, or bone, unspecified site

L89.95 **Pressure ulcer of unspecified site, unstageable**

✓4th **L90 Atrophic disorders of skin**

L90.0 **Lichen sclerosus et atrophicus**
EXCLUDES 2 lichen sclerosus of external female genital organs (N90.4)
lichen sclerosus of external male genital organs (N48.0)

L90.1 **Anetoderma of Schweninger-Buzzi**

L90.2 **Anetoderma of Jadassohn-Pellizzari**

L90.3 **Atrophoderma of Pasini and Pierini**

L90.4 **Acrodermatitis chronica atrophicans**

L90.5 **Scar conditions and fibrosis of skin**
Adherent scar (skin)
Cicatrix
Disfigurement of skin due to scar
Fibrosis of skin NOS
Scar NOS
EXCLUDES 2 hypertrophic scar (L91.0)
keloid scar (L91.0)

L90.6 **Striae atrophicae**

L90.8 **Other atrophic disorders of skin**

L90.9 **Atrophic disorder of skin, unspecified**

✓4th **L91 Hypertrophic disorders of skin**

L91.0 **Hypertrophic scar**
Keloid
Keloid scar
EXCLUDES 2 acne keloid (L73.0)
scar NOS (L90.5)

L91.8 **Other hypertrophic disorders of the skin**

L91.9 **Hypertrophic disorder of the skin, unspecified**

✓4th **L92 Granulomatous disorders of skin and subcutaneous tissue**
EXCLUDES 2 actinic granuloma (L57.5)

L92.0 **Granuloma annulare**
Perforating granuloma annulare

L92.1 **Necrobiosis lipoidica, not elsewhere classified**
EXCLUDES 1 necrobiosis lipoidica associated with diabetes mellitus (E08-E13 with .620)

L92.2 **Granuloma faciale [eosinophilic granuloma of skin]**

L92.3   **Foreign body granuloma of the skin and subcutaneous tissue**
Use additional code to identify the type of retained foreign body (Z18.-)

L92.8   **Other granulomatous disorders of the skin and subcutaneous tissue**

L92.9   **Granulomatous disorder of the skin and subcutaneous tissue, unspecified**

☑4ᵗʰ **L93**   **Lupus erythematosus**
Use additional code for adverse effect, if applicable, to identify drug (T36-T50 with fifth or sixth character 5)
EXCLUDES 1   *lupus exedens (A18.4)*
lupus vulgaris (A18.4)
scleroderma (M34.-)
systemic lupus erythematosus (M32.-)

L93.0   **Discoid lupus erythematosus**
Lupus erythematosus NOS

L93.1   **Subacute cutaneous lupus erythematosus**

L93.2   **Other local lupus erythematosus**
Lupus erythematosus profundus
Lupus panniculitis

☑4ᵗʰ **L94**   **Other localized connective tissue disorders**
EXCLUDES 1   *systemic connective tissue disorders (M30-M36)*

L94.0   **Localized scleroderma [morphea]**
Circumscribed scleroderma

L94.1   **Linear scleroderma**
En coup de sabre lesion

L94.2   **Calcinosis cutis**

L94.3   **Sclerodactyly**

L94.4   **Gottron's papules**

L94.5   **Poikiloderma vasculare atrophicans**

L94.6   **Ainhum**

L94.8   **Other specified localized connective tissue disorders**

L94.9   **Localized connective tissue disorder, unspecified**

☑4ᵗʰ **L95**   **Vasculitis limited to skin, not elsewhere classified**
EXCLUDES 1   *angioma serpiginosum (L81.7)*
Henoch(-Schönlein) purpura (D69.0)
hypersensitivity angiitis (M31.0)
lupus panniculitis (L93.2)
panniculitis NOS (M79.3)
panniculitis of neck and back (M54.0-)
polyarteritis nodosa (M30.0)
relapsing panniculitis (M35.6)
rheumatoid vasculitis (M05.2)
serum sickness (T80.6-)
urticaria (L50.-)
Wegener's granulomatosis (M31.3-)

L95.0   **Livedoid vasculitis**
Atrophie blanche (en plaque)

L95.1   **Erythema elevatum diutinum**

L95.8   **Other vasculitis limited to the skin**

L95.9   **Vasculitis limited to the skin, unspecified**

☑4ᵗʰ **L97**   **Non-pressure chronic ulcer of lower limb, not elsewhere classified**
INCLUDES   chronic ulcer of skin of lower limb NOS
non-healing ulcer of skin
non-infected sinus of skin
trophic ulcer NOS
tropical ulcer NOS
ulcer of skin of lower limb NOS
Code first any associated underlying condition, such as:
atherosclerosis of the lower extremities (I70.23-, I70.24-, I70.33-, I70.34-, I70.43-, I70.44-, I70.53-, I70.54-, I70.63-, I70.64-, I70.73-, I70.74-)
chronic venous hypertension (I87.31-, I87.33-)
diabetic ulcers (E08.621, E08.622, E09.621, E09.622, E10.621, E10.622, E11.621, E11.622, E13.621, E13.622)
postphlebitic syndrome (I87.01-, I87.03-)
postthrombotic syndrome (I87.01-, I87.03-)
varicose ulcer (I83.0-, I83.2-)
Code first any associated gangrene (I96)
EXCLUDES 2   *pressure ulcer (pressure area) (L89.-)*
skin infections (L00-L08)
specific infections classified to A00-B99

☑5ᵗʰ **L97.1**   **Non-pressure chronic ulcer of thigh**

☑6ᵗʰ **L97.10**   **Non-pressure chronic ulcer of unspecified thigh**

L97.101   **Non-pressure chronic ulcer of unspecified thigh limited to breakdown of skin**

L97.102   **Non-pressure chronic ulcer of unspecified thigh with fat layer exposed**

L97.103   **Non-pressure chronic ulcer of unspecified thigh with necrosis of muscle**

L97.104   **Non-pressure chronic ulcer of unspecified thigh with necrosis of bone**

L97.109   **Non-pressure chronic ulcer of unspecified thigh with unspecified severity**

☑6ᵗʰ **L97.11**   **Non-pressure chronic ulcer of right thigh**

L97.111   **Non-pressure chronic ulcer of right thigh limited to breakdown of skin**

L97.112   **Non-pressure chronic ulcer of right thigh with fat layer exposed**

L97.113   **Non-pressure chronic ulcer of right thigh with necrosis of muscle**

L97.114   **Non-pressure chronic ulcer of right thigh with necrosis of bone**

L97.119   **Non-pressure chronic ulcer of right thigh with unspecified severity**

☑6ᵗʰ **L97.12**   **Non-pressure chronic ulcer of left thigh**

L97.121   **Non-pressure chronic ulcer of left thigh limited to breakdown of skin**

L97.122   **Non-pressure chronic ulcer of left thigh with fat layer exposed**

L97.123   **Non-pressure chronic ulcer of left thigh with necrosis of muscle**

L97.124   **Non-pressure chronic ulcer of left thigh with necrosis of bone**

L97.129   **Non-pressure chronic ulcer of left thigh with unspecified severity**

☑5ᵗʰ **L97.2**   **Non-pressure chronic ulcer of calf**

☑6ᵗʰ **L97.20**   **Non-pressure chronic ulcer of unspecified calf**

L97.201   **Non-pressure chronic ulcer of unspecified calf limited to breakdown of skin**

L97.202   **Non-pressure chronic ulcer of unspecified calf with fat layer exposed**

L97.203   **Non-pressure chronic ulcer of unspecified calf with necrosis of muscle**

L97.204   **Non-pressure chronic ulcer of unspecified calf with necrosis of bone**

L97.209   **Non-pressure chronic ulcer of unspecified calf with unspecified severity**

☑6ᵗʰ **L97.21**   **Non-pressure chronic ulcer of right calf**

L97.211   **Non-pressure chronic ulcer of right calf limited to breakdown of skin**

L97.212   **Non-pressure chronic ulcer of right calf with fat layer exposed**

L97.213   **Non-pressure chronic ulcer of right calf with necrosis of muscle**

L97.214   **Non-pressure chronic ulcer of right calf with necrosis of bone**

L97.219   **Non-pressure chronic ulcer of right calf with unspecified severity**

☑6ᵗʰ **L97.22**   **Non-pressure chronic ulcer of left calf**

L97.221   **Non-pressure chronic ulcer of left calf limited to breakdown of skin**

L97.222   **Non-pressure chronic ulcer of left calf with fat layer exposed**

L97.223   **Non-pressure chronic ulcer of left calf with necrosis of muscle**

L97.224   **Non-pressure chronic ulcer of left calf with necrosis of bone**

L97.229   **Non-pressure chronic ulcer of left calf with unspecified severity**

☑5ᵗʰ **L97.3**   **Non-pressure chronic ulcer of ankle**

☑6ᵗʰ **L97.30**   **Non-pressure chronic ulcer of unspecified ankle**

L97.301   **Non-pressure chronic ulcer of unspecified ankle limited to breakdown of skin**

L97.302   **Non-pressure chronic ulcer of unspecified ankle with fat layer exposed**

L97.303   **Non-pressure chronic ulcer of unspecified ankle with necrosis of muscle**

L97.304   **Non-pressure chronic ulcer of unspecified ankle with necrosis of bone**

L97.309   **Non-pressure chronic ulcer of unspecified ankle with unspecified severity**

EXCLUDES 1 Not coded here   **EXCLUDES 2** Not included here   N Newborn Age: 0   P Pediatric Age: 0-17   M Maternity Age: 12-55   A Adult Age: 15-124

642   ICD-10-CM Draft (2015)

✓6ᵗʰ **L97.31 Non-pressure chronic ulcer of** right ankle
- L97.311 **Non-pressure chronic ulcer of right ankle** limited to breakdown of skin
- L97.312 **Non-pressure chronic ulcer of right ankle** with fat layer exposed
- L97.313 **Non-pressure chronic ulcer of right ankle** with necrosis of muscle
- L97.314 **Non-pressure chronic ulcer of right ankle** with necrosis of bone
- L97.319 **Non-pressure chronic ulcer of right ankle with unspecified severity**

✓6ᵗʰ **L97.32 Non-pressure chronic ulcer of** left ankle
- L97.321 **Non-pressure chronic ulcer of left ankle** limited to breakdown of skin
- L97.322 **Non-pressure chronic ulcer of left ankle** with fat layer exposed
- L97.323 **Non-pressure chronic ulcer of left ankle** with necrosis of muscle
- L97.324 **Non-pressure chronic ulcer of left ankle** with necrosis of bone
- L97.329 **Non-pressure chronic ulcer of left ankle with unspecified severity**

✓5ᵗʰ **L97.4 Non-pressure chronic ulcer of** heel and midfoot
Non-pressure chronic ulcer of plantar surface of midfoot

✓6ᵗʰ **L97.40 Non-pressure chronic ulcer of** unspecified heel and midfoot
- L97.401 **Non-pressure chronic ulcer of unspecified heel and midfoot** limited to breakdown of skin
- L97.402 **Non-pressure chronic ulcer of unspecified heel and midfoot** with fat layer exposed
- L97.403 **Non-pressure chronic ulcer of unspecified heel and midfoot** with necrosis of muscle
- L97.404 **Non-pressure chronic ulcer of unspecified heel and midfoot** with necrosis of bone
- L97.409 **Non-pressure chronic ulcer of unspecified heel and midfoot with unspecified severity**

✓6ᵗʰ **L97.41 Non-pressure chronic ulcer of** right heel and midfoot
- L97.411 **Non-pressure chronic ulcer of right heel and midfoot** limited to breakdown of skin
- L97.412 **Non-pressure chronic ulcer of right heel and midfoot** with fat layer exposed
- L97.413 **Non-pressure chronic ulcer of right heel and midfoot** with necrosis of muscle
- L97.414 **Non-pressure chronic ulcer of right heel and midfoot** with necrosis of bone
- L97.419 **Non-pressure chronic ulcer of right heel and midfoot with unspecified severity**

✓6ᵗʰ **L97.42 Non-pressure chronic ulcer of** left heel and midfoot
- L97.421 **Non-pressure chronic ulcer of left heel and midfoot** limited to breakdown of skin
- L97.422 **Non-pressure chronic ulcer of left heel and midfoot** with fat layer exposed
- L97.423 **Non-pressure chronic ulcer of left heel and midfoot** with necrosis of muscle
- L97.424 **Non-pressure chronic ulcer of left heel and midfoot** with necrosis of bone
- L97.429 **Non-pressure chronic ulcer of left heel and midfoot with unspecified severity**

✓5ᵗʰ **L97.5 Non-pressure chronic ulcer of** other part of foot
Non-pressure chronic ulcer of toe

✓6ᵗʰ **L97.50 Non-pressure chronic ulcer of** other part of unspecified foot
- L97.501 **Non-pressure chronic ulcer of other part of unspecified foot** limited to breakdown of skin
- L97.502 **Non-pressure chronic ulcer of other part of unspecified foot** with fat layer exposed
- L97.503 **Non-pressure chronic ulcer of other part of unspecified foot** with necrosis of muscle
- L97.504 **Non-pressure chronic ulcer of other part of unspecified foot** with necrosis of bone
- L97.509 **Non-pressure chronic ulcer of other part of unspecified foot with unspecified severity**

✓6ᵗʰ **L97.51 Non-pressure chronic ulcer of** other part of right foot
- L97.511 **Non-pressure chronic ulcer of other part of right foot** limited to breakdown of skin

- L97.512 **Non-pressure chronic ulcer of other part of right foot** with fat layer exposed
- L97.513 **Non-pressure chronic ulcer of other part of right foot** with necrosis of muscle
- L97.514 **Non-pressure chronic ulcer of other part of right foot** with necrosis of bone
- L97.519 **Non-pressure chronic ulcer of other part of right foot with unspecified severity**

✓6ᵗʰ **L97.52 Non-pressure chronic ulcer of** other part of left foot
- L97.521 **Non-pressure chronic ulcer of other part of left foot** limited to breakdown of skin
- L97.522 **Non-pressure chronic ulcer of other part of left foot** with fat layer exposed
- L97.523 **Non-pressure chronic ulcer of other part of left foot** with necrosis of muscle
- L97.524 **Non-pressure chronic ulcer of other part of left foot** with necrosis of bone
- L97.529 **Non-pressure chronic ulcer of other part of left foot with unspecified severity**

✓5ᵗʰ **L97.8 Non-pressure chronic ulcer of** other part of lower leg

✓6ᵗʰ **L97.80 Non-pressure chronic ulcer of other part of** unspecified lower leg
- L97.801 **Non-pressure chronic ulcer of other part of unspecified lower leg** limited to breakdown of skin
- L97.802 **Non-pressure chronic ulcer of other part of unspecified lower leg** with fat layer exposed
- L97.803 **Non-pressure chronic ulcer of other part of unspecified lower leg** with necrosis of muscle
- L97.804 **Non-pressure chronic ulcer of other part of unspecified lower leg** with necrosis of bone
- L97.809 **Non-pressure chronic ulcer of other part of unspecified lower leg with unspecified severity**

✓6ᵗʰ **L97.81 Non-pressure chronic ulcer of** other part of right lower leg
- L97.811 **Non-pressure chronic ulcer of other part of right lower leg** limited to breakdown of skin
- L97.812 **Non-pressure chronic ulcer of other part of right lower leg** with fat layer exposed
- L97.813 **Non-pressure chronic ulcer of other part of right lower leg** with necrosis of muscle
- L97.814 **Non-pressure chronic ulcer of other part of right lower leg** with necrosis of bone
- L97.819 **Non-pressure chronic ulcer of other part of right lower leg with unspecified severity**

✓6ᵗʰ **L97.82 Non-pressure chronic ulcer of** other part of left lower leg
- L97.821 **Non-pressure chronic ulcer of other part of left lower leg** limited to breakdown of skin
- L97.822 **Non-pressure chronic ulcer of other part of left lower leg** with fat layer exposed
- L97.823 **Non-pressure chronic ulcer of other part of left lower leg** with necrosis of muscle
- L97.824 **Non-pressure chronic ulcer of other part of left lower leg** with necrosis of bone
- L97.829 **Non-pressure chronic ulcer of other part of left lower leg with unspecified severity**

✓5ᵗʰ **L97.9 Non-pressure chronic ulcer of** unspecified part of lower leg

✓6ᵗʰ **L97.90 Non-pressure chronic ulcer of** unspecified part of unspecified lower leg
- L97.901 **Non-pressure chronic ulcer of unspecified part of unspecified lower leg** limited to breakdown of skin
- L97.902 **Non-pressure chronic ulcer of unspecified part of unspecified lower leg** with fat layer exposed
- L97.903 **Non-pressure chronic ulcer of unspecified part of unspecified lower leg** with necrosis of muscle
- L97.904 **Non-pressure chronic ulcer of unspecified part of unspecified lower leg** with necrosis of bone

Diseases of the Skin and Subcutaneous Tissue

L97.909–L99

L97.909   Non-pressure chronic ulcer of unspecified part of unspecified lower leg with unspecified severity

✓6th **L97.91**   Non-pressure chronic ulcer of unspecified part of right lower leg

L97.911   Non-pressure chronic ulcer of unspecified part of right lower leg limited to breakdown of skin

L97.912   Non-pressure chronic ulcer of unspecified part of right lower leg with fat layer exposed

L97.913   Non-pressure chronic ulcer of unspecified part of right lower leg with necrosis of muscle

L97.914   Non-pressure chronic ulcer of unspecified part of right lower leg with necrosis of bone

L97.919   Non-pressure chronic ulcer of unspecified part of right lower leg with unspecified severity

✓6th **L97.92**   Non-pressure chronic ulcer of unspecified part of left lower leg

L97.921   Non-pressure chronic ulcer of unspecified part of left lower leg limited to breakdown of skin

L97.922   Non-pressure chronic ulcer of unspecified part of left lower leg with fat layer exposed

L97.923   Non-pressure chronic ulcer of unspecified part of left lower leg with necrosis of muscle

L97.924   Non-pressure chronic ulcer of unspecified part of left lower leg with necrosis of bone

L97.929   Non-pressure chronic ulcer of unspecified part of left lower leg with unspecified severity

✓4th **L98**   **Other disorders of skin and subcutaneous tissue, not elsewhere classified**

L98.0   **Pyogenic granuloma**
     EXCLUDES 2   pyogenic granuloma of gingiva (K06.8)
                 pyogenic granuloma of maxillary alveolar ridge (K04.5)
                 pyogenic granuloma of oral mucosa (K13.4)

L98.1   **Factitial dermatitis**
     Neurotic excoriation

L98.2   **Febrile neutrophilic dermatosis [Sweet]**

L98.3   **Eosinophilic cellulitis [Wells]**

✓5th **L98.4**   **Non-pressure chronic ulcer of skin, not elsewhere classified**
     Chronic ulcer of skin NOS
     Tropical ulcer NOS
     Ulcer of skin NOS
     EXCLUDES 2   pressure ulcer (pressure area) (L89.-)
                 gangrene (I96)
                 skin infections (L00-L08)
                 specific infections classified to A00-B99
                 ulcer of lower limb NEC (L97.-)
                 varicose ulcer (I83.0-I82.2)

✓6th **L98.41**   **Non-pressure chronic ulcer of buttock**

L98.411   Non-pressure chronic ulcer of buttock limited to breakdown of skin

L98.412   Non-pressure chronic ulcer of buttock with fat layer exposed

L98.413   Non-pressure chronic ulcer of buttock with necrosis of muscle

L98.414   Non-pressure chronic ulcer of buttock with necrosis of bone

L98.419   Non-pressure chronic ulcer of buttock with unspecified severity

✓6th **L98.42**   Non-pressure chronic ulcer of back

L98.421   Non-pressure chronic ulcer of back limited to breakdown of skin

L98.422   Non-pressure chronic ulcer of back with fat layer exposed

L98.423   Non-pressure chronic ulcer of back with necrosis of muscle

L98.424   Non-pressure chronic ulcer of back with necrosis of bone

L98.429   Non-pressure chronic ulcer of back with unspecified severity

✓6th **L98.49**   Non-pressure chronic ulcer of skin of other sites
     Non-pressure chronic ulcer of skin NOS

L98.491   Non-pressure chronic ulcer of skin of other sites limited to breakdown of skin

L98.492   Non-pressure chronic ulcer of skin of other sites with fat layer exposed

L98.493   Non-pressure chronic ulcer of skin of other sites with necrosis of muscle

L98.494   Non-pressure chronic ulcer of skin of other sites with necrosis of bone

L98.499   Non-pressure chronic ulcer of skin of other sites with unspecified severity

L98.5   **Mucinosis of the skin**
     Focal mucinosis
     Lichen myxedematosus
     Reticular erythematous mucinosis
     EXCLUDES 1   focal oral mucinosis (K13.79)
                 myxedema (E03.9)

L98.6   **Other infiltrative disorders of the skin and subcutaneous tissue**
     EXCLUDES 1   hyalinosis cutis et mucosae (E78.89)

L98.8   **Other specified disorders of the skin and subcutaneous tissue**
     AHA: 2013, 2Q, 32

L98.9   **Disorder of the skin and subcutaneous tissue, unspecified**

L99   *Other disorders of skin and subcutaneous tissue in diseases classified elsewhere*
     Code first underlying disease, such as:
       amyloidosis (E85.-)
     EXCLUDES 1   skin disorders in diabetes (E08-E13 with .62)
                 skin disorders in gonorrhea (A54.89)
                 skin disorders in syphilis (A51.31, A52.79)

EXCLUDES 1 Not coded here   EXCLUDES 2 Not included here   N Newborn Age: 0   P Pediatric Age: 0-17   M Maternity Age: 12-55   A Adult Age: 15-124

644   ICD-10-CM Draft (2015)

Chapter 13. Diseases of the Musculoskeletal System and Connective Tissue (M00-M99)

NOTE Use an external cause code following the code for the musculoskeletal condition, if applicable, to identify the cause of the musculoskeletal condition.

EXCLUDES 2 *arthropathic psoriasis (L40.5-)*
certain conditions originating in the perinatal period (P04-P96)
certain infectious and parasitic diseases (A00-B99)
compartment syndrome (traumatic) (T79.A-)
complications of pregnancy, childbirth and the puerperium (O00-O9A)
congenital malformations, deformations, and chromosomal abnormalities (Q00-Q99)
endocrine, nutritional and metabolic diseases (E00-E88)
injury, poisoning and certain other consequences of external causes (S00-T88)
neoplasms (C00-D49)
symptoms, signs and abnormal clinical and laboratory findings, not elsewhere classified (R00-R94)

This chapter contains the following blocks:

M00-M02	Infectious arthropathies
M05-M14	Inflammatory polyarthropathies
M15-M19	Osteoarthritis
M20-M25	Other joint disorders
M26-M27	Dentofacial anomalies [including malocclusion] and other disorders of jaw
M30-M36	Systemic connective tissue disorders
M40-M43	Deforming dorsopathies
M45-M49	Spondylopathies
M50-M54	Other dorsopathies
M60-M63	Disorders of muscles
M65-M67	Disorders of synovium and tendon
M70-M79	Other soft tissue disorders
M80-M85	Disorders of bone density and structure
M86-M90	Other osteopathies
M91-M94	Chondropathies
M95	Other disorders of the musculoskeletal system and connective tissue
M96	Intraoperative and postprocedural complications and disorders of musculoskeletal system, not elsewhere classified
M99	Biomechanical lesions, not elsewhere classified

ARTHROPATHIES (M00-M25)

INCLUDES disorders affecting predominantly peripheral (limb) joints

Infectious arthropathies (M00-M02)

NOTE This block comprises arthropathies due to microbiological agents. Distinction is made between the following types of etiological relationship:

a) direct infection of joint, where organisms invade synovial tissue and microbial antigen is present in the joint;

b) indirect infection, which may be of two types: a reactive arthropathy, where microbial infection of the body is established but neither organisms nor antigens can be identified in the joint, and a postinfective arthropathy, where microbial antigen is present but recovery of an organism is inconstant and evidence of local multiplication is lacking.

✓4th **M00 Pyogenic arthritis**

✓5th **M00.0 Staphylococcal arthritis and polyarthritis**
Use additional code (B95.61-B95.8) to identify bacterial agent
EXCLUDES 2 *infection and inflammatory reaction due to internal joint prosthesis (T84.5-)*

   M00.00 Staphylococcal arthritis, unspecified joint

✓6th **M00.01 Staphylococcal arthritis, shoulder**
   M00.011 Staphylococcal arthritis, right shoulder
   M00.012 Staphylococcal arthritis, left shoulder
   M00.019 Staphylococcal arthritis, unspecified shoulder

✓6th **M00.02 Staphylococcal arthritis, elbow**
   M00.021 Staphylococcal arthritis, right elbow
   M00.022 Staphylococcal arthritis, left elbow
   M00.029 Staphylococcal arthritis, unspecified elbow

✓6th **M00.03 Staphylococcal arthritis, wrist**
   Staphylococcal arthritis of carpal bones
   M00.031 Staphylococcal arthritis, right wrist
   M00.032 Staphylococcal arthritis, left wrist
   M00.039 Staphylococcal arthritis, unspecified wrist

✓6th **M00.04 Staphylococcal arthritis, hand**
   Staphylococcal arthritis of metacarpus and phalanges
   M00.041 Staphylococcal arthritis, right hand
   M00.042 Staphylococcal arthritis, left hand
   M00.049 Staphylococcal arthritis, unspecified hand

✓6th **M00.05 Staphylococcal arthritis, hip**
   M00.051 Staphylococcal arthritis, right hip
   M00.052 Staphylococcal arthritis, left hip
   M00.059 Staphylococcal arthritis, unspecified hip

✓6th **M00.06 Staphylococcal arthritis, knee**
   M00.061 Staphylococcal arthritis, right knee
   M00.062 Staphylococcal arthritis, left knee
   M00.069 Staphylococcal arthritis, unspecified knee

✓6th **M00.07 Staphylococcal arthritis, ankle and foot**
   Staphylococcal arthritis, tarsus, metatarsus and phalanges
   M00.071 Staphylococcal arthritis, right ankle and foot
   M00.072 Staphylococcal arthritis, left ankle and foot
   M00.079 Staphylococcal arthritis, unspecified ankle and foot

   M00.08 Staphylococcal arthritis, vertebrae

   M00.09 Staphylococcal polyarthritis

✓5th **M00.1 Pneumococcal arthritis and polyarthritis**

   M00.10 Pneumococcal arthritis, unspecified joint

✓6th **M00.11 Pneumococcal arthritis, shoulder**
   M00.111 Pneumococcal arthritis, right shoulder
   M00.112 Pneumococcal arthritis, left shoulder
   M00.119 Pneumococcal arthritis, unspecified shoulder

✓6th **M00.12 Pneumococcal arthritis, elbow**
   M00.121 Pneumococcal arthritis, right elbow
   M00.122 Pneumococcal arthritis, left elbow
   M00.129 Pneumococcal arthritis, unspecified elbow

✓6th **M00.13 Pneumococcal arthritis, wrist**
   Pneumococcal arthritis of carpal bones
   M00.131 Pneumococcal arthritis, right wrist
   M00.132 Pneumococcal arthritis, left wrist
   M00.139 Pneumococcal arthritis, unspecified wrist

✓6th **M00.14 Pneumococcal arthritis, hand**
   Pneumococcal arthritis of metacarpus and phalanges
   M00.141 Pneumococcal arthritis, right hand
   M00.142 Pneumococcal arthritis, left hand
   M00.149 Pneumococcal arthritis, unspecified hand

✓6th **M00.15 Pneumococcal arthritis, hip**
   M00.151 Pneumococcal arthritis, right hip
   M00.152 Pneumococcal arthritis, left hip
   M00.159 Pneumococcal arthritis, unspecified hip

✓6th **M00.16 Pneumococcal arthritis, knee**
   M00.161 Pneumococcal arthritis, right knee
   M00.162 Pneumococcal arthritis, left knee
   M00.169 Pneumococcal arthritis, unspecified knee

✓6th **M00.17 Pneumococcal arthritis, ankle and foot**
   Pneumococcal arthritis, tarsus, metatarsus and phalanges
   M00.171 Pneumococcal arthritis, right ankle and foot
   M00.172 Pneumococcal arthritis, left ankle and foot
   M00.179 Pneumococcal arthritis, unspecified ankle and foot

   M00.18 Pneumococcal arthritis, vertebrae

   M00.19 Pneumococcal polyarthritis

✓5th **M00.2 Other streptococcal arthritis and polyarthritis**
Use additional code (B95.0-B95.2, B95.4-B95.5) to identify bacterial agent

   M00.20 Other streptococcal arthritis, unspecified joint

✓6th **M00.21 Other streptococcal arthritis, shoulder**
   M00.211 Other streptococcal arthritis, right shoulder
   M00.212 Other streptococcal arthritis, left shoulder

✓ Additional Character Required   ✓x7th Xtension Alert   Unspecified Dx   Other Specified Dx   Manifestation   ►◄ Revised Text   ● New Code   ▲ Revised Code Title

Diseases of the Musculoskeletal System and Connective Tissue

M00.219–M01.X42

M00.219 **Other streptococcal arthritis, unspecified shoulder**

√6ᵗʰ M00.22 **Other streptococcal arthritis,** elbow

    M00.221 Other streptococcal arthritis, right **elbow**

    M00.222 Other streptococcal arthritis, left **elbow**

    M00.229 **Other streptococcal arthritis, unspecified elbow**

√6ᵗʰ M00.23 **Other streptococcal arthritis,** wrist

    Other streptococcal arthritis of carpal bones

    M00.231 Other streptococcal arthritis, right **wrist**

    M00.232 Other streptococcal arthritis, left **wrist**

    M00.239 **Other streptococcal arthritis, unspecified wrist**

√6ᵗʰ M00.24 **Other streptococcal arthritis,** hand

    Other streptococcal arthritis metacarpus and phalanges

    M00.241 Other streptococcal arthritis, right **hand**

    M00.242 Other streptococcal arthritis, left **hand**

    M00.249 **Other streptococcal arthritis, unspecified hand**

√6ᵗʰ M00.25 **Other streptococcal arthritis,** hip

    M00.251 Other streptococcal arthritis, right **hip**

    M00.252 Other streptococcal arthritis, left **hip**

    M00.259 **Other streptococcal arthritis, unspecified hip**

√6ᵗʰ M00.26 **Other streptococcal arthritis,** knee

    M00.261 Other streptococcal arthritis, right **knee**

    M00.262 Other streptococcal arthritis, left **knee**

    M00.269 **Other streptococcal arthritis, unspecified knee**

√6ᵗʰ M00.27 **Other streptococcal arthritis,** ankle and foot

    Other streptococcal arthritis, tarsus, metatarsus and phalanges

    M00.271 Other streptococcal arthritis, right **ankle and foot**

    M00.272 Other streptococcal arthritis, left **ankle and foot**

    M00.279 **Other streptococcal arthritis, unspecified ankle and foot**

M00.28 **Other streptococcal arthritis,** vertebrae

M00.29 **Other streptococcal polyarthritis**

√5ᵗʰ M00.8 **Arthritis and polyarthritis due to other bacteria**

    Use additional code (B96) to identify bacteria

    M00.80 **Arthritis due to other bacteria, unspecified joint**

√6ᵗʰ M00.81 **Arthritis due to other bacteria,** shoulder

    M00.811 Arthritis due to other bacteria, right **shoulder**

    M00.812 Arthritis due to other bacteria, left **shoulder**

    M00.819 **Arthritis due to other bacteria, unspecified shoulder**

√6ᵗʰ M00.82 **Arthritis due to other bacteria,** elbow

    M00.821 Arthritis due to other bacteria, right **elbow**

    M00.822 Arthritis due to other bacteria, left **elbow**

    M00.829 **Arthritis due to other bacteria, unspecified elbow**

√6ᵗʰ M00.83 **Arthritis due to other bacteria,** wrist

    Arthritis due to other bacteria, carpal bones

    M00.831 Arthritis due to other bacteria, right **wrist**

    M00.832 Arthritis due to other bacteria, left **wrist**

    M00.839 **Arthritis due to other bacteria, unspecified wrist**

√6ᵗʰ M00.84 **Arthritis due to other bacteria,** hand

    Arthritis due to other bacteria, metacarpus and phalanges

    M00.841 Arthritis due to other bacteria, right **hand**

    M00.842 Arthritis due to other bacteria, left **hand**

    M00.849 **Arthritis due to other bacteria, unspecified hand**

√6ᵗʰ M00.85 **Arthritis due to other bacteria,** hip

    M00.851 Arthritis due to other bacteria, right **hip**

    M00.852 Arthritis due to other bacteria, left **hip**

    M00.859 **Arthritis due to other bacteria, unspecified hip**

√6ᵗʰ M00.86 **Arthritis due to other bacteria,** knee

    M00.861 Arthritis due to other bacteria, right **knee**

    M00.862 Arthritis due to other bacteria, left **knee**

    M00.869 **Arthritis due to other bacteria, unspecified knee**

√6ᵗʰ M00.87 **Arthritis due to other bacteria,** ankle and foot

    Arthritis due to other bacteria, tarsus, metatarsus, and phalanges

    M00.871 Arthritis due to other bacteria, right **ankle and foot**

    M00.872 Arthritis due to other bacteria, left **ankle and foot**

    M00.879 **Arthritis due to other bacteria, unspecified ankle and foot**

M00.88 **Arthritis due to other bacteria,** vertebrae

M00.89 **Polyarthritis due to other bacteria**

M00.9 **Pyogenic arthritis, unspecified**

    Infective arthritis NOS

√4ᵗʰ **M01 Direct infections of joint in infectious and parasitic diseases classified elsewhere**

    Code first underlying disease, such as:

      leprosy [Hansen's disease] (A30.-)

      mycoses (B35-B49)

      O'nyong-nyong fever (A92.1)

      paratyphoid fever (A01.1-A01.4)

    EXCLUDES 1 *arthropathy in Lyme disease (A69.23)*

      gonococcal arthritis (A54.42)

      meningococcal arthritis (A39.83)

      mumps arthritis (B26.85)

      postinfective arthropathy (M02.-)

      postmeningococcal arthritis (A39.84)

      reactive arthritis (M02.3)

      rubella arthritis (B06.82)

      sarcoidosis arthritis (D86.86)

      typhoid fever arthritis (A01.04)

      tuberculosis arthritis (A18.01-A18.02)

√5ᵗʰ M01.X **Direct infection of joint in infectious and parasitic diseases classified elsewhere**

    M01.X0 Direct infection of unspecified *joint in infectious and parasitic diseases classified elsewhere*

√6ᵗʰ *M01.X1 Direct infection of* shoulder *joint in infectious and parasitic diseases classified elsewhere*

    M01.X11 Direct infection of right *shoulder in infectious and parasitic diseases classified elsewhere*

    M01.X12 Direct infection of left *shoulder in infectious and parasitic diseases classified elsewhere*

    M01.X19 Direct infection of unspecified *shoulder in infectious and parasitic diseases classified elsewhere*

√6ᵗʰ *M01.X2 Direct infection of* elbow *in infectious and parasitic diseases classified elsewhere*

    M01.X21 Direct infection of right *elbow in infectious and parasitic diseases classified elsewhere*

    M01.X22 Direct infection of left *elbow in infectious and parasitic diseases classified elsewhere*

    M01.X29 Direct infection of unspecified *elbow in infectious and parasitic diseases classified elsewhere*

√6ᵗʰ *M01.X3 Direct infection of* wrist *in infectious and parasitic diseases classified elsewhere*

    Direct infection of carpal bones in infectious and parasitic diseases classified elsewhere

    M01.X31 Direct infection of right *wrist in infectious and parasitic diseases classified elsewhere*

    M01.X32 Direct infection of left *wrist in infectious and parasitic diseases classified elsewhere*

    M01.X39 Direct infection of unspecified *wrist in infectious and parasitic diseases classified elsewhere*

√6ᵗʰ *M01.X4 Direct infection of* hand *in infectious and parasitic diseases classified elsewhere*

    Direct infection of metacarpus and phalanges in infectious and parasitic diseases classified elsewhere

    M01.X41 Direct infection of right *hand in infectious and parasitic diseases classified elsewhere*

    M01.X42 Direct infection of left *hand in infectious and parasitic diseases classified elsewhere*

EXCLUDES 1 Not coded here   **EXCLUDES 2** Not included here   N Newborn Age: 0   P Pediatric Age: 0-17   M Maternity Age: 12-55   A Adult Age: 15-124

646   ICD-10-CM Draft (2015)

M01.X49   *Direct infection of* unspecified *hand in infectious and parasitic diseases classified elsewhere*

✓6ᵗʰ M01.X5   **Direct infection of** hip **in infectious and parasitic diseases classified elsewhere**
   M01.X51   *Direct infection of* right *hip in infectious and parasitic diseases classified elsewhere*
   M01.X52   *Direct infection of* left *hip in infectious and parasitic diseases classified elsewhere*
   M01.X59   *Direct infection of* unspecified *hip in infectious and parasitic diseases classified elsewhere*

✓6ᵗʰ M01.X6   **Direct infection of** knee **in infectious and parasitic diseases classified elsewhere**
   M01.X61   *Direct infection of* right *knee in infectious and parasitic diseases classified elsewhere*
   M01.X62   *Direct infection of* left *knee in infectious and parasitic diseases classified elsewhere*
   M01.X69   *Direct infection of* unspecified *knee in infectious and parasitic diseases classified elsewhere*

✓6ᵗʰ M01.X7   **Direct infection of** ankle and foot **in infectious and parasitic diseases classified elsewhere**
   Direct infection of tarsus, metatarsus and phalanges in infectious and parasitic diseases classified elsewhere
   M01.X71   *Direct infection of* right *ankle and foot in infectious and parasitic diseases classified elsewhere*
   M01.X72   *Direct infection of* left *ankle and foot in infectious and parasitic diseases classified elsewhere*
   M01.X79   *Direct infection of* unspecified *ankle and foot in infectious and parasitic diseases classified elsewhere*

M01.X8   *Direct infection of* vertebrae *in infectious and parasitic diseases classified elsewhere*

M01.X9   *Direct infection of* multiple joints *in infectious and parasitic diseases classified elsewhere*

✓4ᵗʰ **M02 Postinfective and reactive arthropathies**
   Code first underlying disease, such as:
      congenital syphilis [Clutton's joints] (A50.5)
      enteritis due to Yersinia enterocolitica (A04.6)
      infective endocarditis (I33.0)
      viral hepatitis (B15-B19)
   EXCLUDES 1 *Behçet's disease (M35.2)*
      direct infections of joint in infectious and parasitic diseases classified elsewhere (M01.-)
      postmeningococcal arthritis (A39.84)
      mumps arthritis (B26.85)
      rheumatic fever (I00)
      rubella arthritis (B06.82)
      syphilis arthritis (late) (A52.77)
      tabetic arthropathy [Charcôt's] (A52.16)

✓5ᵗʰ **M02.0 Arthropathy** following intestinal bypass
   M02.00   **Arthropathy following intestinal bypass, unspecified site**
   ✓6ᵗʰ M02.01   **Arthropathy following intestinal bypass,** shoulder
      M02.011   **Arthropathy following intestinal bypass,** right shoulder
      M02.012   **Arthropathy following intestinal bypass,** left shoulder
      M02.019   **Arthropathy following intestinal bypass, unspecified shoulder**
   ✓6ᵗʰ M02.02   **Arthropathy following intestinal bypass,** elbow
      M02.021   **Arthropathy following intestinal bypass,** right elbow
      M02.022   **Arthropathy following intestinal bypass,** left elbow
      M02.029   **Arthropathy following intestinal bypass, unspecified elbow**
   ✓6ᵗʰ M02.03   **Arthropathy following intestinal bypass,** wrist
      Arthropathy following intestinal bypass, carpal bones
      M02.031   **Arthropathy following intestinal bypass,** right wrist
      M02.032   **Arthropathy following intestinal bypass,** left wrist
      M02.039   **Arthropathy following intestinal bypass, unspecified wrist**

✓6ᵗʰ M02.04   **Arthropathy following intestinal bypass,** hand
   Arthropathy following intestinal bypass, metacarpals and phalanges
   M02.041   **Arthropathy following intestinal bypass,** right hand
   M02.042   **Arthropathy following intestinal bypass,** left hand
   M02.049   **Arthropathy following intestinal bypass, unspecified hand**
✓6ᵗʰ M02.05   **Arthropathy following intestinal bypass,** hip
   M02.051   **Arthropathy following intestinal bypass,** right hip
   M02.052   **Arthropathy following intestinal bypass,** left hip
   M02.059   **Arthropathy following intestinal bypass, unspecified hip**
✓6ᵗʰ M02.06   **Arthropathy following intestinal bypass,** knee
   M02.061   **Arthropathy following intestinal bypass,** right knee
   M02.062   **Arthropathy following intestinal bypass,** left knee
   M02.069   **Arthropathy following intestinal bypass, unspecified knee**
✓6ᵗʰ M02.07   **Arthropathy following intestinal bypass,** ankle and foot
   Arthropathy following intestinal bypass, tarsus, metatarsus and phalanges
   M02.071   **Arthropathy following intestinal bypass,** right ankle and foot
   M02.072   **Arthropathy following intestinal bypass,** left ankle and foot
   M02.079   **Arthropathy following intestinal bypass, unspecified ankle and foot**
M02.08   **Arthropathy following intestinal bypass,** vertebrae
M02.09   **Arthropathy following intestinal bypass,** multiple sites

✓5ᵗʰ **M02.1 Postdysenteric** arthropathy
   M02.10   **Postdysenteric arthropathy, unspecified site**
   ✓6ᵗʰ M02.11   **Postdysenteric arthropathy,** shoulder
      M02.111   **Postdysenteric arthropathy,** right shoulder
      M02.112   **Postdysenteric arthropathy,** left shoulder
      M02.119   **Postdysenteric arthropathy, unspecified shoulder**
   ✓6ᵗʰ M02.12   **Postdysenteric arthropathy,** elbow
      M02.121   **Postdysenteric arthropathy,** right elbow
      M02.122   **Postdysenteric arthropathy,** left elbow
      M02.129   **Postdysenteric arthropathy, unspecified elbow**
   ✓6ᵗʰ M02.13   **Postdysenteric arthropathy,** wrist
      Postdysenteric arthropathy, carpal bones
      M02.131   **Postdysenteric arthropathy,** right wrist
      M02.132   **Postdysenteric arthropathy,** left wrist
      M02.139   **Postdysenteric arthropathy, unspecified wrist**
   ✓6ᵗʰ M02.14   **Postdysenteric arthropathy,** hand
      Postdysenteric arthropathy, metacarpus and phalanges
      M02.141   **Postdysenteric arthropathy,** right hand
      M02.142   **Postdysenteric arthropathy,** left hand
      M02.149   **Postdysenteric arthropathy, unspecified hand**
   ✓6ᵗʰ M02.15   **Postdysenteric arthropathy,** hip
      M02.151   **Postdysenteric arthropathy,** right hip
      M02.152   **Postdysenteric arthropathy,** left hip
      M02.159   **Postdysenteric arthropathy, unspecified hip**
   ✓6ᵗʰ M02.16   **Postdysenteric arthropathy,** knee
      M02.161   **Postdysenteric arthropathy,** right knee
      M02.162   **Postdysenteric arthropathy,** left knee
      M02.169   **Postdysenteric arthropathy, unspecified knee**

✓6ᵗʰ **M02.17** **Postdysenteric arthropathy,** ankle and foot
Postdysenteric arthropathy, tarsus, metatarsus and phalanges

     M02.171 **Postdysenteric arthropathy,** right ankle and foot

     M02.172 **Postdysenteric arthropathy,** left ankle and foot

     M02.179 **Postdysenteric arthropathy, unspecified ankle and foot**

   M02.18 **Postdysenteric arthropathy,** vertebrae

   M02.19 **Postdysenteric arthropathy,** multiple sites

✓5ᵗʰ **M02.2** **Postimmunization** arthropathy

   M02.20 **Postimmunization arthropathy, unspecified site**

✓6ᵗʰ **M02.21** **Postimmunization arthropathy,** shoulder

     M02.211 **Postimmunization arthropathy,** right shoulder

     M02.212 **Postimmunization arthropathy,** left shoulder

     M02.219 **Postimmunization arthropathy, unspecified shoulder**

✓6ᵗʰ **M02.22** **Postimmunization arthropathy,** elbow

     M02.221 **Postimmunization arthropathy,** right elbow

     M02.222 **Postimmunization arthropathy,** left elbow

     M02.229 **Postimmunization arthropathy, unspecified elbow**

✓6ᵗʰ **M02.23** **Postimmunization arthropathy,** wrist
Postimmunization arthropathy, carpal bones

     M02.231 **Postimmunization arthropathy,** right wrist

     M02.232 **Postimmunization arthropathy,** left wrist

     M02.239 **Postimmunization arthropathy, unspecified wrist**

✓6ᵗʰ **M02.24** **Postimmunization arthropathy,** hand
Postimmunization arthropathy, metacarpus and phalanges

     M02.241 **Postimmunization arthropathy,** right hand

     M02.242 **Postimmunization arthropathy,** left hand

     M02.249 **Postimmunization arthropathy, unspecified hand**

✓6ᵗʰ **M02.25** **Postimmunization arthropathy,** hip

     M02.251 **Postimmunization arthropathy,** right hip

     M02.252 **Postimmunization arthropathy,** left hip

     M02.259 **Postimmunization arthropathy, unspecified hip**

✓6ᵗʰ **M02.26** **Postimmunization arthropathy,** knee

     M02.261 **Postimmunization arthropathy,** right knee

     M02.262 **Postimmunization arthropathy,** left knee

     M02.269 **Postimmunization arthropathy, unspecified knee**

✓6ᵗʰ **M02.27** **Postimmunization arthropathy,** ankle and foot
Postimmunization arthropathy, tarsus, metatarsus and phalanges

     M02.271 **Postimmunization arthropathy,** right ankle and foot

     M02.272 **Postimmunization arthropathy,** left ankle and foot

     M02.279 **Postimmunization arthropathy, unspecified ankle and foot**

   M02.28 **Postimmunization arthropathy,** vertebrae

   M02.29 **Postimmunization arthropathy,** multiple sites

✓5ᵗʰ **M02.3** Reiter's disease
Reactive arthritis

   M02.30 **Reiter's disease, unspecified site**

✓6ᵗʰ **M02.31** **Reiter's disease,** shoulder

     M02.311 **Reiter's disease,** right shoulder

     M02.312 **Reiter's disease,** left shoulder

     M02.319 **Reiter's disease, unspecified shoulder**

✓6ᵗʰ **M02.32** **Reiter's disease,** elbow

     M02.321 **Reiter's disease,** right elbow

     M02.322 **Reiter's disease,** left elbow

     M02.329 **Reiter's disease, unspecified elbow**

✓6ᵗʰ **M02.33** **Reiter's disease,** wrist
Reiter's disease, carpal bones

     M02.331 **Reiter's disease,** right wrist

     M02.332 **Reiter's disease,** left wrist

     M02.339 **Reiter's disease, unspecified wrist**

✓6ᵗʰ **M02.34** **Reiter's disease,** hand
Reiter's disease, metacarpus and phalanges

     M02.341 **Reiter's disease,** right hand

     M02.342 **Reiter's disease,** left hand

     M02.349 **Reiter's disease, unspecified hand**

✓6ᵗʰ **M02.35** **Reiter's disease,** hip

     M02.351 **Reiter's disease,** right hip

     M02.352 **Reiter's disease,** left hip

     M02.359 **Reiter's disease, unspecified hip**

✓6ᵗʰ **M02.36** **Reiter's disease,** knee

     M02.361 **Reiter's disease,** right knee

     M02.362 **Reiter's disease,** left knee

     M02.369 **Reiter's disease, unspecified knee**

✓6ᵗʰ **M02.37** **Reiter's disease,** ankle and foot
Reiter's disease, tarsus, metatarsus and phalanges

     M02.371 **Reiter's disease,** right ankle and foot

     M02.372 **Reiter's disease,** left ankle and foot

     M02.379 **Reiter's disease, unspecified ankle and foot**

   M02.38 **Reiter's disease,** vertebrae

   M02.39 **Reiter's disease,** multiple sites

✓5ᵗʰ **M02.8** Other reactive arthropathies

   M02.80 **Other reactive arthropathies, unspecified site**

✓6ᵗʰ **M02.81** **Other reactive arthropathies,** shoulder

     M02.811 **Other reactive arthropathies,** right shoulder

     M02.812 **Other reactive arthropathies,** left shoulder

     M02.819 **Other reactive arthropathies, unspecified shoulder**

✓6ᵗʰ **M02.82** **Other reactive arthropathies,** elbow

     M02.821 **Other reactive arthropathies,** right elbow

     M02.822 **Other reactive arthropathies,** left elbow

     M02.829 **Other reactive arthropathies, unspecified elbow**

✓6ᵗʰ **M02.83** **Other reactive arthropathies,** wrist
Other reactive arthropathies, carpal bones

     M02.831 **Other reactive arthropathies,** right wrist

     M02.832 **Other reactive arthropathies,** left wrist

     M02.839 **Other reactive arthropathies, unspecified wrist**

✓6ᵗʰ **M02.84** **Other reactive arthropathies,** hand
Other reactive arthropathies, metacarpus and phalanges

     M02.841 **Other reactive arthropathies,** right hand

     M02.842 **Other reactive arthropathies,** left hand

     M02.849 **Other reactive arthropathies, unspecified hand**

✓6ᵗʰ **M02.85** **Other reactive arthropathies,** hip

     M02.851 **Other reactive arthropathies,** right hip

     M02.852 **Other reactive arthropathies,** left hip

     M02.859 **Other reactive arthropathies, unspecified hip**

✓6ᵗʰ **M02.86** **Other reactive arthropathies,** knee

     M02.861 **Other reactive arthropathies,** right knee

     M02.862 **Other reactive arthropathies,** left knee

     M02.869 **Other reactive arthropathies, unspecified knee**

✓6ᵗʰ **M02.87** **Other reactive arthropathies,** ankle and foot
Other reactive arthropathies, tarsus, metatarsus and phalanges

     M02.871 **Other reactive arthropathies,** right ankle and foot

     M02.872 **Other reactive arthropathies,** left ankle and foot

     M02.879 **Other reactive arthropathies, unspecified ankle and foot**

   M02.88 **Other reactive arthropathies,** vertebrae

   M02.89 **Other reactive arthropathies,** multiple sites

M02.9 **Reactive arthropathy,** unspecified

EXCLUDES 1 Not coded here   EXCLUDES 2 Not included here   N Newborn Age: 0   P Pediatric Age: 0-17   M Maternity Age: 12-55   A Adult Age: 15-124

648   ICD-10-CM Draft (2015)

Inflammatory polyarthropathies (M05-M14)

✓4th **M05 Rheumatoid arthritis with rheumatoid factor**

EXCLUDES 1 rheumatic fever (I00)
juvenile rheumatoid arthritis (M08.-)
rheumatoid arthritis of spine (M45.-)

✓5th **M05.0 Felty's syndrome**
Rheumatoid arthritis with splenoadenomegaly and leukopenia

M05.00 **Felty's syndrome, unspecified site**

✓6th M05.01 **Felty's syndrome, shoulder**
M05.011 **Felty's syndrome, right shoulder**
M05.012 **Felty's syndrome, left shoulder**
M05.019 **Felty's syndrome, unspecified shoulder**

✓6th M05.02 **Felty's syndrome, elbow**
M05.021 **Felty's syndrome, right elbow**
M05.022 **Felty's syndrome, left elbow**
M05.029 **Felty's syndrome, unspecified elbow**

✓6th M05.03 **Felty's syndrome, wrist**
Felty's syndrome, carpal bones
M05.031 **Felty's syndrome, right wrist**
M05.032 **Felty's syndrome, left wrist**
M05.039 **Felty's syndrome, unspecified wrist**

✓6th M05.04 **Felty's syndrome, hand**
Felty's syndrome, metacarpus and phalanges
M05.041 **Felty's syndrome, right hand**
M05.042 **Felty's syndrome, left hand**
M05.049 **Felty's syndrome, unspecified hand**

✓6th M05.05 **Felty's syndrome, hip**
M05.051 **Felty's syndrome, right hip**
M05.052 **Felty's syndrome, left hip**
M05.059 **Felty's syndrome, unspecified hip**

✓6th M05.06 **Felty's syndrome, knee**
M05.061 **Felty's syndrome, right knee**
M05.062 **Felty's syndrome, left knee**
M05.069 **Felty's syndrome, unspecified knee**

✓6th M05.07 **Felty's syndrome, ankle and foot**
Felty's syndrome, tarsus, metatarsus and phalanges
M05.071 **Felty's syndrome, right ankle and foot**
M05.072 **Felty's syndrome, left ankle and foot**
M05.079 **Felty's syndrome, unspecified ankle and foot**

M05.09 **Felty's syndrome, multiple sites**

✓5th **M05.1 Rheumatoid lung disease with rheumatoid arthritis**

M05.10 **Rheumatoid lung disease with rheumatoid arthritis of unspecified site**

✓6th M05.11 **Rheumatoid lung disease with rheumatoid arthritis of shoulder**
M05.111 **Rheumatoid lung disease with rheumatoid arthritis of right shoulder**
M05.112 **Rheumatoid lung disease with rheumatoid arthritis of left shoulder**
M05.119 **Rheumatoid lung disease with rheumatoid arthritis of unspecified shoulder**

✓6th M05.12 **Rheumatoid lung disease with rheumatoid arthritis of elbow**
M05.121 **Rheumatoid lung disease with rheumatoid arthritis of right elbow**
M05.122 **Rheumatoid lung disease with rheumatoid arthritis of left elbow**
M05.129 **Rheumatoid lung disease with rheumatoid arthritis of unspecified elbow**

✓6th M05.13 **Rheumatoid lung disease with rheumatoid arthritis of wrist**
Rheumatoid lung disease with rheumatoid arthritis, carpal bones
M05.131 **Rheumatoid lung disease with rheumatoid arthritis of right wrist**
M05.132 **Rheumatoid lung disease with rheumatoid arthritis of left wrist**
M05.139 **Rheumatoid lung disease with rheumatoid arthritis of unspecified wrist**

✓6th **M05.14 Rheumatoid lung disease with rheumatoid arthritis of hand**
Rheumatoid lung disease with rheumatoid arthritis, metacarpus and phalanges
M05.141 **Rheumatoid lung disease with rheumatoid arthritis of right hand**
M05.142 **Rheumatoid lung disease with rheumatoid arthritis of left hand**
M05.149 **Rheumatoid lung disease with rheumatoid arthritis of unspecified hand**

✓6th M05.15 **Rheumatoid lung disease with rheumatoid arthritis of hip**
M05.151 **Rheumatoid lung disease with rheumatoid arthritis of right hip**
M05.152 **Rheumatoid lung disease with rheumatoid arthritis of left hip**
M05.159 **Rheumatoid lung disease with rheumatoid arthritis of unspecified hip**

✓6th M05.16 **Rheumatoid lung disease with rheumatoid arthritis of knee**
M05.161 **Rheumatoid lung disease with rheumatoid arthritis of right knee**
M05.162 **Rheumatoid lung disease with rheumatoid arthritis of left knee**
M05.169 **Rheumatoid lung disease with rheumatoid arthritis of unspecified knee**

✓6th M05.17 **Rheumatoid lung disease with rheumatoid arthritis of ankle and foot**
Rheumatoid lung disease with rheumatoid arthritis, tarsus, metatarsus and phalanges
M05.171 **Rheumatoid lung disease with rheumatoid arthritis of right ankle and foot**
M05.172 **Rheumatoid lung disease with rheumatoid arthritis of left ankle and foot**
M05.179 **Rheumatoid lung disease with rheumatoid arthritis of unspecified ankle and foot**

M05.19 **Rheumatoid lung disease with rheumatoid arthritis of multiple sites**

✓5th **M05.2 Rheumatoid vasculitis with rheumatoid arthritis**

M05.20 **Rheumatoid vasculitis with rheumatoid arthritis of unspecified site**

✓6th M05.21 **Rheumatoid vasculitis with rheumatoid arthritis of shoulder**
M05.211 **Rheumatoid vasculitis with rheumatoid arthritis of right shoulder**
M05.212 **Rheumatoid vasculitis with rheumatoid arthritis of left shoulder**
M05.219 **Rheumatoid vasculitis with rheumatoid arthritis of unspecified shoulder**

✓6th M05.22 **Rheumatoid vasculitis with rheumatoid arthritis of elbow**
M05.221 **Rheumatoid vasculitis with rheumatoid arthritis of right elbow**
M05.222 **Rheumatoid vasculitis with rheumatoid arthritis of left elbow**
M05.229 **Rheumatoid vasculitis with rheumatoid arthritis of unspecified elbow**

✓6th M05.23 **Rheumatoid vasculitis with rheumatoid arthritis of wrist**
Rheumatoid vasculitis with rheumatoid arthritis, carpal bones
M05.231 **Rheumatoid vasculitis with rheumatoid arthritis of right wrist**
M05.232 **Rheumatoid vasculitis with rheumatoid arthritis of left wrist**
M05.239 **Rheumatoid vasculitis with rheumatoid arthritis of unspecified wrist**

✓6th M05.24 **Rheumatoid vasculitis with rheumatoid arthritis of hand**
Rheumatoid vasculitis with rheumatoid arthritis, metacarpus and phalanges
M05.241 **Rheumatoid vasculitis with rheumatoid arthritis of right hand**
M05.242 **Rheumatoid vasculitis with rheumatoid arthritis of left hand**
M05.249 **Rheumatoid vasculitis with rheumatoid arthritis of unspecified hand**

✓ Additional Character Required ✓x7th Xtension Alert Unspecified Dx Other Specified Dx Manifestation ►◄ Revised Text ● New Code ▲ Revised Code Title

ICD-10-CM Draft (2015) 649

✓6th **M05.25** **Rheumatoid vasculitis with rheumatoid arthritis of hip**
- **M05.251** Rheumatoid vasculitis with rheumatoid arthritis of right hip
- **M05.252** Rheumatoid vasculitis with rheumatoid arthritis of left hip
- **M05.259** Rheumatoid vasculitis with rheumatoid arthritis of unspecified hip

✓6th **M05.26** **Rheumatoid vasculitis with rheumatoid arthritis of knee**
- **M05.261** Rheumatoid vasculitis with rheumatoid arthritis of right knee
- **M05.262** Rheumatoid vasculitis with rheumatoid arthritis of left knee
- **M05.269** Rheumatoid vasculitis with rheumatoid arthritis of unspecified knee

✓6th **M05.27** **Rheumatoid vasculitis with rheumatoid arthritis of ankle and foot**
Rheumatoid vasculitis with rheumatoid arthritis, tarsus, metatarsus and phalanges
- **M05.271** Rheumatoid vasculitis with rheumatoid arthritis of right ankle and foot
- **M05.272** Rheumatoid vasculitis with rheumatoid arthritis of left ankle and foot
- **M05.279** Rheumatoid vasculitis with rheumatoid arthritis of unspecified ankle and foot

M05.29 **Rheumatoid vasculitis with rheumatoid arthritis of multiple sites**

✓5th **M05.3** **Rheumatoid heart disease with rheumatoid arthritis**
Rheumatoid carditis   Rheumatoid myocarditis
Rheumatoid endocarditis   Rheumatoid pericarditis

M05.30 **Rheumatoid heart disease with rheumatoid arthritis of unspecified site**

✓6th **M05.31** **Rheumatoid heart disease with rheumatoid arthritis of shoulder**
- **M05.311** Rheumatoid heart disease with rheumatoid arthritis of right shoulder
- **M05.312** Rheumatoid heart disease with rheumatoid arthritis of left shoulder
- **M05.319** Rheumatoid heart disease with rheumatoid arthritis of unspecified shoulder

✓6th **M05.32** **Rheumatoid heart disease with rheumatoid arthritis of elbow**
- **M05.321** Rheumatoid heart disease with rheumatoid arthritis of right elbow
- **M05.322** Rheumatoid heart disease with rheumatoid arthritis of left elbow
- **M05.329** Rheumatoid heart disease with rheumatoid arthritis of unspecified elbow

✓6th **M05.33** **Rheumatoid heart disease with rheumatoid arthritis of wrist**
Rheumatoid heart disease with rheumatoid arthritis, carpal bones
- **M05.331** Rheumatoid heart disease with rheumatoid arthritis of right wrist
- **M05.332** Rheumatoid heart disease with rheumatoid arthritis of left wrist
- **M05.339** Rheumatoid heart disease with rheumatoid arthritis of unspecified wrist

✓6th **M05.34** **Rheumatoid heart disease with rheumatoid arthritis of hand**
Rheumatoid heart disease with rheumatoid arthritis, metacarpus and phalanges
- **M05.341** Rheumatoid heart disease with rheumatoid arthritis of right hand
- **M05.342** Rheumatoid heart disease with rheumatoid arthritis of left hand
- **M05.349** Rheumatoid heart disease with rheumatoid arthritis of unspecified hand

✓6th **M05.35** **Rheumatoid heart disease with rheumatoid arthritis of hip**
- **M05.351** Rheumatoid heart disease with rheumatoid arthritis of right hip
- **M05.352** Rheumatoid heart disease with rheumatoid arthritis of left hip
- **M05.359** Rheumatoid heart disease with rheumatoid arthritis of unspecified hip

✓6th **M05.36** **Rheumatoid heart disease with rheumatoid arthritis of knee**
- **M05.361** Rheumatoid heart disease with rheumatoid arthritis of right knee
- **M05.362** Rheumatoid heart disease with rheumatoid arthritis of left knee
- **M05.369** Rheumatoid heart disease with rheumatoid arthritis of unspecified knee

✓6th **M05.37** **Rheumatoid heart disease with rheumatoid arthritis of ankle and foot**
Rheumatoid heart disease with rheumatoid arthritis, tarsus, metatarsus and phalanges
- **M05.371** Rheumatoid heart disease with rheumatoid arthritis of right ankle and foot
- **M05.372** Rheumatoid heart disease with rheumatoid arthritis of left ankle and foot
- **M05.379** Rheumatoid heart disease with rheumatoid arthritis of unspecified ankle and foot

M05.39 **Rheumatoid heart disease with rheumatoid arthritis of multiple sites**

✓5th **M05.4** **Rheumatoid myopathy with rheumatoid arthritis**

M05.40 **Rheumatoid myopathy with rheumatoid arthritis of unspecified site**

✓6th **M05.41** **Rheumatoid myopathy with rheumatoid arthritis of shoulder**
- **M05.411** Rheumatoid myopathy with rheumatoid arthritis of right shoulder
- **M05.412** Rheumatoid myopathy with rheumatoid arthritis of left shoulder
- **M05.419** Rheumatoid myopathy with rheumatoid arthritis of unspecified shoulder

✓6th **M05.42** **Rheumatoid myopathy with rheumatoid arthritis of elbow**
- **M05.421** Rheumatoid myopathy with rheumatoid arthritis of right elbow
- **M05.422** Rheumatoid myopathy with rheumatoid arthritis of left elbow
- **M05.429** Rheumatoid myopathy with rheumatoid arthritis of unspecified elbow

✓6th **M05.43** **Rheumatoid myopathy with rheumatoid arthritis of wrist**
Rheumatoid myopathy with rheumatoid arthritis, carpal bones
- **M05.431** Rheumatoid myopathy with rheumatoid arthritis of right wrist
- **M05.432** Rheumatoid myopathy with rheumatoid arthritis of left wrist
- **M05.439** Rheumatoid myopathy with rheumatoid arthritis of unspecified wrist

✓6th **M05.44** **Rheumatoid myopathy with rheumatoid arthritis of hand**
Rheumatoid myopathy with rheumatoid arthritis, metacarpus and phalanges
- **M05.441** Rheumatoid myopathy with rheumatoid arthritis of right hand
- **M05.442** Rheumatoid myopathy with rheumatoid arthritis of left hand
- **M05.449** Rheumatoid myopathy with rheumatoid arthritis of unspecified hand

✓6th **M05.45** **Rheumatoid myopathy with rheumatoid arthritis of hip**
- **M05.451** Rheumatoid myopathy with rheumatoid arthritis of right hip
- **M05.452** Rheumatoid myopathy with rheumatoid arthritis of left hip
- **M05.459** Rheumatoid myopathy with rheumatoid arthritis of unspecified hip

✓6th **M05.46** **Rheumatoid myopathy with rheumatoid arthritis of knee**
- **M05.461** Rheumatoid myopathy with rheumatoid arthritis of right knee
- **M05.462** Rheumatoid myopathy with rheumatoid arthritis of left knee
- **M05.469** Rheumatoid myopathy with rheumatoid arthritis of unspecified knee

---

EXCLUDES 1 Not coded here   EXCLUDES 2 Not included here   N Newborn Age: 0   P Pediatric Age: 0-17   M Maternity Age: 12-55   A Adult Age: 15-124

☑6ᵗʰ **M05.47 Rheumatoid myopathy with rheumatoid arthritis of ankle and foot**
Rheumatoid myopathy with rheumatoid arthritis, tarsus, metatarsus and phalanges

M05.471 Rheumatoid myopathy with rheumatoid arthritis of right ankle and foot

M05.472 Rheumatoid myopathy with rheumatoid arthritis of left ankle and foot

M05.479 Rheumatoid myopathy with rheumatoid arthritis of unspecified ankle and foot

M05.49 Rheumatoid myopathy with rheumatoid arthritis of multiple sites

☑5ᵗʰ **M05.5 Rheumatoid polyneuropathy with rheumatoid arthritis**

M05.50 Rheumatoid polyneuropathy with rheumatoid arthritis of unspecified site

☑6ᵗʰ **M05.51 Rheumatoid polyneuropathy with rheumatoid arthritis of shoulder**

M05.511 Rheumatoid polyneuropathy with rheumatoid arthritis of right shoulder

M05.512 Rheumatoid polyneuropathy with rheumatoid arthritis of left shoulder

M05.519 Rheumatoid polyneuropathy with rheumatoid arthritis of unspecified shoulder

☑6ᵗʰ **M05.52 Rheumatoid polyneuropathy with rheumatoid arthritis of elbow**

M05.521 Rheumatoid polyneuropathy with rheumatoid arthritis of right elbow

M05.522 Rheumatoid polyneuropathy with rheumatoid arthritis of left elbow

M05.529 Rheumatoid polyneuropathy with rheumatoid arthritis of unspecified elbow

☑6ᵗʰ **M05.53 Rheumatoid polyneuropathy with rheumatoid arthritis of wrist**
Rheumatoid polyneuropathy with rheumatoid arthritis, carpal bones

M05.531 Rheumatoid polyneuropathy with rheumatoid arthritis of right wrist

M05.532 Rheumatoid polyneuropathy with rheumatoid arthritis of left wrist

M05.539 Rheumatoid polyneuropathy with rheumatoid arthritis of unspecified wrist

☑6ᵗʰ **M05.54 Rheumatoid polyneuropathy with rheumatoid arthritis of hand**
Rheumatoid polyneuropathy with rheumatoid arthritis, metacarpus and phalanges

M05.541 Rheumatoid polyneuropathy with rheumatoid arthritis of right hand

M05.542 Rheumatoid polyneuropathy with rheumatoid arthritis of left hand

M05.549 Rheumatoid polyneuropathy with rheumatoid arthritis of unspecified hand

☑6ᵗʰ **M05.55 Rheumatoid polyneuropathy with rheumatoid arthritis of hip**

M05.551 Rheumatoid polyneuropathy with rheumatoid arthritis of right hip

M05.552 Rheumatoid polyneuropathy with rheumatoid arthritis of left hip

M05.559 Rheumatoid polyneuropathy with rheumatoid arthritis of unspecified hip

☑6ᵗʰ **M05.56 Rheumatoid polyneuropathy with rheumatoid arthritis of knee**

M05.561 Rheumatoid polyneuropathy with rheumatoid arthritis of right knee

M05.562 Rheumatoid polyneuropathy with rheumatoid arthritis of left knee

M05.569 Rheumatoid polyneuropathy with rheumatoid arthritis of unspecified knee

☑6ᵗʰ **M05.57 Rheumatoid polyneuropathy with rheumatoid arthritis of ankle and foot**
Rheumatoid polyneuropathy with rheumatoid arthritis, tarsus, metatarsus and phalanges

M05.571 Rheumatoid polyneuropathy with rheumatoid arthritis of right ankle and foot

M05.572 Rheumatoid polyneuropathy with rheumatoid arthritis of left ankle and foot

M05.579 Rheumatoid polyneuropathy with rheumatoid arthritis of unspecified ankle and foot

M05.59 Rheumatoid polyneuropathy with rheumatoid arthritis of multiple sites

☑5ᵗʰ **M05.6 Rheumatoid arthritis with involvement of other organs and systems**

M05.60 Rheumatoid arthritis of unspecified site with involvement of other organs and systems

☑6ᵗʰ **M05.61 Rheumatoid arthritis of shoulder with involvement of other organs and systems**

M05.611 Rheumatoid arthritis of right shoulder with involvement of other organs and systems

M05.612 Rheumatoid arthritis of left shoulder with involvement of other organs and systems

M05.619 Rheumatoid arthritis of unspecified shoulder with involvement of other organs and systems

☑6ᵗʰ **M05.62 Rheumatoid arthritis of elbow with involvement of other organs and systems**

M05.621 Rheumatoid arthritis of right elbow with involvement of other organs and systems

M05.622 Rheumatoid arthritis of left elbow with involvement of other organs and systems

M05.629 Rheumatoid arthritis of unspecified elbow with involvement of other organs and systems

☑6ᵗʰ **M05.63 Rheumatoid arthritis of wrist with involvement of other organs and systems**
Rheumatoid arthritis of carpal bones with involvement of other organs and systems

M05.631 Rheumatoid arthritis of right wrist with involvement of other organs and systems

M05.632 Rheumatoid arthritis of left wrist with involvement of other organs and systems

M05.639 Rheumatoid arthritis of unspecified wrist with involvement of other organs and systems

☑6ᵗʰ **M05.64 Rheumatoid arthritis of hand with involvement of other organs and systems**
Rheumatoid arthritis of metacarpus and phalanges with involvement of other organs and systems

M05.641 Rheumatoid arthritis of right hand with involvement of other organs and systems

M05.642 Rheumatoid arthritis of left hand with involvement of other organs and systems

M05.649 Rheumatoid arthritis of unspecified hand with involvement of other organs and systems

☑6ᵗʰ **M05.65 Rheumatoid arthritis of hip with involvement of other organs and systems**

M05.651 Rheumatoid arthritis of right hip with involvement of other organs and systems

M05.652 Rheumatoid arthritis of left hip with involvement of other organs and systems

M05.659 Rheumatoid arthritis of unspecified hip with involvement of other organs and systems

☑6ᵗʰ **M05.66 Rheumatoid arthritis of knee with involvement of other organs and systems**

M05.661 Rheumatoid arthritis of right knee with involvement of other organs and systems

M05.662 Rheumatoid arthritis of left knee with involvement of other organs and systems

M05.669 Rheumatoid arthritis of unspecified knee with involvement of other organs and systems

☑6ᵗʰ **M05.67 Rheumatoid arthritis of ankle and foot with involvement of other organs and systems**
Rheumatoid arthritis of tarsus, metatarsus and phalanges with involvement of other organs and systems

M05.671 Rheumatoid arthritis of right ankle and foot with involvement of other organs and systems

M05.672 Rheumatoid arthritis of left ankle and foot with involvement of other organs and systems

---

☑ Additional Character Required   ✓ₓ7ᵗʰ Xtension Alert   Unspecified Dx   Other Specified Dx   Manifestation   ▶◀ Revised Text   ● New Code   ▲ Revised Code Title

ICD-10-CM Draft (2015)   **651**

M05.679 Rheumatoid arthritis of unspecified ankle and foot with involvement of other organs and systems

M05.69 Rheumatoid arthritis of multiple sites with involvement of other organs and systems

✓5th **M05.7** Rheumatoid arthritis with rheumatoid factor without organ or systems involvement

    M05.70 Rheumatoid arthritis with rheumatoid factor of unspecified site without organ or systems involvement

✓6th **M05.71** Rheumatoid arthritis with rheumatoid factor of shoulder without organ or systems involvement

    M05.711 Rheumatoid arthritis with rheumatoid factor of right shoulder without organ or systems involvement

    M05.712 Rheumatoid arthritis with rheumatoid factor of left shoulder without organ or systems involvement

    M05.719 Rheumatoid arthritis with rheumatoid factor of unspecified shoulder without organ or systems involvement

✓6th **M05.72** Rheumatoid arthritis with rheumatoid factor of elbow without organ or systems involvement

    M05.721 Rheumatoid arthritis with rheumatoid factor of right elbow without organ or systems involvement

    M05.722 Rheumatoid arthritis with rheumatoid factor of left elbow without organ or systems involvement

    M05.729 Rheumatoid arthritis with rheumatoid factor of unspecified elbow without organ or systems involvement

✓6th **M05.73** Rheumatoid arthritis with rheumatoid factor of wrist without organ or systems involvement

    M05.731 Rheumatoid arthritis with rheumatoid factor of right wrist without organ or systems involvement

    M05.732 Rheumatoid arthritis with rheumatoid factor of left wrist without organ or systems involvement

    M05.739 Rheumatoid arthritis with rheumatoid factor of unspecified wrist without organ or systems involvement

✓6th **M05.74** Rheumatoid arthritis with rheumatoid factor of hand without organ or systems involvement

    M05.741 Rheumatoid arthritis with rheumatoid factor of right hand without organ or systems involvement

    M05.742 Rheumatoid arthritis with rheumatoid factor of left hand without organ or systems involvement

    M05.749 Rheumatoid arthritis with rheumatoid factor of unspecified hand without organ or systems involvement

✓6th **M05.75** Rheumatoid arthritis with rheumatoid factor of hip without organ or systems involvement

    M05.751 Rheumatoid arthritis with rheumatoid factor of right hip without organ or systems involvement

    M05.752 Rheumatoid arthritis with rheumatoid factor of left hip without organ or systems involvement

    M05.759 Rheumatoid arthritis with rheumatoid factor of unspecified hip without organ or systems involvement

✓6th **M05.76** Rheumatoid arthritis with rheumatoid factor of knee without organ or systems involvement

    M05.761 Rheumatoid arthritis with rheumatoid factor of right knee without organ or systems involvement

    M05.762 Rheumatoid arthritis with rheumatoid factor of left knee without organ or systems involvement

    M05.769 Rheumatoid arthritis with rheumatoid factor of unspecified knee without organ or systems involvement

✓6th **M05.77** Rheumatoid arthritis with rheumatoid factor of ankle and foot without organ or systems involvement

    M05.771 Rheumatoid arthritis with rheumatoid factor of right ankle and foot without organ or systems involvement

    M05.772 Rheumatoid arthritis with rheumatoid factor of left ankle and foot without organ or systems involvement

    M05.779 Rheumatoid arthritis with rheumatoid factor of unspecified ankle and foot without organ or systems involvement

M05.79 Rheumatoid arthritis with rheumatoid factor of multiple sites without organ or systems involvement

✓5th **M05.8** Other rheumatoid arthritis with rheumatoid factor

    M05.80 Other rheumatoid arthritis with rheumatoid factor of unspecified site

✓6th **M05.81** Other rheumatoid arthritis with rheumatoid factor of shoulder

    M05.811 Other rheumatoid arthritis with rheumatoid factor of right shoulder

    M05.812 Other rheumatoid arthritis with rheumatoid factor of left shoulder

    M05.819 Other rheumatoid arthritis with rheumatoid factor of unspecified shoulder

✓6th **M05.82** Other rheumatoid arthritis with rheumatoid factor of elbow

    M05.821 Other rheumatoid arthritis with rheumatoid factor of right elbow

    M05.822 Other rheumatoid arthritis with rheumatoid factor of left elbow

    M05.829 Other rheumatoid arthritis with rheumatoid factor of unspecified elbow

✓6th **M05.83** Other rheumatoid arthritis with rheumatoid factor of wrist

    M05.831 Other rheumatoid arthritis with rheumatoid factor of right wrist

    M05.832 Other rheumatoid arthritis with rheumatoid factor of left wrist

    M05.839 Other rheumatoid arthritis with rheumatoid factor of unspecified wrist

✓6th **M05.84** Other rheumatoid arthritis with rheumatoid factor of hand

    M05.841 Other rheumatoid arthritis with rheumatoid factor of right hand

    M05.842 Other rheumatoid arthritis with rheumatoid factor of left hand

    M05.849 Other rheumatoid arthritis with rheumatoid factor of unspecified hand

✓6th **M05.85** Other rheumatoid arthritis with rheumatoid factor of hip

    M05.851 Other rheumatoid arthritis with rheumatoid factor of right hip

    M05.852 Other rheumatoid arthritis with rheumatoid factor of left hip

    M05.859 Other rheumatoid arthritis with rheumatoid factor of unspecified hip

✓6th **M05.86** Other rheumatoid arthritis with rheumatoid factor of knee

    M05.861 Other rheumatoid arthritis with rheumatoid factor of right knee

    M05.862 Other rheumatoid arthritis with rheumatoid factor of left knee

    M05.869 Other rheumatoid arthritis with rheumatoid factor of unspecified knee

✓6th **M05.87** Other rheumatoid arthritis with rheumatoid factor of ankle and foot

    M05.871 Other rheumatoid arthritis with rheumatoid factor of right ankle and foot

    M05.872 Other rheumatoid arthritis with rheumatoid factor of left ankle and foot

    M05.879 Other rheumatoid arthritis with rheumatoid factor of unspecified ankle and foot

M05.89 Other rheumatoid arthritis with rheumatoid factor of multiple sites

M05.9 Rheumatoid arthritis with rheumatoid factor, unspecified

EXCLUDES 1 Not coded here   **EXCLUDES 2** Not included here   **N** Newborn Age: 0   **P** Pediatric Age: 0-17   **M** Maternity Age: 12-55   **A** Adult Age: 15-124

652   ICD-10-CM Draft (2015)

☑4ᵗʰ **M06** Other **rheumatoid arthritis**

☑5ᵗʰ **M06.0** Rheumatoid arthritis without rheumatoid factor

M06.00 **Rheumatoid arthritis without rheumatoid factor, unspecified site**

☑6ᵗʰ **M06.01** Rheumatoid arthritis without rheumatoid factor, shoulder

M06.011 Rheumatoid arthritis without rheumatoid factor, right shoulder

M06.012 Rheumatoid arthritis without rheumatoid factor, left shoulder

M06.019 **Rheumatoid arthritis without rheumatoid factor, unspecified shoulder**

☑6ᵗʰ **M06.02** Rheumatoid arthritis without rheumatoid factor, elbow

M06.021 Rheumatoid arthritis without rheumatoid factor, right elbow

M06.022 Rheumatoid arthritis without rheumatoid factor, left elbow

M06.029 **Rheumatoid arthritis without rheumatoid factor, unspecified elbow**

☑6ᵗʰ **M06.03** Rheumatoid arthritis without rheumatoid factor, wrist

M06.031 Rheumatoid arthritis without rheumatoid factor, right wrist

M06.032 Rheumatoid arthritis without rheumatoid factor, left wrist

M06.039 **Rheumatoid arthritis without rheumatoid factor, unspecified wrist**

☑6ᵗʰ **M06.04** Rheumatoid arthritis without rheumatoid factor, hand

M06.041 Rheumatoid arthritis without rheumatoid factor, right hand

M06.042 Rheumatoid arthritis without rheumatoid factor, left hand

M06.049 **Rheumatoid arthritis without rheumatoid factor, unspecified hand**

☑6ᵗʰ **M06.05** Rheumatoid arthritis without rheumatoid factor, hip

M06.051 Rheumatoid arthritis without rheumatoid factor, right hip

M06.052 Rheumatoid arthritis without rheumatoid factor, left hip

M06.059 **Rheumatoid arthritis without rheumatoid factor, unspecified hip**

☑6ᵗʰ **M06.06** Rheumatoid arthritis without rheumatoid factor, knee

M06.061 Rheumatoid arthritis without rheumatoid factor, right knee

M06.062 Rheumatoid arthritis without rheumatoid factor, left knee

M06.069 **Rheumatoid arthritis without rheumatoid factor, unspecified knee**

☑6ᵗʰ **M06.07** Rheumatoid arthritis without rheumatoid factor, ankle and foot

M06.071 Rheumatoid arthritis without rheumatoid factor, right ankle and foot

M06.072 Rheumatoid arthritis without rheumatoid factor, left ankle and foot

M06.079 **Rheumatoid arthritis without rheumatoid factor, unspecified ankle and foot**

M06.08 Rheumatoid arthritis without rheumatoid factor, vertebrae

M06.09 Rheumatoid arthritis without rheumatoid factor, multiple sites

M06.1 Adult-onset Still's disease　　　　　Ⓐ

EXCLUDES 1　*Still's disease NOS (M08.2-)*

☑5ᵗʰ **M06.2** Rheumatoid bursitis

M06.20 **Rheumatoid bursitis, unspecified site**

☑6ᵗʰ **M06.21** Rheumatoid bursitis, shoulder

M06.211 Rheumatoid bursitis, right shoulder

M06.212 Rheumatoid bursitis, left shoulder

M06.219 **Rheumatoid bursitis, unspecified shoulder**

☑6ᵗʰ **M06.22** Rheumatoid bursitis, elbow

M06.221 Rheumatoid bursitis, right elbow

M06.222 Rheumatoid bursitis, left elbow

M06.229 **Rheumatoid bursitis, unspecified elbow**

☑6ᵗʰ **M06.23** Rheumatoid bursitis, wrist

M06.231 Rheumatoid bursitis, right wrist

M06.232 Rheumatoid bursitis, left wrist

M06.239 **Rheumatoid bursitis, unspecified wrist**

☑6ᵗʰ **M06.24** Rheumatoid bursitis, hand

M06.241 Rheumatoid bursitis, right hand

M06.242 Rheumatoid bursitis, left hand

M06.249 **Rheumatoid bursitis, unspecified hand**

☑6ᵗʰ **M06.25** Rheumatoid bursitis, hip

M06.251 Rheumatoid bursitis, right hip

M06.252 Rheumatoid bursitis, left hip

M06.259 **Rheumatoid bursitis, unspecified hip**

☑6ᵗʰ **M06.26** Rheumatoid bursitis, knee

M06.261 Rheumatoid bursitis, right knee

M06.262 Rheumatoid bursitis, left knee

M06.269 **Rheumatoid bursitis, unspecified knee**

☑6ᵗʰ **M06.27** Rheumatoid bursitis, ankle and foot

M06.271 Rheumatoid bursitis, right ankle and foot

M06.272 Rheumatoid bursitis, left ankle and foot

M06.279 **Rheumatoid bursitis, unspecified ankle and foot**

M06.28 Rheumatoid bursitis, vertebrae

M06.29 Rheumatoid bursitis, multiple sites

☑5ᵗʰ **M06.3** Rheumatoid nodule

M06.30 **Rheumatoid nodule, unspecified site**

☑6ᵗʰ **M06.31** Rheumatoid nodule, shoulder

M06.311 Rheumatoid nodule, right shoulder

M06.312 Rheumatoid nodule, left shoulder

M06.319 **Rheumatoid nodule, unspecified shoulder**

☑6ᵗʰ **M06.32** Rheumatoid nodule, elbow

M06.321 Rheumatoid nodule, right elbow

M06.322 Rheumatoid nodule, left elbow

M06.329 **Rheumatoid nodule, unspecified elbow**

☑6ᵗʰ **M06.33** Rheumatoid nodule, wrist

M06.331 Rheumatoid nodule, right wrist

M06.332 Rheumatoid nodule, left wrist

M06.339 **Rheumatoid nodule, unspecified wrist**

☑6ᵗʰ **M06.34** Rheumatoid nodule, hand

M06.341 Rheumatoid nodule, right hand

M06.342 Rheumatoid nodule, left hand

M06.349 **Rheumatoid nodule, unspecified hand**

☑6ᵗʰ **M06.35** Rheumatoid nodule, hip

M06.351 Rheumatoid nodule, right hip

M06.352 Rheumatoid nodule, left hip

M06.359 **Rheumatoid nodule, unspecified hip**

☑6ᵗʰ **M06.36** Rheumatoid nodule, knee

M06.361 Rheumatoid nodule, right knee

M06.362 Rheumatoid nodule, left knee

M06.369 **Rheumatoid nodule, unspecified knee**

☑6ᵗʰ **M06.37** Rheumatoid nodule, ankle and foot

M06.371 Rheumatoid nodule, right ankle and foot

M06.372 Rheumatoid nodule, left ankle and foot

M06.379 **Rheumatoid nodule, unspecified ankle and foot**

M06.38 Rheumatoid nodule, vertebrae

M06.39 Rheumatoid nodule, multiple sites

M06.4 Inflammatory polyarthropathy

EXCLUDES 1　*polyarthritis NOS (M13.0)*

☑5ᵗʰ **M06.8** Other specified rheumatoid arthritis

M06.80 **Other specified rheumatoid arthritis, unspecified site**

☑6ᵗʰ **M06.81** Other specified rheumatoid arthritis, shoulder

M06.811 **Other specified rheumatoid arthritis, right shoulder**

M06.812 **Other specified rheumatoid arthritis, left shoulder**

M06.819 **Other specified rheumatoid arthritis, unspecified shoulder**

☑6ᵗʰ **M06.82** Other specified rheumatoid arthritis, elbow

M06.821 **Other specified rheumatoid arthritis, right elbow**

☑ Additional Character Required　　　✓ₓ7ᵗʰ Xtension Alert　　Unspecified Dx　　Other Specified Dx　　Manifestation　　►◄ Revised Text　　● New Code　　▲ Revised Code Title

ICD-10-CM Draft (2015)　　　　　　　　　　　　　　　　　　　　　　　　　　　　　　　　　　　　**653**

M06.822   Other specified rheumatoid arthritis, left elbow

M06.829   Other specified rheumatoid arthritis, unspecified elbow

✓6th M06.83   Other specified rheumatoid arthritis, wrist

M06.831   Other specified rheumatoid arthritis, right wrist

M06.832   Other specified rheumatoid arthritis, left wrist

M06.839   Other specified rheumatoid arthritis, unspecified wrist

✓6th M06.84   Other specified rheumatoid arthritis, hand

M06.841   Other specified rheumatoid arthritis, right hand

M06.842   Other specified rheumatoid arthritis, left hand

M06.849   Other specified rheumatoid arthritis, unspecified hand

✓6th M06.85   Other specified rheumatoid arthritis, hip

M06.851   Other specified rheumatoid arthritis, right hip

M06.852   Other specified rheumatoid arthritis, left hip

M06.859   Other specified rheumatoid arthritis, unspecified hip

✓6th M06.86   Other specified rheumatoid arthritis, knee

M06.861   Other specified rheumatoid arthritis, right knee

M06.862   Other specified rheumatoid arthritis, left knee

M06.869   Other specified rheumatoid arthritis, unspecified knee

✓6th M06.87   Other specified rheumatoid arthritis, ankle and foot

M06.871   Other specified rheumatoid arthritis, right ankle and foot

M06.872   Other specified rheumatoid arthritis, left ankle and foot

M06.879   Other specified rheumatoid arthritis, unspecified ankle and foot

M06.88   Other specified rheumatoid arthritis, vertebrae

M06.89   Other specified rheumatoid arthritis, multiple sites

M06.9   Rheumatoid arthritis, unspecified

✓4th **M07 Enteropathic arthropathies**

Code also associated enteropathy, such as:
regional enteritis [Crohn's disease] (K50.-)
ulcerative colitis (K51.-)

EXCLUDES 1   psoriatic arthropathies (L40.5-)

✓5th M07.6   Enteropathic arthropathies

M07.60   Enteropathic arthropathies, unspecified site

✓6th M07.61   Enteropathic arthropathies, shoulder

M07.611   Enteropathic arthropathies, right shoulder

M07.612   Enteropathic arthropathies, left shoulder

M07.619   Enteropathic arthropathies, unspecified shoulder

✓6th M07.62   Enteropathic arthropathies, elbow

M07.621   Enteropathic arthropathies, right elbow

M07.622   Enteropathic arthropathies, left elbow

M07.629   Enteropathic arthropathies, unspecified elbow

✓6th M07.63   Enteropathic arthropathies, wrist

M07.631   Enteropathic arthropathies, right wrist

M07.632   Enteropathic arthropathies, left wrist

M07.639   Enteropathic arthropathies, unspecified wrist

✓6th M07.64   Enteropathic arthropathies, hand

M07.641   Enteropathic arthropathies, right hand

M07.642   Enteropathic arthropathies, left hand

M07.649   Enteropathic arthropathies, unspecified hand

✓6th M07.65   Enteropathic arthropathies, hip

M07.651   Enteropathic arthropathies, right hip

M07.652   Enteropathic arthropathies, left hip

M07.659   Enteropathic arthropathies, unspecified hip

✓6th M07.66   Enteropathic arthropathies, knee

M07.661   Enteropathic arthropathies, right knee

M07.662   Enteropathic arthropathies, left knee

M07.669   Enteropathic arthropathies, unspecified knee

✓6th M07.67   Enteropathic arthropathies, ankle and foot

M07.671   Enteropathic arthropathies, right ankle and foot

M07.672   Enteropathic arthropathies, left ankle and foot

M07.679   Enteropathic arthropathies, unspecified ankle and foot

M07.68   Enteropathic arthropathies, vertebrae

M07.69   Enteropathic arthropathies, multiple sites

✓4th **M08 Juvenile arthritis**

Code also any associated underlying condition, such as:
regional enteritis [Crohn's disease] (K50.-)
ulcerative colitis (K51.-)

EXCLUDES 1   arthropathy in Whipple's disease (M14.8)
Felty's syndrome (M05.0)
juvenile dermatomyositis (M33.0-)
psoriatic juvenile arthropathy (L40.54)

✓5th M08.0   Unspecified juvenile rheumatoid arthritis

Juvenile rheumatoid arthritis with or without rheumatoid factor

M08.00   Unspecified juvenile rheumatoid arthritis of unspecified site

✓6th M08.01   Unspecified juvenile rheumatoid arthritis, shoulder

M08.011   Unspecified juvenile rheumatoid arthritis, right shoulder

M08.012   Unspecified juvenile rheumatoid arthritis, left shoulder

M08.019   Unspecified juvenile rheumatoid arthritis, unspecified shoulder

✓6th M08.02   Unspecified juvenile rheumatoid arthritis of elbow

M08.021   Unspecified juvenile rheumatoid arthritis, right elbow

M08.022   Unspecified juvenile rheumatoid arthritis, left elbow

M08.029   Unspecified juvenile rheumatoid arthritis, unspecified elbow

✓6th M08.03   Unspecified juvenile rheumatoid arthritis, wrist

M08.031   Unspecified juvenile rheumatoid arthritis, right wrist

M08.032   Unspecified juvenile rheumatoid arthritis, left wrist

M08.039   Unspecified juvenile rheumatoid arthritis, unspecified wrist

✓6th M08.04   Unspecified juvenile rheumatoid arthritis, hand

M08.041   Unspecified juvenile rheumatoid arthritis, right hand

M08.042   Unspecified juvenile rheumatoid arthritis, left hand

M08.049   Unspecified juvenile rheumatoid arthritis, unspecified hand

✓6th M08.05   Unspecified juvenile rheumatoid arthritis, hip

M08.051   Unspecified juvenile rheumatoid arthritis, right hip

M08.052   Unspecified juvenile rheumatoid arthritis, left hip

M08.059   Unspecified juvenile rheumatoid arthritis, unspecified hip

✓6th M08.06   Unspecified juvenile rheumatoid arthritis, knee

M08.061   Unspecified juvenile rheumatoid arthritis, right knee

M08.062   Unspecified juvenile rheumatoid arthritis, left knee

M08.069   Unspecified juvenile rheumatoid arthritis, unspecified knee

✓6th M08.07   Unspecified juvenile rheumatoid arthritis, ankle and foot

M08.071   Unspecified juvenile rheumatoid arthritis, right ankle and foot

M08.072   Unspecified juvenile rheumatoid arthritis, left ankle and foot

M08.079   Unspecified juvenile rheumatoid arthritis, unspecified ankle and foot

M08.08   Unspecified juvenile rheumatoid arthritis, vertebrae

EXCLUDES 1 Not coded here   EXCLUDES 2 Not included here   N Newborn Age: 0   P Pediatric Age: 0-17   M Maternity Age: 12-55   A Adult Age: 15-124

654   ICD-10-CM Draft (2015)

M08.09 **Unspecified juvenile rheumatoid arthritis,** multiple sites

M08.1 **Juvenile ankylosing spondylitis**
> EXCLUDES 1 *ankylosing spondylitis in adults (M45.0-)*

✓5th M08.2 **Juvenile rheumatoid arthritis** with systemic onset
Still's disease NOS
> EXCLUDES 1 *adult-onset Still's disease (M06.1-)*

M08.20 **Juvenile rheumatoid arthritis with systemic onset, unspecified site**

✓6th M08.21 **Juvenile rheumatoid arthritis with systemic onset,** shoulder
M08.211 Juvenile rheumatoid arthritis with systemic onset, right shoulder
M08.212 Juvenile rheumatoid arthritis with systemic onset, left shoulder
M08.219 **Juvenile rheumatoid arthritis with systemic onset, unspecified shoulder**

✓6th M08.22 **Juvenile rheumatoid arthritis with systemic onset,** elbow
M08.221 Juvenile rheumatoid arthritis with systemic onset, right elbow
M08.222 Juvenile rheumatoid arthritis with systemic onset, left elbow
M08.229 **Juvenile rheumatoid arthritis with systemic onset, unspecified elbow**

✓6th M08.23 **Juvenile rheumatoid arthritis with systemic onset,** wrist
M08.231 Juvenile rheumatoid arthritis with systemic onset, right wrist
M08.232 Juvenile rheumatoid arthritis with systemic onset, left wrist
M08.239 **Juvenile rheumatoid arthritis with systemic onset, unspecified wrist**

✓6th M08.24 **Juvenile rheumatoid arthritis with systemic onset,** hand
M08.241 Juvenile rheumatoid arthritis with systemic onset, right hand
M08.242 Juvenile rheumatoid arthritis with systemic onset, left hand
M08.249 **Juvenile rheumatoid arthritis with systemic onset, unspecified hand**

✓6th M08.25 **Juvenile rheumatoid arthritis with systemic onset,** hip
M08.251 Juvenile rheumatoid arthritis with systemic onset, right hip
M08.252 Juvenile rheumatoid arthritis with systemic onset, left hip
M08.259 **Juvenile rheumatoid arthritis with systemic onset, unspecified hip**

✓6th M08.26 **Juvenile rheumatoid arthritis with systemic onset,** knee
M08.261 Juvenile rheumatoid arthritis with systemic onset, right knee
M08.262 Juvenile rheumatoid arthritis with systemic onset, left knee
M08.269 **Juvenile rheumatoid arthritis with systemic onset, unspecified knee**

✓6th M08.27 **Juvenile rheumatoid arthritis with systemic onset,** ankle and foot
M08.271 Juvenile rheumatoid arthritis with systemic onset, right ankle and foot
M08.272 Juvenile rheumatoid arthritis with systemic onset, left ankle and foot
M08.279 **Juvenile rheumatoid arthritis with systemic onset, unspecified ankle and foot**

M08.28 **Juvenile rheumatoid arthritis with systemic onset,** vertebrae

M08.29 **Juvenile rheumatoid arthritis with systemic onset,** multiple sites

M08.3 **Juvenile rheumatoid** polyarthritis (seronegative)

✓5th M08.4 Pauciarticular **juvenile rheumatoid arthritis**

M08.40 **Pauciarticular juvenile rheumatoid arthritis, unspecified site**

✓6th M08.41 **Pauciarticular juvenile rheumatoid arthritis,** shoulder
M08.411 Pauciarticular juvenile rheumatoid arthritis, right shoulder

M08.412 Pauciarticular juvenile rheumatoid arthritis, left shoulder
M08.419 **Pauciarticular juvenile rheumatoid arthritis, unspecified shoulder**

✓6th M08.42 Pauciarticular juvenile rheumatoid arthritis, elbow
M08.421 Pauciarticular juvenile rheumatoid arthritis, right elbow
M08.422 Pauciarticular juvenile rheumatoid arthritis, left elbow
M08.429 **Pauciarticular juvenile rheumatoid arthritis, unspecified elbow**

✓6th M08.43 Pauciarticular juvenile rheumatoid arthritis, wrist
M08.431 Pauciarticular juvenile rheumatoid arthritis, right wrist
M08.432 Pauciarticular juvenile rheumatoid arthritis, left wrist
M08.439 **Pauciarticular juvenile rheumatoid arthritis, unspecified wrist**

✓6th M08.44 Pauciarticular juvenile rheumatoid arthritis, hand
M08.441 Pauciarticular juvenile rheumatoid arthritis, right hand
M08.442 Pauciarticular juvenile rheumatoid arthritis, left hand
M08.449 **Pauciarticular juvenile rheumatoid arthritis, unspecified hand**

✓6th M08.45 Pauciarticular juvenile rheumatoid arthritis, hip
M08.451 Pauciarticular juvenile rheumatoid arthritis, right hip
M08.452 Pauciarticular juvenile rheumatoid arthritis, left hip
M08.459 **Pauciarticular juvenile rheumatoid arthritis, unspecified hip**

✓6th M08.46 Pauciarticular juvenile rheumatoid arthritis, knee
M08.461 Pauciarticular juvenile rheumatoid arthritis, right knee
M08.462 Pauciarticular juvenile rheumatoid arthritis, left knee
M08.469 **Pauciarticular juvenile rheumatoid arthritis, unspecified knee**

✓6th M08.47 Pauciarticular juvenile rheumatoid arthritis, ankle and foot
M08.471 Pauciarticular juvenile rheumatoid arthritis, right ankle and foot
M08.472 Pauciarticular juvenile rheumatoid arthritis, left ankle and foot
M08.479 **Pauciarticular juvenile rheumatoid arthritis, unspecified ankle and foot**

M08.48 Pauciarticular juvenile rheumatoid arthritis, vertebrae

✓5th M08.8 Other juvenile arthritis
M08.80 **Other juvenile arthritis, unspecified site**

✓6th M08.81 Other juvenile arthritis, shoulder
M08.811 **Other juvenile arthritis, right shoulder**
M08.812 **Other juvenile arthritis, left shoulder**
M08.819 **Other juvenile arthritis, unspecified shoulder**

✓6th M08.82 Other juvenile arthritis, elbow
M08.821 **Other juvenile arthritis, right elbow**
M08.822 **Other juvenile arthritis, left elbow**
M08.829 **Other juvenile arthritis, unspecified elbow**

✓6th M08.83 Other juvenile arthritis, wrist
M08.831 **Other juvenile arthritis, right wrist**
M08.832 **Other juvenile arthritis, left wrist**
M08.839 **Other juvenile arthritis, unspecified wrist**

✓6th M08.84 Other juvenile arthritis, hand
M08.841 **Other juvenile arthritis, right hand**
M08.842 **Other juvenile arthritis, left hand**
M08.849 **Other juvenile arthritis, unspecified hand**

✓6th M08.85 Other juvenile arthritis, hip
M08.851 **Other juvenile arthritis, right hip**
M08.852 **Other juvenile arthritis, left hip**
M08.859 **Other juvenile arthritis, unspecified hip**

✓6th M08.86 Other juvenile arthritis, knee
M08.861 **Other juvenile arthritis, right knee**
M08.862 **Other juvenile arthritis, left knee**

☑ Additional Character Required   ✓x7th Xtension Alert   Unspecified Dx   Other Specified Dx   Manifestation   ►◄ Revised Text   ● New Code   ▲ Revised Code Title

M08.869 Other juvenile arthritis, unspecified knee

✓6ᵗʰ M08.87 Other juvenile arthritis, ankle and foot

M08.871 Other juvenile arthritis, right ankle and foot

M08.872 Other juvenile arthritis, left ankle and foot

M08.879 Other juvenile arthritis, unspecified ankle and foot

M08.88 Other juvenile arthritis, other specified site
Other juvenile arthritis, vertebrae

M08.89 Other juvenile arthritis, multiple sites

✓5ᵗʰ M08.9 Juvenile arthritis, unspecified
EXCLUDES 1   juvenile rheumatoid arthritis, unspecified (M08.0-)

M08.90 Juvenile arthritis, unspecified, unspecified site

✓6ᵗʰ M08.91 Juvenile arthritis, unspecified, shoulder

M08.911 Juvenile arthritis, unspecified, right shoulder

M08.912 Juvenile arthritis, unspecified, left shoulder

M08.919 Juvenile arthritis, unspecified, unspecified shoulder

✓6ᵗʰ M08.92 Juvenile arthritis, unspecified, elbow

M08.921 Juvenile arthritis, unspecified, right elbow

M08.922 Juvenile arthritis, unspecified, left elbow

M08.929 Juvenile arthritis, unspecified, unspecified elbow

✓6ᵗʰ M08.93 Juvenile arthritis, unspecified, wrist

M08.931 Juvenile arthritis, unspecified, right wrist

M08.932 Juvenile arthritis, unspecified, left wrist

M08.939 Juvenile arthritis, unspecified, unspecified wrist

✓6ᵗʰ M08.94 Juvenile arthritis, unspecified, hand

M08.941 Juvenile arthritis, unspecified, right hand

M08.942 Juvenile arthritis, unspecified, left hand

M08.949 Juvenile arthritis, unspecified, unspecified hand

✓6ᵗʰ M08.95 Juvenile arthritis, unspecified, hip

M08.951 Juvenile arthritis, unspecified, right hip

M08.952 Juvenile arthritis, unspecified, left hip

M08.959 Juvenile arthritis, unspecified, unspecified hip

✓6ᵗʰ M08.96 Juvenile arthritis, unspecified, knee

M08.961 Juvenile arthritis, unspecified, right knee

M08.962 Juvenile arthritis, unspecified, left knee

M08.969 Juvenile arthritis, unspecified, unspecified knee

✓6ᵗʰ M08.97 Juvenile arthritis, unspecified, ankle and foot

M08.971 Juvenile arthritis, unspecified, right ankle and foot

M08.972 Juvenile arthritis, unspecified, left ankle and foot

M08.979 Juvenile arthritis, unspecified, unspecified ankle and foot

M08.98 Juvenile arthritis, unspecified, vertebrae

M08.99 Juvenile arthritis, unspecified, multiple sites

✓4ᵗʰ **M1A Chronic gout**
Use additional code to identify:
autonomic neuropathy in diseases classified elsewhere (G99.0)
calculus of urinary tract in diseases classified elsewhere (N22)
cardiomyopathy in diseases classified elsewhere (I43)
disorders of external ear in diseases classified elsewhere (H61.1-, H62.8-)
disorders of iris and ciliary body in diseases classified elsewhere (H22)
glomerular disorders in diseases classified elsewhere (N08)
EXCLUDES 1   acute gout (M10.-)
gout NOS (M10.-)

The appropriate 7th character is to be added to each code from category M1A.
0   without tophus (tophi)
1   with tophus (tophi)

✓5ᵗʰ M1A.0 Idiopathic chronic gout
Chronic gouty bursitis   Primary chronic gout

✓x7ᵗʰ M1A.00 Idiopathic chronic gout, unspecified site

✓6ᵗʰ M1A.01 Idiopathic chronic gout, shoulder

✓7ᵗʰ M1A.011 Idiopathic chronic gout, right shoulder

✓7ᵗʰ M1A.012 Idiopathic chronic gout, left shoulder

✓7ᵗʰ M1A.019 Idiopathic chronic gout, unspecified shoulder

✓6ᵗʰ M1A.02 Idiopathic chronic gout, elbow

✓7ᵗʰ M1A.021 Idiopathic chronic gout, right elbow

✓7ᵗʰ M1A.022 Idiopathic chronic gout, left elbow

✓7ᵗʰ M1A.029 Idiopathic chronic gout, unspecified elbow

✓6ᵗʰ M1A.03 Idiopathic chronic gout, wrist

✓7ᵗʰ M1A.031 Idiopathic chronic gout, right wrist

✓7ᵗʰ M1A.032 Idiopathic chronic gout, left wrist

✓7ᵗʰ M1A.039 Idiopathic chronic gout, unspecified wrist

✓6ᵗʰ M1A.04 Idiopathic chronic gout, hand

✓7ᵗʰ M1A.041 Idiopathic chronic gout, right hand

✓7ᵗʰ M1A.042 Idiopathic chronic gout, left hand

✓7ᵗʰ M1A.049 Idiopathic chronic gout, unspecified hand

✓6ᵗʰ M1A.05 Idiopathic chronic gout, hip

✓7ᵗʰ M1A.051 Idiopathic chronic gout, right hip

✓7ᵗʰ M1A.052 Idiopathic chronic gout, left hip

✓7ᵗʰ M1A.059 Idiopathic chronic gout, unspecified hip

✓6ᵗʰ M1A.06 Idiopathic chronic gout, knee

✓7ᵗʰ M1A.061 Idiopathic chronic gout, right knee

✓7ᵗʰ M1A.062 Idiopathic chronic gout, left knee

✓7ᵗʰ M1A.069 Idiopathic chronic gout, unspecified knee

✓6ᵗʰ M1A.07 Idiopathic chronic gout, ankle and foot

✓7ᵗʰ M1A.071 Idiopathic chronic gout, right ankle and foot

✓7ᵗʰ M1A.072 Idiopathic chronic gout, left ankle and foot

✓7ᵗʰ M1A.079 Idiopathic chronic gout, unspecified ankle and foot

✓x7ᵗʰ M1A.08 Idiopathic chronic gout, vertebrae

✓x7ᵗʰ M1A.09 Idiopathic chronic gout, multiple sites

✓5ᵗʰ M1A.1 Lead-induced chronic gout
Code first toxic effects of lead and its compounds (T56.0-)

✓x7ᵗʰ M1A.10 Lead-induced chronic gout, unspecified site

✓6ᵗʰ M1A.11 Lead-induced chronic gout, shoulder

✓7ᵗʰ M1A.111 Lead-induced chronic gout, right shoulder

✓7ᵗʰ M1A.112 Lead-induced chronic gout, left shoulder

✓7ᵗʰ M1A.119 Lead-induced chronic gout, unspecified shoulder

✓6ᵗʰ M1A.12 Lead-induced chronic gout, elbow

✓7ᵗʰ M1A.121 Lead-induced chronic gout, right elbow

✓7ᵗʰ M1A.122 Lead-induced chronic gout, left elbow

✓7ᵗʰ M1A.129 Lead-induced chronic gout, unspecified elbow

✓6ᵗʰ M1A.13 Lead-induced chronic gout, wrist

✓7ᵗʰ M1A.131 Lead-induced chronic gout, right wrist

✓7ᵗʰ M1A.132 Lead-induced chronic gout, left wrist

✓7ᵗʰ M1A.139 Lead-induced chronic gout, unspecified wrist

✓6ᵗʰ M1A.14 Lead-induced chronic gout, hand

✓7ᵗʰ M1A.141 Lead-induced chronic gout, right hand

✓7ᵗʰ M1A.142 Lead-induced chronic gout, left hand

✓7ᵗʰ M1A.149 Lead-induced chronic gout, unspecified hand

✓6ᵗʰ M1A.15 Lead-induced chronic gout, hip

✓7ᵗʰ M1A.151 Lead-induced chronic gout, right hip

✓7ᵗʰ M1A.152 Lead-induced chronic gout, left hip

✓7ᵗʰ M1A.159 Lead-induced chronic gout, unspecified hip

✓6ᵗʰ M1A.16 Lead-induced chronic gout, knee

✓7ᵗʰ M1A.161 Lead-induced chronic gout, right knee

✓7ᵗʰ M1A.162 Lead-induced chronic gout, left knee

✓7ᵗʰ M1A.169 Lead-induced chronic gout, unspecified knee

✓6ᵗʰ M1A.17 Lead-induced chronic gout, ankle and foot

✓7ᵗʰ M1A.171 Lead-induced chronic gout, right ankle and foot

EXCLUDES 1 Not coded here   EXCLUDES 2 Not included here   N Newborn Age: 0   P Pediatric Age: 0-17   M Maternity Age: 12-55   A Adult Age: 15-124

656   ICD-10-CM Draft (2015)

☑7ᵗʰ **M1A.172** Lead-induced chronic gout, left ankle and foot

☑7ᵗʰ **M1A.179** Lead-induced chronic gout, unspecified ankle and foot

☑x7ᵗʰ **M1A.18** Lead-induced chronic gout, vertebrae

☑x7ᵗʰ **M1A.19** Lead-induced chronic gout, multiple sites

☑5ᵗʰ **M1A.2** Drug-induced chronic gout

Use additional code for adverse effect, if applicable, to identify drug (T36-T50 with fifth or sixth character 5)

☑x7ᵗʰ **M1A.20** Drug-induced chronic gout, unspecified site

☑6ᵗʰ **M1A.21** Drug-induced chronic gout, shoulder

  ☑7ᵗʰ **M1A.211** Drug-induced chronic gout, right shoulder

  ☑7ᵗʰ **M1A.212** Drug-induced chronic gout, left shoulder

  ☑7ᵗʰ **M1A.219** Drug-induced chronic gout, unspecified shoulder

☑6ᵗʰ **M1A.22** Drug-induced chronic gout, elbow

  ☑7ᵗʰ **M1A.221** Drug-induced chronic gout, right elbow

  ☑7ᵗʰ **M1A.222** Drug-induced chronic gout, left elbow

  ☑7ᵗʰ **M1A.229** Drug-induced chronic gout, unspecified elbow

☑6ᵗʰ **M1A.23** Drug-induced chronic gout, wrist

  ☑7ᵗʰ **M1A.231** Drug-induced chronic gout, right wrist

  ☑7ᵗʰ **M1A.232** Drug-induced chronic gout, left wrist

  ☑7ᵗʰ **M1A.239** Drug-induced chronic gout, unspecified wrist

☑6ᵗʰ **M1A.24** Drug-induced chronic gout, hand

  ☑7ᵗʰ **M1A.241** Drug-induced chronic gout, right hand

  ☑7ᵗʰ **M1A.242** Drug-induced chronic gout, left hand

  ☑7ᵗʰ **M1A.249** Drug-induced chronic gout, unspecified hand

☑6ᵗʰ **M1A.25** Drug-induced chronic gout, hip

  ☑7ᵗʰ **M1A.251** Drug-induced chronic gout, right hip

  ☑7ᵗʰ **M1A.252** Drug-induced chronic gout, left hip

  ☑7ᵗʰ **M1A.259** Drug-induced chronic gout, unspecified hip

☑6ᵗʰ **M1A.26** Drug-induced chronic gout, knee

  ☑7ᵗʰ **M1A.261** Drug-induced chronic gout, right knee

  ☑7ᵗʰ **M1A.262** Drug-induced chronic gout, left knee

  ☑7ᵗʰ **M1A.269** Drug-induced chronic gout, unspecified knee

☑6ᵗʰ **M1A.27** Drug-induced chronic gout, ankle and foot

  ☑7ᵗʰ **M1A.271** Drug-induced chronic gout, right ankle and foot

  ☑7ᵗʰ **M1A.272** Drug-induced chronic gout, left ankle and foot

  ☑7ᵗʰ **M1A.279** Drug-induced chronic gout, unspecified ankle and foot

☑x7ᵗʰ **M1A.28** Drug-induced chronic gout, vertebrae

☑x7ᵗʰ **M1A.29** Drug-induced chronic gout, multiple sites

☑5ᵗʰ **M1A.3** Chronic gout due to renal impairment

Code first associated renal disease

☑x7ᵗʰ **M1A.30** Chronic gout due to renal impairment, unspecified site

☑6ᵗʰ **M1A.31** Chronic gout due to renal impairment, shoulder

  ☑7ᵗʰ **M1A.311** Chronic gout due to renal impairment, right shoulder

  ☑7ᵗʰ **M1A.312** Chronic gout due to renal impairment, left shoulder

  ☑7ᵗʰ **M1A.319** Chronic gout due to renal impairment, unspecified shoulder

☑6ᵗʰ **M1A.32** Chronic gout due to renal impairment, elbow

  ☑7ᵗʰ **M1A.321** Chronic gout due to renal impairment, right elbow

  ☑7ᵗʰ **M1A.322** Chronic gout due to renal impairment, left elbow

  ☑7ᵗʰ **M1A.329** Chronic gout due to renal impairment, unspecified elbow

☑6ᵗʰ **M1A.33** Chronic gout due to renal impairment, wrist

  ☑7ᵗʰ **M1A.331** Chronic gout due to renal impairment, right wrist

  ☑7ᵗʰ **M1A.332** Chronic gout due to renal impairment, left wrist

  ☑7ᵗʰ **M1A.339** Chronic gout due to renal impairment, unspecified wrist

☑6ᵗʰ **M1A.34** Chronic gout due to renal impairment, hand

  ☑7ᵗʰ **M1A.341** Chronic gout due to renal impairment, right hand

  ☑7ᵗʰ **M1A.342** Chronic gout due to renal impairment, left hand

  ☑7ᵗʰ **M1A.349** Chronic gout due to renal impairment, unspecified hand

☑6ᵗʰ **M1A.35** Chronic gout due to renal impairment, hip

  ☑7ᵗʰ **M1A.351** Chronic gout due to renal impairment, right hip

  ☑7ᵗʰ **M1A.352** Chronic gout due to renal impairment, left hip

  ☑7ᵗʰ **M1A.359** Chronic gout due to renal impairment, unspecified hip

☑6ᵗʰ **M1A.36** Chronic gout due to renal impairment, knee

  ☑7ᵗʰ **M1A.361** Chronic gout due to renal impairment, right knee

  ☑7ᵗʰ **M1A.362** Chronic gout due to renal impairment, left knee

  ☑7ᵗʰ **M1A.369** Chronic gout due to renal impairment, unspecified knee

☑6ᵗʰ **M1A.37** Chronic gout due to renal impairment, ankle and foot

  ☑7ᵗʰ **M1A.371** Chronic gout due to renal impairment, right ankle and foot

  ☑7ᵗʰ **M1A.372** Chronic gout due to renal impairment, left ankle and foot

  ☑7ᵗʰ **M1A.379** Chronic gout due to renal impairment, unspecified ankle and foot

☑x7ᵗʰ **M1A.38** Chronic gout due to renal impairment, vertebrae

☑x7ᵗʰ **M1A.39** Chronic gout due to renal impairment, multiple sites

☑5ᵗʰ **M1A.4** Other secondary chronic gout

Code first associated condition

☑x7ᵗʰ **M1A.40** Other secondary chronic gout, unspecified site

☑6ᵗʰ **M1A.41** Other secondary chronic gout, shoulder

  ☑7ᵗʰ **M1A.411** Other secondary chronic gout, right shoulder

  ☑7ᵗʰ **M1A.412** Other secondary chronic gout, left shoulder

  ☑7ᵗʰ **M1A.419** Other secondary chronic gout, unspecified shoulder

☑6ᵗʰ **M1A.42** Other secondary chronic gout, elbow

  ☑7ᵗʰ **M1A.421** Other secondary chronic gout, right elbow

  ☑7ᵗʰ **M1A.422** Other secondary chronic gout, left elbow

  ☑7ᵗʰ **M1A.429** Other secondary chronic gout, unspecified elbow

☑6ᵗʰ **M1A.43** Other secondary chronic gout, wrist

  ☑7ᵗʰ **M1A.431** Other secondary chronic gout, right wrist

  ☑7ᵗʰ **M1A.432** Other secondary chronic gout, left wrist

  ☑7ᵗʰ **M1A.439** Other secondary chronic gout, unspecified wrist

☑6ᵗʰ **M1A.44** Other secondary chronic gout, hand

  ☑7ᵗʰ **M1A.441** Other secondary chronic gout, right hand

  ☑7ᵗʰ **M1A.442** Other secondary chronic gout, left hand

  ☑7ᵗʰ **M1A.449** Other secondary chronic gout, unspecified hand

☑6ᵗʰ **M1A.45** Other secondary chronic gout, hip

  ☑7ᵗʰ **M1A.451** Other secondary chronic gout, right hip

  ☑7ᵗʰ **M1A.452** Other secondary chronic gout, left hip

  ☑7ᵗʰ **M1A.459** Other secondary chronic gout, unspecified hip

☑6ᵗʰ **M1A.46** Other secondary chronic gout, knee

  ☑7ᵗʰ **M1A.461** Other secondary chronic gout, right knee

  ☑7ᵗʰ **M1A.462** Other secondary chronic gout, left knee

  ☑7ᵗʰ **M1A.469** Other secondary chronic gout, unspecified knee

---

☑ Additional Character Required   ☑x7ᵗʰ Xtension Alert   Unspecified Dx   Other Specified Dx   Manifestation   ▶◀ Revised Text   ● New Code   ▲ Revised Code Title

✓6ᵗʰ **M1A.47** Other secondary chronic gout, ankle and foot

     ✓7ᵗʰ **M1A.471** Other secondary chronic gout, right ankle and foot

     ✓7ᵗʰ **M1A.472** Other secondary chronic gout, left ankle and foot

     ✓7ᵗʰ **M1A.479** Other secondary chronic gout, unspecified ankle and foot

✓x7ᵗʰ **M1A.48** Other secondary chronic gout, vertebrae

✓x7ᵗʰ **M1A.49** Other secondary chronic gout, multiple sites

✓x7ᵗʰ **M1A.9** Chronic gout, unspecified

✓4ᵗʰ **M10 Gout**

     Acute gout   Gout NOS
     Gout attack   Podagra
     Gout flare

     Use additional code to identify:
     autonomic neuropathy in diseases classified elsewhere (G99.0)
     calculus of urinary tract in diseases classified elsewhere (N22)
     cardiomyopathy in diseases classified elsewhere (I43)
     disorders of external ear in diseases classified elsewhere (H61.1-, H62.8-)
     disorders of iris and ciliary body in diseases classified elsewhere (H22)
     glomerular disorders in diseases classified elsewhere (N08)

     EXCLUDES 1   chronic gout (M1A.-)

✓5ᵗʰ **M10.0** Idiopathic gout
     Gouty bursitis
     Primary gout

     M10.00 Idiopathic gout, unspecified site

     ✓6ᵗʰ **M10.01** Idiopathic gout, shoulder
         M10.011 Idiopathic gout, right shoulder
         M10.012 Idiopathic gout, left shoulder
         M10.019 Idiopathic gout, unspecified shoulder

     ✓6ᵗʰ **M10.02** Idiopathic gout, elbow
         M10.021 Idiopathic gout, right elbow
         M10.022 Idiopathic gout, left elbow
         M10.029 Idiopathic gout, unspecified elbow

     ✓6ᵗʰ **M10.03** Idiopathic gout, wrist
         M10.031 Idiopathic gout, right wrist
         M10.032 Idiopathic gout, left wrist
         M10.039 Idiopathic gout, unspecified wrist

     ✓6ᵗʰ **M10.04** Idiopathic gout, hand
         M10.041 Idiopathic gout, right hand
         M10.042 Idiopathic gout, left hand
         M10.049 Idiopathic gout, unspecified hand

     ✓6ᵗʰ **M10.05** Idiopathic gout, hip
         M10.051 Idiopathic gout, right hip
         M10.052 Idiopathic gout, left hip
         M10.059 Idiopathic gout, unspecified hip

     ✓6ᵗʰ **M10.06** Idiopathic gout, knee
         M10.061 Idiopathic gout, right knee
         M10.062 Idiopathic gout, left knee
         M10.069 Idiopathic gout, unspecified knee

     ✓6ᵗʰ **M10.07** Idiopathic gout, ankle and foot
         M10.071 Idiopathic gout, right ankle and foot
         M10.072 Idiopathic gout, left ankle and foot
         M10.079 Idiopathic gout, unspecified ankle and foot

     M10.08 Idiopathic gout, vertebrae
     M10.09 Idiopathic gout, multiple sites

✓5ᵗʰ **M10.1** Lead-induced gout
     Code first toxic effects of lead and its compounds (T56.0-)

     M10.10 Lead-induced gout, unspecified site

     ✓6ᵗʰ **M10.11** Lead-induced gout, shoulder
         M10.111 Lead-induced gout, right shoulder
         M10.112 Lead-induced gout, left shoulder
         M10.119 Lead-induced gout, unspecified shoulder

     ✓6ᵗʰ **M10.12** Lead-induced gout, elbow
         M10.121 Lead-induced gout, right elbow
         M10.122 Lead-induced gout, left elbow
         M10.129 Lead-induced gout, unspecified elbow

     ✓6ᵗʰ **M10.13** Lead-induced gout, wrist
         M10.131 Lead-induced gout, right wrist
         M10.132 Lead-induced gout, left wrist
         M10.139 Lead-induced gout, unspecified wrist

✓6ᵗʰ **M10.14** Lead-induced gout, hand
     M10.141 Lead-induced gout, right hand
     M10.142 Lead-induced gout, left hand
     M10.149 Lead-induced gout, unspecified hand

✓6ᵗʰ **M10.15** Lead-induced gout, hip
     M10.151 Lead-induced gout, right hip
     M10.152 Lead-induced gout, left hip
     M10.159 Lead-induced gout, unspecified hip

✓6ᵗʰ **M10.16** Lead-induced gout, knee
     M10.161 Lead-induced gout, right knee
     M10.162 Lead-induced gout, left knee
     M10.169 Lead-induced gout, unspecified knee

✓6ᵗʰ **M10.17** Lead-induced gout, ankle and foot
     M10.171 Lead-induced gout, right ankle and foot
     M10.172 Lead-induced gout, left ankle and foot
     M10.179 Lead-induced gout, unspecified ankle and foot

✓6ᵗʰ **M10.18** Lead-induced gout, vertebrae

✓6ᵗʰ **M10.19** Lead-induced gout, multiple sites

✓5ᵗʰ **M10.2** Drug-induced gout
     Use additional code for adverse effect, if applicable, to identify drug (T36-T50 with fifth or sixth character 5)

     M10.20 Drug-induced gout, unspecified site

     ✓6ᵗʰ **M10.21** Drug-induced gout, shoulder
         M10.211 Drug-induced gout, right shoulder
         M10.212 Drug-induced gout, left shoulder
         M10.219 Drug-induced gout, unspecified shoulder

     ✓6ᵗʰ **M10.22** Drug-induced gout, elbow
         M10.221 Drug-induced gout, right elbow
         M10.222 Drug-induced gout, left elbow
         M10.229 Drug-induced gout, unspecified elbow

     ✓6ᵗʰ **M10.23** Drug-induced gout, wrist
         M10.231 Drug-induced gout, right wrist
         M10.232 Drug-induced gout, left wrist
         M10.239 Drug-induced gout, unspecified wrist

     ✓6ᵗʰ **M10.24** Drug-induced gout, hand
         M10.241 Drug-induced gout, right hand
         M10.242 Drug-induced gout, left hand
         M10.249 Drug-induced gout, unspecified hand

     ✓6ᵗʰ **M10.25** Drug-induced gout, hip
         M10.251 Drug-induced gout, right hip
         M10.252 Drug-induced gout, left hip
         M10.259 Drug-induced gout, unspecified hip

     ✓6ᵗʰ **M10.26** Drug-induced gout, knee
         M10.261 Drug-induced gout, right knee
         M10.262 Drug-induced gout, left knee
         M10.269 Drug-induced gout, unspecified knee

     ✓6ᵗʰ **M10.27** Drug-induced gout, ankle and foot
         M10.271 Drug-induced gout, right ankle and foot
         M10.272 Drug-induced gout, left ankle and foot
         M10.279 Drug-induced gout, unspecified ankle and foot

     M10.28 Drug-induced gout, vertebrae
     M10.29 Drug-induced gout, multiple sites

✓5ᵗʰ **M10.3** Gout due to renal impairment
     Code first associated renal disease

     M10.30 Gout due to renal impairment, unspecified site

     ✓6ᵗʰ **M10.31** Gout due to renal impairment, shoulder
         M10.311 Gout due to renal impairment, right shoulder
         M10.312 Gout due to renal impairment, left shoulder
         M10.319 Gout due to renal impairment, unspecified shoulder

     ✓6ᵗʰ **M10.32** Gout due to renal impairment, elbow
         M10.321 Gout due to renal impairment, right elbow
         M10.322 Gout due to renal impairment, left elbow
         M10.329 Gout due to renal impairment, unspecified elbow

     ✓6ᵗʰ **M10.33** Gout due to renal impairment, wrist
         M10.331 Gout due to renal impairment, right wrist
         M10.332 Gout due to renal impairment, left wrist

EXCLUDES 1 Not coded here   EXCLUDES 2 Not included here   N Newborn Age: 0   P Pediatric Age: 0-17   M Maternity Age: 12-55   A Adult Age: 15-124

658   ICD-10-CM Draft (2015)

M10.339 **Gout due to renal impairment, unspecified wrist**

√6ᵗʰ M10.34 Gout due to renal impairment, hand
 M10.341 Gout due to renal impairment, right hand
 M10.342 Gout due to renal impairment, left hand
 M10.349 **Gout due to renal impairment, unspecified hand**

√6ᵗʰ M10.35 Gout due to renal impairment, hip
 M10.351 Gout due to renal impairment, right hip
 M10.352 Gout due to renal impairment, left hip
 M10.359 **Gout due to renal impairment, unspecified hip**

√6ᵗʰ M10.36 Gout due to renal impairment, knee
 M10.361 Gout due to renal impairment, right knee
 M10.362 Gout due to renal impairment, left knee
 M10.369 **Gout due to renal impairment, unspecified knee**

√6ᵗʰ M10.37 Gout due to renal impairment, ankle and foot
 M10.371 Gout due to renal impairment, right ankle and foot
 M10.372 Gout due to renal impairment, left ankle and foot
 M10.379 **Gout due to renal impairment, unspecified ankle and foot**

M10.38 Gout due to renal impairment, vertebrae
M10.39 Gout due to renal impairment, multiple sites

√5ᵗʰ M10.4 Other secondary gout
 Code first associated condition
 M10.40 **Other secondary gout, unspecified site**

√6ᵗʰ M10.41 Other secondary gout, shoulder
 M10.411 **Other secondary gout, right shoulder**
 M10.412 **Other secondary gout, left shoulder**
 M10.419 **Other secondary gout, unspecified shoulder**

√6ᵗʰ M10.42 Other secondary gout, elbow
 M10.421 **Other secondary gout, right elbow**
 M10.422 **Other secondary gout, left elbow**
 M10.429 **Other secondary gout, unspecified elbow**

√6ᵗʰ M10.43 Other secondary gout, wrist
 M10.431 **Other secondary gout, right wrist**
 M10.432 **Other secondary gout, left wrist**
 M10.439 **Other secondary gout, unspecified wrist**

√6ᵗʰ M10.44 Other secondary gout, hand
 M10.441 **Other secondary gout, right hand**
 M10.442 **Other secondary gout, left hand**
 M10.449 **Other secondary gout, unspecified hand**

√6ᵗʰ M10.45 Other secondary gout, hip
 M10.451 **Other secondary gout, right hip**
 M10.452 **Other secondary gout, left hip**
 M10.459 **Other secondary gout, unspecified hip**

√6ᵗʰ M10.46 Other secondary gout, knee
 M10.461 **Other secondary gout, right knee**
 M10.462 **Other secondary gout, left knee**
 M10.469 **Other secondary gout, unspecified knee**

√6ᵗʰ M10.47 Other secondary gout, ankle and foot
 M10.471 **Other secondary gout, right ankle and foot**
 M10.472 **Other secondary gout, left ankle and foot**
 M10.479 **Other secondary gout, unspecified ankle and foot**

M10.48 **Other secondary gout, vertebrae**
M10.49 **Other secondary gout, multiple sites**

M10.9 **Gout, unspecified**
 Gout NOS

√4ᵗʰ **M11 Other crystal arthropathies**

√5ᵗʰ M11.0 Hydroxyapatite deposition disease
 M11.00 **Hydroxyapatite deposition disease, unspecified site**

√6ᵗʰ M11.01 Hydroxyapatite deposition disease, shoulder
 M11.011 **Hydroxyapatite deposition disease, right shoulder**
 M11.012 **Hydroxyapatite deposition disease, left shoulder**

 M11.019 **Hydroxyapatite deposition disease, unspecified shoulder**

√6ᵗʰ M11.02 Hydroxyapatite deposition disease, elbow
 M11.021 **Hydroxyapatite deposition disease, right elbow**
 M11.022 **Hydroxyapatite deposition disease, left elbow**
 M11.029 **Hydroxyapatite deposition disease, unspecified elbow**

√6ᵗʰ M11.03 Hydroxyapatite deposition disease, wrist
 M11.031 **Hydroxyapatite deposition disease, right wrist**
 M11.032 **Hydroxyapatite deposition disease, left wrist**
 M11.039 **Hydroxyapatite deposition disease, unspecified wrist**

√6ᵗʰ M11.04 Hydroxyapatite deposition disease, hand
 M11.041 **Hydroxyapatite deposition disease, right hand**
 M11.042 **Hydroxyapatite deposition disease, left hand**
 M11.049 **Hydroxyapatite deposition disease, unspecified hand**

√6ᵗʰ M11.05 Hydroxyapatite deposition disease, hip
 M11.051 **Hydroxyapatite deposition disease, right hip**
 M11.052 **Hydroxyapatite deposition disease, left hip**
 M11.059 **Hydroxyapatite deposition disease, unspecified hip**

√6ᵗʰ M11.06 Hydroxyapatite deposition disease, knee
 M11.061 **Hydroxyapatite deposition disease, right knee**
 M11.062 **Hydroxyapatite deposition disease, left knee**
 M11.069 **Hydroxyapatite deposition disease, unspecified knee**

√6ᵗʰ M11.07 Hydroxyapatite deposition disease, ankle and foot
 M11.071 **Hydroxyapatite deposition disease, right ankle and foot**
 M11.072 **Hydroxyapatite deposition disease, left ankle and foot**
 M11.079 **Hydroxyapatite deposition disease, unspecified ankle and foot**

M11.08 Hydroxyapatite deposition disease, vertebrae
M11.09 Hydroxyapatite deposition disease, multiple sites

√5ᵗʰ M11.1 Familial chondrocalcinosis
 M11.10 **Familial chondrocalcinosis, unspecified site**

√6ᵗʰ M11.11 Familial chondrocalcinosis, shoulder
 M11.111 Familial chondrocalcinosis, right shoulder
 M11.112 Familial chondrocalcinosis, left shoulder
 M11.119 **Familial chondrocalcinosis, unspecified shoulder**

√6ᵗʰ M11.12 Familial chondrocalcinosis, elbow
 M11.121 Familial chondrocalcinosis, right elbow
 M11.122 Familial chondrocalcinosis, left elbow
 M11.129 **Familial chondrocalcinosis, unspecified elbow**

√6ᵗʰ M11.13 Familial chondrocalcinosis, wrist
 M11.131 Familial chondrocalcinosis, right wrist
 M11.132 Familial chondrocalcinosis, left wrist
 M11.139 **Familial chondrocalcinosis, unspecified wrist**

√6ᵗʰ M11.14 Familial chondrocalcinosis, hand
 M11.141 Familial chondrocalcinosis, right hand
 M11.142 Familial chondrocalcinosis, left hand
 M11.149 **Familial chondrocalcinosis, unspecified hand**

√6ᵗʰ M11.15 Familial chondrocalcinosis, hip
 M11.151 Familial chondrocalcinosis, right hip
 M11.152 Familial chondrocalcinosis, left hip
 M11.159 **Familial chondrocalcinosis, unspecified hip**

√6ᵗʰ M11.16 Familial chondrocalcinosis, knee
 M11.161 Familial chondrocalcinosis, right knee

✔ Additional Character Required   √x7ᵗʰ Xtension Alert   Unspecified Dx   Other Specified Dx   Manifestation   ►◄ Revised Text   ● New Code   ▲ Revised Code Title

ICD-10-CM Draft (2015)

659

M11.162 **Familial chondrocalcinosis,** left **knee**

M11.169 **Familial chondrocalcinosis, unspecified knee**

✓6ᵗʰ M11.17 **Familial chondrocalcinosis,** ankle and foot

M11.171 **Familial chondrocalcinosis,** right **ankle and foot**

M11.172 **Familial chondrocalcinosis,** left **ankle and foot**

M11.179 **Familial chondrocalcinosis, unspecified ankle and foot**

M11.18 **Familial chondrocalcinosis,** vertebrae

M11.19 **Familial chondrocalcinosis,** multiple sites

✓5ᵗʰ M11.2 **Other chondrocalcinosis**

Chondrocalcinosis NOS

M11.20 **Other chondrocalcinosis, unspecified site**

✓6ᵗʰ M11.21 **Other chondrocalcinosis,** shoulder

M11.211 **Other chondrocalcinosis,** right **shoulder**
M11.212 **Other chondrocalcinosis,** left **shoulder**
M11.219 **Other chondrocalcinosis, unspecified shoulder**

✓6ᵗʰ M11.22 **Other chondrocalcinosis,** elbow

M11.221 **Other chondrocalcinosis,** right **elbow**
M11.222 **Other chondrocalcinosis,** left **elbow**
M11.229 **Other chondrocalcinosis, unspecified elbow**

✓6ᵗʰ M11.23 **Other chondrocalcinosis,** wrist

M11.231 **Other chondrocalcinosis,** right **wrist**
M11.232 **Other chondrocalcinosis,** left **wrist**
M11.239 **Other chondrocalcinosis, unspecified wrist**

✓6ᵗʰ M11.24 **Other chondrocalcinosis,** hand

M11.241 **Other chondrocalcinosis,** right **hand**
M11.242 **Other chondrocalcinosis,** left **hand**
M11.249 **Other chondrocalcinosis, unspecified hand**

✓6ᵗʰ M11.25 **Other chondrocalcinosis,** hip

M11.251 **Other chondrocalcinosis,** right **hip**
M11.252 **Other chondrocalcinosis,** left **hip**
M11.259 **Other chondrocalcinosis, unspecified hip**

✓6ᵗʰ M11.26 **Other chondrocalcinosis,** knee

M11.261 **Other chondrocalcinosis,** right **knee**
M11.262 **Other chondrocalcinosis,** left **knee**
M11.269 **Other chondrocalcinosis, unspecified knee**

✓6ᵗʰ M11.27 **Other chondrocalcinosis,** ankle and foot

M11.271 **Other chondrocalcinosis,** right **ankle and foot**
M11.272 **Other chondrocalcinosis,** left **ankle and foot**
M11.279 **Other chondrocalcinosis, unspecified ankle and foot**

M11.28 **Other chondrocalcinosis,** vertebrae
M11.29 **Other chondrocalcinosis,** multiple sites

✓5ᵗʰ M11.8 **Other specified crystal arthropathies**

M11.80 **Other specified crystal arthropathies, unspecified site**

✓6ᵗʰ M11.81 **Other specified crystal arthropathies,** shoulder

M11.811 **Other specified crystal arthropathies,** right **shoulder**
M11.812 **Other specified crystal arthropathies,** left **shoulder**
M11.819 **Other specified crystal arthropathies, unspecified shoulder**

✓6ᵗʰ M11.82 **Other specified crystal arthropathies,** elbow

M11.821 **Other specified crystal arthropathies,** right **elbow**
M11.822 **Other specified crystal arthropathies,** left **elbow**
M11.829 **Other specified crystal arthropathies, unspecified elbow**

✓6ᵗʰ M11.83 **Other specified crystal arthropathies,** wrist

M11.831 **Other specified crystal arthropathies,** right **wrist**
M11.832 **Other specified crystal arthropathies,** left **wrist**

M11.839 **Other specified crystal arthropathies, unspecified wrist**

✓6ᵗʰ M11.84 **Other specified crystal arthropathies,** hand

M11.841 **Other specified crystal arthropathies,** right **hand**
M11.842 **Other specified crystal arthropathies,** left **hand**
M11.849 **Other specified crystal arthropathies, unspecified hand**

✓6ᵗʰ M11.85 **Other specified crystal arthropathies,** hip

M11.851 **Other specified crystal arthropathies,** right **hip**
M11.852 **Other specified crystal arthropathies,** left **hip**
M11.859 **Other specified crystal arthropathies, unspecified hip**

✓6ᵗʰ M11.86 **Other specified crystal arthropathies,** knee

M11.861 **Other specified crystal arthropathies,** right **knee**
M11.862 **Other specified crystal arthropathies,** left **knee**
M11.869 **Other specified crystal arthropathies, unspecified knee**

✓6ᵗʰ M11.87 **Other specified crystal arthropathies,** ankle and foot

M11.871 **Other specified crystal arthropathies,** right **ankle and foot**
M11.872 **Other specified crystal arthropathies,** left **ankle and foot**
M11.879 **Other specified crystal arthropathies, unspecified ankle and foot**

M11.88 **Other specified crystal arthropathies,** vertebrae
M11.89 **Other specified crystal arthropathies,** multiple sites

M11.9 **Crystal arthropathy, unspecified**

✓4ᵗʰ M12 **Other and unspecified arthropathy**

EXCLUDES 1 arthrosis (M15-M19)
cricoarytenoid arthropathy (J38.7)

✓5ᵗʰ M12.0 **Chronic postrheumatic arthropathy [Jaccoud]**

M12.00 **Chronic postrheumatic arthropathy [Jaccoud], unspecified site**

✓6ᵗʰ M12.01 **Chronic postrheumatic arthropathy [Jaccoud],** shoulder

M12.011 **Chronic postrheumatic arthropathy [Jaccoud],** right **shoulder**
M12.012 **Chronic postrheumatic arthropathy [Jaccoud],** left **shoulder**
M12.019 **Chronic postrheumatic arthropathy [Jaccoud], unspecified shoulder**

✓6ᵗʰ M12.02 **Chronic postrheumatic arthropathy [Jaccoud],** elbow

M12.021 **Chronic postrheumatic arthropathy [Jaccoud],** right **elbow**
M12.022 **Chronic postrheumatic arthropathy [Jaccoud],** left **elbow**
M12.029 **Chronic postrheumatic arthropathy [Jaccoud], unspecified elbow**

✓6ᵗʰ M12.03 **Chronic postrheumatic arthropathy [Jaccoud],** wrist

M12.031 **Chronic postrheumatic arthropathy [Jaccoud],** right **wrist**
M12.032 **Chronic postrheumatic arthropathy [Jaccoud],** left **wrist**
M12.039 **Chronic postrheumatic arthropathy [Jaccoud], unspecified wrist**

✓6ᵗʰ M12.04 **Chronic postrheumatic arthropathy [Jaccoud],** hand

M12.041 **Chronic postrheumatic arthropathy [Jaccoud],** right **hand**
M12.042 **Chronic postrheumatic arthropathy [Jaccoud],** left **hand**
M12.049 **Chronic postrheumatic arthropathy [Jaccoud], unspecified hand**

✓6ᵗʰ M12.05 **Chronic postrheumatic arthropathy [Jaccoud],** hip

M12.051 **Chronic postrheumatic arthropathy [Jaccoud],** right **hip**
M12.052 **Chronic postrheumatic arthropathy [Jaccoud],** left **hip**
M12.059 **Chronic postrheumatic arthropathy [Jaccoud], unspecified hip**

EXCLUDES 1 Not coded here   EXCLUDES 2 Not included here   N Newborn Age: 0   P Pediatric Age: 0-17   M Maternity Age: 12-55   A Adult Age: 15-124

660   ICD-10-CM Draft (2015)

✓6ᵗʰ **M12.06** Chronic postrheumatic arthropathy [Jaccoud], knee

    M12.061 Chronic postrheumatic arthropathy [Jaccoud], right knee

    M12.062 Chronic postrheumatic arthropathy [Jaccoud], left knee

    M12.069 Chronic postrheumatic arthropathy [Jaccoud], unspecified knee

✓6ᵗʰ **M12.07** Chronic postrheumatic arthropathy [Jaccoud], ankle and foot

    M12.071 Chronic postrheumatic arthropathy [Jaccoud], right ankle and foot

    M12.072 Chronic postrheumatic arthropathy [Jaccoud], left ankle and foot

    M12.079 Chronic postrheumatic arthropathy [Jaccoud], unspecified ankle and foot

   M12.08 Chronic postrheumatic arthropathy [Jaccoud], other specified site

      Chronic postrheumatic arthropathy [Jaccoud], vertebrae

   M12.09 Chronic postrheumatic arthropathy [Jaccoud], multiple sites

✓5ᵗʰ **M12.1** Kaschin-Beck disease

      Osteochondroarthrosis deformans endemica

   M12.10 Kaschin-Beck disease, unspecified site

✓6ᵗʰ **M12.11** Kaschin-Beck disease, shoulder

    M12.111 Kaschin-Beck disease, right shoulder

    M12.112 Kaschin-Beck disease, left shoulder

    M12.119 Kaschin-Beck disease, unspecified shoulder

✓6ᵗʰ **M12.12** Kaschin-Beck disease, elbow

    M12.121 Kaschin-Beck disease, right elbow

    M12.122 Kaschin-Beck disease, left elbow

    M12.129 Kaschin-Beck disease, unspecified elbow

✓6ᵗʰ **M12.13** Kaschin-Beck disease, wrist

    M12.131 Kaschin-Beck disease, right wrist

    M12.132 Kaschin-Beck disease, left wrist

    M12.139 Kaschin-Beck disease, unspecified wrist

✓6ᵗʰ **M12.14** Kaschin-Beck disease, hand

    M12.141 Kaschin-Beck disease, right hand

    M12.142 Kaschin-Beck disease, left hand

    M12.149 Kaschin-Beck disease, unspecified hand

✓6ᵗʰ **M12.15** Kaschin-Beck disease, hip

    M12.151 Kaschin-Beck disease, right hip

    M12.152 Kaschin-Beck disease, left hip

    M12.159 Kaschin-Beck disease, unspecified hip

✓6ᵗʰ **M12.16** Kaschin-Beck disease, knee

    M12.161 Kaschin-Beck disease, right knee

    M12.162 Kaschin-Beck disease, left knee

    M12.169 Kaschin-Beck disease, unspecified knee

✓6ᵗʰ **M12.17** Kaschin-Beck disease, ankle and foot

    M12.171 Kaschin-Beck disease, right ankle and foot

    M12.172 Kaschin-Beck disease, left ankle and foot

    M12.179 Kaschin-Beck disease, unspecified ankle and foot

   M12.18 Kaschin-Beck disease, vertebrae

   M12.19 Kaschin-Beck disease, multiple sites

✓5ᵗʰ **M12.2** Villonodular synovitis (pigmented)

   M12.20 Villonodular synovitis (pigmented), unspecified site

✓6ᵗʰ **M12.21** Villonodular synovitis (pigmented), shoulder

    M12.211 Villonodular synovitis (pigmented), right shoulder

    M12.212 Villonodular synovitis (pigmented), left shoulder

    M12.219 Villonodular synovitis (pigmented), unspecified shoulder

✓6ᵗʰ **M12.22** Villonodular synovitis (pigmented), elbow

    M12.221 Villonodular synovitis (pigmented), right elbow

    M12.222 Villonodular synovitis (pigmented), left elbow

    M12.229 Villonodular synovitis (pigmented), unspecified elbow

✓6ᵗʰ **M12.23** Villonodular synovitis (pigmented), wrist

    M12.231 Villonodular synovitis (pigmented), right wrist

    M12.232 Villonodular synovitis (pigmented), left wrist

    M12.239 Villonodular synovitis (pigmented), unspecified wrist

✓6ᵗʰ **M12.24** Villonodular synovitis (pigmented), hand

    M12.241 Villonodular synovitis (pigmented), right hand

    M12.242 Villonodular synovitis (pigmented), left hand

    M12.249 Villonodular synovitis (pigmented), unspecified hand

✓6ᵗʰ **M12.25** Villonodular synovitis (pigmented), hip

    M12.251 Villonodular synovitis (pigmented), right hip

    M12.252 Villonodular synovitis (pigmented), left hip

    M12.259 Villonodular synovitis (pigmented), unspecified hip

✓6ᵗʰ **M12.26** Villonodular synovitis (pigmented), knee

    M12.261 Villonodular synovitis (pigmented), right knee

    M12.262 Villonodular synovitis (pigmented), left knee

    M12.269 Villonodular synovitis (pigmented), unspecified knee

✓6ᵗʰ **M12.27** Villonodular synovitis (pigmented), ankle and foot

    M12.271 Villonodular synovitis (pigmented), right ankle and foot

    M12.272 Villonodular synovitis (pigmented), left ankle and foot

    M12.279 Villonodular synovitis (pigmented), unspecified ankle and foot

   M12.28 Villonodular synovitis (pigmented), other specified site

      Villonodular synovitis (pigmented), vertebrae

   M12.29 Villonodular synovitis (pigmented), multiple sites

✓5ᵗʰ **M12.3** Palindromic rheumatism

   M12.30 Palindromic rheumatism, unspecified site

✓6ᵗʰ **M12.31** Palindromic rheumatism, shoulder

    M12.311 Palindromic rheumatism, right shoulder

    M12.312 Palindromic rheumatism, left shoulder

    M12.319 Palindromic rheumatism, unspecified shoulder

✓6ᵗʰ **M12.32** Palindromic rheumatism, elbow

    M12.321 Palindromic rheumatism, right elbow

    M12.322 Palindromic rheumatism, left elbow

    M12.329 Palindromic rheumatism, unspecified elbow

✓6ᵗʰ **M12.33** Palindromic rheumatism, wrist

    M12.331 Palindromic rheumatism, right wrist

    M12.332 Palindromic rheumatism, left wrist

    M12.339 Palindromic rheumatism, unspecified wrist

✓6ᵗʰ **M12.34** Palindromic rheumatism, hand

    M12.341 Palindromic rheumatism, right hand

    M12.342 Palindromic rheumatism, left hand

    M12.349 Palindromic rheumatism, unspecified hand

✓6ᵗʰ **M12.35** Palindromic rheumatism, hip

    M12.351 Palindromic rheumatism, right hip

    M12.352 Palindromic rheumatism, left hip

    M12.359 Palindromic rheumatism, unspecified hip

✓6ᵗʰ **M12.36** Palindromic rheumatism, knee

    M12.361 Palindromic rheumatism, right knee

    M12.362 Palindromic rheumatism, left knee

    M12.369 Palindromic rheumatism, unspecified knee

✓6ᵗʰ **M12.37** Palindromic rheumatism, ankle and foot

    M12.371 Palindromic rheumatism, right ankle and foot

    M12.372 Palindromic rheumatism, left ankle and foot

☑ Additional Character Required   ✓ₓ7ᵗʰ Xtension Alert   Unspecified Dx   Other Specified Dx   Manifestation   ▶◀ Revised Text   ● New Code   ▲ Revised Code Title

ICD-10-CM Draft (2015)

661

M12.379 **Palindromic rheumatism, unspecified ankle and foot**

M12.38 **Palindromic rheumatism, other specified site**
Palindromic rheumatism, vertebrae

M12.39 **Palindromic rheumatism, multiple sites**

✓5th M12.4 **Intermittent hydrarthrosis**

M12.40 **Intermittent hydrarthrosis, unspecified site**

✓6th M12.41 **Intermittent hydrarthrosis, shoulder**
M12.411 **Intermittent hydrarthrosis, right shoulder**
M12.412 **Intermittent hydrarthrosis, left shoulder**
M12.419 **Intermittent hydrarthrosis, unspecified shoulder**

✓6th M12.42 **Intermittent hydrarthrosis, elbow**
M12.421 **Intermittent hydrarthrosis, right elbow**
M12.422 **Intermittent hydrarthrosis, left elbow**
M12.429 **Intermittent hydrarthrosis, unspecified elbow**

✓6th M12.43 **Intermittent hydrarthrosis, wrist**
M12.431 **Intermittent hydrarthrosis, right wrist**
M12.432 **Intermittent hydrarthrosis, left wrist**
M12.439 **Intermittent hydrarthrosis, unspecified wrist**

✓6th M12.44 **Intermittent hydrarthrosis, hand**
M12.441 **Intermittent hydrarthrosis, right hand**
M12.442 **Intermittent hydrarthrosis, left hand**
M12.449 **Intermittent hydrarthrosis, unspecified hand**

✓6th M12.45 **Intermittent hydrarthrosis, hip**
M12.451 **Intermittent hydrarthrosis, right hip**
M12.452 **Intermittent hydrarthrosis, left hip**
M12.459 **Intermittent hydrarthrosis, unspecified hip**

✓6th M12.46 **Intermittent hydrarthrosis, knee**
M12.461 **Intermittent hydrarthrosis, right knee**
M12.462 **Intermittent hydrarthrosis, left knee**
M12.469 **Intermittent hydrarthrosis, unspecified knee**

✓6th M12.47 **Intermittent hydrarthrosis, ankle and foot**
M12.471 **Intermittent hydrarthrosis, right ankle and foot**
M12.472 **Intermittent hydrarthrosis, left ankle and foot**
M12.479 **Intermittent hydrarthrosis, unspecified ankle and foot**

M12.48 **Intermittent hydrarthrosis, other site**

M12.49 **Intermittent hydrarthrosis, multiple sites**

✓5th M12.5 **Traumatic arthropathy**
EXCLUDES 1 *current injury-see Alphabetic Index*
post-traumatic osteoarthritis NOS (M19.1-)
post-traumatic osteoarthritis of first carpometacarpal joint (M18.2-M18.3)
post-traumatic osteoarthritis of hip (M16.4-M16.5)
post-traumatic osteoarthritis of knee (M17.2-M17.3)
post-traumatic osteoarthritis of other single joints (M19.1-)

M12.50 **Traumatic arthropathy, unspecified site**

✓6th M12.51 **Traumatic arthropathy, shoulder**
M12.511 **Traumatic arthropathy, right shoulder**
M12.512 **Traumatic arthropathy, left shoulder**
M12.519 **Traumatic arthropathy, unspecified shoulder**

✓6th M12.52 **Traumatic arthropathy, elbow**
M12.521 **Traumatic arthropathy, right elbow**
M12.522 **Traumatic arthropathy, left elbow**
M12.529 **Traumatic arthropathy, unspecified elbow**

✓6th M12.53 **Traumatic arthropathy, wrist**
M12.531 **Traumatic arthropathy, right wrist**
M12.532 **Traumatic arthropathy, left wrist**
M12.539 **Traumatic arthropathy, unspecified wrist**

✓6th M12.54 **Traumatic arthropathy, hand**
M12.541 **Traumatic arthropathy, right hand**
M12.542 **Traumatic arthropathy, left hand**
M12.549 **Traumatic arthropathy, unspecified hand**

✓6th M12.55 **Traumatic arthropathy, hip**

M12.551 **Traumatic arthropathy, right hip**
M12.552 **Traumatic arthropathy, left hip**
M12.559 **Traumatic arthropathy, unspecified hip**

✓6th M12.56 **Traumatic arthropathy, knee**
M12.561 **Traumatic arthropathy, right knee**
M12.562 **Traumatic arthropathy, left knee**
M12.569 **Traumatic arthropathy, unspecified knee**

✓6th M12.57 **Traumatic arthropathy, ankle and foot**
M12.571 **Traumatic arthropathy, right ankle and foot**
M12.572 **Traumatic arthropathy, left ankle and foot**
M12.579 **Traumatic arthropathy, unspecified ankle and foot**

M12.58 **Traumatic arthropathy, other specified site**
Traumatic arthropathy, vertebrae

M12.59 **Traumatic arthropathy, multiple sites**

✓5th M12.8 **Other specific arthropathies, not elsewhere classified**
Transient arthropathy

M12.80 **Other specific arthropathies, not elsewhere classified, unspecified site**

✓6th M12.81 **Other specific arthropathies, not elsewhere classified, shoulder**
M12.811 **Other specific arthropathies, not elsewhere classified, right shoulder**
M12.812 **Other specific arthropathies, not elsewhere classified, left shoulder**
M12.819 **Other specific arthropathies, not elsewhere classified, unspecified shoulder**

✓6th M12.82 **Other specific arthropathies, not elsewhere classified, elbow**
M12.821 **Other specific arthropathies, not elsewhere classified, right elbow**
M12.822 **Other specific arthropathies, not elsewhere classified, left elbow**
M12.829 **Other specific arthropathies, not elsewhere classified, unspecified elbow**

✓6th M12.83 **Other specific arthropathies, not elsewhere classified, wrist**
M12.831 **Other specific arthropathies, not elsewhere classified, right wrist**
M12.832 **Other specific arthropathies, not elsewhere classified, left wrist**
M12.839 **Other specific arthropathies, not elsewhere classified, unspecified wrist**

✓6th M12.84 **Other specific arthropathies, not elsewhere classified, hand**
M12.841 **Other specific arthropathies, not elsewhere classified, right hand**
M12.842 **Other specific arthropathies, not elsewhere classified, left hand**
M12.849 **Other specific arthropathies, not elsewhere classified, unspecified hand**

✓6th M12.85 **Other specific arthropathies, not elsewhere classified, hip**
M12.851 **Other specific arthropathies, not elsewhere classified, right hip**
M12.852 **Other specific arthropathies, not elsewhere classified, left hip**
M12.859 **Other specific arthropathies, not elsewhere classified, unspecified hip**

✓6th M12.86 **Other specific arthropathies, not elsewhere classified, knee**
M12.861 **Other specific arthropathies, not elsewhere classified, right knee**
M12.862 **Other specific arthropathies, not elsewhere classified, left knee**
M12.869 **Other specific arthropathies, not elsewhere classified, unspecified knee**

✓6th M12.87 **Other specific arthropathies, not elsewhere classified, ankle and foot**
M12.871 **Other specific arthropathies, not elsewhere classified, right ankle and foot**
M12.872 **Other specific arthropathies, not elsewhere classified, left ankle and foot**
M12.879 **Other specific arthropathies, not elsewhere classified, unspecified ankle and foot**

EXCLUDES 1 Not coded here   EXCLUDES 2 Not included here   N Newborn Age: 0   P Pediatric Age: 0-17   M Maternity Age: 12-55   A Adult Age: 15-124

662   ICD-10-CM Draft (2015)

M12.88　Other specific arthropathies, not elsewhere classified, other specified site
　　　Other specific arthropathies, not elsewhere classified, vertebrae

M12.89　Other specific arthropathies, not elsewhere classified, multiple sites

M12.9　Arthropathy, unspecified

✓4th **M13** **Other arthritis**
　　EXCLUDES 1　arthrosis (M15-M19)
　　　　　　osteoarthritis (M15-M19)

M13.0　Polyarthritis, unspecified

✓5th M13.1　Monoarthritis, not elsewhere classified

　　M13.10　Monoarthritis, not elsewhere classified, unspecified site

✓6th M13.11　Monoarthritis, not elsewhere classified, shoulder
　　M13.111　Monoarthritis, not elsewhere classified, right shoulder
　　M13.112　Monoarthritis, not elsewhere classified, left shoulder
　　M13.119　Monoarthritis, not elsewhere classified, unspecified shoulder

✓6th M13.12　Monoarthritis, not elsewhere classified, elbow
　　M13.121　Monoarthritis, not elsewhere classified, right elbow
　　M13.122　Monoarthritis, not elsewhere classified, left elbow
　　M13.129　Monoarthritis, not elsewhere classified, unspecified elbow

✓6th M13.13　Monoarthritis, not elsewhere classified, wrist
　　M13.131　Monoarthritis, not elsewhere classified, right wrist
　　M13.132　Monoarthritis, not elsewhere classified, left wrist
　　M13.139　Monoarthritis, not elsewhere classified, unspecified wrist

✓6th M13.14　Monoarthritis, not elsewhere classified, hand
　　M13.141　Monoarthritis, not elsewhere classified, right hand
　　M13.142　Monoarthritis, not elsewhere classified, left hand
　　M13.149　Monoarthritis, not elsewhere classified, unspecified hand

✓6th M13.15　Monoarthritis, not elsewhere classified, hip
　　M13.151　Monoarthritis, not elsewhere classified, right hip
　　M13.152　Monoarthritis, not elsewhere classified, left hip
　　M13.159　Monoarthritis, not elsewhere classified, unspecified hip

✓6th M13.16　Monoarthritis, not elsewhere classified, knee
　　M13.161　Monoarthritis, not elsewhere classified, right knee
　　M13.162　Monoarthritis, not elsewhere classified, left knee
　　M13.169　Monoarthritis, not elsewhere classified, unspecified knee

✓6th M13.17　Monoarthritis, not elsewhere classified, ankle and foot
　　M13.171　Monoarthritis, not elsewhere classified, right ankle and foot
　　M13.172　Monoarthritis, not elsewhere classified, left ankle and foot
　　M13.179　Monoarthritis, not elsewhere classified, unspecified ankle and foot

✓5th M13.8　Other specified arthritis
　　　Allergic arthritis
　　EXCLUDES 1　osteoarthritis (M15-M19)

　　M13.80　Other specified arthritis, unspecified site

✓6th M13.81　Other specified arthritis, shoulder
　　M13.811　Other specified arthritis, right shoulder
　　M13.812　Other specified arthritis, left shoulder
　　M13.819　Other specified arthritis, unspecified shoulder

✓6th M13.82　Other specified arthritis, elbow
　　M13.821　Other specified arthritis, right elbow
　　M13.822　Other specified arthritis, left elbow

M13.829　Other specified arthritis, unspecified elbow

✓6th M13.83　Other specified arthritis, wrist
　　M13.831　Other specified arthritis, right wrist
　　M13.832　Other specified arthritis, left wrist
　　M13.839　Other specified arthritis, unspecified wrist

✓6th M13.84　Other specified arthritis, hand
　　M13.841　Other specified arthritis, right hand
　　M13.842　Other specified arthritis, left hand
　　M13.849　Other specified arthritis, unspecified hand

✓6th M13.85　Other specified arthritis, hip
　　M13.851　Other specified arthritis, right hip
　　M13.852　Other specified arthritis, left hip
　　M13.859　Other specified arthritis, unspecified hip

✓6th M13.86　Other specified arthritis, knee
　　M13.861　Other specified arthritis, right knee
　　M13.862　Other specified arthritis, left knee
　　M13.869　Other specified arthritis, unspecified knee

✓6th M13.87　Other specified arthritis, ankle and foot
　　M13.871　Other specified arthritis, right ankle and foot
　　M13.872　Other specified arthritis, left ankle and foot
　　M13.879　Other specified arthritis, unspecified ankle and foot

M13.88　Other specified arthritis, other site

M13.89　Other specified arthritis, multiple sites

✓4th **M14** **Arthropathies in other diseases classified elsewhere**
　　EXCLUDES 1　arthropathy in:
　　　　diabetes mellitus (E08-E13 with .61-)
　　　　hematological disorders (M36.2-M36.3)
　　　　hypersensitivity reactions (M36.4)
　　　　neoplastic disease (M36.1)
　　　　neurosyphillis (A52.16)
　　　　sarcoidosis (D86.86)
　　　　enteropathic arthropathies (M07.-)
　　　　juvenile psoriatic arthropathy (L40.54)
　　　　lipoid dermatoarthritis (E78.81)

✓5th M14.6　Charcôt's joint
　　　Neuropathic arthropathy
　　EXCLUDES 1　Charcôt's joint in diabetes mellitus (E08-E13 with .610)
　　　　　Charcôt's joint in tabes dorsalis (A52.16)

　　M14.60　Charcôt's joint, unspecified site

✓6th M14.61　Charcôt's joint, shoulder
　　M14.611　Charcôt's joint, right shoulder
　　M14.612　Charcôt's joint, left shoulder
　　M14.619　Charcôt's joint, unspecified shoulder

✓6th M14.62　Charcôt's joint, elbow
　　M14.621　Charcôt's joint, right elbow
　　M14.622　Charcôt's joint, left elbow
　　M14.629　Charcôt's joint, unspecified elbow

✓6th M14.63　Charcôt's joint, wrist
　　M14.631　Charcôt's joint, right wrist
　　M14.632　Charcôt's joint, left wrist
　　M14.639　Charcôt's joint, unspecified wrist

✓6th M14.64　Charcôt's joint, hand
　　M14.641　Charcôt's joint, right hand
　　M14.642　Charcôt's joint, left hand
　　M14.649　Charcôt's joint, unspecified hand

✓6th M14.65　Charcôt's joint, hip
　　M14.651　Charcôt's joint, right hip
　　M14.652　Charcôt's joint, left hip
　　M14.659　Charcôt's joint, unspecified hip

✓6th M14.66　Charcôt's joint, knee
　　M14.661　Charcôt's joint, right knee
　　M14.662　Charcôt's joint, left knee
　　M14.669　Charcôt's joint, unspecified knee

✓6th M14.67　Charcôt's joint, ankle and foot
　　M14.671　Charcôt's joint, right ankle and foot
　　M14.672　Charcôt's joint, left ankle and foot
　　M14.679　Charcôt's joint, unspecified ankle and foot

M14.68　Charcôt's joint, vertebrae

M14.69　Charcôt's joint, multiple sites

☑ Additional Character Required　　✓x7th Xtension Alert　　Unspecified Dx　　Other Specified Dx　　Manifestation　　►◄ Revised Text　　● New Code　　▲ Revised Code Title

Diseases of the Musculoskeletal System and Connective Tissue

M14.8–M18.12

✓5ᵗʰ **M14.8 Arthropathies in other specified diseases classified elsewhere**

Code first underlying disease, such as:
    amyloidosis (E85.-)
    erythema multiforme (L51.-)
    erythema nodosum (L52)
    hemochromatosis (E83.11-)
    hyperparathyroidism (E21.-)
    hypothyroidism (E00-E03)
    sickle-cell disorders (D57.-)
    thyrotoxicosis [hyperthyroidism] (E05.-)
    Whipple's disease (K90.81)

M14.80 **Arthropathies in other specified diseases classified elsewhere,** *unspecified site*

✓6ᵗʰ *M14.81* **Arthropathies in other specified diseases classified elsewhere,** *shoulder*

    M14.811 **Arthropathies in other specified diseases classified elsewhere,** *right* **shoulder**

    M14.812 **Arthropathies in other specified diseases classified elsewhere,** *left* **shoulder**

    M14.819 **Arthropathies in other specified diseases classified elsewhere,** *unspecified* **shoulder**

✓6ᵗʰ *M14.82* **Arthropathies in other specified diseases classified elsewhere,** *elbow*

    M14.821 **Arthropathies in other specified diseases classified elsewhere,** *right* **elbow**

    M14.822 **Arthropathies in other specified diseases classified elsewhere,** *left* **elbow**

    M14.829 **Arthropathies in other specified diseases classified elsewhere,** *unspecified* **elbow**

✓6ᵗʰ *M14.83* **Arthropathies in other specified diseases classified elsewhere,** *wrist*

    M14.831 **Arthropathies in other specified diseases classified elsewhere,** *right* **wrist**

    M14.832 **Arthropathies in other specified diseases classified elsewhere,** *left* **wrist**

    M14.839 **Arthropathies in other specified diseases classified elsewhere,** *unspecified* **wrist**

✓6ᵗʰ *M14.84* **Arthropathies in other specified diseases classified elsewhere,** *hand*

    M14.841 **Arthropathies in other specified diseases classified elsewhere,** *right* **hand**

    M14.842 **Arthropathies in other specified diseases classified elsewhere,** *left* **hand**

    M14.849 **Arthropathies in other specified diseases classified elsewhere,** *unspecified* **hand**

✓6ᵗʰ *M14.85* **Arthropathies in other specified diseases classified elsewhere,** *hip*

    M14.851 **Arthropathies in other specified diseases classified elsewhere,** *right* **hip**

    M14.852 **Arthropathies in other specified diseases classified elsewhere,** *left* **hip**

    M14.859 **Arthropathies in other specified diseases classified elsewhere,** *unspecified* **hip**

✓6ᵗʰ *M14.86* **Arthropathies in other specified diseases classified elsewhere,** *knee*

    M14.861 **Arthropathies in other specified diseases classified elsewhere,** *right* **knee**

    M14.862 **Arthropathies in other specified diseases classified elsewhere,** *left* **knee**

    M14.869 **Arthropathies in other specified diseases classified elsewhere,** *unspecified* **knee**

✓6ᵗʰ *M14.87* **Arthropathies in other specified diseases classified elsewhere,** *ankle and foot*

    M14.871 **Arthropathies in other specified diseases classified elsewhere,** *right* **ankle and foot**

    M14.872 **Arthropathies in other specified diseases classified elsewhere,** *left* **ankle and foot**

    M14.879 **Arthropathies in other specified diseases classified elsewhere,** *unspecified* **ankle and foot**

M14.88 **Arthropathies in other specified diseases classified elsewhere,** *vertebrae*

M14.89 **Arthropathies in other specified diseases classified elsewhere,** *multiple sites*

Osteoarthritis (M15-M19)

EXCLUDES 2   *osteoarthritis of spine (M47.-)*

✓4ᵗʰ **M15 Polyosteoarthritis**

    INCLUDES   arthritis of multiple sites
    EXCLUDES 1   bilateral involvement of single joint (M16-M19)

    M15.0 Primary generalized (osteo)arthritis

    M15.1 Heberden's nodes (with arthropathy)
        Interphalangeal distal osteoarthritis

    M15.2 Bouchard's nodes (with arthropathy)
        Juxtaphalangeal distal osteoarthritis

    M15.3 Secondary multiple arthritis
        Post-traumatic polyosteoarthritis

    M15.4 Erosive (osteo)arthritis

    M15.8 Other polyosteoarthritis

    M15.9 Polyosteoarthritis, unspecified
        Generalized osteoarthritis NOS

✓4ᵗʰ **M16 Osteoarthritis of hip**

    M16.0 Bilateral primary osteoarthritis of hip

✓5ᵗʰ   **M16.1 Unilateral primary osteoarthritis of hip**
        Primary osteoarthritis of hip NOS

      M16.10 Unilateral primary osteoarthritis, unspecified hip

      M16.11 Unilateral primary osteoarthritis, right hip

      M16.12 Unilateral primary osteoarthritis, left hip

    M16.2 Bilateral osteoarthritis resulting from hip dysplasia

✓5ᵗʰ   **M16.3 Unilateral osteoarthritis resulting from hip dysplasia**
        Dysplastic osteoarthritis of hip NOS

      M16.30 Unilateral osteoarthritis resulting from hip dysplasia, unspecified hip

      M16.31 Unilateral osteoarthritis resulting from hip dysplasia, right hip

      M16.32 Unilateral osteoarthritis resulting from hip dysplasia, left hip

    M16.4 Bilateral post-traumatic osteoarthritis of hip

✓5ᵗʰ   **M16.5 Unilateral post-traumatic osteoarthritis of hip**
        Post-traumatic osteoarthritis of hip NOS

      M16.50 Unilateral post-traumatic osteoarthritis, unspecified hip

      M16.51 Unilateral post-traumatic osteoarthritis, right hip

      M16.52 Unilateral post-traumatic osteoarthritis, left hip

    M16.6 Other bilateral secondary osteoarthritis of hip

    M16.7 Other unilateral secondary osteoarthritis of hip
        Secondary osteoarthritis of hip NOS

    M16.9 Osteoarthritis of hip, unspecified

✓4ᵗʰ **M17 Osteoarthritis of knee**

    M17.0 Bilateral primary osteoarthritis of knee

✓5ᵗʰ   **M17.1 Unilateral primary osteoarthritis of knee**
        Primary osteoarthritis of knee NOS

      M17.10 Unilateral primary osteoarthritis, unspecified knee

      M17.11 Unilateral primary osteoarthritis, right knee

      M17.12 Unilateral primary osteoarthritis, left knee

    M17.2 Bilateral post-traumatic osteoarthritis of knee

✓5ᵗʰ   **M17.3 Unilateral post-traumatic osteoarthritis of knee**
        Post-traumatic osteoarthritis of knee NOS

      M17.30 Unilateral post-traumatic osteoarthritis, unspecified knee

      M17.31 Unilateral post-traumatic osteoarthritis, right knee

      M17.32 Unilateral post-traumatic osteoarthritis, left knee

    M17.4 Other bilateral secondary osteoarthritis of knee

    M17.5 Other unilateral secondary osteoarthritis of knee
        Secondary osteoarthritis of knee NOS

    M17.9 Osteoarthritis of knee, unspecified

✓4ᵗʰ **M18 Osteoarthritis of first carpometacarpal joint**

    M18.0 Bilateral primary osteoarthritis of first carpometacarpal joints

✓5ᵗʰ   **M18.1 Unilateral primary osteoarthritis of first carpometacarpal joint**
        Primary osteoarthritis of first carpometacarpal joint NOS

      M18.10 Unilateral primary osteoarthritis of first carpometacarpal joint, unspecified hand

      M18.11 Unilateral primary osteoarthritis of first carpometacarpal joint, right hand

      M18.12 Unilateral primary osteoarthritis of first carpometacarpal joint, left hand

---

EXCLUDES 1 Not coded here   *EXCLUDES 2* Not included here   N Newborn Age: 0   P Pediatric Age: 0-17   M Maternity Age: 12-55   A Adult Age: 15-124

664   ICD-10-CM Draft (2015)

M18.2 Bilateral post-traumatic osteoarthritis of first carpometacarpal joints

✓5ᵗʰ M18.3 Unilateral post-traumatic osteoarthritis of first carpometacarpal joint
Post-traumatic osteoarthritis of first carpometacarpal joint NOS

M18.30 Unilateral post-traumatic osteoarthritis of first carpometacarpal joint, unspecified hand

M18.31 Unilateral post-traumatic osteoarthritis of first carpometacarpal joint, right hand

M18.32 Unilateral post-traumatic osteoarthritis of first carpometacarpal joint, left hand

M18.4 Other bilateral secondary osteoarthritis of first carpometacarpal joints

✓5ᵗʰ M18.5 Other unilateral secondary osteoarthritis of first carpometacarpal joint
Secondary osteoarthritis of first carpometacarpal joint NOS

M18.50 Other unilateral secondary osteoarthritis of first carpometacarpal joint, unspecified hand

M18.51 Other unilateral secondary osteoarthritis of first carpometacarpal joint, right hand

M18.52 Other unilateral secondary osteoarthritis of first carpometacarpal joint, left hand

M18.9 Osteoarthritis of first carpometacarpal joint, unspecified

✓4ᵗʰ M19 Other and unspecified osteoarthritis
EXCLUDES1 polyarthritis (M15.-)
EXCLUDES2 arthrosis of spine (M47.-)
hallux rigidus (M20.2)
osteoarthritis of spine (M47.-)

✓5ᵗʰ M19.0 Primary osteoarthritis of other joints

✓6ᵗʰ M19.01 Primary osteoarthritis, shoulder
M19.011 Primary osteoarthritis, right shoulder
M19.012 Primary osteoarthritis, left shoulder
M19.019 Primary osteoarthritis, unspecified shoulder

✓6ᵗʰ M19.02 Primary osteoarthritis, elbow
M19.021 Primary osteoarthritis, right elbow
M19.022 Primary osteoarthritis, left elbow
M19.029 Primary osteoarthritis, unspecified elbow

✓6ᵗʰ M19.03 Primary osteoarthritis, wrist
M19.031 Primary osteoarthritis, right wrist
M19.032 Primary osteoarthritis, left wrist
M19.039 Primary osteoarthritis, unspecified wrist

✓6ᵗʰ M19.04 Primary osteoarthritis, hand
EXCLUDES2 primary osteoarthritis of first carpometacarpal joint (M18.0-, M18.1-)
M19.041 Primary osteoarthritis, right hand
M19.042 Primary osteoarthritis, left hand
M19.049 Primary osteoarthritis, unspecified hand

✓6ᵗʰ M19.07 Primary osteoarthritis ankle and foot
M19.071 Primary osteoarthritis, right ankle and foot
M19.072 Primary osteoarthritis, left ankle and foot
M19.079 Primary osteoarthritis, unspecified ankle and foot

✓5ᵗʰ M19.1 Post-traumatic osteoarthritis of other joints

✓6ᵗʰ M19.11 Post-traumatic osteoarthritis, shoulder
M19.111 Post-traumatic osteoarthritis, right shoulder
M19.112 Post-traumatic osteoarthritis, left shoulder
M19.119 Post-traumatic osteoarthritis, unspecified shoulder

✓6ᵗʰ M19.12 Post-traumatic osteoarthritis, elbow
M19.121 Post-traumatic osteoarthritis, right elbow
M19.122 Post-traumatic osteoarthritis, left elbow
M19.129 Post-traumatic osteoarthritis, unspecified elbow

✓6ᵗʰ M19.13 Post-traumatic osteoarthritis, wrist
M19.131 Post-traumatic osteoarthritis, right wrist
M19.132 Post-traumatic osteoarthritis, left wrist
M19.139 Post-traumatic osteoarthritis, unspecified wrist

✓6ᵗʰ M19.14 Post-traumatic osteoarthritis, hand
EXCLUDES2 post-traumatic osteoarthritis of first carpometacarpal joint (M18.2-, M18.3-)
M19.141 Post-traumatic osteoarthritis, right hand
M19.142 Post-traumatic osteoarthritis, left hand
M19.149 Post-traumatic osteoarthritis, unspecified hand

✓6ᵗʰ M19.17 Post-traumatic osteoarthritis, ankle and foot
M19.171 Post-traumatic osteoarthritis, right ankle and foot
M19.172 Post-traumatic osteoarthritis, left ankle and foot
M19.179 Post-traumatic osteoarthritis, unspecified ankle and foot

✓5ᵗʰ M19.2 Secondary osteoarthritis of other joints

✓6ᵗʰ M19.21 Secondary osteoarthritis, shoulder
M19.211 Secondary osteoarthritis, right shoulder
M19.212 Secondary osteoarthritis, left shoulder
M19.219 Secondary osteoarthritis, unspecified shoulder

✓6ᵗʰ M19.22 Secondary osteoarthritis, elbow
M19.221 Secondary osteoarthritis, right elbow
M19.222 Secondary osteoarthritis, left elbow
M19.229 Secondary osteoarthritis, unspecified elbow

✓6ᵗʰ M19.23 Secondary osteoarthritis, wrist
M19.231 Secondary osteoarthritis, right wrist
M19.232 Secondary osteoarthritis, left wrist
M19.239 Secondary osteoarthritis, unspecified wrist

✓6ᵗʰ M19.24 Secondary osteoarthritis, hand
M19.241 Secondary osteoarthritis, right hand
M19.242 Secondary osteoarthritis, left hand
M19.249 Secondary osteoarthritis, unspecified hand

✓6ᵗʰ M19.27 Secondary osteoarthritis, ankle and foot
M19.271 Secondary osteoarthritis, right ankle and foot
M19.272 Secondary osteoarthritis, left ankle and foot
M19.279 Secondary osteoarthritis, unspecified ankle and foot

✓5ᵗʰ M19.9 Osteoarthritis, unspecified site
M19.90 Unspecified osteoarthritis, unspecified site
Arthrosis NOS   Osteoarthritis NOS
Arthritis NOS
M19.91 Primary osteoarthritis, unspecified site
Primary osteoarthritis NOS
M19.92 Post-traumatic osteoarthritis, unspecified site
Post-traumatic osteoarthritis NOS
M19.93 Secondary osteoarthritis, unspecified site
Secondary osteoarthritis NOS

Other joint disorders (M20-M25)
EXCLUDES2 joints of the spine (M40-M54)

✓4ᵗʰ M20 Acquired deformities of fingers and toes
EXCLUDES1 acquired absence of fingers and toes (Z89.-)
congenital absence of fingers and toes (Q71.3-, Q72.3-)
congenital deformities and malformations of fingers and toes (Q66-, Q68-Q70, Q74-)

✓5ᵗʰ M20.0 Deformity of finger(s)
EXCLUDES1 clubbing of fingers (R68.3)
palmar fascial fibromatosis [Dupuytren] (M72.0)
trigger finger (M65.3)

✓6ᵗʰ M20.00 Unspecified deformity of finger(s)
M20.001 Unspecified deformity of right finger(s)
M20.002 Unspecified deformity of left finger(s)
M20.009 Unspecified deformity of unspecified finger(s)

✓6ᵗʰ M20.01 Mallet finger
M20.011 Mallet finger of right finger(s)
M20.012 Mallet finger of left finger(s)
M20.019 Mallet finger of unspecified finger(s)

✓6ᵗʰ M20.02 Boutonnière deformity
M20.021 Boutonnière deformity of right finger(s)

M20.022   Boutonnière deformity of left finger(s)
M20.029   Boutonnière deformity of unspecified finger(s)
✓6th **M20.03**   Swan-neck deformity
M20.031   Swan-neck deformity of right finger(s)
M20.032   Swan-neck deformity of left finger(s)
M20.039   Swan-neck deformity of unspecified finger(s)
✓6th **M20.09**   Other deformity of finger(s)
M20.091   Other deformity of right finger(s)
M20.092   Other deformity of left finger(s)
M20.099   Other deformity of finger(s), unspecified finger(s)

✓5th **M20.1**   Hallux valgus (acquired)
   Bunion
M20.10   Hallux valgus (acquired), unspecified foot
M20.11   Hallux valgus (acquired), right foot
M20.12   Hallux valgus (acquired), left foot

✓5th **M20.2**   Hallux rigidus
M20.20   Hallux rigidus, unspecified foot
M20.21   Hallux rigidus, right foot
M20.22   Hallux rigidus, left foot

✓5th **M20.3**   Hallux varus (acquired)
M20.30   Hallux varus (acquired), unspecified foot
M20.31   Hallux varus (acquired), right foot
M20.32   Hallux varus (acquired), left foot

✓5th **M20.4**   Other hammer toe(s) (acquired)
M20.40   Other hammer toe(s) (acquired), unspecified foot
M20.41   Other hammer toe(s) (acquired), right foot
M20.42   Other hammer toe(s) (acquired), left foot

✓5th **M20.5**   Other deformities of toe(s) (acquired)
✓6th **M20.5X**   Other deformities of toe(s) (acquired)
M20.5X1   Other deformities of toe(s) (acquired), right foot
M20.5X2   Other deformities of toe(s) (acquired), left foot
M20.5X9   Other deformities of toe(s) (acquired), unspecified foot

✓5th **M20.6**   Acquired deformities of toe(s), unspecified
M20.60   Acquired deformities of toe(s), unspecified, unspecified foot
M20.61   Acquired deformities of toe(s), unspecified, right foot
M20.62   Acquired deformities of toe(s), unspecified, left foot

✓4th **M21**   Other acquired deformities of limbs
   EXCLUDES1   acquired absence of limb (Z89.-)
     congenital absence of limbs (Q71-Q73)
     congenital deformities and malformations of limbs (Q65-Q66, Q68-Q74)
   EXCLUDES2   acquired deformities of fingers or toes (M20.-)
     coxa plana (M91.2)

✓5th **M21.0**   Valgus deformity, not elsewhere classified
   EXCLUDES1   metatarsus valgus (Q66.6)
     talipes calcaneovalgus (Q66.4)
M21.00   Valgus deformity, not elsewhere classified, unspecified site
✓6th **M21.02**   Valgus deformity, not elsewhere classified, elbow
   Cubitus valgus
M21.021   Valgus deformity, not elsewhere classified, right elbow
M21.022   Valgus deformity, not elsewhere classified, left elbow
M21.029   Valgus deformity, not elsewhere classified, unspecified elbow
✓6th **M21.05**   Valgus deformity, not elsewhere classified, hip
M21.051   Valgus deformity, not elsewhere classified, right hip
M21.052   Valgus deformity, not elsewhere classified, left hip
M21.059   Valgus deformity, not elsewhere classified, unspecified hip

✓6th **M21.06**   Valgus deformity, not elsewhere classified, knee
   Genu valgum   Knock knee
M21.061   Valgus deformity, not elsewhere classified, right knee
M21.062   Valgus deformity, not elsewhere classified, left knee
M21.069   Valgus deformity, not elsewhere classified, unspecified knee
✓6th **M21.07**   Valgus deformity, not elsewhere classified, ankle
M21.071   Valgus deformity, not elsewhere classified, right ankle
M21.072   Valgus deformity, not elsewhere classified, left ankle
M21.079   Valgus deformity, not elsewhere classified, unspecified ankle

✓5th **M21.1**   Varus deformity, not elsewhere classified
   EXCLUDES1   metatarsus varus (Q66.2)
     tibia vara (M92.5)
M21.10   Varus deformity, not elsewhere classified, unspecified site
✓6th **M21.12**   Varus deformity, not elsewhere classified, elbow
   Cubitus varus, elbow
M21.121   Varus deformity, not elsewhere classified, right elbow
M21.122   Varus deformity, not elsewhere classified, left elbow
M21.129   Varus deformity, not elsewhere classified, unspecified elbow
✓6th **M21.15**   Varus deformity, not elsewhere classified, hip
M21.151   Varus deformity, not elsewhere classified, right hip
M21.152   Varus deformity, not elsewhere classified, left hip
M21.159   Varus deformity, not elsewhere classified, unspecified
✓6th **M21.16**   Varus deformity, not elsewhere classified, knee
   Bow leg
   Genu varum
M21.161   Varus deformity, not elsewhere classified, right knee
M21.162   Varus deformity, not elsewhere classified, left knee
M21.169   Varus deformity, not elsewhere classified, unspecified knee
✓6th **M21.17**   Varus deformity, not elsewhere classified, ankle
M21.171   Varus deformity, not elsewhere classified, right ankle
M21.172   Varus deformity, not elsewhere classified, left ankle
M21.179   Varus deformity, not elsewhere classified, unspecified ankle

✓5th **M21.2**   Flexion deformity
M21.20   Flexion deformity, unspecified site
✓6th **M21.21**   Flexion deformity, shoulder
M21.211   Flexion deformity, right shoulder
M21.212   Flexion deformity, left shoulder
M21.219   Flexion deformity, unspecified shoulder
✓6th **M21.22**   Flexion deformity, elbow
M21.221   Flexion deformity, right elbow
M21.222   Flexion deformity, left elbow
M21.229   Flexion deformity, unspecified elbow
✓6th **M21.23**   Flexion deformity, wrist
M21.231   Flexion deformity, right wrist
M21.232   Flexion deformity, left wrist
M21.239   Flexion deformity, unspecified wrist
✓6th **M21.24**   Flexion deformity, finger joints
M21.241   Flexion deformity, right finger joints
M21.242   Flexion deformity, left finger joints
M21.249   Flexion deformity, unspecified finger joints
✓6th **M21.25**   Flexion deformity, hip
M21.251   Flexion deformity, right hip
M21.252   Flexion deformity, left hip
M21.259   Flexion deformity, unspecified hip

✓6ᵗʰ **M21.26 Flexion deformity,** knee
　　M21.261 Flexion deformity, right **knee**
　　M21.262 Flexion deformity, left **knee**
　　M21.269 Flexion deformity, unspecified knee

✓6ᵗʰ **M21.27 Flexion deformity,** ankle and toes
　　M21.271 Flexion deformity, right **ankle and toes**
　　M21.272 Flexion deformity, left **ankle and toes**
　　M21.279 Flexion deformity, unspecified ankle and toes

✓5ᵗʰ **M21.3** Wrist or foot drop (acquired)

✓6ᵗʰ **M21.33** Wrist drop (acquired)
　　M21.331 Wrist drop, right **wrist**
　　M21.332 Wrist drop, left **wrist**
　　M21.339 Wrist drop, unspecified wrist

✓6ᵗʰ **M21.37** Foot drop (acquired)
　　M21.371 Foot drop, right **foot**
　　M21.372 Foot drop, left **foot**
　　M21.379 Foot drop, unspecified foot

✓5ᵗʰ **M21.4** Flat foot [pes planus] (acquired)
　　EXCLUDES 1　congenital pes planus (Q66.5-)
　　M21.40 Flat foot [pes planus] (acquired), unspecified foot
　　M21.41 Flat foot [pes planus] (acquired), right **foot**
　　M21.42 Flat foot [pes planus] (acquired), left **foot**

✓5ᵗʰ **M21.5 Acquired** clawhand, clubhand, clawfoot and clubfoot
　　EXCLUDES 1　clubfoot, not specified as acquired (Q66.89)

✓6ᵗʰ **M21.51 Acquired** clawhand
　　M21.511 Acquired clawhand, right **hand**
　　M21.512 Acquired clawhand, left **hand**
　　M21.519 Acquired clawhand, unspecified hand

✓6ᵗʰ **M21.52 Acquired** clubhand
　　M21.521 Acquired clubhand, right **hand**
　　M21.522 Acquired clubhand, left **hand**
　　M21.529 Acquired clubhand, unspecified hand

✓6ᵗʰ **M21.53 Acquired** clawfoot
　　M21.531 Acquired clawfoot, right **foot**
　　M21.532 Acquired clawfoot, left **foot**
　　M21.539 Acquired clawfoot, unspecified foot

✓6ᵗʰ **M21.54 Acquired** clubfoot
　　M21.541 Acquired clubfoot, right **foot**
　　M21.542 Acquired clubfoot, left **foot**
　　M21.549 Acquired clubfoot, unspecified foot

✓5ᵗʰ **M21.6 Other** acquired deformities of foot
　　EXCLUDES 2　deformities of toe (acquired) (M20.1-M20.6)

✓6ᵗʰ **M21.6X Other acquired deformities of** foot
　　M21.6X1 Other acquired deformities of right **foot**
　　M21.6X2 Other acquired deformities of left **foot**
　　M21.6X9 Other acquired deformities of unspecified foot

✓5ᵗʰ **M21.7** Unequal limb length (acquired)
　　NOTE　The site used should correspond to the shorter limb.
　　M21.70 Unequal limb length (acquired), unspecified site

✓6ᵗʰ **M21.72 Unequal limb length (acquired),** humerus
　　M21.721 Unequal limb length (acquired), right **humerus**
　　M21.722 Unequal limb length (acquired), left **humerus**
　　M21.729 Unequal limb length (acquired), unspecified humerus

✓6ᵗʰ **M21.73 Unequal limb length (acquired),** ulna and radius
　　M21.731 Unequal limb length (acquired), right **ulna**
　　M21.732 Unequal limb length (acquired), left **ulna**
　　M21.733 Unequal limb length (acquired), right **radius**
　　M21.734 Unequal limb length (acquired), left **radius**
　　M21.739 Unequal limb length (acquired), unspecified ulna and radius

✓6ᵗʰ **M21.75 Unequal limb length (acquired),** femur
　　M21.751 Unequal limb length (acquired), right **femur**
　　M21.752 Unequal limb length (acquired), left **femur**
　　M21.759 Unequal limb length (acquired), unspecified femur

✓6ᵗʰ **M21.76 Unequal limb length (acquired),** tibia and fibula
　　M21.761 Unequal limb length (acquired), right **tibia**
　　M21.762 Unequal limb length (acquired), left **tibia**
　　M21.763 Unequal limb length (acquired), right **fibula**
　　M21.764 Unequal limb length (acquired), left **fibula**
　　M21.769 Unequal limb length (acquired), unspecified tibia and fibula

✓5ᵗʰ **M21.8** Other specified acquired deformities of limbs
　　EXCLUDES 2　coxa plana (M91.2)
　　M21.80 Other specified acquired deformities of unspecified limb

✓6ᵗʰ **M21.82 Other specified acquired deformities of** upper arm
　　M21.821 Other specified acquired deformities of right **upper arm**
　　M21.822 Other specified acquired deformities of left **upper arm**
　　M21.829 Other specified acquired deformities of unspecified upper arm

✓6ᵗʰ **M21.83 Other specified acquired deformities of** forearm
　　M21.831 Other specified acquired deformities of right **forearm**
　　M21.832 Other specified acquired deformities of left **forearm**
　　M21.839 Other specified acquired deformities of unspecified forearm

✓6ᵗʰ **M21.85 Other specified acquired deformities of** thigh
　　M21.851 Other specified acquired deformities of right **thigh**
　　M21.852 Other specified acquired deformities of left **thigh**
　　M21.859 Other specified acquired deformities of unspecified thigh

✓6ᵗʰ **M21.86 Other specified acquired deformities of** lower leg
　　M21.861 Other specified acquired deformities of right **lower leg**
　　M21.862 Other specified acquired deformities of left **lower leg**
　　M21.869 Other specified acquired deformities of unspecified lower leg

✓5ᵗʰ **M21.9 Unspecified acquired deformity of** limb and hand
　　M21.90 Unspecified acquired deformity of unspecified limb

✓6ᵗʰ **M21.92 Unspecified acquired deformity of** upper arm
　　M21.921 Unspecified acquired deformity of right **upper arm**
　　M21.922 Unspecified acquired deformity of left **upper arm**
　　M21.929 Unspecified acquired deformity of unspecified upper arm

✓6ᵗʰ **M21.93 Unspecified acquired deformity of** forearm
　　M21.931 Unspecified acquired deformity of right **forearm**
　　M21.932 Unspecified acquired deformity of left **forearm**
　　M21.939 Unspecified acquired deformity of unspecified forearm

✓6ᵗʰ **M21.94 Unspecified acquired deformity of** hand
　　M21.941 Unspecified acquired deformity of hand, right **hand**
　　M21.942 Unspecified acquired deformity of hand, left **hand**
　　M21.949 Unspecified acquired deformity of hand, unspecified hand

✓6ᵗʰ **M21.95 Unspecified acquired deformity of** thigh
　　M21.951 Unspecified acquired deformity of right **thigh**
　　M21.952 Unspecified acquired deformity of left **thigh**
　　M21.959 Unspecified acquired deformity of unspecified thigh

✓6ᵗʰ **M21.96 Unspecified acquired deformity of** lower leg
　　M21.961 Unspecified acquired deformity of right **lower leg**
　　M21.962 Unspecified acquired deformity of left **lower leg**

M21.969   Unspecified acquired deformity of unspecified lower leg

✓4ᵗʰ **M22**   **Disorder of patella**
> **EXCLUDES 1**   *traumatic dislocation of patella (S83.0-)*

✓5ᵗʰ **M22.0**   **Recurrent dislocation of patella**
- **M22.00**   Recurrent dislocation of patella, unspecified knee
- **M22.01**   Recurrent dislocation of patella, right knee
- **M22.02**   Recurrent dislocation of patella, left knee

✓5ᵗʰ **M22.1**   **Recurrent subluxation of patella**
> Incomplete dislocation of patella
- **M22.10**   Recurrent subluxation of patella, unspecified knee
- **M22.11**   Recurrent subluxation of patella, right knee
- **M22.12**   Recurrent subluxation of patella, left knee

✓5ᵗʰ **M22.2**   **Patellofemoral disorders**
- ✓6ᵗʰ **M22.2X**   **Patellofemoral disorders**
  - **M22.2X1**   Patellofemoral disorders, right knee
  - **M22.2X2**   Patellofemoral disorders, left knee
  - **M22.2X9**   Patellofemoral disorders, unspecified knee

✓5ᵗʰ **M22.3**   **Other derangements of patella**
- ✓6ᵗʰ **M22.3X**   **Other derangements of patella**
  - **M22.3X1**   Other derangements of patella, right knee
  - **M22.3X2**   Other derangements of patella, left knee
  - **M22.3X9**   Other derangements of patella, unspecified knee

✓5ᵗʰ **M22.4**   **Chondromalacia patellae**
- **M22.40**   Chondromalacia patellae, unspecified knee
- **M22.41**   Chondromalacia patellae, right knee
- **M22.42**   Chondromalacia patellae, left knee

✓5ᵗʰ **M22.8**   **Other disorders of patella**
- ✓6ᵗʰ **M22.8X**   **Other disorders of patella**
  - **M22.8X1**   Other disorders of patella, right knee
  - **M22.8X2**   Other disorders of patella, left knee
  - **M22.8X9**   Other disorders of patella, unspecified knee

✓5ᵗʰ **M22.9**   **Unspecified disorder of patella**
- **M22.90**   Unspecified disorder of patella, unspecified knee
- **M22.91**   Unspecified disorder of patella, right knee
- **M22.92**   Unspecified disorder of patella, left knee

✓4ᵗʰ **M23**   **Internal derangement of knee**
> **EXCLUDES 1**   *ankylosis (M24.66)*
> *current injury—see injury of knee and lower leg (S80-S89)*
> *deformity of knee (M21.-)*
> *osteochondritis dissecans (M93.2)*
> *recurrent dislocation or subluxation of joints (M24.4)*
> *recurrent dislocation or subluxation of patella (M22.0-M22.1)*

✓5ᵗʰ **M23.0**   **Cystic meniscus**
- ✓6ᵗʰ **M23.00**   **Cystic meniscus, unspecified meniscus**
  > Cystic meniscus, unspecified lateral meniscus
  > Cystic meniscus, unspecified medial meniscus
  - **M23.000**   Cystic meniscus, unspecified lateral meniscus, right knee
  - **M23.001**   Cystic meniscus, unspecified lateral meniscus, left knee
  - **M23.002**   Cystic meniscus, unspecified lateral meniscus, unspecified knee
  - **M23.003**   Cystic meniscus, unspecified medial meniscus, right knee
  - **M23.004**   Cystic meniscus, unspecified medial meniscus, left knee
  - **M23.005**   Cystic meniscus, unspecified medial meniscus, unspecified knee
  - **M23.006**   Cystic meniscus, unspecified meniscus, right knee
  - **M23.007**   Cystic meniscus, unspecified meniscus, left knee
  - **M23.009**   Cystic meniscus, unspecified meniscus, unspecified knee
- ✓6ᵗʰ **M23.01**   **Cystic meniscus, anterior horn of medial meniscus**
  - **M23.011**   Cystic meniscus, anterior horn of medial meniscus, right knee
  - **M23.012**   Cystic meniscus, anterior horn of medial meniscus, left knee

- **M23.019**   Cystic meniscus, anterior horn of medial meniscus, unspecified knee

- ✓6ᵗʰ **M23.02**   **Cystic meniscus, posterior horn of medial meniscus**
  - **M23.021**   Cystic meniscus, posterior horn of medial meniscus, right knee
  - **M23.022**   Cystic meniscus, posterior horn of medial meniscus, left knee
  - **M23.029**   Cystic meniscus, posterior horn of medial meniscus, unspecified knee

- ✓6ᵗʰ **M23.03**   **Cystic meniscus, other medial meniscus**
  - **M23.031**   Cystic meniscus, other medial meniscus, right knee
  - **M23.032**   Cystic meniscus, other medial meniscus, left knee
  - **M23.039**   Cystic meniscus, other medial meniscus, unspecified knee

- ✓6ᵗʰ **M23.04**   **Cystic meniscus, anterior horn of lateral meniscus**
  - **M23.041**   Cystic meniscus, anterior horn of lateral meniscus, right knee
  - **M23.042**   Cystic meniscus, anterior horn of lateral meniscus, left knee
  - **M23.049**   Cystic meniscus, anterior horn of lateral meniscus, unspecified knee

- ✓6ᵗʰ **M23.05**   **Cystic meniscus, posterior horn of lateral meniscus**
  - **M23.051**   Cystic meniscus, posterior horn of lateral meniscus, right knee
  - **M23.052**   Cystic meniscus, posterior horn of lateral meniscus, left knee
  - **M23.059**   Cystic meniscus, posterior horn of lateral meniscus, unspecified knee

- ✓6ᵗʰ **M23.06**   **Cystic meniscus, other lateral meniscus**
  - **M23.061**   Cystic meniscus, other lateral meniscus, right knee
  - **M23.062**   Cystic meniscus, other lateral meniscus, left knee
  - **M23.069**   Cystic meniscus, other lateral meniscus, unspecified knee

✓5ᵗʰ **M23.2**   **Derangement of meniscus due to old tear or injury**
> Old bucket-handle tear
- ✓6ᵗʰ **M23.20**   **Derangement of unspecified meniscus due to old tear or injury**
  > Derangement of unspecified lateral meniscus due to old tear or injury
  > Derangement of unspecified medial meniscus due to old tear or injury
  - **M23.200**   Derangement of unspecified lateral meniscus due to old tear or injury, right knee
  - **M23.201**   Derangement of unspecified lateral meniscus due to old tear or injury, left knee
  - **M23.202**   Derangement of unspecified lateral meniscus due to old tear or injury, unspecified knee
  - **M23.203**   Derangement of unspecified medial meniscus due to old tear or injury, right knee
  - **M23.204**   Derangement of unspecified medial meniscus due to old tear or injury, left knee
  - **M23.205**   Derangement of unspecified medial meniscus due to old tear or injury, unspecified knee
  - **M23.206**   Derangement of unspecified meniscus due to old tear or injury, right knee
  - **M23.207**   Derangement of unspecified meniscus due to old tear or injury, left knee
  - **M23.209**   Derangement of unspecified meniscus due to old tear or injury, unspecified knee

- ✓6ᵗʰ **M23.21**   **Derangement of anterior horn of medial meniscus due to old tear or injury**
  - **M23.211**   Derangement of anterior horn of medial meniscus due to old tear or injury, right knee
  - **M23.212**   Derangement of anterior horn of medial meniscus due to old tear or injury, left knee

EXCLUDES 1 Not coded here   **EXCLUDES 2** Not included here   N Newborn Age: 0   P Pediatric Age: 0-17   M Maternity Age: 12-55   A Adult Age: 15-124

668   ICD-10-CM Draft (2015)

M23.219　Derangement of anterior horn of medial meniscus due to old tear or injury, unspecified knee

✓6ᵗʰ M23.22　Derangement of posterior horn of medial meniscus due to old tear or injury

M23.221　Derangement of posterior horn of medial meniscus due to old tear or injury, right knee

M23.222　Derangement of posterior horn of medial meniscus due to old tear or injury, left knee

M23.229　Derangement of posterior horn of medial meniscus due to old tear or injury, unspecified knee

✓6ᵗʰ M23.23　Derangement of other medial meniscus due to old tear or injury

M23.231　Derangement of other medial meniscus due to old tear or injury, right knee

M23.232　Derangement of other medial meniscus due to old tear or injury, left knee

M23.239　Derangement of other medial meniscus due to old tear or injury, unspecified knee

✓6ᵗʰ M23.24　Derangement of anterior horn of lateral meniscus due to old tear or injury

M23.241　Derangement of anterior horn of lateral meniscus due to old tear or injury, right knee

M23.242　Derangement of anterior horn of lateral meniscus due to old tear or injury, left knee

M23.249　Derangement of anterior horn of lateral meniscus due to old tear or injury, unspecified knee

✓6ᵗʰ M23.25　Derangement of posterior horn of lateral meniscus due to old tear or injury

M23.251　Derangement of posterior horn of lateral meniscus due to old tear or injury, right knee

M23.252　Derangement of posterior horn of lateral meniscus due to old tear or injury, left knee

M23.259　Derangement of posterior horn of lateral meniscus due to old tear or injury, unspecified knee

✓6ᵗʰ M23.26　Derangement of other lateral meniscus due to old tear or injury

M23.261　Derangement of other lateral meniscus due to old tear or injury, right knee

M23.262　Derangement of other lateral meniscus due to old tear or injury, left knee

M23.269　Derangement of other lateral meniscus due to old tear or injury, unspecified knee

✓5ᵗʰ M23.3　Other meniscus derangements
　　Degenerate meniscus
　　Detached meniscus
　　Retained meniscus

✓6ᵗʰ M23.30　Other meniscus derangements, unspecified meniscus
　　Other meniscus derangements, unspecified lateral meniscus
　　Other meniscus derangements, unspecified medial meniscus

M23.300　Other meniscus derangements, unspecified lateral meniscus, right knee

M23.301　Other meniscus derangements, unspecified lateral meniscus, left knee

M23.302　Other meniscus derangements, unspecified lateral meniscus, unspecified knee

M23.303　Other meniscus derangements, unspecified medial meniscus, right knee

M23.304　Other meniscus derangements, unspecified medial meniscus, left knee

M23.305　Other meniscus derangements, unspecified medial meniscus, unspecified knee

M23.306　Other meniscus derangements, unspecified meniscus, right knee

M23.307　Other meniscus derangements, unspecified meniscus, left knee

M23.309　Other meniscus derangements, unspecified meniscus, unspecified knee

✓6ᵗʰ M23.31　Other meniscus derangements, anterior horn of medial meniscus

M23.311　Other meniscus derangements, anterior horn of medial meniscus, right knee

M23.312　Other meniscus derangements, anterior horn of medial meniscus, left knee

M23.319　Other meniscus derangements, anterior horn of medial meniscus, unspecified knee

✓6ᵗʰ M23.32　Other meniscus derangements, posterior horn of medial meniscus

M23.321　Other meniscus derangements, posterior horn of medial meniscus, right knee

M23.322　Other meniscus derangements, posterior horn of medial meniscus, left knee

M23.329　Other meniscus derangements, posterior horn of medial meniscus, unspecified knee

✓6ᵗʰ M23.33　Other meniscus derangements, other medial meniscus

M23.331　Other meniscus derangements, other medial meniscus, right knee

M23.332　Other meniscus derangements, other medial meniscus, left knee

M23.339　Other meniscus derangements, other medial meniscus, unspecified knee

✓6ᵗʰ M23.34　Other meniscus derangements, anterior horn of lateral meniscus

M23.341　Other meniscus derangements, anterior horn of lateral meniscus, right knee

M23.342　Other meniscus derangements, anterior horn of lateral meniscus, left knee

M23.349　Other meniscus derangements, anterior horn of lateral meniscus, unspecified knee

✓6ᵗʰ M23.35　Other meniscus derangements, posterior horn of lateral meniscus

M23.351　Other meniscus derangements, posterior horn of lateral meniscus, right knee

M23.352　Other meniscus derangements, posterior horn of lateral meniscus, left knee

M23.359　Other meniscus derangements, posterior horn of lateral meniscus, unspecified knee

✓6ᵗʰ M23.36　Other meniscus derangements, other lateral meniscus

M23.361　Other meniscus derangements, other lateral meniscus, right knee

M23.362　Other meniscus derangements, other lateral meniscus, left knee

M23.369　Other meniscus derangements, other lateral meniscus, unspecified knee

✓5ᵗʰ M23.4　Loose body in knee

M23.40　Loose body in knee, unspecified knee

M23.41　Loose body in knee, right knee

M23.42　Loose body in knee, left knee

✓5ᵗʰ M23.5　Chronic instability of knee

M23.50　Chronic instability of knee, unspecified knee

M23.51　Chronic instability of knee, right knee

M23.52　Chronic instability of knee, left knee

✓5ᵗʰ M23.6　Other spontaneous disruption of ligament(s) of knee

✓6ᵗʰ M23.60　Other spontaneous disruption of unspecified ligament of knee

M23.601　Other spontaneous disruption of unspecified ligament of right knee

M23.602　Other spontaneous disruption of unspecified ligament of left knee

M23.609　Other spontaneous disruption of unspecified ligament of unspecified knee

✓6ᵗʰ M23.61　Other spontaneous disruption of anterior cruciate ligament of knee

M23.611　Other spontaneous disruption of anterior cruciate ligament of right knee

M23.612　Other spontaneous disruption of anterior cruciate ligament of left knee

M23.619　Other spontaneous disruption of anterior cruciate ligament of unspecified knee

☑ Additional Character Required　　✓×7ᵗʰ Xtension Alert　　Unspecified Dx　　Other Specified Dx　　Manifestation　　▶◀ Revised Text　　● New Code　　▲ Revised Code Title

ICD-10-CM Draft (2015)　　　669

√6th **M23.62 Other spontaneous disruption of** posterior cruciate **ligament of knee**
 M23.621 Other spontaneous disruption of posterior cruciate ligament of right **knee**
 M23.622 Other spontaneous disruption of posterior cruciate ligament of left **knee**
 M23.629 Other spontaneous disruption of posterior cruciate ligament of unspecified knee

√6th **M23.63 Other spontaneous disruption of** medial collateral **ligament of knee**
 M23.631 Other spontaneous disruption of medial collateral ligament of right **knee**
 M23.632 Other spontaneous disruption of medial collateral ligament of left **knee**
 M23.639 Other spontaneous disruption of medial collateral ligament of unspecified knee

√6th **M23.64 Other spontaneous disruption of** lateral collateral **ligament of knee**
 M23.641 Other spontaneous disruption of lateral collateral ligament of right **knee**
 M23.642 Other spontaneous disruption of lateral collateral ligament of left **knee**
 M23.649 Other spontaneous disruption of lateral collateral ligament of unspecified knee

√6th **M23.67 Other spontaneous disruption of** capsular **ligament of knee**
 M23.671 Other spontaneous disruption of capsular ligament of right **knee**
 M23.672 Other spontaneous disruption of capsular ligament of left **knee**
 M23.679 Other spontaneous disruption of capsular ligament of unspecified knee

√5th **M23.8 Other internal derangements of knee**
 Laxity of ligament of knee
 Snapping knee

√6th **M23.8X Other internal derangements of knee**
 M23.8X1 Other internal derangements of right **knee**
 M23.8X2 Other internal derangements of left **knee**
 M23.8X9 Other internal derangements of unspecified knee

√5th **M23.9 Unspecified internal derangement of knee**
 M23.90 Unspecified internal derangement of unspecified knee
 M23.91 Unspecified internal derangement of right **knee**
 M23.92 Unspecified internal derangement of left **knee**

√4th **M24 Other specific joint derangements**
 EXCLUDES 1 current injury—see injury of joint by body region
 EXCLUDES 2 ganglion (M67.4)
 snapping knee (M23.8-)
 temporomandibular joint disorders (M26.6-)

√5th **M24.0 Loose body in joint**
 EXCLUDES 2 loose body in knee (M23.4)
 M24.00 Loose body in unspecified joint

√6th **M24.01 Loose body in** shoulder
 M24.011 Loose body in right **shoulder**
 M24.012 Loose body in left **shoulder**
 M24.019 Loose body in unspecified shoulder

√6th **M24.02 Loose body in** elbow
 M24.021 Loose body in right **elbow**
 M24.022 Loose body in left **elbow**
 M24.029 Loose body in unspecified elbow

√6th **M24.03 Loose body in** wrist
 M24.031 Loose body in right **wrist**
 M24.032 Loose body in left **wrist**
 M24.039 Loose body in unspecified wrist

√6th **M24.04 Loose body in** finger joints
 M24.041 Loose body in right **finger joint(s)**
 M24.042 Loose body in left **finger joint(s)**
 M24.049 Loose body in unspecified finger joint(s)

√6th **M24.05 Loose body in** hip
 M24.051 Loose body in right **hip**
 M24.052 Loose body in left **hip**
 M24.059 Loose body in unspecified hip

√6th **M24.07 Loose body in** ankle and toe joints
 M24.071 Loose body in right **ankle**
 M24.072 Loose body in left **ankle**
 M24.073 Loose body in unspecified ankle
 M24.074 Loose body in right **toe joint(s)**
 M24.075 Loose body in left **toe joint(s)**
 M24.076 Loose body in unspecified toe joints

M24.08 Loose body, other site

√5th **M24.1 Other articular cartilage disorders**
 EXCLUDES 2 chondrocalcinosis (M11.1, M11.2-)
 internal derangement of knee (M23.-)
 metastatic calcification (E83.5)
 ochronosis (E70.2)

M24.10 Other articular cartilage disorders, unspecified site

√6th **M24.11 Other articular cartilage disorders,** shoulder
 M24.111 Other articular cartilage disorders, right **shoulder**
 M24.112 Other articular cartilage disorders, left **shoulder**
 M24.119 Other articular cartilage disorders, unspecified shoulder

√6th **M24.12 Other articular cartilage disorders,** elbow
 M24.121 Other articular cartilage disorders, right **elbow**
 M24.122 Other articular cartilage disorders, left **elbow**
 M24.129 Other articular cartilage disorders, unspecified elbow

√6th **M24.13 Other articular cartilage disorders,** wrist
 M24.131 Other articular cartilage disorders, right **wrist**
 M24.132 Other articular cartilage disorders, left **wrist**
 M24.139 Other articular cartilage disorders, unspecified wrist

√6th **M24.14 Other articular cartilage disorders,** hand
 M24.141 Other articular cartilage disorders, right **hand**
 M24.142 Other articular cartilage disorders, left **hand**
 M24.149 Other articular cartilage disorders, unspecified hand

√6th **M24.15 Other articular cartilage disorders,** hip
 M24.151 Other articular cartilage disorders, right **hip**
 M24.152 Other articular cartilage disorders, left **hip**
 M24.159 Other articular cartilage disorders, unspecified hip

√6th **M24.17 Other articular cartilage disorders,** ankle and foot
 M24.171 Other articular cartilage disorders, right **ankle**
 M24.172 Other articular cartilage disorders, left **ankle**
 M24.173 Other articular cartilage disorders, unspecified ankle
 M24.174 Other articular cartilage disorders, right **foot**
 M24.175 Other articular cartilage disorders, left **foot**
 M24.176 Other articular cartilage disorders, unspecified foot

√5th **M24.2 Disorder of ligament**
 Instability secondary to old ligament injury
 Ligamentous laxity NOS
 EXCLUDES 1 familial ligamentous laxity (M35.7)
 EXCLUDES 2 internal derangement of knee (M23.5-M23.89)

M24.20 Disorder of ligament, unspecified site

√6th **M24.21 Disorder of ligament,** shoulder
 M24.211 Disorder of ligament, right shoulder
 M24.212 Disorder of ligament, left **shoulder**
 M24.219 Disorder of ligament, unspecified shoulder

√6th **M24.22 Disorder of ligament,** elbow
 M24.221 Disorder of ligament, right elbow
 M24.222 Disorder of ligament, left **elbow**
 M24.229 Disorder of ligament, unspecified elbow

EXCLUDES 1 Not coded here EXCLUDES 2 Not included here N Newborn Age: 0 P Pediatric Age: 0-17 M Maternity Age: 12-55 A Adult Age: 15-124

670 ICD-10-CM Draft (2015)

✓6ᵗʰ **M24.23 Disorder of ligament, wrist**
    M24.231 Disorder of ligament, right wrist
    M24.232 Disorder of ligament, left wrist
    M24.239 **Disorder of ligament, unspecified wrist**

✓6ᵗʰ **M24.24 Disorder of ligament, hand**
    M24.241 Disorder of ligament, right hand
    M24.242 Disorder of ligament, left hand
    M24.249 **Disorder of ligament, unspecified hand**

✓6ᵗʰ **M24.25 Disorder of ligament, hip**
    M24.251 Disorder of ligament, right hip
    M24.252 Disorder of ligament, left hip
    M24.259 **Disorder of ligament, unspecified hip**

✓6ᵗʰ **M24.27 Disorder of ligament, ankle and foot**
    M24.271 Disorder of ligament, right ankle
    M24.272 Disorder of ligament, left ankle
    M24.273 **Disorder of ligament, unspecified ankle**
    M24.274 Disorder of ligament, right foot
    M24.275 Disorder of ligament, left foot
    M24.276 **Disorder of ligament, unspecified foot**

    M24.28 Disorder of ligament, vertebrae

✓5ᵗʰ **M24.3 Pathological dislocation of joint, not elsewhere classified**
    EXCLUDES 1 *congenital dislocation or displacement of joint—see congenital malformations and deformations of the musculoskeletal system (Q65-Q79)*
        current injury—see injury of joints and ligaments by body region
        recurrent dislocation of joint (M24.4-)

    M24.30 **Pathological dislocation of unspecified joint, not elsewhere classified**

✓6ᵗʰ **M24.31 Pathological dislocation of shoulder, not elsewhere classified**
    M24.311 Pathological dislocation of right shoulder, not elsewhere classified
    M24.312 Pathological dislocation of left shoulder, not elsewhere classified
    M24.319 **Pathological dislocation of unspecified shoulder, not elsewhere classified**

✓6ᵗʰ **M24.32 Pathological dislocation of elbow, not elsewhere classified**
    M24.321 Pathological dislocation of right elbow, not elsewhere classified
    M24.322 Pathological dislocation of left elbow, not elsewhere classified
    M24.329 **Pathological dislocation of unspecified elbow, not elsewhere classified**

✓6ᵗʰ **M24.33 Pathological dislocation of wrist, not elsewhere classified**
    M24.331 **Pathological dislocation of right wrist, not elsewhere classified**
    M24.332 **Pathological dislocation of left wrist, not elsewhere classified**
    M24.339 **Pathological dislocation of unspecified wrist, not elsewhere classified**

✓6ᵗʰ **M24.34 Pathological dislocation of hand, not elsewhere classified**
    M24.341 **Pathological dislocation of right hand, not elsewhere classified**
    M24.342 **Pathological dislocation of left hand, not elsewhere classified**
    M24.349 **Pathological dislocation of unspecified hand, not elsewhere classified**

✓6ᵗʰ **M24.35 Pathological dislocation of hip, not elsewhere classified**
    M24.351 **Pathological dislocation of right hip, not elsewhere classified**
    M24.352 **Pathological dislocation of left hip, not elsewhere classified**
    M24.359 **Pathological dislocation of unspecified hip, not elsewhere classified**

✓6ᵗʰ **M24.36 Pathological dislocation of knee, not elsewhere classified**
    M24.361 **Pathological dislocation of right knee, not elsewhere classified**
    M24.362 **Pathological dislocation of left knee, not elsewhere classified**

    M24.369 **Pathological dislocation of unspecified knee, not elsewhere classified**

✓6ᵗʰ **M24.37 Pathological dislocation of ankle and foot, not elsewhere classified**
    M24.371 Pathological dislocation of right ankle, not elsewhere classified
    M24.372 Pathological dislocation of left ankle, not elsewhere classified
    M24.373 **Pathological dislocation of unspecified ankle, not elsewhere classified**
    M24.374 Pathological dislocation of right foot, not elsewhere classified
    M24.375 Pathological dislocation of left foot, not elsewhere classified
    M24.376 **Pathological dislocation of unspecified foot, not elsewhere classified**

✓5ᵗʰ **M24.4 Recurrent dislocation of joint**
    Recurrent subluxation of joint
    EXCLUDES 2 *recurrent dislocation of patella (M22.0-M22.1)*
        recurrent vertebral dislocation (M43.3-, M43.4, M43.5-)

    M24.40 **Recurrent dislocation, unspecified joint**

✓6ᵗʰ **M24.41 Recurrent dislocation, shoulder**
    M24.411 Recurrent dislocation, right shoulder
    M24.412 Recurrent dislocation, left shoulder
    M24.419 **Recurrent dislocation, unspecified shoulder**

✓6ᵗʰ **M24.42 Recurrent dislocation, elbow**
    M24.421 Recurrent dislocation, right elbow
    M24.422 Recurrent dislocation, left elbow
    M24.429 **Recurrent dislocation, unspecified elbow**

✓6ᵗʰ **M24.43 Recurrent dislocation, wrist**
    M24.431 Recurrent dislocation, right wrist
    M24.432 Recurrent dislocation, left wrist
    M24.439 **Recurrent dislocation, unspecified wrist**

✓6ᵗʰ **M24.44 Recurrent dislocation, hand and finger(s)**
    M24.441 Recurrent dislocation, right hand
    M24.442 Recurrent dislocation, left hand
    M24.443 **Recurrent dislocation, unspecified hand**
    M24.444 Recurrent dislocation, right finger
    M24.445 Recurrent dislocation, left finger
    M24.446 **Recurrent dislocation, unspecified finger**

✓6ᵗʰ **M24.45 Recurrent dislocation, hip**
    M24.451 Recurrent dislocation, right hip
    M24.452 Recurrent dislocation, left hip
    M24.459 **Recurrent dislocation, unspecified hip**

✓6ᵗʰ **M24.46 Recurrent dislocation, knee**
    M24.461 Recurrent dislocation, right knee
    M24.462 Recurrent dislocation, left knee
    M24.469 **Recurrent dislocation, unspecified knee**

✓6ᵗʰ **M24.47 Recurrent dislocation, ankle, foot and toes**
    M24.471 Recurrent dislocation, right ankle
    M24.472 Recurrent dislocation, left ankle
    M24.473 **Recurrent dislocation, unspecified ankle**
    M24.474 Recurrent dislocation, right foot
    M24.475 Recurrent dislocation, left foot
    M24.476 **Recurrent dislocation, unspecified foot**
    M24.477 Recurrent dislocation, right toe(s)
    M24.478 Recurrent dislocation, left toe(s)
    M24.479 **Recurrent dislocation, unspecified toe(s)**

✓5ᵗʰ **M24.5 Contracture of joint**
    EXCLUDES 1 *contracture of muscle without contracture of joint (M62.4-)*
        contracture of tendon (sheath) without contracture of joint (M62.4-)
        Dupuytren's contracture (M72.0)
    EXCLUDES 2 *acquired deformities of limbs (M20-M21)*

    M24.50 **Contracture, unspecified joint**

✓6ᵗʰ **M24.51 Contracture, shoulder**
    M24.511 Contracture, right shoulder
    M24.512 Contracture, left shoulder
    M24.519 **Contracture, unspecified shoulder**

✓6ᵗʰ **M24.52 Contracture, elbow**
    M24.521 Contracture, right elbow
    M24.522 Contracture, left elbow

☑ Additional Character Required   ✓ˣ⁷ᵗʰ Xtension Alert   Unspecified Dx   Other Specified Dx   Manifestation   ▶◀ Revised Text   ● New Code   ▲ Revised Code Title

ICD-10-CM Draft (2015)   671

M24.529 **Contracture, unspecified elbow**

✓6ᵗʰ M24.53 Contracture, wrist
    M24.531 **Contracture, right wrist**
    M24.532 **Contracture, left wrist**
    M24.539 **Contracture, unspecified wrist**

✓6ᵗʰ M24.54 Contracture, hand
    M24.541 **Contracture, right hand**
    M24.542 **Contracture, left hand**
    M24.549 **Contracture, unspecified hand**

✓6ᵗʰ M24.55 Contracture, hip
    M24.551 **Contracture, right hip**
    M24.552 **Contracture, left hip**
    M24.559 **Contracture, unspecified hip**

✓6ᵗʰ M24.56 Contracture, knee
    M24.561 **Contracture, right knee**
    M24.562 **Contracture, left knee**
    M24.569 **Contracture, unspecified knee**

✓6ᵗʰ M24.57 Contracture, ankle and foot
    M24.571 **Contracture, right ankle**
    M24.572 **Contracture, left ankle**
    M24.573 **Contracture, unspecified ankle**
    M24.574 **Contracture, right foot**
    M24.575 **Contracture, left foot**
    M24.576 **Contracture, unspecified foot**

✓5ᵗʰ M24.6 Ankylosis of joint
    EXCLUDES 1 *stiffness of joint without ankylosis (M25.6-)*
    EXCLUDES 2 *spine (M43.2-)*

    M24.60 **Ankylosis, unspecified joint**

✓6ᵗʰ M24.61 Ankylosis, shoulder
    M24.611 **Ankylosis, right shoulder**
    M24.612 **Ankylosis, left shoulder**
    M24.619 **Ankylosis, unspecified shoulder**

✓6ᵗʰ M24.62 Ankylosis, elbow
    M24.621 **Ankylosis, right elbow**
    M24.622 **Ankylosis, left elbow**
    M24.629 **Ankylosis, unspecified elbow**

✓6ᵗʰ M24.63 Ankylosis, wrist
    M24.631 **Ankylosis, right wrist**
    M24.632 **Ankylosis, left wrist**
    M24.639 **Ankylosis, unspecified wrist**

✓6ᵗʰ M24.64 Ankylosis, hand
    M24.641 **Ankylosis, right hand**
    M24.642 **Ankylosis, left hand**
    M24.649 **Ankylosis, unspecified hand**

✓6ᵗʰ M24.65 Ankylosis, hip
    M24.651 **Ankylosis, right hip**
    M24.652 **Ankylosis, left hip**
    M24.659 **Ankylosis, unspecified hip**

✓6ᵗʰ M24.66 Ankylosis, knee
    M24.661 **Ankylosis, right knee**
    M24.662 **Ankylosis, left knee**
    M24.669 **Ankylosis, unspecified knee**

✓6ᵗʰ M24.67 Ankylosis, ankle and foot
    M24.671 **Ankylosis, right ankle**
    M24.672 **Ankylosis, left ankle**
    M24.673 **Ankylosis, unspecified ankle**
    M24.674 **Ankylosis, right foot**
    M24.675 **Ankylosis, left foot**
    M24.676 **Ankylosis, unspecified foot**

    M24.7 **Protrusio acetabuli**

✓5ᵗʰ M24.8 Other specific joint derangements, not elsewhere classified
    EXCLUDES 2 *iliotibial band syndrome (M76.3)*

    M24.80 **Other specific joint derangements of unspecified joint, not elsewhere classified**

✓6ᵗʰ M24.81 Other specific joint derangements of shoulder, not elsewhere classified
    M24.811 **Other specific joint derangements of right shoulder, not elsewhere classified**
    M24.812 **Other specific joint derangements of left shoulder, not elsewhere classified**

M24.819 **Other specific joint derangements of unspecified shoulder, not elsewhere classified**

✓6ᵗʰ M24.82 Other specific joint derangements of elbow, not elsewhere classified
    M24.821 **Other specific joint derangements of right elbow, not elsewhere classified**
    M24.822 **Other specific joint derangements of left elbow, not elsewhere classified**
    M24.829 **Other specific joint derangements of unspecified elbow, not elsewhere classified**

✓6ᵗʰ M24.83 Other specific joint derangements of wrist, not elsewhere classified
    M24.831 **Other specific joint derangements of right wrist, not elsewhere classified**
    M24.832 **Other specific joint derangements of left wrist, not elsewhere classified**
    M24.839 **Other specific joint derangements of unspecified wrist, not elsewhere classified**

✓6ᵗʰ M24.84 Other specific joint derangements of hand, not elsewhere classified
    M24.841 **Other specific joint derangements of right hand, not elsewhere classified**
    M24.842 **Other specific joint derangements of left hand, not elsewhere classified**
    M24.849 **Other specific joint derangements of unspecified hand, not elsewhere classified**

✓6ᵗʰ M24.85 Other specific joint derangements of hip, not elsewhere classified
    Irritable hip
    M24.851 **Other specific joint derangements of right hip, not elsewhere classified**
    M24.852 **Other specific joint derangements of left hip, not elsewhere classified**
    M24.859 **Other specific joint derangements of unspecified hip, not elsewhere classified**

✓6ᵗʰ M24.87 Other specific joint derangements of ankle and foot, not elsewhere classified
    M24.871 **Other specific joint derangements of right ankle, not elsewhere classified**
    M24.872 **Other specific joint derangements of left ankle, not elsewhere classified**
    M24.873 **Other specific joint derangements of unspecified ankle, not elsewhere classified**
    M24.874 **Other specific joint derangements of right foot, not elsewhere classified**
    M24.875 **Other specific joint derangements of left foot, not elsewhere classified**
    M24.876 **Other specific joint derangements of unspecified foot, not elsewhere classified**

    M24.9 **Joint derangement, unspecified**

M25 **Other joint disorder, not elsewhere classified**
    EXCLUDES 2 *abnormality of gait and mobility (R26.-)*
        acquired deformities of limb (M20-M21)
        calcification of bursa (M71.4-)
        calcification of shoulder (joint) (M75.3)
        calcification of tendon (M65.2-)
        difficulty in walking (R26.2)
        temporomandibular joint disorder (M26.6-)

✓5ᵗʰ M25.0 Hemarthrosis
    EXCLUDES 1 *current injury—see injury of joint by body region*
        hemophilic arthropathy (M36.2)

    M25.00 **Hemarthrosis, unspecified joint**

✓6ᵗʰ M25.01 Hemarthrosis, shoulder
    M25.011 **Hemarthrosis, right shoulder**
    M25.012 **Hemarthrosis, left shoulder**
    M25.019 **Hemarthrosis, unspecified shoulder**

✓6ᵗʰ M25.02 Hemarthrosis, elbow
    M25.021 **Hemarthrosis, right elbow**
    M25.022 **Hemarthrosis, left elbow**
    M25.029 **Hemarthrosis, unspecified elbow**

✓6ᵗʰ M25.03 Hemarthrosis, wrist
    M25.031 **Hemarthrosis, right wrist**
    M25.032 **Hemarthrosis, left wrist**
    M25.039 **Hemarthrosis, unspecified wrist**

EXCLUDES 1 Not coded here   EXCLUDES 2 Not included here   N Newborn Age: 0   P Pediatric Age: 0-17   M Maternity Age: 12-55   A Adult Age: 15-124

672   ICD-10-CM Draft (2015)

√6ᵗʰ **M25.04　Hemarthrosis,** hand
　　　　M25.041　Hemarthrosis, right hand
　　　　M25.042　Hemarthrosis, left hand
　　　　M25.049　Hemarthrosis, unspecified hand

√6ᵗʰ **M25.05　Hemarthrosis,** hip
　　　　M25.051　Hemarthrosis, right hip
　　　　M25.052　Hemarthrosis, left hip
　　　　M25.059　Hemarthrosis, unspecified hip

√6ᵗʰ **M25.06　Hemarthrosis,** knee
　　　　M25.061　Hemarthrosis, right knee
　　　　M25.062　Hemarthrosis, left knee
　　　　M25.069　Hemarthrosis, unspecified knee

√6ᵗʰ **M25.07　Hemarthrosis,** ankle and foot
　　　　M25.071　Hemarthrosis, right ankle
　　　　M25.072　Hemarthrosis, left ankle
　　　　M25.073　Hemarthrosis, unspecified ankle
　　　　M25.074　Hemarthrosis, right foot
　　　　M25.075　Hemarthrosis, left foot
　　　　M25.076　Hemarthrosis, unspecified foot

　　　M25.08　Hemarthrosis, other specified site
　　　　　　Hemarthrosis, vertebrae

√5ᵗʰ **M25.1　Fistula of joint**
　　　M25.10　Fistula, unspecified joint

√6ᵗʰ **M25.11　Fistula,** shoulder
　　　　M25.111　Fistula, right shoulder
　　　　M25.112　Fistula, left shoulder
　　　　M25.119　Fistula, unspecified shoulder

√6ᵗʰ **M25.12　Fistula,** elbow
　　　　M25.121　Fistula, right elbow
　　　　M25.122　Fistula, left elbow
　　　　M25.129　Fistula, unspecified elbow

√6ᵗʰ **M25.13　Fistula,** wrist
　　　　M25.131　Fistula, right wrist
　　　　M25.132　Fistula, left wrist
　　　　M25.139　Fistula, unspecified wrist

√6ᵗʰ **M25.14　Fistula,** hand
　　　　M25.141　Fistula, right hand
　　　　M25.142　Fistula, left hand
　　　　M25.149　Fistula, unspecified hand

√6ᵗʰ **M25.15　Fistula,** hip
　　　　M25.151　Fistula, right hip
　　　　M25.152　Fistula, left hip
　　　　M25.159　Fistula, unspecified hip

√6ᵗʰ **M25.16　Fistula,** knee
　　　　M25.161　Fistula, right knee
　　　　M25.162　Fistula, left knee
　　　　M25.169　Fistula, unspecified knee

√6ᵗʰ **M25.17　Fistula,** ankle and foot
　　　　M25.171　Fistula, right ankle
　　　　M25.172　Fistula, left ankle
　　　　M25.173　Fistula, unspecified ankle
　　　　M25.174　Fistula, right foot
　　　　M25.175　Fistula, left foot
　　　　M25.176　Fistula, unspecified foot

　　　M25.18　Fistula, other specified site
　　　　　　Fistula, vertebrae

√5ᵗʰ **M25.2　Flail joint**
　　　M25.20　Flail joint, unspecified joint

√6ᵗʰ **M25.21　Flail joint,** shoulder
　　　　M25.211　Flail joint, right shoulder
　　　　M25.212　Flail joint, left shoulder
　　　　M25.219　Flail joint, unspecified shoulder

√6ᵗʰ **M25.22　Flail joint,** elbow
　　　　M25.221　Flail joint, right elbow
　　　　M25.222　Flail joint, left elbow
　　　　M25.229　Flail joint, unspecified elbow

√6ᵗʰ **M25.23　Flail joint,** wrist
　　　　M25.231　Flail joint, right wrist
　　　　M25.232　Flail joint, left wrist
　　　　M25.239　Flail joint, unspecified wrist

√6ᵗʰ **M25.24　Flail joint,** hand
　　　　M25.241　Flail joint, right hand
　　　　M25.242　Flail joint, left hand
　　　　M25.249　Flail joint, unspecified hand

√6ᵗʰ **M25.25　Flail joint,** hip
　　　　M25.251　Flail joint, right hip
　　　　M25.252　Flail joint, left hip
　　　　M25.259　Flail joint, unspecified hip

√6ᵗʰ **M25.26　Flail joint,** knee
　　　　M25.261　Flail joint, right knee
　　　　M25.262　Flail joint, left knee
　　　　M25.269　Flail joint, unspecified knee

√6ᵗʰ **M25.27　Flail joint,** ankle and foot
　　　　M25.271　Flail joint, right ankle and foot
　　　　M25.272　Flail joint, left ankle and foot
　　　　M25.279　Flail joint, unspecified ankle and foot

　　　M25.28　Flail joint, other site

√5ᵗʰ **M25.3　Other instability of joint**
　　　EXCLUDES 1　*instability of joint secondary to old ligament injury (M24.2-)*
　　　　　instability of joint secondary to removal of joint prosthesis (M96.8-)
　　　EXCLUDES 2　*spinal instabilities (M53.2-)*

　　　M25.30　Other instability, unspecified joint

√6ᵗʰ **M25.31　Other instability,** shoulder
　　　　M25.311　Other instability, right shoulder
　　　　M25.312　Other instability, left shoulder
　　　　M25.319　Other instability, unspecified shoulder

√6ᵗʰ **M25.32　Other instability,** elbow
　　　　M25.321　Other instability, right elbow
　　　　M25.322　Other instability, left elbow
　　　　M25.329　Other instability, unspecified elbow

√6ᵗʰ **M25.33　Other instability,** wrist
　　　　M25.331　Other instability, right wrist
　　　　M25.332　Other instability, left wrist
　　　　M25.339　Other instability, unspecified wrist

√6ᵗʰ **M25.34　Other instability,** hand
　　　　M25.341　Other instability, right hand
　　　　M25.342　Other instability, left hand
　　　　M25.349　Other instability, unspecified hand

√6ᵗʰ **M25.35　Other instability,** hip
　　　　M25.351　Other instability, right hip
　　　　M25.352　Other instability, left hip
　　　　M25.359　Other instability, unspecified hip

√6ᵗʰ **M25.36　Other instability,** knee
　　　　M25.361　Other instability, right knee
　　　　M25.362　Other instability, left knee
　　　　M25.369　Other instability, unspecified knee

√6ᵗʰ **M25.37　Other instability,** ankle and foot
　　　　M25.371　Other instability, right ankle
　　　　M25.372　Other instability, left ankle
　　　　M25.373　Other instability, unspecified ankle
　　　　M25.374　Other instability, right foot
　　　　M25.375　Other instability, left foot
　　　　M25.376　Other instability, unspecified foot

√5ᵗʰ **M25.4　Effusion of joint**
　　　EXCLUDES 1　*hydrarthrosis in yaws (A66.6)*
　　　　　intermittent hydrarthrosis (M12.4-)
　　　　　other infective (teno)synovitis (M65.1-)

　　　M25.40　Effusion, unspecified joint

√6ᵗʰ **M25.41　Effusion,** shoulder
　　　　M25.411　Effusion, right shoulder
　　　　M25.412　Effusion, left shoulder
　　　　M25.419　Effusion, unspecified shoulder

√6ᵗʰ **M25.42　Effusion,** elbow
　　　　M25.421　Effusion, right elbow
　　　　M25.422　Effusion, left elbow
　　　　M25.429　Effusion, unspecified elbow

√6ᵗʰ **M25.43　Effusion,** wrist
　　　　M25.431　Effusion, right wrist
　　　　M25.432　Effusion, left wrist
　　　　M25.439　Effusion, unspecified wrist

✔ Additional Character Required　　√x7ᵗʰ Xtension Alert　　Unspecified Dx　　Other Specified Dx　　Manifestation　　▶◀ Revised Text　　● New Code　　▲ Revised Code Title

ICD-10-CM Draft (2015)　　　　　　　　　　　　　　　　　　　673

✓6ᵗʰ **M25.44 Effusion, hand**
     M25.441 **Effusion, right hand**
     M25.442 **Effusion, left hand**
     M25.449 **Effusion, unspecified hand**

✓6ᵗʰ **M25.45 Effusion, hip**
     M25.451 **Effusion, right hip**
     M25.452 **Effusion, left hip**
     M25.459 **Effusion, unspecified hip**

✓6ᵗʰ **M25.46 Effusion, knee**
     M25.461 **Effusion, right knee**
     M25.462 **Effusion, left knee**
     M25.469 **Effusion, unspecified knee**

✓6ᵗʰ **M25.47 Effusion, ankle and foot**
     M25.471 **Effusion, right ankle**
     M25.472 **Effusion, left ankle**
     M25.473 **Effusion, unspecified ankle**
     M25.474 **Effusion, right foot**
     M25.475 **Effusion, left foot**
     M25.476 **Effusion, unspecified foot**

     M25.48 **Effusion, other site**

✓5ᵗʰ **M25.5 Pain in joint**
     EXCLUDES 2   *pain in hand (M79.64-)*
          pain in fingers (M79.64-)
          pain in foot (M79.67-)
          pain in limb (M79.6-)
          pain in toes (M79.67-)

     M25.50 **Pain in unspecified joint**

✓6ᵗʰ **M25.51 Pain in shoulder**
     M25.511 **Pain in right shoulder**
     M25.512 **Pain in left shoulder**
     M25.519 **Pain in unspecified shoulder**

✓6ᵗʰ **M25.52 Pain in elbow**
     M25.521 **Pain in right elbow**
     M25.522 **Pain in left elbow**
     M25.529 **Pain in unspecified elbow**

✓6ᵗʰ **M25.53 Pain in wrist**
     M25.531 **Pain in right wrist**
     M25.532 **Pain in left wrist**
     M25.539 **Pain in unspecified wrist**

✓6ᵗʰ **M25.55 Pain in hip**
     M25.551 **Pain in right hip**
     M25.552 **Pain in left hip**
     M25.559 **Pain in unspecified hip**

✓6ᵗʰ **M25.56 Pain in knee**
     M25.561 **Pain in right knee**
     M25.562 **Pain in left knee**
     M25.569 **Pain in unspecified knee**

✓6ᵗʰ **M25.57 Pain in ankle and joints of foot**
     M25.571 **Pain in right ankle and joints of right foot**
     M25.572 **Pain in left ankle and joints of left foot**
     M25.579 **Pain in unspecified ankle and joints of unspecified foot**

✓5ᵗʰ **M25.6 Stiffness of joint, not elsewhere classified**
     EXCLUDES 1   *ankylosis of joint (M24.6-)*
          contracture of joint (M24.5-)

     M25.60 **Stiffness of unspecified joint, not elsewhere classified**

✓6ᵗʰ **M25.61 Stiffness of shoulder, not elsewhere classified**
     M25.611 **Stiffness of right shoulder, not elsewhere classified**
     M25.612 **Stiffness of left shoulder, not elsewhere classified**
     M25.619 **Stiffness of unspecified shoulder, not elsewhere classified**

✓6ᵗʰ **M25.62 Stiffness of elbow, not elsewhere classified**
     M25.621 **Stiffness of right elbow, not elsewhere classified**
     M25.622 **Stiffness of left elbow, not elsewhere classified**
     M25.629 **Stiffness of unspecified elbow, not elsewhere classified**

✓6ᵗʰ **M25.63 Stiffness of wrist, not elsewhere classified**
     M25.631 **Stiffness of right wrist, not elsewhere classified**
     M25.632 **Stiffness of left wrist, not elsewhere classified**
     M25.639 **Stiffness of unspecified wrist, not elsewhere classified**

✓6ᵗʰ **M25.64 Stiffness of hand, not elsewhere classified**
     M25.641 **Stiffness of right hand, not elsewhere classified**
     M25.642 **Stiffness of left hand, not elsewhere classified**
     M25.649 **Stiffness of unspecified hand, not elsewhere classified**

✓6ᵗʰ **M25.65 Stiffness of hip, not elsewhere classified**
     M25.651 **Stiffness of right hip, not elsewhere classified**
     M25.652 **Stiffness of left hip, not elsewhere classified**
     M25.659 **Stiffness of unspecified hip, not elsewhere classified**

✓6ᵗʰ **M25.66 Stiffness of knee, not elsewhere classified**
     M25.661 **Stiffness of right knee, not elsewhere classified**
     M25.662 **Stiffness of left knee, not elsewhere classified**
     M25.669 **Stiffness of unspecified knee, not elsewhere classified**

✓6ᵗʰ **M25.67 Stiffness of ankle and foot, not elsewhere classified**
     M25.671 **Stiffness of right ankle, not elsewhere classified**
     M25.672 **Stiffness of left ankle, not elsewhere classified**
     M25.673 **Stiffness of unspecified ankle, not elsewhere classified**
     M25.674 **Stiffness of right foot, not elsewhere classified**
     M25.675 **Stiffness of left foot, not elsewhere classified**
     M25.676 **Stiffness of unspecified foot, not elsewhere classified**

✓5ᵗʰ **M25.7 Osteophyte**
     M25.70 **Osteophyte, unspecified joint**

✓6ᵗʰ **M25.71 Osteophyte, shoulder**
     M25.711 **Osteophyte, right shoulder**
     M25.712 **Osteophyte, left shoulder**
     M25.719 **Osteophyte, unspecified shoulder**

✓6ᵗʰ **M25.72 Osteophyte, elbow**
     M25.721 **Osteophyte, right elbow**
     M25.722 **Osteophyte, left elbow**
     M25.729 **Osteophyte, unspecified elbow**

✓6ᵗʰ **M25.73 Osteophyte, wrist**
     M25.731 **Osteophyte, right wrist**
     M25.732 **Osteophyte, left wrist**
     M25.739 **Osteophyte, unspecified wrist**

✓6ᵗʰ **M25.74 Osteophyte, hand**
     M25.741 **Osteophyte, right hand**
     M25.742 **Osteophyte, left hand**
     M25.749 **Osteophyte, unspecified hand**

✓6ᵗʰ **M25.75 Osteophyte, hip**
     M25.751 **Osteophyte, right hip**
     M25.752 **Osteophyte, left hip**
     M25.759 **Osteophyte, unspecified hip**

✓6ᵗʰ **M25.76 Osteophyte, knee**
     M25.761 **Osteophyte, right knee**
     M25.762 **Osteophyte, left knee**
     M25.769 **Osteophyte, unspecified knee**

✓6ᵗʰ **M25.77 Osteophyte, ankle and foot**
     M25.771 **Osteophyte, right ankle**
     M25.772 **Osteophyte, left ankle**
     M25.773 **Osteophyte, unspecified ankle**
     M25.774 **Osteophyte, right foot**
     M25.775 **Osteophyte, left foot**
     M25.776 **Osteophyte, unspecified foot**

EXCLUDES 1 Not coded here   EXCLUDES 2 Not included here   N Newborn Age: 0   P Pediatric Age: 0-17   M Maternity Age: 12-55   A Adult Age: 15-124

674   ICD-10-CM Draft (2015)

M25.78　Osteophyte, vertebrae
✓5th　M25.8　Other specified joint disorders
　　　M25.80　Other specified joint disorders, unspecified joint
　　✓6th　M25.81　Other specified joint disorders, shoulder
　　　　　M25.811　Other specified joint disorders, right shoulder
　　　　　M25.812　Other specified joint disorders, left shoulder
　　　　　M25.819　Other specified joint disorders, unspecified shoulder
　　✓6th　M25.82　Other specified joint disorders, elbow
　　　　　M25.821　Other specified joint disorders, right elbow
　　　　　M25.822　Other specified joint disorders, left elbow
　　　　　M25.829　Other specified joint disorders, unspecified elbow
　　✓6th　M25.83　Other specified joint disorders, wrist
　　　　　M25.831　Other specified joint disorders, right wrist
　　　　　M25.832　Other specified joint disorders, left wrist
　　　　　M25.839　Other specified joint disorders, unspecifiedwrist
　　✓6th　M25.84　Other specified joint disorders, hand
　　　　　M25.841　Other specified joint disorders, right hand
　　　　　M25.842　Other specified joint disorders, left hand
　　　　　M25.849　Other specified joint disorders, unspecified hand
　　✓6th　M25.85　Other specified joint disorders, hip
　　　　　M25.851　Other specified joint disorders, right hip
　　　　　M25.852　Other specified joint disorders, left hip
　　　　　M25.859　Other specified joint disorders, unspecified hip
　　✓6th　M25.86　Other specified joint disorders, knee
　　　　　M25.861　Other specified joint disorders, right knee
　　　　　M25.862　Other specified joint disorders, left knee
　　　　　M25.869　Other specified joint disorders, unspecified knee
　　✓6th　M25.87　Other specified joint disorders, ankle and foot
　　　　　M25.871　Other specified joint disorders, right ankle and foot
　　　　　M25.872　Other specified joint disorders, left ankle and foot
　　　　　M25.879　Other specified joint disorders, unspecified ankle and foot
　　　M25.9　Joint disorder, unspecified

Dentofacial anomalies [including malocclusion] and other disorders of jaw (M26-M27)

EXCLUDES 1　hemifacial atrophy or hypertrophy (Q67.4)
　　　　　unilateral condylar hyperplasia or hypoplasia (M27.8)

✓4th　M26　Dentofacial anomalies [including malocclusion]
　✓5th　M26.0　Major anomalies of jaw size
　　　　EXCLUDES 1　acromegaly (E22.0)
　　　　　　　　　Robin's syndrome (Q87.0)
　　　M26.00　Unspecified anomaly of jaw size
　　　M26.01　Maxillary hyperplasia
　　　M26.02　Maxillary hypoplasia
　　　M26.03　Mandibular hyperplasia
　　　M26.04　Mandibular hypoplasia
　　　M26.05　Macrogenia
　　　M26.06　Microgenia
　　　M26.07　Excessive tuberosity of jaw
　　　　　　Entire maxillary tuberosity
　　　M26.09　Other specified anomalies of jaw size
　✓5th　M26.1　Anomalies of jaw-cranial base relationship
　　　M26.10　Unspecified anomaly of jaw-cranial base relationship
　　　M26.11　Maxillary asymmetry
　　　M26.12　Other jaw asymmetry
　　　M26.19　Other specified anomalies of jaw-cranial base relationship
　✓5th　M26.2　Anomalies of dental arch relationship
　　　M26.20　Unspecified anomaly of dental arch relationship

　✓6th　M26.21　Malocclusion, Angle's class
　　　　　M26.211　Malocclusion, Angle's class I
　　　　　　　　Neutro-occlusion
　　　　　M26.212　Malocclusion, Angle's class II
　　　　　　　　Disto-occlusion Division I
　　　　　　　　Disto-occlusion Division II
　　　　　M26.213　Malocclusion, Angle's class III
　　　　　　　　Mesio-occlusion
　　　　　M26.219　Malocclusion, Angle's class, unspecified
　✓6th　M26.22　Open occlusal relationship
　　　　　M26.220　Open anterior occlusal relationship
　　　　　　　　Anterior openbite
　　　　　M26.221　Open posterior occlusal relationship
　　　　　　　　Posterior openbite
　　　M26.23　Excessive horizontal overlap
　　　　　　Excessive horizontal overjet
　　　M26.24　Reverse articulation
　　　　　　Crossbite (anterior) (posterior)
　　　M26.25　Anomalies of interarch distance
　　　M26.29　Other anomalies of dental arch relationship
　　　　　　Midline deviation of dental arch
　　　　　　Overbite (excessive) deep
　　　　　　Overbite (excessive) horizontal
　　　　　　Overbite (excessive) vertical
　　　　　　Posterior lingual occlusion of mandibular teeth
　✓5th　M26.3　Anomalies of tooth position of fully erupted tooth or teeth
　　　　EXCLUDES 2　embedded and impacted teeth (K01.-)
　　　M26.30　Unspecified anomaly of tooth position of fully erupted tooth or teeth
　　　　　　Abnormal spacing of fully erupted tooth or teeth NOS
　　　　　　Displacement of fully erupted tooth or teeth NOS
　　　　　　Transposition of fully erupted tooth or teeth NOS
　　　M26.31　Crowding of fully erupted teeth
　　　M26.32　Excessive spacing of fully erupted teeth
　　　　　　Diastema of fully erupted tooth or teeth NOS
　　　M26.33　Horizontal displacement of fully erupted tooth or teeth
　　　　　　Tipped tooth or teeth
　　　　　　Tipping of fully erupted tooth
　　　M26.34　Vertical displacement of fully erupted tooth or teeth
　　　　　　Extruded tooth
　　　　　　Infraeruption of tooth or teeth
　　　　　　Supraeruption of tooth or teeth
　　　M26.35　Rotation of fully erupted tooth or teeth
　　　M26.36　Insufficient interocclusal distance of fully erupted teeth (ridge)
　　　　　　Lack of adequate intermaxillary vertical dimension of fully erupted teeth
　　　M26.37　Excessive interocclusal distance of fully erupted teeth
　　　　　　Excessive intermaxillary vertical dimension of fully erupted teeth
　　　　　　Loss of occlusal vertical dimension of fully erupted teeth
　　　M26.39　Other anomalies of tooth position of fully erupted tooth or teeth
　　　M26.4　Malocclusion, unspecified
　✓5th　M26.5　Dentofacial functional abnormalities
　　　　EXCLUDES 1　bruxism (F45.8)
　　　　　　　　　teeth-grinding NOS (F45.8)
　　　M26.50　Dentofacial functional abnormalities, unspecified
　　　M26.51　Abnormal jaw closure
　　　M26.52　Limited mandibular range of motion
　　　M26.53　Deviation in opening and closing of the mandible
　　　M26.54　Insufficient anterior guidance
　　　　　　Insufficient anterior occlusal guidance
　　　M26.55　Centric occlusion maximum intercuspation discrepancy
　　　　　　EXCLUDES 1　centric occlusion NOS (M26.59)
　　　M26.56　Non-working side interference
　　　　　　Balancing side interference
　　　M26.57　Lack of posterior occlusal support
　　　M26.59　Other dentofacial functional abnormalities
　　　　　　Centric occlusion (of teeth) NOS
　　　　　　Malocclusion due to abnormal swallowing
　　　　　　Malocclusion due to mouth breathing
　　　　　　Malocclusion due to tongue, lip or finger habits

✓5ᵗʰ **M26.6 Temporomandibular joint disorders**
> *EXCLUDES 2*   *current temporomandibular joint dislocation (S03.0)*
> *current temporomandibular joint sprain (S03.4)*

    M26.60 Temporomandibular joint disorder, unspecified

    M26.61 Adhesions and ankylosis of temporomandibular joint

    M26.62 Arthralgia of temporomandibular joint

    M26.63 Articular disc disorder of temporomandibular joint

    M26.69 Other specified disorders of temporomandibular joint

✓5ᵗʰ **M26.7 Dental alveolar anomalies**

    M26.70 Unspecified alveolar anomaly

    M26.71 Alveolar maxillary hyperplasia

    M26.72 Alveolar mandibular hyperplasia

    M26.73 Alveolar maxillary hypoplasia

    M26.74 Alveolar mandibular hypoplasia

    M26.79 Other specified alveolar anomalies

✓5ᵗʰ **M26.8 Other dentofacial anomalies**

    M26.81 Anterior soft tissue impingement
       Anterior soft tissue impingement on teeth

    M26.82 Posterior soft tissue impingement
       Posterior soft tissue impingement on teeth

    M26.89 Other dentofacial anomalies

M26.9 Dentofacial anomaly, unspecified

✓4ᵗʰ **M27 Other diseases of jaws**

M27.0 Developmental disorders of jaws
    Latent bone cyst of jaw   Torus mandibularis
    Stafne's cyst   Torus palatinus

M27.1 Giant cell granuloma, central
    Giant cell granuloma NOS
> *EXCLUDES 1*   *peripheral giant cell granuloma (K06.8)*

M27.2 Inflammatory conditions of jaws
    Osteitis of jaw(s)   Periostitis jaw(s)
    Osteomyelitis (neonatal) jaw(s)   Sequestrum of jaw bone
    Osteoradionecrosis jaw(s)
    Use additional code (W88-W90, X39.0) to identify radiation, if radiation-induced
> *EXCLUDES 2*   *osteonecrosis of jaw due to drug (M87.180)*

M27.3 Alveolitis of jaws
    Alveolar osteitis
    Dry socket

✓5ᵗʰ **M27.4 Other and unspecified cysts of jaw**
> *EXCLUDES 1*   *cysts of oral region (K09.-)*
> *latent bone cyst of jaw (M27.0)*
> *Stafne's cyst (M27.0)*

    M27.40 Unspecified cyst of jaw
       Cyst of jaw NOS

    M27.49 Other cysts of jaw
       Aneurysmal cyst of jaw
       Hemorrhagic cyst of jaw
       Traumatic cyst of jaw

✓5ᵗʰ **M27.5 Periradicular pathology associated with previous endodontic treatment**

    M27.51 Perforation of root canal space due to endodontic treatment

    M27.52 Endodontic overfill

    M27.53 Endodontic underfill

    M27.59 Other periradicular pathology associated with previous endodontic treatment

✓5ᵗʰ **M27.6 Endosseous dental implant failure**

    M27.61 Osseointegration failure of dental implant
       Hemorrhagic complications of dental implant placement
       Iatrogenic osseointegration failure of dental implant
       Osseointegration failure of dental implant due to complications of systemic disease
       Osseointegration failure of dental implant due to poor bone quality
       Pre-integration failure of dental implant NOS
       Pre-osseointegration failure of dental implant

    M27.62 Post-osseointegration biological failure of dental implant
       Failure of dental implant due to lack of attached gingiva
       Failure of dental implant due to occlusal trauma (caused by poor prosthetic design)
       Failure of dental implant due to parafunctional habits
       Failure of dental implant due to periodontal infection (peri-implantitis)
       Failure of dental implant due to poor oral hygiene
       Iatrogenic post-osseointegration failure of dental implant
       Post-osseointegration failure of dental implant due to complications of systemic disease

    M27.63 Post-osseointegration mechanical failure of dental implant
       Failure of dental prosthesis causing loss of dental implant
       Fracture of dental implant
> *EXCLUDES 2*   *cracked tooth (K03.81)*
> *fractured dental restorative material with loss of material (K08.531)*
> *fractured dental restorative material without loss of material (K08.530)*
> *fractured tooth (S02.5)*

    M27.69 Other endosseous dental implant failure
       Dental implant failure NOS

M27.8 Other specified diseases of jaws
    Cherubism   Unilateral condylar hyperplasia
    Exostosis   Unilateral condylar hypoplasia
    Fibrous dysplasia
> *EXCLUDES 1*   *jaw pain (R68.84)*

M27.9 Disease of jaws, unspecified

Systemic connective tissue disorders (M30-M36)

INCLUDES   autoimmune disease NOS
         collagen (vascular) disease NOS
         systemic autoimmune disease
         systemic collagen (vascular) disease
> *EXCLUDES 1*   *autoimmune disease, single organ or single cell-type—code to relevant condition category*

✓4ᵗʰ **M30 Polyarteritis nodosa and related conditions**
> *EXCLUDES 1*   *microscopic polyarteritis (M31.7)*

M30.0 Polyarteritis nodosa

M30.1 Polyarteritis with lung involvement [Churg-Strauss]
    Allergic granulomatous angiitis

M30.2 Juvenile polyarteritis

M30.3 Mucocutaneous lymph node syndrome [Kawasaki]

M30.8 Other conditions related to polyarteritis nodosa
    Polyangiitis overlap syndrome

✓4ᵗʰ **M31 Other necrotizing vasculopathies**

M31.0 Hypersensitivity angiitis
    Goodpasture's syndrome

M31.1 Thrombotic microangiopathy
    Thrombotic thrombocytopenic purpura

M31.2 Lethal midline granuloma

✓5ᵗʰ **M31.3 Wegener's granulomatosis**
    Necrotizing respiratory granulomatosis

    M31.30 Wegener's granulomatosis without renal involvement
       Wegener's granulomatosis NOS

    M31.31 Wegener's granulomatosis with renal involvement

M31.4 Aortic arch syndrome [Takayasu]

M31.5 Giant cell arteritis with polymyalgia rheumatica

M31.6 Other giant cell arteritis

M31.7 Microscopic polyangiitis
    Microscopic polyarteritis
> *EXCLUDES 1*   *polyarteritis nodosa (M30.0)*

M31.8 Other specified necrotizing vasculopathies
    Hypocomplementemic vasculitis
    Septic vasculitis

M31.9 Necrotizing vasculopathy, unspecified

✓4ᵗʰ **M32 Systemic lupus erythematosus (SLE)**
> *EXCLUDES 1*   *lupus erythematosus (discoid) (NOS) (L93.0)*

M32.0 Drug-induced systemic lupus erythematosus
    Use additional code for adverse effect, if applicable, to identify drug (T36-T50 with fifth or sixth character 5)

EXCLUDES 1 Not coded here   *EXCLUDES 2* Not included here   N Newborn Age: 0   P Pediatric Age: 0-17   M Maternity Age: 12-55   A Adult Age: 15-124

676   ICD-10-CM Draft (2015)

Diseases of the Musculoskeletal System and Connective Tissue

M32.1–M40.14

✓5th **M32.1** Systemic lupus erythematosus with organ or system involvement

    M32.10 **Systemic lupus erythematosus, organ or system involvement unspecified**

    M32.11 Endocarditis in systemic lupus erythematosus
        Libman-Sacks disease

    M32.12 Pericarditis in systemic lupus erythematosus
        Lupus pericarditis

    M32.13 Lung involvement in systemic lupus erythematosus
        Pleural effusion due to systemic lupus erythematosus

    M32.14 Glomerular disease in systemic lupus erythematosus
        Lupus renal disease NOS
        AHA: 2013, 4Q, 125

    M32.15 Tubulo-interstitial nephropathy in systemic lupus erythematosus

    M32.19 **Other** organ or system **involvement in systemic lupus erythematosus**

  M32.8 **Other forms of systemic lupus erythematosus**

  M32.9 **Systemic lupus erythematosus, unspecified**
    SLE NOS
    Systemic lupus erythematosus NOS
    Systemic lupus erythematosus without organ involvement

✓4th **M33** **Dermatopolymyositis**

✓5th **M33.0** Juvenile dermatopolymyositis

    M33.00 **Juvenile dermatopolymyositis, organ involvement unspecified**

    M33.01 **Juvenile dermatopolymyositis with** respiratory **involvement**

    M33.02 **Juvenile dermatopolymyositis with** myopathy

    M33.09 **Juvenile dermatopolymyositis with** other organ **involvement**

✓5th **M33.1** Other dermatopolymyositis

    M33.10 **Other dermatopolymyositis, organ involvement unspecified**

    M33.11 **Other dermatopolymyositis with** respiratory **involvement**

    M33.12 **Other dermatopolymyositis with** myopathy

    M33.19 **Other dermatopolymyositis with other organ involvement**

✓5th **M33.2** Polymyositis

    M33.20 **Polymyositis, organ involvement unspecified**

    M33.21 **Polymyositis with** respiratory **involvement**

    M33.22 **Polymyositis with** myopathy

    M33.29 **Polymyositis with** other organ **involvement**

✓5th **M33.9** Dermatopolymyositis, unspecified

    M33.90 **Dermatopolymyositis, unspecified, organ involvement unspecified**

    M33.91 **Dermatopolymyositis, unspecified with** respiratory **involvement**

    M33.92 **Dermatopolymyositis, unspecified with** myopathy

    M33.99 **Dermatopolymyositis, unspecified with other organ involvement**

✓4th **M34** **Systemic sclerosis [scleroderma]**
    EXCLUDES 1 circumscribed scleroderma (L94.0)
        neonatal scleroderma (P83.8)

  M34.0 Progressive systemic sclerosis

  M34.1 CR(E)ST syndrome
    Combination of calcinosis, Raynaud's phenomenon, esophageal dysfunction, sclerodactyly, telangiectasia

  M34.2 **Systemic sclerosis** induced by drug and chemical
    Code first poisoning due to drug or toxin, if applicable (T36-T65 with fifth or sixth character 1-4 or 6)
    Use additional code for adverse effect, if applicable, to identify drug (T36-T50 with fifth or sixth character 5)

✓5th **M34.8** Other forms of systemic sclerosis

    M34.81 **Systemic sclerosis with** lung **involvement**

    M34.82 **Systemic sclerosis with** myopathy

    M34.83 **Systemic sclerosis with** polyneuropathy

    M34.89 **Other systemic sclerosis**

  M34.9 **Systemic sclerosis, unspecified**

✓4th **M35** **Other systemic involvement of connective tissue**
    EXCLUDES 1 reactive perforating collagenosis (L87.1)

✓5th **M35.0** Sicca syndrome [Sjögren]

    M35.00 **Sicca syndrome, unspecified**

    M35.01 **Sicca syndrome with** keratoconjunctivitis

    M35.02 **Sicca syndrome with** lung **involvement**

    M35.03 **Sicca syndrome with** myopathy

    M35.04 **Sicca syndrome with** tubulo-interstitial nephropathy
        Renal tubular acidosis in sicca syndrome

    M35.09 **Sicca syndrome with other organ involvement**

  M35.1 **Other overlap syndromes**
    Mixed connective tissue disease
    EXCLUDES 1 polyangiitis overlap syndrome (M30.8)

  M35.2 **Behçet's disease**

  M35.3 **Polymyalgia rheumatica**
    EXCLUDES 1 polymyalgia rheumatica with giant cell arteritis (M31.5)

  M35.4 **Diffuse (eosinophilic) fasciitis**

  M35.5 **Multifocal fibrosclerosis**

  M35.6 **Relapsing panniculitis [Weber-Christian]**
    EXCLUDES 1 lupus panniculitis (L93.2)
        panniculitis NOS (M79.3-)

  M35.7 **Hypermobility syndrome**
    Familial ligamentous laxity
    EXCLUDES 1 Ehlers-Danlos syndrome (Q79.6)
        ligamentous laxity, NOS (M24.2-)

  M35.8 **Other specified systemic involvement of connective tissue**

  M35.9 **Systemic involvement of connective tissue, unspecified**
    Autoimmune disease (systemic) NOS
    Collagen (vascular) disease NOS

✓4th **M36** **Systemic disorders of connective tissue in diseases classified elsewhere**
    EXCLUDES 2 arthropathies in diseases classified elsewhere (M14.-)

  M36.0 *Dermato(poly)myositis in neoplastic disease*
    Code first underlying neoplasm (C00-D49)

  M36.1 *Arthropathy in neoplastic disease*
    Code first underlying neoplasm, such as:
        leukemia (C91-C95)
        malignant histiocytosis (C96.A)
        multiple myeloma (C90.0)

  M36.2 *Hemophilic arthropathy*
    Hemarthrosis in hemophilic arthropathy
    Code first underlying disease, such as:
        factor VIII deficiency (D66)
        with vascular defect (D68.0)
        factor IX deficiency (D67)
        hemophilia (classical) (D66)
        hemophilia B (D67)
        hemophilia C (D68.1)

  M36.3 *Arthropathy in other blood disorders*

  M36.4 *Arthropathy in hypersensitivity reactions classified elsewhere*
    Code first underlying disease, such as:
        Henoch (-Schönlein) purpura (D69.0)
        serum sickness (T80.6-)

  M36.8 *Systemic disorders of connective tissue in other diseases classified elsewhere*
    Code first underlying disease, such as:
        alkaptonuria (E70.2)
        hypogammaglobulinemia (D80.-)
        ochronosis (E70.2)

DORSOPATHIES (M40-M54)

Deforming dorsopathies (M40-M43)

✓4th **M40** **Kyphosis and lordosis**
    EXCLUDES 1 congenital kyphosis and lordosis (Q76.4)
        kyphoscoliosis (M41.-)
        postprocedural kyphosis and lordosis (M96.-)

✓5th **M40.0** Postural kyphosis
    EXCLUDES 1 osteochondrosis of spine (M42.-)

    M40.00 **Postural kyphosis, site unspecified**

    M40.03 **Postural kyphosis,** cervicothoracic **region**

    M40.04 **Postural kyphosis,** thoracic **region**

    M40.05 **Postural kyphosis,** thoracolumbar **region**

✓5th **M40.1** Other secondary kyphosis

    M40.10 **Other secondary kyphosis, site unspecified**

    M40.12 **Other secondary kyphosis,** cervical **region**

    M40.13 **Other secondary kyphosis,** cervicothoracic **region**

    M40.14 **Other secondary kyphosis,** thoracic **region**

✓ Additional Character Required   ✓x7th Xtension Alert   Unspecified Dx   Other Specified Dx   Manifestation   ▶◀ Revised Text   ● New Code   ▲ Revised Code Title

Diseases of the Musculoskeletal System and Connective Tissue

M40.15–M42.10

     M40.15   **Other secondary kyphosis,** thoracolumbar **region**

✓5ᵗʰ **M40.2** Other and unspecified kyphosis

    ✓6ᵗʰ **M40.20** Unspecified kyphosis
      M40.202   **Unspecified kyphosis,** cervical **region**
      M40.203   **Unspecified kyphosis,** cervicothoracic **region**
      M40.204   **Unspecified kyphosis,** thoracic **region**
      M40.205   **Unspecified kyphosis,** thoracolumbar **region**
      M40.209   **Unspecified kyphosis, site unspecified**

    ✓6ᵗʰ **M40.29** Other kyphosis
      M40.292   **Other kyphosis,** cervical **region**
      M40.293   **Other kyphosis,** cervicothoracic **region**
      M40.294   **Other kyphosis,** thoracic **region**
      M40.295   **Other kyphosis,** thoracolumbar **region**
      M40.299   **Other kyphosis, site unspecified**

✓5ᵗʰ **M40.3** Flatback syndrome
     M40.30   **Flatback syndrome, site unspecified**
     M40.35   **Flatback syndrome,** thoracolumbar **region**
     M40.36   **Flatback syndrome,** lumbar **region**
     M40.37   **Flatback syndrome,** lumbosacral **region**

✓5ᵗʰ **M40.4** Postural lordosis
     Acquired lordosis
     M40.40   **Postural lordosis, site unspecified**
     M40.45   **Postural lordosis,** thoracolumbar **region**
     M40.46   **Postural lordosis,** lumbar **region**
     M40.47   **Postural lordosis,** lumbosacral **region**

✓5ᵗʰ **M40.5** Lordosis, unspecified
     M40.50   **Lordosis, unspecified, site unspecified**
     M40.55   **Lordosis, unspecified,** thoracolumbar **region**
     M40.56   **Lordosis, unspecified,** lumbar **region**
     M40.57   **Lordosis, unspecified,** lumbosacral **region**

✓4ᵗʰ **M41 Scoliosis**
    INCLUDES   kyphoscoliosis
    EXCLUDES 1   *congenital scoliosis due to bony malformation (Q76.3)*
      congenital scoliosis NOS (Q67.5)
      kyphoscoliotic heart disease (I27.1)
      postprocedural scoliosis (M96.-)
      postural congenital scoliosis (Q67.5)

✓5ᵗʰ **M41.0** Infantile idiopathic scoliosis
     M41.00   **Infantile idiopathic scoliosis, site unspecified**
     M41.02   **Infantile idiopathic scoliosis,** cervical **region**
     M41.03   **Infantile idiopathic scoliosis,** cervicothoracic **region**
     M41.04   **Infantile idiopathic scoliosis,** thoracic **region**
     M41.05   **Infantile idiopathic scoliosis,** thoracolumbar **region**
     M41.06   **Infantile idiopathic scoliosis,** lumbar **region**
     M41.07   **Infantile idiopathic scoliosis,** lumbosacral **region**
     M41.08   **Infantile idiopathic scoliosis,** sacral and sacrococcygeal **region**

✓5ᵗʰ **M41.1** Juvenile and adolescent idiopathic scoliosis

    ✓6ᵗʰ **M41.11** Juvenile idiopathic scoliosis
      M41.112   **Juvenile idiopathic scoliosis,** cervical **region**
      M41.113   **Juvenile idiopathic scoliosis,** cervicothoracic **region**
      M41.114   **Juvenile idiopathic scoliosis,** thoracic **region**
      M41.115   **Juvenile idiopathic scoliosis,** thoracolumbar **region**
      M41.116   **Juvenile idiopathic scoliosis,** lumbar **region**
      M41.117   **Juvenile idiopathic scoliosis,** lumbosacral **region**
      M41.119   **Juvenile idiopathic scoliosis, site unspecified**

    ✓6ᵗʰ **M41.12** Adolescent scoliosis
      M41.122   **Adolescent idiopathic scoliosis,** cervical **region**
      M41.123   **Adolescent idiopathic scoliosis,** cervicothoracic **region**
      M41.124   **Adolescent idiopathic scoliosis,** thoracic **region**
      M41.125   **Adolescent idiopathic scoliosis,** thoracolumbar **region**
      M41.126   **Adolescent idiopathic scoliosis,** lumbar **region**
      M41.127   **Adolescent idiopathic scoliosis,** lumbosacral **region**
      M41.129   **Adolescent idiopathic scoliosis, site unspecified**

✓5ᵗʰ **M41.2** Other idiopathic scoliosis
     M41.20   **Other idiopathic scoliosis, site unspecified**
     M41.22   **Other idiopathic scoliosis,** cervical **region**
     M41.23   **Other idiopathic scoliosis,** cervicothoracic **region**
     M41.24   **Other idiopathic scoliosis,** thoracic **region**
     M41.25   **Other idiopathic scoliosis,** thoracolumbar **region**
     M41.26   **Other idiopathic scoliosis,** lumbar **region**
     M41.27   **Other idiopathic scoliosis,** lumbosacral **region**

✓5ᵗʰ **M41.3** Thoracogenic scoliosis
     M41.30   **Thoracogenic scoliosis, site unspecified**
     M41.34   **Thoracogenic scoliosis,** thoracic **region**
     M41.35   **Thoracogenic scoliosis,** thoracolumbar **region**

✓5ᵗʰ **M41.4** Neuromuscular scoliosis
     Scoliosis secondary to cerebral palsy, Friedreich's ataxia, poliomyelitis and other neuromuscular disorders
     Code also underlying condition
     M41.40   **Neuromuscular scoliosis, site unspecified**
     M41.41   **Neuromuscular scoliosis,** occipito-atlanto-axial **region**
     M41.42   **Neuromuscular scoliosis,** cervical **region**
     M41.43   **Neuromuscular scoliosis,** cervicothoracic **region**
     M41.44   **Neuromuscular scoliosis,** thoracic **region**
     M41.45   **Neuromuscular scoliosis,** thoracolumbar **region**
     M41.46   **Neuromuscular scoliosis,** lumbar **region**
     M41.47   **Neuromuscular scoliosis,** lumbosacral **region**

✓5ᵗʰ **M41.5** Other secondary scoliosis
     M41.50   **Other secondary scoliosis, site unspecified**
     M41.52   **Other secondary scoliosis,** cervical **region**
     M41.53   **Other secondary scoliosis,** cervicothoracic **region**
     M41.54   **Other secondary scoliosis,** thoracic **region**
     M41.55   **Other secondary scoliosis,** thoracolumbar **region**
     M41.56   **Other secondary scoliosis,** lumbar **region**
     M41.57   **Other secondary scoliosis,** lumbosacral **region**

✓5ᵗʰ **M41.8** Other forms of scoliosis
     M41.80   **Other forms of scoliosis, site unspecified**
     M41.82   **Other forms of scoliosis,** cervical **region**
     M41.83   **Other forms of scoliosis,** cervicothoracic **region**
     M41.84   **Other forms of scoliosis,** thoracic **region**
     M41.85   **Other forms of scoliosis,** thoracolumbar **region**
     M41.86   **Other forms of scoliosis,** lumbar **region**
     M41.87   **Other forms of scoliosis,** lumbosacral **region**

     M41.9   **Scoliosis, unspecified**

✓4ᵗʰ **M42 Spinal osteochondrosis**

✓5ᵗʰ **M42.0** Juvenile osteochondrosis of spine
     Calvé's disease
     Scheuermann's disease
    EXCLUDES 1   *postural kyphosis (M40.0)*
     M42.00   **Juvenile osteochondrosis of spine, site unspecified**
     M42.01   **Juvenile osteochondrosis of spine,** occipito-atlanto-axial **region**
     M42.02   **Juvenile osteochondrosis of spine,** cervical **region**
     M42.03   **Juvenile osteochondrosis of spine,** cervicothoracic **region**
     M42.04   **Juvenile osteochondrosis of spine,** thoracic **region**
     M42.05   **Juvenile osteochondrosis of spine,** thoracolumbar **region**
     M42.06   **Juvenile osteochondrosis of spine,** lumbar **region**
     M42.07   **Juvenile osteochondrosis of spine,** lumbosacral **region**
     M42.08   **Juvenile osteochondrosis of spine,** sacral and sacrococcygeal **region**
     M42.09   **Juvenile osteochondrosis of spine,** multiple sites in **spine**

✓5ᵗʰ **M42.1** Adult osteochondrosis of spine
     M42.10   **Adult osteochondrosis of spine, site unspecified** 🄰

EXCLUDES 1 Not coded here   **EXCLUDES 2** Not included here   🄽 Newborn Age: 0   🄿 Pediatric Age: 0-17   🄼 Maternity Age: 12-55   🄰 Adult Age: 15-124

678   ICD-10-CM Draft (2015)

M42.11 **Adult osteochondrosis of spine, occipito-atlanto-axial region**   Ⓐ

M42.12 **Adult osteochondrosis of spine,** cervical **region**   Ⓐ

M42.13 **Adult osteochondrosis of spine,** cervicothoracic **region**   Ⓐ

M42.14 **Adult osteochondrosis of spine,** thoracic **region**   Ⓐ

M42.15 **Adult osteochondrosis of spine,** thoracolumbar **region**   Ⓐ

M42.16 **Adult osteochondrosis of spine,** lumbar **region**   Ⓐ

M42.17 **Adult osteochondrosis of spine,** lumbosacral **region**   Ⓐ

M42.18 **Adult osteochondrosis of spine,** sacral and sacrococcygeal **region**   Ⓐ

M42.19 **Adult osteochondrosis of spine,** multiple sites in spine   Ⓐ

M42.9 **Spinal osteochondrosis, unspecified**

✓4ᵗʰ **M43 Other deforming dorsopathies**

     EXCLUDES 1 *congenital spondylolysis and spondylolisthesis (Q76.2)*
hemivertebra (Q76.3-Q76.4)
Klippel-Feil syndrome (Q76.1)
lumbarization and sacralization (Q76.4)
platyspondylisis (Q76.4)
spina bifida occulta (Q76.0)
spinal curvature in osteoporosis (M80.-)
spinal curvature in Paget's disease of bone [osteitis deformans] (M88.-)

✓5ᵗʰ **M43.0 Spondylolysis**

     EXCLUDES 1 *congenital spondylolysis (Q76.2)*
spondylolisthesis (M43.1)

M43.00 **Spondylolysis, site unspecified**

M43.01 **Spondylolysis,** occipito-atlanto-axial **region**

M43.02 **Spondylolysis,** cervical **region**

M43.03 **Spondylolysis,** cervicothoracic **region**

M43.04 **Spondylolysis,** thoracic **region**

M43.05 **Spondylolysis,** thoracolumbar **region**

M43.06 **Spondylolysis,** lumbar **region**

M43.07 **Spondylolysis,** lumbosacral **region**

M43.08 **Spondylolysis,** sacral and sacrococcygeal **region**

M43.09 **Spondylolysis,** multiple sites in spine

✓5ᵗʰ **M43.1 Spondylolisthesis**

     EXCLUDES 1 *acute traumatic of lumbosacral region (S33.1)*
acute traumatic of sites other than lumbosacral— code to Fracture, vertebra, by region
congenital spondylolisthesis (Q76.2)

M43.10 **Spondylolisthesis, site unspecified**

M43.11 **Spondylolisthesis,** occipito-atlanto-axial **region**

M43.12 **Spondylolisthesis,** cervical **region**

M43.13 **Spondylolisthesis,** cervicothoracic **region**

M43.14 **Spondylolisthesis,** thoracic **region**

M43.15 **Spondylolisthesis,** thoracolumbar **region**

M43.16 **Spondylolisthesis,** lumbar **region**

M43.17 **Spondylolisthesis,** lumbosacral **region**

M43.18 **Spondylolisthesis,** sacral and sacrococcygeal **region**

M43.19 **Spondylolisthesis,** multiple sites in spine

✓5ᵗʰ **M43.2 Fusion of spine**

     Ankylosis of spinal joint

     EXCLUDES 1 *ankylosing spondylitis (M45.0-)*
congenital fusion of spine (Q76.4)

     EXCLUDES 2 *arthrodesis status (Z98.1)*
pseudoarthrosis after fusion or arthrodesis (M96.0)

M43.20 **Fusion of spine, site unspecified**

M43.21 **Fusion of spine,** occipito-atlanto-axial **region**

M43.22 **Fusion of spine,** cervical **region**

M43.23 **Fusion of spine,** cervicothoracic **region**

M43.24 **Fusion of spine,** thoracic **region**

M43.25 **Fusion of spine,** thoracolumbar **region**

M43.26 **Fusion of spine,** lumbar **region**

M43.27 **Fusion of spine,** lumbosacral **region**

M43.28 **Fusion of spine,** sacral and sacrococcygeal **region**

M43.3 **Recurrent atlantoaxial dislocation with myelopathy**

M43.4 **Other recurrent atlantoaxial dislocation**

✓5ᵗʰ **M43.5 Other recurrent vertebral dislocation**

     EXCLUDES 1 *biomechanical lesions NEC (M99.-)*

✓6ᵗʰ **M43.5X Other recurrent vertebral dislocation**

M43.5X2 **Other recurrent vertebral dislocation,** cervical **region**

M43.5X3 **Other recurrent vertebral dislocation,** cervicothoracic **region**

M43.5X4 **Other recurrent vertebral dislocation,** thoracic **region**

M43.5X5 **Other recurrent vertebral dislocation,** thoracolumbar **region**

M43.5X6 **Other recurrent vertebral dislocation,** lumbar **region**

M43.5X7 **Other recurrent vertebral dislocation,** lumbosacral **region**

M43.5X8 **Other recurrent vertebral dislocation,** sacral and sacrococcygeal **region**

M43.5X9 **Other recurrent vertebral dislocation, site unspecified**

M43.6 **Torticollis**

     EXCLUDES 1 *congenital (sternomastoid) torticollis (Q68.0)*
current injury—see Injury, of spine, by body region
ocular torticollis (R29.891)
psychogenic torticollis (F45.8)
spasmodic torticollis (G24.3)
torticollis due to birth injury (P15.2)

✓5ᵗʰ **M43.8 Other specified deforming dorsopathies**

     EXCLUDES 2 *kyphosis and lordosis (M40.-)*
scoliosis (M41.-)

✓6ᵗʰ **M43.8X Other specified deforming dorsopathies**

M43.8X1 **Other specified deforming dorsopathies,** occipito-atlanto-axial **region**

M43.8X2 **Other specified deforming dorsopathies,** cervical **region**

M43.8X3 **Other specified deforming dorsopathies,** cervicothoracic **region**

M43.8X4 **Other specified deforming dorsopathies,** thoracic **region**

M43.8X5 **Other specified deforming dorsopathies,** thoracolumbar **region**

M43.8X6 **Other specified deforming dorsopathies,** lumbar **region**

M43.8X7 **Other specified deforming dorsopathies,** lumbosacral **region**

M43.8X8 **Other specified deforming dorsopathies,** sacral and sacrococcygeal **region**

M43.8X9 **Other specified deforming dorsopathies, site unspecified**

M43.9 **Deforming dorsopathy, unspecified**
     Curvature of spine NOS

Spondylopathies (M45-M49)

✓4ᵗʰ **M45 Ankylosing spondylitis**
     Rheumatoid arthritis of spine

     EXCLUDES 1 *arthropathy in Reiter's disease (M02.3-)*
juvenile (ankylosing) spondylitis (M08.1)

     EXCLUDES 2 *Behçet's disease (M35.2)*

M45.0 **Ankylosing spondylitis of** multiple sites in spine

M45.1 **Ankylosing spondylitis of** occipito-atlanto-axial **region**

M45.2 **Ankylosing spondylitis of** cervical **region**

M45.3 **Ankylosing spondylitis of** cervicothoracic **region**

M45.4 **Ankylosing spondylitis of** thoracic **region**

M45.5 **Ankylosing spondylitis of** thoracolumbar **region**

M45.6 **Ankylosing spondylitis** lumbar **region**

M45.7 **Ankylosing spondylitis of** lumbosacral **region**

M45.8 **Ankylosing spondylitis** sacral and sacrococcygeal **region**

M45.9 **Ankylosing spondylitis of** unspecified sites in spine

✓4ᵗʰ **M46 Other inflammatory spondylopathies**

✓5ᵗʰ **M46.0 Spinal enthesopathy**
     Disorder of ligamentous or muscular attachments of spine

M46.00 **Spinal enthesopathy, site unspecified**

M46.01 **Spinal enthesopathy,** occipito-atlanto-axial **region**

M46.02 **Spinal enthesopathy,** cervical **region**

M46.03 **Spinal enthesopathy,** cervicothoracic **region**

M46.04 **Spinal enthesopathy,** thoracic **region**

☑ Additional Character Required   √x7ᵗʰ Xtension Alert   Unspecified Dx   Other Specified Dx   Manifestation   ►◄ Revised Text   ● New Code   ▲ Revised Code Title

ICD-10-CM Draft (2015)   **679**

M46.05 Spinal enthesopathy, thoracolumbar region
M46.06 Spinal enthesopathy, lumbar region
M46.07 Spinal enthesopathy, lumbosacral region
M46.08 Spinal enthesopathy, sacral and sacrococcygeal region
M46.09 Spinal enthesopathy, multiple sites in spine

M46.1 Sacroiliitis, not elsewhere classified

√5ᵗʰ M46.2 Osteomyelitis of vertebra
M46.20 Osteomyelitis of vertebra, site unspecified
M46.21 Osteomyelitis of vertebra, occipito-atlanto-axial region
M46.22 Osteomyelitis of vertebra, cervical region
M46.23 Osteomyelitis of vertebra, cervicothoracic region
M46.24 Osteomyelitis of vertebra, thoracic region
M46.25 Osteomyelitis of vertebra, thoracolumbar region
M46.26 Osteomyelitis of vertebra, lumbar region
M46.27 Osteomyelitis of vertebra, lumbosacral region
M46.28 Osteomyelitis of vertebra, sacral and sacrococcygeal region

√5ᵗʰ M46.3 Infection of intervertebral disc (pyogenic)
Use additional code (B95-B97) to identify infectious agent
M46.30 Infection of intervertebral disc (pyogenic), site unspecified
M46.31 Infection of intervertebral disc (pyogenic), occipito-atlanto-axial region
M46.32 Infection of intervertebral disc (pyogenic), cervical region
M46.33 Infection of intervertebral disc (pyogenic), cervicothoracic region
M46.34 Infection of intervertebral disc (pyogenic), thoracic region
M46.35 Infection of intervertebral disc (pyogenic), thoracolumbar region
M46.36 Infection of intervertebral disc (pyogenic), lumbar region
M46.37 Infection of intervertebral disc (pyogenic), lumbosacral region
M46.38 Infection of intervertebral disc (pyogenic), sacral and sacrococcygeal region
M46.39 Infection of intervertebral disc (pyogenic), multiple sites in spine

√5ᵗʰ M46.4 Discitis, unspecified
M46.40 Discitis, unspecified, site unspecified
M46.41 Discitis, unspecified, occipito-atlanto-axial region
M46.42 Discitis, unspecified, cervical region
M46.43 Discitis, unspecified, cervicothoracic region
M46.44 Discitis, unspecified, thoracic region
M46.45 Discitis, unspecified, thoracolumbar region
M46.46 Discitis, unspecified, lumbar region
M46.47 Discitis, unspecified, lumbosacral region
M46.48 Discitis, unspecified, sacral and sacrococcygeal region
M46.49 Discitis, unspecified, multiple sites in spine

√5ᵗʰ M46.5 Other infective spondylopathies
M46.50 Other infective spondylopathies, site unspecified
M46.51 Other infective spondylopathies, occipito-atlanto-axial region
M46.52 Other infective spondylopathies, cervical region
M46.53 Other infective spondylopathies, cervicothoracic region
M46.54 Other infective spondylopathies, thoracic region
M46.55 Other infective spondylopathies, thoracolumbar region
M46.56 Other infective spondylopathies, lumbar region
M46.57 Other infective spondylopathies, lumbosacral region
M46.58 Other infective spondylopathies, sacral and sacrococcygeal region
M46.59 Other infective spondylopathies, multiple sites in spine

√5ᵗʰ M46.8 Other specified inflammatory spondylopathies
M46.80 Other specified inflammatory spondylopathies, site unspecified

M46.81 Other specified inflammatory spondylopathies, occipito-atlanto-axial region
M46.82 Other specified inflammatory spondylopathies, cervical region
M46.83 Other specified inflammatory spondylopathies, cervicothoracic region
M46.84 Other specified inflammatory spondylopathies, thoracic region
M46.85 Other specified inflammatory spondylopathies, thoracolumbar region
M46.86 Other specified inflammatory spondylopathies, lumbar region
M46.87 Other specified inflammatory spondylopathies, lumbosacral region
M46.88 Other specified inflammatory spondylopathies, sacral and sacrococcygeal region
M46.89 Other specified inflammatory spondylopathies, multiple sites in spine

√5ᵗʰ M46.9 Unspecified inflammatory spondylopathy
M46.90 Unspecified inflammatory spondylopathy, site unspecified
M46.91 Unspecified inflammatory spondylopathy, occipito-atlanto-axial region
M46.92 Unspecified inflammatory spondylopathy, cervical region
M46.93 Unspecified inflammatory spondylopathy, cervicothoracic region
M46.94 Unspecified inflammatory spondylopathy, thoracic region
M46.95 Unspecified inflammatory spondylopathy, thoracolumbar region
M46.96 Unspecified inflammatory spondylopathy, lumbar region
M46.97 Unspecified inflammatory spondylopathy, lumbosacral region
M46.98 Unspecified inflammatory spondylopathy, sacral and sacrococcygeal region
M46.99 Unspecified inflammatory spondylopathy, multiple sites in spine

√4ᵗʰ M47 Spondylosis
INCLUDES arthrosis or osteoarthritis of spine
degeneration of facet joints

√5ᵗʰ M47.0 Anterior spinal and vertebral artery compression syndromes
√6ᵗʰ M47.01 Anterior spinal artery compression syndromes
M47.011 Anterior spinal artery compression syndromes, occipito-atlanto-axial region
M47.012 Anterior spinal artery compression syndromes, cervical region
M47.013 Anterior spinal artery compression syndromes, cervicothoracic region
M47.014 Anterior spinal artery compression syndromes, thoracic region
M47.015 Anterior spinal artery compression syndromes, thoracolumbar region
M47.016 Anterior spinal artery compression syndromes, lumbar region
M47.019 Anterior spinal artery compression syndromes, site unspecified

√6ᵗʰ M47.02 Vertebral artery compression syndromes
M47.021 Vertebral artery compression syndromes, occipito-atlanto-axial region
M47.022 Vertebral artery compression syndromes, cervical region
M47.029 Vertebral artery compression syndromes, site unspecified

√5ᵗʰ M47.1 Other spondylosis with myelopathy
Spondylogenic compression of spinal cord
EXCLUDES 1 vertebral subluxation (M43.3-M43.5X9)
M47.10 Other spondylosis with myelopathy, site unspecified
M47.11 Other spondylosis with myelopathy, occipito-atlanto-axial region
M47.12 Other spondylosis with myelopathy, cervical region
M47.13 Other spondylosis with myelopathy, cervicothoracic region
M47.14 Other spondylosis with myelopathy, thoracic region

EXCLUDES 1 Not coded here   EXCLUDES 2 Not included here   N Newborn Age: 0   P Pediatric Age: 0-17   M Maternity Age: 12-55   A Adult Age: 15-124

680   ICD-10-CM Draft (2015)

M47.15 **Other spondylosis with myelopathy,** thoracolumbar region

M47.16 **Other spondylosis with myelopathy,** lumbar **region**

✓5ᵗʰ M47.2 **Other spondylosis** with radiculopathy

M47.20 **Other spondylosis with radiculopathy, site unspecified**

M47.21 **Other spondylosis with radiculopathy,** occipito-atlanto-axial **region**

M47.22 **Other spondylosis with radiculopathy,** cervical **region**

M47.23 **Other spondylosis with radiculopathy,** cervicothoracic **region**

M47.24 **Other spondylosis with radiculopathy,** thoracic **region**

M47.25 **Other spondylosis with radiculopathy,** thoracolumbar **region**

M47.26 **Other spondylosis with radiculopathy,** lumbar **region**

M47.27 **Other spondylosis with radiculopathy,** lumbosacral **region**

M47.28 **Other spondylosis with radiculopathy,** sacral and sacrococcygeal **region**

✓5ᵗʰ M47.8 **Other spondylosis**

✓6ᵗʰ M47.81 **Spondylosis** without myelopathy or radiculopathy

M47.811 **Spondylosis without myelopathy or radiculopathy,** occipito-atlanto-axial region

M47.812 **Spondylosis without myelopathy or radiculopathy,** cervical **region**

M47.813 **Spondylosis without myelopathy or radiculopathy,** cervicothoracic **region**

M47.814 **Spondylosis without myelopathy or radiculopathy,** thoracic **region**

M47.815 **Spondylosis without myelopathy or radiculopathy,** thoracolumbar **region**

M47.816 **Spondylosis without myelopathy or radiculopathy,** lumbar **region**

M47.817 **Spondylosis without myelopathy or radiculopathy,** lumbosacral **region**

M47.818 **Spondylosis without myelopathy or radiculopathy,** sacral and sacrococcygeal region

M47.819 **Spondylosis without myelopathy or radiculopathy, site unspecified**

✓6ᵗʰ M47.89 **Other** spondylosis

M47.891 **Other spondylosis,** occipito-atlanto- axial region

M47.892 **Other spondylosis,** cervical **region**

M47.893 **Other spondylosis,** cervicothoracic **region**

M47.894 **Other spondylosis,** thoracic **region**

M47.895 **Other spondylosis,** thoracolumbar **region**

M47.896 **Other spondylosis,** lumbar **region**

M47.897 **Other spondylosis,** lumbosacral **region**

M47.898 **Other spondylosis,** sacral and sacrococcygeal **region**

M47.899 **Other spondylosis, site unspecified**

M47.9 **Spondylosis, unspecified**

✓4ᵗʰ **M48 Other spondylopathies**

✓5ᵗʰ M48.0 **Spinal stenosis**
Caudal stenosis

M48.00 **Spinal stenosis, site unspecified**

M48.01 **Spinal stenosis,** occipito-atlanto-axial **region**

M48.02 **Spinal stenosis,** cervical **region**

M48.03 **Spinal stenosis,** cervicothoracic **region**

M48.04 **Spinal stenosis,** thoracic **region**

M48.05 **Spinal stenosis,** thoracolumbar **region**

M48.06 **Spinal stenosis,** lumbar **region**

M48.07 **Spinal stenosis,** lumbosacral **region**

M48.08 **Spinal stenosis,** sacral and sacrococcygeal **region**

✓5ᵗʰ M48.1 **Ankylosing hyperostosis [Forestier]**
Diffuse idiopathic skeletal hyperostosis [DISH]

M48.10 **Ankylosing hyperostosis [Forestier], site unspecified**

M48.11 **Ankylosing hyperostosis [Forestier],** occipito-atlanto-axial **region**

M48.12 **Ankylosing hyperostosis [Forestier],** cervical **region**

M48.13 **Ankylosing hyperostosis [Forestier],** cervicothoracic region

M48.14 **Ankylosing hyperostosis [Forestier],** thoracic **region**

M48.15 **Ankylosing hyperostosis [Forestier],** thoracolumbar region

M48.16 **Ankylosing hyperostosis [Forestier],** lumbar **region**

M48.17 **Ankylosing hyperostosis [Forestier],** lumbosacral **region**

M48.18 **Ankylosing hyperostosis [Forestier],** sacral and sacrococcygeal **region**

M48.19 **Ankylosing hyperostosis [Forestier],** multiple sites in spine

✓5ᵗʰ M48.2 **Kissing spine**

M48.20 **Kissing spine, site unspecified**

M48.21 **Kissing spine,** occipito-atlanto-axial **region**

M48.22 **Kissing spine,** cervical **region**

M48.23 **Kissing spine,** cervicothoracic **region**

M48.24 **Kissing spine,** thoracic **region**

M48.25 **Kissing spine,** thoracolumbar **region**

M48.26 **Kissing spine,** lumbar **region**

M48.27 **Kissing spine,** lumbosacral **region**

✓5ᵗʰ M48.3 **Traumatic spondylopathy**

M48.30 **Traumatic spondylopathy, site unspecified**

M48.31 **Traumatic spondylopathy,** occipito-atlanto-axial region

M48.32 **Traumatic spondylopathy,** cervical **region**

M48.33 **Traumatic spondylopathy,** cervicothoracic **region**

M48.34 **Traumatic spondylopathy,** thoracic **region**

M48.35 **Traumatic spondylopathy,** thoracolumbar **region**

M48.36 **Traumatic spondylopathy,** lumbar **region**

M48.37 **Traumatic spondylopathy,** lumbosacral **region**

M48.38 **Traumatic spondylopathy,** sacral and sacrococcygeal region

✓5ᵗʰ M48.4 **Fatigue fracture of vertebra**
Stress fracture of vertebra
EXCLUDES 1 *pathological fracture NOS (M84.4-)*
pathological fracture of vertebra due to neoplasm (M84.58)
pathological fracture of vertebra due to other diagnosis (M84.68)
pathological fracture of vertebra due to osteoporosis (M80.-)
traumatic fracture of vertebrae (S12.0-S12.3-, S22.0-, S32.0-)

The appropriate 7th character is to be added to each code from subcategory M48.4.
A   initial encounter for fracture
D   subsequent encounter for fracture with routine healing
G   subsequent encounter for fracture with delayed healing
S   sequela of fracture

✓x7ᵗʰ M48.40 **Fatigue fracture of vertebra, site unspecified**

✓x7ᵗʰ M48.41 **Fatigue fracture of vertebra,** occipito-atlanto-axial region

✓x7ᵗʰ M48.42 **Fatigue fracture of vertebra,** cervical **region**

✓x7ᵗʰ M48.43 **Fatigue fracture of vertebra,** cervicothoracic **region**

✓x7ᵗʰ M48.44 **Fatigue fracture of vertebra,** thoracic **region**

✓x7ᵗʰ M48.45 **Fatigue fracture of vertebra,** thoracolumbar **region**

✓x7ᵗʰ M48.46 **Fatigue fracture of vertebra,** lumbar **region**

✓x7ᵗʰ M48.47 **Fatigue fracture of vertebra,** lumbosacral **region**

✓x7ᵗʰ M48.48 **Fatigue fracture of vertebra,** sacral and sacrococcygeal **region**

☑5ᵗʰ **M48.5　Collapsed vertebra, not elsewhere classified**
Collapsed vertebra NOS
Wedging of vertebra NOS
EXCLUDES 1　*current injury—see Injury of spine, by body region*
fatigue fracture of vertebra (M48.4)
pathological fracture of vertebra due to neoplasm
(M84.58)
pathological fracture of vertebra due to other diagnosis
(M84.68)
pathological fracture of vertebra due to osteoporosis
(M80.-)
pathological fracture NOS (M84.4-)
stress fracture of vertebra (M48.4-)
traumatic fracture of vertebra (S12-, S22-, S32-)

> The appropriate 7th character is to be added to each code
> from subcategory M48.5.
> A　initial encounter for fracture
> D　subsequent encounter for fracture with routine healing
> G　subsequent encounter for fracture with delayed healing
> S　sequela of fracture

☑x7ᵗʰ **M48.50　Collapsed vertebra, not elsewhere classified, site
unspecified**

☑x7ᵗʰ **M48.51　Collapsed vertebra, not elsewhere classified,
occipito-atlanto-axial region**

☑x7ᵗʰ **M48.52　Collapsed vertebra, not elsewhere classified, cervical
region**

☑x7ᵗʰ **M48.53　Collapsed vertebra, not elsewhere classified,
cervicothoracic region**

☑x7ᵗʰ **M48.54　Collapsed vertebra, not elsewhere classified,
thoracic region**

☑x7ᵗʰ **M48.55　Collapsed vertebra, not elsewhere classified,
thoracolumbar region**

☑x7ᵗʰ **M48.56　Collapsed vertebra, not elsewhere classified, lumbar
region**

☑x7ᵗʰ **M48.57　Collapsed vertebra, not elsewhere classified,
lumbosacral region**

☑x7ᵗʰ **M48.58　Collapsed vertebra, not elsewhere classified, sacral
and sacrococcygeal region**

☑5ᵗʰ **M48.8　Other specified spondylopathies**
Ossification of posterior longitudinal ligament

☑6ᵗʰ **M48.8X　Other specified spondylopathies**

**M48.8X1　Other specified spondylopathies,
occipito-atlanto-axial region**

**M48.8X2　Other specified spondylopathies, cervical
region**

**M48.8X3　Other specified spondylopathies,
cervicothoracic region**

**M48.8X4　Other specified spondylopathies, thoracic
region**

**M48.8X5　Other specified spondylopathies,
thoracolumbar region**

**M48.8X6　Other specified spondylopathies, lumbar
region**

**M48.8X7　Other specified spondylopathies,
lumbosacral region**

**M48.8X8　Other specified spondylopathies, sacral
and sacrococcygeal region**

**M48.8X9　Other specified spondylopathies, site
unspecified**

M48.9　Spondylopathy, unspecified

☑4ᵗʰ **M49　Spondylopathies in diseases classified elsewhere**
INCLUDES　curvature of spine in diseases classified elsewhere
deformity of spine in diseases classified elsewhere
kyphosis in diseases classified elsewhere
scoliosis in diseases classified elsewhere
spondylopathy in diseases classified elsewhere
Code first underlying disease, such as:
brucellosis (A23.-)
Charcôt-Marie-Tooth disease (G60.0)
enterobacterial infections (A01-A04)
osteitis fibrosa cystica (E21.0)
EXCLUDES 1　*curvature of spine in tuberculosis [Pott's] (A18.01)*
enteropathic arthropathies (M07.-)
gonococcal spondylitis (A54.41)
neuropathic [tabes dorsalis] spondylitis (A52.11)
neuropathic spondylopathy in syringomyelia (G95.0)
neuropathic spondylopathy in tabes dorsalis (A52.11)
nonsyphilitic neuropathic spondylopathy NEC (G98.0)
spondylitis in syphilis (acquired) (A52.77)
tuberculous spondylitis (A18.01)
typhoid fever spondylitis (A01.05)

☑5ᵗʰ **M49.8　Spondylopathy in diseases classified elsewhere**

*M49.80　Spondylopathy in diseases classified elsewhere,
site unspecified*

*M49.81　Spondylopathy in diseases classified elsewhere,
occipito-atlanto-axial region*

*M49.82　Spondylopathy in diseases classified elsewhere,
cervical region*

*M49.83　Spondylopathy in diseases classified elsewhere,
cervicothoracic region*

*M49.84　Spondylopathy in diseases classified elsewhere,
thoracic region*

*M49.85　Spondylopathy in diseases classified elsewhere,
thoracolumbar region*

*M49.86　Spondylopathy in diseases classified elsewhere,
lumbar region*

*M49.87　Spondylopathy in diseases classified elsewhere,
lumbosacral region*

*M49.88　Spondylopathy in diseases classified elsewhere,
sacral and sacrococcygeal region*

*M49.89　Spondylopathy in diseases classified elsewhere,
multiple sites in spine*

Other dorsopathies (M50-M54)

EXCLUDES 1　*current injury—see injury of spine by body region*
discitis NOS (M46.4-)

☑4ᵗʰ **M50　Cervical disc disorders**
NOTE　Code to the most superior level of disorder.
INCLUDES　cervicothoracic disc disorders with cervicalgia
cervicothoracic disc disorders

☑5ᵗʰ **M50.0　Cervical disc disorder with myelopathy**

**M50.00　Cervical disc disorder with myelopathy,
unspecified cervical region**

**M50.01　Cervical disc disorder with myelopathy, high cervical
region**
C2-C3 disc disorder with myelopathy
C3-C4 disc disorder with myelopathy

**M50.02　Cervical disc disorder with myelopathy, mid-cervical
region**
C4-C5 disc disorder with myelopathy
C5-C6 disc disorder with myelopathy
C6-C7 disc disorder with myelopathy

**M50.03　Cervical disc disorder with myelopathy,
cervicothoracic region**
C7-T1 disc disorder with myelopathy

☑5ᵗʰ **M50.1　Cervical disc disorder with radiculopathy**
EXCLUDES 2　*brachial radiculitis NOS (M54.13)*

**M50.10　Cervical disc disorder with radiculopathy,
unspecified cervical region**

**M50.11　Cervical disc disorder with radiculopathy, high
cervical region**
C2-C3 disc disorder with radiculopathy
C3 radiculopathy due to disc disorder
C3-C4 disc disorder with radiculopathy
C4 radiculopathy due to disc disorder

EXCLUDES 1 Not coded here　　　*EXCLUDES 2* Not included here　　　Ⓝ Newborn Age: 0　　　Ⓟ Pediatric Age: 0-17　　　Ⓜ Maternity Age: 12-55　　　Ⓐ Adult Age: 15-124

682　　ICD-10-CM Draft (2015)

M50.12 Cervical disc disorder with radiculopathy, mid-cervical region
C4-C5 disc disorder with radiculopathy
C5 radiculopathy due to disc disorder
C5-C6 disc disorder with radiculopathy
C6 radiculopathy due to disc disorder
C6-C7 disc disorder with radiculopathy
C7 radiculopathy due to disc disorder

M50.13 Cervical disc disorder with radiculopathy, cervicothoracic region
C7-T1 disc disorder with radiculopathy
C8 radiculopathy due to disc disorder

√5th **M50.2 Other cervical disc displacement**

M50.20 Other cervical disc displacement, unspecified cervical region

M50.21 Other cervical disc displacement, high cervical region
Other C2-C3 cervical disc displacement
Other C3-C4 cervical disc displacement

M50.22 Other cervical disc displacement, mid-cervical region
Other C4-C5 cervical disc displacement
Other C5-C6 cervical disc displacement
Other C6-C7 cervical disc displacement

M50.23 Other cervical disc displacement, cervicothoracic region
Other C7-T1 cervical disc displacement

√5th **M50.3 Other cervical disc degeneration**

M50.30 Other cervical disc degeneration, unspecified cervical region

M50.31 Other cervical disc degeneration, high cervical region
Other C2-C3 cervical disc degeneration
Other C3-C4 cervical disc degeneration

M50.32 Other cervical disc degeneration, mid-cervical region
Other C4-C5 cervical disc degeneration
Other C5-C6 cervical disc degeneration
Other C6-C7 cervical disc degeneration

M50.33 Other cervical disc degeneration, cervicothoracic region
Other C7-T1 cervical disc degeneration

√5th **M50.8 Other cervical disc disorders**

M50.80 Other cervical disc disorders, unspecified cervical region

M50.81 Other cervical disc disorders, high cervical region
Other C2-C3 cervical disc disorders
Other C3-C4 cervical disc disorders

M50.82 Other cervical disc disorders, mid-cervical region
Other C4-C5 cervical disc disorders
Other C5-C6 cervical disc disorders
Other C6-C7 cervical disc disorders

M50.83 Other cervical disc disorders, cervicothoracic region
Other C7-T1 cervical disc disorders

√5th **M50.9 Cervical disc disorder, unspecified**

M50.90 Cervical disc disorder, unspecified, unspecified cervical region

M50.91 Cervical disc disorder, unspecified, high cervical region
C2-C3 cervical disc disorder, unspecified
C3-C4 cervical disc disorder, unspecified

M50.92 Cervical disc disorder, unspecified, mid-cervical region
C4-C5 cervical disc disorder, unspecified
C5-C6 cervical disc disorder, unspecified
C6-C7 cervical disc disorder, unspecified

M50.93 Cervical disc disorder, unspecified, cervicothoracic region
C7-T1 cervical disc disorder, unspecified

√4th **M51 Thoracic, thoracolumbar, and lumbosacral intervertebral disc disorders**
EXCLUDES 2 *cervical and cervicothoracic disc disorders (M50.-)*
sacral and sacrococcygeal disorders (M53.3)

√5th **M51.0 Thoracic, thoracolumbar and lumbosacral intervertebral disc disorders with myelopathy**

M51.04 Intervertebral disc disorders with myelopathy, thoracic region

M51.05 Intervertebral disc disorders with myelopathy, thoracolumbar region

M51.06 Intervertebral disc disorders with myelopathy, lumbar region

√5th **M51.1 Thoracic, thoracolumbar and lumbosacral intervertebral disc disorders with radiculopathy**
Sciatica due to intervertebral disc disorder
EXCLUDES 1 *lumbar radiculitis NOS (M54.16)*
sciatica NOS (M54.3)

M51.14 Intervertebral disc disorders with radiculopathy, thoracic region

M51.15 Intervertebral disc disorders with radiculopathy, thoracolumbar region

M51.16 Intervertebral disc disorders with radiculopathy, lumbar region

M51.17 Intervertebral disc disorders with radiculopathy, lumbosacral region

√5th **M51.2 Other thoracic, thoracolumbar and lumbosacral intervertebral disc displacement**
Lumbago due to displacement of intervertebral disc

M51.24 Other intervertebral disc displacement, thoracic region

M51.25 Other intervertebral disc displacement, thoracolumbar region

M51.26 Other intervertebral disc displacement, lumbar region

M51.27 Other intervertebral disc displacement, lumbosacral region

√5th **M51.3 Other thoracic, thoracolumbar and lumbosacral intervertebral disc degeneration**
AHA: 2013, 3Q, 22

M51.34 Other intervertebral disc degeneration, thoracic region

M51.35 Other intervertebral disc degeneration, thoracolumbar region

M51.36 Other intervertebral disc degeneration, lumbar region

M51.37 Other intervertebral disc degeneration, lumbosacral region

√5th **M51.4 Schmorl's nodes**

M51.44 Schmorl's nodes, thoracic region

M51.45 Schmorl's nodes, thoracolumbar region

M51.46 Schmorl's nodes, lumbar region

M51.47 Schmorl's nodes, lumbosacral region

√5th **M51.8 Other thoracic, thoracolumbar and lumbosacral intervertebral disc disorders**

M51.84 Other intervertebral disc disorders, thoracic region

M51.85 Other intervertebral disc disorders, thoracolumbar region

M51.86 Other intervertebral disc disorders, lumbar region

M51.87 Other intervertebral disc disorders, lumbosacral region

M51.9 Unspecified thoracic, thoracolumbar and lumbosacral intervertebral disc disorder

√4th **M53 Other and unspecified dorsopathies, not elsewhere classified**

M53.0 Cervicocranial syndrome
Posterior cervical sympathetic syndrome

M53.1 Cervicobrachial syndrome
EXCLUDES 2 *cervical disc disorder (M50.-)*
thoracic outlet syndrome (G54.0)

√5th **M53.2 Spinal instabilities**

√6th **M53.2X Spinal instabilities**

M53.2X1 Spinal instabilities, occipito-atlanto-axial region

M53.2X2 Spinal instabilities, cervical region

M53.2X3 Spinal instabilities, cervicothoracic region

M53.2X4 Spinal instabilities, thoracic region

M53.2X5 Spinal instabilities, thoracolumbar region

M53.2X6 Spinal instabilities, lumbar region

M53.2X7 Spinal instabilities, lumbosacral region

M53.2X8 Spinal instabilities, sacral and sacrococcygeal region

M53.2X9 Spinal instabilities, site unspecified

M53.3 Sacrococcygeal disorders, not elsewhere classified
Coccygodynia

√5th **M53.8 Other specified dorsopathies**

M53.80 Other specified dorsopathies, site unspecified

Diseases of the Musculoskeletal System and Connective Tissue

M53.81–M60.069

M53.81 **Other specified dorsopathies,** occipito-atlanto-axial **region**

M53.82 **Other specified dorsopathies,** cervical **region**

M53.83 **Other specified dorsopathies,** cervicothoracic **region**

M53.84 **Other specified dorsopathies,** thoracic **region**

M53.85 **Other specified dorsopathies,** thoracolumbar **region**

M53.86 **Other specified dorsopathies,** lumbar **region**

M53.87 **Other specified dorsopathies,** lumbosacral **region**

M53.88 **Other specified dorsopathies,** sacral and sacrococcygeal **region**

M53.9 **Dorsopathy, unspecified**

✓4ᵗʰ **M54 Dorsalgia**
> EXCLUDES 1   psychogenic dorsalgia (F45.41)

  ✓5ᵗʰ **M54.0 Panniculitis affecting regions of neck and back**
> EXCLUDES 1   lupus panniculitis (L93.2)
> panniculitis NOS (M79.3)
> relapsing [Weber-Christian] panniculitis (M35.6)

M54.00 **Panniculitis affecting regions of neck and back, site unspecified**

M54.01 **Panniculitis affecting regions of neck and back,** occipito-atlanto-axial **region**

M54.02 **Panniculitis affecting regions of neck and back,** cervical **region**

M54.03 **Panniculitis affecting regions of neck and back,** cervicothoracic **region**

M54.04 **Panniculitis affecting regions of neck and back,** thoracic **region**

M54.05 **Panniculitis affecting regions of neck and back,** thoracolumbar **region**

M54.06 **Panniculitis affecting regions of neck and back,** lumbar **region**

M54.07 **Panniculitis affecting regions of neck and back,** lumbosacral **region**

M54.08 **Panniculitis affecting regions of neck and back,** sacral and sacrococcygeal **region**

M54.09 **Panniculitis affecting regions, neck and back,** multiple sites **in spine**

  ✓5ᵗʰ **M54.1 Radiculopathy**
> Brachial neuritis or radiculitis NOS
> Lumbar neuritis or radiculitis NOS
> Lumbosacral neuritis or radiculitis NOS
> Thoracic neuritis or radiculitis NOS
> Radiculitis NOS
> EXCLUDES 1   neuralgia and neuritis NOS (M79.2)
> radiculopathy with cervical disc disorder (M50.1)
> radiculopathy with lumbar and other intervertebral disc disorder (M51.1-)
> radiculopathy with spondylosis (M47.2-)

M54.10 **Radiculopathy, site unspecified**

M54.11 **Radiculopathy,** occipito-atlanto-axial **region**

M54.12 **Radiculopathy,** cervical **region**

M54.13 **Radiculopathy,** cervicothoracic **region**

M54.14 **Radiculopathy,** thoracic **region**

M54.15 **Radiculopathy,** thoracolumbar **region**

M54.16 **Radiculopathy,** lumbar **region**

M54.17 **Radiculopathy,** lumbosacral **region**

M54.18 **Radiculopathy,** sacral and sacrococcygeal **region**

M54.2 **Cervicalgia**
> EXCLUDES 1   cervicalgia due to intervertebral cervical disc disorder (M50.-)

  ✓5ᵗʰ **M54.3 Sciatica**
> EXCLUDES 1   lesion of sciatic nerve (G57.0)
> sciatica due to intervertebral disc disorder (M51.1-)
> sciatica with lumbago (M54.4-)

M54.30 **Sciatica, unspecified side**

M54.31 **Sciatica,** right **side**

M54.32 **Sciatica,** left **side**

  ✓5ᵗʰ **M54.4 Lumbago with sciatica**
> EXCLUDES 1   lumbago with sciatica due to intervertebral disc disorder (M51.1-)

M54.40 **Lumbago with sciatica, unspecified side**

M54.41 **Lumbago with sciatica,** right **side**

M54.42 **Lumbago with sciatica,** left **side**

M54.5 Low back pain
> Loin pain
> Lumbago NOS
> EXCLUDES 1   low back strain (S39.012)
> lumbago due to intervertebral disc displacement (M51.2-)
> lumbago with sciatica (M54.4-)

M54.6 Pain in thoracic spine
> EXCLUDES 1   pain in thoracic spine due to intervertebral disc disorder (M51.-)

✓5ᵗʰ **M54.8 Other dorsalgia**
> EXCLUDES 1   dorsalgia in thoracic region (M54.6)
> low back pain (M54.5)

M54.81 **Occipital neuralgia**

M54.89 **Other dorsalgia**

M54.9 Dorsalgia, unspecified
> Backache NOS   Back pain NOS

SOFT TISSUE DISORDERS (M60-M79)

Disorders of muscles (M60-M63)

> EXCLUDES 1   dermatopolymyositis (M33.-)
> muscular dystrophies and myopathies (G71-G72)
> myopathy in amyloidosis (E85.-)
> myopathy in polyarteritis nodosa (M30.0)
> myopathy in rheumatoid arthritis (M05.32)
> myopathy in scleroderma (M34.-)
> myopathy in Sjögren's syndrome (M35.03)
> myopathy in systemic lupus erythematosus (M32.-)

✓4ᵗʰ **M60 Myositis**
> EXCLUDES 2   inclusion body myositis [IBM] (G72.41)

  ✓5ᵗʰ **M60.0 Infective myositis**
> Tropical pyomyositis
> Use additional code (B95-B97) to identify infectious agent

   ✓6ᵗʰ **M60.00 Infective myositis,** unspecified site

M60.000 **Infective myositis, unspecified** right **arm**
> Infective myositis, right upper limb NOS

M60.001 **Infective myositis, unspecified** left **arm**
> Infective myositis, left upper limb NOS

M60.002 **Infective myositis, unspecified** arm
> Infective myositis, upper limb NOS

M60.003 **Infective myositis, unspecified** right **leg**
> Infective myositis, right lower limb NOS

M60.004 **Infective myositis, unspecified** left **leg**
> Infective myositis, left lower limb NOS

M60.005 **Infective myositis, unspecified** leg
> Infective myositis, lower limb NOS

M60.009 **Infective myositis, unspecified site**

   ✓6ᵗʰ **M60.01 Infective myositis,** shoulder

M60.011 **Infective myositis,** right **shoulder**

M60.012 **Infective myositis,** left **shoulder**

M60.019 **Infective myositis, unspecified shoulder**

   ✓6ᵗʰ **M60.02 Infective myositis,** upper arm

M60.021 **Infective myositis,** right **upper arm**

M60.022 **Infective myositis,** left **upper arm**

M60.029 **Infective myositis, unspecified upper arm**

   ✓6ᵗʰ **M60.03 Infective myositis,** forearm

M60.031 **Infective myositis,** right **forearm**

M60.032 **Infective myositis,** left **forearm**

M60.039 **Infective myositis, unspecified forearm**

   ✓6ᵗʰ **M60.04 Infective myositis,** hand and fingers

M60.041 **Infective myositis,** right **hand**

M60.042 **Infective myositis,** left **hand**

M60.043 **Infective myositis, unspecified hand**

M60.044 **Infective myositis,** right **finger(s)**

M60.045 **Infective myositis,** left **finger(s)**

M60.046 **Infective myositis, unspecified finger(s)**

   ✓6ᵗʰ **M60.05 Infective myositis,** thigh

M60.051 **Infective myositis,** right **thigh**

M60.052 **Infective myositis,** left **thigh**

M60.059 **Infective myositis, unspecified thigh**

   ✓6ᵗʰ **M60.06 Infective myositis,** lower leg

M60.061 **Infective myositis,** right **lower leg**

M60.062 **Infective myositis,** left **lower leg**

M60.069 **Infective myositis, unspecified lower leg**

EXCLUDES 1 Not coded here   EXCLUDES 2 Not included here   N Newborn Age: 0   P Pediatric Age: 0-17   M Maternity Age: 12-55   A Adult Age: 15-124

684   ICD-10-CM Draft (2015)

√6ᵗʰ **M60.07** Infective myositis, ankle, foot and toes
     M60.070 Infective myositis, right ankle
     M60.071 Infective myositis, left ankle
     M60.072 Infective myositis, unspecified ankle
     M60.073 Infective myositis, right foot
     M60.074 Infective myositis, left foot
     M60.075 Infective myositis, unspecified foot
     M60.076 Infective myositis, right toe(s)
     M60.077 Infective myositis, left toe(s)
     M60.078 Infective myositis, unspecified toe(s)
   M60.08 Infective myositis, other site
   M60.09 Infective myositis, multiple sites
√5ᵗʰ **M60.1** Interstitial myositis
   M60.10 Interstitial myositis of unspecified site
√6ᵗʰ **M60.11** Interstitial myositis, shoulder
     M60.111 Interstitial myositis, right shoulder
     M60.112 Interstitial myositis, left shoulder
     M60.119 Interstitial myositis, unspecified shoulder
√6ᵗʰ **M60.12** Interstitial myositis, upper arm
     M60.121 Interstitial myositis, right upper arm
     M60.122 Interstitial myositis, left upper arm
     M60.129 Interstitial myositis, unspecified upper arm
√6ᵗʰ **M60.13** Interstitial myositis, forearm
     M60.131 Interstitial myositis, right forearm
     M60.132 Interstitial myositis, left forearm
     M60.139 Interstitial myositis, unspecified forearm
√6ᵗʰ **M60.14** Interstitial myositis, hand
     M60.141 Interstitial myositis, right hand
     M60.142 Interstitial myositis, left hand
     M60.149 Interstitial myositis, unspecified hand
√6ᵗʰ **M60.15** Interstitial myositis, thigh
     M60.151 Interstitial myositis, right thigh
     M60.152 Interstitial myositis, left thigh
     M60.159 Interstitial myositis, unspecified thigh
√6ᵗʰ **M60.16** Interstitial myositis, lower leg
     M60.161 Interstitial myositis, right lower leg
     M60.162 Interstitial myositis, left lower leg
     M60.169 Interstitial myositis, unspecified lower leg
√6ᵗʰ **M60.17** Interstitial myositis, ankle and foot
     M60.171 Interstitial myositis, right ankle and foot
     M60.172 Interstitial myositis, left ankle and foot
     M60.179 Interstitial myositis, unspecified ankle and foot
   M60.18 Interstitial myositis, other site
   M60.19 Interstitial myositis, multiple sites
√5ᵗʰ **M60.2** Foreign body granuloma of soft tissue, not elsewhere classified
     Use additional code to identify the type of retained foreign body (Z18.-)
     EXCLUDES 1 *foreign body granuloma of skin and subcutaneous tissue (L92.3)*
   M60.20 Foreign body granuloma of soft tissue, not elsewhere classified, unspecified site
√6ᵗʰ **M60.21** Foreign body granuloma of soft tissue, not elsewhere classified, shoulder
     M60.211 Foreign body granuloma of soft tissue, not elsewhere classified, right shoulder
     M60.212 Foreign body granuloma of soft tissue, not elsewhere classified, left shoulder
     M60.219 Foreign body granuloma of soft tissue, not elsewhere classified, unspecified shoulder
√6ᵗʰ **M60.22** Foreign body granuloma of soft tissue, not elsewhere classified, upper arm
     M60.221 Foreign body granuloma of soft tissue, not elsewhere classified, right upper arm
     M60.222 Foreign body granuloma of soft tissue, not elsewhere classified, left upper arm
     M60.229 Foreign body granuloma of soft tissue, not elsewhere classified, unspecified upper arm

√6ᵗʰ **M60.23** Foreign body granuloma of soft tissue, not elsewhere classified, forearm
     M60.231 Foreign body granuloma of soft tissue, not elsewhere classified, right forearm
     M60.232 Foreign body granuloma of soft tissue, not elsewhere classified, left forearm
     M60.239 Foreign body granuloma of soft tissue, not elsewhere classified, unspecified forearm
√6ᵗʰ **M60.24** Foreign body granuloma of soft tissue, not elsewhere classified, hand
     M60.241 Foreign body granuloma of soft tissue, not elsewhere classified, right hand
     M60.242 Foreign body granuloma of soft tissue, not elsewhere classified, left hand
     M60.249 Foreign body granuloma of soft tissue, not elsewhere classified, unspecified hand
√6ᵗʰ **M60.25** Foreign body granuloma of soft tissue, not elsewhere classified, thigh
     M60.251 Foreign body granuloma of soft tissue, not elsewhere classified, right thigh
     M60.252 Foreign body granuloma of soft tissue, not elsewhere classified, left thigh
     M60.259 Foreign body granuloma of soft tissue, not elsewhere classified, unspecified thigh
√6ᵗʰ **M60.26** Foreign body granuloma of soft tissue, not elsewhere classified, lower leg
     M60.261 Foreign body granuloma of soft tissue, not elsewhere classified, right lower leg
     M60.262 Foreign body granuloma of soft tissue, not elsewhere classified, left lower leg
     M60.269 Foreign body granuloma of soft tissue, not elsewhere classified, unspecified lower leg
√6ᵗʰ **M60.27** Foreign body granuloma of soft tissue, not elsewhere classified, ankle and foot
     M60.271 Foreign body granuloma of soft tissue, not elsewhere classified, right ankle and foot
     M60.272 Foreign body granuloma of soft tissue, not elsewhere classified, left ankle and foot
     M60.279 Foreign body granuloma of soft tissue, not elsewhere classified, unspecified ankle and foot
   M60.28 Foreign body granuloma of soft tissue, not elsewhere classified, other site
√5ᵗʰ **M60.8** Other myositis
   M60.80 Other myositis, unspecified site
√6ᵗʰ **M60.81** Other myositis shoulder
     M60.811 Other myositis, right shoulder
     M60.812 Other myositis, left shoulder
     M60.819 Other myositis, unspecified shoulder
√6ᵗʰ **M60.82** Other myositis, upper arm
     M60.821 Other myositis, right upper arm
     M60.822 Other myositis, left upper arm
     M60.829 Other myositis, unspecified upper arm
√6ᵗʰ **M60.83** Other myositis, forearm
     M60.831 Other myositis, right forearm
     M60.832 Other myositis, left forearm
     M60.839 Other myositis, unspecified forearm
√6ᵗʰ **M60.84** Other myositis, hand
     M60.841 Other myositis, right hand
     M60.842 Other myositis, left hand
     M60.849 Other myositis, unspecified hand
√6ᵗʰ **M60.85** Other myositis, thigh
     M60.851 Other myositis, right thigh
     M60.852 Other myositis, left thigh
     M60.859 Other myositis, unspecified thigh
√6ᵗʰ **M60.86** Other myositis, lower leg
     M60.861 Other myositis, right lower leg
     M60.862 Other myositis, left lower leg
     M60.869 Other myositis, unspecified lower leg
√6ᵗʰ **M60.87** Other myositis, ankle and foot
     M60.871 Other myositis, right ankle and foot
     M60.872 Other myositis, left ankle and foot
     M60.879 Other myositis, unspecified ankle and foot
   M60.88 Other myositis, other site
   M60.89 Other myositis, multiple sites

☑ Additional Character Required   √ˣᵗʰ Xtension Alert   Unspecified Dx   Other Specified Dx   Manifestation   ▶◀ Revised Text   ● New Code   ▲ Revised Code Title

M60.9   Myositis, unspecified

✓4ᵗʰ M61   **Calcification and ossification of muscle**

    ✓5ᵗʰ M61.0   Myositis ossificans traumatica

       M61.00   Myositis ossificans traumatica, unspecified site

       ✓6ᵗʰ M61.01   Myositis ossificans traumatica, shoulder

          M61.011   Myositis ossificans traumatica, right shoulder

          M61.012   Myositis ossificans traumatica, left shoulder

          M61.019   Myositis ossificans traumatica, unspecified shoulder

       ✓6ᵗʰ M61.02   Myositis ossificans traumatica, upper arm

          M61.021   Myositis ossificans traumatica, right upper arm

          M61.022   Myositis ossificans traumatica, left upper arm

          M61.029   Myositis ossificans traumatica, unspecified upper arm

       ✓6ᵗʰ M61.03   Myositis ossificans traumatica, forearm

          M61.031   Myositis ossificans traumatica, right forearm

          M61.032   Myositis ossificans traumatica, left forearm

          M61.039   Myositis ossificans traumatica, unspecified forearm

       ✓6ᵗʰ M61.04   Myositis ossificans traumatica, hand

          M61.041   Myositis ossificans traumatica, right hand

          M61.042   Myositis ossificans traumatica, left hand

          M61.049   Myositis ossificans traumatica, unspecified hand

       ✓6ᵗʰ M61.05   Myositis ossificans traumatica, thigh

          M61.051   Myositis ossificans traumatica, right thigh

          M61.052   Myositis ossificans traumatica, left thigh

          M61.059   Myositis ossificans traumatica, unspecified thigh

       ✓6ᵗʰ M61.06   Myositis ossificans traumatica, lower leg

          M61.061   Myositis ossificans traumatica, right lower leg

          M61.062   Myositis ossificans traumatica, left lower leg

          M61.069   Myositis ossificans traumatica, unspecified lower leg

       ✓6ᵗʰ M61.07   Myositis ossificans traumatica, ankle and foot

          M61.071   Myositis ossificans traumatica, right ankle and foot

          M61.072   Myositis ossificans traumatica, left ankle and foot

          M61.079   Myositis ossificans traumatica, unspecified ankle and foot

       M61.08   Myositis ossificans traumatica, other site

       M61.09   Myositis ossificans traumatica, multiple sites

    ✓5ᵗʰ M61.1   Myositis ossificans progressiva

       Fibrodysplasia ossificans progressiva

       M61.10   Myositis ossificans progressiva, unspecified site

       ✓6ᵗʰ M61.11   Myositis ossificans progressiva, shoulder

          M61.111   Myositis ossificans progressiva, right shoulder

          M61.112   Myositis ossificans progressiva, left shoulder

          M61.119   Myositis ossificans progressiva, unspecified shoulder

       ✓6ᵗʰ M61.12   Myositis ossificans progressiva, upper arm

          M61.121   Myositis ossificans progressiva, right upper arm

          M61.122   Myositis ossificans progressiva, left upper arm

          M61.129   Myositis ossificans progressiva, unspecified arm

       ✓6ᵗʰ M61.13   Myositis ossificans progressiva, forearm

          M61.131   Myositis ossificans progressiva, right forearm

          M61.132   Myositis ossificans progressiva, left forearm

          M61.139   Myositis ossificans progressiva, unspecified forearm

       ✓6ᵗʰ M61.14   Myositis ossificans progressiva, hand and finger(s)

          M61.141   Myositis ossificans progressiva, right hand

          M61.142   Myositis ossificans progressiva, left hand

          M61.143   Myositis ossificans progressiva, unspecified hand

          M61.144   Myositis ossificans progressiva, right finger(s)

          M61.145   Myositis ossificans progressiva, left finger(s)

          M61.146   Myositis ossificans progressiva, unspecified finger(s)

       ✓6ᵗʰ M61.15   Myositis ossificans progressiva, thigh

          M61.151   Myositis ossificans progressiva, right thigh

          M61.152   Myositis ossificans progressiva, left thigh

          M61.159   Myositis ossificans progressiva, unspecified thigh

       ✓6ᵗʰ M61.16   Myositis ossificans progressiva, lower leg

          M61.161   Myositis ossificans progressiva, right lower leg

          M61.162   Myositis ossificans progressiva, left lower leg

          M61.169   Myositis ossificans progressiva, unspecified lower leg

       ✓6ᵗʰ M61.17   Myositis ossificans progressiva, ankle, foot and toe(s)

          M61.171   Myositis ossificans progressiva, right ankle

          M61.172   Myositis ossificans progressiva, left ankle

          M61.173   Myositis ossificans progressiva, unspecified ankle

          M61.174   Myositis ossificans progressiva, right foot

          M61.175   Myositis ossificans progressiva, left foot

          M61.176   Myositis ossificans progressiva, unspecified foot

          M61.177   Myositis ossificans progressiva, right toe(s)

          M61.178   Myositis ossificans progressiva, left toe(s)

          M61.179   Myositis ossificans progressiva, unspecified toe(s)

       M61.18   Myositis ossificans progressiva, other site

       M61.19   Myositis ossificans progressiva, multiple sites

    ✓5ᵗʰ M61.2   Paralytic calcification and ossification of muscle

       Myositis ossificans associated with quadriplegia or paraplegia

       M61.20   Paralytic calcification and ossification of muscle, unspecified site

       ✓6ᵗʰ M61.21   Paralytic calcification and ossification of muscle, shoulder

          M61.211   Paralytic calcification and ossification of muscle, right shoulder

          M61.212   Paralytic calcification and ossification of muscle, left shoulder

          M61.219   Paralytic calcification and ossification of muscle, unspecified shoulder

       ✓6ᵗʰ M61.22   Paralytic calcification and ossification of muscle, upper arm

          M61.221   Paralytic calcification and ossification of muscle, right upper arm

          M61.222   Paralytic calcification and ossification of muscle, left upper arm

          M61.229   Paralytic calcification and ossification of muscle, unspecified upper arm

       ✓6ᵗʰ M61.23   Paralytic calcification and ossification of muscle, forearm

          M61.231   Paralytic calcification and ossification of muscle, right forearm

          M61.232   Paralytic calcification and ossification of muscle, left forearm

          M61.239   Paralytic calcification and ossification of muscle, unspecified forearm

       ✓6ᵗʰ M61.24   Paralytic calcification and ossification of muscle, hand

          M61.241   Paralytic calcification and ossification of muscle, right hand

EXCLUDES 1 Not coded here   **EXCLUDES 2** Not included here   **N** Newborn Age: 0   **P** Pediatric Age: 0-17   **M** Maternity Age: 12-55   **A** Adult Age: 15-124

686   ICD-10-CM Draft (2015)

M61.242 Paralytic calcification and ossification of muscle, left hand

M61.249 Paralytic calcification and ossification of muscle, unspecified hand

✓6ᵗʰ M61.25 Paralytic calcification and ossification of muscle, thigh

M61.251 Paralytic calcification and ossification of muscle, right thigh

M61.252 Paralytic calcification and ossification of muscle, left thigh

M61.259 Paralytic calcification and ossification of muscle, unspecified thigh

✓6ᵗʰ M61.26 Paralytic calcification and ossification of muscle, lower leg

M61.261 Paralytic calcification and ossification of muscle, right lower leg

M61.262 Paralytic calcification and ossification of muscle, left lower leg

M61.269 Paralytic calcification and ossification of muscle, unspecified lower leg

✓6ᵗʰ M61.27 Paralytic calcification and ossification of muscle, ankle and foot

M61.271 Paralytic calcification and ossification of muscle, right ankle and foot

M61.272 Paralytic calcification and ossification of muscle, left ankle and foot

M61.279 Paralytic calcification and ossification of muscle, unspecified ankle and foot

M61.28 Paralytic calcification and ossification of muscle, other site

M61.29 Paralytic calcification and ossification of muscle, multiple sites

✓5ᵗʰ M61.3 Calcification and ossification of muscles associated with burns

Myositis ossificans associated with burns

M61.30 Calcification and ossification of muscles associated with burns, unspecified site

✓6ᵗʰ M61.31 Calcification and ossification of muscles associated with burns, shoulder

M61.311 Calcification and ossification of muscles associated with burns, right shoulder

M61.312 Calcification and ossification of muscles associated with burns, left shoulder

M61.319 Calcification and ossification of muscles associated with burns, unspecified shoulder

✓6ᵗʰ M61.32 Calcification and ossification of muscles associated with burns, upper arm

M61.321 Calcification and ossification of muscles associated with burns, right upper arm

M61.322 Calcification and ossification of muscles associated with burns, left upper arm

M61.329 Calcification and ossification of muscles associated with burns, unspecified upper arm

✓6ᵗʰ M61.33 Calcification and ossification of muscles associated with burns, forearm

M61.331 Calcification and ossification of muscles associated with burns, right forearm

M61.332 Calcification and ossification of muscles associated with burns, left forearm

M61.339 Calcification and ossification of muscles associated with burns, unspecified forearm

✓6ᵗʰ M61.34 Calcification and ossification of muscles associated with burns, hand

M61.341 Calcification and ossification of muscles associated with burns, right hand

M61.342 Calcification and ossification of muscles associated with burns, left hand

M61.349 Calcification and ossification of muscles associated with burns, unspecified hand

✓6ᵗʰ M61.35 Calcification and ossification of muscles associated with burns, thigh

M61.351 Calcification and ossification of muscles associated with burns, right thigh

M61.352 Calcification and ossification of muscles associated with burns, left thigh

M61.359 Calcification and ossification of muscles associated with burns, unspecified thigh

✓6ᵗʰ M61.36 Calcification and ossification of muscles associated with burns, lower leg

M61.361 Calcification and ossification of muscles associated with burns, right lower leg

M61.362 Calcification and ossification of muscles associated with burns, left lower leg

M61.369 Calcification and ossification of muscles associated with burns, unspecified lower leg

✓6ᵗʰ M61.37 Calcification and ossification of muscles associated with burns, ankle and foot

M61.371 Calcification and ossification of muscles associated with burns, right ankle and foot

M61.372 Calcification and ossification of muscles associated with burns, left ankle and foot

M61.379 Calcification and ossification of muscles associated with burns, unspecified ankle and foot

M61.38 Calcification and ossification of muscles associated with burns, other site

M61.39 Calcification and ossification of muscles associated with burns, multiple sites

✓5ᵗʰ M61.4 Other calcification of muscle

EXCLUDES 1 calcific tendinitis NOS (M65.2-)
calcific tendinitis of shoulder (M75.3)

M61.40 Other calcification of muscle, unspecified site

✓6ᵗʰ M61.41 Other calcification of muscle, shoulder

M61.411 Other calcification of muscle, right shoulder

M61.412 Other calcification of muscle, left shoulder

M61.419 Other calcification of muscle, unspecified shoulder

✓6ᵗʰ M61.42 Other calcification of muscle, upper arm

M61.421 Other calcification of muscle, right upper arm

M61.422 Other calcification of muscle, left upper arm

M61.429 Other calcification of muscle, unspecified upper arm

✓6ᵗʰ M61.43 Other calcification of muscle, forearm

M61.431 Other calcification of muscle, right forearm

M61.432 Other calcification of muscle, left forearm

M61.439 Other calcification of muscle, unspecified forearm

✓6ᵗʰ M61.44 Other calcification of muscle, hand

M61.441 Other calcification of muscle, right hand

M61.442 Other calcification of muscle, left hand

M61.449 Other calcification of muscle, unspecified hand

✓6ᵗʰ M61.45 Other calcification of muscle, thigh

M61.451 Other calcification of muscle, right thigh

M61.452 Other calcification of muscle, left thigh

M61.459 Other calcification of muscle, unspecified thigh

✓6ᵗʰ M61.46 Other calcification of muscle, lower leg

M61.461 Other calcification of muscle, right lower leg

M61.462 Other calcification of muscle, left lower leg

M61.469 Other calcification of muscle, unspecified lower leg

✓6ᵗʰ M61.47 Other calcification of muscle, ankle and foot

M61.471 Other calcification of muscle, right ankle and foot

M61.472 Other calcification of muscle, left ankle and foot

M61.479 Other calcification of muscle, unspecified ankle and foot

M61.48 Other calcification of muscle, other site

M61.49 Other calcification of muscle, multiple sites

✓5ᵗʰ M61.5 Other ossification of muscle

M61.50 Other ossification of muscle, unspecified site

✔ Additional Character Required ✔x7ᵗʰ Xtension Alert Unspecified Dx Other Specified Dx Manifestation ►◄ Revised Text ● New Code ▲ Revised Code Title

ICD-10-CM Draft (2015) 687

Diseases of the Musculoskeletal System and Connective Tissue

M61.51–M62.161

✓6ᵗʰ **M61.51 Other ossification of muscle,** shoulder
- **M61.511 Other ossification of muscle,** right shoulder
- **M61.512 Other ossification of muscle,** left shoulder
- **M61.519 Other ossification of muscle, unspecified** shoulder

✓6ᵗʰ **M61.52 Other ossification of muscle,** upper arm
- **M61.521 Other ossification of muscle,** right upper arm
- **M61.522 Other ossification of muscle,** left upper arm
- **M61.529 Other ossification of muscle, unspecified** upper arm

✓6ᵗʰ **M61.53 Other ossification of muscle,** forearm
- **M61.531 Other ossification of muscle,** right forearm
- **M61.532 Other ossification of muscle,** left forearm
- **M61.539 Other ossification of muscle, unspecified** forearm

✓6ᵗʰ **M61.54 Other ossification of muscle,** hand
- **M61.541 Other ossification of muscle,** right hand
- **M61.542 Other ossification of muscle,** left hand
- **M61.549 Other ossification of muscle, unspecified** hand

✓6ᵗʰ **M61.55 Other ossification of muscle,** thigh
- **M61.551 Other ossification of muscle,** right thigh
- **M61.552 Other ossification of muscle,** left thigh
- **M61.559 Other ossification of muscle, unspecified** thigh

✓6ᵗʰ **M61.56 Other ossification of muscle,** lower leg
- **M61.561 Other ossification of muscle,** right lower leg
- **M61.562 Other ossification of muscle,** left lower leg
- **M61.569 Other ossification of muscle, unspecified** lower leg

✓6ᵗʰ **M61.57 Other ossification of muscle,** ankle and foot
- **M61.571 Other ossification of muscle,** right ankle and foot
- **M61.572 Other ossification of muscle,** left ankle and foot
- **M61.579 Other ossification of muscle, unspecified** ankle and foot

M61.58 Other ossification of muscle, other site

M61.59 Other ossification of muscle, multiple sites

M61.9 Calcification and ossification of muscle, unspecified

✓4ᵗʰ **M62 Other disorders of muscle**

EXCLUDES 1   *alcoholic myopathy (G72.1)*
cramp and spasm (R25.2)
drug-induced myopathy (G72.0)
myalgia (M79.1)
stiff-man syndrome (G25.82)

EXCLUDES 2   *nontraumatic hematoma of muscle (M79.81)*

✓5ᵗʰ **M62.0 Separation of muscle (nontraumatic)**
Diastasis of muscle

EXCLUDES 1   *diastasis recti complicating pregnancy, labor and delivery (O71.8)*
traumatic separation of muscle—see strain of muscle by body region

M62.00 Separation of muscle (nontraumatic), unspecified site

✓6ᵗʰ **M62.01 Separation of muscle (nontraumatic),** shoulder
- **M62.011 Separation of muscle (nontraumatic),** right shoulder
- **M62.012 Separation of muscle (nontraumatic),** left shoulder
- **M62.019 Separation of muscle (nontraumatic), unspecified** shoulder

✓6ᵗʰ **M62.02 Separation of muscle (nontraumatic),** upper arm
- **M62.021 Separation of muscle (nontraumatic),** right upper arm
- **M62.022 Separation of muscle (nontraumatic),** left upper arm
- **M62.029 Separation of muscle (nontraumatic), unspecified** upper arm

✓6ᵗʰ **M62.03 Separation of muscle (nontraumatic),** forearm
- **M62.031 Separation of muscle (nontraumatic),** right forearm

---

- **M62.032 Separation of muscle (nontraumatic),** left forearm
- **M62.039 Separation of muscle (nontraumatic), unspecified** forearm

✓6ᵗʰ **M62.04 Separation of muscle (nontraumatic),** hand
- **M62.041 Separation of muscle (nontraumatic),** right hand
- **M62.042 Separation of muscle (nontraumatic),** left hand
- **M62.049 Separation of muscle (nontraumatic), unspecified** hand

✓6ᵗʰ **M62.05 Separation of muscle (nontraumatic),** thigh
- **M62.051 Separation of muscle (nontraumatic),** right thigh
- **M62.052 Separation of muscle (nontraumatic),** left thigh
- **M62.059 Separation of muscle (nontraumatic), unspecified** thigh

✓6ᵗʰ **M62.06 Separation of muscle (nontraumatic),** lower leg
- **M62.061 Separation of muscle (nontraumatic),** right lower leg
- **M62.062 Separation of muscle (nontraumatic),** left lower leg
- **M62.069 Separation of muscle (nontraumatic), unspecified** lower leg

✓6ᵗʰ **M62.07 Separation of muscle (nontraumatic),** ankle and foot
- **M62.071 Separation of muscle (nontraumatic),** right ankle and foot
- **M62.072 Separation of muscle (nontraumatic),** left ankle and foot
- **M62.079 Separation of muscle (nontraumatic), unspecified** ankle and foot

M62.08 Separation of muscle (nontraumatic), other site

✓5ᵗʰ **M62.1 Other rupture of muscle (nontraumatic)**

EXCLUDES 1   *traumatic rupture of muscle—see strain of muscle by body region*

EXCLUDES 2   *rupture of tendon (M66.-)*

M62.10 Other rupture of muscle (nontraumatic), unspecified site

✓6ᵗʰ **M62.11 Other rupture of muscle (nontraumatic),** shoulder
- **M62.111 Other rupture of muscle (nontraumatic),** right shoulder
- **M62.112 Other rupture of muscle (nontraumatic),** left shoulder
- **M62.119 Other rupture of muscle (nontraumatic), unspecified** shoulder

✓6ᵗʰ **M62.12 Other rupture of muscle (nontraumatic),** upper arm
- **M62.121 Other rupture of muscle (nontraumatic),** right upper arm
- **M62.122 Other rupture of muscle (nontraumatic),** left upper arm
- **M62.129 Other rupture of muscle (nontraumatic), unspecified** upper arm

✓6ᵗʰ **M62.13 Other rupture of muscle (nontraumatic),** forearm
- **M62.131 Other rupture of muscle (nontraumatic),** right forearm
- **M62.132 Other rupture of muscle (nontraumatic),** left forearm
- **M62.139 Other rupture of muscle (nontraumatic), unspecified** forearm

✓6ᵗʰ **M62.14 Other rupture of muscle (nontraumatic),** hand
- **M62.141 Other rupture of muscle (nontraumatic),** right hand
- **M62.142 Other rupture of muscle (nontraumatic),** left hand
- **M62.149 Other rupture of muscle (nontraumatic), unspecified** hand

✓6ᵗʰ **M62.15 Other rupture of muscle (nontraumatic),** thigh
- **M62.151 Other rupture of muscle (nontraumatic),** right thigh
- **M62.152 Other rupture of muscle (nontraumatic),** left thigh
- **M62.159 Other rupture of muscle (nontraumatic), unspecified** thigh

✓6ᵗʰ **M62.16 Other rupture of muscle (nontraumatic),** lower leg
- **M62.161 Other rupture of muscle (nontraumatic),** right lower leg

---

| EXCLUDES 1 Not coded here | EXCLUDES 2 Not included here | N Newborn Age: 0 | P Pediatric Age: 0-17 | M Maternity Age: 12-55 | A Adult Age: 15-124 |

688   ICD-10-CM Draft (2015)

M62.162 Other rupture of muscle (nontraumatic), left lower leg
M62.169 Other rupture of muscle (nontraumatic), unspecified lower leg

✓6th M62.17 Other rupture of muscle (nontraumatic), ankle and foot
M62.171 Other rupture of muscle (nontraumatic), right ankle and foot
M62.172 Other rupture of muscle (nontraumatic), left ankle and foot
M62.179 Other rupture of muscle (nontraumatic), unspecified ankle and foot

M62.18 Other rupture of muscle (nontraumatic), other site

✓5th M62.2 Nontraumatic ischemic infarction of muscle
EXCLUDES 1 compartment syndrome (traumatic) (T79.A-)
nontraumatic compartment syndrome (M79.A-)
rhabdomyolysis (M62.82)
traumatic ischemia of muscle (T79.6)
Volkmann's ischemic contracture (T79.6)

M62.20 Nontraumatic ischemic infarction of muscle, unspecified site

✓6th M62.21 Nontraumatic ischemic infarction of muscle, shoulder
M62.211 Nontraumatic ischemic infarction of muscle, right shoulder
M62.212 Nontraumatic ischemic infarction of muscle, left shoulder
M62.219 Nontraumatic ischemic infarction of muscle, unspecified shoulder

✓6th M62.22 Nontraumatic ischemic infarction of muscle, upper arm
M62.221 Nontraumatic ischemic infarction of muscle, right upper arm
M62.222 Nontraumatic ischemic infarction of muscle, left upper arm
M62.229 Nontraumatic ischemic infarction of muscle, unspecified upper arm

✓6th M62.23 Nontraumatic ischemic infarction of muscle, forearm
M62.231 Nontraumatic ischemic infarction of muscle, right forearm
M62.232 Nontraumatic ischemic infarction of muscle, left forearm
M62.239 Nontraumatic ischemic infarction of muscle, unspecified forearm

✓6th M62.24 Nontraumatic ischemic infarction of muscle, hand
M62.241 Nontraumatic ischemic infarction of muscle, right hand
M62.242 Nontraumatic ischemic infarction of muscle, left hand
M62.249 Nontraumatic ischemic infarction of muscle, unspecified hand

✓6th M62.25 Nontraumatic ischemic infarction of muscle, thigh
M62.251 Nontraumatic ischemic infarction of muscle, right thigh
M62.252 Nontraumatic ischemic infarction of muscle, left thigh
M62.259 Nontraumatic ischemic infarction of muscle, unspecified thigh

✓6th M62.26 Nontraumatic ischemic infarction of muscle, lower leg
M62.261 Nontraumatic ischemic infarction of muscle, right lower leg
M62.262 Nontraumatic ischemic infarction of muscle, left lower leg
M62.269 Nontraumatic ischemic infarction of muscle, unspecified lower leg

✓6th M62.27 Nontraumatic ischemic infarction of muscle, ankle and foot
M62.271 Nontraumatic ischemic infarction of muscle, right ankle and foot
M62.272 Nontraumatic ischemic infarction of muscle, left ankle and foot
M62.279 Nontraumatic ischemic infarction of muscle, unspecified ankle and foot

M62.28 Nontraumatic ischemic infarction of muscle, other site

M62.3 Immobility syndrome (paraplegic)

✓5th M62.4 Contracture of muscle
Contracture of tendon (sheath)
EXCLUDES 1 contracture of joint (M24.5-)

M62.40 Contracture of muscle, unspecified site

✓6th M62.41 Contracture of muscle, shoulder
M62.411 Contracture of muscle, right shoulder
M62.412 Contracture of muscle, left shoulder
M62.419 Contracture of muscle, unspecified shoulder

✓6th M62.42 Contracture of muscle, upper arm
M62.421 Contracture of muscle, right upper arm
M62.422 Contracture of muscle, left upper arm
M62.429 Contracture of muscle, unspecified upper arm

✓6th M62.43 Contracture of muscle, forearm
M62.431 Contracture of muscle, right forearm
M62.432 Contracture of muscle, left forearm
M62.439 Contracture of muscle, unspecified forearm

✓6th M62.44 Contracture of muscle, hand
M62.441 Contracture of muscle, right hand
M62.442 Contracture of muscle, left hand
M62.449 Contracture of muscle, unspecified hand

✓6th M62.45 Contracture of muscle, thigh
M62.451 Contracture of muscle, right thigh
M62.452 Contracture of muscle, left thigh
M62.459 Contracture of muscle, unspecified thigh

✓6th M62.46 Contracture of muscle, lower leg
M62.461 Contracture of muscle, right lower leg
M62.462 Contracture of muscle, left lower leg
M62.469 Contracture of muscle, unspecified lower leg

✓6th M62.47 Contracture of muscle, ankle and foot
M62.471 Contracture of muscle, right ankle and foot
M62.472 Contracture of muscle, left ankle and foot
M62.479 Contracture of muscle, unspecified ankle and foot

M62.48 Contracture of muscle, other site
M62.49 Contracture of muscle, multiple sites

✓5th M62.5 Muscle wasting and atrophy, not elsewhere classified
Disuse atrophy NEC
EXCLUDES 1 neuralgic amyotrophy (G54.5)
progressive muscular atrophy (G12.29)
EXCLUDES 2 pelvic muscle wasting (N81.84)

M62.50 Muscle wasting and atrophy, not elsewhere classified, unspecified site

✓6th M62.51 Muscle wasting and atrophy, not elsewhere classified, shoulder
M62.511 Muscle wasting and atrophy, not elsewhere classified, right shoulder
M62.512 Muscle wasting and atrophy, not elsewhere classified, left shoulder
M62.519 Muscle wasting and atrophy, not elsewhere classified, unspecified shoulder

✓6th M62.52 Muscle wasting and atrophy, not elsewhere classified, upper arm
M62.521 Muscle wasting and atrophy, not elsewhere classified, right upper arm
M62.522 Muscle wasting and atrophy, not elsewhere classified, left upper arm
M62.529 Muscle wasting and atrophy, not elsewhere classified, unspecified upper arm

✓6th M62.53 Muscle wasting and atrophy, not elsewhere classified, forearm
M62.531 Muscle wasting and atrophy, not elsewhere classified, right forearm
M62.532 Muscle wasting and atrophy, not elsewhere classified, left forearm
M62.539 Muscle wasting and atrophy, not elsewhere classified, unspecified forearm

✓6ᵗʰ **M62.54** Muscle wasting and atrophy, not elsewhere classified, hand

M62.541 Muscle wasting and atrophy, not elsewhere classified, right hand

M62.542 Muscle wasting and atrophy, not elsewhere classified, left hand

M62.549 Muscle wasting and atrophy, not elsewhere classified, unspecified hand

✓6ᵗʰ **M62.55** Muscle wasting and atrophy, not elsewhere classified, thigh

M62.551 Muscle wasting and atrophy, not elsewhere classified, right thigh

M62.552 Muscle wasting and atrophy, not elsewhere classified, left thigh

M62.559 Muscle wasting and atrophy, not elsewhere classified, unspecified thigh

✓6ᵗʰ **M62.56** Muscle wasting and atrophy, not elsewhere classified, lower leg

M62.561 Muscle wasting and atrophy, not elsewhere classified, right lower leg

M62.562 Muscle wasting and atrophy, not elsewhere classified, left lower leg

M62.569 Muscle wasting and atrophy, not elsewhere classified, unspecified lower leg

✓6ᵗʰ **M62.57** Muscle wasting and atrophy, not elsewhere classified, ankle and foot

M62.571 Muscle wasting and atrophy, not elsewhere classified, right ankle and foot

M62.572 Muscle wasting and atrophy, not elsewhere classified, left ankle and foot

M62.579 Muscle wasting and atrophy, not elsewhere classified, unspecified ankle and foot

M62.58 Muscle wasting and atrophy, not elsewhere classified, other site

M62.59 Muscle wasting and atrophy, not elsewhere classified, multiple sites

✓5ᵗʰ **M62.8** Other specified disorders of muscle

EXCLUDES 2　nontraumatic hematoma of muscle (M79.81)

M62.81 Muscle weakness (generalized)

M62.82 Rhabdomyolysis

EXCLUDES 1　traumatic rhabdomyolysis (T79.6)

✓6ᵗʰ **M62.83** Muscle spasm

M62.830 Muscle spasm of back

M62.831 Muscle spasm of calf
Charley-horse

M62.838 Other muscle spasm

M62.89 Other specified disorders of muscle
Muscle (sheath) hernia

M62.9 Disorder of muscle, unspecified

✓4ᵗʰ **M63** Disorders of muscle in diseases classified elsewhere

Code first underlying disease, such as:
leprosy (A30.-)
neoplasm (C49-, C79.89, D21-, D48.1)
schistosomiasis (B65.-)
trichinellosis (B75)

EXCLUDES 1　myopathy in cysticercosis (B69.81)
myopathy in endocrine diseases (G73.7)
myopathy in metabolic diseases (G73.7)
myopathy in sarcoidosis (D86.87)
myopathy in secondary syphilis (A51.49)
myopathy in syphilis (late) (A52.78)
myopathy in toxoplasmosis (B58.82)
myopathy in tuberculosis (A18.09)

✓5ᵗʰ **M63.8** Disorders of muscle in diseases classified elsewhere

M63.80 *Disorders of muscle in diseases classified elsewhere, unspecified site*

✓6ᵗʰ **M63.81** Disorders of muscle in diseases classified elsewhere, shoulder

M63.811 *Disorders of muscle in diseases classified elsewhere, right shoulder*

M63.812 *Disorders of muscle in diseases classified elsewhere, left shoulder*

M63.819 *Disorders of muscle in diseases classified elsewhere, unspecified shoulder*

✓6ᵗʰ **M63.82** Disorders of muscle in diseases classified elsewhere, upper arm

M63.821 *Disorders of muscle in diseases classified elsewhere, right upper arm*

M63.822 *Disorders of muscle in diseases classified elsewhere, left upper arm*

M63.829 *Disorders of muscle in diseases classified elsewhere, unspecified upper arm*

✓6ᵗʰ **M63.83** Disorders of muscle in diseases classified elsewhere, forearm

M63.831 *Disorders of muscle in diseases classified elsewhere, right forearm*

M63.832 *Disorders of muscle in diseases classified elsewhere, left forearm*

M63.839 *Disorders of muscle in diseases classified elsewhere, unspecified forearm*

✓6ᵗʰ **M63.84** Disorders of muscle in diseases classified elsewhere, hand

M63.841 *Disorders of muscle in diseases classified elsewhere, right hand*

M63.842 *Disorders of muscle in diseases classified elsewhere, left hand*

M63.849 *Disorders of muscle in diseases classified elsewhere, unspecified hand*

✓6ᵗʰ **M63.85** Disorders of muscle in diseases classified elsewhere, thigh

M63.851 *Disorders of muscle in diseases classified elsewhere, right thigh*

M63.852 *Disorders of muscle in diseases classified elsewhere, left thigh*

M63.859 *Disorders of muscle in diseases classified elsewhere, unspecified thigh*

✓6ᵗʰ **M63.86** Disorders of muscle in diseases classified elsewhere, lower leg

M63.861 *Disorders of muscle in diseases classified elsewhere, right lower leg*

M63.862 *Disorders of muscle in diseases classified elsewhere, left lower leg*

M63.869 *Disorders of muscle in diseases classified elsewhere, unspecified lower leg*

✓6ᵗʰ **M63.87** Disorders of muscle in diseases classified elsewhere, ankle and foot

M63.871 *Disorders of muscle in diseases classified elsewhere, right ankle and foot*

M63.872 *Disorders of muscle in diseases classified elsewhere, left ankle and foot*

M63.879 *Disorders of muscle in diseases classified elsewhere, unspecified ankle and foot*

M63.88 *Disorders of muscle in diseases classified elsewhere, other site*

M63.89 *Disorders of muscle in diseases classified elsewhere, multiple sites*

Disorders of synovium and tendon (M65-M67)

✓4ᵗʰ **M65** Synovitis and tenosynovitis

EXCLUDES 1　chronic crepitant synovitis of hand and wrist (M70.0-)
current injury—see injury of ligament or tendon by body region
soft tissue disorders related to use, overuse and pressure (M70.-)

✓5ᵗʰ **M65.0** Abscess of tendon sheath

Use additional code (B95-B96) to identify bacterial agent.

M65.00 Abscess of tendon sheath, unspecified site

✓6ᵗʰ **M65.01** Abscess of tendon sheath, shoulder

M65.011 Abscess of tendon sheath, right shoulder

M65.012 Abscess of tendon sheath, left shoulder

M65.019 Abscess of tendon sheath, unspecified shoulder

✓6ᵗʰ **M65.02** Abscess of tendon sheath, upper arm

M65.021 Abscess of tendon sheath, right upper arm

M65.022 Abscess of tendon sheath, left upper arm

M65.029 Abscess of tendon sheath, unspecified upper arm

✓6ᵗʰ **M65.03** Abscess of tendon sheath, forearm

M65.031 Abscess of tendon sheath, right forearm

M65.032 Abscess of tendon sheath, left forearm

M65.039 Abscess of tendon sheath, unspecified forearm

EXCLUDES 1 Not coded here　　　EXCLUDES 2 Not included here　　　N Newborn Age: 0　　　P Pediatric Age: 0-17　　　M Maternity Age: 12-55　　　A Adult Age: 15-124

690　　　ICD-10-CM Draft (2015)

✓6ᵗʰ **M65.04** Abscess of tendon sheath, hand
    M65.041 Abscess of tendon sheath, right hand
    M65.042 Abscess of tendon sheath, left hand
    M65.049 Abscess of tendon sheath, unspecified hand

✓6ᵗʰ **M65.05** Abscess of tendon sheath, thigh
    M65.051 Abscess of tendon sheath, right thigh
    M65.052 Abscess of tendon sheath, left thigh
    M65.059 Abscess of tendon sheath, unspecified thigh

✓6ᵗʰ **M65.06** Abscess of tendon sheath, lower leg
    M65.061 Abscess of tendon sheath, right lower leg
    M65.062 Abscess of tendon sheath, left lower leg
    M65.069 Abscess of tendon sheath, unspecified lower leg

✓6ᵗʰ **M65.07** Abscess of tendon sheath, ankle and foot
    M65.071 Abscess of tendon sheath, right ankle and foot
    M65.072 Abscess of tendon sheath, left ankle and foot
    M65.079 Abscess of tendon sheath, unspecified ankle and foot

  M65.08 Abscess of tendon sheath, other site

✓5ᵗʰ **M65.1** Other infective (teno)synovitis
  M65.10 Other infective (teno)synovitis, unspecified site

✓6ᵗʰ **M65.11** Other infective (teno)synovitis, shoulder
    M65.111 Other infective (teno)synovitis, right shoulder
    M65.112 Other infective (teno)synovitis, left shoulder
    M65.119 Other infective (teno)synovitis, unspecified shoulder

✓6ᵗʰ **M65.12** Other infective (teno)synovitis, elbow
    M65.121 Other infective (teno)synovitis, right elbow
    M65.122 Other infective (teno)synovitis, left elbow
    M65.129 Other infective (teno)synovitis, unspecified elbow

✓6ᵗʰ **M65.13** Other infective (teno)synovitis, wrist
    M65.131 Other infective (teno)synovitis, right wrist
    M65.132 Other infective (teno)synovitis, left wrist
    M65.139 Other infective (teno)synovitis, unspecified wrist

✓6ᵗʰ **M65.14** Other infective (teno)synovitis, hand
    M65.141 Other infective (teno)synovitis, right hand
    M65.142 Other infective (teno)synovitis, left hand
    M65.149 Other infective (teno)synovitis, unspecified hand

✓6ᵗʰ **M65.15** Other infective (teno)synovitis, hip
    M65.151 Other infective (teno)synovitis, right hip
    M65.152 Other infective (teno)synovitis, left hip
    M65.159 Other infective (teno)synovitis, unspecified hip

✓6ᵗʰ **M65.16** Other infective (teno)synovitis, knee
    M65.161 Other infective (teno)synovitis, right knee
    M65.162 Other infective (teno)synovitis, left knee
    M65.169 Other infective (teno)synovitis, unspecified knee

✓6ᵗʰ **M65.17** Other infective (teno)synovitis, ankle and foot
    M65.171 Other infective (teno)synovitis, right ankle and foot
    M65.172 Other infective (teno)synovitis, left ankle and foot
    M65.179 Other infective (teno)synovitis, unspecified ankle and foot

  M65.18 Other infective (teno)synovitis, other site
  M65.19 Other infective (teno)synovitis, multiple sites

✓5ᵗʰ **M65.2** Calcific tendinitis
  EXCLUDES 1 tendinitis as classified in M75-M77
            calcified tendinitis of shoulder (M75.3)

  M65.20 Calcific tendinitis, unspecified site

✓6ᵗʰ **M65.22** Calcific tendinitis, upper arm
    M65.221 Calcific tendinitis, right upper arm
    M65.222 Calcific tendinitis, left upper arm

    M65.229 Calcific tendinitis, unspecified upper arm

✓6ᵗʰ **M65.23** Calcific tendinitis, forearm
    M65.231 Calcific tendinitis, right forearm
    M65.232 Calcific tendinitis, left forearm
    M65.239 Calcific tendinitis, unspecified forearm

✓6ᵗʰ **M65.24** Calcific tendinitis, hand
    M65.241 Calcific tendinitis, right hand
    M65.242 Calcific tendinitis, left hand
    M65.249 Calcific tendinitis, unspecified hand

✓6ᵗʰ **M65.25** Calcific tendinitis, thigh
    M65.251 Calcific tendinitis, right thigh
    M65.252 Calcific tendinitis, left thigh
    M65.259 Calcific tendinitis, unspecified thigh

✓6ᵗʰ **M65.26** Calcific tendinitis, lower leg
    M65.261 Calcific tendinitis, right lower leg
    M65.262 Calcific tendinitis, left lower leg
    M65.269 Calcific tendinitis, unspecified lower leg

✓6ᵗʰ **M65.27** Calcific tendinitis, ankle and foot
    M65.271 Calcific tendinitis, right ankle and foot
    M65.272 Calcific tendinitis, left ankle and foot
    M65.279 Calcific tendinitis, unspecified ankle and foot

  M65.28 Calcific tendinitis, other site
  M65.29 Calcific tendinitis, multiple sites

M65.3 Trigger finger
  Nodular tendinous disease
  M65.30 Trigger finger, unspecified finger

✓6ᵗʰ **M65.31** Trigger thumb
    M65.311 Trigger thumb, right thumb
    M65.312 Trigger thumb, left thumb
    M65.319 Trigger thumb, unspecified thumb

✓6ᵗʰ **M65.32** Trigger finger, index finger
    M65.321 Trigger finger, right index finger
    M65.322 Trigger finger, left index finger
    M65.329 Trigger finger, unspecified index finger

✓6ᵗʰ **M65.33** Trigger finger, middle finger
    M65.331 Trigger finger, right middle finger
    M65.332 Trigger finger, left middle finger
    M65.339 Trigger finger, unspecified middle finger

✓6ᵗʰ **M65.34** Trigger finger, ring finger
    M65.341 Trigger finger, right ring finger
    M65.342 Trigger finger, left ring finger
    M65.349 Trigger finger, unspecified ring finger

✓6ᵗʰ **M65.35** Trigger finger, little finger
    M65.351 Trigger finger, right little finger
    M65.352 Trigger finger, left little finger
    M65.359 Trigger finger, unspecified little finger

M65.4 Radial styloid tenosynovitis [de Quervain]

✓5ᵗʰ **M65.8** Other synovitis and tenosynovitis
  M65.80 Other synovitis and tenosynovitis, unspecified site

✓6ᵗʰ **M65.81** Other synovitis and tenosynovitis, shoulder
    M65.811 Other synovitis and tenosynovitis, right shoulder
    M65.812 Other synovitis and tenosynovitis, left shoulder
    M65.819 Other synovitis and tenosynovitis, unspecified shoulder

✓6ᵗʰ **M65.82** Other synovitis and tenosynovitis, upper arm
    M65.821 Other synovitis and tenosynovitis, right upper arm
    M65.822 Other synovitis and tenosynovitis, left upper arm
    M65.829 Other synovitis and tenosynovitis, unspecified upper arm

✓6ᵗʰ **M65.83** Other synovitis and tenosynovitis, forearm
    M65.831 Other synovitis and tenosynovitis, right forearm
    M65.832 Other synovitis and tenosynovitis, left forearm
    M65.839 Other synovitis and tenosynovitis, unspecified forearm

---

✓ Additional Character Required   ✓x7ᵗʰ Xtension Alert   Unspecified Dx   Other Specified Dx   Manifestation   ►◄ Revised Text   ● New Code   ▲ Revised Code Title

Diseases of the Musculoskeletal System and Connective Tissue

M65.84–M66.322

√6ᵗʰ **M65.84** Other synovitis and tenosynovitis, hand
- **M65.841** Other synovitis and tenosynovitis, right hand
- **M65.842** Other synovitis and tenosynovitis, left hand
- **M65.849** Other synovitis and tenosynovitis, unspecified hand

√6ᵗʰ **M65.85** Other synovitis and tenosynovitis, thigh
- **M65.851** Other synovitis and tenosynovitis, right thigh
- **M65.852** Other synovitis and tenosynovitis, left thigh
- **M65.859** Other synovitis and tenosynovitis, unspecified thigh

√6ᵗʰ **M65.86** Other synovitis and tenosynovitis, lower leg
- **M65.861** Other synovitis and tenosynovitis, right lower leg
- **M65.862** Other synovitis and tenosynovitis, left lower leg
- **M65.869** Other synovitis and tenosynovitis, unspecified lower leg

√6ᵗʰ **M65.87** Other synovitis and tenosynovitis, ankle and foot
- **M65.871** Other synovitis and tenosynovitis, right ankle and foot
- **M65.872** Other synovitis and tenosynovitis, left ankle and foot
- **M65.879** Other synovitis and tenosynovitis, unspecified ankle and foot

M65.88 Other synovitis and tenosynovitis, other site

M65.89 Other synovitis and tenosynovitis, multiple sites

M65.9 Synovitis and tenosynovitis, unspecified

√4ᵗʰ **M66** Spontaneous rupture of synovium and tendon

INCLUDES rupture that occurs when a normal force is applied to tissues that are inferred to have less than normal strength

EXCLUDES 2 rotator cuff syndrome (M75.1-)
rupture where an abnormal force is applied to normal tissue—see injury of tendon by body region

M66.0 Rupture of popliteal cyst

√5ᵗʰ **M66.1** Rupture of synovium
Rupture of synovial cyst
EXCLUDES 2 rupture of popliteal cyst (M66.0)

- **M66.10** Rupture of synovium, unspecified joint

√6ᵗʰ **M66.11** Rupture of synovium, shoulder
- **M66.111** Rupture of synovium, right shoulder
- **M66.112** Rupture of synovium, left shoulder
- **M66.119** Rupture of synovium, unspecified shoulder

√6ᵗʰ **M66.12** Rupture of synovium, elbow
- **M66.121** Rupture of synovium, right elbow
- **M66.122** Rupture of synovium, left elbow
- **M66.129** Rupture of synovium, unspecified elbow

√6ᵗʰ **M66.13** Rupture of synovium, wrist
- **M66.131** Rupture of synovium, right wrist
- **M66.132** Rupture of synovium, left wrist
- **M66.139** Rupture of synovium, unspecified wrist

√6ᵗʰ **M66.14** Rupture of synovium, hand and fingers
- **M66.141** Rupture of synovium, right hand
- **M66.142** Rupture of synovium, left hand
- **M66.143** Rupture of synovium, unspecified hand
- **M66.144** Rupture of synovium, right finger(s)
- **M66.145** Rupture of synovium, left finger(s)
- **M66.146** Rupture of synovium, unspecified finger(s)

√6ᵗʰ **M66.15** Rupture of synovium, hip
- **M66.151** Rupture of synovium, right hip
- **M66.152** Rupture of synovium, left hip
- **M66.159** Rupture of synovium, unspecified hip

√6ᵗʰ **M66.17** Rupture of synovium, ankle, foot and toes
- **M66.171** Rupture of synovium, right ankle
- **M66.172** Rupture of synovium, left ankle
- **M66.173** Rupture of synovium, unspecified ankle
- **M66.174** Rupture of synovium, right foot
- **M66.175** Rupture of synovium, left foot
- **M66.176** Rupture of synovium, unspecified foot

- **M66.177** Rupture of synovium, right toe(s)
- **M66.178** Rupture of synovium, left toe(s)
- **M66.179** Rupture of synovium, unspecified toe(s)

M66.18 Rupture of synovium, other site

√5ᵗʰ **M66.2** Spontaneous rupture of extensor tendons
- **M66.20** Spontaneous rupture of extensor tendons, unspecified site

√6ᵗʰ **M66.21** Spontaneous rupture of extensor tendons, shoulder
- **M66.211** Spontaneous rupture of extensor tendons, right shoulder
- **M66.212** Spontaneous rupture of extensor tendons, left shoulder
- **M66.219** Spontaneous rupture of extensor tendons, unspecified shoulder

√6ᵗʰ **M66.22** Spontaneous rupture of extensor tendons, upper arm
- **M66.221** Spontaneous rupture of extensor tendons, right upper arm
- **M66.222** Spontaneous rupture of extensor tendons, left upper arm
- **M66.229** Spontaneous rupture of extensor tendons, unspecified upper arm

√6ᵗʰ **M66.23** Spontaneous rupture of extensor tendons, forearm
- **M66.231** Spontaneous rupture of extensor tendons, right forearm
- **M66.232** Spontaneous rupture of extensor tendons, left forearm
- **M66.239** Spontaneous rupture of extensor tendons, unspecified forearm

√6ᵗʰ **M66.24** Spontaneous rupture of extensor tendons, hand
- **M66.241** Spontaneous rupture of extensor tendons, right hand
- **M66.242** Spontaneous rupture of extensor tendons, left hand
- **M66.249** Spontaneous rupture of extensor tendons, unspecified hand

√6ᵗʰ **M66.25** Spontaneous rupture of extensor tendons, thigh
- **M66.251** Spontaneous rupture of extensor tendons, right thigh
- **M66.252** Spontaneous rupture of extensor tendons, left thigh
- **M66.259** Spontaneous rupture of extensor tendons, unspecified thigh

√6ᵗʰ **M66.26** Spontaneous rupture of extensor tendons, lower leg
- **M66.261** Spontaneous rupture of extensor tendons, right lower leg
- **M66.262** Spontaneous rupture of extensor tendons, left lower leg
- **M66.269** Spontaneous rupture of extensor tendons, unspecified lower leg

√6ᵗʰ **M66.27** Spontaneous rupture of extensor tendons, ankle and foot
- **M66.271** Spontaneous rupture of extensor tendons, right ankle and foot
- **M66.272** Spontaneous rupture of extensor tendons, left ankle and foot
- **M66.279** Spontaneous rupture of extensor tendons, unspecified ankle and foot

M66.28 Spontaneous rupture of extensor tendons, other site

M66.29 Spontaneous rupture of extensor tendons, multiple sites

√5ᵗʰ **M66.3** Spontaneous rupture of flexor tendons
- **M66.30** Spontaneous rupture of flexor tendons, unspecified site

√6ᵗʰ **M66.31** Spontaneous rupture of flexor tendons, shoulder
- **M66.311** Spontaneous rupture of flexor tendons, right shoulder
- **M66.312** Spontaneous rupture of flexor tendons, left shoulder
- **M66.319** Spontaneous rupture of flexor tendons, unspecified shoulder

√6ᵗʰ **M66.32** Spontaneous rupture of flexor tendons, upper arm
- **M66.321** Spontaneous rupture of flexor tendons, right upper arm
- **M66.322** Spontaneous rupture of flexor tendons, left upper arm

EXCLUDES 1 Not coded here   EXCLUDES 2 Not included here   N Newborn Age: 0   P Pediatric Age: 0-17   M Maternity Age: 12-55   A Adult Age: 15-124

692   ICD-10-CM Draft (2015)

M66.329 **Spontaneous rupture of flexor tendons, unspecified upper arm**

√6ᵗʰ M66.33 Spontaneous rupture of flexor tendons, forearm

M66.331 Spontaneous rupture of flexor tendons, right forearm

M66.332 Spontaneous rupture of flexor tendons, left forearm

M66.339 **Spontaneous rupture of flexor tendons, unspecified forearm**

√6ᵗʰ M66.34 Spontaneous rupture of flexor tendons, hand

M66.341 Spontaneous rupture of flexor tendons, right hand

M66.342 Spontaneous rupture of flexor tendons, left hand

M66.349 **Spontaneous rupture of flexor tendons, unspecified hand**

√6ᵗʰ M66.35 Spontaneous rupture of flexor tendons, thigh

M66.351 Spontaneous rupture of flexor tendons, right thigh

M66.352 Spontaneous rupture of flexor tendons, left thigh

M66.359 **Spontaneous rupture of flexor tendons, unspecified thigh**

√6ᵗʰ M66.36 Spontaneous rupture of flexor tendons, lower leg

M66.361 Spontaneous rupture of flexor tendons, right lower leg

M66.362 Spontaneous rupture of flexor tendons, left lower leg

M66.369 **Spontaneous rupture of flexor tendons, unspecified lower leg**

√6ᵗʰ M66.37 Spontaneous rupture of flexor tendons, ankle and foot

M66.371 Spontaneous rupture of flexor tendons, right ankle and foot

M66.372 Spontaneous rupture of flexor tendons, left ankle and foot

M66.379 **Spontaneous rupture of flexor tendons, unspecified ankle and foot**

M66.38 **Spontaneous rupture of flexor tendons, other site**

M66.39 Spontaneous rupture of flexor tendons, multiple sites

√5ᵗʰ M66.8 Spontaneous rupture of other tendons

M66.80 **Spontaneous rupture of other tendons, unspecified site**

√6ᵗʰ M66.81 Spontaneous rupture of other tendons, shoulder

M66.811 Spontaneous rupture of other tendons, right shoulder

M66.812 Spontaneous rupture of other tendons, left shoulder

M66.819 **Spontaneous rupture of other tendons, unspecified shoulder**

√6ᵗʰ M66.82 Spontaneous rupture of other tendons, upper arm

M66.821 Spontaneous rupture of other tendons, right upper arm

M66.822 Spontaneous rupture of other tendons, left upper arm

M66.829 **Spontaneous rupture of other tendons, unspecified upper arm**

√6ᵗʰ M66.83 Spontaneous rupture of other tendons, forearm

M66.831 Spontaneous rupture of other tendons, right forearm

M66.832 Spontaneous rupture of other tendons, left forearm

M66.839 **Spontaneous rupture of other tendons, unspecified forearm**

√6ᵗʰ M66.84 Spontaneous rupture of other tendons, hand

M66.841 Spontaneous rupture of other tendons, right hand

M66.842 Spontaneous rupture of other tendons, left hand

M66.849 **Spontaneous rupture of other tendons, unspecified hand**

√6ᵗʰ M66.85 Spontaneous rupture of other tendons, thigh

M66.851 Spontaneous rupture of other tendons, right thigh

M66.852 Spontaneous rupture of other tendons, left thigh

M66.859 **Spontaneous rupture of other tendons, unspecified thigh**

√6ᵗʰ M66.86 Spontaneous rupture of other tendons, lower leg

M66.861 Spontaneous rupture of other tendons, right lower leg

M66.862 Spontaneous rupture of other tendons, left lower leg

M66.869 **Spontaneous rupture of other tendons, unspecified lower leg**

√6ᵗʰ M66.87 Spontaneous rupture of other tendons, ankle and foot

M66.871 Spontaneous rupture of other tendons, right ankle and foot

M66.872 Spontaneous rupture of other tendons, left ankle and foot

M66.879 **Spontaneous rupture of other tendons, unspecified ankle and foot**

M66.88 **Spontaneous rupture of other tendons, other**

M66.89 Spontaneous rupture of other tendons, multiple sites

M66.9 **Spontaneous rupture of unspecified tendon**
Rupture at musculotendinous junction, nontraumatic

√4ᵗʰ **M67 Other disorders of synovium and tendon**
EXCLUDES 1 *palmar fascial fibromatosis [Dupuytren] (M72.0)*
tendinitis NOS (M77.9-)
xanthomatosis localized to tendons (E78.2)

√5ᵗʰ M67.0 Short Achilles tendon (acquired)

M67.00 **Short Achilles tendon (acquired), unspecified ankle**

M67.01 **Short Achilles tendon (acquired), right ankle**

M67.02 **Short Achilles tendon (acquired), left ankle**

√5ᵗʰ M67.2 Synovial hypertrophy, not elsewhere classified
EXCLUDES 1 *villonodular synovitis (pigmented) (M12.2-)*

M67.20 **Synovial hypertrophy, not elsewhere classified, unspecified site**

√6ᵗʰ M67.21 Synovial hypertrophy, not elsewhere classified, shoulder

M67.211 Synovial hypertrophy, not elsewhere classified, right shoulder

M67.212 Synovial hypertrophy, not elsewhere classified, left shoulder

M67.219 **Synovial hypertrophy, not elsewhere classified, unspecified shoulder**

√6ᵗʰ M67.22 Synovial hypertrophy, not elsewhere classified, upper arm

M67.221 Synovial hypertrophy, not elsewhere classified, right upper arm

M67.222 Synovial hypertrophy, not elsewhere classified, left upper arm

M67.229 **Synovial hypertrophy, not elsewhere classified, unspecified upper arm**

√6ᵗʰ M67.23 Synovial hypertrophy, not elsewhere classified, forearm

M67.231 Synovial hypertrophy, not elsewhere classified, right forearm

M67.232 Synovial hypertrophy, not elsewhere classified, left forearm

M67.239 **Synovial hypertrophy, not elsewhere classified, unspecified forearm**

√6ᵗʰ M67.24 Synovial hypertrophy, not elsewhere classified, hand

M67.241 Synovial hypertrophy, not elsewhere classified, right hand

M67.242 Synovial hypertrophy, not elsewhere classified, left hand

M67.249 **Synovial hypertrophy, not elsewhere classified, unspecified hand**

√6ᵗʰ M67.25 Synovial hypertrophy, not elsewhere classified, thigh

M67.251 Synovial hypertrophy, not elsewhere classified, right thigh

M67.252 Synovial hypertrophy, not elsewhere classified, left thigh

M67.259 **Synovial hypertrophy, not elsewhere classified, unspecified thigh**

✓6ᵗʰ **M67.26** **Synovial hypertrophy, not elsewhere classified, lower leg**

    M67.261 **Synovial hypertrophy, not elsewhere classified, right lower leg**

    M67.262 **Synovial hypertrophy, not elsewhere classified, left lower leg**

    M67.269 **Synovial hypertrophy, not elsewhere classified, unspecified lower leg**

✓6ᵗʰ **M67.27** **Synovial hypertrophy, not elsewhere classified, ankle and foot**

    M67.271 **Synovial hypertrophy, not elsewhere classified, right ankle and foot**

    M67.272 **Synovial hypertrophy, not elsewhere classified, left ankle and foot**

    M67.279 **Synovial hypertrophy, not elsewhere classified, unspecified ankle and foot**

    M67.28 **Synovial hypertrophy, not elsewhere classified, other site**

    M67.29 **Synovial hypertrophy, not elsewhere classified, multiple sites**

✓5ᵗʰ **M67.3** **Transient synovitis**

    Toxic synovitis

    EXCLUDES 1   *palindromic rheumatism (M12.3-)*

    M67.30 **Transient synovitis, unspecified site**

✓6ᵗʰ **M67.31** **Transient synovitis, shoulder**

    M67.311 **Transient synovitis, right shoulder**

    M67.312 **Transient synovitis, left shoulder**

    M67.319 **Transient synovitis, unspecified shoulder**

✓6ᵗʰ **M67.32** **Transient synovitis, elbow**

    M67.321 **Transient synovitis, right elbow**

    M67.322 **Transient synovitis, left elbow**

    M67.329 **Transient synovitis, unspecified elbow**

✓6ᵗʰ **M67.33** **Transient synovitis, wrist**

    M67.331 **Transient synovitis, right wrist**

    M67.332 **Transient synovitis, left wrist**

    M67.339 **Transient synovitis, unspecified wrist**

✓6ᵗʰ **M67.34** **Transient synovitis, hand**

    M67.341 **Transient synovitis, right hand**

    M67.342 **Transient synovitis, left hand**

    M67.349 **Transient synovitis, unspecified hand**

✓6ᵗʰ **M67.35** **Transient synovitis, hip**

    M67.351 **Transient synovitis, right hip**

    M67.352 **Transient synovitis, left hip**

    M67.359 **Transient synovitis, unspecified hip**

✓6ᵗʰ **M67.36** **Transient synovitis, knee**

    M67.361 **Transient synovitis, right knee**

    M67.362 **Transient synovitis, left knee**

    M67.369 **Transient synovitis, unspecified knee**

✓6ᵗʰ **M67.37** **Transient synovitis, ankle and foot**

    M67.371 **Transient synovitis, right ankle and foot**

    M67.372 **Transient synovitis, left ankle and foot**

    M67.379 **Transient synovitis, unspecified ankle and foot**

    M67.38 **Transient synovitis, other site**

    M67.39 **Transient synovitis, multiple sites**

✓5ᵗʰ **M67.4** **Ganglion**

    Ganglion of joint or tendon (sheath)

    EXCLUDES 1   *ganglion in yaws (A66.6)*

    EXCLUDES 2   *cyst of bursa (M71.2-M71.3)*
                 cyst of synovium (M71.2-M71.3)

    M67.40 **Ganglion, unspecified site**

✓6ᵗʰ **M67.41** **Ganglion, shoulder**

    M67.411 **Ganglion, right shoulder**

    M67.412 **Ganglion, left shoulder**

    M67.419 **Ganglion, unspecified shoulder**

✓6ᵗʰ **M67.42** **Ganglion, elbow**

    M67.421 **Ganglion, right elbow**

    M67.422 **Ganglion, left elbow**

    M67.429 **Ganglion, unspecified elbow**

✓6ᵗʰ **M67.43** **Ganglion, wrist**

    M67.431 **Ganglion, right wrist**

    M67.432 **Ganglion, left wrist**

    M67.439 **Ganglion, unspecified wrist**

✓6ᵗʰ **M67.44** **Ganglion, hand**

    M67.441 **Ganglion, right hand**

    M67.442 **Ganglion, left hand**

    M67.449 **Ganglion, unspecified hand**

✓6ᵗʰ **M67.45** **Ganglion, hip**

    M67.451 **Ganglion, right hip**

    M67.452 **Ganglion, left hip**

    M67.459 **Ganglion, unspecified hip**

✓6ᵗʰ **M67.46** **Ganglion, knee**

    M67.461 **Ganglion, right knee**

    M67.462 **Ganglion, left knee**

    M67.469 **Ganglion, unspecified knee**

✓6ᵗʰ **M67.47** **Ganglion, ankle and foot**

    M67.471 **Ganglion, right ankle and foot**

    M67.472 **Ganglion, left ankle and foot**

    M67.479 **Ganglion, unspecified ankle and foot**

    M67.48 **Ganglion, other site**

    M67.49 **Ganglion, multiple sites**

✓5ᵗʰ **M67.5** **Plica syndrome**

    Plica knee

    M67.50 **Plica syndrome, unspecified knee**

    M67.51 **Plica syndrome, right knee**

    M67.52 **Plica syndrome, left knee**

✓5ᵗʰ **M67.8** **Other specified disorders of synovium and tendon**

    M67.80 **Other specified disorders of synovium and tendon, unspecified site**

✓6ᵗʰ **M67.81** **Other specified disorders of synovium and tendon, shoulder**

    M67.811 **Other specified disorders of synovium, right shoulder**

    M67.812 **Other specified disorders of synovium, left shoulder**

    M67.813 **Other specified disorders of tendon, right shoulder**

    M67.814 **Other specified disorders of tendon, left shoulder**

    M67.819 **Other specified disorders of synovium and tendon, unspecified shoulder**

✓6ᵗʰ **M67.82** **Other specified disorders of synovium and tendon, elbow**

    M67.821 **Other specified disorders of synovium, right elbow**

    M67.822 **Other specified disorders of synovium, left elbow**

    M67.823 **Other specified disorders of tendon, right elbow**

    M67.824 **Other specified disorders of tendon, left elbow**

    M67.829 **Other specified disorders of synovium and tendon, unspecified elbow**

✓6ᵗʰ **M67.83** **Other specified disorders of synovium and tendon, wrist**

    M67.831 **Other specified disorders of synovium, right wrist**

    M67.832 **Other specified disorders of synovium, left wrist**

    M67.833 **Other specified disorders of tendon, right wrist**

    M67.834 **Other specified disorders of tendon, left wrist**

    M67.839 **Other specified disorders of synovium and tendon, unspecified forearm**

✓6ᵗʰ **M67.84** **Other specified disorders of synovium and tendon, hand**

    M67.841 **Other specified disorders of synovium, right hand**

    M67.842 **Other specified disorders of synovium, left hand**

    M67.843 **Other specified disorders of tendon, right hand**

    M67.844 **Other specified disorders of tendon, left hand**

    M67.849 **Other specified disorders of synovium and tendon, unspecified hand**

EXCLUDES 1 Not coded here   EXCLUDES 2 Not included here   N Newborn Age: 0   P Pediatric Age: 0-17   M Maternity Age: 12-55   A Adult Age: 15-124

694   ICD-10-CM Draft (2015)

✓6th **M67.85** Other specified disorders of synovium and tendon, hip

   M67.851 Other specified disorders of synovium, right hip

   M67.852 Other specified disorders of synovium, left hip

   M67.853 Other specified disorders of tendon, right hip

   M67.854 Other specified disorders of tendon, left hip

   M67.859 Other specified disorders of synovium and tendon, unspecified hip

✓6th **M67.86** Other specified disorders of synovium and tendon, knee

   M67.861 Other specified disorders of synovium, right knee

   M67.862 Other specified disorders of synovium, left knee

   M67.863 Other specified disorders of tendon, right knee

   M67.864 Other specified disorders of tendon, left knee

   M67.869 Other specified disorders of synovium and tendon, unspecified knee

✓6th **M67.87** Other specified disorders of synovium and tendon, ankle and foot

   M67.871 Other specified disorders of synovium, right ankle and foot

   M67.872 Other specified disorders of synovium, left ankle and foot

   M67.873 Other specified disorders of tendon, right ankle and foot

   M67.874 Other specified disorders of tendon, left ankle and foot

   M67.879 Other specified disorders of synovium and tendon, unspecified ankle and foot

   M67.88 Other specified disorders of synovium and tendon, other site

   M67.89 Other specified disorders of synovium and tendon, multiple sites

✓5th **M67.9** Unspecified disorder of synovium and tendon

   M67.90 Unspecified disorder of synovium and tendon, unspecified site

✓6th **M67.91** Unspecified disorder of synovium and tendon, shoulder

   M67.911 Unspecified disorder of synovium and tendon, right shoulder

   M67.912 Unspecified disorder of synovium and tendon, left shoulder

   M67.919 Unspecified disorder of synovium and tendon, unspecified shoulder

✓6th **M67.92** Unspecified disorder of synovium and tendon, upper arm

   M67.921 Unspecified disorder of synovium and tendon, right upper arm

   M67.922 Unspecified disorder of synovium and tendon, left upper arm

   M67.929 Unspecified disorder of synovium and tendon, unspecified upper arm

✓6th **M67.93** Unspecified disorder of synovium and tendon, forearm

   M67.931 Unspecified disorder of synovium and tendon, right forearm

   M67.932 Unspecified disorder of synovium and tendon, left forearm

   M67.939 Unspecified disorder of synovium and tendon, unspecified forearm

✓6th **M67.94** Unspecified disorder of synovium and tendon, hand

   M67.941 Unspecified disorder of synovium and tendon, right hand

   M67.942 Unspecified disorder of synovium and tendon, left hand

   M67.949 Unspecified disorder of synovium and tendon, unspecified hand

✓6th **M67.95** Unspecified disorder of synovium and tendon, thigh

   M67.951 Unspecified disorder of synovium and tendon, right thigh

   M67.952 Unspecified disorder of synovium and tendon, left thigh

   M67.959 Unspecified disorder of synovium and tendon, unspecified thigh

✓6th **M67.96** Unspecified disorder of synovium and tendon, lower leg

   M67.961 Unspecified disorder of synovium and tendon, right lower leg

   M67.962 Unspecified disorder of synovium and tendon, left lower leg

   M67.969 Unspecified disorder of synovium and tendon, unspecified lower leg

✓6th **M67.97** Unspecified disorder of synovium and tendon, ankle and foot

   M67.971 Unspecified disorder of synovium and tendon, right ankle and foot

   M67.972 Unspecified disorder of synovium and tendon, left ankle and foot

   M67.979 Unspecified disorder of synovium and tendon, unspecified ankle and foot

   M67.98 Unspecified disorder of synovium and tendon, other site

   M67.99 Unspecified disorder of synovium and tendon, multiple sites

Other soft tissue disorders (M70-M79)

✓4th **M70** **Soft tissue disorders related to use, overuse and pressure**

   INCLUDES soft tissue disorders of occupational origin

   Use additional external cause code to identify activity causing disorder (Y93.-)

   EXCLUDES 1 bursitis NOS (M71.9-)

   EXCLUDES 2 bursitis of shoulder (M75.5)
      enthesopathies (M76-M77)
      pressure ulcer (pressure area) (L89.-)

✓5th **M70.0** Crepitant synovitis (acute) (chronic) of hand and wrist

   ✓6th **M70.03** Crepitant synovitis (acute) (chronic), wrist

      M70.031 Crepitant synovitis (acute) (chronic), right wrist

      M70.032 Crepitant synovitis (acute) (chronic), left wrist

      M70.039 Crepitant synovitis (acute) (chronic), unspecified wrist

   ✓6th **M70.04** Crepitant synovitis (acute) (chronic), hand

      M70.041 Crepitant synovitis (acute) (chronic), right hand

      M70.042 Crepitant synovitis (acute) (chronic), left hand

      M70.049 Crepitant synovitis (acute) (chronic), unspecified hand

✓5th **M70.1** Bursitis of hand

   M70.10 Bursitis, unspecified hand

   M70.11 Bursitis, right hand

   M70.12 Bursitis, left hand

✓5th **M70.2** Olecranon bursitis

   M70.20 Olecranon bursitis, unspecified elbow

   M70.21 Olecranon bursitis, right elbow

   M70.22 Olecranon bursitis, left elbow

✓5th **M70.3** Other bursitis of elbow

   M70.30 Other bursitis of elbow, unspecified elbow

   M70.31 Other bursitis of elbow, right elbow

   M70.32 Other bursitis of elbow, left elbow

✓5th **M70.4** Prepatellar bursitis

   M70.40 Prepatellar bursitis, unspecified knee

   M70.41 Prepatellar bursitis, right knee

   M70.42 Prepatellar bursitis, left knee

✓5th **M70.5** Other bursitis of knee

   M70.50 Other bursitis of knee, unspecified knee

   M70.51 Other bursitis of knee, right knee

   M70.52 Other bursitis of knee, left knee

✓5th **M70.6** Trochanteric bursitis

   Trochanteric tendinitis

   M70.60 Trochanteric bursitis, unspecified hip

   M70.61 Trochanteric bursitis, right hip

   M70.62 Trochanteric bursitis, left hip

✓ Additional Character Required   ✓x7th Xtension Alert   Unspecified Dx   Other Specified Dx   Manifestation   ►◄ Revised Text   ● New Code   ▲ Revised Code Title

ICD-10-CM Draft (2015)   695

Diseases of the Musculoskeletal System and Connective Tissue

M70.7–M71.00

☑5ᵗʰ **M70.7** **Other bursitis of** hip
       Ischial bursitis
     M70.70 **Other bursitis of hip, unspecified hip**
     M70.71 **Other bursitis of hip,** right **hip**
     M70.72 **Other bursitis of hip,** left **hip**

☑5ᵗʰ **M70.8** **Other soft tissue disorders related to use, overuse and pressure**
     M70.80 **Other soft tissue disorders related to use, overuse and pressure of unspecified site**
     ☑6ᵗʰ **M70.81** **Other soft tissue disorders related to use, overuse and pressure of** shoulder
         M70.811 **Other soft tissue disorders related to use, overuse and pressure,** right **shoulder**
         M70.812 **Other soft tissue disorders related to use, overuse and pressure,** left **shoulder**
         M70.819 **Other soft tissue disorders related to use, overuse and pressure, unspecified shoulder**
     ☑6ᵗʰ **M70.82** **Other soft tissue disorders related to use, overuse and pressure of** upper arm
         M70.821 **Other soft tissue disorders related to use, overuse and pressure,** right **upper arm**
         M70.822 **Other soft tissue disorders related to use, overuse and pressure,** left **upper arm**
         M70.829 **Other soft tissue disorders related to use, overuse and pressure, unspecified upper arms**
     ☑6ᵗʰ **M70.83** **Other soft tissue disorders related to use, overuse and pressure of** forearm
         M70.831 **Other soft tissue disorders related to use, overuse and pressure,** right **forearm**
         M70.832 **Other soft tissue disorders related to use, overuse and pressure,** left **forearm**
         M70.839 **Other soft tissue disorders related to use, overuse and pressure, unspecified forearm**
     ☑6ᵗʰ **M70.84** **Other soft tissue disorders related to use, overuse and pressure of** hand
         M70.841 **Other soft tissue disorders related to use, overuse and pressure,** right **hand**
         M70.842 **Other soft tissue disorders related to use, overuse and pressure,** left **hand**
         M70.849 **Other soft tissue disorders related to use, overuse and pressure, unspecified hand**
     ☑6ᵗʰ **M70.85** **Other soft tissue disorders related to use, overuse and pressure of** thigh
         M70.851 **Other soft tissue disorders related to use, overuse and pressure,** right **thigh**
         M70.852 **Other soft tissue disorders related to use, overuse and pressure,** left **thigh**
         M70.859 **Other soft tissue disorders related to use, overuse and pressure, unspecified thigh**
     ☑6ᵗʰ **M70.86** **Other soft tissue disorders related to use, overuse and pressure** lower leg
         M70.861 **Other soft tissue disorders related to use, overuse and pressure,** right **lower leg**
         M70.862 **Other soft tissue disorders related to use, overuse and pressure,** left **lower leg**
         M70.869 **Other soft tissue disorders related to use, overuse and pressure, unspecified leg**
     ☑6ᵗʰ **M70.87** **Other soft tissue disorders related to use, overuse and pressure of** ankle and foot
         M70.871 **Other soft tissue disorders related to use, overuse and pressure,** right **ankle and foot**
         M70.872 **Other soft tissue disorders related to use, overuse and pressure,** left **ankle and foot**
         M70.879 **Other soft tissue disorders related to use, overuse and pressure, unspecified ankle and foot**
     M70.88 **Other soft tissue disorders related to use, overuse and pressure other site**
     M70.89 **Other soft tissue disorders related to use, overuse and pressure** multiple sites

☑5ᵗʰ **M70.9** **Unspecified soft tissue disorder related to use, overuse and pressure**
     M70.90 **Unspecified soft tissue disorder related to use, overuse and pressure of unspecified site**

☑6ᵗʰ **M70.91** **Unspecified soft tissue disorder related to use, overuse and pressure of** shoulder
     M70.911 **Unspecified soft tissue disorder related to use, overuse and pressure,** right **shoulder**
     M70.912 **Unspecified soft tissue disorder related to use, overuse and pressure,** left **shoulder**
     M70.919 **Unspecified soft tissue disorder related to use, overuse and pressure, unspecified shoulder**

☑6ᵗʰ **M70.92** **Unspecified soft tissue disorder related to use, overuse and pressure of** upper arm
     M70.921 **Unspecified soft tissue disorder related to use, overuse and pressure,** right **upper arm**
     M70.922 **Unspecified soft tissue disorder related to use, overuse and pressure,** left **upper arm**
     M70.929 **Unspecified soft tissue disorder related to use, overuse and pressure, unspecified upper arm**

☑6ᵗʰ **M70.93** **Unspecified soft tissue disorder related to use, overuse and pressure of** forearm
     M70.931 **Unspecified soft tissue disorder related to use, overuse and pressure,** right **forearm**
     M70.932 **Unspecified soft tissue disorder related to use, overuse and pressure,** left **forearm**
     M70.939 **Unspecified soft tissue disorder related to use, overuse and pressure, unspecified forearm**

☑6ᵗʰ **M70.94** **Unspecified soft tissue disorder related to use, overuse and pressure of** hand
     M70.941 **Unspecified soft tissue disorder related to use, overuse and pressure,** right **hand**
     M70.942 **Unspecified soft tissue disorder related to use, overuse and pressure,** left **hand**
     M70.949 **Unspecified soft tissue disorder related to use, overuse and pressure, unspecified hand**

☑6ᵗʰ **M70.95** **Unspecified soft tissue disorder related to use, overuse and pressure of** thigh
     M70.951 **Unspecified soft tissue disorder related to use, overuse and pressure,** right **thigh**
     M70.952 **Unspecified soft tissue disorder related to use, overuse and pressure,** left **thigh**
     M70.959 **Unspecified soft tissue disorder related to use, overuse and pressure, unspecified thigh**

☑6ᵗʰ **M70.96** **Unspecified soft tissue disorder related to use, overuse and pressure** lower leg
     M70.961 **Unspecified soft tissue disorder related to use, overuse and pressure,** right **lower leg**
     M70.962 **Unspecified soft tissue disorder related to use, overuse and pressure,** left **lower leg**
     M70.969 **Unspecified soft tissue disorder related to use, overuse and pressure, unspecified lower leg**

☑6ᵗʰ **M70.97** **Unspecified soft tissue disorder related to use, overuse and pressure of** ankle and foot
     M70.971 **Unspecified soft tissue disorder related to use, overuse and pressure,** right **ankle and foot**
     M70.972 **Unspecified soft tissue disorder related to use, overuse and pressure,** left **ankle and foot**
     M70.979 **Unspecified soft tissue disorder related to use, overuse and pressure, unspecified ankle and foot**

     M70.98 **Unspecified soft tissue disorder related to use, overuse and pressure other**
     M70.99 **Unspecified soft tissue disorder related to use, overuse and pressure** multiple sites

☑4ᵗʰ **M71** **Other bursopathies**
     EXCLUDES 1   bunion (M20.1)
         bursitis related to use, overuse or pressure (M70.-)
         enthesopathies (M76-M77)

☑5ᵗʰ **M71.0** **Abscess of bursa**
     Use additional code (B95.-, B96.-) to identify causative organism
     M71.00 **Abscess of bursa, unspecified site**

EXCLUDES 1 Not coded here   **EXCLUDES 2** Not included here   N Newborn Age: 0   P Pediatric Age: 0-17   M Maternity Age: 12-55   A Adult Age: 15-124

696   ICD-10-CM Draft (2015)

☑6ᵗʰ **M71.01 Abscess of bursa,** shoulder
　　M71.011 Abscess of bursa, right shoulder
　　M71.012 Abscess of bursa, left shoulder
　　M71.019 Abscess of bursa, unspecified shoulder
☑6ᵗʰ **M71.02 Abscess of bursa,** elbow
　　M71.021 Abscess of bursa, right elbow
　　M71.022 Abscess of bursa, left elbow
　　M71.029 Abscess of bursa, unspecified elbow
☑6ᵗʰ **M71.03 Abscess of bursa,** wrist
　　M71.031 Abscess of bursa, right wrist
　　M71.032 Abscess of bursa, left wrist
　　M71.039 Abscess of bursa, unspecified wrist
☑6ᵗʰ **M71.04 Abscess of bursa,** hand
　　M71.041 Abscess of bursa, right hand
　　M71.042 Abscess of bursa, left hand
　　M71.049 Abscess of bursa, unspecified hand
☑6ᵗʰ **M71.05 Abscess of bursa,** hip
　　M71.051 Abscess of bursa, right hip
　　M71.052 Abscess of bursa, left hip
　　M71.059 Abscess of bursa, unspecified hip
☑6ᵗʰ **M71.06 Abscess of bursa,** knee
　　M71.061 Abscess of bursa, right knee
　　M71.062 Abscess of bursa, left knee
　　M71.069 Abscess of bursa, unspecified knee
☑6ᵗʰ **M71.07 Abscess of bursa,** ankle and foot
　　M71.071 Abscess of bursa, right ankle and foot
　　M71.072 Abscess of bursa, left ankle and foot
　　M71.079 Abscess of bursa, unspecified ankle and foot
　M71.08 Abscess of bursa, other site
　M71.09 Abscess of bursa, multiple sites
☑5ᵗʰ **M71.1 Other infective bursitis**
　　Use additional code (B95.-, B96.-) to identify causative organism
　M71.10 Other infective bursitis, unspecified site
☑6ᵗʰ **M71.11 Other infective bursitis,** shoulder
　　M71.111 Other infective bursitis, right shoulder
　　M71.112 Other infective bursitis, left shoulder
　　M71.119 Other infective bursitis, unspecified shoulder
☑6ᵗʰ **M71.12 Other infective bursitis,** elbow
　　M71.121 Other infective bursitis, right elbow
　　M71.122 Other infective bursitis, left elbow
　　M71.129 Other infective bursitis, unspecified elbow
☑6ᵗʰ **M71.13 Other infective bursitis,** wrist
　　M71.131 Other infective bursitis, right wrist
　　M71.132 Other infective bursitis, left wrist
　　M71.139 Other infective bursitis, unspecified wrist
☑6ᵗʰ **M71.14 Other infective bursitis,** hand
　　M71.141 Other infective bursitis, right hand
　　M71.142 Other infective bursitis, left hand
　　M71.149 Other infective bursitis, unspecified hand
☑6ᵗʰ **M71.15 Other infective bursitis,** hip
　　M71.151 Other infective bursitis, right hip
　　M71.152 Other infective bursitis, left hip
　　M71.159 Other infective bursitis, unspecified hip
☑6ᵗʰ **M71.16 Other infective bursitis,** knee
　　M71.161 Other infective bursitis, right knee
　　M71.162 Other infective bursitis, left knee
　　M71.169 Other infective bursitis, unspecified knee
☑6ᵗʰ **M71.17 Other infective bursitis,** ankle and foot
　　M71.171 Other infective bursitis, right ankle and foot
　　M71.172 Other infective bursitis, left ankle and foot
　　M71.179 Other infective bursitis, unspecified ankle and foot
　M71.18 Other infective bursitis, other site
　M71.19 Other infective bursitis, multiple sites
☑5ᵗʰ **M71.2 Synovial cyst of popliteal space [Baker]**
　　EXCLUDES 1 synovial cyst of popliteal space with rupture (M66.0)
　M71.20 Synovial cyst of popliteal space [Baker], unspecified knee
　M71.21 Synovial cyst of popliteal space [Baker], right knee

　M71.22 Synovial cyst of popliteal space [Baker], left knee
☑5ᵗʰ **M71.3 Other bursal cyst**
　　Synovial cyst NOS
　　EXCLUDES 1 synovial cyst with rupture (M66.1-)
　M71.30 Other bursal cyst, unspecified site
☑6ᵗʰ **M71.31 Other bursal cyst,** shoulder
　　M71.311 Other bursal cyst, right shoulder
　　M71.312 Other bursal cyst, left shoulder
　　M71.319 Other bursal cyst, unspecified shoulder
☑6ᵗʰ **M71.32 Other bursal cyst,** elbow
　　M71.321 Other bursal cyst, right elbow
　　M71.322 Other bursal cyst, left elbow
　　M71.329 Other bursal cyst, unspecified elbow
☑6ᵗʰ **M71.33 Other bursal cyst,** wrist
　　M71.331 Other bursal cyst, right wrist
　　M71.332 Other bursal cyst, left wrist
　　M71.339 Other bursal cyst, unspecified wrist
☑6ᵗʰ **M71.34 Other bursal cyst,** hand
　　M71.341 Other bursal cyst, right hand
　　M71.342 Other bursal cyst, left hand
　　M71.349 Other bursal cyst, unspecified hand
☑6ᵗʰ **M71.35 Other bursal cyst,** hip
　　M71.351 Other bursal cyst, right hip
　　M71.352 Other bursal cyst, left hip
　　M71.359 Other bursal cyst, unspecified hip
☑6ᵗʰ **M71.37 Other bursal cyst,** ankle and foot
　　M71.371 Other bursal cyst, right ankle and foot
　　M71.372 Other bursal cyst, left ankle and foot
　　M71.379 Other bursal cyst, unspecified ankle and foot
　M71.38 Other bursal cyst, other site
　M71.39 Other bursal cyst, multiple sites
☑5ᵗʰ **M71.4 Calcium deposit in bursa**
　　EXCLUDES 2 calcium deposit in bursa of shoulder (M75.3)
　M71.40 Calcium deposit in bursa, unspecified site
☑6ᵗʰ **M71.42 Calcium deposit in bursa,** elbow
　　M71.421 Calcium deposit in bursa, right elbow
　　M71.422 Calcium deposit in bursa, left elbow
　　M71.429 Calcium deposit in bursa, unspecified elbow
☑6ᵗʰ **M71.43 Calcium deposit in bursa,** wrist
　　M71.431 Calcium deposit in bursa, right wrist
　　M71.432 Calcium deposit in bursa, left wrist
　　M71.439 Calcium deposit in bursa, unspecified wrist
☑6ᵗʰ **M71.44 Calcium deposit in bursa,** hand
　　M71.441 Calcium deposit in bursa, right hand
　　M71.442 Calcium deposit in bursa, left hand
　　M71.449 Calcium deposit in bursa, unspecified hand
☑6ᵗʰ **M71.45 Calcium deposit in bursa,** hip
　　M71.451 Calcium deposit in bursa, right hip
　　M71.452 Calcium deposit in bursa, left hip
　　M71.459 Calcium deposit in bursa, unspecified hip
☑6ᵗʰ **M71.46 Calcium deposit in bursa,** knee
　　M71.461 Calcium deposit in bursa, right knee
　　M71.462 Calcium deposit in bursa, left knee
　　M71.469 Calcium deposit in bursa, unspecified knee
☑6ᵗʰ **M71.47 Calcium deposit in bursa,** ankle and foot
　　M71.471 Calcium deposit in bursa, right ankle and foot
　　M71.472 Calcium deposit in bursa, left ankle and foot
　　M71.479 Calcium deposit in bursa, unspecified ankle and foot
　M71.48 Calcium deposit in bursa, other site
　M71.49 Calcium deposit in bursa, multiple sites

Diseases of the Musculoskeletal System and Connective Tissue

M71.5–M75.112

✓5ᵗʰ **M71.5 Other bursitis, not elsewhere classified**
    EXCLUDES 1   bursitis NOS (M71.9-)
    EXCLUDES 2   bursitis of shoulder (M75.5)
                  bursitis of tibial collateral [Pellegrini-Stieda] (M76.4)

    M71.50 Other bursitis, not elsewhere classified, unspecified site

✓6ᵗʰ   **M71.52 Other bursitis, not elsewhere classified, elbow**
        M71.521 Other bursitis, not elsewhere classified, right elbow
        M71.522 Other bursitis, not elsewhere classified, left elbow
        M71.529 Other bursitis, not elsewhere classified, unspecified elbow

✓6ᵗʰ   **M71.53 Other bursitis, not elsewhere classified, wrist**
        M71.531 Other bursitis, not elsewhere classified, right wrist
        M71.532 Other bursitis, not elsewhere classified, left wrist
        M71.539 Other bursitis, not elsewhere classified, unspecified wrist

✓6ᵗʰ   **M71.54 Other bursitis, not elsewhere classified, hand**
        M71.541 Other bursitis, not elsewhere classified, right hand
        M71.542 Other bursitis, not elsewhere classified, left hand
        M71.549 Other bursitis, not elsewhere classified, unspecified hand

✓6ᵗʰ   **M71.55 Other bursitis, not elsewhere classified, hip**
        M71.551 Other bursitis, not elsewhere classified, right hip
        M71.552 Other bursitis, not elsewhere classified, left hip
        M71.559 Other bursitis, not elsewhere classified, unspecified hip

✓6ᵗʰ   **M71.56 Other bursitis, not elsewhere classified, knee**
        M71.561 Other bursitis, not elsewhere classified, right knee
        M71.562 Other bursitis, not elsewhere classified, left knee
        M71.569 Other bursitis, not elsewhere classified, unspecified knee

✓6ᵗʰ   **M71.57 Other bursitis, not elsewhere classified, ankle and foot**
        M71.571 Other bursitis, not elsewhere classified, right ankle and foot
        M71.572 Other bursitis, not elsewhere classified, left ankle and foot
        M71.579 Other bursitis, not elsewhere classified, unspecified ankle and foot

    M71.58 Other bursitis, not elsewhere classified, other site

✓5ᵗʰ **M71.8 Other specified bursopathies**
    M71.80 Other specified bursopathies, unspecified site

✓6ᵗʰ   **M71.81 Other specified bursopathies, shoulder**
        M71.811 Other specified bursopathies, right shoulder
        M71.812 Other specified bursopathies, left shoulder
        M71.819 Other specified bursopathies, unspecified shoulder

✓6ᵗʰ   **M71.82 Other specified bursopathies, elbow**
        M71.821 Other specified bursopathies, right elbow
        M71.822 Other specified bursopathies, left elbow
        M71.829 Other specified bursopathies, unspecified elbow

✓6ᵗʰ   **M71.83 Other specified bursopathies, wrist**
        M71.831 Other specified bursopathies, right wrist
        M71.832 Other specified bursopathies, left wrist
        M71.839 Other specified bursopathies, unspecified wrist

✓6ᵗʰ   **M71.84 Other specified bursopathies, hand**
        M71.841 Other specified bursopathies, right hand
        M71.842 Other specified bursopathies, left hand
        M71.849 Other specified bursopathies, unspecified hand

✓6ᵗʰ   **M71.85 Other specified bursopathies, hip**
        M71.851 Other specified bursopathies, right hip

        M71.852 Other specified bursopathies, left hip
        M71.859 Other specified bursopathies, unspecified hip

✓6ᵗʰ   **M71.86 Other specified bursopathies, knee**
        M71.861 Other specified bursopathies, right knee
        M71.862 Other specified bursopathies, left knee
        M71.869 Other specified bursopathies, unspecified knee

✓6ᵗʰ   **M71.87 Other specified bursopathies, ankle and foot**
        M71.871 Other specified bursopathies, right ankle and foot
        M71.872 Other specified bursopathies, left ankle and foot
        M71.879 Other specified bursopathies, unspecified ankle and foot

    M71.88 Other specified bursopathies, other site
    M71.89 Other specified bursopathies, multiple sites

M71.9 Bursopathy, unspecified
    Bursitis NOS

✓4ᵗʰ **M72 Fibroblastic disorders**
    EXCLUDES 2   retroperitoneal fibromatosis (D48.3)

M72.0 Palmar fascial fibromatosis [Dupuytren] Ⓐ

M72.1 Knuckle pads

M72.2 Plantar fascial fibromatosis
    Plantar fasciitis

M72.4 Pseudosarcomatous fibromatosis
    Nodular fasciitis

M72.6 Necrotizing fasciitis
    Use additional code (B95.-, B96.-) to identify causative organism

M72.8 Other fibroblastic disorders
    Abscess of fascia
    Fasciitis NEC
    Other infective fasciitis
    Use additional code to (B95.-, B96.-) identify causative organism
    EXCLUDES 1   diffuse (eosinophilic) fasciitis (M35.4)
                  necrotizing fasciitis (M72.6)
                  nodular fasciitis (M72.4)
                  perirenal fasciitis NOS (N13.5)
                  perirenal fasciitis with infection (N13.6)
                  plantar fasciitis (M72.2)

M72.9 Fibroblastic disorder, unspecified
    Fasciitis NOS
    Fibromatosis NOS

✓4ᵗʰ **M75 Shoulder lesions**
    EXCLUDES 2   shoulder-hand syndrome (M89.0-)

✓5ᵗʰ **M75.0 Adhesive capsulitis of shoulder**
    Frozen shoulder
    Periarthritis of shoulder

    M75.00 Adhesive capsulitis of unspecified shoulder
    M75.01 Adhesive capsulitis of right shoulder
    M75.02 Adhesive capsulitis of left shoulder

✓5ᵗʰ **M75.1 Rotator cuff tear or rupture, not specified as traumatic**
    Rotator cuff syndrome
    Supraspinatus syndrome
    Supraspinatus tear or rupture, not specified as traumatic
    EXCLUDES 1   tear of rotator cuff, traumatic (S46.01-)

✓6ᵗʰ   **M75.10 Unspecified rotator cuff tear or rupture, not specified as traumatic**
        M75.100 Unspecified rotator cuff tear or rupture of unspecified shoulder, not specified as traumatic
        M75.101 Unspecified rotator cuff tear or rupture of right shoulder, not specified as traumatic
        M75.102 Unspecified rotator cuff tear or rupture of left shoulder, not specified as traumatic

✓6ᵗʰ   **M75.11 Incomplete rotator cuff tear or rupture not specified as traumatic**
        M75.110 Incomplete rotator cuff tear or rupture of unspecified shoulder, not specified as traumatic
        M75.111 Incomplete rotator cuff tear or rupture of right shoulder, not specified as traumatic
        M75.112 Incomplete rotator cuff tear or rupture of left shoulder, not specified as traumatic

EXCLUDES 1 Not coded here   *EXCLUDES 2* Not included here   Ⓝ Newborn Age: 0   Ⓟ Pediatric Age: 0-17   Ⓜ Maternity Age: 12-55   Ⓐ Adult Age: 15-124

698   ICD-10-CM Draft (2015)

✓6th **M75.12** Complete **rotator cuff tear or rupture not specified as traumatic**

　　M75.120 Complete rotator cuff tear or rupture of unspecified shoulder, not specified as traumatic

　　M75.121 Complete rotator cuff tear or rupture of right shoulder, not specified as traumatic

　　M75.122 Complete rotator cuff tear or rupture of left shoulder, not specified as traumatic

✓5th **M75.2** **Bicipital** tendinitis

　　M75.20 **Bicipital tendinitis, unspecified shoulder**

　　M75.21 Bicipital tendinitis, right shoulder

　　M75.22 Bicipital tendinitis, left shoulder

✓5th **M75.3** **Calcific** tendinitis of shoulder

　　Calcified bursa of shoulder

　　M75.30 **Calcific tendinitis of unspecified shoulder**

　　M75.31 Calcific tendinitis of right shoulder

　　M75.32 Calcific tendinitis of left shoulder

✓5th **M75.4** **Impingement syndrome** of shoulder

　　M75.40 **Impingement syndrome of unspecified shoulder**

　　M75.41 Impingement syndrome of right shoulder

　　M75.42 Impingement syndrome of left shoulder

✓5th **M75.5** **Bursitis** of shoulder

　　M75.50 **Bursitis of unspecified shoulder**

　　M75.51 Bursitis of right shoulder

　　M75.52 Bursitis of left shoulder

✓5th **M75.8** **Other** shoulder lesions

　　M75.80 **Other shoulder lesions, unspecified shoulder**

　　M75.81 **Other shoulder lesions, right shoulder**

　　M75.82 **Other shoulder lesions, left shoulder**

✓5th **M75.9** **Shoulder lesion,** unspecified

　　M75.90 **Shoulder lesion, unspecified, unspecified shoulder**

　　M75.91 Shoulder lesion, unspecified, right shoulder

　　M75.92 Shoulder lesion, unspecified, left shoulder

✓4th **M76** **Enthesopathies, lower limb, excluding foot**

　　EXCLUDES 2　bursitis due to use, overuse and pressure (M70.-)
　　　　enthesopathies of ankle and foot (M77.5-)

✓5th **M76.0** **Gluteal** tendinitis

　　M76.00 **Gluteal tendinitis, unspecified hip**

　　M76.01 Gluteal tendinitis, right hip

　　M76.02 Gluteal tendinitis, left hip

✓5th **M76.1** **Psoas** tendinitis

　　M76.10 **Psoas tendinitis, unspecified hip**

　　M76.11 Psoas tendinitis, right hip

　　M76.12 Psoas tendinitis, left hip

✓5th **M76.2** **Iliac crest** spur

　　M76.20 **Iliac crest spur, unspecified hip**

　　M76.21 Iliac crest spur, right hip

　　M76.22 Iliac crest spur, left hip

✓5th **M76.3** **Iliotibial band** syndrome

　　M76.30 **Iliotibial band syndrome, unspecified leg**

　　M76.31 Iliotibial band syndrome, right leg

　　M76.32 Iliotibial band syndrome, left leg

✓5th **M76.4** **Tibial collateral** bursitis [Pellegrini-Stieda]

　　M76.40 **Tibial collateral bursitis [Pellegrini-Stieda], unspecified leg**

　　M76.41 Tibial collateral bursitis [Pellegrini-Stieda], right leg

　　M76.42 Tibial collateral bursitis [Pellegrini-Stieda], left leg

✓5th **M76.5** **Patellar** tendinitis

　　M76.50 **Patellar tendinitis, unspecified knee**

　　M76.51 Patellar tendinitis, right knee

　　M76.52 Patellar tendinitis, left knee

✓5th **M76.6** **Achilles** tendinitis

　　Achilles bursitis

　　M76.60 **Achilles tendinitis, unspecified leg**

　　M76.61 Achilles tendinitis, right leg

　　M76.62 Achilles tendinitis, left leg

✓5th **M76.7** **Peroneal** tendinitis

　　M76.70 **Peroneal tendinitis, unspecified leg**

　　M76.71 Peroneal tendinitis, right leg

M76.72 Peroneal tendinitis, left leg

✓5th **M76.8** **Other** specified enthesopathies of lower limb, excluding foot

✓6th **M76.81** **Anterior tibial syndrome**

　　M76.811 Anterior tibial syndrome, right leg

　　M76.812 Anterior tibial syndrome, left leg

　　M76.819 Anterior tibial syndrome, unspecified leg

✓6th **M76.82** **Posterior tibial tendinitis**

　　M76.821 Posterior tibial tendinitis, right leg

　　M76.822 Posterior tibial tendinitis, left leg

　　M76.829 Posterior tibial tendinitis, unspecified leg

✓6th **M76.89** **Other specified enthesopathies of** lower limb, excluding foot

　　M76.891 **Other specified enthesopathies of right lower limb, excluding foot**

　　M76.892 **Other specified enthesopathies of left lower limb, excluding foot**

　　M76.899 Other specified enthesopathies of unspecified lower limb, excluding foot

M76.9 **Unspecified enthesopathy, lower limb, excluding foot**

✓4th **M77** **Other enthesopathies**

　　EXCLUDES 1　bursitis NOS (M71.9-)

　　EXCLUDES 2　bursitis due to use, overuse and pressure (M70.-)
　　　　osteophyte (M25.7)
　　　　spinal enthesopathy (M46.0-)

✓5th **M77.0** **Medial** epicondylitis

　　M77.00 **Medial epicondylitis, unspecified elbow**

　　M77.01 Medial epicondylitis, right elbow

　　M77.02 Medial epicondylitis, left elbow

✓5th **M77.1** **Lateral** epicondylitis

　　Tennis elbow

　　M77.10 **Lateral epicondylitis, unspecified elbow**

　　M77.11 Lateral epicondylitis, right elbow

　　M77.12 Lateral epicondylitis, left elbow

✓5th **M77.2** **Periarthritis** of wrist

　　M77.20 **Periarthritis, unspecified wrist**

　　M77.21 Periarthritis, right wrist

　　M77.22 Periarthritis, left wrist

✓5th **M77.3** **Calcaneal spur**

　　M77.30 **Calcaneal spur, unspecified foot**

　　M77.31 Calcaneal spur, right foot

　　M77.32 Calcaneal spur, left foot

✓5th **M77.4** **Metatarsalgia**

　　EXCLUDES 1　Morton's metatarsalgia (G57.6)

　　M77.40 **Metatarsalgia, unspecified foot**

　　M77.41 Metatarsalgia, right foot

　　M77.42 Metatarsalgia, left foot

✓5th **M77.5** **Other** enthesopathy of foot

　　M77.50 **Other enthesopathy of unspecified foot**

　　M77.51 Other enthesopathy of right foot

　　M77.52 Other enthesopathy of left foot

M77.8 **Other enthesopathies, not elsewhere classified**

M77.9 **Enthesopathy, unspecified**

　　Bone spur NOS　　　Periarthritis NOS
　　Capsulitis NOS　　　Tendinitis NOS

✓4th **M79** **Other and unspecified soft tissue disorders, not elsewhere classified**

　　EXCLUDES 1　psychogenic rheumatism (F45.8)
　　　　soft tissue pain, psychogenic (F45.41)

M79.0 **Rheumatism, unspecified**

　　EXCLUDES 1　fibromyalgia (M79.7)
　　　　palindromic rheumatism (M12.3-)

M79.1 **Myalgia**

　　Myofascial pain syndrome

　　EXCLUDES 1　fibromyalgia (M79.7)
　　　　myositis (M60.-)

M79.2 **Neuralgia and neuritis, unspecified**

　　EXCLUDES 1　brachial radiculitis NOS (M54.1)
　　　　lumbosacral radiculitis NOS (M54.1)
　　　　mononeuropathies (G56-G58)
　　　　radiculitis NOS (M54.1)
　　　　sciatica (M54.3-M54.4)

M79.3 Panniculitis, unspecified
> EXCLUDES 1   lupus panniculitis (L93.2)
> neck and back panniculitis (M54.0-)
> relapsing [Weber-Christian] panniculitis (M35.6)

M79.4 Hypertrophy of (infrapatellar) fat pad

M79.5 Residual foreign body in soft tissue
> EXCLUDES 1   foreign body granuloma of skin and subcutaneous
> tissue (L92.3)
> foreign body granuloma of soft tissue (M60.2-)

✓5th **M79.6 Pain in limb, hand, foot, fingers and toes**
> EXCLUDES 2   pain in joint (M25.5-)

   ✓6th **M79.60 Pain in limb, unspecified**
     M79.601 Pain in right arm
       Pain in right upper limb NOS
     M79.602 Pain in left arm
       Pain in left upper limb NOS
     M79.603 Pain in arm, unspecified
       Pain in upper limb NOS
     M79.604 Pain in right leg
       Pain in right lower limb NOS
     M79.605 Pain in left leg
       Pain in left lower limb NOS
     M79.606 Pain in leg, unspecified
       Pain in lower limb NOS
     M79.609 Pain in unspecified limb
       Pain in limb NOS

   ✓6th **M79.62 Pain in upper arm**
     Pain in axillary region
     M79.621 Pain in right upper arm
     M79.622 Pain in left upper arm
     M79.629 Pain in unspecified upper arm

   ✓6th **M79.63 Pain in forearm**
     M79.631 Pain in right forearm
     M79.632 Pain in left forearm
     M79.639 Pain in unspecified forearm

   ✓6th **M79.64 Pain in hand and fingers**
     M79.641 Pain in right hand
     M79.642 Pain in left hand
     M79.643 Pain in unspecified hand
     M79.644 Pain in right finger(s)
     M79.645 Pain in left finger(s)
     M79.646 Pain in unspecified finger(s)

   ✓6th **M79.65 Pain in thigh**
     M79.651 Pain in right thigh
     M79.652 Pain in left thigh
     M79.659 Pain in unspecified thigh

   ✓6th **M79.66 Pain in lower leg**
     M79.661 Pain in right lower leg
     M79.662 Pain in left lower leg
     M79.669 Pain in unspecified lower leg

   ✓6th **M79.67 Pain in foot and toes**
     M79.671 Pain in right foot
     M79.672 Pain in left foot
     M79.673 Pain in unspecified foot
     M79.674 Pain in right toe(s)
     M79.675 Pain in left toe(s)
     M79.676 Pain in unspecified toe(s)

M79.7 Fibromyalgia
   Fibromyositis   Myofibrositis
   Fibrositis

✓5th **M79.A Nontraumatic compartment syndrome**
   Code first, if applicable, associated postprocedural complication
> EXCLUDES 1   compartment syndrome NOS (T79.A-)
> fibromyalgia (M79.7)
> nontraumatic ischemic infarction of muscle (M62.2-)
> traumatic compartment syndrome (T79.A-)

   ✓6th **M79.A1 Nontraumatic compartment syndrome of upper extremity**
     Nontraumatic compartment syndrome of shoulder,
     arm, forearm, wrist, hand, and fingers
     M79.A11 Nontraumatic compartment syndrome of right upper extremity
     M79.A12 Nontraumatic compartment syndrome of left upper extremity

     M79.A19 Nontraumatic compartment syndrome of unspecified upper extremity

   ✓6th **M79.A2 Nontraumatic compartment syndrome of lower extremity**
     Nontraumatic compartment syndrome of hip, buttock,
     thigh, leg, foot, and toes
     M79.A21 Nontraumatic compartment syndrome of right lower extremity
     M79.A22 Nontraumatic compartment syndrome of left lower extremity
     M79.A29 Nontraumatic compartment syndrome of unspecified lower extremity

     M79.A3 Nontraumatic compartment syndrome of abdomen
     M79.A9 Nontraumatic compartment syndrome of other sites

✓5th **M79.8 Other specified soft tissue disorders**
     M79.81 Nontraumatic hematoma of soft tissue
       Nontraumatic hematoma of muscle
       Nontraumatic seroma of muscle and soft tissue

     M79.89 Other specified soft tissue disorders
       Polyalgia

M79.9 Soft tissue disorder, unspecified

OSTEOPATHIES AND CHONDROPATHIES (M80-M94)

Disorders of bone density and structure (M80-M85)

✓4th **M80 Osteoporosis with current pathological fracture**
> INCLUDES   osteoporosis with current fragility fracture

Use additional code to identify major osseous defect, if applicable
(M89.7-)
> EXCLUDES 1   collapsed vertebra NOS (M48.5)
> pathological fracture NOS (M84.4)
> wedging of vertebra NOS (M48.5)
> EXCLUDES 2   personal history of (healed) osteoporosis fracture (Z87.310)

The appropriate 7th character is to be added to each code from
category M80.
A   initial encounter for fracture
D   subsequent encounter for fracture with routine healing
G   subsequent encounter for fracture with delayed healing
K   subsequent encounter for fracture with nonunion
P   subsequent encounter for fracture with malunion
S   sequela

✓5th **M80.0 Age-related osteoporosis with current pathological fracture**
   Involutional osteoporosis with current pathological fracture
   Osteoporosis NOS with current pathological fracture
   Postmenopausal osteoporosis with current pathological fracture
   Senile osteoporosis with current pathological fracture

   ✓x7th **M80.00 Age-related osteoporosis with current pathological fracture, unspecified site** [A]

   ✓6th **M80.01 Age-related osteoporosis with current pathological fracture, shoulder**
     ✓7th **M80.011 Age-related osteoporosis with current pathological fracture, right shoulder** [A]
     ✓7th **M80.012 Age-related osteoporosis with current pathological fracture, left shoulder** [A]
     ✓7th **M80.019 Age-related osteoporosis with current pathological fracture, unspecified shoulder** [A]

   ✓6th **M80.02 Age-related osteoporosis with current pathological fracture, humerus**
     ✓7th **M80.021 Age-related osteoporosis with current pathological fracture, right humerus** [A]
     ✓7th **M80.022 Age-related osteoporosis with current pathological fracture, left humerus** [A]
     ✓7th **M80.029 Age-related osteoporosis with current pathological fracture, unspecified humerus** [A]

   ✓6th **M80.03 Age-related osteoporosis with current pathological fracture, forearm**
     Age-related osteoporosis with current pathological
     fracture of wrist
     ✓7th **M80.031 Age-related osteoporosis with current pathological fracture, right forearm** [A]
     ✓7th **M80.032 Age-related osteoporosis with current pathological fracture, left forearm** [A]
     ✓7th **M80.039 Age-related osteoporosis with current pathological fracture, unspecified forearm** [A]

EXCLUDES 1 Not coded here   EXCLUDES 2 Not included here   N Newborn Age: 0   P Pediatric Age: 0-17   M Maternity Age: 12-55   A Adult Age: 15-124

700   ICD-10-CM Draft (2015)

√6th **M80.04 Age-related osteoporosis with current pathological fracture, hand**

- √7th M80.041 Age-related osteoporosis with current pathological fracture, right hand Ⓐ
- √7th M80.042 Age-related osteoporosis with current pathological fracture, left hand Ⓐ
- √7th M80.049 Age-related osteoporosis with current pathological fracture, unspecified hand Ⓐ

√6th **M80.05 Age-related osteoporosis with current pathological fracture, femur**

Age-related osteoporosis with current pathological fracture of hip

- √7th M80.051 Age-related osteoporosis with current pathological fracture, right femur
- √7th M80.052 Age-related osteoporosis with current pathological fracture, left femur
- √7th M80.059 Age-related osteoporosis with current pathological fracture, unspecified femur

√6th **M80.06 Age-related osteoporosis with current pathological fracture, lower leg**

- √7th M80.061 Age-related osteoporosis with current pathological fracture, right lower leg
- √7th M80.062 Age-related osteoporosis with current pathological fracture, left lower leg
- √7th M80.069 Age-related osteoporosis with current pathological fracture, unspecified lower leg

√6th **M80.07 Age-related osteoporosis with current pathological fracture, ankle and foot**

- √7th M80.071 Age-related osteoporosis with current pathological fracture, right ankle and foot
- √7th M80.072 Age-related osteoporosis with current pathological fracture, left ankle and foot
- √7th M80.079 Age-related osteoporosis with current pathological fracture, unspecified ankle and foot

√x7th **M80.08 Age-related osteoporosis with current pathological fracture, vertebra(e)** Ⓐ

√5th **M80.8 Other osteoporosis with current pathological fracture**

Drug-induced osteoporosis with current pathological fracture
Idiopathic osteoporosis with current pathological fracture
Osteoporosis of disuse with current pathological fracture
Postoophorectomy osteoporosis with current pathological fracture
Postsurgical malabsorption osteoporosis with current pathological fracture
Post-traumatic osteoporosis with current pathological fracture
Use additional code for adverse effect, if applicable, to identify drug (T36-T50 with fifth or sixth character 5)

√x7th **M80.80 Other osteoporosis with current pathological fracture, unspecified site**

√6th **M80.81 Other osteoporosis with pathological fracture, shoulder**

- √7th M80.811 Other osteoporosis with current pathological fracture, right shoulder
- √7th M80.812 Other osteoporosis with current pathological fracture, left shoulder
- √7th M80.819 Other osteoporosis with current pathological fracture, unspecified shoulder

√6th **M80.82 Other osteoporosis with current pathological fracture, humerus**

- √7th M80.821 Other osteoporosis with current pathological fracture, right humerus
- √7th M80.822 Other osteoporosis with current pathological fracture, left humerus
- √7th M80.829 Other osteoporosis with current pathological fracture, unspecified humerus

√6th **M80.83 Other osteoporosis with current pathological fracture, forearm**

Other osteoporosis with current pathological fracture of wrist

- √7th M80.831 Other osteoporosis with current pathological fracture, right forearm
- √7th M80.832 Other osteoporosis with current pathological fracture, left forearm

- √7th M80.839 Other osteoporosis with current pathological fracture, unspecified forearm

√6th **M80.84 Other osteoporosis with current pathological fracture, hand**

- √7th M80.841 Other osteoporosis with current pathological fracture, right hand
- √7th M80.842 Other osteoporosis with current pathological fracture, left hand
- √7th M80.849 Other osteoporosis with current pathological fracture, unspecified hand

√6th **M80.85 Other osteoporosis with current pathological fracture, femur**

Other osteoporosis with current pathological fracture of hip

- √7th M80.851 Other osteoporosis with current pathological fracture, right femur
- √7th M80.852 Other osteoporosis with current pathological fracture, left femur
- √7th M80.859 Other osteoporosis with current pathological fracture, unspecified femur

√6th **M80.86 Other osteoporosis with current pathological fracture, lower leg**

- √7th M80.861 Other osteoporosis with current pathological fracture, right lower leg
- √7th M80.862 Other osteoporosis with current pathological fracture, left lower leg
- √7th M80.869 Other osteoporosis with current pathological fracture, unspecified lower leg

√6th **M80.87 Other osteoporosis with current pathological fracture, ankle and foot**

- √7th M80.871 Other osteoporosis with current pathological fracture, right ankle and foot
- √7th M80.872 Other osteoporosis with current pathological fracture, left ankle and foot
- √7th M80.879 Other osteoporosis with current pathological fracture, unspecified ankle and foot

√x7th **M80.88 Other osteoporosis with current pathological fracture, vertebra(e)**

√4th **M81 Osteoporosis without current pathological fracture**

Use additional code to identify:
major osseous defect, if applicable (M89.7-)
personal history of (healed) osteoporosis fracture, if applicable (Z87.310)

EXCLUDES 1 *osteoporosis with current pathological fracture (M80.-)*
Sudeck's atrophy (M89.0)

M81.0 Age-related osteoporosis without current pathological fracture Ⓐ

Involutional osteoporosis without current pathological fracture
Osteoporosis NOS
Postmenopausal osteoporosis without current pathological fracture
Senile osteoporosis without current pathological fracture

M81.6 Localized osteoporosis [Lequesne]

EXCLUDES 1 *Sudeck's atrophy (M89.0)*

M81.8 Other osteoporosis without current pathological fracture

Drug-induced osteoporosis without current pathological fracture
Idiopathic osteoporosis without current pathological fracture
Osteoporosis of disuse without current pathological fracture
Postoophorectomy osteoporosis without current pathological fracture
Postsurgical malabsorption osteoporosis without current pathological fracture
Post-traumatic osteoporosis without current pathological fracture
Use additional code for adverse effect, if applicable, to identify drug (T36-T50 with fifth or sixth character 5)

√4th **M83 Adult osteomalacia**

EXCLUDES 1 *infantile and juvenile osteomalacia (E55.0)*
renal osteodystrophy (N25.0)
rickets (active) (E55.0)
rickets (active) sequelae (E64.3)
vitamin D-resistant osteomalacia (E83.3)
vitamin D-resistant rickets (active) (E83.3)

M83.0 Puerperal osteomalacia Ⓜ♀

M83.1 Senile osteomalacia Ⓐ

✓ Additional Character Required   √x7th Xtension Alert   Unspecified Dx   Other Specified Dx   Manifestation   ►◄ Revised Text   ● New Code   ▲ Revised Code Title

M83.2 Adult osteomalacia due to malabsorption ▢A
    Postsurgical malabsorption osteomalacia in adults

M83.3 Adult osteomalacia due to malnutrition ▢A

M83.4 Aluminum bone disease

M83.5 Other drug-induced **osteomalacia in adults** ▢A
    Use additional code for adverse effect, if applicable, to identify
        drug (T36-T50 with fifth or sixth character 5)

M83.8 Other adult osteomalacia ▢A

M83.9 Adult osteomalacia, unspecified ▢A

✓4ᵗʰ **M84 Disorder of continuity of bone**
    EXCLUDES 2 traumatic fracture of bone-see fracture, by site

✓5ᵗʰ **M84.3 Stress fracture**
    Fatigue fracture   Stress fracture NOS
    March fracture   Stress reaction
    Use additional external cause code(s) to identify the cause of the
        stress fracture
    EXCLUDES 1 pathological fracture NOS (M84.4-)
        pathological fracture due to osteoporosis (M80.-)
        traumatic fracture (S12-, S22-, S32-, S42-, S52-, S62-,
            S72-, S82-, S92-)
    EXCLUDES 2 personal history of (healed) stress (fatigue) fracture
        (Z87.312)
        stress fracture of vertebra (M48.4-)

    The appropriate 7th character is to be added to each code
    from subcategory M84.3.
    A   initial encounter for fracture
    D   subsequent encounter for fracture with routine healing
    G   subsequent encounter for fracture with delayed healing
    K   subsequent encounter for fracture with nonunion
    P   subsequent encounter for fracture with malunion
    S   sequela

✓x7ᵗʰ **M84.30 Stress fracture, unspecified site**
✓6ᵗʰ **M84.31 Stress fracture,** shoulder
    ✓7ᵗʰ **M84.311 Stress fracture,** right **shoulder**
    ✓7ᵗʰ **M84.312 Stress fracture,** left **shoulder**
    ✓7ᵗʰ **M84.319 Stress fracture, unspecified shoulder**
✓6ᵗʰ **M84.32 Stress fracture,** humerus
    ✓7ᵗʰ **M84.321 Stress fracture,** right **humerus**
    ✓7ᵗʰ **M84.322 Stress fracture,** left **humerus**
    ✓7ᵗʰ **M84.329 Stress fracture, unspecified humerus**
✓6ᵗʰ **M84.33 Stress fracture,** ulna and radius
    ✓7ᵗʰ **M84.331 Stress fracture,** right **ulna**
    ✓7ᵗʰ **M84.332 Stress fracture,** left **ulna**
    ✓7ᵗʰ **M84.333 Stress fracture,** right **radius**
    ✓7ᵗʰ **M84.334 Stress fracture,** left **radius**
    ✓7ᵗʰ **M84.339 Stress fracture, unspecified ulna and
        radius**
✓6ᵗʰ **M84.34 Stress fracture,** hand and fingers
    ✓7ᵗʰ **M84.341 Stress fracture,** right **hand**
    ✓7ᵗʰ **M84.342 Stress fracture,** left **hand**
    ✓7ᵗʰ **M84.343 Stress fracture, unspecified hand**
    ✓7ᵗʰ **M84.344 Stress fracture,** right **finger(s)**
    ✓7ᵗʰ **M84.345 Stress fracture,** left **finger(s)**
    ✓7ᵗʰ **M84.346 Stress fracture, unspecified finger(s)**
✓6ᵗʰ **M84.35 Stress fracture,** pelvis and femur
    Stress fracture, hip
    ✓7ᵗʰ **M84.350 Stress fracture,** pelvis
    ✓7ᵗʰ **M84.351 Stress fracture,** right **femur**
    ✓7ᵗʰ **M84.352 Stress fracture,** left **femur**
    ✓7ᵗʰ **M84.353 Stress fracture, unspecified femur**
    ✓7ᵗʰ **M84.359 Stress fracture, hip, unspecified**
✓6ᵗʰ **M84.36 Stress fracture,** tibia and fibula
    ✓7ᵗʰ **M84.361 Stress fracture,** right **tibia**
    ✓7ᵗʰ **M84.362 Stress fracture,** left **tibia**
    ✓7ᵗʰ **M84.363 Stress fracture,** right **fibula**
    ✓7ᵗʰ **M84.364 Stress fracture,** left **fibula**
    ✓7ᵗʰ **M84.369 Stress fracture, unspecified tibia and
        fibula**
✓6ᵗʰ **M84.37 Stress fracture,** ankle, foot and toes
    ✓7ᵗʰ **M84.371 Stress fracture,** right **ankle**
    ✓7ᵗʰ **M84.372 Stress fracture,** left **ankle**

✓7ᵗʰ **M84.373 Stress fracture, unspecified ankle**
✓7ᵗʰ **M84.374 Stress fracture,** right **foot**
✓7ᵗʰ **M84.375 Stress fracture,** left **foot**
✓7ᵗʰ **M84.376 Stress fracture, unspecified foot**
✓7ᵗʰ **M84.377 Stress fracture,** right **toe(s)**
✓7ᵗʰ **M84.378 Stress fracture,** left **toe(s)**
✓7ᵗʰ **M84.379 Stress fracture, unspecified toe(s)**
✓x7ᵗʰ **M84.38 Stress fracture, other site**
    EXCLUDES 2 stress fracture of vertebra (M48.4-)

✓5ᵗʰ **M84.4 Pathological fracture,** not elsewhere classified
    Chronic fracture
    Pathological fracture NOS
    EXCLUDES 1 collapsed vertebra NEC (M48.5)
        pathological fracture in neoplastic disease (M84.5-)
        pathological fracture in osteoporosis (M80.-)
        pathological fracture in other disease (M84.6-)
        stress fracture (M84.3-)
        traumatic fracture (S12.-, S22.-, S32.-, S42.-, S52.-, S62.-,
            S72.-, S82.-, S92.-)
    EXCLUDES 2 personal history of (healed) pathological fracture
        (Z87.311)

    The appropriate 7th character is to be added to each code
    from subcategory M84.4.
    A   initial encounter for fracture
    D   subsequent encounter for fracture with routine healing
    G   subsequent encounter for fracture with delayed healing
    K   subsequent encounter for fracture with nonunion
    P   subsequent encounter for fracture with malunion
    S   sequela

✓x7ᵗʰ **M84.40 Pathological fracture, unspecified site**
✓6ᵗʰ **M84.41 Pathological fracture,** shoulder
    ✓7ᵗʰ **M84.411 Pathological fracture,** right **shoulder**
    ✓7ᵗʰ **M84.412 Pathological fracture,** left **shoulder**
    ✓7ᵗʰ **M84.419 Pathological fracture, unspecified
        shoulder**
✓6ᵗʰ **M84.42 Pathological fracture,** humerus
    ✓7ᵗʰ **M84.421 Pathological fracture,** right **humerus**
    ✓7ᵗʰ **M84.422 Pathological fracture,** left **humerus**
    ✓7ᵗʰ **M84.429 Pathological fracture, unspecified
        humerus**
✓6ᵗʰ **M84.43 Pathological fracture,** ulna and radius
    ✓7ᵗʰ **M84.431 Pathological fracture,** right **ulna**
    ✓7ᵗʰ **M84.432 Pathological fracture,** left **ulna**
    ✓7ᵗʰ **M84.433 Pathological fracture,** right **radius**
    ✓7ᵗʰ **M84.434 Pathological fracture,** left **radius**
    ✓7ᵗʰ **M84.439 Pathological fracture, unspecified ulna
        and radius**
✓6ᵗʰ **M84.44 Pathological fracture,** hand and fingers
    ✓7ᵗʰ **M84.441 Pathological fracture,** right **hand**
    ✓7ᵗʰ **M84.442 Pathological fracture,** left **hand**
    ✓7ᵗʰ **M84.443 Pathological fracture, unspecified hand**
    ✓7ᵗʰ **M84.444 Pathological fracture,** right **finger(s)**
    ✓7ᵗʰ **M84.445 Pathological fracture,** left **finger(s)**
    ✓7ᵗʰ **M84.446 Pathological fracture, unspecified
        finger(s)**
✓6ᵗʰ **M84.45 Pathological fracture,** femur and pelvis
    ✓7ᵗʰ **M84.451 Pathological fracture,** right **femur**
    ✓7ᵗʰ **M84.452 Pathological fracture,** left **femur**
    ✓7ᵗʰ **M84.453 Pathological fracture, unspecified femur**
    ✓7ᵗʰ **M84.454 Pathological fracture,** pelvis
    ✓7ᵗʰ **M84.459 Pathological fracture, hip, unspecified**
✓6ᵗʰ **M84.46 Pathological fracture,** tibia and fibula
    ✓7ᵗʰ **M84.461 Pathological fracture,** right **tibia**
    ✓7ᵗʰ **M84.462 Pathological fracture,** left **tibia**
    ✓7ᵗʰ **M84.463 Pathological fracture,** right **fibula**
    ✓7ᵗʰ **M84.464 Pathological fracture,** left **fibula**
    ✓7ᵗʰ **M84.469 Pathological fracture, unspecified tibia
        and fibula**
✓6ᵗʰ **M84.47 Pathological fracture,** ankle, foot and toes
    ✓7ᵗʰ **M84.471 Pathological fracture,** right **ankle**
    ✓7ᵗʰ **M84.472 Pathological fracture,** left **ankle**

EXCLUDES 1 Not coded here   *EXCLUDES 2* Not included here   ▢N Newborn Age: 0   ▢P Pediatric Age: 0-17   ▢M Maternity Age: 12-55   ▢A Adult Age: 15-124

702   ICD-10-CM Draft (2015)

√7ʰ **M84.473 Pathological fracture, unspecified ankle**

√7ʰ **M84.474 Pathological fracture,** right foot

√7ʰ **M84.475 Pathological fracture,** left foot

√7ʰ **M84.476 Pathological fracture, unspecified foot**

√7ʰ **M84.477 Pathological fracture,** right toe(s)

√7ʰ **M84.478 Pathological fracture,** left toe(s)

√7ʰ **M84.479 Pathological fracture, unspecified toe(s)**

√x7ʰ **M84.48 Pathological fracture, other site**

√5ʰ **M84.5 Pathological fracture in** neoplastic disease
Code also underlying neoplasm

The appropriate 7th character is to be added to each code from subcategory M84.5.
A   initial encounter for fracture
D   subsequent encounter for fracture with routine healing
G   subsequent encounter for fracture with delayed healing
K   subsequent encounter for fracture with nonunion
P   subsequent encounter for fracture with malunion
S   sequela

√x7ʰ **M84.50 Pathological fracture in neoplastic disease, unspecified site**

√6ʰ **M84.51 Pathological fracture in neoplastic disease,** shoulder

√7ʰ **M84.511 Pathological fracture in neoplastic disease,** right **shoulder**

√7ʰ **M84.512 Pathological fracture in neoplastic disease,** left **shoulder**

√7ʰ **M84.519 Pathological fracture in neoplastic disease, unspecified shoulder**

√6ʰ **M84.52 Pathological fracture in neoplastic disease,** humerus

√7ʰ **M84.521 Pathological fracture in neoplastic disease,** right **humerus**

√7ʰ **M84.522 Pathological fracture in neoplastic disease,** left **humerus**

√7ʰ **M84.529 Pathological fracture in neoplastic disease, unspecified humerus**

√6ʰ **M84.53 Pathological fracture in neoplastic disease,** ulna and radius

√7ʰ **M84.531 Pathological fracture in neoplastic disease,** right ulna

√7ʰ **M84.532 Pathological fracture in neoplastic disease,** left ulna

√7ʰ **M84.533 Pathological fracture in neoplastic disease,** right radius

√7ʰ **M84.534 Pathological fracture in neoplastic disease,** left radius

√7ʰ **M84.539 Pathological fracture in neoplastic disease, unspecified ulna and radius**

√6ʰ **M84.54 Pathological fracture in neoplastic disease,** hand

√7ʰ **M84.541 Pathological fracture in neoplastic disease,** right **hand**

√7ʰ **M84.542 Pathological fracture in neoplastic disease,** left **hand**

√7ʰ **M84.549 Pathological fracture in neoplastic disease, unspecified hand**

√6ʰ **M84.55 Pathological fracture in neoplastic disease,** pelvis and femur

√7ʰ **M84.550 Pathological fracture in neoplastic disease,** pelvis

√7ʰ **M84.551 Pathological fracture in neoplastic disease,** right femur

√7ʰ **M84.552 Pathological fracture in neoplastic disease,** left femur

√7ʰ **M84.553 Pathological fracture in neoplastic disease, unspecified femur**

√7ʰ **M84.559 Pathological fracture in neoplastic disease,** hip, **unspecified**

√6ʰ **M84.56 Pathological fracture in neoplastic disease,** tibia and fibula

√7ʰ **M84.561 Pathological fracture in neoplastic disease,** right tibia

√7ʰ **M84.562 Pathological fracture in neoplastic disease,** left tibia

√7ʰ **M84.563 Pathological fracture in neoplastic disease,** right fibula

√7ʰ **M84.564 Pathological fracture in neoplastic disease,** left fibula

√7ʰ **M84.569 Pathological fracture in neoplastic disease, unspecified tibia and fibula**

√6ʰ **M84.57 Pathological fracture in neoplastic disease,** ankle and foot

√7ʰ **M84.571 Pathological fracture in neoplastic disease,** right ankle

√7ʰ **M84.572 Pathological fracture in neoplastic disease,** left ankle

√7ʰ **M84.573 Pathological fracture in neoplastic disease, unspecified ankle**

√7ʰ **M84.574 Pathological fracture in neoplastic disease,** right foot

√7ʰ **M84.575 Pathological fracture in neoplastic disease,** left foot

√7ʰ **M84.576 Pathological fracture in neoplastic disease, unspecified foot**

√x7ʰ **M84.58 Pathological fracture in neoplastic disease, other specified site**
Pathological fracture in neoplastic disease, vertebrae

√5ʰ **M84.6 Pathological fracture** in other disease
Code also underlying condition
EXCLUDES 1   pathological fracture in osteoporosis (M80.-)

The appropriate 7th character is to be added to each code from subcategory M84.6.
A   initial encounter for fracture
D   subsequent encounter for fracture with routine healing
G   subsequent encounter for fracture with delayed healing
K   subsequent encounter for fracture with nonunion
P   subsequent encounter for fracture with malunion
S   sequela

√x7ʰ **M84.60 Pathological fracture in other disease, unspecified site**

√6ʰ **M84.61 Pathological fracture in other disease,** shoulder

√7ʰ **M84.611 Pathological fracture in other disease,** right **shoulder**

√7ʰ **M84.612 Pathological fracture in other disease,** left **shoulder**

√7ʰ **M84.619 Pathological fracture in other disease, unspecified shoulder**

√6ʰ **M84.62 Pathological fracture in other disease,** humerus

√7ʰ **M84.621 Pathological fracture in other disease,** right **humerus**

√7ʰ **M84.622 Pathological fracture in other disease,** left **humerus**

√7ʰ **M84.629 Pathological fracture in other disease, unspecified humerus**

√6ʰ **M84.63 Pathological fracture in other disease,** ulna and radius

√7ʰ **M84.631 Pathological fracture in other disease,** right ulna

√7ʰ **M84.632 Pathological fracture in other disease,** left ulna

√7ʰ **M84.633 Pathological fracture in other disease,** right radius

√7ʰ **M84.634 Pathological fracture in other disease,** left radius

√7ʰ **M84.639 Pathological fracture in other disease, unspecified ulna and radius**

√6ʰ **M84.64 Pathological fracture in other disease,** hand

√7ʰ **M84.641 Pathological fracture in other disease,** right **hand**

√7ʰ **M84.642 Pathological fracture in other disease,** left **hand**

√7ʰ **M84.649 Pathological fracture in other disease, unspecified hand**

√6ʰ **M84.65 Pathological fracture in other disease,** pelvis and femur

√7ʰ **M84.650 Pathological fracture in other disease,** pelvis

√7ʰ **M84.651 Pathological fracture in other disease,** right femur

√7ʰ **M84.652 Pathological fracture in other disease,** left femur

√7ᵗʰ **M84.653 Pathological fracture in other disease, unspecified femur**

√7ᵗʰ **M84.659 Pathological fracture in other disease, hip, unspecified**

√6ᵗʰ **M84.66 Pathological fracture in other disease, tibia and fibula**

√7ᵗʰ **M84.661 Pathological fracture in other disease, right tibia**

√7ᵗʰ **M84.662 Pathological fracture in other disease, left tibia**

√7ᵗʰ **M84.663 Pathological fracture in other disease, right fibula**

√7ᵗʰ **M84.664 Pathological fracture in other disease, left fibula**

√7ᵗʰ **M84.669 Pathological fracture in other disease, unspecified tibia and fibula**

√6ᵗʰ **M84.67 Pathological fracture in other disease, ankle and foot**

√7ᵗʰ **M84.671 Pathological fracture in other disease, right ankle**

√7ᵗʰ **M84.672 Pathological fracture in other disease, left ankle**

√7ᵗʰ **M84.673 Pathological fracture in other disease, unspecified ankle**

√7ᵗʰ **M84.674 Pathological fracture in other disease, right foot**

√7ᵗʰ **M84.675 Pathological fracture in other disease, left foot**

√7ᵗʰ **M84.676 Pathological fracture in other disease, unspecified foot**

√x7ᵗʰ **M84.68 Pathological fracture in other disease, other site**

√5ᵗʰ **M84.8 Other disorders of continuity of bone**

M84.80 Other disorders of continuity of bone, unspecified site

√6ᵗʰ **M84.81 Other disorders of continuity of bone, shoulder**

M84.811 Other disorders of continuity of bone, right shoulder

M84.812 Other disorders of continuity of bone, left shoulder

M84.819 Other disorders of continuity of bone, unspecified shoulder

√6ᵗʰ **M84.82 Other disorders of continuity of bone, humerus**

M84.821 Other disorders of continuity of bone, right humerus

M84.822 Other disorders of continuity of bone, left humerus

M84.829 Other disorders of continuity of bone, unspecified humerus

√6ᵗʰ **M84.83 Other disorders of continuity of bone, ulna and radius**

M84.831 Other disorders of continuity of bone, right ulna

M84.832 Other disorders of continuity of bone, left ulna

M84.833 Other disorders of continuity of bone, right radius

M84.834 Other disorders of continuity of bone, left radius

M84.839 Other disorders of continuity of bone, unspecified ulna and radius

√6ᵗʰ **M84.84 Other disorders of continuity of bone, hand**

M84.841 Other disorders of continuity of bone, right hand

M84.842 Other disorders of continuity of bone, left hand

M84.849 Other disorders of continuity of bone, unspecified hand

√6ᵗʰ **M84.85 Other disorders of continuity of bone, pelvic region and thigh**

M84.851 Other disorders of continuity of bone, right pelvic region and thigh

M84.852 Other disorders of continuity of bone, left pelvic region and thigh

M84.859 Other disorders of continuity of bone, unspecified pelvic region and thigh

√6ᵗʰ **M84.86 Other disorders of continuity of bone, tibia and fibula**

M84.861 Other disorders of continuity of bone, right tibia

M84.862 Other disorders of continuity of bone, left tibia

M84.863 Other disorders of continuity of bone, right fibula

M84.864 Other disorders of continuity of bone, left fibula

M84.869 Other disorders of continuity of bone, unspecified tibia and fibula

√6ᵗʰ **M84.87 Other disorders of continuity of bone, ankle and foot**

M84.871 Other disorders of continuity of bone, right ankle and foot

M84.872 Other disorders of continuity of bone, left ankle and foot

M84.879 Other disorders of continuity of bone, unspecified ankle and foot

M84.88 Other disorders of continuity of bone, other site

M84.9 Disorder of continuity of bone, unspecified

√4ᵗʰ **M85 Other disorders of bone density and structure**

EXCLUDES 1 osteogenesis imperfecta (Q78.0)
osteopetrosis (Q78.2)
osteopoikilosis (Q78.8)
polyostotic fibrous dysplasia (Q78.1)

√5ᵗʰ **M85.0 Fibrous dysplasia (monostotic)**

EXCLUDES 2 fibrous dysplasia of jaw (M27.8)

M85.00 Fibrous dysplasia (monostotic), unspecified site

√6ᵗʰ **M85.01 Fibrous dysplasia (monostotic), shoulder**

M85.011 Fibrous dysplasia (monostotic), right shoulder

M85.012 Fibrous dysplasia (monostotic), left shoulder

M85.019 Fibrous dysplasia (monostotic), unspecified shoulder

√6ᵗʰ **M85.02 Fibrous dysplasia (monostotic), upper arm**

M85.021 Fibrous dysplasia (monostotic), right upper arm

M85.022 Fibrous dysplasia (monostotic), left upper arm

M85.029 Fibrous dysplasia (monostotic), unspecified upper arm

√6ᵗʰ **M85.03 Fibrous dysplasia (monostotic), forearm**

M85.031 Fibrous dysplasia (monostotic), right forearm

M85.032 Fibrous dysplasia (monostotic), left forearm

M85.039 Fibrous dysplasia (monostotic), unspecified forearm

√6ᵗʰ **M85.04 Fibrous dysplasia (monostotic), hand**

M85.041 Fibrous dysplasia (monostotic), right hand

M85.042 Fibrous dysplasia (monostotic), left hand

M85.049 Fibrous dysplasia (monostotic), unspecified hand

√6ᵗʰ **M85.05 Fibrous dysplasia (monostotic), thigh**

M85.051 Fibrous dysplasia (monostotic), right thigh

M85.052 Fibrous dysplasia (monostotic), left thigh

M85.059 Fibrous dysplasia (monostotic), unspecified thigh

√6ᵗʰ **M85.06 Fibrous dysplasia (monostotic), lower leg**

M85.061 Fibrous dysplasia (monostotic), right lower leg

M85.062 Fibrous dysplasia (monostotic), left lower leg

M85.069 Fibrous dysplasia (monostotic), unspecified lower leg

√6ᵗʰ **M85.07 Fibrous dysplasia (monostotic), ankle and foot**

M85.071 Fibrous dysplasia (monostotic), right ankle and foot

M85.072 Fibrous dysplasia (monostotic), left ankle and foot

M85.079 Fibrous dysplasia (monostotic), unspecified ankle and foot

M85.08 Fibrous dysplasia (monostotic), other site

EXCLUDES 1 Not coded here   EXCLUDES 2 Not included here   N Newborn Age: 0   P Pediatric Age: 0-17   M Maternity Age: 12-55   A Adult Age: 15-124

704   ICD-10-CM Draft (2015)

M85.09   **Fibrous dysplasia (monostotic)**, multiple sites

√5ᵗʰ   **M85.1   Skeletal fluorosis**

    M85.10   **Skeletal fluorosis, unspecified site**

    √6ᵗʰ   M85.11   Skeletal fluorosis, shoulder

      M85.111   Skeletal fluorosis, right shoulder

      M85.112   Skeletal fluorosis, left shoulder

      M85.119   **Skeletal fluorosis, unspecified shoulder**

    √6ᵗʰ   M85.12   Skeletal fluorosis, upper arm

      M85.121   Skeletal fluorosis, right upper arm

      M85.122   Skeletal fluorosis, left upper arm

      M85.129   **Skeletal fluorosis, unspecified upper arm**

    √6ᵗʰ   M85.13   Skeletal fluorosis, forearm

      M85.131   Skeletal fluorosis, right forearm

      M85.132   Skeletal fluorosis, left forearm

      M85.139   **Skeletal fluorosis, unspecified forearm**

    √6ᵗʰ   M85.14   Skeletal fluorosis, hand

      M85.141   Skeletal fluorosis, right hand

      M85.142   Skeletal fluorosis, left hand

      M85.149   **Skeletal fluorosis, unspecified hand**

    √6ᵗʰ   M85.15   Skeletal fluorosis, thigh

      M85.151   Skeletal fluorosis, right thigh

      M85.152   Skeletal fluorosis, left thigh

      M85.159   **Skeletal fluorosis, unspecified thigh**

    √6ᵗʰ   M85.16   Skeletal fluorosis, lower leg

      M85.161   Skeletal fluorosis, right lower leg

      M85.162   Skeletal fluorosis, left lower leg

      M85.169   **Skeletal fluorosis, unspecified lower leg**

    √6ᵗʰ   M85.17   Skeletal fluorosis, ankle and foot

      M85.171   Skeletal fluorosis, right ankle and foot

      M85.172   Skeletal fluorosis, left ankle and foot

      M85.179   **Skeletal fluorosis, unspecified ankle and foot**

    M85.18   **Skeletal fluorosis, other site**

    M85.19   Skeletal fluorosis, multiple sites

M85.2   **Hyperostosis of skull**

√5ᵗʰ   **M85.3   Osteitis condensans**

    M85.30   **Osteitis condensans, unspecified site**

    √6ᵗʰ   M85.31   Osteitis condensans, shoulder

      M85.311   Osteitis condensans, right shoulder

      M85.312   Osteitis condensans, left shoulder

      M85.319   **Osteitis condensans, unspecified shoulder**

    √6ᵗʰ   M85.32   Osteitis condensans, upper arm

      M85.321   Osteitis condensans, right upper arm

      M85.322   Osteitis condensans, left upper arm

      M85.329   **Osteitis condensans, unspecified upper arm**

    √6ᵗʰ   M85.33   Osteitis condensans, forearm

      M85.331   Osteitis condensans, right forearm

      M85.332   Osteitis condensans, left forearm

      M85.339   **Osteitis condensans, unspecified forearm**

    √6ᵗʰ   M85.34   Osteitis condensans, hand

      M85.341   Osteitis condensans, right hand

      M85.342   Osteitis condensans, left hand

      M85.349   **Osteitis condensans, unspecified hand**

    √6ᵗʰ   M85.35   Osteitis condensans, thigh

      M85.351   Osteitis condensans, right thigh

      M85.352   Osteitis condensans, left thigh

      M85.359   **Osteitis condensans, unspecified thigh**

    √6ᵗʰ   M85.36   Osteitis condensans, lower leg

      M85.361   Osteitis condensans, right lower leg

      M85.362   Osteitis condensans, left lower leg

      M85.369   **Osteitis condensans, unspecified lower leg**

    √6ᵗʰ   M85.37   Osteitis condensans, ankle and foot

      M85.371   Osteitis condensans, right ankle and foot

      M85.372   Osteitis condensans, left ankle and foot

      M85.379   **Osteitis condensans, unspecified ankle and foot**

    M85.38   **Osteitis condensans, other site**

    M85.39   Osteitis condensans, multiple sites

√5ᵗʰ   **M85.4   Solitary bone cyst**

    EXCLUDES 2   solitary cyst of jaw (M27.4)

    M85.40   **Solitary bone cyst, unspecified site**

    √6ᵗʰ   M85.41   Solitary bone cyst, shoulder

      M85.411   Solitary bone cyst, right shoulder

      M85.412   Solitary bone cyst, left shoulder

      M85.419   **Solitary bone cyst, unspecified shoulder**

    √6ᵗʰ   M85.42   Solitary bone cyst, humerus

      M85.421   Solitary bone cyst, right humerus

      M85.422   Solitary bone cyst, left humerus

      M85.429   **Solitary bone cyst, unspecified humerus**

    √6ᵗʰ   M85.43   Solitary bone cyst, ulna and radius

      M85.431   Solitary bone cyst, right ulna and radius

      M85.432   Solitary bone cyst, left ulna and radius

      M85.439   **Solitary bone cyst, unspecified ulna and radius**

    √6ᵗʰ   M85.44   Solitary bone cyst, hand

      M85.441   Solitary bone cyst, right hand

      M85.442   Solitary bone cyst, left hand

      M85.449   **Solitary bone cyst, unspecified hand**

    √6ᵗʰ   M85.45   Solitary bone cyst, pelvis

      M85.451   Solitary bone cyst, right pelvis

      M85.452   Solitary bone cyst, left pelvis

      M85.459   **Solitary bone cyst, unspecified pelvis**

    √6ᵗʰ   M85.46   Solitary bone cyst, tibia and fibula

      M85.461   Solitary bone cyst, right tibia and fibula

      M85.462   Solitary bone cyst, left tibia and fibula

      M85.469   **Solitary bone cyst, unspecified tibia and fibula**

    √6ᵗʰ   M85.47   Solitary bone cyst, ankle and foot

      M85.471   Solitary bone cyst, right ankle and foot

      M85.472   Solitary bone cyst, left ankle and foot

      M85.479   **Solitary bone cyst, unspecified ankle and foot**

    M85.48   **Solitary bone cyst, other site**

√5ᵗʰ   **M85.5   Aneurysmal bone cyst**

    EXCLUDES 2   aneurysmal cyst of jaw (M27.4)

    M85.50   **Aneurysmal bone cyst, unspecified site**

    √6ᵗʰ   M85.51   Aneurysmal bone cyst, shoulder

      M85.511   Aneurysmal bone cyst, right shoulder

      M85.512   Aneurysmal bone cyst, left shoulder

      M85.519   **Aneurysmal bone cyst, unspecified shoulder**

    √6ᵗʰ   M85.52   Aneurysmal bone cyst, upper arm

      M85.521   Aneurysmal bone cyst, right upper arm

      M85.522   Aneurysmal bone cyst, left upper arm

      M85.529   **Aneurysmal bone cyst, unspecified upper arm**

    √6ᵗʰ   M85.53   Aneurysmal bone cyst, forearm

      M85.531   Aneurysmal bone cyst, right forearm

      M85.532   Aneurysmal bone cyst, left forearm

      M85.539   **Aneurysmal bone cyst, unspecified forearm**

    √6ᵗʰ   M85.54   Aneurysmal bone cyst, hand

      M85.541   Aneurysmal bone cyst, right hand

      M85.542   Aneurysmal bone cyst, left hand

      M85.549   **Aneurysmal bone cyst, unspecified hand**

    √6ᵗʰ   M85.55   Aneurysmal bone cyst, thigh

      M85.551   Aneurysmal bone cyst, right thigh

      M85.552   Aneurysmal bone cyst, left thigh

      M85.559   **Aneurysmal bone cyst, unspecified thigh**

    √6ᵗʰ   M85.56   Aneurysmal bone cyst, lower leg

      M85.561   Aneurysmal bone cyst, right lower leg

      M85.562   Aneurysmal bone cyst, left lower leg

      M85.569   **Aneurysmal bone cyst, unspecified lower leg**

    √6ᵗʰ   M85.57   Aneurysmal bone cyst, ankle and foot

      M85.571   Aneurysmal bone cyst, right ankle and foot

      M85.572   Aneurysmal bone cyst, left ankle and foot

      M85.579   **Aneurysmal bone cyst, unspecified ankle and foot**

✓ Additional Character Required   ᵛˣ⁷ᵗʰ Xtension Alert   Unspecified Dx   Other Specified Dx   Manifestation   ►◄ Revised Text   ● New Code   ▲ Revised Code Title

M85.58 **Aneurysmal bone cyst, other site**

M85.59 **Aneurysmal bone cyst,** multiple sites

✓5ᵗʰ **M85.6** Other cyst of bone

    EXCLUDES 1   cyst of jaw NEC (M27.4)
           osteitis fibrosa cystica generalisata [von
            Recklinghausen's disease of bone] (E21.0)

M85.60 **Other cyst of bone, unspecified site**

✓6ᵗʰ M85.61 **Other cyst of bone,** shoulder

     M85.611 **Other cyst of bone,** right **shoulder**

     M85.612 **Other cyst of bone,** left **shoulder**

     M85.619 **Other cyst of bone, unspecified shoulder**

✓6ᵗʰ M85.62 **Other cyst of bone,** upper arm

     M85.621 **Other cyst of bone,** right **upper arm**

     M85.622 **Other cyst of bone,** left **upper arm**

     M85.629 **Other cyst of bone, unspecified upper arm**

✓6ᵗʰ M85.63 **Other cyst of bone,** forearm

     M85.631 **Other cyst of bone,** right **forearm**

     M85.632 **Other cyst of bone,** left **forearm**

     M85.639 **Other cyst of bone, unspecified forearm**

✓6ᵗʰ M85.64 **Other cyst of bone,** hand

     M85.641 **Other cyst of bone,** right **hand**

     M85.642 **Other cyst of bone,** left **hand**

     M85.649 **Other cyst of bone, unspecified hand**

✓6ᵗʰ M85.65 **Other cyst of bone,** thigh

     M85.651 **Other cyst of bone,** right **thigh**

     M85.652 **Other cyst of bone,** left **thigh**

     M85.659 **Other cyst of bone, unspecified thigh**

✓6ᵗʰ M85.66 **Other cyst of bone,** lower leg

     M85.661 **Other cyst of bone,** right **lower leg**

     M85.662 **Other cyst of bone,** left **lower leg**

     M85.669 **Other cyst of bone, unspecified lower leg**

✓6ᵗʰ M85.67 **Other cyst of bone,** ankle and foot

     M85.671 **Other cyst of bone,** right **ankle and foot**

     M85.672 **Other cyst of bone,** left **ankle and foot**

     M85.679 **Other cyst of bone, unspecified ankle and foot**

M85.68 **Other cyst of bone, other site**

M85.69 **Other cyst of bone,** multiple sites

✓5ᵗʰ **M85.8** Other specified disorders of bone density and structure

     Hyperostosis of bones, except skull
     Osteosclerosis, acquired

    EXCLUDES 1   diffuse idiopathic skeletal hyperostosis [DISH] (M48.1)
           osteosclerosis congenita (Q77.4)
           osteosclerosis fragilitas (generalista) (Q78.2)
           osteosclerosis myelofibrosis (D75.81)

M85.80 **Other specified disorders of bone density and structure, unspecified site**

✓6ᵗʰ M85.81 **Other specified disorders of bone density and structure,** shoulder

     M85.811 **Other specified disorders of bone density and structure,** right **shoulder**

     M85.812 **Other specified disorders of bone density and structure,** left **shoulder**

     M85.819 **Other specified disorders of bone density and structure, unspecified shoulder**

✓6ᵗʰ M85.82 **Other specified disorders of bone density and structure,** upper arm

     M85.821 **Other specified disorders of bone density and structure,** right **upper arm**

     M85.822 **Other specified disorders of bone density and structure,** left **upper arm**

     M85.829 **Other specified disorders of bone density and structure, unspecified upper arm**

✓6ᵗʰ M85.83 **Other specified disorders of bone density and structure,** forearm

     M85.831 **Other specified disorders of bone density and structure,** right **forearm**

     M85.832 **Other specified disorders of bone density and structure,** left **forearm**

     M85.839 **Other specified disorders of bone density and structure, unspecified forearm**

✓6ᵗʰ M85.84 **Other specified disorders of bone density and structure,** hand

     M85.841 **Other specified disorders of bone density and structure,** right **hand**

M85.842 **Other specified disorders of bone density and structure,** left **hand**

M85.849 **Other specified disorders of bone density and structure, unspecified hand**

✓6ᵗʰ M85.85 **Other specified disorders of bone density and structure,** thigh

     M85.851 **Other specified disorders of bone density and structure,** right **thigh**

     M85.852 **Other specified disorders of bone density and structure,** left **thigh**

     M85.859 **Other specified disorders of bone density and structure, unspecified thigh**

✓6ᵗʰ M85.86 **Other specified disorders of bone density and structure,** lower leg

     M85.861 **Other specified disorders of bone density and structure,** right **lower leg**

     M85.862 **Other specified disorders of bone density and structure,** left **lower leg**

     M85.869 **Other specified disorders of bone density and structure, unspecified lower leg**

✓6ᵗʰ M85.87 **Other specified disorders of bone density and structure,** ankle and foot

     M85.871 **Other specified disorders of bone density and structure,** right **ankle and foot**

     M85.872 **Other specified disorders of bone density and structure,** left **ankle and foot**

     M85.879 **Other specified disorders of bone density and structure, unspecified ankle and foot**

M85.88 **Other specified disorders of bone density and structure, other site**

M85.89 **Other specified disorders of bone density and structure,** multiple sites

M85.9 **Disorder of bone density and structure, unspecified**

Other osteopathies (M86-M90)

EXCLUDES 1   postprocedural osteopathies (M96.-)

✓4ᵗʰ **M86 Osteomyelitis**

     Use additional code (B95-B97) to identify infectious agent
     Use additional code to identify major osseous defect, if applicable (M89.7-)

    EXCLUDES 1   osteomyelitis due to:
           echinococcus (B67.2)
           gonococcus (A54.43)
           salmonella (A02.24)

    EXCLUDES 2   osteomyelitis of:
           orbit (H05.0-)
           petrous bone (H70.2-)
           vertebra (M46.2-)

✓5ᵗʰ **M86.0** Acute hematogenous osteomyelitis

M86.00 **Acute hematogenous osteomyelitis, unspecified site**

✓6ᵗʰ M86.01 **Acute hematogenous osteomyelitis,** shoulder

     M86.011 **Acute hematogenous osteomyelitis,** right **shoulder**

     M86.012 **Acute hematogenous osteomyelitis,** left **shoulder**

     M86.019 **Acute hematogenous osteomyelitis, unspecified shoulder**

✓6ᵗʰ M86.02 **Acute hematogenous osteomyelitis,** humerus

     M86.021 **Acute hematogenous osteomyelitis,** right **humerus**

     M86.022 **Acute hematogenous osteomyelitis,** left **humerus**

     M86.029 **Acute hematogenous osteomyelitis, unspecified humerus**

✓6ᵗʰ M86.03 **Acute hematogenous osteomyelitis,** radius and ulna

     M86.031 **Acute hematogenous osteomyelitis,** right **radius and ulna**

     M86.032 **Acute hematogenous osteomyelitis,** left **radius and ulna**

     M86.039 **Acute hematogenous osteomyelitis, unspecified radius and ulna**

✓6ᵗʰ M86.04 **Acute hematogenous osteomyelitis,** hand

     M86.041 **Acute hematogenous osteomyelitis,** right **hand**

     M86.042 **Acute hematogenous osteomyelitis,** left **hand**

EXCLUDES 1 Not coded here   EXCLUDES 2 Not included here   N Newborn Age: 0   P Pediatric Age: 0-17   M Maternity Age: 12-55   A Adult Age: 15-124

706   ICD-10-CM Draft (2015)

M86.049 **Acute hematogenous osteomyelitis, unspecified hand**

☑6ᵗʰ M86.05 Acute hematogenous osteomyelitis, femur

M86.051 Acute hematogenous osteomyelitis, right femur

M86.052 Acute hematogenous osteomyelitis, left femur

M86.059 **Acute hematogenous osteomyelitis, unspecified femur**

☑6ᵗʰ M86.06 Acute hematogenous osteomyelitis, tibia and fibula

M86.061 Acute hematogenous osteomyelitis, right tibia and fibula

M86.062 Acute hematogenous osteomyelitis, left tibia and fibula

M86.069 **Acute hematogenous osteomyelitis, unspecified tibia and fibula**

☑6ᵗʰ M86.07 Acute hematogenous osteomyelitis, ankle and foot

M86.071 Acute hematogenous osteomyelitis, right ankle and foot

M86.072 Acute hematogenous osteomyelitis, left ankle and foot

M86.079 **Acute hematogenous osteomyelitis, unspecified ankle and foot**

M86.08 **Acute hematogenous osteomyelitis, other sites**

M86.09 Acute hematogenous osteomyelitis, multiple sites

☑5ᵗʰ M86.1 Other acute osteomyelitis

M86.10 **Other acute osteomyelitis, unspecified site**

☑6ᵗʰ M86.11 Other acute osteomyelitis, shoulder

M86.111 Other acute osteomyelitis, right shoulder

M86.112 Other acute osteomyelitis, left shoulder

M86.119 **Other acute osteomyelitis, unspecified shoulder**

☑6ᵗʰ M86.12 Other acute osteomyelitis, humerus

M86.121 Other acute osteomyelitis, right humerus

M86.122 Other acute osteomyelitis, left humerus

M86.129 **Other acute osteomyelitis, unspecified humerus**

☑6ᵗʰ M86.13 Other acute osteomyelitis, radius and ulna

M86.131 Other acute osteomyelitis, right radius and ulna

M86.132 Other acute osteomyelitis, left radius and ulna

M86.139 **Other acute osteomyelitis, unspecified radius and ulna**

☑6ᵗʰ M86.14 Other acute osteomyelitis, hand

M86.141 Other acute osteomyelitis, right hand

M86.142 Other acute osteomyelitis, left hand

M86.149 **Other acute osteomyelitis, unspecified hand**

☑6ᵗʰ M86.15 Other acute osteomyelitis, femur

M86.151 Other acute osteomyelitis, right femur

M86.152 Other acute osteomyelitis, left femur

M86.159 **Other acute osteomyelitis, unspecified femur**

☑6ᵗʰ M86.16 Other acute osteomyelitis, tibia and fibula

M86.161 Other acute osteomyelitis, right tibia and fibula

M86.162 Other acute osteomyelitis, left tibia and fibula

M86.169 **Other acute osteomyelitis, unspecified tibia and fibula**

☑6ᵗʰ M86.17 Other acute osteomyelitis, ankle and foot

M86.171 Other acute osteomyelitis, right ankle and foot

M86.172 Other acute osteomyelitis, left ankle and foot

M86.179 **Other acute osteomyelitis, unspecified ankle and foot**

M86.18 **Other acute osteomyelitis, other site**

M86.19 Other acute osteomyelitis, multiple sites

☑5ᵗʰ M86.2 Subacute osteomyelitis

M86.20 **Subacute osteomyelitis, unspecified site**

☑6ᵗʰ M86.21 Subacute osteomyelitis, shoulder

M86.211 Subacute osteomyelitis, right shoulder

M86.212 Subacute osteomyelitis, left shoulder

M86.219 **Subacute osteomyelitis, unspecified shoulder**

☑6ᵗʰ M86.22 Subacute osteomyelitis, humerus

M86.221 Subacute osteomyelitis, right humerus

M86.222 Subacute osteomyelitis, left humerus

M86.229 **Subacute osteomyelitis, unspecified humerus**

☑6ᵗʰ M86.23 Subacute osteomyelitis, radius and ulna

M86.231 Subacute osteomyelitis, right radius and ulna

M86.232 Subacute osteomyelitis, left radius and ulna

M86.239 **Subacute osteomyelitis, unspecified radius and ulna**

☑6ᵗʰ M86.24 Subacute osteomyelitis, hand

M86.241 Subacute osteomyelitis, right hand

M86.242 Subacute osteomyelitis, left hand

M86.249 **Subacute osteomyelitis, unspecified hand**

☑6ᵗʰ M86.25 Subacute osteomyelitis, femur

M86.251 Subacute osteomyelitis, right femur

M86.252 Subacute osteomyelitis, left femur

M86.259 **Subacute osteomyelitis, unspecified femur**

☑6ᵗʰ M86.26 Subacute osteomyelitis, tibia and fibula

M86.261 Subacute osteomyelitis, right tibia and fibula

M86.262 Subacute osteomyelitis, left tibia and fibula

M86.269 **Subacute osteomyelitis, unspecified tibia and fibula**

☑6ᵗʰ M86.27 Subacute osteomyelitis, ankle and foot

M86.271 Subacute osteomyelitis, right ankle and foot

M86.272 Subacute osteomyelitis, left ankle and foot

M86.279 **Subacute osteomyelitis, unspecified ankle and foot**

M86.28 **Subacute osteomyelitis, other site**

M86.29 Subacute osteomyelitis, multiple sites

☑5ᵗʰ M86.3 Chronic multifocal osteomyelitis

M86.30 **Chronic multifocal osteomyelitis, unspecified site**

☑6ᵗʰ M86.31 Chronic multifocal osteomyelitis, shoulder

M86.311 Chronic multifocal osteomyelitis, right shoulder

M86.312 Chronic multifocal osteomyelitis, left shoulder

M86.319 **Chronic multifocal osteomyelitis, unspecified shoulder**

☑6ᵗʰ M86.32 Chronic multifocal osteomyelitis, humerus

M86.321 Chronic multifocal osteomyelitis, right humerus

M86.322 Chronic multifocal osteomyelitis, left humerus

M86.329 **Chronic multifocal osteomyelitis, unspecified humerus**

☑6ᵗʰ M86.33 Chronic multifocal osteomyelitis, radius and ulna

M86.331 Chronic multifocal osteomyelitis, right radius and ulna

M86.332 Chronic multifocal osteomyelitis, left radius and ulna

M86.339 **Chronic multifocal osteomyelitis, unspecified radius and ulna**

☑6ᵗʰ M86.34 Chronic multifocal osteomyelitis, hand

M86.341 Chronic multifocal osteomyelitis, right hand

M86.342 Chronic multifocal osteomyelitis, left hand

M86.349 **Chronic multifocal osteomyelitis, unspecified hand**

☑6ᵗʰ M86.35 Chronic multifocal osteomyelitis, femur

M86.351 Chronic multifocal osteomyelitis, right femur

M86.352 Chronic multifocal osteomyelitis, left femur

M86.359 **Chronic multifocal osteomyelitis, unspecified femur**

☑ Additional Character Required   ✗x7ᵗʰ Xtension Alert   Unspecified Dx   Other Specified Dx   Manifestation   ►◄ Revised Text   ● New Code   ▲ Revised Code Title

ICD-10-CM Draft (2015)   **707**

√6ᵗʰ **M86.36** Chronic multifocal osteomyelitis, tibia and fibula

     M86.361 Chronic multifocal osteomyelitis, right tibia and fibula

     M86.362 Chronic multifocal osteomyelitis, left tibia and fibula

     M86.369 Chronic multifocal osteomyelitis, unspecified tibia and fibula

√6ᵗʰ **M86.37** Chronic multifocal osteomyelitis, ankle and foot

     M86.371 Chronic multifocal osteomyelitis, right ankle and foot

     M86.372 Chronic multifocal osteomyelitis, left ankle and foot

     M86.379 Chronic multifocal osteomyelitis, unspecified ankle and foot

M86.38 Chronic multifocal osteomyelitis, other site

M86.39 Chronic multifocal osteomyelitis, multiple sites

√5ᵗʰ **M86.4** Chronic osteomyelitis with draining sinus

     M86.40 Chronic osteomyelitis with draining sinus, unspecified site

√6ᵗʰ **M86.41** Chronic osteomyelitis with draining sinus, shoulder

     M86.411 Chronic osteomyelitis with draining sinus, right shoulder

     M86.412 Chronic osteomyelitis with draining sinus, left shoulder

     M86.419 Chronic osteomyelitis with draining sinus, unspecified shoulder

√6ᵗʰ **M86.42** Chronic osteomyelitis with draining sinus, humerus

     M86.421 Chronic osteomyelitis with draining sinus, right humerus

     M86.422 Chronic osteomyelitis with draining sinus, left humerus

     M86.429 Chronic osteomyelitis with draining sinus, unspecified humerus

√6ᵗʰ **M86.43** Chronic osteomyelitis with draining sinus, radius and ulna

     M86.431 Chronic osteomyelitis with draining sinus, right radius and ulna

     M86.432 Chronic osteomyelitis with draining sinus, left radius and ulna

     M86.439 Chronic osteomyelitis with draining sinus, unspecified radius and ulna

√6ᵗʰ **M86.44** Chronic osteomyelitis with draining sinus, hand

     M86.441 Chronic osteomyelitis with draining sinus, right hand

     M86.442 Chronic osteomyelitis with draining sinus, left hand

     M86.449 Chronic osteomyelitis with draining sinus, unspecified hand

√6ᵗʰ **M86.45** Chronic osteomyelitis with draining sinus, femur

     M86.451 Chronic osteomyelitis with draining sinus, right femur

     M86.452 Chronic osteomyelitis with draining sinus, left femur

     M86.459 Chronic osteomyelitis with draining sinus, unspecified femur

√6ᵗʰ **M86.46** Chronic osteomyelitis with draining sinus, tibia and fibula

     M86.461 Chronic osteomyelitis with draining sinus, right tibia and fibula

     M86.462 Chronic osteomyelitis with draining sinus, left tibia and fibula

     M86.469 Chronic osteomyelitis with draining sinus, unspecified tibia and fibula

√6ᵗʰ **M86.47** Chronic osteomyelitis with draining sinus, ankle and foot

     M86.471 Chronic osteomyelitis with draining sinus, right ankle and foot

     M86.472 Chronic osteomyelitis with draining sinus, left ankle and foot

     M86.479 Chronic osteomyelitis with draining sinus, unspecified ankle and foot

M86.48 Chronic osteomyelitis with draining sinus, other site

M86.49 Chronic osteomyelitis with draining sinus, multiple sites

√5ᵗʰ **M86.5** Other chronic hematogenous osteomyelitis

     M86.50 Other chronic hematogenous osteomyelitis, unspecified site

√6ᵗʰ **M86.51** Other chronic hematogenous osteomyelitis, shoulder

     M86.511 Other chronic hematogenous osteomyelitis, right shoulder

     M86.512 Other chronic hematogenous osteomyelitis, left shoulder

     M86.519 Other chronic hematogenous osteomyelitis, unspecified shoulder

√6ᵗʰ **M86.52** Other chronic hematogenous osteomyelitis, humerus

     M86.521 Other chronic hematogenous osteomyelitis, right humerus

     M86.522 Other chronic hematogenous osteomyelitis, left humerus

     M86.529 Other chronic hematogenous osteomyelitis, unspecified humerus

√6ᵗʰ **M86.53** Other chronic hematogenous osteomyelitis, radius and ulna

     M86.531 Other chronic hematogenous osteomyelitis, right radius and ulna

     M86.532 Other chronic hematogenous osteomyelitis, left radius and ulna

     M86.539 Other chronic hematogenous osteomyelitis, unspecified radius and ulna

√6ᵗʰ **M86.54** Other chronic hematogenous osteomyelitis, hand

     M86.541 Other chronic hematogenous osteomyelitis, right hand

     M86.542 Other chronic hematogenous osteomyelitis, left hand

     M86.549 Other chronic hematogenous osteomyelitis, unspecified hand

√6ᵗʰ **M86.55** Other chronic hematogenous osteomyelitis, femur

     M86.551 Other chronic hematogenous osteomyelitis, right femur

     M86.552 Other chronic hematogenous osteomyelitis, left femur

     M86.559 Other chronic hematogenous osteomyelitis, unspecified femur

√6ᵗʰ **M86.56** Other chronic hematogenous osteomyelitis, tibia and fibula

     M86.561 Other chronic hematogenous osteomyelitis, right tibia and fibula

     M86.562 Other chronic hematogenous osteomyelitis, left tibia and fibula

     M86.569 Other chronic hematogenous osteomyelitis, unspecified tibia and fibula

√6ᵗʰ **M86.57** Other chronic hematogenous osteomyelitis, ankle and foot

     M86.571 Other chronic hematogenous osteomyelitis, right ankle and foot

     M86.572 Other chronic hematogenous osteomyelitis, left ankle and foot

     M86.579 Other chronic hematogenous osteomyelitis, unspecified ankle and foot

M86.58 Other chronic hematogenous osteomyelitis, other site

M86.59 Other chronic hematogenous osteomyelitis, multiple sites

√5ᵗʰ **M86.6** Other chronic osteomyelitis

     M86.60 Other chronic osteomyelitis, unspecified site

√6ᵗʰ **M86.61** Other chronic osteomyelitis, shoulder

     M86.611 Other chronic osteomyelitis, right shoulder

     M86.612 Other chronic osteomyelitis, left shoulder

     M86.619 Other chronic osteomyelitis, unspecified shoulder

√6ᵗʰ **M86.62** Other chronic osteomyelitis, humerus

     M86.621 Other chronic osteomyelitis, right humerus

     M86.622 Other chronic osteomyelitis, left humerus

     M86.629 Other chronic osteomyelitis, unspecified humerus

√6ᵗʰ **M86.63** Other chronic osteomyelitis, radius and ulna

     M86.631 Other chronic osteomyelitis, right radius and ulna

     M86.632 Other chronic osteomyelitis, left radius and ulna

EXCLUDES 1 Not coded here   **EXCLUDES 2** Not included here   N Newborn Age: 0   P Pediatric Age: 0-17   M Maternity Age: 12-55   A Adult Age: 15-124

708   ICD-10-CM Draft (2015)

M86.639 **Other chronic osteomyelitis, unspecified radius and ulna**

✓6ᵗʰ M86.64 Other chronic osteomyelitis, hand

M86.641 **Other chronic osteomyelitis, right hand**

M86.642 **Other chronic osteomyelitis, left hand**

M86.649 **Other chronic osteomyelitis, unspecified hand**

✓6ᵗʰ M86.65 Other chronic osteomyelitis, thigh

M86.651 **Other chronic osteomyelitis, right thigh**

M86.652 **Other chronic osteomyelitis, left thigh**

M86.659 **Other chronic osteomyelitis, unspecified thigh**

✓6ᵗʰ M86.66 Other chronic osteomyelitis, tibia and fibula

M86.661 **Other chronic osteomyelitis, right tibia and fibula**

M86.662 **Other chronic osteomyelitis, left tibia and fibula**

M86.669 **Other chronic osteomyelitis, unspecified tibia and fibula**

✓6ᵗʰ M86.67 Other chronic osteomyelitis, ankle and foot

M86.671 **Other chronic osteomyelitis, right ankle and foot**

M86.672 **Other chronic osteomyelitis, left ankle and foot**

M86.679 **Other chronic osteomyelitis, unspecified ankle and foot**

M86.68 **Other chronic osteomyelitis, other site**

M86.69 **Other chronic osteomyelitis, multiple sites**

✓5ᵗʰ M86.8 Other osteomyelitis
Brodie's abscess

✓6ᵗʰ M86.8X Other osteomyelitis

M86.8X0 **Other osteomyelitis, multiple sites**

M86.8X1 **Other osteomyelitis, shoulder**

M86.8X2 **Other osteomyelitis, upper arm**

M86.8X3 **Other osteomyelitis, forearm**

M86.8X4 **Other osteomyelitis, hand**

M86.8X5 **Other osteomyelitis, thigh**

M86.8X6 **Other osteomyelitis, lower leg**

M86.8X7 **Other osteomyelitis, ankle and foot**

M86.8X8 **Other osteomyelitis, other site**

M86.8X9 **Other osteomyelitis, unspecified sites**

M86.9 **Osteomyelitis, unspecified**
Infection of bone NOS   Periostitis without osteomyelitis

✓4ᵗʰ **M87 Osteonecrosis**
INCLUDES avascular necrosis of bone
Use additional code to identify major osseous defect, if applicable (M89.7-)
EXCLUDES 1 juvenile osteonecrosis (M91-M92)
osteochondropathies (M90-M93)

✓5ᵗʰ M87.0 Idiopathic aseptic necrosis of bone

M87.00 **Idiopathic aseptic necrosis of unspecified bone**

✓6ᵗʰ M87.01 Idiopathic aseptic necrosis of shoulder
Idiopathic aseptic necrosis of clavicle and scapula

M87.011 **Idiopathic aseptic necrosis of right shoulder**

M87.012 **Idiopathic aseptic necrosis of left shoulder**

M87.019 **Idiopathic aseptic necrosis of unspecified shoulder**

✓6ᵗʰ M87.02 Idiopathic aseptic necrosis of humerus

M87.021 **Idiopathic aseptic necrosis of right humerus**

M87.022 **Idiopathic aseptic necrosis of left humerus**

M87.029 **Idiopathic aseptic necrosis of unspecified humerus**

✓6ᵗʰ M87.03 Idiopathic aseptic necrosis of radius, ulna and carpus

M87.031 **Idiopathic aseptic necrosis of right radius**

M87.032 **Idiopathic aseptic necrosis of left radius**

M87.033 **Idiopathic aseptic necrosis of unspecified radius**

M87.034 **Idiopathic aseptic necrosis of right ulna**

M87.035 **Idiopathic aseptic necrosis of left ulna**

M87.036 **Idiopathic aseptic necrosis of unspecified ulna**

M87.037 **Idiopathic aseptic necrosis of right carpus**

M87.038 **Idiopathic aseptic necrosis of left carpus**

M87.039 **Idiopathic aseptic necrosis of unspecified carpus**

✓6ᵗʰ M87.04 Idiopathic aseptic necrosis of hand and fingers
Idiopathic aseptic necrosis of metacarpals and phalanges of hands

M87.041 **Idiopathic aseptic necrosis of right hand**

M87.042 **Idiopathic aseptic necrosis of left hand**

M87.043 **Idiopathic aseptic necrosis of unspecified hand**

M87.044 **Idiopathic aseptic necrosis of right finger(s)**

M87.045 **Idiopathic aseptic necrosis of left finger(s)**

M87.046 **Idiopathic aseptic necrosis of unspecified finger(s)**

✓6ᵗʰ M87.05 Idiopathic aseptic necrosis of pelvis and femur

M87.050 **Idiopathic aseptic necrosis of pelvis**

M87.051 **Idiopathic aseptic necrosis of right femur**

M87.052 **Idiopathic aseptic necrosis of left femur**

M87.059 **Idiopathic aseptic necrosis of unspecified femur**
Idiopathic aseptic necrosis of hip NOS

✓6ᵗʰ M87.06 Idiopathic aseptic necrosis of tibia and fibula

M87.061 **Idiopathic aseptic necrosis of right tibia**

M87.062 **Idiopathic aseptic necrosis of left tibia**

M87.063 **Idiopathic aseptic necrosis of unspecified tibia**

M87.064 **Idiopathic aseptic necrosis of right fibula**

M87.065 **Idiopathic aseptic necrosis of left fibula**

M87.066 **Idiopathic aseptic necrosis of unspecified fibula**

✓6ᵗʰ M87.07 Idiopathic aseptic necrosis of ankle, foot and toes
Idiopathic aseptic necrosis of metatarsus, tarsus, and phalanges of toes

M87.071 **Idiopathic aseptic necrosis of right ankle**

M87.072 **Idiopathic aseptic necrosis of left ankle**

M87.073 **Idiopathic aseptic necrosis of unspecified ankle**

M87.074 **Idiopathic aseptic necrosis of right foot**

M87.075 **Idiopathic aseptic necrosis of left foot**

M87.076 **Idiopathic aseptic necrosis of unspecified foot**

M87.077 **Idiopathic aseptic necrosis of right toe(s)**

M87.078 **Idiopathic aseptic necrosis of left toe(s)**

M87.079 **Idiopathic aseptic necrosis of unspecified toe(s)**

M87.08 **Idiopathic aseptic necrosis of bone, other site**

M87.09 **Idiopathic aseptic necrosis of bone, multiple sites**

✓5ᵗʰ M87.1 Osteonecrosis due to drugs
Use additional code for adverse effect, if applicable, to identify drug (T36-T50 with fifth or sixth character 5)

M87.10 **Osteonecrosis due to drugs, unspecified bone**

✓6ᵗʰ M87.11 Osteonecrosis due to drugs, shoulder

M87.111 **Osteonecrosis due to drugs, right shoulder**

M87.112 **Osteonecrosis due to drugs, left shoulder**

M87.119 **Osteonecrosis due to drugs, unspecified shoulder**

✓6ᵗʰ M87.12 Osteonecrosis due to drugs, humerus

M87.121 **Osteonecrosis due to drugs, right humerus**

M87.122 **Osteonecrosis due to drugs, left humerus**

M87.129 **Osteonecrosis due to drugs, unspecified humerus**

✓6ᵗʰ M87.13 Osteonecrosis due to drugs of radius, ulna and carpus

M87.131 **Osteonecrosis due to drugs of right radius**

M87.132 **Osteonecrosis due to drugs of left radius**

M87.133 **Osteonecrosis due to drugs of unspecified radius**

M87.134 **Osteonecrosis due to drugs of right ulna**

M87.135 **Osteonecrosis due to drugs of left ulna**

M87.136 **Osteonecrosis due to drugs of unspecified ulna**

M87.137 **Osteonecrosis due to drugs of right carpus**

M87.138 **Osteonecrosis due to drugs of left carpus**

M87.139 **Osteonecrosis due to drugs of unspecified carpus**

✓6th **M87.14** Osteonecrosis due to drugs, hand and fingers
　　M87.141 Osteonecrosis due to drugs, right hand
　　M87.142 Osteonecrosis due to drugs, left hand
　　M87.143 **Osteonecrosis due to drugs, unspecified hand**
　　M87.144 Osteonecrosis due to drugs, right finger(s)
　　M87.145 Osteonecrosis due to drugs, left finger(s)
　　M87.146 **Osteonecrosis due to drugs, unspecified finger(s)**

✓6th **M87.15** Osteonecrosis due to drugs, pelvis and femur
　　M87.150 Osteonecrosis due to drugs, pelvis
　　M87.151 Osteonecrosis due to drugs, right femur
　　M87.152 Osteonecrosis due to drugs, left femur
　　M87.159 **Osteonecrosis due to drugs, unspecified femur**

✓6th **M87.16** Osteonecrosis due to drugs, tibia and fibula
　　M87.161 Osteonecrosis due to drugs, right tibia
　　M87.162 Osteonecrosis due to drugs, left tibia
　　M87.163 **Osteonecrosis due to drugs, unspecified tibia**
　　M87.164 Osteonecrosis due to drugs, right fibula
　　M87.165 Osteonecrosis due to drugs, left fibula
　　M87.166 **Osteonecrosis due to drugs, unspecified fibula**

✓6th **M87.17** Osteonecrosis due to drugs, ankle, foot and toes
　　M87.171 Osteonecrosis due to drugs, right ankle
　　M87.172 Osteonecrosis due to drugs, left ankle
　　M87.173 **Osteonecrosis due to drugs, unspecified ankle**
　　M87.174 Osteonecrosis due to drugs, right foot
　　M87.175 Osteonecrosis due to drugs, left foot
　　M87.176 **Osteonecrosis due to drugs, unspecified foot**
　　M87.177 Osteonecrosis due to drugs, right toe(s)
　　M87.178 Osteonecrosis due to drugs, left toe(s)
　　M87.179 **Osteonecrosis due to drugs, unspecified toe(s)**

✓6th **M87.18** Osteonecrosis due to drugs, other site
　　M87.180 Osteonecrosis due to drugs, jaw
　　M87.188 **Osteonecrosis due to drugs, other site**

　　M87.19 Osteonecrosis due to drugs, multiple sites

✓5th **M87.2** Osteonecrosis due to previous trauma
　　M87.20 Osteonecrosis due to previous trauma, unspecified bone

✓6th **M87.21** Osteonecrosis due to previous trauma, shoulder
　　M87.211 **Osteonecrosis due to previous trauma, right shoulder**
　　M87.212 **Osteonecrosis due to previous trauma, left shoulder**
　　M87.219 **Osteonecrosis due to previous trauma, unspecified shoulder**

✓6th **M87.22** Osteonecrosis due to previous trauma, humerus
　　M87.221 **Osteonecrosis due to previous trauma, right humerus**
　　M87.222 **Osteonecrosis due to previous trauma, left humerus**
　　M87.229 **Osteonecrosis due to previous trauma, unspecified humerus**

✓6th **M87.23** Osteonecrosis due to previous trauma of radius, ulna and carpus
　　M87.231 Osteonecrosis due to previous trauma of right radius
　　M87.232 Osteonecrosis due to previous trauma of left radius
　　M87.233 **Osteonecrosis due to previous trauma of unspecified radius**
　　M87.234 Osteonecrosis due to previous trauma of right ulna
　　M87.235 Osteonecrosis due to previous trauma of left ulna
　　M87.236 **Osteonecrosis due to previous trauma of unspecified ulna**
　　M87.237 Osteonecrosis due to previous trauma of right carpus
　　M87.238 Osteonecrosis due to previous trauma of left carpus

　　M87.239 **Osteonecrosis due to previous trauma of unspecified carpus**

✓6th **M87.24** Osteonecrosis due to previous trauma, hand and fingers
　　M87.241 Osteonecrosis due to previous trauma, right hand
　　M87.242 Osteonecrosis due to previous trauma, left hand
　　M87.243 **Osteonecrosis due to previous trauma, unspecified hand**
　　M87.244 Osteonecrosis due to previous trauma, right finger(s)
　　M87.245 Osteonecrosis due to previous trauma, left finger(s)
　　M87.246 **Osteonecrosis due to previous trauma, unspecified finger(s)**

✓6th **M87.25** Osteonecrosis due to previous trauma, pelvis and femur
　　M87.250 **Osteonecrosis due to previous trauma, pelvis**
　　M87.251 **Osteonecrosis due to previous trauma, right femur**
　　M87.252 **Osteonecrosis due to previous trauma, left femur**
　　M87.256 **Osteonecrosis due to previous trauma, unspecified femur**

✓6th **M87.26** Osteonecrosis due to previous trauma, tibia and fibula
　　M87.261 **Osteonecrosis due to previous trauma, right tibia**
　　M87.262 **Osteonecrosis due to previous trauma, left tibia**
　　M87.263 **Osteonecrosis due to previous trauma, unspecified tibia**
　　M87.264 Osteonecrosis due to previous trauma, right fibula
　　M87.265 Osteonecrosis due to previous trauma, left fibula
　　M87.266 **Osteonecrosis due to previous trauma, unspecified fibula**

✓6th **M87.27** Osteonecrosis due to previous trauma, ankle, foot and toes
　　M87.271 Osteonecrosis due to previous trauma, right ankle
　　M87.272 Osteonecrosis due to previous trauma, left ankle
　　M87.273 **Osteonecrosis due to previous trauma, unspecified ankle**
　　M87.274 Osteonecrosis due to previous trauma, right foot
　　M87.275 Osteonecrosis due to previous trauma, left foot
　　M87.276 **Osteonecrosis due to previous trauma, unspecified foot**
　　M87.277 Osteonecrosis due to previous trauma, right toe(s)
　　M87.278 Osteonecrosis due to previous trauma, left toe(s)
　　M87.279 **Osteonecrosis due to previous trauma, unspecified toe(s)**

　　M87.28 Osteonecrosis due to previous trauma, other site
　　M87.29 Osteonecrosis due to previous trauma, multiple sites

✓5th **M87.3** Other secondary osteonecrosis
　　M87.30 Other secondary osteonecrosis, unspecified bone

✓6th **M87.31** Other secondary osteonecrosis, shoulder
　　M87.311 **Other secondary osteonecrosis, right shoulder**
　　M87.312 **Other secondary osteonecrosis, left shoulder**
　　M87.319 **Other secondary osteonecrosis, unspecified shoulder**

✓6th **M87.32** Other secondary osteonecrosis, humerus
　　M87.321 **Other secondary osteonecrosis, right humerus**
　　M87.322 **Other secondary osteonecrosis, left humerus**
　　M87.329 **Other secondary osteonecrosis, unspecified humerus**

EXCLUDES 1 Not coded here　　EXCLUDES 2 Not included here　　N Newborn Age: 0　　P Pediatric Age: 0-17　　M Maternity Age: 12-55　　A Adult Age: 15-124

710　　ICD-10-CM Draft (2015)

☑6ᵗʰ **M87.33** Other secondary osteonecrosis of radius, ulna and carpus

　　M87.331 Other secondary osteonecrosis of right radius

　　M87.332 Other secondary osteonecrosis of left radius

　　M87.333 Other secondary osteonecrosis of unspecified radius

　　M87.334 Other secondary osteonecrosis of right ulna

　　M87.335 Other secondary osteonecrosis of left ulna

　　M87.336 Other secondary osteonecrosis of unspecified ulna

　　M87.337 Other secondary osteonecrosis of right carpus

　　M87.338 Other secondary osteonecrosis of left carpus

　　M87.339 Other secondary osteonecrosis of unspecified carpus

☑6ᵗʰ **M87.34** Other secondary osteonecrosis, hand and fingers

　　M87.341 Other secondary osteonecrosis, right hand

　　M87.342 Other secondary osteonecrosis, left hand

　　M87.343 Other secondary osteonecrosis, unspecified hand

　　M87.344 Other secondary osteonecrosis, right finger(s)

　　M87.345 Other secondary osteonecrosis, left finger(s)

　　M87.346 Other secondary osteonecrosis, unspecified finger(s)

☑6ᵗʰ **M87.35** Other secondary osteonecrosis, pelvis and femur

　　M87.350 Other secondary osteonecrosis, pelvis

　　M87.351 Other secondary osteonecrosis, right femur

　　M87.352 Other secondary osteonecrosis, left femur

　　M87.353 Other secondary osteonecrosis, unspecified femur

☑6ᵗʰ **M87.36** Other secondary osteonecrosis, tibia and fibula

　　M87.361 Other secondary osteonecrosis, right tibia

　　M87.362 Other secondary osteonecrosis, left tibia

　　M87.363 Other secondary osteonecrosis, unspecified tibia

　　M87.364 Other secondary osteonecrosis, right fibula

　　M87.365 Other secondary osteonecrosis, left fibula

　　M87.366 Other secondary osteonecrosis, unspecified fibula

☑6ᵗʰ **M87.37** Other secondary osteonecrosis, ankle and foot

　　M87.371 Other secondary osteonecrosis, right ankle

　　M87.372 Other secondary osteonecrosis, left ankle

　　M87.373 Other secondary osteonecrosis, unspecified ankle

　　M87.374 Other secondary osteonecrosis, right foot

　　M87.375 Other secondary osteonecrosis, left foot

　　M87.376 Other secondary osteonecrosis, unspecified foot

　　M87.377 Other secondary osteonecrosis, right toe(s)

　　M87.378 Other secondary osteonecrosis, left toe(s)

　　M87.379 Other secondary osteonecrosis, unspecified toe(s)

　M87.38 Other secondary osteonecrosis, other site

　M87.39 Other secondary osteonecrosis, multiple sites

☑5ᵗʰ **M87.8** Other osteonecrosis

　M87.80 Other osteonecrosis, unspecified bone

☑6ᵗʰ **M87.81** Other osteonecrosis, shoulder

　　M87.811 Other osteonecrosis, right shoulder

　　M87.812 Other osteonecrosis, left shoulder

　　M87.819 Other osteonecrosis, unspecified shoulder

☑6ᵗʰ **M87.82** Other osteonecrosis, humerus

　　M87.821 Other osteonecrosis, right humerus

　　M87.822 Other osteonecrosis, left humerus

　　M87.829 Other osteonecrosis, unspecified humerus

☑6ᵗʰ **M87.83** Other osteonecrosis of radius, ulna and carpus

　　M87.831 Other osteonecrosis of right radius

　　M87.832 Other osteonecrosis of left radius

　　M87.833 Other osteonecrosis of unspecified radius

　　M87.834 Other osteonecrosis of right ulna

　　M87.835 Other osteonecrosis of left ulna

　　M87.836 Other osteonecrosis of unspecified ulna

　　M87.837 Other osteonecrosis of right carpus

　　M87.838 Other osteonecrosis of left carpus

　　M87.839 Other osteonecrosis of unspecified carpus

☑6ᵗʰ **M87.84** Other osteonecrosis, hand and fingers

　　M87.841 Other osteonecrosis, right hand

　　M87.842 Other osteonecrosis, left hand

　　M87.843 Other osteonecrosis, unspecified hand

　　M87.844 Other osteonecrosis, right finger(s)

　　M87.845 Other osteonecrosis, left finger(s)

　　M87.849 Other osteonecrosis, unspecified finger(s)

☑6ᵗʰ **M87.85** Other osteonecrosis, pelvis and femur

　　M87.850 Other osteonecrosis, pelvis

　　M87.851 Other osteonecrosis, right femur

　　M87.852 Other osteonecrosis, left femur

　　M87.859 Other osteonecrosis, unspecified femur

☑6ᵗʰ **M87.86** Other osteonecrosis, tibia and fibula

　　M87.861 Other osteonecrosis, right tibia

　　M87.862 Other osteonecrosis, left tibia

　　M87.863 Other osteonecrosis, unspecified tibia

　　M87.864 Other osteonecrosis, right fibula

　　M87.865 Other osteonecrosis, left fibula

　　M87.869 Other osteonecrosis, unspecified fibula

☑6ᵗʰ **M87.87** Other osteonecrosis, ankle, foot and toes

　　M87.871 Other osteonecrosis, right ankle

　　M87.872 Other osteonecrosis, left ankle

　　M87.873 Other osteonecrosis, unspecified ankle

　　M87.874 Other osteonecrosis, right foot

　　M87.875 Other osteonecrosis, left foot

　　M87.876 Other osteonecrosis, unspecified foot

　　M87.877 Other osteonecrosis, right toe(s)

　　M87.878 Other osteonecrosis, left toe(s)

　　M87.879 Other osteonecrosis, unspecified toe(s)

　M87.88 Other osteonecrosis, other site

　M87.89 Other osteonecrosis, multiple sites

M87.9 Osteonecrosis, unspecified
　Necrosis of bone NOS

☑4ᵗʰ **M88** Osteitis deformans [Paget's disease of bone]
　EXCLUDES 1 osteitis deformans in neoplastic disease (M90.6)

　M88.0 Osteitis deformans of skull

　M88.1 Osteitis deformans of vertebrae

☑5ᵗʰ **M88.8** Osteitis deformans of other bones

☑6ᵗʰ **M88.81** Osteitis deformans of shoulder

　　M88.811 Osteitis deformans of right shoulder

　　M88.812 Osteitis deformans of left shoulder

　　M88.819 Osteitis deformans of unspecified shoulder

☑6ᵗʰ **M88.82** Osteitis deformans of upper arm

　　M88.821 Osteitis deformans of right upper arm

　　M88.822 Osteitis deformans of left upper arm

　　M88.829 Osteitis deformans of unspecified upper arm

☑6ᵗʰ **M88.83** Osteitis deformans of forearm

　　M88.831 Osteitis deformans of right forearm

　　M88.832 Osteitis deformans of left forearm

　　M88.839 Osteitis deformans of unspecified forearm

☑6ᵗʰ **M88.84** Osteitis deformans of hand

　　M88.841 Osteitis deformans of right hand

　　M88.842 Osteitis deformans of left hand

　　M88.849 Osteitis deformans of unspecified hand

☑6ᵗʰ **M88.85** Osteitis deformans of thigh

　　M88.851 Osteitis deformans of right thigh

　　M88.852 Osteitis deformans of left thigh

　　M88.859 Osteitis deformans of unspecified thigh

☑ Additional Character Required　☑x7ᵗʰ Xtension Alert　Unspecified Dx　Other Specified Dx　Manifestation　►◄ Revised Text　● New Code　▲ Revised Code Title

ICD-10-CM Draft (2015)　　　　711

✓6ᵗʰ **M88.86** Osteitis deformans of lower leg
    M88.861 Osteitis deformans of right lower leg
    M88.862 Osteitis deformans of left lower leg
    M88.869 Osteitis deformans of unspecified lower leg

✓6ᵗʰ **M88.87** Osteitis deformans of ankle and foot
    M88.871 Osteitis deformans of right ankle and foot
    M88.872 Osteitis deformans of left ankle and foot
    M88.879 Osteitis deformans of unspecified ankle and foot

M88.88 Osteitis deformans of other bones
    EXCLUDES 2　osteitis deformans of skull (M88.0)
                 osteitis deformans of vertebrae (M88.1)

M88.89 Osteitis deformans of multiple sites

M88.9 Osteitis deformans of unspecified bone

✓4ᵗʰ **M89** Other disorders of bone

✓5ᵗʰ **M89.0** Algoneurodystrophy
    Shoulder-hand syndrome
    Sudeck's atrophy
    EXCLUDES 1　causalgia, lower limb (G57.7-)
                 causalgia, upper limb (G56.4-)
                 complex regional pain syndrome II, lower limb (G57.7-)
                 complex regional pain syndrome II, upper limb (G56.4-)
                 reflex sympathetic dystrophy (G90.5-)

M89.00 Algoneurodystrophy, unspecified site

✓6ᵗʰ **M89.01** Algoneurodystrophy, shoulder
    M89.011 Algoneurodystrophy, right shoulder
    M89.012 Algoneurodystrophy, left shoulder
    M89.019 Algoneurodystrophy, unspecified shoulder

✓6ᵗʰ **M89.02** Algoneurodystrophy, upper arm
    M89.021 Algoneurodystrophy, right upper arm
    M89.022 Algoneurodystrophy, left upper arm
    M89.029 Algoneurodystrophy, unspecified upper arm

✓6ᵗʰ **M89.03** Algoneurodystrophy, forearm
    M89.031 Algoneurodystrophy, right forearm
    M89.032 Algoneurodystrophy, left forearm
    M89.039 Algoneurodystrophy, unspecified forearm

✓6ᵗʰ **M89.04** Algoneurodystrophy, hand
    M89.041 Algoneurodystrophy, right hand
    M89.042 Algoneurodystrophy, left hand
    M89.049 Algoneurodystrophy, unspecified hand

✓6ᵗʰ **M89.05** Algoneurodystrophy, thigh
    M89.051 Algoneurodystrophy, right thigh
    M89.052 Algoneurodystrophy, left thigh
    M89.059 Algoneurodystrophy, unspecified thigh

✓6ᵗʰ **M89.06** Algoneurodystrophy, lower leg
    M89.061 Algoneurodystrophy, right lower leg
    M89.062 Algoneurodystrophy, left lower leg
    M89.069 Algoneurodystrophy, unspecified lower leg

✓6ᵗʰ **M89.07** Algoneurodystrophy, ankle and foot
    M89.071 Algoneurodystrophy, right ankle and foot
    M89.072 Algoneurodystrophy, left ankle and foot
    M89.079 Algoneurodystrophy, unspecified ankle and foot

M89.08 Algoneurodystrophy, other site

M89.09 Algoneurodystrophy, multiple sites

✓5ᵗʰ **M89.1** Physeal arrest
    Arrest of growth plate　　　Growth plate arrest
    Epiphyseal arrest

✓6ᵗʰ **M89.12** Physeal arrest, humerus
    M89.121 Complete physeal arrest, right proximal humerus
    M89.122 Complete physeal arrest, left proximal humerus
    M89.123 Partial physeal arrest, right proximal humerus
    M89.124 Partial physeal arrest, left proximal humerus
    M89.125 Complete physeal arrest, right distal humerus

    M89.126 Complete physeal arrest, left distal humerus
    M89.127 Partial physeal arrest, right distal humerus
    M89.128 Partial physeal arrest, left distal humerus
    M89.129 Physeal arrest, humerus, unspecified

✓6ᵗʰ **M89.13** Physeal arrest, forearm
    M89.131 Complete physeal arrest, right distal radius
    M89.132 Complete physeal arrest, left distal radius
    M89.133 Partial physeal arrest, right distal radius
    M89.134 Partial physeal arrest, left distal radius
    M89.138 Other physeal arrest of forearm
    M89.139 Physeal arrest, forearm, unspecified

✓6ᵗʰ **M89.15** Physeal arrest, femur
    M89.151 Complete physeal arrest, right proximal femur
    M89.152 Complete physeal arrest, left proximal femur
    M89.153 Partial physeal arrest, right proximal femur
    M89.154 Partial physeal arrest, left proximal femur
    M89.155 Complete physeal arrest, right distal femur
    M89.156 Complete physeal arrest, left distal femur
    M89.157 Partial physeal arrest, right distal femur
    M89.158 Partial physeal arrest, left distal femur
    M89.159 Physeal arrest, femur, unspecified

✓6ᵗʰ **M89.16** Physeal arrest, lower leg
    M89.160 Complete physeal arrest, right proximal tibia
    M89.161 Complete physeal arrest, left proximal tibia
    M89.162 Partial physeal arrest, right proximal tibia
    M89.163 Partial physeal arrest, left proximal tibia
    M89.164 Complete physeal arrest, right distal tibia
    M89.165 Complete physeal arrest, left distal tibia
    M89.166 Partial physeal arrest, right distal tibia
    M89.167 Partial physeal arrest, left distal tibia
    M89.168 Other physeal arrest of lower leg
    M89.169 Physeal arrest, lower leg, unspecified

M89.18 Physeal arrest, other site

✓5ᵗʰ **M89.2** Other disorders of bone development and growth
    M89.20 Other disorders of bone development and growth, unspecified site

✓6ᵗʰ **M89.21** Other disorders of bone development and growth, shoulder
    M89.211 Other disorders of bone development and growth, right shoulder
    M89.212 Other disorders of bone development and growth, left shoulder
    M89.219 Other disorders of bone development and growth, unspecified shoulder

✓6ᵗʰ **M89.22** Other disorders of bone development and growth, humerus
    M89.221 Other disorders of bone development and growth, right humerus
    M89.222 Other disorders of bone development and growth, left humerus
    M89.229 Other disorders of bone development and growth, unspecified humerus

✓6ᵗʰ **M89.23** Other disorders of bone development and growth, ulna and radius
    M89.231 Other disorders of bone development and growth, right ulna
    M89.232 Other disorders of bone development and growth, left ulna
    M89.233 Other disorders of bone development and growth, right radius
    M89.234 Other disorders of bone development and growth, left radius
    M89.239 Other disorders of bone development and growth, unspecified ulna and radius

EXCLUDES 1 Not coded here　　　EXCLUDES 2 Not included here　　　N Newborn Age: 0　　　P Pediatric Age: 0-17　　　M Maternity Age: 12-55　　　A Adult Age: 15-124

712　　　ICD-10-CM Draft (2015)

✓6ᵗʰ **M89.24** Other disorders of bone development and growth, hand
  M89.241 Other disorders of bone development and growth, right hand
  M89.242 Other disorders of bone development and growth, left hand
  M89.249 Other disorders of bone development and growth, unspecified hand

✓6ᵗʰ **M89.25** Other disorders of bone development and growth, femur
  M89.251 Other disorders of bone development and growth, right femur
  M89.252 Other disorders of bone development and growth, left femur
  M89.259 Other disorders of bone development and growth, unspecified femur

✓6ᵗʰ **M89.26** Other disorders of bone development and growth, tibia and fibula
  M89.261 Other disorders of bone development and growth, right tibia
  M89.262 Other disorders of bone development and growth, left tibia
  M89.263 Other disorders of bone development and growth, right fibula
  M89.264 Other disorders of bone development and growth, left fibula
  M89.269 Other disorders of bone development and growth, unspecified lower leg

✓6ᵗʰ **M89.27** Other disorders of bone development and growth, ankle and foot
  M89.271 Other disorders of bone development and growth, right ankle and foot
  M89.272 Other disorders of bone development and growth, left ankle and foot
  M89.279 Other disorders of bone development and growth, unspecified ankle and foot

M89.28 Other disorders of bone development and growth, other site

M89.29 Other disorders of bone development and growth, multiple sites

✓5ᵗʰ **M89.3** Hypertrophy of bone
 M89.30 Hypertrophy of bone, unspecified site

✓6ᵗʰ **M89.31** Hypertrophy of bone, shoulder
  M89.311 Hypertrophy of bone, right shoulder
  M89.312 Hypertrophy of bone, left shoulder
  M89.319 Hypertrophy of bone, unspecified shoulder

✓6ᵗʰ **M89.32** Hypertrophy of bone, humerus
  M89.321 Hypertrophy of bone, right humerus
  M89.322 Hypertrophy of bone, left humerus
  M89.329 Hypertrophy of bone, unspecified humerus

✓6ᵗʰ **M89.33** Hypertrophy of bone, ulna and radius
  M89.331 Hypertrophy of bone, right ulna
  M89.332 Hypertrophy of bone, left ulna
  M89.333 Hypertrophy of bone, right radius
  M89.334 Hypertrophy of bone, left radius
  M89.339 Hypertrophy of bone, unspecified ulna and radius

✓6ᵗʰ **M89.34** Hypertrophy of bone, hand
  M89.341 Hypertrophy of bone, right hand
  M89.342 Hypertrophy of bone, left hand
  M89.349 Hypertrophy of bone, unspecified hand

✓6ᵗʰ **M89.35** Hypertrophy of bone, femur
  M89.351 Hypertrophy of bone, right femur
  M89.352 Hypertrophy of bone, left femur
  M89.359 Hypertrophy of bone, unspecified femur

✓6ᵗʰ **M89.36** Hypertrophy of bone, tibia and fibula
  M89.361 Hypertrophy of bone, right tibia
  M89.362 Hypertrophy of bone, left tibia
  M89.363 Hypertrophy of bone, right fibula
  M89.364 Hypertrophy of bone, left fibula
  M89.369 Hypertrophy of bone, unspecified tibia and fibula

✓6ᵗʰ **M89.37** Hypertrophy of bone, ankle and foot
  M89.371 Hypertrophy of bone, right ankle and foot
  M89.372 Hypertrophy of bone, left ankle and foot
  M89.379 Hypertrophy of bone, unspecified ankle and foot

M89.38 Hypertrophy of bone, other site

M89.39 Hypertrophy of bone, multiple sites

✓5ᵗʰ **M89.4** Other hypertrophic osteoarthropathy
 Marie-Bamberger disease   Pachydermoperiostosis

 M89.40 Other hypertrophic osteoarthropathy, unspecified site

✓6ᵗʰ **M89.41** Other hypertrophic osteoarthropathy, shoulder
  M89.411 Other hypertrophic osteoarthropathy, right shoulder
  M89.412 Other hypertrophic osteoarthropathy, left shoulder
  M89.419 Other hypertrophic osteoarthropathy, unspecified shoulder

✓6ᵗʰ **M89.42** Other hypertrophic osteoarthropathy, upper arm
  M89.421 Other hypertrophic osteoarthropathy, right upper arm
  M89.422 Other hypertrophic osteoarthropathy, left upper arm
  M89.429 Other hypertrophic osteoarthropathy, unspecified upper arm

✓6ᵗʰ **M89.43** Other hypertrophic osteoarthropathy, forearm
  M89.431 Other hypertrophic osteoarthropathy, right forearm
  M89.432 Other hypertrophic osteoarthropathy, left forearm
  M89.439 Other hypertrophic osteoarthropathy, unspecified forearm

✓6ᵗʰ **M89.44** Other hypertrophic osteoarthropathy, hand
  M89.441 Other hypertrophic osteoarthropathy, right hand
  M89.442 Other hypertrophic osteoarthropathy, left hand
  M89.449 Other hypertrophic osteoarthropathy, unspecified hand

✓6ᵗʰ **M89.45** Other hypertrophic osteoarthropathy, thigh
  M89.451 Other hypertrophic osteoarthropathy, right thigh
  M89.452 Other hypertrophic osteoarthropathy, left thigh
  M89.459 Other hypertrophic osteoarthropathy, unspecified thigh

✓6ᵗʰ **M89.46** Other hypertrophic osteoarthropathy, lower leg
  M89.461 Other hypertrophic osteoarthropathy, right lower leg
  M89.462 Other hypertrophic osteoarthropathy, left lower leg
  M89.469 Other hypertrophic osteoarthropathy, unspecified lower leg

✓6ᵗʰ **M89.47** Other hypertrophic osteoarthropathy, ankle and foot
  M89.471 Other hypertrophic osteoarthropathy, right ankle and foot
  M89.472 Other hypertrophic osteoarthropathy, left ankle and foot
  M89.479 Other hypertrophic osteoarthropathy, unspecified ankle and foot

M89.48 Other hypertrophic osteoarthropathy, other site

M89.49 Other hypertrophic osteoarthropathy, multiple sites

✓5ᵗʰ **M89.5** Osteolysis
 Use additional code to identify major osseous defect, if applicable (M89.7-)
 EXCLUDES 2 periprosthetic osteolysis of internal prosthetic joint (T84.05-)

 M89.50 Osteolysis, unspecified site

✓6ᵗʰ **M89.51** Osteolysis, shoulder
  M89.511 Osteolysis, right shoulder
  M89.512 Osteolysis, left shoulder
  M89.519 Osteolysis, unspecified shoulder

✓6ᵗʰ **M89.52** Osteolysis, upper arm
  M89.521 Osteolysis, right upper arm
  M89.522 Osteolysis, left upper arm

☑ Additional Character Required ✓ₓ7ᵗʰ Xtension Alert Unspecified Dx Other Specified Dx Manifestation ▶◀ Revised Text ● New Code ▲ Revised Code Title

ICD-10-CM Draft (2015)   713

      M89.529 **Osteolysis, unspecified upper arm**

✓6th M89.53 Osteolysis, forearm
- M89.531 Osteolysis, **right forearm**
- M89.532 Osteolysis, **left forearm**
- M89.539 **Osteolysis, unspecified forearm**

✓6th M89.54 Osteolysis, hand
- M89.541 Osteolysis, **right hand**
- M89.542 Osteolysis, **left hand**
- M89.549 **Osteolysis, unspecified hand**

✓6th M89.55 Osteolysis, thigh
- M89.551 Osteolysis, **right thigh**
- M89.552 Osteolysis, **left thigh**
- M89.559 **Osteolysis, unspecified thigh**

✓6th M89.56 Osteolysis, lower leg
- M89.561 Osteolysis, **right lower leg**
- M89.562 Osteolysis, **left lower leg**
- M89.569 **Osteolysis, unspecified lower leg**

✓6th M89.57 Osteolysis, ankle and foot
- M89.571 Osteolysis, **right ankle and foot**
- M89.572 Osteolysis, **left ankle and foot**
- M89.579 **Osteolysis, unspecified ankle and foot**

M89.58 **Osteolysis, other site**
M89.59 Osteolysis, multiple sites

✓5th M89.6 **Osteopathy after poliomyelitis**
Use additional code (B91) to identify previous poliomyelitis
EXCLUDES 1 postpolio syndrome (G14)

M89.60 **Osteopathy after poliomyelitis, unspecified site**

✓6th M89.61 Osteopathy after poliomyelitis, shoulder
- M89.611 **Osteopathy after poliomyelitis, right shoulder**
- M89.612 **Osteopathy after poliomyelitis, left shoulder**
- M89.619 **Osteopathy after poliomyelitis, unspecified shoulder**

✓6th M89.62 Osteopathy after poliomyelitis, upper arm
- M89.621 **Osteopathy after poliomyelitis, right upper arm**
- M89.622 **Osteopathy after poliomyelitis, left upper arm**
- M89.629 **Osteopathy after poliomyelitis, unspecified upper arm**

✓6th M89.63 Osteopathy after poliomyelitis, forearm
- M89.631 **Osteopathy after poliomyelitis, right forearm**
- M89.632 **Osteopathy after poliomyelitis, left forearm**
- M89.639 **Osteopathy after poliomyelitis, unspecified forearm**

✓6th M89.64 Osteopathy after poliomyelitis, hand
- M89.641 **Osteopathy after poliomyelitis, right hand**
- M89.642 **Osteopathy after poliomyelitis, left hand**
- M89.649 **Osteopathy after poliomyelitis, unspecified hand**

✓6th M89.65 Osteopathy after poliomyelitis, thigh
- M89.651 **Osteopathy after poliomyelitis, right thigh**
- M89.652 **Osteopathy after poliomyelitis, left thigh**
- M89.659 **Osteopathy after poliomyelitis, unspecified thigh**

✓6th M89.66 Osteopathy after poliomyelitis, lower leg
- M89.661 **Osteopathy after poliomyelitis, right lower leg**
- M89.662 **Osteopathy after poliomyelitis, left lower leg**
- M89.669 **Osteopathy after poliomyelitis, unspecified lower leg**

✓6th M89.67 Osteopathy after poliomyelitis, ankle and foot
- M89.671 **Osteopathy after poliomyelitis, right ankle and foot**
- M89.672 **Osteopathy after poliomyelitis, left ankle and foot**
- M89.679 **Osteopathy after poliomyelitis, unspecified ankle and foot**

M89.68 **Osteopathy after poliomyelitis, other site**
M89.69 Osteopathy after poliomyelitis, multiple sites

✓5th M89.7 **Major osseous defect**
Code first underlying disease, if known, such as:
- aseptic necrosis of bone (M87.-)
- malignant neoplasm of bone (C40.-)
- osteolysis (M89.5)
- osteomyelitis (M86.-)
- osteonecrosis (M87.-)
- osteoporosis (M80.-, M81.-)
- periprosthetic osteolysis (T84.05-)

M89.70 **Major osseous defect, unspecified site**

✓6th M89.71 Major osseous defect, shoulder region
Major osseous defect clavicle or scapula
- M89.711 Major osseous defect, **right shoulder region**
- M89.712 Major osseous defect, **left shoulder region**
- M89.719 **Major osseous defect, unspecified shoulder region**

✓6th M89.72 Major osseous defect, humerus
- M89.721 Major osseous defect, **right humerus**
- M89.722 Major osseous defect, **left humerus**
- M89.729 **Major osseous defect, unspecified humerus**

✓6th M89.73 Major osseous defect, forearm
Major osseous defect of radius and ulna
- M89.731 Major osseous defect, **right forearm**
- M89.732 Major osseous defect, **left forearm**
- M89.739 **Major osseous defect, unspecified forearm**

✓6th M89.74 Major osseous defect, hand
Major osseous defect of carpus, fingers, metacarpus
- M89.741 Major osseous defect, **right hand**
- M89.742 Major osseous defect, **left hand**
- M89.749 **Major osseous defect, unspecified hand**

✓6th M89.75 Major osseous defect, pelvic region and thigh
Major osseous defect of femur and pelvis
- M89.751 Major osseous defect, **right pelvic region and thigh**
- M89.752 Major osseous defect, **left pelvic region and thigh**
- M89.759 **Major osseous defect, unspecified pelvic region and thigh**

✓6th M89.76 Major osseous defect, lower leg
Major osseous defect of fibula and tibia
- M89.761 Major osseous defect, **right lower leg**
- M89.762 Major osseous defect, **left lower leg**
- M89.769 **Major osseous defect, unspecified lower leg**

✓6th M89.77 Major osseous defect, ankle and foot
Major osseous defect of metatarsus, tarsus, toes
- M89.771 Major osseous defect, **right ankle and foot**
- M89.772 Major osseous defect, **left ankle and foot**
- M89.779 **Major osseous defect, unspecified ankle and foot**

M89.78 **Major osseous defect, other site**
M89.79 Major osseous defect, multiple sites

✓5th M89.8 **Other specified disorders of bone**
Infantile cortical hyperostoses
Post-traumatic subperiosteal ossification

✓6th M89.8X Other specified disorders of bone
- M89.8X0 **Other specified disorders of bone, multiple sites**
- M89.8X1 **Other specified disorders of bone, shoulder**
- M89.8X2 **Other specified disorders of bone, upper arm**
- M89.8X3 **Other specified disorders of bone, forearm**
- M89.8X4 **Other specified disorders of bone, hand**
- M89.8X5 **Other specified disorders of bone, thigh**
- M89.8X6 **Other specified disorders of bone, lower leg**
- M89.8X7 **Other specified disorders of bone, ankle and foot**
- M89.8X8 **Other specified disorders of bone, other site**
- M89.8X9 **Other specified disorders of bone, unspecified site**

M89.9 **Disorder of bone, unspecified**

EXCLUDES 1 Not coded here   *EXCLUDES 2* Not included here   N Newborn Age: 0   P Pediatric Age: 0-17   M Maternity Age: 12-55   A Adult Age: 15-124

714   ICD-10-CM Draft (2015)

✓4ᵗʰ **M90　Osteopathies in diseases classified elsewhere**

　　EXCLUDES 1 osteochondritis, osteomyelitis, and osteopathy (in):
　　　　　cryptococcosis (B45.3)
　　　　　diabetes mellitus (E08-E13 with .61-)
　　　　　gonococcal (A54.43)
　　　　　neurogenic syphilis (A52.11)
　　　　　renal osteodystrophy (N25.0)
　　　　　salmonellosis (A02.24)
　　　　　secondary syphilis (A51.46)
　　　　　syphilis (late) (A52.77)

✓5ᵗʰ **M90.5　Osteonecrosis in diseases classified elsewhere**

　　Code first underlying disease, such as:
　　　caisson disease (T70.3)
　　　hemoglobinopathy (D50-D64)

　　M90.50　*Osteonecrosis in diseases classified elsewhere, unspecified site*

✓6ᵗʰ 　**M90.51　Osteonecrosis in diseases classified elsewhere, shoulder**

　　　M90.511　Osteonecrosis in diseases classified elsewhere, right shoulder

　　　M90.512　Osteonecrosis in diseases classified elsewhere, left shoulder

　　　M90.519　Osteonecrosis in diseases classified elsewhere, unspecified shoulder

✓6ᵗʰ 　**M90.52　Osteonecrosis in diseases classified elsewhere, upper arm**

　　　M90.521　Osteonecrosis in diseases classified elsewhere, right upper arm

　　　M90.522　Osteonecrosis in diseases classified elsewhere, left upper arm

　　　M90.529　Osteonecrosis in diseases classified elsewhere, unspecified upper arm

✓6ᵗʰ 　**M90.53　Osteonecrosis in diseases classified elsewhere, forearm**

　　　M90.531　Osteonecrosis in diseases classified elsewhere, right forearm

　　　M90.532　Osteonecrosis in diseases classified elsewhere, left forearm

　　　M90.539　Osteonecrosis in diseases classified elsewhere, unspecified forearm

✓6ᵗʰ 　**M90.54　Osteonecrosis in diseases classified elsewhere, hand**

　　　M90.541　Osteonecrosis in diseases classified elsewhere, right hand

　　　M90.542　Osteonecrosis in diseases classified elsewhere, left hand

　　　M90.549　Osteonecrosis in diseases classified elsewhere, unspecified hand

✓6ᵗʰ 　**M90.55　Osteonecrosis in diseases classified elsewhere, thigh**

　　　M90.551　Osteonecrosis in diseases classified elsewhere, right thigh

　　　M90.552　Osteonecrosis in diseases classified elsewhere, left thigh

　　　M90.559　Osteonecrosis in diseases classified elsewhere, unspecified thigh

✓6ᵗʰ 　**M90.56　Osteonecrosis in diseases classified elsewhere, lower leg**

　　　M90.561　Osteonecrosis in diseases classified elsewhere, right lower leg

　　　M90.562　Osteonecrosis in diseases classified elsewhere, left lower leg

　　　M90.569　Osteonecrosis in diseases classified elsewhere, unspecified lower leg

✓6ᵗʰ 　**M90.57　Osteonecrosis in diseases classified elsewhere, ankle and foot**

　　　M90.571　Osteonecrosis in diseases classified elsewhere, right ankle and foot

　　　M90.572　Osteonecrosis in diseases classified elsewhere, left ankle and foot

　　　M90.579　Osteonecrosis in diseases classified elsewhere, unspecified ankle and foot

　　M90.58　*Osteonecrosis in diseases classified elsewhere, other site*

　　M90.59　*Osteonecrosis in diseases classified elsewhere, multiple sites*

✓5ᵗʰ **M90.6　Osteitis deformans in neoplastic diseases**

　　Osteitis deformans in malignant neoplasm of bone
　　Code first the neoplasm (C40-, C41-)

　　　EXCLUDES 1 osteitis deformans [Paget's disease of bone] (M88.-)

　　M90.60　*Osteitis deformans in neoplastic diseases, unspecified site*

✓6ᵗʰ 　**M90.61　Osteitis deformans in neoplastic diseases, shoulder**

　　　M90.611　Osteitis deformans in neoplastic diseases, right shoulder

　　　M90.612　Osteitis deformans in neoplastic diseases, left shoulder

　　　M90.619　Osteitis deformans in neoplastic diseases, unspecified shoulder

✓6ᵗʰ 　**M90.62　Osteitis deformans in neoplastic diseases, upper arm**

　　　M90.621　Osteitis deformans in neoplastic diseases, right upper arm

　　　M90.622　Osteitis deformans in neoplastic diseases, left upper arm

　　　M90.629　Osteitis deformans in neoplastic diseases, unspecified upper arm

✓6ᵗʰ 　**M90.63　Osteitis deformans in neoplastic diseases, forearm**

　　　M90.631　Osteitis deformans in neoplastic diseases, right forearm

　　　M90.632　Osteitis deformans in neoplastic diseases, left forearm

　　　M90.639　Osteitis deformans in neoplastic diseases, unspecified forearm

✓6ᵗʰ 　**M90.64　Osteitis deformans in neoplastic diseases, hand**

　　　M90.641　Osteitis deformans in neoplastic diseases, right hand

　　　M90.642　Osteitis deformans in neoplastic diseases, left hand

　　　M90.649　Osteitis deformans in neoplastic diseases, unspecified hand

✓6ᵗʰ 　**M90.65　Osteitis deformans in neoplastic diseases, thigh**

　　　M90.651　Osteitis deformans in neoplastic diseases, right thigh

　　　M90.652　Osteitis deformans in neoplastic diseases, left thigh

　　　M90.659　Osteitis deformans in neoplastic diseases, unspecified thigh

✓6ᵗʰ 　**M90.66　Osteitis deformans in neoplastic diseases, lower leg**

　　　M90.661　Osteitis deformans in neoplastic diseases, right lower leg

　　　M90.662　Osteitis deformans in neoplastic diseases, left lower leg

　　　M90.669　Osteitis deformans in neoplastic diseases, unspecified lower leg

✓6ᵗʰ 　**M90.67　Osteitis deformans in neoplastic diseases, ankle and foot**

　　　M90.671　Osteitis deformans in neoplastic diseases, right ankle and foot

　　　M90.672　Osteitis deformans in neoplastic diseases, left ankle and foot

　　　M90.679　Osteitis deformans in neoplastic diseases, unspecified ankle and foot

　　M90.68　*Osteitis deformans in neoplastic diseases, other site*

　　M90.69　*Osteitis deformans in neoplastic diseases, multiple sites*

✓5ᵗʰ **M90.8　Osteopathy in diseases classified elsewhere**

　　Code first underlying disease, such as:
　　　rickets (E55.0)
　　　vitamin-D-resistant rickets (E83.3)

　　M90.80　*Osteopathy in diseases classified elsewhere, unspecified site*

✓6ᵗʰ 　**M90.81　Osteopathy in diseases classified elsewhere, shoulder**

　　　M90.811　Osteopathy in diseases classified elsewhere, right shoulder

　　　M90.812　Osteopathy in diseases classified elsewhere, left shoulder

　　　M90.819　Osteopathy in diseases classified elsewhere, unspecified shoulder

✓6ᵗʰ 　**M90.82　Osteopathy in diseases classified elsewhere, upper arm**

　　　M90.821　Osteopathy in diseases classified elsewhere, right upper arm

　　　M90.822　Osteopathy in diseases classified elsewhere, left upper arm

　　　M90.829　Osteopathy in diseases classified elsewhere, unspecified upper arm

---

✔ Additional Character Required　　✓x7ᵗʰ Xtension Alert　　Unspecified Dx　　Other Specified Dx　　Manifestation　　►◄ Revised Text　　● New Code　　▲ Revised Code Title

Diseases of the Musculoskeletal System and Connective Tissue

M90.83–M92.42

✓6ᵗʰ **M90.83** Osteopathy in diseases classified elsewhere, forearm

    M90.831   *Osteopathy in diseases classified elsewhere, right forearm*

    M90.832   *Osteopathy in diseases classified elsewhere, left forearm*

    M90.839   *Osteopathy in diseases classified elsewhere, unspecified forearm*

✓6ᵗʰ **M90.84** Osteopathy in diseases classified elsewhere, hand

    M90.841   *Osteopathy in diseases classified elsewhere, right hand*

    M90.842   *Osteopathy in diseases classified elsewhere, left hand*

    M90.849   *Osteopathy in diseases classified elsewhere, unspecified hand*

✓6ᵗʰ **M90.85** Osteopathy in diseases classified elsewhere, thigh

    M90.851   *Osteopathy in diseases classified elsewhere, right thigh*

    M90.852   *Osteopathy in diseases classified elsewhere, left thigh*

    M90.859   *Osteopathy in diseases classified elsewhere, unspecified thigh*

✓6ᵗʰ **M90.86** Osteopathy in diseases classified elsewhere, lower leg

    M90.861   *Osteopathy in diseases classified elsewhere, right lower leg*

    M90.862   *Osteopathy in diseases classified elsewhere, left lower leg*

    M90.869   *Osteopathy in diseases classified elsewhere, unspecified lower leg*

✓6ᵗʰ **M90.87** Osteopathy in diseases classified elsewhere, ankle and foot

    M90.871   *Osteopathy in diseases classified elsewhere, right ankle and foot*

    M90.872   *Osteopathy in diseases classified elsewhere, left ankle and foot*

    M90.879   *Osteopathy in diseases classified elsewhere, unspecified ankle and foot*

    M90.88 Osteopathy in diseases classified elsewhere, other site

    M90.89 Osteopathy in diseases classified elsewhere, multiple sites

Chondropathies (M91-M94)

EXCLUDES 1 *postprocedural chondropathies (M96.-)*

✓4ᵗʰ **M91 Juvenile osteochondrosis of hip and pelvis**

    EXCLUDES 1 *slipped upper femoral epiphysis (nontraumatic) (M93.0)*

  M91.0 Juvenile osteochondrosis of pelvis

    Osteochondrosis (juvenile) of acetabulum

    Osteochondrosis (juvenile) of iliac crest [Buchanan]

    Osteochondrosis (juvenile) of ischiopubic synchondrosis [van Neck]

    Osteochondrosis (juvenile) of symphysis pubis [Pierson]

✓5ᵗʰ **M91.1** Juvenile osteochondrosis of head of femur [Legg-Calvé-Perthes]

    M91.10 Juvenile osteochondrosis of head of femur [Legg-Calvé-Perthes], unspecified leg

    M91.11 Juvenile osteochondrosis of head of femur [Legg-Calvé-Perthes], right leg

    M91.12 Juvenile osteochondrosis of head of femur [Legg-Calvé-Perthes], left leg

✓5ᵗʰ **M91.2** Coxa plana

    Hip deformity due to previous juvenile osteochondrosis

    M91.20 Coxa plana, unspecified hip

    M91.21 Coxa plana, right hip

    M91.22 Coxa plana, left hip

✓5ᵗʰ **M91.3** Pseudocoxalgia

    M91.30 Pseudocoxalgia, unspecified hip

    M91.31 Pseudocoxalgia, right hip

    M91.32 Pseudocoxalgia, left hip

✓5ᵗʰ **M91.4** Coxa magna

    M91.40 Coxa magna, unspecified hip

    M91.41 Coxa magna, right hip

    M91.42 Coxa magna, left hip

✓5ᵗʰ **M91.8** Other juvenile osteochondrosis of hip and pelvis

    Juvenile osteochondrosis after reduction of congenital dislocation of hip

    M91.80 Other juvenile osteochondrosis of hip and pelvis, unspecified leg

    M91.81 Other juvenile osteochondrosis of hip and pelvis, right leg

    M91.82 Other juvenile osteochondrosis of hip and pelvis, left leg

✓5ᵗʰ **M91.9** Juvenile osteochondrosis of hip and pelvis, unspecified

    M91.90 Juvenile osteochondrosis of hip and pelvis, unspecified, unspecified leg

    M91.91 Juvenile osteochondrosis of hip and pelvis, unspecified, right leg

    M91.92 Juvenile osteochondrosis of hip and pelvis, unspecified, left leg

✓4ᵗʰ **M92 Other juvenile osteochondrosis**

✓5ᵗʰ **M92.0** Juvenile osteochondrosis of humerus

    Osteochondrosis (juvenile) of capitulum of humerus [Panner]

    Osteochondrosis (juvenile) of head of humerus [Haas]

    M92.00 Juvenile osteochondrosis of humerus, unspecified arm

    M92.01 Juvenile osteochondrosis of humerus, right arm

    M92.02 Juvenile osteochondrosis of humerus, left arm

✓5ᵗʰ **M92.1** Juvenile osteochondrosis of radius and ulna

    Osteochondrosis (juvenile) of lower ulna [Burns]

    Osteochondrosis (juvenile) of radial head [Brailsford]

    M92.10 Juvenile osteochondrosis of radius and ulna, unspecified arm

    M92.11 Juvenile osteochondrosis of radius and ulna, right arm

    M92.12 Juvenile osteochondrosis of radius and ulna, left arm

✓5ᵗʰ **M92.2** Juvenile osteochondrosis, hand

  ✓6ᵗʰ **M92.20** Unspecified juvenile osteochondrosis, hand

    M92.201 Unspecified juvenile osteochondrosis, right hand

    M92.202 Unspecified juvenile osteochondrosis, left hand

    M92.209 Unspecified juvenile osteochondrosis, unspecified hand

  ✓6ᵗʰ **M92.21** Osteochondrosis (juvenile) of carpal lunate [Kienböck]

    M92.211 Osteochondrosis (juvenile) of carpal lunate [Kienböck], right hand

    M92.212 Osteochondrosis (juvenile) of carpal lunate [Kienböck], left hand

    M92.219 Osteochondrosis (juvenile) of carpal lunate [Kienböck], unspecified hand

  ✓6ᵗʰ **M92.22** Osteochondrosis (juvenile) of metacarpal heads [Mauclaire]

    M92.221 Osteochondrosis (juvenile) of metacarpal heads [Mauclaire], right hand

    M92.222 Osteochondrosis (juvenile) of metacarpal heads [Mauclaire], left hand

    M92.229 Osteochondrosis (juvenile) of metacarpal heads [Mauclaire], unspecified hand

  ✓6ᵗʰ **M92.29** Other juvenile osteochondrosis, hand

    M92.291 Other juvenile osteochondrosis, right hand

    M92.292 Other juvenile osteochondrosis, left hand

    M92.299 Other juvenile osteochondrosis, unspecified hand

✓5ᵗʰ **M92.3** Other juvenile osteochondrosis, upper limb

    M92.30 Other juvenile osteochondrosis, unspecified upper limb

    M92.31 Other juvenile osteochondrosis, right upper limb

    M92.32 Other juvenile osteochondrosis, left upper limb

✓5ᵗʰ **M92.4** Juvenile osteochondrosis of patella

    Osteochondrosis (juvenile) of primary patellar center [Köhler]

    Osteochondrosis (juvenile) of secondary patellar centre [Sinding Larsen]

    M92.40 Juvenile osteochondrosis of patella, unspecified knee

    M92.41 Juvenile osteochondrosis of patella, right knee

    M92.42 Juvenile osteochondrosis of patella, left knee

EXCLUDES 1 Not coded here   **EXCLUDES 2** Not included here   **N** Newborn Age: 0   **P** Pediatric Age: 0-17   **M** Maternity Age: 12-55   **A** Adult Age: 15-124

✓5th **M92.5 Juvenile osteochondrosis of** tibia and fibula
Osteochondrosis (juvenile) of proximal tibia [Blount]
Osteochondrosis (juvenile) of tibial tubercle [Osgood-Schlatter]
Tibia vara

    M92.50 Juvenile osteochondrosis of tibia and fibula, unspecified leg

    M92.51 Juvenile osteochondrosis of tibia and fibula, right **leg**

    M92.52 Juvenile osteochondrosis of tibia and fibula, left **leg**

✓5th **M92.6 Juvenile osteochondrosis of** tarsus
Osteochondrosis (juvenile) of calcaneum [Sever]
Osteochondrosis (juvenile) of os tibiale externum [Haglund]
Osteochondrosis (juvenile) of talus [Diaz]
Osteochondrosis (juvenile) of tarsal navicular [Köhler]

    M92.60 Juvenile osteochondrosis of tarsus, unspecified ankle

    M92.61 Juvenile osteochondrosis of tarsus, right **ankle**

    M92.62 Juvenile osteochondrosis of tarsus, left **ankle**

✓5th **M92.7 Juvenile osteochondrosis of** metatarsus
Osteochondrosis (juvenile) of fifth metatarsus [Iselin]
Osteochondrosis (juvenile) of second metatarsus [Freiberg]

    M92.70 Juvenile osteochondrosis of metatarsus, unspecified foot

    M92.71 Juvenile osteochondrosis of metatarsus, right **foot**

    M92.72 Juvenile osteochondrosis of metatarsus, left **foot**

M92.8 Other specified juvenile osteochondrosis
Calcaneal apophysitis

M92.9 Juvenile osteochondrosis, unspecified
Juvenile apophysitis NOS
Juvenile epiphysitis NOS
Juvenile osteochondritis NOS
Juvenile osteochondrosis NOS

✓4th **M93 Other osteochondropathies**
    EXCLUDES 2 osteochondrosis of spine (M42.-)

✓5th **M93.0 Slipped upper femoral epiphysis (nontraumatic)**
Use additional code for associated chondrolysis (M94.3)

    ✓6th **M93.00** Unspecified **slipped upper femoral epiphysis (nontraumatic)**

        M93.001 Unspecified slipped upper femoral epiphysis (nontraumatic), right **hip**

        M93.002 Unspecified slipped upper femoral epiphysis (nontraumatic), left **hip**

        M93.003 Unspecified slipped upper femoral epiphysis (nontraumatic), unspecified hip

    ✓6th **M93.01** Acute **slipped upper femoral epiphysis (nontraumatic)**

        M93.011 Acute slipped upper femoral epiphysis (nontraumatic), right **hip**

        M93.012 Acute slipped upper femoral epiphysis (nontraumatic), left **hip**

        M93.013 Acute slipped upper femoral epiphysis (nontraumatic), unspecified hip

    ✓6th **M93.02** Chronic **slipped upper femoral epiphysis (nontraumatic)**

        M93.021 Chronic slipped upper femoral epiphysis (nontraumatic), right **hip**

        M93.022 Chronic slipped upper femoral epiphysis (nontraumatic), left **hip**

        M93.023 Chronic slipped upper femoral epiphysis (nontraumatic), unspecified hip

    ✓6th **M93.03** Acute on chronic **slipped upper femoral epiphysis (nontraumatic)**

        M93.031 Acute on chronic slipped upper femoral epiphysis (nontraumatic), right **hip**

        M93.032 Acute on chronic slipped upper femoral epiphysis (nontraumatic), left **hip**

        M93.033 Acute on chronic slipped upper femoral epiphysis (nontraumatic), unspecified hip

M93.1 Kienböck's disease of adults A
Adult osteochondrosis of carpal lunates

✓5th **M93.2 Osteochondritis dissecans**

    M93.20 Osteochondritis dissecans of unspecified site

    ✓6th **M93.21 Osteochondritis dissecans of** shoulder

        M93.211 Osteochondritis dissecans, right **shoulder**

        M93.212 Osteochondritis dissecans, left **shoulder**

        M93.219 Osteochondritis dissecans, unspecified shoulder

✓6th **M93.22 Osteochondritis dissecans of** elbow

    M93.221 Osteochondritis dissecans, right **elbow**

    M93.222 Osteochondritis dissecans, left **elbow**

    M93.229 Osteochondritis dissecans, unspecified elbow

✓6th **M93.23 Osteochondritis dissecans of** wrist

    M93.231 Osteochondritis dissecans, right **wrist**

    M93.232 Osteochondritis dissecans, left **wrist**

    M93.239 Osteochondritis dissecans, unspecified wrist

✓6th **M93.24 Osteochondritis dissecans of joints of** hand

    M93.241 Osteochondritis dissecans, joints of right **hand**

    M93.242 Osteochondritis dissecans, joints of left **hand**

    M93.249 Osteochondritis dissecans, joints of unspecified hand

✓6th **M93.25 Osteochondritis dissecans of** hip

    M93.251 Osteochondritis dissecans, right **hip**

    M93.252 Osteochondritis dissecans, left **hip**

    M93.259 Osteochondritis dissecans, unspecified hip

✓6th **M93.26 Osteochondritis dissecans** knee

    M93.261 Osteochondritis dissecans, right **knee**

    M93.262 Osteochondritis dissecans, left **knee**

    M93.269 Osteochondritis dissecans, unspecified knee

✓6th **M93.27 Osteochondritis dissecans of** ankle and joints of foot

    M93.271 Osteochondritis dissecans, right **ankle and joints of** right **foot**

    M93.272 Osteochondritis dissecans, left **ankle and joints of** left **foot**

    M93.279 Osteochondritis dissecans, unspecified ankle and joints of foot

M93.28 Osteochondritis dissecans other site

M93.29 Osteochondritis dissecans multiple sites

✓5th **M93.8 Other specified osteochondropathies**

    M93.80 Other specified osteochondropathies of unspecified site

    ✓6th **M93.81 Other specified osteochondropathies of** shoulder

        M93.811 Other specified osteochondropathies, right **shoulder**

        M93.812 Other specified osteochondropathies, left **shoulder**

        M93.819 Other specified osteochondropathies, unspecified shoulder

    ✓6th **M93.82 Other specified osteochondropathies of** upper arm

        M93.821 Other specified osteochondropathies, right **upper arm**

        M93.822 Other specified osteochondropathies, left **upper arm**

        M93.829 Other specified osteochondropathies, unspecified upper arm

    ✓6th **M93.83 Other specified osteochondropathies of** forearm

        M93.831 Other specified osteochondropathies, right **forearm**

        M93.832 Other specified osteochondropathies, left forearm

        M93.839 Other specified osteochondropathies, unspecified forearm

    ✓6th **M93.84 Other specified osteochondropathies of** hand

        M93.841 Other specified osteochondropathies, right **hand**

        M93.842 Other specified osteochondropathies, left **hand**

        M93.849 Other specified osteochondropathies, unspecified hand

    ✓6th **M93.85 Other specified osteochondropathies of** thigh

        M93.851 Other specified osteochondropathies, right **thigh**

        M93.852 Other specified osteochondropathies, left **thigh**

        M93.859 Other specified osteochondropathies, unspecified thigh

☑ Additional Character Required   ✓x7th Xtension Alert   Unspecified Dx   Other Specified Dx   Manifestation   ►◄ Revised Text   ● New Code   ▲ Revised Code Title

ICD-10-CM Draft (2015)   717

M93.86 ✓6th Other specified osteochondropathies lower leg

    M93.861 Other specified osteochondropathies, right lower leg

    M93.862 Other specified osteochondropathies, left lower leg

    M93.869 Other specified osteochondropathies, unspecified lower leg

M93.87 ✓6th Other specified osteochondropathies of ankle and foot

    M93.871 Other specified osteochondropathies, right ankle and foot

    M93.872 Other specified osteochondropathies, left ankle and foot

    M93.879 Other specified osteochondropathies, unspecified ankle and foot

M93.88 Other specified osteochondropathies other site

M93.89 Other specified osteochondropathies multiple sites

M93.9 ✓5th Osteochondropathy, unspecified

    Apophysitis NOS   Osteochondritis NOS
    Epiphysitis NOS   Osteochondrosis NOS

    M93.90 Osteochondropathy, unspecified of unspecified site

    M93.91 ✓6th Osteochondropathy, unspecified of shoulder

        M93.911 Osteochondropathy, unspecified, right shoulder

        M93.912 Osteochondropathy, unspecified, left shoulder

        M93.919 Osteochondropathy, unspecified, unspecified shoulder

    M93.92 ✓6th Osteochondropathy, unspecified of upper arm

        M93.921 Osteochondropathy, unspecified, right upper arm

        M93.922 Osteochondropathy, unspecified, left upper arm

        M93.929 Osteochondropathy, unspecified, unspecified upper arm

    M93.93 ✓6th Osteochondropathy, unspecified of forearm

        M93.931 Osteochondropathy, unspecified, right forearm

        M93.932 Osteochondropathy, unspecified, left forearm

        M93.939 Osteochondropathy, unspecified, unspecified forearm

    M93.94 ✓6th Osteochondropathy, unspecified of hand

        M93.941 Osteochondropathy, unspecified, right hand

        M93.942 Osteochondropathy, unspecified, left hand

        M93.949 Osteochondropathy, unspecified, unspecified hand

    M93.95 ✓6th Osteochondropathy, unspecified of thigh

        M93.951 Osteochondropathy, unspecified, right thigh

        M93.952 Osteochondropathy, unspecified, left thigh

        M93.959 Osteochondropathy, unspecified, unspecified thigh

    M93.96 ✓6th Osteochondropathy, unspecified lower leg

        M93.961 Osteochondropathy, unspecified, right lower leg

        M93.962 Osteochondropathy, unspecified, left lower leg

        M93.969 Osteochondropathy, unspecified, unspecified lower leg

    M93.97 ✓6th Osteochondropathy, unspecified of ankle and foot

        M93.971 Osteochondropathy, unspecified, right ankle and foot

        M93.972 Osteochondropathy, unspecified, left ankle and foot

        M93.979 Osteochondropathy, unspecified, unspecified ankle and foot

    M93.98 Osteochondropathy, unspecified other site

    M93.99 Osteochondropathy, unspecified multiple sites

M94 ✓4th Other disorders of cartilage

M94.0 Chondrocostal junction syndrome [Tietze]
    Costochondritis

M94.1 Relapsing polychondritis

M94.2 ✓5th Chondromalacia

    EXCLUDES 1 chondromalacia patellae (M22.4)

    M94.20 Chondromalacia, unspecified site

    M94.21 ✓6th Chondromalacia, shoulder

        M94.211 Chondromalacia, right shoulder

        M94.212 Chondromalacia, left shoulder

        M94.219 Chondromalacia, unspecified shoulder

    M94.22 ✓6th Chondromalacia, elbow

        M94.221 Chondromalacia, right elbow

        M94.222 Chondromalacia, left elbow

        M94.229 Chondromalacia, unspecified elbow

    M94.23 ✓6th Chondromalacia, wrist

        M94.231 Chondromalacia, right wrist

        M94.232 Chondromalacia, left wrist

        M94.239 Chondromalacia, unspecified wrist

    M94.24 ✓6th Chondromalacia, joints of hand

        M94.241 Chondromalacia, joints of right hand

        M94.242 Chondromalacia, joints of left hand

        M94.249 Chondromalacia, joints of unspecified hand

    M94.25 ✓6th Chondromalacia, hip

        M94.251 Chondromalacia, right hip

        M94.252 Chondromalacia, left hip

        M94.259 Chondromalacia, unspecified hip

    M94.26 ✓6th Chondromalacia, knee

        M94.261 Chondromalacia, right knee

        M94.262 Chondromalacia, left knee

        M94.269 Chondromalacia, unspecified knee

    M94.27 ✓6th Chondromalacia, ankle and joints of foot

        M94.271 Chondromalacia, right ankle and joints of right foot

        M94.272 Chondromalacia, left ankle and joints of left foot

        M94.279 Chondromalacia, unspecified ankle and joints of foot

    M94.28 Chondromalacia, other site

    M94.29 Chondromalacia, multiple sites

M94.3 ✓5th Chondrolysis

    Code first any associated slipped upper femoral epiphysis (nontraumatic) (M93.0-)

    M94.35 ✓6th Chondrolysis, hip

        M94.351 Chondrolysis, right hip

        M94.352 Chondrolysis, left hip

        M94.359 Chondrolysis, unspecified hip

M94.8 ✓5th Other specified disorders of cartilage

    M94.8X ✓6th Other specified disorders of cartilage

        M94.8X0 Other specified disorders of cartilage, multiple sites

        M94.8X1 Other specified disorders of cartilage, shoulder

        M94.8X2 Other specified disorders of cartilage, upper arm

        M94.8X3 Other specified disorders of cartilage, forearm

        M94.8X4 Other specified disorders of cartilage, hand

        M94.8X5 Other specified disorders of cartilage, thigh

        M94.8X6 Other specified disorders of cartilage, lower leg

        M94.8X7 Other specified disorders of cartilage, ankle and foot

        M94.8X8 Other specified disorders of cartilage, other site

        M94.8X9 Other specified disorders of cartilage, unspecified sites

M94.9 Disorder of cartilage, unspecified

EXCLUDES 1 Not coded here   EXCLUDES 2 Not included here   N Newborn Age: 0   P Pediatric Age: 0-17   M Maternity Age: 12-55   A Adult Age: 15-124

718   ICD-10-CM Draft (2015)

Other disorders of the musculoskeletal system and connective tissue (M95)

☑4ᵗʰ **M95 Other acquired deformities of musculoskeletal system and connective tissue**
- EXCLUDES 2 *acquired absence of limbs and organs (Z89-Z90)*
  acquired deformities of limbs (M20-M21)
  congenital malformations and deformations of the musculoskeletal system (Q65-Q79)
  deforming dorsopathies (M40-M43)
  dentofacial anomalies [including malocclusion] (M26.-)
  postprocedural musculoskeletal disorders (M96.-)

M95.0 Acquired deformity of nose
- EXCLUDES 2 *deviated nasal septum (J34.2)*

☑5ᵗʰ **M95.1 Cauliflower ear**
- EXCLUDES 2 *other acquired deformities of ear (H61.1)*

    M95.10 Cauliflower ear, unspecified ear
    M95.11 Cauliflower ear, right ear
    M95.12 Cauliflower ear, left ear

M95.2 Other acquired deformity of head
M95.3 Acquired deformity of neck
M95.4 Acquired deformity of chest and rib
M95.5 Acquired deformity of pelvis
- EXCLUDES 1 *maternal care for known or suspected disproportion (O33.-)*

M95.8 Other specified acquired deformities of musculoskeletal system
M95.9 Acquired deformity of musculoskeletal system, unspecified

Intraoperative and postprocedural complications and disorders of musculoskeletal system, not elsewhere classified (M96)

☑4ᵗʰ **M96 Intraoperative and postprocedural complications and disorders of musculoskeletal system, not elsewhere classified**
- EXCLUDES 2 *arthropathy following intestinal bypass (M02.0-)*
  complications of internal orthopedic prosthetic devices, implants and grafts (T84.-)
  disorders associated with osteoporosis (M80)
  presence of functional implants and other devices (Z96-Z97)

M96.0 Pseudarthrosis after fusion or arthrodesis
M96.1 Postlaminectomy syndrome, not elsewhere classified
M96.2 Postradiation kyphosis
M96.3 Postlaminectomy kyphosis
M96.4 Postsurgical lordosis
M96.5 Postradiation scoliosis

☑5ᵗʰ **M96.6 Fracture of bone following insertion of orthopedic implant, joint prosthesis, or bone plate**
    Intraoperative fracture of bone during insertion of orthopedic implant, joint prosthesis, or bone plate
- EXCLUDES 2 *complication of internal orthopedic devices, implants or grafts (T84.-)*

☑6ᵗʰ **M96.62 Fracture of humerus following insertion of orthopedic implant, joint prosthesis, or bone plate**
    M96.621 Fracture of humerus following insertion of orthopedic implant, joint prosthesis, or bone plate, right arm
    M96.622 Fracture of humerus following insertion of orthopedic implant, joint prosthesis, or bone plate, left arm
    M96.629 Fracture of humerus following insertion of orthopedic implant, joint prosthesis, or bone plate, unspecified arm

☑6ᵗʰ **M96.63 Fracture of radius or ulna following insertion of orthopedic implant, joint prosthesis, or bone plate**
    M96.631 Fracture of radius or ulna following insertion of orthopedic implant, joint prosthesis, or bone plate, right arm
    M96.632 Fracture of radius or ulna following insertion of orthopedic implant, joint prosthesis, or bone plate, left arm
    M96.639 Fracture of radius or ulna following insertion of orthopedic implant, joint prosthesis, or bone plate, unspecified arm

    M96.65 Fracture of pelvis following insertion of orthopedic implant, joint prosthesis, or bone plate

☑6ᵗʰ **M96.66 Fracture of femur following insertion of orthopedic implant, joint prosthesis, or bone plate**
    M96.661 Fracture of femur following insertion of orthopedic implant, joint prosthesis, or bone plate, right leg
    M96.662 Fracture of femur following insertion of orthopedic implant, joint prosthesis, or bone plate, left leg
    M96.669 Fracture of femur following insertion of orthopedic implant, joint prosthesis, or bone plate, unspecified leg

☑6ᵗʰ **M96.67 Fracture of tibia or fibula following insertion of orthopedic implant, joint prosthesis, or bone plate**
    M96.671 Fracture of tibia or fibula following insertion of orthopedic implant, joint prosthesis, or bone plate, right leg
    M96.672 Fracture of tibia or fibula following insertion of orthopedic implant, joint prosthesis, or bone plate, left leg
    M96.679 Fracture of tibia or fibula following insertion of orthopedic implant, joint prosthesis, or bone plate, unspecified leg

    M96.69 Fracture of other bone following insertion of orthopedic implant, joint prosthesis, or bone plate

☑5ᵗʰ **M96.8 Other intraoperative and postprocedural complications and disorders of musculoskeletal system, not elsewhere classified**

☑6ᵗʰ **M96.81 Intraoperative hemorrhage and hematoma of a musculoskeletal structure complicating a procedure**
- EXCLUDES 1 *intraoperative hemorrhage and hematoma of a musculoskeletal structure due to accidental puncture and laceration during a procedure (M96.82-)*

    M96.810 Intraoperative hemorrhage and hematoma of a musculoskeletal structure complicating a musculoskeletal system procedure
    M96.811 Intraoperative hemorrhage and hematoma of a musculoskeletal structure complicating other procedure

☑6ᵗʰ **M96.82 Accidental puncture and laceration of a musculoskeletal structure during a procedure**
    M96.820 Accidental puncture and laceration of a musculoskeletal structure during a musculoskeletal system procedure
    M96.821 Accidental puncture and laceration of a musculoskeletal structure during other procedure

☑6ᵗʰ **M96.83 Postprocedural hemorrhage and hematoma of a musculoskeletal structure following a procedure**
    M96.830 Postprocedural hemorrhage and hematoma of a musculoskeletal structure following a musculoskeletal system procedure
    M96.831 Postprocedural hemorrhage and hematoma of a musculoskeletal structure following other procedure

    M96.89 Other intraoperative and postprocedural complications and disorders of the musculoskeletal system
    Instability of joint secondary to removal of joint prosthesis
    Use additional code, if applicable, to further specify disorder

Biomechanical lesions, not elsewhere classified (M99)

☑4ᵗʰ **M99 Biomechanical lesions, not elsewhere classified**
- NOTE This category should not be used if the condition can be classified elsewhere.

☑5ᵗʰ **M99.0 Segmental and somatic dysfunction**
    M99.00 Segmental and somatic dysfunction of head region
    M99.01 Segmental and somatic dysfunction of cervical region
    M99.02 Segmental and somatic dysfunction of thoracic region
    M99.03 Segmental and somatic dysfunction of lumbar region
    M99.04 Segmental and somatic dysfunction of sacral region
    M99.05 Segmental and somatic dysfunction of pelvic region

☑ Additional Character Required   ✓x7ᵗʰ Xtension Alert   Unspecified Dx   Other Specified Dx   Manifestation   ►◄ Revised Text   ● New Code   ▲ Revised Code Title

ICD-10-CM Draft (2015)   719

M99.06 Segmental and somatic dysfunction of lower extremity

M99.07 Segmental and somatic dysfunction of upper extremity

M99.08 Segmental and somatic dysfunction of rib cage

M99.09 Segmental and somatic dysfunction of abdomen and other regions

✓5ᵗʰ **M99.1** Subluxation complex (vertebral)

M99.10 Subluxation complex (vertebral) of head region

M99.11 Subluxation complex (vertebral) of cervical region

M99.12 Subluxation complex (vertebral) of thoracic region

M99.13 Subluxation complex (vertebral) of lumbar region

M99.14 Subluxation complex (vertebral) of sacral region

M99.15 Subluxation complex (vertebral) of pelvic region

M99.16 Subluxation complex (vertebral) of lower extremity

M99.17 Subluxation complex (vertebral) of upper extremity

M99.18 Subluxation complex (vertebral) of rib cage

M99.19 Subluxation complex (vertebral) of abdomen and other regions

✓5ᵗʰ **M99.2** Subluxation stenosis of neural canal

M99.20 Subluxation stenosis of neural canal of head region

M99.21 Subluxation stenosis of neural canal of cervical region

M99.22 Subluxation stenosis of neural canal of thoracic region

M99.23 Subluxation stenosis of neural canal of lumbar region

M99.24 Subluxation stenosis of neural canal of sacral region

M99.25 Subluxation stenosis of neural canal of pelvic region

M99.26 Subluxation stenosis of neural canal of lower extremity

M99.27 Subluxation stenosis of neural canal of upper extremity

M99.28 Subluxation stenosis of neural canal of rib cage

M99.29 Subluxation stenosis of neural canal of abdomen and other regions

✓5ᵗʰ **M99.3** Osseous stenosis of neural canal

M99.30 Osseous stenosis of neural canal of head region

M99.31 Osseous stenosis of neural canal of cervical region

M99.32 Osseous stenosis of neural canal of thoracic region

M99.33 Osseous stenosis of neural canal of lumbar region

M99.34 Osseous stenosis of neural canal of sacral region

M99.35 Osseous stenosis of neural canal of pelvic region

M99.36 Osseous stenosis of neural canal of lower extremity

M99.37 Osseous stenosis of neural canal of upper extremity

M99.38 Osseous stenosis of neural canal of rib cage

M99.39 Osseous stenosis of neural canal of abdomen and other regions

✓5ᵗʰ **M99.4** Connective tissue stenosis of neural canal

M99.40 Connective tissue stenosis of neural canal of head region

M99.41 Connective tissue stenosis of neural canal of cervical region

M99.42 Connective tissue stenosis of neural canal of thoracic region

M99.43 Connective tissue stenosis of neural canal of lumbar region

M99.44 Connective tissue stenosis of neural canal of sacral region

M99.45 Connective tissue stenosis of neural canal of pelvic region

M99.46 Connective tissue stenosis of neural canal of lower extremity

M99.47 Connective tissue stenosis of neural canal of upper extremity

M99.48 Connective tissue stenosis of neural canal of rib cage

M99.49 Connective tissue stenosis of neural canal of abdomen and other regions

✓5ᵗʰ **M99.5** Intervertebral disc stenosis of neural canal

M99.50 Intervertebral disc stenosis of neural canal of head region

M99.51 Intervertebral disc stenosis of neural canal of cervical region

M99.52 Intervertebral disc stenosis of neural canal of thoracic region

M99.53 Intervertebral disc stenosis of neural canal of lumbar region

M99.54 Intervertebral disc stenosis of neural canal of sacral region

M99.55 Intervertebral disc stenosis of neural canal of pelvic region

M99.56 Intervertebral disc stenosis of neural canal of lower extremity

M99.57 Intervertebral disc stenosis of neural canal of upper extremity

M99.58 Intervertebral disc stenosis of neural canal of rib cage

M99.59 Intervertebral disc stenosis of neural canal of abdomen and other regions

✓5ᵗʰ **M99.6** Osseous and subluxation stenosis of intervertebral foramina

M99.60 Osseous and subluxation stenosis of intervertebral foramina of head region

M99.61 Osseous and subluxation stenosis of intervertebral foramina of cervical region

M99.62 Osseous and subluxation stenosis of intervertebral foramina of thoracic region

M99.63 Osseous and subluxation stenosis of intervertebral foramina of lumbar region

M99.64 Osseous and subluxation stenosis of intervertebral foramina of sacral region

M99.65 Osseous and subluxation stenosis of intervertebral foramina of pelvic region

M99.66 Osseous and subluxation stenosis of intervertebral foramina of lower extremity

M99.67 Osseous and subluxation stenosis of intervertebral foramina of upper extremity

M99.68 Osseous and subluxation stenosis of intervertebral foramina of rib cage

M99.69 Osseous and subluxation stenosis of intervertebral foramina of abdomen and other regions

✓5ᵗʰ **M99.7** Connective tissue and disc stenosis of intervertebral foramina

M99.70 Connective tissue and disc stenosis of intervertebral foramina of head region

M99.71 Connective tissue and disc stenosis of intervertebral foramina of cervical region

M99.72 Connective tissue and disc stenosis of intervertebral foramina of thoracic region

M99.73 Connective tissue and disc stenosis of intervertebral foramina of lumbar region

M99.74 Connective tissue and disc stenosis of intervertebral foramina of sacral region

M99.75 Connective tissue and disc stenosis of intervertebral foramina of pelvic region

M99.76 Connective tissue and disc stenosis of intervertebral foramina of lower extremity

M99.77 Connective tissue and disc stenosis of intervertebral foramina of upper extremity

M99.78 Connective tissue and disc stenosis of intervertebral foramina of rib cage

M99.79 Connective tissue and disc stenosis of intervertebral foramina of abdomen and other regions

✓5ᵗʰ **M99.8** Other biomechanical lesions

M99.80 Other biomechanical lesions of head region

M99.81 Other biomechanical lesions of cervical region

M99.82 Other biomechanical lesions of thoracic region

M99.83 Other biomechanical lesions of lumbar region

M99.84 Other biomechanical lesions of sacral region

M99.85 Other biomechanical lesions of pelvic region

M99.86 Other biomechanical lesions of lower extremity

M99.87 Other biomechanical lesions of upper extremity

M99.88 Other biomechanical lesions of rib cage

M99.89 Other biomechanical lesions of abdomen and other regions

M99.9 Biomechanical lesion, unspecified

EXCLUDES 1 Not coded here   **EXCLUDES 2** Not included here   N Newborn Age: 0   P Pediatric Age: 0-17   M Maternity Age: 12-55   A Adult Age: 15-124

720   ICD-10-CM Draft (2015)

Chapter 14. Diseases of the Genitourinary System (N00-N99)

> EXCLUDES 2 certain conditions originating in the perinatal period (P04-P96)
> certain infectious and parasitic diseases (A00-B99)
> complications of pregnancy, childbirth and the puerperium (O00-O9A)
> congenital malformations, deformations and chromosomal abnormalities (Q00-Q99)
> endocrine, nutritional and metabolic diseases (E00-E88)
> injury, poisoning and certain other consequences of external causes (S00-T88)
> neoplasms (C00-D49)
> symptoms, signs and abnormal clinical and laboratory findings, not elsewhere classified (R00-R94)

This chapter contains the following blocks:

N00-N08	Glomerular diseases
N10-N16	Renal tubulo-interstitial diseases
N17-N19	Acute kidney failure and chronic kidney disease
N20-N23	Urolithiasis
N25-N29	Other disorders of kidney and ureter
N30-N39	Other diseases of the urinary system
N40-N53	Diseases of male genital organs
N60-N65	Disorders of breast
N70-N77	Inflammatory diseases of female pelvic organs
N80-N98	Noninflammatory disorders of female genital tract
N99	Intraoperative and postprocedural complications and disorders of genitourinary system, not elsewhere classified

Glomerular diseases (N00-N08)

Code also any associated kidney failure (N17-N19).

> EXCLUDES 1 hypertensive chronic kidney disease (I12.-)

☑4ᵗʰ **N00 Acute nephritic syndrome**

> INCLUDES acute glomerular disease
> acute glomerulonephritis
> acute nephritis

> EXCLUDES 1 acute tubulo-interstitial nephritis (N10)
> nephritic syndrome NOS (N05.-)

N00.0 Acute nephritic syndrome with minor glomerular abnormality
Acute nephritic syndrome with minimal change lesion

N00.1 Acute nephritic syndrome with focal and segmental glomerular lesions
Acute nephritic syndrome with focal and segmental hyalinosis
Acute nephritic syndrome with focal and segmental sclerosis
Acute nephritic syndrome with focal glomerulonephritis

N00.2 Acute nephritic syndrome with diffuse membranous glomerulonephritis

N00.3 Acute nephritic syndrome with diffuse mesangial proliferative glomerulonephritis

N00.4 Acute nephritic syndrome with diffuse endocapillary proliferative glomerulonephritis

N00.5 Acute nephritic syndrome with diffuse mesangiocapillary glomerulonephritis
Acute nephritic syndrome with membranoproliferative glomerulonephritis, types 1 and 3, or NOS

N00.6 Acute nephritic syndrome with dense deposit disease
Acute nephritic syndrome with membranoproliferative glomerulonephritis, type 2

N00.7 Acute nephritic syndrome with diffuse crescentic glomerulonephritis
Acute nephritic syndrome with extracapillary glomerulonephritis

N00.8 Acute nephritic syndrome with other morphologic changes
Acute nephritic syndrome with proliferative glomerulonephritis NOS

N00.9 Acute nephritic syndrome with unspecified morphologic changes

☑4ᵗʰ **N01 Rapidly progressive nephritic syndrome**

> INCLUDES rapidly progressive glomerular disease
> rapidly progressive glomerulonephritis
> rapidly progressive nephritis

> EXCLUDES 1 nephritic syndrome NOS (N05.-)

N01.0 Rapidly progressive nephritic syndrome with minor glomerular abnormality
Rapidly progressive nephritic syndrome with minimal change lesion

N01.1 Rapidly progressive nephritic syndrome with focal and segmental glomerular lesions
Rapidly progressive nephritic syndrome with focal and segmental hyalinosis
Rapidly progressive nephritic syndrome with focal and segmental sclerosis
Rapidly progressive nephritic syndrome with focal glomerulonephritis

N01.2 Rapidly progressive nephritic syndrome with diffuse membranous glomerulonephritis

N01.3 Rapidly progressive nephritic syndrome with diffuse mesangial proliferative glomerulonephritis

N01.4 Rapidly progressive nephritic syndrome with diffuse endocapillary proliferative glomerulonephritis

N01.5 Rapidly progressive nephritic syndrome with diffuse mesangiocapillary glomerulonephritis
Rapidly progressive nephritic syndrome with membranoproliferative glomerulonephritis, types 1 and 3, or NOS

N01.6 Rapidly progressive nephritic syndrome with dense deposit disease
Rapidly progressive nephritic syndrome with membranoproliferative glomerulonephritis, type 2

N01.7 Rapidly progressive nephritic syndrome with diffuse crescentic glomerulonephritis
Rapidly progressive nephritic syndrome with extracapillary glomerulonephritis

N01.8 Rapidly progressive nephritic syndrome with other morphologic changes
Rapidly progressive nephritic syndrome with proliferative glomerulonephritis NOS

N01.9 Rapidly progressive nephritic syndrome with unspecified morphologic changes

☑4ᵗʰ **N02 Recurrent and persistent hematuria**

> EXCLUDES 1 acute cystitis with hematuria (N30.01)
> hematuria NOS (R31.9)
> hematuria not associated with specified morphologic lesions (R31.-)

N02.0 Recurrent and persistent hematuria with minor glomerular abnormality
Recurrent and persistent hematuria with minimal change lesion

N02.1 Recurrent and persistent hematuria with focal and segmental glomerular lesions
Recurrent and persistent hematuria with focal and segmental hyalinosis
Recurrent and persistent hematuria with focal and segmental sclerosis
Recurrent and persistent hematuria with focal glomerulonephritis

N02.2 Recurrent and persistent hematuria with diffuse membranous glomerulonephritis

N02.3 Recurrent and persistent hematuria with diffuse mesangial proliferative glomerulonephritis

N02.4 Recurrent and persistent hematuria with diffuse endocapillary proliferative glomerulonephritis

N02.5 Recurrent and persistent hematuria with diffuse mesangiocapillary glomerulonephritis
Recurrent and persistent hematuria with membranoproliferative glomerulonephritis, types 1 and 3, or NOS

N02.6 Recurrent and persistent hematuria with dense deposit disease
Recurrent and persistent hematuria with membranoproliferative glomerulonephritis, type 2

N02.7 Recurrent and persistent hematuria with diffuse crescentic glomerulonephritis
Recurrent and persistent hematuria with extracapillary glomerulonephritis

N02.8 Recurrent and persistent hematuria with other morphologic changes
Recurrent and persistent hematuria with proliferative glomerulonephritis NOS

N02.9 Recurrent and persistent hematuria with unspecified morphologic changes

☑ Additional Character Required   ✗7ᵗʰ Xtension Alert   Unspecified Dx   Other Specified Dx   Manifestation   ►◄ Revised Text   ● New Code   ▲ Revised Code Title

ICD-10-CM Draft (2015)   **721**

Diseases of the Genitourinary System

N03–N07.3

✓4ᵗʰ **N03 Chronic nephritic syndrome**
> INCLUDES   chronic glomerular disease
> chronic glomerulonephritis
> chronic nephritis
> EXCLUDES 1   *chronic tubulo-interstitial nephritis (N11.-)*
> *diffuse sclerosing glomerulonephritis (N05.8-)*
> *nephritic syndrome NOS (N05.-)*

N03.0 Chronic nephritic syndrome with minor glomerular abnormality
> Chronic nephritic syndrome with minimal change lesion

N03.1 Chronic nephritic syndrome with focal and segmental glomerular lesions
> Chronic nephritic syndrome with focal and segmental hyalinosis
> Chronic nephritic syndrome with focal and segmental sclerosis
> Chronic nephritic syndrome with focal glomerulonephritis

N03.2 Chronic nephritic syndrome with diffuse membranous glomerulonephritis

N03.3 Chronic nephritic syndrome with diffuse mesangial proliferative glomerulonephritis

N03.4 Chronic nephritic syndrome with diffuse endocapillary proliferative glomerulonephritis

N03.5 Chronic nephritic syndrome with diffuse mesangiocapillary glomerulonephritis
> Chronic nephritic syndrome with membranoproliferative glomerulonephritis, types 1 and 3, or NOS

N03.6 Chronic nephritic syndrome with dense deposit disease
> Chronic nephritic syndrome with membranoproliferative glomerulonephritis, type 2

N03.7 Chronic nephritic syndrome with diffuse crescentic glomerulonephritis
> Chronic nephritic syndrome with extracapillary glomerulonephritis

N03.8 Chronic nephritic syndrome with other morphologic changes
> Chronic nephritic syndrome with proliferative glomerulonephritis NOS

N03.9 Chronic nephritic syndrome with unspecified morphologic changes

✓4ᵗʰ **N04 Nephrotic syndrome**
> INCLUDES   congenital nephrotic syndrome
> lipoid nephrosis

N04.0 Nephrotic syndrome with minor glomerular abnormality
> Nephrotic syndrome with minimal change lesion

N04.1 Nephrotic syndrome with focal and segmental glomerular lesions
> Nephrotic syndrome with focal and segmental hyalinosis
> Nephrotic syndrome with focal and segmental sclerosis
> Nephrotic syndrome with focal glomerulonephritis

N04.2 Nephrotic syndrome with diffuse membranous glomerulonephritis

N04.3 Nephrotic syndrome with diffuse mesangial proliferative glomerulonephritis

N04.4 Nephrotic syndrome with diffuse endocapillary proliferative glomerulonephritis

N04.5 Nephrotic syndrome with diffuse mesangiocapillary glomerulonephritis
> Nephrotic syndrome with membranoproliferative glomerulonephritis, types 1 and 3, or NOS

N04.6 Nephrotic syndrome with dense deposit disease
> Nephrotic syndrome with membranoproliferative glomerulonephritis, type 2

N04.7 Nephrotic syndrome with diffuse crescentic glomerulonephritis
> Nephrotic syndrome with extracapillary glomerulonephritis

N04.8 Nephrotic syndrome with other morphologic changes
> Nephrotic syndrome with proliferative glomerulonephritis NOS

N04.9 Nephrotic syndrome with unspecified morphologic changes

✓4ᵗʰ **N05 Unspecified nephritic syndrome**
> INCLUDES   glomerular disease NOS
> glomerulonephritis NOS
> nephritis NOS
> nephropathy NOS and renal disease NOS with morphological lesion specified in .0-.8
> EXCLUDES 1   *nephropathy NOS with no stated morphological lesion (N28.9)*
> *renal disease NOS with no stated morphological lesion (N28.9)*
> *tubulo-interstitial nephritis NOS (N12)*

N05.0 Unspecified nephritic syndrome with minor glomerular abnormality
> Unspecified nephritic syndrome with minimal change lesion

N05.1 Unspecified nephritic syndrome with focal and segmental glomerular lesions
> Unspecified nephritic syndrome with focal and segmental hyalinosis
> Unspecified nephritic syndrome with focal and segmental sclerosis
> Unspecified nephritic syndrome with focal glomerulonephritis

N05.2 Unspecified nephritic syndrome with diffuse membranous glomerulonephritis

N05.3 Unspecified nephritic syndrome with diffuse mesangial proliferative glomerulonephritis

N05.4 Unspecified nephritic syndrome with diffuse endocapillary proliferative glomerulonephritis

N05.5 Unspecified nephritic syndrome with diffuse mesangiocapillary glomerulonephritis
> Unspecified nephritic syndrome with membranoproliferative glomerulonephritis, types 1 and 3, or NOS

N05.6 Unspecified nephritic syndrome with dense deposit disease
> Unspecified nephritic syndrome with membranoproliferative glomerulonephritis, type 2

N05.7 Unspecified nephritic syndrome with diffuse crescentic glomerulonephritis
> Unspecified nephritic syndrome with extracapillary glomerulonephritis

N05.8 Unspecified nephritic syndrome with other morphologic changes
> Unspecified nephritic syndrome with proliferative glomerulonephritis NOS

N05.9 Unspecified nephritic syndrome with unspecified morphologic changes

✓4ᵗʰ **N06 Isolated proteinuria with specified morphological lesion**
> EXCLUDES 1   *proteinuria not associated with specific morphologic lesions (R80.0)*

N06.0 Isolated proteinuria with minor glomerular abnormality
> Isolated proteinuria with minimal change lesion

N06.1 Isolated proteinuria with focal and segmental glomerular lesions
> Isolated proteinuria with focal and segmental hyalinosis
> Isolated proteinuria with focal and segmental sclerosis
> Isolated proteinuria with focal glomerulonephritis

N06.2 Isolated proteinuria with diffuse membranous glomerulonephritis

N06.3 Isolated proteinuria with diffuse mesangial proliferative glomerulonephritis

N06.4 Isolated proteinuria with diffuse endocapillary proliferative glomerulonephritis

N06.5 Isolated proteinuria with diffuse mesangiocapillary glomerulonephritis
> Isolated proteinuria with membranoproliferative glomerulonephritis, types 1 and 3, or NOS

N06.6 Isolated proteinuria with dense deposit disease
> Isolated proteinuria with membranoproliferative glomerulonephritis, type 2

N06.7 Isolated proteinuria with diffuse crescentic glomerulonephritis
> Isolated proteinuria with extracapillary glomerulonephritis

N06.8 Isolated proteinuria with other morphologic lesion
> Isolated proteinuria with proliferative glomerulonephritis NOS

N06.9 Isolated proteinuria with unspecified morphologic lesion

✓4ᵗʰ **N07 Hereditary nephropathy, not elsewhere classified**
> EXCLUDES 2   *Alport's syndrome (Q87.81-)*
> *hereditary amyloid nephropathy (E85.-)*
> *nail patella syndrome (Q87.2)*
> *non-neuropathic heredofamilial amyloidosis (E85.-)*

N07.0 Hereditary nephropathy, not elsewhere classified with minor glomerular abnormality
> Hereditary nephropathy, not elsewhere classified with minimal change lesion

N07.1 Hereditary nephropathy, not elsewhere classified with focal and segmental glomerular lesions
> Hereditary nephropathy, not elsewhere classified with focal and segmental hyalinosis
> Hereditary nephropathy, not elsewhere classified with focal and segmental sclerosis
> Hereditary nephropathy, not elsewhere classified with focal glomerulonephritis

N07.2 Hereditary nephropathy, not elsewhere classified with diffuse membranous glomerulonephritis

N07.3 Hereditary nephropathy, not elsewhere classified with diffuse mesangial proliferative glomerulonephritis

EXCLUDES 1 Not coded here   EXCLUDES 2 Not included here   N Newborn Age: 0   P Pediatric Age: 0-17   M Maternity Age: 12-55   A Adult Age: 15-124

722   ICD-10-CM Draft (2015)

N07.4 **Hereditary nephropathy, not elsewhere classified with** diffuse endocapillary proliferative glomerulonephritis

N07.5 **Hereditary nephropathy, not elsewhere classified with** diffuse mesangiocapillary glomerulonephritis
Hereditary nephropathy, not elsewhere classified with membranoproliferative glomerulonephritis, types 1 and 3, or NOS

N07.6 **Hereditary nephropathy, not elsewhere classified with** dense deposit disease
Hereditary nephropathy, not elsewhere classified with membranoproliferative glomerulonephritis, type 2

N07.7 **Hereditary nephropathy, not elsewhere classified with** diffuse crescentic glomerulonephritis
Hereditary nephropathy, not elsewhere classified with extracapillary glomerulonephritis

N07.8 **Hereditary nephropathy, not elsewhere classified with other morphologic lesions**
Hereditary nephropathy, not elsewhere classified with proliferative glomerulonephritis NOS

N07.9 **Hereditary nephropathy, not elsewhere classified with unspecified morphologic lesions**

N08 *Glomerular disorders in diseases classified elsewhere*
Glomerulonephritis
Nephritis
Nephropathy
Code first underlying disease, such as:
amyloidosis (E85.-)
congenital syphilis (A50.5)
cryoglobulinemia (D89.1)
disseminated intravascular coagulation (D65)
gout (M1A.-, M10.-)
microscopic polyangiitis (M31.7)
multiple myeloma (C90.0-)
sepsis (A40.0-A41.9)
sickle-cell disease (D57.0-D57.8)
EXCLUDES 1 *glomerulonephritis, nephritis and nephropathy (in):*
antiglomerular basement membrane disease (M31.0)
diabetes (E08-E13 with .21)
gonococcal (A54.21)
Goodpasture's syndrome (M31.0)
hemolytic-uremic syndrome (D59.3)
lupus (M32.14)
mumps (B26.83)
syphilis (A52.75)
systemic lupus erythematosus (M32.14)
Wegener's granulomatosis (M31.31)
pyelonephritis in diseases classified elsewhere (N16)
renal tubulo-interstitial disorders classified elsewhere (N16)

Renal tubulo-interstitial diseases (N10-N16)
INCLUDES pyelonephritis
EXCLUDES 1 *pyeloureteritis cystica (N28.85)*

N10 Acute **tubulo-interstitial nephritis**
Acute infectious interstitial nephritis
Acute pyelitis
Acute pyelonephritis
Hemoglobin nephrosis
Myoglobin nephrosis
Use additional code (B95-B97), to identify infectious agent

✓4th **N11** Chronic **tubulo-interstitial nephritis**
INCLUDES chronic infectious interstitial nephritis
chronic pyelitis
chronic pyelonephritis
Use additional code (B95-B97), to identify infectious agent

N11.0 Nonobstructive reflux-associated **chronic pyelonephritis**
Pyelonephritis (chronic) associated with (vesicoureteral) reflux
EXCLUDES 1 *vesicoureteral reflux NOS (N13.70)*

N11.1 Chronic obstructive **pyelonephritis**
Pyelonephritis (chronic) associated with anomaly of pelviureteric junction
Pyelonephritis (chronic) associated with anomaly of pyeloureteric junction
Pyelonephritis (chronic) associated with crossing of vessel
Pyelonephritis (chronic) associated with kinking of ureter
Pyelonephritis (chronic) associated with obstruction of ureter
Pyelonephritis (chronic) associated with stricture of pelviureteric junction
Pyelonephritis (chronic) associated with stricture of ureter
EXCLUDES 1 *calculous pyelonephritis (N20.9)*
obstructive uropathy (N13.-)

N11.8 **Other chronic tubulo-interstitial nephritis**
Nonobstructive chronic pyelonephritis NOS

N11.9 **Chronic tubulo-interstitial nephritis, unspecified**
Chronic interstitial nephritis NOS
Chronic pyelitis NOS
Chronic pyelonephritis NOS

N12 **Tubulo-interstitial nephritis,** not specified as acute or chronic
Interstitial nephritis NOS
Pyelitis NOS
Pyelonephritis NOS
EXCLUDES 1 *calculous pyelonephritis (N20.9)*

✓4th **N13** **Obstructive and reflux uropathy**
EXCLUDES 2 *calculus of kidney and ureter without hydronephrosis (N20.-)*
congenital obstructive defects of renal pelvis and ureter (Q62.0-Q62.3)
hydronephrosis with ureteropelvic junction obstruction (Q62.1)
obstructive pyelonephritis (N11.1)

N13.1 **Hydronephrosis with ureteral stricture, not elsewhere classified**
EXCLUDES 1 *hydronephrosis with ureteral stricture with infection (N13.6)*

N13.2 **Hydronephrosis with renal and ureteral calculous obstruction**
EXCLUDES 1 *hydronephrosis with renal and ureteral calculous obstruction with infection (N13.6)*

✓5th **N13.3** **Other and unspecified hydronephrosis**
EXCLUDES 1 *hydronephrosis with infection (N13.6)*
N13.30 **Unspecified hydronephrosis**
N13.39 **Other hydronephrosis**

N13.4 **Hydroureter**
EXCLUDES 1 *congenital hydroureter (Q62.3-)*
hydroureter with infection (N13.6)
vesicoureteral-reflux with hydroureter (N13.73-)

N13.5 **Crossing vessel and stricture of ureter without hydronephrosis**
Kinking and stricture of ureter without hydronephrosis
EXCLUDES 1 *crossing vessel and stricture of ureter without hydronephrosis with infection (N13.6)*

N13.6 **Pyonephrosis**
Conditions in N13.1-N13.5 with infection
Obstructive uropathy with infection
Use additional code (B95-B97), to identify infectious agent

✓5th **N13.7** **Vesicoureteral-reflux**
EXCLUDES 1 *reflux-associated pyelonephritis (N11.0)*
N13.70 **Vesicoureteral-reflux, unspecified**
Vesicoureteral-reflux NOS
N13.71 **Vesicoureteral-reflux** without reflux nephropathy
✓6th **N13.72** **Vesicoureteral-reflux** with reflux nephropathy without hydroureter
N13.721 **Vesicoureteral-reflux with reflux nephropathy without hydroureter, unilateral**
N13.722 **Vesicoureteral-reflux with reflux nephropathy without hydroureter, bilateral**
N13.729 **Vesicoureteral-reflux with reflux nephropathy without hydroureter, unspecified**
✓6th **N13.73** **Vesicoureteral-reflux** with reflux nephropathy with hydroureter
N13.731 **Vesicoureteral-reflux with reflux nephropathy with hydroureter,** unilateral
N13.732 **Vesicoureteral-reflux with reflux nephropathy with hydroureter,** bilateral
N13.739 **Vesicoureteral-reflux with reflux nephropathy with hydroureter, unspecified**

N13.8 **Other obstructive and reflux uropathy**
Urinary tract obstruction due to specified cause
Code first, if applicable, any causal condition, such as:
enlarged prostate (N40.1)

N13.9 **Obstructive and reflux uropathy, unspecified**
Urinary tract obstruction NOS

✓4th **N14** **Drug- and heavy-metal-induced tubulo-interstitial and tubular conditions**
Code first poisoning due to drug or toxin, if applicable (T36-T65 with fifth or sixth character 1-4 or 6)
Use additional code for adverse effect, if applicable, to identify drug (T36-T50 with fifth or sixth character 5)

N14.0 **Analgesic nephropathy**

N14.1 Nephropathy induced by other drugs, medicaments and biological substances

N14.2 Nephropathy induced by unspecified drug, medicament or biological substance

N14.3 Nephropathy induced by heavy metals

N14.4 Toxic nephropathy, not elsewhere classified

✓4ᵗʰ **N15 Other renal tubulo-interstitial diseases**

N15.0 Balkan nephropathy
Balkan endemic nephropathy

N15.1 Renal and perinephric abscess

N15.8 Other specified renal tubulo-interstitial diseases

N15.9 Renal tubulo-interstitial disease, unspecified
Infection of kidney NOS
EXCLUDES 1   *urinary tract infection NOS (N39.0)*

N16 Renal tubulo-interstitial disorders in diseases classified elsewhere
Pyelonephritis
Tubulo-interstitial nephritis
Code first underlying disease, such as:
brucellosis (A23.0-A23.9)
cryoglobulinemia (D89.1)
glycogen storage disease (E74.0)
leukemia (C91-C95)
lymphoma (C81.0-C85.9, C96.0-C96.9)
multiple myeloma (C90.0-)
sepsis (A40.0-A41.9)
Wilson's disease (E83.0)
EXCLUDES 1   *diphtheritic pyelonephritis and tubulo-interstitial nephritis (A36.84)*
pyelonephritis and tubulo-interstitial nephritis in candidiasis (B37.49)
pyelonephritis and tubulo-interstitial nephritis in cystinosis (E72.04)
pyelonephritis and tubulo-interstitial nephritis in salmonella infection (A02.25)
pyelonephritis and tubulo-interstitial nephritis in sarcoidosis (D86.84)
pyelonephritis and tubulo-interstitial nephritis in sicca syndrome [Sjogren's] (M35.04)
pyelonephritis and tubulo-interstitial nephritis in systemic lupus erythematosus (M32.15)
pyelonephritis and tubulo-interstitial nephritis in toxoplasmosis (B58.83)
renal tubular degeneration in diabetes (E08-E13 with .29)
syphilitic pyelonephritis and tubulo-interstitial nephritis (A52.75)

Acute kidney failure and chronic kidney disease (N17-N19)
EXCLUDES 2   *congenital renal failure (P96.0)*
drug- and heavy-metal-induced tubulo-interstitial and tubular conditions (N14.-)
extrarenal uremia (R39.2)
hemolytic-uremic syndrome (D59.3)
hepatorenal syndrome (K76.7)
postpartum hepatorenal syndrome (O90.4)
posttraumatic renal failure (T79.5)
prerenal uremia (R39.2)
renal failure complicating abortion or ectopic or molar pregnancy (O00-O07, O08.4)
renal failure following labor and delivery (O90.4)
renal failure postprocedural (N99.0)

✓4ᵗʰ **N17 Acute kidney failure**
Code also associated underlying condition
EXCLUDES 1   *posttraumatic renal failure (T79.5)*
AHA: 2013, 4Q, 124

N17.0 Acute kidney failure with tubular necrosis
Acute tubular necrosis
Renal tubular necrosis
Tubular necrosis NOS

N17.1 Acute kidney failure with acute cortical necrosis
Acute cortical necrosis
Cortical necrosis NOS
Renal cortical necrosis

N17.2 Acute kidney failure with medullary necrosis
Medullary [papillary] necrosis NOS
Acute medullary [papillary] necrosis
Renal medullary [papillary] necrosis

N17.8 Other acute kidney failure

N17.9 Acute kidney failure, unspecified
Acute kidney injury (nontraumatic)
EXCLUDES 2   *traumatic kidney injury (S37.0-)*

✓4ᵗʰ **N18 Chronic kidney disease (CKD)**
Code first any associated:
diabetic chronic kidney disease (E08.22, E09.22, E10.22, E11.22, E13.22)
hypertensive chronic kidney disease (I12-, I13-)
Use additional code to identify kidney transplant status, if applicable, (Z94.0)
AHA: 2013, 1Q, 24

N18.1 Chronic kidney disease, stage 1

N18.2 Chronic kidney disease, stage 2 (mild)

N18.3 Chronic kidney disease, stage 3 (moderate)

N18.4 Chronic kidney disease, stage 4 (severe)

N18.5 Chronic kidney disease, stage 5
EXCLUDES 1   *chronic kidney disease, stage 5 requiring chronic dialysis (N18.6)*

N18.6 End stage renal disease
Chronic kidney disease requiring chronic dialysis
Use additional code to identify dialysis status (Z99.2)
AHA: 2013, 4Q, 124-125

N18.9 Chronic kidney disease, unspecified
Chronic renal disease
Chronic renal failure NOS
Chronic renal insufficiency
Chronic uremia

N19 Unspecified kidney failure
Uremia NOS
EXCLUDES 1   *acute kidney failure (N17.-)*
chronic kidney disease (N18.-)
chronic uremia (N18.9)
extrarenal uremia (R39.2)
prerenal uremia (R39.2)
renal insufficiency (acute) (N28.9)
uremia of newborn (P96.0)

Urolithiasis (N20-N23)

✓4ᵗʰ **N20 Calculus of kidney and ureter**
Calculous pyelonephritis
EXCLUDES 1   *nephrocalcinosis (E83.5)*
that with hydronephrosis (N13.2)

N20.0 Calculus of kidney
Nephrolithiasis NOS
Renal calculus
Renal stone
Staghorn calculus
Stone in kidney

N20.1 Calculus of ureter
Ureteric stone

N20.2 Calculus of kidney with calculus of ureter

N20.9 Urinary calculus, unspecified

✓4ᵗʰ **N21 Calculus of lower urinary tract**
Calculus of lower urinary tract with cystitis and urethritis

N21.0 Calculus in bladder
Calculus in diverticulum of bladder
Urinary bladder stone
EXCLUDES 2   *staghorn calculus (N20.0)*

N21.1 Calculus in urethra
EXCLUDES 2   *calculus of prostate (N42.0)*

N21.8 Other lower urinary tract calculus

N21.9 Calculus of lower urinary tract, unspecified
EXCLUDES 1   *calculus of urinary tract NOS (N20.9)*

N22 Calculus of urinary tract in diseases classified elsewhere
Code first underlying disease, such as:
gout (M1A.-, M10.-)
schistosomiasis (B65.0-B65.9)

N23 Unspecified renal colic

Other disorders of kidney and ureter (N25-N29)
EXCLUDES 2   *disorders of kidney and ureter with urolithiasis (N20-N23)*

✓4ᵗʰ **N25 Disorders resulting from impaired renal tubular function**
EXCLUDES 1   *metabolic disorders classifiable to E70-E88*

N25.0 Renal osteodystrophy
Azotemic osteodystrophy
Phosphate-losing tubular disorders
Renal rickets
Renal short stature

EXCLUDES 1 Not coded here   EXCLUDES 2 Not included here   N Newborn Age: 0   P Pediatric Age: 0-17   M Maternity Age: 12-55   A Adult Age: 15-124

724   ICD-10-CM Draft (2015)

N25.1 Nephrogenic diabetes insipidus
> EXCLUDES 1 *diabetes insipidus NOS (E23.2)*

✓5th **N25.8 Other disorders resulting from impaired renal tubular function**

N25.81 Secondary hyperparathyroidism of renal origin
> EXCLUDES 1 *secondary hyperparathyroidism, non-renal (E21.1)*

N25.89 Other disorders resulting from impaired renal tubular function
> Hypokalemic nephropathy
> Lightwood-Albright syndrome
> Renal tubular acidosis NOS

N25.9 Disorder resulting from impaired renal tubular function, unspecified

✓4th **N26 Unspecified contracted kidney**
> EXCLUDES 1 *contracted kidney due to hypertension (I12.-)*
> *diffuse sclerosing glomerulonephritis (N05.8-)*
> *hypertensive nephrosclerosis (arteriolar) (arteriosclerotic) (I12.-)*
> *small kidney of unknown cause (N27.-)*

N26.1 Atrophy of kidney (terminal)

N26.2 Page kidney

N26.9 Renal sclerosis, unspecified

✓4th **N27 Small kidney of unknown cause**
> INCLUDES oligonephronia

N27.0 Small kidney, unilateral

N27.1 Small kidney, bilateral

N27.9 Small kidney, unspecified

✓4th **N28 Other disorders of kidney and ureter, not elsewhere classified**

N28.0 Ischemia and infarction of kidney
> Renal artery embolism   Renal artery thrombosis
> Renal artery obstruction   Renal infarct
> Renal artery occlusion
> EXCLUDES 1 *atherosclerosis of renal artery (extrarenal part) (I70.1)*
> *congenital stenosis of renal artery (Q27.1)*
> *Goldblatt's kidney (I70.1)*

N28.1 Cyst of kidney, acquired
> Cyst (multiple)(solitary) of kidney, acquired
> EXCLUDES 1 *cystic kidney disease (congenital) (Q61.-)*

✓5th **N28.8 Other specified disorders of kidney and ureter**
> EXCLUDES 1 *hydroureter (N13.4)*
> *ureteric stricture with hydronephrosis (N13.1)*
> *ureteric stricture without hydronephrosis (N13.5)*

N28.81 Hypertrophy of kidney

N28.82 Megaloureter

N28.83 Nephroptosis

N28.84 Pyelitis cystica

N28.85 Pyeloureteritis cystica

N28.86 Ureteritis cystica

N28.89 Other specified disorders of kidney and ureter

N28.9 Disorder of kidney and ureter, unspecified
> Nephropathy NOS
> Renal disease (acute) NOS
> Renal insufficiency (acute)
> EXCLUDES 1 *chronic renal insufficiency (N18.9)*
> *unspecified nephritic syndrome (N05.-)*

N29 Other disorders of kidney and ureter in diseases classified elsewhere
> *Code first underlying disease, such as:*
> *amyloidosis (E85.-)*
> *nephrocalcinosis (E83.5)*
> *schistosomiasis (B65.0-B65.9)*
> EXCLUDES 1 *disorders of kidney and ureter in:*
> *cystinosis (E72.0)*
> *gonorrhea (A54.21)*
> *syphilis (A52.75)*
> *tuberculosis (A18.11)*

Other diseases of the urinary system (N30-N39)
> EXCLUDES 1 *urinary infection (complicating):*
> *abortion or ectopic or molar pregnancy (O00-O07, O08.8)*
> *pregnancy, childbirth and the puerperium (O23-, O75.3, O86.2-)*

✓4th **N30 Cystitis**
> Use additional code to identify infectious agent (B95-B97)
> EXCLUDES 1 *prostatocystitis (N41.3)*

✓5th **N30.0 Acute cystitis**
> EXCLUDES 1 *irradiation cystitis (N30.4-)*
> *trigonitis (N30.3-)*

N30.00 Acute cystitis without hematuria

N30.01 Acute cystitis with hematuria

✓5th **N30.1 Interstitial cystitis (chronic)**

N30.10 Interstitial cystitis (chronic) without hematuria

N30.11 Interstitial cystitis (chronic) with hematuria

✓5th **N30.2 Other chronic cystitis**

N30.20 Other chronic cystitis without hematuria

N30.21 Other chronic cystitis with hematuria

✓5th **N30.3 Trigonitis**
> Urethrotrigonitis

N30.30 Trigonitis without hematuria

N30.31 Trigonitis with hematuria

✓5th **N30.4 Irradiation cystitis**

N30.40 Irradiation cystitis without hematuria

N30.41 Irradiation cystitis with hematuria

✓5th **N30.8 Other cystitis**
> Abscess of bladder

N30.80 Other cystitis without hematuria

N30.81 Other cystitis with hematuria

✓5th **N30.9 Cystitis, unspecified**

N30.90 Cystitis, unspecified without hematuria

N30.91 Cystitis, unspecified with hematuria

✓4th **N31 Neuromuscular dysfunction of bladder, not elsewhere classified**
> Use additional code to identify any associated urinary incontinence (N39.3-N39.4-)
> EXCLUDES 1 *cord bladder NOS (G95.89)*
> *neurogenic bladder due to cauda equina syndrome (G83.4)*
> *neuromuscular dysfunction due to spinal cord lesion (G95.89)*

N31.0 Uninhibited neuropathic bladder, not elsewhere classified

N31.1 Reflex neuropathic bladder, not elsewhere classified

N31.2 Flaccid neuropathic bladder, not elsewhere classified
> Atonic (motor) (sensory) neuropathic bladder
> Autonomous neuropathic bladder
> Nonreflex neuropathic bladder

N31.8 Other neuromuscular dysfunction of bladder

N31.9 Neuromuscular dysfunction of bladder, unspecified
> Neurogenic bladder dysfunction NOS

✓4th **N32 Other disorders of bladder**
> EXCLUDES 2 *calculus of bladder (N21.0)*
> *cystocele (N81.1-)*
> *hernia or prolapse of bladder, female (N81.1-)*

N32.0 Bladder-neck obstruction
> Bladder-neck stenosis (acquired)
> EXCLUDES 1 *congenital bladder-neck obstruction (Q64.3-)*

N32.1 Vesicointestinal fistula
> Vesicorectal fistula

N32.2 Vesical fistula, not elsewhere classified
> EXCLUDES 1 *fistula between bladder and female genital tract (N82.0-N82.1)*

N32.3 Diverticulum of bladder
> EXCLUDES 1 *congenital diverticulum of bladder (Q64.6)*
> *diverticulitis of bladder (N30.8-)*

✓5th **N32.8 Other specified disorders of bladder**

N32.81 Overactive bladder
> Detrusor muscle hyperactivity
> EXCLUDES 1 *frequent urination due to specified bladder condition—code to condition*

N32.89 Other specified disorders of bladder
> Bladder hemorrhage
> Bladder hypertrophy
> Calcified bladder
> Contracted bladder

N32.9 Bladder disorder, unspecified

✓ Additional Character Required   ✓x7th Xtension Alert   Unspecified Dx   Other Specified Dx   Manifestation   ▶◀ Revised Text   ● New Code   ▲ Revised Code Title

Diseases of the Genitourinary System   **N33–N39.9**

N33   *Bladder disorders in diseases classified elsewhere*

Code first underlying disease, such as:
   schistosomiasis (B65.0-B65.9)

EXCLUDES 1   bladder disorder in syphilis (A52.76)
       bladder disorder in tuberculosis (A18.12)
       candidal cystitis (B37.41)
       chlamydial cystitis (A56.01)
       cystitis in gonorrhea (A54.01)
       cystitis in neurogenic bladder (N31.-)
       diphtheritic cystitis (A36.85)
       neurogenic bladder (N31.-)
       syphilitic cystitis (A52.76)
       trichomonal cystitis (A59.03)

√4ᵗʰ N34   Urethritis and urethral syndrome

Use additional code (B95-B97), to identify infectious agent

EXCLUDES 2   Reiter's disease (M02.3-)
       urethritis in diseases with a predominantly sexual mode of
         transmission (A50-A64)
       urethrotrigonitis (N30.3-)

N34.0   Urethral abscess
   Abscess (of) Cowper's gland
   Abscess (of) Littrés gland
   Abscess (of) urethral (gland)
   Periurethral abscess
     EXCLUDES 1   urethral caruncle (N36.2)

N34.1   Nonspecific urethritis
   Nongonococcal urethritis
   Nonvenereal urethritis

N34.2   Other urethritis
   Meatitis, urethral
   Postmenopausal urethritis
   Ulcer of urethra (meatus)
   Urethritis NOS

N34.3   Urethral syndrome, unspecified

√4ᵗʰ N35   Urethral stricture

EXCLUDES 1   congenital urethral stricture (Q64.3-)
       postprocedural urethral stricture (N99.1-)

√5ᵗʰ N35.0   Post-traumatic urethral stricture
   Urethral stricture due to injury
     EXCLUDES 1   postprocedural urethral stricture (N99.1-)

   √6ᵗʰ N35.01   Post-traumatic urethral stricture, male

     N35.010   Post-traumatic urethral stricture, male, meatal   ♂

     N35.011   Post-traumatic bulbous urethral stricture

     N35.012   Post-traumatic membranous urethral stricture

     N35.013   Post-traumatic anterior urethral stricture

     N35.014   Post-traumatic urethral stricture, male, unspecified   ♂

   √6ᵗʰ N35.02   Post-traumatic urethral stricture, female

     N35.021   Urethral stricture due to childbirth   ♀

     N35.028   Other post-traumatic urethral stricture, female   ♀

√5ᵗʰ N35.1   Postinfective urethral stricture, not elsewhere classified
     EXCLUDES 1   urethral stricture associated with schistosomiasis (B65-, N29)
       gonococcal urethral stricture (A54.01)
       syphilitic urethral stricture (A52.76)

   √6ᵗʰ N35.11   Postinfective urethral stricture, not elsewhere classified, male

     N35.111   Postinfective urethral stricture, not elsewhere classified, male, meatal   ♂

     N35.112   Postinfective bulbous urethral stricture, not elsewhere classified

     N35.113   Postinfective membranous urethral stricture, not elsewhere classified

     N35.114   Postinfective anterior urethral stricture, not elsewhere classified

     N35.119   Postinfective urethral stricture, not elsewhere classified, male, unspecified   ♂

   N35.12   Postinfective urethral stricture, not elsewhere classified, female   ♀

N35.8   Other urethral stricture
     EXCLUDES 1   postprocedural urethral stricture (N99.1-)

N35.9   Urethral stricture, unspecified

√4ᵗʰ N36   Other disorders of urethra

N36.0   Urethral fistula
   Urethroperineal fistula
   Urethrorectal fistula
   Urinary fistula NOS
     EXCLUDES 1   urethroscrotal fistula (N50.8)
       urethrovaginal fistula (N82.1)
       urethrovesicovaginal fistula (N82.1)

N36.1   Urethral diverticulum

N36.2   Urethral caruncle

√5ᵗʰ N36.4   Urethral functional and muscular disorders
   Use additional code to identify associated urinary stress
     incontinence (N39.3)

   N36.41   Hypermobility of urethra

   N36.42   Intrinsic sphincter deficiency (ISD)

   N36.43   Combined hypermobility of urethra and intrinsic sphincter deficiency

   N36.44   Muscular disorders of urethra
     Bladder sphincter dyssynergy

N36.5   Urethral false passage

N36.8   Other specified disorders of urethra

N36.9   Urethral disorder, unspecified

N37   *Urethral disorders in diseases classified elsewhere*

Code first underlying disease

EXCLUDES 1   urethritis (in):
       candidal infection (B37.41)
       chlamydial (A56.01)
       gonorrhea (A54.01)
       syphilis (A52.76)
       trichomonal infection (A59.03)
       tuberculosis (A18.13)

√4ᵗʰ N39   Other disorders of urinary system

EXCLUDES 2   hematuria NOS (R31.-)
       recurrent or persistent hematuria (N02.-)
       recurrent or persistent hematuria with specified morphological
         lesion (N02.-)
       proteinuria NOS (R80.-)

N39.0   Urinary tract infection, site not specified
   Use additional code (B95-B97), to identify infectious agent
     EXCLUDES 1   candidiasis of urinary tract (B37.4-)
       neonatal urinary tract infection (P39.3)
       urinary tract infection of specified site, such as:
         cystitis (N30.-)
         urethritis (N34.-)
     AHA: 2012, 4Q, 94

N39.3   Stress incontinence (female) (male)
   Code also any associated overactive bladder (N32.81)
     EXCLUDES 1   mixed incontinence (N39.46)

√5ᵗʰ N39.4   Other specified urinary incontinence
   Code also any associated overactive bladder (N32.81)
     EXCLUDES 1   enuresis NOS (R32)
       functional urinary incontinence (R39.81)
       urinary incontinence associated with cognitive
         impairment (R39.81)
       urinary incontinence NOS (R32)
       urinary incontinence of nonorganic origin (F98.0)

   N39.41   Urge incontinence
     EXCLUDES 1   mixed incontinence (N39.46)

   N39.42   Incontinence without sensory awareness

   N39.43   Post-void dribbling

   N39.44   Nocturnal enuresis

   N39.45   Continuous leakage

   N39.46   Mixed incontinence
     Urge and stress incontinence

   √6ᵗʰ N39.49   Other specified urinary incontinence

     N39.490   Overflow incontinence

     N39.498   Other specified urinary incontinence
       Reflex incontinence
       Total incontinence

N39.8   Other specified disorders of urinary system

N39.9   Disorder of urinary system, unspecified

EXCLUDES 1 Not coded here   EXCLUDES 2 Not included here   N Newborn Age: 0   P Pediatric Age: 0-17   M Maternity Age: 12-55   A Adult Age: 15-124

726   ICD-10-CM Draft (2015)

Diseases of male genital organs (N40-N53)

☑4ᵗʰ N40 Enlarged prostate
Adenofibromatous hypertrophy of prostate
Benign hypertrophy of the prostate
Benign prostatic hyperplasia
Benign prostatic hypertrophy
BPH
Nodular prostate
Polyp of prostate

EXCLUDES 1 benign neoplasms of prostate (adenoma, benign) (fibroadenoma) (fibroma) (myoma) (D29.1)
EXCLUDES 2 malignant neoplasm of prostate (C61)

N40.0 Enlarged prostate without lower urinary tract symptoms 🄰♂
Enlarged prostate NOS
Enlarged prostate without LUTS

N40.1 Enlarged prostate with lower urinary tract symptoms 🄰♂
Enlarged prostate with LUTS
Use additional code for associated symptoms, when specified:
incomplete bladder emptying (R39.14)
nocturia (R35.1)
straining on urination (R39.16)
urinary frequency (R35.0)
urinary hesitancy (R39.11)
urinary incontinence (N39.4-)
urinary obstruction (N13.8)
urinary retention (R33.8)
urinary urgency (R39.15)
weak urinary stream (R39.12)

N40.2 Nodular prostate without lower urinary tract symptoms 🄰♂
Nodular prostate without LUTS

N40.3 Nodular prostate with lower urinary tract symptoms 🄰♂
Use additional code for associated symptoms, when specified:
incomplete bladder emptying (R39.14)
nocturia (R35.1)
straining on urination (R39.16)
urinary frequency (R35.0)
urinary hesitancy (R39.11)
urinary incontinence (N39.4-)
urinary obstruction (N13.8)
urinary retention (R33.8)
urinary urgency (R39.15)
weak urinary stream (R39.12)

☑4ᵗʰ N41 Inflammatory diseases of prostate
Use additional code (B95-B97), to identify infectious agent

N41.0 Acute prostatitis 🄰♂
N41.1 Chronic prostatitis 🄰♂
N41.2 Abscess of prostate 🄰♂
N41.3 Prostatocystitis 🄰♂
N41.4 Granulomatous prostatitis 🄰♂
N41.8 Other inflammatory diseases of prostate 🄰♂
N41.9 Inflammatory disease of prostate, unspecified 🄰♂
Prostatitis NOS

☑4ᵗʰ N42 Other and unspecified disorders of prostate

N42.0 Calculus of prostate 🄰♂
Prostatic stone

N42.1 Congestion and hemorrhage of prostate 🄰♂
EXCLUDES 1 enlarged prostate (N40.-)
hematuria (R31.-)
hyperplasia of prostate (N40.-)
inflammatory diseases of prostate (N41.-)

N42.3 Dysplasia of prostate ♂
Prostatic intraepithelial neoplasia I (PIN I)
Prostatic intraepithelial neoplasia II (PIN II)
EXCLUDES 1 prostatic intraepithelial neoplasia III (PIN III) (D07.5)

☑5ᵗʰ N42.8 Other specified disorders of prostate
N42.81 Prostatodynia syndrome 🄰♂
Painful prostate syndrome
N42.82 Prostatosis syndrome 🄰♂
N42.83 Cyst of prostate 🄰♂
N42.89 Other specified disorders of prostate 🄰♂

N42.9 Disorder of prostate, unspecified 🄰♂

☑4ᵗʰ N43 Hydrocele and spermatocele
INCLUDES hydrocele of spermatic cord, testis or tunica vaginalis
EXCLUDES 1 congenital hydrocele (P83.5)

N43.0 Encysted hydrocele ♂
N43.1 Infected hydrocele ♂
Use additional code (B95-B97), to identify infectious agent

N43.2 Other hydrocele ♂
N43.3 Hydrocele, unspecified ♂

☑5ᵗʰ N43.4 Spermatocele of epididymis ♂
Spermatic cyst
N43.40 Spermatocele of epididymis, unspecified ♂
N43.41 Spermatocele of epididymis, single ♂
N43.42 Spermatocele of epididymis, multiple ♂

☑4ᵗʰ N44 Noninflammatory disorders of testis

☑5ᵗʰ N44.0 Torsion of testis
N44.00 Torsion of testis, unspecified ♂
N44.01 Extravaginal torsion of spermatic cord ♂
N44.02 Intravaginal torsion of spermatic cord ♂
Torsion of spermatic cord NOS
N44.03 Torsion of appendix testis ♂
N44.04 Torsion of appendix epididymis ♂

N44.1 Cyst of tunica albuginea testis ♂
N44.2 Benign cyst of testis ♂
N44.8 Other noninflammatory disorders of the testis ♂

☑4ᵗʰ N45 Orchitis and epididymitis
Use additional code (B95-B97), to identify infectious agent

N45.1 Epididymitis ♂
N45.2 Orchitis ♂
N45.3 Epididymo-orchitis ♂
N45.4 Abscess of epididymis or testis ♂

☑4ᵗʰ N46 Male infertility
EXCLUDES 1 vasectomy status (Z98.52)

☑5ᵗʰ N46.0 Azoospermia
Absolute male infertility
Male infertility due to germinal (cell) aplasia
Male infertility due to spermatogenic arrest (complete)
N46.01 Organic azoospermia 🄰♂
Azoospermia NOS

☑6ᵗʰ N46.02 Azoospermia due to extratesticular causes
Code also associated cause
N46.021 Azoospermia due to drug therapy 🄰♂
N46.022 Azoospermia due to infection 🄰♂
N46.023 Azoospermia due to obstruction of efferent ducts 🄰♂
N46.024 Azoospermia due to radiation 🄰♂
N46.025 Azoospermia due to systemic disease 🄰♂
N46.029 Azoospermia due to other extratesticular causes 🄰♂

☑5ᵗʰ N46.1 Oligospermia
Male infertility due to germinal cell desquamation
Male infertility due to hypospermatogenesis
Male infertility due to incomplete spermatogenic arrest
N46.11 Organic oligospermia 🄰♂
Oligospermia NOS

☑6ᵗʰ N46.12 Oligospermia due to extratesticular causes
Code also associated cause
N46.121 Oligospermia due to drug therapy 🄰♂
N46.122 Oligospermia due to infection 🄰♂
N46.123 Oligospermia due to obstruction of efferent ducts 🄰♂
N46.124 Oligospermia due to radiation 🄰♂
N46.125 Oligospermia due to systemic disease 🄰♂
N46.129 Oligospermia due to other extratesticular causes 🄰♂

N46.8 Other male infertility 🄰♂
N46.9 Male infertility, unspecified 🄰♂

☑4ᵗʰ N47 Disorders of prepuce
N47.0 Adherent prepuce, newborn 🄽♂
N47.1 Phimosis ♂
N47.2 Paraphimosis ♂
N47.3 Deficient foreskin ♂
N47.4 Benign cyst of prepuce ♂
N47.5 Adhesions of prepuce and glans penis ♂
N47.6 Balanoposthitis ♂
Use additional code (B95-B97), to identify infectious agent
EXCLUDES 1 balanitis (N48.1)
N47.7 Other inflammatory diseases of prepuce ♂
Use additional code (B95-B97), to identify infectious agent

☑ Additional Character Required   ☑✗ᵗʰ Xtension Alert   Unspecified Dx   Other Specified Dx   Manifestation   ►◄ Revised Text   ● New Code   ▲ Revised Code Title

Diseases of the Genitourinary System

N47.8–N60.12

N47.8 Other disorders of prepuce ♂

✓4th **N48 Other disorders of penis**

N48.0 Leukoplakia of penis ♂
Balanitis xerotica obliterans
Kraurosis of penis
Lichen sclerosus of external male genital organs
EXCLUDES 1   *carcinoma in situ of penis (D07.4)*

N48.1 Balanitis ♂
Use additional code (B95-B97), to identify infectious agent
EXCLUDES 1   *amebic balanitis (A06.8)*
balanitis xerotica obliterans (N48.0)
candidal balanitis (B37.42)
gonococcal balanitis (A54.23)
herpesviral [herpes simplex] balanitis (A60.01)

✓5th **N48.2 Other inflammatory disorders of penis**
Use additional code (B95-B97), to identify infectious agent
EXCLUDES 1   *balanitis (N48.1)*
balanitis xerotica obliterans (N48.0)
balanoposthitis (N47.6)

N48.21 Abscess of corpus cavernosum and penis ♂
N48.22 Cellulitis of corpus cavernosum and penis ♂
N48.29 Other inflammatory disorders of penis ♂

✓5th **N48.3 Priapism**
Painful erection
Code first underlying cause
N48.30 Priapism, unspecified ♂
N48.31 Priapism due to trauma ♂
N48.32 Priapism due to disease classified elsewhere ♂
N48.33 Priapism, drug-induced ♂
N48.39 Other priapism ♂

N48.5 Ulcer of penis ♂

N48.6 Induration penis plastica ♂
Peyronie's disease
Plastic induration of penis

✓5th **N48.8 Other specified disorders of penis**
N48.81 Thrombosis of superficial vein of penis ♂
N48.82 Acquired torsion of penis ♂
Acquired torsion of penis NOS
EXCLUDES 1   *congenital torsion of penis (Q55.63)*
N48.83 Acquired buried penis
EXCLUDES 1   *congenital hidden penis (Q55.64)*
N48.89 Other specified disorders of penis ♂

N48.9 Disorder of penis, unspecified ♂

✓4th **N49 Inflammatory disorders of male genital organs, not elsewhere classified**
Use additional code (B95-B97), to identify infectious agent
EXCLUDES 1   *inflammation of penis (N48.1, N48.2-)*
orchitis and epididymitis (N45.-)

N49.0 Inflammatory disorders of seminal vesicle ♂
Vesiculitis NOS

N49.1 Inflammatory disorders of spermatic cord, tunica vaginalis and vas deferens ♂
Vasitis

N49.2 Inflammatory disorders of scrotum ♂

N49.3 Fournier gangrene ♂

N49.8 Inflammatory disorders of other specified male genital organs ♂
Inflammation of multiple sites in male genital organs

N49.9 Inflammatory disorder of unspecified male genital organ ♂
Abscess of unspecified male genital organ
Boil of unspecified male genital organ
Carbuncle of unspecified male genital organ
Cellulitis of unspecified male genital organ

✓4th **N50 Other and unspecified disorders of male genital organs**
EXCLUDES 2   *torsion of testis (N44.0-)*

N50.0 Atrophy of testis ♂

N50.1 Vascular disorders of male genital organs ♂
Hematocele, NOS, of male genital organs
Hemorrhage of male genital organs
Thrombosis of male genital organs

N50.3 Cyst of epididymis ♂

N50.8 Other specified disorders of male genital organs ♂
Atrophy of scrotum, seminal vesicle, spermatic cord, tunica vaginalis and vas deferens
Chylocele, tunica vaginalis (nonfilarial) NOS
Edema of scrotum, seminal vesicle, spermatic cord, testis, tunica vaginalis and vas deferens
Hypertrophy of scrotum, seminal vesicle, spermatic cord, testis, tunica vaginalis and vas deferens
Stricture of spermatic cord, tunica vaginalis, and vas deferens
Ulcer of scrotum, seminal vesicle, spermatic cord, testis, tunica vaginalis and vas deferens
Urethroscrotal fistula

N50.9 Disorder of male genital organs, unspecified ♂

N51   *Disorders of male genital organs in diseases classified elsewhere* ♂
Code first underlying disease, such as:
filariasis (B74.0-B74.9)
EXCLUDES 1   *amebic balanitis (A06.8)*
candidal balanitis (B37.42)
gonococcal balanitis (A54.23)
gonococcal prostatitis (A54.22)
herpesviral [herpes simplex] balanitis (A60.01)
trichomonal prostatitis (A59.02)
tuberculous prostatitis (A18.14)

✓4th **N52 Male erectile dysfunction**
EXCLUDES 1   *psychogenic impotence (F52.21)*

✓5th **N52.0 Vasculogenic erectile dysfunction**
N52.01 Erectile dysfunction due to arterial insufficiency A ♂
N52.02 Corporo-venous occlusive erectile dysfunction A ♂
N52.03 Combined arterial insufficiency and corporo-venous occlusive erectile dysfunction A ♂

N52.1 Erectile dysfunction due to diseases classified elsewhere A ♂
Code first underlying disease

N52.2 Drug-induced erectile dysfunction A ♂

✓5th **N52.3 Post-surgical erectile dysfunction**
N52.31 Erectile dysfunction following radical prostatectomy A ♂
N52.32 Erectile dysfunction following radical cystectomy A ♂
N52.33 Erectile dysfunction following urethral surgery A ♂
N52.34 Erectile dysfunction following simple prostatectomy A ♂
N52.39 Other post-surgical erectile dysfunction A ♂

N52.8 Other male erectile dysfunction A ♂

N52.9 Male erectile dysfunction, unspecified A ♂
Impotence NOS

✓4th **N53 Other male sexual dysfunction**
EXCLUDES 1   *psychogenic sexual dysfunction (F52.-)*

✓5th **N53.1 Ejaculatory dysfunction**
EXCLUDES 1   *premature ejaculation (F52.4)*
N53.11 Retarded ejaculation ♂
N53.12 Painful ejaculation ♂
N53.13 Anejaculatory orgasm ♂
N53.14 Retrograde ejaculation ♂
N53.19 Other ejaculatory dysfunction ♂
Ejaculatory dysfunction NOS

N53.8 Other male sexual dysfunction ♂

N53.9 Unspecified male sexual dysfunction ♂

Disorders of breast (N60-N65)

EXCLUDES 1   *disorders of breast associated with childbirth (O91-O92)*

✓4th **N60 Benign mammary dysplasia**
INCLUDES   fibrocystic mastopathy

✓5th **N60.0 Solitary cyst of breast**
Cyst of breast
N60.01 Solitary cyst of right breast
N60.02 Solitary cyst of left breast
N60.09 Solitary cyst of unspecified breast

✓5th **N60.1 Diffuse cystic mastopathy**
Cystic breast
Fibrocystic disease of breast
EXCLUDES 1   *diffuse cystic mastopathy with epithelial proliferation (N60.3-)*
N60.11 Diffuse cystic mastopathy of right breast A
N60.12 Diffuse cystic mastopathy of left breast A

EXCLUDES 1 Not coded here   *EXCLUDES 2* Not included here   N Newborn Age: 0   P Pediatric Age: 0-17   M Maternity Age: 12-55   A Adult Age: 15-124

N60.19 **Diffuse cystic mastopathy of unspecified breast** A

✓5th **N60.2 Fibroadenosis of breast**
Adenofibrosis of breast
EXCLUDES 2 *fibroadenoma of breast (D24.-)*

N60.21 **Fibroadenosis of** right **breast**

N60.22 **Fibroadenosis of** left **breast**

N60.29 **Fibroadenosis of unspecified breast**

✓5th **N60.3 Fibrosclerosis of breast**
Cystic mastopathy with epithelial proliferation

N60.31 **Fibrosclerosis of** right **breast**

N60.32 **Fibrosclerosis of** left **breast**

N60.39 **Fibrosclerosis of unspecified breast**

✓5th **N60.4 Mammary duct ectasia**

N60.41 **Mammary duct ectasia of** right **breast**

N60.42 **Mammary duct ectasia of** left **breast**

N60.49 **Mammary duct ectasia of unspecified breast**

✓5th **N60.8 Other benign mammary dysplasias**

N60.81 Other benign mammary dysplasias of right breast

N60.82 Other benign mammary dysplasias of left breast

N60.89 Other benign mammary dysplasias of unspecified breast

✓5th **N60.9 Unspecified benign mammary dysplasia**

N60.91 **Unspecified benign mammary dysplasia of** right **breast**

N60.92 **Unspecified benign mammary dysplasia of** left **breast**

N60.99 **Unspecified benign mammary dysplasia of unspecified breast**

N61 Inflammatory disorders of breast
Abscess (acute) (chronic) (nonpuerperal) of areola
Abscess (acute) (chronic) (nonpuerperal) of breast
Carbuncle of breast
Infective mastitis (acute) (subacute) (nonpuerperal)
Mastitis (acute) (subacute) (nonpuerperal) NOS
EXCLUDES 1 *inflammatory carcinoma of breast (C50.9)*
inflammatory disorder of breast associated with childbirth (O91.-)
neonatal infective mastitis (P39.0)
thrombophlebitis of breast [Mondor's disease] (I80.8)

N62 Hypertrophy of breast
Gynecomastia
Hypertrophy of breast NOS
Massive pubertal hypertrophy of breast
EXCLUDES 1 *breast engorgement of newborn (P83.4)*
disproportion of reconstructed breast (N65.1)

N63 Unspecified lump in breast
Nodule(s) NOS in breast

✓4th **N64 Other disorders of breast**
EXCLUDES 2 *mechanical complication of breast prosthesis and implant (T85.4-)*

N64.0 **Fissure and fistula of nipple**

N64.1 **Fat necrosis of breast**
Fat necrosis (segmental) of breast
Code first breast necrosis due to breast graft (T85.89)

N64.2 **Atrophy of breast**

N64.3 **Galactorrhea not associated with childbirth**

N64.4 **Mastodynia**

✓5th N64.5 **Other signs and symptoms in breast**
EXCLUDES 2 *abnormal findings on diagnostic imaging of breast (R92.-)*

N64.51 **Induration of breast**

N64.52 **Nipple discharge**
EXCLUDES 1 *abnormal findings in nipple discharge (R89.-)*

N64.53 **Retraction of nipple**

N64.59 Other signs and symptoms in breast

✓5th N64.8 **Other specified disorders of breast**

N64.81 **Ptosis of breast** A
EXCLUDES 1 *ptosis of native breast in relation to reconstructed breast (N65.1)*

N64.82 **Hypoplasia of breast** A
Micromastia
EXCLUDES 1 *congenital absence of breast (Q83.0)*
hypoplasia of native breast in relation to reconstructed breast (N65.1)

N64.89 Other specified disorders of breast
Galactocele
Subinvolution of breast (postlactational)

N64.9 **Disorder of breast, unspecified**

✓4th **N65 Deformity and disproportion of reconstructed breast**

N65.0 **Deformity of reconstructed breast** A
Contour irregularity in reconstructed breast
Excess tissue in reconstructed breast
Misshapen reconstructed breast

N65.1 **Disproportion of reconstructed breast** A
Breast asymmetry between native breast and reconstructed breast
Disproportion between native breast and reconstructed breast

Inflammatory diseases of female pelvic organs (N70-N77)

EXCLUDES 1 *inflammatory diseases of female pelvic organs complicating:*
abortion or ectopic or molar pregnancy (O00-O07, O08.0)
pregnancy, childbirth and the puerperium (O23-, O75.3, O85, O86.-)

✓4th **N70 Salpingitis and oophoritis**
INCLUDES abscess (of) fallopian tube
abscess (of) ovary
pyosalpinx
salpingo-oophoritis
tubo-ovarian abscess
tubo-ovarian inflammatory disease
Use additional code (B95-B97), to identify infectious agent
EXCLUDES 1 *gonococcal infection (A54.24)*
tuberculous infection (A18.17)

✓5th N70.0 **Acute salpingitis and oophoritis**

N70.01 **Acute** salpingitis ♀

N70.02 **Acute** oophoritis ♀

N70.03 **Acute** salpingitis and oophoritis ♀

✓5th N70.1 Chronic **salpingitis and oophoritis**
Hydrosalpinx

N70.11 **Chronic** salpingitis ♀

N70.12 **Chronic** oophoritis ♀

N70.13 **Chronic** salpingitis and oophoritis ♀

✓5th N70.9 **Salpingitis and oophoritis,** unspecified

N70.91 Salpingitis, unspecified ♀

N70.92 Oophoritis, unspecified ♀

N70.93 Salpingitis and oophoritis, **unspecified** ♀

✓4th **N71 Inflammatory disease of uterus, except cervix**

Endo (myo) metritis	Pyometra
Metritis	Uterine abscess
Myometritis	

Use additional code (B95-B97), to identify infectious agent
EXCLUDES 1 *hyperplastic endometritis (N85.0-)*
infection of uterus following delivery (O85, O86.-)

N71.0 Acute **inflammatory disease of uterus** ♀

N71.1 Chronic **inflammatory disease of uterus** ♀

N71.9 **Inflammatory disease of uterus, unspecified** ♀

N72 Inflammatory disease of cervix uteri ♀
Cervicitis (with or without erosion or ectropion)
Endocervicitis (with or without erosion or ectropion)
Exocervicitis (with or without erosion or ectropion)
Use additional code (B95-B97), to identify infectious agent
EXCLUDES 1 *erosion and ectropion of cervix without cervicitis (N86)*

✓4th **N73 Other female pelvic inflammatory diseases**
Use additional code (B95-B97), to identify infectious agent

N73.0 Acute **parametritis and pelvic cellulitis** ♀
Abscess of broad ligament
Abscess of parametrium
Pelvic cellulitis, female

N73.1 Chronic **parametritis and pelvic cellulitis** ♀
Any condition in N73.0 specified as chronic
EXCLUDES 1 *tuberculous parametritis and pelvic cellulitis (A18.17)*

N73.2 **Unspecified parametritis and pelvic cellulitis** ♀
Any condition in N73.0 unspecified whether acute or chronic

N73.3 Female acute **pelvic peritonitis** ♀

N73.4 Female chronic **pelvic peritonitis** ♀
EXCLUDES 1 *tuberculous pelvic (female) peritonitis (A18.17)*

N73.5 **Female pelvic peritonitis, unspecified**

N73.6 **Female pelvic** peritoneal adhesions **(postinfective)** ♀
EXCLUDES 2 *postprocedural pelvic peritoneal adhesions (N99.4)*
AHA: 2014, 1Q, 6

✓ Additional Character Required ✓x7th Xtension Alert Unspecified Dx Other Specified Dx Manifestation ►◄ Revised Text ● New Code ▲ Revised Code Title

Diseases of the Genitourinary System

N73.8–N82.3

N73.8   **Other specified female pelvic inflammatory diseases**   ♀

N73.9   **Female pelvic inflammatory disease, unspecified**   ♀
Female pelvic infection or inflammation NOS

N74   *Female pelvic inflammatory disorders in diseases classified elsewhere*   ♀
Code first underlying disease
EXCLUDES 1   *chlamydial cervicitis (A56.02)*
chlamydial pelvic inflammatory disease (A56.11)
gonococcal cervicitis (A54.03)
gonococcal pelvic inflammatory disease (A54.24)
herpesviral [herpes simplex] cervicitis (A60.03)
herpesviral [herpes simplex] pelvic inflammatory disease (A60.09)
syphilitic cervicitis (A52.76)
syphilitic pelvic inflammatory disease (A52.76)
trichomonal cervicitis (A59.09)
tuberculous cervicitis (A18.16)
tuberculous pelvic inflammatory disease (A18.17)

✓4ᵗʰ **N75**   **Diseases of Bartholin's gland**

N75.0   **Cyst of Bartholin's gland**   ♀

N75.1   **Abscess of Bartholin's gland**   ♀

N75.8   **Other diseases of Bartholin's gland**   ♀
Bartholinitis

N75.9   **Disease of Bartholin's gland, unspecified**   ♀

✓4ᵗʰ **N76**   **Other inflammation of vagina and vulva**
Use additional code (B95-B97), to identify infectious agent
EXCLUDES 2   *senile (atrophic) vaginitis (N95.2)*
vulvar vestibulitis (N94.810)

N76.0   **Acute vaginitis**   ♀
Acute vulvovaginitis
Vaginitis NOS
Vulvovaginitis NOS

N76.1   **Subacute and chronic vaginitis**   ♀
Chronic vulvovaginitis
Subacute vulvovaginitis

N76.2   **Acute vulvitis**   ♀
Vulvitis NOS

N76.3   **Subacute and chronic vulvitis**   ♀

N76.4   **Abscess of vulva**   ♀
Furuncle of vulva

N76.5   **Ulceration of vagina**   ♀

N76.6   **Ulceration of vulva**   ♀

✓5ᵗʰ **N76.8**   **Other specified inflammation of vagina and vulva**

N76.81   **Mucositis (ulcerative) of vagina and vulva**   ♀
Code also type of associated therapy, such as:
antineoplastic and immunosuppressive drugs (T45.1X-)
radiological procedure and radiotherapy (Y84.2)
EXCLUDES 2   *gastrointestinal mucositis (ulcerative) (K92.81)*
nasal mucositis (ulcerative) (J34.81)
oral mucositis (ulcerative) (K12.3-)

N76.89   **Other specified inflammation of vagina and vulva**   ♀

✓4ᵗʰ **N77**   **Vulvovaginal ulceration and inflammation in diseases classified elsewhere**

N77.0   *Ulceration of vulva in diseases classified elsewhere*   ♀
Code first underlying disease, such as:
Behçet's disease (M35.2)
EXCLUDES 1   *ulceration of vulva in gonococcal infection (A54.02)*
ulceration of vulva in herpesviral [herpes simplex] infection (A60.04)
ulceration of vulva in syphilis (A51.0)
ulceration of vulva in tuberculosis (A18.18)

N77.1   *Vaginitis, vulvitis and vulvovaginitis in diseases classified elsewhere*   ♀
Code first underlying disease, such as:
pinworm (B80)
EXCLUDES 1   *candidal vulvovaginitis (B37.3)*
chlamydial vulvovaginitis (A56.02)
gonococcal vulvovaginitis (A54.02)
herpesviral [herpes simplex] vulvovaginitis (A60.04)
trichomonal vulvovaginitis (A59.01)
tuberculous vulvovaginitis (A18.18)
vulvovaginitis in early syphilis (A51.0)
vulvovaginitis in late syphilis (A52.76)

Noninflammatory disorders of female genital tract (N80-N98)

✓4ᵗʰ **N80**   **Endometriosis**

N80.0   **Endometriosis of uterus**   ♀
Adenomyosis
EXCLUDES 1   *stromal endometriosis (D39.0)*

N80.1   **Endometriosis of ovary**   ♀

N80.2   **Endometriosis of fallopian tube**   ♀

N80.3   **Endometriosis of pelvic peritoneum**   ♀

N80.4   **Endometriosis of rectovaginal septum and vagina**   ♀

N80.5   **Endometriosis of intestine**   ♀

N80.6   **Endometriosis in cutaneous scar**   ♀

N80.8   **Other endometriosis**   ♀

N80.9   **Endometriosis, unspecified**   ♀

✓4ᵗʰ **N81**   **Female genital prolapse**
EXCLUDES 1   *genital prolapse complicating pregnancy, labor or delivery (O34.5-)*
prolapse and hernia of ovary and fallopian tube (N83.4)
prolapse of vaginal vault after hysterectomy (N99.3)

N81.0   **Urethrocele**   ♀
EXCLUDES 1   *urethrocele with cystocele (N81.1-)*
urethrocele with prolapse of uterus (N81.2-N81.4)

✓5ᵗʰ **N81.1**   **Cystocele**
Cystocele with urethrocele
Cystourethrocele
EXCLUDES 1   *cystocele with prolapse of uterus (N81.2-N81.4)*

N81.10   **Cystocele, unspecified**   ♀
Prolapse of (anterior) vaginal wall NOS

N81.11   **Cystocele, midline**   ♀

N81.12   **Cystocele, lateral**   ♀
Paravaginal cystocele

N81.2   **Incomplete uterovaginal prolapse**   ♀
First degree uterine prolapse
Prolapse of cervix NOS
Second degree uterine prolapse
EXCLUDES 1   *cervical stump prolapse (N81.85)*

N81.3   **Complete uterovaginal prolapse**   ♀
Procidentia (uteri) NOS
Third degree uterine prolapse

N81.4   **Uterovaginal prolapse, unspecified**   ♀
Prolapse of uterus NOS

N81.5   **Vaginal enterocele**   ♀
EXCLUDES 1   *enterocele with prolapse of uterus (N81.2-N81.4)*

N81.6   **Rectocele**   ♀
Prolapse of posterior vaginal wall
Use additional code for any associated fecal incontinence, if applicable (R15.-)
EXCLUDES 2   *perineocele (N81.81)*
rectal prolapse (K62.3)
rectocele with prolapse of uterus (N81.2-N81.4)

✓5ᵗʰ **N81.8**   **Other female genital prolapse**

N81.81   **Perineocele**   ♀

N81.82   **Incompetence or weakening of pubocervical tissue**   ♀

N81.83   **Incompetence or weakening of rectovaginal tissue**   ♀

N81.84   **Pelvic muscle wasting**   ♀
Disuse atrophy of pelvic muscles and anal sphincter

N81.85   **Cervical stump prolapse**   ♀

N81.89   **Other female genital prolapse**   ♀
Deficient perineum
Old laceration of muscles of pelvic floor

N81.9   **Female genital prolapse, unspecified**   ♀

✓4ᵗʰ **N82**   **Fistulae involving female genital tract**
EXCLUDES 1   *vesicointestinal fistulae (N32.1)*

N82.0   **Vesicovaginal fistula**   ♀

N82.1   **Other female urinary-genital tract fistulae**   ♀
Cervicovesical fistula
Ureterovaginal fistula
Urethrovaginal fistula
Uteroureteric fistula
Uterovesical fistula

N82.2   **Fistula of vagina to small intestine**   ♀

N82.3   **Fistula of vagina to large intestine**   ♀
Rectovaginal fistula

EXCLUDES 1 Not coded here   EXCLUDES 2 Not included here   N Newborn Age: 0   P Pediatric Age: 0-17   M Maternity Age: 12-55   A Adult Age: 15-124

730   ICD-10-CM Draft (2015)

N82.4 **Other female intestinal-genital tract fistulae** ♀
    Intestinouterine fistula

N82.5 **Female** genital tract-skin **fistulae** ♀
    Uterus to abdominal wall fistula
    Vaginoperineal fistula

N82.8 **Other female genital tract fistulae** ♀

N82.9 **Female genital tract fistula, unspecified** ♀

✓4th **N83** **Noninflammatory disorders of ovary, fallopian tube and broad ligament**
    EXCLUDES 2 *hydrosalpinx (N70.1-)*

N83.0 **Follicular cyst of ovary** ♀
    Cyst of graafian follicle
    Hemorrhagic follicular cyst (of ovary)

N83.1 **Corpus luteum cyst** ♀
    Hemorrhagic corpus luteum cyst

✓5th **N83.2** **Other and unspecified ovarian cysts**
    EXCLUDES 1 *developmental ovarian cyst (Q50.1)*
        neoplastic ovarian cyst (D27.-)
        polycystic ovarian syndrome (E28.2)
        Stein-Leventhal syndrome (E28.2)

    N83.20 **Unspecified ovarian cysts** ♀

    N83.29 **Other ovarian cysts** ♀
        Retention cyst of ovary
        Simple cyst of ovary

✓5th **N83.3** **Acquired atrophy of ovary and fallopian tube**
    N83.31 **Acquired atrophy of** ovary ♀
    N83.32 **Acquired atrophy of** fallopian tube ♀
    N83.33 **Acquired atrophy of** ovary and fallopian tube ♀

N83.4 **Prolapse and hernia of ovary and fallopian tube** ♀

✓5th **N83.5** **Torsion of ovary, ovarian pedicle and fallopian tube**
    Torsion of accessory tube

    N83.51 **Torsion of** ovary and ovarian pedicle ♀

    N83.52 **Torsion of** fallopian tube ♀
        Torsion of hydatid of Morgagni

    N83.53 **Torsion of** ovary, ovarian pedicle and fallopian tube ♀

N83.6 **Hematosalpinx** ♀
    EXCLUDES 1 *hematosalpinx (with) (in):*
        hematocolpos (N89.7)
        hematometra (N85.7)
        tubal pregnancy (O00.1)

N83.7 **Hematoma of broad ligament** ♀

N83.8 **Other noninflammatory disorders of ovary, fallopian tube and broad ligament** ♀
    Broad ligament laceration syndrome [Allen-Masters]

N83.9 **Noninflammatory disorder of ovary, fallopian tube and broad ligament, unspecified** ♀

✓4th **N84** **Polyp of female genital tract**
    EXCLUDES 1 *adenomatous polyp (D28.-)*
        placental polyp (O90.89)

N84.0 **Polyp of** corpus uteri ♀
    Polyp of endometrium
    Polyp of uterus NOS
    EXCLUDES 1 *polypoid endometrial hyperplasia (N85.0-)*

N84.1 **Polyp of** cervix uteri ♀
    Mucous polyp of cervix

N84.2 **Polyp of** vagina ♀

N84.3 **Polyp of** vulva ♀
    Polyp of labia

N84.8 **Polyp of other parts of female genital tract** ♀

N84.9 **Polyp of female genital tract, unspecified** ♀

✓4th **N85** **Other noninflammatory disorders of uterus, except cervix**
    EXCLUDES 1 *endometriosis (N80.-)*
        inflammatory diseases of uterus (N71.-)
        noninflammatory disorders of cervix, except malposition (N86-N88)
        polyp of corpus uteri (N84.0)
        uterine prolapse (N81.-)

✓5th **N85.0** **Endometrial hyperplasia**

    N85.00 **Endometrial hyperplasia, unspecified** ♀
        Hyperplasia (adenomatous) (cystic) (glandular) of endometrium
        Hyperplastic endometritis

    N85.01 Benign **endometrial hyperplasia** ♀
        Endometrial hyperplasia (complex) (simple) without atypia

    N85.02 Endometrial intraepithelial neoplasia [EIN] ♀
        Endometrial hyperplasia with atypia
        EXCLUDES 1 *malignant neoplasm of endometrium (with endometrial intraepithelial neoplasia [EIN]) (C54.1)*

N85.2 **Hypertrophy of uterus** ♀
    Bulky or enlarged uterus
    EXCLUDES 1 *puerperal hypertrophy of uterus (O90.89)*

N85.3 **Subinvolution of uterus** ♀
    EXCLUDES 1 *puerperal subinvolution of uterus (O90.89)*

N85.4 **Malposition of uterus** ♀
    Anteversion of uterus   Retroversion of uterus
    Retroflexion of uterus
    EXCLUDES 1 *malposition of uterus complicating pregnancy, labor or delivery (O34.5-, O65.5)*

N85.5 **Inversion of uterus** ♀
    EXCLUDES 1 *current obstetric trauma (O71.2)*
        postpartum inversion of uterus (O71.2)

N85.6 **Intrauterine synechiae** ♀

N85.7 **Hematometra** ♀
    Hematosalpinx with hematometra
    EXCLUDES 1 *hematometra with hematocolpos (N89.7)*

N85.8 **Other specified noninflammatory disorders of uterus** ♀
    Atrophy of uterus, acquired
    Fibrosis of uterus NOS

N85.9 **Noninflammatory disorder of uterus, unspecified** ♀
    Disorder of uterus NOS

N86 **Erosion and ectropion of cervix uteri** ♀
    Decubitus (trophic) ulcer of cervix
    Eversion of cervix
    EXCLUDES 1 *erosion and ectropion of cervix with cervicitis (N72)*

✓4th **N87** **Dysplasia of cervix uteri**
    EXCLUDES 1 *abnormal results from cervical cytologic examination without histologic confirmation (R87.61-)*
        carcinoma in situ of cervix uteri (D06.-)
        cervical intraepithelial neoplasia III [CIN III] (D06.-)
        HGSIL of cervix (R87.613)
        severe dysplasia of cervix uteri (D06.-)

N87.0 Mild **cervical dysplasia** ♀
    Cervical intraepithelial neoplasia I [CIN I]

N87.1 Moderate **cervical dysplasia** ♀
    Cervical intraepithelial neoplasia II [CIN II]

N87.9 **Dysplasia of cervix uteri, unspecified** ♀
    Anaplasia of cervix   Cervical dysplasia NOS
    Cervical atypism

✓4th **N88** **Other noninflammatory disorders of cervix uteri**
    EXCLUDES 2 *inflammatory disease of cervix (N72)*
        polyp of cervix (N84.1)

N88.0 **Leukoplakia of cervix uteri** ♀

N88.1 **Old laceration of cervix uteri** ♀
    Adhesions of cervix
    EXCLUDES 1 *current obstetric trauma (O71.3)*

N88.2 **Stricture and stenosis of cervix uteri** ♀
    EXCLUDES 1 *stricture and stenosis of cervix uteri complicating labor (O65.5)*

N88.3 **Incompetence of cervix uteri** ♀
    Investigation and management of (suspected) cervical incompetence in a nonpregnant woman
    EXCLUDES 1 *cervical incompetence complicating pregnancy (O34.3-)*

N88.4 **Hypertrophic elongation of cervix uteri** ♀

N88.8 **Other specified noninflammatory disorders of cervix uteri** ♀
    EXCLUDES 1 *current obstetric trauma (O71.3)*

N88.9 **Noninflammatory disorder of cervix uteri, unspecified** ♀

✓4th **N89** **Other noninflammatory disorders of vagina**
    EXCLUDES 1 *abnormal results from vaginal cytologic examination without histologic confirmation (R87.62-)*
        carcinoma in situ of vagina (D07.2)
        HGSIL of vagina (R87.623)
        inflammation of vagina (N76.-)
        senile (atrophic) vaginitis (N95.2)
        severe dysplasia of vagina (D07.2)
        trichomonal leukorrhea (A59.00)
        vaginal intraepithelial neoplasia [VAIN], grade III (D07.2)

N89.0 Mild **vaginal dysplasia** ♀
    Vaginal intraepithelial neoplasia [VAIN], grade I

☑ Additional Character Required   √x7th Xtension Alert   Unspecified Dx   Other Specified Dx   Manifestation   ►◄ Revised Text   ● New Code   ▲ Revised Code Title

Diseases of the Genitourinary System

N89.1–N95.0

N89.1 Moderate vaginal dysplasia ♀
Vaginal intraepithelial neoplasia [VAIN], grade II

N89.3 Dysplasia of vagina, unspecified ♀

N89.4 Leukoplakia of vagina ♀

N89.5 Stricture and atresia of vagina ♀
Vaginal adhesions
Vaginal stenosis
  EXCLUDES 1   *congenital atresia or stricture (Q52.4)*
  postprocedural adhesions of vagina (N99.2)

N89.6 Tight hymenal ring ♀
Rigid hymen
Tight introitus
  EXCLUDES 1   *imperforate hymen (Q52.3)*

N89.7 Hematocolpos ♀
Hematocolpos with hematometra or hematosalpinx

N89.8 Other specified noninflammatory disorders of vagina ♀
Leukorrhea NOS
Old vaginal laceration
Pessary ulcer of vagina
  EXCLUDES 1   *current obstetric trauma (O70-, O71.4, O71.7-O71.8)*
  old laceration involving muscles of pelvic floor (N81.8)

N89.9 Noninflammatory disorder of vagina, unspecified ♀

√4ᵗʰ N90 Other noninflammatory disorders of vulva and perineum
  EXCLUDES 1   *anogenital (venereal) warts (A63.0)*
  carcinoma in situ of vulva (D07.1)
  condyloma acuminatum (A63.0)
  current obstetric trauma (O70-, O71.7-O71.8)
  inflammation of vulva (N76.-)
  severe dysplasia of vulva (D07.1)
  vulvar intraepithelial neoplasm III [VIN III] (D07.1)

N90.0 Mild vulvar dysplasia ♀
Vulvar intraepithelial neoplasia [VIN], grade I

N90.1 Moderate vulvar dysplasia ♀
Vulvar intraepithelial neoplasia [VIN], grade II

N90.3 Dysplasia of vulva, unspecified ♀

N90.4 Leukoplakia of vulva ♀
Dystrophy of vulva
Kraurosis of vulva
Lichen sclerosus of external female genital organs

N90.5 Atrophy of vulva ♀
Stenosis of vulva

N90.6 Hypertrophy of vulva ♀
Hypertrophy of labia

N90.7 Vulvar cyst ♀

√5ᵗʰ N90.8 Other specified noninflammatory disorders of vulva and perineum
  √6ᵗʰ N90.81 Female genital mutilation status
  Female genital cutting status
    N90.810 Female genital mutilation status, unspecified ♀
    Female genital cutting status, unspecified
    Female genital mutilation status NOS
    N90.811 Female genital mutilation Type I status ♀
    Clitorectomy status
    Female genital cutting Type I status
    N90.812 Female genital mutilation Type II status ♀
    Clitorectomy with excision of labia minora status
    Female genital cutting Type II status
    N90.813 Female genital mutilation Type III status ♀
    Female genital cutting Type III status
    Infibulation status
    N90.818 Other female genital mutilation status ♀
    Female genital cutting Type IV status
    Female genital mutilation Type IV status
    Other female genital cutting status
  N90.89 Other specified noninflammatory disorders of vulva and perineum ♀
  Adhesions of vulva   Hypertrophy of clitoris

N90.9 Noninflammatory disorder of vulva and perineum, unspecified ♀

√4ᵗʰ N91 Absent, scanty and rare menstruation
  EXCLUDES 1   *ovarian dysfunction (E28.-)*

N91.0 Primary amenorrhea ♀

N91.1 Secondary amenorrhea ♀

N91.2 Amenorrhea, unspecified ♀

N91.3 Primary oligomenorrhea ♀

N91.4 Secondary oligomenorrhea ♀

N91.5 Oligomenorrhea, unspecified ♀
Hypomenorrhea NOS

√4ᵗʰ N92 Excessive, frequent and irregular menstruation
  EXCLUDES 1   *postmenopausal bleeding (N95.0)*
  precocious puberty (menstruation) (E30.1)

N92.0 Excessive and frequent menstruation with regular cycle ♀
Heavy periods NOS
Menorrhagia NOS
Polymenorrhea

N92.1 Excessive and frequent menstruation with irregular cycle ♀
Irregular intermenstrual bleeding
Irregular, shortened intervals between menstrual bleeding
Menometrorrhagia
Metrorrhagia

N92.2 Excessive menstruation at puberty P♀
Excessive bleeding associated with onset of menstrual periods
Pubertal menorrhagia
Puberty bleeding

N92.3 Ovulation bleeding ♀
Regular intermenstrual bleeding

N92.4 Excessive bleeding in the premenopausal period ♀
Climacteric menorrhagia or metrorrhagia
Menopausal menorrhagia or metrorrhagia
Preclimacteric menorrhagia or metrorrhagia
Premenopausal menorrhagia or metrorrhagia

N92.5 Other specified irregular menstruation ♀

N92.6 Irregular menstruation, unspecified ♀
Irregular bleeding NOS
Irregular periods NOS
  EXCLUDES 1   *irregular menstruation with:*
  lengthened intervals or scanty bleeding (N91.3-N91.5)
  shortened intervals or excessive bleeding (N92.1)

√4ᵗʰ N93 Other abnormal uterine and vaginal bleeding
  EXCLUDES 1   *neonatal vaginal hemorrhage (P54.6)*
  precocious puberty (menstruation) (E30.1)
  pseudomenses (P54.6)

N93.0 Postcoital and contact bleeding ♀

N93.8 Other specified abnormal uterine and vaginal bleeding ♀
Dysfunctional or functional uterine or vaginal bleeding NOS

N93.9 Abnormal uterine and vaginal bleeding, unspecified ♀

√4ᵗʰ N94 Pain and other conditions associated with female genital organs and menstrual cycle

N94.0 Mittelschmerz ♀

N94.1 Dyspareunia ♀
  EXCLUDES 1   *psychogenic dyspareunia (F52.6)*

N94.2 Vaginismus ♀
  EXCLUDES 1   *psychogenic vaginismus (F52.5)*

N94.3 Premenstrual tension syndrome ♀
Premenstrual dysphoric disorder
Code also associated menstrual migraine (G43.82-, G43.83-)

N94.4 Primary dysmenorrhea ♀

N94.5 Secondary dysmenorrhea ♀

N94.6 Dysmenorrhea, unspecified ♀
  EXCLUDES 1   *psychogenic dysmenorrhea (F45.8)*

√5ᵗʰ N94.8 Other specified conditions associated with female genital organs and menstrual cycle
  √6ᵗʰ N94.81 Vulvodynia
    N94.810 Vulvar vestibulitis ♀
    N94.818 Other vulvodynia ♀
    N94.819 Vulvodynia, unspecified ♀
    Vulvodynia NOS
  N94.89 Other specified conditions associated with female genital organs and menstrual cycle ♀

N94.9 Unspecified condition associated with female genital organs and menstrual cycle ♀

√4ᵗʰ N95 Menopausal and other perimenopausal disorders
Menopausal and other perimenopausal disorders due to naturally occurring (age-related) menopause and perimenopause
  EXCLUDES 1   *excessive bleeding in the premenopausal period (N92.4)*
  menopausal and perimenopausal disorders due to artificial or premature menopause (E89.4-, E28.31-)
  premature menopause (E28.31-)
  EXCLUDES 2   *postmenopausal osteoporosis (M81.0-)*
  postmenopausal osteoporosis with current pathological fracture (M80.0-)
  postmenopausal urethritis (N34.2)

N95.0 Postmenopausal bleeding ♀

EXCLUDES 1 Not coded here   *EXCLUDES 2* Not included here   N Newborn Age: 0   P Pediatric Age: 0-17   M Maternity Age: 12-55   A Adult Age: 15-124

N95.1 Menopausal and female climacteric states ♀
Symptoms such as flushing, sleeplessness, headache, lack of concentration, associated with natural (age-related) menopause
Use additional code for associated symptoms
EXCLUDES 1 asymptomatic menopausal state (Z78.0)
symptoms associated with artificial menopause (E89.41)
symptoms associated with premature menopause (E28.310)

N95.2 Postmenopausal atrophic vaginitis ♀
Senile (atrophic) vaginitis

N95.8 Other specified menopausal and perimenopausal disorders ♀

N95.9 Unspecified menopausal and perimenopausal disorder ♀

N96 Recurrent pregnancy loss ♀
Investigation or care in a nonpregnant woman with history of recurrent pregnancy loss
EXCLUDES 1 recurrent pregnancy loss with current pregnancy (O26.2-)

☑4ᵗʰ N97 Female infertility
INCLUDES inability to achieve a pregnancy
sterility, female NOS
EXCLUDES 1 female infertility associated with:
hypopituitarism (E23.0)
Stein-Leventhal syndrome (E28.2)
EXCLUDES 2 incompetence of cervix uteri (N88.3)

N97.0 Female infertility associated with anovulation ♀

N97.1 Female infertility of tubal origin ♀
Female infertility associated with congenital anomaly of tube
Female infertility due to tubal block
Female infertility due to tubal occlusion
Female infertility due to tubal stenosis

N97.2 Female infertility of uterine origin ♀
Female infertility associated with congenital anomaly of uterus
Female infertility due to nonimplantation of ovum

N97.8 Female infertility of other origin ♀

N97.9 Female infertility, unspecified ♀

☑4ᵗʰ N98 Complications associated with artificial fertilization

N98.0 Infection associated with artificial insemination ♀

N98.1 Hyperstimulation of ovaries ♀
Hyperstimulation of ovaries NOS
Hyperstimulation of ovaries associated with induced ovulation

N98.2 Complications of attempted introduction of fertilized ovum following in vitro fertilization ♀

N98.3 Complications of attempted introduction of embryo in embryo transfer ♀

N98.8 Other complications associated with artificial fertilization ♀

N98.9 Complication associated with artificial fertilization, unspecified ♀

Intraoperative and postprocedural complications and disorders of genitourinary system, not elsewhere classified (N99)

☑4ᵗʰ N99 Intraoperative and postprocedural complications and disorders of genitourinary system, not elsewhere classified
EXCLUDES 2 irradiation cystitis (N30.4-)
postoophorectomy osteoporosis with current pathological fracture (M80.8-)
postoophorectomy osteoporosis without current pathological fracture (M81.8)

N99.0 Postprocedural (acute) (chronic) kidney failure
Use additional code to type of kidney disease

☑5ᵗʰ N99.1 Postprocedural urethral stricture
Postcatheterization urethral stricture

  ☑6ᵗʰ N99.11 Postprocedural urethral stricture, male

    N99.110 Postprocedural urethral stricture, male, ♂ meatal

    N99.111 Postprocedural bulbous **urethral stricture**

    N99.112 Postprocedural membranous **urethral stricture**

    N99.113 Postprocedural anterior **urethral stricture**

    N99.114 Postprocedural urethral stricture, male unspecified ♂

  N99.12 Postprocedural urethral stricture, female ♀

N99.2 Postprocedural adhesions of vagina ♀

N99.3 Prolapse of vaginal vault after hysterectomy ♀

N99.4 Postprocedural pelvic peritoneal adhesions
EXCLUDES 2 pelvic peritoneal adhesions NOS (N73.6)
postinfective pelvic peritoneal adhesions (N73.6)

☑5ᵗʰ N99.5 Complications of stoma of urinary tract
EXCLUDES 2 mechanical complication of urinary (indwelling) catheter (T83.0-)

  ☑6ᵗʰ N99.51 Complication of cystostomy

    N99.510 Cystostomy hemorrhage

    N99.511 Cystostomy infection

    N99.512 Cystostomy malfunction

    N99.518 Other cystostomy complication

  ☑6ᵗʰ N99.52 Complication of other external stoma of urinary tract

    N99.520 Hemorrhage of other external stoma of urinary tract

    N99.521 Infection of other external stoma of urinary tract

    N99.522 Malfunction of other external stoma of urinary tract

    N99.528 Other complication of other external stoma of urinary tract

  ☑6ᵗʰ N99.53 Complication of other stoma of urinary tract

    N99.530 Hemorrhage of other stoma of urinary tract

    N99.531 Infection of other stoma of urinary tract

    N99.532 Malfunction of other stoma of urinary tract

    N99.538 Other complication of other stoma of urinary tract

☑5ᵗʰ N99.6 Intraoperative hemorrhage and hematoma of a genitourinary system organ or structure complicating a procedure
EXCLUDES 1 intraoperative hemorrhage and hematoma of a genitourinary system organ or structure due to accidental puncture or laceration during a procedure (N99.7-)

  N99.61 Intraoperative hemorrhage and hematoma of a genitourinary system organ or structure complicating a genitourinary system procedure

  N99.62 Intraoperative hemorrhage and hematoma of a genitourinary system organ or structure complicating other procedure

☑5ᵗʰ N99.7 Accidental puncture and laceration of a genitourinary system organ or structure during a procedure

  N99.71 Accidental puncture and laceration of a genitourinary system organ or structure during a genitourinary system procedure

  N99.72 Accidental puncture and laceration of a genitourinary system organ or structure during other procedure

☑5ᵗʰ N99.8 Other intraoperative and postprocedural complications and disorders of genitourinary system

  N99.81 Other intraoperative complications of genitourinary system

  ☑6ᵗʰ N99.82 Postprocedural hemorrhage and hematoma of a genitourinary system organ or structure following a procedure

    N99.820 Postprocedural hemorrhage and hematoma of a genitourinary system organ or structure following a genitourinary system procedure

    N99.821 Postprocedural hemorrhage and hematoma of a genitourinary system organ or structure following other procedure

  N99.83 Residual ovary syndrome ♀

  N99.89 Other postprocedural complications and disorders of genitourinary system

---

☑ Additional Character Required   ☑x7ᵗʰ Xtension Alert   Unspecified Dx   Other Specified Dx   Manifestation   ►◄ Revised Text   ● New Code   ▲ Revised Code Title

Chapter 15. Pregnancy, Childbirth and the Puerperium (O00-O9A)

NOTE CODES FROM THIS CHAPTER ARE FOR USE ONLY ON MATERNAL RECORDS, NEVER ON NEWBORN RECORDS.

Codes from this chapter are for use for conditions related to or aggravated by the pregnancy, childbirth, or by the puerperium (maternal causes or obstetric causes).

NOTE Trimesters are counted from the first day of the last menstrual period. They are defined as follows:

1st trimester- less than 14 weeks 0 days
2nd trimester- 14 weeks 0 days to less than 28 weeks 0 days
3rd trimester- 28 weeks 0 days until delivery.

Use additional code from category Z3A, Weeks of gestation, to identify the specific week of the pregnancy

EXCLUDES 1 *supervision of normal pregnancy (Z34.-)*
EXCLUDES 2 *mental and behavioral disorders associated with the puerperium (F53)*
obstetrical tetanus (A34)
postpartum necrosis of pituitary gland (E23.0)
puerperal osteomalacia (M83.0)

This chapter contains the following blocks:

O00-O08	Pregnancy with abortive outcome
O09	Supervision of high risk pregnancy
O10-O16	Edema, proteinuria and hypertensive disorders in pregnancy, childbirth and the puerperium
O20-O29	Other maternal disorders predominantly related to pregnancy
O30-O48	Maternal care related to the fetus and amniotic cavity and possible delivery problems
O60-O77	Complications of labor and delivery
O80, O82	Encounter for delivery
O85-O92	Complications predominantly related to the puerperium
O94-O9A	Other obstetric conditions, not elsewhere classified

Pregnancy with abortive outcome (O00-O08)

EXCLUDES 1 *continuing pregnancy in multiple gestation after abortion of one fetus or more (O31.1-, O31.3-)*

✓4ᵗʰ O00 Ectopic pregnancy
INCLUDES ruptured ectopic pregnancy
Use additional code from category O08 to identify any associated complication

O00.0 Abdominal pregnancy Ⓜ♀
EXCLUDES 1 *maternal care for viable fetus in abdominal pregnancy (O36.7-)*

O00.1 Tubal pregnancy Ⓜ♀
Fallopian pregnancy
Rupture of (fallopian) tube due to pregnancy
Tubal abortion

O00.2 Ovarian pregnancy Ⓜ♀

O00.8 Other ectopic pregnancy Ⓜ♀
Cervical pregnancy
Cornual pregnancy
Intraligamentous pregnancy
Mural pregnancy

O00.9 Ectopic pregnancy, unspecified Ⓜ♀

✓4ᵗʰ O01 Hydatidiform mole
Use additional code from category O08 to identify any associated complication
EXCLUDES 1 *chorioadenoma (destruens) (D39.2)*
malignant hydatidiform mole (D39.2)

O01.0 Classical hydatidiform mole Ⓜ♀
Complete hydatidiform mole

O01.1 Incomplete and partial hydatidiform mole Ⓜ♀

O01.9 Hydatidiform mole, unspecified Ⓜ♀
Trophoblastic disease NOS
Vesicular mole NOS

✓4ᵗʰ O02 Other abnormal products of conception
Use additional code from category O08 to identify any associated complication
EXCLUDES 1 *papyraceous fetus (O31.0-)*

O02.0 Blighted ovum and nonhydatidiform mole Ⓜ♀
Carneous mole
Fleshy mole
Intrauterine mole NOS
Molar pregnancy NEC
Pathological ovum

O02.1 Missed abortion Ⓜ♀
Early fetal death, before completion of 20 weeks of gestation, with retention of dead fetus
EXCLUDES 1 *failed induced abortion (O07.-)*
fetal death (intrauterine) (late) (O36.4)
missed abortion with blighted ovum (O02.0)
missed abortion with hydatidiform mole (O01.-)
missed abortion with nonhydatidiform (O02.0)
missed abortion with other abnormal products of conception (O02.8-)
missed delivery (O36.4)
stillbirth (P95)

✓5ᵗʰ O02.8 Other specified abnormal products of conception
EXCLUDES 1 *abnormal products of conception with blighted ovum (O02.0)*
abnormal products of conception with hydatidiform mole (O01.-)
abnormal products of conception with nonhydatidiform mole (O02.0)

O02.81 Inappropriate change in quantitative human chorionic gonadotropin (hCG) in early pregnancy Ⓜ♀
Biochemical pregnancy
Chemical pregnancy
Inappropriate level of quantitative human chorionic gonadotropin (hCG) for gestational age in early pregnancy

O02.89 Other abnormal products of conception Ⓜ♀

O02.9 Abnormal product of conception, unspecified Ⓜ♀

✓4ᵗʰ O03 Spontaneous abortion
NOTE Incomplete abortion includes retained products of conception following spontaneous abortion
INCLUDES miscarriage

O03.0 Genital tract and pelvic infection following incomplete spontaneous abortion Ⓜ♀
Endometritis following incomplete spontaneous abortion
Oophoritis following incomplete spontaneous abortion
Parametritis following incomplete spontaneous abortion
Pelvic peritonitis following incomplete spontaneous abortion
Salpingitis following incomplete spontaneous abortion
Salpingo-oophoritis following incomplete spontaneous abortion
EXCLUDES 1 *sepsis following incomplete spontaneous abortion (O03.37)*
urinary tract infection following incomplete spontaneous abortion (O03.38)

O03.1 Delayed or excessive hemorrhage following incomplete spontaneous abortion Ⓜ♀
Afibrinogenemia following incomplete spontaneous abortion
Defibrination syndrome following incomplete spontaneous abortion
Hemolysis following incomplete spontaneous abortion
Intravascular coagulation following incomplete spontaneous abortion

O03.2 Embolism following incomplete spontaneous abortion Ⓜ♀
Air embolism following incomplete spontaneous abortion
Amniotic fluid embolism following incomplete spontaneous abortion
Blood-clot embolism following incomplete spontaneous abortion
Embolism NOS following incomplete spontaneous abortion
Fat embolism following incomplete spontaneous abortion
Pulmonary embolism following incomplete spontaneous abortion
Pyemic embolism following incomplete spontaneous abortion
Septic or septicopyemic embolism following incomplete spontaneous abortion
Soap embolism following incomplete spontaneous abortion

✓5ᵗʰ O03.3 Other and unspecified complications following incomplete spontaneous abortion

O03.30 Unspecified complication following incomplete spontaneous abortion Ⓜ♀

O03.31 Shock following incomplete spontaneous abortion Ⓜ♀
Circulatory collapse following incomplete spontaneous abortion
Shock (postprocedural) following incomplete spontaneous abortion
EXCLUDES 1 *shock due to infection following incomplete spontaneous abortion (O03.37)*

EXCLUDES 1 Not coded here   **EXCLUDES 2** Not included here   Ⓝ Newborn Age: 0   Ⓟ Pediatric Age: 0-17   Ⓜ Maternity Age: 12-55   Ⓐ Adult Age: 15-124

734   ICD-10-CM Draft (2015)

O03.32 Renal failure following incomplete spontaneous abortion   Ⓜ♀

    Kidney failure (acute) following incomplete spontaneous abortion
    Oliguria following incomplete spontaneous abortion
    Renal shutdown following incomplete spontaneous abortion
    Renal tubular necrosis following incomplete spontaneous abortion
    Uremia following incomplete spontaneous abortion

O03.33 Metabolic disorder following incomplete spontaneous abortion   Ⓜ♀

O03.34 Damage to pelvic organs following incomplete spontaneous abortion   Ⓜ♀

    Laceration, perforation, tear or chemical damage of bladder following incomplete spontaneous abortion
    Laceration, perforation, tear or chemical damage of bowel following incomplete spontaneous abortion
    Laceration, perforation, tear or chemical damage of broad ligament following incomplete spontaneous abortion
    Laceration, perforation, tear or chemical damage of cervix following incomplete spontaneous abortion
    Laceration, perforation, tear or chemical damage of periurethral tissue following incomplete spontaneous abortion
    Laceration, perforation, tear or chemical damage of uterus following incomplete spontaneous abortion
    Laceration, perforation, tear or chemical damage of vagina following incomplete spontaneous abortion

O03.35 Other venous complications following incomplete spontaneous abortion   Ⓜ♀

O03.36 Cardiac arrest following incomplete spontaneousabortion   Ⓜ♀

O03.37 Sepsis following incomplete spontaneous abortion   Ⓜ♀

    Use additional code to identify infectious agent (B95-B97)
    Use additional code to identify severe sepsis, if applicable (R65.2-)

    EXCLUDES 1 *septic or septicopyemic embolism following incomplete spontaneous abortion (O03.2)*

O03.38 Urinary tract infection following incomplete spontaneous abortion   Ⓜ♀

    Cystitis following incomplete spontaneous abortion

O03.39 Incomplete spontaneous abortion with other complications   Ⓜ♀

O03.4 Incomplete spontaneous abortion without complication   Ⓜ♀

O03.5 Genital tract and pelvic infection following complete or unspecified spontaneous abortion   Ⓜ♀

    Endometritis following complete or unspecified spontaneous abortion
    Oophoritis following complete or unspecified spontaneous abortion
    Parametritis following complete or unspecified spontaneous abortion
    Pelvic peritonitis following complete or unspecified spontaneous abortion
    Salpingitis following complete or unspecified spontaneous abortion
    Salpingo-oophoritis following complete or unspecified spontaneous abortion

    EXCLUDES 1 *sepsis following complete or unspecified spontaneous abortion (O03.87)*
    urinary tract infection following complete or unspecified spontaneous abortion (O03.88)

O03.6 Delayed or excessive hemorrhage following complete or unspecified spontaneous abortion   Ⓜ♀

    Afibrinogenemia following complete or unspecified spontaneous abortion
    Defibrination syndrome following complete or unspecified spontaneous abortion
    Hemolysis following complete or unspecified spontaneous abortion
    Intravascular coagulation following complete or unspecified spontaneous abortion

O03.7 Embolism following complete or unspecified spontaneous abortion   Ⓜ♀

    Air embolism following complete or unspecified spontaneous abortion
    Amniotic fluid embolism following complete or unspecified spontaneous abortion
    Blood-clot embolism following complete or unspecified spontaneous abortion
    Embolism NOS following complete or unspecified spontaneous abortion
    Fat embolism following complete or unspecified spontaneous abortion
    Pulmonary embolism following complete or unspecified spontaneous abortion
    Pyemic embolism following complete or unspecified spontaneous abortion
    Septic or septicopyemic embolism following complete or unspecified spontaneous abortion
    Soap embolism following complete or unspecified spontaneous abortion

✓5ᵗʰ **O03.8** Other and unspecified complications following complete or unspecified spontaneous abortion

O03.80 Unspecified complication following complete or unspecified spontaneous abortion   Ⓜ♀

O03.81 Shock following complete or unspecified spontaneous abortion   Ⓜ♀

    Circulatory collapse following complete or unspecified spontaneous abortion
    Shock (postprocedural) following complete or unspecified spontaneous abortion

    EXCLUDES 1 *shock due to infection following complete or unspecified spontaneous abortion (O03.87)*

O03.82 Renal failure following complete or unspecified spontaneous abortion   Ⓜ♀

    Kidney failure (acute) following complete or unspecified spontaneous abortion
    Oliguria following complete or unspecified spontaneous abortion
    Renal shutdown following complete or unspecified spontaneous abortion
    Renal tubular necrosis following complete or unspecified spontaneous abortion
    Uremia following complete or unspecified spontaneous abortion

O03.83 Metabolic disorder following complete or unspecified spontaneous abortion   Ⓜ♀

O03.84 Damage to pelvic organs following complete or unspecified spontaneous abortion   Ⓜ♀

    Laceration, perforation, tear or chemical damage of bladder following complete or unspecified spontaneous abortion
    Laceration, perforation, tear or chemical damage of bowel following complete or unspecified spontaneous abortion
    Laceration, perforation, tear or chemical damage of broad ligament following complete or unspecified spontaneous abortion
    Laceration, perforation, tear or chemical damage of cervix following complete or unspecified spontaneous abortion
    Laceration, perforation, tear or chemical damage of periurethral tissue following complete or unspecified spontaneous abortion
    Laceration, perforation, tear or chemical damage of uterus following complete or unspecified spontaneous abortion
    Laceration, perforation, tear or chemical damage of vagina following complete or unspecified spontaneous abortion

O03.85 Other venous complications following complete or unspecified spontaneous abortion   Ⓜ♀

O03.86 Cardiac arrest following complete or unspecified spontaneous abortion   Ⓜ♀

O03.87 Sepsis following complete or unspecified spontaneous abortion   Ⓜ♀

    Use additional code to identify infectious agent (B95-B97)
    Use additional code to identify severe sepsis, if applicable (R65.2-)

    EXCLUDES 1 *septic or septicopyemic embolism following complete or unspecified spontaneous abortion (O03.7)*

✓ Additional Character Required   ✗7ᵗʰ Xtension Alert   Unspecified Dx   Other Specified Dx   Manifestation   ►◄ Revised Text   ● New Code   ▲ Revised Code Title

ICD-10-CM Draft (2015)   **735**

O03.88   **Urinary tract infection following complete or unspecified spontaneous abortion**   Ⓜ♀
  Cystitis following complete or unspecified spontaneous abortion

O03.89   **Complete or unspecified spontaneous abortion with other complications**   Ⓜ♀

O03.9   **Complete or unspecified spontaneous abortion** without complication   Ⓜ♀
  Miscarriage NOS
  Spontaneous abortion NOS

✓4ᵗʰ **O04**   **Complications following (induced) termination of pregnancy**
  [INCLUDES] complications following (induced) termination of pregnancy
  [EXCLUDES 1] encounter for elective termination of pregnancy, uncomplicated (Z33.2)
  failed attempted termination of pregnancy (O07.-)

O04.5   **Genital tract and pelvic infection following (induced) termination of pregnancy**   Ⓜ♀
  Endometritis following (induced) termination of pregnancy
  Oophoritis following (induced) termination of pregnancy
  Parametritis following (induced) termination of pregnancy
  Pelvic peritonitis following (induced) termination of pregnancy
  Salpingitis following (induced) termination of pregnancy
  Salpingo-oophoritis following (induced) termination of pregnancy
  [EXCLUDES 1] sepsis following (induced) termination of pregnancy (O04.87)
  urinary tract infection following (induced) termination of pregnancy (O04.88)

O04.6   **Delayed or excessive hemorrhage following (induced) termination of pregnancy**   Ⓜ♀
  Afibrinogenemia following (induced) termination of pregnancy
  Defibrination syndrome following (induced) termination of pregnancy
  Hemolysis following (induced) termination of pregnancy
  Intravascular coagulation following (induced) termination of pregnancy

O04.7   **Embolism following (induced) termination of pregnancy**   Ⓜ♀
  Air embolism following (induced) termination of pregnancy
  Amniotic fluid embolism following (induced) termination of pregnancy
  Blood-clot embolism following (induced) termination of pregnancy
  Embolism NOS following (induced) termination of pregnancy
  Fat embolism following (induced) termination of pregnancy
  Pulmonary embolism following (induced) termination of pregnancy
  Pyemic embolism following (induced) termination of pregnancy
  Septic or septicopyemic embolism following (induced) termination of pregnancy
  Soap embolism following (induced) termination of pregnancy

✓5ᵗʰ **O04.8**   **(Induced) termination of pregnancy with other and unspecified complications**

O04.80   **(Induced) termination of pregnancy with unspecified complications**   Ⓜ♀

O04.81   **Shock following (induced) termination of pregnancy**   Ⓜ♀
  Circulatory collapse following (induced) termination of pregnancy
  Shock (postprocedural) following (induced) termination of pregnancy
  [EXCLUDES 1] shock due to infection following (induced) termination of pregnancy (O04.87)

O04.82   **Renal failure following (induced) termination of pregnancy**   Ⓜ♀
  Kidney failure (acute) following (induced) termination of pregnancy
  Oliguria following (induced) termination of pregnancy
  Renal shutdown following (induced) termination of pregnancy
  Renal tubular necrosis following (induced) termination of pregnancy
  Uremia following (induced) termination of pregnancy

O04.83   **Metabolic disorder following (induced) termination of pregnancy**   Ⓜ♀

O04.84   **Damage to pelvic organs following (induced) termination of pregnancy**   Ⓜ♀
  Laceration, perforation, tear or chemical damage of bladder following (induced) termination of pregnancy
  Laceration, perforation, tear or chemical damage of bowel following (induced) termination of pregnancy
  Laceration, perforation, tear or chemical damage of broad ligament following (induced) termination of pregnancy
  Laceration, perforation, tear or chemical damage of cervix following (induced) termination of pregnancy
  Laceration, perforation, tear or chemical damage of periurethral tissue following (induced) termination of pregnancy
  Laceration, perforation, tear or chemical damage of uterus following (induced) termination of pregnancy
  Laceration, perforation, tear or chemical damage of vagina following (induced) termination of pregnancy

O04.85   **Other venous complications following (induced) termination of pregnancy**   Ⓜ♀

O04.86   **Cardiac arrest following (induced) termination of pregnancy**   Ⓜ♀

O04.87   **Sepsis following (induced) termination of pregnancy**   Ⓜ♀
  Use additional code to identify infectious agent (B95-B97)
  Use additional code to identify severe sepsis, if applicable (R65.2-)
  [EXCLUDES 1] septic or septicopyemic embolism following (induced) termination of pregnancy (O04.7)

O04.88   **Urinary tract infection following (induced) termination of pregnancy**   Ⓜ♀
  Cystitis following (induced) termination of pregnancy

O04.89   **(Induced) termination of pregnancy with other complications**   Ⓜ♀

✓4ᵗʰ **O07**   **Failed attempted termination of pregnancy**
  [INCLUDES] failure of attempted induction of termination of pregnancy
  incomplete elective abortion
  [EXCLUDES 1] incomplete spontaneous abortion (O03.0-)

O07.0   **Genital tract and pelvic infection following failed attempted termination of pregnancy**   Ⓜ♀
  Endometritis following failed attempted termination of pregnancy
  Oophoritis following failed attempted termination of pregnancy
  Parametritis following failed attempted termination of pregnancy
  Pelvic peritonitis following failed attempted termination of pregnancy
  Salpingitis following failed attempted termination of pregnancy
  Salpingo-oophoritis following failed attempted termination of pregnancy
  [EXCLUDES 1] sepsis following failed attempted termination of pregnancy (O07.37)
  urinary tract infection following failed attempted termination of pregnancy (O07.38)

O07.1   **Delayed or excessive hemorrhage following failed attempted termination of pregnancy**   Ⓜ♀
  Afibrinogenemia following failed attempted termination of pregnancy
  Defibrination syndrome following failed attempted termination of pregnancy
  Hemolysis following failed attempted termination of pregnancy
  Intravascular coagulation following failed attempted termination of pregnancy

---

[EXCLUDES 1] Not coded here   [EXCLUDES 2] Not included here   Ⓝ Newborn Age: 0   Ⓟ Pediatric Age: 0-17   Ⓜ Maternity Age: 12-55   Ⓐ Adult Age: 15-124

736   ICD-10-CM Draft (2015)

O07.2 Embolism following failed attempted termination of pregnancy   Ⓜ♀
  Air embolism following failed attempted termination of pregnancy
  Amniotic fluid embolism following failed attempted termination of pregnancy
  Blood-clot embolism following failed attempted termination of pregnancy
  Embolism NOS following failed attempted termination of pregnancy
  Fat embolism following failed attempted termination of pregnancy
  Pulmonary embolism following failed attempted termination of pregnancy
  Pyemic embolism following failed attempted termination of pregnancy
  Septic or septicopyemic embolism following failed attempted termination of pregnancy
  Soap embolism following failed attempted termination of pregnancy

☑5ᵗʰ O07.3 Failed attempted termination of pregnancy with other and unspecified complications

  O07.30 Failed attempted termination of pregnancy with unspecified complications   Ⓜ♀

  O07.31 Shock following failed attempted termination of pregnancy   Ⓜ♀
    Circulatory collapse following failed attempted termination of pregnancy
    Shock (postprocedural) following failed attempted termination of pregnancy
    EXCLUDES 1 *shock due to infection following failed attempted termination of pregnancy (O07.37)*

  O07.32 Renal failure following failed attempted termination of pregnancy   Ⓜ♀
    Kidney failure (acute) following failed attempted termination of pregnancy
    Oliguria following failed attempted termination of pregnancy
    Renal shutdown following failed attempted termination of pregnancy
    Renal tubular necrosis following failed attempted termination of pregnancy
    Uremia following failed attempted termination of pregnancy

  O07.33 Metabolic disorder following failed attempted termination of pregnancy   Ⓜ♀

  O07.34 Damage to pelvic organs following failed attempted termination of pregnancy   Ⓜ♀
    Laceration, perforation, tear or chemical damage of bladder following failed attempted termination of pregnancy
    Laceration, perforation, tear or chemical damage of bowel following failed attempted termination of pregnancy
    Laceration, perforation, tear or chemical damage of broad ligament following failed attempted termination of pregnancy
    Laceration, perforation, tear or chemical damage of cervix following failed attempted termination of pregnancy
    Laceration, perforation, tear or chemical damage of periurethral tissue following failed attempted termination of pregnancy
    Laceration, perforation, tear or chemical damage of uterus following failed attempted termination of pregnancy
    Laceration, perforation, tear or chemical damage of vagina following failed attempted termination of pregnancy

  O07.35 Other venous complications following failed attempted termination of pregnancy   Ⓜ♀

  O07.36 Cardiac arrest following failed attempted termination of pregnancy   Ⓜ♀

  O07.37 Sepsis following failed attempted termination of pregnancy   Ⓜ♀
    Use additional code to identify infectious agent (B95-B97)
    Use additional code to identify severe sepsis, if applicable (R65.2-)
    EXCLUDES 1 *septic or septicopyemic embolism following failed attempted termination of pregnancy (O07.2)*

  O07.38 Urinary tract infection following failed attempted termination of pregnancy   Ⓜ♀
    Cystitis following failed attempted termination of pregnancy

  O07.39 Failed attempted termination of pregnancy with other complications   Ⓜ♀

O07.4 Failed attempted termination of pregnancy without complication   Ⓜ♀

☑4ᵗʰ O08 Complications following ectopic and molar pregnancy
  This category is for use with categories O00-O02 to identify any associated complications

  O08.0 Genital tract and pelvic infection following ectopic and molar pregnancy   Ⓜ♀
    Endometritis following ectopic and molar pregnancy
    Oophoritis following ectopic and molar pregnancy
    Parametritis following ectopic and molar pregnancy
    Pelvic peritonitis following ectopic and molar pregnancy
    Salpingitis following ectopic and molar pregnancy
    Salpingo-oophoritis following ectopic and molar pregnancy
    EXCLUDES 1 *sepsis following ectopic and molar pregnancy (O08.82)*
    urinary tract infection (O08.83)

  O08.1 Delayed or excessive hemorrhage following ectopic and molar pregnancy   Ⓜ♀
    Afibrinogenemia following ectopic and molar pregnancy
    Defibrination syndrome following ectopic and molar pregnancy
    Hemolysis following ectopic and molar pregnancy
    Intravascular coagulation following ectopic and molar pregnancy
    EXCLUDES 1 *delayed or excessive hemorrhage due to incomplete abortion (O03.1)*

  O08.2 Embolism following ectopic and molar pregnancy   Ⓜ♀
    Air embolism following ectopic and molar pregnancy
    Amniotic fluid embolism following ectopic and molar pregnancy
    Blood-clot embolism following ectopic and molar pregnancy
    Embolism NOS following ectopic and molar pregnancy
    Fat embolism following ectopic and molar pregnancy
    Pulmonary embolism following ectopic and molar pregnancy
    Pyemic embolism following ectopic and molar pregnancy
    Septic or septicopyemic embolism following ectopic and molar pregnancy
    Soap embolism following ectopic and molar pregnancy

  O08.3 Shock following ectopic and molar pregnancy   Ⓜ♀
    Circulatory collapse following ectopic and molar pregnancy
    Shock (postprocedural) following ectopic and molar pregnancy
    EXCLUDES 1 *shock due to infection following ectopic and molar pregnancy (O08.82)*

  O08.4 Renal failure following ectopic and molar pregnancy   Ⓜ♀
    Kidney failure (acute) following ectopic and molar pregnancy
    Oliguria following ectopic and molar pregnancy
    Renal shutdown following ectopic and molar pregnancy
    Renal tubular necrosis following ectopic and molar pregnancy
    Uremia following ectopic and molar pregnancy

  O08.5 Metabolic disorders following an ectopic and molar pregnancy   Ⓜ♀

  O08.6 Damage to pelvic organs and tissues following an ectopic and molar pregnancy   Ⓜ♀
    Laceration, perforation, tear or chemical damage of bladder following an ectopic and molar pregnancy
    Laceration, perforation, tear or chemical damage of bowel following an ectopic and molar pregnancy
    Laceration, perforation, tear or chemical damage of broad ligament following an ectopic and molar pregnancy
    Laceration, perforation, tear or chemical damage of cervix following an ectopic and molar pregnancy
    Laceration, perforation, tear or chemical damage of periurethral tissue following an ectopic and molar pregnancy
    Laceration, perforation, tear or chemical damage of uterus following an ectopic and molar pregnancy
    Laceration, perforation, tear or chemical damage of vagina following an ectopic and molar pregnancy

  O08.7 Other venous complications following an ectopic and molar pregnancy   Ⓜ♀

☑ Additional Character Required   ✓x7ᵗʰ Xtension Alert   Unspecified Dx   Other Specified Dx   Manifestation   ►◄ Revised Text   ● New Code   ▲ Revised Code Title

Pregnancy, Childbirth and the Puerperium

O08.8–O09.812

√5ᵗʰ **O08.8 Other complications following an ectopic and molar pregnancy**

O08.81 **Cardiac arrest following an ectopic and molar pregnancy** Ⓜ♀

O08.82 **Sepsis following ectopic and molar pregnancy** Ⓜ♀
Use additional code to identify infectious agent (B95-B97)
Use additional code to identify severe sepsis, if applicable (R65.2-)
EXCLUDES 1 *septic or septicopyemic embolism following ectopic and molar pregnancy (O08.2)*

O08.83 **Urinary tract infection following an ectopic and molar pregnancy** Ⓜ♀
Cystitis following an ectopic and molar pregnancy

O08.89 **Other complications following an ectopic and molar pregnancy** Ⓜ♀

O08.9 **Unspecified complication following an ectopic and molar pregnancy** Ⓜ♀

Supervision of high risk pregnancy (O09)

√4ᵗʰ **O09 Supervision of high risk pregnancy**

√5ᵗʰ **O09.0 Supervision of pregnancy with history of infertility**

O09.00 **Supervision of pregnancy with history of infertility, unspecified trimester** Ⓜ♀

O09.01 **Supervision of pregnancy with history of infertility, first trimester** Ⓜ♀

O09.02 **Supervision of pregnancy with history of infertility, second trimester** Ⓜ♀

O09.03 **Supervision of pregnancy with history of infertility, third trimester** Ⓜ♀

√5ᵗʰ **O09.1 Supervision of pregnancy with history of ectopic or molar pregnancy**

O09.10 **Supervision of pregnancy with history of ectopic or molar pregnancy, unspecified trimester** Ⓜ♀

O09.11 **Supervision of pregnancy with history of ectopic or molar pregnancy, first trimester** Ⓜ♀

O09.12 **Supervision of pregnancy with history of ectopic or molar pregnancy, second trimester** Ⓜ♀

O09.13 **Supervision of pregnancy with history of ectopic or molar pregnancy, third trimester** Ⓜ♀

√5ᵗʰ **O09.2 Supervision of pregnancy with other poor reproductive or obstetric history**
EXCLUDES 2 *pregnancy care for patient with history of recurrent pregnancy loss (O26.2-)*

√6ᵗʰ **O09.21 Supervision of pregnancy with history of pre-term labor**

O09.211 **Supervision of pregnancy with history of pre-term labor, first trimester** Ⓜ♀

O09.212 **Supervision of pregnancy with history of pre-term labor, second trimester** Ⓜ♀

O09.213 **Supervision of pregnancy with history of pre-term labor, third trimester** Ⓜ♀

O09.219 **Supervision of pregnancy with history of pre-term labor, unspecified trimester** Ⓜ♀

√6ᵗʰ **O09.29 Supervision of pregnancy with other poor reproductive or obstetric history**
Supervision of pregnancy with history of neonatal death
Supervision of pregnancy with history of stillbirth

O09.291 **Supervision of pregnancy with other poor reproductive or obstetric history, first trimester** Ⓜ♀

O09.292 **Supervision of pregnancy with other poor reproductive or obstetric history, second trimester** Ⓜ♀

O09.293 **Supervision of pregnancy with other poor reproductive or obstetric history, third trimester** Ⓜ♀

O09.299 **Supervision of pregnancy with other poor reproductive or obstetric history, unspecified trimester** Ⓜ♀

√5ᵗʰ **O09.3 Supervision of pregnancy with insufficient antenatal care**
Supervision of concealed pregnancy
Supervision of hidden pregnancy

O09.30 **Supervision of pregnancy with insufficient antenatal care, unspecified trimester** Ⓜ♀

O09.31 **Supervision of pregnancy with insufficient antenatal care, first trimester** Ⓜ♀

O09.32 **Supervision of pregnancy with insufficient antenatal care, second trimester** Ⓜ♀

O09.33 **Supervision of pregnancy with insufficient antenatal care, third trimester** Ⓜ♀

√5ᵗʰ **O09.4 Supervision of pregnancy with grand multiparity**

O09.40 **Supervision of pregnancy with grand multiparity, unspecified trimester** Ⓜ♀

O09.41 **Supervision of pregnancy with grand multiparity, first trimester** Ⓜ♀

O09.42 **Supervision of pregnancy with grand multiparity, second trimester** Ⓜ♀

O09.43 **Supervision of pregnancy with grand multiparity, third trimester** Ⓜ♀

√5ᵗʰ **O09.5 Supervision of elderly primigravida and multigravida**
Pregnancy for a female 35 years and older at expected date of delivery

√6ᵗʰ **O09.51 Supervision of elderly primigravida**

O09.511 **Supervision of elderly primigravida, first trimester** Ⓜ♀

O09.512 **Supervision of elderly primigravida, second trimester** Ⓜ♀

O09.513 **Supervision of elderly primigravida, third trimester** Ⓜ♀

O09.519 **Supervision of elderly primigravida, unspecified trimester** Ⓜ♀

√6ᵗʰ **O09.52 Supervision of elderly multigravida**

O09.521 **Supervision of elderly multigravida, first trimester** Ⓜ♀

O09.522 **Supervision of elderly multigravida, second trimester** Ⓜ♀

O09.523 **Supervision of elderly multigravida, third trimester** Ⓜ♀

O09.529 **Supervision of elderly multigravida, unspecified trimester** Ⓜ♀

√5ᵗʰ **O09.6 Supervision of young primigravida and multigravida**
Supervision of pregnancy for a female less than 16 years old at expected date of delivery

√6ᵗʰ **O09.61 Supervision of young primigravida**

O09.611 **Supervision of young primigravida, first trimester** Ⓜ♀

O09.612 **Supervision of young primigravida, second trimester** Ⓜ♀

O09.613 **Supervision of young primigravida, third trimester** Ⓜ♀

O09.619 **Supervision of young primigravida, unspecified trimester** Ⓜ♀

√6ᵗʰ **O09.62 Supervision of young multigravida**

O09.621 **Supervision of young multigravida, first trimester** Ⓜ♀

O09.622 **Supervision of young multigravida, second trimester** Ⓜ♀

O09.623 **Supervision of young multigravida, third trimester** Ⓜ♀

O09.629 **Supervision of young multigravida, unspecified trimester** Ⓜ♀

√5ᵗʰ **O09.7 Supervision of high risk pregnancy due to social problems**

O09.70 **Supervision of high risk pregnancy due to social problems, unspecified trimester** Ⓜ♀

O09.71 **Supervision of high risk pregnancy due to social problems, first trimester** Ⓜ♀

O09.72 **Supervision of high risk pregnancy due to social problems, second trimester** Ⓜ♀

O09.73 **Supervision of high risk pregnancy due to social problems, third trimester** Ⓜ♀

√5ᵗʰ **O09.8 Supervision of other high risk pregnancies**

√6ᵗʰ **O09.81 Supervision of pregnancy resulting from assisted reproductive technology**
Supervision of pregnancy resulting from in-vitro fertilization

O09.811 **Supervision of pregnancy resulting from assisted reproductive technology, first trimester** Ⓜ♀

O09.812 **Supervision of pregnancy resulting from assisted reproductive technology, second trimester** Ⓜ♀

EXCLUDES 1 Not coded here   **EXCLUDES 2** Not included here   Ⓝ Newborn Age: 0   Ⓟ Pediatric Age: 0-17   Ⓜ Maternity Age: 12-55   Ⓐ Adult Age: 15-124

O09.813   Supervision of pregnancy resulting Ⓜ♀ from assisted reproductive technology, third trimester

O09.819   Supervision of pregnancy resulting Ⓜ♀ from assisted reproductive technology, unspecified trimester

✓6ᵗʰ **O09.82**   Supervision of pregnancy with history of in utero procedure during previous pregnancy

O09.821   Supervision of pregnancy with history Ⓜ♀ of in utero procedure during previous pregnancy, first trimester

O09.822   Supervision of pregnancy with history Ⓜ♀ of in utero procedure during previous pregnancy, second trimester

O09.823   Supervision of pregnancy with history Ⓜ♀ of in utero procedure during previous pregnancy, third trimester

O09.829   Supervision of pregnancy with Ⓜ♀ history of in utero procedure during previous pregnancy, unspecified trimester

> EXCLUDES 1   supervision of pregnancy affected by in utero procedure during current pregnancy (O35.7)

✓6ᵗʰ **O09.89**   Supervision of other high risk pregnancies

O09.891   Supervision of other high risk Ⓜ♀ pregnancies, first trimester

O09.892   Supervision of other high risk Ⓜ♀ pregnancies, second trimester

O09.893   Supervision of other high risk Ⓜ♀ pregnancies, third trimester

O09.899   Supervision of other high risk Ⓜ♀ pregnancies, unspecified trimester

✓5ᵗʰ **O09.9**   Supervision of high risk pregnancy, unspecified

O09.90   Supervision of high risk pregnancy, unspecified, Ⓜ♀ unspecified trimester

O09.91   Supervision of high risk pregnancy, unspecified, Ⓜ♀ first trimester

O09.92   Supervision of high risk pregnancy, unspecified, Ⓜ♀ second trimester

O09.93   Supervision of high risk pregnancy, unspecified, Ⓜ♀ third trimester

Edema, proteinuria and hypertensive disorders in pregnancy, childbirth and the puerperium (O10-O16)

✓4ᵗʰ **O10**   Pre-existing hypertension complicating pregnancy, childbirth and the puerperium

Pre-existing hypertension with pre-existing proteinuria complicating pregnancy, childbirth and the puerperium

> EXCLUDES 2   pre-existing hypertension with superimposed pre-eclampsia complicating pregnancy, childbirth and the puerperium (O11.-)

✓5ᵗʰ **O10.0**   Pre-existing essential hypertension complicating pregnancy, childbirth and the puerperium

Any condition in I10 specified as a reason for obstetric care during pregnancy, childbirth or the puerperium

✓6ᵗʰ **O10.01**   Pre-existing essential hypertension complicating pregnancy

O10.011   Pre-existing essential hypertension Ⓜ♀ complicating pregnancy, first trimester

O10.012   Pre-existing essential hypertension Ⓜ♀ complicating pregnancy, second trimester

O10.013   Pre-existing essential hypertension Ⓜ♀ complicating pregnancy, third trimester

O10.019   Pre-existing essential hypertension Ⓜ♀ complicating pregnancy, unspecified trimester

O10.02   Pre-existing essential hypertension Ⓜ♀ complicating childbirth

O10.03   Pre-existing essential hypertension Ⓜ♀ complicating the puerperium

✓5ᵗʰ **O10.1**   Pre-existing hypertensive heart disease complicating pregnancy, childbirth and the puerperium

Any condition in I11 specified as a reason for obstetric care during pregnancy, childbirth or the puerperium

Use additional code from I11 to identify the type of hypertensive heart disease

✓6ᵗʰ **O10.11**   Pre-existing hypertensive heart disease complicating pregnancy

O10.111   Pre-existing hypertensive heart Ⓜ♀ disease complicating pregnancy, first trimester

O10.112   Pre-existing hypertensive heart Ⓜ♀ disease complicating pregnancy, second trimester

O10.113   Pre-existing hypertensive heart Ⓜ♀ disease complicating pregnancy, third trimester

O10.119   Pre-existing hypertensive heart Ⓜ♀ disease complicating pregnancy, unspecified trimester

O10.12   Pre-existing hypertensive heart disease Ⓜ♀ complicating childbirth

O10.13   Pre-existing hypertensive heart disease Ⓜ♀ complicating the puerperium

✓5ᵗʰ **O10.2**   Pre-existing hypertensive chronic kidney disease complicating pregnancy, childbirth and the puerperium

Any condition in I12 specified as a reason for obstetric care during pregnancy, childbirth or the puerperium

Use additional code from I12 to identify the type of hypertensive chronic kidney disease

✓6ᵗʰ **O10.21**   Pre-existing hypertensive chronic kidney disease complicating pregnancy

O10.211   Pre-existing hypertensive chronic Ⓜ♀ kidney disease complicating pregnancy, first trimester

O10.212   Pre-existing hypertensive chronic Ⓜ♀ kidney disease complicating pregnancy, second trimester

O10.213   Pre-existing hypertensive chronic Ⓜ♀ kidney disease complicating pregnancy, third trimester

O10.219   Pre-existing hypertensive chronic Ⓜ♀ kidney disease complicating pregnancy, unspecified trimester

O10.22   Pre-existing hypertensive chronic kidney disease Ⓜ♀ complicating childbirth

O10.23   Pre-existing hypertensive chronic kidney disease Ⓜ♀ complicating the puerperium

✓5ᵗʰ **O10.3**   Pre-existing hypertensive heart and chronic kidney disease complicating pregnancy, childbirth and the puerperium

Any condition in I13 specified as a reason for obstetric care during pregnancy, childbirth or the puerperium

Use additional code from I13 to identify the type of hypertensive heart and chronic kidney disease

✓6ᵗʰ **O10.31**   Pre-existing hypertensive heart and chronic kidney disease complicating pregnancy

O10.311   Pre-existing hypertensive heart and Ⓜ♀ chronic kidney disease complicating pregnancy, first trimester

O10.312   Pre-existing hypertensive heart and Ⓜ♀ chronic kidney disease complicating pregnancy, second trimester

O10.313   Pre-existing hypertensive heart and Ⓜ♀ chronic kidney disease complicating pregnancy, third trimester

O10.319   Pre-existing hypertensive heart and Ⓜ♀ chronic kidney disease complicating pregnancy, unspecified trimester

O10.32   Pre-existing hypertensive heart and chronic Ⓜ♀ kidney disease complicating childbirth

O10.33   Pre-existing hypertensive heart and chronic Ⓜ♀ kidney disease complicating the puerperium

---

✓ Additional Character Required   ✓x7ᵗʰ Xtension Alert   Unspecified Dx   Other Specified Dx   Manifestation   ▶◀ Revised Text   ● New Code   ▲ Revised Code Title

Pregnancy, Childbirth and the Puerperium

O10.4–O21.0

☑5ᵗʰ **O10.4 Pre-existing secondary hypertension complicating pregnancy, childbirth and the puerperium**
Any condition in I15 specified as a reason for obstetric care during pregnancy, childbirth or the puerperium
Use additional code from I15 to identify the type of secondary hypertension

    ☑6ᵗʰ **O10.41 Pre-existing secondary hypertension complicating pregnancy**

       O10.411 Pre-existing secondary hypertension complicating pregnancy, first trimester Ⓜ♀

       O10.412 Pre-existing secondary hypertension complicating pregnancy, second trimester Ⓜ♀

       O10.413 Pre-existing secondary hypertension complicating pregnancy, third trimester Ⓜ♀

       O10.419 Pre-existing secondary hypertension complicating pregnancy, unspecified trimester Ⓜ♀

    O10.42 Pre-existing secondary hypertension complicating childbirth Ⓜ♀

    O10.43 Pre-existing secondary hypertension complicating the puerperium Ⓜ♀

☑5ᵗʰ **O10.9 Unspecified pre-existing hypertension complicating pregnancy, childbirth and the puerperium**

    ☑6ᵗʰ **O10.91 Unspecified pre-existing hypertension complicating pregnancy**

       O10.911 Unspecified pre-existing hypertension complicating pregnancy, first trimester Ⓜ♀

       O10.912 Unspecified pre-existing hypertension complicating pregnancy, second trimester Ⓜ♀

       O10.913 Unspecified pre-existing hypertension complicating pregnancy, third trimester Ⓜ♀

       O10.919 Unspecified pre-existing hypertension complicating pregnancy, unspecified trimester Ⓜ♀

    O10.92 Unspecified pre-existing hypertension complicating childbirth Ⓜ♀

    O10.93 Unspecified pre-existing hypertension complicating the puerperium Ⓜ♀

☑4ᵗʰ **O11 Pre-existing hypertension with pre-eclampsia**
Conditions in O10 complicated by pre-eclampsia
Pre-eclampsia superimposed pre-existing hypertension
Use additional code from O10 to identify the type of hypertension

    O11.1 Pre-existing hypertension with pre-eclampsia, first trimester Ⓜ♀

    O11.2 Pre-existing hypertension with pre-eclampsia, second trimester Ⓜ♀

    O11.3 Pre-existing hypertension with pre-eclampsia, third trimester Ⓜ♀

    O11.9 Pre-existing hypertension with pre-eclampsia, unspecified trimester Ⓜ♀

☑4ᵗʰ **O12 Gestational [pregnancy-induced] edema and proteinuria without hypertension**

    ☑5ᵗʰ **O12.0 Gestational edema**

       O12.00 Gestational edema, unspecified trimester Ⓜ♀

       O12.01 Gestational edema, first trimester Ⓜ♀

       O12.02 Gestational edema, second trimester Ⓜ♀

       O12.03 Gestational edema, third trimester Ⓜ♀

    ☑5ᵗʰ **O12.1 Gestational proteinuria**

       O12.10 Gestational proteinuria, unspecified trimester Ⓜ♀

       O12.11 Gestational proteinuria, first trimester Ⓜ♀

       O12.12 Gestational proteinuria, second trimester Ⓜ♀

       O12.13 Gestational proteinuria, third trimester Ⓜ♀

    ☑5ᵗʰ **O12.2 Gestational edema with proteinuria**

       O12.20 Gestational edema with proteinuria, unspecified trimester Ⓜ♀

       O12.21 Gestational edema with proteinuria, first trimester Ⓜ♀

       O12.22 Gestational edema with proteinuria, second trimester Ⓜ♀

       O12.23 Gestational edema with proteinuria, third trimester Ⓜ♀

☑4ᵗʰ **O13 Gestational [pregnancy-induced] hypertension without significant proteinuria**
INCLUDES gestational hypertension NOS

    O13.1 Gestational [pregnancy-induced] hypertension without significant proteinuria, first trimester Ⓜ♀

    O13.2 Gestational [pregnancy-induced] hypertension without significant proteinuria, second trimester Ⓜ♀

    O13.3 Gestational [pregnancy-induced] hypertension without significant proteinuria, third trimester Ⓜ♀

    O13.9 Gestational [pregnancy-induced] hypertension without significant proteinuria, unspecified trimester Ⓜ♀

☑4ᵗʰ **O14 Pre-eclampsia**
EXCLUDES 1 pre-existing hypertension with pre-eclampsia (O11)

    ☑5ᵗʰ **O14.0 Mild to moderate pre-eclampsia**

       O14.00 Mild to moderate pre-eclampsia, unspecified trimester Ⓜ♀

       O14.02 Mild to moderate pre-eclampsia, second trimester Ⓜ♀

       O14.03 Mild to moderate pre-eclampsia, third trimester Ⓜ♀

    ☑5ᵗʰ **O14.1 Severe pre-eclampsia**
EXCLUDES 1 HELLP syndrome (O14.2-)

       O14.10 Severe pre-eclampsia, unspecified trimester Ⓜ♀

       O14.12 Severe pre-eclampsia, second trimester Ⓜ♀

       O14.13 Severe pre-eclampsia, third trimester Ⓜ♀

    ☑5ᵗʰ **O14.2 HELLP syndrome**
Severe pre-eclampsia with hemolysis, elevated liver enzymes and low platelet count (HELLP)

       O14.20 HELLP syndrome (HELLP), unspecified trimester Ⓜ♀

       O14.22 HELLP syndrome (HELLP), second trimester Ⓜ♀

       O14.23 HELLP syndrome (HELLP), third trimester Ⓜ♀

    ☑5ᵗʰ **O14.9 Unspecified pre-eclampsia**

       O14.90 Unspecified pre-eclampsia, unspecified trimester Ⓜ♀

       O14.92 Unspecified pre-eclampsia, second trimester Ⓜ♀

       O14.93 Unspecified pre-eclampsia, third trimester Ⓜ♀

☑4ᵗʰ **O15 Eclampsia**
INCLUDES convulsions following conditions in O10-O14 and O16

    ☑5ᵗʰ **O15.0 Eclampsia in pregnancy**

       O15.00 Eclampsia in pregnancy, unspecified trimester Ⓜ♀

       O15.02 Eclampsia in pregnancy, second trimester Ⓜ♀

       O15.03 Eclampsia in pregnancy, third trimester Ⓜ♀

    O15.1 Eclampsia in labor Ⓜ♀

    O15.2 Eclampsia in the puerperium Ⓜ♀

    O15.9 Eclampsia, unspecified as to time period Ⓜ♀
Eclampsia NOS

☑4ᵗʰ **O16 Unspecified maternal hypertension**

    O16.1 Unspecified maternal hypertension, first trimester Ⓜ♀

    O16.2 Unspecified maternal hypertension, second trimester Ⓜ♀

    O16.3 Unspecified maternal hypertension, third trimester Ⓜ♀

    O16.9 Unspecified maternal hypertension, unspecified trimester Ⓜ♀

Other maternal disorders predominantly related to pregnancy (O20-O29)

EXCLUDES 2 maternal care related to the fetus and amniotic cavity and possible delivery problems (O30-O48)
maternal diseases classifiable elsewhere but complicating pregnancy, labor and delivery, and the puerperium (O98-O99)

☑4ᵗʰ **O20 Hemorrhage in early pregnancy**
Hemorrhage before completion of 20 weeks gestation
EXCLUDES 1 pregnancy with abortive outcome (O00-O08)

    O20.0 Threatened abortion Ⓜ♀
Hemorrhage specified as due to threatened abortion

    O20.8 Other hemorrhage in early pregnancy Ⓜ♀

    O20.9 Hemorrhage in early pregnancy, unspecified Ⓜ♀

☑4ᵗʰ **O21 Excessive vomiting in pregnancy**

    O21.0 Mild hyperemesis gravidarum Ⓜ♀
Hyperemesis gravidarum, mild or unspecified, starting before the end of the 20th week of gestation

---

EXCLUDES 1 Not coded here   EXCLUDES 2 Not included here   Ⓝ Newborn Age: 0   Ⓟ Pediatric Age: 0-17   Ⓜ Maternity Age: 12-55   Ⓐ Adult Age: 15-124

O21.1 Hyperemesis gravidarum with metabolic disturbance Ⓜ♀
Hyperemesis gravidarum, starting before the end of the 20th week of gestation, with metabolic disturbance such as carbohydrate depletion
Hyperemesis gravidarum, starting before the end of the 20th week of gestation, with metabolic disturbance such as dehydration
Hyperemesis gravidarum, starting before the end of the 20th week of gestation, with metabolic disturbance such as electrolyte imbalance

O21.2 Late vomiting of pregnancy Ⓜ♀
Excessive vomiting starting after 20 completed weeks of gestation

O21.8 Other vomiting complicating pregnancy Ⓜ♀
Vomiting due to diseases classified elsewhere, complicating pregnancy
Use additional code, to identify cause

O21.9 Vomiting of pregnancy, unspecified Ⓜ♀

✓4ᵗʰ **O22 Venous complications and hemorrhoids in pregnancy**
EXCLUDES 1 venous complications of:
abortion NOS (O03.9)
ectopic or molar pregnancy (O08.7)
failed attempted abortion (O07.35)
induced abortion (O04.85)
spontaneous abortion (O03.89)
EXCLUDES 2 obstetric pulmonary embolism (O88.-)
venous complications and hemorrhoids of childbirth and the puerperium (O87.-)

✓5ᵗʰ **O22.0** Varicose veins of lower extremity **in pregnancy**
Varicose veins NOS in pregnancy

O22.00 Varicose veins of lower extremity in pregnancy, unspecified trimester Ⓜ♀

O22.01 Varicose veins of lower extremity in pregnancy, first trimester Ⓜ♀

O22.02 Varicose veins of lower extremity in pregnancy, second trimester Ⓜ♀

O22.03 Varicose veins of lower extremity in pregnancy, third trimester Ⓜ♀

✓5ᵗʰ **O22.1** Genital varices **in pregnancy**
Perineal varices in pregnancy
Vaginal varices in pregnancy
Vulval varices in pregnancy

O22.10 Genital varices in pregnancy, unspecified trimester Ⓜ♀

O22.11 Genital varices in pregnancy, first trimester Ⓜ♀

O22.12 Genital varices in pregnancy, second trimester Ⓜ♀

O22.13 Genital varices in pregnancy, third trimester Ⓜ♀

✓5ᵗʰ **O22.2** Superficial thrombophlebitis **in pregnancy**
Phlebitis in pregnancy NOS
Thrombophlebitis of legs in pregnancy
Thrombosis in pregnancy NOS
Use additional code to identify the superficial thrombophlebitis (I80.0-)

O22.20 Superficial thrombophlebitis in pregnancy, unspecified trimester Ⓜ♀

O22.21 Superficial thrombophlebitis in pregnancy, first trimester Ⓜ♀

O22.22 Superficial thrombophlebitis in pregnancy, second trimester Ⓜ♀

O22.23 Superficial thrombophlebitis in pregnancy, third trimester Ⓜ♀

✓5ᵗʰ **O22.3** Deep phlebothrombosis **in pregnancy**
Deep vein thrombosis, antepartum
Use additional code to identify the deep vein thrombosis (I82.4-, I82.5-, I82.62-. I82.72-)
Use additional code, if applicable, for associated long-term (current) use of anticoagulants (Z79.01)

O22.30 Deep phlebothrombosis in pregnancy, unspecified trimester Ⓜ♀

O22.31 Deep phlebothrombosis in pregnancy, first trimester Ⓜ♀

O22.32 Deep phlebothrombosis in pregnancy, second trimester Ⓜ♀

O22.33 Deep phlebothrombosis in pregnancy, third trimester Ⓜ♀

✓5ᵗʰ **O22.4** Hemorrhoids **in pregnancy**

O22.40 Hemorrhoids in pregnancy, unspecified trimester Ⓜ♀

O22.41 Hemorrhoids in pregnancy, first trimester Ⓜ♀

O22.42 Hemorrhoids in pregnancy, second trimester Ⓜ♀

O22.43 Hemorrhoids in pregnancy, third trimester Ⓜ♀

✓5ᵗʰ **O22.5** Cerebral venous thrombosis **in pregnancy**
Cerebrovenous sinus thrombosis in pregnancy

O22.50 Cerebral venous thrombosis in pregnancy, unspecified trimester Ⓜ♀

O22.51 Cerebral venous thrombosis in pregnancy, first trimester Ⓜ♀

O22.52 Cerebral venous thrombosis in pregnancy, second trimester Ⓜ♀

O22.53 Cerebral venous thrombosis in pregnancy, third trimester Ⓜ♀

✓5ᵗʰ **O22.8** Other venous complications **in pregnancy**

✓6ᵗʰ **O22.8X** Other **venous complications in pregnancy**

O22.8X1 Other venous complications in pregnancy, first trimester Ⓜ♀

O22.8X2 Other venous complications in pregnancy, second trimester Ⓜ♀

O22.8X3 Other venous complications in pregnancy, third trimester Ⓜ♀

O22.8X9 Other venous complications in pregnancy, unspecified trimester Ⓜ♀

✓5ᵗʰ **O22.9** Venous complication **in pregnancy,** unspecified
Gestational phlebitis NOS
Gestational phlebopathy NOS
Gestational thrombosis NOS

O22.90 Venous complication in pregnancy, unspecified, unspecified trimester Ⓜ♀

O22.91 Venous complication in pregnancy, unspecified, first trimester Ⓜ♀

O22.92 Venous complication in pregnancy, unspecified, second trimester Ⓜ♀

O22.93 Venous complication in pregnancy, unspecified, third trimester Ⓜ♀

✓4ᵗʰ **O23 Infections of genitourinary tract in pregnancy**
Use additional code to identify organism (B95.-, B96.-)
EXCLUDES 2 gonococcal infections complicating pregnancy, childbirth and the puerperium (O98.2)
infections with a predominantly sexual mode of transmission NOS complicating pregnancy, childbirth and the puerperium (O98.3)
syphilis complicating pregnancy, childbirth and the puerperium (O98.1)
tuberculosis of genitourinary system complicating pregnancy, childbirth and the puerperium (O98.0)
venereal disease NOS complicating pregnancy, childbirth and the puerperium (O98.3)

✓5ᵗʰ **O23.0** Infections of kidney **in pregnancy**
Pyelonephritis in pregnancy

O23.00 Infections of kidney in pregnancy, unspecified trimester Ⓜ♀

O23.01 Infections of kidney in pregnancy, first trimester Ⓜ♀

O23.02 Infections of kidney in pregnancy, second trimester Ⓜ♀

O23.03 Infections of kidney in pregnancy, third trimester Ⓜ♀

✓5ᵗʰ **O23.1** Infections of bladder **in pregnancy**

O23.10 Infections of bladder in pregnancy, unspecified trimester Ⓜ♀

O23.11 Infections of bladder in pregnancy, first trimester Ⓜ♀

O23.12 Infections of bladder in pregnancy, second trimester Ⓜ♀

O23.13 Infections of bladder in pregnancy, third trimester Ⓜ♀

✓5ᵗʰ **O23.2** Infections of urethra **in pregnancy**

O23.20 Infections of urethra in pregnancy, unspecified trimester Ⓜ♀

O23.21 Infections of urethra in pregnancy, first trimester Ⓜ♀

O23.22 Infections of urethra in pregnancy, second trimester Ⓜ♀

O23.23   **Infections of urethra in pregnancy,** M♀
          third trimester

✓5th O23.3 Infections of other parts of urinary tract in pregnancy

O23.30   **Infections of other parts of urinary tract in** M♀
          pregnancy, unspecified trimester

O23.31   **Infections of other parts of urinary tract in** M♀
          pregnancy, first trimester

O23.32   **Infections of other parts of urinary tract in** M♀
          pregnancy, second trimester

O23.33   **Infections of other parts of urinary tract in** M♀
          pregnancy, third trimester

✓5th O23.4 Unspecified infection of urinary tract in pregnancy

O23.40   **Unspecified infection of urinary tract in** M♀
          pregnancy, unspecified trimester

O23.41   **Unspecified infection of urinary tract in** M♀
          pregnancy, first trimester

O23.42   **Unspecified infection of urinary tract in** M♀
          pregnancy, second trimester

O23.43   **Unspecified infection of urinary tract in** M♀
          pregnancy, third trimester

✓5th O23.5 Infections of the genital tract in pregnancy

✓6th O23.51   Infection of cervix in pregnancy

O23.511   **Infections of cervix in pregnancy,** M♀
          first trimester

O23.512   **Infections of cervix in pregnancy,** M♀
          second trimester

O23.513   **Infections of cervix in pregnancy,** M♀
          third trimester

O23.519   **Infections of cervix in pregnancy,** M♀
          unspecified trimester

✓6th O23.52   Salpingo-oophoritis in pregnancy
          Oophoritis in pregnancy
          Salpingitis in pregnancy

O23.521   **Salpingo-oophoritis in pregnancy,** M♀
          first trimester

O23.522   **Salpingo-oophoritis in pregnancy,** M♀
          second trimester

O23.523   **Salpingo-oophoritis in pregnancy,** M♀
          third trimester

O23.529   **Salpingo-oophoritis in pregnancy,** M♀
          unspecified trimester

✓6th O23.59   Infection of other part of genital tract in pregnancy

O23.591   **Infection of other part of genital tract** M♀
          in pregnancy, first trimester

O23.592   **Infection of other part of genital tract** M♀
          in pregnancy, second trimester

O23.593   **Infection of other part of genital tract** M♀
          in pregnancy, third trimester

O23.599   **Infection of other part of genital tract** M♀
          in pregnancy, unspecified trimester

✓5th O23.9 Unspecified genitourinary tract infection in pregnancy
          Genitourinary tract infection in pregnancy NOS

O23.90   **Unspecified genitourinary tract infection in** M♀
          pregnancy, unspecified trimester

O23.91   **Unspecified genitourinary tract infection in** M♀
          pregnancy, first trimester

O23.92   **Unspecified genitourinary tract infection in** M♀
          pregnancy, second trimester

O23.93   **Unspecified genitourinary tract infection in** M♀
          pregnancy, third trimester

✓4th O24 Diabetes mellitus in pregnancy, childbirth, and the puerperium

✓5th O24.0 Pre-existing diabetes mellitus, type 1, in pregnancy,
          childbirth and the puerperium
          Juvenile onset diabetes mellitus, in pregnancy, childbirth and
          the puerperium
          Ketosis-prone diabetes mellitus in pregnancy, childbirth and the
          puerperium
          Use additional code from category E10 to further identify any
          manifestations

✓6th O24.01   Pre-existing diabetes mellitus, type 1, in pregnancy

O24.011   **Pre-existing diabetes mellitus, type 1,** M♀
          in pregnancy, first trimester

O24.012   **Pre-existing diabetes mellitus, type 1,** M♀
          in pregnancy, second trimester

O24.013   **Pre-existing diabetes mellitus, type 1,** M♀
          in pregnancy, third trimester

O24.019   **Pre-existing diabetes mellitus, type 1,** M♀
          in pregnancy, unspecified trimester

O24.02   **Pre-existing diabetes mellitus, type 1, in** M♀
          childbirth

O24.03   **Pre-existing diabetes mellitus, type 1, in** M♀
          the puerperium

✓5th O24.1 Pre-existing diabetes mellitus, type 2, in pregnancy,
          childbirth and the puerperium
          Insulin-resistant diabetes mellitus in pregnancy, childbirth and
          the puerperium
          Use additional code (for):
          from category E11 to further identify any manifestations
          long-term (current) use of insulin (Z79.4)

✓6th O24.11   Pre-existing diabetes mellitus, type 2, in pregnancy

O24.111   **Pre-existing diabetes mellitus, type 2,** M♀
          in pregnancy, first trimester

O24.112   **Pre-existing diabetes mellitus, type 2,** M♀
          in pregnancy, second trimester

O24.113   **Pre-existing diabetes mellitus, type 2,** M♀
          in pregnancy, third trimester

O24.119   **Pre-existing diabetes mellitus, type 2,** M♀
          in pregnancy, unspecified trimester

O24.12   **Pre-existing diabetes mellitus, type 2, in** M♀
          childbirth

O24.13   **Pre-existing diabetes mellitus, type 2, in the** M♀
          puerperium

✓5th O24.3 Unspecified pre-existing diabetes mellitus in pregnancy,
          childbirth and the puerperium
          Use additional code (for):
          from category E11 to further identify any manifestation
          long-term (current) use of insulin (Z79.4)

✓6th O24.31   Unspecified pre-existing diabetes mellitus in
          pregnancy

O24.311   **Unspecified pre-existing diabetes** M♀
          mellitus in pregnancy, first trimester

O24.312   **Unspecified pre-existing diabetes** M♀
          mellitus in pregnancy, second trimester

O24.313   **Unspecified pre-existing diabetes** M♀
          mellitus in pregnancy, third trimester

O24.319   **Unspecified pre-existing diabetes** M♀
          mellitus in pregnancy, unspecified
          trimester

O24.32   **Unspecified pre-existing diabetes mellitus in** M♀
          childbirth

O24.33   **Unspecified pre-existing diabetes mellitus in** M♀
          the puerperium

✓5th O24.4 Gestational diabetes mellitus
          Diabetes mellitus arising in pregnancy
          Gestational diabetes mellitus NOS

✓6th O24.41   Gestational diabetes mellitus in pregnancy

O24.410   **Gestational diabetes mellitus in** M♀
          pregnancy, diet controlled

O24.414   **Gestational diabetes mellitus in** M♀
          pregnancy, insulin controlled

O24.419   **Gestational diabetes mellitus in** M♀
          pregnancy, unspecified control

✓6th O24.42   Gestational diabetes mellitus in childbirth

O24.420   **Gestational diabetes mellitus in** M♀
          childbirth, diet controlled

O24.424   **Gestational diabetes mellitus in** M♀
          childbirth, insulin controlled

O24.429   **Gestational diabetes mellitus in** M♀
          childbirth, unspecified control

✓6th O24.43   Gestational diabetes mellitus in the puerperium

O24.430   **Gestational diabetes mellitus in the** M♀
          puerperium, diet controlled

O24.434   **Gestational diabetes mellitus in the** M♀
          puerperium, insulin controlled

O24.439   **Gestational diabetes mellitus in the** M♀
          puerperium, unspecified control

EXCLUDES 1 Not coded here   EXCLUDES 2 Not included here   N Newborn Age: 0   P Pediatric Age: 0-17   M Maternity Age: 12-55   A Adult Age: 15-124

742   ICD-10-CM Draft (2015)

√5ᵗʰ **O24.8** Other pre-existing diabetes mellitus in pregnancy, childbirth, and the puerperium
　Use additional code (for):
　　from categories E08, E09 and E13 to further identify any manifestation
　　long-term (current) use of insulin (Z79.4)

√6ᵗʰ **O24.81** Other pre-existing diabetes mellitus in pregnancy
　O24.811 Other pre-existing diabetes mellitus in pregnancy, first trimester Ⓜ♀
　O24.812 Other pre-existing diabetes mellitus in pregnancy, second trimester Ⓜ♀
　O24.813 Other pre-existing diabetes mellitus in pregnancy, third trimester Ⓜ♀
　O24.819 Other pre-existing diabetes mellitus in pregnancy, unspecified trimester Ⓜ♀
O24.82 Other pre-existing diabetes mellitus in childbirth Ⓜ♀
O24.83 Other pre-existing diabetes mellitus in the puerperium Ⓜ♀

√5ᵗʰ **O24.9** Unspecified diabetes mellitus in pregnancy, childbirth and the puerperium
　Use additional code for long-term (current) use of insulin (Z79.4)

√6ᵗʰ **O24.91** Unspecified diabetes mellitus in pregnancy
　O24.911 Unspecified diabetes mellitus in pregnancy, first trimester Ⓜ♀
　O24.912 Unspecified diabetes mellitus in pregnancy, second trimester Ⓜ♀
　O24.913 Unspecified diabetes mellitus in pregnancy, third trimester Ⓜ♀
　O24.919 Unspecified diabetes mellitus in pregnancy, unspecified trimester Ⓜ♀
O24.92 Unspecified diabetes mellitus in childbirth Ⓜ♀
O24.93 Unspecified diabetes mellitus in the puerperium Ⓜ♀

√4ᵗʰ **O25** Malnutrition in pregnancy, childbirth and the puerperium
√5ᵗʰ **O25.1** Malnutrition in pregnancy
　O25.10 Malnutrition in pregnancy, unspecified trimester Ⓜ♀
　O25.11 Malnutrition in pregnancy, first trimester Ⓜ♀
　O25.12 Malnutrition in pregnancy, second trimester Ⓜ♀
　O25.13 Malnutrition in pregnancy, third trimester Ⓜ♀
O25.2 Malnutrition in childbirth Ⓜ♀
O25.3 Malnutrition in the puerperium Ⓜ♀

√4ᵗʰ **O26** Maternal care for other conditions predominantly related to pregnancy
√5ᵗʰ **O26.0** Excessive weight gain in pregnancy
　EXCLUDES 2　gestational edema (O12.0, O12.2)
　O26.00 Excessive weight gain in pregnancy, unspecified trimester Ⓜ♀
　O26.01 Excessive weight gain in pregnancy, first trimester Ⓜ♀
　O26.02 Excessive weight gain in pregnancy, second trimester Ⓜ♀
　O26.03 Excessive weight gain in pregnancy, third trimester Ⓜ♀

√5ᵗʰ **O26.1** Low weight gain in pregnancy
　O26.10 Low weight gain in pregnancy, unspecified trimester Ⓜ♀
　O26.11 Low weight gain in pregnancy, first trimester Ⓜ♀
　O26.12 Low weight gain in pregnancy, second trimester Ⓜ♀
　O26.13 Low weight gain in pregnancy, third trimester Ⓜ♀

√5ᵗʰ **O26.2** Pregnancy care for patient with recurrent pregnancy loss
　O26.20 Pregnancy care for patient with recurrent pregnancy loss, unspecified trimester Ⓜ♀
　O26.21 Pregnancy care for patient with recurrent pregnancy loss, first trimester Ⓜ♀
　O26.22 Pregnancy care for patient with recurrent pregnancy loss, second trimester Ⓜ♀
　O26.23 Pregnancy care for patient with recurrent pregnancy loss, third trimester Ⓜ♀

√5ᵗʰ **O26.3** Retained intrauterine contraceptive device in pregnancy
　O26.30 Retained intrauterine contraceptive device in pregnancy, unspecified trimester Ⓜ♀
　O26.31 Retained intrauterine contraceptive device in pregnancy, first trimester Ⓜ♀
O26.32 Retained intrauterine contraceptive device in pregnancy, second trimester Ⓜ♀
O26.33 Retained intrauterine contraceptive device in pregnancy, third trimester Ⓜ♀

√5ᵗʰ **O26.4** Herpes gestationis
　O26.40 Herpes gestationis, unspecified trimester Ⓜ♀
　O26.41 Herpes gestationis, first trimester Ⓜ♀
　O26.42 Herpes gestationis, second trimester Ⓜ♀
　O26.43 Herpes gestationis, third trimester Ⓜ♀

√5ᵗʰ **O26.5** Maternal hypotension syndrome
　Supine hypotensive syndrome
　O26.50 Maternal hypotension syndrome, unspecified trimester Ⓜ♀
　O26.51 Maternal hypotension syndrome, first trimester Ⓜ♀
　O26.52 Maternal hypotension syndrome, second trimester Ⓜ♀
　O26.53 Maternal hypotension syndrome, third trimester Ⓜ♀

√5ᵗʰ **O26.6** Liver and biliary tract disorders in pregnancy, childbirth and the puerperium
　Use additional code to identify the specific disorder
　EXCLUDES 2　hepatorenal syndrome following labor and delivery (O90.4)

√6ᵗʰ **O26.61** Liver and biliary tract disorders in pregnancy
　O26.611 Liver and biliary tract disorders in pregnancy, first trimester Ⓜ♀
　O26.612 Liver and biliary tract disorders in pregnancy, second trimester Ⓜ♀
　O26.613 Liver and biliary tract disorders in pregnancy, third trimester Ⓜ♀
　O26.619 Liver and biliary tract disorders in pregnancy, unspecified trimester Ⓜ♀
O26.62 Liver and biliary tract disorders in childbirth Ⓜ♀
O26.63 Liver and biliary tract disorders in the puerperium Ⓜ♀

√5ᵗʰ **O26.7** Subluxation of symphysis (pubis) in pregnancy, childbirth and the puerperium
　EXCLUDES 1　traumatic separation of symphysis (pubis) during childbirth (O71.6)

√6ᵗʰ **O26.71** Subluxation of symphysis (pubis) in pregnancy
　O26.711 Subluxation of symphysis (pubis) in pregnancy, first trimester Ⓜ♀
　O26.712 Subluxation of symphysis (pubis) in pregnancy, second trimester Ⓜ♀
　O26.713 Subluxation of symphysis (pubis) in pregnancy, third trimester Ⓜ♀
　O26.719 Subluxation of symphysis (pubis) in pregnancy, unspecified trimester Ⓜ♀
O26.72 Subluxation of symphysis (pubis) in childbirth Ⓜ♀
O26.73 Subluxation of symphysis (pubis) in the puerperium Ⓜ♀

√5ᵗʰ **O26.8** Other specified pregnancy related conditions
√6ᵗʰ **O26.81** Pregnancy related exhaustion and fatigue
　O26.811 Pregnancy related exhaustion and fatigue, first trimester Ⓜ♀
　O26.812 Pregnancy related exhaustion and fatigue, second trimester Ⓜ♀
　O26.813 Pregnancy related exhaustion and fatigue, third trimester Ⓜ♀
　O26.819 Pregnancy related exhaustion and fatigue, unspecified trimester Ⓜ♀
√6ᵗʰ **O26.82** Pregnancy related peripheral neuritis
　O26.821 Pregnancy related peripheral neuritis, first trimester Ⓜ♀
　O26.822 Pregnancy related peripheral neuritis, second trimester Ⓜ♀
　O26.823 Pregnancy related peripheral neuritis, third trimester Ⓜ♀
　O26.829 Pregnancy related peripheral neuritis, unspecified trimester Ⓜ♀
√6ᵗʰ **O26.83** Pregnancy related renal disease
　Use additional code to identify the specific disorder
　O26.831 Pregnancy related renal disease, first trimester Ⓜ♀
　O26.832 Pregnancy related renal disease, second trimester Ⓜ♀

☑ Additional Character Required　　√x7ᵗʰ Xtension Alert　　Unspecified Dx　　Other Specified Dx　　Manifestation　　►◄ Revised Text　　● New Code　　▲ Revised Code Title

O26.833   **Pregnancy related renal disease, third** Ⓜ♀
    trimester

O26.839   **Pregnancy related renal disease,** Ⓜ♀
    unspecified trimester

✓6ᵗʰ   O26.84   **Uterine size-date discrepancy complicating**
    pregnancy
    EXCLUDES 1   *encounter for suspected problem with fetal*
       growth ruled out (Z03.74)

    O26.841   **Uterine size-date discrepancy, first** Ⓜ♀
       trimester

    O26.842   **Uterine size-date discrepancy, second** Ⓜ♀
       trimester

    O26.843   **Uterine size-date discrepancy, third** Ⓜ♀
       trimester

    O26.849   **Uterine size-date discrepancy,** Ⓜ♀
       unspecified trimester

✓6ᵗʰ   O26.85   **Spotting complicating pregnancy**

    O26.851   **Spotting complicating pregnancy,** Ⓜ♀
       first trimester

    O26.852   **Spotting complicating pregnancy,** Ⓜ♀
       second trimester

    O26.853   **Spotting complicating pregnancy,** Ⓜ♀
       third trimester

    O26.859   **Spotting complicating pregnancy,** Ⓜ♀
       unspecified trimester

O26.86   **Pruritic urticarial papules and plaques of** Ⓜ♀
    pregnancy (PUPPP)
    Polymorphic eruption of pregnancy

✓6ᵗʰ   O26.87   **Cervical shortening**
    EXCLUDES 1   *encounter for suspected cervical shortening*
       ruled out (Z03.75)

    O26.872   **Cervical shortening, second trimester** Ⓜ♀
    O26.873   **Cervical shortening, third trimester** Ⓜ♀
    O26.879   **Cervical shortening, unspecified** Ⓜ♀
       trimester

✓6ᵗʰ   O26.89   **Other specified pregnancy related conditions**

    O26.891   **Other specified pregnancy related** Ⓜ♀
       conditions, first trimester

    O26.892   **Other specified pregnancy related** Ⓜ♀
       conditions, second trimester

    O26.893   **Other specified pregnancy related** Ⓜ♀
       conditions, third trimester

    O26.899   **Other specified pregnancy related** Ⓜ♀
       conditions, unspecified trimester

✓5ᵗʰ   O26.9   **Pregnancy related conditions, unspecified**

    O26.90   **Pregnancy related conditions, unspecified,** Ⓜ♀
       unspecified trimester

    O26.91   **Pregnancy related conditions, unspecified,** Ⓜ♀
       first trimester

    O26.92   **Pregnancy related conditions, unspecified,** Ⓜ♀
       second trimester

    O26.93   **Pregnancy related conditions, unspecified,** Ⓜ♀
       third trimester

✓4ᵗʰ   **O28**   **Abnormal findings on antenatal screening of mother**
    EXCLUDES 1   *diagnostic findings classified elsewhere—see Alphabetical*
       Index

O28.0   **Abnormal hematological finding on antenatal screening** Ⓜ♀
    of mother

O28.1   **Abnormal biochemical finding on antenatal screening of** Ⓜ♀
    mother

O28.2   **Abnormal cytological finding on antenatal screening** Ⓜ♀
    of mother

O28.3   **Abnormal ultrasonic finding on antenatal screening** Ⓜ♀
    of mother

O28.4   **Abnormal radiological finding on antenatal screening** Ⓜ♀
    of mother

O28.5   **Abnormal chromosomal and genetic finding on antenatal** Ⓜ♀
    screening of mother

O28.8   **Other abnormal findings on antenatal screening of** Ⓜ♀
    mother

O28.9   **Unspecified abnormal findings on antenatal screening** Ⓜ♀
    of mother

✓4ᵗʰ   **O29**   **Complications of anesthesia during pregnancy**
    INCLUDES   maternal complications arising from the administration of a
       general, regional or local anesthetic, analgesic or other
       sedation during pregnancy
    Use additional code, if necessary, to identify the complication
    EXCLUDES 2   *complications of anesthesia during labor and delivery (O74.-)*
       complications of anesthesia during the puerperium (O89.-)

✓5ᵗʰ   O29.0   **Pulmonary complications of anesthesia during pregnancy**

    ✓6ᵗʰ   O29.01   **Aspiration pneumonitis due to anesthesia during**
       pregnancy
       Inhalation of stomach contents or secretions NOS due
       to anesthesia during pregnancy
       Mendelson's syndrome due to anesthesia during
       pregnancy

       O29.011   **Aspiration pneumonitis due to** Ⓜ♀
          anesthesia during pregnancy, first
          trimester

       O29.012   **Aspiration pneumonitis due to** Ⓜ♀
          anesthesia during pregnancy, second
          trimester

       O29.013   **Aspiration pneumonitis due to** Ⓜ♀
          anesthesia during pregnancy, third
          trimester

       O29.019   **Aspiration pneumonitis due to** Ⓜ♀
          anesthesia during pregnancy,
          unspecified trimester

    ✓6ᵗʰ   O29.02   **Pressure collapse of lung due to anesthesia during**
       pregnancy

       O29.021   **Pressure collapse of lung due to** Ⓜ♀
          anesthesia during pregnancy, first
          trimester

       O29.022   **Pressure collapse of lung due to** Ⓜ♀
          anesthesia during pregnancy, second
          trimester

       O29.023   **Pressure collapse of lung due to** Ⓜ♀
          anesthesia during pregnancy, third
          trimester

       O29.029   **Pressure collapse of lung due to** Ⓜ♀
          anesthesia during pregnancy,
          unspecified trimester

    ✓6ᵗʰ   O29.09   **Other pulmonary complications of anesthesia**
       during pregnancy

       O29.091   **Other pulmonary complications of** Ⓜ♀
          anesthesia during pregnancy, first
          trimester

       O29.092   **Other pulmonary complications of** Ⓜ♀
          anesthesia during pregnancy, second
          trimester

       O29.093   **Other pulmonary complications of** Ⓜ♀
          anesthesia during pregnancy, third
          trimester

       O29.099   **Other pulmonary complications of** Ⓜ♀
          anesthesia during pregnancy,
          unspecified trimester

✓5ᵗʰ   O29.1   **Cardiac complications of anesthesia during pregnancy**

    ✓6ᵗʰ   O29.11   **Cardiac arrest due to anesthesia during pregnancy**

       O29.111   **Cardiac arrest due to anesthesia** Ⓜ♀
          during pregnancy, first trimester

       O29.112   **Cardiac arrest due to anesthesia** Ⓜ♀
          during pregnancy, second trimester

       O29.113   **Cardiac arrest due to anesthesia** Ⓜ♀
          during pregnancy, third trimester

       O29.119   **Cardiac arrest due to anesthesia** Ⓜ♀
          during pregnancy, unspecified trimester

    ✓6ᵗʰ   O29.12   **Cardiac failure due to anesthesia during pregnancy**

       O29.121   **Cardiac failure due to anesthesia** Ⓜ♀
          during pregnancy, first trimester

       O29.122   **Cardiac failure due to anesthesia** Ⓜ♀
          during pregnancy, second trimester

       O29.123   **Cardiac failure due to anesthesia** Ⓜ♀
          during pregnancy, third trimester

       O29.129   **Cardiac failure due to anesthesia** Ⓜ♀
          during pregnancy, unspecified trimester

    ✓6ᵗʰ   O29.19   **Other cardiac complications of anesthesia during**
       pregnancy

       O29.191   **Other cardiac complications of** Ⓜ♀
          anesthesia during pregnancy, first
          trimester

EXCLUDES 1 Not coded here   EXCLUDES 2 Not included here   Ⓝ Newborn Age: 0   Ⓟ Pediatric Age: 0-17   Ⓜ Maternity Age: 12-55   Ⓐ Adult Age: 15-124

744   ICD-10-CM Draft (2015)

O29.192　Other cardiac complications of anesthesia during pregnancy, second trimester　M♀

O29.193　Other cardiac complications of anesthesia during pregnancy, third trimester　M♀

O29.199　Other cardiac complications of anesthesia during pregnancy, unspecified trimester　M♀

☑5th O29.2　Central nervous system complications of anesthesia during pregnancy

☑6th O29.21　Cerebral anoxia due to anesthesia during pregnancy

O29.211　Cerebral anoxia due to anesthesia during pregnancy, first trimester　M♀

O29.212　Cerebral anoxia due to anesthesia during pregnancy, second trimester　M♀

O29.213　Cerebral anoxia due to anesthesia during pregnancy, third trimester　M♀

O29.219　Cerebral anoxia due to anesthesia during pregnancy, unspecified trimester　M♀

☑6th O29.29　Other central nervous system complications of anesthesia during pregnancy

O29.291　Other central nervous system complications of anesthesia during pregnancy, first trimester　M♀

O29.292　Other central nervous system complications of anesthesia during pregnancy, second trimester　M♀

O29.293　Other central nervous system complications of anesthesia during pregnancy, third trimester　M♀

O29.299　Other central nervous system complications of anesthesia during pregnancy, unspecified trimester　M♀

☑5th O29.3　Toxic reaction to local anesthesia during pregnancy

☑6th O29.3X　Toxic reaction to local anesthesia during pregnancy

O29.3X1　Toxic reaction to local anesthesia during pregnancy, first trimester　M♀

O29.3X2　Toxic reaction to local anesthesia during pregnancy, second trimester　M♀

O29.3X3　Toxic reaction to local anesthesia during pregnancy, third trimester　M♀

O29.3X9　Toxic reaction to local anesthesia during pregnancy, unspecified trimester　M♀

☑5th O29.4　Spinal and epidural anesthesia induced headache during pregnancy

O29.40　Spinal and epidural anesthesia induced headacheduring pregnancy, unspecified trimester　M♀

O29.41　Spinal and epidural anesthesia induced headache during pregnancy, first trimester　M♀

O29.42　Spinal and epidural anesthesia induced headache during pregnancy, second trimester　M♀

O29.43　Spinal and epidural anesthesia induced headache during pregnancy, third trimester　M♀

☑5th O29.5　Other complications of spinal and epidural anesthesia during pregnancy

☑6th O29.5X　Other complications of spinal and epidural anesthesia during pregnancy

O29.5X1　Other complications of spinal and epidural anesthesia during pregnancy, first trimester　M♀

O29.5X2　Other complications of spinal and epidural anesthesia during pregnancy, second trimester　M♀

O29.5X3　Other complications of spinal and epidural anesthesia during pregnancy, third trimester　M♀

O29.5X9　Other complications of spinal and epidural anesthesia during pregnancy, unspecified trime ster　M♀

☑5th O29.6　Failed or difficult intubation for anesthesia during pregnancy

O29.60　Failed or difficult intubation for anesthesia during pregnancy, unspecified trimester　M♀

O29.61　Failed or difficult intubation for anesthesia during pregnancy, first trimester　M♀

O29.62　Failed or difficult intubation for anesthesia during pregnancy, second trimester　M♀

O29.63　Failed or difficult intubation for anesthesia during pregnancy, third trimester　M♀

☑5th O29.8　Other complications of anesthesia during pregnancy

☑6th O29.8X　Other complications of anesthesia during pregnancy

O29.8X1　Other complications of anesthesia during pregnancy, first trimester　M♀

O29.8X2　Other complications of anesthesia during pregnancy, second trimester　M♀

O29.8X3　Other complications of anesthesia during pregnancy, third trimester　M♀

O29.8X9　Other complications of anesthesia during pregnancy, unspecified trimester　M♀

☑5th O29.9　Unspecified complication of anesthesia during pregnancy

O29.90　Unspecified complication of anesthesia during pregnancy, unspecified trimester　M♀

O29.91　Unspecified complication of anesthesia during pregnancy, first trimester　M♀

O29.92　Unspecified complication of anesthesia during pregnancy, second trimester　M♀

O29.93　Unspecified complication of anesthesia during pregnancy, third trimester　M♀

Maternal care related to the fetus and amniotic cavity and possible delivery problems (O30-O48)

☑4th O30　Multiple gestation

Code also any complications specific to multiple gestation

☑5th O30.0　Twin pregnancy

☑6th O30.00　Twin pregnancy, unspecified number of placenta and unspecified number of amniotic sacs

O30.001　Twin pregnancy, unspecified number of placenta and unspecified number of amniotic sacs, first trimester　M♀

O30.002　Twin pregnancy, unspecified number of placenta and unspecified number of amniotic sacs, second trimester　M♀

O30.003　Twin pregnancy, unspecified number of placenta and unspecified number of amniotic sacs, third trimester　M♀

O30.009　Twin pregnancy, unspecified number of placenta and unspecified number of amniotic sacs, unspecified trimester　M♀

☑6th O30.01　Twin pregnancy, monochorionic/monoamniotic
Twin pregnancy, one placenta, one amniotic sac
EXCLUDES 1　conjoined twins (O30.02-)

O30.011　Twin pregnancy, monochorionic/monoamniotic, first trimester　M♀

O30.012　Twin pregnancy, monochorionic/monoamniotic, second trimester　M♀

O30.013　Twin pregnancy, monochorionic/monoamniotic, third trimester　M♀

O30.019　Twin pregnancy, monochorionic/monoamniotic, unspecified trimester　M♀

☑6th O30.02　Conjoined twin pregnancy

O30.021　Conjoined twin pregnancy, first trimester　M♀

O30.022　Conjoined twin pregnancy, second trimester　M♀

O30.023　Conjoined twin pregnancy, third trimester　M♀

O30.029　Conjoined twin pregnancy, unspecified trimester　M♀

☑6th O30.03　Twin pregnancy, monochorionic/diamniotic
Twin pregnancy, one placenta, two amniotic sacs

O30.031　Twin pregnancy, monochorionic/diamniotic, first trimester　M♀

O30.032　Twin pregnancy, monochorionic/diamniotic, second trimester　M♀

O30.033　Twin pregnancy, monochorionic/diamniotic, third trimester　M♀

O30.039　Twin pregnancy, monochorionic/diamniotic, unspecified trimester　M♀

☑6th O30.04　Twin pregnancy, dichorionic/diamniotic
Twin pregnancy, two placentae, two amniotic sacs

O30.041　Twin pregnancy, dichorionic/diamniotic, first trimester　M♀

O30.042　Twin pregnancy, dichorionic/diamniotic, second trimester　M♀

O30.043   Twin pregnancy, dichorionic/diamniotic, **third trimester**   M♀

O30.049   Twin pregnancy, dichorionic/diamniotic, **unspecified trimester**   M♀

✓6th O30.09   Twin pregnancy, unable to determine number of placenta and number of amniotic sacs

O30.091   Twin pregnancy, unable to determine number of placenta and number of amniotic sacs, **first trimester**   M♀

O30.092   Twin pregnancy, unable to determine number of placenta and number of amniotic sacs, **second trimester**   M♀

O30.093   Twin pregnancy, unable to determine number of placenta and number of amniotic sacs, **third trimester**   M♀

O30.099   Twin pregnancy, unable to determine number of placenta and number of amniotic sacs, **unspecified trimester**   M♀

✓5th O30.1   Triplet pregnancy

✓6th O30.10   Triplet pregnancy, unspecified number of placenta and unspecified number of amniotic sacs

O30.101   Triplet pregnancy, unspecified number of placenta and unspecified number of amniotic sacs, **first trimester**   M♀

O30.102   Triplet pregnancy, unspecified number of placenta and unspecified number of amniotic sacs, **second trimester**   M♀

O30.103   Triplet pregnancy, unspecified number of placenta and unspecified number of amniotic sacs, **third trimester**   M♀

O30.109   Triplet pregnancy, unspecified number of placenta and unspecified number of amniotic sacs, **unspecified trimester**   M♀

✓6th O30.11   Triplet pregnancy with two or more monochorionic fetuses

O30.111   Triplet pregnancy with two or more monochorionic fetuses, **first trimester**   M♀

O30.112   Triplet pregnancy with two or more monochorionic fetuses, **second trimester**   M♀

O30.113   Triplet pregnancy with two or more monochorionic fetuses, **third trimester**   M♀

O30.119   Triplet pregnancy with two or more monochorionic fetuses, **unspecified trimester**   M♀

✓6th O30.12   Triplet pregnancy with two or more monoamniotic fetuses

O30.121   Triplet pregnancy with two or more monoamniotic fetuses, **first trimester**   M♀

O30.122   Triplet pregnancy with two or more monoamniotic fetuses, **second trimester**   M♀

O30.123   Triplet pregnancy with two or more monoamniotic fetuses, **third trimester**   M♀

O30.129   Triplet pregnancy with two or more monoamniotic fetuses, **unspecified trimester**   M♀

✓6th O30.19   Triplet pregnancy, unable to determine number of placenta and number of amniotic sacs

O30.191   Triplet pregnancy, unable to determine number of placenta and number of amniotic sacs, **first trimester**   M♀

O30.192   Triplet pregnancy, unable to determine number of placenta and number of amniotic sacs, **second trimester**   M♀

O30.193   Triplet pregnancy, unable to determine number of placenta and number of amniotic sacs, **third trimester**   M♀

O30.199   Triplet pregnancy, unable to determine number of placenta and number of amniotic sacs, **unspecified trimester**   M♀

✓6th O30.2   Quadruplet pregnancy

✓6th O30.20   Quadruplet pregnancy, unspecified number of placenta and unspecified number of amniotic sacs

O30.201   Quadruplet pregnancy, unspecified number of placenta and unspecified number of amniotic sacs, **first trimester**   M♀

O30.202   Quadruplet pregnancy, unspecified number of placenta and unspecified number of amniotic sacs, **second trimester**   M♀

O30.203   Quadruplet pregnancy, unspecified number of placenta and unspecified number of amniotic sacs, **third trimester**   M♀

O30.209   Quadruplet pregnancy, unspecified number of placenta and unspecified number of amniotic sacs, **unspecified trimester**   M♀

✓6th O30.21   Quadruplet pregnancy with two or more monochorionic fetuses

O30.211   Quadruplet pregnancy with two or more monochorionic fetuses, **first trimester**   M♀

O30.212   Quadruplet pregnancy with two or more monochorionic fetuses, **second trimester**   M♀

O30.213   Quadruplet pregnancy with two or more monochorionic fetuses, **third trimester**   M♀

O30.219   Quadruplet pregnancy with two or more monochorionic fetuses, **unspecified trimester**   M♀

✓6th O30.22   Quadruplet pregnancy with two or more monoamniotic fetuses

O30.221   Quadruplet pregnancy with two or more monoamniotic fetuses, **first trimester**   M♀

O30.222   Quadruplet pregnancy with two or more monoamniotic fetuses, **second trimester**   M♀

O30.223   Quadruplet pregnancy with two or more monoamniotic fetuses, **third trimester**   M♀

O30.229   Quadruplet pregnancy with two or more monoamniotic fetuses, **unspecified trimester**   M♀

✓6th O30.29   Quadruplet pregnancy, unable to determine number of placenta and number of amniotic sacs

O30.291   Quadruplet pregnancy, unable to determine number of placenta and number of amniotic sacs, **first trimester**   M♀

O30.292   Quadruplet pregnancy, unable to determine number of placenta and number of amniotic sacs, **second trimester**   M♀

O30.293   Quadruplet pregnancy, unable to determine number of placenta and number of amniotic sacs, **third trimester**   M♀

O30.299   Quadruplet pregnancy, unable to determine number of placenta and number of amniotic sacs, **unspecified**   M♀

✓5th O30.8   Other specified multiple gestation
     Multiple gestation pregnancy greater than quadruplets

✓6th O30.80   Other specified multiple gestation, unspecified number of placenta and unspecified number of amniotic sacs

O30.801   Other specified multiple gestation, unspecified number of placenta and unspecified number of amniotic sacs, **first trimester**   M♀

O30.802   Other specified multiple gestation, unspecified number of placenta and unspecified number of amniotic sacs, **second trimester**   M♀

EXCLUDES 1 Not coded here   EXCLUDES 2 Not included here   N Newborn Age: 0   P Pediatric Age: 0–17   M Maternity Age: 12–55   A Adult Age: 15–124

746   ICD-10-CM Draft (2015)

O30.803   Other specified multiple gestation, unspecified number of placenta and unspecified number of amniotic sacs, third trimester   Ⓜ♀

O30.809   Other specified multiple gestation, unspecified number of placenta and unspecified number of amniotic sacs, unspecified trimester   Ⓜ♀

✓6ᵗʰ **O30.81**   Other specified multiple gestation with two or more monochorionic fetuses

O30.811   Other specified multiple gestation with two or more monochorionic fetuses, first trimester   Ⓜ♀

O30.812   Other specified multiple gestation with two or more monochorionic fetuses, second trimester   Ⓜ♀

O30.813   Other specified multiple gestation with two or more monochorionic fetuses, third trimester   Ⓜ♀

O30.819   Other specified multiple gestation with two or more monochorionic fetuses, unspecified trimester   Ⓜ♀

✓6ᵗʰ **O30.82**   Other specified multiple gestation with two or more monoamniotic fetuses

O30.821   Other specified multiple gestation with two or more monoamniotic fetuses, first trimester   Ⓜ♀

O30.822   Other specified multiple gestation with two or more monoamniotic fetuses, second trimester   Ⓜ♀

O30.823   Other specified multiple gestation with two or more monoamniotic fetuses, third trimester   Ⓜ♀

O30.829   Other specified multiple gestation with two or more monoamniotic fetuses, unspecified trimester   Ⓜ♀

✓6ᵗʰ **O30.89**   Other specified multiple gestation, unable to determine number of placenta and number of amniotic sacs

O30.891   Other specified multiple gestation, unable to determine number of placenta and number of amniotic sacs, first trimester   Ⓜ♀

O30.892   Other specified multiple gestation, unable to determine number of placenta and number of amniotic sacs, second trimester   Ⓜ♀

O30.893   Other specified multiple gestation, unable to determine number of placenta and number of amniotic sacs, third trimester   Ⓜ♀

O30.899   Other specified multiple gestation, unable to determine number of placenta and number of amniotic sacs, unspecified trimester   Ⓜ♀

✓5ᵗʰ **O30.9**   Multiple gestation, unspecified
Multiple pregnancy NOS

O30.90   Multiple gestation, unspecified, unspecified trimester   Ⓜ♀

O30.91   Multiple gestation, unspecified, first trimester   Ⓜ♀

O30.92   Multiple gestation, unspecified, second trimester   Ⓜ♀

O30.93   Multiple gestation, unspecified, third trimester   Ⓜ♀

✓4ᵗʰ **O31**   **Complications specific to multiple gestation**

EXCLUDES 2   delayed delivery of second twin, triplet, etc. (O63.2)
malpresentation of one fetus or more (O32.9)
placental transfusion syndromes (O43.0-)

AHA: 2012, 4Q, 107

One of the following 7th characters is to be assigned to each code under category O31. 7th character 0 is for single gestations and multiple gestations where the fetus is unspecified. 7th characters 1 through 9 are for cases of multiple gestations to identify the fetus for which the code applies. The appropriate code from category O30, Multiple gestation, must also be assigned when assigning a code from category O31 that has a 7th character of 1 through 9.

0   not applicable or unspecified   4   fetus 4
1   fetus 1   5   fetus 5
2   fetus 2   9   other fetus
3   fetus 3

✓5ᵗʰ **O31.0**   Papyraceous fetus
Fetus compressus

✓x7ᵗʰ **O31.00**   Papyraceous fetus, unspecified trimester   Ⓜ♀

✓x7ᵗʰ **O31.01**   Papyraceous fetus, first trimester   Ⓜ♀

✓x7ᵗʰ **O31.02**   Papyraceous fetus, second trimester   Ⓜ♀

✓x7ᵗʰ **O31.03**   Papyraceous fetus, third trimester   Ⓜ♀

✓5ᵗʰ **O31.1**   Continuing pregnancy after spontaneous abortion of one fetus or more

✓x7ᵗʰ **O31.10**   Continuing pregnancy after spontaneous abortion of one fetus or more, unspecified trimester   Ⓜ♀

✓x7ᵗʰ **O31.11**   Continuing pregnancy after spontaneous abortion of one fetus or more, first trimester   Ⓜ♀

✓x7ᵗʰ **O31.12**   Continuing pregnancy after spontaneous abortion of one fetus or more, second trimester   Ⓜ♀

✓x7ᵗʰ **O31.13**   Continuing pregnancy after spontaneous abortion of one fetus or more, third trimester   Ⓜ♀

✓5ᵗʰ **O31.2**   Continuing pregnancy after intrauterine death of one fetus or more

✓x7ᵗʰ **O31.20**   Continuing pregnancy after intrauterine death of one fetus or more, unspecified trimester   Ⓜ♀

✓x7ᵗʰ **O31.21**   Continuing pregnancy after intrauterine death of one fetus or more, first trimester   Ⓜ♀

✓x7ᵗʰ **O31.22**   Continuing pregnancy after intrauterine death of one fetus or more, second trimester   Ⓜ♀

✓x7ᵗʰ **O31.23**   Continuing pregnancy after intrauterine death of one fetus or more, third trimester   Ⓜ♀

✓5ᵗʰ **O31.3**   Continuing pregnancy after elective fetal reduction of one fetus or more
Continuing pregnancy after selective termination of one fetus or more

✓x7ᵗʰ **O31.30**   Continuing pregnancy after elective fetal reduction of one fetus or more, unspecified trimester   Ⓜ♀

✓x7ᵗʰ **O31.31**   Continuing pregnancy after elective fetal reduction of one fetus or more, first trimester   Ⓜ♀

✓x7ᵗʰ **O31.32**   Continuing pregnancy after elective fetal reduction of one fetus or more, second trimester   Ⓜ♀

✓x7ᵗʰ **O31.33**   Continuing pregnancy after elective fetal reduction of one fetus or more, third trimester   Ⓜ♀

✓5ᵗʰ **O31.8**   Other complications specific to multiple gestation

✓6ᵗʰ **O31.8X**   Other complications specific to multiple gestation

✓7ᵗʰ **O31.8X1**   Other complications specific to multiple gestation, first trimester   Ⓜ♀

✓7ᵗʰ **O31.8X2**   Other complications specific to multiple gestation, second trimester   Ⓜ♀

✓7ᵗʰ **O31.8X3**   Other complications specific to multiple gestation, third trimester   Ⓜ♀

✓7ᵗʰ **O31.8X9**   Other complications specific to multiple gestation, unspecified trimester   Ⓜ♀

✓ Additional Character Required   ✓x7ᵗʰ Xtension Alert   Unspecified Dx   Other Specified Dx   Manifestation   ►◄ Revised Text   ● New Code   ▲ Revised Code Title

ICD-10-CM Draft (2015)   **747**

Pregnancy, Childbirth and the Puerperium

O32–O34.01

✓4ᵗʰ **O32 Maternal care for malpresentation of fetus**

INCLUDES the listed conditions as a reason for observation, hospitalization or other obstetric care of the mother, or for cesarean delivery before onset of labor

EXCLUDES 1 malpresentation of fetus with obstructed labor (O64.-)

AHA: 2012, 4Q, 107

One of the following 7th characters is to be assigned to each code under category O32. 7th character Ø is for single gestations and multiple gestations where the fetus is unspecified. 7th characters 1 through 9 are for cases of multiple gestations to identify the fetus for which the code applies. The appropriate code from category O3Ø, Multiple gestation, must also be assigned when assigning a code from category O32 that has a 7th character of 1 through 9.

Ø	not applicable or unspecified	4	fetus 4
1	fetus 1	5	fetus 5
2	fetus 2	9	other fetus
3	fetus 3		

✓x7ᵗʰ **O32.Ø Maternal care for unstable lie** Ⓜ♀

✓x7ᵗʰ **O32.1 Maternal care for breech presentation** Ⓜ♀
Maternal care for buttocks presentation
Maternal care for complete breech
Maternal care for frank breech
EXCLUDES 1 footling presentation (O32.8)
incomplete breech (O32.8)

✓x7ᵗʰ **O32.2 Maternal care for transverse and oblique lie** Ⓜ♀
Maternal care for oblique presentation
Maternal care for transverse presentation

✓x7ᵗʰ **O32.3 Maternal care for face, brow and chin presentation** Ⓜ♀

✓x7ᵗʰ **O32.4 Maternal care for high head at term** Ⓜ♀
Maternal care for failure of head to enter pelvic brim

✓x7ᵗʰ **O32.6 Maternal care for compound presentation** Ⓜ♀

✓x7ᵗʰ **O32.8 Maternal care for other malpresentation of fetus** Ⓜ♀
Maternal care for footling presentation
Maternal care for incomplete breech

✓x7ᵗʰ **O32.9 Maternal care for malpresentation of fetus, unspecified** Ⓜ♀

✓4ᵗʰ **O33 Maternal care for disproportion**

INCLUDES the listed conditions as a reason for observation, hospitalization or other obstetric care of the mother, or for cesarean delivery before onset of labor

EXCLUDES 1 disproportion with obstructed labor (O65-O66)

O33.Ø Maternal care for disproportion due to deformity of maternal pelvic bones Ⓜ♀
Maternal care for disproportion due to pelvic deformity causing disproportion NOS

O33.1 Maternal care for disproportion due to generally contracted pelvis Ⓜ♀
Maternal care for disproportion due to contracted pelvis NOS causing disproportion

O33.2 Maternal care for disproportion due to inlet contraction of pelvis Ⓜ♀
Maternal care for disproportion due to inlet contraction (pelvis) causing disproportion

✓x7ᵗʰ **O33.3 Maternal care for disproportion due to outlet contraction of pelvis** Ⓜ♀
Maternal care for disproportion due to mid-cavity contraction (pelvis)
Maternal care for disproportion due to outlet contraction (pelvis)

One of the following 7th characters is to be assigned to code O33.3. 7th character Ø is for single gestations and multiple gestations where the fetus is unspecified. 7th characters 1 through 9 are for cases of multiple gestations to identify the fetus for which the code applies. The appropriate code from category O3Ø, Multiple gestation, must also be assigned when assigning code O33.3 with a 7th character of 1 through 9.

Ø	not applicable or unspecified	4	fetus 4
1	fetus 1	5	fetus 5
2	fetus 2	9	other fetus
3	fetus 3		

✓x7ᵗʰ **O33.4 Maternal care for disproportion of mixed maternal and fetal origin** Ⓜ♀

One of the following 7th characters is to be assigned to code O33.4. 7th character Ø is for single gestations and multiple gestations where the fetus is unspecified. 7th characters 1 through 9 are for cases of multiple gestations to identify the fetus for which the code applies. The appropriate code from category O3Ø, Multiple gestation, must also be assigned when assigning code O33.4 with a 7th character of 1 through 9.

Ø	not applicable or unspecified	4	fetus 4
1	fetus 1	5	fetus 5
2	fetus 2	9	other fetus
3	fetus 3		

✓x7ᵗʰ **O33.5 Maternal care for disproportion due to unusually large fetus** Ⓜ♀
Maternal care for disproportion due to disproportion of fetal origin with normally formed fetus
Maternal care for disproportion due to fetal disproportion NOS

One of the following 7th characters is to be assigned to code O33.5. 7th character Ø is for single gestations and multiple gestations where the fetus is unspecified. 7th characters 1 through 9 are for cases of multiple gestations to identify the fetus for which the code applies. The appropriate code from category O3Ø, Multiple gestation, must also be assigned when assigning code O33.5 with a 7th character of 1 through 9.

Ø	not applicable or unspecified	4	fetus 4
1	fetus 1	5	fetus 5
2	fetus 2	9	other fetus
3	fetus 3		

✓x7ᵗʰ **O33.6 Maternal care for disproportion due to hydrocephalic fetus** Ⓜ♀

One of the following 7th characters is to be assigned to code O33.6. 7th character Ø is for single gestations and multiple gestations where the fetus is unspecified. 7th characters 1 through 9 are for cases of multiple gestations to identify the fetus for which the code applies. The appropriate code from category O3Ø, Multiple gestation, must also be assigned when assigning code O33.6 with a 7th character of 1 through 9.

Ø	not applicable or unspecified	4	fetus 4
1	fetus 1	5	fetus 5
2	fetus 2	9	other fetus
3	fetus 3		

O33.7 Maternal care for disproportion due to other fetal deformities Ⓜ♀
Maternal care for disproportion due to fetal ascites
Maternal care for disproportion due to fetal hydrops
Maternal care for disproportion due to fetal meningomyelocele
Maternal care for disproportion due to fetal sacral teratoma
Maternal care for disproportion due to fetal tumor
EXCLUDES 1 obstructed labor due to other fetal deformities (O66.3)

O33.8 Maternal care for disproportion of other origin Ⓜ♀

O33.9 Maternal care for disproportion, unspecified Ⓜ♀
Maternal care for disproportion due to cephalopelvic disproportion NOS
Maternal care for disproportion due to fetopelvic disproportion NOS

✓4ᵗʰ **O34 Maternal care for abnormality of pelvic organs**

INCLUDES the listed conditions as a reason for hospitalization or other obstetric care of the mother, or for cesarean delivery before onset of labor

Code first any associated obstructed labor (O65.5)

Use additional code for specific condition

✓5ᵗʰ **O34.Ø Maternal care for congenital malformation of uterus**

O34.ØØ Maternal care for unspecified congenital malformation of uterus, unspecified trimester Ⓜ♀

O34.Ø1 Maternal care for unspecified congenital malformation of uterus, first trimester Ⓜ♀

EXCLUDES 1 Not coded here   EXCLUDES 2 Not included here   Ⓝ Newborn Age: Ø   Ⓟ Pediatric Age: Ø-17   Ⓜ Maternity Age: 12-55   Ⓐ Adult Age: 15-124

748   ICD-10-CM Draft (2015)

O34.02 Maternal care for unspecified congenital malformation of uterus, second trimester Ⓜ♀

O34.03 Maternal care for unspecified congenital malformation of uterus, third trimester Ⓜ♀

√5ᵗʰ **O34.1 Maternal care for** benign tumor of corpus uteri
EXCLUDES 2   maternal care for benign tumor of cervix (O34.4-)
maternal care for malignant neoplasm of uterus (O9A.1-)

O34.10 Maternal care for benign tumor of corpus uteri, unspecified trimester Ⓜ♀

O34.11 Maternal care for benign tumor of corpus uteri, first trimester Ⓜ♀

O34.12 Maternal care for benign tumor of corpus uteri, second trimester Ⓜ♀

O34.13 Maternal care for benign tumor of corpus uteri, third trimester Ⓜ♀

√5ᵗʰ **O34.2 Maternal care due to** uterine scar from previous surgery

O34.21 Maternal care for scar from previous cesarean delivery Ⓜ♀

O34.29 Maternal care due to uterine scar from other previous surgery Ⓜ♀

√5ᵗʰ **O34.3 Maternal care for** cervical incompetence
Maternal care for cerclage with or without cervical incompetence
Maternal care for Shirodkar suture with or without cervical incompetence

O34.30 Maternal care for cervical incompetence, unspecified trimester Ⓜ♀

O34.31 Maternal care for cervical incompetence, first trimester Ⓜ♀

O34.32 Maternal care for cervical incompetence, second trimester Ⓜ♀

O34.33 Maternal care for cervical incompetence, third trimester Ⓜ♀

√5ᵗʰ **O34.4 Maternal care for** other abnormalities of cervix

O34.40 Maternal care for other abnormalities of cervix, unspecified trimester Ⓜ♀

O34.41 Maternal care for other abnormalities of cervix, first trimester Ⓜ♀

O34.42 Maternal care for other abnormalities of cervix, second trimester Ⓜ♀

O34.43 Maternal care for other abnormalities of cervix, third trimester Ⓜ♀

√5ᵗʰ **O34.5 Maternal care for** other abnormalities of gravid uterus

√6ᵗʰ **O34.51 Maternal care for** incarceration of gravid uterus

O34.511 Maternal care for incarceration of gravid uterus, first trimester Ⓜ♀

O34.512 Maternal care for incarceration of gravid uterus, second trimester Ⓜ♀

O34.513 Maternal care for incarceration of gravid uterus, third trimester Ⓜ♀

O34.519 Maternal care for incarceration of gravid uterus, unspecified trimester Ⓜ♀

√6ᵗʰ **O34.52 Maternal care for** prolapse of gravid uterus

O34.521 Maternal care for prolapse of gravid uterus, first trimester Ⓜ♀

O34.522 Maternal care for prolapse of gravid uterus, second trimester Ⓜ♀

O34.523 Maternal care for prolapse of gravid uterus, third trimester Ⓜ♀

O34.529 Maternal care for prolapse of gravid uterus, unspecified trimester Ⓜ♀

√6ᵗʰ **O34.53 Maternal care for** retroversion of gravid uterus

O34.531 Maternal care for retroversion of gravid uterus, first trimester Ⓜ♀

O34.532 Maternal care for retroversion of gravid uterus, second trimester Ⓜ♀

O34.533 Maternal care for retroversion of gravid uterus, third trimester Ⓜ♀

O34.539 Maternal care for retroversion of gravid uterus, unspecified trimester Ⓜ♀

√6ᵗʰ **O34.59 Maternal care for** other abnormalities of gravid uterus

O34.591 Maternal care for other abnormalities of gravid uterus, first trimester Ⓜ♀

O34.592 Maternal care for other abnormalities of gravid uterus, second trimester Ⓜ♀

O34.593 Maternal care for other abnormalities of gravid uterus, third trimester Ⓜ♀

O34.599 Maternal care for other abnormalities of gravid uterus, unspecified trimester Ⓜ♀

√5ᵗʰ **O34.6 Maternal care for** abnormality of vagina
EXCLUDES 2   maternal care for vaginal varices in pregnancy (O22.1-)

O34.60 Maternal care for abnormality of vagina, unspecified trimester Ⓜ♀

O34.61 Maternal care for abnormality of vagina, first trimester Ⓜ♀

O34.62 Maternal care for abnormality of vagina, second trimester Ⓜ♀

O34.63 Maternal care for abnormality of vagina, third trimester Ⓜ♀

√5ᵗʰ **O34.7 Maternal care for** abnormality of vulva and perineum
EXCLUDES 2   maternal care for perineal and vulval varices in pregnancy (O22.1-)

O34.70 Maternal care for abnormality of vulva and perineum, unspecified trimester Ⓜ♀

O34.71 Maternal care for abnormality of vulva and perineum, first trimester Ⓜ♀

O34.72 Maternal care for abnormality of vulva and perineum, second trimester Ⓜ♀

O34.73 Maternal care for abnormality of vulva and perineum, third trimester Ⓜ♀

√5ᵗʰ **O34.8 Maternal care for** other abnormalities of pelvic organs

O34.80 Maternal care for other abnormalities of pelvic organs, unspecified trimester Ⓜ♀

O34.81 Maternal care for other abnormalities of pelvic organs, first trimester Ⓜ♀

O34.82 Maternal care for other abnormalities of pelvic organs, second trimester Ⓜ♀

O34.83 Maternal care for other abnormalities of pelvic organs, third trimester Ⓜ♀

√5ᵗʰ **O34.9 Maternal care for abnormality of pelvic organ,** unspecified

O34.90 Maternal care for abnormality of pelvic organ, unspecified, unspecified trimester Ⓜ♀

O34.91 Maternal care for abnormality of pelvic organ, unspecified, first trimester Ⓜ♀

O34.92 Maternal care for abnormality of pelvic organ, unspecified, second trimester Ⓜ♀

O34.93 Maternal care for abnormality of pelvic organ, unspecified, third trimester Ⓜ♀

√4ᵗʰ **O35 Maternal care for known or suspected fetal abnormality and damage**
INCLUDES   the listed conditions in the fetus as a reason for hospitalization or other obstetric care to the mother, or for termination of pregnancy
Code also any associated maternal condition
EXCLUDES 1   encounter for suspected maternal and fetal conditions ruled out (Z03.7-)

One of the following 7th characters is to be assigned to each code under category O35. 7th character Ø is for single gestations and multiple gestations where the fetus is unspecified. 7th characters 1 through 9 are for cases of multiple gestations to identify the fetus for which the code applies. The appropriate code from category O30, Multiple gestation, must also be assigned when assigning a code from category O35 that has a 7th character of 1 through 9.
Ø   not applicable or unspecified   4   fetus 4
1   fetus 1   5   fetus 5
2   fetus 2   9   other fetus
3   fetus 3

√x7ᵗʰ **O35.0 Maternal care for (suspected)** central nervous system malformation in fetus Ⓜ♀
Maternal care for fetal anencephaly
Maternal care for fetal hydrocephalus
Maternal care for fetal spina bifida
EXCLUDES 2   chromosomal abnormality in fetus (O35.1)

√x7ᵗʰ **O35.1 Maternal care for (suspected)** chromosomal abnormality in fetus Ⓜ♀

√x7ᵗʰ **O35.2 Maternal care for (suspected)** hereditary disease in fetus Ⓜ♀
EXCLUDES 2   chromosomal abnormality in fetus (O35.1)

√x7ᵗʰ **O35.3 Maternal care for (suspected)** damage to fetus from viral disease in mother Ⓜ♀
Maternal care for damage to fetus from maternal cytomegalovirus infection
Maternal care for damage to fetus from maternal rubella

Pregnancy, Childbirth and the Puerperium

O35.4–O36.72

√x 7th **O35.4** **Maternal care for (suspected) damage to fetus from alcohol** Ⓜ♀

√x 7th **O35.5** **Maternal care for (suspected) damage to fetus by drugs** Ⓜ♀
Maternal care for damage to fetus from drug addiction

√x 7th **O35.6** **Maternal care for (suspected) damage to fetus by radiation** Ⓜ♀

√x 7th **O35.7** **Maternal care for (suspected) damage to fetus by other medical procedures** Ⓜ♀
Maternal care for damage to fetus by amniocentesis
Maternal care for damage to fetus by biopsy procedures
Maternal care for damage to fetus by hematological investigation
Maternal care for damage to fetus by intrauterine contraceptive device
Maternal care for damage to fetus by intrauterine surgery

√x 7th **O35.8** **Maternal care for other (suspected) fetal abnormality and damage** Ⓜ♀
Maternal care for damage to fetus from maternal listeriosis
Maternal care for damage to fetus from maternal toxoplasmosis

√x 7th **O35.9** **Maternal care for (suspected) fetal abnormality and damage, unspecified** Ⓜ♀

√4th **O36** **Maternal care for other fetal problems**
INCLUDES the listed conditions in the fetus as a reason for hospitalization or other obstetric care of the mother, or for termination of pregnancy
EXCLUDES 1 encounter for suspected maternal and fetal conditions ruled out (Z03.7-)
placental transfusion syndromes (O43.0-)
EXCLUDES 2 labor and delivery complicated by fetal stress (O77.-)

One of the following 7th characters is to be assigned to each code under category O36. 7th character 0 is for single gestations and multiple gestations where the fetus is unspecified. 7th characters 1 through 9 are for cases of multiple gestations to identify the fetus for which the code applies. The appropriate code from category O30, Multiple gestation, must also be assigned when assigning a code from category O36 that has a 7th character of 1 through 9.
0	not applicable or unspecified	4	fetus 4
1	fetus 1	5	fetus 5
2	fetus 2	9	other fetus
3	fetus 3		

√5th **O36.0** **Maternal care for rhesus isoimmunization**
Maternal care for Rh incompatibility (with hydrops fetalis)

   √6th **O36.01** **Maternal care for anti-D [Rh] antibodies**

      √7th **O36.011** **Maternal care for anti-D [Rh] antibodies, first trimester** Ⓜ♀

      √7th **O36.012** **Maternal care for anti-D [Rh] antibodies, second trimester** Ⓜ♀

      √7th **O36.013** **Maternal care for anti-D [Rh] antibodies, third trimester** Ⓜ♀

      √7th **O36.019** **Maternal care for anti-D [Rh] antibodies, unspecified trimester** Ⓜ♀

   √6th **O36.09** **Maternal care for other rhesus isoimmunization**

      √7th **O36.091** **Maternal care for other rhesus isoimmunization, first trimester** Ⓜ♀

      √7th **O36.092** **Maternal care for other rhesus isoimmunization, second trimester** Ⓜ♀

      √7th **O36.093** **Maternal care for other rhesus isoimmunization, third trimester** Ⓜ♀

      √7th **O36.099** **Maternal care for other rhesus isoimmunization, unspecified trimester** Ⓜ♀

√5th **O36.1** **Maternal care for other isoimmunization**
Maternal care for ABO isoimmunization

   √6th **O36.11** **Maternal care for Anti-A sensitization**
Maternal care for isoimmunization NOS (with hydrops fetalis)

      √7th **O36.111** **Maternal care for Anti-A sensitization, first trimester** Ⓜ♀

      √7th **O36.112** **Maternal care for Anti-A sensitization, second trimester** Ⓜ♀

      √7th **O36.113** **Maternal care for Anti-A sensitization, third trimester** Ⓜ♀

      √7th **O36.119** **Maternal care for Anti-A sensitization, unspecified trimester** Ⓜ♀

   √6th **O36.19** **Maternal care for other isoimmunization**
Maternal care for Anti-B sensitization

      √7th **O36.191** **Maternal care for other isoimmunization, first trimester** Ⓜ♀

      √7th **O36.192** **Maternal care for other isoimmunization, second trimester** Ⓜ♀

      √7th **O36.193** **Maternal care for other isoimmunization, third trimester** Ⓜ♀

      √7th **O36.199** **Maternal care for other immunization, unspecified trimester** Ⓜ♀

√5th **O36.2** **Maternal care for hydrops fetalis**
Maternal care for hydrops fetalis NOS
Maternal care for hydrops fetalis not associated with isoimmunization
EXCLUDES 1 hydrops fetalis associated with ABO isoimmunization (O36.1-)
hydrops fetalis associated with rhesus isoimmunization (O36.0-)

   √x 7th **O36.20** **Maternal care for hydrops fetalis, unspecified trimester** Ⓜ♀

   √x 7th **O36.21** **Maternal care for hydrops fetalis, first trimester** Ⓜ♀

   √x 7th **O36.22** **Maternal care for hydrops fetalis, second trimester** Ⓜ♀

   √x 7th **O36.23** **Maternal care for hydrops fetalis, third trimester** Ⓜ♀

√x 7th **O36.4** **Maternal care for intrauterine death** Ⓜ♀
Maternal care for intrauterine fetal death NOS
Maternal care for intrauterine fetal death after completion of 20 weeks of gestation
Maternal care for late fetal death
Maternal care for missed delivery
EXCLUDES 1 missed abortion (O02.1)
stillbirth (P95)

√5th **O36.5** **Maternal care for known or suspected poor fetal growth**

   √6th **O36.51** **Maternal care for known or suspected placental insufficiency**

      √7th **O36.511** **Maternal care for known or suspected placental insufficiency, first trimester** Ⓜ♀

      √7th **O36.512** **Maternal care for known or suspected placental insufficiency, second trimester** Ⓜ♀

      √7th **O36.513** **Maternal care for known or suspected placental insufficiency, third trimester** Ⓜ♀

      √7th **O36.519** **Maternal care for known or suspected placental insufficiency, unspecified trimester** Ⓜ♀

   √6th **O36.59** **Maternal care for other known or suspected poor fetal growth**
Maternal care for known or suspected light-for-dates NOS
Maternal care for known or suspected small-for-dates NOS

      √7th **O36.591** **Maternal care for other known or suspected poor fetal growth, first trimester** Ⓜ♀

      √7th **O36.592** **Maternal care for other known or suspected poor fetal growth, second trimester** Ⓜ♀

      √7th **O36.593** **Maternal care for other known or suspected poor fetal growth, third trimester** Ⓜ♀

      √7th **O36.599** **Maternal care for other known or suspected poor fetal growth, unspecified trimester** Ⓜ♀

√5th **O36.6** **Maternal care for excessive fetal growth**
Maternal care for known or suspected large-for-dates

   √x 7th **O36.60** **Maternal care for excessive fetal growth, unspecified trimester** Ⓜ♀

   √x 7th **O36.61** **Maternal care for excessive fetal growth, first trimester** Ⓜ♀

   √x 7th **O36.62** **Maternal care for excessive fetal growth, second trimester** Ⓜ♀

   √x 7th **O36.63** **Maternal care for excessive fetal growth, third trimester** Ⓜ♀

√5th **O36.7** **Maternal care for viable fetus in abdominal pregnancy**

   √x 7th **O36.70** **Maternal care for viable fetus in abdominal pregnancy, unspecified trimester** Ⓜ♀

   √x 7th **O36.71** **Maternal care for viable fetus in abdominal pregnancy, first trimester** Ⓜ♀

   √x 7th **O36.72** **Maternal care for viable fetus in abdominal pregnancy, second trimester** Ⓜ♀

EXCLUDES 1 Not coded here   **EXCLUDES 2** Not included here   Ⓝ Newborn Age: 0   Ⓟ Pediatric Age: 0-17   Ⓜ Maternity Age: 12-55   Ⓐ Adult Age: 15-124

√x7ᵗʰ **O36.73** **Maternal care for viable fetus in abdominal** Ⓜ♀
pregnancy, third trimester

√5ᵗʰ **O36.8** **Maternal care for other specified fetal problems**

√x7ᵗʰ **O36.80** **Pregnancy with inconclusive fetal viability** Ⓜ♀
Encounter to determine fetal viability of pregnancy

√6ᵗʰ **O36.81** **Decreased fetal movements**

√7ᵗʰ **O36.812** **Decreased fetal movements,** second Ⓜ♀
trimester

√7ᵗʰ **O36.813** **Decreased fetal movements,** third Ⓜ♀
trimester

√7ᵗʰ **O36.819** **Decreased fetal movements,** Ⓜ♀
unspecified trimester

√6ᵗʰ **O36.82** **Fetal anemia and thrombocytopenia**

√7ᵗʰ **O36.821** **Fetal anemia and thrombocytopenia,** Ⓜ♀
first trimester

√7ᵗʰ **O36.822** **Fetal anemia and thrombocytopenia,** Ⓜ♀
second trimester

√7ᵗʰ **O36.823** **Fetal anemia and thrombocytopenia,** Ⓜ♀
third trimester

√7ᵗʰ **O36.829** **Fetal anemia and thrombocytopenia,** Ⓜ♀
unspecified trimester

√6ᵗʰ **O36.89** **Maternal care for other specified fetal problems**

√7ᵗʰ **O36.891** **Maternal care for other specified fetal** Ⓜ♀
problems, first trimester

√7ᵗʰ **O36.892** **Maternal care for other specified fetal** Ⓜ♀
problems, second trimester

√7ᵗʰ **O36.893** **Maternal care for other specified fetal** Ⓜ♀
problems, third trimester

√7ᵗʰ **O36.899** **Maternal care for other specified fetal** Ⓜ♀
problems, unspecified trimester

√5ᵗʰ **O36.9** **Maternal care for fetal problem, unspecified**

√x7ᵗʰ **O36.90** **Maternal care for fetal problem, unspecified,** Ⓜ♀
unspecified trimester

√x7ᵗʰ **O36.91** **Maternal care for fetal problem, unspecified,** Ⓜ♀
first trimester

√x7ᵗʰ **O36.92** **Maternal care for fetal problem, unspecified,** Ⓜ♀
second trimester

√x7ᵗʰ **O36.93** **Maternal care for fetal problem, unspecified,** Ⓜ♀
third trimester

√4ᵗʰ **O40** **Polyhydramnios**
Hydramnios

EXCLUDES 1 *encounter for suspected maternal and fetal conditions ruled out*
(Z03.7-)

One of the following 7th characters is to be assigned to each code
under category O40. 7th character 0 is for single gestations and
multiple gestations where the fetus is unspecified. 7th characters 1
through 9 are for cases of multiple gestations to identify the fetus
for which the code applies. The appropriate code from category
O30, Multiple gestation, must also be assigned when assigning a
code from category O40 that has a 7th character of 1 through 9.

0	not applicable or unspecified	4	fetus 4
1	fetus 1	5	fetus 5
2	fetus 2	9	other fetus
3	fetus 3		

√x7ᵗʰ **O40.1** **Polyhydramnios,** first trimester Ⓜ♀

√x7ᵗʰ **O40.2** **Polyhydramnios,** second trimester Ⓜ♀

√x7ᵗʰ **O40.3** **Polyhydramnios,** third trimester Ⓜ♀

√x7ᵗʰ **O40.9** **Polyhydramnios, unspecified trimester** Ⓜ♀

√4ᵗʰ **O41** **Other disorders of amniotic fluid and membranes**

EXCLUDES 1 *encounter for suspected maternal and fetal conditions ruled out*
(Z03.7-)

One of the following 7th characters is to be assigned to each code
under category O41. 7th character 0 is for single gestations and
multiple gestations where the fetus is unspecified. 7th characters 1
through 9 are for cases of multiple gestations to identify the fetus
for which the code applies. The appropriate code from category
O30, Multiple gestation, must also be assigned when assigning a
code from category O41 that has a 7th character of 1 through 9.

0	not applicable or unspecified	4	fetus 4
1	fetus 1	5	fetus 5
2	fetus 2	9	other fetus
3	fetus 3		

√5ᵗʰ **O41.0** **Oligohydramnios**
Oligohydramnios without rupture of membranes

√x7ᵗʰ **O41.00** **Oligohydramnios, unspecified trimester** Ⓜ♀

√x7ᵗʰ **O41.01** **Oligohydramnios,** first trimester Ⓜ♀

√x7ᵗʰ **O41.02** **Oligohydramnios,** second trimester Ⓜ♀

√x7ᵗʰ **O41.03** **Oligohydramnios,** third trimester Ⓜ♀

√5ᵗʰ **O41.1** **Infection of amniotic sac and membranes**

√6ᵗʰ **O41.10** **Infection of amniotic sac and membranes,**
unspecified

√7ᵗʰ **O41.101** **Infection of amniotic sac and** Ⓜ♀
membranes, unspecified, first
trimester

√7ᵗʰ **O41.102** **Infection of amniotic sac and** Ⓜ♀
membranes, unspecified, second
trimester

√7ᵗʰ **O41.103** **Infection of amniotic sac and** Ⓜ♀
membranes, unspecified, third
trimester

√7ᵗʰ **O41.109** **Infection of amniotic sac and** Ⓜ♀
membranes, unspecified, unspecified
trimester

√6ᵗʰ **O41.12** **Chorioamnionitis**

√7ᵗʰ **O41.121** **Chorioamnionitis,** first trimester Ⓜ♀

√7ᵗʰ **O41.122** **Chorioamnionitis,** second trimester Ⓜ♀

√7ᵗʰ **O41.123** **Chorioamnionitis,** third trimester Ⓜ♀

√7ᵗʰ **O41.129** **Chorioamnionitis,** unspecified Ⓜ♀
trimester

√6ᵗʰ **O41.14** **Placentitis**

√7ᵗʰ **O41.141** **Placentitis,** first trimester Ⓜ♀

√7ᵗʰ **O41.142** **Placentitis,** second trimester Ⓜ♀

√7ᵗʰ **O41.143** **Placentitis,** third trimester Ⓜ♀

√7ᵗʰ **O41.149** **Placentitis,** unspecified trimester Ⓜ♀

√5ᵗʰ **O41.8** **Other specified disorders of amniotic fluid and membranes**

√6ᵗʰ **O41.8X** **Other specified disorders of amniotic fluid and**
membranes

√7ᵗʰ **O41.8X1** **Other specified disorders of amniotic** Ⓜ♀
fluid and membranes, first trimester

√7ᵗʰ **O41.8X2** **Other specified disorders of amniotic** Ⓜ♀
fluid and membranes, second trimester

√7ᵗʰ **O41.8X3** **Other specified disorders of amniotic** Ⓜ♀
fluid and membranes, third trimester

√7ᵗʰ **O41.8X9** **Other specified disorders of amniotic** Ⓜ♀
fluid and membranes, unspecified
trimester

√5ᵗʰ **O41.9** **Disorder of amniotic fluid and membranes, unspecified**

√x7ᵗʰ **O41.90** **Disorder of amniotic fluid and membranes,** Ⓜ♀
unspecified, unspecified trimester

√x7ᵗʰ **O41.91** **Disorder of amniotic fluid and membranes,** Ⓜ♀
unspecified, first trimester

√x7ᵗʰ **O41.92** **Disorder of amniotic fluid and membranes,** Ⓜ♀
unspecified, second trimester

√x7ᵗʰ **O41.93** **Disorder of amniotic fluid and membranes,** Ⓜ♀
unspecified, third trimester

√4ᵗʰ **O42** **Premature rupture of membranes**

√5ᵗʰ **O42.0** **Premature rupture of membranes,** onset of labor within 24
hours of rupture

O42.00 **Premature rupture of membranes, onset of** Ⓜ♀
labor within 24 hours of rupture, unspecified
weeks of gestation

√6ᵗʰ **O42.01** **Preterm premature rupture of membranes,**
onset of labor within 24 hours of rupture
Premature rupture of membranes before 37
completed weeks of gestation

O42.011 **Preterm premature rupture of** Ⓜ♀
membranes, onset of labor within 24
hours of rupture, first trimester

O42.012 **Preterm premature rupture of** Ⓜ♀
membranes, onset of labor within 24
hours of rupture, second trimester

O42.013 **Preterm premature rupture of** Ⓜ♀
membranes, onset of labor within 24
hours of rupture, third trimester

O42.019 **Preterm premature rupture of** Ⓜ♀
membranes, onset of labor within 24
hours of rupture, unspecified trimester

✅ Additional Character Required   √x7ᵗʰ *X*tension Alert   Unspecified Dx   Other Specified Dx   Manifestation   ▶◀ Revised Text   ● New Code   ▲ Revised Code Title

Pregnancy, Childbirth and the Puerperium

O42.02–O43.819

O42.02   **Full-term premature rupture of membranes, onset of labor within 24 hours of rupture**   Ⓜ♀
     Premature rupture of membranes after 37 completed weeks of gestation

✓5th   **O42.1   Premature rupture of membranes, onset of labor more than 24 hours following rupture**

O42.10   **Premature rupture of membranes, onset of labor more than 24 hours following rupture, unspecified weeks of gestation**   Ⓜ♀

✓6th   O42.11   **Preterm premature rupture of membranes, onset of labor more than 24 hours following rupture**
     Premature rupture of membranes before 37 completed weeks of gestation

O42.111   **Preterm premature rupture of membranes, onset of labor more than 24 hours following rupture, first trimester**   Ⓜ♀

O42.112   **Preterm premature rupture of membranes, onset of labor more than 24 hours following rupture, second trimester**   Ⓜ♀

O42.113   **Preterm premature rupture of membranes, onset of labor more than 24 hours following rupture, third trimester**   Ⓜ♀

O42.119   **Preterm premature rupture of membranes, onset of labor more than 24 hours following rupture, unspecified trimester**   Ⓜ♀

O42.12   **Full-term premature rupture of membranes, onset of labor more than 24 hours following rupture**   Ⓜ♀
     Premature rupture of membranes after 37 completed weeks of gestation

✓5th   **O42.9   Premature rupture of membranes, unspecified as to length of time between rupture and onset of labor**

O42.90   **Premature rupture of membranes, unspecified as to length of time between rupture and onset of labor, unspecified weeks of gestation**   Ⓜ♀

✓6th   O42.91   **Preterm premature rupture of membranes, unspecified as to length of time between rupture and onset of labor**
     Premature rupture of membranes before 37 completed weeks of gestation

O42.911   **Preterm premature rupture of membranes, unspecified as to length of time between rupture and onset of labor, first trimester**   Ⓜ♀

O42.912   **Preterm premature rupture of membranes, unspecified as to length of time between rupture and onset of labor, second trimester**   Ⓜ♀

O42.913   **Preterm premature rupture of membranes, unspecified as to length of time between rupture and onset of labor, third trimester**   Ⓜ♀

O42.919   **Preterm premature rupture of membranes, unspecified as to length of time between rupture and onset of labor, unspecified trimester**   Ⓜ♀

O42.92   **Full-term premature rupture of membranes, unspecified as to length of time between rupture and onset of labor**   Ⓜ♀
     Premature rupture of membranes after 37 completed weeks of gestation

✓4th   **O43   Placental disorders**
     EXCLUDES 2   maternal care for poor fetal growth due to placental insufficiency (O36.5-)
        placenta previa (O44.-)
        placental polyp (O90.89)
        placentitis (O41.14-)
        premature separation of placenta [abruptio placentae] (O45.-)

✓5th   **O43.0   Placental transfusion syndromes**

✓6th   O43.01   **Fetomaternal placental transfusion syndrome**
     Maternofetal placental transfusion syndrome

O43.011   **Fetomaternal placental transfusion syndrome, first trimester**   Ⓜ♀

O43.012   **Fetomaternal placental transfusion syndrome, second trimester**   Ⓜ♀

O43.013   **Fetomaternal placental transfusion syndrome, third trimester**   Ⓜ♀

O43.019   **Fetomaternal placental transfusion syndrome, unspecified trimester**   Ⓜ♀

✓6th   O43.02   **Fetus-to-fetus placental transfusion syndrome**

O43.021   **Fetus-to-fetus placental transfusion syndrome, first trimester**   Ⓜ♀

O43.022   **Fetus-to-fetus placental transfusion syndrome, second trimester**   Ⓜ♀

O43.023   **Fetus-to-fetus placental transfusion syndrome, third trimester**   Ⓜ♀

O43.029   **Fetus-to-fetus placental transfusion syndrome, unspecified trimester**   Ⓜ♀

✓5th   **O43.1   Malformation of placenta**

✓6th   O43.10   **Malformation of placenta, unspecified**
     Abnormal placenta NOS

O43.101   **Malformation of placenta, unspecified, first trimester**   Ⓜ♀

O43.102   **Malformation of placenta, unspecified, second trimester**   Ⓜ♀

O43.103   **Malformation of placenta, unspecified, third trimester**   Ⓜ♀

O43.109   **Malformation of placenta, unspecified, unspecified trimester**   Ⓜ♀

✓6th   O43.11   **Circumvallate placenta**

O43.111   **Circumvallate placenta, first trimester**   Ⓜ♀

O43.112   **Circumvallate placenta, second trimester**   Ⓜ♀

O43.113   **Circumvallate placenta, third trimester** Ⓜ♀

O43.119   **Circumvallate placenta, unspecified trimester**   Ⓜ♀

✓6th   O43.12   **Velamentous insertion of umbilical cord**

O43.121   **Velamentous insertion of umbilical cord, first trimester**   Ⓜ♀

O43.122   **Velamentous insertion of umbilical cord, second trimester**   Ⓜ♀

O43.123   **Velamentous insertion of umbilical cord, third trimester**   Ⓜ♀

O43.129   **Velamentous insertion of umbilical cord, unspecified trimester**   Ⓜ♀

✓6th   O43.19   **Other malformation of placenta**

O43.191   **Other malformation of placenta, first trimester**   Ⓜ♀

O43.192   **Other malformation of placenta, second trimester**   Ⓜ♀

O43.193   **Other malformation of placenta, third trimester**   Ⓜ♀

O43.199   **Other malformation of placenta, unspecified trimester**   Ⓜ♀

✓5th   **O43.2   Morbidly adherent placenta**
     Code also associated third stage postpartum hemorrhage, if applicable (O72.0)
     EXCLUDES 1   retained placenta (O73.-)

✓6th   O43.21   **Placenta accreta**

O43.211   **Placenta accreta, first trimester**   Ⓜ♀

O43.212   **Placenta accreta, second trimester**   Ⓜ♀

O43.213   **Placenta accreta, third trimester**   Ⓜ♀

O43.219   **Placenta accreta, unspecified trimester**   Ⓜ♀

✓6th   O43.22   **Placenta increta**

O43.221   **Placenta increta, first trimester**   Ⓜ♀

O43.222   **Placenta increta, second trimester**   Ⓜ♀

O43.223   **Placenta increta, third trimester**   Ⓜ♀

O43.229   **Placenta increta, unspecified trimester**   Ⓜ♀

✓6th   O43.23   **Placenta percreta**

O43.231   **Placenta percreta, first trimester**   Ⓜ♀

O43.232   **Placenta percreta, second trimester**   Ⓜ♀

O43.233   **Placenta percreta, third trimester**   Ⓜ♀

O43.239   **Placenta percreta, unspecified trimester**   Ⓜ♀

✓5th   **O43.8   Other placental disorders**

✓6th   O43.81   **Placental infarction**

O43.811   **Placental infarction, first trimester**   Ⓜ♀

O43.812   **Placental infarction, second trimester**   Ⓜ♀

O43.813   **Placental infarction, third trimester**   ♀

O43.819   **Placental infarction, unspecified trimester**   Ⓜ♀

EXCLUDES 1 Not coded here   **EXCLUDES 2** Not included here   Ⓝ Newborn Age: 0   Ⓟ Pediatric Age: 0-17   Ⓜ Maternity Age: 12-55   Ⓐ Adult Age: 15-124

752   ICD-10-CM Draft (2015)

√6ᵗʰ **O43.89** **Other placental disorders**
Placental dysfunction

O43.891 **Other placental disorders, first trimester** ⓜ♀

O43.892 **Other placental disorders, second trimester** ⓜ♀

O43.893 **Other placental disorders, third trimester** ⓜ♀

O43.899 **Other placental disorders, unspecified trimester** ⓜ♀

√5ᵗʰ **O43.9** **Unspecified placental disorder**

O43.90 **Unspecified placental disorder, unspecified trimester** ⓜ♀

O43.91 **Unspecified placental disorder, first trimester** ⓜ♀

O43.92 **Unspecified placental disorder, second trimester** ⓜ♀

O43.93 **Unspecified placental disorder, third trimester** ⓜ♀

√4ᵗʰ **O44** **Placenta previa**

√5ᵗʰ **O44.0** **Placenta previa specified as without hemorrhage**
Low implantation of placenta specified as without hemorrhage

O44.00 **Placenta previa specified as without hemorrhage, unspecified trimester** ⓜ♀

O44.01 **Placenta previa specified as without hemorrhage, first trimester** ⓜ♀

O44.02 **Placenta previa specified as without hemorrhage, second trimester** ⓜ♀

O44.03 **Placenta previa specified as without hemorrhage, third trimester** ⓜ♀

√5ᵗʰ **O44.1** **Placenta previa with hemorrhage**
Low implantation of placenta, NOS or with hemorrhage
Marginal placenta previa, NOS or with hemorrhage
Partial placenta previa, NOS or with hemorrhage
Total placenta previa, NOS or with hemorrhage

EXCLUDES 1 *labor and delivery complicated by hemorrhage from vasa previa (O69.4)*

O44.10 **Placenta previa with hemorrhage, unspecified trimester** ⓜ♀

O44.11 **Placenta previa with hemorrhage, first trimester** ⓜ♀

O44.12 **Placenta previa with hemorrhage, second trimester** ⓜ♀

O44.13 **Placenta previa with hemorrhage, third trimester** ⓜ♀

√4ᵗʰ **O45** **Premature separation of placenta [abruptio placentae]**

√5ᵗʰ **O45.0** **Premature separation of placenta with coagulation defect**

√6ᵗʰ **O45.00** **Premature separation of placenta with coagulation defect, unspecified**

O45.001 **Premature separation of placenta with coagulation defect, unspecified, first trimester** ⓜ♀

O45.002 **Premature separation of placenta with coagulation defect, unspecified, second trimester** ⓜ♀

O45.003 **Premature separation of placenta with coagulation defect, unspecified, third trimester** ⓜ♀

O45.009 **Premature separation of placenta with coagulation defect, unspecified, unspecified trimester** ⓜ♀

√6ᵗʰ **O45.01** **Premature separation of placenta with afibrinogenemia**
Premature separation of placenta with hypofibrinogenemia

O45.011 **Premature separation of placenta with afibrinogenemia, first trimester** ⓜ♀

O45.012 **Premature separation of placenta with afibrinogenemia, second trimester** ⓜ♀

O45.013 **Premature separation of placenta with afibrinogenemia, third trimester** ⓜ♀

O45.019 **Premature separation of placenta with afibrinogenemia, unspecified trimester** ⓜ♀

√6ᵗʰ **O45.02** **Premature separation of placenta with disseminated intravascular coagulation**

O45.021 **Premature separation of placenta with disseminated intravascular coagulation, first trimester** ⓜ♀

O45.022 **Premature separation of placenta with disseminated intravascular coagulation, second trimester** ⓜ♀

O45.023 **Premature separation of placenta with disseminated intravascular coagulation, third trimester** ⓜ♀

O45.029 **Premature separation of placenta with disseminated intravascular coagulation, unspecified trimester** ⓜ♀

√6ᵗʰ **O45.09** **Premature separation of placenta with other coagulation defect**

O45.091 **Premature separation of placenta with other coagulation defect, first trimester** ⓜ♀

O45.092 **Premature separation of placenta with other coagulation defect, second trimester** ⓜ♀

O45.093 **Premature separation of placenta with other coagulation defect, third trimester** ⓜ♀

O45.099 **Premature separation of placenta with other coagulation defect, unspecified trimester** ⓜ♀

√5ᵗʰ **O45.8** **Other premature separation of placenta**

√6ᵗʰ **O45.8X** **Other premature separation of placenta**

O45.8X1 **Other premature separation of placenta, first trimester** ⓜ♀

O45.8X2 **Other premature separation of placenta, second trimester** ⓜ♀

O45.8X3 **Other premature separation of placenta, third trimester** ⓜ♀

O45.8X9 **Other premature separation of placenta, unspecified trimester** ⓜ♀

√5ᵗʰ **O45.9** **Premature separation of placenta, unspecified**
Abruptio placentae NOS

O45.90 **Premature separation of placenta, unspecified, unspecified trimester** ⓜ♀

O45.91 **Premature separation of placenta, unspecified, first trimester** ⓜ♀

O45.92 **Premature separation of placenta, unspecified, second trimester** ⓜ♀

O45.93 **Premature separation of placenta, unspecified, third trimester** ⓜ♀

√4ᵗʰ **O46** **Antepartum hemorrhage, not elsewhere classified**

EXCLUDES 1 *hemorrhage in early pregnancy (O20.-)*
intrapartum hemorrhage NEC (O67.-)
placenta previa (O44.-)
premature separation of placenta [abruptio placentae] (O45.-)

√5ᵗʰ **O46.0** **Antepartum hemorrhage with coagulation defect**

√6ᵗʰ **O46.00** **Antepartum hemorrhage with coagulation defect, unspecified**

O46.001 **Antepartum hemorrhage with coagulation defect, unspecified, first trimester** ⓜ♀

O46.002 **Antepartum hemorrhage with coagulation defect, unspecified, second trimester** ⓜ♀

O46.003 **Antepartum hemorrhage with coagulation defect, unspecified, third trimester** ⓜ♀

O46.009 **Antepartum hemorrhage with coagulation defect, unspecified, unspecified trimester** ⓜ♀

√6ᵗʰ **O46.01** **Antepartum hemorrhage with afibrinogenemia**
Antepartum hemorrhage with hypofibrinogenemia

O46.011 **Antepartum hemorrhage with afibrinogenemia, first trimester** ⓜ♀

O46.012 **Antepartum hemorrhage with afibrinogenemia, second trimester** ⓜ♀

O46.013 **Antepartum hemorrhage with afibrinogenemia, third trimester** ⓜ♀

O46.019 **Antepartum hemorrhage with afibrinogenemia, unspecified trimester** ⓜ♀

√6ᵗʰ **O46.02** **Antepartum hemorrhage with disseminated intravascular coagulation**

O46.021 **Antepartum hemorrhage with disseminated intravascular coagulation, first trimester** ⓜ♀

☑ Additional Character Required ᵥₓ₇ᵗʰ Xtension Alert Unspecified Dx Other Specified Dx Manifestation ▶◀ Revised Text ● New Code ▲ Revised Code Title

ICD-10-CM Draft (2015) 753

Pregnancy, Childbirth and the Puerperium

O46.022–O62.3

O46.022 **Antepartum hemorrhage with disseminated intravascular coagulation,** second trimester   Ⓜ♀

O46.023 **Antepartum hemorrhage with disseminated intravascular coagulation,** third trimester   Ⓜ♀

O46.029 **Antepartum hemorrhage with disseminated intravascular coagulation,** unspecified trimester   Ⓜ♀

✓6ᵗʰ O46.09 **Antepartum hemorrhage with** other **coagulation defect**

O46.091 **Antepartum hemorrhage with other coagulation defect,** first trimester   Ⓜ♀

O46.092 **Antepartum hemorrhage with other coagulation defect,** second trimester   Ⓜ♀

O46.093 **Antepartum hemorrhage with other coagulation defect,** third trimester   Ⓜ♀

O46.099 **Antepartum hemorrhage with other coagulation defect, unspecified trimester**   Ⓜ♀

✓5ᵗʰ O46.8 Other **antepartum hemorrhage**

✓6ᵗʰ O46.8X Other **antepartum hemorrhage**

O46.8X1 **Other antepartum hemorrhage,** first trimester   Ⓜ♀

O46.8X2 **Other antepartum hemorrhage,** second trimester   Ⓜ♀

O46.8X3 **Other antepartum hemorrhage,** third trimester   Ⓜ♀

O46.8X9 **Other antepartum hemorrhage, unspecified trimester**   Ⓜ♀

✓5ᵗʰ O46.9 **Antepartum hemorrhage,** unspecified

O46.90 **Antepartum hemorrhage, unspecified, unspecified trimester**   Ⓜ♀

O46.91 **Antepartum hemorrhage, unspecified,** first trimester   Ⓜ♀

O46.92 **Antepartum hemorrhage, unspecified,** second trimester   Ⓜ♀

O46.93 **Antepartum hemorrhage, unspecified,** third trimester   Ⓜ♀

✓4ᵗʰ **O47** **False labor**
Braxton Hicks contractions
Threatened labor
EXCLUDES 1   preterm labor (O60.-)

✓5ᵗʰ **O47.0** **False labor** before 37 completed weeks of gestation

O47.00 **False labor before 37 completed weeks of gestation, unspecified trimester**   Ⓜ♀

O47.02 **False labor before 37 completed weeks of gestation,** second trimester   Ⓜ♀

O47.03 **False labor before 37 completed weeks of gestation,** third trimester   Ⓜ♀

O47.1 **False labor** at or after 37 completed weeks of gestation   Ⓜ♀

O47.9 **False labor, unspecified**   Ⓜ♀

✓4ᵗʰ **O48** **Late pregnancy**

O48.0 **Post-term pregnancy**   Ⓜ♀
Pregnancy over 40 completed weeks to 42 completed weeks gestation

O48.1 **Prolonged pregnancy**   Ⓜ♀
Pregnancy which has advanced beyond 42 completed weeks gestation

Complications of labor and delivery (O60-O77)

✓4ᵗʰ **O60** **Preterm labor**
INCLUDES   onset (spontaneous) of labor before 37 completed weeks of gestation
EXCLUDES 1   false labor (O47.0-)
     threatened labor NOS (O47.0-)

✓5ᵗʰ **O60.0** **Preterm labor** without delivery

O60.00 **Preterm labor without delivery, unspecified trimester**   Ⓜ♀

O60.02 **Preterm labor without delivery,** second trimester   Ⓜ♀

O60.03 **Preterm labor without delivery,** third trimester   Ⓜ♀

✓5ᵗʰ **O60.1** **Preterm labor** with preterm delivery

One of the following 7th characters is to be assigned to each code under subcategory O60.1. 7th character Ø is for single gestations and multiple gestations where the fetus is unspecified. 7th characters 1 through 9 are for cases of multiple gestations to identify the fetus for which the code applies. The appropriate code from category O30, Multiple gestation, must also be assigned when assigning a code from subcategory O60.1 that has a 7th character of 1 through 9.

Ø	not applicable or unspecified	4	fetus 4
1	fetus 1	5	fetus 5
2	fetus 2	9	other fetus
3	fetus 3		

✓x7ᵗʰ O60.10 **Preterm labor with preterm delivery, unspecified trimester**   Ⓜ♀
Preterm labor with delivery NOS

✓x7ᵗʰ O60.12 **Preterm labor second trimester with preterm delivery** second trimester   Ⓜ♀

✓x7ᵗʰ O60.13 **Preterm labor second trimester with preterm delivery** third trimester   Ⓜ♀

✓x7ᵗʰ O60.14 **Preterm labor third trimester with preterm delivery** third trimester   Ⓜ♀

✓5ᵗʰ **O60.2** **Term delivery with preterm labor**

One of the following 7th characters is to be assigned to each code under subcategory O60.2. 7th character Ø is for single gestations and multiple gestations where the fetus is unspecified. 7th characters 1 through 9 are for cases of multiple gestations to identify the fetus for which the code applies. The appropriate code from category O30, Multiple gestation, must also be assigned when assigning a code from subcategory O60.2 that has a 7th character of 1 through 9.

Ø	not applicable or unspecified	4	fetus 4
1	fetus 1	5	fetus 5
2	fetus 2	9	other fetus
3	fetus 3		

✓x7ᵗʰ O60.20 **Term delivery with preterm labor, unspecified trimester**   Ⓜ♀

✓x7ᵗʰ O60.22 **Term delivery with preterm labor,** second trimester   Ⓜ♀

✓x7ᵗʰ O60.23 **Term delivery with preterm labor,** third trimester   Ⓜ♀

✓4ᵗʰ **O61** **Failed induction of labor**

O61.0 **Failed** medical **induction of labor**   Ⓜ♀
Failed induction (of labor) by oxytocin
Failed induction (of labor) by prostaglandins

O61.1 **Failed** instrumental **induction of labor**   Ⓜ♀
Failed mechanical induction (of labor)
Failed surgical induction (of labor)

O61.8 **Other failed induction of labor**   Ⓜ♀

O61.9 **Failed induction of labor, unspecified**   Ⓜ♀

✓4ᵗʰ **O62** **Abnormalities of forces of labor**

O62.0 **Primary inadequate contractions**   Ⓜ♀
Failure of cervical dilatation
Primary hypotonic uterine dysfunction
Uterine inertia during latent phase of labor

O62.1 **Secondary uterine inertia**   Ⓜ♀
Arrested active phase of labor
Secondary hypotonic uterine dysfunction

O62.2 **Other uterine inertia**   Ⓜ♀
Atony of uterus without hemorrhage
Atony of uterus NOS
Desultory labor
Hypotonic uterine dysfunction NOS
Irregular labor
Poor contractions
Slow slope active phase of labor
Uterine inertia NOS
EXCLUDES 1   atony of uterus with hemorrhage (postpartum) (O72.1)
     postpartum atony of uterus without hemorrhage (O75.89)

O62.3 **Precipitate labor**   Ⓜ♀

EXCLUDES 1 Not coded here   EXCLUDES 2 Not included here   Ⓝ Newborn Age: 0   Ⓟ Pediatric Age: 0-17   Ⓜ Maternity Age: 12-55   Ⓐ Adult Age: 15-124

754   ICD-10-CM Draft (2015)

O62.4 **Hypertonic, incoordinate, and prolonged uterine contractions** Ⓜ♀

Cervical spasm
Contraction ring dystocia
Dyscoordinate labor
Hour-glass contraction of uterus
Hypertonic uterine dysfunction
Incoordinate uterine action
Tetanic contractions
Uterine dystocia NOS
Uterine spasm

EXCLUDES1 *dystocia (fetal) (maternal) NOS (O66.9)*

O62.8 **Other abnormalities of forces of labor** Ⓜ♀

O62.9 **Abnormality of forces of labor, unspecified** Ⓜ♀

✓4ᵗʰ **O63** **Long labor**

O63.0 **Prolonged first stage** (of labor) Ⓜ♀

O63.1 **Prolonged second stage** (of labor) Ⓜ♀

O63.2 **Delayed delivery** of second twin, triplet, etc. Ⓜ♀

O63.9 **Long labor, unspecified** Ⓜ♀
Prolonged labor NOS

✓4ᵗʰ **O64** **Obstructed labor due to malposition and malpresentation of fetus**

One of the following 7th characters is to be assigned to each code under category O64. 7th character 0 is for single gestations and multiple gestations where the fetus is unspecified. 7th characters 1 through 9 are for cases of multiple gestations to identify the fetus for which the code applies. The appropriate code from category O30, Multiple gestation, must also be assigned when assigning a code from category O64 that has a 7th character of 1 through 9.

0	not applicable or unspecified	4	fetus 4
1	fetus 1	5	fetus 5
2	fetus 2	9	other fetus
3	fetus 3		

✓x7ᵗʰ **O64.0** **Obstructed labor due to incomplete rotation of fetal head** Ⓜ♀

Deep transverse arrest
Obstructed labor due to persistent occipitoiliac (position)
Obstructed labor due to persistent occipitoposterior (position)
Obstructed labor due to persistent occipitosacral (position)
Obstructed labor due to persistent occipitotransverse (position)

✓x7ᵗʰ **O64.1** **Obstructed labor due to breech presentation** Ⓜ♀

Obstructed labor due to buttocks presentation
Obstructed labor due to complete breech presentation
Obstructed labor due to frank breech presentation

✓x7ᵗʰ **O64.2** **Obstructed labor due to face presentation** Ⓜ♀
Obstructed labor due to chin presentation

✓x7ᵗʰ **O64.3** **Obstructed labor due to brow presentation** Ⓜ♀

✓x7ᵗʰ **O64.4** **Obstructed labor due to shoulder presentation** Ⓜ♀
Prolapsed arm
EXCLUDES1 *impacted shoulders (O66.0)*
shoulder dystocia (O66.0)

✓x7ᵗʰ **O64.5** **Obstructed labor due to compound presentation** Ⓜ♀

✓x7ᵗʰ **O64.8** **Obstructed labor due to other malposition and malpresentation** Ⓜ♀
Obstructed labor due to footling presentation
Obstructed labor due to incomplete breech presentation

✓x7ᵗʰ **O64.9** **Obstructed labor due to malposition and malpresentation, unspecified**

✓4ᵗʰ **O65** **Obstructed labor due to maternal pelvic abnormality**

O65.0 **Obstructed labor due to deformed pelvis** Ⓜ♀

O65.1 **Obstructed labor due to generally contracted pelvis** Ⓜ♀

O65.2 **Obstructed labor due to pelvic inlet contraction** Ⓜ♀

O65.3 **Obstructed labor due to pelvic outlet and mid-cavity contraction** Ⓜ♀

O65.4 **Obstructed labor due to fetopelvic disproportion, unspecified** Ⓜ♀
EXCLUDES1 *dystocia due to abnormality of fetus (O66.2-O66.3)*

O65.5 **Obstructed labor due to abnormality of maternal pelvic organs** Ⓜ♀
Obstructed labor due to conditions listed in O34-
Use additional code to identify abnormality of pelvic organs (O34.-)

O65.8 **Obstructed labor due to other maternal pelvic abnormalities** Ⓜ♀

O65.9 **Obstructed labor due to maternal pelvic abnormality, unspecified** Ⓜ♀

✓4ᵗʰ **O66** **Other obstructed labor**

O66.0 **Obstructed labor due to shoulder dystocia** Ⓜ♀
Impacted shoulders

O66.1 **Obstructed labor due to locked twins** Ⓜ♀

O66.2 **Obstructed labor due to unusually large fetus** Ⓜ♀

O66.3 **Obstructed labor due to other abnormalities of fetus** Ⓜ♀
Dystocia due to fetal ascites
Dystocia due to fetal hydrops
Dystocia due to fetal meningomyelocele
Dystocia due to fetal sacral teratoma
Dystocia due to fetal tumor
Dystocia due to hydrocephalic fetus
Use additional code to identify cause of obstruction

✓5ᵗʰ **O66.4** **Failed trial of labor**

O66.40 **Failed trial of labor, unspecified** Ⓜ♀

O66.41 **Failed attempted vaginal birth after previous cesarean delivery** Ⓜ♀
Code first rupture of uterus, if applicable (O71.0-, O71.1)

O66.5 **Attempted application of vacuum extractor and forceps** Ⓜ♀
Attempted application of vacuum or forceps, with subsequent delivery by forceps or cesarean delivery

O66.6 **Obstructed labor due to other multiple fetuses** Ⓜ♀

O66.8 **Other specified obstructed labor** Ⓜ♀
Use additional code to identify cause of obstruction

O66.9 **Obstructed labor, unspecified** Ⓜ♀
Dystocia NOS
Fetal dystocia NOS
Maternal dystocia NOS

✓4ᵗʰ **O67** **Labor and delivery complicated by intrapartum hemorrhage, not elsewhere classified**
EXCLUDES1 *antepartum hemorrhage NEC (O46.-)*
placenta previa (O44.-)
premature separation of placenta [abruptio placentae] (O45.-)
EXCLUDES2 *postpartum hemorrhage (O72.-)*

O67.0 **Intrapartum hemorrhage with coagulation defect** Ⓜ♀
Intrapartum hemorrhage (excessive) associated with afibrinogenemia
Intrapartum hemorrhage (excessive) associated with disseminated intravascular coagulation
Intrapartum hemorrhage (excessive) associated with hyperfibrinolysis
Intrapartum hemorrhage (excessive) associated with hypofibrinogenemia

O67.8 **Other intrapartum hemorrhage** Ⓜ♀
Excessive intrapartum hemorrhage

O67.9 **Intrapartum hemorrhage, unspecified** Ⓜ♀

O68 **Labor and delivery complicated by abnormality of fetal acid-base balance** Ⓜ♀
Fetal acidemia complicating labor and delivery
Fetal acidosis complicating labor and delivery
Fetal alkalosis complicating labor and delivery
Fetal metabolic acidemia complicating labor and delivery
EXCLUDES1 *fetal stress NOS (O77.9)*
labor and delivery complicated by electrocardiographic evidence of fetal stress (O77.8)
labor and delivery complicated by ultrasonic evidence of fetal stress (O77.8)
EXCLUDES2 *abnormality in fetal heart rate or rhythm (O76)*
labor and delivery complicated by meconium in amniotic fluid (O77.0)

✓4ᵗʰ **O69** **Labor and delivery complicated by umbilical cord complications**

One of the following 7th characters is to be assigned to each code under category O69. 7th character 0 is for single gestations and multiple gestations where the fetus is unspecified. 7th characters 1 through 9 are for cases of multiple gestations to identify the fetus for which the code applies. The appropriate code from category O30, Multiple gestation, must also be assigned when assigning a code from category O69 that has a 7th character of 1 through 9.

0	not applicable or unspecified	3	fetus 3
		4	fetus 4
1	fetus 1	5	fetus 5
2	fetus 2	9	other fetus

✓x7ᵗʰ **O69.0** **Labor and delivery complicated by prolapse of cord** Ⓜ♀

✓x7ᵗʰ **O69.1** **Labor and delivery complicated by cord around neck, with compression** Ⓜ♀
EXCLUDES1 *labor and delivery complicated by cord around neck, without compression (O69.81)*

✓ Additional Character Required   ✓x7ᵗʰ Xtension Alert   Unspecified Dx   Other Specified Dx   Manifestation   ▶◀ Revised Text   ● New Code   ▲ Revised Code Title

√x7th **O69.2 Labor and delivery complicated by other cord entanglement, with compression** MQ
Labor and delivery complicated by compression of cord NOS
Labor and delivery complicated by entanglement of cords of twins in monoamniotic sac
Labor and delivery complicated by knot in cord
EXCLUDES 1 labor and delivery complicated by other cord entanglement, without compression (O69.82)

√x7th **O69.3 Labor and delivery complicated by short cord** MQ

√x7th **O69.4 Labor and delivery complicated by vasa previa** MQ
Labor and delivery complicated by hemorrhage from vasa previa

√x7th **O69.5 Labor and delivery complicated by vascular lesion of cord** MQ
Labor and delivery complicated by cord bruising
Labor and delivery complicated by cord hematoma
Labor and delivery complicated by thrombosis of umbilical vessels

√5th **O69.8 Labor and delivery complicated by other cord complications**

√x7th **O69.81 Labor and delivery complicated by cord around neck, without compression** MQ

√x7th **O69.82 Labor and delivery complicated by other cord entanglement, without compression** MQ

√x7th **O69.89 Labor and delivery complicated by other cord complications** MQ

√x7th **O69.9 Labor and delivery complicated by cord complication, unspecified** MQ

√4th **O70 Perineal laceration during delivery**
Episiotomy extended by laceration
EXCLUDES 1 obstetric high vaginal laceration alone (O71.4)

O70.0 First degree perineal laceration during delivery MQ
Perineal laceration, rupture or tear involving fourchette during delivery
Perineal laceration, rupture or tear involving labia during delivery
Perineal laceration, rupture or tear involving skin during delivery
Perineal laceration, rupture or tear involving vagina during delivery
Perineal laceration, rupture or tear involving vulva during delivery
Slight perineal laceration, rupture or tear during delivery

O70.1 Second degree perineal laceration during delivery MQ
Perineal laceration, rupture or tear during delivery as in O70.0, also involving pelvic floor
Perineal laceration, rupture or tear during delivery as in O70.0, also involving perineal muscles
Perineal laceration, rupture or tear during delivery as in O70.0, also involving vaginal muscles
EXCLUDES 1 perineal laceration involving anal sphincter (O70.2)

O70.2 Third degree perineal laceration during delivery MQ
Perineal laceration, rupture or tear during delivery as in O70.1, also involving anal sphincter
Perineal laceration, rupture or tear during delivery as in O70.1, also involving rectovaginal septum
Perineal laceration, rupture or tear during delivery as in O70.1, also involving sphincter NOS
EXCLUDES 1 anal sphincter tear during delivery without third degree perineal laceration (O70.4)
perineal laceration involving anal or rectal mucosa (O70.3)

O70.3 Fourth degree perineal laceration during delivery MQ
Perineal laceration, rupture or tear during delivery as in O70.2, also involving anal mucosa
Perineal laceration, rupture or tear during delivery as in O70.2, also involving rectal mucosa

O70.4 Anal sphincter tear complicating delivery, not associated with third degree laceration MQ
EXCLUDES 1 anal sphincter tear with third degree perineal laceration (O70.2)

O70.9 Perineal laceration during delivery, unspecified MQ

√4th **O71 Other obstetric trauma**
Obstetric damage from instruments

√5th **O71.0 Rupture of uterus (spontaneous) before onset of labor** MQ
EXCLUDES 1 disruption of (current) cesarean delivery wound (O90.0)
laceration of uterus, NEC (O71.81)

O71.00 Rupture of uterus before onset of labor, unspecified trimester MQ

O71.02 Rupture of uterus before onset of labor, second trimester MQ

O71.03 Rupture of uterus before onset of labor, third trimester MQ

O71.1 Rupture of uterus during labor MQ
Rupture of uterus not stated as occurring before onset of labor
EXCLUDES 1 disruption of cesarean delivery wound (O90.0)
laceration of uterus, NEC (O71.81)

O71.2 Postpartum inversion of uterus MQ

O71.3 Obstetric laceration of cervix MQ
Annular detachment of cervix

O71.4 Obstetric high vaginal laceration alone MQ
Laceration of vaginal wall without perineal laceration
EXCLUDES 1 obstetric high vaginal laceration with perineal laceration (O70.-)

O71.5 Other obstetric injury to pelvic organs MQ
Obstetric injury to bladder
Obstetric injury to urethra
EXCLUDES 2 obstetric periurethral trauma (O71.82)

O71.6 Obstetric damage to pelvic joints and ligaments MQ
Obstetric avulsion of inner symphyseal cartilage
Obstetric damage to coccyx
Obstetric traumatic separation of symphysis (pubis)

O71.7 Obstetric hematoma of pelvis MQ
Obstetric hematoma of perineum
Obstetric hematoma of vagina
Obstetric hematoma of vulva

√5th **O71.8 Other specified obstetric trauma**

O71.81 Laceration of uterus, not elsewhere classified MQ

O71.82 Other specified trauma to perineum and vulva MQ
Obstetric periurethral trauma

O71.89 Other specified obstetric trauma MQ

O71.9 Obstetric trauma, unspecified MQ

√4th **O72 Postpartum hemorrhage**
INCLUDES hemorrhage after delivery of fetus or infant

O72.0 Third-stage hemorrhage MQ
Hemorrhage associated with retained, trapped or adherent placenta
Retained placenta NOS
Code also type of adherent placenta (O43.2-)

O72.1 Other immediate postpartum hemorrhage MQ
Hemorrhage following delivery of placenta
Postpartum hemorrhage (atonic) NOS
Uterine atony with hemorrhage
EXCLUDES 1 uterine atony NOS (O62.2)
uterine atony without hemorrhage (O62.2)
postpartum atony of uterus without hemorrhage (O75.89)

O72.2 Delayed and secondary postpartum hemorrhage MQ
Hemorrhage associated with retained portions of placenta or membranes after the first 24 hours following delivery of placenta
Retained products of conception NOS, following delivery

O72.3 Postpartum coagulation defects MQ
Postpartum afibrinogenemia
Postpartum fibrinolysis

√4th **O73 Retained placenta and membranes, without hemorrhage**
EXCLUDES 1 placenta accreta (O43.21-)
placenta increta (O43.22-)
placenta percreta (O43.23-)

O73.0 Retained placenta without hemorrhage MQ
Adherent placenta, without hemorrhage
Trapped placenta without hemorrhage

O73.1 Retained portions of placenta and membranes, without hemorrhage MQ
Retained products of conception following delivery, without hemorrhage

√4th **O74 Complications of anesthesia during labor and delivery**
INCLUDES maternal complications arising from the administration of a general, regional or local anesthetic, analgesic or other sedation during labor and delivery
Use additional code, if applicable, to identify specific complication

O74.0 Aspiration pneumonitis due to anesthesia during labor and delivery Q
Inhalation of stomach contents or secretions NOS due to anesthesia during labor and delivery
Mendelson's syndrome due to anesthesia during labor and delivery

O74.1 Other pulmonary complications of anesthesia during labor and delivery MQ

EXCLUDES 1 Not coded here   *EXCLUDES 2* Not included here   N Newborn Age: 0   P Pediatric Age: 0-17   M Maternity Age: 12-55   A Adult Age: 15-124

756   ICD-10-CM Draft (2015)

O74.2 Cardiac complications of anesthesia during labor and delivery Ⓜ♀

O74.3 Central nervous system complications of anesthesia during labor and delivery Ⓜ♀

O74.4 Toxic reaction to local anesthesia during labor and delivery Ⓜ♀

O74.5 Spinal and epidural anesthesia-induced headache during labor and delivery Ⓜ♀

O74.6 Other complications of spinal and epidural anesthesia during labor and delivery Ⓜ♀

O74.7 Failed or difficult intubation for anesthesia during labor and delivery Ⓜ♀

O74.8 Other complications of anesthesia during labor and delivery Ⓜ♀

O74.9 Complication of anesthesia during labor and delivery, unspecified Ⓜ♀

✓4ᵗʰ **O75** Other complications of labor and delivery, not elsewhere classified

> EXCLUDES 2 puerperal (postpartum) infection (O86.-)
> puerperal (postpartum) sepsis (O85)

O75.0 Maternal distress during labor and delivery Ⓜ♀

O75.1 Shock during or following labor and delivery Ⓜ♀
Obstetric shock following labor and delivery

O75.2 Pyrexia during labor, not elsewhere classified Ⓜ♀

O75.3 Other infection during labor Ⓜ♀
Sepsis during labor
Use additional code (B95-B97), to identify infectious agent

O75.4 Other complications of obstetric surgery and procedures Ⓜ♀
Cardiac arrest following obstetric surgery or procedures
Cardiac failure following obstetric surgery or procedures
Cerebral anoxia following obstetric surgery or procedures
Pulmonary edema following obstetric surgery or procedures
Use additional code to identify specific complication

> EXCLUDES 2 complications of anesthesia during labor and delivery (O74.-)
> disruption of obstetrical (surgical) wound (O90.0-O90.1)
> hematoma of obstetrical (surgical) wound (O90.2)
> infection of obstetrical (surgical) wound (O86.0)

O75.5 Delayed delivery after artificial rupture of membranes Ⓜ♀

✓5ᵗʰ **O75.8** Other specified complications of labor and delivery

O75.81 Maternal exhaustion complicating labor and delivery Ⓜ♀

O75.82 Onset (spontaneous) of labor after 37 completed weeks of gestation but before 39 completed weeks gestation, with delivery by (planned) cesarean section Ⓜ♀
Delivery by (planned) cesarean section occurring after 37 completed weeks of gestation but before 39 completed weeks gestation due to (spontaneous) onset of labor
Code first to specify reason for planned cesarean section such as:
cephalopelvic disproportion (normally formed fetus) (O33.9)
previous cesarean delivery (O34.21)

O75.89 Other specified complications of labor and delivery Ⓜ♀

O75.9 Complication of labor and delivery, unspecified Ⓜ♀

O76 Abnormality in fetal heart rate and rhythm complicating labor and delivery Ⓜ♀
Depressed fetal heart rate tones complicating labor and delivery
Fetal bradycardia complicating labor and delivery
Fetal heart rate abnormal variability complicating labor and delivery
Fetal heart rate decelerations complicating labor and delivery
Fetal heart rate irregularity complicating labor and delivery
Fetal tachycardia complicating labor and delivery
Non-reassuring fetal heart rate or rhythm complicating labor and delivery

> EXCLUDES 1 fetal stress NOS (O77.9)
> labor and delivery complicated by electrocardiographic evidence of fetal stress (O77.8)
> labor and delivery complicated by ultrasonic evidence of fetal stress (O77.8)

> EXCLUDES 2 fetal metabolic acidemia (O68)
> other fetal stress (O77.0-O77.1)

AHA: 2013, 4Q, 118

✓4ᵗʰ **O77** Other fetal stress complicating labor and delivery

O77.0 Labor and delivery complicated by meconium in amniotic fluid Ⓜ♀
AHA: 2013, 4Q, 117-118

O77.1 Fetal stress in labor or delivery due to drug administration Ⓜ♀

O77.8 Labor and delivery complicated by other evidence of fetal stress Ⓜ♀
Labor and delivery complicated by electrocardiographic evidence of fetal stress
Labor and delivery complicated by ultrasonic evidence of fetal stress

> EXCLUDES 1 abnormality in fetal heart rate or rhythm (O76)
> abnormality of fetal acid-base balance (O68)
> fetal metabolic acidemia (O68)

O77.9 Labor and delivery complicated by fetal stress, unspecified Ⓜ♀

> EXCLUDES 1 abnormality in fetal heart rate or rhythm (O76)
> abnormality of fetal acid-base balance (O68)
> fetal metabolic acidemia (O68)

Encounter for delivery (O80, O82)

O80 Encounter for full-term uncomplicated delivery Ⓜ♀
> NOTE Delivery requiring minimal or no assistance, with or without episiotomy, without fetal manipulation [e.g., rotation version] or instrumentation [forceps] of a spontaneous, cephalic, vaginal, full-term, single, live-born infant. This code is for use as a single diagnosis code and is not to be used with any other code from chapter 15.

Use additional code to indicate outcome of delivery (Z37.0)
AHA: 2014, 2Q, 9

O82 Encounter for cesarean delivery without indication Ⓜ♀
Use additional code to indicate outcome of delivery (Z37.0)

Complications predominantly related to the puerperium (O85-O92)

> EXCLUDES 2 mental and behavioral disorders associated with the puerperium (F53)
> obstetrical tetanus (A34)
> puerperal osteomalacia (M83.0)

O85 Puerperal sepsis Ⓜ♀
Postpartum sepsis
Puerperal peritonitis
Puerperal pyemia
Use additional code (B95-B97), to identify infectious agent
Use additional code (R65.2-) to identify severe sepsis, if applicable

> EXCLUDES 1 fever of unknown origin following delivery (O86.4)
> genital tract infection following delivery (O86.1-)
> obstetric pyemic and septic embolism (O88.3-)
> puerperal septic thrombophlebitis (O86.81)
> urinary tract infection following delivery (O86.2-)

> EXCLUDES 2 sepsis during labor (O75.3)

✓4ᵗʰ **O86** Other puerperal infections
Use additional code (B95-B97), to identify infectious agent

> EXCLUDES 2 infection during labor (O75.3)
> obstetrical tetanus (A34)

O86.0 Infection of obstetric surgical wound Ⓜ♀
Infected cesarean delivery wound following delivery
Infected perineal repair following delivery

✓5ᵗʰ **O86.1** Other infection of genital tract following delivery

O86.11 Cervicitis following delivery Ⓜ♀

O86.12 Endometritis following delivery Ⓜ♀

O86.13 Vaginitis following delivery Ⓜ♀

O86.19 Other infection of genital tract following delivery Ⓜ♀

✓5ᵗʰ **O86.2** Urinary tract infection following delivery

O86.20 Urinary tract infection following delivery, unspecified Ⓜ♀
Puerperal urinary tract infection NOS

O86.21 Infection of kidney following delivery Ⓜ♀

O86.22 Infection of bladder following delivery Ⓜ♀
Infection of urethra following delivery

O86.29 Other urinary tract infection following delivery Ⓜ♀

O86.4 Pyrexia of unknown origin following delivery Ⓜ♀
Puerperal infection NOS following delivery
Puerperal pyrexia NOS following delivery

> EXCLUDES 2 pyrexia during labor (O75.2)

✓ Additional Character Required   ✓x7ᵗʰ Xtension Alert   Unspecified Dx   Other Specified Dx   Manifestation   ►◄ Revised Text   ● New Code   ▲ Revised Code Title

ICD-10-CM Draft (2015)   **757**

Pregnancy, Childbirth and the Puerperium

O86.8–O90.6

✓5ᵗʰ **O86.8** Other specified puerperal infections
  O86.81 Puerperal septic thrombophlebitis Ⓜ♀
  O86.89 Other specified puerperal infections Ⓜ♀

✓4ᵗʰ **O87** **Venous complications and hemorrhoids in the puerperium**
Venous complications in labor, delivery and the puerperium
  EXCLUDES 2 obstetric embolism (O88.-)
    puerperal septic thrombophlebitis (O86.81)
    venous complications in pregnancy (O22.-)

O87.0 Superficial thrombophlebitis in the puerperium Ⓜ♀
Puerperal phlebitis NOS
Puerperal thrombosis NOS

O87.1 Deep phlebothrombosis in the puerperium Ⓜ♀
Deep vein thrombosis, postpartum
Pelvic thrombophlebitis, postpartum
Use additional code to identify the deep vein thrombosis (I82.4-, I82.5-, I82.62-. I82.72-)
Use additional code, if applicable, for associated long-term (current) use of anticoagulants (Z79.01)

O87.2 Hemorrhoids in the puerperium Ⓜ♀

O87.3 Cerebral venous thrombosis in the puerperium Ⓜ♀
Cerebrovenous sinus thrombosis in the puerperium

O87.4 Varicose veins of lower extremity in the puerperium Ⓜ♀

O87.8 Other venous complications in the puerperium Ⓜ♀
Genital varices in the puerperium

O87.9 Venous complication in the puerperium, unspecified Ⓜ♀
Puerperal phlebopathy NOS

✓4ᵗʰ **O88** **Obstetric embolism**
  EXCLUDES 1 embolism complicating abortion NOS (O03.2)
    embolism complicating ectopic or molar pregnancy (O08.2)
    embolism complicating failed attempted abortion (O07.2)
    embolism complicating induced abortion (O04.7)
    embolism complicating spontaneous abortion (O03.2, O03.7)

✓5ᵗʰ **O88.0** Obstetric air embolism
  ✓6ᵗʰ **O88.01** Obstetric air embolism in pregnancy
    O88.011 Air embolism in pregnancy, first trimester Ⓜ♀
    O88.012 Air embolism in pregnancy, second trimester Ⓜ♀
    O88.013 Air embolism in pregnancy, third trimester Ⓜ♀
    O88.019 Air embolism in pregnancy, unspecified trimester Ⓜ♀
  O88.02 Air embolism in childbirth Ⓜ♀
  O88.03 Air embolism in the puerperium Ⓜ♀

✓5ᵗʰ **O88.1** Amniotic fluid embolism
Anaphylactoid syndrome in pregnancy
  ✓6ᵗʰ **O88.11** Amniotic fluid embolism in pregnancy
    O88.111 Amniotic fluid embolism in pregnancy, first trimester Ⓜ♀
    O88.112 Amniotic fluid embolism in pregnancy, second trimester Ⓜ♀
    O88.113 Amniotic fluid embolism in pregnancy, third trimester Ⓜ♀
    O88.119 Amniotic fluid embolism in pregnancy, unspecified trimester Ⓜ♀
  O88.12 Amniotic fluid embolism in childbirth Ⓜ♀
  O88.13 Amniotic fluid embolism in the puerperium Ⓜ♀

✓5ᵗʰ **O88.2** Obstetric thromboembolism
  ✓6ᵗʰ **O88.21** Thromboembolism in pregnancy
Obstetric (pulmonary) embolism NOS
    O88.211 Thromboembolism in pregnancy, first trimester Ⓜ♀
    O88.212 Thromboembolism in pregnancy, second trimester Ⓜ♀
    O88.213 Thromboembolism in pregnancy, third trimester Ⓜ♀
    O88.219 Thromboembolism in pregnancy, unspecified trimester Ⓜ♀
  O88.22 Thromboembolism in childbirth Ⓜ♀
  O88.23 Thromboembolism in the puerperium Ⓜ♀
Puerperal (pulmonary) embolism NOS

✓5ᵗʰ **O88.3** Obstetric pyemic and septic embolism
  ✓6ᵗʰ **O88.31** Pyemic and septic embolism in pregnancy
    O88.311 Pyemic and septic embolism in pregnancy, first trimester Ⓜ♀
    O88.312 Pyemic and septic embolism in pregnancy, second trimester Ⓜ♀
    O88.313 Pyemic and septic embolism in pregnancy, third trimester Ⓜ♀
    O88.319 Pyemic and septic embolism in pregnancy, unspecified trimester Ⓜ♀
  O88.32 Pyemic and septic embolism in childbirth Ⓜ♀
  O88.33 Pyemic and septic embolism in the puerperium Ⓜ♀

✓5ᵗʰ **O88.8** Other obstetric embolism
Obstetric fat embolism
  ✓6ᵗʰ **O88.81** Other embolism in pregnancy
    O88.811 Other embolism in pregnancy, first trimester Ⓜ♀
    O88.812 Other embolism in pregnancy, second trimester Ⓜ♀
    O88.813 Other embolism in pregnancy, third trimester Ⓜ♀
    O88.819 Other embolism in pregnancy, unspecified trimester Ⓜ♀
  O88.82 Other embolism in childbirth Ⓜ♀
  O88.83 Other embolism in the puerperium Ⓜ♀

✓4ᵗʰ **O89** **Complications of anesthesia during the puerperium**
  INCLUDES maternal complications arising from the administration of a general, regional or local anesthetic, analgesic or other sedation during the puerperium
Use additional code, if applicable, to identify specific complication

✓5ᵗʰ **O89.0** Pulmonary complications of anesthesia during the puerperium
  O89.01 Aspiration pneumonitis due to anesthesia during the puerperium Ⓜ♀
Inhalation of stomach contents or secretions NOS due to anesthesia during the puerperium
Mendelson's syndrome due to anesthesia during the puerperium
  O89.09 Other pulmonary complications of anesthesia during the puerperium Ⓜ♀

O89.1 Cardiac complications of anesthesia during the puerperium Ⓜ♀

O89.2 Central nervous system complications of anesthesia during the puerperium Ⓜ♀

O89.3 Toxic reaction to local anesthesia during the puerperium Ⓜ♀

O89.4 Spinal and epidural anesthesia-induced headache during the puerperium Ⓜ♀

O89.5 Other complications of spinal and epidural anesthesia during the puerperium Ⓜ♀

O89.6 Failed or difficult intubation for anesthesia during the puerperium Ⓜ♀

O89.8 Other complications of anesthesia during the puerperium Ⓜ♀

O89.9 Complication of anesthesia during the puerperium, unspecified Ⓜ♀

✓4ᵗʰ **O90** **Complications of the puerperium, not elsewhere classified**

O90.0 Disruption of cesarean delivery wound Ⓜ♀
Dehiscence of cesarean delivery wound
  EXCLUDES 1 rupture of uterus (spontaneous) before onset of labor (O71.0-)
    rupture of uterus during labor (O71.1)

O90.1 Disruption of perineal obstetric wound Ⓜ♀
Disruption of wound of episiotomy
Disruption of wound of perineal laceration
Secondary perineal tear

O90.2 Hematoma of obstetric wound Ⓜ♀

O90.3 Peripartum cardiomyopathy Ⓜ♀
Conditions in I42- arising during pregnancy and the puerperium
  EXCLUDES 1 pre-existing heart disease complicating pregnancy and the puerperium (O99.4-)

O90.4 Postpartum acute kidney failure Ⓜ♀
Hepatorenal syndrome following labor and delivery

O90.5 Postpartum thyroiditis Ⓜ♀

O90.6 Postpartum mood disturbance Ⓜ♀
Postpartum blues
Postpartum dysphoria
Postpartum sadness
  EXCLUDES 1 postpartum depression (F53)
    puerperal psychosis (F53)

EXCLUDES 1 Not coded here   EXCLUDES 2 Not included here   Ⓝ Newborn Age: 0   Ⓟ Pediatric Age: 0-17   Ⓜ Maternity Age: 12-55   Ⓐ Adult Age: 15-124

758   ICD-10-CM Draft (2015)

✓5ᵗʰ **O90.8 Other complications of the puerperium, not elsewhere classified**

    O90.81 Anemia of the puerperium Ⓜ♀

        Postpartum anemia NOS

        EXCLUDES 1 *pre-existing anemia complicating the puerperium (O99.03)*

    O90.89 Other complications of the puerperium, not elsewhere classified Ⓜ♀

        Placental polyp

    O90.9 Complication of the puerperium, unspecified Ⓜ♀

✓4ᵗʰ **O91 Infections of breast associated with pregnancy, the puerperium and lactation**

    Use additional code to identify infection

✓5ᵗʰ **O91.0 Infection of nipple associated with pregnancy, the puerperium and lactation**

    ✓6ᵗʰ **O91.01 Infection of nipple associated with pregnancy**

        Gestational abscess of nipple

        O91.011 Infection of nipple associated with pregnancy, first trimester Ⓜ♀

        O91.012 Infection of nipple associated with pregnancy, second trimester Ⓜ♀

        O91.013 Infection of nipple associated with pregnancy, third trimester Ⓜ♀

        O91.019 Infection of nipple associated with pregnancy, unspecified trimester Ⓜ♀

    O91.02 Infection of nipple associated with the puerperium Ⓜ♀

        Puerperal abscess of nipple

    O91.03 Infection of nipple associated with lactation Ⓜ♀

        Abscess of nipple associated with lactation

✓5ᵗʰ **O91.1 Abscess of breast associated with pregnancy, the puerperium and lactation**

    ✓6ᵗʰ **O91.11 Abscess of breast associated with pregnancy**

        Gestational mammary abscess

        Gestational purulent mastitis

        Gestational subareolar abscess

        O91.111 Abscess of breast associated with pregnancy, first trimester Ⓜ♀

        O91.112 Abscess of breast associated with pregnancy, second trimester Ⓜ♀

        O91.113 Abscess of breast associated with pregnancy, third trimester Ⓜ♀

        O91.119 Abscess of breast associated with pregnancy, unspecified trimester Ⓜ♀

    O91.12 Abscess of breast associated with the puerperium Ⓜ♀

        Puerperal mammary abscess

        Puerperal purulent mastitis

        Puerperal subareolar abscess

    O91.13 Abscess of breast associated with lactation Ⓜ♀

        Mammary abscess associated with lactation

        Purulent mastitis associated with lactation

        Subareolar abscess associated with lactation

✓5ᵗʰ **O91.2 Nonpurulent mastitis associated with pregnancy, the puerperium and lactation**

    ✓6ᵗʰ **O91.21 Nonpurulent mastitis associated with pregnancy**

        Gestational interstitial mastitis

        Gestational lymphangitis of breast

        Gestational mastitis NOS

        Gestational parenchymatous mastitis

        O91.211 Nonpurulent mastitis associated with pregnancy, first trimester Ⓜ♀

        O91.212 Nonpurulent mastitis associated with pregnancy, second trimester Ⓜ♀

        O91.213 Nonpurulent mastitis associated with pregnancy, third trimester Ⓜ♀

        O91.219 Nonpurulent mastitis associated with pregnancy, unspecified trimester Ⓜ♀

    O91.22 Nonpurulent mastitis associated with the puerperium Ⓜ♀

        Puerperal interstitial mastitis

        Puerperal lymphangitis of breast

        Puerperal mastitis NOS

        Puerperal parenchymatous mastitis

    O91.23 Nonpurulent mastitis associated with lactation Ⓜ♀

        Interstitial mastitis associated with lactation

        Lymphangitis of breast associated with lactation

        Mastitis NOS associated with lactation

        Parenchymatous mastitis associated with lactation

✓4ᵗʰ **O92 Other disorders of breast and disorders of lactation associated with pregnancy and the puerperium**

✓5ᵗʰ **O92.0 Retracted nipple associated with pregnancy, the puerperium, and lactation**

    ✓6ᵗʰ **O92.01 Retracted nipple associated with pregnancy**

        O92.011 Retracted nipple associated with pregnancy, first trimester Ⓜ♀

        O92.012 Retracted nipple associated with pregnancy, second trimester Ⓜ♀

        O92.013 Retracted nipple associated with pregnancy, third trimester Ⓜ♀

        O92.019 Retracted nipple associated with pregnancy, unspecified trimester Ⓜ♀

    O92.02 Retracted nipple associated with the puerperium Ⓜ♀

    O92.03 Retracted nipple associated with lactation Ⓜ♀

✓5ᵗʰ **O92.1 Cracked nipple associated with pregnancy, the puerperium, and lactation**

    Fissure of nipple, gestational or puerperal

    ✓6ᵗʰ **O92.11 Cracked nipple associated with pregnancy**

        O92.111 Cracked nipple associated with pregnancy, first trimester Ⓜ♀

        O92.112 Cracked nipple associated with pregnancy, second trimester Ⓜ♀

        O92.113 Cracked nipple associated with pregnancy, third trimester Ⓜ♀

        O92.119 Cracked nipple associated with pregnancy, unspecified trimester Ⓜ♀

    O92.12 Cracked nipple associated with the puerperium Ⓜ♀

    O92.13 Cracked nipple associated with lactation Ⓜ♀

✓5ᵗʰ **O92.2 Other and unspecified disorders of breast associated with pregnancy and the puerperium**

    O92.20 Unspecified disorder of breast associated with pregnancy and the puerperium ♀

    O92.29 Other disorders of breast associated with pregnancy and the puerperium Ⓜ♀

    O92.3 Agalactia Ⓜ♀

        Primary agalactia

        EXCLUDES 1 *elective agalactia (O92.5)*

                secondary agalactia (O92.5)

                therapeutic agalactia (O92.5)

    O92.4 Hypogalactia Ⓜ♀

    O92.5 Suppressed lactation Ⓜ♀

        Elective agalactia

        Secondary agalactia

        Therapeutic agalactia

        EXCLUDES 1 *primary agalactia (O92.3)*

    O92.6 Galactorrhea Ⓜ♀

✓5ᵗʰ **O92.7 Other and unspecified disorders of lactation**

    O92.70 Unspecified disorders of lactation Ⓜ♀

    O92.79 Other disorders of lactation Ⓜ♀

        Puerperal galactocele

Other obstetric conditions, not elsewhere classified (O94-O9A)

O94 Sequelae of complication of pregnancy, childbirth, and the puerperium Ⓜ♀

    NOTE This category is to be used to indicate conditions in O00-O77.-, O85-O94 and O98-O9A.- as the cause of late effects. The sequelae include conditions specified as such, or as late effects, which may occur at any time after the puerperium.

    Code first condition resulting from (sequela) of complication of pregnancy, childbirth, and the puerperium

✅ Additional Character Required   ✓7ᵗʰ Xtension Alert   Unspecified Dx   Other Specified Dx   Manifestation   ▶◀ Revised Text   ● New Code   ▲ Revised Code Title

ICD-10-CM Draft (2015)   **759**

Pregnancy, Childbirth and the Puerperium

O98–O98.73

√4ᵗʰ **O98 Maternal infectious and parasitic diseases classifiable elsewhere but complicating pregnancy, childbirth and the puerperium**

> **INCLUDES** the listed conditions when complicating the pregnant state, when aggravated by the pregnancy, or as a reason for obstetric care
>
> Use additional code (Chapter 1), to identify specific infectious or parasitic disease
>
> **EXCLUDES 2** *herpes gestationis (O26.4-)*
> *infectious carrier state (O99.82-, O99.83-)*
> *obstetrical tetanus (A34)*
> *puerperal infection (O86.-)*
> *puerperal sepsis (O85)*
> *when the reason for maternal care is that the disease is known or suspected to have affected the fetus (O35-O36)*

√5ᵗʰ **O98.0 Tuberculosis complicating pregnancy, childbirth and the puerperium**
> Conditions in A15-A19

  √6ᵗʰ **O98.01 Tuberculosis complicating** pregnancy

    O98.011 Tuberculosis complicating pregnancy, first trimester Ⓜ♀

    O98.012 Tuberculosis complicating pregnancy, second trimester Ⓜ♀

    O98.013 Tuberculosis complicating pregnancy, third trimester Ⓜ♀

    O98.019 Tuberculosis complicating pregnancy, unspecified trimester Ⓜ♀

  O98.02 Tuberculosis complicating childbirth Ⓜ♀

  O98.03 Tuberculosis complicating the puerperium Ⓜ♀

√5ᵗʰ **O98.1 Syphilis complicating pregnancy, childbirth and the puerperium**
> Conditions in A50-A53

  √6ᵗʰ **O98.11 Syphilis complicating** pregnancy

    O98.111 Syphilis complicating pregnancy, first trimester Ⓜ♀

    O98.112 Syphilis complicating pregnancy, second trimester Ⓜ♀

    O98.113 Syphilis complicating pregnancy, third trimester Ⓜ♀

    O98.119 Syphilis complicating pregnancy, unspecified trimester Ⓜ♀

  O98.12 Syphilis complicating childbirth Ⓜ♀

  O98.13 Syphilis complicating the puerperium Ⓜ♀

√5ᵗʰ **O98.2 Gonorrhea complicating pregnancy, childbirth and the puerperium**
> Conditions in A54-

  √6ᵗʰ **O98.21 Gonorrhea complicating** pregnancy

    O98.211 Gonorrhea complicating pregnancy, first trimester Ⓜ♀

    O98.212 Gonorrhea complicating pregnancy, second trimester Ⓜ♀

    O98.213 Gonorrhea complicating pregnancy, third trimester Ⓜ♀

    O98.219 Gonorrhea complicating pregnancy, unspecified trimester Ⓜ♀

  O98.22 Gonorrhea complicating childbirth Ⓜ♀

  O98.23 Gonorrhea complicating the puerperium Ⓜ♀

√5ᵗʰ **O98.3 Other infections with a predominantly sexual mode of transmission complicating pregnancy, childbirth and the puerperium**
> Conditions in A55-A64

  √6ᵗʰ **O98.31 Other infections with a predominantly sexual mode of transmission complicating** pregnancy

    O98.311 Other infections with a predominantly sexual mode of transmission complicating pregnancy, first trimester Ⓜ♀

    O98.312 Other infections with a predominantly sexual mode of transmission complicating pregnancy, second trimester Ⓜ♀

    O98.313 Other infections with a predominantly sexual mode of transmission complicating pregnancy, third trimester Ⓜ♀

    O98.319 Other infections with a predominantly sexual mode of transmission complicating pregnancy, unspecified trimester Ⓜ♀

    O98.32 Other infections with a predominantly sexual mode of transmission complicating childbirth Ⓜ♀

    O98.33 Other infections with a predominantly sexual mode of transmission complicating the puerperium Ⓜ♀

√5ᵗʰ **O98.4 Viral hepatitis complicating pregnancy, childbirth and the puerperium**
> Conditions in B15-B19

  √6ᵗʰ **O98.41 Viral hepatitis complicating** pregnancy

    O98.411 Viral hepatitis complicating pregnancy, first trimester Ⓜ♀

    O98.412 Viral hepatitis complicating pregnancy, second trimester Ⓜ♀

    O98.413 Viral hepatitis complicating pregnancy, third trimester Ⓜ♀

    O98.419 Viral hepatitis complicating pregnancy, unspecified trimester Ⓜ♀

  O98.42 Viral hepatitis complicating childbirth Ⓜ♀

  O98.43 Viral hepatitis complicating the puerperium Ⓜ♀

√5ᵗʰ **O98.5 Other viral diseases complicating pregnancy, childbirth and the puerperium**
> Conditions in A80-B09, B25-B34, R87.81-, R87.82-
> **EXCLUDES 1** *human immunodeficiency virus [HIV] disease complicating pregnancy, childbirth and the puerperium (O98.7-)*

  √6ᵗʰ **O98.51 Other viral diseases complicating** pregnancy

    O98.511 Other viral diseases complicating pregnancy, first trimester Ⓜ♀

    O98.512 Other viral diseases complicating pregnancy, second trimester Ⓜ♀

    O98.513 Other viral diseases complicating pregnancy, third trimester Ⓜ♀

    O98.519 Other viral diseases complicating pregnancy, unspecified trimester Ⓜ♀

  O98.52 Other viral diseases complicating childbirth Ⓜ♀

  O98.53 Other viral diseases complicating the puerperium Ⓜ♀

√5ᵗʰ **O98.6 Protozoal diseases complicating pregnancy, childbirth and the puerperium**
> Conditions in B50-B64

  √6ᵗʰ **O98.61 Protozoal diseases complicating** pregnancy

    O98.611 Protozoal diseases complicating pregnancy, first trimester Ⓜ♀

    O98.612 Protozoal diseases complicating pregnancy, second trimester Ⓜ♀

    O98.613 Protozoal diseases complicating pregnancy, third trimester Ⓜ♀

    O98.619 Protozoal diseases complicating pregnancy, unspecified trimester Ⓜ♀

  O98.62 Protozoal diseases complicating childbirth Ⓜ♀

  O98.63 Protozoal diseases complicating the puerperium Ⓜ♀

√5ᵗʰ **O98.7 Human immunodeficiency virus [HIV] disease complicating pregnancy, childbirth and the puerperium**
> Use additional code to identify the type of HIV disease:
> acquired immune deficiency syndrome (AIDS) (B20)
> asymptomatic HIV status (Z21)
> HIV positive NOS (Z21)
> symptomatic HIV disease (B20)

  √6ᵗʰ **O98.71 Human immunodeficiency virus [HIV] disease complicating** pregnancy

    O98.711 Human immunodeficiency virus [HIV] disease complicating pregnancy, first trimester Ⓜ♀

    O98.712 Human immunodeficiency virus [HIV] disease complicating pregnancy, second trimester Ⓜ♀

    O98.713 Human immunodeficiency virus [HIV] disease complicating pregnancy, third trimester Ⓜ♀

    O98.719 Human immunodeficiency virus [HIV] disease complicating pregnancy, unspecified trimester Ⓜ♀

  O98.72 Human immunodeficiency virus [HIV] disease complicating childbirth Ⓜ♀

  O98.73 Human immunodeficiency virus [HIV] disease complicating the puerperium Ⓜ♀

EXCLUDES 1 Not coded here   **EXCLUDES 2** Not included here   Ⓝ Newborn Age: 0   Ⓟ Pediatric Age: 0-17   Ⓜ Maternity Age: 12-55   Ⓐ Adult Age: 15-124

☑5ᵗʰ **O98.8** Other maternal infectious and parasitic diseases complicating pregnancy, childbirth and the puerperium

☑6ᵗʰ **O98.81** Other maternal infectious and parasitic diseases complicating pregnancy

O98.811 Other maternal infectious and parasitic diseases complicating pregnancy, first trimester Ⓜ♀

O98.812 Other maternal infectious and parasitic diseases complicating pregnancy, second trimester Ⓜ♀

O98.813 Other maternal infectious and parasitic diseases complicating pregnancy, third trimester Ⓜ♀

O98.819 Other maternal infectious and parasitic diseases complicating pregnancy, unspecified trimester Ⓜ♀

O98.82 Other maternal infectious and parasitic diseases complicating childbirth Ⓜ♀

O98.83 Other maternal infectious and parasitic diseases complicating the puerperium Ⓜ♀

☑5ᵗʰ **O98.9** Unspecified maternal infectious and parasitic disease complicating pregnancy, childbirth and the puerperium

☑6ᵗʰ **O98.91** Unspecified maternal infectious and parasitic disease complicating pregnancy

O98.911 Unspecified maternal infectious and parasitic disease complicating pregnancy, first trimester Ⓜ♀

O98.912 Unspecified maternal infectious and parasitic disease complicating pregnancy, second trimester Ⓜ♀

O98.913 Unspecified maternal infectious and parasitic disease complicating pregnancy, third trimester Ⓜ♀

O98.919 Unspecified maternal infectious and parasitic disease complicating pregnancy, unspecified trimester Ⓜ♀

O98.92 Unspecified maternal infectious and parasitic disease complicating childbirth Ⓜ♀

O98.93 Unspecified maternal infectious and parasitic disease complicating the puerperium Ⓜ♀

☑4ᵗʰ **O99** Other maternal diseases classifiable elsewhere but complicating pregnancy, childbirth and the puerperium

INCLUDES conditions which complicate the pregnant state, are aggravated by the pregnancy or are a main reason for obstetric care

Use additional code to identify specific condition

EXCLUDES 2 when the reason for maternal care is that the condition is known or suspected to have affected the fetus (O35-O36)

☑5ᵗʰ **O99.0** Anemia complicating pregnancy, childbirth and the puerperium

Conditions in D50-D64

EXCLUDES 1 anemia arising in the puerperium (O90.81)
postpartum anemia NOS (O90.81)

☑6ᵗʰ **O99.01** Anemia complicating pregnancy

O99.011 Anemia complicating pregnancy, first trimester Ⓜ♀

O99.012 Anemia complicating pregnancy, second trimester Ⓜ♀

O99.013 Anemia complicating pregnancy, third trimester Ⓜ♀

O99.019 Anemia complicating pregnancy, unspecified trimester Ⓜ♀

O99.02 Anemia complicating childbirth Ⓜ♀

O99.03 Anemia complicating the puerperium Ⓜ♀

EXCLUDES 1 postpartum anemia not pre-existing prior to delivery (O90.81)

☑5ᵗʰ **O99.1** Other diseases of the blood and blood-forming organs and certain disorders involving the immune mechanism complicating pregnancy, childbirth and the puerperium

Conditions in D65-D89

EXCLUDES 2 hemorrhage with coagulation defects (O45.-, O46.0-, O67.0, O72.3)

☑6ᵗʰ **O99.11** Other diseases of the blood and blood-forming organs and certain disorders involving the immune mechanism complicating pregnancy

O99.111 Other diseases of the blood and blood-forming organs and certain disorders involving the immune mechanism complicating pregnancy, first trimester Ⓜ♀

O99.112 Other diseases of the blood and blood-forming organs and certain disorders involving the immune mechanism complicating pregnancy, second trimester Ⓜ♀

O99.113 Other diseases of the blood and blood-forming organs and certain disorders involving the immune mechanism complicating pregnancy, third trimester Ⓜ♀

O99.119 Other diseases of the blood and blood-forming organs and certain disorders involving the immune mechanism complicating pregnancy, unspecified trimester Ⓜ♀

O99.12 Other diseases of the blood and blood-forming organs and certain disorders involving the immune mechanism complicating childbirth Ⓜ♀

O99.13 Other diseases of the blood and blood-forming organs and certain disorders involving the immune mechanism complicating the puerperium Ⓜ♀

☑5ᵗʰ **O99.2** Endocrine, nutritional and metabolic diseases complicating pregnancy, childbirth and the puerperium

Conditions in E00-E88

EXCLUDES 2 diabetes mellitus (O24.-)
malnutrition (O25.-)
postpartum thyroiditis (O90.5)

☑6ᵗʰ **O99.21** Obesity complicating pregnancy, childbirth, and the puerperium

Use additional code to identify the type of obesity (E66.-)

O99.210 Obesity complicating pregnancy, unspecified trimester Ⓜ♀

O99.211 Obesity complicating pregnancy, first trimester Ⓜ♀

O99.212 Obesity complicating pregnancy, second trimester Ⓜ♀

O99.213 Obesity complicating pregnancy, third trimester Ⓜ♀

O99.214 Obesity complicating childbirth Ⓜ♀

O99.215 Obesity complicating the puerperium Ⓜ♀

☑6ᵗʰ **O99.28** Other endocrine, nutritional and metabolic diseases complicating pregnancy, childbirth and the puerperium

O99.280 Endocrine, nutritional and metabolic diseases complicating pregnancy, unspecified trimester Ⓜ♀

O99.281 Endocrine, nutritional and metabolic diseases complicating pregnancy, first trimester Ⓜ♀

O99.282 Endocrine, nutritional and metabolic diseases complicating pregnancy, second trimester Ⓜ♀

O99.283 Endocrine, nutritional and metabolic diseases complicating pregnancy, third trimester Ⓜ♀

O99.284 Endocrine, nutritional and metabolic diseases complicating childbirth Ⓜ♀

O99.285 Endocrine, nutritional and metabolic diseases complicating the puerperium Ⓜ♀

☑5ᵗʰ **O99.3** Mental disorders and diseases of the nervous system complicating pregnancy, childbirth and the puerperium

☑6ᵗʰ **O99.31** Alcohol use complicating pregnancy, childbirth, and the puerperium

Use additional code(s) from F10 to identify manifestations of the alcohol use

O99.310 Alcohol use complicating pregnancy, unspecified trimester Ⓜ♀

O99.311 Alcohol use complicating pregnancy, first trimester Ⓜ♀

O99.312 Alcohol use complicating pregnancy, second trimester Ⓜ♀

O99.313 Alcohol use complicating pregnancy, third trimester Ⓜ♀

O99.314 Alcohol use complicating childbirth Ⓜ♀

☑ Additional Character Required   ✓x7ᵗʰ Xtension Alert   Unspecified Dx   Other Specified Dx   Manifestation   ▶◀ Revised Text   ● New Code   ▲ Revised Code Title

Pregnancy, Childbirth and the Puerperium

O99.315–O99.7

O99.315 Alcohol use complicating the puerperium Ⓜ♀

✓6ᵗʰ O99.32 Drug use complicating pregnancy, childbirth, and the puerperium
Use additional code(s) from F11-F16 and F18-F19 to identify manifestations of the drug use

O99.320 Drug use complicating pregnancy, unspecified trimester Ⓜ♀

O99.321 Drug use complicating pregnancy, first trimester Ⓜ♀

O99.322 Drug use complicating pregnancy, second trimester Ⓜ♀

O99.323 Drug use complicating pregnancy, third trimester Ⓜ♀

O99.324 Drug use complicating childbirth Ⓜ♀

O99.325 Drug use complicating the puerperium Ⓜ♀

✓6ᵗʰ O99.33 Smoking (tobacco) complicating pregnancy, childbirth, and the puerperium
Use additional code from F17 to identify type of tobacco

O99.330 Smoking (tobacco) complicating pregnancy, unspecified trimester Ⓜ♀

O99.331 Smoking (tobacco) complicating pregnancy, first trimester Ⓜ♀

O99.332 Smoking (tobacco) complicating pregnancy, second trimester Ⓜ♀

O99.333 Smoking (tobacco) complicating pregnancy, third trimester Ⓜ♀

O99.334 Smoking (tobacco) complicating childbirth Ⓜ♀

O99.335 Smoking (tobacco) complicating the puerperium Ⓜ♀

✓6ᵗʰ O99.34 Other mental disorders complicating pregnancy, childbirth, and the puerperium
Conditions in F01-F09 and F20-F99
EXCLUDES 2 postpartum mood disturbance (O90.6)
postnatal psychosis (F53)
puerperal psychosis (F53)

O99.340 Other mental disorders complicating pregnancy, unspecified trimester Ⓜ♀

O99.341 Other mental disorders complicating pregnancy, first trimester Ⓜ♀

O99.342 Other mental disorders complicating pregnancy, second trimester Ⓜ♀

O99.343 Other mental disorders complicating pregnancy, third trimester Ⓜ♀

O99.344 Other mental disorders complicating childbirth Ⓜ♀

O99.345 Other mental disorders complicating the puerperium Ⓜ♀

✓6ᵗʰ O99.35 Diseases of the nervous system complicating pregnancy, childbirth, and the puerperium
Conditions in G00-G99
EXCLUDES 2 pregnancy related peripheral neuritis (O26.8-)

O99.350 Diseases of the nervous system complicating pregnancy, unspecified trimester Ⓜ♀

O99.351 Diseases of the nervous system complicating pregnancy, first trimester Ⓜ♀

O99.352 Diseases of the nervous system complicating pregnancy, second trimester Ⓜ♀

O99.353 Diseases of the nervous system complicating pregnancy, third trimester Ⓜ♀

O99.354 Diseases of the nervous system complicating childbirth Ⓜ♀

O99.355 Diseases of the nervous system complicating the puerperium Ⓜ♀

✓5ᵗʰ O99.4 Diseases of the circulatory system complicating pregnancy, childbirth and the puerperium
Conditions in I00-I99
EXCLUDES 1 peripartum cardiomyopathy (O90.3)
EXCLUDES 2 hypertensive disorders (O10-O16)
obstetric embolism (O88.-)
venous complications and cerebrovenous sinus thrombosis in labor, childbirth and the puerperium (O87.-)
venous complications and cerebrovenous sinus thrombosis in pregnancy (O22.-)

✓6ᵗʰ O99.41 Diseases of the circulatory system complicating pregnancy

O99.411 Diseases of the circulatory system complicating pregnancy, first trimester Ⓜ♀

O99.412 Diseases of the circulatory system complicating pregnancy, second trimester Ⓜ♀

O99.413 Diseases of the circulatory system complicating pregnancy, third trimester Ⓜ♀

O99.419 Diseases of the circulatory system complicating pregnancy, unspecified trimester Ⓜ♀

O99.42 Diseases of the circulatory system complicating childbirth Ⓜ♀

O99.43 Diseases of the circulatory system complicating the puerperium Ⓜ♀

✓5ᵗʰ O99.5 Diseases of the respiratory system complicating pregnancy, childbirth and the puerperium
Conditions in J00-J99

✓6ᵗʰ O99.51 Diseases of the respiratory system complicating pregnancy

O99.511 Diseases of the respiratory system complicating pregnancy, first trimester Ⓜ♀

O99.512 Diseases of the respiratory system complicating pregnancy, second trimester Ⓜ♀

O99.513 Diseases of the respiratory system complicating pregnancy, third trimester Ⓜ♀

O99.519 Diseases of the respiratory system complicating pregnancy, unspecified trimester Ⓜ♀

O99.52 Diseases of the respiratory system complicating childbirth Ⓜ♀

O99.53 Diseases of the respiratory system complicating the puerperium Ⓜ♀

✓5ᵗʰ O99.6 Diseases of the digestive system complicating pregnancy, childbirth and the puerperium
Conditions in K00-K93
EXCLUDES 2 liver and biliary tract disorders in pregnancy, childbirth and the puerperium (O26.6-)

✓6ᵗʰ O99.61 Diseases of the digestive system complicating pregnancy

O99.611 Diseases of the digestive system complicating pregnancy, first trimester Ⓜ♀

O99.612 Diseases of the digestive system complicating pregnancy, second trimester Ⓜ♀

O99.613 Diseases of the digestive system complicating pregnancy, third trimester Ⓜ♀

O99.619 Diseases of the digestive system complicating pregnancy, unspecified trimester Ⓜ♀

O99.62 Diseases of the digestive system complicating childbirth Ⓜ♀

O99.63 Diseases of the digestive system complicating the puerperium Ⓜ♀

✓5ᵗʰ O99.7 Diseases of the skin and subcutaneous tissue complicating pregnancy, childbirth and the puerperium
Conditions in L00-L99
EXCLUDES 2 herpes gestationis (O26.4)
pruritic urticarial papules and plaques of pregnancy (PUPPP) (O26.86)

√6ᵗʰ **O99.71** Diseases of the skin and subcutaneous tissue complicating pregnancy

    O99.711 Diseases of the skin and subcutaneous tissue complicating pregnancy, first trimester ♂♀

    O99.712 Diseases of the skin and subcutaneous tissue complicating pregnancy, second trimester ♂♀

    O99.713 Diseases of the skin and subcutaneous tissue complicating pregnancy, third trimester ♂♀

    O99.719 Diseases of the skin and subcutaneous tissue complicating pregnancy, unspecified trimester ♂♀

O99.72 Diseases of the skin and subcutaneous tissue complicating childbirth ♂♀

O99.73 Diseases of the skin and subcutaneous tissue complicating the puerperium ♂♀

√5ᵗʰ **O99.8** Other specified diseases and conditions complicating pregnancy, childbirth and the puerperium
    Conditions in D00-D48, H00-H95, M00-N99, and Q00-Q99
    Use additional code to identify condition
    EXCLUDES 2 genitourinary infections in pregnancy (O23.-)
        infection of genitourinary tract following delivery (O86.1-O86.3)
        malignant neoplasm complicating pregnancy, childbirth and the puerperium (O9A.1-)
        maternal care for known or suspected abnormality of maternal pelvic organs (O34.-)
        postpartum acute kidney failure (O90.4)
        traumatic injuries in pregnancy (O9A.2)

√6ᵗʰ **O99.81** Abnormal glucose complicating pregnancy, childbirth and the puerperium
    EXCLUDES 1 gestational diabetes (O24.4-)

    O99.810 Abnormal glucose complicating pregnancy ♂♀

    O99.814 Abnormal glucose complicating childbirth ♂♀

    O99.815 Abnormal glucose complicating the puerperium ♂♀

√6ᵗʰ **O99.82** Streptococcus B carrier state complicating pregnancy, childbirth and the puerperium

    O99.820 Streptococcus B carrier state complicating pregnancy ♂♀

    O99.824 Streptococcus B carrier state complicating childbirth ♂♀

    O99.825 Streptococcus B carrier state complicating the puerperium ♂♀

√6ᵗʰ **O99.83** Other infection carrier state complicating pregnancy, childbirth and the puerperium
    Use additional code to identify the carrier state (Z22.-)

    O99.830 Other infection carrier state complicating pregnancy ♂♀

    O99.834 Other infection carrier state complicating childbirth ♂♀

    O99.835 Other infection carrier state complicating the puerperium ♂♀

√6ᵗʰ **O99.84** Bariatric surgery status complicating pregnancy, childbirth and the puerperium
    Gastric banding status complicating pregnancy, childbirth and the puerperium
    Gastric bypass status for obesity complicating pregnancy, childbirth and the puerperium
    Obesity surgery status complicating pregnancy, childbirth and the puerperium

    O99.840 Bariatric surgery status complicating pregnancy, unspecified trimester ♂♀

    O99.841 Bariatric surgery status complicating pregnancy, first trimester ♂♀

    O99.842 Bariatric surgery status complicating pregnancy, second trimester ♂♀

    O99.843 Bariatric surgery status complicating pregnancy, third trimester ♂♀

    O99.844 Bariatric surgery status complicating childbirth ♂♀

    O99.845 Bariatric surgery status complicating the puerperium ♂♀

O99.89 Other specified diseases and conditions complicating pregnancy, childbirth and the puerperium ♂♀

√4ᵗʰ **O9A** Maternal malignant neoplasms, traumatic injuries and abuse classifiable elsewhere but complicating pregnancy, childbirth and the puerperium

√5ᵗʰ **O9A.1** Malignant neoplasm complicating pregnancy, childbirth and the puerperium
    Conditions in C00-C96
    Use additional code to identify neoplasm
    EXCLUDES 2 maternal care for benign tumor of corpus uteri (O34.1-)
        maternal care for benign tumor of cervix (O34.4-)

  √6ᵗʰ **O9A.11** Malignant neoplasm complicating pregnancy

    O9A.111 Malignant neoplasm complicating pregnancy, first trimester ♂♀

    O9A.112 Malignant neoplasm complicating pregnancy, second trimester ♂♀

    O9A.113 Malignant neoplasm complicating pregnancy, third trimester ♂♀

    O9A.119 Malignant neoplasm complicating pregnancy, unspecified trimester ♂♀

  O9A.12 Malignant neoplasm complicating childbirth ♂♀

  O9A.13 Malignant neoplasm complicating the puerperium ♂♀

√5ᵗʰ **O9A.2** Injury, poisoning and certain other consequences of external causes complicating pregnancy, childbirth and the puerperium
    Conditions in S00-T88, except T74 and T76
    Use additional code(s) to identify the injury or poisoning
    EXCLUDES 2 physical, sexual and psychological abuse complicating pregnancy, childbirth and the puerperium (O9A.3-, O9A.4-, O9A.5-)

  √6ᵗʰ **O9A.21** Injury, poisoning and certain other consequences of external causes complicating pregnancy

    O9A.211 Injury, poisoning and certain other consequences of external causes complicating pregnancy, first trimester ♂♀

    O9A.212 Injury, poisoning and certain other consequences of external causes complicating pregnancy, second trimester ♂♀

    O9A.213 Injury, poisoning and certain other consequences of external causes complicating pregnancy, third trimester ♂♀

    O9A.219 Injury, poisoning and certain other consequences of external causes complicating pregnancy, unspecified trimester ♂♀

  O9A.22 Injury, poisoning and certain other consequences of external causes complicating childbirth ♂♀

  O9A.23 Injury, poisoning and certain other consequences of external causes complicating the puerperium ♂♀

√5ᵗʰ **O9A.3** Physical abuse complicating pregnancy, childbirth and the puerperium
    Conditions in T74.11 or T76.11
    Use additional code (if applicable):
        to identify any associated current injury due to physical abuse
        to identify the perpetrator of abuse (Y07.-)
    EXCLUDES 2 sexual abuse complicating pregnancy, childbirth and the puerperium (O9A.4)

  √6ᵗʰ **O9A.31** Physical abuse complicating pregnancy

    O9A.311 Physical abuse complicating pregnancy, first trimester ♂♀

    O9A.312 Physical abuse complicating pregnancy, second trimester ♂♀

    O9A.313 Physical abuse complicating pregnancy, third trimester ♂♀

    O9A.319 Physical abuse complicating pregnancy, unspecified trimester ♂♀

  O9A.32 Physical abuse complicating childbirth ♂♀

  O9A.33 Physical abuse complicating the puerperium ♂♀

☑ Additional Character Required   √x7ᵗʰ Xtension Alert   Unspecified Dx   Other Specified Dx   Manifestation   ►◄ Revised Text   ● New Code   ▲ Revised Code Title

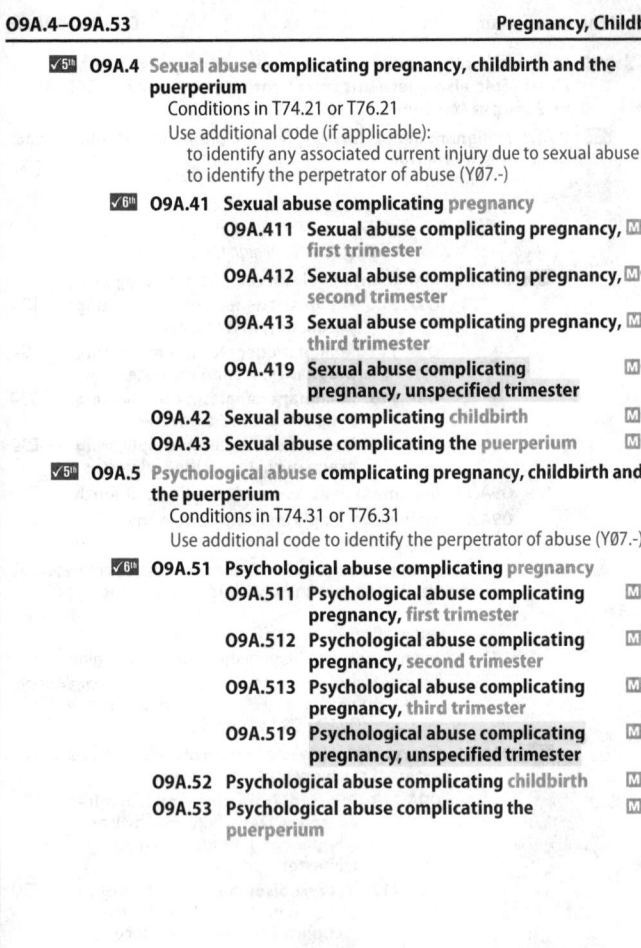

✓5ᵗʰ **O9A.4** Sexual abuse complicating pregnancy, childbirth and the puerperium
Conditions in T74.21 or T76.21
Use additional code (if applicable):
   to identify any associated current injury due to sexual abuse
   to identify the perpetrator of abuse (Y07.-)

✓6ᵗʰ **O9A.41** **Sexual abuse complicating** pregnancy
   O9A.411 **Sexual abuse complicating pregnancy,** Ⓜ♀ first trimester
   O9A.412 **Sexual abuse complicating pregnancy,** Ⓜ♀ second trimester
   O9A.413 **Sexual abuse complicating pregnancy,** Ⓜ♀ third trimester
   O9A.419 **Sexual abuse complicating** Ⓜ♀ **pregnancy, unspecified trimester**
O9A.42 **Sexual abuse complicating** childbirth   Ⓜ♀
O9A.43 **Sexual abuse complicating the** puerperium   Ⓜ♀

✓5ᵗʰ **O9A.5** Psychological abuse complicating pregnancy, childbirth and the puerperium
Conditions in T74.31 or T76.31
Use additional code to identify the perpetrator of abuse (Y07.-)

✓6ᵗʰ **O9A.51** **Psychological abuse complicating** pregnancy
   O9A.511 **Psychological abuse complicating** Ⓜ♀ **pregnancy,** first trimester
   O9A.512 **Psychological abuse complicating** Ⓜ♀ **pregnancy,** second trimester
   O9A.513 **Psychological abuse complicating** Ⓜ♀ **pregnancy,** third trimester
   O9A.519 **Psychological abuse complicating** Ⓜ♀ **pregnancy, unspecified trimester**
O9A.52 **Psychological abuse complicating** childbirth   Ⓜ♀
O9A.53 **Psychological abuse complicating the** Ⓜ♀ **puerperium**

Chapter 16. Certain Conditions Originating in the Perinatal Period (P00-P96)

NOTE　Codes from this chapter are for use on newborn records only, never on maternal records.

INCLUDES　conditions that have their origin in the fetal or perinatal period (before birth through the first 28 days after birth) even if morbidity occurs later

EXCLUDES 2　congenital malformations, deformations and chromosomal abnormalities (Q00-Q99)
endocrine, nutritional and metabolic diseases (E00-E88)
injury, poisoning and certain other consequences of external causes (S00-T88)
neoplasms (C00-D49)
tetanus neonatorum (A33)

This chapter contains the following blocks:

P00-P04　Newborn affected by maternal factors and by complications of pregnancy, labor, and delivery
P05-P08　Disorders of newborn related to length of gestation and fetal growth
P09　Abnormal findings on neonatal screening
P10-P15　Birth trauma
P19-P29　Respiratory and cardiovascular disorders specific to the perinatal period
P35-P39　Infections specific to the perinatal period
P50-P61　Hemorrhagic and hematological disorders of newborn
P70-P74　Transitory endocrine and metabolic disorders specific to newborn
P76-P78　Digestive system disorders of newborn
P80-P83　Conditions involving the integument and temperature regulation of newborn
P84　Other problems with newborn
P90-P96　Other disorders originating in the perinatal period

Newborn affected by maternal factors and by complications of pregnancy, labor, and delivery (P00-P04)

NOTE　These codes are for use when the listed maternal conditions are specified as the cause of confirmed morbidity or potential morbidity which have their origin in the perinatal period (before birth through the first 28 days after birth). Codes from these categories are also for use for newborns who are suspected of having an abnormal condition resulting from exposure from the mother or the birth process, but without signs or symptoms, and, which after examination and observation, is found not to exist. These codes may be used even if treatment is begun for a suspected condition that is ruled out.

✓4ᵗʰ P00　Newborn (suspected to be) affected by maternal conditions that may be unrelated to present pregnancy
Code first any current condition in newborn
EXCLUDES 2　newborn (suspected to be) affected by maternal complications of pregnancy (P01.-)
newborn affected by maternal endocrine and metabolic disorders (P70-P74)
newborn affected by noxious substances transmitted via placenta or breast milk (P04.-)

P00.0　Newborn (suspected to be) affected by maternal hypertensive disorders　N
Newborn (suspected to be) affected by maternal conditions classifiable to O10-O11, O13-O16

P00.1　Newborn (suspected to be) affected by maternal renal and urinary tract diseases　N
Newborn (suspected to be) affected by maternal conditions classifiable to N00-N39

P00.2　Newborn (suspected to be) affected by maternal infectious and parasitic diseases　N
Newborn (suspected to be) affected by maternal infectious disease classifiable to A00-B99, J09 and J10
EXCLUDES 1　infections specific to the perinatal period (P35-P39)
maternal genital tract or other localized infections (P00.8)

P00.3　Newborn (suspected to be) affected by other maternal circulatory and respiratory diseases　N
Newborn (suspected to be) affected by maternal conditions classifiable to I00-I99, J00-J99, Q20-Q34 and not included in P00.0, P00.2

P00.4　Newborn (suspected to be) affected by maternal nutritional disorders　N
Newborn (suspected to be) affected by maternal disorders classifiable to E40-E64
Maternal malnutrition NOS

P00.5　Newborn (suspected to be) affected by maternal injury　N
Newborn (suspected to be) affected by maternal conditions classifiable to O9A.2-

P00.6　Newborn (suspected to be) affected by surgical procedure on mother　N
Newborn (suspected to be) affected by amniocentesis
EXCLUDES 1　Cesarean delivery for present delivery (P03.4)
damage to placenta from amniocentesis, Cesarean delivery or surgical induction (P02.1)
previous surgery to uterus or pelvic organs (P03.89)
EXCLUDES 2　newborn affected by complication of (fetal) intrauterine procedure (P96.5)

P00.7　Newborn (suspected to be) affected by other medical procedures on mother, not elsewhere classified　N
Newborn (suspected to be) affected by radiation to mother
EXCLUDES 1　damage to placenta from amniocentesis, cesarean delivery or surgical induction (P02.1)
newborn affected by other complications of labor and delivery (P03.-)

✓5ᵗʰ P00.8　Newborn (suspected to be) affected by other maternal conditions

P00.81　Newborn (suspected to be) affected by periodontal disease in mother　N

P00.89　Newborn (suspected to be) affected by other maternal conditions　N
Newborn (suspected to be) affected by conditions classifiable to T80-T88
Newborn (suspected to be) affected by maternal genital tract or other localized infections
Newborn (suspected to be) affected by maternal systemic lupus erythematosus

P00.9　Newborn (suspected to be) affected by unspecified maternal condition　N

✓4ᵗʰ P01　Newborn (suspected to be) affected by maternal complications of pregnancy
Code first any current condition in newborn

P01.0　Newborn (suspected to be) affected by incompetent cervix　N

P01.1　Newborn (suspected to be) affected by premature rupture of membranes　N

P01.2　Newborn (suspected to be) affected by oligohydramnios　N
EXCLUDES 1　oligohydramnios due to premature rupture of membranes (P01.1)

P01.3　Newborn (suspected to be) affected by polyhydramnios　N
Newborn (suspected to be) affected by hydramnios

P01.4　Newborn (suspected to be) affected by ectopic pregnancy　N
Newborn (suspected to be) affected by abdominal pregnancy

P01.5　Newborn (suspected to be) affected by multiple pregnancy　N
Newborn (suspected to be) affected by triplet (pregnancy)
Newborn (suspected to be) affected by twin (pregnancy)

P01.6　Newborn (suspected to be) affected by maternal death　N

P01.7　Newborn (suspected to be) affected by malpresentation before labor　N
Newborn (suspected to be) affected by breech presentation before labor
Newborn (suspected to be) affected by external version before labor
Newborn (suspected to be) affected by face presentation before labor
Newborn (suspected to be) affected by transverse lie before labor
Newborn (suspected to be) affected by unstable lie before labor

P01.8　Newborn (suspected to be) affected by other maternal complications of pregnancy　N

P01.9　Newborn (suspected to be) affected by maternal complication of pregnancy, unspecified　N

✓4ᵗʰ P02　Newborn (suspected to be) affected by complications of placenta, cord and membranes
Code first any current condition in newborn

P02.0　Newborn (suspected to be) affected by placenta previa　N

P02.1　Newborn (suspected to be) affected by other forms of placental separation and hemorrhage　N
Newborn (suspected to be) affected by abruptio placenta
Newborn (suspected to be) affected by accidental hemorrhage
Newborn (suspected to be) affected by antepartum hemorrhage
Newborn (suspected to be) affected by damage to placenta from amniocentesis, cesarean delivery or surgical induction
Newborn (suspected to be) affected by maternal blood loss
Newborn (suspected to be) affected by premature separation of placenta

✓5ᵗʰ **P02.2 Newborn (suspected to be) affected by other and unspecified morphological and functional abnormalities of placenta**

    P02.20 Newborn (suspected to be) affected by unspecified morphological and functional abnormalities of placenta N

    P02.29 Newborn (suspected to be) affected by other morphological and functional abnormalities of placenta N
        Newborn (suspected to be) affected by placental dysfunction
        Newborn (suspected to be) affected by placental infarction
        Newborn (suspected to be) affected by placental insufficiency

P02.3 Newborn (suspected to be) affected by placental transfusion syndromes N
    Newborn (suspected to be) affected by placental and cord abnormalities resulting in twin-to-twin or other transplacental transfusion

P02.4 Newborn (suspected to be) affected by prolapsed cord N

P02.5 Newborn (suspected to be) affected by other compression of umbilical cord N
    Newborn (suspected to be) affected by umbilical cord (tightly) around neck
    Newborn (suspected to be) affected by entanglement of umbilical cord
    Newborn (suspected to be) affected by knot in umbilical cord

✓5ᵗʰ **P02.6 Newborn (suspected to be) affected by other and unspecified conditions of umbilical cord**

    P02.60 Newborn (suspected to be) affected by unspecified conditions of umbilical cord N

    P02.69 Newborn (suspected to be) affected by other conditions of umbilical cord N
        Newborn (suspected to be) affected by short umbilical cord
        Newborn (suspected to be) affected by vasa previa
        EXCLUDES 1   newborn affected by single umbilical artery (Q27.0)

P02.7 Newborn (suspected to be) affected by chorioamnionitis N
    Newborn (suspected to be) affected by amnionitis
    Newborn (suspected to be) affected by membranitis
    Newborn (suspected to be) affected by placentitis

P02.8 Newborn (suspected to be) affected by other abnormalities of membranes N

P02.9 Newborn (suspected to be) affected by abnormality of membranes, unspecified N

✓4ᵗʰ **P03 Newborn (suspected to be) affected by other complications of labor and delivery**
    Code first any current condition in newborn

P03.0 Newborn (suspected to be) affected by breech delivery and extraction N

P03.1 Newborn (suspected to be) affected by other malpresentation, malposition and disproportion during labor and delivery N
    Newborn (suspected to be) affected by contracted pelvis
    Newborn (suspected to be) affected by conditions classifiable to O64-O66
    Newborn (suspected to be) affected by persistent occipitoposterior
    Newborn (suspected to be) affected by transverse lie

P03.2 Newborn (suspected to be) affected by forceps delivery N

P03.3 Newborn (suspected to be) affected by delivery by vacuum extractor [ventouse] N

P03.4 Newborn (suspected to be) affected by Cesarean delivery N

P03.5 Newborn (suspected to be) affected by precipitate delivery N
    Newborn (suspected to be) affected by rapid second stage

P03.6 Newborn (suspected to be) affected by abnormal uterine contractions N
    Newborn (suspected to be) affected by conditions classifiable to O62-, except O62.3
    Newborn (suspected to be) affected by hypertonic labor
    Newborn (suspected to be) affected by uterine inertia

✓5ᵗʰ **P03.8 Newborn (suspected to be) affected by other specified complications of labor and delivery**

    ✓6ᵗʰ **P03.81 Newborn (suspected to be) affected by abnormality in fetal (intrauterine) heart rate or rhythm**
        EXCLUDES 1   neonatal cardiac dysrhythmia (P29.1-)

        P03.810 Newborn (suspected to be) affected by abnormality in fetal (intrauterine) heart rate or rhythm before the onset of labor N

        P03.811 Newborn (suspected to be) affected by abnormality in fetal (intrauterine) heart rate or rhythm during labor N

        P03.819 Newborn (suspected to be) affected by abnormality in fetal (intrauterine) heart rate or rhythm, unspecified as to time of onset N

    P03.82 Meconium passage during delivery N
        EXCLUDES 1   meconium aspiration (P24.00, P24.01)
            meconium staining (P96.83)

    P03.89 Newborn (suspected to be) affected by other specified complications of labor and delivery N
        Newborn (suspected to be) affected by abnormality of maternal soft tissues
        Newborn (suspected to be) affected by conditions classifiable to O60-O75 and by procedures used in labor and delivery not included in P02- and P03.0-P03.6
        Newborn (suspected to be) affected by induction of labor

P03.9 Newborn (suspected to be) affected by complication of labor and delivery, unspecified N

✓4ᵗʰ **P04 Newborn (suspected to be) affected by noxious substances transmitted via placenta or breast milk**
    INCLUDES   nonteratogenic effects of substances transmitted via placenta
    EXCLUDES 2   congenital malformations (Q00-Q99)
        neonatal jaundice from excessive hemolysis due to drugs or toxins transmitted from mother (P58.4)
        newborn in contact with and (suspected) exposures hazardous to health not transmitted via placenta or breast milk (Z77.-)

P04.0 Newborn (suspected to be) affected by maternal anesthesia and analgesia in pregnancy, labor and delivery N
    Newborn (suspected to be) affected by reactions and intoxications from maternal opiates and tranquilizers administered during labor and delivery

P04.1 Newborn (suspected to be) affected by other maternal medication N
    Newborn (suspected to be) affected by cancer chemotherapy
    Newborn (suspected to be) affected by cytotoxic drugs
    EXCLUDES 1   dysmorphism due to warfarin (Q86.2)
        fetal hydantoin syndrome (Q86.1)
        maternal use of drugs of addiction (P04.4-)

P04.2 Newborn (suspected to be) affected by maternal use of tobacco N
    Newborn (suspected to be) affected by exposure in utero to tobacco smoke
    EXCLUDES 2   newborn exposure to environmental tobacco smoke (P96.81)

P04.3 Newborn (suspected to be) affected by maternal use of alcohol N
    EXCLUDES 1   fetal alcohol syndrome (Q86.0)

✓5ᵗʰ **P04.4 Newborn (suspected to be) affected by maternal use of drugs of addiction**

    P04.41 Newborn (suspected to be) affected by maternal use of cocaine N
        "Crack baby"

    P04.49 Newborn (suspected to be) affected by maternal use of other drugs of addiction N
        EXCLUDES 2   newborn (suspected to be) affected by maternal anesthesia and analgesia (P04.0)
            withdrawal symptoms from maternal use of drugs of addiction (P96.1)

P04.5 Newborn (suspected to be) affected by maternal use of nutritional chemical substances N

P04.6 Newborn (suspected to be) affected by maternal exposure to environmental chemical substances N

P04.8 Newborn (suspected to be) affected by other maternal noxious substances N

P04.9 Newborn (suspected to be) affected by maternal noxious substance, unspecified N

EXCLUDES 1 Not coded here   **EXCLUDES 2** Not included here   N Newborn Age: 0   P Pediatric Age: 0-17   M Maternity Age: 12-55   A Adult Age: 15-124

766   ICD-10-CM Draft (2015)

Disorders of newborn related to length of gestation and fetal growth (P05-P08)

✓4ᵗʰ **P05　Disorders of newborn related to slow fetal growth and fetal malnutrition**

　✓5ᵗʰ **P05.0　Newborn light for gestational age**
　　　Newborn light-for-dates

　　　P05.00　Newborn light for gestational age, unspecified weight N

　　　P05.01　Newborn light for gestational age, less than 500 grams N

　　　P05.02　Newborn light for gestational age, 500-749 grams N

　　　P05.03　Newborn light for gestational age, 750-999 grams N

　　　P05.04　Newborn light for gestational age, 1000-1249 grams N

　　　P05.05　Newborn light for gestational age, 1250-1499 grams N

　　　P05.06　Newborn light for gestational age, 1500-1749 grams N

　　　P05.07　Newborn light for gestational age, 1750-1999 grams N

　　　P05.08　Newborn light for gestational age, 2000-2499 grams N

　✓5ᵗʰ **P05.1　Newborn small for gestational age**
　　　Newborn small-and-light-for-dates
　　　Newborn small-for-dates

　　　P05.10　Newborn small for gestational age, unspecified weight N

　　　P05.11　Newborn small for gestational age, less than 500 grams N

　　　P05.12　Newborn small for gestational age, 500-749 grams N

　　　P05.13　Newborn small for gestational age, 750-999 grams N

　　　P05.14　Newborn small for gestational age, 1000-1249 grams N

　　　P05.15　Newborn small for gestational age, 1250-1499 grams N

　　　P05.16　Newborn small for gestational age, 1500-1749 grams N

　　　P05.17　Newborn small for gestational age, 1750-1999 grams N

　　　P05.18　Newborn small for gestational age, 2000-2499 grams N

　　P05.2　Newborn affected by fetal (intrauterine) malnutrition not light or small for gestational age N
　　　Infant, not light or small for gestational age, showing signs of fetal malnutrition, such as dry, peeling skin and loss of subcutaneous tissue
　　　EXCLUDES1　*newborn affected by fetal malnutrition with light for gestational age (P05.0-)*
　　　　　　newborn affected by fetal malnutrition with small for gestational age (P05.1-)

　　P05.9　Newborn affected by slow intrauterine growth, unspecified N
　　　Newborn affected by fetal growth retardation NOS

✓4ᵗʰ **P07　Disorders of newborn related to short gestation and low birth weight, not elsewhere classified**
　　NOTE　When both birth weight and gestational age of the newborn are available, both should be coded with birth weight sequenced before gestational age
　　INCLUDES　The listed conditions, without further specification, as the cause of morbidity or additional care, in newborn
　　EXCLUDES1　*low birth weight due to slow fetal growth and fetal malnutrition (P05.-)*

　✓5ᵗʰ **P07.0　Extremely low birth weight newborn**
　　　Newborn birth weight 999 g. or less

　　　P07.00　Extremely low birth weight newborn, unspecified weight N

　　　P07.01　Extremely low birth weight newborn, less than 500 grams N

　　　P07.02　Extremely low birth weight newborn, 500-749 grams N

　　　P07.03　Extremely low birth weight newborn, 750-999 grams N

　✓5ᵗʰ **P07.1　Other low birth weight newborn**
　　　Newborn birth weight 1000-2499 g.

　　　P07.10　Other low birth weight newborn, unspecified weight N

　　　P07.14　Other low birth weight newborn, 1000-1249 grams N

　　　P07.15　Other low birth weight newborn, 1250-1499 grams N

　　　P07.16　Other low birth weight newborn, 1500-1749 grams N

　　　P07.17　Other low birth weight newborn, 1750-1999 grams N

　　　P07.18　Other low birth weight newborn, 2000-2499 grams N

　✓5ᵗʰ **P07.2　Extreme immaturity of newborn**
　　　Less than 28 completed weeks (less than 196 completed days) of gestation.

　　　P07.20　Extreme immaturity of newborn, unspecified weeks of gestation N
　　　　Gestational age less than 28 completed weeks NOS

　　　P07.21　Extreme immaturity of newborn, gestational age less than 23 completed weeks N
　　　　Extreme immaturity of newborn, gestational age less than 23 weeks, 0 days

　　　P07.22　Extreme immaturity of newborn, gestational age 23 completed weeks N
　　　　Extreme immaturity of newborn, gestational age 23 weeks, 0 days through 23 weeks, 6 days

　　　P07.23　Extreme immaturity of newborn, gestational age 24 completed weeks N
　　　　Extreme immaturity of newborn, gestational age 24 weeks, 0 days through 24 weeks, 6 days

　　　P07.24　Extreme immaturity of newborn, gestational age 25 completed weeks N
　　　　Extreme immaturity of newborn, gestational age 25 weeks, 0 days through 25 weeks, 6 days

　　　P07.25　Extreme immaturity of newborn, gestational age 26 completed weeks N
　　　　Extreme immaturity of newborn, gestational age 26 weeks, 0 days through 26 weeks, 6 days

　　　P07.26　Extreme immaturity of newborn, gestational age 27 completed weeks N
　　　　Extreme immaturity of newborn, gestational age 27 weeks, 0 days through 27 weeks, 6 days

　✓5ᵗʰ **P07.3　Preterm [premature] newborn [other]**
　　　28 completed weeks or more but less than 37 completed weeks (196 completed days but less than 259 completed days) of gestation
　　　Prematurity NOS

　　　P07.30　Preterm newborn, unspecified weeks of gestation N

　　　P07.31　Preterm newborn, gestational age 28 completed weeks N
　　　　Preterm newborn, gestational age 28 weeks, 0 days through 28 weeks, 6 days

　　　P07.32　Preterm newborn, gestational age 29 completed weeks N
　　　　Preterm newborn, gestational age 29 weeks, 0 days through 29 weeks, 6 days

　　　P07.33　Preterm newborn, gestational age 30 completed weeks N
　　　　Preterm newborn, gestational age 30 weeks, 0 days through 30 weeks, 6 days

　　　P07.34　Preterm newborn, gestational age 31 completed weeks N
　　　　Preterm newborn, gestational age 31 weeks, 0 days through 31 weeks, 6 days

　　　P07.35　Preterm newborn, gestational age 32 completed weeks N
　　　　Preterm newborn, gestational age 32 weeks, 0 days through 32 weeks, 6 days

　　　P07.36　Preterm newborn, gestational age 33 completed weeks N
　　　　Preterm newborn, gestational age 33 weeks, 0 days through 33 weeks, 6 days

　　　P07.37　Preterm newborn, gestational age 34 completed weeks N
　　　　Preterm newborn, gestational age 34 weeks, 0 days through 34 weeks, 6 days

---

☑ Additional Character Required　　✓x7ᵗʰ Xtension Alert　　Unspecified Dx　　Other Specified Dx　　Manifestation　　▶◀ Revised Text　　● New Code　　▲ Revised Code Title

P07.38   **Preterm newborn, gestational age** 35 completed weeks   N
> Preterm newborn, gestational age 35 weeks, 0 days through 35 weeks, 6 days

P07.39   **Preterm newborn, gestational age** 36 completed weeks   N
> Preterm newborn, gestational age 36 weeks, 0 days through 36 weeks, 6 days

√4ᵗʰ **P08**   **Disorders of newborn related to long gestation and high birth weight**
> **NOTE**   When both birth weight and gestational age of the newborn are available, priority of assignment should be given to birth weight
> **INCLUDES**   the listed conditions, without further specification, as causes of morbidity or additional care, in newborn

P08.0   **Exceptionally large newborn baby**   N
> Usually implies a birth weight of 4500 g. or more
> **EXCLUDES 1**   syndrome of infant of diabetic mother (P70.1)
> syndrome of infant of mother with gestational diabetes (P70.0)

P08.1   **Other heavy for gestational age newborn**   N
> Other newborn heavy- or large-for-dates regardless of period of gestation
> Usually implies a birth weight of 4000 g. to 4499 g.
> **EXCLUDES 1**   newborn with a birth weight of 4500 or more (P08.0)
> syndrome of infant of diabetic mother (P70.1)
> syndrome of infant of mother with gestational diabetes (P70.0).

√5ᵗʰ **P08.2**   **Late newborn, not heavy for gestational age**
> **AHA:** 2014, 1Q, 14

P08.21   **Post-term newborn**   N
> Newborn with gestation period over 40 completed weeks to 42 completed weeks

P08.22   **Prolonged gestation of newborn**   N
> Newborn with gestation period over 42 completed weeks (294 days or more), not heavy- or large-for-dates.
> Postmaturity NOS

Abnormal findings on neonatal screening (P09)

P09   **Abnormal findings on neonatal screening**   N
> Use additional code to identify signs, symptoms and conditions associated with the screening
> **EXCLUDES 2**   nonspecific serologic evidence of human immunodeficiency virus [HIV] (R75)

Birth trauma (P10–P15)

√4ᵗʰ **P10**   **Intracranial laceration and hemorrhage due to birth injury**
> **EXCLUDES 1**   intracranial hemorrhage of newborn NOS (P52.9)
> intracranial hemorrhage of newborn due to anoxia or hypoxia (P52.-)
> nontraumatic intracranial hemorrhage of newborn (P52.-)

P10.0   **Subdural hemorrhage due to birth injury**   N
> Subdural hematoma (localized) due to birth injury
> **EXCLUDES 1**   subdural hemorrhage accompanying tentorial tear (P10.4)

P10.1   **Cerebral hemorrhage due to birth injury**   N
P10.2   **Intraventricular hemorrhage due to birth injury**   N
P10.3   **Subarachnoid hemorrhage due to birth injury**   N
P10.4   **Tentorial tear due to birth injury**   N
P10.8   **Other intracranial lacerations and hemorrhages due to birth injury**   N
P10.9   **Unspecified intracranial laceration and hemorrhage due to birth injury**   N

√4ᵗʰ **P11**   **Other birth injuries to central nervous system**
P11.0   **Cerebral edema due to birth injury**   N
P11.1   **Other specified brain damage due to birth injury**   N
P11.2   **Unspecified brain damage due to birth injury**   N
P11.3   **Birth injury to facial nerve**   N
> Facial palsy due to birth injury
P11.4   **Birth injury to other cranial nerves**   N
P11.5   **Birth injury to spine and spinal cord**   N
> Fracture of spine due to birth injury
P11.9   **Birth injury to central nervous system, unspecified**   N

√4ᵗʰ **P12**   **Birth injury to scalp**
P12.0   **Cephalhematoma due to birth injury**   N
P12.1   **Chignon (from vacuum extraction) due to birth injury**   N
P12.2   **Epicranial subaponeurotic hemorrhage due to birth injury**   N
> Subgaleal hemorrhage
P12.3   **Bruising of scalp due to birth injury**   N
P12.4   **Injury of scalp of newborn due to monitoring equipment**   N
> Sampling incision of scalp of newborn
> Scalp clip (electrode) injury of newborn
√5ᵗʰ **P12.8**   **Other birth injuries to scalp**
P12.81   **Caput succedaneum**   N
P12.89   **Other birth injuries to scalp**   N
P12.9   **Birth injury to scalp, unspecified**   N

√4ᵗʰ **P13**   **Birth injury to skeleton**
> **EXCLUDES 2**   birth injury to spine (P11.5)
P13.0   **Fracture of skull due to birth injury**   N
P13.1   **Other birth injuries to skull**   N
> **EXCLUDES 1**   cephalhematoma (P12.0)
P13.2   **Birth injury to femur**   N
P13.3   **Birth injury to other long bones**   N
P13.4   **Fracture of clavicle due to birth injury**   N
P13.8   **Birth injuries to other parts of skeleton**   N
P13.9   **Birth injury to skeleton, unspecified**   N

√4ᵗʰ **P14**   **Birth injury to peripheral nervous system**
P14.0   **Erb's paralysis due to birth injury**   N
P14.1   **Klumpke's paralysis due to birth injury**   N
P14.2   **Phrenic nerve paralysis due to birth injury**   N
P14.3   **Other brachial plexus birth injuries**   N
P14.8   **Birth injuries to other parts of peripheral nervous system**   N
P14.9   **Birth injury to peripheral nervous system, unspecified**   N

√4ᵗʰ **P15**   **Other birth injuries**
P15.0   **Birth injury to liver**   N
> Rupture of liver due to birth injury
P15.1   **Birth injury to spleen**   N
> Rupture of spleen due to birth injury
P15.2   **Sternomastoid injury due to birth injury**   N
P15.3   **Birth injury to eye**   N
> Subconjunctival hemorrhage due to birth injury
> Traumatic glaucoma due to birth injury
P15.4   **Birth injury to face**   N
> Facial congestion due to birth injury
P15.5   **Birth injury to external genitalia**   N
P15.6   **Subcutaneous fat necrosis due to birth injury**   N
P15.8   **Other specified birth injuries**   N
P15.9   **Birth injury, unspecified**   N

Respiratory and cardiovascular disorders specific to the perinatal period (P19-P29)

√4ᵗʰ **P19**   **Metabolic acidemia in newborn**
> Metabolic acidemia in newborn
P19.0   **Metabolic acidemia in newborn first noted before onset of labor**   N
P19.1   **Metabolic acidemia in newborn first noted during labor**   N
P19.2   **Metabolic acidemia noted at birth**   N
P19.9   **Metabolic acidemia, unspecified**   N

√4ᵗʰ **P22**   **Respiratory distress of newborn**
> **EXCLUDES 1**   respiratory arrest of newborn (P28.81)
> respiratory failure of newborn NOS (P28.5)
P22.0   **Respiratory distress syndrome of newborn**   N
> Cardiorespiratory distress syndrome of newborn
> Hyaline membrane disease
> Idiopathic respiratory distress syndrome [IRDS or RDS] of newborn
> Pulmonary hypoperfusion syndrome
> Respiratory distress syndrome, type I
P22.1   **Transient tachypnea of newborn**   N
> Idiopathic tachypnea of newborn
> Respiratory distress syndrome, type II
> Wet lung syndrome
P22.8   **Other respiratory distress of newborn**   N
P22.9   **Respiratory distress of newborn, unspecified**   N

EXCLUDES 1 Not coded here   **EXCLUDES 2** Not included here   N Newborn Age: 0   P Pediatric Age: 0-17   M Maternity Age: 12-55   A Adult Age: 15-124

768   ICD-10-CM Draft (2015)

☑4ᵗʰ **P23　Congenital pneumonia**
> INCLUDES　infective pneumonia acquired in utero or during birth
> EXCLUDES 1　neonatal pneumonia resulting from aspiration (P24.-)

　P23.0　Congenital pneumonia due to viral agent　Ⓝ
　　　Use additional code (B97) to identify organism
　　　EXCLUDES 1　congenital rubella pneumonitis (P35.0)

　P23.1　Congenital pneumonia due to Chlamydia　Ⓝ

　P23.2　Congenital pneumonia due to staphylococcus　Ⓝ

　P23.3　Congenital pneumonia due to streptococcus, group B　Ⓝ

　P23.4　Congenital pneumonia due to Escherichia coli　Ⓝ

　P23.5　Congenital pneumonia due to Pseudomonas　Ⓝ

　P23.6　Congenital pneumonia due to other bacterial agents　Ⓝ
　　　Congenital pneumonia due to Hemophilus influenzae
　　　Congenital pneumonia due to Klebsiella pneumoniae
　　　Congenital pneumonia due to Mycoplasma
　　　Congenital pneumonia due to Streptococcus, except group B
　　　Use additional code (B95-B96) to identify organism

　P23.8　Congenital pneumonia due to other organisms　Ⓝ

　P23.9　Congenital pneumonia, unspecified　Ⓝ

☑4ᵗʰ **P24　Neonatal aspiration**
> INCLUDES　aspiration in utero and during delivery

　☑5ᵗʰ **P24.0　Meconium aspiration**
　　　EXCLUDES 1　meconium passage (without aspiration) during delivery
　　　　　　　　(P03.82)
　　　　　　　　meconium staining (P96.83)

　　P24.00　Meconium aspiration without respiratory symptoms　Ⓝ
　　　　Meconium aspiration NOS

　　P24.01　Meconium aspiration with respiratory symptoms　Ⓝ
　　　　Meconium aspiration pneumonia
　　　　Meconium aspiration pneumonitis
　　　　Meconium aspiration syndrome NOS
　　　　Use additional code to identify any secondary
　　　　　pulmonary hypertension, if applicable (I27.2)

　☑5ᵗʰ **P24.1　Neonatal aspiration of (clear) amniotic fluid and mucus**
　　　Neonatal aspiration of liquor (amnii)

　　P24.10　Neonatal aspiration of (clear) amniotic fluid and mucus without respiratory symptoms　Ⓝ
　　　　Neonatal aspiration of amniotic fluid and mucus NOS

　　P24.11　Neonatal aspiration of (clear) amniotic fluid and mucus with respiratory symptoms　Ⓝ
　　　　Neonatal aspiration of amniotic fluid and mucus with pneumonia
　　　　Neonatal aspiration of amniotic fluid and mucus with pneumonitis
　　　　Use additional code to identify any secondary
　　　　　pulmonary hypertension, if applicable (I27.2)

　☑5ᵗʰ **P24.2　Neonatal aspiration of blood**

　　P24.20　Neonatal aspiration of blood without respiratory symptoms　Ⓝ
　　　　Neonatal aspiration of blood NOS

　　P24.21　Neonatal aspiration of blood with respiratory symptoms　Ⓝ
　　　　Neonatal aspiration of blood with pneumonia
　　　　Neonatal aspiration of blood with pneumonitis
　　　　Use additional code to identify any secondary
　　　　　pulmonary hypertension, if applicable (I27.2)

　☑5ᵗʰ **P24.3　Neonatal aspiration of milk and regurgitated food**
　　　Neonatal aspiration of stomach contents

　　P24.30　Neonatal aspiration of milk and regurgitated food without respiratory symptoms　Ⓝ
　　　　Neonatal aspiration of milk and regurgitated food NOS

　　P24.31　Neonatal aspiration of milk and regurgitated food with respiratory symptoms　Ⓝ
　　　　Neonatal aspiration of milk and regurgitated food with pneumonia
　　　　Neonatal aspiration of milk and regurgitated food with pneumonitis
　　　　Use additional code to identify any secondary
　　　　　pulmonary hypertension, if applicable (I27.2)

　☑5ᵗʰ **P24.8　Other neonatal aspiration**

　　P24.80　Other neonatal aspiration without respiratory symptoms　Ⓝ
　　　　Neonatal aspiration NEC

　　P24.81　Other neonatal aspiration with respiratory symptoms　Ⓝ
　　　　Neonatal aspiration pneumonia NEC
　　　　Neonatal aspiration with pneumonitis NEC
　　　　Neonatal aspiration with pneumonia NOS
　　　　Neonatal aspiration with pneumonitis NOS
　　　　Use additional code to identify any secondary
　　　　　pulmonary hypertension, if applicable (I27.2)

　P24.9　Neonatal aspiration, unspecified　Ⓝ

☑4ᵗʰ **P25　Interstitial emphysema and related conditions originating in the perinatal period**

　P25.0　Interstitial emphysema originating in the perinatal period　Ⓝ

　P25.1　Pneumothorax originating in the perinatal period　Ⓝ

　P25.2　Pneumomediastinum originating in the perinatal period　Ⓝ

　P25.3　Pneumopericardium originating in the perinatal period　Ⓝ

　P25.8　Other conditions related to interstitial emphysema originating in the perinatal period　Ⓝ

☑4ᵗʰ **P26　Pulmonary hemorrhage originating in the perinatal period**
> EXCLUDES 1　acute idiopathic hemorrhage in infants over 28 days old
> 　　　　　(R04.81)

　P26.0　Tracheobronchial hemorrhage originating in the perinatal period　Ⓝ

　P26.1　Massive pulmonary hemorrhage originating in the perinatal period　Ⓝ

　P26.8　Other pulmonary hemorrhages originating in the perinatal period　Ⓝ

　P26.9　Unspecified pulmonary hemorrhage originating in the perinatal period　Ⓝ

☑4ᵗʰ **P27　Chronic respiratory disease originating in the perinatal period**
> EXCLUDES 1　respiratory distress of newborn (P22.0-P22.9)

　P27.0　Wilson-Mikity syndrome
　　　Pulmonary dysmaturity

　P27.1　Bronchopulmonary dysplasia originating in the perinatal period

　P27.8　Other chronic respiratory diseases originating in the perinatal period
　　　Congenital pulmonary fibrosis
　　　Ventilator lung in newborn

　P27.9　Unspecified chronic respiratory disease originating in the perinatal period

☑4ᵗʰ **P28　Other respiratory conditions originating in the perinatal period**
> EXCLUDES 1　congenital malformations of the respiratory system (Q30-Q34)

　P28.0　Primary atelectasis of newborn
　　　Primary failure to expand terminal respiratory units
　　　Pulmonary hypoplasia associated with short gestation
　　　Pulmonary immaturity NOS

　☑5ᵗʰ **P28.1　Other and unspecified atelectasis of newborn**

　　P28.10　Unspecified atelectasis of newborn　Ⓝ
　　　　Atelectasis of newborn NOS

　　P28.11　Resorption atelectasis without respiratory distress syndrome　Ⓝ
　　　　EXCLUDES 1　resorption atelectasis with respiratory
　　　　　　　　distress syndrome (P22.0)

　　P28.19　Other atelectasis of newborn　Ⓝ
　　　　Partial atelectasis of newborn
　　　　Secondary atelectasis of newborn

　P28.2　Cyanotic attacks of newborn　Ⓝ
　　　EXCLUDES 1　apnea of newborn (P28.3-P28.4)

　P28.3　Primary sleep apnea of newborn　Ⓝ
　　　Central sleep apnea of newborn
　　　Obstructive sleep apnea of newborn
　　　Sleep apnea of newborn NOS

　P28.4　Other apnea of newborn　Ⓝ
　　　Apnea of prematurity
　　　Obstructive apnea of newborn
　　　EXCLUDES 1　obstructive sleep apnea of newborn (P28.3)

　P28.5　Respiratory failure of newborn　Ⓝ
　　　EXCLUDES 1　respiratory arrest of newborn (P28.81)
　　　　　　　　respiratory distress of newborn (P22.0-)

　☑5ᵗʰ **P28.8　Other specified respiratory conditions of newborn**

　　P28.81　Respiratory arrest of newborn　Ⓝ

　　P28.89　Other specified respiratory conditions of newborn　Ⓝ
　　　　Congenital laryngeal stridor
　　　　Sniffles in newborn
　　　　Snuffles in newborn
　　　　EXCLUDES 1　early congenital syphilitic rhinitis (A50.05)

☑ Additional Character Required　☑7ᵗʰ Xtension Alert　Unspecified Dx　Other Specified Dx　Manifestation　►◄ Revised Text　● New Code　▲ Revised Code Title

P28.9 Respiratory condition of newborn, unspecified N
Respiratory depression in newborn

√4ᵗʰ P29 Cardiovascular disorders originating in the perinatal period
EXCLUDES 1 congenital malformations of the circulatory system (Q20-Q28)

P29.0 Neonatal cardiac failure N

√5ᵗʰ P29.1 Neonatal cardiac dysrhythmia
P29.11 Neonatal tachycardia N
P29.12 Neonatal bradycardia N

P29.2 Neonatal hypertension N

P29.3 Persistent fetal circulation N
Delayed closure of ductus arteriosus
(Persistent) pulmonary hypertension of newborn

P29.4 Transient myocardial ischemia in newborn N

√5ᵗʰ P29.8 Other cardiovascular disorders originating in the perinatal period
P29.81 Cardiac arrest of newborn N
P29.89 Other cardiovascular disorders originating in the perinatal period N

P29.9 Cardiovascular disorder originating in the perinatal period, unspecified N

Infections specific to the perinatal period (P35-P39)

Infections acquired in utero, during birth via the umbilicus, or during the first 28 days after birth

EXCLUDES 2 asymptomatic human immunodeficiency virus [HIV] infection status (Z21)
congenital gonococcal infection (A54.-)
congenital pneumonia (P23.-)
congenital syphilis (A50.-)
human immunodeficiency virus [HIV] disease (B20)
infant botulism (A48.51)
infectious diseases not specific to the perinatal period (A00-B99, J09, J10-)
intestinal infectious disease (A00-A09)
laboratory evidence of human immunodeficiency virus [HIV] (R75)
tetanus neonatorum (A33)

√4ᵗʰ P35 Congenital viral diseases
INCLUDES infections acquired in utero or during birth

P35.0 Congenital rubella syndrome N
Congenital rubella pneumonitis

P35.1 Congenital cytomegalovirus infection N
P35.2 Congenital herpesviral [herpes simplex] infection N
P35.3 Congenital viral hepatitis N
P35.8 Other congenital viral diseases N
Congenital varicella [chickenpox]

P35.9 Congenital viral disease, unspecified N

√4ᵗʰ P36 Bacterial sepsis of newborn
INCLUDES congenital sepsis
Use additional code(s), if applicable, to identify severe sepsis (R65.2-) and associated acute organ dysfunction(s)

P36.0 Sepsis of newborn due to streptococcus, group B N

√5ᵗʰ P36.1 Sepsis of newborn due to other and unspecified streptococci
P36.10 Sepsis of newborn due to unspecified streptococci N
P36.19 Sepsis of newborn due to other streptococci N

P36.2 Sepsis of newborn due to Staphylococcus aureus N

√5ᵗʰ P36.3 Sepsis of newborn due to other and unspecified staphylococci
P36.30 Sepsis of newborn due to unspecified staphylococci N
P36.39 Sepsis of newborn due to other staphylococci N

P36.4 Sepsis of newborn due to Escherichia coli N
P36.5 Sepsis of newborn due to anaerobes N
P36.8 Other bacterial sepsis of newborn N
Use additional code from category B96 to identify organism
P36.9 Bacterial sepsis of newborn, unspecified N

√4ᵗʰ P37 Other congenital infectious and parasitic diseases
EXCLUDES 2 congenital syphilis (A50.-)
infectious neonatal diarrhea (A00-A09)
necrotizing enterocolitis in newborn (P77.-)
noninfectious neonatal diarrhea (P78.3)
ophthalmia neonatorum due to gonococcus (A54.31)
tetanus neonatorum (A33)

P37.0 Congenital tuberculosis N
P37.1 Congenital toxoplasmosis N
Hydrocephalus due to congenital toxoplasmosis
P37.2 Neonatal (disseminated) listeriosis N
P37.3 Congenital falciparum malaria N
P37.4 Other congenital malaria N
P37.5 Neonatal candidiasis N
P37.8 Other specified congenital infectious and parasitic diseases N
P37.9 Congenital infectious or parasitic disease, unspecified N

√4ᵗʰ P38 Omphalitis of newborn
EXCLUDES 1 omphalitis not of newborn (L08.82)
tetanus omphalitis (A33)
umbilical hemorrhage of newborn (P51.-)

P38.1 Omphalitis with mild hemorrhage N
P38.9 Omphalitis without hemorrhage N
Omphalitis of newborn NOS

√4ᵗʰ P39 Other infections specific to the perinatal period
Use additional code to identify organism or specific infection

P39.0 Neonatal infective mastitis N
EXCLUDES 1 breast engorgement of newborn (P83.4)
noninfective mastitis of newborn (P83.4)

P39.1 Neonatal conjunctivitis and dacryocystitis N
Neonatal chlamydial conjunctivitis
Ophthalmia neonatorum NOS
EXCLUDES 1 gonococcal conjunctivitis (A54.31)

P39.2 Intra-amniotic infection affecting newborn, not elsewhere classified N
P39.3 Neonatal urinary tract infection N
P39.4 Neonatal skin infection N
Neonatal pyoderma
EXCLUDES 1 pemphigus neonatorum (L00)
staphylococcal scalded skin syndrome (L00)

P39.8 Other specified infections specific to the perinatal period N
P39.9 Infection specific to the perinatal period, unspecified N

Hemorrhagic and hematological disorders of newborn (P50-P61)

EXCLUDES 1 congenital stenosis and stricture of bile ducts (Q44.3)
Crigler-Najjar syndrome (E80.5)
Dubin-Johnson syndrome (E80.6)
Gilbert syndrome (E80.4)
hereditary hemolytic anemias (D55-D58)

√4ᵗʰ P50 Newborn affected by intrauterine (fetal) blood loss
EXCLUDES 1 congenital anemia from intrauterine (fetal) blood loss (P61.3)

P50.0 Newborn affected by intrauterine (fetal) blood loss from vasa previa N
P50.1 Newborn affected by intrauterine (fetal) blood loss from ruptured cord N
P50.2 Newborn affected by intrauterine (fetal) blood loss from placenta N
P50.3 Newborn affected by hemorrhage into co-twin N
P50.4 Newborn affected by hemorrhage into maternal circulation N
P50.5 Newborn affected by intrauterine (fetal) blood loss from cut end of co-twin's cord N
P50.8 Newborn affected by other intrauterine (fetal) blood loss N
P50.9 Newborn affected by intrauterine (fetal) blood loss, unspecified N
Newborn affected by fetal hemorrhage NOS

√4ᵗʰ P51 Umbilical hemorrhage of newborn
EXCLUDES 1 omphalitis with mild hemorrhage (P38.1)
umbilical hemorrhage from cut end of co-twins cord (P50.5)

P51.0 Massive umbilical hemorrhage of newborn N
P51.8 Other umbilical hemorrhages of newborn N
Slipped umbilical ligature NOS
P51.9 Umbilical hemorrhage of newborn, unspecified N

EXCLUDES 1 Not coded here   *EXCLUDES 2* Not included here   N Newborn Age: 0   P Pediatric Age: 0-17   M Maternity Age: 12-55   A Adult Age: 15-124

770   ICD-10-CM Draft (2015)

√4ᵗʰ **P52** Intracranial nontraumatic hemorrhage of newborn
Intracranial hemorrhage due to anoxia or hypoxia
EXCLUDES 1 *intracranial hemorrhage due to birth injury (P10.-)*
intracranial hemorrhage due to other injury (S06.-)

    P52.0 Intraventricular (nontraumatic) hemorrhage, grade 1, of newborn   N
         Subependymal hemorrhage (without intraventricular extension)
         Bleeding into germinal matrix

    P52.1 Intraventricular (nontraumatic) hemorrhage, grade 2, of newborn   N
         Subependymal hemorrhage with intraventricular extension
         Bleeding into ventricle

  √5ᵗʰ **P52.2** Intraventricular (nontraumatic) hemorrhage, grade 3 and grade 4, of newborn

        P52.21 Intraventricular (nontraumatic) hemorrhage, grade 3, of newborn   N
             Subependymal hemorrhage with intraventricular extension with enlargement of ventricle

        P52.22 Intraventricular (nontraumatic) hemorrhage, grade 4, of newborn   N
             Bleeding into cerebral cortex
             Subependymal hemorrhage with intracerebral extension

    P52.3 Unspecified intraventricular (nontraumatic) hemorrhage of newborn   N

    P52.4 Intracerebral (nontraumatic) hemorrhage of newborn   N

    P52.5 Subarachnoid (nontraumatic) hemorrhage of newborn   N

    P52.6 Cerebellar (nontraumatic) and posterior fossa hemorrhage of newborn   N

    P52.8 Other intracranial (nontraumatic) hemorrhages of newborn   N

    P52.9 Intracranial (nontraumatic) hemorrhage of newborn, unspecified   N

  P53 Hemorrhagic disease of newborn   N
       Vitamin K deficiency of newborn

√4ᵗʰ **P54** Other neonatal hemorrhages
EXCLUDES 1 *newborn affected by (intrauterine) blood loss (P50.-)*
pulmonary hemorrhage originating in the perinatal period (P26.-)

    P54.0 Neonatal hematemesis   N
         EXCLUDES 1 *neonatal hematemesis due to swallowed maternal blood (P78.2)*

    P54.1 Neonatal melena   N
         EXCLUDES 1 *neonatal melena due to swallowed maternal blood (P78.2)*

    P54.2 Neonatal rectal hemorrhage   N

    P54.3 Other neonatal gastrointestinal hemorrhage   N

    P54.4 Neonatal adrenal hemorrhage   N

    P54.5 Neonatal cutaneous hemorrhage   N
         Neonatal bruising
         Neonatal ecchymoses
         Neonatal petechiae
         Neonatal superficial hematomata
         EXCLUDES 2 *bruising of scalp due to birth injury (P12.3)*
                 cephalhematoma due to birth injury (P12.0)

    P54.6 Neonatal vaginal hemorrhage   N♀
         Neonatal pseudomenses

    P54.8 Other specified neonatal hemorrhages   N

    P54.9 Neonatal hemorrhage, unspecified   N

√4ᵗʰ **P55** Hemolytic disease of newborn
    P55.0 Rh isoimmunization of newborn   N
    P55.1 ABO isoimmunization of newborn   N
    P55.8 Other hemolytic diseases of newborn   N
    P55.9 Hemolytic disease of newborn, unspecified   N

√4ᵗʰ **P56** Hydrops fetalis due to hemolytic disease
EXCLUDES 1 *hydrops fetalis NOS (P83.2)*

    P56.0 Hydrops fetalis due to isoimmunization   N

  √5ᵗʰ **P56.9** Hydrops fetalis due to other and unspecified hemolytic disease

        P56.90 Hydrops fetalis due to unspecified hemolytic disease   N

        P56.99 Hydrops fetalis due to other hemolytic disease   N

√4ᵗʰ **P57** Kernicterus
    P57.0 Kernicterus due to isoimmunization   N
    P57.8 Other specified kernicterus   N
         EXCLUDES 1 *Crigler-Najjar syndrome (E80.5)*
    P57.9 Kernicterus, unspecified   N

√4ᵗʰ **P58** Neonatal jaundice due to other excessive hemolysis
EXCLUDES 1 *jaundice due to isoimmunization (P55-P57)*

    P58.0 Neonatal jaundice due to bruising   N
    P58.1 Neonatal jaundice due to bleeding   N
    P58.2 Neonatal jaundice due to infection   N
    P58.3 Neonatal jaundice due to polycythemia   N

  √5ᵗʰ **P58.4** Neonatal jaundice due to drugs or toxins transmitted from mother or given to newborn
         Code first poisoning due to drug or toxin, if applicable (T36-T65 with fifth or sixth character 1-4 or 6)
         Use additional code for adverse effect, if applicable, to identify drug (T36-T50 with fifth or sixth character 5)

        P58.41 Neonatal jaundice due to drugs or toxins transmitted from mother   N

        P58.42 Neonatal jaundice due to drugs or toxins given to newborn   N

    P58.5 Neonatal jaundice due to swallowed maternal blood   N

    P58.8 Neonatal jaundice due to other specified excessive hemolysis   N

    P58.9 Neonatal jaundice due to excessive hemolysis, unspecified   N

√4ᵗʰ **P59** Neonatal jaundice from other and unspecified causes
EXCLUDES 1 *jaundice due to inborn errors of metabolism (E70-E88)*
kernicterus (P57.-)

    P59.0 Neonatal jaundice associated with preterm delivery   N
         Hyperbilirubinemia of prematurity
         Jaundice due to delayed conjugation associated with preterm delivery

    P59.1 Inspissated bile syndrome   N

  √5ᵗʰ **P59.2** Neonatal jaundice from other and unspecified hepatocellular damage
         EXCLUDES 1 *congenital viral hepatitis (P35.3)*

        P59.20 Neonatal jaundice from unspecified hepatocellular damage   N

        P59.29 Neonatal jaundice from other hepatocellular damage   N
             Neonatal giant cell hepatitis
             Neonatal (idiopathic) hepatitis

    P59.3 Neonatal jaundice from breast milk inhibitor   N
    P59.8 Neonatal jaundice from other specified causes   N
    P59.9 Neonatal jaundice, unspecified   N
         Neonatal physiological jaundice (intense)(prolonged) NOS

  P60 Disseminated intravascular coagulation of newborn   N
       Defibrination syndrome of newborn

√4ᵗʰ **P61** Other perinatal hematological disorders
EXCLUDES 1 *transient hypogammaglobulinemia of infancy (D80.7)*

    P61.0 Transient neonatal thrombocytopenia   N
         Neonatal thrombocytopenia due to exchange transfusion
         Neonatal thrombocytopenia due to idiopathic maternal thrombocytopenia
         Neonatal thrombocytopenia due to isoimmunization

    P61.1 Polycythemia neonatorum   N
    P61.2 Anemia of prematurity   N
    P61.3 Congenital anemia from fetal blood loss   N
    P61.4 Other congenital anemias, not elsewhere classified   N
         Congenital anemia NOS

    P61.5 Transient neonatal neutropenia   N
         EXCLUDES 1 *congenital neutropenia (nontransient) (D70.0)*

    P61.6 Other transient neonatal disorders of coagulation   N
    P61.8 Other specified perinatal hematological disorders   N
    P61.9 Perinatal hematological disorder, unspecified   N

☑ Additional Character Required   √x7ᵗʰ Xtension Alert   Unspecified Dx   Other Specified Dx   Manifestation   ►◄ Revised Text   ● New Code   ▲ Revised Code Title

ICD-10-CM Draft (2015)   **771**

Certain Conditions Originating in the Perinatal Period

P70–P83.6

Transitory endocrine and metabolic disorders specific to newborn (P70-P74)

INCLUDES   transitory endocrine and metabolic disturbances caused by the infant's response to maternal endocrine and metabolic factors, or its adjustment to extrauterine environment

√4th **P70** **Transitory disorders of carbohydrate metabolism specific to newborn**

     P70.0 **Syndrome of infant of mother with gestational diabetes**   N
       Newborn (with hypoglycemia) affected by maternal gestational diabetes
       EXCLUDES 1   *newborn (with hypoglycemia) affected by maternal (pre-existing) diabetes mellitus (P70.1)*
          syndrome of infant of a diabetic mother (P70.1)

     P70.1 **Syndrome of infant of a diabetic mother**   N
       Newborn (with hypoglycemia) affected by maternal (pre-existing) diabetes mellitus
       EXCLUDES 1   *newborn (with hypoglycemia) affected by maternal gestational diabetes (P70.0)*
          syndrome of infant of mother with gestational diabetes (P70.0)

     P70.2 **Neonatal diabetes mellitus**   N

     P70.3 **Iatrogenic neonatal hypoglycemia**   N

     P70.4 **Other neonatal hypoglycemia**   N
       Transitory neonatal hypoglycemia

     P70.8 **Other transitory disorders of carbohydrate metabolism of newborn**   N

     P70.9 **Transitory disorder of carbohydrate metabolism of newborn, unspecified**   N

√4th **P71** **Transitory neonatal disorders of calcium and magnesium metabolism**

     P71.0 **Cow's milk hypocalcemia in newborn**   N

     P71.1 **Other neonatal hypocalcemia**   N
       EXCLUDES 1   *neonatal hypoparathyroidism (P71.4)*

     P71.2 **Neonatal hypomagnesemia**   N

     P71.3 **Neonatal tetany without calcium or magnesium deficiency**   N
       Neonatal tetany NOS

     P71.4 **Transitory neonatal hypoparathyroidism**   N

     P71.8 **Other transitory neonatal disorders of calcium and magnesium metabolism**   N

     P71.9 **Transitory neonatal disorder of calcium and magnesium metabolism, unspecified**   N

√4th **P72** **Other transitory neonatal endocrine disorders**
     EXCLUDES 1   *congenital hypothyroidism with or without goiter (E03.0-E03.1)*
          dyshormogenetic goiter (E07.1)
          Pendred's syndrome (E07.1)

     P72.0 **Neonatal goiter, not elsewhere classified**   N
       Transitory congenital goiter with normal functioning

     P72.1 **Transitory neonatal hyperthyroidism**   N
       Neonatal thyrotoxicosis

     P72.2 **Other transitory neonatal disorders of thyroid function, not elsewhere classified**   N
       Transitory neonatal hypothyroidism

     P72.8 **Other specified transitory neonatal endocrine disorders**   N

     P72.9 **Transitory neonatal endocrine disorder, unspecified**   N

√4th **P74** **Other transitory neonatal electrolyte and metabolic disturbances**

     P74.0 **Late metabolic acidosis of newborn**   N
       EXCLUDES 1   *(fetal) metabolic acidosis of newborn (P19)*

     P74.1 **Dehydration of newborn**   N

     P74.2 **Disturbances of sodium balance of newborn**   N

     P74.3 **Disturbances of potassium balance of newborn**   N

     P74.4 **Other transitory electrolyte disturbances of newborn**   N

     P74.5 **Transitory tyrosinemia of newborn**   N

     P74.6 **Transitory hyperammonemia of newborn**   N

     P74.8 **Other transitory metabolic disturbances of newborn**   N
       Amino-acid metabolic disorders described as transitory

     P74.9 **Transitory metabolic disturbance of newborn, unspecified**   N

Digestive system disorders of newborn (P76-P78)

√4th **P76** **Other intestinal obstruction of newborn**

     P76.0 **Meconium plug syndrome**   N
       Meconium ileus NOS
       EXCLUDES 1   *meconium ileus in cystic fibrosis (E84.11)*

     P76.1 **Transitory ileus of newborn**   N
       EXCLUDES 1   *Hirschsprung's disease (Q43.1)*

     P76.2 **Intestinal obstruction due to inspissated milk**   N

     P76.8 **Other specified intestinal obstruction of newborn**   N
       EXCLUDES 1   *intestinal obstruction classifiable to K56-*

     P76.9 **Intestinal obstruction of newborn, unspecified**   N

√4th **P77** **Necrotizing enterocolitis of newborn**

     P77.1 **Stage 1 necrotizing enterocolitis in newborn**   N
       Necrotizing enterocolitis without pneumatosis, without perforation

     P77.2 **Stage 2 necrotizing enterocolitis in newborn**   N
       Necrotizing enterocolitis with pneumatosis, without perforation

     P77.3 **Stage 3 necrotizing enterocolitis in newborn**   N
       Necrotizing enterocolitis with perforation
       Necrotizing enterocolitis with pneumatosis and perforation

     P77.9 **Necrotizing enterocolitis in newborn, unspecified**   N
       Necrotizing enterocolitis in newborn, NOS

√4th **P78** **Other perinatal digestive system disorders**
     EXCLUDES 1   *cystic fibrosis (E84.0-E84.9)*
          neonatal gastrointestinal hemorrhages (P54.0-P54.3)

     P78.0 **Perinatal intestinal perforation**   N
       Meconium peritonitis

     P78.1 **Other neonatal peritonitis**   N
       Neonatal peritonitis NOS

     P78.2 **Neonatal hematemesis and melena due to swallowed maternal blood**   N

     P78.3 **Noninfective neonatal diarrhea**   N
       Neonatal diarrhea NOS

     √5th **P78.8** **Other specified perinatal digestive system disorders**

         P78.81 **Congenital cirrhosis (of liver)**   N

         P78.82 **Peptic ulcer of newborn**   N

         P78.83 **Newborn esophageal reflux**   N
            Neonatal esophageal reflux

         P78.89 **Other specified perinatal digestive system disorders**   N

     P78.9 **Perinatal digestive system disorder, unspecified**   N

Conditions involving the integument and temperature regulation of newborn (P80-P83)

√4th **P80** **Hypothermia of newborn**

     P80.0 **Cold injury syndrome**   N
       Severe and usually chronic hypothermia associated with a pink flushed appearance, edema and neurological and biochemical abnormalities.
       EXCLUDES 1   *mild hypothermia of newborn (P80.8)*

     P80.8 **Other hypothermia of newborn**   N
       Mild hypothermia of newborn

     P80.9 **Hypothermia of newborn, unspecified**   N

√4th **P81** **Other disturbances of temperature regulation of newborn**

     P81.0 **Environmental hyperthermia of newborn**   N

     P81.8 **Other specified disturbances of temperature regulation of newborn**   N

     P81.9 **Disturbance of temperature regulation of newborn, unspecified**   N
       Fever of newborn NOS

√4th **P83** **Other conditions of integument specific to newborn**
     EXCLUDES 1   *congenital malformations of skin and integument (Q80-Q84)*
          hydrops fetalis due to hemolytic disease (P56.-)
          neonatal skin infection (P39.4)
          staphylococcal scalded skin syndrome (L00)
     EXCLUDES 2   *cradle cap (L21.0)*
          diaper [napkin] dermatitis (L22)

     P83.0 **Sclerema neonatorum**   N

     P83.1 **Neonatal erythema toxicum**   N

     P83.2 **Hydrops fetalis not due to hemolytic disease**   N
       Hydrops fetalis NOS

     √5th **P83.3** **Other and unspecified edema specific to newborn**

         P83.30 **Unspecified edema specific to newborn**   N

         P83.39 **Other edema specific to newborn**   N

     P83.4 **Breast engorgement of newborn**   N
       Noninfective mastitis of newborn

     P83.5 **Congenital hydrocele**   ♂

     P83.6 **Umbilical polyp of newborn**   N

EXCLUDES 1 Not coded here   EXCLUDES 2 Not included here   N Newborn Age: 0   P Pediatric Age: 0-17   M Maternity Age: 12-55   A Adult Age: 15-124

P83.8 **Other specified conditions of integument specific to newborn**   N
     Bronze baby syndrome
     Neonatal scleroderma
     Urticaria neonatorum

P83.9 **Condition of the integument specific to newborn, unspecified**   N

Other problems with newborn (P84)

P84 **Other problems with newborn**   N
     Acidemia of newborn
     Acidosis of newborn
     Anoxia of newborn NOS
     Asphyxia of newborn NOS
     Hypercapnia of newborn
     Hypoxemia of newborn
     Hypoxia of newborn NOS
     Mixed metabolic and respiratory acidosis of newborn
     EXCLUDES 1   *intracranial hemorrhage due to anoxia or hypoxia (P52.-)*
         hypoxic ischemic encephalopathy [HIE] (P91.6-)
         late metabolic acidosis of newborn (P74.0)

Other disorders originating in the perinatal period (P90-P96)

P90 **Convulsions of newborn**   N
     EXCLUDES 1   *benign myoclonic epilepsy in infancy (G40.3-)*
         benign neonatal convulsions (familial) (G40.3-)

✓4ᵗʰ **P91** **Other disturbances of cerebral status of newborn**

   P91.0 **Neonatal cerebral ischemia**   N

   P91.1 **Acquired periventricular cysts of newborn**   N

   P91.2 **Neonatal cerebral leukomalacia**   N
       Periventricular leukomalacia

   P91.3 **Neonatal cerebral irritability**   N

   P91.4 **Neonatal cerebral depression**   N

   P91.5 **Neonatal coma**   N

   ✓5ᵗʰ **P91.6** **Hypoxic ischemic encephalopathy [HIE]**

     P91.60 **Hypoxic ischemic encephalopathy [HIE], unspecified**   N

     P91.61 **Mild hypoxic ischemic encephalopathy [HIE]**   N

     P91.62 **Moderate hypoxic ischemic encephalopathy [HIE]**   N

     P91.63 **Severe hypoxic ischemic encephalopathy [HIE]**   N

   P91.8 **Other specified disturbances of cerebral status of newborn**   N

   P91.9 **Disturbance of cerebral status of newborn, unspecified**   N

✓4ᵗʰ **P92** **Feeding problems of newborn**
     EXCLUDES 1   *feeding problems in child over 28 days old (R63.3)*

   ✓5ᵗʰ **P92.0** **Vomiting of newborn**
       EXCLUDES 1   *vomiting of child over 28 days old (R11.-)*

     P92.01 **Bilious vomiting of newborn**   N
       EXCLUDES 1   *bilious vomiting in child over 28 days old (R11.14)*

     P92.09 **Other vomiting of newborn**   N
       EXCLUDES 1   *regurgitation of food in newborn (P92.1)*

   P92.1 **Regurgitation and rumination of newborn**   N

   P92.2 **Slow feeding of newborn**   N

   P92.3 **Underfeeding of newborn**   N

   P92.4 **Overfeeding of newborn**   N

   P92.5 **Neonatal difficulty in feeding at breast**   N

   P92.6 **Failure to thrive in newborn**   N
       EXCLUDES 1   *failure to thrive in child over 28 days old (R62.51)*

   P92.8 **Other feeding problems of newborn**   N

   P92.9 **Feeding problem of newborn, unspecified**   N

✓4ᵗʰ **P93** **Reactions and intoxications due to drugs administered to newborn**
     INCLUDES   reactions and intoxications due to drugs administered to fetus affecting newborn
     EXCLUDES 1   *jaundice due to drugs or toxins transmitted from mother or given to newborn (P58.4-)*
         reactions and intoxications from maternal opiates, tranquilizers and other medication (P04.0-P04.1, P04.4)
         withdrawal symptoms from maternal use of drugs of addiction (P96.1)
         withdrawal symptoms from therapeutic use of drugs in newborn (P96.2)

   P93.0 **Grey baby syndrome**   N
       Grey syndrome from chloramphenicol administration in newborn

   P93.8 **Other reactions and intoxications due to drugs administered to newborn**   N
       Use additional code for adverse effect, if applicable, to identify drug (T36-T50 with fifth or sixth character 5)

✓4ᵗʰ **P94** **Disorders of muscle tone of newborn**

   P94.0 **Transient neonatal myasthenia gravis**   N
       EXCLUDES 1   *myasthenia gravis (G70.0)*

   P94.1 **Congenital hypertonia**   N

   P94.2 **Congenital hypotonia**   N
       Floppy baby syndrome, unspecified

   P94.8 **Other disorders of muscle tone of newborn**   N

   P94.9 **Disorder of muscle tone of newborn, unspecified**   N

P95 **Stillbirth**   N
     Deadborn fetus NOS
     Fetal death of unspecified cause
     Stillbirth NOS
     EXCLUDES 1   *maternal care for intrauterine death (O36.4)*
         missed abortion (O02.1)
         outcome of delivery, stillbirth (Z37.1, Z37.3, Z37.4, Z37.7)

✓4ᵗʰ **P96** **Other conditions originating in the perinatal period**

   P96.0 **Congenital renal failure**   N
       Uremia of newborn

   P96.1 **Neonatal withdrawal symptoms from maternal use of drugs of addiction**   N
       Drug withdrawal syndrome in infant of dependent mother
       Neonatal abstinence syndrome
       EXCLUDES 1   *reactions and intoxications from maternal opiates and tranquilizers administered during labor and delivery (P04.0)*

   P96.2 **Withdrawal symptoms from therapeutic use of drugs in newborn**   N

   P96.3 **Wide cranial sutures of newborn**   N
       Neonatal craniotabes

   P96.5 **Complication to newborn due to (fetal) intrauterine procedure**   N
       EXCLUDES 2   *newborn (suspected to be) affected by amniocentesis (P00.6)*

   ✓5ᵗʰ **P96.8** **Other specified conditions originating in the perinatal period**

     P96.81 **Exposure to (parental) (environmental) tobacco smoke in the perinatal period**
       EXCLUDES 2   *newborn affected by in utero exposure to tobacco (P04.2)*
         exposure to environmental tobacco smoke after the perinatal period (Z77.22)

     P96.82 **Delayed separation of umbilical cord**   N

     P96.83 **Meconium staining**   N
       EXCLUDES 1   *meconium aspiration (P24.00, P24.01)*
         meconium passage during delivery (P03.82)

     P96.89 **Other specified conditions originating in the perinatal period**   N
       Use additional code to specify condition

   P96.9 **Condition originating in the perinatal period, unspecified**   N
       Congenital debility NOS

✅ Additional Character Required   ✓x7ᵗʰ Xtension Alert   Unspecified Dx   Other Specified Dx   Manifestation   ►◄ Revised Text   ● New Code   ▲ Revised Code Title

ICD-10-CM Draft (2015)   773

Chapter 17. Congenital Malformations, Deformations and Chromosomal Abnormalities(Q00-Q99)

NOTE   Codes from this chapter are not for use on maternal or fetal records.

EXCLUDES 2 *inborn errors of metabolism (E70-E88)*

This chapter contains the following blocks:

Q00-Q07	Congenital malformations of the nervous system
Q10-Q18	Congenital malformations of eye, ear, face and neck
Q20-Q28	Congenital malformations of the circulatory system
Q30-Q34	Congenital malformations of the respiratory system
Q35-Q37	Cleft lip and cleft palate
Q38-Q45	Other congenital malformations of the digestive system
Q50-Q56	Congenital malformations of genital organs
Q60-Q64	Congenital malformations of the urinary system
Q65-Q79	Congenital malformations and deformations of the musculoskeletal system
Q80-Q89	Other congenital malformations
Q90-Q99	Chromosomal abnormalities, not elsewhere classified

Congenital malformations of the nervous system (Q00-Q07)

✓4ᵗʰ Q00 Anencephaly and similar malformations

    Q00.0 Anencephaly
        Acephaly
        Acrania
        Amyelencephaly
        Hemianencephaly
        Hemicephaly

    Q00.1 Craniorachischisis

    Q00.2 Iniencephaly

✓4ᵗʰ Q01 Encephalocele

    INCLUDES Arnold-Chiari syndrome, type III
        encephalocystocele
        encephalomyelocele
        hydroencephalocele
        hydromeningocele, cranial
        meningocele, cerebral
        meningoencephalocele

    EXCLUDES 1 *Meckel-Gruber syndrome (Q61.9)*

    Q01.0 Frontal encephalocele

    Q01.1 Nasofrontal encephalocele

    Q01.2 Occipital encephalocele

    Q01.8 Encephalocele of other sites

    Q01.9 Encephalocele, unspecified

Q02 Microcephaly

    INCLUDES hydromicrocephaly
        micrencephalon

    EXCLUDES 1 *Meckel-Gruber syndrome (Q61.9)*

✓4ᵗʰ Q03 Congenital hydrocephalus

    INCLUDES hydrocephalus in newborn

    EXCLUDES 1 *Arnold-Chiari syndrome, type II (Q07.0-)*
        acquired hydrocephalus (G91.-)
        hydrocephalus due to congenital toxoplasmosis (P37.1)
        hydrocephalus with spina bifida (Q05.0-Q05.4)

    Q03.0 Malformations of aqueduct of Sylvius
        Anomaly of aqueduct of Sylvius
        Obstruction of aqueduct of Sylvius, congenital
        Stenosis of aqueduct of Sylvius

    Q03.1 Atresia of foramina of Magendie and Luschka
        Dandy-Walker syndrome

    Q03.8 Other congenital hydrocephalus

    Q03.9 Congenital hydrocephalus, unspecified

✓4ᵗʰ Q04 Other congenital malformations of brain

    EXCLUDES 1 *cyclopia (Q87.0)*
        macrocephaly (Q75.3)

    Q04.0 Congenital malformations of corpus callosum
        Agenesis of corpus callosum

    Q04.1 Arhinencephaly

    Q04.2 Holoprosencephaly

    Q04.3 Other reduction deformities of brain
        Absence of part of brain
        Agenesis of part of brain
        Agyria
        Aplasia of part of brain
        Hydranencephaly
        Hypoplasia of part of brain
        Lissencephaly
        Microgyria
        Pachygyria

    EXCLUDES 1 *congenital malformations of corpus callosum (Q04.0)*

    Q04.4 Septo-optic dysplasia of brain

    Q04.5 Megalencephaly

    Q04.6 Congenital cerebral cysts
        Porencephaly
        Schizencephaly

    EXCLUDES 1 *acquired porencephalic cyst (G93.0)*

    Q04.8 Other specified congenital malformations of brain
        Arnold-Chiari syndrome, type IV
        Macrogyria

    Q04.9 Congenital malformation of brain, unspecified
        Congenital anomaly NOS of brain
        Congenital deformity NOS of brain
        Congenital disease or lesion NOS of brain
        Multiple anomalies NOS of brain, congenital

✓4ᵗʰ Q05 Spina bifida

    Hydromeningocele (spinal)
    Meningocele (spinal)
    Meningomyelocele
    Myelocele
    Myelomeningocele
    Rachischisis
    Spina bifida (aperta)(cystica)
    Syringomyelocele
    Use additional code for any associated paraplegia (paraparesis) (G82.2-)

    EXCLUDES 1 *Arnold-Chiari syndrome, type II (Q07.0-)*
        spina bifida occulta (Q76.0)

    Q05.0 Cervical spina bifida with hydrocephalus

    Q05.1 Thoracic spina bifida with hydrocephalus
        Dorsal spina bifida with hydrocephalus
        Thoracolumbar spina bifida with hydrocephalus

    Q05.2 Lumbar spina bifida with hydrocephalus
        Lumbosacral spina bifida with hydrocephalus

    Q05.3 Sacral spina bifida with hydrocephalus

    Q05.4 Unspecified spina bifida with hydrocephalus

    Q05.5 Cervical spina bifida without hydrocephalus

    Q05.6 Thoracic spina bifida without hydrocephalus
        Dorsal spina bifida NOS
        Thoracolumbar spina bifida NOS

    Q05.7 Lumbar spina bifida without hydrocephalus
        Lumbosacral spina bifida NOS

    Q05.8 Sacral spina bifida without hydrocephalus

    Q05.9 Spina bifida, unspecified

✓4ᵗʰ Q06 Other congenital malformations of spinal cord

    Q06.0 Amyelia

    Q06.1 Hypoplasia and dysplasia of spinal cord
        Atelomyelia
        Myelatelia
        Myelodysplasia of spinal cord

    Q06.2 Diastematomyelia

    Q06.3 Other congenital cauda equina malformations

    Q06.4 Hydromyelia
        Hydrorachis

    Q06.8 Other specified congenital malformations of spinal cord

    Q06.9 Congenital malformation of spinal cord, unspecified
        Congenital anomaly NOS of spinal cord
        Congenital deformity NOS of spinal cord
        Congenital disease or lesion NOS of spinal cord

✓4ᵗʰ Q07 Other congenital malformations of nervous system

    EXCLUDES 2 *congenital central alveolar hypoventilation syndrome (G47.35)*
        familial dysautonomia [Riley-Day] (G90.1)
        neurofibromatosis (nonmalignant) (Q85.0-)

    ✓5ᵗʰ Q07.0 Arnold-Chiari syndrome
        Arnold-Chiari syndrome, type II

        EXCLUDES 1 *Arnold-Chiari syndrome, type III (Q01.-)*
            Arnold-Chiari syndrome, type IV (Q04.8)

        Q07.00 Arnold-Chiari syndrome without spina bifida or hydrocephalus

---

EXCLUDES 1 Not coded here   **EXCLUDES 2** Not included here   N Newborn Age: 0   P Pediatric Age: 0-17   M Maternity Age: 12-55   A Adult Age: 15-124

774   ICD-10-CM Draft (2015)

Q07.01   **Arnold-Chiari syndrome** with spina bifida

Q07.02   **Arnold-Chiari syndrome** with hydrocephalus

Q07.03   **Arnold-Chiari syndrome** with spina bifida and hydrocephalus

Q07.8   **Other specified congenital malformations of nervous system**
Agenesis of nerve
Displacement of brachial plexus
Jaw-winking syndrome
Marcus Gunn's syndrome

Q07.9   **Congenital malformation of nervous system, unspecified**
Congenital anomaly NOS of nervous system
Congenital deformity NOS of nervous system
Congenital disease or lesion NOS of nervous system

Congenital malformations of eye, ear, face and neck (Q10-Q18)

EXCLUDES 2   *cleft lip and cleft palate (Q35-Q37)*
congenital malformation of cervical spine (Q05.0, Q05.5, Q67.5, Q76.0-Q76.4)
congenital malformation of larynx (Q31.-)
congenital malformation of lip NEC (Q38.0)
congenital malformation of nose (Q30.-)
congenital malformation of parathyroid gland (Q89.2)
congenital malformation of thyroid gland (Q89.2)

✓4ᵗʰ **Q10 Congenital malformations of** eyelid, lacrimal apparatus and orbit

EXCLUDES 1   *cryptophthalmos NOS (Q11.2)*
cryptophthalmos syndrome (Q87.0)

Q10.0 **Congenital** ptosis

Q10.1 **Congenital** ectropion

Q10.2 **Congenital** entropion

Q10.3 **Other congenital malformations of** eyelid
Ablepharon
Blepharophimosis, congenital
Coloboma of eyelid
Congenital absence or agenesis of cilia
Congenital absence or agenesis of eyelid
Congenital accessory eyelid
Congenital accessory eye muscle
Congenital malformation of eyelid NOS

Q10.4 **Absence and agenesis of lacrimal apparatus**
Congenital absence of punctum lacrimale

Q10.5 **Congenital** stenosis and stricture of lacrimal duct

Q10.6 **Other congenital malformations of** lacrimal apparatus
Congenital malformation of lacrimal apparatus NOS

Q10.7 **Congenital malformation of** orbit

✓4ᵗʰ **Q11 Anophthalmos, microphthalmos and macrophthalmos**

Q11.0 **Cystic eyeball**

Q11.1 **Other anophthalmos**
Anophthalmos NOS
Agenesis of eye
Aplasia of eye

Q11.2 **Microphthalmos**
Cryptophthalmos NOS
Dysplasia of eye
Hypoplasia of eye
Rudimentary eye
EXCLUDES 1 *cryptophthalmos syndrome (Q87.0)*

Q11.3 **Macrophthalmos**
EXCLUDES 1 *macrophthalmos in congenital glaucoma (Q15.0)*

✓4ᵗʰ **Q12 Congenital** lens **malformations**

Q12.0 **Congenital** cataract

Q12.1 **Congenital** displaced lens

Q12.2 **Coloboma of lens**

Q12.3 **Congenital** aphakia

Q12.4 **Spherophakia**

Q12.8 **Other congenital lens malformations**
Microphakia

Q12.9 **Congenital lens malformation, unspecified**

✓4ᵗʰ **Q13 Congenital malformations of** anterior segment of eye

Q13.0 **Coloboma of iris**
Coloboma NOS

Q13.1 **Absence of iris**
Aniridia
Use additional code for associated glaucoma (H42)

Q13.2 **Other congenital malformations of** iris
Anisocoria, congenital
Atresia of pupil
Congenital malformation of iris NOS
Corectopia

Q13.3 **Congenital** corneal opacity

Q13.4 **Other congenital corneal malformations**
Congenital malformation of cornea NOS
Microcornea
Peter's anomaly

Q13.5 Blue sclera

✓5ᵗʰ Q13.8 **Other congenital malformations of anterior segment of eye**

Q13.81 **Rieger's anomaly**
Use additional code for associated glaucoma (H42)

Q13.89 **Other congenital malformations of anterior segment of eye**

Q13.9 **Congenital malformation of anterior segment of eye, unspecified**

✓4ᵗʰ **Q14 Congenital malformations of** posterior segment of eye

EXCLUDES 2 *optic nerve hypoplasia (H47.03-)*

Q14.0 **Congenital malformation of** vitreous humor
Congenital vitreous opacity

Q14.1 **Congenital malformation of** retina
Congenital retinal aneurysm

Q14.2 **Congenital malformation of** optic disc
Coloboma of optic disc

Q14.3 **Congenital malformation of** choroid

Q14.8 **Other congenital malformations of posterior segment of eye**
Coloboma of the fundus

Q14.9 **Congenital malformation of posterior segment of eye, unspecified**

✓4ᵗʰ **Q15 Other congenital malformations of** eye

EXCLUDES 1 *congenital nystagmus (H55.01)*
ocular albinism (E70.31-)
optic nerve hypoplasia (H47.03-)
retinitis pigmentosa (H35.52)

Q15.0 **Congenital glaucoma**
Axenfeld's anomaly
Buphthalmos
Glaucoma of childhood
Glaucoma of newborn
Hydrophthalmos
Keratoglobus, congenital, with glaucoma
Macrocornea with glaucoma
Macrophthalmos in congenital glaucoma
Megalocornea with glaucoma

Q15.8 **Other specified congenital malformations of eye**

Q15.9 **Congenital malformation of eye, unspecified**
Congenital anomaly of eye
Congenital deformity of eye

✓4ᵗʰ **Q16 Congenital malformations of** ear causing impairment of hearing

EXCLUDES 1 *congenital deafness (H90.-)*

Q16.0 **Congenital absence of (ear)** auricle

Q16.1 **Congenital absence,** atresia and stricture of auditory canal **(external)**
Congenital atresia or stricture of osseous meatus

Q16.2 **Absence of** eustachian tube

Q16.3 **Congenital malformation of** ear ossicles
Congenital fusion of ear ossicles

Q16.4 **Other congenital malformations of middle ear**
Congenital malformation of middle ear NOS

Q16.5 **Congenital malformation of** inner ear
Congenital anomaly of membranous labyrinth
Congenital anomaly of organ of Corti

Q16.9 **Congenital malformation of ear causing impairment of hearing, unspecified**
Congenital absence of ear NOS

✓4ᵗʰ **Q17 Other congenital malformations of** ear

EXCLUDES 1 *congenital malformations of ear with impairment of hearing (Q16.0- Q16.9)*
preauricular sinus (Q18.1)

Q17.0 **Accessory auricle**
Accessory tragus
Polyotia
Preauricular appendage or tag
Supernumerary ear
Supernumerary lobule

Q17.1 **Macrotia**

Q17.2 Microtia

Q17.3 Other misshapen ear
Pointed ear

Q17.4 Misplaced ear
Low-set ears
EXCLUDES 1   *cervical auricle (Q18.2)*

Q17.5 Prominent ear
Bat ear

Q17.8 Other specified congenital malformations of ear
Congenital absence of lobe of ear

Q17.9 Congenital malformation of ear, unspecified
Congenital anomaly of ear NOS

✓4ᵗʰ **Q18 Other congenital malformations of face and neck**
EXCLUDES 1   *cleft lip and cleft palate (Q35-Q37)*
conditions classified to Q67.0-Q67.4
congenital malformations of skull and face bones (Q75.-)
cyclopia (Q87.0)
dentofacial anomalies [including malocclusion] (M26.-)
malformation syndromes affecting facial appearance (Q87.0)
persistent thyroglossal duct (Q89.2)

Q18.0 Sinus, fistula and cyst of branchial cleft
Branchial vestige

Q18.1 Preauricular sinus and cyst
Fistula of auricle, congenital
Cervicoaural fistula

Q18.2 Other branchial cleft malformations
Branchial cleft malformation NOS
Cervical auricle
Otocephaly

Q18.3 Webbing of neck
Pterygium colli

Q18.4 Macrostomia

Q18.5 Microstomia

Q18.6 Macrocheilia
Hypertrophy of lip, congenital

Q18.7 Microcheilia

Q18.8 Other specified congenital malformations of face and neck
Medial cyst of face and neck
Medial fistula of face and neck
Medial sinus of face and neck

Q18.9 Congenital malformation of face and neck, unspecified
Congenital anomaly NOS of face and neck

Congenital malformations of the circulatory system (Q20-Q28)

✓4ᵗʰ **Q20 Congenital malformations of cardiac chambers and connections**
EXCLUDES 1   *dextrocardia with situs inversus (Q89.3)*
mirror-image atrial arrangement with situs inversus (Q89.3)

Q20.0 Common arterial trunk
Persistent truncus arteriosus
EXCLUDES 1   *aortic septal defect (Q21.4)*

Q20.1 Double outlet right ventricle
Taussig-Bing syndrome

Q20.2 Double outlet left ventricle

Q20.3 Discordant ventriculoarterial connection
Dextrotransposition of aorta
Transposition of great vessels (complete)

Q20.4 Double inlet ventricle
Common ventricle
Cor triloculare biatriatum
Single ventricle

Q20.5 Discordant atrioventricular connection
Corrected transposition
Levotransposition
Ventricular inversion

Q20.6 Isomerism of atrial appendages
Isomerism of atrial appendages with asplenia or polysplenia

Q20.8 Other congenital malformations of cardiac chambers and connections
Cor binoculare

Q20.9 Congenital malformation of cardiac chambers and connections, unspecified

✓4ᵗʰ **Q21 Congenital malformations of cardiac septa**
EXCLUDES 1   *acquired cardiac septal defect (I51.0)*

Q21.0 Ventricular septal defect
Roger's disease

Q21.1 Atrial septal defect
Coronary sinus defect
Patent or persistent foramen ovale
Patent or persistent ostium secundum defect (type II)
Patent or persistent sinus venosus defect

Q21.2 Atrioventricular septal defect
Common atrioventricular canal
Endocardial cushion defect
Ostium primum atrial septal defect (type I)

Q21.3 Tetralogy of Fallot
Ventricular septal defect with pulmonary stenosis or atresia, dextroposition of aorta and hypertrophy of right ventricle.

Q21.4 Aortopulmonary septal defect
Aortic septal defect
Aortopulmonary window

Q21.8 Other congenital malformations of cardiac septa
Eisenmenger's defect
Pentalogy of Fallot
EXCLUDES 1   *Eisenmenger's complex (I27.8)*
Eisenmenger's syndrome (I27.8)

Q21.9 Congenital malformation of cardiac septum, unspecified
Septal (heart) defect NOS

✓4ᵗʰ **Q22 Congenital malformations of pulmonary and tricuspid valves**

Q22.0 Pulmonary valve atresia

Q22.1 Congenital pulmonary valve stenosis

Q22.2 Congenital pulmonary valve insufficiency
Congenital pulmonary valve regurgitation

Q22.3 Other congenital malformations of pulmonary valve
Congenital malformation of pulmonary valve NOS
Supernumerary cusps of pulmonary valve

Q22.4 Congenital tricuspid stenosis
Congenital tricuspid atresia

Q22.5 Ebstein's anomaly

Q22.6 Hypoplastic right heart syndrome

Q22.8 Other congenital malformations of tricuspid valve

Q22.9 Congenital malformation of tricuspid valve, unspecified

✓4ᵗʰ **Q23 Congenital malformations of aortic and mitral valves**

Q23.0 Congenital stenosis of aortic valve
Congenital aortic atresia
Congenital aortic stenosis NOS
EXCLUDES 1   *congenital stenosis of aortic valve in hypoplastic left heart syndrome (Q23.4)*
congenital subaortic stenosis (Q24.4)
supravalvular aortic stenosis (congenital) (Q25.3)

Q23.1 Congenital insufficiency of aortic valve
Bicuspid aortic valve
Congenital aortic insufficiency

Q23.2 Congenital mitral stenosis
Congenital mitral atresia

Q23.3 Congenital mitral insufficiency

Q23.4 Hypoplastic left heart syndrome

Q23.8 Other congenital malformations of aortic and mitral valves

Q23.9 Congenital malformation of aortic and mitral valves, unspecified

✓4ᵗʰ **Q24 Other congenital malformations of heart**
EXCLUDES 1   *endocardial fibroelastosis (I42.4)*

Q24.0 Dextrocardia
EXCLUDES 1   *dextrocardia with situs inversus (Q89.3)*
isomerism of atrial appendages (with asplenia or polysplenia) (Q20.6)
mirror-image atrial arrangement with situs inversus (Q89.3)

Q24.1 Levocardia

Q24.2 Cor triatriatum

Q24.3 Pulmonary infundibular stenosis
Subvalvular pulmonic stenosis

Q24.4 Congenital subaortic stenosis

Q24.5 Malformation of coronary vessels
Congenital coronary (artery) aneurysm

Q24.6 Congenital heart block

Q24.8 Other specified congenital malformations of heart
Congenital diverticulum of left ventricle
Congenital malformation of myocardium
Congenital malformation of pericardium
Malposition of heart
Uhl's disease

EXCLUDES 1 Not coded here   *EXCLUDES 2* Not included here   N Newborn Age: 0   P Pediatric Age: 0-17   M Maternity Age: 12-55   A Adult Age: 15-124

Q24.9 **Congenital malformation of heart, unspecified**
    Congenital anomaly of heart
    Congenital disease of heart

✓4ᵗʰ **Q25** **Congenital malformations of** great arteries

Q25.0 Patent ductus arteriosus
    Patent ductus Botallo
    Persistent ductus arteriosus

Q25.1 Coarctation **of** aorta
    Coarctation of aorta (preductal) (postductal)

Q25.2 Atresia **of** aorta

Q25.3 Supravalvular **aortic** stenosis
    EXCLUDES 1 *congenital aortic stenosis NOS (Q23.0)*
    congenital stenosis of aortic valve (Q23.0)

Q25.4 **Other congenital malformations of** aorta
    Absence of aorta
    Aneurysm of sinus of Valsalva (ruptured)
    Aplasia of aorta
    Congenital aneurysm of aorta
    Congenital malformations of aorta
    Congenital dilatation of aorta
    Double aortic arch [vascular ring of aorta]
    Hypoplasia of aorta
    Persistent convolutions of aortic arch
    Persistent right aortic arch
    EXCLUDES 1 *hypoplasia of aorta in hypoplastic left heart syndrome (Q23.4)*

Q25.5 Atresia **of** pulmonary **artery**

Q25.6 Stenosis **of** pulmonary **artery**
    Supravalvular pulmonary stenosis

✓5ᵗʰ Q25.7 **Other congenital malformations of** pulmonary **artery**

    Q25.71 Coarctation **of pulmonary artery**

    Q25.72 **Congenital pulmonary** arteriovenous malformation
        Congenital pulmonary arteriovenous aneurysm

    Q25.79 **Other congenital malformations of pulmonary artery**
        Aberrant pulmonary artery
        Agenesis of pulmonary artery
        Congenital aneurysm of pulmonary artery
        Congenital anomaly of pulmonary artery
        Hypoplasia of pulmonary artery

Q25.8 **Other congenital malformations of other great arteries**

Q25.9 **Congenital malformation of great arteries, unspecified**

✓4ᵗʰ **Q26** **Congenital malformations of** great veins

Q26.0 **Congenital** stenosis **of** vena cava
    Congenital stenosis of vena cava (inferior)(superior)

Q26.1 **Persistent** left superior vena cava

Q26.2 Total **anomalous** pulmonary venous connection
    Total anomalous pulmonary venous return [TAPVR], subdiaphragmatic
    Total anomalous pulmonary venous return [TAPVR], supradiaphragmatic

Q26.3 Partial **anomalous** pulmonary venous connection
    Partial anomalous pulmonary venous return

Q26.4 **Anomalous pulmonary venous connection, unspecified**

Q26.5 **Anomalous** portal venous connection

Q26.6 Portal vein-hepatic **artery** fistula

Q26.8 **Other congenital malformations of great veins**
    Absence of vena cava (inferior) (superior)
    Azygos continuation of inferior vena cava
    Persistent left posterior cardinal vein
    Scimitar syndrome

Q26.9 **Congenital malformation of great vein, unspecified**
    Congenital anomaly of vena cava (inferior) (superior) NOS

✓4ᵗʰ **Q27** **Other congenital malformations of** peripheral vascular system
    EXCLUDES 2 *anomalies of cerebral and precerebral vessels (Q28.0-Q28.3)*
    anomalies of coronary vessels (Q24.5)
    anomalies of pulmonary artery (Q25.5-Q25.7)
    congenital retinal aneurysm (Q14.1)
    hemangioma and lymphangioma (D18.-)

Q27.0 **Congenital** absence and hypoplasia **of** umbilical **artery**
    Single umbilical artery

Q27.1 **Congenital** renal **artery** stenosis

Q27.2 **Other congenital malformations of** renal **artery**
    Congenital malformation of renal artery NOS
    Multiple renal arteries

✓5ᵗʰ Q27.3 **Arteriovenous malformation (peripheral)**
    Arteriovenous aneurysm
    EXCLUDES 1 *acquired arteriovenous aneurysm (I77.0)*
    EXCLUDES 2 *arteriovenous malformation of cerebral vessels (Q28.2)*
    arteriovenous malformation of precerebral vessels (Q28.0)

    Q27.30 **Arteriovenous malformation, site unspecified**

    Q27.31 **Arteriovenous malformation of** vessel of upper limb

    Q27.32 **Arteriovenous malformation of** vessel of lower limb

    Q27.33 **Arteriovenous malformation of** digestive system vessel

    Q27.34 **Arteriovenous malformation of** renal vessel

    Q27.39 **Arteriovenous malformation, other site**

Q27.4 **Congenital** phlebectasia

Q27.8 **Other specified congenital malformations of peripheral vascular system**
    Absence of peripheral vascular system
    Atresia of peripheral vascular system
    Congenital aneurysm (peripheral)
    Congenital stricture, artery
    Congenital varix
    EXCLUDES 1 *arteriovenous malformation (Q27.3-)*

Q27.9 **Congenital malformation of peripheral vascular system, unspecified**
    Anomaly of artery or vein NOS

✓4ᵗʰ **Q28** Other **congenital malformations of** circulatory system
    EXCLUDES 1 *congenital aneurysm NOS (Q27.8)*
    congenital coronary aneurysm (Q24.5)
    ruptured cerebral arteriovenous malformation (I60.8)
    ruptured malformation of precerebral vessels (I72.0)
    EXCLUDES 2 *congenital peripheral aneurysm (Q27.8)*
    congenital pulmonary aneurysm (Q25.79)
    congenital retinal aneurysm (Q14.1)

Q28.0 Arteriovenous **malformation of** precerebral **vessels**
    Congenital arteriovenous precerebral aneurysm (nonruptured)

Q28.1 **Other malformations of** precerebral **vessels**
    Congenital malformation of precerebral vessels NOS
    Congenital precerebral aneurysm (nonruptured)

Q28.2 Arteriovenous **malformation of** cerebral **vessels**
    Arteriovenous malformation of brain NOS
    Congenital arteriovenous cerebral aneurysm (nonruptured)

Q28.3 **Other malformations of** cerebral **vessels**
    Congenital cerebral aneurysm (nonruptured)
    Congenital malformation of cerebral vessels NOS
    Developmental venous anomaly

Q28.8 **Other specified congenital malformations of circulatory system**
    Congenital aneurysm, specified site NEC
    Spinal vessel anomaly

Q28.9 **Congenital malformation of circulatory system, unspecified**

Congenital malformations of the respiratory system (Q30-Q34)

✓4ᵗʰ **Q30** **Congenital malformations of** nose
    EXCLUDES 1 *congenital deviation of nasal septum (Q67.4)*

Q30.0 **Choanal** atresia
    Atresia of nares (anterior) (posterior)
    Congenital stenosis of nares (anterior) (posterior)

Q30.1 Agenesis **and underdevelopment of nose**
    Congenital absent of nose

Q30.2 Fissured, notched and cleft **nose**

Q30.3 **Congenital** perforated **nasal septum**

Q30.8 **Other congenital malformations of nose**
    Accessory nose
    Congenital anomaly of nasal sinus wall

Q30.9 **Congenital malformation of nose, unspecified**

✓4ᵗʰ **Q31** **Congenital malformations of** larynx
    EXCLUDES 1 *congenital laryngeal stridor NOS (P28.89)*

Q31.0 Web **of larynx**
    Glottic web of larynx
    Subglottic web of larynx
    Web of larynx NOS

Q31.1 **Congenital** subglottic stenosis

Q31.2 **Laryngeal** hypoplasia

Q31.3 Laryngocele

Q31.5 **Congenital** laryngomalacia

✓ Additional Character Required   ✓x7ᵗʰ Xtension Alert   Unspecified Dx   Other Specified Dx   Manifestation   ▶◀ Revised Text   ● New Code   ▲ Revised Code Title

ICD-10-CM Draft (2015)   **777**

Q31.8 Other congenital malformations of larynx
Absence of larynx
Agenesis of larynx
Atresia of larynx
Congenital cleft thyroid cartilage
Congenital fissure of epiglottis
Congenital stenosis of larynx NEC
Posterior cleft of cricoid cartilage

Q31.9 Congenital malformation of larynx, unspecified

✓4ᵗʰ **Q32 Congenital malformations of trachea and bronchus**
EXCLUDES 1   *congenital bronchiectasis (Q33.4)*

Q32.0 Congenital tracheomalacia

Q32.1 Other congenital malformations of trachea
Atresia of trachea
Congenital anomaly of tracheal cartilage
Congenital dilatation of trachea
Congenital malformation of trachea
Congenital stenosis of trachea
Congenital tracheocele

Q32.2 Congenital bronchomalacia

Q32.3 Congenital stenosis of bronchus

Q32.4 Other congenital malformations of bronchus
Absence of bronchus
Agenesis of bronchus
Atresia of bronchus
Congenital diverticulum of bronchus
Congenital malformation of bronchus NOS

✓4ᵗʰ **Q33 Congenital malformations of lung**

Q33.0 Congenital cystic lung
Congenital cystic lung disease
Congenital honeycomb lung
Congenital polycystic lung disease
EXCLUDES 1   *cystic fibrosis (E84.0)*
cystic lung disease, acquired or unspecified (J98.4)

Q33.1 Accessory lobe of lung
Azygos lobe (fissured), lung

Q33.2 Sequestration of lung

Q33.3 Agenesis of lung
Congenital absence of lung (lobe)

Q33.4 Congenital bronchiectasis

Q33.5 Ectopic tissue in lung

Q33.6 Congenital hypoplasia and dysplasia of lung
EXCLUDES 1   *pulmonary hypoplasia associated with short gestation (P28.0)*

Q33.8 Other congenital malformations of lung

Q33.9 Congenital malformation of lung, unspecified

✓4ᵗʰ **Q34 Other congenital malformations of respiratory system**
EXCLUDES 2   *congenital central alveolar hypoventilation syndrome (G47.35)*

Q34.0 Anomaly of pleura

Q34.1 Congenital cyst of mediastinum

Q34.8 Other specified congenital malformations of respiratory system
Atresia of nasopharynx

Q34.9 Congenital malformation of respiratory system, unspecified
Congenital absence of respiratory system
Congenital anomaly of respiratory system NOS

Cleft lip and cleft palate (Q35-Q37)

Use additional code to identify associated malformation of the nose (Q30.2)
EXCLUDES 1   *Robin's syndrome (Q87.0)*

✓4ᵗʰ **Q35 Cleft palate**
INCLUDES   fissure of palate
palatoschisis
EXCLUDES 1   *cleft palate with cleft lip (Q37.-)*

Q35.1 Cleft hard palate

Q35.3 Cleft soft palate

Q35.5 Cleft hard palate with cleft soft palate

Q35.7 Cleft uvula

Q35.9 Cleft palate, unspecified
Cleft palate NOS

✓4ᵗʰ **Q36 Cleft lip**
Cheiloschisis
Congenital fissure of lip
Harelip
Labium leporinum
EXCLUDES 1   *cleft lip with cleft palate (Q37.-)*

Q36.0 Cleft lip, bilateral

Q36.1 Cleft lip, median

Q36.9 Cleft lip, unilateral
Cleft lip NOS

✓4ᵗʰ **Q37 Cleft palate with cleft lip**
Cheilopalatoschisis

Q37.0 Cleft hard palate with bilateral cleft lip

Q37.1 Cleft hard palate with unilateral cleft lip
Cleft hard palate with cleft lip NOS

Q37.2 Cleft soft palate with bilateral cleft lip

Q37.3 Cleft soft palate with unilateral cleft lip
Cleft soft palate with cleft lip NOS

Q37.4 Cleft hard and soft palate with bilateral cleft lip

Q37.5 Cleft hard and soft palate with unilateral cleft lip
Cleft hard and soft palate with cleft lip NOS

Q37.8 Unspecified cleft palate with bilateral cleft lip

Q37.9 Unspecified cleft palate with unilateral cleft lip
Cleft palate with cleft lip NOS

Other congenital malformations of the digestive system (Q38-Q45)

✓4ᵗʰ **Q38 Other congenital malformations of tongue, mouth and pharynx**
EXCLUDES 1   *dentofacial anomalies (M26.-)*
macrostomia (Q18.4)
microstomia (Q18.5)

Q38.0 Congenital malformations of lips, not elsewhere classified
Congenital fistula of lip
Congenital malformation of lip NOS
Van der Woude's syndrome
EXCLUDES 1   *cleft lip (Q36.-)*
cleft lip with cleft palate (Q37.-)
macrocheilia (Q18.6)
microcheilia (Q18.7)

Q38.1 Ankyloglossia
Tongue tie

Q38.2 Macroglossia
Congenital hypertrophy of tongue

Q38.3 Other congenital malformations of tongue
Aglossia
Bifid tongue
Congenital adhesion of tongue
Congenital fissure of tongue
Congenital malformation of tongue NOS
Double tongue
Hypoglossia
Hypoplasia of tongue
Microglossia

Q38.4 Congenital malformations of salivary glands and ducts
Atresia of salivary glands and ducts
Congenital absence of salivary glands and ducts
Congenital accessory salivary glands and ducts
Congenital fistula of salivary gland

Q38.5 Congenital malformations of palate, not elsewhere classified
Congenital absence of uvula
Congenital malformation of palate NOS
Congenital high arched palate
EXCLUDES 1   *cleft palate (Q35.-)*
cleft palate with cleft lip (Q37.-)

Q38.6 Other congenital malformations of mouth
Congenital malformation of mouth NOS

Q38.7 Congenital pharyngeal pouch
Congenital diverticulum of pharynx
EXCLUDES 1   *pharyngeal pouch syndrome (D82.1)*

Q38.8 Other congenital malformations of pharynx
Congenital malformation of pharynx NOS
Imperforate pharynx

✓4ᵗʰ **Q39 Congenital malformations of esophagus**

Q39.0 Atresia of esophagus without fistula
Atresia of esophagus NOS

Q39.1 Atresia of esophagus with tracheo-esophageal fistula
Atresia of esophagus with broncho-esophageal fistula

EXCLUDES 1 Not coded here   EXCLUDES 2 Not included here   N Newborn Age: 0   P Pediatric Age: 0-17   M Maternity Age: 12-55   A Adult Age: 15-124

778   ICD-10-CM Draft (2015)

Q39.2 Congenital tracheo-esophageal fistula without atresia
Congenital tracheo-esophageal fistula NOS

Q39.3 Congenital stenosis and stricture of esophagus

Q39.4 Esophageal web

Q39.5 Congenital dilatation of esophagus
Congenital cardiospasm

Q39.6 Congenital diverticulum of esophagus
Congenital esophageal pouch

Q39.8 Other congenital malformations of esophagus
Congenital absence of esophagus
Congenital displacement of esophagus
Congenital duplication of esophagus

Q39.9 Congenital malformation of esophagus, unspecified

✓4ᵗʰ Q40 Other congenital malformations of upper alimentary tract

Q40.0 Congenital hypertrophic pyloric stenosis
Congenital or infantile constriction
Congenital or infantile hypertrophy
Congenital or infantile spasm
Congenital or infantile stenosis
Congenital or infantile stricture

Q40.1 Congenital hiatus hernia
Congenital displacement of cardia through esophageal hiatus
EXCLUDES1 *congenital diaphragmatic hernia (Q79.0)*

Q40.2 Other specified congenital malformations of stomach
Congenital displacement of stomach
Congenital diverticulum of stomach
Congenital hourglass stomach
Congenital duplication of stomach
Megalogastria
Microgastria

Q40.3 Congenital malformation of stomach, unspecified

Q40.8 Other specified congenital malformations of upper alimentary tract

Q40.9 Congenital malformation of upper alimentary tract, unspecified
Congenital anomaly of upper alimentary tract
Congenital deformity of upper alimentary tract

✓4ᵗʰ Q41 Congenital absence, atresia and stenosis of small intestine
Congenital obstruction, occlusion or stricture of small intestine or intestine NOS
EXCLUDES1 *cystic fibrosis with intestinal manifestation (E84.11)*
meconium ileus NOS (without cystic fibrosis) (P76.0)

Q41.0 Congenital absence, atresia and stenosis of duodenum

Q41.1 Congenital absence, atresia and stenosis of jejunum
Apple peel syndrome
Imperforate jejunum

Q41.2 Congenital absence, atresia and stenosis of ileum

Q41.8 Congenital absence, atresia and stenosis of other specified parts of small intestine

Q41.9 Congenital absence, atresia and stenosis of small intestine, part unspecified
Congenital absence, atresia and stenosis of intestine NOS

✓4ᵗʰ Q42 Congenital absence, atresia and stenosis of large intestine
Congenital obstruction, occlusion and stricture of large intestine

Q42.0 Congenital absence, atresia and stenosis of rectum with fistula

Q42.1 Congenital absence, atresia and stenosis of rectum without fistula
Imperforate rectum

Q42.2 Congenital absence, atresia and stenosis of anus with fistula

Q42.3 Congenital absence, atresia and stenosis of anus without fistula
Imperforate anus

Q42.8 Congenital absence, atresia and stenosis of other parts of large intestine

Q42.9 Congenital absence, atresia and stenosis of large intestine, part unspecified

✓4ᵗʰ Q43 Other congenital malformations of intestine

Q43.0 Meckel's diverticulum (displaced) (hypertrophic)
Persistent omphalomesenteric duct
Persistent vitelline duct

Q43.1 Hirschsprung's disease
Aganglionosis
Congenital (aganglionic) megacolon

Q43.2 Other congenital functional disorders of colon
Congenital dilatation of colon

Q43.3 Congenital malformations of intestinal fixation
Congenital omental, anomalous adhesions [bands]
Congenital peritoneal adhesions [bands]
Incomplete rotation of cecum and colon
Insufficient rotation of cecum and colon
Jackson's membrane
Malrotation of colon
Rotation failure of cecum and colon
Universal mesentery

Q43.4 Duplication of intestine

Q43.5 Ectopic anus

Q43.6 Congenital fistula of rectum and anus
EXCLUDES1 *congenital fistula of anus with absence, atresia and stenosis (Q42.2)*
congenital fistula of rectum with absence, atresia and stenosis (Q42.0)
congenital rectovaginal fistula (Q52.2)
congenital urethrorectal fistula (Q64.73)
pilonidal fistula or sinus (L05.-)

Q43.7 Persistent cloaca
Cloaca NOS

Q43.8 Other specified congenital malformations of intestine
Congenital blind loop syndrome
Congenital diverticulitis, colon
Congenital diverticulum, intestine
Dolichocolon
Megaloappendix
Megaloduodenum
Microcolon
Transposition of appendix
Transposition of colon
Transposition of intestine
AHA: 2013, 2Q, 31

Q43.9 Congenital malformation of intestine, unspecified

✓4ᵗʰ Q44 Congenital malformations of gallbladder, bile ducts and liver

Q44.0 Agenesis, aplasia and hypoplasia of gallbladder
Congenital absence of gallbladder

Q44.1 Other congenital malformations of gallbladder
Congenital malformation of gallbladder NOS
Intrahepatic gallbladder

Q44.2 Atresia of bile ducts

Q44.3 Congenital stenosis and stricture of bile ducts

Q44.4 Choledochal cyst

Q44.5 Other congenital malformations of bile ducts
Accessory hepatic duct
Biliary duct duplication
Congenital malformation of bile duct NOS
Cystic duct duplication

Q44.6 Cystic disease of liver
Fibrocystic disease of liver

Q44.7 Other congenital malformations of liver
Accessory liver
Alagille's syndrome
Congenital absence of liver
Congenital hepatomegaly
Congenital malformation of liver NOS

✓4ᵗʰ Q45 Other congenital malformations of digestive system
EXCLUDES2 *congenital diaphragmatic hernia (Q79.0)*
congenital hiatus hernia (Q40.1)

Q45.0 Agenesis, aplasia and hypoplasia of pancreas
Congenital absence of pancreas

Q45.1 Annular pancreas

Q45.2 Congenital pancreatic cyst

Q45.3 Other congenital malformations of pancreas and pancreatic duct
Accessory pancreas
Congenital malformation of pancreas or pancreatic duct NOS
EXCLUDES1 *congenital diabetes mellitus (E10.-)*
cystic fibrosis (E84.0-E84.9)
fibrocystic disease of pancreas (E84.-)
neonatal diabetes mellitus (P70.2)

Q45.8 Other specified congenital malformations of digestive system
Absence (complete) (partial) of alimentary tract NOS
Duplication of digestive system
Malposition, congenital of digestive system

Q45.9 Congenital malformation of digestive system, unspecified
Congenital anomaly of digestive system
Congenital deformity of digestive system

☑ Additional Character Required   ✓x7ᵗʰ Xtension Alert   Unspecified Dx   Other Specified Dx   Manifestation   ▶◀ Revised Text   ● New Code   ▲ Revised Code Title

Congenital malformations of genital organs (Q50-Q56)

EXCLUDES 1 *androgen insensitivity syndrome (E34.5-)*
syndromes associated with anomalies in the number and form of chromosomes (Q90-Q99)

☑4ᵗʰ **Q50 Congenital malformations of** ovaries, fallopian tubes and broad ligaments

☑5ᵗʰ **Q50.0 Congenital absence of** ovary

     EXCLUDES 1 *Turner's syndrome (Q96.-)*

     Q50.01 Congenital absence of ovary, unilateral ♀

     Q50.02 Congenital absence of ovary, bilateral ♀

Q50.1 Developmental ovarian cyst ♀

Q50.2 Congenital torsion of ovary ♀

☑5ᵗʰ **Q50.3** Other congenital malformations of ovary

     Q50.31 Accessory ovary ♀

     Q50.32 Ovarian streak ♀
         46, XX with streak gonads

     Q50.39 Other congenital malformation of ovary ♀
         Congenital malformation of ovary NOS

Q50.4 Embryonic cyst of fallopian tube ♀
     Fimbrial cyst

Q50.5 Embryonic cyst of broad ligament ♀
     Epoophoron cyst
     Parovarian cyst

Q50.6 Other congenital malformations of fallopian tube and broad ligament ♀
     Absence of fallopian tube and broad ligament
     Accessory fallopian tube and broad ligament
     Atresia of fallopian tube and broad ligament
     Congenital malformation of fallopian tube or broad ligament NOS

☑4ᵗʰ **Q51 Congenital malformations of** uterus and cervix

Q51.0 Agenesis and aplasia of uterus ♀
     Congenital absence of uterus

☑5ᵗʰ **Q51.1** Doubling of uterus with doubling of cervix and vagina

     Q51.10 Doubling of uterus with doubling of cervix and vagina without obstruction ♀
         Doubling of uterus with doubling of cervix and vagina NOS

     Q51.11 Doubling of uterus with doubling of cervix and vagina with obstruction ♀

Q51.2 Other doubling of uterus ♀
     Doubling of uterus NOS
     Septate uterus, complete or partial

Q51.3 Bicornate uterus ♀
     Bicornate uterus, complete or partial

Q51.4 Unicornate uterus ♀
     Unicornate uterus with or without a separate uterine horn
     Uterus with only one functioning horn

Q51.5 Agenesis and aplasia of cervix ♀
     Congenital absence of cervix

Q51.6 Embryonic cyst of cervix ♀

Q51.7 Congenital fistulae between uterus and digestive and urinary tracts ♀

☑5ᵗʰ **Q51.8** Other congenital malformations of uterus and cervix

     ☑6ᵗʰ **Q51.81 Other congenital malformations of** uterus

         Q51.810 Arcuate uterus ♀
             Arcuatus uterus

         Q51.811 Hypoplasia of uterus ♀

         Q51.818 Other congenital malformations of uterus ♀
             Müllerian anomaly of uterus NEC

     ☑6ᵗʰ **Q51.82 Other congenital malformations of** cervix

         Q51.820 Cervical duplication ♀

         Q51.821 Hypoplasia of cervix ♀

         Q51.828 Other congenital malformations of cervix ♀

Q51.9 Congenital malformation of uterus and cervix, unspecified ♀

☑4ᵗʰ **Q52 Other congenital malformations of** female genitalia

Q52.0 Congenital absence of vagina ♀
     Vaginal agenesis, total or partial

☑5ᵗʰ **Q52.1** Doubling of vagina

     EXCLUDES 1 *doubling of vagina with doubling of uterus and cervix (Q51.1-)*

     Q52.10 Doubling of vagina, unspecified ♀
         Septate vagina NOS

     Q52.11 Transverse vaginal septum ♀

     Q52.12 Longitudinal vaginal septum ♀
         Longitudinal vaginal septum with or without obstruction

Q52.2 Congenital rectovaginal fistula ♀
     EXCLUDES 1 *cloaca (Q43.7)*

Q52.3 Imperforate hymen ♀

Q52.4 Other congenital malformations of vagina ♀
     Canal of Nuck cyst, congenital
     Congenital malformation of vagina NOS
     Embryonic vaginal cyst
     Gartner's duct cyst

Q52.5 Fusion of labia ♀

Q52.6 Congenital malformation of clitoris ♀

☑5ᵗʰ **Q52.7 Other and unspecified congenital malformations of vulva**

     Q52.70 Unspecified congenital malformations of vulva ♀
         Congenital malformation of vulva NOS

     Q52.71 Congenital absence of vulva ♀

     Q52.79 Other congenital malformations of vulva ♀
         Congenital cyst of vulva

Q52.8 Other specified congenital malformations of female genitalia ♀

Q52.9 Congenital malformation of female genitalia, unspecified ♀

☑4ᵗʰ **Q53 Undescended and ectopic** testicle

☑5ᵗʰ **Q53.0** Ectopic testis

     Q53.00 Ectopic testis, unspecified ♂

     Q53.01 Ectopic testis, unilateral ♂

     Q53.02 Ectopic testes, bilateral ♂

☑5ᵗʰ **Q53.1** Undescended testicle, unilateral

     Q53.10 Unspecified undescended testicle, unilateral ♂

     Q53.11 Abdominal testis, unilateral ♂

     Q53.12 Ectopic perineal testis, unilateral ♂

☑5ᵗʰ **Q53.2** Undescended testicle, bilateral

     Q53.20 Undescended testicle, unspecified, bilateral ♂

     Q53.21 Abdominal testis, bilateral ♂

     Q53.22 Ectopic perineal testis, bilateral ♂

Q53.9 Undescended testicle, unspecified ♂
     Cryptorchism NOS

☑4ᵗʰ **Q54 Hypospadias**
     EXCLUDES 1 *epispadias (Q64.0)*

Q54.0 Hypospadias, balanic ♂
     Hypospadias, coronal
     Hypospadias, glandular

Q54.1 Hypospadias, penile ♂

Q54.2 Hypospadias, penoscrotal ♂

Q54.3 Hypospadias, perineal ♂

Q54.4 Congenital chordee ♂
     Chordee without hypospadias

Q54.8 Other hypospadias ♂
     Hypospadias with intersex state

Q54.9 Hypospadias, unspecified ♂

☑4ᵗʰ **Q55 Other congenital malformations of** male genital organs
     EXCLUDES 1 *congenital hydrocele (P83.5)*
         hypospadias (Q54.-)

Q55.0 Absence and aplasia of testis ♂
     Monorchism

Q55.1 Hypoplasia of testis and scrotum ♂
     Fusion of testes

☑5ᵗʰ **Q55.2 Other and unspecified congenital malformations of** testis and scrotum

     Q55.20 Unspecified congenital malformations of testis and scrotum ♂
         Congenital malformation of testis or scrotum NOS

     Q55.21 Polyorchism ♂

     Q55.22 Retractile testis ♂

     Q55.23 Scrotal transposition ♂

     Q55.29 Other congenital malformations of testis and scrotum ♂

Q55.3 Atresia of vas deferens ♂
     Code first any associated cystic fibrosis (E84.-)

EXCLUDES 1 Not coded here   **EXCLUDES 2** Not included here   N Newborn Age: 0   P Pediatric Age: 0-17   M Maternity Age: 12-55   A Adult Age: 15-124

780   ICD-10-CM Draft (2015)

Q55.4 **Other congenital malformations of vas deferens, epididymis, seminal vesicles and prostate** ♂
    Absence or aplasia of prostate
    Absence or aplasia of spermatic cord
    Congenital malformation of vas deferens, epididymis, seminal vesicles or prostate NOS

Q55.5 **Congenital absence and aplasia of penis** ♂

✓5th **Q55.6** **Other congenital malformations of penis**

    Q55.61 **Curvature of penis (lateral)** ♂

    Q55.62 **Hypoplasia of penis** ♂
        Micropenis

    Q55.63 **Congenital torsion of penis** ♂
        EXCLUDES 1 *acquired torsion of penis (N48.82)*

    Q55.64 **Hidden penis** ♂
        Buried penis
        Concealed penis
        EXCLUDES 1 *acquired buried penis (N48.83)*

    Q55.69 **Other congenital malformation of penis** ♂
        Congenital malformation of penis NOS

Q55.7 **Congenital vasocutaneous fistula** ♂

Q55.8 **Other specified congenital malformations of male genital organs** ♂

Q55.9 **Congenital malformation of male genital organ, unspecified** ♂
    Congenital anomaly of male genital organ
    Congenital deformity of male genital organ

✓4th **Q56** **Indeterminate sex and pseudohermaphroditism**
    EXCLUDES 1 *46, XX true hermaphrodite (Q99.1)*
    androgen insensitivity syndrome (E34.5-)
    chimera 46, XX/46, XY true hermaphrodite (Q99.0)
    female pseudohermaphroditism with adrenocortical disorder (E25.-)
    pseudohermaphroditism with specified chromosomal anomaly (Q96-Q99)
    pure gonadal dysgenesis (Q99.1)

    Q56.0 **Hermaphroditism, not elsewhere classified**
        Ovotestis

    Q56.1 **Male pseudohermaphroditism, not elsewhere classified** ♂
        46, XY with streak gonads
        Male pseudohermaphroditism NOS

    Q56.2 **Female pseudohermaphroditism, not elsewhere classified** ♀
        Female pseudohermaphroditism NOS

    Q56.3 **Pseudohermaphroditism, unspecified**

    Q56.4 **Indeterminate sex, unspecified**
        Ambiguous genitalia

Congenital malformations of the urinary system (Q60-Q64)

✓4th **Q60** **Renal agenesis and other reduction defects of kidney**
    Congenital absence of kidney
    Congenital atrophy of kidney
    Infantile atrophy of kidney

    Q60.0 **Renal agenesis, unilateral**

    Q60.1 **Renal agenesis, bilateral**

    Q60.2 **Renal agenesis, unspecified**

    Q60.3 **Renal hypoplasia, unilateral**

    Q60.4 **Renal hypoplasia, bilateral**

    Q60.5 **Renal hypoplasia, unspecified**

    Q60.6 **Potter's syndrome**

✓4th **Q61** **Cystic kidney disease**
    EXCLUDES 1 *acquired cyst of kidney (N28.1)*
    Potter's syndrome (Q60.6)

    ✓5th **Q61.0** **Congenital renal cyst**

        Q61.00 **Congenital renal cyst, unspecified**
            Cyst of kidney NOS (congenital)

        Q61.01 **Congenital single renal cyst**

        Q61.02 **Congenital multiple renal cysts**

    ✓5th **Q61.1** **Polycystic kidney, infantile type**
        Polycystic kidney, autosomal recessive

        Q61.11 **Cystic dilatation of collecting ducts**

        Q61.19 **Other polycystic kidney, infantile type**

    Q61.2 **Polycystic kidney, adult type**
        Polycystic kidney, autosomal dominant

    Q61.3 **Polycystic kidney, unspecified**

Q61.4 **Renal dysplasia**
    Multicystic dysplastic kidney
    Multicystic kidney (development)
    Multicystic kidney disease
    Multicystic renal dysplasia
    EXCLUDES 1 *polycystic kidney disease (Q61.11-Q61.3)*

Q61.5 **Medullary cystic kidney**
    Nephronopthisis
    Sponge kidney NOS

Q61.8 **Other cystic kidney diseases**
    Fibrocystic kidney
    Fibrocystic renal degeneration or disease

Q61.9 **Cystic kidney disease, unspecified**
    Meckel-Gruber syndrome

✓4th **Q62** **Congenital obstructive defects of renal pelvis and congenital malformations of ureter**

    Q62.0 **Congenital hydronephrosis**

    ✓5th **Q62.1** **Congenital occlusion of ureter**
        Atresia and stenosis of ureter

        Q62.10 **Congenital occlusion of ureter, unspecified**

        Q62.11 **Congenital occlusion of ureteropelvic junction**

        Q62.12 **Congenital occlusion of ureterovesical orifice**

    Q62.2 **Congenital megaureter**
        Congenital dilatation of ureter

    ✓5th **Q62.3** **Other obstructive defects of renal pelvis and ureter**

        Q62.31 **Congenital ureterocele, orthotopic**

        Q62.32 **Cecoureterocele**
            Ectopic ureterocele

        Q62.39 **Other obstructive defects of renal pelvis and ureter**
            Ureteropelvic junction obstruction NOS

    Q62.4 **Agenesis of ureter**
        Congenital absence ureter

    Q62.5 **Duplication of ureter**
        Accessory ureter
        Double ureter

    ✓5th **Q62.6** **Malposition of ureter**

        Q62.60 **Malposition of ureter, unspecified**

        Q62.61 **Deviation of ureter**

        Q62.62 **Displacement of ureter**

        Q62.63 **Anomalous implantation of ureter**
            Ectopia of ureter
            Ectopic ureter

        Q62.69 **Other malposition of ureter**

    Q62.7 **Congenital vesico-uretero-renal reflux**

    Q62.8 **Other congenital malformations of ureter**
        Anomaly of ureter NOS

✓4th **Q63** **Other congenital malformations of kidney**
    EXCLUDES 1 *congenital nephrotic syndrome (N04.-)*

    Q63.0 **Accessory kidney**

    Q63.1 **Lobulated, fused and horseshoe kidney**

    Q63.2 **Ectopic kidney**
        Congenital displaced kidney
        Malrotation of kidney

    Q63.3 **Hyperplastic and giant kidney**
        Compensatory hypertrophy of kidney

    Q63.8 **Other specified congenital malformations of kidney**
        Congenital renal calculi

    Q63.9 **Congenital malformation of kidney, unspecified**

✓4th **Q64** **Other congenital malformations of urinary system**

    Q64.0 **Epispadias** ♂
        EXCLUDES 1 *hypospadias (Q54.-)*

    ✓5th **Q64.1** **Exstrophy of urinary bladder**

        Q64.10 **Exstrophy of urinary bladder, unspecified**
            Ectopia vesicae

        Q64.11 **Supravesical fissure of urinary bladder**

        Q64.12 **Cloacal extrophy of urinary bladder**

        Q64.19 **Other exstrophy of urinary bladder**
            Extroversion of bladder

    Q64.2 **Congenital posterior urethral valves**

    ✓5th **Q64.3** **Other atresia and stenosis of urethra and bladder neck**

        Q64.31 **Congenital bladder neck obstruction**
            Congenital obstruction of vesicourethral orifice

        Q64.32 **Congenital stricture of urethra**

        Q64.33 **Congenital stricture of urinary meatus**

✓ Additional Character Required   ✓x7th Xtension Alert   Unspecified Dx   Other Specified Dx   Manifestation   ►◄ Revised Text   ● New Code   ▲ Revised Code Title

Q64.39 Other atresia and stenosis of urethra and bladder neck
Atresia and stenosis of urethra and bladder neck NOS

Q64.4 Malformation of urachus
Cyst of urachus
Patent urachus
Prolapse of urachus

Q64.5 Congenital absence of bladder and urethra

Q64.6 Congenital diverticulum of bladder

✓5th **Q64.7 Other and unspecified congenital malformations of bladder and urethra**
EXCLUDES 1 *congenital prolapse of bladder (mucosa) (Q79.4)*

Q64.70 Unspecified congenital malformation of bladder and urethra
Malformation of bladder or urethra NOS

Q64.71 Congenital prolapse of urethra

Q64.72 Congenital prolapse of urinary meatus

Q64.73 Congenital urethrorectal fistula

Q64.74 Double urethra

Q64.75 Double urinary meatus

Q64.79 Other congenital malformations of bladder and urethra

Q64.8 Other specified congenital malformations of urinary system

Q64.9 Congenital malformation of urinary system, unspecified
Congenital anomaly NOS of urinary system
Congenital deformity NOS of urinary system

Congenital malformations and deformations of the musculoskeletal system (Q65-Q79)

✓4th **Q65 Congenital deformities of** hip
EXCLUDES 1 *clicking hip (R29.4)*

✓5th **Q65.0 Congenital** dislocation of hip, unilateral

Q65.00 Congenital dislocation of unspecified hip, unilateral

Q65.01 Congenital dislocation of right **hip, unilateral**

Q65.02 Congenital dislocation of left **hip, unilateral**

Q65.1 Congenital dislocation of hip, bilateral

Q65.2 Congenital dislocation of hip, unspecified

✓5th **Q65.3 Congenital** partial dislocation of hip, unilateral

Q65.30 Congenital partial dislocation of unspecified hip, unilateral

Q65.31 Congenital partial dislocation of right **hip, unilateral**

Q65.32 Congenital partial dislocation of left **hip, unilateral**

Q65.4 Congenital partial dislocation of hip, bilateral

Q65.5 Congenital partial dislocation of hip, unspecified

Q65.6 Congenital unstable **hip**
Congenital dislocatable hip

✓5th **Q65.8 Other congenital deformities of hip**

Q65.81 Congenital coxa valga

Q65.82 Congenital coxa vara

Q65.89 Other specified congenital deformities of hip
Anteversion of femoral neck
Congenital acetabular dysplasia

Q65.9 Congenital deformity of hip, unspecified

✓4th **Q66 Congenital deformities of** feet
EXCLUDES 1 *reduction defects of feet (Q72.-)*
valgus deformities (acquired) (M21.0-)
varus deformities (acquired) (M21.1-)

Q66.0 Congenital talipes equinovarus

Q66.1 Congenital talipes calcaneovarus

Q66.2 Congenital metatarsus (primus) varus

Q66.3 Other congenital varus deformities of feet
Hallux varus, congenital

Q66.4 Congenital talipes calcaneovalgus

✓5th **Q66.5 Congenital** pes planus
Congenital flat foot
Congenital rigid flat foot
Congenital spastic (everted) flat foot
EXCLUDES 1 *pes planus, acquired (M21.4)*

Q66.50 Congenital pes planus, unspecified foot

Q66.51 Congenital pes planus, right **foot**

Q66.52 Congenital pes planus, left **foot**

Q66.6 Other congenital valgus deformities of feet
Congenital metatarsus valgus

Q66.7 Congenital pes cavus

✓5th **Q66.8 Other congenital deformities of feet**

Q66.80 Congenital vertical talus deformity, unspecified foot

Q66.81 Congenital vertical talus deformity, right **foot**

Q66.82 Congenital vertical talus deformity, left **foot**

Q66.89 Other specified congenital deformities of feet
Congenital asymmetric talipes
Congenital clubfoot NOS
Congenital talipes NOS
Congenital tarsal coalition
Hammer toe, congenital

Q66.9 Congenital deformity of feet, unspecified

✓4th **Q67 Congenital musculoskeletal deformities of** head, face, spine and chest
EXCLUDES 1 *congenital malformation syndromes classified to Q87-*
Potter's syndrome (Q60.6)

Q67.0 Congenital facial asymmetry

Q67.1 Congenital compression facies

Q67.2 Dolichocephaly

Q67.3 Plagiocephaly

Q67.4 Other congenital deformities of skull, face and jaw
Congenital depressions in skull
Congenital hemifacial atrophy or hypertrophy
Deviation of nasal septum, congenital
Squashed or bent nose, congenital
EXCLUDES 1 *dentofacial anomalies [including malocclusion] (M26.-)*
syphilitic saddle nose (A50.5)

Q67.5 Congenital deformity of spine
Congenital postural scoliosis
Congenital scoliosis NOS
EXCLUDES 1 *infantile idiopathic scoliosis (M41.0)*
scoliosis due to congenital bony malformation (Q76.3)

Q67.6 Pectus excavatum
Congenital funnel chest

Q67.7 Pectus carinatum
Congenital pigeon chest

Q67.8 Other congenital deformities of chest
Congenital deformity of chest wall NOS

✓4th **Q68 Other congenital musculoskeletal deformities**
EXCLUDES 1 *reduction defects of limb(s) (Q71-Q73)*
EXCLUDES 2 *congenital myotonic chondrodystrophy (G71.13)*

Q68.0 Congenital deformity of sternocleidomastoid muscle
Congenital contracture of sternocleidomastoid (muscle)
Congenital (sternomastoid) torticollis
Sternomastoid tumor (congenital)

Q68.1 Congenital deformity of finger(s) and hand
Congenital clubfinger
Spade-like hand (congenital)

Q68.2 Congenital deformity of knee
Congenital dislocation of knee
Congenital genu recurvatum

Q68.3 Congenital bowing of femur
EXCLUDES 1 *anteversion of femur (neck) (Q65.89)*

Q68.4 Congenital bowing of tibia and fibula

Q68.5 Congenital bowing of long bones of leg, unspecified

Q68.6 Discoid meniscus

Q68.8 Other specified congenital musculoskeletal deformities
Congenital deformity of clavicle
Congenital deformity of elbow
Congenital deformity of forearm
Congenital deformity of scapula
Congenital deformity of wrist
Congenital dislocation of elbow
Congenital dislocation of shoulder
Congenital dislocation of wrist

✓4th **Q69 Polydactyly**

Q69.0 Accessory finger(s)

Q69.1 Accessory thumb(s)

Q69.2 Accessory toe(s)
Accessory hallux

Q69.9 Polydactyly, unspecified
Supernumerary digit(s) NOS

✓4th **Q70 Syndactyly**

✓5th **Q70.0 Fused fingers**
  Complex syndactly of fingers with synostosis
  Q70.00 Fused fingers, unspecified hand
  Q70.01 Fused fingers, right hand
  Q70.02 Fused fingers, left hand
  Q70.03 Fused fingers, bilateral

✓5th **Q70.1 Webbed fingers**
  Simple syndactyly of fingers without synostosis
  Q70.10 Webbed fingers, unspecified hand
  Q70.11 Webbed fingers, right hand
  Q70.12 Webbed fingers, left hand
  Q70.13 Webbed fingers, bilateral

✓5th **Q70.2 Fused toes**
  Complex syndactyly of toes with synostosis
  Q70.20 Fused toes, unspecified foot
  Q70.21 Fused toes, right foot
  Q70.22 Fused toes, left foot
  Q70.23 Fused toes, bilateral

✓5th **Q70.3 Webbed toes**
  Simpie syndactyly of toes without synostosis
  Q70.30 Webbed toes, unspecified foot
  Q70.31 Webbed toes, right foot
  Q70.32 Webbed toes, left foot
  Q70.33 Webbed toes, bilateral

  Q70.4 Polysyndactyly, unspecified
    EXCLUDES 1 *specified syndactyly of hand and feet—code to specified conditions (Q70.0-Q70.3-)*

  Q70.9 Syndactyly, unspecified
    Symphalangy NOS

✓4th **Q71 Reduction defects of upper limb**

✓5th **Q71.0 Congenital complete absence of upper limb**
  Q71.00 Congenital complete absence of unspecified upper limb
  Q71.01 Congenital complete absence of right upper limb
  Q71.02 Congenital complete absence of left upper limb
  Q71.03 Congenital complete absence of upper limb, bilateral

✓5th **Q71.1 Congenital absence of upper arm and forearm with hand present**
  Q71.10 Congenital absence of unspecified upper arm and forearm with hand present
  Q71.11 Congenital absence of right upper arm and forearm with hand present
  Q71.12 Congenital absence of left upper arm and forearm with hand present
  Q71.13 Congenital absence of upper arm and forearm with hand present, bilateral

✓5th **Q71.2 Congenital absence of both forearm and hand**
  Q71.20 Congenital absence of both forearm and hand, unspecified upper limb
  Q71.21 Congenital absence of both forearm and hand, right upper limb
  Q71.22 Congenital absence of both forearm and hand, left upper limb
  Q71.23 Congenital absence of both forearm and hand, bilateral

✓5th **Q71.3 Congenital absence of hand and finger**
  Q71.30 Congenital absence of unspecified hand and finger
  Q71.31 Congenital absence of right hand and finger
  Q71.32 Congenital absence of left hand and finger
  Q71.33 Congenital absence of hand and finger, bilateral

✓5th **Q71.4 Longitudinal reduction defect of radius**
  Clubhand (congenital)
  Radial clubhand
  Q71.40 Longitudinal reduction defect of unspecified radius
  Q71.41 Longitudinal reduction defect of right radius
  Q71.42 Longitudinal reduction defect of left radius
  Q71.43 Longitudinal reduction defect of radius, bilateral

✓5th **Q71.5 Longitudinal reduction defect of ulna**
  Q71.50 Longitudinal reduction defect of unspecified ulna
  Q71.51 Longitudinal reduction defect of right ulna

  Q71.52 Longitudinal reduction defect of left ulna
  Q71.53 Longitudinal reduction defect of ulna, bilateral

✓5th **Q71.6 Lobster-claw hand**
  Q71.60 Lobster-claw hand, unspecified hand
  Q71.61 Lobster-claw right hand
  Q71.62 Lobster-claw left hand
  Q71.63 Lobster-claw hand, bilateral

✓5th **Q71.8 Other reduction defects of upper limb**
  ✓6th **Q71.81 Congenital shortening of upper limb**
    Q71.811 Congenital shortening of right upper limb
    Q71.812 Congenital shortening of left upper limb
    Q71.813 Congenital shortening of upper limb, bilateral
    Q71.819 Congenital shortening of unspecified upper limb
  ✓6th **Q71.89 Other reduction defects of upper limb**
    Q71.891 Other reduction defects of right upper limb
    Q71.892 Other reduction defects of left upper limb
    Q71.893 Other reduction defects of upper limb, bilateral
    Q71.899 Other reduction defects of unspecified upper limb

✓5th **Q71.9 Unspecified reduction defect of upper limb**
  Q71.90 Unspecified reduction defect of unspecified upper limb
  Q71.91 Unspecified reduction defect of right upper limb
  Q71.92 Unspecified reduction defect of left upper limb
  Q71.93 Unspecified reduction defect of upper limb, bilateral

✓4th **Q72 Reduction defects of lower limb**

✓5th **Q72.0 Congenital complete absence of lower limb**
  Q72.00 Congenital complete absence of unspecified lower limb
  Q72.01 Congenital complete absence of right lower limb
  Q72.02 Congenital complete absence of left lower limb
  Q72.03 Congenital complete absence of lower limb, bilateral

✓5th **Q72.1 Congenital absence of thigh and lower leg with foot present**
  Q72.10 Congenital absence of unspecified thigh and lower leg with foot present
  Q72.11 Congenital absence of right thigh and lower leg with foot present
  Q72.12 Congenital absence of left thigh and lower leg with foot present
  Q72.13 Congenital absence of thigh and lower leg with foot present, bilateral

✓5th **Q72.2 Congenital absence of both lower leg and foot**
  Q72.20 Congenital absence of both lower leg and foot, unspecified lower limb
  Q72.21 Congenital absence of both lower leg and foot, right lower limb
  Q72.22 Congenital absence of both lower leg and foot, left lower limb
  Q72.23 Congenital absence of both lower leg and foot, bilateral

✓5th **Q72.3 Congenital absence of foot and toe(s)**
  Q72.30 Congenital absence of unspecified foot and toe(s)
  Q72.31 Congenital absence of right foot and toe(s)
  Q72.32 Congenital absence of left foot and toe(s)
  Q72.33 Congenital absence of foot and toe(s), bilateral

✓5th **Q72.4 Longitudinal reduction defect of femur**
  Proximal femoral focal deficiency
  Q72.40 Longitudinal reduction defect of unspecified femur
  Q72.41 Longitudinal reduction defect of right femur
  Q72.42 Longitudinal reduction defect of left femur
  Q72.43 Longitudinal reduction defect of femur, bilateral

✓5th **Q72.5 Longitudinal reduction defect of tibia**
  Q72.50 Longitudinal reduction defect of unspecified tibia
  Q72.51 Longitudinal reduction defect of right tibia
  Q72.52 Longitudinal reduction defect of left tibia
  Q72.53 Longitudinal reduction defect of tibia, bilateral

✓5th **Q72.6 Longitudinal reduction defect of fibula**
  Q72.60 Longitudinal reduction defect of unspecified fibula

✓ Additional Character Required   ✓x7th Xtension Alert   Unspecified Dx   Other Specified Dx   Manifestation   ▶◀ Revised Text   ● New Code   ▲ Revised Code Title

Q72.61   Longitudinal reduction defect of right fibula

Q72.62   Longitudinal reduction defect of left fibula

Q72.63   Longitudinal reduction defect of fibula, bilateral

✓5ᵗʰ Q72.7   Split foot

Q72.70   Split foot, unspecified lower limb

Q72.71   Split foot, right lower limb

Q72.72   Split foot, left lower limb

Q72.73   Split foot, bilateral

✓5ᵗʰ Q72.8   Other reduction defects of lower limb

✓6ᵗʰ Q72.81   Congenital shortening of lower limb

Q72.811   Congenital shortening of right lower limb

Q72.812   Congenital shortening of left lower limb

Q72.813   Congenital shortening of lower limb, bilateral

Q72.819   Congenital shortening of unspecified lower limb

✓6ᵗʰ Q72.89   Other reduction defects of lower limb

Q72.891   Other reduction defects of right lower limb

Q72.892   Other reduction defects of left lower limb

Q72.893   Other reduction defects of lower limb, bilateral

Q72.899   Other reduction defects of unspecified lower limb

✓5ᵗʰ Q72.9   Unspecified reduction defect of lower limb

Q72.90   Unspecified reduction defect of unspecified lower limb

Q72.91   Unspecified reduction defect of right lower limb

Q72.92   Unspecified reduction defect of left lower limb

Q72.93   Unspecified reduction defect of lower limb, bilateral

✓4ᵗʰ Q73   Reduction defects of unspecified limb

Q73.0   Congenital absence of unspecified limb(s)

Amelia NOS

Q73.1   Phocomelia, unspecified limb(s)

Phocomelia NOS

Q73.8   Other reduction defects of unspecified limb(s)

Longitudinal reduction deformity of unspecified limb(s)

Ectromelia of limb NOS

Hemimelia of limb NOS

Reduction defect of limb NOS

✓4ᵗʰ Q74   Other congenital malformations of limb(s)

EXCLUDES 1   *polydactyly (Q69.-)*
reduction defect of limb (Q71-Q73)
syndactyly (Q70.-)

Q74.0   Other congenital malformations of upper limb(s), including shoulder girdle

Accessory carpal bones

Cleidocranial dysostosis

Congenital pseudarthrosis of clavicle

Macrodactylia (fingers)

Madelung's deformity

Radioulnar synostosis

Sprengel's deformity

Triphalangeal thumb

Q74.1   Congenital malformation of knee

Congenital absence of patella

Congenital dislocation of patella

Congenital genu valgum

Congenital genu varum

Rudimentary patella

EXCLUDES 1   *congenital dislocation of knee (Q68.2)*
congenital genu recurvatum (Q68.2)
nail patella syndrome (Q87.2)

Q74.2   Other congenital malformations of lower limb(s), including pelvic girdle

Congenital fusion of sacroiliac joint

Congenital malformation of ankle joint

Congenital malformation of sacroiliac joint

EXCLUDES 1   *anteversion of femur (neck) (Q65.89)*

Q74.3   Arthrogryposis multiplex congenita

Q74.8   Other specified congenital malformations of limb(s)

Q74.9   Unspecified congenital malformation of limb(s)

Congenital anomaly of limb(s) NOS

✓4ᵗʰ Q75   Other congenital malformations of skull and face bones

EXCLUDES 1   *congenital malformation of face NOS (Q18.-)*
congenital malformation syndromes classified to Q87.-
dentofacial anomalies [including malocclusion] (M26.-)
musculoskeletal deformities of head and face (Q67.0-Q67.4)
skull defects associated with congenital anomalies of brain such as:
anencephaly (Q00.0)
encephalocele (Q01.-)
hydrocephalus (Q03.-)
microcephaly (Q02)

Q75.0   Craniosynostosis

Acrocephaly

Imperfect fusion of skull

Oxycephaly

Trigonocephaly

Q75.1   Craniofacial dysostosis

Crouzon's disease

Q75.2   Hypertelorism

Q75.3   Macrocephaly

Q75.4   Mandibulofacial dysostosis

Franceschetti syndrome

Treacher Collins syndrome

Q75.5   Oculomandibular dysostosis

Q75.8   Other specified congenital malformations of skull and face bones

Absence of skull bone, congenital

Congenital deformity of forehead

Platybasia

Q75.9   Congenital malformation of skull and face bones, unspecified

Congenital anomaly of face bones NOS

Congenital anomaly of skull NOS

✓4ᵗʰ Q76   Congenital malformations of spine and bony thorax

EXCLUDES 1   *congenital musculoskeletal deformities of spine and chest (Q67.5-Q67.8)*

Q76.0   Spina bifida occulta

EXCLUDES 1   *meningocele (spinal) (Q05.-)*
spina bifida (aperta) (cystica) (Q05.-)

Q76.1   Klippel-Feil syndrome

Cervical fusion syndrome

Q76.2   Congenital spondylolisthesis

Congenital spondylolysis

EXCLUDES 1   *spondylolisthesis (acquired) (M43.1-)*
spondylolysis (acquired) (M43.0-)

Q76.3   Congenital scoliosis due to congenital bony malformation

Hemivertebra fusion or failure of segmentation with scoliosis

✓5ᵗʰ Q76.4   Other congenital malformations of spine, not associated with scoliosis

✓6ᵗʰ Q76.41   Congenital kyphosis

Q76.411   Congenital kyphosis, occipito-atlanto-axial region

Q76.412   Congenital kyphosis, cervical region

Q76.413   Congenital kyphosis, cervicothoracic region

Q76.414   Congenital kyphosis, thoracic region

Q76.415   Congenital kyphosis, thoracolumbar region

Q76.419   Congenital kyphosis, unspecified region

✓6ᵗʰ Q76.42   Congenital lordosis

Q76.425   Congenital lordosis, thoracolumbar region

Q76.426   Congenital lordosis, lumbar region

Q76.427   Congenital lordosis, lumbosacral region

Q76.428   Congenital lordosis, sacral and sacrococcygeal region

Q76.429   Congenital lordosis, unspecified region

Q76.49   Other congenital malformations of spine, not associated with scoliosis

Congenital absence of vertebra NOS

Congenital fusion of spine NOS

Congenital malformation of lumbosacral (joint) (region) NOS

Congenital malformation of spine NOS

Hemivertebra NOS

Malformation of spine NOS

Platyspondylisis NOS

Supernumerary vertebra NOS

Q76.5   Cervical rib

Supernumerary rib in cervical region

EXCLUDES 1 Not coded here   *EXCLUDES 2* Not included here   N Newborn Age: 0   P Pediatric Age: 0-17   M Maternity Age: 12-55   A Adult Age: 15-124

784   ICD-10-CM Draft (2015)

Q76.6 **Other congenital malformations of ribs**
Accessory rib
Congenital absence of rib
Congenital fusion of ribs
Congenital malformation of ribs NOS
EXCLUDES 1 *short rib syndrome (Q77.2)*

Q76.7 **Congenital malformation of sternum**
Congenital absence of sternum
Sternum bifidum

Q76.8 **Other congenital malformations of bony thorax**

Q76.9 **Congenital malformation of bony thorax, unspecified**

✓4th **Q77** **Osteochondrodysplasia with defects of growth of tubular bones and spine**
EXCLUDES 1 *mucopolysaccharidosis (E76.0-E76.3)*
EXCLUDES 2 *congenital myotonic chondrodystrophy (G71.13)*

Q77.0 **Achondrogenesis**
Hypochondrogenesis

Q77.1 **Thanatophoric short stature**

Q77.2 **Short rib syndrome**
Asphyxiating thoracic dysplasia [Jeune]

Q77.3 **Chondrodysplasia punctata**
EXCLUDES 1 *Rhizomelic chondrodysplasia punctata (E71.43)*

Q77.4 **Achondroplasia**
Hypochondroplasia
Osteosclerosis congenita

Q77.5 **Diastrophic dysplasia**

Q77.6 **Chondroectodermal dysplasia**
Ellis-van Creveld syndrome

Q77.7 **Spondyloepiphyseal dysplasia**

Q77.8 **Other osteochondrodysplasia with defects of growth of tubular bones and spine**

Q77.9 **Osteochondrodysplasia with defects of growth of tubular bones and spine, unspecified**

✓4th **Q78** **Other osteochondrodysplasias**
EXCLUDES 2 *congenital myotonic chondrodystrophy (G71.13)*

Q78.0 **Osteogenesis imperfecta**
Fragilitas ossium
Osteopsathyrosis

Q78.1 **Polyostotic fibrous dysplasia**
Albright(-McCune)(-Sternberg) syndrome

Q78.2 **Osteopetrosis**
Albers-Schönberg syndrome
Osteosclerosis NOS

Q78.3 **Progressive diaphyseal dysplasia**
Camurati-Engelmann syndrome

Q78.4 **Enchondromatosis**
Maffucci's syndrome
Ollier's disease

Q78.5 **Metaphyseal dysplasia**
Pyle's syndrome

Q78.6 **Multiple congenital exostoses**
Diaphyseal aclasis

Q78.8 **Other specified osteochondrodysplasias**
Osteopoikilosis

Q78.9 **Osteochondrodysplasia, unspecified**
Chondrodystrophy NOS
Osteodystrophy NOS

✓4th **Q79** **Congenital malformations of musculoskeletal system, not elsewhere classified**
EXCLUDES 2 *congenital (sternomastoid) torticollis (Q68.0)*

Q79.0 **Congenital diaphragmatic hernia**
EXCLUDES 1 *congenital hiatus hernia (Q40.1)*

Q79.1 **Other congenital malformations of diaphragm**
Absence of diaphragm
Congenital malformation of diaphragm NOS
Eventration of diaphragm

Q79.2 **Exomphalos**
Omphalocele
EXCLUDES 1 *umbilical hernia (K42.-)*

Q79.3 **Gastroschisis**

Q79.4 **Prune belly syndrome**
Congenital prolapse of bladder mucosa
Eagle-Barrett syndrome

✓5th **Q79.5** **Other congenital malformations of abdominal wall**
EXCLUDES 1 *umbilical hernia (K42.-)*

   Q79.51 **Congenital hernia of bladder**

   Q79.59 **Other congenital malformations of abdominal wall**

Q79.6 **Ehlers-Danlos syndrome**

Q79.8 **Other congenital malformations of musculoskeletal system**
Absence of muscle
Absence of tendon
Accessory muscle
Amyotrophia congenita
Congenital constricting bands
Congenital shortening of tendon
Poland syndrome

Q79.9 **Congenital malformation of musculoskeletal system, unspecified**
Congenital anomaly of musculoskeletal system NOS
Congenital deformity of musculoskeletal system NOS

Other congenital malformations (Q80-Q89)

✓4th **Q80** **Congenital ichthyosis**
EXCLUDES 1 *Refsum's disease (G60.1)*

Q80.0 **Ichthyosis vulgaris**

Q80.1 **X-linked ichthyosis**

Q80.2 **Lamellar ichthyosis**
Collodion baby

Q80.3 **Congenital bullous ichthyosiform erythroderma**

Q80.4 **Harlequin fetus**

Q80.8 **Other congenital ichthyosis**

Q80.9 **Congenital ichthyosis, unspecified**

✓4th **Q81** **Epidermolysis bullosa**

Q81.0 **Epidermolysis bullosa simplex**
EXCLUDES 1 *Cockayne's syndrome (Q87.1)*

Q81.1 **Epidermolysis bullosa letalis**
Herlitz' syndrome

Q81.2 **Epidermolysis bullosa dystrophica**

Q81.8 **Other epidermolysis bullosa**

Q81.9 **Epidermolysis bullosa, unspecified**

✓4th **Q82** **Other congenital malformations of skin**
EXCLUDES 1 *acrodermatitis enteropathica (E83.2)*
congenital erythropoietic porphyria (E80.0)
pilonidal cyst or sinus (L05.-)
Sturge-Weber (-Dimitri) syndrome (Q85.8)

Q82.0 **Hereditary lymphedema**

Q82.1 **Xeroderma pigmentosum**

Q82.2 **Mastocytosis**
Urticaria pigmentosa
EXCLUDES 1 *malignant mastocytosis (C96.2)*

Q82.3 **Incontinentia pigmenti**

Q82.4 **Ectodermal dysplasia (anhidrotic)**
EXCLUDES 1 *Ellis-van Creveld syndrome (Q77.6)*

Q82.5 **Congenital non-neoplastic nevus**

Birthmark NOS	Strawberry Nevus
Flammeus Nevus	Vascular Nevus NOS
Portwine Nevus	Verrucous Nevus
Sanguineous Nevus	

EXCLUDES 2 *araneus nevus (I78.1)*
café au lait spots (L81.3)
lentigo (L81.4)
melanocytic nevus (D22.-)
nevus NOS (D22.-)
pigmented nevus (D22.-)
spider nevus (I78.1)
stellar nevus (I78.1)

Q82.8 **Other specified congenital malformations of skin**
Abnormal palmar creases
Accessory skin tags
Benign familial pemphigus [Hailey-Hailey]
Congenital poikiloderma
Cutis laxa (hyperelastica)
Dermatoglyphic anomalies
Inherited keratosis palmaris et plantaris
Keratosis follicularis [Darier-White]
EXCLUDES 1 *Ehlers-Danlos syndrome (Q79.6)*

Q82.9 **Congenital malformation of skin, unspecified**

✓4th **Q83** **Congenital malformations of breast**
EXCLUDES 2 *absence of pectoral muscle (Q79.8)*
hypoplasia of breast (N64.82)
micromastia (N64.82)

Q83.0 **Congenital absence of breast with absent nipple**

☑ Additional Character Required   ✓x7th Xtension Alert   Unspecified Dx   Other Specified Dx   Manifestation   ►◄ Revised Text   ● New Code   ▲ Revised Code Title

Q83.1 Accessory breast
    Supernumerary breast

Q83.2 Absent nipple

Q83.3 Accessory nipple
    Supernumerary nipple

Q83.8 **Other congenital malformations of breast**

Q83.9 **Congenital malformation of breast, unspecified**

✓4ᵗʰ **Q84** **Other congenital malformations of integument**

Q84.0 **Congenital alopecia**
    Congenital atrichosis

Q84.1 **Congenital morphological disturbances of hair, not elsewhere classified**
    Beaded hair   Pili annulati
    Monilethrix
    EXCLUDES 1   *Menkes' kinky hair syndrome (E83.0)*

Q84.2 **Other congenital malformations of hair**
    Congenital hypertrichosis
    Congenital malformation of hair NOS
    Persistent lanugo

Q84.3 **Anonychia**
    EXCLUDES 1   *nail patella syndrome (Q87.2)*

Q84.4 **Congenital leukonychia**

Q84.5 **Enlarged and hypertrophic nails**
    Congenital onychauxis   Pachyonychia

Q84.6 **Other congenital malformations of nails**
    Congenital clubnail
    Congenital koilonychia
    Congenital malformation of nail NOS

Q84.8 **Other specified congenital malformations of integument**
    Aplasia cutis congenita

Q84.9 **Congenital malformation of integument, unspecified**
    Congenital anomaly of integument NOS
    Congenital deformity of integument NOS

✓4ᵗʰ **Q85** **Phakomatoses, not elsewhere classified**
    EXCLUDES 1   *ataxia telangiectasia [Louis-Bar] (G11.3)*
            familial dysautonomia [Riley-Day] (G90.1)

✓5ᵗʰ **Q85.0** **Neurofibromatosis (nonmalignant)**

Q85.00 **Neurofibromatosis, unspecified**

Q85.01 **Neurofibromatosis, type 1**
    Von Recklinghausen disease

Q85.02 **Neurofibromatosis, type 2**
    Acoustic neurofibromatosis

Q85.03 **Schwannomatosis**

Q85.09 **Other neurofibromatosis**

Q85.1 **Tuberous sclerosis**
    Bourneville's disease
    Epiloia

Q85.8 **Other phakomatoses, not elsewhere classified**
    Peutz-Jeghers Syndrome
    Sturge-Weber(-Dimitri) syndrome
    von Hippel-Lindau syndrome
    EXCLUDES 1   *Meckel-Gruber syndrome (Q61.9)*

Q85.9 **Phakomatosis, unspecified**
    Hamartosis NOS

✓4ᵗʰ **Q86** **Congenital malformation syndromes due to known exogenous causes, not elsewhere classified**
    EXCLUDES 2   *iodine-deficiency-related hypothyroidism (E00-E02)*
            nonteratogenic effects of substances transmitted via placenta or breast milk (P04.-)

Q86.0 **Fetal alcohol syndrome (dysmorphic)**

Q86.1 **Fetal hydantoin syndrome**   N
    Meadow's syndrome

Q86.2 **Dysmorphism due to warfarin**

Q86.8 **Other congenital malformation syndromes due to known exogenous causes**

✓4ᵗʰ **Q87** **Other specified congenital malformation syndromes affecting multiple systems**
    Use additional code(s) to identify all associated manifestations

Q87.0 **Congenital malformation syndromes predominantly affecting facial appearance**
    Acrocephalopolysyndactyly   Robin syndrome
    Acrocephalosyndactyly [Apert]   Whistling face
    Cryptophthalmos syndrome
    Cyclopia
    Goldenhar syndrome
    Moebius syndrome
    Oro-facial-digital syndrome

Q87.1 **Congenital malformation syndromes predominantly associated with short stature**
    Aarskog syndrome   Robinow-Silverman-Smith
    Cockayne syndrome   syndrome
    De Lange syndrome   Russell-Silver syndrome
    Dubowitz syndrome   Seckel syndrome
    Noonan syndrome
    Prader-Willi syndrome
    EXCLUDES 1   *Ellis-van Creveld syndrome (Q77.6)*
            Smith-Lemli-Opitz syndrome (E78.72)

Q87.2 **Congenital malformation syndromes predominantly involving limbs**
    Holt-Oram syndrome
    Klippel-Trenaunay-Weber syndrome
    Nail patella syndrome
    Rubinstein-Taybi syndrome
    Sirenomelia syndrome
    Thrombocytopenia with absent radius [TAR] syndrome
    VATER syndrome

Q87.3 **Congenital malformation syndromes involving early overgrowth**
    Beckwith-Wiedemann syndrome   Weaver syndrome
    Sotos syndrome

✓5ᵗʰ **Q87.4** **Marfan's syndrome**

Q87.40 **Marfan's syndrome, unspecified**

✓6ᵗʰ **Q87.41** **Marfan's syndrome with cardiovascular manifestations**

Q87.410 **Marfan's syndrome with aortic dilation**

Q87.418 **Marfan's syndrome with other cardiovascular manifestations**

Q87.42 **Marfan's syndrome with ocular manifestations**

Q87.43 **Marfan's syndrome with skeletal manifestation**

Q87.5 **Other congenital malformation syndromes with other skeletal changes**

✓5ᵗʰ **Q87.8** **Other specified congenital malformation syndromes, not elsewhere classified**
    EXCLUDES 1   *Zellweger syndrome (E71.510)*

Q87.81 **Alport syndrome**
    Use additional code to identify stage of chronic kidney disease (N18.1-N18.6)

Q87.89 **Other specified congenital malformation syndromes, not elsewhere classified**
    Laurence-Moon (-Bardet)-Biedl syndrome

✓4ᵗʰ **Q89** **Other congenital malformations, not elsewhere classified**

✓5ᵗʰ **Q89.0** **Congenital absence and malformations of spleen**
    EXCLUDES 1   *isomerism of atrial appendages (with asplenia or polysplenia) (Q20.6)*

Q89.01 **Asplenia (congenital)**

Q89.09 **Congenital malformations of spleen**
    Congenital splenomegaly

Q89.1 **Congenital malformations of adrenal gland**
    EXCLUDES 1   *adrenogenital disorders (E25.-)*
            congenital adrenal hyperplasia (E25.0)

Q89.2 **Congenital malformations of other endocrine glands**
    Congenital malformation of parathyroid or thyroid gland
    Persistent thyroglossal duct
    Thyroglossal cyst
    EXCLUDES 1   *congenital goiter (E03.0)*
            congenital hypothyroidism (E03.1)

Q89.3 **Situs inversus**
    Dextrocardia with situs inversus
    Mirror-image atrial arrangement with situs inversus
    Situs inversus or transversus abdominalis
    Situs inversus or transversus thoracis
    Transposition of abdominal viscera
    Transposition of thoracic viscera
    EXCLUDES 1   *dextrocardia NOS (Q24.0)*

Q89.4 **Conjoined twins**
    Craniopagus   Pygopagus
    Dicephaly   Thoracopagus

Q89.7 **Multiple congenital malformations, not elsewhere classified**
    Multiple congenital anomalies NOS
    Multiple congenital deformities NOS
    EXCLUDES 1   *congenital malformation syndromes affecting multiple systems (Q87.-)*

Q89.8 **Other specified congenital malformations**
    Use additional code(s) to identify all associated manifestations

Q89.9 **Congenital malformation, unspecified**
    Congenital anomaly NOS   Congenital deformity NOS

EXCLUDES 1 Not coded here   *EXCLUDES 2* Not included here   N Newborn Age: 0   P Pediatric Age: 0-17   M Maternity Age: 12-55   A Adult Age: 15-124

Chromosomal abnormalities, not elsewhere classified (Q90-Q99)

EXCLUDES 2 *mitochondrial metabolic disorders (E88.4-)*

✓4ᵗʰ **Q90 Down syndrome**

Use additional code(s) to identify any associated physical conditions and degree of intellectual disabilities (F70-F79)

Q90.0 Trisomy 21, nonmosaicism (meiotic nondisjunction)

Q90.1 Trisomy 21, mosaicism (mitotic nondisjunction)

Q90.2 Trisomy 21, translocation

Q90.9 Down syndrome, unspecified
Trisomy 21 NOS

✓4ᵗʰ **Q91 Trisomy 18 and Trisomy 13**

Q91.0 Trisomy 18, nonmosaicism (meiotic nondisjunction)

Q91.1 Trisomy 18, mosaicism (mitotic nondisjunction)

Q91.2 Trisomy 18, translocation

Q91.3 Trisomy 18, unspecified

Q91.4 Trisomy 13, nonmosaicism (meiotic nondisjunction)

Q91.5 Trisomy 13, mosaicism (mitotic nondisjunction)

Q91.6 Trisomy 13, translocation

Q91.7 Trisomy 13, unspecified

✓4ᵗʰ **Q92 Other trisomies and partial trisomies of the autosomes, not elsewhere classified**

INCLUDES unbalanced translocations and insertions

EXCLUDES 1 *trisomies of chromosomes 13, 18, 21 (Q90-Q91)*

Q92.0 Whole chromosome trisomy, nonmosaicism (meiotic nondisjunction)

Q92.1 Whole chromosome trisomy, mosaicism (mitotic nondisjunction)

Q92.2 Partial trisomy
Less than whole arm duplicated
Whole arm or more duplicated
EXCLUDES 1 *partial trisomy due to unbalanced translocation (Q92.5)*

Q92.5 Duplications with other complex rearrangements
Partial trisomy due to unbalanced translocations
Code also any associated deletions due to unbalanced translocations, inversions and insertions (Q93.7)

✓5ᵗʰ **Q92.6 Marker chromosomes**
Trisomies due to dicentrics
Trisomies due to extra rings
Trisomies due to isochromosomes
Individual with marker heterochromatin

Q92.61 Marker chromosomes in normal individual

Q92.62 Marker chromosomes in abnormal individual

Q92.7 Triploidy and polyploidy

Q92.8 Other specified trisomies and partial trisomies of autosomes
Duplications identified by fluorescence in situ hybridization (FISH)
Duplications identified by in situ hybridization (ISH)
Duplications seen only at prometaphase

Q92.9 Trisomy and partial trisomy of autosomes, unspecified

✓4ᵗʰ **Q93 Monosomies and deletions from the autosomes, not elsewhere classified**

Q93.0 Whole chromosome monosomy, nonmosaicism (meiotic nondisjunction)

Q93.1 Whole chromosome monosomy, mosaicism (mitotic nondisjunction)

Q93.2 Chromosome replaced with ring, dicentric or isochromosome

Q93.3 Deletion of short arm of chromosome 4
Wolff-Hirschorn syndrome

Q93.4 Deletion of short arm of chromosome 5
Cri-du-chat syndrome

Q93.5 Other deletions of part of a chromosome
Angelman syndrome

Q93.7 Deletions with other complex rearrangements
Deletions due to unbalanced translocations, inversions and insertions
Code also any associated duplications due to unbalanced translocations, inversions and insertions (Q92.5)

✓5ᵗʰ **Q93.8 Other deletions from the autosomes**

Q93.81 Velo-cardio-facial syndrome
Deletion 22q11.2

Q93.88 Other microdeletions
Miller-Dieker syndrome
Smith-Magenis syndrome

Q93.89 Other deletions from the autosomes
Deletions identified by fluorescence in situ hybridization (FISH)
Deletions identified by in situ hybridization (ISH)
Deletions seen only at prometaphase

Q93.9 Deletion from autosomes, unspecified

✓4ᵗʰ **Q95 Balanced rearrangements and structural markers, not elsewhere classified**

INCLUDES Robertsonian and balanced reciprocal translocations and insertions

Q95.0 Balanced translocation and insertion in normal individual

Q95.1 Chromosome inversion in normal individual

Q95.2 Balanced autosomal rearrangement in abnormal individual

Q95.3 Balanced sex/autosomal rearrangement in abnormal individual

Q95.5 Individual with autosomal fragile site

Q95.8 Other balanced rearrangements and structural markers

Q95.9 Balanced rearrangement and structural marker, unspecified

✓4ᵗʰ **Q96 Turner's syndrome**

EXCLUDES 1 *Noonan syndrome (Q87.1)*

Q96.0 Karyotype 45, X ♀

Q96.1 Karyotype 46, X iso (Xq) ♀
Karyotype 46, isochromosome Xq

Q96.2 Karyotype 46, X with abnormal sex chromosome, except iso (Xq) ♀
Karyotype 46, X with abnormal sex chromosome, except isochromosome Xq

Q96.3 Mosaicism, 45, X/46, XX or XY ♀

Q96.4 Mosaicism, 45, X/other cell line(s) with abnormal sex chromosome ♀

Q96.8 Other variants of Turner's syndrome ♀

Q96.9 Turner's syndrome, unspecified ♀

✓4ᵗʰ **Q97 Other sex chromosome abnormalities, female phenotype, not elsewhere classified**

EXCLUDES 1 *Turner's syndrome (Q96.-)*

Q97.0 Karyotype 47, XXX ♀

Q97.1 Female with more than three X chromosomes ♀

Q97.2 Mosaicism, lines with various numbers of X chromosomes ♀

Q97.3 Female with 46, XY karyotype ♀

Q97.8 Other specified sex chromosome abnormalities, female phenotype ♀

Q97.9 Sex chromosome abnormality, female phenotype, unspecified ♀

✓4ᵗʰ **Q98 Other sex chromosome abnormalities, male phenotype, not elsewhere classified**

Q98.0 Klinefelter syndrome karyotype 47, XXY ♂

Q98.1 Klinefelter syndrome, male with more than two X chromosomes ♂

Q98.3 Other male with 46, XX karyotype ♂

Q98.4 Klinefelter syndrome, unspecified ♂

Q98.5 Karyotype 47, XYY

Q98.6 Male with structurally abnormal sex chromosome ♂

Q98.7 Male with sex chromosome mosaicism ♂

Q98.8 Other specified sex chromosome abnormalities, male phenotype ♂

Q98.9 Sex chromosome abnormality, male phenotype, unspecified ♂

✓4ᵗʰ **Q99 Other chromosome abnormalities, not elsewhere classified**

Q99.0 Chimera 46, XX/46, XY
Chimera 46, XX/46, XY true hermaphrodite

Q99.1 46, XX true hermaphrodite
46, XX with streak gonads   Pure gonadal dysgenesis
46, XY with streak gonads

Q99.2 Fragile X chromosome
Fragile X syndrome

Q99.8 Other specified chromosome abnormalities

Q99.9 Chromosomal abnormality, unspecified

✓ Additional Character Required   ᵛˣ⁷ᵗʰ Xtension Alert   Unspecified Dx   Other Specified Dx   Manifestation   ▶◀ Revised Text   ● New Code   ▲ Revised Code Title

Chapter 18. Symptoms, Signs and Abnormal Clinical and Laboratory Findings, Not Elsewhere Classified (R00-R99)

NOTE This chapter includes symptoms, signs, abnormal results of clinical or other investigative procedures, and ill-defined conditions regarding which no diagnosis classifiable elsewhere is recorded.

Signs and symptoms that point rather definitely to a given diagnosis have been assigned to a category in other chapters of the classification. In general, categories in this chapter include the less well-defined conditions and symptoms that, without the necessary study of the case to establish a final diagnosis, point perhaps equally to two or more diseases or to two or more systems of the body. Practically all categories in the chapter could be designated "not otherwise specified", "unknown etiology" or "transient". The Alphabetical Index should be consulted to determine which symptoms and signs are to be allocated here and which to other chapters. The residual subcategories, numbered .8, are generally provided for other relevant symptoms that cannot be allocated elsewhere in the classification.

The conditions and signs or symptoms included in categories R00-R94 consist of:

(a) cases for which no more specific diagnosis can be made even after all the facts bearing on the case have been investigated;

(b) signs or symptoms existing at the time of initial encounter that proved to be transient and whose causes could not be determined;

(c) provisional diagnosis in a patient who failed to return for further investigation or care;

(d) cases referred elsewhere for investigation or treatment before the diagnosis was made;

(e) cases in which a more precise diagnosis was not available for any other reason;

(f) certain symptoms, for which supplementary information is provided, that represent important problems in medical care in their own right.

EXCLUDES 2 abnormal findings on antenatal screening of mother (O28.-)
certain conditions originating in the perinatal period (P04-P96)
signs and symptoms classified in the body system chapters
signs and symptoms of breast (N63, N64.5)

This chapter contains the following blocks:

R00-R09 Symptoms and signs involving the circulatory and respiratory systems
R10-R19 Symptoms and signs involving the digestive system and abdomen
R20-R23 Symptoms and signs involving the skin and subcutaneous tissue
R25-R29 Symptoms and signs involving the nervous and musculoskeletal systems
R30-R39 Symptoms and signs involving the genitourinary system
R40-R46 Symptoms and signs involving cognition, perception, emotional state and behavior
R47-R49 Symptoms and signs involving speech and voice
R50-R69 General symptoms and signs
R70-R79 Abnormal findings on examination of blood, without diagnosis
R80-R82 Abnormal findings on examination of urine, without diagnosis
R83-R89 Abnormal findings on examination of other body fluids, substances and tissues, without diagnosis
R90-R94 Abnormal findings on diagnostic imaging and in function studies, without diagnosis
R97 Abnormal tumor markers
R99 Ill-defined and unknown cause of mortality

Symptoms and signs involving the circulatory and respiratory systems (R00-R09)

☑4th R00 Abnormalities of heart beat
EXCLUDES 1 abnormalities originating in the perinatal period (P29.1-)
specified arrhythmias (I47-I49)

R00.0 Tachycardia, unspecified
Rapid heart beat
Sinoauricular tachycardia NOS
Sinus [sinusal] tachycardia NOS
EXCLUDES 1 neonatal tachycardia (P29.11)
paroxysmal tachycardia (I47.-)

R00.1 Bradycardia, unspecified
Sinoatrial bradycardia
Sinus bradycardia
Slow heart beat
Vagal bradycardia
Use additional code for adverse effect, if applicable, to identify drug (T36-T50 with fifth or sixth character 5)
EXCLUDES 1 neonatal bradycardia (P29.12)

R00.2 Palpitations
Awareness of heart beat

R00.8 Other abnormalities of heart beat

R00.9 Unspecified abnormalities of heart beat

☑4th R01 Cardiac murmurs and other cardiac sounds
EXCLUDES 1 cardiac murmurs and sounds originating in the perinatal period (P29.8)

R01.0 Benign and innocent cardiac murmurs
Functional cardiac murmur

R01.1 Cardiac murmur, unspecified
Cardiac bruit NOS
Heart murmur NOS

R01.2 Other cardiac sounds
Cardiac dullness, increased or decreased
Precordial friction

☑4th R03 Abnormal blood-pressure reading, without diagnosis

R03.0 Elevated blood-pressure reading, without diagnosis of hypertension
NOTE This category is to be used to record an episode of elevated blood pressure in a patient in whom no formal diagnosis of hypertension has been made, or as an isolated incidental finding.

R03.1 Nonspecific low blood-pressure reading
EXCLUDES 1 hypotension (I95.-)
maternal hypotension syndrome (O26.5-)
neurogenic orthostatic hypotension (G90.3)

☑4th R04 Hemorrhage from respiratory passages

R04.0 Epistaxis
Hemorrhage from nose
Nosebleed

R04.1 Hemorrhage from throat
EXCLUDES 2 hemoptysis (R04.2)

R04.2 Hemoptysis
Blood-stained sputum
Cough with hemorrhage
AHA: 2013, 4Q, 118

☑5th R04.8 Hemorrhage from other sites in respiratory passages

R04.81 Acute idiopathic pulmonary hemorrhage in infants P
AIPHI
Acute idiopathic hemorrhage in infants over 28 days old
EXCLUDES 1 perinatal pulmonary hemorrhage (P26.-)
von Willebrand's disease (D68.0)

R04.89 Hemorrhage from other sites in respiratory passages
Pulmonary hemorrhage NOS

R04.9 Hemorrhage from respiratory passages, unspecified

R05 Cough
EXCLUDES 1 cough with hemorrhage (R04.2)
smoker's cough (J41.0)

☑4th R06 Abnormalities of breathing
EXCLUDES 1 acute respiratory distress syndrome (J80)
respiratory arrest (R09.2)
respiratory arrest of newborn (P28.81)
respiratory distress syndrome of newborn (P22.-)
respiratory failure (J96.-)
respiratory failure of newborn (P28.5)

☑5th R06.0 Dyspnea
EXCLUDES 1 tachypnea NOS (R06.82)
transient tachypnea of newborn (P22.1)

R06.00 Dyspnea, unspecified

R06.01 Orthopnea

R06.02 Shortness of breath

R06.09 Other forms of dyspnea

R06.1 Stridor
EXCLUDES 1 congenital laryngeal stridor (P28.89)
laryngismus (stridulus) (J38.5)

R06.2 Wheezing
EXCLUDES 1 asthma (J45.-)

R06.3 Periodic breathing
Cheyne-Stokes breathing

R06.4 Hyperventilation
EXCLUDES 1 psychogenic hyperventilation (F45.8)

R06.5 Mouth breathing
EXCLUDES 2 dry mouth NOS (R68.2)

☑ Additional Character Required ✓x7th Xtension Alert Unspecified Dx Other Specified Dx Manifestation ►◄ Revised Text ● New Code ▲ Revised Code Title

R06.6　Hiccough
　　　EXCLUDES 1　psychogenic hiccough (F45.8)

R06.7　Sneezing

✓5ᵗʰ R06.8　Other abnormalities of breathing
　　R06.81　Apnea, not elsewhere classified
　　　　Apnea NOS
　　　　EXCLUDES 1　apnea (of) newborn (P28.4)
　　　　　　sleep apnea (G47.3-)
　　　　　　sleep apnea of newborn (primary) (P28.3)

　　R06.82　Tachypnea, not elsewhere classified
　　　　Tachypnea NOS
　　　　EXCLUDES 1　transitory tachypnea of newborn (P22.1)

　　R06.83　Snoring

　　R06.89　Other abnormalities of breathing
　　　　Breath-holding (spells)
　　　　Sighing

R06.9　Unspecified abnormalities of breathing

✓4ᵗʰ R07　Pain in throat and chest
　　　EXCLUDES 1　epidemic myalgia (B33.0)
　　　EXCLUDES 2　jaw pain (R68.84)
　　　　　pain in breast (N64.4)

R07.0　Pain in throat
　　　EXCLUDES 1　chronic sore throat (J31.2)
　　　　　sore throat (acute) NOS (J02.9)
　　　EXCLUDES 2　dysphagia (R13.1-)
　　　　　pain in neck (M54.2)

R07.1　Chest pain on breathing
　　　Painful respiration

R07.2　Precordial pain

✓5ᵗʰ R07.8　Other chest pain
　　R07.81　Pleurodynia
　　　　Pleurodynia NOS
　　　　EXCLUDES 1　epidemic pleurodynia (B33.0)

　　R07.82　Intercostal pain

　　R07.89　Other chest pain
　　　　Anterior chest-wall pain NOS

R07.9　Chest pain, unspecified

✓4ᵗʰ R09　Other symptoms and signs involving the circulatory and respiratory system
　　　EXCLUDES 1　acute respiratory distress syndrome (J80)
　　　　　respiratory arrest of newborn (P28.81)
　　　　　respiratory distress syndrome of newborn (P22.0)
　　　　　respiratory failure (J96.-)
　　　　　respiratory failure of newborn (P28.5)

✓5ᵗʰ R09.0　Asphyxia and hypoxemia
　　　EXCLUDES 1　asphyxia due to carbon monoxide (T58.-)
　　　　　asphyxia due to foreign body in respiratory tract (T17.-)
　　　　　birth (intrauterine) asphyxia (P84)
　　　　　hypercapnia (R06.4)
　　　　　hyperventilation (R06.4)
　　　　　traumatic asphyxia (T71.-)

　　R09.01　Asphyxia
　　R09.02　Hypoxemia

R09.1　Pleurisy
　　　EXCLUDES 1　pleurisy with effusion (J90)

R09.2　Respiratory arrest
　　　Cardiorespiratory failure
　　　EXCLUDES 1　cardiac arrest (I46.-)
　　　　　respiratory arrest of newborn (P28.81)
　　　　　respiratory distress of newborn (P22.0)
　　　　　respiratory failure (J96.-)
　　　　　respiratory failure of newborn (P28.5)
　　　　　respiratory insufficiency (R06.89)
　　　　　respiratory insufficiency of newborn (P28.5)

R09.3　Abnormal sputum
　　　Abnormal amount of sputum
　　　Abnormal color of sputum
　　　Abnormal odor of sputum
　　　Excessive sputum
　　　EXCLUDES 1　blood-stained sputum (R04.2)

✓5ᵗʰ R09.8　Other specified symptoms and signs involving the circulatory and respiratory systems
　　R09.81　Nasal congestion
　　R09.82　Postnasal drip

R09.89　Other specified symptoms and signs involving the circulatory and respiratory systems
　　　Abnormal chest percussion
　　　Bruit (arterial)
　　　Chest tympany
　　　Choking sensation
　　　Feeling of foreign body in throat
　　　Friction sounds in chest
　　　Rales
　　　Weak pulse
　　　EXCLUDES 2　foreign body in throat (T17.2-)
　　　　　wheezing (R06.2)

Symptoms and signs involving the digestive system and abdomen (R10-R19)

　　EXCLUDES 1　congenital or infantile pylorospasm (Q40.0)
　　　　gastrointestinal hemorrhage (K92.0-K92.2)
　　　　intestinal obstruction (K56.-)
　　　　newborn gastrointestinal hemorrhage (P54.0-P54.3)
　　　　newborn intestinal obstruction (P76.-)
　　　　pylorospasm (K31.3)
　　　　signs and symptoms involving the urinary system (R30-R39)
　　　　symptoms referable to female genital organs (N94.-)
　　　　symptoms referable to male genital organs male (N48-N50)

✓4ᵗʰ R10　Abdominal and pelvic pain
　　　EXCLUDES 1　renal colic (N23)
　　　EXCLUDES 2　dorsalgia (M54.-)
　　　　　flatulence and related conditions (R14.-)

R10.0　Acute abdomen
　　　Severe abdominal pain (generalized) (with abdominal rigidity)
　　　EXCLUDES 1　abdominal rigidity NOS (R19.3)
　　　　　generalized abdominal pain NOS (R10.84)
　　　　　localized abdominal pain (R10.1-R10.3-)

✓5ᵗʰ R10.1　Pain localized to upper abdomen
　　R10.10　Upper abdominal pain, unspecified
　　R10.11　Right upper quadrant pain
　　R10.12　Left upper quadrant pain
　　R10.13　Epigastric pain
　　　　Dyspepsia
　　　　EXCLUDES 1　functional dyspepsia (K30)

R10.2　Pelvic and perineal pain
　　　EXCLUDES 1　vulvodynia (N94.81)

✓5ᵗʰ R10.3　Pain localized to other parts of lower abdomen
　　R10.30　Lower abdominal pain, unspecified
　　R10.31　Right lower quadrant pain
　　R10.32　Left lower quadrant pain
　　R10.33　Periumbilical pain

✓5ᵗʰ R10.8　Other abdominal pain
　　✓6ᵗʰ R10.81　Abdominal tenderness
　　　　Abdominal tenderness NOS
　　　　R10.811　Right upper quadrant abdominal tenderness
　　　　R10.812　Left upper quadrant abdominal tenderness
　　　　R10.813　Right lower quadrant abdominal tenderness
　　　　R10.814　Left lower quadrant abdominal tenderness
　　　　R10.815　Periumbilic abdominal tenderness
　　　　R10.816　Epigastric abdominal tenderness
　　　　R10.817　Generalized abdominal tenderness
　　　　R10.819　Abdominal tenderness, unspecified site
　　✓6ᵗʰ R10.82　Rebound abdominal tenderness
　　　　R10.821　Right upper quadrant rebound abdominal tenderness
　　　　R10.822　Left upper quadrant rebound abdominal tenderness
　　　　R10.823　Right lower quadrant rebound abdominal tenderness
　　　　R10.824　Left lower quadrant rebound abdominal tenderness
　　　　R10.825　Periumbilic rebound abdominal tenderness
　　　　R10.826　Epigastric rebound abdominal tenderness
　　　　R10.827　Generalized rebound abdominal tenderness

EXCLUDES 1 Not coded here　　　EXCLUDES 2 Not included here　　　N Newborn Age: 0　　　P Pediatric Age: 0-17　　　M Maternity Age: 12-55　　　A Adult Age: 15-124

R10.829 **Rebound abdominal tenderness, unspecified site**

R10.83 Colic [P]
Colic NOS
Infantile colic
EXCLUDES 1 *colic in adult and child over 12 months old (R10.84)*

R10.84 Generalized **abdominal pain**
EXCLUDES 1 *generalized abdominal pain associated with acute abdomen (R10.0)*

R10.9 **Unspecified abdominal pain**

✓4th **R11 Nausea and vomiting**
EXCLUDES 1 *cyclical vomiting associated with migraine (G43.A-)*
excessive vomiting in pregnancy (O21.-)
hematemesis (K92.0)
neonatal hematemesis (P54.0)
newborn vomiting (P92.0-)
psychogenic vomiting (F50.8)
vomiting associated with bulimia nervosa (F50.2)
vomiting following gastrointestinal surgery (K91.0)

R11.0 **Nausea**
Nausea NOS
Nausea without vomiting

✓5th R11.1 **Vomiting**
R11.10 **Vomiting, unspecified**
Vomiting NOS
R11.11 **Vomiting** without nausea
R11.12 Projectile **vomiting**
R11.13 **Vomiting of** fecal matter
R11.14 Bilious **vomiting**
Bilious emesis

R11.2 **Nausea with vomiting, unspecified**
Persistent nausea with vomiting NOS

R12 **Heartburn**
EXCLUDES 1 *dyspepsia NOS (R10.13)*
functional dyspepsia (K30)

✓4th **R13 Aphagia and dysphagia**
R13.0 **Aphagia**
Inability to swallow
EXCLUDES 1 *psychogenic aphagia (F50.9)*

✓5th R13.1 **Dysphagia**
Code first, if applicable, dysphagia following cerebrovascular disease (I69. with final characters -91)
EXCLUDES 1 *psychogenic dysphagia (F45.8)*
R13.10 **Dysphagia, unspecified**
Difficulty in swallowing NOS
R13.11 **Dysphagia,** oral phase
R13.12 **Dysphagia,** oropharyngeal phase
R13.13 **Dysphagia,** pharyngeal phase
R13.14 **Dysphagia,** pharyngoesophageal phase
R13.19 **Other dysphagia**
Cervical dysphagia
Neurogenic dysphagia

✓4th **R14 Flatulence and related conditions**
EXCLUDES 1 *psychogenic aerophagy (F45.8)*
R14.0 **Abdominal distension (gaseous)**
Bloating
Tympanites (abdominal) (intestinal)
R14.1 **Gas pain**
R14.2 **Eructation**
R14.3 **Flatulence**

✓4th **R15 Fecal incontinence**
Encopresis NOS
EXCLUDES 1 *fecal incontinence of nonorganic origin (F98.1)*
R15.0 **Incomplete defecation**
EXCLUDES 1 *constipation (K59.0-)*
fecal impaction (K56.41)
R15.1 **Fecal smearing**
Fecal soiling
R15.2 **Fecal urgency**
R15.9 **Full incontinence of feces**
Fecal incontinence NOS

✓4th **R16 Hepatomegaly and splenomegaly, not elsewhere classified**
R16.0 **Hepatomegaly, not elsewhere classified**
Hepatomegaly NOS

R16.1 **Splenomegaly, not elsewhere classified**
Splenomegaly NOS

R16.2 **Hepatomegaly with splenomegaly, not elsewhere classified**
Hepatosplenomegaly NOS

R17 Unspecified jaundice
EXCLUDES 1 *neonatal jaundice (P55, P57-P59)*

✓4th **R18 Ascites**
INCLUDES fluid in peritoneal cavity
EXCLUDES 1 *ascites in alcoholic cirrhosis (K70.31)*
ascites in alcoholic hepatitis (K70.11)
ascites in toxic liver disease with chronic active hepatitis (K71.51)

R18.0 Malignant **ascites**
Code first malignancy, such as:
malignant neoplasm of ovary (C56.-)
secondary malignant neoplasm of retroperitoneum and peritoneum (C78.6)

R18.8 **Other ascites**
Ascites NOS
Peritoneal effusion (chronic)

✓4th **R19 Other symptoms and signs involving the digestive system and abdomen**
EXCLUDES 1 *acute abdomen (R10.0)*

✓5th R19.0 **Intra-abdominal and pelvic swelling, mass and lump**
EXCLUDES 1 *abdominal distension (gaseous) (R14.-)*
ascites (R18.-)
R19.00 **Intra-abdominal and pelvic swelling, mass and lump, unspecified site**
R19.01 Right upper quadrant **abdominal swelling, mass and lump**
R19.02 Left upper quadrant **abdominal swelling, mass and lump**
R19.03 Right lower quadrant **abdominal swelling, mass and lump**
R19.04 Left lower quadrant **abdominal swelling, mass and lump**
R19.05 Periumbilic **swelling, mass or lump**
Diffuse or generalized umbilical swelling or mass
R19.06 Epigastric **swelling, mass or lump**
R19.07 Generalized **intra-abdominal and pelvic swelling, mass and lump**
Diffuse or generalized intra-abdominal swelling or mass NOS
Diffuse or generalized pelvic swelling or mass NOS
R19.09 **Other intra-abdominal and pelvic swelling, mass and lump**

✓5th R19.1 **Abnormal bowel sounds**
R19.11 Absent **bowel sounds**
R19.12 Hyperactive **bowel sounds**
R19.15 **Other abnormal bowel sounds**
Abnormal bowel sounds NOS

R19.2 **Visible peristalsis**
Hyperperistalsis

✓5th R19.3 **Abdominal rigidity**
EXCLUDES 1 *abdominal rigidity with severe abdominal pain (R10.0)*
R19.30 **Abdominal rigidity, unspecified site**
R19.31 Right upper quadrant **abdominal rigidity**
R19.32 Left upper quadrant **abdominal rigidity**
R19.33 Right lower quadrant **abdominal rigidity**
R19.34 Left lower quadrant **abdominal rigidity**
R19.35 Periumbilic **abdominal rigidity**
R19.36 Epigastric **abdominal rigidity**
R19.37 Generalized **abdominal rigidity**

R19.4 **Change in bowel habit**
EXCLUDES 1 *constipation (K59.0-)*
functional diarrhea (K59.1)

R19.5 **Other fecal abnormalities**
Abnormal stool color
Bulky stools
Mucus in stools
Occult blood in feces
Occult blood in stools
EXCLUDES 1 *melena (K92.1)*
neonatal melena (P54.1)

R19.6 **Halitosis**

☑ Additional Character Required   ✓x7th Xtension Alert   Unspecified Dx   Other Specified Dx   Manifestation   ▶◀ Revised Text   ● New Code   ▲ Revised Code Title

Symptoms, Signs and Abnormal Clinical and Laboratory Findings

R19.7–R29.5

R19.7 Diarrhea, unspecified
Diarrhea NOS
EXCLUDES 1   *functional diarrhea (K59.1)*
neonatal diarrhea (P78.3)
psychogenic diarrhea (F45.8)

R19.8 Other specified symptoms and signs involving the digestive system and abdomen

Symptoms and signs involving the skin and subcutaneous tissue (R20-R23)

EXCLUDES 2   *symptoms relating to breast (N64.4-N64.5)*

✓4ᵗʰ **R20 Disturbances of skin sensation**
EXCLUDES 1   *dissociative anesthesia and sensory loss (F44.6)*
psychogenic disturbances (F45.8)

R20.0 Anesthesia of skin

R20.1 Hypoesthesia of skin

R20.2 Paresthesia of skin
Formication
Pins and needles
Tingling skin
EXCLUDES 1   *acroparesthesia (I73.8)*

R20.3 Hyperesthesia

R20.8 Other disturbances of skin sensation

R20.9 Unspecified disturbances of skin sensation

R21 Rash and other nonspecific skin eruption
Rash NOS
EXCLUDES 1   *specified type of rash—code to condition*
vesicular eruption (R23.8)

✓4ᵗʰ **R22 Localized swelling, mass and lump of skin and subcutaneous tissue**
Subcutaneous nodules (localized)(superficial)
EXCLUDES 1   *abnormal findings on diagnostic imaging (R90-R93)*
edema (R60.-)
enlarged lymph nodes (R59.-)
localized adiposity (E65)
swelling of joint (M25.4-)

R22.0 Localized swelling, mass and lump, head

R22.1 Localized swelling, mass and lump, neck

R22.2 Localized swelling, mass and lump, trunk
EXCLUDES 1   *intra-abdominal or pelvic mass and lump (R19.0-)*
intra-abdominal or pelvic swelling (R19.0-)
EXCLUDES 2   *breast mass and lump (N63)*

✓5ᵗʰ **R22.3 Localized swelling, mass and lump, upper limb**

    R22.30 Localized swelling, mass and lump, unspecified upper limb

    R22.31 Localized swelling, mass and lump, right upper limb

    R22.32 Localized swelling, mass and lump, left upper limb

    R22.33 Localized swelling, mass and lump, upper limb, bilateral

✓5ᵗʰ **R22.4 Localized swelling, mass and lump, lower limb**

    R22.40 Localized swelling, mass and lump, unspecified lower limb

    R22.41 Localized swelling, mass and lump, right lower limb

    R22.42 Localized swelling, mass and lump, left lower limb

    R22.43 Localized swelling, mass and lump, lower limb, bilateral

R22.9 Localized swelling, mass and lump, unspecified

✓4ᵗʰ **R23 Other skin changes**

R23.0 Cyanosis
EXCLUDES 1   *acrocyanosis (I73.8)*
cyanotic attacks of newborn (P28.2)

R23.1 Pallor
Clammy skin

R23.2 Flushing
Excessive blushing
Code first, if applicable, menopausal and female climacteric states (N95.1)

R23.3 Spontaneous ecchymoses
Petechiae
EXCLUDES 1   *ecchymoses of newborn (P54.5)*
purpura (D69.-)

R23.4 Changes in skin texture
Desquamation of skin
Induration of skin
Scaling of skin
EXCLUDES 1   *epidermal thickening NOS (L85.9)*

R23.8 Other skin changes

R23.9 Unspecified skin changes

Symptoms and signs involving the nervous and musculoskeletal systems (R25-R29)

✓4ᵗʰ **R25 Abnormal involuntary movements**
EXCLUDES 1   *specific movement disorders (G20-G26)*
stereotyped movement disorders (F98.4)
tic disorders (F95.-)

R25.0 Abnormal head movements

R25.1 Tremor, unspecified
EXCLUDES 1   *chorea NOS (G25.5)*
essential tremor (G25.0)
hysterical tremor (F44.4)
intention tremor (G25.2)

R25.2 Cramp and spasm
EXCLUDES 2   *carpopedal spasm (R29.0)*
charley-horse (M62.831)
infantile spasms (G40.4-)
muscle spasm of back (M62.830)
muscle spasm of calf (M62.831)

R25.3 Fasciculation
Twitching NOS

R25.8 Other abnormal involuntary movements

R25.9 Unspecified abnormal involuntary movements

✓4ᵗʰ **R26 Abnormalities of gait and mobility**
EXCLUDES 1   *ataxia NOS (R27.0)*
hereditary ataxia (G11.-)
locomotor (syphilitic) ataxia (A52.11)
immobility syndrome (paraplegic) (M62.3)

R26.0 Ataxic gait
Staggering gait

R26.1 Paralytic gait
Spastic gait

R26.2 Difficulty in walking, not elsewhere classified
EXCLUDES 1   *falling (R29.6)*
unsteadiness on feet (R26.81)

✓5ᵗʰ **R26.8 Other abnormalities of gait and mobility**

    R26.81 Unsteadiness on feet

    R26.89 Other abnormalities of gait and mobility

R26.9 Unspecified abnormalities of gait and mobility

✓4ᵗʰ **R27 Other lack of coordination**
EXCLUDES 1   *ataxic gait (R26.0)*
hereditary ataxia (G11.-)
vertigo NOS (R42)

R27.0 Ataxia, unspecified
EXCLUDES 1   *ataxia following cerebrovascular disease (I69. with final characters -93)*

R27.8 Other lack of coordination

R27.9 Unspecified lack of coordination

✓4ᵗʰ **R29 Other symptoms and signs involving the nervous and musculoskeletal systems**

R29.0 Tetany
Carpopedal spasm
EXCLUDES 1   *hysterical tetany (F44.5)*
neonatal tetany (P71.3)
parathyroid tetany (E20.9)
post-thyroidectomy tetany (E89.2)

R29.1 Meningismus

R29.2 Abnormal reflex
EXCLUDES 2   *abnormal pupillary reflex (H57.0)*
hyperactive gag reflex (J39.2)
vasovagal reaction or syncope (R55)

R29.3 Abnormal posture

R29.4 Clicking hip
EXCLUDES 1   *congenital deformities of hip (Q65.-)*

R29.5 Transient paralysis
Code first any associated spinal cord injury (S14.0, S14.1-, S24.0, S24.1-, S34.0-, S34.1-)
EXCLUDES 1   *transient ischemic attack (G45.9)*

EXCLUDES 1 Not coded here   *EXCLUDES 2* Not included here   N Newborn Age: 0   P Pediatric Age: 0-17   M Maternity Age: 12-55   A Adult Age: 15-124

R29.6   **Repeated falls**
> Falling
> Tendency to fall
> EXCLUDES 2   at risk for falling (Z91.81)
>   history of falling (Z91.81)

✓5th **R29.8**   **Other symptoms and signs involving the nervous and musculoskeletal systems**

  ✓6th **R29.81**   **Other symptoms and signs involving the nervous system**

    R29.810   **Facial weakness**
> Facial droop
> EXCLUDES 1   Bell's palsy (G51.0)
>   facial weakness following cerebrovascular disease (I69. with final characters -92)

    R29.818   **Other symptoms and signs involving the nervous system**

  ✓6th **R29.89**   **Other symptoms and signs involving the musculoskeletal system**
> EXCLUDES 2   pain in limb (M79.6-)

    R29.890   **Loss of height**
> EXCLUDES 1   osteoporosis (M80-M81)

    R29.891   **Ocular torticollis**
> EXCLUDES 1   congenital (sternomastoid) torticollis Q68.0
>   psychogenic torticollis (F45.8)
>   spasmodic torticollis (G24.3)
>   torticollis due to birth injury (P15.8)
>   torticollis NOS M43.6

    R29.898   **Other symptoms and signs involving the musculoskeletal system**

✓5th **R29.9**   **Unspecified symptoms and signs involving the nervous and musculoskeletal systems**

  R29.90   **Unspecified symptoms and signs involving the nervous system**

  R29.91   **Unspecified symptoms and signs involving the musculoskeletal system**

Symptoms and signs involving the genitourinary system (R30-R39)

✓4th **R30**   **Pain associated with micturition**
> EXCLUDES 1   psychogenic pain associated with micturition (F45.8)

  R30.0   **Dysuria**
> Strangury

  R30.1   **Vesical tenesmus**

  R30.9   **Painful micturition, unspecified**
> Painful urination NOS

✓4th **R31**   **Hematuria**
> EXCLUDES 1   hematuria included with underlying conditions, such as:
>   acute cystitis with hematuria (N30.01)
>   recurrent and persistent hematuria in glomerular diseases (N02.-)

  R31.0   **Gross hematuria**

  R31.1   **Benign essential microscopic hematuria**

  R31.2   **Other microscopic hematuria**

  R31.9   **Hematuria, unspecified**

R32   **Unspecified urinary incontinence**
> Enuresis NOS
> EXCLUDES 1   functional urinary incontinence (R39.81)
>   nonorganic enuresis (F98.0)
>   stress incontinence and other specified urinary incontinence (N39.3-N39.4-)
>   urinary incontinence associated with cognitive impairment (R39.81)

✓4th **R33**   **Retention of urine**
> EXCLUDES 1   psychogenic retention of urine (F45.8)

  R33.0   **Drug induced retention of urine**
> Use additional code for adverse effect, if applicable, to identify drug (T36-T50 with fifth or sixth character 5)

  R33.8   **Other retention of urine**
> Code first, if applicable, any causal condition, such as:
>   enlarged prostate (N40.1)

  R33.9   **Retention of urine, unspecified**

R34   **Anuria and oliguria**
> EXCLUDES 1   anuria and oliguria complicating abortion or ectopic or molar pregnancy (O00-O07, O08.4)
>   anuria and oliguria complicating pregnancy (O26.83-)
>   anuria and oliguria complicating the puerperium (O90.4)

✓4th **R35**   **Polyuria**
> Code first, if applicable, any causal condition, such as:
>   enlarged prostate (N40.1)
> EXCLUDES 1   psychogenic polyuria (F45.8)

  R35.0   **Frequency of micturition**

  R35.1   **Nocturia**

  R35.8   **Other polyuria**
> Polyuria NOS

✓4th **R36**   **Urethral discharge**

  R36.0   **Urethral discharge without blood**

  R36.1   **Hematospermia**   ♂

  R36.9   **Urethral discharge, unspecified**
> Penile discharge NOS
> Urethrorrhea

R37   **Sexual dysfunction, unspecified**

✓4th **R39**   **Other and unspecified symptoms and signs involving the genitourinary system**

  R39.0   **Extravasation of urine**

  ✓5th **R39.1**   **Other difficulties with micturition**
> Code first, if applicable, any causal condition, such as:
>   enlarged prostate (N40.1)

    R39.11   **Hesitancy of micturition**

    R39.12   **Poor urinary stream**
> Weak urinary steam

    R39.13   **Splitting of urinary stream**

    R39.14   **Feeling of incomplete bladder emptying**

    R39.15   **Urgency of urination**
> EXCLUDES 1   urge incontinence (N39.41, N39.46)

    R39.16   **Straining to void**

    R39.19   **Other difficulties with micturition**

  R39.2   **Extrarenal uremia**
> Prerenal uremia
> EXCLUDES 1   uremia NOS (N19)

  ✓5th **R39.8**   **Other symptoms and signs involving the genitourinary system**

    R39.81   **Functional urinary incontinence**
> Urinary incontinence due to cognitive impairment, or severe physical disability or immobility
> EXCLUDES 1   stress incontinence and other specified urinary incontinence (N39.3-N39.4-)
>   urinary incontinence NOS (R32)

    R39.89   **Other symptoms and signs involving the genitourinary system**

  R39.9   **Unspecified symptoms and signs involving the genitourinary system**

Symptoms and signs involving cognition, perception, emotional state and behavior (R40-R46)

> EXCLUDES 1   symptoms and signs constituting part of a pattern of mental disorder (F01-F99)

✓4th **R40**   **Somnolence, stupor and coma**
> EXCLUDES 1   neonatal coma (P91.5)
>   somnolence, stupor and coma in diabetes (E08-E13)
>   somnolence, stupor and coma in hepatic failure (K72.-)
>   somnolence, stupor and coma in hypoglycemia (nondiabetic) (E15)

  R40.0   **Somnolence**
> Drowsiness
> EXCLUDES 1   coma (R40.2-)

  R40.1   **Stupor**
> Catatonic stupor
> Semicoma
> EXCLUDES 1   catatonic schizophrenia (F20.2)
>   coma (R40.2-)
>   depressive stupor (F31-F33)
>   dissociative stupor (F44.2)
>   manic stupor (F30.2)

✓ Additional Character Required   ✓x7th Xtension Alert   Unspecified Dx   Other Specified Dx   Manifestation   ▶◀ Revised Text   ● New Code   ▲ Revised Code Title

ICD-10-CM Draft (2015)   793

Symptoms, Signs and Abnormal Clinical and Laboratory Findings

R29.6–R40.1

✓5ᵗʰ R4Ø.2 **Coma**
     Code first any associated:
        fracture of skull (SØ2.-)
        intracranial injury (SØ6.-)
     NOTE   One code from subcategories R4Ø.21-R4Ø.23 is
            required to complete the coma scale
     AHA: 2Ø14, 1Q, 19

     R4Ø.2Ø **Unspecified coma**
          Coma NOS
          Unconsciousness NOS

     ✓6ᵗʰ R4Ø.21 **Coma scale,** eyes open

          The following appropriate 7th character is to be
          added to subcategory R4Ø.21-.
          Ø   unspecified time
          1   in the field [EMT or ambulance]
          2   at arrival to emergency department
          3   at hospital admission
          4   24 hours or more after hospital admission

         ✓7ᵗʰ R4Ø.211 **Coma scale, eyes open,** never
         ✓7ᵗʰ R4Ø.212 **Coma scale, eyes open,** to pain
         ✓7ᵗʰ R4Ø.213 **Coma scale, eyes open,** to sound
         ✓7ᵗʰ R4Ø.214 **Coma scale, eyes open,** spontaneous

     ✓6ᵗʰ R4Ø.22 **Coma scale,** best verbal response

          The following appropriate 7th character is to be
          added to subcategory R4Ø.22-.
          Ø   unspecified time
          1   in the field [EMT or ambulance]
          2   at arrival to emergency department
          3   at hospital admission
          4   24 hours or more after hospital admission

         ✓7ᵗʰ R4Ø.221 **Coma scale, best verbal response,** none
         ✓7ᵗʰ R4Ø.222 **Coma scale, best verbal response,**
                 incomprehensible words
         ✓7ᵗʰ R4Ø.223 **Coma scale, best verbal response,**
                 inappropriate words
         ✓7ᵗʰ R4Ø.224 **Coma scale, best verbal response,**
                 confused conversation
         ✓7ᵗʰ R4Ø.225 **Coma scale, best verbal response,**
                 oriented

     ✓6ᵗʰ R4Ø.23 **Coma scale,** best motor response

          The following appropriate 7th character is to be
          added to subcategory R4Ø.23-.
          Ø   unspecified time
          1   in the field [EMT or ambulance]
          2   at arrival to emergency department
          3   at hospital admission
          4   24 hours or more after hospital admission

         ✓7ᵗʰ R4Ø.231 **Coma scale, best motor response,** none
         ✓7ᵗʰ R4Ø.232 **Coma scale, best motor response,**
                 extension
         ✓7ᵗʰ R4Ø.233 **Coma scale, best motor response,**
                 abnormal
         ✓7ᵗʰ R4Ø.234 **Coma scale, best motor response,** flexion
                 withdrawal
         ✓7ᵗʰ R4Ø.235 **Coma scale, best motor response,** localizes
                 pain
         ✓7ᵗʰ R4Ø.236 **Coma scale, best motor response,** obeys
                 commands

     ✓6ᵗʰ R4Ø.24 Glasgow coma scale, total score
          Use codes R4Ø.21- through R4Ø.23- only when the
             individual score(s) are documented
         R4Ø.241 **Glasgow coma scale** score 13-15
         R4Ø.242 **Glasgow coma scale** score 9-12
         R4Ø.243 **Glasgow coma scale** score 3-8
         R4Ø.244 **Other coma, without documented**
                 Glasgow coma scale score, or with partial
                 score reported

     R4Ø.3 **Persistent vegetative state**

     R4Ø.4 **Transient alteration of awareness**

✓4ᵗʰ R41 **Other symptoms and signs involving cognitive functions and awareness**
     EXCLUDES 1 *dissociative [conversion] disorders (F44.-)*
              mild cognitive impairment, so stated (G31.84)

     R41.Ø **Disorientation, unspecified**
          Confusion NOS
          Delirium NOS

     R41.1 **Anterograde amnesia**

     R41.2 **Retrograde amnesia**

     R41.3 **Other amnesia**
          Amnesia NOS
          Memory loss NOS
          EXCLUDES 1 *amnestic disorder due to known physiologic condition*
                   (FØ4)
                amnestic syndrome due to psychoactive substance use
                   (F1Ø-F19 with 5th character .6)
                mild memory disturbance due to known physiological
                   condition (FØ6.8)
                transient global amnesia (G45.4)

     R41.4 **Neurologic neglect syndrome**
          Asomatognosia
          Hemi-akinesia
          Hemi-inattention
          Hemispatial neglect
          Left-sided neglect
          Sensory neglect
          Visuospatial neglect
          EXCLUDES 1 *visuospatial deficit (R41.842)*

     ✓5ᵗʰ R41.8 **Other symptoms and signs involving cognitive functions and awareness**
         R41.81 Age-related **cognitive decline**   Ⓐ
             Senility NOS
         R41.82 **Altered mental status, unspecified**
             Change in mental status NOS
             EXCLUDES 1 *altered level of consciousness (R4Ø.-)*
                   altered mental status due to known
                      condition—code to condition
                   delirium NOS (R41.Ø)
             AHA: 2Ø12, 4Q, 97
         R41.83 Borderline intellectual **functioning**
             IQ level 71 to 84
             EXCLUDES 1 *intellectual disabilities (F7Ø-F79)*
         ✓6ᵗʰ R41.84 Other specified cognitive deficit
             R41.84Ø Attention and concentration **deficit**
                 EXCLUDES 1 *attention-deficit hyperactivity*
                      disorders (F9Ø.-)
             R41.841 **Cognitive** communication **deficit**
             R41.842 Visuospatial **deficit**
             R41.843 Psychomotor **deficit**
             R41.844 Frontal lobe and executive function **deficit**
         R41.89 **Other symptoms and signs involving cognitive functions and awareness**
             Anosognosia

     R41.9 **Unspecified symptoms and signs involving cognitive functions and awareness**

R42 **Dizziness and giddiness**
     Light-headedness
     Vertigo NOS
     EXCLUDES 1 *vertiginous syndromes (H81.-)*
              vertigo from infrasound (T75.23)

✓4ᵗʰ R43 **Disturbances of smell and taste**
     R43.Ø **Anosmia**
     R43.1 **Parosmia**
     R43.2 **Parageusia**
     R43.8 **Other disturbances of smell and taste**
          Mixed disturbance of smell and taste
     R43.9 **Unspecified disturbances of smell and taste**

✓4ᵗʰ R44 **Other symptoms and signs involving general sensations and perceptions**
     EXCLUDES 1 *alcoholic hallucinations (F1.5)*
              hallucinations in drug psychosis (F11-F19 with .5)
              hallucinations in mood disorders with psychotic symptoms
                 (F3Ø.2, F31.5, F32.3, F33.3)
              hallucinations in schizophrenia, schizotypal and delusional
                 disorders (F2Ø-F29)
     EXCLUDES 2 *disturbances of skin sensation (R2Ø.-)*
     R44.Ø Auditory **hallucinations**
     R44.1 Visual **hallucinations**

EXCLUDES 1 Not coded here   **EXCLUDES 2** Not included here   Ⓝ Newborn Age: Ø   Ⓟ Pediatric Age: Ø-17   Ⓜ Maternity Age: 12-55   Ⓐ Adult Age: 15-124

794   ICD-1Ø-CM Draft (2Ø15)

R44.2 **Other hallucinations**

R44.3 **Hallucinations, unspecified**

R44.8 **Other symptoms and signs involving general sensations and perceptions**

R44.9 **Unspecified symptoms and signs involving general sensations and perceptions**

✓4ᵗʰ **R45 Symptoms and signs involving emotional state**

R45.0 **Nervousness**
Nervous tension

R45.1 **Restlessness and agitation**

R45.2 **Unhappiness**

R45.3 **Demoralization and apathy**
EXCLUDES 1 anhedonia (R45.84)

R45.4 **Irritability and anger**

R45.5 **Hostility**

R45.6 **Violent behavior**

R45.7 **State of emotional shock and stress, unspecified**

✓5ᵗʰ R45.8 **Other symptoms and signs involving emotional state**

R45.81 **Low self-esteem**

R45.82 **Worries**

R45.83 **Excessive crying of child, adolescent or adult**
EXCLUDES 1 excessive crying of infant (baby) R68.11

R45.84 **Anhedonia**

✓6ᵗʰ R45.85 **Homicidal and suicidal ideations**
EXCLUDES 1 suicide attempt (T14.91)
R45.850 **Homicidal ideations**
R45.851 **Suicidal ideations**

R45.86 **Emotional lability**

R45.87 **Impulsiveness**

R45.89 **Other symptoms and signs involving emotional state**

✓4ᵗʰ **R46 Symptoms and signs involving appearance and behavior**
EXCLUDES 1 appearance and behavior in schizophrenia, schizotypal and delusional disorders (F20-F29)
mental and behavioral disorders (F01-F99)

R46.0 **Very low level of personal hygiene**

R46.1 **Bizarre personal appearance**

R46.2 **Strange and inexplicable behavior**

R46.3 **Overactivity**

R46.4 **Slowness and poor responsiveness**
EXCLUDES 1 stupor (R40.1)

R46.5 **Suspiciousness and marked evasiveness**

R46.6 **Undue concern and preoccupation with stressful events**

R46.7 **Verbosity and circumstantial detail obscuring reason for contact**

✓5ᵗʰ R46.8 **Other symptoms and signs involving appearance and behavior**

R46.81 **Obsessive-compulsive behavior**
EXCLUDES 1 obsessive-compulsive disorder (F42)

R46.89 **Other symptoms and signs involving appearance and behavior**

Symptoms and signs involving speech and voice (R47-R49)

✓4ᵗʰ **R47 Speech disturbances, not elsewhere classified**
EXCLUDES 1 autism (F84.0)
cluttering (F80.81)
specific developmental disorders of speech and language (F80.-)
stuttering (F80.81)

✓5ᵗʰ R47.0 **Dysphasia and aphasia**

R47.01 **Aphasia**
EXCLUDES 1 aphasia following cerebrovascular disease (I69. with final characters -20)
progressive isolated aphasia (G31.01)

R47.02 **Dysphasia**
EXCLUDES 1 dysphasia following cerebrovascular disease (I69. with final characters -21)

R47.1 **Dysarthria and anarthria**
EXCLUDES 1 dysarthria following cerebrovascular disease (I69. with final characters -22)

✓5ᵗʰ R47.8 **Other speech disturbances**
EXCLUDES 1 dysarthria following cerebrovascular disease (I69. with final characters -28)

R47.81 **Slurred speech**

R47.82 *Fluency disorder in conditions classified elsewhere*
Stuttering in conditions classified elsewhere
Code first underlying disease or condition, such as:
Parkinson's disease (G20)
EXCLUDES 1 adult onset fluency disorder (F98.5)
childhood onset fluency disorder (F80.81)
fluency disorder (stuttering) following cerebrovascular disease (I69. with final characters-23)

R47.89 **Other speech disturbances**

R47.9 **Unspecified speech disturbances**

✓4ᵗʰ **R48 Dyslexia and other symbolic dysfunctions, not elsewhere classified**
EXCLUDES 1 specific developmental disorders of scholastic skills (F81.-)

R48.0 **Dyslexia and alexia**

R48.1 **Agnosia**
Astereognosia (astereognosis)
Autotopagnosia
EXCLUDES 1 visual object agnosia (R48.3)

R48.2 **Apraxia**
EXCLUDES 1 apraxia following cerebrovascular disease (I69. with final characters -90)

R48.3 **Visual agnosia**
Prosopagnosia
Simultanagnosia (asimultagnosia)

R48.8 **Other symbolic dysfunctions**
Acalculia
Agraphia

R48.9 **Unspecified symbolic dysfunctions**

✓4ᵗʰ **R49 Voice and resonance disorders**
EXCLUDES 1 psychogenic voice and resonance disorders (F44.4)

R49.0 **Dysphonia**
Hoarseness

R49.1 **Aphonia**
Loss of voice

✓5ᵗʰ R49.2 **Hypernasality and hyponasality**

R49.21 **Hypernasality**

R49.22 **Hyponasality**

R49.8 **Other voice and resonance disorders**

R49.9 **Unspecified voice and resonance disorder**
Change in voice NOS
Resonance disorder NOS

General symptoms and signs (R50-R69)

✓4ᵗʰ **R50 Fever of other and unknown origin**
EXCLUDES 1 chills without fever (R68.83)
febrile convulsions (R56.0-)
fever of unknown origin during labor (O75.2)
fever of unknown origin in newborn (P81.9)
hypothermia due to illness (R68.0)
malignant hyperthermia due to anesthesia (T88.3)
puerperal pyrexia NOS (O86.4)

R50.2 **Drug induced fever**
Use additional code for adverse effect, if applicable, to identify drug (T36-T50 with fifth or sixth character 5)
EXCLUDES 1 postvaccination (postimmunization) fever (R50.83)

✓5ᵗʰ R50.8 **Other specified fever**

R50.81 *Fever presenting with conditions classified elsewhere*
Code first underlying condition when associated fever is present, such as with:
leukemia (C91-C95)
neutropenia (D70.-)
sickle-cell disease (D57.-)

R50.82 **Postprocedural fever**
EXCLUDES 1 postprocedural infection (T81.4)
posttransfusion fever (R50.84)
postvaccination (postimmunization) fever (R50.83)

R50.83 **Postvaccination fever**
Postimmunization fever

R50.84 **Febrile nonhemolytic transfusion reaction**
FNHTR
Posttransfusion fever

☑ Additional Character Required ✓x7ᵗʰ Xtension Alert Unspecified Dx Other Specified Dx Manifestation ►◄ Revised Text ● New Code ▲ Revised Code Title

R50.9 Fever, unspecified
Fever NOS
Fever of unknown origin [FUO]
Fever with chills
Fever with rigors
Hyperpyrexia NOS
Persistent fever
Pyrexia NOS

R51 Headache
Facial pain NOS
EXCLUDES1 atypical face pain (G50.1)
migraine and other headache syndromes (G43-G44)
trigeminal neuralgia (G50.0)

R52 Pain, unspecified
Acute pain NOS
Generalized pain NOS
Pain NOS
EXCLUDES1 acute and chronic pain, not elsewhere classified (G89.-)
localized pain, unspecified type—code to pain by site, such as:
abdomen pain (R10.-)
back pain (M54.9)
breast pain (N64.4)
chest pain (R07.1-R07.9)
ear pain (H92.0-)
eye pain (H57.1)
headache (R51)
joint pain (M25.5-)
limb pain (M79.6-)
lumbar region pain (M54.5)
pelvic and perineal pain (R10.2)
renal colic (N23)
shoulder pain (M25.51-)
spine pain (M54.-)
throat pain (R07.0)
tongue pain (K14.6)
tooth pain (K08.8)
pain disorders exclusively related to psychological factors (F45.41)

R53 Malaise and fatigue
R53.0 Neoplastic (malignant) related fatigue
Code first associated neoplasm
R53.1 Weakness
Asthenia NOS
EXCLUDES1 age-related weakness (R54)
muscle weakness (M62.8-)
senile asthenia (R54)
R53.2 Functional quadriplegia
Complete immobility due to severe physical disability or frailty
EXCLUDES1 frailty NOS (R54)
hysterical paralysis (F44.4)
immobility syndrome (M62.3)
neurologic quadriplegia (G82.5-)
quadriplegia (G82.50)
R53.8 Other malaise and fatigue
EXCLUDES1 combat exhaustion and fatigue (F43.0)
congenital debility (P96.9)
exhaustion and fatigue due to depressive episode (F32.-)
exhaustion and fatigue due to excessive exertion (T73.3)
exhaustion and fatigue due to exposure (T73.2)
exhaustion and fatigue due to heat (T67.-)
exhaustion and fatigue due to pregnancy (O26.8-)
exhaustion and fatigue due to recurrent depressive episode (F33)
exhaustion and fatigue due to senile debility (R54)
R53.81 Other malaise
Chronic debility
Debility NOS
General physical deterioration
Malaise NOS
Nervous debility
EXCLUDES1 age-related physical debility (R54)
R53.82 Chronic fatigue, unspecified
Chronic fatigue syndrome NOS
EXCLUDES1 postviral fatigue syndrome (G93.3)
R53.83 Other fatigue
Fatigue NOS
Lack of energy
Lethargy
Tiredness

R54 Age-related physical debility
Frailty
Old age
Senescence
Senile asthenia
Senile debility
EXCLUDES1 age-related cognitive decline (R41.81)
senile psychosis (F03)
senility NOS (R41.81)

R55 Syncope and collapse
Blackout
Fainting
Vasovagal attack
EXCLUDES1 cardiogenic shock (R57.0)
carotid sinus syncope (G90.01)
heat syncope (T67.1)
neurocirculatory asthenia (F45.8)
neurogenic orthostatic hypotension (G90.3)
orthostatic hypotension (I95.1)
postprocedural shock (T81.1-)
psychogenic syncope (F48.8)
shock NOS (R57.9)
shock complicating or following abortion or ectopic or molar pregnancy (O00-O07, O08.3)
shock complicating or following labor and delivery (O75.1)
Stokes-Adams attack (I45.9)
unconsciousness NOS (R40.2-)

R56 Convulsions, not elsewhere classified
EXCLUDES1 dissociative convulsions and seizures (F44.5)
epileptic convulsions and seizures (G40.-)
newborn convulsions and seizures (P90)
R56.0 Febrile convulsions
R56.00 Simple febrile convulsions
Febrile convulsion NOS
Febrile seizure NOS
R56.01 Complex febrile convulsions
Atypical febrile seizure
Complex febrile seizure
Complicated febrile seizure
EXCLUDES1 status epilepticus (G40.901)
R56.1 Post traumatic seizures
EXCLUDES1 post traumatic epilepsy (G40.-)
R56.9 Unspecified convulsions
Convulsion disorder
Fit NOS
Recurrent convulsions
Seizure(s) (convulsive) NOS

R57 Shock, not elsewhere classified
EXCLUDES1 anaphylactic shock NOS (T78.2)
anaphylactic reaction or shock due to adverse food reaction (T78.0-)
anaphylactic shock due to adverse effect of correct drug or medicament properly administered (T88.6)
anaphylactic shock due to serum (T80.5-)
anesthetic shock (T88.3)
electric shock (T75.4)
obstetric shock (O75.1)
postprocedural shock (T81.1-)
psychic shock (F43.0)
septic shock (R65.21)
shock complicating or following ectopic or molar pregnancy (O00-O07, O08.3)
shock due to lightning (T75.01)
traumatic shock (T79.4)
toxic shock syndrome (A48.3)
R57.0 Cardiogenic shock
R57.1 Hypovolemic shock
R57.8 Other shock
R57.9 Shock, unspecified
Failure of peripheral circulation NOS

R58 Hemorrhage, not elsewhere classified
Hemorrhage NOS
EXCLUDES1 hemorrhage included with underlying conditions, such as:
acute duodenal ulcer with hemorrhage (K26.0)
acute gastritis with bleeding (K29.01)
ulcerative enterocolitis with rectal bleeding (K51.01)

✓4th **R59 Enlarged lymph nodes**
> INCLUDES swollen glands
> EXCLUDES 1 acute lymphadenitis (L04.-)
> chronic lymphadenitis (I88.1)
> lymphadenitis NOS (I88.9)
> mesenteric (acute) (chronic) lymphadenitis (I88.0)

R59.0 Localized enlarged lymph nodes

R59.1 Generalized enlarged lymph nodes
> Lymphadenopathy NOS

R59.9 Enlarged lymph nodes, unspecified

✓4th **R60 Edema, not elsewhere classified**
> EXCLUDES 1 angioneurotic edema (T78.3)
> ascites (R18.-)
> cerebral edema (G93.6)
> cerebral edema due to birth injury (P11.0)
> edema of larynx (J38.4)
> edema of nasopharynx (J39.2)
> edema of pharynx (J39.2)
> gestational edema (O12.0-)
> hereditary edema (Q82.0)
> hydrops fetalis NOS (P83.2)
> hydrothorax (J94.8)
> nutritional edema (E40-E46)
> hydrops fetalis NOS (P83.2)
> newborn edema (P83.3)
> pulmonary edema (J81.-)

R60.0 Localized edema

R60.1 Generalized edema

R60.9 Edema, unspecified
> Fluid retention NOS

R61 Generalized hyperhidrosis
> Excessive sweating
> Night sweats
> Secondary hyperhidrosis
> Code first, if applicable, menopausal and female climacteric states (N95.1)
> EXCLUDES 1 focal (primary) (secondary) hyperhidrosis (L74.5-)
> Frey's syndrome (L74.52)
> localized (primary) (secondary) hyperhidrosis (L74.5-)

✓4th **R62 Lack of expected normal physiological development in childhood and adults**
> EXCLUDES 1 delayed puberty (E30.0)
> gonadal dysgenesis (Q99.1)
> hypopituitarism (E23.0)

R62.0 Delayed milestone in childhood P
> Delayed attainment of expected physiological developmental stage
> Late talker
> Late walker

✓5th **R62.5 Other and unspecified lack of expected normal physiological development in childhood**
> EXCLUDES 1 HIV disease resulting in failure to thrive (B20)
> physical retardation due to malnutrition (E45)

R62.50 Unspecified lack of expected normal physiological development in childhood P
> Infantilism NOS

R62.51 Failure to thrive (child) P
> Failure to gain weight
> EXCLUDES 1 failure to thrive in child under 28 days old (P92.6)

R62.52 Short stature (child) P
> Lack of growth
> Physical retardation
> Short stature NOS
> EXCLUDES 1 short stature due to endocrine disorder (E34.3)

R62.59 Other lack of expected normal physiological development in childhood P

R62.7 Adult failure to thrive A

✓4th **R63 Symptoms and signs concerning food and fluid intake**
> EXCLUDES 1 bulimia NOS (F50.2)
> eating disorders of nonorganic origin (F50.-)
> malnutrition (E40-E46)

R63.0 Anorexia
> Loss of appetite
> EXCLUDES 1 anorexia nervosa (F50.0-)
> loss of appetite of nonorganic origin (F50.8)

R63.1 Polydipsia
> Excessive thirst

R63.2 Polyphagia
> Excessive eating
> Hyperalimentation NOS

R63.3 Feeding difficulties
> Feeding problem (elderly) (infant) NOS
> EXCLUDES 1 feeding problems of newborn (P92.-)
> infant feeding disorder of nonorganic origin (F98.2-)

R63.4 Abnormal weight loss

R63.5 Abnormal weight gain
> EXCLUDES 1 excessive weight gain in pregnancy (O26.0-)
> obesity (E66.-)

R63.6 Underweight
> Use additional code to identify body mass index (BMI), if known (Z68.-)
> EXCLUDES 1 abnormal weight loss (R63.4)
> anorexia nervosa (F50.0-)
> malnutrition (E40-E46)

R63.8 Other symptoms and signs concerning food and fluid intake

R64 Cachexia
> Wasting syndrome
> Code first underlying condition, if known
> EXCLUDES 1 abnormal weight loss (R63.4)
> nutritional marasmus (E41)

✓4th **R65 Symptoms and signs specifically associated with systemic inflammation and infection**

✓5th **R65.1 Systemic inflammatory response syndrome [SIRS] of non-infectious origin**
> Code first underlying condition, such as:
> heatstroke (T67.0)
> injury and trauma (S00-T88)
> EXCLUDES 1 sepsis—code to infection
> severe sepsis (R65.2)

R65.10 Systemic inflammatory response syndrome [SIRS] of non-infectious origin without acute organ dysfunction
> Systemic inflammatory response syndrome (SIRS) NOS

R65.11 Systemic inflammatory response syndrome [SIRS] of non-infectious origin with acute organ dysfunction
> Use additional code to identify specific acute organ dysfunction, such as:
> acute kidney failure (N17.-)
> acute respiratory failure (J96.0-)
> critical illness myopathy (G72.81)
> critical illness polyneuropathy (G62.81)
> disseminated intravascular coagulopathy [DIC] (D65)
> encephalopathy (metabolic) (septic) (G93.41)
> hepatic failure (K72.0-)

✓5th **R65.2 Severe sepsis**
> Infection with associated acute organ dysfunction
> Sepsis with acute organ dysfunction
> Sepsis with multiple organ dysfunction
> Systemic inflammatory response syndrome due to infectious process with acute organ dysfunction
> Code first underlying infection, such as:
> infection following a procedure (T81.4)
> infections following infusion, transfusion and therapeutic injection (T80.2-)
> puerperal sepsis (O85)
> sepsis following complete or unspecified spontaneous abortion (O03.87)
> sepsis following ectopic and molar pregnancy (O08.82)
> sepsis following incomplete spontaneous abortion (O03.37)
> sepsis following (induced) termination of pregnancy (O04.87)
> sepsis NOS (A41.9)
> Use additional code to identify specific acute organ dysfunction, such as:
> acute kidney failure (N17.-)
> acute respiratory failure (J96.0-)
> critical illness myopathy (G72.81)
> critical illness polyneuropathy (G62.81)
> disseminated intravascular coagulopathy [DIC] (D65)
> encephalopathy (metabolic) (septic) (G93.41)
> hepatic failure (K72.0-)

R65.20 Severe sepsis without septic shock
> Severe sepsis NOS
> AHA: 2013, 4Q, 119

R65.21 Severe sepsis with septic shock

Symptoms, Signs and Abnormal Clinical and Laboratory Findings

R68–R77.9

✓4ᵗʰ **R68   Other general symptoms and signs**

     R68.Ø   Hypothermia, not associated with low environmental temperature

         EXCLUDES 1   *hypothermia due to anesthesia (T88.51)*
                 hypothermia due to low environmental temperature (T68)
                 hypothermia NOS (accidental) (T68)
                 newborn hypothermia (P8Ø.-)

     ✓5ᵗʰ **R68.1   Nonspecific symptoms peculiar to infancy**

         EXCLUDES 1   *colic, infantile (R1Ø.83)*
                 neonatal cerebral irritability (P91.3)
                 teething syndrome (KØØ.7)

         R68.11   Excessive crying of infant (baby)   P

                 EXCLUDES 1   *excessive crying of child, adolescent, or adult (R45.83)*

         R68.12   Fussy infant (baby)   P
                 Irritable infant

         R68.13   Apparent life threatening event in infant [ALTE]   P
                 Apparent life threatening event in newborn
                 Code first confirmed diagnosis, if known
                 Use additional code(s) for associated signs and symptoms if no confirmed diagnosis established, or if signs and symptoms are not associated routinely with confirmed diagnosis, or provide additional information for cause of ALTE

         R68.19   Other nonspecific symptoms peculiar to infancy   P

     R68.2   Dry mouth, unspecified

         EXCLUDES 1   *dry mouth due to dehydration (E86.Ø)*
                 dry mouth due to sicca syndrome [Sjögren] (M35.Ø-)
                 salivary gland hyposecretion (K11.7)

     R68.3   Clubbing of fingers
         Clubbing of nails

         EXCLUDES 1   *congenital clubfinger (Q68.1)*

     ✓5ᵗʰ **R68.8   Other general symptoms and signs**

         R68.81   Early satiety

         R68.82   Decreased libido   A
                 Decreased sexual desire

         R68.83   Chills (without fever)
                 Chills NOS

                 EXCLUDES 1   *chills with fever (R5Ø.9)*

         R68.84   Jaw pain
                 Mandibular pain
                 Maxilla pain

                 EXCLUDES 1   *temporomandibular joint arthralgia (M26.62)*

         R68.89   Other general symptoms and signs

  R69   Illness, unspecified
     Unknown and unspecified cases of morbidity

Abnormal findings on examination of blood, without diagnosis (R7Ø-R79)

     EXCLUDES 1   *abnormalities (of)(on):*
            abnormal findings on antenatal screening of mother (O28.-)
            coagulation hemorrhagic disorders (D65-D68)
            lipids (E78.-)
            platelets and thrombocytes (D69.-)
            white blood cells classified elsewhere (D7Ø-D72)
            diagnostic abnormal findings classified elsewhere—see Alphabetical Index
            hemorrhagic and hematological disorders of newborn (P5Ø-P61)

✓4ᵗʰ **R7Ø   Elevated erythrocyte sedimentation rate and abnormality of plasma viscosity**

     R7Ø.Ø   Elevated erythrocyte sedimentation rate

     R7Ø.1   Abnormal plasma viscosity

✓4ᵗʰ **R71   Abnormality of red blood cells**

     EXCLUDES 1   *anemias (D5Ø-D64)*
            anemia of premature infant (P61.2)
            benign (familial) polycythemia (D75.Ø)
            congenital anemias (P61.2-P61.4)
            newborn anemia due to isoimmunization (P55.-)
            polycythemia neonatorum (P61.1)
            polycythemia NOS (D75.1)
            polycythemia vera (D45)
            secondary polycythemia (D75.1)

     R71.Ø   Precipitous drop in hematocrit
         Drop (precipitous) in hemoglobin
         Drop in hematocrit

     R71.8   Other abnormality of red blood cells
         Abnormal red-cell morphology NOS
         Abnormal red-cell volume NOS
         Anisocytosis
         Poikilocytosis

✓4ᵗʰ **R73   Elevated blood glucose level**

     EXCLUDES 1   *diabetes mellitus (EØ8-E13)*
            diabetes mellitus in pregnancy, childbirth and the puerperium (O24.-)
            neonatal disorders (P7Ø.Ø-P7Ø.2)
            postsurgical hypoinsulinemia (E89.1)

     ✓5ᵗʰ **R73.Ø   Abnormal glucose**

         EXCLUDES 1   *abnormal glucose in pregnancy (O99.81-)*
                 diabetes mellitus (EØ8-E13)
                 dysmetabolic syndrome X (E88.81)
                 gestational diabetes (O24.4-)
                 glycosuria (R81)
                 hypoglycemia (E16.2)

         R73.Ø1   Impaired fasting glucose
                 Elevated fasting glucose

         R73.Ø2   Impaired glucose tolerance (oral)
                 Elevated glucose tolerance

         R73.Ø9   Other abnormal glucose
                 Abnormal glucose NOS
                 Abnormal non-fasting glucose tolerance
                 Latent diabetes
                 Prediabetes

     R73.9   Hyperglycemia, unspecified

✓4ᵗʰ **R74   Abnormal serum enzyme levels**

     R74.Ø   Nonspecific elevation of levels of transaminase and lactic acid dehydrogenase [LDH]

     R74.8   Abnormal levels of other serum enzymes
         Abnormal level of acid phosphatase
         Abnormal level of alkaline phosphatase
         Abnormal level of amylase
         Abnormal level of lipase [triacylglycerol lipase]

     R74.9   Abnormal serum enzyme level, unspecified

  R75   Inconclusive laboratory evidence of human immunodeficiency virus [HIV]
     Nonconclusive HIV-test finding in infants

     EXCLUDES 1   *asymptomatic human immunodeficiency virus [HIV] infection status (Z21)*
            human immunodeficiency virus [HIV] disease (B2Ø)

✓4ᵗʰ **R76   Other abnormal immunological findings in serum**

     R76.Ø   Raised antibody titer

         EXCLUDES 1   *isoimmunization in pregnancy (O36.Ø-O36.1)*
                 isoimmunization affecting newborn (P55.-)

     ✓5ᵗʰ **R76.1   Nonspecific reaction to test for tuberculosis**

         R76.11   Nonspecific reaction to tuberculin skin test without active tuberculosis
                 Abnormal result of Mantoux test
                 PPD positive
                 Tuberculin (skin test) positive
                 Tuberculin (skin test) reactor

                 EXCLUDES 1   *nonspecific reaction to cell mediated immunity measurement of gamma interferon antigen response without active tuberculosis (R76.12)*

         R76.12   Nonspecific reaction to cell mediated immunity measurement of gamma interferon antigen response without active tuberculosis
                 Nonspecific reaction to QuantiFERON-TB test (QFT) without active tuberculosis

                 EXCLUDES 1   *nonspecific reaction to tuberculin skin test without active tuberculosis (R76.11)*
                       positive tuberculin skin test (R76.11)

     R76.8   Other specified abnormal immunological findings in serum
         Raised level of immunoglobulins NOS

     R76.9   Abnormal immunological finding in serum, unspecified

✓4ᵗʰ **R77   Other abnormalities of plasma proteins**

     EXCLUDES 1   *disorders of plasma-protein metabolism (E88.Ø)*

     R77.Ø   Abnormality of albumin

     R77.1   Abnormality of globulin
         Hyperglobulinemia NOS

     R77.2   Abnormality of alphafetoprotein

     R77.8   Other specified abnormalities of plasma proteins

     R77.9   Abnormality of plasma protein, unspecified

EXCLUDES 1 Not coded here   *EXCLUDES 2* Not included here   N Newborn Age: Ø   P Pediatric Age: Ø-17   M Maternity Age: 12-55   A Adult Age: 15-124

798   ICD-10-CM Draft (2015)

☑4ᵗʰ **R78 Findings of drugs and other substances, not normally found in blood**

> Use additional code to identify any retained foreign body, if applicable (Z18.-)
>
> *EXCLUDES 1* *mental or behavioral disorders due to psychoactive substance use (F10-F19)*

R78.0 Finding of alcohol in blood

> Use additional external cause code (Y90.-), for detail regarding alcohol level

R78.1 Finding of opiate drug in blood

R78.2 Finding of cocaine in blood

R78.3 Finding of hallucinogen in blood

R78.4 Finding of other drugs of addictive potential in blood

R78.5 Finding of other psychotropic drug in blood

R78.6 Finding of steroid agent in blood

☑5ᵗʰ **R78.7 Finding of abnormal level of heavy metals in blood**

R78.71 Abnormal lead level in blood

> *EXCLUDES 1* *lead poisoning (T56.0-)*

R78.79 Finding of abnormal level of heavy metals in blood

☑5ᵗʰ **R78.8 Finding of other specified substances, not normally found in blood**

R78.81 Bacteremia

> *EXCLUDES 1* *sepsis—code to specified infection (A00-B99)*

R78.89 Finding of other specified substances, not normally found in blood

> Finding of abnormal level of lithium in blood

R78.9 Finding of unspecified substance, not normally found in blood

☑4ᵗʰ **R79 Other abnormal findings of blood chemistry**

> Use additional code to identify any retained foreign body, if applicable (Z18.-)
>
> *EXCLUDES 1* *abnormality of fluid, electrolyte or acid-base balance (E86-E87)*
> *asymptomatic hyperuricemia (E79.0)*
> *hyperglycemia NOS (R73.9)*
> *hypoglycemia NOS (E16.2)*
> *neonatal hypoglycemia (P70.3-P70.4)*
> *specific findings indicating disorder of amino-acid metabolism (E70-E72)*
> *specific findings indicating disorder of carbohydrate metabolism (E73-E74)*
> *specific findings indicating disorder of lipid metabolism (E75.-)*

R79.0 Abnormal level of blood mineral

> Abnormal blood level of cobalt
> Abnormal blood level of copper
> Abnormal blood level of iron
> Abnormal blood level of magnesium
> Abnormal blood level of mineral NEC
> Abnormal blood level of zinc
>
> *EXCLUDES 1* *abnormal level of lithium (R78.89)*
> *disorders of mineral metabolism (E83.-)*
> *neonatal hypomagnesemia (P71.2)*
> *nutritional mineral deficiency (E58-E61)*

R79.1 Abnormal coagulation profile

> Abnormal or prolonged bleeding time
> Abnormal or prolonged coagulation time
> Abnormal or prolonged partial thromboplastin time [PTT]
> Abnormal or prolonged prothrombin time [PT]
>
> *EXCLUDES 1* *coagulation defects (D68.-)*

☑5ᵗʰ **R79.8 Other specified abnormal findings of blood chemistry**

R79.81 Abnormal blood-gas level

R79.82 Elevated C-reactive protein [CRP]

R79.89 Other specified abnormal findings of blood chemistry

R79.9 Abnormal finding of blood chemistry, unspecified

Abnormal findings on examination of urine, without diagnosis (R80-R82)

> *EXCLUDES 1* *abnormal findings on antenatal screening of mother (O28.-)*
> *diagnostic abnormal findings classified elsewhere—see Alphabetical Index*
> *specific findings indicating disorder of amino-acid metabolism (E70-E72)*
> *specific findings indicating disorder of carbohydrate metabolism (E73-E74)*

☑4ᵗʰ **R80 Proteinuria**

> *EXCLUDES 1* *gestational proteinuria (O12.1-)*

R80.0 Isolated proteinuria

> Idiopathic proteinuria
>
> *EXCLUDES 1* *isolated proteinuria with specific morphological lesion (N06.-)*

R80.1 Persistent proteinuria, unspecified

R80.2 Orthostatic proteinuria, unspecified

> Postural proteinuria

R80.3 Bence Jones proteinuria

R80.8 Other proteinuria

R80.9 Proteinuria, unspecified

> Albuminuria NOS

R81 Glycosuria

> *EXCLUDES 1* *renal glycosuria (E74.8)*

☑4ᵗʰ **R82 Other and unspecified abnormal findings in urine**

> Chromoabnormalities in urine
> Use additional code to identify any retained foreign body, if applicable (Z18.-)
>
> *EXCLUDES 2* *hematuria (R31.-)*

R82.0 Chyluria

> *EXCLUDES 1* *filarial chyluria (B74.-)*

R82.1 Myoglobinuria

R82.2 Biliuria

R82.3 Hemoglobinuria

> *EXCLUDES 1* *hemoglobinuria due to hemolysis from external causes NEC (D59.6)*
> *hemoglobinuria due to paroxysmal nocturnal [Marchiafava-Micheli] (D59.5)*

R82.4 Acetonuria

> Ketonuria

R82.5 Elevated urine levels of drugs, medicaments and biological substances

> Elevated urine levels of catecholamines
> Elevated urine levels of indoleacetic acid
> Elevated urine levels of 17-ketosteroids
> Elevated urine levels of steroids

R82.6 Abnormal urine levels of substances chiefly nonmedicinal as to source

> Abnormal urine level of heavy metals

R82.7 Abnormal findings on microbiological examination of urine

> Positive culture findings of urine
>
> *EXCLUDES 1* *colonization status (Z22.-)*

R82.8 Abnormal findings on cytological and histological examination of urine

☑5ᵗʰ **R82.9 Other and unspecified abnormal findings in urine**

R82.90 Unspecified abnormal findings in urine

R82.91 Other chromoabnormalities of urine

> Chromoconversion (dipstick)
> Idiopathic dipstick converts positive for blood with no cellular forms in sediment
>
> *EXCLUDES 1* *hemoglobinuria (R82.3)*
> *myoglobinuria (R82.1)*

R82.99 Other abnormal findings in urine

> Cells and casts in urine
> Crystalluria
> Melanuria

☑ Additional Character Required   ✓x7ᵗʰ Xtension Alert   Unspecified Dx   Other Specified Dx   Manifestation   ►◄ Revised Text   ● New Code   ▲ Revised Code Title

ICD-10-CM Draft (2015)

799

Symptoms, Signs and Abnormal Clinical and Laboratory Findings   R78–R82.99

Abnormal findings on examination of other body fluids, substances and tissues, without diagnosis (R83-R89)

EXCLUDES 1   *abnormal findings on antenatal screening of mother (O28.-)*
diagnostic abnormal findings classified elsewhere—see Alphabetical Index

EXCLUDES 2   *abnormal findings on examination of blood, without diagnosis (R70-R79)*
abnormal findings on examination of urine, without diagnosis (R80-R82)
abnormal tumor markers (R97.-)

✓4th **R83   Abnormal findings in cerebrospinal fluid**

     R83.0   **Abnormal level of enzymes in cerebrospinal fluid**

     R83.1   **Abnormal level of hormones in cerebrospinal fluid**

     R83.2   **Abnormal level of other drugs, medicaments and biological substances in cerebrospinal fluid**

     R83.3   **Abnormal level of substances chiefly nonmedicinal as to source in cerebrospinal fluid**

     R83.4   **Abnormal immunological findings in cerebrospinal fluid**

     R83.5   **Abnormal microbiological findings in cerebrospinal fluid**
         Positive culture findings in cerebrospinal fluid
         EXCLUDES 1   *colonization status (Z22.-)*

     R83.6   **Abnormal cytological findings in cerebrospinal fluid**

     R83.8   **Other abnormal findings in cerebrospinal fluid**
         Abnormal chromosomal findings in cerebrospinal fluid

     R83.9   **Unspecified abnormal finding in cerebrospinal fluid**

✓4th **R84   Abnormal findings in specimens from respiratory organs and thorax**
         Abnormal findings in bronchial washings
         Abnormal findings in nasal secretions
         Abnormal findings in pleural fluid
         Abnormal findings in sputum
         Abnormal findings in throat scrapings
         EXCLUDES 1   *blood-stained sputum (R04.2)*

     R84.0   **Abnormal level of enzymes in specimens from respiratory organs and thorax**

     R84.1   **Abnormal level of hormones in specimens from respiratory organs and thorax**

     R84.2   **Abnormal level of other drugs, medicaments and biological substances in specimens from respiratory organs and thorax**

     R84.3   **Abnormal level of substances chiefly nonmedicinal as to source in specimens from respiratory organs and thorax**

     R84.4   **Abnormal immunological findings in specimens from respiratory organs and thorax**

     R84.5   **Abnormal microbiological findings in specimens from respiratory organs and thorax**
         Positive culture findings in specimens from respiratory organs and thorax
         EXCLUDES 1   *colonization status (Z22.-)*

     R84.6   **Abnormal cytological findings in specimens from respiratory organs and thorax**

     R84.7   **Abnormal histological findings in specimens from respiratory organs and thorax**

     R84.8   **Other abnormal findings in specimens from respiratory organs and thorax**
         Abnormal chromosomal findings in specimens from respiratory organs and thorax

     R84.9   **Unspecified abnormal finding in specimens from respiratory organs and thorax**

✓4th **R85   Abnormal findings in specimens from digestive organs and abdominal cavity**
         INCLUDES   abnormal findings in peritoneal fluid
                 abnormal findings in saliva
         EXCLUDES 1   *cloudy peritoneal dialysis effluent (R88.0)*
                 fecal abnormalities (R19.5)

     R85.0   **Abnormal level of enzymes in specimens from digestive organs and abdominal cavity**

     R85.1   **Abnormal level of hormones in specimens from digestive organs and abdominal cavity**

     R85.2   **Abnormal level of other drugs, medicaments and biological substances in specimens from digestive organs and abdominal cavity**

     R85.3   **Abnormal level of substances chiefly nonmedicinal as to source in specimens from digestive organs and abdominal cavity**

     R85.4   **Abnormal immunological findings in specimens from digestive organs and abdominal cavity**

     R85.5   **Abnormal microbiological findings in specimens from digestive organs and abdominal cavity**
         Positive culture findings in specimens from digestive organs and abdominal cavity
         EXCLUDES 1   *colonization status (Z22.-)*

✓5th   R85.6   **Abnormal cytological findings in specimens from digestive organs and abdominal cavity**

     ✓6th   R85.61   **Abnormal cytologic smear of anus**
         EXCLUDES 1   *abnormal cytological findings in specimens from other digestive organs and abdominal cavity (R85.69)*
                 anal intraepithelial neoplasia I [AIN I] (K62.82)
                 anal intraepithelial neoplasia II [AIN II] (K62.82)
                 anal intraepithelial neoplasia III [AIN III] (D01.3)
                 carcinoma in situ of anus (histologically confirmed) (D01.3)
                 dysplasia (mild) (moderate) of anus (histologically confirmed) (K62.82)
                 severe dysplasia of anus (histologically confirmed) (D01.3)
         EXCLUDES 2   *anal high risk human papillomavirus (HPV) DNA test positive (R85.81)*
                 anal low risk human papillomavirus (HPV) DNA test positive (R85.82)

         R85.610   **Atypical squamous cells of undetermined significance on cytologic smear of anus [ASC-US]**

         R85.611   **Atypical squamous cells cannot exclude high grade squamous intraepithelial lesion on cytologic smear of anus [ASC-H]**

         R85.612   **Low grade squamous intraepithelial lesion on cytologic smear of anus [LGSIL]**

         R85.613   **High grade squamous intraepithelial lesion on cytologic smear of anus [HGSIL]**

         R85.614   **Cytologic evidence of malignancy on smear of anus**

         R85.615   **Unsatisfactory cytologic smear of anus**
         Inadequate sample of cytologic smear of anus

         R85.616   **Satisfactory anal smear but lacking transformation zone**

         R85.618   **Other abnormal cytological findings on specimens from anus**

         R85.619   **Unspecified abnormal cytological findings in specimens from anus**
         Abnormal anal cytology NOS
         Atypical glandular cells of anus NOS

     R85.69   **Abnormal cytological findings in specimens from other digestive organs and abdominal cavity**

     R85.7   **Abnormal histological findings in specimens from digestive organs and abdominal cavity**

✓5th   R85.8   **Other abnormal findings in specimens from digestive organs and abdominal cavity**

     R85.81   **Anal high risk human papillomavirus [HPV] DNA test positive**
         EXCLUDES 1   *anogenital warts due to human papillomavirus (HPV) (A63.0)*
                 condyloma acuminatum (A63.0)

     R85.82   **Anal low risk human papillomavirus [HPV] DNA test positive**
         Use additional code for associated human papillomavirus (B97.7)

     R85.89   **Other abnormal findings in specimens from digestive organs and abdominal cavity**
         Abnormal chromosomal findings in specimens from digestive organs and abdominal cavity

     R85.9   **Unspecified abnormal finding in specimens from digestive organs and abdominal cavity**

✓4th **R86   Abnormal findings in specimens from male genital organs**
         INCLUDES   abnormal findings in prostatic secretions
                 abnormal findings in semen, seminal fluid
                 abnormal spermatozoa
         EXCLUDES 1   *azoospermia (N46.0-)*
                 oligospermia (N46.1-)

     R86.0   **Abnormal level of enzymes in specimens from male genital organs**   ♂

     R86.1   **Abnormal level of hormones in specimens from male genital organs**   ♂

EXCLUDES 1 Not coded here   EXCLUDES 2 Not included here   N Newborn Age: 0   P Pediatric Age: 0-17   M Maternity Age: 12-55   A Adult Age: 15-124

800   ICD-10-CM Draft (2015)

R86.2 **Abnormal level of other drugs, medicants and biological substances in specimens from male genital organs** ♂

R86.3 **Abnormal level of** substances chiefly nonmedicinal **as to source in specimens from male genital organs** ♂

R86.4 **Abnormal** immunological **findings in specimens from male genital organs** ♂

R86.5 **Abnormal** microbiological **findings in specimens from male genital organs** ♂
　　Positive culture findings in specimens from male genital organs
　　EXCLUDES 1 colonization status (Z22.-)

R86.6 **Abnormal** cytological **findings in specimens from male genital organs** ♂

R86.7 **Abnormal** histological **findings in specimens from male genital organs** ♂

R86.8 **Other abnormal findings in specimens from male genital organs** ♂
　　Abnormal chromosomal findings in specimens from male genital organs

R86.9 **Unspecified abnormal finding in specimens from male genital organs** ♂

✓4ᵗʰ **R87 Abnormal findings in specimens from** female genital organs
　　Abnormal findings in secretion and smears from cervix uteri
　　Abnormal findings in secretion and smears from vagina
　　Abnormal findings in secretion and smears from vulva

R87.0 **Abnormal level of** enzymes **in specimens from female genital organs** ♀

R87.1 **Abnormal level of** hormones **in specimens from female genital organs** ♀

R87.2 **Abnormal level of other drugs, medicants and biological substances in specimens from female genital organs** ♀

R87.3 **Abnormal level of** substances chiefly nonmedicinal **as to source in specimens from female genital organs** ♀

R87.4 **Abnormal** immunological **findings in specimens from female genital organs** ♀

R87.5 **Abnormal** microbiological **findings in specimens from female genital organs** ♀
　　Positive culture findings in specimens from female genital organs
　　EXCLUDES 1 colonization status (Z22.-)

✓5ᵗʰ R87.6 **Abnormal** cytological **findings in specimens from female genital organs**

✓6ᵗʰ R87.61 **Abnormal cytological findings in specimens from** cervix uteri
　　EXCLUDES 1 abnormal cytological findings in specimens from other female genital organs (R87.69)
　　abnormal cytological findings in specimens from vagina (R87.62-)
　　carcinoma in situ of cervix uteri (histologically confirmed) (D06.-)
　　cervical intraepithelial neoplasia I [CIN I] (N87.0)
　　cervical intraepithelial neoplasia II [CIN II] (N87.1)
　　cervical intraepithelial neoplasia III [CIN III] (D06.-)
　　dysplasia (mild) (moderate) of cervix uteri (histologically confirmed) (N87.-)
　　severe dysplasia of cervix uteri (histologically confirmed) (D06.-)
　　EXCLUDES 2 cervical high risk human papillomavirus (HPV) DNA test positive (R87.810)
　　cervical low risk human papillomavirus (HPV) DNA test positive (R87.820)

R87.610 Atypical **squamous cells of** undetermined significance **on cytologic smear of cervix [ASC-US]** ♀

R87.611 Atypical **squamous cells cannot exclude** high grade **squamous intraepithelial lesion on cytologic smear of cervix [ASC-H]** ♀

R87.612 Low grade **squamous intraepithelial lesion on cytologic smear of cervix [LGSIL]** ♀

R87.613 High grade **squamous intraepithelial lesion on cytologic smear of cervix [HGSIL]** ♀

R87.614 **Cytologic evidence of** malignancy **on smear of cervix** ♀

R87.615 Unsatisfactory **cytologic smear of cervix** ♀
　　Inadequate sample of cytologic smear of cervix

R87.616 Satisfactory **cervical smear but** lacking transformation zone ♀

R87.618 **Other abnormal cytological findings on specimens from cervix uteri** ♀

R87.619 **Unspecified abnormal cytological findings in specimens from cervix uteri** ♀
　　Abnormal cervical cytology NOS
　　Abnormal Papanicolaou smear of cervix NOS
　　Abnormal thin preparation smear of cervix NOS
　　Atypical endocervical cells of cervix NOS
　　Atypical endometrial cells of cervix NOS
　　Atypical glandular cells of cervix NOS

✓6ᵗʰ R87.62 **Abnormal cytological findings in specimens from** vagina
　　Use additional code to identify acquired absence of uterus and cervix, if applicable (Z90.71-)
　　EXCLUDES 1 abnormal cytological findings in specimens from cervix uteri (R87.61-)
　　abnormal cytological findings in specimens from other female genital organs (R87.69)
　　carcinoma in situ of vagina (histologically confirmed) (D07.2)
　　dysplasia (mild) (moderate) of vagina (histologically confirmed) (N89.-)
　　severe dysplasia of vagina (histologically confirmed) (D07.2)
　　vaginal intraepithelial neoplasia I [VAIN I] (N89.0)
　　vaginal intraepithelial neoplasia II [VAIN II] (N89.1)
　　vaginal intraepithelial neoplasia III [VAIN III] (D07.2)
　　EXCLUDES 2 vaginal high risk human papillomavirus (HPV) DNA test positive (R87.811)
　　vaginal low risk human papillomavirus (HPV) DNA test positive (R87.821)

R87.620 Atypical **squamous cells of** undetermined significance **on cytologic smear of vagina [ASC-US]** ♀

R87.621 Atypical **squamous cells cannot exclude** high grade **squamous intraepithelial lesion on cytologic smear of vagina [ASC-H]** ♀

R87.622 Low grade **squamous intraepithelial lesion on cytologic smear of vagina [LGSIL]** ♀

R87.623 High grade **squamous intraepithelial lesion on cytologic smear of vagina [HGSIL]** ♀

R87.624 **Cytologic evidence of** malignancy **on smear of vagina** ♀

R87.625 Unsatisfactory **cytologic smear of vagina** ♀
　　Inadequate sample of cytologic smear of vagina

R87.628 **Other abnormal cytological findings on specimens from vagina** ♀

R87.629 **Unspecified abnormal cytological findings in specimens from vagina** ♀
　　Abnormal Papanicolaou smear of vagina NOS
　　Abnormal thin preparation smear of vagina NOS
　　Abnormal vaginal cytology NOS
　　Atypical endocervical cells of vagina NOS
　　Atypical endometrial cells of vagina NOS
　　Atypical glandular cells of vagina NOS

R87.69 **Abnormal cytological findings in specimens from other female genital organs** ♀
　　Abnormal cytological findings in specimens from female genital organs NOS
　　EXCLUDES 1 dysplasia of vulva (histologically confirmed) (N90.0-N90.3)

Symptoms, Signs and Abnormal Clinical and Laboratory Findings

R87.7–R93.5

R87.7 **Abnormal histological findings in specimens from female genital organs** ♀

> EXCLUDES 1   *carcinoma in situ (histologically confirmed) of female genital organs (D06-D07.3)*
> *cervical intraepithelial neoplasia I [CIN I] (N87.0)*
> *cervical intraepithelial neoplasia II [CIN II] (N87.1)*
> *cervical intraepithelial neoplasia III [CIN III] (D06.-)*
> *dysplasia (mild) (moderate) of cervix uteri (histologically confirmed) (N87.-)*
> *dysplasia (mild) (moderate) of vagina (histologically confirmed) (N89.-)*
> *severe dysplasia of cervix uteri (histologically confirmed) (D06.-)*
> *severe dysplasia of vagina (histologically confirmed) (D07.2)*
> *vaginal intraepithelial neoplasia I [VAIN I] (N89.0)*
> *vaginal intraepithelial neoplasia II [VAIN II] (N89.1)*
> *vaginal intraepithelial neoplasia III [VAIN III] (D07.2)*

✓5th R87.8 **Other abnormal findings in specimens from female genital organs**

    ✓6th R87.81 **High risk human papillomavirus [HPV] DNA test positive from female genital organs**

> EXCLUDES 1   *anogenital warts due to human papillomavirus (HPV) (A63.0)*
> *condyloma acuminatum (A63.0)*

       R87.810 **Cervical high risk human papillomavirus [HPV] DNA test positive** ♀

       R87.811 **Vaginal high risk human papillomavirus [HPV] DNA test positive** ♀

    ✓6th R87.82 **Low risk human papillomavirus [HPV] DNA test positive from female genital organs**

       Use additional code for associated human papillomavirus (B97.7)

       R87.820 **Cervical low risk human papillomavirus [HPV] DNA test positive** ♀

       R87.821 **Vaginal low risk human papillomavirus [HPV] DNA test positive** ♀

    R87.89 **Other abnormal findings in specimens from female genital organs** ♀

       Abnormal chromosomal findings in specimens from female genital organs

    R87.9 **Unspecified abnormal finding in specimens from female genital organs** ♀

✓4th R88 **Abnormal findings in other body fluids and substances**

    R88.0 **Cloudy (hemodialysis) (peritoneal) dialysis effluent**

    R88.8 **Abnormal findings in other body fluids and substances**

✓4th R89 **Abnormal findings in specimens from other organs, systems and tissues**

> INCLUDES   abnormal findings in nipple discharge
> abnormal findings in synovial fluid
> abnormal findings in wound secretions

    R89.0 **Abnormal level of enzymes in specimens from other organs, systems and tissues**

    R89.1 **Abnormal level of hormones in specimens from other organs, systems and tissues**

    R89.2 **Abnormal level of other drugs, medicaments and biological substances in specimens from other organs, systems and tissues**

    R89.3 **Abnormal level of substances chiefly nonmedicinal as to source in specimens from other organs, systems and tissues**

    R89.4 **Abnormal immunological findings in specimens from other organs, systems and tissues**

    R89.5 **Abnormal microbiological findings in specimens from other organs, systems and tissues**

       Positive culture findings in specimens from other organs, systems and tissues

> EXCLUDES 1   *colonization status (Z22.-)*

    R89.6 **Abnormal cytological findings in specimens from other organs, systems and tissues**

    R89.7 **Abnormal histological findings in specimens from other organs, systems and tissues**

    R89.8 **Other abnormal findings in specimens from other organs, systems and tissues**

       Abnormal chromosomal findings in specimens from other organs, systems and tissues

    R89.9 **Unspecified abnormal finding in specimens from other organs, systems and tissues**

Abnormal findings on diagnostic imaging and in function studies, without diagnosis (R90-R94)

> INCLUDES   nonspecific abnormal findings on diagnostic imaging by computerized axial tomography [CAT scan]
> nonspecific abnormal findings on diagnostic imaging by magnetic resonance imaging [MRI][NMR]
> nonspecific abnormal findings on diagnostic imaging by positron emission tomography [PET scan]
> nonspecific abnormal findings on diagnostic imaging by thermography
> nonspecific abnormal findings on diagnostic imaging by ultrasound [echogram]
> nonspecific abnormal findings on diagnostic imaging by X-ray examination

> EXCLUDES 1   *abnormal findings on antenatal screening of mother (O28.-)*
> *diagnostic abnormal findings classified elsewhere—see Alphabetical Index*

✓4th R90 **Abnormal findings on diagnostic imaging of central nervous system**

    R90.0 **Intracranial space-occupying lesion found on diagnostic imaging of central nervous system**

    ✓5th R90.8 **Other abnormal findings on diagnostic imaging of central nervous system**

       R90.81 **Abnormal echoencephalogram**

       R90.82 **White matter disease, unspecified**

       R90.89 **Other abnormal findings on diagnostic imaging of central nervous system**

          Other cerebrovascular abnormality found on diagnostic imaging of central nervous system

✓4th R91 **Abnormal findings on diagnostic imaging of lung**

    R91.1 **Solitary pulmonary nodule**

       Coin lesion lung
       Solitary pulmonary nodule, subsegmental branch of the bronchial tree

    R91.8 **Other nonspecific abnormal finding of lung field**

       Lung mass NOS found on diagnostic imaging of lung
       Pulmonary infiltrate NOS
       Shadow, lung

✓4th R92 **Abnormal and inconclusive findings on diagnostic imaging of breast**

    R92.0 **Mammographic microcalcification found on diagnostic imaging of breast**

> EXCLUDES 2   *mammographic calcification (calculus) found on diagnostic imaging of breast (R92.1)*

    R92.1 **Mammographic calcification found on diagnostic imaging of breast**

       Mammographic calculus found on diagnostic imaging of breast

    R92.2 **Inconclusive mammogram**

       Dense breasts NOS
       Inconclusive mammogram NEC
       Inconclusive mammography due to dense breasts
       Inconclusive mammography NEC

    R92.8 **Other abnormal and inconclusive findings on diagnostic imaging of breast**

✓4th R93 **Abnormal findings on diagnostic imaging of other body structures**

    R93.0 **Abnormal findings on diagnostic imaging of skull and head, not elsewhere classified**

> EXCLUDES 1   *intracranial space-occupying lesion found on diagnostic imaging (R90.0)*

    R93.1 **Abnormal findings on diagnostic imaging of heart and coronary circulation**

       Abnormal echocardiogram NOS
       Abnormal heart shadow

    R93.2 **Abnormal findings on diagnostic imaging of liver and biliary tract**

       Nonvisualization of gallbladder

    R93.3 **Abnormal findings on diagnostic imaging of other parts of digestive tract**

    R93.4 **Abnormal findings on diagnostic imaging of urinary organs**

       Filling defect of bladder found on diagnostic imaging
       Filling defect of kidney found on diagnostic imaging
       Filling defect of ureter found on diagnostic imaging

> EXCLUDES 1   *hypertrophy of kidney (N28.81)*

    R93.5 **Abnormal findings on diagnostic imaging of other abdominal regions, including retroperitoneum**

EXCLUDES 1 Not coded here   EXCLUDES 2 Not included here   N Newborn Age: 0   P Pediatric Age: 0-17   M Maternity Age: 12-55   A Adult Age: 15-124

802   ICD-10-CM Draft (2015)

R93.6   **Abnormal findings on diagnostic imaging of** limbs
> *EXCLUDES 2* *abnormal finding in skin and subcutaneous tissue (R93.8)*

R93.7   **Abnormal findings on diagnostic imaging of** other parts of musculoskeletal system
> *EXCLUDES 2* *abnormal findings on diagnostic imaging of skull (R93.0)*

R93.8   **Abnormal findings on diagnostic imaging of other specified body structures**
Abnormal finding by radioisotope localization of placenta
Abnormal radiological finding in skin and subcutaneous tissue
Mediastinal shift

R93.9   **Diagnostic imaging inconclusive due to** excess body fat of patient

✓4ᵗʰ **R94   Abnormal results of function studies**
> *INCLUDES* abnormal results of radionuclide [radioisotope] uptake studies
> abnormal results of scintigraphy

✓5ᵗʰ   R94.0   **Abnormal results of function studies of** central nervous system
   R94.01   **Abnormal** electroencephalogram [EEG]
   R94.02   **Abnormal** brain scan
   R94.09   **Abnormal results of other function studies of central nervous system**

✓5ᵗʰ   R94.1   **Abnormal results of function studies of** peripheral nervous system and special senses
   ✓6ᵗʰ   R94.11   **Abnormal results of function studies of** eye
      R94.110   **Abnormal** electro-oculogram [EOG]
      R94.111   **Abnormal** electroretinogram [ERG]
         Abnormal retinal function study
      R94.112   **Abnormal** visually evoked potential [VEP]
      R94.113   **Abnormal** oculomotor study
      R94.118   **Abnormal results of other function studies of eye**
   ✓6ᵗʰ   R94.12   **Abnormal results of function studies of** ear and other special senses
      R94.120   **Abnormal** auditory function study
      R94.121   **Abnormal** vestibular function study
      R94.128   **Abnormal results of other function studies of ear and other special senses**
   ✓6ᵗʰ   R94.13   **Abnormal results of function studies of** peripheral nervous system
      R94.130   **Abnormal response to nerve stimulation, unspecified**
      R94.131   Abnormal electromyogram [EMG]
         > *EXCLUDES 1* *electromyogram of eye (R94.113)*
      R94.138   **Abnormal results of other function studies of peripheral nervous system**

   R94.2   **Abnormal results of** pulmonary function **studies**
      Reduced ventilatory capacity
      Reduced vital capacity

✓5ᵗʰ   R94.3   **Abnormal results of** cardiovascular function **studies**
   R94.30   **Abnormal result of cardiovascular function study, unspecified**
   R94.31   **Abnormal** electrocardiogram [ECG] [EKG]
      > *EXCLUDES 1* *long QT syndrome (I45.81)*
   R94.39   **Abnormal result of other cardiovascular function study**
      Abnormal electrophysiological intracardiac studies
      Abnormal phonocardiogram
      Abnormal vectorcardiogram

   R94.4   **Abnormal results of** kidney function **studies**
      Abnormal renal function test

   R94.5   **Abnormal results of** liver function **studies**

   R94.6   **Abnormal results of** thyroid function **studies**

   R94.7   **Abnormal results of other endocrine function studies**
      > *EXCLUDES 2* *abnormal glucose (R73.0-)*

   R94.8   **Abnormal results of function studies of** other organs and systems
      Abnormal basal metabolic rate [BMR]
      Abnormal bladder function test
      Abnormal splenic function test

Abnormal tumor markers (R97)

✓4ᵗʰ **R97   Abnormal tumor markers**
   Elevated tumor associated antigens [TAA]
   Elevated tumor specific antigens [TSA]
   R97.0   **Elevated carcinoembryonic antigen [CEA]**
   R97.1   **Elevated cancer antigen 125 [CA 125]**   ♀
   R97.2   **Elevated prostate specific antigen [PSA]**   🄰♂
   R97.8   **Other abnormal tumor markers**

Ill-defined and unknown cause of mortality (R99)

R99   Ill-defined and unknown cause of mortality
   Death (unexplained) NOS
   Unspecified cause of mortality

| ✓ Additional Character Required | ✓x7ᵗʰ Xtension Alert | Unspecified Dx | Other Specified Dx | Manifestation | ►◄ Revised Text | ● New Code | ▲ Revised Code Title |

ICD-10-CM Draft (2015)   803

Chapter 19. Injury, Poisoning and Certain Other Consequences of External Causes (S00–T88)

NOTE   Use secondary code(s) from Chapter 20, External causes of morbidity, to indicate cause of injury. Codes within the T section that include the external cause do not require an additional external cause code.

Use additional code to identify any retained foreign body, if applicable (Z18.-)

EXCLUDES 1   birth trauma (P10-P15)
       obstetric trauma (O70-O71)

NOTE   The chapter uses the S-section for coding different types of injuries related to single body regions and the T-section to cover injuries to unspecified body regions as well as poisoning and certain other consequences of external causes.

This chapter contains the following blocks:

S00-S09	Injuries to the head
S10-S19	Injuries to the neck
S20-S29	Injuries to the thorax
S30-S39	Injuries to the abdomen, lower back, lumbar spine, pelvis and external genitals
S40-S49	Injuries to the shoulder and upper arm
S50-S59	Injuries to the elbow and forearm
S60-S69	Injuries to the wrist, hand and fingers
S70-S79	Injuries to the hip and thigh
S80-S89	Injuries to the knee and lower leg
S90-S99	Injuries to the ankle and foot
T07	Injuries involving multiple body regions
T14	Injury of unspecified body region
T15-T19	Effects of foreign body entering through natural orifice
T20-T25	Burns and corrosions of external body surface, specified by site
T26-T28	Burns and corrosions confined to eye and internal organs
T30-T32	Burns and corrosions of multiple and unspecified body regions
T33-T34	Frostbite
T36-T50	Poisoning by, adverse effect of and underdosing of drugs, medicaments and biological substances
T51-T65	Toxic effects of substances chiefly nonmedicinal as to source
T66-T78	Other and unspecified effects of external causes
T79	Certain early complications of trauma
T80-T88	Complications of surgical and medical care, not elsewhere classified

Injuries to the head (S00-S09)

INCLUDES   injuries of ear
       injuries of eye
       injuries of face [any part]
       injuries of gum
       injuries of jaw
       injuries of oral cavity
       injuries of palate
       injuries of periocular area
       injuries of scalp
       injuries of temporomandibular joint area
       injuries of tongue
       injuries of tooth

Code also for any associated infection

EXCLUDES 2   burns and corrosions (T20-T32)
       effects of foreign body in ear (T16)
       effects of foreign body in larynx (T17.3)
       effects of foreign body in mouth NOS (T18.0)
       effects of foreign body in nose (T17.0-T17.1)
       effects of foreign body in pharynx (T17.2)
       effects of foreign body on external eye (T15.-)
       frostbite (T33-T34)
       insect bite or sting, venomous (T63.4)

✓4ᵗʰ S00   Superficial injury of head

EXCLUDES 1   diffuse cerebral contusion (S06.2-)
       focal cerebral contusion (S06.3-)
       injury of eye and orbit (S05.-)
       open wound of head (S01.-)

The appropriate 7th character is to be added to each code from category S00.
A   initial encounter
D   subsequent encounter
S   sequela

✓5ᵗʰ S00.0   Superficial injury of scalp

   ✓x7ᵗʰ   S00.00   **Unspecified superficial injury of scalp**

   ✓x7ᵗʰ   S00.01   Abrasion **of scalp**

   ✓x7ᵗʰ   S00.02   Blister **(nonthermal) of scalp**

   ✓x7ᵗʰ   S00.03   Contusion **of scalp**
             Bruise of scalp
             Hematoma of scalp

   ✓x7ᵗʰ   S00.04   External constriction **of part of scalp**

   ✓x7ᵗʰ   S00.05   Superficial foreign body **of scalp**
             Splinter in the scalp

   ✓x7ᵗʰ   S00.06   Insect bite **(nonvenomous) of scalp**

   ✓x7ᵗʰ   S00.07   Other superficial bite **of scalp**
      EXCLUDES 1   open bite of scalp (S01.05)

✓5ᵗʰ S00.1   Contusion of eyelid and periocular area
     Black eye
     EXCLUDES 2   contusion of eyeball and orbital tissues (S05.1)

   ✓x7ᵗʰ   S00.10   Contusion of **unspecified eyelid and periocular area**

   ✓x7ᵗʰ   S00.11   Contusion of right **eyelid and periocular area**

   ✓x7ᵗʰ   S00.12   Contusion of left **eyelid and periocular area**

✓5ᵗʰ S00.2   Other and unspecified superficial injuries of eyelid and periocular area
     EXCLUDES 2   superficial injury of conjunctiva and cornea (S05.0-)

   ✓6ᵗʰ   S00.20   Unspecified **superficial injury of eyelid and periocular area**

       ✓7ᵗʰ   S00.201   **Unspecified superficial injury of** right **eyelid and periocular area**

       ✓7ᵗʰ   S00.202   **Unspecified superficial injury of** left **eyelid and periocular area**

       ✓7ᵗʰ   S00.209   **Unspecified superficial injury of unspecified eyelid and periocular area**

   ✓6ᵗʰ   S00.21   Abrasion **of eyelid and periocular area**

       ✓7ᵗʰ   S00.211   **Abrasion of** right **eyelid and periocular area**

       ✓7ᵗʰ   S00.212   **Abrasion of** left **eyelid and periocular area**

       ✓7ᵗʰ   S00.219   **Abrasion of unspecified eyelid and periocular area**

   ✓6ᵗʰ   S00.22   Blister **(nonthermal) of eyelid and periocular area**

       ✓7ᵗʰ   S00.221   **Blister (nonthermal) of** right **eyelid and periocular area**

       ✓7ᵗʰ   S00.222   **Blister (nonthermal) of** left **eyelid and periocular area**

       ✓7ᵗʰ   S00.229   **Blister (nonthermal) of unspecified eyelid and periocular area**

   ✓6ᵗʰ   S00.24   External constriction **of eyelid and periocular area**

       ✓7ᵗʰ   S00.241   **External constriction of** right **eyelid and periocular area**

       ✓7ᵗʰ   S00.242   **External constriction of** left **eyelid and periocular area**

       ✓7ᵗʰ   S00.249   **External constriction of unspecified eyelid and periocular area**

   ✓6ᵗʰ   S00.25   Superficial foreign body **of eyelid and periocular area**
         Splinter of eyelid and periocular area
        EXCLUDES 2   retained foreign body in eyelid (H02.81-)

       ✓7ᵗʰ   S00.251   **Superficial foreign body of** right **eyelid and periocular area**

       ✓7ᵗʰ   S00.252   **Superficial foreign body of** left **eyelid and periocular area**

       ✓7ᵗʰ   S00.259   **Superficial foreign body of unspecified eyelid and periocular area**

   ✓6ᵗʰ   S00.26   Insect bite **(nonvenomous) of eyelid and periocular area**

       ✓7ᵗʰ   S00.261   **Insect bite (nonvenomous) of** right **eyelid and periocular area**

       ✓7ᵗʰ   S00.262   **Insect bite (nonvenomous) of** left **eyelid and periocular area**

       ✓7ᵗʰ   S00.269   **Insect bite (nonvenomous) of unspecified eyelid and periocular area**

   ✓6ᵗʰ   S00.27   Other superficial bite **of eyelid and periocular area**
       EXCLUDES 1   open bite of eyelid and periocular area (S01.15)

       ✓7ᵗʰ   S00.271   **Other superficial bite of** right **eyelid and periocular area**

       ✓7ᵗʰ   S00.272   **Other superficial bite of** left **eyelid and periocular area**

       ✓7ᵗʰ   S00.279   **Other superficial bite of unspecified eyelid and periocular area**

✓5ᵗʰ S00.3   Superficial injury of nose

   ✓x7ᵗʰ   S00.30   **Unspecified superficial injury of nose**

   ✓x7ᵗʰ   S00.31   Abrasion **of nose**

   ✓x7ᵗʰ   S00.32   Blister **(nonthermal) of nose**

EXCLUDES 1 Not coded here   **EXCLUDES 2** Not included here   **N** Newborn Age: 0   **P** Pediatric Age: 0-17   **M** Maternity Age: 12-55   **A** Adult Age: 15-124

804   ICD-10-CM Draft (2015)

☑x7ᵗʰ S00.33 Contusion of nose
Bruise of nose
Hematoma of nose

☑x7ᵗʰ S00.34 External constriction of nose

☑x7ᵗʰ S00.35 Superficial foreign body **of nose**
Splinter in the nose

☑x7ᵗʰ S00.36 Insect bite (nonvenomous) of nose

☑x7ᵗʰ S00.37 Other superficial bite of nose
EXCLUDES 1 *open bite of nose (S01.25)*

☑5ᵗʰ S00.4 Superficial injury of ear

☑6ᵗʰ S00.40 Unspecified superficial injury of ear

☑7ᵗʰ S00.401 Unspecified superficial injury of right ear

☑7ᵗʰ S00.402 Unspecified superficial injury of left ear

☑7ᵗʰ S00.409 Unspecified superficial injury of unspecified ear

☑6ᵗʰ S00.41 Abrasion of ear

☑7ᵗʰ S00.411 Abrasion of right ear

☑7ᵗʰ S00.412 Abrasion of left ear

☑7ᵗʰ S00.419 Abrasion of unspecified ear

☑6ᵗʰ S00.42 Blister (nonthermal) of ear

☑7ᵗʰ S00.421 Blister (nonthermal) of right ear

☑7ᵗʰ S00.422 Blister (nonthermal) of left ear

☑7ᵗʰ S00.429 Blister (nonthermal) of unspecified ear

☑6ᵗʰ S00.43 Contusion of ear
Bruise of ear
Hematoma of ear

☑7ᵗʰ S00.431 Contusion of right ear

☑7ᵗʰ S00.432 Contusion of left ear

☑7ᵗʰ S00.439 Contusion of unspecified ear

☑6ᵗʰ S00.44 External constriction of ear

☑7ᵗʰ S00.441 External constriction of right ear

☑7ᵗʰ S00.442 External constriction of left ear

☑7ᵗʰ S00.449 External constriction of unspecified ear

☑6ᵗʰ S00.45 Superficial foreign body of ear
Splinter in the ear

☑7ᵗʰ S00.451 Superficial foreign body of right ear

☑7ᵗʰ S00.452 Superficial foreign body of left ear

☑7ᵗʰ S00.459 Superficial foreign body of unspecified ear

☑6ᵗʰ S00.46 Insect bite (nonvenomous) of ear

☑7ᵗʰ S00.461 Insect bite (nonvenomous) of right ear

☑7ᵗʰ S00.462 Insect bite (nonvenomous) of left ear

☑7ᵗʰ S00.469 Insect bite (nonvenomous) of unspecified ear

☑6ᵗʰ S00.47 Other superficial bite of ear
EXCLUDES 1 *open bite of ear (S01.35)*

☑7ᵗʰ S00.471 Other superficial bite of right ear

☑7ᵗʰ S00.472 Other superficial bite of left ear

☑7ᵗʰ S00.479 Other superficial bite of unspecified ear

☑5ᵗʰ S00.5 Superficial injury of lip and oral cavity

☑6ᵗʰ S00.50 Unspecified superficial injury of lip and oral cavity

☑7ᵗʰ S00.501 Unspecified superficial injury of lip

☑7ᵗʰ S00.502 Unspecified superficial injury of oral cavity

☑6ᵗʰ S00.51 Abrasion of lip and oral cavity

☑7ᵗʰ S00.511 Abrasion of lip

☑7ᵗʰ S00.512 Abrasion of oral cavity

☑6ᵗʰ S00.52 Blister (nonthermal) of lip and oral cavity

☑7ᵗʰ S00.521 Blister (nonthermal) of lip

☑7ᵗʰ S00.522 Blister (nonthermal) of oral cavity

☑6ᵗʰ S00.53 Contusion of lip and oral cavity

☑7ᵗʰ S00.531 Contusion of lip
Bruise of lip
Hematoma of oral cavity

☑7ᵗʰ S00.532 Contusion of oral cavity
Bruise of lip
Hematoma of oral cavity

☑6ᵗʰ S00.54 External constriction of lip and oral cavity

☑7ᵗʰ S00.541 External constriction of lip

☑7ᵗʰ S00.542 External constriction of oral cavity

☑6ᵗʰ S00.55 Superficial foreign body of lip and oral cavity

☑7ᵗʰ S00.551 Superficial foreign body of lip
Splinter of lip and oral cavity

☑7ᵗʰ S00.552 Superficial foreign body of oral cavity
Splinter of lip and oral cavity

☑6ᵗʰ S00.56 Insect bite (nonvenomous) of lip and oral cavity

☑7ᵗʰ S00.561 Insect bite (nonvenomous) of lip

☑7ᵗʰ S00.562 Insect bite (nonvenomous) of oral cavity

☑6ᵗʰ S00.57 Other superficial bite of lip and oral cavity

☑7ᵗʰ S00.571 Other superficial bite of lip
EXCLUDES 1 *open bite of lip (S01.551)*

☑7ᵗʰ S00.572 Other superficial bite of oral cavity
EXCLUDES 1 *open bite of oral cavity (S01.552)*

☑5ᵗʰ S00.8 Superficial injury of other parts of head

☑x7ᵗʰ S00.80 Unspecified superficial injury of other part of head

☑x7ᵗʰ S00.81 Abrasion of other part of head

☑x7ᵗʰ S00.82 Blister (nonthermal) of other part of head

☑x7ᵗʰ S00.83 Contusion of other part of head
Bruise of other part of head
Hematoma of other part of head

☑x7ᵗʰ S00.84 External constriction of other part of head

☑x7ᵗʰ S00.85 Superficial foreign body of other part of head
Splinter in other part of head

☑x7ᵗʰ S00.86 Insect bite (nonvenomous) of other part of head

☑x7ᵗʰ S00.87 Other superficial bite of other part of head
EXCLUDES 1 *open bite of other part of head (S01.85)*

☑5ᵗʰ S00.9 Superficial injury of unspecified part of head

☑x7ᵗʰ S00.90 Unspecified superficial injury of unspecified part of head

☑x7ᵗʰ S00.91 Abrasion of unspecified part of head

☑x7ᵗʰ S00.92 Blister (nonthermal) of unspecified part of head

☑x7ᵗʰ S00.93 Contusion of unspecified part of head
Bruise of head
Hematoma of head

☑x7ᵗʰ S00.94 External constriction of unspecified part of head

☑x7ᵗʰ S00.95 Superficial foreign body of unspecified part of head
Splinter of head

☑x7ᵗʰ S00.96 Insect bite (nonvenomous) of unspecified part of head

☑x7ᵗʰ S00.97 Other superficial bite of unspecified part of head
EXCLUDES 1 *open bite of head (S01.95)*

☑4ᵗʰ S01 Open wound of head
Code also any associated:
injury of cranial nerve (S04.-)
injury of muscle and tendon of head (S09.1-)
intracranial injury (S06.-)
wound infection
EXCLUDES 1 *open skull fracture (S02- with 7th character B)*
EXCLUDES 2 *injury of eye and orbit (S05.-)*
traumatic amputation of part of head (S08.-)

The appropriate 7th character is to be added to each code from category S01.
A   initial encounter
D   subsequent encounter
S   sequela

☑5ᵗʰ S01.0 Open wound of scalp
EXCLUDES 1 *avulsion of scalp (S08.0)*

☑x7ᵗʰ S01.00 Unspecified open wound of scalp

☑x7ᵗʰ S01.01 Laceration without foreign body of scalp

☑x7ᵗʰ S01.02 Laceration with foreign body of scalp

☑x7ᵗʰ S01.03 Puncture wound without foreign body of scalp

☑x7ᵗʰ S01.04 Puncture wound with foreign body of scalp

☑x7ᵗʰ S01.05 Open bite of scalp
Bite of scalp NOS
EXCLUDES 1 *superficial bite of scalp (S00.06, S00.07-)*

☑5ᵗʰ S01.1 Open wound of eyelid and periocular area
Open wound of eyelid and periocular area with or without involvement of lacrimal passages

☑6ᵗʰ S01.10 Unspecified open wound of eyelid and periocular area

☑7ᵗʰ S01.101 Unspecified open wound of right eyelid and periocular area

√7ᵗʰ **S01.102** **Unspecified open wound of** left **eyelid and periocular area**

√7ᵗʰ **S01.109** **Unspecified open wound of unspecified eyelid and periocular area**

√6ᵗʰ **S01.11** Laceration without foreign body **of eyelid and periocular area**

√7ᵗʰ **S01.111** **Laceration without foreign body of** right **eyelid and periocular area**

√7ᵗʰ **S01.112** **Laceration without foreign body of** left **eyelid and periocular area**

√7ᵗʰ **S01.119** **Laceration without foreign body of unspecified eyelid and periocular area**

√6ᵗʰ **S01.12** Laceration with foreign body **of eyelid and periocular area**

√7ᵗʰ **S01.121** **Laceration with foreign body of** right **eyelid and periocular area**

√7ᵗʰ **S01.122** **Laceration with foreign body of** left **eyelid and periocular area**

√7ᵗʰ **S01.129** **Laceration with foreign body of unspecified eyelid and periocular area**

√6ᵗʰ **S01.13** Puncture wound without foreign body **of eyelid and periocular area**

√7ᵗʰ **S01.131** **Puncture wound without foreign body of** right **eyelid and periocular area**

√7ᵗʰ **S01.132** **Puncture wound without foreign body of** left **eyelid and periocular area**

√7ᵗʰ **S01.139** **Puncture wound without foreign body of unspecified eyelid and periocular area**

√6ᵗʰ **S01.14** Puncture wound with foreign body **of eyelid and periocular area**

√7ᵗʰ **S01.141** **Puncture wound with foreign body of** right **eyelid and periocular area**

√7ᵗʰ **S01.142** **Puncture wound with foreign body of** left **eyelid and periocular area**

√7ᵗʰ **S01.149** **Puncture wound with foreign body of unspecified eyelid and periocular area**

√6ᵗʰ **S01.15** Open bite **of eyelid and periocular area**
    Bite of eyelid and periocular area NOS
    EXCLUDES 1   superficial bite of eyelid and periocular area (S00.26, S00.27)

√7ᵗʰ **S01.151** **Open bite of** right **eyelid and periocular area**

√7ᵗʰ **S01.152** **Open bite of** left **eyelid and periocular area**

√7ᵗʰ **S01.159** **Open bite of unspecified eyelid and periocular area**

√5ᵗʰ **S01.2** **Open wound of** nose

√x7ᵗʰ **S01.20** **Unspecified open wound of nose**

√x7ᵗʰ **S01.21** Laceration without foreign body **of nose**

√x7ᵗʰ **S01.22** Laceration with foreign body **of nose**

√x7ᵗʰ **S01.23** Puncture wound without foreign body **of nose**

√x7ᵗʰ **S01.24** Puncture wound with foreign body **of nose**

√x7ᵗʰ **S01.25** Open bite **of nose**
    Bite of nose NOS
    EXCLUDES 1   superficial bite of nose (S00.36, S00.37)

√5ᵗʰ **S01.3** **Open wound of** ear

√6ᵗʰ **S01.30** Unspecified open wound of ear

√7ᵗʰ **S01.301** **Unspecified open wound of** right **ear**

√7ᵗʰ **S01.302** **Unspecified open wound of** left **ear**

√7ᵗʰ **S01.309** **Unspecified open wound of unspecified ear**

√6ᵗʰ **S01.31** Laceration without foreign body **of ear**

√7ᵗʰ **S01.311** **Laceration without foreign body of** right **ear**

√7ᵗʰ **S01.312** **Laceration without foreign body of** left **ear**

√7ᵗʰ **S01.319** **Laceration without foreign body of unspecified ear**

√6ᵗʰ **S01.32** Laceration with foreign body **of ear**

√7ᵗʰ **S01.321** **Laceration with foreign body of** right **ear**

√7ᵗʰ **S01.322** **Laceration with foreign body of** left **ear**

√7ᵗʰ **S01.329** **Laceration with foreign body of unspecified ear**

√6ᵗʰ **S01.33** Puncture wound without foreign body **of ear**

√7ᵗʰ **S01.331** **Puncture wound without foreign body of** right **ear**

√7ᵗʰ **S01.332** **Puncture wound without foreign body of** left **ear**

√7ᵗʰ **S01.339** **Puncture wound without foreign body of unspecified ear**

√6ᵗʰ **S01.34** Puncture wound with foreign body **of ear**

√7ᵗʰ **S01.341** **Puncture wound with foreign body of** right **ear**

√7ᵗʰ **S01.342** **Puncture wound with foreign body of** left **ear**

√7ᵗʰ **S01.349** **Puncture wound with foreign body of unspecified ear**

√6ᵗʰ **S01.35** Open bite **of ear**
    Bite of ear NOS
    EXCLUDES 1   superficial bite of ear (S00.46, S00.47)

√7ᵗʰ **S01.351** **Open bite of** right **ear**

√7ᵗʰ **S01.352** **Open bite of** left **ear**

√7ᵗʰ **S01.359** **Open bite of unspecified ear**

√5ᵗʰ **S01.4** **Open wound of** cheek and temporomandibular area

√6ᵗʰ **S01.40** Unspecified **open wound of cheek and temporomandibular area**

√7ᵗʰ **S01.401** **Unspecified open wound of** right **cheek and temporomandibular area**

√7ᵗʰ **S01.402** **Unspecified open wound of** left **cheek and temporomandibular area**

√7ᵗʰ **S01.409** **Unspecified open wound of unspecified cheek and temporomandibular area**

√6ᵗʰ **S01.41** Laceration without foreign body **of cheek and temporomandibular area**

√7ᵗʰ **S01.411** **Laceration without foreign body of** right **cheek and temporomandibular area**

√7ᵗʰ **S01.412** **Laceration without foreign body of** left **cheek and temporomandibular area**

√7ᵗʰ **S01.419** **Laceration without foreign body of unspecified cheek and temporomandibular area**

√6ᵗʰ **S01.42** Laceration with foreign body **of cheek and temporomandibular area**

√7ᵗʰ **S01.421** **Laceration with foreign body of** right **cheek and temporomandibular area**

√7ᵗʰ **S01.422** **Laceration with foreign body of** left **cheek and temporomandibular area**

√7ᵗʰ **S01.429** **Laceration with foreign body of unspecified cheek and temporomandibular area**

√6ᵗʰ **S01.43** Puncture wound without foreign body **of cheek and temporomandibular area**

√7ᵗʰ **S01.431** **Puncture wound without foreign body of** right **cheek and temporomandibular area**

√7ᵗʰ **S01.432** **Puncture wound without foreign body of** left **cheek and temporomandibular area**

√7ᵗʰ **S01.439** **Puncture wound without foreign body of unspecified cheek and temporomandibular area**

√6ᵗʰ **S01.44** Puncture wound with foreign body **of cheek and temporomandibular area**

√7ᵗʰ **S01.441** **Puncture wound with foreign body of** right **cheek and temporomandibular area**

√7ᵗʰ **S01.442** **Puncture wound with foreign body of** left **cheek and temporomandibular area**

√7ᵗʰ **S01.449** **Puncture wound with foreign body of unspecified cheek and temporomandibular area**

√6ᵗʰ **S01.45** Open bite **of cheek and temporomandibular area**
    Bite of cheek and temporomandibular area NOS
    EXCLUDES 2   superficial bite of cheek and temporomandibular area (S00.86, S00.87)

√7ᵗʰ **S01.451** **Open bite of** right **cheek and temporomandibular area**

√7ᵗʰ **S01.452** **Open bite of** left **cheek and temporomandibular area**

√7ᵗʰ **S01.459** **Open bite of unspecified cheek and temporomandibular area**

EXCLUDES 1 Not coded here   EXCLUDES 2 Not included here   Ⓝ Newborn Age: 0   Ⓟ Pediatric Age: 0-17   Ⓜ Maternity Age: 12-55   Ⓐ Adult Age: 15-124

806   ICD-10-CM Draft (2015)

✓5ᵗʰ S01.5　Open wound of lip and oral cavity
　　EXCLUDES 2　tooth dislocation (S03.2)
　　　　　　　tooth fracture (S02.5)

　✓6ᵗʰ **S01.50　Unspecified open wound of lip and oral cavity**
　　✓7ᵗʰ **S01.501　Unspecified open wound of lip**
　　✓7ᵗʰ **S01.502　Unspecified open wound of oral cavity**

　✓6ᵗʰ **S01.51　Laceration of lip and oral cavity without foreign body**
　　✓7ᵗʰ **S01.511　Laceration without foreign body of lip**
　　✓7ᵗʰ **S01.512　Laceration without foreign body of oral cavity**

　✓6ᵗʰ **S01.52　Laceration of lip and oral cavity with foreign body**
　　✓7ᵗʰ **S01.521　Laceration with foreign body of lip**
　　✓7ᵗʰ **S01.522　Laceration with foreign body of oral cavity**

　✓6ᵗʰ **S01.53　Puncture wound of lip and oral cavity without foreign body**
　　✓7ᵗʰ **S01.531　Puncture wound without foreign body of lip**
　　✓7ᵗʰ **S01.532　Puncture wound without foreign body of oral cavity**

　✓6ᵗʰ **S01.54　Puncture wound of lip and oral cavity with foreign body**
　　✓7ᵗʰ **S01.541　Puncture wound with foreign body of lip**
　　✓7ᵗʰ **S01.542　Puncture wound with foreign body of oral cavity**

　✓6ᵗʰ **S01.55　Open bite of lip and oral cavity**
　　✓7ᵗʰ **S01.551　Open bite of lip**
　　　　Bite of lip NOS
　　　　EXCLUDES 1　superficial bite of lip (S00.571)
　　✓7ᵗʰ **S01.552　Open bite of oral cavity**
　　　　Bite of oral cavity NOS
　　　　EXCLUDES 1　superficial bite of oral cavity (S00.572)

✓5ᵗʰ S01.8　Open wound of other parts of head
　✓x7ᵗʰ **S01.80　Unspecified open wound of other part of head**
　✓x7ᵗʰ **S01.81　Laceration without foreign body of other part of head**
　✓x7ᵗʰ **S01.82　Laceration with foreign body of other part of head**
　✓x7ᵗʰ **S01.83　Puncture wound without foreign body of other part of head**
　✓x7ᵗʰ **S01.84　Puncture wound with foreign body of other part of head**
　✓x7ᵗʰ **S01.85　Open bite of other part of head**
　　　　Bite of other part of head NOS
　　　　EXCLUDES 1　superficial bite of other part of head (S00.85)

✓5ᵗʰ S01.9　Open wound of unspecified part of head
　✓x7ᵗʰ **S01.90　Unspecified open wound of unspecified part of head**
　✓x7ᵗʰ **S01.91　Laceration without foreign body of unspecified part of head**
　✓x7ᵗʰ **S01.92　Laceration with foreign body of unspecified part of head**
　✓x7ᵗʰ **S01.93　Puncture wound without foreign body of unspecified part of head**
　✓x7ᵗʰ **S01.94　Puncture wound with foreign body of unspecified part of head**
　✓x7ᵗʰ **S01.95　Open bite of unspecified part of head**
　　　　Bite of head NOS
　　　　EXCLUDES 1　superficial bite of head NOS (S00.97)

✓4ᵗʰ S02　Fracture of skull and facial bones
　　NOTE　A fracture not indicated as open or closed should be coded to closed.
　　Code also any associated intracranial injury (S06.-).

　　The appropriate 7th character is to be added to each code from category S02.
　　A　initial encounter for closed fracture
　　B　initial encounter for open fracture
　　D　subsequent encounter for fracture with routine healing
　　G　subsequent encounter for fracture with delayed healing
　　K　subsequent encounter for fracture with nonunion
　　S　sequela

　✓x7ᵗʰ **S02.0　Fracture of vault of skull**
　　　　Fracture of frontal bone
　　　　Fracture of parietal bone

✓5ᵗʰ S02.1　Fracture of base of skull
　　EXCLUDES 1　orbit NOS (S02.8)
　　EXCLUDES 2　orbital floor (S02.3-)

　✓x7ᵗʰ **S02.10　Unspecified fracture of base of skull**
　✓6ᵗʰ **S02.11　Fracture of occiput**
　　✓7ᵗʰ **S02.110　Type I occipital condyle fracture**
　　✓7ᵗʰ **S02.111　Type II occipital condyle fracture**
　　✓7ᵗʰ **S02.112　Type III occipital condyle fracture**
　　✓7ᵗʰ **S02.113　Unspecified occipital condyle fracture**
　　✓7ᵗʰ **S02.118　Other fracture of occiput**
　　✓7ᵗʰ **S02.119　Unspecified fracture of occiput**
　✓x7ᵗʰ **S02.19　Other fracture of base of skull**
　　　　Fracture of anterior fossa of base of skull
　　　　Fracture of ethmoid sinus
　　　　Fracture of frontal sinus
　　　　Fracture of middle fossa of base of skull
　　　　Fracture of orbital roof
　　　　Fracture of posterior fossa of base of skull
　　　　Fracture of sphenoid
　　　　Fracture of temporal bone

　✓x7ᵗʰ **S02.2　Fracture of nasal bones**
　✓x7ᵗʰ **S02.3　Fracture of orbital floor**
　　EXCLUDES 1　orbit NOS (S02.8)
　　EXCLUDES 2　orbital roof (S02.1-)

✓5ᵗʰ S02.4　Fracture of malar, maxillary and zygoma bones
　　　Fracture of superior maxilla
　　　Fracture of upper jaw (bone)
　　　Fracture of zygomatic process of temporal bone

　✓6ᵗʰ **S02.40　Fracture of malar, maxillary and zygoma bones, unspecified**
　　✓7ᵗʰ **S02.400　Malar fracture unspecified**
　　✓7ᵗʰ **S02.401　Maxillary fracture, unspecified**
　　✓7ᵗʰ **S02.402　Zygomatic fracture, unspecified**
　✓6ᵗʰ **S02.41　LeFort fracture**
　　✓7ᵗʰ **S02.411　LeFort I fracture**
　　✓7ᵗʰ **S02.412　LeFort II fracture**
　　✓7ᵗʰ **S02.413　LeFort III fracture**
　✓x7ᵗʰ **S02.42　Fracture of alveolus of maxilla**

　✓x7ᵗʰ **S02.5　Fracture of tooth (traumatic)**
　　　Broken tooth
　　　EXCLUDES 1　cracked tooth (nontraumatic) (K03.81)

✓5ᵗʰ S02.6　Fracture of mandible
　　　Fracture of lower jaw (bone)

　✓6ᵗʰ **S02.60　Fracture of mandible, unspecified**
　　✓7ᵗʰ **S02.600　Fracture of unspecified part of body of mandible**
　　✓7ᵗʰ **S02.609　Fracture of mandible, unspecified**
　✓x7ᵗʰ **S02.61　Fracture of condylar process of mandible**
　✓x7ᵗʰ **S02.62　Fracture of subcondylar process of mandible**
　✓x7ᵗʰ **S02.63　Fracture of coronoid process of mandible**
　✓x7ᵗʰ **S02.64　Fracture of ramus of mandible**
　✓x7ᵗʰ **S02.65　Fracture of angle of mandible**
　✓x7ᵗʰ **S02.66　Fracture of symphysis of mandible**
　✓x7ᵗʰ **S02.67　Fracture of alveolus of mandible**
　✓x7ᵗʰ **S02.69　Fracture of mandible of other specified site**

　✓x7ᵗʰ **S02.8　Fractures of other specified skull and facial bones**
　　　Fracture of orbit NOS
　　　Fracture of palate
　　　EXCLUDES 1　fracture of orbital floor (S02.3-)
　　　　　　　　fracture of orbital roof (S02.1-)

✓5ᵗʰ S02.9　Fracture of unspecified skull and facial bones
　✓x7ᵗʰ **S02.91　Unspecified fracture of skull**
　✓x7ᵗʰ **S02.92　Unspecified fracture of facial bones**

√4ᵗʰ **S03** **Dislocation and sprain of joints and ligaments of head**
> INCLUDES   avulsion of joint (capsule) or ligament of head
> laceration of cartilage, joint (capsule) or ligament of head
> sprain of cartilage, joint (capsule) or ligament of head
> traumatic hemarthrosis of joint or ligament of head
> traumatic rupture of joint or ligament of head
> traumatic subluxation of joint or ligament of head
> traumatic tear of joint or ligament of head
>
> Code also any associated open wound
> EXCLUDES 2   *strain of muscle or tendon of head (S09.1)*

> The appropriate 7th character is to be added to each code from category S03.
> A   initial encounter
> D   subsequent encounter
> S   sequela

√x7ᵗʰ **S03.0** **Dislocation of jaw**
> Dislocation of jaw (cartilage) (meniscus)
> Dislocation of mandible
> Dislocation of temporomandibular (joint)

√x7ᵗʰ **S03.1** **Dislocation of septal cartilage of nose**

√x7ᵗʰ **S03.2** **Dislocation of tooth**

√x7ᵗʰ **S03.4** **Sprain of jaw**
> Sprain of temporomandibular (joint) (ligament)

√x7ᵗʰ **S03.8** **Sprain of joints and ligaments of other parts of head**

√x7ᵗʰ **S03.9** **Sprain of joints and ligaments of unspecified parts of head**

√4ᵗʰ **S04** **Injury of cranial nerve**
> The selection of side should be based on the side of the body being affected
> Codes first any associated intracranial injury (S06.-)
> Code also any associated:
> open wound of head (S01.-)
> skull fracture (S02.-)

> The appropriate 7th character is to be added to each code from category S04.
> A   initial encounter
> D   subsequent encounter
> S   sequela

√5ᵗʰ **S04.0** **Injury of optic nerve and pathways**
> Use additional code to identify any visual field defect or blindness (H53.4-, H54)

√6ᵗʰ **S04.01** **Injury of** optic nerve
> Injury of 2nd cranial nerve

√7ᵗʰ **S04.011** **Injury of optic nerve,** right **eye**

√7ᵗʰ **S04.012** **Injury of optic nerve,** left **eye**

√7ᵗʰ **S04.019** **Injury of optic nerve, unspecified eye**
> Injury of optic nerve NOS

√x7ᵗʰ **S04.02** **Injury of optic** chiasm

√6ᵗʰ **S04.03** **Injury of optic** tract and pathways
> Injury of optic radiation

√7ᵗʰ **S04.031** **Injury of optic tract and pathways,** right **eye**

√7ᵗʰ **S04.032** **Injury of optic tract and pathways,** left **eye**

√7ᵗʰ **S04.039** **Injury of optic tract and pathways, unspecified eye**
> Injury of optic tract and pathways NOS

√6ᵗʰ **S04.04** **Injury of** visual cortex

√7ᵗʰ **S04.041** **Injury of visual cortex,** right **eye**

√7ᵗʰ **S04.042** **Injury of visual cortex,** left **eye**

√7ᵗʰ **S04.049** **Injury of visual cortex, unspecified eye**
> Injury of visual cortex NOS

√5ᵗʰ **S04.1** **Injury of** oculomotor nerve
> Injury of 3rd cranial nerve

√x7ᵗʰ **S04.10** **Injury of oculomotor nerve, unspecified side**

√x7ᵗʰ **S04.11** **Injury of oculomotor nerve,** right **side**

√x7ᵗʰ **S04.12** **Injury of oculomotor nerve,** left **side**

√5ᵗʰ **S04.2** **Injury of** trochlear nerve
> Injury of 4th cranial nerve

√x7ᵗʰ **S04.20** **Injury of trochlear nerve, unspecified side**

√x7ᵗʰ **S04.21** **Injury of trochlear nerve,** right **side**

√x7ᵗʰ **S04.22** **Injury of trochlear nerve,** left **side**

√5ᵗʰ **S04.3** **Injury of** trigeminal nerve
> Injury of 5th cranial nerve

√x7ᵗʰ **S04.30** **Injury of trigeminal nerve, unspecified side**

√x7ᵗʰ **S04.31** **Injury of trigeminal nerve,** right **side**

√x7ᵗʰ **S04.32** **Injury of trigeminal nerve,** left **side**

√5ᵗʰ **S04.4** **Injury of** abducent nerve
> Injury of 6th cranial nerve

√x7ᵗʰ **S04.40** **Injury of abducent nerve, unspecified side**

√x7ᵗʰ **S04.41** **Injury of abducent nerve,** right **side**

√x7ᵗʰ **S04.42** **Injury of abducent nerve,** left **side**

√5ᵗʰ **S04.5** **Injury of** facial nerve
> Injury of 7th cranial nerve

√x7ᵗʰ **S04.50** **Injury of facial nerve, unspecified side**

√x7ᵗʰ **S04.51** **Injury of facial nerve,** right **side**

√x7ᵗʰ **S04.52** **Injury of facial nerve,** left **side**

√5ᵗʰ **S04.6** **Injury of** acoustic nerve
> Injury of auditory nerve
> Injury of 8th cranial nerve

√x7ᵗʰ **S04.60** **Injury of acoustic nerve, unspecified side**

√x7ᵗʰ **S04.61** **Injury of acoustic nerve,** right **side**

√x7ᵗʰ **S04.62** **Injury of acoustic nerve,** left **side**

√5ᵗʰ **S04.7** **Injury of** accessory nerve
> Injury of 11th cranial nerve

√x7ᵗʰ **S04.70** **Injury of accessory nerve, unspecified side**

√x7ᵗʰ **S04.71** **Injury of accessory nerve,** right **side**

√x7ᵗʰ **S04.72** **Injury of accessory nerve,** left **side**

√5ᵗʰ **S04.8** **Injury of** other cranial nerves

√6ᵗʰ **S04.81** **Injury of** olfactory [1st] nerve

√7ᵗʰ **S04.811** **Injury of olfactory [1st] nerve,** right **side**

√7ᵗʰ **S04.812** **Injury of olfactory [1st] nerve,** left **side**

√7ᵗʰ **S04.819** **Injury of olfactory [1st] nerve, unspecified side**

√6ᵗʰ **S04.89** **Injury of** other cranial nerves
> Injury of vagus [10th] nerve

√7ᵗʰ **S04.891** **Injury of other cranial nerves,** right **side**

√7ᵗʰ **S04.892** **Injury of other cranial nerves,** left **side**

√7ᵗʰ **S04.899** **Injury of other cranial nerves, unspecified side**

√x7ᵗʰ **S04.9** **Injury of unspecified cranial nerve**

√4ᵗʰ **S05** **Injury of eye and orbit**
> Open wound of eye and orbit
> EXCLUDES 2   *2nd cranial [optic] nerve injury (S04.0-)*
> *3rd cranial [oculomotor] nerve injury (S04.1-)*
> *open wound of eyelid and periocular area (S01.1-)*
> *orbital bone fracture (S02.1-, S02.3-, S02.8-)*
> *superficial injury of eyelid (S00.1-S00.2)*

> The appropriate 7th character is to be added to each code from category S05.
> A   initial encounter
> D   subsequent encounter
> S   sequela

√5ᵗʰ **S05.0** **Injury of conjunctiva and corneal abrasion** without foreign body
> EXCLUDES 1   *foreign body in conjunctival sac (T15.1)*
> *foreign body in cornea (T15.0)*

√x7ᵗʰ **S05.00** **Injury of conjunctiva and corneal abrasion without foreign body, unspecified eye**

√x7ᵗʰ **S05.01** **Injury of conjunctiva and corneal abrasion without foreign body,** right **eye**

√x7ᵗʰ **S05.02** **Injury of conjunctiva and corneal abrasion without foreign body,** left **eye**

√5ᵗʰ **S05.1** **Contusion of eyeball and orbital tissues**
> Traumatic hyphema
> EXCLUDES 2   *black eye NOS (S00.1)*
> *contusion of eyelid and periocular area (S00.1)*

√x7ᵗʰ **S05.10** **Contusion of eyeball and orbital tissues, unspecified eye**

√x7ᵗʰ **S05.11** **Contusion of eyeball and orbital tissues,** right **eye**

√x7ᵗʰ **S05.12** **Contusion of eyeball and orbital tissues,** left **eye**

√5ᵗʰ **S05.2** **Ocular laceration and rupture** with prolapse or loss of intraocular tissue

√x7ᵗʰ **S05.20** **Ocular laceration and rupture with prolapse or loss of intraocular tissue, unspecified eye**

√x7ᵗʰ **S05.21** **Ocular laceration and rupture with prolapse or loss of intraocular tissue,** right **eye**

EXCLUDES 1 Not coded here   EXCLUDES 2 Not included here   N Newborn Age: 0   P Pediatric Age: 0-17   M Maternity Age: 12-55   A Adult Age: 15-124

808   ICD-10-CM Draft (2015)

√x 7ᵗʰ **S05.22** Ocular laceration and rupture with prolapse or loss of intraocular tissue, left eye

✓5ᵗʰ **S05.3** Ocular laceration without prolapse or loss of intraocular tissue
Laceration of eye NOS

√x 7ᵗʰ **S05.30** Ocular laceration without prolapse or loss of intraocular tissue, unspecified eye

√x 7ᵗʰ **S05.31** Ocular laceration without prolapse or loss of intraocular tissue, right eye

√x 7ᵗʰ **S05.32** Ocular laceration without prolapse or loss of intraocular tissue, left eye

✓5ᵗʰ **S05.4** Penetrating wound of orbit with or without foreign body
EXCLUDES 2 retained (old) foreign body following penetrating wound in orbit (H05.5-)

√x 7ᵗʰ **S05.40** Penetrating wound of orbit with or without foreign body, unspecified eye

√x 7ᵗʰ **S05.41** Penetrating wound of orbit with or without foreign body, right eye

√x 7ᵗʰ **S05.42** Penetrating wound of orbit with or without foreign body, left eye

✓5ᵗʰ **S05.5** Penetrating wound with foreign body of eyeball
EXCLUDES 2 retained (old) intraocular foreign body (H44.6-, H44.7)

√x 7ᵗʰ **S05.50** Penetrating wound with foreign body of unspecified eyeball

√x 7ᵗʰ **S05.51** Penetrating wound with foreign body of right eyeball

√x 7ᵗʰ **S05.52** Penetrating wound with foreign body of left eyeball

✓5ᵗʰ **S05.6** Penetrating wound without foreign body of eyeball
Ocular penetration NOS

√x 7ᵗʰ **S05.60** Penetrating wound without foreign body of unspecified eyeball

√x 7ᵗʰ **S05.61** Penetrating wound without foreign body of right eyeball

√x 7ᵗʰ **S05.62** Penetrating wound without foreign body of left eyeball

✓5ᵗʰ **S05.7** Avulsion of eye
Traumatic enucleation

√x 7ᵗʰ **S05.70** Avulsion of unspecified eye

√x 7ᵗʰ **S05.71** Avulsion of right eye

√x 7ᵗʰ **S05.72** Avulsion of left eye

✓5ᵗʰ **S05.8** Other injuries of eye and orbit
Lacrimal duct injury

✓6ᵗʰ **S05.8X** Other injuries of eye and orbit

√7ᵗʰ **S05.8X1** Other injuries of right eye and orbit

√7ᵗʰ **S05.8X2** Other injuries of left eye and orbit

√7ᵗʰ **S05.8X9** Other injuries of unspecified eye and orbit

✓5ᵗʰ **S05.9** Unspecified injury of eye and orbit
Injury of eye NOS

√x 7ᵗʰ **S05.90** Unspecified injury of unspecified eye and orbit

√x 7ᵗʰ **S05.91** Unspecified injury of right eye and orbit

√x 7ᵗʰ **S05.92** Unspecified injury of left eye and orbit

✓4ᵗʰ **S06 Intracranial injury**
Traumatic brain injury
Code also any associated:
open wound of head (S01.-)
skull fracture (S02.-)
EXCLUDES 1 head injury NOS (S09.90)

The appropriate 7th character is to be added to each code from category S06.
A   initial encounter
D   subsequent encounter
S   sequela

✓5ᵗʰ **S06.0 Concussion**
Commotio cerebri
EXCLUDES 1 concussion with other intracranial injuries classified in category S06—code to specified intracranial injury

✓6ᵗʰ **S06.0X** Concussion

√7ᵗʰ **S06.0X0** Concussion without loss of consciousness

√7ᵗʰ **S06.0X1** Concussion with loss of consciousness of 30 minutes or less

√7ᵗʰ **S06.0X2** Concussion with loss of consciousness of 31 minutes to 59 minutes

√7ᵗʰ **S06.0X3** Concussion with loss of consciousness of 1 hour to 5 hours 59 minutes

√7ᵗʰ **S06.0X4** Concussion with loss of consciousness of 6 hours to 24 hours

√7ᵗʰ **S06.0X5** Concussion with loss of consciousness greater than 24 hours with return to pre-existing conscious level

√7ᵗʰ **S06.0X6** Concussion with loss of consciousness greater than 24 hours without return to pre-existing conscious level with patient surviving

√7ᵗʰ **S06.0X7** Concussion with loss of consciousness of any duration with death due to brain injury prior to regaining consciousness

√7ᵗʰ **S06.0X8** Concussion with loss of consciousness of any duration with death due to other cause prior to regaining consciousness

√7ᵗʰ **S06.0X9** Concussion with loss of consciousness of unspecified duration
Concussion NOS

✓5ᵗʰ **S06.1 Traumatic cerebral edema**
Diffuse traumatic cerebral edema
Focal traumatic cerebral edema

✓6ᵗʰ **S06.1X** Traumatic cerebral edema

√7ᵗʰ **S06.1X0** Traumatic cerebral edema without loss of consciousness

√7ᵗʰ **S06.1X1** Traumatic cerebral edema with loss of consciousness of 30 minutes or less

√7ᵗʰ **S06.1X2** Traumatic cerebral edema with loss of consciousness of 31 minutes to 59 minutes

√7ᵗʰ **S06.1X3** Traumatic cerebral edema with loss of consciousness of 1 hour to 5 hours 59 minutes

√7ᵗʰ **S06.1X4** Traumatic cerebral edema with loss of consciousness of 6 hours to 24 hours

√7ᵗʰ **S06.1X5** Traumatic cerebral edema with loss of consciousness greater than 24 hours with return to pre-existing conscious level

√7ᵗʰ **S06.1X6** Traumatic cerebral edema with loss of consciousness greater than 24 hours without return to pre-existing conscious level with patient surviving

√7ᵗʰ **S06.1X7** Traumatic cerebral edema with loss of consciousness of any duration with death due to brain injury prior to regaining consciousness

√7ᵗʰ **S06.1X8** Traumatic cerebral edema with loss of consciousness of any duration with death due to other cause prior to regaining consciousness

√7ᵗʰ **S06.1X9** Traumatic cerebral edema with loss of consciousness of unspecified duration
Traumatic cerebral edema NOS

✓5ᵗʰ **S06.2 Diffuse traumatic brain injury**
Diffuse axonal brain injury
EXCLUDES 1 traumatic diffuse cerebral edema (S06.1X-)

✓6ᵗʰ **S06.2X** Diffuse traumatic brain injury

√7ᵗʰ **S06.2X0** Diffuse traumatic brain injury without loss of consciousness

√7ᵗʰ **S06.2X1** Diffuse traumatic brain injury with loss of consciousness of 30 minutes or less

√7ᵗʰ **S06.2X2** Diffuse traumatic brain injury with loss of consciousness of 31 minutes to 59 minutes

√7ᵗʰ **S06.2X3** Diffuse traumatic brain injury with loss of consciousness of 1 hour to 5 hours 59 minutes

√7ᵗʰ **S06.2X4** Diffuse traumatic brain injury with loss of consciousness of 6 hours to 24 hours

√7ᵗʰ **S06.2X5** Diffuse traumatic brain injury with loss of consciousness greater than 24 hours with return to pre-existing conscious levels

√7ᵗʰ **S06.2X6** Diffuse traumatic brain injury with loss of consciousness greater than 24 hours without return to pre-existing conscious level with patient surviving

Injury, Poisoning and Certain Other Consequences of External Causes

S06.2X7–S06.338

√7ᵗʰ **S06.2X7 Diffuse traumatic brain injury with loss of consciousness of** any duration with death due to brain injury prior to regaining consciousness

√7ᵗʰ **S06.2X8 Diffuse traumatic brain injury with loss of consciousness of** any duration with death due to other cause prior to regaining consciousness

√7ᵗʰ **S06.2X9 Diffuse traumatic brain injury with loss of consciousness of unspecified duration**
     Diffuse traumatic brain injury NOS

√5ᵗʰ **S06.3 Focal traumatic brain injury**
     EXCLUDES 1   any condition classifiable to S06.4-S06.6
                 focal cerebral edema (S06.1)

√6ᵗʰ **S06.30 Unspecified focal traumatic brain injury**

√7ᵗʰ **S06.300 Unspecified focal traumatic brain injury** without loss of consciousness

√7ᵗʰ **S06.301 Unspecified focal traumatic brain injury with loss of consciousness of** 30 minutes or less

√7ᵗʰ **S06.302 Unspecified focal traumatic brain injury with loss of consciousness of** 31 minutes to 59 minutes

√7ᵗʰ **S06.303 Unspecified focal traumatic brain injury with loss of consciousness of** 1 hour to 5 hours 59 minutes

√7ᵗʰ **S06.304 Unspecified focal traumatic brain injury with loss of consciousness of** 6 hours to 24 hours

√7ᵗʰ **S06.305 Unspecified focal traumatic brain injury with loss of consciousness** greater than 24 hours with return to pre-existing conscious level

√7ᵗʰ **S06.306 Unspecified focal traumatic brain injury with loss of consciousness** greater than 24 hours without return to pre-existing conscious level with patient surviving

√7ᵗʰ **S06.307 Unspecified focal traumatic brain injury with loss of consciousness of** any duration with death due to brain injury prior to regaining consciousness

√7ᵗʰ **S06.308 Unspecified focal traumatic brain injury with loss of consciousness of** any duration with death due to other cause prior to regaining consciousness

√7ᵗʰ **S06.309 Unspecified focal traumatic brain injury with loss of consciousness of unspecified duration**
     Unspecified focal traumatic brain injury NOS

√6ᵗʰ **S06.31 Contusion and laceration of** right cerebrum

√7ᵗʰ **S06.310 Contusion and laceration of right cerebrum** without loss of consciousness

√7ᵗʰ **S06.311 Contusion and laceration of right cerebrum with loss of consciousness of** 30 minutes or less

√7ᵗʰ **S06.312 Contusion and laceration of right cerebrum with loss of consciousness of** 31 minutes to 59 minutes

√7ᵗʰ **S06.313 Contusion and laceration of right cerebrum with loss of consciousness of** 1 hour to 5 hours 59 minutes

√7ᵗʰ **S06.314 Contusion and laceration of right cerebrum with loss of consciousness of** 6 hours to 24 hours

√7ᵗʰ **S06.315 Contusion and laceration of right cerebrum with loss of consciousness** greater than 24 hours with return to pre-existing conscious level

√7ᵗʰ **S06.316 Contusion and laceration of right cerebrum with loss of consciousness** greater than 24 hours without return to pre-existing conscious level with patient surviving

√7ᵗʰ **S06.317 Contusion and laceration of right cerebrum with loss of consciousness of** any duration with death due to brain injury prior to regaining consciousness

√7ᵗʰ **S06.318 Contusion and laceration of right cerebrum with loss of consciousness of** any duration with death due to other cause prior to regaining consciousness

√7ᵗʰ **S06.319 Contusion and laceration of right cerebrum with loss of consciousness of unspecified duration**
     Contusion and laceration of right cerebrum NOS

√6ᵗʰ **S06.32 Contusion and laceration of** left cerebrum

√7ᵗʰ **S06.320 Contusion and laceration of left cerebrum** without loss of consciousness

√7ᵗʰ **S06.321 Contusion and laceration of left cerebrum with loss of consciousness of** 30 minutes or less

√7ᵗʰ **S06.322 Contusion and laceration of left cerebrum with loss of consciousness of** 31 minutes to 59 minutes

√7ᵗʰ **S06.323 Contusion and laceration of left cerebrum with loss of consciousness of** 1 hour to 5 hours 59 minutes

√7ᵗʰ **S06.324 Contusion and laceration of left cerebrum with loss of consciousness of** 6 hours to 24 hours

√7ᵗʰ **S06.325 Contusion and laceration of left cerebrum with loss of consciousness** greater than 24 hours with return to pre-existing conscious level

√7ᵗʰ **S06.326 Contusion and laceration of left cerebrum with loss of consciousness** greater than 24 hours without return to pre-existing conscious level with patient surviving

√7ᵗʰ **S06.327 Contusion and laceration of left cerebrum with loss of consciousness of** any duration with death due to brain injury prior to regaining consciousness

√7ᵗʰ **S06.328 Contusion and laceration of left cerebrum with loss of consciousness of** any duration with death due to other cause prior to regaining consciousness

√7ᵗʰ **S06.329 Contusion and laceration of left cerebrum with loss of consciousness of unspecified duration**
     Contusion and laceration of left cerebrum NOS

√6ᵗʰ **S06.33 Contusion and laceration of** cerebrum, unspecified

√7ᵗʰ **S06.330 Contusion and laceration of cerebrum, unspecified,** without loss of consciousness

√7ᵗʰ **S06.331 Contusion and laceration of cerebrum, unspecified, with loss of consciousness of** 30 minutes or less

√7ᵗʰ **S06.332 Contusion and laceration of cerebrum, unspecified, with loss of consciousness of** 31 minutes to 59 minutes

√7ᵗʰ **S06.333 Contusion and laceration of cerebrum, unspecified, with loss of consciousness of** 1 hour to 5 hours 59 minutes

√7ᵗʰ **S06.334 Contusion and laceration of cerebrum, unspecified, with loss of consciousness of** 6 hours to 24 hours

√7ᵗʰ **S06.335 Contusion and laceration of cerebrum, unspecified, with loss of consciousness** greater than 24 hours with return to pre-existing conscious level

√7ᵗʰ **S06.336 Contusion and laceration of cerebrum, unspecified, with loss of consciousness** greater than 24 hours without return to pre-existing conscious level with patient surviving

√7ᵗʰ **S06.337 Contusion and laceration of cerebrum, unspecified, with loss of consciousness of** any duration with death due to brain injury prior to regaining consciousness

√7ᵗʰ **S06.338 Contusion and laceration of cerebrum, unspecified, with loss of consciousness of** any duration with death due to other cause prior to regaining consciousness

EXCLUDES 1 Not coded here   EXCLUDES 2 Not included here   N Newborn Age: 0   P Pediatric Age: 0-17   M Maternity Age: 12-55   A Adult Age: 15-124

810   ICD-10-CM Draft (2015)

☑7ᵗʰ **S06.339 Contusion and laceration of cerebrum, unspecified, with loss of consciousness of unspecified duration**
Contusion and laceration of cerebrum NOS

☑6ᵗʰ **S06.34 Traumatic hemorrhage of** right cerebrum
Traumatic intracerebral hemorrhage and hematoma of right cerebrum

☑7ᵗʰ **S06.340 Traumatic hemorrhage of right cerebrum** without loss of consciousness

☑7ᵗʰ **S06.341 Traumatic hemorrhage of right cerebrum with loss of consciousness of** 30 minutes or less

☑7ᵗʰ **S06.342 Traumatic hemorrhage of right cerebrum with loss of consciousness of** 31 minutes to 59 minutes

☑7ᵗʰ **S06.343 Traumatic hemorrhage of right cerebrum with loss of consciousness of** 1 hours to 5 hours 59 minutes

☑7ᵗʰ **S06.344 Traumatic hemorrhage of right cerebrum with loss of consciousness of** 6 hours to 24 hours

☑7ᵗʰ **S06.345 Traumatic hemorrhage of right cerebrum with loss of consciousness** greater than 24 hours with return to pre-existing conscious level

☑7ᵗʰ **S06.346 Traumatic hemorrhage of right cerebrum with loss of consciousness** greater than 24 hours without return to pre-existing conscious level with patient surviving

☑7ᵗʰ **S06.347 Traumatic hemorrhage of right cerebrum with loss of consciousness of** any duration with death due to brain injury prior to regaining consciousness

☑7ᵗʰ **S06.348 Traumatic hemorrhage of right cerebrum with loss of consciousness of** any duration with death due to **other** cause prior to regaining consciousness

☑7ᵗʰ **S06.349 Traumatic hemorrhage of right cerebrum with loss of consciousness of unspecified duration**
Traumatic hemorrhage of right cerebrum NOS

☑6ᵗʰ **S06.35 Traumatic hemorrhage of** left cerebrum
Traumatic intracerebral hemorrhage and hematoma of left cerebrum

☑7ᵗʰ **S06.350 Traumatic hemorrhage of left cerebrum** without loss of consciousness

☑7ᵗʰ **S06.351 Traumatic hemorrhage of left cerebrum with loss of consciousness of** 30 minutes or less

☑7ᵗʰ **S06.352 Traumatic hemorrhage of left cerebrum with loss of consciousness of** 31 minutes to 59 minutes

☑7ᵗʰ **S06.353 Traumatic hemorrhage of left cerebrum with loss of consciousness of** 1 hours to 5 hours 59 minutes

☑7ᵗʰ **S06.354 Traumatic hemorrhage of left cerebrum with loss of consciousness of** 6 hours to 24 hours

☑7ᵗʰ **S06.355 Traumatic hemorrhage of left cerebrum with loss of consciousness** greater than 24 hours with return to pre-existing conscious level

☑7ᵗʰ **S06.356 Traumatic hemorrhage of left cerebrum with loss of consciousness** greater than 24 hours without return to pre-existing conscious level with patient surviving

☑7ᵗʰ **S06.357 Traumatic hemorrhage of left cerebrum with loss of consciousness of** any duration with death due to brain injury prior to regaining consciousness

☑7ᵗʰ **S06.358 Traumatic hemorrhage of left cerebrum with loss of consciousness of** any duration with death due to **other** cause prior to regaining consciousness

☑7ᵗʰ **S06.359 Traumatic hemorrhage of left cerebrum with loss of consciousness of unspecified duration**
Traumatic hemorrhage of left cerebrum NOS

☑6ᵗʰ **S06.36 Traumatic hemorrhage of** cerebrum, unspecified
Traumatic intracerebral hemorrhage and hematoma, unspecified

☑7ᵗʰ **S06.360 Traumatic hemorrhage of cerebrum, unspecified,** without loss of consciousness

☑7ᵗʰ **S06.361 Traumatic hemorrhage of cerebrum, unspecified, with loss of consciousness of** 30 minutes or less

☑7ᵗʰ **S06.362 Traumatic hemorrhage of cerebrum, unspecified, with loss of consciousness of** 31 minutes to 59 minutes

☑7ᵗʰ **S06.363 Traumatic hemorrhage of cerebrum, unspecified, with loss of consciousness of** 1 hours to 5 hours 59 minutes

☑7ᵗʰ **S06.364 Traumatic hemorrhage of cerebrum, unspecified, with loss of consciousness of** 6 hours to 24 hours

☑7ᵗʰ **S06.365 Traumatic hemorrhage of cerebrum, unspecified, with loss of consciousness** greater than 24 hours with return to pre-existing conscious level

☑7ᵗʰ **S06.366 Traumatic hemorrhage of cerebrum, unspecified, with loss of consciousness** greater than 24 hours without return to pre-existing conscious level with patient surviving

☑7ᵗʰ **S06.367 Traumatic hemorrhage of cerebrum, unspecified, with loss of consciousness of** any duration with death due to brain injury prior to regaining consciousness

☑7ᵗʰ **S06.368 Traumatic hemorrhage of cerebrum, unspecified, with loss of consciousness of** any duration with death due to **other** cause prior to regaining consciousness

☑7ᵗʰ **S06.369 Traumatic hemorrhage of cerebrum, unspecified, with loss of consciousness of unspecified duration**
Traumatic hemorrhage of cerebrum NOS

☑6ᵗʰ **S06.37 Contusion, laceration, and hemorrhage of** cerebellum

☑7ᵗʰ **S06.370 Contusion, laceration, and hemorrhage of cerebellum** without loss of consciousness

☑7ᵗʰ **S06.371 Contusion, laceration, and hemorrhage of cerebellum with loss of consciousness of** 30 minutes or less

☑7ᵗʰ **S06.372 Contusion, laceration, and hemorrhage of cerebellum with loss of consciousness of** 31 minutes to 59 minutes

☑7ᵗʰ **S06.373 Contusion, laceration, and hemorrhage of cerebellum with loss of consciousness of** 1 hour to 5 hours 59 minutes

☑7ᵗʰ **S06.374 Contusion, laceration, and hemorrhage of cerebellum with loss of consciousness of** 6 hours to 24 hours

☑7ᵗʰ **S06.375 Contusion, laceration, and hemorrhage of cerebellum with loss of consciousness** greater than 24 hours with return to pre-existing conscious level

☑7ᵗʰ **S06.376 Contusion, laceration, and hemorrhage of cerebellum with loss of consciousness** greater than 24 hours without return to pre-existing conscious level with patient surviving

☑7ᵗʰ **S06.377 Contusion, laceration, and hemorrhage of cerebellum with loss of consciousness of** any duration with death due to brain injury prior to regaining consciousness

☑7ᵗʰ **S06.378 Contusion, laceration, and hemorrhage of cerebellum with loss of consciousness of** any duration with death due to **other** cause prior to regaining consciousness

☑7ᵗʰ **S06.379 Contusion, laceration, and hemorrhage of cerebellum with loss of consciousness of unspecified duration**
Contusion, laceration, and hemorrhage of cerebellum NOS

☑6ᵗʰ **S06.38 Contusion, laceration, and hemorrhage of** brainstem

☑7ᵗʰ **S06.380 Contusion, laceration, and hemorrhage of brainstem** without loss of consciousness

---

☑ Additional Character Required   ☑ˣ⁷ᵗʰ Xtension Alert   Unspecified Dx   Other Specified Dx   Manifestation   ►◄ Revised Text   ● New Code   ▲ Revised Code Title

√7th **S06.381** Contusion, laceration, and hemorrhage of brainstem with loss of consciousness of 30 minutes or less

√7th **S06.382** Contusion, laceration, and hemorrhage of brainstem with loss of consciousness of 31 minutes to 59 minutes

√7th **S06.383** Contusion, laceration, and hemorrhage of brainstem with loss of consciousness of 1 hour to 5 hours 59 minutes

√7th **S06.384** Contusion, laceration, and hemorrhage of brainstem with loss of consciousness of 6 hours to 24 hours

√7th **S06.385** Contusion, laceration, and hemorrhage of brainstem with loss of consciousness greater than 24 hours with return to pre-existing conscious level

√7th **S06.386** Contusion, laceration, and hemorrhage of brainstem with loss of consciousness greater than 24 hours without return to pre-existing conscious level with patient surviving

√7th **S06.387** Contusion, laceration, and hemorrhage of brainstem with loss of consciousness of any duration with death due to brain injury prior to regaining consciousness

√7th **S06.388** Contusion, laceration, and hemorrhage of brainstem with loss of consciousness of any duration with death due to other cause prior to regaining consciousness

√7th **S06.389** Contusion, laceration, and hemorrhage of brainstem with loss of consciousness of unspecified duration
Contusion, laceration, and hemorrhage of brainstem NOS

√5th **S06.4** **Epidural hemorrhage**
Extradural hemorrhage NOS
Extradural hemorrhage (traumatic)

√6th **S06.4X** **Epidural hemorrhage**

√7th **S06.4X0** Epidural hemorrhage without loss of consciousness

√7th **S06.4X1** Epidural hemorrhage with loss of consciousness of 30 minutes or less

√7th **S06.4X2** Epidural hemorrhage with loss of consciousness of 31 minutes to 59 minutes

√7th **S06.4X3** Epidural hemorrhage with loss of consciousness of 1 hour to 5 hours 59 minutes

√7th **S06.4X4** Epidural hemorrhage with loss of consciousness of 6 hours to 24 hours

√7th **S06.4X5** Epidural hemorrhage with loss of consciousness greater than 24 hours with return to pre-existing conscious level

√7th **S06.4X6** Epidural hemorrhage with loss of consciousness greater than 24 hours without return to pre-existing conscious level with patient surviving

√7th **S06.4X7** Epidural hemorrhage with loss of consciousness of any duration with death due to brain injury prior to regaining consciousness

√7th **S06.4X8** Epidural hemorrhage with loss of consciousness of any duration with death due to other causes prior to regaining consciousness

√7th **S06.4X9** Epidural hemorrhage with loss of consciousness of unspecified duration
Epidural hemorrhage NOS

√5th **S06.5** **Traumatic subdural hemorrhage**

√6th **S06.5X** **Traumatic subdural hemorrhage**

√7th **S06.5X0** Traumatic subdural hemorrhage without loss of consciousness

√7th **S06.5X1** Traumatic subdural hemorrhage with loss of consciousness of 30 minutes or less

√7th **S06.5X2** Traumatic subdural hemorrhage with loss of consciousness of 31 minutes to 59 minutes

√7th **S06.5X3** Traumatic subdural hemorrhage with loss of consciousness of 1 hour to 5 hours 59 minutes

√7th **S06.5X4** Traumatic subdural hemorrhage with loss of consciousness of 6 hours to 24 hours

√7th **S06.5X5** Traumatic subdural hemorrhage with loss of consciousness greater than 24 hours with return to pre-existing conscious level

√7th **S06.5X6** Traumatic subdural hemorrhage with loss of consciousness greater than 24 hours without return to pre-existing conscious level with patient surviving

√7th **S06.5X7** Traumatic subdural hemorrhage with loss of consciousness of any duration with death due to brain injury before regaining consciousness

√7th **S06.5X8** Traumatic subdural hemorrhage with loss of consciousness of any duration with death due to other cause before regaining consciousness

√7th **S06.5X9** Traumatic subdural hemorrhage with loss of consciousness of unspecified duration
Traumatic subdural hemorrhage NOS

√5th **S06.6** **Traumatic subarachnoid hemorrhage**

√6th **S06.6X** **Traumatic subarachnoid hemorrhage**

√7th **S06.6X0** Traumatic subarachnoid hemorrhage without loss of consciousness

√7th **S06.6X1** Traumatic subarachnoid hemorrhage with loss of consciousness of 30 minutes or less

√7th **S06.6X2** Traumatic subarachnoid hemorrhage with loss of consciousness of 31 minutes to 59 minutes

√7th **S06.6X3** Traumatic subarachnoid hemorrhage with loss of consciousness of 1 hour to 5 hours 59 minutes

√7th **S06.6X4** Traumatic subarachnoid hemorrhage with loss of consciousness of 6 hours to 24 hours

√7th **S06.6X5** Traumatic subarachnoid hemorrhage with loss of consciousness greater than 24 hours with return to pre-existing conscious level

√7th **S06.6X6** Traumatic subarachnoid hemorrhage with loss of consciousness greater than 24 hours without return to pre-existing conscious level with patient surviving

√7th **S06.6X7** Traumatic subarachnoid hemorrhage with loss of consciousness of any duration with death due to brain injury prior to regaining consciousness

√7th **S06.6X8** Traumatic subarachnoid hemorrhage with loss of consciousness of any duration with death due to other cause prior to regaining consciousness

√7th **S06.6X9** Traumatic subarachnoid hemorrhage with loss of consciousness of unspecified duration
Traumatic subarachnoid hemorrhage NOS

√5th **S06.8** **Other specified intracranial injuries**

√6th **S06.81** **Injury of right internal carotid artery, intracranial portion, not elsewhere classified**

√7th **S06.810** Injury of right internal carotid artery, intracranial portion, not elsewhere classified without loss of consciousness

√7th **S06.811** Injury of right internal carotid artery, intracranial portion, not elsewhere classified with loss of consciousness of 30 minutes or less

√7th **S06.812** Injury of right internal carotid artery, intracranial portion, not elsewhere classified with loss of consciousness of 31 minutes to 59 minutes

√7th **S06.813** Injury of right internal carotid artery, intracranial portion, not elsewhere classified with loss of consciousness of 1 hour to 5 hours 59 minutes

√7th **S06.814** Injury of right internal carotid artery, intracranial portion, not elsewhere classified with loss of consciousness of 6 hours to 24 hours

EXCLUDES 1 Not coded here   EXCLUDES 2 Not included here   N Newborn Age: 0   P Pediatric Age: 0-17   M Maternity Age: 12-55   A Adult Age: 15-124

812   ICD-10-CM Draft (2015)

√7ᵗʰ **S06.815** **Injury of right internal carotid artery, intracranial portion, not elsewhere classified with loss of consciousness** greater than 24 hours with return to pre-existing conscious level

√7ᵗʰ **S06.816** **Injury of right internal carotid artery, intracranial portion, not elsewhere classified with loss of consciousness** greater than 24 hours without return to pre-existing conscious level with patient surviving

√7ᵗʰ **S06.817** **Injury of right internal carotid artery, intracranial portion, not elsewhere classified with loss of consciousness of** any duration with death due to brain injury prior to regaining consciousness

√7ᵗʰ **S06.818** **Injury of right internal carotid artery, intracranial portion, not elsewhere classified with loss of consciousness of** any duration with death due to **other** cause prior to regaining consciousness

√7ᵗʰ **S06.819** **Injury of right internal carotid artery, intracranial portion, not elsewhere classified with loss of consciousness of unspecified duration**
    Injury of right internal carotid artery, intracranial portion, not elsewhere classified NOS

√6ᵗʰ **S06.82** **Injury of** left internal carotid artery, **intracranial portion, not elsewhere classified**

√7ᵗʰ **S06.820** **Injury of left internal carotid artery, intracranial portion, not elsewhere classified** without loss of consciousness

√7ᵗʰ **S06.821** **Injury of left internal carotid artery, intracranial portion, not elsewhere classified with loss of consciousness of** 30 minutes or less

√7ᵗʰ **S06.822** **Injury of left internal carotid artery, intracranial portion, not elsewhere classified with loss of consciousness of** 31 minutes to 59 minutes

√7ᵗʰ **S06.823** **Injury of left internal carotid artery, intracranial portion, not elsewhere classified with loss of consciousness of** 1 hour to 5 hours 59 minutes

√7ᵗʰ **S06.824** **Injury of left internal carotid artery, intracranial portion, not elsewhere classified with loss of consciousness of** 6 hours to 24 hours

√7ᵗʰ **S06.825** **Injury of left internal carotid artery, intracranial portion, not elsewhere classified with loss of consciousness** greater than 24 hours with return to pre-existing conscious level

√7ᵗʰ **S06.826** **Injury of left internal carotid artery, intracranial portion, not elsewhere classified with loss of consciousness** greater than 24 hours without return to pre-existing conscious level with patient surviving

√7ᵗʰ **S06.827** **Injury of left internal carotid artery, intracranial portion, not elsewhere classified with loss of consciousness of** any duration with death due to brain injury prior to regaining consciousness

√7ᵗʰ **S06.828** **Injury of left internal carotid artery, intracranial portion, not elsewhere classified with loss of consciousness of** any duration with death due to **other** cause prior to regaining consciousness

√7ᵗʰ **S06.829** **Injury of left internal carotid artery, intracranial portion, not elsewhere classified with loss of consciousness of unspecified duration**
    Injury of left internal carotid artery, intracranial portion, not elsewhere classified NOS

√6ᵗʰ **S06.89** **Other** specified intracranial injury

√7ᵗʰ **S06.890** **Other specified intracranial injury** without loss of consciousness

√7ᵗʰ **S06.891** **Other specified intracranial injury with loss of consciousness of** 30 minutes or less

√7ᵗʰ **S06.892** **Other specified intracranial injury with loss of consciousness of** 31 minutes to 59 minutes

√7ᵗʰ **S06.893** **Other specified intracranial injury with loss of consciousness of** 1 hour to 5 hours 59 minutes

√7ᵗʰ **S06.894** **Other specified intracranial injury with loss of consciousness of** 6 hours to 24 hours

√7ᵗʰ **S06.895** **Other specified intracranial injury with loss of consciousness** greater than 24 hours with return to pre-existing conscious level

√7ᵗʰ **S06.896** **Other specified intracranial injury with loss of consciousness** greater than 24 hours without return to pre-existing conscious level with patient surviving

√7ᵗʰ **S06.897** **Other specified intracranial injury with loss of consciousness of** any duration with death due to brain injury prior to regaining consciousness

√7ᵗʰ **S06.898** **Other specified intracranial injury with loss of consciousness of** any duration with death due to **other** cause prior to regaining consciousness

√7ᵗʰ **S06.899** **Other specified intracranial injury with loss of consciousness of unspecified duration**

√5ᵗʰ **S06.9** **Unspecified intracranial injury**
    Brain injury NOS
    Head injury NOS with loss of consciousness
    EXCLUDES 1   head injury NOS (S09.90)

√6ᵗʰ **S06.9X** Unspecified intracranial injury

√7ᵗʰ **S06.9X0** **Unspecified intracranial injury** without loss of consciousness

√7ᵗʰ **S06.9X1** **Unspecified intracranial injury with loss of consciousness of** 30 minutes or less

√7ᵗʰ **S06.9X2** **Unspecified intracranial injury with loss of consciousness of** 31 minutes to 59 minutes

√7ᵗʰ **S06.9X3** **Unspecified intracranial injury with loss of consciousness of** 1 hour to 5 hours 59 minutes

√7ᵗʰ **S06.9X4** **Unspecified intracranial injury with loss of consciousness of** 6 hours to 24 hours

√7ᵗʰ **S06.9X5** **Unspecified intracranial injury with loss of consciousness** greater than 24 hours with return to pre-existing conscious level

√7ᵗʰ **S06.9X6** **Unspecified intracranial injury with loss of consciousness** greater than 24 hours without return to pre-existing conscious level with patient surviving

√7ᵗʰ **S06.9X7** **Unspecified intracranial injury with loss of consciousness of** any duration with death due to brain injury prior to regaining consciousness

√7ᵗʰ **S06.9X8** **Unspecified intracranial injury with loss of consciousness of** any duration with death due to **other** cause prior to regaining consciousness

√7ᵗʰ **S06.9X9** **Unspecified intracranial injury with loss of consciousness of unspecified duration**

√4ᵗʰ **S07** **Crushing injury of head**
    Use additional code for all associated injuries, such as:
      intracranial injuries (S06.-)
      skull fractures (S02.-)

> The appropriate 7th character is to be added to each code from category S07.
> A   initial encounter
> D   subsequent encounter
> S   sequela

√x7ᵗʰ **S07.0** **Crushing injury of** face

√x7ᵗʰ **S07.1** **Crushing injury of** skull

√x7ᵗʰ **S07.8** **Crushing injury of other parts of head**

√x7ᵗʰ **S07.9** **Crushing injury of** head, **part unspecified**

✓ Additional Character Required   √x7ᵗʰ Xtension Alert   Unspecified Dx   Other Specified Dx   Manifestation   ►◄ Revised Text   ● New Code   ▲ Revised Code Title

Injury, Poisoning and Certain Other Consequences of External Causes   S08–S10.95

✓4th S08   Avulsion and traumatic amputation of part of head

> **NOTE**   An amputation not identified as partial or complete should be coded to complete

> The appropriate 7th character is to be added to each code from category S08.
> A   initial encounter
> D   subsequent encounter
> S   sequela

✓x7th **S08.0**   Avulsion of scalp

✓5th **S08.1**   Traumatic amputation of ear

     ✓6th **S08.11**   Complete traumatic amputation of ear

       ✓7th **S08.111**   Complete traumatic amputation of right ear

       ✓7th **S08.112**   Complete traumatic amputation of left ear

       ✓7th **S08.119**   Complete traumatic amputation of unspecified ear

     ✓6th **S08.12**   Partial traumatic amputation of ear

       ✓7th **S08.121**   Partial traumatic amputation of right ear

       ✓7th **S08.122**   Partial traumatic amputation of left ear

       ✓7th **S08.129**   Partial traumatic amputation of unspecified ear

✓5th **S08.8**   Traumatic amputation of other parts of head

     ✓6th **S08.81**   Traumatic amputation of nose

       ✓7th **S08.811**   Complete traumatic amputation of nose

       ✓7th **S08.812**   Partial traumatic amputation of nose

     ✓x7th **S08.89**   Traumatic amputation of other parts of head

✓4th S09   Other and unspecified injuries of head

> The appropriate 7th character is to be added to each code from category S09.
> A   initial encounter
> D   subsequent encounter
> S   sequela

✓x7th **S09.0**   Injury of blood vessels of head, not elsewhere classified

> **EXCLUDES 1**   injury of cerebral blood vessels (S06.-)
> injury of precerebral blood vessels (S15.-)

✓5th **S09.1**   Injury of muscle and tendon of head

     Code also any associated open wound (S01.-)

     EXCLUDES 2   sprain to joints and ligament of head (S03.9)

     ✓x7th **S09.10**   Unspecified injury of muscle and tendon of head
       Injury of muscle and tendon of head NOS

     ✓x7th **S09.11**   Strain of muscle and tendon of head

     ✓x7th **S09.12**   Laceration of muscle and tendon of head

     ✓x7th **S09.19**   Other specified injury of muscle and tendon of head

✓5th **S09.2**   Traumatic rupture of ear drum

     EXCLUDES 1   traumatic rupture of ear drum due to blast injury (S09.31-)

     ✓x7th **S09.20**   Traumatic rupture of unspecified ear drum

     ✓x7th **S09.21**   Traumatic rupture of right ear drum

     ✓x7th **S09.22**   Traumatic rupture of left ear drum

✓5th **S09.3**   Other specified and unspecified injury of middle and inner ear

     EXCLUDES 1   injury to ear NOS (S09.91-)
     EXCLUDES 2   injury to external ear (S00.4-, S01.3-, S08.1-)

     ✓6th **S09.30**   Unspecified injury of middle and inner ear

       ✓7th **S09.301**   Unspecified injury of right middle and inner ear

       ✓7th **S09.302**   Unspecified injury of left middle and inner ear

       ✓7th **S09.309**   Unspecified injury of unspecified middle and inner ear

     ✓6th **S09.31**   Primary blast injury of ear
       Blast injury of ear NOS

       ✓7th **S09.311**   Primary blast injury of right ear

       ✓7th **S09.312**   Primary blast injury of left ear

       ✓7th **S09.313**   Primary blast injury of ear, bilateral

       ✓7th **S09.319**   Primary blast injury of unspecified ear

     ✓6th **S09.39**   Other specified injury of middle and inner ear
       Secondary blast injury to ear

       ✓7th **S09.391**   Other specified injury of right middle and inner ear

       ✓7th **S09.392**   Other specified injury of left middle and inner ear

       ✓7th **S09.399**   Other specified injury of unspecified middle and inner ear

✓x7th **S09.8**   Other specified injuries of head

✓5th **S09.9**   Unspecified injury of face and head

     ✓x7th **S09.90**   Unspecified injury of head
       Head injury NOS

       EXCLUDES 1   brain injury NOS (S06.9-)
       head injury NOS with loss of consciousness (S06.9-)
       intracranial injury NOS (S06.9-)

     ✓x7th **S09.91**   Unspecified injury of ear
       Injury of ear NOS

     ✓x7th **S09.92**   Unspecified injury of nose
       Injury of nose NOS

     ✓x7th **S09.93**   Unspecified injury of face
       Injury of face NOS

Injuries to the neck (S10-S19)

> **INCLUDES**   injuries of nape
> injuries of supraclavicular region
> injuries of throat
> **EXCLUDES 2**   burns and corrosions (T20-T32)
> effects of foreign body in esophagus (T18.1)
> effects of foreign body in larynx (T17.3)
> effects of foreign body in pharynx (T17.2)
> effects of foreign body in trachea (T17.4)
> frostbite (T33-T34)
> insect bite or sting, venomous (T63.4)

✓4th S10   Superficial injury of neck

> The appropriate 7th character is to be added to each code from category S10.
> A   initial encounter
> D   subsequent encounter
> S   sequela

✓x7th **S10.0**   Contusion of throat
     Contusion of cervical esophagus
     Contusion of larynx
     Contusion of pharynx
     Contusion of trachea

✓5th **S10.1**   Other and unspecified superficial injuries of throat

     ✓x7th **S10.10**   Unspecified superficial injuries of throat

     ✓x7th **S10.11**   Abrasion of throat

     ✓x7th **S10.12**   Blister (nonthermal) of throat

     ✓x7th **S10.14**   External constriction of part of throat

     ✓x7th **S10.15**   Superficial foreign body of throat
       Splinter in the throat

     ✓x7th **S10.16**   Insect bite (nonvenomous) of throat

     ✓x7th **S10.17**   Other superficial bite of throat
       EXCLUDES 1   open bite of throat (S11.85)

✓5th **S10.8**   Superficial injury of other specified parts of neck

     ✓x7th **S10.80**   Unspecified superficial injury of other specified part of neck

     ✓x7th **S10.81**   Abrasion of other specified part of neck

     ✓x7th **S10.82**   Blister (nonthermal) of other specified part of neck

     ✓x7th **S10.83**   Contusion of other specified part of neck

     ✓x7th **S10.84**   External constriction of other specified part of neck

     ✓x7th **S10.85**   Superficial foreign body of other specified part of neck
       Splinter in other specified part of neck

     ✓x7th **S10.86**   Insect bite of other specified part of neck

     ✓x7th **S10.87**   Other superficial bite of other specified part of neck
       EXCLUDES 1   open bite of other specified parts of neck (S11.85)

✓5th **S10.9**   Superficial injury of unspecified part of neck

     ✓x7th **S10.90**   Unspecified superficial injury of unspecified part of neck

     ✓x7th **S10.91**   Abrasion of unspecified part of neck

     ✓x7th **S10.92**   Blister (nonthermal) of unspecified part of neck

     ✓x7th **S10.93**   Contusion of unspecified part of neck

     ✓x7th **S10.94**   External constriction of unspecified part of neck

     ✓x7th **S10.95**   Superficial foreign body of unspecified part of neck

EXCLUDES 1 Not coded here   **EXCLUDES 2** Not included here   N Newborn Age: 0   P Pediatric Age: 0-17   M Maternity Age: 12-55   A Adult Age: 15-124

814   ICD-10-CM Draft (2015)

√x7ᵗʰ **S10.96** Insect bite of unspecified part of neck

√x7ᵗʰ **S10.97** **Other superficial** bite of unspecified part of neck

√4ᵗʰ **S11** **Open wound of neck**

Code also any associated:
spinal cord injury (S14.0, S14.1-)
wound infection

EXCLUDES 2   open fracture of vertebra (S12- with 7th character B)

The appropriate 7th character is to be added to each code from category S11.
A   initial encounter
D   subsequent encounter
S   sequela

√5ᵗʰ **S11.0** **Open wound of larynx and trachea**

√6ᵗʰ **S11.01** **Open wound of** larynx

EXCLUDES 2   open wound of vocal cord (S11.03)

√7ᵗʰ **S11.011** Laceration without foreign body of larynx

√7ᵗʰ **S11.012** Laceration with foreign body of larynx

√7ᵗʰ **S11.013** Puncture wound without foreign body of larynx

√7ᵗʰ **S11.014** Puncture wound with foreign body of larynx

√7ᵗʰ **S11.015** Open bite of larynx
Bite of larynx NOS

√7ᵗʰ **S11.019** **Unspecified open wound of larynx**

√6ᵗʰ **S11.02** **Open wound of** trachea
Open wound of cervical trachea
Open wound of trachea NOS

EXCLUDES 2   open wound of thoracic trachea (S27.5-)

√7ᵗʰ **S11.021** Laceration without foreign body of trachea

√7ᵗʰ **S11.022** Laceration with foreign body of trachea

√7ᵗʰ **S11.023** Puncture wound without foreign body of trachea

√7ᵗʰ **S11.024** Puncture wound with foreign body of trachea

√7ᵗʰ **S11.025** Open bite of trachea
Bite of trachea NOS

√7ᵗʰ **S11.029** **Unspecified open wound of trachea**

√6ᵗʰ **S11.03** **Open wound of** vocal cord

√7ᵗʰ **S11.031** Laceration without foreign body of vocal cord

√7ᵗʰ **S11.032** Laceration with foreign body of vocal cord

√7ᵗʰ **S11.033** Puncture wound without foreign body of vocal cord

√7ᵗʰ **S11.034** Puncture wound with foreign body of vocal cord

√7ᵗʰ **S11.035** Open bite of vocal cord
Bite of vocal cord NOS

√7ᵗʰ **S11.039** **Unspecified open wound of vocal cord**

√5ᵗʰ **S11.1** **Open wound of** thyroid gland

√x7ᵗʰ **S11.10** **Unspecified open wound of thyroid gland**

√x7ᵗʰ **S11.11** Laceration without foreign body of thyroid gland

√x7ᵗʰ **S11.12** Laceration with foreign body of thyroid gland

√x7ᵗʰ **S11.13** Puncture wound without foreign body of thyroid gland

√x7ᵗʰ **S11.14** Puncture wound with foreign body of thyroid gland

√x7ᵗʰ **S11.15** Open bite of thyroid gland
Bite of thyroid gland NOS

√5ᵗʰ **S11.2** **Open wound of** pharynx and cervical esophagus

EXCLUDES 1   open wound of esophagus NOS (S27.8-)

√x7ᵗʰ **S11.20** **Unspecified open wound of pharynx and cervical esophagus**

√x7ᵗʰ **S11.21** Laceration without foreign body of pharynx and cervical esophagus

√x7ᵗʰ **S11.22** Laceration with foreign body of pharynx and cervical esophagus

√x7ᵗʰ **S11.23** Puncture wound without foreign body of pharynx and cervical esophagus

√x7ᵗʰ **S11.24** Puncture wound with foreign body of pharynx and cervical esophagus

√x7ᵗʰ **S11.25** Open bite of pharynx and cervical esophagus
Bite of pharynx and cervical esophagus NOS

√5ᵗʰ **S11.8** **Open wound of** other specified parts of neck

√x7ᵗʰ **S11.80** **Unspecified open wound of other specified part of neck**

√x7ᵗʰ **S11.81** Laceration without foreign body of other specified part of neck

√x7ᵗʰ **S11.82** Laceration with foreign body of other specified part of neck

√x7ᵗʰ **S11.83** Puncture wound without foreign body of other specified part of neck

√x7ᵗʰ **S11.84** Puncture wound with foreign body of other specified part of neck

√x7ᵗʰ **S11.85** Open bite of other specified part of neck
Bite of other specified part of neck NOS

EXCLUDES 1   superficial bite of other specified part of neck (S10.87)

√x7ᵗʰ **S11.89** **Other open wound of other specified part of neck**

√5ᵗʰ **S11.9** **Open wound of** unspecified part of neck

√x7ᵗʰ **S11.90** **Unspecified open wound of unspecified part of neck**

√x7ᵗʰ **S11.91** Laceration without foreign body of unspecified part of neck

√x7ᵗʰ **S11.92** Laceration with foreign body of unspecified part of neck

√x7ᵗʰ **S11.93** Puncture wound without foreign body of unspecified part of neck

√x7ᵗʰ **S11.94** Puncture wound with foreign body of unspecified part of neck

√x7ᵗʰ **S11.95** Open bite of unspecified part of neck
Bite of neck NOS

EXCLUDES 1   superficial bite of neck (S10.97)

√4ᵗʰ **S12** **Fracture of cervical vertebra and other parts of neck**

NOTE   A fracture not indicated as nondisplaced or displaced should be coded to displaced.
A fracture not indicated as open or closed should be coded to closed.

INCLUDES   fracture of cervical neural arch
fracture of cervical spine
fracture of cervical spinous process
fracture of cervical transverse process
fracture of cervical vertebral arch
fracture of neck

Code first any associated cervical spinal cord injury (S14.0, S14.1-)

The appropriate 7th character is to be added to all codes from subcategories S12.0-S12.6.
A   initial encounter for closed fracture
B   initial encounter for open fracture
D   subsequent encounter for fracture with routine healing
G   subsequent encounter for fracture with delayed healing
K   subsequent encounter for fracture with nonunion
S   sequela

√5ᵗʰ **S12.0** **Fracture of** first cervical vertebra
Atlas

√6ᵗʰ **S12.00** **Unspecified fracture of first cervical vertebra**

√7ᵗʰ **S12.000** **Unspecified** displaced **fracture of first cervical vertebra**

√7ᵗʰ **S12.001** **Unspecified** nondisplaced **fracture of first cervical vertebra**

√x7ᵗʰ **S12.01** Stable burst **fracture of first cervical vertebra**

√x7ᵗʰ **S12.02** Unstable burst **fracture of first cervical vertebra**

√6ᵗʰ **S12.03** Posterior arch **fracture of first cervical vertebra**

√7ᵗʰ **S12.030** Displaced posterior arch fracture of first cervical vertebra

√7ᵗʰ **S12.031** Nondisplaced posterior arch fracture of first cervical vertebra

√6ᵗʰ **S12.04** Lateral mass **fracture of first cervical vertebra**

√7ᵗʰ **S12.040** Displaced lateral mass fracture of first cervical vertebra

√7ᵗʰ **S12.041** Nondisplaced lateral mass fracture of first cervical vertebra

√6ᵗʰ **S12.09** Other **fracture of first cervical vertebra**

√7ᵗʰ **S12.090** **Other** displaced **fracture of first cervical vertebra**

√7ᵗʰ **S12.091** **Other** nondisplaced **fracture of first cervical vertebra**

✔ Additional Character Required   √x7ᵗʰ Xtension Alert   Unspecified Dx   Other Specified Dx   Manifestation   ►◄ Revised Text   ● New Code   ▲ Revised Code Title

ICD-10-CM Draft (2015)   **815**

Injury, Poisoning and Certain Other Consequences of External Causes

S12.1–S12.590

√5ᵗʰ **S12.1** Fracture of second cervical vertebra
     Axis

   √6ᵗʰ **S12.10** Unspecified fracture of second cervical vertebra

     √7ᵗʰ **S12.100** Unspecified displaced fracture of second cervical vertebra

     √7ᵗʰ **S12.101** Unspecified nondisplaced fracture of second cervical vertebra

   √6ᵗʰ **S12.11** Type II dens fracture

     √7ᵗʰ **S12.110** Anterior displaced Type II dens fracture

     √7ᵗʰ **S12.111** Posterior displaced Type II dens fracture

     √7ᵗʰ **S12.112** Nondisplaced Type II dens fracture

   √6ᵗʰ **S12.12** Other dens fracture

     √7ᵗʰ **S12.120** Other displaced dens fracture

     √7ᵗʰ **S12.121** Other nondisplaced dens fracture

   √6ᵗʰ **S12.13** Unspecified traumatic spondylolisthesis of second cervical vertebra

     √7ᵗʰ **S12.130** Unspecified traumatic displaced spondylolisthesis of second cervical vertebra

     √7ᵗʰ **S12.131** Unspecified traumatic nondisplaced spondylolisthesis of second cervical vertebra

   √x7ᵗʰ **S12.14** Type III traumatic spondylolisthesis of second cervical vertebra

   √6ᵗʰ **S12.15** Other traumatic spondylolisthesis of second cervical vertebra

     √7ᵗʰ **S12.150** Other traumatic displaced spondylolisthesis of second cervical vertebra

     √7ᵗʰ **S12.151** Other traumatic nondisplaced spondylolisthesis of second cervical vertebra

   √6ᵗʰ **S12.19** Other fracture of second cervical vertebra

     √7ᵗʰ **S12.190** Other displaced fracture of second cervical vertebra

     √7ᵗʰ **S12.191** Other nondisplaced fracture of second cervical vertebra

√5ᵗʰ **S12.2** Fracture of third cervical vertebra

   √6ᵗʰ **S12.20** Unspecified fracture of third cervical vertebra

     √7ᵗʰ **S12.200** Unspecified displaced fracture of third cervical vertebra

     √7ᵗʰ **S12.201** Unspecified nondisplaced fracture of third cervical vertebra

   √6ᵗʰ **S12.23** Unspecified traumatic spondylolisthesis of third cervical vertebra

     √7ᵗʰ **S12.230** Unspecified traumatic displaced spondylolisthesis of third cervical vertebra

     √7ᵗʰ **S12.231** Unspecified traumatic nondisplaced spondylolisthesis of third cervical vertebra

   √x7ᵗʰ **S12.24** Type III traumatic spondylolisthesis of third cervical vertebra

   √6ᵗʰ **S12.25** Other traumatic spondylolisthesis of third cervical vertebra

     √7ᵗʰ **S12.250** Other traumatic displaced spondylolisthesis of third cervical vertebra

     √7ᵗʰ **S12.251** Other traumatic nondisplaced spondylolisthesis of third cervical vertebra

   √6ᵗʰ **S12.29** Other fracture of third cervical vertebra

     √7ᵗʰ **S12.290** Other displaced fracture of third cervical vertebra

     √7ᵗʰ **S12.291** Other nondisplaced fracture of third cervical vertebra

√5ᵗʰ **S12.3** Fracture of fourth cervical vertebra

   √6ᵗʰ **S12.30** Unspecified fracture of fourth cervical vertebra

     √7ᵗʰ **S12.300** Unspecified displaced fracture of fourth cervical vertebra

     √7ᵗʰ **S12.301** Unspecified nondisplaced fracture of fourth cervical vertebra

   √6ᵗʰ **S12.33** Unspecified traumatic spondylolisthesis of fourth cervical vertebra

     √7ᵗʰ **S12.330** Unspecified traumatic displaced spondylolisthesis of fourth cervical vertebra

     √7ᵗʰ **S12.331** Unspecified traumatic nondisplaced spondylolisthesis of fourth cervical vertebra

   √x7ᵗʰ **S12.34** Type III traumatic spondylolisthesis of fourth cervical vertebra

   √6ᵗʰ **S12.35** Other traumatic spondylolisthesis of fourth cervical vertebra

     √7ᵗʰ **S12.350** Other traumatic displaced spondylolisthesis of fourth cervical vertebra

     √7ᵗʰ **S12.351** Other traumatic nondisplaced spondylolisthesis of fourth cervical vertebra

   √6ᵗʰ **S12.39** Other fracture of fourth cervical vertebra

     √7ᵗʰ **S12.390** Other displaced fracture of fourth cervical vertebra

     √7ᵗʰ **S12.391** Other nondisplaced fracture of fourth cervical vertebra

√5ᵗʰ **S12.4** Fracture of fifth cervical vertebra

   √6ᵗʰ **S12.40** Unspecified fracture of fifth cervical vertebra

     √7ᵗʰ **S12.400** Unspecified displaced fracture of fifth cervical vertebra

     √7ᵗʰ **S12.401** Unspecified nondisplaced fracture of fifth cervical vertebra

   √6ᵗʰ **S12.43** Unspecified traumatic spondylolisthesis of fifth cervical vertebra

     √7ᵗʰ **S12.430** Unspecified traumatic displaced spondylolisthesis of fifth cervical vertebra

     √7ᵗʰ **S12.431** Unspecified traumatic nondisplaced spondylolisthesis of fifth cervical vertebra

   √x7ᵗʰ **S12.44** Type III traumatic spondylolisthesis of fifth cervical vertebra

   √6ᵗʰ **S12.45** Other traumatic spondylolisthesis of fifth cervical vertebra

     √7ᵗʰ **S12.450** Other traumatic displaced spondylolisthesis of fifth cervical vertebra

     √7ᵗʰ **S12.451** Other traumatic nondisplaced spondylolisthesis of fifth cervical vertebra

   √6ᵗʰ **S12.49** Other fracture of fifth cervical vertebra

     √7ᵗʰ **S12.490** Other displaced fracture of fifth cervical vertebra

     √7ᵗʰ **S12.491** Other nondisplaced fracture of fifth cervical vertebra

√5ᵗʰ **S12.5** Fracture of sixth cervical vertebra

   √6ᵗʰ **S12.50** Unspecified fracture of sixth cervical vertebra

     √7ᵗʰ **S12.500** Unspecified displaced fracture of sixth cervical vertebra

     √7ᵗʰ **S12.501** Unspecified nondisplaced fracture of sixth cervical vertebra

   √6ᵗʰ **S12.53** Unspecified traumatic spondylolisthesis of sixth cervical vertebra

     √7ᵗʰ **S12.530** Unspecified traumatic displaced spondylolisthesis of sixth cervical vertebra

     √7ᵗʰ **S12.531** Unspecified traumatic nondisplaced spondylolisthesis of sixth cervical vertebra

   √x7ᵗʰ **S12.54** Type III traumatic spondylolisthesis of sixth cervical vertebra

   √6ᵗʰ **S12.55** Other traumatic spondylolisthesis of sixth cervical vertebra

     √7ᵗʰ **S12.550** Other traumatic displaced spondylolisthesis of sixth cervical vertebra

     √7ᵗʰ **S12.551** Other traumatic nondisplaced spondylolisthesis of sixth cervical vertebra

   √6ᵗʰ **S12.59** Other fracture of sixth cervical vertebra

     √7ᵗʰ **S12.590** Other displaced fracture of sixth cervical vertebra

---

EXCLUDES 1 Not coded here   **EXCLUDES 2** Not included here   N Newborn Age: 0   P Pediatric Age: 0–17   M Maternity Age: 12–55   A Adult Age: 15–124

√7ᵗʰ S12.591 **Other** nondisplaced **fracture of sixth cervical vertebra**

√5ᵗʰ S12.6 **Fracture of** seventh **cervical vertebra**

√6ᵗʰ S12.60 Unspecified **fracture of seventh cervical vertebra**

√7ᵗʰ S12.600 **Unspecified** displaced **fracture of seventh cervical vertebra**

√7ᵗʰ S12.601 **Unspecified** nondisplaced **fracture of seventh cervical vertebra**

√6ᵗʰ S12.63 Unspecified **traumatic** spondylolisthesis **of seventh cervical vertebra**

√7ᵗʰ S12.630 **Unspecified traumatic** displaced **spondylolisthesis of seventh cervical vertebra**

√7ᵗʰ S12.631 **Unspecified traumatic** nondisplaced **spondylolisthesis of seventh cervical vertebra**

√x7ᵗʰ S12.64 Type III **traumatic** spondylolisthesis **of seventh cervical vertebra**

√6ᵗʰ S12.65 Other **traumatic** spondylolisthesis **of seventh cervical vertebra**

√7ᵗʰ S12.650 **Other traumatic** displaced **spondylolisthesis of seventh cervical vertebra**

√7ᵗʰ S12.651 **Other traumatic** nondisplaced **spondylolisthesis of seventh cervical vertebra**

√6ᵗʰ S12.69 Other **fracture of seventh cervical vertebra**

√7ᵗʰ S12.690 **Other** displaced **fracture of seventh cervical vertebra**

√7ᵗʰ S12.691 **Other** nondisplaced **fracture of seventh cervical vertebra**

√x S12.8 **Fracture of other parts of neck**
Hyoid bone
Larynx
Thyroid cartilage
Trachea

The appropriate 7th character is to be added to code S12.8.
A   initial encounter
D   subsequent encounter
S   sequela

√x7ᵗʰ S12.9 **Fracture of neck, unspecified**
Fracture of cervical spine NOS
Fracture of cervical vertebra NOS
Fracture of neck NOS

The appropriate 7th character is to be added to code S12.9.
A   initial encounter
D   subsequent encounter
S   sequela

√4ᵗʰ **S13   Dislocation and sprain of joints and ligaments at neck level**
INCLUDES   avulsion of joint or ligament at neck level
laceration of cartilage, joint or ligament at neck level
sprain of cartilage, joint or ligament at neck level
traumatic hemarthrosis of joint or ligament at neck level
traumatic rupture of joint or ligament at neck level
traumatic subluxation of joint or ligament at neck level
traumatic tear of joint or ligament at neck level

Code also any associated open wound
EXCLUDES 2   strain of muscle or tendon at neck level (S16.1)

The appropriate 7th character is to be added to each code from category S13.
A   initial encounter
D   subsequent encounter
S   sequela

√x7ᵗʰ S13.0 **Traumatic rupture of cervical intervertebral disc**
EXCLUDES 1   rupture or displacement (nontraumatic) of cervical intervertebral disc NOS (M50.-)

√5ᵗʰ S13.1 **Subluxation and dislocation of cervical vertebrae**
Code also any associated:
open wound of neck (S11.-)
spinal cord injury (S14.1-)
EXCLUDES 2   fracture of cervical vertebrae (S12.0--S12.3-)

√6ᵗʰ S13.10 **Subluxation and dislocation of** unspecified **cervical vertebrae**

√7ᵗʰ S13.100 Subluxation **of unspecified cervical vertebrae**

√7ᵗʰ S13.101 Dislocation **of unspecified cervical vertebrae**

√6ᵗʰ S13.11 **Subluxation and dislocation of** C0/C1 **cervical vertebrae**
Subluxation and dislocation of atlantooccipital joint
Subluxation and dislocation of atloidooccipital joint
Subluxation and dislocation of occipitoatloid joint

√7ᵗʰ S13.110 Subluxation **of C0/C1 cervical vertebrae**

√7ᵗʰ S13.111 Dislocation **of C0/C1 cervical vertebrae**

√6ᵗʰ S13.12 **Subluxation and dislocation of** C1/C2 **cervical vertebrae**
Subluxation and dislocation of atlantoaxial joint

√7ᵗʰ S13.120 Subluxation **of C1/C2 cervical vertebrae**

√7ᵗʰ S13.121 Dislocation **of C1/C2 cervical vertebrae**

√6ᵗʰ S13.13 **Subluxation and dislocation of** C2/C3 **cervical vertebrae**

√7ᵗʰ S13.130 Subluxation **of C2/C3 cervical vertebrae**

√7ᵗʰ S13.131 Dislocation **of C2/C3 cervical vertebrae**

√6ᵗʰ S13.14 **Subluxation and dislocation of** C3/C4 **cervical vertebrae**

√7ᵗʰ S13.140 Subluxation **of C3/C4 cervical vertebrae**

√7ᵗʰ S13.141 Dislocation **of C3/C4 cervical vertebrae**

√6ᵗʰ S13.15 **Subluxation and dislocation of** C4/C5 **cervical vertebrae**

√7ᵗʰ S13.150 Subluxation **of C4/C5 cervical vertebrae**

√7ᵗʰ S13.151 Dislocation **of C4/C5 cervical vertebrae**

√6ᵗʰ S13.16 **Subluxation and dislocation of** C5/C6 **cervical vertebrae**

√7ᵗʰ S13.160 Subluxation **of C5/C6 cervical vertebrae**

√7ᵗʰ S13.161 Dislocation **of C5/C6 cervical vertebrae**

√6ᵗʰ S13.17 **Subluxation and dislocation of** C6/C7 **cervical vertebrae**

√7ᵗʰ S13.170 Subluxation **of C6/C7 cervical vertebrae**

√7ᵗʰ S13.171 Dislocation **of C6/C7 cervical vertebrae**

√6ᵗʰ S13.18 **Subluxation and dislocation of** C7/T1 **cervical vertebrae**

√7ᵗʰ S13.180 Subluxation **of C7/T1 cervical vertebrae**

√7ᵗʰ S13.181 Dislocation **of C7/T1 cervical vertebrae**

√5ᵗʰ S13.2 **Dislocation of other and unspecified parts of neck**

√x7ᵗʰ S13.20 **Dislocation of unspecified parts of neck**

√x7ᵗʰ S13.29 **Dislocation of other parts of neck**

√x7ᵗʰ S13.4 **Sprain of ligaments of cervical spine**
Sprain of anterior longitudinal (ligament), cervical
Sprain of atlanto-axial (joints)
Sprain of atlanto-occipital (joints)
Whiplash injury of cervical spine

√x7ᵗʰ S13.5 **Sprain of thyroid region**
Sprain of cricoarytenoid (joint) (ligament)
Sprain of cricothyroid (joint) (ligament)
Sprain of thyroid cartilage

√x7ᵗʰ S13.8 **Sprain of joints and ligaments of other parts of neck**

√x7ᵗʰ S13.9 **Sprain of joints and ligaments of unspecified parts of neck**

√4ᵗʰ **S14   Injury of nerves and spinal cord at neck level**
NOTE   Code to highest level of cervical cord injury.
Code also any associated:
fracture of cervical vertebra (S12.0- -S12.6-)
open wound of neck (S11.-)
transient paralysis (R29.5)

The appropriate 7th character is to be added to each code from category S14.
A   initial encounter
D   subsequent encounter
S   sequela

√x7ᵗʰ S14.0 **Concussion and edema of cervical spinal cord**

√5ᵗʰ S14.1 **Other and unspecified injuries of cervical spinal cord**

√6ᵗʰ S14.10 Unspecified injury **of cervical spinal cord**

√7ᵗʰ S14.101 **Unspecified injury at** C1 level **of cervical spinal cord**

√7ᵗʰ S14.102 **Unspecified injury at** C2 level **of cervical spinal cord**

√7ᵗʰ S14.103 **Unspecified injury at** C3 level **of cervical spinal cord**

☑ Additional Character Required   √x7ᵗʰ Xtension Alert   Unspecified Dx   Other Specified Dx   Manifestation   ►◄ Revised Text   ● New Code   ▲ Revised Code Title

√7th **S14.104** **Unspecified injury at** C4 level **of cervical spinal cord**

√7th **S14.105** **Unspecified injury at** C5 level **of cervical spinal cord**

√7th **S14.106** **Unspecified injury at** C6 level **of cervical spinal cord**

√7th **S14.107** **Unspecified injury at** C7 level **of cervical spinal cord**

√7th **S14.108** **Unspecified injury at** C8 level **of cervical spinal cord**

√7th **S14.109** **Unspecified injury at unspecified level of cervical spinal cord**
    Injury of cervical spinal cord NOS

√6th **S14.11** Complete lesion **of cervical spinal cord**

√7th **S14.111** **Complete lesion at** C1 level **of cervical spinal cord**

√7th **S14.112** **Complete lesion at** C2 level **of cervical spinal cord**

√7th **S14.113** **Complete lesion at** C3 level **of cervical spinal cord**

√7th **S14.114** **Complete lesion at** C4 level **of cervical spinal cord**

√7th **S14.115** **Complete lesion at** C5 level **of cervical spinal cord**

√7th **S14.116** **Complete lesion at** C6 level **of cervical spinal cord**

√7th **S14.117** **Complete lesion at** C7 level **of cervical spinal cord**

√7th **S14.118** **Complete lesion at** C8 level **of cervical spinal cord**

√7th **S14.119** **Complete lesion at unspecified level of cervical spinal cord**

√6th **S14.12** Central cord syndrome **of cervical spinal cord**

√7th **S14.121** **Central cord syndrome at** C1 level **of cervical spinal cord**

√7th **S14.122** **Central cord syndrome at** C2 level **of cervical spinal cord**

√7th **S14.123** **Central cord syndrome at** C3 level **of cervical spinal cord**

√7th **S14.124** **Central cord syndrome at** C4 level **of cervical spinal cord**

√7th **S14.125** **Central cord syndrome at** C5 level **of cervical spinal cord**

√7th **S14.126** **Central cord syndrome at** C6 level **of cervical spinal cord**

√7th **S14.127** **Central cord syndrome at** C7 level **of cervical spinal cord**

√7th **S14.128** **Central cord syndrome at** C8 level **of cervical spinal cord**

√7th **S14.129** **Central cord syndrome at unspecified level of cervical spinal cord**

√6th **S14.13** Anterior cord syndrome **of cervical spinal cord**

√7th **S14.131** **Anterior cord syndrome at** C1 level **of cervical spinal cord**

√7th **S14.132** **Anterior cord syndrome at** C2 level **of cervical spinal cord**

√7th **S14.133** **Anterior cord syndrome at** C3 level **of cervical spinal cord**

√7th **S14.134** **Anterior cord syndrome at** C4 level **of cervical spinal cord**

√7th **S14.135** **Anterior cord syndrome at** C5 level **of cervical spinal cord**

√7th **S14.136** **Anterior cord syndrome at** C6 level **of cervical spinal cord**

√7th **S14.137** **Anterior cord syndrome at** C7 level **of cervical spinal cord**

√7th **S14.138** **Anterior cord syndrome at** C8 level **of cervical spinal cord**

√7th **S14.139** **Anterior cord syndrome at unspecified level of cervical spinal cord**

√6th **S14.14** Brown-Séquard syndrome **of cervical spinal cord**

√7th **S14.141** **Brown-Séquard syndrome at** C1 level **of cervical spinal cord**

√7th **S14.142** **Brown-Séquard syndrome at** C2 level **of cervical spinal cord**

√7th **S14.143** **Brown-Séquard syndrome at** C3 level **of cervical spinal cord**

√7th **S14.144** **Brown-Séquard syndrome at** C4 level **of cervical spinal cord**

√7th **S14.145** **Brown-Séquard syndrome at** C5 level **of cervical spinal cord**

√7th **S14.146** **Brown-Séquard syndrome at** C6 level **of cervical spinal cord**

√7th **S14.147** **Brown-Séquard syndrome at** C7 level **of cervical spinal cord**

√7th **S14.148** **Brown-Séquard syndrome at** C8 level **of cervical spinal cord**

√7th **S14.149** **Brown-Séquard syndrome at unspecified level of cervical spinal cord**

√6th **S14.15** Other incomplete lesions **of cervical spinal cord**
    Incomplete lesion of cervical spinal cord NOS
    Posterior cord syndrome of cervical spinal cord

√7th **S14.151** **Other incomplete lesion at** C1 level **of cervical spinal cord**

√7th **S14.152** **Other incomplete lesion at** C2 level **of cervical spinal cord**

√7th **S14.153** **Other incomplete lesion at** C3 level **of cervical spinal cord**

√7th **S14.154** **Other incomplete lesion at** C4 level **of cervical spinal cord**

√7th **S14.155** **Other incomplete lesion at** C5 level **of cervical spinal cord**

√7th **S14.156** **Other incomplete lesion at** C6 level **of cervical spinal cord**

√7th **S14.157** **Other incomplete lesion at** C7 level **of cervical spinal cord**

√7th **S14.158** **Other incomplete lesion at** C8 level **of cervical spinal cord**

√7th **S14.159** **Other incomplete lesion at unspecified level of cervical spinal cord**

√x7th **S14.2** **Injury of** nerve root of cervical spine

√x7th **S14.3** **Injury of** brachial plexus

√x7th **S14.4** **Injury of** peripheral nerves of neck

√x7th **S14.5** **Injury of** cervical sympathetic nerves

√x7th **S14.8** **Injury of other specified nerves of neck**

√x7th **S14.9** **Injury of unspecified nerves of neck**

√4th **S15** **Injury of blood vessels at neck level**
    Code also any associated open wound (S11.-)

    The appropriate 7th character is to be added to each code from category S15.
    A   initial encounter
    D   subsequent encounter
    S   sequela

√5th **S15.0** **Injury of** carotid artery **of neck**
    Injury of carotid artery (common) (external) (internal, extracranial portion)
    Injury of carotid artery NOS
    EXCLUDES 1   injury of internal carotid artery, intracranial portion (S06.8)

√6th **S15.00** Unspecified **injury of carotid artery**

√7th **S15.001** **Unspecified injury of** right **carotid artery**

√7th **S15.002** **Unspecified injury of** left **carotid artery**

√7th **S15.009** **Unspecified injury of unspecified carotid artery**

√6th **S15.01** Minor laceration **of carotid artery**
    Incomplete transection of carotid artery
    Laceration of carotid artery NOS
    Superficial laceration of carotid artery

√7th **S15.011** **Minor laceration of** right **carotid artery**

√7th **S15.012** **Minor laceration of** left **carotid artery**

√7th **S15.019** **Minor laceration of unspecified carotid artery**

√6th **S15.02** Major laceration **of carotid artery**
    Complete transection of carotid artery
    Traumatic rupture of carotid artery

√7th **S15.021** **Major laceration of** right **carotid artery**

√7th **S15.022** **Major laceration of** left **carotid artery**

√7th **S15.029** **Major laceration of unspecified carotid artery**

EXCLUDES 1 Not coded here   **EXCLUDES 2** Not included here   **N** Newborn Age: 0   **P** Pediatric Age: 0-17   **M** Maternity Age: 12-55   **A** Adult Age: 15-124

√6ᵗʰ **S15.09** Other specified injury of carotid artery

  √7ᵗʰ **S15.091** **Other specified injury of** right **carotid artery**

  √7ᵗʰ **S15.092** **Other specified injury of** left **carotid artery**

  √7ᵗʰ **S15.099** **Other specified injury of unspecified carotid artery**

√5ᵗʰ **S15.1** **Injury of** vertebral artery

 √6ᵗʰ **S15.10** Unspecified **injury of vertebral artery**

  √7ᵗʰ **S15.101** **Unspecified injury of** right **vertebral artery**

  √7ᵗʰ **S15.102** **Unspecified injury of** left **vertebral artery**

  √7ᵗʰ **S15.109** **Unspecified injury of unspecified vertebral artery**

 √6ᵗʰ **S15.11** Minor laceration **of vertebral artery**
    Incomplete transection of vertebral artery
    Laceration of vertebral artery NOS
    Superficial laceration of vertebral artery

  √7ᵗʰ **S15.111** **Minor laceration of** right **vertebral artery**

  √7ᵗʰ **S15.112** **Minor laceration of** left **vertebral artery**

  √7ᵗʰ **S15.119** **Minor laceration of unspecified vertebral artery**

 √6ᵗʰ **S15.12** Major laceration **of vertebral artery**
    Complete transection of vertebral artery
    Traumatic rupture of vertebral artery

  √7ᵗʰ **S15.121** **Major laceration of** right **vertebral artery**

  √7ᵗʰ **S15.122** **Major laceration of** left **vertebral artery**

  √7ᵗʰ **S15.129** **Major laceration of unspecified vertebral artery**

 √6ᵗʰ **S15.19** Other specified **injury of vertebral artery**

  √7ᵗʰ **S15.191** **Other specified injury of** right **vertebral artery**

  √7ᵗʰ **S15.192** **Other specified injury of** left **vertebral artery**

  √7ᵗʰ **S15.199** **Other specified injury of unspecified vertebral artery**

√5ᵗʰ **S15.2** **Injury of** external jugular vein

 √6ᵗʰ **S15.20** Unspecified **injury of external jugular vein**

  √7ᵗʰ **S15.201** **Unspecified injury of** right **external jugular vein**

  √7ᵗʰ **S15.202** **Unspecified injury of** left **external jugular vein**

  √7ᵗʰ **S15.209** **Unspecified injury of unspecified external jugular vein**

 √6ᵗʰ **S15.21** Minor laceration **of external jugular vein**
    Incomplete transection of external jugular vein
    Laceration of external jugular vein NOS
    Superficial laceration of external jugular vein

  √7ᵗʰ **S15.211** **Minor laceration of** right **external jugular vein**

  √7ᵗʰ **S15.212** **Minor laceration of** left **external jugular vein**

  √7ᵗʰ **S15.219** **Minor laceration of unspecified external jugular vein**

 √6ᵗʰ **S15.22** Major laceration **of external jugular vein**
    Complete transection of external jugular vein
    Traumatic rupture of external jugular vein

  √7ᵗʰ **S15.221** **Major laceration of** right **external jugular vein**

  √7ᵗʰ **S15.222** **Major laceration of** left **external jugular vein**

  √7ᵗʰ **S15.229** **Major laceration of unspecified external jugular vein**

 √6ᵗʰ **S15.29** Other specified **injury of external jugular vein**

  √7ᵗʰ **S15.291** **Other specified injury of** right **external jugular vein**

  √7ᵗʰ **S15.292** **Other specified injury of** left **external jugular vein**

  √7ᵗʰ **S15.299** **Other specified injury of unspecified external jugular vein**

√5ᵗʰ **S15.3** **Injury of** internal jugular vein

 √6ᵗʰ **S15.30** Unspecified **injury of internal jugular vein**

  √7ᵗʰ **S15.301** **Unspecified injury of** right **internal jugular vein**

  √7ᵗʰ **S15.302** **Unspecified injury of** left **internal jugular vein**

  √7ᵗʰ **S15.309** **Unspecified injury of unspecified internal jugular vein**

 √6ᵗʰ **S15.31** Minor laceration **of internal jugular vein**
    Incomplete transection of internal jugular vein
    Laceration of internal jugular vein NOS
    Superficial laceration of internal jugular vein

  √7ᵗʰ **S15.311** **Minor laceration of** right **internal jugular vein**

  √7ᵗʰ **S15.312** **Minor laceration of** left **internal jugular vein**

  √7ᵗʰ **S15.319** **Minor laceration of unspecified internal jugular vein**

 √6ᵗʰ **S15.32** Major laceration **of internal jugular vein**
    Complete transection of internal jugular vein
    Traumatic rupture of internal jugular vein

  √7ᵗʰ **S15.321** **Major laceration of** right **internal jugular vein**

  √7ᵗʰ **S15.322** **Major laceration of** left **internal jugular vein**

  √7ᵗʰ **S15.329** **Major laceration of unspecified internal jugular vein**

 √6ᵗʰ **S15.39** Other specified **injury of internal jugular vein**

  √7ᵗʰ **S15.391** **Other specified injury of** right **internal jugular vein**

  √7ᵗʰ **S15.392** **Other specified injury of** left **internal jugular vein**

  √7ᵗʰ **S15.399** **Other specified injury of unspecified internal jugular vein**

√x7ᵗʰ **S15.8** **Injury of other specified blood vessels at neck level**

√x7ᵗʰ **S15.9** **Injury of unspecified blood vessel at neck level**

√4ᵗʰ **S16** **Injury of muscle, fascia and tendon at neck level**
    Code also any associated open wound (S11.-)
    EXCLUDES 2 sprain of joint or ligament at neck level (S13.9)

    The appropriate 7th character is to be added to each code from category S16.
    A   initial encounter
    D   subsequent encounter
    S   sequela

 √x7ᵗʰ **S16.1** **Strain of muscle, fascia and tendon at neck level**

 √x7ᵗʰ **S16.2** **Laceration of muscle, fascia and tendon at neck level**

 √x7ᵗʰ **S16.8** **Other specified injury of muscle, fascia and tendon at neck level**

 √x7ᵗʰ **S16.9** **Unspecified injury of muscle, fascia and tendon at neck level**

√4ᵗʰ **S17** **Crushing injury of neck**
    Use additional code for all associated injuries, such as:
      injury of blood vessels (S15.-)
      open wound of neck (S11.-)
      spinal cord injury (S14.0, S14.1-)
      vertebral fracture (S12.0- -S12.3-)

    The appropriate 7th character is to be added to each code from category S17.
    A   initial encounter
    D   subsequent encounter
    S   sequela

 √x7ᵗʰ **S17.0** **Crushing injury of larynx and trachea**

 √x7ᵗʰ **S17.8** **Crushing injury of other specified parts of neck**

 √x7ᵗʰ **S17.9** **Crushing injury of neck, part unspecified**

√4ᵗʰ **S19** **Other specified and unspecified injuries of neck**

    The appropriate 7th character is to be added to each code from category S19.
    A   initial encounter
    D   subsequent encounter
    S   sequela

 √5ᵗʰ **S19.8** **Other specified injuries of neck**

  √x7ᵗʰ **S19.80** **Other specified injuries of unspecified part of neck**

  √x7ᵗʰ **S19.81** **Other specified injuries of** larynx

  √x7ᵗʰ **S19.82** **Other specified injuries of cervical** trachea
      EXCLUDES 2 other specified injury of thoracic trachea (S27.5-)

  √x7ᵗʰ **S19.83** **Other specified injuries of** vocal cord

  √x7ᵗʰ **S19.84** **Other specified injuries of** thyroid gland

---

☑ Additional Character Required   √x7ᵗʰ *X*tension Alert   Unspecified Dx   Other Specified Dx   Manifestation   ▶◀ Revised Text   ● New Code   ▲ Revised Code Title

ICD-10-CM Draft (2015)   819

√x7ᵗʰ **S19.85** **Other specified injuries of** pharynx and cervical esophagus

√x7ᵗʰ **S19.89** **Other specified injuries of other specified part of neck**

√x7ᵗʰ **S19.9** **Unspecified injury of neck**

Injuries to the thorax (S20-S29)

INCLUDES   injuries of breast
injuries of chest (wall)
injuries of interscapular area

EXCLUDES 2   burns and corrosions (T20-T32)
effects of foreign body in bronchus (T17.5)
effects of foreign body in esophagus (T18.1)
effects of foreign body in lung (T17.8)
effects of foreign body in trachea (T17.4)
frostbite (T33-T34)
injuries of axilla
injuries of clavicle
injuries of scapular region
injuries of shoulder
insect bite or sting, venomous (T63.4)

√4ᵗʰ **S20** **Superficial injury of thorax**

The appropriate 7th character is to be added to each code from category S20.
A   initial encounter
D   subsequent encounter
S   sequela

√5ᵗʰ **S20.0** Contusion of breast

√x7ᵗʰ **S20.00** **Contusion of breast, unspecified breast**

√x7ᵗʰ **S20.01** **Contusion of** right **breast**

√x7ᵗʰ **S20.02** **Contusion of** left **breast**

√5ᵗʰ **S20.1** **Other and unspecified superficial injuries of breast**

√6ᵗʰ **S20.10** Unspecified **superficial injuries of breast**

√7ᵗʰ **S20.101** **Unspecified superficial injuries of breast,** right **breast**

√7ᵗʰ **S20.102** **Unspecified superficial injuries of breast,** left **breast**

√7ᵗʰ **S20.109** **Unspecified superficial injuries of breast, unspecified breast**

√6ᵗʰ **S20.11** Abrasion **of breast**

√7ᵗʰ **S20.111** **Abrasion of breast,** right **breast**

√7ᵗʰ **S20.112** **Abrasion of breast,** left **breast**

√7ᵗʰ **S20.119** **Abrasion of breast, unspecified breast**

√6ᵗʰ **S20.12** Blister **(nonthermal) of breast**

√7ᵗʰ **S20.121** **Blister (nonthermal) of breast,** right **breast**

√7ᵗʰ **S20.122** **Blister (nonthermal) of breast,** left **breast**

√7ᵗʰ **S20.129** **Blister (nonthermal) of breast, unspecified breast**

√6ᵗʰ **S20.14** External constriction **of part of breast**

√7ᵗʰ **S20.141** **External constriction of part of breast,** right **breast**

√7ᵗʰ **S20.142** **External constriction of part of breast,** left **breast**

√7ᵗʰ **S20.149** **External constriction of part of breast, unspecified breast**

√6ᵗʰ **S20.15** **Superficial** foreign body **of breast**
Splinter in the breast

√7ᵗʰ **S20.151** **Superficial foreign body of breast,** right **breast**

√7ᵗʰ **S20.152** **Superficial foreign body of breast,** left **breast**

√7ᵗʰ **S20.159** **Superficial foreign body of breast, unspecified breast**

√6ᵗʰ **S20.16** Insect bite **(nonvenomous) of breast**

√7ᵗʰ **S20.161** **Insect bite (nonvenomous) of breast,** right **breast**

√7ᵗʰ **S20.162** **Insect bite (nonvenomous) of breast,** left **breast**

√7ᵗʰ **S20.169** **Insect bite (nonvenomous) of breast, unspecified breast**

√6ᵗʰ **S20.17** Other **superficial** bite **of breast**
EXCLUDES 1   open bite of breast (S21.05-)

√7ᵗʰ **S20.171** **Other superficial bite of breast,** right **breast**

√7ᵗʰ **S20.172** **Other superficial bite of breast,** left **breast**

√7ᵗʰ **S20.179** **Other superficial bite of breast, unspecified breast**

√5ᵗʰ **S20.2** **Contusion of thorax**

√x7ᵗʰ **S20.20** **Contusion of thorax, unspecified**

√6ᵗʰ **S20.21** **Contusion of** front wall **of thorax**

√7ᵗʰ **S20.211** **Contusion of** right **front wall of thorax**

√7ᵗʰ **S20.212** **Contusion of** left **front wall of thorax**

√7ᵗʰ **S20.219** **Contusion of unspecified front wall of thorax**

√6ᵗʰ **S20.22** **Contusion of** back wall **of thorax**

√7ᵗʰ **S20.221** **Contusion of** right **back wall of thorax**

√7ᵗʰ **S20.222** **Contusion of** left **back wall of thorax**

√7ᵗʰ **S20.229** **Contusion of unspecified back wall of thorax**

√5ᵗʰ **S20.3** **Other and unspecified superficial injuries of** front wall of thorax

√6ᵗʰ **S20.30** Unspecified **superficial injuries of front wall of thorax**

√7ᵗʰ **S20.301** **Unspecified superficial injuries of** right **front wall of thorax**

√7ᵗʰ **S20.302** **Unspecified superficial injuries of** left **front wall of thorax**

√7ᵗʰ **S20.309** **Unspecified superficial injuries of unspecified front wall of thorax**

√6ᵗʰ **S20.31** Abrasion **of front wall of thorax**

√7ᵗʰ **S20.311** **Abrasion of** right **front wall of thorax**

√7ᵗʰ **S20.312** **Abrasion of** left **front wall of thorax**

√7ᵗʰ **S20.319** **Abrasion of unspecified front wall of thorax**

√6ᵗʰ **S20.32** Blister **(nonthermal) of front wall of thorax**

√7ᵗʰ **S20.321** **Blister (nonthermal) of** right **front wall of thorax**

√7ᵗʰ **S20.322** **Blister (nonthermal) of** left **front wall of thorax**

√7ᵗʰ **S20.329** **Blister (nonthermal) of unspecified front wall of thorax**

√6ᵗʰ **S20.34** External constriction **of front wall of thorax**

√7ᵗʰ **S20.341** **External constriction of** right **front wall of thorax**

√7ᵗʰ **S20.342** **External constriction of** left **front wall of thorax**

√7ᵗʰ **S20.349** **External constriction of unspecified front wall of thorax**

√6ᵗʰ **S20.35** **Superficial** foreign body **of front wall of thorax**
Splinter in front wall of thorax

√7ᵗʰ **S20.351** **Superficial foreign body of** right **front wall of thorax**

√7ᵗʰ **S20.352** **Superficial foreign body of** left **front wall of thorax**

√7ᵗʰ **S20.359** **Superficial foreign body of unspecified front wall of thorax**

√6ᵗʰ **S20.36** Insect bite **(nonvenomous) of front wall of thorax**

√7ᵗʰ **S20.361** **Insect bite (nonvenomous) of** right **front wall of thorax**

√7ᵗʰ **S20.362** **Insect bite (nonvenomous) of** left **front wall of thorax**

√7ᵗʰ **S20.369** **Insect bite (nonvenomous) of unspecified front wall of thorax**

√6ᵗʰ **S20.37** Other **superficial** bite **of front wall of thorax**
EXCLUDES 1   open bite of front wall of thorax (S21.14)

√7ᵗʰ **S20.371** **Other superficial bite of** right **front wall of thorax**

√7ᵗʰ **S20.372** **Other superficial bite of** left **front wall of thorax**

√7ᵗʰ **S20.379** **Other superficial bite of unspecified front wall of thorax**

√5ᵗʰ **S20.4** **Other and unspecified superficial injuries of** back wall of thorax

√6ᵗʰ **S20.40** Unspecified **superficial injuries of back wall of thorax**

√7ᵗʰ **S20.401** **Unspecified superficial injuries of** right **back wall of thorax**

EXCLUDES 1 Not coded here   EXCLUDES 2 Not included here   N Newborn Age: 0   P Pediatric Age: 0-17   M Maternity Age: 12-55   A Adult Age: 15-124

820   ICD-10-CM Draft (2015)

☑7ᵗʰ **S20.402** Unspecified superficial injuries of left back wall of thorax

☑7ᵗʰ **S20.409** Unspecified superficial injuries of unspecified back wall of thorax

✓6ᵗʰ **S20.41** Abrasion of back wall of thorax

☑7ᵗʰ **S20.411** Abrasion of right back wall of thorax

☑7ᵗʰ **S20.412** Abrasion of left back wall of thorax

☑7ᵗʰ **S20.419** Abrasion of unspecified back wall of thorax

✓6ᵗʰ **S20.42** Blister (nonthermal) of back wall of thorax

☑7ᵗʰ **S20.421** Blister (nonthermal) of right back wall of thorax

☑7ᵗʰ **S20.422** Blister (nonthermal) of left back wall of thorax

☑7ᵗʰ **S20.429** Blister (nonthermal) of unspecified back wall of thorax

✓6ᵗʰ **S20.44** External constriction of back wall of thorax

☑7ᵗʰ **S20.441** External constriction of right back wall of thorax

☑7ᵗʰ **S20.442** External constriction of left back wall of thorax

☑7ᵗʰ **S20.449** External constriction of unspecified back wall of thorax

✓6ᵗʰ **S20.45** Superficial foreign body of back wall of thorax
Splinter of back wall of thorax

☑7ᵗʰ **S20.451** Superficial foreign body of right back wall of thorax

☑7ᵗʰ **S20.452** Superficial foreign body of left back wall of thorax

☑7ᵗʰ **S20.459** Superficial foreign body of unspecified back wall of thorax

✓6ᵗʰ **S20.46** Insect bite (nonvenomous) of back wall of thorax

☑7ᵗʰ **S20.461** Insect bite (nonvenomous) of right back wall of thorax

☑7ᵗʰ **S20.462** Insect bite (nonvenomous) of left back wall of thorax

☑7ᵗʰ **S20.469** Insect bite (nonvenomous) of unspecified back wall of thorax

✓6ᵗʰ **S20.47** Other superficial bite of back wall of thorax
EXCLUDES 1 open bite of back wall of thorax (S21.24)

☑7ᵗʰ **S20.471** Other superficial bite of right back wall of thorax

☑7ᵗʰ **S20.472** Other superficial bite of left back wall of thorax

☑7ᵗʰ **S20.479** Other superficial bite of unspecified back wall of thorax

✓5ᵗʰ **S20.9** Superficial injury of unspecified parts of thorax
EXCLUDES 1 contusion of thorax NOS (S20.20)

☑x7ᵗʰ **S20.90** Unspecified superficial injury of unspecified parts of thorax
Superficial injury of thoracic wall NOS

☑x7ᵗʰ **S20.91** Abrasion of unspecified parts of thorax

☑x7ᵗʰ **S20.92** Blister (nonthermal) of unspecified parts of thorax

☑x7ᵗʰ **S20.94** External constriction of unspecified parts of thorax

☑x7ᵗʰ **S20.95** Superficial foreign body of unspecified parts of thorax
Splinter in thorax NOS

☑x7ᵗʰ **S20.96** Insect bite (nonvenomous) of unspecified parts of thorax

☑x7ᵗʰ **S20.97** Other superficial bite of unspecified parts of thorax
EXCLUDES 1 open bite of thorax NOS (S21.95)

✓4ᵗʰ **S21 Open wound of thorax**
Code also any associated injury, such as:
injury of heart (S26.-)
injury of intrathoracic organs (S27.-)
rib fracture (S22.3-, S22.4-)
spinal cord injury (S24.0-, S24.1-)
traumatic hemopneumothorax (S27.3)
traumatic hemothorax (S27.1)
traumatic pneumothorax (S27.0)
wound infection
EXCLUDES 1 traumatic amputation (partial) of thorax (S28.1)

The appropriate 7th character is to be added to each code from category S21.
A   initial encounter
D   subsequent encounter
S   sequela

✓6ᵗʰ **S21.0** Open wound of breast

✓6ᵗʰ **S21.00** Unspecified open wound of breast

☑7ᵗʰ **S21.001** Unspecified open wound of right breast

☑7ᵗʰ **S21.002** Unspecified open wound of left breast

☑7ᵗʰ **S21.009** Unspecified open wound of unspecified breast

✓6ᵗʰ **S21.01** Laceration without foreign body of breast

☑7ᵗʰ **S21.011** Laceration without foreign body of right breast

☑7ᵗʰ **S21.012** Laceration without foreign body of left breast

☑7ᵗʰ **S21.019** Laceration without foreign body of unspecified breast

✓6ᵗʰ **S21.02** Laceration with foreign body of breast

☑7ᵗʰ **S21.021** Laceration with foreign body of right breast

☑7ᵗʰ **S21.022** Laceration with foreign body of left breast

☑7ᵗʰ **S21.029** Laceration with foreign body of unspecified breast

✓6ᵗʰ **S21.03** Puncture wound without foreign body of breast

☑7ᵗʰ **S21.031** Puncture wound without foreign body of right breast

☑7ᵗʰ **S21.032** Puncture wound without foreign body of left breast

☑7ᵗʰ **S21.039** Puncture wound without foreign body of unspecified breast

✓6ᵗʰ **S21.04** Puncture wound with foreign body of breast

☑7ᵗʰ **S21.041** Puncture wound with foreign body of right breast

☑7ᵗʰ **S21.042** Puncture wound with foreign body of left breast

☑7ᵗʰ **S21.049** Puncture wound with foreign body of unspecified breast

✓6ᵗʰ **S21.05** Open bite of breast
Bite of breast NOS
EXCLUDES 1 superficial bite of breast (S20.17)

☑7ᵗʰ **S21.051** Open bite of right breast

☑7ᵗʰ **S21.052** Open bite of left breast

☑7ᵗʰ **S21.059** Open bite of unspecified breast

✓5ᵗʰ **S21.1** Open wound of front wall of thorax without penetration into thoracic cavity
Open wound of chest without penetration into thoracic cavity

✓6ᵗʰ **S21.10** Unspecified open wound of front wall of thorax without penetration into thoracic cavity

☑7ᵗʰ **S21.101** Unspecified open wound of right front wall of thorax without penetration into thoracic cavity

☑7ᵗʰ **S21.102** Unspecified open wound of left front wall of thorax without penetration into thoracic cavity

☑7ᵗʰ **S21.109** Unspecified open wound of unspecified front wall of thorax without penetration into thoracic cavity

✓6ᵗʰ **S21.11** Laceration without foreign body of front wall of thorax without penetration into thoracic cavity

☑7ᵗʰ **S21.111** Laceration without foreign body of right front wall of thorax without penetration into thoracic cavity

✓7ᵗʰ **S21.112** Laceration without foreign body of left front wall of thorax without penetration into thoracic cavity

✓7ᵗʰ **S21.119** Laceration without foreign body of unspecified front wall of thorax without penetration into thoracic cavity

✓6ᵗʰ **S21.12** Laceration with foreign body of front wall of thorax without penetration into thoracic cavity

✓7ᵗʰ **S21.121** Laceration with foreign body of right front wall of thorax without penetration into thoracic cavity

✓7ᵗʰ **S21.122** Laceration with foreign body of left front wall of thorax without penetration into thoracic cavity

✓7ᵗʰ **S21.129** Laceration with foreign body of unspecified front wall of thorax without penetration into thoracic cavity

✓6ᵗʰ **S21.13** Puncture wound without foreign body of front wall of thorax without penetration into thoracic cavity

✓7ᵗʰ **S21.131** Puncture wound without foreign body of right front wall of thorax without penetration into thoracic cavity

✓7ᵗʰ **S21.132** Puncture wound without foreign body of left front wall of thorax without penetration into thoracic cavity

✓7ᵗʰ **S21.139** Puncture wound without foreign body of unspecified front wall of thorax without penetration into thoracic cavity

✓6ᵗʰ **S21.14** Puncture wound with foreign body of front wall of thorax without penetration into thoracic cavity

✓7ᵗʰ **S21.141** Puncture wound with foreign body of right front wall of thorax without penetration into thoracic cavity

✓7ᵗʰ **S21.142** Puncture wound with foreign body of left front wall of thorax without penetration into thoracic cavity

✓7ᵗʰ **S21.149** Puncture wound with foreign body of unspecified front wall of thorax without penetration into thoracic cavity

✓6ᵗʰ **S21.15** Open bite of front wall of thorax without penetration into thoracic cavity
Bite of front wall of thorax NOS
EXCLUDES 1   superficial bite of front wall of thorax (S20.37)

✓7ᵗʰ **S21.151** Open bite of right front wall of thorax without penetration into thoracic cavity

✓7ᵗʰ **S21.152** Open bite of left front wall of thorax without penetration into thoracic cavity

✓7ᵗʰ **S21.159** Open bite of unspecified front wall of thorax without penetration into thoracic cavity

✓5ᵗʰ **S21.2** Open wound of back wall of thorax without penetration into thoracic cavity

✓6ᵗʰ **S21.20** Unspecified open wound of back wall of thorax without penetration into thoracic cavity

✓7ᵗʰ **S21.201** Unspecified open wound of right back wall of thorax without penetration into thoracic cavity

✓7ᵗʰ **S21.202** Unspecified open wound of left back wall of thorax without penetration into thoracic cavity

✓7ᵗʰ **S21.209** Unspecified open wound of unspecified back wall of thorax without penetration into thoracic cavity

✓6ᵗʰ **S21.21** Laceration without foreign body of back wall of thorax without penetration into thoracic cavity

✓7ᵗʰ **S21.211** Laceration without foreign body of right back wall of thorax without penetration into thoracic cavity

✓7ᵗʰ **S21.212** Laceration without foreign body of left back wall of thorax without penetration into thoracic cavity

✓7ᵗʰ **S21.219** Laceration without foreign body of unspecified back wall of thorax without penetration into thoracic cavity

✓6ᵗʰ **S21.22** Laceration with foreign body of back wall of thorax without penetration into thoracic cavity

✓7ᵗʰ **S21.221** Laceration with foreign body of right back wall of thorax without penetration into thoracic cavity

✓7ᵗʰ **S21.222** Laceration with foreign body of left back wall of thorax without penetration into thoracic cavity

✓7ᵗʰ **S21.229** Laceration with foreign body of unspecified back wall of thorax without penetration into thoracic cavity

✓6ᵗʰ **S21.23** Puncture wound without foreign body of back wall of thorax without penetration into thoracic cavity

✓7ᵗʰ **S21.231** Puncture wound without foreign body of right back wall of thorax without penetration into thoracic cavity

✓7ᵗʰ **S21.232** Puncture wound without foreign body of left back wall of thorax without penetration into thoracic cavity

✓7ᵗʰ **S21.239** Puncture wound without foreign body of unspecified back wall of thorax without penetration into thoracic cavity

✓6ᵗʰ **S21.24** Puncture wound with foreign body of back wall of thorax without penetration into thoracic cavity

✓7ᵗʰ **S21.241** Puncture wound with foreign body of right back wall of thorax without penetration into thoracic cavity

✓7ᵗʰ **S21.242** Puncture wound with foreign body of left back wall of thorax without penetration into thoracic cavity

✓7ᵗʰ **S21.249** Puncture wound with foreign body of unspecified back wall of thorax without penetration into thoracic cavity

✓6ᵗʰ **S21.25** Open bite of back wall of thorax without penetration into thoracic cavity
Bite of back wall of thorax NOS
EXCLUDES 1   superficial bite of back wall of thorax (S20.47)

✓7ᵗʰ **S21.251** Open bite of right back wall of thorax without penetration into thoracic cavity

✓7ᵗʰ **S21.252** Open bite of left back wall of thorax without penetration into thoracic cavity

✓7ᵗʰ **S21.259** Open bite of unspecified back wall of thorax without penetration into thoracic cavity

✓5ᵗʰ **S21.3** Open wound of front wall of thorax with penetration into thoracic cavity
Open wound of chest with penetration into thoracic cavity

✓6ᵗʰ **S21.30** Unspecified open wound of front wall of thorax with penetration into thoracic cavity

✓7ᵗʰ **S21.301** Unspecified open wound of right front wall of thorax with penetration into thoracic cavity

✓7ᵗʰ **S21.302** Unspecified open wound of left front wall of thorax with penetration into thoracic cavity

✓7ᵗʰ **S21.309** Unspecified open wound of unspecified front wall of thorax with penetration into thoracic cavity

✓6ᵗʰ **S21.31** Laceration without foreign body of front wall of thorax with penetration into thoracic cavity

✓7ᵗʰ **S21.311** Laceration without foreign body of right front wall of thorax with penetration into thoracic cavity

✓7ᵗʰ **S21.312** Laceration without foreign body of left front wall of thorax with penetration into thoracic cavity

✓7ᵗʰ **S21.319** Laceration without foreign body of unspecified front wall of thorax with penetration into thoracic cavity

✓6ᵗʰ **S21.32** Laceration with foreign body of front wall of thorax with penetration into thoracic cavity

✓7ᵗʰ **S21.321** Laceration with foreign body of right front wall of thorax with penetration into thoracic cavity

✓7ᵗʰ **S21.322** Laceration with foreign body of left front wall of thorax with penetration into thoracic cavity

EXCLUDES 1 Not coded here   EXCLUDES 2 Not included here   N Newborn Age: 0   P Pediatric Age: 0-17   M Maternity Age: 12-55   A Adult Age: 15-124

822   ICD-10-CM Draft (2015)

√7ᵗʰ **S21.329** Laceration with foreign body of unspecified front wall of thorax with penetration into thoracic cavity

√6ᵗʰ **S21.33** Puncture wound without foreign body of front wall of thorax with penetration into thoracic cavity

√7ᵗʰ **S21.331** Puncture wound without foreign body of right front wall of thorax with penetration into thoracic cavity

√7ᵗʰ **S21.332** Puncture wound without foreign body of left front wall of thorax with penetration into thoracic cavity

√7ᵗʰ **S21.339** Puncture wound without foreign body of unspecified front wall of thorax with penetration into thoracic cavity

√6ᵗʰ **S21.34** Puncture wound with foreign body of front wall of thorax with penetration into thoracic cavity

√7ᵗʰ **S21.341** Puncture wound with foreign body of right front wall of thorax with penetration into thoracic cavity

√7ᵗʰ **S21.342** Puncture wound with foreign body of left front wall of thorax with penetration into thoracic cavity

√7ᵗʰ **S21.349** Puncture wound with foreign body of unspecified front wall of thorax with penetration into thoracic cavity

√6ᵗʰ **S21.35** Open bite of front wall of thorax with penetration into thoracic cavity
  EXCLUDES 1 superficial bite of front wall of thorax (S20.37)

√7ᵗʰ **S21.351** Open bite of right front wall of thorax with penetration into thoracic cavity

√7ᵗʰ **S21.352** Open bite of left front wall of thorax with penetration into thoracic cavity

√7ᵗʰ **S21.359** Open bite of unspecified front wall of thorax with penetration into thoracic cavity

√5ᵗʰ **S21.4** Open wound of back wall of thorax with penetration into thoracic cavity

√6ᵗʰ **S21.40** Unspecified open wound of back wall of thorax with penetration into thoracic cavity

√7ᵗʰ **S21.401** Unspecified open wound of right back wall of thorax with penetration into thoracic cavity

√7ᵗʰ **S21.402** Unspecified open wound of left back wall of thorax with penetration into thoracic cavity

√7ᵗʰ **S21.409** Unspecified open wound of unspecified back wall of thorax with penetration into thoracic cavity

√6ᵗʰ **S21.41** Laceration without foreign body of back wall of thorax with penetration into thoracic cavity

√7ᵗʰ **S21.411** Laceration without foreign body of right back wall of thorax with penetration into thoracic cavity

√7ᵗʰ **S21.412** Laceration without foreign body of left back wall of thorax with penetration into thoracic cavity

√7ᵗʰ **S21.419** Laceration without foreign body of unspecified back wall of thorax with penetration into thoracic cavity

√6ᵗʰ **S21.42** Laceration with foreign body of back wall of thorax with penetration into thoracic cavity

√7ᵗʰ **S21.421** Laceration with foreign body of right back wall of thorax with penetration into thoracic cavity

√7ᵗʰ **S21.422** Laceration with foreign body of left back wall of thorax with penetration into thoracic cavity

√7ᵗʰ **S21.429** Laceration with foreign body of unspecified back wall of thorax with penetration into thoracic cavity

√6ᵗʰ **S21.43** Puncture wound without foreign body of back wall of thorax with penetration into thoracic cavity

√7ᵗʰ **S21.431** Puncture wound without foreign body of right back wall of thorax with penetration into thoracic cavity

√7ᵗʰ **S21.432** Puncture wound without foreign body of left back wall of thorax with penetration into thoracic cavity

√7ᵗʰ **S21.439** Puncture wound without foreign body of unspecified back wall of thorax with penetration into thoracic cavity

√6ᵗʰ **S21.44** Puncture wound with foreign body of back wall of thorax with penetration into thoracic cavity

√7ᵗʰ **S21.441** Puncture wound with foreign body of right back wall of thorax with penetration into thoracic cavity

√7ᵗʰ **S21.442** Puncture wound with foreign body of left back wall of thorax with penetration into thoracic cavity

√7ᵗʰ **S21.449** Puncture wound with foreign body of unspecified back wall of thorax with penetration into thoracic cavity

√6ᵗʰ **S21.45** Open bite of back wall of thorax with penetration into thoracic cavity
  Bite of back wall of thorax NOS
  EXCLUDES 1 superficial bite of back wall of thorax (S20.47)

√7ᵗʰ **S21.451** Open bite of right back wall of thorax with penetration into thoracic cavity

√7ᵗʰ **S21.452** Open bite of left back wall of thorax with penetration into thoracic cavity

√7ᵗʰ **S21.459** Open bite of unspecified back wall of thorax with penetration into thoracic cavity

√5ᵗʰ **S21.9** Open wound of unspecified part of thorax
  Open wound of thoracic wall NOS

√x7ᵗʰ **S21.90** Unspecified open wound of unspecified part of thorax

√x7ᵗʰ **S21.91** Laceration without foreign body of unspecified part of thorax

√x7ᵗʰ **S21.92** Laceration with foreign body of unspecified part of thorax

√x7ᵗʰ **S21.93** Puncture wound without foreign body of unspecified part of thorax

√x7ᵗʰ **S21.94** Puncture wound with foreign body of unspecified part of thorax

√x7ᵗʰ **S21.95** Open bite of unspecified part of thorax
  EXCLUDES 1 superficial bite of thorax (S20.97)

√4ᵗʰ **S22 Fracture of rib(s), sternum and thoracic spine**
  NOTE A fracture not indicated as nondisplaced or displaced should be coded to displaced.
  A fracture not indicated as open or closed should be coded to closed.
  INCLUDES fracture of thoracic neural arch
  fracture of thoracic spinous process
  fracture of thoracic transverse process
  fracture of thoracic vertebra
  fracture of thoracic vertebral arch
  Code first any associated:
    injury of intrathoracic organ (S27.-)
    spinal cord injury (S24.0-, S24.1-)
  EXCLUDES 1 transection of thorax (S28.1)
  EXCLUDES 2 fracture of clavicle (S42.0-)
    fracture of scapula (S42.1-)

The appropriate 7th character is to be added to each code from category S22.
A initial encounter for closed fracture
B initial encounter for open fracture
D subsequent encounter for fracture with routine healing
G subsequent encounter for fracture with delayed healing
K subsequent encounter for fracture with nonunion
S sequela

√5ᵗʰ **S22.0 Fracture of thoracic vertebra**

√6ᵗʰ **S22.00** Fracture of unspecified thoracic vertebra

√7ᵗʰ **S22.000** Wedge compression fracture of unspecified thoracic vertebra

√7ᵗʰ **S22.001** Stable burst fracture of unspecified thoracic vertebra

√7ᵗʰ **S22.002** Unstable burst fracture of unspecified thoracic vertebra

√7ᵗʰ **S22.008** Other fracture of unspecified thoracic vertebra

√7ᵗʰ **S22.009** Unspecified fracture of unspecified thoracic vertebra

☑ Additional Character Required √x7ᵗʰ Xtension Alert Unspecified Dx Other Specified Dx Manifestation ►◄ Revised Text ● New Code ▲ Revised Code Title

ICD-10-CM Draft (2015) 823

Injury, Poisoning and Certain Other Consequences of External Causes

S22.01–S23.143

✓6th **S22.01** Fracture of first thoracic vertebra
- ✓7th **S22.010** Wedge compression fracture of first thoracic vertebra
- ✓7th **S22.011** Stable burst fracture of first thoracic vertebra
- ✓7th **S22.012** Unstable burst fracture of first thoracic vertebra
- ✓7th **S22.018** Other fracture of first thoracic vertebra
- ✓7th **S22.019** Unspecified fracture of first thoracic vertebra

✓6th **S22.02** Fracture of second thoracic vertebra
- ✓7th **S22.020** Wedge compression fracture of second thoracic vertebra
- ✓7th **S22.021** Stable burst fracture of second thoracic vertebra
- ✓7th **S22.022** Unstable burst fracture of second thoracic vertebra
- ✓7th **S22.028** Other fracture of second thoracic vertebra
- ✓7th **S22.029** Unspecified fracture of second thoracic vertebra

✓6th **S22.03** Fracture of third thoracic vertebra
- ✓7th **S22.030** Wedge compression fracture of third thoracic vertebra
- ✓7th **S22.031** Stable burst fracture of third thoracic vertebra
- ✓7th **S22.032** Unstable burst fracture of third thoracic vertebra
- ✓7th **S22.038** Other fracture of third thoracic vertebra
- ✓7th **S22.039** Unspecified fracture of third thoracic vertebra

✓6th **S22.04** Fracture of fourth thoracic vertebra
- ✓7th **S22.040** Wedge compression fracture of fourth thoracic vertebra
- ✓7th **S22.041** Stable burst fracture of fourth thoracic vertebra
- ✓7th **S22.042** Unstable burst fracture of fourth thoracic vertebra
- ✓7th **S22.048** Other fracture of fourth thoracic vertebra
- ✓7th **S22.049** Unspecified fracture of fourth thoracic vertebra

✓6th **S22.05** Fracture of T5-T6 vertebra
- ✓7th **S22.050** Wedge compression fracture of T5-T6 vertebra
- ✓7th **S22.051** Stable burst fracture of T5-T6 vertebra
- ✓7th **S22.052** Unstable burst fracture of T5-T6 vertebra
- ✓7th **S22.058** Other fracture of T5-T6 vertebra
- ✓7th **S22.059** Unspecified fracture of T5-T6 vertebra

✓6th **S22.06** Fracture of T7-T8 vertebra
- ✓7th **S22.060** Wedge compression fracture of T7-T8 vertebra
- ✓7th **S22.061** Stable burst fracture of T7-T8 vertebra
- ✓7th **S22.062** Unstable burst fracture of T7-T8 vertebra
- ✓7th **S22.068** Other fracture of T7-T8 thoracic vertebra
- ✓7th **S22.069** Unspecified fracture of T7-T8 vertebra

✓6th **S22.07** Fracture of T9-T10 vertebra
- ✓7th **S22.070** Wedge compression fracture of T9-T10 vertebra
- ✓7th **S22.071** Stable burst fracture of T9-T10 vertebra
- ✓7th **S22.072** Unstable burst fracture of T9-T10 vertebra
- ✓7th **S22.078** Other fracture of T9-T10 vertebra
- ✓7th **S22.079** Unspecified fracture of T9-T10 vertebra

✓6th **S22.08** Fracture of T11-T12 vertebra
- ✓7th **S22.080** Wedge compression fracture of T11-T12 vertebra
- ✓7th **S22.081** Stable burst fracture of T11-T12 vertebra
- ✓7th **S22.082** Unstable burst fracture of T11-T12 vertebra
- ✓7th **S22.088** Other fracture of T11-T12 vertebra
- ✓7th **S22.089** Unspecified fracture of T11-T12 vertebra

✓5th **S22.2** Fracture of sternum
- ✓x7th **S22.20** Unspecified fracture of sternum

- ✓x7th **S22.21** Fracture of manubrium
- ✓x7th **S22.22** Fracture of body of sternum
- ✓x7th **S22.23** Sternal manubrial dissociation
- ✓x7th **S22.24** Fracture of xiphoid process

✓5th **S22.3** Fracture of one rib
- ✓x7th **S22.31** Fracture of one rib, right side
- ✓x7th **S22.32** Fracture of one rib, left side
- ✓x7th **S22.39** Fracture of one rib, unspecified side

✓5th **S22.4** Multiple fractures of ribs
Fractures of two or more ribs
> EXCLUDES 1   flail chest (S22.5-)
- ✓x7th **S22.41** Multiple fractures of ribs, right side
- ✓x7th **S22.42** Multiple fractures of ribs, left side
- ✓x7th **S22.43** Multiple fractures of ribs, bilateral
- ✓x7th **S22.49** Multiple fractures of ribs, unspecified side

✓x7th **S22.5** Flail chest

✓x7th **S22.9** Fracture of bony thorax, part unspecified

✓4th **S23** Dislocation and sprain of joints and ligaments of thorax
> INCLUDES   avulsion of joint or ligament of thorax
> laceration of cartilage, joint or ligament of thorax
> sprain of cartilage, joint or ligament of thorax
> traumatic hemarthrosis of joint or ligament of thorax
> traumatic rupture of joint or ligament of thorax
> traumatic subluxation of joint or ligament of thorax
> traumatic tear of joint or ligament of thorax

Code also any associated open wound
> EXCLUDES 2   dislocation, sprain of sternoclavicular joint (S43.2, S43.6)
> strain of muscle or tendon of thorax (S29.01-)

The appropriate 7th character is to be added to each code from category S23.
- A   initial encounter
- D   subsequent encounter
- S   sequela

✓x7th **S23.0** Traumatic rupture of thoracic intervertebral disc
> EXCLUDES 1   rupture or displacement (nontraumatic) of thoracic intervertebral disc NOS (M51- with fifth character 4)

✓5th **S23.1** Subluxation and dislocation of thoracic vertebra
Code also any associated
open wound of thorax (S21.-)
spinal cord injury (S24.0-, S24.1-)
> EXCLUDES 2   fracture of thoracic vertebrae (S22.0-)

  ✓6th **S23.10** Subluxation and dislocation of unspecified thoracic vertebra
- ✓7th **S23.100** Subluxation of unspecified thoracic vertebra
- ✓7th **S23.101** Dislocation of unspecified thoracic vertebra

  ✓6th **S23.11** Subluxation and dislocation of T1/T2 thoracic vertebra
- ✓7th **S23.110** Subluxation of T1/T2 thoracic vertebra
- ✓7th **S23.111** Dislocation of T1/T2 thoracic vertebra

  ✓6th **S23.12** Subluxation and dislocation of T2/T3-T3/T4 thoracic vertebra
- ✓7th **S23.120** Subluxation of T2/T3 thoracic vertebra
- ✓7th **S23.121** Dislocation of T2/T3 thoracic vertebra
- ✓7th **S23.122** Subluxation of T3/T4 thoracic vertebra
- ✓7th **S23.123** Dislocation of T3/T4 thoracic vertebra

  ✓6th **S23.13** Subluxation and dislocation of T4/T5-T5/T6 thoracic vertebra
- ✓7th **S23.130** Subluxation of T4/T5 thoracic vertebra
- ✓7th **S23.131** Dislocation of T4/T5 thoracic vertebra
- ✓7th **S23.132** Subluxation of T5/T6 thoracic vertebra
- ✓7th **S23.133** Dislocation of T5/T6 thoracic vertebra

  ✓6th **S23.14** Subluxation and dislocation of T6/T7-T7/T8 thoracic vertebra
- ✓7th **S23.140** Subluxation of T6/T7 thoracic vertebra
- ✓7th **S23.141** Dislocation of T6/T7 thoracic vertebra
- ✓7th **S23.142** Subluxation of T7/T8 thoracic vertebra
- ✓7th **S23.143** Dislocation of T7/T8 thoracic vertebra

EXCLUDES 1 Not coded here   EXCLUDES 2 Not included here   N Newborn Age: 0   P Pediatric Age: 0-17   M Maternity Age: 12-55   A Adult Age: 15-124

824   ICD-10-CM Draft (2015)

✓6ᵗʰ **S23.15** Subluxation and dislocation of T8/T9-T9/T10 thoracic vertebra
- ✓7ᵗʰ **S23.150** Subluxation of T8/T9 thoracic vertebra
- ✓7ᵗʰ **S23.151** Dislocation of T8/T9 thoracic vertebra
- ✓7ᵗʰ **S23.152** Subluxation of T9/T10 thoracic vertebra
- ✓7ᵗʰ **S23.153** Dislocation of T9/T10 thoracic vertebra

✓6ᵗʰ **S23.16** Subluxation and dislocation of T10/T11-T11/T12 thoracic vertebra
- ✓7ᵗʰ **S23.160** Subluxation of T10/T11 thoracic vertebra
- ✓7ᵗʰ **S23.161** Dislocation of T10/T11 thoracic vertebra
- ✓7ᵗʰ **S23.162** Subluxation of T11/T12 thoracic vertebra
- ✓7ᵗʰ **S23.163** Dislocation of T11/T12 thoracic vertebra

✓6ᵗʰ **S23.17** Subluxation and dislocation of T12/L1 thoracic vertebra
- ✓7ᵗʰ **S23.170** Subluxation of T12/L1 thoracic vertebra
- ✓7ᵗʰ **S23.171** Dislocation of T12/L1 thoracic vertebra

✓5ᵗʰ **S23.2** Dislocation of other and unspecified parts of thorax
- ✓x7ᵗʰ **S23.20** Dislocation of unspecified part of thorax
- ✓x7ᵗʰ **S23.29** Dislocation of other parts of thorax

✓x7ᵗʰ **S23.3** Sprain of ligaments of thoracic spine

✓5ᵗʰ **S23.4** Sprain of ribs and sternum
- ✓x7ᵗʰ **S23.41** Sprain of ribs
- ✓6ᵗʰ **S23.42** Sprain of sternum
  - ✓7ᵗʰ **S23.420** Sprain of sternoclavicular (joint) (ligament)
  - ✓7ᵗʰ **S23.421** Sprain of chondrosternal joint
  - ✓7ᵗʰ **S23.428** Other sprain of sternum
  - ✓7ᵗʰ **S23.429** Unspecified sprain of sternum

✓x7ᵗʰ **S23.8** Sprain of other specified parts of thorax

✓x7ᵗʰ **S23.9** Sprain of unspecified parts of thorax

✓4ᵗʰ **S24** Injury of nerves and spinal cord at thorax level

> **NOTE** Code to highest level of thoracic spinal cord injury.
> Injuries to the spinal cord (S24.0 and S24.1) refer to the cord level and not bone level injury, and can affect nerve roots at and below the level given.

Code also any associated:
- fracture of thoracic vertebra (S22.0-)
- open wound of thorax (S21.-)
- transient paralysis (R29.5)

EXCLUDES 2 injury of brachial plexus (S14.3)

The appropriate 7th character is to be added to each code from category S24.
- A   initial encounter
- D   subsequent encounter
- S   sequela

✓x7ᵗʰ **S24.0** Concussion and edema of thoracic spinal cord

✓5ᵗʰ **S24.1** Other and unspecified injuries of thoracic spinal cord
- ✓6ᵗʰ **S24.10** Unspecified injury of thoracic spinal cord
  - ✓7ᵗʰ **S24.101** Unspecified injury at T1 level of thoracic spinal cord
  - ✓7ᵗʰ **S24.102** Unspecified injury at T2-T6 level of thoracic spinal cord
  - ✓7ᵗʰ **S24.103** Unspecified injury at T7-T10 level of thoracic spinal cord
  - ✓7ᵗʰ **S24.104** Unspecified injury at T11-T12 level of thoracic spinal cord
  - ✓7ᵗʰ **S24.109** Unspecified injury at unspecified level of thoracic spinal cord
    Injury of thoracic spinal cord NOS
- ✓6ᵗʰ **S24.11** Complete lesion of thoracic spinal cord
  - ✓7ᵗʰ **S24.111** Complete lesion at T1 level of thoracic spinal cord
  - ✓7ᵗʰ **S24.112** Complete lesion at T2-T6 level of thoracic spinal cord
  - ✓7ᵗʰ **S24.113** Complete lesion at T7-T10 level of thoracic spinal cord
  - ✓7ᵗʰ **S24.114** Complete lesion at T11-T12 level of thoracic spinal cord
  - ✓7ᵗʰ **S24.119** Complete lesion at unspecified level of thoracic spinal cord

✓6ᵗʰ **S24.13** Anterior cord syndrome of thoracic spinal cord
- ✓7ᵗʰ **S24.131** Anterior cord syndrome at T1 level of thoracic spinal cord
- ✓7ᵗʰ **S24.132** Anterior cord syndrome at T2-T6 level of thoracic spinal cord
- ✓7ᵗʰ **S24.133** Anterior cord syndrome at T7-T10 level of thoracic spinal cord
- ✓7ᵗʰ **S24.134** Anterior cord syndrome at T11-T12 level of thoracic spinal cord
- ✓7ᵗʰ **S24.139** Anterior cord syndrome at unspecified level of thoracic spinal cord

✓6ᵗʰ **S24.14** Brown-Séquard syndrome of thoracic spinal cord
- ✓7ᵗʰ **S24.141** Brown-Séquard syndrome at T1 level of thoracic spinal cord
- ✓7ᵗʰ **S24.142** Brown-Séquard syndrome at T2-T6 level of thoracic spinal cord
- ✓7ᵗʰ **S24.143** Brown-Séquard syndrome at T7-T10 level of thoracic spinal cord
- ✓7ᵗʰ **S24.144** Brown-Séquard syndrome at T11-T12 level of thoracic spinal cord
- ✓7ᵗʰ **S24.149** Brown-Séquard syndrome at unspecified level of thoracic spinal cord

✓6ᵗʰ **S24.15** Other incomplete lesions of thoracic spinal cord
  Incomplete lesion of thoracic spinal cord NOS
  Posterior cord syndrome of thoracic spinal cord
- ✓7ᵗʰ **S24.151** Other incomplete lesion at T1 level of thoracic spinal cord
- ✓7ᵗʰ **S24.152** Other incomplete lesion at T2-T6 level of thoracic spinal cord
- ✓7ᵗʰ **S24.153** Other incomplete lesion at T7-T10 level of thoracic spinal cord
- ✓7ᵗʰ **S24.154** Other incomplete lesion at T11-T12 level of thoracic spinal cord
- ✓7ᵗʰ **S24.159** Other incomplete lesion at unspecified level of thoracic spinal cord

✓x7ᵗʰ **S24.2** Injury of nerve root of thoracic spine

✓x7ᵗʰ **S24.3** Injury of peripheral nerves of thorax

✓x7ᵗʰ **S24.4** Injury of thoracic sympathetic nervous system
  Injury of cardiac plexus
  Injury of esophageal plexus
  Injury of pulmonary plexus
  Injury of stellate ganglion
  Injury of thoracic sympathetic ganglion

✓x7ᵗʰ **S24.8** Injury of other specified nerves of thorax

✓x7ᵗʰ **S24.9** Injury of unspecified nerve of thorax

✓4ᵗʰ **S25** Injury of blood vessels of thorax
  Code also any associated open wound (S21.-)

The appropriate 7th character is to be added to each code from category S25.
- A   initial encounter
- D   subsequent encounter
- S   sequela

✓5ᵗʰ **S25.0** Injury of thoracic aorta
  Injury of aorta NOS
- ✓x7ᵗʰ **S25.00** Unspecified injury of thoracic aorta
- ✓x7ᵗʰ **S25.01** Minor laceration of thoracic aorta
    Incomplete transection of thoracic aorta
    Laceration of thoracic aorta NOS
    Superficial laceration of thoracic aorta
- ✓x7ᵗʰ **S25.02** Major laceration of thoracic aorta
    Complete transection of thoracic aorta
    Traumatic rupture of thoracic aorta
- ✓x7ᵗʰ **S25.09** Other specified injury of thoracic aorta

✓5ᵗʰ **S25.1** Injury of innominate or subclavian artery
- ✓6ᵗʰ **S25.10** Unspecified injury of innominate or subclavian artery
  - ✓7ᵗʰ **S25.101** Unspecified injury of right innominate or subclavian artery
  - ✓7ᵗʰ **S25.102** Unspecified injury of left innominate or subclavian artery
  - ✓7ᵗʰ **S25.109** Unspecified injury of unspecified innominate or subclavian artery

✓ Additional Character Required   ✓x7ᵗʰ Xtension Alert   Unspecified Dx   Other Specified Dx   Manifestation   ►◄ Revised Text   ● New Code   ▲ Revised Code Title

ICD-10-CM Draft (2015)   825

Injury, Poisoning and Certain Other Consequences of External Causes   S23.15–S25.109

Injury, Poisoning and Certain Other Consequences of External Causes

S25.11–S25.819

✓6th **S25.11** Minor laceration of innominate or subclavian artery
Incomplete transection of innominate or subclavian artery
Laceration of innominate or subclavian artery NOS
Superficial laceration of innominate or subclavian artery

    ✓7th **S25.111** Minor laceration of right innominate or subclavian artery

    ✓7th **S25.112** Minor laceration of left innominate or subclavian artery

    ✓7th **S25.119** Minor laceration of unspecified innominate or subclavian artery

✓6th **S25.12** Major laceration of innominate or subclavian artery
Complete transection of innominate or subclavian artery
Traumatic rupture of innominate or subclavian artery

    ✓7th **S25.121** Major laceration of right innominate or subclavian artery

    ✓7th **S25.122** Major laceration of left innominate or subclavian artery

    ✓7th **S25.129** Major laceration of unspecified innominate or subclavian artery

✓6th **S25.19** Other specified injury of innominate or subclavian artery

    ✓7th **S25.191** Other specified injury of right innominate or subclavian artery

    ✓7th **S25.192** Other specified injury of left innominate or subclavian artery

    ✓7th **S25.199** Other specified injury of unspecified innominate or subclavian artery

✓5th **S25.2** Injury of superior vena cava
Injury of vena cava NOS

    ✓x7th **S25.20** Unspecified injury of superior vena cava

    ✓x7th **S25.21** Minor laceration of superior vena cava
Incomplete transection of superior vena cava
Laceration of superior vena cava NOS
Superficial laceration of superior vena cava

    ✓x7th **S25.22** Major laceration of superior vena cava
Complete transection of superior vena cava
Traumatic rupture of superior vena cava

    ✓x7th **S25.29** Other specified injury of superior vena cava

✓5th **S25.3** Injury of innominate or subclavian vein

    ✓6th **S25.30** Unspecified injury of innominate or subclavian vein

      ✓7th **S25.301** Unspecified injury of right innominate or subclavian vein

      ✓7th **S25.302** Unspecified injury of left innominate or subclavian vein

      ✓7th **S25.309** Unspecified injury of unspecified innominate or subclavian vein

    ✓6th **S25.31** Minor laceration of innominate or subclavian vein
Incomplete transection of innominate or subclavian vein
Laceration of innominate or subclavian vein NOS
Superficial laceration of innominate or subclavian vein

      ✓7th **S25.311** Minor laceration of right innominate or subclavian vein

      ✓7th **S25.312** Minor laceration of left innominate or subclavian vein

      ✓7th **S25.319** Minor laceration of unspecified innominate or subclavian vein

    ✓6th **S25.32** Major laceration of innominate or subclavian vein
Complete transection of innominate or subclavian vein
Traumatic rupture of innominate or subclavian vein

      ✓7th **S25.321** Major laceration of right innominate or subclavian vein

      ✓7th **S25.322** Major laceration of left innominate or subclavian vein

      ✓7th **S25.329** Major laceration of unspecified innominate or subclavian vein

    ✓6th **S25.39** Other specified injury of innominate or subclavian vein

      ✓7th **S25.391** Other specified injury of right innominate or subclavian vein

      ✓7th **S25.392** Other specified injury of left innominate or subclavian vein

      ✓7th **S25.399** Other specified injury of unspecified innominate or subclavian vein

✓5th **S25.4** Injury of pulmonary blood vessels

    ✓6th **S25.40** Unspecified injury of pulmonary blood vessels

      ✓7th **S25.401** Unspecified injury of right pulmonary blood vessels

      ✓7th **S25.402** Unspecified injury of left pulmonary blood vessels

      ✓7th **S25.409** Unspecified injury of unspecified pulmonary blood vessels

    ✓6th **S25.41** Minor laceration of pulmonary blood vessels
Incomplete transection of pulmonary blood vessels
Laceration of pulmonary blood vessels NOS
Superficial laceration of pulmonary blood vessels

      ✓7th **S25.411** Minor laceration of right pulmonary blood vessels

      ✓7th **S25.412** Minor laceration of left pulmonary blood vessels

      ✓7th **S25.419** Minor laceration of unspecified pulmonary blood vessels

    ✓6th **S25.42** Major laceration of pulmonary blood vessels
Complete transection of pulmonary blood vessels
Traumatic rupture of pulmonary blood vessels

      ✓7th **S25.421** Major laceration of right pulmonary blood vessels

      ✓7th **S25.422** Major laceration of left pulmonary blood vessels

      ✓7th **S25.429** Major laceration of unspecified pulmonary blood vessels

    ✓6th **S25.49** Other specified injury of pulmonary blood vessels

      ✓7th **S25.491** Other specified injury of right pulmonary blood vessels

      ✓7th **S25.492** Other specified injury of left pulmonary blood vessels

      ✓7th **S25.499** Other specified injury of unspecified pulmonary blood vessels

✓5th **S25.5** Injury of intercostal blood vessels

    ✓6th **S25.50** Unspecified injury of intercostal blood vessels

      ✓7th **S25.501** Unspecified injury of intercostal blood vessels, right side

      ✓7th **S25.502** Unspecified injury of intercostal blood vessels, left side

      ✓7th **S25.509** Unspecified injury of intercostal blood vessels, unspecified side

    ✓6th **S25.51** Laceration of intercostal blood vessels

      ✓7th **S25.511** Laceration of intercostal blood vessels, right side

      ✓7th **S25.512** Laceration of intercostal blood vessels, left side

      ✓7th **S25.519** Laceration of intercostal blood vessels, unspecified side

    ✓6th **S25.59** Other specified injury of intercostal blood vessels

      ✓7th **S25.591** Other specified injury of intercostal blood vessels, right side

      ✓7th **S25.592** Other specified injury of intercostal blood vessels, left side

      ✓7th **S25.599** Other specified injury of intercostal blood vessels, unspecified side

✓5th **S25.8** Injury of other blood vessels of thorax
Injury of azygos vein   Injury of mammary artery or vein

    ✓6th **S25.80** Unspecified injury of other blood vessels of thorax

      ✓7th **S25.801** Unspecified injury of other blood vessels of thorax, right side

      ✓7th **S25.802** Unspecified injury of other blood vessels of thorax, left side

      ✓7th **S25.809** Unspecified injury of other blood vessels of thorax, unspecified side

    ✓6th **S25.81** Laceration of other blood vessels of thorax

      ✓7th **S25.811** Laceration of other blood vessels of thorax, right side

      ✓7th **S25.812** Laceration of other blood vessels of thorax, left side

      ✓7th **S25.819** Laceration of other blood vessels of thorax, unspecified side

EXCLUDES 1 Not coded here   **EXCLUDES 2** Not included here   **N** Newborn Age: 0   **P** Pediatric Age: 0-17   **M** Maternity Age: 12-55   **A** Adult Age: 15-124

826

ICD-10-CM Draft (2015)

✓6ᵗʰ **S25.89** Other specified injury of other blood vessels of thorax

    ✓7ᵗʰ **S25.891** Other specified injury of other blood vessels of thorax, right side

    ✓7ᵗʰ **S25.892** Other specified injury of other blood vessels of thorax, left side

    ✓7ᵗʰ **S25.899** Other specified injury of other blood vessels of thorax, unspecified side

✓5ᵗʰ **S25.9** Injury of unspecified blood vessel of thorax

    ✓x7ᵗʰ **S25.90** Unspecified injury of unspecified blood vessel of thorax

    ✓x7ᵗʰ **S25.91** Laceration of unspecified blood vessel of thorax

    ✓x7ᵗʰ **S25.99** Other specified injury of unspecified blood vessel of thorax

✓4ᵗʰ **S26** **Injury of heart**

    Code also any associated:
      open wound of thorax (S21.-)
      traumatic hemopneumothorax (S27.2)
      traumatic hemothorax (S27.1)
      traumatic pneumothorax (S27.0)

    The appropriate 7th character is to be added to each code from category S26.
    A   initial encounter
    D   subsequent encounter
    S   sequela

✓5ᵗʰ **S26.0** Injury of heart with hemopericardium

    ✓x7ᵗʰ **S26.00** Unspecified injury of heart with hemopericardium

    ✓x7ᵗʰ **S26.01** Contusion of heart with hemopericardium

    ✓6ᵗʰ **S26.02** Laceration of heart with hemopericardium

      ✓7ᵗʰ **S26.020** Mild laceration of heart with hemopericardium
        Laceration of heart without penetration of heart chamber

      ✓7ᵗʰ **S26.021** Moderate laceration of heart with hemopericardium
        Laceration of heart with penetration of heart chamber

      ✓7ᵗʰ **S26.022** Major laceration of heart with hemopericardium
        Laceration of heart with penetration of multiple heart chambers

    ✓x7ᵗʰ **S26.09** Other injury of heart with hemopericardium

✓5ᵗʰ **S26.1** Injury of heart without hemopericardium

    ✓x7ᵗʰ **S26.10** Unspecified injury of heart without hemopericardium

    ✓x7ᵗʰ **S26.11** Contusion of heart without hemopericardium

    ✓x7ᵗʰ **S26.12** Laceration of heart without hemopericardium

    ✓x7ᵗʰ **S26.19** Other injury of heart without hemopericardium

✓5ᵗʰ **S26.9** Injury of heart, unspecified with or without hemopericardium

    ✓x7ᵗʰ **S26.90** Unspecified injury of heart, unspecified with or without hemopericardium

    ✓x7ᵗʰ **S26.91** Contusion of heart, unspecified with or without hemopericardium

    ✓x7ᵗʰ **S26.92** Laceration of heart, unspecified with or without hemopericardium
      Laceration of heart NOS

    ✓x7ᵗʰ **S26.99** Other injury of heart, unspecified with or without hemopericardium

✓4ᵗʰ **S27** **Injury of other and unspecified intrathoracic organs**

    Code also any associated open wound of thorax (S21.-)
    EXCLUDES 2   injury of cervical esophagus (S10-S19)
            injury of trachea (cervical) (S10-S19)

    The appropriate 7th character is to be added to each code from category S27.
    A   initial encounter
    D   subsequent encounter
    S   sequela

    ✓x7ᵗʰ **S27.0** **Traumatic pneumothorax**
      EXCLUDES 1   spontaneous pneumothorax (J93.-)

    ✓x7ᵗʰ **S27.1** **Traumatic hemothorax**

    ✓x7ᵗʰ **S27.2** **Traumatic hemopneumothorax**

    ✓5ᵗʰ **S27.3** **Other and unspecified injuries of lung**

      ✓6ᵗʰ **S27.30** Unspecified injury of lung

        ✓7ᵗʰ **S27.301** Unspecified injury of lung, unilateral

        ✓7ᵗʰ **S27.302** Unspecified injury of lung, bilateral

        ✓7ᵗʰ **S27.309** Unspecified injury of lung, unspecified

      ✓6ᵗʰ **S27.31** Primary blast injury of lung
        Blast injury of lung NOS

        ✓7ᵗʰ **S27.311** Primary blast injury of lung, unilateral

        ✓7ᵗʰ **S27.312** Primary blast injury of lung, bilateral

        ✓7ᵗʰ **S27.319** Primary blast injury of lung, unspecified

      ✓6ᵗʰ **S27.32** Contusion of lung

        ✓7ᵗʰ **S27.321** Contusion of lung, unilateral

        ✓7ᵗʰ **S27.322** Contusion of lung, bilateral

        ✓7ᵗʰ **S27.329** Contusion of lung, unspecified

      ✓6ᵗʰ **S27.33** Laceration of lung

        ✓7ᵗʰ **S27.331** Laceration of lung, unilateral

        ✓7ᵗʰ **S27.332** Laceration of lung, bilateral

        ✓7ᵗʰ **S27.339** Laceration of lung, unspecified

      ✓6ᵗʰ **S27.39** Other injuries of lung
        Secondary blast injury of lung

        ✓7ᵗʰ **S27.391** Other injuries of lung, unilateral

        ✓7ᵗʰ **S27.392** Other injuries of lung, bilateral

        ✓7ᵗʰ **S27.399** Other injuries of lung, unspecified

    ✓5ᵗʰ **S27.4** Injury of bronchus

      ✓6ᵗʰ **S27.40** Unspecified injury of bronchus

        ✓7ᵗʰ **S27.401** Unspecified injury of bronchus, unilateral

        ✓7ᵗʰ **S27.402** Unspecified injury of bronchus, bilateral

        ✓7ᵗʰ **S27.409** Unspecified injury of bronchus, unspecified

      ✓6ᵗʰ **S27.41** Primary blast injury of bronchus
        Blast injury of bronchus NOS

        ✓7ᵗʰ **S27.411** Primary blast injury of bronchus, unilateral

        ✓7ᵗʰ **S27.412** Primary blast injury of bronchus, bilateral

        ✓7ᵗʰ **S27.419** Primary blast injury of bronchus, unspecified

      ✓6ᵗʰ **S27.42** Contusion of bronchus

        ✓7ᵗʰ **S27.421** Contusion of bronchus, unilateral

        ✓7ᵗʰ **S27.422** Contusion of bronchus, bilateral

        ✓7ᵗʰ **S27.429** Contusion of bronchus, unspecified

      ✓6ᵗʰ **S27.43** Laceration of bronchus

        ✓7ᵗʰ **S27.431** Laceration of bronchus, unilateral

        ✓7ᵗʰ **S27.432** Laceration of bronchus, bilateral

        ✓7ᵗʰ **S27.439** Laceration of bronchus, unspecified

      ✓6ᵗʰ **S27.49** Other injury of bronchus
        Secondary blast injury of bronchus

        ✓7ᵗʰ **S27.491** Other injury of bronchus, unilateral

        ✓7ᵗʰ **S27.492** Other injury of bronchus, bilateral

        ✓7ᵗʰ **S27.499** Other injury of bronchus, unspecified

    ✓5ᵗʰ **S27.5** Injury of thoracic trachea

      ✓x7ᵗʰ **S27.50** Unspecified injury of thoracic trachea

      ✓x7ᵗʰ **S27.51** Primary blast injury of thoracic trachea
        Blast injury of thoracic trachea NOS

      ✓x7ᵗʰ **S27.52** Contusion of thoracic trachea

      ✓x7ᵗʰ **S27.53** Laceration of thoracic trachea

      ✓x7ᵗʰ **S27.59** Other injury of thoracic trachea
        Secondary blast injury of thoracic trachea

    ✓5ᵗʰ **S27.6** Injury of pleura

      ✓x7ᵗʰ **S27.60** Unspecified injury of pleura

      ✓x7ᵗʰ **S27.63** Laceration of pleura

      ✓x7ᵗʰ **S27.69** Other injury of pleura

    ✓5ᵗʰ **S27.8** Injury of other specified intrathoracic organs

      ✓6ᵗʰ **S27.80** Injury of diaphragm

        ✓7ᵗʰ **S27.802** Contusion of diaphragm

        ✓7ᵗʰ **S27.803** Laceration of diaphragm

        ✓7ᵗʰ **S27.808** Other injury of diaphragm

        ✓7ᵗʰ **S27.809** Unspecified injury of diaphragm

      ✓6ᵗʰ **S27.81** Injury of esophagus (thoracic part)

        ✓7ᵗʰ **S27.812** Contusion of esophagus (thoracic part)

        ✓7ᵗʰ **S27.813** Laceration of esophagus (thoracic part)

✓ Additional Character Required   ✓x7ᵗʰ Xtension Alert   Unspecified Dx   Other Specified Dx   Manifestation   ▶◀ Revised Text   ● New Code   ▲ Revised Code Title

ICD-10-CM Draft (2015)   **827**

Injury, Poisoning and Certain Other Consequences of External Causes

S27.818–S30.825

√7ᵗʰ **S27.818** Other injury of esophagus (thoracic part)

√7ᵗʰ **S27.819** Unspecified injury of esophagus (thoracic part)

√6ᵗʰ **S27.89** Injury of other specified intrathoracic organs
Injury of lymphatic thoracic duct
Injury of thymus gland

√7ᵗʰ **S27.892** Contusion of other specified intrathoracic organs

√7ᵗʰ **S27.893** Laceration of other specified intrathoracic organs

√7ᵗʰ **S27.898** Other injury of other specified intrathoracic organs

√7ᵗʰ **S27.899** Unspecified injury of other specified intrathoracic organs

√x7ᵗʰ **S27.9** Injury of unspecified intrathoracic organ

√4ᵗʰ **S28** Crushing injury of thorax, and traumatic amputation of part of thorax

The appropriate 7th character is to be added to each code from category S28.
A   initial encounter
D   subsequent encounter
S   sequela

√x7ᵗʰ **S28.0** Crushed chest
Use additional code for all associated injuries
EXCLUDES 1   flail chest (S22.5)

√x7ᵗʰ **S28.1** Traumatic amputation (partial) of part of thorax, except breast

√5ᵗʰ **S28.2** Traumatic amputation of breast

√6ᵗʰ **S28.21** Complete traumatic amputation of breast
Traumatic amputation of breast NOS

√7ᵗʰ **S28.211** Complete traumatic amputation of right breast

√7ᵗʰ **S28.212** Complete traumatic amputation of left breast

√7ᵗʰ **S28.219** Complete traumatic amputation of unspecified breast

√6ᵗʰ **S28.22** Partial traumatic amputation of breast

√7ᵗʰ **S28.221** Partial traumatic amputation of right breast

√7ᵗʰ **S28.222** Partial traumatic amputation of left breast

√7ᵗʰ **S28.229** Partial traumatic amputation of unspecified breast

√4ᵗʰ **S29** Other and unspecified injuries of thorax
Code also any associated open wound (S21.-)

The appropriate 7th character is to be added to each code from category S29.
A   initial encounter
D   subsequent encounter
S   sequela

√5ᵗʰ **S29.0** Injury of muscle and tendon at thorax level

√6ᵗʰ **S29.00** Unspecified injury of muscle and tendon of thorax

√7ᵗʰ **S29.001** Unspecified injury of muscle and tendon of front wall of thorax

√7ᵗʰ **S29.002** Unspecified injury of muscle and tendon of back wall of thorax

√7ᵗʰ **S29.009** Unspecified injury of muscle and tendon of unspecified wall of thorax

√6ᵗʰ **S29.01** Strain of muscle and tendon of thorax

√7ᵗʰ **S29.011** Strain of muscle and tendon of front wall of thorax

√7ᵗʰ **S29.012** Strain of muscle and tendon of back wall of thorax

√7ᵗʰ **S29.019** Strain of muscle and tendon of unspecified wall of thorax

√6ᵗʰ **S29.02** Laceration of muscle and tendon of thorax

√7ᵗʰ **S29.021** Laceration of muscle and tendon of front wall of thorax

√7ᵗʰ **S29.022** Laceration of muscle and tendon of back wall of thorax

√7ᵗʰ **S29.029** Laceration of muscle and tendon of unspecified wall of thorax

√6ᵗʰ **S29.09** Other injury of muscle and tendon of thorax

√7ᵗʰ **S29.091** Other injury of muscle and tendon of front wall of thorax

√7ᵗʰ **S29.092** Other injury of muscle and tendon of back wall of thorax

√7ᵗʰ **S29.099** Other injury of muscle and tendon of unspecified wall of thorax

√x7ᵗʰ **S29.8** Other specified injuries of thorax

√x7ᵗʰ **S29.9** Unspecified injury of thorax

Injuries to the abdomen, lower back, lumbar spine, pelvis and external genitals (S30-S39)

INCLUDES   injuries to the abdominal wall
injuries to the anus
injuries to the buttock
injuries to the external genitalia
injuries to the flank
injuries to the groin

EXCLUDES 2   burns and corrosions (T20-T32)
effects of foreign body in anus and rectum (T18.5)
effects of foreign body in genitourinary tract (T19.-)
effects of foreign body in stomach, small intestine and colon (T18.2-T18.4)
frostbite (T33-T34)
insect bite or sting, venomous (T63.4)

√4ᵗʰ **S30** Superficial injury of abdomen, lower back, pelvis and external genitals

EXCLUDES 2   superficial injury of hip (S70.-)

The appropriate 7th character is to be added to each code from category S30.
A   initial encounter
D   subsequent encounter
S   sequela

√x7ᵗʰ **S30.0** Contusion of lower back and pelvis
Contusion of buttock

√x7ᵗʰ **S30.1** Contusion of abdominal wall
Contusion of flank   Contusion of groin

√5ᵗʰ **S30.2** Contusion of external genital organs

√6ᵗʰ **S30.20** Contusion of unspecified external genital organ

√7ᵗʰ **S30.201** Contusion of unspecified external genital organ, male   ♂

√7ᵗʰ **S30.202** Contusion of unspecified external genital organ, female   ♀

√x7ᵗʰ **S30.21** Contusion of penis   ♂

√x7ᵗʰ **S30.22** Contusion of scrotum and testes   ♂

√x7ᵗʰ **S30.23** Contusion of vagina and vulva   ♀

√x7ᵗʰ **S30.3** Contusion of anus

√5ᵗʰ **S30.8** Other superficial injuries of abdomen, lower back, pelvis and external genitals

√6ᵗʰ **S30.81** Abrasion of abdomen, lower back, pelvis and external genitals

√7ᵗʰ **S30.810** Abrasion of lower back and pelvis

√7ᵗʰ **S30.811** Abrasion of abdominal wall

√7ᵗʰ **S30.812** Abrasion of penis   ♂

√7ᵗʰ **S30.813** Abrasion of scrotum and testes   ♂

√7ᵗʰ **S30.814** Abrasion of vagina and vulva   ♀

√7ᵗʰ **S30.815** Abrasion of unspecified external genital organs, male   ♂

√7ᵗʰ **S30.816** Abrasion of unspecified external genital organs, female   ♀

√7ᵗʰ **S30.817** Abrasion of anus

√6ᵗʰ **S30.82** Blister (nonthermal) of abdomen, lower back, pelvis and external genitals

√7ᵗʰ **S30.820** Blister (nonthermal) of lower back and pelvis

√7ᵗʰ **S30.821** Blister (nonthermal) of abdominal wall

√7ᵗʰ **S30.822** Blister (nonthermal) of penis   ♂

√7ᵗʰ **S30.823** Blister (nonthermal) of scrotum and testes   ♂

√7ᵗʰ **S30.824** Blister (nonthermal) of vagina and vulva   ♀

√7ᵗʰ **S30.825** Blister (nonthermal) of unspecified external genital organs, male   ♂

EXCLUDES 1 Not coded here   **EXCLUDES 2** Not included here   N Newborn Age: 0   P Pediatric Age: 0-17   M Maternity Age: 12-55   A Adult Age: 15-124

828   ICD-10-CM Draft (2015)

☑7ᵗʰ **S30.826** **Blister (nonthermal) of** unspecified external genital organs, female ♀

☑7ᵗʰ **S30.827** **Blister (nonthermal) of** anus

✓6ᵗʰ **S30.84** External constriction **of abdomen, lower back, pelvis and external genitals**

☑7ᵗʰ **S30.840** **External constriction of** lower back and pelvis

☑7ᵗʰ **S30.841** **External constriction of** abdominal wall

☑7ᵗʰ **S30.842** **External constriction of** penis ♂
Hair tourniquet syndrome of penis
Use additional cause code to identify the constricting item (W49.0-)

☑7ᵗʰ **S30.843** **External constriction of** scrotum and testes ♂

☑7ᵗʰ **S30.844** **External constriction of** vagina and vulva ♀

☑7ᵗʰ **S30.845** **External constriction of unspecified** external genital organs, male ♂

☑7ᵗʰ **S30.846** **External constriction of unspecified** external genital organs, female ♀

✓6ᵗʰ **S30.85** **Superficial** foreign body **of abdomen, lower back, pelvis and external genitals**
Splinter in the abdomen, lower back, pelvis and external genitals

☑7ᵗʰ **S30.850** **Superficial foreign body of** lower back and pelvis

☑7ᵗʰ **S30.851** **Superficial foreign body of** abdominal wall

☑7ᵗʰ **S30.852** **Superficial foreign body of** penis ♂

☑7ᵗʰ **S30.853** **Superficial foreign body of** scrotum and testes ♂

☑7ᵗʰ **S30.854** **Superficial foreign body of** vagina and vulva ♀

☑7ᵗʰ **S30.855** **Superficial foreign body of unspecified** external genital organs, male ♂

☑7ᵗʰ **S30.856** **Superficial foreign body of unspecified** external genital organs, female ♀

☑7ᵗʰ **S30.857** **Superficial foreign body of** anus

✓6ᵗʰ **S30.86** Insect bite **(nonvenomous) of abdomen, lower back, pelvis and external genitals**

☑7ᵗʰ **S30.860** **Insect bite (nonvenomous) of** lower back and pelvis

☑7ᵗʰ **S30.861** **Insect bite (nonvenomous) of** abdominal wall

☑7ᵗʰ **S30.862** **Insect bite (nonvenomous) of** penis ♂

☑7ᵗʰ **S30.863** **Insect bite (nonvenomous) of** scrotum and testes ♂

☑7ᵗʰ **S30.864** **Insect bite (nonvenomous) of** vagina and vulva ♀

☑7ᵗʰ **S30.865** **Insect bite (nonvenomous) of unspecified** external genital organs, male ♂

☑7ᵗʰ **S30.866** **Insect bite (nonvenomous) of unspecified** external genital organs, female ♀

☑7ᵗʰ **S30.867** **Insect bite (nonvenomous) of** anus

✓6ᵗʰ **S30.87** Other superficial **bite of abdomen, lower back, pelvis and external genitals**
EXCLUDES 1 open bite of abdomen, lower back, pelvis and external genitals (S31.05, S31.15, S31.25, S31.35, S31.45, S31.55)

☑7ᵗʰ **S30.870** **Other superficial bite of** lower back and pelvis

☑7ᵗʰ **S30.871** **Other superficial bite of** abdominal wall

☑7ᵗʰ **S30.872** **Other superficial bite of** penis ♂

☑7ᵗʰ **S30.873** **Other superficial bite of** scrotum and testes ♂

☑7ᵗʰ **S30.874** **Other superficial bite of** vagina and vulva ♀

☑7ᵗʰ **S30.875** **Other superficial bite of unspecified** external genital organs, male ♂

☑7ᵗʰ **S30.876** **Other superficial bite of unspecified** external genital organs, female ♀

☑7ᵗʰ **S30.877** **Other superficial bite of** anus

✓5ᵗʰ **S30.9** Unspecified **superficial injury of abdomen, lower back, pelvis and external genitals**

√x7ᵗʰ **S30.91** **Unspecified superficial injury of** lower back and pelvis

√x7ᵗʰ **S30.92** **Unspecified superficial injury of** abdominal wall

√x7ᵗʰ **S30.93** **Unspecified superficial injury of** penis ♂

√x7ᵗʰ **S30.94** **Unspecified superficial injury of** scrotum and testes ♂

√x7ᵗʰ **S30.95** **Unspecified superficial injury of** vagina and vulva ♀

√x7ᵗʰ **S30.96** **Unspecified superficial injury of unspecified** external genital organs, male ♂

√x7ᵗʰ **S30.97** **Unspecified superficial injury of unspecified** external genital organs, female ♀

√x7ᵗʰ **S30.98** **Unspecified superficial injury of** anus

✓4ᵗʰ **S31** **Open wound of abdomen, lower back, pelvis and external genitals**
Code also any associated:
spinal cord injury (S24.0, S24.1-, S34.0-, S34.1-)
wound infection
EXCLUDES 1 traumatic amputation of part of abdomen, lower back and pelvis (S38.2-, S38.3)
EXCLUDES 2 open wound of hip (S71.00-S71.02)
open fracture of pelvis (S32.1- -S32.9 with 7th character B)

The appropriate 7th character is to be added to each code from category S31.
A   initial encounter
D   subsequent encounter
S   sequela

✓5ᵗʰ **S31.0** **Open wound of** lower back and pelvis

✓6ᵗʰ **S31.00** Unspecified open wound **of lower back and pelvis**

☑7ᵗʰ **S31.000** **Unspecified open wound of lower back and pelvis** without penetration into retroperitoneum
Unspecified open wound of lower back and pelvis NOS

☑7ᵗʰ **S31.001** **Unspecified open wound of lower back and pelvis** with penetration into retroperitoneum

✓6ᵗʰ **S31.01** Laceration without foreign body **of lower back and pelvis**

☑7ᵗʰ **S31.010** **Laceration without foreign body of lower back and pelvis** without penetration into retroperitoneum
Laceration without foreign body of lower back and pelvis NOS

☑7ᵗʰ **S31.011** **Laceration without foreign body of lower back and pelvis** with penetration into retroperitoneum

✓6ᵗʰ **S31.02** Laceration with foreign body **of lower back and pelvis**

☑7ᵗʰ **S31.020** **Laceration with foreign body of lower back and pelvis** without penetration into retroperitoneum
Laceration with foreign body of lower back and pelvis NOS

☑7ᵗʰ **S31.021** **Laceration with foreign body of lower back and pelvis** with penetration into retroperitoneum

✓6ᵗʰ **S31.03** Puncture wound without foreign body **of lower back and pelvis**

☑7ᵗʰ **S31.030** **Puncture wound without foreign body of lower back and pelvis** without penetration into retroperitoneum
Puncture wound without foreign body of lower back and pelvis NOS

☑7ᵗʰ **S31.031** **Puncture wound without foreign body of lower back and pelvis** with penetration into retroperitoneum

✓6ᵗʰ **S31.04** Puncture wound with foreign body **of lower back and pelvis**

☑7ᵗʰ **S31.040** **Puncture wound with foreign body of lower back and pelvis** without penetration into retroperitoneum
Puncture wound with foreign body of lower back and pelvis NOS

☑ Additional Character Required   √x7ᵗʰ Xtension Alert   Unspecified Dx   Other Specified Dx   Manifestation   ►◄ Revised Text   ● New Code   ▲ Revised Code Title

☑7ᵗʰ **S31.041** **Puncture wound with foreign body of lower back and pelvis** with penetration into retroperitoneum

☑6ᵗʰ **S31.05** Open bite **of lower back and pelvis**
Bite of lower back and pelvis NOS
EXCLUDES 1 *superficial bite of lower back and pelvis (S30.860, S30.870)*

☑7ᵗʰ **S31.050** **Open bite of lower back and pelvis** without penetration into retroperitoneum
Open bite of lower back and pelvis NOS

☑7ᵗʰ **S31.051** **Open bite of lower back and pelvis** with penetration into retroperitoneum

☑5ᵗʰ **S31.1** **Open wound of** abdominal wall without penetration into peritoneal cavity
Open wound of abdominal wall NOS
EXCLUDES 2 *open wound of abdominal wall with penetration into peritoneal cavity (S31.6-)*

☑6ᵗʰ **S31.10** Unspecified **open wound of abdominal wall without penetration into peritoneal cavity**

☑7ᵗʰ **S31.100** **Unspecified open wound of abdominal wall,** right upper quadrant **without penetration into peritoneal cavity**

☑7ᵗʰ **S31.101** **Unspecified open wound of abdominal wall,** left upper quadrant **without penetration into peritoneal cavity**

☑7ᵗʰ **S31.102** **Unspecified open wound of abdominal wall,** epigastric region **without penetration into peritoneal cavity**

☑7ᵗʰ **S31.103** **Unspecified open wound of abdominal wall,** right lower quadrant **without penetration into peritoneal cavity**

☑7ᵗʰ **S31.104** **Unspecified open wound of abdominal wall,** left lower quadrant **without penetration into peritoneal cavity**

☑7ᵗʰ **S31.105** **Unspecified open wound of abdominal wall,** periumbilic region **without penetration into peritoneal cavity**

☑7ᵗʰ **S31.109** **Unspecified open wound of abdominal wall, unspecified quadrant without penetration into peritoneal cavity**
Unspecified open wound of abdominal wall NOS

☑6ᵗʰ **S31.11** Laceration without foreign body **of abdominal wall without penetration into peritoneal cavity**

☑7ᵗʰ **S31.110** **Laceration without foreign body of abdominal wall,** right upper quadrant **without penetration into peritoneal cavity**

☑7ᵗʰ **S31.111** **Laceration without foreign body of abdominal wall,** left upper quadrant **without penetration into peritoneal cavity**

☑7ᵗʰ **S31.112** **Laceration without foreign body of abdominal wall,** epigastric region **without penetration into peritoneal cavity**

☑7ᵗʰ **S31.113** **Laceration without foreign body of abdominal wall,** right lower quadrant **without penetration into peritoneal cavity**

☑7ᵗʰ **S31.114** **Laceration without foreign body of abdominal wall,** left lower quadrant **without penetration into peritoneal cavity**

☑7ᵗʰ **S31.115** **Laceration without foreign body of abdominal wall,** periumbilic region **without penetration into peritoneal cavity**

☑7ᵗʰ **S31.119** **Laceration without foreign body of abdominal wall, unspecified quadrant without penetration into peritoneal cavity**

☑6ᵗʰ **S31.12** Laceration with foreign body **of abdominal wall without penetration into peritoneal cavity**

☑7ᵗʰ **S31.120** **Laceration of abdominal wall with foreign body,** right upper quadrant **without penetration into peritoneal cavity**

☑7ᵗʰ **S31.121** **Laceration of abdominal wall with foreign body,** left upper quadrant **without penetration into peritoneal cavity**

☑7ᵗʰ **S31.122** **Laceration of abdominal wall with foreign body,** epigastric region **without penetration into peritoneal cavity**

☑7ᵗʰ **S31.123** **Laceration of abdominal wall with foreign body,** right lower quadrant **without penetration into peritoneal cavity**

☑7ᵗʰ **S31.124** **Laceration of abdominal wall with foreign body,** left lower quadrant **without penetration into peritoneal cavity**

☑7ᵗʰ **S31.125** **Laceration of abdominal wall with foreign body,** periumbilic region **without penetration into peritoneal cavity**

☑7ᵗʰ **S31.129** **Laceration of abdominal wall with foreign body, unspecified quadrant without penetration into peritoneal cavity**

☑6ᵗʰ **S31.13** Puncture wound **of abdominal wall without foreign body without penetration into peritoneal cavity**

☑7ᵗʰ **S31.130** **Puncture wound of abdominal wall without foreign body,** right upper quadrant **without penetration into peritoneal cavity**

☑7ᵗʰ **S31.131** **Puncture wound of abdominal wall without foreign body,** left upper quadrant **without penetration into peritoneal cavity**

☑7ᵗʰ **S31.132** **Puncture wound of abdominal wall without foreign body,** epigastric region **without penetration into peritoneal cavity**

☑7ᵗʰ **S31.133** **Puncture wound of abdominal wall without foreign body,** right lower quadrant **without penetration into peritoneal cavity**

☑7ᵗʰ **S31.134** **Puncture wound of abdominal wall without foreign body,** left lower quadrant **without penetration into peritoneal cavity**

☑7ᵗʰ **S31.135** **Puncture wound of abdominal wall without foreign body,** periumbilic region **without penetration into peritoneal cavity**

☑7ᵗʰ **S31.139** **Puncture wound of abdominal wall without foreign body, unspecified quadrant without penetration into peritoneal cavity**

☑6ᵗʰ **S31.14** Puncture wound **of abdominal wall with foreign body without penetration into peritoneal cavity**

☑7ᵗʰ **S31.140** **Puncture wound of abdominal wall with foreign body,** right upper quadrant **without penetration into peritoneal cavity**

☑7ᵗʰ **S31.141** **Puncture wound of abdominal wall with foreign body,** left upper quadrant **without penetration into peritoneal cavity**

☑7ᵗʰ **S31.142** **Puncture wound of abdominal wall with foreign body,** epigastric region **without penetration into peritoneal cavity**

☑7ᵗʰ **S31.143** **Puncture wound of abdominal wall with foreign body,** right lower quadrant **without penetration into peritoneal cavity**

☑7ᵗʰ **S31.144** **Puncture wound of abdominal wall with foreign body,** left lower quadrant **without penetration into peritoneal cavity**

☑7ᵗʰ **S31.145** **Puncture wound of abdominal wall with foreign body,** periumbilic region **without penetration into peritoneal cavity**

☑7ᵗʰ **S31.149** **Puncture wound of abdominal wall with foreign body, unspecified quadrant without penetration into peritoneal cavity**

☑6ᵗʰ **S31.15** Open bite **of abdominal wall without penetration into peritoneal cavity**
Bite of abdominal wall NOS
EXCLUDES 1 *superficial bite of abdominal wall (S30.871)*

☑7ᵗʰ **S31.150** **Open bite of abdominal wall,** right upper quadrant **without penetration into peritoneal cavity**

☑7ᵗʰ **S31.151** **Open bite of abdominal wall,** left upper quadrant **without penetration into peritoneal cavity**

☑7ᵗʰ **S31.152** **Open bite of abdominal wall,** epigastric region **without penetration into peritoneal cavity**

☑7ᵗʰ **S31.153** **Open bite of abdominal wall,** right lower quadrant **without penetration into peritoneal cavity**

☑7ᵗʰ **S31.154** **Open bite of abdominal wall,** left lower quadrant **without penetration into peritoneal cavity**

EXCLUDES 1 Not coded here   EXCLUDES 2 Not included here   N Newborn Age: 0   P Pediatric Age: 0-17   M Maternity Age: 12-55   A Adult Age: 15-124

830   ICD-10-CM Draft (2015)

√7ᵗʰ **S31.155** **Open bite of abdominal wall,** periumbilic region **without penetration into peritoneal cavity**

√7ᵗʰ **S31.159** **Open bite of abdominal wall, unspecified quadrant without penetration into peritoneal cavity**

√5ᵗʰ **S31.2** **Open wound of** penis

   √x7ᵗʰ **S31.20** **Unspecified open wound of penis** ♂

   √x7ᵗʰ **S31.21** Laceration without foreign body **of penis** ♂

   √x7ᵗʰ **S31.22** Laceration with foreign body **of penis** ♂

   √x7ᵗʰ **S31.23** Puncture wound without foreign body **of penis** ♂

   √x7ᵗʰ **S31.24** Puncture wound with foreign body **of penis** ♂

   √x7ᵗʰ **S31.25** Open bite **of penis** ♂
       Bite of penis NOS
       EXCLUDES 1 *superficial bite of penis (S30.862, S30.872)*

√5ᵗʰ **S31.3** **Open wound of** scrotum and testes

   √x7ᵗʰ **S31.30** **Unspecified open wound of scrotum and testes** ♂

   √x7ᵗʰ **S31.31** Laceration without foreign body **of scrotum and testes** ♂

   √x7ᵗʰ **S31.32** Laceration with foreign body **of scrotum and testes** ♂

   √x7ᵗʰ **S31.33** Puncture wound without foreign body **of scrotum and testes** ♂

   √x7ᵗʰ **S31.34** Puncture wound with foreign body **of scrotum and testes** ♂

   √x7ᵗʰ **S31.35** Open bite **of scrotum and testes** ♂
       Bite of scrotum and testes NOS
       EXCLUDES 1 *superficial bite of scrotum and testes (S30.863, S30.873)*

√5ᵗʰ **S31.4** **Open wound of** vagina and vulva
     EXCLUDES 1 *injury to vagina and vulva during delivery (O70-, O71.4)*

   √x7ᵗʰ **S31.40** **Unspecified open wound of vagina and vulva** ♀

   √x7ᵗʰ **S31.41** Laceration without foreign body **of vagina and vulva** ♀

   √x7ᵗʰ **S31.42** Laceration with foreign body **of vagina and vulva** ♀

   √x7ᵗʰ **S31.43** Puncture wound without foreign body **of vagina and vulva** ♀

   √x7ᵗʰ **S31.44** Puncture wound with foreign body **of vagina and vulva** ♀

   √x7ᵗʰ **S31.45** Open bite **of vagina and vulva** ♀
       Bite of vagina and vulva NOS
       EXCLUDES 1 *superficial bite of vagina and vulva (S30.864, S30.874)*

√5ᵗʰ **S31.5** **Open wound of** unspecified external genital organs
     EXCLUDES 1 *traumatic amputation of external genital organs (S38.21, S38.22)*

   √6ᵗʰ **S31.50** Unspecified **open wound of unspecified external genital organs**

     √7ᵗʰ **S31.501** **Unspecified open wound of unspecified** ♂ **external genital organs,** male

     √7ᵗʰ **S31.502** **Unspecified open wound of unspecified** ♀ **external genital organs,** female

   √6ᵗʰ **S31.51** Laceration without foreign body **of unspecified external genital organs**

     √7ᵗʰ **S31.511** **Laceration without foreign body of** ♂ **unspecified external genital organs,** male

     √7ᵗʰ **S31.512** **Laceration without foreign body of** ♀ **unspecified external genital organs,** female

   √6ᵗʰ **S31.52** Laceration with foreign body **of unspecified external genital organs**

     √7ᵗʰ **S31.521** **Laceration with foreign body of** ♂ **unspecified external genital organs,** male

     √7ᵗʰ **S31.522** **Laceration with foreign body of** ♀ **unspecified external genital organs,** female

   √6ᵗʰ **S31.53** Puncture wound without foreign body **of unspecified external genital organs**

     √7ᵗʰ **S31.531** **Puncture wound without foreign body** ♂ **of unspecified external genital organs,** male

√7ᵗʰ **S31.532** **Puncture wound without foreign body** ♀ **of unspecified external genital organs,** female

√6ᵗʰ **S31.54** Puncture wound with foreign body **of unspecified external genital organs**

   √7ᵗʰ **S31.541** **Puncture wound with foreign body of** ♂ **unspecified external genital organs,** male

   √7ᵗʰ **S31.542** **Puncture wound with foreign body of** ♀ **unspecified external genital organs,** female

√6ᵗʰ **S31.55** Open bite **of unspecified external genital organs**
     Bite of unspecified external genital organs NOS
     EXCLUDES 1 *superficial bite of unspecified external genital organs (S30.865, S30.866, S30.875, S30.876)*

   √7ᵗʰ **S31.551** **Open bite of unspecified external** ♂ **genital organs,** male

   √7ᵗʰ **S31.552** **Open bite of unspecified external** ♀ **genital organs,** female

√5ᵗʰ **S31.6** **Open wound of** abdominal wall with penetration into peritoneal cavity

   √6ᵗʰ **S31.60** Unspecified **open wound of abdominal wall with penetration into peritoneal cavity**

     √7ᵗʰ **S31.600** **Unspecified open wound of abdominal wall,** right upper quadrant **with penetration into peritoneal cavity**

     √7ᵗʰ **S31.601** **Unspecified open wound of abdominal wall,** left upper quadrant **with penetration into peritoneal cavity**

     √7ᵗʰ **S31.602** **Unspecified open wound of abdominal wall,** epigastric region **with penetration into peritoneal cavity**

     √7ᵗʰ **S31.603** **Unspecified open wound of abdominal wall,** right lower quadrant **with penetration into peritoneal cavity**

     √7ᵗʰ **S31.604** **Unspecified open wound of abdominal wall,** left lower quadrant **with penetration into peritoneal cavity**

     √7ᵗʰ **S31.605** **Unspecified open wound of abdominal wall,** periumbilic region **with penetration into peritoneal cavity**

     √7ᵗʰ **S31.609** **Unspecified open wound of abdominal wall, unspecified quadrant with penetration into peritoneal cavity**

   √6ᵗʰ **S31.61** Laceration without foreign body **of abdominal wall with penetration into peritoneal cavity**

     √7ᵗʰ **S31.610** **Laceration without foreign body of abdominal wall,** right upper quadrant **with penetration into peritoneal cavity**

     √7ᵗʰ **S31.611** **Laceration without foreign body of abdominal wall,** left upper quadrant **with penetration into peritoneal cavity**

     √7ᵗʰ **S31.612** **Laceration without foreign body of abdominal wall,** epigastric region **with penetration into peritoneal cavity**

     √7ᵗʰ **S31.613** **Laceration without foreign body of abdominal wall,** right lower quadrant **with penetration into peritoneal cavity**

     √7ᵗʰ **S31.614** **Laceration without foreign body of abdominal wall,** left lower quadrant **with penetration into peritoneal cavity**

     √7ᵗʰ **S31.615** **Laceration without foreign body of abdominal wall,** periumbilic region **with penetration into peritoneal cavity**

     √7ᵗʰ **S31.619** **Laceration without foreign body of abdominal wall, unspecified quadrant with penetration into peritoneal cavity**

   √6ᵗʰ **S31.62** Laceration with foreign body **of abdominal wall with penetration into peritoneal cavity**

     √7ᵗʰ **S31.620** **Laceration with foreign body of abdominal wall,** right upper quadrant **with penetration into peritoneal cavity**

     √7ᵗʰ **S31.621** **Laceration with foreign body of abdominal wall,** left upper quadrant **with penetration into peritoneal cavity**

✔️ Additional Character Required   √x7ᵗʰ Xtension Alert   Unspecified Dx   Other Specified Dx   Manifestation   ▶◀ Revised Text   ● New Code   ▲ Revised Code Title

✓7ᵗʰ **S31.622** Laceration with foreign body of abdominal wall, epigastric region with penetration into peritoneal cavity

✓7ᵗʰ **S31.623** Laceration with foreign body of abdominal wall, right lower quadrant with penetration into peritoneal cavity

✓7ᵗʰ **S31.624** Laceration with foreign body of abdominal wall, left lower quadrant with penetration into peritoneal cavity

✓7ᵗʰ **S31.625** Laceration with foreign body of abdominal wall, periumbilic region with penetration into peritoneal cavity

✓7ᵗʰ **S31.629** Laceration with foreign body of abdominal wall, unspecified quadrant with penetration into peritoneal cavity

✓6ᵗʰ **S31.63** Puncture wound without foreign body of abdominal wall with penetration into peritoneal cavity

✓7ᵗʰ **S31.630** Puncture wound without foreign body of abdominal wall, right upper quadrant with penetration into peritoneal cavity

✓7ᵗʰ **S31.631** Puncture wound without foreign body of abdominal wall, left upper quadrant with penetration into peritoneal cavity

✓7ᵗʰ **S31.632** Puncture wound without foreign body of abdominal wall, epigastric region with penetration into peritoneal cavity

✓7ᵗʰ **S31.633** Puncture wound without foreign body of abdominal wall, right lower quadrant with penetration into peritoneal cavity

✓7ᵗʰ **S31.634** Puncture wound without foreign body of abdominal wall, left lower quadrant with penetration into peritoneal cavity

✓7ᵗʰ **S31.635** Puncture wound without foreign body of abdominal wall, periumbilic region with penetration into peritoneal cavity

✓7ᵗʰ **S31.639** Puncture wound without foreign body of abdominal wall, unspecified quadrant with penetration into peritoneal cavity

✓6ᵗʰ **S31.64** Puncture wound with foreign body of abdominal wall with penetration into peritoneal cavity

✓7ᵗʰ **S31.640** Puncture wound with foreign body of abdominal wall, right upper quadrant with penetration into peritoneal cavity

✓7ᵗʰ **S31.641** Puncture wound with foreign body of abdominal wall, left upper quadrant with penetration into peritoneal cavity

✓7ᵗʰ **S31.642** Puncture wound with foreign body of abdominal wall, epigastric region with penetration into peritoneal cavity

✓7ᵗʰ **S31.643** Puncture wound with foreign body of abdominal wall, right lower quadrant with penetration into peritoneal cavity

✓7ᵗʰ **S31.644** Puncture wound with foreign body of abdominal wall, left lower quadrant with penetration into peritoneal cavity

✓7ᵗʰ **S31.645** Puncture wound with foreign body of abdominal wall, periumbilic region with penetration into peritoneal cavity

✓7ᵗʰ **S31.649** Puncture wound with foreign body of abdominal wall, unspecified quadrant with penetration into peritoneal cavity

✓6ᵗʰ **S31.65** Open bite of abdominal wall with penetration into peritoneal cavity
EXCLUDES 1 superficial bite of abdominal wall (S30.861, S30.871)

✓7ᵗʰ **S31.650** Open bite of abdominal wall, right upper quadrant with penetration into peritoneal cavity

✓7ᵗʰ **S31.651** Open bite of abdominal wall, left upper quadrant with penetration into peritoneal cavity

✓7ᵗʰ **S31.652** Open bite of abdominal wall, epigastric region with penetration into peritoneal cavity

✓7ᵗʰ **S31.653** Open bite of abdominal wall, right lower quadrant with penetration into peritoneal cavity

✓7ᵗʰ **S31.654** Open bite of abdominal wall, left lower quadrant with penetration into peritoneal cavity

✓7ᵗʰ **S31.655** Open bite of abdominal wall, periumbilic region with penetration into peritoneal cavity

✓7ᵗʰ **S31.659** Open bite of abdominal wall, unspecified quadrant with penetration into peritoneal cavity

✓5ᵗʰ **S31.8** Open wound of other parts of abdomen, lower back and pelvis

✓6ᵗʰ **S31.80** Open wound of unspecified buttock

✓7ᵗʰ **S31.801** Laceration without foreign body of unspecified buttock

✓7ᵗʰ **S31.802** Laceration with foreign body of unspecified buttock

✓7ᵗʰ **S31.803** Puncture wound without foreign body of unspecified buttock

✓7ᵗʰ **S31.804** Puncture wound with foreign body of unspecified buttock

✓7ᵗʰ **S31.805** Open bite of unspecified buttock
Bite of buttock NOS
EXCLUDES 1 superficial bite of buttock (S30.870)

✓7ᵗʰ **S31.809** Unspecified open wound of unspecified buttock

✓6ᵗʰ **S31.81** Open wound of right buttock

✓7ᵗʰ **S31.811** Laceration without foreign body of right buttock

✓7ᵗʰ **S31.812** Laceration with foreign body of right buttock

✓7ᵗʰ **S31.813** Puncture wound without foreign body of right buttock

✓7ᵗʰ **S31.814** Puncture wound with foreign body of right buttock

✓7ᵗʰ **S31.815** Open bite of right buttock
Bite of right buttock NOS
EXCLUDES 1 superficial bite of buttock (S30.870)

✓7ᵗʰ **S31.819** Unspecified open wound of right buttock

✓6ᵗʰ **S31.82** Open wound of left buttock

✓7ᵗʰ **S31.821** Laceration without foreign body of left buttock

✓7ᵗʰ **S31.822** Laceration with foreign body of left buttock

✓7ᵗʰ **S31.823** Puncture wound without foreign body of left buttock

✓7ᵗʰ **S31.824** Puncture wound with foreign body of left buttock

✓7ᵗʰ **S31.825** Open bite of left buttock
Bite of left buttock NOS
EXCLUDES 1 superficial bite of buttock (S30.870)

✓7ᵗʰ **S31.829** Unspecified open wound of left buttock

✓6ᵗʰ **S31.83** Open wound of anus

✓7ᵗʰ **S31.831** Laceration without foreign body of anus

✓7ᵗʰ **S31.832** Laceration with foreign body of anus

✓7ᵗʰ **S31.833** Puncture wound without foreign body of anus

✓7ᵗʰ **S31.834** Puncture wound with foreign body of anus

✓7ᵗʰ **S31.835** Open bite of anus
Bite of anus NOS
EXCLUDES 1 superficial bite of anus (S30.877)

✓7ᵗʰ **S31.839** Unspecified open wound of anus

EXCLUDES 1 Not coded here   EXCLUDES 2 Not included here   N Newborn Age: 0   P Pediatric Age: 0-17   M Maternity Age: 12-55   A Adult Age: 15-124

832   ICD-10-CM Draft (2015)

✓4th S32 Fracture of lumbar spine and pelvis

> **NOTE** A fracture not indicated as displaced or nondisplaced should be coded to displaced.
> A fracture not indicated as opened or closed should be coded to closed.
>
> **INCLUDES** fracture of lumbosacral neural arch
> fracture of lumbosacral spinous process
> fracture of lumbosacral transverse process
> fracture of lumbosacral vertebra
> fracture of lumbosacral vertebral arch

Code first any associated spinal cord and spinal nerve injury (S34.-)

EXCLUDES 1 transection of abdomen (S38.3)

EXCLUDES 2 fracture of hip NOS (S72.0-)

AHA: 2012, 4Q, 93

The appropriate 7th character is to be added to each code from category S32.
A   initial encounter for closed fracture
B   initial encounter for open fracture
D   subsequent encounter for fracture with routine healing
G   subsequent encounter for fracture with delayed healing
K   subsequent encounter for fracture with nonunion
S   sequela

✓5th S32.0 Fracture of lumbar vertebra
Fracture of lumbar spine NOS

   ✓6th S32.00 Fracture of unspecified lumbar vertebra

     ✓7th S32.000 Wedge compression fracture of unspecified lumbar vertebra

     ✓7th S32.001 Stable burst fracture of unspecified lumbar vertebra

     ✓7th S32.002 Unstable burst fracture of unspecified lumbar vertebra

     ✓7th S32.008 Other fracture of unspecified lumbar vertebra

     ✓7th S32.009 Unspecified fracture of unspecified lumbar vertebra

   ✓6th S32.01 Fracture of first lumbar vertebra

     ✓7th S32.010 Wedge compression fracture of first lumbar vertebra

     ✓7th S32.011 Stable burst fracture of first lumbar vertebra

     ✓7th S32.012 Unstable burst fracture of first lumbar vertebra

     ✓7th S32.018 Other fracture of first lumbar vertebra

     ✓7th S32.019 Unspecified fracture of first lumbar vertebra

   ✓6th S32.02 Fracture of second lumbar vertebra

     ✓7th S32.020 Wedge compression fracture of second lumbar vertebra

     ✓7th S32.021 Stable burst fracture of second lumbar vertebra

     ✓7th S32.022 Unstable burst fracture of second lumbar vertebra

     ✓7th S32.028 Other fracture of second lumbar vertebra

     ✓7th S32.029 Unspecified fracture of second lumbar vertebra

   ✓6th S32.03 Fracture of third lumbar vertebra

     ✓7th S32.030 Wedge compression fracture of third lumbar vertebra

     ✓7th S32.031 Stable burst fracture of third lumbar vertebra

     ✓7th S32.032 Unstable burst fracture of third lumbar vertebra

     ✓7th S32.038 Other fracture of third lumbar vertebra

     ✓7th S32.039 Unspecified fracture of third lumbar vertebra

   ✓6th S32.04 Fracture of fourth lumbar vertebra

     ✓7th S32.040 Wedge compression fracture of fourth lumbar vertebra

     ✓7th S32.041 Stable burst fracture of fourth lumbar vertebra

     ✓7th S32.042 Unstable burst fracture of fourth lumbar vertebra

     ✓7th S32.048 Other fracture of fourth lumbar vertebra

     ✓7th S32.049 Unspecified fracture of fourth lumbar vertebra

   ✓6th S32.05 Fracture of fifth lumbar vertebra

     ✓7th S32.050 Wedge compression fracture of fifth lumbar vertebra

     ✓7th S32.051 Stable burst fracture of fifth lumbar vertebra

     ✓7th S32.052 Unstable burst fracture of fifth lumbar vertebra

     ✓7th S32.058 Other fracture of fifth lumbar vertebra

     ✓7th S32.059 Unspecified fracture of fifth lumbar vertebra

✓5th S32.1 Fracture of sacrum

> **NOTE** For vertical fractures, code to most medial fracture extension.
> Use two codes if both a vertical and transverse fracture are present.

Code also any associated fracture of pelvic ring (S32.8-)

   ✓x7th S32.10 Unspecified fracture of sacrum

   ✓6th S32.11 Zone I fracture of sacrum
      Vertical sacral ala fracture of sacrum

     ✓7th S32.110 Nondisplaced Zone I fracture of sacrum

     ✓7th S32.111 Minimally displaced Zone I fracture of sacrum

     ✓7th S32.112 Severely displaced Zone I fracture of sacrum

     ✓7th S32.119 Unspecified Zone I fracture of sacrum

   ✓6th S32.12 Zone II fracture of sacrum
      Vertical foraminal region fracture of sacrum

     ✓7th S32.120 Nondisplaced Zone II fracture of sacrum

     ✓7th S32.121 Minimally displaced Zone II fracture of sacrum

     ✓7th S32.122 Severely displaced Zone II fracture of sacrum

     ✓7th S32.129 Unspecified Zone II fracture of sacrum

   ✓6th S32.13 Zone III fracture of sacrum
      Vertical fracture into spinal canal region of sacrum

     ✓7th S32.130 Nondisplaced Zone III fracture of sacrum

     ✓7th S32.131 Minimally displaced Zone III fracture of sacrum

     ✓7th S32.132 Severely displaced Zone III fracture of sacrum

     ✓7th S32.139 Unspecified Zone III fracture of sacrum

   ✓x7th S32.14 Type 1 fracture of sacrum
      Transverse flexion fracture of sacrum without displacement

   ✓x7th S32.15 Type 2 fracture of sacrum
      Transverse flexion fracture of sacrum with posterior displacement

   ✓x7th S32.16 Type 3 fracture of sacrum
      Transverse extension fracture of sacrum with anterior displacement

   ✓x7th S32.17 Type 4 fracture of sacrum
      Transverse segmental comminution of upper sacrum

   ✓x7th S32.19 Other fracture of sacrum

✓x7th S32.2 Fracture of coccyx

✓5th S32.3 Fracture of ilium

> **EXCLUDES 1** fracture of ilium with associated disruption of pelvic ring (S32.8-)

   ✓6th S32.30 Unspecified fracture of ilium

     ✓7th S32.301 Unspecified fracture of right ilium

     ✓7th S32.302 Unspecified fracture of left ilium

     ✓7th S32.309 Unspecified fracture of unspecified ilium

   ✓6th S32.31 Avulsion fracture of ilium

     ✓7th S32.311 Displaced avulsion fracture of right ilium

     ✓7th S32.312 Displaced avulsion fracture of left ilium

     ✓7th S32.313 Displaced avulsion fracture of unspecified ilium

     ✓7th S32.314 Nondisplaced avulsion fracture of right ilium

     ✓7th S32.315 Nondisplaced avulsion fracture of left ilium

     ✓7th S32.316 Nondisplaced avulsion fracture of unspecified ilium

✓ Additional Character Required   ✓x7th Xtension Alert   Unspecified Dx   Other Specified Dx   Manifestation   ▶◀ Revised Text   ● New Code   ▲ Revised Code Title

ICD-10-CM Draft (2015)   833

✓6ᵗʰ **S32.39** Other fracture of ilium
    ✓7ᵗʰ **S32.391** Other fracture of right ilium
    ✓7ᵗʰ **S32.392** Other fracture of left ilium
    ✓7ᵗʰ **S32.399** Other fracture of unspecified ilium

✓5ᵗʰ **S32.4** Fracture of acetabulum
    Code also any associated fracture of pelvic ring (S32.8-)

✓6ᵗʰ **S32.40** Unspecified fracture of acetabulum
    ✓7ᵗʰ **S32.401** Unspecified fracture of right acetabulum
    ✓7ᵗʰ **S32.402** Unspecified fracture of left acetabulum
    ✓7ᵗʰ **S32.409** Unspecified fracture of unspecified acetabulum

✓6ᵗʰ **S32.41** Fracture of anterior wall of acetabulum
    ✓7ᵗʰ **S32.411** Displaced fracture of anterior wall of right acetabulum
    ✓7ᵗʰ **S32.412** Displaced fracture of anterior wall of left acetabulum
    ✓7ᵗʰ **S32.413** Displaced fracture of anterior wall of unspecified acetabulum
    ✓7ᵗʰ **S32.414** Nondisplaced fracture of anterior wall of right acetabulum
    ✓7ᵗʰ **S32.415** Nondisplaced fracture of anterior wall of left acetabulum
    ✓7ᵗʰ **S32.416** Nondisplaced fracture of anterior wall of unspecified acetabulum

✓6ᵗʰ **S32.42** Fracture of posterior wall of acetabulum
    ✓7ᵗʰ **S32.421** Displaced fracture of posterior wall of right acetabulum
    ✓7ᵗʰ **S32.422** Displaced fracture of posterior wall of left acetabulum
    ✓7ᵗʰ **S32.423** Displaced fracture of posterior wall of unspecified acetabulum
    ✓7ᵗʰ **S32.424** Nondisplaced fracture of posterior wall of right acetabulum
    ✓7ᵗʰ **S32.425** Nondisplaced fracture of posterior wall of left acetabulum
    ✓7ᵗʰ **S32.426** Nondisplaced fracture of posterior wall of unspecified acetabulum

✓6ᵗʰ **S32.43** Fracture of anterior column [iliopubic] of acetabulum
    ✓7ᵗʰ **S32.431** Displaced fracture of anterior column [iliopubic] of right acetabulum
    ✓7ᵗʰ **S32.432** Displaced fracture of anterior column [iliopubic] of left acetabulum
    ✓7ᵗʰ **S32.433** Displaced fracture of anterior column [iliopubic] of unspecified acetabulum
    ✓7ᵗʰ **S32.434** Nondisplaced fracture of anterior column [iliopubic] of right acetabulum
    ✓7ᵗʰ **S32.435** Nondisplaced fracture of anterior column [iliopubic] of left acetabulum
    ✓7ᵗʰ **S32.436** Nondisplaced fracture of anterior column [iliopubic] of unspecified acetabulum

✓6ᵗʰ **S32.44** Fracture of posterior column [ilioischial] of acetabulum
    ✓7ᵗʰ **S32.441** Displaced fracture of posterior column [ilioischial] of right acetabulum
    ✓7ᵗʰ **S32.442** Displaced fracture of posterior column [ilioischial] of left acetabulum
    ✓7ᵗʰ **S32.443** Displaced fracture of posterior column [ilioischial] of unspecified acetabulum
    ✓7ᵗʰ **S32.444** Nondisplaced fracture of posterior column [ilioischial] of right acetabulum
    ✓7ᵗʰ **S32.445** Nondisplaced fracture of posterior column [ilioischial] of left acetabulum
    ✓7ᵗʰ **S32.446** Nondisplaced fracture of posterior column [ilioischial] of unspecified acetabulum

✓6ᵗʰ **S32.45** Transverse fracture of acetabulum
    ✓7ᵗʰ **S32.451** Displaced transverse fracture of right acetabulum
    ✓7ᵗʰ **S32.452** Displaced transverse fracture of left acetabulum
    ✓7ᵗʰ **S32.453** Displaced transverse fracture of unspecified acetabulum
    ✓7ᵗʰ **S32.454** Nondisplaced transverse fracture of right acetabulum

✓7ᵗʰ **S32.455** Nondisplaced transverse fracture of left acetabulum
✓7ᵗʰ **S32.456** Nondisplaced transverse fracture of unspecified acetabulum

✓6ᵗʰ **S32.46** Associated transverse-posterior fracture of acetabulum
    ✓7ᵗʰ **S32.461** Displaced associated transverse-posterior fracture of right acetabulum
    ✓7ᵗʰ **S32.462** Displaced associated transverse-posterior fracture of left acetabulum
    ✓7ᵗʰ **S32.463** Displaced associated transverse-posterior fracture of unspecified acetabulum
    ✓7ᵗʰ **S32.464** Nondisplaced associated transverse-posterior fracture of right acetabulum
    ✓7ᵗʰ **S32.465** Nondisplaced associated transverse-posterior fracture of left acetabulum
    ✓7ᵗʰ **S32.466** Nondisplaced associated transverse-posterior fracture of unspecified acetabulum

✓6ᵗʰ **S32.47** Fracture of medial wall of acetabulum
    ✓7ᵗʰ **S32.471** Displaced fracture of medial wall of right acetabulum
    ✓7ᵗʰ **S32.472** Displaced fracture of medial wall of left acetabulum
    ✓7ᵗʰ **S32.473** Displaced fracture of medial wall of unspecified acetabulum
    ✓7ᵗʰ **S32.474** Nondisplaced fracture of medial wall of right acetabulum
    ✓7ᵗʰ **S32.475** Nondisplaced fracture of medial wall of left acetabulum
    ✓7ᵗʰ **S32.476** Nondisplaced fracture of medial wall of unspecified acetabulum

✓6ᵗʰ **S32.48** Dome fracture of acetabulum
    ✓7ᵗʰ **S32.481** Displaced dome fracture of right acetabulum
    ✓7ᵗʰ **S32.482** Displaced dome fracture of left acetabulum
    ✓7ᵗʰ **S32.483** Displaced dome fracture of unspecified acetabulum
    ✓7ᵗʰ **S32.484** Nondisplaced dome fracture of right acetabulum
    ✓7ᵗʰ **S32.485** Nondisplaced dome fracture of left acetabulum
    ✓7ᵗʰ **S32.486** Nondisplaced dome fracture of unspecified acetabulum

✓6ᵗʰ **S32.49** Other specified fracture of acetabulum
    ✓7ᵗʰ **S32.491** Other specified fracture of right acetabulum
    ✓7ᵗʰ **S32.492** Other specified fracture of left acetabulum
    ✓7ᵗʰ **S32.499** Other specified fracture of unspecified acetabulum

✓5ᵗʰ **S32.5** Fracture of pubis
    EXCLUDES 1 fracture of pubis with associated disruption of pelvic ring (S32.8-)

✓6ᵗʰ **S32.50** Unspecified fracture of pubis
    ✓7ᵗʰ **S32.501** Unspecified fracture of right pubis
    ✓7ᵗʰ **S32.502** Unspecified fracture of left pubis
    ✓7ᵗʰ **S32.509** Unspecified fracture of unspecified pubis

✓6ᵗʰ **S32.51** Fracture of superior rim of pubis
    ✓7ᵗʰ **S32.511** Fracture of superior rim of right pubis
    ✓7ᵗʰ **S32.512** Fracture of superior rim of left pubis
    ✓7ᵗʰ **S32.519** Fracture of superior rim of unspecified pubis

✓6ᵗʰ **S32.59** Other specified fracture of pubis
    ✓7ᵗʰ **S32.591** Other specified fracture of right pubis
    ✓7ᵗʰ **S32.592** Other specified fracture of left pubis
    ✓7ᵗʰ **S32.599** Other specified fracture of unspecified pubis

---

EXCLUDES 1 Not coded here   **EXCLUDES 2** Not included here   N Newborn Age: 0   P Pediatric Age: 0-17   M Maternity Age: 12-55   A Adult Age: 15-124

834   ICD-10-CM Draft (2015)

✓5th **S32.6   Fracture of** ischium

EXCLUDES1   *fracture of ischium with associated disruption of pelvic ring (S32.8-)*

✓6th **S32.60   Unspecified fracture of ischium**

✓7th   **S32.601   Unspecified fracture of** right **ischium**

✓7th   **S32.602   Unspecified fracture of** left **ischium**

✓7th   **S32.609   Unspecified fracture of unspecified ischium**

✓6th **S32.61   Avulsion fracture of ischium**

✓7th   **S32.611   Displaced avulsion fracture of** right **ischium**

✓7th   **S32.612   Displaced avulsion fracture of** left **ischium**

✓7th   **S32.613   Displaced avulsion fracture of unspecified ischium**

✓7th   **S32.614   Nondisplaced avulsion fracture of** right **ischium**

✓7th   **S32.615   Nondisplaced avulsion fracture of** left **ischium**

✓7th   **S32.616   Nondisplaced avulsion fracture of unspecified ischium**

✓6th **S32.69   Other specified fracture of ischium**

✓7th   **S32.691   Other specified fracture of** right **ischium**

✓7th   **S32.692   Other specified fracture of** left **ischium**

✓7th   **S32.699   Other specified fracture of unspecified ischium**

✓5th **S32.8   Fracture of** other parts **of pelvis**

Code also any associated:
    fracture of acetabulum (S32.4-)
    sacral fracture (S32.1-)

✓6th **S32.81   Multiple fractures of pelvis with disruption of pelvic ring**

Multiple pelvic fractures with disruption of pelvic circle

✓7th   **S32.810   Multiple fractures of pelvis with** stable **disruption of pelvic ring**

✓7th   **S32.811   Multiple fractures of pelvis with** unstable **disruption of pelvic ring**

✓x7th **S32.82   Multiple fractures of pelvis without disruption of pelvic ring**

Multiple pelvic fractures without disruption of pelvic circle

✓x7th **S32.89   Fracture of other parts of pelvis**

✓x7th **S32.9   Fracture of unspecified parts of lumbosacral spine and pelvis**

Fracture of lumbosacral spine NOS
Fracture of pelvis NOS
AHA: 2012, 4Q, 93

✓4th **S33   Dislocation and sprain of joints and ligaments of lumbar spine and pelvis**

INCLUDES   avulsion of joint or ligament of lumbar spine and pelvis
laceration of cartilage, joint or ligament of lumbar spine and pelvis
sprain of cartilage, joint or ligament of lumbar spine and pelvis
traumatic hemarthrosis of joint or ligament of lumbar spine and pelvis
traumatic rupture of joint or ligament of lumbar spine and pelvis
traumatic subluxation of joint or ligament of lumbar spine and pelvis
traumatic tear of joint or ligament of lumbar spine and pelvis

Code also any associated open wound

EXCLUDES1   *nontraumatic rupture or displacement of lumbar intervertebral disc NOS (M51.-)*
    obstetric damage to pelvic joints and ligaments (O71.6)

EXCLUDES2   *dislocation and sprain of joints and ligaments of hip (S73.-)*
    strain of muscle of lower back and pelvis (S39.01-)

The appropriate 7th character is to be added to each code from category S33.
A   initial encounter
D   subsequent encounter
S   sequela

✓x7th **S33.0   Traumatic rupture of lumbar intervertebral disc**

EXCLUDES1   *rupture or displacement (nontraumatic) of lumbar intervertebral disc NOS (M51- with fifth character 6)*

✓5th **S33.1   Subluxation and dislocation of** lumbar vertebra

Code also any associated:
    open wound of abdomen, lower back and pelvis (S31)
    spinal cord injury (S24.0, S24.1-, S34.0-, S34.1-)

EXCLUDES2   *fracture of lumbar vertebrae (S32.0-)*

✓6th **S33.10   Subluxation and dislocation of** unspecified **lumbar vertebra**

✓7th   **S33.100   Subluxation of unspecified lumbar vertebra**

✓7th   **S33.101   Dislocation of unspecified lumbar vertebra**

✓6th **S33.11   Subluxation and dislocation of** L1/L2 **lumbar vertebra**

✓7th   **S33.110   Subluxation of L1/L2 lumbar vertebra**

✓7th   **S33.111   Dislocation of L1/L2 lumbar vertebra**

✓6th **S33.12   Subluxation and dislocation of** L2/L3 **lumbar vertebra**

✓7th   **S33.120   Subluxation of L2/L3 lumbar vertebra**

✓7th   **S33.121   Dislocation of L2/L3 lumbar vertebra**

✓6th **S33.13   Subluxation and dislocation of** L3/L4 **lumbar vertebra**

✓7th   **S33.130   Subluxation of L3/L4 lumbar vertebra**

✓7th   **S33.131   Dislocation of L3/L4 lumbar vertebra**

✓6th **S33.14   Subluxation and dislocation of** L4/L5 **lumbar vertebra**

✓7th   **S33.140   Subluxation of L4/L5 lumbar vertebra**

✓7th   **S33.141   Dislocation of L4/L5 lumbar vertebra**

✓x7th **S33.2   Dislocation of** sacroiliac **and** sacrococcygeal **joint**

✓5th **S33.3   Dislocation of** other and unspecified parts **of lumbar spine and pelvis**

✓x7th **S33.30   Dislocation of unspecified parts of lumbar spine and pelvis**

✓x7th **S33.39   Dislocation of other parts of lumbar spine and pelvis**

✓x7th **S33.4   Traumatic rupture of** symphysis pubis

✓x7th **S33.5   Sprain of ligaments of** lumbar spine

✓x7th **S33.6   Sprain of** sacroiliac joint

✓x7th **S33.8   Sprain of other parts of lumbar spine and pelvis**

✓x7th **S33.9   Sprain of unspecified parts of lumbar spine and pelvis**

✓4th **S34   Injury of lumbar and sacral spinal cord and nerves at abdomen, lower back and pelvis level**

NOTE   Code to highest level of lumbar cord injury.
    Injuries to the spinal cord (S34.0 and S34.1) refer to the cord level and not bone level injury, and can affect nerve roots at and below the level given.

Code also any associated:
    fracture of vertebra (S22.0-, S32.0-)
    open wound of abdomen, lower back and pelvis (S31.-)
    transient paralysis (R29.5)

The appropriate 7th character is to be added to each code from category S34.
A   initial encounter
D   subsequent encounter
S   sequela

✓5th **S34.0   Concussion and edema of lumbar and sacral spinal cord**

✓x7th **S34.01   Concussion and edema of** lumbar **spinal cord**

✓x7th **S34.02   Concussion and edema of** sacral **spinal cord**

Concussion and edema of conus medullaris

✓5th **S34.1   Other and unspecified injury of lumbar and sacral spinal cord**

✓6th **S34.10   Unspecified injury to lumbar spinal cord**

✓7th   **S34.101   Unspecified injury to** L1 level **of lumbar spinal cord**

✓7th   **S34.102   Unspecified injury to** L2 level **of lumbar spinal cord**

✓7th   **S34.103   Unspecified injury to** L3 level **of lumbar spinal cord**

✓7th   **S34.104   Unspecified injury to** L4 level **of lumbar spinal cord**

✓7th   **S34.105   Unspecified injury to** L5 level **of lumbar spinal cord**

✓7th   **S34.109   Unspecified injury to unspecified level of lumbar spinal cord**

✓ Additional Character Required   ✓x7th Xtension Alert   Unspecified Dx   Other Specified Dx   Manifestation   ►◄ Revised Text   ● New Code   ▲ Revised Code Title

Injury, Poisoning and Certain Other Consequences of External Causes   **S34.11–S35.299**

☑6ᵗʰ **S34.11** Complete lesion of lumbar spinal cord

     ☑7ᵗʰ **S34.111** Complete lesion of L1 level of lumbar spinal cord

     ☑7ᵗʰ **S34.112** Complete lesion of L2 level of lumbar spinal cord

     ☑7ᵗʰ **S34.113** Complete lesion of L3 level of lumbar spinal cord

     ☑7ᵗʰ **S34.114** Complete lesion of L4 level of lumbar spinal cord

     ☑7ᵗʰ **S34.115** Complete lesion of L5 level of lumbar spinal cord

     ☑7ᵗʰ **S34.119** Complete lesion of unspecified level of lumbar spinal cord

☑6ᵗʰ **S34.12** Incomplete lesion of lumbar spinal cord

     ☑7ᵗʰ **S34.121** Incomplete lesion of L1 level of lumbar spinal cord

     ☑7ᵗʰ **S34.122** Incomplete lesion of L2 level of lumbar spinal cord

     ☑7ᵗʰ **S34.123** Incomplete lesion of L3 level of lumbar spinal cord

     ☑7ᵗʰ **S34.124** Incomplete lesion of L4 level of lumbar spinal cord

     ☑7ᵗʰ **S34.125** Incomplete lesion of L5 level of lumbar spinal cord

     ☑7ᵗʰ **S34.129** Incomplete lesion of unspecified level of lumbar spinal cord

☑6ᵗʰ **S34.13** Other and unspecified injury to sacral spinal cord
     Other injury to conus medullaris

     ☑7ᵗʰ **S34.131** Complete lesion of sacral spinal cord
         Complete lesion of conus medullaris

     ☑7ᵗʰ **S34.132** Incomplete lesion of sacral spinal cord
         Incomplete lesion of conus medullaris

     ☑7ᵗʰ **S34.139** Unspecified injury to sacral spinal cord
         Unspecified injury of conus medullaris

☑5ᵗʰ **S34.2** Injury of nerve root of lumbar and sacral spine

     ☑x7ᵗʰ **S34.21** Injury of nerve root of lumbar spine

     ☑x7ᵗʰ **S34.22** Injury of nerve root of sacral spine

☑x7ᵗʰ **S34.3** Injury of cauda equina

☑x7ᵗʰ **S34.4** Injury of lumbosacral plexus

☑x7ᵗʰ **S34.5** Injury of lumbar, sacral and pelvic sympathetic nerves
     Injury of celiac ganglion or plexus
     Injury of hypogastric plexus
     Injury of mesenteric plexus (inferior) (superior)
     Injury of splanchnic nerve

☑x7ᵗʰ **S34.6** Injury of peripheral nerve(s) at abdomen, lower back and pelvis level

☑x7ᵗʰ **S34.8** Injury of other nerves at abdomen, lower back and pelvis level

☑x7ᵗʰ **S34.9** Injury of unspecified nerves at abdomen, lower back and pelvis level

☑4ᵗʰ **S35** Injury of blood vessels at abdomen, lower back and pelvis level
     Code also any associated open wound (S31.-)

     The appropriate 7th character is to be added to each code from category S35.
     A   initial encounter
     D   subsequent encounter
     S   sequela

☑5ᵗʰ **S35.0** Injury of abdominal aorta
     EXCLUDES 1   injury of aorta NOS (S25.0)

     ☑x7ᵗʰ **S35.00** Unspecified injury of abdominal aorta

     ☑x7ᵗʰ **S35.01** Minor laceration of abdominal aorta
         Incomplete transection of abdominal aorta
         Laceration of abdominal aorta NOS
         Superficial laceration of abdominal aorta

     ☑x7ᵗʰ **S35.02** Major laceration of abdominal aorta
         Complete transection of abdominal aorta
         Traumatic rupture of abdominal aorta

     ☑x7ᵗʰ **S35.09** Other injury of abdominal aorta

☑5ᵗʰ **S35.1** Injury of inferior vena cava
     Injury of hepatic vein
     EXCLUDES 1   injury of vena cava NOS (S25.2)

     ☑x7ᵗʰ **S35.10** Unspecified injury of inferior vena cava

☑x7ᵗʰ **S35.11** Minor laceration of inferior vena cava
     Incomplete transection of inferior vena cava
     Laceration of inferior vena cava NOS
     Superficial laceration of inferior vena cava

☑x7ᵗʰ **S35.12** Major laceration of inferior vena cava
     Complete transection of inferior vena cava
     Traumatic rupture of inferior vena cava

☑x7ᵗʰ **S35.19** Other injury of inferior vena cava

☑5ᵗʰ **S35.2** Injury of celiac or mesenteric artery and branches

     ☑6ᵗʰ **S35.21** Injury of celiac artery

         ☑7ᵗʰ **S35.211** Minor laceration of celiac artery
             Incomplete transection of celiac artery
             Laceration of celiac artery NOS
             Superficial laceration of celiac artery

         ☑7ᵗʰ **S35.212** Major laceration of celiac artery
             Complete transection of celiac artery
             Traumatic rupture of celiac artery

         ☑7ᵗʰ **S35.218** Other injury of celiac artery

         ☑7ᵗʰ **S35.219** Unspecified injury of celiac artery

     ☑6ᵗʰ **S35.22** Injury of superior mesenteric artery

         ☑7ᵗʰ **S35.221** Minor laceration of superior mesenteric artery
             Incomplete transection of superior mesenteric artery
             Laceration of superior mesenteric artery NOS
             Superficial laceration of superior mesenteric artery

         ☑7ᵗʰ **S35.222** Major laceration of superior mesenteric artery
             Complete transection of superior mesenteric artery
             Traumatic rupture of superior mesenteric artery

         ☑7ᵗʰ **S35.228** Other injury of superior mesenteric artery

         ☑7ᵗʰ **S35.229** Unspecified injury of superior mesenteric artery

     ☑6ᵗʰ **S35.23** Injury of inferior mesenteric artery

         ☑7ᵗʰ **S35.231** Minor laceration of inferior mesenteric artery
             Incomplete transection of inferior mesenteric artery
             Laceration of inferior mesenteric artery NOS
             Superficial laceration of inferior mesenteric artery

         ☑7ᵗʰ **S35.232** Major laceration of inferior mesenteric artery
             Complete transection of inferior mesenteric artery
             Traumatic rupture of inferior mesenteric artery

         ☑7ᵗʰ **S35.238** Other injury of inferior mesenteric artery

         ☑7ᵗʰ **S35.239** Unspecified injury of inferior mesenteric artery

     ☑6ᵗʰ **S35.29** Injury of branches of celiac and mesenteric artery
         Injury of gastric artery
         Injury of gastroduodenal artery
         Injury of hepatic artery
         Injury of splenic artery

         ☑7ᵗʰ **S35.291** Minor laceration of branches of celiac and mesenteric artery
             Incomplete transection of branches of celiac and mesenteric artery
             Laceration of branches of celiac and mesenteric artery NOS
             Superficial laceration of branches of celiac and mesenteric artery

         ☑7ᵗʰ **S35.292** Major laceration of branches of celiac and mesenteric artery
             Complete transection of branches of celiac and mesenteric artery
             Traumatic rupture of branches of celiac and mesenteric artery

         ☑7ᵗʰ **S35.298** Other injury of branches of celiac and mesenteric artery

         ☑7ᵗʰ **S35.299** Unspecified injury of branches of celiac and mesenteric artery

EXCLUDES 1 Not coded here   **EXCLUDES 2** Not included here   N Newborn Age: 0   P Pediatric Age: 0-17   M Maternity Age: 12-55   A Adult Age: 15-124

836   ICD-10-CM Draft (2015)

✓5ᵗʰ **S35.3** Injury of portal or splenic vein and branches
- ✓6ᵗʰ **S35.31** Injury of portal vein
  - ✓7ᵗʰ **S35.311** Laceration of portal vein
  - ✓7ᵗʰ **S35.318** Other specified injury of portal vein
  - ✓7ᵗʰ **S35.319** Unspecified injury of portal vein
- ✓6ᵗʰ **S35.32** Injury of splenic vein
  - ✓7ᵗʰ **S35.321** Laceration of splenic vein
  - ✓7ᵗʰ **S35.328** Other specified injury of splenic vein
  - ✓7ᵗʰ **S35.329** Unspecified injury of splenic vein
- ✓6ᵗʰ **S35.33** Injury of superior mesenteric vein
  - ✓7ᵗʰ **S35.331** Laceration of superior mesenteric vein
  - ✓7ᵗʰ **S35.338** Other specified injury of superior mesenteric vein
  - ✓7ᵗʰ **S35.339** Unspecified injury of superior mesenteric vein
- ✓6ᵗʰ **S35.34** Injury of inferior mesenteric vein
  - ✓7ᵗʰ **S35.341** Laceration of inferior mesenteric vein
  - ✓7ᵗʰ **S35.348** Other specified injury of inferior mesenteric vein
  - ✓7ᵗʰ **S35.349** Unspecified injury of inferior mesenteric vein

✓5ᵗʰ **S35.4** Injury of renal blood vessels
- ✓6ᵗʰ **S35.40** Unspecified injury of renal blood vessel
  - ✓7ᵗʰ **S35.401** Unspecified injury of right renal artery
  - ✓7ᵗʰ **S35.402** Unspecified injury of left renal artery
  - ✓7ᵗʰ **S35.403** Unspecified injury of unspecified renal artery
  - ✓7ᵗʰ **S35.404** Unspecified injury of right renal vein
  - ✓7ᵗʰ **S35.405** Unspecified injury of left renal vein
  - ✓7ᵗʰ **S35.406** Unspecified injury of unspecified renal vein
- ✓6ᵗʰ **S35.41** Laceration of renal blood vessel
  - ✓7ᵗʰ **S35.411** Laceration of right renal artery
  - ✓7ᵗʰ **S35.412** Laceration of left renal artery
  - ✓7ᵗʰ **S35.413** Laceration of unspecified renal artery
  - ✓7ᵗʰ **S35.414** Laceration of right renal vein
  - ✓7ᵗʰ **S35.415** Laceration of left renal vein
  - ✓7ᵗʰ **S35.416** Laceration of unspecified renal vein
- ✓6ᵗʰ **S35.49** Other specified injury of renal blood vessel
  - ✓7ᵗʰ **S35.491** Other specified injury of right renal artery
  - ✓7ᵗʰ **S35.492** Other specified injury of left renal artery
  - ✓7ᵗʰ **S35.493** Other specified injury of unspecified renal artery
  - ✓7ᵗʰ **S35.494** Other specified injury of right renal vein
  - ✓7ᵗʰ **S35.495** Other specified injury of left renal vein
  - ✓7ᵗʰ **S35.496** Other specified injury of unspecified renal vein

✓5ᵗʰ **S35.5** Injury of iliac blood vessels
- ✓ₓ7ᵗʰ **S35.50** Injury of unspecified iliac blood vessel(s)
- ✓6ᵗʰ **S35.51** Injury of iliac artery or vein
  - Injury of hypogastric artery or vein
  - ✓7ᵗʰ **S35.511** Injury of right iliac artery
  - ✓7ᵗʰ **S35.512** Injury of left iliac artery
  - ✓7ᵗʰ **S35.513** Injury of unspecified iliac artery
  - ✓7ᵗʰ **S35.514** Injury of right iliac vein
  - ✓7ᵗʰ **S35.515** Injury of left iliac vein
  - ✓7ᵗʰ **S35.516** Injury of unspecified iliac vein
- ✓6ᵗʰ **S35.53** Injury of uterine artery or vein
  - ✓7ᵗʰ **S35.531** Injury of right uterine artery ♀
  - ✓7ᵗʰ **S35.532** Injury of left uterine artery ♀
  - ✓7ᵗʰ **S35.533** Injury of unspecified uterine artery ♀
  - ✓7ᵗʰ **S35.534** Injury of right uterine vein ♀
  - ✓7ᵗʰ **S35.535** Injury of left uterine vein ♀
  - ✓7ᵗʰ **S35.536** Injury of unspecified uterine vein ♀
- ✓ₓ7ᵗʰ **S35.59** Injury of other iliac blood vessels

✓5ᵗʰ **S35.8** Injury of other blood vessels at abdomen, lower back and pelvis level
- Injury of ovarian artery or vein
- ✓6ᵗʰ **S35.8X** Injury of other blood vessels at abdomen, lower back and pelvis level
  - ✓7ᵗʰ **S35.8X1** Laceration of other blood vessels at abdomen, lower back and pelvis level
  - ✓7ᵗʰ **S35.8X8** Other specified injury of other blood vessels at abdomen, lower back and pelvis level
  - ✓7ᵗʰ **S35.8X9** Unspecified injury of other blood vessels at abdomen, lower back and pelvis level

✓5ᵗʰ **S35.9** Injury of unspecified blood vessel at abdomen, lower back and pelvis level
- ✓ₓ7ᵗʰ **S35.90** Unspecified injury of unspecified blood vessel at abdomen, lower back and pelvis level
- ✓ₓ7ᵗʰ **S35.91** Laceration of unspecified blood vessel at abdomen, lower back and pelvis level
- ✓ₓ7ᵗʰ **S35.99** Other specified injury of unspecified blood vessel at abdomen, lower back and pelvis level

✓4ᵗʰ **S36 Injury of intra-abdominal organs**
Code also any associated open wound (S31.-)

> The appropriate 7th character is to be added to each code from category S36.
> A initial encounter
> D subsequent encounter
> S sequela

✓5ᵗʰ **S36.0** Injury of spleen
- ✓ₓ7ᵗʰ **S36.00** Unspecified injury of spleen
- ✓6ᵗʰ **S36.02** Contusion of spleen
  - ✓7ᵗʰ **S36.020** Minor contusion of spleen
    - Contusion of spleen less than 2 cm
  - ✓7ᵗʰ **S36.021** Major contusion of spleen
    - Contusion of spleen greater than 2 cm
  - ✓7ᵗʰ **S36.029** Unspecified contusion of spleen
- ✓6ᵗʰ **S36.03** Laceration of spleen
  - ✓7ᵗʰ **S36.030** Superficial (capsular) laceration of spleen
    - Laceration of spleen less than 1cm
    - Minor laceration of spleen
  - ✓7ᵗʰ **S36.031** Moderate laceration of spleen
    - Laceration of spleen 1 to 3 cm
  - ✓7ᵗʰ **S36.032** Major laceration of spleen
    - Avulsion of spleen
    - Laceration of spleen greater than 3 cm
    - Massive laceration of spleen
    - Multiple moderate lacerations of spleen
    - Stellate laceration of spleen
  - ✓7ᵗʰ **S36.039** Unspecified laceration of spleen
- ✓ₓ7ᵗʰ **S36.09** Other injury of spleen

✓5ᵗʰ **S36.1** Injury of liver and gallbladder and bile duct
- ✓6ᵗʰ **S36.11** Injury of liver
  - ✓7ᵗʰ **S36.112** Contusion of liver
  - ✓7ᵗʰ **S36.113** Laceration of liver, unspecified degree
  - ✓7ᵗʰ **S36.114** Minor laceration of liver
    - Laceration involving capsule only, or, without significant involvement of hepatic parenchyma [i.e., less than 1cm deep]
  - ✓7ᵗʰ **S36.115** Moderate laceration of liver
    - Laceration involving parenchyma but without major disruption of parenchyma [i.e., less than 10 cm long and less than 3 cm deep]
  - ✓7ᵗʰ **S36.116** Major laceration of liver
    - Laceration with significant disruption of hepatic parenchyma [i.e., greater than 10 cm long and 3 cm deep]
    - Multiple moderate lacerations, with or without hematoma
    - Stellate laceration of liver
  - ✓7ᵗʰ **S36.118** Other injury of liver
  - ✓7ᵗʰ **S36.119** Unspecified injury of liver
- ✓6ᵗʰ **S36.12** Injury of gallbladder
  - ✓7ᵗʰ **S36.122** Contusion of gallbladder
  - ✓7ᵗʰ **S36.123** Laceration of gallbladder

      √7th **S36.128** Other injury of gallbladder
      √7th **S36.129** Unspecified injury of gallbladder
   √x7th **S36.13** Injury of bile duct
  √5th **S36.2** Injury of pancreas
    √6th **S36.20** Unspecified injury of pancreas
      √7th **S36.200** Unspecified injury of head of pancreas
      √7th **S36.201** Unspecified injury of body of pancreas
      √7th **S36.202** Unspecified injury of tail of pancreas
      √7th **S36.209** Unspecified injury of unspecified part of pancreas
    √6th **S36.22** Contusion of pancreas
      √7th **S36.220** Contusion of head of pancreas
      √7th **S36.221** Contusion of body of pancreas
      √7th **S36.222** Contusion of tail of pancreas
      √7th **S36.229** Contusion of unspecified part of pancreas
    √6th **S36.23** Laceration of pancreas, unspecified degree
      √7th **S36.230** Laceration of head of pancreas, unspecified degree
      √7th **S36.231** Laceration of body of pancreas, unspecified degree
      √7th **S36.232** Laceration of tail of pancreas, unspecified degree
      √7th **S36.239** Laceration of unspecified part of pancreas, unspecified degree
    √6th **S36.24** Minor laceration of pancreas
      √7th **S36.240** Minor laceration of head of pancreas
      √7th **S36.241** Minor laceration of body of pancreas
      √7th **S36.242** Minor laceration of tail of pancreas
      √7th **S36.249** Minor laceration of unspecified part of pancreas
    √6th **S36.25** Moderate laceration of pancreas
      √7th **S36.250** Moderate laceration of head of pancreas
      √7th **S36.251** Moderate laceration of body of pancreas
      √7th **S36.252** Moderate laceration of tail of pancreas
      √7th **S36.259** Moderate laceration of unspecified part of pancreas
    √6th **S36.26** Major laceration of pancreas
      √7th **S36.260** Major laceration of head of pancreas
      √7th **S36.261** Major laceration of body of pancreas
      √7th **S36.262** Major laceration of tail of pancreas
      √7th **S36.269** Major laceration of unspecified part of pancreas
    √6th **S36.29** Other injury of pancreas
      √7th **S36.290** Other injury of head of pancreas
      √7th **S36.291** Other injury of body of pancreas
      √7th **S36.292** Other injury of tail of pancreas
      √7th **S36.299** Other injury of unspecified part of pancreas
  √5th **S36.3** Injury of stomach
    √x7th **S36.30** Unspecified injury of stomach
    √x7th **S36.32** Contusion of stomach
    √x7th **S36.33** Laceration of stomach
    √x7th **S36.39** Other injury of stomach
  √5th **S36.4** Injury of small intestine
    √6th **S36.40** Unspecified injury of small intestine
      √7th **S36.400** Unspecified injury of duodenum
      √7th **S36.408** Unspecified injury of other part of small intestine
      √7th **S36.409** Unspecified injury of unspecified part of small intestine
    √6th **S36.41** Primary blast injury of small intestine
      Blast injury of small intestine NOS
      √7th **S36.410** Primary blast injury of duodenum
      √7th **S36.418** Primary blast injury of other part of small intestine
      √7th **S36.419** Primary blast injury of unspecified part of small intestine
    √6th **S36.42** Contusion of small intestine
      √7th **S36.420** Contusion of duodenum
      √7th **S36.428** Contusion of other part of small intestine

      √7th **S36.429** Contusion of unspecified part of small intestine
    √6th **S36.43** Laceration of small intestine
      √7th **S36.430** Laceration of duodenum
      √7th **S36.438** Laceration of other part of small intestine
      √7th **S36.439** Laceration of unspecified part of small intestine
    √6th **S36.49** Other injury of small intestine
      √7th **S36.490** Other injury of duodenum
      √7th **S36.498** Other injury of other part of small intestine
      √7th **S36.499** Other injury of unspecified part of small intestine
  √5th **S36.5** Injury of colon
    EXCLUDES 2 injury of rectum (S36.6-)
    √6th **S36.50** Unspecified injury of colon
      √7th **S36.500** Unspecified injury of ascending [right] colon
      √7th **S36.501** Unspecified injury of transverse colon
      √7th **S36.502** Unspecified injury of descending [left] colon
      √7th **S36.503** Unspecified injury of sigmoid colon
      √7th **S36.508** Unspecified injury of other part of colon
      √7th **S36.509** Unspecified injury of unspecified part of colon
    √6th **S36.51** Primary blast injury of colon
      Blast injury of colon NOS
      √7th **S36.510** Primary blast injury of ascending [right] colon
      √7th **S36.511** Primary blast injury of transverse colon
      √7th **S36.512** Primary blast injury of descending [left] colon
      √7th **S36.513** Primary blast injury of sigmoid colon
      √7th **S36.518** Primary blast injury of other part of colon
      √7th **S36.519** Primary blast injury of unspecified part of colon
    √6th **S36.52** Contusion of colon
      √7th **S36.520** Contusion of ascending [right] colon
      √7th **S36.521** Contusion of transverse colon
      √7th **S36.522** Contusion of descending [left] colon
      √7th **S36.523** Contusion of sigmoid colon
      √7th **S36.528** Contusion of other part of colon
      √7th **S36.529** Contusion of unspecified part of colon
    √6th **S36.53** Laceration of colon
      √7th **S36.530** Laceration of ascending [right] colon
      √7th **S36.531** Laceration of transverse colon
      √7th **S36.532** Laceration of descending [left] colon
      √7th **S36.533** Laceration of sigmoid colon
      √7th **S36.538** Laceration of other part of colon
      √7th **S36.539** Laceration of unspecified part of colon
    √6th **S36.59** Other injury of colon
      Secondary blast injury of colon
      √7th **S36.590** Other injury of ascending [right] colon
      √7th **S36.591** Other injury of transverse colon
      √7th **S36.592** Other injury of descending [left] colon
      √7th **S36.593** Other injury of sigmoid colon
      √7th **S36.598** Other injury of other part of colon
      √7th **S36.599** Other injury of unspecified part of colon
  √5th **S36.6** Injury of rectum
    √x7th **S36.60** Unspecified injury of rectum
    √x7th **S36.61** Primary blast injury of rectum
      Blast injury of rectum NOS
    √x7th **S36.62** Contusion of rectum
    √x7th **S36.63** Laceration of rectum
    √x7th **S36.69** Other injury of rectum
      Secondary blast injury of rectum
  √5th **S36.8** Injury of other intra-abdominal organs
    √x7th **S36.81** Injury of peritoneum
    √6th **S36.89** Injury of other intra-abdominal organs
      Injury of retroperitoneum

EXCLUDES 1 Not coded here   **EXCLUDES 2** Not included here   **N** Newborn Age: 0   **P** Pediatric Age: 0-17   **M** Maternity Age: 12-55   **A** Adult Age: 15-124

838   ICD-10-CM Draft (2015)

✓7th **S36.892** Contusion of other intra-abdominal organs

✓7th **S36.893** Laceration of other intra-abdominal organs

✓7th **S36.898** Other injury of other intra-abdominal organs

✓7th **S36.899** Unspecified injury of other intra-abdominal organs

✓5th **S36.9 Injury of unspecified intra-abdominal organ**

✓x7th **S36.90** Unspecified injury of unspecified intra-abdominal organ

✓x7th **S36.92** Contusion of unspecified intra-abdominal organ

✓x7th **S36.93** Laceration of unspecified intra-abdominal organ

✓x7th **S36.99** Other injury of unspecified intra-abdominal organ

✓4th **S37 Injury of urinary and pelvic organs**

Code also any associated open wound (S31.-)

EXCLUDES 1 obstetric trauma to pelvic organs (O71.-)

EXCLUDES 2 injury of peritoneum (S36.81)
injury of retroperitoneum (S36.89-)

The appropriate 7th character is to be added to each code from category S37.
A   initial encounter
D   subsequent encounter
S   sequela

✓5th **S37.0 Injury of kidney**

EXCLUDES 2 acute kidney injury (nontraumatic) (N17.9)

✓6th **S37.00** Unspecified injury of kidney

✓7th **S37.001** Unspecified injury of right kidney

✓7th **S37.002** Unspecified injury of left kidney

✓7th **S37.009** Unspecified injury of unspecified kidney

✓6th **S37.01** Minor contusion of kidney
Contusion of kidney less than 2 cm
Contusion of kidney NOS

✓7th **S37.011** Minor contusion of right kidney

✓7th **S37.012** Minor contusion of left kidney

✓7th **S37.019** Minor contusion of unspecified kidney

✓6th **S37.02** Major contusion of kidney
Contusion of kidney greater than 2 cm

✓7th **S37.021** Major contusion of right kidney

✓7th **S37.022** Major contusion of left kidney

✓7th **S37.029** Major contusion of unspecified kidney

✓6th **S37.03** Laceration of kidney, unspecified degree

✓7th **S37.031** Laceration of right kidney, unspecified degree

✓7th **S37.032** Laceration of left kidney, unspecified degree

✓7th **S37.039** Laceration of unspecified kidney, unspecified degree

✓6th **S37.04** Minor laceration of kidney
Laceration of kidney less than 1 cm

✓7th **S37.041** Minor laceration of right kidney

✓7th **S37.042** Minor laceration of left kidney

✓7th **S37.049** Minor laceration of unspecified kidney

✓6th **S37.05** Moderate laceration of kidney
Laceration of kidney 1 to 3 cm

✓7th **S37.051** Moderate laceration of right kidney

✓7th **S37.052** Moderate laceration of left kidney

✓7th **S37.059** Moderate laceration of unspecified kidney

✓6th **S37.06** Major laceration of kidney
Avulsion of kidney
Laceration of kidney greater than 3 cm
Massive laceration of kidney
Multiple moderate lacerations of kidney
Stellate laceration of kidney

✓7th **S37.061** Major laceration of right kidney

✓7th **S37.062** Major laceration of left kidney

✓7th **S37.069** Major laceration of unspecified kidney

✓6th **S37.09** Other injury of kidney

✓7th **S37.091** Other injury of right kidney

✓7th **S37.092** Other injury of left kidney

✓7th **S37.099** Other injury of unspecified kidney

✓5th **S37.1 Injury of ureter**

✓x7th **S37.10** Unspecified injury of ureter

✓x7th **S37.12** Contusion of ureter

✓x7th **S37.13** Laceration of ureter

✓x7th **S37.19** Other injury of ureter

✓5th **S37.2 Injury of bladder**

✓x7th **S37.20** Unspecified injury of bladder

✓x7th **S37.22** Contusion of bladder

✓x7th **S37.23** Laceration of bladder

✓x7th **S37.29** Other injury of bladder

✓5th **S37.3 Injury of urethra**

✓x7th **S37.30** Unspecified injury of urethra

✓x7th **S37.32** Contusion of urethra

✓x7th **S37.33** Laceration of urethra

✓x7th **S37.39** Other injury of urethra

✓5th **S37.4 Injury of ovary**

✓6th **S37.40** Unspecified injury of ovary

✓7th **S37.401** Unspecified injury of ovary, unilateral ♀

✓7th **S37.402** Unspecified injury of ovary, bilateral ♀

✓7th **S37.409** Unspecified injury of ovary, unspecified ♀

✓6th **S37.42** Contusion of ovary

✓7th **S37.421** Contusion of ovary, unilateral ♀

✓7th **S37.422** Contusion of ovary, bilateral ♀

✓7th **S37.429** Contusion of ovary, unspecified ♀

✓6th **S37.43** Laceration of ovary

✓7th **S37.431** Laceration of ovary, unilateral ♀

✓7th **S37.432** Laceration of ovary, bilateral ♀

✓7th **S37.439** Laceration of ovary, unspecified ♀

✓6th **S37.49** Other injury of ovary

✓7th **S37.491** Other injury of ovary, unilateral ♀

✓7th **S37.492** Other injury of ovary, bilateral ♀

✓7th **S37.499** Other injury of ovary, unspecified ♀

✓5th **S37.5 Injury of fallopian tube**

S37.50 Unspecified injury of fallopian tube

✓7th **S37.501** Unspecified injury of fallopian tube, unilateral ♀

✓7th **S37.502** Unspecified injury of fallopian tube, bilateral ♀

✓7th **S37.509** Unspecified injury of fallopian tube, unspecified ♀

✓6th **S37.51** Primary blast injury of fallopian tube
Blast injury of fallopian tube NOS

✓7th **S37.511** Primary blast injury of fallopian tube, unilateral ♀

✓7th **S37.512** Primary blast injury of fallopian tube, bilateral ♀

✓7th **S37.519** Primary blast injury of fallopian tube, unspecified ♀

✓6th **S37.52** Contusion of fallopian tube

✓7th **S37.521** Contusion of fallopian tube, unilateral ♀

✓7th **S37.522** Contusion of fallopian tube, bilateral ♀

✓7th **S37.529** Contusion of fallopian tube, unspecified ♀

✓6th **S37.53** Laceration of fallopian tube

✓7th **S37.531** Laceration of fallopian tube, unilateral ♀

✓7th **S37.532** Laceration of fallopian tube, bilateral ♀

✓7th **S37.539** Laceration of fallopian tube, unspecified ♀

✓6th **S37.59** Other injury of fallopian tube
Secondary blast injury of fallopian tube

✓7th **S37.591** Other injury of fallopian tube, unilateral ♀

✓7th **S37.592** Other injury of fallopian tube, bilateral ♀

✓7th **S37.599** Other injury of fallopian tube, unspecified ♀

✓5th **S37.6 Injury of uterus**

EXCLUDES 1 injury to gravid uterus (O9A.2-)
injury to uterus during delivery (O71.-)

✓x7th **S37.60** Unspecified injury of uterus ♀

✓x7th **S37.62** Contusion of uterus ♀

✓x7th **S37.63** Laceration of uterus ♀

✓ Additional Character Required   ✓x7th Xtension Alert   Unspecified Dx   Other Specified Dx   Manifestation   ▶◀ Revised Text   ● New Code   ▲ Revised Code Title

ICD-10-CM Draft (2015)   839

√x7th **S37.69** **Other injury of uterus** ♀

√5th **S37.8** **Injury of other urinary and pelvic organs**

     √6th **S37.81** **Injury of** adrenal gland

         √7th **S37.812** Contusion of adrenal gland

         √7th **S37.813** Laceration of adrenal gland

         √7th **S37.818** **Other injury of adrenal gland**

         √7th **S37.819** **Unspecified injury of adrenal gland**

     √6th **S37.82** **Injury of** prostate

         √7th **S37.822** Contusion of prostate ♂

         √7th **S37.823** Laceration of prostate ♂

         √7th **S37.828** **Other injury of prostate** ♂

         √7th **S37.829** **Unspecified injury of prostate** ♂

     √6th **S37.89** **Injury of** other urinary and pelvic organ

         √7th **S37.892** Contusion of other urinary and pelvic organ

         √7th **S37.893** Laceration of other urinary and pelvic organ

         √7th **S37.898** **Other injury of other urinary and pelvic organ**

         √7th **S37.899** **Unspecified injury of other urinary and pelvic organ**

√5th **S37.9** **Injury of unspecified urinary and pelvic organ**

     √x7th **S37.90** **Unspecified injury of unspecified urinary and pelvic organ**

     √x7th **S37.92** Contusion of unspecified urinary and pelvic organ

     √x7th **S37.93** Laceration of unspecified urinary and pelvic organ

     √x7th **S37.99** **Other injury of unspecified urinary and pelvic organ**

√4th **S38** **Crushing injury and traumatic amputation of abdomen, lower back, pelvis and external genitals**

> **NOTE** An amputation not identified as partial or complete should be coded to complete.

> The appropriate 7th character is to be added to each code from category S38.
> A   initial encounter
> D   subsequent encounter
> S   sequela

√5th **S38.0** **Crushing injury of** external genital organs

     Use additional code for any associated injuries

     √6th **S38.00** **Crushing injury of** unspecified external genital organs

         √7th **S38.001** **Crushing injury of unspecified external genital organs,** male ♂

         √7th **S38.002** **Crushing injury of unspecified external genital organs,** female ♀

     √x7th **S38.01** **Crushing injury of** penis ♂

     √x7th **S38.02** **Crushing injury of** scrotum and testis ♂

     √x7th **S38.03** **Crushing injury of** vulva ♀

√x7th **S38.1** **Crushing injury of abdomen, lower back, and pelvis**

     Use additional code for all associated injuries, such as:
     fracture of thoracic or lumbar spine and pelvis (S22.0-, S32-)
     injury to intra-abdominal organs (S36.-)
     injury to urinary and pelvic organs (S37.-)
     open wound of abdominal wall (S31.-)
     spinal cord injury (S34.0, S34.1-)

     EXCLUDES 2   crushing injury of external genital organs (S38.0-)

√5th **S38.2** Traumatic amputation of external genital organs

     √6th **S38.21** **Traumatic amputation of** female **external genital organs**

         Traumatic amputation of clitoris
         Traumatic amputation of labium (majus) (minus)
         Traumatic amputation of vulva

         √7th **S38.211** Complete **traumatic amputation of female external genital organs** ♀

         √7th **S38.212** Partial **traumatic amputation of female external genital organs** ♀

     √6th **S38.22** **Traumatic amputation of** penis

         √7th **S38.221** Complete **traumatic amputation of penis** ♂

         √7th **S38.222** Partial **traumatic amputation of penis** ♂

     √6th **S38.23** **Traumatic amputation of** scrotum and testis

         √7th **S38.231** Complete **traumatic amputation of scrotum and testis** ♂

√x7th **S38.232** Partial **traumatic amputation of scrotum and testis** ♂

√x7th **S38.3** **Transection (partial) of abdomen**

√4th **S39** **Other and unspecified injuries of abdomen, lower back, pelvis and external genitals**

     Code also any associated open wound (S31.-)

     EXCLUDES 2   sprain of joints and ligaments of lumbar spine and pelvis (S33.-)

> The appropriate 7th character is to be added to each code from category S39.
> A   initial encounter
> D   subsequent encounter
> S   sequela

√5th **S39.0** **Injury of muscle, fascia and tendon of abdomen, lower back and pelvis**

     √6th **S39.00** Unspecified injury of muscle, fascia and tendon of abdomen, lower back and pelvis

         √7th **S39.001** **Unspecified injury of muscle, fascia and tendon of** abdomen

         √7th **S39.002** **Unspecified injury of muscle, fascia and tendon of** lower back

         √7th **S39.003** **Unspecified injury of muscle, fascia and tendon of** pelvis

     √6th **S39.01** Strain of muscle, fascia and tendon of abdomen, lower back and pelvis

         √7th **S39.011** **Strain of muscle, fascia and tendon of** abdomen

         √7th **S39.012** **Strain of muscle, fascia and tendon of** lower back

         √7th **S39.013** **Strain of muscle, fascia and tendon of** pelvis

     √6th **S39.02** Laceration of muscle, fascia and tendon of abdomen, lower back and pelvis

         √7th **S39.021** **Laceration of muscle, fascia and tendon of** abdomen

         √7th **S39.022** **Laceration of muscle, fascia and tendon of** lower back

         √7th **S39.023** **Laceration of muscle, fascia and tendon of** pelvis

     √6th **S39.09** Other injury of muscle, fascia and tendon of abdomen, lower back and pelvis

         √7th **S39.091** **Other injury of muscle, fascia and tendon of** abdomen

         √7th **S39.092** **Other injury of muscle, fascia and tendon of** lower back

         √7th **S39.093** **Other injury of muscle, fascia and tendon of** pelvis

√5th **S39.8** Other specified injuries of abdomen, lower back, pelvis and external genitals

     √x7th **S39.81** **Other specified injuries of** abdomen

     √x7th **S39.82** **Other specified injuries of** lower back

     √x7th **S39.83** **Other specified injuries of** pelvis

     √6th **S39.84** **Other specified injuries of** external genitals

         √7th **S39.840** **Fracture of** corpus cavernosum penis ♂

         √7th **S39.848** **Other specified injuries of external genitals**

√5th **S39.9** Unspecified injury of abdomen, lower back, pelvis and external genitals

     √x7th **S39.91** **Unspecified injury of** abdomen

     √x7th **S39.92** **Unspecified injury of** lower back

     √x7th **S39.93** **Unspecified injury of** pelvis

     √x7th **S39.94** **Unspecified injury of** external genitals

EXCLUDES 1 Not coded here   EXCLUDES 2 Not included here   N Newborn Age: 0   P Pediatric Age: 0-17   M Maternity Age: 12-55   A Adult Age: 15-124

840   ICD-10-CM Draft (2015)

Injuries to the shoulder and upper arm (S40-S49)

INCLUDES   injuries of axilla
injuries of scapular region
EXCLUDES 2   burns and corrosions (T20-T32)
frostbite (T33-T34)
injuries of elbow (S50-S59)
insect bite or sting, venomous (T63.4)

✓4ᵗʰ S40   Superficial injury of shoulder and upper arm

The appropriate 7th character is to be added to each code from category S40.
A   initial encounter
D   subsequent encounter
S   sequela

✓5ᵗʰ **S40.0**   Contusion of shoulder and upper arm
✓6ᵗʰ **S40.01**   Contusion of shoulder
✓7ᵗʰ   **S40.011**   Contusion of right shoulder
✓7ᵗʰ   **S40.012**   Contusion of left shoulder
✓7ᵗʰ   **S40.019**   Contusion of unspecified shoulder
✓6ᵗʰ **S40.02**   Contusion of upper arm
✓7ᵗʰ   **S40.021**   Contusion of right upper arm
✓7ᵗʰ   **S40.022**   Contusion of left upper arm
✓7ᵗʰ   **S40.029**   Contusion of unspecified upper arm

✓5ᵗʰ **S40.2**   Other superficial injuries of shoulder
✓6ᵗʰ **S40.21**   Abrasion of shoulder
✓7ᵗʰ   **S40.211**   Abrasion of right shoulder
✓7ᵗʰ   **S40.212**   Abrasion of left shoulder
✓7ᵗʰ   **S40.219**   Abrasion of unspecified shoulder
✓6ᵗʰ **S40.22**   Blister (nonthermal) of shoulder
✓7ᵗʰ   **S40.221**   Blister (nonthermal) of right shoulder
✓7ᵗʰ   **S40.222**   Blister (nonthermal) of left shoulder
✓7ᵗʰ   **S40.229**   Blister (nonthermal) of unspecified shoulder
✓6ᵗʰ **S40.24**   External constriction of shoulder
✓7ᵗʰ   **S40.241**   External constriction of right shoulder
✓7ᵗʰ   **S40.242**   External constriction of left shoulder
✓7ᵗʰ   **S40.249**   External constriction of unspecified shoulder
✓6ᵗʰ **S40.25**   Superficial foreign body of shoulder
Splinter in the shoulder
✓7ᵗʰ   **S40.251**   Superficial foreign body of right shoulder
✓7ᵗʰ   **S40.252**   Superficial foreign body of left shoulder
✓7ᵗʰ   **S40.259**   Superficial foreign body of unspecified shoulder
✓6ᵗʰ **S40.26**   Insect bite (nonvenomous) of shoulder
✓7ᵗʰ   **S40.261**   Insect bite (nonvenomous) of right shoulder
✓7ᵗʰ   **S40.262**   Insect bite (nonvenomous) of left shoulder
✓7ᵗʰ   **S40.269**   Insect bite (nonvenomous) of unspecified shoulder
✓6ᵗʰ **S40.27**   Other superficial bite of shoulder
EXCLUDES 1   open bite of shoulder (S41.05)
✓7ᵗʰ   **S40.271**   Other superficial bite of right shoulder
✓7ᵗʰ   **S40.272**   Other superficial bite of left shoulder
✓7ᵗʰ   **S40.279**   Other superficial bite of unspecified shoulder

✓5ᵗʰ **S40.8**   Other superficial injuries of upper arm
✓6ᵗʰ **S40.81**   Abrasion of upper arm
✓7ᵗʰ   **S40.811**   Abrasion of right upper arm
✓7ᵗʰ   **S40.812**   Abrasion of left upper arm
✓7ᵗʰ   **S40.819**   Abrasion of unspecified upper arm
✓6ᵗʰ **S40.82**   Blister (nonthermal) of upper arm
✓7ᵗʰ   **S40.821**   Blister (nonthermal) of right upper arm
✓7ᵗʰ   **S40.822**   Blister (nonthermal) of left upper arm
✓7ᵗʰ   **S40.829**   Blister (nonthermal) of unspecified upper arm
✓6ᵗʰ **S40.84**   External constriction of upper arm
✓7ᵗʰ   **S40.841**   External constriction of right upper arm
✓7ᵗʰ   **S40.842**   External constriction of left upper arm
✓7ᵗʰ   **S40.849**   External constriction of unspecified upper arm

✓6ᵗʰ **S40.85**   Superficial foreign body of upper arm
Splinter in the upper arm
✓7ᵗʰ   **S40.851**   Superficial foreign body of right upper arm
✓7ᵗʰ   **S40.852**   Superficial foreign body of left upper arm
✓7ᵗʰ   **S40.859**   Superficial foreign body of unspecified upper arm
✓6ᵗʰ **S40.86**   Insect bite (nonvenomous) of upper arm
✓7ᵗʰ   **S40.861**   Insect bite (nonvenomous) of right upper arm
✓7ᵗʰ   **S40.862**   Insect bite (nonvenomous) of left upper arm
✓7ᵗʰ   **S40.869**   Insect bite (nonvenomous) of unspecified upper arm
✓6ᵗʰ **S40.87**   Other superficial bite of upper arm
EXCLUDES 1   open bite of upper arm (S41.14)
EXCLUDES 2   other superficial bite of shoulder (S40.27-)
✓7ᵗʰ   **S40.871**   Other superficial bite of right upper arm
✓7ᵗʰ   **S40.872**   Other superficial bite of left upper arm
✓7ᵗʰ   **S40.879**   Other superficial bite of unspecified upper arm

✓5ᵗʰ **S40.9**   Unspecified superficial injury of shoulder and upper arm
✓6ᵗʰ **S40.91**   Unspecified superficial injury of shoulder
✓7ᵗʰ   **S40.911**   Unspecified superficial injury of right shoulder
✓7ᵗʰ   **S40.912**   Unspecified superficial injury of left shoulder
✓7ᵗʰ   **S40.919**   Unspecified superficial injury of unspecified shoulder
✓6ᵗʰ **S40.92**   Unspecified superficial injury of upper arm
✓7ᵗʰ   **S40.921**   Unspecified superficial injury of right upper arm
✓7ᵗʰ   **S40.922**   Unspecified superficial injury of left upper arm
✓7ᵗʰ   **S40.929**   Unspecified superficial injury of unspecified upper arm

✓4ᵗʰ S41   Open wound of shoulder and upper arm

Code also any associated wound infection
EXCLUDES 1   traumatic amputation of shoulder and upper arm (S48.-)
EXCLUDES 2   open fracture of shoulder and upper arm (S42.- with 7th character B or C)

The appropriate 7th character is to be added to each code from category S41.
A   initial encounter
D   subsequent encounter
S   sequela

✓5ᵗʰ **S41.0**   Open wound of shoulder
✓6ᵗʰ **S41.00**   Unspecified open wound of shoulder
✓7ᵗʰ   **S41.001**   Unspecified open wound of right shoulder
✓7ᵗʰ   **S41.002**   Unspecified open wound of left shoulder
✓7ᵗʰ   **S41.009**   Unspecified open wound of unspecified shoulder
✓6ᵗʰ **S41.01**   Laceration without foreign body of shoulder
✓7ᵗʰ   **S41.011**   Laceration without foreign body of right shoulder
✓7ᵗʰ   **S41.012**   Laceration without foreign body of left shoulder
✓7ᵗʰ   **S41.019**   Laceration without foreign body of unspecified shoulder
✓6ᵗʰ **S41.02**   Laceration with foreign body of shoulder
✓7ᵗʰ   **S41.021**   Laceration with foreign body of right shoulder
✓7ᵗʰ   **S41.022**   Laceration with foreign body of left shoulder
✓7ᵗʰ   **S41.029**   Laceration with foreign body of unspecified shoulder
✓6ᵗʰ **S41.03**   Puncture wound without foreign body of shoulder
✓7ᵗʰ   **S41.031**   Puncture wound without foreign body of right shoulder
✓7ᵗʰ   **S41.032**   Puncture wound without foreign body of left shoulder
✓7ᵗʰ   **S41.039**   Puncture wound without foreign body of unspecified shoulder

---

✓ Additional Character Required   ✓x7ᵗʰ Xtension Alert   Unspecified Dx   Other Specified Dx   Manifestation   ►◄ Revised Text   ● New Code   ▲ Revised Code Title

✓6ᵗʰ **S41.04** Puncture wound with foreign body of shoulder
  ✓7ᵗʰ **S41.041** Puncture wound with foreign body of right shoulder
  ✓7ᵗʰ **S41.042** Puncture wound with foreign body of left shoulder
  ✓7ᵗʰ **S41.049** Puncture wound with foreign body of unspecified shoulder

✓6ᵗʰ **S41.05** Open bite of shoulder
  Bite of shoulder NOS
  EXCLUDES 1   superficial bite of shoulder (S40.27)
  ✓7ᵗʰ **S41.051** Open bite of right shoulder
  ✓7ᵗʰ **S41.052** Open bite of left shoulder
  ✓7ᵗʰ **S41.059** Open bite of unspecified shoulder

✓5ᵗʰ **S41.1** Open wound of upper arm
✓6ᵗʰ **S41.10** Unspecified open wound of upper arm
  ✓7ᵗʰ **S41.101** Unspecified open wound of right upper arm
  ✓7ᵗʰ **S41.102** Unspecified open wound of left upper arm
  ✓7ᵗʰ **S41.109** Unspecified open wound of unspecified upper arm

✓6ᵗʰ **S41.11** Laceration without foreign body of upper arm
  ✓7ᵗʰ **S41.111** Laceration without foreign body of right upper arm
  ✓7ᵗʰ **S41.112** Laceration without foreign body of left upper arm
  ✓7ᵗʰ **S41.119** Laceration without foreign body of unspecified upper arm

✓6ᵗʰ **S41.12** Laceration with foreign body of upper arm
  ✓7ᵗʰ **S41.121** Laceration with foreign body of right upper arm
  ✓7ᵗʰ **S41.122** Laceration with foreign body of left upper arm
  ✓7ᵗʰ **S41.129** Laceration with foreign body of unspecified upper arm

✓6ᵗʰ **S41.13** Puncture wound without foreign body of upper arm
  ✓7ᵗʰ **S41.131** Puncture wound without foreign body of right upper arm
  ✓7ᵗʰ **S41.132** Puncture wound without foreign body of left upper arm
  ✓7ᵗʰ **S41.139** Puncture wound without foreign body of unspecified upper arm

✓6ᵗʰ **S41.14** Puncture wound with foreign body of upper arm
  ✓7ᵗʰ **S41.141** Puncture wound with foreign body of right upper arm
  ✓7ᵗʰ **S41.142** Puncture wound with foreign body of left upper arm
  ✓7ᵗʰ **S41.149** Puncture wound with foreign body of unspecified upper arm

✓6ᵗʰ **S41.15** Open bite of upper arm
  Bite of upper arm NOS
  EXCLUDES 1   superficial bite of upper arm (S40.87)
  ✓7ᵗʰ **S41.151** Open bite of right upper arm
  ✓7ᵗʰ **S41.152** Open bite of left upper arm
  ✓7ᵗʰ **S41.159** Open bite of unspecified upper arm

✓4ᵗʰ **S42** Fracture of shoulder and upper arm
  NOTE A fracture not indicated as displaced or nondisplaced should be coded to displaced.
  A fracture not indicated as open or closed should be coded to closed.
  EXCLUDES 1   traumatic amputation of shoulder and upper arm (S48.-)

  The appropriate 7th character is to be added to all codes from category S42 [unless otherwise indicated].
  A   initial encounter for closed fracture
  B   initial encounter for open fracture
  D   subsequent encounter for fracture with routine healing
  G   subsequent encounter for fracture with delayed healing
  K   subsequent encounter for fracture with nonunion
  P   subsequent encounter for fracture with malunion
  S   sequela

✓5ᵗʰ **S42.0** Fracture of clavicle
✓6ᵗʰ **S42.00** Fracture of unspecified part of clavicle
  ✓7ᵗʰ **S42.001** Fracture of unspecified part of right clavicle
  ✓7ᵗʰ **S42.002** Fracture of unspecified part of left clavicle

  ✓7ᵗʰ **S42.009** Fracture of unspecified part of unspecified clavicle
    AHA: 2012, 4Q, 93

✓6ᵗʰ **S42.01** Fracture of sternal end of clavicle
  ✓7ᵗʰ **S42.011** Anterior displaced fracture of sternal end of right clavicle
  ✓7ᵗʰ **S42.012** Anterior displaced fracture of sternal end of left clavicle
  ✓7ᵗʰ **S42.013** Anterior displaced fracture of sternal end of unspecified clavicle
    Displaced fracture of sternal end of clavicle NOS
  ✓7ᵗʰ **S42.014** Posterior displaced fracture of sternal end of right clavicle
  ✓7ᵗʰ **S42.015** Posterior displaced fracture of sternal end of left clavicle
  ✓7ᵗʰ **S42.016** Posterior displaced fracture of sternal end of unspecified clavicle
  ✓7ᵗʰ **S42.017** Nondisplaced fracture of sternal end of right clavicle
  ✓7ᵗʰ **S42.018** Nondisplaced fracture of sternal end of left clavicle
  ✓7ᵗʰ **S42.019** Nondisplaced fracture of sternal end of unspecified clavicle

✓6ᵗʰ **S42.02** Fracture of shaft of clavicle
  ✓7ᵗʰ **S42.021** Displaced fracture of shaft of right clavicle
  ✓7ᵗʰ **S42.022** Displaced fracture of shaft of left clavicle
  ✓7ᵗʰ **S42.023** Displaced fracture of shaft of unspecified clavicle
  ✓7ᵗʰ **S42.024** Nondisplaced fracture of shaft of right clavicle
  ✓7ᵗʰ **S42.025** Nondisplaced fracture of shaft of left clavicle
  ✓7ᵗʰ **S42.026** Nondisplaced fracture of shaft of unspecified clavicle

✓6ᵗʰ **S42.03** Fracture of lateral end of clavicle
  Fracture of acromial end of clavicle
  ✓7ᵗʰ **S42.031** Displaced fracture of lateral end of right clavicle
  ✓7ᵗʰ **S42.032** Displaced fracture of lateral end of left clavicle
  ✓7ᵗʰ **S42.033** Displaced fracture of lateral end of unspecified clavicle
  ✓7ᵗʰ **S42.034** Nondisplaced fracture of lateral end of right clavicle
  ✓7ᵗʰ **S42.035** Nondisplaced fracture of lateral end of left clavicle
  ✓7ᵗʰ **S42.036** Nondisplaced fracture of lateral end of unspecified clavicle

✓5ᵗʰ **S42.1** Fracture of scapula
✓6ᵗʰ **S42.10** Fracture of unspecified part of scapula
  ✓7ᵗʰ **S42.101** Fracture of unspecified part of scapula, right shoulder
  ✓7ᵗʰ **S42.102** Fracture of unspecified part of scapula, left shoulder
  ✓7ᵗʰ **S42.109** Fracture of unspecified part of scapula, unspecified shoulder

✓6ᵗʰ **S42.11** Fracture of body of scapula
  ✓7ᵗʰ **S42.111** Displaced fracture of body of scapula, right shoulder
  ✓7ᵗʰ **S42.112** Displaced fracture of body of scapula, left shoulder
  ✓7ᵗʰ **S42.113** Displaced fracture of body of scapula, unspecified shoulder
  ✓7ᵗʰ **S42.114** Nondisplaced fracture of body of scapula, right shoulder
  ✓7ᵗʰ **S42.115** Nondisplaced fracture of body of scapula, left shoulder
  ✓7ᵗʰ **S42.116** Nondisplaced fracture of body of scapula, unspecified shoulder

✓6ᵗʰ **S42.12** Fracture of acromial process
  ✓7ᵗʰ **S42.121** Displaced fracture of acromial process, right shoulder
  ✓7ᵗʰ **S42.122** Displaced fracture of acromial process, left shoulder

☑7ᵗʰ **S42.123** Displaced fracture of acromial process, unspecified shoulder

☑7ᵗʰ **S42.124** Nondisplaced fracture of acromial process, right shoulder

☑7ᵗʰ **S42.125** Nondisplaced fracture of acromial process, left shoulder

☑7ᵗʰ **S42.126** Nondisplaced fracture of acromial process, unspecified shoulder

☑6ᵗʰ **S42.13** Fracture of coracoid process

☑7ᵗʰ **S42.131** Displaced fracture of coracoid process, right shoulder

☑7ᵗʰ **S42.132** Displaced fracture of coracoid process, left shoulder

☑7ᵗʰ **S42.133** Displaced fracture of coracoid process, unspecified shoulder

☑7ᵗʰ **S42.134** Nondisplaced fracture of coracoid process, right shoulder

☑7ᵗʰ **S42.135** Nondisplaced fracture of coracoid process, left shoulder

☑7ᵗʰ **S42.136** Nondisplaced fracture of coracoid process, unspecified shoulder

☑6ᵗʰ **S42.14** Fracture of glenoid cavity of scapula

☑7ᵗʰ **S42.141** Displaced fracture of glenoid cavity of scapula, right shoulder

☑7ᵗʰ **S42.142** Displaced fracture of glenoid cavity of scapula, left shoulder

☑7ᵗʰ **S42.143** Displaced fracture of glenoid cavity of scapula, unspecified shoulder

☑7ᵗʰ **S42.144** Nondisplaced fracture of glenoid cavity of scapula, right shoulder

☑7ᵗʰ **S42.145** Nondisplaced fracture of glenoid cavity of scapula, left shoulder

☑7ᵗʰ **S42.146** Nondisplaced fracture of glenoid cavity of scapula, unspecified shoulder

☑6ᵗʰ **S42.15** Fracture of neck of scapula

☑7ᵗʰ **S42.151** Displaced fracture of neck of scapula, right shoulder

☑7ᵗʰ **S42.152** Displaced fracture of neck of scapula, left shoulder

☑7ᵗʰ **S42.153** Displaced fracture of neck of scapula, unspecified shoulder

☑7ᵗʰ **S42.154** Nondisplaced fracture of neck of scapula, right shoulder

☑7ᵗʰ **S42.155** Nondisplaced fracture of neck of scapula, left shoulder

☑7ᵗʰ **S42.156** Nondisplaced fracture of neck of scapula, unspecified shoulder

☑6ᵗʰ **S42.19** Fracture of other part of scapula

☑7ᵗʰ **S42.191** Fracture of other part of scapula, right shoulder

☑7ᵗʰ **S42.192** Fracture of other part of scapula, left shoulder

☑7ᵗʰ **S42.199** Fracture of other part of scapula, unspecified shoulder

☑5ᵗʰ **S42.2** **Fracture of upper end of humerus**
Fracture of proximal end of humerus
EXCLUDES 2 *fracture of shaft of humerus (S42.3-)*
physeal fracture of upper end of humerus (S49.0-)

☑6ᵗʰ **S42.20** Unspecified fracture of upper end of humerus

☑7ᵗʰ **S42.201** Unspecified fracture of upper end of right humerus

☑7ᵗʰ **S42.202** Unspecified fracture of upper end of left humerus

☑7ᵗʰ **S42.209** Unspecified fracture of upper end of unspecified humerus

☑6ᵗʰ **S42.21** Unspecified fracture of surgical neck of humerus
Fracture of neck of humerus NOS

☑7ᵗʰ **S42.211** Unspecified displaced fracture of surgical neck of right humerus

☑7ᵗʰ **S42.212** Unspecified displaced fracture of surgical neck of left humerus

☑7ᵗʰ **S42.213** Unspecified displaced fracture of surgical neck of unspecified humerus

☑7ᵗʰ **S42.214** Unspecified nondisplaced fracture of surgical neck of right humerus

☑7ᵗʰ **S42.215** Unspecified nondisplaced fracture of surgical neck of left humerus

☑7ᵗʰ **S42.216** Unspecified nondisplaced fracture of surgical neck of unspecified humerus

☑6ᵗʰ **S42.22** 2-part fracture of surgical neck of humerus

☑7ᵗʰ **S42.221** 2-part displaced fracture of surgical neck of right humerus

☑7ᵗʰ **S42.222** 2-part displaced fracture of surgical neck of left humerus

☑7ᵗʰ **S42.223** 2-part displaced fracture of surgical neck of unspecified humerus

☑7ᵗʰ **S42.224** 2-part nondisplaced fracture of surgical neck of right humerus

☑7ᵗʰ **S42.225** 2-part nondisplaced fracture of surgical neck of left humerus

☑7ᵗʰ **S42.226** 2-part nondisplaced fracture of surgical neck of unspecified humerus

☑6ᵗʰ **S42.23** 3-part fracture of surgical neck of humerus

☑7ᵗʰ **S42.231** 3-part fracture of surgical neck of right humerus

☑7ᵗʰ **S42.232** 3-part fracture of surgical neck of left humerus

☑7ᵗʰ **S42.239** 3-part fracture of surgical neck of unspecified humerus

☑6ᵗʰ **S42.24** 4-part fracture of surgical neck of humerus

☑7ᵗʰ **S42.241** 4-part fracture of surgical neck of right humerus

☑7ᵗʰ **S42.242** 4-part fracture of surgical neck of left humerus

☑7ᵗʰ **S42.249** 4-part fracture of surgical neck of unspecified humerus

☑6ᵗʰ **S42.25** Fracture of greater tuberosity of humerus

☑7ᵗʰ **S42.251** Displaced fracture of greater tuberosity of right humerus

☑7ᵗʰ **S42.252** Displaced fracture of greater tuberosity of left humerus

☑7ᵗʰ **S42.253** Displaced fracture of greater tuberosity of unspecified humerus

☑7ᵗʰ **S42.254** Nondisplaced fracture of greater tuberosity of right humerus

☑7ᵗʰ **S42.255** Nondisplaced fracture of greater tuberosity of left humerus

☑7ᵗʰ **S42.256** Nondisplaced fracture of greater tuberosity of unspecified humerus

☑6ᵗʰ **S42.26** Fracture of lesser tuberosity of humerus

☑7ᵗʰ **S42.261** Displaced fracture of lesser tuberosity of right humerus

☑7ᵗʰ **S42.262** Displaced fracture of lesser tuberosity of left humerus

☑7ᵗʰ **S42.263** Displaced fracture of lesser tuberosity of unspecified humerus

☑7ᵗʰ **S42.264** Nondisplaced fracture of lesser tuberosity of right humerus

☑7ᵗʰ **S42.265** Nondisplaced fracture of lesser tuberosity of left humerus

☑7ᵗʰ **S42.266** Nondisplaced fracture of lesser tuberosity of unspecified humerus

☑6ᵗʰ **S42.27** Torus fracture of upper end of humerus

The appropriate 7th character is to be added to all codes in subcategory S42.27.
A   initial encounter for closed fracture
D   subsequent encounter for fracture with routine healing
G   subsequent encounter for fracture with delayed healing
K   subsequent encounter for fracture with nonunion
P   subsequent encounter for fracture with malunion
S   sequela

☑7ᵗʰ **S42.271** Torus fracture of upper end of right humerus

☑7ᵗʰ **S42.272** Torus fracture of upper end of left humerus

☑ Additional Character Required   ☑7ᵗʰ Xtension Alert   Unspecified Dx   Other Specified Dx   Manifestation   ▶◀ Revised Text   ● New Code   ▲ Revised Code Title

ICD-10-CM Draft (2015)   **843**

√7ᵗʰ **S42.279** **Torus fracture of upper end of unspecified humerus**

√6ᵗʰ **S42.29** Other fracture of upper end of humerus
Fracture of anatomical neck of humerus
Fracture of articular head of humerus

√7ᵗʰ **S42.291** **Other displaced fracture of upper end of right humerus**

√7ᵗʰ **S42.292** **Other displaced fracture of upper end of left humerus**

√7ᵗʰ **S42.293** **Other displaced fracture of upper end of unspecified humerus**

√7ᵗʰ **S42.294** **Other nondisplaced fracture of upper end of right humerus**

√7ᵗʰ **S42.295** **Other nondisplaced fracture of upper end of left humerus**

√7ᵗʰ **S42.296** **Other nondisplaced fracture of upper end of unspecified humerus**

√5ᵗʰ **S42.3** Fracture of shaft of humerus
Fracture of humerus NOS
Fracture of upper arm NOS
EXCLUDES 2 physeal fractures of upper end of humerus (S49.0-)
physeal fractures of lower end of humerus (S49.1-)

√6ᵗʰ **S42.30** Unspecified fracture of shaft of humerus

√7ᵗʰ **S42.301** **Unspecified fracture of shaft of humerus, right arm**

√7ᵗʰ **S42.302** **Unspecified fracture of shaft of humerus, left arm**

√7ᵗʰ **S42.309** **Unspecified fracture of shaft of humerus, unspecified arm**

√6ᵗʰ **S42.31** Greenstick fracture of shaft of humerus

The appropriate 7th character is to be added to all codes in subcategory S42.31.
A initial encounter for closed fracture
D subsequent encounter for fracture with routine healing
G subsequent encounter for fracture with delayed healing
K subsequent encounter for fracture with nonunion
P subsequent encounter for fracture with malunion
S sequela

√7ᵗʰ **S42.311** **Greenstick fracture of shaft of humerus, right arm**

√7ᵗʰ **S42.312** **Greenstick fracture of shaft of humerus, left arm**

√7ᵗʰ **S42.319** **Greenstick fracture of shaft of humerus, unspecified arm**

√6ᵗʰ **S42.32** Transverse fracture of shaft of humerus

√7ᵗʰ **S42.321** **Displaced transverse fracture of shaft of humerus, right arm**

√7ᵗʰ **S42.322** **Displaced transverse fracture of shaft of humerus, left arm**

√7ᵗʰ **S42.323** **Displaced transverse fracture of shaft of humerus, unspecified arm**

√7ᵗʰ **S42.324** **Nondisplaced transverse fracture of shaft of humerus, right arm**

√7ᵗʰ **S42.325** **Nondisplaced transverse fracture of shaft of humerus, left arm**

√7ᵗʰ **S42.326** **Nondisplaced transverse fracture of shaft of humerus, unspecified arm**

√6ᵗʰ **S42.33** Oblique fracture of shaft of humerus

√7ᵗʰ **S42.331** **Displaced oblique fracture of shaft of humerus, right arm**

√7ᵗʰ **S42.332** **Displaced oblique fracture of shaft of humerus, left arm**

√7ᵗʰ **S42.333** **Displaced oblique fracture of shaft of humerus, unspecified arm**

√7ᵗʰ **S42.334** **Nondisplaced oblique fracture of shaft of humerus, right arm**

√7ᵗʰ **S42.335** **Nondisplaced oblique fracture of shaft of humerus, left arm**

√7ᵗʰ **S42.336** **Nondisplaced oblique fracture of shaft of humerus, unspecified arm**

√6ᵗʰ **S42.34** Spiral fracture of shaft of humerus

√7ᵗʰ **S42.341** **Displaced spiral fracture of shaft of humerus, right arm**

√7ᵗʰ **S42.342** **Displaced spiral fracture of shaft of humerus, left arm**

√7ᵗʰ **S42.343** **Displaced spiral fracture of shaft of humerus, unspecified arm**

√7ᵗʰ **S42.344** **Nondisplaced spiral fracture of shaft of humerus, right arm**

√7ᵗʰ **S42.345** **Nondisplaced spiral fracture of shaft of humerus, left arm**

√7ᵗʰ **S42.346** **Nondisplaced spiral fracture of shaft of humerus, unspecified arm**

√6ᵗʰ **S42.35** Comminuted fracture of shaft of humerus

√7ᵗʰ **S42.351** **Displaced comminuted fracture of shaft of humerus, right arm**

√7ᵗʰ **S42.352** **Displaced comminuted fracture of shaft of humerus, left arm**

√7ᵗʰ **S42.353** **Displaced comminuted fracture of shaft of humerus, unspecified arm**

√7ᵗʰ **S42.354** **Nondisplaced comminuted fracture of shaft of humerus, right arm**

√7ᵗʰ **S42.355** **Nondisplaced comminuted fracture of shaft of humerus, left arm**

√7ᵗʰ **S42.356** **Nondisplaced comminuted fracture of shaft of humerus, unspecified arm**

√6ᵗʰ **S42.36** Segmental fracture of shaft of humerus

√7ᵗʰ **S42.361** **Displaced segmental fracture of shaft of humerus, right arm**

√7ᵗʰ **S42.362** **Displaced segmental fracture of shaft of humerus, left arm**

√7ᵗʰ **S42.363** **Displaced segmental fracture of shaft of humerus, unspecified arm**

√7ᵗʰ **S42.364** **Nondisplaced segmental fracture of shaft of humerus, right arm**

√7ᵗʰ **S42.365** **Nondisplaced segmental fracture of shaft of humerus, left arm**

√7ᵗʰ **S42.366** **Nondisplaced segmental fracture of shaft of humerus, unspecified arm**

√6ᵗʰ **S42.39** Other fracture of shaft of humerus

√7ᵗʰ **S42.391** **Other fracture of shaft of right humerus**

√7ᵗʰ **S42.392** **Other fracture of shaft of left humerus**

√7ᵗʰ **S42.399** **Other fracture of shaft of unspecified humerus**

√5ᵗʰ **S42.4** Fracture of lower end of humerus
Fracture of distal end of humerus
EXCLUDES 2 fracture of shaft of humerus (S42.3-)
physeal fracture of lower end of humerus (S49.1-)

√6ᵗʰ **S42.40** Unspecified fracture of lower end of humerus
Fracture of elbow NOS

√7ᵗʰ **S42.401** **Unspecified fracture of lower end of right humerus**

√7ᵗʰ **S42.402** **Unspecified fracture of lower end of left humerus**

√7ᵗʰ **S42.409** **Unspecified fracture of lower end of unspecified humerus**

√6ᵗʰ **S42.41** Simple supracondylar fracture without intercondylar fracture of humerus

√7ᵗʰ **S42.411** **Displaced simple supracondylar fracture without intercondylar fracture of right humerus**

√7ᵗʰ **S42.412** **Displaced simple supracondylar fracture without intercondylar fracture of left humerus**

√7ᵗʰ **S42.413** **Displaced simple supracondylar fracture without intercondylar fracture of unspecified humerus**

√7ᵗʰ **S42.414** **Nondisplaced simple supracondylar fracture without intercondylar fracture of right humerus**

√7ᵗʰ **S42.415** **Nondisplaced simple supracondylar fracture without intercondylar fracture of left humerus**

√7ᵗʰ **S42.416** **Nondisplaced simple supracondylar fracture without intercondylar fracture of unspecified humerus**

√6th **S42.42** Comminuted supracondylar fracture without intercondylar **fracture of humerus**

√7th **S42.421** Displaced comminuted supracondylar fracture without intercondylar fracture of right humerus

√7th **S42.422** Displaced comminuted supracondylar fracture without intercondylar fracture of left humerus

√7th **S42.423** Displaced comminuted supracondylar fracture without intercondylar fracture of unspecified humerus

√7th **S42.424** Nondisplaced comminuted supracondylar fracture without intercondylar fracture of right humerus

√7th **S42.425** Nondisplaced comminuted supracondylar fracture without intercondylar fracture of left humerus

√7th **S42.426** Nondisplaced comminuted supracondylar fracture without intercondylar fracture of unspecified humerus

√6th **S42.43** Fracture (avulsion) of lateral epicondyle **of humerus**

√7th **S42.431** Displaced fracture (avulsion) of lateral epicondyle of right humerus

√7th **S42.432** Displaced fracture (avulsion) of lateral epicondyle of left humerus

√7th **S42.433** Displaced fracture (avulsion) of lateral epicondyle of unspecified humerus

√7th **S42.434** Nondisplaced fracture (avulsion) of lateral epicondyle of right humerus

√7th **S42.435** Nondisplaced fracture (avulsion) of lateral epicondyle of left humerus

√7th **S42.436** Nondisplaced fracture (avulsion) of lateral epicondyle of unspecified humerus

√6th **S42.44** Fracture (avulsion) of medial epicondyle **of humerus**

S42.441 Displaced fracture (avulsion) of medial epicondyle of right humerus

√7th **S42.442** Displaced fracture (avulsion) of medial epicondyle of left humerus

√7th **S42.443** Displaced fracture (avulsion) of medial epicondyle of unspecified humerus

√7th **S42.444** Nondisplaced fracture (avulsion) of medial epicondyle of right humerus

√7th **S42.445** Nondisplaced fracture (avulsion) of medial epicondyle of left humerus

√7th **S42.446** Nondisplaced fracture (avulsion) of medial epicondyle of unspecified humerus

√7th **S42.447** Incarcerated fracture (avulsion) of medial epicondyle of right humerus

√7th **S42.448** Incarcerated fracture (avulsion) of medial epicondyle of left humerus

√7th **S42.449** Incarcerated fracture (avulsion) of medial epicondyle of unspecified humerus

√6th **S42.45** Fracture of lateral condyle **of humerus**
Fracture of capitellum of humerus

√7th **S42.451** Displaced fracture of lateral condyle of right humerus

√7th **S42.452** Displaced fracture of lateral condyle of left humerus

√7th **S42.453** Displaced fracture of lateral condyle of unspecified humerus

√7th **S42.454** Nondisplaced fracture of lateral condyle of right humerus

√7th **S42.455** Nondisplaced fracture of lateral condyle of left humerus

√7th **S42.456** Nondisplaced fracture of lateral condyle of unspecified humerus

√6th **S42.46** Fracture of medial condyle **of humerus**
Trochlea fracture of humerus

√7th **S42.461** Displaced fracture of medial condyle of right humerus

√7th **S42.462** Displaced fracture of medial condyle of left humerus

√7th **S42.463** Displaced fracture of medial condyle of unspecified humerus

√7th **S42.464** Nondisplaced fracture of medial condyle of right humerus

√7th **S42.465** Nondisplaced fracture of medial condyle of left humerus

√7th **S42.466** Nondisplaced fracture of medial condyle of unspecified humerus

√6th **S42.47** Transcondylar fracture **of humerus**

√7th **S42.471** Displaced transcondylar fracture of right humerus

√7th **S42.472** Displaced transcondylar fracture of left humerus

√7th **S42.473** Displaced transcondylar fracture of unspecified humerus

√7th **S42.474** Nondisplaced transcondylar fracture of right humerus

√7th **S42.475** Nondisplaced transcondylar fracture of left humerus

√7th **S42.476** Nondisplaced transcondylar fracture of unspecified humerus

√6th **S42.48** Torus fracture of lower end of humerus

The appropriate 7th character is to be added to all codes in subcategory S42.48.
A   initial encounter for closed fracture
D   subsequent encounter for fracture with routine healing
G   subsequent encounter for fracture with delayed healing
K   subsequent encounter for fracture with nonunion
P   subsequent encounter for fracture with malunion
S   sequela

√7th **S42.481** Torus fracture of lower end of right humerus

√7th **S42.482** Torus fracture of lower end of left humerus

√7th **S42.489** Torus fracture of lower end of unspecified humerus

√6th **S42.49** Other fracture of lower end of humerus

√7th **S42.491** Other displaced fracture of lower end of right humerus

√7th **S42.492** Other displaced fracture of lower end of left humerus

√7th **S42.493** Other displaced fracture of lower end of unspecified humerus

√7th **S42.494** Other nondisplaced fracture of lower end of right humerus

√7th **S42.495** Other nondisplaced fracture of lower end of left humerus

√7th **S42.496** Other nondisplaced fracture of lower end of unspecified humerus

√5th **S42.9** Fracture of shoulder girdle, part unspecified
Fracture of shoulder NOS

√x7th **S42.90** Fracture of unspecified shoulder girdle, part unspecified

√x7th **S42.91** Fracture of right shoulder girdle, part unspecified

√x7th **S42.92** Fracture of left shoulder girdle, part unspecified

✓4ᵗʰ S43 Dislocation and sprain of joints and ligaments of shoulder girdle

> INCLUDES
> avulsion of joint or ligament of shoulder girdle
> laceration of cartilage, joint or ligament of shoulder girdle
> sprain of cartilage, joint or ligament of shoulder girdle
> traumatic hemarthrosis of joint or ligament of shoulder girdle
> traumatic rupture of joint or ligament of shoulder girdle
> traumatic subluxation of joint or ligament of shoulder girdle
> traumatic tear of joint or ligament of shoulder girdle

Code also any associated open wound

> EXCLUDES 2 strain of muscle, fascia and tendon of shoulder and upper arm (S46.-)

> The appropriate 7th character is to be added to each code from category S43.
> A   initial encounter
> D   subsequent encounter
> S   sequela

✓5ᵗʰ S43.0 Subluxation and dislocation of shoulder joint
> Dislocation of glenohumeral joint
> Subluxation of glenohumeral joint

✓6ᵗʰ S43.00 Unspecified subluxation and dislocation of shoulder joint
> Dislocation of humerus NOS
> Subluxation of humerus NOS

- ✓7ᵗʰ **S43.001 Unspecified subluxation of right shoulder joint**
- ✓7ᵗʰ **S43.002 Unspecified subluxation of left shoulder joint**
- ✓7ᵗʰ **S43.003 Unspecified subluxation of unspecified shoulder joint**
- ✓7ᵗʰ **S43.004 Unspecified dislocation of right shoulder joint**
- ✓7ᵗʰ **S43.005 Unspecified dislocation of left shoulder joint**
- ✓7ᵗʰ **S43.006 Unspecified dislocation of unspecified shoulder joint**

✓6ᵗʰ S43.01 Anterior subluxation and dislocation of humerus
- ✓7ᵗʰ **S43.011 Anterior subluxation of right humerus**
- ✓7ᵗʰ **S43.012 Anterior subluxation of left humerus**
- ✓7ᵗʰ **S43.013 Anterior subluxation of unspecified humerus**
- ✓7ᵗʰ **S43.014 Anterior dislocation of right humerus**
- ✓7ᵗʰ **S43.015 Anterior dislocation of left humerus**
- ✓7ᵗʰ **S43.016 Anterior dislocation of unspecified humerus**

✓6ᵗʰ S43.02 Posterior subluxation and dislocation of humerus
- ✓7ᵗʰ **S43.021 Posterior subluxation of right humerus**
- ✓7ᵗʰ **S43.022 Posterior subluxation of left humerus**
- ✓7ᵗʰ **S43.023 Posterior subluxation of unspecified humerus**
- ✓7ᵗʰ **S43.024 Posterior dislocation of right humerus**
- ✓7ᵗʰ **S43.025 Posterior dislocation of left humerus**
- ✓7ᵗʰ **S43.026 Posterior dislocation of unspecified humerus**

✓6ᵗʰ S43.03 Inferior subluxation and dislocation of humerus
- ✓7ᵗʰ **S43.031 Inferior subluxation of right humerus**
- ✓7ᵗʰ **S43.032 Inferior subluxation of left humerus**
- ✓7ᵗʰ **S43.033 Inferior subluxation of unspecified humerus**
- ✓7ᵗʰ **S43.034 Inferior dislocation of right humerus**
- ✓7ᵗʰ **S43.035 Inferior dislocation of left humerus**
- ✓7ᵗʰ **S43.036 Inferior dislocation of unspecified humerus**

✓6ᵗʰ S43.08 Other subluxation and dislocation of shoulder joint
- ✓7ᵗʰ **S43.081 Other subluxation of right shoulder joint**
- ✓7ᵗʰ **S43.082 Other subluxation of left shoulder joint**
- ✓7ᵗʰ **S43.083 Other subluxation of unspecified shoulder joint**
- ✓7ᵗʰ **S43.084 Other dislocation of right shoulder joint**
- ✓7ᵗʰ **S43.085 Other dislocation of left shoulder joint**
- ✓7ᵗʰ **S43.086 Other dislocation of unspecified shoulder joint**

✓5ᵗʰ S43.1 Subluxation and dislocation of acromioclavicular joint

✓6ᵗʰ S43.10 Unspecified dislocation of acromioclavicular joint
- ✓7ᵗʰ **S43.101 Unspecified dislocation of right acromioclavicular joint**
- ✓7ᵗʰ **S43.102 Unspecified dislocation of left acromioclavicular joint**
- ✓7ᵗʰ **S43.109 Unspecified dislocation of unspecified acromioclavicular joint**

✓6ᵗʰ S43.11 Subluxation of acromioclavicular joint
- ✓7ᵗʰ **S43.111 Subluxation of right acromioclavicular joint**
- ✓7ᵗʰ **S43.112 Subluxation of left acromioclavicular joint**
- ✓7ᵗʰ **S43.119 Subluxation of unspecified acromioclavicular joint**

✓6ᵗʰ S43.12 Dislocation of acromioclavicular joint, 100%-200% displacement
- ✓7ᵗʰ **S43.121 Dislocation of right acromioclavicular joint, 100%-200% displacement**
- ✓7ᵗʰ **S43.122 Dislocation of left acromioclavicular joint, 100%-200% displacement**
- ✓7ᵗʰ **S43.129 Dislocation of unspecified acromioclavicular joint, 100%-200% displacement**

✓6ᵗʰ S43.13 Dislocation of acromioclavicular joint, greater than 200% displacement
- ✓7ᵗʰ **S43.131 Dislocation of right acromioclavicular joint, greater than 200% displacement**
- ✓7ᵗʰ **S43.132 Dislocation of left acromioclavicular joint, greater than 200% displacement**
- ✓7ᵗʰ **S43.139 Dislocation of unspecified acromioclavicular joint, greater than 200% displacement**

✓6ᵗʰ S43.14 Inferior dislocation of acromioclavicular joint
- ✓7ᵗʰ **S43.141 Inferior dislocation of right acromioclavicular joint**
- ✓7ᵗʰ **S43.142 Inferior dislocation of left acromioclavicular joint**
- ✓7ᵗʰ **S43.149 Inferior dislocation of unspecified acromioclavicular joint**

✓6ᵗʰ S43.15 Posterior dislocation of acromioclavicular joint
- ✓7ᵗʰ **S43.151 Posterior dislocation of right acromioclavicular joint**
- ✓7ᵗʰ **S43.152 Posterior dislocation of left acromioclavicular joint**
- ✓7ᵗʰ **S43.159 Posterior dislocation of unspecified acromioclavicular joint**

✓5ᵗʰ S43.2 Subluxation and dislocation of sternoclavicular joint

✓6ᵗʰ S43.20 Unspecified subluxation and dislocation of sternoclavicular joint
- ✓7ᵗʰ **S43.201 Unspecified subluxation of right sternoclavicular joint**
- ✓7ᵗʰ **S43.202 Unspecified subluxation of left sternoclavicular joint**
- ✓7ᵗʰ **S43.203 Unspecified subluxation of unspecified sternoclavicular joint**
- ✓7ᵗʰ **S43.204 Unspecified dislocation of right sternoclavicular joint**
- ✓7ᵗʰ **S43.205 Unspecified dislocation of left sternoclavicular joint**
- ✓7ᵗʰ **S43.206 Unspecified dislocation of unspecified sternoclavicular joint**

✓6ᵗʰ S43.21 Anterior subluxation and dislocation of sternoclavicular joint
- ✓7ᵗʰ **S43.211 Anterior subluxation of right sternoclavicular joint**
- ✓7ᵗʰ **S43.212 Anterior subluxation of left sternoclavicular joint**
- ✓7ᵗʰ **S43.213 Anterior subluxation of unspecified sternoclavicular joint**
- ✓7ᵗʰ **S43.214 Anterior dislocation of right sternoclavicular joint**
- ✓7ᵗʰ **S43.215 Anterior dislocation of left sternoclavicular joint**
- ✓7ᵗʰ **S43.216 Anterior dislocation of unspecified sternoclavicular joint**

EXCLUDES 1 Not coded here   EXCLUDES 2 Not included here   N Newborn Age: 0   P Pediatric Age: 0-17   M Maternity Age: 12-55   A Adult Age: 15-124

846   ICD-10-CM Draft (2015)

√6th **S43.22** Posterior **subluxation and dislocation of sternoclavicular joint**

    √7th **S43.221** Posterior subluxation of right **sternoclavicular joint**

    √7th **S43.222** Posterior subluxation of left **sternoclavicular joint**

    √7th **S43.223** Posterior subluxation of unspecified **sternoclavicular joint**

    √7th **S43.224** Posterior dislocation of right **sternoclavicular joint**

    √7th **S43.225** Posterior dislocation of left **sternoclavicular joint**

    √7th **S43.226** Posterior dislocation of unspecified **sternoclavicular joint**

√5th **S43.3** **Subluxation and dislocation of other and unspecified parts of shoulder girdle**

  √6th **S43.30** **Subluxation and dislocation of** unspecified parts **of shoulder girdle**

    Dislocation of shoulder girdle NOS
    Subluxation of shoulder girdle NOS

    √7th **S43.301** Subluxation of unspecified parts of right **shoulder girdle**

    √7th **S43.302** Subluxation of unspecified parts of left **shoulder girdle**

    √7th **S43.303** Subluxation of unspecified parts of **unspecified shoulder girdle**

    √7th **S43.304** Dislocation of unspecified parts of right **shoulder girdle**

    √7th **S43.305** Dislocation of unspecified parts of left **shoulder girdle**

    √7th **S43.306** Dislocation of unspecified parts of **unspecified shoulder girdle**

  √6th **S43.31** **Subluxation and dislocation of** scapula

    √7th **S43.311** Subluxation of right scapula

    √7th **S43.312** Subluxation of left scapula

    √7th **S43.313** Subluxation of unspecified scapula

    √7th **S43.314** Dislocation of right scapula

    √7th **S43.315** Dislocation of left scapula

    √7th **S43.316** Dislocation of unspecified scapula

  √6th **S43.39** **Subluxation and dislocation of** other parts **of shoulder girdle**

    √7th **S43.391** Subluxation of other parts of right **shoulder girdle**

    √7th **S43.392** Subluxation of other parts of left **shoulder girdle**

    √7th **S43.393** Subluxation of other parts of unspecified **shoulder girdle**

    √7th **S43.394** Dislocation of other parts of right **shoulder girdle**

    √7th **S43.395** Dislocation of other parts of left **shoulder girdle**

    √7th **S43.396** Dislocation of other parts of unspecified **shoulder girdle**

√5th **S43.4** **Sprain of** shoulder joint

  √6th **S43.40** Unspecified **sprain of shoulder joint**

    √7th **S43.401** Unspecified sprain of right **shoulder joint**

    √7th **S43.402** Unspecified sprain of left **shoulder joint**

    √7th **S43.409** Unspecified sprain of unspecified **shoulder joint**

  √6th **S43.41** **Sprain of** coracohumeral (ligament)

    √7th **S43.411** Sprain of right coracohumeral (ligament)

    √7th **S43.412** Sprain of left coracohumeral (ligament)

    √7th **S43.419** Sprain of unspecified coracohumeral (ligament)

  √6th **S43.42** **Sprain of** rotator cuff capsule

    EXCLUDES 1 rotator cuff syndrome (complete) (incomplete), not specified as traumatic (M75.1-)

    EXCLUDES 2 injury of tendon of rotator cuff (S46.0-)

    √7th **S43.421** Sprain of right rotator cuff capsule

    √7th **S43.422** Sprain of left rotator cuff capsule

    √7th **S43.429** Sprain of unspecified rotator cuff capsule

√6th **S43.43** Superior glenoid labrum **lesion**

    SLAP lesion

    √7th **S43.431** Superior glenoid labrum lesion of right **shoulder**

    √7th **S43.432** Superior glenoid labrum lesion of left **shoulder**

    √7th **S43.439** Superior glenoid labrum lesion of **unspecified shoulder**

  √6th **S43.49** Other **sprain of shoulder joint**

    √7th **S43.491** Other sprain of right shoulder joint

    √7th **S43.492** Other sprain of left shoulder joint

    √7th **S43.499** Other sprain of unspecified shoulder joint

√5th **S43.5** **Sprain of** acromioclavicular **joint**

    Sprain of acromioclavicular ligament

  √x7th **S43.50** **Sprain of unspecified acromioclavicular joint**

  √x7th **S43.51** **Sprain of** right **acromioclavicular joint**

  √x7th **S43.52** **Sprain of** left **acromioclavicular joint**

√5th **S43.6** **Sprain of** sternoclavicular **joint**

  √x7th **S43.60** **Sprain of unspecified sternoclavicular joint**

  √x7th **S43.61** **Sprain of** right **sternoclavicular joint**

  √x7th **S43.62** **Sprain of** left **sternoclavicular joint**

√5th **S43.8** **Sprain of** other **specified parts of shoulder girdle**

  √x7th **S43.80** **Sprain of other specified parts of unspecified shoulder girdle**

  √x7th **S43.81** **Sprain of other specified parts of** right **shoulder girdle**

  √x7th **S43.82** **Sprain of other specified parts of** left **shoulder girdle**

√5th **S43.9** **Sprain of** unspecified **parts of shoulder girdle**

  √x7th **S43.90** **Sprain of unspecified parts of unspecified shoulder girdle**

    Sprain of shoulder girdle NOS

  √x7th **S43.91** **Sprain of unspecified parts of** right **shoulder girdle**

  √x7th **S43.92** **Sprain of unspecified parts of** left **shoulder girdle**

√4th **S44** **Injury of nerves at shoulder and upper arm level**

  Code also any associated open wound (S41.-)

  EXCLUDES 2 injury of brachial plexus (S14.3-)

  The appropriate 7th character is to be added to each code from category S44.
  A   initial encounter
  D   subsequent encounter
  S   sequela

√5th **S44.0** **Injury of** ulnar nerve **at upper arm level**

    EXCLUDES 1 ulnar nerve NOS (S54.0)

  √x7th **S44.00** **Injury of ulnar nerve at upper arm level, unspecified arm**

  √x7th **S44.01** **Injury of ulnar nerve at upper arm level,** right **arm**

  √x7th **S44.02** **Injury of ulnar nerve at upper arm level,** left **arm**

√5th **S44.1** **Injury of** median nerve **at upper arm level**

    EXCLUDES 1 median nerve NOS (S54.1)

  √x7th **S44.10** **Injury of median nerve at upper arm level, unspecified arm**

  √x7th **S44.11** **Injury of median nerve at upper arm level,** right **arm**

  √x7th **S44.12** **Injury of median nerve at upper arm level,** left **arm**

√5th **S44.2** **Injury of** radial nerve **at upper arm level**

    EXCLUDES 1 radial nerve NOS (S54.2)

  √x7th **S44.20** **Injury of radial nerve at upper arm level, unspecified arm**

  √x7th **S44.21** **Injury of radial nerve at upper arm level,** right **arm**

  √x7th **S44.22** **Injury of radial nerve at upper arm level,** left **arm**

√5th **S44.3** **Injury of** axillary nerve

  √x7th **S44.30** **Injury of axillary nerve, unspecified arm**

  √x7th **S44.31** **Injury of axillary nerve,** right **arm**

  √x7th **S44.32** **Injury of axillary nerve,** left **arm**

√5th **S44.4** **Injury of** musculocutaneous nerve

  √x7th **S44.40** **Injury of musculocutaneous nerve, unspecified arm**

  √x7th **S44.41** **Injury of musculocutaneous nerve,** right **arm**

  √x7th **S44.42** **Injury of musculocutaneous nerve,** left **arm**

✔ Additional Character Required   √x7th Xtension Alert   Unspecified Dx   Other Specified Dx   Manifestation   ►◄ Revised Text   ● New Code   ▲ Revised Code Title

ICD-10-CM Draft (2015)   **847**

Injury, Poisoning and Certain Other Consequences of External Causes

S44.5–S45.891

✓5ᵗʰ **S44.5** **Injury of** cutaneous sensory nerve **at shoulder and upper arm level**

     ✓x7ᵗʰ **S44.50** **Injury of cutaneous sensory nerve at shoulder and upper arm level, unspecified arm**

     ✓x7ᵗʰ **S44.51** **Injury of cutaneous sensory nerve at shoulder and upper arm level,** right **arm**

     ✓x7ᵗʰ **S44.52** **Injury of cutaneous sensory nerve at shoulder and upper arm level,** left **arm**

✓5ᵗʰ **S44.8** **Injury of other nerves at shoulder and upper arm level**

     ✓6ᵗʰ **S44.8X** **Injury of** other nerves **at shoulder and upper arm level**

         ✓7ᵗʰ **S44.8X1** **Injury of other nerves at shoulder and upper arm level,** right **arm**

         ✓7ᵗʰ **S44.8X2** **Injury of other nerves at shoulder and upper arm level,** left **arm**

         ✓7ᵗʰ **S44.8X9** **Injury of other nerves at shoulder and upper arm level, unspecified arm**

✓5ᵗʰ **S44.9** **Injury of** unspecified **nerve at shoulder and upper arm level**

     ✓x7ᵗʰ **S44.90** **Injury of unspecified nerve at shoulder and upper arm level, unspecified arm**

     ✓x7ᵗʰ **S44.91** **Injury of unspecified nerve at shoulder and upper arm level,** right **arm**

     ✓x7ᵗʰ **S44.92** **Injury of unspecified nerve at shoulder and upper arm level,** left **arm**

✓4ᵗʰ **S45** **Injury of blood vessels at shoulder and upper arm level**

     Code also any associated open wound (S41.-)

     EXCLUDES 2   injury of subclavian artery (S25.1)
                    injury of subclavian vein (S25.3)

     The appropriate 7th character is to be added to each code from category S45.
     A   initial encounter
     D   subsequent encounter
     S   sequela

     ✓5ᵗʰ **S45.0** **Injury of** axillary artery

         ✓6ᵗʰ **S45.00** **Unspecified injury of axillary artery**

             ✓7ᵗʰ **S45.001** **Unspecified injury of axillary artery,** right **side**

             ✓7ᵗʰ **S45.002** **Unspecified injury of axillary artery,** left **side**

             ✓7ᵗʰ **S45.009** **Unspecified injury of axillary artery, unspecified side**

         ✓6ᵗʰ **S45.01** **Laceration of axillary artery**

             ✓7ᵗʰ **S45.011** **Laceration of axillary artery,** right **side**

             ✓7ᵗʰ **S45.012** **Laceration of axillary artery,** left **side**

             ✓7ᵗʰ **S45.019** **Laceration of axillary artery, unspecified side**

         ✓6ᵗʰ **S45.09** **Other** specified injury of axillary artery

             ✓7ᵗʰ **S45.091** **Other specified injury of axillary artery,** right **side**

             ✓7ᵗʰ **S45.092** **Other specified injury of axillary artery,** left **side**

             ✓7ᵗʰ **S45.099** **Other specified injury of axillary artery, unspecified side**

     ✓5ᵗʰ **S45.1** **Injury of** brachial artery

         ✓6ᵗʰ **S45.10** **Unspecified injury of brachial artery**

             ✓7ᵗʰ **S45.101** **Unspecified injury of brachial artery,** right **side**

             ✓7ᵗʰ **S45.102** **Unspecified injury of brachial artery,** left **side**

             ✓7ᵗʰ **S45.109** **Unspecified injury of brachial artery, unspecified side**

         ✓6ᵗʰ **S45.11** **Laceration of brachial artery**

             ✓7ᵗʰ **S45.111** **Laceration of brachial artery,** right **side**

             ✓7ᵗʰ **S45.112** **Laceration of brachial artery,** left **side**

             ✓7ᵗʰ **S45.119** **Laceration of brachial artery, unspecified side**

         ✓6ᵗʰ **S45.19** **Other** specified injury of brachial artery

             ✓7ᵗʰ **S45.191** **Other specified injury of brachial artery,** right **side**

             ✓7ᵗʰ **S45.192** **Other specified injury of brachial artery,** left **side**

             ✓7ᵗʰ **S45.199** **Other specified injury of brachial artery, unspecified side**

✓5ᵗʰ **S45.2** **Injury of** axillary or brachial vein

     ✓6ᵗʰ **S45.20** **Unspecified** injury of axillary or brachial vein

         ✓7ᵗʰ **S45.201** **Unspecified injury of axillary or brachial vein,** right **side**

         ✓7ᵗʰ **S45.202** **Unspecified injury of axillary or brachial vein,** left **side**

         ✓7ᵗʰ **S45.209** **Unspecified injury of axillary or brachial vein, unspecified side**

     ✓6ᵗʰ **S45.21** **Laceration** of axillary or brachial vein

         ✓7ᵗʰ **S45.211** **Laceration of axillary or brachial vein,** right **side**

         ✓7ᵗʰ **S45.212** **Laceration of axillary or brachial vein,** left **side**

         ✓7ᵗʰ **S45.219** **Laceration of axillary or brachial vein, unspecified side**

     ✓6ᵗʰ **S45.29** **Other** specified injury of axillary or brachial vein

         ✓7ᵗʰ **S45.291** **Other specified injury of axillary or brachial vein,** right **side**

         ✓7ᵗʰ **S45.292** **Other specified injury of axillary or brachial vein,** left **side**

         ✓7ᵗʰ **S45.299** **Other specified injury of axillary or brachial vein, unspecified side**

✓5ᵗʰ **S45.3** **Injury of** superficial vein **at shoulder and upper arm level**

     ✓6ᵗʰ **S45.30** **Unspecified** injury of superficial vein at shoulder and upper arm level

         ✓7ᵗʰ **S45.301** **Unspecified injury of superficial vein at shoulder and upper arm level,** right **arm**

         ✓7ᵗʰ **S45.302** **Unspecified injury of superficial vein at shoulder and upper arm level,** left **arm**

         ✓7ᵗʰ **S45.309** **Unspecified injury of superficial vein at shoulder and upper arm level, unspecified arm**

     ✓6ᵗʰ **S45.31** **Laceration** of superficial vein at shoulder and upper arm level

         ✓7ᵗʰ **S45.311** **Laceration of superficial vein at shoulder and upper arm level,** right **arm**

         ✓7ᵗʰ **S45.312** **Laceration of superficial vein at shoulder and upper arm level,** left **arm**

         ✓7ᵗʰ **S45.319** **Laceration of superficial vein at shoulder and upper arm level, unspecified arm**

     ✓6ᵗʰ **S45.39** **Other** specified injury of superficial vein at shoulder and upper arm level

         ✓7ᵗʰ **S45.391** **Other specified injury of superficial vein at shoulder and upper arm level,** right **arm**

         ✓7ᵗʰ **S45.392** **Other specified injury of superficial vein at shoulder and upper arm level,** left **arm**

         ✓7ᵗʰ **S45.399** **Other specified injury of superficial vein at shoulder and upper arm level, unspecified arm**

✓5ᵗʰ **S45.8** **Injury of** other specified blood vessels **at shoulder and upper arm level**

     ✓6ᵗʰ **S45.80** **Unspecified** injury of other specified blood vessels at shoulder and upper arm level

         ✓7ᵗʰ **S45.801** **Unspecified injury of other specified blood vessels at shoulder and upper arm level,** right **arm**

         ✓7ᵗʰ **S45.802** **Unspecified injury of other specified blood vessels at shoulder and upper arm level,** left **arm**

         ✓7ᵗʰ **S45.809** **Unspecified injury of other specified blood vessels at shoulder and upper arm level, unspecified arm**

     ✓6ᵗʰ **S45.81** **Laceration** of other specified blood vessels at shoulder and upper arm level

         ✓7ᵗʰ **S45.811** **Laceration of other specified blood vessels at shoulder and upper arm level,** right **arm**

         ✓7ᵗʰ **S45.812** **Laceration of other specified blood vessels at shoulder and upper arm level,** left **arm**

         ✓7ᵗʰ **S45.819** **Laceration of other specified blood vessels at shoulder and upper arm level, unspecified arm**

     ✓6ᵗʰ **S45.89** **Other** specified injury of other specified blood vessels at shoulder and upper arm level

         ✓7ᵗʰ **S45.891** **Other specified injury of other specified blood vessels at shoulder and upper arm level,** right **arm**

EXCLUDES 1 Not coded here   EXCLUDES 2 Not included here   N Newborn Age: 0   P Pediatric Age: 0-17   M Maternity Age: 12-55   A Adult Age: 15-124

√7ᵗʰ **S45.892** Other specified injury of other specified blood vessels at shoulder and upper arm level, left arm

√7ᵗʰ **S45.899** Other specified injury of other specified blood vessels at shoulder and upper arm level, unspecified arm

√5ᵗʰ **S45.9** Injury of unspecified blood vessel at shoulder and upper arm level

√6ᵗʰ **S45.90** Unspecified injury of unspecified blood vessel at shoulder and upper arm level

√7ᵗʰ **S45.901** Unspecified injury of unspecified blood vessel at shoulder and upper arm level, right arm

√7ᵗʰ **S45.902** Unspecified injury of unspecified blood vessel at shoulder and upper arm level, left arm

√7ᵗʰ **S45.909** Unspecified injury of unspecified blood vessel at shoulder and upper arm level, unspecified arm

√6ᵗʰ **S45.91** Laceration of unspecified blood vessel at shoulder and upper arm level

√7ᵗʰ **S45.911** Laceration of unspecified blood vessel at shoulder and upper arm level, right arm

√7ᵗʰ **S45.912** Laceration of unspecified blood vessel at shoulder and upper arm level, left arm

√7ᵗʰ **S45.919** Laceration of unspecified blood vessel at shoulder and upper arm level, unspecified arm

√6ᵗʰ **S45.99** Other specified injury of unspecified blood vessel at shoulder and upper arm level

√7ᵗʰ **S45.991** Other specified injury of unspecified blood vessel at shoulder and upper arm level, right arm

√7ᵗʰ **S45.992** Other specified injury of unspecified blood vessel at shoulder and upper arm level, left arm

√7ᵗʰ **S45.999** Other specified injury of unspecified blood vessel at shoulder and upper arm level, unspecified arm

√4ᵗʰ **S46** Injury of muscle, fascia and tendon at shoulder and upper arm level

Code also any associated open wound (S41.-)

EXCLUDES 2   injury of muscle, fascia and tendon at elbow (S56.-)
sprain of joints and ligaments of shoulder girdle (S43.9)

The appropriate 7th character is to be added to each code from category S46.
A   initial encounter
D   subsequent encounter
S   sequela

√5ᵗʰ **S46.0** Injury of muscle(s) and tendon(s) of the rotator cuff of shoulder

√6ᵗʰ **S46.00** Unspecified injury of muscle(s) and tendon(s) of the rotator cuff of shoulder

√7ᵗʰ **S46.001** Unspecified injury of muscle(s) and tendon(s) of the rotator cuff of right shoulder

√7ᵗʰ **S46.002** Unspecified injury of muscle(s) and tendon(s) of the rotator cuff of left shoulder

√7ᵗʰ **S46.009** Unspecified injury of muscle(s) and tendon(s) of the rotator cuff of unspecified shoulder

√6ᵗʰ **S46.01** Strain of muscle(s) and tendon(s) of the rotator cuff of shoulder

√7ᵗʰ **S46.011** Strain of muscle(s) and tendon(s) of the rotator cuff of right shoulder

√7ᵗʰ **S46.012** Strain of muscle(s) and tendon(s) of the rotator cuff of left shoulder

√7ᵗʰ **S46.019** Strain of muscle(s) and tendon(s) of the rotator cuff of unspecified shoulder

√6ᵗʰ **S46.02** Laceration of muscle(s) and tendon(s) of the rotator cuff of shoulder

√7ᵗʰ **S46.021** Laceration of muscle(s) and tendon(s) of the rotator cuff of right shoulder

√7ᵗʰ **S46.022** Laceration of muscle(s) and tendon(s) of the rotator cuff of left shoulder

√7ᵗʰ **S46.029** Laceration of muscle(s) and tendon(s) of the rotator cuff of unspecified shoulder

√6ᵗʰ **S46.09** Other injury of muscle(s) and tendon(s) of the rotator cuff of shoulder

√7ᵗʰ **S46.091** Other injury of muscle(s) and tendon(s) of the rotator cuff of right shoulder

√7ᵗʰ **S46.092** Other injury of muscle(s) and tendon(s) of the rotator cuff of left shoulder

√7ᵗʰ **S46.099** Other injury of muscle(s) and tendon(s) of the rotator cuff of unspecified shoulder

√5ᵗʰ **S46.1** Injury of muscle, fascia and tendon of long head of biceps

√6ᵗʰ **S46.10** Unspecified injury of muscle, fascia and tendon of long head of biceps

√7ᵗʰ **S46.101** Unspecified injury of muscle, fascia and tendon of long head of biceps, right arm

√7ᵗʰ **S46.102** Unspecified injury of muscle, fascia and tendon of long head of biceps, left arm

√7ᵗʰ **S46.109** Unspecified injury of muscle, fascia and tendon of long head of biceps, unspecified arm

√6ᵗʰ **S46.11** Strain of muscle, fascia and tendon of long head of biceps

√7ᵗʰ **S46.111** Strain of muscle, fascia and tendon of long head of biceps, right arm

√7ᵗʰ **S46.112** Strain of muscle, fascia and tendon of long head of biceps, left arm

√7ᵗʰ **S46.119** Strain of muscle, fascia and tendon of long head of biceps, unspecified arm

√6ᵗʰ **S46.12** Laceration of muscle, fascia and tendon of long head of biceps

√7ᵗʰ **S46.121** Laceration of muscle, fascia and tendon of long head of biceps, right arm

√7ᵗʰ **S46.122** Laceration of muscle, fascia and tendon of long head of biceps, left arm

√7ᵗʰ **S46.129** Laceration of muscle, fascia and tendon of long head of biceps, unspecified arm

√6ᵗʰ **S46.19** Other injury of muscle, fascia and tendon of long head of biceps

√7ᵗʰ **S46.191** Other injury of muscle, fascia and tendon of long head of biceps, right arm

√7ᵗʰ **S46.192** Other injury of muscle, fascia and tendon of long head of biceps, left arm

√7ᵗʰ **S46.199** Other injury of muscle, fascia and tendon of long head of biceps, unspecified arm

√5ᵗʰ **S46.2** Injury of muscle, fascia and tendon of other parts of biceps

√6ᵗʰ **S46.20** Unspecified injury of muscle, fascia and tendon of other parts of biceps

√7ᵗʰ **S46.201** Unspecified injury of muscle, fascia and tendon of other parts of biceps, right arm

√7ᵗʰ **S46.202** Unspecified injury of muscle, fascia and tendon of other parts of biceps, left arm

√7ᵗʰ **S46.209** Unspecified injury of muscle, fascia and tendon of other parts of biceps, unspecified arm

√6ᵗʰ **S46.21** Strain of muscle, fascia and tendon of other parts of biceps

√7ᵗʰ **S46.211** Strain of muscle, fascia and tendon of other parts of biceps, right arm

√7ᵗʰ **S46.212** Strain of muscle, fascia and tendon of other parts of biceps, left arm

√7ᵗʰ **S46.219** Strain of muscle, fascia and tendon of other parts of biceps, unspecified arm

√6ᵗʰ **S46.22** Laceration of muscle, fascia and tendon of other parts of biceps

√7ᵗʰ **S46.221** Laceration of muscle, fascia and tendon of other parts of biceps, right arm

√7ᵗʰ **S46.222** Laceration of muscle, fascia and tendon of other parts of biceps, left arm

√7ᵗʰ **S46.229** Laceration of muscle, fascia and tendon of other parts of biceps, unspecified arm

√6ᵗʰ **S46.29** Other injury of muscle, fascia and tendon of other parts of biceps

√7ᵗʰ **S46.291** Other injury of muscle, fascia and tendon of other parts of biceps, right arm

☑ Additional Character Required   √x7ᵗʰ Xtension Alert   Unspecified Dx   Other Specified Dx   Manifestation   ►◄ Revised Text   ● New Code   ▲ Revised Code Title

ICD-10-CM Draft (2015)   849

✓7ᵗʰ **S46.292** Other injury of muscle, fascia and tendon of other parts of biceps, left arm

✓7ᵗʰ **S46.299** Other injury of muscle, fascia and tendon of other parts of biceps, unspecified arm

✓5ᵗʰ **S46.3** Injury of muscle, fascia and tendon of triceps

  ✓6ᵗʰ **S46.30** Unspecified injury of muscle, fascia and tendon of triceps

    ✓7ᵗʰ **S46.301** Unspecified injury of muscle, fascia and tendon of triceps, right arm

    ✓7ᵗʰ **S46.302** Unspecified injury of muscle, fascia and tendon of triceps, left arm

    ✓7ᵗʰ **S46.309** Unspecified injury of muscle, fascia and tendon of triceps, unspecified arm

  ✓6ᵗʰ **S46.31** Strain of muscle, fascia and tendon of triceps

    ✓7ᵗʰ **S46.311** Strain of muscle, fascia and tendon of triceps, right arm

    ✓7ᵗʰ **S46.312** Strain of muscle, fascia and tendon of triceps, left arm

    ✓7ᵗʰ **S46.319** Strain of muscle, fascia and tendon of triceps, unspecified arm

  ✓6ᵗʰ **S46.32** Laceration of muscle, fascia and tendon of triceps

    ✓7ᵗʰ **S46.321** Laceration of muscle, fascia and tendon of triceps, right arm

    ✓7ᵗʰ **S46.322** Laceration of muscle, fascia and tendon of triceps, left arm

    ✓7ᵗʰ **S46.329** Laceration of muscle, fascia and tendon of triceps, unspecified arm

  ✓6ᵗʰ **S46.39** Other injury of muscle, fascia and tendon of triceps

    ✓7ᵗʰ **S46.391** Other injury of muscle, fascia and tendon of triceps, right arm

    ✓7ᵗʰ **S46.392** Other injury of muscle, fascia and tendon of triceps, left arm

    ✓7ᵗʰ **S46.399** Other injury of muscle, fascia and tendon of triceps, unspecified arm

✓5ᵗʰ **S46.8** Injury of other muscles, fascia and tendons at shoulder and upper arm level

  ✓6ᵗʰ **S46.80** Unspecified injury of other muscles, fascia and tendons at shoulder and upper arm level

    ✓7ᵗʰ **S46.801** Unspecified injury of other muscles, fascia and tendons at shoulder and upper arm level, right arm

    ✓7ᵗʰ **S46.802** Unspecified injury of other muscles, fascia and tendons at shoulder and upper arm level, left arm

    ✓7ᵗʰ **S46.809** Unspecified injury of other muscles, fascia and tendons at shoulder and upper arm level, unspecified arm

  ✓6ᵗʰ **S46.81** Strain of other muscles, fascia and tendons at shoulder and upper arm level

    ✓7ᵗʰ **S46.811** Strain of other muscles, fascia and tendons at shoulder and upper arm level, right arm

    ✓7ᵗʰ **S46.812** Strain of other muscles, fascia and tendons at shoulder and upper arm level, left arm

    ✓7ᵗʰ **S46.819** Strain of other muscles, fascia and tendons at shoulder and upper arm level, unspecified arm

  ✓6ᵗʰ **S46.82** Laceration of other muscles, fascia and tendons at shoulder and upper arm level

    ✓7ᵗʰ **S46.821** Laceration of other muscles, fascia and tendons at shoulder and upper arm level, right arm

    ✓7ᵗʰ **S46.822** Laceration of other muscles, fascia and tendons at shoulder and upper arm level, left arm

    ✓7ᵗʰ **S46.829** Laceration of other muscles, fascia and tendons at shoulder and upper arm level, unspecified arm

  ✓6ᵗʰ **S46.89** Other injury of other muscles, fascia and tendons at shoulder and upper arm level

    ✓7ᵗʰ **S46.891** Other injury of other muscles, fascia and tendons at shoulder and upper arm level, right arm

✓7ᵗʰ **S46.892** Other injury of other muscles, fascia and tendons at shoulder and upper arm level, left arm

✓7ᵗʰ **S46.899** Other injury of other muscles, fascia and tendons at shoulder and upper arm level, unspecified arm

✓5ᵗʰ **S46.9** Injury of unspecified muscle, fascia and tendon at shoulder and upper arm level

  ✓6ᵗʰ **S46.90** Unspecified injury of unspecified muscle, fascia and tendon at shoulder and upper arm level

    ✓7ᵗʰ **S46.901** Unspecified injury of unspecified muscle, fascia and tendon at shoulder and upper arm level, right arm

    ✓7ᵗʰ **S46.902** Unspecified injury of unspecified muscle, fascia and tendon at shoulder and upper arm level, left arm

    ✓7ᵗʰ **S46.909** Unspecified injury of unspecified muscle, fascia and tendon at shoulder and upper arm level, unspecified arm

  ✓6ᵗʰ **S46.91** Strain of unspecified muscle, fascia and tendon at shoulder and upper arm level

    ✓7ᵗʰ **S46.911** Strain of unspecified muscle, fascia and tendon at shoulder and upper arm level, right arm

    ✓7ᵗʰ **S46.912** Strain of unspecified muscle, fascia and tendon at shoulder and upper arm level, left arm

    ✓7ᵗʰ **S46.919** Strain of unspecified muscle, fascia and tendon at shoulder and upper arm level, unspecified arm

  ✓6ᵗʰ **S46.92** Laceration of unspecified muscle, fascia and tendon at shoulder and upper arm level

    ✓7ᵗʰ **S46.921** Laceration of unspecified muscle, fascia and tendon at shoulder and upper arm level, right arm

    ✓7ᵗʰ **S46.922** Laceration of unspecified muscle, fascia and tendon at shoulder and upper arm level, left arm

    ✓7ᵗʰ **S46.929** Laceration of unspecified muscle, fascia and tendon at shoulder and upper arm level, unspecified arm

  ✓6ᵗʰ **S46.99** Other injury of unspecified muscle, fascia and tendon at shoulder and upper arm level

    ✓7ᵗʰ **S46.991** Other injury of unspecified muscle, fascia and tendon at shoulder and upper arm level, right arm

    ✓7ᵗʰ **S46.992** Other injury of unspecified muscle, fascia and tendon at shoulder and upper arm level, left arm

    ✓7ᵗʰ **S46.999** Other injury of unspecified muscle, fascia and tendon at shoulder and upper arm level, unspecified arm

✓4ᵗʰ **S47** **Crushing injury** of shoulder and upper arm

  Use additional code for all associated injuries

  EXCLUDES 2 crushing injury of elbow (S57.0-)

  The appropriate 7th character is to be added to each code from category S47.
  A   initial encounter
  D   subsequent encounter
  S   sequela

  ✓x7ᵗʰ **S47.1** Crushing injury of right shoulder and upper arm

  ✓x7ᵗʰ **S47.2** Crushing injury of left shoulder and upper arm

  ✓x7ᵗʰ **S47.9** Crushing injury of shoulder and upper arm, unspecified arm

✓4ᵗʰ **S48** **Traumatic amputation of shoulder and upper arm**

  NOTE An amputation not identified as partial or complete should be coded to complete.

  EXCLUDES 1 traumatic amputation at elbow level (S58.0)

  The appropriate 7th character is to be added to each code from category S48.
  A   initial encounter
  D   subsequent encounter
  S   sequela

  ✓5ᵗʰ **S48.0** Traumatic amputation at shoulder joint

    ✓6ᵗʰ **S48.01** Complete traumatic amputation at shoulder joint

      ✓7ᵗʰ **S48.011** Complete traumatic amputation at right shoulder joint

---

EXCLUDES 1 Not coded here   **EXCLUDES 2** Not included here   **N** Newborn Age: 0   **P** Pediatric Age: 0-17   **M** Maternity Age: 12-55   **A** Adult Age: 15-124

850   ICD-10-CM Draft (2015)

√7ᵗʰ **S48.012** Complete traumatic amputation at left shoulder joint

√7ᵗʰ **S48.019** Complete traumatic amputation at unspecified shoulder joint

√6ᵗʰ **S48.02** Partial traumatic amputation at shoulder joint

√7ᵗʰ **S48.021** Partial traumatic amputation at right shoulder joint

√7ᵗʰ **S48.022** Partial traumatic amputation at left shoulder joint

√7ᵗʰ **S48.029** Partial traumatic amputation at unspecified shoulder joint

√5ᵗʰ **S48.1** Traumatic amputation at level between shoulder and elbow

√6ᵗʰ **S48.11** Complete traumatic amputation at level between shoulder and elbow

√7ᵗʰ **S48.111** Complete traumatic amputation at level between right shoulder and elbow

√7ᵗʰ **S48.112** Complete traumatic amputation at level between left shoulder and elbow

√7ᵗʰ **S48.119** Complete traumatic amputation at level between unspecified shoulder and elbow

√6ᵗʰ **S48.12** Partial traumatic amputation at level between shoulder and elbow

√7ᵗʰ **S48.121** Partial traumatic amputation at level between right shoulder and elbow

√7ᵗʰ **S48.122** Partial traumatic amputation at level between left shoulder and elbow

√7ᵗʰ **S48.129** Partial traumatic amputation at level between unspecified shoulder and elbow

√5ᵗʰ **S48.9** Traumatic amputation of shoulder and upper arm, level unspecified

√6ᵗʰ **S48.91** Complete traumatic amputation of shoulder and upper arm, level unspecified

√7ᵗʰ **S48.911** Complete traumatic amputation of right shoulder and upper arm, level unspecified

√7ᵗʰ **S48.912** Complete traumatic amputation of left shoulder and upper arm, level unspecified

√7ᵗʰ **S48.919** Complete traumatic amputation of unspecified shoulder and upper arm, level unspecified

√6ᵗʰ **S48.92** Partial traumatic amputation of shoulder and upper arm, level unspecified

√7ᵗʰ **S48.921** Partial traumatic amputation of right shoulder and upper arm, level unspecified

√7ᵗʰ **S48.922** Partial traumatic amputation of left shoulder and upper arm, level unspecified

√7ᵗʰ **S48.929** Partial traumatic amputation of unspecified shoulder and upper arm, level unspecified

√4ᵗʰ **S49** Other and unspecified injuries of shoulder and upper arm

The appropriate 7th character is to be added to each code from subcategories S49.0 and S49.1.
A   initial encounter for closed fracture
D   subsequent encounter for fracture with routine healing
G   subsequent encounter for fracture with delayed healing
K   subsequent encounter for fracture with nonunion
P   subsequent encounter for fracture with malunion
S   sequela

√5ᵗʰ **S49.0** Physeal fracture of upper end of humerus

√6ᵗʰ **S49.00** Unspecified physeal fracture of upper end of humerus

√7ᵗʰ **S49.001** Unspecified physeal fracture of upper end of humerus, right arm

√7ᵗʰ **S49.002** Unspecified physeal fracture of upper end of humerus, left arm

√7ᵗʰ **S49.009** Unspecified physeal fracture of upper end of humerus, unspecified arm

√6ᵗʰ **S49.01** Salter-Harris Type I physeal fracture of upper end of humerus

√7ᵗʰ **S49.011** Salter-Harris Type I physeal fracture of upper end of humerus, right arm

√7ᵗʰ **S49.012** Salter-Harris Type I physeal fracture of upper end of humerus, left arm

√7ᵗʰ **S49.019** Salter-Harris Type I physeal fracture of upper end of humerus, unspecified arm

√6ᵗʰ **S49.02** Salter-Harris Type II physeal fracture of upper end of humerus

√7ᵗʰ **S49.021** Salter-Harris Type II physeal fracture of upper end of humerus, right arm

√7ᵗʰ **S49.022** Salter-Harris Type II physeal fracture of upper end of humerus, left arm

√7ᵗʰ **S49.029** Salter-Harris Type II physeal fracture of upper end of humerus, unspecified arm

√6ᵗʰ **S49.03** Salter-Harris Type III physeal fracture of upper end of humerus

√7ᵗʰ **S49.031** Salter Harris Type III physeal fracture of upper end of humerus, right arm

√7ᵗʰ **S49.032** Salter Harris Type III physeal fracture of upper end of humerus, left arm

√7ᵗʰ **S49.039** Salter Harris Type III physeal fracture of upper end of humerus, unspecified arm

√6ᵗʰ **S49.04** Salter-Harris Type IV physeal fracture of upper end of humerus

√7ᵗʰ **S49.041** Salter-Harris Type IV physeal fracture of upper end of humerus, right arm

√7ᵗʰ **S49.042** Salter-Harris Type IV physeal fracture of upper end of humerus, left arm

√7ᵗʰ **S49.049** Salter-Harris Type IV physeal fracture of upper end of humerus, unspecified arm

√6ᵗʰ **S49.09** Other physeal fracture of upper end of humerus

√7ᵗʰ **S49.091** Other physeal fracture of upper end of humerus, right arm

√7ᵗʰ **S49.092** Other physeal fracture of upper end of humerus, left arm

√7ᵗʰ **S49.099** Other physeal fracture of upper end of humerus, unspecified arm

√5ᵗʰ **S49.1** Physeal fracture of lower end of humerus

√6ᵗʰ **S49.10** Unspecified physeal fracture of lower end of humerus

√7ᵗʰ **S49.101** Unspecified physeal fracture of lower end of humerus, right arm

√7ᵗʰ **S49.102** Unspecified physeal fracture of lower end of humerus, left arm

√7ᵗʰ **S49.109** Unspecified physeal fracture of lower end of humerus, unspecified arm

√6ᵗʰ **S49.11** Salter-Harris Type I physeal fracture of lower end of humerus

√7ᵗʰ **S49.111** Salter-Harris Type I physeal fracture of lower end of humerus, right arm

√7ᵗʰ **S49.112** Salter-Harris Type I physeal fracture of lower end of humerus, left arm

√7ᵗʰ **S49.119** Salter-Harris Type I physeal fracture of lower end of humerus, unspecified arm

√6ᵗʰ **S49.12** Salter-Harris Type II physeal fracture of lower end of humerus

√7ᵗʰ **S49.121** Salter-Harris Type II physeal fracture of lower end of humerus, right arm

√7ᵗʰ **S49.122** Salter-Harris Type II physeal fracture of lower end of humerus, left arm

√7ᵗʰ **S49.129** Salter-Harris Type II physeal fracture of lower end of humerus, unspecified arm

√6ᵗʰ **S49.13** Salter Harris Type III physeal fracture of lower end of humerus

√7ᵗʰ **S49.131** Salter Harris Type III physeal fracture of lower end of humerus, right arm

√7ᵗʰ **S49.132** Salter Harris Type III physeal fracture of lower end of humerus, left arm

√7ᵗʰ **S49.139** Salter Harris Type III physeal fracture of lower end of humerus, unspecified arm

√6ᵗʰ **S49.14** Salter-Harris Type IV physeal fracture of lower end of humerus

√7ᵗʰ **S49.141** Salter-Harris Type IV physeal fracture of lower end of humerus, right arm

√7ᵗʰ **S49.142** Salter-Harris Type IV physeal fracture of lower end of humerus, left arm

√7ᵗʰ **S49.149** Salter-Harris Type IV physeal fracture of lower end of humerus, unspecified arm

√6ᵗʰ **S49.19** Other physeal fracture of lower end of humerus

√7ᵗʰ **S49.191** Other physeal fracture of lower end of humerus, right arm

☑ Additional Character Required   √x7ᵗʰ Xtension Alert   Unspecified Dx   Other Specified Dx   Manifestation   ►◄ Revised Text   ● New Code   ▲ Revised Code Title

ICD-10-CM Draft (2015)   851

✓7th **S49.192** **Other physeal fracture of lower end of humerus, left arm**

✓7th **S49.199** **Other physeal fracture of lower end of humerus, unspecified arm**

✓5th **S49.8** **Other specified injuries of shoulder and upper arm**

The appropriate 7th character is to be added to each code in subcategory S49.8.
A   initial encounter
D   subsequent encounter
S   sequela

✓x7th **S49.80** **Other specified injuries of shoulder and upper arm, unspecified arm**

✓x7th **S49.81** **Other specified injuries of right shoulder and upper arm**

✓x7th **S49.82** **Other specified injuries of left shoulder and upper arm**

✓5th **S49.9** **Unspecified injury of shoulder and upper arm**

The appropriate 7th character is to be added to each code in subcategory S49.9.
A   initial encounter
D   subsequent encounter
S   sequela

✓x7th **S49.90** **Unspecified injury of shoulder and upper arm, unspecified arm**

✓x7th **S49.91** **Unspecified injury of right shoulder and upper arm**

✓x7th **S49.92** **Unspecified injury of left shoulder and upper arm**

Injuries to the elbow and forearm (S50-S59)

EXCLUDES 2   burns and corrosions (T20-T32)
frostbite (T33-T34)
injuries of wrist and hand (S60-S69)
insect bite or sting, venomous (T63.4)

✓4th **S50** **Superficial injury of elbow and forearm**

EXCLUDES 2   superficial injury of wrist and hand (S60.-)

The appropriate 7th character is to be added to each code from category S50.
A   initial encounter
D   subsequent encounter
S   sequela

✓5th **S50.0** **Contusion of elbow**

✓x7th **S50.00** **Contusion of unspecified elbow**

✓x7th **S50.01** **Contusion of right elbow**

✓x7th **S50.02** **Contusion of left elbow**

✓5th **S50.1** **Contusion of forearm**

✓x7th **S50.10** **Contusion of unspecified forearm**

✓x7th **S50.11** **Contusion of right forearm**

✓x7th **S50.12** **Contusion of left forearm**

✓5th **S50.3** **Other superficial injuries of elbow**

✓6th **S50.31** **Abrasion of elbow**

✓7th **S50.311** **Abrasion of right elbow**

✓7th **S50.312** **Abrasion of left elbow**

✓7th **S50.319** **Abrasion of unspecified elbow**

✓6th **S50.32** **Blister (nonthermal) of elbow**

✓7th **S50.321** **Blister (nonthermal) of right elbow**

✓7th **S50.322** **Blister (nonthermal) of left elbow**

✓7th **S50.329** **Blister (nonthermal) of unspecified elbow**

✓6th **S50.34** **External constriction of elbow**

✓7th **S50.341** **External constriction of right elbow**

✓7th **S50.342** **External constriction of left elbow**

✓7th **S50.349** **External constriction of unspecified elbow**

✓6th **S50.35** **Superficial foreign body of elbow**
Splinter in the elbow

✓7th **S50.351** **Superficial foreign body of right elbow**

✓7th **S50.352** **Superficial foreign body of left elbow**

✓7th **S50.359** **Superficial foreign body of unspecified elbow**

✓6th **S50.36** **Insect bite (nonvenomous) of elbow**

✓7th **S50.361** **Insect bite (nonvenomous) of right elbow**

✓7th **S50.362** **Insect bite (nonvenomous) of left elbow**

✓7th **S50.369** **Insect bite (nonvenomous) of unspecified elbow**

✓6th **S50.37** **Other superficial bite of elbow**

EXCLUDES 1   open bite of elbow (S51.05)

✓7th **S50.371** **Other superficial bite of right elbow**

✓7th **S50.372** **Other superficial bite of left elbow**

✓7th **S50.379** **Other superficial bite of unspecified elbow**

✓5th **S50.8** **Other superficial injuries of forearm**

✓6th **S50.81** **Abrasion of forearm**

✓7th **S50.811** **Abrasion of right forearm**

✓7th **S50.812** **Abrasion of left forearm**

✓7th **S50.819** **Abrasion of unspecified forearm**

✓6th **S50.82** **Blister (nonthermal) of forearm**

✓7th **S50.821** **Blister (nonthermal) of right forearm**

✓7th **S50.822** **Blister (nonthermal) of left forearm**

✓7th **S50.829** **Blister (nonthermal) of unspecified forearm**

✓6th **S50.84** **External constriction of forearm**

✓7th **S50.841** **External constriction of right forearm**

✓7th **S50.842** **External constriction of left forearm**

✓7th **S50.849** **External constriction of unspecified forearm**

✓6th **S50.85** **Superficial foreign body of forearm**
Splinter in the forearm

✓7th **S50.851** **Superficial foreign body of right forearm**

✓7th **S50.852** **Superficial foreign body of left forearm**

✓7th **S50.859** **Superficial foreign body of unspecified forearm**

✓6th **S50.86** **Insect bite (nonvenomous) of forearm**

✓7th **S50.861** **Insect bite (nonvenomous) of right forearm**

✓7th **S50.862** **Insect bite (nonvenomous) of left forearm**

✓7th **S50.869** **Insect bite (nonvenomous) of unspecified forearm**

✓6th **S50.87** **Other superficial bite of forearm**

EXCLUDES 1   open bite of forearm (S51.85)

✓7th **S50.871** **Other superficial bite of right forearm**

✓7th **S50.872** **Other superficial bite of left forearm**

✓7th **S50.879** **Other superficial bite of unspecified forearm**

✓5th **S50.9** **Unspecified superficial injury of elbow and forearm**

✓6th **S50.90** **Unspecified superficial injury of elbow**

✓7th **S50.901** **Unspecified superficial injury of right elbow**

✓7th **S50.902** **Unspecified superficial injury of left elbow**

✓7th **S50.909** **Unspecified superficial injury of unspecified elbow**

✓6th **S50.91** **Unspecified superficial injury of forearm**

✓7th **S50.911** **Unspecified superficial injury of right forearm**

✓7th **S50.912** **Unspecified superficial injury of left forearm**

✓7th **S50.919** **Unspecified superficial injury of unspecified forearm**

✓4th **S51** **Open wound of elbow and forearm**

Code also any associated wound infection

EXCLUDES 1   open fracture of elbow and forearm (S52- with open fracture 7th character)
traumatic amputation of elbow and forearm (S58.-)

EXCLUDES 2   open wound of wrist and hand (S61.-)

The appropriate 7th character is to be added to each code from category S51.
A   initial encounter
D   subsequent encounter
S   sequela

✓5th **S51.0** **Open wound of elbow**

✓6th **S51.00** **Unspecified open wound of elbow**

✓7th **S51.001** **Unspecified open wound of right elbow**
AHA: 2012, 4Q, 108

✓7th **S51.002** **Unspecified open wound of left elbow**

EXCLUDES 1 Not coded here   EXCLUDES 2 Not included here   N Newborn Age: 0   P Pediatric Age: 0-17   M Maternity Age: 12-55   A Adult Age: 15-124

852   ICD-10-CM Draft (2015)

√7ᵗʰ **S51.009** **Unspecified open wound of unspecified elbow**
Open wound of elbow NOS

√6ᵗʰ **S51.01** Laceration without foreign body of elbow

√7ᵗʰ **S51.011** **Laceration without foreign body of** right **elbow**

√7ᵗʰ **S51.012** **Laceration without foreign body of** left **elbow**

√7ᵗʰ **S51.019** **Laceration without foreign body of unspecified elbow**

√6ᵗʰ **S51.02** Laceration with foreign body of elbow

√7ᵗʰ **S51.021** **Laceration with foreign body of** right **elbow**

√7ᵗʰ **S51.022** **Laceration with foreign body of** left **elbow**

√7ᵗʰ **S51.029** **Laceration with foreign body of unspecified elbow**

√6ᵗʰ **S51.03** Puncture wound without foreign body of elbow

√7ᵗʰ **S51.031** **Puncture wound without foreign body of** right **elbow**

√7ᵗʰ **S51.032** **Puncture wound without foreign body of** left **elbow**

√7ᵗʰ **S51.039** **Puncture wound without foreign body of unspecified elbow**

√6ᵗʰ **S51.04** Puncture wound with foreign body of elbow

√7ᵗʰ **S51.041** **Puncture wound with foreign body of** right **elbow**

√7ᵗʰ **S51.042** **Puncture wound with foreign body of** left **elbow**

√7ᵗʰ **S51.049** **Puncture wound with foreign body of unspecified elbow**

√6ᵗʰ **S51.05** Open bite of elbow
Bite of elbow NOS
EXCLUDES 1 superficial bite of elbow (S50.36, S50.37)

√7ᵗʰ **S51.051** **Open bite,** right **elbow**

√7ᵗʰ **S51.052** **Open bite,** left **elbow**

√7ᵗʰ **S51.059** **Open bite, unspecified elbow**

√5ᵗʰ **S51.8** **Open wound of** forearm
EXCLUDES 2 open wound of elbow (S51.0-)

√6ᵗʰ **S51.80** Unspecified open wound of forearm

√7ᵗʰ **S51.801** **Unspecified open wound of** right **forearm**

√7ᵗʰ **S51.802** **Unspecified open wound of** left **forearm**

√7ᵗʰ **S51.809** **Unspecified open wound of unspecified forearm**
Open wound of forearm NOS

√6ᵗʰ **S51.81** Laceration without foreign body of forearm

√7ᵗʰ **S51.811** **Laceration without foreign body of** right **forearm**

√7ᵗʰ **S51.812** **Laceration without foreign body of** left **forearm**

√7ᵗʰ **S51.819** **Laceration without foreign body of unspecified forearm**

√6ᵗʰ **S51.82** Laceration with foreign body of forearm

√7ᵗʰ **S51.821** **Laceration with foreign body of** right **forearm**

√7ᵗʰ **S51.822** **Laceration with foreign body of** left **forearm**

√7ᵗʰ **S51.829** **Laceration with foreign body of unspecified forearm**

√6ᵗʰ **S51.83** Puncture wound without foreign body of forearm

√7ᵗʰ **S51.831** **Puncture wound without foreign body of** right **forearm**

√7ᵗʰ **S51.832** **Puncture wound without foreign body of** left **forearm**

√7ᵗʰ **S51.839** **Puncture wound without foreign body of unspecified forearm**

√6ᵗʰ **S51.84** Puncture wound with foreign body of forearm

√7ᵗʰ **S51.841** **Puncture wound with foreign body of** right **forearm**

√7ᵗʰ **S51.842** **Puncture wound with foreign body of** left **forearm**

√7ᵗʰ **S51.849** **Puncture wound with foreign body of unspecified forearm**

√6ᵗʰ **S51.85** Open bite of forearm
Bite of forearm NOS
EXCLUDES 1 superficial bite of forearm (S50.86, S50.87)

√7ᵗʰ **S51.851** **Open bite of** right **forearm**

√7ᵗʰ **S51.852** **Open bite of** left **forearm**

√7ᵗʰ **S51.859** **Open bite of unspecified forearm**

√4ᵗʰ **S52** **Fracture of forearm**
NOTE A fracture not indicated as displaced or nondisplaced should be coded to displaced.
A fracture not indicated as open or closed should be coded to closed.
The open fracture designations are based on the Gustilo open fracture classification.
EXCLUDES 1 traumatic amputation of forearm (S58.-)
EXCLUDES 2 fracture at wrist and hand level (S62.-)

The appropriate 7th character is to be added to all codes from category S52 [unless otherwise indicated].
A　initial encounter for closed fracture
B　initial encounter for open fracture type I or II
　　initial encounter for open fracture NOS
C　initial encounter for open fracture type IIIA, IIIB, or IIIC
D　subsequent encounter for closed fracture with routine healing
E　subsequent encounter for open fracture type I or II with routine healing
F　subsequent encounter for open fracture type IIIA, IIIB, or IIIC with routine healing
G　subsequent encounter for closed fracture with delayed healing
H　subsequent encounter for open fracture type I or II with delayed healing
J　subsequent encounter for open fracture type IIIA, IIIB, or IIIC with delayed healing
K　subsequent encounter for closed fracture with nonunion
M　subsequent encounter for open fracture type I or II with nonunion
N　subsequent encounter for open fracture type IIIA, IIIB, or IIIC with nonunion
P　subsequent encounter for closed fracture with malunion
Q　subsequent encounter for open fracture type I or II with malunion
R　subsequent encounter for open fracture type IIIA, IIIB, or IIIC with malunion
S　sequela

√5ᵗʰ **S52.0** **Fracture of** upper end of ulna
Fracture of proximal end of ulna
EXCLUDES 2 fracture of elbow NOS (S42.40-)
fractures of shaft of ulna (S52.2-)

√6ᵗʰ **S52.00** Unspecified fracture of upper end of ulna

√7ᵗʰ **S52.001** **Unspecified fracture of upper end of** right **ulna**

√7ᵗʰ **S52.002** **Unspecified fracture of upper end of** left **ulna**

√7ᵗʰ **S52.009** **Unspecified fracture of upper end of unspecified ulna**

√6ᵗʰ **S52.01** Torus fracture of upper end of ulna

The appropriate 7th character is to be added to all codes in subcategory S52.01.
A　initial encounter for closed fracture
D　subsequent encounter for fracture with routine healing
G　subsequent encounter for fracture with delayed healing
K　subsequent encounter for fracture with nonunion
P　subsequent encounter for fracture with malunion
S　sequela

√7ᵗʰ **S52.011** **Torus fracture of upper end of** right **ulna**

√7ᵗʰ **S52.012** **Torus fracture of upper end of** left **ulna**

√7ᵗʰ **S52.019** **Torus fracture of upper end of unspecified ulna**

√6ᵗʰ **S52.02** Fracture of olecranon process without intraarticular extension of ulna

√7ᵗʰ **S52.021** **Displaced fracture of olecranon process without intraarticular extension of** right **ulna**

☑ Additional Character Required　　√x7ᵗʰ *X*tension Alert　　Unspecified Dx　　Other Specified Dx　　Manifestation　　▶◀ Revised Text　　● New Code　　▲ Revised Code Title

ICD-10-CM Draft (2015)

853

S52.022–S52.232

Injury, Poisoning and Certain Other Consequences of External Causes

√7ᵗʰ **S52.022** Displaced fracture of olecranon process without intraarticular extension of left ulna

√7ᵗʰ **S52.023** Displaced fracture of olecranon process without intraarticular extension of unspecified ulna

√7ᵗʰ **S52.024** Nondisplaced fracture of olecranon process without intraarticular extension of right ulna

√7ᵗʰ **S52.025** Nondisplaced fracture of olecranon process without intraarticular extension of left ulna

√7ᵗʰ **S52.026** Nondisplaced fracture of olecranon process without intraarticular extension of unspecified ulna

√6ᵗʰ **S52.03** Fracture of olecranon process with intraarticular extension of ulna

√7ᵗʰ **S52.031** Displaced fracture of olecranon process with intraarticular extension of right ulna

√7ᵗʰ **S52.032** Displaced fracture of olecranon process with intraarticular extension of left ulna

√7ᵗʰ **S52.033** Displaced fracture of olecranon process with intraarticular extension of unspecified ulna

√7ᵗʰ **S52.034** Nondisplaced fracture of olecranon process with intraarticular extension of right ulna

√7ᵗʰ **S52.035** Nondisplaced fracture of olecranon process with intraarticular extension of left ulna

√7ᵗʰ **S52.036** Nondisplaced fracture of olecranon process with intraarticular extension of unspecified ulna

√6ᵗʰ **S52.04** Fracture of coronoid process of ulna

√7ᵗʰ **S52.041** Displaced fracture of coronoid process of right ulna

√7ᵗʰ **S52.042** Displaced fracture of coronoid process of left ulna

√7ᵗʰ **S52.043** Displaced fracture of coronoid process of unspecified ulna

√7ᵗʰ **S52.044** Nondisplaced fracture of coronoid process of right ulna

√7ᵗʰ **S52.045** Nondisplaced fracture of coronoid process of left ulna

√7ᵗʰ **S52.046** Nondisplaced fracture of coronoid process of unspecified ulna

√6ᵗʰ **S52.09** Other fracture of upper end of ulna

√7ᵗʰ **S52.091** Other fracture of upper end of right ulna

√7ᵗʰ **S52.092** Other fracture of upper end of left ulna

√7ᵗʰ **S52.099** Other fracture of upper end of unspecified ulna

√5ᵗʰ **S52.1** Fracture of upper end of radius
Fracture of proximal end of radius

EXCLUDES 2 physeal fractures of upper end of radius (S59.2-)
fracture of shaft of radius (S52.3-)

√6ᵗʰ **S52.10** Unspecified fracture of upper end of radius

√7ᵗʰ **S52.101** Unspecified fracture of upper end of right radius

√7ᵗʰ **S52.102** Unspecified fracture of upper end of left radius

√7ᵗʰ **S52.109** Unspecified fracture of upper end of unspecified radius

√6ᵗʰ **S52.11** Torus fracture of upper end of radius

The appropriate 7th character is to be added to all codes in subcategory S52.11.
A   initial encounter for closed fracture
D   subsequent encounter for fracture with routine healing
G   subsequent encounter for fracture with delayed healing
K   subsequent encounter for fracture with nonunion
P   subsequent encounter for fracture with malunion
S   sequela

√7ᵗʰ **S52.111** Torus fracture of upper end of right radius

√7ᵗʰ **S52.112** Torus fracture of upper end of left radius

√7ᵗʰ **S52.119** Torus fracture of upper end of unspecified radius

√6ᵗʰ **S52.12** Fracture of head of radius

√7ᵗʰ **S52.121** Displaced fracture of head of right radius

√7ᵗʰ **S52.122** Displaced fracture of head of left radius

√7ᵗʰ **S52.123** Displaced fracture of head of unspecified radius

√7ᵗʰ **S52.124** Nondisplaced fracture of head of right radius

√7ᵗʰ **S52.125** Nondisplaced fracture of head of left radius

√7ᵗʰ **S52.126** Nondisplaced fracture of head of unspecified radius

√6ᵗʰ **S52.13** Fracture of neck of radius

√7ᵗʰ **S52.131** Displaced fracture of neck of right radius

√7ᵗʰ **S52.132** Displaced fracture of neck of left radius

√7ᵗʰ **S52.133** Displaced fracture of neck of unspecified radius

√7ᵗʰ **S52.134** Nondisplaced fracture of neck of right radius

√7ᵗʰ **S52.135** Nondisplaced fracture of neck of left radius

√7ᵗʰ **S52.136** Nondisplaced fracture of neck of unspecified radius

√6ᵗʰ **S52.18** Other fracture of upper end of radius

√7ᵗʰ **S52.181** Other fracture of upper end of right radius

√7ᵗʰ **S52.182** Other fracture of upper end of left radius

√7ᵗʰ **S52.189** Other fracture of upper end of unspecified radius

√5ᵗʰ **S52.2** Fracture of shaft of ulna

√6ᵗʰ **S52.20** Unspecified fracture of shaft of ulna
Fracture of ulna NOS

√7ᵗʰ **S52.201** Unspecified fracture of shaft of right ulna

√7ᵗʰ **S52.202** Unspecified fracture of shaft of left ulna

√7ᵗʰ **S52.209** Unspecified fracture of shaft of unspecified ulna

√6ᵗʰ **S52.21** Greenstick fracture of shaft of ulna

The appropriate 7th character is to be added to all codes in subcategory S52.21.
A   initial encounter for closed fracture
D   subsequent encounter for fracture with routine healing
G   subsequent encounter for fracture with delayed healing
K   subsequent encounter for fracture with nonunion
P   subsequent encounter for fracture with malunion
S   sequela

√7ᵗʰ **S52.211** Greenstick fracture of shaft of right ulna

√7ᵗʰ **S52.212** Greenstick fracture of shaft of left ulna

√7ᵗʰ **S52.219** Greenstick fracture of shaft of unspecified ulna

√6ᵗʰ **S52.22** Transverse fracture of shaft of ulna

√7ᵗʰ **S52.221** Displaced transverse fracture of shaft of right ulna

√7ᵗʰ **S52.222** Displaced transverse fracture of shaft of left ulna

√7ᵗʰ **S52.223** Displaced transverse fracture of shaft of unspecified ulna

√7ᵗʰ **S52.224** Nondisplaced transverse fracture of shaft of right ulna

√7ᵗʰ **S52.225** Nondisplaced transverse fracture of shaft of left ulna

√7ᵗʰ **S52.226** Nondisplaced transverse fracture of shaft of unspecified ulna

√6ᵗʰ **S52.23** Oblique fracture of shaft of ulna

√7ᵗʰ **S52.231** Displaced oblique fracture of shaft of right ulna

√7ᵗʰ **S52.232** Displaced oblique fracture of shaft of left ulna

EXCLUDES 1 Not coded here   EXCLUDES 2 Not included here   N Newborn Age: 0   P Pediatric Age: 0-17   M Maternity Age: 12-55   A Adult Age: 15-124

854   ICD-10-CM Draft (2015)

√7ᵗʰ **S52.233** Displaced oblique fracture of shaft of unspecified ulna

√7ᵗʰ **S52.234** Nondisplaced oblique fracture of shaft of right ulna

√7ᵗʰ **S52.235** Nondisplaced oblique fracture of shaft of left ulna

√7ᵗʰ **S52.236** Nondisplaced oblique fracture of shaft of unspecified ulna

√6ᵗʰ **S52.24** Spiral fracture of shaft of ulna

√7ᵗʰ **S52.241** Displaced spiral fracture of shaft of ulna, right arm

√7ᵗʰ **S52.242** Displaced spiral fracture of shaft of ulna, left arm

√7ᵗʰ **S52.243** Displaced spiral fracture of shaft of ulna, unspecified arm

√7ᵗʰ **S52.244** Nondisplaced spiral fracture of shaft of ulna, right arm

√7ᵗʰ **S52.245** Nondisplaced spiral fracture of shaft of ulna, left arm

√7ᵗʰ **S52.246** Nondisplaced spiral fracture of shaft of ulna, unspecified arm

√6ᵗʰ **S52.25** Comminuted fracture of shaft of ulna

√7ᵗʰ **S52.251** Displaced comminuted fracture of shaft of ulna, right arm

√7ᵗʰ **S52.252** Displaced comminuted fracture of shaft of ulna, left arm

√7ᵗʰ **S52.253** Displaced comminuted fracture of shaft of ulna, unspecified arm

√7ᵗʰ **S52.254** Nondisplaced comminuted fracture of shaft of ulna, right arm

√7ᵗʰ **S52.255** Nondisplaced comminuted fracture of shaft of ulna, left arm

√7ᵗʰ **S52.256** Nondisplaced comminuted fracture of shaft of ulna, unspecified arm

√6ᵗʰ **S52.26** Segmental fracture of shaft of ulna

√7ᵗʰ **S52.261** Displaced segmental fracture of shaft of ulna, right arm

√7ᵗʰ **S52.262** Displaced segmental fracture of shaft of ulna, left arm

√7ᵗʰ **S52.263** Displaced segmental fracture of shaft of ulna, unspecified arm

√7ᵗʰ **S52.264** Nondisplaced segmental fracture of shaft of ulna, right arm

√7ᵗʰ **S52.265** Nondisplaced segmental fracture of shaft of ulna, left arm

√7ᵗʰ **S52.266** Nondisplaced segmental fracture of shaft of ulna, unspecified arm

√6ᵗʰ **S52.27** Monteggia's fracture of ulna
Fracture of upper shaft of ulna with dislocation of radial head

√7ᵗʰ **S52.271** Monteggia's fracture of right ulna

√7ᵗʰ **S52.272** Monteggia's fracture of left ulna

√7ᵗʰ **S52.279** Monteggia's fracture of unspecified ulna

√6ᵗʰ **S52.28** Bent bone of ulna

√7ᵗʰ **S52.281** Bent bone of right ulna

√7ᵗʰ **S52.282** Bent bone of left ulna

√7ᵗʰ **S52.283** Bent bone of unspecified ulna

√6ᵗʰ **S52.29** Other fracture of shaft of ulna

√7ᵗʰ **S52.291** Other fracture of shaft of right ulna

√7ᵗʰ **S52.292** Other fracture of shaft of left ulna

√7ᵗʰ **S52.299** Other fracture of shaft of unspecified ulna

√5ᵗʰ **S52.3** Fracture of shaft of radius

√6ᵗʰ **S52.30** Unspecified fracture of shaft of radius

√7ᵗʰ **S52.301** Unspecified fracture of shaft of right radius

√7ᵗʰ **S52.302** Unspecified fracture of shaft of left radius

√7ᵗʰ **S52.309** Unspecified fracture of shaft of unspecified radius

√6ᵗʰ **S52.31** Greenstick fracture of shaft of radius

The appropriate 7th character is to be added to all codes in subcategory S52.31.
A initial encounter for closed fracture
D subsequent encounter for fracture with routine healing
G subsequent encounter for fracture with delayed healing
K subsequent encounter for fracture with nonunion
P subsequent encounter for fracture with malunion
S sequela

√7ᵗʰ **S52.311** Greenstick fracture of shaft of radius, right arm

√7ᵗʰ **S52.312** Greenstick fracture of shaft of radius, left arm

√7ᵗʰ **S52.319** Greenstick fracture of shaft of radius, unspecified arm

√6ᵗʰ **S52.32** Transverse fracture of shaft of radius

√7ᵗʰ **S52.321** Displaced transverse fracture of shaft of right radius

√7ᵗʰ **S52.322** Displaced transverse fracture of shaft of left radius

√7ᵗʰ **S52.323** Displaced transverse fracture of shaft of unspecified radius

√7ᵗʰ **S52.324** Nondisplaced transverse fracture of shaft of right radius

√7ᵗʰ **S52.325** Nondisplaced transverse fracture of shaft of left radius

√7ᵗʰ **S52.326** Nondisplaced transverse fracture of shaft of unspecified radius

√6ᵗʰ **S52.33** Oblique fracture of shaft of radius

√7ᵗʰ **S52.331** Displaced oblique fracture of shaft of right radius

√7ᵗʰ **S52.332** Displaced oblique fracture of shaft of left radius

√7ᵗʰ **S52.333** Displaced oblique fracture of shaft of unspecified radius

√7ᵗʰ **S52.334** Nondisplaced oblique fracture of shaft of right radius

√7ᵗʰ **S52.335** Nondisplaced oblique fracture of shaft of left radius

√7ᵗʰ **S52.336** Nondisplaced oblique fracture of shaft of unspecified radius

√6ᵗʰ **S52.34** Spiral fracture of shaft of radius

√7ᵗʰ **S52.341** Displaced spiral fracture of shaft of radius, right arm

√7ᵗʰ **S52.342** Displaced spiral fracture of shaft of radius, left arm

√7ᵗʰ **S52.343** Displaced spiral fracture of shaft of radius, unspecified arm

√7ᵗʰ **S52.344** Nondisplaced spiral fracture of shaft of radius, right arm

√7ᵗʰ **S52.345** Nondisplaced spiral fracture of shaft of radius, left arm

√7ᵗʰ **S52.346** Nondisplaced spiral fracture of shaft of radius, unspecified arm

√6ᵗʰ **S52.35** Comminuted fracture of shaft of radius

√7ᵗʰ **S52.351** Displaced comminuted fracture of shaft of radius, right arm

√7ᵗʰ **S52.352** Displaced comminuted fracture of shaft of radius, left arm

√7ᵗʰ **S52.353** Displaced comminuted fracture of shaft of radius, unspecified arm

√7ᵗʰ **S52.354** Nondisplaced comminuted fracture of shaft of radius, right arm

√7ᵗʰ **S52.355** Nondisplaced comminuted fracture of shaft of radius, left arm

√7ᵗʰ **S52.356** Nondisplaced comminuted fracture of shaft of radius, unspecified arm

√6ᵗʰ **S52.36** Segmental fracture of shaft of radius

√7ᵗʰ **S52.361** Displaced segmental fracture of shaft of radius, right arm

☑ Additional Character Required   √ₓ7ᵗʰ Xtension Alert   Unspecified Dx   Other Specified Dx   Manifestation   ►◄ Revised Text   ● New Code   ▲ Revised Code Title

✓7ᵗʰ **S52.362** Displaced **segmental fracture of shaft of radius,** left **arm**

✓7ᵗʰ **S52.363** Displaced **segmental fracture of shaft of radius, unspecified arm**

✓7ᵗʰ **S52.364** Nondisplaced **segmental fracture of shaft of radius,** right **arm**

✓7ᵗʰ **S52.365** Nondisplaced **segmental fracture of shaft of radius,** left **arm**

✓7ᵗʰ **S52.366** Nondisplaced **segmental fracture of shaft of radius, unspecified arm**

✓6ᵗʰ **S52.37** Galeazzi's **fracture**
Fracture of lower shaft of radius with radioulnar joint dislocation

    ✓7ᵗʰ **S52.371** **Galeazzi's fracture of** right **radius**

    ✓7ᵗʰ **S52.372** **Galeazzi's fracture of** left **radius**

    ✓7ᵗʰ **S52.379** **Galeazzi's fracture of unspecified radius**

✓6ᵗʰ **S52.38** Bent bone **of radius**

    ✓7ᵗʰ **S52.381** **Bent bone of** right **radius**

    ✓7ᵗʰ **S52.382** **Bent bone of** left **radius**

    ✓7ᵗʰ **S52.389** **Bent bone of unspecified radius**

✓6ᵗʰ **S52.39** Other **fracture of shaft of radius**

    ✓7ᵗʰ **S52.391** **Other fracture of shaft of radius,** right **arm**

    ✓7ᵗʰ **S52.392** **Other fracture of shaft of radius,** left **arm**

    ✓7ᵗʰ **S52.399** **Other fracture of shaft of radius, unspecified arm**

✓5ᵗʰ **S52.5** **Fracture of** lower end of radius
Fracture of distal end of radius
EXCLUDES 2   physeal fractures of lower end of radius (S59.2-)

✓6ᵗʰ **S52.50** Unspecified **fracture of the lower end of radius**

    ✓7ᵗʰ **S52.501** **Unspecified fracture of the lower end of** right **radius**

    ✓7ᵗʰ **S52.502** **Unspecified fracture of the lower end of** left **radius**

    ✓7ᵗʰ **S52.509** **Unspecified fracture of the lower end of unspecified radius**

✓6ᵗʰ **S52.51** **Fracture of** radial styloid process

    ✓7ᵗʰ **S52.511** Displaced **fracture of** right **radial styloid process**

    ✓7ᵗʰ **S52.512** Displaced **fracture of** left **radial styloid process**

    ✓7ᵗʰ **S52.513** Displaced **fracture of unspecified radial styloid process**

    ✓7ᵗʰ **S52.514** Nondisplaced **fracture of** right **radial styloid process**

    ✓7ᵗʰ **S52.515** Nondisplaced **fracture of** left **radial styloid process**

    ✓7ᵗʰ **S52.516** Nondisplaced **fracture of unspecified radial styloid process**

✓6ᵗʰ **S52.52** Torus **fracture of lower end of radius**

> The appropriate 7th character is to be added to all codes in subcategory S52.52.
> A   initial encounter for closed fracture
> D   subsequent encounter for fracture with routine healing
> G   subsequent encounter for fracture with delayed healing
> K   subsequent encounter for fracture with nonunion
> P   subsequent encounter for fracture with malunion
> S   sequela

    ✓7ᵗʰ **S52.521** **Torus fracture of lower end of** right **radius**

    ✓7ᵗʰ **S52.522** **Torus fracture of lower end of** left **radius**

    ✓7ᵗʰ **S52.529** **Torus fracture of lower end of unspecified radius**

✓6ᵗʰ **S52.53** Colles' **fracture**

    ✓7ᵗʰ **S52.531** **Colles' fracture of** right **radius**

    ✓7ᵗʰ **S52.532** **Colles' fracture of** left **radius**

    ✓7ᵗʰ **S52.539** **Colles' fracture of unspecified radius**

✓6ᵗʰ **S52.54** Smith's **fracture**

    ✓7ᵗʰ **S52.541** **Smith's fracture of** right **radius**

    ✓7ᵗʰ **S52.542** **Smith's fracture of** left **radius**

    ✓7ᵗʰ **S52.549** **Smith's fracture of unspecified radius**

✓6ᵗʰ **S52.55** Other extraarticular **fracture of lower end of radius**

    ✓7ᵗʰ **S52.551** **Other extraarticular fracture of lower end of** right **radius**

    ✓7ᵗʰ **S52.552** **Other extraarticular fracture of lower end of** left **radius**

    ✓7ᵗʰ **S52.559** **Other extraarticular fracture of lower end of unspecified radius**

✓6ᵗʰ **S52.56** Barton's **fracture**

    ✓7ᵗʰ **S52.561** **Barton's fracture of** right **radius**

    ✓7ᵗʰ **S52.562** **Barton's fracture of** left **radius**

    ✓7ᵗʰ **S52.569** **Barton's fracture of unspecified radius**

✓6ᵗʰ **S52.57** Other intraarticular **fracture of lower end of radius**

    ✓7ᵗʰ **S52.571** **Other intraarticular fracture of lower end of** right **radius**

    ✓7ᵗʰ **S52.572** **Other intraarticular fracture of lower end of** left **radius**

    ✓7ᵗʰ **S52.579** **Other intraarticular fracture of lower end of unspecified radius**

✓6ᵗʰ **S52.59** Other **fractures of lower end of radius**

    ✓7ᵗʰ **S52.591** **Other fractures of lower end of** right **radius**

    ✓7ᵗʰ **S52.592** **Other fractures of lower end of** left **radius**

    ✓7ᵗʰ **S52.599** **Other fractures of lower end of unspecified radius**

✓5ᵗʰ **S52.6** **Fracture of** lower end of ulna

✓6ᵗʰ **S52.60** Unspecified **fracture of lower end of ulna**

    ✓7ᵗʰ **S52.601** **Unspecified fracture of lower end of** right **ulna**

    ✓7ᵗʰ **S52.602** **Unspecified fracture of lower end of** left **ulna**

    ✓7ᵗʰ **S52.609** **Unspecified fracture of lower end of unspecified ulna**

✓6ᵗʰ **S52.61** **Fracture of ulna** styloid process

    ✓7ᵗʰ **S52.611** Displaced **fracture of** right **ulna styloid process**

    ✓7ᵗʰ **S52.612** Displaced **fracture of** left **ulna styloid process**

    ✓7ᵗʰ **S52.613** Displaced **fracture of unspecified ulna styloid process**

    ✓7ᵗʰ **S52.614** Nondisplaced **fracture of** right **ulna styloid process**

    ✓7ᵗʰ **S52.615** Nondisplaced **fracture of** left **ulna styloid process**

    ✓7ᵗʰ **S52.616** Nondisplaced **fracture of unspecified ulna styloid process**

✓6ᵗʰ **S52.62** Torus **fracture of lower end of ulna**

> The appropriate 7th character is to be added to all codes in subcategory S52.62.
> A   initial encounter for closed fracture
> D   subsequent encounter for fracture with routine healing
> G   subsequent encounter for fracture with delayed healing
> K   subsequent encounter for fracture with nonunion
> P   subsequent encounter for fracture with malunion
> S   sequela

    ✓7ᵗʰ **S52.621** **Torus fracture of lower end of** right **ulna**

    ✓7ᵗʰ **S52.622** **Torus fracture of lower end of** left **ulna**

    ✓7ᵗʰ **S52.629** **Torus fracture of lower end of unspecified ulna**

✓6ᵗʰ **S52.69** Other **fracture of lower end of ulna**

    ✓7ᵗʰ **S52.691** **Other fracture of lower end of** right **ulna**

    ✓7ᵗʰ **S52.692** **Other fracture of lower end of** left **ulna**

    ✓7ᵗʰ **S52.699** **Other fracture of lower end of unspecified ulna**

✓5ᵗʰ **S52.9** **Unspecified fracture of** forearm

    ✓x7ᵗʰ **S52.90** **Unspecified fracture of unspecified forearm**

    ✓x7ᵗʰ **S52.91** **Unspecified fracture of** right **forearm**

    ✓x7ᵗʰ **S52.92** **Unspecified fracture of** left **forearm**

EXCLUDES 1 Not coded here   *EXCLUDES 2* Not included here   **N** Newborn Age: 0   **P** Pediatric Age: 0-17   **M** Maternity Age: 12-55   **A** Adult Age: 15-124

✓4ᵗʰ S53 Dislocation and sprain of joints and ligaments of elbow

INCLUDES avulsion of joint or ligament of elbow
laceration of cartilage, joint or ligament of elbow
sprain of cartilage, joint or ligament of elbow
traumatic hemarthrosis of joint or ligament of elbow
traumatic rupture of joint or ligament of elbow
traumatic subluxation of joint or ligament of elbow
traumatic tear of joint or ligament of elbow

Code also any associated open wound

EXCLUDES 2 *strain of muscle, fascia and tendon at forearm level (S56.-)*

The appropriate 7th character is to be added to each code from category S53.
- A initial encounter
- D subsequent encounter
- S sequela

✓5ᵗʰ S53.0 Subluxation and dislocation of radial head
Dislocation of radiohumeral joint
Subluxation of radiohumeral joint

EXCLUDES 1 *Monteggia's fracture-dislocation (S52.27-)*

✓6ᵗʰ S53.00 Unspecified subluxation and dislocation of radial head
- ✓7ᵗʰ **S53.001** Unspecified subluxation of right radial head
- ✓7ᵗʰ **S53.002** Unspecified subluxation of left radial head
- ✓7ᵗʰ **S53.003** Unspecified subluxation of unspecified radial head
- ✓7ᵗʰ **S53.004** Unspecified dislocation of right radial head
- ✓7ᵗʰ **S53.005** Unspecified dislocation of left radial head
- ✓7ᵗʰ **S53.006** Unspecified dislocation of unspecified radial head

✓6ᵗʰ S53.01 Anterior subluxation and dislocation of radial head
Anteriomedial subluxation and dislocation of radial head
- ✓7ᵗʰ **S53.011** Anterior subluxation of right radial head
- ✓7ᵗʰ **S53.012** Anterior subluxation of left radial head
- ✓7ᵗʰ **S53.013** Anterior subluxation of unspecified radial head
- ✓7ᵗʰ **S53.014** Anterior dislocation of right radial head
- ✓7ᵗʰ **S53.015** Anterior dislocation of left radial head
- ✓7ᵗʰ **S53.016** Anterior dislocation of unspecified radial head

✓6ᵗʰ S53.02 Posterior subluxation and dislocation of radial head
Posteriolateral subluxation and dislocation of radial head
- ✓7ᵗʰ **S53.021** Posterior subluxation of right radial head
- ✓7ᵗʰ **S53.022** Posterior subluxation of left radial head
- ✓7ᵗʰ **S53.023** Posterior subluxation of unspecified radial head
- ✓7ᵗʰ **S53.024** Posterior dislocation of right radial head
- ✓7ᵗʰ **S53.025** Posterior dislocation of left radial head
- ✓7ᵗʰ **S53.026** Posterior dislocation of unspecified radial head

✓6ᵗʰ S53.03 Nursemaid's elbow
- ✓7ᵗʰ **S53.031** Nursemaid's elbow, right elbow
- ✓7ᵗʰ **S53.032** Nursemaid's elbow, left elbow
- ✓7ᵗʰ **S53.033** Nursemaid's elbow, unspecified elbow

✓6ᵗʰ S53.09 Other subluxation and dislocation of radial head
- ✓7ᵗʰ **S53.091** Other subluxation of right radial head
- ✓7ᵗʰ **S53.092** Other subluxation of left radial head
- ✓7ᵗʰ **S53.093** Other subluxation of unspecified radial head
- ✓7ᵗʰ **S53.094** Other dislocation of right radial head
- ✓7ᵗʰ **S53.095** Other dislocation of left radial head
- ✓7ᵗʰ **S53.096** Other dislocation of unspecified radial head

✓5ᵗʰ S53.1 Subluxation and dislocation of ulnohumeral joint
Subluxation and dislocation of elbow NOS

EXCLUDES 1 *dislocation of radial head alone (S53.0-)*

✓6ᵗʰ S53.10 Unspecified subluxation and dislocation of ulnohumeral joint
- ✓7ᵗʰ **S53.101** Unspecified subluxation of right ulnohumeral joint
- ✓7ᵗʰ **S53.102** Unspecified subluxation of left ulnohumeral joint
- ✓7ᵗʰ **S53.103** Unspecified subluxation of unspecified ulnohumeral joint
- ✓7ᵗʰ **S53.104** Unspecified dislocation of right ulnohumeral joint
- ✓7ᵗʰ **S53.105** Unspecified dislocation of left ulnohumeral joint
- ✓7ᵗʰ **S53.106** Unspecified dislocation of unspecified ulnohumeral joint

✓6ᵗʰ S53.11 Anterior subluxation and dislocation of ulnohumeral joint
- ✓7ᵗʰ **S53.111** Anterior subluxation of right ulnohumeral joint
- ✓7ᵗʰ **S53.112** Anterior subluxation of left ulnohumeral joint
- ✓7ᵗʰ **S53.113** Anterior subluxation of unspecified ulnohumeral joint
- ✓7ᵗʰ **S53.114** Anterior dislocation of right ulnohumeral joint
  - AHA: 2012, 4Q, 108
- ✓7ᵗʰ **S53.115** Anterior dislocation of left ulnohumeral joint
- ✓7ᵗʰ **S53.116** Anterior dislocation of unspecified ulnohumeral joint

✓6ᵗʰ S53.12 Posterior subluxation and dislocation of ulnohumeral joint
- ✓7ᵗʰ **S53.121** Posterior subluxation of right ulnohumeral joint
- ✓7ᵗʰ **S53.122** Posterior subluxation of left ulnohumeral joint
- ✓7ᵗʰ **S53.123** Posterior subluxation of unspecified ulnohumeral joint
- ✓7ᵗʰ **S53.124** Posterior dislocation of right ulnohumeral joint
- ✓7ᵗʰ **S53.125** Posterior dislocation of left ulnohumeral joint
- ✓7ᵗʰ **S53.126** Posterior dislocation of unspecified ulnohumeral joint

✓6ᵗʰ S53.13 Medial subluxation and dislocation of ulnohumeral joint
- ✓7ᵗʰ **S53.131** Medial subluxation of right ulnohumeral joint
- ✓7ᵗʰ **S53.132** Medial subluxation of left ulnohumeral joint
- ✓7ᵗʰ **S53.133** Medial subluxation of unspecified ulnohumeral joint
- ✓7ᵗʰ **S53.134** Medial dislocation of right ulnohumeral joint
- ✓7ᵗʰ **S53.135** Medial dislocation of left ulnohumeral joint
- ✓7ᵗʰ **S53.136** Medial dislocation of unspecified ulnohumeral joint

✓6ᵗʰ S53.14 Lateral subluxation and dislocation of ulnohumeral joint
- ✓7ᵗʰ **S53.141** Lateral subluxation of right ulnohumeral joint
- ✓7ᵗʰ **S53.142** Lateral subluxation of left ulnohumeral joint
- ✓7ᵗʰ **S53.143** Lateral subluxation of unspecified ulnohumeral joint
- ✓7ᵗʰ **S53.144** Lateral dislocation of right ulnohumeral joint
- ✓7ᵗʰ **S53.145** Lateral dislocation of left ulnohumeral joint
- ✓7ᵗʰ **S53.146** Lateral dislocation of unspecified ulnohumeral joint

✓6ᵗʰ S53.19 Other subluxation and dislocation of ulnohumeral joint
- ✓7ᵗʰ **S53.191** Other subluxation of right ulnohumeral joint
- ✓7ᵗʰ **S53.192** Other subluxation of left ulnohumeral joint
- ✓7ᵗʰ **S53.193** Other subluxation of unspecified ulnohumeral joint

✓ Additional Character Required   ✓x7ᵗʰ Xtension Alert   Unspecified Dx   Other Specified Dx   Manifestation   ►◄ Revised Text   ● New Code   ▲ Revised Code Title

ICD-10-CM Draft (2015)   857

Injury, Poisoning and Certain Other Consequences of External Causes

S53.194–S55.111

✓7ᵗʰ **S53.194 Other** dislocation of **right ulnohumeral joint**

✓7ᵗʰ **S53.195 Other** dislocation of **left ulnohumeral joint**

✓7ᵗʰ **S53.196 Other** dislocation **of unspecified ulnohumeral joint**

✓5ᵗʰ **S53.2 Traumatic rupture of** radial collateral ligament
    EXCLUDES 1   *sprain of radial collateral ligament NOS (S53.43-)*

✓7ᵗʰ **S53.20 Traumatic rupture of unspecified radial collateral ligament**

✓7ᵗʰ **S53.21 Traumatic rupture of** right **radial collateral ligament**

✓7ᵗʰ **S53.22 Traumatic rupture of** left **radial collateral ligament**

✓5ᵗʰ **S53.3 Traumatic rupture of** ulnar collateral ligament
    EXCLUDES 1   *sprain of ulnar collateral ligament (S53.44-)*

✓7ᵗʰ **S53.30 Traumatic rupture of unspecified ulnar collateral ligament**

✓7ᵗʰ **S53.31 Traumatic rupture of** right **ulnar collateral ligament**

✓7ᵗʰ **S53.32 Traumatic rupture of** left **ulnar collateral ligament**

✓5ᵗʰ **S53.4 Sprain of** elbow
    EXCLUDES 2   *traumatic rupture of radial collateral ligament (S53.2-)*
                traumatic rupture of ulnar collateral ligament (S53.3-)

✓6ᵗʰ **S53.40** Unspecified **sprain of elbow**

✓7ᵗʰ **S53.401 Unspecified sprain of** right **elbow**

✓7ᵗʰ **S53.402 Unspecified sprain of** left **elbow**

✓7ᵗʰ **S53.409 Unspecified sprain of unspecified elbow**
         Sprain of elbow NOS

✓6ᵗʰ **S53.41** Radiohumeral **(joint) sprain**

✓7ᵗʰ **S53.411 Radiohumeral (joint) sprain of** right **elbow**

✓7ᵗʰ **S53.412 Radiohumeral (joint) sprain of** left **elbow**

✓7ᵗʰ **S53.419 Radiohumeral (joint) sprain of unspecified elbow**

✓6ᵗʰ **S53.42** Ulnohumeral **(joint) sprain**

✓7ᵗʰ **S53.421 Ulnohumeral (joint) sprain of** right **elbow**

✓7ᵗʰ **S53.422 Ulnohumeral (joint) sprain of** left **elbow**

✓7ᵗʰ **S53.429 Ulnohumeral (joint) sprain of unspecified elbow**

✓6ᵗʰ **S53.43** Radial collateral ligament **sprain**

✓7ᵗʰ **S53.431 Radial collateral ligament sprain of** right **elbow**

✓7ᵗʰ **S53.432 Radial collateral ligament sprain of** left **elbow**

✓7ᵗʰ **S53.439 Radial collateral ligament sprain of unspecified elbow**

✓6ᵗʰ **S53.44** Ulnar collateral ligament **sprain**

✓7ᵗʰ **S53.441 Ulnar collateral ligament sprain of** right **elbow**

✓7ᵗʰ **S53.442 Ulnar collateral ligament sprain of** left **elbow**

✓7ᵗʰ **S53.449 Ulnar collateral ligament sprain of unspecified elbow**

✓6ᵗʰ **S53.49** Other **sprain of elbow**

✓7ᵗʰ **S53.491 Other sprain of** right **elbow**

✓7ᵗʰ **S53.492 Other sprain of** left **elbow**

✓7ᵗʰ **S53.499 Other sprain of unspecified elbow**

✓4ᵗʰ **S54 Injury of nerves at forearm level**
    Code also any associated open wound (S51.-)
    EXCLUDES 2   *injury of nerves at wrist and hand level (S64.-)*

The appropriate 7th character is to be added to each code from category S54.
A   initial encounter
D   subsequent encounter
S   sequela

✓5ᵗʰ **S54.0 Injury of** ulnar **nerve at forearm level**
    Injury of ulnar nerve NOS

✓ₓ7ᵗʰ **S54.00 Injury of ulnar nerve at forearm level, unspecified arm**

✓ₓ7ᵗʰ **S54.01 Injury of ulnar nerve at forearm level,** right **arm**

✓ₓ7ᵗʰ **S54.02 Injury of ulnar nerve at forearm level,** left **arm**

✓5ᵗʰ **S54.1 Injury of** median **nerve at forearm level**
    Injury of median nerve NOS

✓ₓ7ᵗʰ **S54.10 Injury of median nerve at forearm level, unspecified arm**

✓ₓ7ᵗʰ **S54.11 Injury of median nerve at forearm level,** right **arm**

✓ₓ7ᵗʰ **S54.12 Injury of median nerve at forearm level,** left **arm**

✓5ᵗʰ **S54.2 Injury of** radial **nerve at forearm level**
    Injury of radial nerve NOS

✓ₓ7ᵗʰ **S54.20 Injury of radial nerve at forearm level, unspecified arm**

✓ₓ7ᵗʰ **S54.21 Injury of radial nerve at forearm level,** right **arm**

✓ₓ7ᵗʰ **S54.22 Injury of radial nerve at forearm level,** left **arm**

✓5ᵗʰ **S54.3 Injury of** cutaneous sensory **nerve at forearm level**

✓ₓ7ᵗʰ **S54.30 Injury of cutaneous sensory nerve at forearm level, unspecified arm**

✓ₓ7ᵗʰ **S54.31 Injury of cutaneous sensory nerve at forearm level,** right **arm**

✓ₓ7ᵗʰ **S54.32 Injury of cutaneous sensory nerve at forearm level,** left **arm**

✓5ᵗʰ **S54.8 Injury of** other **nerves at forearm level**

✓6ᵗʰ **S54.8X Unspecified injury of other nerves at forearm level**

✓7ᵗʰ **S54.8X1 Unspecified injury of other nerves at forearm level,** right **arm**

✓7ᵗʰ **S54.8X2 Unspecified injury of other nerves at forearm level,** left **arm**

✓7ᵗʰ **S54.8X9 Unspecified injury of other nerves at forearm level, unspecified arm**

✓5ᵗʰ **S54.9 Injury of** unspecified **nerve at forearm level**

✓ₓ7ᵗʰ **S54.90 Injury of unspecified nerve at forearm level, unspecified arm**

✓ₓ7ᵗʰ **S54.91 Injury of unspecified nerve at forearm level,** right **arm**

✓ₓ7ᵗʰ **S54.92 Injury of unspecified nerve at forearm level,** left **arm**

✓4ᵗʰ **S55 Injury of blood vessels at forearm level**
    Code also any associated open wound (S51.-)
    EXCLUDES 2   *injury of blood vessels at wrist and hand level (S65.-)*
                injury of brachial vessels (S45.1-S45.2)

The appropriate 7th character is to be added to each code from category S55.
A   initial encounter
D   subsequent encounter
S   sequela

✓5ᵗʰ **S55.0 Injury of** ulnar artery **at forearm level**

✓6ᵗʰ **S55.00** Unspecified **injury of ulnar artery at forearm level**

✓7ᵗʰ **S55.001 Unspecified injury of ulnar artery at forearm level,** right **arm**

✓7ᵗʰ **S55.002 Unspecified injury of ulnar artery at forearm level,** left **arm**

✓7ᵗʰ **S55.009 Unspecified injury of ulnar artery at forearm level, unspecified arm**

✓6ᵗʰ **S55.01** Laceration **of ulnar artery at forearm level**

✓7ᵗʰ **S55.011 Laceration of ulnar artery at forearm level,** right **arm**

✓7ᵗʰ **S55.012 Laceration of ulnar artery at forearm level,** left **arm**

✓7ᵗʰ **S55.019 Laceration of ulnar artery at forearm level, unspecified arm**

✓6ᵗʰ **S55.09** Other **specified injury of ulnar artery at forearm level**

✓7ᵗʰ **S55.091 Other specified injury of ulnar artery at forearm level,** right **arm**

✓7ᵗʰ **S55.092 Other specified injury of ulnar artery at forearm level,** left **arm**

✓7ᵗʰ **S55.099 Other specified injury of ulnar artery at forearm level, unspecified arm**

✓5ᵗʰ **S55.1 Injury of** radial artery **at forearm level**

✓6ᵗʰ **S55.10** Unspecified **injury of radial artery at forearm level**

✓7ᵗʰ **S55.101 Unspecified injury of radial artery at forearm level,** right **arm**

✓7ᵗʰ **S55.102 Unspecified injury of radial artery at forearm level,** left **arm**

✓7ᵗʰ **S55.109 Unspecified injury of radial artery at forearm level, unspecified arm**

✓6ᵗʰ **S55.11** Laceration **of radial artery at forearm level**

✓7ᵗʰ **S55.111 Laceration of radial artery at forearm level,** right **arm**

EXCLUDES 1 Not coded here   EXCLUDES 2 Not included here   N Newborn Age: 0   P Pediatric Age: 0-17   M Maternity Age: 12-55   A Adult Age: 15-124

√7th **S55.112** Laceration of radial artery at forearm level, left arm

√7th **S55.119** Laceration of radial artery at forearm level, unspecified arm

√6th **S55.19** Other specified injury of radial artery at forearm level

√7th **S55.191** Other specified injury of radial artery at forearm level, right arm

√7th **S55.192** Other specified injury of radial artery at forearm level, left arm

√7th **S55.199** Other specified injury of radial artery at forearm level, unspecified arm

√5th **S55.2** Injury of vein at forearm level

√6th **S55.20** Unspecified injury of vein at forearm level

√7th **S55.201** Unspecified injury of vein at forearm level, right arm

√7th **S55.202** Unspecified injury of vein at forearm level, left arm

√7th **S55.209** Unspecified injury of vein at forearm level, unspecified arm

√6th **S55.21** Laceration of vein at forearm level

√7th **S55.211** Laceration of vein at forearm level, right arm

√7th **S55.212** Laceration of vein at forearm level, left arm

√7th **S55.219** Laceration of vein at forearm level, unspecified arm

√6th **S55.29** Other specified injury of vein at forearm level

√7th **S55.291** Other specified injury of vein at forearm level, right arm

√7th **S55.292** Other specified injury of vein at forearm level, left arm

√7th **S55.299** Other specified injury of vein at forearm level, unspecified arm

√5th **S55.8** Injury of other blood vessels at forearm level

√6th **S55.80** Unspecified injury of other blood vessels at forearm level

√7th **S55.801** Unspecified injury of other blood vessels at forearm level, right arm

√7th **S55.802** Unspecified injury of other blood vessels at forearm level, left arm

√7th **S55.809** Unspecified injury of other blood vessels at forearm level, unspecified arm

√6th **S55.81** Laceration of other blood vessels at forearm level

√7th **S55.811** Laceration of other blood vessels at forearm level, right arm

√7th **S55.812** Laceration of other blood vessels at forearm level, left arm

√7th **S55.819** Laceration of other blood vessels at forearm level, unspecified arm

√6th **S55.89** Other specified injury of other blood vessels at forearm level

√7th **S55.891** Other specified injury of other blood vessels at forearm level, right arm

√7th **S55.892** Other specified injury of other blood vessels at forearm level, left arm

√7th **S55.899** Other specified injury of other blood vessels at forearm level, unspecified arm

√5th **S55.9** Injury of unspecified blood vessel at forearm level

√6th **S55.90** Unspecified injury of unspecified blood vessel at forearm level

√7th **S55.901** Unspecified injury of unspecified blood vessel at forearm level, right arm

√7th **S55.902** Unspecified injury of unspecified blood vessel at forearm level, left arm

√7th **S55.909** Unspecified injury of unspecified blood vessel at forearm level, unspecified arm

√6th **S55.91** Laceration of unspecified blood vessel at forearm level

√7th **S55.911** Laceration of unspecified blood vessel at forearm level, right arm

√7th **S55.912** Laceration of unspecified blood vessel at forearm level, left arm

√7th **S55.919** Laceration of unspecified blood vessel at forearm level, unspecified arm

√6th **S55.99** Other specified injury of unspecified blood vessel at forearm level

√7th **S55.991** Other specified injury of unspecified blood vessel at forearm level, right arm

√7th **S55.992** Other specified injury of unspecified blood vessel at forearm level, left arm

√7th **S55.999** Other specified injury of unspecified blood vessel at forearm level, unspecified arm

√4th **S56** **Injury of muscle, fascia and tendon at forearm level**

Code also any associated open wound (S51.-)

EXCLUDES 2 injury of muscle, fascia and tendon at or below wrist (S66.-)
sprain of joints and ligaments of elbow (S53.4-)

The appropriate 7th character is to be added to each code from category S56.
A   initial encounter
D   subsequent encounter
S   sequela

√5th **S56.0** Injury of flexor muscle, fascia and tendon of thumb at forearm level

√6th **S56.00** Unspecified injury of flexor muscle, fascia and tendon of thumb at forearm level

√7th **S56.001** Unspecified injury of flexor muscle, fascia and tendon of right thumb at forearm level

√7th **S56.002** Unspecified injury of flexor muscle, fascia and tendon of left thumb at forearm level

√7th **S56.009** Unspecified injury of flexor muscle, fascia and tendon of unspecified thumb at forearm level

√6th **S56.01** Strain of flexor muscle, fascia and tendon of thumb at forearm level

√7th **S56.011** Strain of flexor muscle, fascia and tendon of right thumb at forearm level

√7th **S56.012** Strain of flexor muscle, fascia and tendon of left thumb at forearm level

√7th **S56.019** Strain of flexor muscle, fascia and tendon of unspecified thumb at forearm level

√6th **S56.02** Laceration of flexor muscle, fascia and tendon of thumb at forearm level

√7th **S56.021** Laceration of flexor muscle, fascia and tendon of right thumb at forearm level

√7th **S56.022** Laceration of flexor muscle, fascia and tendon of left thumb at forearm level

√7th **S56.029** Laceration of flexor muscle, fascia and tendon of unspecified thumb at forearm level

√6th **S56.09** Other injury of flexor muscle, fascia and tendon of thumb at forearm level

√7th **S56.091** Other injury of flexor muscle, fascia and tendon of right thumb at forearm level

√7th **S56.092** Other injury of flexor muscle, fascia and tendon of left thumb at forearm level

√7th **S56.099** Other injury of flexor muscle, fascia and tendon of unspecified thumb at forearm level

√5th **S56.1** Injury of flexor muscle, fascia and tendon of other and unspecified finger at forearm level

√6th **S56.10** Unspecified injury of flexor muscle, fascia and tendon of other and unspecified finger at forearm level

√7th **S56.101** Unspecified injury of flexor muscle, fascia and tendon of right index finger at forearm level

√7th **S56.102** Unspecified injury of flexor muscle, fascia and tendon of left index finger at forearm level

√7th **S56.103** Unspecified injury of flexor muscle, fascia and tendon of right middle finger at forearm level

√7th **S56.104** Unspecified injury of flexor muscle, fascia and tendon of left middle finger at forearm level

✓7th **S56.105** Unspecified injury of flexor muscle, fascia and tendon of right ring finger at forearm level

✓7th **S56.106** Unspecified injury of flexor muscle, fascia and tendon of left ring finger at forearm level

✓7th **S56.107** Unspecified injury of flexor muscle, fascia and tendon of right little finger at forearm level

✓7th **S56.108** Unspecified injury of flexor muscle, fascia and tendon of left little finger at forearm level

✓7th **S56.109** Unspecified injury of flexor muscle, fascia and tendon of unspecified finger at forearm level

✓6th **S56.11** Strain of flexor muscle, fascia and tendon of other and unspecified finger at forearm level

✓7th **S56.111** Strain of flexor muscle, fascia and tendon of right index finger at forearm level

✓7th **S56.112** Strain of flexor muscle, fascia and tendon of left index finger at forearm level

✓7th **S56.113** Strain of flexor muscle, fascia and tendon of right middle finger at forearm level

✓7th **S56.114** Strain of flexor muscle, fascia and tendon of left middle finger at forearm level

✓7th **S56.115** Strain of flexor muscle, fascia and tendon of right ring finger at forearm level

✓7th **S56.116** Strain of flexor muscle, fascia and tendon of left ring finger at forearm level

✓7th **S56.117** Strain of flexor muscle, fascia and tendon of right little finger at forearm level

✓7th **S56.118** Strain of flexor muscle, fascia and tendon of left little finger at forearm level

✓7th **S56.119** Strain of flexor muscle, fascia and tendon of finger of unspecified finger at forearm level

✓6th **S56.12** Laceration of flexor muscle, fascia and tendon of other and unspecified finger at forearm level

✓7th **S56.121** Laceration of flexor muscle, fascia and tendon of right index finger at forearm level

✓7th **S56.122** Laceration of flexor muscle, fascia and tendon of left index finger at forearm level

✓7th **S56.123** Laceration of flexor muscle, fascia and tendon of right middle finger at forearm level

✓7th **S56.124** Laceration of flexor muscle, fascia and tendon of left middle finger at forearm level

✓7th **S56.125** Laceration of flexor muscle, fascia and tendon of right ring finger at forearm level

✓7th **S56.126** Laceration of flexor muscle, fascia and tendon of left ring finger at forearm level

✓7th **S56.127** Laceration of flexor muscle, fascia and tendon of right little finger at forearm level

✓7th **S56.128** Laceration of flexor muscle, fascia and tendon of left little finger at forearm level

✓7th **S56.129** Laceration of flexor muscle, fascia and tendon of unspecified finger at forearm level

✓6th **S56.19** Other injury of flexor muscle, fascia and tendon of other and unspecified finger at forearm level

✓7th **S56.191** Other injury of flexor muscle, fascia and tendon of right index finger at forearm level

✓7th **S56.192** Other injury of flexor muscle, fascia and tendon of left index finger at forearm level

✓7th **S56.193** Other injury of flexor muscle, fascia and tendon of right middle finger at forearm level

✓7th **S56.194** Other injury of flexor muscle, fascia and tendon of left middle finger at forearm level

✓7th **S56.195** Other injury of flexor muscle, fascia and tendon of right ring finger at forearm level

✓7th **S56.196** Other injury of flexor muscle, fascia and tendon of left ring finger at forearm level

✓7th **S56.197** Other injury of flexor muscle, fascia and tendon of right little finger at forearm level

✓7th **S56.198** Other injury of flexor muscle, fascia and tendon of left little finger at forearm level

✓7th **S56.199** Other injury of flexor muscle, fascia and tendon of unspecified finger at forearm level

✓5th **S56.2** Injury of other flexor muscle, fascia and tendon at forearm level

✓6th **S56.20** Unspecified injury of other flexor muscle, fascia and tendon at forearm level

✓7th **S56.201** Unspecified injury of other flexor muscle, fascia and tendon at forearm level, right arm

✓7th **S56.202** Unspecified injury of other flexor muscle, fascia and tendon at forearm level, left arm

✓7th **S56.209** Unspecified injury of other flexor muscle, fascia and tendon at forearm level, unspecified arm

✓6th **S56.21** Strain of other flexor muscle, fascia and tendon at forearm level

✓7th **S56.211** Strain of other flexor muscle, fascia and tendon at forearm level, right arm

✓7th **S56.212** Strain of other flexor muscle, fascia and tendon at forearm level, left arm

✓7th **S56.219** Strain of other flexor muscle, fascia and tendon at forearm level, unspecified arm

✓6th **S56.22** Laceration of other flexor muscle, fascia and tendon at forearm level

✓7th **S56.221** Laceration of other flexor muscle, fascia and tendon at forearm level, right arm

✓7th **S56.222** Laceration of other flexor muscle, fascia and tendon at forearm level, left arm

✓7th **S56.229** Laceration of other flexor muscle, fascia and tendon at forearm level, unspecified arm

✓6th **S56.29** Other injury of other flexor muscle, fascia and tendon at forearm level

✓7th **S56.291** Other injury of other flexor muscle, fascia and tendon at forearm level, right arm

✓7th **S56.292** Other injury of other flexor muscle, fascia and tendon at forearm level, left arm

✓7th **S56.299** Other injury of other flexor muscle, fascia and tendon at forearm level, unspecified arm

✓5th **S56.3** Injury of extensor or abductor muscles, fascia and tendons of thumb at forearm level

✓6th **S56.30** Unspecified injury of extensor or abductor muscles, fascia and tendons of thumb at forearm level

✓7th **S56.301** Unspecified injury of extensor or abductor muscles, fascia and tendons of right thumb at forearm level

✓7th **S56.302** Unspecified injury of extensor or abductor muscles, fascia and tendons of left thumb at forearm level

✓7th **S56.309** Unspecified injury of extensor or abductor muscles, fascia and tendons of unspecified thumb at forearm level

✓6th **S56.31** Strain of extensor or abductor muscles, fascia and tendons of thumb at forearm level

✓7th **S56.311** Strain of extensor or abductor muscles, fascia and tendons of right thumb at forearm level

✓7th **S56.312** Strain of extensor or abductor muscles, fascia and tendons of left thumb at forearm level

✓7th **S56.319** Strain of extensor or abductor muscles, fascia and tendons of unspecified thumb at forearm level

✓6th **S56.32** Laceration of extensor or abductor muscles, fascia and tendons of thumb at forearm level

EXCLUDES 1 Not coded here   **EXCLUDES 2** Not included here   **N** Newborn Age: 0   **P** Pediatric Age: 0-17   **M** Maternity Age: 12-55   **A** Adult Age: 15-124

860   ICD-10-CM Draft (2015)

✓7ᵗʰ **S56.321** Laceration of extensor or abductor muscles, fascia and tendons of right thumb at forearm level

✓7ᵗʰ **S56.322** Laceration of extensor or abductor muscles, fascia and tendons of left thumb at forearm level

✓7ᵗʰ **S56.329** Laceration of extensor or abductor muscles, fascia and tendons of unspecified thumb at forearm level

✓6ᵗʰ **S56.39** Other injury of extensor or abductor muscles, fascia and tendons of thumb at forearm level

✓7ᵗʰ **S56.391** Other injury of extensor or abductor muscles, fascia and tendons of right thumb at forearm level

✓7ᵗʰ **S56.392** Other injury of extensor or abductor muscles, fascia and tendons of left thumb at forearm level

✓7ᵗʰ **S56.399** Other injury of extensor or abductor muscles, fascia and tendons of unspecified thumb at forearm level

✓5ᵗʰ **S56.4** Injury of extensor muscle and tendon of other and unspecified finger at forearm level

✓6ᵗʰ **S56.40** Unspecified injury of extensor muscle, fascia and tendon of other and unspecified finger at forearm level

✓7ᵗʰ **S56.401** Unspecified injury of extensor muscle, fascia and tendon of right index finger at forearm level

✓7ᵗʰ **S56.402** Unspecified injury of extensor muscle, fascia and tendon of left index finger at forearm level

✓7ᵗʰ **S56.403** Unspecified injury of extensor muscle, fascia and tendon of right middle finger at forearm level

✓7ᵗʰ **S56.404** Unspecified injury of extensor muscle, fascia and tendon of left middle finger at forearm level

✓7ᵗʰ **S56.405** Unspecified injury of extensor muscle, fascia and tendon of right ring finger at forearm level

✓7ᵗʰ **S56.406** Unspecified injury of extensor muscle, fascia and tendon of left ring finger at forearm level

✓7ᵗʰ **S56.407** Unspecified injury of extensor muscle, fascia and tendon of right little finger at forearm level

✓7ᵗʰ **S56.408** Unspecified injury of extensor muscle, fascia and tendon of left little finger at forearm level

✓7ᵗʰ **S56.409** Unspecified injury of extensor muscle, fascia and tendon of unspecified finger at forearm level

✓6ᵗʰ **S56.41** Strain of extensor muscle, fascia and tendon of other and unspecified finger at forearm level

✓7ᵗʰ **S56.411** Strain of extensor muscle, fascia and tendon of right index finger at forearm level

✓7ᵗʰ **S56.412** Strain of extensor muscle, fascia and tendon of left index finger at forearm level

✓7ᵗʰ **S56.413** Strain of extensor muscle, fascia and tendon of right middle finger at forearm level

✓7ᵗʰ **S56.414** Strain of extensor muscle, fascia and tendon of left middle finger at forearm level

✓7ᵗʰ **S56.415** Strain of extensor muscle, fascia and tendon of right ring finger at forearm level

✓7ᵗʰ **S56.416** Strain of extensor muscle, fascia and tendon of left ring finger at forearm level

✓7ᵗʰ **S56.417** Strain of extensor muscle, fascia and tendon of right little finger at forearm level

✓7ᵗʰ **S56.418** Strain of extensor muscle, fascia and tendon of left little finger at forearm level

✓7ᵗʰ **S56.419** Strain of extensor muscle, fascia and tendon of finger, unspecified finger at forearm level

✓6ᵗʰ **S56.42** Laceration of extensor muscle, fascia and tendon of other and unspecified finger at forearm level

✓7ᵗʰ **S56.421** Laceration of extensor muscle, fascia and tendon of right index finger at forearm level

✓7ᵗʰ **S56.422** Laceration of extensor muscle, fascia and tendon of left index finger at forearm level

✓7ᵗʰ **S56.423** Laceration of extensor muscle, fascia and tendon of right middle finger at forearm level

✓7ᵗʰ **S56.424** Laceration of extensor muscle, fascia and tendon of left middle finger at forearm level

✓7ᵗʰ **S56.425** Laceration of extensor muscle, fascia and tendon of right ring finger at forearm level

✓7ᵗʰ **S56.426** Laceration of extensor muscle, fascia and tendon of left ring finger at forearm level

✓7ᵗʰ **S56.427** Laceration of extensor muscle, fascia and tendon of right little finger at forearm level

✓7ᵗʰ **S56.428** Laceration of extensor muscle, fascia and tendon of left little finger at forearm level

✓7ᵗʰ **S56.429** Laceration of extensor muscle, fascia and tendon of unspecified finger at forearm level

✓6ᵗʰ **S56.49** Other injury of extensor muscle, fascia and tendon of other and unspecified finger at forearm level

✓7ᵗʰ **S56.491** Other injury of extensor muscle, fascia and tendon of right index finger at forearm level

✓7ᵗʰ **S56.492** Other injury of extensor muscle, fascia and tendon of left index finger at forearm level

✓7ᵗʰ **S56.493** Other injury of extensor muscle, fascia and tendon of right middle finger at forearm level

✓7ᵗʰ **S56.494** Other injury of extensor muscle, fascia and tendon of left middle finger at forearm level

✓7ᵗʰ **S56.495** Other injury of extensor muscle, fascia and tendon of right ring finger at forearm level

✓7ᵗʰ **S56.496** Other injury of extensor muscle, fascia and tendon of left ring finger at forearm level

✓7ᵗʰ **S56.497** Other injury of extensor muscle, fascia and tendon of right little finger at forearm level

✓7ᵗʰ **S56.498** Other injury of extensor muscle, fascia and tendon of left little finger at forearm level

✓7ᵗʰ **S56.499** Other injury of extensor muscle, fascia and tendon of unspecified finger at forearm level

✓5ᵗʰ **S56.5** Injury of other extensor muscle, fascia and tendon at forearm level

✓6ᵗʰ **S56.50** Unspecified injury of other extensor muscle, fascia and tendon at forearm level

✓7ᵗʰ **S56.501** Unspecified injury of other extensor muscle, fascia and tendon at forearm level, right arm

✓7ᵗʰ **S56.502** Unspecified injury of other extensor muscle, fascia and tendon at forearm level, left arm

✓7ᵗʰ **S56.509** Unspecified injury of other extensor muscle, fascia and tendon at forearm level, unspecified arm

✓6ᵗʰ **S56.51** Strain of other extensor muscle, fascia and tendon at forearm level

✓7ᵗʰ **S56.511** Strain of other extensor muscle, fascia and tendon at forearm level, right arm

✓7ᵗʰ **S56.512** Strain of other extensor muscle, fascia and tendon at forearm level, left arm

✓7ᵗʰ **S56.519** Strain of other extensor muscle, fascia and tendon at forearm level, unspecified arm

✓6ᵗʰ **S56.52** Laceration of other extensor muscle, fascia and tendon at forearm level

---

☑ Additional Character Required   ✓×7ᵗʰ Xtension Alert   Unspecified Dx   Other Specified Dx   Manifestation   ►◄ Revised Text   ● New Code   ▲ Revised Code Title

ICD-10-CM Draft (2015)   861

√7ᵗʰ **S56.521** **Laceration of other extensor muscle, fascia and tendon at forearm level,** right arm

√7ᵗʰ **S56.522** **Laceration of other extensor muscle, fascia and tendon at forearm level,** left arm

√7ᵗʰ **S56.529** **Laceration of other extensor muscle, fascia and tendon at forearm level, unspecified arm**

√6ᵗʰ **S56.59** Other **injury of other extensor muscle, fascia and tendon at forearm level**

√7ᵗʰ **S56.591** **Other injury of other extensor muscle, fascia and tendon at forearm level,** right arm

√7ᵗʰ **S56.592** **Other injury of other extensor muscle, fascia and tendon at forearm level,** left arm

√7ᵗʰ **S56.599** **Other injury of other extensor muscle, fascia and tendon at forearm level, unspecified arm**

√5ᵗʰ **S56.8** **Injury of** other **muscles, fascia and tendons at forearm level**

√6ᵗʰ **S56.80** Unspecified **injury of other muscles, fascia and tendons at forearm level**

√7ᵗʰ **S56.801** **Unspecified injury of other muscles, fascia and tendons at forearm level,** right arm

√7ᵗʰ **S56.802** **Unspecified injury of other muscles, fascia and tendons at forearm level,** left arm

√7ᵗʰ **S56.809** **Unspecified injury of other muscles, fascia and tendons at forearm level, unspecified arm**

√6ᵗʰ **S56.81** Strain **of other muscles, fascia and tendons at forearm level**

√7ᵗʰ **S56.811** **Strain of other muscles, fascia and tendons at forearm level,** right arm

√7ᵗʰ **S56.812** **Strain of other muscles, fascia and tendons at forearm level,** left arm

√7ᵗʰ **S56.819** **Strain of other muscles, fascia and tendons at forearm level, unspecified arm**

√6ᵗʰ **S56.82** Laceration **of other muscles, fascia and tendons at forearm level**

√7ᵗʰ **S56.821** **Laceration of other muscles, fascia and tendons at forearm level,** right arm

√7ᵗʰ **S56.822** **Laceration of other muscles, fascia and tendons at forearm level,** left arm

√7ᵗʰ **S56.829** **Laceration of other muscles, fascia and tendons at forearm level, unspecified arm**

√6ᵗʰ **S56.89** Other **injury of other muscles, fascia and tendons at forearm level**

√7ᵗʰ **S56.891** **Other injury of other muscles, fascia and tendons at forearm level,** right arm

√7ᵗʰ **S56.892** **Other injury of other muscles, fascia and tendons at forearm level,** left arm

√7ᵗʰ **S56.899** **Other injury of other muscles, fascia and tendons at forearm level, unspecified arm**

√5ᵗʰ **S56.9** **Injury of** unspecified **muscles, fascia and tendons at** forearm **level**

√6ᵗʰ **S56.90** Unspecified **injury of unspecified muscles, fascia and tendons at forearm level**

√7ᵗʰ **S56.901** **Unspecified injury of unspecified muscles, fascia and tendons at forearm level,** right arm

√7ᵗʰ **S56.902** **Unspecified injury of unspecified muscles, fascia and tendons at forearm level,** left arm

√7ᵗʰ **S56.909** **Unspecified injury of unspecified muscles, fascia and tendons at forearm level, unspecified arm**

√6ᵗʰ **S56.91** Strain **of unspecified muscles, fascia and tendons at forearm level**

√7ᵗʰ **S56.911** **Strain of unspecified muscles, fascia and tendons at forearm level,** right arm

√7ᵗʰ **S56.912** **Strain of unspecified muscles, fascia and tendons at forearm level,** left arm

√7ᵗʰ **S56.919** **Strain of unspecified muscles, fascia and tendons at forearm level, unspecified arm**

√6ᵗʰ **S56.92** Laceration **of unspecified muscles, fascia and tendons at forearm level**

√7ᵗʰ **S56.921** **Laceration of unspecified muscles, fascia and tendons at forearm level,** right arm

√7ᵗʰ **S56.922** **Laceration of unspecified muscles, fascia and tendons at forearm level,** left arm

√7ᵗʰ **S56.929** **Laceration of unspecified muscles, fascia and tendons at forearm level, unspecified arm**

√6ᵗʰ **S56.99** Other **injury of unspecified muscles, fascia and tendons at forearm level**

√7ᵗʰ **S56.991** **Other injury of unspecified muscles, fascia and tendons at forearm level,** right arm

√7ᵗʰ **S56.992** **Other injury of unspecified muscles, fascia and tendons at forearm level,** left arm

√7ᵗʰ **S56.999** **Other injury of unspecified muscles, fascia and tendons at forearm level, unspecified arm**

√4ᵗʰ **S57** **Crushing injury of elbow and forearm**
Use additional code(s) for all associated injuries
EXCLUDES 2 crushing injury of wrist and hand (S67.-)

The appropriate 7th character is to be added to each code from category S57.
A   initial encounter
D   subsequent encounter
S   sequela

√5ᵗʰ **S57.0** **Crushing injury of** elbow

√x 7ᵗʰ **S57.00** **Crushing injury of unspecified elbow**

√x 7ᵗʰ **S57.01** **Crushing injury of** right **elbow**

√x 7ᵗʰ **S57.02** **Crushing injury of** left **elbow**

√5ᵗʰ **S57.8** **Crushing injury of** forearm

√x 7ᵗʰ **S57.80** **Crushing injury of unspecified forearm**

√x 7ᵗʰ **S57.81** **Crushing injury of** right **forearm**

√x 7ᵗʰ **S57.82** **Crushing injury of** left **forearm**

√4ᵗʰ **S58** **Traumatic amputation of elbow and forearm**
NOTE   An amputation not identified as partial or complete should be coded to complete.
EXCLUDES 1 traumatic amputation of wrist and hand (S68.-)

The appropriate 7th character is to be added to each code from category S58.
A   initial encounter
D   subsequent encounter
S   sequela

√5ᵗʰ **S58.0** **Traumatic amputation at** elbow **level**

√6ᵗʰ **S58.01** Complete **traumatic amputation at elbow level**

√7ᵗʰ **S58.011** **Complete traumatic amputation at elbow level,** right arm

√7ᵗʰ **S58.012** **Complete traumatic amputation at elbow level,** left arm

√7ᵗʰ **S58.019** **Complete traumatic amputation at elbow level, unspecified arm**

√6ᵗʰ **S58.02** Partial **traumatic amputation at elbow level**

√7ᵗʰ **S58.021** **Partial traumatic amputation at elbow level,** right arm

√7ᵗʰ **S58.022** **Partial traumatic amputation at elbow level,** left arm

√7ᵗʰ **S58.029** **Partial traumatic amputation at elbow level, unspecified arm**

√5ᵗʰ **S58.1** **Traumatic amputation at level** between elbow and wrist

√6ᵗʰ **S58.11** Complete **traumatic amputation at level between elbow and wrist**

√7ᵗʰ **S58.111** **Complete traumatic amputation at level between elbow and wrist,** right arm

√7ᵗʰ **S58.112** **Complete traumatic amputation at level between elbow and wrist,** left arm

√7ᵗʰ **S58.119** **Complete traumatic amputation at level between elbow and wrist, unspecified arm**

√6ᵗʰ **S58.12** Partial **traumatic amputation at level between elbow and wrist**

√7ᵗʰ **S58.121** **Partial traumatic amputation at level between elbow and wrist,** right arm

EXCLUDES 1 Not coded here   EXCLUDES 2 Not included here   N Newborn Age: 0   P Pediatric Age: 0-17   M Maternity Age: 12-55   A Adult Age: 15-124

862   ICD-10-CM Draft (2015)

☑7ᵗʰ **S58.122**   Partial traumatic amputation at level between elbow and wrist, left arm

☑7ᵗʰ **S58.129**   Partial traumatic amputation at level between elbow and wrist, unspecified arm

☑5ᵗʰ **S58.9**   Traumatic amputation of forearm, level unspecified

    EXCLUDES 1   *traumatic amputation of wrist (S68.-)*

☑6ᵗʰ **S58.91**   Complete traumatic amputation of forearm, level unspecified

☑7ᵗʰ **S58.911**   Complete traumatic amputation of right forearm, level unspecified

☑7ᵗʰ **S58.912**   Complete traumatic amputation of left forearm, level unspecified

☑7ᵗʰ **S58.919**   Complete traumatic amputation of unspecified forearm, level unspecified

☑6ᵗʰ **S58.92**   Partial traumatic amputation of forearm, level unspecified

☑7ᵗʰ **S58.921**   Partial traumatic amputation of right forearm, level unspecified

☑7ᵗʰ **S58.922**   Partial traumatic amputation of left forearm, level unspecified

☑7ᵗʰ **S58.929**   Partial traumatic amputation of unspecified forearm, level unspecified

☑4ᵗʰ **S59**   **Other and unspecified injuries of elbow and forearm**

    EXCLUDES 2   *other and unspecified injuries of wrist and hand (S69.-)*

The appropriate 7th character is to be added to each code from subcategories S59.0, S59.1, and S59.2.
A   initial encounter for closed fracture
D   subsequent encounter for fracture with routine healing
G   subsequent encounter for fracture with delayed healing
K   subsequent encounter for fracture with nonunion
P   subsequent encounter for fracture with malunion
S   sequela

☑5ᵗʰ **S59.0**   Physeal fracture of lower end of ulna

☑6ᵗʰ **S59.00**   Unspecified physeal fracture of lower end of ulna

☑7ᵗʰ **S59.001**   Unspecified physeal fracture of lower end of ulna, right arm

☑7ᵗʰ **S59.002**   Unspecified physeal fracture of lower end of ulna, left arm

☑7ᵗʰ **S59.009**   Unspecified physeal fracture of lower end of ulna, unspecified arm

☑6ᵗʰ **S59.01**   Salter-Harris Type I physeal fracture of lower end of ulna

☑7ᵗʰ **S59.011**   Salter-Harris Type I physeal fracture of lower end of ulna, right arm

☑7ᵗʰ **S59.012**   Salter-Harris Type I physeal fracture of lower end of ulna, left arm

☑7ᵗʰ **S59.019**   Salter-Harris Type I physeal fracture of lower end of ulna, unspecified arm

☑6ᵗʰ **S59.02**   Salter-Harris Type II physeal fracture of lower end of ulna

☑7ᵗʰ **S59.021**   Salter-Harris Type II physeal fracture of lower end of ulna, right arm

☑7ᵗʰ **S59.022**   Salter-Harris Type II physeal fracture of lower end of ulna, left arm

☑7ᵗʰ **S59.029**   Salter-Harris Type II physeal fracture of lower end of ulna, unspecified arm

☑6ᵗʰ **S59.03**   Salter-Harris Type III physeal fracture of lower end of ulna

☑7ᵗʰ **S59.031**   Salter-Harris Type III physeal fracture of lower end of ulna, right arm

☑7ᵗʰ **S59.032**   Salter-Harris Type III physeal fracture of lower end of ulna, left arm

☑7ᵗʰ **S59.039**   Salter-Harris Type III physeal fracture of lower end of ulna, unspecified arm

☑6ᵗʰ **S59.04**   Salter-Harris Type IV physeal fracture of lower end of ulna

☑7ᵗʰ **S59.041**   Salter-Harris Type IV physeal fracture of lower end of ulna, right arm

☑7ᵗʰ **S59.042**   Salter-Harris Type IV physeal fracture of lower end of ulna, left arm

☑7ᵗʰ **S59.049**   Salter-Harris Type IV physeal fracture of lower end of ulna, unspecified arm

☑6ᵗʰ **S59.09**   Other physeal fracture of lower end of ulna

☑7ᵗʰ **S59.091**   Other physeal fracture of lower end of ulna, right arm

☑7ᵗʰ **S59.092**   Other physeal fracture of lower end of ulna, left arm

☑7ᵗʰ **S59.099**   Other physeal fracture of lower end of ulna, unspecified arm

☑5ᵗʰ **S59.1**   Physeal fracture of upper end of radius

☑6ᵗʰ **S59.10**   Unspecified physeal fracture of upper end of radius

☑7ᵗʰ **S59.101**   Unspecified physeal fracture of upper end of radius, right arm

☑7ᵗʰ **S59.102**   Unspecified physeal fracture of upper end of radius, left arm

☑7ᵗʰ **S59.109**   Unspecified physeal fracture of upper end of radius, unspecified arm

☑6ᵗʰ **S59.11**   Salter-Harris Type I physeal fracture of upper end of radius

☑7ᵗʰ **S59.111**   Salter-Harris Type I physeal fracture of upper end of radius, right arm

☑7ᵗʰ **S59.112**   Salter-Harris Type I physeal fracture of upper end of radius, left arm

☑7ᵗʰ **S59.119**   Salter-Harris Type I physeal fracture of upper end of radius, unspecified arm

☑6ᵗʰ **S59.12**   Salter-Harris Type II physeal fracture of upper end of radius

☑7ᵗʰ **S59.121**   Salter-Harris Type II physeal fracture of upper end of radius, right arm

☑7ᵗʰ **S59.122**   Salter-Harris Type II physeal fracture of upper end of radius, left arm

☑7ᵗʰ **S59.129**   Salter-Harris Type II physeal fracture of upper end of radius, unspecified arm

☑6ᵗʰ **S59.13**   Salter-Harris Type III physeal fracture of upper end of radius

☑7ᵗʰ **S59.131**   Salter-Harris Type III physeal fracture of upper end of radius, right arm

☑7ᵗʰ **S59.132**   Salter-Harris Type III physeal fracture of upper end of radius, left arm

☑7ᵗʰ **S59.139**   Salter-Harris Type III physeal fracture of upper end of radius, unspecified arm

☑6ᵗʰ **S59.14**   Salter-Harris Type IV physeal fracture of upper end of radius

☑7ᵗʰ **S59.141**   Salter-Harris Type IV physeal fracture of upper end of radius, right arm

☑7ᵗʰ **S59.142**   Salter-Harris Type IV physeal fracture of upper end of radius, left arm

☑7ᵗʰ **S59.149**   Salter-Harris Type IV physeal fracture of upper end of radius, unspecified arm

☑6ᵗʰ **S59.19**   Other physeal fracture of upper end of radius

☑7ᵗʰ **S59.191**   Other physeal fracture of upper end of radius, right arm

☑7ᵗʰ **S59.192**   Other physeal fracture of upper end of radius, left arm

☑7ᵗʰ **S59.199**   Other physeal fracture of upper end of radius, unspecified arm

☑5ᵗʰ **S59.2**   Physeal fracture of lower end of radius

☑6ᵗʰ **S59.20**   Unspecified physeal fracture of lower end of radius

☑7ᵗʰ **S59.201**   Unspecified physeal fracture of lower end of radius, right arm

☑7ᵗʰ **S59.202**   Unspecified physeal fracture of lower end of radius, left arm

☑7ᵗʰ **S59.209**   Unspecified physeal fracture of lower end of radius, unspecified arm

☑6ᵗʰ **S59.21**   Salter-Harris Type I physeal fracture of lower end of radius

☑7ᵗʰ **S59.211**   Salter-Harris Type I physeal fracture of lower end of radius, right arm

☑7ᵗʰ **S59.212**   Salter-Harris Type I physeal fracture of lower end of radius, left arm

☑7ᵗʰ **S59.219**   Salter-Harris Type I physeal fracture of lower end of radius, unspecified arm

☑6ᵗʰ **S59.22**   Salter-Harris Type II physeal fracture of lower end of radius

☑7ᵗʰ **S59.221**   Salter-Harris Type II physeal fracture of lower end of radius, right arm

☑7ᵗʰ **S59.222**   Salter-Harris Type II physeal fracture of lower end of radius, left arm

☑7ᵗʰ **S59.229**   Salter-Harris Type II physeal fracture of lower end of radius, unspecified arm

---

☑ Additional Character Required   ☑x7ᵗʰ Xtension Alert   Unspecified Dx   Other Specified Dx   Manifestation   ▶◀ Revised Text   ● New Code   ▲ Revised Code Title

  ✓6ᵗʰ **S59.23** Salter-Harris Type III physeal fracture of lower end of radius

    ✓7ᵗʰ **S59.231** Salter-Harris Type III physeal fracture of lower end of radius, right arm

    ✓7ᵗʰ **S59.232** Salter-Harris Type III physeal fracture of lower end of radius, left arm

    ✓7ᵗʰ **S59.239** Salter-Harris Type III physeal fracture of lower end of radius, unspecified arm

  ✓6ᵗʰ **S59.24** Salter-Harris Type IV physeal fracture of lower end of radius

    ✓7ᵗʰ **S59.241** Salter-Harris Type IV physeal fracture of lower end of radius, right arm

    ✓7ᵗʰ **S59.242** Salter-Harris Type IV physeal fracture of lower end of radius, left arm

    ✓7ᵗʰ **S59.249** Salter-Harris Type IV physeal fracture of lower end of radius, unspecified arm

  ✓6ᵗʰ **S59.29** Other physeal fracture of lower end of radius

    ✓7ᵗʰ **S59.291** Other physeal fracture of lower end of radius, right arm

    ✓7ᵗʰ **S59.292** Other physeal fracture of lower end of radius, left arm

    ✓7ᵗʰ **S59.299** Other physeal fracture of lower end of radius, unspecified arm

 ✓5ᵗʰ **S59.8** Other specified injuries of elbow and forearm

> The appropriate 7th character is to be added to each code in subcategory S59.8.
> A   initial encounter
> D   subsequent encounter
> S   sequela

  ✓6ᵗʰ **S59.80** Other specified injuries of elbow

    ✓7ᵗʰ **S59.801** Other specified injuries of right elbow

    ✓7ᵗʰ **S59.802** Other specified injuries of left elbow

    ✓7ᵗʰ **S59.809** Other specified injuries of unspecified elbow

  ✓6ᵗʰ **S59.81** Other specified injuries of forearm

    ✓7ᵗʰ **S59.811** Other specified injuries right forearm

    ✓7ᵗʰ **S59.812** Other specified injuries left forearm

    ✓7ᵗʰ **S59.819** Other specified injuries unspecified forearm

 ✓5ᵗʰ **S59.9** Unspecified injury of elbow and forearm

> The appropriate 7th character is to be added to each code in subcategory S59.9.
> A   initial encounter
> D   subsequent encounter
> S   sequela

  ✓6ᵗʰ **S59.90** Unspecified injury of elbow

    ✓7ᵗʰ **S59.901** Unspecified injury of right elbow

    ✓7ᵗʰ **S59.902** Unspecified injury of left elbow

    ✓7ᵗʰ **S59.909** Unspecified injury of unspecified elbow

  ✓6ᵗʰ **S59.91** Unspecified injury of forearm

    ✓7ᵗʰ **S59.911** Unspecified injury of right forearm

    ✓7ᵗʰ **S59.912** Unspecified injury of left forearm

    ✓7ᵗʰ **S59.919** Unspecified injury of unspecified forearm

Injuries to the wrist, hand and fingers (S60-S69)

EXCLUDES 2   burns and corrosions (T20-T32)
frostbite (T33-T34)
insect bite or sting, venomous (T63.4)

✓4ᵗʰ **S60** Superficial injury of wrist, hand and fingers

> The appropriate 7th character is to be added to each code from category S60.
> A   initial encounter
> D   subsequent encounter
> S   sequela

 ✓5ᵗʰ **S60.0** Contusion of finger without damage to nail

> EXCLUDES 1   contusion involving nail (matrix) (S60.1)

  ✓x7ᵗʰ **S60.00** Contusion of unspecified finger without damage to nail

> Contusion of finger(s) NOS

  ✓6ᵗʰ **S60.01** Contusion of thumb without damage to nail

    ✓7ᵗʰ **S60.011** Contusion of right thumb without damage to nail

    ✓7ᵗʰ **S60.012** Contusion of left thumb without damage to nail

    ✓7ᵗʰ **S60.019** Contusion of unspecified thumb without damage to nail

  ✓6ᵗʰ **S60.02** Contusion of index finger without damage to nail

    ✓7ᵗʰ **S60.021** Contusion of right index finger without damage to nail

    ✓7ᵗʰ **S60.022** Contusion of left index finger without damage to nail

    ✓7ᵗʰ **S60.029** Contusion of unspecified index finger without damage to nail

  ✓6ᵗʰ **S60.03** Contusion of middle finger without damage to nail

    ✓7ᵗʰ **S60.031** Contusion of right middle finger without damage to nail

    ✓7ᵗʰ **S60.032** Contusion of left middle finger without damage to nail

    ✓7ᵗʰ **S60.039** Contusion of unspecified middle finger without damage to nail

  ✓6ᵗʰ **S60.04** Contusion of ring finger without damage to nail

    ✓7ᵗʰ **S60.041** Contusion of right ring finger without damage to nail

    ✓7ᵗʰ **S60.042** Contusion of left ring finger without damage to nail

    ✓7ᵗʰ **S60.049** Contusion of unspecified ring finger without damage to nail

  ✓6ᵗʰ **S60.05** Contusion of little finger without damage to nail

    ✓7ᵗʰ **S60.051** Contusion of right little finger without damage to nail

    ✓7ᵗʰ **S60.052** Contusion of left little finger without damage to nail

    ✓7ᵗʰ **S60.059** Contusion of unspecified little finger without damage to nail

 ✓5ᵗʰ **S60.1** Contusion of finger with damage to nail

  ✓x7ᵗʰ **S60.10** Contusion of unspecified finger with damage to nail

  ✓6ᵗʰ **S60.11** Contusion of thumb with damage to nail

    ✓7ᵗʰ **S60.111** Contusion of right thumb with damage to nail

    ✓7ᵗʰ **S60.112** Contusion of left thumb with damage to nail

    ✓7ᵗʰ **S60.119** Contusion of unspecified thumb with damage to nail

  ✓6ᵗʰ **S60.12** Contusion of index finger with damage to nail

    ✓7ᵗʰ **S60.121** Contusion of right index finger with damage to nail

    ✓7ᵗʰ **S60.122** Contusion of left index finger with damage to nail

    ✓7ᵗʰ **S60.129** Contusion of unspecified index finger with damage to nail

  ✓6ᵗʰ **S60.13** Contusion of middle finger with damage to nail

    ✓7ᵗʰ **S60.131** Contusion of right middle finger with damage to nail

    ✓7ᵗʰ **S60.132** Contusion of left middle finger with damage to nail

    ✓7ᵗʰ **S60.139** Contusion of unspecified middle finger with damage to nail

  ✓6ᵗʰ **S60.14** Contusion of ring finger with damage to nail

    ✓7ᵗʰ **S60.141** Contusion of right ring finger with damage to nail

    ✓7ᵗʰ **S60.142** Contusion of left ring finger with damage to nail

    ✓7ᵗʰ **S60.149** Contusion of unspecified ring finger with damage to nail

  ✓6ᵗʰ **S60.15** Contusion of little finger with damage to nail

    ✓7ᵗʰ **S60.151** Contusion of right little finger with damage to nail

    ✓7ᵗʰ **S60.152** Contusion of left little finger with damage to nail

    ✓7ᵗʰ **S60.159** Contusion of unspecified little finger with damage to nail

 ✓5ᵗʰ **S60.2** Contusion of wrist and hand

> EXCLUDES 2   contusion of fingers (S60.0-, S60.1-)

EXCLUDES 1 Not coded here   EXCLUDES 2 Not included here   Ⓝ Newborn Age: 0   Ⓟ Pediatric Age: 0-17   Ⓜ Maternity Age: 12-55   Ⓐ Adult Age: 15-124

✓6th **S60.21** Contusion of wrist
　✓7th **S60.211** Contusion of right wrist
　✓7th **S60.212** Contusion of left wrist
　✓7th **S60.219** Contusion of unspecified wrist
✓6th **S60.22** Contusion of hand
　✓7th **S60.221** Contusion of right hand
　✓7th **S60.222** Contusion of left hand
　✓7th **S60.229** Contusion of unspecified hand
✓5th **S60.3** Other superficial injuries of thumb
　✓6th **S60.31** Abrasion of thumb
　　✓7th **S60.311** Abrasion of right thumb
　　✓7th **S60.312** Abrasion of left thumb
　　✓7th **S60.319** Abrasion of unspecified thumb
　✓6th **S60.32** Blister (nonthermal) of thumb
　　✓7th **S60.321** Blister (nonthermal) of right thumb
　　✓7th **S60.322** Blister (nonthermal) of left thumb
　　✓7th **S60.329** Blister (nonthermal) of unspecified thumb
　✓6th **S60.34** External constriction of thumb
　　　Hair tourniquet syndrome of thumb
　　　Use additional cause code to identify the constricting item (W49.0-)
　　✓7th **S60.341** External constriction of right thumb
　　✓7th **S60.342** External constriction of left thumb
　　✓7th **S60.349** External constriction of unspecified thumb
　✓6th **S60.35** Superficial foreign body of thumb
　　　Splinter in the thumb
　　✓7th **S60.351** Superficial foreign body of right thumb
　　✓7th **S60.352** Superficial foreign body of left thumb
　　✓7th **S60.359** Superficial foreign body of unspecified thumb
　✓6th **S60.36** Insect bite (nonvenomous) of thumb
　　✓7th **S60.361** Insect bite (nonvenomous) of right thumb
　　✓7th **S60.362** Insect bite (nonvenomous) of left thumb
　　✓7th **S60.369** Insect bite (nonvenomous) of unspecified thumb
　✓6th **S60.37** Other superficial bite of thumb
　　　EXCLUDES 1　open bite of thumb (S61.05-, S61.15-)
　　✓7th **S60.371** Other superficial bite of right thumb
　　✓7th **S60.372** Other superficial bite of left thumb
　　✓7th **S60.379** Other superficial bite of unspecified thumb
　✓6th **S60.39** Other superficial injuries of thumb
　　✓7th **S60.391** Other superficial injuries of right thumb
　　✓7th **S60.392** Other superficial injuries of left thumb
　　✓7th **S60.399** Other superficial injuries of unspecified thumb
✓5th **S60.4** Other superficial injuries of other fingers
　✓6th **S60.41** Abrasion of fingers
　　✓7th **S60.410** Abrasion of right index finger
　　✓7th **S60.411** Abrasion of left index finger
　　✓7th **S60.412** Abrasion of right middle finger
　　✓7th **S60.413** Abrasion of left middle finger
　　✓7th **S60.414** Abrasion of right ring finger
　　✓7th **S60.415** Abrasion of left ring finger
　　✓7th **S60.416** Abrasion of right little finger
　　✓7th **S60.417** Abrasion of left little finger
　　✓7th **S60.418** Abrasion of other finger
　　　　Abrasion of specified finger with unspecified laterality
　　✓7th **S60.419** Abrasion of unspecified finger
　✓6th **S60.42** Blister (nonthermal) of fingers
　　✓7th **S60.420** Blister (nonthermal) of right index finger
　　✓7th **S60.421** Blister (nonthermal) of left index finger
　　✓7th **S60.422** Blister (nonthermal) of right middle finger
　　✓7th **S60.423** Blister (nonthermal) of left middle finger
　　✓7th **S60.424** Blister (nonthermal) of right ring finger
　　✓7th **S60.425** Blister (nonthermal) of left ring finger
　　✓7th **S60.426** Blister (nonthermal) of right little finger

　　✓7th **S60.427** Blister (nonthermal) of left little finger
　　✓7th **S60.428** Blister (nonthermal) of other finger
　　　　Blister (nonthermal) of specified finger with unspecified laterality
　　✓7th **S60.429** Blister (nonthermal) of unspecified finger
　✓6th **S60.44** External constriction of fingers
　　　Hair tourniquet syndrome of finger
　　　Use additional cause code to identify the constricting item (W49.0-)
　　✓7th **S60.440** External constriction of right index finger
　　✓7th **S60.441** External constriction of left index finger
　　✓7th **S60.442** External constriction of right middle finger
　　✓7th **S60.443** External constriction of left middle finger
　　✓7th **S60.444** External constriction of right ring finger
　　✓7th **S60.445** External constriction of left ring finger
　　✓7th **S60.446** External constriction of right little finger
　　✓7th **S60.447** External constriction of left little finger
　　✓7th **S60.448** External constriction of other finger
　　　　External constriction of specified finger with unspecified laterality
　　✓7th **S60.449** External constriction of unspecified finger
　✓6th **S60.45** Superficial foreign body of fingers
　　　Splinter in the finger(s)
　　✓7th **S60.450** Superficial foreign body of right index finger
　　✓7th **S60.451** Superficial foreign body of left index finger
　　✓7th **S60.452** Superficial foreign body of right middle finger
　　✓7th **S60.453** Superficial foreign body of left middle finger
　　✓7th **S60.454** Superficial foreign body of right ring finger
　　✓7th **S60.455** Superficial foreign body of left ring finger
　　✓7th **S60.456** Superficial foreign body of right little finger
　　✓7th **S60.457** Superficial foreign body of left little finger
　　✓7th **S60.458** Superficial foreign body of other finger
　　　　Superficial foreign body of specified finger with unspecified laterality
　　✓7th **S60.459** Superficial foreign body of unspecified finger
　✓6th **S60.46** Insect bite (nonvenomous) of fingers
　　✓7th **S60.460** Insect bite (nonvenomous) of right index finger
　　✓7th **S60.461** Insect bite (nonvenomous) of left index finger
　　✓7th **S60.462** Insect bite (nonvenomous) of right middle finger
　　✓7th **S60.463** Insect bite (nonvenomous) of left middle finger
　　✓7th **S60.464** Insect bite (nonvenomous) of right ring finger
　　✓7th **S60.465** Insect bite (nonvenomous) of left ring finger
　　✓7th **S60.466** Insect bite (nonvenomous) of right little finger
　　✓7th **S60.467** Insect bite (nonvenomous) of left little finger
　　✓7th **S60.468** Insect bite (nonvenomous) of other finger
　　　　Insect bite (nonvenomous) of specified finger with unspecified laterality
　　✓7th **S60.469** Insect bite (nonvenomous) of unspecified finger
　✓6th **S60.47** Other superficial bite of fingers
　　　EXCLUDES 1　open bite of fingers (S61.25-, S61.35-)
　　✓7th **S60.470** Other superficial bite of right index finger
　　✓7th **S60.471** Other superficial bite of left index finger
　　✓7th **S60.472** Other superficial bite of right middle finger
　　✓7th **S60.473** Other superficial bite of left middle finger
　　✓7th **S60.474** Other superficial bite of right ring finger
　　✓7th **S60.475** Other superficial bite of left ring finger

√7ᵗʰ **S60.476** Other superficial bite of right little finger
√7ᵗʰ **S60.477** Other superficial bite of left little finger
√7ᵗʰ **S60.478** Other superficial bite of other finger
Other superficial bite of specified finger with unspecified laterality
√7ᵗʰ **S60.479** Other superficial bite of unspecified finger

√5ᵗʰ **S60.5** **Other superficial injuries of** hand
    EXCLUDES 2 *superficial injuries of fingers (S60.3-, S60.4-)*

√6ᵗʰ **S60.51** **Abrasion** of hand
√7ᵗʰ **S60.511** Abrasion of right hand
√7ᵗʰ **S60.512** Abrasion of left hand
√7ᵗʰ **S60.519** Abrasion of unspecified hand

√6ᵗʰ **S60.52** **Blister** (nonthermal) of hand
√7ᵗʰ **S60.521** Blister (nonthermal) of right hand
√7ᵗʰ **S60.522** Blister (nonthermal) of left hand
√7ᵗʰ **S60.529** Blister (nonthermal) of unspecified hand

√6ᵗʰ **S60.54** **External constriction** of hand
√7ᵗʰ **S60.541** External constriction of right hand
√7ᵗʰ **S60.542** External constriction of left hand
√7ᵗʰ **S60.549** External constriction of unspecified hand

√6ᵗʰ **S60.55** **Superficial** foreign body of hand
Splinter in the hand
√7ᵗʰ **S60.551** Superficial foreign body of right hand
√7ᵗʰ **S60.552** Superficial foreign body of left hand
√7ᵗʰ **S60.559** Superficial foreign body of unspecified hand

√6ᵗʰ **S60.56** **Insect bite** (nonvenomous) of hand
√7ᵗʰ **S60.561** Insect bite (nonvenomous) of right hand
√7ᵗʰ **S60.562** Insect bite (nonvenomous) of left hand
√7ᵗʰ **S60.569** Insect bite (nonvenomous) of unspecified hand

√6ᵗʰ **S60.57** **Other superficial** bite of hand
    EXCLUDES 1 *open bite of hand (S61.45-)*
√7ᵗʰ **S60.571** Other superficial bite of hand of right hand
√7ᵗʰ **S60.572** Other superficial bite of hand of left hand
√7ᵗʰ **S60.579** Other superficial bite of hand of unspecified hand

√5ᵗʰ **S60.8** **Other superficial injuries of** wrist

√6ᵗʰ **S60.81** **Abrasion** of wrist
√7ᵗʰ **S60.811** Abrasion of right wrist
√7ᵗʰ **S60.812** Abrasion of left wrist
√7ᵗʰ **S60.819** Abrasion of unspecified wrist

√6ᵗʰ **S60.82** **Blister** (nonthermal) of wrist
√7ᵗʰ **S60.821** Blister (nonthermal) of right wrist
√7ᵗʰ **S60.822** Blister (nonthermal) of left wrist
√7ᵗʰ **S60.829** Blister (nonthermal) of unspecified wrist

√6ᵗʰ **S60.84** **External constriction** of wrist
√7ᵗʰ **S60.841** External constriction of right wrist
√7ᵗʰ **S60.842** External constriction of left wrist
√7ᵗʰ **S60.849** External constriction of unspecified wrist

√6ᵗʰ **S60.85** **Superficial** foreign body of wrist
Splinter in the wrist
√7ᵗʰ **S60.851** Superficial foreign body of right wrist
√7ᵗʰ **S60.852** Superficial foreign body of left wrist
√7ᵗʰ **S60.859** Superficial foreign body of unspecified wrist

√6ᵗʰ **S60.86** **Insect bite** (nonvenomous) of wrist
√7ᵗʰ **S60.861** Insect bite (nonvenomous) of right wrist
√7ᵗʰ **S60.862** Insect bite (nonvenomous) of left wrist
√7ᵗʰ **S60.869** Insect bite (nonvenomous) of unspecified wrist

√6ᵗʰ **S60.87** **Other superficial** bite of wrist
    EXCLUDES 1 *open bite of wrist (S61.55)*
√7ᵗʰ **S60.871** Other superficial bite of right wrist
√7ᵗʰ **S60.872** Other superficial bite of left wrist
√7ᵗʰ **S60.879** Other superficial bite of unspecified wrist

√5ᵗʰ **S60.9** **Unspecified** superficial injury of wrist, hand and fingers

√6ᵗʰ **S60.91** **Unspecified superficial injury of** wrist

√7ᵗʰ **S60.911** Unspecified superficial injury of right wrist
√7ᵗʰ **S60.912** Unspecified superficial injury of left wrist
√7ᵗʰ **S60.919** Unspecified superficial injury of unspecified wrist

√6ᵗʰ **S60.92** **Unspecified superficial injury of** hand
√7ᵗʰ **S60.921** Unspecified superficial injury of right hand
√7ᵗʰ **S60.922** Unspecified superficial injury of left hand
√7ᵗʰ **S60.929** Unspecified superficial injury of unspecified hand

√6ᵗʰ **S60.93** **Unspecified superficial injury of** thumb
√7ᵗʰ **S60.931** Unspecified superficial injury of right thumb
√7ᵗʰ **S60.932** Unspecified superficial injury of left thumb
√7ᵗʰ **S60.939** Unspecified superficial injury of unspecified thumb

√6ᵗʰ **S60.94** **Unspecified superficial injury of other** fingers
√7ᵗʰ **S60.940** Unspecified superficial injury of right index finger
√7ᵗʰ **S60.941** Unspecified superficial injury of left index finger
√7ᵗʰ **S60.942** Unspecified superficial injury of right middle finger
√7ᵗʰ **S60.943** Unspecified superficial injury of left middle finger
√7ᵗʰ **S60.944** Unspecified superficial injury of right ring finger
√7ᵗʰ **S60.945** Unspecified superficial injury of left ring finger
√7ᵗʰ **S60.946** Unspecified superficial injury of right little finger
√7ᵗʰ **S60.947** Unspecified superficial injury of left little finger
√7ᵗʰ **S60.948** Unspecified superficial injury of other finger
Unspecified superficial injury of specified finger with unspecified laterality
√7ᵗʰ **S60.949** Unspecified superficial injury of unspecified finger

√4ᵗʰ **S61** **Open wound of wrist, hand and fingers**
Code also any associated wound infection
    EXCLUDES 1 *open fracture of wrist, hand and finger (S62- with 7th character B)*
       traumatic amputation of wrist and hand (S68.-)

The appropriate 7th character is to be added to each code from category S61.
A   initial encounter
D   subsequent encounter
S   sequela

√5ᵗʰ **S61.0** **Open wound of** thumb without damage to nail
    EXCLUDES 1 *open wound of thumb with damage to nail (S61.1-)*

√6ᵗʰ **S61.00** **Unspecified** open wound of thumb without damage to nail
√7ᵗʰ **S61.001** Unspecified open wound of right thumb without damage to nail
√7ᵗʰ **S61.002** Unspecified open wound of left thumb without damage to nail
√7ᵗʰ **S61.009** Unspecified open wound of unspecified thumb without damage to nail

√6ᵗʰ **S61.01** **Laceration without foreign body** of thumb without damage to nail
√7ᵗʰ **S61.011** Laceration without foreign body of right thumb without damage to nail
√7ᵗʰ **S61.012** Laceration without foreign body of left thumb without damage to nail
√7ᵗʰ **S61.019** Laceration without foreign body of unspecified thumb without damage to nail

√6ᵗʰ **S61.02** **Laceration with foreign body** of thumb without damage to nail
√7ᵗʰ **S61.021** Laceration with foreign body of right thumb without damage to nail

☑7ᵗʰ **S61.022** Laceration with foreign body of left thumb without damage to nail

☑7ᵗʰ **S61.029** Laceration with foreign body of unspecified thumb without damage to nail

☑6ᵗʰ **S61.03** Puncture wound without foreign body of thumb without damage to nail

☑7ᵗʰ **S61.031** Puncture wound without foreign body of right thumb without damage to nail

☑7ᵗʰ **S61.032** Puncture wound without foreign body of left thumb without damage to nail

☑7ᵗʰ **S61.039** Puncture wound without foreign body of unspecified thumb without damage to nail

☑6ᵗʰ **S61.04** Puncture wound with foreign body of thumb without damage to nail

☑7ᵗʰ **S61.041** Puncture wound with foreign body of right thumb without damage to nail

☑7ᵗʰ **S61.042** Puncture wound with foreign body of left thumb without damage to nail

☑7ᵗʰ **S61.049** Puncture wound with foreign body of unspecified thumb without damage to nail

☑6ᵗʰ **S61.05** Open bite of thumb without damage to nail
Bite of thumb NOS
EXCLUDES 1 *superficial bite of thumb (S60.36-, S60.37-)*

☑7ᵗʰ **S61.051** Open bite of right thumb without damage to nail

☑7ᵗʰ **S61.052** Open bite of left thumb without damage to nail

☑7ᵗʰ **S61.059** Open bite of unspecified thumb without damage to nail

☑5ᵗʰ **S61.1** Open wound of thumb with damage to nail

☑6ᵗʰ **S61.10** Unspecified open wound of thumb with damage to nail

☑7ᵗʰ **S61.101** Unspecified open wound of right thumb with damage to nail

☑7ᵗʰ **S61.102** Unspecified open wound of left thumb with damage to nail

☑7ᵗʰ **S61.109** Unspecified open wound of unspecified thumb with damage to nail

☑6ᵗʰ **S61.11** Laceration without foreign body of thumb with damage to nail

☑7ᵗʰ **S61.111** Laceration without foreign body of right thumb with damage to nail

☑7ᵗʰ **S61.112** Laceration without foreign body of left thumb with damage to nail

☑7ᵗʰ **S61.119** Laceration without foreign body of unspecified thumb with damage to nail

☑6ᵗʰ **S61.12** Laceration with foreign body of thumb with damage to nail

☑7ᵗʰ **S61.121** Laceration with foreign body of right thumb with damage to nail

☑7ᵗʰ **S61.122** Laceration with foreign body of left thumb with damage to nail

☑7ᵗʰ **S61.129** Laceration with foreign body of unspecified thumb with damage to nail

☑6ᵗʰ **S61.13** Puncture wound without foreign body of thumb with damage to nail

☑7ᵗʰ **S61.131** Puncture wound without foreign body of right thumb with damage to nail

☑7ᵗʰ **S61.132** Puncture wound without foreign body of left thumb with damage to nail

☑7ᵗʰ **S61.139** Puncture wound without foreign body of unspecified thumb with damage to nail

☑6ᵗʰ **S61.14** Puncture wound with foreign body of thumb with damage to nail

☑7ᵗʰ **S61.141** Puncture wound with foreign body of right thumb with damage to nail

☑7ᵗʰ **S61.142** Puncture wound with foreign body of left thumb with damage to nail

☑7ᵗʰ **S61.149** Puncture wound with foreign body of unspecified thumb with damage to nail

☑6ᵗʰ **S61.15** Open bite of thumb with damage to nail
Bite of thumb with damage to nail NOS
EXCLUDES 1 *superficial bite of thumb (S60.36-, S60.37-)*

☑7ᵗʰ **S61.151** Open bite of right thumb with damage to nail

☑7ᵗʰ **S61.152** Open bite of left thumb with damage to nail

☑7ᵗʰ **S61.159** Open bite of unspecified thumb with damage to nail

☑5ᵗʰ **S61.2** Open wound of other finger without damage to nail
EXCLUDES 1 *open wound of finger involving nail (matrix) (S61.3-)*
EXCLUDES 2 *open wound of thumb without damage to nail (S61.0-)*

☑6ᵗʰ **S61.20** Unspecified open wound of other finger without damage to nail

☑7ᵗʰ **S61.200** Unspecified open wound of right index finger without damage to nail

☑7ᵗʰ **S61.201** Unspecified open wound of left index finger without damage to nail

☑7ᵗʰ **S61.202** Unspecified open wound of right middle finger without damage to nail

☑7ᵗʰ **S61.203** Unspecified open wound of left middle finger without damage to nail

☑7ᵗʰ **S61.204** Unspecified open wound of right ring finger without damage to nail

☑7ᵗʰ **S61.205** Unspecified open wound of left ring finger without damage to nail

☑7ᵗʰ **S61.206** Unspecified open wound of right little finger without damage to nail

☑7ᵗʰ **S61.207** Unspecified open wound of left little finger without damage to nail

☑7ᵗʰ **S61.208** Unspecified open wound of other finger without damage to nail
Unspecified open wound of specified finger with unspecified laterality without damage to nail

☑7ᵗʰ **S61.209** Unspecified open wound of unspecified finger without damage to nail

☑6ᵗʰ **S61.21** Laceration without foreign body of finger without damage to nail

☑7ᵗʰ **S61.210** Laceration without foreign body of right index finger without damage to nail

☑7ᵗʰ **S61.211** Laceration without foreign body of left index finger without damage to nail

☑7ᵗʰ **S61.212** Laceration without foreign body of right middle finger without damage to nail

☑7ᵗʰ **S61.213** Laceration without foreign body of left middle finger without damage to nail

☑7ᵗʰ **S61.214** Laceration without foreign body of right ring finger without damage to nail

☑7ᵗʰ **S61.215** Laceration without foreign body of left ring finger without damage to nail

☑7ᵗʰ **S61.216** Laceration without foreign body of right little finger without damage to nail

☑7ᵗʰ **S61.217** Laceration without foreign body of left little finger without damage to nail

☑7ᵗʰ **S61.218** Laceration without foreign body of other finger without damage to nail
Laceration without foreign body of specified finger with unspecified laterality without damage to nail

☑7ᵗʰ **S61.219** Laceration without foreign body of unspecified finger without damage to nail

☑6ᵗʰ **S61.22** Laceration with foreign body of finger without damage to nail

☑7ᵗʰ **S61.220** Laceration with foreign body of right index finger without damage to nail

☑7ᵗʰ **S61.221** Laceration with foreign body of left index finger without damage to nail

☑7ᵗʰ **S61.222** Laceration with foreign body of right middle finger without damage to nail

☑7ᵗʰ **S61.223** Laceration with foreign body of left middle finger without damage to nail

☑7ᵗʰ **S61.224** Laceration with foreign body of right ring finger without damage to nail

☑7ᵗʰ **S61.225** Laceration with foreign body of left ring finger without damage to nail

☑7ᵗʰ **S61.226** Laceration with foreign body of right little finger without damage to nail

☑ Additional Character Required   ☑7ᵗʰ Xtension Alert   Unspecified Dx   Other Specified Dx   Manifestation   ▶◀ Revised Text   ● New Code   ▲ Revised Code Title

ICD-10-CM Draft (2015)   **867**

✓7ᵗʰ S61.227 Laceration with foreign body of left little finger without damage to nail

✓7ᵗʰ S61.228 Laceration with foreign body of other finger without damage to nail
Laceration with foreign body of specified finger with unspecified laterality without damage to nail

✓7ᵗʰ S61.229 Laceration with foreign body of unspecified finger without damage to nail

✓6ᵗʰ S61.23 Puncture wound without foreign body of finger without damage to nail

✓7ᵗʰ S61.230 Puncture wound without foreign body of right index finger without damage to nail

✓7ᵗʰ S61.231 Puncture wound without foreign body of left index finger without damage to nail

✓7ᵗʰ S61.232 Puncture wound without foreign body of right middle finger without damage to nail

✓7ᵗʰ S61.233 Puncture wound without foreign body of left middle finger without damage to nail

✓7ᵗʰ S61.234 Puncture wound without foreign body of right ring finger without damage to nail

✓7ᵗʰ S61.235 Puncture wound without foreign body of left ring finger without damage to nail

✓7ᵗʰ S61.236 Puncture wound without foreign body of right little finger without damage to nail

✓7ᵗʰ S61.237 Puncture wound without foreign body of left little finger without damage to nail

✓7ᵗʰ S61.238 Puncture wound without foreign body of other finger without damage to nail
Puncture wound without foreign body of specified finger with unspecified laterality without damage to nail

✓7ᵗʰ S61.239 Puncture wound without foreign body of unspecified finger without damage to nail

✓6ᵗʰ S61.24 Puncture wound with foreign body of finger without damage to nail

✓7ᵗʰ S61.240 Puncture wound with foreign body of right index finger without damage to nail

✓7ᵗʰ S61.241 Puncture wound with foreign body of left index finger without damage to nail

✓7ᵗʰ S61.242 Puncture wound with foreign body of right middle finger without damage to nail

✓7ᵗʰ S61.243 Puncture wound with foreign body of left middle finger without damage to nail

✓7ᵗʰ S61.244 Puncture wound with foreign body of right ring finger without damage to nail

✓7ᵗʰ S61.245 Puncture wound with foreign body of left ring finger without damage to nail

✓7ᵗʰ S61.246 Puncture wound with foreign body of right little finger without damage to nail

✓7ᵗʰ S61.247 Puncture wound with foreign body of left little finger without damage to nail

✓7ᵗʰ S61.248 Puncture wound with foreign body of other finger without damage to nail
Puncture wound with foreign body of specified finger with unspecified laterality without damage to nail

✓7ᵗʰ S61.249 Puncture wound with foreign body of unspecified finger without damage to nail

✓6ᵗʰ S61.25 Open bite of finger without damage to nail
Bite of finger without damage to nail NOS
EXCLUDES 1 superficial bite of finger (S60.46-, S60.47-)

✓7ᵗʰ S61.250 Open bite of right index finger without damage to nail

✓7ᵗʰ S61.251 Open bite of left index finger without damage to nail

✓7ᵗʰ S61.252 Open bite of right middle finger without damage to nail

✓7ᵗʰ S61.253 Open bite of left middle finger without damage to nail

✓7ᵗʰ S61.254 Open bite of right ring finger without damage to nail

✓7ᵗʰ S61.255 Open bite of left ring finger without damage to nail

✓7ᵗʰ S61.256 Open bite of right little finger without damage to nail

✓7ᵗʰ S61.257 Open bite of left little finger without damage to nail

✓7ᵗʰ S61.258 Open bite of other finger without damage to nail
Open bite of specified finger with unspecified laterality without damage to nail

✓7ᵗʰ S61.259 Open bite of unspecified finger without damage to nail

✓5ᵗʰ S61.3 Open wound of other finger with damage to nail

✓6ᵗʰ S61.30 Unspecified open wound of finger with damage to nail

✓7ᵗʰ S61.300 Unspecified open wound of right index finger with damage to nail

✓7ᵗʰ S61.301 Unspecified open wound of left index finger with damage to nail

✓7ᵗʰ S61.302 Unspecified open wound of right middle finger with damage to nail

✓7ᵗʰ S61.303 Unspecified open wound of left middle finger with damage to nail

✓7ᵗʰ S61.304 Unspecified open wound of right ring finger with damage to nail

✓7ᵗʰ S61.305 Unspecified open wound of left ring finger with damage to nail

✓7ᵗʰ S61.306 Unspecified open wound of right little finger with damage to nail

✓7ᵗʰ S61.307 Unspecified open wound of left little finger with damage to nail

✓7ᵗʰ S61.308 Unspecified open wound of other finger with damage to nail
Unspecified open wound of specified finger with unspecified laterality with damage to nail

✓7ᵗʰ S61.309 Unspecified open wound of unspecified finger with damage to nail

✓6ᵗʰ S61.31 Laceration without foreign body of finger with damage to nail

✓7ᵗʰ S61.310 Laceration without foreign body of right index finger with damage to nail

✓7ᵗʰ S61.311 Laceration without foreign body of left index finger with damage to nail

✓7ᵗʰ S61.312 Laceration without foreign body of right middle finger with damage to nail

✓7ᵗʰ S61.313 Laceration without foreign body of left middle finger with damage to nail

✓7ᵗʰ S61.314 Laceration without foreign body of right ring finger with damage to nail

✓7ᵗʰ S61.315 Laceration without foreign body of left ring finger with damage to nail

✓7ᵗʰ S61.316 Laceration without foreign body of right little finger with damage to nail

✓7ᵗʰ S61.317 Laceration without foreign body of left little finger with damage to nail

✓7ᵗʰ S61.318 Laceration without foreign body of other finger with damage to nail
Laceration without foreign body of specified finger with unspecified laterality with damage to nail

✓7ᵗʰ S61.319 Laceration without foreign body of unspecified finger with damage to nail

✓6ᵗʰ S61.32 Laceration with foreign body of finger with damage to nail

✓7ᵗʰ S61.320 Laceration with foreign body of right index finger with damage to nail

✓7ᵗʰ S61.321 Laceration with foreign body of left index finger with damage to nail

✓7ᵗʰ S61.322 Laceration with foreign body of right middle finger with damage to nail

✓7ᵗʰ S61.323 Laceration with foreign body of left middle finger with damage to nail

✓7ᵗʰ S61.324 Laceration with foreign body of right ring finger with damage to nail

✓7ᵗʰ S61.325 Laceration with foreign body of left ring finger with damage to nail

---

EXCLUDES 1 Not coded here   **EXCLUDES 2** Not included here   **N** Newborn Age: 0   **P** Pediatric Age: 0-17   **M** Maternity Age: 12-55   **A** Adult Age: 15-124

868   ICD-10-CM Draft (2015)

✓7ᵗʰ **S61.326** **Laceration with foreign body of** right little **finger with damage to nail**

✓7ᵗʰ **S61.327** **Laceration with foreign body of** left little **finger with damage to nail**

✓7ᵗʰ **S61.328** **Laceration with foreign body of other finger with damage to nail**
Laceration with foreign body of specified finger with unspecified laterality with damage to nail

✓7ᵗʰ **S61.329** **Laceration with foreign body of unspecified finger with damage to nail**

✓6ᵗʰ **S61.33** Puncture wound without foreign body **of finger with damage to nail**

✓7ᵗʰ **S61.330** **Puncture wound without foreign body of** right index **finger with damage to nail**

✓7ᵗʰ **S61.331** **Puncture wound without foreign body of** left index **finger with damage to nail**

✓7ᵗʰ **S61.332** **Puncture wound without foreign body of** right middle **finger with damage to nail**

✓7ᵗʰ **S61.333** **Puncture wound without foreign body of** left middle **finger with damage to nail**

✓7ᵗʰ **S61.334** **Puncture wound without foreign body of** right ring **finger with damage to nail**

✓7ᵗʰ **S61.335** **Puncture wound without foreign body of** left ring **finger with damage to nail**

✓7ᵗʰ **S61.336** **Puncture wound without foreign body of** right little **finger with damage to nail**

✓7ᵗʰ **S61.337** **Puncture wound without foreign body of** left little **finger with damage to nail**

✓7ᵗʰ **S61.338** **Puncture wound without foreign body of other finger with damage to nail**
Puncture wound without foreign body of specified finger with unspecified laterality with damage to nail

✓7ᵗʰ **S61.339** **Puncture wound without foreign body of unspecified finger with damage to nail**

✓6ᵗʰ **S61.34** Puncture wound with foreign body **of finger with damage to nail**

✓7ᵗʰ **S61.340** **Puncture wound with foreign body of** right index **finger with damage to nail**

✓7ᵗʰ **S61.341** **Puncture wound with foreign body of** left index **finger with damage to nail**

✓7ᵗʰ **S61.342** **Puncture wound with foreign body of** right middle **finger with damage to nail**

✓7ᵗʰ **S61.343** **Puncture wound with foreign body of** left middle **finger with damage to nail**

✓7ᵗʰ **S61.344** **Puncture wound with foreign body of** right ring **finger with damage to nail**

✓7ᵗʰ **S61.345** **Puncture wound with foreign body of** left ring **finger with damage to nail**

✓7ᵗʰ **S61.346** **Puncture wound with foreign body of** right little **finger with damage to nail**

✓7ᵗʰ **S61.347** **Puncture wound with foreign body of** left little **finger with damage to nail**

✓7ᵗʰ **S61.348** **Puncture wound with foreign body of other finger with damage to nail**
Puncture wound with foreign body of specified finger with unspecified laterality with damage to nail

✓7ᵗʰ **S61.349** **Puncture wound with foreign body of unspecified finger with damage to nail**

✓6ᵗʰ **S61.35** Open bite **of finger with damage to nail**
Bite of finger with damage to nail NOS
EXCLUDES 1 superficial bite of finger (S60.46-, S60.47-)

✓7ᵗʰ **S61.350** **Open bite of** right index **finger with damage to nail**

✓7ᵗʰ **S61.351** **Open bite of** left index **finger with damage to nail**

✓7ᵗʰ **S61.352** **Open bite of** right middle **finger with damage to nail**

✓7ᵗʰ **S61.353** **Open bite of** left middle **finger with damage to nail**

✓7ᵗʰ **S61.354** **Open bite of** right ring **finger with damage to nail**

✓7ᵗʰ **S61.355** **Open bite of** left ring **finger with damage to nail**

✓7ᵗʰ **S61.356** **Open bite of** right little **finger with damage to nail**

✓7ᵗʰ **S61.357** **Open bite of** left little **finger with damage to nail**

✓7ᵗʰ **S61.358** **Open bite of other finger with damage to nail**
Open bite of specified finger with unspecified laterality with damage to nail

✓7ᵗʰ **S61.359** **Open bite of unspecified finger with damage to nail**

✓5ᵗʰ **S61.4** **Open wound of** hand

✓6ᵗʰ **S61.40** Unspecified **open wound of hand**

✓7ᵗʰ **S61.401** **Unspecified open wound of** right **hand**

✓7ᵗʰ **S61.402** **Unspecified open wound of** left **hand**

✓7ᵗʰ **S61.409** **Unspecified open wound of unspecified hand**

✓6ᵗʰ **S61.41** Laceration without foreign body **of hand**

✓7ᵗʰ **S61.411** **Laceration without foreign body of** right **hand**

✓7ᵗʰ **S61.412** **Laceration without foreign body of** left **hand**

✓7ᵗʰ **S61.419** **Laceration without foreign body of unspecified hand**

✓6ᵗʰ **S61.42** Laceration with foreign body **of hand**

✓7ᵗʰ **S61.421** **Laceration with foreign body of** right **hand**

✓7ᵗʰ **S61.422** **Laceration with foreign body of** left **hand**

✓7ᵗʰ **S61.429** **Laceration with foreign body of unspecified hand**

✓6ᵗʰ **S61.43** Puncture wound without foreign body **of hand**

✓7ᵗʰ **S61.431** **Puncture wound without foreign body of** right **hand**

✓7ᵗʰ **S61.432** **Puncture wound without foreign body of** left **hand**

✓7ᵗʰ **S61.439** **Puncture wound without foreign body of unspecified hand**

✓6ᵗʰ **S61.44** Puncture wound with foreign body **of hand**

✓7ᵗʰ **S61.441** **Puncture wound with foreign body of** right **hand**

✓7ᵗʰ **S61.442** **Puncture wound with foreign body of** left **hand**

✓7ᵗʰ **S61.449** **Puncture wound with foreign body of unspecified hand**

✓6ᵗʰ **S61.45** Open bite **of hand**
Bite of hand NOS
EXCLUDES 1 superficial bite of hand (S60.56-, S60.57-)

✓7ᵗʰ **S61.451** **Open bite of** right **hand**

✓7ᵗʰ **S61.452** **Open bite of** left **hand**

✓7ᵗʰ **S61.459** **Open bite of unspecified hand**

✓5ᵗʰ **S61.5** **Open wound of** wrist

✓6ᵗʰ **S61.50** Unspecified **open wound of wrist**

✓7ᵗʰ **S61.501** **Unspecified open wound of** right **wrist**

✓7ᵗʰ **S61.502** **Unspecified open wound of** left **wrist**

✓7ᵗʰ **S61.509** **Unspecified open wound of unspecified wrist**

✓6ᵗʰ **S61.51** Laceration without foreign body **of wrist**

✓7ᵗʰ **S61.511** **Laceration without foreign body of** right **wrist**

✓7ᵗʰ **S61.512** **Laceration without foreign body of** left **wrist**

✓7ᵗʰ **S61.519** **Laceration without foreign body of unspecified wrist**

✓6ᵗʰ **S61.52** Laceration with foreign body **of wrist**

✓7ᵗʰ **S61.521** **Laceration with foreign body of** right **wrist**

✓7ᵗʰ **S61.522** **Laceration with foreign body of** left **wrist**

✓7ᵗʰ **S61.529** **Laceration with foreign body of unspecified wrist**

✓6ᵗʰ **S61.53** Puncture wound without foreign body **of wrist**

✓7ᵗʰ **S61.531** **Puncture wound without foreign body of** right **wrist**

✓7ᵗʰ **S61.532** **Puncture wound without foreign body of** left **wrist**

✓ Additional Character Required	✓₇ₜₕ Xtension Alert	Unspecified Dx	Other Specified Dx	Manifestation	▶◀ Revised Text ● New Code ▲ Revised Code Title

Injury, Poisoning and Certain Other Consequences of External Causes

S61.539–S62.143

√7ᵗʰ **S61.539 Puncture wound without foreign body of unspecified wrist**

√6ᵗʰ **S61.54** Puncture wound with foreign body of wrist

  √7ᵗʰ **S61.541 Puncture wound with foreign body of** right **wrist**

  √7ᵗʰ **S61.542 Puncture wound with foreign body of** left **wrist**

  √7ᵗʰ **S61.549 Puncture wound with foreign body of unspecified wrist**

√6ᵗʰ **S61.55** Open bite **of wrist**
     Bite of wrist NOS
     EXCLUDES 1   *superficial bite of wrist (S60.86-, S60.87-)*

  √7ᵗʰ **S61.551 Open bite of** right **wrist**

  √7ᵗʰ **S61.552 Open bite of** left **wrist**

  √7ᵗʰ **S61.559 Open bite of unspecified wrist**

√4ᵗʰ **S62 Fracture at wrist and hand level**

  NOTE   A fracture not indicated as displaced or nondisplaced should be coded to displaced.
         A fracture not indicated as open or closed should be coded to closed.

  EXCLUDES 1   *traumatic amputation of wrist and hand (S68.-)*
  EXCLUDES 2   *fracture of distal parts of ulna and radius (S52.-)*

  The appropriate 7th character is to be added to each code from category S62.
  A   initial encounter for closed fracture
  B   initial encounter for open fracture
  D   subsequent encounter for fracture with routine healing
  G   subsequent encounter for fracture with delayed healing
  K   subsequent encounter for fracture with nonunion
  P   subsequent encounter for fracture with malunion
  S   sequela

√5ᵗʰ **S62.0** Fracture of navicular [scaphoid] **bone of wrist**

  √6ᵗʰ **S62.00** Unspecified fracture of navicular [scaphoid] bone of wrist

    √7ᵗʰ **S62.001 Unspecified fracture of navicular [scaphoid] bone of** right **wrist**

    √7ᵗʰ **S62.002 Unspecified fracture of navicular [scaphoid] bone of** left **wrist**
         AHA: 2012, 4Q, 106

    √7ᵗʰ **S62.009 Unspecified fracture of navicular [scaphoid] bone of unspecified wrist**

  √6ᵗʰ **S62.01** Fracture of distal pole of navicular [scaphoid] bone of wrist
     Fracture of volar tuberosity of navicular [scaphoid] bone of wrist

    √7ᵗʰ **S62.011** Displaced **fracture of distal pole of navicular [scaphoid] bone of** right **wrist**

    √7ᵗʰ **S62.012** Displaced **fracture of distal pole of navicular [scaphoid] bone of** left **wrist**

    √7ᵗʰ **S62.013** Displaced **fracture of distal pole of navicular [scaphoid] bone of unspecified wrist**

    √7ᵗʰ **S62.014** Nondisplaced **fracture of distal pole of navicular [scaphoid] bone of** right **wrist**

    √7ᵗʰ **S62.015** Nondisplaced **fracture of distal pole of navicular [scaphoid] bone of** left **wrist**

    √7ᵗʰ **S62.016** Nondisplaced **fracture of distal pole of navicular [scaphoid] bone of unspecified wrist**

  √6ᵗʰ **S62.02** Fracture of middle third of navicular [scaphoid] bone of wrist

    √7ᵗʰ **S62.021** Displaced **fracture of middle third of navicular [scaphoid] bone of** right **wrist**

    √7ᵗʰ **S62.022** Displaced **fracture of middle third of navicular [scaphoid] bone of** left **wrist**

    √7ᵗʰ **S62.023** Displaced **fracture of middle third of navicular [scaphoid] bone of unspecified wrist**

    √7ᵗʰ **S62.024** Nondisplaced **fracture of middle third of navicular [scaphoid] bone of** right **wrist**

    √7ᵗʰ **S62.025** Nondisplaced **fracture of middle third of navicular [scaphoid] bone of** left **wrist**

    √7ᵗʰ **S62.026** Nondisplaced **fracture of middle third of navicular [scaphoid] bone of unspecified wrist**

√6ᵗʰ **S62.03** Fracture of proximal third of navicular [scaphoid] bone of wrist

  √7ᵗʰ **S62.031** Displaced **fracture of proximal third of navicular [scaphoid] bone of** right **wrist**

  √7ᵗʰ **S62.032** Displaced **fracture of proximal third of navicular [scaphoid] bone of** left **wrist**

  √7ᵗʰ **S62.033** Displaced **fracture of proximal third of navicular [scaphoid] bone of unspecified wrist**

  √7ᵗʰ **S62.034** Nondisplaced **fracture of proximal third of navicular [scaphoid] bone of** right **wrist**

  √7ᵗʰ **S62.035** Nondisplaced **fracture of proximal third of navicular [scaphoid] bone of** left **wrist**

  √7ᵗʰ **S62.036** Nondisplaced **fracture of proximal third of navicular [scaphoid] bone of unspecified wrist**

√5ᵗʰ **S62.1** Fracture of other and unspecified carpal bone(s)
    EXCLUDES 2   *fracture of scaphoid of wrist (S62.0-)*

  √6ᵗʰ **S62.10** Fracture of unspecified carpal bone
     Fracture of wrist NOS

    √7ᵗʰ **S62.101 Fracture of unspecified carpal bone,** right **wrist**

    √7ᵗʰ **S62.102 Fracture of unspecified carpal bone,** left **wrist**
         AHA: 2012, 4Q, 95

    √7ᵗʰ **S62.109 Fracture of unspecified carpal bone, unspecified wrist**

  √6ᵗʰ **S62.11** Fracture of triquetrum [cuneiform] bone of wrist

    √7ᵗʰ **S62.111** Displaced **fracture of triquetrum [cuneiform] bone,** right **wrist**

    √7ᵗʰ **S62.112** Displaced **fracture of triquetrum [cuneiform] bone,** left **wrist**

    √7ᵗʰ **S62.113** Displaced **fracture of triquetrum [cuneiform] bone, unspecified wrist**

    √7ᵗʰ **S62.114** Nondisplaced **fracture of triquetrum [cuneiform] bone,** right **wrist**

    √7ᵗʰ **S62.115** Nondisplaced **fracture of triquetrum [cuneiform] bone,** left **wrist**

    √7ᵗʰ **S62.116** Nondisplaced **fracture of triquetrum [cuneiform] bone, unspecified wrist**

  √6ᵗʰ **S62.12** Fracture of lunate [semilunar]

    √7ᵗʰ **S62.121** Displaced **fracture of lunate [semilunar],** right **wrist**

    √7ᵗʰ **S62.122** Displaced **fracture of lunate [semilunar],** left **wrist**

    √7ᵗʰ **S62.123** Displaced **fracture of lunate [semilunar], unspecified wrist**

    √7ᵗʰ **S62.124** Nondisplaced **fracture of lunate [semilunar],** right **wrist**

    √7ᵗʰ **S62.125** Nondisplaced **fracture of lunate [semilunar],** left **wrist**

    √7ᵗʰ **S62.126** Nondisplaced **fracture of lunate [semilunar], unspecified wrist**

  √6ᵗʰ **S62.13** Fracture of capitate [os magnum] bone

    √7ᵗʰ **S62.131** Displaced **fracture of capitate [os magnum] bone,** right **wrist**

    √7ᵗʰ **S62.132** Displaced **fracture of capitate [os magnum] bone,** left **wrist**

    √7ᵗʰ **S62.133** Displaced **fracture of capitate [os magnum] bone, unspecified wrist**

    √7ᵗʰ **S62.134** Nondisplaced **fracture of capitate [os magnum] bone,** right **wrist**

    √7ᵗʰ **S62.135** Nondisplaced **fracture of capitate [os magnum] bone,** left **wrist**

    √7ᵗʰ **S62.136** Nondisplaced **fracture of capitate [os magnum] bone, unspecified wrist**

  √6ᵗʰ **S62.14** Fracture of body of hamate [unciform] bone
     Fracture of hamate [unciform] bone NOS

    √7ᵗʰ **S62.141** Displaced **fracture of body of hamate [unciform] bone,** right **wrist**

    √7ᵗʰ **S62.142** Displaced **fracture of body of hamate [unciform] bone,** left **wrist**

    √7ᵗʰ **S62.143** Displaced **fracture of body of hamate [unciform] bone, unspecified wrist**

EXCLUDES 1 Not coded here   *EXCLUDES 2* Not included here   N Newborn Age: 0   P Pediatric Age: 0-17   M Maternity Age: 12-55   A Adult Age: 15-124

870   ICD-10-CM Draft (2015)

✓7ᵗʰ **S62.144** Nondisplaced fracture of body of hamate [unciform] bone, right wrist

✓7ᵗʰ **S62.145** Nondisplaced fracture of body of hamate [unciform] bone, left wrist

✓7ᵗʰ **S62.146** Nondisplaced fracture of body of hamate [unciform] bone, unspecified wrist

✓6ᵗʰ **S62.15** Fracture of hook process of hamate [unciform] bone
Fracture of unciform process of hamate [unciform] bone

✓7ᵗʰ **S62.151** Displaced fracture of hook process of hamate [unciform] bone, right wrist

✓7ᵗʰ **S62.152** Displaced fracture of hook process of hamate [unciform] bone, left wrist

✓7ᵗʰ **S62.153** Displaced fracture of hook process of hamate [unciform] bone, unspecified wrist

✓7ᵗʰ **S62.154** Nondisplaced fracture of hook process of hamate [unciform] bone, right wrist

✓7ᵗʰ **S62.155** Nondisplaced fracture of hook process of hamate [unciform] bone, left wrist

✓7ᵗʰ **S62.156** Nondisplaced fracture of hook process of hamate [unciform] bone, unspecified wrist

✓6ᵗʰ **S62.16** Fracture of pisiform

✓7ᵗʰ **S62.161** Displaced fracture of pisiform, right wrist

✓7ᵗʰ **S62.162** Displaced fracture of pisiform, left wrist

✓7ᵗʰ **S62.163** Displaced fracture of pisiform, unspecified wrist

✓7ᵗʰ **S62.164** Nondisplaced fracture of pisiform, right wrist

✓7ᵗʰ **S62.165** Nondisplaced fracture of pisiform, left wrist

✓7ᵗʰ **S62.166** Nondisplaced fracture of pisiform, unspecified wrist

✓6ᵗʰ **S62.17** Fracture of trapezium [larger multangular]

✓7ᵗʰ **S62.171** Displaced fracture of trapezium [larger multangular], right wrist

✓7ᵗʰ **S62.172** Displaced fracture of trapezium [larger multangular], left wrist

✓7ᵗʰ **S62.173** Displaced fracture of trapezium [larger multangular], unspecified wrist

✓7ᵗʰ **S62.174** Nondisplaced fracture of trapezium [larger multangular], right wrist

✓7ᵗʰ **S62.175** Nondisplaced fracture of trapezium [larger multangular], left wrist

✓7ᵗʰ **S62.176** Nondisplaced fracture of trapezium [larger multangular], unspecified wrist

✓6ᵗʰ **S62.18** Fracture of trapezoid [smaller multangular]

✓7ᵗʰ **S62.181** Displaced fracture of trapezoid [smaller multangular], right wrist

✓7ᵗʰ **S62.182** Displaced fracture of trapezoid [smaller multangular], left wrist

✓7ᵗʰ **S62.183** Displaced fracture of trapezoid [smaller multangular], unspecified wrist

✓7ᵗʰ **S62.184** Nondisplaced fracture of trapezoid [smaller multangular], right wrist

✓7ᵗʰ **S62.185** Nondisplaced fracture of trapezoid [smaller multangular], left wrist

✓7ᵗʰ **S62.186** Nondisplaced fracture of trapezoid [smaller multangular], unspecified wrist

✓5ᵗʰ **S62.2** Fracture of first metacarpal bone

✓6ᵗʰ **S62.20** Unspecified fracture of first metacarpal bone

✓7ᵗʰ **S62.201** Unspecified fracture of first metacarpal bone, right hand

✓7ᵗʰ **S62.202** Unspecified fracture of first metacarpal bone, left hand

✓7ᵗʰ **S62.209** Unspecified fracture of first metacarpal bone, unspecified hand

✓6ᵗʰ **S62.21** Bennett's fracture

✓7ᵗʰ **S62.211** Bennett's fracture, right hand

✓7ᵗʰ **S62.212** Bennett's fracture, left hand

✓7ᵗʰ **S62.213** Bennett's fracture, unspecified hand

✓6ᵗʰ **S62.22** Rolando's fracture

✓7ᵗʰ **S62.221** Displaced Rolando's fracture, right hand

✓7ᵗʰ **S62.222** Displaced Rolando's fracture, left hand

✓7ᵗʰ **S62.223** Displaced Rolando's fracture, unspecified hand

✓7ᵗʰ **S62.224** Nondisplaced Rolando's fracture, right hand

✓7ᵗʰ **S62.225** Nondisplaced Rolando's fracture, left hand

✓7ᵗʰ **S62.226** Nondisplaced Rolando's fracture, unspecified hand

✓6ᵗʰ **S62.23** Other fracture of base of first metacarpal bone

✓7ᵗʰ **S62.231** Other displaced fracture of base of first metacarpal bone, right hand

✓7ᵗʰ **S62.232** Other displaced fracture of base of first metacarpal bone, left hand

✓7ᵗʰ **S62.233** Other displaced fracture of base of first metacarpal bone, unspecified hand

✓7ᵗʰ **S62.234** Other nondisplaced fracture of base of first metacarpal bone, right hand

✓7ᵗʰ **S62.235** Other nondisplaced fracture of base of first metacarpal bone, left hand

✓7ᵗʰ **S62.236** Other nondisplaced fracture of base of first metacarpal bone, unspecified hand

✓6ᵗʰ **S62.24** Fracture of shaft of first metacarpal bone

✓7ᵗʰ **S62.241** Displaced fracture of shaft of first metacarpal bone, right hand

✓7ᵗʰ **S62.242** Displaced fracture of shaft of first metacarpal bone, left hand

✓7ᵗʰ **S62.243** Displaced fracture of shaft of first metacarpal bone, unspecified hand

✓7ᵗʰ **S62.244** Nondisplaced fracture of shaft of first metacarpal bone, right hand

✓7ᵗʰ **S62.245** Nondisplaced fracture of shaft of first metacarpal bone, left hand

✓7ᵗʰ **S62.246** Nondisplaced fracture of shaft of first metacarpal bone, unspecified hand

✓6ᵗʰ **S62.25** Fracture of neck of first metacarpal bone

✓7ᵗʰ **S62.251** Displaced fracture of neck of first metacarpal bone, right hand

✓7ᵗʰ **S62.252** Displaced fracture of neck of first metacarpal bone, left hand

✓7ᵗʰ **S62.253** Displaced fracture of neck of first metacarpal bone, unspecified hand

✓7ᵗʰ **S62.254** Nondisplaced fracture of neck of first metacarpal bone, right hand

✓7ᵗʰ **S62.255** Nondisplaced fracture of neck of first metacarpal bone, left hand

✓7ᵗʰ **S62.256** Nondisplaced fracture of neck of first metacarpal bone, unspecified hand

✓6ᵗʰ **S62.29** Other fracture of first metacarpal bone

✓7ᵗʰ **S62.291** Other fracture of first metacarpal bone, right hand

✓7ᵗʰ **S62.292** Other fracture of first metacarpal bone, left hand

✓7ᵗʰ **S62.299** Other fracture of first metacarpal bone, unspecified hand

✓5ᵗʰ **S62.3** Fracture of other and unspecified metacarpal bone
EXCLUDES 2 fracture of first metacarpal bone (S62.2-)

✓6ᵗʰ **S62.30** Unspecified fracture of other metacarpal bone

✓7ᵗʰ **S62.300** Unspecified fracture of second metacarpal bone, right hand

✓7ᵗʰ **S62.301** Unspecified fracture of second metacarpal bone, left hand

✓7ᵗʰ **S62.302** Unspecified fracture of third metacarpal bone, right hand

✓7ᵗʰ **S62.303** Unspecified fracture of third metacarpal bone, left hand

✓7ᵗʰ **S62.304** Unspecified fracture of fourth metacarpal bone, right hand

✓7ᵗʰ **S62.305** Unspecified fracture of fourth metacarpal bone, left hand

✓7ᵗʰ **S62.306** Unspecified fracture of fifth metacarpal bone, right hand

✓7ᵗʰ **S62.307** Unspecified fracture of fifth metacarpal bone, left hand

---

✓ Additional Character Required   ✓ₓ7ᵗʰ Xtension Alert   Unspecified Dx   Other Specified Dx   Manifestation   ▶◀ Revised Text   ● New Code   ▲ Revised Code Title

√7th **S62.308 Unspecified fracture of other metacarpal bone**
Unspecified fracture of specified metacarpal bone with unspecified laterality

√7th **S62.309 Unspecified fracture of unspecified metacarpal bone**

√6th **S62.31** Displaced fracture of base of other metacarpal bone

√7th **S62.310 Displaced fracture of base of** second **metacarpal bone,** right **hand**

√7th **S62.311 Displaced fracture of base of** second **metacarpal bone,** left **hand**

√7th **S62.312 Displaced fracture of base of** third **metacarpal bone,** right **hand**

√7th **S62.313 Displaced fracture of base of** third **metacarpal bone,** left **hand**

√7th **S62.314 Displaced fracture of base of** fourth **metacarpal bone,** right **hand**

√7th **S62.315 Displaced fracture of base of** fourth **metacarpal bone,** left **hand**

√7th **S62.316 Displaced fracture of base of** fifth **metacarpal bone,** right **hand**

√7th **S62.317 Displaced fracture of base of** fifth **metacarpal bone,** left **hand**

√7th **S62.318 Displaced fracture of base of other metacarpal bone**
Displaced fracture of base of specified metacarpal bone with unspecified laterality

√7th **S62.319 Displaced fracture of base of unspecified metacarpal bone**

√6th **S62.32** Displaced fracture of shaft of other metacarpal bone

√7th **S62.320 Displaced fracture of shaft of** second **metacarpal bone,** right **hand**

√7th **S62.321 Displaced fracture of shaft of** second **metacarpal bone,** left **hand**

√7th **S62.322 Displaced fracture of shaft of** third **metacarpal bone,** right **hand**

√7th **S62.323 Displaced fracture of shaft of** third **metacarpal bone,** left **hand**

√7th **S62.324 Displaced fracture of shaft of** fourth **metacarpal bone,** right **hand**

√7th **S62.325 Displaced fracture of shaft of** fourth **metacarpal bone,** left **hand**

√7th **S62.326 Displaced fracture of shaft of** fifth **metacarpal bone,** right **hand**

√7th **S62.327 Displaced fracture of shaft of** fifth **metacarpal bone,** left **hand**

√7th **S62.328 Displaced fracture of shaft of other metacarpal bone**
Displaced fracture of shaft of specified metacarpal bone with unspecified laterality

√7th **S62.329 Displaced fracture of shaft of unspecified metacarpal bone**

√6th **S62.33** Displaced fracture of neck of other metacarpal bone

√7th **S62.330 Displaced fracture of neck of** second **metacarpal bone,** right **hand**

√7th **S62.331 Displaced fracture of neck of** second **metacarpal bone,** left **hand**

√7th **S62.332 Displaced fracture of neck of** third **metacarpal bone,** right **hand**

√7th **S62.333 Displaced fracture of neck of** third **metacarpal bone,** left **hand**

√7th **S62.334 Displaced fracture of neck of** fourth **metacarpal bone,** right **hand**

√7th **S62.335 Displaced fracture of neck of** fourth **metacarpal bone,** left **hand**

√7th **S62.336 Displaced fracture of neck of** fifth **metacarpal bone,** right **hand**

√7th **S62.337 Displaced fracture of neck of** fifth **metacarpal bone,** left **hand**

√7th **S62.338 Displaced fracture of neck of other metacarpal bone**
Displaced fracture of neck of specified metacarpal bone with unspecified laterality

√7th **S62.339 Displaced fracture of neck of unspecified metacarpal bone**

√6th **S62.34** Nondisplaced fracture of base of other metacarpal bone

√7th **S62.340 Nondisplaced fracture of base of** second **metacarpal bone,** right **hand**

√7th **S62.341 Nondisplaced fracture of base of** second **metacarpal bone,** left **hand**

√7th **S62.342 Nondisplaced fracture of base of** third **metacarpal bone,** right **hand**

√7th **S62.343 Nondisplaced fracture of base of** third **metacarpal bone,** left **hand**

√7th **S62.344 Nondisplaced fracture of base of** fourth **metacarpal bone,** right **hand**

√7th **S62.345 Nondisplaced fracture of base of** fourth **metacarpal bone,** left **hand**

√7th **S62.346 Nondisplaced fracture of base of** fifth **metacarpal bone,** right **hand**

√7th **S62.347 Nondisplaced fracture of base of** fifth **metacarpal bone,** left **hand**

√7th **S62.348 Nondisplaced fracture of base of other metacarpal bone**
Nondisplaced fracture of base of specified metacarpal bone with unspecified laterality

√7th **S62.349 Nondisplaced fracture of base of unspecified metacarpal bone**

√6th **S62.35** Nondisplaced fracture of shaft of other metacarpal bone

√7th **S62.350 Nondisplaced fracture of shaft of** second **metacarpal bone,** right **hand**

√7th **S62.351 Nondisplaced fracture of shaft of** second **metacarpal bone,** left **hand**

√7th **S62.352 Nondisplaced fracture of shaft of** third **metacarpal bone,** right **hand**

√7th **S62.353 Nondisplaced fracture of shaft of** third **metacarpal bone,** left **hand**

√7th **S62.354 Nondisplaced fracture of shaft of** fourth **metacarpal bone,** right **hand**

√7th **S62.355 Nondisplaced fracture of shaft of** fourth **metacarpal bone,** left **hand**

√7th **S62.356 Nondisplaced fracture of shaft of** fifth **metacarpal bone,** right **hand**

√7th **S62.357 Nondisplaced fracture of shaft of** fifth **metacarpal bone,** left **hand**

√7th **S62.358 Nondisplaced fracture of shaft of other metacarpal bone**
Nondisplaced fracture of shaft of specified metacarpal bone with unspecified laterality

√7th **S62.359 Nondisplaced fracture of shaft of unspecified metacarpal bone**

√6th **S62.36** Nondisplaced fracture of neck of other metacarpal bone

√7th **S62.360 Nondisplaced fracture of neck of** second **metacarpal bone,** right **hand**

√7th **S62.361 Nondisplaced fracture of neck of** second **metacarpal bone,** left **hand**

√7th **S62.362 Nondisplaced fracture of neck of** third **metacarpal bone,** right **hand**

√7th **S62.363 Nondisplaced fracture of neck of** third **metacarpal bone,** left **hand**

√7th **S62.364 Nondisplaced fracture of neck of** fourth **metacarpal bone,** right **hand**

√7th **S62.365 Nondisplaced fracture of neck of** fourth **metacarpal bone,** left **hand**

√7th **S62.366 Nondisplaced fracture of neck of** fifth **metacarpal bone,** right **hand**

√7th **S62.367 Nondisplaced fracture of neck of** fifth **metacarpal bone,** left **hand**

EXCLUDES 1 Not coded here   EXCLUDES 2 Not included here   N Newborn Age: 0   P Pediatric Age: 0-17   M Maternity Age: 12-55   A Adult Age: 15-124

872   ICD-10-CM Draft (2015)

✓7th **S62.368** **Nondisplaced fracture of neck of other metacarpal bone**
Nondisplaced fracture of neck of specified metacarpal bone with unspecified laterality

✓7th **S62.369** **Nondisplaced fracture of neck of unspecified metacarpal bone**

✓6th **S62.39** Other **fracture of** other **metacarpal bone**

✓7th **S62.390** **Other fracture of** second **metacarpal bone,** right **hand**

✓7th **S62.391** **Other fracture of** second **metacarpal bone,** left **hand**

✓7th **S62.392** **Other fracture of** third **metacarpal bone,** right **hand**

✓7th **S62.393** **Other fracture of** third **metacarpal bone,** left **hand**

✓7th **S62.394** **Other fracture of** fourth **metacarpal bone,** right **hand**

✓7th **S62.395** **Other fracture of** fourth **metacarpal bone,** left **hand**

✓7th **S62.396** **Other fracture of** fifth **metacarpal bone,** right **hand**

✓7th **S62.397** **Other fracture of** fifth **metacarpal bone,** left **hand**

✓7th **S62.398** **Other fracture of other metacarpal bone**
Other fracture of specified metacarpal bone with unspecified laterality

✓7th **S62.399** **Other fracture of unspecified metacarpal bone**

✓5th **S62.5** **Fracture of** thumb

✓6th **S62.50** **Fracture of** unspecified phalanx **of thumb**

✓7th **S62.501** **Fracture of unspecified phalanx of** right **thumb**

✓7th **S62.502** **Fracture of unspecified phalanx of** left **thumb**

✓7th **S62.509** **Fracture of unspecified phalanx of unspecified thumb**

✓6th **S62.51** **Fracture of** proximal phalanx **of thumb**

✓7th **S62.511** Displaced **fracture of proximal phalanx of** right **thumb**

✓7th **S62.512** Displaced **fracture of proximal phalanx of** left **thumb**

✓7th **S62.513** Displaced **fracture of proximal phalanx of unspecified thumb**

✓7th **S62.514** Nondisplaced **fracture of proximal phalanx of** right **thumb**

✓7th **S62.515** Nondisplaced **fracture of proximal phalanx of** left **thumb**

✓7th **S62.516** Nondisplaced **fracture of proximal phalanx of unspecified thumb**

✓6th **S62.52** **Fracture of** distal phalanx **of thumb**

✓7th **S62.521** Displaced **fracture of distal phalanx of** right **thumb**

✓7th **S62.522** Displaced **fracture of distal phalanx of** left **thumb**

✓7th **S62.523** Displaced **fracture of distal phalanx of unspecified thumb**

✓7th **S62.524** Nondisplaced **fracture of distal phalanx of** right **thumb**

✓7th **S62.525** Nondisplaced **fracture of distal phalanx of** left **thumb**

✓7th **S62.526** Nondisplaced **fracture of distal phalanx of unspecified thumb**

✓5th **S62.6** **Fracture of other and unspecified** finger(s)
EXCLUDES 2 *fracture of thumb (S62.5-)*

✓6th **S62.60** **Fracture of** unspecified phalanx **of finger**

✓7th **S62.600** **Fracture of unspecified phalanx of** right index **finger**

✓7th **S62.601** **Fracture of unspecified phalanx of** left index **finger**

✓7th **S62.602** **Fracture of unspecified phalanx of** right middle **finger**

✓7th **S62.603** **Fracture of unspecified phalanx of** left middle **finger**

✓7th **S62.604** **Fracture of unspecified phalanx of** right ring **finger**

✓7th **S62.605** **Fracture of unspecified phalanx of** left ring **finger**

✓7th **S62.606** **Fracture of unspecified phalanx of** right little **finger**

✓7th **S62.607** **Fracture of unspecified phalanx of** left little **finger**

✓7th **S62.608** **Fracture of unspecified phalanx of other finger**
Fracture of unspecified phalanx of specified finger with unspecified laterality

✓7th **S62.609** **Fracture of unspecified phalanx of unspecified finger**

✓6th **S62.61** Displaced **fracture of** proximal phalanx **of finger**

✓7th **S62.610** **Displaced fracture of proximal phalanx of** right index **finger**

✓7th **S62.611** **Displaced fracture of proximal phalanx of** left index **finger**

✓7th **S62.612** **Displaced fracture of proximal phalanx of** right middle **finger**

✓7th **S62.613** **Displaced fracture of proximal phalanx of** left middle **finger**

✓7th **S62.614** **Displaced fracture of proximal phalanx of** right ring **finger**

✓7th **S62.615** **Displaced fracture of proximal phalanx of** left ring **finger**

✓7th **S62.616** **Displaced fracture of proximal phalanx of** right little **finger**

✓7th **S62.617** **Displaced fracture of proximal phalanx of** left little **finger**

✓7th **S62.618** **Displaced fracture of proximal phalanx of other finger**
Displaced fracture of proximal phalanx of specified finger with unspecified laterality

✓7th **S62.619** **Displaced fracture of proximal phalanx of unspecified finger**

✓6th **S62.62** Displaced **fracture of** medial phalanx **of finger**

✓7th **S62.620** **Displaced fracture of medial phalanx of** right index **finger**

✓7th **S62.621** **Displaced fracture of medial phalanx of** left index **finger**

✓7th **S62.622** **Displaced fracture of medial phalanx of** right middle **finger**

✓7th **S62.623** **Displaced fracture of medial phalanx of** left middle **finger**

✓7th **S62.624** **Displaced fracture of medial phalanx of** right ring **finger**

✓7th **S62.625** **Displaced fracture of medial phalanx of** left ring **finger**

✓7th **S62.626** **Displaced fracture of medial phalanx of** right little **finger**

✓7th **S62.627** **Displaced fracture of medial phalanx of** left little **finger**

✓7th **S62.628** **Displaced fracture of medial phalanx of other finger**
Displaced fracture of medial phalanx of specified finger with unspecified laterality

✓7th **S62.629** **Displaced fracture of medial phalanx of unspecified finger**

✓6th **S62.63** Displaced **fracture of** distal phalanx **of finger**

✓7th **S62.630** **Displaced fracture of distal phalanx of** right index **finger**

✓7th **S62.631** **Displaced fracture of distal phalanx of** left index **finger**

✓7th **S62.632** **Displaced fracture of distal phalanx of** right middle **finger**

✓7th **S62.633** **Displaced fracture of distal phalanx of** left middle **finger**

✓7th **S62.634** **Displaced fracture of distal phalanx of** right ring **finger**

✓7th **S62.635** **Displaced fracture of distal phalanx of** left ring **finger**

✓ Additional Character Required | ✓x7th Xtension Alert | Unspecified Dx | Other Specified Dx | Manifestation | ▶◀ Revised Text | ● New Code | ▲ Revised Code Title

ICD-10-CM Draft (2015)

873

√7ᵗʰ **S62.636** Displaced fracture of distal phalanx of right little finger

√7ᵗʰ **S62.637** Displaced fracture of distal phalanx of left little finger

√7ᵗʰ **S62.638** Displaced fracture of distal phalanx of other finger
Displaced fracture of distal phalanx of specified finger with unspecified laterality

√7ᵗʰ **S62.639** Displaced fracture of distal phalanx of unspecified finger

√6ᵗʰ **S62.64** Nondisplaced fracture of proximal phalanx of finger

√7ᵗʰ **S62.640** Nondisplaced fracture of proximal phalanx of right index finger

√7ᵗʰ **S62.641** Nondisplaced fracture of proximal phalanx of left index finger

√7ᵗʰ **S62.642** Nondisplaced fracture of proximal phalanx of right middle finger

√7ᵗʰ **S62.643** Nondisplaced fracture of proximal phalanx of left middle finger

√7ᵗʰ **S62.644** Nondisplaced fracture of proximal phalanx of right ring finger

√7ᵗʰ **S62.645** Nondisplaced fracture of proximal phalanx of left ring finger

√7ᵗʰ **S62.646** Nondisplaced fracture of proximal phalanx of right little finger

√7ᵗʰ **S62.647** Nondisplaced fracture of proximal phalanx of left little finger

√7ᵗʰ **S62.648** Nondisplaced fracture of proximal phalanx of other finger
Nondisplaced fracture of proximal phalanx of specified finger with unspecified laterality

√7ᵗʰ **S62.649** Nondisplaced fracture of proximal phalanx of unspecified finger

√6ᵗʰ **S62.65** Nondisplaced fracture of medial phalanx of finger

√7ᵗʰ **S62.650** Nondisplaced fracture of medial phalanx of right index finger

√7ᵗʰ **S62.651** Nondisplaced fracture of medial phalanx of left index finger

√7ᵗʰ **S62.652** Nondisplaced fracture of medial phalanx of right middle finger

√7ᵗʰ **S62.653** Nondisplaced fracture of medial phalanx of left middle finger

√7ᵗʰ **S62.654** Nondisplaced fracture of medial phalanx of right ring finger

√7ᵗʰ **S62.655** Nondisplaced fracture of medial phalanx of left ring finger

√7ᵗʰ **S62.656** Nondisplaced fracture of medial phalanx of right little finger

√7ᵗʰ **S62.657** Nondisplaced fracture of medial phalanx of left little finger

√7ᵗʰ **S62.658** Nondisplaced fracture of medial phalanx of other finger
Nondisplaced fracture of medial phalanx of specified finger with unspecified laterality

√7ᵗʰ **S62.659** Nondisplaced fracture of medial phalanx of unspecified finger

√6ᵗʰ **S62.66** Nondisplaced fracture of distal phalanx of finger

√7ᵗʰ **S62.660** Nondisplaced fracture of distal phalanx of right index finger

√7ᵗʰ **S62.661** Nondisplaced fracture of distal phalanx of left index finger

√7ᵗʰ **S62.662** Nondisplaced fracture of distal phalanx of right middle finger

√7ᵗʰ **S62.663** Nondisplaced fracture of distal phalanx of left middle finger

√7ᵗʰ **S62.664** Nondisplaced fracture of distal phalanx of right ring finger

√7ᵗʰ **S62.665** Nondisplaced fracture of distal phalanx of left ring finger

√7ᵗʰ **S62.666** Nondisplaced fracture of distal phalanx of right little finger

√7ᵗʰ **S62.667** Nondisplaced fracture of distal phalanx of left little finger

√7ᵗʰ **S62.668** Nondisplaced fracture of distal phalanx of other finger
Nondisplaced fracture of distal phalanx of specified finger with unspecified laterality

√7ᵗʰ **S62.669** Nondisplaced fracture of distal phalanx of unspecified finger

√5ᵗʰ **S62.9** Unspecified fracture of wrist and hand

√x7ᵗʰ **S62.90** Unspecified fracture of unspecified wrist and hand

√x7ᵗʰ **S62.91** Unspecified fracture of right wrist and hand

√x7ᵗʰ **S62.92** Unspecified fracture of left wrist and hand

√4ᵗʰ **S63** Dislocation and sprain of joints and ligaments at wrist and hand level

INCLUDES   avulsion of joint or ligament at wrist and hand level
laceration of cartilage, joint or ligament at wrist and hand level
sprain of cartilage, joint or ligament at wrist and hand level
traumatic hemarthrosis of joint or ligament at wrist and hand level
traumatic rupture of joint or ligament at wrist and hand level
traumatic subluxation of joint or ligament at wrist and hand level
traumatic tear of joint or ligament at wrist and hand level

Code also any associated open wound

EXCLUDES 2   strain of muscle, fascia and tendon of wrist and hand (S66.-)

The appropriate 7th character is to be added to each code from category S63.
A   initial encounter
D   subsequent encounter
S   sequela

√5ᵗʰ **S63.0** Subluxation and dislocation of wrist and hand joints

√6ᵗʰ **S63.00** Unspecified subluxation and dislocation of wrist and hand
Dislocation of carpal bone NOS
Dislocation of distal end of radius NOS
Subluxation of carpal bone NOS
Subluxation of distal end of radius NOS

√7ᵗʰ **S63.001** Unspecified subluxation of right wrist and hand

√7ᵗʰ **S63.002** Unspecified subluxation of left wrist and hand

√7ᵗʰ **S63.003** Unspecified subluxation of unspecified wrist and hand

√7ᵗʰ **S63.004** Unspecified dislocation of right wrist and hand

√7ᵗʰ **S63.005** Unspecified dislocation of left wrist and hand

√7ᵗʰ **S63.006** Unspecified dislocation of unspecified wrist and hand

√6ᵗʰ **S63.01** Subluxation and dislocation of distal radioulnar joint

√7ᵗʰ **S63.011** Subluxation of distal radioulnar joint of right wrist

√7ᵗʰ **S63.012** Subluxation of distal radioulnar joint of left wrist

√7ᵗʰ **S63.013** Subluxation of distal radioulnar joint of unspecified wrist

√7ᵗʰ **S63.014** Dislocation of distal radioulnar joint of right wrist

√7ᵗʰ **S63.015** Dislocation of distal radioulnar joint of left wrist

√7ᵗʰ **S63.016** Dislocation of distal radioulnar joint of unspecified wrist

√6ᵗʰ **S63.02** Subluxation and dislocation of radiocarpal joint

√7ᵗʰ **S63.021** Subluxation of radiocarpal joint of right wrist

√7ᵗʰ **S63.022** Subluxation of radiocarpal joint of left wrist

√7ᵗʰ **S63.023** Subluxation of radiocarpal joint of unspecified wrist

√7ᵗʰ **S63.024** Dislocation of radiocarpal joint of right wrist

√7ᵗʰ **S63.025** Dislocation of radiocarpal joint of left wrist

EXCLUDES 1 Not coded here   EXCLUDES 2 Not included here   N Newborn Age: 0   P Pediatric Age: 0-17   M Maternity Age: 12-55   A Adult Age: 15-124

874   ICD-10-CM Draft (2015)

√7ᵗʰ **S63.026** Dislocation of radiocarpal joint of unspecified wrist

√6ᵗʰ **S63.03** Subluxation and dislocation of midcarpal joint

√7ᵗʰ **S63.031** Subluxation of midcarpal joint of right wrist

√7ᵗʰ **S63.032** Subluxation of midcarpal joint of left wrist

√7ᵗʰ **S63.033** Subluxation of midcarpal joint of unspecified wrist

√7ᵗʰ **S63.034** Dislocation of midcarpal joint of right wrist

√7ᵗʰ **S63.035** Dislocation of midcarpal joint of left wrist

√7ᵗʰ **S63.036** Dislocation of midcarpal joint of unspecified wrist

√6ᵗʰ **S63.04** Subluxation and dislocation of carpometacarpal joint of thumb

EXCLUDES 2 interphalangeal subluxation and dislocation of thumb (S63.1-)

√7ᵗʰ **S63.041** Subluxation of carpometacarpal joint of right thumb

√7ᵗʰ **S63.042** Subluxation of carpometacarpal joint of left thumb

√7ᵗʰ **S63.043** Subluxation of carpometacarpal joint of unspecified thumb

√7ᵗʰ **S63.044** Dislocation of carpometacarpal joint of right thumb

√7ᵗʰ **S63.045** Dislocation of carpometacarpal joint of left thumb

√7ᵗʰ **S63.046** Dislocation of carpometacarpal joint of unspecified thumb

√6ᵗʰ **S63.05** Subluxation and dislocation of other carpometacarpal joint

EXCLUDES 2 subluxation and dislocation of carpometacarpal joint of thumb (S63.04-)

√7ᵗʰ **S63.051** Subluxation of other carpometacarpal joint of right hand

√7ᵗʰ **S63.052** Subluxation of other carpometacarpal joint of left hand

√7ᵗʰ **S63.053** Subluxation of other carpometacarpal joint of unspecified hand

√7ᵗʰ **S63.054** Dislocation of other carpometacarpal joint of right hand

√7ᵗʰ **S63.055** Dislocation of other carpometacarpal joint of left hand

√7ᵗʰ **S63.056** Dislocation of other carpometacarpal joint of unspecified hand

√6ᵗʰ **S63.06** Subluxation and dislocation of metacarpal (bone), proximal end

√7ᵗʰ **S63.061** Subluxation of metacarpal (bone), proximal end of right hand

√7ᵗʰ **S63.062** Subluxation of metacarpal (bone), proximal end of left hand

√7ᵗʰ **S63.063** Subluxation of metacarpal (bone), proximal end of unspecified hand

√7ᵗʰ **S63.064** Dislocation of metacarpal (bone), proximal end of right hand

√7ᵗʰ **S63.065** Dislocation of metacarpal (bone), proximal end of left hand

√7ᵗʰ **S63.066** Dislocation of metacarpal (bone), proximal end of unspecified hand

√6ᵗʰ **S63.07** Subluxation and dislocation of distal end of ulna

√7ᵗʰ **S63.071** Subluxation of distal end of right ulna

√7ᵗʰ **S63.072** Subluxation of distal end of left ulna

√7ᵗʰ **S63.073** Subluxation of distal end of unspecified ulna

√7ᵗʰ **S63.074** Dislocation of distal end of right ulna

√7ᵗʰ **S63.075** Dislocation of distal end of left ulna

√7ᵗʰ **S63.076** Dislocation of distal end of unspecified ulna

√6ᵗʰ **S63.09** Other subluxation and dislocation of wrist and hand

√7ᵗʰ **S63.091** Other subluxation of right wrist and hand

√7ᵗʰ **S63.092** Other subluxation of left wrist and hand

√7ᵗʰ **S63.093** Other subluxation of unspecified wrist and hand

√7ᵗʰ **S63.094** Other dislocation of right wrist and hand

√7ᵗʰ **S63.095** Other dislocation of left wrist and hand

√7ᵗʰ **S63.096** Other dislocation of unspecified wrist and hand

√5ᵗʰ **S63.1** Subluxation and dislocation of thumb

√6ᵗʰ **S63.10** Unspecified subluxation and dislocation of thumb

√7ᵗʰ **S63.101** Unspecified subluxation of right thumb

√7ᵗʰ **S63.102** Unspecified subluxation of left thumb

√7ᵗʰ **S63.103** Unspecified subluxation of unspecified thumb

√7ᵗʰ **S63.104** Unspecified dislocation of right thumb

√7ᵗʰ **S63.105** Unspecified dislocation of left thumb

√7ᵗʰ **S63.106** Unspecified dislocation of unspecified thumb

√6ᵗʰ **S63.11** Subluxation and dislocation of metacarpophalangeal joint of thumb

√7ᵗʰ **S63.111** Subluxation of metacarpophalangeal joint of right thumb

√7ᵗʰ **S63.112** Subluxation of metacarpophalangeal joint of left thumb

√7ᵗʰ **S63.113** Subluxation of metacarpophalangeal joint of unspecified thumb

√7ᵗʰ **S63.114** Dislocation of metacarpophalangeal joint of right thumb

√7ᵗʰ **S63.115** Dislocation of metacarpophalangeal joint of left thumb

√7ᵗʰ **S63.116** Dislocation of metacarpophalangeal joint of unspecified thumb

√6ᵗʰ **S63.12** Subluxation and dislocation of unspecified interphalangeal joint of thumb

√7ᵗʰ **S63.121** Subluxation of unspecified interphalangeal joint of right thumb

√7ᵗʰ **S63.122** Subluxation of unspecified interphalangeal joint of left thumb

√7ᵗʰ **S63.123** Subluxation of unspecified interphalangeal joint of unspecified thumb

√7ᵗʰ **S63.124** Dislocation of unspecified interphalangeal joint of right thumb

√7ᵗʰ **S63.125** Dislocation of unspecified interphalangeal joint of left thumb

√7ᵗʰ **S63.126** Dislocation of unspecified interphalangeal joint of unspecified thumb

√6ᵗʰ **S63.13** Subluxation and dislocation of proximal interphalangeal joint of thumb

√7ᵗʰ **S63.131** Subluxation of proximal interphalangeal joint of right thumb

√7ᵗʰ **S63.132** Subluxation of proximal interphalangeal joint of left thumb

√7ᵗʰ **S63.133** Subluxation of proximal interphalangeal joint of unspecified thumb

√7ᵗʰ **S63.134** Dislocation of proximal interphalangeal joint of right thumb

√7ᵗʰ **S63.135** Dislocation of proximal interphalangeal joint of left thumb

√7ᵗʰ **S63.136** Dislocation of proximal interphalangeal joint of unspecified thumb

√6ᵗʰ **S63.14** Subluxation and dislocation of distal interphalangeal joint of thumb

√7ᵗʰ **S63.141** Subluxation of distal interphalangeal joint of right thumb

√7ᵗʰ **S63.142** Subluxation of distal interphalangeal joint of left thumb

√7ᵗʰ **S63.143** Subluxation of distal interphalangeal joint of unspecified thumb

√7ᵗʰ **S63.144** Dislocation of distal interphalangeal joint of right thumb

√7ᵗʰ **S63.145** Dislocation of distal interphalangeal joint of left thumb

√7ᵗʰ **S63.146** Dislocation of distal interphalangeal joint of unspecified thumb

√5ᵗʰ **S63.2** Subluxation and dislocation of other finger(s)

EXCLUDES 2 subluxation and dislocation of thumb (S63.1-)

√6ᵗʰ **S63.20** Unspecified subluxation of other finger

√ Additional Character Required   √x7ᵗʰ Xtension Alert   Unspecified Dx   Other Specified Dx   Manifestation   ▶◀ Revised Text   ● New Code   ▲ Revised Code Title

√7th **S63.200 Unspecified subluxation of** right index finger

√7th **S63.201 Unspecified subluxation of** left index finger

√7th **S63.202 Unspecified subluxation of** right middle finger

√7th **S63.203 Unspecified subluxation of** left middle finger

√7th **S63.204 Unspecified subluxation of** right ring finger

√7th **S63.205 Unspecified subluxation of** left ring finger

√7th **S63.206 Unspecified subluxation of** right little finger

√7th **S63.207 Unspecified subluxation of** left little finger

√7th **S63.208 Unspecified subluxation of other finger**
Unspecified subluxation of specified finger with unspecified laterality

√7th **S63.209 Unspecified subluxation of unspecified finger**

√6th **S63.21 Subluxation of** metacarpophalangeal joint **of finger**

√7th **S63.210 Subluxation of metacarpophalangeal joint of** right index finger

√7th **S63.211 Subluxation of metacarpophalangeal joint of** left index finger

√7th **S63.212 Subluxation of metacarpophalangeal joint of** right middle finger

√7th **S63.213 Subluxation of metacarpophalangeal joint of** left middle finger

√7th **S63.214 Subluxation of metacarpophalangeal joint of** right ring finger

√7th **S63.215 Subluxation of metacarpophalangeal joint of** left ring finger

√7th **S63.216 Subluxation of metacarpophalangeal joint of** right little finger

√7th **S63.217 Subluxation of metacarpophalangeal joint of** left little finger

√7th **S63.218 Subluxation of metacarpophalangeal joint of other finger**
Subluxation of metacarpophalangeal joint of specified finger with unspecified laterality

√7th **S63.219 Subluxation of metacarpophalangeal joint of unspecified finger**

√6th **S63.22 Subluxation of unspecified** interphalangeal joint **of finger**

√7th **S63.220 Subluxation of unspecified interphalangeal joint of** right index finger

√7th **S63.221 Subluxation of unspecified interphalangeal joint of** left index finger

√7th **S63.222 Subluxation of unspecified interphalangeal joint of** right middle finger

√7th **S63.223 Subluxation of unspecified interphalangeal joint of** left middle finger

√7th **S63.224 Subluxation of unspecified interphalangeal joint of** right ring finger

√7th **S63.225 Subluxation of unspecified interphalangeal joint of** left ring finger

√7th **S63.226 Subluxation of unspecified interphalangeal joint of** right little finger

√7th **S63.227 Subluxation of unspecified interphalangeal joint of** left little finger

√7th **S63.228 Subluxation of unspecified interphalangeal joint of other finger**
Subluxation of unspecified interphalangeal joint of specified finger with unspecified laterality

√7th **S63.229 Subluxation of unspecified interphalangeal joint of unspecified finger**

√6th **S63.23 Subluxation of** proximal interphalangeal joint of finger

√7th **S63.230 Subluxation of proximal interphalangeal joint of** right index finger

√7th **S63.231 Subluxation of proximal interphalangeal joint of** left index finger

√7th **S63.232 Subluxation of proximal interphalangeal joint of** right middle finger

√7th **S63.233 Subluxation of proximal interphalangeal joint of** left middle finger

√7th **S63.234 Subluxation of proximal interphalangeal joint of** right ring finger

√7th **S63.235 Subluxation of proximal interphalangeal joint of** left ring finger

√7th **S63.236 Subluxation of proximal interphalangeal joint of** right little finger

√7th **S63.237 Subluxation of proximal interphalangeal joint of** left little finger

√7th **S63.238 Subluxation of proximal interphalangeal joint of other finger**
Subluxation of proximal interphalangeal joint of specified finger with unspecified laterality

√7th **S63.239 Subluxation of proximal interphalangeal joint of unspecified finger**

√6th **S63.24 Subluxation of** distal interphalangeal **joint of finger**

√7th **S63.240 Subluxation of distal interphalangeal joint of** right index finger

√7th **S63.241 Subluxation of distal interphalangeal joint of** left index finger

√7th **S63.242 Subluxation of distal interphalangeal joint of** right middle finger

√7th **S63.243 Subluxation of distal interphalangeal joint of** left middle finger

√7th **S63.244 Subluxation of distal interphalangeal joint of** right ring finger

√7th **S63.245 Subluxation of distal interphalangeal joint of** left ring finger

√7th **S63.246 Subluxation of distal interphalangeal joint of** right little finger

√7th **S63.247 Subluxation of distal interphalangeal joint of** left little finger

√7th **S63.248 Subluxation of distal interphalangeal joint of other finger**
Subluxation of distal interphalangeal joint of specified finger with unspecified laterality

√7th **S63.249 Subluxation of distal interphalangeal joint of unspecified finger**

√6th **S63.25 Unspecified dislocation of** other finger

√7th **S63.250 Unspecified dislocation of** right index finger

√7th **S63.251 Unspecified dislocation of** left index finger

√7th **S63.252 Unspecified dislocation of** right middle finger

√7th **S63.253 Unspecified dislocation of** left middle finger

√7th **S63.254 Unspecified dislocation of** right ring finger

√7th **S63.255 Unspecified dislocation of** left ring finger

√7th **S63.256 Unspecified dislocation of** right little finger

√7th **S63.257 Unspecified dislocation of** left little finger

√7th **S63.258 Unspecified dislocation of other finger**
Unspecified dislocation of specified finger with unspecified laterality

√7th **S63.259 Unspecified dislocation of unspecified finger**
Unspecified dislocation of specified finger with unspecified laterality

√6th **S63.26 Dislocation of** metacarpophalangeal joint **of finger**

√7th **S63.260 Dislocation of metacarpophalangeal joint of** right index finger

√7th **S63.261 Dislocation of metacarpophalangeal joint of** left index finger

√7th **S63.262 Dislocation of metacarpophalangeal joint of** right middle finger

√7th **S63.263 Dislocation of metacarpophalangeal joint of** left middle finger

√7th **S63.264 Dislocation of metacarpophalangeal joint of** right ring finger

√7th **S63.265 Dislocation of metacarpophalangeal joint of** left ring finger

---

EXCLUDES 1 Not coded here   EXCLUDES 2 Not included here   N Newborn Age: 0   P Pediatric Age: 0-17   M Maternity Age: 12-55   A Adult Age: 15-124

876
ICD-10-CM Draft (2015)

✓7th **S63.266** Dislocation of metacarpophalangeal joint of right little finger

✓7th **S63.267** Dislocation of metacarpophalangeal joint of left little finger

✓7th **S63.268** Dislocation of metacarpophalangeal joint of other finger
Dislocation of metacarpophalangeal joint of specified finger with unspecified laterality

✓7th **S63.269** Dislocation of metacarpophalangeal joint of unspecified finger

✓6th **S63.27** Dislocation of unspecified interphalangeal joint of finger

✓7th **S63.270** Dislocation of unspecified interphalangeal joint of right index finger

✓7th **S63.271** Dislocation of unspecified interphalangeal joint of left index finger

✓7th **S63.272** Dislocation of unspecified interphalangeal joint of right middle finger

✓7th **S63.273** Dislocation of unspecified interphalangeal joint of left middle finger

✓7th **S63.274** Dislocation of unspecified interphalangeal joint of right ring finger

✓7th **S63.275** Dislocation of unspecified interphalangeal joint of left ring finger

✓7th **S63.276** Dislocation of unspecified interphalangeal joint of right little finger

✓7th **S63.277** Dislocation of unspecified interphalangeal joint of left little finger

✓7th **S63.278** Dislocation of unspecified interphalangeal joint of other finger
Dislocation of unspecified interphalangeal joint of specified finger with unspecified laterality

✓7th **S63.279** Dislocation of unspecified interphalangeal joint of unspecified finger
Dislocation of unspecified interphalangeal joint of specified finger without specified laterality

✓6th **S63.28** Dislocation of proximal interphalangeal joint of finger

✓7th **S63.280** Dislocation of proximal interphalangeal joint of right index finger

✓7th **S63.281** Dislocation of proximal interphalangeal joint of left index finger

✓7th **S63.282** Dislocation of proximal interphalangeal joint of right middle finger

✓7th **S63.283** Dislocation of proximal interphalangeal joint of left middle finger

✓7th **S63.284** Dislocation of proximal interphalangeal joint of right ring finger

✓7th **S63.285** Dislocation of proximal interphalangeal joint of left ring finger

✓7th **S63.286** Dislocation of proximal interphalangeal joint of right little finger

✓7th **S63.287** Dislocation of proximal interphalangeal joint of left little finger

✓7th **S63.288** Dislocation of proximal interphalangeal joint of other finger
Dislocation of proximal interphalangeal joint of specified finger with unspecified laterality

✓7th **S63.289** Dislocation of proximal interphalangeal joint of unspecified finger

✓6th **S63.29** Dislocation of distal interphalangeal joint of finger

✓7th **S63.290** Dislocation of distal interphalangeal joint of right index finger

✓7th **S63.291** Dislocation of distal interphalangeal joint of left index finger

✓7th **S63.292** Dislocation of distal interphalangeal joint of right middle finger

✓7th **S63.293** Dislocation of distal interphalangeal joint of left middle finger

✓7th **S63.294** Dislocation of distal interphalangeal joint of right ring finger

✓7th **S63.295** Dislocation of distal interphalangeal joint of left ring finger

✓7th **S63.296** Dislocation of distal interphalangeal joint of right little finger

✓7th **S63.297** Dislocation of distal interphalangeal joint of left little finger

✓7th **S63.298** Dislocation of distal interphalangeal joint of other finger
Dislocation of distal interphalangeal joint of specified finger with unspecified laterality

✓7th **S63.299** Dislocation of distal interphalangeal joint of unspecified finger

✓5th **S63.3** Traumatic rupture of ligament of wrist

✓6th **S63.30** Traumatic rupture of unspecified ligament of wrist

✓7th **S63.301** Traumatic rupture of unspecified ligament of right wrist

✓7th **S63.302** Traumatic rupture of unspecified ligament of left wrist

✓7th **S63.309** Traumatic rupture of unspecified ligament of unspecified wrist

✓6th **S63.31** Traumatic rupture of collateral ligament of wrist

✓7th **S63.311** Traumatic rupture of collateral ligament of right wrist

✓7th **S63.312** Traumatic rupture of collateral ligament of left wrist

✓7th **S63.319** Traumatic rupture of collateral ligament of unspecified wrist

✓6th **S63.32** Traumatic rupture of radiocarpal ligament

✓7th **S63.321** Traumatic rupture of right radiocarpal ligament

✓7th **S63.322** Traumatic rupture of left radiocarpal ligament

✓7th **S63.329** Traumatic rupture of unspecified radiocarpal ligament

✓6th **S63.33** Traumatic rupture of ulnocarpal (palmar) ligament

✓7th **S63.331** Traumatic rupture of right ulnocarpal (palmar) ligament

✓7th **S63.332** Traumatic rupture of left ulnocarpal (palmar) ligament

✓7th **S63.339** Traumatic rupture of unspecified ulnocarpal (palmar) ligament

✓6th **S63.39** Traumatic rupture of other ligament of wrist

✓7th **S63.391** Traumatic rupture of other ligament of right wrist

✓7th **S63.392** Traumatic rupture of other ligament of left wrist

✓7th **S63.399** Traumatic rupture of other ligament of unspecified wrist

✓5th **S63.4** Traumatic rupture of ligament of finger at metacarpophalangeal and interphalangeal joint(s)

✓6th **S63.40** Traumatic rupture of unspecified ligament of finger at metacarpophalangeal and interphalangeal joint

✓7th **S63.400** Traumatic rupture of unspecified ligament of right index finger at metacarpophalangeal and interphalangeal joint

✓7th **S63.401** Traumatic rupture of unspecified ligament of left index finger at metacarpophalangeal and interphalangeal joint

✓7th **S63.402** Traumatic rupture of unspecified ligament of right middle finger at metacarpophalangeal and interphalangeal joint

✓7th **S63.403** Traumatic rupture of unspecified ligament of left middle finger at metacarpophalangeal and interphalangeal joint

✓7th **S63.404** Traumatic rupture of unspecified ligament of right ring finger at metacarpophalangeal and interphalangeal joint

✓7th **S63.405** Traumatic rupture of unspecified ligament of left ring finger at metacarpophalangeal and interphalangeal joint

✓7th **S63.406** Traumatic rupture of unspecified ligament of right little finger at metacarpophalangeal and interphalangeal joint

---

✓ Additional Character Required   ✓x7th Xtension Alert   Unspecified Dx   Other Specified Dx   Manifestation   ▶◀ Revised Text   ● New Code   ▲ Revised Code Title

√7th **S63.407** **Traumatic rupture of unspecified ligament of left little finger at metacarpophalangeal and interphalangeal joint**

√7th **S63.408** **Traumatic rupture of unspecified ligament of other finger at metacarpophalangeal and interphalangeal joint**

Traumatic rupture of unspecified ligament of specified finger with unspecified laterality at metacarpophalangeal and interphalangeal joint

√7th **S63.409** **Traumatic rupture of unspecified ligament of unspecified finger at metacarpophalangeal and interphalangeal joint**

√6th **S63.41** **Traumatic rupture of** collateral ligament **of finger at metacarpophalangeal and interphalangeal joint**

√7th **S63.410** **Traumatic rupture of collateral ligament of** right index **finger at metacarpophalangeal and interphalangeal joint**

√7th **S63.411** **Traumatic rupture of collateral ligament of** left index **finger at metacarpophalangeal and interphalangeal joint**

√7th **S63.412** **Traumatic rupture of collateral ligament of** right middle **finger at metacarpophalangeal and interphalangeal joint**

√7th **S63.413** **Traumatic rupture of collateral ligament of** left middle **finger at metacarpophalangeal and interphalangeal joint**

√7th **S63.414** **Traumatic rupture of collateral ligament of** right ring **finger at metacarpophalangeal and interphalangeal joint**

√7th **S63.415** **Traumatic rupture of collateral ligament of** left ring **finger at metacarpophalangeal and interphalangeal joint**

√7th **S63.416** **Traumatic rupture of collateral ligament of** right little **finger at metacarpophalangeal and interphalangeal joint**

√7th **S63.417** **Traumatic rupture of collateral ligament of** left little **finger at metacarpophalangeal and interphalangeal joint**

√7th **S63.418** **Traumatic rupture of collateral ligament of other finger at metacarpophalangeal and interphalangeal joint**

Traumatic rupture of collateral ligament of specified finger with unspecified laterality at metacarpophalangeal and interphalangeal joint

√7th **S63.419** **Traumatic rupture of collateral ligament of unspecified finger at metacarpophalangeal and interphalangeal joint**

√6th **S63.42** **Traumatic rupture of** palmar ligament **of finger at metacarpophalangeal and interphalangeal joint**

√7th **S63.420** **Traumatic rupture of palmar ligament of** right index **finger at metacarpophalangeal and interphalangeal joint**

√7th **S63.421** **Traumatic rupture of palmar ligament of** left index **finger at metacarpophalangeal and interphalangeal joint**

√7th **S63.422** **Traumatic rupture of palmar ligament of** right middle **finger at metacarpophalangeal and interphalangeal joint**

√7th **S63.423** **Traumatic rupture of palmar ligament of** left middle **finger at metacarpophalangeal and interphalangeal joint**

√7th **S63.424** **Traumatic rupture of palmar ligament of** right ring **finger at metacarpophalangeal and interphalangeal joint**

√7th **S63.425** **Traumatic rupture of palmar ligament of** left ring **finger at metacarpophalangeal and interphalangeal joint**

√7th **S63.426** **Traumatic rupture of palmar ligament of** right little **finger at metacarpophalangeal and interphalangeal joint**

√7th **S63.427** **Traumatic rupture of palmar ligament of** left little **finger at metacarpophalangeal and interphalangeal joint**

√7th **S63.428** **Traumatic rupture of palmar ligament of other finger at metacarpophalangeal and interphalangeal joint**

Traumatic rupture of palmar ligament of specified finger with unspecified laterality at metacarpophalangeal and interphalangeal joint

√7th **S63.429** **Traumatic rupture of palmar ligament of unspecified finger at metacarpophalangeal and interphalangeal joint**

√6th **S63.43** **Traumatic rupture of** volar plate **of finger at metacarpophalangeal and interphalangeal joint**

√7th **S63.430** **Traumatic rupture of volar plate of** right index **finger at metacarpophalangeal and interphalangeal joint**

√7th **S63.431** **Traumatic rupture of volar plate of** left index **finger at metacarpophalangeal and interphalangeal joint**

√7th **S63.432** **Traumatic rupture of volar plate of** right middle **finger at metacarpophalangeal and interphalangeal joint**

√7th **S63.433** **Traumatic rupture of volar plate of** left middle **finger at metacarpophalangeal and interphalangeal joint**

√7th **S63.434** **Traumatic rupture of volar plate of** right ring **finger at metacarpophalangeal and interphalangeal joint**

√7th **S63.435** **Traumatic rupture of volar plate of** left ring **finger at metacarpophalangeal and interphalangeal joint**

√7th **S63.436** **Traumatic rupture of volar plate of** right little **finger at metacarpophalangeal and interphalangeal joint**

√7th **S63.437** **Traumatic rupture of volar plate of** left little **finger at metacarpophalangeal and interphalangeal joint**

√7th **S63.438** **Traumatic rupture of volar plate of other finger at metacarpophalangeal and interphalangeal joint**

Traumatic rupture of volar plate of specified finger with unspecified laterality at metacarpophalangeal and interphalangeal joint

√7th **S63.439** **Traumatic rupture of volar plate of unspecified finger at metacarpophalangeal and interphalangeal joint**

√6th **S63.49** **Traumatic rupture of** other ligament **of finger at metacarpophalangeal and interphalangeal joint**

√7th **S63.490** **Traumatic rupture of other ligament of** right index **finger at metacarpophalangeal and interphalangeal joint**

√7th **S63.491** **Traumatic rupture of other ligament of** left index **finger at metacarpophalangeal and interphalangeal joint**

√7th **S63.492** **Traumatic rupture of other ligament of** right middle **finger at metacarpophalangeal and interphalangeal joint**

√7th **S63.493** **Traumatic rupture of other ligament of** left middle **finger at metacarpophalangeal and interphalangeal joint**

√7th **S63.494** **Traumatic rupture of other ligament of** right ring **finger at metacarpophalangeal and interphalangeal joint**

√7th **S63.495** **Traumatic rupture of other ligament of** left ring **finger at metacarpophalangeal and interphalangeal joint**

√7th **S63.496** **Traumatic rupture of other ligament of** right little **finger at metacarpophalangeal and interphalangeal joint**

√7th **S63.497** **Traumatic rupture of other ligament of** left little **finger at metacarpophalangeal and interphalangeal joint**

√7th **S63.498** **Traumatic rupture of other ligament of other finger at metacarpophalangeal and interphalangeal joint**

Traumatic rupture of ligament of specified finger with unspecified laterality at metacarpophalangeal and interphalangeal joint

EXCLUDES 1 Not coded here   **EXCLUDES 2** Not included here   **N** Newborn Age: 0   **P** Pediatric Age: 0-17   **M** Maternity Age: 12-55   **A** Adult Age: 15-124

878   ICD-10-CM Draft (2015)

√7ᵗʰ **S63.499 Traumatic rupture of other ligament of unspecified finger at metacarpo-phalangeal and interphalangeal joint**

√5ᵗʰ **S63.5 Other and unspecified** sprain of wrist

√6ᵗʰ **S63.50 Unspecified** sprain of wrist

√7ᵗʰ **S63.501 Unspecified sprain of** right **wrist**

√7ᵗʰ **S63.502 Unspecified sprain of** left **wrist**

√7ᵗʰ **S63.509 Unspecified sprain of unspecified wrist**

√6ᵗʰ **S63.51 Sprain of** carpal **(joint)**

√7ᵗʰ **S63.511 Sprain of carpal joint of** right **wrist**

√7ᵗʰ **S63.512 Sprain of carpal joint of** left **wrist**

√7ᵗʰ **S63.519 Sprain of carpal joint of unspecified wrist**

√6ᵗʰ **S63.52 Sprain of** radiocarpal **joint**

EXCLUDES 1 *traumatic rupture of radiocarpal ligament (S63.32-)*

√7ᵗʰ **S63.521 Sprain of radiocarpal joint of** right **wrist**

√7ᵗʰ **S63.522 Sprain of radiocarpal joint of** left **wrist**

√7ᵗʰ **S63.529 Sprain of radiocarpal joint of unspecified wrist**

√6ᵗʰ **S63.59 Other** specified sprain of wrist

√7ᵗʰ **S63.591 Other specified sprain of** right **wrist**

√7ᵗʰ **S63.592 Other specified sprain of** left **wrist**

√7ᵗʰ **S63.599 Other specified sprain of unspecified wrist**

√5ᵗʰ **S63.6 Other and unspecified sprain of finger(s)**

EXCLUDES 1 *traumatic rupture of ligament of finger at metacarpophalangeal and interphalangeal joint(s) (S63.4-)*

√6ᵗʰ **S63.60 Unspecified sprain of** thumb

√7ᵗʰ **S63.601 Unspecified sprain of** right **thumb**

√7ᵗʰ **S63.602 Unspecified sprain of** left **thumb**

√7ᵗʰ **S63.609 Unspecified sprain of unspecified thumb**

√6ᵗʰ **S63.61 Unspecified sprain of** other and unspecified finger(s)

√7ᵗʰ **S63.610 Unspecified sprain of** right index **finger**

√7ᵗʰ **S63.611 Unspecified sprain of** left index **finger**

√7ᵗʰ **S63.612 Unspecified sprain of** right middle **finger**

√7ᵗʰ **S63.613 Unspecified sprain of** left middle **finger**

√7ᵗʰ **S63.614 Unspecified sprain of** right ring **finger**

√7ᵗʰ **S63.615 Unspecified sprain of** left ring **finger**

√7ᵗʰ **S63.616 Unspecified sprain of** right little **finger**

√7ᵗʰ **S63.617 Unspecified sprain of** left little **finger**

√7ᵗʰ **S63.618 Unspecified sprain of other finger**

Unspecified sprain of specified finger with unspecified laterality

√7ᵗʰ **S63.619 Unspecified sprain of unspecified finger**

√6ᵗʰ **S63.62 Sprain of** interphalangeal joint of thumb

√7ᵗʰ **S63.621 Sprain of interphalangeal joint of** right **thumb**

√7ᵗʰ **S63.622 Sprain of interphalangeal joint of** left **thumb**

√7ᵗʰ **S63.629 Sprain of interphalangeal joint of unspecified thumb**

√6ᵗʰ **S63.63 Sprain of** interphalangeal joint of other and unspecified finger(s)

√7ᵗʰ **S63.630 Sprain of interphalangeal joint of** right index **finger**

√7ᵗʰ **S63.631 Sprain of interphalangeal joint of** left index **finger**

√7ᵗʰ **S63.632 Sprain of interphalangeal joint of** right middle **finger**

√7ᵗʰ **S63.633 Sprain of interphalangeal joint of** left middle **finger**

√7ᵗʰ **S63.634 Sprain of interphalangeal joint of** right ring **finger**

√7ᵗʰ **S63.635 Sprain of interphalangeal joint of** left ring **finger**

√7ᵗʰ **S63.636 Sprain of interphalangeal joint of** right little **finger**

√7ᵗʰ **S63.637 Sprain of interphalangeal joint of** left little **finger**

√7ᵗʰ **S63.638 Sprain of interphalangeal joint of other finger**

√7ᵗʰ **S63.639 Sprain of interphalangeal joint of unspecified finger**

√6ᵗʰ **S63.64 Sprain of** metacarpophalangeal joint of thumb

√7ᵗʰ **S63.641 Sprain of metacarpophalangeal joint of** right **thumb**

√7ᵗʰ **S63.642 Sprain of metacarpophalangeal joint of** left **thumb**

√7ᵗʰ **S63.649 Sprain of metacarpophalangeal joint of unspecified thumb**

√6ᵗʰ **S63.65 Sprain of** metacarpophalangeal joint of other and unspecified finger(s)

√7ᵗʰ **S63.650 Sprain of metacarpophalangeal joint of** right index **finger**

√7ᵗʰ **S63.651 Sprain of metacarpophalangeal joint of** left index **finger**

√7ᵗʰ **S63.652 Sprain of metacarpophalangeal joint of** right middle **finger**

√7ᵗʰ **S63.653 Sprain of metacarpophalangeal joint of** left middle **finger**

√7ᵗʰ **S63.654 Sprain of metacarpophalangeal joint of** right ring **finger**

√7ᵗʰ **S63.655 Sprain of metacarpophalangeal joint of** left ring **finger**

√7ᵗʰ **S63.656 Sprain of metacarpophalangeal joint of** right little **finger**

√7ᵗʰ **S63.657 Sprain of metacarpophalangeal joint of** left little **finger**

√7ᵗʰ **S63.658 Sprain of metacarpophalangeal joint of other finger**

Sprain of metacarpophalangeal joint of specified finger with unspecified laterality

√7ᵗʰ **S63.659 Sprain of metacarpophalangeal joint of unspecified finger**

√6ᵗʰ **S63.68 Other sprain of** thumb

√7ᵗʰ **S63.681 Other sprain of** right **thumb**

√7ᵗʰ **S63.682 Other sprain of** left **thumb**

√7ᵗʰ **S63.689 Other sprain of unspecified thumb**

√6ᵗʰ **S63.69 Other sprain of** other and unspecified finger(s)

√7ᵗʰ **S63.690 Other sprain of** right index **finger**

√7ᵗʰ **S63.691 Other sprain of** left index **finger**

√7ᵗʰ **S63.692 Other sprain of** right middle **finger**

√7ᵗʰ **S63.693 Other sprain of** left middle **finger**

√7ᵗʰ **S63.694 Other sprain of** right ring **finger**

√7ᵗʰ **S63.695 Other sprain of** left ring **finger**

√7ᵗʰ **S63.696 Other sprain of** right little **finger**

√7ᵗʰ **S63.697 Other sprain of** left little **finger**

√7ᵗʰ **S63.698 Other sprain of other finger**

Other sprain of specified finger with unspecified laterality

√7ᵗʰ **S63.699 Other sprain of unspecified finger**

√5ᵗʰ **S63.8 Sprain of other part of wrist and hand**

√6ᵗʰ **S63.8X Sprain of other part of wrist and hand**

√7ᵗʰ **S63.8X1 Sprain of other part of** right **wrist and hand**

√7ᵗʰ **S63.8X2 Sprain of other part of** left **wrist and hand**

√7ᵗʰ **S63.8X9 Sprain of other part of unspecified wrist and hand**

√5ᵗʰ **S63.9 Sprain of unspecified part of wrist and hand**

√x7ᵗʰ **S63.90 Sprain of unspecified part of unspecified wrist and hand**

√x7ᵗʰ **S63.91 Sprain of unspecified part of** right **wrist and hand**

√x7ᵗʰ **S63.92 Sprain of unspecified part of** left **wrist and hand**

√4ᵗʰ **S64 Injury of nerves at wrist and hand level**

Code also any associated open wound (S61.-)

> The appropriate 7th character is to be added to each code from category S64.
> A   initial encounter
> D   subsequent encounter
> S   sequela

√5ᵗʰ **S64.0 Injury of** ulnar **nerve at wrist and hand level**

☑ Additional Character Required   √x7ᵗʰ Xtension Alert   Unspecified Dx   Other Specified Dx   Manifestation   ►◄ Revised Text   ● New Code   ▲ Revised Code Title

ICD-10-CM Draft (2015)

879

√x7ᵗʰ **S64.00** Injury of ulnar nerve at wrist and hand level of unspecified arm
√x7ᵗʰ **S64.01** Injury of ulnar nerve at wrist and hand level of right arm
√x7ᵗʰ **S64.02** Injury of ulnar nerve at wrist and hand level of left arm

√5ᵗʰ **S64.1** Injury of median nerve at wrist and hand level
√x7ᵗʰ **S64.10** Injury of median nerve at wrist and hand level of unspecified arm
√x7ᵗʰ **S64.11** Injury of median nerve at wrist and hand level of right arm
√x7ᵗʰ **S64.12** Injury of median nerve at wrist and hand level of left arm

√5ᵗʰ **S64.2** Injury of radial nerve at wrist and hand level
√x7ᵗʰ **S64.20** Injury of radial nerve at wrist and hand level of unspecified arm
√x7ᵗʰ **S64.21** Injury of radial nerve at wrist and hand level of right arm
√x7ᵗʰ **S64.22** Injury of radial nerve at wrist and hand level of left arm

√5ᵗʰ **S64.3** Injury of digital nerve of thumb
√x7ᵗʰ **S64.30** Injury of digital nerve of unspecified thumb
√x7ᵗʰ **S64.31** Injury of digital nerve of right thumb
√x7ᵗʰ **S64.32** Injury of digital nerve of left thumb

√5ᵗʰ **S64.4** Injury of digital nerve of other and unspecified finger
√x7ᵗʰ **S64.40** Injury of digital nerve of unspecified finger
√6ᵗʰ **S64.49** Injury of digital nerve of other finger
√7ᵗʰ **S64.490** Injury of digital nerve of right index finger
√7ᵗʰ **S64.491** Injury of digital nerve of left index finger
√7ᵗʰ **S64.492** Injury of digital nerve of right middle finger
√7ᵗʰ **S64.493** Injury of digital nerve of left middle finger
√7ᵗʰ **S64.494** Injury of digital nerve of right ring finger
√7ᵗʰ **S64.495** Injury of digital nerve of left ring finger
√7ᵗʰ **S64.496** Injury of digital nerve of right little finger
√7ᵗʰ **S64.497** Injury of digital nerve of left little finger
√7ᵗʰ **S64.498** Injury of digital nerve of other finger
Injury of digital nerve of specified finger with unspecified laterality

√5ᵗʰ **S64.8** Injury of other nerves at wrist and hand level
√6ᵗʰ **S64.8X** Injury of other nerves at wrist and hand level
√7ᵗʰ **S64.8X1** Injury of other nerves at wrist and hand level of right arm
√7ᵗʰ **S64.8X2** Injury of other nerves at wrist and hand level of left arm
√7ᵗʰ **S64.8X9** Injury of other nerves at wrist and hand level of unspecified arm

√5ᵗʰ **S64.9** Injury of unspecified nerve at wrist and hand level
√x7ᵗʰ **S64.90** Injury of unspecified nerve at wrist and hand level of unspecified arm
√x7ᵗʰ **S64.91** Injury of unspecified nerve at wrist and hand level of right arm
√x7ᵗʰ **S64.92** Injury of unspecified nerve at wrist and hand level of left arm

√4ᵗʰ **S65** Injury of blood vessels at wrist and hand level
Code also any associated open wound (S61.-)

The appropriate 7th character is to be added to each code from category S65.
A   initial encounter
D   subsequent encounter
S   sequela

√5ᵗʰ **S65.0** Injury of ulnar artery at wrist and hand level
√6ᵗʰ **S65.00** Unspecified injury of ulnar artery at wrist and hand level
√7ᵗʰ **S65.001** Unspecified injury of ulnar artery at wrist and hand level of right arm
√7ᵗʰ **S65.002** Unspecified injury of ulnar artery at wrist and hand level of left arm
√7ᵗʰ **S65.009** Unspecified injury of ulnar artery at wrist and hand level of unspecified arm

√6ᵗʰ **S65.01** Laceration of ulnar artery at wrist and hand level
√7ᵗʰ **S65.011** Laceration of ulnar artery at wrist and hand level of right arm
√7ᵗʰ **S65.012** Laceration of ulnar artery at wrist and hand level of left arm
√7ᵗʰ **S65.019** Laceration of ulnar artery at wrist and hand level of unspecified arm

√6ᵗʰ **S65.09** Other specified injury of ulnar artery at wrist and hand level
√7ᵗʰ **S65.091** Other specified injury of ulnar artery at wrist and hand level of right arm
√7ᵗʰ **S65.092** Other specified injury of ulnar artery at wrist and hand level of left arm
√7ᵗʰ **S65.099** Other specified injury of ulnar artery at wrist and hand level of unspecified arm

√5ᵗʰ **S65.1** Injury of radial artery at wrist and hand level
√6ᵗʰ **S65.10** Unspecified injury of radial artery at wrist and hand level
√7ᵗʰ **S65.101** Unspecified injury of radial artery at wrist and hand level of right arm
√7ᵗʰ **S65.102** Unspecified injury of radial artery at wrist and hand level of left arm
√7ᵗʰ **S65.109** Unspecified injury of radial artery at wrist and hand level of unspecified arm

√6ᵗʰ **S65.11** Laceration of radial artery at wrist and hand level
√7ᵗʰ **S65.111** Laceration of radial artery at wrist and hand level of right arm
√7ᵗʰ **S65.112** Laceration of radial artery at wrist and hand level of left arm
√7ᵗʰ **S65.119** Laceration of radial artery at wrist and hand level of unspecified arm

√6ᵗʰ **S65.19** Other specified injury of radial artery at wrist and hand level
√7ᵗʰ **S65.191** Other specified injury of radial artery at wrist and hand level of right arm
√7ᵗʰ **S65.192** Other specified injury of radial artery at wrist and hand level of left arm
√7ᵗʰ **S65.199** Other specified injury of radial artery at wrist and hand level of unspecified arm

√5ᵗʰ **S65.2** Injury of superficial palmar arch
√6ᵗʰ **S65.20** Unspecified injury of superficial palmar arch
√7ᵗʰ **S65.201** Unspecified injury of superficial palmar arch of right hand
√7ᵗʰ **S65.202** Unspecified injury of superficial palmar arch of left hand
√7ᵗʰ **S65.209** Unspecified injury of superficial palmar arch of unspecified hand

√6ᵗʰ **S65.21** Laceration of superficial palmar arch
√7ᵗʰ **S65.211** Laceration of superficial palmar arch of right hand
√7ᵗʰ **S65.212** Laceration of superficial palmar arch of left hand
√7ᵗʰ **S65.219** Laceration of superficial palmar arch of unspecified hand

√6ᵗʰ **S65.29** Other specified injury of superficial palmar arch
√7ᵗʰ **S65.291** Other specified injury of superficial palmar arch of right hand
√7ᵗʰ **S65.292** Other specified injury of superficial palmar arch of left hand
√7ᵗʰ **S65.299** Other specified injury of superficial palmar arch of unspecified hand

√5ᵗʰ **S65.3** Injury of deep palmar arch
√6ᵗʰ **S65.30** Unspecified injury of deep palmar arch
√7ᵗʰ **S65.301** Unspecified injury of deep palmar arch of right hand
√7ᵗʰ **S65.302** Unspecified injury of deep palmar arch of left hand
√7ᵗʰ **S65.309** Unspecified injury of deep palmar arch of unspecified hand

√6ᵗʰ **S65.31** Laceration of deep palmar arch
√7ᵗʰ **S65.311** Laceration of deep palmar arch of right hand
√7ᵗʰ **S65.312** Laceration of deep palmar arch of left hand

✓7th **S65.319** Laceration of deep palmar arch of unspecified hand

✓6th **S65.39** Other specified injury of deep palmar arch

✓7th **S65.391** Other specified injury of deep palmar arch of right hand

✓7th **S65.392** Other specified injury of deep palmar arch of left hand

✓7th **S65.399** Other specified injury of deep palmar arch of unspecified hand

✓5th **S65.4** Injury of blood vessel of thumb

✓6th **S65.40** Unspecified injury of blood vessel of thumb

✓7th **S65.401** Unspecified injury of blood vessel of right thumb

✓7th **S65.402** Unspecified injury of blood vessel of left thumb

✓7th **S65.409** Unspecified injury of blood vessel of unspecified thumb

✓6th **S65.41** Laceration of blood vessel of thumb

✓7th **S65.411** Laceration of blood vessel of right thumb

✓7th **S65.412** Laceration of blood vessel of left thumb

✓7th **S65.419** Laceration of blood vessel of unspecified thumb

✓6th **S65.49** Other specified injury of blood vessel of thumb

✓7th **S65.491** Other specified injury of blood vessel of right thumb

✓7th **S65.492** Other specified injury of blood vessel of left thumb

✓7th **S65.499** Other specified injury of blood vessel of unspecified thumb

✓5th **S65.5** Injury of blood vessel of other and unspecified finger

✓6th **S65.50** Unspecified injury of blood vessel of other and unspecified finger

✓7th **S65.500** Unspecified injury of blood vessel of right index finger

✓7th **S65.501** Unspecified injury of blood vessel of left index finger

✓7th **S65.502** Unspecified injury of blood vessel of right middle finger

✓7th **S65.503** Unspecified injury of blood vessel of left middle finger

✓7th **S65.504** Unspecified injury of blood vessel of right ring finger

✓7th **S65.505** Unspecified injury of blood vessel of left ring finger

✓7th **S65.506** Unspecified injury of blood vessel of right little finger

✓7th **S65.507** Unspecified injury of blood vessel of left little finger

✓7th **S65.508** Unspecified injury of blood vessel of other finger
Unspecified injury of blood vessel of specified finger with unspecified laterality

✓7th **S65.509** Unspecified injury of blood vessel of unspecified finger

✓6th **S65.51** Laceration of blood vessel of other and unspecified finger

✓7th **S65.510** Laceration of blood vessel of right index finger

✓7th **S65.511** Laceration of blood vessel of left index finger

✓7th **S65.512** Laceration of blood vessel of right middle finger

✓7th **S65.513** Laceration of blood vessel of left middle finger

✓7th **S65.514** Laceration of blood vessel of right ring finger

✓7th **S65.515** Laceration of blood vessel of left ring finger

✓7th **S65.516** Laceration of blood vessel of right little finger

✓7th **S65.517** Laceration of blood vessel of left little finger

✓7th **S65.518** Laceration of blood vessel of other finger
Laceration of blood vessel of specified finger with unspecified laterality

✓7th **S65.519** Laceration of blood vessel of unspecified finger

✓6th **S65.59** Other specified injury of blood vessel of other and unspecified finger

✓7th **S65.590** Other specified injury of blood vessel of right index finger

✓7th **S65.591** Other specified injury of blood vessel of left index finger

✓7th **S65.592** Other specified injury of blood vessel of right middle finger

✓7th **S65.593** Other specified injury of blood vessel of left middle finger

✓7th **S65.594** Other specified injury of blood vessel of right ring finger

✓7th **S65.595** Other specified injury of blood vessel of left ring finger

✓7th **S65.596** Other specified injury of blood vessel of right little finger

✓7th **S65.597** Other specified injury of blood vessel of left little finger

✓7th **S65.598** Other specified injury of blood vessel of other finger
Other specified injury of blood vessel of specified finger with unspecified laterality

✓7th **S65.599** Other specified injury of blood vessel of unspecified finger

✓5th **S65.8** Injury of other blood vessels at wrist and hand level

✓6th **S65.80** Unspecified injury of other blood vessels at wrist and hand level

✓7th **S65.801** Unspecified injury of other blood vessels at wrist and hand level of right arm

✓7th **S65.802** Unspecified injury of other blood vessels at wrist and hand level of left arm

✓7th **S65.809** Unspecified injury of other blood vessels at wrist and hand level of unspecified arm

✓6th **S65.81** Laceration of other blood vessels at wrist and hand level

✓7th **S65.811** Laceration of other blood vessels at wrist and hand level of right arm

✓7th **S65.812** Laceration of other blood vessels at wrist and hand level of left arm

✓7th **S65.819** Laceration of other blood vessels at wrist and hand level of unspecified arm

✓6th **S65.89** Other specified injury of other blood vessels at wrist and hand level

✓7th **S65.891** Other specified injury of other blood vessels at wrist and hand level of right arm

✓7th **S65.892** Other specified injury of other blood vessels at wrist and hand level of left arm

✓7th **S65.899** Other specified injury of other blood vessels at wrist and hand level of unspecified arm

✓5th **S65.9** Injury of unspecified blood vessel at wrist and hand level

✓6th **S65.90** Unspecified injury of unspecified blood vessel at wrist and hand level

✓7th **S65.901** Unspecified injury of unspecified blood vessel at wrist and hand level of right arm

✓7th **S65.902** Unspecified injury of unspecified blood vessel at wrist and hand level of left arm

✓7th **S65.909** Unspecified injury of unspecified blood vessel at wrist and hand level of unspecified arm

✓6th **S65.91** Laceration of unspecified blood vessel at wrist and hand level

✓7th **S65.911** Laceration of unspecified blood vessel at wrist and hand level of right arm

✓7th **S65.912** Laceration of unspecified blood vessel at wrist and hand level of left arm

✓7th **S65.919** Laceration of unspecified blood vessel at wrist and hand level of unspecified arm

✓ Additional Character Required   ✓x7th Xtension Alert   Unspecified Dx   Other Specified Dx   Manifestation   ►◄ Revised Text   ● New Code   ▲ Revised Code Title

ICD-10-CM Draft (2015)   881

√6ᵗʰ **S65.99** Other specified injury of unspecified blood vessel at wrist and hand level

  √7ᵗʰ **S65.991** Other specified injury of unspecified blood vessel at wrist and hand of right arm

  √7ᵗʰ **S65.992** Other specified injury of unspecified blood vessel at wrist and hand of left arm

  √7ᵗʰ **S65.999** Other specified injury of unspecified blood vessel at wrist and hand of unspecified arm

√4ᵗʰ **S66 Injury of muscle, fascia and tendon at wrist and hand level**

Code also any associated open wound (S61.-)

EXCLUDES 2   sprain of joints and ligaments of wrist and hand (S63.-)

The appropriate 7th character is to be added to each code from category S66.
A   initial encounter
D   subsequent encounter
S   sequela

√5ᵗʰ **S66.0** Injury of long flexor muscle, fascia and tendon of thumb at wrist and hand level

 √6ᵗʰ **S66.00** Unspecified injury of long flexor muscle, fascia and tendon of thumb at wrist and hand level

  √7ᵗʰ **S66.001** Unspecified injury of long flexor muscle, fascia and tendon of right thumb at wrist and hand level

  √7ᵗʰ **S66.002** Unspecified injury of long flexor muscle, fascia and tendon of left thumb at wrist and hand level

  √7ᵗʰ **S66.009** Unspecified injury of long flexor muscle, fascia and tendon of unspecified thumb at wrist and hand level

 √6ᵗʰ **S66.01** Strain of long flexor muscle, fascia and tendon of thumb at wrist and hand level

  √7ᵗʰ **S66.011** Strain of long flexor muscle, fascia and tendon of right thumb at wrist and hand level

  √7ᵗʰ **S66.012** Strain of long flexor muscle, fascia and tendon of left thumb at wrist and hand level

  √7ᵗʰ **S66.019** Strain of long flexor muscle, fascia and tendon of unspecified thumb at wrist and hand level

 √6ᵗʰ **S66.02** Laceration of long flexor muscle, fascia and tendon of thumb at wrist and hand level

  √7ᵗʰ **S66.021** Laceration of long flexor muscle, fascia and tendon of right thumb at wrist and hand level

  √7ᵗʰ **S66.022** Laceration of long flexor muscle, fascia and tendon of left thumb at wrist and hand level

  √7ᵗʰ **S66.029** Laceration of long flexor muscle, fascia and tendon of unspecified thumb at wrist and hand level

 √6ᵗʰ **S66.09** Other specified injury of long flexor muscle, fascia and tendon of thumb at wrist and hand level

  √7ᵗʰ **S66.091** Other specified injury of long flexor muscle, fascia and tendon of right thumb at wrist and hand level

  √7ᵗʰ **S66.092** Other specified injury of long flexor muscle, fascia and tendon of left thumb at wrist and hand level

  √7ᵗʰ **S66.099** Other specified injury of long flexor muscle, fascia and tendon of unspecified thumb at wrist and hand level

√5ᵗʰ **S66.1** Injury of flexor muscle, fascia and tendon of other and unspecified finger at wrist and hand level

EXCLUDES 2   Injury of long flexor muscle, fascia and tendon of thumb at wrist and hand level (S66.0-)

 √6ᵗʰ **S66.10** Unspecified injury of flexor muscle, fascia and tendon of other and unspecified finger at wrist and hand level

  √7ᵗʰ **S66.100** Unspecified injury of flexor muscle, fascia and tendon of right index finger at wrist and hand level

  √7ᵗʰ **S66.101** Unspecified injury of flexor muscle, fascia and tendon of left index finger at wrist and hand level

  √7ᵗʰ **S66.102** Unspecified injury of flexor muscle, fascia and tendon of right middle finger at wrist and hand level

  √7ᵗʰ **S66.103** Unspecified injury of flexor muscle, fascia and tendon of left middle finger at wrist and hand level

  √7ᵗʰ **S66.104** Unspecified injury of flexor muscle, fascia and tendon of right ring finger at wrist and hand level

  √7ᵗʰ **S66.105** Unspecified injury of flexor muscle, fascia and tendon of left ring finger at wrist and hand level

  √7ᵗʰ **S66.106** Unspecified injury of flexor muscle, fascia and tendon of right little finger at wrist and hand level

  √7ᵗʰ **S66.107** Unspecified injury of flexor muscle, fascia and tendon of left little finger at wrist and hand level

  √7ᵗʰ **S66.108** Unspecified injury of flexor muscle, fascia and tendon of other finger at wrist and hand level

Unspecified injury of flexor muscle, fascia and tendon of specified finger with unspecified laterality at wrist and hand level

  √7ᵗʰ **S66.109** Unspecified injury of flexor muscle, fascia and tendon of unspecified finger at wrist and hand level

 √6ᵗʰ **S66.11** Strain of flexor muscle, fascia and tendon of other and unspecified finger at wrist and hand level

  √7ᵗʰ **S66.110** Strain of flexor muscle, fascia and tendon of right index finger at wrist and hand level

  √7ᵗʰ **S66.111** Strain of flexor muscle, fascia and tendon of left index finger at wrist and hand level

  √7ᵗʰ **S66.112** Strain of flexor muscle, fascia and tendon of right middle finger at wrist and hand level

  √7ᵗʰ **S66.113** Strain of flexor muscle, fascia and tendon of left middle finger at wrist and hand level

  √7ᵗʰ **S66.114** Strain of flexor muscle, fascia and tendon of right ring finger at wrist and hand level

  √7ᵗʰ **S66.115** Strain of flexor muscle, fascia and tendon of left ring finger at wrist and hand level

  √7ᵗʰ **S66.116** Strain of flexor muscle, fascia and tendon of right little finger at wrist and hand level

  √7ᵗʰ **S66.117** Strain of flexor muscle, fascia and tendon of left little finger at wrist and hand level

  √7ᵗʰ **S66.118** Strain of flexor muscle, fascia and tendon of other finger at wrist and hand level

Strain of flexor muscle, fascia and tendon of specified finger with unspecified laterality at wrist and hand level

  √7ᵗʰ **S66.119** Strain of flexor muscle, fascia and tendon of unspecified finger at wrist and hand level

 √6ᵗʰ **S66.12** Laceration of flexor muscle, fascia and tendon of other and unspecified finger at wrist and hand level

  √7ᵗʰ **S66.120** Laceration of flexor muscle, fascia and tendon of right index finger at wrist and hand level

  √7ᵗʰ **S66.121** Laceration of flexor muscle, fascia and tendon of left index finger at wrist and hand level

  √7ᵗʰ **S66.122** Laceration of flexor muscle, fascia and tendon of right middle finger at wrist and hand level

  √7ᵗʰ **S66.123** Laceration of flexor muscle, fascia and tendon of left middle finger at wrist and hand level

  √7ᵗʰ **S66.124** Laceration of flexor muscle, fascia and tendon of right ring finger at wrist and hand level

  √7ᵗʰ **S66.125** Laceration of flexor muscle, fascia and tendon of left ring finger at wrist and hand level

---

EXCLUDES 1 Not coded here   EXCLUDES 2 Not included here   N Newborn Age: 0   P Pediatric Age: 0-17   M Maternity Age: 12-55   A Adult Age: 15-124

✓7th **S66.126** Laceration of flexor muscle, fascia and tendon of right little finger at wrist and hand level

✓7th **S66.127** Laceration of flexor muscle, fascia and tendon of left little finger at wrist and hand level

✓7th **S66.128** Laceration of flexor muscle, fascia and tendon of other finger at wrist and hand level

Laceration of flexor muscle, fascia and tendon of specified finger with unspecified laterality at wrist and hand level

✓7th **S66.129** Laceration of flexor muscle, fascia and tendon of unspecified finger at wrist and hand level

✓6th **S66.19** Other injury of flexor muscle, fascia and tendon of other and unspecified finger at wrist and hand level

✓7th **S66.190** Other injury of flexor muscle, fascia and tendon of right index finger at wrist and hand level

✓7th **S66.191** Other injury of flexor muscle, fascia and tendon of left index finger at wrist and hand level

✓7th **S66.192** Other injury of flexor muscle, fascia and tendon of right middle finger at wrist and hand level

✓7th **S66.193** Other injury of flexor muscle, fascia and tendon of left middle finger at wrist and hand level

✓7th **S66.194** Other injury of flexor muscle, fascia and tendon of right ring finger at wrist and hand level

✓7th **S66.195** Other injury of flexor muscle, fascia and tendon of left ring finger at wrist and hand level

✓7th **S66.196** Other injury of flexor muscle, fascia and tendon of right little finger at wrist and hand level

✓7th **S66.197** Other injury of flexor muscle, fascia and tendon of left little finger at wrist and hand level

✓7th **S66.198** Other injury of flexor muscle, fascia and tendon of other finger at wrist and hand level

Other injury of flexor muscle, fascia and tendon of specified finger with unspecified laterality at wrist and hand level

✓7th **S66.199** Other injury of flexor muscle, fascia and tendon of unspecified finger at wrist and hand level

✓5th **S66.2** Injury of extensor muscle, fascia and tendon of thumb at wrist and hand level

✓6th **S66.20** Unspecified injury of extensor muscle, fascia and tendon of thumb at wrist and hand level

✓7th **S66.201** Unspecified injury of extensor muscle, fascia and tendon of right thumb at wrist and hand level

✓7th **S66.202** Unspecified injury of extensor muscle, fascia and tendon of left thumb at wrist and hand level

✓7th **S66.209** Unspecified injury of extensor muscle, fascia and tendon of unspecified thumb at wrist and hand level

✓6th **S66.21** Strain of extensor muscle, fascia and tendon of thumb at wrist and hand level

✓7th **S66.211** Strain of extensor muscle, fascia and tendon of right thumb at wrist and hand level

✓7th **S66.212** Strain of extensor muscle, fascia and tendon of left thumb at wrist and hand level

✓7th **S66.219** Strain of extensor muscle, fascia and tendon of unspecified thumb at wrist and hand level

✓6th **S66.22** Laceration of extensor muscle, fascia and tendon of thumb at wrist and hand level

✓7th **S66.221** Laceration of extensor muscle, fascia and tendon of right thumb at wrist and hand level

✓7th **S66.222** Laceration of extensor muscle, fascia and tendon of left thumb at wrist and hand level

✓7th **S66.229** Laceration of extensor muscle, fascia and tendon of unspecified thumb at wrist and hand level

✓6th **S66.29** Other specified injury of extensor muscle, fascia and tendon of thumb at wrist and hand level

✓7th **S66.291** Other specified injury of extensor muscle, fascia and tendon of right thumb at wrist and hand level

✓7th **S66.292** Other specified injury of extensor muscle, fascia and tendon of left thumb at wrist and hand level

✓7th **S66.299** Other specified injury of extensor muscle, fascia and tendon of unspecified thumb at wrist and hand level

✓5th **S66.3** Injury of extensor muscle, fascia and tendon of other and unspecified finger at wrist and hand level

EXCLUDES 2 Injury of extensor muscle, fascia and tendon of thumb at wrist and hand level (S66.2-)

✓6th **S66.30** Unspecified injury of extensor muscle, fascia and tendon of other and unspecified finger at wrist and hand level

✓7th **S66.300** Unspecified injury of extensor muscle, fascia and tendon of right index finger at wrist and hand level

✓7th **S66.301** Unspecified injury of extensor muscle, fascia and tendon of left index finger at wrist and hand level

✓7th **S66.302** Unspecified injury of extensor muscle, fascia and tendon of right middle finger at wrist and hand level

✓7th **S66.303** Unspecified injury of extensor muscle, fascia and tendon of left middle finger at wrist and hand level

✓7th **S66.304** Unspecified injury of extensor muscle, fascia and tendon of right ring finger at wrist and hand level

✓7th **S66.305** Unspecified injury of extensor muscle, fascia and tendon of left ring finger at wrist and hand level

✓7th **S66.306** Unspecified injury of extensor muscle, fascia and tendon of right little finger at wrist and hand level

✓7th **S66.307** Unspecified injury of extensor muscle, fascia and tendon of left little finger at wrist and hand level

✓7th **S66.308** Unspecified injury of extensor muscle, fascia and tendon of other finger at wrist and hand level

Unspecified injury of extensor muscle, fascia and tendon of specified finger with unspecified laterality at wrist and hand level

✓7th **S66.309** Unspecified injury of extensor muscle, fascia and tendon of unspecified finger at wrist and hand level

✓6th **S66.31** Strain of extensor muscle, fascia and tendon of other and unspecified finger at wrist and hand level

✓7th **S66.310** Strain of extensor muscle, fascia and tendon of right index finger at wrist and hand level

✓7th **S66.311** Strain of extensor muscle, fascia and tendon of left index finger at wrist and hand level

✓7th **S66.312** Strain of extensor muscle, fascia and tendon of right middle finger at wrist and hand level

✓7th **S66.313** Strain of extensor muscle, fascia and tendon of left middle finger at wrist and hand level

✓7th **S66.314** Strain of extensor muscle, fascia and tendon of right ring finger at wrist and hand level

☑ Additional Character Required   ✓x7th Xtension Alert   Unspecified Dx   Other Specified Dx   Manifestation   ►◄ Revised Text   ● New Code   ▲ Revised Code Title

ICD-10-CM Draft (2015)   883

√7ᵗʰ **S66.315** Strain of extensor muscle, fascia and tendon of left ring finger at wrist and hand level

√7ᵗʰ **S66.316** Strain of extensor muscle, fascia and tendon of right little finger at wrist and hand level

√7ᵗʰ **S66.317** Strain of extensor muscle, fascia and tendon of left little finger at wrist and hand level

√7ᵗʰ **S66.318** Strain of extensor muscle, fascia and tendon of other finger at wrist and hand level

Strain of extensor muscle, fascia and tendon of specified finger with unspecified laterality at wrist and hand level

√7ᵗʰ **S66.319** Strain of extensor muscle, fascia and tendon of unspecified finger at wrist and hand level

√6ᵗʰ **S66.32** Laceration of extensor muscle, fascia and tendon of other and unspecified finger at wrist and hand level

√7ᵗʰ **S66.320** Laceration of extensor muscle, fascia and tendon of right index finger at wrist and hand level

√7ᵗʰ **S66.321** Laceration of extensor muscle, fascia and tendon of left index finger at wrist and hand level

√7ᵗʰ **S66.322** Laceration of extensor muscle, fascia and tendon of right middle finger at wrist and hand level

√7ᵗʰ **S66.323** Laceration of extensor muscle, fascia and tendon of left middle finger at wrist and hand level

√7ᵗʰ **S66.324** Laceration of extensor muscle, fascia and tendon of right ring finger at wrist and hand level

√7ᵗʰ **S66.325** Laceration of extensor muscle, fascia and tendon of left ring finger at wrist and hand level

√7ᵗʰ **S66.326** Laceration of extensor muscle, fascia and tendon of right little finger at wrist and hand level

√7ᵗʰ **S66.327** Laceration of extensor muscle, fascia and tendon of left little finger at wrist and hand level

√7ᵗʰ **S66.328** Laceration of extensor muscle, fascia and tendon of other finger at wrist and hand level

Laceration of extensor muscle, fascia and tendon of specified finger with unspecified laterality at wrist and hand level

√7ᵗʰ **S66.329** Laceration of extensor muscle, fascia and tendon of unspecified finger at wrist and hand level

√6ᵗʰ **S66.39** Other injury of extensor muscle, fascia and tendon of other and unspecified finger at wrist and hand level

√7ᵗʰ **S66.390** Other injury of extensor muscle, fascia and tendon of right index finger at wrist and hand level

√7ᵗʰ **S66.391** Other injury of extensor muscle, fascia and tendon of left index finger at wrist and hand level

√7ᵗʰ **S66.392** Other injury of extensor muscle, fascia and tendon of right middle finger at wrist and hand level

√7ᵗʰ **S66.393** Other injury of extensor muscle, fascia and tendon of left middle finger at wrist and hand level

√7ᵗʰ **S66.394** Other injury of extensor muscle, fascia and tendon of right ring finger at wrist and hand level

√7ᵗʰ **S66.395** Other injury of extensor muscle, fascia and tendon of left ring finger at wrist and hand level

√7ᵗʰ **S66.396** Other injury of extensor muscle, fascia and tendon of right little finger at wrist and hand level

√7ᵗʰ **S66.397** Other injury of extensor muscle, fascia and tendon of left little finger at wrist and hand level

√7ᵗʰ **S66.398** Other injury of extensor muscle, fascia and tendon of other finger at wrist and hand level

Other injury of extensor muscle, fascia and tendon of specified finger with unspecified laterality at wrist and hand level

√7ᵗʰ **S66.399** Other injury of extensor muscle, fascia and tendon of unspecified finger at wrist and hand level

√5ᵗʰ **S66.4** Injury of intrinsic muscle, fascia and tendon of thumb at wrist and hand level

√6ᵗʰ **S66.40** Unspecified injury of intrinsic muscle, fascia and tendon of thumb at wrist and hand level

√7ᵗʰ **S66.401** Unspecified injury of intrinsic muscle, fascia and tendon of right thumb at wrist and hand level

√7ᵗʰ **S66.402** Unspecified injury of intrinsic muscle, fascia and tendon of left thumb at wrist and hand level

√7ᵗʰ **S66.409** Unspecified injury of intrinsic muscle, fascia and tendon of unspecified thumb at wrist and hand level

√6ᵗʰ **S66.41** Strain of intrinsic muscle, fascia and tendon of thumb at wrist and hand level

√7ᵗʰ **S66.411** Strain of intrinsic muscle, fascia and tendon of right thumb at wrist and hand level

√7ᵗʰ **S66.412** Strain of intrinsic muscle, fascia and tendon of left thumb at wrist and hand level

√7ᵗʰ **S66.419** Strain of intrinsic muscle, fascia and tendon of unspecified thumb at wrist and hand level

√6ᵗʰ **S66.42** Laceration of intrinsic muscle, fascia and tendon of thumb at wrist and hand level

√7ᵗʰ **S66.421** Laceration of intrinsic muscle, fascia and tendon of right thumb at wrist and hand level

√7ᵗʰ **S66.422** Laceration of intrinsic muscle, fascia and tendon of left thumb at wrist and hand level

√7ᵗʰ **S66.429** Laceration of intrinsic muscle, fascia and tendon of unspecified thumb at wrist and hand level

√6ᵗʰ **S66.49** Other specified injury of intrinsic muscle, fascia and tendon of thumb at wrist and hand level

√7ᵗʰ **S66.491** Other specified injury of intrinsic muscle, fascia and tendon of right thumb at wrist and hand level

√7ᵗʰ **S66.492** Other specified injury of intrinsic muscle, fascia and tendon of left thumb at wrist and hand level

√7ᵗʰ **S66.499** Other specified injury of intrinsic muscle, fascia and tendon of unspecified thumb at wrist and hand level

√5ᵗʰ **S66.5** Injury of intrinsic muscle, fascia and tendon of other and unspecified finger at wrist and hand level

EXCLUDES 2 injury of intrinsic muscle, fascia and tendon of thumb at wrist and hand level (S66.4-)

√6ᵗʰ **S66.50** Unspecified injury of intrinsic muscle, fascia and tendon of other and unspecified finger at wrist and hand level

√7ᵗʰ **S66.500** Unspecified injury of intrinsic muscle, fascia and tendon of right index finger at wrist and hand level

√7ᵗʰ **S66.501** Unspecified injury of intrinsic muscle, fascia and tendon of left index finger at wrist and hand level

√7ᵗʰ **S66.502** Unspecified injury of intrinsic muscle, fascia and tendon of right middle finger at wrist and hand level

√7ᵗʰ **S66.503** Unspecified injury of intrinsic muscle, fascia and tendon of left middle finger at wrist and hand level

EXCLUDES 1 Not coded here   *EXCLUDES 2* Not included here   N Newborn Age: 0   P Pediatric Age: 0-17   M Maternity Age: 12-55   A Adult Age: 15-124

884   ICD-10-CM Draft (2015)

√7th **S66.504** **Unspecified injury of intrinsic muscle, fascia and tendon of** right ring **finger at wrist and hand level**

√7th **S66.505** **Unspecified injury of intrinsic muscle, fascia and tendon of** left ring **finger at wrist and hand level**

√7th **S66.506** **Unspecified injury of intrinsic muscle, fascia and tendon of** right little **finger at wrist and hand level**

√7th **S66.507** **Unspecified injury of intrinsic muscle, fascia and tendon of** left little **finger at wrist and hand level**

√7th **S66.508** **Unspecified injury of intrinsic muscle, fascia and tendon of other finger at wrist and hand level**

Unspecified injury of intrinsic muscle, fascia and tendon of specified finger with unspecified laterality at wrist and hand level

√7th **S66.509** **Unspecified injury of intrinsic muscle, fascia and tendon of unspecified finger at wrist and hand level**

√6th **S66.51** Strain **of intrinsic muscle, fascia and tendon of** other and unspecified finger **at wrist and hand level**

√7th **S66.510** **Strain of intrinsic muscle, fascia and tendon of** right index **finger at wrist and hand level**

√7th **S66.511** **Strain of intrinsic muscle, fascia and tendon of** left index **finger at wrist and hand level**

√7th **S66.512** **Strain of intrinsic muscle, fascia and tendon of** right middle **finger at wrist and hand level**

√7th **S66.513** **Strain of intrinsic muscle, fascia and tendon of** left middle **finger at wrist and hand level**

√7th **S66.514** **Strain of intrinsic muscle, fascia and tendon of** right ring **finger at wrist and hand level**

√7th **S66.515** **Strain of intrinsic muscle, fascia and tendon of** left ring **finger at wrist and hand level**

√7th **S66.516** **Strain of intrinsic muscle, fascia and tendon of** right little **finger at wrist and hand level**

√7th **S66.517** **Strain of intrinsic muscle, fascia and tendon of** left little **finger at wrist and hand level**

√7th **S66.518** **Strain of intrinsic muscle, fascia and tendon of other finger at wrist and hand level**

Strain of intrinsic muscle, fascia and tendon of specified finger with unspecified laterality at wrist and hand level

√7th **S66.519** **Strain of intrinsic muscle, fascia and tendon of unspecified finger at wrist and hand level**

√6th **S66.52** Laceration **of intrinsic muscle, fascia and tendon of other and unspecified finger at wrist and hand level**

√7th **S66.520** **Laceration of intrinsic muscle, fascia and tendon of** right index **finger at wrist and hand level**

√7th **S66.521** **Laceration of intrinsic muscle, fascia and tendon of** left index **finger at wrist and hand level**

√7th **S66.522** **Laceration of intrinsic muscle, fascia and tendon of** right middle **finger at wrist and hand level**

√7th **S66.523** **Laceration of intrinsic muscle, fascia and tendon of** left middle **finger at wrist and hand level**

√7th **S66.524** **Laceration of intrinsic muscle, fascia and tendon of** right ring **finger at wrist and hand level**

√7th **S66.525** **Laceration of intrinsic muscle, fascia and tendon of** left ring **finger at wrist and hand level**

√7th **S66.526** **Laceration of intrinsic muscle, fascia and tendon of** right little **finger at wrist and hand level**

√7th **S66.527** **Laceration of intrinsic muscle, fascia and tendon of** left little **finger at wrist and hand level**

√7th **S66.528** **Laceration of intrinsic muscle, fascia and tendon of other finger at wrist and hand level**

Laceration of intrinsic muscle, fascia and tendon of specified finger with unspecified laterality at wrist and hand level

√7th **S66.529** **Laceration of intrinsic muscle, fascia and tendon of unspecified finger at wrist and hand level**

√6th **S66.59** Other **injury of intrinsic muscle, fascia and tendon of other and unspecified finger at wrist and hand level**

√7th **S66.590** **Other injury of intrinsic muscle, fascia and tendon of** right index **finger at wrist and hand level**

√7th **S66.591** **Other injury of intrinsic muscle, fascia and tendon of** left index **finger at wrist and hand level**

√7th **S66.592** **Other injury of intrinsic muscle, fascia and tendon of** right middle **finger at wrist and hand level**

√7th **S66.593** **Other injury of intrinsic muscle, fascia and tendon of** left middle **finger at wrist and hand level**

√7th **S66.594** **Other injury of intrinsic muscle, fascia and tendon of** right ring **finger at wrist and hand level**

√7th **S66.595** **Other injury of intrinsic muscle, fascia and tendon of** left ring **finger at wrist and hand level**

√7th **S66.596** **Other injury of intrinsic muscle, fascia and tendon of** right little **finger at wrist and hand level**

√7th **S66.597** **Other injury of intrinsic muscle, fascia and tendon of** left little **finger at wrist and hand level**

√7th **S66.598** **Other injury of intrinsic muscle, fascia and tendon of other finger at wrist and hand level**

Other injury of intrinsic muscle, fascia and tendon of specified finger with unspecified laterality at wrist and hand level

√7th **S66.599** **Other injury of intrinsic muscle, fascia and tendon of unspecified finger at wrist and hand level**

√5th **S66.8** **Injury of** other specified muscles**, fascia and tendons at wrist and hand level**

√6th **S66.80** Unspecified **injury of other specified muscles, fascia and tendons at wrist and hand level**

√7th **S66.801** **Unspecified injury of other specified muscles, fascia and tendons at wrist and hand level,** right **hand**

√7th **S66.802** **Unspecified injury of other specified muscles, fascia and tendons at wrist and hand level,** left **hand**

√7th **S66.809** **Unspecified injury of other specified muscles, fascia and tendons at wrist and hand level, unspecified hand**

√6th **S66.81** Strain **of other specified muscles, fascia and tendons at wrist and hand level**

√7th **S66.811** **Strain of other specified muscles, fascia and tendons at wrist and hand level,** right **hand**

√7th **S66.812** **Strain of other specified muscles, fascia and tendons at wrist and hand level,** left **hand**

√7th **S66.819** **Strain of other specified muscles, fascia and tendons at wrist and hand level, unspecified hand**

√6th **S66.82** Laceration **of other specified muscles, fascia and tendons at wrist and hand level**

√7th **S66.821** **Laceration of other specified muscles, fascia and tendons at wrist and hand level,** right **hand**

☑ Additional Character Required   √x7th Xtension Alert   Unspecified Dx   Other Specified Dx   Manifestation   ►◄ Revised Text   ● New Code   ▲ Revised Code Title

ICD-10-CM Draft (2015)   885

√7ᵗʰ **S66.822** Laceration of other specified muscles, fascia and tendons at wrist and hand level, left hand

√7ᵗʰ **S66.829** Laceration of other specified muscles, fascia and tendons at wrist and hand level, unspecified hand

√6ᵗʰ **S66.89** Other injury of other specified muscles, fascia and tendons at wrist and hand level

√7ᵗʰ **S66.891** Other injury of other specified muscles, fascia and tendons at wrist and hand level, right hand

√7ᵗʰ **S66.892** Other injury of other specified muscles, fascia and tendons at wrist and hand level, left hand

√7ᵗʰ **S66.899** Other injury of other specified muscles, fascia and tendons at wrist and hand level, unspecified hand

√5ᵗʰ **S66.9** Injury of unspecified muscle, fascia and tendon at wrist and hand level

√6ᵗʰ **S66.90** Unspecified injury of unspecified muscle, fascia and tendon at wrist and hand level

√7ᵗʰ **S66.901** Unspecified injury of unspecified muscle, fascia and tendon at wrist and hand level, right hand

√7ᵗʰ **S66.902** Unspecified injury of unspecified muscle, fascia and tendon at wrist and hand level, left hand

√7ᵗʰ **S66.909** Unspecified injury of unspecified muscle, fascia and tendon at wrist and hand level, unspecified hand

√6ᵗʰ **S66.91** Strain of unspecified muscle, fascia and tendon at wrist and hand level

√7ᵗʰ **S66.911** Strain of unspecified muscle, fascia and tendon at wrist and hand level, right hand

√7ᵗʰ **S66.912** Strain of unspecified muscle, fascia and tendon at wrist and hand level, left hand

√7ᵗʰ **S66.919** Strain of unspecified muscle, fascia and tendon at wrist and hand level, unspecified hand

√ᵗʰ **S66.92** Laceration of unspecified muscle, fascia and tendon at wrist and hand level

√7ᵗʰ **S66.921** Laceration of unspecified muscle, fascia and tendon at wrist and hand level, right hand

√7ᵗʰ **S66.922** Laceration of unspecified muscle, fascia and tendon at wrist and hand level, left hand

√7ᵗʰ **S66.929** Laceration of unspecified muscle, fascia and tendon at wrist and hand level, unspecified hand

√6ᵗʰ **S66.99** Other injury of unspecified muscle, fascia and tendon at wrist and hand level

√7ᵗʰ **S66.991** Other injury of unspecified muscle, fascia and tendon at wrist and hand level, right hand

√7ᵗʰ **S66.992** Other injury of unspecified muscle, fascia and tendon at wrist and hand level, left hand

√7ᵗʰ **S66.999** Other injury of unspecified muscle, fascia and tendon at wrist and hand level, unspecified hand

√4ᵗʰ **S67** Crushing injury of wrist, hand and fingers

Use additional code for all associated injuries, such as:
fracture of wrist and hand (S62.-)
open wound of wrist and hand (S61.-)

The appropriate 7th character is to be added to each code from category S67.
A   initial encounter
D   subsequent encounter
S   sequela

√5ᵗʰ **S67.0** Crushing injury of thumb

√x7ᵗʰ **S67.00** Crushing injury of unspecified thumb

√x7ᵗʰ **S67.01** Crushing injury of right thumb

√x7ᵗʰ **S67.02** Crushing injury of left thumb

√5ᵗʰ **S67.1** Crushing injury of other and unspecified finger(s)

EXCLUDES 2   crushing injury of thumb (S67.0-)

√x7ᵗʰ **S67.10** Crushing injury of unspecified finger(s)

√6ᵗʰ **S67.19** Crushing injury of other finger(s)

√7ᵗʰ **S67.190** Crushing injury of right index finger

√7ᵗʰ **S67.191** Crushing injury of left index finger

√7ᵗʰ **S67.192** Crushing injury of right middle finger

√7ᵗʰ **S67.193** Crushing injury of left middle finger

√7ᵗʰ **S67.194** Crushing injury of right ring finger

√7ᵗʰ **S67.195** Crushing injury of left ring finger

√7ᵗʰ **S67.196** Crushing injury of right little finger

√7ᵗʰ **S67.197** Crushing injury of left little finger

√7ᵗʰ **S67.198** Crushing injury of other finger
Crushing injury of specified finger with unspecified laterality

√5ᵗʰ **S67.2** Crushing injury of hand

EXCLUDES 2   crushing injury of fingers (S67.1-)
crushing injury of thumb (S67.0-)

√x7ᵗʰ **S67.20** Crushing injury of unspecified hand

√x7ᵗʰ **S67.21** Crushing injury of right hand

√x7ᵗʰ **S67.22** Crushing injury of left hand

√5ᵗʰ **S67.3** Crushing injury of wrist

√x7ᵗʰ **S67.30** Crushing injury of unspecified wrist

√x7ᵗʰ **S67.31** Crushing injury of right wrist

√x7ᵗʰ **S67.32** Crushing injury of left wrist

√5ᵗʰ **S67.4** Crushing injury of wrist and hand

EXCLUDES 1   crushing injury of hand alone (S67.2-)
crushing injury of wrist alone (S67.3-)

EXCLUDES 2   crushing injury of fingers (S67.1-)
crushing injury of thumb (S67.0-)

√x7ᵗʰ **S67.40** Crushing injury of unspecified wrist and hand

√x7ᵗʰ **S67.41** Crushing injury of right wrist and hand

√x7ᵗʰ **S67.42** Crushing injury of left wrist and hand

√5ᵗʰ **S67.9** Crushing injury of unspecified part(s) of wrist, hand and fingers

√x7ᵗʰ **S67.90** Crushing injury of unspecified part(s) of unspecified wrist, hand and fingers

√x7ᵗʰ **S67.91** Crushing injury of unspecified part(s) of right wrist, hand and fingers

√x7ᵗʰ **S67.92** Crushing injury of unspecified part(s) of left wrist, hand and fingers

√4ᵗʰ **S68** Traumatic amputation of wrist, hand and fingers

NOTE   An amputation not identified as partial or complete should be coded to complete.

The appropriate 7th character is to be added to each code from category S68.
A   initial encounter
D   subsequent encounter
S   sequela

√5ᵗʰ **S68.0** Traumatic metacarpophalangeal amputation of thumb
Traumatic amputation of thumb NOS

√6ᵗʰ **S68.01** Complete traumatic metacarpophalangeal amputation of thumb

√7ᵗʰ **S68.011** Complete traumatic metacarpophalangeal amputation of right thumb

√7ᵗʰ **S68.012** Complete traumatic metacarpophalangeal amputation of left thumb

√7ᵗʰ **S68.019** Complete traumatic metacarpophalangeal amputation of unspecified thumb

√6ᵗʰ **S68.02** Partial traumatic metacarpophalangeal amputation of thumb

√7ᵗʰ **S68.021** Partial traumatic metacarpophalangeal amputation of right thumb

√7ᵗʰ **S68.022** Partial traumatic metacarpophalangeal amputation of left thumb

√7ᵗʰ **S68.029** Partial traumatic metacarpophalangeal amputation of unspecified thumb

EXCLUDES 1 Not coded here   EXCLUDES 2 Not included here   N Newborn Age: 0   P Pediatric Age: 0-17   M Maternity Age: 12-55   A Adult Age: 15-124

886   ICD-10-CM Draft (2015)

√5ᵗʰ **S68.1** **Traumatic** metacarpophalangeal **amputation of** other and unspecified finger

Traumatic amputation of finger NOS

> EXCLUDES 2   *traumatic metacarpophalangeal amputation of thumb (S68.0-)*

√6ᵗʰ **S68.11** Complete **traumatic metacarpophalangeal amputation of other and unspecified finger**

√7ᵗʰ **S68.110** **Complete traumatic metacarpophalangeal amputation of** right **index finger**

√7ᵗʰ **S68.111** **Complete traumatic metacarpophalangeal amputation of** left index finger

√7ᵗʰ **S68.112** **Complete traumatic metacarpophalangeal amputation of** right middle finger

√7ᵗʰ **S68.113** **Complete traumatic metacarpophalangeal amputation of** left middle finger

√7ᵗʰ **S68.114** **Complete traumatic metacarpophalangeal amputation of** right ring finger

√7ᵗʰ **S68.115** **Complete traumatic metacarpophalangeal amputation of** left ring **finger**

√7ᵗʰ **S68.116** **Complete traumatic metacarpophalangeal amputation of** right little finger

√7ᵗʰ **S68.117** **Complete traumatic metacarpophalangeal amputation of** left little **finger**

√7ᵗʰ **S68.118** **Complete traumatic metacarpophalangeal amputation of other finger**

> Complete traumatic metacarpophalangeal amputation of specified finger with unspecified laterality

√7ᵗʰ **S68.119** **Complete traumatic metacarpophalangeal amputation of unspecified finger**

√6ᵗʰ **S68.12** Partial **traumatic metacarpophalangeal amputation of other and unspecified finger**

√7ᵗʰ **S68.120** **Partial traumatic metacarpophalangeal amputation of** right index **finger**

√7ᵗʰ **S68.121** **Partial traumatic metacarpophalangeal amputation of** left index **finger**

√7ᵗʰ **S68.122** **Partial traumatic metacarpophalangeal amputation of** right middle **finger**

√7ᵗʰ **S68.123** **Partial traumatic metacarpophalangeal amputation of** left middle **finger**

√7ᵗʰ **S68.124** **Partial traumatic metacarpophalangeal amputation of** right ring **finger**

√7ᵗʰ **S68.125** **Partial traumatic metacarpophalangeal amputation of** left ring **finger**

√7ᵗʰ **S68.126** **Partial traumatic metacarpophalangeal amputation of** right little **finger**

√7ᵗʰ **S68.127** **Partial traumatic metacarpophalangeal amputation of** left little **finger**

√7ᵗʰ **S68.128** **Partial traumatic metacarpophalangeal amputation of other finger**

> Partial traumatic metacarpophalangeal amputation of specified finger with unspecified laterality

√7ᵗʰ **S68.129** **Partial traumatic metacarpophalangeal amputation of unspecified finger**

√5ᵗʰ **S68.4** **Traumatic amputation of** hand at wrist level

Traumatic amputation of hand NOS
Traumatic amputation of wrist

√6ᵗʰ **S68.41** Complete **traumatic amputation of hand at wrist level**

√7ᵗʰ **S68.411** **Complete traumatic amputation of** right **hand at wrist level**

√7ᵗʰ **S68.412** **Complete traumatic amputation of** left **hand at wrist level**

√7ᵗʰ **S68.419** **Complete traumatic amputation of unspecified hand at wrist level**

√6ᵗʰ **S68.42** Partial **traumatic amputation of hand at wrist level**

√7ᵗʰ **S68.421** **Partial traumatic amputation of** right **hand at wrist level**

√7ᵗʰ **S68.422** **Partial traumatic amputation of** left **hand at wrist level**

√7ᵗʰ **S68.429** **Partial traumatic amputation of unspecified hand at wrist level**

√5ᵗʰ **S68.5** **Traumatic** transphalangeal **amputation of** thumb

Traumatic interphalangeal joint amputation of thumb

√6ᵗʰ **S68.51** Complete **traumatic transphalangeal amputation of thumb**

√7ᵗʰ **S68.511** **Complete traumatic transphalangeal amputation of** right **thumb**

√7ᵗʰ **S68.512** **Complete traumatic transphalangeal amputation of** left **thumb**

√7ᵗʰ **S68.519** **Complete traumatic transphalangeal amputation of unspecified thumb**

√6ᵗʰ **S68.52** Partial **traumatic transphalangeal amputation of thumb**

√7ᵗʰ **S68.521** **Partial traumatic transphalangeal amputation of** right **thumb**

√7ᵗʰ **S68.522** **Partial traumatic transphalangeal amputation of** left **thumb**

√7ᵗʰ **S68.529** **Partial traumatic transphalangeal amputation of unspecified thumb**

√5ᵗʰ **S68.6** **Traumatic** transphalangeal **amputation of** other and unspecified finger

√6ᵗʰ **S68.61** Complete **traumatic transphalangeal amputation of other and unspecified finger(s)**

√7ᵗʰ **S68.610** **Complete traumatic transphalangeal amputation of** right index **finger**

√7ᵗʰ **S68.611** **Complete traumatic transphalangeal amputation of** left index **finger**

√7ᵗʰ **S68.612** **Complete traumatic transphalangeal amputation of** right middle **finger**

√7ᵗʰ **S68.613** **Complete traumatic transphalangeal amputation of** left middle **finger**

√7ᵗʰ **S68.614** **Complete traumatic transphalangeal amputation of** right ring **finger**

√7ᵗʰ **S68.615** **Complete traumatic transphalangeal amputation of** left ring **finger**

√7ᵗʰ **S68.616** **Complete traumatic transphalangeal amputation of** right little **finger**

√7ᵗʰ **S68.617** **Complete traumatic transphalangeal amputation of** left little **finger**

√7ᵗʰ **S68.618** **Complete traumatic transphalangeal amputation of other finger**

> Complete traumatic transphalangeal amputation of specified finger with unspecified laterality

√7ᵗʰ **S68.619** **Complete traumatic transphalangeal amputation of unspecified finger**

√6ᵗʰ **S68.62** Partial **traumatic transphalangeal amputation of other and unspecified finger**

√7ᵗʰ **S68.620** **Partial traumatic transphalangeal amputation of** right index **finger**

√7ᵗʰ **S68.621** **Partial traumatic transphalangeal amputation of** left index **finger**

√7ᵗʰ **S68.622** **Partial traumatic transphalangeal amputation of** right middle **finger**

√7ᵗʰ **S68.623** **Partial traumatic transphalangeal amputation of** left middle **finger**

√7ᵗʰ **S68.624** **Partial traumatic transphalangeal amputation of** right ring **finger**

√7ᵗʰ **S68.625** **Partial traumatic transphalangeal amputation of** left ring **finger**

√7ᵗʰ **S68.626** **Partial traumatic transphalangeal amputation of** right little **finger**

√7ᵗʰ **S68.627** **Partial traumatic transphalangeal amputation of** left little **finger**

√7ᵗʰ **S68.628** **Partial traumatic transphalangeal amputation of other finger**

> Partial traumatic transphalangeal amputation of specified finger with unspecified laterality

√7ᵗʰ **S68.629** **Partial traumatic transphalangeal amputation of unspecified finger**

√5ᵗʰ **S68.7** **Traumatic** transmetacarpal **amputation of** hand

√6ᵗʰ **S68.71** Complete **traumatic transmetacarpal amputation of hand**

☑ Additional Character Required   √x7ᵗʰ Xtension Alert   Unspecified Dx   Other Specified Dx   Manifestation   ►◄ Revised Text   ● New Code   ▲ Revised Code Title

√7th **S68.711 Complete traumatic transmetacarpal amputation of** right **hand**

√7th **S68.712 Complete traumatic transmetacarpal amputation of** left **hand**

√7th **S68.719 Complete traumatic transmetacarpal amputation of unspecified hand**

√6th **S68.72** Partial **traumatic transmetacarpal amputation of hand**

√7th **S68.721 Partial traumatic transmetacarpal amputation of** right **hand**

√7th **S68.722 Partial traumatic transmetacarpal amputation of** left **hand**

√7th **S68.729 Partial traumatic transmetacarpal amputation of unspecified hand**

√4th **S69 Other and unspecified injuries of wrist, hand and finger(s)**

The appropriate 7th character is to be added to each code from category S69.
A   initial encounter
D   subsequent encounter
S   sequela

√5th **S69.8 Other specified injuries of wrist, hand and finger(s)**

√x7th **S69.80 Other specified injuries of unspecified wrist, hand and finger(s)**

√x7th **S69.81 Other specified injuries of** right **wrist, hand and finger(s)**

√x7th **S69.82 Other specified injuries of** left **wrist, hand and finger(s)**

√5th **S69.9 Unspecified injury of wrist, hand and finger(s)**

√x7th **S69.90 Unspecified injury of unspecified wrist, hand and finger(s)**

√x7th **S69.91 Unspecified injury of** right **wrist, hand and finger(s)**

√x7th **S69.92 Unspecified injury of** left **wrist, hand and finger(s)**

Injuries to the hip and thigh (S70-S79)

EXCLUDES 2   burns and corrosions (T20-T32)
frostbite (T33-T34)
snake bite (T63.0-)
venomous insect bite or sting (T63.4-)

√4th **S70 Superficial injury of hip and thigh**

The appropriate 7th character is to be added to each code from category S70.
A   initial encounter
D   subsequent encounter
S   sequela

√5th **S70.0 Contusion of** hip

√x7th **S70.00 Contusion of unspecified hip**

√x7th **S70.01 Contusion of** right **hip**

√x7th **S70.02 Contusion of** left **hip**

√5th **S70.1 Contusion of** thigh

√x7th **S70.10 Contusion of unspecified thigh**

√x7th **S70.11 Contusion of** right **thigh**

√x7th **S70.12 Contusion of** left **thigh**

√5th **S70.2** Other **superficial injuries of** hip

√6th **S70.21** Abrasion **of hip**

√7th **S70.211 Abrasion,** right **hip**

√7th **S70.212 Abrasion,** left **hip**

√7th **S70.219 Abrasion, unspecified hip**

√6th **S70.22** Blister **(nonthermal) of hip**

√7th **S70.221 Blister (nonthermal),** right **hip**

√7th **S70.222 Blister (nonthermal),** left **hip**

√7th **S70.229 Blister (nonthermal), unspecified hip**

√6th **S70.24** External constriction **of hip**

√7th **S70.241 External constriction,** right **hip**

√7th **S70.242 External constriction,** left **hip**

√7th **S70.249 External constriction, unspecified hip**

√6th **S70.25** Superficial foreign body **of hip**
Splinter in the hip

√7th **S70.251 Superficial foreign body,** right **hip**

√7th **S70.252 Superficial foreign body,** left **hip**

√7th **S70.259 Superficial foreign body, unspecified hip**

√6th **S70.26** Insect bite **(nonvenomous) of hip**

√7th **S70.261 Insect bite (nonvenomous),** right **hip**

√7th **S70.262 Insect bite (nonvenomous),** left **hip**

√7th **S70.269 Insect bite (nonvenomous), unspecified hip**

√6th **S70.27** Other superficial **bite of hip**
EXCLUDES 1   open bite of hip (S71.05-)

√7th **S70.271 Other superficial bite of hip,** right **hip**

√7th **S70.272 Other superficial bite of hip,** left **hip**

√7th **S70.279 Other superficial bite of hip, unspecified hip**

√5th **S70.3 Other superficial injuries of** thigh

√6th **S70.31** Abrasion **of thigh**

√7th **S70.311 Abrasion,** right **thigh**

√7th **S70.312 Abrasion,** left **thigh**

√7th **S70.319 Abrasion, unspecified thigh**

√6th **S70.32** Blister **(nonthermal) of thigh**

√7th **S70.321 Blister (nonthermal),** right **thigh**

√7th **S70.322 Blister (nonthermal),** left **thigh**

√7th **S70.329 Blister (nonthermal), unspecified thigh**

√6th **S70.34** External constriction **of thigh**

√7th **S70.341 External constriction,** right **thigh**

√7th **S70.342 External constriction,** left **thigh**

√7th **S70.349 External constriction, unspecified thigh**

√6th **S70.35** Superficial foreign body **of thigh**
Splinter in the thigh

√7th **S70.351 Superficial foreign body,** right **thigh**

√7th **S70.352 Superficial foreign body,** left **thigh**

√7th **S70.359 Superficial foreign body, unspecified thigh**

√6th **S70.36** Insect bite **(nonvenomous) of thigh**

√7th **S70.361 Insect bite (nonvenomous),** right **thigh**

√7th **S70.362 Insect bite (nonvenomous),** left **thigh**

√7th **S70.369 Insect bite (nonvenomous), unspecified thigh**

√6th **S70.37** Other superficial **bite of thigh**
EXCLUDES 1   open bite of thigh (S71.15)

√7th **S70.371 Other superficial bite of** right **thigh**

√7th **S70.372 Other superficial bite of** left **thigh**

√7th **S70.379 Other superficial bite of unspecified thigh**

√5th **S70.9 Unspecified superficial injury of** hip and thigh

√6th **S70.91 Unspecified superficial injury of** hip

√7th **S70.911 Unspecified superficial injury of** right **hip**

√7th **S70.912 Unspecified superficial injury of** left **hip**

√7th **S70.919 Unspecified superficial injury of unspecified hip**

√6th **S70.92 Unspecified superficial injury of** thigh

√7th **S70.921 Unspecified superficial injury of** right **thigh**

√7th **S70.922 Unspecified superficial injury of** left **thigh**

√7th **S70.929 Unspecified superficial injury of unspecified thigh**

√4th **S71 Open wound of hip and thigh**
Code also any associated wound infection
EXCLUDES 1   open fracture of hip and thigh (S72.-)
traumatic amputation of hip and thigh (S78.-)
EXCLUDES 2   bite of venomous animal (T63.-)
open wound of ankle, foot and toes (S91.-)
open wound of knee and lower leg (S81.-)

The appropriate 7th character is to be added to each code from category S71.
A   initial encounter
D   subsequent encounter
S   sequela

√5th **S71.0 Open wound of** hip

√6th **S71.00** Unspecified **open wound of hip**

√7th **S71.001 Unspecified open wound,** right **hip**

√7th **S71.002 Unspecified open wound,** left **hip**

EXCLUDES 1 Not coded here   EXCLUDES 2 Not included here   N Newborn Age: 0   P Pediatric Age: 0-17   M Maternity Age: 12-55   A Adult Age: 15-124

888   ICD-10-CM Draft (2015)

✓7th **S71.009** Unspecified open wound, unspecified hip

✓6th **S71.01** Laceration without foreign body of hip
  ✓7th **S71.011** Laceration without foreign body, right hip
  ✓7th **S71.012** Laceration without foreign body, left hip
  ✓7th **S71.019** Laceration without foreign body, unspecified hip

✓6th **S71.02** Laceration with foreign body of hip
  ✓7th **S71.021** Laceration with foreign body, right hip
  ✓7th **S71.022** Laceration with foreign body, left hip
  ✓7th **S71.029** Laceration with foreign body, unspecified hip

✓6th **S71.03** Puncture wound without foreign body of hip
  ✓7th **S71.031** Puncture wound without foreign body, right hip
  ✓7th **S71.032** Puncture wound without foreign body, left hip
  ✓7th **S71.039** Puncture wound without foreign body, unspecified hip

✓6th **S71.04** Puncture wound with foreign body of hip
  ✓7th **S71.041** Puncture wound with foreign body, right hip
  ✓7th **S71.042** Puncture wound with foreign body, left hip
  ✓7th **S71.049** Puncture wound with foreign body, unspecified hip

✓6th **S71.05** Open bite of hip
    Bite of hip NOS
    EXCLUDES 1 *superficial bite of hip (S70.26, S70.27)*
  ✓7th **S71.051** Open bite, right hip
  ✓7th **S71.052** Open bite, left hip
  ✓7th **S71.059** Open bite, unspecified hip

✓5th **S71.1** Open wound of thigh

✓6th **S71.10** Unspecified open wound of thigh
  ✓7th **S71.101** Unspecified open wound, right thigh
  ✓7th **S71.102** Unspecified open wound, left thigh
  ✓7th **S71.109** Unspecified open wound, unspecified thigh

✓6th **S71.11** Laceration without foreign body of thigh
  ✓7th **S71.111** Laceration without foreign body, right thigh
  ✓7th **S71.112** Laceration without foreign body, left thigh
  ✓7th **S71.119** Laceration without foreign body, unspecified thigh

✓6th **S71.12** Laceration with foreign body of thigh
  ✓7th **S71.121** Laceration with foreign body, right thigh
  ✓7th **S71.122** Laceration with foreign body, left thigh
  ✓7th **S71.129** Laceration with foreign body, unspecified thigh

✓6th **S71.13** Puncture wound without foreign body of thigh
  ✓7th **S71.131** Puncture wound without foreign body, right thigh
  ✓7th **S71.132** Puncture wound without foreign body, left thigh
  ✓7th **S71.139** Puncture wound without foreign body, unspecified thigh

✓6th **S71.14** Puncture wound with foreign body of thigh
  ✓7th **S71.141** Puncture wound with foreign body, right thigh
  ✓7th **S71.142** Puncture wound with foreign body, left thigh
  ✓7th **S71.149** Puncture wound with foreign body, unspecified thigh

✓6th **S71.15** Open bite of thigh
    Bite of thigh NOS
    EXCLUDES 1 *superficial bite of thigh (S70.37-)*
  ✓7th **S71.151** Open bite, right thigh
  ✓7th **S71.152** Open bite, left thigh
  ✓7th **S71.159** Open bite, unspecified thigh

✓4th **S72** Fracture of femur
    NOTE   A fracture not indicated as displaced or nondisplaced should be coded to displaced.
    The open fracture designations are based on the Gustilo open fracture classification.
    A fracture not indicated as open or closed should be coded to closed.
    EXCLUDES 1 *traumatic amputation of hip and thigh (S78.-)*
    EXCLUDES 2 *fracture of foot (S92.-)*
    fracture of lower leg and ankle (S82.-)
    periprosthetic fracture of prosthetic implant of hip (T84.040, T84.041)
    AHA: 2013, 4Q, 128

The appropriate 7th character is to be added to all codes from category S72 [unless otherwise indicated].
A   initial encounter for closed fracture
B   initial encounter for open fracture type I or II
    initial encounter for open fracture NOS
C   initial encounter for open fracture type IIIA, IIIB, or IIIC
D   subsequent encounter for closed fracture with routine healing
E   subsequent encounter for open fracture type I or II with routine healing
F   subsequent encounter for open fracture type IIIA, IIIB, or IIIC with routine healing
G   subsequent encounter for closed fracture with delayed healing
H   subsequent encounter for open fracture type I or II with delayed healing
J   subsequent encounter for open fracture type IIIA, IIIB, or IIIC with delayed healing
K   subsequent encounter for closed fracture with nonunion
M   subsequent encounter for open fracture type I or II with nonunion
N   subsequent encounter for open fracture type IIIA, IIIB, or IIIC with nonunion
P   subsequent encounter for closed fracture with malunion
Q   subsequent encounter for open fracture type I or II with malunion
R   subsequent encounter for open fracture type IIIA, IIIB, or IIIC with malunion
S   sequela

✓5th **S72.0** Fracture of head and neck of femur
    EXCLUDES 2 *physeal fracture of upper end of femur (S79.0-)*

✓6th **S72.00** Fracture of unspecified part of neck of femur
    Fracture of hip NOS   Fracture of neck of femur NOS
  ✓7th **S72.001** Fracture of unspecified part of neck of right femur
  ✓7th **S72.002** Fracture of unspecified part of neck of left femur
  ✓7th **S72.009** Fracture of unspecified part of neck of unspecified femur

✓6th **S72.01** Unspecified intracapsular fracture of femur
    Subcapital fracture of femur
  ✓7th **S72.011** Unspecified intracapsular fracture of right femur
  ✓7th **S72.012** Unspecified intracapsular fracture of left femur
  ✓7th **S72.019** Unspecified intracapsular fracture of unspecified femur

✓6th **S72.02** Fracture of epiphysis (separation) (upper) of femur
    Transepiphyseal fracture of femur
    EXCLUDES 1 *capital femoral epiphyseal fracture (pediatric) of femur (S79.01-)*
    Salter-Harris Type I physeal fracture of upper end of femur (S79.01-)
  ✓7th **S72.021** Displaced fracture of epiphysis (separation) (upper) of right femur
  ✓7th **S72.022** Displaced fracture of epiphysis (separation) (upper) of left femur
  ✓7th **S72.023** Displaced fracture of epiphysis (separation) (upper) of unspecified femur
  ✓7th **S72.024** Nondisplaced fracture of epiphysis (separation) (upper) of right femur
  ✓7th **S72.025** Nondisplaced fracture of epiphysis (separation) (upper) of left femur
  ✓7th **S72.026** Nondisplaced fracture of epiphysis (separation) (upper) of unspecified femur

✓6th **S72.03** Midcervical fracture of femur
    Transcervical fracture of femur NOS

✓7th **S72.031** Displaced midcervical fracture of right femur

✓7th **S72.032** Displaced midcervical fracture of left femur

✓7th **S72.033** Displaced midcervical fracture of unspecified femur

✓7th **S72.034** Nondisplaced midcervical fracture of right femur

✓7th **S72.035** Nondisplaced midcervical fracture of left femur

✓7th **S72.036** Nondisplaced midcervical fracture of unspecified femur

✓6th **S72.04** Fracture of base of neck of femur
Cervicotrochanteric fracture of femur

✓7th **S72.041** Displaced fracture of base of neck of right femur

✓7th **S72.042** Displaced fracture of base of neck of left femur

✓7th **S72.043** Displaced fracture of base of neck of unspecified femur

✓7th **S72.044** Nondisplaced fracture of base of neck of right femur

✓7th **S72.045** Nondisplaced fracture of base of neck of left femur

✓7th **S72.046** Nondisplaced fracture of base of neck of unspecified femur

✓6th **S72.05** Unspecified fracture of head of femur
Fracture of head of femur NOS

✓7th **S72.051** Unspecified fracture of head of right femur

✓7th **S72.052** Unspecified fracture of head of left femur

✓7th **S72.059** Unspecified fracture of head of unspecified femur

✓6th **S72.06** Articular fracture of head of femur

✓7th **S72.061** Displaced articular fracture of head of right femur

✓7th **S72.062** Displaced articular fracture of head of left femur

✓7th **S72.063** Displaced articular fracture of head of unspecified femur

✓7th **S72.064** Nondisplaced articular fracture of head of right femur

✓7th **S72.065** Nondisplaced articular fracture of head of left femur

✓7th **S72.066** Nondisplaced articular fracture of head of unspecified femur

✓6th **S72.09** Other fracture of head and neck of femur

✓7th **S72.091** Other fracture of head and neck of right femur

✓7th **S72.092** Other fracture of head and neck of left femur

✓7th **S72.099** Other fracture of head and neck of unspecified femur

✓5th **S72.1** Pertrochanteric fracture

✓6th **S72.10** Unspecified trochanteric fracture of femur
Fracture of trochanter NOS

✓7th **S72.101** Unspecified trochanteric fracture of right femur

✓7th **S72.102** Unspecified trochanteric fracture of left femur

✓7th **S72.109** Unspecified trochanteric fracture of unspecified femur

✓6th **S72.11** Fracture of greater trochanter of femur

✓7th **S72.111** Displaced fracture of greater trochanter of right femur

✓7th **S72.112** Displaced fracture of greater trochanter of left femur

✓7th **S72.113** Displaced fracture of greater trochanter of unspecified femur

✓7th **S72.114** Nondisplaced fracture of greater trochanter of right femur

✓7th **S72.115** Nondisplaced fracture of greater trochanter of left femur

✓7th **S72.116** Nondisplaced fracture of greater trochanter of unspecified femur

✓6th **S72.12** Fracture of lesser trochanter of femur

✓7th **S72.121** Displaced fracture of lesser trochanter of right femur

✓7th **S72.122** Displaced fracture of lesser trochanter of left femur

✓7th **S72.123** Displaced fracture of lesser trochanter of unspecified femur

✓7th **S72.124** Nondisplaced fracture of lesser trochanter of right femur

✓7th **S72.125** Nondisplaced fracture of lesser trochanter of left femur

✓7th **S72.126** Nondisplaced fracture of lesser trochanter of unspecified femur

✓6th **S72.13** Apophyseal fracture of femur
EXCLUDES 1 chronic (nontraumatic) slipped upper femoral epiphysis (M93.0-)

✓7th **S72.131** Displaced apophyseal fracture of right femur

✓7th **S72.132** Displaced apophyseal fracture of left femur

✓7th **S72.133** Displaced apophyseal fracture of unspecified femur

✓7th **S72.134** Nondisplaced apophyseal fracture of right femur

✓7th **S72.135** Nondisplaced apophyseal fracture of left femur

✓7th **S72.136** Nondisplaced apophyseal fracture of unspecified femur

✓6th **S72.14** Intertrochanteric fracture of femur

✓7th **S72.141** Displaced intertrochanteric fracture of right femur

✓7th **S72.142** Displaced intertrochanteric fracture of left femur

✓7th **S72.143** Displaced intertrochanteric fracture of unspecified femur

✓7th **S72.144** Nondisplaced intertrochanteric fracture of right femur

✓7th **S72.145** Nondisplaced intertrochanteric fracture of left femur

✓7th **S72.146** Nondisplaced intertrochanteric fracture of unspecified femur

✓5th **S72.2** Subtrochanteric fracture of femur

✓x7th **S72.21** Displaced subtrochanteric fracture of right femur

✓x7th **S72.22** Displaced subtrochanteric fracture of left femur

✓x7th **S72.23** Displaced subtrochanteric fracture of unspecified femur

✓x7th **S72.24** Nondisplaced subtrochanteric fracture of right femur

✓x7th **S72.25** Nondisplaced subtrochanteric fracture of left femur

✓x7th **S72.26** Nondisplaced subtrochanteric fracture of unspecified femur

✓5th **S72.3** Fracture of shaft of femur

✓6th **S72.30** Unspecified fracture of shaft of femur

✓7th **S72.301** Unspecified fracture of shaft of right femur

✓7th **S72.302** Unspecified fracture of shaft of left femur

✓7th **S72.309** Unspecified fracture of shaft of unspecified femur

✓6th **S72.32** Transverse fracture of shaft of femur

✓7th **S72.321** Displaced transverse fracture of shaft of right femur

✓7th **S72.322** Displaced transverse fracture of shaft of left femur

✓7th **S72.323** Displaced transverse fracture of shaft of unspecified femur

✓7th **S72.324** Nondisplaced transverse fracture of shaft of right femur

✓7th **S72.325** Nondisplaced transverse fracture of shaft of left femur

✓7th **S72.326** Nondisplaced transverse fracture of shaft of unspecified femur

✓6th **S72.33** Oblique fracture of shaft of femur

✓7th **S72.331** Displaced oblique fracture of shaft of right femur

√7ᵗʰ **S72.332** Displaced oblique fracture of shaft of left femur

√7ᵗʰ **S72.333** Displaced oblique fracture of shaft of unspecified femur

√7ᵗʰ **S72.334** Nondisplaced oblique fracture of shaft of right femur

√7ᵗʰ **S72.335** Nondisplaced oblique fracture of shaft of left femur

√7ᵗʰ **S72.336** Nondisplaced oblique fracture of shaft of unspecified femur

√6ᵗʰ **S72.34** Spiral fracture of shaft of femur

√7ᵗʰ **S72.341** Displaced spiral fracture of shaft of right femur

√7ᵗʰ **S72.342** Displaced spiral fracture of shaft of left femur

√7ᵗʰ **S72.343** Displaced spiral fracture of shaft of unspecified femur

√7ᵗʰ **S72.344** Nondisplaced spiral fracture of shaft of right femur

√7ᵗʰ **S72.345** Nondisplaced spiral fracture of shaft of left femur

√7ᵗʰ **S72.346** Nondisplaced spiral fracture of shaft of unspecified femur

√6ᵗʰ **S72.35** Comminuted fracture of shaft of femur

√7ᵗʰ **S72.351** Displaced comminuted fracture of shaft of right femur

√7ᵗʰ **S72.352** Displaced comminuted fracture of shaft of left femur

√7ᵗʰ **S72.353** Displaced comminuted fracture of shaft of unspecified femur

√7ᵗʰ **S72.354** Nondisplaced comminuted fracture of shaft of right femur

√7ᵗʰ **S72.355** Nondisplaced comminuted fracture of shaft of left femur

√7ᵗʰ **S72.356** Nondisplaced comminuted fracture of shaft of unspecified femur

√6ᵗʰ **S72.36** Segmental fracture of shaft of femur

√7ᵗʰ **S72.361** Displaced segmental fracture of shaft of right femur

√7ᵗʰ **S72.362** Displaced segmental fracture of shaft of left femur

√7ᵗʰ **S72.363** Displaced segmental fracture of shaft of unspecified femur

√7ᵗʰ **S72.364** Nondisplaced segmental fracture of shaft of right femur

√7ᵗʰ **S72.365** Nondisplaced segmental fracture of shaft of left femur

√7ᵗʰ **S72.366** Nondisplaced segmental fracture of shaft of unspecified femur

√6ᵗʰ **S72.39** Other fracture of shaft of femur

√7ᵗʰ **S72.391** Other fracture of shaft of right femur

√7ᵗʰ **S72.392** Other fracture of shaft of left femur

√7ᵗʰ **S72.399** Other fracture of shaft of unspecified femur

√5ᵗʰ **S72.4** Fracture of lower end of femur
Fracture of distal end of femur
EXCLUDES 2 fracture of shaft of femur (S72.3-)
physeal fracture of lower end of femur (S79.1-)

√6ᵗʰ **S72.40** Unspecified fracture of lower end of femur

√7ᵗʰ **S72.401** Unspecified fracture of lower end of right femur

√7ᵗʰ **S72.402** Unspecified fracture of lower end of left femur

√7ᵗʰ **S72.409** Unspecified fracture of lower end of unspecified femur

√6ᵗʰ **S72.41** Unspecified condyle fracture of lower end of femur
Condyle fracture of femur NOS

√7ᵗʰ **S72.411** Displaced unspecified condyle fracture of lower end of right femur

√7ᵗʰ **S72.412** Displaced unspecified condyle fracture of lower end of left femur

√7ᵗʰ **S72.413** Displaced unspecified condyle fracture of lower end of unspecified femur

√7ᵗʰ **S72.414** Nondisplaced unspecified condyle fracture of lower end of right femur

√7ᵗʰ **S72.415** Nondisplaced unspecified condyle fracture of lower end of left femur

√7ᵗʰ **S72.416** Nondisplaced unspecified condyle fracture of lower end of unspecified femur

√6ᵗʰ **S72.42** Fracture of lateral condyle of femur

√7ᵗʰ **S72.421** Displaced fracture of lateral condyle of right femur

√7ᵗʰ **S72.422** Displaced fracture of lateral condyle of left femur

√7ᵗʰ **S72.423** Displaced fracture of lateral condyle of unspecified femur

√7ᵗʰ **S72.424** Nondisplaced fracture of lateral condyle of right femur

√7ᵗʰ **S72.425** Nondisplaced fracture of lateral condyle of left femur

√7ᵗʰ **S72.426** Nondisplaced fracture of lateral condyle of unspecified femur

√6ᵗʰ **S72.43** Fracture of medial condyle of femur

√7ᵗʰ **S72.431** Displaced fracture of medial condyle of right femur

√7ᵗʰ **S72.432** Displaced fracture of medial condyle of left femur

√7ᵗʰ **S72.433** Displaced fracture of medial condyle of unspecified femur

√7ᵗʰ **S72.434** Nondisplaced fracture of medial condyle of right femur

√7ᵗʰ **S72.435** Nondisplaced fracture of medial condyle of left femur

√7ᵗʰ **S72.436** Nondisplaced fracture of medial condyle of unspecified femur

√6ᵗʰ **S72.44** Fracture of lower epiphysis (separation) of femur
EXCLUDES 1 Salter-Harris Type I physeal fracture of lower end of femur (S79.11-)

√7ᵗʰ **S72.441** Displaced fracture of lower epiphysis (separation) of right femur

√7ᵗʰ **S72.442** Displaced fracture of lower epiphysis (separation) of left femur

√7ᵗʰ **S72.443** Displaced fracture of lower epiphysis (separation) of unspecified femur

√7ᵗʰ **S72.444** Nondisplaced fracture of lower epiphysis (separation) of right femur

√7ᵗʰ **S72.445** Nondisplaced fracture of lower epiphysis (separation) of left femur

√7ᵗʰ **S72.446** Nondisplaced fracture of lower epiphysis (separation) of unspecified femur

√6ᵗʰ **S72.45** Supracondylar fracture without intracondylar extension of lower end of femur
Supracondylar fracture of lower end of femur NOS
EXCLUDES 1 supracondylar fracture with intracondylar extension of lower end of femur (S72.46-)

√7ᵗʰ **S72.451** Displaced supracondylar fracture without intracondylar extension of lower end of right femur

√7ᵗʰ **S72.452** Displaced supracondylar fracture without intracondylar extension of lower end of left femur

√7ᵗʰ **S72.453** Displaced supracondylar fracture without intracondylar extension of lower end of unspecified femur

√7ᵗʰ **S72.454** Nondisplaced supracondylar fracture without intracondylar extension of lower end of right femur

√7ᵗʰ **S72.455** Nondisplaced supracondylar fracture without intracondylar extension of lower end of left femur

√7ᵗʰ **S72.456** Nondisplaced supracondylar fracture without intracondylar extension of lower end of unspecified femur

√6ᵗʰ **S72.46** Supracondylar fracture with intracondylar extension of lower end of femur
EXCLUDES 1 supracondylar fracture without intracondylar extension of lower end of femur (S72.45-)

√7ᵗʰ **S72.461** Displaced supracondylar fracture with intracondylar extension of lower end of right femur

---

√ Additional Character Required   √x7ᵗʰ X'tension Alert   Unspecified Dx   Other Specified Dx   Manifestation   ►◄ Revised Text   ● New Code   ▲ Revised Code Title

Injury, Poisoning and Certain Other Consequences of External Causes

S72.462–S74.02

✓7th **S72.462** Displaced supracondylar fracture with intracondylar extension of lower end of left femur

✓7th **S72.463** Displaced supracondylar fracture with intracondylar extension of lower end of unspecified femur

✓7th **S72.464** Nondisplaced supracondylar fracture with intracondylar extension of lower end of right femur

✓7th **S72.465** Nondisplaced supracondylar fracture with intracondylar extension of lower end of left femur

✓7th **S72.466** Nondisplaced supracondylar fracture with intracondylar extension of lower end of unspecified femur

✓6th **S72.47** Torus fracture of lower end of femur

> The appropriate 7th character is to be added to all codes in subcategory S72.47.
> A   initial encounter for closed fracture
> D   subsequent encounter for fracture with routine healing
> G   subsequent encounter for fracture with delayed healing
> K   subsequent encounter for fracture with nonunion
> P   subsequent encounter for fracture with malunion
> S   sequela

✓7th **S72.471** Torus fracture of lower end of right femur

✓7th **S72.472** Torus fracture of lower end of left femur

✓7th **S72.479** Torus fracture of lower end of unspecified femur

✓6th **S72.49** Other fracture of lower end of femur

✓7th **S72.491** Other fracture of lower end of right femur

✓7th **S72.492** Other fracture of lower end of left femur

✓7th **S72.499** Other fracture of lower end of unspecified femur

✓5th **S72.8 Other fracture of femur**

✓6th **S72.8X** Other fracture of femur

✓7th **S72.8X1** Other fracture of right femur

✓7th **S72.8X2** Other fracture of left femur

✓7th **S72.8X9** Other fracture of unspecified femur

✓5th **S72.9 Unspecified fracture of femur**
Fracture of thigh NOS
Fracture of upper leg NOS
> **EXCLUDES 1** fracture of hip NOS (S72.00-, S72.01-)

✓x7th **S72.90** Unspecified fracture of unspecified femur
AHA: 2012, 4Q, 93

✓x7th **S72.91** Unspecified fracture of right femur

✓x7th **S72.92** Unspecified fracture of left femur

✓4th **S73 Dislocation and sprain of joint and ligaments of hip**

> **INCLUDES** avulsion of joint or ligament of hip
> laceration of cartilage, joint or ligament of hip
> sprain of cartilage, joint or ligament of hip
> traumatic hemarthrosis of joint or ligament of hip
> traumatic rupture of joint or ligament of hip
> traumatic subluxation of joint or ligament of hip
> traumatic tear of joint or ligament of hip

Code also any associated open wound
> **EXCLUDES 2** strain of muscle, fascia and tendon of hip and thigh (S76.-)

> The appropriate 7th character is to be added to each code from category S73.
> A   initial encounter
> D   subsequent encounter
> S   sequela

✓5th **S73.0 Subluxation and dislocation of hip**
> **EXCLUDES 2** dislocation and subluxation of hip prosthesis (T84.020, T84.021)

✓6th **S73.00** Unspecified subluxation and dislocation of hip
Dislocation of hip NOS
Subluxation of hip NOS

✓7th **S73.001** Unspecified subluxation of right hip

✓7th **S73.002** Unspecified subluxation of left hip

✓7th **S73.003** Unspecified subluxation of unspecified hip

✓7th **S73.004** Unspecified dislocation of right hip

✓7th **S73.005** Unspecified dislocation of left hip

✓7th **S73.006** Unspecified dislocation of unspecified hip

✓6th **S73.01** Posterior subluxation and dislocation of hip

✓7th **S73.011** Posterior subluxation of right hip

✓7th **S73.012** Posterior subluxation of left hip

✓7th **S73.013** Posterior subluxation of unspecified hip

✓7th **S73.014** Posterior dislocation of right hip

✓7th **S73.015** Posterior dislocation of left hip

✓7th **S73.016** Posterior dislocation of unspecified hip

✓6th **S73.02** Obturator subluxation and dislocation of hip

✓7th **S73.021** Obturator subluxation of right hip

✓7th **S73.022** Obturator subluxation of left hip

✓7th **S73.023** Obturator subluxation of unspecified hip

✓7th **S73.024** Obturator dislocation of right hip

✓7th **S73.025** Obturator dislocation of left hip

✓7th **S73.026** Obturator dislocation of unspecified hip

✓6th **S73.03** Other anterior dislocation of hip

✓7th **S73.031** Other anterior subluxation of right hip

✓7th **S73.032** Other anterior subluxation of left hip

✓7th **S73.033** Other anterior subluxation of unspecified hip

✓7th **S73.034** Other anterior dislocation of right hip

✓7th **S73.035** Other anterior dislocation of left hip

✓7th **S73.036** Other anterior dislocation of unspecified hip

✓6th **S73.04** Central dislocation of hip

✓7th **S73.041** Central subluxation of right hip

✓7th **S73.042** Central subluxation of left hip

✓7th **S73.043** Central subluxation of unspecified hip

✓7th **S73.044** Central dislocation of right hip

✓7th **S73.045** Central dislocation of left hip

✓7th **S73.046** Central dislocation of unspecified hip

✓5th **S73.1 Sprain of hip**

✓6th **S73.10** Unspecified sprain of hip

✓7th **S73.101** Unspecified sprain of right hip

✓7th **S73.102** Unspecified sprain of left hip

✓7th **S73.109** Unspecified sprain of unspecified hip

✓6th **S73.11** Iliofemoral ligament sprain of hip

✓7th **S73.111** Iliofemoral ligament sprain of right hip

✓7th **S73.112** Iliofemoral ligament sprain of left hip

✓7th **S73.119** Iliofemoral ligament sprain of unspecified hip

✓6th **S73.12** Ischiocapsular (ligament) sprain of hip

✓7th **S73.121** Ischiocapsular ligament sprain of right hip

✓7th **S73.122** Ischiocapsular ligament sprain of left hip

✓7th **S73.129** Ischiocapsular ligament sprain of unspecified hip

✓6th **S73.19** Other sprain of hip

✓7th **S73.191** Other sprain of right hip

✓7th **S73.192** Other sprain of left hip

✓7th **S73.199** Other sprain of unspecified hip

✓4th **S74 Injury of nerves at hip and thigh level**
Code also any associated open wound (S71.-)
> **EXCLUDES 2** injury of nerves at ankle and foot level (S94.-)
> injury of nerves at lower leg level (S84.-)

> The appropriate 7th character is to be added to each code from category S74.
> A   initial encounter
> D   subsequent encounter
> S   sequela

✓5th **S74.0 Injury of sciatic nerve at hip and thigh level**

✓x7th **S74.00** Injury of sciatic nerve at hip and thigh level, unspecified leg

✓x7th **S74.01** Injury of sciatic nerve at hip and thigh level, right leg

✓x7th **S74.02** Injury of sciatic nerve at hip and thigh level, left leg

EXCLUDES 1 Not coded here   **EXCLUDES 2** Not included here   N Newborn Age: 0   P Pediatric Age: 0-17   M Maternity Age: 12-55   A Adult Age: 15-124

892   ICD-10-CM Draft (2015)

☑5ᵗʰ **S74.1** Injury of femoral nerve at hip and thigh level

    ☑x7ᵗʰ **S74.10** **Injury of femoral nerve at hip and thigh level, unspecified leg**

    ☑x7ᵗʰ **S74.11** **Injury of femoral nerve at hip and thigh level, right leg**

    ☑x7ᵗʰ **S74.12** **Injury of femoral nerve at hip and thigh level, left leg**

☑5ᵗʰ **S74.2** Injury of cutaneous sensory nerve at hip and thigh level

    ☑x7ᵗʰ **S74.20** **Injury of cutaneous sensory nerve at hip and thigh level, unspecified leg**

    ☑x7ᵗʰ **S74.21** **Injury of cutaneous sensory nerve at hip and high level, right leg**

    ☑x7ᵗʰ **S74.22** **Injury of cutaneous sensory nerve at hip and thigh level, left leg**

☑5ᵗʰ **S74.8** Injury of other nerves at hip and thigh level

    ☑6ᵗʰ **S74.8X** **Injury of other nerves at hip and thigh level**

        ☑7ᵗʰ **S74.8X1** **Injury of other nerves at hip and thigh level, right leg**

        ☑7ᵗʰ **S74.8X2** **Injury of other nerves at hip and thigh level, left leg**

        ☑7ᵗʰ **S74.8X9** **Injury of other nerves at hip and thigh level, unspecified leg**

☑5ᵗʰ **S74.9** Injury of unspecified nerve at hip and thigh level

    ☑x7ᵗʰ **S74.90** **Injury of unspecified nerve at hip and thigh level, unspecified leg**

    ☑x7ᵗʰ **S74.91** **Injury of unspecified nerve at hip and thigh level, right leg**

    ☑x7ᵗʰ **S74.92** **Injury of unspecified nerve at hip and thigh level, left leg**

☑4ᵗʰ **S75** **Injury of blood vessels at hip and thigh level**

    Code also any associated open wound (S71.-)

    EXCLUDES 2   injury of blood vessels at lower leg level (S85.-)
                 injury of popliteal artery (S85.0)

    The appropriate 7th character is to be added to each code from category S75.
    A   initial encounter
    D   subsequent encounter
    S   sequela

☑5ᵗʰ **S75.0** Injury of femoral artery

    ☑6ᵗʰ **S75.00** Unspecified injury of femoral artery

        ☑7ᵗʰ **S75.001** **Unspecified injury of femoral artery, right leg**

        ☑7ᵗʰ **S75.002** **Unspecified injury of femoral artery, left leg**

        ☑7ᵗʰ **S75.009** **Unspecified injury of femoral artery, unspecified leg**

    ☑6ᵗʰ **S75.01** Minor laceration of femoral artery

        Incomplete transection of femoral artery
        Laceration of femoral artery NOS
        Superficial laceration of femoral artery

        ☑7ᵗʰ **S75.011** **Minor laceration of femoral artery, right leg**

        ☑7ᵗʰ **S75.012** **Minor laceration of femoral artery, left leg**

        ☑7ᵗʰ **S75.019** **Minor laceration of femoral artery, unspecified leg**

    ☑6ᵗʰ **S75.02** Major laceration of femoral artery

        Complete transection of femoral artery
        Traumatic rupture of femoral artery

        ☑7ᵗʰ **S75.021** **Major laceration of femoral artery, right leg**

        ☑7ᵗʰ **S75.022** **Major laceration of femoral artery, left leg**

        ☑7ᵗʰ **S75.029** **Major laceration of femoral artery, unspecified leg**

    ☑6ᵗʰ **S75.09** Other specified injury of femoral artery

        ☑7ᵗʰ **S75.091** **Other specified injury of femoral artery, right leg**

        ☑7ᵗʰ **S75.092** **Other specified injury of femoral artery, left leg**

        ☑7ᵗʰ **S75.099** **Other specified injury of femoral artery, unspecified leg**

☑5ᵗʰ **S75.1** Injury of femoral vein at hip and thigh level

    ☑6ᵗʰ **S75.10** Unspecified injury of femoral vein at hip and thigh level

        ☑7ᵗʰ **S75.101** **Unspecified injury of femoral vein at hip and thigh level, right leg**

        ☑7ᵗʰ **S75.102** **Unspecified injury of femoral vein at hip and thigh level, left leg**

        ☑7ᵗʰ **S75.109** **Unspecified injury of femoral vein at hip and thigh level, unspecified leg**

    ☑6ᵗʰ **S75.11** Minor laceration of femoral vein at hip and thigh level

        Incomplete transection of femoral vein at hip and thigh level
        Laceration of femoral vein at hip and thigh level NOS
        Superficial laceration of femoral vein at hip and thigh level

        ☑7ᵗʰ **S75.111** **Minor laceration of femoral vein at hip and thigh level, right leg**

        ☑7ᵗʰ **S75.112** **Minor laceration of femoral vein at hip and thigh level, left leg**

        ☑7ᵗʰ **S75.119** **Minor laceration of femoral vein at hip and thigh level, unspecified leg**

    ☑6ᵗʰ **S75.12** Major laceration of femoral vein at hip and thigh level

        Complete transection of femoral vein at hip and thigh level
        Traumatic rupture of femoral vein at hip and thigh level

        ☑7ᵗʰ **S75.121** **Major laceration of femoral vein at hip and thigh level, right leg**

        ☑7ᵗʰ **S75.122** **Major laceration of femoral vein at hip and thigh level, left leg**

        ☑7ᵗʰ **S75.129** **Major laceration of femoral vein at hip and thigh level, unspecified leg**

    ☑6ᵗʰ **S75.19** Other specified injury of femoral vein at hip and thigh level

        ☑7ᵗʰ **S75.191** **Other specified injury of femoral vein at hip and thigh level, right leg**

        ☑7ᵗʰ **S75.192** **Other specified injury of femoral vein at hip and thigh level, left leg**

        ☑7ᵗʰ **S75.199** **Other specified injury of femoral vein at hip and thigh level, unspecified leg**

☑5ᵗʰ **S75.2** Injury of greater saphenous vein at hip and thigh level

    EXCLUDES 1   greater saphenous vein NOS (S85.3)

    ☑6ᵗʰ **S75.20** Unspecified injury of greater saphenous vein at hip and thigh level

        ☑7ᵗʰ **S75.201** **Unspecified injury of greater saphenous vein at hip and thigh level, right leg**

        ☑7ᵗʰ **S75.202** **Unspecified injury of greater saphenous vein at hip and thigh level, left leg**

        ☑7ᵗʰ **S75.209** **Unspecified injury of greater saphenous vein at hip and thigh level, unspecified leg**

    ☑6ᵗʰ **S75.21** Minor laceration of greater saphenous vein at hip and thigh level

        Incomplete transection of greater saphenous vein at hip and thigh level
        Laceration of greater saphenous vein at hip and thigh level NOS
        Superficial laceration of greater saphenous vein at hip and thigh level

        ☑7ᵗʰ **S75.211** **Minor laceration of greater saphenous vein at hip and thigh level, right leg**

        ☑7ᵗʰ **S75.212** **Minor laceration of greater saphenous vein at hip and thigh level, left leg**

        ☑7ᵗʰ **S75.219** **Minor laceration of greater saphenous vein at hip and thigh level, unspecified leg**

    ☑6ᵗʰ **S75.22** Major laceration of greater saphenous vein at hip and thigh level

        Complete transection of greater saphenous vein at hip and thigh level
        Traumatic rupture of greater saphenous vein at hip and thigh level

        ☑7ᵗʰ **S75.221** **Major laceration of greater saphenous vein at hip and thigh level, right leg**

☑ Additional Character Required   ☑x7ᵗʰ Xtension Alert   Unspecified Dx   Other Specified Dx   Manifestation   ►◄ Revised Text   ● New Code   ▲ Revised Code Title

ICD-10-CM Draft (2015)   **893**

√7ᵗʰ **S75.222 Major laceration of greater saphenous vein at hip and thigh level,** left **leg**

√7ᵗʰ **S75.229 Major laceration of greater saphenous vein at hip and thigh level, unspecified leg**

√6ᵗʰ **S75.29 Other** specified injury of greater saphenous vein at hip and thigh level

√7ᵗʰ **S75.291 Other specified injury of greater saphenous vein at hip and thigh level,** right **leg**

√7ᵗʰ **S75.292 Other specified injury of greater saphenous vein at hip and thigh level,** left **leg**

√7ᵗʰ **S75.299 Other specified injury of greater saphenous vein at hip and thigh level, unspecified leg**

√5ᵗʰ **S75.8 Injury of** other blood vessels **at hip and thigh level**

√6ᵗʰ **S75.80 Unspecified** injury of other blood vessels at hip and thigh level

√7ᵗʰ **S75.801 Unspecified injury of other blood vessels at hip and thigh level,** right **leg**

√7ᵗʰ **S75.802 Unspecified injury of other blood vessels at hip and thigh level,** left **leg**

√7ᵗʰ **S75.809 Unspecified injury of other blood vessels at hip and thigh level, unspecified leg**

√6ᵗʰ **S75.81 Laceration** of other blood vessels at hip and thigh level

√7ᵗʰ **S75.811 Laceration of other blood vessels at hip and thigh level,** right **leg**

√7ᵗʰ **S75.812 Laceration of other blood vessels at hip and thigh level,** left **leg**

√7ᵗʰ **S75.819 Laceration of other blood vessels at hip and thigh level, unspecified leg**

√6ᵗʰ **S75.89 Other** specified injury of other blood vessels at hip and thigh level

√7ᵗʰ **S75.891 Other specified injury of other blood vessels at hip and thigh level,** right **leg**

√7ᵗʰ **S75.892 Other specified injury of other blood vessels at hip and thigh level,** left **leg**

√7ᵗʰ **S75.899 Other specified injury of other blood vessels at hip and thigh level, unspecified leg**

√5ᵗʰ **S75.9 Injury of unspecified blood vessel at hip and thigh level**

√6ᵗʰ **S75.90 Unspecified** injury of unspecified blood vessel at hip and thigh level

√7ᵗʰ **S75.901 Unspecified injury of unspecified blood vessel at hip and thigh level,** right **leg**

√7ᵗʰ **S75.902 Unspecified injury of unspecified blood vessel at hip and thigh level,** left **leg**

√7ᵗʰ **S75.909 Unspecified injury of unspecified blood vessel at hip and thigh level, unspecified leg**

√6ᵗʰ **S75.91 Laceration** of unspecified blood vessel at hip and thigh level

√7ᵗʰ **S75.911 Laceration of unspecified blood vessel at hip and thigh level,** right **leg**

√7ᵗʰ **S75.912 Laceration of unspecified blood vessel at hip and thigh level,** left **leg**

√7ᵗʰ **S75.919 Laceration of unspecified blood vessel at hip and thigh level, unspecified leg**

√6ᵗʰ **S75.99 Other** specified injury of unspecified blood vessel at hip and thigh level

√7ᵗʰ **S75.991 Other specified injury of unspecified blood vessel at hip and thigh level,** right **leg**

√7ᵗʰ **S75.992 Other specified injury of unspecified blood vessel at hip and thigh level,** left **leg**

√7ᵗʰ **S75.999 Other specified injury of unspecified blood vessel at hip and thigh level, unspecified leg**

√4ᵗʰ **S76 Injury of muscle, fascia and tendon at hip and thigh level**

Code also any associated open wound (S71.-)

EXCLUDES 2   injury of muscle, fascia and tendon at lower leg level (S86)
sprain of joint and ligament of hip (S73.1)

The appropriate 7th character is to be added to each code from category S76.
A   initial encounter
D   subsequent encounter
S   sequela

√5ᵗʰ **S76.0 Injury of muscle, fascia and tendon of hip**

√6ᵗʰ **S76.00 Unspecified** injury of muscle, fascia and tendon of hip

√7ᵗʰ **S76.001 Unspecified injury of muscle, fascia and tendon of** right **hip**

√7ᵗʰ **S76.002 Unspecified injury of muscle, fascia and tendon of** left **hip**

√7ᵗʰ **S76.009 Unspecified injury of muscle, fascia and tendon of unspecified hip**

√6ᵗʰ **S76.01 Strain** of muscle, fascia and tendon of hip

√7ᵗʰ **S76.011 Strain of muscle, fascia and tendon of** right **hip**

√7ᵗʰ **S76.012 Strain of muscle, fascia and tendon of** left **hip**

√7ᵗʰ **S76.019 Strain of muscle, fascia and tendon of unspecified hip**

√6ᵗʰ **S76.02 Laceration** of muscle, fascia and tendon of hip

√7ᵗʰ **S76.021 Laceration of muscle, fascia and tendon of** right **hip**

√7ᵗʰ **S76.022 Laceration of muscle, fascia and tendon of** left **hip**

√7ᵗʰ **S76.029 Laceration of muscle, fascia and tendon of unspecified hip**

√6ᵗʰ **S76.09 Other** specified injury of muscle, fascia and tendon of hip

√7ᵗʰ **S76.091 Other specified injury of muscle, fascia and tendon of** right **hip**

√7ᵗʰ **S76.092 Other specified injury of muscle, fascia and tendon of** left **hip**

√7ᵗʰ **S76.099 Other specified injury of muscle, fascia and tendon of unspecified hip**

√5ᵗʰ **S76.1 Injury of** quadriceps **muscle, fascia and tendon**

Injury of patellar ligament (tendon)

√6ᵗʰ **S76.10 Unspecified** injury of quadriceps muscle, fascia and tendon

√7ᵗʰ **S76.101 Unspecified injury of** right **quadriceps muscle, fascia and tendon**

√7ᵗʰ **S76.102 Unspecified injury of** left **quadriceps muscle, fascia and tendon**

√7ᵗʰ **S76.109 Unspecified injury of unspecified quadriceps muscle, fascia and tendon**

√6ᵗʰ **S76.11 Strain** of quadriceps muscle, fascia and tendon

√7ᵗʰ **S76.111 Strain of** right **quadriceps muscle, fascia and tendon**

√7ᵗʰ **S76.112 Strain of** left **quadriceps muscle, fascia and tendon**

√7ᵗʰ **S76.119 Strain of unspecified quadriceps muscle, fascia and tendon**

√6ᵗʰ **S76.12 Laceration** of quadriceps muscle, fascia and tendon

√7ᵗʰ **S76.121 Laceration of** right **quadriceps muscle, fascia and tendon**

√7ᵗʰ **S76.122 Laceration of** left **quadriceps muscle, fascia and tendon**

√7ᵗʰ **S76.129 Laceration of unspecified quadriceps muscle, fascia and tendon**

√6ᵗʰ **S76.19 Other** specified injury of quadriceps muscle, fascia and tendon

√7ᵗʰ **S76.191 Other specified injury of** right **quadriceps muscle, fascia and tendon**

√7ᵗʰ **S76.192 Other specified injury of** left **quadriceps muscle, fascia and tendon**

√7ᵗʰ **S76.199 Other specified injury of unspecified quadriceps muscle, fascia and tendon**

EXCLUDES 1 Not coded here   EXCLUDES 2 Not included here   N Newborn Age: 0   P Pediatric Age: 0–17   M Maternity Age: 12–55   A Adult Age: 15–124

894   ICD-10-CM Draft (2015)

✓5ᵗʰ **S76.2** Injury of adductor muscle, fascia and tendon of thigh

  ✓6ᵗʰ **S76.20** Unspecified injury of adductor muscle, fascia and tendon of thigh

    ✓7ᵗʰ **S76.201** Unspecified injury of adductor muscle, fascia and tendon of right thigh

    ✓7ᵗʰ **S76.202** Unspecified injury of adductor muscle, fascia and tendon of left thigh

    ✓7ᵗʰ **S76.209** Unspecified injury of adductor muscle, fascia and tendon of unspecified thigh

  ✓6ᵗʰ **S76.21** Strain of adductor muscle, fascia and tendon of thigh

    ✓7ᵗʰ **S76.211** Strain of adductor muscle, fascia and tendon of right thigh

    ✓7ᵗʰ **S76.212** Strain of adductor muscle, fascia and tendon of left thigh

    ✓7ᵗʰ **S76.219** Strain of adductor muscle, fascia and tendon of unspecified thigh

  ✓6ᵗʰ **S76.22** Laceration of adductor muscle, fascia and tendon of thigh

    ✓7ᵗʰ **S76.221** Laceration of adductor muscle, fascia and tendon of right thigh

    ✓7ᵗʰ **S76.222** Laceration of adductor muscle, fascia and tendon of left thigh

    ✓7ᵗʰ **S76.229** Laceration of adductor muscle, fascia and tendon of unspecified thigh

  ✓6ᵗʰ **S76.29** Other injury of adductor muscle, fascia and tendon of thigh

    ✓7ᵗʰ **S76.291** Other injury of adductor muscle, fascia and tendon of right thigh

    ✓7ᵗʰ **S76.292** Other injury of adductor muscle, fascia and tendon of left thigh

    ✓7ᵗʰ **S76.299** Other injury of adductor muscle, fascia and tendon of unspecified thigh

✓5ᵗʰ **S76.3** Injury of muscle, fascia and tendon of the posterior muscle group at thigh level

  ✓6ᵗʰ **S76.30** Unspecified injury of muscle, fascia and tendon of the posterior muscle group at thigh level

    ✓7ᵗʰ **S76.301** Unspecified injury of muscle, fascia and tendon of the posterior muscle group at thigh level, right thigh

    ✓7ᵗʰ **S76.302** Unspecified injury of muscle, fascia and tendon of the posterior muscle group at thigh level, left thigh

    ✓7ᵗʰ **S76.309** Unspecified injury of muscle, fascia and tendon of the posterior muscle group at thigh level, unspecified thigh

  ✓6ᵗʰ **S76.31** Strain of muscle, fascia and tendon of the posterior muscle group at thigh level

    ✓7ᵗʰ **S76.311** Strain of muscle, fascia and tendon of the posterior muscle group at thigh level, right thigh

    ✓7ᵗʰ **S76.312** Strain of muscle, fascia and tendon of the posterior muscle group at thigh level, left thigh

    ✓7ᵗʰ **S76.319** Strain of muscle, fascia and tendon of the posterior muscle group at thigh level, unspecified thigh

  ✓6ᵗʰ **S76.32** Laceration of muscle, fascia and tendon of the posterior muscle group at thigh level

    ✓7ᵗʰ **S76.321** Laceration of muscle, fascia and tendon of the posterior muscle group at thigh level, right thigh

    ✓7ᵗʰ **S76.322** Laceration of muscle, fascia and tendon of the posterior muscle group at thigh level, left thigh

    ✓7ᵗʰ **S76.329** Laceration of muscle, fascia and tendon of the posterior muscle group at thigh level, unspecified thigh

  ✓6ᵗʰ **S76.39** Other specified injury of muscle, fascia and tendon of the posterior muscle group at thigh level

    ✓7ᵗʰ **S76.391** Other specified injury of muscle, fascia and tendon of the posterior muscle group at thigh level, right thigh

    ✓7ᵗʰ **S76.392** Other specified injury of muscle, fascia and tendon of the posterior muscle group at thigh level, left thigh

    ✓7ᵗʰ **S76.399** Other specified injury of muscle, fascia and tendon of the posterior muscle group at thigh level, unspecified thigh

✓5ᵗʰ **S76.8** Injury of other specified muscles, fascia and tendons at thigh level

  ✓6ᵗʰ **S76.80** Unspecified injury of other specified muscles, fascia and tendons at thigh level

    ✓7ᵗʰ **S76.801** Unspecified injury of other specified muscles, fascia and tendons at thigh level, right thigh

    ✓7ᵗʰ **S76.802** Unspecified injury of other specified muscles, fascia and tendons at thigh level, left thigh

    ✓7ᵗʰ **S76.809** Unspecified injury of other specified muscles, fascia and tendons at thigh level, unspecified thigh

  ✓6ᵗʰ **S76.81** Strain of other specified muscles, fascia and tendons at thigh level

    ✓7ᵗʰ **S76.811** Strain of other specified muscles, fascia and tendons at thigh level, right thigh

    ✓7ᵗʰ **S76.812** Strain of other specified muscles, fascia and tendons at thigh level, left thigh

    ✓7ᵗʰ **S76.819** Strain of other specified muscles, fascia and tendons at thigh level, unspecified thigh

  ✓6ᵗʰ **S76.82** Laceration of other specified muscles, fascia and tendons at thigh level

    ✓7ᵗʰ **S76.821** Laceration of other specified muscles, fascia and tendons at thigh level, right thigh

    ✓7ᵗʰ **S76.822** Laceration of other specified muscles, fascia and tendons at thigh level, left thigh

    ✓7ᵗʰ **S76.829** Laceration of other specified muscles, fascia and tendons at thigh level, unspecified thigh

  ✓6ᵗʰ **S76.89** Other injury of other specified muscles, fascia and tendons at thigh level

    ✓7ᵗʰ **S76.891** Other injury of other specified muscles, fascia and tendons at thigh level, right thigh

    ✓7ᵗʰ **S76.892** Other injury of other specified muscles, fascia and tendons at thigh level, left thigh

    ✓7ᵗʰ **S76.899** Other injury of other specified muscles, fascia and tendons at thigh level, unspecified thigh

✓5ᵗʰ **S76.9** Injury of unspecified muscles, fascia and tendons at thigh level

  ✓6ᵗʰ **S76.90** Unspecified injury of unspecified muscles, fascia and tendons at thigh level

    ✓7ᵗʰ **S76.901** Unspecified injury of unspecified muscles, fascia and tendons at thigh level, right thigh

    ✓7ᵗʰ **S76.902** Unspecified injury of unspecified muscles, fascia and tendons at thigh level, left thigh

    ✓7ᵗʰ **S76.909** Unspecified injury of unspecified muscles, fascia and tendons at thigh level, unspecified thigh

  ✓6ᵗʰ **S76.91** Strain of unspecified muscles, fascia and tendons at thigh level

    ✓7ᵗʰ **S76.911** Strain of unspecified muscles, fascia and tendons at thigh level, right thigh

    ✓7ᵗʰ **S76.912** Strain of unspecified muscles, fascia and tendons at thigh level, left thigh

    ✓7ᵗʰ **S76.919** Strain of unspecified muscles, fascia and tendons at thigh level, unspecified thigh

  ✓6ᵗʰ **S76.92** Laceration of unspecified muscles, fascia and tendons at thigh level

    ✓7ᵗʰ **S76.921** Laceration of unspecified muscles, fascia and tendons at thigh level, right thigh

    ✓7ᵗʰ **S76.922** Laceration of unspecified muscles, fascia and tendons at thigh level, left thigh

    ✓7ᵗʰ **S76.929** Laceration of unspecified muscles, fascia and tendons at thigh level, unspecified thigh

---

✓ Additional Character Required   ✓x7ᵗʰ Xtension Alert   Unspecified Dx   Other Specified Dx   Manifestation   ►◄ Revised Text   ● New Code   ▲ Revised Code Title

✓6ᵗʰ **S76.99** Other specified injury of unspecified muscles, fascia and tendons at thigh level

- ✓7ᵗʰ **S76.991** Other specified injury of unspecified muscles, fascia and tendons at thigh level, right thigh
- ✓7ᵗʰ **S76.992** Other specified injury of unspecified muscles, fascia and tendons at thigh level, left thigh
- ✓7ᵗʰ **S76.999** Other specified injury of unspecified muscles, fascia and tendons at thigh level, unspecified thigh

✓4ᵗʰ **S77 Crushing injury of hip and thigh**

Use additional code(s) for all associated injuries

EXCLUDES 2 crushing injury of ankle and foot (S97.-)
crushing injury of lower leg (S87.-)

The appropriate 7th character is to be added to each code from category S77.
A   initial encounter
D   subsequent encounter
S   sequela

✓5ᵗʰ **S77.Ø Crushing injury of hip**
- ✓x7ᵗʰ **S77.ØØ** Crushing injury of unspecified hip
- ✓x7ᵗʰ **S77.Ø1** Crushing injury of right hip
- ✓x7ᵗʰ **S77.Ø2** Crushing injury of left hip

✓5ᵗʰ **S77.1 Crushing injury of thigh**
- ✓x7ᵗʰ **S77.1Ø** Crushing injury of unspecified thigh
- ✓x7ᵗʰ **S77.11** Crushing injury of right thigh
- ✓x7ᵗʰ **S77.12** Crushing injury of left thigh

✓5ᵗʰ **S77.2 Crushing injury of hip with thigh**
- ✓x7ᵗʰ **S77.2Ø** Crushing injury of unspecified hip with thigh
- ✓x7ᵗʰ **S77.21** Crushing injury of right hip with thigh
- ✓x7ᵗʰ **S77.22** Crushing injury of left hip with thigh

✓4ᵗʰ **S78 Traumatic amputation of hip and thigh**

NOTE An amputation not identified as partial or complete should be coded to complete.

EXCLUDES 1 traumatic amputation of knee (S88.Ø-)

The appropriate 7th character is to be added to each code from category S78.
A   initial encounter
D   subsequent encounter
S   sequela

✓5ᵗʰ **S78.Ø Traumatic amputation at hip joint**
- ✓6ᵗʰ **S78.Ø1** Complete traumatic amputation at hip joint
  - ✓7ᵗʰ **S78.Ø11** Complete traumatic amputation at right hip joint
  - ✓7ᵗʰ **S78.Ø12** Complete traumatic amputation at left hip joint
  - ✓7ᵗʰ **S78.Ø19** Complete traumatic amputation at unspecified hip joint
- ✓6ᵗʰ **S78.Ø2** Partial traumatic amputation at hip joint
  - ✓7ᵗʰ **S78.Ø21** Partial traumatic amputation at right hip joint
  - ✓7ᵗʰ **S78.Ø22** Partial traumatic amputation at left hip joint
  - ✓7ᵗʰ **S78.Ø29** Partial traumatic amputation at unspecified hip joint

✓5ᵗʰ **S78.1 Traumatic amputation at level between hip and knee**

EXCLUDES 1 traumatic amputation of knee (S88.Ø-)

- ✓6ᵗʰ **S78.11** Complete traumatic amputation at level between hip and knee
  - ✓7ᵗʰ **S78.111** Complete traumatic amputation at level between right hip and knee
  - ✓7ᵗʰ **S78.112** Complete traumatic amputation at level between left hip and knee
  - ✓7ᵗʰ **S78.119** Complete traumatic amputation at level between unspecified hip and knee
- ✓6ᵗʰ **S78.12** Partial traumatic amputation at level between hip and knee
  - ✓7ᵗʰ **S78.121** Partial traumatic amputation at level between right hip and knee
  - ✓7ᵗʰ **S78.122** Partial traumatic amputation at level between left hip and knee

- ✓7ᵗʰ **S78.129** Partial traumatic amputation at level between unspecified hip and knee

✓5ᵗʰ **S78.9 Traumatic amputation of hip and thigh, level unspecified**
- ✓6ᵗʰ **S78.91** Complete traumatic amputation of hip and thigh, level unspecified
  - ✓7ᵗʰ **S78.911** Complete traumatic amputation of right hip and thigh, level unspecified
  - ✓7ᵗʰ **S78.912** Complete traumatic amputation of left hip and thigh, level unspecified
  - ✓7ᵗʰ **S78.919** Complete traumatic amputation of unspecified hip and thigh, level unspecified
- ✓6ᵗʰ **S78.92** Partial traumatic amputation of hip and thigh, level unspecified
  - ✓7ᵗʰ **S78.921** Partial traumatic amputation of right hip and thigh, level unspecified
  - ✓7ᵗʰ **S78.922** Partial traumatic amputation of left hip and thigh, level unspecified
  - ✓7ᵗʰ **S78.929** Partial traumatic amputation of unspecified hip and thigh, level unspecified

✓4ᵗʰ **S79 Other and unspecified injuries of hip and thigh**

✓5ᵗʰ **S79.Ø Physeal fracture of upper end of femur**

NOTE A fracture not indicated as open or closed should be coded to closed.

EXCLUDES 1 apophyseal fracture of upper end of femur (S72.13-)
nontraumatic slipped upper femoral epiphysis (M93.Ø-)

The appropriate 7th character is to be added to each code from subcategory S79.Ø.
A   initial encounter for closed fracture
D   subsequent encounter for fracture with routine healing
G   subsequent encounter for fracture with delayed healing
K   subsequent encounter for fracture with nonunion
P   subsequent encounter for fracture with malunion
S   sequela

✓6ᵗʰ **S79.ØØ** Unspecified physeal fracture of upper end of femur
- ✓7ᵗʰ **S79.ØØ1** Unspecified physeal fracture of upper end of right femur
- ✓7ᵗʰ **S79.ØØ2** Unspecified physeal fracture of upper end of left femur
- ✓7ᵗʰ **S79.ØØ9** Unspecified physeal fracture of upper end of unspecified femur

✓6ᵗʰ **S79.Ø1** Salter-Harris Type I physeal fracture of upper end of femur

Acute on chronic slipped capital femoral epiphysis (traumatic)
Acute slipped capital femoral epiphysis (traumatic)
Capital femoral epiphyseal fracture

EXCLUDES 1 chronic slipped upper femoral epiphysis (nontraumatic) (M93.Ø2-)

- ✓7ᵗʰ **S79.Ø11** Salter-Harris Type I physeal fracture of upper end of right femur
- ✓7ᵗʰ **S79.Ø12** Salter-Harris Type I physeal fracture of upper end of left femur
- ✓7ᵗʰ **S79.Ø19** Salter-Harris Type I physeal fracture of upper end of unspecified femur

✓6ᵗʰ **S79.Ø9** Other physeal fracture of upper end of femur
- ✓7ᵗʰ **S79.Ø91** Other physeal fracture of upper end of right femur
- ✓7ᵗʰ **S79.Ø92** Other physeal fracture of upper end of left femur
- ✓7ᵗʰ **S79.Ø99** Other physeal fracture of upper end of unspecified femur

EXCLUDES 1 Not coded here   **EXCLUDES 2** Not included here   N Newborn Age: Ø   P Pediatric Age: Ø-17   M Maternity Age: 12-55   A Adult Age: 15-124

896

ICD-1Ø-CM Draft (2Ø15)

✓5th **S79.1** Physeal **fracture of** lower end of femur

> **NOTE**   A fracture not indicated as open or closed should be coded to closed.

> The appropriate 7th character is to be added to each code from subcategory S79.1.
> A   initial encounter for closed fracture
> D   subsequent encounter for fracture with routine healing
> G   subsequent encounter for fracture with delayed healing
> K   subsequent encounter for fracture with nonunion
> P   subsequent encounter for fracture with malunion
> S   sequela

✓6th **S79.10** Unspecified physeal fracture of lower end of femur

✓7th **S79.101** Unspecified physeal fracture of lower end of right femur

✓7th **S79.102** Unspecified physeal fracture of lower end of left femur

✓7th **S79.109** Unspecified physeal fracture of lower end of unspecified femur

✓6th **S79.11** Salter-Harris Type I physeal fracture of lower end of femur

✓7th **S79.111** Salter-Harris Type I physeal fracture of lower end of right femur

✓7th **S79.112** Salter-Harris Type I physeal fracture of lower end of left femur

✓7th **S79.119** Salter-Harris Type I physeal fracture of lower end of unspecified femur

✓6th **S79.12** Salter-Harris Type II physeal fracture of lower end of femur

✓7th **S79.121** Salter-Harris Type II physeal fracture of lower end of right femur

✓7th **S79.122** Salter-Harris Type II physeal fracture of lower end of left femur

✓7th **S79.129** Salter-Harris Type II physeal fracture of lower end of unspecified femur

✓6th **S79.13** Salter-Harris Type III physeal fracture of lower end of femur

✓7th **S79.131** Salter-Harris Type III physeal fracture of lower end of right femur

✓7th **S79.132** Salter-Harris Type III physeal fracture of lower end of left femur

✓7th **S79.139** Salter-Harris Type III physeal fracture of lower end of unspecified femur

✓6th **S79.14** Salter-Harris Type IV physeal fracture of lower end of femur

✓7th **S79.141** Salter-Harris Type IV physeal fracture of lower end of right femur

✓7th **S79.142** Salter-Harris Type IV physeal fracture of lower end of left femur

✓7th **S79.149** Salter-Harris Type IV physeal fracture of lower end of unspecified femur

✓6th **S79.19** Other physeal fracture of lower end of femur

✓7th **S79.191** Other physeal fracture of lower end of right femur

✓7th **S79.192** Other physeal fracture of lower end of left femur

✓7th **S79.199** Other physeal fracture of lower end of unspecified femur

✓5th **S79.8** Other specified injuries of hip and thigh

> The appropriate 7th character is to be added to each code in subcategory S79.8.
> A   initial encounter
> D   subsequent encounter
> S   sequela

✓6th **S79.81** Other specified injuries of hip

✓7th **S79.811** Other specified injuries of right hip

✓7th **S79.812** Other specified injuries of left hip

✓7th **S79.819** Other specified injuries of unspecified hip

✓6th **S79.82** Other specified injuries of thigh

✓7th **S79.821** Other specified injuries of right thigh

✓7th **S79.822** Other specified injuries of left thigh

✓7th **S79.829** Other specified injuries of unspecified thigh

✓5th **S79.9** Unspecified injury of hip and thigh

> The appropriate 7th character is to be added to each code in subcategory S79.9.
> A   initial encounter
> D   subsequent encounter
> S   sequela

✓6th **S79.91** Unspecified injury of hip

✓7th **S79.911** Unspecified injury of right hip

✓7th **S79.912** Unspecified injury of left hip

✓7th **S79.919** Unspecified injury of unspecified hip

✓6th **S79.92** Unspecified injury of thigh

✓7th **S79.921** Unspecified injury of right thigh

✓7th **S79.922** Unspecified injury of left thigh

✓7th **S79.929** Unspecified injury of unspecified thigh

Injuries to the knee and lower leg (S80-S89)

EXCLUDES 2 burns and corrosions (T20-T32)
frostbite (T33-T34)
injuries of ankle and foot, except fracture of ankle and malleolus (S90-S99)
insect bite or sting, venomous (T63.4)

✓4th **S80** **Superficial injury of knee and lower leg**

> **EXCLUDES 2** superficial injury of ankle and foot (S90.-)

> The appropriate 7th character is to be added to each code from category S80.
> A   initial encounter
> D   subsequent encounter
> S   sequela

✓5th **S80.0** Contusion of knee

✓x7th **S80.00** Contusion of unspecified knee

✓x7th **S80.01** Contusion of right knee

✓x7th **S80.02** Contusion of left knee

✓5th **S80.1** Contusion of lower leg

✓x7th **S80.10** Contusion of unspecified lower leg

✓x7th **S80.11** Contusion of right lower leg

✓x7th **S80.12** Contusion of left lower leg

✓5th **S80.2** Other superficial injuries of knee

✓6th **S80.21** Abrasion of knee

✓7th **S80.211** Abrasion, right knee

✓7th **S80.212** Abrasion, left knee

✓7th **S80.219** Abrasion, unspecified knee

✓6th **S80.22** Blister (nonthermal) of knee

✓7th **S80.221** Blister (nonthermal), right knee

✓7th **S80.222** Blister (nonthermal), left knee

✓7th **S80.229** Blister (nonthermal), unspecified knee

✓6th **S80.24** External constriction of knee

✓7th **S80.241** External constriction, right knee

✓7th **S80.242** External constriction, left knee

✓7th **S80.249** External constriction, unspecified knee

✓6th **S80.25** Superficial foreign body of knee
Splinter in the knee

✓7th **S80.251** Superficial foreign body, right knee

✓7th **S80.252** Superficial foreign body, left knee

✓7th **S80.259** Superficial foreign body, unspecified knee

✓6th **S80.26** Insect bite (nonvenomous) of knee

✓7th **S80.261** Insect bite (nonvenomous), right knee

✓7th **S80.262** Insect bite (nonvenomous), left knee

✓7th **S80.269** Insect bite (nonvenomous), unspecified knee

✓6th **S80.27** Other superficial bite of knee

> **EXCLUDES 1** open bite of knee (S81.05-)

✓7th **S80.271** Other superficial bite of right knee

✓7th **S80.272** Other superficial bite of left knee

✓7th **S80.279** Other superficial bite of unspecified knee

✓5th **S80.8** Other superficial injuries of lower leg

✓6th **S80.81** Abrasion of lower leg

✓7th **S80.811** Abrasion, right lower leg

✓7th **S80.812** Abrasion, left lower leg

✓7th **S80.819** Abrasion, unspecified lower leg

(left margin) Injury, Poisoning and Certain Other Consequences of External Causes

(left margin) S80.82–S81.859

√6ᵗʰ **S80.82** Blister (nonthermal) of lower leg
- √7ᵗʰ **S80.821** Blister (nonthermal), right lower leg
- √7ᵗʰ **S80.822** Blister (nonthermal), left lower leg
- √7ᵗʰ **S80.829** Blister (nonthermal), unspecified lower leg

√6ᵗʰ **S80.84** External constriction of lower leg
- √7ᵗʰ **S80.841** External constriction, right lower leg
- √7ᵗʰ **S80.842** External constriction, left lower leg
- √7ᵗʰ **S80.849** External constriction, unspecified lower leg

√6ᵗʰ **S80.85** Superficial foreign body of lower leg
Splinter in the lower leg
- √7ᵗʰ **S80.851** Superficial foreign body, right lower leg
- √7ᵗʰ **S80.852** Superficial foreign body, left lower leg
- √7ᵗʰ **S80.859** Superficial foreign body, unspecified lower leg

√6ᵗʰ **S80.86** Insect bite (nonvenomous) of lower leg
- √7ᵗʰ **S80.861** Insect bite (nonvenomous), right lower leg
- √7ᵗʰ **S80.862** Insect bite (nonvenomous), left lower leg
- √7ᵗʰ **S80.869** Insect bite (nonvenomous), unspecified lower leg

√6ᵗʰ **S80.87** Other superficial bite of lower leg
EXCLUDES 1   open bite of lower leg (S81.85-)
- √7ᵗʰ **S80.871** Other superficial bite, right lower leg
- √7ᵗʰ **S80.872** Other superficial bite, left lower leg
- √7ᵗʰ **S80.879** Other superficial bite, unspecified lower leg

√5ᵗʰ **S80.9** Unspecified superficial injury of knee and lower leg

√6ᵗʰ **S80.91** Unspecified superficial injury of knee
- √7ᵗʰ **S80.911** Unspecified superficial injury of right knee
- √7ᵗʰ **S80.912** Unspecified superficial injury of left knee
- √7ᵗʰ **S80.919** Unspecified superficial injury of unspecified knee

√6ᵗʰ **S80.92** Unspecified superficial injury of lower leg
- √7ᵗʰ **S80.921** Unspecified superficial injury of right lower leg
- √7ᵗʰ **S80.922** Unspecified superficial injury of left lower leg
- √7ᵗʰ **S80.929** Unspecified superficial injury of unspecified lower leg

√4ᵗʰ **S81** Open wound of knee and lower leg
Code also any associated wound infection
EXCLUDES 1   open fracture of knee and lower leg (S82.-)
             traumatic amputation of lower leg (S88.-)
EXCLUDES 2   open wound of ankle and foot (S91.-)

The appropriate 7th character is to be added to each code from category S81.
A   initial encounter
D   subsequent encounter
S   sequela

√5ᵗʰ **S81.0** Open wound of knee

√6ᵗʰ **S81.00** Unspecified open wound of knee
- √7ᵗʰ **S81.001** Unspecified open wound, right knee
- √7ᵗʰ **S81.002** Unspecified open wound, left knee
- √7ᵗʰ **S81.009** Unspecified open wound, unspecified knee

√6ᵗʰ **S81.01** Laceration without foreign body of knee
- √7ᵗʰ **S81.011** Laceration without foreign body, right knee
- √7ᵗʰ **S81.012** Laceration without foreign body, left knee
- √7ᵗʰ **S81.019** Laceration without foreign body, unspecified knee

√6ᵗʰ **S81.02** Laceration with foreign body of knee
- √7ᵗʰ **S81.021** Laceration with foreign body, right knee
- √7ᵗʰ **S81.022** Laceration with foreign body, left knee
- √7ᵗʰ **S81.029** Laceration with foreign body, unspecified knee

√6ᵗʰ **S81.03** Puncture wound without foreign body of knee
- √7ᵗʰ **S81.031** Puncture wound without foreign body, right knee

√7ᵗʰ **S81.032** Puncture wound without foreign body, left knee
√7ᵗʰ **S81.039** Puncture wound without foreign body, unspecified knee

√6ᵗʰ **S81.04** Puncture wound with foreign body of knee
- √7ᵗʰ **S81.041** Puncture wound with foreign body, right knee
- √7ᵗʰ **S81.042** Puncture wound with foreign body, left knee
- √7ᵗʰ **S81.049** Puncture wound with foreign body, unspecified knee

√6ᵗʰ **S81.05** Open bite of knee
Bite of knee NOS
EXCLUDES 1   superficial bite of knee (S80.27-)
- √7ᵗʰ **S81.051** Open bite, right knee
- √7ᵗʰ **S81.052** Open bite, left knee
- √7ᵗʰ **S81.059** Open bite, unspecified knee

√5ᵗʰ **S81.8** Open wound of lower leg

√6ᵗʰ **S81.80** Unspecified open wound of lower leg
- √7ᵗʰ **S81.801** Unspecified open wound, right lower leg
- √7ᵗʰ **S81.802** Unspecified open wound, left lower leg
- √7ᵗʰ **S81.809** Unspecified open wound, unspecified lower leg

√6ᵗʰ **S81.81** Laceration without foreign body of lower leg
- √7ᵗʰ **S81.811** Laceration without foreign body, right lower leg
- √7ᵗʰ **S81.812** Laceration without foreign body, left lower leg
- √7ᵗʰ **S81.819** Laceration without foreign body, unspecified lower leg

√6ᵗʰ **S81.82** Laceration with foreign body of lower leg
- √7ᵗʰ **S81.821** Laceration with foreign body, right lower leg
- √7ᵗʰ **S81.822** Laceration with foreign body, left lower leg
- √7ᵗʰ **S81.829** Laceration with foreign body, unspecified lower leg

√6ᵗʰ **S81.83** Puncture wound without foreign body of lower leg
- √7ᵗʰ **S81.831** Puncture wound without foreign body, right lower leg
- √7ᵗʰ **S81.832** Puncture wound without foreign body, left lower leg
- √7ᵗʰ **S81.839** Puncture wound without foreign body, unspecified lower leg

√6ᵗʰ **S81.84** Puncture wound with foreign body of lower leg
- √7ᵗʰ **S81.841** Puncture wound with foreign body, right lower leg
- √7ᵗʰ **S81.842** Puncture wound with foreign body, left lower leg
- √7ᵗʰ **S81.849** Puncture wound with foreign body, unspecified lower leg

√6ᵗʰ **S81.85** Open bite of lower leg
Bite of lower leg NOS
EXCLUDES 1   superficial bite of lower leg (S80.86-, S80.87-)
- √7ᵗʰ **S81.851** Open bite, right lower leg
- √7ᵗʰ **S81.852** Open bite, left lower leg
- √7ᵗʰ **S81.859** Open bite, unspecified lower leg

EXCLUDES 1 Not coded here   EXCLUDES 2 Not included here   N Newborn Age: 0   P Pediatric Age: 0-17   M Maternity Age: 12-55   A Adult Age: 15-124

898   ICD-10-CM Draft (2015)

☑4ᵗʰ S82   Fracture of lower leg, including ankle

> **NOTE**   A fracture not indicated as displaced or nondisplaced should be coded to displaced.
> A fracture not designated as open or closed should be coded to closed.
> The open fracture designations are based on the Gustilo open fracture classification.
>
> **INCLUDES**   fracture of malleolus
> **EXCLUDES 1**   traumatic amputation of lower leg (S88.-)
> **EXCLUDES 2**   fracture of foot, except ankle (S92.-)
> periprosthetic fracture of prosthetic implant of knee (T84.042, T84.043)

> The appropriate 7th character is to be added to all codes from category S82 [unless otherwise indicated].
> A   initial encounter for closed fracture
> B   initial encounter for open fracture type I or II
>   initial encounter for open fracture NOS
> C   initial encounter for open fracture type IIIA, IIIB, or IIIC
> D   subsequent encounter for closed fracture with routine healing
> E   subsequent encounter for open fracture type I or II with routine healing
> F   subsequent encounter for open fracture type IIIA, IIIB, or IIIC with routine healing
> G   subsequent encounter for closed fracture with delayed healing
> H   subsequent encounter for open fracture type I or II with delayed healing
> J   subsequent encounter for open fracture type IIIA, IIIB or IIIC with delayed healing
> K   subsequent encounter for closed fracture with nonunion
> M   subsequent encounter for open fracture type I or II with nonunion
> N   subsequent encounter for open fracture type IIIA, IIIB or IIIC with nonunion
> P   subsequent encounter for closed fracture with malunion
> Q   subsequent encounter for open fracture type I or II with malunion
> R   subsequent encounter for open fracture type IIIA, IIIB or IIIC with malunion
> S   sequela

☑5ᵗʰ S82.0   Fracture of patella
Knee cap
- **☑6ᵗʰ S82.00   Unspecified fracture of patella**
  - ☑7ᵗʰ S82.001   Unspecified fracture of right patella
  - ☑7ᵗʰ S82.002   Unspecified fracture of left patella
  - ☑7ᵗʰ S82.009   Unspecified fracture of unspecified patella
- **☑6ᵗʰ S82.01   Osteochondral fracture of patella**
  - ☑7ᵗʰ S82.011   Displaced osteochondral fracture of right patella
  - ☑7ᵗʰ S82.012   Displaced osteochondral fracture of left patella
  - ☑7ᵗʰ S82.013   Displaced osteochondral fracture of unspecified patella
  - ☑7ᵗʰ S82.014   Nondisplaced osteochondral fracture of right patella
  - ☑7ᵗʰ S82.015   Nondisplaced osteochondral fracture of left patella
  - ☑7ᵗʰ S82.016   Nondisplaced osteochondral fracture of unspecified patella
- **☑6ᵗʰ S82.02   Longitudinal fracture of patella**
  - ☑7ᵗʰ S82.021   Displaced longitudinal fracture of right patella
  - ☑7ᵗʰ S82.022   Displaced longitudinal fracture of left patella
  - ☑7ᵗʰ S82.023   Displaced longitudinal fracture of unspecified patella
  - ☑7ᵗʰ S82.024   Nondisplaced longitudinal fracture of right patella
  - ☑7ᵗʰ S82.025   Nondisplaced longitudinal fracture of left patella
  - ☑7ᵗʰ S82.026   Nondisplaced longitudinal fracture of unspecified patella
- **☑6ᵗʰ S82.03   Transverse fracture of patella**
  - ☑7ᵗʰ S82.031   Displaced transverse fracture of right patella
  - ☑7ᵗʰ S82.032   Displaced transverse fracture of left patella
  - ☑7ᵗʰ S82.033   Displaced transverse fracture of unspecified patella
  - ☑7ᵗʰ S82.034   Nondisplaced transverse fracture of right patella
  - ☑7ᵗʰ S82.035   Nondisplaced transverse fracture of left patella
  - ☑7ᵗʰ S82.036   Nondisplaced transverse fracture of unspecified patella
- **☑6ᵗʰ S82.04   Comminuted fracture of patella**
  - ☑7ᵗʰ S82.041   Displaced comminuted fracture of right patella
  - ☑7ᵗʰ S82.042   Displaced comminuted fracture of left patella
  - ☑7ᵗʰ S82.043   Displaced comminuted fracture of unspecified patella
  - ☑7ᵗʰ S82.044   Nondisplaced comminuted fracture of right patella
  - ☑7ᵗʰ S82.045   Nondisplaced comminuted fracture of left patella
  - ☑7ᵗʰ S82.046   Nondisplaced comminuted fracture of unspecified patella
- **☑6ᵗʰ S82.09   Other fracture of patella**
  - ☑7ᵗʰ S82.091   Other fracture of right patella
  - ☑7ᵗʰ S82.092   Other fracture of left patella
  - ☑7ᵗʰ S82.099   Other fracture of unspecified patella

☑5ᵗʰ S82.1   Fracture of upper end of tibia
Fracture of proximal end of tibia
> **EXCLUDES 2**   fracture of shaft of tibia (S82.2-)
> physeal fracture of upper end of tibia (S89.0-)
- **☑6ᵗʰ S82.10   Unspecified fracture of upper end of tibia**
  - ☑7ᵗʰ S82.101   Unspecified fracture of upper end of right tibia
  - ☑7ᵗʰ S82.102   Unspecified fracture of upper end of left tibia
  - ☑7ᵗʰ S82.109   Unspecified fracture of upper end of unspecified tibia
- **☑6ᵗʰ S82.11   Fracture of tibial spine**
  - ☑7ᵗʰ S82.111   Displaced fracture of right tibial spine
  - ☑7ᵗʰ S82.112   Displaced fracture of left tibial spine
  - ☑7ᵗʰ S82.113   Displaced fracture of unspecified tibial spine
  - ☑7ᵗʰ S82.114   Nondisplaced fracture of right tibial spine
  - ☑7ᵗʰ S82.115   Nondisplaced fracture of left tibial spine
  - ☑7ᵗʰ S82.116   Nondisplaced fracture of unspecified tibial spine
- **☑6ᵗʰ S82.12   Fracture of lateral condyle of tibia**
  - ☑7ᵗʰ S82.121   Displaced fracture of lateral condyle of right tibia
  - ☑7ᵗʰ S82.122   Displaced fracture of lateral condyle of left tibia
  - ☑7ᵗʰ S82.123   Displaced fracture of lateral condyle of unspecified tibia
  - ☑7ᵗʰ S82.124   Nondisplaced fracture of lateral condyle of right tibia
  - ☑7ᵗʰ S82.125   Nondisplaced fracture of lateral condyle of left tibia
  - ☑7ᵗʰ S82.126   Nondisplaced fracture of lateral condyle of unspecified tibia
- **☑6ᵗʰ S82.13   Fracture of medial condyle of tibia**
  - ☑7ᵗʰ S82.131   Displaced fracture of medial condyle of right tibia
  - ☑7ᵗʰ S82.132   Displaced fracture of medial condyle of left tibia
  - ☑7ᵗʰ S82.133   Displaced fracture of medial condyle of unspecified tibia
  - ☑7ᵗʰ S82.134   Nondisplaced fracture of medial condyle of right tibia
  - ☑7ᵗʰ S82.135   Nondisplaced fracture of medial condyle of left tibia
  - ☑7ᵗʰ S82.136   Nondisplaced fracture of medial condyle of unspecified tibia
- **☑6ᵗʰ S82.14   Bicondylar fracture of tibia**
  Fracture of tibial plateau NOS
  - ☑7ᵗʰ S82.141   Displaced bicondylar fracture of right tibia

√7ᵗʰ **S82.142** Displaced bicondylar fracture of left tibia

√7ᵗʰ **S82.143** Displaced bicondylar fracture of unspecified tibia

√7ᵗʰ **S82.144** Nondisplaced bicondylar fracture of right tibia

√7ᵗʰ **S82.145** Nondisplaced bicondylar fracture of left tibia

√7ᵗʰ **S82.146** Nondisplaced bicondylar fracture of unspecified tibia

√6ᵗʰ **S82.15** Fracture of tibial tuberosity

√7ᵗʰ **S82.151** Displaced fracture of right tibial tuberosity

√7ᵗʰ **S82.152** Displaced fracture of left tibial tuberosity

√7ᵗʰ **S82.153** Displaced fracture of unspecified tibial tuberosity

√7ᵗʰ **S82.154** Nondisplaced fracture of right tibial tuberosity

√7ᵗʰ **S82.155** Nondisplaced fracture of left tibial tuberosity

√7ᵗʰ **S82.156** Nondisplaced fracture of unspecified tibial tuberosity

√6ᵗʰ **S82.16** Torus fracture of upper end of tibia

> The appropriate 7th character is to be added to all codes in subcategory S82.16.
> A　initial encounter for closed fracture
> D　subsequent encounter for fracture with routine healing
> G　subsequent encounter for fracture with delayed healing
> K　subsequent encounter for fracture with nonunion
> P　subsequent encounter for fracture with malunion
> S　sequela

√7ᵗʰ **S82.161** Torus fracture of upper end of right tibia

√7ᵗʰ **S82.162** Torus fracture of upper end of left tibia

√7ᵗʰ **S82.169** Torus fracture of upper end of unspecified tibia

√6ᵗʰ **S82.19** Other fracture of upper end of tibia

√7ᵗʰ **S82.191** Other fracture of upper end of right tibia

√7ᵗʰ **S82.192** Other fracture of upper end of left tibia

√7ᵗʰ **S82.199** Other fracture of upper end of unspecified tibia

√5ᵗʰ **S82.2** Fracture of shaft of tibia

√6ᵗʰ **S82.20** Unspecified fracture of shaft of tibia
Fracture of tibia NOS

√7ᵗʰ **S82.201** Unspecified fracture of shaft of right tibia

√7ᵗʰ **S82.202** Unspecified fracture of shaft of left tibia

√7ᵗʰ **S82.209** Unspecified fracture of shaft of unspecified tibia

√6ᵗʰ **S82.22** Transverse fracture of shaft of tibia

√7ᵗʰ **S82.221** Displaced transverse fracture of shaft of right tibia

√7ᵗʰ **S82.222** Displaced transverse fracture of shaft of left tibia

√7ᵗʰ **S82.223** Displaced transverse fracture of shaft of unspecified tibia

√7ᵗʰ **S82.224** Nondisplaced transverse fracture of shaft of right tibia

√7ᵗʰ **S82.225** Nondisplaced transverse fracture of shaft of left tibia

√7ᵗʰ **S82.226** Nondisplaced transverse fracture of shaft of unspecified tibia

√6ᵗʰ **S82.23** Oblique fracture of shaft of tibia

√7ᵗʰ **S82.231** Displaced oblique fracture of shaft of right tibia

√7ᵗʰ **S82.232** Displaced oblique fracture of shaft of left tibia

√7ᵗʰ **S82.233** Displaced oblique fracture of shaft of unspecified tibia

√7ᵗʰ **S82.234** Nondisplaced oblique fracture of shaft of right tibia

√7ᵗʰ **S82.235** Nondisplaced oblique fracture of shaft of left tibia

√7ᵗʰ **S82.236** Nondisplaced oblique fracture of shaft of unspecified tibia

√6ᵗʰ **S82.24** Spiral fracture of shaft of tibia
Toddler fracture

√7ᵗʰ **S82.241** Displaced spiral fracture of shaft of right tibia

√7ᵗʰ **S82.242** Displaced spiral fracture of shaft of left tibia

√7ᵗʰ **S82.243** Displaced spiral fracture of shaft of unspecified tibia

√7ᵗʰ **S82.244** Nondisplaced spiral fracture of shaft of right tibia

√7ᵗʰ **S82.245** Nondisplaced spiral fracture of shaft of left tibia

√7ᵗʰ **S82.246** Nondisplaced spiral fracture of shaft of unspecified tibia

√6ᵗʰ **S82.25** Comminuted fracture of shaft of tibia

√7ᵗʰ **S82.251** Displaced comminuted fracture of shaft of right tibia

√7ᵗʰ **S82.252** Displaced comminuted fracture of shaft of left tibia

√7ᵗʰ **S82.253** Displaced comminuted fracture of shaft of unspecified tibia

√7ᵗʰ **S82.254** Nondisplaced comminuted fracture of shaft of right tibia

√7ᵗʰ **S82.255** Nondisplaced comminuted fracture of shaft of left tibia

√7ᵗʰ **S82.256** Nondisplaced comminuted fracture of shaft of unspecified tibia

√6ᵗʰ **S82.26** Segmental fracture of shaft of tibia

√7ᵗʰ **S82.261** Displaced segmental fracture of shaft of right tibia

√7ᵗʰ **S82.262** Displaced segmental fracture of shaft of left tibia

√7ᵗʰ **S82.263** Displaced segmental fracture of shaft of unspecified tibia

√7ᵗʰ **S82.264** Nondisplaced segmental fracture of shaft of right tibia

√7ᵗʰ **S82.265** Nondisplaced segmental fracture of shaft of left tibia

√7ᵗʰ **S82.266** Nondisplaced segmental fracture of shaft of unspecified tibia

√6ᵗʰ **S82.29** Other fracture of shaft of tibia

√7ᵗʰ **S82.291** Other fracture of shaft of right tibia

√7ᵗʰ **S82.292** Other fracture of shaft of left tibia

√7ᵗʰ **S82.299** Other fracture of shaft of unspecified tibia

√5ᵗʰ **S82.3** Fracture of lower end of tibia

> **EXCLUDES 1**　bimalleolar fracture of lower leg (S82.84-)
> fracture of medial malleolus alone (S82.5-)
> Maisonneuve's fracture (S82.86-)
> pilon fracture of distal tibia (S82.87-)
> trimalleolar fractures of lower leg (S82.85-)

√6ᵗʰ **S82.30** Unspecified fracture of lower end of tibia

√7ᵗʰ **S82.301** Unspecified fracture of lower end of right tibia

√7ᵗʰ **S82.302** Unspecified fracture of lower end of left tibia

√7ᵗʰ **S82.309** Unspecified fracture of lower end of unspecified tibia

√6ᵗʰ **S82.31** Torus fracture of lower end of tibia

> The appropriate 7th character is to be added to all codes in subcategory S82.31.
> A　initial encounter for closed fracture
> D　subsequent encounter for fracture with routine healing
> G　subsequent encounter for fracture with delayed healing
> K　subsequent encounter for fracture with nonunion
> P　subsequent encounter for fracture with malunion
> S　sequela

√7ᵗʰ **S82.311** Torus fracture of lower end of right tibia

√7ᵗʰ **S82.312** Torus fracture of lower end of left tibia

EXCLUDES 1 Not coded here　　**EXCLUDES 2** Not included here　　Ⓝ Newborn Age: 0　　Ⓟ Pediatric Age: 0-17　　Ⓜ Maternity Age: 12-55　　Ⓐ Adult Age: 15-124

900　　　　ICD-10-CM Draft (2015)

√7ᵗʰ **S82.319** **Torus fracture of lower end of unspecified tibia**

√6ᵗʰ **S82.39** Other fracture of lower end of tibia

√7ᵗʰ **S82.391** Other fracture of lower end of right tibia

√7ᵗʰ **S82.392** Other fracture of lower end of left tibia

√7ᵗʰ **S82.399** **Other fracture of lower end of unspecified tibia**

√5ᵗʰ **S82.4** Fracture of shaft of fibula

> EXCLUDES 2   fracture of lateral malleolus alone (S82.6-)

√6ᵗʰ **S82.40** Unspecified fracture of shaft of fibula

√7ᵗʰ **S82.401** **Unspecified fracture of shaft of right fibula**

√7ᵗʰ **S82.402** **Unspecified fracture of shaft of left fibula**

√7ᵗʰ **S82.409** **Unspecified fracture of shaft of unspecified fibula**

√6ᵗʰ **S82.42** Transverse fracture of shaft of fibula

√7ᵗʰ **S82.421** Displaced transverse fracture of shaft of right fibula

√7ᵗʰ **S82.422** Displaced transverse fracture of shaft of left fibula

√7ᵗʰ **S82.423** Displaced transverse fracture of shaft of unspecified fibula

√7ᵗʰ **S82.424** Nondisplaced transverse fracture of shaft of right fibula

√7ᵗʰ **S82.425** Nondisplaced transverse fracture of shaft of left fibula

√7ᵗʰ **S82.426** Nondisplaced transverse fracture of shaft of unspecified fibula

√6ᵗʰ **S82.43** Oblique fracture of shaft of fibula

√7ᵗʰ **S82.431** Displaced oblique fracture of shaft of right fibula

√7ᵗʰ **S82.432** Displaced oblique fracture of shaft of left fibula

√7ᵗʰ **S82.433** Displaced oblique fracture of shaft of unspecified fibula

√7ᵗʰ **S82.434** Nondisplaced oblique fracture of shaft of right fibula

√7ᵗʰ **S82.435** Nondisplaced oblique fracture of shaft of left fibula

√7ᵗʰ **S82.436** Nondisplaced oblique fracture of shaft of unspecified fibula

√6ᵗʰ **S82.44** Spiral fracture of shaft of fibula

√7ᵗʰ **S82.441** Displaced spiral fracture of shaft of right fibula

√7ᵗʰ **S82.442** Displaced spiral fracture of shaft of left fibula

√7ᵗʰ **S82.443** Displaced spiral fracture of shaft of unspecified fibula

√7ᵗʰ **S82.444** Nondisplaced spiral fracture of shaft of right fibula

√7ᵗʰ **S82.445** Nondisplaced spiral fracture of shaft of left fibula

√7ᵗʰ **S82.446** Nondisplaced spiral fracture of shaft of unspecified fibula

√6ᵗʰ **S82.45** Comminuted fracture of shaft of fibula

√7ᵗʰ **S82.451** Displaced comminuted fracture of shaft of right fibula

√7ᵗʰ **S82.452** Displaced comminuted fracture of shaft of left fibula

√7ᵗʰ **S82.453** Displaced comminuted fracture of shaft of unspecified fibula

√7ᵗʰ **S82.454** Nondisplaced comminuted fracture of shaft of right fibula

√7ᵗʰ **S82.455** Nondisplaced comminuted fracture of shaft of left fibula

√7ᵗʰ **S82.456** Nondisplaced comminuted fracture of shaft of unspecified fibula

√6ᵗʰ **S82.46** Segmental fracture of shaft of fibula

√7ᵗʰ **S82.461** Displaced segmental fracture of shaft of right fibula

√7ᵗʰ **S82.462** Displaced segmental fracture of shaft of left fibula

√7ᵗʰ **S82.463** Displaced segmental fracture of shaft of unspecified fibula

√7ᵗʰ **S82.464** Nondisplaced segmental fracture of shaft of right fibula

√7ᵗʰ **S82.465** Nondisplaced segmental fracture of shaft of left fibula

√7ᵗʰ **S82.466** Nondisplaced segmental fracture of shaft of unspecified fibula

√6ᵗʰ **S82.49** Other fracture of shaft of fibula

√7ᵗʰ **S82.491** Other fracture of shaft of right fibula

√7ᵗʰ **S82.492** Other fracture of shaft of left fibula

√7ᵗʰ **S82.499** **Other fracture of shaft of unspecified fibula**

√5ᵗʰ **S82.5** Fracture of medial malleolus

> EXCLUDES 1   pilon fracture of distal tibia (S82.87-)
> Salter-Harris type III of lower end of tibia (S89.13-)
> Salter-Harris type IV of lower end of tibia (S89.14-)

√x7ᵗʰ **S82.51** Displaced fracture of medial malleolus of right tibia

√x7ᵗʰ **S82.52** Displaced fracture of medial malleolus of left tibia

√x7ᵗʰ **S82.53** Displaced fracture of medial malleolus of unspecified tibia

√x7ᵗʰ **S82.54** Nondisplaced fracture of medial malleolus of right tibia

√x7ᵗʰ **S82.55** Nondisplaced fracture of medial malleolus of left tibia

√x7ᵗʰ **S82.56** Nondisplaced fracture of medial malleolus of unspecified tibia

√5ᵗʰ **S82.6** Fracture of lateral malleolus

> EXCLUDES 1   pilon fracture of distal tibia (S82.87-)

√x7ᵗʰ **S82.61** Displaced fracture of lateral malleolus of right fibula

√x7ᵗʰ **S82.62** Displaced fracture of lateral malleolus of left fibula

√x7ᵗʰ **S82.63** Displaced fracture of lateral malleolus of unspecified fibula

√x7ᵗʰ **S82.64** Nondisplaced fracture of lateral malleolus of right fibula

√x7ᵗʰ **S82.65** Nondisplaced fracture of lateral malleolus of left fibula

√x7ᵗʰ **S82.66** Nondisplaced fracture of lateral malleolus of unspecified fibula

√5ᵗʰ **S82.8** Other fractures of lower leg

√6ᵗʰ **S82.81** Torus fracture of upper end of fibula

> The appropriate 7th character is to be added to all codes in subcategory S82.81.
> A   initial encounter for closed fracture
> D   subsequent encounter for fracture with routine healing
> G   subsequent encounter for fracture with delayed healing
> K   subsequent encounter for fracture with nonunion
> P   subsequent encounter for fracture with malunion
> S   sequela

√7ᵗʰ **S82.811** Torus fracture of upper end of right fibula

√7ᵗʰ **S82.812** Torus fracture of upper end of left fibula

√7ᵗʰ **S82.819** Torus fracture of upper end of unspecified fibula

√6ᵗʰ **S82.82** Torus fracture of lower end of fibula

> The appropriate 7th character is to be added to all codes in subcategory S82.82.
> A   initial encounter for closed fracture
> D   subsequent encounter for fracture with routine healing
> G   subsequent encounter for fracture with delayed healing
> K   subsequent encounter for fracture with nonunion
> P   subsequent encounter for fracture with malunion
> S   sequela

√7ᵗʰ **S82.821** Torus fracture of lower end of right fibula

√7ᵗʰ **S82.822** Torus fracture of lower end of left fibula

√7ᵗʰ **S82.829** **Torus fracture of lower end of unspecified fibula**

✔ Additional Character Required   √x7ᵗʰ Xtension Alert   Unspecified Dx   Other Specified Dx   Manifestation   ▶◀ Revised Text   ● New Code   ▲ Revised Code Title

ICD-10-CM Draft (2015)   901

Injury, Poisoning and Certain Other Consequences of External Causes   S82.83–S83.116

✓6th S82.83 Other fracture of upper and lower end of fibula

- **✓7th S82.831** Other fracture of upper and lower end of right fibula
- **✓7th S82.832** Other fracture of upper and lower end of left fibula
- **✓7th S82.839** Other fracture of upper and lower end of unspecified fibula

✓6th S82.84 Bimalleolar fracture of lower leg

- **✓7th S82.841** Displaced bimalleolar fracture of right lower leg
- **✓7th S82.842** Displaced bimalleolar fracture of left lower leg
- **✓7th S82.843** Displaced bimalleolar fracture of unspecified lower leg
- **✓7th S82.844** Nondisplaced bimalleolar fracture of right lower leg
- **✓7th S82.845** Nondisplaced bimalleolar fracture of left lower leg
- **✓7th S82.846** Nondisplaced bimalleolar fracture of unspecified lower leg

✓6th S82.85 Trimalleolar fracture of lower leg

- **✓7th S82.851** Displaced trimalleolar fracture of right lower leg
- **✓7th S82.852** Displaced trimalleolar fracture of left lower leg
- **✓7th S82.853** Displaced trimalleolar fracture of unspecified lower leg
- **✓7th S82.854** Nondisplaced trimalleolar fracture of right lower leg
- **✓7th S82.855** Nondisplaced trimalleolar fracture of left lower leg
- **✓7th S82.856** Nondisplaced trimalleolar fracture of unspecified lower leg

✓6th S82.86 Maisonneuve's fracture

- **✓7th S82.861** Displaced Maisonneuve's fracture of right leg
- **✓7th S82.862** Displaced Maisonneuve's fracture of left leg
- **✓7th S82.863** Displaced Maisonneuve's fracture of unspecified leg
- **✓7th S82.864** Nondisplaced Maisonneuve's fracture of right leg
- **✓7th S82.865** Nondisplaced Maisonneuve's fracture of left leg
- **✓7th S82.866** Nondisplaced Maisonneuve's fracture of unspecified leg

✓6th S82.87 Pilon fracture of tibia

- **✓7th S82.871** Displaced pilon fracture of right tibia
- **✓7th S82.872** Displaced pilon fracture of left tibia
- **✓7th S82.873** Displaced pilon fracture of unspecified tibia
- **✓7th S82.874** Nondisplaced pilon fracture of right tibia
- **✓7th S82.875** Nondisplaced pilon fracture of left tibia
- **✓7th S82.876** Nondisplaced pilon fracture of unspecified tibia

✓6th S82.89 Other fractures of lower leg

Fracture of ankle NOS

- **✓7th S82.891** Other fracture of right lower leg
- **✓7th S82.892** Other fracture of left lower leg
- **✓7th S82.899** Other fracture of unspecified lower leg

✓5th S82.9 Unspecified fracture of lower leg

- **✓x 7th S82.90** Unspecified fracture of unspecified lower leg
- **✓x 7th S82.91** Unspecified fracture of right lower leg
- **✓x 7th S82.92** Unspecified fracture of left lower leg

✓4th S83 Dislocation and sprain of joints and ligaments of knee

INCLUDES
- avulsion of joint or ligament of knee
- laceration of cartilage, joint or ligament of knee
- sprain of cartilage, joint or ligament of knee
- traumatic hemarthrosis of joint or ligament of knee
- traumatic rupture of joint or ligament of knee
- traumatic subluxation of joint or ligament of knee
- traumatic tear of joint or ligament of knee

Code also any associated open wound

EXCLUDES 1
- derangement of patella (M22.0-M22.3)
- injury of patellar ligament (tendon) (S76.1-)
- internal derangement of knee (M23.-)
- old dislocation of knee (M24.36)
- pathological dislocation of knee (M24.36)
- recurrent dislocation of knee (M22.0)

EXCLUDES 2 strain of muscle, fascia and tendon of lower leg (S86.-)

The appropriate 7th character is to be added to each code from category S83.

- A   initial encounter
- D   subsequent encounter
- S   sequela

✓5th S83.0 Subluxation and dislocation of patella

✓6th S83.00 Unspecified subluxation and dislocation of patella

- **✓7th S83.001** Unspecified subluxation of right patella
- **✓7th S83.002** Unspecified subluxation of left patella
- **✓7th S83.003** Unspecified subluxation of unspecified patella
- **✓7th S83.004** Unspecified dislocation of right patella
- **✓7th S83.005** Unspecified dislocation of left patella
- **✓7th S83.006** Unspecified dislocation of unspecified patella

✓6th S83.01 Lateral subluxation and dislocation of patella

- **✓7th S83.011** Lateral subluxation of right patella
- **✓7th S83.012** Lateral subluxation of left patella
- **✓7th S83.013** Lateral subluxation of unspecified patella
- **✓7th S83.014** Lateral dislocation of right patella
- **✓7th S83.015** Lateral dislocation of left patella
- **✓7th S83.016** Lateral dislocation of unspecified patella

✓6th S83.09 Other subluxation and dislocation of patella

- **✓7th S83.091** Other subluxation of right patella
- **✓7th S83.092** Other subluxation of left patella
- **✓7th S83.093** Other subluxation of unspecified patella
- **✓7th S83.094** Other dislocation of right patella
- **✓7th S83.095** Other dislocation of left patella
- **✓7th S83.096** Other dislocation of unspecified patella

✓5th S83.1 Subluxation and dislocation of knee

EXCLUDES 2 instability of knee prosthesis (T84.022, T84.023)

✓6th S83.10 Unspecified subluxation and dislocation of knee

- **✓7th S83.101** Unspecified subluxation of right knee
- **✓7th S83.102** Unspecified subluxation of left knee
- **✓7th S83.103** Unspecified subluxation of unspecified knee
- **✓7th S83.104** Unspecified dislocation of right knee
- **✓7th S83.105** Unspecified dislocation of left knee
- **✓7th S83.106** Unspecified dislocation of unspecified knee

✓6th S83.11 Anterior subluxation and dislocation of proximal end of tibia

Posterior subluxation and dislocation of distal end of femur

- **✓7th S83.111** Anterior subluxation of proximal end of tibia, right knee
- **✓7th S83.112** Anterior subluxation of proximal end of tibia, left knee
- **✓7th S83.113** Anterior subluxation of proximal end of tibia, unspecified knee
- **✓7th S83.114** Anterior dislocation of proximal end of tibia, right knee
- **✓7th S83.115** Anterior dislocation of proximal end of tibia, left knee
- **✓7th S83.116** Anterior dislocation of proximal end of tibia, unspecified knee

EXCLUDES 1 Not coded here   **EXCLUDES 2** Not included here   **N** Newborn Age: 0   **P** Pediatric Age: 0-17   **M** Maternity Age: 12-55   **A** Adult Age: 15-124

902   ICD-10-CM Draft (2015)

√6ᵗʰ **S83.12** Posterior subluxation and dislocation of proximal end of tibia
Anterior dislocation of distal end of femur

√7ᵗʰ **S83.121** Posterior subluxation of proximal end of tibia, right knee

√7ᵗʰ **S83.122** Posterior subluxation of proximal end of tibia, left knee

√7ᵗʰ **S83.123** Posterior subluxation of proximal end of tibia, unspecified knee

√7ᵗʰ **S83.124** Posterior dislocation of proximal end of tibia, right knee

√7ᵗʰ **S83.125** Posterior dislocation of proximal end of tibia, left knee

√7ᵗʰ **S83.126** Posterior dislocation of proximal end of tibia, unspecified knee

√6ᵗʰ **S83.13** Medial subluxation and dislocation of proximal end of tibia

√7ᵗʰ **S83.131** Medial subluxation of proximal end of tibia, right knee

√7ᵗʰ **S83.132** Medial subluxation of proximal end of tibia, left knee

√7ᵗʰ **S83.133** Medial subluxation of proximal end of tibia, unspecified knee

√7ᵗʰ **S83.134** Medial dislocation of proximal end of tibia, right knee

√7ᵗʰ **S83.135** Medial dislocation of proximal end of tibia, left knee

√7ᵗʰ **S83.136** Medial dislocation of proximal end of tibia, unspecified knee

√6ᵗʰ **S83.14** Lateral subluxation and dislocation of proximal end of tibia

√7ᵗʰ **S83.141** Lateral subluxation of proximal end of tibia, right knee

√7ᵗʰ **S83.142** Lateral subluxation of proximal end of tibia, left knee

√7ᵗʰ **S83.143** Lateral subluxation of proximal end of tibia, unspecified knee

√7ᵗʰ **S83.144** Lateral dislocation of proximal end of tibia, right knee

√7ᵗʰ **S83.145** Lateral dislocation of proximal end of tibia, left knee

√7ᵗʰ **S83.146** Lateral dislocation of proximal end of tibia, unspecified knee

√6ᵗʰ **S83.19** Other subluxation and dislocation of knee

√7ᵗʰ **S83.191** Other subluxation of right knee

√7ᵗʰ **S83.192** Other subluxation of left knee

√7ᵗʰ **S83.193** Other subluxation of unspecified knee

√7ᵗʰ **S83.194** Other dislocation of right knee

√7ᵗʰ **S83.195** Other dislocation of left knee

√7ᵗʰ **S83.196** Other dislocation of unspecified knee

√5ᵗʰ **S83.2** Tear of meniscus, current injury
EXCLUDES 1 old bucket-handle tear (M23.2)

√6ᵗʰ **S83.20** Tear of unspecified meniscus, current injury
Tear of meniscus of knee NOS

√7ᵗʰ **S83.200** Bucket-handle tear of unspecified meniscus, current injury, right knee

√7ᵗʰ **S83.201** Bucket-handle tear of unspecified meniscus, current injury, left knee

√7ᵗʰ **S83.202** Bucket-handle tear of unspecified meniscus, current injury, unspecified knee

√7ᵗʰ **S83.203** Other tear of unspecified meniscus, current injury, right knee

√7ᵗʰ **S83.204** Other tear of unspecified meniscus, current injury, left knee

√7ᵗʰ **S83.205** Other tear of unspecified meniscus, current injury, unspecified knee

√7ᵗʰ **S83.206** Unspecified tear of unspecified meniscus, current injury, right knee

√7ᵗʰ **S83.207** Unspecified tear of unspecified meniscus, current injury, left knee

√7ᵗʰ **S83.209** Unspecified tear of unspecified meniscus, current injury, unspecified knee

√6ᵗʰ **S83.21** Bucket-handle tear of medial meniscus, current injury

√7ᵗʰ **S83.211** Bucket-handle tear of medial meniscus, current injury, right knee

√7ᵗʰ **S83.212** Bucket-handle tear of medial meniscus, current injury, left knee

√7ᵗʰ **S83.219** Bucket-handle tear of medial meniscus, current injury, unspecified knee

√6ᵗʰ **S83.22** Peripheral tear of medial meniscus, current injury

√7ᵗʰ **S83.221** Peripheral tear of medial meniscus, current injury, right knee

√7ᵗʰ **S83.222** Peripheral tear of medial meniscus, current injury, left knee

√7ᵗʰ **S83.229** Peripheral tear of medial meniscus, current injury, unspecified knee

√6ᵗʰ **S83.23** Complex tear of medial meniscus, current injury

√7ᵗʰ **S83.231** Complex tear of medial meniscus, current injury, right knee

√7ᵗʰ **S83.232** Complex tear of medial meniscus, current injury, left knee

√7ᵗʰ **S83.239** Complex tear of medial meniscus, current injury, unspecified knee

√6ᵗʰ **S83.24** Other tear of medial meniscus, current injury

√7ᵗʰ **S83.241** Other tear of medial meniscus, current injury, right knee

√7ᵗʰ **S83.242** Other tear of medial meniscus, current injury, left knee

√7ᵗʰ **S83.249** Other tear of medial meniscus, current injury, unspecified knee

√6ᵗʰ **S83.25** Bucket-handle tear of lateral meniscus, current injury

√7ᵗʰ **S83.251** Bucket-handle tear of lateral meniscus, current injury, right knee

√7ᵗʰ **S83.252** Bucket-handle tear of lateral meniscus, current injury, left knee

√7ᵗʰ **S83.259** Bucket-handle tear of lateral meniscus, current injury, unspecified knee

√6ᵗʰ **S83.26** Peripheral tear of lateral meniscus, current injury

√7ᵗʰ **S83.261** Peripheral tear of lateral meniscus, current injury, right knee

√7ᵗʰ **S83.262** Peripheral tear of lateral meniscus, current injury, left knee

√7ᵗʰ **S83.269** Peripheral tear of lateral meniscus, current injury, unspecified knee

√6ᵗʰ **S83.27** Complex tear of lateral meniscus, current injury

√7ᵗʰ **S83.271** Complex tear of lateral meniscus, current injury, right knee

√7ᵗʰ **S83.272** Complex tear of lateral meniscus, current injury, left knee

√7ᵗʰ **S83.279** Complex tear of lateral meniscus, current injury, unspecified knee

√6ᵗʰ **S83.28** Other tear of lateral meniscus, current injury

√7ᵗʰ **S83.281** Other tear of lateral meniscus, current injury, right knee

√7ᵗʰ **S83.282** Other tear of lateral meniscus, current injury, left knee

√7ᵗʰ **S83.289** Other tear of lateral meniscus, current injury, unspecified knee

√5ᵗʰ **S83.3** Tear of articular cartilage of knee, current

√x7ᵗʰ **S83.30** Tear of articular cartilage of unspecified knee, current

√x7ᵗʰ **S83.31** Tear of articular cartilage of right knee, current

√x7ᵗʰ **S83.32** Tear of articular cartilage of left knee, current

√5ᵗʰ **S83.4** Sprain of collateral ligament of knee

√6ᵗʰ **S83.40** Sprain of unspecified collateral ligament of knee

√7ᵗʰ **S83.401** Sprain of unspecified collateral ligament of right knee

√7ᵗʰ **S83.402** Sprain of unspecified collateral ligament of left knee

√7ᵗʰ **S83.409** Sprain of unspecified collateral ligament of unspecified knee

Injury, Poisoning and Certain Other Consequences of External Causes

S83.41–S85.122

✓6th S83.41 Sprain of medial collateral ligament of knee
Sprain of tibial collateral ligament
- ✓7th **S83.411** Sprain of medial collateral ligament of right knee
- ✓7th **S83.412** Sprain of medial collateral ligament of left knee
- ✓7th **S83.419** Sprain of medial collateral ligament of unspecified knee

✓6th S83.42 Sprain of lateral collateral ligament of knee
Sprain of fibular collateral ligament
- ✓7th **S83.421** Sprain of lateral collateral ligament of right knee
- ✓7th **S83.422** Sprain of lateral collateral ligament of left knee
- ✓7th **S83.429** Sprain of lateral collateral ligament of unspecified knee

✓5th S83.5 Sprain of cruciate ligament of knee
- **✓6th S83.50 Sprain of unspecified cruciate ligament of knee**
  - ✓7th **S83.501** Sprain of unspecified cruciate ligament of right knee
  - ✓7th **S83.502** Sprain of unspecified cruciate ligament of left knee
  - ✓7th **S83.509** Sprain of unspecified cruciate ligament of unspecified knee
- **✓6th S83.51 Sprain of anterior cruciate ligament of knee**
  - ✓7th **S83.511** Sprain of anterior cruciate ligament of right knee
  - ✓7th **S83.512** Sprain of anterior cruciate ligament of left knee
  - ✓7th **S83.519** Sprain of anterior cruciate ligament of unspecified knee
- **✓6th S83.52 Sprain of posterior cruciate ligament of knee**
  - ✓7th **S83.521** Sprain of posterior cruciate ligament of right knee
  - ✓7th **S83.522** Sprain of posterior cruciate ligament of left knee
  - ✓7th **S83.529** Sprain of posterior cruciate ligament of unspecified knee

✓5th S83.6 Sprain of the superior tibiofibular joint and ligament
- ✓x7th **S83.60** Sprain of the superior tibiofibular joint and ligament, unspecified knee
- ✓x7th **S83.61** Sprain of the superior tibiofibular joint and ligament, right knee
- ✓x7th **S83.62** Sprain of the superior tibiofibular joint and ligament, left knee

✓5th S83.8 Sprain of other specified parts of knee
- **✓6th S83.8X Sprain of other specified parts of knee**
  - ✓7th **S83.8X1** Sprain of other specified parts of right knee
  - ✓7th **S83.8X2** Sprain of other specified parts of left knee
  - ✓7th **S83.8X9** Sprain of other specified parts of unspecified knee

✓5th S83.9 Sprain of unspecified site of knee
- ✓x7th **S83.90** Sprain of unspecified site of unspecified knee
- ✓x7th **S83.91** Sprain of unspecified site of right knee
- ✓x7th **S83.92** Sprain of unspecified site of left knee

✓4th S84 Injury of nerves at lower leg level
Code also any associated open wound (S81.-)
EXCLUDES 2 injury of nerves at ankle and foot level (S94.-)

The appropriate 7th character is to be added to each code from category S84.
A   initial encounter
D   subsequent encounter
S   sequela

✓5th S84.0 Injury of tibial nerve at lower leg level
- ✓x7th **S84.00** Injury of tibial nerve at lower leg level, unspecified leg
- ✓x7th **S84.01** Injury of tibial nerve at lower leg level, right leg
- ✓x7th **S84.02** Injury of tibial nerve at lower leg level, left leg

✓5th S84.1 Injury of peroneal nerve at lower leg level
- ✓x7th **S84.10** Injury of peroneal nerve at lower leg level, unspecified leg

- ✓x7th **S84.11** Injury of peroneal nerve at lower leg level, right leg
- ✓x7th **S84.12** Injury of peroneal nerve at lower leg level, left leg

✓5th S84.2 Injury of cutaneous sensory nerve at lower leg level
- ✓x7th **S84.20** Injury of cutaneous sensory nerve at lower leg level, unspecified leg
- ✓x7th **S84.21** Injury of cutaneous sensory nerve at lower leg level, right leg
- ✓x7th **S84.22** Injury of cutaneous sensory nerve at lower leg level, left leg

✓5th S84.8 Injury of other nerves at lower leg level
- **✓6th S84.80 Injury of other nerves at lower leg level**
  - ✓7th **S84.801** Injury of other nerves at lower leg level, right leg
  - ✓7th **S84.802** Injury of other nerves at lower leg level, left leg
  - ✓7th **S84.809** Injury of other nerves at lower leg level, unspecified leg

✓5th S84.9 Injury of unspecified nerve at lower leg level
- ✓x7th **S84.90** Injury of unspecified nerve at lower leg level, unspecified leg
- ✓x7th **S84.91** Injury of unspecified nerve at lower leg level, right leg
- ✓x7th **S84.92** Injury of unspecified nerve at lower leg level, left leg

✓4th S85 Injury of blood vessels at lower leg level
Code also any associated open wound (S81.-)
EXCLUDES 2 injury of blood vessels at ankle and foot level (S95.-)

The appropriate 7th character is to be added to each code from category S85.
A   initial encounter
D   subsequent encounter
S   sequela

✓5th S85.0 Injury of popliteal artery
- **✓6th S85.00 Unspecified injury of popliteal artery**
  - ✓7th **S85.001** Unspecified injury of popliteal artery, right leg
  - ✓7th **S85.002** Unspecified injury of popliteal artery, left leg
  - ✓7th **S85.009** Unspecified injury of popliteal artery, unspecified leg
- **✓6th S85.01 Laceration of popliteal artery**
  - ✓7th **S85.011** Laceration of popliteal artery, right leg
  - ✓7th **S85.012** Laceration of popliteal artery, left leg
  - ✓7th **S85.019** Laceration of popliteal artery, unspecified leg
- **✓6th S85.09 Other specified injury of popliteal artery**
  - ✓7th **S85.091** Other specified injury of popliteal artery, right leg
  - ✓7th **S85.092** Other specified injury of popliteal artery, left leg
  - ✓7th **S85.099** Other specified injury of popliteal artery, unspecified leg

✓5th S85.1 Injury of tibial artery
- **✓6th S85.10 Unspecified injury of unspecified tibial artery**
  Injury of tibial artery NOS
  - ✓7th **S85.101** Unspecified injury of unspecified tibial artery, right leg
  - ✓7th **S85.102** Unspecified injury of unspecified tibial artery, left leg
  - ✓7th **S85.109** Unspecified injury of unspecified tibial artery, unspecified leg
- **✓6th S85.11 Laceration of unspecified tibial artery**
  - ✓7th **S85.111** Laceration of unspecified tibial artery, right leg
  - ✓7th **S85.112** Laceration of unspecified tibial artery, left leg
  - ✓7th **S85.119** Laceration of unspecified tibial artery, unspecified leg
- **✓6th S85.12 Other specified injury of unspecified tibial artery**
  - ✓7th **S85.121** Other specified injury of unspecified tibial artery, right leg
  - ✓7th **S85.122** Other specified injury of unspecified tibial artery, left leg

EXCLUDES 1 Not coded here   *EXCLUDES 2* Not included here   **N** Newborn Age: 0   **P** Pediatric Age: 0-17   **M** Maternity Age: 12-55   **A** Adult Age: 15-124

904   ICD-10-CM Draft (2015)

✓7ᵗʰ **S85.129** Other specified injury of unspecified tibial artery, unspecified leg

✓6ᵗʰ **S85.13** Unspecified injury of anterior tibial artery

  ✓7ᵗʰ **S85.131** Unspecified injury of anterior tibial artery, right leg

  ✓7ᵗʰ **S85.132** Unspecified injury of anterior tibial artery, left leg

  ✓7ᵗʰ **S85.139** Unspecified injury of anterior tibial artery, unspecified leg

✓6ᵗʰ **S85.14** Laceration of anterior tibial artery

  ✓7ᵗʰ **S85.141** Laceration of anterior tibial artery, right leg

  ✓7ᵗʰ **S85.142** Laceration of anterior tibial artery, left leg

  ✓7ᵗʰ **S85.149** Laceration of anterior tibial artery, unspecified leg

✓6ᵗʰ **S85.15** Other specified injury of anterior tibial artery

  ✓7ᵗʰ **S85.151** Other specified injury of anterior tibial artery, right leg

  ✓7ᵗʰ **S85.152** Other specified injury of anterior tibial artery, left leg

  ✓7ᵗʰ **S85.159** Other specified injury of anterior tibial artery, unspecified leg

✓6ᵗʰ **S85.16** Unspecified injury of posterior tibial artery

  ✓7ᵗʰ **S85.161** Unspecified injury of posterior tibial artery, right leg

  ✓7ᵗʰ **S85.162** Unspecified injury of posterior tibial artery, left leg

  ✓7ᵗʰ **S85.169** Unspecified injury of posterior tibial artery, unspecified leg

✓6ᵗʰ **S85.17** Laceration of posterior tibial artery

  ✓7ᵗʰ **S85.171** Laceration of posterior tibial artery, right leg

  ✓7ᵗʰ **S85.172** Laceration of posterior tibial artery, left leg

  ✓7ᵗʰ **S85.179** Laceration of posterior tibial artery, unspecified leg

✓6ᵗʰ **S85.18** Other specified injury of posterior tibial artery

  ✓7ᵗʰ **S85.181** Other specified injury of posterior tibial artery, right leg

  ✓7ᵗʰ **S85.182** Other specified injury of posterior tibial artery, left leg

  ✓7ᵗʰ **S85.189** Other specified injury of posterior tibial artery, unspecified leg

✓5ᵗʰ **S85.2** Injury of peroneal artery

✓6ᵗʰ **S85.20** Unspecified injury of peroneal artery

  ✓7ᵗʰ **S85.201** Unspecified injury of peroneal artery, right leg

  ✓7ᵗʰ **S85.202** Unspecified injury of peroneal artery, left leg

  ✓7ᵗʰ **S85.209** Unspecified injury of peroneal artery, unspecified leg

✓6ᵗʰ **S85.21** Laceration of peroneal artery

  ✓7ᵗʰ **S85.211** Laceration of peroneal artery, right leg

  ✓7ᵗʰ **S85.212** Laceration of peroneal artery, left leg

  ✓7ᵗʰ **S85.219** Laceration of peroneal artery, unspecified leg

✓6ᵗʰ **S85.29** Other specified injury of peroneal artery

  ✓7ᵗʰ **S85.291** Other specified injury of peroneal artery, right leg

  ✓7ᵗʰ **S85.292** Other specified injury of peroneal artery, left leg

  ✓7ᵗʰ **S85.299** Other specified injury of peroneal artery, unspecified leg

✓5ᵗʰ **S85.3** Injury of greater saphenous vein at lower leg level
Injury of greater saphenous vein NOS
Injury of saphenous vein NOS

✓6ᵗʰ **S85.30** Unspecified injury of greater saphenous vein at lower leg level

  ✓7ᵗʰ **S85.301** Unspecified injury of greater saphenous vein at lower leg level, right leg

  ✓7ᵗʰ **S85.302** Unspecified injury of greater saphenous vein at lower leg level, left leg

  ✓7ᵗʰ **S85.309** Unspecified injury of greater saphenous vein at lower leg level, unspecified leg

✓6ᵗʰ **S85.31** Laceration of greater saphenous vein at lower leg level

  ✓7ᵗʰ **S85.311** Laceration of greater saphenous vein at lower leg level, right leg

  ✓7ᵗʰ **S85.312** Laceration of greater saphenous vein at lower leg level, left leg

  ✓7ᵗʰ **S85.319** Laceration of greater saphenous vein at lower leg level, unspecified leg

✓6ᵗʰ **S85.39** Other specified injury of greater saphenous vein at lower leg level

  ✓7ᵗʰ **S85.391** Other specified injury of greater saphenous vein at lower leg level, right leg

  ✓7ᵗʰ **S85.392** Other specified injury of greater saphenous vein at lower leg level, left leg

  ✓7ᵗʰ **S85.399** Other specified injury of greater saphenous vein at lower leg level, unspecified leg

✓5ᵗʰ **S85.4** Injury of lesser saphenous vein at lower leg level

✓6ᵗʰ **S85.40** Unspecified injury of lesser saphenous vein at lower leg level

  ✓7ᵗʰ **S85.401** Unspecified injury of lesser saphenous vein at lower leg level, right leg

  ✓7ᵗʰ **S85.402** Unspecified injury of lesser saphenous vein at lower leg level, left leg

  ✓7ᵗʰ **S85.409** Unspecified injury of lesser saphenous vein at lower leg level, unspecified leg

✓6ᵗʰ **S85.41** Laceration of lesser saphenous vein at lower leg level

  ✓7ᵗʰ **S85.411** Laceration of lesser saphenous vein at lower leg level, right leg

  ✓7ᵗʰ **S85.412** Laceration of lesser saphenous vein at lower leg level, left leg

  ✓7ᵗʰ **S85.419** Laceration of lesser saphenous vein at lower leg level, unspecified leg

✓6ᵗʰ **S85.49** Other specified injury of lesser saphenous vein at lower leg level

  ✓7ᵗʰ **S85.491** Other specified injury of lesser saphenous vein at lower leg level, right leg

  ✓7ᵗʰ **S85.492** Other specified injury of lesser saphenous vein at lower leg level, left leg

  ✓7ᵗʰ **S85.499** Other specified injury of lesser saphenous vein at lower leg level, unspecified leg

✓5ᵗʰ **S85.5** Injury of popliteal vein

✓6ᵗʰ **S85.50** Unspecified injury of popliteal vein

  ✓7ᵗʰ **S85.501** Unspecified injury of popliteal vein, right leg

  ✓7ᵗʰ **S85.502** Unspecified injury of popliteal vein, left leg

  ✓7ᵗʰ **S85.509** Unspecified injury of popliteal vein, unspecified leg

✓6ᵗʰ **S85.51** Laceration of popliteal vein

  ✓7ᵗʰ **S85.511** Laceration of popliteal vein, right leg

  ✓7ᵗʰ **S85.512** Laceration of popliteal vein, left leg

  ✓7ᵗʰ **S85.519** Laceration of popliteal vein, unspecified leg

✓6ᵗʰ **S85.59** Other specified injury of popliteal vein

  ✓7ᵗʰ **S85.591** Other specified injury of popliteal vein, right leg

  ✓7ᵗʰ **S85.592** Other specified injury of popliteal vein, left leg

  ✓7ᵗʰ **S85.599** Other specified injury of popliteal vein, unspecified leg

✓5ᵗʰ **S85.8** Injury of other blood vessels at lower leg level

✓6ᵗʰ **S85.80** Unspecified injury of other blood vessels at lower leg level

  ✓7ᵗʰ **S85.801** Unspecified injury of other blood vessels at lower leg level, right leg

  ✓7ᵗʰ **S85.802** Unspecified injury of other blood vessels at lower leg level, left leg

  ✓7ᵗʰ **S85.809** Unspecified injury of other blood vessels at lower leg level, unspecified leg

---

✓ Additional Character Required　　✓ˣ⁷ᵗʰ Xtension Alert　　Unspecified Dx　　Other Specified Dx　　Manifestation　　▶◀ Revised Text　　● New Code　　▲ Revised Code Title

Injury, Poisoning and Certain Other Consequences of External Causes

S85.81–S86.222

✓6ᵗʰ **S85.81** Laceration of other blood vessels at lower leg level

     ✓7ᵗʰ **S85.811** **Laceration of other blood vessels at lower leg level, right leg**

     ✓7ᵗʰ **S85.812** **Laceration of other blood vessels at lower leg level, left leg**

     ✓7ᵗʰ **S85.819** **Laceration of other blood vessels at lower leg level, unspecified leg**

✓6ᵗʰ **S85.89** Other specified injury of other blood vessels at lower leg level

     ✓7ᵗʰ **S85.891** **Other specified injury of other blood vessels at lower leg level, right leg**

     ✓7ᵗʰ **S85.892** **Other specified injury of other blood vessels at lower leg level, left leg**

     ✓7ᵗʰ **S85.899** **Other specified injury of other blood vessels at lower leg level, unspecified leg**

✓5ᵗʰ **S85.9** Injury of unspecified blood vessel at lower leg level

     ✓6ᵗʰ **S85.90** Unspecified injury of unspecified blood vessel at lower leg level

         ✓7ᵗʰ **S85.901** **Unspecified injury of unspecified blood vessel at lower leg level, right leg**

         ✓7ᵗʰ **S85.902** **Unspecified injury of unspecified blood vessel at lower leg level, left leg**

         ✓7ᵗʰ **S85.909** **Unspecified injury of unspecified blood vessel at lower leg level, unspecified leg**

     ✓6ᵗʰ **S85.91** Laceration of unspecified blood vessel at lower leg level

         ✓7ᵗʰ **S85.911** **Laceration of unspecified blood vessel at lower leg level, right leg**

         ✓7ᵗʰ **S85.912** **Laceration of unspecified blood vessel at lower leg level, left leg**

         ✓7ᵗʰ **S85.919** **Laceration of unspecified blood vessel at lower leg level, unspecified leg**

     ✓6ᵗʰ **S85.99** Other specified injury of unspecified blood vessel at lower leg level

         ✓7ᵗʰ **S85.991** **Other specified injury of unspecified blood vessel at lower leg level, right leg**

         ✓7ᵗʰ **S85.992** **Other specified injury of unspecified blood vessel at lower leg level, left leg**

         ✓7ᵗʰ **S85.999** **Other specified injury of unspecified blood vessel at lower leg level, unspecified leg**

✓4ᵗʰ **S86** **Injury of muscle, fascia and tendon at lower leg level**

     Code also any associated open wound (S81.-)

     EXCLUDES 2   injury of muscle, fascia and tendon at ankle (S96.-)
            injury of patellar ligament (tendon) (S76.1-)
            sprain of joints and ligaments of knee (S83.-)

     The appropriate 7th character is to be added to each code from category S86.
     A   initial encounter
     D   subsequent encounter
     S   sequela

     ✓5ᵗʰ **S86.0** Injury of Achilles tendon

         ✓6ᵗʰ **S86.00** Unspecified injury of Achilles tendon

            ✓7ᵗʰ **S86.001** **Unspecified injury of right Achilles tendon**

            ✓7ᵗʰ **S86.002** **Unspecified injury of left Achilles tendon**

            ✓7ᵗʰ **S86.009** **Unspecified injury of unspecified Achilles tendon**

         ✓6ᵗʰ **S86.01** Strain of Achilles tendon

            ✓7ᵗʰ **S86.011** **Strain of right Achilles tendon**

            ✓7ᵗʰ **S86.012** **Strain of left Achilles tendon**

            ✓7ᵗʰ **S86.019** **Strain of unspecified Achilles tendon**

         ✓6ᵗʰ **S86.02** Laceration of Achilles tendon

            ✓7ᵗʰ **S86.021** **Laceration of right Achilles tendon**

            ✓7ᵗʰ **S86.022** **Laceration of left Achilles tendon**

            ✓7ᵗʰ **S86.029** **Laceration of unspecified Achilles tendon**

         ✓6ᵗʰ **S86.09** Other specified injury of Achilles tendon

            ✓7ᵗʰ **S86.091** **Other specified injury of right Achilles tendon**

            ✓7ᵗʰ **S86.092** **Other specified injury of left Achilles tendon**

            ✓7ᵗʰ **S86.099** **Other specified injury of unspecified Achilles tendon**

✓5ᵗʰ **S86.1** Injury of other muscle(s) and tendon(s) of posterior muscle group at lower leg level

     ✓6ᵗʰ **S86.10** Unspecified injury of other muscle(s) and tendon(s) of posterior muscle group at lower leg level

         ✓7ᵗʰ **S86.101** **Unspecified injury of other muscle(s) and tendon(s) of posterior muscle group at lower leg level, right leg**

         ✓7ᵗʰ **S86.102** **Unspecified injury of other muscle(s) and tendon(s) of posterior muscle group at lower leg level, left leg**

         ✓7ᵗʰ **S86.109** **Unspecified injury of other muscle(s) and tendon(s) of posterior muscle group at lower leg level, unspecified leg**

     ✓6ᵗʰ **S86.11** Strain of other muscle(s) and tendon(s) of posterior muscle group at lower leg level

         ✓7ᵗʰ **S86.111** **Strain of other muscle(s) and tendon(s) of posterior muscle group at lower leg level, right leg**

         ✓7ᵗʰ **S86.112** **Strain of other muscle(s) and tendon(s) of posterior muscle group at lower leg level, left leg**

         ✓7ᵗʰ **S86.119** **Strain of other muscle(s) and tendon(s) of posterior muscle group at lower leg level, unspecified leg**

     ✓6ᵗʰ **S86.12** Laceration of other muscle(s) and tendon(s) of posterior muscle group at lower leg level

         ✓7ᵗʰ **S86.121** **Laceration of other muscle(s) and tendon(s) of posterior muscle group at lower leg level, right leg**

         ✓7ᵗʰ **S86.122** **Laceration of other muscle(s) and tendon(s) of posterior muscle group at lower leg level, left leg**

         ✓7ᵗʰ **S86.129** **Laceration of other muscle(s) and tendon(s) of posterior muscle group at lower leg level, unspecified leg**

     ✓6ᵗʰ **S86.19** Other injury of other muscle(s) and tendon(s) of posterior muscle group at lower leg level

         ✓7ᵗʰ **S86.191** **Other injury of other muscle(s) and tendon(s) of posterior muscle group at lower leg level, right leg**

         ✓7ᵗʰ **S86.192** **Other injury of other muscle(s) and tendon(s) of posterior muscle group at lower leg level, left leg**

         ✓7ᵗʰ **S86.199** **Other injury of other muscle(s) and tendon(s) of posterior muscle group at lower leg level, unspecified leg**

✓5ᵗʰ **S86.2** Injury of muscle(s) and tendon(s) of anterior muscle group at lower leg level

     ✓6ᵗʰ **S86.20** Unspecified injury of muscle(s) and tendon(s) of anterior muscle group at lower leg level

         ✓7ᵗʰ **S86.201** **Unspecified injury of muscle(s) and tendon(s) of anterior muscle group at lower leg level, right leg**

         ✓7ᵗʰ **S86.202** **Unspecified injury of muscle(s) and tendon(s) of anterior muscle group at lower leg level, left leg**

         ✓7ᵗʰ **S86.209** **Unspecified injury of muscle(s) and tendon(s) of anterior muscle group at lower leg level, unspecified leg**

     ✓6ᵗʰ **S86.21** Strain of muscle(s) and tendon(s) of anterior muscle group at lower leg level

         ✓7ᵗʰ **S86.211** **Strain of muscle(s) and tendon(s) of anterior muscle group at lower leg level, right leg**

         ✓7ᵗʰ **S86.212** **Strain of muscle(s) and tendon(s) of anterior muscle group at lower leg level, left leg**

         ✓7ᵗʰ **S86.219** **Strain of muscle(s) and tendon(s) of anterior muscle group at lower leg level, unspecified leg**

     ✓6ᵗʰ **S86.22** Laceration of muscle(s) and tendon(s) of anterior muscle group at lower leg level

         ✓7ᵗʰ **S86.221** **Laceration of muscle(s) and tendon(s) of anterior muscle group at lower leg level, right leg**

         ✓7ᵗʰ **S86.222** **Laceration of muscle(s) and tendon(s) of anterior muscle group at lower leg level, left leg**

EXCLUDES 1 Not coded here   *EXCLUDES 2* Not included here   N Newborn Age: 0   P Pediatric Age: 0-17   M Maternity Age: 12-55   A Adult Age: 15-124

906   ICD-10-CM Draft (2015)

☑7ᵗʰ **S86.229** Laceration of muscle(s) and tendon(s) of anterior muscle group at lower leg level, unspecified leg

☑6ᵗʰ **S86.29** Other injury of muscle(s) and tendon(s) of anterior muscle group at lower leg level

    ☑7ᵗʰ **S86.291** Other injury of muscle(s) and tendon(s) of anterior muscle group at lower leg level, right leg

    ☑7ᵗʰ **S86.292** Other injury of muscle(s) and tendon(s) of anterior muscle group at lower leg level, left leg

    ☑7ᵗʰ **S86.299** Other injury of muscle(s) and tendon(s) of anterior muscle group at lower leg level, unspecified leg

☑5ᵗʰ **S86.3** Injury of muscle(s) and tendon(s) of peroneal muscle group at lower leg level

   ☑6ᵗʰ **S86.30** Unspecified injury of muscle(s) and tendon(s) of peroneal muscle group at lower leg level

    ☑7ᵗʰ **S86.301** Unspecified injury of muscle(s) and tendon(s) of peroneal muscle group at lower leg level, right leg

    ☑7ᵗʰ **S86.302** Unspecified injury of muscle(s) and tendon(s) of peroneal muscle group at lower leg level, left leg

    ☑7ᵗʰ **S86.309** Unspecified injury of muscle(s) and tendon(s) of peroneal muscle group at lower leg level, unspecified leg

   ☑6ᵗʰ **S86.31** Strain of muscle(s) and tendon(s) of peroneal muscle group at lower leg level

    ☑7ᵗʰ **S86.311** Strain of muscle(s) and tendon(s) of peroneal muscle group at lower leg level, right leg

    ☑7ᵗʰ **S86.312** Strain of muscle(s) and tendon(s) of peroneal muscle group at lower leg level, left leg

    ☑7ᵗʰ **S86.319** Strain of muscle(s) and tendon(s) of peroneal muscle group at lower leg level, unspecified leg

   ☑6ᵗʰ **S86.32** Laceration of muscle(s) and tendon(s) of peroneal muscle group at lower leg level

    ☑7ᵗʰ **S86.321** Laceration of muscle(s) and tendon(s) of peroneal muscle group at lower leg level, right leg

    ☑7ᵗʰ **S86.322** Laceration of muscle(s) and tendon(s) of peroneal muscle group at lower leg level, left leg

    ☑7ᵗʰ **S86.329** Laceration of muscle(s) and tendon(s) of peroneal muscle group at lower leg level, unspecified leg

   ☑6ᵗʰ **S86.39** Other injury of muscle(s) and tendon(s) of peroneal muscle group at lower leg level

    ☑7ᵗʰ **S86.391** Other injury of muscle(s) and tendon(s) of peroneal muscle group at lower leg level, right leg

    ☑7ᵗʰ **S86.392** Other injury of muscle(s) and tendon(s) of peroneal muscle group at lower leg level, left leg

    ☑7ᵗʰ **S86.399** Other injury of muscle(s) and tendon(s) of peroneal muscle group at lower leg level, unspecified leg

☑5ᵗʰ **S86.8** Injury of other muscles and tendons at lower leg level

   ☑6ᵗʰ **S86.80** Unspecified injury of other muscles and tendons at lower leg level

    ☑7ᵗʰ **S86.801** Unspecified injury of other muscle(s) and tendon(s) at lower leg level, right leg

    ☑7ᵗʰ **S86.802** Unspecified injury of other muscle(s) and tendon(s) at lower leg level, left leg

    ☑7ᵗʰ **S86.809** Unspecified injury of other muscle(s) and tendon(s) at lower leg level, unspecified leg

   ☑6ᵗʰ **S86.81** Strain of other muscles and tendons at lower leg level

    ☑7ᵗʰ **S86.811** Strain of other muscle(s) and tendon(s) at lower leg level, right leg

    ☑7ᵗʰ **S86.812** Strain of other muscle(s) and tendon(s) at lower leg level, left leg

    ☑7ᵗʰ **S86.819** Strain of other muscle(s) and tendon(s) at lower leg level, unspecified leg

   ☑6ᵗʰ **S86.82** Laceration of other muscles and tendons at lower leg level

    ☑7ᵗʰ **S86.821** Laceration of other muscle(s) and tendon(s) at lower leg level, right leg

    ☑7ᵗʰ **S86.822** Laceration of other muscle(s) and tendon(s) at lower leg level, left leg

    ☑7ᵗʰ **S86.829** Laceration of other muscle(s) and tendon(s) at lower leg level, unspecified leg

   ☑6ᵗʰ **S86.89** Other injury of other muscles and tendons at lower leg level

    ☑7ᵗʰ **S86.891** Other injury of other muscle(s) and tendon(s) at lower leg level, right leg

    ☑7ᵗʰ **S86.892** Other injury of other muscle(s) and tendon(s) at lower leg level, left leg

    ☑7ᵗʰ **S86.899** Other injury of other muscle(s) and tendon(s) at lower leg level, unspecified leg

☑5ᵗʰ **S86.9** Injury of unspecified muscle and tendon at lower leg level

   ☑6ᵗʰ **S86.90** Unspecified injury of unspecified muscle and tendon at lower leg level

    ☑7ᵗʰ **S86.901** Unspecified injury of unspecified muscle(s) and tendon(s) at lower leg level, right leg

    ☑7ᵗʰ **S86.902** Unspecified injury of unspecified muscle(s) and tendon(s) at lower leg level, left leg

    ☑7ᵗʰ **S86.909** Unspecified injury of unspecified muscle(s) and tendon(s) at lower leg level, unspecified leg

   ☑6ᵗʰ **S86.91** Strain of unspecified muscle and tendon at lower leg level

    ☑7ᵗʰ **S86.911** Strain of unspecified muscle(s) and tendon(s) at lower leg level, right leg

    ☑7ᵗʰ **S86.912** Strain of unspecified muscle(s) and tendon(s) at lower leg level, left leg

    ☑7ᵗʰ **S86.919** Strain of unspecified muscle(s) and tendon(s) at lower leg level, unspecified leg

   ☑6ᵗʰ **S86.92** Laceration of unspecified muscle and tendon at lower leg level

    ☑7ᵗʰ **S86.921** Laceration of unspecified muscle(s) and tendon(s) at lower leg level, right leg

    ☑7ᵗʰ **S86.922** Laceration of unspecified muscle(s) and tendon(s) at lower leg level, left leg

    ☑7ᵗʰ **S86.929** Laceration of unspecified muscle(s) and tendon(s) at lower leg level, unspecified leg

   ☑6ᵗʰ **S86.99** Other injury of unspecified muscle and tendon at lower leg level

    ☑7ᵗʰ **S86.991** Other injury of unspecified muscle(s) and tendon(s) at lower leg level, right leg

    ☑7ᵗʰ **S86.992** Other injury of unspecified muscle(s) and tendon(s) at lower leg level, left leg

    ☑7ᵗʰ **S86.999** Other injury of unspecified muscle(s) and tendon(s) at lower leg level, unspecified leg

☑4ᵗʰ **S87** Crushing injury of lower leg

   Use additional code(s) for all associated injuries

   EXCLUDES 2   crushing injury of ankle and foot (S97.-)

   The appropriate 7th character is to be added to each code from category S87.
   A   initial encounter
   D   subsequent encounter
   S   sequela

   ☑5ᵗʰ **S87.0** Crushing injury of knee

    ☑x7ᵗʰ **S87.00** Crushing injury of unspecified knee

    ☑x7ᵗʰ **S87.01** Crushing injury of right knee

    ☑x7ᵗʰ **S87.02** Crushing injury of left knee

   ☑5ᵗʰ **S87.8** Crushing injury of lower leg

    ☑x7ᵗʰ **S87.80** Crushing injury of unspecified lower leg

    ☑x7ᵗʰ **S87.81** Crushing injury of right lower leg

☑ Additional Character Required   ☑x7ᵗʰ Xtension Alert   Unspecified Dx   Other Specified Dx   Manifestation   ▶◀ Revised Text   ● New Code   ▲ Revised Code Title

Injury, Poisoning and Certain Other Consequences of External Causes

S87.82–S89.129

✓x7th **S87.82** Crushing injury of left lower leg

✓4th **S88** **Traumatic amputation of lower leg**

> **NOTE** An amputation not identified as partial or complete should be coded to complete.

> **EXCLUDES 1** traumatic amputation of ankle and foot (S98.-)

> The appropriate 7th character is to be added to each code from category S88.
> A   initial encounter
> D   subsequent encounter
> S   sequela

✓5th **S88.0** **Traumatic amputation at knee level**

✓6th **S88.01** Complete traumatic amputation at knee level

✓7th **S88.011** Complete traumatic amputation at knee level, right lower leg

✓7th **S88.012** Complete traumatic amputation at knee level, left lower leg

✓7th **S88.019** Complete traumatic amputation at knee level, unspecified lower leg

✓6th **S88.02** Partial traumatic amputation at knee level

✓7th **S88.021** Partial traumatic amputation at knee level, right lower leg

✓7th **S88.022** Partial traumatic amputation at knee level, left lower leg

✓7th **S88.029** Partial traumatic amputation at knee level, unspecified lower leg

✓5th **S88.1** **Traumatic amputation at level between knee and ankle**

✓6th **S88.11** Complete traumatic amputation at level between knee and ankle

✓7th **S88.111** Complete traumatic amputation at level between knee and ankle, right lower leg

✓7th **S88.112** Complete traumatic amputation at level between knee and ankle, left lower leg

✓7th **S88.119** Complete traumatic amputation at level between knee and ankle, unspecified lower leg

✓6th **S88.12** Partial traumatic amputation at level between knee and ankle

✓7th **S88.121** Partial traumatic amputation at level between knee and ankle, right lower leg

✓7th **S88.122** Partial traumatic amputation at level between knee and ankle, left lower leg

✓7th **S88.129** Partial traumatic amputation at level between knee and ankle, unspecified lower leg

✓5th **S88.9** **Traumatic amputation of lower leg, level unspecified**

✓6th **S88.91** Complete traumatic amputation of lower leg, level unspecified

✓7th **S88.911** Complete traumatic amputation of right lower leg, level unspecified

✓7th **S88.912** Complete traumatic amputation of left lower leg, level unspecified

✓7th **S88.919** Complete traumatic amputation of unspecified lower leg, level unspecified

✓6th **S88.92** Partial traumatic amputation of lower leg, level unspecified

✓7th **S88.921** Partial traumatic amputation of right lower leg, level unspecified

✓7th **S88.922** Partial traumatic amputation of left lower leg, level unspecified

✓7th **S88.929** Partial traumatic amputation of unspecified lower leg, level unspecified

✓4th **S89** **Other and unspecified injuries of lower leg**

> **NOTE** A fracture not indicated as open or closed should be coded to closed.

> **EXCLUDES 2** other and unspecified injuries of ankle and foot (S99.-)

> The appropriate 7th character is to be added to each code from subcategories S89.0, S89.1, S89.2, and S89.3.
> A   initial encounter for closed fracture
> D   subsequent encounter for fracture with routine healing
> G   subsequent encounter for fracture with delayed healing
> K   subsequent encounter for fracture with nonunion
> P   subsequent encounter for fracture with malunion
> S   sequela

✓5th **S89.0** Physeal fracture of upper end of tibia

✓6th **S89.00** Unspecified physeal fracture of upper end of tibia

✓7th **S89.001** Unspecified physeal fracture of upper end of right tibia

✓7th **S89.002** Unspecified physeal fracture of upper end of left tibia

✓7th **S89.009** Unspecified physeal fracture of upper end of unspecified tibia

✓6th **S89.01** Salter-Harris Type I physeal fracture of upper end of tibia

✓7th **S89.011** Salter-Harris Type I physeal fracture of upper end of right tibia

✓7th **S89.012** Salter-Harris Type I physeal fracture of upper end of left tibia

✓7th **S89.019** Salter-Harris Type I physeal fracture of upper end of unspecified tibia

✓6th **S89.02** Salter-Harris Type II physeal fracture of upper end of tibia

✓7th **S89.021** Salter-Harris Type II physeal fracture of upper end of right tibia

✓7th **S89.022** Salter-Harris Type II physeal fracture of upper end of left tibia

✓7th **S89.029** Salter-Harris Type II physeal fracture of upper end of unspecified tibia

✓6th **S89.03** Salter-Harris Type III physeal fracture of upper end of tibia

✓7th **S89.031** Salter-Harris Type III physeal fracture of upper end of right tibia

✓7th **S89.032** Salter-Harris Type III physeal fracture of upper end of left tibia

✓7th **S89.039** Salter-Harris Type III physeal fracture of upper end of unspecified tibia

✓6th **S89.04** Salter-Harris Type IV physeal fracture of upper end of tibia

✓7th **S89.041** Salter-Harris Type IV physeal fracture of upper end of right tibia

✓7th **S89.042** Salter-Harris Type IV physeal fracture of upper end of left tibia

✓7th **S89.049** Salter-Harris Type IV physeal fracture of upper end of unspecified tibia

✓6th **S89.09** Other physeal fracture of upper end of tibia

✓7th **S89.091** Other physeal fracture of upper end of right tibia

✓7th **S89.092** Other physeal fracture of upper end of left tibia

✓7th **S89.099** Other physeal fracture of upper end of unspecified tibia

✓5th **S89.1** Physeal fracture of lower end of tibia

✓6th **S89.10** Unspecified physeal fracture of lower end of tibia

✓7th **S89.101** Unspecified physeal fracture of lower end of right tibia

✓7th **S89.102** Unspecified physeal fracture of lower end of left tibia

✓7th **S89.109** Unspecified physeal fracture of lower end of unspecified tibia

✓6th **S89.11** Salter-Harris Type I physeal fracture of ower end of tibia

✓7th **S89.111** Salter-Harris Type I physeal fracture of lower end of right tibia

✓7th **S89.112** Salter-Harris Type I physeal fracture of lower end of left tibia

✓7th **S89.119** Salter-Harris Type I physeal fracture of lower end of unspecified tibia

✓6th **S89.12** Salter-Harris Type II physeal fracture of lower end of tibia

✓7th **S89.121** Salter-Harris Type II physeal fracture of lower end of right tibia

✓7th **S89.122** Salter-Harris Type II physeal fracture of lower end of left tibia

✓7th **S89.129** Salter-Harris Type II physeal fracture of lower end of unspecified tibia

EXCLUDES 1 Not coded here   **EXCLUDES 2** Not included here   N Newborn Age: 0   P Pediatric Age: 0-17   M Maternity Age: 12-55   A Adult Age: 15-124

908   ICD-10-CM Draft (2015)

✓6ᵗʰ **S89.13**   Salter-Harris Type III physeal fracture of lower end of tibia
> **EXCLUDES 1**   *fracture of medial malleolus (adult) (S82.5-)*

✓7ᵗʰ **S89.131**   Salter-Harris Type III physeal fracture of lower end of right tibia

✓7ᵗʰ **S89.132**   Salter-Harris Type III physeal fracture of lower end of left tibia

✓7ᵗʰ **S89.139**   Salter-Harris Type III physeal fracture of lower end of unspecified tibia

✓6ᵗʰ **S89.14**   Salter-Harris Type IV physeal fracture of lower end of tibia
> **EXCLUDES 1**   *fracture of medial malleolus (adult) (S82.5-)*

✓7ᵗʰ **S89.141**   Salter-Harris Type IV physeal fracture of lower end of right tibia

✓7ᵗʰ **S89.142**   Salter-Harris Type IV physeal fracture of lower end of left tibia

✓7ᵗʰ **S89.149**   Salter-Harris Type IV physeal fracture of lower end of unspecified tibia

✓6ᵗʰ **S89.19**   Other physeal fracture of lower end of tibia

✓7ᵗʰ **S89.191**   Other physeal fracture of lower end of right tibia

✓7ᵗʰ **S89.192**   Other physeal fracture of lower end of left tibia

✓7ᵗʰ **S89.199**   Other physeal fracture of lower end of unspecified tibia

✓5ᵗʰ **S89.2**   Physeal fracture of upper end of fibula

✓6ᵗʰ **S89.20**   Unspecified physeal fracture of upper end of fibula

✓7ᵗʰ **S89.201**   Unspecified physeal fracture of upper end of right fibula

✓7ᵗʰ **S89.202**   Unspecified physeal fracture of upper end of left fibula

✓7ᵗʰ **S89.209**   Unspecified physeal fracture of upper end of unspecified fibula

✓6ᵗʰ **S89.21**   Salter-Harris Type I physeal fracture of upper end of fibula

✓7ᵗʰ **S89.211**   Salter-Harris Type I physeal fracture of upper end of right fibula

✓7ᵗʰ **S89.212**   Salter-Harris Type I physeal fracture of upper end of left fibula

✓7ᵗʰ **S89.219**   Salter-Harris Type I physeal fracture of upper end of unspecified fibula

✓6ᵗʰ **S89.22**   Salter-Harris Type II physeal fracture of upper end of fibula

✓7ᵗʰ **S89.221**   Salter-Harris Type II physeal fracture of upper end of right fibula

✓7ᵗʰ **S89.222**   Salter-Harris Type II physeal fracture of upper end of left fibula

✓7ᵗʰ **S89.229**   Salter-Harris Type II physeal fracture of upper end of unspecified fibula

✓6ᵗʰ **S89.29**   Other physeal fracture of upper end of fibula

✓7ᵗʰ **S89.291**   Other physeal fracture of upper end of right fibula

✓7ᵗʰ **S89.292**   Other physeal fracture of upper end of left fibula

✓7ᵗʰ **S89.299**   Other physeal fracture of upper end of unspecified fibula

✓5ᵗʰ **S89.3**   Physeal fracture of lower end of fibula

✓6ᵗʰ **S89.30**   Unspecified physeal fracture of lower end of fibula

✓7ᵗʰ **S89.301**   Unspecified physeal fracture of lower end of right fibula

✓7ᵗʰ **S89.302**   Unspecified physeal fracture of lower end of left fibula

✓7ᵗʰ **S89.309**   Unspecified physeal fracture of lower end of unspecified fibula

✓6ᵗʰ **S89.31**   Salter-Harris Type I physeal fracture of lower end of fibula

✓7ᵗʰ **S89.311**   Salter-Harris Type I physeal fracture of lower end of right fibula

✓7ᵗʰ **S89.312**   Salter-Harris Type I physeal fracture of lower end of left fibula

✓7ᵗʰ **S89.319**   Salter-Harris Type I physeal fracture of lower end of unspecified fibula

✓6ᵗʰ **S89.32**   Salter-Harris Type II physeal fracture of lower end of fibula

✓7ᵗʰ **S89.321**   Salter-Harris Type II physeal fracture of lower end of right fibula

✓7ᵗʰ **S89.322**   Salter-Harris Type II physeal fracture of lower end of left fibula

✓7ᵗʰ **S89.329**   Salter-Harris Type II physeal fracture of lower end of unspecified fibula

✓6ᵗʰ **S89.39**   Other physeal fracture of lower end of fibula

✓7ᵗʰ **S89.391**   Other physeal fracture of lower end of right fibula

✓7ᵗʰ **S89.392**   Other physeal fracture of lower end of left fibula

✓7ᵗʰ **S89.399**   Other physeal fracture of lower end of unspecified fibula

✓5ᵗʰ **S89.8**   Other specified injuries of lower leg

> The appropriate 7th character is to be added to each code in subcategory S89.8.
> A   initial encounter
> D   subsequent encounter
> S   sequela

✓×7ᵗʰ **S89.80**   Other specified injuries of unspecified lower leg

✓×7ᵗʰ **S89.81**   Other specified injuries of right lower leg

✓×7ᵗʰ **S89.82**   Other specified injuries of left lower leg

✓5ᵗʰ **S89.9**   Unspecified injury of lower leg

> The appropriate 7th character is to be added to each code in subcategory S89.9.
> A   initial encounter
> D   subsequent encounter
> S   sequela

✓×7ᵗʰ **S89.90**   Unspecified injury of unspecified lower leg

✓×7ᵗʰ **S89.91**   Unspecified injury of right lower leg

✓×7ᵗʰ **S89.92**   Unspecified injury of left lower leg

Injuries to the ankle and foot (S90-S99)

EXCLUDES 2   *burns and corrosions (T20-T32)*
fracture of ankle and malleolus (S82.-)
frostbite (T33-T34)
insect bite or sting, venomous (T63.4)

✓4ᵗʰ **S90**   **Superficial injury of ankle, foot and toes**

> The appropriate 7th character is to be added to each code from category S90.
> A   initial encounter
> D   subsequent encounter
> S   sequela

✓5ᵗʰ **S90.0**   Contusion of ankle

✓×7ᵗʰ **S90.00**   Contusion of unspecified ankle

✓×7ᵗʰ **S90.01**   Contusion of right ankle

✓×7ᵗʰ **S90.02**   Contusion of left ankle

✓5ᵗʰ **S90.1**   Contusion of toe without damage to nail

✓6ᵗʰ **S90.11**   Contusion of great toe without damage to nail

✓7ᵗʰ **S90.111**   Contusion of right great toe without damage to nail

✓7ᵗʰ **S90.112**   Contusion of left great toe without damage to nail

✓7ᵗʰ **S90.119**   Contusion of unspecified great toe without damage to nail

✓6ᵗʰ **S90.12**   Contusion of lesser toe without damage to nail

✓7ᵗʰ **S90.121**   Contusion of right lesser toe(s) without damage to nail

✓7ᵗʰ **S90.122**   Contusion of left lesser toe(s) without damage to nail

✓7ᵗʰ **S90.129**   Contusion of unspecified lesser toe(s) without damage to nail
Contusion of toe NOS

✓5ᵗʰ **S90.2**   Contusion of toe with damage to nail

✓6ᵗʰ **S90.21**   Contusion of great toe with damage to nail

✓7ᵗʰ **S90.211**   Contusion of right great toe with damage to nail

✓7ᵗʰ **S90.212**   Contusion of left great toe with damage to nail

✓ Additional Character Required   ✓×7ᵗʰ Xtension Alert   Unspecified Dx   Other Specified Dx   Manifestation   ►◄ Revised Text   ● New Code   ▲ Revised Code Title

ICD-10-CM Draft (2015)   **909**

✓7ᵗʰ **S90.219** **Contusion of unspecified great toe with damage to nail**

✓6ᵗʰ **S90.22** Contusion of lesser toe with damage to nail

     ✓7ᵗʰ **S90.221** **Contusion of right lesser toe(s) with damage to nail**

     ✓7ᵗʰ **S90.222** **Contusion of left lesser toe(s) with damage to nail**

     ✓7ᵗʰ **S90.229** **Contusion of unspecified lesser toe(s) with damage to nail**

✓5ᵗʰ **S90.3** **Contusion of foot**

     EXCLUDES 2   contusion of toes (S90.1-, S90.2-)

✓x7ᵗʰ **S90.30** **Contusion of unspecified foot**
     Contusion of foot NOS

✓x7ᵗʰ **S90.31** **Contusion of right foot**

✓x7ᵗʰ **S90.32** **Contusion of left foot**

✓5ᵗʰ **S90.4** **Other superficial injuries of toe**

✓6ᵗʰ **S90.41** Abrasion of toe

     ✓7ᵗʰ **S90.411** **Abrasion, right great toe**

     ✓7ᵗʰ **S90.412** **Abrasion, left great toe**

     ✓7ᵗʰ **S90.413** **Abrasion, unspecified great toe**

     ✓7ᵗʰ **S90.414** **Abrasion, right lesser toe(s)**

     ✓7ᵗʰ **S90.415** **Abrasion, left lesser toe(s)**

     ✓7ᵗʰ **S90.416** **Abrasion, unspecified lesser toe(s)**

✓6ᵗʰ **S90.42** Blister (nonthermal) of toe

     ✓7ᵗʰ **S90.421** **Blister (nonthermal), right great toe**

     ✓7ᵗʰ **S90.422** **Blister (nonthermal), left great toe**

     ✓7ᵗʰ **S90.423** **Blister (nonthermal), unspecified great toe**

     ✓7ᵗʰ **S90.424** **Blister (nonthermal), right lesser toe(s)**

     ✓7ᵗʰ **S90.425** **Blister (nonthermal), left lesser toe(s)**

     ✓7ᵗʰ **S90.426** **Blister (nonthermal), unspecified lesser toe(s)**

✓6ᵗʰ **S90.44** External constriction of toe
     Hair tourniquet syndrome of toe

     ✓7ᵗʰ **S90.441** **External constriction, right great toe**

     ✓7ᵗʰ **S90.442** **External constriction, left great toe**

     ✓7ᵗʰ **S90.443** **External constriction, unspecified great toe**

     ✓7ᵗʰ **S90.444** **External constriction, right lesser toe(s)**

     ✓7ᵗʰ **S90.445** **External constriction, left lesser toe(s)**

     ✓7ᵗʰ **S90.446** **External constriction, unspecified lesser toe(s)**

✓6ᵗʰ **S90.45** Superficial foreign body of toe
     Splinter in the toe

     ✓7ᵗʰ **S90.451** **Superficial foreign body, right great toe**

     ✓7ᵗʰ **S90.452** **Superficial foreign body, left great toe**

     ✓7ᵗʰ **S90.453** **Superficial foreign body, unspecified great toe**

     ✓7ᵗʰ **S90.454** **Superficial foreign body, right lesser toe(s)**

     ✓7ᵗʰ **S90.455** **Superficial foreign body, left lesser toe(s)**

     ✓7ᵗʰ **S90.456** **Superficial foreign body, unspecified lesser toe(s)**

✓6ᵗʰ **S90.46** Insect bite (nonvenomous) of toe

     ✓7ᵗʰ **S90.461** **Insect bite (nonvenomous), right great toe**

     ✓7ᵗʰ **S90.462** **Insect bite (nonvenomous), left great toe**

     ✓7ᵗʰ **S90.463** **Insect bite (nonvenomous), unspecified great toe**

     ✓7ᵗʰ **S90.464** **Insect bite (nonvenomous), right lesser toe(s)**

     ✓7ᵗʰ **S90.465** **Insect bite (nonvenomous), left lesser toe(s)**

     ✓7ᵗʰ **S90.466** **Insect bite (nonvenomous), unspecified lesser toe(s)**

✓6ᵗʰ **S90.47** Other superficial bite of toe
     EXCLUDES 1   open bite of toe (S91.15-, S91.25-)

     ✓7ᵗʰ **S90.471** **Other superficial bite of right great toe**

     ✓7ᵗʰ **S90.472** **Other superficial bite of left great toe**

     ✓7ᵗʰ **S90.473** **Other superficial bite of unspecified great toe**

     ✓7ᵗʰ **S90.474** **Other superficial bite of right lesser toe(s)**

     ✓7ᵗʰ **S90.475** **Other superficial bite of left lesser toe(s)**

     ✓7ᵗʰ **S90.476** **Other superficial bite of unspecified lesser toe(s)**

✓5ᵗʰ **S90.5** **Other superficial injuries of ankle**

✓6ᵗʰ **S90.51** Abrasion of ankle

     ✓7ᵗʰ **S90.511** **Abrasion, right ankle**

     ✓7ᵗʰ **S90.512** **Abrasion, left ankle**

     ✓7ᵗʰ **S90.519** **Abrasion, unspecified ankle**

✓6ᵗʰ **S90.52** Blister (nonthermal) of ankle

     ✓7ᵗʰ **S90.521** **Blister (nonthermal), right ankle**

     ✓7ᵗʰ **S90.522** **Blister (nonthermal), left ankle**

     ✓7ᵗʰ **S90.529** **Blister (nonthermal), unspecified ankle**

✓6ᵗʰ **S90.54** External constriction of ankle

     ✓7ᵗʰ **S90.541** **External constriction, right ankle**

     ✓7ᵗʰ **S90.542** **External constriction, left ankle**

     ✓7ᵗʰ **S90.549** **External constriction, unspecified ankle**

✓6ᵗʰ **S90.55** Superficial foreign body of ankle
     Splinter in the ankle

     ✓7ᵗʰ **S90.551** **Superficial foreign body, right ankle**

     ✓7ᵗʰ **S90.552** **Superficial foreign body, left ankle**

     ✓7ᵗʰ **S90.559** **Superficial foreign body, unspecified ankle**

✓6ᵗʰ **S90.56** Insect bite (nonvenomous) of ankle

     ✓7ᵗʰ **S90.561** **Insect bite (nonvenomous), right ankle**

     ✓7ᵗʰ **S90.562** **Insect bite (nonvenomous), left ankle**

     ✓7ᵗʰ **S90.569** **Insect bite (nonvenomous), unspecified ankle**

✓6ᵗʰ **S90.57** Other superficial bite of ankle
     EXCLUDES 1   open bite of ankle (S91.05-)

     ✓7ᵗʰ **S90.571** **Other superficial bite of ankle, right ankle**

     ✓7ᵗʰ **S90.572** **Other superficial bite of ankle, left ankle**

     ✓7ᵗʰ **S90.579** **Other superficial bite of ankle, unspecified ankle**

✓5ᵗʰ **S90.8** **Other superficial injuries of foot**

✓6ᵗʰ **S90.81** Abrasion of foot

     ✓7ᵗʰ **S90.811** **Abrasion, right foot**

     ✓7ᵗʰ **S90.812** **Abrasion, left foot**

     ✓7ᵗʰ **S90.819** **Abrasion, unspecified foot**

✓6ᵗʰ **S90.82** Blister (nonthermal) of foot

     ✓7ᵗʰ **S90.821** **Blister (nonthermal), right foot**

     ✓7ᵗʰ **S90.822** **Blister (nonthermal), left foot**

     ✓7ᵗʰ **S90.829** **Blister (nonthermal), unspecified foot**

✓6ᵗʰ **S90.84** External constriction of foot

     ✓7ᵗʰ **S90.841** **External constriction, right foot**

     ✓7ᵗʰ **S90.842** **External constriction, left foot**

     ✓7ᵗʰ **S90.849** **External constriction, unspecified foot**

✓6ᵗʰ **S90.85** Superficial foreign body of foot
     Splinter in the foot

     ✓7ᵗʰ **S90.851** **Superficial foreign body, right foot**

     ✓7ᵗʰ **S90.852** **Superficial foreign body, left foot**

     ✓7ᵗʰ **S90.859** **Superficial foreign body, unspecified foot**

✓6ᵗʰ **S90.86** Insect bite (nonvenomous) of foot

     ✓7ᵗʰ **S90.861** **Insect bite (nonvenomous), right foot**

     ✓7ᵗʰ **S90.862** **Insect bite (nonvenomous), left foot**

     ✓7ᵗʰ **S90.869** **Insect bite (nonvenomous), unspecified foot**

✓6ᵗʰ **S90.87** Other superficial bite of foot
     EXCLUDES 1   open bite of foot (S91.35-)

     ✓7ᵗʰ **S90.871** **Other superficial bite of right foot**

     ✓7ᵗʰ **S90.872** **Other superficial bite of left foot**

     ✓7ᵗʰ **S90.879** **Other superficial bite of unspecified foot**

✓5ᵗʰ **S90.9** **Unspecified superficial injury of ankle, foot and toe**

✓6ᵗʰ **S90.91** Unspecified superficial injury of ankle

     ✓7ᵗʰ **S90.911** **Unspecified superficial injury of right ankle**

     ✓7ᵗʰ **S90.912** **Unspecified superficial injury of left ankle**

     ✓7ᵗʰ **S90.919** **Unspecified superficial injury of unspecified ankle**

✓6ᵗʰ **S90.92** Unspecified superficial injury of foot

     ✓7ᵗʰ **S90.921** **Unspecified superficial injury of right foot**

EXCLUDES 1 Not coded here   EXCLUDES 2 Not included here   N Newborn Age: 0   P Pediatric Age: 0-17   M Maternity Age: 12-55   A Adult Age: 15-124

910   ICD-10-CM Draft (2015)

☑7ᵗʰ **S90.922** Unspecified superficial injury of left foot

☑7ᵗʰ **S90.929** Unspecified superficial injury of unspecified foot

☑6ᵗʰ **S90.93** Unspecified superficial injury of toes

☑7ᵗʰ **S90.931** Unspecified superficial injury of right great toe

☑7ᵗʰ **S90.932** Unspecified superficial injury of left great toe

☑7ᵗʰ **S90.933** Unspecified superficial injury of unspecified great toe

☑7ᵗʰ **S90.934** Unspecified superficial injury of right lesser toe(s)

☑7ᵗʰ **S90.935** Unspecified superficial injury of left lesser toe(s)

☑7ᵗʰ **S90.936** Unspecified superficial injury of unspecified lesser toe(s)

☑4ᵗʰ **S91** Open wound of ankle, foot and toes

Code also any associated wound infection

EXCLUDES 1 open fracture of ankle, foot and toes (S92-with 7th character B)
traumatic amputation of ankle and foot (S98.-)

The appropriate 7th character is to be added to each code from category S91.
A   initial encounter
D   subsequent encounter
S   sequela

☑5ᵗʰ **S91.0** Open wound of ankle

☑6ᵗʰ **S91.00** Unspecified open wound of ankle

☑7ᵗʰ **S91.001** Unspecified open wound, right ankle

☑7ᵗʰ **S91.002** Unspecified open wound, left ankle

☑7ᵗʰ **S91.009** Unspecified open wound, unspecified ankle

☑6ᵗʰ **S91.01** Laceration without foreign body of ankle

☑7ᵗʰ **S91.011** Laceration without foreign body, right ankle

☑7ᵗʰ **S91.012** Laceration without foreign body, left ankle

☑7ᵗʰ **S91.019** Laceration without foreign body, unspecified ankle

☑6ᵗʰ **S91.02** Laceration with foreign body of ankle

☑7ᵗʰ **S91.021** Laceration with foreign body, right ankle

☑7ᵗʰ **S91.022** Laceration with foreign body, left ankle

☑7ᵗʰ **S91.029** Laceration with foreign body, unspecified ankle

☑6ᵗʰ **S91.03** Puncture wound without foreign body of ankle

☑7ᵗʰ **S91.031** Puncture wound without foreign body, right ankle

☑7ᵗʰ **S91.032** Puncture wound without foreign body, left ankle

☑7ᵗʰ **S91.039** Puncture wound without foreign body, unspecified ankle

☑6ᵗʰ **S91.04** Puncture wound with foreign body of ankle

☑7ᵗʰ **S91.041** Puncture wound with foreign body, right ankle

☑7ᵗʰ **S91.042** Puncture wound with foreign body, left ankle

☑7ᵗʰ **S91.049** Puncture wound with foreign body, unspecified ankle

☑6ᵗʰ **S91.05** Open bite of ankle

EXCLUDES 1 superficial bite of ankle (S90.56-, S90.57-)

☑7ᵗʰ **S91.051** Open bite, right ankle

☑7ᵗʰ **S91.052** Open bite, left ankle

☑7ᵗʰ **S91.059** Open bite, unspecified ankle

☑5ᵗʰ **S91.1** Open wound of toe without damage to nail

☑6ᵗʰ **S91.10** Unspecified open wound of toe without damage to nail

☑7ᵗʰ **S91.101** Unspecified open wound of right great toe without damage to nail

☑7ᵗʰ **S91.102** Unspecified open wound of left great toe without damage to nail

☑7ᵗʰ **S91.103** Unspecified open wound of unspecified great toe without damage to nail

☑7ᵗʰ **S91.104** Unspecified open wound of right lesser toe(s) without damage to nail

☑7ᵗʰ **S91.105** Unspecified open wound of left lesser toe(s) without damage to nail

☑7ᵗʰ **S91.106** Unspecified open wound of unspecified lesser toe(s) without damage to nail

☑7ᵗʰ **S91.109** Unspecified open wound of unspecified toe(s) without damage to nail

☑6ᵗʰ **S91.11** Laceration without foreign body of toe without damage to nail

☑7ᵗʰ **S91.111** Laceration without foreign body of right great toe without damage to nail

☑7ᵗʰ **S91.112** Laceration without foreign body of left great toe without damage to nail

☑7ᵗʰ **S91.113** Laceration without foreign body of unspecified great toe without damage to nail

☑7ᵗʰ **S91.114** Laceration without foreign body of right lesser toe(s) without damage to nail

☑7ᵗʰ **S91.115** Laceration without foreign body of left lesser toe(s) without damage to nail

☑7ᵗʰ **S91.116** Laceration without foreign body of unspecified lesser toe(s) without damage to nail

☑7ᵗʰ **S91.119** Laceration without foreign body of unspecified toe without damage to nail

☑6ᵗʰ **S91.12** Laceration with foreign body of toe without damage to nail

☑7ᵗʰ **S91.121** Laceration with foreign body of right great toe without damage to nail

☑7ᵗʰ **S91.122** Laceration with foreign body of left great toe without damage to nail

☑7ᵗʰ **S91.123** Laceration with foreign body of unspecified great toe without damage to nail

☑7ᵗʰ **S91.124** Laceration with foreign body of right lesser toe(s) without damage to nail

☑7ᵗʰ **S91.125** Laceration with foreign body of left lesser toe(s) without damage to nail

☑7ᵗʰ **S91.126** Laceration with foreign body of unspecified lesser toe(s) without damage to nail

☑7ᵗʰ **S91.129** Laceration with foreign body of unspecified toe(s) without damage to nail

☑6ᵗʰ **S91.13** Puncture wound without foreign body of toe without damage to nail

☑7ᵗʰ **S91.131** Puncture wound without foreign body of right great toe without damage to nail

☑7ᵗʰ **S91.132** Puncture wound without foreign body of left great toe without damage to nail

☑7ᵗʰ **S91.133** Puncture wound without foreign body of unspecified great toe without damage to nail

☑7ᵗʰ **S91.134** Puncture wound without foreign body of right lesser toe(s) without damage to nail

☑7ᵗʰ **S91.135** Puncture wound without foreign body of left lesser toe(s) without damage to nail

☑7ᵗʰ **S91.136** Puncture wound without foreign body of unspecified lesser toe(s) without damage to nail

☑7ᵗʰ **S91.139** Puncture wound without foreign body of unspecified toe(s) without damage to nail

☑6ᵗʰ **S91.14** Puncture wound with foreign body of toe without damage to nail

☑7ᵗʰ **S91.141** Puncture wound with foreign body of right great toe without damage to nail

☑7ᵗʰ **S91.142** Puncture wound with foreign body of left great toe without damage to nail

☑7ᵗʰ **S91.143** Puncture wound with foreign body of unspecified great toe without damage to nail

☑7ᵗʰ **S91.144** Puncture wound with foreign body of right lesser toe(s) without damage to nail

☑7ᵗʰ **S91.145** Puncture wound with foreign body of left lesser toe(s) without damage to nail

☑7ᵗʰ **S91.146** Puncture wound with foreign body of unspecified lesser toe(s) without damage to nail

---

☑ Additional Character Required   ☑ⅹ7ᵗʰ Xtension Alert   Unspecified Dx   Other Specified Dx   Manifestation   ►◄ Revised Text   ● New Code   ▲ Revised Code Title

√7ᵗʰ **S91.149** Puncture wound with foreign body of unspecified toe(s) without damage to nail

√6ᵗʰ **S91.15** Open bite of toe without damage to nail
   Bite of toe NOS
   EXCLUDES 1 *superficial bite of toe (S90.46-, S90.47-)*

  √7ᵗʰ **S91.151** Open bite of right great toe without damage to nail

  √7ᵗʰ **S91.152** Open bite of left great toe without damage to nail

  √7ᵗʰ **S91.153** Open bite of unspecified great toe without damage to nail

  √7ᵗʰ **S91.154** Open bite of right lesser toe(s) without damage to nail

  √7ᵗʰ **S91.155** Open bite of left lesser toe(s) without damage to nail

  √7ᵗʰ **S91.156** Open bite of unspecified lesser toe(s) without damage to nail

  √7ᵗʰ **S91.159** Open bite of unspecified toe(s) without damage to nail

√5ᵗʰ **S91.2** Open wound of toe with damage to nail

 √6ᵗʰ **S91.20** Unspecified open wound of toe with damage to nail

  √7ᵗʰ **S91.201** Unspecified open wound of right great toe with damage to nail

  √7ᵗʰ **S91.202** Unspecified open wound of left great toe with damage to nail

  √7ᵗʰ **S91.203** Unspecified open wound of unspecified great toe with damage to nail

  √7ᵗʰ **S91.204** Unspecified open wound of right lesser toe(s) with damage to nail

  √7ᵗʰ **S91.205** Unspecified open wound of left lesser toe(s) with damage to nail

  √7ᵗʰ **S91.206** Unspecified open wound of unspecified lesser toe(s) with damage to nail

  √7ᵗʰ **S91.209** Unspecified open wound of unspecified toe(s) with damage to nail

 √6ᵗʰ **S91.21** Laceration without foreign body of toe with damage to nail

  √7ᵗʰ **S91.211** Laceration without foreign body of right great toe with damage to nail

  √7ᵗʰ **S91.212** Laceration without foreign body of left great toe with damage to nail

  √7ᵗʰ **S91.213** Laceration without foreign body of unspecified great toe with damage to nail

  √7ᵗʰ **S91.214** Laceration without foreign body of right lesser toe(s) with damage to nail

  √7ᵗʰ **S91.215** Laceration without foreign body of left lesser toe(s) with damage to nail

  √7ᵗʰ **S91.216** Laceration without foreign body of unspecified lesser toe(s) with damage to nail

  √7ᵗʰ **S91.219** Laceration without foreign body of unspecified toe(s) with damage to nail

 √6ᵗʰ **S91.22** Laceration with foreign body of toe with damage to nail

  √7ᵗʰ **S91.221** Laceration with foreign body of right great toe with damage to nail

  √7ᵗʰ **S91.222** Laceration with foreign body of left great toe with damage to nail

  √7ᵗʰ **S91.223** Laceration with foreign body of unspecified great toe with damage to nail

  √7ᵗʰ **S91.224** Laceration with foreign body of right lesser toe(s) with damage to nail

  √7ᵗʰ **S91.225** Laceration with foreign body of left lesser toe(s) with damage to nail

  √7ᵗʰ **S91.226** Laceration with foreign body of unspecified lesser toe(s) with damage to nail

  √7ᵗʰ **S91.229** Laceration with foreign body of unspecified toe(s) with damage to nail

 √6ᵗʰ **S91.23** Puncture wound without foreign body of toe with damage to nail

  √7ᵗʰ **S91.231** Puncture wound without foreign body of right great toe with damage to nail

  √7ᵗʰ **S91.232** Puncture wound without foreign body of left great toe with damage to nail

  √7ᵗʰ **S91.233** Puncture wound without foreign body of unspecified great toe with damage to nail

  √7ᵗʰ **S91.234** Puncture wound without foreign body of right lesser toe(s) with damage to nail

  √7ᵗʰ **S91.235** Puncture wound without foreign body of left lesser toe(s) with damage to nail

  √7ᵗʰ **S91.236** Puncture wound without foreign body of unspecified lesser toe(s) with damage to nail

  √7ᵗʰ **S91.239** Puncture wound without foreign body of unspecified toe(s) with damage to nail

 √6ᵗʰ **S91.24** Puncture wound with foreign body of toe with damage to nail

  √7ᵗʰ **S91.241** Puncture wound with foreign body of right great toe with damage to nail

  √7ᵗʰ **S91.242** Puncture wound with foreign body of left great toe with damage to nail

  √7ᵗʰ **S91.243** Puncture wound with foreign body of unspecified great toe with damage to nail

  √7ᵗʰ **S91.244** Puncture wound with foreign body of right lesser toe(s) with damage to nail

  √7ᵗʰ **S91.245** Puncture wound with foreign body of left lesser toe(s) with damage to nail

  √7ᵗʰ **S91.246** Puncture wound with foreign body of unspecified lesser toe(s) with damage to nail

  √7ᵗʰ **S91.249** Puncture wound with foreign body of unspecified toe(s) with damage to nail

 √6ᵗʰ **S91.25** Open bite of toe with damage to nail
   Bite of toe with damage to nail NOS
   EXCLUDES 1 *superficial bite of toe (S90.46-, S90.47-)*

  √7ᵗʰ **S91.251** Open bite of right great toe with damage to nail

  √7ᵗʰ **S91.252** Open bite of left great toe with damage to nail

  √7ᵗʰ **S91.253** Open bite of unspecified great toe with damage to nail

  √7ᵗʰ **S91.254** Open bite of right lesser toe(s) with damage to nail

  √7ᵗʰ **S91.255** Open bite of left lesser toe(s) with damage to nail

  √7ᵗʰ **S91.256** Open bite of unspecified lesser toe(s) with damage to nail

  √7ᵗʰ **S91.259** Open bite of unspecified toe(s) with damage to nail

√5ᵗʰ **S91.3** Open wound of foot

 √6ᵗʰ **S91.30** Unspecified open wound of foot

  √7ᵗʰ **S91.301** Unspecified open wound, right foot

  √7ᵗʰ **S91.302** Unspecified open wound, left foot

  √7ᵗʰ **S91.309** Unspecified open wound, unspecified foot

 √6ᵗʰ **S91.31** Laceration without foreign body of foot

  √7ᵗʰ **S91.311** Laceration without foreign body, right foot

  √7ᵗʰ **S91.312** Laceration without foreign body, left foot

  √7ᵗʰ **S91.319** Laceration without foreign body, unspecified foot

 √6ᵗʰ **S91.32** Laceration with foreign body of foot

  √7ᵗʰ **S91.321** Laceration with foreign body, right foot

  √7ᵗʰ **S91.322** Laceration with foreign body, left foot

  √7ᵗʰ **S91.329** Laceration with foreign body, unspecified foot

 √6ᵗʰ **S91.33** Puncture wound without foreign body of foot

  √7ᵗʰ **S91.331** Puncture wound without foreign body, right foot

  √7ᵗʰ **S91.332** Puncture wound without foreign body, left foot

  √7ᵗʰ **S91.339** Puncture wound without foreign body, unspecified foot

 √6ᵗʰ **S91.34** Puncture wound with foreign body of foot

  √7ᵗʰ **S91.341** Puncture wound with foreign body, right foot

  √7ᵗʰ **S91.342** Puncture wound with foreign body, left foot

---

EXCLUDES 1 Not coded here   EXCLUDES 2 Not included here   N Newborn Age: 0   P Pediatric Age: 0-17   M Maternity Age: 12-55   A Adult Age: 15-124

☑7ᵗʰ **S91.349** Puncture wound with foreign body, unspecified foot

☑6ᵗʰ **S91.35** Open bite of foot

    EXCLUDES 1 superficial bite of foot (S90.86-, S90.87-)

☑7ᵗʰ **S91.351** Open bite, right foot

☑7ᵗʰ **S91.352** Open bite, left foot

☑7ᵗʰ **S91.359** Open bite, unspecified foot

☑4ᵗʰ **S92** Fracture of foot and toe, except ankle

NOTE A fracture not indicated as displaced or nondisplaced should be coded to displaced.
A fracture not indicated as open or closed should be coded to closed.

EXCLUDES 1 traumatic amputation of ankle and foot (S98.-)

EXCLUDES 2 fracture of ankle (S82.-)
fracture of malleolus (S82.-)

The appropriate 7th character is to be added to each code from category S92.
A   initial encounter for closed fracture
B   initial encounter for open fracture
D   subsequent encounter for fracture with routine healing
G   subsequent encounter for fracture with delayed healing
K   subsequent encounter for fracture with nonunion
P   subsequent encounter for fracture with malunion
S   sequela

☑5ᵗʰ **S92.0** Fracture of calcaneus
Heel bone
Os calcis

☑6ᵗʰ **S92.00** Unspecified fracture of calcaneus

☑7ᵗʰ **S92.001** Unspecified fracture of right calcaneus

☑7ᵗʰ **S92.002** Unspecified fracture of left calcaneus

☑7ᵗʰ **S92.009** Unspecified fracture of unspecified calcaneus

☑6ᵗʰ **S92.01** Fracture of body of calcaneus

☑7ᵗʰ **S92.011** Displaced fracture of body of right calcaneus

☑7ᵗʰ **S92.012** Displaced fracture of body of left calcaneus

☑7ᵗʰ **S92.013** Displaced fracture of body of unspecified calcaneus

☑7ᵗʰ **S92.014** Nondisplaced fracture of body of right calcaneus

☑7ᵗʰ **S92.015** Nondisplaced fracture of body of left calcaneus

☑7ᵗʰ **S92.016** Nondisplaced fracture of body of unspecified calcaneus

☑6ᵗʰ **S92.02** Fracture of anterior process of calcaneus

☑7ᵗʰ **S92.021** Displaced fracture of anterior process of right calcaneus

☑7ᵗʰ **S92.022** Displaced fracture of anterior process of left calcaneus

☑7ᵗʰ **S92.023** Displaced fracture of anterior process of unspecified calcaneus

☑7ᵗʰ **S92.024** Nondisplaced fracture of anterior process of right calcaneus

☑7ᵗʰ **S92.025** Nondisplaced fracture of anterior process of left calcaneus

☑7ᵗʰ **S92.026** Nondisplaced fracture of anterior process of unspecified calcaneus

☑6ᵗʰ **S92.03** Avulsion fracture of tuberosity of calcaneus

☑7ᵗʰ **S92.031** Displaced avulsion fracture of tuberosity of right calcaneus

☑7ᵗʰ **S92.032** Displaced avulsion fracture of tuberosity of left calcaneus

☑7ᵗʰ **S92.033** Displaced avulsion fracture of tuberosity of unspecified calcaneus

☑7ᵗʰ **S92.034** Nondisplaced avulsion fracture of tuberosity of right calcaneus

☑7ᵗʰ **S92.035** Nondisplaced avulsion fracture of tuberosity of left calcaneus

☑7ᵗʰ **S92.036** Nondisplaced avulsion fracture of tuberosity of unspecified calcaneus

☑6ᵗʰ **S92.04** Other fracture of tuberosity of calcaneus

☑7ᵗʰ **S92.041** Displaced other fracture of tuberosity of right calcaneus

☑7ᵗʰ **S92.042** Displaced other fracture of tuberosity of left calcaneus

☑7ᵗʰ **S92.043** Displaced other fracture of tuberosity of unspecified calcaneus

☑7ᵗʰ **S92.044** Nondisplaced other fracture of tuberosity of right calcaneus

☑7ᵗʰ **S92.045** Nondisplaced other fracture of tuberosity of left calcaneus

☑7ᵗʰ **S92.046** Nondisplaced other fracture of tuberosity of unspecified calcaneus

☑6ᵗʰ **S92.05** Other extraarticular fracture of calcaneus

☑7ᵗʰ **S92.051** Displaced other extraarticular fracture of right calcaneus

☑7ᵗʰ **S92.052** Displaced other extraarticular fracture of left calcaneus

☑7ᵗʰ **S92.053** Displaced other extraarticular fracture of unspecified calcaneus

☑7ᵗʰ **S92.054** Nondisplaced other extraarticular fracture of right calcaneus

☑7ᵗʰ **S92.055** Nondisplaced other extraarticular fracture of left calcaneus

☑7ᵗʰ **S92.056** Nondisplaced other extraarticular fracture of unspecified calcaneus

☑6ᵗʰ **S92.06** Intraarticular fracture of calcaneus

☑7ᵗʰ **S92.061** Displaced intraarticular fracture of right calcaneus

☑7ᵗʰ **S92.062** Displaced intraarticular fracture of left calcaneus

☑7ᵗʰ **S92.063** Displaced intraarticular fracture of unspecified calcaneus

☑7ᵗʰ **S92.064** Nondisplaced intraarticular fracture of right calcaneus

☑7ᵗʰ **S92.065** Nondisplaced intraarticular fracture of left calcaneus

☑7ᵗʰ **S92.066** Nondisplaced intraarticular fracture of unspecified calcaneus

☑5ᵗʰ **S92.1** Fracture of talus
Astragalus

☑6ᵗʰ **S92.10** Unspecified fracture of talus

S92.101 Unspecified fracture of right talus

S92.102 Unspecified fracture of left talus

S92.109 Unspecified fracture of unspecified talus

☑6ᵗʰ **S92.11** Fracture of neck of talus

S92.111 Displaced fracture of neck of right talus

S92.112 Displaced fracture of neck of left talus

☑7ᵗʰ **S92.113** Displaced fracture of neck of unspecified talus

☑7ᵗʰ **S92.114** Nondisplaced fracture of neck of right talus

☑7ᵗʰ **S92.115** Nondisplaced fracture of neck of left talus

☑7ᵗʰ **S92.116** Nondisplaced fracture of neck of unspecified talus

☑6ᵗʰ **S92.12** Fracture of body of talus

☑7ᵗʰ **S92.121** Displaced fracture of body of right talus

☑7ᵗʰ **S92.122** Displaced fracture of body of left talus

☑7ᵗʰ **S92.123** Displaced fracture of body of unspecified talus

☑7ᵗʰ **S92.124** Nondisplaced fracture of body of right talus

☑7ᵗʰ **S92.125** Nondisplaced fracture of body of left talus

☑7ᵗʰ **S92.126** Nondisplaced fracture of body of unspecified talus

☑6ᵗʰ **S92.13** Fracture of posterior process of talus

☑7ᵗʰ **S92.131** Displaced fracture of posterior process of right talus

☑7ᵗʰ **S92.132** Displaced fracture of posterior process of left talus

☑7ᵗʰ **S92.133** Displaced fracture of posterior process of unspecified talus

☑7ᵗʰ **S92.134** Nondisplaced fracture of posterior process of right talus

☑7ᵗʰ **S92.135** Nondisplaced fracture of posterior process of left talus

☑ Additional Character Required   ✓ₓ7ᵗʰ Xtension Alert   Unspecified Dx   Other Specified Dx   Manifestation   ▶◀ Revised Text   ● New Code   ▲ Revised Code Title

ICD-10-CM Draft (2015)

913

Injury, Poisoning and Certain Other Consequences of External Causes   **S92.136–S92.336**

✓7th **S92.136** Nondisplaced fracture of posterior process of unspecified talus

✓6th **S92.14** Dome fracture of talus
> EXCLUDES 1   *osteochondritis dissecans (M93.2)*

   ✓7th **S92.141** Displaced dome fracture of right talus

   ✓7th **S92.142** Displaced dome fracture of left talus

   ✓7th **S92.143** Displaced dome fracture of unspecified talus

   ✓7th **S92.144** Nondisplaced dome fracture of right talus

   ✓7th **S92.145** Nondisplaced dome fracture of left talus

   ✓7th **S92.146** Nondisplaced dome fracture of unspecified talus

✓6th **S92.15** Avulsion fracture (chip fracture) of talus

   ✓7th **S92.151** Displaced avulsion fracture (chip fracture) of right talus

   ✓7th **S92.152** Displaced avulsion fracture (chip fracture) of left talus

   ✓7th **S92.153** Displaced avulsion fracture (chip fracture) of unspecified talus

   ✓7th **S92.154** Nondisplaced avulsion fracture (chip fracture) of right talus

   ✓7th **S92.155** Nondisplaced avulsion fracture (chip fracture) of left talus

   ✓7th **S92.156** Nondisplaced avulsion fracture (chip fracture) of unspecified talus

✓6th **S92.19** Other fracture of talus

   ✓7th **S92.191** Other fracture of right talus

   ✓7th **S92.192** Other fracture of left talus

   ✓7th **S92.199** Other fracture of unspecified talus

✓5th **S92.2** Fracture of other and unspecified tarsal bone(s)

  ✓6th **S92.20** Fracture of unspecified tarsal bone(s)

   ✓7th **S92.201** Fracture of unspecified tarsal bone(s) of right foot

   ✓7th **S92.202** Fracture of unspecified tarsal bone(s) of left foot

   ✓7th **S92.209** Fracture of unspecified tarsal bone(s) of unspecified foot

  ✓6th **S92.21** Fracture of cuboid bone

   ✓7th **S92.211** Displaced fracture of cuboid bone of right foot

   ✓7th **S92.212** Displaced fracture of cuboid bone of left foot

   ✓7th **S92.213** Displaced fracture of cuboid bone of unspecified foot

   ✓7th **S92.214** Nondisplaced fracture of cuboid bone of right foot

   ✓7th **S92.215** Nondisplaced fracture of cuboid bone of left foot

   ✓7th **S92.216** Nondisplaced fracture of cuboid bone of unspecified foot

  ✓6th **S92.22** Fracture of lateral cuneiform

   ✓7th **S92.221** Displaced fracture of lateral cuneiform of right foot

   ✓7th **S92.222** Displaced fracture of lateral cuneiform of left foot

   ✓7th **S92.223** Displaced fracture of lateral cuneiform of unspecified foot

   ✓7th **S92.224** Nondisplaced fracture of lateral cuneiform of right foot

   ✓7th **S92.225** Nondisplaced fracture of lateral cuneiform of left foot

   ✓7th **S92.226** Nondisplaced fracture of lateral cuneiform of unspecified foot

  ✓6th **S92.23** Fracture of intermediate cuneiform

   ✓7th **S92.231** Displaced fracture of intermediate cuneiform of right foot

   ✓7th **S92.232** Displaced fracture of intermediate cuneiform of left foot

   ✓7th **S92.233** Displaced fracture of intermediate cuneiform of unspecified foot

   ✓7th **S92.234** Nondisplaced fracture of intermediate cuneiform of right foot

   ✓7th **S92.235** Nondisplaced fracture of intermediate cuneiform of left foot

   ✓7th **S92.236** Nondisplaced fracture of intermediate cuneiform of unspecified foot

  ✓6th **S92.24** Fracture of medial cuneiform

   ✓7th **S92.241** Displaced fracture of medial cuneiform of right foot

   ✓7th **S92.242** Displaced fracture of medial cuneiform of left foot

   ✓7th **S92.243** Displaced fracture of medial cuneiform of unspecified foot

   ✓7th **S92.244** Nondisplaced fracture of medial cuneiform of right foot

   ✓7th **S92.245** Nondisplaced fracture of medial cuneiform of left foot

   ✓7th **S92.246** Nondisplaced fracture of medial cuneiform of unspecified foot

  ✓6th **S92.25** Fracture of navicular [scaphoid] of foot

   ✓7th **S92.251** Displaced fracture of navicular [scaphoid] of right foot

   ✓7th **S92.252** Displaced fracture of navicular [scaphoid] of left foot

   ✓7th **S92.253** Displaced fracture of navicular [scaphoid] of unspecified foot

   ✓7th **S92.254** Nondisplaced fracture of navicular [scaphoid] of right foot

   ✓7th **S92.255** Nondisplaced fracture of navicular [scaphoid] of left foot

   ✓7th **S92.256** Nondisplaced fracture of navicular [scaphoid] of unspecified foot

✓5th **S92.3** Fracture of metatarsal bone(s)

  ✓6th **S92.30** Fracture of unspecified metatarsal bone(s)

   ✓7th **S92.301** Fracture of unspecified metatarsal bone(s), right foot

   ✓7th **S92.302** Fracture of unspecified metatarsal bone(s), left foot

   ✓7th **S92.309** Fracture of unspecified metatarsal bone(s), unspecified foot

  ✓6th **S92.31** Fracture of first metatarsal bone

   ✓7th **S92.311** Displaced fracture of first metatarsal bone, right foot

   ✓7th **S92.312** Displaced fracture of first metatarsal bone, left foot

   ✓7th **S92.313** Displaced fracture of first metatarsal bone, unspecified foot

   ✓7th **S92.314** Nondisplaced fracture of first metatarsal bone, right foot

   ✓7th **S92.315** Nondisplaced fracture of first metatarsal bone, left foot

   ✓7th **S92.316** Nondisplaced fracture of first metatarsal bone, unspecified foot

  ✓6th **S92.32** Fracture of second metatarsal bone

   ✓7th **S92.321** Displaced fracture of second metatarsal bone, right foot

   ✓7th **S92.322** Displaced fracture of second metatarsal bone, left foot

   ✓7th **S92.323** Displaced fracture of second metatarsal bone, unspecified foot

   ✓7th **S92.324** Nondisplaced fracture of second metatarsal bone, right foot

   ✓7th **S92.325** Nondisplaced fracture of second metatarsal bone, left foot

   ✓7th **S92.326** Nondisplaced fracture of second metatarsal bone, unspecified foot

  ✓6th **S92.33** Fracture of third metatarsal bone

   ✓7th **S92.331** Displaced fracture of third metatarsal bone, right foot

   ✓7th **S92.332** Displaced fracture of third metatarsal bone, left foot

   ✓7th **S92.333** Displaced fracture of third metatarsal bone, unspecified foot

   ✓7th **S92.334** Nondisplaced fracture of third metatarsal bone, right foot

   ✓7th **S92.335** Nondisplaced fracture of third metatarsal bone, left foot

   ✓7th **S92.336** Nondisplaced fracture of third metatarsal bone, unspecified foot

---

EXCLUDES 1 Not coded here   EXCLUDES 2 Not included here   N Newborn Age: 0   P Pediatric Age: 0-17   M Maternity Age: 12-55   A Adult Age: 15-124

Injury, Poisoning and Certain Other Consequences of External Causes   S92.34–S92.919

✓6th **S92.34** Fracture of fourth metatarsal bone
- ✓7th **S92.341** Displaced fracture of fourth metatarsal bone, right foot
- ✓7th **S92.342** Displaced fracture of fourth metatarsal bone, left foot
- ✓7th **S92.343** Displaced fracture of fourth metatarsal bone, unspecified foot
- ✓7th **S92.344** Nondisplaced fracture of fourth metatarsal bone, right foot
- ✓7th **S92.345** Nondisplaced fracture of fourth metatarsal bone, left foot
- ✓7th **S92.346** Nondisplaced fracture of fourth metatarsal bone, unspecified foot

✓6th **S92.35** Fracture of fifth metatarsal bone
- ✓7th **S92.351** Displaced fracture of fifth metatarsal bone, right foot
- ✓7th **S92.352** Displaced fracture of fifth metatarsal bone, left foot
- ✓7th **S92.353** Displaced fracture of fifth metatarsal bone, unspecified foot
- ✓7th **S92.354** Nondisplaced fracture of fifth metatarsal bone, right foot
- ✓7th **S92.355** Nondisplaced fracture of fifth metatarsal bone, left foot
- ✓7th **S92.356** Nondisplaced fracture of fifth metatarsal bone, unspecified foot

✓5th **S92.4** Fracture of great toe
- ✓6th **S92.40** Unspecified fracture of great toe
  - ✓7th **S92.401** Displaced unspecified fracture of right great toe
  - ✓7th **S92.402** Displaced unspecified fracture of left great toe
  - ✓7th **S92.403** Displaced unspecified fracture of unspecified great toe
  - ✓7th **S92.404** Nondisplaced unspecified fracture of right great toe
  - ✓7th **S92.405** Nondisplaced unspecified fracture of left great toe
  - ✓7th **S92.406** Nondisplaced unspecified fracture of unspecified great toe
- ✓6th **S92.41** Fracture of proximal phalanx of great toe
  - ✓7th **S92.411** Displaced fracture of proximal phalanx of right great toe
  - ✓7th **S92.412** Displaced fracture of proximal phalanx of left great toe
  - ✓7th **S92.413** Displaced fracture of proximal phalanx of unspecified great toe
  - ✓7th **S92.414** Nondisplaced fracture of proximal phalanx of right great toe
  - ✓7th **S92.415** Nondisplaced fracture of proximal phalanx of left great toe
  - ✓7th **S92.416** Nondisplaced fracture of proximal phalanx of unspecified great toe
- ✓6th **S92.42** Fracture of distal phalanx of great toe
  - ✓7th **S92.421** Displaced fracture of distal phalanx of right great toe
  - ✓7th **S92.422** Displaced fracture of distal phalanx of left great toe
  - ✓7th **S92.423** Displaced fracture of distal phalanx of unspecified great toe
  - ✓7th **S92.424** Nondisplaced fracture of distal phalanx of right great toe
  - ✓7th **S92.425** Nondisplaced fracture of distal phalanx of left great toe
  - ✓7th **S92.426** Nondisplaced fracture of distal phalanx of unspecified great toe
- ✓6th **S92.49** Other fracture of great toe
  - ✓7th **S92.491** Other fracture of right great toe
  - ✓7th **S92.492** Other fracture of left great toe
  - ✓7th **S92.499** Other fracture of unspecified great toe

✓5th **S92.5** Fracture of lesser toe(s)
- ✓6th **S92.50** Unspecified fracture of lesser toe(s)
  - ✓7th **S92.501** Displaced unspecified fracture of right lesser toe(s)
  - ✓7th **S92.502** Displaced unspecified fracture of left lesser toe(s)
  - ✓7th **S92.503** Displaced unspecified fracture of unspecified lesser toe(s)
  - ✓7th **S92.504** Nondisplaced unspecified fracture of right lesser toe(s)
  - ✓7th **S92.505** Nondisplaced unspecified fracture of left lesser toe(s)
  - ✓7th **S92.506** Nondisplaced unspecified fracture of unspecified lesser toe(s)
- ✓6th **S92.51** Fracture of proximal phalanx of lesser toe(s)
  - ✓7th **S92.511** Displaced fracture of proximal phalanx of right lesser toe(s)
  - ✓7th **S92.512** Displaced fracture of proximal phalanx of left lesser toe(s)
  - ✓7th **S92.513** Displaced fracture of proximal phalanx of unspecified lesser toe(s)
  - ✓7th **S92.514** Nondisplaced fracture of proximal phalanx of right lesser toe(s)
  - ✓7th **S92.515** Nondisplaced fracture of proximal phalanx of left lesser toe(s)
  - ✓7th **S92.516** Nondisplaced fracture of proximal phalanx of unspecified lesser toe(s)
- ✓6th **S92.52** Fracture of medial phalanx of lesser toe(s)
  - ✓7th **S92.521** Displaced fracture of medial phalanx of right lesser toe(s)
  - ✓7th **S92.522** Displaced fracture of medial phalanx of left lesser toe(s)
  - ✓7th **S92.523** Displaced fracture of medial phalanx of unspecified lesser toe(s)
  - ✓7th **S92.524** Nondisplaced fracture of medial phalanx of right lesser toe(s)
  - ✓7th **S92.525** Nondisplaced fracture of medial phalanx of left lesser toe(s)
  - ✓7th **S92.526** Nondisplaced fracture of medial phalanx of unspecified lesser toe(s)
- ✓6th **S92.53** Fracture of distal phalanx of lesser toe(s)
  - ✓7th **S92.531** Displaced fracture of distal phalanx of right lesser toe(s)
  - ✓7th **S92.532** Displaced fracture of distal phalanx of left lesser toe(s)
  - ✓7th **S92.533** Displaced fracture of distal phalanx of unspecified lesser toe(s)
  - ✓7th **S92.534** Nondisplaced fracture of distal phalanx of right lesser toe(s)
  - ✓7th **S92.535** Nondisplaced fracture of distal phalanx of left lesser toe(s)
  - ✓7th **S92.536** Nondisplaced fracture of distal phalanx of unspecified lesser toe(s)
- ✓6th **S92.59** Other fracture of lesser toe(s)
  - ✓7th **S92.591** Other fracture of right lesser toe(s)
  - ✓7th **S92.592** Other fracture of left lesser toe(s)
  - ✓7th **S92.599** Other fracture of unspecified lesser toe(s)

✓5th **S92.9** Unspecified fracture of foot and toe
- ✓6th **S92.90** Unspecified fracture of foot
  - ✓7th **S92.901** Unspecified fracture of right foot
  - ✓7th **S92.902** Unspecified fracture of left foot
  - ✓7th **S92.909** Unspecified fracture of unspecified foot
- ✓6th **S92.91** Unspecified fracture of toe
  - ✓7th **S92.911** Unspecified fracture of right toe(s)
  - ✓7th **S92.912** Unspecified fracture of left toe(s)
  - ✓7th **S92.919** Unspecified fracture of unspecified toe(s)

☑ Additional Character Required   ✓x7th Xtension Alert   Unspecified Dx   Other Specified Dx   Manifestation   ▶◀ Revised Text   ● New Code   ▲ Revised Code Title

Injury, Poisoning and Certain Other Consequences of External Causes

S93–S93.336

√4th **S93** **Dislocation and sprain of joints and ligaments at ankle, foot and toe level**

INCLUDES   avulsion of joint or ligament of ankle, foot and toe
laceration of cartilage, joint or ligament of ankle, foot and toe
sprain of cartilage, joint or ligament of ankle, foot and toe
traumatic hemarthrosis of joint or ligament of ankle, foot and toe
traumatic rupture of joint or ligament of ankle, foot and toe
traumatic subluxation of joint or ligament of ankle, foot and toe
traumatic tear of joint or ligament of ankle, foot and toe

Code also any associated open wound

EXCLUDES 2   strain of muscle and tendon of ankle and foot (S96.-)

The appropriate 7th character is to be added to each code from category S93.
A   initial encounter
D   subsequent encounter
S   sequela

√5th **S93.0 Subluxation and dislocation of** ankle joint
Subluxation and dislocation of astragalus
Subluxation and dislocation of fibula, lower end
Subluxation and dislocation of talus
Subluxation and dislocation of tibia, lower end

√x7th   **S93.01** Subluxation of right ankle joint
√x7th   **S93.02** Subluxation of left ankle joint
√x7th   **S93.03** Subluxation of unspecified ankle joint
√x7th   **S93.04** Dislocation of right ankle joint
√x7th   **S93.05** Dislocation of left ankle joint
√x7th   **S93.06** Dislocation of unspecified ankle joint

√5th **S93.1 Subluxation and dislocation of** toe

√6th   **S93.10** Unspecified subluxation and dislocation of toe
Dislocation of toe NOS
Subluxation of toe NOS

√7th   **S93.101** Unspecified subluxation of right toe(s)
√7th   **S93.102** Unspecified subluxation of left toe(s)
√7th   **S93.103** Unspecified subluxation of unspecified toe(s)
√7th   **S93.104** Unspecified dislocation of right toe(s)
√7th   **S93.105** Unspecified dislocation of left toe(s)
√7th   **S93.106** Unspecified dislocation of unspecified toe(s)

√6th   **S93.11** Dislocation of interphalangeal joint

√7th   **S93.111** Dislocation of interphalangeal joint of right great toe
√7th   **S93.112** Dislocation of interphalangeal joint of left great toe
√7th   **S93.113** Dislocation of interphalangeal joint of unspecified great toe
√7th   **S93.114** Dislocation of interphalangeal joint of right lesser toe(s)
√7th   **S93.115** Dislocation of interphalangeal joint of left lesser toe(s)
√7th   **S93.116** Dislocation of interphalangeal joint of unspecified lesser toe(s)
√7th   **S93.119** Dislocation of interphalangeal joint of unspecified toe(s)

√6th   **S93.12** Dislocation of metatarsophalangeal joint

√7th   **S93.121** Dislocation of metatarsophalangeal joint of right great toe
√7th   **S93.122** Dislocation of metatarsophalangeal joint of left great toe
√7th   **S93.123** Dislocation of metatarsophalangeal joint of unspecified great toe
√7th   **S93.124** Dislocation of metatarsophalangeal joint of right lesser toe(s)
√7th   **S93.125** Dislocation of metatarsophalangeal joint of left lesser toe(s)
√7th   **S93.126** Dislocation of metatarsophalangeal joint of unspecified lesser toe(s)
√7th   **S93.129** Dislocation of metatarsophalangeal joint of unspecified toe(s)

√6th   **S93.13** Subluxation of interphalangeal joint

√7th   **S93.131** Subluxation of interphalangeal joint of right great toe
√7th   **S93.132** Subluxation of interphalangeal joint of left great toe
√7th   **S93.133** Subluxation of interphalangeal joint of unspecified great toe
√7th   **S93.134** Subluxation of interphalangeal joint of right lesser toe(s)
√7th   **S93.135** Subluxation of interphalangeal joint of left lesser toe(s)
√7th   **S93.136** Subluxation of interphalangeal joint of unspecified lesser toe(s)
√7th   **S93.139** Subluxation of interphalangeal joint of unspecified toe(s)

√6th   **S93.14** Subluxation of metatarsophalangeal joint

√7th   **S93.141** Subluxation of metatarsophalangeal joint of right great toe
√7th   **S93.142** Subluxation of metatarsophalangeal joint of left great toe
√7th   **S93.143** Subluxation of metatarsophalangeal joint of unspecified great toe
√7th   **S93.144** Subluxation of metatarsophalangeal joint of right lesser toe(s)
√7th   **S93.145** Subluxation of metatarsophalangeal joint of left lesser toe(s)
√7th   **S93.146** Subluxation of metatarsophalangeal joint of unspecified lesser toe(s)
√7th   **S93.149** Subluxation of metatarsophalangeal joint of unspecified toe(s)

√5th **S93.3 Subluxation and dislocation of** foot
EXCLUDES 2   dislocation of toe (S93.1-)

√6th   **S93.30** Unspecified subluxation and dislocation of foot
Dislocation of foot NOS
Subluxation of foot NOS

√7th   **S93.301** Unspecified subluxation of right foot
√7th   **S93.302** Unspecified subluxation of left foot
√7th   **S93.303** Unspecified subluxation of unspecified foot
√7th   **S93.304** Unspecified dislocation of right foot
√7th   **S93.305** Unspecified dislocation of left foot
√7th   **S93.306** Unspecified dislocation of unspecified foot

√6th   **S93.31** Subluxation and dislocation of tarsal joint

√7th   **S93.311** Subluxation of tarsal joint of right foot
√7th   **S93.312** Subluxation of tarsal joint of left foot
√7th   **S93.313** Subluxation of tarsal joint of unspecified foot
√7th   **S93.314** Dislocation of tarsal joint of right foot
√7th   **S93.315** Dislocation of tarsal joint of left foot
√7th   **S93.316** Dislocation of tarsal joint of unspecified foot

√6th   **S93.32** Subluxation and dislocation of tarsometatarsal joint

√7th   **S93.321** Subluxation of tarsometatarsal joint of right foot
√7th   **S93.322** Subluxation of tarsometatarsal joint of left foot
√7th   **S93.323** Subluxation of tarsometatarsal joint of unspecified foot
√7th   **S93.324** Dislocation of tarsometatarsal joint of right foot
√7th   **S93.325** Dislocation of tarsometatarsal joint of left foot
√7th   **S93.326** Dislocation of tarsometatarsal joint of unspecified foot

√6th   **S93.33** Other subluxation and dislocation of foot

√7th   **S93.331** Other subluxation of right foot
√7th   **S93.332** Other subluxation of left foot
√7th   **S93.333** Other subluxation of unspecified foot
√7th   **S93.334** Other dislocation of right foot
√7th   **S93.335** Other dislocation of left foot
√7th   **S93.336** Other dislocation of unspecified foot

EXCLUDES 1 Not coded here   **EXCLUDES 2** Not included here   **N** Newborn Age: 0   **P** Pediatric Age: 0-17   **M** Maternity Age: 12-55   **A** Adult Age: 15-124

916   ICD-10-CM Draft (2015)

✓5th **S93.4 Sprain of** ankle

    EXCLUDES 2 *injury of Achilles tendon (S86.0-)*

  ✓6th **S93.40 Sprain of** unspecified **ligament of ankle**
      Sprain of ankle NOS
      Sprained ankle NOS

    ✓7th **S93.401 Sprain of unspecified ligament of** right **ankle**

    ✓7th **S93.402 Sprain of unspecified ligament of** left **ankle**

    ✓7th **S93.409 Sprain of unspecified ligament of unspecified ankle**

  ✓6th **S93.41 Sprain of** calcaneofibular **ligament**

    ✓7th **S93.411 Sprain of calcaneofibular ligament of** right **ankle**

    ✓7th **S93.412 Sprain of calcaneofibular ligament of** left **ankle**

    ✓7th **S93.419 Sprain of calcaneofibular ligament of unspecified ankle**

  ✓6th **S93.42 Sprain of** deltoid **ligament**

    ✓7th **S93.421 Sprain of deltoid ligament of** right **ankle**

    ✓7th **S93.422 Sprain of deltoid ligament of** left **ankle**

    ✓7th **S93.429 Sprain of deltoid ligament of unspecified ankle**

  ✓6th **S93.43 Sprain of** tibiofibular **ligament**

    ✓7th **S93.431 Sprain of tibiofibular ligament of** right **ankle**

    ✓7th **S93.432 Sprain of tibiofibular ligament of** left **ankle**

    ✓7th **S93.439 Sprain of tibiofibular ligament of unspecified ankle**

  ✓6th **S93.49 Sprain of** other **ligament of ankle**
      Sprain of internal collateral ligament
      Sprain of talofibular ligament

    ✓7th **S93.491 Sprain of other ligament of** right **ankle**

    ✓7th **S93.492 Sprain of other ligament of** left **ankle**

    ✓7th **S93.499 Sprain of other ligament of unspecified ankle**

✓5th **S93.5 Sprain of** toe

  ✓6th **S93.50 Unspecified sprain of toe**

    ✓7th **S93.501 Unspecified sprain of** right great **toe**

    ✓7th **S93.502 Unspecified sprain of** left great **toe**

    ✓7th **S93.503 Unspecified sprain of unspecified great toe**

    ✓7th **S93.504 Unspecified sprain of** right lesser **toe(s)**

    ✓7th **S93.505 Unspecified sprain of** left lesser **toe(s)**

    ✓7th **S93.506 Unspecified sprain of unspecified lesser toe(s)**

    ✓7th **S93.509 Unspecified sprain of unspecified toe(s)**

  ✓6th **S93.51 Sprain of** interphalangeal joint **of toe**

    ✓7th **S93.511 Sprain of interphalangeal joint of** right **great toe**

    ✓7th **S93.512 Sprain of interphalangeal joint of** left **great toe**

    ✓7th **S93.513 Sprain of interphalangeal joint of unspecified great toe**

    ✓7th **S93.514 Sprain of interphalangeal joint of** right **lesser toe(s)**

    ✓7th **S93.515 Sprain of interphalangeal joint of** left **lesser toe(s)**

    ✓7th **S93.516 Sprain of interphalangeal joint of unspecified lesser toe(s)**

    ✓7th **S93.519 Sprain of interphalangeal joint of unspecified toe(s)**

  ✓6th **S93.52 Sprain of** metatarsophalangeal joint **of toe**

    ✓7th **S93.521 Sprain of metatarsophalangeal joint of** right great **toe**

    ✓7th **S93.522 Sprain of metatarsophalangeal joint of** left great **toe**

    ✓7th **S93.523 Sprain of metatarsophalangeal joint of unspecified great toe**

    ✓7th **S93.524 Sprain of metatarsophalangeal joint of** right lesser **toe(s)**

    ✓7th **S93.525 Sprain of metatarsophalangeal joint of** left lesser **toe(s)**

    ✓7th **S93.526 Sprain of metatarsophalangeal joint of unspecified lesser toe(s)**

    ✓7th **S93.529 Sprain of metatarsophalangeal joint of unspecified toe(s)**

✓5th **S93.6 Sprain of** foot

    EXCLUDES 2 *sprain of metatarsophalangeal joint of toe (S93.52-)*
              sprain of toe (S93.5-)

  ✓6th **S93.60 Unspecified sprain of foot**

    ✓7th **S93.601 Unspecified sprain of** right **foot**

    ✓7th **S93.602 Unspecified sprain of** left **foot**

    ✓7th **S93.609 Unspecified sprain of unspecified foot**

  ✓6th **S93.61 Sprain of** tarsal ligament **of foot**

    ✓7th **S93.611 Sprain of tarsal ligament of** right **foot**

    ✓7th **S93.612 Sprain of tarsal ligament of** left **foot**

    ✓7th **S93.619 Sprain of tarsal ligament of unspecified foot**

  ✓6th **S93.62 Sprain of** tarsometatarsal ligament **of foot**

    ✓7th **S93.621 Sprain of tarsometatarsal ligament of** right **foot**

    ✓7th **S93.622 Sprain of tarsometatarsal ligament of** left **foot**

    ✓7th **S93.629 Sprain of tarsometatarsal ligament of unspecified foot**

  ✓6th **S93.69 Other sprain of foot**

    ✓7th **S93.691 Other sprain of** right **foot**

    ✓7th **S93.692 Other sprain of** left **foot**

    ✓7th **S93.699 Other sprain of unspecified foot**

✓4th **S94 Injury of nerves at ankle and foot level**
    Code also any associated open wound (S91.-)

    The appropriate 7th character is to be added to each code from category S94.
    A   initial encounter
    D   subsequent encounter
    S   sequela

  ✓5th **S94.0 Injury of** lateral plantar **nerve**

    ✓x7th **S94.00 Injury of lateral plantar nerve, unspecified leg**

    ✓x7th **S94.01 Injury of lateral plantar nerve,** right **leg**

    ✓x7th **S94.02 Injury of lateral plantar nerve,** left **leg**

  ✓5th **S94.1 Injury of** medial plantar **nerve**

    ✓x7th **S94.10 Injury of medial plantar nerve, unspecified leg**

    ✓x7th **S94.11 Injury of medial plantar nerve,** right **leg**

    ✓x7th **S94.12 Injury of medial plantar nerve,** left **leg**

  ✓5th **S94.2 Injury of** deep peroneal **nerve at ankle and foot level**
      Injury of terminal, lateral branch of deep peroneal nerve

    ✓x7th **S94.20 Injury of deep peroneal nerve at ankle and foot level, unspecified leg**

    ✓x7th **S94.21 Injury of deep peroneal nerve at ankle and foot level,** right **leg**

    ✓x7th **S94.22 Injury of deep peroneal nerve at ankle and foot level,** left **leg**

  ✓5th **S94.3 Injury of** cutaneous sensory **nerve at ankle and foot level**

    ✓x7th **S94.30 Injury of cutaneous sensory nerve at ankle and foot level, unspecified leg**

    ✓x7th **S94.31 Injury of cutaneous sensory nerve at ankle and foot level,** right **leg**

    ✓x7th **S94.32 Injury of cutaneous sensory nerve at ankle and foot level,** left **leg**

  ✓5th **S94.8 Injury of** other **nerves at ankle and foot level**

    ✓6th **S94.8X Injury of other nerves at ankle and foot level**

      ✓7th **S94.8X1 Injury of other nerves at ankle and foot level,** right **leg**

      ✓7th **S94.8X2 Injury of other nerves at ankle and foot level,** left **leg**

      ✓7th **S94.8X9 Injury of other nerves at ankle and foot level, unspecified leg**

  ✓5th **S94.9 Injury of** unspecified **nerve at ankle and foot level**

✓ Additional Character Required   ✓x7th Xtension Alert   Unspecified Dx   Other Specified Dx   Manifestation   ▶◀ Revised Text   ● New Code   ▲ Revised Code Title

√×7ᵗʰ **S94.90** **Injury of unspecified nerve at ankle and foot level, unspecified leg**

√×7ᵗʰ **S94.91** **Injury of unspecified nerve at ankle and foot level, right leg**

√×7ᵗʰ **S94.92** **Injury of unspecified nerve at ankle and foot level, left leg**

√4ᵗʰ **S95** **Injury of blood vessels at ankle and foot level**

Code also any associated open wound (S91.-)

EXCLUDES 2   injury of posterior tibial artery and vein (S85.1-, S85.8-)

> The appropriate 7th character is to be added to each code from category S95.
> A   initial encounter
> D   subsequent encounter
> S   sequela

√5ᵗʰ **S95.0** **Injury of dorsal artery of foot**

√6ᵗʰ **S95.00** **Unspecified injury of dorsal artery of foot**

√7ᵗʰ **S95.001** **Unspecified injury of dorsal artery of right foot**

√7ᵗʰ **S95.002** **Unspecified injury of dorsal artery of left foot**

√7ᵗʰ **S95.009** **Unspecified injury of dorsal artery of unspecified foot**

√6ᵗʰ **S95.01** **Laceration of dorsal artery of foot**

√7ᵗʰ **S95.011** **Laceration of dorsal artery of right foot**

√7ᵗʰ **S95.012** **Laceration of dorsal artery of left foot**

√7ᵗʰ **S95.019** **Laceration of dorsal artery of unspecified foot**

√6ᵗʰ **S95.09** **Other specified injury of dorsal artery of foot**

√7ᵗʰ **S95.091** **Other specified injury of dorsal artery of right foot**

√7ᵗʰ **S95.092** **Other specified injury of dorsal artery of left foot**

√7ᵗʰ **S95.099** **Other specified injury of dorsal artery of unspecified foot**

√5ᵗʰ **S95.1** **Injury of plantar artery of foot**

√6ᵗʰ **S95.10** **Unspecified injury of plantar artery of foot**

√7ᵗʰ **S95.101** **Unspecified injury of plantar artery of right foot**

√7ᵗʰ **S95.102** **Unspecified injury of plantar artery of left foot**

√7ᵗʰ **S95.109** **Unspecified injury of plantar artery of unspecified foot**

√6ᵗʰ **S95.11** **Laceration of plantar artery of foot**

√7ᵗʰ **S95.111** **Laceration of plantar artery of right foot**

√7ᵗʰ **S95.112** **Laceration of plantar artery of left foot**

√7ᵗʰ **S95.119** **Laceration of plantar artery of unspecified foot**

√6ᵗʰ **S95.19** **Other specified injury of plantar artery of foot**

√7ᵗʰ **S95.191** **Other specified injury of plantar artery of right foot**

√7ᵗʰ **S95.192** **Other specified injury of plantar artery of left foot**

√7ᵗʰ **S95.199** **Other specified injury of plantar artery of unspecified foot**

√5ᵗʰ **S95.2** **Injury of dorsal vein of foot**

√6ᵗʰ **S95.20** **Unspecified injury of dorsal vein of foot**

√7ᵗʰ **S95.201** **Unspecified injury of dorsal vein of right foot**

√7ᵗʰ **S95.202** **Unspecified injury of dorsal vein of left foot**

√7ᵗʰ **S95.209** **Unspecified injury of dorsal vein of unspecified foot**

√6ᵗʰ **S95.21** **Laceration of dorsal vein of foot**

√7ᵗʰ **S95.211** **Laceration of dorsal vein of right foot**

√7ᵗʰ **S95.212** **Laceration of dorsal vein of left foot**

√7ᵗʰ **S95.219** **Laceration of dorsal vein of unspecified foot**

√6ᵗʰ **S95.29** **Other specified injury of dorsal vein of foot**

√7ᵗʰ **S95.291** **Other specified injury of dorsal vein of right foot**

√7ᵗʰ **S95.292** **Other specified injury of dorsal vein of left foot**

√7ᵗʰ **S95.299** **Other specified injury of dorsal vein of unspecified foot**

√5ᵗʰ **S95.8** **Injury of other blood vessels at ankle and foot level**

√6ᵗʰ **S95.80** **Unspecified injury of other blood vessels at ankle and foot level**

√7ᵗʰ **S95.801** **Unspecified injury of other blood vessels at ankle and foot level, right leg**

√7ᵗʰ **S95.802** **Unspecified injury of other blood vessels at ankle and foot level, left leg**

√7ᵗʰ **S95.809** **Unspecified injury of other blood vessels at ankle and foot level, unspecified leg**

√6ᵗʰ **S95.81** **Laceration of other blood vessels at ankle and foot level**

√7ᵗʰ **S95.811** **Laceration of other blood vessels at ankle and foot level, right leg**

√7ᵗʰ **S95.812** **Laceration of other blood vessels at ankle and foot level, left leg**

√7ᵗʰ **S95.819** **Laceration of other blood vessels at ankle and foot level, unspecified leg**

√6ᵗʰ **S95.89** **Other specified injury of other blood vessels at ankle and foot level**

√7ᵗʰ **S95.891** **Other specified injury of other blood vessels at ankle and foot level, right leg**

√7ᵗʰ **S95.892** **Other specified injury of other blood vessels at ankle and foot level, left leg**

√7ᵗʰ **S95.899** **Other specified injury of other blood vessels at ankle and foot level, unspecified leg**

√5ᵗʰ **S95.9** **Injury of unspecified blood vessel at ankle and foot level**

√6ᵗʰ **S95.90** **Unspecified injury of unspecified blood vessel at ankle and foot level**

√7ᵗʰ **S95.901** **Unspecified injury of unspecified blood vessel at ankle and foot level, right leg**

√7ᵗʰ **S95.902** **Unspecified injury of unspecified blood vessel at ankle and foot level, left leg**

√7ᵗʰ **S95.909** **Unspecified injury of unspecified blood vessel at ankle and foot level, unspecified leg**

√6ᵗʰ **S95.91** **Laceration of unspecified blood vessel at ankle and foot level**

√7ᵗʰ **S95.911** **Laceration of unspecified blood vessel at ankle and foot level, right leg**

√7ᵗʰ **S95.912** **Laceration of unspecified blood vessel at ankle and foot level, left leg**

√7ᵗʰ **S95.919** **Laceration of unspecified blood vessel at ankle and foot level, unspecified leg**

√6ᵗʰ **S95.99** **Other specified injury of unspecified blood vessel at ankle and foot level**

√7ᵗʰ **S95.991** **Other specified injury of unspecified blood vessel at ankle and foot level, right leg**

√7ᵗʰ **S95.992** **Other specified injury of unspecified blood vessel at ankle and foot level, left leg**

√7ᵗʰ **S95.999** **Other specified injury of unspecified blood vessel at ankle and foot level, unspecified leg**

√4ᵗʰ **S96** **Injury of muscle and tendon at ankle and foot level**

Code also any associated open wound (S91.-)

EXCLUDES 2   injury of Achilles tendon (S86.0-)
               sprain of joints and ligaments of ankle and foot (S93.-)

> The appropriate 7th character is to be added to each code from category S96.
> A   initial encounter
> D   subsequent encounter
> S   sequela

√5ᵗʰ **S96.0** **Injury of muscle and tendon of long flexor muscle of toe at ankle and foot level**

√6ᵗʰ **S96.00** **Unspecified injury of muscle and tendon of long flexor muscle of toe at ankle and foot level**

√7ᵗʰ **S96.001** **Unspecified injury of muscle and tendon of long flexor muscle of toe at ankle and foot level, right foot**

√7ᵗʰ **S96.002** **Unspecified injury of muscle and tendon of long flexor muscle of toe at ankle and foot level, left foot**

EXCLUDES 1 Not coded here   EXCLUDES 2 Not included here   N Newborn Age: 0   P Pediatric Age: 0-17   M Maternity Age: 12-55   A Adult Age: 15-124

918   ICD-10-CM Draft (2015)

√7th **S96.009** Unspecified injury of muscle and tendon of long flexor muscle of toe at ankle and foot level, unspecified foot

√6th **S96.01** Strain of muscle and tendon of long flexor muscle of toe at ankle and foot level

√7th **S96.011** Strain of muscle and tendon of long flexor muscle of toe at ankle and foot level, right foot

√7th **S96.012** Strain of muscle and tendon of long flexor muscle of toe at ankle and foot level, left foot

√7th **S96.019** Strain of muscle and tendon of long flexor muscle of toe at ankle and foot level, unspecified foot

√6th **S96.02** Laceration of muscle and tendon of long flexor muscle of toe at ankle and foot level

√7th **S96.021** Laceration of muscle and tendon of long flexor muscle of toe at ankle and foot level, right foot

√7th **S96.022** Laceration of muscle and tendon of long flexor muscle of toe at ankle and foot level, left foot

√7th **S96.029** Laceration of muscle and tendon of long flexor muscle of toe at ankle and foot level, unspecified foot

√6th **S96.09** Other injury of muscle and tendon of long flexor muscle of toe at ankle and foot level

√7th **S96.091** Other injury of muscle and tendon of long flexor muscle of toe at ankle and foot level, right foot

√7th **S96.092** Other injury of muscle and tendon of long flexor muscle of toe at ankle and foot level, left foot

√7th **S96.099** Other injury of muscle and tendon of long flexor muscle of toe at ankle and foot level, unspecified foot

√5th **S96.1** Injury of muscle and tendon of long extensor muscle of toe at ankle and foot level

√6th **S96.10** Unspecified injury of muscle and tendon of long extensor muscle of toe at ankle and foot level

√7th **S96.101** Unspecified injury of muscle and tendon of long extensor muscle of toe at ankle and foot level, right foot

√7th **S96.102** Unspecified injury of muscle and tendon of long extensor muscle of toe at ankle and foot level, left foot

√7th **S96.109** Unspecified injury of muscle and tendon of long extensor muscle of toe at ankle and foot level, unspecified foot

√6th **S96.11** Strain of muscle and tendon of long extensor muscle of toe at ankle and foot level

√7th **S96.111** Strain of muscle and tendon of long extensor muscle of toe at ankle and foot level, right foot

√7th **S96.112** Strain of muscle and tendon of long extensor muscle of toe at ankle and foot level, left foot

√7th **S96.119** Strain of muscle and tendon of long extensor muscle of toe at ankle and foot level, unspecified foot

√6th **S96.12** Laceration of muscle and tendon of long extensor muscle of toe at ankle and foot level

√7th **S96.121** Laceration of muscle and tendon of long extensor muscle of toe at ankle and foot level, right foot

√7th **S96.122** Laceration of muscle and tendon of long extensor muscle of toe at ankle and foot level, left foot

√7th **S96.129** Laceration of muscle and tendon of long extensor muscle of toe at ankle and foot level, unspecified foot

√6th **S96.19** Other specified injury of muscle and tendon of long extensor muscle of toe at ankle and foot level

√7th **S96.191** Other specified injury of muscle and tendon of long extensor muscle of toe at ankle and foot level, right foot

√7th **S96.192** Other specified injury of muscle and tendon of long extensor muscle of toe at ankle and foot level, left foot

√7th **S96.199** Other specified injury of muscle and tendon of long extensor muscle of toe at ankle and foot level, unspecified foot

√5th **S96.2** Injury of intrinsic muscle and tendon at ankle and foot level

√6th **S96.20** Unspecified injury of intrinsic muscle and tendon at ankle and foot level

√7th **S96.201** Unspecified injury of intrinsic muscle and tendon at ankle and foot level, right foot

√7th **S96.202** Unspecified injury of intrinsic muscle and tendon at ankle and foot level, left foot

√7th **S96.209** Unspecified injury of intrinsic muscle and tendon at ankle and foot level, unspecified foot

√6th **S96.21** Strain of intrinsic muscle and tendon at ankle and foot level

√7th **S96.211** Strain of intrinsic muscle and tendon at ankle and foot level, right foot

√7th **S96.212** Strain of intrinsic muscle and tendon at ankle and foot level, left foot

√7th **S96.219** Strain of intrinsic muscle and tendon at ankle and foot level, unspecified foot

√6th **S96.22** Laceration of intrinsic muscle and tendon at ankle and foot level

√7th **S96.221** Laceration of intrinsic muscle and tendon at ankle and foot level, right foot

√7th **S96.222** Laceration of intrinsic muscle and tendon at ankle and foot level, left foot

√7th **S96.229** Laceration of intrinsic muscle and tendon at ankle and foot level, unspecified foot

√6th **S96.29** Other specified injury of intrinsic muscle and tendon at ankle and foot level

√7th **S96.291** Other specified injury of intrinsic muscle and tendon at ankle and foot level, right foot

√7th **S96.292** Other specified injury of intrinsic muscle and tendon at ankle and foot level, left foot

√7th **S96.299** Other specified injury of intrinsic muscle and tendon at ankle and foot level, unspecified foot

√5th **S96.8** Injury of other specified muscles and tendons at ankle and foot level

√6th **S96.80** Unspecified injury of other specified muscles and tendons at ankle and foot level

√7th **S96.801** Unspecified injury of other specified muscles and tendons at ankle and foot level, right foot

√7th **S96.802** Unspecified injury of other specified muscles and tendons at ankle and foot level, left foot

√7th **S96.809** Unspecified injury of other specified muscles and tendons at ankle and foot level, unspecified foot

√6th **S96.81** Strain of other specified muscles and tendons at ankle and foot level

√7th **S96.811** Strain of other specified muscles and tendons at ankle and foot level, right foot

√7th **S96.812** Strain of other specified muscles and tendons at ankle and foot level, left foot

√7th **S96.819** Strain of other specified muscles and tendons at ankle and foot level, unspecified foot

√6th **S96.82** Laceration of other specified muscles and tendons at ankle and foot level

√7th **S96.821** Laceration of other specified muscles and tendons at ankle and foot level, right foot

√7th **S96.822** Laceration of other specified muscles and tendons at ankle and foot level, left foot

√7th **S96.829** Laceration of other specified muscles and tendons at ankle and foot level, unspecified foot

✓6ᵗʰ **S96.89** **Other** specified injury of other specified muscles and tendons at ankle and foot level

✓7ᵗʰ **S96.891** **Other specified injury of other specified muscles and tendons at ankle and foot level, right foot**

✓7ᵗʰ **S96.892** **Other specified injury of other specified muscles and tendons at ankle and foot level, left foot**

✓7ᵗʰ **S96.899** **Other specified injury of other specified muscles and tendons at ankle and foot level, unspecified foot**

✓5ᵗʰ **S96.9** **Injury of** unspecified **muscle and tendon at ankle and foot level**

✓6ᵗʰ **S96.90** **Unspecified** injury of unspecified muscle and tendon at ankle and foot level

✓7ᵗʰ **S96.901** **Unspecified injury of unspecified muscle and tendon at ankle and foot level, right foot**

✓7ᵗʰ **S96.902** **Unspecified injury of unspecified muscle and tendon at ankle and foot level, left foot**

✓7ᵗʰ **S96.909** **Unspecified injury of unspecified muscle and tendon at ankle and foot level, unspecified foot**

✓6ᵗʰ **S96.91** **Strain** of unspecified muscle and tendon at ankle and foot level

✓7ᵗʰ **S96.911** **Strain of unspecified muscle and tendon at ankle and foot level, right foot**

✓7ᵗʰ **S96.912** **Strain of unspecified muscle and tendon at ankle and foot level, left foot**

✓7ᵗʰ **S96.919** **Strain of unspecified muscle and tendon at ankle and foot level, unspecified foot**

✓6ᵗʰ **S96.92** **Laceration** of unspecified muscle and tendon at ankle and foot level

✓7ᵗʰ **S96.921** **Laceration of unspecified muscle and tendon at ankle and foot level, right foot**

✓7ᵗʰ **S96.922** **Laceration of unspecified muscle and tendon at ankle and foot level, left foot**

✓7ᵗʰ **S96.929** **Laceration of unspecified muscle and tendon at ankle and foot level, unspecified foot**

✓6ᵗʰ **S96.99** **Other** specified injury of unspecified muscle and tendon at ankle and foot level

✓7ᵗʰ **S96.991** **Other specified injury of unspecified muscle and tendon at ankle and foot level, right foot**

✓7ᵗʰ **S96.992** **Other specified injury of unspecified muscle and tendon at ankle and foot level, left foot**

✓7ᵗʰ **S96.999** **Other specified injury of unspecified muscle and tendon at ankle and foot level, unspecified foot**

✓4ᵗʰ **S97** **Crushing injury of ankle and foot**

Use additional code(s) for all associated injuries

The appropriate 7th character is to be added to each code from category S97.
A   initial encounter
D   subsequent encounter
S   sequela

✓5ᵗʰ **S97.0** **Crushing injury of** ankle

✓x7ᵗʰ **S97.00** **Crushing injury of unspecified ankle**

✓x7ᵗʰ **S97.01** **Crushing injury of** right **ankle**

✓x7ᵗʰ **S97.02** **Crushing injury of** left **ankle**

✓5ᵗʰ **S97.1** **Crushing injury of** toe

✓6ᵗʰ **S97.10** **Crushing injury of** unspecified **toe(s)**

✓7ᵗʰ **S97.101** **Crushing injury of unspecified** right **toe(s)**

✓7ᵗʰ **S97.102** **Crushing injury of unspecified** left **toe(s)**

✓7ᵗʰ **S97.109** **Crushing injury of unspecified toe(s)**
Crushing injury of toe NOS

✓6ᵗʰ **S97.11** **Crushing injury of** great **toe**

✓7ᵗʰ **S97.111** **Crushing injury of** right **great toe**

✓7ᵗʰ **S97.112** **Crushing injury of** left **great toe**

✓7ᵗʰ **S97.119** **Crushing injury of unspecified great toe**

✓6ᵗʰ **S97.12** **Crushing injury of** lesser **toe(s)**

✓7ᵗʰ **S97.121** **Crushing injury of** right **lesser toe(s)**

✓7ᵗʰ **S97.122** **Crushing injury of** left **lesser toe(s)**

✓7ᵗʰ **S97.129** **Crushing injury of unspecified lesser toe(s)**

✓5ᵗʰ **S97.8** **Crushing injury of** foot

✓x7ᵗʰ **S97.80** **Crushing injury of unspecified foot**
Crushing injury of foot NOS

✓x7ᵗʰ **S97.81** **Crushing injury of** right **foot**

✓x7ᵗʰ **S97.82** **Crushing injury of** left **foot**

✓4ᵗʰ **S98** **Traumatic amputation of ankle and foot**

An amputation not identified as partial or complete should be coded to complete

The appropriate 7th character is to be added to each code from category S98.
A   initial encounter
D   subsequent encounter
S   sequela

✓5ᵗʰ **S98.0** **Traumatic amputation of** foot at ankle level

✓6ᵗʰ **S98.01** **Complete** traumatic amputation of foot at ankle level

✓7ᵗʰ **S98.011** **Complete traumatic amputation of** right **foot at ankle level**

✓7ᵗʰ **S98.012** **Complete traumatic amputation of** left **foot at ankle level**

✓7ᵗʰ **S98.019** **Complete traumatic amputation of unspecified foot at ankle level**

✓6ᵗʰ **S98.02** **Partial** traumatic amputation of foot at ankle level

✓7ᵗʰ **S98.021** **Partial traumatic amputation of** right **foot at ankle level**

✓7ᵗʰ **S98.022** **Partial traumatic amputation of** left **foot at ankle level**

✓7ᵗʰ **S98.029** **Partial traumatic amputation of unspecified foot at ankle level**

✓5ᵗʰ **S98.1** **Traumatic amputation of** one toe

✓6ᵗʰ **S98.11** **Complete** traumatic amputation of great toe

✓7ᵗʰ **S98.111** **Complete traumatic amputation of** right **great toe**

✓7ᵗʰ **S98.112** **Complete traumatic amputation of** left **great toe**

✓7ᵗʰ **S98.119** **Complete traumatic amputation of unspecified great toe**

✓6ᵗʰ **S98.12** **Partial** traumatic amputation of great toe

✓7ᵗʰ **S98.121** **Partial traumatic amputation of** right **great toe**

✓7ᵗʰ **S98.122** **Partial traumatic amputation of** left **great toe**

✓7ᵗʰ **S98.129** **Partial traumatic amputation of unspecified great toe**

✓6ᵗʰ **S98.13** **Complete** traumatic amputation of one lesser toe
Traumatic amputation of toe NOS

✓7ᵗʰ **S98.131** **Complete traumatic amputation of one** right **lesser toe**

✓7ᵗʰ **S98.132** **Complete traumatic amputation of one** left **lesser toe**

✓7ᵗʰ **S98.139** **Complete traumatic amputation of one unspecified lesser toe**

✓6ᵗʰ **S98.14** **Partial** traumatic amputation of one lesser toe

✓7ᵗʰ **S98.141** **Partial traumatic amputation of one** right **lesser toe**

✓7ᵗʰ **S98.142** **Partial traumatic amputation of one** left **lesser toe**

✓7ᵗʰ **S98.149** **Partial traumatic amputation of one unspecified lesser toe**

✓5ᵗʰ **S98.2** **Traumatic amputation of** two or more lesser toes

✓6ᵗʰ **S98.21** **Complete** traumatic amputation of two or more lesser toes

✓7ᵗʰ **S98.211** **Complete traumatic amputation of two or more** right **lesser toes**

✓7ᵗʰ **S98.212** **Complete traumatic amputation of two or more** left **lesser toes**

✓7ᵗʰ **S98.219** **Complete traumatic amputation of two or more unspecified lesser toes**

EXCLUDES 1 Not coded here   EXCLUDES 2 Not included here   N Newborn Age: 0   P Pediatric Age: 0-17   M Maternity Age: 12-55   A Adult Age: 15-124

920   ICD-10-CM Draft (2015)

☑6ᵗʰ **S98.22** Partial traumatic amputation of two or more lesser toes

    ☑7ᵗʰ **S98.221** Partial traumatic amputation of two or more right lesser toes

    ☑7ᵗʰ **S98.222** Partial traumatic amputation of two or more left lesser toes

    ☑7ᵗʰ **S98.229** Partial traumatic amputation of two or more unspecified lesser toes

☑5ᵗʰ **S98.3** Traumatic amputation of midfoot

   ☑6ᵗʰ **S98.31** Complete traumatic amputation of midfoot

    ☑7ᵗʰ **S98.311** Complete traumatic amputation of right midfoot

    ☑7ᵗʰ **S98.312** Complete traumatic amputation of left midfoot

    ☑7ᵗʰ **S98.319** Complete traumatic amputation of unspecified midfoot

   ☑6ᵗʰ **S98.32** Partial traumatic amputation of midfoot

    ☑7ᵗʰ **S98.321** Partial traumatic amputation of right midfoot

    ☑7ᵗʰ **S98.322** Partial traumatic amputation of left midfoot

    ☑7ᵗʰ **S98.329** Partial traumatic amputation of unspecified midfoot

☑5ᵗʰ **S98.9** Traumatic amputation of foot, level unspecified

   ☑6ᵗʰ **S98.91** Complete traumatic amputation of foot, level unspecified

    ☑7ᵗʰ **S98.911** Complete traumatic amputation of right foot, level unspecified

    ☑7ᵗʰ **S98.912** Complete traumatic amputation of left foot, level unspecified

    ☑7ᵗʰ **S98.919** Complete traumatic amputation of unspecified foot, level unspecified

   ☑6ᵗʰ **S98.92** Partial traumatic amputation of foot, level unspecified

    ☑7ᵗʰ **S98.921** Partial traumatic amputation of right foot, level unspecified

    ☑7ᵗʰ **S98.922** Partial traumatic amputation of left foot, level unspecified

    ☑7ᵗʰ **S98.929** Partial traumatic amputation of unspecified foot, level unspecified

☑4ᵗʰ **S99 Other and unspecified injuries of ankle and foot**

> The appropriate 7th character is to be added to each code from category S99.
> A   initial encounter
> D   subsequent encounter
> S   sequela

☑5ᵗʰ **S99.8** Other specified injuries of ankle and foot

   ☑6ᵗʰ **S99.81** Other specified injuries of ankle

    ☑7ᵗʰ **S99.811** Other specified injuries of right ankle

    ☑7ᵗʰ **S99.812** Other specified injuries of left ankle

    ☑7ᵗʰ **S99.819** Other specified injuries of unspecified ankle

   ☑6ᵗʰ **S99.82** Other specified injuries of foot

    ☑7ᵗʰ **S99.821** Other specified injuries of right foot

    ☑7ᵗʰ **S99.822** Other specified injuries of left foot

    ☑7ᵗʰ **S99.829** Other specified injuries of unspecified foot

☑5ᵗʰ **S99.9** Unspecified injury of ankle and foot

   ☑6ᵗʰ **S99.91** Unspecified injury of ankle

    ☑7ᵗʰ **S99.911** Unspecified injury of right ankle

    ☑7ᵗʰ **S99.912** Unspecified injury of left ankle

    ☑7ᵗʰ **S99.919** Unspecified injury of unspecified ankle

   ☑6ᵗʰ **S99.92** Unspecified injury of foot

    ☑7ᵗʰ **S99.921** Unspecified injury of right foot

    ☑7ᵗʰ **S99.922** Unspecified injury of left foot

    ☑7ᵗʰ **S99.929** Unspecified injury of unspecified foot

Injury, Poisoning And Certain Other Consequences Of External Causes (T07-T88)

Injuries involving multiple body regions (T07)

> **EXCLUDES 1**   burns and corrosions (T20-T32)
> frostbite (T33-T34)
> insect bite or sting, venomous (T63.4)
> sunburn (L55.-)

T07 Unspecified multiple injuries

> **EXCLUDES 1**   injury NOS (T14)

Injury of unspecified body region (T14)

☑4ᵗʰ **T14 Injury of unspecified body region**

> **EXCLUDES 1**   multiple unspecified injuries (T07)

   T14.8 Other injury of unspecified body region
> Abrasion NOS
> Contusion NOS
> Crush injury NOS
> Fracture NOS
> Skin injury NOS
> Vascular injury NOS

  ☑5ᵗʰ **T14.9 Unspecified injury**

   T14.90 Injury, unspecified
> Injury NOS

   T14.91 Suicide attempt
> Attempted suicide NOS

Effects of foreign body entering through natural orifice (T15-T19)

> **EXCLUDES 2**   foreign body accidentally left in operation wound (T81.5-)
> foreign body in penetrating wound—See open wound by body region
> residual foreign body in soft tissue (M79.5)
> splinter, without open wound—See superficial injury by body region

☑4ᵗʰ **T15 Foreign body on external eye**

> **EXCLUDES 2**   foreign body in penetrating wound of orbit and eye ball (S05.4-, S05.5-)
> open wound of eyelid and periocular area (S01.1-)
> retained foreign body in eyelid (H02.8-)
> retained (old) foreign body in penetrating wound of orbit and eye ball (H05.5-, H44.6-, H44.7-)
> superficial foreign body of eyelid and periocular area (S00.25-)

> The appropriate 7th character is to be added to each code from category T15.
> A   initial encounter
> D   subsequent encounter
> S   sequela

  ☑5ᵗʰ **T15.0** Foreign body in cornea

   ☑x7ᵗʰ **T15.00 Foreign body in cornea, unspecified eye**

   ☑x7ᵗʰ **T15.01 Foreign body in cornea, right eye**

   ☑x7ᵗʰ **T15.02 Foreign body in cornea, left eye**

  ☑5ᵗʰ **T15.1** Foreign body in conjunctival sac

   ☑x7ᵗʰ **T15.10 Foreign body in conjunctival sac, unspecified eye**

   ☑x7ᵗʰ **T15.11 Foreign body in conjunctival sac, right eye**

   ☑x7ᵗʰ **T15.12 Foreign body in conjunctival sac, left eye**

  ☑5ᵗʰ **T15.8** Foreign body in other and multiple parts of external eye
> Foreign body in lacrimal punctum

   ☑x7ᵗʰ **T15.80 Foreign body in other and multiple parts of external eye, unspecified eye**

   ☑x7ᵗʰ **T15.81 Foreign body in other and multiple parts of external eye, right eye**

   ☑x7ᵗʰ **T15.82 Foreign body in other and multiple parts of external eye, left eye**

  ☑5ᵗʰ **T15.9** Foreign body on external eye, part unspecified

   ☑x7ᵗʰ **T15.90 Foreign body on external eye, part unspecified, unspecified eye**

   ☑x7ᵗʰ **T15.91 Foreign body on external eye, part unspecified, right eye**

   ☑x7ᵗʰ **T15.92 Foreign body on external eye, part unspecified, left eye**

☑ Additional Character Required   ☑x7ᵗʰ Xtension Alert   Unspecified Dx   Other Specified Dx   Manifestation   ►◄ Revised Text   ● New Code   ▲ Revised Code Title

ICD-10-CM Draft (2015)   921

Injury, Poisoning and Certain Other Consequences of External Causes   T16–T17.900

☑4ᵗʰ **T16**   **Foreign body in** ear
     Foreign body in auditory canal

> The appropriate 7th character is to be added to each code from category T16.
> A   initial encounter
> D   subsequent encounter
> S   sequela

☑x7ᵗʰ **T16.1**   **Foreign body in** right **ear**

☑x7ᵗʰ **T16.2**   **Foreign body in** left **ear**

☑x7ᵗʰ **T16.9**   **Foreign body in ear,** unspecified **ear**

☑4ᵗʰ **T17**   **Foreign body in respiratory tract**

> The appropriate 7th character is to be added to each code from category T17.
> A   initial encounter
> D   subsequent encounter
> S   sequela

☑x7ᵗʰ **T17.0**   **Foreign body in** nasal sinus

☑x7ᵗʰ **T17.1**   **Foreign body in** nostril
     Foreign body in nose NOS

☑5ᵗʰ **T17.2**   **Foreign body in** pharynx
     Foreign body in nasopharynx
     Foreign body in throat NOS

    ☑6ᵗʰ **T17.20**   Unspecified **foreign body in pharynx**

       ☑7ᵗʰ **T17.200**   **Unspecified foreign body in pharynx** causing asphyxiation

       ☑7ᵗʰ **T17.208**   **Unspecified foreign body in pharynx** causing other injury

    ☑6ᵗʰ **T17.21**   Gastric contents **in pharynx**
       Aspiration of gastric contents into pharynx
       Vomitus in pharynx

       ☑7ᵗʰ **T17.210**   **Gastric contents in pharynx** causing asphyxiation

       ☑7ᵗʰ **T17.218**   **Gastric contents in pharynx** causing other injury

    ☑6ᵗʰ **T17.22**   Food **in pharynx**
       Bones in pharynx
       Seeds in pharynx

       ☑7ᵗʰ **T17.220**   **Food in pharynx** causing asphyxiation

       ☑7ᵗʰ **T17.228**   **Food in pharynx** causing other injury

    ☑6ᵗʰ **T17.29**   Other **foreign object in pharynx**

       ☑7ᵗʰ **T17.290**   **Other foreign object in pharynx** causing asphyxiation

       ☑7ᵗʰ **T17.298**   **Other foreign object in pharynx** causing other injury

☑5ᵗʰ **T17.3**   **Foreign body in** larynx

    ☑6ᵗʰ **T17.30**   Unspecified **foreign body in larynx**

       ☑7ᵗʰ **T17.300**   **Unspecified foreign body in larynx causing asphyxiation**

       ☑7ᵗʰ **T17.308**   **Unspecified foreign body in larynx** causing other injury

    ☑6ᵗʰ **T17.31**   Gastric contents **in larynx**
       Aspiration of gastric contents into larynx
       Vomitus in larynx

       ☑7ᵗʰ **T17.310**   **Gastric contents in larynx** causing asphyxiation

       ☑7ᵗʰ **T17.318**   **Gastric contents in larynx** causing other injury

    ☑6ᵗʰ **T17.32**   Food **in larynx**
       Bones in larynx
       Seeds in larynx

       ☑7ᵗʰ **T17.320**   **Food in larynx** causing asphyxiation

       ☑7ᵗʰ **T17.328**   **Food in larynx** causing other injury

    ☑6ᵗʰ **T17.39**   Other **foreign object in larynx**

       ☑7ᵗʰ **T17.390**   **Other foreign object in larynx** causing asphyxiation

       ☑7ᵗʰ **T17.398**   **Other foreign object in larynx** causing other injury

☑5ᵗʰ **T17.4**   **Foreign body in** trachea

    ☑6ᵗʰ **T17.40**   Unspecified **foreign body in trachea**

       ☑7ᵗʰ **T17.400**   **Unspecified foreign body in trachea causing asphyxiation**

       ☑7ᵗʰ **T17.408**   **Unspecified foreign body in trachea causing other injury**

    ☑6ᵗʰ **T17.41**   Gastric contents **in trachea**
       Aspiration of gastric contents into trachea
       Vomitus in trachea

       ☑7ᵗʰ **T17.410**   **Gastric contents in trachea** causing asphyxiation

       ☑7ᵗʰ **T17.418**   **Gastric contents in trachea** causing other injury

    ☑6ᵗʰ **T17.42**   Food **in trachea**
       Bones in trachea
       Seeds in trachea

       ☑7ᵗʰ **T17.420**   **Food in trachea** causing asphyxiation

       ☑7ᵗʰ **T17.428**   **Food in trachea** causing other injury

    ☑6ᵗʰ **T17.49**   Other **foreign object in trachea**

       ☑7ᵗʰ **T17.490**   **Other foreign object in trachea** causing asphyxiation

       ☑7ᵗʰ **T17.498**   **Other foreign object in trachea** causing other injury

☑5ᵗʰ **T17.5**   **Foreign body in** bronchus

    ☑6ᵗʰ **T17.50**   Unspecified **foreign body in bronchus**

       ☑7ᵗʰ **T17.500**   **Unspecified foreign body in bronchus causing asphyxiation**

       ☑7ᵗʰ **T17.508**   **Unspecified foreign body in bronchus causing other injury**

    ☑6ᵗʰ **T17.51**   Gastric contents **in bronchus**
       Aspiration of gastric contents into bronchus
       Vomitus in bronchus

       ☑7ᵗʰ **T17.510**   **Gastric contents in bronchus** causing asphyxiation

       ☑7ᵗʰ **T17.518**   **Gastric contents in bronchus** causing other injury

    ☑6ᵗʰ **T17.52**   Food **in bronchus**
       Bones in bronchus   Seeds in bronchus

       ☑7ᵗʰ **T17.520**   **Food in bronchus** causing asphyxiation

       ☑7ᵗʰ **T17.528**   **Food in bronchus** causing other injury

    ☑6ᵗʰ **T17.59**   Other **foreign object in bronchus**

       ☑7ᵗʰ **T17.590**   **Other foreign object in bronchus** causing asphyxiation

       ☑7ᵗʰ **T17.598**   **Other foreign object in bronchus** causing other injury

☑5ᵗʰ **T17.8**   **Foreign body in** other parts **of respiratory tract**
     Foreign body in bronchioles
     Foreign body in lung

    ☑6ᵗʰ **T17.80**   Unspecified **foreign body in other parts of respiratory tract**

       ☑7ᵗʰ **T17.800**   **Unspecified foreign body in other parts of respiratory tract** causing asphyxiation

       ☑7ᵗʰ **T17.808**   **Unspecified foreign body in other parts of respiratory tract** causing other injury

    ☑6ᵗʰ **T17.81**   Gastric contents **in other parts of respiratory tract**
       Aspiration of gastric contents into other parts of respiratory tract
       Vomitus in other parts of respiratory tract

       ☑7ᵗʰ **T17.810**   **Gastric contents in other parts of respiratory tract** causing asphyxiation

       ☑7ᵗʰ **T17.818**   **Gastric contents in other parts of respiratory tract** causing other injury

    ☑6ᵗʰ **T17.82**   Food **in other parts of respiratory tract**
       Bones in other parts of respiratory tract
       Seeds in other parts of respiratory tract

       ☑7ᵗʰ **T17.820**   **Food in other parts of respiratory tract** causing asphyxiation

       ☑7ᵗʰ **T17.828**   **Food in other parts of respiratory tract** causing other injury

    ☑6ᵗʰ **T17.89**   Other **foreign object in other parts of respiratory tract**

       ☑7ᵗʰ **T17.890**   **Other foreign object in other parts of respiratory tract** causing asphyxiation

       ☑7ᵗʰ **T17.898**   **Other foreign object in other parts of respiratory tract** causing other injury

☑5ᵗʰ **T17.9**   **Foreign body in respiratory tract,** part unspecified

    ☑6ᵗʰ **T17.90**   Unspecified **foreign body in respiratory tract, part unspecified**

       ☑7ᵗʰ **T17.900**   **Unspecified foreign body in respiratory tract, part unspecified** causing asphyxiation

---

EXCLUDES 1 Not coded here   **EXCLUDES 2** Not included here   N Newborn Age: 0   P Pediatric Age: 0-17   M Maternity Age: 12-55   A Adult Age: 15-124

☑7th **T17.908** **Unspecified foreign body in respiratory tract, part unspecified** causing other injury

☑6th **T17.91** Gastric contents **in respiratory tract, part unspecified**
Aspiration of gastric contents into respiratory tract, part unspecified
Vomitus in trachea respiratory tract, part unspecified

☑7th **T17.910** **Gastric contents in respiratory tract, part unspecified** causing asphyxiation

☑7th **T17.918** **Gastric contents in respiratory tract, part unspecified** causing other injury

☑6th **T17.92** Food **in respiratory tract, part unspecified**
Bones in respiratory tract, part unspecified
Seeds in respiratory tract, part unspecified

☑7th **T17.920** **Food in respiratory tract, part unspecified** causing asphyxiation

☑7th **T17.928** **Food in respiratory tract, part unspecified** causing other injury

☑6th **T17.99** Other **foreign object in respiratory tract, part unspecified**

☑7th **T17.990** **Other foreign object in respiratory tract, part unspecified in** causing asphyxiation

☑7th **T17.998** **Other foreign object in respiratory tract, part unspecified** causing other injury

☑4th **T18** **Foreign body in alimentary tract**
EXCLUDES 2 *foreign body in pharynx (T17.2-)*

The appropriate 7th character is to be added to each code from category T18.
A   initial encounter
D   subsequent encounter
S   sequela

☑x7th **T18.0** **Foreign body in** mouth

☑5th **T18.1** **Foreign body in** esophagus
EXCLUDES 2 *foreign body in respiratory tract (T17.-)*

☑6th **T18.10** Unspecified **foreign body in esophagus**

☑7th **T18.100** **Unspecified foreign body in esophagus** causing compression of trachea
Unspecified foreign body in esophagus causing obstruction of respiration

☑7th **T18.108** **Unspecified foreign body in esophagus** causing other injury

☑6th **T18.11** Gastric contents **in esophagus**
Vomitus in esophagus

☑7th **T18.110** **Gastric contents in esophagus** causing compression of trachea
Gastric contents in esophagus causing obstruction of respiration

☑7th **T18.118** **Gastric contents in esophagus** causing other injury

☑6th **T18.12** Food **in esophagus**
Bones in esophagus
Seeds in esophagus

☑7th **T18.120** **Food in esophagus** causing compression of trachea
Food in esophagus causing obstruction of respiration

☑7th **T18.128** **Food in esophagus** causing other injury

☑6th **T18.19** Other **foreign object in esophagus**

☑7th **T18.190** **Other foreign object in esophagus** causing compression of trachea
Other foreign body in esophagus causing obstruction of respiration

☑7th **T18.198** **Other foreign object in esophagus** causing other injury

☑x7th **T18.2** **Foreign body in** stomach

☑x7th **T18.3** **Foreign body in** small intestine

☑x7th **T18.4** **Foreign body in** colon

☑x7th **T18.5** **Foreign body in** anus and rectum
Foreign body in rectosigmoid (junction)

☑x7th **T18.8** **Foreign body in other** parts of alimentary tract

☑x7th **T18.9** **Foreign body of alimentary tract, part unspecified**
Foreign body in digestive system NOS
Swallowed foreign body NOS

☑4th **T19** **Foreign body in genitourinary tract**
EXCLUDES 2 *complications due to implanted mesh (T83.7-)*
mechanical complications of contraceptive device (intrauterine) (vaginal) (T83.3-)
presence of contraceptive device (intrauterine) (vaginal) (Z97.5)

The appropriate 7th character is to be added to each code from category T19.
A   initial encounter
D   subsequent encounter
S   sequela

☑x7th **T19.0** **Foreign body in** urethra

☑x7th **T19.1** **Foreign body in** bladder

☑x7th **T19.2** **Foreign body in** vulva and vagina   ♀

☑x7th **T19.3** **Foreign body in** uterus   ♀

☑x7th **T19.4** **Foreign body in** penis   ♂

☑x7th **T19.8** **Foreign body in other parts of genitourinary tract**

☑x7th **T19.9** **Foreign body in genitourinary tract, part unspecified**

Burns and corrosions (T20-T32)

INCLUDES   burns (thermal) from electrical heating appliances
burns (thermal) from electricity
burns (thermal) from flame
burns (thermal) from friction
burns (thermal) from hot air and hot gases
burns (thermal) from hot objects
burns (thermal) from lightning
burns (thermal) from radiation
chemical burn [corrosion] (external) (internal)
scalds

EXCLUDES 2   *erythema [dermatitis] ab igne (L59.0)*
radiation-related disorders of the skin and subcutaneous tissue (L55-L59)
sunburn (L55.-)

Burns and corrosions of external body surface, specified by site (T20-T25)

INCLUDES   burns and corrosions of first degree [erythema]
burns and corrosions of second degree [blisters] [epidermal loss]
burns and corrosions of third degree [deep necrosis of underlying tissue] [full-thickness skin loss]

Use additional code from category T31 or T32 to identify extent of body surface involved

☑4th **T20** **Burn and corrosion of head, face, and neck**
EXCLUDES 2   *burn and corrosion of ear drum (T28.41, T28.91)*
burn and corrosion of eye and adnexa (T26.-)
burn and corrosion of mouth and pharynx (T28.0)

The appropriate 7th character is to be added to each code from category T20.
A   initial encounter
D   subsequent encounter
S   sequela

☑5th **T20.0** **Burn of** unspecified degree **of head, face, and neck**
Use additional external cause code to identify the source, place and intent of the burn (X00-X19, X75-X77, X96-X98, Y92)

☑x7th **T20.00** **Burn of unspecified degree of head, face, and neck, unspecified site**

☑6th **T20.01** **Burn of unspecified degree of** ear [any part, except ear drum]
EXCLUDES 2 *burn of ear drum (T28.41-)*

☑7th **T20.011** **Burn of unspecified degree of** right **ear [any part, except ear drum]**

☑7th **T20.012** **Burn of unspecified degree of** left **ear [any part, except ear drum]**

☑7th **T20.019** **Burn of unspecified degree of unspecified ear [any part, except ear drum]**

☑x7th **T20.02** **Burn of unspecified degree of** lip(s)

☑x7th **T20.03** **Burn of unspecified degree of** chin

☑x7th **T20.04** **Burn of unspecified degree of** nose (septum)

☑x7th **T20.05** **Burn of unspecified degree of** scalp [any part]

☑x7th **T20.06** **Burn of unspecified degree of** forehead and cheek

☑x7th **T20.07** **Burn of unspecified degree of** neck

☑x7th **T20.09** **Burn of unspecified degree of** multiple sites **of head, face, and neck**

Injury, Poisoning and Certain Other Consequences of External Causes

T20.1–T20.70

√5ᵗʰ **T20.1** Burn of first degree of head, face, and neck
Use additional external cause code to identify the source, place and intent of the burn (X00-X19, X75-X77, X96-X98, Y92)

√x7ᵗʰ **T20.10** Burn of first degree of head, face, and neck, unspecified site

√6ᵗʰ **T20.11** Burn of first degree of ear [any part, except ear drum]
EXCLUDES 2 *burn of ear drum (T28.41-)*

√7ᵗʰ **T20.111** Burn of first degree of right ear [any part, except ear drum]

√7ᵗʰ **T20.112** Burn of first degree of left ear [any part, except ear drum]

√7ᵗʰ **T20.119** Burn of first degree of unspecified ear [any part, except ear drum]

√x7ᵗʰ **T20.12** Burn of first degree of lip(s)

√x7ᵗʰ **T20.13** Burn of first degree of chin

√x7ᵗʰ **T20.14** Burn of first degree of nose (septum)

√x7ᵗʰ **T20.15** Burn of first degree of scalp [any part]

√x7ᵗʰ **T20.16** Burn of first degree of forehead and cheek

√x7ᵗʰ **T20.17** Burn of first degree of neck

√x7ᵗʰ **T20.19** Burn of first degree of multiple sites of head, face, and neck

√5ᵗʰ **T20.2** Burn of second degree of head, face, and neck
Use additional external cause code to identify the source, place and intent of the burn (X00-X19, X75-X77, X96-X98, Y92)

√x7ᵗʰ **T20.20** Burn of second degree of head, face, and neck, unspecified site

√6ᵗʰ **T20.21** Burn of second degree of ear [any part, except ear drum]
EXCLUDES 2 *burn of ear drum (T28.41-)*

√7ᵗʰ **T20.211** Burn of second degree of right ear [any part, except ear drum]

√7ᵗʰ **T20.212** Burn of second degree of left ear [any part, except ear drum]

√7ᵗʰ **T20.219** Burn of second degree of unspecified ear [any part, except ear drum]

√x7ᵗʰ **T20.22** Burn of second degree of lip(s)

√x7ᵗʰ **T20.23** Burn of second degree of chin

√x7ᵗʰ **T20.24** Burn of second degree of nose (septum)

√x7ᵗʰ **T20.25** Burn of second degree of scalp [any part]

√x7ᵗʰ **T20.26** Burn of second degree of forehead and cheek

√x7ᵗʰ **T20.27** Burn of second degree of neck

√x7ᵗʰ **T20.29** Burn of second degree of multiple sites of head, face, and neck

√5ᵗʰ **T20.3** Burn of third degree of head, face, and neck
Use additional external cause code to identify the source, place and intent of the burn (X00-X19, X75-X77, X96-X98, Y92)

√x7ᵗʰ **T20.30** Burn of third degree of head, face, and neck, unspecified site

√6ᵗʰ **T20.31** Burn of third degree of ear [any part, except ear drum]
EXCLUDES 2 *burn of ear drum (T28.41-)*

√7ᵗʰ **T20.311** Burn of third degree of right ear [any part, except ear drum]

√7ᵗʰ **T20.312** Burn of third degree of left ear [any part, except ear drum]

√7ᵗʰ **T20.319** Burn of third degree of unspecified ear [any part, except ear drum]

√x7ᵗʰ **T20.32** Burn of third degree of lip(s)

√x7ᵗʰ **T20.33** Burn of third degree of chin

√x7ᵗʰ **T20.34** Burn of third degree of nose (septum)

√x7ᵗʰ **T20.35** Burn of third degree of scalp [any part]

√x7ᵗʰ **T20.36** Burn of third degree of forehead and cheek

√x7ᵗʰ **T20.37** Burn of third degree of neck

√x7ᵗʰ **T20.39** Burn of third degree of multiple sites of head, face, and neck

√5ᵗʰ **T20.4** Corrosion of unspecified degree of head, face, and neck
Code first (T51-T65) to identify chemical and intent
Use additional external cause code to identify place (Y92)

√x7ᵗʰ **T20.40** Corrosion of unspecified degree of head, face, and neck, unspecified site

√6ᵗʰ **T20.41** Corrosion of unspecified degree of ear [any part, except ear drum]
EXCLUDES 2 *corrosion of ear drum (T28.91-)*

√7ᵗʰ **T20.411** Corrosion of unspecified degree of right ear [any part, except ear drum]

√7ᵗʰ **T20.412** Corrosion of unspecified degree of left ear [any part, except ear drum]

√7ᵗʰ **T20.419** Corrosion of unspecified degree of unspecified ear [any part, except ear drum]

√x7ᵗʰ **T20.42** Corrosion of unspecified degree of lip(s)

√x7ᵗʰ **T20.43** Corrosion of unspecified degree of chin

√x7ᵗʰ **T20.44** Corrosion of unspecified degree of nose (septum)

√x7ᵗʰ **T20.45** Corrosion of unspecified degree of scalp [any part]

√x7ᵗʰ **T20.46** Corrosion of unspecified degree of forehead and cheek

√x7ᵗʰ **T20.47** Corrosion of unspecified degree of neck

√x7ᵗʰ **T20.49** Corrosion of unspecified degree of multiple sites of head, face, and neck

√5ᵗʰ **T20.5** Corrosion of first degree of head, face, and neck
Code first (T51-T65) to identify chemical and intent
Use additional external cause code to identify place (Y92)

√x7ᵗʰ **T20.50** Corrosion of first degree of head, face, and neck, unspecified site

√6ᵗʰ **T20.51** Corrosion of first degree of ear [any part, except ear drum]
EXCLUDES 2 *corrosion of ear drum (T28.91-)*

√7ᵗʰ **T20.511** Corrosion of first degree of right ear [any part, except ear drum]

√7ᵗʰ **T20.512** Corrosion of first degree of left ear [any part, except ear drum]

√7ᵗʰ **T20.519** Corrosion of first degree of unspecified ear [any part, except ear drum]

√x7ᵗʰ **T20.52** Corrosion of first degree of lip(s)

√x7ᵗʰ **T20.53** Corrosion of first degree of chin

√x7ᵗʰ **T20.54** Corrosion of first degree of nose (septum)

√x7ᵗʰ **T20.55** Corrosion of first degree of scalp [any part]

√x7ᵗʰ **T20.56** Corrosion of first degree of forehead and cheek

√x7ᵗʰ **T20.57** Corrosion of first degree of neck

√x7ᵗʰ **T20.59** Corrosion of first degree of multiple sites of head, face, and neck

√5ᵗʰ **T20.6** Corrosion of second degree of head, face, and neck
Code first (T51-T65) to identify chemical and intent
Use additional external cause code to identify place (Y92)

√x7ᵗʰ **T20.60** Corrosion of second degree of head, face, and neck, unspecified site

√6ᵗʰ **T20.61** Corrosion of second degree of ear [any part, except ear drum]
EXCLUDES 2 *corrosion of ear drum (T28.91-)*

√7ᵗʰ **T20.611** Corrosion of second degree of right ear [any part, except ear drum]

√7ᵗʰ **T20.612** Corrosion of second degree of left ear [any part, except ear drum]

√7ᵗʰ **T20.619** Corrosion of second degree of unspecified ear [any part, except ear drum]

√x7ᵗʰ **T20.62** Corrosion of second degree of lip(s)

√x7ᵗʰ **T20.63** Corrosion of second degree of chin

√x7ᵗʰ **T20.64** Corrosion of second degree of nose (septum)

√x7ᵗʰ **T20.65** Corrosion of second degree of scalp [any part]

√x7ᵗʰ **T20.66** Corrosion of second degree of forehead and cheek

√x7ᵗʰ **T20.67** Corrosion of second degree of neck

√x7ᵗʰ **T20.69** Corrosion of second degree of multiple sites of head, face, and neck

√5ᵗʰ **T20.7** Corrosion of third degree of head, face, and neck
Code first (T51-T65) to identify chemical and intent
Use additional external cause code to identify place (Y92)

√x7ᵗʰ **T20.70** Corrosion of third degree of head, face, and neck, unspecified site

EXCLUDES 1 Not coded here   EXCLUDES 2 Not included here   N Newborn Age: 0   P Pediatric Age: 0-17   M Maternity Age: 12-55   A Adult Age: 15-124

924   ICD-10-CM Draft (2015)

√6ᵗʰ **T20.71** **Corrosion of third degree of** ear [any part, except ear drum]
　　EXCLUDES 2　*corrosion of ear drum (T28.91-)*

√7ᵗʰ **T20.711** **Corrosion of third degree of** right ear [any part, except ear drum]

√7ᵗʰ **T20.712** **Corrosion of third degree of** left ear [any part, except ear drum]

√7ᵗʰ **T20.719** **Corrosion of third degree of unspecified ear [any part, except ear drum]**

√x7ᵗʰ **T20.72** **Corrosion of third degree of** lip(s)

√x7ᵗʰ **T20.73** **Corrosion of third degree of** chin

√x7ᵗʰ **T20.74** **Corrosion of third degree of** nose (septum)

√x7ᵗʰ **T20.75** **Corrosion of third degree of** scalp [any part]

√x7ᵗʰ **T20.76** **Corrosion of third degree of** forehead and cheek

√x7ᵗʰ **T20.77** **Corrosion of third degree of** neck

√x7ᵗʰ **T20.79** **Corrosion of third degree of** multiple sites **of head, face, and neck**

√4ᵗʰ **T21** **Burn and corrosion of trunk**
　　Burns and corrosion of hip region
　　EXCLUDES 2　*burns and corrosion of axilla (T22.- with fifth character 4)*
　　　　burns and corrosion of scapular region (T22.- with fifth character 6)
　　　　burns and corrosion of shoulder (T22.- with fifth character 5)

The appropriate 7th character is to be added to each code from category T21.
　A　initial encounter
　D　subsequent encounter
　S　sequela

√5ᵗʰ **T21.0** **Burn of** unspecified degree **of trunk**
　　Use additional external cause code to identify the source, place and intent of the burn (X00-X19, X75-X77, X96-X98, Y92)

√7ᵗʰ **T21.00** **Burn of unspecified degree of trunk, unspecified site**

√7ᵗʰ **T21.01** **Burn of unspecified degree of** chest wall
　　Burn of of unspecified degree of breast

√7ᵗʰ **T21.02** **Burn of unspecified degree of** abdominal wall
　　Burn of unspecified degree of flank
　　Burn of unspecified degree of groin

√7ᵗʰ **T21.03** **Burn of unspecified degree of** upper back
　　Burn of unspecified degree of interscapular region

√7ᵗʰ **T21.04** **Burn of unspecified degree of** lower back

√7ᵗʰ **T21.05** **Burn of unspecified degree of** buttock
　　Burn of unspecified degree of anus

√7ᵗʰ **T21.06** **Burn of unspecified degree of** male genital region ♂
　　Burn of unspecified degree of penis
　　Burn of unspecified degree of scrotum
　　Burn of unspecified degree of testis

√7ᵗʰ **T21.07** **Burn of unspecified degree of** female genital region ♀
　　Burn of unspecified degree of labium (majus) (minus)
　　Burn of unspecified degree of perineum
　　Burn of unspecified degree of vulva
　　EXCLUDES 2　*burn of vagina (T28.3)*

√7ᵗʰ **T21.09** **Burn of unspecified degree of other site of trunk**

√5ᵗʰ **T21.1** **Burn of** first degree **of trunk**
　　Use additional external cause code to identify the source, place and intent of the burn (X00-X19, X75-X77, X96-X98, Y92)

√7ᵗʰ **T21.10** **Burn of first degree of trunk, unspecified site**

√7ᵗʰ **T21.11** **Burn of first degree of** chest wall
　　Burn of first degree of breast

√7ᵗʰ **T21.12** **Burn of first degree of** abdominal wall
　　Burn of first degree of flank
　　Burn of first degree of groin

√7ᵗʰ **T21.13** **Burn of first degree of** upper back
　　Burn of first degree of interscapular region

√7ᵗʰ **T21.14** **Burn of first degree of** lower back

√7ᵗʰ **T21.15** **Burn of first degree of** buttock
　　Burn of first degree of anus

√7ᵗʰ **T21.16** **Burn of first degree of** male genital region ♂
　　Burn of first degree of penis
　　Burn of first degree of scrotum
　　Burn of first degree of testis

√7ᵗʰ **T21.17** **Burn of first degree of** female genital region ♀
　　Burn of first degree of labium (majus) (minus)
　　Burn of first degree of perineum
　　Burn of first degree of vulva
　　EXCLUDES 2　*burn of vagina (T28.3)*

√7ᵗʰ **T21.19** **Burn of first degree of other site of trunk**

√5ᵗʰ **T21.2** **Burn of** second degree **of trunk**
　　Use additional external cause code to identify the source, place and intent of the burn (X00-X19, X75-X77, X96-X98, Y92)

√7ᵗʰ **T21.20** **Burn of second degree of trunk, unspecified site**

√7ᵗʰ **T21.21** **Burn of second degree of** chest wall
　　Burn of second degree of breast

√7ᵗʰ **T21.22** **Burn of second degree of** abdominal wall
　　Burn of second degree of flank
　　Burn of second degree of groin

√7ᵗʰ **T21.23** **Burn of second degree of** upper back
　　Burn of second degree of interscapular region

√7ᵗʰ **T21.24** **Burn of second degree of** lower back

√7ᵗʰ **T21.25** **Burn of second degree of** buttock
　　Burn of second degree of anus

√7ᵗʰ **T21.26** **Burn of second degree of** male genital region ♂
　　Burn of second degree of penis
　　Burn of second degree of scrotum
　　Burn of second degree of testis

√7ᵗʰ **T21.27** **Burn of second degree of** female genital region ♀
　　Burn of second degree of labium (majus) (minus)
　　Burn of second degree of perineum
　　Burn of second degree of vulva
　　EXCLUDES 2　*burn of vagina (T28.3)*

√7ᵗʰ **T21.29** **Burn of second degree of other site of trunk**

√5ᵗʰ **T21.3** **Burn of** third degree **of trunk**
　　Use additional external cause code to identify the source, place and intent of the burn (X00-X19, X75-X77, X96-X98, Y92)

√7ᵗʰ **T21.30** **Burn of third degree of trunk, unspecified site**

√7ᵗʰ **T21.31** **Burn of third degree of** chest wall
　　Burn of third degree of breast

√7ᵗʰ **T21.32** **Burn of third degree of** abdominal wall
　　Burn of third degree of flank
　　Burn of third degree of groin

√7ᵗʰ **T21.33** **Burn of third degree of** upper back
　　Burn of third degree of interscapular region

√7ᵗʰ **T21.34** **Burn of third degree of** lower back

√7ᵗʰ **T21.35** **Burn of third degree of** buttock
　　Burn of third degree of anus

√7ᵗʰ **T21.36** **Burn of third degree of** male genital region ♂
　　Burn of third degree of penis
　　Burn of third degree of scrotum
　　Burn of third degree of testis

√7ᵗʰ **T21.37** **Burn of third degree of** female genital region ♀
　　Burn of third degree of labium (majus) (minus)
　　Burn of third degree of perineum
　　Burn of third degree of vulva
　　EXCLUDES 2　*burn of vagina (T28.3)*

√7ᵗʰ **T21.39** **Burn of third degree of other site of trunk**

√5ᵗʰ **T21.4** **Corrosion of** unspecified degree **of trunk**
　　Code first (T51-T65) to identify chemical and intent
　　Use additional external cause code to identify place (Y92)

√7ᵗʰ **T21.40** **Corrosion of unspecified degree of trunk, unspecified site**

√7ᵗʰ **T21.41** **Corrosion of unspecified degree of** chest wall
　　Corrosion of unspecified degree of breast

√7ᵗʰ **T21.42** **Corrosion of unspecified degree of** abdominal wall
　　Corrosion of unspecified degree of flank
　　Corrosion of unspecified degree of groin

√7ᵗʰ **T21.43** **Corrosion of unspecified degree of** upper back
　　Corrosion of unspecified degree of interscapular region

√7ᵗʰ **T21.44** **Corrosion of unspecified degree of** lower back

√7ᵗʰ **T21.45** **Corrosion of unspecified degree of** buttock
　　Corrosion of unspecified degree of anus

√7ᵗʰ **T21.46** **Corrosion of unspecified degree of** male genital region ♂
　　Corrosion of unspecified degree of penis
　　Corrosion of unspecified degree of scrotum
　　Corrosion of unspecified degree of testis

Injury, Poisoning and Certain Other Consequences of External Causes   **T21.47–T22.099**

√x7ᵗʰ **T21.47 Corrosion of unspecified degree of** female genital region ♀
Corrosion of unspecified degree of labium (majus) (minus)
Corrosion of unspecified degree of perineum
Corrosion of unspecified degree of vulva
EXCLUDES 2   *corrosion of vagina (T28.8)*

√x7ᵗʰ **T21.49 Corrosion of unspecified degree of other site of trunk**

√5ᵗʰ **T21.5 Corrosion of** first degree **of trunk**
Code first (T51-T65) to identify chemical and intent
Use additional external cause code to identify place (Y92)

√x7ᵗʰ **T21.50 Corrosion of first degree of trunk, unspecified site**

√x7ᵗʰ **T21.51 Corrosion of first degree of** chest wall
Corrosion of first degree of breast

√x7ᵗʰ **T21.52 Corrosion of first degree of** abdominal wall
Corrosion of first degree of flank
Corrosion of first degree of groin

√x7ᵗʰ **T21.53 Corrosion of first degree of** upper back
Corrosion of first degree of interscapular region

√x7ᵗʰ **T21.54 Corrosion of first degree of** lower back

√x7ᵗʰ **T21.55 Corrosion of first degree of** buttock
Corrosion of first degree of anus

√x7ᵗʰ **T21.56 Corrosion of first degree of** male genital region ♂
Corrosion of first degree of penis
Corrosion of first degree of scrotum
Corrosion of first degree of testis

√x7ᵗʰ **T21.57 Corrosion of first degree of** female genital region ♀
Corrosion of first degree of labium (majus) (minus)
Corrosion of first degree of perineum
Corrosion of first degree of vulva
EXCLUDES 2   *corrosion of vagina (T28.8)*

√x7ᵗʰ **T21.59 Corrosion of first degree of other site of trunk**

√5ᵗʰ **T21.6 Corrosion of** second degree **of trunk**
Code first (T51-T65) to identify chemical and intent
Use additional external cause code to identify place (Y92)

√x7ᵗʰ **T21.60 Corrosion of second degree of trunk, unspecified site**

√x7ᵗʰ **T21.61 Corrosion of second degree of** chest wall
Corrosion of second degree of breast

√x7ᵗʰ **T21.62 Corrosion of second degree of** abdominal wall
Corrosion of second degree of flank
Corrosion of second degree of groin

√x7ᵗʰ **T21.63 Corrosion of second degree of** upper back
Corrosion of second degree of interscapular region

√x7ᵗʰ **T21.64 Corrosion of second degree of** lower back

√x7ᵗʰ **T21.65 Corrosion of second degree of** buttock
Corrosion of second degree of anus

√x7ᵗʰ **T21.66 Corrosion of second degree of** male genital region ♂
Corrosion of second degree of penis
Corrosion of second degree of scrotum
Corrosion of second degree of testis

√x7ᵗʰ **T21.67 Corrosion of second degree of** female genital region ♀
Corrosion of second degree of labium (majus) (minus)
Corrosion of second degree of perineum
Corrosion of second degree of vulva
EXCLUDES 2   *corrosion of vagina (T28.8)*

√x7ᵗʰ **T21.69 Corrosion of second degree of other site of trunk**

√5ᵗʰ **T21.7 Corrosion of** third degree **of trunk**
Code first (T51-T65) to identify chemical and intent
Use additional external cause code to identify place (Y92)

√x7ᵗʰ **T21.70 Corrosion of third degree of trunk, unspecified site**

√x7ᵗʰ **T21.71 Corrosion of third degree of** chest wall
Corrosion of third degree of breast

√x7ᵗʰ **T21.72 Corrosion of third degree of** abdominal wall
Corrosion of third degree of flank
Corrosion of third degree of groin

√x7ᵗʰ **T21.73 Corrosion of third degree of** upper back
Corrosion of third degree of interscapular region

√x7ᵗʰ **T21.74 Corrosion of third degree of** lower back

√x7ᵗʰ **T21.75 Corrosion of third degree of** buttock
Corrosion of third degree of anus

√x7ᵗʰ **T21.76 Corrosion of third degree of** male genital region ♂
Corrosion of third degree of penis
Corrosion of third degree of scrotum
Corrosion of third degree of testis

√x7ᵗʰ **T21.77 Corrosion of third degree of** female genital region ♀
Corrosion of third degree of labium (majus) (minus)
Corrosion of third degree of perineum
Corrosion of third degree of vulva
EXCLUDES 2   *corrosion of vagina (T28.8)*

√x7ᵗʰ **T21.79 Corrosion of third degree of other site of trunk**

√4ᵗʰ **T22 Burn and corrosion of shoulder and upper limb, except wrist and hand**
EXCLUDES 2   *burn and corrosion of interscapular region (T21.-)*
              burn and corrosion of wrist and hand (T23.-)

The appropriate 7th character is to be added to each code from category T22.
A   initial encounter
D   subsequent encounter
S   sequela

√5ᵗʰ **T22.0 Burn of** unspecified degree **of shoulder and upper limb, except wrist and hand**
Use additional external cause code to identify the source, place and intent of the burn (X00-X19, X75-X77, X96-X98, Y92)

√x7ᵗʰ **T22.00 Burn of unspecified degree of shoulder and upper limb, except wrist and hand, unspecified site**

√6ᵗʰ **T22.01 Burn of unspecified degree of** forearm

√7ᵗʰ **T22.011 Burn of unspecified degree of** right **forearm**

√7ᵗʰ **T22.012 Burn of unspecified degree of** left **forearm**

√7ᵗʰ **T22.019 Burn of unspecified degree of unspecified forearm**

√6ᵗʰ **T22.02 Burn of unspecified degree of** elbow

√7ᵗʰ **T22.021 Burn of unspecified degree of** right **elbow**

√7ᵗʰ **T22.022 Burn of unspecified degree of** left **elbow**

√7ᵗʰ **T22.029 Burn of unspecified degree of unspecified elbow**

√6ᵗʰ **T22.03 Burn of unspecified degree of** upper arm

√7ᵗʰ **T22.031 Burn of unspecified degree of** right **upper arm**

√7ᵗʰ **T22.032 Burn of unspecified degree of** left **upper arm**

√7ᵗʰ **T22.039 Burn of unspecified degree of unspecified upper arm**

√6ᵗʰ **T22.04 Burn of unspecified degree of** axilla

√7ᵗʰ **T22.041 Burn of unspecified degree of** right **axilla**

√7ᵗʰ **T22.042 Burn of unspecified degree of** left **axilla**

√7ᵗʰ **T22.049 Burn of unspecified degree of unspecified axilla**

√6ᵗʰ **T22.05 Burn of unspecified degree of** shoulder

√7ᵗʰ **T22.051 Burn of unspecified degree of** right **shoulder**

√7ᵗʰ **T22.052 Burn of unspecified degree of** left **shoulder**

√7ᵗʰ **T22.059 Burn of unspecified degree of unspecified shoulder**

√6ᵗʰ **T22.06 Burn of unspecified degree of** scapular region

√7ᵗʰ **T22.061 Burn of unspecified degree of** right **scapular region**

√7ᵗʰ **T22.062 Burn of unspecified degree of** left **scapular region**

√7ᵗʰ **T22.069 Burn of unspecified degree of unspecified scapular region**

√6ᵗʰ **T22.09 Burn of unspecified degree of** multiple sites **of shoulder and upper limb, except wrist and hand**

√7ᵗʰ **T22.091 Burn of unspecified degree of multiple sites of** right **shoulder and upper limb, except wrist and hand**

√7ᵗʰ **T22.092 Burn of unspecified degree of multiple sites of** left **shoulder and upper limb, except wrist and hand**

√7ᵗʰ **T22.099 Burn of unspecified degree of multiple sites of unspecified shoulder and upper limb, except wrist and hand**

EXCLUDES 1 Not coded here   *EXCLUDES 2* Not included here   N Newborn Age: 0   P Pediatric Age: 0-17   M Maternity Age: 12-55   A Adult Age: 15-124

926   ICD-10-CM Draft (2015)

√5ᵗʰ **T22.1** **Burn of** first degree **of shoulder and upper limb, except wrist and hand**

Use additional external cause code to identify the source, place and intent of the burn (X00-X19, X75-X77, X96-X98, Y92)

√x7ᵗʰ **T22.10** **Burn of first degree of shoulder and upper limb, except wrist and hand,** unspecified site

√6ᵗʰ **T22.11** **Burn of first degree of** forearm

√7ᵗʰ T22.111 Burn of first degree of right forearm
√7ᵗʰ T22.112 Burn of first degree of left forearm
√7ᵗʰ T22.119 **Burn of first degree of unspecified forearm**

√6ᵗʰ **T22.12** **Burn of first degree of** elbow

√7ᵗʰ T22.121 Burn of first degree of right elbow
√7ᵗʰ T22.122 Burn of first degree of left elbow
√7ᵗʰ T22.129 **Burn of first degree of unspecified elbow**

√6ᵗʰ **T22.13** **Burn of first degree of** upper arm

√7ᵗʰ T22.131 Burn of first degree of right upper arm
√7ᵗʰ T22.132 Burn of first degree of left upper arm
√7ᵗʰ T22.139 **Burn of first degree of unspecified upper arm**

√6ᵗʰ **T22.14** **Burn of first degree of** axilla

√7ᵗʰ T22.141 Burn of first degree of right axilla
√7ᵗʰ T22.142 Burn of first degree of left axilla
√7ᵗʰ T22.149 **Burn of first degree of unspecified axilla**

√6ᵗʰ **T22.15** **Burn of first degree of** shoulder

√7ᵗʰ T22.151 Burn of first degree of right shoulder
√7ᵗʰ T22.152 Burn of first degree of left shoulder
√7ᵗʰ T22.159 **Burn of first degree of unspecified shoulder**

√6ᵗʰ **T22.16** **Burn of first degree of** scapular region

√7ᵗʰ T22.161 Burn of first degree of right scapular region
√7ᵗʰ T22.162 Burn of first degree of left scapular region
√7ᵗʰ T22.169 **Burn of first degree of unspecified scapular region**

√6ᵗʰ **T22.19** **Burn of first degree of** multiple sites **of shoulder and upper limb, except wrist and hand**

√7ᵗʰ T22.191 Burn of first degree of multiple sites of right shoulder and upper limb, except wrist and hand
√7ᵗʰ T22.192 Burn of first degree of multiple sites of left shoulder and upper limb, except wrist and hand
√7ᵗʰ T22.199 **Burn of first degree of multiple sites of unspecified shoulder and upper limb, except wrist and hand**

√5ᵗʰ **T22.2** **Burn of** second degree **of shoulder and upper limb, except wrist and hand**

Use additional external cause code to identify the source, place and intent of the burn (X00-X19, X75-X77, X96-X98, Y92)

√x7ᵗʰ **T22.20** **Burn of second degree of shoulder and upper limb, except wrist and hand,** unspecified site

√6ᵗʰ **T22.21** **Burn of second degree of** forearm

√7ᵗʰ T22.211 Burn of second degree of right forearm
√7ᵗʰ T22.212 Burn of second degree of left forearm
√7ᵗʰ T22.219 **Burn of second degree of unspecified forearm**

√6ᵗʰ **T22.22** **Burn of second degree of** elbow

√7ᵗʰ T22.221 Burn of second degree of right elbow
√7ᵗʰ T22.222 Burn of second degree of left elbow
√7ᵗʰ T22.229 **Burn of second degree of unspecified elbow**

√6ᵗʰ **T22.23** **Burn of second degree of** upper arm

√7ᵗʰ T22.231 Burn of second degree of right upper arm
√7ᵗʰ T22.232 Burn of second degree of left upper arm
√7ᵗʰ T22.239 **Burn of second degree of unspecified upper arm**

√6ᵗʰ **T22.24** **Burn of second degree of** axilla

√7ᵗʰ T22.241 Burn of second degree of right axilla
√7ᵗʰ T22.242 Burn of second degree of left axilla
√7ᵗʰ T22.249 **Burn of second degree of unspecified axilla**

√6ᵗʰ **T22.25** **Burn of second degree of** shoulder

√7ᵗʰ T22.251 Burn of second degree of right shoulder
√7ᵗʰ T22.252 Burn of second degree of left shoulder
√7ᵗʰ T22.259 **Burn of second degree of unspecified shoulder**

√6ᵗʰ **T22.26** **Burn of second degree of** scapular region

√7ᵗʰ T22.261 Burn of second degree of right scapular region
√7ᵗʰ T22.262 Burn of second degree of left scapular region
√7ᵗʰ T22.269 **Burn of second degree of unspecified scapular region**

√6ᵗʰ **T22.29** **Burn of second degree of** multiple sites **of shoulder and upper limb, except wrist and hand**

√7ᵗʰ T22.291 Burn of second degree of multiple sites of right shoulder and upper limb, except wrist and hand
√7ᵗʰ T22.292 Burn of second degree of multiple sites of left shoulder and upper limb, except wrist and hand
√7ᵗʰ T22.299 **Burn of second degree of multiple sites of unspecified shoulder and upper limb, except wrist and hand**

√5ᵗʰ **T22.3** **Burn of** third degree **of shoulder and upper limb, except wrist and hand**

Use additional external cause code to identify the source, place and intent of the burn (X00-X19, X75-X77, X96-X98, Y92)

√x7ᵗʰ **T22.30** **Burn of third degree of shoulder and upper limb, except wrist and hand, unspecified site**

√6ᵗʰ **T22.31** **Burn of third degree of** forearm

√7ᵗʰ T22.311 Burn of third degree of right forearm
√7ᵗʰ T22.312 Burn of third degree of left forearm
√7ᵗʰ T22.319 **Burn of third degree of unspecified forearm**

√6ᵗʰ **T22.32** **Burn of third degree of** elbow

√7ᵗʰ T22.321 Burn of third degree of right elbow
√7ᵗʰ T22.322 Burn of third degree of left elbow
√7ᵗʰ T22.329 **Burn of third degree of unspecified elbow**

√6ᵗʰ **T22.33** **Burn of third degree of** upper arm

√7ᵗʰ T22.331 Burn of third degree of right upper arm
√7ᵗʰ T22.332 Burn of third degree of left upper arm
√7ᵗʰ T22.339 **Burn of third degree of unspecified upper arm**

√6ᵗʰ **T22.34** **Burn of third degree of** axilla

√7ᵗʰ T22.341 Burn of third degree of right axilla
√7ᵗʰ T22.342 Burn of third degree of left axilla
√7ᵗʰ T22.349 **Burn of third degree of unspecified axilla**

√6ᵗʰ **T22.35** **Burn of third degree of** shoulder

√7ᵗʰ T22.351 Burn of third degree of right shoulder
√7ᵗʰ T22.352 Burn of third degree of left shoulder
√7ᵗʰ T22.359 **Burn of third degree of unspecified shoulder**

√6ᵗʰ **T22.36** **Burn of third degree of** scapular region

√7ᵗʰ T22.361 Burn of third degree of right scapular region
√7ᵗʰ T22.362 Burn of third degree of left scapular region
√7ᵗʰ T22.369 **Burn of third degree of unspecified scapular region**

√6ᵗʰ **T22.39** **Burn of third degree of** multiple sites **of shoulder and upper limb, except wrist and hand**

√7ᵗʰ T22.391 Burn of third degree of multiple sites of right shoulder and upper limb, except wrist and hand
√7ᵗʰ T22.392 Burn of third degree of multiple sites of left shoulder and upper limb, except wrist and hand
√7ᵗʰ T22.399 **Burn of third degree of multiple sites of unspecified shoulder and upper limb, except wrist and hand**

Injury, Poisoning and Certain Other Consequences of External Causes

T22.4–T22.659

✓5ᵗʰ **T22.4** **Corrosion of** unspecified degree **of shoulder and upper limb, except wrist and hand**
     Code first (T51-T65) to identify chemical and intent
     Use additional external cause code to identify place (Y92)

   ✓x7ᵗʰ **T22.40** **Corrosion of unspecified degree of shoulder and upper limb, except wrist and hand, unspecified site**

   ✓6ᵗʰ **T22.41** **Corrosion of unspecified degree of** forearm

     ✓7ᵗʰ **T22.411** **Corrosion of unspecified degree of** right **forearm**

     ✓7ᵗʰ **T22.412** **Corrosion of unspecified degree of** left **forearm**

     ✓7ᵗʰ **T22.419** **Corrosion of unspecified degree of unspecified forearm**

   ✓6ᵗʰ **T22.42** **Corrosion of unspecified degree of** elbow

     ✓7ᵗʰ **T22.421** **Corrosion of unspecified degree of** right **elbow**

     ✓7ᵗʰ **T22.422** **Corrosion of unspecified degree of** left **elbow**

     ✓7ᵗʰ **T22.429** **Corrosion of unspecified degree of unspecified elbow**

   ✓6ᵗʰ **T22.43** **Corrosion of unspecified degree of** upper arm

     ✓7ᵗʰ **T22.431** **Corrosion of unspecified degree of** right **upper arm**

     ✓7ᵗʰ **T22.432** **Corrosion of unspecified degree of** left **upper arm**

     ✓7ᵗʰ **T22.439** **Corrosion of unspecified degree of unspecified upper arm**

   ✓6ᵗʰ **T22.44** **Corrosion of unspecified degree of** axilla

     ✓7ᵗʰ **T22.441** **Corrosion of unspecified degree of** right **axilla**

     ✓7ᵗʰ **T22.442** **Corrosion of unspecified degree of** left **axilla**

     ✓7ᵗʰ **T22.449** **Corrosion of unspecified degree of unspecified axilla**

   ✓6ᵗʰ **T22.45** **Corrosion of unspecified degree of** shoulder

     ✓7ᵗʰ **T22.451** **Corrosion of unspecified degree of** right **shoulder**

     ✓7ᵗʰ **T22.452** **Corrosion of unspecified degree of** left **shoulder**

     ✓7ᵗʰ **T22.459** **Corrosion of unspecified degree of unspecified shoulder**

   ✓6ᵗʰ **T22.46** **Corrosion of unspecified degree of** scapular region

     ✓7ᵗʰ **T22.461** **Corrosion of unspecified degree of** right **scapular region**

     ✓7ᵗʰ **T22.462** **Corrosion of unspecified degree of** left **scapular region**

     ✓7ᵗʰ **T22.469** **Corrosion of unspecified degree of unspecified scapular region**

   ✓6ᵗʰ **T22.49** **Corrosion of unspecified degree of** multiple sites **of shoulder and upper limb, except wrist and hand**

     ✓7ᵗʰ **T22.491** **Corrosion of unspecified degree of multiple sites of** right **shoulder and upper limb, except wrist and hand**

     ✓7ᵗʰ **T22.492** **Corrosion of unspecified degree of multiple sites of** left **shoulder and upper limb, except wrist and hand**

     ✓7ᵗʰ **T22.499** **Corrosion of unspecified degree of multiple sites of unspecified shoulder and upper limb, except wrist and hand**

✓5ᵗʰ **T22.5** **Corrosion of** first degree **of shoulder and upper limb, except wrist and hand**
     Code first (T51-T65) to identify chemical and intent
     Use additional external cause code to identify place (Y92)

   ✓x7ᵗʰ **T22.50** **Corrosion of first degree of shoulder and upper limb, except wrist and hand unspecified site**

   ✓6ᵗʰ **T22.51** **Corrosion of first degree of** forearm

     ✓7ᵗʰ **T22.511** **Corrosion of first degree of** right **forearm**

     ✓7ᵗʰ **T22.512** **Corrosion of first degree of** left **forearm**

     ✓7ᵗʰ **T22.519** **Corrosion of first degree of unspecified forearm**

   ✓6ᵗʰ **T22.52** **Corrosion of first degree of** elbow

     ✓7ᵗʰ **T22.521** **Corrosion of first degree of** right **elbow**

     ✓7ᵗʰ **T22.522** **Corrosion of first degree of** left **elbow**

     ✓7ᵗʰ **T22.529** **Corrosion of first degree of unspecified elbow**

   ✓6ᵗʰ **T22.53** **Corrosion of first degree of** upper arm

     ✓7ᵗʰ **T22.531** **Corrosion of first degree of** right **upper arm**

     ✓7ᵗʰ **T22.532** **Corrosion of first degree of** left **upper arm**

     ✓7ᵗʰ **T22.539** **Corrosion of first degree of unspecified upper arm**

   ✓6ᵗʰ **T22.54** **Corrosion of first degree of** axilla

     ✓7ᵗʰ **T22.541** **Corrosion of first degree of** right **axilla**

     ✓7ᵗʰ **T22.542** **Corrosion of first degree of** left **axilla**

     ✓7ᵗʰ **T22.549** **Corrosion of first degree of unspecified axilla**

   ✓6ᵗʰ **T22.55** **Corrosion of first degree of** shoulder

     ✓7ᵗʰ **T22.551** **Corrosion of first degree of** right **shoulder**

     ✓7ᵗʰ **T22.552** **Corrosion of first degree of** left **shoulder**

     ✓7ᵗʰ **T22.559** **Corrosion of first degree of unspecified shoulder**

   ✓6ᵗʰ **T22.56** **Corrosion of first degree of** scapular region

     ✓7ᵗʰ **T22.561** **Corrosion of first degree of** right **scapular region**

     ✓7ᵗʰ **T22.562** **Corrosion of first degree of** left **scapular region**

     ✓7ᵗʰ **T22.569** **Corrosion of first degree of unspecified scapular region**

   ✓6ᵗʰ **T22.59** **Corrosion of first degree of** multiple sites **of shoulder and upper limb, except wrist and hand**

     ✓7ᵗʰ **T22.591** **Corrosion of first degree of multiple sites of** right **shoulder and upper limb, except wrist and hand**

     ✓7ᵗʰ **T22.592** **Corrosion of first degree of multiple sites of** left **shoulder and upper limb, except wrist and hand**

     ✓7ᵗʰ **T22.599** **Corrosion of first degree of multiple sites of unspecified shoulder and upper limb, except wrist and hand**

✓5ᵗʰ **T22.6** **Corrosion of** second degree **of shoulder and upper limb, except wrist and hand**
     Code first (T51-T65) to identify chemical and intent
     Use additional external cause code to identify place (Y92)

   ✓x7ᵗʰ **T22.60** **Corrosion of second degree of shoulder and upper limb, except wrist and hand, unspecified site**

   ✓6ᵗʰ **T22.61** **Corrosion of second degree of** forearm

     ✓7ᵗʰ **T22.611** **Corrosion of second degree of** right **forearm**

     ✓7ᵗʰ **T22.612** **Corrosion of second degree of** left **forearm**

     ✓7ᵗʰ **T22.619** **Corrosion of second degree of unspecified forearm**

   ✓6ᵗʰ **T22.62** **Corrosion of second degree of** elbow

     ✓7ᵗʰ **T22.621** **Corrosion of second degree of** right **elbow**

     ✓7ᵗʰ **T22.622** **Corrosion of second degree of** left **elbow**

     ✓7ᵗʰ **T22.629** **Corrosion of second degree of unspecified elbow**

   ✓6ᵗʰ **T22.63** **Corrosion of second degree of** upper arm

     ✓7ᵗʰ **T22.631** **Corrosion of second degree of** right **upper arm**

     ✓7ᵗʰ **T22.632** **Corrosion of second degree of** left **upper arm**

     ✓7ᵗʰ **T22.639** **Corrosion of second degree of unspecified upper arm**

   ✓6ᵗʰ **T22.64** **Corrosion of second degree of** axilla

     ✓7ᵗʰ **T22.641** **Corrosion of second degree of** right **axilla**

     ✓7ᵗʰ **T22.642** **Corrosion of second degree of** left **axilla**

     ✓7ᵗʰ **T22.649** **Corrosion of second degree of unspecified axilla**

   ✓6ᵗʰ **T22.65** **Corrosion of second degree of** shoulder

     ✓7ᵗʰ **T22.651** **Corrosion of second degree of** right **shoulder**

     ✓7ᵗʰ **T22.652** **Corrosion of second degree of** left **shoulder**

     ✓7ᵗʰ **T22.659** **Corrosion of second degree of unspecified shoulder**

EXCLUDES 1 Not coded here   EXCLUDES 2 Not included here   N Newborn Age: 0   P Pediatric Age: 0-17   M Maternity Age: 12-55   A Adult Age: 15-124

928   ICD-10-CM Draft (2015)

☑6th **T22.66** Corrosion of second degree of scapular region
- ☑7th **T22.661** Corrosion of second degree of right scapular region
- ☑7th **T22.662** Corrosion of second degree of left scapular region
- ☑7th **T22.669** Corrosion of second degree of unspecified scapular region

☑6th **T22.69** Corrosion of second degree of multiple sites of shoulder and upper limb, except wrist and hand
- ☑7th **T22.691** Corrosion of second degree of multiple sites of right shoulder and upper limb, except wrist and hand
- ☑7th **T22.692** Corrosion of second degree of multiple sites of left shoulder and upper limb, except wrist and hand
- ☑7th **T22.699** Corrosion of second degree of multiple sites of unspecified shoulder and upper limb, except wrist and hand

☑5th **T22.7** Corrosion of third degree of shoulder and upper limb, except wrist and hand
  Code first (T51-T65) to identify chemical and intent
  Use additional external cause code to identify place (Y92)

☑x7th **T22.70** Corrosion of third degree of shoulder and upper limb, except wrist and hand, unspecified site

☑6th **T22.71** Corrosion of third degree of forearm
- ☑7th **T22.711** Corrosion of third degree of right forearm
- ☑7th **T22.712** Corrosion of third degree of left forearm
- ☑7th **T22.719** Corrosion of third degree of unspecified forearm

☑6th **T22.72** Corrosion of third degree of elbow
- ☑7th **T22.721** Corrosion of third degree of right elbow
- ☑7th **T22.722** Corrosion of third degree of left elbow
- ☑7th **T22.729** Corrosion of third degree of unspecified elbow

☑6th **T22.73** Corrosion of third degree of upper arm
- ☑7th **T22.731** Corrosion of third degree of right upper arm
- ☑7th **T22.732** Corrosion of third degree of left upper arm
- ☑7th **T22.739** Corrosion of third degree of unspecified upper arm

☑6th **T22.74** Corrosion of third degree of axilla
- ☑7th **T22.741** Corrosion of third degree of right axilla
- ☑7th **T22.742** Corrosion of third degree of left axilla
- ☑7th **T22.749** Corrosion of third degree of unspecified axilla

☑6th **T22.75** Corrosion of third degree of shoulder
- ☑7th **T22.751** Corrosion of third degree of right shoulder
- ☑7th **T22.752** Corrosion of third degree of left shoulder
- ☑7th **T22.759** Corrosion of third degree of unspecified shoulder

☑6th **T22.76** Corrosion of third degree of scapular region
- ☑7th **T22.761** Corrosion of third degree of right scapular region
- ☑7th **T22.762** Corrosion of third degree of left scapular region
- ☑7th **T22.769** Corrosion of third degree of unspecified scapular region

☑6th **T22.79** Corrosion of third degree of multiple sites of shoulder and upper limb, except wrist and hand
- ☑7th **T22.791** Corrosion of third degree of multiple sites of right shoulder and upper limb, except wrist and hand
- ☑7th **T22.792** Corrosion of third degree of multiple sites of left shoulder and upper limb, except wrist and hand
- ☑7th **T22.799** Corrosion of third degree of multiple sites of unspecified shoulder and upper limb, except wrist and hand

☑4th **T23** Burn and corrosion of wrist and hand

The appropriate 7th character is to be added to each code from category T23.
A initial encounter
D subsequent encounter
S sequela

☑5th **T23.0** Burn of unspecified degree of wrist and hand
  Use additional external cause code to identify the source, place and intent of the burn (X00-X19, X75-X77, X96-X98, Y92)

☑6th **T23.00** Burn of unspecified degree of hand, unspecified site
- ☑7th **T23.001** Burn of unspecified degree of right hand, unspecified site
- ☑7th **T23.002** Burn of unspecified degree of left hand, unspecified site
- ☑7th **T23.009** Burn of unspecified degree of unspecified hand, unspecified site

☑6th **T23.01** Burn of unspecified degree of thumb (nail)
- ☑7th **T23.011** Burn of unspecified degree of right thumb (nail)
- ☑7th **T23.012** Burn of unspecified degree of left thumb (nail)
- ☑7th **T23.019** Burn of unspecified degree of unspecified thumb (nail)

☑6th **T23.02** Burn of unspecified degree of single finger (nail) except thumb
- ☑7th **T23.021** Burn of unspecified degree of single right finger (nail) except thumb
- ☑7th **T23.022** Burn of unspecified degree of single left finger (nail) except thumb
- ☑7th **T23.029** Burn of unspecified degree of unspecified single finger (nail) except thumb

☑6th **T23.03** Burn of unspecified degree of multiple fingers (nail), not including thumb
- ☑7th **T23.031** Burn of unspecified degree of multiple right fingers (nail), not including thumb
- ☑7th **T23.032** Burn of unspecified degree of multiple left fingers (nail), not including thumb
- ☑7th **T23.039** Burn of unspecified degree of unspecified multiple fingers (nail), not including thumb

☑6th **T23.04** Burn of unspecified degree of multiple fingers (nail), including thumb
- ☑7th **T23.041** Burn of unspecified degree of multiple right fingers (nail), including thumb
- ☑7th **T23.042** Burn of unspecified degree of multiple left fingers (nail), including thumb
- ☑7th **T23.049** Burn of unspecified degree of unspecified multiple fingers (nail), including thumb

☑6th **T23.05** Burn of unspecified degree of palm
- ☑7th **T23.051** Burn of unspecified degree of right palm
- ☑7th **T23.052** Burn of unspecified degree of left palm
- ☑7th **T23.059** Burn of unspecified degree of unspecified palm

☑6th **T23.06** Burn of unspecified degree of back of hand
- ☑7th **T23.061** Burn of unspecified degree of back of right hand
- ☑7th **T23.062** Burn of unspecified degree of back of left hand
- ☑7th **T23.069** Burn of unspecified degree of back of unspecified hand

☑6th **T23.07** Burn of unspecified degree of wrist
- ☑7th **T23.071** Burn of unspecified degree of right wrist
- ☑7th **T23.072** Burn of unspecified degree of left wrist
- ☑7th **T23.079** Burn of unspecified degree of unspecified wrist

☑6th **T23.09** Burn of unspecified degree of multiple sites of wrist and hand
- ☑7th **T23.091** Burn of unspecified degree of multiple sites of right wrist and hand
- ☑7th **T23.092** Burn of unspecified degree of multiple sites of left wrist and hand
- ☑7th **T23.099** Burn of unspecified degree of multiple sites of unspecified wrist and hand

---

☑ Additional Character Required   ☑x7th Xtension Alert   Unspecified Dx   Other Specified Dx   Manifestation   ►◄ Revised Text   ● New Code   ▲ Revised Code Title

Injury, Poisoning and Certain Other Consequences of External Causes

T23.1–T23.321

✓5ᵗʰ **T23.1** **Burn of first degree of wrist and hand**
Use additional external cause code to identify the source, place and intent of the burn (X00-X19, X75-X77, X96-X98, Y92)

✓6ᵗʰ **T23.10** **Burn of first degree of hand, unspecified site**

- ✓7ᵗʰ **T23.101** Burn of first degree of right hand, unspecified site
- ✓7ᵗʰ **T23.102** Burn of first degree of left hand, unspecified site
- ✓7ᵗʰ **T23.109** Burn of first degree of unspecified hand, unspecified site

✓6ᵗʰ **T23.11** **Burn of first degree of thumb (nail)**

- ✓7ᵗʰ **T23.111** Burn of first degree of right thumb (nail)
- ✓7ᵗʰ **T23.112** Burn of first degree of left thumb (nail)
- ✓7ᵗʰ **T23.119** Burn of first degree of unspecified thumb (nail)

✓6ᵗʰ **T23.12** **Burn of first degree of single finger (nail) except thumb**

- ✓7ᵗʰ **T23.121** Burn of first degree of single right finger (nail) except thumb
- ✓7ᵗʰ **T23.122** Burn of first degree of single left finger (nail) except thumb
- ✓7ᵗʰ **T23.129** Burn of first degree of unspecified single finger (nail) except thumb

✓6ᵗʰ **T23.13** **Burn of first degree of multiple fingers (nail), not including thumb**

- ✓7ᵗʰ **T23.131** Burn of first degree of multiple right fingers (nail), not including thumb
- ✓7ᵗʰ **T23.132** Burn of first degree of multiple left fingers (nail), not including thumb
- ✓7ᵗʰ **T23.139** Burn of first degree of unspecified multiple fingers (nail), not including thumb

✓6ᵗʰ **T23.14** **Burn of first degree of multiple fingers (nail), including thumb**

- ✓7ᵗʰ **T23.141** Burn of first degree of multiple right fingers (nail), including thumb
- ✓7ᵗʰ **T23.142** Burn of first degree of multiple left fingers (nail), including thumb
- ✓7ᵗʰ **T23.149** Burn of first degree of unspecified multiple fingers (nail), including thumb

✓6ᵗʰ **T23.15** **Burn of first degree of palm**

- ✓7ᵗʰ **T23.151** Burn of first degree of right palm
- ✓7ᵗʰ **T23.152** Burn of first degree of left palm
- ✓7ᵗʰ **T23.159** Burn of first degree of unspecified palm

✓6ᵗʰ **T23.16** **Burn of first degree of back of hand**

- ✓7ᵗʰ **T23.161** Burn of first degree of back of right hand
- ✓7ᵗʰ **T23.162** Burn of first degree of back of left hand
- ✓7ᵗʰ **T23.169** Burn of first degree of back of unspecified hand

✓6ᵗʰ **T23.17** **Burn of first degree of wrist**

- ✓7ᵗʰ **T23.171** Burn of first degree of right wrist
- ✓7ᵗʰ **T23.172** Burn of first degree of left wrist
- ✓7ᵗʰ **T23.179** Burn of first degree of unspecified wrist

✓6ᵗʰ **T23.19** **Burn of first degree of multiple sites of wrist and hand**

- ✓7ᵗʰ **T23.191** Burn of first degree of multiple sites of right wrist and hand
- ✓7ᵗʰ **T23.192** Burn of first degree of multiple sites of left wrist and hand
- ✓7ᵗʰ **T23.199** Burn of first degree of multiple sites of unspecified wrist and hand

✓5ᵗʰ **T23.2** **Burn of second degree of wrist and hand**
Use additional external cause code to identify the source, place and intent of the burn (X00-X19, X75-X77, X96-X98, Y92)

✓6ᵗʰ **T23.20** **Burn of second degree of hand, unspecified site**

- ✓7ᵗʰ **T23.201** Burn of second degree of right hand, unspecified site
- ✓7ᵗʰ **T23.202** Burn of second degree of left hand, unspecified site
- ✓7ᵗʰ **T23.209** Burn of second degree of unspecified hand, unspecified site

✓6ᵗʰ **T23.21** **Burn of second degree of thumb (nail)**

- ✓7ᵗʰ **T23.211** Burn of second degree of right thumb (nail)
- ✓7ᵗʰ **T23.212** Burn of second degree of left thumb (nail)
- ✓7ᵗʰ **T23.219** Burn of second degree of unspecified thumb (nail)

✓6ᵗʰ **T23.22** **Burn of second degree of single finger (nail) except thumb**

- ✓7ᵗʰ **T23.221** Burn of second degree of single right finger (nail) except thumb
- ✓7ᵗʰ **T23.222** Burn of second degree of single left finger (nail) except thumb
- ✓7ᵗʰ **T23.229** Burn of second degree of unspecified single finger (nail) except thumb

✓6ᵗʰ **T23.23** **Burn of second degree of multiple fingers (nail), not including thumb**

- ✓7ᵗʰ **T23.231** Burn of second degree of multiple right fingers (nail), not including thumb
- ✓7ᵗʰ **T23.232** Burn of second degree of multiple left fingers (nail), not including thumb
- ✓7ᵗʰ **T23.239** Burn of second degree of unspecified multiple fingers (nail), not including thumb

✓6ᵗʰ **T23.24** **Burn of second degree of multiple fingers (nail), including thumb**

- ✓7ᵗʰ **T23.241** Burn of second degree of multiple right fingers (nail), including thumb
- ✓7ᵗʰ **T23.242** Burn of second degree of multiple left fingers (nail), including thumb
- ✓7ᵗʰ **T23.249** Burn of second degree of unspecified multiple fingers (nail), including thumb

✓6ᵗʰ **T23.25** **Burn of second degree of palm**

- ✓7ᵗʰ **T23.251** Burn of second degree of right palm
- ✓7ᵗʰ **T23.252** Burn of second degree of left palm
- ✓7ᵗʰ **T23.259** Burn of second degree of unspecified palm

✓6ᵗʰ **T23.26** **Burn of second degree of back of hand**

- ✓7ᵗʰ **T23.261** Burn of second degree of back of right hand
- ✓7ᵗʰ **T23.262** Burn of second degree of back of left hand
- ✓7ᵗʰ **T23.269** Burn of second degree of back of unspecified hand

✓6ᵗʰ **T23.27** **Burn of second degree of wrist**

- ✓7ᵗʰ **T23.271** Burn of second degree of right wrist
- ✓7ᵗʰ **T23.272** Burn of second degree of left wrist
- ✓7ᵗʰ **T23.279** Burn of second degree of unspecified wrist

✓6ᵗʰ **T23.29** **Burn of second degree of multiple sites of wrist and hand**

- ✓7ᵗʰ **T23.291** Burn of second degree of multiple sites of right wrist and hand
- ✓7ᵗʰ **T23.292** Burn of second degree of multiple sites of left wrist and hand
- ✓7ᵗʰ **T23.299** Burn of second degree of multiple sites of unspecified wrist and hand

✓5ᵗʰ **T23.3** **Burn of third degree of wrist and hand**
Use additional external cause code to identify the source, place and intent of the burn (X00-X19, X75-X77, X96-X98, Y92)

✓6ᵗʰ **T23.30** **Burn of third degree of hand, unspecified site**

- ✓7ᵗʰ **T23.301** Burn of third degree of right hand, unspecified site
- ✓7ᵗʰ **T23.302** Burn of third degree of left hand, unspecified site
- ✓7ᵗʰ **T23.309** Burn of third degree of unspecified hand, unspecified site

✓6ᵗʰ **T23.31** **Burn of third degree of thumb (nail)**

- ✓7ᵗʰ **T23.311** Burn of third degree of right thumb (nail)
- ✓7ᵗʰ **T23.312** Burn of third degree of left thumb (nail)
- ✓7ᵗʰ **T23.319** Burn of third degree of unspecified thumb (nail)

✓6ᵗʰ **T23.32** **Burn of third degree of single finger (nail) except thumb**

- ✓7ᵗʰ **T23.321** Burn of third degree of single right finger (nail) except thumb

EXCLUDES 1 Not coded here   EXCLUDES 2 Not included here   N Newborn Age: 0   P Pediatric Age: 0-17   M Maternity Age: 12-55   A Adult Age: 15-124

930   ICD-10-CM Draft (2015)

☑7ᵗʰ **T23.322** Burn of third degree of single left finger (nail) except thumb

☑7ᵗʰ **T23.329 Burn of third degree of unspecified single finger (nail) except thumb**

☑6ᵗʰ **T23.33** Burn of third degree of multiple fingers (nail), not including thumb

    ☑7ᵗʰ **T23.331** Burn of third degree of multiple right fingers (nail), not including thumb

    ☑7ᵗʰ **T23.332** Burn of third degree of multiple left fingers (nail), not including thumb

    ☑7ᵗʰ **T23.339 Burn of third degree of unspecified multiple fingers (nail), not including thumb**

☑6ᵗʰ **T23.34** Burn of third degree of multiple fingers (nail), including thumb

    ☑7ᵗʰ **T23.341** Burn of third degree of multiple right fingers (nail), including thumb

    ☑7ᵗʰ **T23.342** Burn of third degree of multiple left fingers (nail), including thumb

    ☑7ᵗʰ **T23.349 Burn of third degree of unspecified multiple fingers (nail), including thumb**

☑6ᵗʰ **T23.35** Burn of third degree of palm

    ☑7ᵗʰ **T23.351** Burn of third degree of right palm

    ☑7ᵗʰ **T23.352** Burn of third degree of left palm

    ☑7ᵗʰ **T23.359 Burn of third degree of unspecified palm**

☑6ᵗʰ **T23.36** Burn of third degree of back of hand

    ☑7ᵗʰ **T23.361** Burn of third degree of back of right hand

    ☑7ᵗʰ **T23.362** Burn of third degree of back of left hand

    ☑7ᵗʰ **T23.369 Burn of third degree of back of unspecified hand**

☑6ᵗʰ **T23.37** Burn of third degree of wrist

    ☑7ᵗʰ **T23.371** Burn of third degree of right wrist

    ☑7ᵗʰ **T23.372** Burn of third degree of left wrist

    ☑7ᵗʰ **T23.379 Burn of third degree of unspecified wrist**

☑6ᵗʰ **T23.39** Burn of third degree of multiple sites of wrist and hand

    ☑7ᵗʰ **T23.391** Burn of third degree of multiple sites of right wrist and hand

    ☑7ᵗʰ **T23.392** Burn of third degree of multiple sites of left wrist and hand

    ☑7ᵗʰ **T23.399 Burn of third degree of multiple sites of unspecified wrist and hand**

☑5ᵗʰ **T23.4 Corrosion of** unspecified degree **of wrist and hand**
    Code first (T51-T65) to identify chemical and intent
    Use additional external cause code to identify place (Y92)

☑6ᵗʰ **T23.40** Corrosion of unspecified degree of hand, unspecified site

    ☑7ᵗʰ **T23.401 Corrosion of unspecified degree of right hand, unspecified site**

    ☑7ᵗʰ **T23.402 Corrosion of unspecified degree of left hand, unspecified site**

    ☑7ᵗʰ **T23.409 Corrosion of unspecified degree of unspecified hand, unspecified site**

☑6ᵗʰ **T23.41** Corrosion of unspecified degree of thumb (nail)

    ☑7ᵗʰ **T23.411 Corrosion of unspecified degree of right thumb (nail)**

    ☑7ᵗʰ **T23.412 Corrosion of unspecified degree of left thumb (nail)**

    ☑7ᵗʰ **T23.419 Corrosion of unspecified degree of unspecified thumb (nail)**

☑6ᵗʰ **T23.42** Corrosion of unspecified degree of single finger (nail) except thumb

    ☑7ᵗʰ **T23.421 Corrosion of unspecified degree of single right finger (nail) except thumb**

    ☑7ᵗʰ **T23.422 Corrosion of unspecified degree of single left finger (nail) except thumb**

    ☑7ᵗʰ **T23.429 Corrosion of unspecified degree of unspecified single finger (nail) except thumb**

☑6ᵗʰ **T23.43** Corrosion of unspecified degree of multiple fingers (nail), not including thumb

    ☑7ᵗʰ **T23.431 Corrosion of unspecified degree of multiple right fingers (nail), not including thumb**

☑7ᵗʰ **T23.432 Corrosion of unspecified degree of multiple left fingers (nail), not including thumb**

☑7ᵗʰ **T23.439 Corrosion of unspecified degree of unspecified multiple fingers (nail), not including thumb**

☑6ᵗʰ **T23.44** Corrosion of unspecified degree of multiple fingers (nail), including thumb

    ☑7ᵗʰ **T23.441 Corrosion of unspecified degree of multiple right fingers (nail), including thumb**

    ☑7ᵗʰ **T23.442 Corrosion of unspecified degree of multiple left fingers (nail), including thumb**

    ☑7ᵗʰ **T23.449 Corrosion of unspecified degree of unspecified multiple fingers (nail), including thumb**

☑6ᵗʰ **T23.45** Corrosion of unspecified degree of palm

    ☑7ᵗʰ **T23.451 Corrosion of unspecified degree of right palm**

    ☑7ᵗʰ **T23.452 Corrosion of unspecified degree of left palm**

    ☑7ᵗʰ **T23.459 Corrosion of unspecified degree of unspecified palm**

☑6ᵗʰ **T23.46** Corrosion of unspecified degree of back of hand

    ☑7ᵗʰ **T23.461 Corrosion of unspecified degree of back of right hand**

    ☑7ᵗʰ **T23.462 Corrosion of unspecified degree of back of left hand**

    ☑7ᵗʰ **T23.469 Corrosion of unspecified degree of back of unspecified hand**

☑6ᵗʰ **T23.47** Corrosion of unspecified degree of wrist

    ☑7ᵗʰ **T23.471 Corrosion of unspecified degree of right wrist**

    ☑7ᵗʰ **T23.472 Corrosion of unspecified degree of left wrist**

    ☑7ᵗʰ **T23.479 Corrosion of unspecified degree of unspecified wrist**

☑6ᵗʰ **T23.49** Corrosion of unspecified degree of multiple sites of wrist and hand

    ☑7ᵗʰ **T23.491 Corrosion of unspecified degree of multiple sites of right wrist and hand**

    ☑7ᵗʰ **T23.492 Corrosion of unspecified degree of multiple sites of left wrist and hand**

    ☑7ᵗʰ **T23.499 Corrosion of unspecified degree of multiple sites of unspecified wrist and hand**

☑5ᵗʰ **T23.5 Corrosion of** first degree **of wrist and hand**
    Code first (T51-T65) to identify chemical and intent
    Use additional external cause code to identify place (Y92)

☑6ᵗʰ **T23.50** Corrosion of first degree of hand, unspecified site

    ☑7ᵗʰ **T23.501 Corrosion of first degree of right hand, unspecified site**

    ☑7ᵗʰ **T23.502 Corrosion of first degree of left hand, unspecified site**

    ☑7ᵗʰ **T23.509 Corrosion of first degree of unspecified hand, unspecified site**

☑6ᵗʰ **T23.51** Corrosion of first degree of thumb (nail)

    ☑7ᵗʰ **T23.511 Corrosion of first degree of right thumb (nail)**

    ☑7ᵗʰ **T23.512 Corrosion of first degree of left thumb (nail)**

    ☑7ᵗʰ **T23.519 Corrosion of first degree of unspecified thumb (nail)**

☑6ᵗʰ **T23.52** Corrosion of first degree of single finger (nail) except thumb

    ☑7ᵗʰ **T23.521 Corrosion of first degree of single right finger (nail) except thumb**

    ☑7ᵗʰ **T23.522 Corrosion of first degree of single left finger (nail) except thumb**

    ☑7ᵗʰ **T23.529 Corrosion of first degree of unspecified single finger (nail) except thumb**

☑ Additional Character Required   ✓x7ᵗʰ Xtension Alert   Unspecified Dx   Other Specified Dx   Manifestation   ►◄ Revised Text   ● New Code   ▲ Revised Code Title

ICD-10-CM Draft (2015)   931

Injury, Poisoning and Certain Other Consequences of External Causes

T23.53–T23.741

✓6th **T23.53** Corrosion of first degree of multiple fingers (nail), not including thumb

     ✓7th **T23.531** Corrosion of first degree of multiple right fingers (nail), not including thumb

     ✓7th **T23.532** Corrosion of first degree of multiple left fingers (nail), not including thumb

     ✓7th **T23.539 Corrosion of first degree of unspecified multiple fingers (nail), not including thumb**

✓6th **T23.54** Corrosion of first degree of multiple fingers (nail), including thumb

     ✓7th **T23.541** Corrosion of first degree of multiple right fingers (nail), including thumb

     ✓7th **T23.542** Corrosion of first degree of multiple left fingers (nail), including thumb

     ✓7th **T23.549 Corrosion of first degree of unspecified multiple fingers (nail), including thumb**

✓6th **T23.55** Corrosion of first degree of palm

     ✓7th **T23.551** Corrosion of first degree of right palm

     ✓7th **T23.552** Corrosion of first degree of left palm

     ✓7th **T23.559 Corrosion of first degree of unspecified palm**

✓6th **T23.56** Corrosion of first degree of back of hand

     ✓7th **T23.561** Corrosion of first degree of back of right hand

     ✓7th **T23.562** Corrosion of first degree of back of left hand

     ✓7th **T23.569 Corrosion of first degree of back of unspecified hand**

✓6th **T23.57** Corrosion of first degree of wrist

     ✓7th **T23.571** Corrosion of first degree of right wrist

     ✓7th **T23.572** Corrosion of first degree of left wrist

     ✓7th **T23.579 Corrosion of first degree of unspecified wrist**

✓6th **T23.59** Corrosion of first degree of multiple sites of wrist and hand

     ✓7th **T23.591** Corrosion of first degree of multiple sites of right wrist and hand

     ✓7th **T23.592** Corrosion of first degree of multiple sites of left wrist and hand

     ✓7th **T23.599 Corrosion of first degree of multiple sites of unspecified wrist and hand**

✓5th **T23.6** Corrosion of second degree of wrist and hand

     Code first (T51-T65) to identify chemical and intent

     Use additional external cause code to identify place (Y92)

     ✓6th **T23.60** Corrosion of second degree of hand, unspecified site

         ✓7th **T23.601 Corrosion of second degree of right hand, unspecified site**

         ✓7th **T23.602 Corrosion of second degree of left hand, unspecified site**

         ✓7th **T23.609 Corrosion of second degree of unspecified hand, unspecified site**

     ✓6th **T23.61** Corrosion of second degree of thumb (nail)

         ✓7th **T23.611 Corrosion of second degree of right thumb (nail)**

         ✓7th **T23.612 Corrosion of second degree of left thumb (nail)**

         ✓7th **T23.619 Corrosion of second degree of unspecified thumb (nail)**

     ✓6th **T23.62** Corrosion of second degree of single finger (nail) except thumb

         ✓7th **T23.621** Corrosion of second degree of single right finger (nail) except thumb

         ✓7th **T23.622** Corrosion of second degree of single left finger (nail) except thumb

         ✓7th **T23.629 Corrosion of second degree of unspecified single finger (nail) except thumb**

     ✓6th **T23.63** Corrosion of second degree of multiple fingers (nail), not including thumb

         ✓7th **T23.631** Corrosion of second degree of multiple right fingers (nail), not including thumb

         ✓7th **T23.632** Corrosion of second degree of multiple left fingers (nail), not including thumb

         ✓7th **T23.639 Corrosion of second degree of unspecified multiple fingers (nail), not including thumb**

✓6th **T23.64** Corrosion of second degree of multiple fingers (nail), including thumb

     ✓7th **T23.641** Corrosion of second degree of multiple right fingers (nail), including thumb

     ✓7th **T23.642** Corrosion of second degree of multiple left fingers (nail), including thumb

     ✓7th **T23.649 Corrosion of second degree of unspecified multiple fingers (nail), including thumb**

✓6th **T23.65** Corrosion of second degree of palm

     ✓7th **T23.651** Corrosion of second degree of right palm

     ✓7th **T23.652** Corrosion of second degree of left palm

     ✓7th **T23.659 Corrosion of second degree of unspecified palm**

✓6th **T23.66** Corrosion of second degree of back of hand

     ✓7th **T23.661** Corrosion of second degree back of right hand

     ✓7th **T23.662** Corrosion of second degree back of left hand

     ✓7th **T23.669 Corrosion of second degree back of unspecified hand**

✓6th **T23.67** Corrosion of second degree of wrist

     ✓7th **T23.671** Corrosion of second degree of right wrist

     ✓7th **T23.672** Corrosion of second degree of left wrist

     ✓7th **T23.679 Corrosion of second degree of unspecified wrist**

✓6th **T23.69** Corrosion of second degree of multiple sites of wrist and hand

     ✓7th **T23.691** Corrosion of second degree of multiple sites of right wrist and hand

     ✓7th **T23.692** Corrosion of second degree of multiple sites of left wrist and hand

     ✓7th **T23.699 Corrosion of second degree of multiple sites of unspecified wrist and hand**

✓5th **T23.7** Corrosion of third degree of wrist and hand

     Code first (T51-T65) to identify chemical and intent

     Use additional external cause code to identify place (Y92)

     ✓6th **T23.70** Corrosion of third degree of hand, unspecified site

         ✓7th **T23.701** Corrosion of third degree of right hand, unspecified site

         ✓7th **T23.702** Corrosion of third degree of left hand, unspecified site

         ✓7th **T23.709 Corrosion of third degree of unspecified hand, unspecified site**

     ✓6th **T23.71** Corrosion of third degree of thumb (nail)

         ✓7th **T23.711** Corrosion of third degree of right thumb (nail)

         ✓7th **T23.712** Corrosion of third degree of left thumb (nail)

         ✓7th **T23.719 Corrosion of third degree of unspecified thumb (nail)**

     ✓6th **T23.72** Corrosion of third degree of single finger (nail) except thumb

         ✓7th **T23.721** Corrosion of third degree of single right finger (nail) except thumb

         ✓7th **T23.722** Corrosion of third degree of single left finger (nail) except thumb

         ✓7th **T23.729 Corrosion of third degree of unspecified single finger (nail) except thumb**

     ✓6th **T23.73** Corrosion of third degree of multiple fingers (nail), not including thumb

         ✓7th **T23.731** Corrosion of third degree of multiple right fingers (nail), not including thumb

         ✓7th **T23.732** Corrosion of third degree of multiple left fingers (nail), not including thumb

         ✓7th **T23.739 Corrosion of third degree of unspecified multiple fingers (nail), not including thumb**

     ✓6th **T23.74** Corrosion of third degree of multiple fingers (nail), including thumb

         ✓7th **T23.741** Corrosion of third degree of multiple right fingers (nail), including thumb

EXCLUDES 1 Not coded here   EXCLUDES 2 Not included here   N Newborn Age: 0   P Pediatric Age: 0-17   M Maternity Age: 12-55   A Adult Age: 15-124

932   ICD-10-CM Draft (2015)

√7th T23.742 Corrosion of third degree of multiple left fingers (nail), including thumb

√7th T23.749 Corrosion of third degree of unspecified multiple fingers (nail), including thumb

√6th T23.75 Corrosion of third degree of palm

   √7th T23.751 Corrosion of third degree of right palm

   √7th T23.752 Corrosion of third degree of left palm

   √7th T23.759 Corrosion of third degree of unspecified palm

√6th T23.76 Corrosion of third degree of back of hand

   √7th T23.761 Corrosion of third degree of back of right hand

   √7th T23.762 Corrosion of third degree of back of left hand

   √7th T23.769 Corrosion of third degree back of unspecified hand

√6th T23.77 Corrosion of third degree of wrist

   √7th T23.771 Corrosion of third degree of right wrist

   √7th T23.772 Corrosion of third degree of left wrist

   √7th T23.779 Corrosion of third degree of unspecified wrist

√6th T23.79 Corrosion of third degree of multiple sites of wrist and hand

   √7th T23.791 Corrosion of third degree of multiple sites of right wrist and hand

   √7th T23.792 Corrosion of third degree of multiple sites of left wrist and hand

   √7th T23.799 Corrosion of third degree of multiple sites of unspecified wrist and hand

√4th T24 Burn and corrosion of lower limb, except ankle and foot

> *EXCLUDES 2*   burn and corrosion of ankle and foot (T25.-)
>   burn and corrosion of hip region (T21.-)

> The appropriate 7th character is to be added to each code from category T24.
> A   initial encounter
> D   subsequent encounter
> S   sequela

√5th T24.0 Burn of unspecified degree of lower limb, except ankle and foot

> Use additional external cause code to identify the source, place and intent of the burn (X00-X19, X75-X77, X96-X98, Y92)

√6th T24.00 Burn of unspecified degree of unspecified site of lower limb, except ankle and foot

   √7th T24.001 Burn of unspecified degree of unspecified site of right lower limb, except ankle and foot

   √7th T24.002 Burn of unspecified degree of unspecified site of left lower limb, except ankle and foot

   √7th T24.009 Burn of unspecified degree of unspecified site of unspecified lower limb, except ankle and foot

√6th T24.01 Burn of unspecified degree of thigh

   √7th T24.011 Burn of unspecified degree of right thigh

   √7th T24.012 Burn of unspecified degree of left thigh

   √7th T24.019 Burn of unspecified degree of unspecified thigh

√6th T24.02 Burn of unspecified degree of knee

   √7th T24.021 Burn of unspecified degree of right knee

   √7th T24.022 Burn of unspecified degree of left knee

   √7th T24.029 Burn of unspecified degree of unspecified knee

√6th T24.03 Burn of unspecified degree of lower leg

   √7th T24.031 Burn of unspecified degree of right lower leg

   √7th T24.032 Burn of unspecified degree of left lower leg

   √7th T24.039 Burn of unspecified degree of unspecified lower leg

√6th T24.09 Burn of unspecified degree of multiple sites of lower limb, except ankle and foot

   √7th T24.091 Burn of unspecified degree of multiple sites of right lower limb, except ankle and foot

   √7th T24.092 Burn of unspecified degree of multiple sites of left lower limb, except ankle and foot

   √7th T24.099 Burn of unspecified degree of multiple sites of unspecified lower limb, except ankle and foot

√5th T24.1 Burn of first degree of lower limb, except ankle and foot

> Use additional external cause code to identify the source, place and intent of the burn (X00-X19, X75-X77, X96-X98, Y92)

√6th T24.10 Burn of first degree of unspecified site of lower limb, except ankle and foot

   √7th T24.101 Burn of first degree of unspecified site of right lower limb, except ankle and foot

   √7th T24.102 Burn of first degree of unspecified site of left lower limb, except ankle and foot

   √7th T24.109 Burn of first degree of unspecified site of unspecified lower limb, except ankle and foot

√6th T24.11 Burn of first degree of thigh

   √7th T24.111 Burn of first degree of right thigh

   √7th T24.112 Burn of first degree of left thigh

   √7th T24.119 Burn of first degree of unspecified thigh

√6th T24.12 Burn of first degree of knee

   √7th T24.121 Burn of first degree of right knee

   √7th T24.122 Burn of first degree of left knee

   √7th T24.129 Burn of first degree of unspecified knee

√6th T24.13 Burn of first degree of lower leg

   √7th T24.131 Burn of first degree of right lower leg

   √7th T24.132 Burn of first degree of left lower leg

   √7th T24.139 Burn of first degree of unspecified lower leg

√6th T24.19 Burn of first degree of multiple sites of lower limb, except ankle and foot

   √7th T24.191 Burn of first degree of multiple sites of right lower limb, except ankle and foot

   √7th T24.192 Burn of first degree of multiple sites of left lower limb, except ankle and foot

   √7th T24.199 Burn of first degree of multiple sites of unspecified lower limb, except ankle and foot

√5th T24.2 Burn of second degree of lower limb, except ankle and foot

> Use additional external cause code to identify the source, place and intent of the burn (X00-X19, X75-X77, X96-X98, Y92)

√6th T24.20 Burn of second degree of unspecified site of lower limb, except ankle and foot

   √7th T24.201 Burn of second degree of unspecified site of right lower limb, except ankle and foot

   √7th T24.202 Burn of second degree of unspecified site of left lower limb, except ankle and foot

   √7th T24.209 Burn of second degree of unspecified site of unspecified lower limb, except ankle and foot

√6th T24.21 Burn of second degree of thigh

   √7th T24.211 Burn of second degree of right thigh

   √7th T24.212 Burn of second degree of left thigh

   √7th T24.219 Burn of second degree of unspecified thigh

√6th T24.22 Burn of second degree of knee

   √7th T24.221 Burn of second degree of right knee

   √7th T24.222 Burn of second degree of left knee

   √7th T24.229 Burn of second degree of unspecified knee

√6th T24.23 Burn of second degree of lower leg

   √7th T24.231 Burn of second degree of right lower leg

   √7th T24.232 Burn of second degree of left lower leg

   √7th T24.239 Burn of second degree of unspecified lower leg

√6th T24.29 Burn of second degree of multiple sites of lower limb, except ankle and foot

   √7th T24.291 Burn of second degree of multiple sites of right lower limb, except ankle and foot

   √7th T24.292 Burn of second degree of multiple sites of left lower limb, except ankle and foot

☑ Additional Character Required   √x7th Xtension Alert   Unspecified Dx   Other Specified Dx   Manifestation   ►◄ Revised Text   ● New Code   ▲ Revised Code Title

ICD-10-CM Draft (2015)   **933**

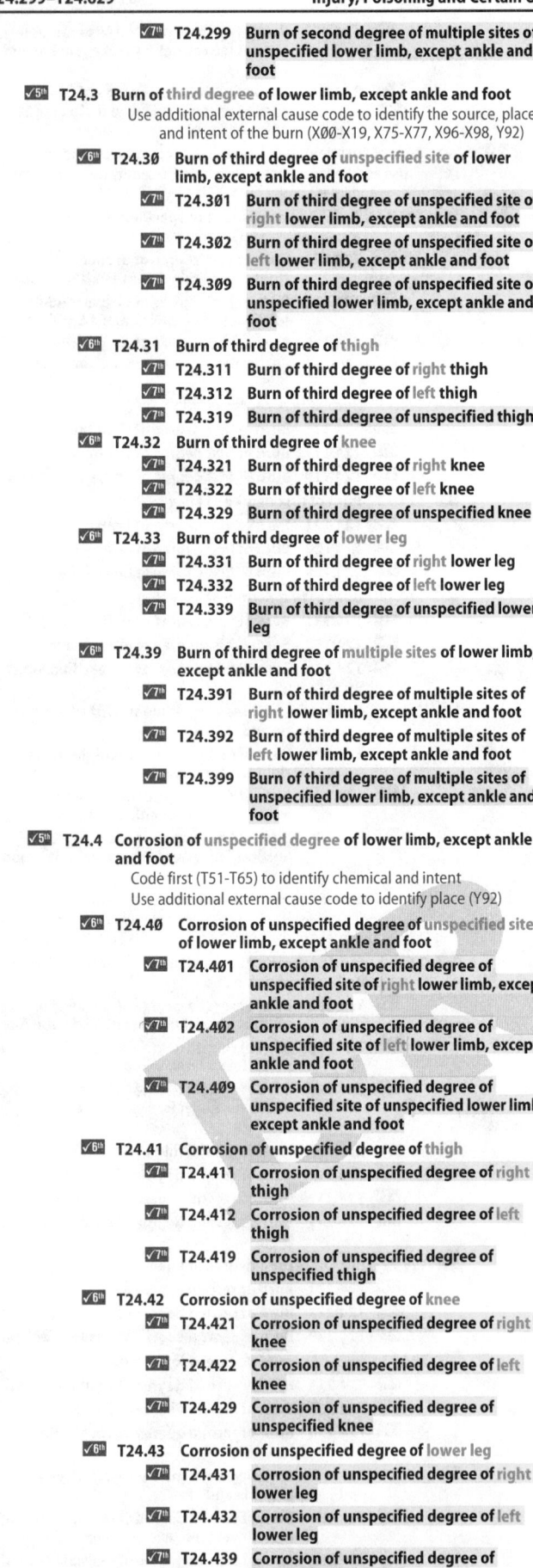

√7th **T24.299** Burn of second degree of multiple sites of unspecified lower limb, except ankle and foot

√5th **T24.3** Burn of third degree of lower limb, except ankle and foot
Use additional external cause code to identify the source, place and intent of the burn (X00-X19, X75-X77, X96-X98, Y92)

√6th **T24.30** Burn of third degree of unspecified site of lower limb, except ankle and foot

√7th **T24.301** Burn of third degree of unspecified site of right lower limb, except ankle and foot

√7th **T24.302** Burn of third degree of unspecified site of left lower limb, except ankle and foot

√7th **T24.309** Burn of third degree of unspecified site of unspecified lower limb, except ankle and foot

√6th **T24.31** Burn of third degree of thigh

√7th **T24.311** Burn of third degree of right thigh

√7th **T24.312** Burn of third degree of left thigh

√7th **T24.319** Burn of third degree of unspecified thigh

√6th **T24.32** Burn of third degree of knee

√7th **T24.321** Burn of third degree of right knee

√7th **T24.322** Burn of third degree of left knee

√7th **T24.329** Burn of third degree of unspecified knee

√6th **T24.33** Burn of third degree of lower leg

√7th **T24.331** Burn of third degree of right lower leg

√7th **T24.332** Burn of third degree of left lower leg

√7th **T24.339** Burn of third degree of unspecified lower leg

√6th **T24.39** Burn of third degree of multiple sites of lower limb, except ankle and foot

√7th **T24.391** Burn of third degree of multiple sites of right lower limb, except ankle and foot

√7th **T24.392** Burn of third degree of multiple sites of left lower limb, except ankle and foot

√7th **T24.399** Burn of third degree of multiple sites of unspecified lower limb, except ankle and foot

√5th **T24.4** Corrosion of unspecified degree of lower limb, except ankle and foot
Code first (T51-T65) to identify chemical and intent
Use additional external cause code to identify place (Y92)

√6th **T24.40** Corrosion of unspecified degree of unspecified site of lower limb, except ankle and foot

√7th **T24.401** Corrosion of unspecified degree of unspecified site of right lower limb, except ankle and foot

√7th **T24.402** Corrosion of unspecified degree of unspecified site of left lower limb, except ankle and foot

√7th **T24.409** Corrosion of unspecified degree of unspecified site of unspecified lower limb, except ankle and foot

√6th **T24.41** Corrosion of unspecified degree of thigh

√7th **T24.411** Corrosion of unspecified degree of right thigh

√7th **T24.412** Corrosion of unspecified degree of left thigh

√7th **T24.419** Corrosion of unspecified degree of unspecified thigh

√6th **T24.42** Corrosion of unspecified degree of knee

√7th **T24.421** Corrosion of unspecified degree of right knee

√7th **T24.422** Corrosion of unspecified degree of left knee

√7th **T24.429** Corrosion of unspecified degree of unspecified knee

√6th **T24.43** Corrosion of unspecified degree of lower leg

√7th **T24.431** Corrosion of unspecified degree of right lower leg

√7th **T24.432** Corrosion of unspecified degree of left lower leg

√7th **T24.439** Corrosion of unspecified degree of unspecified lower leg

√6th **T24.49** Corrosion of unspecified degree of multiple sites of lower limb, except ankle and foot

√7th **T24.491** Corrosion of unspecified degree of multiple sites of right lower limb, except ankle and foot

√7th **T24.492** Corrosion of unspecified degree of multiple sites of left lower limb, except ankle and foot

√7th **T24.499** Corrosion of unspecified degree of multiple sites of unspecified lower limb, except ankle and foot

√5th **T24.5** Corrosion of first degree of lower limb, except ankle and foot
Code first (T51-T65) to identify chemical and intent
Use additional external cause code to identify place (Y92)

√6th **T24.50** Corrosion of first degree of unspecified site of lower limb, except ankle and foot

√7th **T24.501** Corrosion of first degree of unspecified site of right lower limb, except ankle and foot

√7th **T24.502** Corrosion of first degree of unspecified site of left lower limb, except ankle and foot

√7th **T24.509** Corrosion of first degree of unspecified site of unspecified lower limb, except ankle and foot

√6th **T24.51** Corrosion of first degree of thigh

√7th **T24.511** Corrosion of first degree of right thigh

√7th **T24.512** Corrosion of first degree of left thigh

√7th **T24.519** Corrosion of first degree of unspecified thigh

√6th **T24.52** Corrosion of first degree of knee

√7th **T24.521** Corrosion of first degree of right knee

√7th **T24.522** Corrosion of first degree of left knee

√7th **T24.529** Corrosion of first degree of unspecified knee

√6th **T24.53** Corrosion of first degree of lower leg

√7th **T24.531** Corrosion of first degree of right lower leg

√7th **T24.532** Corrosion of first degree of left lower leg

√7th **T24.539** Corrosion of first degree of unspecified lower leg

√6th **T24.59** Corrosion of first degree of multiple sites of lower limb, except ankle and foot

√7th **T24.591** Corrosion of first degree of multiple sites of right lower limb, except ankle and foot

√7th **T24.592** Corrosion of first degree of multiple sites of left lower limb, except ankle and foot

√7th **T24.599** Corrosion of first degree of multiple sites of unspecified lower limb, except ankle and foot

√5th **T24.6** Corrosion of second degree of lower limb, except ankle and foot
Code first (T51-T65) to identify chemical and intent
Use additional external cause code to identify place (Y92)

√6th **T24.60** Corrosion of second degree of unspecified site of lower limb, except ankle and foot

√7th **T24.601** Corrosion of second degree of unspecified site of right lower limb, except ankle and foot

√7th **T24.602** Corrosion of second degree of unspecified site of left lower limb, except ankle and foot

√7th **T24.609** Corrosion of second degree of unspecified site of unspecified lower limb, except ankle and foot

√6th **T24.61** Corrosion of second degree of thigh

√7th **T24.611** Corrosion of second degree of right thigh

√7th **T24.612** Corrosion of second degree of left thigh

√7th **T24.619** Corrosion of second degree of unspecified thigh

√6th **T24.62** Corrosion of second degree of knee

√7th **T24.621** Corrosion of second degree of right knee

√7th **T24.622** Corrosion of second degree of left knee

√7th **T24.629** Corrosion of second degree of unspecified knee

EXCLUDES 1 Not coded here   **EXCLUDES 2** Not included here   N Newborn Age: 0   P Pediatric Age: 0-17   M Maternity Age: 12-55   A Adult Age: 15-124

934   ICD-10-CM Draft (2015)

√6ᵗʰ **T24.63 Corrosion of second degree of** lower leg

  √7ᵗʰ **T24.631 Corrosion of second degree of** right **lower leg**

  √7ᵗʰ **T24.632 Corrosion of second degree of** left **lower leg**

  √7ᵗʰ **T24.639 Corrosion of second degree of unspecified lower leg**

√6ᵗʰ **T24.69 Corrosion of second degree of** multiple sites **of lower limb, except ankle and foot**

  √7ᵗʰ **T24.691 Corrosion of second degree of multiple sites of** right **lower limb, except ankle and foot**

  √7ᵗʰ **T24.692 Corrosion of second degree of multiple sites of** left **lower limb, except ankle and foot**

  √7ᵗʰ **T24.699 Corrosion of second degree of multiple sites of unspecified lower limb, except ankle and foot**

√5ᵗʰ **T24.7 Corrosion of** third degree **of lower limb, except ankle and foot**

Code first (T51-T65) to identify chemical and intent
Use additional external cause code to identify place (Y92)

√6ᵗʰ **T24.70 Corrosion of third degree of** unspecified site **of lower limb, except ankle and foot**

  √7ᵗʰ **T24.701 Corrosion of third degree of unspecified site of** right **lower limb, except ankle and foot**

  √7ᵗʰ **T24.702 Corrosion of third degree of unspecified site of** left **lower limb, except ankle and foot**

  √7ᵗʰ **T24.709 Corrosion of third degree of unspecified site of unspecified lower limb, except ankle and foot**

√6ᵗʰ **T24.71 Corrosion of third degree of** thigh

  √7ᵗʰ **T24.711 Corrosion of third degree of** right **thigh**

  √7ᵗʰ **T24.712 Corrosion of third degree of** left **thigh**

  √7ᵗʰ **T24.719 Corrosion of third degree of unspecified thigh**

√6ᵗʰ **T24.72 Corrosion of third degree of** knee

  √7ᵗʰ **T24.721 Corrosion of third degree of** right **knee**

  √7ᵗʰ **T24.722 Corrosion of third degree of** left **knee**

  √7ᵗʰ **T24.729 Corrosion of third degree of unspecified knee**

√6ᵗʰ **T24.73 Corrosion of third degree of** lower leg

  √7ᵗʰ **T24.731 Corrosion of third degree of** right **lower leg**

  √7ᵗʰ **T24.732 Corrosion of third degree of** left **lower leg**

  √7ᵗʰ **T24.739 Corrosion of third degree of unspecified lower leg**

√6ᵗʰ **T24.79 Corrosion of third degree of** multiple sites **of lower limb, except ankle and foot**

  √7ᵗʰ **T24.791 Corrosion of third degree of multiple sites of** right **lower limb, except ankle and foot**

  √7ᵗʰ **T24.792 Corrosion of third degree of multiple sites of** left **lower limb, except ankle and foot**

  √7ᵗʰ **T24.799 Corrosion of third degree of multiple sites of unspecified lower limb, except ankle and foot**

√4ᵗʰ **T25 Burn and corrosion of ankle and foot**

The appropriate 7th character is to be added to each code from category T25.
A   initial encounter
D   subsequent encounter
S   sequela

√5ᵗʰ **T25.0 Burn of** unspecified degree **of ankle and foot**

Use additional external cause code to identify the source, place and intent of the burn (X00-X19, X75-X77, X96-X98, Y92)

√6ᵗʰ **T25.01 Burn of unspecified degree of** ankle

  √7ᵗʰ **T25.011 Burn of unspecified degree of** right **ankle**

  √7ᵗʰ **T25.012 Burn of unspecified degree of** left **ankle**

  √7ᵗʰ **T25.019 Burn of unspecified degree of unspecified ankle**

√6ᵗʰ **T25.02 Burn of unspecified degree of** foot

  EXCLUDES 2 *burn of unspecified degree of toe(s) (nail) (T25.03-)*

√7ᵗʰ **T25.021 Burn of unspecified degree of** right **foot**

√7ᵗʰ **T25.022 Burn of unspecified degree of** left **foot**

√7ᵗʰ **T25.029 Burn of unspecified degree of unspecified foot**

√6ᵗʰ **T25.03 Burn of unspecified degree of** toe(s) (nail)

  √7ᵗʰ **T25.031 Burn of unspecified degree of** right **toe(s) (nail)**

  √7ᵗʰ **T25.032 Burn of unspecified degree of** left **toe(s) (nail)**

  √7ᵗʰ **T25.039 Burn of unspecified degree of unspecified toe(s) (nail)**

√6ᵗʰ **T25.09 Burn of unspecified degree of** multiple sites **of ankle and foot**

  √7ᵗʰ **T25.091 Burn of unspecified degree of multiple sites of** right **ankle and foot**

  √7ᵗʰ **T25.092 Burn of unspecified degree of multiple sites of** left **ankle and foot**

  √7ᵗʰ **T25.099 Burn of unspecified degree of multiple sites of unspecified ankle and foot**

√5ᵗʰ **T25.1 Burn of** first degree **of ankle and foot**

Use additional external cause code to identify the source, place and intent of the burn (X00-X19, X75-X77, X96-X98, Y92)

√6ᵗʰ **T25.11 Burn of first degree of** ankle

  √7ᵗʰ **T25.111 Burn of first degree of** right **ankle**

  √7ᵗʰ **T25.112 Burn of first degree of** left **ankle**

  √7ᵗʰ **T25.119 Burn of first degree of unspecified ankle**

√6ᵗʰ **T25.12 Burn of first degree of** foot

  EXCLUDES 2 *burn of first degree of toe(s) (nail) (T25.13-)*

  √7ᵗʰ **T25.121 Burn of first degree of** right **foot**

  √7ᵗʰ **T25.122 Burn of first degree of** left **foot**

  √7ᵗʰ **T25.129 Burn of first degree of unspecified foot**

√6ᵗʰ **T25.13 Burn of first degree of** toe(s) (nail)

  √7ᵗʰ **T25.131 Burn of first degree of** right **toe(s) (nail)**

  √7ᵗʰ **T25.132 Burn of first degree of** left **toe(s) (nail)**

  √7ᵗʰ **T25.139 Burn of first degree of unspecified toe(s) (nail)**

√6ᵗʰ **T25.19 Burn of first degree of** multiple sites **of ankle and foot**

  √7ᵗʰ **T25.191 Burn of first degree of multiple sites of** right **ankle and foot**

  √7ᵗʰ **T25.192 Burn of first degree of multiple sites of** left **ankle and foot**

  √7ᵗʰ **T25.199 Burn of first degree of multiple sites of unspecified ankle and foot**

√5ᵗʰ **T25.2 Burn of** second degree **of ankle and foot**

Use additional external cause code to identify the source, place and intent of the burn (X00-X19, X75-X77, X96-X98, Y92)

√6ᵗʰ **T25.21 Burn of second degree of** ankle

  √7ᵗʰ **T25.211 Burn of second degree of** right **ankle**

  √7ᵗʰ **T25.212 Burn of second degree of** left **ankle**

  √7ᵗʰ **T25.219 Burn of second degree of unspecified ankle**

√6ᵗʰ **T25.22 Burn of second degree of** foot

  EXCLUDES 2 *burn of second degree of toe(s) (nail) (T25.23-)*

  √7ᵗʰ **T25.221 Burn of second degree of** right **foot**

  √7ᵗʰ **T25.222 Burn of second degree of** left **foot**

  √7ᵗʰ **T25.229 Burn of second degree of unspecified foot**

√6ᵗʰ **T25.23 Burn of second degree of** toe(s) (nail)

  √7ᵗʰ **T25.231 Burn of second degree of** right **toe(s) (nail)**

  √7ᵗʰ **T25.232 Burn of second degree of** left **toe(s) (nail)**

  √7ᵗʰ **T25.239 Burn of second degree of unspecified toe(s) (nail)**

√6ᵗʰ **T25.29 Burn of second degree of** multiple sites **of ankle and foot**

  √7ᵗʰ **T25.291 Burn of second degree of multiple sites of** right **ankle and foot**

  √7ᵗʰ **T25.292 Burn of second degree of multiple sites of** left **ankle and foot**

  √7ᵗʰ **T25.299 Burn of second degree of multiple sites of unspecified ankle and foot**

☑ Additional Character Required   √x7ᵗʰ Xtension Alert   Unspecified Dx   Other Specified Dx   Manifestation   ▶◀ Revised Text   ● New Code   ▲ Revised Code Title

Injury, Poisoning and Certain Other Consequences of External Causes

T25.3–T25.792

✓5ᵗʰ **T25.3 Burn of** third degree **of ankle and foot**
Use additional external cause code to identify the source, place and intent of the burn (X00-X19, X75-X77, X96-X98, Y92)

  ✓6ᵗʰ **T25.31 Burn of third degree of** ankle
    ✓7ᵗʰ **T25.311 Burn of third degree of** right **ankle**
    ✓7ᵗʰ **T25.312 Burn of third degree of** left **ankle**
    ✓7ᵗʰ **T25.319 Burn of third degree of unspecified ankle**

  ✓6ᵗʰ **T25.32 Burn of third degree of** foot
    EXCLUDES 2 *burn of third degree of toe(s) (nail) (T25.33-)*
    ✓7ᵗʰ **T25.321 Burn of third degree of** right **foot**
    ✓7ᵗʰ **T25.322 Burn of third degree of** left **foot**
    ✓7ᵗʰ **T25.329 Burn of third degree of unspecified foot**

  ✓6ᵗʰ **T25.33 Burn of third degree of** toe(s) (nail)
    ✓7ᵗʰ **T25.331 Burn of third degree of** right **toe(s) (nail)**
    ✓7ᵗʰ **T25.332 Burn of third degree of** left **toe(s) (nail)**
    ✓7ᵗʰ **T25.339 Burn of third degree of unspecified toe(s) (nail)**

  ✓6ᵗʰ **T25.39 Burn of third degree of** multiple sites **of ankle and foot**
    ✓7ᵗʰ **T25.391 Burn of third degree of multiple sites of** right **ankle and foot**
    ✓7ᵗʰ **T25.392 Burn of third degree of multiple sites of** left **ankle and foot**
    ✓7ᵗʰ **T25.399 Burn of third degree of multiple sites of unspecified ankle and foot**

✓5ᵗʰ **T25.4 Corrosion of** unspecified degree **of ankle and foot**
Code first (T51-T65) to identify chemical and intent
Use additional external cause code to identify place (Y92)

  ✓6ᵗʰ **T25.41 Corrosion of unspecified degree of** ankle
    ✓7ᵗʰ **T25.411 Corrosion of unspecified degree of** right **ankle**
    ✓7ᵗʰ **T25.412 Corrosion of unspecified degree of** left **ankle**
    ✓7ᵗʰ **T25.419 Corrosion of unspecified degree of unspecified ankle**

  ✓6ᵗʰ **T25.42 Corrosion of unspecified degree of** foot
    EXCLUDES 2 *corrosion of unspecified degree of toe(s) (nail) (T25.43-)*
    ✓7ᵗʰ **T25.421 Corrosion of unspecified degree of** right **foot**
    ✓7ᵗʰ **T25.422 Corrosion of unspecified degree of** left **foot**
    ✓7ᵗʰ **T25.429 Corrosion of unspecified degree of unspecified foot**

  ✓6ᵗʰ **T25.43 Corrosion of unspecified degree of** toe(s) (nail)
    ✓7ᵗʰ **T25.431 Corrosion of unspecified degree of** right **toe(s) (nail)**
    ✓7ᵗʰ **T25.432 Corrosion of unspecified degree of** left **toe(s) (nail)**
    ✓7ᵗʰ **T25.439 Corrosion of unspecified degree of unspecified toe(s) (nail)**

  ✓6ᵗʰ **T25.49 Corrosion of unspecified degree of** multiple sites **of ankle and foot**
    ✓7ᵗʰ **T25.491 Corrosion of unspecified degree of multiple sites of** right **ankle and foot**
    ✓7ᵗʰ **T25.492 Corrosion of unspecified degree of multiple sites of** left **ankle and foot**
    ✓7ᵗʰ **T25.499 Corrosion of unspecified degree of multiple sites of unspecified ankle and foot**

✓5ᵗʰ **T25.5 Corrosion of** first degree **of ankle and foot**
Code first (T51-T65) to identify chemical and intent
Use additional external cause code to identify place (Y92)

  ✓6ᵗʰ **T25.51 Corrosion of first degree of** ankle
    ✓7ᵗʰ **T25.511 Corrosion of first degree of** right **ankle**
    ✓7ᵗʰ **T25.512 Corrosion of first degree of** left **ankle**
    ✓7ᵗʰ **T25.519 Corrosion of first degree of unspecified ankle**

  ✓6ᵗʰ **T25.52 Corrosion of first degree of** foot
    EXCLUDES 2 *corrosion of first degree of toe(s) (nail) (T25.53-)*
    ✓7ᵗʰ **T25.521 Corrosion of first degree of** right **foot**
    ✓7ᵗʰ **T25.522 Corrosion of first degree of** left **foot**

    ✓7ᵗʰ **T25.529 Corrosion of first degree of unspecified foot**

  ✓6ᵗʰ **T25.53 Corrosion of first degree of** toe(s) (nail)
    ✓7ᵗʰ **T25.531 Corrosion of first degree of** right **toe(s) (nail)**
    ✓7ᵗʰ **T25.532 Corrosion of first degree of** left **toe(s) (nail)**
    ✓7ᵗʰ **T25.539 Corrosion of first degree of unspecified toe(s) (nail)**

  ✓6ᵗʰ **T25.59 Corrosion of first degree of** multiple sites **of ankle and foot**
    ✓7ᵗʰ **T25.591 Corrosion of first degree of multiple sites of** right **ankle and foot**
    ✓7ᵗʰ **T25.592 Corrosion of first degree of multiple sites of** left **ankle and foot**
    ✓7ᵗʰ **T25.599 Corrosion of first degree of multiple sites of unspecified ankle and foot**

✓5ᵗʰ **T25.6 Corrosion of** second degree **of ankle and foot**
Code first (T51-T65) to identify chemical and intent
Use additional external cause code to identify place (Y92)

  ✓6ᵗʰ **T25.61 Corrosion of second degree of** ankle
    ✓7ᵗʰ **T25.611 Corrosion of second degree of** right **ankle**
    ✓7ᵗʰ **T25.612 Corrosion of second degree of** left **ankle**
    ✓7ᵗʰ **T25.619 Corrosion of second degree of unspecified ankle**

  ✓6ᵗʰ **T25.62 Corrosion of second degree of** foot
    EXCLUDES 2 *corrosion of second degree of toe(s) (nail) (T25.63-)*
    ✓7ᵗʰ **T25.621 Corrosion of second degree of** right **foot**
    ✓7ᵗʰ **T25.622 Corrosion of second degree of** left **foot**
    ✓7ᵗʰ **T25.629 Corrosion of second degree of unspecified foot**

  ✓6ᵗʰ **T25.63 Corrosion of second degree of** toe(s) (nail)
    ✓7ᵗʰ **T25.631 Corrosion of second degree of** right **toe(s) (nail)**
    ✓7ᵗʰ **T25.632 Corrosion of second degree of** left **toe(s) (nail)**
    ✓7ᵗʰ **T25.639 Corrosion of second degree of unspecified toe(s) (nail)**

  ✓6ᵗʰ **T25.69 Corrosion of second degree of** multiple sites **of ankle and foot**
    ✓7ᵗʰ **T25.691 Corrosion of second degree of multiple sites of** right **ankle and foot**
    ✓7ᵗʰ **T25.692 Corrosion of second degree of multiple sites of** left **ankle and foot**
    ✓7ᵗʰ **T25.699 Corrosion of second degree of multiple sites of unspecified ankle and foot**

✓5ᵗʰ **T25.7 Corrosion of** third degree **of ankle and foot**
Code first (T51-T65) to identify chemical and intent
Use additional external cause code to identify place (Y92)

  ✓6ᵗʰ **T25.71 Corrosion of third degree of** ankle
    ✓7ᵗʰ **T25.711 Corrosion of third degree of** right **ankle**
    ✓7ᵗʰ **T25.712 Corrosion of third degree of** left **ankle**
    ✓7ᵗʰ **T25.719 Corrosion of third degree of unspecified ankle**

  ✓6ᵗʰ **T25.72 Corrosion of third degree of** foot
    EXCLUDES 2 *corrosion of third degree of toe(s) (nail) (T25.73-)*
    ✓7ᵗʰ **T25.721 Corrosion of third degree of** right **foot**
    ✓7ᵗʰ **T25.722 Corrosion of third degree of** left **foot**
    ✓7ᵗʰ **T25.729 Corrosion of third degree of unspecified foot**

  ✓6ᵗʰ **T25.73 Corrosion of third degree of** toe(s) (nail)
    ✓7ᵗʰ **T25.731 Corrosion of third degree of** right **toe(s) (nail)**
    ✓7ᵗʰ **T25.732 Corrosion of third degree of** left **toe(s) (nail)**
    ✓7ᵗʰ **T25.739 Corrosion of third degree of unspecified toe(s) (nail)**

  ✓6ᵗʰ **T25.79 Corrosion of third degree of** multiple sites **of ankle and foot**
    ✓7ᵗʰ **T25.791 Corrosion of third degree of multiple sites of** right **ankle and foot**
    ✓7ᵗʰ **T25.792 Corrosion of third degree of multiple sites of** left **ankle and foot**

EXCLUDES 1 Not coded here   EXCLUDES 2 Not included here   N Newborn Age: 0   P Pediatric Age: 0-17   M Maternity Age: 12-55   A Adult Age: 15-124

936   ICD-10-CM Draft (2015)

☑7ᵗʰ **T25.799**   **Corrosion of third degree of multiple sites of unspecified ankle and foot**

Burns and corrosions confined to eye and internal organs (T26-T28)

☑4ᵗʰ **T26**   **Burn and corrosion confined to eye and adnexa**

> The appropriate 7th character is to be added to each code from category T26.
> A   initial encounter
> D   subsequent encounter
> S   sequela

☑5ᵗʰ **T26.0**   **Burn of** eyelid and periocular area
> Use additional external cause code to identify the source, place and intent of the burn (X00-X19, X75-X77, X96-X98, Y92)

    ☑x7ᵗʰ **T26.00**   Burn of unspecified eyelid and periocular area

    ☑x7ᵗʰ **T26.01**   Burn of right eyelid and periocular area

    ☑x7ᵗʰ **T26.02**   Burn of left eyelid and periocular area

☑5ᵗʰ **T26.1**   **Burn of** cornea and conjunctival sac
> Use additional external cause code to identify the source, place and intent of the burn (X00-X19, X75-X77, X96-X98, Y92)

    ☑x7ᵗʰ **T26.10**   **Burn of cornea and conjunctival sac, unspecified eye**

    ☑x7ᵗʰ **T26.11**   **Burn of cornea and conjunctival sac, right eye**

    ☑x7ᵗʰ **T26.12**   **Burn of cornea and conjunctival sac, left eye**

☑5ᵗʰ **T26.2**   **Burn with resulting** rupture and destruction of eyeball
> Use additional external cause code to identify the source, place and intent of the burn (X00-X19, X75-X77, X96-X98, Y92)

    ☑x7ᵗʰ **T26.20**   **Burn with resulting rupture and destruction of unspecified eyeball**

    ☑x7ᵗʰ **T26.21**   **Burn with resulting rupture and destruction of** right **eyeball**

    ☑x7ᵗʰ **T26.22**   **Burn with resulting rupture and destruction of** left **eyeball**

☑5ᵗʰ **T26.3**   **Burns of** other specified parts **of eye and adnexa**
> Use additional external cause code to identify the source, place and intent of the burn (X00-X19, X75-X77, X96-X98, Y92)

    ☑x7ᵗʰ **T26.30**   **Burns of other specified parts of unspecified eye and adnexa**

    ☑x7ᵗʰ **T26.31**   **Burns of other specified parts of** right **eye and adnexa**

    ☑x7ᵗʰ **T26.32**   **Burns of other specified parts of** left **eye and adnexa**

☑5ᵗʰ **T26.4**   **Burn of eye and adnexa,** part unspecified
> Use additional external cause code to identify the source, place and intent of the burn (X00-X19, X75-X77, X96-X98, Y92)

    ☑x7ᵗʰ **T26.40**   **Burn of unspecified eye and adnexa, part unspecified**

    ☑x7ᵗʰ **T26.41**   **Burn of** right **eye and adnexa, part unspecified**

    ☑x7ᵗʰ **T26.42**   **Burn of** left **eye and adnexa, part unspecified**

☑5ᵗʰ **T26.5**   **Corrosion of** eyelid and periocular area
> Code first (T51-T65) to identify chemical and intent
> Use additional external cause code to identify place (Y92)

    ☑x7ᵗʰ **T26.50**   **Corrosion of unspecified eyelid and periocular area**

    ☑x7ᵗʰ **T26.51**   **Corrosion of** right **eyelid and periocular area**

    ☑x7ᵗʰ **T26.52**   **Corrosion of** left **eyelid and periocular area**

☑5ᵗʰ **T26.6**   **Corrosion of** cornea and conjunctival sac
> Code first (T51-T65) to identify chemical and intent
> Use additional external cause code to identify place (Y92)

    ☑x7ᵗʰ **T26.60**   **Corrosion of cornea and conjunctival sac, unspecified eye**

    ☑x7ᵗʰ **T26.61**   **Corrosion of cornea and conjunctival sac,** right **eye**

    ☑x7ᵗʰ **T26.62**   **Corrosion of cornea and conjunctival sac,** left **eye**

☑5ᵗʰ **T26.7**   **Corrosion with resulting** rupture and destruction of eyeball
> Code first (T51-T65) to identify chemical and intent
> Use additional external cause code to identify place (Y92)

    ☑x7ᵗʰ **T26.70**   **Corrosion with resulting rupture and destruction of unspecified eyeball**

    ☑x7ᵗʰ **T26.71**   **Corrosion with resulting rupture and destruction of** right **eyeball**

    ☑x7ᵗʰ **T26.72**   **Corrosion with resulting rupture and destruction of** left **eyeball**

☑5ᵗʰ **T26.8**   **Corrosions of** other specified parts **of eye and adnexa**
> Code first (T51-T65) to identify chemical and intent
> Use additional external cause code to identify place (Y92)

    ☑x7ᵗʰ **T26.80**   **Corrosions of other specified parts of unspecified eye and adnexa**

    ☑x7ᵗʰ **T26.81**   **Corrosions of other specified parts of** right **eye and adnexa**

    ☑x7ᵗʰ **T26.82**   **Corrosions of other specified parts of** left **eye and adnexa**

☑5ᵗʰ **T26.9**   **Corrosion of eye and adnexa,** part unspecified
> Code first (T51-T65) to identify chemical and intent
> Use additional external cause code to identify place (Y92)

    ☑x7ᵗʰ **T26.90**   **Corrosion of unspecified eye and adnexa, part unspecified**

    ☑x7ᵗʰ **T26.91**   **Corrosion of** right **eye and adnexa, part unspecified**

    ☑x7ᵗʰ **T26.92**   **Corrosion of** left **eye and adnexa, part unspecified**

☑4ᵗʰ **T27**   **Burn and corrosion of respiratory tract**
> Use additional external cause code to identify the source and intent of the burn (X00-X19, X75-X77, X96-X98)
> Use additional external cause code to identify place (Y92)

> The appropriate 7th character is to be added to each code from category T27.
> A   initial encounter
> D   subsequent encounter
> S   sequela

☑x7ᵗʰ **T27.0**   **Burn of** larynx and trachea

☑x7ᵗʰ **T27.1**   **Burn involving** larynx and trachea with lung

☑x7ᵗʰ **T27.2**   **Burn of other** parts **of respiratory tract**
> Burn of thoracic cavity

☑x7ᵗʰ **T27.3**   **Burn of respiratory tract, part unspecified**
> Code first (T51-T65) to identify chemical and intent for codes T27.4-T27.7

☑x7ᵗʰ **T27.4**   **Corrosion of** larynx and trachea

☑x7ᵗʰ **T27.5**   **Corrosion involving** larynx and trachea with lung

☑x7ᵗʰ **T27.6**   **Corrosion of other** parts **of respiratory tract**

☑x7ᵗʰ **T27.7**   **Corrosion of respiratory tract, part unspecified**

☑4ᵗʰ **T28**   **Burn and corrosion of other internal organs**
> Use additional external cause code to identify the source and intent of the burn (X00- X19, X75-X77, X96-X98)
> Use additional external cause code to identify place (Y92)

> The appropriate 7th character is to be added to each code from category T28.
> A   initial encounter
> D   subsequent encounter
> S   sequela

☑x7ᵗʰ **T28.0**   **Burn of** mouth and pharynx

☑x7ᵗʰ **T28.1**   **Burn of** esophagus

☑x7ᵗʰ **T28.2**   **Burn of other parts of** alimentary tract

☑x7ᵗʰ **T28.3**   **Burn of** internal genitourinary organs

☑5ᵗʰ **T28.4**   **Burns of other and unspecified internal organs**

    ☑x7ᵗʰ **T28.40**   **Burn of unspecified internal organ**

    ☑6ᵗʰ **T28.41**   **Burn of** ear drum

       ☑7ᵗʰ **T28.411**   **Burn of** right **ear drum**

       ☑7ᵗʰ **T28.412**   **Burn of** left **ear drum**

       ☑7ᵗʰ **T28.419**   **Burn of unspecified ear drum**

    ☑x7ᵗʰ **T28.49**   **Burn of other internal organ**
> Code first (T51-T65) to identify chemical and intent for T28.5-T28.9-

☑x7ᵗʰ **T28.5**   **Corrosion of** mouth and pharynx

☑x7ᵗʰ **T28.6**   **Corrosion of** esophagus

☑x7ᵗʰ **T28.7**   **Corrosion of other parts of** alimentary tract

☑x7ᵗʰ **T28.8**   **Corrosion of internal** genitourinary organs

☑5ᵗʰ **T28.9**   **Corrosions of other and unspecified internal organs**

    ☑x7ᵗʰ **T28.90**   **Corrosions of unspecified internal organs**

    ☑6ᵗʰ **T28.91**   **Corrosions of** ear drum

       ☑7ᵗʰ **T28.911**   **Corrosions of** right **ear drum**

       ☑7ᵗʰ **T28.912**   **Corrosions of** left **ear drum**

       ☑7ᵗʰ **T28.919**   **Corrosions of unspecified ear drum**

    ☑x7ᵗʰ **T28.99**   **Corrosions of other internal organs**

☑ Additional Character Required   ☑x7ᵗʰ Xtension Alert   Unspecified Dx   Other Specified Dx   Manifestation   ►◄ Revised Text   ● New Code   ▲ Revised Code Title

Injury, Poisoning and Certain Other Consequences of External Causes

T30–T32.0

Burns and corrosions of multiple and unspecified body regions (T30–T32)

✓4ᵗʰ T30   Burn and corrosion, body region unspecified

    T30.0   Burn of unspecified body region, unspecified degree
        NOTE   This code is not for inpatient use. Code to specified site and degree of burns.
        Burn NOS
        Multiple burns NOS

    T30.4   Corrosion of unspecified body region, unspecified degree
        NOTE   This code is not for inpatient use. Code to specified site and degree of corrosion.
        Corrosion NOS
        Multiple corrosion NOS

✓4ᵗʰ T31   Burns classified according to extent of body surface involved
    NOTE   This category is to be used as the primary code only when the site of the burn is unspecified. It should be used as a supplementary code with categories T20-T25 when the site is specified.

    T31.0   Burns involving less than 10% of body surface

    ✓5ᵗʰ T31.1   Burns involving 10-19% of body surface
        T31.10   Burns involving 10-19% of body surface with 0% to 9% third degree burns
            Burns involving 10-19% of body surface NOS
        T31.11   Burns involving 10-19% of body surface with 10-19% third degree burns

    ✓5ᵗʰ T31.2   Burns involving 20-29% of body surface
        T31.20   Burns involving 20-29% of body surface with 0% to 9% third degree burns
            Burns involving 20-29% of body surface NOS
        T31.21   Burns involving 20-29% of body surface with 10-19% third degree burns
        T31.22   Burns involving 20-29% of body surface with 20-29% third degree burns

    ✓5ᵗʰ T31.3   Burns involving 30-39% of body surface
        T31.30   Burns involving 30-39% of body surface with 0% to 9% third degree burns
            Burns involving 30-39% of body surface NOS
        T31.31   Burns involving 30-39% of body surface with 10-19% third degree burns
        T31.32   Burns involving 30-39% of body surface with 20-29% third degree burns
        T31.33   Burns involving 30-39% of body surface with 30-39% third degree burns

    ✓5ᵗʰ T31.4   Burns involving 40-49% of body surface
        T31.40   Burns involving 40-49% of body surface with 0% to 9% third degree burns
            Burns involving 40-49% of body surface NOS
        T31.41   Burns involving 40-49% of body surface with 10-19% third degree burns
        T31.42   Burns involving 40-49% of body surface with 20-29% third degree burns
        T31.43   Burns involving 40-49% of body surface with 30-39% third degree burns
        T31.44   Burns involving 40-49% of body surface with 40-49% third degree burns

    ✓5ᵗʰ T31.5   Burns involving 50-59% of body surface
        T31.50   Burns involving 50-59% of body surface with 0% to 9% third degree burns
            Burns involving 50-59% of body surface NOS
        T31.51   Burns involving 50-59% of body surface with 10-19% third degree burns
        T31.52   Burns involving 50-59% of body surface with 20-29% third degree burns
        T31.53   Burns involving 50-59% of body surface with 30-39% third degree burns
        T31.54   Burns involving 50-59% of body surface with 40-49% third degree burns
        T31.55   Burns involving 50-59% of body surface with 50-59% third degree burns

    ✓5ᵗʰ T31.6   Burns involving 60-69% of body surface
        T31.60   Burns involving 60-69% of body surface with 0% to 9% third degree burns
            Burns involving 60-69% of body surface NOS
        T31.61   Burns involving 60-69% of body surface with 10-19% third degree burns

        T31.62   Burns involving 60-69% of body surface with 20-29% third degree burns
        T31.63   Burns involving 60-69% of body surface with 30-39% third degree burns
        T31.64   Burns involving 60-69% of body surface with 40-49% third degree burns
        T31.65   Burns involving 60-69% of body surface with 50-59% third degree burns
        T31.66   Burns involving 60-69% of body surface with 60-69% third degree burns

    ✓5ᵗʰ T31.7   Burns involving 70-79% of body surface
        T31.70   Burns involving 70-79% of body surface with 0% to 9% third degree burns
            Burns involving 70-79% of body surface NOS
        T31.71   Burns involving 70-79% of body surface with 10-19% third degree burns
        T31.72   Burns involving 70-79% of body surface with 20-29% third degree burns
        T31.73   Burns involving 70-79% of body surface with 30-39% third degree burns
        T31.74   Burns involving 70-79% of body surface with 40-49% third degree burns
        T31.75   Burns involving 70-79% of body surface with 50-59% third degree burns
        T31.76   Burns involving 70-79% of body surface with 60-69% third degree burns
        T31.77   Burns involving 70-79% of body surface with 70-79% third degree burns

    ✓5ᵗʰ T31.8   Burns involving 80-89% of body surface
        T31.80   Burns involving 80-89% of body surface with 0% to 9% third degree burns
            Burns involving 80-89% of body surface NOS
        T31.81   Burns involving 80-89% of body surface with 10-19% third degree burns
        T31.82   Burns involving 80-89% of body surface with 20-29% third degree burns
        T31.83   Burns involving 80-89% of body surface with 30-39% third degree burns
        T31.84   Burns involving 80-89% of body surface with 40-49% third degree burns
        T31.85   Burns involving 80-89% of body surface with 50-59% third degree burns
        T31.86   Burns involving 80-89% of body surface with 60-69% third degree burns
        T31.87   Burns involving 80-89% of body surface with 70-79% third degree burns
        T31.88   Burns involving 80-89% of body surface with 80-89% third degree burns

    ✓5ᵗʰ T31.9   Burns involving 90% or more of body surface
        T31.90   Burns involving 90% or more of body surface with 0% to 9% third degree burns
            Burns involving 90% or more of body surface NOS
        T31.91   Burns involving 90% or more of body surface with 10-19% third degree burns
        T31.92   Burns involving 90% or more of body surface with 20-29% third degree burns
        T31.93   Burns involving 90% or more of body surface with 30-39% third degree burns
        T31.94   Burns involving 90% or more of body surface with 40-49% third degree burns
        T31.95   Burns involving 90% or more of body surface with 50-59% third degree burns
        T31.96   Burns involving 90% or more of body surface with 60-69% third degree burns
        T31.97   Burns involving 90% or more of body surface with 70-79% third degree burns
        T31.98   Burns involving 90% or more of body surface with 80-89% third degree burns
        T31.99   Burns involving 90% or more of body surface with 90% or more third degree burns

✓4ᵗʰ T32   Corrosions classified according to extent of body surface involved
    NOTE   This category is to be used as the primary code only when the site of the corrosion is unspecified. It may be used as a supplementary code with categories T20-T25 when the site is specified.

    T32.0   Corrosions involving less than 10% of body surface

EXCLUDES1 Not coded here   **EXCLUDES2** Not included here   **N** Newborn Age: 0   **P** Pediatric Age: 0-17   **M** Maternity Age: 12-55   **A** Adult Age: 15-124

938   ICD-10-CM Draft (2015)

✓5ᵗʰ **T32.1**   Corrosions involving 10-19% of body surface

     T32.10   Corrosions involving 10-19% of body surface with 0% to 9% third degree **corrosion**
          Corrosions involving 10-19% of body surface NOS

     T32.11   Corrosions involving 10-19% of body surface with 10-19% third degree **corrosion**

✓5ᵗʰ **T32.2**   Corrosions involving 20-29% of body surface

     T32.20   Corrosions involving 20-29% of body surface with 0% to 9% third degree **corrosion**

     T32.21   Corrosions involving 20-29% of body surface with 10-19% third degree **corrosion**

     T32.22   Corrosions involving 20-29% of body surface with 20-29% third degree **corrosion**

✓5ᵗʰ **T32.3**   Corrosions involving 30-39% of body surface

     T32.30   Corrosions involving 30-39% of body surface with 0% to 9% third degree **corrosion**

     T32.31   Corrosions involving 30-39% of body surface with 10-19% third degree **corrosion**

     T32.32   Corrosions involving 30-39% of body surface with 20-29% third degree **corrosion**

     T32.33   Corrosions involving 30-39% of body surface with 30-39% third degree **corrosion**

✓5ᵗʰ **T32.4**   Corrosions involving 40-49% of body surface

     T32.40   Corrosions involving 40-49% of body surface with 0% to 9% third degree **corrosion**

     T32.41   Corrosions involving 40-49% of body surface with 10-19% third degree **corrosion**

     T32.42   Corrosions involving 40-49% of body surface with 20-29% third degree **corrosion**

     T32.43   Corrosions involving 40-49% of body surface with 30-39% third degree **corrosion**

     T32.44   Corrosions involving 40-49% of body surface with 40-49% third degree **corrosion**

✓5ᵗʰ **T32.5**   Corrosions involving 50-59% of body surface

     T32.50   Corrosions involving 50-59% of body surface with 0% to 9% third degree **corrosion**

     T32.51   Corrosions involving 50-59% of body surface with 10-19% third degree **corrosion**

     T32.52   Corrosions involving 50-59% of body surface with 20-29% third degree **corrosion**

     T32.53   Corrosions involving 50-59% of body surface with 30-39% third degree **corrosion**

     T32.54   Corrosions involving 50-59% of body surface with 40-49% third degree **corrosion**

     T32.55   Corrosions involving 50-59% of body surface with 50-59% third degree **corrosion**

✓5ᵗʰ **T32.6**   Corrosions involving 60-69% of body surface

     T32.60   Corrosions involving 60-69% of body surface with 0% to 9% third degree **corrosion**

     T32.61   Corrosions involving 60-69% of body surface with 10-19% third degree **corrosion**

     T32.62   Corrosions involving 60-69% of body surface with 20-29% third degree **corrosion**

     T32.63   Corrosions involving 60-69% of body surface with 30-39% third degree **corrosion**

     T32.64   Corrosions involving 60-69% of body surface with 40-49% third degree **corrosion**

     T32.65   Corrosions involving 60-69% of body surface with 50-59% third degree **corrosion**

     T32.66   Corrosions involving 60-69% of body surface with 60-69% third degree **corrosion**

✓5ᵗʰ **T32.7**   Corrosions involving 70-79% of body surface

     T32.70   Corrosions involving 70-79% of body surface with 0% to 9% third degree **corrosion**

     T32.71   Corrosions involving 70-79% of body surface with 10-19% third degree **corrosion**

     T32.72   Corrosions involving 70-79% of body surface with 20-29% third degree **corrosion**

     T32.73   Corrosions involving 70-79% of body surface with 30-39% third degree **corrosion**

     T32.74   Corrosions involving 70-79% of body surface with 40-49% third degree **corrosion**

     T32.75   Corrosions involving 70-79% of body surface with 50-59% third degree **corrosion**

     T32.76   Corrosions involving 70-79% of body surface with 60-69% third degree **corrosion**

     T32.77   Corrosions involving 70-79% of body surface with 70-79% third degree **corrosion**

✓5ᵗʰ **T32.8**   Corrosions involving 80-89% of body surface

     T32.80   Corrosions involving 80-89% of body surface with 0% to 9% third degree **corrosion**

     T32.81   Corrosions involving 80-89% of body surface with 10-19% third degree **corrosion**

     T32.82   Corrosions involving 80-89% of body surface with 20-29% third degree **corrosion**

     T32.83   Corrosions involving 80-89% of body surface with 30-39% third degree **corrosion**

     T32.84   Corrosions involving 80-89% of body surface with 40-49% third degree **corrosion**

     T32.85   Corrosions involving 80-89% of body surface with 50-59% third degree **corrosion**

     T32.86   Corrosions involving 80-89% of body surface with 60-69% third degree **corrosion**

     T32.87   Corrosions involving 80-89% of body surface with 70-79% third degree **corrosion**

     T32.88   Corrosions involving 80-89% of body surface with 80-89% third degree **corrosion**

✓5ᵗʰ **T32.9**   Corrosions involving 90% or more of body surface

     T32.90   Corrosions involving 90% or more of body surface with 0% to 9% third degree **corrosion**

     T32.91   Corrosions involving 90% or more of body surface with 10-19% third degree **corrosion**

     T32.92   Corrosions involving 90% or more of body surface with 20-29% third degree **corrosion**

     T32.93   Corrosions involving 90% or more of body surface with 30-39% third degree **corrosion**

     T32.94   Corrosions involving 90% or more of body surface with 40-49% third degree **corrosion**

     T32.95   Corrosions involving 90% or more of body surface with 50-59% third degree **corrosion**

     T32.96   Corrosions involving 90% or more of body surface with 60-69% third degree **corrosion**

     T32.97   Corrosions involving 90% or more of body surface with 70-79% third degree **corrosion**

     T32.98   Corrosions involving 90% or more of body surface with 80-89% third degree **corrosion**

     T32.99   Corrosions involving 90% or more of body surface with 90% or more third degree **corrosion**

Frostbite (T33-T34)

EXCLUDES 2   *hypothermia and other effects of reduced temperature (T68, T69-)*

✓4ᵗʰ **T33**   **Superficial frostbite**

     INCLUDES   frostbite with partial thickness skin loss

> The appropriate 7th character is to be added to each code from category T33.
> A   initial encounter
> D   subsequent encounter
> S   sequela

✓5ᵗʰ **T33.0**   Superficial frostbite of head

     ✓6ᵗʰ **T33.01**   Superficial frostbite of ear

         ✓7ᵗʰ **T33.011**   Superficial frostbite of right ear

         ✓7ᵗʰ **T33.012**   Superficial frostbite of left ear

         ✓7ᵗʰ **T33.019**   Superficial frostbite of unspecified ear

     ✓x7ᵗʰ **T33.02**   Superficial frostbite of nose

     ✓x7ᵗʰ **T33.09**   Superficial frostbite of other part of head

✓x7ᵗʰ **T33.1**   Superficial frostbite of neck

✓x7ᵗʰ **T33.2**   Superficial frostbite of thorax

✓x7ᵗʰ **T33.3**   Superficial frostbite of abdominal wall, lower back and pelvis

✓5ᵗʰ **T33.4**   Superficial frostbite of arm

     EXCLUDES 2   *superficial frostbite of wrist and hand (T33.5-)*

     ✓x7ᵗʰ **T33.40**   Superficial frostbite of unspecified arm

     ✓x7ᵗʰ **T33.41**   Superficial frostbite of right arm

     ✓x7ᵗʰ **T33.42**   Superficial frostbite of left arm

✓5ᵗʰ **T33.5**   Superficial frostbite of wrist, hand, and fingers

     ✓6ᵗʰ **T33.51**   Superficial frostbite of wrist

         ✓7ᵗʰ **T33.511**   Superficial frostbite of right wrist

         ✓7ᵗʰ **T33.512**   Superficial frostbite of left wrist

---

✓ Additional Character Required   ✓x7ᵗʰ *Xtension Alert*   Unspecified Dx   Other Specified Dx   Manifestation   ▶◀ Revised Text   ● New Code   ▲ Revised Code Title

Injury, Poisoning and Certain Other Consequences of External Causes

T33.519–T34.99

☑7ᵗʰ **T33.519** **Superficial frostbite of unspecified wrist**

☑6ᵗʰ **T33.52** **Superficial frostbite of** hand
    EXCLUDES 2 *superficial frostbite of fingers (T33.53-)*

    ☑7ᵗʰ **T33.521** **Superficial frostbite of** right **hand**

    ☑7ᵗʰ **T33.522** **Superficial frostbite of** left **hand**

    ☑7ᵗʰ **T33.529** **Superficial frostbite of unspecified hand**

☑6ᵗʰ **T33.53** **Superficial frostbite of** finger(s)

    ☑7ᵗʰ **T33.531** **Superficial frostbite of** right **finger(s)**

    ☑7ᵗʰ **T33.532** **Superficial frostbite of** left **finger(s)**

    ☑7ᵗʰ **T33.539** **Superficial frostbite of unspecified finger(s)**

☑5ᵗʰ **T33.6** **Superficial frostbite of** hip and thigh

    ☑x7ᵗʰ **T33.60** **Superficial frostbite of unspecified hip and thigh**

    ☑x7ᵗʰ **T33.61** **Superficial frostbite of** right **hip and thigh**

    ☑x7ᵗʰ **T33.62** **Superficial frostbite of** left **hip and thigh**

☑5ᵗʰ **T33.7** **Superficial frostbite of** knee and lower leg
    EXCLUDES 2 *superficial frostbite of ankle and foot (T33.8-)*

    ☑x7ᵗʰ **T33.70** **Superficial frostbite of unspecified knee and lower leg**

    ☑x7ᵗʰ **T33.71** **Superficial frostbite of** right **knee and lower leg**

    ☑x7ᵗʰ **T33.72** **Superficial frostbite of** left **knee and lower leg**

☑5ᵗʰ **T33.8** **Superficial frostbite of** ankle, foot, and toe(s)

    ☑6ᵗʰ **T33.81** **Superficial frostbite of** ankle

        ☑7ᵗʰ **T33.811** **Superficial frostbite of** right **ankle**

        ☑7ᵗʰ **T33.812** **Superficial frostbite of** left **ankle**

        ☑7ᵗʰ **T33.819** **Superficial frostbite of unspecified ankle**

    ☑6ᵗʰ **T33.82** **Superficial frostbite of** foot

        ☑7ᵗʰ **T33.821** **Superficial frostbite of** right **foot**

        ☑7ᵗʰ **T33.822** **Superficial frostbite of** left **foot**

        ☑7ᵗʰ **T33.829** **Superficial frostbite of unspecified foot**

    ☑6ᵗʰ **T33.83** **Superficial frostbite of** toe(s)

        ☑7ᵗʰ **T33.831** **Superficial frostbite of** right **toe(s)**

        ☑7ᵗʰ **T33.832** **Superficial frostbite of** left **toe(s)**

        ☑7ᵗʰ **T33.839** **Superficial frostbite of unspecified toe(s)**

☑5ᵗʰ **T33.9** **Superficial frostbite of other and unspecified sites**

    ☑x7ᵗʰ **T33.90** **Superficial frostbite of unspecified sites**
        Superficial frostbite NOS

    ☑x7ᵗʰ **T33.99** **Superficial frostbite of other sites**
        Superficial frostbite of leg NOS
        Superficial frostbite of trunk NOS

☑4ᵗʰ **T34** **Frostbite** with tissue necrosis

> The appropriate 7th character is to be added to each code from category T34.
> A   initial encounter
> D   subsequent encounter
> S   sequela

☑5ᵗʰ **T34.0** **Frostbite with tissue necrosis of** head

    ☑6ᵗʰ **T34.01** **Frostbite with tissue necrosis of** ear

        ☑7ᵗʰ **T34.011** **Frostbite with tissue necrosis of** right **ear**

        ☑7ᵗʰ **T34.012** **Frostbite with tissue necrosis of** left **ear**

        ☑7ᵗʰ **T34.019** **Frostbite with tissue necrosis of unspecified ear**

    ☑x7ᵗʰ **T34.02** **Frostbite with tissue necrosis of** nose

    ☑x7ᵗʰ **T34.09** **Frostbite with tissue necrosis of other part of head**

☑x7ᵗʰ **T34.1** **Frostbite with tissue necrosis of** neck

☑x7ᵗʰ **T34.2** **Frostbite with tissue necrosis of** thorax

☑x7ᵗʰ **T34.3** **Frostbite with tissue necrosis of** abdominal wall, lower back and pelvis

☑5ᵗʰ **T34.4** **Frostbite with tissue necrosis of** arm
    EXCLUDES 2 *frostbite with tissue necrosis of wrist and hand (T34.5-)*

    ☑x7ᵗʰ **T34.40** **Frostbite with tissue necrosis of unspecified arm**

    ☑x7ᵗʰ **T34.41** **Frostbite with tissue necrosis of** right **arm**

    ☑x7ᵗʰ **T34.42** **Frostbite with tissue necrosis of** left **arm**

☑5ᵗʰ **T34.5** **Frostbite with tissue necrosis of** wrist, hand, and finger(s)

    ☑6ᵗʰ **T34.51** **Frostbite with tissue necrosis of** wrist

        ☑7ᵗʰ **T34.511** **Frostbite with tissue necrosis of** right **wrist**

        ☑7ᵗʰ **T34.512** **Frostbite with tissue necrosis of** left **wrist**

☑7ᵗʰ **T34.519** **Frostbite with tissue necrosis of unspecified wrist**

☑6ᵗʰ **T34.52** **Frostbite with tissue necrosis of** hand
    EXCLUDES 2 *frostbite with tissue necrosis of finger(s) (T34.53-)*

    ☑7ᵗʰ **T34.521** **Frostbite with tissue necrosis of** right **hand**

    ☑7ᵗʰ **T34.522** **Frostbite with tissue necrosis of** left **hand**

    ☑7ᵗʰ **T34.529** **Frostbite with tissue necrosis of unspecified hand**

☑6ᵗʰ **T34.53** **Frostbite with tissue necrosis of** finger(s)

    ☑7ᵗʰ **T34.531** **Frostbite with tissue necrosis of** right **finger(s)**

    ☑7ᵗʰ **T34.532** **Frostbite with tissue necrosis of** left **finger(s)**

    ☑7ᵗʰ **T34.539** **Frostbite with tissue necrosis of unspecified finger(s)**

☑5ᵗʰ **T34.6** **Frostbite with tissue necrosis of** hip and thigh

    ☑x7ᵗʰ **T34.60** **Frostbite with tissue necrosis of unspecified hip and thigh**

    ☑x7ᵗʰ **T34.61** **Frostbite with tissue necrosis of** right **hip and thigh**

    ☑x7ᵗʰ **T34.62** **Frostbite with tissue necrosis of** left **hip and thigh**

☑5ᵗʰ **T34.7** **Frostbite with tissue necrosis of** knee and lower leg
    EXCLUDES 2 *frostbite with tissue necrosis of ankle and foot (T34.8-)*

    ☑x7ᵗʰ **T34.70** **Frostbite with tissue necrosis of unspecified knee and lower leg**

    ☑x7ᵗʰ **T34.71** **Frostbite with tissue necrosis of** right **knee and lower leg**

    ☑x7ᵗʰ **T34.72** **Frostbite with tissue necrosis of** left **knee and lower leg**

☑5ᵗʰ **T34.8** **Frostbite with tissue necrosis of** ankle, foot, and toe(s)

    ☑6ᵗʰ **T34.81** **Frostbite with tissue necrosis of** ankle

        ☑7ᵗʰ **T34.811** **Frostbite with tissue necrosis of** right **ankle**

        ☑7ᵗʰ **T34.812** **Frostbite with tissue necrosis of** left **ankle**

        ☑7ᵗʰ **T34.819** **Frostbite with tissue necrosis of unspecified ankle**

    ☑6ᵗʰ **T34.82** **Frostbite with tissue necrosis of** foot

        ☑7ᵗʰ **T34.821** **Frostbite with tissue necrosis of** right **foot**

        ☑7ᵗʰ **T34.822** **Frostbite with tissue necrosis of** left **foot**

        ☑7ᵗʰ **T34.829** **Frostbite with tissue necrosis of unspecified foot**

    ☑6ᵗʰ **T34.83** **Frostbite with tissue necrosis of** toe(s)

        ☑7ᵗʰ **T34.831** **Frostbite with tissue necrosis of** right **toe(s)**

        ☑7ᵗʰ **T34.832** **Frostbite with tissue necrosis of** left **toe(s)**

        ☑7ᵗʰ **T34.839** **Frostbite with tissue necrosis of unspecified toe(s)**

☑5ᵗʰ **T34.9** **Frostbite with tissue necrosis of other and unspecified sites**

    ☑x7ᵗʰ **T34.90** **Frostbite with tissue necrosis of unspecified sites**
        Frostbite with tissue necrosis NOS

    ☑x7ᵗʰ **T34.99** **Frostbite with tissue necrosis of other sites**
        Frostbite with tissue necrosis of leg NOS
        Frostbite with tissue necrosis of trunk NOS

EXCLUDES 1 Not coded here   **EXCLUDES 2** Not included here   N Newborn Age: 0   P Pediatric Age: 0-17   M Maternity Age: 12-55   A Adult Age: 15-124

940   ICD-10-CM Draft (2015)

Poisoning by, adverse effects of and underdosing of drugs, medicaments and biological substances (T36-T50)

INCLUDES adverse effect of correct substance properly administered
poisoning by overdose of substance
poisoning by wrong substance given or taken in error
underdosing by (inadvertently) (deliberately) taking less substance than prescribed or instructed

Code first, for adverse effects, the nature of the adverse effect, such as:
adverse effect NOS (T88.7)
aspirin gastritis (K29.-)
blood disorders (D56-D76)
contact dermatitis (L23-L25)
dermatitis due to substances taken internally (L27.-)
nephropathy (N14.0-N14.2)

NOTE The drug giving rise to the adverse effect should be identified by use of codes from categories T36-T50 with fifth or sixth character 5.

Use additional code(s) to specify:
manifestations of poisoning
underdosing or failure in dosage during medical and surgical care (Y63.6, Y63.8-Y63.9)
underdosing of medication regimen (Z91.12-, Z91.13-)

EXCLUDES 1 toxic reaction to local anesthesia in pregnancy (O29.3-)
EXCLUDES 2 abuse and dependence of psychoactive substances (F10-F19)
abuse of non-dependence-producing substances (F55.-)
drug reaction and poisoning affecting newborn (P00-P96)
pathological drug intoxication (inebriation) (F10-F19)

√4th **T36 Poisoning by, adverse effect of and underdosing of systemic antibiotics**

EXCLUDES 1 antineoplastic antibiotics (T45.1-)
locally applied antibiotic NEC (T49.0)
topically used antibiotic for ear, nose and throat (T49.6)
topically used antibiotic for eye (T49.5)

The appropriate 7th character is to be added to each code from category T36.
A   initial encounter
D   subsequent encounter
S   sequela

√5th **T36.0 Poisoning by, adverse effect of and underdosing of penicillins**

√6th **T36.0X Poisoning by, adverse effect of and underdosing of penicillins**

√7th T36.0X1 **Poisoning by penicillins,** accidental (unintentional)
Poisoning by penicillins NOS

√7th T36.0X2 **Poisoning by penicillins,** intentional self-harm

√7th T36.0X3 **Poisoning by penicillins,** assault

√7th T36.0X4 **Poisoning by penicillins,** undetermined

√7th T36.0X5 Adverse effect **of penicillins**

√7th T36.0X6 Underdosing **of penicillins**

√5th **T36.1 Poisoning by, adverse effect of and underdosing of cephalosporins and other beta-lactam antibiotics**

√6th **T36.1X Poisoning by, adverse effect of and underdosing of cephalosporins and other beta-lactam antibiotics**

√7th T36.1X1 **Poisoning by cephalosporins and other beta-lactam antibiotics,** accidental (unintentional)
Poisoning by cephalosporins and other beta-lactam antibiotics NOS

√7th T36.1X2 **Poisoning by cephalosporins and other beta-lactam antibiotics,** intentional self-harm

√7th T36.1X3 **Poisoning by cephalosporins and other beta-lactam antibiotics,** assault

√7th T36.1X4 **Poisoning by cephalosporins and other beta-lactam antibiotics,** undetermined

√7th T36.1X5 Adverse effect **of cephalosporins and other beta-lactam antibiotics**

√7th T36.1X6 Underdosing **of cephalosporins and other beta-lactam antibiotics**

√5th **T36.2 Poisoning by, adverse effect of and underdosing of chloramphenicol group**

√6th **T36.2X Poisoning by, adverse effect of and underdosing of chloramphenicol group**

√7th T36.2X1 **Poisoning by chloramphenicol group,** accidental (unintentional)
Poisoning by chloramphenicol group NOS

√7th T36.2X2 **Poisoning by chloramphenicol group,** intentional self-harm

√7th T36.2X3 **Poisoning by chloramphenicol group,** assault

√7th T36.2X4 **Poisoning by chloramphenicol group,** undetermined

√7th T36.2X5 Adverse effect **of chloramphenicol group**

√7th T36.2X6 Underdosing **of chloramphenicol group**

√5th **T36.3 Poisoning by, adverse effect of and underdosing of macrolides**

√6th **T36.3X Poisoning by, adverse effect of and underdosing of macrolides**

√7th T36.3X1 **Poisoning by macrolides,** accidental (unintentional)
Poisoning by macrolides NOS

√7th T36.3X2 **Poisoning by macrolides,** intentional self-harm

√7th T36.3X3 **Poisoning by macrolides,** assault

√7th T36.3X4 **Poisoning by macrolides,** undetermined

√7th T36.3X5 Adverse effect **of macrolides**

√7th T36.3X6 Underdosing **of macrolides**

√5th **T36.4 Poisoning by, adverse effect of and underdosing of tetracyclines**

√6th **T36.4X Poisoning by, adverse effect of and underdosing of tetracyclines**

√7th T36.4X1 **Poisoning by tetracyclines,** accidental (unintentional)
Poisoning by tetracyclines NOS

√7th T36.4X2 **Poisoning by tetracyclines,** intentional self-harm

√7th T36.4X3 **Poisoning by tetracyclines,** assault

√7th T36.4X4 **Poisoning by tetracyclines,** undetermined

√7th T36.4X5 Adverse effect **of tetracyclines**

√7th T36.4X6 Underdosing **of tetracyclines**

√5th **T36.5 Poisoning by, adverse effect of and underdosing of aminoglycosides**
Poisoning by, adverse effect of and underdosing of streptomycin

√6th **T36.5X Poisoning by, adverse effect of and underdosing of aminoglycosides**

√7th T36.5X1 **Poisoning by aminoglycosides,** accidental (unintentional)
Poisoning by aminoglycosides NOS

√7th T36.5X2 **Poisoning by aminoglycosides,** intentional self-harm

√7th T36.5X3 **Poisoning by aminoglycosides,** assault

√7th T36.5X4 **Poisoning by aminoglycosides,** undetermined

√7th T36.5X5 Adverse effect **of aminoglycosides**

√7th T36.5X6 Underdosing **of aminoglycosides**

√5th **T36.6 Poisoning by, adverse effect of and underdosing of rifampicins**

√6th **T36.6X Poisoning by, adverse effect of and underdosing of rifampicins**

√7th T36.6X1 **Poisoning by rifampicins,** accidental (unintentional)
Poisoning by rifampicins NOS

√7th T36.6X2 **Poisoning by rifampicins,** intentional self-harm

√7th T36.6X3 **Poisoning by rifampicins,** assault

√7th T36.6X4 **Poisoning by rifampicins,** undetermined

√7th T36.6X5 Adverse effect **of rifampicins**

√7th T36.6X6 Underdosing **of rifampicins**

√5th **T36.7 Poisoning by, adverse effect of and underdosing of antifungal antibiotics, systemically used**

√6th **T36.7X Poisoning by, adverse effect of and underdosing of antifungal antibiotics, systemically used**

√7th T36.7X1 **Poisoning by antifungal antibiotics, systemically used,** accidental (unintentional)
Poisoning by antifungal antibiotics, systemically used NOS

√7th T36.7X2 **Poisoning by antifungal antibiotics, systemically used,** intentional self-harm

✓7th **T36.7X3** Poisoning by antifungal antibiotics, systemically used, assault

✓7th **T36.7X4** Poisoning by antifungal antibiotics, systemically used, undetermined

✓7th **T36.7X5** Adverse effect of antifungal antibiotics, systemically used

✓7th **T36.7X6** Underdosing of antifungal antibiotics, systemically used

✓5th **T36.8** Poisoning by, adverse effect of and underdosing of other systemic antibiotics

    ✓6th **T36.8X** Poisoning by, adverse effect of and underdosing of other systemic antibiotics

       ✓7th **T36.8X1** Poisoning by other systemic antibiotics, accidental (unintentional)
          Poisoning by other systemic antibiotics NOS

       ✓7th **T36.8X2** Poisoning by other systemic antibiotics, intentional self-harm

       ✓7th **T36.8X3** Poisoning by other systemic antibiotics, assault

       ✓7th **T36.8X4** Poisoning by other systemic antibiotics, undetermined

       ✓7th **T36.8X5** Adverse effect of other systemic antibiotics

       ✓7th **T36.8X6** Underdosing of other systemic antibiotics

✓5th **T36.9** Poisoning by, adverse effect of and underdosing of unspecified systemic antibiotic

    ✓x7th **T36.91** Poisoning by unspecified systemic antibiotic, accidental (unintentional)
       Poisoning by systemic antibiotic NOS

    ✓x7th **T36.92** Poisoning by unspecified systemic antibiotic, intentional self-harm

    ✓x7th **T36.93** Poisoning by unspecified systemic antibiotic, assault

    ✓x7th **T36.94** Poisoning by unspecified systemic antibiotic, undetermined

    ✓x7th **T36.95** Adverse effect of unspecified systemic antibiotic

    ✓x7th **T36.96** Underdosing of unspecified systemic antibiotic

✓4th **T37** Poisoning by, adverse effect of and underdosing of other systemic anti-infectives and antiparasitics

    EXCLUDES 1   anti-infectives topically used for ear, nose and throat (T49.6-)
       anti-infectives topically used for eye (T49.5-)
       locally applied anti-infectives NEC (T49.0-)

    The appropriate 7th character is to be added to each code from category T37.
    A   initial encounter
    D   subsequent encounter
    S   sequela

✓5th **T37.0** Poisoning by, adverse effect of and underdosing of sulfonamides

    ✓6th **T37.0X** Poisoning by, adverse effect of and underdosing of sulfonamides

       ✓7th **T37.0X1** Poisoning by sulfonamides, accidental (unintentional)
          Poisoning by sulfonamides NOS

       ✓7th **T37.0X2** Poisoning by sulfonamides, intentional self-harm

       ✓7th **T37.0X3** Poisoning by sulfonamides, assault

       ✓7th **T37.0X4** Poisoning by sulfonamides, undetermined

       ✓7th **T37.0X5** Adverse effect of sulfonamides

       ✓7th **T37.0X6** Underdosing of sulfonamides

✓5th **T37.1** Poisoning by, adverse effect of and underdosing of antimycobacterial drugs

    EXCLUDES 1   rifampicins (T36.6-)
       streptomycin (T36.5-)

    ✓6th **T37.1X** Poisoning by, adverse effect of and underdosing of antimycobacterial drugs

       ✓7th **T37.1X1** Poisoning by antimycobacterial drugs, accidental (unintentional)
          Poisoning by antimycobacterial drugs NOS

       ✓7th **T37.1X2** Poisoning by antimycobacterial drugs, intentional self-harm

       ✓7th **T37.1X3** Poisoning by antimycobacterial drugs, assault

✓7th **T37.1X4** Poisoning by antimycobacterial drugs, undetermined

✓7th **T37.1X5** Adverse effect of antimycobacterial drugs

✓7th **T37.1X6** Underdosing of antimycobacterial drugs

✓5th **T37.2** Poisoning by, adverse effect of and underdosing of antimalarials and drugs acting on other blood protozoa

    EXCLUDES 1   hydroxyquinoline derivatives (T37.8-)

    ✓6th **T37.2X** Poisoning by, adverse effect of and underdosing of antimalarials and drugs acting on other blood protozoa

       ✓7th **T37.2X1** Poisoning by antimalarials and drugs acting on other blood protozoa, accidental (unintentional)
          Poisoning by antimalarials and drugs acting on other blood protozoa NOS

       ✓7th **T37.2X2** Poisoning by antimalarials and drugs acting on other blood protozoa, intentional self-harm

       ✓7th **T37.2X3** Poisoning by antimalarials and drugs acting on other blood protozoa, assault

       ✓7th **T37.2X4** Poisoning by antimalarials and drugs acting on other blood protozoa, undetermined

       ✓7th **T37.2X5** Adverse effect of antimalarials and drugs acting on other blood protozoa

       ✓7th **T37.2X6** Underdosing of antimalarials and drugs acting on other blood protozoa

✓5th **T37.3** Poisoning by, adverse effect of and underdosing of other antiprotozoal drugs

    ✓6th **T37.3X** Poisoning by, adverse effect of and underdosing of other antiprotozoal drugs

       ✓7th **T37.3X1** Poisoning by other antiprotozoal drugs, accidental (unintentional)
          Poisoning by other antiprotozoal drugs NOS

       ✓7th **T37.3X2** Poisoning by other antiprotozoal drugs, intentional self-harm

       ✓7th **T37.3X3** Poisoning by other antiprotozoal drugs, assault

       ✓7th **T37.3X4** Poisoning by other antiprotozoal drugs, undetermined

       ✓7th **T37.3X5** Adverse effect of other antiprotozoal drugs

       ✓7th **T37.3X6** Underdosing of other antiprotozoal drugs

✓5th **T37.4** Poisoning by, adverse effect of and underdosing of anthelminthics

    ✓6th **T37.4X** Poisoning by, adverse effect of and underdosing of anthelminthics

       ✓7th **T37.4X1** Poisoning by anthelminthics, accidental (unintentional)
          Poisoning by anthelminthics NOS

       ✓7th **T37.4X2** Poisoning by anthelminthics, intentional self-harm

       ✓7th **T37.4X3** Poisoning by anthelminthics, assault

       ✓7th **T37.4X4** Poisoning by anthelminthics, undetermined

       ✓7th **T37.4X5** Adverse effect of anthelminthics

       ✓7th **T37.4X6** Underdosing of anthelminthics

✓5th **T37.5** Poisoning by, adverse effect of and underdosing of antiviral drugs

    EXCLUDES 1   amantadine (T42.8-)
       cytarabine (T45.1-)

    ✓6th **T37.5X** Poisoning by, adverse effect of and underdosing of antiviral drugs

       ✓7th **T37.5X1** Poisoning by antiviral drugs, accidental (unintentional)
          Poisoning by antiviral drugs NOS

       ✓7th **T37.5X2** Poisoning by antiviral drugs, intentional self-harm

       ✓7th **T37.5X3** Poisoning by antiviral drugs, assault

       ✓7th **T37.5X4** Poisoning by antiviral drugs, undetermined

       ✓7th **T37.5X5** Adverse effect of antiviral drugs

       ✓7th **T37.5X6** Underdosing of antiviral drugs

EXCLUDES 1 Not coded here   EXCLUDES 2 Not included here   N Newborn Age: 0   P Pediatric Age: 0-17   M Maternity Age: 12-55   A Adult Age: 15-124

√5ᵗʰ **T37.8 Poisoning by, adverse effect of and underdosing of other specified systemic anti-infectives and antiparasitics**
Poisoning by, adverse effect of and underdosing of hydroxyquinoline derivatives
EXCLUDES 1 *antimalarial drugs (T37.2-)*

√6ᵗʰ **T37.8X Poisoning by, adverse effect of and underdosing of other specified** systemic anti-infectives and antiparasitics

√7ᵗʰ **T37.8X1 Poisoning by other specified systemic anti-infectives and antiparasitics, accidental (unintentional)**
Poisoning by other specified systemic anti-infectives and antiparasitics NOS

√7ᵗʰ **T37.8X2 Poisoning by other specified systemic anti-infectives and antiparasitics, intentional self-harm**

√7ᵗʰ **T37.8X3 Poisoning by other specified systemic anti-infectives and antiparasitics, assault**

√7ᵗʰ **T37.8X4 Poisoning by other specified systemic anti-infectives and antiparasitics, undetermined**

√7ᵗʰ **T37.8X5 Adverse effect of other specified systemic anti-infectives and antiparasitics**

√7ᵗʰ **T37.8X6 Underdosing of other specified systemic anti-infectives and antiparasitics**

√5ᵗʰ **T37.9 Poisoning by, adverse effect of and underdosing of unspecified systemic anti-infective and antiparasitics**

√x7ᵗʰ **T37.91 Poisoning by unspecified systemic anti-infective and antiparasitics, accidental (unintentional)**
Poisoning by, adverse effect of and underdosing of systemic anti-infective and antiparasitics NOS

√x7ᵗʰ **T37.92 Poisoning by unspecified systemic anti-infective and antiparasitics, intentional self-harm**

√x7ᵗʰ **T37.93 Poisoning by unspecified systemic anti-infective and antiparasitics, assault**

√x7ᵗʰ **T37.94 Poisoning by unspecified systemic anti-infective and antiparasitics, undetermined**

√x7ᵗʰ **T37.95 Adverse effect of unspecified systemic anti-infective and antiparasitic**

√x7ᵗʰ **T37.96 Underdosing of unspecified systemic anti-infectives and antiparasitics**

√4ᵗʰ **T38 Poisoning by, adverse effect of and underdosing of hormones and their synthetic substitutes and antagonists, not elsewhere classified**
EXCLUDES 1 *mineralocorticoids and their antagonists (T50.0-)*
oxytocic hormones (T48.0-)
parathyroid hormones and derivatives (T50.9-)

The appropriate 7th character is to be added to each code from category T38.
A   initial encounter
D   subsequent encounter
S   sequela

√5ᵗʰ **T38.0 Poisoning by, adverse effect of and underdosing of glucocorticoids and synthetic analogues**
EXCLUDES 1 *glucocorticoids, topically used (T49.-)*

√6ᵗʰ **T38.0X Poisoning by, adverse effect of and underdosing of glucocorticoids and synthetic analogues**

√7ᵗʰ **T38.0X1 Poisoning by glucocorticoids and synthetic analogues, accidental (unintentional)**
Poisoning by glucocorticoids and synthetic analogues NOS

√7ᵗʰ **T38.0X2 Poisoning by glucocorticoids and synthetic analogues, intentional self-harm**

√7ᵗʰ **T38.0X3 Poisoning by glucocorticoids and synthetic analogues, assault**

√7ᵗʰ **T38.0X4 Poisoning by glucocorticoids and synthetic analogues, undetermined**

√7ᵗʰ **T38.0X5 Adverse effect of glucocorticoids and synthetic analogues**

√7ᵗʰ **T38.0X6 Underdosing of glucocorticoids and synthetic analogues**

√5ᵗʰ **T38.1 Poisoning by, adverse effect of and underdosing of thyroid hormones and substitutes**

√6ᵗʰ **T38.1X Poisoning by, adverse effect of and underdosing of thyroid hormones and substitutes**

√7ᵗʰ **T38.1X1 Poisoning by thyroid hormones and substitutes, accidental (unintentional)**
Poisoning by thyroid hormones and substitutes NOS

√7ᵗʰ **T38.1X2 Poisoning by thyroid hormones and substitutes, intentional self-harm**

√7ᵗʰ **T38.1X3 Poisoning by thyroid hormones and substitutes, assault**

√7ᵗʰ **T38.1X4 Poisoning by thyroid hormones and substitutes, undetermined**

√7ᵗʰ **T38.1X5 Adverse effect of thyroid hormones and substitutes**

√7ᵗʰ **T38.1X6 Underdosing of thyroid hormones and substitutes**

√5ᵗʰ **T38.2 Poisoning by, adverse effect of and underdosing of antithyroid drugs**

√6ᵗʰ **T38.2X Poisoning by, adverse effect of and underdosing of antithyroid drugs**

√7ᵗʰ **T38.2X1 Poisoning by antithyroid drugs, accidental (unintentional)**
Poisoning by antithyroid drugs NOS

√7ᵗʰ **T38.2X2 Poisoning by antithyroid drugs, intentional self-harm**

√7ᵗʰ **T38.2X3 Poisoning by antithyroid drugs, assault**

√7ᵗʰ **T38.2X4 Poisoning by antithyroid drugs, undetermined**

√7ᵗʰ **T38.2X5 Adverse effect of antithyroid drugs**

√7ᵗʰ **T38.2X6 Underdosing of antithyroid drugs**

√5ᵗʰ **T38.3 Poisoning by, adverse effect of and underdosing of insulin and oral hypoglycemic [antidiabetic] drugs**

√6ᵗʰ **T38.3X Poisoning by, adverse effect of and underdosing of insulin and oral hypoglycemic [antidiabetic] drugs**

√7ᵗʰ **T38.3X1 Poisoning by insulin and oral hypoglycemic [antidiabetic] drugs, accidental (unintentional)**
Poisoning by insulin and oral hypoglycemic [antidiabetic] drugs NOS

√7ᵗʰ **T38.3X2 Poisoning by insulin and oral hypoglycemic [antidiabetic] drugs, intentional self-harm**

√7ᵗʰ **T38.3X3 Poisoning by insulin and oral hypoglycemic [antidiabetic] drugs, assault**

√7ᵗʰ **T38.3X4 Poisoning by insulin and oral hypoglycemic [antidiabetic] drugs, undetermined**

√7ᵗʰ **T38.3X5 Adverse effect of insulin and oral hypoglycemic [antidiabetic] drugs**

√7ᵗʰ **T38.3X6 Underdosing of insulin and oral hypoglycemic [antidiabetic] drugs**

√5ᵗʰ **T38.4 Poisoning by, adverse effect of and underdosing of oral contraceptives**
Poisoning by, adverse effect of and underdosing of multiple- and single-ingredient oral contraceptive preparations

√6ᵗʰ **T38.4X Poisoning by, adverse effect of and underdosing of oral contraceptives**

√7ᵗʰ **T38.4X1 Poisoning by oral contraceptives, accidental (unintentional)**
Poisoning by oral contraceptives NOS

√7ᵗʰ **T38.4X2 Poisoning by oral contraceptives, intentional self-harm**

√7ᵗʰ **T38.4X3 Poisoning by oral contraceptives, assault**

√7ᵗʰ **T38.4X4 Poisoning by oral contraceptives, undetermined**

√7ᵗʰ **T38.4X5 Adverse effect of oral contraceptives**

√7ᵗʰ **T38.4X6 Underdosing of oral contraceptives**

☑ Additional Character Required   √x7ᵗʰ Xtension Alert   Unspecified Dx   Other Specified Dx   Manifestation   ►◄ Revised Text   ● New Code   ▲ Revised Code Title

ICD-10-CM Draft (2015)   943

Injury, Poisoning and Certain Other Consequences of External Causes

T38.5–T38.993

✓5ᵗʰ **T38.5** **Poisoning by, adverse effect of and underdosing of other estrogens and progestogens**
Poisoning by, adverse effect of and underdosing of estrogens and progestogens mixtures and substitutes

  ✓6ᵗʰ **T38.5X** **Poisoning by, adverse effect of and underdosing of other** estrogens and progestogens

    ✓7ᵗʰ **T38.5X1** **Poisoning by other estrogens and progestogens,** accidental **(unintentional)**
Poisoning by other estrogens and progestogens NOS

    ✓7ᵗʰ **T38.5X2** **Poisoning by other estrogens and progestogens,** intentional self-harm

    ✓7ᵗʰ **T38.5X3** **Poisoning by other estrogens and progestogens,** assault

    ✓7ᵗʰ **T38.5X4** **Poisoning by other estrogens and progestogens,** undetermined

    ✓7ᵗʰ **T38.5X5** Adverse effect **of other estrogens and progestogens**

    ✓7ᵗʰ **T38.5X6** Underdosing **of other estrogens and progestogens**

✓5ᵗʰ **T38.6** **Poisoning by, adverse effect of and underdosing of antigonadotrophins, antiestrogens, antiandrogens, not elsewhere classified**
Poisoning by, adverse effect of and underdosing of tamoxifen

  ✓6ᵗʰ **T38.6X** **Poisoning by, adverse effect of and underdosing of** antigonadotrophins, antiestrogens, antiandrogens, **not elsewhere classified**

    ✓7ᵗʰ **T38.6X1** **Poisoning by antigonadotrophins, antiestrogens, antiandrogens, not elsewhere classified,** accidental **(unintentional)**
Poisoning by antigonadotrophins, antiestrogens, antiandrogens, not elsewhere classified NOS

    ✓7ᵗʰ **T38.6X2** **Poisoning by antigonadotrophins, antiestrogens, antiandrogens, not elsewhere classified,** intentional self-harm

    ✓7ᵗʰ **T38.6X3** **Poisoning by antigonadotrophins, antiestrogens, antiandrogens, not elsewhere classified,** assault

    ✓7ᵗʰ **T38.6X4** **Poisoning by antigonadotrophins, antiestrogens, antiandrogens, not elsewhere classified,** undetermined

    ✓7ᵗʰ **T38.6X5** Adverse effect **of antigonadotrophins, antiestrogens, antiandrogens, not elsewhere classified**

    ✓7ᵗʰ **T38.6X6** Underdosing **of antigonadotrophins, antiestrogens, antiandrogens, not elsewhere classified**

✓5ᵗʰ **T38.7** **Poisoning by, adverse effect of and underdosing of androgens and anabolic congeners**

  ✓6ᵗʰ **T38.7X** **Poisoning by, adverse effect of and underdosing of** androgens and anabolic congeners

    ✓7ᵗʰ **T38.7X1** **Poisoning by androgens and anabolic congeners,** accidental **(unintentional)**
Poisoning by androgens and anabolic congeners NOS

    ✓7ᵗʰ **T38.7X2** **Poisoning by androgens and anabolic congeners,** intentional self-harm

    ✓7ᵗʰ **T38.7X3** **Poisoning by androgens and anabolic congeners,** assault

    ✓7ᵗʰ **T38.7X4** **Poisoning by androgens and anabolic congeners,** undetermined

    ✓7ᵗʰ **T38.7X5** Adverse effect **of androgens and anabolic congeners**

    ✓7ᵗʰ **T38.7X6** Underdosing **of androgens and anabolic congeners**

✓5ᵗʰ **T38.8** **Poisoning by, adverse effect of and underdosing of other and unspecified hormones and synthetic substitutes**

  ✓6ᵗʰ **T38.80** **Poisoning by, adverse effect of and underdosing of** unspecified hormones and synthetic substitutes

    ✓7ᵗʰ **T38.801** **Poisoning by unspecified hormones and synthetic substitutes,** accidental **(unintentional)**
Poisoning by unspecified hormones and synthetic substitutes NOS

    ✓7ᵗʰ **T38.802** **Poisoning by unspecified hormones and synthetic substitutes,** intentional self-harm

    ✓7ᵗʰ **T38.803** **Poisoning by unspecified hormones and synthetic substitutes,** assault

    ✓7ᵗʰ **T38.804** **Poisoning by unspecified hormones and synthetic substitutes,** undetermined

    ✓7ᵗʰ **T38.805** Adverse effect **of unspecified hormones and synthetic substitutes**

    ✓7ᵗʰ **T38.806** Underdosing **of unspecified hormones and synthetic substitutes**

  ✓6ᵗʰ **T38.81** **Poisoning by, adverse effect of and underdosing of** anterior pituitary [adenohypophyseal] hormones

    ✓7ᵗʰ **T38.811** **Poisoning by anterior pituitary [adenohypophyseal] hormones,** accidental **(unintentional)**
Poisoning by anterior pituitary [adenohypophyseal] hormones NOS

    ✓7ᵗʰ **T38.812** **Poisoning by anterior pituitary [adenohypophyseal] hormones,** intentional self-harm

    ✓7ᵗʰ **T38.813** **Poisoning by anterior pituitary [adenohypophyseal] hormones,** assault

    ✓7ᵗʰ **T38.814** **Poisoning by anterior pituitary [adenohypophyseal] hormones,** undetermined

    ✓7ᵗʰ **T38.815** Adverse effect **of anterior pituitary [adenohypophyseal] hormones**

    ✓7ᵗʰ **T38.816** Underdosing **of anterior pituitary [adenohypophyseal] hormones**

  ✓6ᵗʰ **T38.89** **Poisoning by, adverse effect of and underdosing of** other hormones and synthetic substitutes

    ✓7ᵗʰ **T38.891** **Poisoning by other hormones and synthetic substitutes,** accidental **(unintentional)**
Poisoning by other hormones and synthetic substitutes NOS

    ✓7ᵗʰ **T38.892** **Poisoning by other hormones and synthetic substitutes,** intentional self-harm

    ✓7ᵗʰ **T38.893** **Poisoning by other hormones and synthetic substitutes,** assault

    ✓7ᵗʰ **T38.894** **Poisoning by other hormones and synthetic substitutes,** undetermined

    ✓7ᵗʰ **T38.895** Adverse effect **of other hormones and synthetic substitutes**

    ✓7ᵗʰ **T38.896** Underdosing **of other hormones and synthetic substitutes**

✓5ᵗʰ **T38.9** **Poisoning by, adverse effect of and underdosing of other and unspecified hormone antagonists**

  ✓6ᵗʰ **T38.90** **Poisoning by, adverse effect of and underdosing of** unspecified hormone antagonists

    ✓7ᵗʰ **T38.901** **Poisoning by unspecified hormone antagonists,** accidental **(unintentional)**
Poisoning by unspecified hormone antagonists NOS

    ✓7ᵗʰ **T38.902** **Poisoning by unspecified hormone antagonists,** intentional self-harm

    ✓7ᵗʰ **T38.903** **Poisoning by unspecified hormone antagonists,** assault

    ✓7ᵗʰ **T38.904** **Poisoning by unspecified hormone antagonists,** undetermined

    ✓7ᵗʰ **T38.905** Adverse effect **of unspecified hormone antagonists**

    ✓7ᵗʰ **T38.906** Underdosing **of unspecified hormone antagonists**

  ✓6ᵗʰ **T38.99** **Poisoning by, adverse effect of and underdosing of** other hormone antagonists

    ✓7ᵗʰ **T38.991** **Poisoning by other hormone antagonists,** accidental **(unintentional)**
Poisoning by other hormone antagonists NOS

    ✓7ᵗʰ **T38.992** **Poisoning by other hormone antagonists,** intentional self-harm

    ✓7ᵗʰ **T38.993** **Poisoning by other hormone antagonists,** assault

EXCLUDES 1 Not coded here   EXCLUDES 2 Not included here   N Newborn Age: 0   P Pediatric Age: 0-17   M Maternity Age: 12-55   A Adult Age: 15-124

944   ICD-10-CM Draft (2015)

☑7th **T38.994** **Poisoning by other hormone antagonists,** undetermined

☑7th **T38.995** Adverse effect **of other hormone antagonists**

☑7th **T38.996** Underdosing **of other hormone antagonists**

☑4th **T39** **Poisoning by, adverse effect of and underdosing of nonopioid analgesics, antipyretics and antirheumatics**

> The appropriate 7th character is to be added to each code from category T39.
> A   initial encounter
> D   subsequent encounter
> S   sequela

☑5th **T39.0** **Poisoning by, adverse effect of and underdosing of** salicylates

☑6th **T39.01** **Poisoning by, adverse effect of and underdosing of** aspirin

Poisoning by, adverse effect of and underdosing of acetylsalicylic acid

☑7th **T39.011** **Poisoning by aspirin,** accidental **(unintentional)**

☑7th **T39.012** **Poisoning by aspirin,** intentional self-harm

☑7th **T39.013** **Poisoning by aspirin,** assault

☑7th **T39.014** **Poisoning by aspirin,** undetermined

☑7th **T39.015** Adverse effect **of aspirin**

☑7th **T39.016** Underdosing **of aspirin**

☑6th **T39.09** **Poisoning by, adverse effect of and underdosing of** other salicylates

☑7th **T39.091** **Poisoning by salicylates,** accidental **(unintentional)**

Poisoning by salicylates NOS

☑7th **T39.092** **Poisoning by salicylates,** intentional self-harm

☑7th **T39.093** **Poisoning by salicylates,** assault

☑7th **T39.094** **Poisoning by salicylates,** undetermined

☑7th **T39.095** Adverse effect **of salicylates**

☑7th **T39.096** Underdosing **of salicylates**

☑5th **T39.1** **Poisoning by, adverse effect of and underdosing of 4-Aminophenol derivatives**

☑6th **T39.1X** **Poisoning by, adverse effect of and underdosing of** 4-Aminophenol derivatives

☑7th **T39.1X1** **Poisoning by 4-Aminophenol derivatives,** accidental (unintentional)

Poisoning by 4-Aminophenol derivatives NOS

☑7th **T39.1X2** **Poisoning by 4-Aminophenol derivatives,** intentional self-harm

☑7th **T39.1X3** **Poisoning by 4-Aminophenol derivatives,** assault

☑7th **T39.1X4** **Poisoning by 4-Aminophenol derivatives,** undetermined

☑7th **T39.1X5** Adverse effect **of 4-Aminophenol derivatives**

☑7th **T39.1X6** Underdosing **of 4-Aminophenol derivatives**

☑5th **T39.2** **Poisoning by, adverse effect of and underdosing of pyrazolone derivatives**

☑6th **T39.2X** **Poisoning by, adverse effect of and underdosing of** pyrazolone derivatives

☑7th **T39.2X1** **Poisoning by pyrazolone derivatives,** accidental **(unintentional)**

Poisoning by pyrazolone derivatives NOS

☑7th **T39.2X2** **Poisoning by pyrazolone derivatives,** intentional self-harm

☑7th **T39.2X3** **Poisoning by pyrazolone derivatives,** assault

☑7th **T39.2X4** **Poisoning by pyrazolone derivatives,** undetermined

☑7th **T39.2X5** Adverse effect **of pyrazolone derivatives**

☑7th **T39.2X6** Underdosing **of pyrazolone derivatives**

☑5th **T39.3** **Poisoning by, adverse effect of and underdosing of other nonsteroidal anti-inflammatory drugs [NSAID]**

☑6th **T39.31** **Poisoning by, adverse effect of and underdosing of** propionic acid derivatives

Poisoning by, adverse effect of and underdosing of fenoprofen

Poisoning by, adverse effect of and underdosing of flurbiprofen

Poisoning by, adverse effect of and underdosing of ibuprofen

Poisoning by, adverse effect of and underdosing of ketoprofen

Poisoning by, adverse effect of and underdosing of naproxen

Poisoning by, adverse effect of and underdosing of oxaprozin

☑7th **T39.311** **Poisoning by propionic acid derivatives,** accidental **(unintentional)**

☑7th **T39.312** **Poisoning by propionic acid derivatives,** intentional self-harm

☑7th **T39.313** **Poisoning by propionic acid derivatives,** assault

☑7th **T39.314** **Poisoning by propionic acid derivatives,** undetermined

☑7th **T39.315** Adverse effect **of propionic acid derivatives**

☑7th **T39.316** Underdosing **of propionic acid derivatives**

☑6th **T39.39** **Poisoning by, adverse effect of and underdosing of** other nonsteroidal anti-inflammatory drugs [NSAID]

☑7th **T39.391** **Poisoning by other nonsteroidal anti-inflammatory drugs [NSAID],** accidental **(unintentional)**

Poisoning by other nonsteroidal anti-inflammatory drugs NOS

☑7th **T39.392** **Poisoning by other nonsteroidal anti-inflammatory drugs [NSAID],** intentional self-harm

☑7th **T39.393** **Poisoning by other nonsteroidal anti-inflammatory drugs [NSAID],** assault

☑7th **T39.394** **Poisoning by other nonsteroidal anti-inflammatory drugs [NSAID],** undetermined

☑7th **T39.395** Adverse effect **of other nonsteroidal anti-inflammatory drugs [NSAID]**

☑7th **T39.396** Underdosing **of other nonsteroidal anti-inflammatory drugs [NSAID]**

☑5th **T39.4** **Poisoning by, adverse effect of and underdosing of antirheumatics, not elsewhere classified**

> **EXCLUDES 1**   poisoning by, adverse effect of and underdosing of glucocorticoids (T38.0-)
> poisoning by, adverse effect of and underdosing of salicylates (T39.0-)

☑6th **T39.4X** **Poisoning by, adverse effect of and underdosing of** antirheumatics, **not elsewhere classified**

☑7th **T39.4X1** **Poisoning by antirheumatics, not elsewhere classified,** accidental **(unintentional)**

Poisoning by antirheumatics, not elsewhere classified NOS

☑7th **T39.4X2** **Poisoning by antirheumatics, not elsewhere classified,** intentional self-harm

☑7th **T39.4X3** **Poisoning by antirheumatics, not elsewhere classified,** assault

☑7th **T39.4X4** **Poisoning by antirheumatics, not elsewhere classified,** undetermined

☑7th **T39.4X5** Adverse effect **of antirheumatics, not elsewhere classified**

☑7th **T39.4X6** Underdosing **of antirheumatics, not elsewhere classified**

☑ Additional Character Required   ☑7th Xtension Alert   Unspecified Dx   Other Specified Dx   Manifestation   ►◄ Revised Text   ● New Code   ▲ Revised Code Title

Injury, Poisoning and Certain Other Consequences of External Causes

T39.8–T40.691

✓5th **T39.8** **Poisoning by, adverse effect of and underdosing of other nonopioid analgesics and antipyretics, not elsewhere classified**

     ✓6th **T39.8X** **Poisoning by, adverse effect of and underdosing of** other nonopioid analgesics and antipyretics, **not elsewhere classified**

         ✓7th **T39.8X1** **Poisoning by other nonopioid analgesics and antipyretics, not elsewhere classified,** accidental **(unintentional)**
             Poisoning by other nonopioid analgesics and antipyretics, not elsewhere classified NOS

         ✓7th **T39.8X2** **Poisoning by other nonopioid analgesics and antipyretics, not elsewhere classified,** intentional self-harm

         ✓7th **T39.8X3** **Poisoning by other nonopioid analgesics and antipyretics, not elsewhere classified,** assault

         ✓7th **T39.8X4** **Poisoning by other nonopioid analgesics and antipyretics, not elsewhere classified,** undetermined

         ✓7th **T39.8X5** Adverse effect **of other nonopioid analgesics and antipyretics, not elsewhere classified**

         ✓7th **T39.8X6** Underdosing **of other nonopioid analgesics and antipyretics, not elsewhere classified**

✓5th **T39.9** **Poisoning by, adverse effect of and underdosing of** unspecified nonopioid analgesic, antipyretic and antirheumatic

     ✓x7th **T39.91** **Poisoning by unspecified nonopioid analgesic, antipyretic and antirheumatic,** accidental **(unintentional)**
         Poisoning by nonopioid analgesic, antipyretic and antirheumatic NOS

     ✓x7th **T39.92** **Poisoning by unspecified nonopioid analgesic, antipyretic and antirheumatic,** intentional self-harm

     ✓x7th **T39.93** **Poisoning by unspecified nonopioid analgesic, antipyretic and antirheumatic,** assault

     ✓x7th **T39.94** **Poisoning by unspecified nonopioid analgesic, antipyretic and antirheumatic,** undetermined

     ✓x7th **T39.95** Adverse effect **of unspecified nonopioid analgesic, antipyretic and antirheumatic**

     ✓x7th **T39.96** Underdosing **of unspecified nonopioid analgesic, antipyretic and antirheumatic**

✓4th **T40** **Poisoning by, adverse effect of and underdosing of narcotics and psychodysleptics [hallucinogens]**

     EXCLUDES 2   *drug dependence and related mental and behavioral disorders due to psychoactive substance use (F10-F19-)*

     The appropriate 7th character is to be added to each code from category T40.
     A   initial encounter
     D   subsequent encounter
     S   sequela

✓5th **T40.0** **Poisoning by, adverse effect of and underdosing of opium**

     ✓6th **T40.0X** **Poisoning by, adverse effect of and underdosing of** opium

         ✓7th **T40.0X1** **Poisoning by opium,** accidental **(unintentional)**
             Poisoning by opium NOS

         ✓7th **T40.0X2** **Poisoning by opium,** intentional self-harm

         ✓7th **T40.0X3** **Poisoning by opium,** assault

         ✓7th **T40.0X4** **Poisoning by opium,** undetermined

         ✓7th **T40.0X5** Adverse effect **of opium**

         ✓7th **T40.0X6** Underdosing **of opium**

✓5th **T40.1** **Poisoning by and adverse effect of** heroin

     ✓6th **T40.1X** **Poisoning by and adverse effect of heroin**

         ✓7th **T40.1X1** **Poisoning by heroin,** accidental **(unintentional)**
             Poisoning by heroin NOS

         ✓7th **T40.1X2** **Poisoning by heroin,** intentional self-harm

         ✓7th **T40.1X3** **Poisoning by heroin,** assault

         ✓7th **T40.1X4** **Poisoning by heroin,** undetermined

---

✓5th **T40.2** **Poisoning by, adverse effect of and underdosing of other opioids**

     ✓6th **T40.2X** **Poisoning by, adverse effect of and underdosing of** other opioids

         ✓7th **T40.2X1** **Poisoning by other opioids,** accidental **(unintentional)**
             Poisoning by other opioids NOS

         ✓7th **T40.2X2** **Poisoning by other opioids,** intentional self-harm

         ✓7th **T40.2X3** **Poisoning by other opioids,** assault

         ✓7th **T40.2X4** **Poisoning by other opioids,** undetermined

         ✓7th **T40.2X5** Adverse effect **of other opioids**

         ✓7th **T40.2X6** Underdosing **of other opioids**

✓5th **T40.3** **Poisoning by, adverse effect of and underdosing of methadone**

     ✓6th **T40.3X** **Poisoning by, adverse effect of and underdosing of** methadone

         ✓7th **T40.3X1** **Poisoning by methadone,** accidental **(unintentional)**
             Poisoning by methadone NOS

         ✓7th **T40.3X2** **Poisoning by methadone,** intentional self-harm

         ✓7th **T40.3X3** **Poisoning by methadone,** assault

         ✓7th **T40.3X4** **Poisoning by methadone,** undetermined

         ✓7th **T40.3X5** Adverse effect **of methadone**

         ✓7th **T40.3X6** Underdosing **of methadone**

✓5th **T40.4** **Poisoning by, adverse effect of and underdosing of other synthetic narcotics**

     ✓6th **T40.4X** **Poisoning by, adverse effect of and underdosing of** other synthetic narcotics

         ✓7th **T40.4X1** **Poisoning by other synthetic narcotics,** accidental **(unintentional)**
             Poisoning by other synthetic narcotics NOS

         ✓7th **T40.4X2** **Poisoning by other synthetic narcotics,** intentional self-harm

         ✓7th **T40.4X3** **Poisoning by other synthetic narcotics,** assault

         ✓7th **T40.4X4** **Poisoning by other synthetic narcotics,** undetermined

         ✓7th **T40.4X5** Adverse effect **of other synthetic narcotics**

         ✓7th **T40.4X6** Underdosing **of other synthetic narcotics**

✓5th **T40.5** **Poisoning by, adverse effect of and underdosing of cocaine**

     ✓6th **T40.5X** **Poisoning by, adverse effect of and underdosing of** cocaine

         ✓7th **T40.5X1** **Poisoning by cocaine,** accidental **(unintentional)**
             Poisoning by cocaine NOS

         ✓7th **T40.5X2** **Poisoning by cocaine,** intentional self-harm

         ✓7th **T40.5X3** **Poisoning by cocaine,** assault

         ✓7th **T40.5X4** **Poisoning by cocaine,** undetermined

         ✓7th **T40.5X5** Adverse effect **of cocaine**

         ✓7th **T40.5X6** Underdosing **of cocaine**

✓5th **T40.6** **Poisoning by, adverse effect of and underdosing of other and unspecified narcotics**

     ✓6th **T40.60** **Poisoning by, adverse effect of and underdosing of** unspecified narcotics

         ✓7th **T40.601** **Poisoning by unspecified narcotics,** accidental **(unintentional)**
             Poisoning by narcotics NOS

         ✓7th **T40.602** **Poisoning by unspecified narcotics,** intentional self-harm

         ✓7th **T40.603** **Poisoning by unspecified narcotics,** assault

         ✓7th **T40.604** **Poisoning by unspecified narcotics,** undetermined

         ✓7th **T40.605** Adverse effect **of unspecified narcotics**

         ✓7th **T40.606** Underdosing **of unspecified narcotics**

     ✓6th **T40.69** **Poisoning by, adverse effect of and underdosing of** other narcotics

         ✓7th **T40.691** **Poisoning by other narcotics,** accidental **(unintentional)**
             Poisoning by other narcotics NOS

EXCLUDES 1 Not coded here   EXCLUDES 2 Not included here   N Newborn Age: 0   P Pediatric Age: 0-17   M Maternity Age: 12-55   A Adult Age: 15-124

946   ICD-10-CM Draft (2015)

☑7ᵗʰ **T40.692** Poisoning by other narcotics, intentional self-harm

☑7ᵗʰ **T40.693** Poisoning by other narcotics, assault

☑7ᵗʰ **T40.694** Poisoning by other narcotics, undetermined

☑7ᵗʰ **T40.695** Adverse effect of other narcotics

☑7ᵗʰ **T40.696** Underdosing of other narcotics

☑5ᵗʰ **T40.7** Poisoning by, adverse effect of and underdosing of cannabis (derivatives)

☑6ᵗʰ **T40.7X** Poisoning by, adverse effect of and underdosing of cannabis (derivatives)

☑7ᵗʰ **T40.7X1** Poisoning by cannabis (derivatives), accidental (unintentional)
Poisoning by cannabis NOS

☑7ᵗʰ **T40.7X2** Poisoning by cannabis (derivatives), intentional self-harm

☑7ᵗʰ **T40.7X3** Poisoning by cannabis (derivatives), assault

☑7ᵗʰ **T40.7X4** Poisoning by cannabis (derivatives), undetermined

☑7ᵗʰ **T40.7X5** Adverse effect of cannabis (derivatives)

☑7ᵗʰ **T40.7X6** Underdosing of cannabis (derivatives)

☑5ᵗʰ **T40.8** Poisoning by and adverse effect of lysergide [LSD]

☑6ᵗʰ **T40.8X** Poisoning by and adverse effect of lysergide [LSD]

☑7ᵗʰ **T40.8X1** Poisoning by lysergide [LSD], accidental (unintentional)
Poisoning by lysergide [LSD]NOS

☑7ᵗʰ **T40.8X2** Poisoning by lysergide [LSD], intentional self-harm

☑7ᵗʰ **T40.8X3** Poisoning by lysergide [LSD], assault

☑7ᵗʰ **T40.8X4** Poisoning by lysergide [LSD], undetermined

☑5ᵗʰ **T40.9** Poisoning by, adverse effect of and underdosing of other and unspecified psychodysleptics [hallucinogens]

☑6ᵗʰ **T40.90** Poisoning by, adverse effect of and underdosing of unspecified psychodysleptics [hallucinogens]

☑7ᵗʰ **T40.901** Poisoning by unspecified psychodysleptics [hallucinogens], accidental (unintentional)

☑7ᵗʰ **T40.902** Poisoning by unspecified psychodysleptics [hallucinogens], intentional self-harm

☑7ᵗʰ **T40.903** Poisoning by unspecified psychodysleptics [hallucinogens], assault

☑7ᵗʰ **T40.904** Poisoning by unspecified psychodysleptics [hallucinogens], undetermined

☑7ᵗʰ **T40.905** Adverse effect of unspecified psychodysleptics [hallucinogens]

☑7ᵗʰ **T40.906** Underdosing of unspecified psychodysleptics

☑6ᵗʰ **T40.99** Poisoning by, adverse effect of and underdosing of other psychodysleptics [hallucinogens]

☑7ᵗʰ **T40.991** Poisoning by other psychodysleptics [hallucinogens], accidental (unintentional)
Poisoning by other psychodysleptics [hallucinogens] NOS

☑7ᵗʰ **T40.992** Poisoning by other psychodysleptics [hallucinogens], intentional self-harm

☑7ᵗʰ **T40.993** Poisoning by other psychodysleptics [hallucinogens], assault

☑7ᵗʰ **T40.994** Poisoning by other psychodysleptics [hallucinogens], undetermined

☑7ᵗʰ **T40.995** Adverse effect of other psychodysleptics [hallucinogens]

☑7ᵗʰ **T40.996** Underdosing of other psychodysleptics

☑4ᵗʰ **T41** Poisoning by, adverse effect of and underdosing of anesthetics and therapeutic gases

EXCLUDES 1 benzodiazepines (T42.4-)
cocaine (T40.5-)
complications of anesthesia during labor and delivery (O74.-)
complications of anesthesia during pregnancy (O29.-)
complications of anesthesia during the puerperium (O89.-)
opioids (T40.0-T40.2-)

The appropriate 7th character is to be added to each code from category T41.
A   initial encounter
D   subsequent encounter
S   sequela

☑5ᵗʰ **T41.0** Poisoning by, adverse effect of and underdosing of inhaled anesthetics

EXCLUDES 1 oxygen (T41.5-)

☑6ᵗʰ **T41.0X** Poisoning by, adverse effect of and underdosing of inhaled anesthetics

☑7ᵗʰ **T41.0X1** Poisoning by inhaled anesthetics, accidental (unintentional)
Poisoning by inhaled anesthetics NOS

☑7ᵗʰ **T41.0X2** Poisoning by inhaled anesthetics, intentional self-harm

☑7ᵗʰ **T41.0X3** Poisoning by inhaled anesthetics, assault

☑7ᵗʰ **T41.0X4** Poisoning by inhaled anesthetics, undetermined

☑7ᵗʰ **T41.0X5** Adverse effect of inhaled anesthetics

☑7ᵗʰ **T41.0X6** Underdosing of inhaled anesthetics

☑5ᵗʰ **T41.1** Poisoning by, adverse effect of and underdosing of intravenous anesthetics
Poisoning by, adverse effect of and underdosing of thiobarbiturates

☑6ᵗʰ **T41.1X** Poisoning by, adverse effect of and underdosing of intravenous anesthetics

☑7ᵗʰ **T41.1X1** Poisoning by intravenous anesthetics, accidental (unintentional)
Poisoning by intravenous anesthetics NOS

☑7ᵗʰ **T41.1X2** Poisoning by intravenous anesthetics, intentional self-harm

☑7ᵗʰ **T41.1X3** Poisoning by intravenous anesthetics, assault

☑7ᵗʰ **T41.1X4** Poisoning by intravenous anesthetics, undetermined

☑7ᵗʰ **T41.1X5** Adverse effect of intravenous anesthetics

☑7ᵗʰ **T41.1X6** Underdosing of intravenous anesthetics

☑5ᵗʰ **T41.2** Poisoning by, adverse effect of and underdosing of other and unspecified general anesthetics

☑6ᵗʰ **T41.20** Poisoning by, adverse effect of and underdosing of unspecified general anesthetics

☑7ᵗʰ **T41.201** Poisoning by unspecified general anesthetics, accidental (unintentional)
Poisoning by general anesthetics NOS

☑7ᵗʰ **T41.202** Poisoning by unspecified general anesthetics, intentional self-harm

☑7ᵗʰ **T41.203** Poisoning by unspecified general anesthetics, assault

☑7ᵗʰ **T41.204** Poisoning by unspecified general anesthetics, undetermined

☑7ᵗʰ **T41.205** Adverse effect of unspecified general anesthetics

☑7ᵗʰ **T41.206** Underdosing of unspecified general anesthetics

☑6ᵗʰ **T41.29** Poisoning by, adverse effect of and underdosing of other general anesthetics

☑7ᵗʰ **T41.291** Poisoning by other general anesthetics, accidental (unintentional)
Poisoning by other general anesthetics NOS

☑7ᵗʰ **T41.292** Poisoning by other general anesthetics, intentional self-harm

☑7ᵗʰ **T41.293** Poisoning by other general anesthetics, assault

☑7ᵗʰ **T41.294** Poisoning by other general anesthetics, undetermined

☑7ᵗʰ **T41.295** Adverse effect of other general anesthetics

☑ Additional Character Required   ☑7ᵗʰ Xtension Alert   Unspecified Dx   Other Specified Dx   Manifestation   ►◄ Revised Text   ● New Code   ▲ Revised Code Title
ICD-10-CM Draft (2015)

947

✓7ᵗʰ **T41.296** Underdosing of other general anesthetics

✓5ᵗʰ **T41.3 Poisoning by, adverse effect of and underdosing of local anesthetics**
Cocaine (topical)
> EXCLUDES 2   poisoning by cocaine used as a central nervous system stimulant (T40.5X1-T40.5X4)

✓6ᵗʰ **T41.3X Poisoning by, adverse effect of and underdosing of local anesthetics**

✓7ᵗʰ **T41.3X1 Poisoning by local anesthetics, accidental (unintentional)**
Poisoning by local anesthetics NOS

✓7ᵗʰ **T41.3X2 Poisoning by local anesthetics, intentional self-harm**

✓7ᵗʰ **T41.3X3 Poisoning by local anesthetics, assault**

✓7ᵗʰ **T41.3X4 Poisoning by local anesthetics, undetermined**

✓7ᵗʰ **T41.3X5 Adverse effect of local anesthetics**

✓7ᵗʰ **T41.3X6 Underdosing of local anesthetics**

✓5ᵗʰ **T41.4 Poisoning by, adverse effect of and underdosing of unspecified anesthetic**

✓x7ᵗʰ **T41.41 Poisoning by unspecified anesthetic, accidental (unintentional)**
Poisoning by anesthetic NOS

✓x7ᵗʰ **T41.42 Poisoning by unspecified anesthetic, intentional self-harm**

✓x7ᵗʰ **T41.43 Poisoning by unspecified anesthetic, assault**

✓x7ᵗʰ **T41.44 Poisoning by unspecified anesthetic, undetermined**

✓x7ᵗʰ **T41.45 Adverse effect of unspecified anesthetic**

✓x7ᵗʰ **T41.46 Underdosing of unspecified anesthetics**

✓5ᵗʰ **T41.5 Poisoning by, adverse effect of and underdosing of therapeutic gases**

✓6ᵗʰ **T41.5X Poisoning by, adverse effect of and underdosing of therapeutic gases**

✓7ᵗʰ **T41.5X1 Poisoning by therapeutic gases, accidental (unintentional)**
Poisoning by therapeutic gases NOS

✓7ᵗʰ **T41.5X2 Poisoning by therapeutic gases, intentional self-harm**

✓7ᵗʰ **T41.5X3 Poisoning by therapeutic gases, assault**

✓7ᵗʰ **T41.5X4 Poisoning by therapeutic gases, undetermined**

✓7ᵗʰ **T41.5X5 Adverse effect of therapeutic gases**

✓7ᵗʰ **T41.5X6 Underdosing of therapeutic gases**

✓4ᵗʰ **T42 Poisoning by, adverse effect of and underdosing of antiepileptic, sedative- hypnotic and antiparkinsonism drugs**
> EXCLUDES 2   drug dependence and related mental and behavioral disorders due to psychoactive substance use (F10.- -F19.-)

The appropriate 7th character is to be added to each code from category T42.
A   initial encounter
D   subsequent encounter
S   sequela

✓5ᵗʰ **T42.0 Poisoning by, adverse effect of and underdosing of hydantoin derivatives**

✓6ᵗʰ **T42.0X Poisoning by, adverse effect of and underdosing of hydantoin derivatives**

✓7ᵗʰ **T42.0X1 Poisoning by hydantoin derivatives, accidental (unintentional)**
Poisoning by hydantoin derivatives NOS

✓7ᵗʰ **T42.0X2 Poisoning by hydantoin derivatives, intentional self-harm**

✓7ᵗʰ **T42.0X3 Poisoning by hydantoin derivatives, assault**

✓7ᵗʰ **T42.0X4 Poisoning by hydantoin derivatives, undetermined**

✓7ᵗʰ **T42.0X5 Adverse effect of hydantoin derivatives**

✓7ᵗʰ **T42.0X6 Underdosing of hydantoin derivatives**

✓5ᵗʰ **T42.1 Poisoning by, adverse effect of and underdosing of iminostilbenes**
Poisoning by, adverse effect of and underdosing of carbamazepine

✓6ᵗʰ **T42.1X Poisoning by, adverse effect of and underdosing of iminostilbenes**

✓7ᵗʰ **T42.1X1 Poisoning by iminostilbenes, accidental (unintentional)**
Poisoning by iminostilbenes NOS

✓7ᵗʰ **T42.1X2 Poisoning by iminostilbenes, intentional self-harm**

✓7ᵗʰ **T42.1X3 Poisoning by iminostilbenes, assault**

✓7ᵗʰ **T42.1X4 Poisoning by iminostilbenes, undetermined**

✓7ᵗʰ **T42.1X5 Adverse effect of iminostilbenes**

✓7ᵗʰ **T42.1X6 Underdosing of iminostilbenes**

✓5ᵗʰ **T42.2 Poisoning by, adverse effect of and underdosing of succinimides and oxazolidinediones**

✓6ᵗʰ **T42.2X Poisoning by, adverse effect of and underdosing of succinimides and oxazolidinediones**

✓7ᵗʰ **T42.2X1 Poisoning by succinimides and oxazolidinediones, accidental (unintentional)**
Poisoning by succinimides and oxazolidinediones NOS

✓7ᵗʰ **T42.2X2 Poisoning by succinimides and oxazolidinediones, intentional self-harm**

✓7ᵗʰ **T42.2X3 Poisoning by succinimides and oxazolidinediones, assault**

✓7ᵗʰ **T42.2X4 Poisoning by succinimides and oxazolidinediones, undetermined**

✓7ᵗʰ **T42.2X5 Adverse effect of succinimides and oxazolidinediones**

✓7ᵗʰ **T42.2X6 Underdosing of succinimides and oxazolidinediones**

✓5ᵗʰ **T42.3 Poisoning by, adverse effect of and underdosing of barbiturates**
> EXCLUDES 1   poisoning by, adverse effect of and underdosing of thiobarbiturates (T41.1-)

✓6ᵗʰ **T42.3X Poisoning by, adverse effect of and underdosing of barbiturates**

✓7ᵗʰ **T42.3X1 Poisoning by barbiturates, accidental (unintentional)**
Poisoning by barbiturates NOS

✓7ᵗʰ **T42.3X2 Poisoning by barbiturates, intentional self-harm**

✓7ᵗʰ **T42.3X3 Poisoning by barbiturates, assault**

✓7ᵗʰ **T42.3X4 Poisoning by barbiturates, undetermined**

✓7ᵗʰ **T42.3X5 Adverse effect of barbiturates**

✓7ᵗʰ **T42.3X6 Underdosing of barbiturates**

✓5ᵗʰ **T42.4 Poisoning by, adverse effect of and underdosing of benzodiazepines**

✓6ᵗʰ **T42.4X Poisoning by, adverse effect of and underdosing of benzodiazepines**

✓7ᵗʰ **T42.4X1 Poisoning by benzodiazepines, accidental (unintentional)**
Poisoning by benzodiazepines NOS

✓7ᵗʰ **T42.4X2 Poisoning by benzodiazepines, intentional self-harm**

✓7ᵗʰ **T42.4X3 Poisoning by benzodiazepines, assault**

✓7ᵗʰ **T42.4X4 Poisoning by benzodiazepines, undetermined**

✓7ᵗʰ **T42.4X5 Adverse effect of benzodiazepines**

✓7ᵗʰ **T42.4X6 Underdosing of benzodiazepines**

✓5ᵗʰ **T42.5 Poisoning by, adverse effect of and underdosing of mixed antiepileptics**

✓6ᵗʰ **T42.5X Poisoning by, adverse effect of and underdosing of antiepileptics**

✓7ᵗʰ **T42.5X1 Poisoning by mixed antiepileptics, accidental (unintentional)**
Poisoning by mixed antiepileptics NOS

✓7ᵗʰ **T42.5X2 Poisoning by mixed antiepileptics, intentional self-harm**

✓7ᵗʰ **T42.5X3 Poisoning by mixed antiepileptics, assault**

EXCLUDES 1 Not coded here   EXCLUDES 2 Not included here   N Newborn Age: 0   P Pediatric Age: 0-17   M Maternity Age: 12-55   A Adult Age: 15-124

948   ICD-10-CM Draft (2015)

☑7ᵗʰ **T42.5X4** Poisoning by mixed antiepileptics, undetermined

☑7ᵗʰ **T42.5X5** Adverse effect of mixed antiepileptics

☑7ᵗʰ **T42.5X6** Underdosing of mixed antiepileptics

☑5ᵗʰ **T42.6** Poisoning by, adverse effect of and underdosing of other antiepileptic and sedative-hypnotic drugs

Poisoning by, adverse effect of and underdosing of methaqualone

Poisoning by, adverse effect of and underdosing of valproic acid

EXCLUDES 1 *poisoning by, adverse effect of and underdosing of carbamazepine (T42.1-)*

☑6ᵗʰ **T42.6X** Poisoning by, adverse effect of and underdosing of other antiepileptic and sedative-hypnotic drugs

☑7ᵗʰ **T42.6X1** Poisoning by other antiepileptic and sedative-hypnotic drugs, accidental (unintentional)

Poisoning by other antiepileptic and sedative-hypnotic drugs NOS

☑7ᵗʰ **T42.6X2** Poisoning by other antiepileptic and sedative-hypnotic drugs, intentional self-harm

☑7ᵗʰ **T42.6X3** Poisoning by other antiepileptic and sedative-hypnotic drugs, assault

☑7ᵗʰ **T42.6X4** Poisoning by other antiepileptic and sedative-hypnotic drugs, undetermined

☑7ᵗʰ **T42.6X5** Adverse effect of other antiepileptic and sedative-hypnotic drugs

☑7ᵗʰ **T42.6X6** Underdosing of other antiepileptic and sedative-hypnotic drugs

☑5ᵗʰ **T42.7** Poisoning by, adverse effect of and underdosing of unspecified antiepileptic and sedative-hypnotic drugs

☑x7ᵗʰ **T42.71** Poisoning by unspecified antiepileptic and sedative-hypnotic drugs, accidental (unintentional)

Poisoning by antiepileptic and sedative-hypnotic drugs NOS

☑x7ᵗʰ **T42.72** Poisoning by unspecified antiepileptic and sedative-hypnotic drugs, intentional self-harm

☑x7ᵗʰ **T42.73** Poisoning by unspecified antiepileptic and sedative-hypnotic drugs, assault

☑x7ᵗʰ **T42.74** Poisoning by unspecified antiepileptic and sedative-hypnotic drugs, undetermined

☑x7ᵗʰ **T42.75** Adverse effect of unspecified antiepileptic and sedative-hypnotic drugs

☑x7ᵗʰ **T42.76** Underdosing of unspecified antiepileptic and sedative-hypnotic drugs

☑5ᵗʰ **T42.8** Poisoning by, adverse effect of and underdosing of antiparkinsonism drugs and other central muscle-tone depressants

Poisoning by, adverse effect of and underdosing of amantadine

☑6ᵗʰ **T42.8X** Poisoning by, adverse effect of and underdosing of antiparkinsonism drugs and other central muscle-tone depressants

☑7ᵗʰ **T42.8X1** Poisoning by antiparkinsonism drugs and other central muscle-tone depressants, accidental (unintentional)

Poisoning by antiparkinsonism drugs and other central muscle-tone depressants NOS

☑7ᵗʰ **T42.8X2** Poisoning by antiparkinsonism drugs and other central muscle-tone depressants, intentional self-harm

☑7ᵗʰ **T42.8X3** Poisoning by antiparkinsonism drugs and other central muscle-tone depressants, assault

☑7ᵗʰ **T42.8X4** Poisoning by antiparkinsonism drugs and other central muscle-tone depressants, undetermined

☑7ᵗʰ **T42.8X5** Adverse effect of antiparkinsonism drugs and other central muscle-tone depressants

☑7ᵗʰ **T42.8X6** Underdosing of antiparkinsonism drugs and other central muscle-tone depressants

☑4ᵗʰ **T43** Poisoning by, adverse effect of and underdosing of psychotropic drugs, not elsewhere classified

EXCLUDES 1 appetite depressants (T50.5-)
barbiturates (T42.3-)
benzodiazepines (T42.4-)
methaqualone (T42.6-)
psychodysleptics [hallucinogens] (T40.7-T40.9-)

EXCLUDES 2 drug dependence and related mental and behavioral disorders due to psychoactive substance use (F10.--F19.-)

The appropriate 7th character is to be added to each code from category T43.
A   initial encounter
D   subsequent encounter
S   sequela

☑5ᵗʰ **T43.0** Poisoning by, adverse effect of and underdosing of tricyclic and tetracyclic antidepressants

☑6ᵗʰ **T43.01** Poisoning by, adverse effect of and underdosing of tricyclic antidepressants

☑7ᵗʰ **T43.011** Poisoning by tricyclic antidepressants, accidental (unintentional)

Poisoning by tricyclic antidepressants NOS

☑7ᵗʰ **T43.012** Poisoning by tricyclic antidepressants, intentional self-harm

☑7ᵗʰ **T43.013** Poisoning by tricyclic antidepressants, assault

☑7ᵗʰ **T43.014** Poisoning by tricyclic antidepressants, undetermined

☑7ᵗʰ **T43.015** Adverse effect of tricyclic antidepressants

☑7ᵗʰ **T43.016** Underdosing of tricyclic antidepressants

☑6ᵗʰ **T43.02** Poisoning by, adverse effect of and underdosing of tetracyclic antidepressants

☑7ᵗʰ **T43.021** Poisoning by tetracyclic antidepressants, accidental (unintentional)

Poisoning by tetracyclic antidepressants NOS

☑7ᵗʰ **T43.022** Poisoning by tetracyclic antidepressants, intentional self-harm

☑7ᵗʰ **T43.023** Poisoning by tetracyclic antidepressants, assault

☑7ᵗʰ **T43.024** Poisoning by tetracyclic antidepressants, undetermined

☑7ᵗʰ **T43.025** Adverse effect of tetracyclic antidepressants

☑7ᵗʰ **T43.026** Underdosing of tetracyclic antidepressants

☑5ᵗʰ **T43.1** Poisoning by, adverse effect of and underdosing of monoamine-oxidase-inhibitor antidepressants

☑6ᵗʰ **T43.1X** Poisoning by, adverse effect of and underdosing of monoamine-oxidase-inhibitor antidepressants

☑7ᵗʰ **T43.1X1** Poisoning by monoamine-oxidase-inhibitor antidepressants, accidental (unintentional)

Poisoning by monoamine-oxidase-inhibitor antidepressants NOS

☑7ᵗʰ **T43.1X2** Poisoning by monoamine-oxidase-inhibitor antidepressants, intentional self-harm

☑7ᵗʰ **T43.1X3** Poisoning by monoamine-oxidase-inhibitor antidepressants, assault

☑7ᵗʰ **T43.1X4** Poisoning by monoamine-oxidase-inhibitor antidepressants, undetermined

☑7ᵗʰ **T43.1X5** Adverse effect of monoamine-oxidase-inhibitor antidepressants

☑7ᵗʰ **T43.1X6** Underdosing of monoamine-oxidase-inhibitor antidepressants

☑5ᵗʰ **T43.2** Poisoning by, adverse effect of and underdosing of other and unspecified antidepressants

☑6ᵗʰ **T43.20** Poisoning by, adverse effect of and underdosing of unspecified antidepressants

☑7ᵗʰ **T43.201** Poisoning by unspecified antidepressants, accidental (unintentional)

Poisoning by antidepressants NOS

☑7ᵗʰ **T43.202** Poisoning by unspecified antidepressants, intentional self-harm

☑7ᵗʰ **T43.203** Poisoning by unspecified antidepressants, assault

☑ Additional Character Required   ☑x7ᵗʰ Xtension Alert   Unspecified Dx   Other Specified Dx   Manifestation   ►◄ Revised Text   ● New Code   ▲ Revised Code Title

ICD-10-CM Draft (2015)   949

√7th **T43.204 Poisoning by unspecified antidepressants, undetermined**

√7th **T43.205 Adverse effect of unspecified antidepressants**

√7th **T43.206 Underdosing of unspecified antidepressants**

√6th **T43.21 Poisoning by, adverse effect of and underdosing of selective serotonin and norepinephrine reuptake inhibitors**
Poisoning by, adverse effect of and underdosing of SSNRI antidepressants

√7th **T43.211 Poisoning by selective serotonin and norepinephrine reuptake inhibitors, accidental (unintentional)**

√7th **T43.212 Poisoning by selective serotonin and norepinephrine reuptake inhibitors, intentional self-harm**

√7th **T43.213 Poisoning by selective serotonin and norepinephrine reuptake inhibitors, assault**

√7th **T43.214 Poisoning by selective serotonin and norepinephrine reuptake inhibitors, undetermined**

√7th **T43.215 Adverse effect of selective serotonin and norepinephrine reuptake inhibitors**

√7th **T43.216 Underdosing of selective serotonin and norepinephrine reuptake inhibitors**

√6th **T43.22 Poisoning by, adverse effect of and underdosing of selective serotonin reuptake inhibitors**
Poisoning by, adverse effect of and underdosing of SSRI antidepressants

√7th **T43.221 Poisoning by selective serotonin reuptake inhibitors, accidental (unintentional)**

√7th **T43.222 Poisoning by selective serotonin reuptake inhibitors, intentional self-harm**

√7th **T43.223 Poisoning by selective serotonin reuptake inhibitors, assault**

√7th **T43.224 Poisoning by selective serotonin reuptake inhibitors, undetermined**

√7th **T43.225 Adverse effect of selective serotonin reuptake inhibitors**

√7th **T43.226 Underdosing of selective serotonin reuptake inhibitors**

√6th **T43.29 Poisoning by, adverse effect of and underdosing of other antidepressants**

√7th **T43.291 Poisoning by other antidepressants, accidental (unintentional)**
Poisoning by other antidepressants NOS

√7th **T43.292 Poisoning by other antidepressants, intentional self-harm**

√7th **T43.293 Poisoning by other antidepressants, assault**

√7th **T43.294 Poisoning by other antidepressants, undetermined**

√7th **T43.295 Adverse effect of other antidepressants**

√7th **T43.296 Underdosing of other antidepressants**

√5th **T43.3 Poisoning by, adverse effect of and underdosing of phenothiazine antipsychotics and neuroleptics**

√6th **T43.3X Poisoning by, adverse effect of and underdosing of phenothiazine antipsychotics and neuroleptics**

√7th **T43.3X1 Poisoning by phenothiazine antipsychotics and neuroleptics, accidental (unintentional)**
Poisoning by phenothiazine antipsychotics and neuroleptics NOS

√7th **T43.3X2 Poisoning by phenothiazine antipsychotics and neuroleptics, intentional self-harm**

√7th **T43.3X3 Poisoning by phenothiazine antipsychotics and neuroleptics, assault**

√7th **T43.3X4 Poisoning by phenothiazine antipsychotics and neuroleptics, undetermined**

√7th **T43.3X5 Adverse effect of phenothiazine antipsychotics and neuroleptics**

√7th **T43.3X6 Underdosing of phenothiazine antipsychotics and neuroleptics**

√5th **T43.4 Poisoning by, adverse effect of and underdosing of butyrophenone and thiothixene neuroleptics**

√6th **T43.4X Poisoning by, adverse effect of and underdosing of butyrophenone and thiothixene neuroleptics**

√7th **T43.4X1 Poisoning by butyrophenone and thiothixene neuroleptics, accidental (unintentional)**
Poisoning by butyrophenone and thiothixene neuroleptics NOS

√7th **T43.4X2 Poisoning by butyrophenone and thiothixene neuroleptics, intentional self-harm**

√7th **T43.4X3 Poisoning by butyrophenone and thiothixene neuroleptics, assault**

√7th **T43.4X4 Poisoning by butyrophenone and thiothixene neuroleptics, undetermined**

√7th **T43.4X5 Adverse effect of butyrophenone and thiothixene neuroleptics**

√7th **T43.4X6 Underdosing of butyrophenone and thiothixene neuroleptics**

√5th **T43.5 Poisoning by, adverse effect of and underdosing of other and unspecified antipsychotics and neuroleptics**
EXCLUDES 1 poisoning by, adverse effect of and underdosing of rauwolfia (T46.5-)

√6th **T43.50 Poisoning by, adverse effect of and underdosing of unspecified antipsychotics and neuroleptics**

√7th **T43.501 Poisoning by unspecified antipsychotics and neuroleptics, accidental (unintentional)**
Poisoning by antipsychotics and neuroleptics NOS

√7th **T43.502 Poisoning by unspecified antipsychotics and neuroleptics, intentional self-harm**

√7th **T43.503 Poisoning by unspecified antipsychotics and neuroleptics, assault**

√7th **T43.504 Poisoning by unspecified antipsychotics and neuroleptics, undetermined**

√7th **T43.505 Adverse effect of unspecified antipsychotics and neuroleptics**

√7th **T43.506 Underdosing of unspecified antipsychotics and neuroleptics**

√6th **T43.59 Poisoning by, adverse effect of and underdosing of other antipsychotics and neuroleptics**

√7th **T43.591 Poisoning by other antipsychotics and neuroleptics, accidental (unintentional)**
Poisoning by other antipsychotics and neuroleptics NOS

√7th **T43.592 Poisoning by other antipsychotics and neuroleptics, intentional self-harm**

√7th **T43.593 Poisoning by other antipsychotics and neuroleptics, assault**

√7th **T43.594 Poisoning by other antipsychotics and neuroleptics, undetermined**

√7th **T43.595 Adverse effect of other antipsychotics and neuroleptics**

√7th **T43.596 Underdosing of other antipsychotics and neuroleptics**

√5th **T43.6 Poisoning by, adverse effect of and underdosing of psychostimulants**
EXCLUDES 1 poisoning by, adverse effect of and underdosing of cocaine (T40.5-)

√6th **T43.60 Poisoning by, adverse effect of and underdosing of unspecified psychostimulant**

√7th **T43.601 Poisoning by unspecified psychostimulants, accidental (unintentional)**
Poisoning by psychostimulants NOS

√7th **T43.602 Poisoning by unspecified psychostimulants, intentional self-harm**

√7th **T43.603 Poisoning by unspecified psychostimulants, assault**

√7th **T43.604 Poisoning by unspecified psychostimulants, undetermined**

√7th **T43.605 Adverse effect of unspecified psychostimulants**

√7th **T43.606 Underdosing of unspecified psychostimulants**

EXCLUDES 1 Not coded here   EXCLUDES 2 Not included here   N Newborn Age: 0   P Pediatric Age: 0-17   M Maternity Age: 12-55   A Adult Age: 15-124

950   ICD-10-CM Draft (2015)

√6ᵗʰ **T43.61** Poisoning by, adverse effect of and underdosing of caffeine

√7ᵗʰ **T43.611** **Poisoning by caffeine,** accidental **(unintentional)**
Poisoning by caffeine NOS

√7ᵗʰ **T43.612** **Poisoning by caffeine,** intentional **self-harm**

√7ᵗʰ **T43.613** **Poisoning by caffeine,** assault

√7ᵗʰ **T43.614** **Poisoning by caffeine,** undetermined

√7ᵗʰ **T43.615** Adverse effect of caffeine

√7ᵗʰ **T43.616** Underdosing of caffeine

√6ᵗʰ **T43.62** Poisoning by, adverse effect of and underdosing of amphetamines
Poisoning by, adverse effect of and underdosing of methamphetamines

√7ᵗʰ **T43.621** **Poisoning by amphetamines,** accidental **(unintentional)**
Poisoning by amphetamines NOS

√7ᵗʰ **T43.622** **Poisoning by amphetamines,** intentional **self-harm**

√7ᵗʰ **T43.623** **Poisoning by amphetamines,** assault

√7ᵗʰ **T43.624** **Poisoning by amphetamines,** undetermined

√7ᵗʰ **T43.625** Adverse effect of amphetamines

√7ᵗʰ **T43.626** Underdosing of amphetamines

√6ᵗʰ **T43.63** Poisoning by, adverse effect of and underdosing of methylphenidate

√7ᵗʰ **T43.631** **Poisoning by methylphenidate,** accidental **(unintentional)**
Poisoning by methylphenidate NOS

√7ᵗʰ **T43.632** **Poisoning by methylphenidate,** intentional self-harm

√7ᵗʰ **T43.633** **Poisoning by methylphenidate,** assault

√7ᵗʰ **T43.634** **Poisoning by methylphenidate,** undetermined

√7ᵗʰ **T43.635** Adverse effect of methylphenidate

√7ᵗʰ **T43.636** Underdosing of methylphenidate

√6ᵗʰ **T43.69** Poisoning by, adverse effect of and underdosing of other psychostimulants

√7ᵗʰ **T43.691** **Poisoning by other psychostimulants, accidental (unintentional)**
Poisoning by other psychostimulants NOS

√7ᵗʰ **T43.692** **Poisoning by other psychostimulants, intentional self-harm**

√7ᵗʰ **T43.693** **Poisoning by other psychostimulants, assault**

√7ᵗʰ **T43.694** **Poisoning by other psychostimulants, undetermined**

√7ᵗʰ **T43.695** Adverse effect of other psychostimulants

√7ᵗʰ **T43.696** Underdosing of other psychostimulants

√5ᵗʰ **T43.8** Poisoning by, adverse effect of and underdosing of other psychotropic drugs

√6ᵗʰ **T43.8X** Poisoning by, adverse effect of and underdosing of other psychotropic drugs

√7ᵗʰ **T43.8X1** **Poisoning by other psychotropic drugs, accidental (unintentional)**
Poisoning by other psychotropic drugs NOS

√7ᵗʰ **T43.8X2** **Poisoning by other psychotropic drugs, intentional self-harm**

√7ᵗʰ **T43.8X3** **Poisoning by other psychotropic drugs, assault**

√7ᵗʰ **T43.8X4** **Poisoning by other psychotropic drugs, undetermined**

√7ᵗʰ **T43.8X5** Adverse effect of other psychotropic drugs

√7ᵗʰ **T43.8X6** Underdosing of other psychotropic drugs

√5ᵗʰ **T43.9** Poisoning by, adverse effect of and underdosing of unspecified psychotropic drug

√x7ᵗʰ **T43.91** **Poisoning by unspecified psychotropic drug, accidental (unintentional)**
Poisoning by psychotropic drug NOS

√x7ᵗʰ **T43.92** **Poisoning by unspecified psychotropic drug, intentional self-harm**

√x7ᵗʰ **T43.93** **Poisoning by unspecified psychotropic drug,** assault

√x7ᵗʰ **T43.94** **Poisoning by unspecified psychotropic drug,** undetermined

√x7ᵗʰ **T43.95** Adverse effect of unspecified psychotropic drug

√x7ᵗʰ **T43.96** Underdosing of unspecified psychotropic drug

√4ᵗʰ **T44** Poisoning by, adverse effect of and underdosing of drugs primarily affecting the autonomic nervous system

The appropriate 7th character is to be added to each code from category T44.
A initial encounter
D subsequent encounter
S sequela

√5ᵗʰ **T44.0** Poisoning by, adverse effect of and underdosing of anticholinesterase agents

√6ᵗʰ **T44.0X** Poisoning by, adverse effect of and underdosing of anticholinesterase agents

√7ᵗʰ **T44.0X1** **Poisoning by anticholinesterase agents,** accidental **(unintentional)**
Poisoning by anticholinesterase agents NOS

√7ᵗʰ **T44.0X2** **Poisoning by anticholinesterase agents,** intentional self-harm

√7ᵗʰ **T44.0X3** **Poisoning by anticholinesterase agents,** assault

√7ᵗʰ **T44.0X4** **Poisoning by anticholinesterase agents,** undetermined

√7ᵗʰ **T44.0X5** Adverse effect of anticholinesterase agents

√7ᵗʰ **T44.0X6** Underdosing of anticholinesterase agents

√5ᵗʰ **T44.1** Poisoning by, adverse effect of and underdosing of other parasympathomimetics [cholinergics]

√6ᵗʰ **T44.1X** Poisoning by, adverse effect of and underdosing of other parasympathomimetics [cholinergics]

√7ᵗʰ **T44.1X1** **Poisoning by other parasympathomimetics [cholinergics], accidental (unintentional)**
Poisoning by other parasympathomimetics [cholinergics] NOS

√7ᵗʰ **T44.1X2** **Poisoning by other parasympathomimetics [cholinergics], intentional self-harm**

√7ᵗʰ **T44.1X3** **Poisoning by other parasympathomimetics [cholinergics], assault**

√7ᵗʰ **T44.1X4** **Poisoning by other parasympathomimetics [cholinergics], undetermined**

√7ᵗʰ **T44.1X5** Adverse effect of other parasympathomimetics [cholinergics]

√7ᵗʰ **T44.1X6** Underdosing of other parasympathomimetics

√5ᵗʰ **T44.2** Poisoning by, adverse effect of and underdosing of ganglionic blocking drugs

√6ᵗʰ **T44.2X** Poisoning by, adverse effect of and underdosing of ganglionic blocking drugs

√7ᵗʰ **T44.2X1** **Poisoning by ganglionic blocking drugs,** accidental **(unintentional)**
Poisoning by ganglionic blocking drugs NOS

√7ᵗʰ **T44.2X2** **Poisoning by ganglionic blocking drugs,** intentional self-harm

√7ᵗʰ **T44.2X3** **Poisoning by ganglionic blocking drugs,** assault

√7ᵗʰ **T44.2X4** **Poisoning by ganglionic blocking drugs,** undetermined

√7ᵗʰ **T44.2X5** Adverse effect of ganglionic blocking drugs

√7ᵗʰ **T44.2X6** Underdosing of ganglionic blocking drugs

☑ Additional Character Required   √7ᵗʰ Xtension Alert   Unspecified Dx   Other Specified Dx   Manifestation   ►◄ Revised Text   ● New Code   ▲ Revised Code Title

Injury, Poisoning and Certain Other Consequences of External Causes

T44.3–T44.8X6

✓5ᵗʰ **T44.3 Poisoning by, adverse effect of and underdosing of other parasympatholytics [anticholinergics and antimuscarinics] and spasmolytics**

Poisoning by, adverse effect of and underdosing of papaverine

✓6ᵗʰ **T44.3X Poisoning by, adverse effect of and underdosing of other parasympatholytics [anticholinergics and antimuscarinics] and spasmolytics**

✓7ᵗʰ **T44.3X1 Poisoning by other parasympatholytics [anticholinergics and antimuscarinics] and spasmolytics, accidental (unintentional)**

Poisoning by other parasympatholytics [anticholinergics and antimuscarinics] and spasmolytics NOS

✓7ᵗʰ **T44.3X2 Poisoning by other parasympatholytics [anticholinergics and antimuscarinics] and spasmolytics, intentional self-harm**

✓7ᵗʰ **T44.3X3 Poisoning by other parasympatholytics [anticholinergics and antimuscarinics] and spasmolytics, assault**

✓7ᵗʰ **T44.3X4 Poisoning by other parasympatholytics [anticholinergics and antimuscarinics] and spasmolytics, undetermined**

✓7ᵗʰ **T44.3X5 Adverse effect of other parasympatholytics [anticholinergics and antimuscarinics] and spasmolytics**

✓7ᵗʰ **T44.3X6 Underdosing of other parasympatholytics [anticholinergics and antimuscarinics] and spasmolytics**

✓5ᵗʰ **T44.4 Poisoning by, adverse effect of and underdosing of predominantly alpha-adrenoreceptor agonists**

Poisoning by, adverse effect of and underdosing of metaraminol

✓6ᵗʰ **T44.4X Poisoning by, adverse effect of and underdosing of predominantly alpha-adrenoreceptor agonists**

✓7ᵗʰ **T44.4X1 Poisoning by predominantly alpha-adrenoreceptor agonists, accidental (unintentional)**

Poisoning by predominantly alpha-adrenoreceptor agonists NOS

✓7ᵗʰ **T44.4X2 Poisoning by predominantly alpha-adrenoreceptor agonists, intentional self-harm**

✓7ᵗʰ **T44.4X3 Poisoning by predominantly alpha-adrenoreceptor agonists, assault**

✓7ᵗʰ **T44.4X4 Poisoning by predominantly alpha-adrenoreceptor agonists, undetermined**

✓7ᵗʰ **T44.4X5 Adverse effect of predominantly alpha-adrenoreceptor agonists**

✓7ᵗʰ **T44.4X6 Underdosing of predominantly alpha-adrenoreceptor agonists**

✓5ᵗʰ **T44.5 Poisoning by, adverse effect of and underdosing of predominantly beta-adrenoreceptor agonists**

EXCLUDES 1   poisoning by, adverse effect of and underdosing of beta-adrenoreceptor agonists used in asthma therapy (T48.6-)

✓6ᵗʰ **T44.5X Poisoning by, adverse effect of and underdosing of predominantly beta-adrenoreceptor agonists**

✓7ᵗʰ **T44.5X1 Poisoning by predominantly beta-adrenoreceptor agonists, accidental (unintentional)**

Poisoning by predominantly beta-adrenoreceptor agonists NOS

✓7ᵗʰ **T44.5X2 Poisoning by predominantly beta-adrenoreceptor agonists, intentional self-harm**

✓7ᵗʰ **T44.5X3 Poisoning by predominantly beta-adrenoreceptor agonists, assault**

✓7ᵗʰ **T44.5X4 Poisoning by predominantly beta-adrenoreceptor agonists, undetermined**

✓7ᵗʰ **T44.5X5 Adverse effect of predominantly beta-adrenoreceptor agonists**

✓7ᵗʰ **T44.5X6 Underdosing of predominantly beta-adrenoreceptor agonists**

✓5ᵗʰ **T44.6 Poisoning by, adverse effect of and underdosing of alpha-adrenoreceptor antagonists**

EXCLUDES 1   poisoning by, adverse effect of and underdosing of ergot alkaloids (T48.0)

✓6ᵗʰ **T44.6X Poisoning by, adverse effect of and underdosing of alpha-adrenoreceptor antagonists**

✓7ᵗʰ **T44.6X1 Poisoning by alpha-adrenoreceptor antagonists, accidental (unintentional)**

Poisoning by alpha-adrenoreceptor antagonists NOS

✓7ᵗʰ **T44.6X2 Poisoning by alpha-adrenoreceptor antagonists, intentional self-harm**

✓7ᵗʰ **T44.6X3 Poisoning by alpha-adrenoreceptor antagonists, assault**

✓7ᵗʰ **T44.6X4 Poisoning by alpha-adrenoreceptor antagonists, undetermined**

✓7ᵗʰ **T44.6X5 Adverse effect of alpha-adrenoreceptor antagonists**

✓7ᵗʰ **T44.6X6 Underdosing of alpha-adrenoreceptor antagonists**

✓5ᵗʰ **T44.7 Poisoning by, adverse effect of and underdosing of beta-adrenoreceptor antagonists**

✓6ᵗʰ **T44.7X Poisoning by, adverse effect of and underdosing of beta-adrenoreceptor antagonists**

✓7ᵗʰ **T44.7X1 Poisoning by beta-adrenoreceptor antagonists, accidental (unintentional)**

Poisoning by beta-adrenoreceptor antagonists NOS

✓7ᵗʰ **T44.7X2 Poisoning by beta-adrenoreceptor antagonists, intentional self-harm**

✓7ᵗʰ **T44.7X3 Poisoning by beta-adrenoreceptor antagonists, assault**

✓7ᵗʰ **T44.7X4 Poisoning by beta-adrenoreceptor antagonists, undetermined**

✓7ᵗʰ **T44.7X5 Adverse effect of beta-adrenoreceptor antagonists**

✓7ᵗʰ **T44.7X6 Underdosing of beta-adrenoreceptor antagonists**

✓5ᵗʰ **T44.8 Poisoning by, adverse effect of and underdosing of centrally-acting and adrenergic-neuron- blocking agents**

EXCLUDES 1   poisoning by, adverse effect of and underdosing of clonidine (T46.5)

poisoning by, adverse effect of and underdosing of guanethidine (T46.5)

✓6ᵗʰ **T44.8X Poisoning by, adverse effect of and underdosing of centrally-acting and adrenergic-neuron-blocking agents**

✓7ᵗʰ **T44.8X1 Poisoning by centrally-acting and adrenergic-neuron-blocking agents, accidental (unintentional)**

Poisoning by centrally-acting and adrenergic-neuron-blocking agents NOS

✓7ᵗʰ **T44.8X2 Poisoning by centrally-acting and adrenergic-neuron-blocking agents, intentional self-harm**

✓7ᵗʰ **T44.8X3 Poisoning by centrally-acting and adrenergic-neuron-blocking agents, assault**

✓7ᵗʰ **T44.8X4 Poisoning by centrally-acting and adrenergic-neuron-blocking agents, undetermined**

✓7ᵗʰ **T44.8X5 Adverse effect of centrally-acting and adrenergic-neuron-blocking agents**

✓7ᵗʰ **T44.8X6 Underdosing of centrally-acting and adrenergic-neuron-blocking agents**

EXCLUDES 1 Not coded here   EXCLUDES 2 Not included here   N Newborn Age: 0   P Pediatric Age: 0-17   M Maternity Age: 12-55   A Adult Age: 15-124

952   ICD-10-CM Draft (2015)

✓5ᵗʰ **T44.9 Poisoning by, adverse effect of and underdosing of other and unspecified drugs** primarily affecting the autonomic nervous system
  Poisoning by, adverse effect of and underdosing of drug stimulating both alpha and beta-adrenoreceptors

✓6ᵗʰ **T44.90 Poisoning by, adverse effect of and underdosing of** unspecified **drugs primarily affecting the autonomic nervous system**

✓7ᵗʰ **T44.901 Poisoning by unspecified drugs primarily affecting the autonomic nervous system,** accidental **(unintentional)**
  Poisoning by unspecified drugs primarily affecting the autonomic nervous system NOS

✓7ᵗʰ **T44.902 Poisoning by unspecified drugs primarily affecting the autonomic nervous system,** intentional self-harm

✓7ᵗʰ **T44.903 Poisoning by unspecified drugs primarily affecting the autonomic nervous system,** assault

✓7ᵗʰ **T44.904 Poisoning by unspecified drugs primarily affecting the autonomic nervous system,** undetermined

✓7ᵗʰ **T44.905** Adverse effect **of unspecified drugs primarily affecting the autonomic nervous system**

✓7ᵗʰ **T44.906** Underdosing **of unspecified drugs primarily affecting the autonomic nervous system**

✓6ᵗʰ **T44.99 Poisoning by, adverse effect of and underdosing of** other **drugs primarily affecting the autonomic nervous system**

✓7ᵗʰ **T44.991 Poisoning by other drug primarily affecting the autonomic nervous system,** accidental **(unintentional)**
  Poisoning by other drugs primarily affecting the autonomic nervous system NOS

✓7ᵗʰ **T44.992 Poisoning by other drug primarily affecting the autonomic nervous system,** intentional self-harm

✓7ᵗʰ **T44.993 Poisoning by other drug primarily affecting the autonomic nervous system,** assault

✓7ᵗʰ **T44.994 Poisoning by other drug primarily affecting the autonomic nervous system,** undetermined

✓7ᵗʰ **T44.995** Adverse effect **of other drug primarily affecting the autonomic nervous system**

✓7ᵗʰ **T44.996** Underdosing **of other drug primarily affecting the autonomic nervous system**

✓4ᵗʰ **T45 Poisoning by, adverse effect of and underdosing of primarily systemic and hematological agents, not elsewhere classified**

The appropriate 7th character is to be added to each code from category T45.
A initial encounter
D subsequent encounter
S sequela

✓5ᵗʰ **T45.0 Poisoning by, adverse effect of and underdosing of antiallergic and antiemetic drugs**
EXCLUDES 1 *poisoning by, adverse effect of and underdosing of phenothiazine-based neuroleptics (T43.3)*

✓6ᵗʰ **T45.0X Poisoning by, adverse effect of and underdosing of** antiallergic and antiemetic **drugs**

✓7ᵗʰ **T45.0X1 Poisoning by antiallergic and antiemetic drugs,** accidental **(unintentional)**
  Poisoning by antiallergic and antiemetic drugs NOS

✓7ᵗʰ **T45.0X2 Poisoning by antiallergic and antiemetic drugs,** intentional self-harm

✓7ᵗʰ **T45.0X3 Poisoning by antiallergic and antiemetic drugs,** assault

✓7ᵗʰ **T45.0X4 Poisoning by antiallergic and antiemetic drugs,** undetermined

✓7ᵗʰ **T45.0X5** Adverse effect **of antiallergic and antiemetic drugs**

✓7ᵗʰ **T45.0X6** Underdosing **of antiallergic and antiemetic drugs**

✓5ᵗʰ **T45.1 Poisoning by, adverse effect of and underdosing of antineoplastic and immunosuppressive drugs**
EXCLUDES 1 *poisoning by, adverse effect of and underdosing of tamoxifen (T38.6)*

✓6ᵗʰ **T45.1X Poisoning by, adverse effect of and underdosing of** antineoplastic and immunosuppressive **drugs**

✓7ᵗʰ **T45.1X1 Poisoning by antineoplastic and immunosuppressive drugs,** accidental **(unintentional)**
  Poisoning by antineoplastic and immunosuppressive drugs NOS

✓7ᵗʰ **T45.1X2 Poisoning by antineoplastic and immunosuppressive drugs,** intentional self-harm

✓7ᵗʰ **T45.1X3 Poisoning by antineoplastic and immunosuppressive drugs,** assault

✓7ᵗʰ **T45.1X4 Poisoning by antineoplastic and immunosuppressive drugs,** undetermined

✓7ᵗʰ **T45.1X5** Adverse effect **of antineoplastic and immunosuppressive drugs**

✓7ᵗʰ **T45.1X6** Underdosing **of antineoplastic and immunosuppressive drugs**

✓5ᵗʰ **T45.2 Poisoning by, adverse effect of and underdosing of vitamins**
EXCLUDES 2 *poisoning by, adverse effect of and underdosing of iron (T45.4)*
poisoning by, adverse effect of and underdosing of nicotinic acid (derivatives) (T46.7)
poisoning by, adverse effect of and underdosing of vitamin K (T45.7)

✓6ᵗʰ **T45.2X Poisoning by, adverse effect of and underdosing of** vitamins

✓7ᵗʰ **T45.2X1 Poisoning by vitamins,** accidental **(unintentional)**
  Poisoning by vitamins NOS

✓7ᵗʰ **T45.2X2 Poisoning by vitamins,** intentional self-harm

✓7ᵗʰ **T45.2X3 Poisoning by vitamins,** assault

✓7ᵗʰ **T45.2X4 Poisoning by vitamins,** undetermined

✓7ᵗʰ **T45.2X5** Adverse effect **of vitamins**

✓7ᵗʰ **T45.2X6** Underdosing **of vitamins**
EXCLUDES 1 *vitamin deficiencies (E50-E56)*

✓5ᵗʰ **T45.3 Poisoning by, adverse effect of and underdosing of enzymes**

✓6ᵗʰ **T45.3X Poisoning by, adverse effect of and underdosing of** enzymes

✓7ᵗʰ **T45.3X1 Poisoning by enzymes,** accidental **(unintentional)**
  Poisoning by enzymes NOS

✓7ᵗʰ **T45.3X2 Poisoning by enzymes,** intentional self-harm

✓7ᵗʰ **T45.3X3 Poisoning by enzymes,** assault

✓7ᵗʰ **T45.3X4 Poisoning by enzymes,** undetermined

✓7ᵗʰ **T45.3X5** Adverse effect **of enzymes**

✓7ᵗʰ **T45.3X6** Underdosing **of enzymes**

✓5ᵗʰ **T45.4 Poisoning by, adverse effect of and underdosing of iron and its compounds**

✓6ᵗʰ **T45.4X Poisoning by, adverse effect of and underdosing of** iron **and its compounds**

T45.4X1 Poisoning by iron and its compounds, accidental **(unintentional)**
  Poisoning by iron and its compounds NOS

✓7ᵗʰ **T45.4X2 Poisoning by iron and its compounds,** intentional self-harm

✓7ᵗʰ **T45.4X3 Poisoning by iron and its compounds,** assault

✓7ᵗʰ **T45.4X4 Poisoning by iron and its compounds,** undetermined

✓7ᵗʰ **T45.4X5** Adverse effect **of iron and its compounds**

✓7ᵗʰ **T45.4X6** Underdosing **of iron and its compounds**
EXCLUDES 1 *iron deficiency (E61.1)*

✓5ᵗʰ **T45.5 Poisoning by, adverse effect of and underdosing of** anticoagulants and antithrombotic **drugs**

✓6ᵗʰ **T45.51 Poisoning by, adverse effect of and underdosing of** anticoagulants

✓7ᵗʰ **T45.511 Poisoning by anticoagulants,** accidental **(unintentional)**
  Poisoning by anticoagulants NOS

√7ᵗʰ **T45.512** **Poisoning by anticoagulants,** intentional self-harm

√7ᵗʰ **T45.513** **Poisoning by anticoagulants,** assault

√7ᵗʰ **T45.514** **Poisoning by anticoagulants,** undetermined

√7ᵗʰ **T45.515** Adverse effect **of anticoagulants**
AHA: 2013, 2Q, 34

√7ᵗʰ **T45.516** Underdosing **of anticoagulants**

√6ᵗʰ **T45.52** **Poisoning by, adverse effect of and underdosing of** antithrombotic **drugs**
Poisoning by, adverse effect of and underdosing of antiplatelet drugs
EXCLUDES 2   poisoning by, adverse effect of and underdosing of aspirin (T39.01-)
poisoning by, adverse effect of and underdosing of acetylsalicylic acid (T39.01-)

√7ᵗʰ **T45.521** **Poisoning by antithrombotic drugs,** accidental (unintentional)
Poisoning by antithrombotic drug NOS

√7ᵗʰ **T45.522** **Poisoning by antithrombotic drugs,** intentional self-harm

√7ᵗʰ **T45.523** **Poisoning by antithrombotic drugs,** assault

√7ᵗʰ **T45.524** **Poisoning by antithrombotic drugs,** undetermined

√7ᵗʰ **T45.525** Adverse effect **of antithrombotic drugs**

√7ᵗʰ **T45.526** Underdosing **of antithrombotic drugs**

√5ᵗʰ **T45.6** **Poisoning by, adverse effect of and underdosing of fibrinolysis-affecting drugs**

√6ᵗʰ **T45.60** **Poisoning by, adverse effect of and underdosing of unspecified** fibrinolysis-affecting **drugs**

√7ᵗʰ **T45.601** **Poisoning by unspecified fibrinolysis-affecting drugs,** accidental (unintentional)
Poisoning by fibrinolysis-affecting drug NOS

√7ᵗʰ **T45.602** **Poisoning by unspecified fibrinolysis-affecting drugs,** intentional self-harm

√7ᵗʰ **T45.603** **Poisoning by unspecified fibrinolysis-affecting drugs,** assault

√7ᵗʰ **T45.604** **Poisoning by unspecified fibrinolysis-affecting drugs,** undetermined

√7ᵗʰ **T45.605** Adverse effect **of unspecified fibrinolysis-affecting drugs**

√7ᵗʰ **T45.606** Underdosing **of unspecified fibrinolysis-affecting drugs**

√6ᵗʰ **T45.61** **Poisoning by, adverse effect of and underdosing of** thrombolytic **drugs**

√7ᵗʰ **T45.611** **Poisoning by thrombolytic drug,** accidental (unintentional)
Poisoning by thrombolytic drug NOS

√7ᵗʰ **T45.612** **Poisoning by thrombolytic drug,** intentional self-harm

√7ᵗʰ **T45.613** **Poisoning by thrombolytic drug,** assault

√7ᵗʰ **T45.614** **Poisoning by thrombolytic drug,** undetermined

√7ᵗʰ **T45.615** Adverse effect **of thrombolytic drugs**

√7ᵗʰ **T45.616** Underdosing **of thrombolytic drugs**

√6ᵗʰ **T45.62** **Poisoning by, adverse effect of and underdosing of** hemostatic **drugs**

√7ᵗʰ **T45.621** **Poisoning by hemostatic drug,** accidental (unintentional)
Poisoning by hemostatic drug NOS

√7ᵗʰ **T45.622** **Poisoning by hemostatic drug,** intentional self-harm

√7ᵗʰ **T45.623** **Poisoning by hemostatic drug,** assault

√7ᵗʰ **T45.624** **Poisoning by hemostatic drug,** undetermined

√7ᵗʰ **T45.625** Adverse effect **of hemostatic drug**

√7ᵗʰ **T45.626** Underdosing **of hemostatic drugs**

√6ᵗʰ **T45.69** **Poisoning by, adverse effect of and underdosing of** other fibrinolysis-affecting **drugs**

√7ᵗʰ **T45.691** **Poisoning by other fibrinolysis-affecting drugs,** accidental (unintentional)
Poisoning by other fibrinolysis-affecting drug NOS

√7ᵗʰ **T45.692** **Poisoning by other fibrinolysis-affecting drugs,** intentional self-harm

√7ᵗʰ **T45.693** **Poisoning by other fibrinolysis-affecting drugs,** assault

√7ᵗʰ **T45.694** **Poisoning by other fibrinolysis-affecting drugs,** undetermined

√7ᵗʰ **T45.695** Adverse effect **of other fibrinolysis-affecting drugs**

√7ᵗʰ **T45.696** Underdosing **of other fibrinolysis-affecting drugs**

√5ᵗʰ **T45.7** **Poisoning by, adverse effect of and underdosing of anticoagulant antagonists, vitamin K and other coagulants**

√6ᵗʰ **T45.7X** **Poisoning by, adverse effect of and underdosing of** anticoagulant antagonists, vitamin K and other coagulants

√7ᵗʰ **T45.7X1** **Poisoning by anticoagulant antagonists, vitamin K and other coagulants,** accidental (unintentional)
Poisoning by anticoagulant antagonists, vitamin K and other coagulants NOS

√7ᵗʰ **T45.7X2** **Poisoning by anticoagulant antagonists, vitamin K and other coagulants,** intentional self-harm

√7ᵗʰ **T45.7X3** **Poisoning by anticoagulant antagonists, vitamin K and other coagulants,** assault

√7ᵗʰ **T45.7X4** **Poisoning by anticoagulant antagonists, vitamin K and other coagulants,** undetermined

√7ᵗʰ **T45.7X5** Adverse effect **of anticoagulant antagonists, vitamin K and other coagulants**

√7ᵗʰ **T45.7X6** Underdosing **of anticoagulant antagonist, vitamin K and other coagulants**
EXCLUDES 1   vitamin K deficiency (E56.1)

√5ᵗʰ **T45.8** **Poisoning by, adverse effect of and underdosing of other** primarily systemic and hematological agents
Poisoning by, adverse effect of and underdosing of liver preparations and other antianemic agents
Poisoning by, adverse effect of and underdosing of natural blood and blood products
Poisoning by, adverse effect of and underdosing of plasma substitute
EXCLUDES 2   poisoning by, adverse effect of and underdosing of immunoglobulin (T50.Z1)
poisoning by, adverse effect of and underdosing of iron (T45.4)
transfusion reactions (T80.-)

√6ᵗʰ **T45.8X** **Poisoning by, adverse effect of and underdosing of** other primarily systemic and hematological agents

√7ᵗʰ **T45.8X1** **Poisoning by other primarily systemic and hematological agents,** accidental (unintentional)
Poisoning by other primarily systemic and hematological agents NOS

√7ᵗʰ **T45.8X2** **Poisoning by other primarily systemic and hematological agents,** intentional self-harm

√7ᵗʰ **T45.8X3** **Poisoning by other primarily systemic and hematological agents,** assault

√7ᵗʰ **T45.8X4** **Poisoning by other primarily systemic and hematological agents,** undetermined

√7ᵗʰ **T45.8X5** Adverse effect **of other primarily systemic and hematological agents**

√7ᵗʰ **T45.8X6** Underdosing **of other primarily systemic and hematological agents**

√5ᵗʰ **T45.9** **Poisoning by, adverse effect of and underdosing of** unspecified primarily systemic and hematological agent

√x7ᵗʰ **T45.91** **Poisoning by unspecified primarily systemic and hematological agent,** accidental (unintentional)
Poisoning by primarily systemic and hematological agent NOS

√x7ᵗʰ **T45.92** **Poisoning by unspecified primarily systemic and hematological agent,** intentional self-harm

√x7ᵗʰ **T45.93** **Poisoning by unspecified primarily systemic and hematological agent,** assault

√x7ᵗʰ **T45.94** **Poisoning by unspecified primarily systemic and hematological agent,** undetermined

✓x7ᵗʰ **T45.95** Adverse effect of unspecified primarily systemic and hematological agent

✓x7ᵗʰ **T45.96** Underdosing of unspecified primarily systemic and hematological agent

✓4ᵗʰ **T46** **Poisoning by, adverse effect of and underdosing of agents primarily affecting the cardiovascular system**
> **EXCLUDES 1** *poisoning by, adverse effect of and underdosing of metaraminol (T44.4)*

> The appropriate 7th character is to be added to each code from category T46.
> A　initial encounter
> D　subsequent encounter
> S　sequela

✓5ᵗʰ **T46.0** Poisoning by, adverse effect of and underdosing of cardiac-stimulant glycosides and drugs of similar action

  ✓6ᵗʰ **T46.0X** Poisoning by, adverse effect of and underdosing of cardiac-stimulant glycosides and drugs of similar action

    ✓7ᵗʰ **T46.0X1** Poisoning by cardiac-stimulant glycosides and drugs of similar action, accidental (unintentional)
      Poisoning by cardiac-stimulant glycosides and drugs of similar action NOS

    ✓7ᵗʰ **T46.0X2** Poisoning by cardiac-stimulant glycosides and drugs of similar action, intentional self-harm

    ✓7ᵗʰ **T46.0X3** Poisoning by cardiac-stimulant glycosides and drugs of similar action, assault

    ✓7ᵗʰ **T46.0X4** Poisoning by cardiac-stimulant glycosides and drugs of similar action, undetermined

    ✓7ᵗʰ **T46.0X5** Adverse effect of cardiac-stimulant glycosides and drugs of similar action

    ✓7ᵗʰ **T46.0X6** Underdosing of cardiac-stimulant glycosides and drugs of similar action

✓5ᵗʰ **T46.1** Poisoning by, adverse effect of and underdosing of calcium-channel blockers

  ✓6ᵗʰ **T46.1X** Poisoning by, adverse effect of and underdosing of calcium-channel blockers

    ✓7ᵗʰ **T46.1X1** Poisoning by calcium-channel blockers, accidental (unintentional)
      Poisoning by calcium-channel blockers NOS

    ✓7ᵗʰ **T46.1X2** Poisoning by calcium-channel blockers, intentional self-harm

    ✓7ᵗʰ **T46.1X3** Poisoning by calcium-channel blockers, assault

    ✓7ᵗʰ **T46.1X4** Poisoning by calcium-channel blockers, undetermined

    ✓7ᵗʰ **T46.1X5** Adverse effect of calcium-channel blockers

    ✓7ᵗʰ **T46.1X6** Underdosing of calcium-channel blockers

✓5ᵗʰ **T46.2** Poisoning by, adverse effect of and underdosing of other antidysrhythmic drugs, not elsewhere classified
> **EXCLUDES 1** *poisoning by, adverse effect of and underdosing of beta-adrenoreceptor antagonists (T44.7-)*

  ✓6ᵗʰ **T46.2X** Poisoning by, adverse effect of and underdosing of other antidysrhythmic drugs

    ✓7ᵗʰ **T46.2X1** Poisoning by other antidysrhythmic drugs, accidental (unintentional)
      Poisoning by other antidysrhythmic drugs NOS

    ✓7ᵗʰ **T46.2X2** Poisoning by other antidysrhythmic drugs, intentional self-harm

    ✓7ᵗʰ **T46.2X3** Poisoning by other antidysrhythmic drugs, assault

    ✓7ᵗʰ **T46.2X4** Poisoning by other antidysrhythmic drugs, undetermined

    ✓7ᵗʰ **T46.2X5** Adverse effect of other antidysrhythmic drugs

    ✓7ᵗʰ **T46.2X6** Underdosing of other antidysrhythmic drugs

✓5ᵗʰ **T46.3** Poisoning by, adverse effect of and underdosing of coronary vasodilators
  Poisoning by, adverse effect of and underdosing of dipyridamole
> **EXCLUDES 1** *poisoning by, adverse effect of and underdosing of calcium-channel blockers (T46.1)*

  ✓6ᵗʰ **T46.3X** Poisoning by, adverse effect of and underdosing of coronary vasodilators

    ✓7ᵗʰ **T46.3X1** Poisoning by coronary vasodilators, accidental (unintentional)
      Poisoning by coronary vasodilators NOS

    ✓7ᵗʰ **T46.3X2** Poisoning by coronary vasodilators, intentional self-harm

    ✓7ᵗʰ **T46.3X3** Poisoning by coronary vasodilators, assault

    ✓7ᵗʰ **T46.3X4** Poisoning by coronary vasodilators, undetermined

    ✓7ᵗʰ **T46.3X5** Adverse effect of coronary vasodilators

    ✓7ᵗʰ **T46.3X6** Underdosing of coronary vasodilators

✓5ᵗʰ **T46.4** Poisoning by, adverse effect of and underdosing of angiotensin-converting-enzyme inhibitors

  ✓6ᵗʰ **T46.4X** Poisoning by, adverse effect of and underdosing of angiotensin-converting-enzyme inhibitors

    ✓7ᵗʰ **T46.4X1** Poisoning by angiotensin-converting-enzyme inhibitors, accidental (unintentional)
      Poisoning by angiotensin-converting-enzyme inhibitors NOS

    ✓7ᵗʰ **T46.4X2** Poisoning by angiotensin-converting-enzyme inhibitors, intentional self-harm

    ✓7ᵗʰ **T46.4X3** Poisoning by angiotensin-converting-enzyme inhibitors, assault

    ✓7ᵗʰ **T46.4X4** Poisoning by angiotensin-converting-enzyme inhibitors, undetermined

    ✓7ᵗʰ **T46.4X5** Adverse effect of angiotensin-converting-enzyme inhibitors

    ✓7ᵗʰ **T46.4X6** Underdosing of angiotensin-converting-enzyme inhibitors

✓5ᵗʰ **T46.5** Poisoning by, adverse effect of and underdosing of other antihypertensive drugs
> **EXCLUDES 2** *poisoning by, adverse effect of and underdosing of beta-adrenoreceptor antagonists (T44.7)*
> *poisoning by, adverse effect of and underdosing of calcium-channel blockers (T46.1)*
> *poisoning by, adverse effect of and underdosing of diuretics (T50.0-T50.2)*

  ✓6ᵗʰ **T46.5X** Poisoning by, adverse effect of and underdosing of other antihypertensive drugs

    ✓7ᵗʰ **T46.5X1** Poisoning by other antihypertensive drugs, accidental (unintentional)
      Poisoning by other antihypertensive drugs NOS

    ✓7ᵗʰ **T46.5X2** Poisoning by other antihypertensive drugs, intentional self-harm

    ✓7ᵗʰ **T46.5X3** Poisoning by other antihypertensive drugs, assault

    ✓7ᵗʰ **T46.5X4** Poisoning by other antihypertensive drugs, undetermined

    ✓7ᵗʰ **T46.5X5** Adverse effect of other antihypertensive drugs

    ✓7ᵗʰ **T46.5X6** Underdosing of other antihypertensive drugs

✓5ᵗʰ **T46.6** Poisoning by, adverse effect of and underdosing of antihyperlipidemic and antiarteriosclerotic drugs

  ✓6ᵗʰ **T46.6X** Poisoning by, adverse effect of and underdosing of antihyperlipidemic and antiarteriosclerotic drugs

    ✓7ᵗʰ **T46.6X1** Poisoning by antihyperlipidemic and antiarteriosclerotic drugs, accidental (unintentional)
      Poisoning by antihyperlipidemic and antiarteriosclerotic drugs NOS

    ✓7ᵗʰ **T46.6X2** Poisoning by antihyperlipidemic and antiarteriosclerotic drugs, intentional self-harm

    ✓7ᵗʰ **T46.6X3** Poisoning by antihyperlipidemic and antiarteriosclerotic drugs, assault

---

✓7th   **T46.6X4**   **Poisoning by antihyperlipidemic and antiarteriosclerotic drugs,** undetermined

✓7th   **T46.6X5**   Adverse effect **of antihyperlipidemic and antiarteriosclerotic drugs**

✓7th   **T46.6X6**   Underdosing **of antihyperlipidemic and antiarteriosclerotic drugs**

✓5th   **T46.7**   **Poisoning by, adverse effect of and underdosing of peripheral vasodilators**

     Poisoning by, adverse effect of and underdosing of nicotinic acid (derivatives)

     EXCLUDES 1   *poisoning by, adverse effect of and underdosing of papaverine (T44.3)*

✓6th   **T46.7X**   **Poisoning by, adverse effect of and underdosing of** peripheral vasodilators

    ✓7th   **T46.7X1**   **Poisoning by peripheral vasodilators,** accidental **(unintentional)**

       Poisoning by peripheral vasodilators NOS

    ✓7th   **T46.7X2**   **Poisoning by peripheral vasodilators,** intentional self-harm

    ✓7th   **T46.7X3**   **Poisoning by peripheral vasodilators,** assault

    ✓7th   **T46.7X4**   **Poisoning by peripheral vasodilators,** undetermined

    ✓7th   **T46.7X5**   Adverse effect **of peripheral vasodilators**

    ✓7th   **T46.7X6**   Underdosing **of peripheral vasodilators**

✓5th   **T46.8**   **Poisoning by, adverse effect of and underdosing of antivaricose drugs, including sclerosing agents**

✓6th   **T46.8X**   **Poisoning by, adverse effect of and underdosing of** antivaricose **drugs, including sclerosing agents**

    ✓7th   **T46.8X1**   **Poisoning by antivaricose drugs, including sclerosing agents,** accidental **(unintentional)**

       Poisoning by antivaricose drugs, including sclerosing agents NOS

    ✓7th   **T46.8X2**   **Poisoning by antivaricose drugs, including sclerosing agents,** intentional self-harm

    ✓7th   **T46.8X3**   **Poisoning by antivaricose drugs, including sclerosing agents,** assault

    ✓7th   **T46.8X4**   **Poisoning by antivaricose drugs, including sclerosing agents,** undetermined

    ✓7th   **T46.8X5**   Adverse effect **of antivaricose drugs, including sclerosing agents**

    ✓7th   **T46.8X6**   Underdosing **of antivaricose drugs, including sclerosing agents**

✓5th   **T46.9**   **Poisoning by, adverse effect of and underdosing of other and unspecified** agents primarily affecting the cardiovascular system

✓6th   **T46.90**   **Poisoning by, adverse effect of and underdosing of** unspecified **agents primarily affecting the cardiovascular system**

    ✓7th   **T46.901**   **Poisoning by unspecified agents primarily affecting the cardiovascular system,** accidental **(unintentional)**

    ✓7th   **T46.902**   **Poisoning by unspecified agents primarily affecting the cardiovascular system,** intentional self-harm

    ✓7th   **T46.903**   **Poisoning by unspecified agents primarily affecting the cardiovascular system,** assault

    ✓7th   **T46.904**   **Poisoning by unspecified agents primarily affecting the cardiovascular system,** undetermined

    ✓7th   **T46.905**   Adverse effect **of unspecified agents primarily affecting the cardiovascular system**

    ✓7th   **T46.906**   Underdosing **of unspecified agents primarily affecting the cardiovascular system**

✓6th   **T46.99**   **Poisoning by, adverse effect of and underdosing of** other **agents primarily affecting the cardiovascular system**

    ✓7th   **T46.991**   **Poisoning by other agents primarily affecting the cardiovascular system,** accidental **(unintentional)**

    ✓7th   **T46.992**   **Poisoning by other agents primarily affecting the cardiovascular system,** intentional self-harm

    ✓7th   **T46.993**   **Poisoning by other agents primarily affecting the cardiovascular system,** assault

    ✓7th   **T46.994**   **Poisoning by other agents primarily affecting the cardiovascular system,** undetermined

    ✓7th   **T46.995**   Adverse effect **of other agents primarily affecting the cardiovascular system**

    ✓7th   **T46.996**   Underdosing **of other agents primarily affecting the cardiovascular system**

✓4th   **T47**   **Poisoning by, adverse effect of and underdosing of agents primarily affecting the gastrointestinal system**

    The appropriate 7th character is to be added to each code from category T47.
    A   initial encounter
    D   subsequent encounter
    S   sequela

✓5th   **T47.0**   **Poisoning by, adverse effect of and underdosing of histamine H2-receptor blockers**

✓6th   **T47.0X**   **Poisoning by, adverse effect of and underdosing of** histamine H2-receptor blockers

    ✓7th   **T47.0X1**   **Poisoning by histamine H2-receptor blockers,** accidental **(unintentional)**

       Poisoning by histamine H2-receptor blockers NOS

    ✓7th   **T47.0X2**   **Poisoning by histamine H2-receptor blockers,** intentional self-harm

    ✓7th   **T47.0X3**   **Poisoning by histamine H2-receptor blockers,** assault

    ✓7th   **T47.0X4**   **Poisoning by histamine H2-receptor blockers,** undetermined

    ✓7th   **T47.0X5**   Adverse effect **of histamine H2-receptor blockers**

    ✓7th   **T47.0X6**   Underdosing **of histamine H2-receptor blockers**

✓5th   **T47.1**   **Poisoning by, adverse effect of and underdosing of other antacids and anti-gastric-secretion drugs**

✓6th   **T47.1X**   **Poisoning by, adverse effect of and underdosing of** other antacids and anti-gastric-secretion **drugs**

    ✓7th   **T47.1X1**   **Poisoning by other antacids and anti-gastric-secretion drugs,** accidental **(unintentional)**

       Poisoning by other antacids and anti-gastric-secretion drugs NOS

    ✓7th   **T47.1X2**   **Poisoning by other antacids and anti-gastric-secretion drugs,** intentional self-harm

    ✓7th   **T47.1X3**   **Poisoning by other antacids and anti-gastric-secretion drugs,** assault

    ✓7th   **T47.1X4**   **Poisoning by other antacids and anti-gastric-secretion drugs,** undetermined

    ✓7th   **T47.1X5**   Adverse effect **of other antacids and anti-gastric-secretion drugs**

    ✓7th   **T47.1X6**   Underdosing **of other antacids and anti-gastric-secretion drugs**

✓5th   **T47.2**   **Poisoning by, adverse effect of and underdosing of stimulant laxatives**

✓6th   **T47.2X**   **Poisoning by, adverse effect of and underdosing of** stimulant laxatives

    ✓7th   **T47.2X1**   **Poisoning by stimulant laxatives,** accidental **(unintentional)**

       Poisoning by stimulant laxatives NOS

    ✓7th   **T47.2X2**   **Poisoning by stimulant laxatives,** intentional self-harm

    ✓7th   **T47.2X3**   **Poisoning by stimulant laxatives,** assault

    ✓7th   **T47.2X4**   **Poisoning by stimulant laxatives,** undetermined

    ✓7th   **T47.2X5**   Adverse effect **of stimulant laxatives**

    ✓7th   **T47.2X6**   Underdosing **of stimulant laxatives**

EXCLUDES 1 Not coded here   EXCLUDES 2 Not included here   N Newborn Age: 0   P Pediatric Age: 0-17   M Maternity Age: 12-55   A Adult Age: 15-124

956   ICD-10-CM Draft (2015)

✓5ᵗʰ T47.3 Poisoning by, adverse effect of and underdosing of saline and osmotic laxatives

     ✓6ᵗʰ T47.3X Poisoning by and adverse effect of saline and osmotic laxatives

         ✓7ᵗʰ T47.3X1 Poisoning by saline and osmotic laxatives, accidental **(unintentional)**
            Poisoning by saline and osmotic laxatives NOS

         ✓7ᵗʰ T47.3X2 Poisoning by saline and osmotic laxatives, intentional self-harm

         ✓7ᵗʰ T47.3X3 Poisoning by saline and osmotic laxatives, assault

         ✓7ᵗʰ T47.3X4 Poisoning by saline and osmotic laxatives, undetermined

         ✓7ᵗʰ T47.3X5 Adverse effect **of saline and osmotic laxatives**

         ✓7ᵗʰ T47.3X6 Underdosing **of saline and osmotic laxatives**

✓5ᵗʰ T47.4 Poisoning by, adverse effect of and underdosing of other laxatives

     ✓6ᵗʰ T47.4X Poisoning by, adverse effect of and underdosing of other laxatives

         ✓7ᵗʰ T47.4X1 Poisoning by other laxatives, accidental **(unintentional)**
            Poisoning by other laxatives NOS

         ✓7ᵗʰ T47.4X2 Poisoning by other laxatives, intentional self-harm

         ✓7ᵗʰ T47.4X3 Poisoning by other laxatives, assault

         ✓7ᵗʰ T47.4X4 Poisoning by other laxatives, undetermined

         ✓7ᵗʰ T47.4X5 Adverse effect **of other laxatives**

         ✓7ᵗʰ T47.4X6 Underdosing **of other laxatives**

✓5ᵗʰ T47.5 Poisoning by, adverse effect of and underdosing of digestants

     ✓6ᵗʰ T47.5X Poisoning by, adverse effect of and underdosing of digestants

         ✓7ᵗʰ T47.5X1 Poisoning by digestants, accidental **(unintentional)**
            Poisoning by digestants NOS

         ✓7ᵗʰ T47.5X2 Poisoning by digestants, intentional self-harm

         ✓7ᵗʰ T47.5X3 Poisoning by digestants, assault

         ✓7ᵗʰ T47.5X4 Poisoning by digestants, undetermined

         ✓7ᵗʰ T47.5X5 Adverse effect **of digestants**

         ✓7ᵗʰ T47.5X6 Underdosing **of digestants**

✓5ᵗʰ T47.6 Poisoning by, adverse effect of and underdosing of antidiarrheal drugs

         EXCLUDES 2 *poisoning by, adverse effect of and underdosing of systemic antibiotics and other anti-infectives (T36-T37)*

     ✓6ᵗʰ T47.6X Poisoning by, adverse effect of and underdosing of antidiarrheal **drugs**

         ✓7ᵗʰ T47.6X1 Poisoning by antidiarrheal drugs, accidental **(unintentional)**
            Poisoning by antidiarrheal drugs NOS

         ✓7ᵗʰ T47.6X2 Poisoning by antidiarrheal drugs, intentional self-harm

         ✓7ᵗʰ T47.6X3 Poisoning by antidiarrheal drugs, assault

         ✓7ᵗʰ T47.6X4 Poisoning by antidiarrheal drugs, undetermined

         ✓7ᵗʰ T47.6X5 Adverse effect **of antidiarrheal drugs**

         ✓7ᵗʰ T47.6X6 Underdosing **of antidiarrheal drugs**

✓5ᵗʰ T47.7 Poisoning by, adverse effect of and underdosing of emetics

     ✓6ᵗʰ T47.7X Poisoning by, adverse effect of and underdosing of emetics

         ✓7ᵗʰ T47.7X1 Poisoning by emetics, accidental **(unintentional)**
            Poisoning by emetics NOS

         ✓7ᵗʰ T47.7X2 Poisoning by emetics, intentional self-harm

         ✓7ᵗʰ T47.7X3 Poisoning by emetics, assault

         ✓7ᵗʰ T47.7X4 Poisoning by emetics, undetermined

         ✓7ᵗʰ T47.7X5 Adverse effect **of emetics**

         ✓7ᵗʰ T47.7X6 Underdosing **of emetics**

✓5ᵗʰ T47.8 Poisoning by, adverse effect of and underdosing of other agents primarily affecting gastrointestinal system

     ✓6ᵗʰ T47.8X Poisoning by, adverse effect of and underdosing of other **agents primarily affecting gastrointestinal system**

         ✓7ᵗʰ T47.8X1 Poisoning by other agents primarily affecting gastrointestinal system, accidental **(unintentional)**
            Poisoning by other agents primarily affecting gastrointestinal system NOS

         ✓7ᵗʰ T47.8X2 Poisoning by other agents primarily affecting gastrointestinal system, intentional self-harm

         ✓7ᵗʰ T47.8X3 Poisoning by other agents primarily affecting gastrointestinal system, assault

         ✓7ᵗʰ T47.8X4 Poisoning by other agents primarily affecting gastrointestinal system, undetermined

         ✓7ᵗʰ T47.8X5 Adverse effect **of other agents primarily affecting gastrointestinal system**

         ✓7ᵗʰ T47.8X6 Underdosing **of other agents primarily affecting gastrointestinal system**

✓5ᵗʰ T47.9 Poisoning by, adverse effect of and underdosing of unspecified **agents primarily affecting the gastrointestinal system**

     ✓×7ᵗʰ T47.91 Poisoning by unspecified agents primarily affecting the gastrointestinal system, accidental **(unintentional)**
         Poisoning by agents primarily affecting the gastrointestinal system NOS

     ✓×7ᵗʰ T47.92 Poisoning by unspecified agents primarily affecting the gastrointestinal system, intentional self-harm

     ✓×7ᵗʰ T47.93 Poisoning by unspecified agents primarily affecting the gastrointestinal system, assault

     ✓×7ᵗʰ T47.94 Poisoning by unspecified agents primarily affecting the gastrointestinal system, undetermined

     ✓×7ᵗʰ T47.95 Adverse effect **of unspecified agents primarily affecting the gastrointestinal system**

     ✓×7ᵗʰ T47.96 Underdosing **of unspecified agents primarily affecting the gastrointestinal system**

✓4ᵗʰ T48 Poisoning by, adverse effect of and underdosing of agents primarily acting on smooth and skeletal muscles and the respiratory system

     The appropriate 7th character is to be added to each code from category T48.
     A   initial encounter
     D   subsequent encounter
     S   sequela

✓5ᵗʰ T48.0 Poisoning by, adverse effect of and underdosing of oxytocic drugs

     EXCLUDES 1 *poisoning by, adverse effect of and underdosing of estrogens, progestogens and antagonists (T38.4-T38.6)*

     ✓6ᵗʰ T48.0X Poisoning by, adverse effect of and underdosing of oxytocic **drugs**

         ✓7ᵗʰ T48.0X1 Poisoning by oxytocic drugs, accidental **(unintentional)**
            Poisoning by oxytocic drugs NOS

         ✓7ᵗʰ T48.0X2 Poisoning by oxytocic drugs, intentional self-harm

         ✓7ᵗʰ T48.0X3 Poisoning by oxytocic drugs, assault

         ✓7ᵗʰ T48.0X4 Poisoning by oxytocic drugs, undetermined

         ✓7ᵗʰ T48.0X5 Adverse effect **of oxytocic drugs**

         ✓7ᵗʰ T48.0X6 Underdosing **of oxytocic drugs**

✓5ᵗʰ T48.1 Poisoning by, adverse effect of and underdosing of skeletal muscle relaxants [neuromuscular blocking agents]

     ✓6ᵗʰ T48.1X Poisoning by, adverse effect of and underdosing of skeletal muscle relaxants **[neuromuscular blocking agents]**

         ✓7ᵗʰ T48.1X1 Poisoning by skeletal muscle relaxants [neuromuscular blocking agents], accidental **(unintentional)**
            Poisoning by skeletal muscle relaxants [neuromuscular blocking agents] NOS

✓ Additional Character Required   ✓×7ᵗʰ Xtension Alert   Unspecified Dx   Other Specified Dx   Manifestation   ►◄ Revised Text   ● New Code   ▲ Revised Code Title

✓7ᵗʰ **T48.1X2 Poisoning by skeletal muscle relaxants [neuromuscular blocking agents], intentional self-harm**

✓7ᵗʰ **T48.1X3 Poisoning by skeletal muscle relaxants [neuromuscular blocking agents], assault**

✓7ᵗʰ **T48.1X4 Poisoning by skeletal muscle relaxants [neuromuscular blocking agents], undetermined**

✓7ᵗʰ **T48.1X5 Adverse effect of skeletal muscle relaxants [neuromuscular blocking agents]**

✓7ᵗʰ **T48.1X6 Underdosing of skeletal muscle relaxants [neuromuscular blocking agents]**

✓5ᵗʰ **T48.2 Poisoning by, adverse effect of and underdosing of other and unspecified drugs acting on muscles**

  ✓6ᵗʰ **T48.20 Poisoning by, adverse effect of and underdosing of unspecified drugs acting on muscles**

    ✓7ᵗʰ **T48.201 Poisoning by unspecified drugs acting on muscles, accidental (unintentional)**
Poisoning by unspecified drugs acting on muscles NOS

    ✓7ᵗʰ **T48.202 Poisoning by unspecified drugs acting on muscles, intentional self-harm**

    ✓7ᵗʰ **T48.203 Poisoning by unspecified drugs acting on muscles, assault**

    ✓7ᵗʰ **T48.204 Poisoning by unspecified drugs acting on muscles, undetermined**

    ✓7ᵗʰ **T48.205 Adverse effect of unspecified drugs acting on muscles**

    ✓7ᵗʰ **T48.206 Underdosing of unspecified drugs acting on muscles**

  ✓6ᵗʰ **T48.29 Poisoning by, adverse effect of and underdosing of other drugs acting on muscles**

    ✓7ᵗʰ **T48.291 Poisoning by other drugs acting on muscles, accidental (unintentional)**
Poisoning by other drugs acting on muscles NOS

    ✓7ᵗʰ **T48.292 Poisoning by other drugs acting on muscles, intentional self-harm**

    ✓7ᵗʰ **T48.293 Poisoning by other drugs acting on muscles, assault**

    ✓7ᵗʰ **T48.294 Poisoning by other drugs acting on muscles, undetermined**

    ✓7ᵗʰ **T48.295 Adverse effect of other drugs acting on muscles**

    ✓7ᵗʰ **T48.296 Underdosing of other drugs acting on muscles**

✓5ᵗʰ **T48.3 Poisoning by, adverse effect of and underdosing of antitussives**

  ✓6ᵗʰ **T48.3X Poisoning by, adverse effect of and underdosing of antitussives**

    ✓7ᵗʰ **T48.3X1 Poisoning by antitussives, accidental (unintentional)**
Poisoning by antitussives NOS

    ✓7ᵗʰ **T48.3X2 Poisoning by antitussives, intentional self-harm**

    ✓7ᵗʰ **T48.3X3 Poisoning by antitussives, assault**

    ✓7ᵗʰ **T48.3X4 Poisoning by antitussives, undetermined**

    ✓7ᵗʰ **T48.3X5 Adverse effect of antitussives**

    ✓7ᵗʰ **T48.3X6 Underdosing of antitussives**

✓5ᵗʰ **T48.4 Poisoning by, adverse effect of and underdosing of expectorants**

  ✓6ᵗʰ **T48.4X Poisoning by, adverse effect of and underdosing of expectorants**

    ✓7ᵗʰ **T48.4X1 Poisoning by expectorants, accidental (unintentional)**
Poisoning by expectorants NOS

    ✓7ᵗʰ **T48.4X2 Poisoning by expectorants, intentional self-harm**

    ✓7ᵗʰ **T48.4X3 Poisoning by expectorants, assault**

    ✓7ᵗʰ **T48.4X4 Poisoning by expectorants, undetermined**

    ✓7ᵗʰ **T48.4X5 Adverse effect of expectorants**

    ✓7ᵗʰ **T48.4X6 Underdosing of expectorants**

✓5ᵗʰ **T48.5 Poisoning by, adverse effect of and underdosing of other anti-common-cold drugs**
Poisoning by, adverse effect of and underdosing of decongestants

  EXCLUDES 2   poisoning by, adverse effect of and underdosing of antipyretics, NEC (T39.9-)
      poisoning by, adverse effect of and underdosing of non-steroidal antiinflammatory drugs (T39.3-)
      poisoning by, adverse effect of and underdosing of salicylates (T39.0-)

  ✓6ᵗʰ **T48.5X Poisoning by, adverse effect of and underdosing of other anti-common-cold drugs**

    ✓7ᵗʰ **T48.5X1 Poisoning by other anti-common-cold drugs, accidental (unintentional)**
Poisoning by other anti-common-cold drugs NOS

    ✓7ᵗʰ **T48.5X2 Poisoning by other anti-common-cold drugs, intentional self-harm**

    ✓7ᵗʰ **T48.5X3 Poisoning by other anti-common-cold drugs, assault**

    ✓7ᵗʰ **T48.5X4 Poisoning by other anti-common-cold drugs, undetermined**

    ✓7ᵗʰ **T48.5X5 Adverse effect of other anti-common-cold drugs**

    ✓7ᵗʰ **T48.5X6 Underdosing of other anti-common-cold drugs**

✓5ᵗʰ **T48.6 Poisoning by, adverse effect of and underdosing of antiasthmatics, not elsewhere classified**
Poisoning by, adverse effect of and underdosing of beta-adrenoreceptor agonists used in asthma therapy

  EXCLUDES 1   poisoning by, adverse effect of and underdosing of anterior pituitary [adenohypophyseal] hormones (T38.8)
      poisoning by, adverse effect of and underdosing of beta-adrenoreceptor agonists not used in asthma therapy (T44.5)

  ✓6ᵗʰ **T48.6X Poisoning by, adverse effect of and underdosing of antiasthmatics**

    ✓7ᵗʰ **T48.6X1 Poisoning by antiasthmatics, accidental (unintentional)**
Poisoning by antiasthmatics NOS

    ✓7ᵗʰ **T48.6X2 Poisoning by antiasthmatics, intentional self-harm**

    ✓7ᵗʰ **T48.6X3 Poisoning by antiasthmatics, assault**

    ✓7ᵗʰ **T48.6X4 Poisoning by antiasthmatics, undetermined**

    ✓7ᵗʰ **T48.6X5 Adverse effect of antiasthmatics**

    ✓7ᵗʰ **T48.6X6 Underdosing of antiasthmatics**

✓5ᵗʰ **T48.9 Poisoning by, adverse effect of and underdosing of other and unspecified agents primarily acting on the respiratory system**

  ✓6ᵗʰ **T48.90 Poisoning by, adverse effect of and underdosing of unspecified agents primarily acting on the respiratory system**

    ✓7ᵗʰ **T48.901 Poisoning by unspecified agents primarily acting on the respiratory system, accidental (unintentional)**

    ✓7ᵗʰ **T48.902 Poisoning by unspecified agents primarily acting on the respiratory system, intentional self-harm**

    ✓7ᵗʰ **T48.903 Poisoning by unspecified agents primarily acting on the respiratory system, assault**

    ✓7ᵗʰ **T48.904 Poisoning by unspecified agents primarily acting on the respiratory system, undetermined**

    ✓7ᵗʰ **T48.905 Adverse effect of unspecified agents primarily acting on the respiratory system**

    ✓7ᵗʰ **T48.906 Underdosing of unspecified agents primarily acting on the respiratory system**

  ✓6ᵗʰ **T48.99 Poisoning by, adverse effect of and underdosing of other agents primarily acting on the respiratory system**

    ✓7ᵗʰ **T48.991 Poisoning by other agents primarily acting on the respiratory system, accidental (unintentional)**

    ✓7ᵗʰ **T48.992 Poisoning by other agents primarily acting on the respiratory system, intentional self-harm**

EXCLUDES 1 Not coded here   *EXCLUDES 2* Not included here   N Newborn Age: 0   P Pediatric Age: 0-17   M Maternity Age: 12-55   A Adult Age: 15-124

958   ICD-10-CM Draft (2015)

√7th **T48.993** **Poisoning by other agents primarily acting on the respiratory system, assault**

√7th **T48.994** **Poisoning by other agents primarily acting on the respiratory system, undetermined**

√7th **T48.995** Adverse effect **of other agents primarily acting on the respiratory system**

√7th **T48.996** Underdosing **of other agents primarily acting on the respiratory system**

√4th **T49** **Poisoning by, adverse effect of and underdosing of topical agents primarily affecting skin and mucous membrane and by ophthalmological, otorhinolaryngological and dental drugs**

Poisoning by, adverse effect of and underdosing of glucocorticoids, topically used

The appropriate 7th character is to be added to each code from category T49.
A   initial encounter
D   subsequent encounter
S   sequela

√5th **T49.0** **Poisoning by, adverse effect of and underdosing of local antifungal, anti-infective and anti-inflammatory drugs**

√6th **T49.0X** **Poisoning by, adverse effect of and underdosing of** local antifungal, anti-infective and anti-inflammatory **drugs**

√7th **T49.0X1** **Poisoning by local antifungal, anti-infective and anti-inflammatory drugs,** accidental **(unintentional)**
Poisoning by local antifungal, anti-infective and anti-inflammatory drugs NOS

√7th **T49.0X2** **Poisoning by local antifungal, anti-infective and anti-inflammatory drugs,** intentional self-harm

√7th **T49.0X3** **Poisoning by local antifungal, anti-infective and anti-inflammatory drugs,** assault

√7th **T49.0X4** **Poisoning by local antifungal, anti-infective and anti-inflammatory drugs,** undetermined

√7th **T49.0X5** Adverse effect **of local antifungal, anti-infective and anti-inflammatory drugs**

√7th **T49.0X6** Underdosing **of local antifungal, anti-infective and anti-inflammatory drugs**

√5th **T49.1** **Poisoning by, adverse effect of and underdosing of antipruritics**

√6th **T49.1X** **Poisoning by, adverse effect of and underdosing of** antipruritics

√7th **T49.1X1** **Poisoning by antipruritics,** accidental **(unintentional)**
Poisoning by antipruritics NOS

√7th **T49.1X2** **Poisoning by antipruritics,** intentional self-harm

√7th **T49.1X3** **Poisoning by antipruritics,** assault

√7th **T49.1X4** **Poisoning by antipruritics,** undetermined

√7th **T49.1X5** Adverse effect **of antipruritics**

√7th **T49.1X6** Underdosing **of antipruritics**

√5th **T49.2** **Poisoning by, adverse effect of and underdosing of local astringents and local detergents**

√6th **T49.2X** **Poisoning by, adverse effect of and underdosing of** local astringents and local detergents

√7th **T49.2X1** **Poisoning by local astringents and local detergents,** accidental **(unintentional)**
Poisoning by local astringents and local detergents NOS

√7th **T49.2X2** **Poisoning by local astringents and local detergents,** intentional self-harm

√7th **T49.2X3** **Poisoning by local astringents and local detergents,** assault

√7th **T49.2X4** **Poisoning by local astringents and local detergents,** undetermined

√7th **T49.2X5** Adverse effect **of local astringents and local detergents**

√7th **T49.2X6** Underdosing **of local astringents and local detergents**

√5th **T49.3** **Poisoning by, adverse effect of and underdosing of emollients, demulcents and protectants**

√6th **T49.3X** **Poisoning by, adverse effect of and underdosing of** emollients, demulcents and protectants

√7th **T49.3X1** **Poisoning by emollients, demulcents and protectants,** accidental **(unintentional)**
Poisoning by emollients, demulcents and protectants NOS

√7th **T49.3X2** **Poisoning by emollients, demulcents and protectants,** intentional self-harm

√7th **T49.3X3** **Poisoning by emollients, demulcents and protectants,** assault

√7th **T49.3X4** **Poisoning by emollients, demulcents and protectants,** undetermined

√7th **T49.3X5** Adverse effect **of emollients, demulcents and protectants**

√7th **T49.3X6** Underdosing **of emollients, demulcents and protectants**

√5th **T49.4** **Poisoning by, adverse effect of and underdosing of keratolytics, keratoplastics, and other hair treatment drugs and preparations**

√6th **T49.4X** **Poisoning by, adverse effect of and underdosing of** keratolytics, keratoplastics, and other hair treatment drugs and preparations

√7th **T49.4X1** **Poisoning by keratolytics, keratoplastics, and other hair treatment drugs and preparations,** accidental **(unintentional)**
Poisoning by keratolytics, keratoplastics, and other hair treatment drugs and preparations NOS

√7th **T49.4X2** **Poisoning by keratolytics, keratoplastics, and other hair treatment drugs and preparations,** intentional self-harm

√7th **T49.4X3** **Poisoning by keratolytics, keratoplastics, and other hair treatment drugs and preparations,** assault

√7th **T49.4X4** **Poisoning by keratolytics, keratoplastics, and other hair treatment drugs and preparations,** undetermined

√7th **T49.4X5** Adverse effect **of keratolytics, keratoplastics, and other hair treatment drugs and preparations**

√7th **T49.4X6** Underdosing **of keratolytics, keratoplastics, and other hair treatment drugs and preparations**

√5th **T49.5** **Poisoning by, adverse effect of and underdosing of ophthalmological drugs and preparations**

√6th **T49.5X** **Poisoning by, adverse effect of and underdosing of** ophthalmological **drugs and preparations**

√7th **T49.5X1** **Poisoning by ophthalmological drugs and preparations,** accidental **(unintentional)**
Poisoning by ophthalmological drugs and preparations NOS

√7th **T49.5X2** **Poisoning by ophthalmological drugs and preparations,** intentional self-harm

√7th **T49.5X3** **Poisoning by ophthalmological drugs and preparations,** assault

√7th **T49.5X4** **Poisoning by ophthalmological drugs and preparations,** undetermined

√7th **T49.5X5** Adverse effect **of ophthalmological drugs and preparations**

√7th **T49.5X6** Underdosing **of ophthalmological drugs and preparations**

√5th **T49.6** **Poisoning by, adverse effect of and underdosing of otorhinolaryngological drugs and preparations**

√6th **T49.6X** **Poisoning by, adverse effect of and underdosing of** otorhinolaryngological **drugs and preparations**

√7th **T49.6X1** **Poisoning by otorhinolaryngological drugs and preparations,** accidental **(unintentional)**
Poisoning by otorhinolaryngological drugs and preparations NOS

√7th **T49.6X2** **Poisoning by otorhinolaryngological drugs and preparations,** intentional self-harm

√7th **T49.6X3** **Poisoning by otorhinolaryngological drugs and preparations,** assault

T49.6X4 Poisoning by otorhinolaryngological drugs and preparations, undetermined

T49.6X5 Adverse effect of otorhinolaryngological drugs and preparations

T49.6X6 Underdosing of otorhinolaryngological drugs and preparations

T49.7 Poisoning by, adverse effect of and underdosing of dental drugs, topically applied

   T49.7X Poisoning by, adverse effect of and underdosing of dental drugs, topically applied

     T49.7X1 Poisoning by dental drugs, topically applied, accidental (unintentional)
       Poisoning by dental drugs, topically applied NOS

     T49.7X2 Poisoning by dental drugs, topically applied, intentional self-harm

     T49.7X3 Poisoning by dental drugs, topically applied, assault

     T49.7X4 Poisoning by dental drugs, topically applied, undetermined

     T49.7X5 Adverse effect of dental drugs, topically applied

     T49.7X6 Underdosing of dental drugs, topically applied

T49.8 Poisoning by, adverse effect of and underdosing of other topical agents
   Poisoning by, adverse effect of and underdosing of spermicides

   T49.8X Poisoning by, adverse effect of and underdosing of other topical agents

     T49.8X1 Poisoning by other topical agents, accidental (unintentional)
       Poisoning by other topical agents NOS

     T49.8X2 Poisoning by other topical agents, intentional self-harm

     T49.8X3 Poisoning by other topical agents, assault
     T49.8X4 Poisoning by other topical agents, undetermined

     T49.8X5 Adverse effect of other topical agents

     T49.8X6 Underdosing of other topical agents

T49.9 Poisoning by, adverse effect of and underdosing of unspecified topical agent

   T49.91 Poisoning by unspecified topical agent, accidental (unintentional)

   T49.92 Poisoning by unspecified topical agent, intentional self-harm

   T49.93 Poisoning by unspecified topical agent, assault

   T49.94 Poisoning by unspecified topical agent, undetermined

   T49.95 Adverse effect of unspecified topical agent

   T49.96 Underdosing of unspecified topical agent

T50 Poisoning by, adverse effect of and underdosing of diuretics and other and unspecified drugs, medicaments and biological substances

> The appropriate 7th character is to be added to each code from category T50.
> A   initial encounter
> D   subsequent encounter
> S   sequela

T50.0 Poisoning by, adverse effect of and underdosing of mineralocorticoids and their antagonists

   T50.0X Poisoning by, adverse effect of and underdosing of mineralocorticoids and their antagonists

     T50.0X1 Poisoning by mineralocorticoids and their antagonists, accidental (unintentional)
       Poisoning by mineralocorticoids and their antagonists NOS

     T50.0X2 Poisoning by mineralocorticoids and their antagonists, intentional self-harm

     T50.0X3 Poisoning by mineralocorticoids and their antagonists, assault

     T50.0X4 Poisoning by mineralocorticoids and their antagonists, undetermined

     T50.0X5 Adverse effect of mineralocorticoids and their antagonists

T50.0X6 Underdosing of mineralocorticoids and their antagonists

T50.1 Poisoning by, adverse effect of and underdosing of loop [high-ceiling] diuretics

   T50.1X Poisoning by, adverse effect of and underdosing of loop [high-ceiling] diuretics

     T50.1X1 Poisoning by loop [high-ceiling] diuretics, accidental (unintentional)
       Poisoning by loop [high-ceiling] diuretics NOS

     T50.1X2 Poisoning by loop [high-ceiling] diuretics, intentional self-harm

     T50.1X3 Poisoning by loop [high-ceiling] diuretics, assault

     T50.1X4 Poisoning by loop [high-ceiling] diuretics, undetermined

     T50.1X5 Adverse effect of loop [high-ceiling] diuretics

     T50.1X6 Underdosing of loop [high-ceiling] diuretics

T50.2 Poisoning by, adverse effect of and underdosing of carbonic-anhydrase inhibitors, benzothiadiazides and other diuretics
   Poisoning by, adverse effect of and underdosing of acetazolamide

   T50.2X Poisoning by, adverse effect of and underdosing of carbonic-anhydrase inhibitors, benzothiadiazides and other diuretics

     T50.2X1 Poisoning by carbonic-anhydrase inhibitors, benzothiadiazides and other diuretics, accidental (unintentional)
       Poisoning by carbonic-anhydrase inhibitors, benzothiadiazides and other diuretics NOS

     T50.2X2 Poisoning by carbonic-anhydrase inhibitors, benzothiadiazides and other diuretics, intentional self-harm

     T50.2X3 Poisoning by carbonic-anhydrase inhibitors, benzothiadiazides and other diuretics, assault

     T50.2X4 Poisoning by carbonic-anhydrase inhibitors, benzothiadiazides and other diuretics, undetermined

     T50.2X5 Adverse effect of carbonic-anhydrase inhibitors, benzothiadiazides and other diuretics

     T50.2X6 Underdosing of carbonic-anhydrase inhibitors, benzothiadiazides and other diuretics

T50.3 Poisoning by, adverse effect of and underdosing of electrolytic, caloric and water-balance agents
   Poisoning by, adverse effect of and underdosing of oral rehydration salts

   T50.3X Poisoning by, adverse effect of and underdosing of electrolytic, caloric and water-balance agents

     T50.3X1 Poisoning by electrolytic, caloric and water-balance agents, accidental (unintentional)
       Poisoning by electrolytic, caloric and water-balance agents NOS

     T50.3X2 Poisoning by electrolytic, caloric and water-balance agents, intentional self-harm

     T50.3X3 Poisoning by electrolytic, caloric and water-balance agents, assault

     T50.3X4 Poisoning by electrolytic, caloric and water-balance agents, undetermined

     T50.3X5 Adverse effect of electrolytic, caloric and water-balance agents

     T50.3X6 Underdosing of electrolytic, caloric and water-balance agents

EXCLUDES 1 Not coded here   **EXCLUDES 2** Not included here   **N** Newborn Age: 0   **P** Pediatric Age: 0-17   **M** Maternity Age: 12-55   **A** Adult Age: 15-124

960   ICD-10-CM Draft (2015)

✓5th **T50.4** Poisoning by, adverse effect of and underdosing of drugs affecting uric acid metabolism

  ✓6th **T50.4X** Poisoning by, adverse effect of and underdosing of drugs affecting uric acid metabolism

    ✓7th **T50.4X1** Poisoning by drugs affecting uric acid metabolism, accidental (unintentional)
      Poisoning by drugs affecting uric acid metabolism NOS

    ✓7th **T50.4X2** Poisoning by drugs affecting uric acid metabolism, intentional self-harm

    ✓7th **T50.4X3** Poisoning by drugs affecting uric acid metabolism, assault

    ✓7th **T50.4X4** Poisoning by drugs affecting uric acid metabolism, undetermined

    ✓7th **T50.4X5** Adverse effect of drugs affecting uric acid metabolism

    ✓7th **T50.4X6** Underdosing of drugs affecting uric acid metabolism

✓5th **T50.5** Poisoning by, adverse effect of and underdosing of appetite depressants

  ✓6th **T50.5X** Poisoning by, adverse effect of and underdosing of appetite depressants

    ✓7th **T50.5X1** Poisoning by appetite depressants, accidental (unintentional)
      Poisoning by appetite depressants NOS

    ✓7th **T50.5X2** Poisoning by appetite depressants, intentional self-harm

    ✓7th **T50.5X3** Poisoning by appetite depressants, assault

    ✓7th **T50.5X4** Poisoning by appetite depressants, undetermined

    ✓7th **T50.5X5** Adverse effect of appetite depressants

    ✓7th **T50.5X6** Underdosing of appetite depressants

✓5th **T50.6** Poisoning by, adverse effect of and underdosing of antidotes and chelating agents
  Poisoning by, adverse effect of and underdosing of alcohol deterrents

  ✓6th **T50.6X** Poisoning by, adverse effect of and underdosing of antidotes and chelating agents

    ✓7th **T50.6X1** Poisoning by antidotes and chelating agents, accidental (unintentional)
      Poisoning by antidotes and chelating agents NOS

    ✓7th **T50.6X2** Poisoning by antidotes and chelating agents, intentional self-harm

    ✓7th **T50.6X3** Poisoning by antidotes and chelating agents, assault

    ✓7th **T50.6X4** Poisoning by antidotes and chelating agents, undetermined

    ✓7th **T50.6X5** Adverse effect of antidotes and chelating agents

    ✓7th **T50.6X6** Underdosing of antidotes and chelating agents

✓5th **T50.7** Poisoning by, adverse effect of and underdosing of analeptics and opioid receptor antagonists

  ✓6th **T50.7X** Poisoning by, adverse effect of and underdosing of analeptics and opioid receptor antagonists

    ✓7th **T50.7X1** Poisoning by analeptics and opioid receptor antagonists, accidental (unintentional)
      Poisoning by analeptics and opioid receptor antagonists NOS

    ✓7th **T50.7X2** Poisoning by analeptics and opioid receptor antagonists, intentional self-harm

    ✓7th **T50.7X3** Poisoning by analeptics and opioid receptor antagonists, assault

    ✓7th **T50.7X4** Poisoning by analeptics and opioid receptor antagonists, undetermined

    ✓7th **T50.7X5** Adverse effect of analeptics and opioid receptor antagonists

    ✓7th **T50.7X6** Underdosing of analeptics and opioid receptor antagonists

✓5th **T50.8** Poisoning by, adverse effect of and underdosing of diagnostic agents

  ✓6th **T50.8X** Poisoning by, adverse effect of and underdosing of diagnostic agents

    ✓7th **T50.8X1** Poisoning by diagnostic agents, accidental (unintentional)
      Poisoning by diagnostic agents NOS

    ✓7th **T50.8X2** Poisoning by diagnostic agents, intentional self-harm

    ✓7th **T50.8X3** Poisoning by diagnostic agents, assault

    ✓7th **T50.8X4** Poisoning by diagnostic agents, undetermined

    ✓7th **T50.8X5** Adverse effect of diagnostic agents

    ✓7th **T50.8X6** Underdosing of diagnostic agents

✓5th **T50.A** Poisoning by, adverse effect of and underdosing of bacterial vaccines

  ✓6th **T50.A1** Poisoning by, adverse effect of and underdosing of pertussis vaccine, including combinations with a pertussis component

    ✓7th **T50.A11** Poisoning by pertussis vaccine, including combinations with a pertussis component, accidental (unintentional)

    ✓7th **T50.A12** Poisoning by pertussis vaccine, including combinations with a pertussis component, intentional self-harm

    ✓7th **T50.A13** Poisoning by pertussis vaccine, including combinations with a pertussis component, assault

    ✓7th **T50.A14** Poisoning by pertussis vaccine, including combinations with a pertussis component, undetermined

    ✓7th **T50.A15** Adverse effect of pertussis vaccine, including combinations with a pertussis component

    ✓7th **T50.A16** Underdosing of pertussis vaccine, including combinations with a pertussis component

  ✓6th **T50.A2** Poisoning by, adverse effect of and underdosing of mixed bacterial vaccines without a pertussis component

    ✓7th **T50.A21** Poisoning by mixed bacterial vaccines without a pertussis component, accidental (unintentional)

    ✓7th **T50.A22** Poisoning by mixed bacterial vaccines without a pertussis component, intentional self-harm

    ✓7th **T50.A23** Poisoning by mixed bacterial vaccines without a pertussis component, assault

    ✓7th **T50.A24** Poisoning by mixed bacterial vaccines without a pertussis component, undetermined

    ✓7th **T50.A25** Adverse effect of mixed bacterial vaccines without a pertussis component

    ✓7th **T50.A26** Underdosing of mixed bacterial vaccines without a pertussis component

  ✓6th **T50.A9** Poisoning by, adverse effect of and underdosing of other bacterial vaccines

    ✓7th **T50.A91** Poisoning by other bacterial vaccines, accidental (unintentional)

    ✓7th **T50.A92** Poisoning by other bacterial vaccines, intentional self-harm

    ✓7th **T50.A93** Poisoning by other bacterial vaccines, assault

    ✓7th **T50.A94** Poisoning by other bacterial vaccines, undetermined

    ✓7th **T50.A95** Adverse effect of other bacterial vaccines

    ✓7th **T50.A96** Underdosing of other bacterial vaccines

✓5th **T50.B** Poisoning by, adverse effect of and underdosing of viral vaccines

  ✓6th **T50.B1** Poisoning by, adverse effect of and underdosing of smallpox vaccines

    ✓7th **T50.B11** Poisoning by smallpox vaccines, accidental (unintentional)

    ✓7th **T50.B12** Poisoning by smallpox vaccines, intentional self-harm

    ✓7th **T50.B13** Poisoning by smallpox vaccines, assault

✓ Additional Character Required   ✓x7th Xtension Alert   Unspecified Dx   Other Specified Dx   Manifestation   ►◄ Revised Text   ● New Code   ▲ Revised Code Title

ICD-10-CM Draft (2015)   **961**

✓7th **T50.B14** **Poisoning by smallpox vaccines, undetermined**

✓7th **T50.B15** Adverse effect of smallpox vaccines

✓7th **T50.B16** Underdosing of smallpox vaccines

✓6th **T50.B9** **Poisoning by, adverse effect of and underdosing of** other viral vaccines

     ✓7th **T50.B91** **Poisoning by other viral vaccines, accidental (unintentional)**

     ✓7th **T50.B92** **Poisoning by other viral vaccines, intentional self-harm**

     ✓7th **T50.B93** **Poisoning by other viral vaccines, assault**

     ✓7th **T50.B94** **Poisoning by other viral vaccines, undetermined**

     ✓7th **T50.B95** Adverse effect of other viral vaccines

     ✓7th **T50.B96** Underdosing of other viral vaccines

✓5th **T50.Z** **Poisoning by, adverse effect of and underdosing of** other vaccines and biological substances

   ✓6th **T50.Z1** **Poisoning by, adverse effect of and underdosing of** immunoglobulin

     ✓7th **T50.Z11** **Poisoning by immunoglobulin, accidental (unintentional)**

     ✓7th **T50.Z12** **Poisoning by immunoglobulin, intentional self-harm**

     ✓7th **T50.Z13** **Poisoning by immunoglobulin, assault**

     ✓7th **T50.Z14** **Poisoning by immunoglobulin, undetermined**

     ✓7th **T50.Z15** Adverse effect of immunoglobulin

     ✓7th **T50.Z16** Underdosing of immunoglobulin

   ✓6th **T50.Z9** **Poisoning by, adverse effect of and underdosing of** other vaccines and biological substances

     ✓7th **T50.Z91** **Poisoning by other vaccines and biological substances, accidental (unintentional)**

     ✓7th **T50.Z92** **Poisoning by other vaccines and biological substances, intentional self-harm**

     ✓7th **T50.Z93** **Poisoning by other vaccines and biological substances, assault**

     ✓7th **T50.Z94** **Poisoning by other vaccines and biological substances, undetermined**

     ✓7th **T50.Z95** Adverse effect of other vaccines and biological substances

     ✓7th **T50.Z96** Underdosing of other vaccines and biological substances

✓5th **T50.9** **Poisoning by, adverse effect of and underdosing of** other and unspecified drugs, medicaments and biological substances

   ✓6th **T50.90** **Poisoning by, adverse effect of and underdosing of** unspecified drugs, medicaments and biological substances

     ✓7th **T50.901** **Poisoning by unspecified drugs, medicaments and biological substances, accidental (unintentional)**

     ✓7th **T50.902** **Poisoning by unspecified drugs, medicaments and biological substances, intentional self-harm**

     ✓7th **T50.903** **Poisoning by unspecified drugs, medicaments and biological substances, assault**

     ✓7th **T50.904** **Poisoning by unspecified drugs, medicaments and biological substances, undetermined**

     ✓7th **T50.905** Adverse effect of unspecified drugs, medicaments and biological substances

     ✓7th **T50.906** Underdosing of unspecified drugs, medicaments and biological substances

   ✓6th **T50.99** **Poisoning by, adverse effect of and underdosing of** other drugs, medicaments and biological substances

     ✓7th **T50.991** **Poisoning by other drugs, medicaments and biological substances, accidental (unintentional)**

     ✓7th **T50.992** **Poisoning by other drugs, medicaments and biological substances, intentional self-harm**

     ✓7th **T50.993** **Poisoning by other drugs, medicaments and biological substances, assault**

     ✓7th **T50.994** **Poisoning by other drugs, medicaments and biological substances, undetermined**

     ✓7th **T50.995** Adverse effect of other drugs, medicaments and biological substances

     ✓7th **T50.996** Underdosing of other drugs, medicaments and biological substances

Toxic effects of substances chiefly nonmedicinal as to source (T51-T65)

NOTE   When no intent is indicated code to accidental. Undetermined intent is only for use when there is specific documentation in the record that the intent of the toxic effect cannot be determined.

Use additional code(s) for all associated manifestations of toxic effect, such as:
    personal history of foreign body fully removed (Z87.821)
    respiratory conditions due to external agents (J60-J70)
    to identify any retained foreign body, if applicable (Z18.-)

EXCLUDES 1   contact with and (suspected) exposure to toxic substances (Z77.-)

✓4th **T51** **Toxic effect of alcohol**

> The appropriate 7th character is to be added to each code from category T51.
> A   initial encounter
> D   subsequent encounter
> S   sequela

   ✓5th **T51.0** **Toxic effect of ethanol**
     Toxic effect of ethyl alcohol

     EXCLUDES 2   acute alcohol intoxication or 'hangover' effects (F10.129, F10.229, F10.929)
       drunkenness (F10.129, F10.229, F10.929)
       pathological alcohol intoxication (F10.129, F10.229, F10.929)

    ✓6th **T51.0X** **Toxic effect of ethanol**

     ✓7th **T51.0X1** **Toxic effect of ethanol, accidental (unintentional)**
       Toxic effect of ethanol NOS

     ✓7th **T51.0X2** **Toxic effect of ethanol, intentional self-harm**

     ✓7th **T51.0X3** **Toxic effect of ethanol, assault**

     ✓7th **T51.0X4** **Toxic effect of ethanol, undetermined**

   ✓5th **T51.1** **Toxic effect of methanol**
     Toxic effect of methyl alcohol

    ✓6th **T51.1X** **Toxic effect of methanol**

     ✓7th **T51.1X1** **Toxic effect of methanol, accidental (unintentional)**
       Toxic effect of methanol NOS

     ✓7th **T51.1X2** **Toxic effect of methanol, intentional self-harm**

     ✓7th **T51.1X3** **Toxic effect of methanol, assault**

     ✓7th **T51.1X4** **Toxic effect of methanol, undetermined**

   ✓5th **T51.2** **Toxic effect of 2-Propanol**
     Toxic effect of isopropyl alcohol

    ✓6th **T51.2X** **Toxic effect of 2-Propanol**

     ✓7th **T51.2X1** **Toxic effect of 2-Propanol, accidental (unintentional)**
       Toxic effect of 2-Propanol NOS

     ✓7th **T51.2X2** **Toxic effect of 2-Propanol, intentional self-harm**

     ✓7th **T51.2X3** **Toxic effect of 2-Propanol, assault**

     ✓7th **T51.2X4** **Toxic effect of 2-Propanol, undetermined**

   ✓5th **T51.3** **Toxic effect of fusel oil**
     Toxic effect of amyl alcohol
     Toxic effect of butyl [1-butanol] alcohol
     Toxic effect of propyl [1-propanol] alcohol

    ✓6th **T51.3X** **Toxic effect of fusel oil**

     ✓7th **T51.3X1** **Toxic effect of fusel oil, accidental (unintentional)**
       Toxic effect of fusel oil NOS

     ✓7th **T51.3X2** **Toxic effect of fusel oil, intentional self-harm**

     ✓7th **T51.3X3** **Toxic effect of fusel oil, assault**

     ✓7th **T51.3X4** **Toxic effect of fusel oil, undetermined**

   ✓5th **T51.8** **Toxic effect of other alcohols**

    ✓6th **T51.8X** **Toxic effect of other alcohols**

     ✓7th **T51.8X1** **Toxic effect of other alcohols, accidental (unintentional)**
       Toxic effect of other alcohols NOS

EXCLUDES 1 Not coded here   **EXCLUDES 2** Not included here   **N** Newborn Age: 0   **P** Pediatric Age: 0-17   **M** Maternity Age: 12-55   **A** Adult Age: 15-124

962   ICD-10-CM Draft (2015)

☑7ᵗʰ **T51.8X2** **Toxic effect of other alcohols, intentional self-harm**

☑7ᵗʰ **T51.8X3** **Toxic effect of other alcohols, assault**

☑7ᵗʰ **T51.8X4** **Toxic effect of other alcohols, undetermined**

☑5ᵗʰ **T51.9** **Toxic effect of unspecified alcohol**

✓ₓ7ᵗʰ **T51.91** **Toxic effect of unspecified alcohol, accidental (unintentional)**

✓ₓ7ᵗʰ **T51.92** **Toxic effect of unspecified alcohol, intentional self-harm**

✓ₓ7ᵗʰ **T51.93** **Toxic effect of unspecified alcohol, assault**

✓ₓ7ᵗʰ **T51.94** **Toxic effect of unspecified alcohol, undetermined**

☑4ᵗʰ **T52** **Toxic effect of organic solvents**

> EXCLUDES 1   *halogen derivatives of aliphatic and aromatic hydrocarbons (T53.-)*

> The appropriate 7th character is to be added to each code from category T52.
> A   initial encounter
> D   subsequent encounter
> S   sequela

☑5ᵗʰ **T52.0** **Toxic effects of petroleum products**
Toxic effects of ether petroleum
Toxic effects of gasoline [petrol]
Toxic effects of kerosene [paraffin oil]
Toxic effects of naphtha petroleum
Toxic effects of paraffin wax
Toxic effects of spirit petroleum

☑6ᵗʰ **T52.0X** **Toxic effects of petroleum products**

☑7ᵗʰ **T52.0X1** **Toxic effect of petroleum products, accidental (unintentional)**
Toxic effects of petroleum products NOS

☑7ᵗʰ **T52.0X2** **Toxic effect of petroleum products, intentional self-harm**

☑7ᵗʰ **T52.0X3** **Toxic effect of petroleum products, assault**

☑7ᵗʰ **T52.0X4** **Toxic effect of petroleum products, undetermined**

☑5ᵗʰ **T52.1** **Toxic effects of benzene**

> EXCLUDES 1   *homologues of benzene (T52.2)*
> *nitroderivatives and aminoderivatives of benzene and its homologues (T65.3)*

☑6ᵗʰ **T52.1X** **Toxic effects of benzene**

☑7ᵗʰ **T52.1X1** **Toxic effect of benzene, accidental (unintentional)**
Toxic effects of benzene NOS

☑7ᵗʰ **T52.1X2** **Toxic effect of benzene, intentional self-harm**

☑7ᵗʰ **T52.1X3** **Toxic effect of benzene, assault**

☑7ᵗʰ **T52.1X4** **Toxic effect of benzene, undetermined**

☑5ᵗʰ **T52.2** **Toxic effects of homologues of benzene**
Toxic effects of toluene [methylbenzene]
Toxic effects of xylene [dimethylbenzene]

☑6ᵗʰ **T52.2X** **Toxic effects of homologues of benzene**

☑7ᵗʰ **T52.2X1** **Toxic effect of homologues of benzene, accidental (unintentional)**
Toxic effects of homologues of benzene NOS

☑7ᵗʰ **T52.2X2** **Toxic effect of homologues of benzene, intentional self-harm**

☑7ᵗʰ **T52.2X3** **Toxic effect of homologues of benzene, assault**

☑7ᵗʰ **T52.2X4** **Toxic effect of homologues of benzene, undetermined**

☑5ᵗʰ **T52.3** **Toxic effects of glycols**

☑6ᵗʰ **T52.3X** **Toxic effects of glycols**

☑7ᵗʰ **T52.3X1** **Toxic effect of glycols, accidental (unintentional)**
Toxic effects of glycols NOS

☑7ᵗʰ **T52.3X2** **Toxic effect of glycols, intentional self-harm**

☑7ᵗʰ **T52.3X3** **Toxic effect of glycols, assault**

☑7ᵗʰ **T52.3X4** **Toxic effect of glycols, undetermined**

☑5ᵗʰ **T52.4** **Toxic effects of ketones**

☑6ᵗʰ **T52.4X** **Toxic effects of ketones**

☑7ᵗʰ **T52.4X1** **Toxic effect of ketones, accidental (unintentional)**
Toxic effects of ketones NOS

☑7ᵗʰ **T52.4X2** **Toxic effect of ketones, intentional self-harm**

☑7ᵗʰ **T52.4X3** **Toxic effect of ketones, assault**

☑7ᵗʰ **T52.4X4** **Toxic effect of ketones, undetermined**

☑5ᵗʰ **T52.8** **Toxic effects of other organic solvents**

☑6ᵗʰ **T52.8X** **Toxic effects of other organic solvents**

☑7ᵗʰ **T52.8X1** **Toxic effect of other organic solvents, accidental (unintentional)**
Toxic effects of other organic solvents NOS

☑7ᵗʰ **T52.8X2** **Toxic effect of other organic solvents, intentional self-harm**

☑7ᵗʰ **T52.8X3** **Toxic effect of other organic solvents, assault**

☑7ᵗʰ **T52.8X4** **Toxic effect of other organic solvents, undetermined**

☑5ᵗʰ **T52.9** **Toxic effects of unspecified organic solvent**

✓ₓ7ᵗʰ **T52.91** **Toxic effect of unspecified organic solvent, accidental (unintentional)**

✓ₓ7ᵗʰ **T52.92** **Toxic effect of unspecified organic solvent, intentional self-harm**

✓ₓ7ᵗʰ **T52.93** **Toxic effect of unspecified organic solvent, assault**

✓ₓ7ᵗʰ **T52.94** **Toxic effect of unspecified organic solvent, undetermined**

☑4ᵗʰ **T53** **Toxic effect of halogen derivatives of aliphatic and aromatic hydrocarbons**

> The appropriate 7th character is to be added to each code from category T53.
> A   initial encounter
> D   subsequent encounter
> S   sequela

☑5ᵗʰ **T53.0** **Toxic effects of carbon tetrachloride**
Toxic effects of tetrachloromethane

☑6ᵗʰ **T53.0X** **Toxic effects of carbon tetrachloride**

☑7ᵗʰ **T53.0X1** **Toxic effect of carbon tetrachloride, accidental (unintentional)**
Toxic effects of carbon tetrachloride NOS

☑7ᵗʰ **T53.0X2** **Toxic effect of carbon tetrachloride, intentional self-harm**

☑7ᵗʰ **T53.0X3** **Toxic effect of carbon tetrachloride, assault**

☑7ᵗʰ **T53.0X4** **Toxic effect of carbon tetrachloride, undetermined**

☑5ᵗʰ **T53.1** **Toxic effects of chloroform**
Toxic effects of trichloromethane

☑6ᵗʰ **T53.1X** **Toxic effects of chloroform**

☑7ᵗʰ **T53.1X1** **Toxic effect of chloroform, accidental (unintentional)**
Toxic effects of chloroform NOS

☑7ᵗʰ **T53.1X2** **Toxic effect of chloroform, intentional self-harm**

☑7ᵗʰ **T53.1X3** **Toxic effect of chloroform, assault**

☑7ᵗʰ **T53.1X4** **Toxic effect of chloroform, undetermined**

☑5ᵗʰ **T53.2** **Toxic effects of trichloroethylene**
Toxic effects of trichloroethene

☑6ᵗʰ **T53.2X** **Toxic effects of trichloroethylene**

☑7ᵗʰ **T53.2X1** **Toxic effect of trichloroethylene, accidental (unintentional)**
Toxic effects of trichloroethylene NOS

☑7ᵗʰ **T53.2X2** **Toxic effect of trichloroethylene, intentional self-harm**

☑7ᵗʰ **T53.2X3** **Toxic effect of trichloroethylene, assault**

☑7ᵗʰ **T53.2X4** **Toxic effect of trichloroethylene, undetermined**

☑ Additional Character Required   ✓ₓ7ᵗʰ *Xtension Alert*   Unspecified Dx   Other Specified Dx   Manifestation   ►◄ Revised Text   ● New Code   ▲ Revised Code Title

ICD-10-CM Draft (2015)   **963**

√5ᵗʰ **T53.3** **Toxic effects of tetrachloroethylene**
Toxic effects of perchloroethylene
Toxic effect of tetrachloroethene

√6ᵗʰ **T53.3X** **Toxic effects of** tetrachloroethylene

√7ᵗʰ **T53.3X1** **Toxic effect of tetrachloroethylene, accidental (unintentional)**
Toxic effects of tetrachloroethylene NOS

√7ᵗʰ **T53.3X2** **Toxic effect of tetrachloroethylene, intentional self-harm**

√7ᵗʰ **T53.3X3** **Toxic effect of tetrachloroethylene, assault**

√7ᵗʰ **T53.3X4** **Toxic effect of tetrachloroethylene, undetermined**

√5ᵗʰ **T53.4** **Toxic effects of dichloromethane**
Toxic effects of methylene chloride

√6ᵗʰ **T53.4X** **Toxic effects of** dichloromethane

√7ᵗʰ **T53.4X1** **Toxic effect of dichloromethane, accidental (unintentional)**
Toxic effects of dichloromethane NOS

√7ᵗʰ **T53.4X2** **Toxic effect of dichloromethane, intentional self-harm**

√7ᵗʰ **T53.4X3** **Toxic effect of dichloromethane, assault**

√7ᵗʰ **T53.4X4** **Toxic effect of dichloromethane, undetermined**

√5ᵗʰ **T53.5** **Toxic effects of chlorofluorocarbons**

√6ᵗʰ **T53.5X** **Toxic effects of** chlorofluorocarbons

√7ᵗʰ **T53.5X1** **Toxic effect of chlorofluorocarbons, accidental (unintentional)**
Toxic effects of chlorofluorocarbons NOS

√7ᵗʰ **T53.5X2** **Toxic effect of chlorofluorocarbons, intentional self-harm**

√7ᵗʰ **T53.5X3** **Toxic effect of chlorofluorocarbons, assault**

√7ᵗʰ **T53.5X4** **Toxic effect of chlorofluorocarbons, undetermined**

√5ᵗʰ **T53.6** **Toxic effects of other halogen derivatives of aliphatic hydrocarbons**

√6ᵗʰ **T53.6X** **Toxic effects of other** halogen derivatives of aliphatic hydrocarbons

√7ᵗʰ **T53.6X1** **Toxic effect of other halogen derivatives of aliphatic hydrocarbons, accidental (unintentional)**
Toxic effects of other halogen derivatives of aliphatic hydrocarbons NOS

√7ᵗʰ **T53.6X2** **Toxic effect of other halogen derivatives of aliphatic hydrocarbons, intentional self-harm**

√7ᵗʰ **T53.6X3** **Toxic effect of other halogen derivatives of aliphatic hydrocarbons, assault**

√7ᵗʰ **T53.6X4** **Toxic effect of other halogen derivatives of aliphatic hydrocarbons, undetermined**

√5ᵗʰ **T53.7** **Toxic effects of other halogen derivatives of aromatic hydrocarbons**

√6ᵗʰ **T53.7X** **Toxic effects of other** halogen derivatives of aromatic hydrocarbons

√7ᵗʰ **T53.7X1** **Toxic effect of other halogen derivatives of aromatic hydrocarbons, accidental (unintentional)**
Toxic effects of other halogen derivatives of aromatic hydrocarbons NOS

√7ᵗʰ **T53.7X2** **Toxic effect of other halogen derivatives of aromatic hydrocarbons, intentional self-harm**

√7ᵗʰ **T53.7X3** **Toxic effect of other halogen derivatives of aromatic hydrocarbons, assault**

√7ᵗʰ **T53.7X4** **Toxic effect of other halogen derivatives of aromatic hydrocarbons, undetermined**

√5ᵗʰ **T53.9** **Toxic effects of** unspecified halogen derivatives of aliphatic and aromatic hydrocarbons

√x7ᵗʰ **T53.91** **Toxic effect of unspecified halogen derivatives of aliphatic and aromatic hydrocarbons, accidental (unintentional)**

√x7ᵗʰ **T53.92** **Toxic effect of unspecified halogen derivatives of aliphatic and aromatic hydrocarbons, intentional self-harm**

√x7ᵗʰ **T53.93** **Toxic effect of unspecified halogen derivatives of aliphatic and aromatic hydrocarbons, assault**

√x7ᵗʰ **T53.94** **Toxic effect of unspecified halogen derivatives of aliphatic and aromatic hydrocarbons, undetermined**

√4ᵗʰ **T54** **Toxic effect of corrosive substances**

> The appropriate 7th character is to be added to each code from category T54.
> A   initial encounter
> D   subsequent encounter
> S   sequela

√5ᵗʰ **T54.0** **Toxic effects of phenol and phenol homologues**

√6ᵗʰ **T54.0X** **Toxic effects of** phenol and phenol homologues

√7ᵗʰ **T54.0X1** **Toxic effect of phenol and phenol homologues, accidental (unintentional)**
Toxic effects of phenol and phenol homologues NOS

√7ᵗʰ **T54.0X2** **Toxic effect of phenol and phenol homologues, intentional self-harm**

√7ᵗʰ **T54.0X3** **Toxic effect of phenol and phenol homologues, assault**

√7ᵗʰ **T54.0X4** **Toxic effect of phenol and phenol homologues, undetermined**

√5ᵗʰ **T54.1** **Toxic effects of other corrosive organic compounds**

√6ᵗʰ **T54.1X** **Toxic effects of** other corrosive organic compounds

√7ᵗʰ **T54.1X1** **Toxic effect of other corrosive organic compounds, accidental (unintentional)**
Toxic effects of other corrosive organic compounds NOS

√7ᵗʰ **T54.1X2** **Toxic effect of other corrosive organic compounds, intentional self-harm**

√7ᵗʰ **T54.1X3** **Toxic effect of other corrosive organic compounds, assault**

√7ᵗʰ **T54.1X4** **Toxic effect of other corrosive organic compounds, undetermined**

√5ᵗʰ **T54.2** **Toxic effects of corrosive acids and acid-like substances**
Toxic effects of hydrochloric acid
Toxic effects of sulfuric acid

√6ᵗʰ **T54.2X** **Toxic effects of corrosive** acids and acid-like substances

√7ᵗʰ **T54.2X1** **Toxic effect of corrosive acids and acid-like substances, accidental (unintentional)**
Toxic effects of corrosive acids and acid-like substances NOS

√7ᵗʰ **T54.2X2** **Toxic effect of corrosive acids and acid-like substances, intentional self-harm**

√7ᵗʰ **T54.2X3** **Toxic effect of corrosive acids and acid-like substances, assault**

√7ᵗʰ **T54.2X4** **Toxic effect of corrosive acids and acid-like substances, undetermined**

√5ᵗʰ **T54.3** **Toxic effects of corrosive alkalis and alkali-like substances**
Toxic effects of potassium hydroxide
Toxic effects of sodium hydroxide

√6ᵗʰ **T54.3X** **Toxic effects of corrosive** alkalis and alkali-like substances

√7ᵗʰ **T54.3X1** **Toxic effect of corrosive alkalis and alkali-like substances, accidental (unintentional)**
Toxic effects of corrosive alkalis and alkali-like substances NOS

√7ᵗʰ **T54.3X2** **Toxic effect of corrosive alkalis and alkali-like substances, intentional self-harm**

√7ᵗʰ **T54.3X3** **Toxic effect of corrosive alkalis and alkali-like substances, assault**

√7ᵗʰ **T54.3X4** **Toxic effect of corrosive alkalis and alkali-like substances, undetermined**

√5ᵗʰ **T54.9** **Toxic effects of** unspecified corrosive substance

√x7ᵗʰ **T54.91** **Toxic effect of unspecified corrosive substance, accidental (unintentional)**

√x7ᵗʰ **T54.92** **Toxic effect of unspecified corrosive substance, intentional self-harm**

√x7ᵗʰ **T54.93** **Toxic effect of unspecified corrosive substance, assault**

√x7ᵗʰ **T54.94** **Toxic effect of unspecified corrosive substance, undetermined**

EXCLUDES 1 Not coded here   **EXCLUDES 2** Not included here   **N** Newborn Age: 0   **P** Pediatric Age: 0-17   **M** Maternity Age: 12-55   **A** Adult Age: 15-124

964   ICD-10-CM Draft (2015)

√4th **T55   Toxic effect of soaps and detergents**

> The appropriate 7th character is to be added to each code from category T55.
> A   initial encounter
> D   subsequent encounter
> S   sequela

√5th   **T55.0   Toxic effect of soaps**

√6th   **T55.0X   Toxic effect of soaps**

√7th   **T55.0X1   Toxic effect of soaps, accidental (unintentional)**
                    Toxic effect of soaps NOS

√7th   **T55.0X2   Toxic effect of soaps, intentional self-harm**

√7th   **T55.0X3   Toxic effect of soaps, assault**

√7th   **T55.0X4   Toxic effect of soaps, undetermined**

√5th   **T55.1   Toxic effect of detergents**

√6th   **T55.1X   Toxic effect of detergents**

√7th   **T55.1X1   Toxic effect of detergents, accidental (unintentional)**
                    Toxic effect of detergents NOS

√7th   **T55.1X2   Toxic effect of detergents, intentional self-harm**

√7th   **T55.1X3   Toxic effect of detergents, assault**

√7th   **T55.1X4   Toxic effect of detergents, undetermined**

√4th **T56   Toxic effect of metals**

> INCLUDES   toxic effects of fumes and vapors of metals
> toxic effects of metals from all sources, except medicinal substances
> Use additional code to identify any retained metal foreign body, if applicable (Z18.0-, T18.1-)
> EXCLUDES 1   arsenic and its compounds (T57.0)
> manganese and its compounds (T57.2)

> The appropriate 7th character is to be added to each code from category T56.
> A   initial encounter
> D   subsequent encounter
> S   sequela

√5th   **T56.0   Toxic effects of lead and its compounds**

√6th   **T56.0X   Toxic effects of lead and its compounds**

√7th   **T56.0X1   Toxic effect of lead and its compounds, accidental (unintentional)**
                    Toxic effects of lead and its compounds NOS

√7th   **T56.0X2   Toxic effect of lead and its compounds, intentional self-harm**

√7th   **T56.0X3   Toxic effect of lead and its compounds, assault**

√7th   **T56.0X4   Toxic effect of lead and its compounds, undetermined**

√5th   **T56.1   Toxic effects of mercury and its compounds**

√6th   **T56.1X   Toxic effects of mercury and its compounds**

√7th   **T56.1X1   Toxic effect of mercury and its compounds, accidental (unintentional)**
                    Toxic effects of mercury and its compounds NOS

√7th   **T56.1X2   Toxic effect of mercury and its compounds, intentional self-harm**

√7th   **T56.1X3   Toxic effect of mercury and its compounds, assault**

√7th   **T56.1X4   Toxic effect of mercury and its compounds, undetermined**

√5th   **T56.2   Toxic effects of chromium and its compounds**

√6th   **T56.2X   Toxic effects of chromium and its compounds**

√7th   **T56.2X1   Toxic effect of chromium and its compounds, accidental (unintentional)**
                    Toxic effects of chromium and its compounds NOS

√7th   **T56.2X2   Toxic effect of chromium and its compounds, intentional self-harm**

√7th   **T56.2X3   Toxic effect of chromium and its compounds, assault**

√7th   **T56.2X4   Toxic effect of chromium and its compounds, undetermined**

√5th   **T56.3   Toxic effects of cadmium and its compounds**

√6th   **T56.3X   Toxic effects of cadmium and its compounds**

√7th   **T56.3X1   Toxic effect of cadmium and its compounds, accidental (unintentional)**
                    Toxic effects of cadmium and its compounds NOS

√7th   **T56.3X2   Toxic effect of cadmium and its compounds, intentional self-harm**

√7th   **T56.3X3   Toxic effect of cadmium and its compounds, assault**

√7th   **T56.3X4   Toxic effect of cadmium and its compounds, undetermined**

√5th   **T56.4   Toxic effects of copper and its compounds**

√6th   **T56.4X   Toxic effects of copper and its compounds**

√7th   **T56.4X1   Toxic effect of copper and its compounds, accidental (unintentional)**
                    Toxic effects of copper and its compounds NOS

√7th   **T56.4X2   Toxic effect of copper and its compounds, intentional self-harm**

√7th   **T56.4X3   Toxic effect of copper and its compounds, assault**

√7th   **T56.4X4   Toxic effect of copper and its compounds, undetermined**

√5th   **T56.5   Toxic effects of zinc and its compounds**

√6th   **T56.5X   Toxic effects of zinc and its compounds**

√7th   **T56.5X1   Toxic effect of zinc and its compounds, accidental (unintentional)**
                    Toxic effects of zinc and its compounds NOS

√7th   **T56.5X2   Toxic effect of zinc and its compounds, intentional self-harm**

√7th   **T56.5X3   Toxic effect of zinc and its compounds, assault**

√7th   **T56.5X4   Toxic effect of zinc and its compounds, undetermined**

√5th   **T56.6   Toxic effects of tin and its compounds**

√6th   **T56.6X   Toxic effects of tin and its compounds**

√7th   **T56.6X1   Toxic effect of tin and its compounds, accidental (unintentional)**
                    Toxic effects of tin and its compounds NOS

√7th   **T56.6X2   Toxic effect of tin and its compounds, intentional self-harm**

√7th   **T56.6X3   Toxic effect of tin and its compounds, assault**

√7th   **T56.6X4   Toxic effect of tin and its compounds, undetermined**

√5th   **T56.7   Toxic effects of beryllium and its compounds**

√6th   **T56.7X   Toxic effects of beryllium and its compounds**

√7th   **T56.7X1   Toxic effect of beryllium and its compounds, accidental (unintentional)**
                    Toxic effects of beryllium and its compounds NOS

√7th   **T56.7X2   Toxic effect of beryllium and its compounds, intentional self-harm**

√7th   **T56.7X3   Toxic effect of beryllium and its compounds, assault**

√7th   **T56.7X4   Toxic effect of beryllium and its compounds, undetermined**

√5th   **T56.8   Toxic effects of other metals**

√6th   **T56.81   Toxic effect of thallium**

√7th   **T56.811   Toxic effect of thallium, accidental (unintentional)**
                    Toxic effect of thallium NOS

√7th   **T56.812   Toxic effect of thallium, intentional self-harm**

√7th   **T56.813   Toxic effect of thallium, assault**

√7th   **T56.814   Toxic effect of thallium, undetermined**

√6th   **T56.89   Toxic effects of other metals**

√7th   **T56.891   Toxic effect of other metals, accidental (unintentional)**
                    Toxic effects of other metals NOS

√7th   **T56.892   Toxic effect of other metals, intentional self-harm**

√7th   **T56.893   Toxic effect of other metals, assault**

T56.894 **Toxic effect of other metals, undetermined**

✓5ᵗʰ **T56.9** **Toxic effects of unspecified metal**

    ✓ₓ7ᵗʰ **T56.91** **Toxic effect of unspecified metal, accidental (unintentional)**

    ✓ₓ7ᵗʰ **T56.92** **Toxic effect of unspecified metal, intentional self-harm**

    ✓ₓ7ᵗʰ **T56.93** **Toxic effect of unspecified metal, assault**

    ✓ₓ7ᵗʰ **T56.94** **Toxic effect of unspecified metal, undetermined**

✓4ᵗʰ **T57** **Toxic effect of other inorganic substances**

> The appropriate 7th character is to be added to each code from category T57.
> A   initial encounter
> D   subsequent encounter
> S   sequela

✓5ᵗʰ **T57.0** **Toxic effect of arsenic and its compounds**

    ✓6ᵗʰ **T57.0X** **Toxic effect of arsenic and its compounds**

       ✓7ᵗʰ **T57.0X1** **Toxic effect of arsenic and its compounds, accidental (unintentional)**
          Toxic effect of arsenic and its compounds NOS

       ✓7ᵗʰ **T57.0X2** **Toxic effect of arsenic and its compounds, intentional self-harm**

       ✓7ᵗʰ **T57.0X3** **Toxic effect of arsenic and its compounds, assault**

       ✓7ᵗʰ **T57.0X4** **Toxic effect of arsenic and its compounds, undetermined**

✓5ᵗʰ **T57.1** **Toxic effect of phosphorus and its compounds**
    EXCLUDES 1   organophosphate insecticides (T60.0)

    ✓6ᵗʰ **T57.1X** **Toxic effect of phosphorus and its compounds**

       ✓7ᵗʰ **T57.1X1** **Toxic effect of phosphorus and its compounds, accidental (unintentional)**
          Toxic effect of phosphorus and its compounds NOS

       ✓7ᵗʰ **T57.1X2** **Toxic effect of phosphorus and its compounds, intentional self-harm**

       ✓7ᵗʰ **T57.1X3** **Toxic effect of phosphorus and its compounds, assault**

       ✓7ᵗʰ **T57.1X4** **Toxic effect of phosphorus and its compounds, undetermined**

✓5ᵗʰ **T57.2** **Toxic effect of manganese and its compounds**

    ✓6ᵗʰ **T57.2X** **Toxic effect of manganese and its compounds**

       ✓7ᵗʰ **T57.2X1** **Toxic effect of manganese and its compounds, accidental (unintentional)**
          Toxic effect of manganese and its compounds NOS

       ✓7ᵗʰ **T57.2X2** **Toxic effect of manganese and its compounds, intentional self-harm**

       ✓7ᵗʰ **T57.2X3** **Toxic effect of manganese and its compounds, assault**

       ✓7ᵗʰ **T57.2X4** **Toxic effect of manganese and its compounds, undetermined**

✓5ᵗʰ **T57.3** **Toxic effect of hydrogen cyanide**

    ✓6ᵗʰ **T57.3X** **Toxic effect of hydrogen cyanide**

       ✓7ᵗʰ **T57.3X1** **Toxic effect of hydrogen cyanide, accidental (unintentional)**
          Toxic effect of hydrogen cyanide NOS

       ✓7ᵗʰ **T57.3X2** **Toxic effect of hydrogen cyanide, intentional self-harm**

       ✓7ᵗʰ **T57.3X3** **Toxic effect of hydrogen cyanide, assault**

       ✓7ᵗʰ **T57.3X4** **Toxic effect of hydrogen cyanide, undetermined**

✓5ᵗʰ **T57.8** **Toxic effect of other specified inorganic substances**

    ✓6ᵗʰ **T57.8X** **Toxic effect of other specified inorganic substances**

       ✓7ᵗʰ **T57.8X1** **Toxic effect of other specified inorganic substances, accidental (unintentional)**
          Toxic effect of other specified inorganic substances NOS

       ✓7ᵗʰ **T57.8X2** **Toxic effect of other specified inorganic substances, intentional self-harm**

       ✓7ᵗʰ **T57.8X3** **Toxic effect of other specified inorganic substances, assault**

       ✓7ᵗʰ **T57.8X4** **Toxic effect of other specified inorganic substances, undetermined**

✓5ᵗʰ **T57.9** **Toxic effect of unspecified inorganic substance**

    ✓ₓ7ᵗʰ **T57.91** **Toxic effect of unspecified inorganic substance, accidental (unintentional)**

    ✓ₓ7ᵗʰ **T57.92** **Toxic effect of unspecified inorganic substance, intentional self-harm**

    ✓ₓ7ᵗʰ **T57.93** **Toxic effect of unspecified inorganic substance, assault**

    ✓ₓ7ᵗʰ **T57.94** **Toxic effect of unspecified inorganic substance, undetermined**

✓4ᵗʰ **T58** **Toxic effect of carbon monoxide**
    INCLUDES   asphyxiation from carbon monoxide
            toxic effect of carbon monoxide from all sources

> The appropriate 7th character is to be added to each code from category T58.
> A   initial encounter
> D   subsequent encounter
> S   sequela

✓5ᵗʰ **T58.0** **Toxic effect of carbon monoxide from motor vehicle exhaust**
    Toxic effect of exhaust gas from gas engine
    Toxic effect of exhaust gas from motor pump

    ✓ₓ7ᵗʰ **T58.01** **Toxic effect of carbon monoxide from motor vehicle exhaust, accidental (unintentional)**

    ✓ₓ7ᵗʰ **T58.02** **Toxic effect of carbon monoxide from motor vehicle exhaust, intentional self-harm**

    ✓ₓ7ᵗʰ **T58.03** **Toxic effect of carbon monoxide from motor vehicle exhaust, assault**

    ✓ₓ7ᵗʰ **T58.04** **Toxic effect of carbon monoxide from motor vehicle exhaust, undetermined**

✓5ᵗʰ **T58.1** **Toxic effect of carbon monoxide from utility gas**
    Toxic effect of acetylene
    Toxic effect of gas NOS used for lighting, heating, cooking
    Toxic effect of water gas

    ✓ₓ7ᵗʰ **T58.11** **Toxic effect of carbon monoxide from utility gas, accidental (unintentional)**

    ✓ₓ7ᵗʰ **T58.12** **Toxic effect of carbon monoxide from utility gas, intentional self-harm**

    ✓ₓ7ᵗʰ **T58.13** **Toxic effect of carbon monoxide from utility gas, assault**

    ✓ₓ7ᵗʰ **T58.14** **Toxic effect of carbon monoxide from utility gas, undetermined**

✓5ᵗʰ **T58.2** **Toxic effect of carbon monoxide from incomplete combustion of other domestic fuels**
    Toxic effect of carbon monoxide from incomplete combustion of coal, coke, kerosene, wood

    ✓6ᵗʰ **T58.2X** **Toxic effect of carbon monoxide from incomplete combustion of other domestic fuels**

       ✓7ᵗʰ **T58.2X1** **Toxic effect of carbon monoxide from incomplete combustion of other domestic fuels, accidental (unintentional)**

       ✓7ᵗʰ **T58.2X2** **Toxic effect of carbon monoxide from incomplete combustion of other domestic fuels, intentional self-harm**

       ✓7ᵗʰ **T58.2X3** **Toxic effect of carbon monoxide from incomplete combustion of other domestic fuels, assault**

       ✓7ᵗʰ **T58.2X4** **Toxic effect of carbon monoxide from incomplete combustion of other domestic fuels, undetermined**

✓5ᵗʰ **T58.8** **Toxic effect of carbon monoxide from other source**
    Toxic effect of carbon monoxide from blast furnace gas
    Toxic effect of carbon monoxide from fuels in industrial use
    Toxic effect of carbon monoxide from kiln vapor

    ✓6ᵗʰ **T58.8X** **Toxic effect of carbon monoxide from other source**

       ✓7ᵗʰ **T58.8X1** **Toxic effect of carbon monoxide from other source, accidental (unintentional)**

       ✓7ᵗʰ **T58.8X2** **Toxic effect of carbon monoxide from other source, intentional self-harm**

       ✓7ᵗʰ **T58.8X3** **Toxic effect of carbon monoxide from other source, assault**

       ✓7ᵗʰ **T58.8X4** **Toxic effect of carbon monoxide from other source, undetermined**

✓5ᵗʰ **T58.9** **Toxic effect of carbon monoxide from unspecified source**

    ✓ₓ7ᵗʰ **T58.91** **Toxic effect of carbon monoxide from unspecified source, accidental (unintentional)**

EXCLUDES 1 Not coded here   EXCLUDES 2 Not included here   N Newborn Age: 0   P Pediatric Age: 0-17   M Maternity Age: 12-55   A Adult Age: 15-124

966   ICD-10-CM Draft (2015)

√x7ᵗʰ **T58.92** **Toxic effect of carbon monoxide from unspecified source,** intentional self-harm

√x7ᵗʰ **T58.93** **Toxic effect of carbon monoxide from unspecified source,** assault

√x7ᵗʰ **T58.94** **Toxic effect of carbon monoxide from unspecified source,** undetermined

√4ᵗʰ **T59** **Toxic effect of other gases, fumes and vapors**
INCLUDES aerosol propellants
EXCLUDES 1 chlorofluorocarbons (T53.5)

The appropriate 7th character is to be added to each code from category T59.
A initial encounter
D subsequent encounter
S sequela

√5ᵗʰ **T59.0** **Toxic effect of nitrogen oxides**

√6ᵗʰ **T59.0X** **Toxic effect of** nitrogen oxides

√7ᵗʰ **T59.0X1** **Toxic effect of nitrogen oxides,** accidental (unintentional)
Toxic effect of nitrogen oxides NOS

√7ᵗʰ **T59.0X2** **Toxic effect of nitrogen oxides,** intentional self-harm

√7ᵗʰ **T59.0X3** **Toxic effect of nitrogen oxides,** assault

√7ᵗʰ **T59.0X4** **Toxic effect of nitrogen oxides,** undetermined

√5ᵗʰ **T59.1** **Toxic effect of sulfur dioxide**

√6ᵗʰ **T59.1X** **Toxic effect of** sulfur dioxide

√7ᵗʰ **T59.1X1** **Toxic effect of sulfur dioxide,** accidental (unintentional)
Toxic effect of sulfur dioxide NOS

√7ᵗʰ **T59.1X2** **Toxic effect of sulfur dioxide,** intentional self-harm

√7ᵗʰ **T59.1X3** **Toxic effect of sulfur dioxide,** assault

√7ᵗʰ **T59.1X4** **Toxic effect of sulfur dioxide,** undetermined

√5ᵗʰ **T59.2** **Toxic effect of formaldehyde**

√6ᵗʰ **T59.2X** **Toxic effect of** formaldehyde

√7ᵗʰ **T59.2X1** **Toxic effect of formaldehyde,** accidental (unintentional)
Toxic effect of formaldehyde NOS

√7ᵗʰ **T59.2X2** **Toxic effect of formaldehyde,** intentional self-harm

√7ᵗʰ **T59.2X3** **Toxic effect of formaldehyde,** assault

√7ᵗʰ **T59.2X4** **Toxic effect of formaldehyde,** undetermined

√5ᵗʰ **T59.3** **Toxic effect of lacrimogenic gas**
Toxic effect of tear gas

√6ᵗʰ **T59.3X** **Toxic effect of** lacrimogenic gas

√7ᵗʰ **T59.3X1** **Toxic effect of lacrimogenic gas,** accidental (unintentional)
Toxic effect of lacrimogenic gas NOS

√7ᵗʰ **T59.3X2** **Toxic effect of lacrimogenic gas,** intentional self-harm

√7ᵗʰ **T59.3X3** **Toxic effect of lacrimogenic gas,** assault

√7ᵗʰ **T59.3X4** **Toxic effect of lacrimogenic gas,** undetermined

√5ᵗʰ **T59.4** **Toxic effect of chlorine gas**

√6ᵗʰ **T59.4X** **Toxic effect of** chlorine gas

√7ᵗʰ **T59.4X1** **Toxic effect of chlorine gas,** accidental (unintentional)
Toxic effect of chlorine gas NOS

√7ᵗʰ **T59.4X2** **Toxic effect of chlorine gas,** intentional self-harm

√7ᵗʰ **T59.4X3** **Toxic effect of chlorine gas,** assault

√7ᵗʰ **T59.4X4** **Toxic effect of chlorine gas,** undetermined

√5ᵗʰ **T59.5** **Toxic effect of fluorine gas and hydrogen fluoride**

√6ᵗʰ **T59.5X** **Toxic effect of** fluorine gas **and** hydrogen fluoride

√7ᵗʰ **T59.5X1** **Toxic effect of fluorine gas and hydrogen fluoride,** accidental (unintentional)
Toxic effect of fluorine gas and hydrogen fluoride NOS

√7ᵗʰ **T59.5X2** **Toxic effect of fluorine gas and hydrogen fluoride,** intentional self-harm

√7ᵗʰ **T59.5X3** **Toxic effect of fluorine gas and hydrogen fluoride,** assault

√7ᵗʰ **T59.5X4** **Toxic effect of fluorine gas and hydrogen fluoride,** undetermined

√5ᵗʰ **T59.6** **Toxic effect of hydrogen sulfide**

√6ᵗʰ **T59.6X** **Toxic effect of** hydrogen sulfide

√7ᵗʰ **T59.6X1** **Toxic effect of hydrogen sulfide,** accidental (unintentional)
Toxic effect of hydrogen sulfide NOS

√7ᵗʰ **T59.6X2** **Toxic effect of hydrogen sulfide,** intentional self-harm

√7ᵗʰ **T59.6X3** **Toxic effect of hydrogen sulfide,** assault

√7ᵗʰ **T59.6X4** **Toxic effect of hydrogen sulfide,** undetermined

√5ᵗʰ **T59.7** **Toxic effect of carbon dioxide**

√6ᵗʰ **T59.7X** **Toxic effect of** carbon dioxide

√7ᵗʰ **T59.7X1** **Toxic effect of carbon dioxide,** accidental (unintentional)
Toxic effect of carbon dioxide NOS

√7ᵗʰ **T59.7X2** **Toxic effect of carbon dioxide,** intentional self-harm

√7ᵗʰ **T59.7X3** **Toxic effect of carbon dioxide,** assault

√7ᵗʰ **T59.7X4** **Toxic effect of carbon dioxide,** undetermined

√5ᵗʰ **T59.8** **Toxic effect of** other **specified gases, fumes and vapors**

√6ᵗʰ **T59.81** **Toxic effect of** smoke
Smoke inhalation
EXCLUDES 2 toxic effect of cigarette (tobacco) smoke (T65.22-)

√7ᵗʰ **T59.811** **Toxic effect of smoke,** accidental (unintentional)
Toxic effect of smoke NOS
AHA: 2013, 4Q, 121

√7ᵗʰ **T59.812** **Toxic effect of smoke,** intentional self-harm

√7ᵗʰ **T59.813** **Toxic effect of smoke,** assault

√7ᵗʰ **T59.814** **Toxic effect of smoke,** undetermined

√6ᵗʰ **T59.89** **Toxic effect of** other **specified gases, fumes and vapors**

√7ᵗʰ **T59.891** **Toxic effect of other specified gases, fumes and vapors,** accidental (unintentional)

√7ᵗʰ **T59.892** **Toxic effect of other specified gases, fumes and vapors,** intentional self-harm

√7ᵗʰ **T59.893** **Toxic effect of other specified gases, fumes and vapors,** assault

√7ᵗʰ **T59.894** **Toxic effect of other specified gases, fumes and vapors,** undetermined

√5ᵗʰ **T59.9** **Toxic effect of** unspecified **gases, fumes and vapors**

√x7ᵗʰ **T59.91** **Toxic effect of unspecified gases, fumes and vapors,** accidental (unintentional)

√x7ᵗʰ **T59.92** **Toxic effect of unspecified gases, fumes and vapors,** intentional self-harm

√x7ᵗʰ **T59.93** **Toxic effect of unspecified gases, fumes and vapors,** assault

√x7ᵗʰ **T59.94** **Toxic effect of unspecified gases, fumes and vapors,** undetermined

√4ᵗʰ **T60** **Toxic effect of pesticides**
INCLUDES toxic effect of wood preservatives

The appropriate 7th character is to be added to each code from category T60.
A initial encounter
D subsequent encounter
S sequela

√5ᵗʰ **T60.0** **Toxic effect of organophosphate and carbamate insecticides**

√6ᵗʰ **T60.0X** **Toxic effect of** organophosphate and carbamate insecticides

√7ᵗʰ **T60.0X1** **Toxic effect of organophosphate and carbamate insecticides,** accidental (unintentional)
Toxic effect of organophosphate and carbamate insecticides NOS

√7ᵗʰ **T60.0X2** **Toxic effect of organophosphate and carbamate insecticides,** intentional self-harm

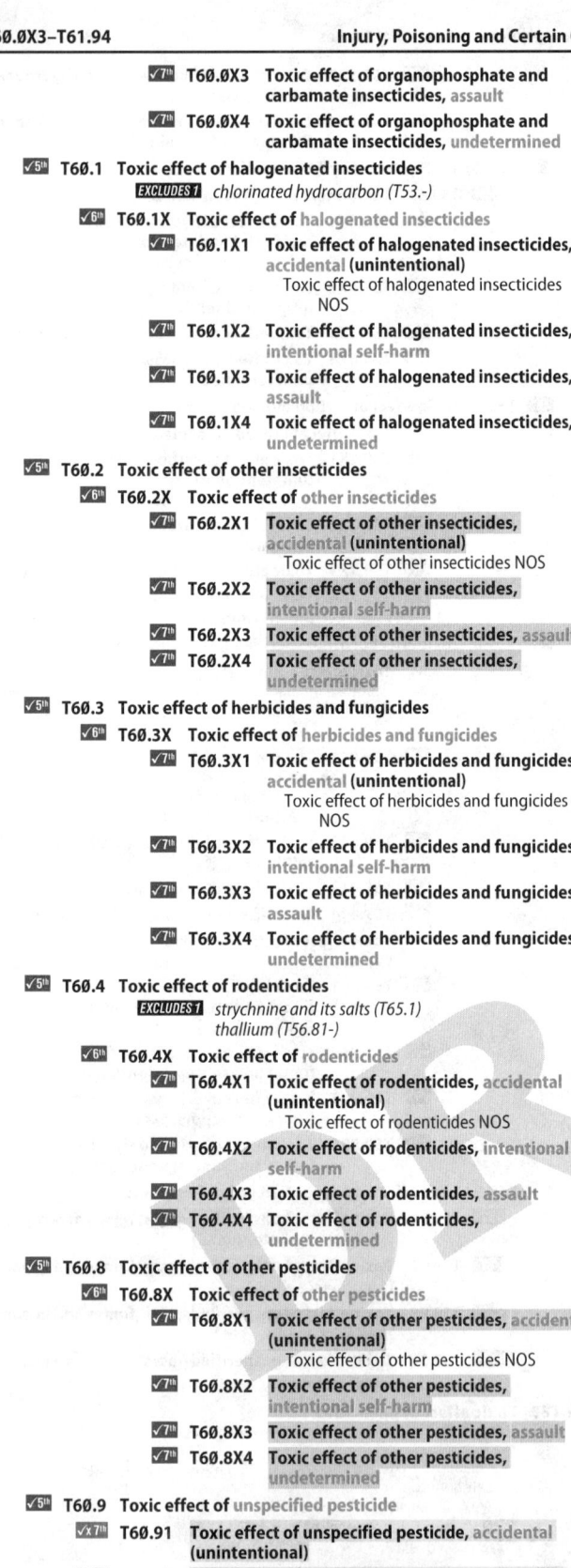

✓7ᵗʰ **T60.0X3** **Toxic effect of organophosphate and carbamate insecticides,** assault

✓7ᵗʰ **T60.0X4** **Toxic effect of organophosphate and carbamate insecticides,** undetermined

✓5ᵗʰ **T60.1** **Toxic effect of halogenated insecticides**
  EXCLUDES 1 *chlorinated hydrocarbon (T53.-)*

✓6ᵗʰ **T60.1X** **Toxic effect of** halogenated insecticides

✓7ᵗʰ **T60.1X1** **Toxic effect of halogenated insecticides,** accidental (unintentional)
  Toxic effect of halogenated insecticides NOS

✓7ᵗʰ **T60.1X2** **Toxic effect of halogenated insecticides,** intentional self-harm

✓7ᵗʰ **T60.1X3** **Toxic effect of halogenated insecticides,** assault

✓7ᵗʰ **T60.1X4** **Toxic effect of halogenated insecticides,** undetermined

✓5ᵗʰ **T60.2** **Toxic effect of other insecticides**

✓6ᵗʰ **T60.2X** **Toxic effect of** other insecticides

✓7ᵗʰ **T60.2X1** **Toxic effect of other insecticides,** accidental (unintentional)
  Toxic effect of other insecticides NOS

✓7ᵗʰ **T60.2X2** **Toxic effect of other insecticides,** intentional self-harm

✓7ᵗʰ **T60.2X3** **Toxic effect of other insecticides,** assault

✓7ᵗʰ **T60.2X4** **Toxic effect of other insecticides,** undetermined

✓5ᵗʰ **T60.3** **Toxic effect of herbicides and fungicides**

✓6ᵗʰ **T60.3X** **Toxic effect of** herbicides and fungicides

✓7ᵗʰ **T60.3X1** **Toxic effect of herbicides and fungicides,** accidental (unintentional)
  Toxic effect of herbicides and fungicides NOS

✓7ᵗʰ **T60.3X2** **Toxic effect of herbicides and fungicides,** intentional self-harm

✓7ᵗʰ **T60.3X3** **Toxic effect of herbicides and fungicides,** assault

✓7ᵗʰ **T60.3X4** **Toxic effect of herbicides and fungicides,** undetermined

✓5ᵗʰ **T60.4** **Toxic effect of rodenticides**
  EXCLUDES 1 *strychnine and its salts (T65.1)*
            thallium (T56.81-)

✓6ᵗʰ **T60.4X** **Toxic effect of** rodenticides

✓7ᵗʰ **T60.4X1** **Toxic effect of rodenticides,** accidental (unintentional)
  Toxic effect of rodenticides NOS

✓7ᵗʰ **T60.4X2** **Toxic effect of rodenticides,** intentional self-harm

✓7ᵗʰ **T60.4X3** **Toxic effect of rodenticides,** assault

✓7ᵗʰ **T60.4X4** **Toxic effect of rodenticides,** undetermined

✓5ᵗʰ **T60.8** **Toxic effect of other pesticides**

✓6ᵗʰ **T60.8X** **Toxic effect of** other pesticides

✓7ᵗʰ **T60.8X1** **Toxic effect of other pesticides,** accidental (unintentional)
  Toxic effect of other pesticides NOS

✓7ᵗʰ **T60.8X2** **Toxic effect of other pesticides,** intentional self-harm

✓7ᵗʰ **T60.8X3** **Toxic effect of other pesticides,** assault

✓7ᵗʰ **T60.8X4** **Toxic effect of other pesticides,** undetermined

✓5ᵗʰ **T60.9** **Toxic effect of unspecified pesticide**

✓x7ᵗʰ **T60.91** **Toxic effect of unspecified pesticide,** accidental (unintentional)

✓x7ᵗʰ **T60.92** **Toxic effect of unspecified pesticide,** intentional self-harm

✓x7ᵗʰ **T60.93** **Toxic effect of unspecified pesticide,** assault

✓x7ᵗʰ **T60.94** **Toxic effect of unspecified pesticide,** undetermined

✓4ᵗʰ **T61** **Toxic effect of noxious substances eaten as seafood**
  EXCLUDES 1 *allergic reaction to food, such as:*
    anaphylactic reaction or shock due to adverse food reaction (T78.0-)
    dermatitis (L23.6, L25.4, L27.2)
    gastroenteritis (noninfective) (K52.2)
    bacterial foodborne intoxications (A05.-)
    toxic effect of aflatoxin and other mycotoxins (T64)
    toxic effect of cyanides (T65.0-)
    toxic effect of harmful algae bloom (T65.82-)
    toxic effect of hydrogen cyanide (T57.3-)
    toxic effect of mercury (T56.1-)
    toxic effect of red tide (T65.82-)

The appropriate 7th character is to be added to each code from category T61.
A	initial encounter
D	subsequent encounter
S	sequela

✓5ᵗʰ **T61.0** Ciguatera fish poisoning

✓x7ᵗʰ **T61.01** **Ciguatera fish poisoning,** accidental (unintentional)

✓x7ᵗʰ **T61.02** **Ciguatera fish poisoning,** intentional self-harm

✓x7ᵗʰ **T61.03** **Ciguatera fish poisoning,** assault

✓x7ᵗʰ **T61.04** **Ciguatera fish poisoning,** undetermined

✓5ᵗʰ **T61.1** Scombroid fish poisoning
  Histamine-like syndrome

✓x7ᵗʰ **T61.11** **Scombroid fish poisoning,** accidental (unintentional)

✓x7ᵗʰ **T61.12** **Scombroid fish poisoning,** intentional self-harm

✓x7ᵗʰ **T61.13** **Scombroid fish poisoning,** assault

✓x7ᵗʰ **T61.14** **Scombroid fish poisoning,** undetermined

✓5ᵗʰ **T61.7** Other fish and shellfish poisoning

✓6ᵗʰ **T61.77** **Other** fish poisoning

✓7ᵗʰ **T61.771** **Other fish poisoning,** accidental (unintentional)

✓7ᵗʰ **T61.772** **Other fish poisoning,** intentional self-harm

✓7ᵗʰ **T61.773** **Other fish poisoning,** assault

✓7ᵗʰ **T61.774** **Other fish poisoning,** undetermined

✓6ᵗʰ **T61.78** **Other** shellfish poisoning

✓7ᵗʰ **T61.781** **Other shellfish poisoning,** accidental (unintentional)

✓7ᵗʰ **T61.782** **Other shellfish poisoning,** intentional self-harm

✓7ᵗʰ **T61.783** **Other shellfish poisoning,** assault

✓7ᵗʰ **T61.784** **Other shellfish poisoning,** undetermined

✓5ᵗʰ **T61.8** **Toxic effect of other seafood**

✓6ᵗʰ **T61.8X** **Toxic effect of** other seafood

✓7ᵗʰ **T61.8X1** **Toxic effect of other seafood,** accidental (unintentional)

✓7ᵗʰ **T61.8X2** **Toxic effect of other seafood,** intentional self-harm

✓7ᵗʰ **T61.8X3** **Toxic effect of other seafood,** assault

✓7ᵗʰ **T61.8X4** **Toxic effect of other seafood,** undetermined

✓5ᵗʰ **T61.9** **Toxic effect of** unspecified seafood

✓x7ᵗʰ **T61.91** **Toxic effect of unspecified seafood,** accidental (unintentional)

✓x7ᵗʰ **T61.92** **Toxic effect of unspecified seafood,** intentional self-harm

✓x7ᵗʰ **T61.93** **Toxic effect of unspecified seafood,** assault

✓x7ᵗʰ **T61.94** **Toxic effect of unspecified seafood,** undetermined

✓4th **T62　Toxic effect of other noxious substances eaten as food**

　　EXCLUDES 1　*allergic reaction to food, such as:*
　　　　　anaphylactic shock (reaction) due to adverse food reaction
　　　　　　(T78.0-)
　　　　　dermatitis (L23.6, L25.4, L27.2)
　　　　　gastroenteritis (noninfective) (K52.2)
　　　　bacterial food borne intoxications (A05.-)
　　　　toxic effect of aflatoxin and other mycotoxins (T64)
　　　　toxic effect of cyanides (T65.0-)
　　　　toxic effect of hydrogen cyanide (T57.3-)
　　　　toxic effect of mercury (T56.1-)

　　The appropriate 7th character is to be added to each code from category T62.
　　A　initial encounter
　　D　subsequent encounter
　　S　sequela

✓5th **T62.0　Toxic effect of ingested mushrooms**

　✓6th **T62.0X　Toxic effect of** ingested mushrooms

　　✓7th **T62.0X1　Toxic effect of ingested mushrooms, accidental (unintentional)**
　　　　　Toxic effect of ingested mushrooms NOS

　　✓7th **T62.0X2　Toxic effect of ingested mushrooms, intentional self-harm**

　　✓7th **T62.0X3　Toxic effect of ingested mushrooms, assault**

　　✓7th **T62.0X4　Toxic effect of ingested mushrooms, undetermined**

✓5th **T62.1　Toxic effect of ingested berries**

　✓6th **T62.1X　Toxic effect of** ingested berries

　　✓7th **T62.1X1　Toxic effect of ingested berries, accidental (unintentional)**
　　　　　Toxic effect of ingested berries NOS

　　✓7th **T62.1X2　Toxic effect of ingested berries, intentional self-harm**

　　✓7th **T62.1X3　Toxic effect of ingested berries, assault**

　　✓7th **T62.1X4　Toxic effect of ingested berries, undetermined**

✓5th **T62.2　Toxic effect of other ingested (parts of) plant(s)**

　✓6th **T62.2X　Toxic effect of** other ingested **(parts of)** plant**(s)**

　　✓7th **T62.2X1　Toxic effect of other ingested (parts of) plant(s), accidental (unintentional)**
　　　　　Toxic effect of other ingested (parts of) plant(s) NOS

　　✓7th **T62.2X2　Toxic effect of other ingested (parts of) plant(s), intentional self-harm**

　　✓7th **T62.2X3　Toxic effect of other ingested (parts of) plant(s), assault**

　　✓7th **T62.2X4　Toxic effect of other ingested (parts of) plant(s), undetermined**

✓5th **T62.8　Toxic effect of other specified** noxious substances eaten as food

　✓6th **T62.8X　Toxic effect of** other **specified noxious substances eaten as food**

　　✓7th **T62.8X1　Toxic effect of other specified noxious substances eaten as food, accidental (unintentional)**
　　　　　Toxic effect of other specified noxious substances eaten as food NOS

　　✓7th **T62.8X2　Toxic effect of other specified noxious substances eaten as food, intentional self-harm**

　　✓7th **T62.8X3　Toxic effect of other specified noxious substances eaten as food, assault**

　　✓7th **T62.8X4　Toxic effect of other specified noxious substances eaten as food, undetermined**

✓5th **T62.9　Toxic effect of** unspecified **noxious substance eaten as food**

　✓x7th **T62.91　Toxic effect of unspecified noxious substance eaten as food, accidental (unintentional)**
　　　　Toxic effect of unspecified noxious substance eaten as food NOS

　✓x7th **T62.92　Toxic effect of unspecified noxious substance eaten as food, intentional self-harm**

　✓x7th **T62.93　Toxic effect of unspecified noxious substance eaten as food, assault**

　✓x7th **T62.94　Toxic effect of unspecified noxious substance eaten as food, undetermined**

✓4th **T63　Toxic effect of contact with venomous animals and plants**

　　INCLUDES　bite or touch of venomous animal
　　　　　pricked or stuck by thorn or leaf
　　EXCLUDES 2　*ingestion of toxic animal or plant (T61.-, T62.-)*

　　The appropriate 7th character is to be added to each code from category T63.
　　A　initial encounter
　　D　subsequent encounter
　　S　sequela

✓5th **T63.0　Toxic effect of** snake venom

　✓6th **T63.00　Toxic effect of** unspecified **snake venom**

　　✓7th **T63.001　Toxic effect of unspecified snake venom, accidental (unintentional)**
　　　　　Toxic effect of unspecified snake venom NOS

　　✓7th **T63.002　Toxic effect of unspecified snake venom, intentional self-harm**

　　✓7th **T63.003　Toxic effect of unspecified snake venom, assault**

　　✓7th **T63.004　Toxic effect of unspecified snake venom, undetermined**

　✓6th **T63.01　Toxic effect of** rattlesnake **venom**

　　✓7th **T63.011　Toxic effect of rattlesnake venom, accidental (unintentional)**
　　　　　Toxic effect of rattlesnake venom NOS

　　✓7th **T63.012　Toxic effect of rattlesnake venom, intentional self-harm**

　　✓7th **T63.013　Toxic effect of rattlesnake venom, assault**

　　✓7th **T63.014　Toxic effect of rattlesnake venom, undetermined**

　✓6th **T63.02　Toxic effect of** coral snake **venom**

　　✓7th **T63.021　Toxic effect of coral snake venom, accidental (unintentional)**
　　　　　Toxic effect of coral snake venom NOS

　　✓7th **T63.022　Toxic effect of coral snake venom, intentional self-harm**

　　✓7th **T63.023　Toxic effect of coral snake venom, assault**

　　✓7th **T63.024　Toxic effect of coral snake venom, undetermined**

　✓6th **T63.03　Toxic effect of** taipan **venom**

　　✓7th **T63.031　Toxic effect of taipan venom, accidental (unintentional)**
　　　　　Toxic effect of taipan venom NOS

　　✓7th **T63.032　Toxic effect of taipan venom, intentional self-harm**

　　✓7th **T63.033　Toxic effect of taipan venom, assault**

　　✓7th **T63.034　Toxic effect of taipan venom, undetermined**

　✓6th **T63.04　Toxic effect of** cobra **venom**

　　✓7th **T63.041　Toxic effect of cobra venom, accidental (unintentional)**
　　　　　Toxic effect of cobra venom NOS

　　✓7th **T63.042　Toxic effect of cobra venom, intentional self-harm**

　　✓7th **T63.043　Toxic effect of cobra venom, assault**

　　✓7th **T63.044　Toxic effect of cobra venom, undetermined**

　✓6th **T63.06　Toxic effect of venom of** other North and South American snake

　　✓7th **T63.061　Toxic effect of venom of other North and South American snake, accidental (unintentional)**
　　　　　Toxic effect of venom of other North and South American snake NOS

　　✓7th **T63.062　Toxic effect of venom of other North and South American snake, intentional self-harm**

　　✓7th **T63.063　Toxic effect of venom of other North and South American snake, assault**

　　✓7th **T63.064　Toxic effect of venom of other North and South American snake, undetermined**

√6ᵗʰ **T63.07** Toxic effect of venom of other Australian snake

- √7ᵗʰ **T63.071** Toxic effect of venom of other Australian snake, accidental (unintentional)
  Toxic effect of venom of other Australian snake NOS
- √7ᵗʰ **T63.072** Toxic effect of venom of other Australian snake, intentional self-harm
- √7ᵗʰ **T63.073** Toxic effect of venom of other Australian snake, assault
- √7ᵗʰ **T63.074** Toxic effect of venom of other Australian snake, undetermined

√6ᵗʰ **T63.08** Toxic effect of venom of other African and Asian snake

- √7ᵗʰ **T63.081** Toxic effect of venom of other African and Asian snake, accidental (unintentional)
  Toxic effect of venom of other African and Asian snake NOS
- √7ᵗʰ **T63.082** Toxic effect of venom of other African and Asian snake, intentional self-harm
- √7ᵗʰ **T63.083** Toxic effect of venom of other African and Asian snake, assault
- √7ᵗʰ **T63.084** Toxic effect of venom of other African and Asian snake, undetermined

√6ᵗʰ **T63.09** Toxic effect of venom of other snake

- √7ᵗʰ **T63.091** Toxic effect of venom of other snake, accidental (unintentional)
  Toxic effect of venom of other snake NOS
- √7ᵗʰ **T63.092** Toxic effect of venom of other snake, intentional self-harm
- √7ᵗʰ **T63.093** Toxic effect of venom of other snake, assault
- √7ᵗʰ **T63.094** Toxic effect of venom of other snake, undetermined

√5ᵗʰ **T63.1** Toxic effect of venom of other reptiles

√6ᵗʰ **T63.11** Toxic effect of venom of gila monster

- √7ᵗʰ **T63.111** Toxic effect of venom of gila monster, accidental (unintentional)
  Toxic effect of venom of gila monster NOS
- √7ᵗʰ **T63.112** Toxic effect of venom of gila monster, intentional self-harm
- √7ᵗʰ **T63.113** Toxic effect of venom of gila monster, assault
- √7ᵗʰ **T63.114** Toxic effect of venom of gila monster, undetermined

√6ᵗʰ **T63.12** Toxic effect of venom of other venomous lizard

- √7ᵗʰ **T63.121** Toxic effect of venom of other venomous lizard, accidental (unintentional)
  Toxic effect of venom of other venomous lizard NOS
- √7ᵗʰ **T63.122** Toxic effect of venom of other venomous lizard, intentional self-harm
- √7ᵗʰ **T63.123** Toxic effect of venom of other venomous lizard, assault
- √7ᵗʰ **T63.124** Toxic effect of venom of other venomous lizard, undetermined

√6ᵗʰ **T63.19** Toxic effect of venom of other reptiles

- √7ᵗʰ **T63.191** Toxic effect of venom of other reptiles, accidental (unintentional)
  Toxic effect of venom of other reptiles NOS
- √7ᵗʰ **T63.192** Toxic effect of venom of other reptiles, intentional self-harm
- √7ᵗʰ **T63.193** Toxic effect of venom of other reptiles, assault
- √7ᵗʰ **T63.194** Toxic effect of venom of other reptiles, undetermined

√5ᵗʰ **T63.2** Toxic effect of venom of scorpion

√6ᵗʰ **T63.2X** Toxic effect of venom of scorpion

- √7ᵗʰ **T63.2X1** Toxic effect of venom of scorpion, accidental (unintentional)
  Toxic effect of venom of scorpion NOS
- √7ᵗʰ **T63.2X2** Toxic effect of venom of scorpion, intentional self-harm
- √7ᵗʰ **T63.2X3** Toxic effect of venom of scorpion, assault
- √7ᵗʰ **T63.2X4** Toxic effect of venom of scorpion, undetermined

√5ᵗʰ **T63.3** Toxic effect of venom of spider

√6ᵗʰ **T63.30** Toxic effect of unspecified spider venom

- √7ᵗʰ **T63.301** Toxic effect of unspecified spider venom, accidental (unintentional)
- √7ᵗʰ **T63.302** Toxic effect of unspecified spider venom, intentional self-harm
- √7ᵗʰ **T63.303** Toxic effect of unspecified spider venom, assault
- √7ᵗʰ **T63.304** Toxic effect of unspecified spider venom, undetermined

√6ᵗʰ **T63.31** Toxic effect of venom of black widow spider

- √7ᵗʰ **T63.311** Toxic effect of venom of black widow spider, accidental (unintentional)
- √7ᵗʰ **T63.312** Toxic effect of venom of black widow spider, intentional self-harm
- √7ᵗʰ **T63.313** Toxic effect of venom of black widow spider, assault
- √7ᵗʰ **T63.314** Toxic effect of venom of black widow spider, undetermined

√6ᵗʰ **T63.32** Toxic effect of venom of tarantula

- √7ᵗʰ **T63.321** Toxic effect of venom of tarantula, accidental (unintentional)
- √7ᵗʰ **T63.322** Toxic effect of venom of tarantula, intentional self-harm
- √7ᵗʰ **T63.323** Toxic effect of venom of tarantula, assault
- √7ᵗʰ **T63.324** Toxic effect of venom of tarantula, undetermined

√6ᵗʰ **T63.33** Toxic effect of venom of brown recluse spider

- √7ᵗʰ **T63.331** Toxic effect of venom of brown recluse spider, accidental (unintentional)
- √7ᵗʰ **T63.332** Toxic effect of venom of brown recluse spider, intentional self-harm
- √7ᵗʰ **T63.333** Toxic effect of venom of brown recluse spider, assault
- √7ᵗʰ **T63.334** Toxic effect of venom of brown recluse spider, undetermined

√6ᵗʰ **T63.39** Toxic effect of venom of other spider

- √7ᵗʰ **T63.391** Toxic effect of venom of other spider, accidental (unintentional)
- √7ᵗʰ **T63.392** Toxic effect of venom of other spider, intentional self-harm
- √7ᵗʰ **T63.393** Toxic effect of venom of other spider, assault
- √7ᵗʰ **T63.394** Toxic effect of venom of other spider, undetermined

√5ᵗʰ **T63.4** Toxic effect of venom of other arthropods

√6ᵗʰ **T63.41** Toxic effect of venom of centipedes and venomous millipedes

- √7ᵗʰ **T63.411** Toxic effect of venom of centipedes and venomous millipedes, accidental (unintentional)
- √7ᵗʰ **T63.412** Toxic effect of venom of centipedes and venomous millipedes, intentional self-harm
- √7ᵗʰ **T63.413** Toxic effect of venom of centipedes and venomous millipedes, assault
- √7ᵗʰ **T63.414** Toxic effect of venom of centipedes and venomous millipedes, undetermined

√6ᵗʰ **T63.42** Toxic effect of venom of ants

- √7ᵗʰ **T63.421** Toxic effect of venom of ants, accidental (unintentional)
- √7ᵗʰ **T63.422** Toxic effect of venom of ants, intentional self-harm
- √7ᵗʰ **T63.423** Toxic effect of venom of ants, assault
- √7ᵗʰ **T63.424** Toxic effect of venom of ants, undetermined

√6ᵗʰ **T63.43** Toxic effect of venom of caterpillars

- √7ᵗʰ **T63.431** Toxic effect of venom of caterpillars, accidental (unintentional)
- √7ᵗʰ **T63.432** Toxic effect of venom of caterpillars, intentional self-harm
- √7ᵗʰ **T63.433** Toxic effect of venom of caterpillars, assault

---

EXCLUDES 1 Not coded here   EXCLUDES 2 Not included here   N Newborn Age: 0   P Pediatric Age: 0-17   M Maternity Age: 12-55   A Adult Age: 15-124

√7ᵗʰ **T63.434** Toxic effect of venom of caterpillars, undetermined

√6ᵗʰ **T63.44** Toxic effect of venom of bees
   √7ᵗʰ **T63.441** Toxic effect of venom of bees, accidental (unintentional)
   √7ᵗʰ **T63.442** Toxic effect of venom of bees, intentional self-harm
   √7ᵗʰ **T63.443** Toxic effect of venom of bees, assault
   √7ᵗʰ **T63.444** Toxic effect of venom of bees, undetermined

√6ᵗʰ **T63.45** Toxic effect of venom of hornets
   √7ᵗʰ **T63.451** Toxic effect of venom of hornets, accidental (unintentional)
   √7ᵗʰ **T63.452** Toxic effect of venom of hornets, intentional self-harm
   √7ᵗʰ **T63.453** Toxic effect of venom of hornets, assault
   √7ᵗʰ **T63.454** Toxic effect of venom of hornets, undetermined

√6ᵗʰ **T63.46** Toxic effect of venom of wasps
      Toxic effect of yellow jacket
   √7ᵗʰ **T63.461** Toxic effect of venom of wasps, accidental (unintentional)
   √7ᵗʰ **T63.462** Toxic effect of venom of wasps, intentional self-harm
   √7ᵗʰ **T63.463** Toxic effect of venom of wasps, assault
   √7ᵗʰ **T63.464** Toxic effect of venom of wasps, undetermined

√6ᵗʰ **T63.48** Toxic effect of venom of other arthropod
   √7ᵗʰ **T63.481** Toxic effect of venom of other arthropod, accidental (unintentional)
   √7ᵗʰ **T63.482** Toxic effect of venom of other arthropod, intentional self-harm
   √7ᵗʰ **T63.483** Toxic effect of venom of other arthropod, assault
   √7ᵗʰ **T63.484** Toxic effect of venom of other arthropod, undetermined

√5ᵗʰ **T63.5** Toxic effect of contact with venomous fish
   EXCLUDES 2 poisoning by ingestion of fish (T61.-)

√6ᵗʰ **T63.51** Toxic effect of contact with stingray
   √7ᵗʰ **T63.511** Toxic effect of contact with stingray, accidental (unintentional)
   √7ᵗʰ **T63.512** Toxic effect of contact with stingray, intentional self-harm
   √7ᵗʰ **T63.513** Toxic effect of contact with stingray, assault
   √7ᵗʰ **T63.514** Toxic effect of contact with stingray, undetermined

√6ᵗʰ **T63.59** Toxic effect of contact with other venomous fish
   √7ᵗʰ **T63.591** Toxic effect of contact with other venomous fish, accidental (unintentional)
   √7ᵗʰ **T63.592** Toxic effect of contact with other venomous fish, intentional self-harm
   √7ᵗʰ **T63.593** Toxic effect of contact with other venomous fish, assault
   √7ᵗʰ **T63.594** Toxic effect of contact with other venomous fish, undetermined

√5ᵗʰ **T63.6** Toxic effect of contact with other venomous marine animals
   EXCLUDES 1 sea-snake venom (T63.09)
   EXCLUDES 2 poisoning by ingestion of shellfish (T61.78-)

√6ᵗʰ **T63.61** Toxic effect of contact with Portugese Man-o-war
      Toxic effect of contact with bluebottle
   √7ᵗʰ **T63.611** Toxic effect of contact with Portugese Man-o-war, accidental (unintentional)
   √7ᵗʰ **T63.612** Toxic effect of contact with Portugese Man-o-war, intentional self-harm
   √7ᵗʰ **T63.613** Toxic effect of contact with Portugese Man-o-war, assault
   √7ᵗʰ **T63.614** Toxic effect of contact with Portugese Man-o-war, undetermined

√6ᵗʰ **T63.62** Toxic effect of contact with other jellyfish
   √7ᵗʰ **T63.621** Toxic effect of contact with other jellyfish, accidental (unintentional)
   √7ᵗʰ **T63.622** Toxic effect of contact with other jellyfish, intentional self-harm
   √7ᵗʰ **T63.623** Toxic effect of contact with other jellyfish, assault
   √7ᵗʰ **T63.624** Toxic effect of contact with other jellyfish, undetermined

√6ᵗʰ **T63.63** Toxic effect of contact with sea anemone
   √7ᵗʰ **T63.631** Toxic effect of contact with sea anemone, accidental (unintentional)
   √7ᵗʰ **T63.632** Toxic effect of contact with sea anemone, intentional self-harm
   √7ᵗʰ **T63.633** Toxic effect of contact with sea anemone, assault
   √7ᵗʰ **T63.634** Toxic effect of contact with sea anemone, undetermined

√6ᵗʰ **T63.69** Toxic effect of contact with other venomous marine animals
   √7ᵗʰ **T63.691** Toxic effect of contact with other venomous marine animals, accidental (unintentional)
   √7ᵗʰ **T63.692** Toxic effect of contact with other venomous marine animals, intentional self-harm
   √7ᵗʰ **T63.693** Toxic effect of contact with other venomous marine animals, assault
   √7ᵗʰ **T63.694** Toxic effect of contact with other venomous marine animals, undetermined

√5ᵗʰ **T63.7** Toxic effect of contact with venomous plant

√6ᵗʰ **T63.71** Toxic effect of contact with venomous marine plant
   √7ᵗʰ **T63.711** Toxic effect of contact with venomous marine plant, accidental (unintentional)
   √7ᵗʰ **T63.712** Toxic effect of contact with venomous marine plant, intentional self-harm
   √7ᵗʰ **T63.713** Toxic effect of contact with venomous marine plant, assault
   √7ᵗʰ **T63.714** Toxic effect of contact with venomous marine plant, undetermined

√6ᵗʰ **T63.79** Toxic effect of contact with other venomous plant
   √7ᵗʰ **T63.791** Toxic effect of contact with other venomous plant, accidental (unintentional)
   √7ᵗʰ **T63.792** Toxic effect of contact with other venomous plant, intentional self-harm
   √7ᵗʰ **T63.793** Toxic effect of contact with other venomous plant, assault
   √7ᵗʰ **T63.794** Toxic effect of contact with other venomous plant, undetermined

√5ᵗʰ **T63.8** Toxic effect of contact with other venomous animals

√6ᵗʰ **T63.81** Toxic effect of contact with venomous frog
   EXCLUDES 1 contact with nonvenomous frog (W62.0)
   √7ᵗʰ **T63.811** Toxic effect of contact with venomous frog, accidental (unintentional)
   √7ᵗʰ **T63.812** Toxic effect of contact with venomous frog, intentional self-harm
   √7ᵗʰ **T63.813** Toxic effect of contact with venomous frog, assault
   √7ᵗʰ **T63.814** Toxic effect of contact with venomous frog, undetermined

√6ᵗʰ **T63.82** Toxic effect of contact with venomous toad
   EXCLUDES 1 contact with nonvenomous toad (W62.1)
   √7ᵗʰ **T63.821** Toxic effect of contact with venomous toad, accidental (unintentional)
   √7ᵗʰ **T63.822** Toxic effect of contact with venomous toad, intentional self-harm
   √7ᵗʰ **T63.823** Toxic effect of contact with venomous toad, assault
   √7ᵗʰ **T63.824** Toxic effect of contact with venomous toad, undetermined

√6ᵗʰ **T63.83** Toxic effect of contact with other venomous amphibian
   EXCLUDES 1 contact with nonvenomous amphibian (W62.9)
   √7ᵗʰ **T63.831** Toxic effect of contact with other venomous amphibian, accidental (unintentional)

√ Additional Character Required   √ˣ⁷ᵗʰ Xtension Alert   Unspecified Dx   Other Specified Dx   Manifestation   ▶◀ Revised Text   ● New Code   ▲ Revised Code Title

✓7ᵗʰ   **T63.832   Toxic effect of contact with other venomous amphibian,** intentional self-harm

✓7ᵗʰ   **T63.833   Toxic effect of contact with other venomous amphibian,** assault

✓7ᵗʰ   **T63.834   Toxic effect of contact with other venomous amphibian,** undetermined

✓6ᵗʰ   **T63.89   Toxic effect of contact with** other **venomous** animals

✓7ᵗʰ   **T63.891   Toxic effect of contact with other venomous animals,** accidental **(unintentional)**

✓7ᵗʰ   **T63.892   Toxic effect of contact with other venomous animals,** intentional self-harm

✓7ᵗʰ   **T63.893   Toxic effect of contact with other venomous animals,** assault

✓7ᵗʰ   **T63.894   Toxic effect of contact with other venomous animals,** undetermined

✓5ᵗʰ   **T63.9   Toxic effect of contact with** unspecified **venomous** animal

✓x7ᵗʰ   **T63.91   Toxic effect of contact with unspecified venomous animal,** accidental **(unintentional)**

✓x7ᵗʰ   **T63.92   Toxic effect of contact with unspecified venomous animal,** intentional self-harm

✓x7ᵗʰ   **T63.93   Toxic effect of contact with unspecified venomous animal,** assault

✓x7ᵗʰ   **T63.94   Toxic effect of contact with unspecified venomous animal,** undetermined

✓4ᵗʰ   **T64   Toxic effect of aflatoxin and other mycotoxin food contaminants**

The appropriate 7th character is to be added to each code from category T64.
A   initial encounter
D   subsequent encounter
S   sequela

✓5ᵗʰ   **T64.0   Toxic effect of** aflatoxin

✓x7ᵗʰ   **T64.01   Toxic effect of aflatoxin,** accidental (unintentional)

✓x7ᵗʰ   **T64.02   Toxic effect of aflatoxin,** intentional self-harm

✓x7ᵗʰ   **T64.03   Toxic effect of aflatoxin,** assault

✓x7ᵗʰ   **T64.04   Toxic effect of aflatoxin,** undetermined

✓5ᵗʰ   **T64.8   Toxic effect of** other mycotoxin **food contaminants**

✓x7ᵗʰ   **T64.81   Toxic effect of other mycotoxin food contaminants,** accidental **(unintentional)**

✓x7ᵗʰ   **T64.82   Toxic effect of other mycotoxin food contaminants,** intentional self-harm

✓x7ᵗʰ   **T64.83   Toxic effect of other mycotoxin food contaminants,** assault

✓x7ᵗʰ   **T64.84   Toxic effect of other mycotoxin food contaminants,** undetermined

✓4ᵗʰ   **T65   Toxic effect of other and unspecified substances**

The appropriate 7th character is to be added to each code from category T65.
A   initial encounter
D   subsequent encounter
S   sequela

✓5ᵗʰ   **T65.0   Toxic effect of** cyanides

EXCLUDES 1   hydrogen cyanide (T57.3-)

✓6ᵗʰ   **T65.0X   Toxic effect of cyanides**

✓7ᵗʰ   **T65.0X1   Toxic effect of cyanides,** accidental **(unintentional)**
Toxic effect of cyanides NOS

✓7ᵗʰ   **T65.0X2   Toxic effect of cyanides,** intentional self-harm

✓7ᵗʰ   **T65.0X3   Toxic effect of cyanides,** assault

✓7ᵗʰ   **T65.0X4   Toxic effect of cyanides,** undetermined

✓5ᵗʰ   **T65.1   Toxic effect of** strychnine **and its salts**

✓6ᵗʰ   **T65.1X   Toxic effect of strychnine and its salts**

✓7ᵗʰ   **T65.1X1   Toxic effect of strychnine and its salts,** accidental **(unintentional)**
Toxic effect of strychnine and its salts NOS

✓7ᵗʰ   **T65.1X2   Toxic effect of strychnine and its salts,** intentional self-harm

✓7ᵗʰ   **T65.1X3   Toxic effect of strychnine and its salts,** assault

✓7ᵗʰ   **T65.1X4   Toxic effect of strychnine and its salts,** undetermined

✓5ᵗʰ   **T65.2   Toxic effect of** tobacco and nicotine

EXCLUDES 2   nicotine dependence (F17.-)

✓6ᵗʰ   **T65.21   Toxic effect of** chewing tobacco

✓7ᵗʰ   **T65.211   Toxic effect of chewing tobacco,** accidental **(unintentional)**
Toxic effect of chewing tobacco NOS

✓7ᵗʰ   **T65.212   Toxic effect of chewing tobacco,** intentional self-harm

✓7ᵗʰ   **T65.213   Toxic effect of chewing tobacco,** assault

✓7ᵗʰ   **T65.214   Toxic effect of chewing tobacco,** undetermined

✓6ᵗʰ   **T65.22   Toxic effect of** tobacco cigarettes
Toxic effect of tobacco smoke
Use additional code for exposure to second hand tobacco smoke (Z57.31, Z77.22)

✓7ᵗʰ   **T65.221   Toxic effect of tobacco cigarettes,** accidental **(unintentional)**
Toxic effect of tobacco cigarettes NOS

✓7ᵗʰ   **T65.222   Toxic effect of tobacco cigarettes,** intentional self-harm

✓7ᵗʰ   **T65.223   Toxic effect of tobacco cigarettes,** assault

✓7ᵗʰ   **T65.224   Toxic effect of tobacco cigarettes,** undetermined

✓6ᵗʰ   **T65.29   Toxic effect of** other tobacco and nicotine

✓7ᵗʰ   **T65.291   Toxic effect of other tobacco and nicotine,** accidental **(unintentional)**
Toxic effect of other tobacco and nicotine NOS

✓7ᵗʰ   **T65.292   Toxic effect of other tobacco and nicotine,** intentional self-harm

✓7ᵗʰ   **T65.293   Toxic effect of other tobacco and nicotine,** assault

✓7ᵗʰ   **T65.294   Toxic effect of other tobacco and nicotine,** undetermined

✓5ᵗʰ   **T65.3   Toxic effect of** nitroderivatives and aminoderivatives of benzene and its homologues
Toxic effect of anilin [benzenamine]
Toxic effect of nitrobenzene
Toxic effect of trinitrotoluene

✓6ᵗʰ   **T65.3X   Toxic effect of nitroderivatives and aminoderivatives of benzene and its homologues**

✓7ᵗʰ   **T65.3X1   Toxic effect of nitroderivatives and aminoderivatives of benzene and its homologues,** accidental **(unintentional)**
Toxic effect of nitroderivatives and aminoderivatives of benzene and its homologues NOS

✓7ᵗʰ   **T65.3X2   Toxic effect of nitroderivatives and aminoderivatives of benzene and its homologues,** intentional self-harm

✓7ᵗʰ   **T65.3X3   Toxic effect of nitroderivatives and aminoderivatives of benzene and its homologues,** assault

✓7ᵗʰ   **T65.3X4   Toxic effect of nitroderivatives and aminoderivatives of benzene and its homologues,** undetermined

✓5ᵗʰ   **T65.4   Toxic effect of** carbon disulfide

✓6ᵗʰ   **T65.4X   Toxic effect of carbon disulfide**

✓7ᵗʰ   **T65.4X1   Toxic effect of carbon disulfide,** accidental **(unintentional)**
Toxic effect of carbon disulfide NOS

✓7ᵗʰ   **T65.4X2   Toxic effect of carbon disulfide,** intentional self-harm

✓7ᵗʰ   **T65.4X3   Toxic effect of carbon disulfide,** assault

✓7ᵗʰ   **T65.4X4   Toxic effect of carbon disulfide,** undetermined

✓5ᵗʰ   **T65.5   Toxic effect of** nitroglycerin and other nitric acids and esters
Toxic effect of 1,2,3-Propanetriol trinitrate

✓6ᵗʰ   **T65.5X   Toxic effect of nitroglycerin and other nitric acids and esters**

✓7ᵗʰ   **T65.5X1   Toxic effect of nitroglycerin and other nitric acids and esters,** accidental **(unintentional)**
Toxic effect of nitroglycerin and other nitric acids and esters NOS

EXCLUDES 1 Not coded here   **EXCLUDES 2** Not included here   **N** Newborn Age: 0   **P** Pediatric Age: 0-17   **M** Maternity Age: 12-55   **A** Adult Age: 15-124

972   ICD-10-CM Draft (2015)

√7ᵗʰ **T65.5X2 Toxic effect of nitroglycerin and other nitric acids and esters,** intentional self-harm

√7ᵗʰ **T65.5X3 Toxic effect of nitroglycerin and other nitric acids and esters,** assault

√7ᵗʰ **T65.5X4 Toxic effect of nitroglycerin and other nitric acids and esters,** undetermined

√5ᵗʰ **T65.6 Toxic effect of** paints and dyes, **not elsewhere classified**

√6ᵗʰ **T65.6X Toxic effect of paints and dyes, not elsewhere classified**

√7ᵗʰ **T65.6X1 Toxic effect of paints and dyes, not elsewhere classified,** accidental (unintentional)
Toxic effect of paints and dyes NOS

√7ᵗʰ **T65.6X2 Toxic effect of paints and dyes, not elsewhere classified,** intentional self-harm

√7ᵗʰ **T65.6X3 Toxic effect of paints and dyes, not elsewhere classified,** assault

√7ᵗʰ **T65.6X4 Toxic effect of paints and dyes, not elsewhere classified,** undetermined

√5ᵗʰ **T65.8 Toxic effect of** other specified substances

√6ᵗʰ **T65.81 Toxic effect of** latex

√7ᵗʰ **T65.811 Toxic effect of latex,** accidental (unintentional)
Toxic effect of latex NOS

√7ᵗʰ **T65.812 Toxic effect of latex,** intentional self-harm

√7ᵗʰ **T65.813 Toxic effect of latex,** assault

√7ᵗʰ **T65.814 Toxic effect of latex,** undetermined

√6ᵗʰ **T65.82 Toxic effect of harmful** algae **and algae toxins**
Toxic effect of (harmful) algae bloom NOS
Toxic effect of blue-green algae bloom
Toxic effect of brown tide
Toxic effect of cyanobacteria bloom
Toxic effect of Florida red tide
Toxic effect of pfiesteria piscicida
Toxic effect of red tide

√7ᵗʰ **T65.821 Toxic effect of harmful algae and algae toxins,** accidental (unintentional)
Toxic effect of harmful algae and algae toxins NOS

√7ᵗʰ **T65.822 Toxic effect of harmful algae and algae toxins,** intentional self-harm

√7ᵗʰ **T65.823 Toxic effect of harmful algae and algae toxins,** assault

√7ᵗʰ **T65.824 Toxic effect of harmful algae and algae toxins,** undetermined

√6ᵗʰ **T65.83 Toxic effect of** fiberglass

√7ᵗʰ **T65.831 Toxic effect of fiberglass,** accidental (unintentional)
Toxic effect of fiberglass NOS

√7ᵗʰ **T65.832 Toxic effect of fiberglass,** intentional self-harm

√7ᵗʰ **T65.833 Toxic effect of fiberglass,** assault

√7ᵗʰ **T65.834 Toxic effect of fiberglass,** undetermined

√6ᵗʰ **T65.89 Toxic effect of** other **specified substances**

√7ᵗʰ **T65.891 Toxic effect of other specified substances, accidental (unintentional)**
Toxic effect of other specified substances NOS

√7ᵗʰ **T65.892 Toxic effect of other specified substances, intentional self-harm**

√7ᵗʰ **T65.893 Toxic effect of other specified substances, assault**

√7ᵗʰ **T65.894 Toxic effect of other specified substances, undetermined**

√5ᵗʰ **T65.9 Toxic effect of** unspecified **substance**

√x7ᵗʰ **T65.91 Toxic effect of unspecified substance,** accidental (unintentional)
Poisoning NOS

√x7ᵗʰ **T65.92 Toxic effect of unspecified substance,** intentional self-harm

√x7ᵗʰ **T65.93 Toxic effect of unspecified substance,** assault

√x7ᵗʰ **T65.94 Toxic effect of unspecified substance,** undetermined

Other and unspecified effects of external causes (T66-T78)

√x7ᵗʰ **T66 Radiation sickness, unspecified**

EXCLUDES 1 specified adverse effects of radiation, such as:
burns (T20-T31)
leukemia (C91-C95)
radiation gastroenteritis and colitis (K52.0)
radiation pneumonitis (J70.0)
radiation related disorders of the skin and subcutaneous tissue (L55-L59)
radiation sunburn (L55.-)

The appropriate 7th character is to be added to code T66.
A   initial encounter
D   subsequent encounter
S   sequela

√4ᵗʰ **T67 Effects of heat and light**

EXCLUDES 1 erythema [dermatitis] ab igne (L59.0)
malignant hyperpyrexia due to anesthesia (T88.3)
radiation-related disorders of the skin and subcutaneous tissue (L55-L59)

EXCLUDES 2 burns (T20-T31)
sunburn (L55.-)
sweat disorder due to heat (L74-L75)

The appropriate 7th character is to be added to each code from category T67.
A   initial encounter
D   subsequent encounter
S   sequela

√x7ᵗʰ **T67.0 Heatstroke and sunstroke**
Heat apoplexy   Siriasis
Heat pyrexia   Thermoplegia
Use additional code(s) to identify any associated complications of heatstroke, such as:
coma and stupor (R40.-)
systemic inflammatory response syndrome (R65.1-)

√x7ᵗʰ **T67.1 Heat** syncope
Heat collapse

√x7ᵗʰ **T67.2 Heat** cramp

√x7ᵗʰ **T67.3 Heat exhaustion,** anhydrotic
Heat prostration due to water depletion
EXCLUDES 1 heat exhaustion due to salt depletion (T67.4)

√x7ᵗʰ **T67.4 Heat exhaustion** due to salt depletion
Heat prostration due to salt (and water) depletion

√x7ᵗʰ **T67.5 Heat exhaustion, unspecified**
Heat prostration NOS

√x7ᵗʰ **T67.6 Heat** fatigue, **transient**

√x7ᵗʰ **T67.7 Heat** edema

√x7ᵗʰ **T67.8 Other effects of heat and light**

√x7ᵗʰ **T67.9 Effect of heat and light, unspecified**

√x7ᵗʰ **T68 Hypothermia**
Accidental hypothermia   Hypothermia NOS
Use additional code to identify source of exposure:
exposure to excessive cold of man-made origin (W93)
exposure to excessive cold of natural origin (X31)
EXCLUDES 1 hypothermia following anesthesia (T88.51)
hypothermia not associated with low environmental temperature (R68.0)
hypothermia of newborn (P80.-)
EXCLUDES 2 frostbite (T33-T34)

The appropriate 7th character is to be added to code T68.
A   initial encounter
D   subsequent encounter
S   sequela

√4ᵗʰ **T69 Other effects of reduced temperature**
Use additional code to identify source of exposure:
exposure to excessive cold of man-made origin (W93)
exposure to excessive cold of natural origin (X31)
EXCLUDES 2 frostbite (T33-T34)

The appropriate 7th character is to be added to each code from category T69.
A   initial encounter
D   subsequent encounter
S   sequela

√5ᵗʰ **T69.0 Immersion hand and foot**

√6ᵗʰ **T69.01 Immersion** hand

√7ᵗʰ **T69.011 Immersion hand,** right **hand**

☑ Additional Character Required   √x7ᵗʰ Xtension Alert   Unspecified Dx   Other Specified Dx   Manifestation   ►◄ Revised Text   ● New Code   ▲ Revised Code Title

Injury, Poisoning and Certain Other Consequences of External Causes

T69.012–T71.221

    √7ᵗʰ **T69.012** **Immersion hand,** left **hand**

    √7ᵗʰ **T69.019** **Immersion hand, unspecified hand**

   √6ᵗʰ **T69.02** **Immersion** foot
      Trench foot

    √7ᵗʰ **T69.021** **Immersion foot,** right **foot**

    √7ᵗʰ **T69.022** **Immersion foot,** left **foot**

    √7ᵗʰ **T69.029** **Immersion foot, unspecified foot**

√x7ᵗʰ **T69.1** **Chilblains**

√x7ᵗʰ **T69.8** **Other specified effects of reduced temperature**

√x7ᵗʰ **T69.9** **Effect of reduced temperature, unspecified**

√4ᵗʰ **T70** **Effects of air pressure and water pressure**

> The appropriate 7th character is to be added to each code from category T70.
> A   initial encounter
> D   subsequent encounter
> S   sequela

√x7ᵗʰ **T70.0** **Otitic barotrauma**
     Aero-otitis media
     Effects of change in ambient atmospheric pressure or water pressure on ears

√x7ᵗʰ **T70.1** **Sinus barotrauma**
     Aerosinusitis
     Effects of change in ambient atmospheric pressure on sinuses

√5ᵗʰ **T70.2** **Other and unspecified effects of high altitude**
     EXCLUDES 2   polycythemia due to high altitude (D75.1)

   √x7ᵗʰ **T70.20** **Unspecified effects of high altitude**

   √x7ᵗʰ **T70.29** **Other effects of high altitude**
      Alpine sickness
      Anoxia due to high altitude
      Barotrauma NOS
      Hypobaropathy
      Mountain sickness

√x7ᵗʰ **T70.3** **Caisson disease [decompression sickness]**
     Compressed-air disease
     Diver's palsy or paralysis

√x7ᵗʰ **T70.4** **Effects of high-pressure fluids**
     Hydraulic jet injection (industrial)
     Pneumatic jet injection (industrial)
     Traumatic jet injection (industrial)

√x7ᵗʰ **T70.8** **Other effects of air pressure and water pressure**

√x7ᵗʰ **T70.9** **Effect of air pressure and water pressure, unspecified**

√4ᵗʰ **T71** **Asphyxiation**
     Mechanical suffocation
     Traumatic suffocation
     EXCLUDES 1   acute respiratory distress (syndrome) (J80)
             anoxia due to high altitude (T70.2)
             asphyxia NOS (R09.01)
             asphyxia from carbon monoxide (T58.-)
             asphyxia from inhalation of food or foreign body (T17.-)
             asphyxia from other gases, fumes and vapors (T59.-)
             respiratory distress (syndrome) in newborn (P22.-)

> The appropriate 7th character is to be added to each code from category T71.
> A   initial encounter
> D   subsequent encounter
> S   sequela

√5ᵗʰ **T71.1** **Asphyxiation due to** mechanical threat to breathing
     Suffocation due to mechanical threat to breathing

   √6ᵗʰ **T71.11** **Asphyxiation due to** smothering under pillow

    √7ᵗʰ **T71.111** **Asphyxiation due to smothering under pillow,** accidental
        Asphyxiation due to smothering under pillow NOS

    √7ᵗʰ **T71.112** **Asphyxiation due to smothering under pillow,** intentional self-harm

    √7ᵗʰ **T71.113** **Asphyxiation due to smothering under pillow,** assault

    √7ᵗʰ **T71.114** **Asphyxiation due to smothering under pillow,** undetermined

   √6ᵗʰ **T71.12** **Asphyxiation due to** plastic bag

    √7ᵗʰ **T71.121** **Asphyxiation due to plastic bag,** accidental
        Asphyxiation due to plastic bag NOS

    √7ᵗʰ **T71.122** **Asphyxiation due to plastic bag,** intentional self-harm

    √7ᵗʰ **T71.123** **Asphyxiation due to plastic bag,** assault

    √7ᵗʰ **T71.124** **Asphyxiation due to plastic bag,** undetermined

   √6ᵗʰ **T71.13** **Asphyxiation due to being** trapped in bed linens

    √7ᵗʰ **T71.131** **Asphyxiation due to being trapped in bed linens,** accidental
        Asphyxiation due to being trapped in bed linens NOS

    √7ᵗʰ **T71.132** **Asphyxiation due to being trapped in bed linens,** intentional self-harm

    √7ᵗʰ **T71.133** **Asphyxiation due to being trapped in bed linens,** assault

    √7ᵗʰ **T71.134** **Asphyxiation due to being trapped in bed linens,** undetermined

   √6ᵗʰ **T71.14** **Asphyxiation due to** smothering under another person's body **(in bed)**

    √7ᵗʰ **T71.141** **Asphyxiation due to smothering under another person's body (in bed),** accidental
        Asphyxiation due to smothering under another person's body (in bed) NOS

    √7ᵗʰ **T71.143** **Asphyxiation due to smothering under another person's body (in bed),** assault

    √7ᵗʰ **T71.144** **Asphyxiation due to smothering under another person's body (in bed),** undetermined

   √6ᵗʰ **T71.15** **Asphyxiation due to** smothering in furniture

    √7ᵗʰ **T71.151** **Asphyxiation due to smothering in furniture,** accidental
        Asphyxiation due to smothering in furniture NOS

    √7ᵗʰ **T71.152** **Asphyxiation due to smothering in furniture,** intentional self-harm

    √7ᵗʰ **T71.153** **Asphyxiation due to smothering in furniture,** assault

    √7ᵗʰ **T71.154** **Asphyxiation due to smothering in furniture,** undetermined

   √6ᵗʰ **T71.16** **Asphyxiation due to** hanging
      Hanging by window shade cord
      Use additional code for any associated injuries, such as:
        crushing injury of neck (S17.-)
        fracture of cervical vertebrae (S12.0-S12.2-)
        open wound of neck (S11.-)

    √7ᵗʰ **T71.161** **Asphyxiation due to hanging,** accidental
        Asphyxiation due to hanging NOS
        Hanging NOS

    √7ᵗʰ **T71.162** **Asphyxiation due to hanging,** intentional self-harm

    √7ᵗʰ **T71.163** **Asphyxiation due to hanging,** assault

    √7ᵗʰ **T71.164** **Asphyxiation due to hanging,** undetermined

   √6ᵗʰ **T71.19** **Asphyxiation due to mechanical threat to breathing** due to other causes

    √7ᵗʰ **T71.191** **Asphyxiation due to mechanical threat to breathing due to other causes,** accidental
        Asphyxiation due to other causes NOS

    √7ᵗʰ **T71.192** **Asphyxiation due to mechanical threat to breathing due to other causes,** intentional self-harm

    √7ᵗʰ **T71.193** **Asphyxiation due to mechanical threat to breathing due to other causes,** assault

    √7ᵗʰ **T71.194** **Asphyxiation due to mechanical threat to breathing due to other causes,** undetermined

√5ᵗʰ **T71.2** **Asphyxiation due to** systemic oxygen deficiency due to low oxygen content in ambient air
     Suffocation due to systemic oxygen deficiency due to low oxygen content in ambient air

   √x7ᵗʰ **T71.20** **Asphyxiation due to systemic oxygen deficiency due to low oxygen content in ambient air due to unspecified cause**

   √x7ᵗʰ **T71.21** **Asphyxiation due to** cave-in or falling earth
      Use additional code for any associated cataclysm (X34-X38)

   √6ᵗʰ **T71.22** **Asphyxiation due to** being trapped in a car trunk

    √7ᵗʰ **T71.221** **Asphyxiation due to being trapped in a car trunk,** accidental

EXCLUDES 1 Not coded here   EXCLUDES 2 Not included here   N Newborn Age: 0   P Pediatric Age: 0-17   M Maternity Age: 12-55   A Adult Age: 15-124

974   ICD-10-CM Draft (2015)

√7ᵗʰ **T71.222** **Asphyxiation due to being trapped in a car trunk,** intentional self-harm

√7ᵗʰ **T71.223** **Asphyxiation due to being trapped in a car trunk,** assault

√7ᵗʰ **T71.224** **Asphyxiation due to being trapped in a car trunk,** undetermined

√6ᵗʰ **T71.23** **Asphyxiation due to being** trapped in a (discarded) refrigerator

√7ᵗʰ **T71.231** **Asphyxiation due to being trapped in a (discarded) refrigerator,** accidental

√7ᵗʰ **T71.232** **Asphyxiation due to being trapped in a (discarded) refrigerator,** intentional self-harm

√7ᵗʰ **T71.233** **Asphyxiation due to being trapped in a (discarded) refrigerator,** assault

√7ᵗʰ **T71.234** **Asphyxiation due to being trapped in a (discarded) refrigerator,** undetermined

√x7ᵗʰ **T71.29** **Asphyxiation due to being trapped in other low oxygen environment**

√x7ᵗʰ **T71.9** **Asphyxiation due to unspecified cause**
Suffocation (by strangulation) due to unspecified cause
Suffocation NOS
Systemic oxygen deficiency due to low oxygen content in ambient air due to unspecified cause
Systemic oxygen deficiency due to mechanical threat to breathing due to unspecified cause
Traumatic asphyxia NOS

√4ᵗʰ **T73** **Effects of other deprivation**

The appropriate 7th character is to be added to each code from category T73.
A   initial encounter
D   subsequent encounter
S   sequela

√x7ᵗʰ **T73.0** **Starvation**
Deprivation of food

√x7ᵗʰ **T73.1** **Deprivation of water**

√x7ᵗʰ **T73.2** **Exhaustion due to exposure**

√x7ᵗʰ **T73.3** **Exhaustion due to excessive exertion**
Exhaustion due to overexertion

√x7ᵗʰ **T73.8** **Other effects of deprivation**

√x7ᵗʰ **T73.9** **Effect of deprivation, unspecified**

√4ᵗʰ **T74** **Adult and child abuse, neglect and other maltreatment, confirmed**
Use additional code, if applicable, to identify any associated current injury
Use additional external cause code to identify perpetrator, if known (Y07.-)
EXCLUDES 1 abuse and maltreatment in pregnancy (O9A.3-, O9A.4-, O9A.5-)
adult and child maltreatment, suspected (T76.-)

The appropriate 7th character is to be added to each code from category T74.
A   initial encounter
D   subsequent encounter
S   sequela

√5ᵗʰ **T74.0** **Neglect or abandonment, confirmed**

√x7ᵗʰ **T74.01** **Adult** neglect or abandonment, confirmed 🅐

√x7ᵗʰ **T74.02** **Child** neglect or abandonment, confirmed 🅟

√5ᵗʰ **T74.1** **Physical abuse, confirmed**
EXCLUDES 2 sexual abuse (T74.2-)

√x7ᵗʰ **T74.11** **Adult** physical abuse, confirmed 🅐

√x7ᵗʰ **T74.12** **Child** physical abuse, confirmed 🅟
EXCLUDES 2 shaken infant syndrome (T74.4)

√5ᵗʰ **T74.2** **Sexual abuse, confirmed**
Rape, confirmed
Sexual assault, confirmed

√x7ᵗʰ **T74.21** **Adult** sexual abuse, confirmed 🅐

√x7ᵗʰ **T74.22** **Child** sexual abuse, confirmed 🅟

√5ᵗʰ **T74.3** **Psychological abuse, confirmed**

√x7ᵗʰ **T74.31** **Adult** psychological abuse, confirmed 🅐

√x7ᵗʰ **T74.32** **Child** psychological abuse, confirmed 🅟

√x7ᵗʰ **T74.4** **Shaken infant syndrome** 🅟

√5ᵗʰ **T74.9** **Unspecified maltreatment, confirmed**

√x7ᵗʰ **T74.91** **Unspecified** adult maltreatment, confirmed 🅐

√x7ᵗʰ **T74.92** **Unspecified** child maltreatment, confirmed 🅟

√4ᵗʰ **T75** **Other and unspecified effects of other external causes**
EXCLUDES 1 adverse effects NEC (T78.-)
EXCLUDES 2 burns (electric) (T20-T31)

The appropriate 7th character is to be added to each code from category T75.
A   initial encounter
D   subsequent encounter
S   sequela

√5ᵗʰ **T75.0** **Effects of lightning**
Struck by lightning

√x7ᵗʰ **T75.00** **Unspecified effects of lightning**
Struck by lightning NOS

√x7ᵗʰ **T75.01** **Shock due to being struck by lightning**

√x7ᵗʰ **T75.09** **Other effects of lightning**
Use additional code for other effects of lightning

√x7ᵗʰ **T75.1** **Unspecified effects of drowning and nonfatal submersion**
Immersion
EXCLUDES 1 specified effects of drowning—code to effects

√5ᵗʰ **T75.2** **Effects of vibration**

√x7ᵗʰ **T75.20** **Unspecified effects of vibration**

√x7ᵗʰ **T75.21** **Pneumatic hammer syndrome**

√x7ᵗʰ **T75.22** **Traumatic vasospastic syndrome**

√x7ᵗʰ **T75.23** **Vertigo from infrasound**
EXCLUDES 1 vertigo NOS (R42)

√x7ᵗʰ **T75.29** **Other effects of vibration**

√x7ᵗʰ **T75.3** **Motion sickness**
Airsickness
Seasickness
Travel sickness
Use additional external cause code to identify vehicle or type of motion (Y92.81-, Y93.5-)

√x7ᵗʰ **T75.4** **Electrocution**
Shock from electric current
Shock from electroshock gun (taser)

√5ᵗʰ **T75.8** **Other specified effects of external causes**

√x7ᵗʰ **T75.81** **Effects of abnormal gravitation [G] forces**

√x7ᵗʰ **T75.82** **Effects of weightlessness**

√x7ᵗʰ **T75.89** **Other specified effects of external causes**

√4ᵗʰ **T76** **Adult and child abuse, neglect and other maltreatment, suspected**
Use additional code, if applicable, to identify any associated current injury
EXCLUDES 1 adult and child maltreatment, confirmed (T74.-)
suspected abuse and maltreatment in pregnancy (O9A.3-, O9A.4-, O9A.5-)
suspected adult physical abuse, ruled out (Z04.71)
suspected adult sexual abuse, ruled out (Z04.41)
suspected child physical abuse, ruled out (Z04.72)
suspected child sexual abuse, ruled out (Z04.42)

The appropriate 7th character is to be added to each code from category T76.
A   initial encounter
D   subsequent encounter
S   sequela

√5ᵗʰ **T76.0** **Neglect or abandonment, suspected**

√x7ᵗʰ **T76.01** **Adult** neglect or abandonment, suspected 🅐

√x7ᵗʰ **T76.02** **Child** neglect or abandonment, suspected 🅟

√5ᵗʰ **T76.1** **Physical abuse, suspected**

√x7ᵗʰ **T76.11** **Adult** physical abuse, suspected 🅐

√x7ᵗʰ **T76.12** **Child** physical abuse, suspected 🅟

√5ᵗʰ **T76.2** **Sexual abuse, suspected**
Rape, suspected
Sexual abuse, suspected
EXCLUDES 1 alleged abuse, ruled out (Z04.7)

√x7ᵗʰ **T76.21** **Adult** sexual abuse, suspected 🅐

√x7ᵗʰ **T76.22** **Child** sexual abuse, suspected 🅟

√5ᵗʰ **T76.3** **Psychological abuse, suspected**

√x7ᵗʰ **T76.31** **Adult** psychological abuse, suspected 🅐

√x7ᵗʰ **T76.32** **Child** psychological abuse, suspected 🅟

Injury, Poisoning and Certain Other Consequences of External Causes   T76.9–T79.A19

√5ᵗʰ **T76.9 Unspecified maltreatment, suspected**

     √x7ᵗʰ **T76.91 Unspecified adult maltreatment, suspected**   Ⓐ

     √x7ᵗʰ **T76.92 Unspecified child maltreatment, suspected**   Ⓟ

√4ᵗʰ **T78 Adverse effects, not elsewhere classified**

     EXCLUDES 2   *complications of surgical and medical care NEC (T80-T88)*

> The appropriate 7th character is to be added to each code from category T78.
> A   initial encounter
> D   subsequent encounter
> S   sequela

√5ᵗʰ **T78.0 Anaphylactic reaction due to food**

     Anaphylactic reaction due to adverse food reaction
     Anaphylactic shock or reaction due to nonpoisonous foods
     Anaphylactoid reaction due to food

     √x7ᵗʰ **T78.00 Anaphylactic reaction due to unspecified food**

     √x7ᵗʰ **T78.01 Anaphylactic reaction due to peanuts**

     √x7ᵗʰ **T78.02 Anaphylactic reaction due to shellfish (crustaceans)**

     √x7ᵗʰ **T78.03 Anaphylactic reaction due to other fish**

     √x7ᵗʰ **T78.04 Anaphylactic reaction due to fruits and vegetables**

     √x7ᵗʰ **T78.05 Anaphylactic reaction due to tree nuts and seeds**

         EXCLUDES 1   *anaphylactic reaction due to peanuts (T78.01)*

     √x7ᵗʰ **T78.06 Anaphylactic reaction due to food additives**

     √x7ᵗʰ **T78.07 Anaphylactic reaction due to milk and dairy products**

     √x7ᵗʰ **T78.08 Anaphylactic reaction due to eggs**

     √x7ᵗʰ **T78.09 Anaphylactic reaction due to other food products**

√x7ᵗʰ **T78.1 Other adverse food reactions, not elsewhere classified**

     Use additional code to identify the type of reaction

     EXCLUDES 1   *anaphylactic reaction or shock due to adverse food reaction (T78.0-)*
                 anaphylactic reaction due to food (T78.0-)
                 bacterial food borne intoxications (A05.-)

     EXCLUDES 2   *allergic and dietetic gastroenteritis and colitis (K52.2)*
                 allergic rhinitis due to food (J30.5)
                 dermatitis due to food in contact with skin (L23.6, L24.6, L25.4)
                 dermatitis due to ingested food (L27.2)

√x7ᵗʰ **T78.2 Anaphylactic shock, unspecified**

     Allergic shock
     Anaphylactic reaction
     Anaphylaxis

     EXCLUDES 1   *anaphylactic reaction or shock due to adverse effect of correct medicinal substance properly administered (T88.6)*
                 anaphylactic reaction or shock due to adverse food reaction (T78.0-)
                 anaphylactic reaction or shock due to serum (T80.5-)

√x7ᵗʰ **T78.3 Angioneurotic edema**

     Allergic angioedema
     Giant urticaria
     Quincke's edema

     EXCLUDES 1   *serum urticaria (T80.6-)*
                 urticaria (L50.-)

√5ᵗʰ **T78.4 Other and unspecified allergy**

     EXCLUDES 1   *specified types of allergic reaction such as:*
                 allergic diarrhea (K52.2)
                 allergic gastroenteritis and colitis (K52.2)
                 dermatitis (L23-L25, L27-)
                 hay fever (J30.1)

     √x7ᵗʰ **T78.40 Allergy, unspecified**

         Allergic reaction NOS
         Hypersensitivity NOS

     √x7ᵗʰ **T78.41 Arthus phenomenon**

         Arthus reaction

     √x7ᵗʰ **T78.49 Other allergy**

√x7ᵗʰ **T78.8 Other adverse effects, not elsewhere classified**

Certain early complications of trauma (T79)

√4ᵗʰ **T79 Certain early complications of trauma, not elsewhere classified**

     EXCLUDES 2   *acute respiratory distress syndrome (J80)*
                 complications occurring during or following medical procedures (T80-T88)
                 complications of surgical and medical care NEC (T80-T88)
                 newborn respiratory distress syndrome (P22.0)

> The appropriate 7th character is to be added to each code from category T79.
> A   initial encounter
> D   subsequent encounter
> S   sequela

√x7ᵗʰ **T79.0 Air embolism (traumatic)**

     EXCLUDES 1   *air embolism complicating abortion or ectopic or molar pregnancy (O00-O07, O08.2)*
                 air embolism complicating pregnancy, childbirth and the puerperium (O88.0)
                 air embolism following infusion, transfusion, and therapeutic injection (T80.0)
                 air embolism following procedure NEC (T81.7-)

√x7ᵗʰ **T79.1 Fat embolism (traumatic)**

     EXCLUDES 1   *fat embolism complicating:*
                 abortion or ectopic or molar pregnancy (O00-O07, O08.2)
                 pregnancy, childbirth and the puerperium (O88.8)

√x7ᵗʰ **T79.2 Traumatic secondary and recurrent hemorrhage and seroma**

√x7ᵗʰ **T79.4 Traumatic shock**

     Shock (immediate) (delayed) following injury

     EXCLUDES 1   *anaphylactic shock due to adverse food reaction (T78.0-)*
                 anaphylactic shock due to correct medicinal substance properly administered (T88.6)
                 anaphylactic shock due to serum (T80.5-)
                 anaphylactic shock NOS (T78.2)
                 anesthetic shock (T88.2)
                 electric shock (T75.4)
                 nontraumatic shock NEC (R57.-)
                 obstetric shock (O75.1)
                 postprocedural shock (T81.1-)
                 septic shock (R65.21)
                 shock complicating abortion or ectopic or molar pregnancy (O00-O07, O08.3)
                 shock due to lightning (T75.01)
                 shock NOS (R57.9)

√x7ᵗʰ **T79.5 Traumatic anuria**

     Crush syndrome
     Renal failure following crushing

√x7ᵗʰ **T79.6 Traumatic ischemia of muscle**

     Traumatic rhabdomyolysis
     Volkmann's ischemic contracture

     EXCLUDES 2   *anterior tibial syndrome (M76.8)*
                 compartment syndrome (traumatic) (T79.A-)
                 nontraumatic ischemia of muscle (M62.2-)

√x7ᵗʰ **T79.7 Traumatic subcutaneous emphysema**

     EXCLUDES 1   *emphysema NOS (J43)*
                 emphysema (subcutaneous) resulting from a procedure (T81.82)

√5ᵗʰ **T79.A Traumatic compartment syndrome**

     EXCLUDES 1   *fibromyalgia (M79.7)*
                 nontraumatic compartment syndrome (M79.A-)
                 traumatic ischemic infarction of muscle (T79.6)

     √x7ᵗʰ **T79.A0 Compartment syndrome, unspecified**

         Compartment syndrome NOS

     √6ᵗʰ **T79.A1 Traumatic compartment syndrome of upper extremity**

         Traumatic compartment syndrome of shoulder, arm, forearm, wrist, hand, and fingers

         √7ᵗʰ **T79.A11 Traumatic compartment syndrome of right upper extremity**

         √7ᵗʰ **T79.A12 Traumatic compartment syndrome of left upper extremity**

         √7ᵗʰ **T79.A19 Traumatic compartment syndrome of unspecified upper extremity**

EXCLUDES 1 Not coded here   EXCLUDES 2 Not included here   Ⓝ Newborn Age: 0   Ⓟ Pediatric Age: 0-17   Ⓜ Maternity Age: 12-55   Ⓐ Adult Age: 15-124

976   ICD-10-CM Draft (2015)

√6ᵗʰ **T79.A2 Traumatic compartment syndrome of** lower extremity

Traumatic compartment syndrome of hip, buttock, thigh, leg, foot, and toes

√7ᵗʰ **T79.A21 Traumatic compartment syndrome of** right **lower extremity**

√7ᵗʰ **T79.A22 Traumatic compartment syndrome of** left lower extremity

√7ᵗʰ **T79.A29 Traumatic compartment syndrome of unspecified lower extremity**

√x7ᵗʰ **T79.A3 Traumatic compartment syndrome of** abdomen

√x7ᵗʰ **T79.A9 Traumatic compartment syndrome of other sites**

√x7ᵗʰ **T79.8 Other early complications of trauma**

√x7ᵗʰ **T79.9 Unspecified early complication of trauma**

Complications of surgical and medical care, not elsewhere classified (T80-T88)

Use additional code for adverse effect, if applicable, to identify drug (T36-T50 with fifth or sixth character 5)

Use additional code(s) to identify the specified condition resulting from the complication

Use additional code to identify devices involved and details of circumstances (Y62-Y82)

EXCLUDES 2 *any encounters with medical care for postprocedural conditions in which no complications are present, such as:*
artificial opening status (Z93.-)
closure of external stoma (Z43.-)
fitting and adjustment of external prosthetic device (Z44.-)
burns and corrosions from local applications and irradiation (T20-T32)
complications of surgical procedures during pregnancy, childbirth and the puerperium (O00-O9A)
mechanical complication of respirator [ventilator] (J95.850)
poisoning and toxic effects of drugs and chemicals (T36-T65 with fifth or sixth character 1-4 or 6)
postprocedural fever (R50.82)
specified complications classified elsewhere, such as:
cerebrospinal fluid leak from spinal puncture (G97.0)
colostomy malfunction (K94.0-)
disorders of fluid and electrolyte imbalance (E86-E87)
functional disturbances following cardiac surgery (I97.0-I97.1)
intraoperative and postprocedural complications of specified body systems (D78.-, E36.-, E89.-, G97.3-, G97.4, H59.3-, H59.-, H95.2-, H95.3, I97.4-, I97.5, J95.6-, J95.7, K91.6-, L76.-, M96.-, N99.-)
ostomy complications (J95.0-, K94.-, N99.5-)
postgastric surgery syndromes (K91.1)
postlaminectomy syndrome NEC (M96.1)
postmastectomy lymphedema syndrome (I97.2)
postsurgical blind-loop syndrome (K91.2)
ventilator associated pneumonia (J95.851)

√4ᵗʰ **T80 Complications following infusion, transfusion and therapeutic injection**

INCLUDES complications following perfusion

EXCLUDES 2 *bone marrow transplant rejection (T86.01)*
febrile nonhemolytic transfusion reaction (R50.84)
fluid overload due to transfusion (E87.71)
posttransfusion purpura (D69.51)
transfusion associated circulatory overload (TACO) (E87.71)
transfusion (red blood cell) associated hemochromatosis (E83.111)
transfusion related acute lung injury (TRALI) (J95.84)

The appropriate 7th character is to be added to each code from category T80.
A   initial encounter
D   subsequent encounter
S   sequela

√x7ᵗʰ **T80.0** Air embolism **following infusion, transfusion and therapeutic injection**

√x7ᵗʰ **T80.1** Vascular complications **following infusion, transfusion and therapeutic injection**

Use additional code to identify the vascular complication

EXCLUDES 2 *extravasation of vesicant agent (T80.81-)*
infiltration of vesicant agent (T80.81-)
postprocedural vascular complications (T81.7-)
vascular complications specified as due to prosthetic devices, implants and grafts (T82.8-, T83.8, T84.8-, T85.8)

√5ᵗʰ **T80.2 Infections following infusion, transfusion and therapeutic injection**

Use additional code to identify the specific infection, such as: sepsis (A41.9)

Use additional code (R65.2-) to identify severe sepsis, if applicable

EXCLUDES 2 *infections specified as due to prosthetic devices, implants and grafts (T82.6-T82.7, T83.5-T83.6, T84.5-T84.7, T85.7)*
postprocedural infections (T81.4)

√6ᵗʰ **T80.21 Infection** due to central venous catheter

√7ᵗʰ **T80.211** Bloodstream infection **due to central venous catheter**

Catheter-related bloodstream infection (CRBSI) NOS

Central line-associated bloodstream infection (CLABSI)

Bloodstream infection due to Hickman catheter

Bloodstream infection due to peripherally inserted central catheter (PICC)

Bloodstream infection due to portacath (port-a-cath)

Bloodstream infection due to triple lumen catheter

Bloodstream infection due to umbilical venous catheter

√7ᵗʰ **T80.212** Local infection **due to central venous catheter**

Exit or insertion site infection

Local infection due to Hickman catheter

Local infection due to peripherally inserted central catheter (PICC)

Local infection due to portacath (port-a-cath)

Local infection due to triple lumen catheter

Local infection due to umbilical venous catheter

Port or reservoir infection

Tunnel infection

√7ᵗʰ **T80.218 Other infection due to central venous catheter**

Other central line-associated infection

Other infection due to Hickman catheter

Other infection due to peripherally inserted central catheter (PICC)

Other infection due to portacath (port-a-cath)

Other infection due to triple lumen catheter

Other infection due to umbilical venous catheter

√7ᵗʰ **T80.219 Unspecified infection due to central venous catheter**

Central line-associated infection NOS

Unspecified infection due to Hickman catheter

Unspecified infection due to peripherally inserted central catheter (PICC)

Unspecified infection due to portacath (port-a-cath)

Unspecified infection due to triple lumen catheter

Unspecified infection due to umbilical venous catheter

√x7ᵗʰ **T80.22 Acute infection following transfusion, infusion, or injection of blood and blood products**

√x7ᵗʰ **T80.29 Infection following other infusion, transfusion and therapeutic injection**

☑ Additional Character Required   √x7ᵗʰ Xtension Alert   Unspecified Dx   Other Specified Dx   Manifestation   ►◄ Revised Text   ● New Code   ▲ Revised Code Title

ICD-10-CM Draft (2015)   **977**

Injury, Poisoning and Certain Other Consequences of External Causes   T79.A2–T80.29

☑5ᵗʰ **T80.3** ABO incompatibility **reaction due to transfusion of blood or blood products**

> EXCLUDES 1   *minor blood group antigens reactions (Duffy) (E) (K(ell)) (Kidd) (Lewis) (M) (N) (P) (S) (T80.A)*

     ☑x7ᵗʰ **T80.30** **ABO incompatibility reaction due to transfusion of blood or blood products, unspecified**

> ABO incompatibility blood transfusion NOS
> Reaction to ABO incompatibility from transfusion NOS

     ☑6ᵗʰ **T80.31** **ABO incompatibility** with hemolytic transfusion reaction

         ☑7ᵗʰ **T80.310** **ABO incompatibility with** acute **hemolytic transfusion reaction**

> ABO incompatibility with hemolytic transfusion reaction less than 24 hours after transfusion
> Acute hemolytic transfusion reaction (AHTR) due to ABO incompatibility

         ☑7ᵗʰ **T80.311** **ABO incompatibility with** delayed **hemolytic transfusion reaction**

> ABO incompatibility with hemolytic transfusion reaction 24 hours or more after transfusion
> Delayed hemolytic transfusion reaction (DHTR) due to ABO incompatibility

         ☑7ᵗʰ **T80.319** **ABO incompatibility with hemolytic transfusion reaction, unspecified**

> ABO incompatibility with hemolytic transfusion reaction at unspecified time after transfusion
> Hemolytic transfusion reaction (HTR) due to ABO incompatibility NOS

     ☑x7ᵗʰ **T80.39** **Other ABO incompatibility reaction due to transfusion of blood or blood products**

> Delayed serologic transfusion reaction (DSTR) from ABO incompatibility
> Other ABO incompatible blood transfusion
> Other reaction to ABO incompatible blood transfusion

☑x7ᵗʰ **T80.4** Rh incompatibility **reaction due to transfusion of blood or blood products**

> Reaction due to incompatibility of Rh antigens (C) (c) (D) (E) (e)

     ☑x7ᵗʰ **T80.40** **Rh incompatibility reaction due to transfusion of blood or blood products, unspecified**

> Reaction due to Rh factor in transfusion NOS
> Rh incompatible blood transfusion NOS

     ☑6ᵗʰ **T80.41** **Rh incompatibility** with hemolytic transfusion reaction

         ☑7ᵗʰ **T80.410** **Rh incompatibility with** acute **transfusion reaction**

> Acute hemolytic transfusion reaction (AHTR) due to Rh incompatibility
> Rh incompatibility with hemolytic transfusion reaction less than 24 hours after transfusion

         ☑7ᵗʰ **T80.411** **Rh incompatibility with** delayed **hemolytic transfusion reaction**

> Delayed hemolytic transfusion reaction (DHTR) due to Rh incompatibility
> Rh incompatibility with hemolytic transfusion reaction 24 hours or more after transfusion

         ☑7ᵗʰ **T80.419** **Rh incompatibility with hemolytic transfusion reaction, unspecified**

> Hemolytic transfusion reaction (HTR) due to Rh incompatibility NOS
> Rh incompatibility with hemolytic transfusion reaction at unspecified time after transfusion

     ☑x7ᵗʰ **T80.49** **Other Rh incompatibility reaction due to transfusion of blood or blood products**

> Delayed serologic transfusion reaction (DSTR) from Rh incompatibility
> Other reaction to Rh incompatible blood transfusion

☑5ᵗʰ **T80.A** Non-ABO incompatibility **reaction due to transfusion of blood or blood products**

> Reaction due to incompatibility of minor antigens (Duffy) (Kell) (Kidd) (Lewis) (M) (N) (P) (S)

     ☑x7ᵗʰ **T80.A0** **Non-ABO incompatibility reaction due to transfusion of blood or blood products, unspecified**

> Non-ABO antigen incompatibility reaction from transfusion NOS

☑6ᵗʰ **T80.A1** **Non-ABO incompatibility** with hemolytic transfusion reaction

     ☑7ᵗʰ **T80.A10** **Non-ABO incompatibility with** acute **hemolytic transfusion reaction**

> Acute hemolytic transfusion reaction (AHTR) due to non-ABO incompatibility
> Non-ABO incompatibility with hemolytic transfusion reaction less than 24 hours after transfusion

     ☑7ᵗʰ **T80.A11** **Non-ABO incompatibility with** delayed **hemolytic transfusion reaction**

> Delayed hemolytic transfusion reaction (DHTR) due to non-ABO incompatibility
> Non-ABO incompatibility with hemolytic transfusion reaction 24 or more hours after transfusion

     ☑7ᵗʰ **T80.A19** **Non-ABO incompatibility with hemolytic transfusion reaction, unspecified**

> Hemolytic transfusion reaction (HTR) due to non-ABO incompatibility NOS
> Non-ABO incompatibility with hemolytic transfusion reaction at unspecified time after transfusion

☑x7ᵗʰ **T80.A9** **Other non-ABO incompatibility reaction due to transfusion of blood or blood products**

> Delayed serologic transfusion reaction (DSTR) from non-ABO incompatibility
> Other reaction to non-ABO incompatible blood transfusion

☑5ᵗʰ **T80.5** **Anaphylactic reaction due to serum**

> Allergic shock due to serum
> Anaphylactic shock due to serum
> Anaphylactoid reaction due to serum
> Anaphylaxis due to serum

> EXCLUDES 1   *ABO incompatibility reaction due to transfusion of blood or blood products (T80.3-)*
> *allergic reaction or shock NOS (T78.2)*
> *anaphylactic reaction or shock NOS (T78.2)*
> *anaphylactic reaction or shock due to adverse effect of correct medicinal substance properly administered (T88.6)*
> *other serum reaction (T80.6-)*

     ☑x7ᵗʰ **T80.51** **Anaphylactic reaction due to** administration of blood and blood products

     ☑x7ᵗʰ **T80.52** **Anaphylactic reaction due to** vaccination

     ☑x7ᵗʰ **T80.59** **Anaphylactic reaction due to other serum**

☑5ᵗʰ **T80.6** **Other serum reactions**

> Intoxication by serum
> Protein sickness
> Serum rash
> Serum sickness
> Serum urticaria

> EXCLUDES 2   *serum hepatitis (B16.-)*

     ☑x7ᵗʰ **T80.61** **Other serum reaction** due to administration of blood and blood products

     ☑x7ᵗʰ **T80.62** **Other serum reaction** due to vaccination

     ☑x7ᵗʰ **T80.69** **Other serum reaction due to other** serum

☑5ᵗʰ **T80.8** **Other complications following infusion, transfusion and therapeutic injection**

     ☑6ᵗʰ **T80.81** **Extravasation of vesicant agent**

> Infiltration of vesicant agent

         ☑7ᵗʰ **T80.810** **Extravasation of vesicant antineoplastic chemotherapy**

> Infiltration of vesicant antineoplastic chemotherapy

         ☑7ᵗʰ **T80.818** **Extravasation of other vesicant agent**

> Infiltration of other vesicant agent

     ☑x7ᵗʰ **T80.89** **Other complications following infusion, transfusion and therapeutic injection**

> Delayed serologic transfusion reaction (DSTR), unspecified incompatibility
> Use additional code to identify graft-versus-host reaction, if applicable, (D89.81-)

☑5ᵗʰ **T80.9** **Unspecified complication following infusion, transfusion and therapeutic injection**

     ☑x7ᵗʰ **T80.90** **Unspecified complication** following infusion and therapeutic injection

---

EXCLUDES 1 Not coded here   EXCLUDES 2 Not included here   Ⓝ Newborn Age: 0   Ⓟ Pediatric Age: 0-17   Ⓜ Maternity Age: 12-55   Ⓐ Adult Age: 15-124

978   ICD-10-CM Draft (2015)

✓6ᵗʰ **T80.91** Hemolytic transfusion reaction, unspecified incompatibility

  EXCLUDES 1 *ABO incompatibility with hemolytic transfusion reaction (T80.31-)*
     Non-ABO incompatibility with hemolytic transfusion reaction (T80.A1-)
     Rh incompatibility with hemolytic transfusion reaction (T80.41-)

 ✓7ᵗʰ **T80.910** Acute hemolytic transfusion reaction, unspecified incompatibility

 ✓7ᵗʰ **T80.911** Delayed hemolytic transfusion reaction, unspecified incompatibility

 ✓7ᵗʰ **T80.919** Hemolytic transfusion reaction, unspecified incompatibility, unspecified as acute or delayed
    Hemolytic transfusion reaction NOS

✓x7ᵗʰ **T80.92** Unspecified transfusion reaction
  Transfusion reaction NOS

✓4ᵗʰ **T81** **Complications of procedures, not elsewhere classified**

 Use additional code for adverse effect, if applicable, to identify drug (T36-T50 with fifth or sixth character 5)

 EXCLUDES 2 *complications following immunization (T88.0-T88.1)*
   complications following infusion, transfusion and therapeutic injection (T80.-)
   complications of transplanted organs and tissue (T86.-)
   specified complications classified elsewhere, such as:
    complication of prosthetic devices, implants and grafts (T82-T85)
    dermatitis due to drugs and medicaments (L23.3, L24.4, L25.1, L27.0-L27.1)
    endosseous dental implant failure (M27.6-)
    floppy iris syndrome (IFIS) (intraoperative) (H21.81)
    intraoperative and postprocedural complications of specific body system (D78.-, E36.-, E89.-, G97.3-, G97.4, H59.3-, H59.-, H95.2-, H95.3, I97.4-, I97.5, J95, K91.-, L76.-, M96.-, N99.-)
    ostomy complications (J95.0-, K94.-, N99.5-)
    plateau iris syndrome (post-iridectomy) (postprocedural) (H21.82)
    poisoning and toxic effects of drugs and chemicals (T36-T65 with fifth or sixth character 1-4 or 6)

 The appropriate 7th character is to be added to each code from category T81.
  A initial encounter
  D subsequent encounter
  S sequela

 ✓5ᵗʰ **T81.1** **Postprocedural shock**
  Shock during or resulting from a procedure, not elsewhere classified

  EXCLUDES 1 *anaphylactic shock due to correct substance properly administered (T88.6)*
    anaphylactic shock due to serum (T80.5-)
    anaphylactic shock NOS (T78.2)
    anesthetic shock (T88.2)
    electric shock (T75.4)
    obstetric shock (O75.1)
    septic shock (R65.21)
    shock following abortion or ectopic or molar pregnancy (O00-O07, O08.3)
    traumatic shock (T79.4)

  ✓x7ᵗʰ **T81.10** Postprocedural shock unspecified
   Collapse NOS during or resulting from a procedure, not elsewhere classified
   Postprocedural failure of peripheral circulation
   Postprocedural shock NOS

  ✓x7ᵗʰ **T81.11** Postprocedural cardiogenic shock

  ✓x7ᵗʰ **T81.12** Postprocedural septic shock
   Postprocedural endotoxic shock during or resulting from a procedure, not elsewhere classified
   Postprocedural gram-negative shock during or resulting from a procedure, not elsewhere classified
   Code first underlying infection
   Use additional code, to identify any associated acute organ dysfunction, if applicable

  ✓x7ᵗʰ **T81.19** Other postprocedural shock
   Postprocedural hypovolemic shock

✓5ᵗʰ **T81.3** **Disruption of wound, not elsewhere classified**
 Disruption of any suture materials or other closure methods

 EXCLUDES 1 *breakdown (mechanical) of permanent sutures (T85.612)*
   displacement of permanent sutures (T85.622)
   disruption of cesarean delivery wound (O90.0)
   disruption of perineal obstetric wound (O90.1)
   mechanical complication of permanent sutures NEC (T85.692)

 AHA: 2014, 1Q, 23

 ✓x7ᵗʰ **T81.30** Disruption of wound, unspecified
  Disruption of wound NOS

 ✓x7ᵗʰ **T81.31** Disruption of external operation (surgical) wound, not elsewhere classified
  Dehiscence of operation wound NOS
  Disruption of operation wound NOS
  Disruption or dehiscence of closure of cornea
  Disruption or dehiscence of closure of mucosa
  Disruption or dehiscence of closure of skin and subcutaneous tissue
  Full-thickness skin disruption or dehiscence
  Superficial disruption or dehiscence of operation wound

  EXCLUDES 1 *dehiscence of amputation stump (T87.81)*

 ✓x7ᵗʰ **T81.32** Disruption of internal operation (surgical) wound, not elsewhere classified
  Deep disruption or dehiscence of operation wound NOS
  Disruption or dehiscence of closure of internal organ or other internal tissue
  Disruption or dehiscence of closure of muscle or muscle flap
  Disruption or dehiscence of closure of ribs or rib cage
  Disruption or dehiscence of closure of skull or craniotomy
  Disruption or dehiscence of closure of sternum or sternotomy
  Disruption or dehiscence of closure of tendon or ligament
  Disruption or dehiscence of closure of superficial or muscular fascia

 ✓x7ᵗʰ **T81.33** Disruption of traumatic injury wound repair
  Disruption or dehiscence of closure of traumatic laceration (external) (internal)

 ✓x7ᵗʰ **T81.4** **Infection following a procedure**
  Intra-abdominal abscess following a procedure
  Postprocedural infection, not elsewhere classified
  Sepsis following a procedure
  Stitch abscess following a procedure
  Subphrenic abscess following a procedure
  Wound abscess following a procedure
  Use additional code to identify infection
  Use additional code (R65.2-) to identify severe sepsis, if applicable

  EXCLUDES 1 *obstetric surgical wound infection (O86.0)*
   postprocedural fever NOS (R50.82)
   postprocedural retroperitoneal abscess (K68.11)

  EXCLUDES 2 *bleb associated endophthalmitis (H59.4-)*
   infection due to infusion, transfusion and therapeutic injection (T80.2-)
   infection due to prosthetic devices, implants and grafts (T82.6-T82.7, T83.5-T83.6, T84.5-T84.7, T85.7)

  AHA: 2014, 1Q, 23

✓5ᵗʰ **T81.5** **Complications of foreign body accidentally left in body following procedure**

 ✓6ᵗʰ **T81.50** Unspecified complication of foreign body accidentally left in body following procedure

  ✓7ᵗʰ **T81.500** Unspecified complication of foreign body accidentally left in body following surgical operation

  ✓7ᵗʰ **T81.501** Unspecified complication of foreign body accidentally left in body following infusion or transfusion

  ✓7ᵗʰ **T81.502** Unspecified complication of foreign body accidentally left in body following kidney dialysis

  ✓7ᵗʰ **T81.503** Unspecified complication of foreign body accidentally left in body following injection or immunization

  ✓7ᵗʰ **T81.504** Unspecified complication of foreign body accidentally left in body following endoscopic examination

☑ Additional Character Required ✓x7ᵗʰ Xtension Alert Unspecified Dx Other Specified Dx Manifestation ►◄ Revised Text ● New Code ▲ Revised Code Title

ICD-10-CM Draft (2015)   **979**

Injury, Poisoning and Certain Other Consequences of External Causes

T81.505–T81.599

√7th **T81.505** **Unspecified complication of foreign body accidentally left in body following** heart catheterization

√7th **T81.506** **Unspecified complication of foreign body accidentally left in body following** aspiration, puncture or other catheterization

√7th **T81.507** **Unspecified complication of foreign body accidentally left in body following** removal of catheter or packing

√7th **T81.508** **Unspecified complication of foreign body accidentally left in body following other procedure**

√7th **T81.509** **Unspecified complication of foreign body accidentally left in body following unspecified procedure**

√6th **T81.51** Adhesions **due to foreign body accidentally left in body following procedure**

√7th **T81.510** **Adhesions due to foreign body accidentally left in body following** surgical operation

√7th **T81.511** **Adhesions due to foreign body accidentally left in body following** infusion or transfusion

√7th **T81.512** **Adhesions due to foreign body accidentally left in body following** kidney dialysis

√7th **T81.513** **Adhesions due to foreign body accidentally left in body following** injection or immunization

√7th **T81.514** **Adhesions due to foreign body accidentally left in body following** endoscopic examination

√7th **T81.515** **Adhesions due to foreign body accidentally left in body following** heart catheterization

√7th **T81.516** **Adhesions due to foreign body accidentally left in body following** aspiration, puncture or other catheterization

√7th **T81.517** **Adhesions due to foreign body accidentally left in body following** removal of catheter or packing

√7th **T81.518** **Adhesions due to foreign body accidentally left in body following other procedure**

√7th **T81.519** **Adhesions due to foreign body accidentally left in body following unspecified procedure**

√6th **T81.52** Obstruction **due to foreign body accidentally left in body following procedure**

√7th **T81.520** **Obstruction due to foreign body accidentally left in body following** surgical operation

√7th **T81.521** **Obstruction due to foreign body accidentally left in body following** infusion or transfusion

√7th **T81.522** **Obstruction due to foreign body accidentally left in body following** kidney dialysis

√7th **T81.523** **Obstruction due to foreign body accidentally left in body following** injection or immunization

√7th **T81.524** **Obstruction due to foreign body accidentally left in body following** endoscopic examination

√7th **T81.525** **Obstruction due to foreign body accidentally left in body following** heart catheterization

√7th **T81.526** **Obstruction due to foreign body accidentally left in body following** aspiration, puncture or other catheterization

√7th **T81.527** **Obstruction due to foreign body accidentally left in body following** removal of catheter or packing

√7th **T81.528** **Obstruction due to foreign body accidentally left in body following other procedure**

√7th **T81.529** **Obstruction due to foreign body accidentally left in body following unspecified procedure**

√6th **T81.53** Perforation **due to foreign body accidentally left in body following procedure**

√7th **T81.530** **Perforation due to foreign body accidentally left in body following** surgical operation

√7th **T81.531** **Perforation due to foreign body accidentally left in body following** infusion or transfusion

√7th **T81.532** **Perforation due to foreign body accidentally left in body following** kidney dialysis

√7th **T81.533** **Perforation due to foreign body accidentally left in body following** injection or immunization

√7th **T81.534** **Perforation due to foreign body accidentally left in body following** endoscopic examination

√7th **T81.535** **Perforation due to foreign body accidentally left in body following** heart catheterization

√7th **T81.536** **Perforation due to foreign body accidentally left in body following** aspiration, puncture or other catheterization

√7th **T81.537** **Perforation due to foreign body accidentally left in body following** removal of catheter or packing

√7th **T81.538** **Perforation due to foreign body accidentally left in body following other procedure**

√7th **T81.539** **Perforation due to foreign body accidentally left in body following unspecified procedure**

√6th **T81.59** Other **complications of foreign body accidentally left in body following procedure**

EXCLUDES 2   *obstruction or perforation due to prosthetic devices and implants intentionally left in body (T82.0-T82.5, T83.0-T83.4, T83.7, T84.0-T84.4, T85.0-T85.6)*

√7th **T81.590** **Other complications of foreign body accidentally left in body following** surgical operation

√7th **T81.591** **Other complications of foreign body accidentally left in body following** infusion or transfusion

√7th **T81.592** **Other complications of foreign body accidentally left in body following** kidney dialysis

√7th **T81.593** **Other complications of foreign body accidentally left in body following** injection or immunization

√7th **T81.594** **Other complications of foreign body accidentally left in body following** endoscopic examination

√7th **T81.595** **Other complications of foreign body accidentally left in body following** heart catheterization

√7th **T81.596** **Other complications of foreign body accidentally left in body following** aspiration, puncture or other catheterization

√7th **T81.597** **Other complications of foreign body accidentally left in body following** removal of catheter or packing

√7th **T81.598** **Other complications of foreign body accidentally left in body following other procedure**

√7th **T81.599** **Other complications of foreign body accidentally left in body following unspecified procedure**

EXCLUDES 1 Not coded here   EXCLUDES 2 Not included here   N Newborn Age: 0   P Pediatric Age: 0-17   M Maternity Age: 12-55   A Adult Age: 15-124

980   ICD-10-CM Draft (2015)

√5ᵗʰ **T81.6** **Acute reaction to foreign substance accidentally left during a procedure**
> EXCLUDES 2   *complications of foreign body accidentally left in body cavity or operation wound following procedure (T81.5-)*

√x7ᵗʰ **T81.60** **Unspecified acute reaction to foreign substance accidentally left during a procedure**

√x7ᵗʰ **T81.61** **Aseptic peritonitis** **due to foreign substance accidentally left during a procedure**
> Chemical peritonitis

√x7ᵗʰ **T81.69** **Other acute reaction to foreign substance accidentally left during a procedure**

√5ᵗʰ **T81.7** **Vascular complications following a procedure, not elsewhere classified**
> Air embolism following procedure NEC
> Phlebitis or thrombophlebitis resulting from a procedure
> EXCLUDES 1   *embolism complicating abortion or ectopic or molar pregnancy (O00-O07, O08.2)*
> *embolism complicating pregnancy, childbirth and the puerperium (O88.-)*
> *traumatic embolism (T79.0)*
> EXCLUDES 2   *embolism due to prosthetic devices, implants and grafts (T82.8-, T83.8, T84.8-, T85.8)*
> *embolism following infusion, transfusion and therapeutic injection (T80.0)*

√6ᵗʰ **T81.71** **Complication of artery following a procedure, not elsewhere classified**

√7ᵗʰ **T81.710** **Complication of mesenteric artery following a procedure, not elsewhere classified**

√7ᵗʰ **T81.711** **Complication of renal artery following a procedure, not elsewhere classified**

√7ᵗʰ **T81.718** **Complication of other artery following a procedure, not elsewhere classified**

√7ᵗʰ **T81.719** **Complication of unspecified artery following a procedure, not elsewhere classified**

√x7ᵗʰ **T81.72** **Complication of vein following a procedure, not elsewhere classified**

√5ᵗʰ **T81.8** **Other complications of procedures, not elsewhere classified**
> EXCLUDES 2   *hypothermia following anesthesia (T88.51)*
> *malignant hyperpyrexia due to anesthesia (T88.3)*

√x7ᵗʰ **T81.81** **Complication of inhalation therapy**

√x7ᵗʰ **T81.82** **Emphysema (subcutaneous) resulting from a procedure**

√x7ᵗʰ **T81.83** **Persistent postprocedural fistula**

√x7ᵗʰ **T81.89** **Other complications of procedures, not elsewhere classified**
> Use additional code to specify complication, such as: postprocedural delirium (F05)
> AHA: 2014, 1Q, 23

√x7ᵗʰ **T81.9** **Unspecified complication of procedure**

√4ᵗʰ **T82** **Complications of cardiac and vascular prosthetic devices, implants and grafts**
> EXCLUDES 2   *failure and rejection of transplanted organs and tissue (T86.-)*

> The appropriate 7th character is to be added to each code from category T82.
> A   initial encounter
> D   subsequent encounter
> S   sequela

√5ᵗʰ **T82.0** **Mechanical complication of heart valve prosthesis**
> Mechanical complication of artificial heart valve
> EXCLUDES 1   *mechanical complication of biological heart valve graft (T82.22-)*

√x7ᵗʰ **T82.01** **Breakdown (mechanical) of heart valve prosthesis**

√x7ᵗʰ **T82.02** **Displacement of heart valve prosthesis**
> Malposition of heart valve prosthesis

√x7ᵗʰ **T82.03** **Leakage of heart valve prosthesis**

√x7ᵗʰ **T82.09** **Other mechanical complication of heart valve prosthesis**
> Obstruction (mechanical) of heart valve prosthesis
> Perforation of heart valve prosthesis
> Protrusion of heart valve prosthesis

√5ᵗʰ **T82.1** **Mechanical complication of cardiac electronic device**

√6ᵗʰ **T82.11** **Breakdown (mechanical) of cardiac electronic device**

√7ᵗʰ **T82.110** **Breakdown (mechanical) of cardiac electrode**

√7ᵗʰ **T82.111** **Breakdown (mechanical) of cardiac pulse generator (battery)**

√7ᵗʰ **T82.118** **Breakdown (mechanical) of other cardiac electronic device**

√7ᵗʰ **T82.119** **Breakdown (mechanical) of unspecified cardiac electronic device**

√6ᵗʰ **T82.12** **Displacement of cardiac electronic device**
> Malposition of cardiac electronic device

√7ᵗʰ **T82.120** **Displacement of cardiac electrode**

√7ᵗʰ **T82.121** **Displacement of cardiac pulse generator (battery)**

√7ᵗʰ **T82.128** **Displacement of other cardiac electronic device**

√7ᵗʰ **T82.129** **Displacement of unspecified cardiac electronic device**

√6ᵗʰ **T82.19** **Other mechanical complication of cardiac electronic device**
> Leakage of cardiac electronic device
> Obstruction of cardiac electronic device
> Perforation of cardiac electronic device
> Protrusion of cardiac electronic device

√7ᵗʰ **T82.190** **Other mechanical complication of cardiac electrode**

√7ᵗʰ **T82.191** **Other mechanical complication of cardiac pulse generator (battery)**

√7ᵗʰ **T82.198** **Other mechanical complication of other cardiac electronic device**

√7ᵗʰ **T82.199** **Other mechanical complication of unspecified cardiac device**

√5ᵗʰ **T82.2** **Mechanical complication of coronary artery bypass graft and biological heart valve graft**
> EXCLUDES 1   *mechanical complication of artificial heart valve prosthesis (T82.0-)*

√6ᵗʰ **T82.21** **Mechanical complication of coronary artery bypass graft**

√7ᵗʰ **T82.211** **Breakdown (mechanical) of coronary artery bypass graft**

√7ᵗʰ **T82.212** **Displacement of coronary artery bypass graft**
> Malposition of coronary artery bypass graft

√7ᵗʰ **T82.213** **Leakage of coronary artery bypass graft**

√7ᵗʰ **T82.218** **Other mechanical complication of coronary artery bypass graft**
> Obstruction, mechanical of coronary artery bypass graft
> Perforation of coronary artery bypass graft
> Protrusion of coronary artery bypass graft

√6ᵗʰ **T82.22** **Mechanical complication of biological heart valve graft**

√7ᵗʰ **T82.221** **Breakdown (mechanical) of biological heart valve graft**

√7ᵗʰ **T82.222** **Displacement of biological heart valve graft**
> Malposition of biological heart valve graft

√7ᵗʰ **T82.223** **Leakage of biological heart valve graft**

√7ᵗʰ **T82.228** **Other mechanical complication of biological heart valve graft**
> Obstruction of biological heart valve graft
> Perforation of biological heart valve graft
> Protrusion of biological heart valve graft

√5ᵗʰ **T82.3** **Mechanical complication of other vascular grafts**

√6ᵗʰ **T82.31** **Breakdown (mechanical) of other vascular grafts**

√7ᵗʰ **T82.310** **Breakdown (mechanical) of aortic (bifurcation) graft (replacement)**

√7ᵗʰ **T82.311** **Breakdown (mechanical) of carotid arterial graft (bypass)**

√7ᵗʰ **T82.312** **Breakdown (mechanical) of femoral arterial graft (bypass)**

√7ᵗʰ **T82.318** **Breakdown (mechanical) of other vascular grafts**

√7ᵗʰ **T82.319** **Breakdown (mechanical) of unspecified vascular grafts**

✓6ᵗʰ **T82.32** Displacement of other vascular grafts
Malposition of other vascular grafts

  ✓7ᵗʰ **T82.320** Displacement of aortic (bifurcation) graft (replacement)

  ✓7ᵗʰ **T82.321** Displacement of carotid arterial graft (bypass)

  ✓7ᵗʰ **T82.322** Displacement of femoral arterial graft (bypass)

  ✓7ᵗʰ **T82.328** Displacement of other vascular grafts

  ✓7ᵗʰ **T82.329** Displacement of unspecified vascular grafts

✓6ᵗʰ **T82.33** Leakage of other vascular grafts

  ✓7ᵗʰ **T82.330** Leakage of aortic (bifurcation) graft (replacement)

  ✓7ᵗʰ **T82.331** Leakage of carotid arterial graft (bypass)

  ✓7ᵗʰ **T82.332** Leakage of femoral arterial graft (bypass)

  ✓7ᵗʰ **T82.338** Leakage of other vascular grafts

  ✓7ᵗʰ **T82.339** Leakage of unspecified vascular graft

✓6ᵗʰ **T82.39** Other mechanical complication of other vascular grafts
Obstruction (mechanical) of other vascular grafts
Perforation of other vascular grafts
Protrusion of other vascular grafts

  ✓7ᵗʰ **T82.390** Other mechanical complication of aortic (bifurcation) graft (replacement)

  ✓7ᵗʰ **T82.391** Other mechanical complication of carotid arterial graft (bypass)

  ✓7ᵗʰ **T82.392** Other mechanical complication of femoral arterial graft (bypass)

  ✓7ᵗʰ **T82.398** Other mechanical complication of other vascular grafts

  ✓7ᵗʰ **T82.399** Other mechanical complication of unspecified vascular grafts

✓5ᵗʰ **T82.4** Mechanical complication of vascular dialysis catheter
Mechanical complication of hemodialysis catheter
EXCLUDES 1   mechanical complication of intraperitoneal dialysis catheter (T85.62)

  ✓x7ᵗʰ **T82.41** Breakdown (mechanical) of vascular dialysis catheter

  ✓x7ᵗʰ **T82.42** Displacement of vascular dialysis catheter
Malposition of vascular dialysis catheter

  ✓x7ᵗʰ **T82.43** Leakage of vascular dialysis catheter

  ✓x7ᵗʰ **T82.49** Other complication of vascular dialysis catheter
Obstruction (mechanical) of vascular dialysis catheter
Perforation of vascular dialysis catheter
Protrusion of vascular dialysis catheter

✓5ᵗʰ **T82.5** Mechanical complication of other cardiac and vascular devices and implants
EXCLUDES 2   mechanical complication of epidural and subdural infusion catheter (T85.61)

✓6ᵗʰ **T82.51** Breakdown (mechanical) of other cardiac and vascular devices and implants

  ✓7ᵗʰ **T82.510** Breakdown (mechanical) of surgically created arteriovenous fistula

  ✓7ᵗʰ **T82.511** Breakdown (mechanical) of surgically created arteriovenous shunt

  ✓7ᵗʰ **T82.512** Breakdown (mechanical) of artificial heart

  ✓7ᵗʰ **T82.513** Breakdown (mechanical) of balloon (counterpulsation) device

  ✓7ᵗʰ **T82.514** Breakdown (mechanical) of infusion catheter

  ✓7ᵗʰ **T82.515** Breakdown (mechanical) of umbrella device

  ✓7ᵗʰ **T82.518** Breakdown (mechanical) of other cardiac and vascular devices and implants

  ✓7ᵗʰ **T82.519** Breakdown (mechanical) of unspecified cardiac and vascular devices and implants

✓6ᵗʰ **T82.52** Displacement of other cardiac and vascular devices and implants
Malposition of other cardiac and vascular devices and implants

  ✓7ᵗʰ **T82.520** Displacement of surgically created arteriovenous fistula

  ✓7ᵗʰ **T82.521** Displacement of surgically created arteriovenous shunt

  ✓7ᵗʰ **T82.522** Displacement of artificial heart

  ✓7ᵗʰ **T82.523** Displacement of balloon (counterpulsation) device

  ✓7ᵗʰ **T82.524** Displacement of infusion catheter

  ✓7ᵗʰ **T82.525** Displacement of umbrella device

  ✓7ᵗʰ **T82.528** Displacement of other cardiac and vascular devices and implants

  ✓7ᵗʰ **T82.529** Displacement of unspecified cardiac and vascular devices and implants

✓6ᵗʰ **T82.53** Leakage of other cardiac and vascular devices and implants

  ✓7ᵗʰ **T82.530** Leakage of surgically created arteriovenous fistula

  ✓7ᵗʰ **T82.531** Leakage of surgically created arteriovenous shunt

  ✓7ᵗʰ **T82.532** Leakage of artificial heart

  ✓7ᵗʰ **T82.533** Leakage of balloon (counterpulsation) device

  ✓7ᵗʰ **T82.534** Leakage of infusion catheter

  ✓7ᵗʰ **T82.535** Leakage of umbrella device

  ✓7ᵗʰ **T82.538** Leakage of other cardiac and vascular devices and implants

  ✓7ᵗʰ **T82.539** Leakage of unspecified cardiac and vascular devices and implants

✓6ᵗʰ **T82.59** Other mechanical complication of other cardiac and vascular devices and implants
Obstruction (mechanical) of other cardiac and vascular devices and implants
Perforation of other cardiac and vascular devices and implants
Protrusion of other cardiac and vascular devices and implants

  ✓7ᵗʰ **T82.590** Other mechanical complication of surgically created arteriovenous fistula

  ✓7ᵗʰ **T82.591** Other mechanical complication of surgically created arteriovenous shunt

  ✓7ᵗʰ **T82.592** Other mechanical complication of artificial heart

  ✓7ᵗʰ **T82.593** Other mechanical complication of balloon (counterpulsation) device

  ✓7ᵗʰ **T82.594** Other mechanical complication of infusion catheter

  ✓7ᵗʰ **T82.595** Other mechanical complication of umbrella device

  ✓7ᵗʰ **T82.598** Other mechanical complication of other cardiac and vascular devices and implants

  ✓7ᵗʰ **T82.599** Other mechanical complication of unspecified cardiac and vascular devices and implants

✓x7ᵗʰ **T82.6** Infection and inflammatory reaction due to cardiac valve prosthesis
Use additional code to identify infection

✓x7ᵗʰ **T82.7** Infection and inflammatory reaction due to other cardiac and vascular devices, implants and grafts
Use additional code to identify infection

✓5ᵗʰ **T82.8** Other specified complications of cardiac and vascular prosthetic devices, implants and grafts

✓6ᵗʰ **T82.81** Embolism of cardiac and vascular prosthetic devices, implants and grafts

  ✓7ᵗʰ **T82.817** Embolism of cardiac prosthetic devices, implants and grafts

  ✓7ᵗʰ **T82.818** Embolism of vascular prosthetic devices, implants and grafts

✓6ᵗʰ **T82.82** Fibrosis of cardiac and vascular prosthetic devices, implants and grafts

  ✓7ᵗʰ **T82.827** Fibrosis of cardiac prosthetic devices, implants and grafts

  ✓7ᵗʰ **T82.828** Fibrosis of vascular prosthetic devices, implants and grafts

✓6ᵗʰ **T82.83** Hemorrhage of cardiac and vascular prosthetic devices, implants and grafts

  ✓7ᵗʰ **T82.837** Hemorrhage of cardiac prosthetic devices, implants and grafts

  ✓7ᵗʰ **T82.838** Hemorrhage of vascular prosthetic devices, implants and grafts

EXCLUDES 1 Not coded here   *EXCLUDES 2* Not included here   N Newborn Age: 0   P Pediatric Age: 0-17   M Maternity Age: 12-55   A Adult Age: 15-124

982   ICD-10-CM Draft (2015)

√6ᵗʰ **T82.84** Pain from cardiac and vascular prosthetic devices, implants and grafts

    √7ᵗʰ **T82.847** Pain from cardiac prosthetic devices, implants and grafts

    √7ᵗʰ **T82.848** Pain from vascular prosthetic devices, implants and grafts

√6ᵗʰ **T82.85** Stenosis of cardiac and vascular prosthetic devices, implants and grafts

    √7ᵗʰ **T82.857** Stenosis of cardiac prosthetic devices, implants and grafts

    √7ᵗʰ **T82.858** Stenosis of vascular prosthetic devices, implants and grafts

√6ᵗʰ **T82.86** Thrombosis of cardiac and vascular prosthetic devices, implants and grafts

    √7ᵗʰ **T82.867** Thrombosis of cardiac prosthetic devices, implants and grafts

    √7ᵗʰ **T82.868** Thrombosis of vascular prosthetic devices, implants and grafts

√6ᵗʰ **T82.89** Other specified complication of cardiac and vascular prosthetic devices, implants and grafts

    √7ᵗʰ **T82.897** Other specified complication of cardiac prosthetic devices, implants and grafts

    √7ᵗʰ **T82.898** Other specified complication of vascular prosthetic devices, implants and grafts

√×7ᵗʰ **T82.9** Unspecified complication of cardiac and vascular prosthetic device, implant and graft

√4ᵗʰ **T83** **Complications of genitourinary prosthetic devices, implants and grafts**

    EXCLUDES 2 *failure and rejection of transplanted organs and tissue (T86.-)*

    The appropriate 7th character is to be added to each code from category T83.
    A   initial encounter
    D   subsequent encounter
    S   sequela

√5ᵗʰ **T83.0** Mechanical complication of urinary (indwelling) catheter

    EXCLUDES 2 *complications of stoma of urinary tract (N99.5-)*

   √6ᵗʰ **T83.01** Breakdown (mechanical) of urinary (indwelling) catheter

    √7ᵗʰ **T83.010** Breakdown (mechanical) of cystostomy catheter

    √7ᵗʰ **T83.018** Breakdown (mechanical) of other indwelling urethral catheter

   √6ᵗʰ **T83.02** Displacement of urinary (indwelling) catheter
      Malposition of urinary (indwelling) catheter

    √7ᵗʰ **T83.020** Displacement of cystostomy catheter

    √7ᵗʰ **T83.028** Displacement of other indwelling urethral catheter

   √6ᵗʰ **T83.03** Leakage of urinary (indwelling) catheter

    √7ᵗʰ **T83.030** Leakage of cystostomy catheter

    √7ᵗʰ **T83.038** Leakage of other indwelling urethral catheter

   √6ᵗʰ **T83.09** Other mechanical complication of urinary (indwelling) catheter
      Obstruction (mechanical) of urinary (indwelling) catheter
      Perforation of urinary (indwelling) catheter
      Protrusion of urinary (indwelling) catheter

    √7ᵗʰ **T83.090** Other mechanical complication of cystostomy catheter

    √7ᵗʰ **T83.098** Other mechanical complication of other indwelling urethral catheter

√5ᵗʰ **T83.1** Mechanical complication of other urinary devices and implants

   √6ᵗʰ **T83.11** Breakdown (mechanical) of other urinary devices and implants

    √7ᵗʰ **T83.110** Breakdown (mechanical) of urinary electronic stimulator device

    √7ᵗʰ **T83.111** Breakdown (mechanical) of urinary sphincter implant

    √7ᵗʰ **T83.112** Breakdown (mechanical) of urinary stent

    √7ᵗʰ **T83.118** Breakdown (mechanical) of other urinary devices and implants

√6ᵗʰ **T83.12** Displacement of other urinary devices and implants
    Malposition of other urinary devices and implants

   √7ᵗʰ **T83.120** Displacement of urinary electronic stimulator device

   √7ᵗʰ **T83.121** Displacement of urinary sphincter implant

   √7ᵗʰ **T83.122** Displacement of urinary stent

   √7ᵗʰ **T83.128** Displacement of other urinary devices and implants

√6ᵗʰ **T83.19** Other mechanical complication of other urinary devices and implants
    Leakage of other urinary devices and implants
    Obstruction (mechanical) of other urinary devices and implants
    Perforation of other urinary devices and implants
    Protrusion of other urinary devices and implants

   √7ᵗʰ **T83.190** Other mechanical complication of urinary electronic stimulator device

   √7ᵗʰ **T83.191** Other mechanical complication of urinary sphincter implant

   √7ᵗʰ **T83.192** Other mechanical complication of urinary stent

   √7ᵗʰ **T83.198** Other mechanical complication of other urinary devices and implants

√5ᵗʰ **T83.2** Mechanical complication of graft of urinary organ

   √×7ᵗʰ **T83.21** Breakdown (mechanical) of graft of urinary organ

   √×7ᵗʰ **T83.22** Displacement of graft of urinary organ
    Malposition of graft of urinary organ

   √×7ᵗʰ **T83.23** Leakage of graft of urinary organ

   √×7ᵗʰ **T83.29** Other mechanical complication of graft of urinary organ
    Obstruction (mechanical) of graft of urinary organ
    Perforation of graft of urinary organ
    Protrusion of graft of urinary organ

√5ᵗʰ **T83.3** Mechanical complication of intrauterine contraceptive device

   √×7ᵗʰ **T83.31** Breakdown (mechanical) of intrauterine contraceptive device ♀

   √×7ᵗʰ **T83.32** Displacement of intrauterine contraceptive device ♀
    Malposition of intrauterine contraceptive device

   √×7ᵗʰ **T83.39** Other mechanical complication of intrauterine contraceptive device ♀
    Leakage of intrauterine contraceptive device
    Obstruction (mechanical) of intrauterine contraceptive device
    Perforation of intrauterine contraceptive device
    Protrusion of intrauterine contraceptive device

√5ᵗʰ **T83.4** Mechanical complication of other prosthetic devices, implants and grafts of genital tract

   √6ᵗʰ **T83.41** Breakdown (mechanical) of other prosthetic devices, implants and grafts of genital tract

    √7ᵗʰ **T83.410** Breakdown (mechanical) of penile (implanted) prosthesis ♂

    √7ᵗʰ **T83.418** Breakdown (mechanical) of other prosthetic devices, implants and grafts of genital tract

   √6ᵗʰ **T83.42** Displacement of other prosthetic devices, implants and grafts of genital tract
    Malposition of other prosthetic devices, implants and grafts of genital tract

    √7ᵗʰ **T83.420** Displacement of penile (implanted) prosthesis ♂

    √7ᵗʰ **T83.428** Displacement of other prosthetic devices, implants and grafts of genital tract

   √6ᵗʰ **T83.49** Other mechanical complication of other prosthetic devices, implants and grafts of genital tract
    Leakage of other prosthetic devices, implants and grafts of genital tract
    Obstruction, mechanical of other prosthetic devices, implants and grafts of genital tract
    Perforation of other prosthetic devices, implants and grafts of genital tract
    Protrusion of other prosthetic devices, implants and grafts of genital tract

    √7ᵗʰ **T83.490** Other mechanical complication of penile (implanted) prosthesis ♂

    √7ᵗʰ **T83.498** Other mechanical complication of other prosthetic devices, implants and grafts of genital tract

---

✔ Additional Character Required   √×7ᵗʰ Xtension Alert   Unspecified Dx   Other Specified Dx   Manifestation   ►◄ Revised Text   ● New Code   ▲ Revised Code Title

ICD-10-CM Draft (2015)

983

√5ᵗʰ **T83.5** **Infection and inflammatory reaction due to prosthetic device, implant and graft in** urinary system
Use additional code to identify infection

√x7ᵗʰ **T83.51** **Infection and inflammatory reaction due to** indwelling urinary catheter
EXCLUDES 2 *complications of stoma of urinary tract (N99.5-)*

√x7ᵗʰ **T83.59** **Infection and inflammatory reaction due to** prosthetic device, implant and graft in urinary system

√x7ᵗʰ **T83.6** **Infection and inflammatory reaction due to prosthetic device, implant and graft in** genital tract
Use additional code to identify infection

√5ᵗʰ **T83.7** **Complications due to** implanted mesh and other prosthetic materials

√6ᵗʰ **T83.71** Erosion **of implanted mesh and other prosthetic materials to surrounding organ or tissue**

√7ᵗʰ **T83.711** **Erosion of implanted** vaginal **mesh and other prosthetic materials to surrounding organ or tissue** ♀
Erosion of implanted vaginal mesh and other prosthetic materials into pelvic floor muscles

√7ᵗʰ **T83.718** **Erosion of other implanted mesh and other prosthetic materials to surrounding organ or tissue**

√6ᵗʰ **T83.72** Exposure **of implanted mesh and other prosthetic materials into surrounding organ or tissue**

√7ᵗʰ **T83.721** **Exposure of implanted** vaginal **mesh and other prosthetic materials into** vagina ♀
Exposure of implanted vaginal mesh and other prosthetic materials through vaginal wall

√7ᵗʰ **T83.728** **Exposure of** other **implanted mesh and other prosthetic materials to surrounding organ or tissue**

√5ᵗʰ **T83.8** **Other specified complications of** genitourinary prosthetic devices, implants and grafts

√x7ᵗʰ **T83.81** Embolism **of genitourinary prosthetic devices, implants and grafts**

√x7ᵗʰ **T83.82** Fibrosis **of genitourinary prosthetic devices, implants and grafts**

√x7ᵗʰ **T83.83** Hemorrhage **of genitourinary prosthetic devices, implants and grafts**

√x7ᵗʰ **T83.84** Pain **from genitourinary prosthetic devices, implants and grafts**

√x7ᵗʰ **T83.85** Stenosis **of genitourinary prosthetic devices, implants and grafts**

√x7ᵗʰ **T83.86** Thrombosis **of genitourinary prosthetic devices, implants and grafts**

√x7ᵗʰ **T83.89** **Other specified complication of genitourinary prosthetic devices, implants and grafts**

√x7ᵗʰ **T83.9** **Unspecified complication of genitourinary prosthetic device, implant and graft**

√4ᵗʰ **T84** **Complications of internal orthopedic prosthetic devices, implants and grafts**
EXCLUDES 2 *failure and rejection of transplanted organs and tissues (T86.-)*
fracture of bone following insertion of orthopedic implant, joint prosthesis or bone plate (M96.6)

The appropriate 7th character is to be added to each code from category T84.
A   initial encounter
D   subsequent encounter
S   sequela

√5ᵗʰ **T84.0** **Mechanical complication of** internal joint prosthesis

√6ᵗʰ **T84.01** Broken **internal joint prosthesis**
Breakage (fracture) of prosthetic joint
Broken prosthetic joint implant
EXCLUDES 1 *periprosthetic joint implant fracture (T84.04)*

√7ᵗʰ **T84.010** **Broken internal** right hip **prosthesis**
√7ᵗʰ **T84.011** **Broken internal** left hip **prosthesis**
√7ᵗʰ **T84.012** **Broken internal** right knee **prosthesis**
√7ᵗʰ **T84.013** **Broken internal** left knee **prosthesis**

√7ᵗʰ **T84.018** **Broken internal joint prosthesis, other site**
Use additional code to identify the joint (Z96.-)

√7ᵗʰ **T84.019** **Broken internal joint prosthesis, unspecified site**

√6ᵗʰ **T84.02** Dislocation **of internal joint prosthesis**
Instability of internal joint prosthesis
Subluxation of internal joint prosthesis

√7ᵗʰ **T84.020** **Dislocation of internal** right hip **prosthesis**
√7ᵗʰ **T84.021** **Dislocation of internal** left hip **prosthesis**
√7ᵗʰ **T84.022** Instability **of internal** right knee **prosthesis**
√7ᵗʰ **T84.023** Instability **of internal** left knee **prosthesis**
√7ᵗʰ **T84.028** **Dislocation of other internal joint prosthesis**
Use additional code to identify the joint (Z96.6-)
√7ᵗʰ **T84.029** **Dislocation of unspecified internal joint prosthesis**

√6ᵗʰ **T84.03** Mechanical loosening **of internal prosthetic joint**
Aseptic loosening of prosthetic joint

√7ᵗʰ **T84.030** **Mechanical loosening of internal** right hip **prosthetic joint**
√7ᵗʰ **T84.031** **Mechanical loosening of internal** left hip **prosthetic joint**
√7ᵗʰ **T84.032** **Mechanical loosening of internal** right knee **prosthetic joint**
√7ᵗʰ **T84.033** **Mechanical loosening of internal** left knee **prosthetic joint**
√7ᵗʰ **T84.038** **Mechanical loosening of other internal prosthetic joint**
Use additional code to identify the joint (Z96.6-)
√7ᵗʰ **T84.039** **Mechanical loosening of unspecified internal prosthetic joint**

√6ᵗʰ **T84.04** Periprosthetic fracture **around internal prosthetic joint**
EXCLUDES 2 *breakage (fracture) of prosthetic joint (T84.01)*

√7ᵗʰ **T84.040** **Periprosthetic fracture around internal prosthetic** right hip joint
√7ᵗʰ **T84.041** **Periprosthetic fracture around internal prosthetic** left hip joint
√7ᵗʰ **T84.042** **Periprosthetic fracture around internal prosthetic** right knee joint
√7ᵗʰ **T84.043** **Periprosthetic fracture around internal prosthetic** left knee joint
√7ᵗʰ **T84.048** **Periprosthetic fracture around other internal prosthetic joint**
Use additional code to identify the joint (Z96.6-)
√7ᵗʰ **T84.049** **Periprosthetic fracture around unspecified internal prosthetic joint**

√6ᵗʰ **T84.05** Periprosthetic osteolysis **of internal prosthetic joint**
Use additional code to identify major osseous defect, if applicable (M89.7-)

√7ᵗʰ **T84.050** **Periprosthetic osteolysis of internal prosthetic** right hip joint
√7ᵗʰ **T84.051** **Periprosthetic osteolysis of internal prosthetic** left hip joint
√7ᵗʰ **T84.052** **Periprosthetic osteolysis of internal prosthetic** right knee joint
√7ᵗʰ **T84.053** **Periprosthetic osteolysis of internal prosthetic** left knee joint
√7ᵗʰ **T84.058** **Periprosthetic osteolysis of other internal prosthetic joint**
Use additional code to identify the joint (Z96.6-)
√7ᵗʰ **T84.059** **Periprosthetic osteolysis of unspecified internal prosthetic joint**

√6ᵗʰ **T84.06** Wear of articular bearing surface **of internal prosthetic joint**

√7ᵗʰ **T84.060** **Wear of articular bearing surface of internal prosthetic** right hip joint
√7ᵗʰ **T84.061** **Wear of articular bearing surface of internal prosthetic** left hip joint

---

EXCLUDES 1 Not coded here   EXCLUDES 2 Not included here   N Newborn Age: 0   P Pediatric Age: 0-17   M Maternity Age: 12-55   A Adult Age: 15-124

984   ICD-10-CM Draft (2015)

√7ᵗʰ **T84.062** Wear of articular bearing surface of internal prosthetic right knee joint

√7ᵗʰ **T84.063** Wear of articular bearing surface of internal prosthetic left knee joint

√7ᵗʰ **T84.068** Wear of articular bearing surface of other internal prosthetic joint
Use additional code to identify the joint (Z96.6-)

√7ᵗʰ **T84.069** Wear of articular bearing surface of unspecified internal prosthetic joint

√6ᵗʰ **T84.09** Other mechanical complication of internal joint prosthesis
Prosthetic joint implant failure NOS

√7ᵗʰ **T84.090** Other mechanical complication of internal right hip prosthesis

√7ᵗʰ **T84.091** Other mechanical complication of internal left hip prosthesis

√7ᵗʰ **T84.092** Other mechanical complication of internal right knee prosthesis

√7ᵗʰ **T84.093** Other mechanical complication of internal left knee prosthesis

√7ᵗʰ **T84.098** Other mechanical complication of other internal joint prosthesis
Use additional code to identify the joint (Z96.6-)

√7ᵗʰ **T84.099** Other mechanical complication of unspecified internal joint prosthesis

√5ᵗʰ **T84.1** Mechanical complication of internal fixation device of bones of limb
EXCLUDES 2   *mechanical complication of internal fixation device of bones of feet (T84.2-)*
mechanical complication of internal fixation device of bones of fingers (T84.2-)
mechanical complication of internal fixation device of bones of hands (T84.2-)
mechanical complication of internal fixation device of bones of toes (T84.2-)

√6ᵗʰ **T84.11** Breakdown (mechanical) of internal fixation device of bones of limb

√7ᵗʰ **T84.110** Breakdown (mechanical) of internal fixation device of right humerus

√7ᵗʰ **T84.111** Breakdown (mechanical) of internal fixation device of left humerus

√7ᵗʰ **T84.112** Breakdown (mechanical) of internal fixation device of bone of right forearm

√7ᵗʰ **T84.113** Breakdown (mechanical) of internal fixation device of bone of left forearm

√7ᵗʰ **T84.114** Breakdown (mechanical) of internal fixation device of right femur

√7ᵗʰ **T84.115** Breakdown (mechanical) of internal fixation device of left femur

√7ᵗʰ **T84.116** Breakdown (mechanical) of internal fixation device of bone of right lower leg

√7ᵗʰ **T84.117** Breakdown (mechanical) of internal fixation device of bone of left lower leg

√7ᵗʰ **T84.119** Breakdown (mechanical) of internal fixation device of unspecified bone of limb

√6ᵗʰ **T84.12** Displacement of internal fixation device of bones of limb
Malposition of internal fixation device of bones of limb

√7ᵗʰ **T84.120** Displacement of internal fixation device of right humerus

√7ᵗʰ **T84.121** Displacement of internal fixation device of left humerus

√7ᵗʰ **T84.122** Displacement of internal fixation device of bone of right forearm

√7ᵗʰ **T84.123** Displacement of internal fixation device of bone of left forearm

√7ᵗʰ **T84.124** Displacement of internal fixation device of right femur

√7ᵗʰ **T84.125** Displacement of internal fixation device of left femur

√7ᵗʰ **T84.126** Displacement of internal fixation device of bone of right lower leg

√7ᵗʰ **T84.127** Displacement of internal fixation device of bone of left lower leg

√7ᵗʰ **T84.129** Displacement of internal fixation device of unspecified bone of limb

√6ᵗʰ **T84.19** Other mechanical complication of internal fixation device of bones of limb
Obstruction (mechanical) of internal fixation device of bones of limb
Perforation of internal fixation device of bones of limb
Protrusion of internal fixation device of bones of limb

√7ᵗʰ **T84.190** Other mechanical complication of internal fixation device of right humerus

√7ᵗʰ **T84.191** Other mechanical complication of internal fixation device of left humerus

√7ᵗʰ **T84.192** Other mechanical complication of internal fixation device of bone of right forearm

√7ᵗʰ **T84.193** Other mechanical complication of internal fixation device of bone of left forearm

√7ᵗʰ **T84.194** Other mechanical complication of internal fixation device of right femur

√7ᵗʰ **T84.195** Other mechanical complication of internal fixation device of left femur

√7ᵗʰ **T84.196** Other mechanical complication of internal fixation device of bone of right lower leg

√7ᵗʰ **T84.197** Other mechanical complication of internal fixation device of bone of left lower leg

√7ᵗʰ **T84.199** Other mechanical complication of internal fixation device of unspecified bone of limb

√5ᵗʰ **T84.2** Mechanical complication of internal fixation device of other bones

√6ᵗʰ **T84.21** Breakdown (mechanical) of internal fixation device of other bones

√7ᵗʰ **T84.210** Breakdown (mechanical) of internal fixation device of bones of hand and fingers

√7ᵗʰ **T84.213** Breakdown (mechanical) of internal fixation device of bones of foot and toes

√7ᵗʰ **T84.216** Breakdown (mechanical) of internal fixation device of vertebrae

√7ᵗʰ **T84.218** Breakdown (mechanical) of internal fixation device of other bones

√6ᵗʰ **T84.22** Displacement of internal fixation device of other bones
Malposition of internal fixation device of other bones

√7ᵗʰ **T84.220** Displacement of internal fixation device of bones of hand and fingers

√7ᵗʰ **T84.223** Displacement of internal fixation device of bones of foot and toes

√7ᵗʰ **T84.226** Displacement of internal fixation device of vertebrae

√7ᵗʰ **T84.228** Displacement of internal fixation device of other bones

√6ᵗʰ **T84.29** Other mechanical complication of internal fixation device of other bones
Obstruction (mechanical) of internal fixation device of other bones
Perforation of internal fixation device of other bones
Protrusion of internal fixation device of other bones

√7ᵗʰ **T84.290** Other mechanical complication of internal fixation device of bones of hand and fingers

√7ᵗʰ **T84.293** Other mechanical complication of internal fixation device of bones of foot and toes

√7ᵗʰ **T84.296** Other mechanical complication of internal fixation device of vertebrae

√7ᵗʰ **T84.298** Other mechanical complication of internal fixation device of other bones

√5ᵗʰ **T84.3** Mechanical complication of other bone devices, implants and grafts
EXCLUDES 2   *other complications of bone graft (T86.83-)*

√6ᵗʰ **T84.31** Breakdown (mechanical) of other bone devices, implants and grafts

√7ᵗʰ **T84.310** Breakdown (mechanical) of electronic bone stimulator

√7ᵗʰ **T84.318** Breakdown (mechanical) of other bone devices, implants and grafts

√6ᵗʰ **T84.32** Displacement of other bone devices, implants and grafts
Malposition of other bone devices, implants and grafts

☑ Additional Character Required   √ₓ7ᵗʰ Xtension Alert   Unspecified Dx   Other Specified Dx   Manifestation   ►◄ Revised Text   ● New Code   ▲ Revised Code Title

Injury, Poisoning and Certain Other Consequences of External Causes

T84.320–T85.09

√7ᵗʰ **T84.320** **Displacement of** electronic bone stimulator

√7ᵗʰ **T84.328** **Displacement of other bone devices, implants and grafts**

√6ᵗʰ **T84.39** Other **mechanical complication of other bone devices, implants and grafts**
Obstruction (mechanical) of other bone devices, implants and grafts
Perforation of other bone devices, implants and grafts
Protrusion of other bone devices, implants and grafts

√7ᵗʰ **T84.390** **Other mechanical complication of** electronic bone stimulator

√7ᵗʰ **T84.398** **Other mechanical complication of other bone devices, implants and grafts**

√5ᵗʰ **T84.4** **Mechanical complication of** other internal orthopedic devices, implants and grafts

√6ᵗʰ **T84.41** Breakdown **(mechanical) of other internal orthopedic devices, implants and grafts**

√7ᵗʰ **T84.410** **Breakdown (mechanical) of** muscle and tendon graft

√7ᵗʰ **T84.418** **Breakdown (mechanical) of other internal orthopedic devices, implants and grafts**

√6ᵗʰ **T84.42** Displacement **of other internal orthopedic devices, implants and grafts**
Malposition of other internal orthopedic devices, implants and grafts

√7ᵗʰ **T84.420** **Displacement of** muscle and tendon graft

√7ᵗʰ **T84.428** **Displacement of other internal orthopedic devices, implants and grafts**

√6ᵗʰ **T84.49** Other **mechanical complication of other internal orthopedic devices, implants and grafts**
Mechanical complication of other internal orthopedic devices, implants and grafts NOS
Obstruction (mechanical) of other internal orthopedic devices, implants and grafts
Perforation of other internal orthopedic devices, implants and grafts
Protrusion of other internal orthopedic devices, implants and grafts

√7ᵗʰ **T84.490** **Other mechanical complication of** muscle and tendon graft

√7ᵗʰ **T84.498** **Other mechanical complication of other internal orthopedic devices, implants and grafts**

√5ᵗʰ **T84.5** **Infection and inflammatory reaction due to** internal joint prosthesis
Use additional code to identify infection

√x7ᵗʰ **T84.50** **Infection and inflammatory reaction due to unspecified internal joint prosthesis**

√x7ᵗʰ **T84.51** **Infection and inflammatory reaction due to internal** right hip **prosthesis**

√x7ᵗʰ **T84.52** **Infection and inflammatory reaction due to internal** left hip **prosthesis**

√x7ᵗʰ **T84.53** **Infection and inflammatory reaction due to internal** right knee **prosthesis**

√x7ᵗʰ **T84.54** **Infection and inflammatory reaction due to internal** left knee **prosthesis**

√x7ᵗʰ **T84.59** **Infection and inflammatory reaction due to other internal joint prosthesis**

√5ᵗʰ **T84.6** **Infection and inflammatory reaction due to** internal fixation device
Use additional code to identify infection

√x7ᵗʰ **T84.60** **Infection and inflammatory reaction due to internal fixation device of unspecified site**

√6ᵗʰ **T84.61** **Infection and inflammatory reaction due to internal fixation device of** arm

√7ᵗʰ **T84.610** **Infection and inflammatory reaction due to internal fixation device of** right humerus

√7ᵗʰ **T84.611** **Infection and inflammatory reaction due to internal fixation device of** left humerus

√7ᵗʰ **T84.612** **Infection and inflammatory reaction due to internal fixation device of** right radius

√7ᵗʰ **T84.613** **Infection and inflammatory reaction due to internal fixation device of** left radius

√7ᵗʰ **T84.614** **Infection and inflammatory reaction due to internal fixation device of** right ulna

√7ᵗʰ **T84.615** **Infection and inflammatory reaction due to internal fixation device of** left ulna

√7ᵗʰ **T84.619** **Infection and inflammatory reaction due to internal fixation device of unspecified** bone **of arm**

√6ᵗʰ **T84.62** **Infection and inflammatory reaction due to internal fixation device of** leg

√7ᵗʰ **T84.620** **Infection and inflammatory reaction due to internal fixation device of** right femur

√7ᵗʰ **T84.621** **Infection and inflammatory reaction due to internal fixation device of** left femur

√7ᵗʰ **T84.622** **Infection and inflammatory reaction due to internal fixation device of** right tibia

√7ᵗʰ **T84.623** **Infection and inflammatory reaction due to internal fixation device of** left tibia

√7ᵗʰ **T84.624** **Infection and inflammatory reaction due to internal fixation device of** right fibula

√7ᵗʰ **T84.625** **Infection and inflammatory reaction due to internal fixation device of** left fibula

√7ᵗʰ **T84.629** **Infection and inflammatory reaction due to internal fixation device of unspecified** bone **of leg**

√x7ᵗʰ **T84.63** **Infection and inflammatory reaction due to internal fixation device of** spine

√x7ᵗʰ **T84.69** **Infection and inflammatory reaction due to internal fixation device of other site**

√x7ᵗʰ **T84.7** **Infection and inflammatory reaction due to other internal orthopedic prosthetic devices, implants and grafts**
Use additional code to identify infection

√5ᵗʰ **T84.8** **Other specified complications of internal orthopedic prosthetic devices, implants and grafts**

√x7ᵗʰ **T84.81** Embolism **due to internal orthopedic prosthetic devices, implants and grafts**

√x7ᵗʰ **T84.82** Fibrosis **due to internal orthopedic prosthetic devices, implants and grafts**

√x7ᵗʰ **T84.83** Hemorrhage **due to internal orthopedic prosthetic devices, implants and grafts**

√x7ᵗʰ **T84.84** Pain **due to internal orthopedic prosthetic devices, implants and grafts**

√x7ᵗʰ **T84.85** Stenosis **due to internal orthopedic prosthetic devices, implants and grafts**

√x7ᵗʰ **T84.86** Thrombosis **due to internal orthopedic prosthetic devices, implants and grafts**

√x7ᵗʰ **T84.89** **Other specified complication of internal orthopedic prosthetic devices, implants and grafts**

√x7ᵗʰ **T84.9** **Unspecified complication of internal orthopedic prosthetic device, implant and graft**

√4ᵗʰ **T85** **Complications of other internal prosthetic devices, implants and grafts**

EXCLUDES 2 *failure and rejection of transplanted organs and tissue (T86.-)*

The appropriate 7th character is to be added to each code from category T85.
A   initial encounter
D   subsequent encounter
S   sequela

√5ᵗʰ **T85.0** **Mechanical complication of** ventricular intracranial (communicating) shunt

√x7ᵗʰ **T85.01** Breakdown **(mechanical) of ventricular intracranial (communicating) shunt**

√x7ᵗʰ **T85.02** Displacement **of ventricular intracranial (communicating) shunt**
Malposition of ventricular intracranial (communicating) shunt

√x7ᵗʰ **T85.03** Leakage **of ventricular intracranial (communicating) shunt**

√x7ᵗʰ **T85.09** **Other mechanical complication of ventricular intracranial (communicating) shunt**
Obstruction (mechanical) of ventricular intracranial (communicating) shunt
Perforation of ventricular intracranial (communicating) shunt
Protrusion of ventricular intracranial (communicating) shunt

EXCLUDES 1 Not coded here   **EXCLUDES 2** Not included here   N Newborn Age: 0   P Pediatric Age: 0-17   M Maternity Age: 12-55   A Adult Age: 15-124

986   ICD-10-CM Draft (2015)

☑5ᵗʰ **T85.1** Mechanical complication of implanted electronic stimulator of nervous system

  ☑6ᵗʰ **T85.11** Breakdown (mechanical) of implanted electronic stimulator of nervous system

    ☑7ᵗʰ **T85.110** Breakdown (mechanical) of implanted electronic neurostimulator (electrode) of brain

    ☑7ᵗʰ **T85.111** Breakdown (mechanical) of implanted electronic neurostimulator (electrode) of peripheral nerve

    ☑7ᵗʰ **T85.112** Breakdown (mechanical) of implanted electronic neurostimulator (electrode) of spinal cord

    ☑7ᵗʰ **T85.118** Breakdown (mechanical) of other implanted electronic stimulator of nervous system

  ☑6ᵗʰ **T85.12** Displacement of implanted electronic stimulator of nervous system

    Malposition of implanted electronic stimulator of nervous system

    ☑7ᵗʰ **T85.120** Displacement of implanted electronic neurostimulator (electrode) of brain

    ☑7ᵗʰ **T85.121** Displacement of implanted electronic neurostimulator (electrode) of peripheral nerve

    ☑7ᵗʰ **T85.122** Displacement of implanted electronic neurostimulator (electrode) of spinal cord

    ☑7ᵗʰ **T85.128** Displacement of other implanted electronic stimulator of nervous system

  ☑6ᵗʰ **T85.19** Other mechanical complication of implanted electronic stimulator of nervous system

    Leakage of implanted electronic stimulator of nervous system

    Obstruction (mechanical) of implanted electronic stimulator of nervous system

    Perforation of implanted electronic stimulator of nervous system

    Protrusion of implanted electronic stimulator of nervous system

    ☑7ᵗʰ **T85.190** Other mechanical complication of implanted electronic neurostimulator (electrode) of brain

    ☑7ᵗʰ **T85.191** Other mechanical complication of implanted electronic neurostimulator (electrode) of peripheral nerve

    ☑7ᵗʰ **T85.192** Other mechanical complication of implanted electronic neurostimulator (electrode) of spinal cord

    ☑7ᵗʰ **T85.199** Other mechanical complication of other implanted electronic stimulator of nervous system

☑5ᵗʰ **T85.2** Mechanical complication of intraocular lens

  ☑x7ᵗʰ **T85.21** Breakdown (mechanical) of intraocular lens

  ☑x7ᵗʰ **T85.22** Displacement of intraocular lens

    Malposition of intraocular lens

  ☑x7ᵗʰ **T85.29** Other mechanical complication of intraocular lens

    Obstruction (mechanical) of intraocular lens

    Perforation of intraocular lens

    Protrusion of intraocular lens

☑5ᵗʰ **T85.3** Mechanical complication of other ocular prosthetic devices, implants and grafts

    EXCLUDES 2 other complications of corneal graft (T86.84-)

  ☑6ᵗʰ **T85.31** Breakdown (mechanical) of other ocular prosthetic devices, implants and grafts

    ☑7ᵗʰ **T85.310** Breakdown (mechanical) of prosthetic orbit of right eye

    ☑7ᵗʰ **T85.311** Breakdown (mechanical) of prosthetic orbit of left eye

    ☑7ᵗʰ **T85.318** Breakdown (mechanical) of other ocular prosthetic devices, implants and grafts

  ☑6ᵗʰ **T85.32** Displacement of other ocular prosthetic devices, implants and grafts

    Malposition of other ocular prosthetic devices, implants and grafts

    ☑7ᵗʰ **T85.320** Displacement of prosthetic orbit of right eye

    ☑7ᵗʰ **T85.321** Displacement of prosthetic orbit of left eye

    ☑7ᵗʰ **T85.328** Displacement of other ocular prosthetic devices, implants and grafts

  ☑6ᵗʰ **T85.39** Other mechanical complication of other ocular prosthetic devices, implants and grafts

    Obstruction (mechanical) of other ocular prosthetic devices, implants and grafts

    Perforation of other ocular prosthetic devices, implants and grafts

    Protrusion of other ocular prosthetic devices, implants and grafts

    ☑7ᵗʰ **T85.390** Other mechanical complication of prosthetic orbit of right eye

    ☑7ᵗʰ **T85.391** Other mechanical complication of prosthetic orbit of left eye

    ☑7ᵗʰ **T85.398** Other mechanical complication of other ocular prosthetic devices, implants and grafts

☑5ᵗʰ **T85.4** Mechanical complication of breast prosthesis and implant

  ☑x7ᵗʰ **T85.41** Breakdown (mechanical) of breast prosthesis and implant

  ☑x7ᵗʰ **T85.42** Displacement of breast prosthesis and implant

    Malposition of breast prosthesis and implant

  ☑x7ᵗʰ **T85.43** Leakage of breast prosthesis and implant

  ☑x7ᵗʰ **T85.44** Capsular contracture of breast implant

  ☑x7ᵗʰ **T85.49** Other mechanical complication of breast prosthesis and implant

    Obstruction (mechanical) of breast prosthesis and implant

    Perforation of breast prosthesis and implant

    Protrusion of breast prosthesis and implant

☑5ᵗʰ **T85.5** Mechanical complication of gastrointestinal prosthetic devices, implants and grafts

  ☑6ᵗʰ **T85.51** Breakdown (mechanical) of gastrointestinal prosthetic devices, implants and grafts

    ☑7ᵗʰ **T85.510** Breakdown (mechanical) of bile duct prosthesis

    ☑7ᵗʰ **T85.511** Breakdown (mechanical) of esophageal anti-reflux device

    ☑7ᵗʰ **T85.518** Breakdown (mechanical) of other gastrointestinal prosthetic devices, implants and grafts

  ☑6ᵗʰ **T85.52** Displacement of gastrointestinal prosthetic devices, implants and grafts

    Malposition of gastrointestinal prosthetic devices, implants and grafts

    ☑7ᵗʰ **T85.520** Displacement of bile duct prosthesis

    ☑7ᵗʰ **T85.521** Displacement of esophageal anti-reflux device

    ☑7ᵗʰ **T85.528** Displacement of other gastrointestinal prosthetic devices, implants and grafts

  ☑6ᵗʰ **T85.59** Other mechanical complication of gastrointestinal prosthetic devices, implants and

    Obstruction, mechanical of gastrointestinal prosthetic devices, implants and grafts

    Perforation of gastrointestinal prosthetic devices, implants and grafts

    Protrusion of gastrointestinal prosthetic devices, implants and grafts

    ☑7ᵗʰ **T85.590** Other mechanical complication of bile duct prosthesis

    ☑7ᵗʰ **T85.591** Other mechanical complication of esophageal anti-reflux device

    ☑7ᵗʰ **T85.598** Other mechanical complication of other gastrointestinal prosthetic devices, implants and grafts

☑5ᵗʰ **T85.6** Mechanical complication of other specified internal and external prosthetic devices, implants and grafts

  ☑6ᵗʰ **T85.61** Breakdown (mechanical) of other specified internal prosthetic devices, implants and grafts

    ☑7ᵗʰ **T85.610** Breakdown (mechanical) of epidural and subdural infusion catheter

    ☑7ᵗʰ **T85.611** Breakdown (mechanical) of intraperitoneal dialysis catheter

      EXCLUDES 1 mechanical complication of vascular dialysis catheter (T82.4-)

☑ Additional Character Required ☑x7ᵗʰ Xtension Alert Unspecified Dx Other Specified Dx Manifestation ►◄ Revised Text ● New Code ▲ Revised Code Title

ICD-10-CM Draft (2015)   **987**

Injury, Poisoning and Certain Other Consequences of External Causes *(left margin)*

T85.612–T86.31 *(left margin)*

√7th **T85.612 Breakdown (mechanical) of permanent sutures**
- EXCLUDES 1 *mechanical complication of permanent (wire) suture used in bone repair (T84.1-T84.2)*

√7th **T85.613 Breakdown (mechanical) of artificial skin graft and decellularized allodermis**
- Failure of artificial skin graft and decellularized allodermis
- Non-adherence of artificial skin graft and decellularized allodermis
- Poor incorporation of artificial skin graft and decellularized allodermis
- Shearing of artificial skin graft and decellularized allodermis

√7th **T85.614 Breakdown (mechanical) of insulin pump**

√7th **T85.618 Breakdown (mechanical) of other specified internal prosthetic devices, implants and grafts**

√6th **T85.62 Displacement of other specified internal prosthetic devices, implants and grafts**
- Malposition of other specified internal prosthetic devices, implants and grafts

√7th **T85.620 Displacement of epidural and subdural infusion catheter**

√7th **T85.621 Displacement of intraperitoneal dialysis catheter**
- EXCLUDES 1 *mechanical complication of vascular dialysis catheter (T82.4-)*

√7th **T85.622 Displacement of permanent sutures**
- EXCLUDES 1 *mechanical complication of permanent (wire) suture used in bone repair (T84.1-T84.2)*

√7th **T85.623 Displacement of artificial skin graft and decellularized allodermis**
- Dislodgement of artificial skin graft and decellularized allodermis
- Displacement of artificial skin graft and decellularized allodermis

√7th **T85.624 Displacement of insulin pump**

√7th **T85.628 Displacement of other specified internal prosthetic devices, implants and grafts**

√6th **T85.63 Leakage of other specified internal prosthetic devices, implants and grafts**

√7th **T85.630 Leakage of epidural and subdural infusion catheter**

√7th **T85.631 Leakage of intraperitoneal dialysis catheter**
- EXCLUDES 1 *mechanical complication of vascular dialysis catheter (T82.4)*

√7th **T85.633 Leakage of insulin pump**

√7th **T85.638 Leakage of other specified internal prosthetic devices, implants and grafts**

√6th **T85.69 Other mechanical complication of other specified internal prosthetic devices, implants and grafts**
- Obstruction, mechanical of other specified internal prosthetic devices, implants and grafts
- Perforation of other specified internal prosthetic devices, implants and grafts
- Protrusion of other specified internal prosthetic devices, implants and grafts

√7th **T85.690 Other mechanical complication of epidural and subdural infusion catheter**

√7th **T85.691 Other mechanical complication of intraperitoneal dialysis catheter**
- EXCLUDES 1 *mechanical complication of vascular dialysis catheter (T82.4)*

√7th **T85.692 Other mechanical complication of permanent sutures**
- EXCLUDES 1 *mechanical complication of permanent (wire) suture used in bone repair (T84.1-T84.2)*

√7th **T85.693 Other mechanical complication of artificial skin graft and decellularized allodermis**

√7th **T85.694 Other mechanical complication of insulin pump**

√7th **T85.698 Other mechanical complication of other specified internal prosthetic devices, implants and grafts**
- Mechanical complication of nonabsorbable surgical material NOS

√5th **T85.7 Infection and inflammatory reaction due to other internal prosthetic devices, implants and grafts**
- Use additional code to identify infection

√x7th **T85.71 Infection and inflammatory reaction due to peritoneal dialysis catheter**

√x7th **T85.72 Infection and inflammatory reaction due to insulin pump**

√x7th **T85.79 Infection and inflammatory reaction due to other internal prosthetic devices, implants and grafts**

√5th **T85.8 Other specified complications of internal prosthetic devices, implants and grafts, not elsewhere classified**

√x7th **T85.81 Embolism due to internal prosthetic devices, implants and grafts, not elsewhere classified**

√x7th **T85.82 Fibrosis due to internal prosthetic devices, implants and grafts, not elsewhere classified**

√x7th **T85.83 Hemorrhage due to internal prosthetic devices, implants and grafts, not elsewhere classified**

√x7th **T85.84 Pain due to internal prosthetic devices, implants and grafts, not elsewhere classified**

√x7th **T85.85 Stenosis due to internal prosthetic devices, implants and grafts, not elsewhere classified**

√x7th **T85.86 Thrombosis due to internal prosthetic devices, implants and grafts, not elsewhere classified**

√x7th **T85.89 Other specified complication of internal prosthetic devices, implants and grafts, not elsewhere classified**

√x7th **T85.9 Unspecified complication of internal prosthetic device, implant and graft**
- Complication of internal prosthetic device, implant and graft NOS

√4th **T86 Complications of transplanted organs and tissue**
- Use additional code to identify other transplant complications, such as:
- graft-versus-host disease (D89.81-)
- malignancy associated with organ transplant (C80.2)
- post-transplant lymphoproliferative disorders (PTLD) (D47.Z1)

√5th **T86.0 Complications of bone marrow transplant**

T86.00 Unspecified complication of bone marrow transplant

T86.01 Bone marrow transplant rejection

T86.02 Bone marrow transplant failure

T86.03 Bone marrow transplant infection

T86.09 Other complications of bone marrow transplant

√5th **T86.1 Complications of kidney transplant**

T86.10 Unspecified complication of kidney transplant

T86.11 Kidney transplant rejection

T86.12 Kidney transplant failure
- AHA: 2013, 1Q, 24

T86.13 Kidney transplant infection
- Use additional code to specify infection

T86.19 Other complication of kidney transplant

√5th **T86.2 Complications of heart transplant**
- EXCLUDES 1 *complication of:*
  artificial heart device (T82.5)
  heart-lung transplant (T86.3)

T86.20 Unspecified complication of heart transplant

T86.21 Heart transplant rejection

T86.22 Heart transplant failure

T86.23 Heart transplant infection
- Use additional code to specify infection

√6th **T86.29 Other complications of heart transplant**

T86.290 Cardiac allograft vasculopathy
- EXCLUDES 1 *atherosclerosis of coronary arteries (I25.75-, I25.76-, I25.81-)*

T86.298 Other complications of heart transplant

√5th **T86.3 Complications of heart-lung transplant**

T86.30 Unspecified complication of heart-lung transplant

T86.31 Heart-lung transplant rejection

EXCLUDES 1 Not coded here   EXCLUDES 2 Not included here   N Newborn Age: 0   P Pediatric Age: 0-17   M Maternity Age: 12-55   A Adult Age: 15-124

988   ICD-10-CM Draft (2015)

T86.32   **Heart-lung transplant** failure

T86.33   **Heart-lung transplant** infection
     Use additional code to specify infection

T86.39   **Other complications of heart-lung transplant**

☑5ᵗʰ   **T86.4**   **Complications of** liver **transplant**

T86.40   **Unspecified complication of liver transplant**

T86.41   **Liver transplant** rejection

T86.42   **Liver transplant** failure

T86.43   **Liver transplant** infection
     Use additional code to identify infection, such as:
     cytomegalovirus (CMV) infection (B25.-)

T86.49   **Other complications of liver transplant**

T86.5   **Complications of** stem cell **transplant**
     Complications from stem cells from peripheral blood
     Complications from stem cells from umbilical cord

☑6ᵗʰ   **T86.8**   **Complications of** other **transplanted organs and tissues**

☑6ᵗʰ   T86.81   **Complications of** lung **transplant**
     EXCLUDES 1   complication of heart-lung transplant (T86.3-)

T86.810   **Lung transplant** rejection

T86.811   **Lung transplant** failure

T86.812   **Lung transplant** infection
     Use additional code to specify infection

T86.818   **Other complications of lung transplant**

T86.819   **Unspecified complication of lung transplant**

☑6ᵗʰ   T86.82   **Complications of** skin graft (allograft) (autograft)
     EXCLUDES 2   complication of artificial skin graft (T85.693)

T86.820   **Skin graft (allograft)** rejection

T86.821   **Skin graft (allograft) (autograft)** failure

T86.822   **Skin graft (allograft) (autograft)** infection
     Use additional code to specify infection

T86.828   **Other complications of skin graft (allograft) (autograft)**

T86.829   **Unspecified complication of skin graft (allograft) (autograft)**

☑6ᵗʰ   T86.83   **Complications of** bone graft
     EXCLUDES 2   mechanical complications of bone graft (T84.3-)

T86.830   **Bone graft** rejection

T86.831   **Bone graft** failure

T86.832   **Bone graft** infection
     Use additional code to specify infection

T86.838   **Other complications of bone graft**

T86.839   **Unspecified complication of bone graft**

☑6ᵗʰ   T86.84   **Complications of** corneal **transplant**
     EXCLUDES 2   mechanical complications of corneal graft (T85.3-)

T86.840   **Corneal transplant** rejection

T86.841   **Corneal transplant** failure

T86.842   **Corneal transplant** infection
     Use additional code to specify infection

T86.848   **Other complications of corneal transplant**

T86.849   **Unspecified complication of corneal transplant**

☑6ᵗʰ   T86.85   **Complication of** intestine **transplant**

T86.850   **Intestine transplant** rejection

T86.851   **Intestine transplant** failure

T86.852   **Intestine transplant** infection
     Use additional code to specify infection

T86.858   **Other complications of intestine transplant**

T86.859   **Unspecified complication of intestine transplant**

☑6ᵗʰ   T86.89   **Complications of** other **transplanted** tissue
     Transplant failure or rejection of pancreas

T86.890   **Other transplanted tissue** rejection

T86.891   **Other transplanted tissue** failure

T86.892   **Other transplanted tissue** infection
     Use additional code to specify infection

T86.898   **Other complications of other transplanted tissue**

T86.899   **Unspecified complication of other transplanted tissue**

☑5ᵗʰ   **T86.9**   **Complication of** unspecified **transplanted** organ and tissue

T86.90   **Unspecified complication of unspecified transplanted organ and tissue**

T86.91   **Unspecified transplanted organ and tissue** rejection

T86.92   **Unspecified transplanted organ and tissue** failure

T86.93   **Unspecified transplanted organ and tissue** infection
     Use additional code to specify infection

T86.99   **Other complications of unspecified transplanted organ and tissue**

☑4ᵗʰ   **T87**   **Complications peculiar to reattachment and amputation**

☑5ᵗʰ   **T87.0**   **Complications of reattached (part of)** upper extremity

☑6ᵗʰ   T87.0X   **Complications of reattached (part of) upper extremity**

T87.0X1   **Complications of reattached (part of)** right upper extremity

T87.0X2   **Complications of reattached (part of)** left upper extremity

T87.0X9   **Complications of reattached (part of) unspecified upper extremity**

☑5ᵗʰ   **T87.1**   **Complications of reattached (part of)** lower extremity

☑6ᵗʰ   T87.1X   **Complications of reattached (part of) lower extremity**

T87.1X1   **Complications of reattached (part of)** right lower extremity

T87.1X2   **Complications of reattached (part of)** left lower extremity

T87.1X9   **Complications of reattached (part of) unspecified lower extremity**

T87.2   **Complications of other reattached body part**

☑5ᵗʰ   **T87.3**   Neuroma **of amputation stump**

T87.30   **Neuroma of amputation stump, unspecified extremity**

T87.31   **Neuroma of amputation stump,** right upper extremity

T87.32   **Neuroma of amputation stump,** left upper **extremity**

T87.33   **Neuroma of amputation stump,** right lower extremity

T87.34   **Neuroma of amputation stump,** left lower **extremity**

☑5ᵗʰ   **T87.4**   Infection **of amputation stump**

T87.40   **Infection of amputation stump, unspecified extremity**

T87.41   **Infection of amputation stump,** right upper extremity

T87.42   **Infection of amputation stump,** left upper **extremity**

T87.43   **Infection of amputation stump,** right lower extremity

T87.44   **Infection of amputation stump,** left lower **extremity**

☑5ᵗʰ   **T87.5**   Necrosis **of amputation stump**

T87.50   **Necrosis of amputation stump, unspecified extremity**

T87.51   **Necrosis of amputation stump,** right upper extremity

T87.52   **Necrosis of amputation stump,** left upper **extremity**

T87.53   **Necrosis of amputation stump,** right lower **extremity**

T87.54   **Necrosis of amputation stump,** left lower **extremity**

☑5ᵗʰ   **T87.8**   Other **complications of amputation stump**

T87.81   Dehiscence **of amputation stump**

T87.89   **Other complications of amputation stump**
     Amputation stump contracture
     Amputation stump contracture of next proximal joint
     Amputation stump flexion
     Amputation stump edema
     Amputation stump hematoma
     EXCLUDES 2   phantom limb syndrome (G54.6-G54.7)

T87.9   **Unspecified complications of amputation stump**

☑ Additional Character Required   ☑x7ᵗʰ Xtension Alert   Unspecified Dx   Other Specified Dx   Manifestation   ▶◀ Revised Text   ● New Code   ▲ Revised Code Title

ICD-10-CM Draft (2015)   **989**

Injury, Poisoning and Certain Other Consequences of External Causes *(left margin)*

T88–T88.9 *(left margin)*

√4ᵗʰ **T88 Other complications of surgical and medical care, not elsewhere classified**

EXCLUDES 2 complication following infusion, transfusion and therapeutic injection (T80.-)
complication following procedure NEC (T81.-)
complications of anesthesia in labor and delivery (O74.-)
complications of anesthesia in pregnancy (O29.-)
complications of anesthesia in puerperium (O89.-)
complications of devices, implants and grafts (T82-T85)
complications of obstetric surgery and procedure (O75.4)
dermatitis due to drugs and medicaments (L23.3, L24.4, L25.1, L27.0-L27.1)
poisoning and toxic effects of drugs and chemicals (T36-T65 with fifth or sixth character 1-4 or 6)
specified complications classified elsewhere

The appropriate 7th character is to be added to each code from category T88.
A   initial encounter
D   subsequent encounter
S   sequela

√x7ᵗʰ **T88.0 Infection following immunization**
Sepsis following immunization

√x7ᵗʰ **T88.1 Other complications following immunization, not elsewhere classified**
Generalized vaccinia
Rash following immunization
EXCLUDES 1 vaccinia not from vaccine (B08.011)
EXCLUDES 2 anaphylactic shock due to serum (T80.5-)
other serum reactions (T80.6-)
postimmunization arthropathy (M02.2)
postimmunization encephalitis (G04.02)
postimmunization fever (R50.83)

√x7ᵗʰ **T88.2 Shock due to anesthesia**
Use additional code for adverse effect, if applicable, to identify drug (T41.- with fifth or sixth character 5)
EXCLUDES 1 complications of anesthesia (in):
labor and delivery (O74.-)
postprocedural shock NOS (T81.1-)
pregnancy (O29.-)
puerperium (O89.-)

√x7ᵗʰ **T88.3 Malignant hyperthermia due to anesthesia**
Use additional code for adverse effect, if applicable, to identify drug (T41.- with fifth or sixth character 5)

√x7ᵗʰ **T88.4 Failed or difficult intubation**

√5ᵗʰ **T88.5 Other complications of anesthesia**
Use additional code for adverse effect, if applicable, to identify drug (T41.- with fifth or sixth character 5)

√x7ᵗʰ **T88.51 Hypothermia following anesthesia**

√x7ᵗʰ **T88.52 Failed moderate sedation during procedure**
Failed conscious sedation during procedure
EXCLUDES 2 personal history of failed moderate sedation (Z92.83)

√x7ᵗʰ **T88.59 Other complications of anesthesia**

√x7ᵗʰ **T88.6 Anaphylactic reaction due to adverse effect of correct drug or medicament properly administered**
Anaphylactic shock due to adverse effect of correct drug or medicament properly administered
Anaphylactoid reaction NOS
Use additional code for adverse effect, if applicable, to identify drug (T36-T50 with fifth or sixth character 5)
EXCLUDES 1 anaphylactic reaction due to serum (T80.5-)
anaphylactic shock or reaction due to adverse food reaction (T78.0-)

√x7ᵗʰ **T88.7 Unspecified adverse effect of drug or medicament**
Drug hypersensitivity NOS
Drug reaction NOS
Use additional code for adverse effect, if applicable, to identify drug (T36-T50 with fifth or sixth character 5)
EXCLUDES 1 specified adverse effects of drugs and medicaments (A00-R94 and T80-T88.6, T88.8)

√x7ᵗʰ **T88.8 Other specified complications of surgical and medical care, not elsewhere classified**
Use additional code to identify the complication

√x7ᵗʰ **T88.9 Complication of surgical and medical care, unspecified**

Chapter 20. External Causes of Morbidity (V00–Y99)

> **NOTE**   This chapter permits the classification of environmental events and circumstances as the cause of injury, and other adverse effects. Where a code from this section is applicable, it is intended that it shall be used secondary to a code from another chapter of the Classification indicating the nature of the condition. Most often, the condition will be classifiable to Chapter 19, Injury, poisoning and certain other consequences of external causes (S00–T88). Other conditions that may be stated to be due to external causes are classified in Chapters I to XVIII. For these conditions, codes from Chapter 20 should be used to provide additional information as to the cause of the condition.

This chapter contains the following blocks:

V00–V09	Pedestrian injured in transport accident
V10–V19	Pedal cycle rider injured in transport accident
V20–V29	Motorcycle rider injured in transport accident
V30–V39	Occupant of three-wheeled motor vehicle injured in transport accident
V40–V49	Car occupant injured in transport accident
V50–V59	Occupant of pick-up truck or van injured in transport accident
V60–V69	Occupant of heavy transport vehicle injured in transport accident
V70–V79	Bus occupant injured in transport accident
V80–V89	Other land transport accidents
V90–V94	Water transport accidents
V95–V97	Air and space transport accidents
V98–V99	Other and unspecified transport accidents
W00–X58	Other external causes of accidental injury
W00–W19	Slipping, tripping, stumbling and falls
W20–W49	Exposure to inanimate mechanical forces
W50–W64	Exposure to animate mechanical forces
W65–W74	Accidental non-transport drowning and submersion
W85–W99	Exposure to electric current, radiation and extreme ambient air temperature and pressure
X00–X08	Exposure to smoke, fire and flames
X10–X19	Contact with heat and hot substances
X30–X39	Exposure to forces of nature
X52, X58	Accidental exposure to other specified factors
X71–X83	Intentional self-harm
X92–Y08	Assault
Y21–Y33	Event of undetermined intent
Y35–Y38	Legal intervention, operations of war, military operations, and terrorism
Y62–Y84	Complications of medical and surgical care
Y62–Y69	Misadventures to patients during surgical and medical care
Y70–Y82	Medical devices associated with adverse incidents in diagnostic and therapeutic use
Y83–Y84	Surgical and other medical procedures as the cause of abnormal reaction of the patient, or of later complication, without mention of misadventure at the time of the procedure
Y90–Y99	Supplementary factors related to causes of morbidity classified elsewhere

Accidents (V00–X58)

Transport accidents (V00–V99)

Use additional code to identify:
  airbag injury (W22.1)
  type of street or road (Y92.4-)
  use of cellular telephone and other electronic equipment at the time of the transport accident (Y93.C-)

> **EXCLUDES 1**   agricultural vehicles in stationary use or maintenance (W31.-)
> assault by crashing of motor vehicle (Y03.-)
> automobile or motor cycle in stationary use or maintenance—code to type of accident
> crashing of motor vehicle, undetermined intent (Y32)
> intentional self-harm by crashing of motor vehicle (X82)

> **EXCLUDES 2**   transport accidents due to cataclysm (X34–X38)

This section is structured in 12 groups. Those relating to land transport accidents (V01–V89) reflect the victim's mode of transport and are subdivided to identify the victim's 'counterpart' or the type of event. The vehicle of which the injured person is an occupant is identified in the first two characters since it is seen as the most important factor to identify for prevention purposes. A transport accident is one in which the vehicle involved must be moving or running or in use for transport purposes at the time of the accident.

Pedestrian injured in transport accident (V00–V09)

> **INCLUDES**   person changing tire on transport vehicle
> person examining engine of vehicle broken down in (on side of) road

> **EXCLUDES 1**   fall due to non-transport collision with other person (W03)
> pedestrian on foot falling (slipping) on ice and snow (W00.-)
> struck or bumped by another person (W51)

✓4ᵗʰ **V00   Pedestrian conveyance accident**

Use additional place of occurrence and activity external cause codes, if known (Y92-, Y93-)

> **EXCLUDES 1**   collision with another person without fall (W51)
> fall due to person on foot colliding with another person on foot (W03)
> fall from non-moving wheelchair, nonmotorized scooter and motorized mobility scooter without collision (W05.-)
> pedestrian (conveyance) collision with other land transport vehicle (V01-V09)
> pedestrian on foot falling (slipping) on ice and snow (W00.-)

> The appropriate 7th character is to be added to each code from category V00.
> A   initial encounter
> D   subsequent encounter
> S   sequela

✓5ᵗʰ **V00.0   Pedestrian on foot injured in collision with pedestrian conveyance**

  ✓x7ᵗʰ **V00.01   Pedestrian on foot injured in collision with roller-skater**

  ✓x7ᵗʰ **V00.02   Pedestrian on foot injured in collision with skateboarder**

  ✓x7ᵗʰ **V00.09   Pedestrian on foot injured in collision with other pedestrian conveyance**

✓5ᵗʰ **V00.1   Rolling-type pedestrian conveyance accident**

> **EXCLUDES 1**   accident with babystroller (V00.82-)
> accident with motorized mobility scooter (V00.83-)
> accident with wheelchair (powered) (V00.81-)

  ✓6ᵗʰ **V00.11   In-line roller-skate accident**

    ✓7ᵗʰ **V00.111   Fall from in-line roller-skates**

    ✓7ᵗʰ **V00.112   In-line roller-skater colliding with stationary object**

    ✓7ᵗʰ **V00.118   Other in-line roller-skate accident**
> **EXCLUDES 1**   roller-skater collision with other land transport vehicle (V01-V09 with 5th character 1)

  ✓6ᵗʰ **V00.12   Non-in- line roller-skate accident**

    ✓7ᵗʰ **V00.121   Fall from non-in-line roller-skates**

    ✓7ᵗʰ **V00.122   Non-in-line roller-skater colliding with stationary object**

    ✓7ᵗʰ **V00.128   Other non-in-line roller-skating accident**
> **EXCLUDES 1**   roller-skater collision with other land transport vehicle (V01-V09 with 5th character 1)

  ✓6ᵗʰ **V00.13   Skateboard accident**

    ✓7ᵗʰ **V00.131   Fall from skateboard**

    ✓7ᵗʰ **V00.132   Skateboarder colliding with stationary object**

    ✓7ᵗʰ **V00.138   Other skateboard accident**
> **EXCLUDES 1**   skateboarder collision with other land transport vehicle (V01-V09 with 5th character 2)

  ✓6ᵗʰ **V00.14   Scooter (nonmotorized) accident**
> **EXCLUDES 1**   motorscooter accident (V20-V29)

    ✓7ᵗʰ **V00.141   Fall from scooter (nonmotorized)**

    ✓7ᵗʰ **V00.142   Scooter (nonmotorized) colliding with stationary object**

    ✓7ᵗʰ **V00.148   Other scooter (nonmotorized) accident**
> **EXCLUDES 1**   scooter (nonmotorized) collision with other land transport vehicle (V01-V09 with fifth character 9)

  ✓6ᵗʰ **V00.15   Heelies accident**
    Rolling shoe
    Wheeled shoe
    Wheelies accident

    ✓7ᵗʰ **V00.151   Fall from heelies**

✓ Additional Character Required   ✓x7ᵗʰ Xtension Alert   Unspecified Dx   Other Specified Dx   Manifestation   ►◄ Revised Text   ● New Code   ▲ Revised Code Title

ICD-10-CM Draft (2015)   **991**

☑7ᵗʰ **V00.152** Heelies colliding with stationary object

☑7ᵗʰ **V00.158** Other heelies accident

☑6ᵗʰ **V00.18** Accident on other rolling-type pedestrian conveyance

☑7ᵗʰ **V00.181** Fall from other rolling-type pedestrian conveyance

☑7ᵗʰ **V00.182** Pedestrian on other rolling-type pedestrian conveyance colliding with stationary object

☑7ᵗʰ **V00.188** Other accident on other rolling-type pedestrian conveyance

☑5ᵗʰ **V00.2** Gliding-type pedestrian conveyance accident

☑6ᵗʰ **V00.21** Ice-skates accident

☑7ᵗʰ **V00.211** Fall from ice-skates

☑7ᵗʰ **V00.212** Ice-skater colliding with stationary object

☑7ᵗʰ **V00.218** Other ice-skates accident
EXCLUDES 1 ice-skater collision with other land transport vehicle (V01-V09 with 5th digit 9)

☑6ᵗʰ **V00.22** Sled accident

☑7ᵗʰ **V00.221** Fall from sled

☑7ᵗʰ **V00.222** Sledder colliding with stationary object

☑7ᵗʰ **V00.228** Other sled accident
EXCLUDES 1 sled collision with other land transport vehicle (V01-V09 with 5th digit 9)

☑6ᵗʰ **V00.28** Other gliding-type pedestrian conveyance accident

☑7ᵗʰ **V00.281** Fall from other gliding-type pedestrian conveyance

☑7ᵗʰ **V00.282** Pedestrian on other gliding-type pedestrian conveyance colliding with stationary object

☑7ᵗʰ **V00.288** Other accident on other gliding-type pedestrian conveyance
EXCLUDES 1 gliding-type pedestrian conveyance collision with other land transport vehicle (V01-V09 with 5th digit 9)

☑5ᵗʰ **V00.3** Flat-bottomed pedestrian conveyance accident

☑6ᵗʰ **V00.31** Snowboard accident

☑7ᵗʰ **V00.311** Fall from snowboard

☑7ᵗʰ **V00.312** Snowboarder colliding with stationary object

☑7ᵗʰ **V00.318** Other snowboard accident
EXCLUDES 1 snowboarder collision with other land transport vehicle (V01-V09 with 5th digit 9)

☑6ᵗʰ **V00.32** Snow-ski accident

☑7ᵗʰ **V00.321** Fall from snow-skis

☑7ᵗʰ **V00.322** Snow-skier colliding with stationary object

☑7ᵗʰ **V00.328** Other snow-ski accident
EXCLUDES 1 snow-skier collision with other land transport vehicle (V01-V09 with 5th digit 9)

☑6ᵗʰ **V00.38** Other flat-bottomed pedestrian conveyance accident

☑7ᵗʰ **V00.381** Fall from other flat-bottomed pedestrian conveyance

☑7ᵗʰ **V00.382** Pedestrian on other flat-bottomed pedestrian conveyance colliding with stationary object

☑7ᵗʰ **V00.388** Other accident on other flat-bottomed pedestrian conveyance

☑5ᵗʰ **V00.8** Accident on other pedestrian conveyance

☑6ᵗʰ **V00.81** Accident with wheelchair (powered)

☑7ᵗʰ **V00.811** Fall from moving wheelchair (powered)
EXCLUDES 1 fall from non-moving wheelchair (W05.0)

☑7ᵗʰ **V00.812** Wheelchair (powered) colliding with stationary object

☑7ᵗʰ **V00.818** Other accident with wheelchair (powered)

☑6ᵗʰ **V00.82** Accident with babystroller

☑7ᵗʰ **V00.821** Fall from babystroller

☑7ᵗʰ **V00.822** Babystroller colliding with stationary object

☑7ᵗʰ **V00.828** Other accident with babystroller

☑6ᵗʰ **V00.83** Accident with motorized mobility scooter

V00.831 Fall from motorized mobility scooter
EXCLUDES 1 fall from non-moving motorized mobility scooter (W05.2)

V00.832 Motorized mobility scooter colliding with stationary object

V00.838 Other accident with motorized mobility scooter

☑6ᵗʰ **V00.89** Accident on other pedestrian conveyance

☑7ᵗʰ **V00.891** Fall from other pedestrian conveyance

☑7ᵗʰ **V00.892** Pedestrian on other pedestrian conveyance colliding with stationary object

☑7ᵗʰ **V00.898** Other accident on other pedestrian conveyance
EXCLUDES 1 other pedestrian (conveyance) collision with other land transport vehicle (V01-V09 with 5th digit 9)

☑4ᵗʰ **V01** Pedestrian injured in collision with pedal cycle

The appropriate 7th character is to be added to each code from category V01.
A   initial encounter
D   subsequent encounter
S   sequela

☑5ᵗʰ **V01.0** Pedestrian injured in collision with pedal cycle in nontraffic accident

√x7ᵗʰ **V01.00** Pedestrian on foot injured in collision with pedal cycle in nontraffic accident
Pedestrian NOS injured in collision with pedal cycle in nontraffic accident

√x7ᵗʰ **V01.01** Pedestrian on roller-skates injured in collision with pedal cycle in nontraffic accident

√x7ᵗʰ **V01.02** Pedestrian on skateboard injured in collision with pedal cycle in nontraffic accident

√x7ᵗʰ **V01.09** Pedestrian with other conveyance injured in collision with pedal cycle in nontraffic accident
Pedestrian with babystroller injured in collision with pedal cycle in nontraffic accident
Pedestrian on ice-skates injured in collision with pedal cycle in nontraffic accident
Pedestrian on nonmotorized scooter injured in collision with pedal cycle in nontraffic accident
Pedestrian on sled injured in collision with pedal cycle in nontraffic accident
Pedestrian on snowboard injured in collision with pedal cycle in nontraffic accident
Pedestrian on snow-skis injured in collision with pedal cycle in nontraffic accident
Pedestrian in wheelchair (powered) injured in collision with pedal cycle in nontraffic accident
Pedestrian in motorized mobility scooter injured in collision with pedal cycle in nontraffic accident

☑5ᵗʰ **V01.1** Pedestrian injured in collision with pedal cycle in traffic accident

√x7ᵗʰ **V01.10** Pedestrian on foot injured in collision with pedal cycle in traffic accident
Pedestrian NOS injured in collision with pedal cycle in traffic accident

√x7ᵗʰ **V01.11** Pedestrian on roller-skates injured in collision with pedal cycle in traffic accident

√x7ᵗʰ **V01.12** Pedestrian on skateboard injured in collision with pedal cycle in traffic accident

✓x7th V01.19 Pedestrian with other conveyance injured in collision with pedal cycle in traffic accident
Pedestrian with babystroller injured in collision with pedal cycle in traffic accident
Pedestrian on ice-skates injured in collision with pedal cycle in traffic accident
Pedestrian on nonmotorized scooter injured in collision with pedal cycle in traffic accident
Pedestrian on sled injured in collision with pedal cycle in traffic accident
Pedestrian on snowboard injured in collision with pedal cycle in traffic accident
Pedestrian on snow-skis injured in collision with pedal cycle in traffic accident
Pedestrian in wheelchair (powered) injured in collision with pedal cycle in traffic accident
Pedestrian in motorized mobility scooter injured in collision with pedal cycle in traffic accident

✓5th V01.9 Pedestrian injured in collision with pedal cycle, unspecified whether traffic or nontraffic accident

✓x7th V01.90 Pedestrian on foot injured in collision with pedal cycle, unspecified whether traffic or nontraffic accident
Pedestrian NOS injured in collision with pedal cycle, unspecified whether traffic or nontraffic accident

✓x7th V01.91 Pedestrian on roller-skates injured in collision with pedal cycle, unspecified whether traffic or nontraffic accident

✓x7th V01.92 Pedestrian on skateboard injured in collision with pedal cycle, unspecified whether traffic or nontraffic accident

✓x7th V01.99 Pedestrian with other conveyance injured in collision with pedal cycle, unspecified whether traffic or nontraffic accident
Pedestrian with babystroller injured in collision with pedal cycle, unspecified whether traffic or nontraffic accident
Pedestrian on ice-skates injured in collision with pedal cycle unspecified, whether traffic or nontraffic accident
Pedestrian on nonmotorized scooter injured in collision with pedal cycle, unspecified whether traffic or nontraffic accident
Pedestrian on sled injured in collision with pedal cycle unspecified, whether traffic or nontraffic accident
Pedestrian on snowboard injured in collision with pedal cycle, unspecified whether traffic or nontraffic accident
Pedestrian on snow-skis injured in collision with pedal cycle, unspecified whether traffic or nontraffic accident
Pedestrian in wheelchair (powered) injured in collision with pedal cycle, unspecified whether traffic or nontraffic accident
Pedestrian in motorized mobility scooter injured in collision with pedal cycle, unspecified whether traffic or nontraffic accident

✓4th V02 Pedestrian injured in collision with two- or three-wheeled motor vehicle

The appropriate 7th character is to be added to each code from category V02.
A	initial encounter
D	subsequent encounter
S	sequela

✓5th V02.0 Pedestrian injured in collision with two- or three-wheeled motor vehicle in nontraffic accident

✓x7th V02.00 Pedestrian on foot injured in collision with two- or three-wheeled motor vehicle in nontraffic accident
Pedestrian NOS injured in collision with two- or three-wheeled motor vehicle in nontraffic accident

✓x7th V02.01 Pedestrian on roller-skates injured in collision with two- or three-wheeled motor vehicle in nontraffic accident

✓x7th V02.02 Pedestrian on skateboard injured in collision with two- or three-wheeled motor vehicle in nontraffic accident

✓x7th V02.09 Pedestrian with other conveyance injured in collision with two- or three-wheeled motor vehicle in nontraffic accident
Pedestrian with babystroller injured in collision with two- or three-wheeled motor vehicle in nontraffic accident
Pedestrian on ice-skates injured in collision with two- or three-wheeled motor vehicle in nontraffic accident
Pedestrian on nonmotorized scooter injured in collision with two- or three-wheeled motor vehicle in nontraffic accident
Pedestrian on sled injured in collision with two- or three-wheeled motor vehicle in nontraffic accident
Pedestrian on snowboard injured in collision with two- or three-wheeled motor vehicle in nontraffic accident
Pedestrian on snow-skis injured in collision with two- or three-wheeled motor vehicle in nontraffic accident
Pedestrian in wheelchair (powered) injured in collision with two- or three-wheeled motor vehicle in nontraffic accident
Pedestrian in motorized mobility scooter injured in collision with two- or three-wheeled motor vehicle in nontraffic accident

✓5th V02.1 Pedestrian injured in collision with two- or three-wheeled motor vehicle in traffic accident

✓x7th V02.10 Pedestrian on foot injured in collision with two- or three-wheeled motor vehicle in traffic accident
Pedestrian NOS injured in collision with two- or three-wheeled motor vehicle in traffic accident

✓x7th V02.11 Pedestrian on roller-skates injured in collision with two- or three-wheeled motor vehicle in traffic accident

✓x7th V02.12 Pedestrian on skateboard injured in collision with two- or three-wheeled motor vehicle in traffic accident

✓x7th V02.19 Pedestrian with other conveyance injured in collision with two- or three-wheeled motor vehicle in traffic accident
Pedestrian with babystroller injured in collision with two- or three-wheeled motor vehicle in traffic accident
Pedestrian on ice-skates injured in collision with two- or three-wheeled motor vehicle in traffic accident
Pedestrian on nonmotorized scooter injured in collision with two- or three-wheeled motor vehicle in traffic accident
Pedestrian on sled injured in collision with two- or three-wheeled motor vehicle in traffic accident
Pedestrian on snowboard injured in collision with two- or three-wheeled motor vehicle in traffic accident
Pedestrian on snow-skis injured in collision with two- or three-wheeled motor vehicle in traffic accident
Pedestrian in wheelchair (powered) injured in collision with two- or three-wheeled motor vehicle in traffic accident
Pedestrian in motorized mobility scooter injured in collision with two- or three-wheeled motor vehicle in traffic accident

✓5th V02.9 Pedestrian injured in collision with two- or three-wheeled motor vehicle, unspecified whether traffic or nontraffic accident

✓x7th V02.90 Pedestrian on foot injured in collision with two- or three-wheeled motor vehicle, unspecified whether traffic or nontraffic accident
Pedestrian NOS injured in collision with two- or three-wheeled motor vehicle, unspecified whether traffic or nontraffic accident

✓x7th V02.91 Pedestrian on roller-skates injured in collision with two- or three-wheeled motor vehicle, unspecified whether traffic or nontraffic accident

✓x7th V02.92 Pedestrian on skateboard injured in collision with two- or three-wheeled motor vehicle, unspecified whether traffic or nontraffic accident

✓x7ᵗʰ **V02.99** **Pedestrian with other** conveyance **injured in collision with two- or three-wheeled motor vehicle, unspecified whether traffic or nontraffic accident**

Pedestrian with babystroller injured in collision with two- or three-wheeled motor vehicle, unspecified whether traffic or nontraffic accident

Pedestrian on ice-skates injured in collision with two- or three-wheeled motor vehicle, unspecified whether traffic or nontraffic accident

Pedestrian on nonmotorized scooter injured in collision with two- or three-wheeled motor vehicle, unspecified whether traffic or nontraffic accident

Pedestrian on sled injured in collision with two- or three-wheeled motor vehicle, unspecified whether traffic or nontraffic accident

Pedestrian on snowboard injured in collision with two- or three-wheeled motor vehicle, unspecified whether traffic or nontraffic accident

Pedestrian on snow-skis injured in collision with two- or three-wheeled motor vehicle, unspecified whether traffic or nontraffic accident

Pedestrian in wheelchair (powered) injured in collision with two- or three-wheeled motor vehicle, unspecified whether traffic or nontraffic accident

Pedestrian in motorized mobility scooter injured in collision with two- or three-wheeled motor vehicle, unspecified whether traffic or nontraffic accident

✓4ᵗʰ **V03** **Pedestrian injured in collision with car, pick-up truck or van**

The appropriate 7th character is to be added to each code from category V03.
A   initial encounter
D   subsequent encounter
S   sequela

✓5ᵗʰ **V03.0** **Pedestrian injured in collision with car, pick-up truck or van in nontraffic accident**

✓x7ᵗʰ **V03.00** **Pedestrian on foot injured in collision with car, pick-up truck or van in nontraffic accident**

Pedestrian NOS injured in collision with car, pick-up truck or van in nontraffic accident

✓x7ᵗʰ **V03.01** **Pedestrian on roller-skates injured in collision with car, pick-up truck or van in nontraffic accident**

✓x7ᵗʰ **V03.02** **Pedestrian on skateboard injured in collision with car, pick-up truck or van in nontraffic accident**

✓x7ᵗʰ **V03.09** **Pedestrian with other** conveyance **injured in collision with car, pick-up truck or van in nontraffic accident**

Pedestrian with babystroller injured in collision with car, pick-up truck or van in nontraffic accident

Pedestrian on ice-skates injured in collision with car, pick-up truck or van in nontraffic accident

Pedestrian on nonmotorized scooter injured in collision with car, pick-up truck or van in nontraffic accident

Pedestrian on sled injured in collision with car, pick-up truck or van in nontraffic accident

Pedestrian on snowboard injured in collision with car, pick-up truck or van in nontraffic accident

Pedestrian on snow-skis injured in collision with car, pick-up truck or van in nontraffic accident

Pedestrian in wheelchair (powered) injured in collision with car, pick-up truck or van in nontraffic accident

Pedestrian in motorized mobility scooter injured in collision with car, pick-up truck or van in nontraffic accident

✓5ᵗʰ **V03.1** **Pedestrian injured in collision with car, pick-up truck or van in traffic accident**

✓x7ᵗʰ **V03.10** **Pedestrian on foot injured in collision with car, pick-up truck or van in traffic accident**

Pedestrian NOS injured in collision with car, pick-up truck or van in traffic accident

✓x7ᵗʰ **V03.11** **Pedestrian on roller-skates injured in collision with car, pick-up truck or van in traffic accident**

✓x7ᵗʰ **V03.12** **Pedestrian on skateboard injured in collision with car, pick-up truck or van in traffic accident**

✓x7ᵗʰ **V03.19** **Pedestrian with other** conveyance **injured in collision with car, pick-up truck or van in traffic accident**

Pedestrian with babystroller injured in collision with car, pick-up truck or van in traffic accident

Pedestrian on ice-skates injured in collision with car, pick-up truck or van in traffic accident

Pedestrian on nonmotorized scooter injured in collision with car, pick-up truck or van in traffic accident

Pedestrian on sled injured in collision with car, pick-up truck or van in traffic accident

Pedestrian on snowboard injured in collision with car, pick-up truck or van in traffic accident

Pedestrian on snow-skis injured in collision with car, pick-up truck or van in traffic accident

Pedestrian in wheelchair (powered) injured in collision with car, pick-up truck or van in traffic accident

Pedestrian in motorized mobility scooter injured in collision with car, pick-up truck or van in traffic accident

✓5ᵗʰ **V03.9** **Pedestrian injured in collision with car, pick-up truck or van, unspecified whether traffic or nontraffic accident**

✓x7ᵗʰ **V03.90** **Pedestrian on foot injured in collision with car, pick-up truck or van, unspecified whether traffic or nontraffic accident**

Pedestrian NOS injured in collision with car, pick-up truck or van, unspecified whether traffic or nontraffic accident

✓x7ᵗʰ **V03.91** **Pedestrian on roller-skates injured in collision with car, pick-up truck or van, unspecified whether traffic or nontraffic accident**

✓x7ᵗʰ **V03.92** **Pedestrian on skateboard injured in collision with car, pick-up truck or van, unspecified whether traffic or nontraffic accident**

✓x7ᵗʰ **V03.99** **Pedestrian with other** conveyance **injured in collision with car, pick-up truck or van, unspecified whether traffic or nontraffic accident**

Pedestrian with babystroller injured in collision with car, pick-up truck or van, unspecified whether traffic or nontraffic accident

Pedestrian on ice-skates injured in collision with car, pick-up truck or van, unspecified whether traffic or nontraffic accident

Pedestrian on nonmotorized scooter injured in collision with car, pick-up truck or van, unspecified whether traffic or nontraffic accident

Pedestrian on sled injured in collision with car, pick-up truck or van in nontraffic accident

Pedestrian on snowboard injured in collision with car, pick-up truck or van, unspecified whether traffic or nontraffic accident

Pedestrian on snow-skis injured in collision with car, pick-up truck or van, unspecified whether traffic or nontraffic accident

Pedestrian in wheelchair (powered) injured in collision with car, pick-up truck or van, unspecified whether traffic or nontraffic accident

Pedestrian in motorized mobility scooter injured in collision with car, pick-up truck or van, unspecified whether traffic or nontraffic accident

✓4ᵗʰ **V04** **Pedestrian injured in collision with heavy transport vehicle or bus**

EXCLUDES1   pedestrian injured in collision with military vehicle (V09.01, V09.21)

The appropriate 7th character is to be added to each code from category V04.
A   initial encounter
D   subsequent encounter
S   sequela

✓5ᵗʰ **V04.0** **Pedestrian injured in collision with heavy transport vehicle or bus in nontraffic accident**

✓x7ᵗʰ **V04.00** **Pedestrian on foot injured in collision with heavy transport vehicle or bus in nontraffic accident**

Pedestrian NOS injured in collision with heavy transport vehicle or bus in nontraffic accident

✓x7ᵗʰ **V04.01** **Pedestrian on roller-skates injured in collision with heavy transport vehicle or bus in nontraffic accident**

✓x7ᵗʰ **V04.02** **Pedestrian on skateboard injured in collision with heavy transport vehicle or bus in nontraffic accident**

EXCLUDES1 Not coded here   EXCLUDES2 Not included here   N Newborn Age: 0   P Pediatric Age: 0-17   M Maternity Age: 12-55   A Adult Age: 15-124

994   ICD-10-CM Draft (2015)

✓x 7th **V04.09** **Pedestrian with other** conveyance **injured in collision with heavy transport vehicle or bus in nontraffic accident**

> Pedestrian with babystroller injured in collision with heavy transport vehicle or bus in nontraffic accident
> Pedestrian on ice-skates injured in collision with heavy transport vehicle or bus in nontraffic accident
> Pedestrian on nonmotorized scooter injured in collision with heavy transport vehicle or bus in nontraffic accident
> Pedestrian on sled injured in collision with heavy transport vehicle or bus in nontraffic accident
> Pedestrian on snowboard injured in collision with heavy transport vehicle or bus in nontraffic accident
> Pedestrian on snow-skis injured in collision with heavy transport vehicle or bus in nontraffic accident
> Pedestrian in wheelchair (powered) injured in collision with heavy transport vehicle or bus in nontraffic accident
> Pedestrian in motorized mobility scooter injured in collision with heavy transport vehicle or bus in nontraffic accident

✓5th **V04.1** **Pedestrian injured in collision with heavy transport vehicle or bus** in traffic accident

✓x 7th **V04.10** **Pedestrian** on foot **injured in collision with heavy transport vehicle or bus in traffic accident**

> Pedestrian NOS injured in collision with heavy transport vehicle or bus in traffic accident

✓x 7th **V04.11** **Pedestrian** on roller-skates **injured in collision with heavy transport vehicle or bus in traffic accident**

✓x 7th **V04.12** **Pedestrian** on skateboard **injured in collision with heavy transport vehicle or bus in traffic accident**

✓x 7th **V04.19** **Pedestrian with other** conveyance **injured in collision with heavy transport vehicle or bus in traffic accident**

> Pedestrian with babystroller injured in collision with heavy transport vehicle or bus in traffic accident
> Pedestrian on ice-skates injured in collision with heavy transport vehicle or bus in traffic accident
> Pedestrian on nonmotorized scooter injured in collision with heavy transport vehicle or bus in traffic accident
> Pedestrian on sled injured in collision with heavy transport vehicle or bus in traffic accident
> Pedestrian on snowboard injured in collision with heavy transport vehicle or bus in traffic accident
> Pedestrian on snow-skis injured in collision with heavy transport vehicle or bus in traffic accident
> Pedestrian in wheelchair (powered) injured in collision with heavy transport vehicle or bus in traffic accident
> Pedestrian in motorized mobility scooter injured in collision with heavy transport vehicle or bus in traffic accident

✓5th **V04.9** **Pedestrian injured in collision with heavy transport vehicle or bus,** unspecified whether traffic or nontraffic accident

✓x 7th **V04.90** **Pedestrian** on foot **injured in collision with heavy transport vehicle or bus, unspecified whether traffic or nontraffic accident**

> Pedestrian NOS injured in collision with heavy transport vehicle or bus, unspecified whether traffic or nontraffic accident

✓x 7th **V04.91** **Pedestrian** on roller-skates **injured in collision with heavy transport vehicle or bus, unspecified whether traffic or nontraffic accident**

✓x 7th **V04.92** **Pedestrian** on skateboard **injured in collision with heavy transport vehicle or bus, unspecified whether traffic or nontraffic accident**

✓x 7th **V04.99** **Pedestrian with other** conveyance **injured in collision with heavy transport vehicle or bus, unspecified whether traffic or nontraffic accident**

> Pedestrian with babystroller injured in collision with heavy transport vehicle or bus, unspecified whether traffic or nontraffic accident
> Pedestrian on ice-skates injured in collision with heavy transport vehicle or bus, unspecified whether traffic or nontraffic accident
> Pedestrian on nonmotorized scooter injured in collision with heavy transport vehicle or bus, unspecified whether traffic or nontraffic accident
> Pedestrian on sled injured in collision with heavy transport vehicle or bus, unspecified whether traffic or nontraffic accident
> Pedestrian on snowboard injured in collision with heavy transport vehicle or bus, unspecified whether traffic or nontraffic accident
> Pedestrian on snow-skis injured in collision with heavy transport vehicle or bus, unspecified whether traffic or nontraffic accident
> Pedestrian in wheelchair (powered) injured in collision with heavy transport vehicle or bus, unspecified whether traffic or nontraffic accident
> Pedestrian in motorized mobility scooter injured in collision with heavy transport vehicle or bus, unspecified whether traffic or nontraffic accident

✓4th **V05** **Pedestrian injured in collision with railway train or railway vehicle**

> The appropriate 7th character is to be added to each code from category V05.
> A　　initial encounter
> D　　subsequent encounter
> S　　sequela

✓5th **V05.0** **Pedestrian injured in collision with railway train or railway vehicle** in nontraffic accident

✓x 7th **V05.00** **Pedestrian** on foot **injured in collision with railway train or railway vehicle in nontraffic accident**

> Pedestrian NOS injured in collision with railway train or railway vehicle in nontraffic accident

✓x 7th **V05.01** **Pedestrian** on roller-skates **injured in collision with railway train or railway vehicle in nontraffic accident**

✓x 7th **V05.02** **Pedestrian** on skateboard **injured in collision with railway train or railway vehicle in nontraffic accident**

✓x 7th **V05.09** **Pedestrian with other** conveyance **injured in collision with railway train or railway vehicle in nontraffic accident**

> Pedestrian with babystroller injured in collision with railway train or railway vehicle in nontraffic accident
> Pedestrian on ice-skates injured in collision with railway train or railway vehicle in nontraffic accident
> Pedestrian on nonmotorized scooter injured in collision with railway train or railway vehicle in nontraffic accident
> Pedestrian on sled injured in collision with railway train or railway vehicle in nontraffic accident
> Pedestrian on snowboard injured in collision with railway train or railway vehicle in nontraffic accident
> Pedestrian on snow-skis injured in collision with railway train or railway vehicle in nontraffic accident
> Pedestrian in wheelchair (powered) injured in collision with railway train or railway vehicle in nontraffic accident
> Pedestrian in motorized mobility scooter injured in collision with railway train or railway vehicle in nontraffic accident

✓5th **V05.1** **Pedestrian injured in collision with railway train or railway vehicle** in traffic accident

✓x 7th **V05.10** **Pedestrian** on foot **injured in collision with railway train or railway vehicle in traffic accident**

> Pedestrian NOS injured in collision with railway train or railway vehicle in traffic accident

✓x 7th **V05.11** **Pedestrian** on roller-skates **injured in collision with railway train or railway vehicle in traffic accident**

✓x 7th **V05.12** **Pedestrian** on skateboard **injured in collision with railway train or railway vehicle in traffic accident**

✓ Additional Character Required　　✓x 7th Xtension Alert　　Unspecified Dx　　Other Specified Dx　　Manifestation　　▶◀ Revised Text　　● New Code　　▲ Revised Code Title

√x7ᵗʰ **V05.19** **Pedestrian with other conveyance injured in collision with railway train or railway vehicle in traffic accident**
> Pedestrian with babystroller injured in collision with railway train or railway vehicle in traffic accident
> Pedestrian on ice-skates injured in collision with railway train or railway vehicle in traffic accident
> Pedestrian on nonmotorized scooter injured in collision with railway train or railway vehicle in traffic accident
> Pedestrian on sled injured in collision with railway train or railway vehicle in traffic accident
> Pedestrian on snowboard injured in collision with railway train or railway vehicle in traffic accident
> Pedestrian on snow-skis injured in collision with railway train or railway vehicle in traffic accident
> Pedestrian in wheelchair (powered) injured in collision with railway train or railway vehicle in traffic accident
> Pedestrian in motorized mobility scooter injured in collision with railway train or railway vehicle in traffic accident

√5ᵗʰ **V05.9** **Pedestrian injured in collision with railway train or railway vehicle, unspecified whether traffic or nontraffic accident**

√x7ᵗʰ **V05.90** **Pedestrian on foot injured in collision with railway train or railway vehicle, unspecified whether traffic or nontraffic accident**
> Pedestrian NOS injured in collision with railway train or railway vehicle, unspecified whether traffic or nontraffic accident

√x7ᵗʰ **V05.91** **Pedestrian on roller-skates injured in collision with railway train or railway vehicle, unspecified whether traffic or nontraffic accident**

√x7ᵗʰ **V05.92** **Pedestrian on skateboard injured in collision with railway train or railway vehicle, unspecified whether traffic or nontraffic accident**

√x7ᵗʰ **V05.99** **Pedestrian with other conveyance injured in collision with railway train or railway vehicle, unspecified whether traffic or nontraffic accident**
> Pedestrian with babystroller injured in collision with railway train or railway vehicle, unspecified whether traffic or nontraffic
> Pedestrian on ice-skates injured in collision with railway train or railway vehicle, unspecified whether traffic or nontraffic
> Pedestrian on nonmotorized scooter injured in collision with railway train or railway vehicle, unspecified whether traffic or nontraffic
> Pedestrian on sled injured in collision with railway train or railway vehicle, unspecified whether traffic or nontraffic
> Pedestrian on snowboard injured in collision with railway train or railway vehicle, unspecified whether traffic or nontraffic
> Pedestrian on snow-skis injured in collision with railway train or railway vehicle, unspecified whether traffic or nontraffic
> Pedestrian in wheelchair (powered) injured in collision with railway train or railway vehicle, unspecified whether traffic or nontraffic
> Pedestrian in motorized mobility scooter injured in collision with railway train or railway vehicle, unspecified whether traffic or nontraffic

√4ᵗʰ **V06** **Pedestrian injured in collision with other nonmotor vehicle**
> INCLUDES collision with animal-drawn vehicle, animal being ridden, nonpowered streetcar
> EXCLUDES 1 pedestrian injured in collision with pedestrian conveyance (V00.0-)

The appropriate 7th character is to be added to each code from category V06.
A   initial encounter
D   subsequent encounter
S   sequela

√5ᵗʰ **V06.0** **Pedestrian injured in collision with other nonmotor vehicle in nontraffic accident**

√x7ᵗʰ **V06.00** **Pedestrian on foot injured in collision with other nonmotor vehicle in nontraffic accident**
> Pedestrian NOS injured in collision with other nonmotor vehicle in nontraffic accident

√x7ᵗʰ **V06.01** **Pedestrian on roller-skates injured in collision with other nonmotor vehicle in nontraffic accident**

√x7ᵗʰ **V06.02** **Pedestrian on skateboard injured in collision with other nonmotor vehicle in nontraffic accident**

√x7ᵗʰ **V06.09** **Pedestrian with other conveyance injured in collision with other nonmotor vehicle in nontraffic accident**
> Pedestrian with babystroller injured in collision with other nonmotor vehicle in nontraffic accident
> Pedestrian on ice-skates injured in collision with other nonmotor vehicle in nontraffic accident
> Pedestrian on nonmotorized scooter injured in collision with other nonmotor vehicle in nontraffic accident
> Pedestrian on sled injured in collision with other nonmotor vehicle in nontraffic accident
> Pedestrian on snowboard injured in collision with other nonmotor vehicle in nontraffic accident
> Pedestrian on snow-skis injured in collision with other nonmotor vehicle in nontraffic accident
> Pedestrian in wheelchair (powered) injured in collision with other nonmotor vehicle in nontraffic accident
> Pedestrian in motorized mobility scooter injured in collision with other nonmotor vehicle in nontraffic accident

√5ᵗʰ **V06.1** **Pedestrian injured in collision with other nonmotor vehicle in traffic accident**

√x7ᵗʰ **V06.10** **Pedestrian on foot injured in collision with other nonmotor vehicle in traffic accident**
> Pedestrian NOS injured in collision with other nonmotor vehicle in traffic accident

√x7ᵗʰ **V06.11** **Pedestrian on roller-skates injured in collision with other nonmotor vehicle in traffic accident**

√x7ᵗʰ **V06.12** **Pedestrian on skateboard injured in collision with other nonmotor vehicle in traffic accident**

√x7ᵗʰ **V06.19** **Pedestrian with other conveyance injured in collision with other nonmotor vehicle in traffic accident**
> Pedestrian with babystroller injured in collision with other nonmotor vehicle in nontraffic accident
> Pedestrian on ice-skates injured in collision with other nonmotor vehicle in traffic accident
> Pedestrian on nonmotorized scooter injured in collision with other nonmotor vehicle in traffic accident
> Pedestrian on sled injured in collision with other nonmotor vehicle in traffic accident
> Pedestrian on snowboard injured in collision with other nonmotor vehicle in traffic accident
> Pedestrian on snow-skis injured in collision with other nonmotor vehicle in traffic accident
> Pedestrian in wheelchair (powered) injured in collision with other nonmotor vehicle in traffic accident
> Pedestrian in motorized mobility scooter injured in collision with other nonmotor vehicle in traffic accident

√5ᵗʰ **V06.9** **Pedestrian injured in collision with other nonmotor vehicle, unspecified whether traffic or nontraffic accident**

√x7ᵗʰ **V06.90** **Pedestrian on foot injured in collision with other nonmotor vehicle, unspecified whether traffic or nontraffic accident**
> Pedestrian NOS injured in collision with other nonmotor vehicle, unspecified whether traffic or nontraffic accident

√x7ᵗʰ **V06.91** **Pedestrian on roller-skates injured in collision with other nonmotor vehicle, unspecified whether traffic or nontraffic accident**

√x7ᵗʰ **V06.92** **Pedestrian on skateboard injured in collision with other nonmotor vehicle, unspecified whether traffic or nontraffic accident**

√x7ᵗʰ **V06.99** **Pedestrian with other** conveyance **injured in collision with other nonmotor vehicle, unspecified whether traffic or nontraffic accident**

Pedestrian with babystroller injured in collision with other nonmotor vehicle, unspecified whether traffic or nontraffic accident

Pedestrian on ice-skates injured in collision with other nonmotor vehicle, unspecified whether traffic or nontraffic accident

Pedestrian on nonmotorized scooter injured in collision with other nonmotor vehicle, unspecified whether traffic or nontraffic accident

Pedestrian on sled injured in collision with other nonmotor vehicle, unspecified whether traffic or nontraffic accident

Pedestrian on snowboard injured in collision with other nonmotor vehicle, unspecified whether traffic or nontraffic accident

Pedestrian on snow-skis injured in collision with other nonmotor vehicle, unspecified whether traffic or nontraffic accident

Pedestrian in wheelchair (powered) injured in collision with other nonmotor vehicle, unspecified whether traffic or nontraffic accident

Pedestrian in motorized mobility scooter injured in collision with other nonmotor vehicle, unspecified whether traffic or nontraffic accident

√4ᵗʰ **V09** **Pedestrian injured in other and unspecified transport accidents**

The appropriate 7th character is to be added to each code from category V09.
A   initial encounter
D   subsequent encounter
S   sequela

√5ᵗʰ **V09.0** **Pedestrian injured in** nontraffic **accident involving** other **and unspecified motor vehicles**

√x7ᵗʰ **V09.00** **Pedestrian injured in nontraffic accident involving unspecified motor vehicles**

√x7ᵗʰ **V09.01** **Pedestrian injured in nontraffic accident involving** military **vehicle**

√x7ᵗʰ **V09.09** **Pedestrian injured in nontraffic accident involving other motor vehicles**

Pedestrian injured in nontraffic accident by special vehicle

√x7ᵗʰ **V09.1** **Pedestrian injured in unspecified** nontraffic **accident**

√5ᵗʰ **V09.2** **Pedestrian injured in** traffic accident **involving other and unspecified motor vehicles**

√x7ᵗʰ **V09.20** **Pedestrian injured in traffic accident involving unspecified motor vehicles**

√x7ᵗʰ **V09.21** **Pedestrian injured in traffic accident involving** military vehicle

√x7ᵗʰ **V09.29** **Pedestrian injured in traffic accident involving other motor vehicles**

√x7ᵗʰ **V09.3** **Pedestrian injured in unspecified** traffic **accident**

√x7ᵗʰ **V09.9** **Pedestrian injured in unspecified** transport **accident**

Pedal cycle rider injured in transport accident (V10-V19)

INCLUDES   any non-motorized vehicle, excluding an animal-drawn vehicle, or a sidecar or trailer attached to the pedal cycle
EXCLUDES 2   rupture of pedal cycle tire (W37.0)

√4ᵗʰ **V10** **Pedal cycle rider injured in collision with pedestrian or animal**

EXCLUDES 1   pedal cycle rider collision with animal-drawn vehicle or animal being ridden (V16.-)

The appropriate 7th character is to be added to each code from category V10.
A   initial encounter
D   subsequent encounter
S   sequela

√x7ᵗʰ **V10.0** **Pedal cycle** driver **injured in collision with pedestrian or animal** in nontraffic accident

√x7ᵗʰ **V10.1** **Pedal cycle** passenger **injured in collision with pedestrian or animal** in nontraffic accident

√x7ᵗʰ **V10.2** **Unspecified pedal cyclist injured in collision with pedestrian or animal** in nontraffic accident

√x7ᵗʰ **V10.3** Person boarding or alighting **a pedal cycle injured in collision with pedestrian or animal**

√x7ᵗʰ **V10.4** **Pedal cycle** driver **injured in collision with pedestrian or animal** in traffic accident

√x7ᵗʰ **V10.5** **Pedal cycle** passenger **injured in collision with pedestrian or animal** in traffic accident

√x7ᵗʰ **V10.9** **Unspecified pedal cyclist injured in collision with pedestrian or animal** in traffic accident

√4ᵗʰ **V11** **Pedal cycle rider injured in collision with other pedal cycle**

The appropriate 7th character is to be added to each code from category V11.
A   initial encounter
D   subsequent encounter
S   sequela

√x7ᵗʰ **V11.0** **Pedal cycle** driver **injured in collision with other pedal cycle in** nontraffic accident

√x7ᵗʰ **V11.1** **Pedal cycle** passenger **injured in collision with other pedal cycle in** nontraffic accident

√x7ᵗʰ **V11.2** **Unspecified pedal cyclist injured in collision with other pedal cycle in** nontraffic accident

√x7ᵗʰ **V11.3** Person boarding or alighting **a pedal cycle injured in collision with other pedal cycle**

√x7ᵗʰ **V11.4** **Pedal cycle** driver **injured in collision with other pedal cycle in** traffic accident

√x7ᵗʰ **V11.5** **Pedal cycle** passenger **injured in collision with other pedal cycle in** traffic accident

√x7ᵗʰ **V11.9** **Unspecified pedal cyclist injured in collision with other pedal cycle** in traffic accident

√4ᵗʰ **V12** **Pedal cycle rider injured in collision with two- or three-wheeled motor vehicle**

The appropriate 7th character is to be added to each code from category V12.
A   initial encounter
D   subsequent encounter
S   sequela

√x7ᵗʰ **V12.0** **Pedal cycle** driver **injured in collision with two- or three-wheeled motor vehicle** in nontraffic accident

√x7ᵗʰ **V12.1** **Pedal cycle** passenger **injured in collision with two- or three-wheeled motor vehicle** in nontraffic accident

√x7ᵗʰ **V12.2** **Unspecified pedal cyclist injured in collision with two- or three-wheeled motor vehicle** in nontraffic accident

√x7ᵗʰ **V12.3** Person boarding or alighting **a pedal cycle injured in collision with two- or three-wheeled motor vehicle**

√x7ᵗʰ **V12.4** **Pedal cycle** driver **injured in collision with two- or three-wheeled motor vehicle** in traffic accident

√x7ᵗʰ **V12.5** **Pedal cycle** passenger **injured in collision with two- or three-wheeled motor vehicle** in traffic accident

√x7ᵗʰ **V12.9** **Unspecified pedal cyclist injured in collision with two- or three-wheeled motor vehicle** in traffic accident

√4ᵗʰ **V13** **Pedal cycle rider injured in collision with car, pick-up truck or van**

The appropriate 7th character is to be added to each code from category V13.
A   initial encounter
D   subsequent encounter
S   sequela

√x7ᵗʰ **V13.0** **Pedal cycle** driver **injured in collision with car, pick-up truck or van** in nontraffic accident

√x7ᵗʰ **V13.1** **Pedal cycle** passenger **injured in collision with car, pick-up truck or van** in nontraffic accident

√x7ᵗʰ **V13.2** **Unspecified pedal cyclist injured in collision with car, pick-up truck or van** in nontraffic accident

√x7ᵗʰ **V13.3** Person boarding or alighting **a pedal cycle injured in collision with car, pick-up truck or van**

√x7ᵗʰ **V13.4** **Pedal cycle** driver **injured in collision with car, pick-up truck or van** in traffic accident

√x7ᵗʰ **V13.5** **Pedal cycle** passenger **injured in collision with car, pick-up truck or van** in traffic accident

√x7ᵗʰ **V13.9** **Unspecified pedal cyclist injured in collision with car, pick-up truck or van** in traffic accident

---

✓ Additional Character Required   √x7ᵗʰ Xtension Alert   Unspecified Dx   Other Specified Dx   Manifestation   ▶◀ Revised Text   ● New Code   ▲ Revised Code Title

External Causes of Morbidity

V14–V19.29

√4th **V14 Pedal cycle rider injured in collision with heavy transport vehicle or bus**

> EXCLUDES 1   *pedal cycle rider injured in collision with military vehicle (V19.81)*

> The appropriate 7th character is to be added to each code from category V14.
> A   initial encounter
> D   subsequent encounter
> S   sequela

√x7th **V14.0 Pedal cycle driver injured in collision with heavy transport vehicle or bus in nontraffic accident**

√x7th **V14.1 Pedal cycle passenger injured in collision with heavy transport vehicle or bus in nontraffic accident**

√x7th **V14.2 Unspecified pedal cyclist injured in collision with heavy transport vehicle or bus in nontraffic accident**

√x7th **V14.3 Person boarding or alighting a pedal cycle injured in collision with heavy transport vehicle or bus**

√x7th **V14.4 Pedal cycle driver injured in collision with heavy transport vehicle or bus in traffic accident**

√x7th **V14.5 Pedal cycle passenger injured in collision with heavy transport vehicle or bus in traffic accident**

√x7th **V14.9 Unspecified pedal cyclist injured in collision with heavy transport vehicle or bus in traffic accident**

√4th **V15 Pedal cycle rider injured in collision with railway train or railway vehicle**

> The appropriate 7th character is to be added to each code from category V15.
> A   initial encounter
> D   subsequent encounter
> S   sequela

√x7th **V15.0 Pedal cycle driver injured in collision with railway train or railway vehicle in nontraffic accident**

√x7th **V15.1 Pedal cycle passenger injured in collision with railway train or railway vehicle in nontraffic accident**

√x7th **V15.2 Unspecified pedal cyclist injured in collision with railway train or railway vehicle in nontraffic accident**

√x7th **V15.3 Person boarding or alighting a pedal cycle injured in collision with railway train or railway vehicle**

√x7th **V15.4 Pedal cycle driver injured in collision with railway train or railway vehicle in traffic accident**

√x7th **V15.5 Pedal cycle passenger injured in collision with railway train or railway vehicle in traffic accident**

√x7th **V15.9 Unspecified pedal cyclist injured in collision with railway train or railway vehicle in traffic accident**

√4th **V16 Pedal cycle rider injured in collision with other nonmotor vehicle**

> INCLUDES   collision with animal-drawn vehicle, animal being ridden, streetcar

> The appropriate 7th character is to be added to each code from category V16.
> A   initial encounter
> D   subsequent encounter
> S   sequela

√x7th **V16.0 Pedal cycle driver injured in collision with other nonmotor vehicle in nontraffic accident**

√x7th **V16.1 Pedal cycle passenger injured in collision with other nonmotor vehicle in nontraffic accident**

√x7th **V16.2 Unspecified pedal cyclist injured in collision with other nonmotor vehicle in nontraffic accident**

√x7th **V16.3 Person boarding or alighting a pedal cycle injured in collision with other nonmotor vehicle in nontraffic accident**

√x7th **V16.4 Pedal cycle driver injured in collision with other nonmotor vehicle in traffic accident**

√x7th **V16.5 Pedal cycle passenger injured in collision with other nonmotor vehicle in traffic accident**

√x7th **V16.9 Unspecified pedal cyclist injured in collision with other nonmotor vehicle in traffic accident**

√4th **V17 Pedal cycle rider injured in collision with fixed or stationary object**

> The appropriate 7th character is to be added to each code from category V17.
> A   initial encounter
> D   subsequent encounter
> S   sequela

√x7th **V17.0 Pedal cycle driver injured in collision with fixed or stationary object in nontraffic accident**

√x7th **V17.1 Pedal cycle passenger injured in collision with fixed or stationary object in nontraffic accident**

√x7th **V17.2 Unspecified pedal cyclist injured in collision with fixed or stationary object in nontraffic accident**

√x7th **V17.3 Person boarding or alighting a pedal cycle injured in collision with fixed or stationary object**

√x7th **V17.4 Pedal cycle driver injured in collision with fixed or stationary object in traffic accident**

√x7th **V17.5 Pedal cycle passenger injured in collision with fixed or stationary object in traffic accident**

√x7th **V17.9 Unspecified pedal cyclist injured in collision with fixed or stationary object in traffic accident**

√4th **V18 Pedal cycle rider injured in noncollision transport accident**

> INCLUDES   fall or thrown from pedal cycle (without antecedent collision)
> overturning pedal cycle NOS
> overturning pedal cycle without collision

> The appropriate 7th character is to be added to each code from category V18.
> A   initial encounter
> D   subsequent encounter
> S   sequela

√x7th **V18.0 Pedal cycle driver injured in noncollision transport accident in nontraffic accident**

√x7th **V18.1 Pedal cycle passenger injured in noncollision transport accident in nontraffic accident**

√x7th **V18.2 Unspecified pedal cyclist injured in noncollision transport accident in nontraffic accident**

√x7th **V18.3 Person boarding or alighting a pedal cycle injured in noncollision transport accident**

√x7th **V18.4 Pedal cycle driver injured in noncollision transport accident in traffic accident**

√x7th **V18.5 Pedal cycle passenger injured in noncollision transport accident in traffic accident**

√x7th **V18.9 Unspecified pedal cyclist injured in noncollision transport accident in traffic accident**

√4th **V19 Pedal cycle rider injured in other and unspecified transport accidents**

> The appropriate 7th character is to be added to each code from category V19.
> A   initial encounter
> D   subsequent encounter
> S   sequela

√5th **V19.0 Pedal cycle driver injured in collision with other and unspecified motor vehicles in nontraffic accident**

√x7th **V19.00 Pedal cycle driver injured in collision with unspecified motor vehicles in nontraffic accident**

√x7th **V19.09 Pedal cycle driver injured in collision with other motor vehicles in nontraffic accident**

√5th **V19.1 Pedal cycle passenger injured in collision with other and unspecified motor vehicles in nontraffic accident**

√x7th **V19.10 Pedal cycle passenger injured in collision with unspecified motor vehicles in nontraffic accident**

√x7th **V19.19 Pedal cycle passenger injured in collision with other motor vehicles in nontraffic accident**

√5th **V19.2 Unspecified pedal cyclist injured in collision with other and unspecified motor vehicles in nontraffic accident**

√x7th **V19.20 Unspecified pedal cyclist injured in collision with unspecified motor vehicles in nontraffic accident**
Pedal cycle collision NOS, nontraffic

√x7th **V19.29 Unspecified pedal cyclist injured in collision with other motor vehicles in nontraffic accident**

EXCLUDES 1 Not coded here   EXCLUDES 2 Not included here   N Newborn Age: 0   P Pediatric Age: 0-17   M Maternity Age: 12-55   A Adult Age: 15-124

998   ICD-10-CM Draft (2015)

☑x7ᵗʰ **V19.3** **Pedal cyclist (driver) (passenger) injured in unspecified nontraffic accident**
     Pedal cycle accident NOS, nontraffic
     Pedal cyclist injured in nontraffic accident NOS

☑5ᵗʰ **V19.4** **Pedal cycle** driver **injured in collision with other and unspecified motor vehicles in traffic accident**

     ☑x7ᵗʰ **V19.40** **Pedal cycle driver injured in collision with unspecified motor vehicles in traffic accident**

     ☑x7ᵗʰ **V19.49** **Pedal cycle driver injured in collision with other motor vehicles in traffic accident**

☑5ᵗʰ **V19.5** **Pedal cycle** passenger **injured in collision with other and unspecified motor vehicles in traffic accident**

     ☑x7ᵗʰ **V19.50** **Pedal cycle passenger injured in collision with unspecified motor vehicles in traffic accident**

     ☑x7ᵗʰ **V19.59** **Pedal cycle passenger injured in collision with other motor vehicles in traffic accident**

☑5ᵗʰ **V19.6** Unspecified **pedal cyclist injured in collision with** other and unspecified motor vehicles in traffic accident

     ☑x7ᵗʰ **V19.60** **Unspecified pedal cyclist injured in collision with unspecified motor vehicles in traffic accident**
         Pedal cycle collision NOS (traffic)

     ☑x7ᵗʰ **V19.69** **Unspecified pedal cyclist injured in collision with other motor vehicles in traffic accident**

☑5ᵗʰ **V19.8** **Pedal cyclist (driver) (passenger) injured in** other specified transport accidents

     ☑x7ᵗʰ **V19.81** **Pedal cyclist (driver) (passenger) injured in transport accident with** military vehicle

     ☑x7ᵗʰ **V19.88** **Pedal cyclist (driver) (passenger) injured in other specified transport accidents**

☑x7ᵗʰ **V19.9** **Pedal cyclist (driver) (passenger) injured in unspecified traffic accident**
     Pedal cycle accident NOS

Motorcycle rider injured in transport accident (V20-V29)

INCLUDES   moped
         motorcycle with sidecar
         motorized bicycle
         motor scooter
EXCLUDES 1   *three-wheeled motor vehicle (V30-V39)*

☑4ᵗʰ **V20** **Motorcycle rider injured in collision with pedestrian or animal**
     EXCLUDES 1   *motorcycle rider collision with animal-drawn vehicle or animal being ridden (V26.-)*

     The appropriate 7th character is to be added to each code from category V20.
     A   initial encounter
     D   subsequent encounter
     S   sequela

☑x7ᵗʰ **V20.0** **Motorcycle** driver **injured in collision with pedestrian or animal** in nontraffic accident

☑x7ᵗʰ **V20.1** **Motorcycle** passenger **injured in collision with pedestrian or animal** in nontraffic accident

☑x7ᵗʰ **V20.2** **Unspecified motorcycle rider injured in collision with pedestrian or animal** in nontraffic accident

☑x7ᵗʰ **V20.3** Person boarding or alighting **a motorcycle injured in collision with pedestrian or animal**

☑x7ᵗʰ **V20.4** **Motorcycle** driver **injured in collision with pedestrian or animal** in traffic accident

☑x7ᵗʰ **V20.5** **Motorcycle** passenger **injured in collision with pedestrian or animal** in traffic accident

☑x7ᵗʰ **V20.9** **Unspecified motorcycle rider injured in collision with pedestrian or animal** in traffic accident

☑4ᵗʰ **V21** **Motorcycle rider injured in collision with pedal cycle**

     The appropriate 7th character is to be added to each code from category V21.
     A   initial encounter
     D   subsequent encounter
     S   sequela

☑x7ᵗʰ **V21.0** **Motorcycle** driver **injured in collision with pedal cycle** in nontraffic accident

☑x7ᵗʰ **V21.1** **Motorcycle** passenger **injured in collision with pedal cycle** in nontraffic accident

☑x7ᵗʰ **V21.2** **Unspecified motorcycle rider injured in collision with pedal cycle** in nontraffic accident

☑x7ᵗʰ **V21.3** Person boarding or alighting **a motorcycle injured in collision with pedal cycle**

☑x7ᵗʰ **V21.4** **Motorcycle** driver **injured in collision with pedal cycle** in traffic accident

☑x7ᵗʰ **V21.5** **Motorcycle** passenger **injured in collision with pedal cycle** in traffic accident

☑x7ᵗʰ **V21.9** **Unspecified motorcycle rider injured in collision with pedal cycle** in traffic accident

☑4ᵗʰ **V22** **Motorcycle rider injured in collision with two- or three-wheeled motor vehicle**

     The appropriate 7th character is to be added to each code from category V22.
     A   initial encounter
     D   subsequent encounter
     S   sequela

☑x7ᵗʰ **V22.0** **Motorcycle** driver **injured in collision with two- or three-wheeled motor vehicle** in nontraffic accident

☑x7ᵗʰ **V22.1** **Motorcycle** passenger **injured in collision with two- or three-wheeled motor vehicle** in nontraffic accident

☑x7ᵗʰ **V22.2** **Unspecified motorcycle rider injured in collision with two- or three-wheeled motor vehicle** in nontraffic accident

☑x7ᵗʰ **V22.3** Person boarding or alighting **a motorcycle injured in collision with two- or three-wheeled motor vehicle**

☑x7ᵗʰ **V22.4** **Motorcycle** driver **injured in collision with two- or three-wheeled motor vehicle** in traffic accident

☑x7ᵗʰ **V22.5** **Motorcycle** passenger **injured in collision with two- or three-wheeled motor vehicle** in traffic accident

☑x7ᵗʰ **V22.9** **Unspecified motorcycle rider injured in collision with two- or three-wheeled motor vehicle** in traffic accident

☑4ᵗʰ **V23** **Motorcycle rider injured in collision with car, pick-up truck or van**

     The appropriate 7th character is to be added to each code from category V23.
     A   initial encounter
     D   subsequent encounter
     S   sequela

☑x7ᵗʰ **V23.0** **Motorcycle** driver **injured in collision with car, pick-up truck or van** in nontraffic accident

☑x7ᵗʰ **V23.1** **Motorcycle** passenger **injured in collision with car, pick-up truck or van** in nontraffic accident

☑x7ᵗʰ **V23.2** **Unspecified motorcycle rider injured in collision with car, pick-up truck or van** in nontraffic accident

☑x7ᵗʰ **V23.3** Person boarding or alighting **a motorcycle injured in collision with car, pick-up truck or van**

☑x7ᵗʰ **V23.4** **Motorcycle** driver **injured in collision with car, pick-up truck or van** in traffic accident

☑x7ᵗʰ **V23.5** **Motorcycle** passenger **injured in collision with car, pick-up truck or van** in traffic accident

☑x7ᵗʰ **V23.9** **Unspecified motorcycle rider injured in collision with car, pick-up truck or van** in traffic accident

☑4ᵗʰ **V24** **Motorcycle rider injured in collision with heavy transport vehicle or bus**
     EXCLUDES 1   *motorcycle rider injured in collision with military vehicle (V29.81)*

     The appropriate 7th character is to be added to each code from category V24.
     A   initial encounter
     D   subsequent encounter
     S   sequela

☑x7ᵗʰ **V24.0** **Motorcycle** driver **injured in collision with heavy transport vehicle or bus** in nontraffic accident

☑x7ᵗʰ **V24.1** **Motorcycle** passenger **injured in collision with heavy transport vehicle or bus** in nontraffic accident

☑x7ᵗʰ **V24.2** **Unspecified motorcycle rider injured in collision with heavy transport vehicle or bus** in nontraffic accident

☑x7ᵗʰ **V24.3** Person boarding or alighting **a motorcycle injured in collision with heavy transport vehicle or bus**

☑x7ᵗʰ **V24.4** **Motorcycle** driver **injured in collision with heavy transport vehicle or bus** in traffic accident

☑x7ᵗʰ **V24.5** **Motorcycle** passenger **injured in collision with heavy transport vehicle or bus** in traffic accident

☑x7ᵗʰ **V24.9** **Unspecified motorcycle rider injured in collision with heavy transport vehicle or bus** in traffic accident

☑ Additional Character Required   ☑x7ᵗʰ Xtension Alert   Unspecified Dx   Other Specified Dx   Manifestation   ►◄ Revised Text   ● New Code   ▲ Revised Code Title

ICD-10-CM Draft (2015)   **999**

External Causes of Morbidity

V25–V29.69

☑4ᵗʰ **V25 Motorcycle rider injured in collision with railway train or railway vehicle**

> The appropriate 7th character is to be added to each code from category V25.
> A   initial encounter
> D   subsequent encounter
> S   sequela

✓x7ᵗʰ **V25.0** Motorcycle driver injured in collision with railway train or railway vehicle in nontraffic accident

✓x7ᵗʰ **V25.1** Motorcycle passenger injured in collision with railway train or railway vehicle in nontraffic accident

✓x7ᵗʰ **V25.2 Unspecified motorcycle rider injured in collision with railway train or railway vehicle in nontraffic accident**

✓x7ᵗʰ **V25.3** Person boarding or alighting a motorcycle injured in collision with railway train or railway vehicle

✓x7ᵗʰ **V25.4** Motorcycle driver injured in collision with railway train or railway vehicle in traffic accident

✓x7ᵗʰ **V25.5** Motorcycle passenger injured in collision with railway train or railway vehicle in traffic accident

✓x7ᵗʰ **V25.9 Unspecified motorcycle rider injured in collision with railway train or railway vehicle in traffic accident**

☑4ᵗʰ **V26 Motorcycle rider injured in collision with other nonmotor vehicle**

> INCLUDES   collision with animal-drawn vehicle, animal being ridden, streetcar

> The appropriate 7th character is to be added to each code from category V26.
> A   initial encounter
> D   subsequent encounter
> S   sequela

✓x7ᵗʰ **V26.0** Motorcycle driver injured in collision with other nonmotor vehicle in nontraffic accident

✓x7ᵗʰ **V26.1** Motorcycle passenger injured in collision with other nonmotor vehicle in nontraffic accident

✓x7ᵗʰ **V26.2 Unspecified motorcycle rider injured in collision with other nonmotor vehicle in nontraffic accident**

✓x7ᵗʰ **V26.3** Person boarding or alighting a motorcycle injured in collision with other nonmotor vehicle

✓x7ᵗʰ **V26.4** Motorcycle driver injured in collision with other nonmotor vehicle in traffic accident

✓x7ᵗʰ **V26.5** Motorcycle passenger injured in collision with other nonmotor vehicle in traffic accident

✓x7ᵗʰ **V26.9 Unspecified motorcycle rider injured in collision with other nonmotor vehicle in traffic accident**

☑4ᵗʰ **V27 Motorcycle rider injured in collision with fixed or stationary object**

> The appropriate 7th character is to be added to each code from category V27.
> A   initial encounter
> D   subsequent encounter
> S   sequela

✓x7ᵗʰ **V27.0** Motorcycle driver injured in collision with fixed or stationary object in nontraffic accident

✓x7ᵗʰ **V27.1** Motorcycle passenger injured in collision with fixed or stationary object in nontraffic accident

✓x7ᵗʰ **V27.2 Unspecified motorcycle rider injured in collision with fixed or stationary object in nontraffic accident**

✓x7ᵗʰ **V27.3** Person boarding or alighting a motorcycle injured in collision with fixed or stationary object

✓x7ᵗʰ **V27.4** Motorcycle driver injured in collision with fixed or stationary object in traffic accident

✓x7ᵗʰ **V27.5** Motorcycle passenger injured in collision with fixed or stationary object in traffic accident

✓x7ᵗʰ **V27.9 Unspecified motorcycle rider injured in collision with fixed or stationary object in traffic accident**

☑4ᵗʰ **V28 Motorcycle rider injured in noncollision transport accident**

> INCLUDES   fall or thrown from motorcycle (without antecedent collision)
> overturning motorcycle NOS
> overturning motorcycle without collision

> The appropriate 7th character is to be added to each code from category V28.
> A   initial encounter
> D   subsequent encounter
> S   sequela

✓x7ᵗʰ **V28.0** Motorcycle driver injured in noncollision transport accident in nontraffic accident

✓x7ᵗʰ **V28.1** Motorcycle passenger injured in noncollision transport accident in nontraffic accident

✓x7ᵗʰ **V28.2 Unspecified motorcycle rider injured in noncollision transport accident in nontraffic accident**

✓x7ᵗʰ **V28.3** Person boarding or alighting a motorcycle injured in noncollision transport accident

✓x7ᵗʰ **V28.4** Motorcycle driver injured in noncollision transport accident in traffic accident

✓x7ᵗʰ **V28.5** Motorcycle passenger injured in noncollision transport accident in traffic accident

✓x7ᵗʰ **V28.9 Unspecified motorcycle rider injured in noncollision transport accident in traffic accident**

☑4ᵗʰ **V29 Motorcycle rider injured in other and unspecified transport accidents**

> The appropriate 7th character is to be added to each code from category V29.
> A   initial encounter
> D   subsequent encounter
> S   sequela

✓5ᵗʰ **V29.0** Motorcycle driver injured in collision with other and unspecified motor vehicles in nontraffic accident

    ✓x7ᵗʰ **V29.00 Motorcycle driver injured in collision with unspecified motor vehicles in nontraffic accident**

    ✓x7ᵗʰ **V29.09 Motorcycle driver injured in collision with other motor vehicles in nontraffic accident**

✓5ᵗʰ **V29.1** Motorcycle passenger injured in collision with other and unspecified motor vehicles in nontraffic accident

    ✓x7ᵗʰ **V29.10 Motorcycle passenger injured in collision with unspecified motor vehicles in nontraffic accident**

    ✓x7ᵗʰ **V29.19 Motorcycle passenger injured in collision with other motor vehicles in nontraffic accident**

✓5ᵗʰ **V29.2** Unspecified motorcycle rider injured in collision with other and unspecified motor vehicles in nontraffic accident

    ✓x7ᵗʰ **V29.20 Unspecified motorcycle rider injured in collision with unspecified motor vehicles in nontraffic accident**
        Motorcycle collision NOS, nontraffic

    ✓x7ᵗʰ **V29.29 Unspecified motorcycle rider injured in collision with other motor vehicles in nontraffic accident**

✓x7ᵗʰ **V29.3** Motorcycle rider (driver) (passenger) injured in unspecified nontraffic accident
    Motorcycle accident NOS, nontraffic
    Motorcycle rider injured in nontraffic accident NOS

✓5ᵗʰ **V29.4** Motorcycle driver injured in collision with other and unspecified motor vehicles in traffic accident

    ✓x7ᵗʰ **V29.40 Motorcycle driver injured in collision with unspecified motor vehicles in traffic accident**

    ✓x7ᵗʰ **V29.49 Motorcycle driver injured in collision with other motor vehicles in traffic accident**

✓5ᵗʰ **V29.5** Motorcycle passenger injured in collision with other and unspecified motor vehicles in traffic accident

    ✓x7ᵗʰ **V29.50 Motorcycle passenger injured in collision with unspecified motor vehicles in traffic accident**

    ✓x7ᵗʰ **V29.59 Motorcycle passenger injured in collision with other motor vehicles in traffic accident**

✓5ᵗʰ **V29.6** Unspecified motorcycle rider injured in collision with other and unspecified motor vehicles in traffic accident

    ✓x7ᵗʰ **V29.60 Unspecified motorcycle rider injured in collision with unspecified motor vehicles in traffic accident**
        Motorcycle collision NOS (traffic)

    ✓x7ᵗʰ **V29.69 Unspecified motorcycle rider injured in collision with other motor vehicles in traffic accident**

EXCLUDES 1 Not coded here   EXCLUDES 2 Not included here   N Newborn Age: 0   P Pediatric Age: 0-17   M Maternity Age: 12-55   A Adult Age: 15-124

1000   ICD-10-CM Draft (2015)

√5ᵗʰ **V29.8** **Motorcycle rider (driver) (passenger) injured in** other specified transport accidents

    √x 7ᵗʰ **V29.81** **Motorcycle rider (driver) (passenger) injured in transport accident with** military vehicle

    √x 7ᵗʰ **V29.88** **Motorcycle rider (driver) (passenger) injured in other specified transport accidents**

√x 7ᵗʰ **V29.9** **Motorcycle rider (driver) (passenger) injured in unspecified traffic accident**

        Motorcycle accident NOS

Occupant of three-wheeled motor vehicle injured in transport accident (V30-V39)

INCLUDES   motorized tricycle
            motorized rickshaw
            three-wheeled motor car

EXCLUDES 1   *all-terrain vehicles (V86.-)*
            motorcycle with sidecar (V20-V29)
            vehicle designed primarily for off-road use (V86.-)

√4ᵗʰ **V30** **Occupant of three-wheeled motor vehicle injured in collision with pedestrian or animal**

     EXCLUDES 1   *three-wheeled motor vehicle collision with animal-drawn vehicle or animal being ridden (V36.-)*

> The appropriate 7th character is to be added to each code from category V30.
> A   initial encounter
> D   subsequent encounter
> S   sequela

√x 7ᵗʰ **V30.0** Driver **of three-wheeled motor vehicle injured in collision with pedestrian or animal** in nontraffic accident

√x 7ᵗʰ **V30.1** Passenger **in three-wheeled motor vehicle injured in collision with pedestrian or animal** in nontraffic accident

√x 7ᵗʰ **V30.2** Person on outside **of three-wheeled motor vehicle injured in collision with pedestrian or animal** in nontraffic accident

√x 7ᵗʰ **V30.3** **Unspecified occupant of three-wheeled motor vehicle injured in collision with pedestrian or animal** in nontraffic accident

√x 7ᵗʰ **V30.4** Person boarding or alighting **a three-wheeled motor vehicle injured in collision with pedestrian or animal**

√x 7ᵗʰ **V30.5** Driver **of three-wheeled motor vehicle injured in collision with pedestrian or animal** in traffic accident

√x 7ᵗʰ **V30.6** Passenger **in three-wheeled motor vehicle injured in collision with pedestrian or animal** in traffic accident

√x 7ᵗʰ **V30.7** Person on outside **of three-wheeled motor vehicle injured in collision with pedestrian or animal** in traffic accident

√x 7ᵗʰ **V30.9** **Unspecified occupant of three-wheeled motor vehicle injured in collision with pedestrian or animal** in traffic accident

√4ᵗʰ **V31** **Occupant of three-wheeled motor vehicle injured in collision with pedal cycle**

> The appropriate 7th character is to be added to each code from category V31.
> A   initial encounter
> D   subsequent encounter
> S   sequela

√x 7ᵗʰ **V31.0** Driver **of three-wheeled motor vehicle injured in collision with pedal cycle** in nontraffic accident

√x 7ᵗʰ **V31.1** Passenger **in three-wheeled motor vehicle injured in collision with pedal cycle** in nontraffic accident

√x 7ᵗʰ **V31.2** Person on outside **of three-wheeled motor vehicle injured in collision with pedal cycle** in nontraffic accident

√x 7ᵗʰ **V31.3** **Unspecified occupant of three-wheeled motor vehicle injured in collision with pedal cycle** in nontraffic accident

√x 7ᵗʰ **V31.4** Person boarding or alighting **a three-wheeled motor vehicle injured in collision with pedal cycle**

√x 7ᵗʰ **V31.5** Driver **of three-wheeled motor vehicle injured in collision with pedal cycle** in traffic accident

√x 7ᵗʰ **V31.6** Passenger **in three-wheeled motor vehicle injured in collision with pedal cycle** in traffic accident

√x 7ᵗʰ **V31.7** Person on outside **of three-wheeled motor vehicle injured in collision with pedal cycle** in traffic accident

√x 7ᵗʰ **V31.9** **Unspecified occupant of three-wheeled motor vehicle injured in collision with pedal cycle** in traffic accident

√4ᵗʰ **V32** **Occupant of three-wheeled motor vehicle injured in collision with two- or three-wheeled motor vehicle**

> The appropriate 7th character is to be added to each code from category V32.
> A   initial encounter
> D   subsequent encounter
> S   sequela

√x 7ᵗʰ **V32.0** Driver **of three-wheeled motor vehicle injured in collision with two- or three-wheeled motor vehicle** in nontraffic accident

√x 7ᵗʰ **V32.1** Passenger **in three-wheeled motor vehicle injured in collision with two- or three-wheeled motor vehicle** in nontraffic accident

√x 7ᵗʰ **V32.2** Person on outside **of three-wheeled motor vehicle injured in collision with two- or three-wheeled motor vehicle** in nontraffic accident

√x 7ᵗʰ **V32.3** **Unspecified occupant of three-wheeled motor vehicle injured in collision with two- or three-wheeled motor vehicle** in nontraffic accident

√x 7ᵗʰ **V32.4** Person boarding or alighting **a three-wheeled motor vehicle injured in collision with two- or three-wheeled motor vehicle**

√x 7ᵗʰ **V32.5** Driver **of three-wheeled motor vehicle injured in collision with two- or three-wheeled motor vehicle** in traffic accident

√x 7ᵗʰ **V32.6** Passenger **in three-wheeled motor vehicle injured in collision with two- or three-wheeled motor vehicle** in traffic accident

√x 7ᵗʰ **V32.7** Person on outside **of three-wheeled motor vehicle injured in collision with two- or three-wheeled motor vehicle** in traffic accident

√x 7ᵗʰ **V32.9** **Unspecified occupant of three-wheeled motor vehicle injured in collision with two- or three-wheeled motor vehicle** in traffic accident

√4ᵗʰ **V33** **Occupant of three-wheeled motor vehicle injured in collision with car, pick-up truck or van**

> The appropriate 7th character is to be added to each code from category V33.
> A   initial encounter
> D   subsequent encounter
> S   sequela

√x 7ᵗʰ **V33.0** Driver **of three-wheeled motor vehicle injured in collision with car, pick-up truck or van** in nontraffic accident

√x 7ᵗʰ **V33.1** Passenger **in three-wheeled motor vehicle injured in collision with car, pick-up truck or van** in nontraffic accident

√x 7ᵗʰ **V33.2** Person on outside **of three-wheeled motor vehicle injured in collision with car, pick-up truck or van** in nontraffic accident

√x 7ᵗʰ **V33.3** **Unspecified occupant of three-wheeled motor vehicle injured in collision with car, pick-up truck or van** in nontraffic accident

√x 7ᵗʰ **V33.4** Person boarding or alighting **a three-wheeled motor vehicle injured in collision with car, pick-up truck or van**

√x 7ᵗʰ **V33.5** Driver **of three-wheeled motor vehicle injured in collision with car, pick-up truck or van** in traffic accident

√x 7ᵗʰ **V33.6** Passenger **in three-wheeled motor vehicle injured in collision with car, pick-up truck or van** in traffic accident

√x 7ᵗʰ **V33.7** Person on outside **of three-wheeled motor vehicle injured in collision with car, pick-up truck or van** in traffic accident

√x 7ᵗʰ **V33.9** **Unspecified occupant of three-wheeled motor vehicle injured in collision with car, pick-up truck or van** in traffic accident

√4ᵗʰ **V34** **Occupant of three-wheeled motor vehicle injured in collision with heavy transport vehicle or bus**

     EXCLUDES 1   *occupant of three-wheeled motor vehicle injured in collision with military vehicle (V39.81)*

> The appropriate 7th character is to be added to each code from category V34.
> A   initial encounter
> D   subsequent encounter
> S   sequela

√x 7ᵗʰ **V34.0** Driver **of three-wheeled motor vehicle injured in collision with heavy transport vehicle or bus** in nontraffic accident

√x 7ᵗʰ **V34.1** Passenger **in three-wheeled motor vehicle injured in collision with heavy transport vehicle or bus** in nontraffic accident

√x 7ᵗʰ **V34.2** Person on outside **of three-wheeled motor vehicle injured in collision with heavy transport vehicle or bus** in nontraffic accident

✓ Additional Character Required   √x 7ᵗʰ Xtension Alert   Unspecified Dx   Other Specified Dx   Manifestation   ►◄ Revised Text   ● New Code   ▲ Revised Code Title

ICD-10-CM Draft (2015)   1001

√x7th **V34.3** Unspecified occupant of three-wheeled motor vehicle injured in collision with heavy transport vehicle or bus in nontraffic accident

√x7th **V34.4** Person boarding or alighting a three-wheeled motor vehicle injured in collision with heavy transport vehicle or bus

√x7th **V34.5** Driver of three-wheeled motor vehicle injured in collision with heavy transport vehicle or bus in traffic accident

√x7th **V34.6** Passenger in three-wheeled motor vehicle injured in collision with heavy transport vehicle or bus in traffic accident

√x7th **V34.7** Person on outside of three-wheeled motor vehicle injured in collision with heavy transport vehicle or bus in traffic accident

√x7th **V34.9** Unspecified occupant of three-wheeled motor vehicle injured in collision with heavy transport vehicle or bus in traffic accident

✓4th **V35 Occupant of three-wheeled motor vehicle injured in collision with railway train or railway vehicle**

The appropriate 7th character is to be added to each code from category V35.
A   initial encounter
D   subsequent encounter
S   sequela

√x7th **V35.0** Driver of three-wheeled motor vehicle injured in collision with railway train or railway vehicle in nontraffic accident

√x7th **V35.1** Passenger in three-wheeled motor vehicle injured in collision with railway train or railway vehicle in nontraffic accident

√x7th **V35.2** Person on outside of three-wheeled motor vehicle injured in collision with railway train or railway vehicle in nontraffic accident

√x7th **V35.3** Unspecified occupant of three-wheeled motor vehicle injured in collision with railway train or railway vehicle in nontraffic accident

√x7th **V35.4** Person boarding or alighting a three-wheeled motor vehicle injured in collision with railway train or railway vehicle

√x7th **V35.5** Driver of three-wheeled motor vehicle injured in collision with railway train or railway vehicle in traffic accident

√x7th **V35.6** Passenger in three-wheeled motor vehicle injured in collision with railway train or railway vehicle in traffic accident

√x7th **V35.7** Person on outside of three-wheeled motor vehicle injured in collision with railway train or railway vehicle in traffic accident

√x7th **V35.9** Unspecified occupant of three-wheeled motor vehicle injured in collision with railway train or railway vehicle in traffic accident

✓4th **V36 Occupant of three-wheeled motor vehicle injured in collision with other nonmotor vehicle**

INCLUDES   collision with animal-drawn vehicle, animal being ridden, streetcar

The appropriate 7th character is to be added to each code from category V36.
A   initial encounter
D   subsequent encounter
S   sequela

√x7th **V36.0** Driver of three-wheeled motor vehicle injured in collision with other nonmotor vehicle in nontraffic accident

√x7th **V36.1** Passenger in three-wheeled motor vehicle injured in collision with other nonmotor vehicle in nontraffic accident

√x7th **V36.2** Person on outside of three-wheeled motor vehicle injured in collision with other nonmotor vehicle in nontraffic accident

√x7th **V36.3** Unspecified occupant of three-wheeled motor vehicle injured in collision with other nonmotor vehicle in nontraffic accident

√x7th **V36.4** Person boarding or alighting a three-wheeled motor vehicle injured in collision with other nonmotor vehicle

√x7th **V36.5** Driver of three-wheeled motor vehicle injured in collision with other nonmotor vehicle in traffic accident

√x7th **V36.6** Passenger in three-wheeled motor vehicle injured in collision with other nonmotor vehicle in traffic accident

√x7th **V36.7** Person on outside of three-wheeled motor vehicle injured in collision with other nonmotor vehicle in traffic accident

√x7th **V36.9** Unspecified occupant of three-wheeled motor vehicle injured in collision with other nonmotor vehicle in traffic accident

✓4th **V37 Occupant of three-wheeled motor vehicle injured in collision with fixed or stationary object**

The appropriate 7th character is to be added to each code from category V37.
A   initial encounter
D   subsequent encounter
S   sequela

√x7th **V37.0** Driver of three-wheeled motor vehicle injured in collision with fixed or stationary object in nontraffic accident

√x7th **V37.1** Passenger in three-wheeled motor vehicle injured in collision with fixed or stationary object in nontraffic accident

√x7th **V37.2** Person on outside of three-wheeled motor vehicle injured in collision with fixed or stationary object in nontraffic accident

√x7th **V37.3** Unspecified occupant of three-wheeled motor vehicle injured in collision with fixed or stationary object in nontraffic accident

√x7th **V37.4** Person boarding or alighting a three-wheeled motor vehicle injured in collision with fixed or stationary object

√x7th **V37.5** Driver of three-wheeled motor vehicle injured in collision with fixed or stationary object in traffic accident

√x7th **V37.6** Passenger in three-wheeled motor vehicle injured in collision with fixed or stationary object in traffic accident

√x7th **V37.7** Person on outside of three-wheeled motor vehicle injured in collision with fixed or stationary object in traffic accident

√x7th **V37.9** Unspecified occupant of three-wheeled motor vehicle injured in collision with fixed or stationary object in traffic accident

V38 Occupant of three-wheeled motor vehicle injured in noncollision transport accident

INCLUDES   fall or thrown from three-wheeled motor vehicle
overturning of three-wheeled motor vehicle NOS
overturning of three-wheeled motor vehicle without collision

The appropriate 7th character is to be added to each code from category V38.
A   initial encounter
D   subsequent encounter
S   sequela

√x7th **V38.0** Driver of three-wheeled motor vehicle injured in noncollision transport accident in nontraffic accident

√x7th **V38.1** Passenger in three-wheeled motor vehicle injured in noncollision transport accident in nontraffic accident

√x7th **V38.2** Person on outside of three-wheeled motor vehicle injured in noncollision transport accident in nontraffic accident

√x7th **V38.3** Unspecified occupant of three-wheeled motor vehicle injured in noncollision transport accident in nontraffic accident

√x7th **V38.4** Person boarding or alighting a three-wheeled motor vehicle injured in noncollision transport accident

√x7th **V38.5** Driver of three-wheeled motor vehicle injured in noncollision transport accident in traffic accident

√x7th **V38.6** Passenger in three-wheeled motor vehicle injured in noncollision transport accident in traffic accident

√x7th **V38.7** Person on outside of three-wheeled motor vehicle injured in noncollision transport accident in traffic accident

√x7th **V38.9** Unspecified occupant of three-wheeled motor vehicle injured in noncollision transport accident in traffic accident

✓4th **V39 Occupant of three-wheeled motor vehicle injured in other and unspecified transport accidents**

The appropriate 7th character is to be added to each code from category V39.
A   initial encounter
D   subsequent encounter
S   sequela

√5th **V39.0** Driver of three-wheeled motor vehicle injured in collision with other and unspecified motor vehicles in nontraffic accident

√x7th **V39.00** Driver of three-wheeled motor vehicle injured in collision with unspecified motor vehicles in nontraffic accident

√x7th **V39.09** Driver of three-wheeled motor vehicle injured in collision with other motor vehicles in nontraffic accident

---

EXCLUDES1 Not coded here   EXCLUDES2 Not included here   N Newborn Age: 0   P Pediatric Age: 0-17   M Maternity Age: 12-55   A Adult Age: 15-124

☑5ᵗʰ **V39.1** Passenger in three-wheeled motor vehicle injured in collision with other and unspecified motor vehicles in nontraffic accident

     ☑x7ᵗʰ **V39.10** Passenger in three-wheeled motor vehicle injured in collision with unspecified motor vehicles in nontraffic accident

     ☑x7ᵗʰ **V39.19** Passenger in three-wheeled motor vehicle injured in collision with other motor vehicles in nontraffic accident

☑5ᵗʰ **V39.2** Unspecified occupant of three-wheeled motor vehicle injured in collision with other and unspecified motor vehicles in nontraffic accident

     ☑x7ᵗʰ **V39.20** Unspecified occupant of three-wheeled motor vehicle injured in collision with unspecified motor vehicles in nontraffic accident

        Collision NOS involving three-wheeled motor vehicle, nontraffic

     ☑x7ᵗʰ **V39.29** Unspecified occupant of three-wheeled motor vehicle injured in collision with other motor vehicles in nontraffic accident

☑x7ᵗʰ **V39.3** Occupant (driver) (passenger) of three-wheeled motor vehicle injured in unspecified nontraffic accident

        Accident NOS involving three-wheeled motor vehicle, nontraffic

        Occupant of three-wheeled motor vehicle injured in nontraffic accident NOS

☑5ᵗʰ **V39.4** Driver of three-wheeled motor vehicle injured in collision with other and unspecified motor vehicles in traffic accident

     ☑x7ᵗʰ **V39.40** Driver of three-wheeled motor vehicle injured in collision with unspecified motor vehicles in traffic accident

     ☑x7ᵗʰ **V39.49** Driver of three-wheeled motor vehicle injured in collision with other motor vehicles in traffic accident

☑5ᵗʰ **V39.5** Passenger in three-wheeled motor vehicle injured in collision with other and unspecified motor vehicles in traffic accident

     ☑x7ᵗʰ **V39.50** Passenger in three-wheeled motor vehicle injured in collision with unspecified motor vehicles in traffic accident

     ☑x7ᵗʰ **V39.59** Passenger in three-wheeled motor vehicle injured in collision with other motor vehicles in traffic accident

☑5ᵗʰ **V39.6** Unspecified occupant of three-wheeled motor vehicle injured in collision with other and unspecified motor vehicles in traffic accident

     ☑x7ᵗʰ **V39.60** Unspecified occupant of three-wheeled motor vehicle injured in collision with unspecified motor vehicles in traffic accident

        Collision NOS involving three-wheeled motor vehicle (traffic)

     ☑x7ᵗʰ **V39.69** Unspecified occupant of three-wheeled motor vehicle injured in collision with other motor vehicles in traffic accident

☑5ᵗʰ **V39.8** Occupant (driver) (passenger) of three-wheeled motor vehicle injured in other specified transport accidents

     ☑x7ᵗʰ **V39.81** Occupant (driver) (passenger) of three-wheeled motor vehicle injured in transport accident with military vehicle

     ☑x7ᵗʰ **V39.89** Occupant (driver) (passenger) of three-wheeled motor vehicle injured in other specified transport accidents

☑x7ᵗʰ **V39.9** Occupant (driver) (passenger) of three-wheeled motor vehicle injured in unspecified traffic accident

        Accident NOS involving three-wheeled motor vehicle

Car occupant injured in transport accident (V40-V49)

INCLUDES   a four-wheeled motor vehicle designed primarily for carrying passengers

        automobile (pulling a trailer or camper)

EXCLUDES 1   bus (V50-V59)

        minibus (V50-V59)

        minivan (V50-V59)

        motorcoach (V70-V79)

        pick-up truck (V50-V59)

        sport utility vehicle (SUV) (V50-V59)

☑4ᵗʰ **V40** Car occupant injured in collision with pedestrian or animal

     EXCLUDES 1   car collision with animal-drawn vehicle or animal being ridden (V46.-)

     The appropriate 7th character is to be added to each code from category V40.
     A   initial encounter
     D   subsequent encounter
     S   sequela

     ☑x7ᵗʰ **V40.0** Car driver injured in collision with pedestrian or animal in nontraffic accident

     ☑x7ᵗʰ **V40.1** Car passenger injured in collision with pedestrian or animal in nontraffic accident

     ☑x7ᵗʰ **V40.2** Person on outside of car injured in collision with pedestrian or animal in nontraffic accident

     ☑x7ᵗʰ **V40.3** Unspecified car occupant injured in collision with pedestrian or animal in nontraffic accident

     ☑x7ᵗʰ **V40.4** Person boarding or alighting a car injured in collision with pedestrian or animal

     ☑x7ᵗʰ **V40.5** Car driver injured in collision with pedestrian or animal in traffic accident

     ☑x7ᵗʰ **V40.6** Car passenger injured in collision with pedestrian or animal in traffic accident

     ☑x7ᵗʰ **V40.7** Person on outside of car injured in collision with pedestrian or animal in traffic accident

     ☑x7ᵗʰ **V40.9** Unspecified car occupant injured in collision with pedestrian or animal in traffic accident

☑4ᵗʰ **V41** Car occupant injured in collision with pedal cycle

     The appropriate 7th character is to be added to each code from category V41.
     A   initial encounter
     D   subsequent encounter
     S   sequela

     ☑x7ᵗʰ **V41.0** Car driver injured in collision with pedal cycle in nontraffic accident

     ☑x7ᵗʰ **V41.1** Car passenger injured in collision with pedal cycle in nontraffic accident

     ☑x7ᵗʰ **V41.2** Person on outside of car injured in collision with pedal cycle in nontraffic accident

     ☑x7ᵗʰ **V41.3** Unspecified car occupant injured in collision with pedal cycle in nontraffic accident

     ☑x7ᵗʰ **V41.4** Person boarding or alighting a car injured in collision with pedal cycle

     ☑x7ᵗʰ **V41.5** Car driver injured in collision with pedal cycle in traffic accident

     ☑x7ᵗʰ **V41.6** Car passenger injured in collision with pedal cycle in traffic accident

     ☑x7ᵗʰ **V41.7** Person on outside of car injured in collision with pedal cycle in traffic accident

     ☑x7ᵗʰ **V41.9** Unspecified car occupant injured in collision with pedal cycle in traffic accident

☑4ᵗʰ **V42** Car occupant injured in collision with two- or three-wheeled motor vehicle

     The appropriate 7th character is to be added to each code from category V42.
     A   initial encounter
     D   subsequent encounter
     S   sequela

     ☑x7ᵗʰ **V42.0** Car driver injured in collision with two- or three-wheeled motor vehicle in nontraffic accident

     ☑x7ᵗʰ **V42.1** Car passenger injured in collision with two- or three-wheeled motor vehicle in nontraffic accident

     ☑x7ᵗʰ **V42.2** Person on outside of car injured in collision with two- or three-wheeled motor vehicle in nontraffic accident

☑ Additional Character Required   ☑x7ᵗʰ Xtension Alert   Unspecified Dx   Other Specified Dx   Manifestation   ▶◀ Revised Text   ● New Code   ▲ Revised Code Title

ICD-10-CM Draft (2015)   1003

External Causes of Morbidity

V42.3–V45.1

✓x7th **V42.3** Unspecified car occupant injured in collision with two- or three-wheeled motor vehicle in nontraffic accident

✓x7th **V42.4** Person boarding or alighting a car injured in collision with two- or three-wheeled motor vehicle

✓x7th **V42.5** Car driver injured in collision with two- or three-wheeled motor vehicle in traffic accident

✓x7th **V42.6** Car passenger injured in collision with two- or three-wheeled motor vehicle in traffic accident

✓x7th **V42.7** Person on outside of car injured in collision with two- or three-wheeled motor vehicle in traffic accident

✓x7th **V42.9** Unspecified car occupant injured in collision with two- or three-wheeled motor vehicle in traffic accident

✓4th **V43** Car occupant injured in collision with car, pick-up truck or van

> The appropriate 7th character is to be added to each code from category V43.
> A   initial encounter
> D   subsequent encounter
> S   sequela

✓5th **V43.0** Car driver injured in collision with car, pick-up truck or van in nontraffic accident

     ✓x7th **V43.01** Car driver injured in collision with sport utility vehicle in nontraffic accident

     ✓x7th **V43.02** Car driver injured in collision with other type car in nontraffic accident

     ✓x7th **V43.03** Car driver injured in collision with pick-up truck in nontraffic accident

     ✓x7th **V43.04** Car driver injured in collision with van in nontraffic accident

✓5th **V43.1** Car passenger injured in collision with car, pick-up truck or van in nontraffic accident

     ✓x7th **V43.11** Car passenger injured in collision with sport utility vehicle in nontraffic accident

     ✓x7th **V43.12** Car passenger injured in collision with other type car in nontraffic accident

     ✓x7th **V43.13** Car passenger injured in collision with pick-up in nontraffic accident

     ✓x7th **V43.14** Car passenger injured in collision with van in nontraffic accident

✓5th **V43.2** Person on outside of car injured in collision with car, pick-up truck or van in nontraffic accident

     ✓x7th **V43.21** Person on outside of car injured in collision with sport utility vehicle in nontraffic accident

     ✓x7th **V43.22** Person on outside of car injured in collision with other type car in nontraffic accident

     ✓x7th **V43.23** Person on outside of car injured in collision with pick-up truck in nontraffic accident

     ✓x7th **V43.24** Person on outside of car injured in collision with van in nontraffic accident

✓5th **V43.3** Unspecified car occupant injured in collision with car, pick-up truck or van in nontraffic accident

     ✓x7th **V43.31** Unspecified car occupant injured in collision with sport utility vehicle in nontraffic accident

     ✓x7th **V43.32** Unspecified car occupant injured in collision with other type car in nontraffic accident

     ✓x7th **V43.33** Unspecified car occupant injured in collision with pick-up truck in nontraffic accident

     ✓x7th **V43.34** Unspecified car occupant injured in collision with van in nontraffic accident

✓5th **V43.4** Person boarding or alighting a car injured in collision with car, pick-up truck or van

     ✓x7th **V43.41** Person boarding or alighting a car injured in collision with sport utility vehicle

     ✓x7th **V43.42** Person boarding or alighting a car injured in collision with other type car

     ✓x7th **V43.43** Person boarding or alighting a car injured in collision with pick-up truck

     ✓x7th **V43.44** Person boarding or alighting a car injured in collision with van

✓5th **V43.5** Car driver injured in collision with car, pick-up truck or van in traffic accident

     ✓x7th **V43.51** Car driver injured in collision with sport utility vehicle in traffic accident

✓x7th **V43.52** Car driver injured in collision with other type car in traffic accident

✓x7th **V43.53** Car driver injured in collision with pick-up truck in traffic accident

✓x7th **V43.54** Car driver injured in collision with van in traffic accident

✓5th **V43.6** Car passenger injured in collision with car, pick-up truck or van in traffic accident

     ✓x7th **V43.61** Car passenger injured in collision with sport utility vehicle in traffic accident

     ✓x7th **V43.62** Car passenger injured in collision with other type car in traffic accident

     ✓x7th **V43.63** Car passenger injured in collision with pick-up truck in traffic accident

     ✓x7th **V43.64** Car passenger injured in collision with van in traffic accident

✓5th **V43.7** Person on outside of car injured in collision with car, pick-up truck or van in traffic accident

     ✓x7th **V43.71** Person on outside of car injured in collision with sport utility vehicle in traffic accident

     ✓x7th **V43.72** Person on outside of car injured in collision with other type car in traffic accident

     ✓x7th **V43.73** Person on outside of car injured in collision with pick-up truck in traffic accident

     ✓x7th **V43.74** Person on outside of car injured in collision with van in traffic accident

✓5th **V43.9** Unspecified car occupant injured in collision with car, pick-up truck or van in traffic accident

     ✓x7th **V43.91** Unspecified car occupant injured in collision with sport utility vehicle in traffic accident

     ✓x7th **V43.92** Unspecified car occupant injured in collision with other type car in traffic accident

     ✓x7th **V43.93** Unspecified car occupant injured in collision with pick-up truck in traffic accident

     ✓x7th **V43.94** Unspecified car occupant injured in collision with van in traffic accident

✓4th **V44** Car occupant injured in collision with heavy transport vehicle or bus

> **EXCLUDES 1**   car occupant injured in collision with military vehicle (V49.81)

> The appropriate 7th character is to be added to each code from category V44.
> A   initial encounter
> D   subsequent encounter
> S   sequela

✓x7th **V44.0** Car driver injured in collision with heavy transport vehicle or bus in nontraffic accident

✓x7th **V44.1** Car passenger injured in collision with heavy transport vehicle or bus in nontraffic accident

✓x7th **V44.2** Person on outside of car injured in collision with heavy transport vehicle or bus in nontraffic accident

✓x7th **V44.3** Unspecified car occupant injured in collision with heavy transport vehicle or bus in nontraffic accident

✓x7th **V44.4** Person boarding or alighting a car injured in collision with heavy transport vehicle or bus

✓x7th **V44.5** Car driver injured in collision with heavy transport vehicle or bus in traffic accident

✓x7th **V44.6** Car passenger injured in collision with heavy transport vehicle or bus in traffic accident

✓x7th **V44.7** Person on outside of car injured in collision with heavy transport vehicle or bus in traffic accident

✓x7th **V44.9** Unspecified car occupant injured in collision with heavy transport vehicle or bus in traffic accident

✓4th **V45** Car occupant injured in collision with railway train or railway vehicle

> The appropriate 7th character is to be added to each code from category V45.
> A   initial encounter
> D   subsequent encounter
> S   sequela

✓x7th **V45.0** Car driver injured in collision with railway train or railway vehicle in nontraffic accident

✓x7th **V45.1** Car passenger injured in collision with railway train or railway vehicle in nontraffic accident

---

EXCLUDES 1 Not coded here   **EXCLUDES 2** Not included here   N Newborn Age: 0   P Pediatric Age: 0-17   M Maternity Age: 12-55   A Adult Age: 15-124

1004   ICD-10-CM Draft (2015)

✓x7th **V45.2** Person on outside of car injured in collision with railway train or railway vehicle in nontraffic accident

✓x7th **V45.3** Unspecified car occupant injured in collision with railway train or railway vehicle in nontraffic accident

✓x7th **V45.4** Person boarding or alighting a car injured in collision with railway train or railway vehicle

✓x7th **V45.5** Car driver injured in collision with railway train or railway vehicle in traffic accident

✓x7th **V45.6** Car passenger injured in collision with railway train or railway vehicle in traffic accident

✓x7th **V45.7** Person on outside of car injured in collision with railway train or railway vehicle in traffic accident

✓x7th **V45.9** Unspecified car occupant injured in collision with railway train or railway vehicle in traffic accident

✓4th **V46 Car occupant injured in collision with other nonmotor vehicle**
    INCLUDES collision with animal-drawn vehicle, animal being ridden, streetcar

> The appropriate 7th character is to be added to each code from category V46.
> A initial encounter
> D subsequent encounter
> S sequela

✓x7th **V46.0** Car driver injured in collision with other nonmotor vehicle in nontraffic accident

✓x7th **V46.1** Car passenger injured in collision with other nonmotor vehicle in nontraffic accident

✓x7th **V46.2** Person on outside of car injured in collision with other nonmotor vehicle in nontraffic accident

✓x7th **V46.3** Unspecified car occupant injured in collision with other nonmotor vehicle in nontraffic accident

✓x7th **V46.4** Person boarding or alighting a car injured in collision with other nonmotor vehicle

✓x7th **V46.5** Car driver injured in collision with other nonmotor vehicle in traffic accident

✓x7th **V46.6** Car passenger injured in collision with other nonmotor vehicle in traffic accident

✓x7th **V46.7** Person on outside of car injured in collision with other nonmotor vehicle in traffic accident

✓x7th **V46.9** Unspecified car occupant injured in collision with other nonmotor vehicle in traffic accident

✓4th **V47 Car occupant injured in collision with fixed or stationary object**

> The appropriate 7th character is to be added to each code from category V47.
> A initial encounter
> D subsequent encounter
> S sequela

✓5th **V47.0** Car driver injured in collision with fixed or stationary object in nontraffic accident

    ✓x7th **V47.01** Driver of sport utility vehicle injured in collision with fixed or stationary object in nontraffic accident

    ✓x7th **V47.02** Driver of other type car injured in collision with fixed or stationary object in nontraffic accident

✓5th **V47.1** Car passenger injured in collision with fixed or stationary object in nontraffic accident

    ✓x7th **V47.11** Passenger of sport utility vehicle injured in collision with fixed or stationary object in nontraffic accident

    ✓x7th **V47.12** Passenger of other type car injured in collision with fixed or stationary object in nontraffic accident

✓x7th **V47.2** Person on outside of car injured in collision with fixed or stationary object in nontraffic accident

✓5th **V47.3** Unspecified car occupant injured in collision with fixed or stationary object in nontraffic accident

    ✓x7th **V47.31** Unspecified occupant of sport utility vehicle injured in collision with fixed or stationary object in nontraffic accident

    ✓x7th **V47.32** Unspecified occupant of other type car injured in collision with fixed or stationary object in nontraffic accident

✓x7th **V47.4** Person boarding or alighting a car injured in collision with fixed or stationary object

✓5th **V47.5** Car driver injured in collision with fixed or stationary object in traffic accident

    ✓x7th **V47.51** Driver of sport utility vehicle injured in collision with fixed or stationary object in traffic accident

    ✓x7th **V47.52** Driver of other type car injured in collision with fixed or stationary object in traffic accident

✓5th **V47.6** Car passenger injured in collision with fixed or stationary object in traffic accident

    ✓x7th **V47.61** Passenger of sport utility vehicle injured in collision with fixed or stationary object in traffic accident

    ✓x7th **V47.62** Passenger of other type car injured in collision with fixed or stationary object in traffic accident

✓x7th **V47.7** Person on outside of car injured in collision with fixed or stationary object in traffic accident

✓5th **V47.9** Unspecified car occupant injured in collision with fixed or stationary object in traffic accident

    ✓x7th **V47.91** Unspecified occupant of sport utility vehicle injured in collision with fixed or stationary object in traffic accident

    ✓x7th **V47.92** Unspecified occupant of other type car injured in collision with fixed or stationary object in traffic accident

✓4th **V48 Car occupant injured in noncollision transport accident**
    INCLUDES overturning car NOS
               overturning car without collision

> The appropriate 7th character is to be added to each code from category V48.
> A initial encounter
> D subsequent encounter
> S sequela

✓x7th **V48.0** Car driver injured in noncollision transport accident in nontraffic accident

✓x7th **V48.1** Car passenger injured in noncollision transport accident in nontraffic accident

✓x7th **V48.2** Person on outside of car injured in noncollision transport accident in nontraffic accident

✓x7th **V48.3** Unspecified car occupant injured in noncollision transport accident in nontraffic accident

✓x7th **V48.4** Person boarding or alighting a car injured in noncollision transport accident

✓x7th **V48.5** Car driver injured in noncollision transport accident in traffic accident

✓x7th **V48.6** Car passenger injured in noncollision transport accident in traffic accident

✓x7th **V48.7** Person on outside of car injured in noncollision transport accident in traffic accident

✓x7th **V48.9** Unspecified car occupant injured in noncollision transport accident in traffic accident

✓4th **V49 Car occupant injured in other and unspecified transport accidents**

> The appropriate 7th character is to be added to each code from category V49.
> A initial encounter
> D subsequent encounter
> S sequela

✓5th **V49.0** Driver injured in collision with other and unspecified motor vehicles in nontraffic accident

    ✓x7th **V49.00** Driver injured in collision with unspecified motor vehicles in nontraffic accident

    ✓x7th **V49.09** Driver injured in collision with other motor vehicles in nontraffic accident

✓5th **V49.1** Passenger injured in collision with other and unspecified motor vehicles in nontraffic accident

    ✓x7th **V49.10** Passenger injured in collision with unspecified motor vehicles in nontraffic accident

    ✓x7th **V49.19** Passenger injured in collision with other motor vehicles in nontraffic accident

✓5th **V49.2** Unspecified car occupant injured in collision with other and unspecified motor vehicles in nontraffic accident

    ✓x7th **V49.20** Unspecified car occupant injured in collision with unspecified motor vehicles in nontraffic accident
        Car collision NOS, nontraffic

    ✓x7th **V49.29** Unspecified car occupant injured in collision with other motor vehicles in nontraffic accident

✓x7th **V49.3** Car occupant (driver) (passenger) injured in unspecified nontraffic accident
    Car accident NOS, nontraffic
    Car occupant injured in nontraffic accident NOS

✓ Additional Character Required   ✓x7th Xtension Alert   Unspecified Dx   Other Specified Dx   Manifestation   ►◄ Revised Text   ● New Code   ▲ Revised Code Title

External Causes of Morbidity

V49.4–V53.6

√5th **V49.4** Driver injured in collision with other and unspecified motor vehicles in traffic accident

√x7th **V49.40** Driver injured in collision with unspecified motor vehicles in traffic accident

√x7th **V49.49** Driver injured in collision with other motor vehicles in traffic accident

√5th **V49.5** Passenger injured in collision with other and unspecified motor vehicles in traffic accident

√x7th **V49.50** Passenger injured in collision with unspecified motor vehicles in traffic accident

√x7th **V49.59** Passenger injured in collision with other motor vehicles in traffic accident

√5th **V49.6** Unspecified car occupant injured in collision with other and unspecified motor vehicles in traffic accident

√x7th **V49.60** Unspecified car occupant injured in collision with unspecified motor vehicles in traffic accident
Car collision NOS (traffic)

√x7th **V49.69** Unspecified car occupant injured in collision with other motor vehicles in traffic accident

√5th **V49.8** Car occupant (driver) (passenger) injured in other specified transport accidents

√x7th **V49.81** Car occupant (driver) (passenger) injured in transport accident with military vehicle

√x7th **V49.88** Car occupant (driver) (passenger) injured in other specified transport accidents

√x7th **V49.9** Car occupant (driver) (passenger) injured in unspecified traffic accident
Car accident NOS

Occupant of pick-up truck or van injured in transport accident (V50-V59)

INCLUDES   a four or six wheel motor vehicle designed primarily for carrying passengers and property but weighing less than the local limit for classification as a heavy goods vehicle
minibus
minivan
sport utility vehicle (SUV)
truck
van

EXCLUDES 1   heavy transport vehicle (V60-V69)

√4th **V50** Occupant of pick-up truck or van injured in collision with pedestrian or animal

EXCLUDES 1   pick-up truck or van collision with animal-drawn vehicle or animal being ridden (V56.-)

The appropriate 7th character is to be added to each code from category V50.
A   initial encounter
D   subsequent encounter
S   sequela

√x7th **V50.0** Driver of pick-up truck or van injured in collision with pedestrian or animal in nontraffic accident

√x7th **V50.1** Passenger in pick-up truck or van injured in collision with pedestrian or animal in nontraffic accident

√x7th **V50.2** Person on outside of pick-up truck or van injured in collision with pedestrian or animal in nontraffic accident

√x7th **V50.3** Unspecified occupant of pick-up truck or van injured in collision with pedestrian or animal in nontraffic accident

√x7th **V50.4** Person boarding or alighting a pick-up truck or van injured in collision with pedestrian or animal

√x7th **V50.5** Driver of pick-up truck or van injured in collision with pedestrian or animal in traffic accident

√x7th **V50.6** Passenger in pick-up truck or van injured in collision with pedestrian or animal in traffic accident

√x7th **V50.7** Person on outside of pick-up truck or van injured in collision with pedestrian or animal in traffic accident

√x7th **V50.9** Unspecified occupant of pick-up truck or van injured in collision with pedestrian or animal in traffic accident

√4th **V51** Occupant of pick-up truck or van injured in collision with pedal cycle

The appropriate 7th character is to be added to each code from category V51.
A   initial encounter
D   subsequent encounter
S   sequela

√x7th **V51.0** Driver of pick-up truck or van injured in collision with pedal cycle in nontraffic accident

√x7th **V51.1** Passenger in pick-up truck or van injured in collision with pedal cycle in nontraffic accident

√x7th **V51.2** Person on outside of pick-up truck or van injured in collision with pedal cycle in nontraffic accident

√x7th **V51.3** Unspecified occupant of pick-up truck or van injured in collision with pedal cycle in nontraffic accident

√x7th **V51.4** Person boarding or alighting a pick-up truck or van injured in collision with pedal cycle

√x7th **V51.5** Driver of pick-up truck or van injured in collision with pedal cycle in traffic accident

√x7th **V51.6** Passenger in pick-up truck or van injured in collision with pedal cycle in traffic accident

√x7th **V51.7** Person on outside of pick-up truck or van injured in collision with pedal cycle in traffic accident

√x7th **V51.9** Unspecified occupant of pick-up truck or van injured in collision with pedal cycle in traffic accident

√4th **V52** Occupant of pick-up truck or van injured in collision with two- or three-wheeled motor vehicle

The appropriate 7th character is to be added to each code from category V52.
A   initial encounter
D   subsequent encounter
S   sequela

√x7th **V52.0** Driver of pick-up truck or van injured in collision with two- or three-wheeled motor vehicle in nontraffic accident

√x7th **V52.1** Passenger in pick-up truck or van injured in collision with two- or three-wheeled motor vehicle in nontraffic accident

√x7th **V52.2** Person on outside of pick-up truck or van injured in collision with two- or three-wheeled motor vehicle in nontraffic accident

√x7th **V52.3** Unspecified occupant of pick-up truck or van injured in collision with two- or three-wheeled motor vehicle in nontraffic accident

√x7th **V52.4** Person boarding or alighting a pick-up truck or van injured in collision with two- or three-wheeled motor vehicle

√x7th **V52.5** Driver of pick-up truck or van injured in collision with two- or three-wheeled motor vehicle in traffic accident

√x7th **V52.6** Passenger in pick-up truck or van injured in collision with two- or three-wheeled motor vehicle in traffic accident

√x7th **V52.7** Person on outside of pick-up truck or van injured in collision with two- or three-wheeled motor vehicle in traffic accident

√x7th **V52.9** Unspecified occupant of pick-up truck or van injured in collision with two- or three-wheeled motor vehicle in traffic accident

√4th **V53** Occupant of pick-up truck or van injured in collision with car, pick-up truck or van

The appropriate 7th character is to be added to each code from category V53.
A   initial encounter
D   subsequent encounter
S   sequela

√x7th **V53.0** Driver of pick-up truck or van injured in collision with car, pick-up truck or van in nontraffic accident

√x7th **V53.1** Passenger in pick-up truck or van injured in collision with car, pick-up truck or van in nontraffic accident

√x7th **V53.2** Person on outside of pick-up truck or van injured in collision with car, pick-up truck or van in nontraffic accident

√x7th **V53.3** Unspecified occupant of pick-up truck or van injured in collision with car, pick-up truck or van in nontraffic accident

√x7th **V53.4** Person boarding or alighting a pick-up truck or van injured in collision with car, pick-up truck or van

√x7th **V53.5** Driver of pick-up truck or van injured in collision with car, pick-up truck or van in traffic accident

√x7th **V53.6** Passenger in pick-up truck or van injured in collision with car, pick-up truck or van in traffic accident

EXCLUDES 1 Not coded here   EXCLUDES 2 Not included here   N Newborn Age: 0   P Pediatric Age: 0-17   M Maternity Age: 12-55   A Adult Age: 15-124

1006   ICD-10-CM Draft (2015)

☑x7ᵗʰ **V53.7** Person on outside of pick-up truck or van injured in collision with car, pick-up truck or van in traffic accident

☑x7ᵗʰ **V53.9** Unspecified occupant of pick-up truck or van injured in collision with car, pick-up truck or van in traffic accident

☑4ᵗʰ **V54 Occupant of pick-up truck or van injured in collision with heavy transport vehicle or bus**

> EXCLUDES 1   occupant of pick-up truck or van injured in collision with military vehicle (V59.81)

> The appropriate 7th character is to be added to each code from category V54.
> A   initial encounter
> D   subsequent encounter
> S   sequela

☑x7ᵗʰ **V54.0** Driver of pick-up truck or van injured in collision with heavy transport vehicle or bus in nontraffic accident

☑x7ᵗʰ **V54.1** Passenger in pick-up truck or van injured in collision with heavy transport vehicle or bus in nontraffic accident

☑x7ᵗʰ **V54.2** Person on outside of pick-up truck or van injured in collision with heavy transport vehicle or bus in nontraffic accident

☑x7ᵗʰ **V54.3** Unspecified occupant of pick-up truck or van injured in collision with heavy transport vehicle or bus in nontraffic accident

☑x7ᵗʰ **V54.4** Person boarding or alighting a pick-up truck or van injured in collision with heavy transport vehicle or bus

☑x7ᵗʰ **V54.5** Driver of pick-up truck or van injured in collision with heavy transport vehicle or bus in traffic accident

☑x7ᵗʰ **V54.6** Passenger in pick-up truck or van injured in collision with heavy transport vehicle or bus in traffic accident

☑x7ᵗʰ **V54.7** Person on outside of pick-up truck or van injured in collision with heavy transport vehicle or bus in traffic accident

☑x7ᵗʰ **V54.9** Unspecified occupant of pick-up truck or van injured in collision with heavy transport vehicle or bus in traffic accident

☑4ᵗʰ **V55 Occupant of pick-up truck or van injured in collision with railway train or railway vehicle**

> The appropriate 7th character is to be added to each code from category V55.
> A   initial encounter
> D   subsequent encounter
> S   sequela

☑x7ᵗʰ **V55.0** Driver of pick-up truck or van injured in collision with railway train or railway vehicle in nontraffic accident

☑x7ᵗʰ **V55.1** Passenger in pick-up truck or van injured in collision with railway train or railway vehicle in nontraffic accident

☑x7ᵗʰ **V55.2** Person on outside of pick-up truck or van injured in collision with railway train or railway vehicle in nontraffic accident

☑x7ᵗʰ **V55.3** Unspecified occupant of pick-up truck or van injured in collision with railway train or railway vehicle in nontraffic accident

☑x7ᵗʰ **V55.4** Person boarding or alighting a pick-up truck or van injured in collision with railway train or railway vehicle

☑x7ᵗʰ **V55.5** Driver of pick-up truck or van injured in collision with railway train or railway vehicle in traffic accident

☑x7ᵗʰ **V55.6** Passenger in pick-up truck or van injured in collision with railway train or railway vehicle in traffic accident

☑x7ᵗʰ **V55.7** Person on outside of pick-up truck or van injured in collision with railway train or railway vehicle in traffic accident

☑x7ᵗʰ **V55.9** Unspecified occupant of pick-up truck or van injured in collision with railway train or railway vehicle in traffic accident

☑4ᵗʰ **V56 Occupant of pick-up truck or van injured in collision with other nonmotor vehicle**

> INCLUDES   collision with animal-drawn vehicle, animal being ridden, streetcar

> The appropriate 7th character is to be added to each code from category V56.
> A   initial encounter
> D   subsequent encounter
> S   sequela

☑x7ᵗʰ **V56.0** Driver of pick-up truck or van injured in collision with other nonmotor vehicle in nontraffic accident

☑x7ᵗʰ **V56.1** Passenger in pick-up truck or van injured in collision with other nonmotor vehicle in nontraffic accident

☑x7ᵗʰ **V56.2** Person on outside of pick-up truck or van injured in collision with other nonmotor vehicle in nontraffic accident

☑x7ᵗʰ **V56.3** Unspecified occupant of pick-up truck or van injured in collision with other nonmotor vehicle in nontraffic accident

☑x7ᵗʰ **V56.4** Person boarding or alighting a pick-up truck or van injured in collision with other nonmotor vehicle

☑x7ᵗʰ **V56.5** Driver of pick-up truck or van injured in collision with other nonmotor vehicle in traffic accident

☑x7ᵗʰ **V56.6** Passenger in pick-up truck or van injured in collision with other nonmotor vehicle in traffic accident

☑x7ᵗʰ **V56.7** Person on outside of pick-up truck or van injured in collision with other nonmotor vehicle in traffic accident

☑x7ᵗʰ **V56.9** Unspecified occupant of pick-up truck or van injured in collision with other nonmotor vehicle in traffic accident

☑4ᵗʰ **V57 Occupant of pick-up truck or van injured in collision with fixed or stationary object**

> The appropriate 7th character is to be added to each code from category V57.
> A   initial encounter
> D   subsequent encounter
> S   sequela

☑x7ᵗʰ **V57.0** Driver of pick-up truck or van injured in collision with fixed or stationary object in nontraffic accident

☑x7ᵗʰ **V57.1** Passenger in pick-up truck or van injured in collision with fixed or stationary object in nontraffic accident

☑x7ᵗʰ **V57.2** Person on outside of pick-up truck or van injured in collision with fixed or stationary object in nontraffic accident

☑x7ᵗʰ **V57.3** Unspecified occupant of pick-up truck or van injured in collision with fixed or stationary object in nontraffic accident

☑x7ᵗʰ **V57.4** Person boarding or alighting a pick-up truck or van injured in collision with fixed or stationary object

☑x7ᵗʰ **V57.5** Driver of pick-up truck or van injured in collision with fixed or stationary object in traffic accident

☑x7ᵗʰ **V57.6** Passenger in pick-up truck or van injured in collision with fixed or stationary object in traffic accident

☑x7ᵗʰ **V57.7** Person on outside of pick-up truck or van injured in collision with fixed or stationary object in traffic accident

☑x7ᵗʰ **V57.9** Unspecified occupant of pick-up truck or van injured in collision with fixed or stationary object in traffic accident

☑4ᵗʰ **V58 Occupant of pick-up truck or van injured in noncollision transport accident**

> INCLUDES   overturning pick-up truck or van NOS
> overturning pick-up truck or van without collision

> The appropriate 7th character is to be added to each code from category V58.
> A   initial encounter
> D   subsequent encounter
> S   sequela

☑x7ᵗʰ **V58.0** Driver of pick-up truck or van injured in noncollision transport accident in nontraffic accident

☑x7ᵗʰ **V58.1** Passenger in pick-up truck or van injured in noncollision transport accident in nontraffic accident

☑x7ᵗʰ **V58.2** Person on outside of pick-up truck or van injured in noncollision transport accident in nontraffic accident

☑x7ᵗʰ **V58.3** Unspecified occupant of pick-up truck or van injured in noncollision transport accident in nontraffic accident

☑x7ᵗʰ **V58.4** Person boarding or alighting a pick-up truck or van injured in noncollision transport accident

☑x7ᵗʰ **V58.5** Driver of pick-up truck or van injured in noncollision transport accident in traffic accident

☑x7ᵗʰ **V58.6** Passenger in pick-up truck or van injured in noncollision transport accident in traffic accident

☑x7ᵗʰ **V58.7** Person on outside of pick-up truck or van injured in noncollision transport accident in traffic accident

☑x7ᵗʰ **V58.9** Unspecified occupant of pick-up truck or van injured in noncollision transport accident in traffic accident

---

☑ Additional Character Required   ☑x7ᵗʰ Xtension Alert   Unspecified Dx   Other Specified Dx   Manifestation   ►◄ Revised Text   ● New Code   ▲ Revised Code Title

External Causes of Morbidity

V59–V62.2

✓4ᵗʰ **V59 Occupant of pick-up truck or van injured in other and unspecified transport accidents**

> The appropriate 7th character is to be added to each code from category V59.
> A   initial encounter
> D   subsequent encounter
> S   sequela

✓5ᵗʰ **V59.0** Driver of pick-up truck or van injured in collision with other and unspecified motor vehicles in nontraffic accident

  ✓x7ᵗʰ **V59.00** Driver of pick-up truck or van injured in collision with unspecified motor vehicles in nontraffic accident

  ✓x7ᵗʰ **V59.09** Driver of pick-up truck or van injured in collision with other motor vehicles in nontraffic accident

✓5ᵗʰ **V59.1** Passenger in pick-up truck or van injured in collision with other and unspecified motor vehicles in nontraffic accident

  ✓x7ᵗʰ **V59.10** Passenger in pick-up truck or van injured in collision with unspecified motor vehicles in nontraffic accident

  ✓x7ᵗʰ **V59.19** Passenger in pick-up truck or van injured in collision with other motor vehicles in nontraffic accident

✓5ᵗʰ **V59.2** Unspecified occupant of pick-up truck or van injured in collision with other and unspecified motor vehicles in nontraffic accident

  ✓x7ᵗʰ **V59.20** Unspecified occupant of pick-up truck or van injured in collision with unspecified motor vehicles in nontraffic accident
> Collision NOS involving pick-up truck or van, nontraffic

  ✓x7ᵗʰ **V59.29** Unspecified occupant of pick-up truck or van injured in collision with other motor vehicles in nontraffic accident

✓x7ᵗʰ **V59.3** Occupant (driver) (passenger) of pick-up truck or van injured in unspecified nontraffic accident
> Accident NOS involving pick-up truck or van, nontraffic
> Occupant of pick-up truck or van injured in nontraffic accident NOS

✓5ᵗʰ **V59.4** Driver of pick-up truck or van injured in collision with other and unspecified motor vehicles in traffic accident

  ✓x7ᵗʰ **V59.40** Driver of pick-up truck or van injured in collision with unspecified motor vehicles in traffic accident

  ✓x7ᵗʰ **V59.49** Driver of pick-up truck or van injured in collision with other motor vehicles in traffic accident

✓5ᵗʰ **V59.5** Passenger in pick-up truck or van injured in collision with other and unspecified motor vehicles in traffic accident

  ✓x7ᵗʰ **V59.50** Passenger in pick-up truck or van injured in collision with unspecified motor vehicles in traffic accident

  ✓x7ᵗʰ **V59.59** Passenger in pick-up truck or van injured in collision with other motor vehicles in traffic accident

✓5ᵗʰ **V59.6** Unspecified occupant of pick-up truck or van injured in collision with other and unspecified motor vehicles in traffic accident

  ✓x7ᵗʰ **V59.60** Unspecified occupant of pick-up truck or van injured in collision with unspecified motor vehicles in traffic accident
> Collision NOS involving pick-up truck or van (traffic)

  ✓x7ᵗʰ **V59.69** Unspecified occupant of pick-up truck or van injured in collision with other motor vehicles in traffic accident

✓5ᵗʰ **V59.8** Occupant (driver) (passenger) of pick-up truck or van injured in other specified transport accidents

  ✓x7ᵗʰ **V59.81** Occupant (driver) (passenger) of pick-up truck or van injured in transport accident with military vehicle

  ✓x7ᵗʰ **V59.88** Occupant (driver) (passenger) of pick-up truck or van injured in other specified transport accidents

✓x7ᵗʰ **V59.9** Occupant (driver) (passenger) of pick-up truck or van injured in unspecified traffic accident
> Accident NOS involving pick-up truck or van

Occupant of heavy transport vehicle injured in transport accident (V60-V69)

> INCLUDES   18 wheeler
> armored car
> panel truck
> EXCLUDES 1   bus
> motorcoach

✓4ᵗʰ **V60 Occupant of heavy transport vehicle injured in collision with pedestrian or animal**

> EXCLUDES 1   heavy transport vehicle collision with animal-drawn vehicle or animal being ridden (V66.-)

> The appropriate 7th character is to be added to each code from category V60.
> A   initial encounter
> D   subsequent encounter
> S   sequela

✓x7ᵗʰ **V60.0** Driver of heavy transport vehicle injured in collision with pedestrian or animal in nontraffic accident

✓x7ᵗʰ **V60.1** Passenger in heavy transport vehicle injured in collision with pedestrian or animal in nontraffic accident

✓x7ᵗʰ **V60.2** Person on outside of heavy transport vehicle injured in collision with pedestrian or animal in nontraffic accident

✓x7ᵗʰ **V60.3** Unspecified occupant of heavy transport vehicle injured in collision with pedestrian or animal in nontraffic accident

✓x7ᵗʰ **V60.4** Person boarding or alighting a heavy transport vehicle injured in collision with pedestrian or animal

✓x7ᵗʰ **V60.5** Driver of heavy transport vehicle injured in collision with pedestrian or animal in traffic accident

✓x7ᵗʰ **V60.6** Passenger in heavy transport vehicle injured in collision with pedestrian or animal in traffic accident

✓x7ᵗʰ **V60.7** Person on outside of heavy transport vehicle injured in collision with pedestrian or animal in traffic accident

✓x7ᵗʰ **V60.9** Unspecified occupant of heavy transport vehicle injured in collision with pedestrian or animal in traffic accident

✓4ᵗʰ **V61 Occupant of heavy transport vehicle injured in collision with pedal cycle**

> The appropriate 7th character is to be added to each code from category V61.
> A   initial encounter
> D   subsequent encounter
> S   sequela

✓x7ᵗʰ **V61.0** Driver of heavy transport vehicle injured in collision with pedal cycle in nontraffic accident

✓x7ᵗʰ **V61.1** Passenger in heavy transport vehicle injured in collision with pedal cycle in nontraffic accident

✓x7ᵗʰ **V61.2** Person on outside of heavy transport vehicle injured in collision with pedal cycle in nontraffic accident

✓x7ᵗʰ **V61.3** Unspecified occupant of heavy transport vehicle injured in collision with pedal cycle in nontraffic accident

✓x7ᵗʰ **V61.4** Person boarding or alighting a heavy transport vehicle injured in collision with pedal cycle while boarding or alighting

✓x7ᵗʰ **V61.5** Driver of heavy transport vehicle injured in collision with pedal cycle in traffic accident

✓x7ᵗʰ **V61.6** Passenger in heavy transport vehicle injured in collision with pedal cycle in traffic accident

✓x7ᵗʰ **V61.7** Person on outside of heavy transport vehicle injured in collision with pedal cycle in traffic accident

✓x7ᵗʰ **V61.9** Unspecified occupant of heavy transport vehicle injured in collision with pedal cycle in traffic accident

✓4ᵗʰ **V62 Occupant of heavy transport vehicle injured in collision with two- or three-wheeled motor vehicle**

> The appropriate 7th character is to be added to each code from category V62.
> A   initial encounter
> D   subsequent encounter
> S   sequela

✓x7ᵗʰ **V62.0** Driver of heavy transport vehicle injured in collision with two- or three-wheeled motor vehicle in nontraffic accident

✓x7ᵗʰ **V62.1** Passenger in heavy transport vehicle injured in collision with two- or three-wheeled motor vehicle in nontraffic accident

✓x7ᵗʰ **V62.2** Person on outside of heavy transport vehicle injured in collision with two- or three-wheeled motor vehicle in nontraffic accident

---

EXCLUDES 1 Not coded here   EXCLUDES 2 Not included here   N Newborn Age: 0   P Pediatric Age: 0-17   M Maternity Age: 12-55   A Adult Age: 15-124

√x7th **V62.3** Unspecified occupant of heavy transport vehicle injured in collision with two- or three-wheeled motor vehicle in nontraffic accident

√x7th **V62.4** Person boarding or alighting a heavy transport vehicle injured in collision with two- or three-wheeled motor vehicle

√x7th **V62.5** Driver of heavy transport vehicle injured in collision with two- or three-wheeled motor vehicle in traffic accident

√x7th **V62.6** Passenger in heavy transport vehicle injured in collision with two- or three-wheeled motor vehicle in traffic accident

√x7th **V62.7** Person on outside of heavy transport vehicle injured in collision with two- or three-wheeled motor vehicle in traffic accident

√x7th **V62.9** Unspecified occupant of heavy transport vehicle injured in collision with two- or three-wheeled motor vehicle in traffic accident

√4th **V63** Occupant of heavy transport vehicle injured in collision with car, pick-up truck or van

The appropriate 7th character is to be added to each code from category V63.
A   initial encounter
D   subsequent encounter
S   sequela

√x7th **V63.0** Driver of heavy transport vehicle injured in collision with car, pick-up truck or van in nontraffic accident

√x7th **V63.1** Passenger in heavy transport vehicle injured in collision with car, pick-up truck or van in nontraffic accident

√x7th **V63.2** Person on outside of heavy transport vehicle injured in collision with car, pick-up truck or van in nontraffic accident

√x7th **V63.3** Unspecified occupant of heavy transport vehicle injured in collision with car, pick-up truck or van in nontraffic accident

√x7th **V63.4** Person boarding or alighting a heavy transport vehicle injured in collision with car, pick-up truck or van

√x7th **V63.5** Driver of heavy transport vehicle injured in collision with car, pick-up truck or van in traffic accident

√x7th **V63.6** Passenger in heavy transport vehicle injured in collision with car, pick-up truck or van in traffic accident

√x7th **V63.7** Person on outside of heavy transport vehicle injured in collision with car, pick-up truck or van in traffic accident

√x7th **V63.9** Unspecified occupant of heavy transport vehicle injured in collision with car, pick-up truck or van in traffic accident

√4th **V64** Occupant of heavy transport vehicle injured in collision with heavy transport vehicle or bus

EXCLUDES 1   occupant of heavy transport vehicle injured in collision with military vehicle (V69.81)

The appropriate 7th character is to be added to each code from category V64.
A   initial encounter
D   subsequent encounter
S   sequela

√x7th **V64.0** Driver of heavy transport vehicle injured in collision with heavy transport vehicle or bus in nontraffic accident

√x7th **V64.1** Passenger in heavy transport vehicle injured in collision with heavy transport vehicle or bus in nontraffic accident

√x7th **V64.2** Person on outside of heavy transport vehicle injured in collision with heavy transport vehicle or bus in nontraffic accident

√x7th **V64.3** Unspecified occupant of heavy transport vehicle injured in collision with heavy transport vehicle or bus in nontraffic accident

√x7th **V64.4** Person boarding or alighting a heavy transport vehicle injured in collision with heavy transport vehicle or bus while boarding or alighting

√x7th **V64.5** Driver of heavy transport vehicle injured in collision with heavy transport vehicle or bus in traffic accident

√x7th **V64.6** Passenger in heavy transport vehicle injured in collision with heavy transport vehicle or bus in traffic accident

√x7th **V64.7** Person on outside of heavy transport vehicle injured in collision with heavy transport vehicle or bus in traffic accident

√x7th **V64.9** Unspecified occupant of heavy transport vehicle injured in collision with heavy transport vehicle or bus in traffic accident

√4th **V65** Occupant of heavy transport vehicle injured in collision with railway train or railway vehicle

The appropriate 7th character is to be added to each code from category V65.
A   initial encounter
D   subsequent encounter
S   sequela

√x7th **V65.0** Driver of heavy transport vehicle injured in collision with railway train or railway vehicle in nontraffic accident

√x7th **V65.1** Passenger in heavy transport vehicle injured in collision with railway train or railway vehicle in nontraffic accident

√x7th **V65.2** Person on outside of heavy transport vehicle injured in collision with railway train or railway vehicle in nontraffic accident

√x7th **V65.3** Unspecified occupant of heavy transport vehicle injured in collision with railway train or railway vehicle in nontraffic accident

√x7th **V65.4** Person boarding or alighting a heavy transport vehicle injured in collision with railway train or railway vehicle

√x7th **V65.5** Driver of heavy transport vehicle injured in collision with railway train or railway vehicle in traffic accident

√x7th **V65.6** Passenger in heavy transport vehicle injured in collision with railway train or railway vehicle in traffic accident

√x7th **V65.7** Person on outside of heavy transport vehicle injured in collision with railway train or railway vehicle in traffic accident

√x7th **V65.9** Unspecified occupant of heavy transport vehicle injured in collision with railway train or railway vehicle in traffic accident

√4th **V66** Occupant of heavy transport vehicle injured in collision with other nonmotor vehicle

INCLUDES   collision with animal-drawn vehicle, animal being ridden, streetcar

The appropriate 7th character is to be added to each code from category V66.
A   initial encounter
D   subsequent encounter
S   sequela

√x7th **V66.0** Driver of heavy transport vehicle injured in collision with other nonmotor vehicle in nontraffic accident

√x7th **V66.1** Passenger in heavy transport vehicle injured in collision with other nonmotor vehicle in nontraffic accident

√x7th **V66.2** Person on outside of heavy transport vehicle injured in collision with other nonmotor vehicle in nontraffic accident

√x7th **V66.3** Unspecified occupant of heavy transport vehicle injured in collision with other nonmotor vehicle in nontraffic accident

√x7th **V66.4** Person boarding or alighting a heavy transport vehicle injured in collision with other nonmotor vehicle

√x7th **V66.5** Driver of heavy transport vehicle injured in collision with other nonmotor vehicle in traffic accident

√x7th **V66.6** Passenger in heavy transport vehicle injured in collision with other nonmotor vehicle in traffic accident

√x7th **V66.7** Person on outside of heavy transport vehicle injured in collision with other nonmotor vehicle in traffic accident

√x7th **V66.9** Unspecified occupant of heavy transport vehicle injured in collision with other nonmotor vehicle in traffic accident

√4th **V67** Occupant of heavy transport vehicle injured in collision with fixed or stationary object

The appropriate 7th character is to be added to each code from category V67.
A   initial encounter
D   subsequent encounter
S   sequela

√x7th **V67.0** Driver of heavy transport vehicle injured in collision with fixed or stationary object in nontraffic accident

√x7th **V67.1** Passenger in heavy transport vehicle injured in collision with fixed or stationary object in nontraffic accident

√x7th **V67.2** Person on outside of heavy transport vehicle injured in collision with fixed or stationary object in nontraffic accident

√x7th **V67.3** Unspecified occupant of heavy transport vehicle injured in collision with fixed or stationary object in nontraffic accident

√x7th **V67.4** Person boarding or alighting a heavy transport vehicle injured in collision with fixed or stationary object

√x7ᵗʰ **V67.5** Driver of heavy transport vehicle injured in collision with fixed or stationary object in traffic accident

√x7ᵗʰ **V67.6** Passenger in heavy transport vehicle injured in collision with fixed or stationary object in traffic accident

√x7ᵗʰ **V67.7** Person on outside of heavy transport vehicle injured in collision with fixed or stationary object in traffic accident

√x7ᵗʰ **V67.9** Unspecified occupant of heavy transport vehicle injured in collision with fixed or stationary object in traffic accident

√4ᵗʰ **V68 Occupant of heavy transport vehicle injured in noncollision transport accident**

> INCLUDES overturning heavy transport vehicle NOS
> overturning heavy transport vehicle without collision

> The appropriate 7th character is to be added to each code from category V68.
> A   initial encounter
> D   subsequent encounter
> S   sequela

√x7ᵗʰ **V68.0** Driver of heavy transport vehicle injured in noncollision transport accident in nontraffic accident

√x7ᵗʰ **V68.1** Passenger in heavy transport vehicle injured in noncollision transport accident in nontraffic accident

√x7ᵗʰ **V68.2** Person on outside of heavy transport vehicle injured in noncollision transport accident in nontraffic accident

√x7ᵗʰ **V68.3** Unspecified occupant of heavy transport vehicle injured in noncollision transport accident in nontraffic accident

√x7ᵗʰ **V68.4** Person boarding or alighting a heavy transport vehicle injured in noncollision transport accident

√x7ᵗʰ **V68.5** Driver of heavy transport vehicle injured in noncollision transport accident in traffic accident

√x7ᵗʰ **V68.6** Passenger in heavy transport vehicle injured in noncollision transport accident in traffic accident

√x7ᵗʰ **V68.7** Person on outside of heavy transport vehicle injured in noncollision transport accident in traffic accident

√x7ᵗʰ **V68.9** Unspecified occupant of heavy transport vehicle injured in noncollision transport accident in traffic accident

√4ᵗʰ **V69 Occupant of heavy transport vehicle injured in other and unspecified transport accidents**

> The appropriate 7th character is to be added to each code from category V69.
> A   initial encounter
> D   subsequent encounter
> S   sequela

√5ᵗʰ **V69.0** Driver of heavy transport vehicle injured in collision with other and unspecified motor vehicles in nontraffic accident

√x7ᵗʰ **V69.00** Driver of heavy transport vehicle injured in collision with unspecified motor vehicles in nontraffic accident

√x7ᵗʰ **V69.09** Driver of heavy transport vehicle injured in collision with other motor vehicles in nontraffic accident

√5ᵗʰ **V69.1** Passenger in heavy transport vehicle injured in collision with other and unspecified motor vehicles in nontraffic accident

√x7ᵗʰ **V69.10** Passenger in heavy transport vehicle injured in collision with unspecified motor vehicles in nontraffic accident

√x7ᵗʰ **V69.19** Passenger in heavy transport vehicle injured in collision with other motor vehicles in nontraffic accident

√5ᵗʰ **V69.2** Unspecified occupant of heavy transport vehicle injured in collision with other and unspecified motor vehicles in nontraffic accident

√x7ᵗʰ **V69.20** Unspecified occupant of heavy transport vehicle injured in collision with unspecified motor vehicles in nontraffic accident

> Collision NOS involving heavy transport vehicle, nontraffic

√x7ᵗʰ **V69.29** Unspecified occupant of heavy transport vehicle injured in collision with other motor vehicles in nontraffic accident

√x7ᵗʰ **V69.3** Occupant (driver) (passenger) of heavy transport vehicle injured in unspecified nontraffic accident

> Accident NOS involving heavy transport vehicle, nontraffic
> Occupant of heavy transport vehicle injured in nontraffic accident NOS

√5ᵗʰ **V69.4** Driver of heavy transport vehicle injured in collision with other and unspecified motor vehicles in traffic accident

√x7ᵗʰ **V69.40** Driver of heavy transport vehicle injured in collision with unspecified motor vehicles in traffic accident

√x7ᵗʰ **V69.49** Driver of heavy transport vehicle injured in collision with other motor vehicles in traffic accident

√5ᵗʰ **V69.5** Passenger in heavy transport vehicle injured in collision with other and unspecified motor vehicles in traffic accident

√x7ᵗʰ **V69.50** Passenger in heavy transport vehicle injured in collision with unspecified motor vehicles in traffic accident

√x7ᵗʰ **V69.59** Passenger in heavy transport vehicle injured in collision with other motor vehicles in traffic accident

√5ᵗʰ **V69.6** Unspecified occupant of heavy transport vehicle injured in collision with other and unspecified motor vehicles in traffic accident

√x7ᵗʰ **V69.60** Unspecified occupant of heavy transport vehicle injured in collision with unspecified motor vehicles in traffic accident

> Collision NOS involving heavy transport vehicle (traffic)

√x7ᵗʰ **V69.69** Unspecified occupant of heavy transport vehicle injured in collision with other motor vehicles in traffic accident

√5ᵗʰ **V69.8** Occupant (driver) (passenger) of heavy transport vehicle injured in other specified transport accidents

√x7ᵗʰ **V69.81** Occupant (driver) (passenger) of heavy transport vehicle injured in transport accidents with military vehicle

√x7ᵗʰ **V69.88** Occupant (driver) (passenger) of heavy transport vehicle injured in other specified transport accidents

√x7ᵗʰ **V69.9** Occupant (driver) (passenger) of heavy transport vehicle injured in unspecified traffic accident

> Accident NOS involving heavy transport vehicle

Bus occupant injured in transport accident (V70-V79)

> INCLUDES motorcoach
> EXCLUDES 1 minibus (V50-V59)

√4ᵗʰ **V70 Bus occupant injured in collision with pedestrian or animal**

> EXCLUDES 1 bus collision with animal-drawn vehicle or animal being ridden (V76.-)

> The appropriate 7th character is to be added to each code from category V70.
> A   initial encounter
> D   subsequent encounter
> S   sequela

√x7ᵗʰ **V70.0** Driver of bus injured in collision with pedestrian or animal in nontraffic accident

√x7ᵗʰ **V70.1** Passenger on bus injured in collision with pedestrian or animal in nontraffic accident

√x7ᵗʰ **V70.2** Person on outside of bus injured in collision with pedestrian or animal in nontraffic accident

√x7ᵗʰ **V70.3** Unspecified occupant of bus injured in collision with pedestrian or animal in nontraffic accident

√x7ᵗʰ **V70.4** Person boarding or alighting from bus injured in collision with pedestrian or animal

√x7ᵗʰ **V70.5** Driver of bus injured in collision with pedestrian or animal in traffic accident

√x7ᵗʰ **V70.6** Passenger on bus injured in collision with pedestrian or animal in traffic accident

√x7ᵗʰ **V70.7** Person on outside of bus injured in collision with pedestrian or animal in traffic accident

√x7ᵗʰ **V70.9** Unspecified occupant of bus injured in collision with pedestrian or animal in traffic accident

√4ᵗʰ **V71 Bus occupant injured in collision with pedal cycle**

> The appropriate 7th character is to be added to each code from category V71.
> A   initial encounter
> D   subsequent encounter
> S   sequela

√x7ᵗʰ **V71.0** Driver of bus injured in collision with pedal cycle in nontraffic accident

√x7ᵗʰ **V71.1** Passenger on bus injured in collision with pedal cycle in nontraffic accident

EXCLUDES 1 Not coded here   EXCLUDES 2 Not included here   N Newborn Age: 0   P Pediatric Age: 0-17   M Maternity Age: 12-55   A Adult Age: 15-124

1010   ICD-10-CM Draft (2015)

√x7ᵗʰ **V71.2** Person on outside of bus injured in collision with pedal cycle in nontraffic accident

√x7ᵗʰ **V71.3** Unspecified occupant of bus injured in collision with pedal cycle in nontraffic accident

√x7ᵗʰ **V71.4** Person boarding or alighting from bus injured in collision with pedal cycle

√x7ᵗʰ **V71.5** Driver of bus injured in collision with pedal cycle in traffic accident

√x7ᵗʰ **V71.6** Passenger on bus injured in collision with pedal cycle in traffic accident

√x7ᵗʰ **V71.7** Person on outside of bus injured in collision with pedal cycle in traffic accident

√x7ᵗʰ **V71.9** Unspecified occupant of bus injured in collision with pedal cycle in traffic accident

✓4ᵗʰ **V72** **Bus occupant injured in collision with two- or three-wheeled motor vehicle**

> The appropriate 7th character is to be added to each code from category V72.
> A   initial encounter
> D   subsequent encounter
> S   sequela

√x7ᵗʰ **V72.0** Driver of bus injured in collision with two- or three-wheeled motor vehicle in nontraffic accident

√x7ᵗʰ **V72.1** Passenger on bus injured in collision with two- or three-wheeled motor vehicle in nontraffic accident

√x7ᵗʰ **V72.2** Person on outside of bus injured in collision with two- or three-wheeled motor vehicle in nontraffic accident

√x7ᵗʰ **V72.3** Unspecified occupant of bus injured in collision with two- or three-wheeled motor vehicle in nontraffic accident

√x7ᵗʰ **V72.4** Person boarding or alighting from bus injured in collision with two- or three-wheeled motor vehicle

√x7ᵗʰ **V72.5** Driver of bus injured in collision with two- or three-wheeled motor vehicle in traffic accident

√x7ᵗʰ **V72.6** Passenger on bus injured in collision with two- or three-wheeled motor vehicle in traffic accident

√x7ᵗʰ **V72.7** Person on outside of bus injured in collision with two- or three-wheeled motor vehicle in traffic accident

√x7ᵗʰ **V72.9** Unspecified occupant of bus injured in collision with two- or three-wheeled motor vehicle in traffic accident

✓4ᵗʰ **V73** **Bus occupant injured in collision with car, pick-up truck or van**

> The appropriate 7th character is to be added to each code from category V73.
> A   initial encounter
> D   subsequent encounter
> S   sequela

√x7ᵗʰ **V73.0** Driver of bus injured in collision with car, pick-up truck or van in nontraffic accident

√x7ᵗʰ **V73.1** Passenger on bus injured in collision with car, pick-up truck or van in nontraffic accident

√x7ᵗʰ **V73.2** Person on outside of bus injured in collision with car, pick-up truck or van in nontraffic accident

√x7ᵗʰ **V73.3** Unspecified occupant of bus injured in collision with car, pick-up truck or van in nontraffic accident

√x7ᵗʰ **V73.4** Person boarding or alighting from bus injured in collision with car, pick-up truck or van

√x7ᵗʰ **V73.5** Driver of bus injured in collision with car, pick-up truck or van in traffic accident

√x7ᵗʰ **V73.6** Passenger on bus injured in collision with car, pick-up truck or van in traffic accident

√x7ᵗʰ **V73.7** Person on outside of bus injured in collision with car, pick-up truck or van in traffic accident

√x7ᵗʰ **V73.9** Unspecified occupant of bus injured in collision with car, pick-up truck or van in traffic accident

✓4ᵗʰ **V74** **Bus occupant injured in collision with heavy transport vehicle or bus**

> **EXCLUDES 1**   bus occupant injured in collision with military vehicle (V79.81)

> The appropriate 7th character is to be added to each code from category V74.
> A   initial encounter
> D   subsequent encounter
> S   sequela

√x7ᵗʰ **V74.0** Driver of bus injured in collision with heavy transport vehicle or bus in nontraffic accident

√x7ᵗʰ **V74.1** Passenger on bus injured in collision with heavy transport vehicle or bus in nontraffic accident

√x7ᵗʰ **V74.2** Person on outside of bus injured in collision with heavy transport vehicle or bus in nontraffic accident

√x7ᵗʰ **V74.3** Unspecified occupant of bus injured in collision with heavy transport vehicle or bus in nontraffic accident

√x7ᵗʰ **V74.4** Person boarding or alighting from bus injured in collision with heavy transport vehicle or bus

√x7ᵗʰ **V74.5** Driver of bus injured in collision with heavy transport vehicle or bus in traffic accident

√x7ᵗʰ **V74.6** Passenger on bus injured in collision with heavy transport vehicle or bus in traffic accident

√x7ᵗʰ **V74.7** Person on outside of bus injured in collision with heavy transport vehicle or bus in traffic accident

√x7ᵗʰ **V74.9** Unspecified occupant of bus injured in collision with heavy transport vehicle or bus in traffic accident

✓4ᵗʰ **V75** **Bus occupant injured in collision with railway train or railway vehicle**

> The appropriate 7th character is to be added to each code from category V75.
> A   initial encounter
> D   subsequent encounter
> S   sequela

√x7ᵗʰ **V75.0** Driver of bus injured in collision with railway train or railway vehicle in nontraffic accident

√x7ᵗʰ **V75.1** Passenger on bus injured in collision with railway train or railway vehicle in nontraffic accident

√x7ᵗʰ **V75.2** Person on outside of bus injured in collision with railway train or railway vehicle in nontraffic accident

√x7ᵗʰ **V75.3** Unspecified occupant of bus injured in collision with railway train or railway vehicle in nontraffic accident

√x7ᵗʰ **V75.4** Person boarding or alighting from bus injured in collision with railway train or railway vehicle

√x7ᵗʰ **V75.5** Driver of bus injured in collision with railway train or railway vehicle in traffic accident

√x7ᵗʰ **V75.6** Passenger on bus injured in collision with railway train or railway vehicle in traffic accident

√x7ᵗʰ **V75.7** Person on outside of bus injured in collision with railway train or railway vehicle in traffic accident

√x7ᵗʰ **V75.9** Unspecified occupant of bus injured in collision with railway train or railway vehicle in traffic accident

✓4ᵗʰ **V76** **Bus occupant injured in collision with other nonmotor vehicle**

> **INCLUDES**   collision with animal-drawn vehicle, animal being ridden, streetcar

> The appropriate 7th character is to be added to each code from category V76.
> A   initial encounter
> D   subsequent encounter
> S   sequela

√x7ᵗʰ **V76.0** Driver of bus injured in collision with other nonmotor vehicle in nontraffic accident

√x7ᵗʰ **V76.1** Passenger on bus injured in collision with other nonmotor vehicle in nontraffic accident

√x7ᵗʰ **V76.2** Person on outside of bus injured in collision with other nonmotor vehicle in nontraffic accident

√x7ᵗʰ **V76.3** Unspecified occupant of bus injured in collision with other nonmotor vehicle in nontraffic accident

√x7ᵗʰ **V76.4** Person boarding or alighting from bus injured in collision with other nonmotor vehicle

√x7ᵗʰ **V76.5** Driver of bus injured in collision with other nonmotor vehicle in traffic accident

√x7ᵗʰ **V76.6** Passenger on bus injured in collision with other nonmotor vehicle in traffic accident

√x7ᵗʰ **V76.7** Person on outside of bus injured in collision with other nonmotor vehicle in traffic accident

√x7ᵗʰ **V76.9** Unspecified occupant of bus injured in collision with other nonmotor vehicle in traffic accident

---

✓ Additional Character Required   √x7ᵗʰ Xtension Alert   Unspecified Dx   Other Specified Dx   Manifestation   ►◄ Revised Text   ● New Code   ▲ Revised Code Title

√4ᵗʰ **V77   Bus occupant injured in collision with fixed or stationary object**

> The appropriate 7th character is to be added to each code from category V77.
> A   initial encounter
> D   subsequent encounter
> S   sequela

√x7ᵗʰ **V77.0**   Driver of bus injured in collision with fixed or stationary object in nontraffic accident

√x7ᵗʰ **V77.1**   Passenger on bus injured in collision with fixed or stationary object in nontraffic accident

√x7ᵗʰ **V77.2**   Person on outside of bus injured in collision with fixed or stationary object in nontraffic accident

√x7ᵗʰ **V77.3**   Unspecified occupant of bus injured in collision with fixed or stationary object in nontraffic accident

√x7ᵗʰ **V77.4**   Person boarding or alighting from bus injured in collision with fixed or stationary object

√x7ᵗʰ **V77.5**   Driver of bus injured in collision with fixed or stationary object in traffic accident

√x7ᵗʰ **V77.6**   Passenger on bus injured in collision with fixed or stationary object in traffic accident

√x7ᵗʰ **V77.7**   Person on outside of bus injured in collision with fixed or stationary object in traffic accident

√x7ᵗʰ **V77.9**   Unspecified occupant of bus injured in collision with fixed or stationary object in traffic accident

√4ᵗʰ **V78   Bus occupant injured in noncollision transport accident**

> INCLUDES   overturning bus NOS
> overturning bus without collision

> The appropriate 7th character is to be added to each code from category V78.
> A   initial encounter
> D   subsequent encounter
> S   sequela

√x7ᵗʰ **V78.0**   Driver of bus injured in noncollision transport accident in nontraffic accident

√x7ᵗʰ **V78.1**   Passenger on bus injured in noncollision transport accident in nontraffic accident

√x7ᵗʰ **V78.2**   Person on outside of bus injured in noncollision transport accident in nontraffic accident

√x7ᵗʰ **V78.3**   Unspecified occupant of bus injured in noncollision transport accident in nontraffic accident

√x7ᵗʰ **V78.4**   Person boarding or alighting from bus injured in noncollision transport accident

√x7ᵗʰ **V78.5**   Driver of bus injured in noncollision transport accident in traffic accident

√x7ᵗʰ **V78.6**   Passenger on bus injured in noncollision transport accident in traffic accident

√x7ᵗʰ **V78.7**   Person on outside of bus injured in noncollision transport accident in traffic accident

√x7ᵗʰ **V78.9**   Unspecified occupant of bus injured in noncollision transport accident in traffic accident

√4ᵗʰ **V79   Bus occupant injured in other and unspecified transport accidents**

> The appropriate 7th character is to be added to each code from category V79.
> A   initial encounter
> D   subsequent encounter
> S   sequela

√5ᵗʰ **V79.0**   Driver of bus injured in collision with other and unspecified motor vehicles in nontraffic accident

√x7ᵗʰ **V79.00**   Driver of bus injured in collision with unspecified motor vehicles in nontraffic accident

√x7ᵗʰ **V79.09**   Driver of bus injured in collision with other motor vehicles in nontraffic accident

√5ᵗʰ **V79.1**   Passenger on bus injured in collision with other and unspecified motor vehicles in nontraffic accident

√x7ᵗʰ **V79.10**   Passenger on bus injured in collision with unspecified motor vehicles in nontraffic accident

√x7ᵗʰ **V79.19**   Passenger on bus injured in collision with other motor vehicles in nontraffic accident

√5ᵗʰ **V79.2**   Unspecified bus occupant injured in collision with other and unspecified motor vehicles in nontraffic accident

√x7ᵗʰ **V79.20**   Unspecified bus occupant injured in collision with unspecified motor vehicles in nontraffic accident
> Bus collision NOS, nontraffic

√x7ᵗʰ **V79.29**   Unspecified bus occupant injured in collision with other motor vehicles in nontraffic accident

√x7ᵗʰ **V79.3**   Bus occupant (driver) (passenger) injured in unspecified nontraffic accident
> Bus accident NOS, nontraffic
> Bus occupant injured in nontraffic accident NOS

√5ᵗʰ **V79.4**   Driver of bus injured in collision with other and unspecified motor vehicles in traffic accident

√x7ᵗʰ **V79.40**   Driver of bus injured in collision with unspecified motor vehicles in traffic accident

√x7ᵗʰ **V79.49**   Driver of bus injured in collision with other motor vehicles in traffic accident

√5ᵗʰ **V79.5**   Passenger on bus injured in collision with other and unspecified motor vehicles in traffic accident

√x7ᵗʰ **V79.50**   Passenger on bus injured in collision with unspecified motor vehicles in traffic accident

√x7ᵗʰ **V79.59**   Passenger on bus injured in collision with other motor vehicles in traffic accident

√5ᵗʰ **V79.6**   Unspecified bus occupant injured in collision with other and unspecified motor vehicles in traffic accident

√x7ᵗʰ **V79.60**   Unspecified bus occupant injured in collision with unspecified motor vehicles in traffic accident
> Bus collision NOS (traffic)

√x7ᵗʰ **V79.69**   Unspecified bus occupant injured in collision with other motor vehicles in traffic accident

√5ᵗʰ **V79.8**   Bus occupant (driver) (passenger) injured in other specified transport accidents

√x7ᵗʰ **V79.81**   Bus occupant (driver) (passenger) injured in transport accidents with military vehicle

√x7ᵗʰ **V79.88**   Bus occupant (driver) (passenger) injured in other specified transport accidents

√x7ᵗʰ **V79.9**   Bus occupant (driver) (passenger) injured in unspecified traffic accident
> Bus accident NOS

Other land transport accidents (V80-V89)

√4ᵗʰ **V80   Animal-rider or occupant of animal-drawn vehicle injured in transport accident**

> The appropriate 7th character is to be added to each code from category V80.
> A   initial encounter
> D   subsequent encounter
> S   sequela

√5ᵗʰ **V80.0**   Animal-rider or occupant of animal drawn vehicle injured by fall from or being thrown from animal or animal-drawn vehicle in noncollision accident

√6ᵗʰ **V80.01**   Animal-rider injured by fall from or being thrown from animal in noncollision accident

√7ᵗʰ **V80.010**   Animal-rider injured by fall from or being thrown from horse in noncollision accident

√7ᵗʰ **V80.018**   Animal-rider injured by fall from or being thrown from other animal in noncollision accident

√x7ᵗʰ **V80.02**   Occupant of animal-drawn vehicle injured by fall from or being thrown from animal-drawn vehicle in noncollision accident
> Overturning animal-drawn vehicle NOS
> Overturning animal-drawn vehicle without collision

√5ᵗʰ **V80.1**   Animal-rider or occupant of animal-drawn vehicle injured in collision with pedestrian or animal

> EXCLUDES 1   animal-rider or animal-drawn vehicle collision with animal-drawn vehicle or animal being ridden (V80.7)

√x7ᵗʰ **V80.11**   Animal-rider injured in collision with pedestrian or animal

√x7ᵗʰ **V80.12**   Occupant of animal-drawn vehicle injured in collision with pedestrian or animal

---

EXCLUDES 1 Not coded here   EXCLUDES 2 Not included here   N Newborn Age: 0   P Pediatric Age: 0-17   M Maternity Age: 12-55   A Adult Age: 15-124

√5ᵗʰ **V80.2** Animal-rider or occupant of animal-drawn vehicle injured in collision with pedal cycle

  √x7ᵗʰ **V80.21** Animal-rider injured in collision with pedal cycle

  √x7ᵗʰ **V80.22** Occupant of animal-drawn vehicle injured in collision with pedal cycle

√5ᵗʰ **V80.3** Animal-rider or occupant of animal-drawn vehicle injured in collision with two- or three-wheeled motor vehicle

  √x7ᵗʰ **V80.31** Animal-rider injured in collision with two- or three-wheeled motor vehicle

  √x7ᵗʰ **V80.32** Occupant of animal-drawn vehicle injured in collision with two- or three-wheeled motor vehicle

√5ᵗʰ **V80.4** Animal-rider or occupant of animal-drawn vehicle injured in collision with car, pick-up truck, van, heavy transport vehicle or bus

  EXCLUDES 1 animal-rider injured in collision with military vehicle (V80.910)

  occupant of animal-drawn vehicle injured in collision with military vehicle (V80.920)

  √x7ᵗʰ **V80.41** Animal-rider injured in collision with car, pick-up truck, van, heavy transport vehicle or bus

  √x7ᵗʰ **V80.42** Occupant of animal-drawn vehicle injured in collision with car, pick-up truck, van, heavy transport vehicle or bus

√5ᵗʰ **V80.5** Animal-rider or occupant of animal-drawn vehicle injured in collision with other specified motor vehicle

  √x7ᵗʰ **V80.51** Animal-rider injured in collision with other specified motor vehicle

  √x7ᵗʰ **V80.52** Occupant of animal-drawn vehicle injured in collision with other specified motor vehicle

√5ᵗʰ **V80.6** Animal-rider or occupant of animal-drawn vehicle injured in collision with railway train or railway vehicle

  √x7ᵗʰ **V80.61** Animal-rider injured in collision with railway train or railway vehicle

  √x7ᵗʰ **V80.62** Occupant of animal-drawn vehicle injured in collision with railway train or railway vehicle

√5ᵗʰ **V80.7** Animal-rider or occupant of animal-drawn vehicle injured in collision with other nonmotor vehicles

  √6ᵗʰ **V80.71** Animal-rider or occupant of animal-drawn vehicle injured in collision with animal being ridden

    √7ᵗʰ **V80.710** Animal-rider injured in collision with other animal being ridden

    √7ᵗʰ **V80.711** Occupant of animal-drawn vehicle injured in collision with animal being ridden

  √6ᵗʰ **V80.72** Animal-rider or occupant of animal-drawn vehicle injured in collision with other animal-drawn vehicle

    √7ᵗʰ **V80.720** Animal-rider injured in collision with animal-drawn vehicle

    √7ᵗʰ **V80.721** Occupant of animal-drawn vehicle injured in collision with other animal-drawn vehicle

  √6ᵗʰ **V80.73** Animal-rider or occupant of animal-drawn vehicle injured in collision with streetcar

    √7ᵗʰ **V80.730** Animal-rider injured in collision with streetcar

    √7ᵗʰ **V80.731** Occupant of animal-drawn vehicle injured in collision with streetcar

  √6ᵗʰ **V80.79** Animal-rider or occupant of animal-drawn vehicle injured in collision with other nonmotor vehicles

    √7ᵗʰ **V80.790** Animal-rider injured in collision with other nonmotor vehicles

    √7ᵗʰ **V80.791** Occupant of animal-drawn vehicle injured in collision with other nonmotor vehicles

√5ᵗʰ **V80.8** Animal-rider or occupant of animal-drawn vehicle injured in collision with fixed or stationary object

  √x7ᵗʰ **V80.81** Animal-rider injured in collision with fixed or stationary object

  √x7ᵗʰ **V80.82** Occupant of animal-drawn vehicle injured in collision with fixed or stationary object

√5ᵗʰ **V80.9** Animal-rider or occupant of animal-drawn vehicle injured in other and unspecified transport accidents

  √6ᵗʰ **V80.91** Animal-rider injured in other and unspecified transport accidents

    √7ᵗʰ **V80.910** Animal-rider injured in transport accident with military vehicle

    √7ᵗʰ **V80.918** Animal-rider injured in other transport accident

    √7ᵗʰ **V80.919** Animal-rider injured in unspecified transport accident

      Animal rider accident NOS

  √6ᵗʰ **V80.92** Occupant of animal-drawn vehicle injured in other and unspecified transport accidents

    √7ᵗʰ **V80.920** Occupant of animal-drawn vehicle injured in transport accident with military vehicle

    √7ᵗʰ **V80.928** Occupant of animal-drawn vehicle injured in other transport accident

    √7ᵗʰ **V80.929** Occupant of animal-drawn vehicle injured in unspecified transport accident

      Animal-drawn vehicle accident NOS

√4ᵗʰ **V81** Occupant of railway train or railway vehicle injured in transport accident

  INCLUDES derailment of railway train or railway vehicle

  person on outside of train

  EXCLUDES 1 streetcar (V82.-)

  The appropriate 7th character is to be added to each code from category V81.
  A initial encounter
  D subsequent encounter
  S sequela

√x7ᵗʰ **V81.0** Occupant of railway train or railway vehicle injured in collision with motor vehicle in nontraffic accident

  EXCLUDES 1 occupant of railway train or railway vehicle injured due to collision with military vehicle (V81.83)

√x7ᵗʰ **V81.1** Occupant of railway train or railway vehicle injured in collision with motor vehicle in traffic accident

  EXCLUDES 1 occupant of railway train or railway vehicle injured due to collision with military vehicle (V81.83)

√x7ᵗʰ **V81.2** Occupant of railway train or railway vehicle injured in collision with or hit by rolling stock

√x7ᵗʰ **V81.3** Occupant of railway train or railway vehicle injured in collision with other object

  Railway collision NOS

√x7ᵗʰ **V81.4** Person injured while boarding or alighting from railway train or railway vehicle

√x7ᵗʰ **V81.5** Occupant of railway train or railway vehicle injured by fall in railway train or railway vehicle

√x7ᵗʰ **V81.6** Occupant of railway train or railway vehicle injured by fall from railway train or railway vehicle

√x7ᵗʰ **V81.7** Occupant of railway train or railway vehicle injured in derailment without antecedent collision

√5ᵗʰ **V81.8** Occupant of railway train or railway vehicle injured in other specified railway accidents

  √x7ᵗʰ **V81.81** Occupant of railway train or railway vehicle injured due to explosion or fire on train

  √x7ᵗʰ **V81.82** Occupant of railway train or railway vehicle injured due to object falling onto train

    Occupant of railway train or railway vehicle injured due to falling earth onto train
    Occupant of railway train or railway vehicle injured due to falling rocks onto train
    Occupant of railway train or railway vehicle injured due to falling snow onto train
    Occupant of railway train or railway vehicle injured due to falling trees onto train

  √x7ᵗʰ **V81.83** Occupant of railway train or railway vehicle injured due to collision with military vehicle

  √x7ᵗʰ **V81.89** Occupant of railway train or railway vehicle injured due to other specified railway accident

√x7ᵗʰ **V81.9** Occupant of railway train or railway vehicle injured in unspecified railway accident

  Railway accident NOS

✓ Additional Character Required   √x7ᵗʰ Xtension Alert   Unspecified Dx   Other Specified Dx   Manifestation   ▶◀ Revised Text   ● New Code   ▲ Revised Code Title

ICD-10-CM Draft (2015)   1013

External Causes of Morbidity

V82–V85.9

✓4ᵗʰ V82 Occupant of powered streetcar injured in transport accident

INCLUDES   interurban electric car
person on outside of streetcar
tram (car)
trolley (car)

EXCLUDES 1   bus (V70-V79)
motorcoach (V70-V79)
nonpowered streetcar (V76.-)
train (V81.-)

> The appropriate 7th character is to be added to each code from category V82.
> A   initial encounter
> D   subsequent encounter
> S   sequela

✓x7ᵗʰ **V82.0 Occupant of streetcar injured in collision with motor vehicle in nontraffic accident**

✓x7ᵗʰ **V82.1 Occupant of streetcar injured in collision with motor vehicle in traffic accident**

✓x7ᵗʰ **V82.2 Occupant of streetcar injured in collision with or hit by rolling stock**

✓x7ᵗʰ **V82.3 Occupant of streetcar injured in collision with other object**

EXCLUDES 1   collision with animal-drawn vehicle or animal being ridden (V82.8)

✓x7ᵗʰ **V82.4 Person injured while boarding or alighting from streetcar**

✓x7ᵗʰ **V82.5 Occupant of streetcar injured by fall in streetcar**

EXCLUDES 1   fall in streetcar:
while boarding or alighting (V82.4)
with antecedent collision (V82.0-V82.3)

✓x7ᵗʰ **V82.6 Occupant of streetcar injured by fall from streetcar**

EXCLUDES 1   fall from streetcar:
while boarding or alighting (V82.4)
with antecedent collision (V82.0-V82.3)

✓x7ᵗʰ **V82.7 Occupant of streetcar injured in derailment without antecedent collision**

EXCLUDES 1   occupant of streetcar injured in derailment with antecedent collision (V82.0-V82.3)

✓x7ᵗʰ **V82.8 Occupant of streetcar injured in other specified transport accidents**

Streetcar collision with military vehicle
Streetcar collision with train or nonmotor vehicles

✓x7ᵗʰ **V82.9 Occupant of streetcar injured in unspecified traffic accident**

Streetcar accident NOS

✓4ᵗʰ V83 Occupant of special vehicle mainly used on industrial premises injured in transport accident

INCLUDES   battery-powered airport passenger vehicle
battery-powered truck (baggage) (mail)
coal-car in mine
forklift (truck)
logging car
self-propelled industrial truck
station baggage truck (powered)
tram, truck, or tub (powered) in mine or quarry

EXCLUDES 1   special construction vehicles (V85.-)
special industrial vehicle in stationary use or maintenance (W31.-)

> The appropriate 7th character is to be added to each code from category V83.
> A   initial encounter
> D   subsequent encounter
> S   sequela

✓x7ᵗʰ **V83.0 Driver of special industrial vehicle injured in traffic accident**

✓x7ᵗʰ **V83.1 Passenger of special industrial vehicle injured in traffic accident**

✓x7ᵗʰ **V83.2 Person on outside of special industrial vehicle injured in traffic accident**

✓x7ᵗʰ **V83.3 Unspecified occupant of special industrial vehicle injured in traffic accident**

✓x7ᵗʰ **V83.4 Person injured while boarding or alighting from special industrial vehicle**

✓x7ᵗʰ **V83.5 Driver of special industrial vehicle injured in nontraffic accident**

✓x7ᵗʰ **V83.6 Passenger of special industrial vehicle injured in nontraffic accident**

✓x7ᵗʰ **V83.7 Person on outside of special industrial vehicle injured in nontraffic accident**

✓x7ᵗʰ **V83.9 Unspecified occupant of special industrial vehicle injured in nontraffic accident**

Special-industrial-vehicle accident NOS

✓4ᵗʰ V84 Occupant of special vehicle mainly used in agriculture injured in transport accident

INCLUDES   self-propelled farm machinery
tractor (and trailer)

EXCLUDES 1   animal-powered farm machinery accident (W30.8-)
contact with combine harvester (W30.0)
special agricultural vehicle in stationary use or maintenance (W30.-)

> The appropriate 7th character is to be added to each code from category V84.
> A   initial encounter
> D   subsequent encounter
> S   sequela

✓x7ᵗʰ **V84.0 Driver of special agricultural vehicle injured in traffic accident**

✓x7ᵗʰ **V84.1 Passenger of special agricultural vehicle injured in traffic accident**

✓x7ᵗʰ **V84.2 Person on outside of special agricultural vehicle injured in traffic accident**

✓x7ᵗʰ **V84.3 Unspecified occupant of special agricultural vehicle injured in traffic accident**

✓x7ᵗʰ **V84.4 Person injured while boarding or alighting from special agricultural vehicle**

✓x7ᵗʰ **V84.5 Driver of special agricultural vehicle injured in nontraffic accident**

✓x7ᵗʰ **V84.6 Passenger of special agricultural vehicle injured in nontraffic accident**

✓x7ᵗʰ **V84.7 Person on outside of special agricultural vehicle injured in nontraffic accident**

✓x7ᵗʰ **V84.9 Unspecified occupant of special agricultural vehicle injured in nontraffic accident**

Special-agricultural vehicle accident NOS

✓4ᵗʰ V85 Occupant of special construction vehicle injured in transport accident

INCLUDES   bulldozer
digger
dump truck
earth-leveller
mechanical shovel
road-roller

EXCLUDES 1   special industrial vehicle (V83.-)
special construction vehicle in stationary use or maintenance (W31.-)

> The appropriate 7th character is to be added to each code from category V85.
> A   initial encounter
> D   subsequent encounter
> S   sequela

✓x7ᵗʰ **V85.0 Driver of special construction vehicle injured in traffic accident**

✓x7ᵗʰ **V85.1 Passenger of special construction vehicle injured in traffic accident**

✓x7ᵗʰ **V85.2 Person on outside of special construction vehicle injured in traffic accident**

✓x7ᵗʰ **V85.3 Unspecified occupant of special construction vehicle injured in traffic accident**

✓x7ᵗʰ **V85.4 Person injured while boarding or alighting from special construction vehicle**

✓x7ᵗʰ **V85.5 Driver of special construction vehicle injured in nontraffic accident**

✓x7ᵗʰ **V85.6 Passenger of special construction vehicle injured in nontraffic accident**

✓x7ᵗʰ **V85.7 Person on outside of special construction vehicle injured in nontraffic accident**

✓x7ᵗʰ **V85.9 Unspecified occupant of special construction vehicle injured in nontraffic accident**

Special-construction-vehicle accident NOS

EXCLUDES 1 Not coded here   EXCLUDES 2 Not included here   N Newborn Age: 0   P Pediatric Age: 0-17   M Maternity Age: 12-55   A Adult Age: 15-124

✓4th **V86** **Occupant of special all-terrain or other off-road motor vehicle, injured in transport accident**

> **EXCLUDES 1**　special all-terrain vehicle in stationary use or maintenance (W31.-)
> sport-utility vehicle (V50-V59)
> three-wheeled motor vehicle designed for on-road use (V30-V39)

> The appropriate 7th character is to be added to each code from category V86.
> A　initial encounter
> D　subsequent encounter
> S　sequela

✓5th **V86.0** **Driver** of special all-terrain or other off-road motor vehicle **injured** in traffic accident

　✓x7th **V86.01**　**Driver of** ambulance **or** fire engine **injured in traffic accident**

　✓x7th **V86.02**　**Driver of** snowmobile **injured in traffic accident**

　✓x7th **V86.03**　**Driver of** dune buggy **injured in traffic accident**

　✓x7th **V86.04**　**Driver of** military vehicle **injured in traffic accident**

　✓x7th **V86.09**　**Driver of** other special all-terrain or other off-road motor vehicle injured in traffic accident
　　Driver of dirt bike injured in traffic accident
　　Driver of go cart injured in traffic accident
　　Driver of golf cart injured in traffic accident

✓5th **V86.1** **Passenger** of special all-terrain or other off-road motor vehicle injured in traffic accident

　✓x7th **V86.11**　**Passenger of** ambulance **or** fire engine **injured in traffic accident**

　✓x7th **V86.12**　**Passenger of** snowmobile **injured in traffic accident**

　✓x7th **V86.13**　**Passenger of** dune buggy **injured in traffic accident**

　✓x7th **V86.14**　**Passenger of** military vehicle **injured in traffic accident**

　✓x7th **V86.19**　**Passenger of other special all-terrain or other off-road motor vehicle injured in traffic accident**
　　Passenger of dirt bike injured in traffic accident
　　Passenger of go cart injured in traffic accident
　　Passenger of golf cart injured in traffic accident

✓5th **V86.2** **Person on outside** of special all-terrain or other off-road motor vehicle injured in traffic accident

　✓x7th **V86.21**　**Person on outside of** ambulance **or** fire engine **injured in traffic accident**

　✓x7th **V86.22**　**Person on outside of** snowmobile **injured in traffic accident**

　✓x7th **V86.23**　**Person on outside of** dune buggy **injured in traffic accident**

　✓x7th **V86.24**　**Person on outside of** military vehicle **injured in traffic accident**

　✓x7th **V86.29**　**Person on outside of other special all-terrain or other off-road motor vehicle injured in traffic accident**
　　Person on outside of dirt bike injured in traffic accident
　　Person on outside of go cart in traffic accident
　　Person on outside of golf cart injured in traffic accident

✓5th **V86.3** **Unspecified occupant** of special all-terrain or other off-road motor vehicle injured in traffic accident

　✓x7th **V86.31**　**Unspecified occupant of** ambulance **or** fire engine **injured in traffic accident**

　✓x7th **V86.32**　**Unspecified occupant of** snowmobile **injured in traffic accident**

　✓x7th **V86.33**　**Unspecified occupant of** dune buggy **injured in traffic accident**

　✓x7th **V86.34**　**Unspecified occupant of** military vehicle **injured in traffic accident**

　✓x7th **V86.39**　**Unspecified occupant of other special all-terrain or other off-road motor vehicle injured in traffic accident**
　　Unspecified occupant of dirt bike injured in traffic accident
　　Unspecified occupant of go cart injured in traffic accident
　　Unspecified occupant of golf cart injured in traffic accident

✓5th **V86.4** **Person injured while** boarding or alighting **from special all-terrain or other off-road motor vehicle**

　✓x7th **V86.41**　**Person injured while boarding or alighting from** ambulance **or** fire engine

　✓x7th **V86.42**　**Person injured while boarding or alighting from** snowmobile

　✓x7th **V86.43**　**Person injured while boarding or alighting from** dune buggy

　✓x7th **V86.44**　**Person injured while boarding or alighting from** military vehicle

　✓x7th **V86.49**　**Person injured while boarding or alighting from other special all-terrain or other off-road motor vehicle**
　　Person injured while boarding or alighting from dirt bike
　　Person injured while boarding or alighting from go cart
　　Person injured while boarding or alighting from golf cart

✓5th **V86.5** **Driver** of special all-terrain or other off-road motor vehicle injured in nontraffic accident

　✓x7th **V86.51**　**Driver of** ambulance **or** fire engine **injured in nontraffic accident**

　✓x7th **V86.52**　**Driver of** snowmobile **injured in nontraffic accident**

　✓x7th **V86.53**　**Driver of** dune buggy **injured in nontraffic accident**

　✓x7th **V86.54**　**Driver of** military vehicle **injured in nontraffic accident**

　✓x7th **V86.59**　**Driver of other special all-terrain or other off-road motor vehicle injured in nontraffic accident**
　　Driver of dirt bike injured in nontraffic accident
　　Driver of go cart injured in nontraffic accident
　　Driver of golf cart injured in nontraffic accident

✓5th **V86.6** **Passenger** of special all-terrain or other off-road motor vehicle injured in nontraffic accident

　✓x7th **V86.61**　**Passenger of** ambulance **or** fire engine **injured in nontraffic accident**

　✓x7th **V86.62**　**Passenger of** snowmobile **injured in nontraffic accident**

　✓x7th **V86.63**　**Passenger of** dune buggy **injured in nontraffic accident**

　✓x7th **V86.64**　**Passenger of** military vehicle **injured in nontraffic accident**

　✓x7th **V86.69**　**Passenger of other special all-terrain or other off-road motor vehicle injured in nontraffic accident**
　　Passenger of dirt bike injured in nontraffic accident
　　Passenger of go cart injured in nontraffic accident
　　Passenger of golf cart injured in nontraffic accident

✓5th **V86.7** **Person on outside** of special all-terrain or other off-road motor vehicle injured in nontraffic accident

　✓x7th **V86.71**　**Person on outside of** ambulance **or** fire engine **injured in nontraffic accident**

　✓x7th **V86.72**　**Person on outside of** snowmobile **injured in nontraffic accident**

　✓x7th **V86.73**　**Person on outside of** dune buggy **injured in nontraffic accident**

　✓x7th **V86.74**　**Person on outside of** military vehicle **injured in nontraffic accident**

　✓x7th **V86.79**　**Person on outside of other special all-terrain or other off-road motor vehicles injured in nontraffic accident**
　　Person on outside of dirt bike injured in nontraffic accident
　　Person on outside of go cart injured in nontraffic accident
　　Person on outside of golf cart injured in nontraffic accident

✓5th **V86.9** **Unspecified occupant** of special all-terrain or other off-road motor vehicle injured in nontraffic accident

　✓x7th **V86.91**　**Unspecified occupant of** ambulance **or** fire engine **injured in nontraffic accident**

　✓x7th **V86.92**　**Unspecified occupant of** snowmobile **injured in nontraffic accident**

　✓x7th **V86.93**　**Unspecified occupant of** dune buggy **injured in nontraffic accident**

　✓x7th **V86.94**　**Unspecified occupant of** military vehicle **injured in nontraffic accident**

✓ Additional Character Required　　✓x7th Xtension Alert　　Unspecified Dx　　Other Specified Dx　　Manifestation　　►◄ Revised Text　　● New Code　　▲ Revised Code Title

√x7th **V86.99 Unspecified occupant of other special all-terrain or other off-road motor vehicle injured in nontraffic accident**
    All-terrain motor-vehicle accident NOS
    Off-road motor-vehicle accident NOS
    Other motor-vehicle accident NOS
    Unspecified occupant of dirt bike injured in nontraffic accident
    Unspecified occupant of go cart injured in nontraffic accident
    Unspecified occupant of golf cart injured in nontraffic accident

√4th **V87 Traffic accident of specified type but victim's mode of transport unknown**

EXCLUDES 1   collision involving:
    pedal cycle (V10-V19)
    pedestrian (V01-V09)

The appropriate 7th character is to be added to each code from category V87.
  A   initial encounter
  D   subsequent encounter
  S   sequela

√x7th **V87.0 Person injured in collision between car and two- or three-wheeled powered vehicle (traffic)**

√x7th **V87.1 Person injured in collision between other motor vehicle and two- or three-wheeled motor vehicle (traffic)**

√x7th **V87.2 Person injured in collision between car and pick-up truck or van (traffic)**

√x7th **V87.3 Person injured in collision between car and bus (traffic)**

√x7th **V87.4 Person injured in collision between car and heavy transport vehicle (traffic)**

√x7th **V87.5 Person injured in collision between heavy transport vehicle and bus (traffic)**

√x7th **V87.6 Person injured in collision between railway train or railway vehicle and car (traffic)**

√x7th **V87.7 Person injured in collision between other specified motor vehicles (traffic)**

√x7th **V87.8 Person injured in other specified noncollision transport accidents involving motor vehicle (traffic)**

√x7th **V87.9 Person injured in other specified (collision)(noncollision) transport accidents involving nonmotor vehicle (traffic)**

√4th **V88 Nontraffic accident of specified type but victim's mode of transport unknown**

EXCLUDES 1   collision involving:
    pedal cycle (V10-V19)
    pedestrian (V01-V09)

The appropriate 7th character is to be added to each code from category V88.
  A   initial encounter
  D   subsequent encounter
  S   sequela

√x7th **V88.0 Person injured in collision between car and two- or three-wheeled motor vehicle, nontraffic**

√x7th **V88.1 Person injured in collision between other motor vehicle and two- or three-wheeled motor vehicle, nontraffic**

√x7th **V88.2 Person injured in collision between car and pick-up truck or van, nontraffic**

√x7th **V88.3 Person injured in collision between car and bus, nontraffic**

√x7th **V88.4 Person injured in collision between car and heavy transport vehicle, nontraffic**

√x7th **V88.5 Person injured in collision between heavy transport vehicle and bus, nontraffic**

√x7th **V88.6 Person injured in collision between railway train or railway vehicle and car, nontraffic**

√x7th **V88.7 Person injured in collision between other specified motor vehicle, nontraffic**

√x7th **V88.8 Person injured in other specified noncollision transport accidents involving motor vehicle, nontraffic**

√x7th **V88.9 Person injured in other specified (collision)(noncollision) transport accidents involving nonmotor vehicle, nontraffic**

√4th **V89 Motor- or nonmotor-vehicle accident, type of vehicle unspecified**

The appropriate 7th character is to be added to each code from category V89.
  A   initial encounter
  D   subsequent encounter
  S   sequela

√x7th **V89.0 Person injured in unspecified motor-vehicle accident, nontraffic**
    Motor-vehicle accident NOS, nontraffic

√x7th **V89.1 Person injured in unspecified nonmotor-vehicle accident, nontraffic**
    Nonmotor-vehicle accident NOS (nontraffic)

√x7th **V89.2 Person injured in unspecified motor-vehicle accident, traffic**
    Motor-vehicle accident [MVA] NOS
    Road (traffic) accident [RTA] NOS

√x7th **V89.3 Person injured in unspecified nonmotor-vehicle accident, traffic**
    Nonmotor-vehicle traffic accident NOS

√x7th **V89.9 Person injured in unspecified vehicle accident**
    Collision NOS

Water transport accidents (V90-V94)

√4th **V90 Drowning and submersion due to accident to watercraft**

EXCLUDES 1   civilian water transport accident involving military watercraft (V94.81-)
    fall into water not from watercraft (W16.-)
    military watercraft accident in military or war operations (Y36.0-, Y37.0-)
    water-transport-related drowning or submersion without accident to watercraft (V92.-)

The appropriate 7th character is to be added to each code from category V90.
  A   initial encounter
  D   subsequent encounter
  S   sequela

√5th **V90.0 Drowning and submersion due to watercraft overturning**

√x7th **V90.00 Drowning and submersion due to merchant ship overturning**

√x7th **V90.01 Drowning and submersion due to passenger ship overturning**
    Drowning and submersion due to Ferry-boat overturning
    Drowning and submersion due to Liner overturning

√x7th **V90.02 Drowning and submersion due to fishing boat overturning**

√x7th **V90.03 Drowning and submersion due to other powered watercraft overturning**
    Drowning and submersion due to Hovercraft (on open water) overturning
    Drowning and submersion due to Jet ski overturning

√x7th **V90.04 Drowning and submersion due to sailboat overturning**

√x7th **V90.05 Drowning and submersion due to canoe or kayak overturning**

√x7th **V90.06 Drowning and submersion due to (nonpowered) inflatable craft overturning**

√x7th **V90.08 Drowning and submersion due to other unpowered watercraft overturning**
    Drowning and submersion due to windsurfer overturning

√x7th **V90.09 Drowning and submersion due to unspecified watercraft overturning**
    Drowning and submersion due to boat NOS overturning
    Drowning and submersion due to ship NOS overturning
    Drowning and submersion due to watercraft NOS overturning

√5th **V90.1 Drowning and submersion due to watercraft sinking**

√x7th **V90.10 Drowning and submersion due to merchant ship sinking**

√x7th **V90.11 Drowning and submersion due to passenger ship sinking**
    Drowning and submersion due to Ferry-boat sinking
    Drowning and submersion due to Liner sinking

√x7th **V90.12 Drowning and submersion due to fishing boat sinking**

EXCLUDES 1 Not coded here   EXCLUDES 2 Not included here   N Newborn Age: 0   P Pediatric Age: 0-17   M Maternity Age: 12-55   A Adult Age: 15-124

1016   ICD-10-CM Draft (2015)

✓x7ᵗʰ **V90.13** **Drowning and submersion due to other** powered **watercraft sinking**
- Drowning and submersion due to Hovercraft (on open water) sinking
- Drowning and submersion due to Jet ski sinking

✓x7ᵗʰ **V90.14** **Drowning and submersion due to** sailboat **sinking**

✓x7ᵗʰ **V90.15** **Drowning and submersion due to** canoe or kayak **sinking**

✓x7ᵗʰ **V90.16** **Drowning and submersion due to (nonpowered)** inflatable craft **sinking**

✓x7ᵗʰ **V90.18** **Drowning and submersion due to other** unpowered **watercraft sinking**

✓x7ᵗʰ **V90.19** **Drowning and submersion due to unspecified watercraft sinking**
- Drowning and submersion due to boat NOS sinking
- Drowning and submersion due to ship NOS sinking
- Drowning and submersion due to watercraft NOS sinking

✓5ᵗʰ **V90.2** **Drowning and submersion due to** falling or jumping from burning **watercraft**

✓x7ᵗʰ **V90.20** **Drowning and submersion due to falling or jumping from burning** merchant ship

✓x7ᵗʰ **V90.21** **Drowning and submersion due to falling or jumping from burning** passenger ship
- Drowning and submersion due to falling or jumping from burning Ferry-boat
- Drowning and submersion due to falling or jumping from burning Liner

✓x7ᵗʰ **V90.22** **Drowning and submersion due to falling or jumping from burning** fishing boat

✓x7ᵗʰ **V90.23** **Drowning and submersion due to falling or jumping from other burning** powered **watercraft**
- Drowning and submersion due to falling and jumping from burning Hovercraft (on open water)
- Drowning and submersion due to falling and jumping from burning Jet ski

✓x7ᵗʰ **V90.24** **Drowning and submersion due to falling or jumping from burning** sailboat

✓x7ᵗʰ **V90.25** **Drowning and submersion due to falling or jumping from burning** canoe or kayak

✓x7ᵗʰ **V90.26** **Drowning and submersion due to falling or jumping from burning (nonpowered)** inflatable craft

✓x7ᵗʰ **V90.27** **Drowning and submersion due to falling or jumping from burning** water-skis

✓x7ᵗʰ **V90.28** **Drowning and submersion due to falling or jumping from other burning** unpowered **watercraft**
- Drowning and submersion due to falling and jumping from burning surf-board
- Drowning and submersion due to falling and jumping from burning windsurfer

✓x7ᵗʰ **V90.29** **Drowning and submersion due to falling or jumping from unspecified burning watercraft**
- Drowning and submersion due to falling or jumping from burning boat NOS
- Drowning and submersion due to falling or jumping from burning ship NOS
- Drowning and submersion due to falling or jumping from burning watercraft NOS

✓5ᵗʰ **V90.3** **Drowning and submersion due to** falling or jumping from crushed watercraft

✓x7ᵗʰ **V90.30** **Drowning and submersion due to falling or jumping from crushed** merchant ship

✓x7ᵗʰ **V90.31** **Drowning and submersion due to falling or jumping from crushed** passenger ship
- Drowning and submersion due to falling and jumping from crushed Ferry boat
- Drowning and submersion due to falling and jumping from crushed Liner

✓x7ᵗʰ **V90.32** **Drowning and submersion due to falling or jumping from crushed** fishing boat

✓x7ᵗʰ **V90.33** **Drowning and submersion due to falling or jumping from other crushed** powered **watercraft**
- Drowning and submersion due to falling and jumping from crushed Hovercraft
- Drowning and submersion due to falling and jumping from crushed Jet ski

✓x7ᵗʰ **V90.34** **Drowning and submersion due to falling or jumping from crushed** sailboat

✓x7ᵗʰ **V90.35** **Drowning and submersion due to falling or jumping from crushed** canoe or kayak

✓x7ᵗʰ **V90.36** **Drowning and submersion due to falling or jumping from crushed (nonpowered)** inflatable craft

✓x7ᵗʰ **V90.37** **Drowning and submersion due to falling or jumping from crushed** water-skis

✓x7ᵗʰ **V90.38** **Drowning and submersion due to falling or jumping from other crushed** unpowered **watercraft**
- Drowning and submersion due to falling and jumping from crushed surf-board
- Drowning and submersion due to falling and jumping from crushed windsurfer

✓x7ᵗʰ **V90.39** **Drowning and submersion due to falling or jumping from crushed unspecified watercraft**
- Drowning and submersion due to falling and jumping from crushed boat NOS
- Drowning and submersion due to falling and jumping from crushed ship NOS
- Drowning and submersion due to falling and jumping from crushed watercraft NOS

✓5ᵗʰ **V90.8** **Drowning and submersion due to** other accident to watercraft

✓x7ᵗʰ **V90.80** **Drowning and submersion due to other accident to** merchant ship

✓x7ᵗʰ **V90.81** **Drowning and submersion due to other accident to** passenger ship
- Drowning and submersion due to other accident to Ferry-boat
- Drowning and submersion due to other accident to Liner

✓x7ᵗʰ **V90.82** **Drowning and submersion due to other accident to** fishing boat

✓x7ᵗʰ **V90.83** **Drowning and submersion due to other accident to other** powered **watercraft**
- Drowning and submersion due to other accident to Hovercraft (on open water)
- Drowning and submersion due to other accident to Jet ski

✓x7ᵗʰ **V90.84** **Drowning and submersion due to other accident to** sailboat

✓x7ᵗʰ **V90.85** **Drowning and submersion due to other accident to** canoe or kayak

✓x7ᵗʰ **V90.86** **Drowning and submersion due to other accident to (nonpowered)** inflatable craft

✓x7ᵗʰ **V90.87** **Drowning and submersion due to other accident to** water-skis

✓x7ᵗʰ **V90.88** **Drowning and submersion due to other accident to other** unpowered **watercraft**
- Drowning and submersion due to other accident to surf-board
- Drowning and submersion due to other accident to windsurfer

✓x7ᵗʰ **V90.89** **Drowning and submersion due to other accident to unspecified watercraft**
- Drowning and submersion due to other accident to boat NOS
- Drowning and submersion due to other accident to ship NOS
- Drowning and submersion due to other accident to watercraft NOS

✓4ᵗʰ **V91** **Other injury due to accident to watercraft**

INCLUDES   any injury except drowning and submersion as a result of an accident to watercraft

EXCLUDES 1   *civilian water transport accident involving military watercraft (V94.81-)*
military watercraft accident in military or war operations (Y36, Y37.-)

EXCLUDES 2   *drowning and submersion due to accident to watercraft (V90.-)*

The appropriate 7th character is to be added to each code from category V91.
A	initial encounter
D	subsequent encounter
S	sequela

✓5ᵗʰ **V91.0** **Burn due to watercraft on fire**

EXCLUDES 1   *burn from localized fire or explosion on board ship without accident to watercraft (V93.-)*

✓x7ᵗʰ **V91.00** **Burn due to** merchant ship **on fire**

✓ Additional Character Required   ✓x7ᵗʰ Xtension Alert   Unspecified Dx   Other Specified Dx   Manifestation   ►◄ Revised Text   ● New Code   ▲ Revised Code Title

ICD-10-CM Draft (2015)   **1017**

√x7ᵗʰ **V91.01**   **Burn due to passenger ship on fire**
     Burn due to Ferry-boat on fire
     Burn due to Liner on fire

√x7ᵗʰ **V91.02**   **Burn due to fishing boat on fire**

√x7ᵗʰ **V91.03**   **Burn due to other powered watercraft on fire**
     Burn due to Hovercraft (on open water) on fire
     Burn due to Jet ski on fire

√x7ᵗʰ **V91.04**   **Burn due to sailboat on fire**

√x7ᵗʰ **V91.05**   **Burn due to canoe or kayak on fire**

√x7ᵗʰ **V91.06**   **Burn due to (nonpowered) inflatable craft on fire**

√x7ᵗʰ **V91.07**   **Burn due to water-skis on fire**

√x7ᵗʰ **V91.08**   **Burn due to other unpowered watercraft on fire**

√x7ᵗʰ **V91.09**   **Burn due to unspecified watercraft on fire**
     Burn due to boat NOS on fire
     Burn due to ship NOS on fire
     Burn due to watercraft NOS on fire

√5ᵗʰ **V91.1**   **Crushed between watercraft and other watercraft or other object due to collision**
     Crushed by lifeboat after abandoning ship in a collision
     NOTE   Select the specified type of watercraft that the victim was on at the time of the collision

√x7ᵗʰ **V91.10**   **Crushed between merchant ship and other watercraft or other object due to collision**

√x7ᵗʰ **V91.11**   **Crushed between passenger ship and other watercraft or other object due to collision**
     Crushed between Ferry-boat and other watercraft or other object due to collision
     Crushed between Liner and other watercraft or other object due to collision

√x7ᵗʰ **V91.12**   **Crushed between fishing boat and other watercraft or other object due to collision**

√x7ᵗʰ **V91.13**   **Crushed between other powered watercraft and other watercraft or other object due to collision**
     Crushed between Hovercraft (on open water) and other watercraft or other object due to collision
     Crushed between Jet ski and other watercraft or other object due to collision

√x7ᵗʰ **V91.14**   **Crushed between sailboat and other watercraft or other object due to collision**

√x7ᵗʰ **V91.15**   **Crushed between canoe or kayak and other watercraft or other object due to collision**

√x7ᵗʰ **V91.16**   **Crushed between (nonpowered) inflatable craft and other watercraft or other object due to collision**

√x7ᵗʰ **V91.18**   **Crushed between other unpowered watercraft and other watercraft or other object due to collision**
     Crushed between surfboard and other watercraft or other object due to collision
     Crushed between windsurfer and other watercraft or other object due to collision

√x7ᵗʰ **V91.19**   **Crushed between unspecified watercraft and other watercraft or other object due to collision**
     Crushed between boat NOS and other watercraft or other object due to collision
     Crushed between ship NOS and other watercraft or other object due to collision
     Crushed between watercraft NOS and other watercraft or other object due to collision

√5ᵗʰ **V91.2**   **Fall due to collision between watercraft and other watercraft or other object**
     Fall while remaining on watercraft after collision
     NOTE   Select the specified type of watercraft that the victim was on at the time of the collision.
     EXCLUDES 1   crushed between watercraft and other watercraft and other object due to collision (V91.1-)
         drowning and submersion due to falling from crushed watercraft (V90.3-)

√x7ᵗʰ **V91.20**   **Fall due to collision between merchant ship and other watercraft or other object**

√x7ᵗʰ **V91.21**   **Fall due to collision between passenger ship and other watercraft or other object**
     Fall due to collision between Ferry-boat and other watercraft or other object
     Fall due to collision between Liner and other watercraft or other object

√x7ᵗʰ **V91.22**   **Fall due to collision between fishing boat and other watercraft or other object**

√x7ᵗʰ **V91.23**   **Fall due to collision between other powered watercraft and other watercraft or other object**
     Fall due to collision between Hovercraft (on open water) and other watercraft or other object
     Fall due to collision between Jet ski and other watercraft or other object

√x7ᵗʰ **V91.24**   **Fall due to collision between sailboat and other watercraft or other object**

√x7ᵗʰ **V91.25**   **Fall due to collision between canoe or kayak and other watercraft or other object**

√x7ᵗʰ **V91.26**   **Fall due to collision between (nonpowered) inflatable craft and other watercraft or other object**

√x7ᵗʰ **V91.29**   **Fall due to collision between unspecified watercraft and other watercraft or other object**
     Fall due to collision between boat NOS and other watercraft or other object
     Fall due to collision between ship NOS and other watercraft or other object
     Fall due to collision between watercraft NOS and other watercraft or other object

√5ᵗʰ **V91.3**   **Hit or struck by falling object due to accident to watercraft**
     Hit or struck by falling object (part of damaged watercraft or other object) after falling or jumping from damaged watercraft
     EXCLUDES 2   drowning or submersion due to fall or jumping from damaged watercraft (V90.2-, V90.3-)

√x7ᵗʰ **V91.30**   **Hit or struck by falling object due to accident to merchant ship**

√x7ᵗʰ **V91.31**   **Hit or struck by falling object due to accident to passenger ship**
     Hit or struck by falling object due to accident to Ferry-boat
     Hit or struck by falling object due to accident to Liner

√x7ᵗʰ **V91.32**   **Hit or struck by falling object due to accident to fishing boat**

√x7ᵗʰ **V91.33**   **Hit or struck by falling object due to accident to other powered watercraft**
     Hit or struck by falling object due to accident to Hovercraft (on open water)
     Hit or struck by falling object due to accident to Jet ski

√x7ᵗʰ **V91.34**   **Hit or struck by falling object due to accident to sailboat**

√x7ᵗʰ **V91.35**   **Hit or struck by falling object due to accident to canoe or kayak**

√x7ᵗʰ **V91.36**   **Hit or struck by falling object due to accident to (nonpowered) inflatable craft**

√x7ᵗʰ **V91.37**   **Hit or struck by falling object due to accident to water-skis**
     Hit by water-skis after jumping off of waterskis

√x7ᵗʰ **V91.38**   **Hit or struck by falling object due to accident to other unpowered watercraft**
     Hit or struck by surf-board after falling off damaged surf-board
     Hit or struck by object after falling off damaged windsurfer

√x7ᵗʰ **V91.39**   **Hit or struck by falling object due to accident to unspecified watercraft**
     Hit or struck by falling object due to accident to boat NOS
     Hit or struck by falling object due to accident to ship NOS
     Hit or struck by falling object due to accident to watercraft NOS

√5ᵗʰ **V91.8**   **Other injury due to other accident to watercraft**

√x7ᵗʰ **V91.80**   **Other injury due to other accident to merchant ship**

√x7ᵗʰ **V91.81**   **Other injury due to other accident to passenger ship**
     Other injury due to other accident to Ferry-boat
     Other injury due to other accident to Liner

√x7ᵗʰ **V91.82**   **Other injury due to other accident to fishing boat**

√x7ᵗʰ **V91.83**   **Other injury due to other accident to other powered watercraft**
     Other injury due to other accident to Hovercraft (on open water)
     Other injury due to other accident to Jet ski

√x7ᵗʰ **V91.84**   **Other injury due to other accident to sailboat**

√x7ᵗʰ **V91.85**   **Other injury due to other accident to canoe or kayak**

√x7ᵗʰ **V91.86**   **Other injury due to other accident to (nonpowered) inflatable craft**

EXCLUDES 1 Not coded here   **EXCLUDES 2** Not included here   **N** Newborn Age: 0   **P** Pediatric Age: 0-17   **M** Maternity Age: 12-55   **A** Adult Age: 15-124

1018   ICD-10-CM Draft (2015)

✓x7th **V91.87 Other injury due to other accident to** water-skis

✓x7th **V91.88 Other injury due to other accident to other** unpowered **watercraft**
> Other injury due to other accident to surf-board
> Other injury due to other accident to windsurfer

✓x7th **V91.89 Other injury due to other accident to unspecified watercraft**
> Other injury due to other accident to boat NOS
> Other injury due to other accident to ship NOS
> Other injury due to other accident to watercraft NOS

✓4th **V92 Drowning and submersion due to accident on board watercraft, without accident to watercraft**
> EXCLUDES 1   civilian water transport accident involving military watercraft (V94.81-)
> drowning or submersion due to accident to watercraft (V90-V91)
> drowning or submersion of diver who voluntarily jumps from boat not involved in an accident (W16.711, W16.721)
> fall into water without watercraft (W16.-)
> military watercraft accident in military or war operations (Y36, Y37)

> The appropriate 7th character is to be added to each code from category V92.
> A   initial encounter
> D   subsequent encounter
> S   sequela

✓5th **V92.0 Drowning and submersion due to** fall off **watercraft**
> Drowning and submersion due to fall from gangplank of watercraft
> Drowning and submersion due to fall overboard watercraft
> EXCLUDES 2   hitting head on object or bottom of body of water due to fall from watercraft (V94.0-)

✓x7th **V92.00 Drowning and submersion due to fall off** merchant ship

✓x7th **V92.01 Drowning and submersion due to fall off** passenger ship
> Drowning and submersion due to fall off Ferry-boat
> Drowning and submersion due to fall off Liner

✓x7th **V92.02 Drowning and submersion due to fall off** fishing boat

✓x7th **V92.03 Drowning and submersion due to fall off other** powered **watercraft**
> Drowning and submersion due to fall off Hovercraft (on open water)
> Drowning and submersion due to fall off Jet ski

✓x7th **V92.04 Drowning and submersion due to fall off** sailboat

✓x7th **V92.05 Drowning and submersion due to fall off** canoe or kayak

✓x7th **V92.06 Drowning and submersion due to fall off** (nonpowered) inflatable craft

✓x7th **V92.07 Drowning and submersion due to fall off** water-skis
> EXCLUDES 1   drowning and submersion due to falling off burning water-skis (V90.27)
> drowning and submersion due to falling off crushed water-skis (V90.37)
> hit by boat while water-skiing NOS (V94.X)

✓x7th **V92.08 Drowning and submersion due to fall off other** unpowered **watercraft**
> Drowning and submersion due to fall off surf-board
> Drowning and submersion due to fall off windsurfer
> EXCLUDES 1   drowning and submersion due to fall off burning unpowered watercraft (V90.28)
> drowning and submersion due to fall off crushed unpowered watercraft (V90.38)
> drowning and submersion due to fall off damaged unpowered watercraft (V90.88)
> drowning and submersion due to rider of nonpowered watercraft being hit by other watercraft (V94.-)
> other injury due to rider of nonpowered watercraft being hit by other watercraft (V94.-)

✓x7th **V92.09 Drowning and submersion due to fall off unspecified watercraft**
> Drowning and submersion due to fall off boat NOS
> Drowning and submersion due to fall off ship
> Drowning and submersion due to fall off watercraft NOS

✓5th **V92.1 Drowning and submersion due to being** thrown overboard **by motion of watercraft**
> EXCLUDES 1   drowning and submersion due to fall off surf-board (V92.08)
> drowning and submersion due to fall off water-skis (V92.07)
> drowning and submersion due to fall off windsurfer (V92.08)

✓x7th **V92.10 Drowning and submersion due to being thrown overboard by motion of** merchant ship

✓x7th **V92.11 Drowning and submersion due to being thrown overboard by motion of** passenger ship
> Drowning and submersion due to being thrown overboard by motion of Ferry-boat
> Drowning and submersion due to being thrown overboard by motion of Liner

✓x7th **V92.12 Drowning and submersion due to being thrown overboard by motion of** fishing boat

✓x7th **V92.13 Drowning and submersion due to being thrown overboard by motion of other** powered **watercraft**
> Drowning and submersion due to being thrown overboard by motion of Hovercraft

✓x7th **V92.14 Drowning and submersion due to being thrown overboard by motion of** sailboat

✓x7th **V92.15 Drowning and submersion due to being thrown overboard by motion of** canoe or kayak

✓x7th **V92.16 Drowning and submersion due to being thrown overboard by motion of** (nonpowered) inflatable craft

✓x7th **V92.19 Drowning and submersion due to being thrown overboard by motion of unspecified watercraft**
> Drowning and submersion due to being thrown overboard by motion of boat NOS
> Drowning and submersion due to being thrown overboard by motion of ship NOS
> Drowning and submersion due to being thrown overboard by motion of watercraft NOS

✓5th **V92.2 Drowning and submersion due to being** washed overboard **from watercraft**
> Code first any associated cataclysm (X37.0-)

✓x7th **V92.20 Drowning and submersion due to being washed overboard from** merchant ship

✓x7th **V92.21 Drowning and submersion due to being washed overboard from** passenger ship
> Drowning and submersion due to being washed overboard from Ferry-boat
> Drowning and submersion due to being washed overboard from Liner

✓x7th **V92.22 Drowning and submersion due to being washed overboard from** fishing boat

✓x7th **V92.23 Drowning and submersion due to being washed overboard from other** powered **watercraft**
> Drowning and submersion due to being washed overboard from Hovercraft (on open water)
> Drowning and submersion due to being washed overboard from Jet ski

✓x7th **V92.24 Drowning and submersion due to being washed overboard from** sailboat

✓x7th **V92.25 Drowning and submersion due to being washed overboard from** canoe or kayak

✓x7th **V92.26 Drowning and submersion due to being washed overboard from** (nonpowered) inflatable craft

✓x7th **V92.27 Drowning and submersion due to being washed overboard from** water-skis
> EXCLUDES 1   drowning and submersion due to fall off water-skis (V92.07)

✓x7th **V92.28 Drowning and submersion due to being washed overboard from other** unpowered **watercraft**
> Drowning and submersion due to being washed overboard from surf-board
> Drowning and submersion due to being washed overboard from windsurfer

✓x7th **V92.29 Drowning and submersion due to being washed overboard from unspecified watercraft**
> Drowning and submersion due to being washed overboard from boat NOS
> Drowning and submersion due to being washed overboard from ship NOS
> Drowning and submersion due to being washed overboard from watercraft NOS

External Causes of Morbidity

V91.87–V92.29

External Causes of Morbidity

V93–V93.84

✓4ᵗʰ **V93** **Other injury due to accident on board watercraft, without accident to watercraft**

> EXCLUDES 1   civilian water transport accident involving military watercraft (V94.81-)
> other injury due to accident to watercraft (V91.-)
> military watercraft accident in military or war operations (Y36, Y37.-)
>
> EXCLUDES 2   drowning and submersion due to accident on board watercraft, without accident to watercraft (V92.-)

> The appropriate 7th character is to be added to each code from category V93.
> A   initial encounter
> D   subsequent encounter
> S   sequela

✓5ᵗʰ **V93.0** **Burn due to localized fire on board watercraft**

> EXCLUDES 1   burn due to watercraft on fire (V91.0-)

✓x7ᵗʰ **V93.00** **Burn due to localized fire on board merchant vessel**

✓x7ᵗʰ **V93.01** **Burn due to localized fire on board passenger vessel**
Burn due to localized fire on board Ferry-boat
Burn due to localized fire on board Liner

✓x7ᵗʰ **V93.02** **Burn due to localized fire on board fishing boat**

✓x7ᵗʰ **V93.03** **Burn due to localized fire on board other powered watercraft**
Burn due to localized fire on board Hovercraft
Burn due to localized fire on board Jet ski

✓x7ᵗʰ **V93.04** **Burn due to localized fire on board sailboat**

✓x7ᵗʰ **V93.09** **Burn due to localized fire on board unspecified watercraft**
Burn due to localized fire on board boat NOS
Burn due to localized fire on board ship NOS
Burn due to localized fire on board watercraft NOS

✓5ᵗʰ **V93.1** **Other burn on board watercraft**
Burn due to source other than fire on board watercraft

> EXCLUDES 1   burn due to watercraft on fire (V91.0-)

✓x7ᵗʰ **V93.10** **Other burn on board merchant vessel**

✓x7ᵗʰ **V93.11** **Other burn on board passenger vessel**
Other burn on board Ferry-boat
Other burn on board Liner

✓x7ᵗʰ **V93.12** **Other burn on board fishing boat**

✓x7ᵗʰ **V93.13** **Other burn on board other powered watercraft**
Other burn on board Hovercraft
Other burn on board Jet ski

✓x7ᵗʰ **V93.14** **Other burn on board sailboat**

✓x7ᵗʰ **V93.19** **Other burn on board unspecified watercraft**
Other burn on board boat NOS
Other burn on board ship NOS
Other burn on board watercraft NOS

✓5ᵗʰ **V93.2** **Heat exposure on board watercraft**

> EXCLUDES 1   exposure to man-made heat not aboard watercraft (W92)
> exposure to natural heat while on board watercraft (X30)
> exposure to sunlight while on board watercraft (X32)
>
> EXCLUDES 2   burn due to fire on board watercraft (V93.0-)

✓x7ᵗʰ **V93.20** **Heat exposure on board merchant ship**

✓x7ᵗʰ **V93.21** **Heat exposure on board passenger ship**
Heat exposure on board Ferry-boat
Heat exposure on board Liner

✓x7ᵗʰ **V93.22** **Heat exposure on board fishing boat**

✓x7ᵗʰ **V93.23** **Heat exposure on board other powered watercraft**
Heat exposure on board hovercraft

✓x7ᵗʰ **V93.24** **Heat exposure on board sailboat**

✓x7ᵗʰ **V93.29** **Heat exposure on board unspecified watercraft**
Heat exposure on board boat NOS
Heat exposure on board ship NOS
Heat exposure on board watercraft NOS

✓5ᵗʰ **V93.3** **Fall on board watercraft**

> EXCLUDES 1   fall due to collision of watercraft (V91.2-)

✓x7ᵗʰ **V93.30** **Fall on board merchant ship**

✓x7ᵗʰ **V93.31** **Fall on board passenger ship**
Fall on board Ferry-boat
Fall on board Liner

✓x7ᵗʰ **V93.32** **Fall on board fishing boat**

✓x7ᵗʰ **V93.33** **Fall on board other powered watercraft**
Fall on board Hovercraft (on open water)
Fall on board Jet ski

✓x7ᵗʰ **V93.34** **Fall on board sailboat**

✓x7ᵗʰ **V93.35** **Fall on board canoe or kayak**

✓x7ᵗʰ **V93.36** **Fall on board (nonpowered) inflatable craft**

✓x7ᵗʰ **V93.38** **Fall on board other unpowered watercraft**

✓x7ᵗʰ **V93.39** **Fall on board unspecified watercraft**
Fall on board boat NOS
Fall on board ship NOS
Fall on board watercraft NOS

✓5ᵗʰ **V93.4** **Struck by falling object on board watercraft**
Hit by falling object on board watercraft

> EXCLUDES 1   struck by falling object due to accident to watercraft (V91.3)

✓x7ᵗʰ **V93.40** **Struck by falling object on merchant ship**

✓x7ᵗʰ **V93.41** **Struck by falling object on passenger ship**
Struck by falling object on Ferry-boat
Struck by falling object on Liner

✓x7ᵗʰ **V93.42** **Struck by falling object on fishing boat**

✓x7ᵗʰ **V93.43** **Struck by falling object on other powered watercraft**
Struck by falling object on Hovercraft

✓x7ᵗʰ **V93.44** **Struck by falling object on sailboat**

✓x7ᵗʰ **V93.48** **Struck by falling object on other unpowered watercraft**

✓x7ᵗʰ **V93.49** **Struck by falling object on unspecified watercraft**

✓5ᵗʰ **V93.5** **Explosion on board watercraft**
Boiler explosion on steamship

> EXCLUDES 2   fire on board watercraft (V93.0-)

✓x7ᵗʰ **V93.50** **Explosion on board merchant ship**

✓x7ᵗʰ **V93.51** **Explosion on board passenger ship**
Explosion on board Ferry-boat
Explosion on board Liner

✓x7ᵗʰ **V93.52** **Explosion on board fishing boat**

✓x7ᵗʰ **V93.53** **Explosion on board other powered watercraft**
Explosion on board Hovercraft
Explosion on board Jet ski

✓x7ᵗʰ **V93.54** **Explosion on board sailboat**

✓x7ᵗʰ **V93.59** **Explosion on board unspecified watercraft**
Explosion on board boat NOS
Explosion on board ship NOS
Explosion on board watercraft NOS

✓5ᵗʰ **V93.6** **Machinery accident on board watercraft**

> EXCLUDES 1   machinery explosion on board watercraft (V93.4-)
> machinery fire on board watercraft (V93.0-)

✓x7ᵗʰ **V93.60** **Machinery accident on board merchant ship**

✓x7ᵗʰ **V93.61** **Machinery accident on board passenger ship**
Machinery accident on board Ferry-boat
Machinery accident on board Liner

✓x7ᵗʰ **V93.62** **Machinery accident on board fishing boat**

✓x7ᵗʰ **V93.63** **Machinery accident on board other powered watercraft**
Machinery accident on board Hovercraft

✓x7ᵗʰ **V93.64** **Machinery accident on board sailboat**

✓x7ᵗʰ **V93.69** **Machinery accident on board unspecified watercraft**
Machinery accident on board boat NOS
Machinery accident on board ship NOS
Machinery accident on board watercraft NOS

✓5ᵗʰ **V93.8** **Other injury due to other accident on board watercraft**
Accidental poisoning by gases or fumes on watercraft

✓x7ᵗʰ **V93.80** **Other injury due to other accident on board merchant ship**

✓x7ᵗʰ **V93.81** **Other injury due to other accident on board passenger ship**
Other injury due to other accident on board Ferry-boat
Other injury due to other accident on board Liner

✓x7ᵗʰ **V93.82** **Other injury due to other accident on board fishing boat**

✓x7ᵗʰ **V93.83** **Other injury due to other accident on board other powered watercraft**
Other injury due to other accident on board Hovercraft
Other injury due to other accident on board Jet ski

✓x7ᵗʰ **V93.84** **Other injury due to other accident on board sailboat**

EXCLUDES 1 Not coded here   EXCLUDES 2 Not included here   N Newborn Age: 0   P Pediatric Age: 0–17   M Maternity Age: 12–55   A Adult Age: 15–124

1020   ICD-10-CM Draft (2015)

✓x7ᵗʰ V93.85 Other injury due to other accident on board canoe or kayak

✓x7ᵗʰ V93.86 Other injury due to other accident on board (nonpowered) inflatable craft

✓x7ᵗʰ V93.87 Other injury due to other accident on board water-skis
Hit or struck by object while waterskiing

✓x7ᵗʰ V93.88 Other injury due to other accident on board other unpowered **watercraft**
Hit or struck by object while surfing
Hit or struck by object while on board windsurfer

✓x7ᵗʰ V93.89 Other injury due to other accident on board unspecified watercraft
Other injury due to other accident on board boat NOS
Other injury due to other accident on board ship NOS
Other injury due to other accident on board watercraft NOS

✓4ᵗʰ V94 Other and unspecified water transport accidents

EXCLUDES 1 military watercraft accidents in military or war operations (Y36, Y37)

The appropriate 7th character is to be added to each code from category V94.
A   initial encounter
D   subsequent encounter
S   sequela

✓x7ᵗʰ V94.0 Hitting object or bottom of body of water due to fall from watercraft

EXCLUDES 2 drowning and submersion due to fall from watercraft (V92.0-)

✓5ᵗʰ V94.1 Bather struck by watercraft
Swimmer hit by watercraft

✓x7ᵗʰ V94.11 Bather struck by powered **watercraft**

✓x7ᵗʰ V94.12 Bather struck by nonpowered **watercraft**

✓5ᵗʰ V94.2 Rider of nonpowered watercraft struck by other watercraft

✓x7ᵗʰ V94.21 Rider of nonpowered watercraft struck by other nonpowered **watercraft**
Canoer hit by other nonpowered watercraft
Surfer hit by other nonpowered watercraft
Windsurfer hit by other nonpowered watercraft

✓x7ᵗʰ V94.22 Rider of nonpowered watercraft struck by powered **watercraft**
Canoer hit by motorboat
Surfer hit by motorboat
Windsurfer hit by motorboat

✓5ᵗʰ V94.3 Injury to rider of (inflatable) watercraft being pulled behind other watercraft

✓x7ᵗʰ V94.31 Injury to rider of (inflatable) recreational **watercraft being pulled behind other watercraft**
Injury to rider of inner-tube pulled behind motor boat

✓x7ᵗʰ V94.32 Injury to rider of non-recreational **watercraft being pulled behind other watercraft**
Injury to occupant of dingy being pulled behind boat or ship
Injury to occupant of life-raft being pulled behind boat or ship

✓x7ᵗʰ V94.4 Injury to barefoot water-skier
Injury to person being pulled behind boat or ship

✓5ᵗʰ V94.8 Other water transport accident

✓6ᵗʰ V94.81 Water transport accident involving military watercraft

✓7ᵗʰ V94.810 Civilian watercraft involved in water transport accident with military watercraft
Passenger on civilian watercraft injured due to accident with military watercraft

✓7ᵗʰ V94.811 Civilian in water injured by military watercraft

✓7ᵗʰ V94.818 Other water transport accident involving military watercraft

✓x7ᵗʰ V94.89 Other water transport accident

✓x7ᵗʰ V94.9 Unspecified water transport accident
Water transport accident NOS

Air and space transport accidents (V95-V97)

EXCLUDES 1 military aircraft accidents in military or war operations (Y36, Y37)

✓4ᵗʰ V95 Accident to powered aircraft causing injury to occupant

The appropriate 7th character is to be added to each code from category V95.
A   initial encounter
D   subsequent encounter
S   sequela

✓5ᵗʰ V95.0 Helicopter accident injuring occupant

✓x7ᵗʰ V95.00 Unspecified helicopter accident injuring occupant

✓x7ᵗʰ V95.01 Helicopter crash **injuring occupant**

✓x7ᵗʰ V95.02 Forced landing of helicopter injuring occupant

✓x7ᵗʰ V95.03 Helicopter collision **injuring occupant**
Helicopter collision with any object, fixed, movable or moving

✓x7ᵗʰ V95.04 Helicopter fire **injuring occupant**

✓x7ᵗʰ V95.05 Helicopter explosion **injuring occupant**

✓x7ᵗʰ V95.09 Other helicopter accident injuring occupant

✓5ᵗʰ V95.1 Ultralight, microlight or powered-glider accident injuring occupant

✓x7ᵗʰ V95.10 Unspecified ultralight, microlight or powered-glider accident injuring occupant

✓x7ᵗʰ V95.11 Ultralight, microlight or powered-glider crash **injuring occupant**

✓x7ᵗʰ V95.12 Forced landing of ultralight, microlight or powered-glider injuring occupant

✓x7ᵗʰ V95.13 Ultralight, microlight or powered-glider collision **injuring occupant**
Ultralight, microlight or powered-glider collision with any object, fixed, movable or moving

✓x7ᵗʰ V95.14 Ultralight, microlight or powered-glider fire **injuring occupant**

✓x7ᵗʰ V95.15 Ultralight, microlight or powered-glider explosion **injuring occupant**

✓x7ᵗʰ V95.19 Other ultralight, microlight or powered-glider accident injuring occupant

✓5ᵗʰ V95.2 Other private fixed-wing aircraft accident injuring occupant

✓x7ᵗʰ V95.20 Unspecified accident to other private fixed-wing aircraft, injuring occupant

✓x7ᵗʰ V95.21 Other private fixed-wing aircraft crash injuring occupant

✓x7ᵗʰ V95.22 Forced landing of other private fixed-wing aircraft injuring occupant

✓x7ᵗʰ V95.23 Other private fixed-wing aircraft collision **injuring occupant**
Other private fixed-wing aircraft collision with any object, fixed, movable or moving

✓x7ᵗʰ V95.24 Other private fixed-wing aircraft fire **injuring occupant**

✓x7ᵗʰ V95.25 Other private fixed-wing aircraft explosion **injuring occupant**

✓x7ᵗʰ V95.29 Other accident to other private fixed-wing aircraft injuring occupant

✓5ᵗʰ V95.3 Commercial fixed-wing aircraft accident injuring occupant

✓x7ᵗʰ V95.30 Unspecified accident to commercial fixed-wing aircraft injuring occupant

✓x7ᵗʰ V95.31 Commercial fixed-wing aircraft crash **injuring occupant**

✓x7ᵗʰ V95.32 Forced landing of commercial fixed-wing aircraft injuring occupant

✓x7ᵗʰ V95.33 Commercial fixed-wing aircraft collision **injuring occupant**
Commercial fixed-wing aircraft collision with any object, fixed, movable or moving

✓x7ᵗʰ V95.34 Commercial fixed-wing aircraft fire **injuring occupant**

✓x7ᵗʰ V95.35 Commercial fixed-wing aircraft explosion **injuring occupant**

✓x7ᵗʰ V95.39 Other accident to commercial fixed-wing aircraft injuring occupant

✓5ᵗʰ V95.4 Spacecraft accident injuring occupant

✓x7ᵗʰ V95.40 Unspecified spacecraft accident injuring occupant

√x7ᵗʰ **V95.41** **Spacecraft** crash **injuring occupant**

√x7ᵗʰ **V95.42** Forced landing **of spacecraft injuring occupant**

√x7ᵗʰ **V95.43** **Spacecraft** collision **injuring occupant**
       Spacecraft collision with any object, fixed, moveable or moving

√x7ᵗʰ **V95.44** **Spacecraft** fire **injuring occupant**

√x7ᵗʰ **V95.45** **Spacecraft** explosion **injuring occupant**

√x7ᵗʰ **V95.49** **Other spacecraft accident injuring occupant**

√x7ᵗʰ **V95.8** Other powered **aircraft accidents injuring occupant**

√x7ᵗʰ **V95.9** **Unspecified aircraft accident injuring occupant**
       Aircraft accident NOS
       Air transport accident NOS

√4ᵗʰ **V96** **Accident to nonpowered aircraft causing injury to occupant**

The appropriate 7th character is to be added to each code from category V96.
A   initial encounter
D   subsequent encounter
S   sequela

√5ᵗʰ **V96.0** Balloon **accident injuring occupant**

√x7ᵗʰ **V96.00** **Unspecified balloon accident injuring occupant**

√x7ᵗʰ **V96.01** **Balloon** crash **injuring occupant**

√x7ᵗʰ **V96.02** Forced landing **of balloon injuring occupant**

√x7ᵗʰ **V96.03** **Balloon** collision **injuring occupant**
       Balloon collision with any object, fixed, moveable or moving

√x7ᵗʰ **V96.04** **Balloon** fire **injuring occupant**

√x7ᵗʰ **V96.05** **Balloon** explosion **injuring occupant**

√x7ᵗʰ **V96.09** **Other balloon accident injuring occupant**

√5ᵗʰ **V96.1** Hang-glider **accident injuring occupant**

√x7ᵗʰ **V96.10** **Unspecified hang-glider accident injuring occupant**

√x7ᵗʰ **V96.11** **Hang-glider** crash **injuring occupant**

√x7ᵗʰ **V96.12** Forced landing **of hang-glider injuring occupant**

√x7ᵗʰ **V96.13** **Hang-glider** collision **injuring occupant**
       Hang-glider collision with any object, fixed, moveable or moving

√x7ᵗʰ **V96.14** **Hang-glider** fire **injuring occupant**

√x7ᵗʰ **V96.15** **Hang-glider** explosion **injuring occupant**

√x7ᵗʰ **V96.19** **Other hang-glider accident injuring occupant**

√5ᵗʰ **V96.2** Glider (nonpowered) **accident injuring occupant**

√x7ᵗʰ **V96.20** **Unspecified glider (nonpowered) accident injuring occupant**

√x7ᵗʰ **V96.21** **Glider (nonpowered)** crash **injuring occupant**

√x7ᵗʰ **V96.22** Forced landing **of glider (nonpowered) injuring occupant**

√x7ᵗʰ **V96.23** **Glider (nonpowered)** collision **injuring occupant**
       Glider (nonpowered) collision with any object, fixed, moveable or moving

√x7ᵗʰ **V96.24** **Glider (nonpowered)** fire **injuring occupant**

√x7ᵗʰ **V96.25** **Glider (nonpowered)** explosion **injuring occupant**

√x7ᵗʰ **V96.29** **Other glider (nonpowered) accident injuring occupant**

√x7ᵗʰ **V96.8** Other nonpowered-aircraft **accidents injuring occupant**
       Kite carrying a person accident injuring occupant

√x7ᵗʰ **V96.9** **Unspecified nonpowered-aircraft accident injuring occupant**
       Nonpowered-aircraft accident NOS

√4ᵗʰ **V97** **Other specified air transport accidents**

The appropriate 7th character is to be added to each code from category V97.
A   initial encounter
D   subsequent encounter
S   sequela

√x7ᵗʰ **V97.0** **Occupant of aircraft injured in other specified air transport accidents**
       Fall in, on or from aircraft in air transport accident
       EXCLUDES 1   accident while boarding or alighting aircraft (V97.1)

√x7ᵗʰ **V97.1** **Person injured while boarding or alighting from aircraft**

√5ᵗʰ **V97.2** **Parachutist accident**

√x7ᵗʰ **V97.21** **Parachutist entangled in object**
       Parachutist landing in tree

√x7ᵗʰ **V97.22** **Parachutist injured on landing**

√x7ᵗʰ **V97.29** **Other parachutist accident**

√5ᵗʰ **V97.3** **Person on ground injured in air transport accident**

√x7ᵗʰ **V97.31** **Hit by object falling from aircraft**
       Hit by crashing aircraft
       Injured by aircraft hitting house
       Injured by aircraft hitting car

√x7ᵗʰ **V97.32** **Injured by rotating propeller**

√x7ᵗʰ **V97.33** **Sucked into jet engine**

√x7ᵗʰ **V97.39** **Other injury to person on ground due to air transport accident**

√5ᵗʰ **V97.8** **Other air transport accidents, not elsewhere classified**
       EXCLUDES 1   aircraft accident NOS (V95.9)
                exposure to changes in air pressure during ascent or descent (W94.-)

√6ᵗʰ **V97.81** **Air transport accident involving military aircraft**

√7ᵗʰ **V97.810** **Civilian aircraft involved in air transport accident with military aircraft**
       Passenger in civilian aircraft injured due to accident with military aircraft

√7ᵗʰ **V97.811** **Civilian injured by military aircraft**

√7ᵗʰ **V97.818** **Other air transport accident involving military aircraft**

√x7ᵗʰ **V97.89** **Other air transport accidents, not elsewhere classified**
       Injury from machinery on aircraft

Other and unspecified transport accidents (V98-V99)

EXCLUDES 1   vehicle accident, type of vehicle unspecified (V89.-)

√4ᵗʰ **V98** **Other specified transport accidents**

The appropriate 7th character is to be added to each code from category V98.
A   initial encounter
D   subsequent encounter
S   sequela

√x7ᵗʰ **V98.0** **Accident to, on or involving** cable-car, **not on rails**
       Caught or dragged by cable-car, not on rails
       Fall or jump from cable-car, not on rails
       Object thrown from or in cable-car, not on rails

√x7ᵗʰ **V98.1** **Accident to, on or involving** land-yacht

√x7ᵗʰ **V98.2** **Accident to, on or involving** ice yacht

√x7ᵗʰ **V98.3** **Accident to, on or involving** ski lift
       Accident to, on or involving ski chair-lift
       Accident to, on or involving ski-lift with gondola

√x7ᵗʰ **V98.8** **Other specified transport accidents**

√x7ᵗʰ **V99** **Unspecified transport accident**

The appropriate 7th character is to be added to code V99.
A   initial encounter
D   subsequent encounter
S   sequela

OTHER EXTERNAL CAUSES OF ACCIDENTAL INJURY (W00-X58)

Slipping, tripping, stumbling and falls (W00-W19)

EXCLUDES 1   assault involving a fall (Y01-Y02)
               fall from animal (V80.-)
               fall (in) (from) machinery (in operation) (W28-W31)
               fall (in) (from) transport vehicle (V01-V99)
               intentional self-harm involving a fall (X80-X81)
EXCLUDES 2   at risk for fall (history of fall) (Z91.81)
               fall (in) (from) burning building (X00.-)
               fall into fire (X00-X04, X08-X09)

√4ᵗʰ **W00** **Fall due to ice and snow**
       INCLUDES   pedestrian on foot falling (slipping) on ice and snow
       EXCLUDES 1   fall on (from) ice and snow involving pedestrian conveyance (V00.-)
                fall from stairs and steps not due to ice and snow (W10.-)

The appropriate 7th character is to be added to each code from category W00.
A   initial encounter
D   subsequent encounter
S   sequela

√x7ᵗʰ **W00.0** **Fall on** same level **due to ice and snow**

EXCLUDES 1 Not coded here   **EXCLUDES 2** Not included here   N Newborn Age: 0   P Pediatric Age: 0-17   M Maternity Age: 12-55   A Adult Age: 15-124

1022   ICD-10-CM Draft (2015)

√x7ᵗʰ **W00.1** Fall from stairs and steps due to ice and snow

√x7ᵗʰ **W00.2 Other fall from one level to another due to ice and snow**

√x7ᵗʰ **W00.9 Unspecified fall due to ice and snow**

√4ᵗʰ **W01 Fall on same level from slipping, tripping and stumbling**
> INCLUDES fall on moving sidewalk
> EXCLUDES 1 *fall due to bumping (striking) against object (W18.0-)*
> *fall in shower or bathtub (W18.2-)*
> *fall on same level NOS (W18.30)*
> *fall on same level from slipping, tripping and stumbling due to*
> *ice or snow (W00.0)*
> *fall off or from toilet (W18.1-)*
> *slipping, tripping and stumbling NOS (W18.40)*
> *slipping, tripping and stumbling without falling (W18.4-)*

> The appropriate 7th character is to be added to each code from
> category W01.
> A   initial encounter
> D   subsequent encounter
> S   sequela

√x7ᵗʰ **W01.0 Fall on same level from slipping, tripping and stumbling**
without subsequent striking against object
Falling over animal

√5ᵗʰ **W01.1 Fall on same level from slipping, tripping and stumbling** with
subsequent striking against object

√x7ᵗʰ **W01.10 Fall on same level from slipping, tripping and stumbling with subsequent striking against unspecified object**

√6ᵗʰ **W01.11 Fall on same level from slipping, tripping and stumbling with subsequent striking against** sharp object

√7ᵗʰ **W01.110 Fall on same level from slipping, tripping and stumbling with subsequent striking against sharp** glass

√7ᵗʰ **W01.111 Fall on same level from slipping, tripping and stumbling with subsequent striking against** power tool or machine

√7ᵗʰ **W01.118 Fall on same level from slipping, tripping and stumbling with subsequent striking against other sharp object**

√7ᵗʰ **W01.119 Fall on same level from slipping, tripping and stumbling with subsequent striking against unspecified sharp object**

√6ᵗʰ **W01.19 Fall on same level from slipping, tripping and stumbling with subsequent striking against other object**

√7ᵗʰ **W01.190 Fall on same level from slipping, tripping and stumbling with subsequent striking against** furniture

√7ᵗʰ **W01.198 Fall on same level from slipping, tripping and stumbling with subsequent striking against other object**

√x7ᵗʰ **W03 Other fall on same level due to collision with another person**
Fall due to non-transport collision with other person
> EXCLUDES 1 *collision with another person without fall (W51)*
> *crushed or pushed by a crowd or human stampede (W52)*
> *fall involving pedestrian conveyance (V00-V09)*
> *fall due to ice or snow (W00)*
> *fall on same level NOS (W18.30)*
> **AHA:** 2012, 4Q, 108

> The appropriate 7th character is to be added to code W03.
> A   initial encounter
> D   subsequent encounter
> S   sequela

√x7ᵗʰ **W04 Fall while being carried or supported by other persons**
Accidentally dropped while being carried

> The appropriate 7th character is to be added to code W04.
> A   initial encounter
> D   subsequent encounter
> S   sequela

√4ᵗʰ **W05 Fall from non-moving wheelchair, nonmotorized scooter and motorized mobility scooter**
> EXCLUDES 1 *fall from moving wheelchair (powered) (V00.811)*
> *fall from moving motorized mobility scooter (V00.831)*
> *fall from nonmotorized scooter (V00.141)*

> The appropriate 7th character is to be added to each code from
> category W05.
> A   initial encounter
> D   subsequent encounter
> S   sequela

√x7ᵗʰ **W05.0 Fall from non-moving** wheelchair

√x7ᵗʰ **W05.1 Fall from non-moving** nonmotorized scooter

√x7ᵗʰ **W05.2 Fall from non-moving** motorized mobility scooter

√x7ᵗʰ **W06 Fall from bed**

> The appropriate 7th character is to be added to code W06.
> A   initial encounter
> D   subsequent encounter
> S   sequela

√x7ᵗʰ **W07 Fall from chair**

> The appropriate 7th character is to be added to code W07.
> A   initial encounter
> D   subsequent encounter
> S   sequela

√x7ᵗʰ **W08 Fall from other furniture**

> The appropriate 7th character is to be added to code W08.
> A   initial encounter
> D   subsequent encounter
> S   sequela

√4ᵗʰ **W09 Fall on and from playground equipment**
> EXCLUDES 1 *fall involving recreational machinery (W31)*

> The appropriate 7th character is to be added to each code from
> category W09.
> A   initial encounter
> D   subsequent encounter
> S   sequela

√x7ᵗʰ **W09.0 Fall on or from playground slide**

√x7ᵗʰ **W09.1 Fall from playground swing**

√x7ᵗʰ **W09.2 Fall on or from jungle gym**

√x7ᵗʰ **W09.8 Fall on or from other playground equipment**

√4ᵗʰ **W10 Fall on and from stairs and steps**
> EXCLUDES 1 *Fall from stairs and steps due to ice and snow (W00.1)*

> The appropriate 7th character is to be added to each code from
> category W10.
> A   initial encounter
> D   subsequent encounter
> S   sequela

√x7ᵗʰ **W10.0 Fall (on)(from) escalator**

√x7ᵗʰ **W10.1 Fall (on)(from) sidewalk curb**

√x7ᵗʰ **W10.2 Fall (on)(from) incline**
Fall (on) (from) ramp

√x7ᵗʰ **W10.8 Fall (on) (from) other stairs and steps**

√x7ᵗʰ **W10.9 Fall (on) (from) unspecified stairs and steps**

√x7ᵗʰ **W11 Fall on and from ladder**

> The appropriate 7th character is to be added to code W11.
> A   initial encounter
> D   subsequent encounter
> S   sequela

√x7ᵗʰ **W12 Fall on and from scaffolding**

> The appropriate 7th character is to be added to code W12.
> A   initial encounter
> D   subsequent encounter
> S   sequela

☑ Additional Character Required   √x7ᵗʰ Xtension Alert   Unspecified Dx   Other Specified Dx   Manifestation   ▶◀ Revised Text   ● New Code   ▲ Revised Code Title

External Causes of Morbidity

W13–W16.42

√4th **W13 Fall from, out of or through building or structure**

The appropriate 7th character is to be added to each code from category W13.
A   initial encounter
D   subsequent encounter
S   sequela

√x7th **W13.0 Fall from, out of or through balcony**
Fall from, out of or through railing

√x7th **W13.1 Fall from, out of or through bridge**

√x7th **W13.2 Fall from, out of or through roof**

√x7th **W13.3 Fall through floor**

√x7th **W13.4 Fall from, out of or through window**
EXCLUDES 2 *fall with subsequent striking against sharp glass (W01.110)*

√x7th **W13.8 Fall from, out of or through other building or structure**
Fall from, out of or through viaduct
Fall from, out of or through wall
Fall from, out of or through flag-pole

√x7th **W13.9 Fall from, out of or through building, not otherwise specified**
EXCLUDES 1 *collapse of a building or structure (W20.-)*
fall or jump from burning building or structure (X00.-)

√x7th **W14 Fall from tree**

The appropriate 7th character is to be added to code W14.
A   initial encounter
D   subsequent encounter
S   sequela

√x7th **W15 Fall from cliff**

The appropriate 7th character is to be added to code W15.
A   initial encounter
D   subsequent encounter
S   sequela

√4th **W16 Fall, jump or diving into water**
EXCLUDES 1 *accidental non-watercraft drowning and submersion not involving fall (W65-W74)*
effects of air pressure from diving (W94.-)
fall into water from watercraft (V90-V94)
hitting an object or against bottom when falling from watercraft (V94.0)
EXCLUDES 2 *striking or hitting diving board (W21.4)*

The appropriate 7th character is to be added to each code from category W16.
A   initial encounter
D   subsequent encounter
S   sequela

√5th **W16.0 Fall into swimming pool**
Fall into swimming pool NOS
EXCLUDES 1 *fall into empty swimming pool (W17.3)*

√6th **W16.01 Fall into swimming pool striking water surface**

√7th **W16.011 Fall into swimming pool striking water surface causing drowning and submersion**
EXCLUDES 1 *drowning and submersion while in swimming pool without fall (W67)*

√7th **W16.012 Fall into swimming pool striking water surface causing other injury**

√6th **W16.02 Fall into swimming pool striking bottom**

√7th **W16.021 Fall into swimming pool striking bottom causing drowning and submersion**
EXCLUDES 1 *drowning and submersion while in swimming pool without fall (W67)*

√7th **W16.022 Fall into swimming pool striking bottom causing other injury**

√6th **W16.03 Fall into swimming pool striking wall**

√7th **W16.031 Fall into swimming pool striking wall causing drowning and submersion**
EXCLUDES 1 *drowning and submersion while in swimming pool without fall (W67)*

√7th **W16.032 Fall into swimming pool striking wall causing other injury**

√5th **W16.1 Fall into natural body of water**
Fall into lake
Fall into open sea
Fall into river
Fall into stream

√6th **W16.11 Fall into natural body of water striking water surface**

√7th **W16.111 Fall into natural body of water striking water surface causing drowning and submersion**
EXCLUDES 1 *drowning and submersion while in natural body of water without fall (W69)*

√7th **W16.112 Fall into natural body of water striking water surface causing other injury**

√6th **W16.12 Fall into natural body of water striking bottom**

√7th **W16.121 Fall into natural body of water striking bottom causing drowning and submersion**
EXCLUDES 1 *drowning and submersion while in natural body of water without fall (W69)*

√7th **W16.122 Fall into natural body of water striking bottom causing other injury**

√6th **W16.13 Fall into natural body of water striking side**

√7th **W16.131 Fall into natural body of water striking side causing drowning and submersion**
EXCLUDES 1 *drowning and submersion while in natural body of water without fall (W69)*

√7th **W16.132 Fall into natural body of water striking side causing other injury**

√5th **W16.2 Fall in (into) filled bathtub or bucket of water**

√6th **W16.21 Fall in (into) filled bathtub**
EXCLUDES 1 *fall into empty bathtub (W18.2)*

√7th **W16.211 Fall in (into) filled bathtub causing drowning and submersion**
EXCLUDES 1 *drowning and submersion while in filled bathtub without fall (W65)*

√7th **W16.212 Fall in (into) filled bathtub causing other injury**

√6th **W16.22 Fall in (into) bucket of water**

√7th **W16.221 Fall in (into) bucket of water causing drowning and submersion**

√7th **W16.222 Fall in (into) bucket of water causing other injury**

√5th **W16.3 Fall into other water**
Fall into fountain
Fall into reservoir

√6th **W16.31 Fall into other water striking water surface**

√7th **W16.311 Fall into other water striking water surface causing drowning and submersion**
EXCLUDES 1 *drowning and submersion while in other water without fall (W73)*

√7th **W16.312 Fall into other water striking water surface causing other injury**

√6th **W16.32 Fall into other water striking bottom**

√7th **W16.321 Fall into other water striking bottom causing drowning and submersion**
EXCLUDES 1 *drowning and submersion while in other water without fall (W73)*

√7th **W16.322 Fall into other water striking bottom causing other injury**

√6th **W16.33 Fall into other water striking wall**

√7th **W16.331 Fall into other water striking wall causing drowning and submersion**
EXCLUDES 1 *drowning and submersion while in other water without fall (W73)*

√7th **W16.332 Fall into other water striking wall causing other injury**

√5th **W16.4 Fall into unspecified water**

√x7th **W16.41 Fall into unspecified water causing drowning and submersion**

√x7th **W16.42 Fall into unspecified water causing other injury**

EXCLUDES 1 Not coded here   EXCLUDES 2 Not included here   N Newborn Age: 0   P Pediatric Age: 0-17   M Maternity Age: 12-55   A Adult Age: 15-124

☑5ᵗʰ W16.5 Jumping or diving into swimming pool

    ☑6ᵗʰ W16.51 Jumping or diving into swimming pool striking water surface

        ☑7ᵗʰ W16.511 Jumping or diving into swimming pool striking water surface causing drowning **and submersion**

            EXCLUDES 1 *drowning and submersion while in swimming pool without jumping or diving (W67)*

        ☑7ᵗʰ W16.512 Jumping or diving into swimming pool striking water surface causing other injury

    ☑6ᵗʰ W16.52 Jumping or diving into swimming pool striking bottom

        ☑7ᵗʰ W16.521 Jumping or diving into swimming pool striking bottom causing drowning **and submersion**

            EXCLUDES 1 *drowning and submersion while in swimming pool without jumping or diving (W67)*

        ☑7ᵗʰ W16.522 Jumping or diving into swimming pool striking bottom causing other injury

    ☑6ᵗʰ W16.53 Jumping or diving into swimming pool striking wall

        ☑7ᵗʰ W16.531 Jumping or diving into swimming pool striking wall causing drowning **and submersion**

            EXCLUDES 1 *drowning and submersion while in swimming pool without jumping or diving (W67)*

        ☑7ᵗʰ W16.532 Jumping or diving into swimming pool striking wall causing other injury

☑5ᵗʰ W16.6 Jumping or diving into natural body of water
    Jumping or diving into lake
    Jumping or diving into open sea
    Jumping or diving into river
    Jumping or diving into stream

    ☑6ᵗʰ W16.61 Jumping or diving into natural body of water striking water surface

        ☑7ᵗʰ W16.611 Jumping or diving into natural body of water striking water surface causing drowning **and submersion**

            EXCLUDES 1 *drowning and submersion while in natural body of water without jumping or diving (W69)*

        ☑7ᵗʰ W16.612 Jumping or diving into natural body of water striking water surface causing other injury

    ☑6ᵗʰ W16.62 Jumping or diving into natural body of water striking bottom

        ☑7ᵗʰ W16.621 Jumping or diving into natural body of water striking bottom causing drowning **and submersion**

            EXCLUDES 1 *drowning and submersion while in natural body of water without jumping or diving (W69)*

        ☑7ᵗʰ W16.622 Jumping or diving into natural body of water striking bottom causing other injury

☑5ᵗʰ W16.7 Jumping or diving from boat

    EXCLUDES 1 *Fall from boat into water—see watercraft accident (V90-V94)*

    ☑6ᵗʰ W16.71 Jumping or diving from boat striking water surface

        ☑7ᵗʰ W16.711 Jumping or diving from boat striking water surface causing drowning **and submersion**

        ☑7ᵗʰ W16.712 Jumping or diving from boat striking water surface causing other injury

    ☑6ᵗʰ W16.72 Jumping or diving from boat striking bottom

        ☑7ᵗʰ W16.721 Jumping or diving from boat striking bottom causing drowning **and submersion**

        ☑7ᵗʰ W16.722 Jumping or diving from boat striking bottom causing other injury

☑5ᵗʰ W16.8 Jumping or diving into other water
    Jumping or diving into fountain
    Jumping or diving into reservoir

    ☑6ᵗʰ W16.81 Jumping or diving into other water striking water surface

        ☑7ᵗʰ W16.811 Jumping or diving into other water striking water surface causing drowning **and submersion**

            EXCLUDES 1 *drowning and submersion while in other water without jumping or diving (W73)*

        ☑7ᵗʰ W16.812 Jumping or diving into other water striking water surface causing other injury

    ☑6ᵗʰ W16.82 Jumping or diving into other water striking bottom

        ☑7ᵗʰ W16.821 Jumping or diving into other water striking bottom causing drowning **and submersion**

            EXCLUDES 1 *drowning and submersion while in other water without jumping or diving (W73)*

        ☑7ᵗʰ W16.822 Jumping or diving into other water striking bottom causing other injury

    ☑6ᵗʰ W16.83 Jumping or diving into other water striking wall

        ☑7ᵗʰ W16.831 Jumping or diving into other water striking wall causing drowning **and submersion**

            EXCLUDES 1 *drowning and submersion while in other water without jumping or diving (W73)*

        ☑7ᵗʰ W16.832 Jumping or diving into other water striking wall causing other injury

☑5ᵗʰ W16.9 Jumping or diving into unspecified **water**

    ☑x7ᵗʰ W16.91 Jumping or diving into unspecified water causing drowning **and submersion**

    ☑x7ᵗʰ W16.92 Jumping or diving into unspecified water causing other injury

☑4ᵗʰ W17 Other fall from one level to another

    The appropriate 7th character is to be added to each code from category W17.
    A   initial encounter
    D   subsequent encounter
    S   sequela

    ☑x7ᵗʰ W17.0 Fall into well

    ☑x7ᵗʰ W17.1 Fall into storm drain or manhole

    ☑x7ᵗʰ W17.2 Fall into hole
        Fall into pit

    ☑x7ᵗʰ W17.3 Fall into empty swimming pool
        EXCLUDES 1 *fall into filled swimming pool (W16.0-)*

    ☑x7ᵗʰ W17.4 Fall from dock

    ☑5ᵗʰ W17.8 Other fall from one level to another

        ☑x7ᵗʰ W17.81 Fall down embankment (hill)

        ☑x7ᵗʰ W17.82 Fall from (out of) grocery cart
            Fall due to grocery cart tipping over

        ☑x7ᵗʰ W17.89 Other fall from one level to another
            Fall from cherry picker
            Fall from lifting device
            Fall from mobile elevated work platform [MEWP]
            Fall from sky lift

☑4ᵗʰ W18 Other slipping, tripping and stumbling and falls

    The appropriate 7th character is to be added to each code from category W18.
    A   initial encounter
    D   subsequent encounter
    S   sequela

    ☑5ᵗʰ W18.0 Fall due to bumping against object
        Striking against object with subsequent fall
        EXCLUDES 1 *fall on same level due to slipping, tripping, or stumbling with subsequent striking against object (W01.1-)*

        ☑x7ᵗʰ W18.00 Striking against unspecified object with subsequent fall

        ☑x7ᵗʰ W18.01 Striking against sports equipment **with subsequent fall**

        ☑x7ᵗʰ W18.02 Striking against glass **with subsequent fall**

        ☑x7ᵗʰ W18.09 Striking against other object with subsequent fall

---

☑ Additional Character Required   ☑x7ᵗʰ Xtension Alert   Unspecified Dx   Other Specified Dx   Manifestation   ►◄ Revised Text   ● New Code   ▲ Revised Code Title

✓5ᵗʰ **W18.1** Fall from or off toilet

     ✓x7ᵗʰ **W18.11** Fall from or off toilet without subsequent striking against object
         Fall from (off) toilet NOS

     ✓x7ᵗʰ **W18.12** Fall from or off toilet with subsequent striking against object

✓x7ᵗʰ **W18.2** Fall in (into) shower or empty bathtub
     EXCLUDES 1   fall in full bathtub causing drowning or submersion (W16.21-)

✓5ᵗʰ **W18.3** Other and unspecified fall on same level

     ✓x7ᵗʰ **W18.30** Fall on same level, unspecified

     ✓x7ᵗʰ **W18.31** Fall on same level due to stepping on an object
         Fall on same level due to stepping on an animal
         EXCLUDES 1   slipping, tripping and stumbling without fall due to stepping on animal (W18.41)

     ✓x7ᵗʰ **W18.39** Other fall on same level

✓5ᵗʰ **W18.4** Slipping, tripping and stumbling without falling
     EXCLUDES 1   collision with another person without fall (W51)

     ✓x7ᵗʰ **W18.40** Slipping, tripping and stumbling without falling, unspecified

     ✓x7ᵗʰ **W18.41** Slipping, tripping and stumbling without falling due to stepping on object
         Slipping, tripping and stumbling without falling due to stepping on animal
         EXCLUDES 1   slipping, tripping and stumbling with fall due to stepping on animal (W18.31)

     ✓x7ᵗʰ **W18.42** Slipping, tripping and stumbling without falling due to stepping into hole or opening

     ✓x7ᵗʰ **W18.43** Slipping, tripping and stumbling without falling due to stepping from one level to another

     ✓x7ᵗʰ **W18.49** Other slipping, tripping and stumbling without falling

✓x7ᵗʰ **W19 Unspecified fall**
Accidental fall NOS
AHA: 2012, 4Q, 95

The appropriate 7th character is to be added to code W19.
A   initial encounter
D   subsequent encounter
S   sequela

Exposure to inanimate mechanical forces (W20-W49)

EXCLUDES 1   assault (X92-Y08)
     contact or collision with animals or persons (W50-W64)
     exposure to inanimate mechanical forces involving military or war operations (Y36-, Y37-)
     intentional self-harm (X71-X83)

✓4ᵗʰ **W20 Struck by thrown, projected or falling object**
Code first any associated:
     cataclysm (X34-X39)
     lightning strike (T75.00)
EXCLUDES 1   falling object in machinery accident (W24, W28-W31)
     falling object in transport accident (V01-V99)
     object set in motion by explosion (W35-W40)
     object set in motion by firearm (W32-W34)
     struck by thrown sports equipment (W21.-)

The appropriate 7th character is to be added to each code from category W20.
A   initial encounter
D   subsequent encounter
S   sequela

✓x7ᵗʰ **W20.0** Struck by falling object in cave-in
     EXCLUDES 2   asphyxiation due to cave-in (T71.21)

✓x7ᵗʰ **W20.1** Struck by object due to collapse of building
     EXCLUDES 1   struck by object due to collapse of burning building (X00.2, X02.2)

✓x7ᵗʰ **W20.8** Other cause of strike by thrown, projected or falling object
     EXCLUDES 1   struck by thrown sports equipment (W21.-)

✓4ᵗʰ **W21 Striking against or struck by sports equipment**
     EXCLUDES 1   assault with sports equipment (Y08.0-)
         striking against or struck by sports equipment with subsequent fall (W18.01)

The appropriate 7th character is to be added to each code from category W21.
A   initial encounter
D   subsequent encounter
S   sequela

✓5ᵗʰ **W21.0** Struck by hit or thrown ball

     ✓x7ᵗʰ **W21.00** Struck by hit or thrown ball, unspecified type

     ✓x7ᵗʰ **W21.01** Struck by football

     ✓x7ᵗʰ **W21.02** Struck by soccer ball

     ✓x7ᵗʰ **W21.03** Struck by baseball

     ✓x7ᵗʰ **W21.04** Struck by golf ball

     ✓x7ᵗʰ **W21.05** Struck by basketball

     ✓x7ᵗʰ **W21.06** Struck by volleyball

     ✓x7ᵗʰ **W21.07** Struck by softball

     ✓x7ᵗʰ **W21.09** Struck by other hit or thrown ball

✓5ᵗʰ **W21.1** Struck by bat, racquet or club

     ✓x7ᵗʰ **W21.11** Struck by baseball bat

     ✓x7ᵗʰ **W21.12** Struck by tennis racquet

     ✓x7ᵗʰ **W21.13** Struck by golf club

     ✓x7ᵗʰ **W21.19** Struck by other bat, racquet or club

✓5ᵗʰ **W21.2** Struck by hockey stick or puck

     ✓6ᵗʰ **W21.21** Struck by hockey stick

         ✓7ᵗʰ **W21.210** Struck by ice hockey stick

         ✓7ᵗʰ **W21.211** Struck by field hockey stick

     ✓6ᵗʰ **W21.22** Struck by hockey puck

         ✓7ᵗʰ **W21.220** Struck by ice hockey puck

         ✓7ᵗʰ **W21.221** Struck by field hockey puck

✓5ᵗʰ **W21.3** Struck by sports foot wear

     ✓x7ᵗʰ **W21.31** Struck by shoe cleats
         Stepped on by shoe cleats

     ✓x7ᵗʰ **W21.32** Struck by skate blades
         Skated over by skate blades

     ✓x7ᵗʰ **W21.39** Struck by other sports foot wear

✓x7ᵗʰ **W21.4** Striking against diving board
     Use additional code for subsequent falling into water, if applicable (W16.-)

✓5ᵗʰ **W21.8** Striking against or struck by other sports equipment

     ✓x7ᵗʰ **W21.81** Striking against or struck by football helmet

     ✓x7ᵗʰ **W21.89** Striking against or struck by other sports equipment

✓x7ᵗʰ **W21.9** Striking against or struck by unspecified sports equipment

✓4ᵗʰ **W22 Striking against or struck by other objects**
     EXCLUDES 1   striking against or struck by object with subsequent fall (W18.09)

The appropriate 7th character is to be added to each code from category W22.
A   initial encounter
D   subsequent encounter
S   sequela

✓5ᵗʰ **W22.0** Striking against stationary object
     EXCLUDES 1   striking against stationary sports equipment (W21.8)

     ✓x7ᵗʰ **W22.01** Walked into wall

     ✓x7ᵗʰ **W22.02** Walked into lamppost

     ✓x7ᵗʰ **W22.03** Walked into furniture

     ✓6ᵗʰ **W22.04** Striking against wall of swimming pool

         ✓7ᵗʰ **W22.041** Striking against wall of swimming pool causing drowning and submersion
             EXCLUDES 1   drowning and submersion while swimming without striking against wall (W67)

         ✓7ᵗʰ **W22.042** Striking against wall of swimming pool causing other injury

     ✓x7ᵗʰ **W22.09** Striking against other stationary object

✓5ᵗʰ **W22.1** Striking against or struck by automobile airbag

     ✓x7ᵗʰ **W22.10** Striking against or struck by unspecified automobile airbag

---

EXCLUDES 1 Not coded here   EXCLUDES 2 Not included here   N Newborn Age: 0   P Pediatric Age: 0-17   M Maternity Age: 12-55   A Adult Age: 15-124

1026   ICD-10-CM Draft (2015)

√x7ᵗʰ **W22.11 Striking against or struck by** driver side **automobile airbag**

√x7ᵗʰ **W22.12 Striking against or struck by** front passenger **side automobile airbag**

√x7ᵗʰ **W22.19 Striking against or struck by other automobile airbag**

√x7ᵗʰ **W22.8 Striking against or struck by other objects**
Striking against or struck by object NOS
EXCLUDES 1   *struck by thrown, projected or falling object (W20.-)*

✅4ᵗʰ **W23 Caught, crushed, jammed or pinched in or between objects**
EXCLUDES 1   *injury caused by cutting or piercing instruments (W25-W27)*
injury caused by firearms malfunction (W32.1, W33.1-, W34.1-)
injury caused by lifting and transmission devices (W24.-)
injury caused by machinery (W28-W31)
injury caused by nonpowered hand tools (W27.-)
injury caused by transport vehicle being used as a means of transportation (V01-V99)
injury caused by struck by thrown, projected or falling object (W20.-)

The appropriate 7th character is to be added to each code from category W23.
A   initial encounter
D   subsequent encounter
S   sequela

√x7ᵗʰ **W23.0 Caught, crushed, jammed, or pinched between** moving objects

√x7ᵗʰ **W23.1 Caught, crushed, jammed, or pinched between** stationary objects

✅4ᵗʰ **W24 Contact with lifting and transmission devices, not elsewhere classified**
EXCLUDES 1   *transport accidents (V01-V99)*

The appropriate 7th character is to be added to each code from category W24.
A   initial encounter
D   subsequent encounter
S   sequela

√x7ᵗʰ **W24.0 Contact with lifting devices, not elsewhere classified**
Contact with chain hoist
Contact with drive belt
Contact with pulley (block)

√x7ᵗʰ **W24.1 Contact with transmission devices, not elsewhere classified**
Contact with transmission belt or cable

√x7ᵗʰ **W25 Contact with sharp glass**
Code first any associated:
injury due to flying glass from explosion or firearm discharge (W32-W40)
transport accident (V00-V99)
EXCLUDES 1   *fall on same level due to slipping, tripping and stumbling with subsequent striking against sharp glass (W01.10)*
striking against sharp glass with subsequent fall (W18.02)

The appropriate 7th character is to be added to code W25.
A   initial encounter
D   subsequent encounter
S   sequela

✅4ᵗʰ **W26 Contact with knife, sword or dagger**

The appropriate 7th character is to be added to each code from category W26.
A   initial encounter
D   subsequent encounter
S   sequela

√x7ᵗʰ **W26.0 Contact with knife**
EXCLUDES 1   *contact with electric knife (W29.1)*

√x7ᵗʰ **W26.1 Contact with sword or dagger**

✅4ᵗʰ **W27 Contact with nonpowered hand tool**

The appropriate 7th character is to be added to each code from category W27.
A   initial encounter
D   subsequent encounter
S   sequela

√x7ᵗʰ **W27.0 Contact with** workbench tool
Contact with auger
Contact with axe
Contact with chisel
Contact with handsaw
Contact with screwdriver

√x7ᵗʰ **W27.1 Contact with** garden tool
Contact with hoe
Contact with nonpowered lawn mower
Contact with pitchfork
Contact with rake

√x7ᵗʰ **W27.2 Contact with** scissors

√x7ᵗʰ **W27.3 Contact with** needle **(sewing)**
EXCLUDES 1   *contact with hypodermic needle (W46.-)*

√x7ᵗʰ **W27.4 Contact with** kitchen utensil
Contact with fork
Contact with ice-pick
Contact with can-opener NOS

√x7ᵗʰ **W27.5 Contact with** paper-cutter

√x7ᵗʰ **W27.8 Contact with other nonpowered hand tool**
Contact with nonpowered sewing machine
Contact with shovel

√x7ᵗʰ **W28 Contact with powered lawn mower**
Powered lawn mower (commercial) (residential)
EXCLUDES 1   *contact with nonpowered lawn mower (W27.1)*
EXCLUDES 2   *exposure to electric current (W86.-)*

The appropriate 7th character is to be added to code W28.
A   initial encounter
D   subsequent encounter
S   sequela

✅4ᵗʰ **W29 Contact with other powered hand tools and household machinery**
EXCLUDES 1   *contact with commercial machinery (W31.82)*
contact with hot household appliance (X15)
contact with nonpowered hand tool (W27.-)
exposure to electric current (W86)

The appropriate 7th character is to be added to each code from category W29.
A   initial encounter
D   subsequent encounter
S   sequela

√x7ᵗʰ **W29.0 Contact with powered kitchen appliance**
Contact with blender
Contact with can-opener
Contact with garbage disposal
Contact with mixer

√x7ᵗʰ **W29.1 Contact with electric knife**

√x7ᵗʰ **W29.2 Contact with other powered household machinery**
Contact with electric fan
Contact with powered dryer (clothes) (powered) (spin)
Contact with washing-machine
Contact with sewing machine

√x7ᵗʰ **W29.3 Contact with powered garden and outdoor hand tools and machinery**
Contact with chainsaw
Contact with edger
Contact with garden cultivator (tiller)
Contact with hedge trimmer
Contact with other powered garden tool
EXCLUDES 1   *contact with powered lawn mower (W28)*

√x7ᵗʰ **W29.4 Contact with nail gun**

√x7ᵗʰ **W29.8 Contact with other powered hand tools and household machinery**
Contact with do-it-yourself tool NOS

✅4ᵗʰ **W30 Contact with agricultural machinery**
INCLUDES   animal-powered farm machine
EXCLUDES 1   *agricultural transport vehicle accident (V01-V99)*
explosion of grain store (W40.8)
exposure to electric current (W86.-)

The appropriate 7th character is to be added to each code from category W30.
A   initial encounter
D   subsequent encounter
S   sequela

√x7ᵗʰ **W30.0 Contact with combine harvester**
Contact with reaper
Contact with thresher

√x7ᵗʰ **W30.1 Contact with power take-off devices (PTO)**

√x7ᵗʰ **W30.2 Contact with hay derrick**

√x7ᵗʰ **W30.3 Contact with grain storage elevator**
EXCLUDES 1   *explosion of grain store (W40.8)*

✅ Additional Character Required   √x7ᵗʰ Xtension Alert   Unspecified Dx   Other Specified Dx   Manifestation   ▶◀ Revised Text   ● New Code   ▲ Revised Code Title

ICD-10-CM Draft (2015)   1027

External Causes of Morbidity

W30.8–W33.12

√5ᵗʰ **W30.8 Contact with other specified agricultural machinery**

√x7ᵗʰ   **W30.81 Contact with agricultural transport vehicle in stationary use**
Contact with agricultural transport vehicle under repair, not on public roadway
EXCLUDES 1 *agricultural transport vehicle accident (V01-V99)*

√x7ᵗʰ   **W30.89 Contact with other specified agricultural machinery**

√x7ᵗʰ **W30.9 Contact with unspecified agricultural machinery**
Contact with farm machinery NOS

√4ᵗʰ **W31 Contact with other and unspecified machinery**
EXCLUDES 1 *contact with agricultural machinery (W30.-)*
contact with machinery in transport under own power or being towed by a vehicle (V01-V99)
exposure to electric current (W86)

The appropriate 7th character is to be added to each code from category W31.
A   initial encounter
D   subsequent encounter
S   sequela

√x7ᵗʰ **W31.0 Contact with mining and earth-drilling machinery**
Contact with bore or drill (land) (seabed)
Contact with shaft hoist
Contact with shaft lift
Contact with undercutter

√x7ᵗʰ **W31.1 Contact with metalworking machines**
Contact with abrasive wheel
Contact with forging machine
Contact with lathe
Contact with mechanical shears
Contact with metal drilling machine
Contact with milling machine
Contact with power press
Contact with rolling-mill
Contact with metal sawing machine

√x7ᵗʰ **W31.2 Contact with powered woodworking and forming machines**
Contact with band saw
Contact with bench saw
Contact with circular saw
Contact with molding machine
Contact with overhead plane
Contact with powered saw
Contact with radial saw
Contact with sander
EXCLUDES 1 *nonpowered woodworking tools (W27.0)*

√x7ᵗʰ **W31.3 Contact with prime movers**
Contact with gas turbine
Contact with internal combustion engine
Contact with steam engine
Contact with water driven turbine

√5ᵗʰ **W31.8 Contact with other specified machinery**

√x7ᵗʰ   **W31.81 Contact with recreational machinery**
Contact with roller coaster

√x7ᵗʰ   **W31.82 Contact with other commercial machinery**
Contact with commercial electric fan
Contact with commercial kitchen appliances
Contact with commercial powered dryer (clothes) (powered) (spin)
Contact with commercial washing-machine
Contact with commercial sewing machine
EXCLUDES 1 *contact with household machinery (W29.-)*
contact with powered lawn mower (W28)

√x7ᵗʰ   **W31.83 Contact with special construction vehicle in stationary use**
Contact with special construction vehicle under repair, not on public roadway
EXCLUDES 1 *special construction vehicle accident (V01-V99)*

√x7ᵗʰ   **W31.89 Contact with other specified machinery**

√x7ᵗʰ **W31.9 Contact with unspecified machinery**
Contact with machinery NOS

√4ᵗʰ **W32 Accidental handgun discharge and malfunction**
INCLUDES accidental discharge and malfunction of gun for single hand use
accidental discharge and malfunction of pistol
accidental discharge and malfunction of revolver
handgun discharge and malfunction NOS
EXCLUDES 1 *accidental airgun discharge and malfunction (W34.010, W34.110)*
accidental BB gun discharge and malfunction (W34.010, W34.110)
accidental pellet gun discharge and malfunction (W34.010, W34.110)
accidental shotgun discharge and malfunction (W33.01, W33.11)
assault by handgun discharge (X93)
handgun discharge involving legal intervention (Y35.0-)
handgun discharge involving military or war operations (Y36.4-)
intentional self-harm by handgun discharge (X72)
Very pistol discharge and malfunction (W34.09, W34.19)

The appropriate 7th character is to be added to each code from category W32.
A   initial encounter
D   subsequent encounter
S   sequela

√x7ᵗʰ **W32.0 Accidental handgun discharge**

√x7ᵗʰ **W32.1 Accidental handgun malfunction**
Injury due to explosion of handgun (parts)
Injury due to malfunction of mechanism or component of handgun
Injury due to recoil of handgun
Powder burn from handgun

√4ᵗʰ **W33 Accidental rifle, shotgun and larger firearm discharge and malfunction**
INCLUDES rifle, shotgun and larger firearm discharge and malfunction NOS
EXCLUDES 1 *accidental airgun discharge and malfunction (W34.010, W34.110)*
accidental BB gun discharge and malfunction (W34.010, W34.110)
accidental handgun discharge and malfunction (W32.-)
accidental pellet gun discharge and malfunction (W34.010, W34.110)
assault by rifle, shotgun and larger firearm discharge (X94)
firearm discharge involving legal intervention (Y35.0-)
firearm discharge involving military or war operations (Y36.4-)
intentional self-harm by rifle, shotgun and larger firearm discharge (X73)

The appropriate 7th character is to be added to each code from category W33.
A   initial encounter
D   subsequent encounter
S   sequela

√5ᵗʰ **W33.0 Accidental rifle, shotgun and larger firearm discharge**

√x7ᵗʰ   **W33.00 Accidental discharge of unspecified larger firearm**
Discharge of unspecified larger firearm NOS

√x7ᵗʰ   **W33.01 Accidental discharge of shotgun**
Discharge of shotgun NOS

√x7ᵗʰ   **W33.02 Accidental discharge of hunting rifle**
Discharge of hunting rifle NOS

√x7ᵗʰ   **W33.03 Accidental discharge of machine gun**
Discharge of machine gun NOS

√x7ᵗʰ   **W33.09 Accidental discharge of other larger firearm**
Discharge of other larger firearm NOS

√5ᵗʰ **W33.1 Accidental rifle, shotgun and larger firearm malfunction**
Injury due to explosion of rifle, shotgun and larger firearm (parts)
Injury due to malfunction of mechanism or component of rifle, shotgun and larger firearm
Injury due to piercing, cutting, crushing or pinching due to (by) slide trigger mechanism, scope or other gun part
Injury due to recoil of rifle, shotgun and larger firearm
Powder burn from rifle, shotgun and larger firearm

√x7ᵗʰ   **W33.10 Accidental malfunction of unspecified larger firearm**
Malfunction of unspecified larger firearm NOS

√x7ᵗʰ   **W33.11 Accidental malfunction of shotgun**
Malfunction of shotgun NOS

√x7ᵗʰ   **W33.12 Accidental malfunction of hunting rifle**
Malfunction of hunting rifle NOS

EXCLUDES 1 Not coded here   EXCLUDES 2 Not included here   N Newborn Age: 0   P Pediatric Age: 0-17   M Maternity Age: 12-55   A Adult Age: 15-124

1028   ICD-10-CM Draft (2015)

√x7ᵗʰ **W33.13** Accidental malfunction of machine gun
　　　　Malfunction of machine gun NOS

√x7ᵗʰ **W33.19** Accidental malfunction of other larger firearm
　　　　Malfunction of other larger firearm NOS

√4ᵗʰ **W34** Accidental discharge and malfunction from other and unspecified firearms and guns

　　The appropriate 7th character is to be added to each code from category W34.
　　A　initial encounter
　　D　subsequent encounter
　　S　sequela

√5ᵗʰ **W34.0** Accidental discharge from other and unspecified firearms and guns

√x7ᵗʰ **W34.00** Accidental discharge from unspecified firearms or gun
　　　　Discharge from firearm NOS
　　　　Gunshot wound NOS
　　　　Shot NOS

√6ᵗʰ **W34.01** Accidental discharge of gas, air or spring-operated guns

√7ᵗʰ **W34.010** Accidental discharge of airgun
　　　　Accidental discharge of BB gun
　　　　Accidental discharge of pellet gun

√7ᵗʰ **W34.011** Accidental discharge of paintball gun
　　　　Accidental injury due to paintball discharge

√7ᵗʰ **W34.018** Accidental discharge of other gas, air or spring-operated gun

√x7ᵗʰ **W34.09** Accidental discharge from other specified firearms
　　　　Accidental discharge from Very pistol [flare]

√5ᵗʰ **W34.1** Accidental malfunction from other and unspecified firearms and guns

√x7ᵗʰ **W34.10** Accidental malfunction from unspecified firearms or gun
　　　　Firearm malfunction NOS

√6ᵗʰ **W34.11** Accidental malfunction of gas, air or spring-operated guns

√7ᵗʰ **W34.110** Accidental malfunction of airgun
　　　　Accidental malfunction of BB gun
　　　　Accidental malfunction of pellet gun

√7ᵗʰ **W34.111** Accidental malfunction of paintball gun
　　　　Accidental injury due to paintball gun malfunction

√7ᵗʰ **W34.118** Accidental malfunction of other gas, air or spring-operated gun

√x7ᵗʰ **W34.19** Accidental malfunction from other specified firearms
　　　　Accidental malfunction from Very pistol [flare]

√x7ᵗʰ **W35** Explosion and rupture of boiler
　　EXCLUDES 1　explosion and rupture of boiler on watercraft (V93.4)

　　The appropriate 7th character is to be added to code W35.
　　A　initial encounter
　　D　subsequent encounter
　　S　sequela

√4ᵗʰ **W36** Explosion and rupture of gas cylinder

　　The appropriate 7th character is to be added to each code from category W36.
　　A　initial encounter
　　D　subsequent encounter
　　S　sequela

√x7ᵗʰ **W36.1** Explosion and rupture of aerosol can

√x7ᵗʰ **W36.2** Explosion and rupture of air tank

√x7ᵗʰ **W36.3** Explosion and rupture of pressurized-gas tank

√x7ᵗʰ **W36.8** Explosion and rupture of other gas cylinder

√x7ᵗʰ **W36.9** Explosion and rupture of unspecified gas cylinder

√4ᵗʰ **W37** Explosion and rupture of pressurized tire, pipe or hose

　　The appropriate 7th character is to be added to each code from category W37.
　　A　initial encounter
　　D　subsequent encounter
　　S　sequela

√x7ᵗʰ **W37.0** Explosion of bicycle tire

√x7ᵗʰ **W37.8** Explosion and rupture of other pressurized tire, pipe or hose

√x7ᵗʰ **W38** Explosion and rupture of other specified pressurized devices

　　The appropriate 7th character is to be added to code W38.
　　A　initial encounter
　　D　subsequent encounter
　　S　sequela

√x7ᵗʰ **W39** Discharge of firework

　　The appropriate 7th character is to be added to code W39.
　　A　initial encounter
　　D　subsequent encounter
　　S　sequela

√4ᵗʰ **W40** Explosion of other materials
　　EXCLUDES 1　assault by explosive material (X96)
　　　　explosion involving legal intervention (Y35.1-)
　　　　explosion involving military or war operations (Y36.0-, Y36.2-)
　　　　intentional self-harm by explosive material (X75)

　　The appropriate 7th character is to be added to each code from category W40.
　　A　initial encounter
　　D　subsequent encounter
　　S　sequela

√x7ᵗʰ **W40.0** Explosion of blasting material
　　　　Explosion of blasting cap
　　　　Explosion of detonator
　　　　Explosion of dynamite
　　　　Explosion of explosive (any) used in blasting operations

√x7ᵗʰ **W40.1** Explosion of explosive gases
　　　　Explosion of acetylene
　　　　Explosion of butane
　　　　Explosion of coal gas
　　　　Explosion in mine NOS
　　　　Explosion of explosive gas
　　　　Explosion of fire damp
　　　　Explosion of gasoline fumes
　　　　Explosion of methane
　　　　Explosion of propane

√x7ᵗʰ **W40.8** Explosion of other specified explosive materials
　　　　Explosion in dump NOS
　　　　Explosion in factory NOS
　　　　Explosion in grain store
　　　　Explosion in munitions
　　EXCLUDES 1　explosion involving legal intervention (Y35.1-)
　　　　explosion involving military or war operations (Y36.0-, Y36.2-)

√x7ᵗʰ **W40.9** Explosion of unspecified explosive materials
　　　　Explosion NOS

√4ᵗʰ **W42** Exposure to noise

　　The appropriate 7th character is to be added to each code from category W42.
　　A　initial encounter
　　D　subsequent encounter
　　S　sequela

√x7ᵗʰ **W42.0** Exposure to supersonic waves

√x7ᵗʰ **W42.9** Exposure to other noise
　　　　Exposure to sound waves NOS

√4ᵗʰ **W45** Foreign body or object entering through skin
　　EXCLUDES 2　contact with hand tools (nonpowered) (powered) (W27-W29)
　　　　contact with knife, sword or dagger (W26.-)
　　　　contact with sharp glass (W25.-)
　　　　struck by objects (W20-W22)

　　The appropriate 7th character is to be added to each code from category W45.
　　A　initial encounter
　　D　subsequent encounter
　　S　sequela

√x7ᵗʰ **W45.0** Nail entering through skin

√x7ᵗʰ **W45.1** Paper entering through skin
　　　　Paper cut

√x7ᵗʰ **W45.2** Lid of can entering through skin

√x7ᵗʰ **W45.8** Other foreign body or object entering through skin
　　　　Splinter in skin NOS

√ Additional Character Required　　√x7ᵗʰ Xtension Alert　　Unspecified Dx　　Other Specified Dx　　Manifestation　　►◄ Revised Text　　● New Code　　▲ Revised Code Title

External Causes of Morbidity

W46–W55.51

☑4ᵗʰ **W46 Contact with hypodermic needle**

> The appropriate 7th character is to be added to each code from category W46.
> A   initial encounter
> D   subsequent encounter
> S   sequela

   ☑7ᵗʰ **W46.0 Contact with hypodermic needle**
       Hypodermic needle stick NOS

   ☑7ᵗʰ **W46.1 Contact with** contaminated **hypodermic needle**

☑4ᵗʰ **W49 Exposure to other inanimate mechanical forces**
   INCLUDES   exposure to abnormal gravitational [G] forces
            exposure to inanimate mechanical forces NEC
   EXCLUDES 1   exposure to inanimate mechanical forces involving military or
            war operations (Y36.-, Y37.-)

> The appropriate 7th character is to be added to each code from category W49.
> A   initial encounter
> D   subsequent encounter
> S   sequela

   ☑5ᵗʰ **W49.0 Item causing** external constriction

     ☑7ᵗʰ **W49.01 Hair causing external constriction**

     ☑7ᵗʰ **W49.02 String or thread causing external constriction**

     ☑7ᵗʰ **W49.03 Rubber band causing external constriction**

     ☑7ᵗʰ **W49.04 Ring or other jewelry causing external constriction**

     ☑7ᵗʰ **W49.09 Other specified item causing external constriction**

   ☑7ᵗʰ **W49.9 Exposure to other inanimate mechanical forces**

Exposure to animate mechanical forces (W50-W64)

   EXCLUDES 1   *Toxic effect of contact with venomous animals and plants (T63.-)*

☑4ᵗʰ **W50 Accidental hit, strike, kick, twist, bite or scratch by another person**
       Hit, strike, kick, twist, bite, or scratch by another person NOS
   EXCLUDES 1   assault by bodily force (Y04)
            struck by objects (W20-W22)

> The appropriate 7th character is to be added to each code from category W50.
> A   initial encounter
> D   subsequent encounter
> S   sequela

   ☑7ᵗʰ **W50.0 Accidental hit or strike by another person**
       Hit or strike by another person NOS

   ☑7ᵗʰ **W50.1 Accidental kick by another person**
       Kick by another person NOS

   ☑7ᵗʰ **W50.2 Accidental twist by another person**
       Twist by another person NOS

   ☑7ᵗʰ **W50.3 Accidental bite by another person**
       Human bite
       Bite by another person NOS

   ☑7ᵗʰ **W50.4 Accidental scratch by another person**
       Scratch by another person NOS

☑7ᵗʰ **W51 Accidental striking against or bumped into by another person**
   EXCLUDES 1   assault by striking against or bumping into by another person
            (Y04.2)
            fall due to collision with another person (W03)

> The appropriate 7th character is to be added to code W51.
> A   initial encounter
> D   subsequent encounter
> S   sequela

☑7ᵗʰ **W52 Crushed, pushed or stepped on by crowd or human stampede**
       Crushed, pushed or stepped on by crowd or human stampede with or
       without fall

> The appropriate 7th character is to be added to code W52.
> A   initial encounter
> D   subsequent encounter
> S   sequela

☑4ᵗʰ **W53 Contact with rodent**
   INCLUDES   contact with saliva, feces or urine of rodent

> The appropriate 7th character is to be added to each code from category W53.
> A   initial encounter
> D   subsequent encounter
> S   sequela

   ☑5ᵗʰ **W53.0 Contact with** mouse

     ☑7ᵗʰ **W53.01 Bitten by mouse**

     ☑7ᵗʰ **W53.09 Other contact with mouse**

   ☑5ᵗʰ **W53.1 Contact with** rat

     ☑7ᵗʰ **W53.11 Bitten by rat**

     ☑7ᵗʰ **W53.19 Other contact with rat**

   ☑5ᵗʰ **W53.2 Contact with** squirrel

     ☑7ᵗʰ **W53.21 Bitten by squirrel**

     ☑7ᵗʰ **W53.29 Other contact with squirrel**

   ☑5ᵗʰ **W53.8 Contact with** other rodent

     ☑7ᵗʰ **W53.81 Bitten by other rodent**

     ☑7ᵗʰ **W53.89 Other contact with other rodent**

☑4ᵗʰ **W54 Contact with dog**
   INCLUDES   contact with saliva, feces or urine of dog

> The appropriate 7th character is to be added to each code from category W54.
> A   initial encounter
> D   subsequent encounter
> S   sequela

   ☑7ᵗʰ **W54.0 Bitten by dog**

   ☑7ᵗʰ **W54.1 Struck by dog**
       Knocked over by dog

   ☑7ᵗʰ **W54.8 Other contact with dog**

☑4ᵗʰ **W55 Contact with other mammals**
   INCLUDES   contact with saliva, feces or urine of mammal
   EXCLUDES 1   animal being ridden—see transport accidents
            bitten or struck by dog (W54)
            bitten or struck by rodent (W53.-)
            contact with marine mammals (W56.-)

> The appropriate 7th character is to be added to each code from category W55.
> A   initial encounter
> D   subsequent encounter
> S   sequela

   ☑5ᵗʰ **W55.0 Contact with** cat

     ☑7ᵗʰ **W55.01 Bitten by cat**

     ☑7ᵗʰ **W55.03 Scratched by cat**

     ☑7ᵗʰ **W55.09 Other contact with cat**

   ☑5ᵗʰ **W55.1 Contact with** horse

     ☑7ᵗʰ **W55.11 Bitten by horse**

     ☑7ᵗʰ **W55.12 Struck by horse**

     ☑7ᵗʰ **W55.19 Other contact with horse**

   ☑5ᵗʰ **W55.2 Contact with** cow
       Contact with bull

     ☑7ᵗʰ **W55.21 Bitten by cow**

     ☑7ᵗʰ **W55.22 Struck by cow**
         Gored by bull

     ☑7ᵗʰ **W55.29 Other contact with cow**

   ☑5ᵗʰ **W55.3 Contact with other** hoof stock
       Contact with goats
       Contact with sheep

     ☑7ᵗʰ **W55.31 Bitten by other hoof stock**

     ☑7ᵗʰ **W55.32 Struck by other hoof stock**
         Gored by goat
         Gored by ram

     ☑7ᵗʰ **W55.39 Other contact with other hoof stock**

   ☑5ᵗʰ **W55.4 Contact with** pig

     ☑7ᵗʰ **W55.41 Bitten by pig**

     ☑7ᵗʰ **W55.42 Struck by pig**

     ☑7ᵗʰ **W55.49 Other contact with pig**

   ☑5ᵗʰ **W55.5 Contact with** raccoon

     ☑7ᵗʰ **W55.51 Bitten by raccoon**

EXCLUDES 1 Not coded here   EXCLUDES 2 Not included here   N Newborn Age: 0   P Pediatric Age: 0-17   M Maternity Age: 12-55   A Adult Age: 15-124

1030   ICD-10-CM Draft (2015)

✓x7ᵗʰ   **W55.52**   Struck **by raccoon**

✓x7ᵗʰ   **W55.59**   Other contact with raccoon

✓5ᵗʰ   **W55.8 Contact with** other mammals

     ✓x7ᵗʰ   **W55.81**   Bitten **by other mammals**

     ✓x7ᵗʰ   **W55.82**   Struck **by other mammals**

     ✓x7ᵗʰ   **W55.89**   Other contact with other mammals

✓4ᵗʰ   **W56 Contact with nonvenomous marine animal**

     EXCLUDES 1   *contact with venomous marine animal (T63.-)*

     The appropriate 7th character is to be added to each code from category W56.
     A   initial encounter
     D   subsequent encounter
     S   sequela

✓5ᵗʰ   **W56.0 Contact with** dolphin

     ✓x7ᵗʰ   **W56.01**   Bitten **by dolphin**

     ✓x7ᵗʰ   **W56.02**   Struck **by dolphin**

     ✓x7ᵗʰ   **W56.09**   Other contact with dolphin

✓5ᵗʰ   **W56.1 Contact with** sea lion

     ✓x7ᵗʰ   **W56.11**   Bitten **by sea lion**

     ✓x7ᵗʰ   **W56.12**   Struck **by sea lion**

     ✓x7ᵗʰ   **W56.19**   Other contact with sea lion

✓5ᵗʰ   **W56.2 Contact with** orca

     Contact with killer whale

     ✓x7ᵗʰ   **W56.21**   Bitten **by orca**

     ✓x7ᵗʰ   **W56.22**   Struck **by orca**

     ✓x7ᵗʰ   **W56.29**   Other contact with orca

✓5ᵗʰ   **W56.3 Contact with** other marine mammals

     ✓x7ᵗʰ   **W56.31**   Bitten **by other marine mammals**

     ✓x7ᵗʰ   **W56.32**   Struck **by other marine mammals**

     ✓x7ᵗʰ   **W56.39**   Other contact with other marine mammals

✓5ᵗʰ   **W56.4 Contact with** shark

     ✓x7ᵗʰ   **W56.41**   Bitten **by shark**

     ✓x7ᵗʰ   **W56.42**   Struck **by shark**

     ✓x7ᵗʰ   **W56.49**   Other contact with shark

✓5ᵗʰ   **W56.5 Contact with other** fish

     ✓x7ᵗʰ   **W56.51**   Bitten **by other fish**

     ✓x7ᵗʰ   **W56.52**   Struck **by other fish**

     ✓x7ᵗʰ   **W56.59**   Other contact with other fish

✓5ᵗʰ   **W56.8 Contact with** other nonvenomous marine animals

     ✓x7ᵗʰ   **W56.81**   Bitten **by other nonvenomous marine animals**

     ✓x7ᵗʰ   **W56.82**   Struck **by other nonvenomous marine animals**

     ✓x7ᵗʰ   **W56.89**   Other contact with other nonvenomous marine animals

✓x7ᵗʰ   **W57 Bitten or stung by nonvenomous insect and other nonvenomous arthropods**

     EXCLUDES 1   *contact with venomous insects and arthropods (T63.2-, T63.3-, T63.4-)*

     The appropriate 7th character is to be added to code W57.
     A   initial encounter
     D   subsequent encounter
     S   sequela

✓4ᵗʰ   **W58 Contact with crocodile or alligator**

     The appropriate 7th character is to be added to each code from category W58.
     A   initial encounter
     D   subsequent encounter
     S   sequela

✓5ᵗʰ   **W58.0 Contact with** alligator

     ✓x7ᵗʰ   **W58.01**   Bitten **by alligator**

     ✓x7ᵗʰ   **W58.02**   Struck **by alligator**

     ✓x7ᵗʰ   **W58.03**   Crushed **by alligator**

     ✓x7ᵗʰ   **W58.09**   Other contact with alligator

✓5ᵗʰ   **W58.1 Contact with** crocodile

     ✓x7ᵗʰ   **W58.11**   Bitten **by crocodile**

     ✓x7ᵗʰ   **W58.12**   Struck **by crocodile**

     ✓x7ᵗʰ   **W58.13**   Crushed **by crocodile**

     ✓x7ᵗʰ   **W58.19**   Other contact with crocodile

✓4ᵗʰ   **W59 Contact with other nonvenomous reptiles**

     EXCLUDES 1   *contact with venomous reptile (T63.0-, T63.1-)*

     The appropriate 7th character is to be added to each code from category W59.
     A   initial encounter
     D   subsequent encounter
     S   sequela

✓5ᵗʰ   **W59.0 Contact with nonvenomous** lizards

     ✓x7ᵗʰ   **W59.01**   Bitten **by nonvenomous lizards**

     ✓x7ᵗʰ   **W59.02**   Struck **by nonvenomous lizards**

     ✓x7ᵗʰ   **W59.09**   Other contact with nonvenomous lizards

         Exposure to nonvenomous lizards

✓5ᵗʰ   **W59.1 Contact with nonvenomous** snakes

     ✓x7ᵗʰ   **W59.11**   Bitten **by nonvenomous snake**

     ✓x7ᵗʰ   **W59.12**   Struck **by nonvenomous snake**

     ✓x7ᵗʰ   **W59.13**   Crushed **by nonvenomous snake**

     ✓x7ᵗʰ   **W59.19**   Other contact with nonvenomous snake

✓5ᵗʰ   **W59.2 Contact with** turtles

     EXCLUDES 1   *contact with tortoises (W59.8-)*

     ✓x7ᵗʰ   **W59.21**   Bitten **by turtle**

     ✓x7ᵗʰ   **W59.22**   Struck **by turtle**

     ✓x7ᵗʰ   **W59.29**   Other contact with turtle

         Exposure to turtles

✓5ᵗʰ   **W59.8 Contact with** other nonvenomous reptiles

     ✓x7ᵗʰ   **W59.81**   Bitten **by other nonvenomous reptiles**

     ✓x7ᵗʰ   **W59.82**   Struck **by other nonvenomous reptiles**

     ✓x7ᵗʰ   **W59.83**   Crushed **by other nonvenomous reptiles**

     ✓x7ᵗʰ   **W59.89**   Other contact with other nonvenomous reptiles

✓x7ᵗʰ   **W60 Contact with nonvenomous plant thorns and spines and sharp leaves**

     EXCLUDES 1   *contact with venomous plants (T63.7-)*

     The appropriate 7th character is to be added to code W60.
     A   initial encounter
     D   subsequent encounter
     S   sequela

✓4ᵗʰ   **W61 Contact with birds (domestic) (wild)**

     INCLUDES   contact with excreta of birds

     The appropriate 7th character is to be added to each code from category W61.
     A   initial encounter
     D   subsequent encounter
     S   sequela

✓5ᵗʰ   **W61.0 Contact with** parrot

     ✓x7ᵗʰ   **W61.01**   Bitten **by parrot**

     ✓x7ᵗʰ   **W61.02**   Struck **by parrot**

     ✓x7ᵗʰ   **W61.09**   Other contact with parrot

         Exposure to parrots

✓5ᵗʰ   **W61.1 Contact with** macaw

     ✓x7ᵗʰ   **W61.11**   Bitten **by macaw**

     ✓x7ᵗʰ   **W61.12**   Struck **by macaw**

     ✓x7ᵗʰ   **W61.19**   Other contact with macaw

         Exposure to macaws

✓5ᵗʰ   **W61.2 Contact with other** psittacines

     ✓x7ᵗʰ   **W61.21**   Bitten **by other psittacines**

     ✓x7ᵗʰ   **W61.22**   Struck **by other psittacines**

     ✓x7ᵗʰ   **W61.29**   Other contact with other psittacines

         Exposure to other psittacines

✓5ᵗʰ   **W61.3 Contact with** chicken

     ✓x7ᵗʰ   **W61.32**   Struck **by chicken**

     ✓x7ᵗʰ   **W61.33**   Pecked **by chicken**

     ✓x7ᵗʰ   **W61.39**   Other contact with chicken

         Exposure to chickens

✓5ᵗʰ   **W61.4 Contact with** turkey

     ✓x7ᵗʰ   **W61.42**   Struck **by turkey**

     ✓x7ᵗʰ   **W61.43**   Pecked **by turkey**

     ✓x7ᵗʰ   **W61.49**   Other contact with turkey

✓5ᵗʰ   **W61.5 Contact with** goose

     ✓x7ᵗʰ   **W61.51**   Bitten **by goose**

✓ Additional Character Required   ✓x7ᵗʰ Xtension Alert   Unspecified Dx   Other Specified Dx   Manifestation   ▶◀ Revised Text   ● New Code   ▲ Revised Code Title

External Causes of Morbidity

W61.52–W89.9

√x7th   **W61.52**   Struck **by goose**

√x7th   **W61.59**   Other contact with **goose**

√5th   **W61.6 Contact with** duck

√x7th   **W61.61**   Bitten **by duck**

√x7th   **W61.62**   Struck **by duck**

√x7th   **W61.69**   Other contact with **duck**

√5th   **W61.9 Contact with** other **birds**

√x7th   **W61.91**   Bitten **by other birds**

√x7th   **W61.92**   Struck **by other birds**

√x7th   **W61.99**   Other contact with other **birds**
        Contact with bird NOS

√4th   **W62 Contact with nonvenomous amphibians**
     EXCLUDES 1   *contact with venomous amphibians (T63.81-R63.83)*

> The appropriate 7th character is to be added to each code from category W62.
> A   initial encounter
> D   subsequent encounter
> S   sequela

√x7th   **W62.0 Contact with nonvenomous** frogs

√x7th   **W62.1 Contact with nonvenomous** toads

√x7th   **W62.9 Contact with other nonvenomous** amphibians

√x7th   **W64 Exposure to other animate mechanical forces**
     INCLUDES   exposure to nonvenomous animal NOS
     EXCLUDES 1   *contact with venomous animal (T63.-)*

> The appropriate 7th character is to be added to code W64.
> A   initial encounter
> D   subsequent encounter
> S   sequela

Accidental non-transport drowning and submersion (W65-W74)

     EXCLUDES 1   *accidental drowning and submersion due to fall into water (W16.-)*
                  accidental drowning and submersion due to water transport accident (V90.-, V92.-)
     EXCLUDES 2   *accidental drowning and submersion due to cataclysm (X34-X39)*

√x7th   **W65 Accidental drowning and submersion while in** bath-tub
     EXCLUDES 1   *accidental drowning and submersion due to fall in (into) bathtub (W16.211)*

> The appropriate 7th character is to be added to code W65.
> A   initial encounter
> D   subsequent encounter
> S   sequela

√x7th   **W67 Accidental drowning and submersion while in** swimming-pool
     EXCLUDES 1   *accidental drowning and submersion due to fall into swimming pool (W16.011, W16.021, W16.031)*
                  accidental drowning and submersion due to striking into wall of swimming pool (W22.041)

> The appropriate 7th character is to be added to code W67.
> A   initial encounter
> D   subsequent encounter
> S   sequela

√x7th   **W69 Accidental drowning and submersion while in** natural water
     Accidental drowning and submersion while in lake
     Accidental drowning and submersion while in open sea
     Accidental drowning and submersion while in river
     Accidental drowning and submersion while in stream
     EXCLUDES 1   *accidental drowning and submersion due to fall into natural body of water (W16.111, W16.121, W16.131)*

> The appropriate 7th character is to be added to code W69.
> A   initial encounter
> D   subsequent encounter
> S   sequela

√x7th   **W73 Other specified cause of accidental non-transport drowning and submersion**
     Accidental drowning and submersion while in quenching tank
     Accidental drowning and submersion while in reservoir
     EXCLUDES 1   *accidental drowning and submersion due to fall into other water (W16.311, W16.321, W16.331)*

> The appropriate 7th character is to be added to code W73.
> A   initial encounter
> D   subsequent encounter
> S   sequela

√x7th   **W74 Unspecified cause of accidental drowning and submersion**
     Drowning NOS

> The appropriate 7th character is to be added to code W74.
> A   initial encounter
> D   subsequent encounter
> S   sequela

Exposure to electric current, radiation and extreme ambient air temperature and pressure (W85-W99)

     EXCLUDES 1   exposure to:
         failure in dosage of radiation or temperature during surgical and medical care (Y63.2-Y63.5)
         lightning (T75.0-)
         natural cold (X31)
         natural heat (X30)
         natural radiation NOS (X39)
         radiological procedure and radiotherapy (Y84.2)
         sunlight (X32)

√x7th   **W85 Exposure to electric transmission lines**
     Broken power line

> The appropriate 7th character is to be added to code W85.
> A   initial encounter
> D   subsequent encounter
> S   sequela

√4th   **W86 Exposure to other specified electric current**

> The appropriate 7th character is to be added to each code from category W86.
> A   initial encounter
> D   subsequent encounter
> S   sequela

√x7th   **W86.0 Exposure to domestic wiring and appliances**

√x7th   **W86.1 Exposure to industrial wiring, appliances and electrical machinery**
     Exposure to conductors
     Exposure to control apparatus
     Exposure to electrical equipment and machinery
     Exposure to transformers

√x7th   **W86.8 Exposure to other electric current**
     Exposure to wiring and appliances in or on farm (not farmhouse)
     Exposure to wiring and appliances outdoors
     Exposure to wiring and appliances in or on public building
     Exposure to wiring and appliances in or on residential institutions
     Exposure to wiring and appliances in or on schools

√4th   **W88 Exposure to ionizing radiation**
     EXCLUDES 1   *exposure to sunlight (X32)*

> The appropriate 7th character is to be added to each code from category W88.
> A   initial encounter
> D   subsequent encounter
> S   sequela

√x7th   **W88.0 Exposure to** X-rays

√x7th   **W88.1 Exposure to** radioactive isotopes

√x7th   **W88.8 Exposure to other ionizing radiation**

√4th   **W89 Exposure to man-made visible and ultraviolet light**
     INCLUDES   exposure to welding light (arc)
     EXCLUDES 2   *exposure to sunlight (X32)*

> The appropriate 7th character is to be added to each code from category W89.
> A   initial encounter
> D   subsequent encounter
> S   sequela

√x7th   **W89.0 Exposure to** welding light **(arc)**

√x7th   **W89.1 Exposure to** tanning bed

√x7th   **W89.8 Exposure to other man-made visible and ultraviolet light**

√x7th   **W89.9 Exposure to unspecified man-made visible and ultraviolet light**

EXCLUDES 1 Not coded here   *EXCLUDES 2* Not included here   N Newborn Age: 0   P Pediatric Age: 0-17   M Maternity Age: 12-55   A Adult Age: 15-124

1032   ICD-10-CM Draft (2015)

✓4th **W90 Exposure to other nonionizing radiation**
>   EXCLUDES 1   *exposure to sunlight (X32)*
>
>   The appropriate 7th character is to be added to each code from category W90.
>   A   initial encounter
>   D   subsequent encounter
>   S   sequela

✓x7th **W90.0 Exposure to** radiofrequency
✓x7th **W90.1 Exposure to** infrared radiation
✓x7th **W90.2 Exposure to** laser radiation
✓x7th **W90.8 Exposure to other nonionizing radiation**

✓x7th **W92 Exposure to excessive heat of man-made origin**
>   The appropriate 7th character is to be added to code W92.
>   A   initial encounter
>   D   subsequent encounter
>   S   sequela

✓4th **W93 Exposure to excessive cold of man-made origin**
>   The appropriate 7th character is to be added to each code from category W93.
>   A   initial encounter
>   D   subsequent encounter
>   S   sequela

✓5th **W93.0 Contact with or inhalation of** dry ice
   ✓x7th **W93.01 Contact with dry ice**
   ✓x7th **W93.02 Inhalation of dry ice**

✓5th **W93.1 Contact with or inhalation of** liquid air
   ✓x7th **W93.11 Contact with liquid air**
      Contact with liquid hydrogen
      Contact with liquid nitrogen
   ✓x7th **W93.12 Inhalation of liquid air**
      Inhalation of liquid hydrogen
      Inhalation of liquid nitrogen

✓x7th **W93.2 Prolonged exposure in deep freeze unit or refrigerator**
✓x7th **W93.8 Exposure to other excessive cold of man-made origin**

✓4th **W94 Exposure to high and low air pressure and changes in air pressure**
>   The appropriate 7th character is to be added to each code from category W94.
>   A   initial encounter
>   D   subsequent encounter
>   S   sequela

✓x7th **W94.0 Exposure to prolonged high air pressure**
✓5th **W94.1 Exposure to prolonged low air pressure**
   ✓x7th **W94.11 Exposure to residence or prolonged visit at high altitude**
   ✓x7th **W94.12 Exposure to other prolonged low air pressure**
✓5th **W94.2 Exposure to rapid changes in air pressure during** ascent
   ✓x7th **W94.21 Exposure to reduction in atmospheric pressure while surfacing from** deep-water diving
   ✓x7th **W94.22 Exposure to reduction in atmospheric pressure while surfacing from** underground
   ✓x7th **W94.23 Exposure to sudden change in air pressure in** aircraft **during ascent**
   ✓x7th **W94.29 Exposure to other rapid changes in air pressure during ascent**
✓5th **W94.3 Exposure to rapid changes in air pressure during** descent
   ✓x7th **W94.31 Exposure to sudden change in air pressure in** aircraft **during descent**
   ✓x7th **W94.32 Exposure to high air pressure from rapid descent in** water
   ✓x7th **W94.39 Exposure to other rapid changes in air pressure during descent**

✓x7th **W99 Exposure to other man-made environmental factors**
>   The appropriate 7th character is to be added to code W99.
>   A   initial encounter
>   D   subsequent encounter
>   S   sequela

Exposure to smoke, fire and flames (X00-X08)

> EXCLUDES 1   *arson (X97)*
> EXCLUDES 2   *explosions (W35-W40)*
>   *lightning (T75.0-)*
>   *transport accident (V01-V99)*

✓4th **X00 Exposure to** uncontrolled fire **in building or structure**
>   INCLUDES   conflagration in building or structure
>   Code first any associated cataclysm
>   EXCLUDES 2   *exposure to ignition or melting of nightwear (X05)*
>   *exposure to ignition or melting of other clothing and apparel (X06.-)*
>   *exposure to other specified smoke, fire and flames (X08.-)*
>
>   The appropriate 7th character is to be added to each code from category X00.
>   A   initial encounter
>   D   subsequent encounter
>   S   sequela

✓x7th **X00.0 Exposure to** flames **in uncontrolled fire in building or structure**
✓x7th **X00.1 Exposure to** smoke **in uncontrolled fire in building or structure**
✓x7th **X00.2 Injury due to collapse of burning building or structure in uncontrolled fire**
>   EXCLUDES 1   *injury due to collapse of building not on fire (W20.1)*
✓x7th **X00.3 Fall from burning building or structure in uncontrolled fire**
✓x7th **X00.4 Hit by object from burning building or structure in uncontrolled fire**
✓x7th **X00.5 Jump from burning building or structure in uncontrolled fire**
✓x7th **X00.8 Other exposure to uncontrolled fire in building or structure**

✓4th **X01 Exposure to uncontrolled fire, not in building or structure**
>   INCLUDES   exposure to forest fire
>
>   The appropriate 7th character is to be added to each code from category X01.
>   A   initial encounter
>   D   subsequent encounter
>   S   sequela

✓x7th **X01.0 Exposure to** flames **in uncontrolled fire, not in building or structure**
✓x7th **X01.1 Exposure to** smoke **in uncontrolled fire, not in building or structure**
✓x7th **X01.3 Fall due to uncontrolled fire, not in building or structure**
✓x7th **X01.4 Hit by object due to uncontrolled fire, not in building or structure**
✓x7th **X01.8 Other exposure to uncontrolled fire, not in building or structure**

✓4th **X02 Exposure to** controlled fire **in building or structure**
>   INCLUDES   exposure to fire in fireplace
>   exposure to fire in stove
>
>   The appropriate 7th character is to be added to each code from category X02.
>   A   initial encounter
>   D   subsequent encounter
>   S   sequela

✓x7th **X02.0 Exposure to** flames **in controlled fire in building or structure**
✓x7th **X02.1 Exposure to** smoke **in controlled fire in building or structure**
✓x7th **X02.2 Injury due to collapse of burning building or structure in controlled fire**
>   EXCLUDES 1   *injury due to collapse of building not on fire (W20.1)*
✓x7th **X02.3 Fall from burning building or structure in controlled fire**
✓x7th **X02.4 Hit by object from burning building or structure in controlled fire**
✓x7th **X02.5 Jump from burning building or structure in controlled fire**
✓x7th **X02.8 Other exposure to controlled fire in building or structure**

✓ Additional Character Required   ✓x7th Xtension Alert   Unspecified Dx   Other Specified Dx   Manifestation   ▶◀ Revised Text   ● New Code   ▲ Revised Code Title

☑4ᵗʰ **X03** **Exposure to** controlled fire**, not in building or structure**
> INCLUDES   exposure to bon fire
> exposure to camp-fire
> exposure to trash fire

> The appropriate 7th character is to be added to each code from category X03.
> A   initial encounter
> D   subsequent encounter
> S   sequela

☑x7ᵗʰ **X03.0** **Exposure to** flames **in controlled fire, not in building or structure**

☑x7ᵗʰ **X03.1** **Exposure to** smoke **in controlled fire, not in building or structure**

☑x7ᵗʰ **X03.3** Fall due to **controlled fire, not in building or structure**

☑x7ᵗʰ **X03.4** Hit by object **due to controlled fire, not in building or structure**

☑x7ᵗʰ **X03.8** **Other exposure to controlled fire, not in building or structure**

☑x7ᵗʰ **X04** **Exposure to ignition of highly flammable material**
> Exposure to ignition of gasoline
> Exposure to ignition of kerosene
> Exposure to ignition of petrol
> EXCLUDES 2   exposure to ignition or melting of nightwear (X05)
> exposure to ignition or melting of other clothing and apparel (X06)

> The appropriate 7th character is to be added to code X04.
> A   initial encounter
> D   subsequent encounter
> S   sequela

☑x7ᵗʰ **X05** **Exposure to ignition or melting of nightwear**
> EXCLUDES 2   exposure to uncontrolled fire in building or structure (X00.-)
> exposure to uncontrolled fire, not in building or structure (X01.-)
> exposure to controlled fire in building or structure (X02.-)
> exposure to controlled fire, not in building or structure (X03.-)
> exposure to ignition of highly flammable materials (X04.-)

> The appropriate 7th character is to be added to code X05.
> A   initial encounter
> D   subsequent encounter
> S   sequela

☑4ᵗʰ **X06** **Exposure to ignition or melting of other clothing and apparel**
> EXCLUDES 2   exposure to uncontrolled fire in building or structure (X00.-)
> exposure to uncontrolled fire, not in building or structure (X01.-)
> exposure to controlled fire in building or structure (X02.-)
> exposure to controlled fire, not in building or structure (X03.-)
> exposure to ignition of highly flammable materials (X04.-)

> The appropriate 7th character is to be added to each code from category X06.
> A   initial encounter
> D   subsequent encounter
> S   sequela

☑x7ᵗʰ **X06.0** **Exposure to ignition of plastic jewelry**

☑x7ᵗʰ **X06.1** **Exposure to melting of plastic jewelry**

☑x7ᵗʰ **X06.2** **Exposure to ignition of other clothing and apparel**

☑x7ᵗʰ **X06.3** **Exposure to melting of other clothing and apparel**

☑4ᵗʰ **X08** **Exposure to other specified smoke, fire and flames**

> The appropriate 7th character is to be added to each code from category X08.
> A   initial encounter
> D   subsequent encounter
> S   sequela

☑5ᵗʰ **X08.0** **Exposure to** bed **fire**
> Exposure to mattress fire

☑x7ᵗʰ   **X08.00** **Exposure to bed fire due to unspecified burning material**

☑x7ᵗʰ   **X08.01** **Exposure to bed fire due to** burning cigarette

☑x7ᵗʰ   **X08.09** **Exposure to bed fire due to other burning material**

☑5ᵗʰ **X08.1** **Exposure to** sofa **fire**

☑x7ᵗʰ   **X08.10** **Exposure to sofa fire due to unspecified burning material**

☑x7ᵗʰ   **X08.11** **Exposure to sofa fire due to** burning cigarette

☑x7ᵗʰ   **X08.19** **Exposure to sofa fire due to other burning material**

☑5ᵗʰ **X08.2** **Exposure to** other furniture **fire**

☑x7ᵗʰ   **X08.20** **Exposure to other furniture fire due to unspecified burning material**

☑x7ᵗʰ   **X08.21** **Exposure to other furniture fire due to** burning cigarette

☑x7ᵗʰ   **X08.29** **Exposure to other furniture fire due to other burning material**

☑x7ᵗʰ **X08.8** **Exposure to other specified smoke, fire and flames**

Contact with heat and hot substances (X10-X19)

> EXCLUDES 1   exposure to excessive natural heat (X30)
> exposure to fire and flames (X00-X09)

☑4ᵗʰ **X10** **Contact with hot drinks, food, fats and cooking oils**

> The appropriate 7th character is to be added to each code from category X10.
> A   initial encounter
> D   subsequent encounter
> S   sequela

☑x7ᵗʰ **X10.0** **Contact with hot** drinks

☑x7ᵗʰ **X10.1** **Contact with hot** food

☑x7ᵗʰ **X10.2** **Contact with** fats and cooking oils

☑4ᵗʰ **X11** **Contact with hot tap-water**
> INCLUDES   contact with boiling tap-water
> contact with boiling water NOS
> EXCLUDES 1   contact with water heated on stove (X12)

> The appropriate 7th character is to be added to each code from category X11.
> A   initial encounter
> D   subsequent encounter
> S   sequela

☑x7ᵗʰ **X11.0** **Contact with hot water** in bath or tub
> EXCLUDES 1   contact with running hot water in bath or tub (X11.1)

☑x7ᵗʰ **X11.1** **Contact with** running **hot water**
> Contact with hot water running out of hose
> Contact with hot water running out of tap

☑x7ᵗʰ **X11.8** **Contact with other hot tap-water**
> Contact with hot water in bucket
> Contact with hot tap-water NOS

☑x7ᵗʰ **X12** **Contact with other hot fluids**
> Contact with water heated on stove
> EXCLUDES 1   hot (liquid) metals (X18)

> The appropriate 7th character is to be added to code X12.
> A   initial encounter
> D   subsequent encounter
> S   sequela

☑4ᵗʰ **X13** **Contact with steam and other hot vapors**

> The appropriate 7th character is to be added to each code from category X13.
> A   initial encounter
> D   subsequent encounter
> S   sequela

☑x7ᵗʰ **X13.0** **Inhalation of steam and other hot vapors**

☑x7ᵗʰ **X13.1** **Other contact with steam and other hot vapors**

☑4ᵗʰ **X14** **Contact with hot air and other hot gases**

> The appropriate 7th character is to be added to each code from category X14.
> A   initial encounter
> D   subsequent encounter
> S   sequela

☑x7ᵗʰ **X14.0** **Inhalation of hot air and gases**

☑x7ᵗʰ **X14.1** **Other contact with hot air and other hot gases**

☑4ᵗʰ **X15** **Contact with hot household appliances**
> EXCLUDES 1   contact with heating appliances (X16)
> contact with powered household appliances (W29.-)
> exposure to controlled fire in building or structure due to household appliance (X02.8)
> exposure to household appliances electrical current (W86.0)

> The appropriate 7th character is to be added to each code from category X15.
> A   initial encounter
> D   subsequent encounter
> S   sequela

☑x7ᵗʰ **X15.0** **Contact with hot** stove **(kitchen)**

☑x7ᵗʰ **X15.1** **Contact with hot** toaster

EXCLUDES 1 Not coded here   EXCLUDES 2 Not included here   N Newborn Age: 0   P Pediatric Age: 0-17   M Maternity Age: 12-55   A Adult Age: 15-124

1034   ICD-10-CM Draft (2015)

√x7ᵗʰ **X15.2 Contact with** hotplate

√x7ᵗʰ **X15.3 Contact with hot** saucepan or skillet

√x7ᵗʰ **X15.8 Contact with other hot household appliances**
    Contact with cooker   Contact with light bulbs
    Contact with kettle

√x7ᵗʰ **X16 Contact with hot heating appliances, radiators and pipes**
  EXCLUDES 1 *contact with powered appliances (W29.-)*
     exposure to controlled fire in building or structure due to
      appliance (X02.8)
     exposure to industrial appliances electrical current (W86.1)

  The appropriate 7th character is to be added to code X16.
  A initial encounter
  D subsequent encounter
  S sequela

√x7ᵗʰ **X17 Contact with hot engines, machinery and tools**
  EXCLUDES 1 *contact with hot heating appliances, radiators and pipes (X16)*
     contact with hot household appliances (X15)

  The appropriate 7th character is to be added to code X17.
  A initial encounter
  D subsequent encounter
  S sequela

√x7ᵗʰ **X18 Contact with other hot metals**
   Contact with liquid metal

  The appropriate 7th character is to be added to code X18.
  A initial encounter
  D subsequent encounter
  S sequela

√x7ᵗʰ **X19 Contact with other heat and hot substances**
  EXCLUDES 1 *objects that are not normally hot, e.g., an object made hot by a*
     house fire (X00-X09)

  The appropriate 7th character is to be added to code X19.
  A initial encounter
  D subsequent encounter
  S sequela

Exposure to forces of nature (X30-X39)

√x7ᵗʰ **X30 Exposure to excessive** natural heat
   Exposure to excessive heat as the cause of sunstroke
   Exposure to heat NOS
  EXCLUDES 1 *excessive heat of man-made origin (W92)*
     exposure to man-made radiation (W89)
     exposure to sunlight (X32)
     exposure to tanning bed (W89)

  The appropriate 7th character is to be added to code X30.
  A initial encounter
  D subsequent encounter
  S sequela

√x7ᵗʰ **X31 Exposure to excessive** natural cold
   Excessive cold as the cause of chilblains NOS
   Excessive cold as the cause of immersion foot or hand
   Exposure to cold NOS
   Exposure to weather conditions
  EXCLUDES 1 *cold of man-made origin (W93.-)*
     contact with or inhalation of dry ice (W93.-)
     contact with or inhalation of liquefied gas (W93.-)

  The appropriate 7th character is to be added to code X31.
  A initial encounter
  D subsequent encounter
  S sequela

√x7ᵗʰ **X32 Exposure to sunlight**
  EXCLUDES 1 *radiation-related disorders of the skin and subcutaneous tissue*
     (L55-L59)
     man-made radiation (tanning bed) (W89)

  The appropriate 7th character is to be added to code X32.
  A initial encounter
  D subsequent encounter
  S sequela

√x7ᵗʰ **X34 Earthquake**
  EXCLUDES 2 *tidal wave (tsunami) due to earthquake (X37.41)*

  The appropriate 7th character is to be added to code X34.
  A initial encounter
  D subsequent encounter
  S sequela

√x7ᵗʰ **X35 Volcanic eruption**
  EXCLUDES 2 *tidal wave (tsunami) due to volcanic eruption (X37.41)*

  The appropriate 7th character is to be added to code X35.
  A initial encounter
  D subsequent encounter
  S sequela

√4ᵗʰ **X36 Avalanche, landslide and other earth movements**
  INCLUDES victim of mudslide of cataclysmic nature
  EXCLUDES 1 *earthquake (X34)*
  EXCLUDES 2 *transport accident involving collision with avalanche or*
     landslide not in motion (V01-V99)

  The appropriate 7th character is to be added to each code from
  category X36.
  A initial encounter
  D subsequent encounter
  S sequela

√x7ᵗʰ **X36.0 Collapse of dam or man-made structure causing earth
   movement**

√x7ᵗʰ **X36.1 Avalanche, landslide, or mudslide**

√4ᵗʰ **X37 Cataclysmic storm**

  The appropriate 7th character is to be added to each code from
  category X37.
  A initial encounter
  D subsequent encounter
  S sequela

√x7ᵗʰ **X37.0 Hurricane**
   Storm surge
   Typhoon

√x7ᵗʰ **X37.1 Tornado**
   Cyclone
   Twister

√x7ᵗʰ **X37.2 Blizzard (snow)(ice)**

√x7ᵗʰ **X37.3 Dust storm**

√5ᵗʰ **X37.4 Tidalwave**

  √x7ᵗʰ **X37.41 Tidal wave due to** earthquake **or** volcanic eruption
     Tidal wave NOS
     Tsunami

  √x7ᵗʰ **X37.42 Tidal wave due to** storm

  √x7ᵗʰ **X37.43 Tidal wave due to** landslide

√x7ᵗʰ **X37.8 Other cataclysmic storms**
   Cloudburst
   Torrential rain
   EXCLUDES 2 *flood (X38)*

√x7ᵗʰ **X37.9 Unspecified cataclysmic storm**
   Storm NOS
   EXCLUDES 1 *collapse of dam or man-made structure causing earth*
     movement (X39.0)

√x7ᵗʰ **X38 Flood**
   Flood arising from remote storm
   Flood of cataclysmic nature arising from melting snow
   Flood resulting directly from storm
  EXCLUDES 1 *collapse of dam or man-made structure causing earth*
     movement (X39.0)
     tidal wave NOS (X37.41)
     tidal wave caused by storm (X37.2)

  The appropriate 7th character is to be added to code X38.
  A initial encounter
  D subsequent encounter
  S sequela

√4ᵗʰ **X39 Exposure to other forces of nature**

  The appropriate 7th character is to be added to each code from
  category X39.
  A initial encounter
  D subsequent encounter
  S sequela

√5ᵗʰ **X39.0 Exposure to natural radiation**
   EXCLUDES 1 *contact with and (suspected) exposure to radon and*
     other naturally occuring radiation (Z77.122)
     exposure to man-made radiation (W88-W90)
     exposure to sunlight (X32)

  √x7ᵗʰ **X39.01 Exposure to radon**

  √x7ᵗʰ **X39.08 Exposure to other natural radiation**

√x7ᵗʰ **X39.8 Other exposure to forces of nature**

☑ Additional Character Required √x7ᵗʰ Xtension Alert Unspecified Dx Other Specified Dx Manifestation ▶◀ Revised Text ● New Code ▲ Revised Code Title

ICD-10-CM Draft (2015)   1035

Accidental exposure to other specified factors (X52, X58)

√x7ᵗʰ X52 Prolonged stay in weightless environment
Weightlessness in spacecraft (simulator)

The appropriate 7th character is to be added to code X52.
A   initial encounter
D   subsequent encounter
S   sequela

√x7ᵗʰ X58 Exposure to other specified factors
Accident NOS
Exposure NOS

The appropriate 7th character is to be added to code X58.
A   initial encounter
D   subsequent encounter
S   sequela

Intentional self-harm (X71-X83)

Purposely self-inflicted injury
Suicide (attempted)

√4ᵗʰ X71 Intentional self-harm by drowning and submersion

The appropriate 7th character is to be added to each code from category X71.
A   initial encounter
D   subsequent encounter
S   sequela

√x7ᵗʰ X71.0 Intentional self-harm by drowning and submersion while in bathtub

√x7ᵗʰ X71.1 Intentional self-harm by drowning and submersion while in swimming pool

√x7ᵗʰ X71.2 Intentional self-harm by drowning and submersion after jump into swimming pool

√x7ᵗʰ X71.3 Intentional self-harm by drowning and submersion in natural water

√x7ᵗʰ X71.8 Other intentional self-harm by drowning and submersion

√x7ᵗʰ X71.9 Intentional self-harm by drowning and submersion, unspecified

√x7ᵗʰ X72 Intentional self-harm by handgun discharge
Intentional self-harm by gun for single hand use
Intentional self-harm by pistol
Intentional self-harm by revolver
EXCLUDES 1   Very pistol (X74.8)

The appropriate 7th character is to be added to code X72.
A   initial encounter
D   subsequent encounter
S   sequela

√4ᵗʰ X73 Intentional self-harm by rifle, shotgun and larger firearm discharge
EXCLUDES 1   airgun (X74.01)

The appropriate 7th character is to be added to each code from category X73.
A   initial encounter
D   subsequent encounter
S   sequela

√x7ᵗʰ X73.0 Intentional self-harm by shotgun discharge

√x7ᵗʰ X73.1 Intentional self-harm by hunting rifle discharge

√x7ᵗʰ X73.2 Intentional self-harm by machine gun discharge

√x7ᵗʰ X73.8 Intentional self-harm by other larger firearm discharge

√x7ᵗʰ X73.9 Intentional self-harm by unspecified larger firearm discharge

√4ᵗʰ X74 Intentional self-harm by other and unspecified firearm and gun discharge

The appropriate 7th character is to be added to each code from category X74.
A   initial encounter
D   subsequent encounter
S   sequela

√5ᵗʰ X74.0 Intentional self-harm by gas, air or spring-operated guns

√x7ᵗʰ X74.01 Intentional self-harm by airgun
Intentional self-harm by BB gun discharge
Intentional self-harm by pellet gun discharge

√x7ᵗʰ X74.02 Intentional self-harm by paintball gun

√x7ᵗʰ X74.09 Intentional self-harm by other gas, air or spring-operated gun

√x7ᵗʰ X74.8 Intentional self-harm by other firearm discharge
Intentional self-harm by Very pistol [flare] discharge

√x7ᵗʰ X74.9 Intentional self-harm by unspecified firearm discharge

√x7ᵗʰ X75 Intentional self-harm by explosive material

The appropriate 7th character is to be added to code X75.
A   initial encounter
D   subsequent encounter
S   sequela

√x7ᵗʰ X76 Intentional self-harm by smoke, fire and flames

The appropriate 7th character is to be added to code X76.
A   initial encounter
D   subsequent encounter
S   sequela

√4ᵗʰ X77 Intentional self-harm by steam, hot vapors and hot objects

The appropriate 7th character is to be added to each code from category X77.
A   initial encounter
D   subsequent encounter
S   sequela

√x7ᵗʰ X77.0 Intentional self-harm by steam or hot vapors

√x7ᵗʰ X77.1 Intentional self-harm by hot tap water

√x7ᵗʰ X77.2 Intentional self-harm by other hot fluids

√x7ᵗʰ X77.3 Intentional self-harm by hot household appliances

√x7ᵗʰ X77.8 Intentional self-harm by other hot objects

√x7ᵗʰ X77.9 Intentional self-harm by unspecified hot objects

√4ᵗʰ X78 Intentional self-harm by sharp object

The appropriate 7th character is to be added to each code from category X78.
A   initial encounter
D   subsequent encounter
S   sequela

√x7ᵗʰ X78.0 Intentional self-harm by sharp glass

√x7ᵗʰ X78.1 Intentional self-harm by knife

√x7ᵗʰ X78.2 Intentional self-harm by sword or dagger

√x7ᵗʰ X78.8 Intentional self-harm by other sharp object

√x7ᵗʰ X78.9 Intentional self-harm by unspecified sharp object

√x7ᵗʰ X79 Intentional self-harm by blunt object

The appropriate 7th character is to be added to code X79.
A   initial encounter
D   subsequent encounter
S   sequela

√x7ᵗʰ X80 Intentional self-harm by jumping from a high place
Intentional fall from one level to another

The appropriate 7th character is to be added to code X80.
A   initial encounter
D   subsequent encounter
S   sequela

√4ᵗʰ X81 Intentional self-harm by jumping or lying in front of moving object

The appropriate 7th character is to be added to each code from category X81.
A   initial encounter
D   subsequent encounter
S   sequela

√x7ᵗʰ X81.0 Intentional self-harm by jumping or lying in front of motor vehicle

√x7ᵗʰ X81.1 Intentional self-harm by jumping or lying in front of (subway) train

√x7ᵗʰ X81.8 Intentional self-harm by jumping or lying in front of other moving object

√4ᵗʰ X82 Intentional self-harm by crashing of motor vehicle

The appropriate 7th character is to be added to each code from category X82.
A   initial encounter
D   subsequent encounter
S   sequela

√x7ᵗʰ X82.0 Intentional collision of motor vehicle with other motor vehicle

√x7ᵗʰ X82.1 Intentional collision of motor vehicle with train

EXCLUDES 1 Not coded here   **EXCLUDES 2** Not included here   N Newborn Age: 0   P Pediatric Age: 0-17   M Maternity Age: 12-55   A Adult Age: 15-124

1036   ICD-10-CM Draft (2015)

✓x7th X82.2 **Intentional collision of motor vehicle with** tree

✓x7th X82.8 **Other intentional self-harm by crashing of motor vehicle**

✓4th **X83 Intentional self-harm by other specified means**
  EXCLUDES 1 *intentional self-harm by poisoning or contact with toxic substance—see Table of Drugs and Chemicals*

The appropriate 7th character is to be added to each code from category X83.
  A   initial encounter
  D   subsequent encounter
  S   sequela

✓x7th X83.0 **Intentional self-harm by** crashing of aircraft

✓x7th X83.1 **Intentional self-harm by** electrocution

✓x7th X83.2 **Intentional self-harm by** exposure to extremes of cold

✓x7th X83.8 **Intentional self-harm by other specified means**

Assault (X92–Y08)

INCLUDES homicide
  injuries inflicted by another person with intent to injure or kill, by any means
EXCLUDES 1 *injuries due to legal intervention (Y35.-)*
  injuries due to operations of war (Y36.-)
  injuries due to terrorism (Y38.-)

✓4th **X92 Assault by drowning and submersion**

The appropriate 7th character is to be added to each code from category X92.
  A   initial encounter
  D   subsequent encounter
  S   sequela

✓x7th X92.0 **Assault by drowning and submersion while in** bathtub

✓x7th X92.1 **Assault by drowning and submersion while in** swimming pool

✓x7th X92.2 **Assault by drowning and submersion** after push into swimming pool

✓x7th X92.3 **Assault by drowning and submersion** in natural water

✓x7th X92.8 **Other assault by drowning and submersion**

✓x7th X92.9 **Assault by drowning and submersion, unspecified**

✓x7th **X93 Assault by** handgun **discharge**
  Assault by discharge of gun for single hand use
  Assault by discharge of pistol
  Assault by discharge of revolver
  EXCLUDES 1 *Very pistol (X95.8)*

The appropriate 7th character is to be added to code X93.
  A   initial encounter
  D   subsequent encounter
  S   sequela

✓4th **X94 Assault by** rifle, shotgun and larger firearm **discharge**
  EXCLUDES 1 *airgun (X95.01)*

The appropriate 7th character is to be added to each code from category X94.
  A   initial encounter
  D   subsequent encounter
  S   sequela

✓x7th X94.0 **Assault by** shotgun

✓x7th X94.1 **Assault by** hunting rifle

✓x7th X94.2 **Assault by** machine gun

✓x7th X94.8 **Assault by other larger firearm discharge**

✓x7th X94.9 **Assault by unspecified larger firearm discharge**

✓4th **X95 Assault by other and unspecified firearm and gun discharge**

The appropriate 7th character is to be added to each code from category X95.
  A   initial encounter
  D   subsequent encounter
  S   sequela

✓5th X95.0 **Assault by** gas, air or spring-operated guns

  ✓x7th X95.01 **Assault by** airgun **discharge**
    Assault by BB gun discharge
    Assault by pellet gun discharge

  ✓x7th X95.02 **Assault by** paintball gun **discharge**

  ✓x7th X95.09 **Assault by other gas, air or spring-operated gun**

✓x7th X95.8 **Assault by other firearm discharge**
    Assault by Very pistol [flare] discharge

✓x7th X95.9 **Assault by unspecified firearm discharge**

✓4th **X96 Assault by explosive material**
  EXCLUDES 1 *incendiary device (X97)*
    terrorism involving explosive material (Y38.2-)

The appropriate 7th character is to be added to each code from category X96.
  A   initial encounter
  D   subsequent encounter
  S   sequela

✓x7th X96.0 **Assault by** antipersonnel **bomb**
    EXCLUDES 1 *antipersonnel bomb use in military or war (Y36.2-)*

✓x7th X96.1 **Assault by** gasoline **bomb**

✓x7th X96.2 **Assault by** letter **bomb**

✓x7th X96.3 **Assault by** fertilizer **bomb**

✓x7th X96.4 **Assault by** pipe **bomb**

✓x7th X96.8 **Assault by other specified explosive**

✓x7th X96.9 **Assault by unspecified explosive**

✓x7th **X97 Assault by smoke, fire and flames**
    Assault by arson
    Assault by cigarettes
    Assault by incendiary device

The appropriate 7th character is to be added to code X97.
  A   initial encounter
  D   subsequent encounter
  S   sequela

✓4th **X98 Assault by steam, hot vapors and hot objects**

The appropriate 7th character is to be added to each code from category X98.
  A   initial encounter
  D   subsequent encounter
  S   sequela

✓x7th X98.0 **Assault by steam or hot** vapors

✓x7th X98.1 **Assault by hot** tap water

✓x7th X98.2 **Assault by hot** fluids

✓x7th X98.3 **Assault by hot household** appliances

✓x7th X98.8 **Assault by other hot objects**

✓x7th X98.9 **Assault by unspecified hot objects**

✓4th **X99 Assault by sharp object**
  EXCLUDES 1 *assault by strike by sports equipment (Y08.0-)*

The appropriate 7th character is to be added to each code from category X99.
  A   initial encounter
  D   subsequent encounter
  S   sequela

✓x7th X99.0 **Assault by sharp** glass

✓x7th X99.1 **Assault by** knife

✓x7th X99.2 **Assault by** sword **or** dagger

✓x7th X99.8 **Assault by other sharp object**

✓x7th X99.9 **Assault by unspecified sharp object**
    Assault by stabbing NOS

✓x7th **Y00 Assault by blunt object**
  EXCLUDES 1 *assault by strike by sports equipment (Y08.0-)*

The appropriate 7th character is to be added to code Y00.
  A   initial encounter
  D   subsequent encounter
  S   sequela

✓x7th **Y01 Assault by pushing from high place**

The appropriate 7th character is to be added to code Y01.
  A   initial encounter
  D   subsequent encounter
  S   sequela

✓4th **Y02 Assault by pushing or placing victim in front of moving object**

The appropriate 7th character is to be added to each code from category Y02.
  A   initial encounter
  D   subsequent encounter
  S   sequela

✓x7th Y02.0 **Assault by pushing or placing victim in front of** motor vehicle

✓x7th Y02.1 **Assault by pushing or placing victim in front of (subway)** train

✓ Additional Character Required   ✓x7th Xtension Alert   Unspecified Dx   Other Specified Dx   Manifestation   ▶◀ Revised Text   ● New Code   ▲ Revised Code Title

ICD-10-CM Draft (2015)   1037

External Causes of Morbidity

Y02.8–Y09

√x7th **Y02.8 Assault by pushing or placing victim in front of other moving object**

√4th **Y03 Assault by crashing of motor vehicle**

> The appropriate 7th character is to be added to each code from category Y03.
> A   initial encounter
> D   subsequent encounter
> S   sequela

√x7th **Y03.0 Assault by being hit or run over by motor vehicle**

√x7th **Y03.8 Other assault by crashing of motor vehicle**

√4th **Y04 Assault by bodily force**

> EXCLUDES 1   assault by:
>   submersion (X92.-)
>   use of weapon (X93-X95, X99, Y00)

> The appropriate 7th character is to be added to each code from category Y04.
> A   initial encounter
> D   subsequent encounter
> S   sequela

√x7th **Y04.0 Assault by unarmed brawl or fight**

√x7th **Y04.1 Assault by human bite**

√x7th **Y04.2 Assault by strike against or bumped into by another person**

√x7th **Y04.8 Assault by other bodily force**
> Assault by bodily force NOS

√4th **Y07 Perpetrator of assault, maltreatment and neglect**

> NOTE   Codes from this category are for use only in cases of confirmed abuse (T74.-)
> Selection of the correct perpetrator code is based on the relationship between the perpetrator and the victim
> INCLUDES   perpetrator of abandonment
>   perpetrator of emotional neglect
>   perpetrator of mental cruelty
>   perpetrator of physical abuse
>   perpetrator of physical neglect
>   perpetrator of sexual abuse
>   perpetrator of torture

√5th **Y07.0 Spouse or partner, perpetrator of maltreatment and neglect**
> NOTE   Spouse or partner, perpetrator of maltreatment and neglect against spouse or partner

   Y07.01 Husband, perpetrator of maltreatment and neglect

   Y07.02 Wife, perpetrator of maltreatment and neglect

   Y07.03 Male partner, perpetrator of maltreatment and neglect

   Y07.04 Female partner, perpetrator of maltreatment and neglect

√5th **Y07.1 Parent (adoptive) (biological), perpetrator of maltreatment and neglect**

   Y07.11 Biological father, perpetrator of maltreatment and neglect

   Y07.12 Biological mother, perpetrator of maltreatment and neglect

   Y07.13 Adoptive father, perpetrator of maltreatment and neglect

   Y07.14 Adoptive mother, perpetrator of maltreatment and neglect

√5th **Y07.4 Other family member, perpetrator of maltreatment and neglect**

   √6th **Y07.41 Sibling, perpetrator of maltreatment and neglect**
> EXCLUDES 1   stepsibling, perpetrator of maltreatment and neglect (Y07.435, Y07.436)

      Y07.410 Brother, perpetrator of maltreatment and neglect

      Y07.411 Sister, perpetrator of maltreatment and neglect

   √6th **Y07.42 Foster parent, perpetrator of maltreatment and neglect**

      Y07.420 Foster father, perpetrator of maltreatment and neglect

      Y07.421 Foster mother, perpetrator of maltreatment and neglect

   √6th **Y07.43 Stepparent or stepsibling, perpetrator of maltreatment and neglect**

      Y07.430 Stepfather, perpetrator of maltreatment and neglect

      Y07.432 Male friend of parent (co-residing in household), perpetrator of maltreatment and neglect

      Y07.433 Stepmother, perpetrator of maltreatment and neglect

      Y07.434 Female friend of parent (co-residing in household), perpetrator of maltreatment and neglect

      Y07.435 Stepbrother, perpetrator or maltreatment and neglect

      Y07.436 Stepsister, perpetrator of maltreatment and neglect

   √6th **Y07.49 Other family member, perpetrator of maltreatment and neglect**

      Y07.490 Male cousin, perpetrator of maltreatment and neglect

      Y07.491 Female cousin, perpetrator of maltreatment and neglect

      Y07.499 Other family member, perpetrator of maltreatment and neglect

√5th **Y07.5 Non-family member, perpetrator of maltreatment and neglect**

   Y07.50 Unspecified non-family member, perpetrator of maltreatment and neglect

   √6th **Y07.51 Daycare provider, perpetrator of maltreatment and neglect**

      Y07.510 At-home childcare provider, perpetrator of maltreatment and neglect

      Y07.511 Daycare center childcare provider, perpetrator of maltreatment and neglect

      Y07.512 At-home adultcare provider, perpetrator of maltreatment and neglect

      Y07.513 Adultcare center provider, perpetrator of maltreatment and neglect

      Y07.519 Unspecified daycare provider, perpetrator of maltreatment and neglect

   √6th **Y07.52 Healthcare provider, perpetrator of maltreatment and neglect**

      Y07.521 Mental health provider, perpetrator of maltreatment and neglect

      Y07.528 Other therapist or healthcare provider, perpetrator of maltreatment and neglect
> Nurse, perpetrator of maltreatment and neglect
> Occupational therapist, perpetrator of maltreatment and neglect
> Physical therapist, perpetrator of maltreatment and neglect
> Speech therapist, perpetrator of maltreatment and neglect

      Y07.529 Unspecified healthcare provider, perpetrator of maltreatment and neglect

   Y07.53 Teacher or instructor, perpetrator of maltreatment and neglect
> Coach, perpetrator of maltreatment and neglect

   Y07.59 Other non-family member, perpetrator of maltreatment and neglect

   Y07.9 Unspecified perpetrator of maltreatment and neglect

√4th **Y08 Assault by other specified means**

> The appropriate 7th character is to be added to each code from category Y08.
> A   initial encounter
> D   subsequent encounter
> S   sequela

√6th **Y08.0 Assault by strike by sport equipment**

   √x7th **Y08.01 Assault by strike by hockey stick**

   √x7th **Y08.02 Assault by strike by baseball bat**

   √x7th **Y08.09 Assault by strike by other specified type of sport equipment**

√5th **Y08.8 Assault by other specified means**

   √x7th **Y08.81 Assault by crashing of aircraft**

   √x7th **Y08.89 Assault by other specified means**

Y09 Assault by unspecified means
> Assassination (attempted) NOS
> Homicide (attempted) NOS
> Manslaughter (attempted) NOS
> Murder (attempted) NOS

EXCLUDES 1   Not coded here   EXCLUDES 2   Not included here   N Newborn Age: 0   P Pediatric Age: 0-17   M Maternity Age: 12-55   A Adult Age: 15-124

1038   ICD-10-CM Draft (2015)

Event of undetermined intent (Y21-Y33)

Undetermined intent is only for use when there is specific documentation in the record that the intent of the injury cannot be determined. If no such documentation is present, code to accidental (unintentional)

☑4ᵗʰ Y21 Drowning and submersion, undetermined intent

> The appropriate 7th character is to be added to each code from category Y21.
> A   initial encounter
> D   subsequent encounter
> S   sequela

☑x7ᵗʰ **Y21.0** Drowning and submersion while in bathtub, undetermined intent

☑x7ᵗʰ **Y21.1** Drowning and submersion after fall into bathtub, undetermined intent

☑x7ᵗʰ **Y21.2** Drowning and submersion while in swimming pool, undetermined intent

☑x7ᵗʰ **Y21.3** Drowning and submersion after fall into swimming pool, undetermined intent

☑x7ᵗʰ **Y21.4** Drowning and submersion in natural water, undetermined intent

☑x7ᵗʰ **Y21.8** Other drowning and submersion, undetermined intent

☑x7ᵗʰ **Y21.9** Unspecified drowning and submersion, undetermined intent

☑x7ᵗʰ Y22 Handgun discharge, undetermined intent
Discharge of gun for single hand use, undetermined intent
Discharge of pistol, undetermined intent
Discharge of revolver, undetermined intent
> **EXCLUDES 2** Very pistol (Y24.8)

> The appropriate 7th character is to be added to code Y22.
> A   initial encounter
> D   subsequent encounter
> S   sequela

☑4ᵗʰ Y23 Rifle, shotgun and larger firearm discharge, undetermined intent
> **EXCLUDES 2** airgun (Y24.0)

> The appropriate 7th character is to be added to each code from category Y23.
> A   initial encounter
> D   subsequent encounter
> S   sequela

☑x7ᵗʰ **Y23.0** Shotgun discharge, undetermined intent

☑x7ᵗʰ **Y23.1** Hunting rifle discharge, undetermined intent

☑x7ᵗʰ **Y23.2** Military firearm discharge, undetermined intent

☑x7ᵗʰ **Y23.3** Machine gun discharge, undetermined intent

☑x7ᵗʰ **Y23.8** Other larger firearm discharge, undetermined intent

☑x7ᵗʰ **Y23.9** Unspecified larger firearm discharge, undetermined intent

☑4ᵗʰ Y24 Other and unspecified firearm discharge, undetermined intent

> The appropriate 7th character is to be added to each code from category Y24.
> A   initial encounter
> D   subsequent encounter
> S   sequela

☑x7ᵗʰ **Y24.0** Airgun discharge, undetermined intent
BB gun discharge, undetermined intent
Pellet gun discharge, undetermined intent

☑x7ᵗʰ **Y24.8** Other firearm discharge, undetermined intent
Paintball gun discharge, undetermined intent
Very pistol [flare] discharge, undetermined intent

☑x7ᵗʰ **Y24.9** Unspecified firearm discharge, undetermined intent

☑x7ᵗʰ Y25 Contact with explosive material, undetermined intent

> The appropriate 7th character is to be added to code Y25.
> A   initial encounter
> D   subsequent encounter
> S   sequela

☑x7ᵗʰ Y26 Exposure to smoke, fire and flames, undetermined intent

> The appropriate 7th character is to be added to code Y26.
> A   initial encounter
> D   subsequent encounter
> S   sequela

☑4ᵗʰ Y27 Contact with steam, hot vapors and hot objects, undetermined intent

> The appropriate 7th character is to be added to each code from category Y27.
> A   initial encounter
> D   subsequent encounter
> S   sequela

☑x7ᵗʰ **Y27.0** Contact with steam and hot vapors, undetermined intent

☑x7ᵗʰ **Y27.1** Contact with hot tap water, undetermined intent

☑x7ᵗʰ **Y27.2** Contact with hot fluids, undetermined intent

☑x7ᵗʰ **Y27.3** Contact with hot household appliance, undetermined intent

☑x7ᵗʰ **Y27.8** Contact with other hot objects, undetermined intent

☑x7ᵗʰ **Y27.9** Contact with unspecified hot objects, undetermined intent

☑4ᵗʰ Y28 Contact with sharp object, undetermined intent

> The appropriate 7th character is to be added to each code from category Y28.
> A   initial encounter
> D   subsequent encounter
> S   sequela

☑x7ᵗʰ **Y28.0** Contact with sharp glass, undetermined intent

☑x7ᵗʰ **Y28.1** Contact with knife, undetermined intent

☑x7ᵗʰ **Y28.2** Contact with sword or dagger, undetermined intent

☑x7ᵗʰ **Y28.8** Contact with other sharp object, undetermined intent

☑x7ᵗʰ **Y28.9** Contact with unspecified hot objects, undetermined intent

☑x7ᵗʰ Y29 Contact with blunt object, undetermined intent

> The appropriate 7th character is to be added to code Y29.
> A   initial encounter
> D   subsequent encounter
> S   sequela

☑x7ᵗʰ Y30 Falling, jumping or pushed from a high place, undetermined intent
Victim falling from one level to another, undetermined intent

> The appropriate 7th character is to be added to code Y30.
> A   initial encounter
> D   subsequent encounter
> S   sequela

☑x7ᵗʰ Y31 Falling, lying or running before or into moving object, undetermined intent

> The appropriate 7th character is to be added to code Y31.
> A   initial encounter
> D   subsequent encounter
> S   sequela

☑x7ᵗʰ Y32 Crashing of motor vehicle, undetermined intent

> The appropriate 7th character is to be added to code Y32.
> A   initial encounter
> D   subsequent encounter
> S   sequela

☑x7ᵗʰ Y33 Other specified events, undetermined intent

> The appropriate 7th character is to be added to code Y33.
> A   initial encounter
> D   subsequent encounter
> S   sequela

☑ Additional Character Required   ☑x7ᵗʰ Xtension Alert   Unspecified Dx   Other Specified Dx   Manifestation   ►◄ Revised Text   ● New Code   ▲ Revised Code Title

External Causes of Morbidity

Y35–Y35.392

Legal intervention, operations of war, military operations, and terrorism (Y35-Y38)

☑4ᵗʰ **Y35** **Legal intervention**

INCLUDES any injury sustained as a result of an encounter with any law enforcement official, serving in any capacity at the time of the encounter, whether on-duty or off-duty. Includes: injury to law enforcement official, suspect and bystander

☑5ᵗʰ **Y35.0** **Legal intervention involving** firearm discharge

  ☑6ᵗʰ **Y35.00** **Legal intervention involving** unspecified **firearm discharge**

    Legal intervention involving gunshot wound
    Legal intervention involving shot NOS

    ☑7ᵗʰ **Y35.001** **Legal intervention involving unspecified firearm discharge,** law enforcement **official injured**

    ☑7ᵗʰ **Y35.002** **Legal intervention involving unspecified firearm discharge,** bystander **injured**

    ☑7ᵗʰ **Y35.003** **Legal intervention involving unspecified firearm discharge,** suspect **injured**

  ☑6ᵗʰ **Y35.01** **Legal intervention involving injury by** machine gun

    ☑7ᵗʰ **Y35.011** **Legal intervention involving injury by machine gun,** law enforcement **official injured**

    ☑7ᵗʰ **Y35.012** **Legal intervention involving injury by machine gun,** bystander **injured**

    ☑7ᵗʰ **Y35.013** **Legal intervention involving injury by machine gun,** suspect **injured**

  ☑6ᵗʰ **Y35.02** **Legal intervention involving injury by** handgun

    ☑7ᵗʰ **Y35.021** **Legal intervention involving injury by handgun,** law enforcement **official injured**

    ☑7ᵗʰ **Y35.022** **Legal intervention involving injury by handgun,** bystander **injured**

    ☑7ᵗʰ **Y35.023** **Legal intervention involving injury by handgun,** suspect **injured**

  ☑6ᵗʰ **Y35.03** **Legal intervention involving injury by** rifle pellet

    ☑7ᵗʰ **Y35.031** **Legal intervention involving injury by rifle pellet,** law enforcement **official injured**

    ☑7ᵗʰ **Y35.032** **Legal intervention involving injury by rifle pellet,** bystander **injured**

    ☑7ᵗʰ **Y35.033** **Legal intervention involving injury by rifle pellet,** suspect **injured**

  ☑6ᵗʰ **Y35.04** **Legal intervention involving injury by** rubber bullet

    ☑7ᵗʰ **Y35.041** **Legal intervention involving injury by rubber bullet,** law enforcement **official injured**

    ☑7ᵗʰ **Y35.042** **Legal intervention involving injury by rubber bullet,** bystander **injured**

    ☑7ᵗʰ **Y35.043** **Legal intervention involving injury by rubber bullet,** suspect **injured**

  ☑6ᵗʰ **Y35.09** **Legal intervention involving** other **firearm discharge**

    ☑7ᵗʰ **Y35.091** **Legal intervention involving other firearm discharge,** law enforcement **official injured**

    ☑7ᵗʰ **Y35.092** **Legal intervention involving other firearm discharge,** bystander **injured**

    ☑7ᵗʰ **Y35.093** **Legal intervention involving other firearm discharge,** suspect **injured**

☑5ᵗʰ **Y35.1** **Legal intervention involving** explosives

  ☑6ᵗʰ **Y35.10** **Legal intervention involving** unspecified **explosives**

    ☑7ᵗʰ **Y35.101** **Legal intervention involving unspecified explosives,** law enforcement **official injured**

    ☑7ᵗʰ **Y35.102** **Legal intervention involving unspecified explosives,** bystander **injured**

    ☑7ᵗʰ **Y35.103** **Legal intervention involving unspecified explosives,** suspect **injured**

  ☑6ᵗʰ **Y35.11** **Legal intervention involving injury by** dynamite

    ☑7ᵗʰ **Y35.111** **Legal intervention involving injury by dynamite,** law enforcement **official injured**

    ☑7ᵗʰ **Y35.112** **Legal intervention involving injury by dynamite,** bystander **injured**

    ☑7ᵗʰ **Y35.113** **Legal intervention involving injury by dynamite,** suspect **injured**

  ☑6ᵗʰ **Y35.12** **Legal intervention involving injury by** explosive shell

    ☑7ᵗʰ **Y35.121** **Legal intervention involving injury by explosive shell,** law enforcement **official injured**

    ☑7ᵗʰ **Y35.122** **Legal intervention involving injury by explosive shell,** bystander **injured**

    ☑7ᵗʰ **Y35.123** **Legal intervention involving injury by explosive shell,** suspect **injured**

  ☑6ᵗʰ **Y35.19** **Legal intervention involving** other explosives

    Legal intervention involving injury by grenade
    Legal intervention involving injury by mortar bomb

    ☑7ᵗʰ **Y35.191** **Legal intervention involving other explosives,** law enforcement **official injured**

    ☑7ᵗʰ **Y35.192** **Legal intervention involving other explosives,** bystander **injured**

    ☑7ᵗʰ **Y35.193** **Legal intervention involving other explosives,** suspect **injured**

☑5ᵗʰ **Y35.2** **Legal intervention involving** gas

    Legal intervention involving asphyxiation by gas
    Legal intervention involving poisoning by gas

  ☑6ᵗʰ **Y35.20** **Legal intervention involving** unspecified **gas**

    ☑7ᵗʰ **Y35.201** **Legal intervention involving unspecified gas,** law enforcement **official injured**

    ☑7ᵗʰ **Y35.202** **Legal intervention involving unspecified gas,** bystander **injured**

    ☑7ᵗʰ **Y35.203** **Legal intervention involving unspecified gas,** suspect **injured**

  ☑6ᵗʰ **Y35.21** **Legal intervention involving injury by** tear gas

    ☑7ᵗʰ **Y35.211** **Legal intervention involving injury by tear gas,** law enforcement **official injured**

    ☑7ᵗʰ **Y35.212** **Legal intervention involving injury by tear gas,** bystander **injured**

    ☑7ᵗʰ **Y35.213** **Legal intervention involving injury by tear gas,** suspect **injured**

  ☑6ᵗʰ **Y35.29** **Legal intervention involving** other gas

    ☑7ᵗʰ **Y35.291** **Legal intervention involving other gas,** law enforcement **official injured**

    ☑7ᵗʰ **Y35.292** **Legal intervention involving other gas,** bystander **injured**

    ☑7ᵗʰ **Y35.293** **Legal intervention involving other gas,** suspect **injured**

☑5ᵗʰ **Y35.3** **Legal intervention involving** blunt objects

    Legal intervention involving being hit or struck by blunt object

  ☑6ᵗʰ **Y35.30** **Legal intervention involving** unspecified **blunt objects**

    ☑7ᵗʰ **Y35.301** **Legal intervention involving unspecified blunt objects,** law enforcement **official injured**

    ☑7ᵗʰ **Y35.302** **Legal intervention involving unspecified blunt objects,** bystander **injured**

    ☑7ᵗʰ **Y35.303** **Legal intervention involving unspecified blunt objects,** suspect **injured**

  ☑6ᵗʰ **Y35.31** **Legal intervention involving** baton

    ☑7ᵗʰ **Y35.311** **Legal intervention involving baton,** law enforcement **official injured**

    ☑7ᵗʰ **Y35.312** **Legal intervention involving baton,** bystander **injured**

    ☑7ᵗʰ **Y35.313** **Legal intervention involving baton,** suspect **injured**

  ☑6ᵗʰ **Y35.39** **Legal intervention involving** other **blunt objects**

    ☑7ᵗʰ **Y35.391** **Legal intervention involving other blunt objects,** law enforcement **official injured**

    ☑7ᵗʰ **Y35.392** **Legal intervention involving other blunt objects,** bystander **injured**

EXCLUDES 1 Not coded here   EXCLUDES 2 Not included here   N Newborn Age: 0   P Pediatric Age: 0-17   M Maternity Age: 12-55   A Adult Age: 15-124

1040   ICD-10-CM Draft (2015)

✓7th **Y35.393** **Legal intervention involving other blunt objects, suspect injured**

✓5th **Y35.4** **Legal intervention involving sharp objects**
Legal intervention involving being cut by sharp objects
Legal intervention involving being stabbed by sharp objects

✓6th **Y35.40** **Legal intervention involving unspecified sharp objects**

✓7th **Y35.401** **Legal intervention involving unspecified sharp objects, law enforcement official injured**

✓7th **Y35.402** **Legal intervention involving unspecified sharp objects, bystander injured**

✓7th **Y35.403** **Legal intervention involving unspecified sharp objects, suspect injured**

✓6th **Y35.41** **Legal intervention involving bayonet**

✓7th **Y35.411** **Legal intervention involving bayonet, law enforcement official injured**

✓7th **Y35.412** **Legal intervention involving bayonet, bystander injured**

✓7th **Y35.413** **Legal intervention involving bayonet, suspect injured**

✓6th **Y35.49** **Legal intervention involving other sharp objects**

✓7th **Y35.491** **Legal intervention involving other sharp objects, law enforcement official injured**

✓7th **Y35.492** **Legal intervention involving other sharp objects, bystander injured**

✓7th **Y35.493** **Legal intervention involving other sharp objects, suspect injured**

✓5th **Y35.8** **Legal intervention involving other specified means**

✓6th **Y35.81** **Legal intervention involving manhandling**

✓7th **Y35.811** **Legal intervention involving manhandling, law enforcement official injured**

✓7th **Y35.812** **Legal intervention involving manhandling, bystander injured**

✓7th **Y35.813** **Legal intervention involving manhandling, suspect injured**

✓6th **Y35.89** **Legal intervention involving other specified means**

✓7th **Y35.891** **Legal intervention involving other specified means, law enforcement official injured**

✓7th **Y35.892** **Legal intervention involving other specified means, bystander injured**

✓7th **Y35.893** **Legal intervention involving other specified means, suspect injured**

✓5th **Y35.9** **Legal intervention, means unspecified**

✓x7th **Y35.91** **Legal intervention, means unspecified, law enforcement official injured**

✓x7th **Y35.92** **Legal intervention, means unspecified, bystander injured**

✓x7th **Y35.93** **Legal intervention, means unspecified, suspect injured**

✓4th **Y36** **Operations of war**

INCLUDES injuries to military personnel and civilians caused by war, civil insurrection, and peacekeeping missions

EXCLUDES 1 injury to military personnel occurring during peacetime military operations (Y37.-)
military vehicles involved in transport accidents with non-military vehicle during peacetime (V09.01, V09.21, V19.81, V29.81, V39.81, V49.81, V59.81, V69.81, V79.81)

The appropriate 7th character is to be added to each code from category Y36.
A   initial encounter
D   subsequent encounter
S   sequela

✓5th **Y36.0** **War operations involving explosion of marine weapons**

✓6th **Y36.00** **War operations involving explosion of unspecified marine weapon**
War operations involving underwater blast NOS

✓7th **Y36.000** **War operations involving explosion of unspecified marine weapon, military personnel**

✓7th **Y36.001** **War operations involving explosion of unspecified marine weapon, civilian**

✓6th **Y36.01** **War operations involving explosion of depth-charge**

✓7th **Y36.010** **War operations involving explosion of depth-charge, military personnel**

✓7th **Y36.011** **War operations involving explosion of depth-charge, civilian**

✓6th **Y36.02** **War operations involving explosion of marine mine**
War operations involving explosion of marine mine, at sea or in harbor

✓7th **Y36.020** **War operations involving explosion of marine mine, military personnel**

✓7th **Y36.021** **War operations involving explosion of marine mine, civilian**

✓6th **Y36.03** **War operations involving explosion of sea-based artillery shell**

✓7th **Y36.030** **War operations involving explosion of sea-based artillery shell, military personnel**

✓7th **Y36.031** **War operations involving explosion of sea-based artillery shell, civilian**

✓6th **Y36.04** **War operations involving explosion of torpedo**

✓7th **Y36.040** **War operations involving explosion of torpedo, military personnel**

✓7th **Y36.041** **War operations involving explosion of torpedo, civilian**

✓6th **Y36.05** **War operations involving accidental detonation of onboard marine weapons**

✓7th **Y36.050** **War operations involving accidental detonation of onboard marine weapons, military personnel**

✓7th **Y36.051** **War operations involving accidental detonation of onboard marine weapons, civilian**

✓6th **Y36.09** **War operations involving explosion of other marine weapons**

✓7th **Y36.090** **War operations involving explosion of other marine weapons, military personnel**

✓7th **Y36.091** **War operations involving explosion of other marine weapons, civilian**

✓5th **Y36.1** **War operations involving destruction of aircraft**

✓6th **Y36.10** **War operations involving unspecified destruction of aircraft**

✓7th **Y36.100** **War operations involving unspecified destruction of aircraft, military personnel**

✓7th **Y36.101** **War operations involving unspecified destruction of aircraft, civilian**

✓6th **Y36.11** **War operations involving destruction of aircraft due to enemy fire or explosives**
War operations involving destruction of aircraft due to air to air missile
War operations involving destruction of aircraft due to explosive placed on aircraft
War operations involving destruction of aircraft due to rocket propelled grenade [RPG]
War operations involving destruction of aircraft due to small arms fire
War operations involving destruction of aircraft due to surface to air missile

✓7th **Y36.110** **War operations involving destruction of aircraft due to enemy fire or explosives, military personnel**

✓7th **Y36.111** **War operations involving destruction of aircraft due to enemy fire or explosives, civilian**

✓6th **Y36.12** **War operations involving destruction of aircraft due to collision with other aircraft**

✓7th **Y36.120** **War operations involving destruction of aircraft due to collision with other aircraft, military personnel**

✓7th **Y36.121** **War operations involving destruction of aircraft due to collision with other aircraft, civilian**

✓6th **Y36.13** **War operations involving destruction of aircraft due to onboard fire**

✓7th **Y36.130** **War operations involving destruction of aircraft due to onboard fire, military personnel**

✓ Additional Character Required   ✓x7th Xtension Alert   Unspecified Dx   Other Specified Dx   Manifestation   ►◄ Revised Text   ● New Code   ▲ Revised Code Title

ICD-10-CM Draft (2015)   1041

External Causes of Morbidity

Y36.131–Y36.391

☑7th **Y36.131 War operations involving destruction of aircraft due to onboard fire, civilian**

☑6th **Y36.14 War operations involving destruction of aircraft due to** accidental detonation of onboard munitions and explosives

☑7th **Y36.140 War operations involving destruction of aircraft due to accidental detonation of onboard munitions and explosives, military personnel**

☑7th **Y36.141 War operations involving destruction of aircraft due to accidental detonation of onboard munitions and explosives, civilian**

☑6th **Y36.19 War operations involving** other **destruction of aircraft**

☑7th **Y36.190 War operations involving other destruction of aircraft,** military personnel

☑7th **Y36.191 War operations involving other destruction of aircraft,** civilian

☑5th **Y36.2 War operations involving** other **explosions and fragments**

EXCLUDES 1   *war operations involving explosion of aircraft (Y36.1-)*
war operations involving explosion of marine weapons (Y36.0-)
war operations involving explosion of nuclear weapons (Y36.5-)
war operations involving explosion occurring after cessation of hostilities (Y36.8-)

☑6th **Y36.20 War operations involving** unspecified **explosion and fragments**

War operations involving air blast NOS
War operations involving blast NOS
War operations involving blast fragments NOS
War operations involving blast wave NOS
War operations involving blast wind NOS
War operations involving explosion NOS
War operations involving explosion of bomb NOS

☑7th **Y36.200 War operations involving unspecified explosion and fragments,** military personnel

☑7th **Y36.201 War operations involving unspecified explosion and fragments,** civilian

☑6th **Y36.21 War operations involving explosion of** aerial bomb

☑7th **Y36.210 War operations involving explosion of aerial bomb,** military personnel

☑7th **Y36.211 War operations involving explosion of aerial bomb,** civilian

☑6th **Y36.22 War operations involving explosion of** guided missile

☑7th **Y36.220 War operations involving explosion of guided missile,** military personnel

☑7th **Y36.221 War operations involving explosion of guided missile,** civilian

☑6th **Y36.23 War operations involving explosion of** improvised explosive device **[IED]**

War operations involving explosion of person-borne improvised explosive device [IED]
War operations involving explosion of vehicle-borne improvised explosive device [IED]
War operations involving explosion of roadside improvised explosive device [IED]

☑7th **Y36.230 War operations involving explosion of improvised explosive device [IED],** military personnel

☑7th **Y36.231 War operations involving explosion of improvised explosive device [IED],** civilian

☑6th **Y36.24 War operations involving explosion due to** accidental detonation and discharge of own munitions or munitions launch device

☑7th **Y36.240 War operations involving explosion due to accidental detonation and discharge of own munitions or munitions launch device,** military personnel

☑7th **Y36.241 War operations involving explosion due to accidental detonation and discharge of own munitions or munitions launch device,** civilian

☑6th **Y36.25 War operations involving** fragments from munitions

☑7th **Y36.250 War operations involving fragents from munitions,** military personnel

☑7th **Y36.251 War operations involving fragments from munitions,** civilian

☑6th **Y36.26 War operations involving fragments of** improvised explosive device **[IED]**

War operations involving fragments of person-borne improvised explosive device [IED]
War operations involving fragments of vehicle-borne improvised explosive device [IED]
War operations involving fragments of roadside improvised explosive device [IED]

☑7th **Y36.260 War operations involving fragments of improvised explosive device [IED],** military personnel

☑7th **Y36.261 War operations involving fragments of improvised explosive device [IED],** civilian

☑6th **Y36.27 War operations involving** fragments from weapons

☑7th **Y36.270 War operations involving fragments from weapons,** military personnel

☑7th **Y36.271 War operations involving fragments from weapons,** civilian

☑6th **Y36.29 War operations involving** other **explosions and fragments**

War operations involving explosion of grenade
War operations involving explosions of land mine
War operations involving shrapnel NOS

☑7th **Y36.290 War operations involving other explosions and fragments,** military personnel

☑7th **Y36.291 War operations involving other explosions and fragments,** civilian

☑5th **Y36.3 War operations involving** fires, conflagrations and hot substances

War operations involving smoke, fumes, and heat from fires, conflagrations and hot substances

EXCLUDES 1   *war operations involving fires and conflagrations aboard military aircraft (Y36.1-)*
war operations involving fires and conflagrations aboard military watercraft (Y36.0-)
war operations involving fires and conflagrations caused indirectly by conventional weapons (Y36.2-)
war operations involving fires and thermal effects of nuclear weapons (Y36.53-)

☑6th **Y36.30 War operations involving** unspecified **fire, conflagration and hot substance**

☑7th **Y36.300 War operations involving unspecified fire, conflagration and hot substance,** military personnel

☑7th **Y36.301 War operations involving unspecified fire, conflagration and hot substance,** civilian

☑6th **Y36.31 War operations involving** gasoline bomb

War operations involving incendiary bomb
War operations involving petrol bomb

☑7th **Y36.310 War operations involving gasoline bomb,** military personnel

☑7th **Y36.311 War operations involving gasoline bomb,** civilian

☑6th **Y36.32 War operations involving** incendiary bullet

☑7th **Y36.320 War operations involving incendiary bullet,** military personnel

☑7th **Y36.321 War operations involving incendiary bullet,** civilian

☑6th **Y36.33 War operations involving** flamethrower

☑7th **Y36.330 War operations involving flamethrower,** military personnel

☑7th **Y36.331 War operations involving flamethrower,** civilian

☑6th **Y36.39 War operations involving other fires,** conflagrations and hot substances

☑7th **Y36.390 War operations involving other fires, conflagrations and hot substances,** military personnel

☑7th **Y36.391 War operations involving other fires, conflagrations and hot substances,** civilian

---

EXCLUDES 1 Not coded here   EXCLUDES 2 Not included here   N Newborn Age: 0   P Pediatric Age: 0-17   M Maternity Age: 12-55   A Adult Age: 15-124

1042   ICD-10-CM Draft (2015)

✓5ᵗʰ **Y36.4** **War operations involving firearm discharge and other forms of conventional warfare**

  ✓6ᵗʰ **Y36.41** **War operations involving** rubber bullets

    ✓7ᵗʰ **Y36.410** **War operations involving rubber bullets, military personnel**

    ✓7ᵗʰ **Y36.411** **War operations involving rubber bullets, civilian**

  ✓6ᵗʰ **Y36.42** **War operations involving** firearms pellets

    ✓7ᵗʰ **Y36.420** **War operations involving firearms pellets, military personnel**

    ✓7ᵗʰ **Y36.421** **War operations involving firearms pellets, civilian**

  ✓6ᵗʰ **Y36.43** **War operations involving** other **firearms discharge**

    War operations involving bullets NOS

    EXCLUDES 1 *war operations involving munitions fragments (Y36.25-)*

        war operations involving incendiary bullets (Y36.32-)

    ✓7ᵗʰ **Y36.430** **War operations involving other firearms discharge, military personnel**

    ✓7ᵗʰ **Y36.431** **War operations involving other firearms discharge, civilian**

  ✓6ᵗʰ **Y36.44** **War operations involving** unarmed hand to hand combat

    EXCLUDES 1 *war operations involving combat using blunt or piercing object (Y36.45-)*

        war operations involving intentional restriction of air and airway (Y36.46-)

        war operations involving unintentional restriction of air and airway (Y36.47-)

    ✓7ᵗʰ **Y36.440** **War operations involving unarmed hand to hand combat, military personnel**

    ✓7ᵗʰ **Y36.441** **War operations involving unarmed hand to hand combat, civilian**

  ✓6ᵗʰ **Y36.45** **War operations involving combat using blunt or piercing object**

    ✓7ᵗʰ **Y36.450** **War operations involving combat using blunt or piercing object, military personnel**

    ✓7ᵗʰ **Y36.451** **War operations involving combat using blunt or piercing object, civilian**

  ✓6ᵗʰ **Y36.46** **War operations involving** intentional restriction of air and airway

    ✓7ᵗʰ **Y36.460** **War operations involving intentional restriction of air and airway, military personnel**

    ✓7ᵗʰ **Y36.461** **War operations involving intentional restriction of air and airway, civilian**

  ✓6ᵗʰ **Y36.47** **War operations involving** unintentional restriction of air and airway

    ✓7ᵗʰ **Y36.470** **War operations involving unintentional restriction of air and airway, military personnel**

    ✓7ᵗʰ **Y36.471** **War operations involving unintentional restriction of air and airway, civilian**

  ✓6ᵗʰ **Y36.49** **War operations involving** other **forms of conventional warfare**

    ✓7ᵗʰ **Y36.490** **War operations involving other forms of conventional warfare, military personnel**

    ✓7ᵗʰ **Y36.491** **War operations involving other forms of conventional warfare, civilian**

✓5ᵗʰ **Y36.5** **War operations involving** nuclear weapons

  War operations involving dirty bomb NOS

  ✓6ᵗʰ **Y36.50** **War operations involving** unspecified **effect of nuclear weapon**

    ✓7ᵗʰ **Y36.500** **War operations involving unspecified effect of nuclear weapon, military personnel**

    ✓7ᵗʰ **Y36.501** **War operations involving unspecified effect of nuclear weapon, civilian**

  ✓6ᵗʰ **Y36.51** **War operations involving** direct blast **effect of nuclear weapon**

    War operations involving blast pressure of nuclear weapon

    ✓7ᵗʰ **Y36.510** **War operations involving direct blast effect of nuclear weapon, military personnel**

    ✓7ᵗʰ **Y36.511** **War operations involving direct blast effect of nuclear weapon, civilian**

  ✓6ᵗʰ **Y36.52** **War operations involving** indirect blast **effect of nuclear weapon**

    War operations involving being thrown by blast of nuclear weapon

    War operations involving being struck or crushed by blast debris of nuclear weapon

    ✓7ᵗʰ **Y36.520** **War operations involving indirect blast effect of nuclear weapon, military personnel**

    ✓7ᵗʰ **Y36.521** **War operations involving indirect blast effect of nuclear weapon, civilian**

  ✓6ᵗʰ **Y36.53** **War operations involving** thermal radiation **effect of nuclear weapon**

    War operations involving direct heat from nuclear weapon

    War operation involving fireball effects from nuclear weapon

    ✓7ᵗʰ **Y36.530** **War operations involving thermal radiation effect of nuclear weapon, military personnel**

    ✓7ᵗʰ **Y36.531** **War operations involving thermal radiation effect of nuclear weapon, civilian**

  ✓6ᵗʰ **Y36.54** **War operation involving** nuclear radiation **effects of nuclear weapon**

    War operation involving acute radiation exposure from nuclear weapon

    War operation involving exposure to immediate ionizing radiation from nuclear weapon

    War operation involving fallout exposure from nuclear weapon

    War operation involving secondary effects of nuclear weapons

    ✓7ᵗʰ **Y36.540** **War operation involving nuclear radiation effects of nuclear weapon, military personnel**

    ✓7ᵗʰ **Y36.541** **War operation involving nuclear radiation effects of nuclear weapon, civilian**

  ✓6ᵗʰ **Y36.59** **War operation involving** other **effects of nuclear weapons**

    ✓7ᵗʰ **Y36.590** **War operation involving other effects of nuclear weapons, military personnel**

    ✓7ᵗʰ **Y36.591** **War operation involving other effects of nuclear weapons, civilian**

✓5ᵗʰ **Y36.6** **War operations involving biological weapons**

  ✓6ᵗʰ **Y36.6X** **War operations involving** biological weapons

    ✓7ᵗʰ **Y36.6X0** **War operations involving biological weapons, military personnel**

    ✓7ᵗʰ **Y36.6X1** **War operations involving biological weapons, civilian**

✓5ᵗʰ **Y36.7** **War operations involving chemical weapons and other forms of unconventional warfare**

  EXCLUDES 1 *war operations involving incendiary devices (Y36.3-, Y36.5-)*

  ✓6ᵗʰ **Y36.7X** **War operations involving** chemical weapons and other **forms of** unconventional warfare

    ✓7ᵗʰ **Y36.7X0** **War operations involving chemical weapons and other forms of unconventional warfare, military personnel**

    ✓7ᵗʰ **Y36.7X1** **War operations involving chemical weapons and other forms of unconventional warfare, civilian**

✓5ᵗʰ **Y36.8** **War operations occurring** after cessation of hostilities

  War operations classifiable to categories Y36.0-Y36.8 but occurring after cessation of hostilities

  ✓6ᵗʰ **Y36.81** **Explosion of** mine **placed during war operations but exploding after cessation of hostilities**

    ✓7ᵗʰ **Y36.810** **Explosion of mine placed during war operations but exploding after cessation of hostilities, military personnel**

    ✓7ᵗʰ **Y36.811** **Explosion of mine placed during war operations but exploding after cessation of hostilities, civilian**

☑ Additional Character Required   ✓x7ᵗʰ Xtension Alert   Unspecified Dx   Other Specified Dx   Manifestation   ►◄ Revised Text   ● New Code   ▲ Revised Code Title

ICD-10-CM Draft (2015)   1043

√6th **Y36.82** Explosion of bomb placed during war operations but exploding after cessation of hostilities

√7th **Y36.820** Explosion of bomb placed during war operations but exploding after cessation of hostilities, military personnel

√7th **Y36.821** Explosion of bomb placed during war operations but exploding after cessation of hostilities, civilian

√6th **Y36.88** Other war operations occurring after cessation of hostilities

√7th **Y36.880** Other war operations occurring after cessation of hostilities, military personnel

√7th **Y36.881** Other war operations occurring after cessation of hostilities, civilian

√6th **Y36.89** Unspecified war operations occurring after cessation of hostilities

√7th **Y36.890** Unspecified war operations occurring after cessation of hostilities, military personnel

√7th **Y36.891** Unspecified war operations occurring after cessation of hostilities, civilian

√5th **Y36.9** Other and unspecified war operations

√x7th **Y36.90** War operations, unspecified

√x7th **Y36.91** War operations involving unspecified weapon of mass destruction [WMD]

√x7th **Y36.92** War operations involving friendly fire

√4th **Y37 Military operations**

INCLUDES injuries to military personnel and civilians occurring during peacetime on military property and during routine military exercises and operations

EXCLUDES 1 military aircraft involved in aircraft accident with civilian aircraft (V97.81-)

military vehicles involved in transport accident with civilian vehicle (V09.01, V09.21, V19.81, V29.81, V39.81, V49.81, V59.81, V69.81, V79.81)

military watercraft involved in water transport accident with civilian watercraft (V94.81-)

war operations (Y36.-)

The appropriate 7th character is to be added to each code from category Y37.
A initial encounter
D subsequent encounter
S sequela

√5th **Y37.0** Military operations involving explosion of marine weapons

√6th **Y37.00** Military operations involving explosion of unspecified marine weapon

Military operations involving underwater blast NOS

√7th **Y37.000** Military operations involving explosion of unspecified marine weapon, military personnel

√7th **Y37.001** Military operations involving explosion of unspecified marine weapon, civilian

√6th **Y37.01** Military operations involving explosion of depth-charge

√7th **Y37.010** Military operations involving explosion of depth-charge, military personnel

√7th **Y37.011** Military operations involving explosion of depth-charge, civilian

√6th **Y37.02** Military operations involving explosion of marine mine

Military operations involving explosion of marine mine, at sea or in harbor

√7th **Y37.020** Military operations involving explosion of marine mine, military personnel

√7th **Y37.021** Military operations involving explosion of marine mine, civilian

√6th **Y37.03** Military operations involving explosion of sea-based artillery shell

√7th **Y37.030** Military operations involving explosion of sea-based artillery shell, military personnel

√7th **Y37.031** Military operations involving explosion of sea-based artillery shell, civilian

√6th **Y37.04** Military operations involving explosion of torpedo

√7th **Y37.040** Military operations involving explosion of torpedo, military personnel

√7th **Y37.041** Military operations involving explosion of torpedo, civilian

√6th **Y37.05** Military operations involving accidental detonation of onboard marine weapons

√7th **Y37.050** Military operations involving accidental detonation of onboard marine weapons, military personnel

√7th **Y37.051** Military operations involving accidental detonation of onboard marine weapons, civilian

√6th **Y37.09** Military operations involving explosion of other marine weapons

√7th **Y37.090** Military operations involving explosion of other marine weapons, military personnel

√7th **Y37.091** Military operations involving explosion of other marine weapons, civilian

√5th **Y37.1** Military operations involving destruction of aircraft

√6th **Y37.10** Military operations involving unspecified destruction of aircraft

√7th **Y37.100** Military operations involving unspecified destruction of aircraft, military personnel

√7th **Y37.101** Military operations involving unspecified destruction of aircraft, civilian

√6th **Y37.11** Military operations involving destruction of aircraft due to enemy fire or explosives

Military operations involving destruction of aircraft due to air to air missile
Military operations involving destruction of aircraft due to explosive placed on aircraft
Military operations involving destruction of aircraft due to rocket propelled grenade [RPG]
Military operations involving destruction of aircraft due to small arms fire
Military operations involving destruction of aircraft due to surface to air missile

√7th **Y37.110** Military operations involving destruction of aircraft due to enemy fire or explosives, military personnel

√7th **Y37.111** Military operations involving destruction of aircraft due to enemy fire or explosives, civilian

√6th **Y37.12** Military operations involving destruction of aircraft due to collision with other aircraft

√7th **Y37.120** Military operations involving destruction of aircraft due to collision with other aircraft, military personnel

√7th **Y37.121** Military operations involving destruction of aircraft due to collision with other aircraft, civilian

√6th **Y37.13** Military operations involving destruction of aircraft due to onboard fire

√7th **Y37.130** Military operations involving destruction of aircraft due to onboard fire, military personnel

√7th **Y37.131** Military operations involving destruction of aircraft due to onboard fire, civilian

√6th **Y37.14** Military operations involving destruction of aircraft due to accidental detonation of onboard munitions and explosives

√7th **Y37.140** Military operations involving destruction of aircraft due to accidental detonation of onboard munitions and explosives, military personnel

√7th **Y37.141** Military operations involving destruction of aircraft due to accidental detonation of onboard munitions and explosives, civilian

√6th **Y37.19** Military operations involving other destruction of aircraft

√7th **Y37.190** Military operations involving other destruction of aircraft, military personnel

√7th **Y37.191** Military operations involving other destruction of aircraft, civilian

EXCLUDES 1 Not coded here EXCLUDES 2 Not included here N Newborn Age: 0 P Pediatric Age: 0-17 M Maternity Age: 12-55 A Adult Age: 15-124

1044 ICD-10-CM Draft (2015)

✓5ᵗʰ **Y37.2** **Military operations involving** other explosions and fragments
EXCLUDES 1　*military operations involving explosion of aircraft (Y37.1-)*
military operations involving explosion of marine weapons (Y37.0-)
military operations involving explosion of nuclear weapons (Y37.5-)

✓6ᵗʰ **Y37.20** **Military operations involving** unspecified explosion and fragments
Military operations involving air blast NOS
Military operations involving blast NOS
Military operations involving blast fragments NOS
Military operations involving blast wave NOS
Military operations involving blast wind NOS
Military operations involving explosion NOS
Military operations involving explosion of bomb NOS

✓7ᵗʰ **Y37.200** **Military operations involving unspecified explosion and fragments,** military personnel

✓7ᵗʰ **Y37.201** **Military operations involving unspecified explosion and fragments,** civilian

✓6ᵗʰ **Y37.21** **Military operations involving explosion of** aerial bomb

✓7ᵗʰ **Y37.210** **Military operations involving explosion of aerial bomb,** military personnel

✓7ᵗʰ **Y37.211** **Military operations involving explosion of aerial bomb,** civilian

✓6ᵗʰ **Y37.22** **Military operations involving explosion of** guided missile

✓7ᵗʰ **Y37.220** **Military operations involving explosion of guided missile,** military personnel

✓7ᵗʰ **Y37.221** **Military operations involving explosion of guided missile,** civilian

✓6ᵗʰ **Y37.23** **Military operations involving explosion of** improvised explosive device [IED]
Military operations involving explosion of person-borne improvised explosive device [IED]
Military operations involving explosion of vehicle-borne improvised explosive device [IED]
Military operations involving explosion of roadside improvised explosive device [IED]

✓7ᵗʰ **Y37.230** **Military operations involving explosion of improvised explosive device [IED],** military personnel

✓7ᵗʰ **Y37.231** **Military operations involving explosion of improvised explosive device [IED],** civilian

✓6ᵗʰ **Y37.24** **Military operations involving explosion** due to accidental detonation and discharge of own munitions or munitions launch device

✓7ᵗʰ **Y37.240** **Military operations involving explosion due to accidental detonation and discharge of own munitions or munitions launch device,** military personnel

✓7ᵗʰ **Y37.241** **Military operations involving explosion due to accidental detonation and discharge of own munitions or munitions launch device,** civilian

✓6ᵗʰ **Y37.25** **Military operations involving** fragments from munitions

✓7ᵗʰ **Y37.250** **Military operations involving fragments from munitions,** military personnel

✓7ᵗʰ **Y37.251** **Military operations involving fragments from munitions,** civilian

✓6ᵗʰ **Y37.26** **Military operations involving fragments of** improvised explosive device [IED]
Military operations involving fragments of person-borne improvised explosive device [IED]
Military operations involving fragments of vehicle-borne improvised explosive device [IED]
Military operations involving fragments of roadside improvised explosive device [IED]

✓7ᵗʰ **Y37.260** **Military operations involving fragments of improvised explosive device [IED],** military personnel

✓7ᵗʰ **Y37.261** **Military operations involving fragments of improvised explosive device [IED],** civilian

✓6ᵗʰ **Y37.27** **Military operations involving fragments from** weapons

✓7ᵗʰ **Y37.270** **Military operations involving fragments from weapons,** military personnel

✓7ᵗʰ **Y37.271** **Military operations involving fragments from weapons,** civilian

✓6ᵗʰ **Y37.29** **Military operations involving** other explosions and fragments
Military operations involving explosion of grenade
Military operations involving explosions of land mine
Military operations involving shrapnel NOS

✓7ᵗʰ **Y37.290** **Military operations involving other explosions and fragments,** military personnel

✓7ᵗʰ **Y37.291** **Military operations involving other explosions and fragments,** civilian

✓5ᵗʰ **Y37.3** **Military operations involving** fires, conflagrations and hot substances
Military operations involving smoke, fumes, and heat from fires, conflagrations and hot substances
EXCLUDES 1　*military operations involving fires and conflagrations aboard military aircraft (Y37.1-)*
military operations involving fires and conflagrations aboard military watercraft (Y37.0-)
military operations involving fires and conflagrations caused indirectly by conventional weapons (Y37.2-)
military operations involving fires and thermal effects of nuclear weapons (Y36.53-)

✓6ᵗʰ **Y37.30** **Military operations involving** unspecified fire, conflagration and hot substance

✓7ᵗʰ **Y37.300** **Military operations involving unspecified fire, conflagration and hot substance,** military personnel

✓7ᵗʰ **Y37.301** **Military operations involving unspecified fire, conflagration and hot substance,** civilian

✓6ᵗʰ **Y37.31** **Military operations involving** gasoline bomb
Military operations involving incendiary bomb
Military operations involving petrol bomb

✓7ᵗʰ **Y37.310** **Military operations involving gasoline bomb,** military personnel

✓7ᵗʰ **Y37.311** **Military operations involving gasoline bomb,** civilian

✓6ᵗʰ **Y37.32** **Military operations involving** incendiary bullet

✓7ᵗʰ **Y37.320** **Military operations involving incendiary bullet,** military personnel

✓7ᵗʰ **Y37.321** **Military operations involving incendiary bullet,** civilian

✓6ᵗʰ **Y37.33** **Military operations involving** flamethrower

✓7ᵗʰ **Y37.330** **Military operations involving flamethrower,** military personnel

✓7ᵗʰ **Y37.331** **Military operations involving flamethrower,** civilian

✓6ᵗʰ **Y37.39** **Military operations involving** other fires, conflagrations and hot substances

✓7ᵗʰ **Y37.390** **Military operations involving other fires, conflagrations and hot substances,** military personnel

✓7ᵗʰ **Y37.391** **Military operations involving other fires, conflagrations and hot substances,** civilian

✓5ᵗʰ **Y37.4** **Military operations involving firearm discharge and other forms of conventional warfare**

✓6ᵗʰ **Y37.41** **Military operations involving** rubber bullets

✓7ᵗʰ **Y37.410** **Military operations involving rubber bullets,** military personnel

✓7ᵗʰ **Y37.411** **Military operations involving rubber bullets,** civilian

✓6ᵗʰ **Y37.42** **Military operations involving** firearms pellets

✓7ᵗʰ **Y37.420** **Military operations involving firearms pellets,** military personnel

✓7ᵗʰ **Y37.421** **Military operations involving firearms pellets,** civilian

---

✓ Additional Character Required　　✓x7ᵗʰ Xtension Alert　　Unspecified Dx　　Other Specified Dx　　Manifestation　　▶◀ Revised Text　　● New Code　　▲ Revised Code Title

External Causes of Morbidity

Y37.43–Y37.92

✓6ᵗʰ **Y37.43** Military operations involving other firearms discharge

    Military operations involving bullets NOS

    EXCLUDES 1 *military operations involving munitions fragments (Y37.25-)*

        military operations involving incendiary bullets (Y37.32-)

    ✓7ᵗʰ **Y37.430** Military operations involving other firearms discharge, military personnel

    ✓7ᵗʰ **Y37.431** Military operations involving other firearms discharge, civilian

✓6ᵗʰ **Y37.44** Military operations involving unarmed hand to hand combat

    EXCLUDES 1 *military operations involving combat using blunt or piercing object (Y37.45-)*

        military operations involving intentional restriction of air and airway (Y37.46-)

        military operations involving unintentional restriction of air and airway (Y37.47-)

    ✓7ᵗʰ **Y37.440** Military operations involving unarmed hand to hand combat, military personnel

    ✓7ᵗʰ **Y37.441** Military operations involving unarmed hand to hand combat, civilian

✓6ᵗʰ **Y37.45** Military operations involving combat using blunt or piercing object

    ✓7ᵗʰ **Y37.450** Military operations involving combat using blunt or piercing object, military personnel

    ✓7ᵗʰ **Y37.451** Military operations involving combat using blunt or piercing object, civilian

✓6ᵗʰ **Y37.46** Military operations involving intentional restriction of air and airway

    ✓7ᵗʰ **Y37.460** Military operations involving intentional restriction of air and airway, military personnel

    ✓7ᵗʰ **Y37.461** Military operations involving intentional restriction of air and airway, civilian

✓6ᵗʰ **Y37.47** Military operations involving unintentional restriction of air and airway

    ✓7ᵗʰ **Y37.470** Military operations involving unintentional restriction of air and airway, military personnel

    ✓7ᵗʰ **Y37.471** Military operations involving unintentional restriction of air and airway, civilian

✓6ᵗʰ **Y37.49** Military operations involving other forms of conventional warfare

    ✓7ᵗʰ **Y37.490** Military operations involving other forms of conventional warfare, military personnel

    ✓7ᵗʰ **Y37.491** Military operations involving other forms of conventional warfare, civilian

✓5ᵗʰ **Y37.5** Military operations involving nuclear weapons

    Military operation involving dirty bomb NOS

  ✓6ᵗʰ **Y37.50** Military operations involving unspecified effect of nuclear weapon

    ✓7ᵗʰ **Y37.500** Military operations involving unspecified effect of nuclear weapon, military personnel

    ✓7ᵗʰ **Y37.501** Military operations involving unspecified effect of nuclear weapon, civilian

  ✓6ᵗʰ **Y37.51** Military operations involving direct blast effect of nuclear weapon

    Military operations involving blast pressure of nuclear weapon

    ✓7ᵗʰ **Y37.510** Military operations involving direct blast effect of nuclear weapon, military personnel

    ✓7ᵗʰ **Y37.511** Military operations involving direct blast effect of nuclear weapon, civilian

✓6ᵗʰ **Y37.52** Military operations involving indirect blast effect of nuclear weapon

    Military operations involving being thrown by blast of nuclear weapon

    Military operations involving being struck or crushed by blast debris of nuclear weapon

    ✓7ᵗʰ **Y37.520** Military operations involving indirect blast effect of nuclear weapon, military personnel

    ✓7ᵗʰ **Y37.521** Military operations involving indirect blast effect of nuclear weapon, civilian

✓6ᵗʰ **Y37.53** Military operations involving thermal radiation effect of nuclear weapon

    Military operations involving direct heat from nuclear weapon

    Military operation involving fireball effects from nuclear weapon

    ✓7ᵗʰ **Y37.530** Military operations involving thermal radiation effect of nuclear weapon, military personnel

    ✓7ᵗʰ **Y37.531** Military operations involving thermal radiation effect of nuclear weapon, civilian

✓6ᵗʰ **Y37.54** Military operation involving nuclear radiation effects of nuclear weapon

    Military operation involving acute radiation exposure from nuclear weapon

    Military operation involving exposure to immediate ionizing radiation from nuclear weapon

    Military operation involving fallout exposure from nuclear weapon

    Military operation involving secondary effects of nuclear weapons

    ✓7ᵗʰ **Y37.540** Military operation involving nuclear radiation effects of nuclear weapon, military personnel

    ✓7ᵗʰ **Y37.541** Military operation involving nuclear radiation effects of nuclear weapon, civilian

✓6ᵗʰ **Y37.59** Military operation involving other effects of nuclear weapons

    ✓7ᵗʰ **Y37.590** Military operation involving other effects of nuclear weapons, military personnel

    ✓7ᵗʰ **Y37.591** Military operation involving other effects of nuclear weapons, civilian

✓5ᵗʰ **Y37.6** Military operations involving biological weapons

  ✓6ᵗʰ **Y37.6X** Military operations involving biological weapons

    ✓7ᵗʰ **Y37.6X0** Military operations involving biological weapons, military personnel

    ✓7ᵗʰ **Y37.6X1** Military operations involving biological weapons, civilian

✓5ᵗʰ **Y37.7** Military operations involving chemical weapons and other forms of unconventional warfare

    EXCLUDES 1 *military operations involving incendiary devices (Y36.3-, Y36.5-)*

  ✓6ᵗʰ **Y37.7X** Military operations involving chemical weapons and other forms of unconventional warfare

    ✓7ᵗʰ **Y37.7X0** Military operations involving chemical weapons and other forms of unconventional warfare, military personnel

    ✓7ᵗʰ **Y37.7X1** Military operations involving chemical weapons and other forms of unconventional warfare, civilian

✓5ᵗʰ **Y37.9** Other and unspecified military operations

  ✓x7ᵗʰ **Y37.90** Military operations, unspecified

  ✓x7ᵗʰ **Y37.91** Military operations involving unspecified weapon of mass destruction [WMD]

  ✓x7ᵗʰ **Y37.92** Military operations involving friendly fire

---

EXCLUDES 1 Not coded here   **EXCLUDES 2** Not included here   N Newborn Age: 0   P Pediatric Age: 0-17   M Maternity Age: 12-55   A Adult Age: 15-124

1046   ICD-10-CM Draft (2015)

✓4th Y38　Terrorism

NOTE　These codes are for use to identify injuries resulting from the unlawful use of force or violence against persons or property to intimidate or coerce a Government, the civilian population, or any segment thereof, in furtherance of political or social objective.

Use additional code for place of occurrence (Y92.-)

The appropriate 7th character is to be added to each code from category Y38.
A　initial encounter
D　subsequent encounter
S　sequela

✓5th Y38.0　Terrorism involving explosion of marine weapons
Terrorism involving depth-charge
Terrorism involving marine mine
Terrorism involving mine NOS, at sea or in harbor
Terrorism involving sea-based artillery shell
Terrorism involving torpedo
Terrorism involving underwater blast

✓6th Y38.0X　Terrorism involving explosion of marine weapons

✓7th **Y38.0X1**　Terrorism involving explosion of marine weapons, public safety official injured

✓7th **Y38.0X2**　Terrorism involving explosion of marine weapons, civilian injured

✓7th **Y38.0X3**　Terrorism involving explosion of marine weapons, terrorist injured

✓5th Y38.1　Terrorism involving destruction of aircraft
Terrorism involving aircraft burned
Terrorism involving aircraft exploded
Terrorism involving aircraft being shot down
Terrorism involving aircraft used as a weapon

✓6th Y38.1X　Terrorism involving destruction of aircraft

✓7th **Y38.1X1**　Terrorism involving destruction of aircraft, public safety official injured

✓7th **Y38.1X2**　Terrorism involving destruction of aircraft, civilian injured

✓7th **Y38.1X3**　Terrorism involving destruction of aircraft, terrorist injured

✓5th Y38.2　Terrorism involving other explosions and fragments
Terrorism involving antipersonnel (fragments) bomb
Terrorism involving blast NOS
Terrorism involving explosion NOS
Terrorism involving explosion of breech block
Terrorism involving explosion of cannon block
Terrorism involving explosion (fragments) of artillery shell
Terrorism involving explosion (fragments) of bomb
Terrorism involving explosion (fragments) of grenade
Terrorism involving explosion (fragments) of guided missile
Terrorism involving explosion (fragments) of land mine
Terrorism involving explosion of mortar bomb
Terrorism involving explosion of munitions
Terrorism involving explosion (fragments) of rocket
Terrorism involving explosion (fragments) of shell
Terrorism involving shrapnel
Terrorism involving mine NOS, on land

EXCLUDES 1　terrorism involving explosion of nuclear weapon (Y38.5)
terrorism involving suicide bomber (Y38.81)

✓6th Y38.2X　Terrorism involving other explosions and fragments

✓7th **Y38.2X1**　Terrorism involving other explosions and fragments, public safety official injured

✓7th **Y38.2X2**　Terrorism involving other explosions and fragments, civilian injured

✓7th **Y38.2X3**　Terrorism involving other explosions and fragments, terrorist injured

✓5th Y38.3　Terrorism involving fires, conflagration and hot substances
Terrorism involving conflagration NOS
Terrorism involving fire NOS
Terrorism involving petrol bomb

EXCLUDES 1　terrorism involving fire or heat of nuclear weapon (Y38.5)

✓6th Y38.3X　Terrorism involving fires, conflagration and hot substances

✓7th **Y38.3X1**　Terrorism involving fires, conflagration and hot substances, public safety official injured

✓7th **Y38.3X2**　Terrorism involving fires, conflagration and hot substances, civilian injured

✓7th **Y38.3X3**　Terrorism involving fires, conflagration and hot substances, terrorist injured

✓5th Y38.4　Terrorism involving firearms
Terrorism involving carbine bullet
Terrorism involving machine gun bullet
Terrorism involving pellets (shotgun)
Terrorism involving pistol bullet
Terrorism involving rifle bullet
Terrorism involving rubber (rifle) bullet

✓6th Y38.4X　Terrorism involving firearms

✓7th **Y38.4X1**　Terrorism involving firearms, public safety official injured

✓7th **Y38.4X2**　Terrorism involving firearms, civilian injured

✓7th **Y38.4X3**　Terrorism involving firearms, terrorist injured

✓5th Y38.5　Terrorism involving nuclear weapons
Terrorism involving blast effects of nuclear weapon
Terrorism involving exposure to ionizing radiation from nuclear weapon
Terrorism involving fireball effect of nuclear weapon
Terrorism involving heat from nuclear weapon

✓6th Y38.5X　Terrorism involving nuclear weapons

✓7th **Y38.5X1**　Terrorism involving nuclear weapons, public safety official injured

✓7th **Y38.5X2**　Terrorism involving nuclear weapons, civilian injured

✓7th **Y38.5X3**　Terrorism involving nuclear weapons, terrorist injured

✓5th Y38.6　Terrorism involving biological weapons
Terrorism involving anthrax
Terrorism involving cholera
Terrorism involving smallpox

✓6th Y38.6X　Terrorism involving biological weapons

✓7th **Y38.6X1**　Terrorism involving biological weapons, public safety official injured

✓7th **Y38.6X2**　Terrorism involving biological weapons, civilian injured

✓7th **Y38.6X3**　Terrorism involving biological weapons, terrorist injured

✓5th Y38.7　Terrorism involving chemical weapons
Terrorism involving gases, fumes, chemicals
Terrorism involving hydrogen cyanide
Terrorism involving phosgene
Terrorism involving sarin

✓6th Y38.7X　Terrorism involving chemical weapons

✓7th **Y38.7X1**　Terrorism involving chemical weapons, public safety official injured

✓7th **Y38.7X2**　Terrorism involving chemical weapons, civilian injured

✓7th **Y38.7X3**　Terrorism involving chemical weapons, terrorist injured

✓5th Y38.8　Terrorism involving other and unspecified means

Y38.80　Terrorism involving unspecified means
Terrorism NOS

✓6th Y38.81　Terrorism involving suicide bomber

✓7th **Y38.811**　Terrorism involving suicide bomber, public safety official injured

✓7th **Y38.812**　Terrorism involving suicide bomber, civilian injured

✓6th Y38.89　Terrorism involving other means
Terrorism involving drowning and submersion
Terrorism involving lasers
Terrorism involving piercing or stabbing instruments

✓7th **Y38.891**　Terrorism involving other means, public safety official injured

✓7th **Y38.892**　Terrorism involving other means, civilian injured

✓7th **Y38.893**　Terrorism involving other means, terrorist injured

✓5th Y38.9　Terrorism, secondary effects

NOTE　This code is for use to identify injuries occurring subsequent to a terrorist attack, not those that are due to the initial terrorist attack.

✓6th Y38.9X　Terrorism, secondary effects

✓7th **Y38.9X1**　Terrorism, secondary effects, public safety official injured

---

✓ Additional Character Required　　✓x7th Xtension Alert　　Unspecified Dx　　Other Specified Dx　　Manifestation　　►◄ Revised Text　　● New Code　　▲ Revised Code Title

✓7ᵗʰ **Y38.9X2** **Terrorism, secondary effects,** civilian injured

Complications of medical and surgical care (Y62-Y84)

INCLUDES   complications of medical devices
surgical and medical procedures as the cause of abnormal reaction of the patient, or of later complication, without mention of misadventure at the time of the procedure

Misadventures to patients during surgical and medical care (Y62-Y69)

EXCLUDES 2   breakdown or malfunctioning of medical device (during procedure) (after implantation) (ongoing use) (Y70-Y82)
surgical and medical procedures as the cause of abnormal reaction of the patient, without mention of misadventure at the time of the procedure (Y83-Y84)

✓4ᵗʰ **Y62** **Failure of** sterile precautions **during surgical and medical care**

Y62.0 **Failure of sterile precautions during** surgical operation

Y62.1 **Failure of sterile precautions during** infusion or transfusion

Y62.2 **Failure of sterile precautions during** kidney dialysis and other perfusion

Y62.3 **Failure of sterile precautions during** injection or immunization

Y62.4 **Failure of sterile precautions during** endoscopic examination

Y62.5 **Failure of sterile precautions during** heart catheterization

Y62.6 **Failure of sterile precautions during** aspiration, puncture and other catheterization

Y62.8 **Failure of sterile precautions during other surgical and medical care**

Y62.9 **Failure of sterile precautions during unspecified surgical and medical care**

✓4ᵗʰ **Y63** **Failure in** dosage **during surgical and medical care**

EXCLUDES 2   accidental overdose of drug or wrong drug given in error (T36-T50)

Y63.0 **Excessive amount of blood or other fluid given during transfusion or infusion**

Y63.1 **Incorrect dilution of fluid used during infusion**

Y63.2 **Overdose of radiation given during therapy**

Y63.3 **Inadvertent exposure of patient to radiation during medical care**

Y63.4 **Failure in dosage in electroshock or insulin-shock therapy**

Y63.5 **Inappropriate temperature in local application and packing**

Y63.6 **Underdosing and nonadministration of necessary drug, medicament or biological substance**

Y63.8 **Failure in dosage during other surgical and medical care**

Y63.9 **Failure in dosage during unspecified surgical and medical care**

✓4ᵗʰ **Y64** Contaminated **medical or biological** substances

Y64.0 **Contaminated medical or biological substance,** transfused or infused

Y64.1 **Contaminated medical or biological substance,** injected or used for immunization

Y64.8 **Contaminated medical or biological substance administered by other means**

Y64.9 **Contaminated medical or biological substance administered by unspecified means**
Administered contaminated medical or biological substance NOS

✓4ᵗʰ **Y65** Other misadventures **during surgical and medical care**

Y65.0 **Mismatched blood in transfusion**

Y65.1 **Wrong fluid used in infusion**

Y65.2 **Failure in suture or ligature during surgical operation**

Y65.3 **Endotracheal tube wrongly placed during anesthetic procedure**

Y65.4 **Failure to introduce or to remove other tube or instrument**

✓5ᵗʰ **Y65.5** **Performance of** wrong procedure **(operation)**

Y65.51 **Performance of wrong procedure (operation) on** correct patient
Wrong device implanted into correct surgical site
EXCLUDES 1   performance of correct procedure (operation) on wrong side or body part (Y65.53)

Y65.52 **Performance of procedure (operation) on** patient not scheduled for surgery
Performance of procedure (operation) intended for another patient
Performance of procedure (operation) on wrong patient

Y65.53 **Performance of correct procedure (operation) on** wrong side or body part
Performance of correct procedure (operation) on wrong side
Performance of correct procedure (operation) on wrong site

Y65.8 **Other specified** misadventures **during surgical and medical care**

Y66 **Nonadministration of surgical and medical care**
Premature cessation of surgical and medical care
EXCLUDES 1   DNR status (Z66)
palliative care (Z51.5)

Y69 **Unspecified misadventure during surgical and medical care**

Medical devices associated with adverse incidents in diagnostic and therapeutic use (Y70-Y82)

INCLUDES   breakdown or malfunction of medical devices (during use) (after implantation) (ongoing use)

EXCLUDES 1   misadventure to patients during surgical and medical care, classifiable to (Y62-Y69)
later complications following use of medical devices without breakdown or malfunctioning of device (Y83-Y84)

✓4ᵗʰ **Y70** Anesthesiology **devices associated with adverse incidents**

Y70.0 Diagnostic and monitoring **anesthesiology devices associated with adverse incidents**

Y70.1 Therapeutic (nonsurgical) and rehabilitative **anesthesiology devices associated with adverse incidents**

Y70.2 Prosthetic and other implants, **materials and accessory anesthesiology devices associated with adverse incidents**

Y70.3 Surgical instruments, materials **and anesthesiology devices (including sutures) associated with adverse incidents**

Y70.8 **Miscellaneous anesthesiology devices associated with adverse incidents, not elsewhere classified**

✓4ᵗʰ **Y71** Cardiovascular **devices associated with adverse incidents**

Y71.0 Diagnostic and monitoring **cardiovascular devices associated with adverse incidents**

Y71.1 Therapeutic (nonsurgical) and rehabilitative **cardiovascular devices associated with adverse incidents**

Y71.2 Prosthetic and other implants, **materials and accessory cardiovascular devices associated with adverse incidents**

Y71.3 Surgical instruments, materials **and cardiovascular devices (including sutures) associated with adverse incidents**

Y71.8 **Miscellaneous cardiovascular devices associated with adverse incidents, not elsewhere classified**

✓4ᵗʰ **Y72** Otorhinolaryngological **devices associated with adverse incidents**

Y72.0 Diagnostic and monitoring **otorhinolaryngological devices associated with adverse incidents**

Y72.1 Therapeutic (nonsurgical) and rehabilitative **otorhinolaryngological devices associated with adverse incidents**

Y72.2 Prosthetic and other implants, **materials and accessory otorhinolaryngological devices associated with adverse incidents**

Y72.3 Surgical instruments, materials **and otorhinolaryngological devices (including sutures) associated with adverse incidents**

Y72.8 **Miscellaneous otorhinolaryngological devices associated with adverse incidents, not elsewhere classified**

✓4ᵗʰ **Y73** Gastroenterology **and** urology **devices associated with adverse incidents**

Y73.0 Diagnostic and monitoring **gastroenterology and urology devices associated with adverse incidents**

Y73.1 Therapeutic (nonsurgical) and rehabilitative **gastroenterology and urology devices associated with adverse incidents**

Y73.2 Prosthetic and other implants, **materials and accessory gastroenterology and urology devices associated with adverse incidents**

Y73.3 Surgical instruments, materials **and gastroenterology and urology devices (including sutures) associated with adverse incidents**

EXCLUDES 1 Not coded here   EXCLUDES 2 Not included here   N Newborn Age: 0   P Pediatric Age: 0-17   M Maternity Age: 12-55   A Adult Age: 15-124

1048   ICD-10-CM Draft (2015)

Y73.8 Miscellaneous gastroenterology and urology devices associated with adverse incidents, not elsewhere classified

✓4ᵗʰ **Y74** General hospital and personal-use devices associated with adverse incidents

Y74.0 Diagnostic and monitoring general hospital and personal-use devices associated with adverse incidents

Y74.1 Therapeutic (nonsurgical) and rehabilitative general hospital and personal-use devices associated with adverse incidents

Y74.2 Prosthetic and other implants, materials and accessory general hospital and personal-use devices associated with adverse incidents

Y74.3 Surgical instruments, materials and general hospital and personal-use devices (including sutures) associated with adverse incidents

Y74.8 Miscellaneous general hospital and personal-use devices associated with adverse incidents, not elsewhere classified

✓4ᵗʰ **Y75** Neurological devices associated with adverse incidents

Y75.0 Diagnostic and monitoring neurological devices associated with adverse incidents

Y75.1 Therapeutic (nonsurgical) and rehabilitative neurological devices associated with adverse incidents

Y75.2 Prosthetic and other implants, materials and neurological devices associated with adverse incidents

Y75.3 Surgical instruments, materials and neurological devices (including sutures) associated with adverse incidents

Y75.8 Miscellaneous neurological devices associated with adverse incidents, not elsewhere classified

✓4ᵗʰ **Y76** Obstetric and gynecological devices associated with adverse incidents

Y76.0 Diagnostic and monitoring obstetric and gynecological devices associated with adverse incidents ♀

Y76.1 Therapeutic (nonsurgical) and rehabilitative obstetric and gynecological devices associated with adverse incidents ♀

Y76.2 Prosthetic and other implants, materials and accessory obstetric and gynecological devices associated with adverse incidents ♀

Y76.3 Surgical instruments, materials and obstetric and gynecological devices (including sutures) associated with adverse incidents ♀

Y76.8 Miscellaneous obstetric and gynecological devices associated with adverse incidents, not elsewhere classified ♀

✓4ᵗʰ **Y77** Ophthalmic devices associated with adverse incidents

Y77.0 Diagnostic and monitoring ophthalmic devices associated with adverse incidents

Y77.1 Therapeutic (nonsurgical) and rehabilitative ophthalmic devices associated with adverse incidents

Y77.2 Prosthetic and other implants, materials and accessory ophthalmic devices associated with adverse incidents

Y77.3 Surgical instruments, materials and ophthalmic devices (including sutures) associated with adverse incidents

Y77.8 Miscellaneous ophthalmic devices associated with adverse incidents, not elsewhere classified

✓4ᵗʰ **Y78** Radiological devices associated with adverse incidents

Y78.0 Diagnostic and monitoring radiological devices associated with adverse incidents

Y78.1 Therapeutic (nonsurgical) and rehabilitative radiological devices associated with adverse incidents

Y78.2 Prosthetic and other implants, materials and accessory radiological devices associated with adverse incidents

Y78.3 Surgical instruments, materials and radiological devices (including sutures) associated with adverse incidents

Y78.8 Miscellaneous radiological devices associated with adverse incidents, not elsewhere classified

✓4ᵗʰ **Y79** Orthopedic devices associated with adverse incidents

Y79.0 Diagnostic and monitoring orthopedic devices associated with adverse incidents

Y79.1 Therapeutic (nonsurgical) and rehabilitative orthopedic devices associated with adverse incidents

Y79.2 Prosthetic and other implants, materials and accessory orthopedic devices associated with adverse incidents

Y79.3 Surgical instruments, materials and orthopedic devices (including sutures) associated with adverse incidents

Y79.8 Miscellaneous orthopedic devices associated with adverse incidents, not elsewhere classified

✓4ᵗʰ **Y80** Physical medicine devices associated with adverse incidents

Y80.0 Diagnostic and monitoring physical medicine devices associated with adverse incidents

Y80.1 Therapeutic (nonsurgical) and rehabilitative physical medicine devices associated with adverse incidents

Y80.2 Prosthetic and other implants, materials and accessory physical medicine devices associated with adverse incidents

Y80.3 Surgical instruments, materials and physical medicine devices (including sutures) associated with adverse incidents

Y80.8 Miscellaneous physical medicine devices associated with adverse incidents, not elsewhere classified

✓4ᵗʰ **Y81** General- and plastic-surgery devices associated with adverse incidents

Y81.0 Diagnostic and monitoring general- and plastic-surgery devices associated with adverse incidents

Y81.1 Therapeutic (nonsurgical) and rehabilitative general- and plastic-surgery devices associated with adverse incidents

Y81.2 Prosthetic and other implants, materials and accessory general- and plastic-surgery devices associated with adverse incidents

Y81.3 Surgical instruments, materials and general- and plastic-surgery devices (including sutures) associated with adverse incidents

Y81.8 Miscellaneous general- and plastic-surgery devices associated with adverse incidents, not elsewhere classified

✓4ᵗʰ **Y82** Other and unspecified medical devices associated with adverse incidents

Y82.8 Other medical devices associated with adverse incidents

Y82.9 Unspecified medical devices associated with adverse incidents

Surgical and other medical procedures as the cause of abnormal reaction of the patient, or of later complication, without mention of misadventure at the time of the procedure (Y83-Y84)

EXCLUDES 1　misadventures to patients during surgical and medical care, classifiable to (Y62-Y69)

✓4ᵗʰ **Y83** Surgical operation and other surgical procedures as the cause of abnormal reaction of the patient, or of later complication, without mention of misadventure at the time of the procedure

Y83.0 Surgical operation with transplant of whole organ as the cause of abnormal reaction of the patient, or of later complication, without mention of misadventure at the time of the procedure

Y83.1 Surgical operation with implant of artificial internal device as the cause of abnormal reaction of the patient, or of later complication, without mention of misadventure at the time of the procedure

Y83.2 Surgical operation with anastomosis, bypass or graft as the cause of abnormal reaction of the patient, or of later complication, without mention of misadventure at the time of the procedure

Y83.3 Surgical operation with formation of external stoma as the cause of abnormal reaction of the patient, or of later complication, without mention of misadventure at the time of the procedure

Y83.4 Other reconstructive surgery as the cause of abnormal reaction of the patient, or of later complication, without mention of misadventure at the time of the procedure

Y83.5 Amputation of limb(s) as the cause of abnormal reaction of the patient, or of later complication, without mention of misadventure at the time of the procedure

Y83.6 Removal of other organ (partial) (total) as the cause of abnormal reaction of the patient, or of later complication, without mention of misadventure at the time of the procedure

Y83.8 Other surgical procedures as the cause of abnormal reaction of the patient, or of later complication, without mention of misadventure at the time of the procedure

Y83.9 Surgical procedure, unspecified as the cause of abnormal reaction of the patient, or of later complication, without mention of misadventure at the time of the procedure

✓4ᵗʰ **Y84** Other medical procedures as the cause of abnormal reaction of the patient, or of later complication, without mention of misadventure at the time of the procedure

Y84.0 Cardiac catheterization as the cause of abnormal reaction of the patient, or of later complication, without mention of misadventure at the time of the procedure

✓ Additional Character Required　✓7ᵗʰ Xtension Alert　Unspecified Dx　Other Specified Dx　Manifestation　►◄ Revised Text　● New Code　▲ Revised Code Title

ICD-10-CM Draft (2015)　　　　　　　　　　　　　　　　　　　　　　　　　　　　　　1049

External Causes of Morbidity

Y73.8–Y84.0

External Causes of Morbidity

Y84.1–Y92.Ø31

Y84.1   Kidney dialysis as the cause of abnormal reaction of the patient, or of later complication, without mention of misadventure at the time of the procedure

Y84.2   Radiological procedure and radiotherapy as the cause of abnormal reaction of the patient, or of later complication, without mention of misadventure at the time of the procedure

Y84.3   Shock therapy as the cause of abnormal reaction of the patient, or of later complication, without mention of misadventure at the time of the procedure

Y84.4   Aspiration of fluid as the cause of abnormal reaction of the patient, or of later complication, without mention of misadventure at the time of the procedure

Y84.5   Insertion of gastric or duodenal sound as the cause of abnormal reaction of the patient, or of later complication, without mention of misadventure at the time of the procedure

Y84.6   Urinary catheterization as the cause of abnormal reaction of the patient, or of later complication, without mention of misadventure at the time of the procedure

Y84.7   Blood-sampling as the cause of abnormal reaction of the patient, or of later complication, without mention of misadventure at the time of the procedure

Y84.8   Other medical procedures as the cause of abnormal reaction of the patient, or of later complication, without mention of misadventure at the time of the procedure

Y84.9   Medical procedure, unspecified as the cause of abnormal reaction of the patient, or of later complication, without mention of misadventure at the time of the procedure

Supplementary factors related to causes of morbidity classified elsewhere (Y9Ø-Y99)

NOTE   These categories may be used to provide supplementary information concerning causes of morbidity. They are not to be used for single-condition coding.

☑4ᵗʰ **Y9Ø**   **Evidence of alcohol involvement determined by blood alcohol level**

Code first any associated alcohol related disorders (F1Ø)

Y9Ø.Ø   Blood alcohol level of less than 2Ø mg/1ØØ ml

Y9Ø.1   Blood alcohol level of 2Ø-39 mg/1ØØ ml

Y9Ø.2   Blood alcohol level of 4Ø-59 mg/1ØØ ml

Y9Ø.3   Blood alcohol level of 6Ø-79 mg/1ØØ ml

Y9Ø.4   Blood alcohol level of 8Ø-99 mg/1ØØ ml

Y9Ø.5   Blood alcohol level of 1ØØ-119 mg/1ØØ ml

Y9Ø.6   Blood alcohol level of 12Ø-199 mg/1ØØ ml

Y9Ø.7   Blood alcohol level of 2ØØ-239 mg/1ØØ ml

Y9Ø.8   Blood alcohol level of 24Ø mg/1ØØ ml or more

Y9Ø.9   Presence of alcohol in blood, level not specified

☑4ᵗʰ **Y92**   **Place of occurrence of the external cause**

The following category is for use, when relevant, to identify the place of occurrence of the external cause. Use in conjunction with an activity code.

Place of occurrence should be recorded only at the initial encounter for treatment

☑5ᵗʰ **Y92.Ø**   Non-institutional (private) residence as the place of occurrence of the external cause

EXCLUDES 1   abandoned or derelict house (Y92.89)
home under construction but not yet occupied (Y92.6-)
institutional place of residence (Y92.1-)

☑6ᵗʰ **Y92.ØØ**   Unspecified non-institutional (private) residence as the place of occurrence of the external cause

Y92.ØØØ   Kitchen of unspecified non-institutional (private) residence as the place of occurrence of the external cause

Y92.ØØ1   Dining room of unspecified non-institutional (private) residence as the place of occurrence of the external cause

Y92.ØØ2   Bathroom of unspecified non-institutional (private) residence single-family (private) house as the place of occurrence of the external cause

Y92.ØØ3   Bedroom of unspecified non-institutional (private) residence as the place of occurrence of the external cause

Y92.ØØ7   Garden or yard of unspecified non-institutional (private) residence as the place of occurrence of the external cause

Y92.ØØ8   Other place in unspecified non-institutional (private) residence as the place of occurrence of the external cause

Y92.ØØ9   Unspecified place in unspecified non-institutional (private) residence as the place of occurrence of the external cause
Home (NOS) as the place of occurrence of the external cause

☑6ᵗʰ **Y92.Ø1**   Single-family non-institutional (private) house as the place of occurrence of the external cause
Farmhouse as the place of occurrence of the external cause

EXCLUDES 1   barn (Y92.71)
chicken coop or hen house (Y92.72)
farm field (Y92.73)
orchard (Y92.74)
single family mobile home or trailer (Y92.Ø2-)
slaughter house (Y92.86)

Y92.Ø1Ø   Kitchen of single-family (private) house as the place of occurrence of the external cause

Y92.Ø11   Dining room of single-family (private) house as the place of occurrence of the external cause

Y92.Ø12   Bathroom of single-family (private) house as the place of occurrence of the external cause

Y92.Ø13   Bedroom of single-family (private) house as the place of occurrence of the external cause

Y92.Ø14   Private driveway to single-family (private) house as the place of occurrence of the external cause

Y92.Ø15   Private garage of single-family (private) house as the place of occurrence of the external cause

Y92.Ø16   Swimming-pool in single-family (private) house or garden as the place of occurrence of the external cause

Y92.Ø17   Garden or yard in single-family (private) house as the place of occurrence of the external cause

Y92.Ø18   Other place in single-family (private) house as the place of occurrence of the external cause

Y92.Ø19   Unspecified place in single-family (private) house as the place of occurrence of the external cause

☑6ᵗʰ **Y92.Ø2**   Mobile home as the place of occurrence of the external cause

Y92.Ø2Ø   Kitchen in mobile home as the place of occurrence of the external cause

Y92.Ø21   Dining room in mobile home as the place of occurrence of the external cause

Y92.Ø22   Bathroom in mobile home as the place of occurrence of the external cause

Y92.Ø23   Bedroom in mobile home as the place of occurrence of the external cause

Y92.Ø24   Driveway of mobile home as the place of occurrence of the external cause

Y92.Ø25   Garage of mobile home as the place of occurrence of the external cause

Y92.Ø26   Swimming-pool of mobile home as the place of occurrence of the external cause

Y92.Ø27   Garden or yard of mobile home as the place of occurrence of the external cause

Y92.Ø28   Other place in mobile home as the place of occurrence of the external cause

Y92.Ø29   Unspecified place in mobile home as the place of occurrence of the external cause

☑6ᵗʰ **Y92.Ø3**   Apartment as the place of occurrence of the external cause
Condominium as the place of occurrence of the external cause
Co-op apartment as the place of occurrence of the external cause

Y92.Ø3Ø   Kitchen in apartment as the place of occurrence of the external cause

Y92.Ø31   Bathroom in apartment as the place of occurrence of the external cause

EXCLUDES 1 Not coded here   EXCLUDES 2 Not included here   N Newborn Age: Ø   P Pediatric Age: Ø-17   M Maternity Age: 12-55   A Adult Age: 15-124

1Ø5Ø   ICD-1Ø-CM Draft (2Ø15)

Y92.032　Bedroom in apartment as the place of occurrence of the external cause

Y92.038　Other place in apartment as the place of occurrence of the external cause

Y92.039　Unspecified place in apartment as the place of occurrence of the external cause

☑6ᵗʰ Y92.04　Boarding-house as the place of occurrence of the external cause

Y92.040　Kitchen in boarding-house as the place of occurrence of the external cause

Y92.041　Bathroom in boarding-house as the place of occurrence of the external cause

Y92.042　Bedroom in boarding-house as the place of occurrence of the external cause

Y92.043　Driveway of boarding-house as the place of occurrence of the external cause

Y92.044　Garage of boarding-house as the place of occurrence of the external cause

Y92.045　Swimming-pool of boarding-house as the place of occurrence of the external cause

Y92.046　Garden or yard of boarding-house as the place of occurrence of the external cause

Y92.048　Other place in boarding-house as the place of occurrence of the external cause

Y92.049　Unspecified place in boarding-house as the place of occurrence of the external cause

☑6ᵗʰ Y92.09　Other non-institutional residence as the place of occurrence of the external cause

Y92.090　Kitchen in other non-institutional residence as the place of occurrence of the external cause

Y92.091　Bathroom in other non-institutional residence as the place of occurrence of the external cause

Y92.092　Bedroom in other non-institutional residence as the place of occurrence of the external cause

Y92.093　Driveway of other non-institutional residence as the place of occurrence of the external cause

Y92.094　Garage of other non-institutional residence as the place of occurrence of the external cause

Y92.095　Swimming-pool of other non-institutional residence as the place of occurrence of the external cause

Y92.096　Garden or yard of other non-institutional residence as the place of occurrence of the external cause

Y92.098　Other place in other non-institutional residence as the place of occurrence of the external cause

Y92.099　Unspecified place in other non-institutional residence as the place of occurrence of the external cause

☑5ᵗʰ Y92.1　Institutional (nonprivate) residence as the place of occurrence of the external cause

Y92.10　Unspecified residential institution as the place of occurrence of the external cause

☑6ᵗʰ Y92.11　Children's home and orphanage as the place of occurrence of the external cause

Y92.110　Kitchen in children's home and orphanage as the place of occurrence of the external cause

Y92.111　Bathroom in children's home and orphanage as the place of occurrence of the external cause

Y92.112　Bedroom in children's home and orphanage as the place of occurrence of the external cause

Y92.113　Driveway of children's home and orphanage as the place of occurrence of the external cause

Y92.114　Garage of children's home and orphanage as the place of occurrence of the external cause

Y92.115　Swimming-pool of children's home and orphanage as the place of occurrence of the external cause

Y92.116　Garden or yard of children's home and orphanage as the place of occurrence of the external cause

Y92.118　Other place in children's home and orphanage as the place of occurrence of the external cause

Y92.119　Unspecified place in children's home and orphanage as the place of occurrence of the external cause

☑6ᵗʰ Y92.12　Nursing home as the place of occurrence of the external cause

Home for the sick as the place of occurrence of the external cause

Hospice as the place of occurrence of the external cause

Y92.120　Kitchen in nursing home as the place of occurrence of the external cause

Y92.121　Bathroom in nursing home as the place of occurrence of the external cause

Y92.122　Bedroom in nursing home as the place of occurrence of the external cause

Y92.123　Driveway of nursing home as the place of occurrence of the external cause

Y92.124　Garage of nursing home as the place of occurrence of the external cause

Y92.125　Swimming-pool of nursing home as the place of occurrence of the external cause

Y92.126　Garden or yard of nursing home as the place of occurrence of the external cause

Y92.128　Other place in nursing home as the place of occurrence of the external cause

Y92.129　Unspecified place in nursing home as the place of occurrence of the external cause

☑6ᵗʰ Y92.13　Military base as the place of occurrence of the external cause

EXCLUDES 1　military training grounds (Y92.83)

Y92.130　Kitchen on military base as the place of occurrence of the external cause

Y92.131　Mess hall on military base as the place of occurrence of the external cause

Y92.133　Barracks on military base as the place of occurrence of the external cause

Y92.135　Garage on military base as the place of occurrence of the external cause

Y92.136　Swimming-pool on military base as the place of occurrence of the external cause

Y92.137　Garden or yard on military base as the place of occurrence of the external cause

Y92.138　Other place on military base as the place of occurrence of the external cause

Y92.139　Unspecified place military base as the place of occurrence of the external cause

☑6ᵗʰ Y92.14　Prison as the place of occurrence of the external cause

Y92.140　Kitchen in prison as the place of occurrence of the external cause

Y92.141　Dining room in prison as the place of occurrence of the external cause

Y92.142　Bathroom in prison as the place of occurrence of the external cause

Y92.143　Cell of prison as the place of occurrence of the external cause

Y92.146　Swimming-pool of prison as the place of occurrence of the external cause

Y92.147　Courtyard of prison as the place of occurrence of the external cause

Y92.148　Other place in prison as the place of occurrence of the external cause

Y92.149　Unspecified place in prison as the place of occurrence of the external cause

☑6ᵗʰ Y92.15　Reform school as the place of occurrence of the external cause

Y92.150　Kitchen in reform school as the place of occurrence of the external cause

Y92.151　Dining room in reform school as the place of occurrence of the external cause

Y92.152　Bathroom in reform school as the place of occurrence of the external cause

☑ Additional Character Required　　☑x7ᵗʰ Xtension Alert　　Unspecified Dx　　Other Specified Dx　　Manifestation　　▶◀ Revised Text　　● New Code　　▲ Revised Code Title

ICD-10-CM Draft (2015)　　　　　　　　　　　　　　　　　　　　　　　　　　　　　　　　1051

External Causes of Morbidity

Y92.153–Y92.248

Y92.153   **Bedroom** in reform school as the place of occurrence of the external cause

Y92.154   **Driveway** of reform school as the place of occurrence of the external cause

Y92.155   **Garage** of reform school as the place of occurrence of the external cause

Y92.156   **Swimming-pool** of reform school as the place of occurrence of the external cause

Y92.157   **Garden or yard** of reform school as the place of occurrence of the external cause

Y92.158   **Other place in reform school as the place of occurrence of the external cause**

Y92.159   **Unspecified place in reform school as the place of occurrence of the external cause**

✓6ᵗʰ   **Y92.16**   **School dormitory** as the place of occurrence of the external cause

> *EXCLUDES 1*   *reform school as the place of occurrence of the external cause (Y92.15-)*
> *school buildings and grounds as the place of occurrence of the external cause (Y92.2-)*
> *school sports and athletic areas as the place of occurrence of the external cause (Y92.3-)*

Y92.160   **Kitchen** in school dormitory as the place of occurrence of the external cause

Y92.161   **Dining room** in school dormitory as the place of occurrence of the external cause

Y92.162   **Bathroom** in school dormitory as the place of occurrence of the external cause

Y92.163   **Bedroom** in school dormitory as the place of occurrence of the external cause

Y92.168   **Other place in school dormitory as the place of occurrence of the external cause**

Y92.169   **Unspecified place in school dormitory as the place of occurrence of the external cause**

✓6ᵗʰ   **Y92.19**   **Other specified residential institution** as the place of occurrence of the external cause

Y92.190   **Kitchen** in other specified residential institution as the place of occurrence of the external cause

Y92.191   **Dining** room in other specified residential institution as the place of occurrence of the external cause

Y92.192   **Bathroom** in other specified residential institution as the place of occurrence of the external cause

Y92.193   **Bedroom** in other specified residential institution as the place of occurrence of the external cause

Y92.194   **Driveway** of other specified residential institution as the place of occurrence of the external cause

Y92.195   **Garage** of other specified residential institution as the place of occurrence of the external cause

Y92.196   **Pool** of other specified residential institution as the place of occurrence of the external cause

Y92.197   **Garden or yard** of other specified residential institution as the place of occurrence of the external cause

Y92.198   **Other place in other specified residential institution as the place of occurrence of the external cause**

Y92.199   **Unspecified place in other specified residential institution as the place of occurrence of the external cause**

✓5ᵗʰ   **Y92.2**   **School, other institution and public administrative area as the place of occurrence of the external cause**

Building and adjacent grounds used by the general public or by a particular group of the public

> *EXCLUDES 1*   *building under construction as the place of occurrence of the external cause (Y92.6)*
> *residential institution as the place of occurrence of the external cause (Y92.1)*
> *school dormitory as the place of occurrence of the external cause (Y92.16-)*
> *sports and athletics area of schools as the place of occurrence of the external cause (Y92.3-)*

✓6ᵗʰ   **Y92.21**   **School (private) (public) (state)** as the place of occurrence of the external cause

Y92.210   **Daycare** center as the place of occurrence of the external cause

Y92.211   **Elementary school** as the place of occurrence of the external cause
> Kindergarten as the place of occurrence of the external cause

Y92.212   **Middle school** as the place of occurrence of the external cause

Y92.213   **High school** as the place of occurrence of the external cause
> **AHA:** 2012, 4Q, 108

Y92.214   **College** as the place of occurrence of the external cause
> University as the place of occurrence of the external cause

Y92.215   **Trade school** as the place of occurrence of the external cause

Y92.218   **Other school as the place of occurrence of the external cause**

Y92.219   **Unspecified school as the place of occurrence of the external cause**

Y92.22   **Religious institution** as the place of occurrence of the external cause
> Church as the place of occurrence of the external cause
> Mosque as the place of occurrence of the external cause
> Synagogue as the place of occurrence of the external cause

✓6ᵗʰ   **Y92.23**   **Hospital** as the place of occurrence of the external cause

> *EXCLUDES 1*   *ambulatory (outpatient) health services establishments (Y92.53-)*
> *home for the sick as the place of occurrence of the external cause (Y92.12-)*
> *hospice as the place of occurrence of the external cause (Y92.12-)*
> *nursing home as the place of occurrence of the external cause (Y92.12-)*

Y92.230   **Patient room** in hospital as the place of occurrence of the external cause

Y92.231   **Patient bathroom** in hospital as the place of occurrence of the external cause

Y92.232   **Corridor** of hospital as the place of occurrence of the external cause

Y92.233   **Cafeteria** of hospital as the place of occurrence of the external cause

Y92.234   **Operating room** of hospital as the place of occurrence of the external cause

Y92.238   **Other place in hospital as the place of occurrence of the external cause**

Y92.239   **Unspecified place in hospital as the place of occurrence of the external cause**

✓6ᵗʰ   **Y92.24**   **Public administrative building** as the place of occurrence of the external cause

Y92.240   **Courthouse** as the place of occurrence of the external cause

Y92.241   **Library** as the place of occurrence of the external cause

Y92.242   **Post office** as the place of occurrence of the external cause

Y92.243   **City hall** as the place of occurrence of the external cause

Y92.248   **Other public administrative building as the place of occurrence of the external cause**

EXCLUDES 1 Not coded here   *EXCLUDES 2* Not included here   **N** Newborn Age: 0   **P** Pediatric Age: 0-17   **M** Maternity Age: 12-55   **A** Adult Age: 15-124

1052   ICD-10-CM Draft (2015)

✓6ᵗʰ **Y92.25** Cultural building as the place of occurrence of the external cause

    Y92.250 Art Gallery as the place of occurrence of the external cause

    Y92.251 Museum as the place of occurrence of the external cause

    Y92.252 Music hall as the place of occurrence of the external cause

    Y92.253 Opera house as the place of occurrence of the external cause

    Y92.254 Theater (live) as the place of occurrence of the external cause

    Y92.258 Other cultural public building as the place of occurrence of the external cause

Y92.26 Movie house or cinema as the place of occurrence of the external cause

Y92.29 Other specified public building as the place of occurrence of the external cause

    Assembly hall as the place of occurrence of the external cause

    Clubhouse as the place of occurrence of the external cause

✓5ᵗʰ **Y92.3** Sports and athletics area as the place of occurrence of the external cause

✓6ᵗʰ **Y92.31** Athletic court as the place of occurrence of the external cause

    EXCLUDES 1 *tennis court in private home or garden (Y92.09)*

    Y92.310 Basketball court as the place of occurrence of the external cause

    Y92.311 Squash court as the place of occurrence of the external cause

    Y92.312 Tennis court as the place of occurrence of the external cause

    Y92.318 Other athletic court as the place of occurrence of the external cause

✓6ᵗʰ **Y92.32** Athletic field as the place of occurrence of the external cause

    Y92.320 Baseball field as the place of occurrence of the external cause

    Y92.321 Football field as the place of occurrence of the external cause

    Y92.322 Soccer field as the place of occurrence of the external cause

    Y92.328 Other athletic field as the place of occurrence of the external cause

        Cricket field as the place of occurrence of the external cause

        Hockey field as the place of occurrence of the external cause

✓6ᵗʰ **Y92.33** Skating rink as the place of occurrence of the external cause

    Y92.330 Ice skating rink (indoor) (outdoor) as the place of occurrence of the external cause

    Y92.331 Roller skating rink as the place of occurrence of the external cause

Y92.34 Swimming pool (public) as the place of occurrence of the external cause

    EXCLUDES 1 *swimming pool in private home or garden (Y92.016)*

Y92.39 Other specified sports and athletic area as the place of occurrence of the external cause

    Golf-course as the place of occurrence of the external cause

    Gymnasium as the place of occurrence of the external cause

    Riding-school as the place of occurrence of the external cause

    Stadium as the place of occurrence of the external cause

✓5ᵗʰ **Y92.4** Street, highway and other paved roadways as the place of occurrence of the external cause

    EXCLUDES 1 *private driveway of residence (Y92.014, Y92.024, Y92.043, Y92.093, Y92.113, Y92.123, Y92.154, Y92.194)*

✓6ᵗʰ **Y92.41** Street and highway as the place of occurrence of the external cause

    Y92.410 Unspecified street and highway as the place of occurrence of the external cause

        Road NOS as the place of occurrence of the external cause

    Y92.411 Interstate highway as the place of occurrence of the external cause

        Freeway as the place of occurrence of the external cause

        Motorway as the place of occurrence of the external cause

    Y92.412 Parkway as the place of occurrence of the external cause

    Y92.413 State road as the place of occurrence of the external cause

    Y92.414 Local residential or business street as the place of occurrence of the external cause

    Y92.415 Exit ramp or entrance ramp of street or highway as the place of occurrence of the external cause

✓6ᵗʰ **Y92.48** Other paved roadways as the place of occurrence of the external cause

    Y92.480 Sidewalk as the place of occurrence of the external cause

    Y92.481 Parking lot as the place of occurrence of the external cause

    Y92.482 Bike path as the place of occurrence of the external cause

    Y92.488 Other paved roadways as the place of occurrence of the external cause

✓5ᵗʰ **Y92.5** Trade and service area as the place of occurrence of the external cause

    EXCLUDES 1 *garage in private home (Y92.015)*
                schools and other public administration buildings (Y92.2-)

✓6ᵗʰ **Y92.51** Private commercial establishments as the place of occurrence of the external cause

    Y92.510 Bank as the place of occurrence of the external cause

    Y92.511 Restaurant or café as the place of occurrence of the external cause

    Y92.512 Supermarket, store or market as the place of occurrence of the external cause

    Y92.513 Shop (commercial) as the place of occurrence of the external cause

✓6ᵗʰ **Y92.52** Service areas as the place of occurrence of the external cause

    Y92.520 Airport as the place of occurrence of the external cause

    Y92.521 Bus station as the place of occurrence of the external cause

    Y92.522 Railway station as the place of occurrence of the external cause

    Y92.523 Highway rest stop as the place of occurrence of the external cause

    Y92.524 Gas station as the place of occurrence of the external cause

        Petroleum station as the place of occurrence of the external cause

        Service station as the place of occurrence of the external cause

✓6ᵗʰ **Y92.53** Ambulatory health services establishments as the place of occurrence of the external cause

    Y92.530 Ambulatory surgery center as the place of occurrence of the external cause

        Outpatient surgery center, including that connected with a hospital as the place of occurrence of the external cause

        Same day surgery center, including that connected with a hospital as the place of occurrence of the external cause

    Y92.531 Health care provider office as the place of occurrence of the external cause

        Physician office as the place of occurrence of the external cause

    Y92.532 Urgent care center as the place of occurrence of the external cause

---

✓ Additional Character Required   ✓x7ᵗʰ *X*tension Alert   Unspecified Dx   Other Specified Dx   Manifestation   ▶◀ Revised Text   ● New Code   ▲ Revised Code Title

ICD-10-CM Draft (2015)   **1053**

Y92.538 Other ambulatory health services establishments as the place of occurrence of the external cause

Y92.59 Other trade areas as the place of occurrence of the external cause

Office building as the place of occurrence of the external cause

Casino as the place of occurrence of the external cause

Garage (commercial) as the place of occurrence of the external cause

Hotel as the place of occurrence of the external cause

Radio or television station as the place of occurrence of the external cause

Shopping mall as the place of occurrence of the external cause

Warehouse as the place of occurrence of the external cause

✓5ᵗʰ **Y92.6** Industrial and construction area as the place of occurrence of the external cause

Y92.61 Building [any] under construction as the place of occurrence of the external cause

Y92.62 Dock or shipyard as the place of occurrence of the external cause

Dockyard as the place of occurrence of the external cause

Dry dock as the place of occurrence of the external cause

Shipyard as the place of occurrence of the external cause

Y92.63 Factory as the place of occurrence of the external cause

Factory building as the place of occurrence of the external cause

Factory premises as the place of occurrence of the external cause

Industrial yard as the place of occurrence of the external cause

Y92.64 Mine or pit as the place of occurrence of the external cause

Mine as the place of occurrence of the external cause

Y92.65 Oil rig as the place of occurrence of the external cause

Pit (coal) (gravel) (sand) as the place of occurrence of the external cause

Y92.69 Other specified industrial and construction area as the place of occurrence of the external cause

Gasworks as the place of occurrence of the external cause

Power-station (coal) (nuclear) (oil) as the place of occurrence of the external cause

Tunnel under construction as the place of occurrence of the external cause

Workshop as the place of occurrence of the external cause

✓5ᵗʰ **Y92.7** Farm as the place of occurrence of the external cause

Ranch as the place of occurrence of the external cause

EXCLUDES 1   *farmhouse and home premises of farm (Y92.01-)*

Y92.71 Barn as the place of occurrence of the external cause

Y92.72 Chicken coop as the place of occurrence of the external cause

Hen house as the place of occurrence of the external cause

Y92.73 Farm field as the place of occurrence of the external cause

Y92.74 Orchard as the place of occurrence of the external cause

Y92.79 Other farm location as the place of occurrence of the external cause

✓5ᵗʰ **Y92.8** Other places as the place of occurrence of the external cause

✓6ᵗʰ **Y92.81** Transport vehicle as the place of occurrence of the external cause

EXCLUDES 1   *transport accidents (V00-V99)*

Y92.810 Car as the place of occurrence of the external cause

Y92.811 Bus as the place of occurrence of the external cause

Y92.812 Truck as the place of occurrence of the external cause

Y92.813 Airplane as the place of occurrence of the external cause

Y92.814 Boat as the place of occurrence of the external cause

Y92.815 Train as the place of occurrence of the external cause

Y92.816 Subway car as the place of occurrence of the external cause

Y92.818 Other transport vehicle as the place of occurrence of the external cause

✓6ᵗʰ **Y92.82** Wilderness area

Y92.820 Desert as the place of occurrence of the external cause

Y92.821 Forest as the place of occurrence of the external cause

Y92.828 Other wilderness area as the place of occurrence of the external cause

Swamp as the place of occurrence of the external cause

Mountain as the place of occurrence of the external cause

Marsh as the place of occurrence of the external cause

Prairie as the place of occurrence of the external cause

✓6ᵗʰ **Y92.83** Recreation area as the place of occurrence of the external cause

Y92.830 Public park as the place of occurrence of the external cause

Y92.831 Amusement park as the place of occurrence of the external cause

Y92.832 Beach as the place of occurrence of the external cause

Seashore as the place of occurrence of the external cause

Y92.833 Campsite as the place of occurrence of the external cause

Y92.834 Zoological garden (Zoo) as the place of occurrence of the external cause

Y92.838 Other recreation area as the place of occurrence of the external cause

Y92.84 Military training ground as the place of occurrence of the external cause

Y92.85 Railroad track as the place of occurrence of the external cause

Y92.86 Slaughter house as the place of occurrence of the external cause

Y92.89 Other specified places as the place of occurrence of the external cause

Derelict house as the place of occurrence of the external cause

Y92.9 Unspecified place or not applicable

EXCLUDES 1 Not coded here   EXCLUDES 2 Not included here   N Newborn Age: 0   P Pediatric Age: 0-17   M Maternity Age: 12-55   A Adult Age: 15-124

✓4ᵗʰ **Y93   Activity codes**

NOTE   Category Y93 is provided for use to indicate the activity of the person seeking healthcare for an injury or health condition, such as a heart attack while shoveling snow, which resulted from, or was contributed to, by the activity. These codes are appropriate for use for both acute injuries, such as those from chapter 19, and conditions that are due to the long-term, cumulative effects of an activity, such as those from chapter 13. They are also appropriate for use with external cause codes for cause and intent if identifying the activity provides additional information on the event. These codes should be used in conjunction with codes for external cause status (Y99) and place of occurrence (Y92).
This section contains the following broad activity categories:
Y93.0   Activities involving walking and running
Y93.1   Activities involving water and water craft
Y93.2   Activities involving ice and snow
Y93.3   Activities involving climbing, rappelling, and jumping off
Y93.4   Activities involving dancing and other rhythmic movement
Y93.5   Activities involving other sports and athletics played individually
Y93.6   Activities involving other sports and athletics played as a team or group
Y93.7   Activities involving other specified sports and athletics
Y93.A   Activities involving other cardiorespiratory exercise
Y93.B   Activities involving other muscle strengthening exercises
Y93.C   Activities involving computer technology and electronic devices
Y93.D   Activities involving arts and handcrafts
Y93.E   Activities involving personal hygiene and interior property and clothing maintenance
Y93.F   Activities involving caregiving
Y93.G   Activities involving food preparation, cooking and grilling
Y93.H   Activities involving exterior property and land maintenance, building and construction
Y93.I   Activities involving roller coasters and other types of external motion
Y93.J   Activities involving playing musical instrument
Y93.K   Activities involving animal care
Y93.8   Activities, other specified
Y93.9   Activity, unspecified

✓5ᵗʰ **Y93.0   Activities involving walking and running**
EXCLUDES 1   *activity, walking an animal (Y93.K1)*
activity, walking or running on a treadmill (Y93.A1)

Y93.01   Activity, walking, marching and hiking
Activity, walking, marching and hiking on level or elevated terrain
EXCLUDES 1   *activity, mountain climbing (Y93.31)*

Y93.02   Activity, running

✓5ᵗʰ **Y93.1   Activities involving water and water craft**
EXCLUDES 1   *activities involving ice (Y93.2-)*

Y93.11   Activity, swimming
Y93.12   Activity, springboard and platform diving
Y93.13   Activity, water polo
Y93.14   Activity, water aerobics and water exercise
Y93.15   Activity, underwater diving and snorkeling
Activity, SCUBA diving
Y93.16   Activity, rowing, canoeing, kayaking, rafting and tubing
Activity, canoeing, kayaking, rafting and tubing in calm and turbulent water
Y93.17   Activity, water skiing and wake boarding
Y93.18   Activity, surfing, windsurfing and boogie boarding
Activity, water sliding
Y93.19   Activity, other involving water and watercraft
Activity involving water NOS
Activity, parasailing
Activity, water survival training and testing

✓5ᵗʰ **Y93.2   Activities involving ice and snow**
EXCLUDES 1   *activity, shoveling ice and snow (Y93.H1)*

Y93.21   Activity, ice skating
Activity, figure skating (singles) (pairs)
Activity, ice dancing
EXCLUDES 1   *activity, ice hockey (Y93.22)*

Y93.22   Activity, ice hockey

Y93.23   Activity, snow (alpine) (downhill) skiing, snow boarding, sledding, tobogganing and snow tubing
EXCLUDES 1   *activity, cross country skiing (Y93.24)*

Y93.24   Activity, cross country skiing
Activity, nordic skiing

Y93.29   Activity, other involving ice and snow
Activity involving ice and snow NOS

✓5ᵗʰ **Y93.3   Activities involving climbing, rappelling and jumping off**
EXCLUDES 1   *activity, hiking on level or elevated terrain (Y93.01)*
activity, jumping rope (Y93.56)
activity, trampoline jumping (Y93.44)

Y93.31   Activity, mountain climbing, rock climbing and wall climbing
Y93.32   Activity, rappelling
Y93.33   Activity, BASE jumping
Activity, Building, Antenna, Span, Earth jumping
Y93.34   Activity, bungee jumping
Y93.35   Activity, hang gliding
Y93.39   Activity, other involving climbing, rappelling and jumping off

✓5ᵗʰ **Y93.4   Activities involving dancing and other rhythmic movement**
EXCLUDES 1   *activity, martial arts (Y93.75)*

Y93.41   Activity, dancing
AHA: 2012, 4Q, 108
Y93.42   Activity, yoga
Y93.43   Activity, gymnastics
Activity, rhythmic gymnastics
EXCLUDES 1   *activity, trampolining (Y93.44)*
Y93.44   Activity, trampolining
Y93.45   Activity, cheerleading
Y93.49   Activity, other involving dancing and other rhythmic movements

✓5ᵗʰ **Y93.5   Activities involving other sports and athletics played individually**
EXCLUDES 1   *activity, dancing (Y93.41)*
activity, gymnastic (Y93.43)
activity, trampolining (Y93.44)
activity, yoga (Y93.42)
Y93.51   Activity, roller skating (inline) and skateboarding
Y93.52   Activity, horseback riding
Y93.53   Activity, golf
Y93.54   Activity, bowling
Y93.55   Activity, bike riding
Y93.56   Activity, jumping rope
Y93.57   Activity, non-running track and field events
EXCLUDES 1   *activity, running (any form) (Y93.02)*
Y93.59   Activity, other involving other sports and athletics played individually
EXCLUDES 1   *activities involving climbing, rappelling, and jumping (Y93.3-)*
activities involving ice and snow (Y93.2-)
activities involving walking and running (Y93.0-)
activities involving water and watercraft (Y93.1-)

✓5ᵗʰ **Y93.6   Activities involving other sports and athletics played as a team or group**
EXCLUDES 1   *activity, ice hockey (Y93.22)*
activity, water polo (Y93.13)
Y93.61   Activity, American tackle football
Activity, football NOS
Y93.62   Activity, American flag or touch football
Y93.63   Activity, rugby
Y93.64   Activity, baseball
Activity, softball
Y93.65   Activity, lacrosse and field hockey
Y93.66   Activity, soccer
Y93.67   Activity, basketball
Y93.68   Activity, volleyball (beach) (court)
Y93.6A   Activity, physical games generally associated with school recess, summer camp and children   [P]
Activity, capture the flag
Activity, dodge ball
Activity, four square
Activity, kickball

✓ Additional Character Required   ✓7ᵗʰ Xtension Alert   Unspecified Dx   Other Specified Dx   Manifestation   ▶◀ Revised Text   ● New Code   ▲ Revised Code Title
ICD-10-CM Draft (2015)

1055

Y93.69   **Activity, other involving other sports and athletics played as a team or group**
    Activity, cricket

✓5ᵗʰ **Y93.7**   **Activities involving other specified sports and athletics**

Y93.71   **Activity,** boxing

Y93.72   **Activity,** wrestling

Y93.73   **Activity,** racquet and hand **sports**
    Activity, handball
    Activity, racquetball
    Activity, squash
    Activity, tennis

Y93.74   **Activity,** frisbee
    Activity, ultimate frisbee

Y93.75   **Activity,** martial arts
    Activity, combatives

Y93.79   **Activity, other specified sports and athletics**
    EXCLUDES 1   sports and athletics activities specified in categories Y93.0-Y93.6

✓5ᵗʰ **Y93.A**   **Activities involving other cardiorespiratory exercise**
    Activities involving physical training

Y93.A1   **Activity,** exercise machines **primarily for cardiorespiratory conditioning**
    Activity, elliptical and stepper machines
    Activity, stationary bike
    Activity, treadmill

Y93.A2   **Activity,** calisthenics
    Activity, jumping jacks
    Activity, warm up and cool down

Y93.A3   **Activity,** aerobic and step exercise

Y93.A4   **Activity,** circuit training

Y93.A5   **Activity,** obstacle course
    Activity, challenge course
    Activity, confidence course

Y93.A6   **Activity,** grass drills
    Activity, guerilla drills

Y93.A9   **Activity, other involving cardiorespiratory exercise**
    EXCLUDES 1   activities involving cardiorespiratory exercise specified in categories Y93.0-Y93.7

✓5ᵗʰ **Y93.B**   **Activities involving other muscle strengthening exercises**

Y93.B1   **Activity,** exercise machines **primarily for muscle strengthening**

Y93.B2   **Activity,** push-ups, pull-ups, sit-ups

Y93.B3   **Activity,** free weights
    Activity, barbells
    Activity, dumbbells

Y93.B4   **Activity,** pilates

Y93.B9   **Activity, other involving muscle strengthening exercises**
    EXCLUDES 1   activities involving muscle strengthening specified in categories Y93.0-Y93.A

✓5ᵗʰ **Y93.C**   **Activities involving computer technology and electronic devices**
    EXCLUDES 1   activity, electronic musical keyboard or instruments (Y93.J-)

Y93.C1   **Activity,** computer keyboarding
    Activity, electronic game playing using keyboard or other stationary device

Y93.C2   **Activity,** hand held interactive electronic device
    Activity, cellular telephone and communication device
    Activity, electronic game playing using interactive device
    EXCLUDES 1   activity, electronic game playing using keyboard or other stationary device (Y93.C1)

Y93.C9   **Activity, other involving computer technology and electronic devices**

✓5ᵗʰ **Y93.D**   **Activities involving arts and handcrafts**
    EXCLUDES 1   activities involving playing musical instrument (Y93.J-)

Y93.D1   **Activity,** knitting and crocheting

Y93.D2   **Activity,** sewing

Y93.D3   **Activity,** furniture building and finishing
    Activity, furniture repair

Y93.D9   **Activity, other involving arts and handcrafts**

✓5ᵗʰ **Y93.E**   **Activities involving personal hygiene and interior property and clothing maintenance**
    EXCLUDES 1   activities involving cooking and grilling (Y93.G-)
       activities involving exterior property and land maintenance, building and construction (Y93.H-)
       activities involving caregiving (Y93.F-)
       activity, dishwashing (Y93.G1)
       activity, food preparation (Y93.G1)
       activity, gardening (Y93.H2)

Y93.E1   **Activity, personal** bathing and showering

Y93.E2   **Activity,** laundry

Y93.E3   **Activity,** vacuuming

Y93.E4   **Activity,** ironing

Y93.E5   **Activity,** floor mopping and cleaning

Y93.E6   **Activity,** residential relocation
    Activity, packing up and unpacking involved in moving to a new residence

Y93.E8   **Activity, other** personal hygiene

Y93.E9   **Activity, other** interior property and clothing maintenance

✓5ᵗʰ **Y93.F**   **Activities involving** caregiving
    Activity involving the provider of caregiving

Y93.F1   **Activity, caregiving,** bathing

Y93.F2   **Activity, caregiving,** lifting

Y93.F9   **Activity, other caregiving**

✓5ᵗʰ **Y93.G**   **Activities involving food preparation, cooking and grilling**

Y93.G1   **Activity, food** preparation and clean up
    Activity, dishwashing

Y93.G2   **Activity,** grilling and smoking food

Y93.G3   **Activity,** cooking and baking
    Activity, use of stove, oven and microwave oven

Y93.G9   **Activity, other involving cooking and grilling**

✓5ᵗʰ **Y93.H**   **Activities involving exterior property and land maintenance, building and construction**

Y93.H1   **Activity,** digging, shoveling and raking
    Activity, dirt digging
    Activity, raking leaves
    Activity, snow shoveling

Y93.H2   **Activity,** gardening and landscaping
    Activity, pruning, trimming shrubs, weeding

Y93.H3   **Activity,** building and construction

Y93.H9   **Activity, other involving exterior property and land maintenance, building and construction**

✓5ᵗʰ **Y93.I**   **Activities involving roller coasters and other types of external motion**

Y93.I1   **Activity,** rollercoaster riding

Y93.I9   **Activity, other involving external motion**

✓5ᵗʰ **Y93.J**   **Activities involving playing musical instrument**
    Activity involving playing electric musical instrument

Y93.J1   **Activity,** piano playing
    Activity, musical keyboard (electronic) playing

Y93.J2   **Activity,** drum and other percussion instrument **playing**

Y93.J3   **Activity,** string instrument **playing**

Y93.J4   **Activity,** winds and brass instrument **playing**

✓5ᵗʰ **Y93.K**   **Activities involving** animal care
    EXCLUDES 1   activity, horseback riding (Y93.52)

Y93.K1   **Activity,** walking **an animal**

Y93.K2   **Activity,** milking **an animal**

Y93.K3   **Activity,** grooming and shearing **an animal**

Y93.K9   **Activity, other involving animal care**

✓5ᵗʰ **Y93.8**   **Activities, other specified**

Y93.81   **Activity,** refereeing **a sports activity**

Y93.82   **Activity,** spectator **at an event**

Y93.83   **Activity,** rough housing and horseplay

Y93.84   **Activity,** sleeping

Y93.89   **Activity, other specified**

Y93.9   **Activity, unspecified**

Y95   **Nosocomial condition**
    AHA: 2013, 4Q, 119

EXCLUDES 1 Not coded here   EXCLUDES 2 Not included here   N Newborn Age: 0   P Pediatric Age: 0-17   M Maternity Age: 12-55   A Adult Age: 15-124

✓4ᵗʰ **Y99　External cause status**

> **NOTE**　A single code from category Y99 should be used in conjunction with the external cause code(s) assigned to a record to indicate the status of the person at the time the event occurred.

Y99.0　Civilian activity done for income or pay
　　　Civilian activity done for financial or other compensation
> **EXCLUDES 1**　military activity (Y99.1)
> 　　　　　　volunteer activity (Y99.2)

Y99.1　Military activity
> **EXCLUDES 1**　activity of off duty military personnel (Y99.8)

Y99.2　Volunteer activity
> **EXCLUDES 1**　activity of child or other family member assisting in compensated work of other family member (Y99.8)

Y99.8　Other external cause status
　　　Activity NEC
　　　Activity of child or other family member assisting in compensated work of other family member
　　　Hobby not done for income
　　　Leisure activity
　　　Off-duty activity of military personnel
　　　Recreation or sport not for income or while a student
　　　Student activity
> **EXCLUDES 1**　civilian activity done for income or compensation (Y99.0)
> 　　　　　　military activity (Y99.1)

　　　AHA: 2012, 4Q, 108

Y99.9　Unspecified external cause status

✓ Additional Character Required　　✓x7ᵗʰ Xtension Alert　　Unspecified Dx　　Other Specified Dx　　Manifestation　　►◄ Revised Text　　● New Code　　▲ Revised Code Title

ICD-10-CM Draft (2015)　　　　　　　　　　　　　　　　　　　　　　　　　　　　　　1057

Chapter 21. Factors Influencing Health Status and Contact With Health Services (Z00-Z99)

NOTE Z codes represent reasons for encounters. A corresponding procedure code must accompany a Z code if a procedure is performed. Categories Z00-Z99 are provided for occasions when circumstances other than a disease, injury or external cause classifiable to categories A00-Y89 are recorded as "diagnoses" or "problems". This can arise in two main ways:

(a) When a person who may or may not be sick encounters the health services for some specific purpose, such as to receive limited care or service for a current condition, to donate an organ or tissue, to receive prophylactic vaccination (immunization), or to discuss a problem which is in itself not a disease or injury.

(b) When some circumstance or problem is present which influences the person's health status but is not in itself a current illness or injury.

This chapter contains the following blocks:

Z00-Z13	Persons encountering health services for examinations
Z14-Z15	Genetic carrier and genetic susceptibility to disease
Z16	Resistance to antimicrobial drugs
Z17	Estrogen receptor status
Z18	Retained foreign body fragments
Z20-Z28	Persons with potential health hazards related to communicable diseases
Z30-Z39	Persons encountering health services in circumstances related to reproduction
Z40-Z53	Encounters for other specific health care
Z55-Z65	Persons with potential health hazards related to socioeconomic and psychosocial circumstances
Z66	Do not resuscitate status
Z67	Blood type
Z68	Body mass index (BMI)
Z69-Z76	Persons encountering health services in other circumstances
Z77-Z99	Persons with potential health hazards related to family and personal history and certain conditions influencing health status

Persons encountering health services for examinations (Z00-Z13)

NOTE Nonspecific abnormal findings disclosed at the time of these examinations are classified to categories R70-R94.

EXCLUDES 1 examinations related to pregnancy and reproduction (Z30-Z36, Z39-)

✓4ᵗʰ **Z00** **Encounter for general examination without complaint, suspected or reported diagnosis**

EXCLUDES 1 encounter for examination for administrative purposes (Z02.-)

EXCLUDES 2 encounter for pre-procedural examinations (Z01.81-)
special screening examinations (Z11-Z13)

✓5ᵗʰ **Z00.0** **Encounter for general adult medical examination**
Encounter for adult periodic examination (annual) (physical) and any associated laboratory and radiologic examinations

EXCLUDES 1 encounter for examination of sign or symptom—code to sign or symptom
general health check-up of infant or child (Z00.12-)

Z00.00 **Encounter for general adult medical examination without abnormal findings** PDx A
Encounter for adult health check-up NOS

Z00.01 **Encounter for general adult medical examination with abnormal findings** PDx A
Use additional code to identify abnormal findings

✓5ᵗʰ **Z00.1** **Encounter for newborn, infant and child health examinations**

✓6ᵗʰ **Z00.11** **Newborn health examination**
Health check for child under 29 days old
Use additional code to identify any abnormal findings

EXCLUDES 1 health check for child over 28 days old (Z00.12-)

Z00.110 **Health examination for newborn under 8 days old** PDx N
Health check for newborn under 8 days old

Z00.111 **Health examination for newborn 8 to 28 days old** PDx N
Health check for newborn 8 to 28 days old
Newborn weight check

✓6ᵗʰ **Z00.12** **Encounter for routine child health examination**
Encounter for development testing of infant or child
Health check (routine) for child over 28 days old

EXCLUDES 1 health check for child under 29 days old (Z00.11-)
health supervision of foundling or other healthy infant or child (Z76.1-Z76.2)
newborn health examination (Z00.11-)

Z00.121 **Encounter for routine child health examination with abnormal findings** PDx P
Use additional code to identify abnormal findings

Z00.129 **Encounter for routine child health examination without abnormal findings** PDx P
Encounter for routine child health examination NOS

Z00.2 **Encounter for examination for period of rapid growth in childhood** PDx P

Z00.3 **Encounter for examination for adolescent development state** PDx P
Encounter for puberty development state

Z00.5 **Encounter for examination of potential donor of organ and tissue** PDx

Z00.6 **Encounter for examination for normal comparison and control in clinical research program** PDx
Examination of participant or control in clinical research program

✓5ᵗʰ **Z00.7** **Encounter for examination for period of delayed growth in childhood**

Z00.70 **Encounter for examination for period of delayed growth in childhood without abnormal findings** PDx P

Z00.71 **Encounter for examination for period of delayed growth in childhood with abnormal findings** PDx P
Use additional code to identify abnormal findings

Z00.8 **Encounter for other general examination**
Encounter for health examination in population surveys

✓4ᵗʰ **Z01** **Encounter for other special examination without complaint, suspected or reported diagnosis**

INCLUDES routine examination of specific system

NOTE Codes from category Z01 represent the reason for the encounter. A separate procedure code is required to identify any examinations or procedures performed.

EXCLUDES 1 encounter for examination for administrative purposes (Z02.-)
encounter for examination for suspected conditions, proven not to exist (Z03.-)
encounter for laboratory and radiologic examinations as a component of general medical examinations (Z00.0-)
encounter for laboratory, radiologic and imaging examinations for sign(s) and symptom(s)—code to the sign(s) or symptom(s)

EXCLUDES 2 screening examinations (Z11-Z13)

✓5ᵗʰ **Z01.0** **Encounter for examination of eyes and vision**

EXCLUDES 1 examination for driving license (Z02.4)

Z01.00 **Encounter for examination of eyes and vision without abnormal findings** PDx
Encounter for examination of eyes and vision NOS

Z01.01 **Encounter for examination of eyes and vision with abnormal findings** PDx
Use additional code to identify abnormal findings

✓5ᵗʰ **Z01.1** **Encounter for examination of ears and hearing**

Z01.10 **Encounter for examination of ears and hearing without abnormal findings** PDx
Encounter for examination of ears and hearing NOS

✓6ᵗʰ **Z01.11** **Encounter for examination of ears and hearing with abnormal findings**

Z01.110 **Encounter for hearing examination following failed hearing screening** PDx

Z01.118 **Encounter for examination of ears and hearing with other abnormal findings** PDx
Use additional code to identify abnormal findings

Z01.12 **Encounter for hearing conservation and treatment**

✓5ᵗʰ **Z01.2** **Encounter for dental examination and cleaning**

Z01.20 **Encounter for dental examination and cleaning without abnormal findings** PDx
Encounter for dental examination and cleaning NOS

Z01.21 **Encounter for dental examination and cleaning with abnormal findings** PDx
Use additional code to identify abnormal findings

EXCLUDES 1 Not coded here   **EXCLUDES 2** Not included here   PDx Primary Diagnosis Only   N Newborn Age: 0   P Pediatric Age: 0-17   M Maternity Age: 12-55   A Adult Age: 15-124

1058   ICD-10-CM Draft (2015)

☑5ᵗʰ **Z01.3 Encounter for examination of** blood pressure

Z01.30 Encounter for examination of blood pressure `PDx`
without abnormal findings
Encounter for examination of blood pressure NOS

Z01.31 Encounter for examination of blood pressure `PDx`
with abnormal findings
Use additional code to identify abnormal findings

☑5ᵗʰ **Z01.4 Encounter for** gynecological **examination**
EXCLUDES 2   *pregnancy examination or test (Z32.0-)*
routine examination for contraceptive maintenance
(Z30.4-)

☑6ᵗʰ **Z01.41 Encounter for** routine **gynecological examination**
Encounter for general gynecological examination with
or without cervical smear
Encounter for gynecological examination (general)
(routine) NOS
Encounter for pelvic examination (annual) (periodic)
Use additional code:
for screening for human papillomavirus, if
applicable, (Z11.51)
for screening vaginal pap smear, if applicable
(Z12.72)
to identify acquired absence of uterus, if applicable
(Z90.71-)
EXCLUDES 1   *gynecologic examination status-post*
hysterectomy for malignant condition
(Z08)
screening cervical pap smear not a part of a
routine gynecological examination
(Z12.4)

Z01.411 Encounter for gynecological `PDx` ♀
examination (general) (routine) with
abnormal findings

Z01.419 Encounter for gynecological `PDx` ♀
examination (general) (routine) without
abnormal findings
Use additional code to identify abnormal
findings

Z01.42 Encounter for cervical smear to confirm `PDx` ♀
findings **of recent normal smear following initial**
abnormal smear

☑5ᵗʰ **Z01.8 Encounter for** other specified special **examinations**

☑6ᵗʰ **Z01.81 Encounter for** preprocedural **examinations**
Encounter for preoperative examinations
Encounter for radiological and imaging examinations
as part of preprocedural examination

Z01.810 Encounter for preprocedural `PDx`
cardiovascular examination

Z01.811 Encounter for preprocedural `PDx`
respiratory examination

Z01.812 Encounter for preprocedural `PDx`
laboratory examination
Blood and urine tests prior to treatment or
procedure

Z01.818 Encounter for other preprocedural `PDx`
examination
Encounter for preprocedural examination
NOS
Encounter for examinations prior to
antineoplastic chemotherapy

Z01.82 Encounter for allergy testing `PDx`
EXCLUDES 1   *encounter for antibody response*
examination (Z01.84)

Z01.83 Encounter for blood typing `PDx`
Encounter for Rh typing

Z01.84 Encounter for antibody response examination `PDx`
Encounter for immunity status testing
EXCLUDES 1   *encounter for allergy testing (Z01.82)*

Z01.89 Encounter for other specified special `PDx`
examinations

☑4ᵗʰ **Z02 Encounter for** administrative **examination**

Z02.0 Encounter for examination for admission to educational `PDx`
institution
Encounter for examination for admission to preschool
(education)
Encounter for examination for re-admission to school following
illness or medical treatment

Z02.1 Encounter for pre-employment **examination** `PDx`

Z02.2 Encounter for examination for admission to residential `PDx`
institution
EXCLUDES 1   *examination for admission to prison (Z02.89)*

Z02.3 Encounter for examination for recruitment to armed `PDx`
forces

Z02.4 Encounter for examination for driving license `PDx`

Z02.5 Encounter for examination for participation in sport `PDx`
EXCLUDES 1   *blood-alcohol and blood-drug test (Z02.83)*

Z02.6 Encounter for examination for insurance purposes `PDx`

☑5ᵗʰ **Z02.7 Encounter for** issue of medical certificate
EXCLUDES 1   *encounter for general medical examination (Z00-Z01,*
Z02.0-Z02.6, Z02.8-Z02.9)

Z02.71 Encounter for disability determination `PDx`
Encounter for issue of medical certificate of incapacity
Encounter for issue of medical certificate of invalidity

Z02.79 Encounter for issue of other medical certificate `PDx`

☑5ᵗʰ **Z02.8 Encounter for** other administrative **examinations**

Z02.81 Encounter for paternity testing `PDx`

Z02.82 Encounter for adoption services `PDx`

Z02.83 Encounter for blood-alcohol and blood-drug `PDx`
test
Use additional code for findings of alcohol or drugs in
blood (R78.-)

Z02.89 Encounter for other administrative `PDx`
examinations
Encounter for examination for admission to prison
Encounter for examination for admission to summer
camp
Encounter for immigration examination
Encounter for naturalization examination
Encounter for premarital examination
EXCLUDES 1   *health supervision of foundling or other*
healthy infant or child (Z76.1-Z76.2)

Z02.9 Encounter for administrative examinations, unspecified `PDx`

☑4ᵗʰ **Z03 Encounter for** medical observation **for suspected diseases and**
conditions ruled out
NOTE   This category is to be used when a person without a
diagnosis is suspected of having an abnormal condition,
without signs or symptoms, which requires study, but after
examination and observation, is ruled out. This category is
also for use for administrative and legal observation status.
EXCLUDES 1   *contact with and (suspected) exposures hazardous to health*
(Z77.-)
newborn observation for suspected condition, ruled out
(P00-P04)
person with feared complaint in whom no diagnosis is made
(Z71.1)
signs or symptoms under study—code to signs or symptoms

Z03.6 Encounter for observation for suspected toxic effect `PDx`
from ingested substance **ruled out**
Encounter for observation for suspected adverse effect from
drug
Encounter for observation for suspected poisoning

☑5ᵗʰ **Z03.7 Encounter for suspected** maternal and fetal conditions **ruled**
out
Encounter for suspected maternal and fetal conditions not
found
EXCLUDES 1   *known or suspected fetal anomalies affecting*
management of mother, not ruled out (O26-,
O35-, O36-, O40-, O41-)

Z03.71 Encounter for suspected problem with `PDx` M ♀
amniotic cavity and membrane **ruled out**
Encounter for suspected oligohydramnios ruled out
Encounter for suspected polyhydramnios ruled out

Z03.72 Encounter for suspected placental `PDx` M ♀
problem **ruled out**

Z03.73 Encounter for suspected fetal anomaly `PDx` M ♀
ruled out

Z03.74 Encounter for suspected problem with fetal `PDx` M ♀
growth **ruled out**

Z03.75 Encounter for suspected cervical shortening `PDx` M ♀
ruled out

Z03.79 Encounter for other suspected maternal and `PDx` M ♀
fetal conditions ruled out

☑ Additional Character Required   ☑x7ᵗʰ Xtension Alert   Unspecified Dx   Other Specified Dx   Manifestation   ▶◀ Revised Text   ● New Code   ▲ Revised Code Title

✓5ᵗʰ **Z03.8 Encounter for** observation **for other suspected diseases and conditions ruled out**

   ✓6ᵗʰ **Z03.81 Encounter for observation for suspected** exposure to biological agents **ruled out**

     Z03.810 Encounter for observation for suspected exposure to anthrax **ruled out** ᴾᴰˣ

     Z03.818 Encounter for observation for suspected exposure to other biological agents ruled out ᴾᴰˣ

   Z03.89 Encounter for observation for other suspected diseases and conditions ruled out ᴾᴰˣ

✓4ᵗʰ **Z04 Encounter for examination and observation for other reasons**

   INCLUDES encounter for examination for medicolegal reasons

   NOTE This category is to be used when a person without a diagnosis is suspected of having an abnormal condition, without signs or symptoms, which requires study, but after examination and observation, is ruled-out. This category is also for use for administrative and legal observation status.

   Z04.1 Encounter for examination and observation following transport accident ᴾᴰˣ

     EXCLUDES 1 encounter for examination and observation following work accident (Z04.2)

   Z04.2 Encounter for examination and observation following work accident ᴾᴰˣ

   Z04.3 Encounter for examination and observation following other accident ᴾᴰˣ

   ✓5ᵗʰ **Z04.4 Encounter for examination and observation following alleged rape**

     Encounter for examination and observation of victim following alleged rape

     Encounter for examination and observation of victim following alleged sexual abuse

     Z04.41 Encounter for examination and observation following alleged adult **rape** ᴾᴰˣ ᴬ

       Suspected adult rape, ruled out

       Suspected adult sexual abuse, ruled out

     Z04.42 Encounter for examination and observation following alleged child **rape** ᴾᴰˣ ᴾ

       Suspected child rape, ruled out

       Suspected child sexual abuse, ruled out

   Z04.6 Encounter for general psychiatric examination, requested by authority ᴾᴰˣ

   ✓5ᵗʰ **Z04.7 Encounter for examination and observation following alleged physical abuse**

     Z04.71 Encounter for examination and observation following alleged adult **physical abuse** ᴾᴰˣ ᴬ

       Suspected adult physical abuse, ruled out

       EXCLUDES 1 confirmed case of adult physical abuse (T74.-)

         encounter for examination and observation following alleged adult sexual abuse (Z04.41)

         suspected case of adult physical abuse, not ruled out (T76.-)

     Z04.72 Encounter for examination and observation following alleged child **physical abuse** ᴾᴰˣ ᴾ

       Suspected child physical abuse, ruled out

       EXCLUDES 1 confirmed case of child physical abuse (T74.-)

         encounter for examination and observation following alleged child sexual abuse (Z04.42)

         suspected case of child physical abuse, not ruled out (T76.-)

   Z04.8 Encounter for examination and observation for other specified reasons ᴾᴰˣ

     Encounter for examination and observation for request for expert evidence

   Z04.9 Encounter for examination and observation for unspecified reason ᴾᴰˣ

     Encounter for observation NOS

Z08 Encounter for follow-up **examination** after completed treatment **for** malignant neoplasm

   Medical surveillance following completed treatment

   Use additional code to identify any acquired absence of organs (Z90.-)

   Use additional code to identify the personal history of malignant neoplasm (Z85.-)

   EXCLUDES 1 aftercare following medical care (Z43-Z49, Z51)

Z09 Encounter for follow-up **examination** after completed treatment **for conditions** other **than malignant neoplasm**

   Medical surveillance following completed treatment

   Use additional code to identify any applicable history of disease code (Z86-. Z87-)

   EXCLUDES 1 aftercare following medical care (Z43-Z49, Z51)

     surveillance of contraception (Z30.4-)

     surveillance of prosthetic and other medical devices (Z44-Z46)

✓4ᵗʰ **Z11 Encounter for** screening **for** infectious and parasitic diseases

   NOTE Screening is the testing for disease or disease precursors in asymptomatic individuals so that early detection and treatment can be provided for those who test positive for the disease.

   EXCLUDES 1 encounter for diagnostic examination—code to sign or symptom

   Z11.0 Encounter for screening for intestinal **infectious diseases**

   Z11.1 Encounter for screening for respiratory tuberculosis

   Z11.2 Encounter for screening for other bacterial **diseases**

   Z11.3 Encounter for screening for infections with a predominantly sexual mode of transmission

     EXCLUDES 2 encounter for screening for human immunodeficiency virus [HIV] (Z11.4)

       encounter for screening for human papillomavirus (Z11.51)

   Z11.4 Encounter for screening for human immunodeficiency virus **[HIV]**

   ✓5ᵗʰ **Z11.5 Encounter for screening for** other viral **diseases**

     EXCLUDES 2 encounter for screening for viral intestinal disease (Z11.0)

     Z11.51 Encounter for screening for human papillomavirus **(HPV)**

     Z11.59 Encounter for screening for other viral **diseases**

   Z11.6 Encounter for screening for other protozoal diseases and helminthiases

     EXCLUDES 2 encounter for screening for protozoal intestinal disease (Z11.0)

   Z11.8 Encounter for screening for other infectious and parasitic diseases

     Encounter for screening for chlamydia

     Encounter for screening for rickettsial

     Encounter for screening for spirochetal

     Encounter for screening for mycoses

   Z11.9 Encounter for screening for infectious and parasitic diseases, unspecified

✓4ᵗʰ **Z12 Encounter for** screening for malignant neoplasms

   NOTE Screening is the testing for disease or disease precursors in asymptomatic individuals so that early detection and treatment can be provided for those who test positive for the disease.

   Use additional code to identify any family history of malignant neoplasm (Z80.-)

   EXCLUDES 1 encounter for diagnostic examination—code to sign or symptom

   Z12.0 Encounter for screening for malignant neoplasm of stomach

   ✓5ᵗʰ **Z12.1 Encounter for screening for malignant neoplasm of** intestinal tract

     Z12.10 Encounter for screening for malignant neoplasm of intestinal tract, unspecified

     Z12.11 Encounter for screening for malignant neoplasm of colon

       Encounter for screening colonoscopy NOS

     Z12.12 Encounter for screening for malignant neoplasm of rectum

     Z12.13 Encounter for screening for malignant neoplasm of small intestine

   Z12.2 Encounter for screening for malignant neoplasm of respiratory organs

   ✓5ᵗʰ **Z12.3 Encounter for screening for malignant neoplasm of** breast

     Z12.31 Encounter for screening mammogram **for malignant neoplasm of breast**

       EXCLUDES 1 inconclusive mammogram (R92.2)

     Z12.39 Encounter for other screening for malignant neoplasm of breast

EXCLUDES 1 Not coded here   **EXCLUDES 2** Not included here   ᴾᴰˣ Primary Diagnosis Only   ᴺ Newborn Age: 0   ᴾ Pediatric Age: 0-17   ᴹ Maternity Age: 12-55   ᴬ Adult Age: 15-124

1060   ICD-10-CM Draft (2015)

Z12.4 Encounter for screening for malignant neoplasm of cervix ♀
Encounter for screening pap smear for malignant neoplasm of cervix
EXCLUDES 1 *encounter for screening for human papillomavirus (Z11.51)*
when screening is part of general gynecological examination (Z01.4-)

Z12.5 Encounter for screening for malignant neoplasm of prostate ♂

Z12.6 Encounter for screening for malignant neoplasm of bladder

✓5ᵗʰ **Z12.7** Encounter for screening for malignant neoplasm of other genitourinary organs

     Z12.71 Encounter for screening for malignant neoplasm of testis ♂

     Z12.72 Encounter for screening for malignant neoplasm of vagina ♀
Vaginal pap smear status-post hysterectomy for non-malignant condition
Use additional code to identify acquired absence of uterus (Z90.71-)
EXCLUDES 1 *vaginal pap smear status-post hysterectomy for malignant conditions (Z08)*

     Z12.73 Encounter for screening for malignant neoplasm of ovary ♀

     Z12.79 Encounter for screening for malignant neoplasm of other genitourinary organs

✓5ᵗʰ **Z12.8** Encounter for screening for malignant neoplasm of other sites

     Z12.81 Encounter for screening for malignant neoplasm of oral cavity

     Z12.82 Encounter for screening for malignant neoplasm of nervous system

     Z12.83 Encounter for screening for malignant neoplasm of skin

     Z12.89 Encounter for screening for malignant neoplasm of other sites

Z12.9 Encounter for screening for malignant neoplasm, site unspecified

✓4ᵗʰ **Z13** Encounter for screening for other diseases and disorders
NOTE Screening is the testing for disease or disease precursors in asymptomatic individuals so that early detection and treatment can be provided for those who test positive for the disease.
EXCLUDES 1 *encounter for diagnostic examination—code to sign or symptom*

Z13.0 Encounter for screening for diseases of the blood and blood-forming organs and certain disorders involving the immune mechanism

Z13.1 Encounter for screening for diabetes mellitus

✓5ᵗʰ **Z13.2** Encounter for screening for nutritional, metabolic and other endocrine disorders

     Z13.21 Encounter for screening for nutritional disorder

     ✓6ᵗʰ **Z13.22** Encounter for screening for metabolic disorder

         Z13.220 Encounter for screening for lipoid disorders
Encounter for screening for cholesterol level
Encounter for screening for hypercholesterolemia
Encounter for screening for hyperlipidemia

         Z13.228 Encounter for screening for other metabolic disorders

     Z13.29 Encounter for screening for other suspected endocrine disorder
EXCLUDES 1 *encounter for screening for diabetes mellitus (Z13.1)*

Z13.4 Encounter for screening for certain developmental disorders in childhood ℗
Encounter for screening for developmental handicaps in early childhood
EXCLUDES 1 *routine development testing of infant or child (Z00.1-)*

Z13.5 Encounter for screening for eye and ear disorders
EXCLUDES 2 *encounter for general hearing examination (Z01.1-)*
encounter for general vision examination (Z01.0-)

Z13.6 Encounter for screening for cardiovascular disorders

✓5ᵗʰ **Z13.7** Encounter for screening for genetic and chromosomal anomalies
EXCLUDES 1 *genetic testing for procreative management (Z31.4-)*

     Z13.71 Encounter for nonprocreative screening for genetic disease carrier status

     Z13.79 Encounter for other screening for genetic and chromosomal anomalies

✓5ᵗʰ **Z13.8** Encounter for screening for other specified diseases and disorders
EXCLUDES 2 *screening for malignant neoplasms (Z12.-)*

     ✓6ᵗʰ **Z13.81** Encounter for screening for digestive system disorders

         Z13.810 Encounter for screening for upper gastrointestinal disorder

         Z13.811 Encounter for screening for lower gastrointestinal disorder
EXCLUDES 1 *encounter for screening for intestinal infectious disease (Z11.0)*

         Z13.818 Encounter for screening for other digestive system disorders

     ✓6ᵗʰ **Z13.82** Encounter for screening for musculoskeletal disorder

         Z13.820 Encounter for screening for osteoporosis

         Z13.828 Encounter for screening for other musculoskeletal disorder

     Z13.83 Encounter for screening for respiratory disorder NEC
EXCLUDES 1 *encounter for screening for respiratory tuberculosis (Z11.1)*

     Z13.84 Encounter for screening for dental disorders

     ✓6ᵗʰ **Z13.85** Encounter for screening for nervous system disorders

         Z13.850 Encounter for screening for traumatic brain injury

         Z13.858 Encounter for screening for other nervous system disorders

     Z13.88 Encounter for screening for disorder due to exposure to contaminants
EXCLUDES 1 *those exposed to contaminants without suspected disorders (Z57-Z77-)*

     Z13.89 Encounter for screening for other disorder
Encounter for screening for genitourinary disorders

Z13.9 Encounter for screening, unspecified

Genetic carrier and genetic susceptibility to disease (Z14-Z15)

✓4ᵗʰ **Z14** Genetic carrier

     ✓5ᵗʰ **Z14.0** Hemophilia A carrier

         Z14.01 Asymptomatic hemophilia A carrier

         Z14.02 Symptomatic hemophilia A carrier

     Z14.1 Cystic fibrosis carrier

     Z14.8 Genetic carrier of other disease

✓4ᵗʰ **Z15** Genetic susceptibility to disease
Confirmed abnormal gene
Use additional code, if applicable, for any associated family history of the disease (Z80-Z84)
EXCLUDES 1 *chromosomal anomalies (Q90-Q99)*

     ✓5ᵗʰ **Z15.0** Genetic susceptibility to malignant neoplasm
Code first, if applicable, any current malignant neoplasm (C00-C75, C81-C96)
Use additional code, if applicable, for any personal history of malignant neoplasm (Z85.-)

         Z15.01 Genetic susceptibility to malignant neoplasm of breast

         Z15.02 Genetic susceptibility to malignant neoplasm of ovary ♀

         Z15.03 Genetic susceptibility to malignant neoplasm of prostate ♂

         Z15.04 Genetic susceptibility to malignant neoplasm of endometrium ♀

         Z15.09 Genetic susceptibility to other malignant neoplasm

     ✓5ᵗʰ **Z15.8** Genetic susceptibility to other disease

         Z15.81 Genetic susceptibility to multiple endocrine neoplasia [MEN]
EXCLUDES 1 *multiple endocrine neoplasia [MEN] syndromes (E31.2-)*

         Z15.89 Genetic susceptibility to other disease

✓ Additional Character Required   ✓7ᵗʰ Xtension Alert   Unspecified Dx   Other Specified Dx   Manifestation   ▶◀ Revised Text   ● New Code   ▲ Revised Code Title

ICD-10-CM Draft (2015)   1061

Resistance to antimicrobial drugs (Z16)

☑4th Z16　Resistance to antimicrobial drugs
> **NOTE**　The codes in this category are provided for use as additional codes to identify the resistance and non-responsiveness of a condition to antimicrobial drugs.
>
> Code first the infection
> **EXCLUDES 1**　*Methicillin resistant Staphylococcus aureus infection (A49.02)*
> *Methicillin resistant Staphylococcus aureus infection in diseases classified elsewhere (B95.62)*
> *Methicillin resistant Staphylococcus aureus pneumonia (J15.212)*
> *Sepsis due to Methicillin resistant Staphylococcus aureus (A41.02)*

☑5th Z16.1　Resistance to beta lactam antibiotics
- **Z16.10　Resistance to unspecified beta lactam antibiotics**
- **Z16.11　Resistance to penicillins**
  - Resistance to amoxicillin　　Resistance to ampicillin
- **Z16.12　Extended spectrum beta lactamase (ESBL) resistance**
- **Z16.19　Resistance to other specified beta lactam antibiotics**
  - Resistance to cephalosporins

☑5th Z16.2　Resistance to other antibiotics
- **Z16.20　Resistance to unspecified antibiotic**
  - Resistance to antibiotics NOS
- **Z16.21　Resistance to vancomycin**
- **Z16.22　Resistance to vancomycin related antibiotics**
- **Z16.23　Resistance to quinolones and fluoroquinolones**
- **Z16.24　Resistance to multiple antibiotics**
- **Z16.29　Resistance to other single specified antibiotic**
  - Resistance to aminoglycosides
  - Resistance to macrolides
  - Resistance to sulfonamides
  - Resistance to tetracyclines

☑5th Z16.3　Resistance to other antimicrobial drugs
> **EXCLUDES 1**　*resistance to antibiotics (Z16.1-, Z16.2-)*
- **Z16.30　Resistance to unspecified antimicrobial drugs**
  - Drug resistance NOS
- **Z16.31　Resistance to antiparasitic drug(s)**
  - Resistance to quinine and related compounds
- **Z16.32　Resistance to antifungal drug(s)**
- **Z16.33　Resistance to antiviral drug(s)**
- **☑6th Z16.34　Resistance to antimycobacterial drug(s)**
  - Resistance to tuberculostatics
  - **Z16.341　Resistance to single antimycobacterial drug**
    - Resistance to antimycobacterial drug NOS
  - **Z16.342　Resistance to multiple antimycobacterial drugs**
- **Z16.35　Resistance to multiple antimicrobial drugs**
  - **EXCLUDES 1**　*Resistance to multiple antibiotics only (Z16.24)*
- **Z16.39　Resistance to other specified antimicrobial drug**

Estrogen receptor status (Z17)

☑4th Z17　Estrogen receptor status
> Code first malignant neoplasm of breast (C50.-)
- **Z17.0　Estrogen receptor positive status [ER+]**
- **Z17.1　Estrogen receptor negative status [ER-]**

Retained foreign body fragment (Z18)

☑4th Z18　Retained foreign body fragments
> Embedded fragment (status)
> Embedded splinter (status)
> Retained foreign body status
> **EXCLUDES 1**　*artificial joint prosthesis status (Z96.6-)*
> *foreign body accidentally left during a procedure (T81.5-)*
> *foreign body entering through orifice (T15-T19)*
> *in situ cardiac device (Z95.-)*
> *organ or tissue replaced by means other than transplant (Z96.-, Z97.-)*
> *organ or tissue replaced by transplant (Z94.-)*
> *personal history of retained foreign body fully removed (Z87.821)*
> *superficial foreign body (non-embedded splinter)—code to superficial foreign body, by site*

☑5th Z18.0　Retained radioactive fragments
- **Z18.01　Retained depleted uranium fragments**

- **Z18.09　Other retained radioactive fragments**
  - Other retained depleted isotope fragments
  - Retained nontherapeutic radioactive fragments
- **☑5th Z18.1　Retained metal fragments**
  - **EXCLUDES 1**　*retained radioactive metal fragments (Z18.01-Z18.09)*
  - **Z18.10　Retained metal fragments, unspecified**
    - Retained metal fragment NOS
  - **Z18.11　Retained magnetic metal fragments**
  - **Z18.12　Retained nonmagnetic metal fragments**
- **Z18.2　Retained plastic fragments**
  - Acrylics fragments
  - Diethylhexylphthalates fragments
  - Isocyanate fragments
- **☑5th Z18.3　Retained organic fragments**
  - **Z18.31　Retained animal quills or spines**
  - **Z18.32　Retained tooth**
  - **Z18.33　Retained wood fragments**
  - **Z18.39　Other retained organic fragments**
- **☑5th Z18.8　Other specified retained foreign body**
  - **Z18.81　Retained glass fragments**
  - **Z18.83　Retained stone or crystalline fragments**
    - Retained concrete or cement fragments
  - **Z18.89　Other specified retained foreign body fragments**
- **Z18.9　Retained foreign body fragments, unspecified material**

Persons with potential health hazards related to communicable diseases (Z20-Z28)

☑4th Z20　Contact with and (suspected) exposure to communicable diseases
> **EXCLUDES 1**　*carrier of infectious disease (Z22.-)*
> *diagnosed current infectious or parasitic disease—see Alphabetic Index*
> **EXCLUDES 2**　*personal history of infectious and parasitic diseases (Z86.1-)*

☑5th Z20.0　Contact with and (suspected) exposure to intestinal infectious diseases
- **Z20.01　Contact with and (suspected) exposure to intestinal infectious diseases due to Escherichia coli (E. coli)**
- **Z20.09　Contact with and (suspected) exposure to other intestinal infectious diseases**

- **Z20.1　Contact with and (suspected) exposure to tuberculosis**
- **Z20.2　Contact with and (suspected) exposure to infections with a predominantly sexual mode of transmission**
- **Z20.3　Contact with and (suspected) exposure to rabies**
- **Z20.4　Contact with and (suspected) exposure to rubella**
- **Z20.5　Contact with and (suspected) exposure to viral hepatitis**
- **Z20.6　Contact with and (suspected) exposure to human immunodeficiency virus [HIV]**
  - **EXCLUDES 1**　*asymptomatic human immunodeficiency virus [HIV] HIV infection status (Z21)*
- **Z20.7　Contact with and (suspected) exposure to pediculosis, acariasis and other infestations**

☑5th Z20.8　Contact with and (suspected) exposure to other communicable diseases
- **☑6th Z20.81　Contact with and (suspected) exposure to other bacterial communicable diseases**
  - **Z20.810　Contact with and (suspected) exposure to anthrax**
  - **Z20.811　Contact with and (suspected) exposure to meningococcus**
  - **Z20.818　Contact with and (suspected) exposure to other bacterial communicable diseases**
- **☑6th Z20.82　Contact with and (suspected) exposure to other viral communicable diseases**
  - **Z20.820　Contact with and (suspected) exposure to varicella**
  - **Z20.828　Contact with and (suspected) exposure to other viral communicable diseases**
- **Z20.89　Contact with and (suspected) exposure to other communicable diseases**
- **Z20.9　Contact with and (suspected) exposure to unspecified communicable disease**

EXCLUDES 1 Not coded here　**EXCLUDES 2** Not included here　**PDx** Primary Diagnosis Only　**N** Newborn Age: 0　**P** Pediatric Age: 0-17　**M** Maternity Age: 12-55　**A** Adult Age: 15-124

1062　　　　　　　　　　　　　　　　　　　　　　　　　　　　　　　　ICD-10-CM Draft (2015)

Z21   **Asymptomatic human immunodeficiency virus [HIV] infection status**
HIV positive NOS
Code first human immunodeficiency virus [HIV] disease complicating pregnancy, childbirth and the puerperium, if applicable (O98.7-)
EXCLUDES 1   acquired immunodeficiency syndrome (B20)
contact with human immunodeficiency virus [HIV] (Z20.6)
exposure to human immunodeficiency virus [HIV] (Z20.6)
human immunodeficiency virus [HIV] disease (B20)
inconclusive laboratory evidence of human immunodeficiency virus [HIV] (R75)

✓4ᵗʰ Z22   **Carrier of infectious disease**
Colonization status
Suspected carrier

Z22.0   **Carrier of** typhoid

Z22.1   **Carrier of other** intestinal **infectious diseases**

Z22.2   **Carrier of** diphtheria

✓5ᵗʰ Z22.3   **Carrier of** other **specified bacterial diseases**

   Z22.31   **Carrier of bacterial disease due to** meningococci

   ✓6ᵗʰ Z22.32   **Carrier of bacterial disease due to** staphylococci

     Z22.321   **Carrier or suspected carrier of** Methicillin **susceptible Staphylococcus aureus**
MSSA colonization

     Z22.322   **Carrier or suspected carrier of** Methicillin **resistant Staphylococcus aureus**
MRSA colonization

   ✓6ᵗʰ Z22.33   **Carrier of bacterial disease due to** streptococci

     Z22.330   **Carrier of** Group B **streptococcus**

     Z22.338   **Carrier of other streptococcus**

   Z22.39   **Carrier of other specified bacterial diseases**

Z22.4   **Carrier of infections with a predominantly sexual mode of transmission**

✓5ᵗʰ Z22.5   **Carrier of** viral hepatitis

   Z22.50   **Carrier of unspecified viral hepatitis**

   Z22.51   **Carrier of viral hepatitis** B
Hepatitis B surface antigen [HBsAg] carrier

   Z22.52   **Carrier of viral hepatitis** C

   Z22.59   **Carrier of other viral hepatitis**

Z22.6   **Carrier of** human T-lymphotropic virus type-1 [HTLV-1] **infection**

Z22.8   **Carrier of other infectious diseases**

Z22.9   **Carrier of infectious disease, unspecified**

Z23   **Encounter for immunization**
Code first any routine childhood examination
NOTE   Procedure codes are required to identify the types of immunizations given

✓4ᵗʰ Z28   **Immunization not carried out and underimmunization status**
Vaccination not carried out

✓5ᵗʰ Z28.0   **Immunization not carried out because of** contraindication

   Z28.01   **Immunization not carried out because of** acute illness **of patient**

   Z28.02   **Immunization not carried out because of** chronic illness **or condition of patient**

   Z28.03   **Immunization not carried out because of** immune compromised state **of patient**

   Z28.04   **Immunization not carried out because of patient** allergy to vaccine or component

   Z28.09   **Immunization not carried out because of other** contraindication

Z28.1   **Immunization not carried out because of patient decision for** reasons of belief or group pressure
Immunization not carried out because of religious belief

✓5ᵗʰ Z28.2   **Immunization not carried out because of patient decision for** other and unspecified **reason**

   Z28.20   **Immunization not carried out because of patient decision for unspecified reason**

   Z28.21   **Immunization not carried out because of patient refusal**

   Z28.29   **Immunization not carried out because of patient decision for other reason**

Z28.3   **Underimmunization status**
Delinquent immunization status
Lapsed immunization schedule status

✓5ᵗʰ Z28.8   **Immunization not carried out for other reason**

   Z28.81   **Immunization not carried out due to** patient having had the disease

   Z28.82   **Immunization not carried out because of** caregiver refusal
Immunization not carried out because of guardian refusal
Immunization not carried out because of parent refusal
EXCLUDES 1   immunization not carried out because of caregiver refusal because of religious belief (Z28.1)

   Z28.89   **Immunization not carried out for other reason**

Z28.9   **Immunization not carried out for unspecified reason**

Persons encountering health services in circumstances related to reproduction (Z30-Z39)

✓4ᵗʰ Z30   **Encounter for contraceptive management**

✓5ᵗʰ Z30.0   **Encounter for general counseling and advice on** contraception

   ✓6ᵗʰ Z30.01   **Encounter for** initial prescription **of contraceptives**
EXCLUDES 1   encounter for surveillance of contraceptives (Z30.4-)

     Z30.011   **Encounter for** initial prescription **of contraceptive pills**   ♀

     Z30.012   **Encounter for prescription of** emergency **contraception**   ♀
Encounter for postcoital contraception

     Z30.013   **Encounter for initial prescription of** injectable **contraceptive**   ♀

     Z30.014   **Encounter for initial prescription of** intrauterine **contraceptive device**   ♀
EXCLUDES 1   encounter for insertion of intrauterine contraceptive device (Z30.430, Z30.432)

     Z30.018   **Encounter for initial prescription of other contraceptives**   ♀

     Z30.019   **Encounter for initial prescription of contraceptives, unspecified**   ♀

   Z30.02   **Counseling and instruction in** natural family planning **to avoid pregnancy**

   Z30.09   **Encounter for other general counseling and advice on contraception**
Encounter for family planning advice NOS

Z30.2   **Encounter for** sterilization

✓5ᵗʰ Z30.4   **Encounter for** surveillance **of contraceptives**

   Z30.40   **Encounter for surveillance of contraceptives, unspecified**

   Z30.41   **Encounter for surveillance of contraceptive** pills   ♀
Encounter for repeat prescription for contraceptive pill

   Z30.42   **Encounter for surveillance of** injectable **contraceptive**   ♀

   ✓6ᵗʰ Z30.43   **Encounter for surveillance of** intrauterine **contraceptive device**

     Z30.430   **Encounter for** insertion **of intrauterine contraceptive device**   ♀

     Z30.431   **Encounter for** routine checking **of intrauterine contraceptive device**   ♀

     Z30.432   **Encounter for** removal **of intrauterine contraceptive device**   ♀

     Z30.433   **Encounter for** removal and reinsertion **of intrauterine contraceptive device**   ♀
Encounter for replacement of intrauterine contraceptive device

   Z30.49   **Encounter for surveillance of other contraceptives**   ♀

Z30.8   **Encounter for other contraceptive management**
Encounter for postvasectomy sperm count
Encounter for routine examination for contraceptive maintenance
EXCLUDES 1   sperm count following sterilization reversal (Z31.42)
sperm count for fertility testing (Z31.41)

Z30.9   **Encounter for contraceptive management, unspecified**

✓4ᵗʰ Z31   **Encounter for procreative management**
EXCLUDES 1   complications associated with artificial fertilization (N98.-)
female infertility (N97.-)
male infertility (N46.-)

Z31.0   **Encounter for** reversal of previous sterilization

| ✓ Additional Character Required | ✓x7ᵗʰ Xtension Alert | Unspecified Dx | Other Specified Dx | Manifestation | ►◄ Revised Text | ● New Code | ▲ Revised Code Title |

ICD-10-CM Draft (2015)   **1063**

Factors Influencing Health Status and Contact With Health Services

Z31.4–Z3A.29

✓5th **Z31.4 Encounter for procreative investigation and testing**
     EXCLUDES 1   *postvasectomy sperm count (Z30.8)*

  Z31.41 Encounter for fertility testing
       Encounter for fallopian tube patency testing
       Encounter for sperm count for fertility testing

  Z31.42 Aftercare following sterilization reversal
       Sperm count following sterilization reversal

✓6th   **Z31.43 Encounter for genetic testing of female for procreative management**
       Use additional code for recurrent pregnancy loss, if applicable (N96, O26.2-)
       EXCLUDES 1   *nonprocreative genetic testing (Z13.7-)*

    Z31.430 Encounter of female for testing for genetic disease carrier status for procreative management ♀

    Z31.438 Encounter for other genetic testing of female for procreative management ♀

✓6th   **Z31.44 Encounter for genetic testing of male for procreative management**
       EXCLUDES 1   *nonprocreative genetic testing (Z13.7-)*

    Z31.440 Encounter of male for testing for genetic disease carrier status for procreative management ♂

    Z31.441 Encounter for testing of male partner patient with recurrent pregnancy loss Ⓐ♂

    Z31.448 Encounter for other genetic testing of male for procreative management Ⓐ♂

  Z31.49 Encounter for other procreative investigation and testing

Z31.5 Encounter for genetic counseling

✓5th **Z31.6 Encounter for general counseling and advice on procreation**

  Z31.61 Procreative counseling and advice using natural family planning

  Z31.62 Encounter for fertility preservation counseling
       Encounter for fertility preservation counseling prior to cancer therapy
       Encounter for fertility preservation counseling prior to surgical removal of gonads

  Z31.69 Encounter for other general counseling and advice on procreation

✓5th **Z31.8 Encounter for other procreative management**

  Z31.81 Encounter for male factor infertility in female patient PDx♀

  Z31.82 Encounter for Rh incompatibility status PDx♀

  Z31.83 Encounter for assisted reproductive fertility procedure cycle PDx♀
       Patient undergoing in vitro fertilization cycle
       Use additional code to identify the type of infertility
       EXCLUDES 1   *pre-cycle diagnosis and testing—code to reason for encounter*

  Z31.84 Encounter for fertility preservation procedure PDx
       Encounter for fertility preservation procedure prior to cancer therapy
       Encounter for fertility preservation procedure prior to surgical removal of gonads

  Z31.89 Encounter for other procreative management

Z31.9 Encounter for procreative management, unspecified

✓4th **Z32 Encounter for pregnancy test and childbirth and childcare instruction**

✓5th **Z32.0 Encounter for pregnancy test**

  Z32.00 Encounter for pregnancy test, result unknown ♀
       Encounter for pregnancy test NOS

  Z32.01 Encounter for pregnancy test, result positive Ⓜ♀

  Z32.02 Encounter for pregnancy test, result negative ♀

Z32.2 Encounter for childbirth instruction

Z32.3 Encounter for childcare instruction
     Encounter for prenatal or postpartum childcare instruction

✓4th **Z33 Pregnant state**

Z33.1 Pregnant state, incidental Ⓜ♀
     Pregnant state NOS
     EXCLUDES 1   *complications of pregnancy (O00-O9A)*

Z33.2 Encounter for elective termination of pregnancy PDx Ⓜ♀
     EXCLUDES 1   *early fetal death with retention of dead fetus (O02.1)*
                late fetal death (O36.4)
                spontaneous abortion (O03)

✓4th **Z34 Encounter for supervision of normal pregnancy**
     EXCLUDES 1   *any complication of pregnancy (O00-O9A)*
                encounter for pregnancy test (Z32.0-)
                encounter for supervision of high risk pregnancy (O09.-)

✓5th **Z34.0 Encounter for supervision of normal first pregnancy**

  Z34.00 Encounter for supervision of normal first pregnancy, unspecified trimester PDx Ⓜ♀

  Z34.01 Encounter for supervision of normal first pregnancy, first trimester PDx Ⓜ♀

  Z34.02 Encounter for supervision of normal first pregnancy, second trimester PDx Ⓜ♀

  Z34.03 Encounter for supervision of normal first pregnancy, third trimester PDx Ⓜ♀

✓5th **Z34.8 Encounter for supervision of other normal pregnancy**

  Z34.80 Encounter for supervision of other normal pregnancy, unspecified trimester PDx Ⓜ♀

  Z34.81 Encounter for supervision of other normal pregnancy, first trimester PDx Ⓜ♀

  Z34.82 Encounter for supervision of other normal pregnancy, second trimester PDx Ⓜ♀

  Z34.83 Encounter for supervision of other normal pregnancy, third trimester PDx Ⓜ♀

✓5th **Z34.9 Encounter for supervision of normal pregnancy, unspecified**

  Z34.90 Encounter for supervision of normal pregnancy, unspecified, unspecified trimester PDx Ⓜ♀

  Z34.91 Encounter for supervision of normal pregnancy, unspecified, first trimester PDx Ⓜ♀

  Z34.92 Encounter for supervision of normal pregnancy, unspecified, second trimester PDx Ⓜ♀

  Z34.93 Encounter for supervision of normal pregnancy, unspecified, third trimester PDx Ⓜ♀

Z36 Encounter for antenatal screening of mother Ⓜ♀
     EXCLUDES 1   *abnormal findings on antenatal screening of mother (O28.-)*
                diagnostic examination—code to sign or symptom
                encounter for suspected maternal and fetal conditions ruled out (Z03.7-)
                suspected fetal condition affecting management of pregnancy—code to condition in Chapter 15
     EXCLUDES 2   *genetic counseling and testing (Z31.43-, Z31.5)*
                routine prenatal care (Z34)

✓4th **Z3A Weeks of gestation**
     NOTE   Codes from category Z3A are for use, only on the maternal record, to indicate the weeks of gestation of the pregnancy.
     Code first complications of pregnancy, childbirth and the puerperium (O00-O9A)
     AHA: 2014, 2Q, 9; 2013, 2Q, 33

✓5th **Z3A.0 Weeks of gestation of pregnancy, unspecified or less than 10 weeks**

  Z3A.00 Weeks of gestation of pregnancy not specified Ⓜ♀

  Z3A.01 Less than 8 weeks gestation of pregnancy Ⓜ♀

  Z3A.08 8 weeks gestation of pregnancy Ⓜ♀

  Z3A.09 9 weeks gestation of pregnancy Ⓜ♀

✓5th **Z3A.1 Weeks of gestation of pregnancy, weeks 10-19**

  Z3A.10 10 weeks gestation of pregnancy Ⓜ♀

  Z3A.11 11 weeks gestation of pregnancy Ⓜ♀

  Z3A.12 12 weeks gestation of pregnancy Ⓜ♀

  Z3A.13 13 weeks gestation of pregnancy Ⓜ♀

  Z3A.14 14 weeks gestation of pregnancy Ⓜ♀

  Z3A.15 15 weeks gestation of pregnancy Ⓜ♀

  Z3A.16 16 weeks gestation of pregnancy Ⓜ♀

  Z3A.17 17 weeks gestation of pregnancy Ⓜ♀

  Z3A.18 18 weeks gestation of pregnancy Ⓜ♀

  Z3A.19 19 weeks gestation of pregnancy Ⓜ♀

✓5th **Z3A.2 Weeks of gestation of pregnancy, weeks 20-29**

  Z3A.20 20 weeks gestation of pregnancy Ⓜ♀

  Z3A.21 21 weeks gestation of pregnancy Ⓜ♀

  Z3A.22 22 weeks gestation of pregnancy Ⓜ♀

  Z3A.23 23 weeks gestation of pregnancy Ⓜ♀

  Z3A.24 24 weeks gestation of pregnancy Ⓜ♀

  Z3A.25 25 weeks gestation of pregnancy Ⓜ♀

  Z3A.26 26 weeks gestation of pregnancy Ⓜ♀

  Z3A.27 27 weeks gestation of pregnancy Ⓜ♀

  Z3A.28 28 weeks gestation of pregnancy Ⓜ♀

  Z3A.29 29 weeks gestation of pregnancy Ⓜ♀

EXCLUDES 1 Not coded here   EXCLUDES 2 Not included here   PDx Primary Diagnosis Only   Ⓝ Newborn Age: 0   Ⓟ Pediatric Age: 0-17   Ⓜ Maternity Age: 12-55   Ⓐ Adult Age: 15-124

1064   ICD-10-CM Draft (2015)

✓5ᵗʰ **Z3A.3 Weeks of gestation of pregnancy, weeks 30-39**

    Z3A.30 30 weeks gestation of pregnancy   Ⓜ♀

    Z3A.31 31 weeks gestation of pregnancy   Ⓜ♀

    Z3A.32 32 weeks gestation of pregnancy   Ⓜ♀

    Z3A.33 33 weeks gestation of pregnancy   Ⓜ♀

    Z3A.34 34 weeks gestation of pregnancy   Ⓜ♀

    Z3A.35 35 weeks gestation of pregnancy   Ⓜ♀

    Z3A.36 36 weeks gestation of pregnancy   Ⓜ♀

    Z3A.37 37 weeks gestation of pregnancy   Ⓜ♀

    Z3A.38 38 weeks gestation of pregnancy   Ⓜ♀

    Z3A.39 39 weeks gestation of pregnancy   Ⓜ♀

✓5ᵗʰ **Z3A.4 Weeks of gestation of pregnancy, weeks 40 or greater**

    Z3A.40 40 weeks gestation of pregnancy   Ⓜ♀

    Z3A.41 41 weeks gestation of pregnancy   Ⓜ♀

    Z3A.42 42 weeks gestation of pregnancy   Ⓜ♀

    Z3A.49 Greater than 42 weeks gestation of pregnancy   Ⓜ♀

✓4ᵗʰ **Z37 Outcome of delivery**

> **NOTE** This category is intended for use as an additional code to identify the outcome of delivery on the mother's record. It is not for use on the newborn record.
>
> **EXCLUDES 1** *stillbirth (P95)*

  Z37.0 Single live birth   Ⓜ♀
    AHA: 2014, 2Q, 9

  Z37.1 Single stillbirth   Ⓜ♀

  Z37.2 Twins, both liveborn   Ⓜ♀

  Z37.3 Twins, one liveborn and one stillborn   Ⓜ♀

  Z37.4 Twins, both stillborn   Ⓜ♀

✓5ᵗʰ **Z37.5 Other multiple births, all liveborn**

    Z37.50 Multiple births, unspecified, all liveborn   Ⓜ♀

    Z37.51 Triplets, all liveborn   Ⓜ♀

    Z37.52 Quadruplets, all liveborn   Ⓜ♀

    Z37.53 Quintuplets, all liveborn   Ⓜ♀

    Z37.54 Sextuplets, all liveborn   Ⓜ♀

    Z37.59 Other multiple births, all liveborn   Ⓜ♀

✓5ᵗʰ **Z37.6 Other multiple births, some liveborn**

    Z37.60 Multiple births, unspecified, some liveborn   Ⓜ♀

    Z37.61 Triplets, some liveborn   Ⓜ♀

    Z37.62 Quadruplets, some liveborn   Ⓜ♀

    Z37.63 Quintuplets, some liveborn   Ⓜ♀

    Z37.64 Sextuplets, some liveborn   Ⓜ♀

    Z37.69 Other multiple births, some liveborn   Ⓜ♀

  Z37.7 Other multiple births, all stillborn   Ⓜ♀

  Z37.9 Outcome of delivery, unspecified   Ⓜ♀
    Multiple birth NOS
    Single birth NOS

✓4ᵗʰ **Z38 Liveborn infants according to place of birth and type of delivery**

> **NOTE** This category is for use as the principal code on the initial record of a newborn baby. It is to be used for the initial birth record only. It is not to be used on the mother's record.

✓5ᵗʰ **Z38.0 Single liveborn infant, born in hospital**
    Single liveborn infant, born in birthing center or other health care facility

    Z38.00 Single liveborn infant, delivered vaginally   PDx Ⓝ

    Z38.01 Single liveborn infant, delivered by cesarean   PDx Ⓝ

  Z38.1 Single liveborn infant, born outside hospital   PDx Ⓝ

  Z38.2 Single liveborn infant, unspecified as to place of birth   PDx Ⓝ
    Single liveborn infant NOS

✓5ᵗʰ **Z38.3 Twin liveborn infant, born in hospital**

    Z38.30 Twin liveborn infant, delivered vaginally   PDx Ⓝ

    Z38.31 Twin liveborn infant, delivered by cesarean   PDx Ⓝ

  Z38.4 Twin liveborn infant, born outside hospital   PDx Ⓝ

  Z38.5 Twin liveborn infant, unspecified as to place of birth   PDx Ⓝ

✓5ᵗʰ **Z38.6 Other multiple liveborn infant, born in hospital**

    Z38.61 Triplet liveborn infant, delivered vaginally   PDx Ⓝ

    Z38.62 Triplet liveborn infant, delivered by cesarean   PDx Ⓝ

    Z38.63 Quadruplet liveborn infant, delivered vaginally   PDx Ⓝ

    Z38.64 Quadruplet liveborn infant, delivered by cesarean   PDx Ⓝ

    Z38.65 Quintuplet liveborn infant, delivered vaginally   PDx Ⓝ

    Z38.66 Quintuplet liveborn infant, delivered by cesarean   PDx Ⓝ

    Z38.68 Other multiple liveborn infant, delivered vaginally   PDx Ⓝ

    Z38.69 Other multiple liveborn infant, delivered by cesarean   PDx Ⓝ

  Z38.7 Other multiple liveborn infant, born outside hospital   PDx Ⓝ

  Z38.8 Other multiple liveborn infant, unspecified as to place of birth   PDx Ⓝ

✓4ᵗʰ **Z39 Encounter for maternal postpartum care and examination**

  Z39.0 Encounter for care and examination of mother immediately after delivery   PDx Ⓜ♀
    Care and observation in uncomplicated cases when the delivery occurs outside a healthcare facility

>   **EXCLUDES 1** *care for postpartum complication—see Alphabetic index*

  Z39.1 Encounter for care and examination of lactating mother   PDx Ⓜ♀
    Encounter for supervision of lactation

>   **EXCLUDES 1** *disorders of lactation (O92.-)*

  Z39.2 Encounter for routine postpartum follow-up   PDx Ⓜ♀

Encounters for other specific health care (Z40-Z53)

> **NOTE** Categories Z40-Z53 are intended for use to indicate a reason for care. They may be used for patients who have already been treated for a disease or injury, but who are receiving aftercare or prophylactic care, or care to consolidate the treatment, or to deal with a residual state.
>
> **EXCLUDES 2** *follow-up examination for medical surveillance after treatment (Z08-Z09)*

✓4ᵗʰ **Z40 Encounter for prophylactic surgery**

> **EXCLUDES 1** *organ donations (Z52.-)*
>   *therapeutic organ removal—code to condition*

✓5ᵗʰ **Z40.0 Encounter for prophylactic surgery for risk factors related to malignant neoplasms**
    Admission for prophylactic organ removal
    Use additional code to identify risk factor

    Z40.00 Encounter for prophylactic removal of unspecified organ

    Z40.01 Encounter for prophylactic removal of breast

    Z40.02 Encounter for prophylactic removal of ovary   ♀

    Z40.09 Encounter for prophylactic removal of other organ

  Z40.8 Encounter for other prophylactic surgery

  Z40.9 Encounter for prophylactic surgery, unspecified

✓4ᵗʰ **Z41 Encounter for procedures for purposes other than remedying health state**

  Z41.1 Encounter for cosmetic surgery
    Encounter for cosmetic breast implant
    Encounter for cosmetic procedure

>   **EXCLUDES 1** *encounter for plastic and reconstructive surgery following medical procedure or healed injury (Z42.-)*
>   *encounter for post-mastectomy breast implantation (Z42.1)*

  Z41.2 Encounter for routine and ritual male circumcision   ♂

  Z41.3 Encounter for ear piercing

  Z41.8 Encounter for other procedures for purposes other than remedying health state

  Z41.9 Encounter for procedure for purposes other than remedying health state, unspecified

✓4ᵗʰ **Z42 Encounter for plastic and reconstructive surgery following medical procedure or healed injury**

> **EXCLUDES 1** *encounter for cosmetic plastic surgery (Z41.1)*
>   *encounter for plastic surgery for treatment of current injury—code to relevent injury*

  Z42.1 Encounter for breast reconstruction following mastectomy   PDx Ⓐ

>   **EXCLUDES 1** *deformity and disproportion of reconstructed breast (N65.1-)*

  Z42.8 Encounter for other plastic and reconstructive surgery following medical procedure or healed injury   PDx

| ✓ Additional Character Required | ✗7ᵗʰ Xtension Alert | Unspecified Dx | Other Specified Dx | Manifestation | ▶◀ Revised Text | ● New Code | ▲ Revised Code Title |

ICD-10-CM Draft (2015)   **1065**

☑4ᵗʰ **Z43 Encounter for attention to artificial openings**
    INCLUDES   closure of artificial openings
       passage of sounds or bougies through artificial openings
       reforming artificial openings
       removal of catheter from artificial openings
       toilet or cleansing of artificial openings
    EXCLUDES 1   *artificial opening status only, without need for care (Z93.-)*
       complications of external stoma (J95.0-, K94.-, N99.5-)
    EXCLUDES 2   *fitting and adjustment of prosthetic and other devices (Z44-Z46)*

    Z43.0 Encounter for attention to tracheostomy
    Z43.1 Encounter for attention to gastrostomy
    Z43.2 Encounter for attention to ileostomy
    Z43.3 Encounter for attention to colostomy
    Z43.4 Encounter for attention to other artificial openings of digestive tract
    Z43.5 Encounter for attention to cystostomy
    Z43.6 Encounter for attention to other artificial openings of urinary tract
       Encounter for attention to nephrostomy
       Encounter for attention to ureterostomy
       Encounter for attention to urethrostomy
    Z43.7 Encounter for attention to artificial vagina
    Z43.8 Encounter for attention to other artificial openings
    Z43.9 Encounter for attention to unspecified artificial opening

☑4ᵗʰ **Z44 Encounter for fitting and adjustment of external prosthetic device**
    INCLUDES   removal or replacement of external prosthetic device
    EXCLUDES 1   *malfunction or other complications of device—see Alphabetical Index*
       presence of prosthetic device (Z97.-)

    ☑5ᵗʰ **Z44.0 Encounter for fitting and adjustment of** artificial arm
       ☑6ᵗʰ **Z44.00 Encounter for fitting and adjustment of** unspecified artificial arm
          Z44.001 Encounter for fitting and adjustment of unspecified right **artificial arm**
          Z44.002 Encounter for fitting and adjustment of unspecified left **artificial arm**
          Z44.009 Encounter for fitting and adjustment of unspecified artificial arm, unspecified arm
       ☑6ᵗʰ **Z44.01 Encounter for fitting and adjustment of** complete **artificial arm**
          Z44.011 Encounter for fitting and adjustment of complete right **artificial arm**
          Z44.012 Encounter for fitting and adjustment of complete left **artificial arm**
          Z44.019 Encounter for fitting and adjustment of complete artificial arm, unspecified arm
       ☑6ᵗʰ **Z44.02 Encounter for fitting and adjustment of** partial **artificial arm**
          Z44.021 Encounter for fitting and adjustment of partial artificial right **arm**
          Z44.022 Encounter for fitting and adjustment of partial artificial left **arm**
          Z44.029 Encounter for fitting and adjustment of partial artificial arm, unspecified arm

    ☑5ᵗʰ **Z44.1 Encounter for fitting and adjustment of** artificial leg
       ☑6ᵗʰ **Z44.10 Encounter for fitting and adjustment of** unspecified **artificial leg**
          Z44.101 Encounter for fitting and adjustment of unspecified right **artificial leg**
          Z44.102 Encounter for fitting and adjustment of unspecified left **artificial leg**
          Z44.109 Encounter for fitting and adjustment of unspecified artificial leg, unspecified leg
       ☑6ᵗʰ **Z44.11 Encounter for fitting and adjustment of** complete **artificial leg**
          Z44.111 Encounter for fitting and adjustment of complete right **artificial leg**
          Z44.112 Encounter for fitting and adjustment of complete left **artificial leg**
          Z44.119 Encounter for fitting and adjustment of complete artificial leg, unspecified leg
       ☑6ᵗʰ **Z44.12 Encounter for fitting and adjustment of** partial **artificial leg**
          Z44.121 Encounter for fitting and adjustment of partial artificial right **leg**

          Z44.122 Encounter for fitting and adjustment of partial artificial left **leg**
          Z44.129 Encounter for fitting and adjustment of partial artificial leg, unspecified leg

    ☑5ᵗʰ **Z44.2 Encounter for fitting and adjustment of** artificial eye
       EXCLUDES 1   *mechanical complication of ocular prosthesis (T85.3)*
       Z44.20 Encounter for fitting and adjustment of artificial eye, unspecified
       Z44.21 Encounter for fitting and adjustment of artificial right **eye**
       Z44.22 Encounter for fitting and adjustment of artificial left **eye**

    ☑5ᵗʰ **Z44.3 Encounter for fitting and adjustment of** external breast prosthesis
       EXCLUDES 1   *complications of breast implant (T85.4-)*
       encounter for adjustment or removal of breast implant (Z45.81-)
       encounter for initial breast implant insertion for cosmetic breast augmentation (Z41.1)
       encounter for breast reconstruction following mastectomy (Z42.1)
       Z44.30 Encounter for fitting and adjustment of external breast prosthesis, unspecified breast ♀
       Z44.31 Encounter for fitting and adjustment of external right **breast prosthesis** ♀
       Z44.32 Encounter for fitting and adjustment of external left **breast prosthesis** ♀

    Z44.8 Encounter for fitting and adjustment of other external prosthetic devices
    Z44.9 Encounter for fitting and adjustment of unspecified external prosthetic device

☑4ᵗʰ **Z45 Encounter for adjustment and management of implanted device**
    INCLUDES   removal or replacement of implanted device
    EXCLUDES 1   *malfunction or other complications of device—see Alphabetical Index*
       presence of prosthetic and other devices (Z95-Z97)
    EXCLUDES 2   *encounter for fitting and adjustment of non-implanted device (Z46.-)*

    ☑5ᵗʰ **Z45.0 Encounter for adjustment and management of** cardiac device
       ☑6ᵗʰ **Z45.01 Encounter for adjustment and management of cardiac** pacemaker
          EXCLUDES 1   *encounter for adjustment and management of automatic implantable cardiac defibrillator with synchronous cardiac pacemaker (Z45.02)*
          Z45.010 Encounter for checking and testing of cardiac pacemaker pulse generator **[battery]**
             Encounter for replacing cardiac pacemaker pulse generator [battery]
          Z45.018 Encounter for adjustment and management of other part of cardiac pacemaker
       Z45.02 Encounter for adjustment and management of automatic implantable cardiac defibrillator
          Encounter for adjustment and management of automatic implantable cardiac defibrillator with synchronous cardiac pacemaker
       Z45.09 Encounter for adjustment and management of other cardiac device

    Z45.1 Encounter for adjustment and management of infusion pump
    Z45.2 Encounter for adjustment and management of vascular access device
       Encounter for adjustment and management of vascular catheters
       EXCLUDES 1   *encounter for adjustment and management of renal dialysis catheter (Z49.01)*

    ☑5ᵗʰ **Z45.3 Encounter for adjustment and management of implanted** devices of the special senses
       Z45.31 Encounter for adjustment and management of implanted visual substitution device
       ☑6ᵗʰ **Z45.32 Encounter for adjustment and management of implanted** hearing device
          EXCLUDES 1   *Encounter for fitting and adjustment of hearing aide (Z46.1)*
          Z45.320 Encounter for adjustment and management of bone conduction **device**
          Z45.321 Encounter for adjustment and management of cochlear **device**

EXCLUDES 1 Not coded here   EXCLUDES 2 Not included here   PDX Primary Diagnosis Only   N Newborn Age: 0   P Pediatric Age: 0-17   M Maternity Age: 12-55   A Adult Age: 15-124

1066   ICD-10-CM Draft (2015)

Z45.328 **Encounter for adjustment and management of other implanted hearing device**

✓5th Z45.4 **Encounter for adjustment and management of implanted** nervous system device

Z45.41 **Encounter for adjustment and management of** cerebrospinal fluid drainage **device**
Encounter for adjustment and management of cerebral ventricular (communicating) shunt

Z45.42 **Encounter for adjustment and management of** neuropacemaker **(brain) (peripheral nerve) (spinal cord)**

Z45.49 **Encounter for adjustment and management of other implanted nervous system device**

✓5th Z45.8 **Encounter for adjustment and management of** other implanted devices

✓6th Z45.81 **Encounter for adjustment or** removal of breast implant
Encounter for elective implant exchange (different material) (different size)
Encounter removal of tissue expander without synchronous insertion of permanent implant
EXCLUDES1 *complications of breast implant (T85.4-)*
encounter for initial breast implant insertion for cosmetic breast augmentation (Z41.1)
encounter for breast reconstruction following mastectomy (Z42.1)

Z45.811 **Encounter for adjustment or removal of** ♀ right **breast implant**

Z45.812 **Encounter for adjustment or removal of** ♀ left **breast implant**

Z45.819 **Encounter for adjustment or removal of** ♀ unspecified breast implant

Z45.82 **Encounter for adjustment or removal of** myringotomy device **(stent) (tube)**

Z45.89 **Encounter for adjustment and management of other implanted devices**

Z45.9 **Encounter for adjustment and management of unspecified implanted device**

✓4th Z46 **Encounter for fitting and adjustment of other devices**
INCLUDES removal or replacement of other device
EXCLUDES1 *malfunction or other complications of device—see Alphabetical Index*
EXCLUDES2 *encounter for fitting and management of implanted devices (Z45.-)*
issue of repeat prescription only (Z76.0)
presence of prosthetic and other devices (Z95-Z97)

Z46.0 **Encounter for fitting and adjustment of** spectacles and contact lenses

Z46.1 **Encounter for fitting and adjustment of** hearing aid
EXCLUDES1 *encounter for adjustment and management of implanted hearing device (Z45.32-)*

Z46.2 **Encounter for fitting and adjustment of other** devices related to nervous system and special senses
EXCLUDES2 *encounter for adjustment and management of implanted nervous system device (Z45.4-)*
encounter for adjustment and management of implanted visual substitution device (Z45.31)

Z46.3 **Encounter for fitting and adjustment of** dental prosthetic device
Encounter for fitting and adjustment of dentures

Z46.4 **Encounter for fitting and adjustment of** orthodontic device

✓5th Z46.5 **Encounter for fitting and adjustment of other gastrointestinal** appliance and device
EXCLUDES1 *encounter for attention to artificial openings of digestive tract (Z43.1-Z43.4)*

Z46.51 **Encounter for fitting and adjustment of** gastric lap band

Z46.59 **Encounter for fitting and adjustment of other gastrointestinal appliance and device**

Z46.6 **Encounter for fitting and adjustment of** urinary device
EXCLUDES2 *attention to artificial openings of urinary tract (Z43.5, Z43.6)*

✓5th Z46.8 **Encounter for fitting and adjustment of** other specified devices

Z46.81 **Encounter for fitting and adjustment of** insulin pump
Encounter for insulin pump instruction and training
Encounter for insulin pump titration

Z46.82 **Encounter for fitting and adjustment of** non-vascular catheter

Z46.89 **Encounter for fitting and adjustment of other specified devices**
Encounter for fitting and adjustment of wheelchair

Z46.9 **Encounter for fitting and adjustment of unspecified device**

✓4th Z47 **Orthopedic aftercare**
EXCLUDES1 *aftercare for healing fracture—code to fracture with 7th character D*

Z47.1 **Aftercare following** joint replacement surgery
Use additional code to identify the joint (Z96.6-)

Z47.2 **Encounter for removal of** internal fixation device
EXCLUDES1 *encounter for adjustment of internal fixation device for fracture treatment—code to fracture with appropriate 7th character*
encounter for removal of external fixation device—code to fracture with 7th character D
infection or inflammatory reaction to internal fixation device (T84.6-)
mechanical complication of internal fixation device (T84.1-)

✓5th Z47.3 **Aftercare following explantation of** joint prosthesis
Aftercare following explantation of joint prosthesis, staged procedure
Encounter for joint prosthesis insertion following prior explantation of joint prosthesis

Z47.31 **Aftercare following explantation of** shoulder **joint prosthesis**
EXCLUDES1 *acquired absence of shoulder joint following prior explantation of shoulder joint prosthesis (Z89.23-)*
shoulder joint prosthesis explantation status (Z89.23-)

Z47.32 **Aftercare following explantation of** hip **joint prosthesis**
EXCLUDES1 *acquired absence of hip joint following prior explantation of hip joint prosthesis (Z89.62-)*
hip joint prosthesis explantation status (Z89.62-)

Z47.33 **Aftercare following explantation of** knee **joint prosthesis**
EXCLUDES1 *acquired absence of knee joint following prior explantation of knee prosthesis (Z89.52-)*
knee joint prosthesis explantation status (Z89.52-)

✓6th Z47.8 **Encounter for** other orthopedic aftercare

Z47.81 **Encounter for orthopedic aftercare** following surgical amputation
Use additional code to identify the limb amputated (Z89.-)

Z47.82 **Encounter for orthopedic aftercare** following scoliosis surgery

Z47.89 **Encounter for other orthopedic aftercare**

✓4th Z48 **Encounter for other postprocedural aftercare**
EXCLUDES1 *encounter for follow-up examination after completed treatment (Z08-Z09)*
EXCLUDES2 *encounter for attention to artificial openings (Z43.-)*
encounter for fitting and adjustment of prosthetic and other devices (Z44-Z46)

✓5th Z48.0 **Encounter for** attention to dressings, sutures and drains
EXCLUDES1 *encounter for planned postprocedural wound closure (Z48.1)*

Z48.00 **Encounter for change or removal of** nonsurgical wound dressing
Encounter for change or removal of wound dressing NOS

Z48.01 **Encounter for change or removal of** surgical wound dressing

Z48.02 **Encounter for removal of** sutures
Encounter for removal of staples

Z48.03 **Encounter for change or removal of** drains

Z48.1 **Encounter for planned** postprocedural **wound closure**
> EXCLUDES 1 *encounter for attention to dressings and sutures (Z48.0-)*

√5ᵗʰ **Z48.2** **Encounter for aftercare following** organ transplant

Z48.21 **Encounter for aftercare following** heart **transplant**

Z48.22 **Encounter for aftercare following** kidney **transplant**

Z48.23 **Encounter for aftercare following** liver **transplant**

Z48.24 **Encounter for aftercare following** lung **transplant**

√6ᵗʰ **Z48.28** **Encounter for aftercare following** multiple **organ transplant**

Z48.280 **Encounter for aftercare following** heart-lung **transplant**

Z48.288 **Encounter for aftercare following** multiple **organ transplant**

√6ᵗʰ **Z48.29** **Encounter for aftercare following** other **organ transplant**

Z48.290 **Encounter for aftercare following** bone marrow **transplant**

Z48.298 **Encounter for aftercare following other organ transplant**

Z48.3 **Aftercare following** surgery for neoplasm
> Use additional code to identify the neoplasm

√5ᵗʰ **Z48.8** **Encounter for other specified postprocedural aftercare**

√6ᵗʰ **Z48.81** **Encounter for surgical aftercare following** surgery on specified body systems

> NOTE These codes identify the body system requiring aftercare. They are for use in conjunction with other aftercare codes to fully explain the aftercare encounter. The condition treated should also be coded if still present.
> EXCLUDES 1 *aftercare for injury—code the injury with 7th character D*
> *aftercare following surgery for neoplasm (Z48.3)*
> EXCLUDES 2 *aftercare following organ transplant (Z48.2-)*
> *orthopedic aftercare (Z47.-)*

Z48.810 **Encounter for surgical aftercare following surgery on the** sense organs

Z48.811 **Encounter for surgical aftercare following surgery on the** nervous system
> EXCLUDES 2 *encounter for surgical aftercare following surgery on the sense organs (Z48.810)*

Z48.812 **Encounter for surgical aftercare following surgery on the** circulatory system
> AHA: 2012, 4Q, 96

Z48.813 **Encounter for surgical aftercare following surgery on the** respiratory system

Z48.814 **Encounter for surgical aftercare following surgery on the** teeth or oral cavity

Z48.815 **Encounter for surgical aftercare following surgery on the** digestive system

Z48.816 **Encounter for surgical aftercare following surgery on the** genitourinary system
> EXCLUDES 1 *encounter for aftercare following sterilization reversal (Z31.42)*

Z48.817 **Encounter for surgical aftercare following surgery on the** skin and subcutaneous tissue

Z48.89 **Encounter for other specified surgical aftercare**

√4ᵗʰ **Z49** **Encounter for care involving renal dialysis**
> Code also associated end stage renal disease (N18.6)

√5ᵗʰ **Z49.0** Preparatory care **for renal dialysis**
> Encounter for dialysis instruction and training

Z49.01 **Encounter for fitting and adjustment of** extracorporeal dialysis catheter
> Removal or replacement of renal dialysis catheter
> Toilet or cleansing of renal dialysis catheter

Z49.02 **Encounter for fitting and adjustment of** peritoneal dialysis catheter

√5ᵗʰ **Z49.3** **Encounter for** adequacy testing for dialysis

Z49.31 **Encounter for adequacy testing for** hemodialysis

Z49.32 **Encounter for adequacy testing for** peritoneal dialysis
> Encounter for peritoneal equilibration test

√4ᵗʰ **Z51** **Encounter for other aftercare**
> Code also condition requiring care
> EXCLUDES 1 *follow-up examination after treatment (Z08-Z09)*

Z51.0 **Encounter for antineoplastic** radiation therapy   PDx

√5ᵗʰ **Z51.1** **Encounter for antineoplastic chemotherapy and immunotherapy**
> EXCLUDES 2 *encounter for chemotherapy and immunotherapy for nonneoplastic condition—code to condition*

Z51.11 **Encounter for antineoplastic** chemotherapy   PDx

Z51.12 **Encounter for antineoplastic** immunotherapy   PDx

Z51.5 **Encounter for** palliative care

√5ᵗʰ **Z51.8** **Encounter for** other specified aftercare
> EXCLUDES 1 *holiday relief care (Z75.5)*

Z51.81 **Encounter for** therapeutic drug level **monitoring**
> Code also any long-term (current) drug therapy (Z79.-)
> EXCLUDES 1 *encounter for blood-drug test for administrative or medicolegal reasons (Z02.83)*

Z51.89 **Encounter for other specified aftercare**
> AHA: 2012, 4Q, 95-97

√4ᵗʰ **Z52** **Donors of organs and tissues**
> INCLUDES autologous and other living donors
> EXCLUDES 1 *cadaveric donor—omit code*
> *examination of potential donor (Z00.5)*
> AHA: 2012, 4Q, 99

√5ᵗʰ **Z52.0** Blood **donor**

√6ᵗʰ **Z52.00** Unspecified **blood donor**

Z52.000 **Unspecified donor,** whole blood   PDx

Z52.001 **Unspecified donor,** stem cells   PDx

Z52.008 **Unspecified donor, other blood**   PDx

√6ᵗʰ **Z52.01** Autologous **blood donor**

Z52.010 **Autologous donor,** whole blood   PDx

Z52.011 **Autologous donor,** stem cells   PDx

Z52.018 **Autologous donor, other blood**   PDx

√6ᵗʰ **Z52.09** Other **blood donor**
> Volunteer donor

Z52.090 **Other blood donor,** whole blood   PDx

Z52.091 **Other blood donor,** stem cells   PDx

Z52.098 **Other blood donor, other blood**   PDx

√5ᵗʰ **Z52.1** Skin **donor**

Z52.10 **Skin donor, unspecified**   PDx

Z52.11 **Skin donor,** autologous   PDx

Z52.19 **Skin donor, other**   PDx

√5ᵗʰ **Z52.2** Bone **donor**

Z52.20 **Bone donor, unspecified**   PDx

Z52.21 **Bone donor,** autologous   PDx

Z52.29 **Bone donor, other**   PDx

Z52.3 Bone marrow **donor**   PDx

Z52.4 Kidney **donor**   PDx

Z52.5 Cornea **donor**   PDx

Z52.6 Liver **donor**   PDx

√5ᵗʰ **Z52.8** **Donor of** other specified organs or tissues

√6ᵗʰ **Z52.81** Egg (Oocyte) **donor**

Z52.810 **Egg (Oocyte) donor** under age 35, anonymous **recipient**   PDx♀
> Egg donor under age 35 NOS

Z52.811 **Egg (Oocyte) donor** under age 35, designated **recipient**   PDx♀

Z52.812 **Egg (Oocyte) donor** age 35 and over, anonymous **recipient**   PDx♀
> Egg donor age 35 and over NOS

Z52.813 **Egg (Oocyte) donor** age 35 and over, designated **recipient**   PDx♀

Z52.819 **Egg (Oocyte) donor, unspecified**   PDx♀

Z52.89 **Donor of other specified organs or tissues**   PDx

Z52.9 **Donor of unspecified organ or tissue**   PDx
> Donor NOS

√4ᵗʰ **Z53** **Persons encountering health services for specific procedures and treatment, not carried out**

√5ᵗʰ **Z53.0** **Procedure and treatment not carried out because of** contraindication

Z53.01 **Procedure and treatment not carried out due to** patient smoking

EXCLUDES 1 Not coded here   EXCLUDES 2 Not included here   PDx Primary Diagnosis Only   N Newborn Age: 0   P Pediatric Age: 0-17   M Maternity Age: 12-55   A Adult Age: 15-124

1068   ICD-10-CM Draft (2015)

Z53.09   **Procedure and treatment not carried out because of other contraindication**

Z53.1   **Procedure and treatment not carried out because of patient's decision for** reasons of belief and group pressure

✓5ᵗʰ Z53.2   **Procedure and treatment not carried out because of patient's decision for** other and unspecified **reasons**

Z53.20   **Procedure and treatment not carried out because of patient's decision for unspecified reasons**

Z53.21   **Procedure and treatment not carried out due to patient** leaving prior to being seen by health care provider

Z53.29   **Procedure and treatment not carried out because of patient's decision for other reasons**

Z53.8   **Procedure and treatment not carried out for other reasons**

Z53.9   **Procedure and treatment not carried out, unspecified reason**

Persons with potential health hazards related to socioeconomic and psychosocial circumstances (Z55-Z65)

✓4ᵗʰ **Z55   Problems related to education and literacy**
EXCLUDES 1   disorders of psychological development (F80-F89)

Z55.0   **Illiteracy and low-level literacy**

Z55.1   **Schooling unavailable and unattainable**

Z55.2   **Failed school examinations**

Z55.3   **Underachievement in school**

Z55.4   **Educational maladjustment and discord with teachers and classmates**

Z55.8   **Other problems related to education and literacy**
Problems related to inadequate teaching

Z55.9   **Problems related to education and literacy, unspecified**
Academic problems NOS

✓4ᵗʰ **Z56   Problems related to employment and unemployment**
EXCLUDES 2   occupational exposure to risk factors (Z57.-)
problems related to housing and economic circumstances (Z59.-)

Z56.0   **Unemployment, unspecified**

Z56.1   **Change of job**

Z56.2   **Threat of job loss**

Z56.3   **Stressful work schedule**

Z56.4   **Discord with boss and workmates**

Z56.5   **Uncongenial work environment**
Difficult conditions at work

Z56.6   **Other physical and mental strain related to work**

✓5ᵗʰ Z56.8   **Other problems related to employment**

Z56.81   **Sexual harassment on the job**

Z56.82   **Military deployment status**
Individual (civilian or military) currently deployed in theater or in support of military war, peacekeeping and humanitarian operations

Z56.89   **Other problems related to employment**

Z56.9   **Unspecified problems related to employment**
Occupational problems NOS

✓4ᵗʰ **Z57   Occupational exposure to risk factors**

Z57.0   **Occupational exposure to** noise

Z57.1   **Occupational exposure to** radiation

Z57.2   **Occupational exposure to** dust

✓5ᵗʰ Z57.3   **Occupational exposure to** other air contaminants

Z57.31   **Occupational exposure to environmental** tobacco smoke
EXCLUDES 2   exposure to environmental tobacco smoke (Z77.22)

Z57.39   **Occupational exposure to other** air contaminants

Z57.4   **Occupational exposure to** toxic agents in agriculture
Occupational exposure to solids, liquids, gases or vapors in agriculture

Z57.5   **Occupational exposure to** toxic agents in other industries
Occupational exposure to solids, liquids, gases or vapors in other industries

Z57.6   **Occupational exposure to** extreme temperature

Z57.7   **Occupational exposure to** vibration

Z57.8   **Occupational exposure to other risk factors**

Z57.9   **Occupational exposure to unspecified risk factor**

✓4ᵗʰ **Z59   Problems related to housing and economic circumstances**
EXCLUDES 2   problems related to upbringing (Z62.-)

Z59.0   **Homelessness**

Z59.1   **Inadequate housing**
Lack of heating
Restriction of space
Technical defects in home preventing adequate care
Unsatisfactory surroundings
EXCLUDES 1   problems related to the natural and physical environment (Z77.1-)

Z59.2   **Discord with neighbors, lodgers and landlord**

Z59.3   **Problems related to living in residential institution**
Boarding-school resident
EXCLUDES 1   institutional upbringing (Z62.2)

Z59.4   **Lack of adequate food and safe drinking water**
Inadequate drinking water supply
EXCLUDES 1   effects of hunger (T73.0)
inappropriate diet or eating habits (Z72.4)
malnutrition (E40-E46)

Z59.5   **Extreme poverty**

Z59.6   **Low income**

Z59.7   **Insufficient social insurance and welfare support**

Z59.8   **Other problems related to housing and economic circumstances**
Foreclosure on loan
Isolated dwelling
Problems with creditors

Z59.9   **Problem related to housing and economic circumstances, unspecified**

✓4ᵗʰ **Z60   Problems related to social environment**

Z60.0   **Problems of adjustment to life-cycle transitions**
Empty nest syndrome
Phase of life problem
Problem with adjustment to retirement [pension]

Z60.2   **Problems related to living alone**

Z60.3   **Acculturation difficulty**
Problem with migration
Problem with social transplantation

Z60.4   **Social exclusion and rejection**
Exclusion and rejection on the basis of personal characteristics, such as unusual physical appearance, illness or behavior.
EXCLUDES 1   target of adverse discrimination such as for racial or religious reasons (Z60.5)

Z60.5   **Target of (perceived) adverse discrimination and persecution**
EXCLUDES 1   social exclusion and rejection (Z60.4)

Z60.8   **Other problems related to social environment**

Z60.9   **Problem related to social environment, unspecified**

✓4ᵗʰ **Z62   Problems related to upbringing**
Current and past negative life events in childhood
Current and past problems of a child related to upbringing
EXCLUDES 2   maltreatment syndrome (T74.-)
problems related to housing and economic circumstances (Z59.-)

Z62.0   **Inadequate parental supervision and control**

Z62.1   **Parental overprotection**

✓5ᵗʰ Z62.2   **Upbringing away from parents**
EXCLUDES 1   problems with boarding school (Z59.3)

Z62.21   **Child in welfare custody** 🄿
Child in care of non-parental family member
Child in foster care
EXCLUDES 2   problem for parent due to child in welfare custody (Z63.5)

Z62.22   **Institutional upbringing**
Child living in orphanage or group home

Z62.29   **Other upbringing away from parents**

Z62.3   **Hostility towards and scapegoating of child** 🄿

Z62.6   **Inappropriate (excessive) parental pressure**

✓5ᵗʰ Z62.8   **Other specified problems related to upbringing**

✓6ᵗʰ Z62.81   **Personal history of abuse in childhood**

Z62.810   **Personal history of** physical and sexual abuse in childhood
EXCLUDES 1   current child physical abuse (T74.12, T76.12)
current child sexual abuse (T74.22, T76.22)

☑ Additional Character Required   ✓ₓₜₕ Xtension Alert   Unspecified Dx   Other Specified Dx   Manifestation   ►◄ Revised Text   ● New Code   ▲ Revised Code Title

ICD-10-CM Draft (2015)   **1069**

Z62.811 Personal history of psychological abuse in childhood
> EXCLUDES 1 *current child psychological abuse (T74.32, T76.32)*

Z62.812 Personal history of neglect in childhood
> EXCLUDES 1 *current child neglect (T74.02, T76.02)*

Z62.819 Personal history of unspecified abuse in childhood
> EXCLUDES 1 *current child abuse NOS (T74.92, T76.92)*

✓6th **Z62.82** Parent-child conflict

    Z62.820 Parent-biological child conflict
> Parent-child problem NOS

    Z62.821 Parent-adopted child conflict

    Z62.822 Parent-foster child conflict

✓6th **Z62.89** Other specified problems related to upbringing

    Z62.890 Parent-child estrangement NEC

    Z62.891 Sibling rivalry

    Z62.898 Other specified problems related to upbringing

Z62.9 Problem related to upbringing, unspecified

✓4th **Z63** Other problems related to primary support group, including family circumstances
> EXCLUDES 2 *maltreatment syndrome (T74-, T76)*
> *parent-child problems (Z62.-)*
> *problems related to negative life events in childhood (Z62.-)*
> *problems related to upbringing (Z62.-)*

Z63.0 Problems in relationship with spouse or partner
> EXCLUDES 1 *counseling for spousal or partner abuse problems (Z69.1)*
> *counseling related to sexual attitude, behavior, and orientation (Z70.-)*

Z63.1 Problems in relationship with in-laws

✓5th **Z63.3** Absence of family member
> EXCLUDES 1 *absence of family member due to disappearance and death (Z63.4)*
> *absence of family member due to separation and divorce (Z63.5)*

    Z63.31 Absence of family member due to military deployment
> Individual or family affected by other family member being on military deployment
> EXCLUDES 1 *family disruption due to return of family member from military deployment (Z63.71)*

    Z63.32 Other absence of family member

Z63.4 Disappearance and death of family member
> Assumed death of family member
> Bereavement
> **AHA:** 2014, 1Q, 25

Z63.5 Disruption of family by separation and divorce
> Marital estrangement

Z63.6 Dependent relative needing care at home

✓5th **Z63.7** Other stressful life events affecting family and household

    Z63.71 Stress on family due to return of family member from military deployment
> Individual or family affected by family member having returned from military deployment (current or past conflict)

    Z63.72 Alcoholism and drug addiction in family

    Z63.79 Other stressful life events affecting family and household
> Anxiety (normal) about sick person in family
> Health problems within family
> Ill or disturbed family member
> Isolated family

Z63.8 Other specified problems related to primary support group
> Family discord NOS
> Family estrangement NOS
> High expressed emotional level within family
> Inadequate family support NOS
> Inadequate or distorted communication within family

Z63.9 Problem related to primary support group, unspecified
> Relationship disorder NOS

✓4th **Z64** Problems related to certain psychosocial circumstances

Z64.0 Problems related to unwanted pregnancy   M♀

Z64.1 Problems related to multiparity   ♀

Z64.4 Discord with counselors
> Discord with probation officer
> Discord with social worker

✓4th **Z65** Problems related to other psychosocial circumstances

Z65.0 Conviction in civil and criminal proceedings without imprisonment

Z65.1 Imprisonment and other incarceration

Z65.2 Problems related to release from prison

Z65.3 Problems related to other legal circumstances
> Arrest
> Child custody or support proceedings
> Litigation
> Prosecution

Z65.4 Victim of crime and terrorism
> Victim of torture

Z65.5 Exposure to disaster, war and other hostilities
> EXCLUDES 1 *target of perceived discrimination or persecution (Z60.5)*

Z65.8 Other specified problems related to psychosocial circumstances

Z65.9 Problem related to unspecified psychosocial circumstances

Do not resuscitate status (Z66)

Z66 Do not resuscitate
> DNR status

Blood type (Z67)

✓4th **Z67** Blood type

✓5th **Z67.1** Type A blood

    Z67.10 Type A blood, Rh positive

    Z67.11 Type A blood, Rh negative

✓5th **Z67.2** Type B blood

    Z67.20 Type B blood, Rh positive

    Z67.21 Type B blood, Rh negative

✓5th **Z67.3** Type AB blood

    Z67.30 Type AB blood, Rh positive

    Z67.31 Type AB blood, Rh negative

✓5th **Z67.4** Type O blood

    Z67.40 Type O blood, Rh positive

    Z67.41 Type O blood, Rh negative

✓5th **Z67.9** Unspecified blood type

    Z67.90 Unspecified blood type, Rh positive

    Z67.91 Unspecified blood type, Rh negative

Body mass index [BMI] (Z68)

✓4th **Z68** Body mass index [BMI]
> Kilograms per meters squared
> **NOTE** BMI adult codes are for use for persons 21 years of age or older.
> BMI pediatric codes are for use for persons 2-20 years of age. These percentiles are based on the growth charts published by the Centers for Disease Control and Prevention (CDC).

Z68.1 Body mass index [BMI] 19 or less, adult   A

✓5th **Z68.2** Body mass index [BMI] 20-29, adult

    Z68.20 Body mass index [BMI] 20.0-20.9, adult   A

    Z68.21 Body mass index [BMI] 21.0-21.9, adult   A

    Z68.22 Body mass index [BMI] 22.0-22.9, adult   A

    Z68.23 Body mass index [BMI] 23.0-23.9, adult   A

    Z68.24 Body mass index [BMI] 24.0-24.9, adult   A

    Z68.25 Body mass index [BMI] 25.0-25.9, adult   A

    Z68.26 Body mass index [BMI] 26.0-26.9, adult   A

    Z68.27 Body mass index [BMI] 27.0-27.9, adult   A

    Z68.28 Body mass index [BMI] 28.0-28.9, adult   A

    Z68.29 Body mass index [BMI] 29.0-29.9, adult   A

✓5th **Z68.3** Body mass index [BMI] 30-39, adult

    Z68.30 Body mass index [BMI] 30.0-30.9, adult   A

    Z68.31 Body mass index [BMI] 31.0-31.9, adult   A

    Z68.32 Body mass index [BMI] 32.0-32.9, adult   A

    Z68.33 Body mass index [BMI] 33.0-33.9, adult   A

    Z68.34 Body mass index [BMI] 34.0-34.9, adult   A

    Z68.35 Body mass index [BMI] 35.0-35.9, adult   A

EXCLUDES 1 Not coded here   EXCLUDES 2 Not included here   PDX Primary Diagnosis Only   N Newborn Age: 0   P Pediatric Age: 0-17   M Maternity Age: 12-55   A Adult Age: 15-124

1070   ICD-10-CM Draft (2015)

Z68.36	Body mass index [BMI] 36.0-36.9, adult	A
Z68.37	Body mass index [BMI] 37.0-37.9, adult	A
Z68.38	Body mass index [BMI] 38.0-38.9, adult	A
Z68.39	Body mass index [BMI] 39.0-39.9, adult	A

✓5th **Z68.4 Body mass index [BMI] 40 or greater, adult**

Z68.41	Body mass index [BMI] 40.0-44.9, adult	A
Z68.42	Body mass index [BMI] 45.0-49.9, adult	A
Z68.43	Body mass index [BMI] 50-59.9, adult	A
Z68.44	Body mass index [BMI] 60.0-69.9, adult	A
Z68.45	Body mass index [BMI] 70 or greater, adult	A

✓5th **Z68.5 Body mass index [BMI] pediatric**

Z68.51 Body mass index [BMI] pediatric, less than 5th percentile for age P

Z68.52 Body mass index [BMI] pediatric, 5th percentile to less than 85th percentile for age P

Z68.53 Body mass index [BMI] pediatric, 85th percentile to less than 95th percentile for age P

Z68.54 Body mass index [BMI] pediatric, greater than or equal to 95th percentile for age P

Persons encountering health services in other circumstances (Z69-Z76)

✓4th **Z69 Encounter for mental health services for victim and perpetrator of abuse**
Counseling for victims and perpetrators of abuse

✓5th **Z69.0 Encounter for mental health services for child abuse problems**

✓6th **Z69.01 Encounter for mental health services for parental child abuse**

Z69.010 Encounter for mental health services for victim of parental child abuse P

Z69.011 Encounter for mental health services for perpetrator of parental child abuse
EXCLUDES 1 encounter for mental health services for non-parental child abuse (Z69.02-)

✓6th **Z69.02 Encounter for mental health services for non-parental child abuse**

Z69.020 Encounter for mental health services for victim of non-parental child abuse P

Z69.021 Encounter for mental health services for perpetrator of non-parental child abuse

✓5th **Z69.1 Encounter for mental health services for spousal or partner abuse problems**

Z69.11 Encounter for mental health services for victim of spousal or partner abuse

Z69.12 Encounter for mental health services for perpetrator of spousal or partner abuse

✓5th **Z69.8 Encounter for mental health services for victim or perpetrator of other abuse**

Z69.81 Encounter for mental health services for victim of other abuse
Encounter for rape victim counseling

Z69.82 Encounter for mental health services for perpetrator of other abuse

✓4th **Z70 Counseling related to sexual attitude, behavior and orientation**
Encounter for mental health services for sexual attitude, behavior and orientation
EXCLUDES 2 contraceptive or procreative counseling (Z30-Z31)

Z70.0 Counseling related to sexual attitude

Z70.1 Counseling related to patient's sexual behavior and orientation
Patient concerned regarding impotence
Patient concerned regarding non-responsiveness
Patient concerned regarding promiscuity
Patient concerned regarding sexual orientation

Z70.2 Counseling related to sexual behavior and orientation of third party
Advice sought regarding sexual behavior and orientation of child
Advice sought regarding sexual behavior and orientation of partner
Advice sought regarding sexual behavior and orientation of spouse

Z70.3 Counseling related to combined concerns regarding sexual attitude, behavior and orientation

Z70.8 Other sex counseling
Encounter for sex education

Z70.9 Sex counseling, unspecified

✓4th **Z71 Persons encountering health services for other counseling and medical advice, not elsewhere classified**
EXCLUDES 2 contraceptive or procreation counseling (Z30-Z31)
sex counseling (Z70.-)

Z71.0 Person encountering health services to consult on behalf of another person
Person encountering health services to seek advice or treatment for non-attending third party
EXCLUDES 2 anxiety (normal) about sick person in family (Z63.7)
expectant (adoptive) parent(s) pre-birth pediatrician visit (Z76.81)

Z71.1 Person with feared health complaint in whom no diagnosis is made
Person encountering health services with feared condition which was not demonstrated
Person encountering health services in which problem was normal state
"Worried well"
EXCLUDES 1 medical observation for suspected diseases and conditions proven not to exist (Z03.-)

Z71.2 Person consulting for explanation of examination or test findings

Z71.3 Dietary counseling and surveillance
Use additional code for any associated underlying medical condition
Use additional code to identify body mass index (BMI), if known (Z68.-)

✓5th **Z71.4 Alcohol abuse counseling and surveillance**
Use additional code for alcohol abuse or dependence (F10.-)

Z71.41 Alcohol abuse counseling and surveillance of alcoholic

Z71.42 Counseling for family member of alcoholic
Counseling for significant other, partner, or friend of alcoholic

✓5th **Z71.5 Drug abuse counseling and surveillance**
Use additional code for drug abuse or dependence (F11-F16, F18-F19)

Z71.51 Drug abuse counseling and surveillance of drug abuser

Z71.52 Counseling for family member of drug abuser
Counseling for significant other, partner, or friend of drug abuser

Z71.6 Tobacco abuse counseling
Use additional code for nicotine dependence (F17.-)

Z71.7 Human immunodeficiency virus [HIV] counseling

✓5th **Z71.8 Other specified counseling**
EXCLUDES 2 counseling for contraception (Z30.0-)
counseling for genetics (Z31.5)
counseling for procreative management (Z31.6-)

Z71.81 Spiritual or religious counseling

Z71.89 Other specified counseling

Z71.9 Counseling, unspecified
Encounter for medical advice NOS

✓4th **Z72 Problems related to lifestyle**
EXCLUDES 2 problems related to life-management difficulty (Z73.-)
problems related to socioeconomic and psychosocial circumstances (Z55-Z65)

Z72.0 Tobacco use
Tobacco use NOS
EXCLUDES 1 history of tobacco dependence (Z87.891)
nicotine dependence (F17.2-)
tobacco dependence (F17.2-)
tobacco use during pregnancy (O99.33-)

Z72.3 Lack of physical exercise

Z72.4 Inappropriate diet and eating habits
EXCLUDES 1 behavioral eating disorders of infancy or childhood (F98.2- F98.3)
eating disorders (F50.-)
lack of adequate food (Z59.4)
malnutrition and other nutritional deficiencies (E40-E64)

✓5th **Z72.5 High risk sexual behavior**
Promiscuity
EXCLUDES 1 paraphilias (F65)

Z72.51 High risk heterosexual behavior

☑ Additional Character Required   ✓x7th Xtension Alert   Unspecified Dx   Other Specified Dx   Manifestation   ►◄ Revised Text   ● New Code   ▲ Revised Code Title

      Z72.52   **High risk** homosexual **behavior**

      Z72.53   **High risk** bisexual **behavior**

   Z72.6   **Gambling and betting**
      EXCLUDES 1   compulsive or pathological gambling (F63.Ø)

✓5ᵗʰ   Z72.8   **Other problems related to lifestyle**

     ✓6ᵗʰ   Z72.81   **Antisocial behavior**
          EXCLUDES 1   conduct disorders (F91.-)

         Z72.81Ø   **Child and adolescent antisocial**   P
                behavior
                Antisocial behavior (child) (adolescent)
                    without manifest psychiatric disorder
                Delinquency NOS
                Group delinquency
                Offenses in the context of gang
                    membership
                Stealing in company with others
                Truancy from school

         Z72.811   **Adult antisocial behavior**   A
                Adult antisocial behavior without manifest
                    psychiatric disorder

     ✓6ᵗʰ   Z72.82   **Problems related to sleep**

         Z72.82Ø   **Sleep** deprivation
                Lack of adequate sleep
                EXCLUDES 1   insomnia (G47.Ø-)

         Z72.821   **Inadequate sleep hygiene**
                Bad sleep habits
                Irregular sleep habits
                Unhealthy sleep wake schedule
                EXCLUDES 1   insomnia (F51.Ø-, G47.Ø-)

     Z72.89   **Other problems related to lifestyle**
         Self-damaging behavior

   Z72.9   **Problem related to lifestyle, unspecified**

✓4ᵗʰ   **Z73**   **Problems related to life management difficulty**
      EXCLUDES 2   problems related to socioeconomic and psychosocial
                circumstances (Z55-Z65)

   Z73.Ø   **Burn-out**

   Z73.1   **Type A behavior pattern**

   Z73.2   **Lack of relaxation and leisure**

   Z73.3   **Stress, not elsewhere classified**
         Physical and mental strain NOS
      EXCLUDES 1   stress related to employment or unemployment (Z56.-)

   Z73.4   **Inadequate social skills, not elsewhere classified**

   Z73.5   **Social role conflict, not elsewhere classified**

   Z73.6   **Limitation of activities due to disability**
      EXCLUDES 1   care-provider dependency (Z74.-)

✓5ᵗʰ   Z73.8   **Other problems related to life management difficulty**

     ✓6ᵗʰ   Z73.81   **Behavioral insomnia of childhood**

         Z73.81Ø   **Behavioral insomnia of childhood,**   P
                sleep-onset association **type**

         Z73.811   **Behavioral insomnia of childhood,**   P
                limit setting **type**

         Z73.812   **Behavioral insomnia of childhood,**   P
                combined **type**

         Z73.819   **Behavioral insomnia of childhood,**   P
                unspecified **type**

     Z73.82   **Dual sensory impairment**

     Z73.89   **Other problems related to life management**
         difficulty

   Z73.9   **Problem related to life management difficulty, unspecified**

✓4ᵗʰ   **Z74**   **Problems related to care provider dependency**
      EXCLUDES 2   dependence on enabling machines or devices NEC (Z99.-)

✓5ᵗʰ   Z74.Ø   **Reduced mobility**

     Z74.Ø1   **Bed confinement status**
         Bedridden

     Z74.Ø9   **Other reduced mobility**
         Chair ridden
         Reduced mobility NOS
         EXCLUDES 2   wheelchair dependence (Z99.3)

   Z74.1   **Need for assistance with** personal care

   Z74.2   **Need for assistance at home and** no other household member able to render care

   Z74.3   **Need for** continuous supervision

   Z74.8   **Other problems related to care provider dependency**

   Z74.9   **Problem related to care provider dependency, unspecified**

✓4ᵗʰ   **Z75**   **Problems related to medical facilities and other health care**

   Z75.Ø   **Medical services** not available in home
      EXCLUDES 1   no other household member able to render care (Z74.2)

   Z75.1   **Person** awaiting admission **to adequate facility elsewhere**

   Z75.2   **Other** waiting period for investigation **and treatment**

   Z75.3   **Unavailability and inaccessibility of** health-care facilities
      EXCLUDES 1   bed unavailable (Z75.1)

   Z75.4   **Unavailability and inaccessibility of other** helping agencies

   Z75.5   Holiday relief care

   Z75.8   **Other problems related to medical facilities and other health care**

   Z75.9   **Unspecified problem related to medical facilities and other health care**

✓4ᵗʰ   **Z76**   **Persons encountering health services in other circumstances**

   Z76.Ø   **Encounter for issue of repeat prescription**
         Encounter for issue of repeat prescription for appliance
         Encounter for issue of repeat prescription for medicaments
         Encounter for issue of repeat prescription for spectacles
      EXCLUDES 2   issue of medical certificate (ZØ2.7)
                repeat prescription for contraceptive (Z3Ø.4-)

   Z76.1   **Encounter for health supervision and care of foundling**   PDx

   Z76.2   **Encounter for health supervision and care of other**   PDx P
         healthy infant and child
         Encounter for medical or nursing care or supervision of healthy
                infant under circumstances such as adverse socioeconomic
                conditions at home
         Encounter for medical or nursing care or supervision of healthy
                infant under circumstances such as awaiting foster or
                adoptive placement
         Encounter for medical or nursing care or supervision of healthy
                infant under circumstances such as maternal illness
         Encounter for medical or nursing care or supervision of healthy
                infant under circumstances such as number of children at
                home preventing or interfering with normal care

   Z76.3   **Healthy person accompanying sick person**

   Z76.4   **Other boarder to healthcare facility**
      EXCLUDES 1   homelessness (Z59.Ø)

   Z76.5   **Malingerer [conscious simulation]**
         Person feigning illness (with obvious motivation)
      EXCLUDES 1   factitious disorder (F68.1-)
                peregrinating patient (F68.1-)

✓5ᵗʰ   Z76.8   **Persons encountering health services in other specified circumstances**

     Z76.81   **Expectant parent(s) prebirth pediatrician visit**
         Pre-adoption pediatrician visit for adoptive parent(s)

     Z76.82   **Awaiting organ transplant status**
         Patient waiting for organ availability

     Z76.89   **Persons encountering health services in other specified circumstances**
         Persons encountering health services NOS
         AHA: 2Ø14, 2Q, 1Ø

Persons with potential health hazards related to family and personal history and certain conditions influencing health status (Z77-Z99)

Code also any follow-up examination (ZØ8-ZØ9)

✓4ᵗʰ   **Z77**   **Other contact with and (suspected) exposures hazardous to health**
      INCLUDES   contact with and (suspected) exposures to potential hazards
                to health
      EXCLUDES 2   contact with and (suspected) exposure to communicable
                diseases (Z2Ø.-)
                exposure to (parental) (environmental) tobacco smoke in the
                   perinatal period (P96.81)
                newborn (suspected to be) affected by noxious substances
                   transmitted via placenta or breast milk (PØ4.-)
                occupational exposure to risk factors (Z57.-)
                retained foreign body (Z18.-)
                retained foreign body fully removed (Z87.821)
                toxic effects of substances chiefly nonmedicinal as to source
                   (T51-T65)

✓5ᵗʰ   Z77.Ø   **Contact with and (suspected) exposure to** hazardous, chiefly nonmedicinal, chemicals

     ✓6ᵗʰ   Z77.Ø1   **Contact with and (suspected) exposure to hazardous** metals

         Z77.Ø1Ø   **Contact with and (suspected) exposure to** arsenic

---

EXCLUDES 1 Not coded here   *EXCLUDES 2* Not included here   PDx Primary Diagnosis Only   N Newborn Age: Ø   P Pediatric Age: Ø-17   M Maternity Age: 12-55   A Adult Age: 15-124

1Ø72   ICD-1Ø-CM Draft (2Ø15)

Z77.011 **Contact with and (suspected) exposure to** lead

Z77.012 **Contact with and (suspected) exposure to** uranium
EXCLUDES 1 *retained depleted uranium fragments (Z18.01)*

Z77.018 **Contact with and (suspected) exposure to other hazardous metals**
Contact with and (suspected) exposure to chromium compounds
Contact with and (suspected) exposure to nickel dust

✓6th Z77.02 **Contact with and (suspected) exposure to hazardous** aromatic compounds

Z77.020 **Contact with and (suspected) exposure to** aromatic amines

Z77.021 **Contact with and (suspected) exposure to** benzene

Z77.028 **Contact with and (suspected) exposure to other hazardous aromatic compounds**
Aromatic dyes NOS
Polycyclic aromatic hydrocarbons

✓6th Z77.09 **Contact with and (suspected) exposure to other hazardous, chiefly** nonmedicinal, chemicals

Z77.090 **Contact with and (suspected) exposure to** asbestos

Z77.098 **Contact with and (suspected) exposure to other hazardous, chiefly nonmedicinal, chemicals**
Dyes NOS

✓5th Z77.1 **Contact with and (suspected) exposure to environmental pollution and** hazards in the physical environment

✓6th Z77.11 **Contact with and (suspected) exposure to** environmental pollution

Z77.110 **Contact with and (suspected) exposure to** air pollution

Z77.111 **Contact with and (suspected) exposure to** water pollution

Z77.112 **Contact with and (suspected) exposure to** soil pollution

Z77.118 **Contact with and (suspected) exposure to other environmental pollution**

✓6th Z77.12 **Contact with and (suspected) exposure to hazards in the physical environment**

Z77.120 **Contact with and (suspected) exposure to** mold **(toxic)**

Z77.121 **Contact with and (suspected) exposure to** harmful algae and algae toxins
Contact with and (suspected) exposure to (harmful) algae bloom NOS
Contact with and (suspected) exposure to blue-green algae bloom
Contact with and (suspected) exposure to brown tide
Contact with and (suspected) exposure to cyanobacteria bloom
Contact with and (suspected) exposure to Florida red tide
Contact with and (suspected) exposure to pfiesteria piscicida
Contact with and (suspected) exposure to red tide

Z77.122 **Contact with and (suspected) exposure to** noise

Z77.123 **Contact with and (suspected) exposure to** radon and other naturally occuring radiation
EXCLUDES 2 *radiation exposure as the cause of a confirmed condition (W88-W90, X39.0-)*
radiation sickness NOS (T66)

Z77.128 **Contact with and (suspected) exposure to other hazards in the physical environment**

✓5th Z77.2 **Contact with and (suspected) exposure to** other **hazardous substances**

Z77.21 **Contact with and (suspected) exposure to potentially hazardous** body fluids

Z77.22 **Contact with and (suspected) exposure to** environmental tobacco smoke **(acute) (chronic)**
Exposure to second hand tobacco smoke (acute) (chronic)
Passive smoking (acute) (chronic)
EXCLUDES 1 *nicotine dependence (F17.-)*
tobacco use (Z72.0)
EXCLUDES 2 *occupational exposure to environmental tobacco smoke (Z57.31)*

Z77.29 **Contact with and (suspected) exposure to other hazardous substances**

Z77.9 **Other contact with and (suspected) exposures hazardous to health**

✓4th **Z78 Other specified health status**
EXCLUDES 2 *asymptomatic human immunodeficiency virus [HIV] infection status (Z21)*
postprocedural status (Z93- Z99)
sex reassignment status (Z87.890)

Z78.0 **Asymptomatic menopausal state** Ⓐ♀
Menopausal state NOS
Postmenopausal status NOS
EXCLUDES 2 *symptomatic menopausal state (N95.1)*

Z78.1 **Physical restraint status**
EXCLUDES 1 *physical restraint due to a procedure - omit code*

Z78.9 **Other specified health status**

✓4th **Z79 Long term (current) drug therapy**
INCLUDES long term (current) drug use for prophylactic purposes
Code also any therapeutic drug level monitoring (Z51.81)
EXCLUDES 2 *drug abuse and dependence (F11-F19)*
drug use complicating pregnancy, childbirth, and the puerperium (O99.32-)

✓5th Z79.0 **Long term (current) use of anticoagulants and antithrombotics/antiplatelets**
EXCLUDES 2 *long term (current) use of aspirin (Z79.82)*

Z79.01 **Long term (current) use of** anticoagulants

Z79.02 **Long term (current) use of** antithrombotics/antiplatelets

Z79.1 **Long term (current) use of** non-steroidal anti-inflammatories **(NSAID)**
EXCLUDES 2 *long term (current) use of aspirin (Z79.82)*

Z79.2 **Long term (current) use of** antibiotics

Z79.3 **Long term (current) use of** hormonal contraceptives
Long term (current) use of birth control pill or patch

Z79.4 **Long term (current) use of** insulin

✓5th Z79.5 **Long term (current) use of** steroids

Z79.51 **Long term (current) use of** inhaled steroids

Z79.52 **Long term (current) use of** systemic steroids

✓5th Z79.8 **Other long term (current) drug therapy**

✓6th Z79.81 **Long term (current) use of agents affecting estrogen receptors and estrogen levels**
Code first, if applicable:
malignant neoplasm of breast (C50.-)
malignant neoplasm of prostate (C61)
Use additional code, if applicable, to identify:
estrogen receptor positive status (Z17.0)
family history of breast cancer (Z80.3)
genetic susceptibility to malignant neoplasm (cancer) (Z15.0-)
personal history of breast cancer (Z85.3)
personal history of prostate cancer (Z85.46)
postmenopausal status (Z78.0)
EXCLUDES 1 *hormone replacement therapy (postmenopausal) (Z79.890)*

Z79.810 **Long term (current) use of selective** estrogen receptor modulators **(SERMs)**
Long term (current) use of raloxifene (Evista)
Long term (current) use of tamoxifen (Nolvadex)
Long term (current) use of toremifene (Fareston)

Z79.811 **Long term (current) use of** aromatase inhibitors
Long term (current) use of anastrozole (Arimidex)
Long term (current) use of exemestane (Aromasin)
Long term (current) use of letrozole (Femara)

Factors Influencing Health Status and Contact With Health Services

Z79.818–Z83.6

Z79.818   **Long term (current) use of other agents affecting estrogen receptors and estrogen levels**
Long term (current) use of estrogen receptor downregulators
Long term (current) use of fulvestrant (Faslodex)
Long term (current) use of gonadotropin-releasing hormone (GnRH) agonist
Long term (current) use of goserelin acetate (Zoladex)
Long term (current) use of leuprolide acetate (leuprorelin) (Lupron)
Long term (current) use of megestrol acetate (Megace)

Z79.82   **Long term (current) use of aspirin**

Z79.83   **Long term (current) use of bisphosphonates**

✓6ᵗʰ **Z79.89**   **Other long term (current) drug therapy**

    Z79.890   Hormone replacement therapy (postmenopausal)   ♀

    Z79.891   **Long term (current) use of opiate analgesic**
Long term (current) use of methadone for pain management
EXCLUDES 1   methadone use NOS (F11.2-)
use of methadone for treatment of heroin addiction (F11.2-)

    Z79.899   **Other long term (current) drug therapy**

✓4ᵗʰ **Z80**   **Family history of primary malignant neoplasm**

Z80.0   **Family history of malignant neoplasm of digestive organs**
Conditions classifiable to C15-C26

Z80.1   **Family history of malignant neoplasm of trachea, bronchus and lung**
Conditions classifiable to C33-C34

Z80.2   **Family history of malignant neoplasm of other respiratory and intrathoracic organs**
Conditions classifiable to C30-C32, C37-C39

Z80.3   **Family history of malignant neoplasm of breast**
Conditions classifiable to C50-

✓5ᵗʰ **Z80.4**   **Family history of malignant neoplasm of genital organs**
Conditions classifiable to C51-C63

    Z80.41   **Family history of malignant neoplasm of ovary**   ♀

    Z80.42   **Family history of malignant neoplasm of prostate**   ♂

    Z80.43   **Family history of malignant neoplasm of testis**   ♂

    Z80.49   **Family history of malignant neoplasm of other genital organs**

✓5ᵗʰ **Z80.5**   **Family history of malignant neoplasm of urinary tract**
Conditions classifiable to C64-C68

    Z80.51   **Family history of malignant neoplasm of kidney**

    Z80.52   **Family history of malignant neoplasm of bladder**

    Z80.59   **Family history of malignant neoplasm of other urinary tract organ**

Z80.6   **Family history of leukemia**
Conditions classifiable to C91-C95

Z80.7   **Family history of other malignant neoplasms of lymphoid, hematopoietic and related tissues**
Conditions classifiable to C81-C90, C96-

Z80.8   **Family history of malignant neoplasm of other organs or systems**
Conditions classifiable to C00-C14, C40-C49, C69-C79

Z80.9   **Family history of malignant neoplasm, unspecified**
Conditions classifiable to C80.1

✓4ᵗʰ **Z81**   **Family history of mental and behavioral disorders**

Z81.0   **Family history of intellectual disabilities**
Conditions classifiable to F70-F79

Z81.1   **Family history of alcohol abuse and dependence**
Conditions classifiable to F10-

Z81.2   **Family history of tobacco abuse and dependence**
Conditions classifiable to F17-

Z81.3   **Family history of other psychoactive substance abuse and dependence**
Conditions classifiable to F11-F16, F18-F19

Z81.4   **Family history of other substance abuse and dependence**
Conditions classifiable to F55

Z81.8   **Family history of other mental and behavioral disorders**
Conditions classifiable elsewhere in F01-F99

✓4ᵗʰ **Z82**   **Family history of certain disabilities and chronic diseases (leading to disablement)**

Z82.0   **Family history of epilepsy and other diseases of the nervous system**
Conditions classifiable to G00-G99

Z82.1   **Family history of blindness and visual loss**
Conditions classifiable to H54-

Z82.2   **Family history of deafness and hearing loss**
Conditions classifiable to H90-H91

Z82.3   **Family history of stroke**
Conditions classifiable to I60-I64

✓5ᵗʰ **Z82.4**   **Family history of ischemic heart disease and other diseases of the circulatory system**
Conditions classifiable to I00-I52, I65-I99

    Z82.41   **Family history of sudden cardiac death**

    Z82.49   **Family history of ischemic heart disease and other diseases of the circulatory system**

Z82.5   **Family history of asthma and other chronic lower respiratory diseases**
Conditions classifiable to J40-J47
EXCLUDES 2   family history of other diseases of the respiratory system (Z83.6)

✓5ᵗʰ **Z82.6**   **Family history of arthritis and other diseases of the musculoskeletal system and connective tissue**
Conditions classifiable to M00-M99

    Z82.61   **Family history of arthritis**

    Z82.62   **Family history of osteoporosis**

    Z82.69   **Family history of other diseases of the musculoskeletal system and connective tissue**

✓5ᵗʰ **Z82.7**   **Family history of congenital malformations, deformations and chromosomal abnormalities**
Conditions classifiable to Q00-Q99

    Z82.71   **Family history of polycystic kidney**

    Z82.79   **Family history of other congenital malformations, deformations and chromosomal abnormalities**

Z82.8   **Family history of other disabilities and chronic diseases leading to disablement, not elsewhere classified**

✓4ᵗʰ **Z83**   **Family history of other specific disorders**
EXCLUDES 2   contact with and (suspected) exposure to communicable disease in the family (Z20.-)

Z83.0   **Family history of human immunodeficiency virus [HIV] disease**
Conditions classifiable to B20

Z83.1   **Family history of other infectious and parasitic diseases**
Conditions classifiable to A00-B19, B25-B94, B99

Z83.2   **Family history of diseases of the blood and blood-forming organs and certain disorders involving the immune mechanism**
Conditions classifiable to D50-D89

Z83.3   **Family history of diabetes mellitus**
Conditions classifiable to E08-E13

✓5ᵗʰ **Z83.4**   **Family history of other endocrine, nutritional and metabolic diseases**
Conditions classifiable to E00-E07, E15-E88

    Z83.41   **Family history of multiple endocrine neoplasia [MEN] syndrome**

    Z83.49   **Family history of other endocrine, nutritional and metabolic diseases**

✓5ᵗʰ **Z83.5**   **Family history of eye and ear disorders**

    ✓6ᵗʰ **Z83.51**   **Family history of eye disorders**
Conditions classifiable to H00-H53, H55-H59
EXCLUDES 2   family history of blindness and visual loss (Z82.1)

      Z83.511   **Family history of glaucoma**

      Z83.518   **Family history of other specified eye disorder**

    Z83.52   **Family history of ear disorders**
Conditions classifiable to H60-H83, H92-H95
EXCLUDES 2   family history of deafness and hearing loss (Z82.2)

Z83.6   **Family history of other diseases of the respiratory system**
Conditions classifiable to J00-J39, J60-J99
EXCLUDES 2   family history of asthma and other chronic lower respiratory diseases (Z82.5)

EXCLUDES 1 Not coded here   *EXCLUDES 2* Not included here   *PDx* Primary Diagnosis Only   N Newborn Age: 0   P Pediatric Age: 0-17   M Maternity Age: 12-55   A Adult Age: 15-124

1074   ICD-10-CM Draft (2015)

✓5ᵗʰ **Z83.7 Family history of diseases of the digestive system**
Conditions classifiable to K00-K93

    Z83.71 Family history of colonic polyps
        EXCLUDES 1   *family history of malignant neoplasm of digestive organs (Z80.0)*

    Z83.79 Family history of other diseases of the digestive system

✓4ᵗʰ **Z84 Family history of other conditions**

    Z84.0 Family history of diseases of the skin and subcutaneous tissue
        Conditions classifiable to L00-L99

    Z84.1 Family history of disorders of kidney and ureter
        Conditions classifiable to N00-N29

    Z84.2 Family history of other diseases of the genitourinary system
        Conditions classifiable to N30-N99

    Z84.3 Family history of consanguinity

✓5ᵗʰ **Z84.8 Family history of other specified conditions**

    Z84.81 Family history of carrier of genetic disease

    Z84.89 Family history of other specified conditions

✓4ᵗʰ **Z85 Personal history of malignant neoplasm**
Code first any follow-up examination after treatment of malignant neoplasm (Z08)
Use additional code to identify:
    alcohol use and dependence (F10.-)
    exposure to environmental tobacco smoke (Z77.22)
    history of tobacco use (Z87.891)
    occupational exposure to environmental tobacco smoke (Z57.31)
    tobacco dependence (F17.-)
    tobacco use (Z72.0)
    EXCLUDES 2 *personal history of benign neoplasm (Z86.01-)*
                 personal history of carcinoma-in-situ (Z86.00-)

✓5ᵗʰ **Z85.0 Personal history of malignant neoplasm of** digestive organs

    Z85.00 Personal history of malignant neoplasm of unspecified digestive organ

    Z85.01 Personal history of malignant neoplasm of esophagus
        Conditions classifiable to C15

✓6ᵗʰ   **Z85.02 Personal history of malignant neoplasm of** stomach

      Z85.020 Personal history of malignant carcinoid **tumor of stomach**
          Conditions classifiable to C7A.092

      Z85.028 Personal history of other malignant neoplasm of stomach
          Conditions classifiable to C16

✓6ᵗʰ   **Z85.03 Personal history of malignant neoplasm of** large intestine

      Z85.030 Personal history of malignant carcinoid **tumor of large intestine**
          Conditions classifiable to C7A.022-C7A.025, C7A.029

      Z85.038 Personal history of other malignant neoplasm of large intestine
          Conditions classifiable to C18

✓6ᵗʰ   **Z85.04 Personal history of malignant neoplasm of** rectum, rectosigmoid junction, and anus

      Z85.040 Personal history of malignant carcinoid **tumor of rectum**
          Conditions classifiable to C7A.026

      Z85.048 Personal history of other malignant neoplasm of rectum, rectosigmoid junction, and anus
          Conditions classifiable to C19-C21

    Z85.05 Personal history of malignant neoplasm of liver
        Conditions classifiable to C22

✓6ᵗʰ   **Z85.06 Personal history of malignant neoplasm of** small intestine

      Z85.060 Personal history of malignant carcinoid **tumor of small intestine**
          Conditions classifiable to C7A.01-

      Z85.068 Personal history of other malignant neoplasm of small intestine
          Conditions classifiable to C17

    Z85.07 Personal history of malignant neoplasm of pancreas
        Conditions classifiable to C25

    Z85.09 Personal history of malignant neoplasm of other digestive organs

✓5ᵗʰ **Z85.1 Personal history of malignant neoplasm of** trachea, bronchus and lung

✓6ᵗʰ   **Z85.11 Personal history of malignant neoplasm of** bronchus and lung

      Z85.110 Personal history of malignant carcinoid **tumor of bronchus and lung**
          Conditions classifiable to C7A.090

      Z85.118 Personal history of other malignant neoplasm of bronchus and lung
          Conditions classifiable to C34

    Z85.12 Personal history of malignant neoplasm of trachea
        Conditions classifiable to C33

✓5ᵗʰ **Z85.2 Personal history of malignant neoplasm of other** respiratory and intrathoracic organs

    Z85.20 Personal history of malignant neoplasm of unspecified respiratory organ

    Z85.21 Personal history of malignant neoplasm of larynx
        Conditions classifiable to C32

    Z85.22 Personal history of malignant neoplasm of nasal cavities, middle ear, and accessory sinuses
        Conditions classifiable to C30-C31

✓6ᵗʰ   **Z85.23 Personal history of malignant neoplasm of** thymus

      Z85.230 Personal history of malignant carcinoid **tumor of thymus**
          Conditions classifiable to C7A.091

      Z85.238 Personal history of other malignant neoplasm of thymus
          Conditions classifiable to C37

    Z85.29 Personal history of malignant neoplasm of other respiratory and intrathoracic organs

    Z85.3 Personal history of malignant neoplasm of breast
        Conditions classifiable to C50-

✓5ᵗʰ **Z85.4 Personal history of malignant neoplasm of** genital organs
        Conditions classifiable to C51-C63

    Z85.40 Personal history of malignant neoplasm of unspecified female **genital organ** ♀

    Z85.41 Personal history of malignant neoplasm of cervix uteri ♀

    Z85.42 Personal history of malignant neoplasm of other parts of uterus ♀

    Z85.43 Personal history of malignant neoplasm of ovary ♀

    Z85.44 Personal history of malignant neoplasm of other female genital organs ♀

    Z85.45 Personal history of malignant neoplasm of unspecified male **genital organ** ♂

    Z85.46 Personal history of malignant neoplasm of prostate ♂

    Z85.47 Personal history of malignant neoplasm of testis ♂

    Z85.48 Personal history of malignant neoplasm of epididymis ♂

    Z85.49 Personal history of malignant neoplasm of other male **genital organs** ♂

✓5ᵗʰ **Z85.5 Personal history of malignant neoplasm of** urinary tract
        Conditions classifiable to C64-C68

    Z85.50 Personal history of malignant neoplasm of unspecified urinary tract organ

    Z85.51 Personal history of malignant neoplasm of bladder

✓6ᵗʰ   **Z85.52 Personal history of malignant neoplasm of** kidney
        EXCLUDES 1 *personal history of malignant neoplasm of renal pelvis (Z85.53)*

      Z85.520 Personal history of malignant carcinoid **tumor of kidney**
          Conditions classifiable to C7A.093

      Z85.528 Personal history of other malignant neoplasm of kidney
          Conditions classifiable to C64

    Z85.53 Personal history of malignant neoplasm of renal pelvis

    Z85.54 Personal history of malignant neoplasm of ureter

    Z85.59 Personal history of malignant neoplasm of other urinary tract organ

    Z85.6 Personal history of leukemia
        Conditions classifiable to C91-C95
        EXCLUDES 1 *leukemia in remission C91.0-C95.9 with 5th character 1*

✓ Additional Character Required   ✓x7ᵗʰ Xtension Alert   Unspecified Dx   Other Specified Dx   Manifestation   ▶◀ Revised Text   ● New Code   ▲ Revised Code Title

√5th **Z85.7** **Personal history of other malignant neoplasms of lymphoid, hematopoietic and related tissues**

     Z85.71 **Personal history of** Hodgkin lymphoma
         Conditions classifiable to C81

     Z85.72 **Personal history of** non-Hodgkin lymphomas
         Conditions classifiable to C82-C85

     Z85.79 **Personal history of other malignant neoplasms of lymphoid, hematopoietic and related tissues**
         Conditions classifiable to C88-C9Ø, C96
         EXCLUDES 1   multiple myeloma in remission (C9Ø.Ø1)
                 plasma cell leukemia in remission (C9Ø.11)
                 plasmacytoma in remission (C9Ø.21)

√5th **Z85.8** **Personal history of malignant neoplasms of other organs and systems**
     Conditions classifiable to CØØ-C14, C4Ø-C49, C69-C79, C7A.Ø98

√6th **Z85.81** **Personal history of malignant neoplasm of** lip, oral cavity, and pharynx

     Z85.81Ø **Personal history of malignant neoplasm of** tongue

     Z85.818 **Personal history of malignant neoplasm of other sites of** lip, oral cavity, and pharynx

     Z85.819 **Personal history of malignant neoplasm of unspecified site of** lip, oral cavity, and pharynx

√6th **Z85.82** **Personal history of malignant neoplasm of** skin

     Z85.82Ø **Personal history of malignant** melanoma **of skin**
         Conditions classifiable to C43

     Z85.821 **Personal history of** Merkel cell carcinoma
         Conditions classifiable to C4A

     Z85.828 **Personal history of other malignant neoplasm of skin**
         Conditions classifiable to C44

√6th **Z85.83** **Personal history of malignant neoplasm of** bone and soft tissue

     Z85.83Ø **Personal history of malignant neoplasm of bone**

     Z85.831 **Personal history of malignant neoplasm of soft tissue**
         EXCLUDES 2   personal history of malignant neoplasm of skin (Z85.82-)

√6th **Z85.84** **Personal history of malignant neoplasm of** eye and nervous tissue

     Z85.84Ø **Personal history of malignant neoplasm of eye**

     Z85.841 **Personal history of malignant neoplasm of brain**

     Z85.848 **Personal history of malignant neoplasm of other parts of nervous tissue**

√6th **Z85.85** **Personal history of malignant neoplasm of** endocrine glands

     Z85.85Ø **Personal history of malignant neoplasm of thyroid**

     Z85.858 **Personal history of malignant neoplasm of other endocrine glands**

     Z85.89 **Personal history of malignant neoplasm of other organs and systems**

     Z85.9 **Personal history of malignant neoplasm, unspecified**
     Conditions classifiable to C7A.ØØ, C8Ø.1

√4th **Z86** **Personal history of certain other diseases**
     Code first any follow-up examination after treatment (ZØ9)

√5th **Z86.Ø** **Personal history of in-situ and benign neoplasms and neoplasms of uncertain behavior**
     EXCLUDES 2   personal history of malignant neoplasms (Z85.-)

√6th **Z86.ØØ** **Personal history of** in-situ neoplasm

     Z86.ØØØ **Personal history of in-situ neoplasm of** breast

     Z86.ØØ1 **Personal history of in-situ neoplasm of** cervix uteri ♀

     Z86.ØØ8 **Personal history of in-situ neoplasm of other site**

√6th **Z86.Ø1** **Personal history of** benign neoplasm

     Z86.Ø1Ø **Personal history of** colonic polyps

     Z86.Ø11 **Personal history of benign neoplasm of the** brain

     Z86.Ø12 **Personal history of benign** carcinoid tumor

     Z86.Ø18 **Personal history of other benign neoplasm**

     Z86.Ø3 **Personal history of** neoplasm of uncertain behavior

√5th **Z86.1** **Personal history of** infectious and parasitic diseases
     Conditions classifiable to AØØ-B89, B99
     EXCLUDES 1   personal history of infectious diseases specific to a body system
                 sequelae of infectious and parasitic diseases (B9Ø-B94)

     Z86.11 **Personal history of** tuberculosis

     Z86.12 **Personal history of** poliomyelitis

     Z86.13 **Personal history of** malaria

     Z86.14 **Personal history of** Methicillin resistant Staphylococcus aureus **infection**
         Personal history of MRSA infection

     Z86.19 **Personal history of other infectious and parasitic diseases**

     Z86.2 **Personal history of diseases of the** blood and blood-forming organs **and certain disorders involving the** immune mechanism
     Conditions classifiable to D5Ø-D89

√5th **Z86.3** **Personal history of** endocrine, nutritional and metabolic diseases
     Conditions classifiable to EØØ-E88

     Z86.31 **Personal history of** diabetic foot ulcer
         EXCLUDES 2   current diabetic foot ulcer (EØ8.621, EØ9.621, E1Ø.621, E11.621, E13.621)

     Z86.32 **Personal history of** gestational diabetes ♀
         Personal history of conditions classifiable to O24.4-
         EXCLUDES 1   gestational diabetes mellitus in current pregnancy (O24.4-)

     Z86.39 **Personal history of other endocrine, nutritional and metabolic disease**

√5th **Z86.5** **Personal history of** mental and behavioral disorders
     Conditions classifiable to F4Ø-F59

     Z86.51 **Personal history of** combat and operational stress reaction A

     Z86.59 **Personal history of other mental and behavioral disorders**

√5th **Z86.6** **Personal history of diseases of the** nervous system and sense organs
     Conditions classifiable to GØØ-G99, HØØ-H95
     EXCLUDES 2   personal history of anaphylactic shock (Z87.892)

     Z86.61 **Personal history of** infections of the central nervous system
         Personal history of encephalitis
         Personal history of meningitis

     Z86.69 **Personal history of other diseases of the nervous system and sense organs**

√5th **Z86.7** **Personal history of diseases of the** circulatory system
     Conditions classifiable to IØØ-I99
     EXCLUDES 2   old myocardial infarction (I25.2)
                 personal history of anaphylactic shock (Z87.892)
                 postmyocardial infarction syndrome (I24.1)

√6th **Z86.71** **Personal history of** venous thrombosis and embolism

     Z86.711 **Personal history of** pulmonary embolism

     Z86.718 **Personal history of other venous thrombosis and embolism**

     Z86.72 **Personal history of** thrombophlebitis

     Z86.73 **Personal history of** transient ischemic attack **(TIA), and cerebral infarction without residual deficits**
         Personal history of prolonged reversible ischemic neurological deficit (PRIND)
         Personal history of stroke NOS without residual deficits
         EXCLUDES 1   personal history of traumatic brain injury (Z87.82Ø)
                 sequelae of cerebrovascular disease (I69.-)
         AHA: 2Ø12, 4Q, 92

     Z86.74 **Personal history of** sudden cardiac arrest
         Personal history of sudden cardiac death successfully resuscitated

     Z86.79 **Personal history of other diseases of the circulatory system**

√4th **Z87** **Personal history of other diseases and conditions**
     Code first any follow-up examination after treatment (ZØ9)

√5th **Z87.Ø** **Personal history of diseases of the** respiratory system
     Conditions classifiable to JØØ-J99

EXCLUDES 1 Not coded here   EXCLUDES 2 Not included here   PDx Primary Diagnosis Only   N Newborn Age: Ø   P Pediatric Age: Ø-17   M Maternity Age: 12-55   A Adult Age: 15-124

1Ø76   ICD-1Ø-CM Draft (2Ø15)

Z87.01 **Personal history of** pneumonia **(recurrent)**

Z87.09 **Personal history of other diseases of the respiratory system**

✓5th Z87.1 **Personal history of diseases of the** digestive system
Conditions classifiable to K00-K93

Z87.11 **Personal history of** peptic ulcer **disease**

Z87.19 **Personal history of other diseases of the digestive system**

Z87.2 **Personal history of diseases of the** skin and subcutaneous tissue
Conditions classifiable to L00-L99
EXCLUDES 2 *personal history of diabetic foot ulcer (Z86.31)*

✓5th Z87.3 **Personal history of diseases of the** musculoskeletal system and connective tissue
Conditions classifiable to M00-M99
EXCLUDES 2 *personal history of (healed) traumatic fracture (Z87.81)*

✓6th Z87.31 **Personal history of (healed)** nontraumatic fracture

Z87.310 **Personal history of (healed)** osteoporosis **fracture**
Personal history of (healed) fragility fracture
Personal history of (healed) collapsed vertebra due to osteoporosis

Z87.311 **Personal history of (healed) other pathological fracture**
Personal history of (healed) collapsed vertebra NOS
EXCLUDES 2 *personal history of osteoporosis fracture (Z87.310)*

Z87.312 **Personal history of (healed)** stress **fracture**
Personal history of (healed) fatigue fracture

Z87.39 **Personal history of other diseases of the musculoskeletal system and connective tissue**

✓5th Z87.4 **Personal history of diseases of** genitourinary system
Conditions classifiable to N00-N99

✓6th Z87.41 **Personal history of** dysplasia of the female genital tract
EXCLUDES 1 *personal history of malignant neoplasm of female genital tract (Z85.40-Z85.44)*

Z87.410 **Personal history of** cervical **dysplasia** ♀
Z87.411 **Personal history of** vaginal **dysplasia** ♀
Z87.412 **Personal history of** vulvar **dysplasia** ♀

Z87.42 **Personal history of other diseases of the** female **genital tract** ♀

✓6th Z87.43 **Personal history of diseases of the** male genital organs

Z87.430 **Personal history of** prostatic dysplasia
EXCLUDES 1 *personal history of malignant neoplasm of prostate (Z85.46)*

Z87.438 **Personal history of other diseases of** male **genital organs**

✓6th Z87.44 **Personal history of diseases of the** urinary system
EXCLUDES 1 *personal history of malignant neoplasm of cervix uteri (Z85.41)*

Z87.440 **Personal history of urinary (tract) infections**

Z87.441 **Personal history of** nephrotic syndrome

Z87.442 **Personal history of urinary** calculi
Personal history of kidney stones

Z87.448 **Personal history of other diseases of urinary system**

✓5th Z87.5 **Personal history of complications of** pregnancy, childbirth and the puerperium
Conditions classifiable to O00-O9A
EXCLUDES 2 *recurrent pregnancy loss (N96)*

Z87.51 **Personal history of** pre-term labor ♀
EXCLUDES 1 *current pregnancy with history of pre-term labor (O09.21-)*

Z87.59 **Personal history of other** complications of **pregnancy, childbirth and the puerperium** ♀
Personal history of trophoblastic disease

✓5th Z87.7 **Personal history of (corrected)** congenital malformations
Conditions classifiable to Q00-Q89 that have been repaired or corrected
EXCLUDES 1 *congenital malformations that have been partially corrected or repaired but which still require medical treatment—code to condition*
EXCLUDES 2 *other postprocedural states (Z98.-)*
personal history of medical treatment (Z92.-)
presence of cardiac and vascular implants and grafts (Z95.-)
presence of other devices (Z97.-)
presence of other functional implants (Z96.-)
transplanted organ and tissue status (Z94.-)

✓6th Z87.71 **Personal history of (corrected) congenital malformations of** genitourinary system

Z87.710 **Personal history of (corrected)** ♂ **hypospadias**

Z87.718 **Personal history of other specified (corrected) congenital malformations of genitourinary system**

✓6th Z87.72 **Personal history of (corrected) congenital malformations of** nervous system and sense organs

Z87.720 **Personal history of (corrected) congenital malformations of** eye

Z87.721 **Personal history of (corrected) congenital malformations of** ear

Z87.728 **Personal history of other specified (corrected) congenital malformations of nervous system and sense organs**

✓6th Z87.73 **Personal history of (corrected) congenital malformations of** digestive system

Z87.730 **Personal history of (corrected)** cleft lip and palate

Z87.738 **Personal history of other specified (corrected) congenital malformations of digestive system**

Z87.74 **Personal history of (corrected) congenital malformations of** heart and circulatory system

Z87.75 **Personal history of (corrected) congenital malformations of** respiratory system

Z87.76 **Personal history of (corrected) congenital malformations of** integument, limbs and musculoskeletal system

✓6th Z87.79 **Personal history of** other **(corrected) congenital malformations**

Z87.790 **Personal history of (corrected) congenital malformations of** face and neck

Z87.798 **Personal history of other (corrected) congenital malformations**

✓5th Z87.8 **Personal history of other specified conditions**
EXCLUDES 2 *personal history of self harm (Z91.5)*

Z87.81 **Personal history of (healed)** traumatic fracture
EXCLUDES 2 *personal history of (healed) nontraumatic fracture (Z87.31-)*

✓6th Z87.82 **Personal history of other (healed)** physical injury and trauma
Conditions classifiable to S00-T88, except traumatic fractures

Z87.820 **Personal history of traumatic** brain injury
EXCLUDES 1 *personal history of transient ischemic attack (TIA), and cerebral infarction without residual deficits (Z86.73)*

Z87.821 **Personal history of** retained foreign body fully removed

Z87.828 **Personal history of other (healed) physical injury and trauma**

✓6th Z87.89 **Personal history of** other specified conditions

Z87.890 **Personal history of** sex reassignment

Z87.891 **Personal history of** nicotine dependence
EXCLUDES 1 *current nicotine dependence (F17.2-)*

Z87.892 **Personal history of** anaphylaxis
Code also allergy status such as:
allergy status to drugs, medicaments and biological substances (Z88.-)
allergy status, other than to drugs and biological substances (Z91.0-)

Factors Influencing Health Status and Contact With Health Services

Z87.898–Z90.3

Z87.898 **Personal history of other specified conditions**
    AHA: 2013, 1Q, 21

✓4th **Z88 Allergy status to drugs, medicaments and biological substances**
    EXCLUDES 2   *allergy status, other than to drugs and biological substances (Z91.0-)*

Z88.0 **Allergy status to** penicillin

Z88.1 **Allergy status to other** antibiotic **agents status**

Z88.2 **Allergy status to** sulfonamides **status**

Z88.3 **Allergy status to other** anti-infective **agents status**

Z88.4 **Allergy status to** anesthetic **agent status**

Z88.5 **Allergy status to** narcotic **agent status**

Z88.6 **Allergy status to** analgesic **agent status**

Z88.7 **Allergy status to** serum and vaccine **status**

Z88.8 **Allergy status to other drugs, medicaments and biological substances status**

Z88.9 **Allergy status to unspecified drugs, medicaments and biological substances status**

✓4th **Z89 Acquired absence of limb**
    INCLUDES   amputation status
           postprocedural loss of limb
           post-traumatic loss of limb
    EXCLUDES 1   *acquired deformities of limbs (M20-M21)*
           congenital absence of limbs (Q71-Q73)

✓5th Z89.0 **Acquired absence of** thumb and other finger(s)

✓6th Z89.01 **Acquired absence of** thumb

Z89.011 **Acquired absence of** right **thumb**

Z89.012 **Acquired absence of** left **thumb**

Z89.019 **Acquired absence of unspecified thumb**

✓6th Z89.02 **Acquired absence of** other finger(s)
    EXCLUDES 2   *acquired absence of thumb (Z89.01-)*

Z89.021 **Acquired absence of** right **finger(s)**

Z89.022 **Acquired absence of** left **finger(s)**

Z89.029 **Acquired absence of unspecified finger(s)**

✓5th Z89.1 **Acquired absence of** hand and wrist

✓6th Z89.11 **Acquired absence of** hand

Z89.111 **Acquired absence of** right **hand**

Z89.112 **Acquired absence of** left **hand**

Z89.119 **Acquired absence of unspecified hand**

✓6th Z89.12 **Acquired absence of** wrist
    Disarticulation at wrist

Z89.121 **Acquired absence of** right **wrist**

Z89.122 **Acquired absence of** left **wrist**

Z89.129 **Acquired absence of unspecified wrist**

✓5th Z89.2 **Acquired absence of** upper limb above wrist

✓6th Z89.20 **Acquired absence of** upper limb, unspecified level

Z89.201 **Acquired absence of** right **upper limb, unspecified level**

Z89.202 **Acquired absence of** left **upper limb, unspecified level**

Z89.209 **Acquired absence of unspecified upper limb, unspecified level**
    Acquired absence of arm NOS

✓6th Z89.21 **Acquired absence of** upper limb below elbow

Z89.211 **Acquired absence of** right **upper limb below elbow**

Z89.212 **Acquired absence of** left **upper limb below elbow**

Z89.219 **Acquired absence of unspecified upper limb below elbow**

✓6th Z89.22 **Acquired absence of** upper limb above elbow
    Disarticulation at elbow

Z89.221 **Acquired absence of** right **upper limb above elbow**

Z89.222 **Acquired absence of** left **upper limb above elbow**

Z89.229 **Acquired absence of unspecified upper limb above elbow**

✓6th Z89.23 **Acquired absence of** shoulder
    Acquired absence of shoulder joint following explantation of shoulder joint prosthesis, with or without presence of antibiotic-impregnated cement spacer

Z89.231 **Acquired absence of** right **shoulder**

Z89.232 **Acquired absence of** left **shoulder**

Z89.239 **Acquired absence of unspecified shoulder**

✓5th Z89.4 **Acquired absence of** toe(s), foot, and ankle

✓6th Z89.41 **Acquired absence of** great toe

Z89.411 **Acquired absence of** right **great toe**

Z89.412 **Acquired absence of** left **great toe**

Z89.419 **Acquired absence of unspecified great toe**

✓6th Z89.42 **Acquired absence of** other toe(s)
    EXCLUDES 2   *acquired absence of great toe (Z89.41-)*

Z89.421 **Acquired absence of other** right **toe(s)**

Z89.422 **Acquired absence of other** left **toe(s)**

Z89.429 **Acquired absence of other toe(s), unspecified side**

✓6th Z89.43 **Acquired absence of** foot

Z89.431 **Acquired absence of** right **foot**

Z89.432 **Acquired absence of** left **foot**

Z89.439 **Acquired absence of unspecified foot**

✓6th Z89.44 **Acquired absence of** ankle
    Disarticulation of ankle

Z89.441 **Acquired absence of** right **ankle**

Z89.442 **Acquired absence of** left **ankle**

Z89.449 **Acquired absence of unspecified ankle**

✓5th Z89.5 **Acquired absence of leg below knee**

✓6th Z89.51 **Acquired absence of** leg below knee

Z89.511 **Acquired absence of** right **leg below knee**

Z89.512 **Acquired absence of** left **leg below knee**

Z89.519 **Acquired absence of unspecified leg below knee**

✓6th Z89.52 **Acquired absence of** knee
    Acquired absence of knee joint following explantation of knee joint prosthesis, with or without presence of antibiotic-impregnated cement spacer

Z89.521 **Acquired absence of** right **knee**

Z89.522 **Acquired absence of** left **knee**

Z89.529 **Acquired absence of unspecified knee**

✓5th Z89.6 **Acquired absence of leg above knee**

✓6th Z89.61 **Acquired absence of** leg above knee
    Acquired absence of leg NOS
    Disarticulation at knee

Z89.611 **Acquired absence of** right **leg above knee**

Z89.612 **Acquired absence of** left **leg above knee**

Z89.619 **Acquired absence of unspecified leg above knee**

✓6th Z89.62 **Acquired absence of** hip
    Acquired absence of hip joint following explantation of hip joint prosthesis, with or without presence of antibiotic-impregnated cement spacer
    Disarticulation at hip

Z89.621 **Acquired absence of** right **hip joint**

Z89.622 **Acquired absence of** left **hip joint**

Z89.629 **Acquired absence of unspecified hip joint**

Z89.9 **Acquired absence of limb, unspecified**

✓4th **Z90 Acquired absence of organs, not elsewhere classified**
    INCLUDES   postprocedural or post-traumatic loss of body part NEC
    EXCLUDES 1   *congenital absence—see Alphabetical Index*
    EXCLUDES 2   *postprocedural absence of endocrine glands (E89.-)*

✓5th Z90.0 **Acquired absence of part of** head and neck

Z90.01 **Acquired absence of** eye

Z90.02 **Acquired absence of** larynx

Z90.09 **Acquired absence of other part of head and neck**
    Acquired absence of nose
    EXCLUDES 2   *teeth (K08.1)*

✓5th Z90.1 **Acquired absence of** breast and nipple

Z90.10 **Acquired absence of unspecified breast and nipple**

Z90.11 **Acquired absence of** right **breast and nipple**

Z90.12 **Acquired absence of** left **breast and nipple**

Z90.13 **Acquired absence of** bilateral **breasts and nipples**

Z90.2 **Acquired absence of** lung [part of]

Z90.3 **Acquired absence of** stomach [part of]

EXCLUDES 1 Not coded here   EXCLUDES 2 Not included here   PDx Primary Diagnosis Only   N Newborn Age: 0   P Pediatric Age: 0-17   M Maternity Age: 12-55   A Adult Age: 15-124

1078   ICD-10-CM Draft (2015)

√5ᵗʰ **Z90.4** **Acquired absence of** other **specified parts of digestive tract**

    √6ᵗʰ **Z90.41** **Acquired absence of** pancreas
         Use additional code to identify any associated:
         insulin use (Z79.4)
         diabetes mellitus, postpancreatectomy (E13.-)

         Z90.410 **Acquired** total absence **of pancreas**
             Acquired absence of pancreas NOS

         Z90.411 **Acquired** partial absence **of pancreas**

    Z90.49 **Acquired absence of other specified parts of digestive tract**

Z90.5 **Acquired absence of** kidney

Z90.6 **Acquired absence of other** parts of urinary tract
     Acquired absence of bladder

√5ᵗʰ **Z90.7** **Acquired absence of** genital organ(s)
     EXCLUDES 1   *personal history of sex reassignment (Z87.890)*
     EXCLUDES 2   *female genital mutilation status (N90.81-)*

    √6ᵗʰ **Z90.71** **Acquired absence of** cervix and uterus

         Z90.710 **Acquired absence of** both **cervix and uterus**   ♀
             Acquired absence of uterus NOS
             Status post total hysterectomy

         Z90.711 **Acquired absence of uterus** with remaining cervical stump   ♀
             Status post partial hysterectomy with remaining cervical stump

         Z90.712 **Acquired absence of cervix with remaining uterus**   ♀

    √6ᵗʰ **Z90.72** **Acquired absence of** ovaries

         Z90.721 **Acquired absence of ovaries,** unilateral   ♀

         Z90.722 **Acquired absence of ovaries,** bilateral   ♀

    Z90.79 **Acquired absence of other genital organ(s)**

√5ᵗʰ **Z90.8** **Acquired absence of** other **organs**

    Z90.81 **Acquired absence of** spleen

    Z90.89 **Acquired absence of other organs**

√4ᵗʰ **Z91** **Personal risk factors, not elsewhere classified**
     EXCLUDES 2   *contact with and (suspected) exposures hazardous to health (Z77.-)*
         exposure to pollution and other problems related to physical environment (Z77.1-)
         personal history of physical injury and trauma (Z87.81, Z87.82-)
         occupational exposure to risk factors (Z57.-)

√5ᵗʰ **Z91.0** **Allergy status, other than to drugs and biological substances**
     EXCLUDES 2   *allergy status to drugs, medicaments, and biological substances (Z88.-)*

    √6ᵗʰ **Z91.01** **Food** allergy status
         EXCLUDES 2   *food additives allergy status (Z91.02)*

         Z91.010 **Allergy to** peanuts

         Z91.011 **Allergy to** milk products
             EXCLUDES 1   *lactose intolerance (E73.-)*

         Z91.012 **Allergy to** eggs

         Z91.013 **Allergy to** seafood
             Allergy to shellfish
             Allergy to octopus or squid ink

         Z91.018 **Allergy to other foods**
             Allergy to nuts other than peanuts

    Z91.02 **Food additives allergy status**

    √6ᵗʰ **Z91.03** Insect **allergy status**

         Z91.030 Bee **allergy status**

         Z91.038 **Other insect allergy status**

    √6ᵗʰ **Z91.04** **Nonmedicinal substance allergy status**

         Z91.040 Latex **allergy status**
             Latex sensitivity status

         Z91.041 Radiographic dye **allergy status**
             Allergy status to contrast media used for diagnostic X-ray procedure

         Z91.048 **Other nonmedicinal substance allergy status**

    Z91.09 **Other allergy status, other than to drugs and biological substances**

√5ᵗʰ **Z91.1** **Patient's noncompliance with medical treatment and regimen**

    Z91.11 **Patient's noncompliance with** dietary regimen

√6ᵗʰ **Z91.12** **Patient's** intentional underdosing of medication regimen
     Code first underdosing of medication (T36-T50) with fifth or sixth character 6
     EXCLUDES 1   *adverse effect of prescribed drug taken as directed—code to adverse effect poisoning (overdose)—code to poisoning*

    Z91.120 **Patient's intentional underdosing of medication regimen due to** financial hardship

    Z91.128 **Patient's intentional underdosing of medication regimen for other** reason

√6ᵗʰ **Z91.13** **Patient's** unintentional underdosing of medication regimen
     Code first underdosing of medication (T36-T50) with fifth or sixth character 6
     EXCLUDES 1   *adverse effect of prescribed drug taken as directed—code to adverse effect poisoning (overdose)—code to poisoning*

    Z91.130 **Patient's unintentional underdosing of medication regimen due to** age-related debility

    Z91.138 **Patient's unintentional underdosing of medication regimen for other** reason

Z91.14 **Patient's other noncompliance with medication regimen**
     Patient's underdosing of medication NOS

Z91.15 **Patient's noncompliance with** renal dialysis

Z91.19 **Patient's noncompliance with other medical treatment and regimen**

√5ᵗʰ **Z91.4** **Personal history of psychological trauma, not elsewhere classified**

    √6ᵗʰ **Z91.41** **Personal history of** adult abuse
         EXCLUDES 2   *personal history of abuse in childhood (Z62.81-)*

         Z91.410 **Personal history of adult** physical and sexual **abuse**   A
             EXCLUDES 1   *current adult physical abuse (T74.11, T76.11) current adult sexual abuse (T74.21, T76.11)*

         Z91.411 **Personal history of adult** psychological **abuse**   A

         Z91.412 **Personal history of** adult neglect   A
             EXCLUDES 1   *current adult neglect (T74.01, T76.01)*

         Z91.419 **Personal history of unspecified adult abuse**   A

    Z91.49 **Other personal history of psychological trauma, not elsewhere classified**

Z91.5 **Personal history of self-harm**
     Personal history of parasuicide
     Personal history of self-poisoning
     Personal history of suicide attempt

√5ᵗʰ **Z91.8** **Other specified personal risk factors, not elsewhere classified**

    Z91.81 **History of falling**
         At risk for falling

    Z91.82 **Personal history of military deployment**   A
         Individual (civilian or military) with past history of military war, peacekeeping and humanitarian deployment (current or past conflict)
         Returned from military deployment

    Z91.83 *Wandering in diseases classified elsewhere*
         Code first underlying disorder such as:
         Alzheimer's disease (G30.-)
         autism or pervasive developmental disorder (F84.-)
         intellectual disabilities (F70-F79)
         unspecified dementia with behavioral disturbance (F03.9-)

    Z91.89 **Other specified personal risk factors, not elsewhere classified**

√4ᵗʰ **Z92** **Personal history of medical treatment**
     EXCLUDES 2   *postprocedural states (Z98.-)*

    Z92.0 **Personal history of** contraception
         EXCLUDES 1   *counseling or management of current contraceptive practices (Z30.-)*
         long term (current) use of contraception (Z79.3)
         presence of (intrauterine) contraceptive device (Z97.5)

☑ Additional Character Required   √x7ᵗʰ Xtension Alert   Unspecified Dx   Other Specified Dx   Manifestation   ►◄ Revised Text   ● New Code   ▲ Revised Code Title

ICD-10-CM Draft (2015)   **1079**

✓5ᵗʰ **Z92.2** **Personal history of** drug therapy
  EXCLUDES 2 *long term (current) drug therapy (Z79.-)*

Z92.21 **Personal history of** antineoplastic chemotherapy

Z92.22 **Personal history of** monoclonal drug **therapy**

Z92.23 **Personal history of** estrogen **therapy**

✓6ᵗʰ **Z92.24** **Personal history of** steroid **therapy**

  Z92.240 **Personal history of** inhaled steroid **therapy**

  Z92.241 **Personal history of** systemic steroid **therapy**
    Personal history of steroid therapy NOS

Z92.25 **Personal history of** immunosupression **therapy**
  EXCLUDES 2 *personal history of steroid therapy (Z92.24)*

Z92.29 **Personal history of other drug therapy**

Z92.3 **Personal history of** irradiation
  Personal history of exposure to therapeutic radiation
  EXCLUDES 1 *exposure to radiation in the physical environment (Z77.12)*
    occupational exposure to radiation (Z57.1)

✓5ᵗʰ **Z92.8** **Personal history of other medical treatment**

Z92.81 **Personal history of extracorporeal membrane oxygenation (ECMO)**

Z92.82 **Status post administration of tPA (rtPA) in a different facility within the last 24 hours prior to admission to current facility**
  Code first condition requiring tPA administration, such as:
    acute cerebral infarction (I63.-)
    acute myocardial infarction (I21-, I22-)
  AHA: 2013, 4Q, 124

Z92.83 **Personal history of failed moderate sedation**
  Personal history of failed conscious sedation
  EXCLUDES 2 *failed moderate sedation during procedure (T88.52)*

Z92.89 **Personal history of other medical treatment**

✓4ᵗʰ **Z93** **Artificial opening status**
  EXCLUDES 1 *artificial openings requiring attention or management (Z43.-)*
    complications of external stoma (J95.0-, K94.-, N99.5-)

Z93.0 Tracheostomy **status**
  AHA: 2013, 4Q, 129

Z93.1 Gastrostomy **status**

Z93.2 Ileostomy **status**

Z93.3 Colostomy **status**

Z93.4 **Other artificial openings of gastrointestinal tract status**

✓5ᵗʰ **Z93.5** Cystostomy **status**

  Z93.50 **Unspecified cystostomy status**

  Z93.51 Cutaneous-vesicostomy **status**

  Z93.52 Appendico-vesicostomy **status**

  Z93.59 **Other cystostomy status**

Z93.6 **Other artificial openings of** urinary tract **status**
  Nephrostomy status
  Ureterostomy status
  Urethrostomy status

Z93.8 **Other artificial opening status**

Z93.9 **Artificial opening status, unspecified**

✓4ᵗʰ **Z94** **Transplanted organ and tissue status**
  INCLUDES organ or tissue replaced by heterogenous or homogenous transplant
  EXCLUDES 1 *complications of transplanted organ or tissue—see Alphabetical Index*
  EXCLUDES 2 *presence of vascular grafts (Z95.-)*

Z94.0 Kidney **transplant status**

Z94.1 Heart **transplant status**
  EXCLUDES 1 *artificial heart status (Z95.812)*
    heart-valve replacement status (Z95.2-Z95.4)

Z94.2 Lung **transplant status**

Z94.3 Heart and lungs **transplant status**

Z94.4 Liver **transplant status**

Z94.5 Skin **transplant status**
  Autogenous skin transplant status

Z94.6 Bone **transplant status**

Z94.7 Corneal **transplant status**

✓5ᵗʰ **Z94.8** **Other transplanted organ and tissue status**

  Z94.81 Bone marrow **transplant status**

  Z94.82 Intestine **transplant status**

Z94.83 Pancreas **transplant status**

Z94.84 Stem cells **transplant status**

Z94.89 **Other transplanted organ and tissue status**

Z94.9 **Transplanted organ and tissue status, unspecified**

✓4ᵗʰ **Z95** **Presence of cardiac and vascular implants and grafts**
  EXCLUDES 1 *complications of cardiac and vascular devices, implants and grafts (T82.-)*

Z95.0 **Presence of** cardiac pacemaker
  EXCLUDES 1 *adjustment or management of cardiac pacemaker (Z45.0)*
    presence of automatic (implantable) cardiac defibrillator with synchronous cardiac pacemaker (Z95.810)

Z95.1 **Presence of** aortocoronary bypass graft

Z95.2 **Presence of** prosthetic heart valve
  Presence of heart valve NOS

Z95.3 **Presence of** xenogenic heart valve

Z95.4 **Presence of other** heart-valve **replacement**

Z95.5 **Presence of** coronary angioplasty **implant and graft**
  EXCLUDES 1 *coronary angioplasty status without implant and graft (Z98.61)*

✓5ᵗʰ **Z95.8** **Presence of other cardiac and vascular implants and grafts**

✓6ᵗʰ **Z95.81** **Presence of** other **cardiac implants and grafts**

  Z95.810 **Presence of** automatic (implantable) cardiac defibrillator
    Presence of automatic (implantable) cardiac defibrillator with synchronous cardiac pacemaker

  Z95.811 **Presence of** heart assist device

  Z95.812 **Presence of** fully implantable artificial heart

  Z95.818 **Presence of other cardiac implants and grafts**

✓6ᵗʰ **Z95.82** **Presence of other vascular implants and grafts**

  Z95.820 **Peripheral** vascular angioplasty status **with implants and grafts**
    EXCLUDES 1 *peripheral vascular angioplasty without implant and graft (Z98.62)*

  Z95.828 **Presence of other vascular implants and grafts**
    Presence of intravascular prosthesis NEC

Z95.9 **Presence of cardiac and vascular implant and graft, unspecified**

✓4ᵗʰ **Z96** **Presence of other functional implants**
  EXCLUDES 2 *complications of internal prosthetic devices, implants and grafts (T82-T85)*
    fitting and adjustment of prosthetic and other devices (Z44-Z46)

Z96.0 **Presence of** urogenital **implants**

Z96.1 **Presence of** intraocular lens
  Presence of pseudophakia

✓5ᵗʰ **Z96.2** **Presence of** otological and audiological **implants**

  Z96.20 **Presence of otological and audiological implant, unspecified**

  Z96.21 Cochlear implant **status**

  Z96.22 Myringotomy tube(s) **status**

  Z96.29 **Presence of other otological and audiological implants**
    Presence of bone-conduction hearing device
    Presence of eustachian tube stent
    Stapes replacement

Z96.3 **Presence of** artificial larynx

✓5ᵗʰ **Z96.4** **Presence of** endocrine **implants**

  Z96.41 **Presence of** insulin pump (external) (internal)

  Z96.49 **Presence of other endocrine implants**

Z96.5 **Presence of** tooth-root and mandibular **implants**

✓5ᵗʰ **Z96.6** **Presence of** orthopedic joint **implants**

  Z96.60 **Presence of unspecified orthopedic joint implant**

✓6ᵗʰ **Z96.61** **Presence of** artificial shoulder joint

  Z96.611 **Presence of** right **artificial shoulder joint**

  Z96.612 **Presence of** left **artificial shoulder joint**

  Z96.619 **Presence of unspecified artificial shoulder joint**

✓6ᵗʰ **Z96.62** **Presence of** artificial elbow joint

  Z96.621 **Presence of** right **artificial elbow joint**

Z96.622 Presence of left artificial elbow joint
Z96.629 Presence of unspecified artificial elbow joint

√6ᵗʰ Z96.63 Presence of artificial wrist joint
Z96.631 Presence of right artificial wrist joint
Z96.632 Presence of left artificial wrist joint
Z96.639 Presence of unspecified artificial wrist joint

√6ᵗʰ Z96.64 Presence of artificial hip joint
Hip-joint replacement (partial) (total)
Z96.641 Presence of right artificial hip joint
Z96.642 Presence of left artificial hip joint
Z96.643 Presence of artificial hip joint, bilateral
Z96.649 Presence of unspecified artificial hip joint

√6ᵗʰ Z96.65 Presence of artificial knee joint
Z96.651 Presence of right artificial knee joint
Z96.652 Presence of left artificial knee joint
Z96.653 Presence of artificial knee joint, bilateral
Z96.659 Presence of unspecified artificial knee joint

√6ᵗʰ Z96.66 Presence of artificial ankle joint
Z96.661 Presence of right artificial ankle joint
Z96.662 Presence of left artificial ankle joint
Z96.669 Presence of unspecified artificial ankle joint

√6ᵗʰ Z96.69 Presence of other orthopedic joint implants
Z96.691 Finger-joint replacement of right hand
Z96.692 Finger-joint replacement of left hand
Z96.693 Finger-joint replacement, bilateral
Z96.698 Presence of other orthopedic joint implants

Z96.7 Presence of other bone and tendon implants
Presence of skull plate

√5ᵗʰ Z96.8 Presence of other specified functional implants
Z96.81 Presence of artificial skin
Z96.89 Presence of other specified functional implants

Z96.9 Presence of functional implant, unspecified

√4ᵗʰ **Z97 Presence of other devices**
EXCLUDES 1 complications of internal prosthetic devices, implants and grafts (T82-T85)
fitting and adjustment of prosthetic and other devices (Z44-Z46)
EXCLUDES 2 presence of cerebrospinal fluid drainage device (Z98.2)

Z97.0 Presence of artificial eye

√5ᵗʰ Z97.1 Presence of artificial limb (complete) (partial)
Z97.10 Presence of artificial limb (complete) (partial), unspecified
Z97.11 Presence of artificial right arm (complete) (partial)
Z97.12 Presence of artificial left arm (complete) (partial)
Z97.13 Presence of artificial right leg (complete) (partial)
Z97.14 Presence of artificial left leg (complete) (partial)
Z97.15 Presence of artificial arms, bilateral (complete) (partial)
Z97.16 Presence of artificial legs, bilateral (complete) (partial)

Z97.2 Presence of dental prosthetic device (complete) (partial)
Presence of dentures (complete) (partial)

Z97.3 Presence of spectacles and contact lenses

Z97.4 Presence of external hearing-aid

Z97.5 Presence of (intrauterine) contraceptive device ♀
EXCLUDES 1 checking, reinsertion or removal of contraceptive device (Z30.43)

Z97.8 Presence of other specified devices

√4ᵗʰ **Z98 Other postprocedural states**
EXCLUDES 2 aftercare (Z43-Z49, Z51)
follow-up medical care (Z08- Z09)
postprocedural complication—see Alphabetical Index

Z98.0 Intestinal bypass and anastomosis status
EXCLUDES 2 bariatric surgery status (Z98.84)
gastric bypass status (Z98.84)
obesity surgery status (Z98.84)

Z98.1 Arthrodesis status

Z98.2 Presence of cerebrospinal fluid drainage device
Presence of CSF shunt

Z98.3 Post therapeutic collapse of lung status
Code first underlying disease

√5ᵗʰ Z98.4 Cataract extraction status
Use additional code to identify intraocular lens implant status (Z96.1)
EXCLUDES 1 aphakia (H27.0)
Z98.41 Cataract extraction status, right eye
Z98.42 Cataract extraction status, left eye
Z98.49 Cataract extraction status, unspecified eye

√5ᵗʰ Z98.5 Sterilization status
EXCLUDES 1 female infertility (N97.-)
male infertility (N46.-)
Z98.51 Tubal ligation status ♀
Z98.52 Vasectomy status A♂

√5ᵗʰ Z98.6 Angioplasty status
Z98.61 Coronary angioplasty status
EXCLUDES 1 coronary angioplasty status with implant and graft (Z95.5)
Z98.62 Peripheral vascular angioplasty status
EXCLUDES 1 peripheral vascular angioplasty status with implant and graft (Z95.820)

√5ᵗʰ Z98.8 Other specified postprocedural states
√6ᵗʰ Z98.81 Dental procedure status
Z98.810 Dental sealant status
Z98.811 Dental restoration status
Dental crown status
Dental fillings status
Z98.818 Other dental procedure status
Z98.82 Breast implant status
EXCLUDES 1 breast implant removal status (Z98.86)
Z98.83 Filtering (vitreous) bleb after glaucoma surgery status
EXCLUDES 1 inflammation (infection) of postprocedural bleb (H59.4-)
Z98.84 Bariatric surgery status
Gastric banding status
Gastric bypass status for obesity
Obesity surgery status
EXCLUDES 1 bariatric surgery status complicating pregnancy, childbirth, or the puerperium (O99.84)
EXCLUDES 2 intestinal bypass and anastomosis status (Z98.0)
Z98.85 Transplanted organ removal status
Transplanted organ previously removed due to complication, failure, rejection or infection
EXCLUDES 1 encounter for removal of transplanted organ—code to complication of transplanted organ (T86.-)
Z98.86 Personal history of breast implant removal
√6ᵗʰ Z98.87 Personal history of in utero procedure
Z98.870 Personal history of in utero procedure during pregnancy ♀
EXCLUDES 2 complications from in utero procedure for current pregnancy (O35.7)
supervision of current pregnancy with history of in utero procedure during previous pregnancy (O09.82-)
Z98.871 Personal history of in utero procedure while a fetus
Z98.89 Other specified postprocedural states
Personal history of surgery, not elsewhere classified

√4ᵗʰ **Z99 Dependence on enabling machines and devices, not elsewhere classified**
EXCLUDES 1 cardiac pacemaker status (Z95.0)

Z99.0 Dependence on aspirator

√5ᵗʰ Z99.1 Dependence on respirator
Dependence on ventilator
Z99.11 Dependence on respirator [ventilator] status
Z99.12 Encounter for respirator [ventilator] dependence during power failure PDx
EXCLUDES 1 mechanical complication of respirator [ventilator] (J95.850)

Z99.2   Dependence on renal dialysis
  Hemodialysis status
  Peritoneal dialysis status
  Presence of arteriovenous shunt for dialysis
  Renal dialysis status NOS
  EXCLUDES 1 *encounter for fitting and adjustment of dialysis catheter (Z49.0-)*
      noncompliance with renal dialysis (Z91.15)
  AHA: 2013, 4Q, 125

Z99.3   Dependence on wheelchair
  Wheelchair confinement status
  Code first cause of dependence, such as:
    muscular dystrophy (G71.0)
    obesity (E66.-)

✓5ᵗʰ **Z99.8   Dependence on other enabling machines and devices**

  Z99.81   Dependence on supplemental oxygen
    Dependence on long-term oxygen
    AHA: 2013, 4Q, 129

  Z99.89   Dependence on other enabling machines and devices
    Dependence on machine or device NOS

EXCLUDES 1 Not coded here   **EXCLUDES 2** Not included here   **PDx** Primary Diagnosis Only   **N** Newborn Age: 0   **P** Pediatric Age: 0-17   **M** Maternity Age: 12-55   **A** Adult Age: 15-124

1082   ICD-10-CM Draft (2015)

Peripheral Nervous System

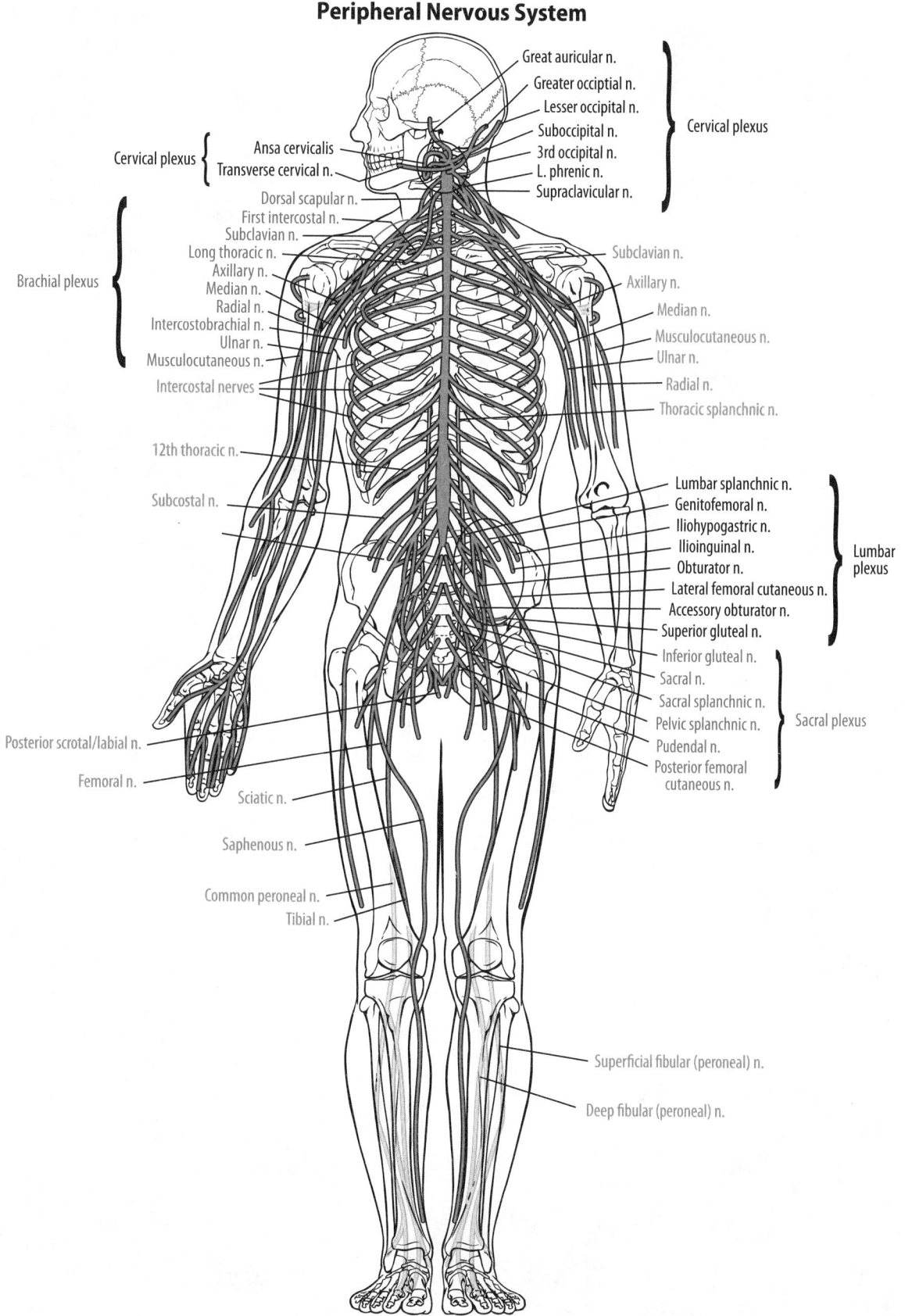

Great auricular n.
Greater occiptial n.
Lesser occipital n.
Suboccipital n.
3rd occipital n.
L. phrenic n.
Supraclavicular n.

Cervical plexus

Cervical plexus {
Ansa cervicalis
Transverse cervical n.

Dorsal scapular n.
First intercostal n.
Subclavian n.
Long thoracic n.
Axillary n.
Median n.
Radial n.
Intercostobrachial n.
Ulnar n.
Musculocutaneous n.
Intercostal nerves

Brachial plexus {

Subclavian n.
Axillary n.
Median n.
Musculocutaneous n.
Ulnar n.
Radial n.
Thoracic splanchnic n.

12th thoracic n.

Subcostal n.

Lumbar splanchnic n.
Genitofemoral n.
Iliohypogastric n.
Ilioinguinal n.
Obturator n.
Lateral femoral cutaneous n.
Accessory obturator n.
Superior gluteal n.

Lumbar plexus

Inferior gluteal n.
Sacral n.
Sacral splanchnic n.
Pelvic splanchnic n.
Pudendal n.
Posterior femoral cutaneous n.

Sacral plexus

Posterior scrotal/labial n.

Femoral n.

Sciatic n.

Saphenous n.

Common peroneal n.
Tibial n.

Superficial fibular (peroneal) n.

Deep fibular (peroneal) n.

Brain

Cranial Nerves

Eye

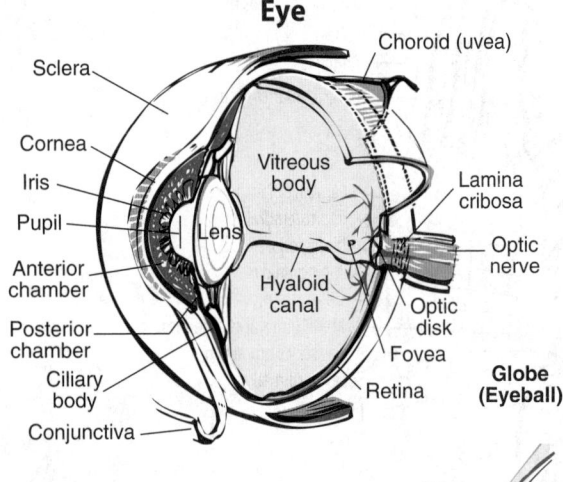

Globe
(Eyeball)

Middle Ear

Exposed view of middle and inner ear

Posterior Pole of Globe

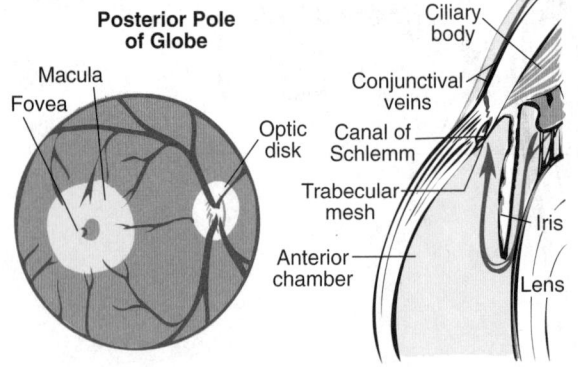

Flow of Aqueous Humor

Lacrimal System

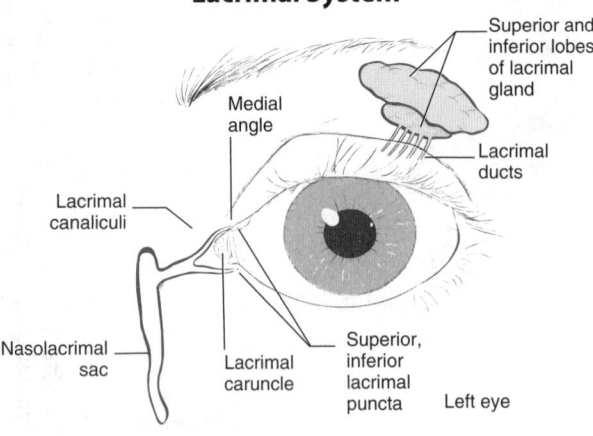

Left eye

Ear and Mastoid

Arteries

Veins

Upper Veins:

Lower Veins:

Superficial temporal v.

Vertebral v.

Internal jugular v.

External jugular v.

Subclavian v.

Innominate v.

Azygos v.

Axillary v.

Hemiazygos v.

Brachial v.

Cephalic v.

Basilic v.

Inferior vena cava

Esophageal v.

Common hepatic v.

L. gastric v.

Portal v.

Splenic v.

R. gastric v.

Renal v.

R. colic v.

Inferior mesenteric v.

Superior mesenteric v.

Radial v.

L. colic v.

Ulnar v.

Common iliac v.

Internal iliac v. (Hypogastric v.)

External iliac v.

Internal pudendal v.

Rectal venous plexus

Femoral v.

Greater saphenous v.

Popliteal v.

Lesser saphenous v.

Anterior tibial v.

Lesser saphenous v.

Posterior tibial v.

Greater saphenous v.

Anatomy of Heart

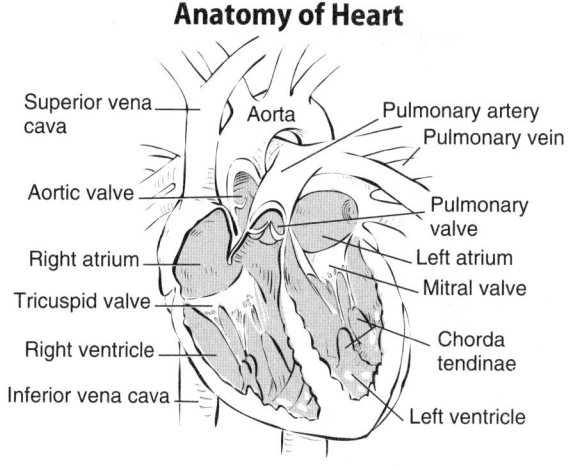

Superior vena cava
Aorta
Pulmonary artery
Pulmonary vein
Aortic valve
Pulmonary valve
Right atrium
Left atrium
Tricuspid valve
Mitral valve
Right ventricle
Chorda tendinae
Inferior vena cava
Left ventricle

Arteries of Heart

Aortic valve
Right coronary artery
Marginal branches
Descending branch (posterior interventricular artery)
Left coronary artery
Circumflex branch
Descending branch (anterior interventricular artery)

Cerebrovascular Arteries

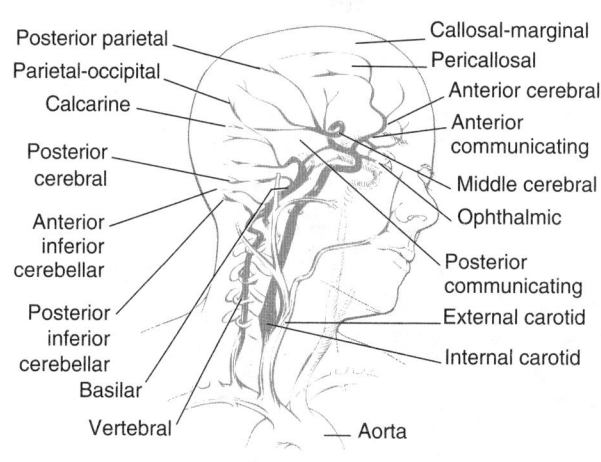

Posterior parietal
Parietal-occipital
Calcarine
Posterior cerebral
Anterior inferior cerebellar
Posterior inferior cerebellar
Basilar
Vertebral
Callosal-marginal
Pericallosal
Anterior cerebral
Anterior communicating
Middle cerebral
Ophthalmic
Posterior communicating
External carotid
Internal carotid
Aorta

Veins of Head and Neck

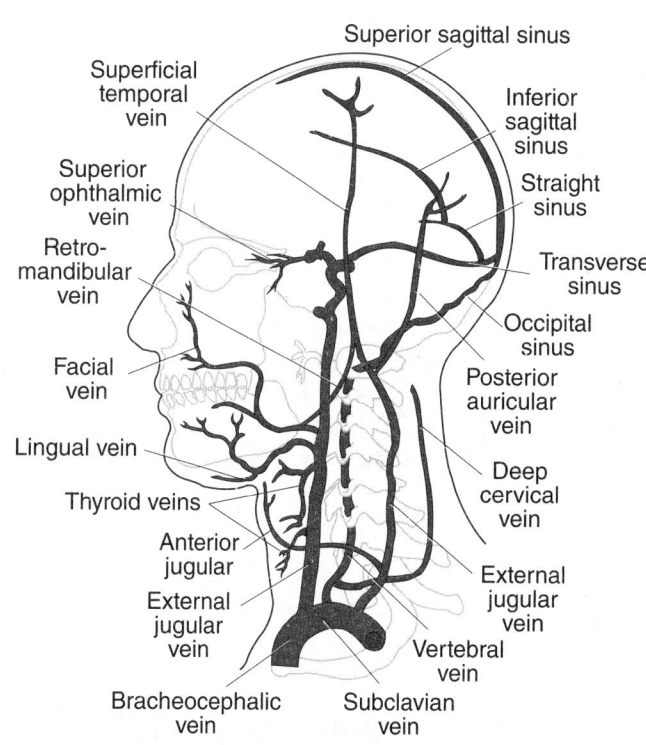

Superficial temporal vein
Superior ophthalmic vein
Retro-mandibular vein
Facial vein
Lingual vein
Thyroid veins
Anterior jugular
External jugular vein
Bracheocephalic vein
Superior sagittal sinus
Inferior sagittal sinus
Straight sinus
Transverse sinus
Occipital sinus
Posterior auricular vein
Deep cervical vein
External jugular vein
Vertebral vein
Subclavian vein

Lymphatic System of Head and Neck

Afferent vessels (in)
Blood vessels
Hilum
Efferent vessel (out)

Schematic of lymph node

Jugulodigastric
Submental
Submandibular
Jugulomyohyoid
Anterior cervical
Superficial parotid
Occipital

Lymphatic drainage of the head, neck, and face

Lymph Nodes

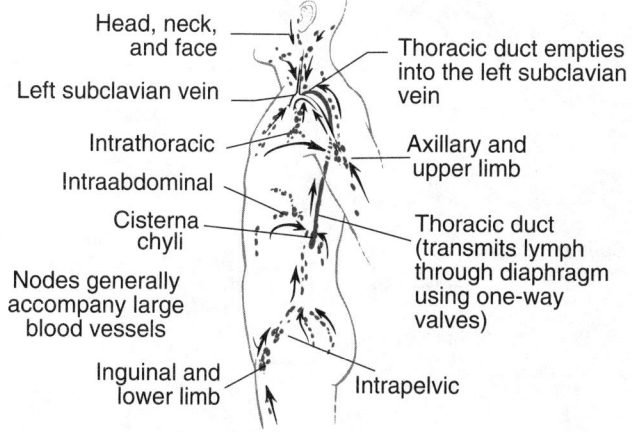

Head, neck, and face
Left subclavian vein
Intrathoracic
Intraabdominal
Cisterna chyli
Nodes generally accompany large blood vessels
Inguinal and lower limb
Thoracic duct empties into the left subclavian vein
Axillary and upper limb
Thoracic duct (transmits lymph through diaphragm using one-way valves)
Intrapelvic

Respiratory System

Paranasal Sinuses

Oral Cavity

Pancreas

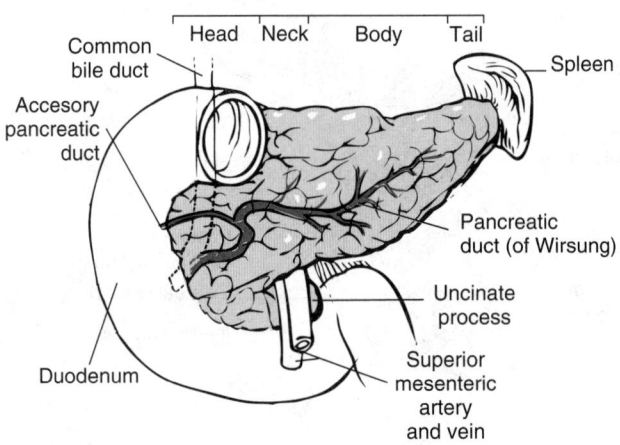

Gallbladder and Bile Ducts

Liver

Gastrointestinal System

Ethmoid sinus

Frontal sinus

Sphenoid sinus

Maxillary sinus

Esophageal region:

Cervical portion

Upper esophagus

Thoracic portion

Lower esophagus

Fundus

Esophagogastric junction

Abdominal portion

Stomach

Diaphragm

Pylorus

Left colic (splenic) flexure

Transverse colon

Right colic (hepatic) flexure

Duodenum

Large intestine

Ascending colon

Descending colon

Jejunum

Ileocecal junction

Cecum

Appendix

Ileum

Small intestine

Rectum

Anus

Sigmoid colon

Anal sphincter

Endocrine System

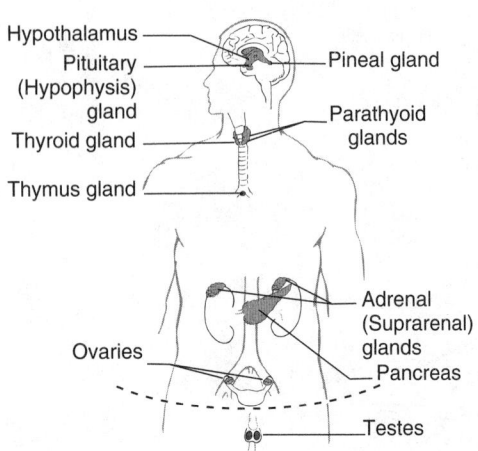

Dorsal View of Parathyroid Gland

Kidney

Urinary System

Male Pelvic Organs

Female Genitourinary System

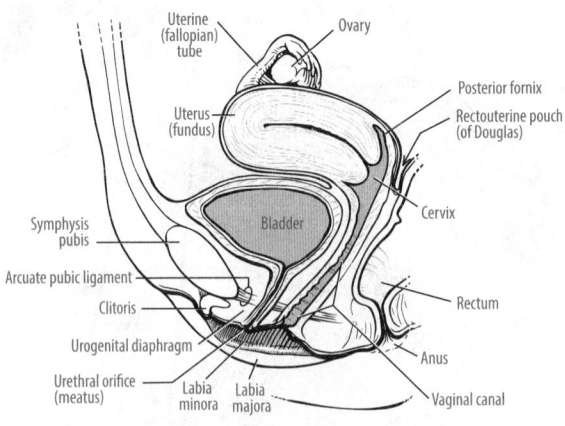

Joints

Shoulder (Anterior View)

Shoulder (Posterior View)

Elbow (Anterior View)

Elbow (Posterior View)

Hand

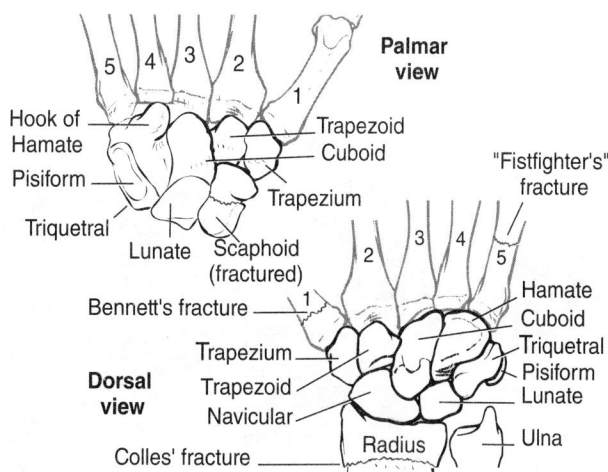

Joints

Hip (Anterior View)

Hip (Posterior View)

Knee (Anterior View)

Knee (Posterior View)

Right Foot

Bones/Joints

Muscles

Frontalis m.
Temporalis m.
Orbicularis oculi m.
Orbicularis oris m.
Masseter m.
Depressor labii inferioris m.
Zygomaticus major m.
Mentalis m.
Splenius m.
Sternocleidomastoid m. (Clavicular head)
Omohyoid m.
Sternocleidomastoid m. (Sternal head)
Levator scapulae m.
Platysma m.
Deltoid m.
Pectoralis major m.
Latissimus dorsi m.
Coracobrachialis m.
Serratus anterior m.
Biceps brachii m. (short head)
Biceps brachii m.
Biceps brachii m. (long head)
Triceps m.
Linea alba
Brachialis m.
Brachioradialis m.
Rectus abdominis m.
Extensor carpi radialis longus m.
Brachioradialis m.
Bicipital aponeurosis
Pronator teres m.
External oblique m.
Flexor carpi radialis m.
Flexor carpi radialis m.
Extensor carpi radialis longus m.
Palmaris longus m.
Extensor carpi radialis brevis m.
Flexor carpi ulnaris m.
Flexor digitorum superficialis m.
Extensor digitorum m.
Extensor digiti minimi m.
Extensor retinaculum
Extensor retinaculum
Anterior
Superior
Iliac Spine
Iliopsoas m.
Pectineus m.
Pubic
tubercle
Adductor longus m.
Pudendal n.
Sartorius m.
Gracilis m.
Tensor fascia latae m.
Rectus femoris m.
Vastus lateralis m.
Vastus medialis m.
Tensor fascia latae m.
Patella
Gastrocnemius m.
Tibia
Tibialis anterior m.
Peroneus longus m.
Soleus m.
Extensor digitorum longus m.
Superior extensor retinaculum
Medial maleolus
Lateral maleolus